CHESTNUT'S

OBSTETRIC ANESTHESIA

PRINCIPLES and PRACTICE

CHESTNUT'S
OBSTETRIC ANESTHESIA
PRINCIPLES and PRACTICE

SEVENTH EDITION

Cynthia A. Wong, MD
Professor and Chair
Department of Anesthesia
University of Iowa
Iowa City, Iowa

Warwick D. Ngan Kee, BHB, MBChB, MD, FANZCA, FHKCA
Clinical Professor (Honorary)
Department of Anaesthesia and Intensive Care
The Chinese University of Hong Kong
Hong Kong, China
Guest Professor
Zhejiang University School of Medicine
Hangzhou, China

Lawrence C. Tsen, MD
Clinical Professor
Department of Anesthesiology
Mass General Brigham
Harvard Medical School
Director, Human Research Office
Mass General Brigham
Boston, Massachusetts

Yaakov Beilin, MD
Professor
Departments of Anesthesiology and Obstetrics, Gynecology and
    Reproductive Science
Vice Chair for Quality
Department of Anesthesiology
Icahn School of Medicine at Mount Sinai
New York, New York

Jill M. Mhyre, MD
The Dola S. Thompson Professor and Chair
Department of Anesthesiology
University of Arkansas for Medical Sciences
Little Rock, Arkansas

Brian T. Bateman, MD, MSc
Professor and Chair
Department of Anesthesiology, Perioperative and Pain Medicine
Stanford University
Stanford, California

Lisa R. Leffert, MD
Professor and Chair
Department of Anesthesiology
Yale University School of Medicine
New Haven, Connecticut

David H. Chestnut, MD
Professor
Department of Anesthesiology
Vanderbilt University Medical Center
Nashville, Tennessee

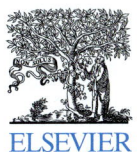

ELSEVIER

Elsevier
1600 John F. Kennedy Blvd.
Ste 1800
Philadelphia, PA 19103-2899

CHESTNUT'S OBSTETRIC ANESTHESIA: PRINCIPLES AND PRACTICE,
SEVENTH EDITION

ISBN: 978-0-443-11184-6

Notice

Previous editions copyrighted 2020, 2014, 2009, 2004, 1999, and 1994.

Executive Content Strategist: Kayla Wolfe
Senior Content Development Specialist: Kevin Travers
Content Development Manager: Meghan Andress
Publishing Services Manager: Deepthi Unni
Senior Project Manager: Beula Christopher
Senior Designer: Patrick Ferguson

Printed in India

Last digit is the print number: 9 8 7 6 5 4 3 2 1

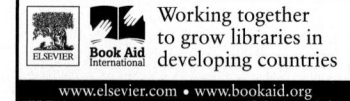

To my wife, **Janet**; our children, **John Mark** and **Catherine**, **Michael** and **Jordan**, **Mary Beth**, **Annie** and **Aaron**, and **Stephen** and **Emily**; and our grandchildren, **Caleb**, Emily, **Hannah**, **Jack**, **Mae**, **William**, **Graham**, and **John**

DHC

In memory of my husband, **Lawrence**, and to our children, **Anna**, **Molly**, **Leah**, and **Sofie**

CAW

To my wife, **Rosemary**, and our children, **Sam**, **Nick**, **Ellie**, and **Katie**

WDNK

To my wife, **Jennifer**, and our children, **Noah**, **Zachary**, **Jeremy**, **London**, **Hamilton**, and **Asher**

LCT

In memory of my mother, **Adelle Beilin**; to my wife, **Karen**; our children, **Yehuda** and **Aliza**, **Shani** and **Nati**, and **Shua** and **Ayelet**; my father, **Isaiah**; my parents-in-law, **Susan** and **Maurice**; and our grandchildren, **Addie, Ozzy, Meir, Yishai, Akiva,** and **Liam**.

YB

To my husband, **Keith**, and our children, **Fiona** and **Rhys**

JMM

To my wife, **Stephanie**, and our children, **Christian** and **Graham**

BTB

To my husband, **Lee**, and my sons, **Sam** and **Eli**.

LRL

ACKNOWLEDGMENT OF CONTRIBUTORS TO PREVIOUS EDITIONS

The editors gratefully acknowledge the work of the following authors who contributed to chapters of previous editions of this book. Their expertise, wisdom, and scholarship have provided the foundation for the seventh edition.

Physiologic Changes of Pregnancy
Kenneth A. Conklin, MD, PhD
Anita Backus Chang, MD
Robert Gaiser, MD

Uteroplacental Blood Flow
James C. Eisenach, MD
Carl P. Weiner, MD
Warwick D. Ngan Kee, BHB, MBChB, MD, FANZCA, FHKCA, FHKAM (Anaesthesiology)

The Placenta: Anatomy, Physiology, and Transfer of Drugs
Norman L. Herman, MD, PhD
Mark I. Zakowski, MD
Andrew Geller, MD

Fetal Physiology
Andrew P. Harris, MD, MHS
Kenneth E. Nelson, MD
Mieke Soens, MD
Lawrence C. Tsen, MD

Antepartum Fetal Assessment and Therapy
Katharine D. Wenstrom, MD
Katherine Campbell, MD
Teresa Marino, MD
George M. Graham III, MD
Joong Shin Park, MD, PhD
Errol R. Norwitz, MD, PhD

Anesthesia for Fetal Surgery and Other Intrauterine Procedures
Mark A. Rosen, MD

Intrapartum Fetal Assessment and Therapy
Elizabeth G. Livingston, MD

Neonatal Assessment and Resuscitation
Rhonda L. Zuckerman, MD
Marvin Cornblath, MD

Fetal and Neonatal Neurologic Injury
Donald H. Penning, MD

Patient Safety and Team Training
Eduardo Salas, PhD

Spinal, Epidural, and Caudal Anesthesia: Anatomy, Physiology, and Technique
David L. Brown, MD
Vijaya Gottumkkala, MBBS, MD, FRCA
Cynthia A. Wong, MD

Local Anesthetics and Opioids
Hilda Pedersen, MD
Mieczyslaw Finster, MD
Brenda Bucklin, MD
Alan Santos, MD, PhD

Pharmacology During Pregnancy and Lactation
Jennifer R. Niebyl, MD
Jerome Yankowitz, MD
Tony Gin, MBChB, MD, FANZCA, FHKAM

***In Vitro* Fertilization and Other Assisted Reproductive Technology**
Robert D. Vincent, Jr., MD
Lawrence C. Tsen, MD

Problems of Early Pregnancy
Robert C. Chantigian, MD
Paula D. M. Chantigian, MD
Katherine W. Arendt, MD

Nonobstetric Surgery during Pregnancy
Sheila E. Cohen, MB, ChB, FRCA
Norah N. Naughton, MD

Obstetric Management of Labor and Vaginal Delivery
Frank J. Zlatnik, MD
Dwight J. Rouse, MD, MSPH

The Pain of Childbirth and Its Effect on the Mother and the Fetus
Theodore G. Cheek, MD
Brett B. Gutsche, MD
Robert R. Gaiser, MD
James C. Eisenach, MD
Jessica L. Booth, MD

Systemic Analgesia: Parenteral and Inhalational Agents
Marsha L. Wakefield, MD
Tanya Jones, MB, ChB, MRCP, FRCA
Niveen El-Wahab, MBBCh, MRCP, FRCA
Thunga Setty, MBChB, FRCA
Roshan Fernando, MD, FRCA

Epidural and Spinal Analgesia/ Anesthesia for Labor and Vaginal Delivery
Beth Glosten, MD
Brian K. Ross, MD, PhD
David H. Chestnut, MD
Edward T. Riley, MD
Linda S. Polley, MD

Alternative Regional Anesthesia Techniques for Labor and Vaginal Delivery
David H. Chestnut, MD

Anesthesia for Cesarean Delivery
Laurence S. Reisner, MD
Dennis Lin, MD
Krzysztof M. Kuczkowski, MD

Postoperative Analgesia
Robert K. Parker, DO
Raymond S. Sinatra, MD, PhD
Chakib M. Ayoub, MD
David Hepner, MD
Sunil Eappen, MD
Pedram Aleshi, MD
Brendan Carvalho, MBBCh, FRCA, MDCH
Alexander J. Butwick, MBBS, FRCA, MS
Pamela Flood, MD

Aspiration: Risk, Prophylaxis, and Treatment
Thomas S. Guyton, MD
Charles P. Gibbs, MD
Geraldine O'Sullivan, MD, FRCA
M. Shankar Hari, Dip. Epi., MD, FRCA, FFICM

The Difficult Airway: Risk, Assessment, Prophylaxis, and Management
Sheila D. Cooper, MD
Jonathan L. Benumof, MD
Laurence S. Reisner, MD
Krzysztof M. Kuczkowski, MD
John A. Thomas, MD
Carin A. Hagberg, MD
Mansukh Popat, MBBS, FRCA
Robin Russell, MBBS, MD, FRCA

Postpartum Headache
Sally K. Weeks, MBBS
Alison MacArthur, BMSc, MD, FRPCP, MSc

Neurologic Complications of Pregnancy and Neuraxial Anesthesia
Philip R. Bromage, MBBS, FRCA, FRCPC
Felicity Reynolds, MD, MBBS, FRCA, FRCOG ad eundem

Medicolegal Issues in Obstetric Anesthesia
William Gild, MB, ChB, JD
H. S. Chadwick, MD
Lisa Vincler Brock, JD
Brian K. Ross, MD, PhD
Mark S. Williams, MD, MBA, JD
Joanna M. Davies, MBBS, FRCA

Shared Decision-Making and Communication
Vilma E. Ortiz, MD
Joshua Abrams, JD
May C. M. Pian-Smith, MD, MS

Preterm Labor and Delivery
Joan M. McGrath, MD
David H. Chestnut, MD
Holly A. Muir, MD, FRCPC
Cynthia A. Wong, MD
Janelle R. Bolden, MD
William A. Grobman, MD, MBA

Abnormal Presentation and Multiple Gestation
BettyLou Koffel, MD
Joy L. Hawkins, MD

Hypertensive Disorders
Desmond Writer, MB, ChB, FRCA, FRCPC
David R. Gambling, MB, BS, FRCPC
Linda S. Polley, MD
Robert A. Dyer, FCA (SA), PhD
Justiaan L. Swanevelder, FCA (SA), FRCA, MMed (Anaesthesiology)
Brian T. Bateman, MD, MSc

Infection
Harvey Carp, PhD, MD
David H. Chestnut, MD
Scott Segal, MD, MHCM
David J. Wlody, MD

Antepartum and Postpartum Hemorrhage
David C. Mayer, MD
Fred J. Spielman, MD
Elizabeth A. Bell, MD, MPH
Kathleen A. Smith, MD
Jennifer E. Hofer, MD
Barbara M. Scavone, MD

Embolic Disorders
Andrew M. Malinow, MD
Kathleen M. Davis, MD

Autoimmune Disorders
Robert W. Reid, MD
David H. Chestnut, MD

Cardiovascular Disease
Marsha L. Thornhill, MD
William R. Camann, MD
Miriam Harnett, MB, FFARCSI
Philip S. Mushlin, MD
Lawrence C. Tsen, MD

Hematologic and Coagulation Disorders
Robert B. Lechner, MD, PhD
Shiv K. Sharma, MD, FRCA

Liver Disease
Robert W. Reid, MD
David H. Chestnut, MD
Michael Frolich, MD, MS
Yaakov Beilin, MD

Malignant Hyperthermia
M. Joanne Douglas, MD, FRCPC

Musculoskeletal Disorders
Edward T. Crosby, MD, FRCPC

Neurologic and Neuromuscular Disease
Angela M. Bader, MD, MPH

Obesity
David Dewan, MD
Robert D'Angelo, MD

Psychiatric Disorders
Warwick D. Ngan Kee, BHB, MBChB, MD, FANZCA, FHKCA, FHKAM (Anaesthesiology)
Vijay J. Roach, MBBS, MRCOG, FRANZCOG, MHKCOG

Renal Disease
Robert W. Reid, MD
David H. Chestnut, MD

Substance Use Disorders
David J. Birnbach, MD

Trauma and Critical Care
B. Wycke Baker, MD
Paul Howell, MBChB, FRCA

CONTRIBUTORS

Catherine M. Albright, MD, MS
Associate Professor, Maternal-Fetal Medicine
Department of Obstetrics and Gynecology
University of Washington Medical Center
Seattle, Washington

Katherine W. Arendt, MD
Professor
Department of Anesthesiology and
 Perioperative Medicine
Mayo Clinic College of Medicine
Rochester, Minnesota

David Arnolds, MD, PhD
Clinical Associate Professor
Departments of Anesthesiology and
 Obstetrics and Gynecology
Section Head, Obstetric Anesthesia
University of Michigan Medical School
Ann Arbor, Michigan

Susan W. Aucott, MD
Adjunct Associate Professor
Department of Pediatrics
Johns Hopkins University
Baltimore, Maryland;
Director
Department of Neonatology
Greater Baltimore Medical Center
Towson, Maryland

Jennifer M. Banayan, MD
Associate Professor
Department of Anesthesiology
Northwestern University Feinberg School of
 Medicine
Chicago, Illinois

Brian T. Bateman, MD, MSc
Professor and Chair
Department of Anesthesiology, Perioperative
 and Pain Medicine
Stanford University
Stanford, California

Jeanette R. Bauchat, MD, MS
Professor
Department of Anesthesiology
Vanderbilt University Medical Center
Nashville, Tennessee

Melissa E. Bauer, DO
Associate Professor
Department of Anesthesiology
Duke University School of Medicine
Durham, North Carolina

Yaakov Beilin, MD
Professor
Departments of Anesthesiology and
 Obstetrics, Gynecology and Reproductive
 Science
Vice Chair for Quality
Department of Anesthesiology
Icahn School of Medicine at Mount Sinai
New York, New York

David J. Birnbach, MD, MPH
Miller Professor and Executive Vice Provost,
 Emeritus
Department of Anesthesiology
University of Miami
Director Emeritus
UM-JMH Center for Patient Safety
Jackson Memorial Hospital
Miami, Florida

Adrianne Rahde Bischoff, MD
Clinical Assistant Professor
Department of Pediatrics
University of Iowa
Iowa City, Iowa

David G. Bishop, MD, PhD, FCA
Associate Professor
Department of Anaesthesiology
University of KwaZulu-Natal
Pietermaritzburg, KwaZulu-Natal, South Africa

Rupsa C. Boelig, MD, MS
Associate Professor
Department of Obstetrics and Gynecology,
 Division of Maternal-Fetal Medicine
Sidney Kimmel Medical College
Thomas Jefferson University
Philadelphia, Pennsylvania

Kaitlyn Brennan, DO, MPH
Assistant Professor
Department of Anesthesiology
Vanderbilt University Medical Center
Nashville, Tennessee

Alexander J. Butwick, MBBS, FRCA, MS
Professor
Department of Anesthesia and Perioperative
 Care
University of California San Francisco
San Francisco, California

Donald Caton, MD
Professor Emeritus
Department of Anesthesiology
University of Florida
Gainesville, Florida

David H. Chestnut, MD
Professor
Department of Anesthesiology
Vanderbilt University Medical Center
Nashville, Tennessee

Jonathan P. W. Collins, MA (Oxon), BM, BCh, FRCPC
Clinical Assistant Professor
Department of Anesthesiology, Pharmacy
 and Therapeutics
University of British Columbia;
Associate Head
Department of Anesthesia
BC Women's Hospital
Vancouver, British Columbia, Canada

Holly B. Ende, MD
Associate Professor
Department of Anesthesiology
Chief, Division of Obstetric Anesthesiology
Vanderbilt University Medical Center
Associate Director
Vanderbilt Anesthesiology and Perioperative
 Informatics Research
Nashville, Tennessee

Tania F. Esakoff, MD
Professor
Department of Obstetrics and Gynecology
Cedars Sinai Medical Center
Los Angeles, California

Sara Eyal, PhD
Professor
Institute for Drug Research
The Hebrew University of Jerusalem
Jerusalem, Israel

Ada Ezihe-Ejiofor, MBBS (Nig), DA, FWACS, FRCA
Department of Anesthesiology
Guys and St. Thomas' NHS Foundation Trust
Honorary Senior Lecturer, King's College
London, United Kingdom

Michaela K. Farber, MD, MS
Associate Professor
Department of Anesthesiology
Chief, Division of Obstetric Anesthesiology
Mass General Brigham
Harvard Medical School
Boston, Massachusetts

Ronald B. George, MD, FRCPC
Professor
Department of Anesthesiology and Pain
  Management
University of Toronto
Director of Obstetric Anesthesia
Mount Sinai Hospital
Toronto, Ontario, Canada

Yehuda Ginosar, BSc, MBBS
Director of Mother and Child Anesthesia Unit
Department of Anesthesiology, Critical Care
  and Pain Medicine
Hadassah Hebrew University Medical Center
Jerusalem, Israel

Ashraf S. Habib, MBBCh, MSc, MHSc, FRCA
Professor
Departments of Anesthesiology and
  Obstetrics and Gynecology
Chief, Division of Women's Anesthesia
Duke University School of Medicine
Durham, North Carolina

Joy L. Hawkins, MD
Professor
Department of Anesthesiology
University of Colorado School of Medicine
Aurora, Colorado

Mai He, MD, PhD
Professor
Director of Pediatric Pathology
Department of Pathology and Immunology
Washington University School of Medicine
Pathologist-in-Chief
Department of Pathology
St. Louis Children's Hospital
St. Louis, Missouri

Philip E. Hess, MD
Associate Professor
Department of Anesthesiology, Critical Care
  and Pain Medicine
Beth Israel Deaconess Medical Center
Boston, Massachusetts

Rachel M. Kacmar, MD
Associate Professor
Residency Program Director
Department of Anesthesiology
University of Colorado School of Medicine
Aurora, Colorado

Anjali Kaimal, MD, MAS
Professor
Department of Obstetrics and Gynecology
University of South Florida Morsani College
  of Medicine
Tampa, Florida

Daniel Katz, MD
Professor
Department of Anesthesiology
Icahn School of Medicine at Mount Sinai
New York, New York

Sarah J. Kilpatrick, MD, PhD
Professor and Chair
Department of Obstetrics and Gynecology
Vice Dean
Diversity and Inclusion
Cedars Sinai Medical Center
Los Angeles, California

Klaus Kjaer, MD, MBA
Professor
Departments of Anesthesiology and
  Healthcare Policy and Research
Weill Cornell Medicine
New York, New York

Joanna A. Kountanis, MD
Associate Professor
Departments of Anesthesiology and
  Obstetrics and Gynecology
University of Michigan
Ann Arbor, Michigan

Ruth Landau, MD
Virginia Apgar Professor in
  Anesthesiology
Department of Anesthesiology
Columbia University
New York, New York

Elizabeth M.S. Lange, MD
Associate Professor
Department of Anesthesiology
Emory University School of Medicine
Atlanta, Georgia

Lisa R. Leffert, MD
Professor and Chair
Department of Anesthesiology
Yale University School of Medicine
New Haven, Connecticut

Grace Lim, MD, MS
Associate Professor
Department of Anesthesiology and
  Perioperative Medicine
University of Pittsburgh
Chief, Obstetric and Women's
  Anesthesiology
UPMC Magee Women's Hospital
UPMC Health System
Pittsburgh, Pennsylvania

Karen S. Lindeman, MD
Associate Professor
Department of Anesthesiology and Critical
  Care Medicine
Johns Hopkins University School of
  Medicine
Baltimore, Maryland

Kathryn J. Lindley, MD
Associate Professor
Departments of Medicine and Obstetrics
  and Gynecology
Vanderbilt University Medical Center
Nashville, Tennessee

Margaret E. Long, MD
Associate Professor
Department of Obstetrics and Gynecology
Mayo Clinic
Rochester, Minnesota

Leena Mathew, MD
Associate Professor
Program Director, Pain Medicine Fellowship
Department of Anesthesiology
Division of Pain Medicine
Columbia University Medical Center
New York, New York

Patrick J. McNamara, MB, BCH, BAO, MRCPCH, DCh, MSc, FASE
Professor
Departments of Pediatrics and Internal
  Medicine
University of Iowa
Iowa City, Iowa

K.A. Kelly McQueen, MD, MPH, FASA
Professor and Chair
Department of Anesthesiology
University of Wisconsin Madison
Madison, Wisconsin

Jessica M. Meister Berger, MD, JD
Assistant Professor
Department of Anesthesiology, Divisions
  of Obstetric Anesthesiology and Pain
  Medicine
Wake Forest University School of Medicine
Winston-Salem, North Carolina

Jill M. Mhyre, MD
The Dola S. Thompson Professor and Chair
Department of Anesthesiology
University of Arkansas for Medical Sciences
Little Rock, Arkansas

Rebecca D. Minehart, MD, MSHPEd
Vice Chair, Faculty Development
Division Chief, Obstetric Anesthesia
Department of Anesthesiology
Brown University Alpert School of Medicine
Providence, Rhode Island

Marie E. Minnich, MD, MMM, MBA, CPE
Associate
Division of Anesthesiology
Geisinger Health System
Danville, Pennsylvania

Jamie D. Murphy, MD
Associate Professor
Department of Anesthesiology and Critical
    Care Medicine
Johns Hopkins University
Baltimore, Maryland

Emily E. Naoum, MD
Clinical Instructor
Department of Anesthesiology
Mass General Brigham
Harvard Medical School
Boston, Massachusetts

Naveen Nathan, MD
Department of Anesthesiology, Critical Care
    and Pain Medicine
Endeavor Health
Evanston, Illinois

David B. Nelson, MD
Associate Professor
Department of Obstetrics and Gynecology
Division Chief
Division of Maternal-Fetal Medicine
University of Texas Southwestern Medical
    Center
Dallas, Texas

D. Michael Nelson, MD, PhD
Virginia S. Lang Emeritus Professor
Department of Obstetrics and Gynecology
Washington University School of Medicine
St. Louis, Missouri

Medge D. Owen, MD
Professor
Department of Anesthesiology
Wake Forest School of Medicine
Winston-Salem, North Carolina
Founder and Director
Kybele, Inc.
Lewisville, North Carolina

Luis D. Pacheco, MD
Professor
Departments of Obstetrics and Gynecology
    and Anesthesiology
University of Texas Medical Branch
Galveston, Texas

Arvind Palanisamy, MBBS, MD, FRCA
Professor
Department of Anesthesiology
Washington University School of Medicine
St. Louis, Missouri

Peter H. Pan, MD, MSEE
Professor
Department of Anesthesiology
Wake Forest School of Medicine
Winston-Salem, North Carolina

Feyce M. Peralta, MD, MS
Professor
Department of Anesthesiology
Northwestern University Feinberg School of
    Medicine
Chicago, Illinois

Emily A. Pinheiro, MD, PhD
Resident Physician
Department of Obstetrics and Gynecology
Mass General Brigham
Harvard Medical School
Boston, Massachusetts

**Phil Popham, BSc, MBBS, FRCA, MD,
PG Cert US**
Consultant (Retired)
Department of Anaesthesia
Royal Women's Hospital
Melbourne, Victoria, Australia

Roanne L. Preston, MD, FRCPC
Professor
Department of Anesthesiology,
    Pharmacology and Therapeutics
University of British Columbia
British Columbia Women's Hospital and
    Health Centre
Vancouver, British Columbia, Canada

Britany L. Raymond, MD
Assistant Professor
Department of Anesthesiology
Vanderbilt University Medical Center
Nashville, Tennessee

Sharon C. Reale, MD
Assistant Professor
Department of Anesthesiology, Perioperative
    and Pain Medicine
Brigham and Women's Hospital
Boston, Massachusetts

Mark D. Rollins, MD, PhD
Professor
Department of Anesthesiology and
    Perioperative Medicine
Mayo Clinic
Rochester, Minnesota

**Joshua I. Rosenbloom, MD, MPH,
FACOG**
Associate Clinical Professor
Department of Obstetrics and Gynecology
Hadassah Medical Center- Hebrew
    University of Jerusalem Medical School
Jerusalem, Israel

Emily E. Sharpe, MD
Associate Professor
Department of Anesthesiology and
    Perioperative Medicine
Mayo Clinic
Rochester, Minnesota

Edward R. Sherwood, MD, PhD
Professor and Vice Chair for Research
Department of Anesthesiology
Vanderbilt University Medical Center
Nashville, Tennessee

Natalie K. Smith, MD
Associate Professor
Department of Anesthesiology, Perioperative
    and Pain Medicine
Icahn School of Medicine at Mount Sinai
New York, New York

**Ban Leong Sng, MBBS, FANZCA,
FFMANZCA, MCI, FAMS**
Professor
Department of Women's Anaesthesia
KK Women's and Children's Hospital
Singapore

Catherine Y. Spong, MD
Tenured Professor and Chair
Department of Obstetrics and Gynecology
UT Southwestern Medical Center
Dallas, Texas

Catherine S. Stika, MD
Clinical Professor
Department of Obstetrics and Gynecology
Northwestern University Feinberg School of
    Medicine
Chicago, Illinois

Akila Subramaniam, MD, MPH
Associate Professor
Department of Obstetrics and Gynecology,
    Division of Maternal-Fetal Medicine
University of Alabama at Birmingham
Birmingham, Alabama

Caitlin D. Sutton, MD
Associate Professor
Department of Anesthesiology,
    Perioperative, and Pain Medicine
Texas Children's Hospital, Baylor College of
    Medicine
Houston, Texas

Hans P. Sviggum, MD
Associate Professor
Department of Anesthesiology and
    Perioperative Medicine
Mayo Clinic
Rochester, Minnesota

Hon Sen Tan, MD, MMed, MHSc
Consultant
Department of Women's Anaesthesia
KK Women's and Children's Hospital
Singapore

Alan T. N. Tita, MD, PhD
Professor
Department of Obstetrics and Gynecology
University of Alabama at Birmingham
Birmingham, Alabama

Roulhac D. Toledano, MD, PhD
Associate Professor
Department of Anesthesiology
Zucker School of Medicine at Hofstra/
    Northwell
Long Island Jewish Medical Center
New Hyde Park, New York

Paloma Toledo, MD, MPH, FASA
Professor
Department of Anesthesiology
University of Miami
Miami, Florida

Alyssa L. Trochtenberg, MD
Fellow
Department of Obstetrics and Gynecology,
    Division of Maternal-Fetal Medicine
Tufts Medical Center
Boston, Massachusetts

Lawrence C. Tsen, MD
Clinical Professor
Department of Anesthesiology
Mass General Brigham
Harvard Medical School
Director, Human Research Office
Mass General Brigham
Boston, Massachusetts

Marc Van de Velde, MD, PhD, EDRA, FESAIC
Professor and Training Coordinator
Department of Anesthesiology
UZLeuven and KULeuven
Leuven, Belgium

Mladen I. Vidovich, MD, FACC, FSCAI
Professor
Department of Medicine, Division of
    Cardiology
University of Illinois at Chicago
Chicago, Illinois

Tracey M. Vogel, MD, FASA
Obstetric Anesthesiologist
Director of the Perinatal Trauma-informed
    Care Clinic
Department of Anesthesiology
West Penn Hospital/Allegheny Health
    Network
Pittsburgh, Pennsylvania

David B. Wax, MD
Professor
Department of Anesthesiology
Icahn School of Medicine at Mount Sinai
New York, New York

Erika F. Werner, MD
Professor
Department of Obstetrics and Gynecology
Tufts University School of Medicine
Boston, Massachusetts

Richard N. Wissler, MD, PhD, FASA
Professor Emeritus
Departments of Anesthesiology and
    Perioperative Medicine and Obstetrics
    and Gynecology
University of Rochester
Director Emeritus of Obstetric Anesthesia
Strong Memorial Hospital/URMC
Rochester, New York

Cynthia A. Wong, MD
Professor and Chair
Department of Anesthesia
University of Iowa
Iowa City, Iowa

Valerie Zaphiratos, MSc, MD, FRCPC
Clinical Associate Professor
Department of Anesthesia
University of Montreal
CHU Sainte-Justine Hospital
Montreal, Quebec, Canada

PREFACE

The first edition of this text was published over 30 years ago (1994). In the preface to the first edition, David Chestnut, then the sole editor, identified two goals: (1) to collate the most important information that anesthesia providers should know about obstetrics and (2) to prepare a thorough and user-friendly review of anesthesia care for obstetric patients. Each contributor was asked to write a thorough, scholarly discussion of the subject and to provide clear, practical recommendations for clinical practice. Those goals remain intact in the seventh edition, and the result is a comprehensive resource for all anesthesia providers (and obstetricians, midwives, and family practitioners) who provide care for pregnant women.

As with every new edition, the seventh edition is an extensive revision with much new content that is highly relevant to clinical practice. Three chapters have been retired; their relevant material has been incorporated into other chapters. Two new chapters discuss racial and ethnic disparities in obstetric anesthesia and obstetric anesthesia in the developing world. Several chapters have been rewritten from start to finish, and most other chapters have undergone substantial revision.

The previous chapter on patient safety and teamwork has been renamed "Quality, Patient Safety, and Medical Error" to reflect that excellent teamwork and communication are but one aspect of quality and patient safety. The chapter on pharmacology during pregnancy and lactation has been completely rewritten to summarize mechanisms of drug disposition and effects during pregnancy, as well as the transfer of maternally administered drugs across the placenta and into breast milk. The neuraxial labor analgesia chapter includes an expanded discussion of the dural puncture epidural analgesia technique as well as an updated discussion of epidural-related maternal fever. Airway disasters remain a major cause of anesthesia-related maternal mortality; the airway chapter provides detailed information about airway management during pregnancy, especially management of the difficult airway during emergency cesarean delivery. The chapter on postoperative analgesia emphasizes the role of enhanced recovery after cesarean and multimodal analgesia in recovery from childbirth.

The updated chapter on shared decision-making in obstetric anesthesia considers many ethical aspects of providing care, including cultural considerations and conflicts that arise from the maternal-fetal relationship. The infection chapter has been updated to include information about the care of pregnant women with SARS-CoV-2 infection, and the revised cardiovascular disease chapter discusses the latest guidelines for the care of pregnant patients with cardiovascular disease. Finally, the chapter on substance use disorder summarizes the latest evidence on the care of pregnant women with this disease.

Our expert **editorial team** from the sixth edition (David H. Chestnut, Cynthia A. Wong, Lawrence C. Tsen, Warwick D. Ngan Kee, Yaakov Beilin, Jill M. Mhyre, and Brian T. Bateman) remains intact and has expanded. We are happy to welcome one outstanding new editor, **Lisa R. Leffert**. Although Dr. Chestnut remains actively involved, Dr. Wong has assumed the senior editor responsibilities, and, along with Dr. Ngan Kee, was responsible for the final seventh edition product. It seems appropriate to note that the major work for both the first and current (seventh) editions was done at the University of Iowa, where the idea and plans for this book were conceived in 1991.

Each chapter in this new edition has been carefully reviewed and edited by at least three editors. The seventh edition also includes 43 new **contributors** from around the world. We have recognized past authors of previous editions in a list in the front matter of the textbook—their superb work in prior editions provided the underpinnings for the current edition. Altogether, the seventh edition reflects the collective wisdom of a diverse group of prominent anesthesiologists and obstetricians from 25 US states and Canadian provinces, 6 other countries, and 5 continents.

The seventh edition **cover** again features a striking maternal-fetal image, which draws attention to the fact that the anesthesia provider (and the obstetrician, family practitioner, and midwife) provide simultaneous care for two (or more) patients—both the mother and her unborn child(ren). The cover image was created by an extraordinarily talented anesthesiologist and artist, Naveen Nathan, who returns as graphics editor for the seventh edition. Dr. Nathan prepared many new illustrations (and revised existing illustrations) for the updated seventh edition.

Language evolves and the terminology used in this textbook has evolved since it was first published. Of note, over the past three decades, the words describing sex and gender have also evolved. We have elected to retain the use of the words *woman*, *women*, and *mother(s)*, although we recognize that these words usually describe gender (a social construct), not sex (a biological construct). Most individuals giving birth identify as women, and almost all published studies and data refer to individuals giving birth as *women*. Thus, our use of the words *women* and *mothers* in this textbook is meant to include all individuals who give birth. Clinicians should ask their individual patients their preferred term(s) and use these words when communicating with them.

It remains gratifying to continue to receive positive feedback on this textbook. The three most common comments that we hear about the first six editions are that the content is *comprehensive*, the material is both *current* and relevant, and the writing is *clear*. Indeed, the editors place high value on clarity. We are especially grateful to our international readers because we know they are using the knowledge gained from reading our book to improve the obstetric anesthesia care of women around the world.

Similar to previous editions, we would like to acknowledge the important roles of four groups of special people.

First, we express our heartfelt thanks to the 88 distinguished and talented contributors to the seventh edition. Second, we gratefully acknowledge the invaluable help provided by our competent and loyal assistants. Third, we acknowledge the encouragement, expertise, and attention to detail provided by the professional production team at Elsevier. And finally, we should like to thank *you*, the readers, not only for your continued confidence in this textbook, but especially for your ongoing commitment to the provision of safe and compassionate care for pregnant women and their unborn children.

Cynthia A. Wong, MD
David H. Chestnut, MD
Micah 6:8

CONTENTS

PART I

Introduction

The History of Obstetric Anesthesia

Donald Caton, MD

For I heard a cry as of a woman in travail, anguish as of one bringing forth her first child, the cry of the daughter of Zion gasping for breath, stretching out her hands, "Woe is me!"

—*Jeremiah 4:31*

CHAPTER OUTLINE

Editor's Note: This chapter has remained intact since written for the first edition of the textbook published in 1994; the material continues to be as relevant today as it was then. Thus, the textbook editors have elected not to make revisions to the chapter, despite its age, but offer the following reflections.

In the last paragraph of the chapter, Dr. Caton noted that "only a fraction of the information available from basic sciences has been used to improve obstetric anesthesia care" and that "realizing the rewards from the clinical use of such information may be the most important lesson from the past and the greatest challenge for the future of obstetric anesthesia."

In the 30 years that have passed since Dr. Caton wrote these words, much has changed in the practice of obstetrics and obstetric anesthesiology. Physicians and scientists have rigorously studied and promoted evidence-based care. Much of the knowledge resulting from this research is documented in the following pages of this textbook. Our understanding of the physiologic changes of pregnancy and their effects on anesthesia care has advanced. So too has our knowledge of the drugs used in pregnancy, including their effects on pregnancy and the effects of pregnancy on drug pharmacokinetics and pharmacodynamics. Ground-breaking research on the role and techniques of neuraxial labor analgesia in the care of parturients has enabled individualized care that minimizes adverse effects on the mother and fetus/neonate. Similarly, incremental, but significant advances in anesthesia for cesarean delivery have made anesthesia care safer. As women with significant comorbid medical conditions and advanced maternal age can now conceive and carry pregnancies past the age of fetal viability, anesthesia providers are extending the depth and duration of their care of these high-risk parturients to include prepartum optimization, and

intra- and postpartum management of pain and stabilization of cardiopulmonary, hematologic, and critical care issues. Multidisciplinary, team-based care is increasingly recognized as an important contributor to patient outcomes, and anesthesia providers contribute significantly to these models of care on labor and delivery units.

But, as noted by Dr. Caton in his parting words, there is still much we do not know. We continue to rely on lessons from the past to improve care for women and their children and advance the science of obstetric anesthesiology.

"The position of woman in any civilization is an index of the advancement of that civilization; the position of woman is gauged best by the care given her at the birth of her child." So wrote Haggard[1] in 1929. If his thesis is true, Western civilization made a giant leap on January 19, 1847, when James Young Simpson used diethyl ether to anesthetize a woman with a deformed pelvis for delivery. This first use of a modern anesthetic for childbirth occurred a scant 3 months after Morton's historic demonstration of the anesthetic properties of ether at the Massachusetts General Hospital in Boston. Strangely enough, Simpson's innovation evoked strong criticism from contemporary obstetricians, who questioned its safety, and from many segments of the lay public, who questioned its wisdom. The debate over these issues lasted more than 5 years and influenced the future of obstetric anesthesia.[2]

JAMES YOUNG SIMPSON

Few people were better equipped than Simpson to deal with controversy. Just 36 years of age, Simpson already had 7 years' tenure as Professor of Midwifery at the University of

Edinburgh, one of the most prestigious medical schools of its day (Fig. 1.1). By that time, he had established a reputation as one of the foremost obstetricians in Great Britain, if not the world. On the day he first used ether for childbirth, he also received a letter of appointment as Queen's Physician in Scotland. Etherization for childbirth was only one of Simpson's contributions. He also designed obstetric forceps (which still bear his name), discovered the anesthetic properties of chloroform, made important innovations in hospital architecture, and wrote a textbook on the practice of witchcraft in Scotland that was used by several generations of anthropologists.[3]

An imposing man, Simpson had a large head, a massive mane of hair, and the pudgy body of an adolescent. Contemporaries described his voice as "commanding," with a wide range of volume and intonation. Clearly Simpson had "presence" and "charisma." These attributes were indispensable to someone in his profession, because in the mid-19th century, the role of science in the development of medical theory and practice was minimal; rhetoric resolved more issues than facts. The medical climate in Edinburgh was particularly contentious and vituperative. In this milieu, Simpson had trained, competed for advancement and recognition, and succeeded. The rigor of this preparation served him well. Initially, virtually every prominent obstetrician, including Montgomery of Dublin, Ramsbotham of London, Dubois of Paris, and Meigs of Philadelphia, opposed etherization for childbirth. Simpson called on all of his professional and personal finesse to sway opinion in the ensuing controversy.

MEDICAL OBJECTIONS TO THE USE OF ETHER FOR CHILDBIRTH

Shortly after Simpson administered the first obstetric anesthetic, he wrote, "It will be necessary to ascertain anesthesia's precise effect, both upon the action of the uterus and on the assistant abdominal muscles; its influence, if any, upon the child; whether it has a tendency to hemorrhage or other complications."[4] With this statement, he identified the issues that would most concern obstetricians who succeeded him and thus shaped the subsequent development of the specialty.

Simpson's most articulate, persistent, and persuasive critic was Charles D. Meigs, Professor of Midwifery at Jefferson Medical College in Philadelphia (Fig. 1.2). In character and stature, Meigs equaled Simpson. Born to a prominent New England family, Meigs's forebears included heroes of the American Revolutionary War, the first governor of the state of Ohio, and the founder of the University of Georgia. His descendants included a prominent pediatrician, an obstetrician, and one son who served the Union Army as Quartermaster General during the Civil War.[5]

At the heart of the dispute between Meigs and Simpson was a difference in their interpretation of the nature of labor and the significance of labor pain. Simpson maintained that all pain, labor pain included, is without physiologic value.

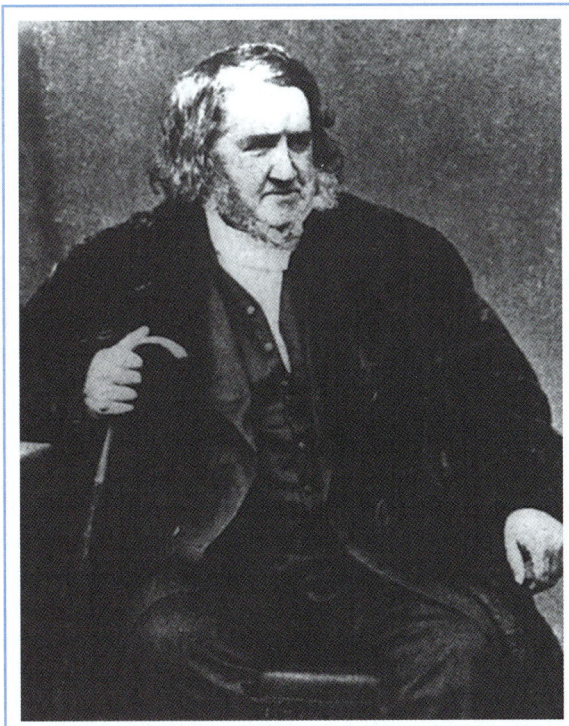

Fig. 1.1 James Young Simpson, the obstetrician who first administered a modern anesthetic for childbirth. He also discovered the anesthetic properties of chloroform. Many believe that he was the most prominent and influential physician of his day. Illustration Yale Medical History Library.

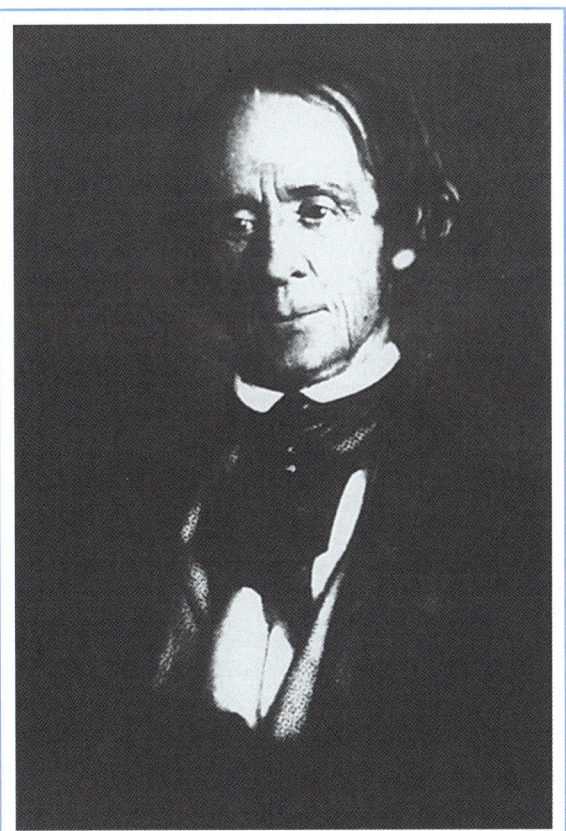

Fig. 1.2 Charles D. Meigs, the American obstetrician who opposed the use of anesthesia for obstetrics. He questioned the safety of anesthesia and said that there was no demonstrated need for it during a normal delivery. Illustration Wood-Library Museum.

He said that pain only degrades and destroys those who experience it. In contrast, Meigs argued that labor pain has purpose, that uterine pain is inseparable from contractions, and that any drug that abolishes pain will alter contractions. Meigs also believed that pregnancy and labor are normal processes that usually end quite well. He said that physicians should therefore not intervene with powerful, potentially disruptive drugs (Fig. 1.3). We must accept the statements of both men as expressions of natural philosophy, because neither had facts to buttress his position. Indeed, in 1847, physicians had little information of any sort about uterine function, pain, or the relationship between them. Studies of the anatomy and physiology of pain had just begun. It was only during the preceding 20 years that investigators had recognized that specific nerves and areas of the brain have different functions and that specialized peripheral receptors for painful stimuli exist.[2]

In 1850, more physicians expressed support for Meigs's views than for Simpson's. For example, Baron Paul Dubois[6] of the Faculty of Paris wondered whether ether, "after having exerted a stupefying action over the cerebrospinal nerves, could not induce paralysis of the muscular element of the uterus?" Similarly, Ramsbotham[7] of London Hospital said that he believed the "treatment of rendering a patient in labor completely insensible through the agency of anesthetic

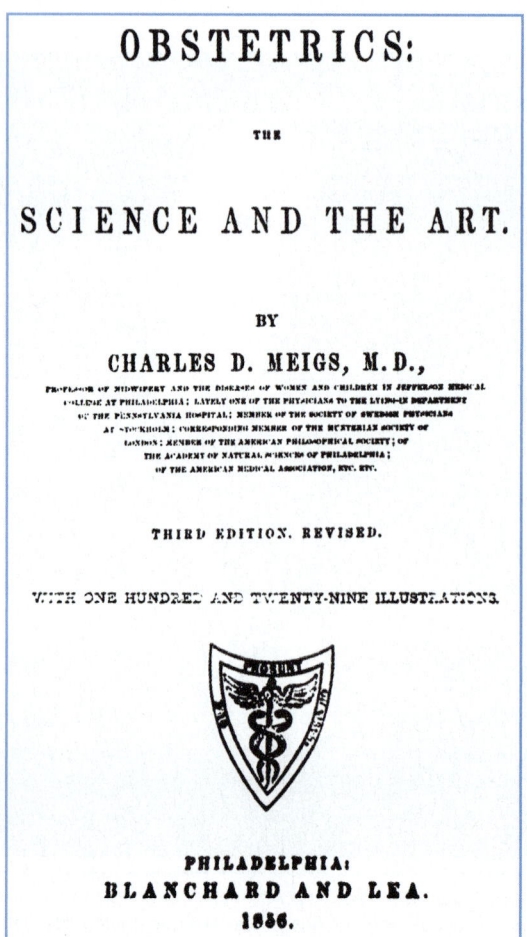

OBSTETRICS:

THE

SCIENCE AND THE ART.

BY

CHARLES D. MEIGS, M. D.,

PROFESSOR OF MIDWIFERY AND THE DISEASES OF WOMEN AND CHILDREN IN JEFFERSON MEDICAL COLLEGE AT PHILADELPHIA; LATELY ONE OF THE PHYSICIANS TO THE LYING-IN DEPARTMENT OF THE PENNSYLVANIA HOSPITAL; MEMBER OF THE SOCIETY OF SWEDISH PHYSICIANS AT STOCKHOLM; CORRESPONDING MEMBER OF THE HUSTERIAN SOCIETY OF LONDON; MEMBER OF THE AMERICAN PHILOSOPHICAL SOCIETY; OF THE ACADEMY OF NATURAL SCIENCES OF PHILADELPHIA; OF THE AMERICAN MEDICAL ASSOCIATION, ETC. ETC.

THIRD EDITION. REVISED.

WITH ONE HUNDRED AND TWENTY-NINE ILLUSTRATIONS.

PHILADELPHIA:
BLANCHARD AND LEA.
1856.

Fig. 1.3 Frontispiece From Meigs's Textbook of Obstetrics.

remedies … is fraught with extreme danger." These physicians' fears gained credence from the report by a special committee of the Royal Medical and Chirurgical Society documenting 123 deaths that "could be positively assigned to the inhalation of chloroform."[8] Although none involved obstetric patients, safety was on the minds of obstetricians.

The reaction to the delivery of Queen Victoria's eighth child in 1853 illustrated the aversion of the medical community to obstetric anesthesia. According to private records, John Snow anesthetized the Queen for the delivery of Prince Leopold at the request of her personal physicians. Although no one made a formal announcement of this fact, rumors surfaced and provoked strong public criticism. Thomas Wakley, the irascible founding editor of *The Lancet*, was particularly incensed. He "could not imagine that anyone had incurred the awful responsibility of advising the administration of chloroform to her Majesty during a perfectly natural labor with a seventh child."[9] (It was her eighth child, but Wakley had apparently lost count—a forgivable error considering the propensity of the Queen to bear children.) Court physicians did not defend their decision to use ether. Perhaps not wanting a public confrontation, they simply denied that the Queen had received an anesthetic. In fact, they first acknowledged a royal anesthetic 4 years later when the Queen delivered her ninth and last child, Princess Beatrice. By that time, however, the issue was no longer controversial.[9]

PUBLIC REACTION TO ETHERIZATION FOR CHILDBIRTH

The controversy surrounding obstetric anesthesia was not resolved by the medical community. Physicians remained skeptical, but public opinion changed. Women lost their reservations, decided they wanted anesthesia, and virtually forced physicians to offer it to them. The change in the public's attitude in favor of obstetric anesthesia marked the culmination of a more general change in social attitudes that had been developing over several centuries.

Before the 19th century, pain meant something quite different from what it does today. Since antiquity, people had believed that all manner of calamities—disease, drought, poverty, and pain—signified divine retribution inflicted as punishment for sin. According to Scripture, childbirth pain originated when God punished Eve and her descendants for Eve's disobedience in the Garden of Eden. Many believed that it was wrong to avoid the pain of divine punishment. This belief was sufficiently prevalent and strong to retard acceptance of even the idea of anesthesia, especially for obstetric patients. Only when this tradition weakened did people seek ways to free themselves from disease and pain. In most Western countries, the transition occurred during the 19th century. Disease and pain lost their theologic connotations for many people and became biologic processes subject to study and control by new methods of science and technology. This evolution of thought facilitated the development of modern medicine and stimulated public acceptance of obstetric anesthesia.[10]

The reluctance that physicians felt about the administration of anesthesia for childbirth pain stands in stark contrast to the enthusiasm expressed by early obstetric patients. In 1847, Fanny Longfellow, wife of the American poet Henry Wadsworth Longfellow and the first woman in the United States anesthetized for childbirth, wrote:

I am very sorry you all thought me so rash and naughty in trying the ether. Henry's faith gave me courage, and I had heard such a thing had succeeded abroad, where the surgeons extend this great blessing more boldly and universally than our timid doctors. … This is certainly the greatest blessing of this age.[11]

Queen Victoria, responding to news of the birth of her first grandchild in 1860 and perhaps remembering her own recent confinement, wrote, "What a blessing she [Victoria, her oldest daughter] had chloroform. Perhaps without it her strength would have suffered very much."[9] The new understanding of pain as a controllable biologic process left no room for Meigs's idea that pain might have physiologic value. The eminent 19th-century social philosopher John Stuart Mill stated that the "hurtful agencies of nature" promote good only by "inciting rational creatures to rise up and struggle against them."[12]

Simpson prophesied the role of public opinion in the acceptance of obstetric anesthesia, a fact not lost on his adversaries. Early in the controversy he predicted, "Medical men may oppose for a time the superinduction of anesthesia in parturition but they will oppose it in vain; for certainly our patients themselves will force use of it upon the profession. The whole question is, even now, one merely of time."[13] By 1860, Simpson's prophecy came true; anesthesia for childbirth became part of medical practice by public acclaim, in large part in response to the demands of women.

OPIOIDS AND OBSTETRICS

The next major innovation in obstetric anesthesia came approximately 50 years later. *Dämmerschlaff*, which means "twilight sleep," was a technique developed by von Steinbüchel[14] of Graz and popularized by Gauss[15] of Freiberg. It combined opioids with scopolamine to make women amnestic and somewhat comfortable during labor (Fig. 1.4). Until that time, opioids had been used sparingly for obstetrics. Although opium had been part of the medical armamentarium since the Roman Empire, it was not used extensively, in part because of the difficulty of obtaining consistent results with the crude extracts available at that time. Therapeutics made a substantial advance in 1809 when Sertürner, a German pharmacologist, isolated codeine and morphine from a crude extract of the poppy seed. Methods for administering the drugs remained unsophisticated. Physicians gave morphine orally or by a method resembling vaccination, in which they placed a drop of solution on the skin and then made multiple small puncture holes with a sharp instrument to facilitate absorption. In 1853, the year Queen Victoria delivered her eighth child, the syringe and hollow metal needle were developed. This technical advance simplified the administration of opioids and facilitated the development of twilight sleep approximately 50 years later.[16]

Although reports of labor pain relief with hypodermic morphine appeared as early as 1868, few physicians favored its use. For example, in an article published in *Transactions of the Obstetrical Society of London*, Sansom[17] listed the following four agents for relief of labor pain: (1) carbon tetrachloride, the use of which he favored; (2) bichloride of methylene, which was under evaluation; (3) nitrous oxide, which had been introduced recently by Klikgowich of Russia; and (4) chloroform. He did not mention opioids, but neither did he mention diethyl ether, which many physicians still favored. Similarly, Gusserow,[18] a prominent German obstetrician, described using salicylic acid but not morphine for labor pain. (Von Baeyer did not introduce acetylsalicylic acid to medical practice until 1899.) In retrospect, von Steinbüchel's and Gauss's descriptions of twilight sleep in the first decade of the century may have been important more for popularizing morphine than for suggesting that scopolamine be given with morphine.

Physicians reacted to twilight sleep as they had reacted to diethyl ether several years earlier. They resisted it, questioning whether the benefits justified the risks. Patients also reacted as they had before. Not aware of, or perhaps not concerned with, the technical considerations that confronted physicians, patients harbored few doubts and persuaded physicians to use it, sometimes against the physicians' better judgment. The confrontation between physicians and patients was particularly strident in the United States. Champions of twilight sleep lectured throughout the country and published articles in popular magazines. Public enthusiasm for the therapy subsided slightly after 1920, when a prominent advocate of the method died during childbirth. She was given twilight sleep, but her physicians said that her death was unrelated to any complication from its use. Whatever anxiety this incident may have created in the minds of patients, it did not seriously diminish their resolve. Confronted by such firm insistence, physicians acquiesced and used twilight sleep with increasing frequency.[19,20]

Vorläufige Mittheilung über die Anwendung von Skopolamin-Morphium-Injektionen in der Geburtshilfe.

Von

Dr. v. Steinbüchel,

Docent für Geburtshilfe und Gynäkologie an der Universität Graz.

(Aus der Frauenklinik in Basel.)

II. Über Medullarnarkose bei Gebärenden.

Von

Oskar Kreis,

Assistenzarzt der geburtshilflichen Abtheilung.

Fig. 1.4 Title Pages From Two Important Papers Published in the First Years of the 20th Century. The paper by von Steinbüchel introduced twilight sleep. The paper by Kreis described the first use of spinal anesthesia for obstetrics.

Although the reaction of physicians to twilight sleep resembled their reaction to etherization, the medical milieu in which the debate over twilight sleep developed was quite different from that in which etherization was deliberated. Between 1850 and 1900, medicine had changed, particularly in Europe. Physiology, chemistry, anatomy, and bacteriology became part of medical theory and practice. Bright students from America traveled to leading clinics in Germany, England, and France. They returned with new facts and methods that they used to examine problems and critique ideas. These developments became the basis for the revolution in American medical education and practice launched by the Flexner report published in 1914.[21]

Obstetrics also changed. During the years preceding World War I, it had earned a reputation as one of the most exciting and scientifically advanced specialties. Obstetricians experimented with new drugs and techniques. They recognized that change entails risk, and they examined each innovation more critically. In addition, they turned to science for information and methods to help them solve problems of medical management. Developments in obstetric anesthesia reflected this change in strategy. New methods introduced during this time stimulated physicians to reexamine two important but unresolved issues, the effects of drugs on the child, and the relationship between pain and labor.

THE EFFECTS OF ANESTHESIA ON THE NEWBORN

Many physicians, Simpson included, worried that anesthetic drugs might cross the placenta and harm the newborn. Available information justified their concern. The idea that gases cross the placenta appeared long before the discovery of oxygen and carbon dioxide. In the 16th century, English physiologist John Mayow[22] suggested that "nitro-aerial" particles from the mother nourish the fetus. By 1847, physiologists had corroborative evidence. Clinical experience gave more support. John Snow[23] observed depressed neonatal breathing and motor activity and smelled ether on the breath of neonates delivered from mothers who had been given ether. In an early paper, he surmised that anesthetic gases cross the placenta. Regardless, some advocates of obstetric anesthesia discounted the possibility. For example, Harvard Professor Walter Channing denied that ether crossed the placenta because he could not detect its odor in the cut ends of the umbilical cord. Oddly enough, he did not attempt to smell ether on the child's exhalations as John Snow had done.[24]

In 1874, Swiss obstetrician Paul Zweifel[25] published an account of work that finally resolved the debate about the placental transfer of drugs (Fig. 1.5). He used a chemical reaction to demonstrate the presence of chloroform in the umbilical blood of neonates. In a separate paper, Zweifel[26] used a light-absorption technique to demonstrate a difference in oxygen content between umbilical arterial and venous blood, thereby establishing the placental transfer of oxygen. Although clinicians recognized the importance of these data, they accepted the implications slowly. Some clinicians pointed to several

decades of clinical use "without problems." For example, Otto Spiegelberg,[27] Professor of Obstetrics at the University of Breslau, wrote in 1887, "as far as the fetus is concerned no unimpeachable clinical observation has yet been published in which a fetus was injured by chloroform administered to its mother." Experience lulled them into complacency, which may explain their failure to appreciate the threat posed by twilight sleep.

Dangers from twilight sleep probably developed insidiously. The originators of the method, von Steinbüchel and Gauss, recommended conservative doses of drugs. They suggested that 0.3 mg of scopolamine be given every 2 to 3 hours to induce amnesia and that no more than 10 mg of morphine be administered subcutaneously for the whole labor. Gauss, who was especially meticulous, even advised physicians to administer a "memory test" to women in labor to evaluate the need for additional scopolamine. However, as other physicians used the technique, they changed it. Some gave larger doses of opioid—as much as 40 or 50 mg of morphine during labor. Others gave additional drugs (e.g., as much as 600 mg of pentobarbital during labor and inhalation agents for delivery). Despite administering these large doses to their patients, some physicians said they had seen no adverse effects on the infants.[28] They probably spoke the truth, but this probability says more about their powers of observation than the safety of the method.

Two situations eventually made physicians confront problems associated with placental transmission of anesthetic

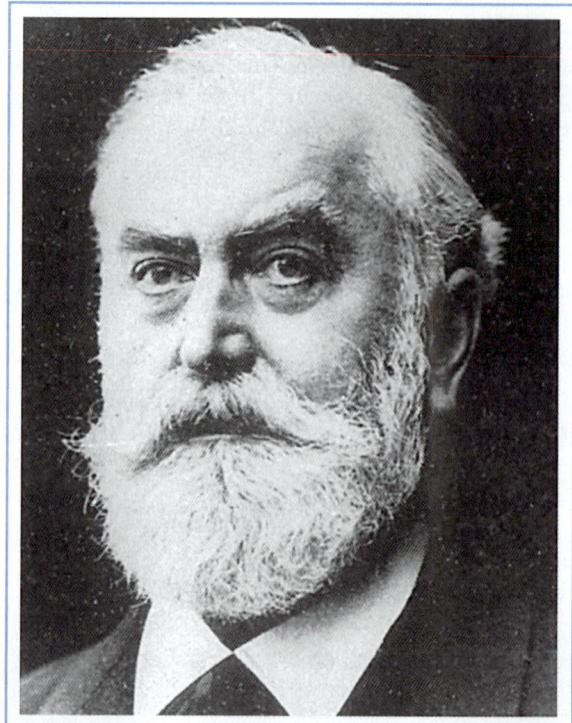

Fig. 1.5 Paul Zweifel, the Swiss-born obstetrician who performed the first experiments that chemically demonstrated the presence of chloroform in the umbilical blood and urine of infants delivered by women who had been anesthetized during labor. Illustration J.F. Bergmann-Verlag, München, Germany.

drugs. The first was the changing use of morphine.[29] In the latter part of the 19th century (before the enactment of laws governing the use of addictive drugs), morphine was a popular ingredient of patent medicines and a drug frequently prescribed by physicians. As addiction became more common, obstetricians saw many pregnant women who were taking large amounts of morphine daily. When they tried to decrease their patients' opioid use, several obstetricians noted unexpected problems (e.g., violent fetal movements, sudden fetal death), which they correctly identified as signs of withdrawal. Second, physiologists and anatomists began extensive studies of placental structure and function. By the turn of the century, they had identified many of the physical and chemical factors that affect rates of drug transfer. Thus, even before twilight sleep became popular, physicians had clinical and laboratory evidence to justify caution. As early as 1877, Gillette[30] described 15 instances of neonatal depression that he attributed to morphine given during labor. Similarly, in a review article published in 1914, Knipe[31] identified stillbirths and neonatal oligopnea and asphyxia as complications of twilight sleep and gave the incidence of each problem as reported by other writers.

When the studies of obstetric anesthesia published between 1880 and 1950 are considered, four characteristics stand out. First, few of them described effects of anesthesia on the newborn. Second, those who did report newborn apnea, oligopnea, or asphyxia seldom defined these words. Third, few used controls or compared one mode of treatment with another. Finally, few writers used their data to evaluate the safety of the practice that they described. In other words, by today's standards, even the best of these papers lacked substance. They did, however, demonstrate a growing concern among physicians about the effects of anesthetic drugs on neonates. Perhaps even more important, their work prepared clinicians for the work of Virginia Apgar (Fig. 1.6).

Apgar became an anesthesiologist when the chairman of the Department of Surgery at the Columbia University College of Physicians and Surgeons dissuaded her from becoming a surgeon. After training in anesthesia with Ralph Waters at the University of Wisconsin and with E.A. Rovenstine at Bellevue Hospital, she returned to Columbia Presbyterian Hospital as director of the Division of Anesthesia. In 1949, she was appointed professor, the first woman to attain that rank at Columbia University.[32]

In 1953, Apgar[33] described a simple, reliable system for evaluating newborns and showed that it was sufficiently sensitive to detect differences among neonates whose mothers had been anesthetized for cesarean delivery by different techniques (Fig. 1.7). Infants delivered of women with spinal anesthesia had higher scores than those delivered with general anesthesia. The Apgar score had three important effects. First, it replaced simple observation of neonates with a reproducible measurement—that is, it substituted a numerical score for the ambiguities of words such as oligopnea and asphyxia. Thus, it established the possibility of the systematic comparison of different treatments. Second, it provided objective criteria for the initiation of neonatal resuscitation. Third, and

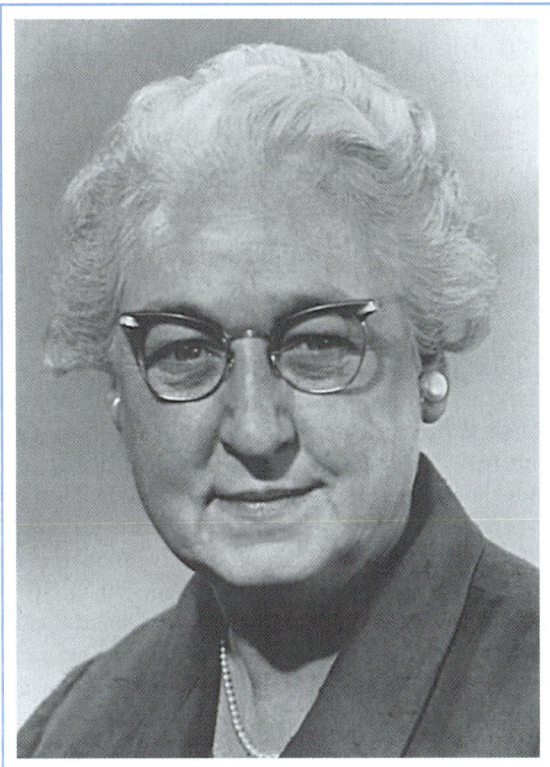

Fig. 1.6 Virginia Apgar, whose scoring system revolutionized the practice of obstetrics and anesthesia. Her work made the well-being of the infant the major criterion for the evaluation of medical management of pregnant women. Illustration Wood-Library Museum.

Current Researches in Anesthesia and Analgesia—July-August, 1953

A Proposal for a New Method of Evaluation of the Newborn Infant.*
Virginia Apgar, M.D., New York, N. Y.
Department of Anesthesiology, Columbia University, College of Physicians and Surgeons and the Anesthesia Service, The Presbyterian Hospital

Fig. 1.7 Title page from the paper in which Virginia Apgar described her new scoring system for evaluating the well-being of a newborn.

most important, it helped change the focus of obstetric care. Until that time, the primary criterion for success or failure had been the survival and well-being of the mother, a natural goal considering the maternal risks of childbirth until that time. After 1900, as maternal risks diminished, the well-being of the mother no longer served as a sensitive measure of outcome. The Apgar score called attention to the child and made its condition the new standard for evaluating obstetric management.

THE EFFECTS OF ANESTHESIA ON LABOR

The effects of anesthesia on labor also worried physicians. Again, their fears were well founded. Diethyl ether and chloroform depress uterine contractions. If given in sufficient amounts, they also abolish reflex pushing with the abdominal muscles during the second stage of labor. These effects are not difficult to detect, even with moderate doses of either inhalation agent.

Simpson's method of obstetric anesthesia used significant amounts of drugs. He started the anesthetic early, and sometimes he rendered patients unconscious during the first stage of labor. In addition, he increased the depth of anesthesia for the delivery.[34] As many people copied his technique, they presumably had ample opportunity to observe uterine atony and postpartum hemorrhage.

Some physicians noticed the effects of anesthetics on uterine function. For example, Meigs[35] said unequivocally that etherization suppressed uterine function, and he described occasions in which he had had to suspend etherization to allow labor to resume. Other physicians waffled, however. For example, Walter Channing,[36] Professor of Midwifery and Medical Jurisprudence at Harvard (seemingly a strange combination of disciplines, but at that time neither of the two was thought sufficiently important to warrant a separate chair), published a book about the use of ether for obstetrics (Fig. 1.8). He endorsed etherization and influenced many others to use it. However, his book contained blatant contradictions. On different pages Channing contended that ether had no effect, that it increased uterine contractility, and that it suspended contractions entirely. Then, in a pronouncement smacking more of panache than reason, Channing swept aside his inconsistencies and said that whatever effect ether may have on the uterus he "welcomes it." Noting similar contradictions among other writers, W.F.H. Montgomery,[37] Professor of Midwifery at the King and Queen's College of Physicians in Ireland, wrote, "By one writer we are told that, if uterine action is excessive, chloroform will abate it; by another that if feeble, it will strengthen it and add new vigor to each parturient effort."

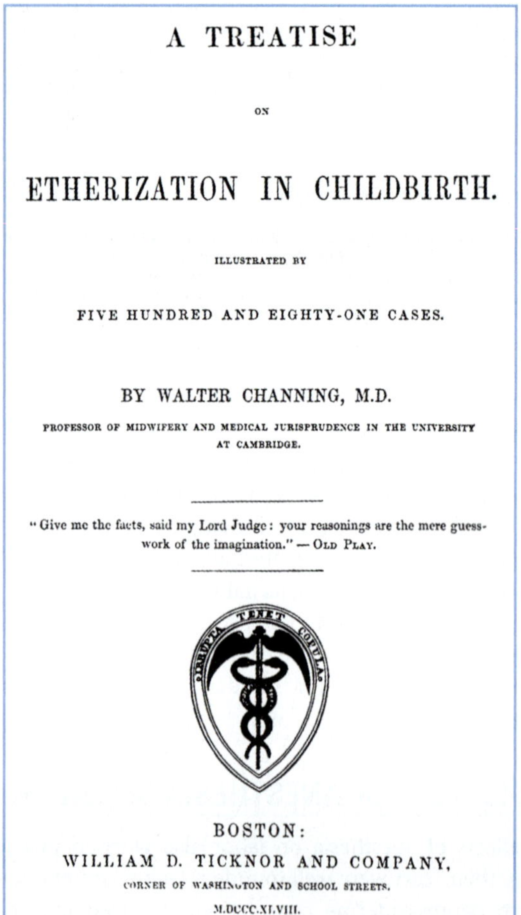

John Snow[23] gave a more balanced review of the effects of anesthesia on labor. Originally a surgeon, Snow became the first physician to restrict his practice to anesthesia. He experimented with ether and chloroform and wrote many insightful papers and books describing his work (Fig. 1.9). Snow's technique differed from Simpson's. Snow withheld anesthesia until the second stage of labor, limited administration to brief periods during contractions, and attempted to keep his patients comfortable but responsive. To achieve better control of the depth of anesthesia, he recommended using the vaporizing apparatus that he had developed for surgical cases. Snow[23] spoke disparagingly of Simpson's technique and the tendency of people to use it simply because of Simpson's reputation:

> The high position of Dr. Simpson and his previous services in this department, more particularly in being the first to administer ether in labour, gave his recommendations very great influence; the consequence of which is that the practice of anesthesia is presently probably in a much less satisfactory state than it would have been if chloroform had never been introduced.

Snow's method, which was the same one he had used to anesthetize Queen Victoria, eventually prevailed over Simpson's. Physicians became more cautious with anesthesia, reserving it for special problems such as cephalic version, the application of forceps, abnormal presentation, and eclampsia. They also became more conservative with dosage, often giving anesthesia only during the second stage of labor. Snow's methods were applied to each new inhalation agent—including nitrous oxide, ethylene, cyclopropane, trichloroethylene, and methoxyflurane—as it was introduced to obstetric anesthesia.

Early physicians modified their use of anesthesia from experience, not from study of normal labor or from learning more about the pharmacology of the drugs. Moreover, they had not yet defined the relationship between uterine pain and contractions. As physicians turned more to science during the latter part of the century, however, their strategies began to change. For example, in 1893, the English physiologist Henry Head[38] published his classic studies of the innervation of abdominal viscera. His work stimulated others to investigate the role of the nervous system in the control of labor. Subsequently, clinical and laboratory studies of pregnancy after spinal cord transection established the independence of labor from nervous control.[39] When regional anesthesia appeared during the first decades of the 20th century, physicians therefore had a conceptual basis from which to explore its effects on labor.

A TREATISE

ON

ETHERIZATION IN CHILDBIRTH.

ILLUSTRATED BY

FIVE HUNDRED AND EIGHTY-ONE CASES.

BY WALTER CHANNING, M.D.

PROFESSOR OF MIDWIFERY AND MEDICAL JURISPRUDENCE IN THE UNIVERSITY AT CAMBRIDGE.

"Give me the facts, said my Lord Judge: your reasonings are the mere guess-work of the imagination." — OLD PLAY.

BOSTON:
WILLIAM D. TICKNOR AND COMPANY,
CORNER OF WASHINGTON AND SCHOOL STREETS.
M.DCCC.XLVIII.

Fig. 1.8 Frontispiece From Walter Channing's Book on the Use of Etherization for Childbirth. Channing favored the use of etherization, and he persuaded others to use it, although evidence ensuring its safety was scant.

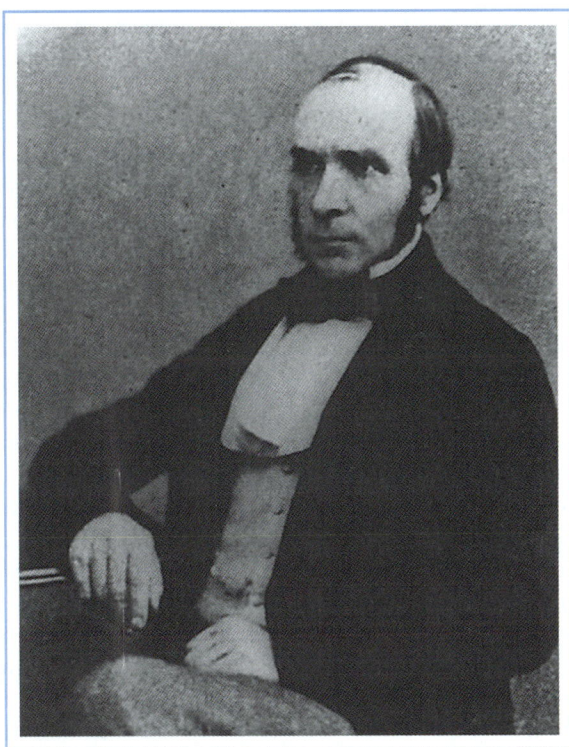

Fig. 1.9 John Snow, a London surgeon who gave up his surgical practice to become the first physician to devote all his time to anesthesia. He wrote many monographs and papers, some of which accurately describe the effects of anesthesia on the infant and mother. Illustration Wood-Library Museum.

Carl Koller[40] introduced regional anesthesia when he used cocaine for eye surgery in 1884. Recognizing the potential of Koller's innovation, surgeons developed techniques for other procedures. Obstetricians quickly adopted many of these techniques for their own use. The first papers describing obstetric applications of spinal, lumbar epidural, caudal, paravertebral, parasacral, and pudendal nerve blocks appeared between 1900 and 1930 (see Fig. 1.4).[41–43] Recognition of the potential effects of regional anesthesia on labor developed more slowly, primarily because obstetricians seldom used it. They continued to rely on inhalation agents and opioids, partly because few drugs and materials were available for regional anesthesia at that time, but also because obstetricians did not appreciate the chief advantage of regional over general anesthesia—the relative absence of drug effects on the infant. Moreover, they rarely used regional anesthesia except for delivery, and then they often used elective forceps anyway. This set of circumstances limited their opportunity and motivation to study the effects of regional anesthesia on labor.

Among early papers dealing with regional anesthesia, one written by Cleland[44] stands out. He described his experience with paravertebral anesthesia, but he also wrote a thoughtful analysis of the nerve pathways mediating labor pain, an analysis he based on information he had gleaned from clinical and laboratory studies. Few investigators were as meticulous or insightful as Cleland. Most of those who studied the effects of anesthesia simply timed the length of the first and second stages of labor. Some timed the duration of individual contractions or estimated changes in the strength of contractions by palpation. None of the investigators measured the intrauterine pressures, even though a German physician had described such a method in 1898 and had used it to evaluate the effects of morphine and ether on the contractions of laboring women.[45]

More detailed and accurate studies of the effects of anesthesia started to appear after 1944. Part of the stimulus was a method for continuous caudal anesthesia introduced by Hingson and Edwards,[46] in which a malleable needle remained in the sacral canal throughout labor. Small, flexible plastic catheters eventually replaced malleable needles and made continuous epidural anesthesia even more popular. With the help of these innovations, obstetricians began using anesthesia earlier in labor. Ensuing problems, real and imagined, stimulated more studies. Although good studies were scarce, the strong interest in the problem represented a marked change from the early days of obstetric anesthesia.

Ironically, "natural childbirth" appeared just as regional anesthesia started to become popular and as clinicians began to understand how to use it without disrupting labor. Dick-Read,[47] the originator of the natural method, recognized "no physiological function in the body which gives rise to pain in the normal course of health." He attributed pain in an otherwise uncomplicated labor to an "activation of the sympathetic nervous system by the emotion of fear." He argued that fear made the uterus contract and become ischemic and therefore painful. He said that women could avoid the pain if they simply learned to abolish their fear of labor. Dick-Read never explained why uterine ischemia that results from fear causes pain, whereas ischemia that results from a normal contraction does not. In other words, Dick-Read, like Simpson a century earlier, claimed no necessary or physiologic relationship between labor pain and contractions. Dick-Read's book, written more for the public than for the medical profession, represented a regression of almost a century in medical thought and practice. It is important to note that contemporary methods of childbirth preparation do not maintain that fear alone causes labor pain. However, they do attempt to reduce fear by education and to help patients manage pain by teaching techniques of self-control. This represents a significant difference from and an important advance over Dick-Read's original theory.

SOME LESSONS

History is important in proportion to the lessons it teaches. With respect to obstetric anesthesia, four lessons stand out. First, every new drug and method entails risks. Physicians who first used obstetric anesthesia seemed reluctant to accept this fact, perhaps because of their inexperience with potent drugs (pharmacology was in its infancy) or because they acceded too quickly to patients, who wanted relief from pain and had little understanding of the technical issues confronting physicians. Whatever the reason, this period of denial lasted almost half a century, until 1900. Almost another half-century passed before obstetricians learned to modify their practice to limit the effects of anesthetics on the child and the labor process.

Second, new drugs or therapies often cause problems in completely unexpected ways. For example, in 1900, physicians noted a rising rate of puerperal fever.[48] The timing was odd. Several decades had passed since Robert Koch had suggested the germ theory of disease and since Semmelweis had recognized that physicians often transmit infection from one woman to the next with their unclean hands. With the adoption of aseptic methods, deaths from puerperal fever had diminished dramatically. During the waning years of the 19th century, however, they increased again. Some physicians attributed this resurgence of puerperal fever to anesthesia. In a presidential address to the Obstetrical Society of Edinburgh in 1900, Murray[49] stated the following:

> I feel sure that an explanation of much of the increase of maternal mortality from 1847 onwards will be found in, first the misuse of anaesthesia and second in the ridiculous parody which, in many hands, stands for the use of antiseptics. … Before the days of anaesthesia, interference was limited and obstetric operations were at a minimum because interference of all kinds increased the conscious suffering of the patient. … When anaesthesia became possible, and interference became more frequent because it involved no additional suffering, operations were undertaken when really unnecessary … and so complications arose and the dangers of the labor increased.

Although it was not a direct complication of the use of anesthesia in obstetric practice, puerperal fever appeared to be an indirect consequence of it.

Changes in obstetric practice also had unexpected effects on anesthetic complications. During the first decades of the 20th century, when cesarean deliveries were rare and obstetricians used only inhalation analgesia for delivery, few women were exposed to the risk of aspiration during deep anesthesia. As obstetric practice changed and cesarean deliveries became more common, this risk rose. The syndrome of aspiration was not identified and labeled until 1946, when obstetrician Curtis Mendelson[50] described and named it. The pathophysiology of the syndrome had already been described by Winternitz et al.,[51] who instilled hydrochloric acid into the lungs of dogs to simulate the lesions found in veterans poisoned by gas during the trench warfare of World War I. Unfortunately, the reports of these studies, although excellent, did not initiate any change in practice. Change occurred only after several deaths of obstetric patients were highly publicized in lay, legal, and medical publications. Of course,

rapid-sequence induction, currently recommended to reduce the risk for aspiration, creates another set of risks—those associated with a failed intubation.

The third lesson offered by the history of obstetric anesthesia concerns the role of basic science. Modern medicine developed during the 19th century after physicians learned to apply principles of anatomy, physiology, and chemistry to the study and treatment of disease. Obstetric anesthesia underwent a similar pattern of development. Studies of placental structure and function called physicians' attention to the transmission of drugs and the potential effects of drugs on the infant. Similarly, studies of the physiology and anatomy of the uterus helped elucidate potential effects of anesthesia on labor. In each instance, lessons from basic science helped improve patient care.

The fourth and perhaps the most important lesson is the role that patients have played in the use of anesthesia for obstetrics. During the 19th century, it was women who pressured cautious physicians to incorporate routine use of anesthesia into their obstetric practice. A century later, it was women again who altered patterns of practice, this time questioning the overuse of anesthesia for routine deliveries. In both instances, the pressure on physicians emanated from prevailing social values regarding pain. In 1900, the public believed that pain, and in particular obstetric pain, was destructive and something that should be avoided. Half a century later, with the advent of the natural childbirth movement, many people began to suggest that the experience of pain during childbirth, perhaps even in other situations, might have some physiologic if not social value. Physicians must recognize and acknowledge the extent to which social values may shape medical "science" and practice.[52,53]

During the past 80 years, scientists have accumulated a wealth of information about many processes integral to normal labor: the processes that initiate and control lactation; neuroendocrine events that initiate and maintain labor; the biochemical maturation of the fetal lung and liver; the metabolic requirements of the normal fetus and the protective mechanisms that it may invoke in times of stress; and the normal mechanisms that regulate the amount and distribution of blood flow to the uterus and placenta. At this point, we have only the most rudimentary understanding of the interaction of anesthesia with any of these processes. Only a fraction of the information available from basic science has been used to improve obstetric anesthesia care. Realizing the rewards from the clinical use of such information may be the most important lesson from the past and the greatest challenge for the future of obstetric anesthesia.

KEY POINTS

- Physicians have debated the safety of obstetric anesthesia since 1847, when James Young Simpson first administered anesthesia for delivery. Two issues have dominated the debate: the effects of anesthesia on labor and the effects of anesthesia on the newborn.

- Despite controversy, physicians quickly incorporated anesthesia into clinical practice, largely because of their patients' desire to avoid childbirth pain.
- Only after obstetric anesthesia was in use for many years did problems become apparent.

- Important milestones in obstetric anesthesia are the introduction of inhalation agents in 1847, the expanded use of opioids in the early decades of the 20th century, and the refinement of regional anesthesia starting in the mid-20th century.
- Outstanding conceptual developments include (1) Zweifel's idea that drugs given to the mother cross the placenta and affect the fetus and (2) Apgar's idea that the condition of the newborn is the most sensitive assay of the quality of anesthetic care of the mother.
- The history of obstetric anesthesia suggests that the major improvements in patient care have followed the application of principles of basic science.

REFERENCES

1. Haggard HW. *Devils, Drugs, and Doctors: The Story of the Science of Healing From Medicine-Man to Doctor*. Harper & Brothers; 1929.
2. Caton D. *What a Blessing She Had Chloroform: The Medical and Social Response to the Pain of Childbirth From 1800 to the Present*. Yale University Press; 1999.
3. Shepherd JA. *Simpson and Syme of Edinburgh*. E & S Livingstone; 1969.
4. Simpson WG, ed. *The Works of Sir JY Simpson. Vol. II. Anaesthesia*. Adam and Charles Black; 1871: 199–200.
5. Levinson A. The three Meigs and their contribution to pediatrics. *Ann Med Hist*. 1928;10:138–148.
6. Dubois P. On the inhalation of ether applied to cases of midwifery. *Lancet*. 1847;49:246–249.
7. Ramsbotham FH. *The Principles and Practice of Obstetric Medicine and Surgery in Reference to the Process of Parturition With Sixty-Four Plates and Numerous Wood-Cuts*. Blanchard and Lea; 1855.
8. Report of the Committee Appointed by the Royal Medical and Chirurgical Society to Inquire into the Uses and the Physiological, Therapeutical, and Toxical Effects of Chloroform, as Well as into the Best Mode of Administering it, and of Obviating Any Ill Consequences Resulting from its Administration. *Med Chir Trans*. 1864;47:323–442.
9. Sykes WS. *Essays on the First Hundred Years of Anaesthesia. Vol. I*. Wood Library Museum of Anesthesiology; 1982.
10. Caton D. The secularization of pain. *Anesthesiology*. 1985;62:493–501.
11. Wagenknecht E, ed. *Mrs. Longfellow: Selected Letters and Journals of Fanny Appleton Longfellow*. Longmans, Green; 1956:1817–1861.
12. Cohen M, ed. *Nature: The Philosophy of John Stuart Mill*. Modern Library; 1961:463–467.
13. Simpson WG, ed. *The Works of Sir JY Simpson. Vol. II. Anaesthesia*. Adam and Charles Black; 1871:177.
14. von Steinbüchel R. Vorläufige Mitteilung über die Anwendung von Skopolamin-Morphium-Injektionen in der Geburtshilfe. *Zentralblatt Gynäkol*. 1902;30:1304–1306.
15. Gauss CJ. Die Anwendung des Skopolamin-Morphium-Dämmerschlafes in der Geburtshilfe. *Med Klin*. 1906;2: 136–138.
16. Macht DI. The history of opium and some of its preparations and alkaloids. *JAMA*. 1915;64:477–481.
17. Sansom AE. On the pain of parturition, and anaesthetics in obstetric practice. *Trans Obstet Soc Lond*. 1868;10:121–140.
18. Gusserow A. Zur Lehre vom Stoffwechsel des Foetus. *Arch Gynäkol*. 1871;3:241.
19. Wertz RW, Wertz DC. *Lying-In: A History of Childbirth in America*. Schocken Books; 1979.
20. Leavitt JW. *Brought to Bed: Childbearing in America*. Oxford University Press; 1986:1750–1950.
21. Kaufman M. *American Medical Education: The Formative Years*. Greenwood Press; 1976:1765–1910.
22. Mayow J. *Tractatus quinque medico-physici*. Quoted in: Needham J. *Chemical Embryology*. Hafner Publishing; 1963.
23. Snow J. On the administration of chloroform during parturition. *Assoc Med J*. 1853;1:500–502.
24. Caton D. Obstetric anesthesia and concepts of placental transport: a historical review of the nineteenth century. *Anesthesiology*. 1977;46:132–137.
25. Zweifel P. Einfluss der Chloroformnarcose Kreissender auf den Fötus. *Klin Wochenschr*. 1874;21:1–2.
26. Zweifel P. Die Respiration des Fotus. *Arch Gynäkol*. 1876;9: 291–305.
27. Spiegelberg O. *A Textbook of Midwifery*. The New Sydenham Society; 1887.
28. Gwathmey JT. A further study, based on more than twenty thousand cases. *Surg Gynecol Obstet*. 1930;51:190–195.
29. Terry CE, Pellens M. *The Opium Problem*. Bureau of Social Hygiene; 1928.
30. Gillette WR. The narcotic effect of morphia on the new-born child, when administered to the mother in labor. *Am J Obstet Dis Women Child*. 1877;10:612–623.
31. Knipe WHW. The Freiburg method of Daemmerschlaf or twilight sleep. *Am J Obstet Gynecol*. 1914;70:884.
32. Calmes SH. Virginia Apgar: a woman physician's career in a developing specialty. *J Am Med Wom Assoc*. 1984;39:184–188.
33. Apgar V. A proposal for a new method of evaluation of the newborn infant. *Curr Res Anesth Analg*. 1953;32:260–267.
34. Thoms H. Anesthesia á la Reine—a chapter in the history of anesthesia. *Am J Obstet Gynecol*. 1940;40:340–346.
35. Meigs CD. *Obstetrics, The Science and the Art*. Blanchard and Lea; 1865:364–376.
36. Channing W. *A Treatise on Etherization in Childbirth*. William D. Ticknor and Company; 1848.
37. Montgomery WFH. *Objections to the Indiscriminate Administration of Anaesthetic Agents in Midwifery*. Hodges and Smith; 1849.
38. Head H. On disturbances of sensation with especial reference to the pain of visceral disease. *Brain*. 1893;16(1–2).
39. Gertsman NM. Über Uterusinnervation an Hand des Falles einer Geburt bei Quersnittslahmung. *Monatsschrift Geburtshuffle Gynäkol*. 1926;73:253–257.
40. Koller C. On the use of cocaine for producing anaesthesia on the eye. *Lancet*. 1884;124:990–992.
41. Kreis O. Über Medullarnarkose bei Gebärenden. *Zentralblatt Gynäkol*. 1900;28:724–727.
42. Bonar BE, Meeker WR. The value of sacral nerve block anesthesia in obstetrics. *JAMA*. 1923;89:1079–1083.
43. Schlimpert H. Concerning sacral anaesthesia. *Surg Gynecol Obstet*. 1913;16:488–492.

44. Cleland JGP. Paravertebral anaesthesia in obstetrics. *Surg Gynecol Obstet.* 1933;57:51–62.

45. Hensen H. Über den Einfluss des Morphiums und des Äthers auf die Wehenthätigkeit des Uterus. *Arch Gynäkol.* 1898;55: 129–177.

46. Hingson RA, Edwards WB. Continuous caudal analgesia: an analysis of the first ten thousand confinements thus managed with the report of the authors' first thousand cases. *JAMA.* 1943;123:538–546.

47. Dick-Read G. *Childbirth Without Fear: The Principles and Practice of Natural Childbirth.* Harper & Row; 1970.

48. Lea AWW. *Puerperal Infection.* Oxford University Press; 1910.

49. Murray M. Presidential address to the Obstetrical Society of Edinburgh, 1900. Quoted in: Cullingworth CJ. Oliver Wendell Holmes and the contagiousness of puerperal fever. *J Obstet Gynaecol Br Emp.* 1905;8:387–388.

50. Mendelson CL. The aspiration of stomach contents into the lungs during obstetric anesthesia. *Am J Obstet Gynecol.* 1946;52:191–205.

51. Winternitz MC, Smith GH, McNamara FP. Effect of intrabronchial insufflation of acid. *J Exp Med.* 1920;32: 199–204.

52. Caton D. "The poem in the pain": the social significance of pain in Western civilization. *Anesthesiology.* 1994;81: 1044–1052.

53. Caton D. Medical science and social values. *Int J Obstet Anesth.* 2004;13:167–173.

PART II

Maternal and Fetal Physiology

Physiologic Changes of Pregnancy

Rachel M. Kacmar, MD

CHAPTER OUTLINE

Marked anatomic and physiologic changes occur during pregnancy to allow the woman to adapt to the developing fetus and its metabolic demands. The enlarging gravid uterus places mechanical strain on the woman's body. Greater hormonal production by the ovaries and the placenta further alters maternal physiology. The hallmark of successful anesthetic management of the pregnant woman is recognition of these changes and appropriate adaptation of anesthetic techniques to account for them. The physiologic alterations of normal pregnancy and their anesthetic implications are reviewed in this chapter.

BODY WEIGHT AND COMPOSITION

The mean maternal weight increase during pregnancy is 17% of the prepregnancy weight or approximately 12 kg. It results from an increase in the size of the uterus and its contents (uterus, 1 kg; amniotic fluid, 1 kg; fetus and placenta, 4 kg), increases in blood volume and interstitial fluid (approximately 1 kg each), and deposition of new fat and protein (approximately 4 kg). Maternal resting metabolic rate increases steadily across pregnancy.[1] The weight gain during pregnancy recommended by the Institute of Medicine is tiered based on prepregnancy body mass index (BMI; Table 2.1) and reflects the increasing incidence of obesity.[2] The expected weight increase during the first trimester in a nonobese individual is 1 to 2 kg, and there is a 5- to 6-kg increase in each of the last two trimesters. The recommended gain is less in individuals with obesity, and recent studies propose weight gain during pregnancy should be restricted to a maximum of 5 kg in patients with preconception BMI $\geq 35 \, kg/m^2$.[1] Excessive weight gain during pregnancy is a risk factor for a long-term increase in BMI.[3]

TABLE 2.1 Recommended Weight Gain During Pregnancy

Prepregnancy Body Mass Index (kg/m²)	Total Weight Gain in kg (lb)	Rate of Weight Gain During Second and Third Trimester in kg/w (lb/w)
<18.5	12.7–18.2 (28–40)	0.45 (1)
18.5–24.9	11.4–15.9 (25–35)	0.45 (1)
25.0–29.9	6.8–11.4 (15–25)	0.27 (0.6)
≥30	5.0–9.1 (11–20)	0.23 (0.5)

Modified from Rasmussen KM, Yaktine AL, eds. *Weight Gain During Pregnancy: Reexamining the Guidelines*. National Academies Press; 2009; CDC. *CDC Guidelines for Weight Gain in Pregnancy*. https://www.cdc.gov/maternal-infant-health/pregnancy-weight/index.html. Accessed 9 March 2024.

BOX 2.1 Changes in the Cardiac Examination in the Pregnant Patient

- Accentuation of first heart sound (S1) and exaggerated splitting of the mitral and tricuspid components
- Typical systolic ejection murmur
- Possible presence of third heart sound (S3) and fourth heart sound (S4); no clinical significance
- Leftward displacement of point of maximal cardiac impulse

CARDIOVASCULAR CHANGES

Physical Examination and Cardiac Studies

Pregnancy causes the heart to increase in size, a result of both greater blood volume and increased stretch and force of contraction.[4] These changes, coupled with the elevation of the diaphragm from the expanding uterus, cause several changes in the physical examination and in cardiac studies.

Changes in heart sounds include accentuation of the first heart sound with exaggerated splitting of the mitral and tricuspid components (Box 2.1).[5] The second heart sound changes little, although the aortic-pulmonic interval tends to vary less with respiration during the third trimester, a finding without clinical significance. A fourth heart sound may be heard in 16% of pregnant women, although typically it disappears at term. A grade II systolic ejection murmur is commonly heard at the left sternal border[6]; the murmur is considered a benign flow murmur, attributable to cardiac enlargement from increased intravascular volume, which causes dilation of the tricuspid annulus and mild tricuspid regurgitation. Elevation of the diaphragm by the growing uterus may shift the mediastinum anteriorly. Evidence of cephalad cardiac displacement varies by study with minimal change in position seen from magnetic resonance imaging[7] and up to 6 cm cranial shift seen on transthoracic echocardiography.[8] No change in hand position for cardiopulmonary resuscitation is recommended for pregnant women compared with nonpregnant women.

Echocardiography demonstrates left ventricular (LV) hypertrophy by 12 weeks' gestation with a 23% increase in LV mass from the first to the third trimester[9] and an overall 50% increase in mass at term.[10] This eccentric hypertrophy results from an increase in the size of the preexisting cardiomyocytes, resembling the changes that occur from repeated, strenuous exercise.[11] Left atrial diameter increases during pregnancy with maximum diameter in the third trimester.[12] The annular diameters of the mitral, tricuspid, and pulmonic valves increase; 94% of term pregnant women exhibit tricuspid and pulmonic regurgitation, and 27% exhibit mitral regurgitation.[13] The aortic annulus does not dilate from normal pregnancy-induced physiologic changes.

The electrocardiogram typically changes, especially during the third trimester. Heart rate steadily increases during the first and second trimesters, and both the PR interval and the uncorrected QT interval are shortened. This has clinical implications for women with long QT syndrome (see Chapter 41). The QRS axis shifts to the right during the first trimester but may shift to the left during the third trimester.[14] Depressed ST segments and isoelectric low-voltage T waves in the left-sided precordial and limb leads are common.[15]

Central Hemodynamics

To accurately determine central hemodynamic values and/or changes during pregnancy, patient position should be considered to minimize the impact of aortocaval compression. Comparisons must be made with an appropriate control, such as prepregnancy values or a matched group of nonpregnant women. If control measurements are made postpartum, a sufficient interval must elapse for parameters to have returned to prepregnancy values; this may take weeks to months.[16] There is significant heterogeneity in cardiac output measurement using different noninvasive devices; these differences should be taken into account when caring for individual patients.[17] There may also be diurnal variation in cardiac output, cardiac index, and heart rate measurements, with the highest measurements occurring in the afternoon.[18]

Cardiac output begins to increase by 5 weeks' gestation and is 35% to 40% above baseline by the end of the first trimester.[10,19] It continues increasing throughout the second trimester to approximately 50% greater than nonpregnant values (Figs. 2.1 and 2.2).[10,16,20,21] Cardiac output does not change further during the third trimester.[22] Some studies have reported a decrease in cardiac output during the third trimester; however, typically this is with measurements made in the supine position and thus likely reflects vena caval compression rather than a true gestational decline.

The initial increase in cardiac output results from an increase in heart rate.[10] Heart rate increases 15% to 25% above baseline by the end of the first trimester and remains relatively stable for the remainder of the pregnancy.[10,16,19–21,23] Cardiac output continues to increase through the second trimester owing to an increase in stroke volume. Stroke volume increases by approximately 20% during the first trimester and by 25% to 30% above baseline during the second trimester.[10,16,19,23] The increased stroke volume correlates with increasing estrogen levels.[11] Stroke volume index decreases over the course of pregnancy, while cardiac index remains slightly increased from prepregnancy values.[22]

LV end-diastolic volume increases during pregnancy, whereas end-systolic volume remains unchanged, resulting in

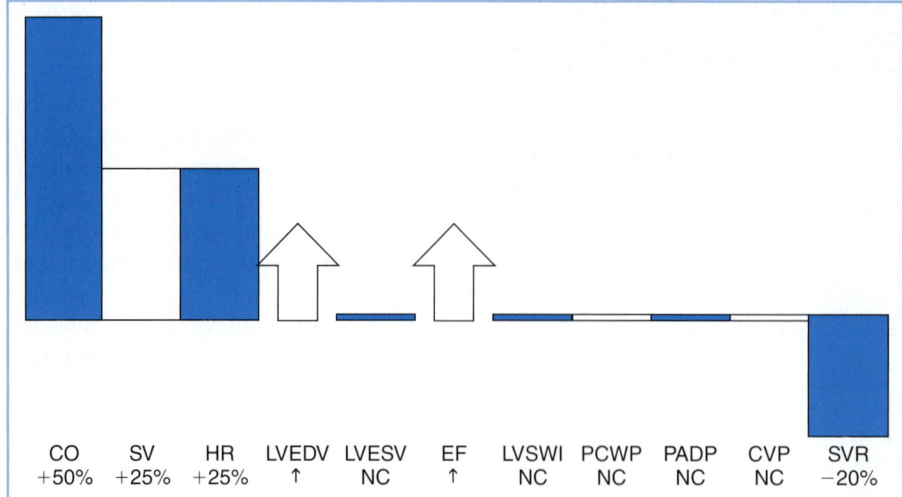

Fig. 2.1 Central Hemodynamic Changes at Term Gestation. Changes are relative to the nonpregnant state. *CO,* Cardiac output; *CVP,* central venous pressure; *EF,* ejection fraction; *HR,* heart rate; *LVEDV,* left ventricular end-diastolic volume; *LVESV,* left ventricular end-systolic volume; *LVSWI,* left ventricular stroke work index; *NC,* no change; *PADP,* pulmonary artery diastolic pressure; *PCWP,* pulmonary capillary wedge pressure; *SV,* stroke volume; *SVR,* systemic vascular resistance. Data from Conklin KA. Maternal physiological adaptations during gestation, labor, and puerperium. *Semin Anesth.* 1991;10:221–234.

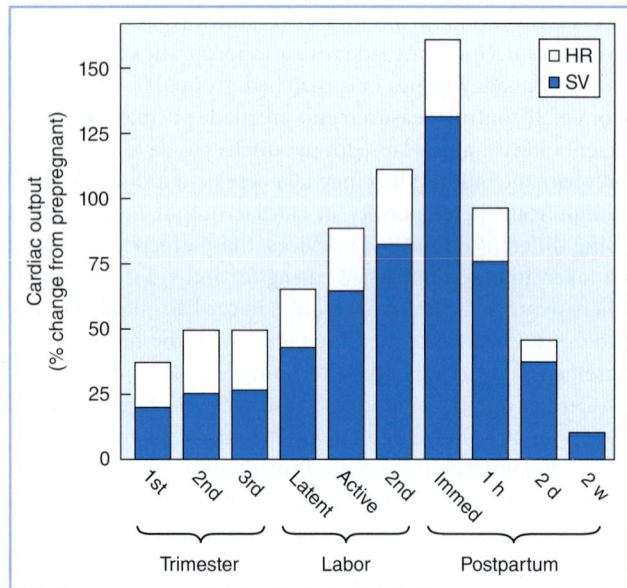

Fig. 2.2 Cardiac Output During Pregnancy, Labor, and the Puerperium. Values during pregnancy are measured at the end of the first, second, and third trimesters. Values during labor are measured between contractions. For each measurement, the relative contributions of heart rate (*HR*) and stroke volume (*SV*) to the change in cardiac output are illustrated.

a larger ejection fraction.[10,16,19,20,23] Central venous, pulmonary artery diastolic, and pulmonary capillary wedge pressures are within the normal nonpregnant range.[21] The apparent discrepancy between LV filling pressure and end-diastolic volume is explained by both hypertrophy and dilation, with the dilated ventricle accommodating a greater volume without an increase in pressure.

Myocardial contractility increases, as demonstrated by a higher velocity of LV circumferential fiber shortening.[10,20,23] Tissue Doppler imaging, which is relatively independent of preload, has been used to assess diastolic function.[24] A mild

degree of diastolic dysfunction may be seen during the third trimester compared with earlier in pregnancy and nonpregnant controls.[22]

The increase in cardiac output during pregnancy results in increased perfusion to the uterus, kidneys, and extremities. Uterine blood flow increases to meet the demands of the developing fetus from a baseline value of approximately 50 mL/min (prepregnancy) to a level at term of 700 to 900 mL/min.[25–27] During the second half of pregnancy, the proportion of cardiac output distributed to the uterine circulation increases from 5% to 12%.[28] Approximately 90% of this flow perfuses the intervillous space, with the balance perfusing the myometrium.[26] At term, skin blood flow is approximately three to four times the nonpregnant level, resulting in higher skin temperature.[29] Renal plasma flow is increased by 80% at 16 to 26 weeks' gestation but is only 50% above the prepregnancy baseline at term.[30]

The US Department of Health and Human Services recommends that pregnant women have at least 150 minutes of moderate-intensity aerobic activity every week,[31] and the American College of Obstetricians and Gynecologists recommends 20 to 30 minutes per day[32]; however, most women do not achieve this goal. Pregnant women are less active, with only half as many meeting guidelines for vigorous activity compared with nonpregnant women.[33] For every two women who exercise before pregnancy, one will not do so during pregnancy. Failure to exercise increases the risk for greater gestational weight gain.[34] Exercise is safe for the fetus[34,35]; in a study of 45 women, exercise on a treadmill of moderate intensity (40% to 59% of heart rate reserve) did not affect fetal heart or umbilical artery Doppler indices.[35]

During exercise, maximal oxygen consumption is greater in pregnancy,[36] especially during cardiovascular exercise. The rate of increase in minute ventilation is greater with exercise during pregnancy.[37] Cardiac output is also greater, primarily from increased stroke volume[38] and oxygen delivery to the fetus.

Blood Pressure and Systemic Vascular Resistance

Positioning, gestational age, and parity affect blood pressure measurements. Brachial sphygmomanometry yields the highest measurements in the supine position and the lowest measurements in the lateral position, especially with the cuff on the nondependent arm.[39] Blood pressure increases with maternal age, and for a given age, nulliparous women have a slightly higher mean pressure than parous women, although with extended interpregnancy intervals that effect is lost.[40–42] Systolic, diastolic, and mean blood pressure decrease during mid-pregnancy and return toward baseline as the pregnancy approaches term.[43] Diastolic blood pressure decreases more than systolic blood pressure, with early- to mid-gestational decreases of approximately 20%.[44]

The changes in blood pressure are consistent with changes in systemic vascular resistance (SVR), which decreases during early gestation, reaches its nadir (35% decline) at 20 weeks' gestation, and increases toward prepregnancy baseline during late gestation. Unlike blood pressure, however, SVR remains approximately 20% below the nonpregnant level at term.[16,21] A postulated explanation for the decreased SVR is the low-resistance uteroplacental vascular bed as well as systemic maternal vasodilation caused by prostacyclin, estrogen, and progesterone. Other contributions may come from elevation in systemic levels of nitric oxide, prostacyclin, endothelium-derived hyperpolarizing factor, progesterone, and relaxin.[45] The trend toward lower blood pressure often persists beyond pregnancy. A longitudinal study of 2304 initially normotensive women over 20 years showed that nulliparous women who subsequently delivered one or more infants maintained a blood pressure that was 1 to 2 mm Hg lower than women who did not have children.[41,44] This finding demonstrates that pregnancy may create long-lasting vascular changes. Advanced maternal age has been associated with higher median SVR during pregnancy, and pregnant women who smoke have demonstrated a lower SVR compared with nonsmoking parturients.[46]

Aortocaval Compression

The extent of compression of the aorta and inferior vena cava by the gravid uterus depends on positioning and gestational age. At term, partial vena caval compression occurs when the woman is in the lateral position, as documented by angiography.[47] This finding is consistent with the 75% elevation above baseline of femoral venous and lower inferior vena caval pressures.[48] Despite caval compression, collateral circulation maintains venous return, as reflected by right ventricular filling pressure, which is unaltered in the lateral position.[21] Intraabdominal pressure is often elevated in term pregnant patients regardless of BMI but is significantly lower in the lateral position compared with supine.[49]

In the supine position, significant and sometimes complete compression of the inferior vena cava is evident at term.[50,51] Blood returns from the lower extremities through the intraosseous, vertebral, paravertebral, and epidural veins.[52] However, this collateral venous return is less than would occur through the inferior vena cava, resulting in a decrease in right atrial pressure.[53] Compression of the inferior vena cava occurs as early as 13 to 16 weeks' gestation and is evident from the 50% increase in femoral venous pressure observed when these women assume the supine position (Fig. 2.3).[54] By term, femoral venous and lower inferior vena caval pressures are approximately 2.5 times the nonpregnant measurements in the supine position.[48,54] Vena cava volume at term is significantly higher with 30-degree left lateral tilt compared with the supine position, whereas there is no difference between

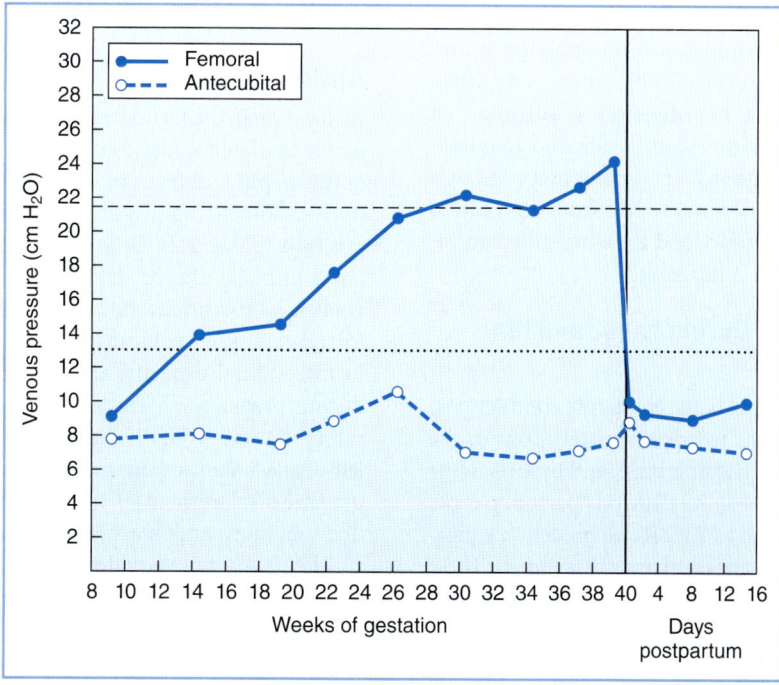

Fig. 2.3 Femoral and Antecubital Venous Pressures in the Supine Position Throughout Normal Pregnancy and the Puerperium. Modified from McLennan CE. Antecubital and femoral venous pressure in normal and toxemic pregnancy. *Am J Obstet Gynecol.* 1943;45:568–591.

women in the supine position and those tilted left at 15 degrees.[51] A minority of women have the highest inferior vena cava volume with 30-degree right lateral tilt.[55]

In the supine position, the aorta may be compressed by the term gravid uterus. This compression could account for lower pressure in the femoral versus the brachial artery in the supine position.[56,57] Angiographic studies in supine pregnant women showed partial obstruction of the aorta at the level of the lumbar lordosis and enhanced compression during periods of maternal hypotension.[58] Conversely, a comparison of magnetic resonance images of healthy women at term in the supine position compared with nonpregnant women showed no difference in aortic volume at the level of the mid- to upper lumbar vertebra.[51]

At term, the left lateral decubitus position is associated with less enhancement of cardiac sympathetic nervous system activity and less suppression of cardiac vagal activity than the supine or right lateral decubitus position.[59] Women who assume the supine position at term gestation experience a 10% to 20% decline in stroke volume and cardiac output,[60,61] consistent with the decrease in right atrial filling pressure. Blood flow in the upper extremities is normal, whereas uterine blood flow decreases by 20% and lower extremity blood flow decreases by 50%.[62] Perfusion of the uterus is less affected than that of the lower extremities because compression of the vena cava does not obstruct venous outflow via the ovarian veins.[63] The adverse hemodynamic effects of aortocaval compression are reduced once the fetal head is engaged.[56,57] The sitting position, especially with neck and hip flexion, has also been shown to rotate the uterus against the vena cava, resulting in aortocaval compression with a decrease in cardiac output of 10%.[64] There is no evidence that short intervals in the sitting position, such as occurs during epidural catheter placement, have any clinically significant impact on uteroplacental blood flow.

Some term pregnant women exhibit an increase in brachial artery blood pressure when they assume the supine position, which is caused by higher SVR from compression of the aorta. Up to 15% of women at term experience bradycardia and a substantial decrease in blood pressure when supine, the so-called **supine hypotension syndrome**.[65] It may take several minutes for the bradycardia and hypotension to develop, and the bradycardia is usually preceded by a period of tachycardia. The syndrome results from a profound decrease in venous return and preload for which the cardiovascular system is not able to compensate.

Hemodynamic Changes During Labor and the Puerperium

Cardiac output during labor (but between uterine contractions) increases from prelabor values by approximately 10% in the early first stage, by 25% in the late first stage, and by 40% in the second stage of labor.[66–68] In the immediate postpartum period, cardiac output may be as much as 75% above predelivery measurements and 150% above prepregnancy baseline.[67] These changes result from an increase in stroke volume caused by greater venous return and increased sympathetic nervous system activity. During labor, uterine contractions displace 300 to 500 mL of blood from the intervillous space through the ovarian venous outflow system into the central circulation (autotransfusion).[69–71] The postpartum increase in cardiac output

results from relief of vena caval compression, diminished lower extremity venous pressure, sustained myometrial contraction, and increased venous return.[68] Cardiac output decreases to just below prelabor values at 24 hours postpartum[69] and returns to prepregnancy levels between 12 and 24 weeks postpartum[16] (see Fig. 2.2). Heart rate decreases rapidly after delivery, reaches prepregnancy levels by 2 weeks postpartum, and is slightly below the prepregnancy rate for the next several months.[16,66]

THE RESPIRATORY SYSTEM

Despite the multiple anatomic and physiologic changes that occur during pregnancy, it is remarkable that pregnancy has a relatively minor impact on lung function.

Anatomy

The thorax undergoes both mechanical and hormonal changes during pregnancy. Relaxin (the hormone responsible for relaxation of the pelvic ligaments) causes relaxation of the ligamentous attachments to the lower ribs.[72] The subcostal angle progressively widens from approximately 69 degrees to 104 degrees. The anteroposterior and transverse diameters of the chest wall each increase by 2 cm, resulting in an increase of 5 to 7 cm in the circumference of the lower rib cage. These changes peak at 37 weeks' gestation. The subcostal angle remains about 20% wider than the baseline value after delivery.[73] The vertical measurement of the chest cavity decreases by as much as 4 cm as a result of the elevated position of the diaphragm (Fig. 2.4). The timing of return to baseline nonpregnant status is unclear.[74]

Capillary engorgement of the larynx and the nasal and oropharyngeal mucosa begins early in the first trimester and increases progressively throughout pregnancy.[75] The effect of estrogen on the nasal mucosa may cause symptoms of rhinitis and epistaxis. Nasal breathing commonly becomes difficult, and nasal congestion may contribute to the perceived shortness of breath of pregnancy.[76]

Airflow Mechanics

Inspiration in the term pregnant woman is almost totally attributable to diaphragmatic excursion[77] because of greater descent of the diaphragm from its elevated resting position and limitation of thoracic cage expansion because of its expanded resting position (Table 2.2). Both large- and small-airway functions are minimally altered during pregnancy. The shape of flow-volume loops, the absolute flow rates at normal lung volumes,[78] forced expiratory volume in 1 second (FEV_1), the ratio of FEV_1 to forced vital capacity, and closing capacity are unchanged during pregnancy.[79] There is no significant change in respiratory muscle strength during pregnancy despite the cephalad displacement of the diaphragm. Furthermore, despite the upward displacement of the diaphragm by the gravid uterus, diaphragm excursion actually increases by 2 cm.[80]

The peak expiratory flow (PEF) rate achieved with a maximal effort after a maximal inspiration is often considered a surrogate for FEV_1 and can be used to monitor asthma therapy. Studies of changes in PEF rate during pregnancy show conflicting results,[81,82] likely reflecting differences in measurement devices and patient position; however, any changes seen are likely not clinically significant and PEF remains a valid

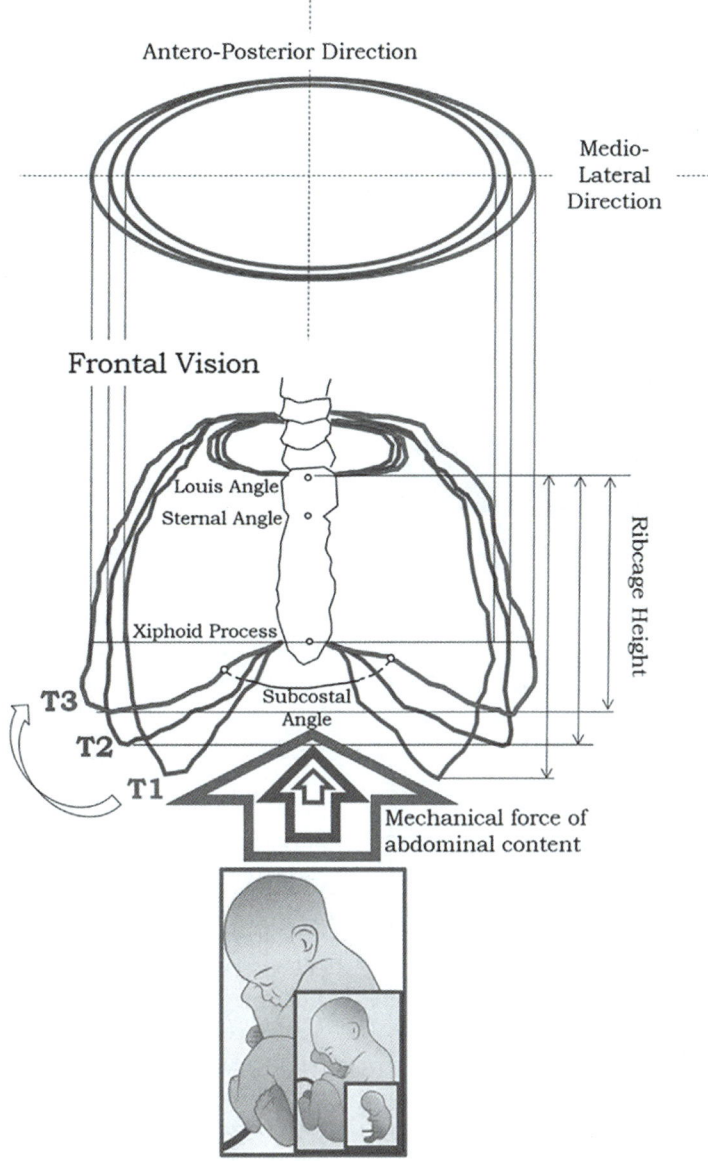

Fig. 2.4 Changes in the Geometry of the Ribcage During Pregnancy. The position of the ribs is depicted for the first (T1), the second (T2), and the third (T3) trimesters of pregnancy. Reproduced from LoMauro A, Aliverti A. Respiratory physiology in pregnancy and assessment of pulmonary function. *Best Pract Res Clin Obstet Gynaecol.* 2022;85(Pt A):3–16.

TABLE 2.2 Effects of Pregnancy on Respiratory Mechanics

Parameter	Change[a]
Diaphragm excursion	Increased
Chest wall excursion	Decreased
Pulmonary resistance	Decreased 50%
FEV_1	No change
FEV_1/FVC	No change
Flow-volume loop	No change
Closing capacity	No change
Peak expiratory force	Slight decrease

FEV_1, Forced expiratory volume in 1 s; *FVC,* forced vital capacity.
[a]Relative to nonpregnant state.
Modified from Conklin KA. Maternal physiological adaptations during gestation, labor, and the puerperium. *Semin Anesth.* 1991;10:221–234.

tool during pregnancy. In the postpartum period, Harirah et al. reported significantly decreased PEF at 6 weeks.[81]

Lung Volumes and Capacities

Lung volumes can be measured by using body plethysmography or inert gas techniques with slightly differing results.[83] By term, total lung capacity is slightly reduced,[84] whereas tidal volume increases by 45%, with approximately half the change occurring during the first trimester (Table 2.3 and Fig. 2.5). The early change in tidal volume is associated with a transient reduction in inspiratory reserve volume. Residual volume tends to decrease slightly, a change that maintains vital capacity. Inspiratory capacity increases by 15% during the third trimester because of increases in tidal volume and inspiratory reserve volume.[85,86] There is a corresponding decrease in expiratory reserve volume.[85,86] The functional residual capacity (FRC) begins to decrease by the fifth month of pregnancy with uterine enlargement and diaphragm elevation and is decreased by 400 to 700 mL to 80% of the prepregnancy value at term.[85,86] The overall reduction is caused by a 25% (200 to 300 mL) reduction in expiratory reserve volume and a 15% (200 to 400 mL) reduction in residual volume. Assumption of the supine position causes the FRC to decrease further to 70% of the prepregnancy value. The supine FRC can be increased by 10% (approximately 188 mL) by placing the patient in a 30-degree head-up position.[87]

Ventilation and Blood Gases

During pregnancy, respiratory patterns remain relatively unchanged. Minute ventilation increases via an increase in tidal volume from 450 to 600 mL and a small increase in

TABLE 2.3 Changes in Respiratory Physiology at Term Gestation

Parameter	Change[a]
Lung Volumes	
Inspiratory reserve volume	+5%
Tidal volume	+45%
Expiratory reserve volume	−25%
Residual volume	−15%
Lung Capacities	
Inspiratory capacity	+15%
Functional residual capacity	−20%
Vital capacity	No change
Total lung capacity	−5%
Ventilation	
Minute ventilation	+45%
Alveolar ventilation	+45%

[a]Relative to nonpregnant state.
From Conklin KA. Maternal physiological adaptations during gestation, labor and the puerperium. *Semin Anesth.* 1991;10:221–234.

respiratory rate of 1 to 2 breaths/min.[88] This occurs primarily during the first 12 weeks of gestation with a minimal increase thereafter. The ratio of total dead space to tidal volume remains constant during pregnancy, resulting in an increase in alveolar ventilation of 30% to 50% above baseline. The increase in minute ventilation results from hormonal changes and from an increase in CO_2 production at rest by approximately 30% to 300 mL/min. The former is closely related to the blood level of progesterone,[89] which acts as a direct respiratory stimulant. The progesterone-induced increase in chemosensitivity also results in a steeper slope and a leftward shift of the CO_2-ventilatory response curve. This change occurs early in pregnancy and remains constant until delivery.[78]

Dyspnea is a common complaint during pregnancy, affecting up to 75% of women.[90] Contributing factors include increased respiratory drive, decreased $Paco_2$, increased oxygen consumption from the enlarging uterus and fetus, larger pulmonary blood volume, anemia, and nasal congestion. Dyspnea typically begins in the first or second trimester but improves as the pregnancy progresses. In a study in which 35 women were observed closely during pregnancy and postpartum, dyspnea was not caused by alterations in central ventilatory control or respiratory mechanical factors but rather by the awareness of the increased ventilation.[91] Exercise has no effect on pregnancy-induced changes in ventilation or alveolar gas exchange.[92] The hypoxic ventilatory response is increased during pregnancy to twice the normal level, secondary to elevations in estrogen and progesterone levels.[93] This increase occurs despite blood and cerebrospinal fluid (CSF) alkalosis.

During pregnancy, Pao_2 increases to 100 to 105 mm Hg (13.3 to 14.0 kPa) as a result of greater alveolar ventilation and a decline in $Paco_2$ (Table 2.4).[94–96] As pregnancy progresses, oxygen consumption continues to increase and cardiac output increases to a lesser extent, resulting in a reduced mixed venous oxygen content and increased arteriovenous oxygen difference. After mid-gestation, pregnant women in the supine position frequently have a $Pao_2 < 100$ mm Hg (13.3 kPa). This occurs because the FRC may be less than closing capacity,

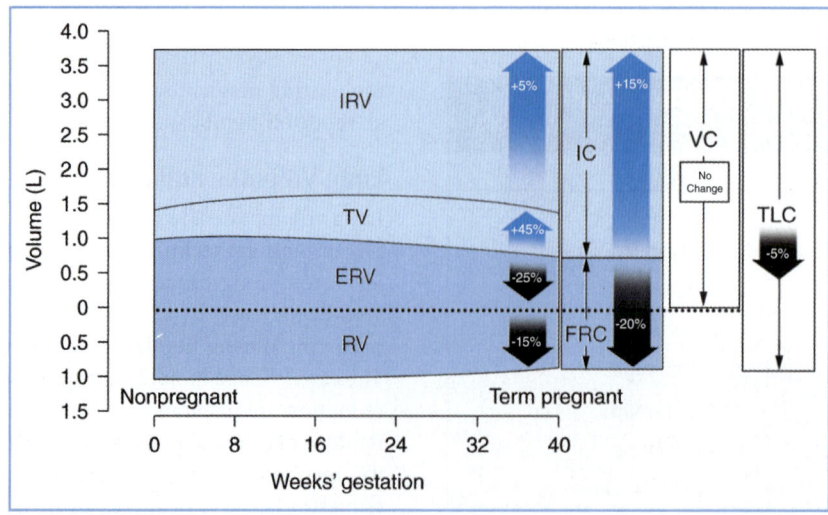

Fig. 2.5 Lung Volumes and Capacities During Pregnancy. *ERV,* Expiratory reserve volume; *FRC,* functional residual capacity; *IC,* inspiratory capacity; *IRV,* inspiratory reserve volume; *RV,* residual volume; *TLC,* total lung capacity; *TV,* tidal volume; *VC,* vital capacity.

TABLE 2.4 Blood Gas Parameters During Pregnancy

Parameter	Nonpregnant	TRIMESTER		
		First	Second	Third
$Paco_2$ in mm Hg (kPa)	40 (5.3)	30 (4.0)	30 (4.0)	30 (4.0)
Pao_2 in mm Hg (kPa)	100 (13.3)	107 (14.3)	105 (14.0)	103 (13.7)
pH	7.40	7.44	7.44	7.44
Bicarbonate (mEq/L)	24	21	20	20

resulting in closure of small airways during normal tidal volume ventilation.[94] Moving a pregnant woman from the supine to the erect or lateral decubitus position improves arterial oxygenation and reduces the alveolar-to-arterial oxygen gradient. The increased oxygen tension facilitates the transfer of oxygen across the placenta to the fetus.

$Paco_2$ declines to approximately 30 mm Hg (4.0 kPa) by 12 weeks' gestation but does not change further during the remainder of the pregnancy. Although a gradient exists between the end-tidal CO_2 tension and $Paco_2$ in nonpregnant women, the two measurements are equivalent during early pregnancy,[97] at term gestation,[98] and in the postpartum period.[99] This is attributable to a reduction in alveolar dead space, which results from an increase in cardiac output and increased basilar atelectasis during pregnancy. The mixed venous Pco_2 is 6 to 8 mm Hg (0.8 to 1.1 kPa) below the nonpregnant level from late in the first trimester until term.[11]

The respiratory alkalosis of pregnancy causes a compensatory increase in renal bicarbonate excretion and a reduction in serum bicarbonate concentration to approximately 20 mEq/L, the base excess by 2 to 3 mEq/L, and the total buffer base by approximately 5 mEq/L.[100] This compensation is incomplete, as demonstrated by the elevation of venous,[101] capillary,[102] and arterial[94] blood pH by 0.02 to 0.06 units (see Table 2.4). The decrease in plasmabicarbonate affects the woman's ability to buffer an acid load while pregnant. The slight respiratory alkalosis would normally shift the oxyhemoglobin saturation curve to the left; however, a concurrent increase in 2,3-bisphosphoglycerate (also known as 2,3-diphosphoglycerate) causes the curve to shift slightly to the right.

Metabolism and Respiration During Labor and the Puerperium

Minute ventilation in the unmedicated parturient increases by 70% to 140% in the first stage of labor and by 120% to 200% in the second stage of labor compared with prepregnancy values.[103] Pain, anxiety, and coached breathing techniques all increase minute ventilation. $Paco_2$ may decrease to as low as 10 to 15 mm Hg (1.3 to 2.0 kPa). Oxygen consumption increases above the prelabor value by 40% in the first stage of labor and by 75% in the second stage, secondary to the increased metabolic demands of hyperventilation, uterine activity, and maternal expulsive efforts.[103,104] The maternal aerobic requirement for oxygen exceeds oxygen consumption during labor, as is evident from the progressive

elevation of blood lactate concentration, an index of anaerobic metabolism.[104–107] Effective neuraxial analgesia prevents these changes during the first stage of labor and mitigates the changes during the second stage of labor.[104,107]

FRC increases after delivery but remains below the prepregnancy volume for 1 to 2 weeks. Although minute ventilation decreases halfway toward nonpregnant values by 72 hours, oxygen consumption, tidal volume, and minute ventilation remain elevated until at least 6 to 8 weeks after delivery. The alveolar and mixed venous Pco_2 values increase slowly after delivery and are still slightly below prepregnancy levels at 6 to 8 weeks postpartum.[11]

THE GASTROINTESTINAL SYSTEM

Anatomy, Barrier Pressure, and Gastroesophageal Reflux

Baseline gastric volume in fasting pregnant nonlaboring patients is not significantly different to that in nonpregnant women.[108] The stomach is displaced upward toward the left side of the diaphragm during pregnancy, and its axis is rotated approximately 45 degrees to the right from its normal vertical position. This altered position displaces the intraabdominal segment of the esophagus into the thorax in most women, causing a reduction in tone of the lower esophageal high-pressure zone (LEHPZ), which normally prevents the reflux of gastric contents. Progestins also may contribute to relaxation of the LEHPZ.[109]

Approximately 30% to 50% of women experience **gastroesophageal reflux disease (GERD)** during pregnancy.[110] The prevalence of GERD is approximately 10% in the first trimester, 40% in the second trimester, and 55% in the third trimester. In the first trimester of pregnancy, basal LEHPZ pressure may not change, but the sphincter is less responsive to physiologic stimuli that usually increase pressure.[111] In the second and third trimesters, LEHPZ pressure gradually decreases to approximately 50% of basal values, reaching a nadir at 36 weeks' gestation and returning to prepregnancy values at 1 to 4 weeks postpartum (Table 2.5). Risk factors for GERD in pregnancy include gestational age, heartburn antecedent to pregnancy, and multiparity. Gravidity, prepregnancy BMI, and weight gain during pregnancy do not correlate with the occurrence of reflux, whereas maternal age has an inverse correlation.[112]

TABLE 2.5   Changes in Gastrointestinal Physiology During Pregnancy[a]

Parameter	TRIMESTER			Labor	Postpartum (18 h)
	First	**Second**	**Third**		
Barrier pressure[b]	Decreased	Decreased	Decreased	Decreased	?
Gastric emptying	No change	No change	No change	Delayed	No change
Gastric acid secretion	No change	No change	No change	?	?
Proportion of women with gastric volume > 25 mL	No change	No change	No change	Increased	No change
Proportion of women with gastric pH < 2.5	No change	No change	No change	No change	No change

[a]Relative to nonpregnant state.
[b]Difference between intragastric pressure and tone of the lower esophageal high-pressure zone.

Gastrointestinal Motility

Gastric emptying is not altered during pregnancy. This has been demonstrated by studies that measured the absorption of orally administered acetaminophen (paracetamol)[113] and by studies that assessed the emptying of a test beverage or meal by radiographic,[114] ultrasonographic,[113] dye dilution,[115] epigastric impedance,[116] and applied potential tomographic[117] techniques. In a study of morbidly obese women at term, no difference was noted between gastric emptying of 300 and 50 mL of water, suggesting that fasting guidelines should not differ for obese versus lean parturients.[118] In fasted pregnant patients who consumed 250 mL of tea with milk, ultrasonographic measurement of the gastric antrum returned to baseline by 90 minutes.[119]

Esophageal peristalsis and intestinal transit are slowed during pregnancy,[120,121] which has been attributed to the inhibition of gastrointestinal contractile activity by progesterone. However, this inhibition may be an indirect action that results from a negative effect of progesterone on the plasma concentration of motilin, which declines during pregnancy.[120] Up to 40% of women suffer from constipation at some time during their pregnancy.[122] The prevalence of constipation is greatest in the first two trimesters of gestation and declines in the third trimester.

Gastric Acid Secretion

Early work suggested that both basal and maximal gastric acid secretion decline in mid-gestation, reaching a nadir at 20 to 30 weeks' gestation.[123] Van Thiel et al.[124] demonstrated no difference in basal or peak gastric acid secretion in four pregnant women studied in each trimester and at 1 to 4 weeks postpartum, although a plasma gastrin level significantly lower than postpartum levels was observed during the first trimester. Levels of gastric pH and serum gastrin concentration were compared in 100 women scheduled for elective cesarean delivery and in 100 nonpregnant women undergoing gynecologic surgery.[125] The mean pH was lower in the pregnant group (2.4 versus 3.0), but serum gastrin levels were not different despite the fact that gastrin is secreted by the placenta from 15 weeks' gestation onward. This may reflect a dilutional effect of increased plasma volume. Other studies

have shown that approximately 80% of both pregnant and nonpregnant women have gastric pH ≤ 2.5, approximately 50% have gastric volume ≥ 25 mL, and 40% to 50% exhibit both low pH and gastric volume > 25 mL.[126]

Nausea and Vomiting

Approximately 80% of pregnant women will experience nausea and vomiting during pregnancy.[127] The symptoms typically start between 4 and 9 weeks' gestation and may last until 12 to 16 weeks' gestation.[128] Of these women, 1% to 5% will develop symptoms that persist throughout the pregnancy, known as **hyperemesis gravidarum** (see Chapter 17).

Gastric Function During Labor and the Puerperium

Gastric emptying is slowed during labor, as shown by ultrasonographic imaging, emptying of a test meal, and the rate of absorption of oral acetaminophen.[129,130] Direct measurements show that the mean gastric volume increases.[131] However, in one study, postpartum gastric volume was found to be no different in parturients who consumed water in labor compared with those who consumed an isotonic sports drink composed of mixed carbohydrates and electrolytes.[132] Gastric acid secretion may decrease during labor because only 25% of parturients who are in labor have a gastric pH ≤ 2.5.[133] Gastric emptying is also delayed during the early postpartum period but returns to prepregnancy levels by 18 hours postpartum.[134] Fasting gastric volume and pH values are similar to nonpregnant patients at 18 hours postpartum.[135–137] The effects of opioids and neuraxial analgesia on gastric emptying are discussed in Chapters 24 and 28.

THE LIVER AND GALLBLADDER

Liver size, morphology, and blood flow patterns do not change during pregnancy, although the liver is displaced upward, posteriorly, and to the right during late pregnancy.

Serum levels of bilirubin, alanine aminotransferase, aspartate aminotransferase, and lactate dehydrogenase increase to the upper limits of the normal range during pregnancy.[138] The total alkaline phosphatase activity increases twofold to fourfold, mostly from production by the placenta. Excretion of sulfobromophthalein into bile decreases, whereas the hepatic extraction and retention of this compound increases.[139]

Biliary stasis and greater secretion of bile with cholesterol increase the risk for gallbladder disease during pregnancy.[140] The incidence of gallstones is 5% to 12% in pregnant women.[141] During pregnancy 1 in 1600 to 1 in 10,000 women undergo cholecystectomy. Progesterone inhibits the contractility of gastrointestinal smooth muscle, leading to gallbladder hypomotility.[142] The size of the total bile acid pool increases by about 50% during pregnancy, and the relative proportions of the various bile acids change.[143] The changes in the composition of bile revert rapidly after delivery, even in patients with gallstones.

THE KIDNEYS

Owing to an increase in total intravascular volume, both renal vascular and interstitial volume increase during pregnancy. These increases are reflected in enlarged kidneys, with renal volume increased by as much as 30%.[144] Vasodilation of the kidneys contributes to the overall decline in SVR during the first trimester. The collecting system, including the renal calyces, pelvis, and ureters, dilates. Hydronephrosis occurs in 80% or more of women by mid-pregnancy.[145]

Glomerular filtration rate (GFR) and renal plasma flow increase markedly during pregnancy secondary to reduced renal vascular resistance.[30] The renal blood flow is 75% greater than nonpregnant values by 16 weeks' gestation and is maintained until 34 weeks, when a slight decline occurs. By the end of the first trimester, the GFR is 50% greater than baseline, and this rate is maintained until the end of pregnancy. The GFR does not return to prepregnancy levels until 3 months postpartum. Because the GFR does not increase as rapidly or as much as the renal blood flow, the filtration fraction decreases from nonpregnant levels until the third trimester.[146] The role of nitric oxide in the renal vasodilation during pregnancy was tested and confirmed in a rat model.[147] Renin and aldosterone also both increase during pregnancy.[148]

Creatinine clearance is increased to 150 to 200 mL/min from the normal baseline value of 120 mL/min.[149] The increase occurs early in pregnancy, reaches a maximum by the end of the first trimester, decreases slightly near term, and returns to the prepregnancy level by 8 to 12 weeks postpartum.[146] These renal hemodynamic alterations are among the earliest and most dramatic maternal adaptations to pregnancy. The increased GFR results in reduced blood concentrations of nitrogenous metabolites. The blood urea nitrogen concentration decreases to 8 to 9 mg/dL (urea concentration 2.9 to 3.2 mmol/L) by the end of the first trimester and remains at that level until term.[149] Serum creatinine concentration is a reflection of skeletal muscle production and urinary excretion. In pregnancy, skeletal muscle production of creatinine remains relatively constant, but the GFR is increased, resulting in reduced serum creatinine concentration. The serum creatinine concentration decreases progressively to 0.5 to 0.6 mg/dL (44 to 53 μmol/L) by the end of pregnancy. The serum uric acid level declines in early pregnancy to 2.0 to 3.0 mg/dL (0.12

to 0.18 mmol/L) by 24 weeks' gestation because of the rise in GFR.[150] Subsequently, the uric acid level begins to increase, reaching the prepregnancy level by the end of pregnancy. Tubular reabsorption of urate accounts for this restored uric acid level during the third trimester.

Total protein excretion and urinary albumin excretion are higher than nonpregnant levels. Average 24-hour total protein and albumin excretion are 200 and 12 mg, respectively (upper limits are 300 and 20 mg, respectively).[151,152] Proteinuria (>300 mg/24 hours) has been described without the diagnosis of preeclampsia.[153] However, women with isolated proteinuria are more likely to progress to preeclampsia than women with isolated hypertension. The protein-to-creatinine (P:C) ratio in a random urine sample correlates well with a 24-hour urine protein measurement, and a value > 0.3 has been defined as the threshold for diagnosing preeclampsia.[154] The degree of proteinuria in normal pregnancy correlates with gestation. Baba et al.[155] suggested that in normotensive patients, a P:C ratio of more than 0.75 may be the "rule-in" threshold for significant proteinuria.[155] Women with twin pregnancy have greater protein excretion compared with those with singleton pregnancy.[156]

Glucose is filtered and almost completely absorbed in the proximal tubule. In the nonpregnant state, a small amount of glucose is excreted. Pregnancy imposes a change in the glucose resorptive capacity of the proximal tubules, so all pregnant women exhibit an elevation of glucose excretion. Of pregnant women who have normal glucose tolerance to an oral load and normal glucose excretion when not pregnant, approximately half will exhibit a doubling of glucose excretion. Most of the remainder have increases of 3 to 10 times the nonpregnant amount, and a small proportion (<10%) excrete as much as 20 times the nonpregnant amount.[157] Overall, the amount of glucose excreted in the third trimester is several times greater than that in the nonpregnant state. The normal nonpregnant pattern of glucose excretion is reestablished within 1 week after delivery.

HEMATOLOGY

Blood Volume

Maternal plasma volume expansion begins as early as 6 weeks' gestation and continues until it reaches a net increase of approximately 50% by 34 weeks' gestation (Table 2.6; Fig. 2.6).[158] After 34 weeks' gestation, the plasma volume stabilizes or decreases slightly. Red blood cell volume decreases during the first 8 weeks of pregnancy, increases to the prepregnancy level by 16 weeks, and undergoes a further rise to 30% above the prepregnancy level at term.[159–161] The red blood cell volume increases in response to elevated erythropoietin concentration[162] and the erythropoietic effects of progesterone, prolactin, and placental lactogen. The increase in plasma volume exceeds the increase in red blood cell volume, resulting in the **physiologic anemia of pregnancy**. Hemoglobin concentration (hematocrit), which typically ranges from 12.0 to 15.8 g/dL (35.4% to 44.4%) in nonpregnant woman, decreases to 11.6 to 13.9 g/dL (31% to 41%) in the first trimester, 9.7 to

TABLE 2.6 Hematologic Parameters at Term Gestation

Parameter	Change[a] or Actual Measurement
Blood volume	+45%[a]
Plasma volume	+55%[a]
Red blood cell volume	+30%[a]
Hemoglobin concentration (g/dL)	11.6
Hematocrit	35.5%

[a]Relative to nonpregnant state.
Modified from Conklin KA. Maternal physiological adaptations during gestation, labor, and puerperium. *Semin Anesth*. 1991;10:221–234.

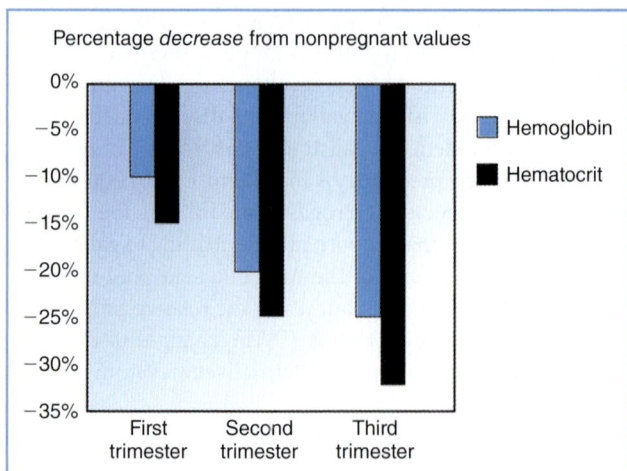

Fig. 2.7 The Decrease in Both Hemoglobin Concentration and Hematocrit During Pregnancy Underlies the Physiologic Anemia of Pregnancy. The decrease is greater for hematocrit, and the greatest decreases occur during the third trimester. Data from Abbassi-Ghanavati M, Greer LG, Cunningham FG. Pregnancy and laboratory studies: a reference table for clinicians. *Obstet Gynecol*. 2009;114:1326–1331.

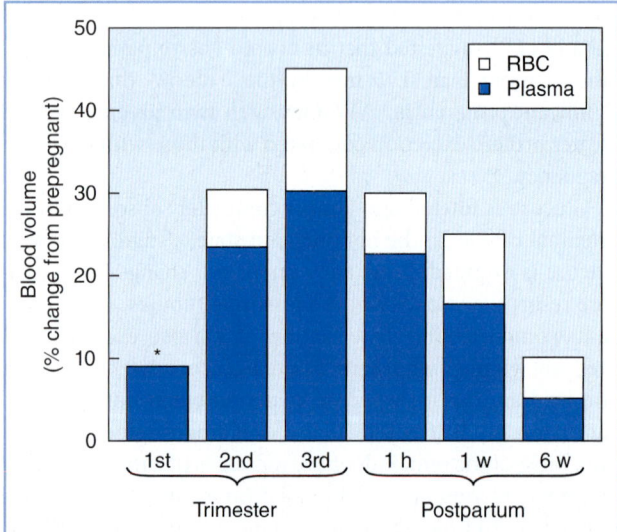

Fig. 2.6 Blood Volume During Pregnancy and the Puerperium. Values during pregnancy measured at the end of the first, second, and third trimesters. Postpartum values measured after a vaginal delivery. The values for red blood cell volume (*RBC*) and plasma volume (*Plasma*) do not represent the actual percentage of change in these parameters but rather reflect the relative contribution of each to the change in blood volume. The asterisk indicates that RBC volume is below the prepregnancy volume at the end of the first trimester.

14.8 g/dL (30% to 39%) in the second trimester, and 9.5 to 15.0 g/dL (28% to 40%) in the third trimester (Fig. 2.7).[159–161,163] Women who do not receive iron supplements during pregnancy have greater decreases in hemoglobin concentration and hematocrit.[160] Iron deficiency anemia in pregnancy is defined by a hemoglobin concentration < 10.5 g/dL in the second and third trimesters.[164]

The increase in plasma volume results from fetal and maternal hormone production, and several systems may play a role. The maternal concentrations of estrogen and progesterone increase nearly 100-fold during pregnancy. Estrogens increase plasma renin activity, enhancing renal sodium absorption and water retention via the renin-angiotensin-aldosterone system. Fetal adrenal production of the estrogen precursor dehydroepiandrosterone may be the underlying

control mechanism. Progesterone also enhances aldosterone production. These changes result in marked increases in plasma renin activity and aldosterone level as well as in retention of approximately 900 mEq of sodium and 7000 mL of total body water. The concentration of plasma adrenomedullin, a potent vasodilating peptide, increases during pregnancy and correlates significantly with blood volume.[165]

Blood volume is positively correlated with the size of the fetus in singleton pregnancies and is greater in multiple gestations.[166] The physiologic hypervolemia facilitates delivery of nutrients to the fetus, protects the mother from hypotension, and reduces the risks associated with hemorrhage at delivery.[161,167] The decrease in blood viscosity associated with the lower hematocrit decreases resistance to blood flow, which may be an essential component of maintaining the patency of the uteroplacental vascular bed.

Circulating blood volume may be overestimated with increasing BMI, and a pragmatic approach to estimating blood volume is based on maternal BMI category in a "mL/kg" calculation. For a parturient with a BMI of 18.5 to 24.9 kg/m² the estimated circulating blood volume is 95 mL/kg, and for patients with a BMI of 25 to 29.9, 30 to 39.9, and more than 40 kg/m² the estimated circulating blood volumes are 85, 75, and 70 mL/kg, respectively.[168]

Plasma Proteins

Plasma albumin concentration decreases from a nonpregnant range of 4.1 to 5.3 g/dL to ranges of 3.1 to 5.1 g/dL in the first trimester, 2.6 to 4.5 g/dL in the second trimester, and 2.3 to 4.2 g/dL in the third trimester (Table 2.7).[163,169,170] The globulin level decreases by 10% in the first trimester and then increases throughout the remainder of pregnancy to 10% above the prepregnancy value at term.[169] The albumin-globulin ratio decreases during pregnancy from 1.4 to 0.9,

TABLE 2.7 Plasma Protein Values During Pregnancy

Protein	Nonpregnant	TRIMESTER		
		First	Second	Third
Total protein (g/dL)	7.8	6.9	6.9	7.0
Albumin (g/dL)	4.5	3.9	3.6	3.3
Globulin (g/dL)	3.3	3.0	3.3	3.7
Albumin/globulin ratio	1.4	1.3	1.1	0.9
Change in plasma cholinesterase activity (%)		−25	−25	−25
Colloid osmotic pressure (mm Hg)	27	25	23	22

Adapted from Avram MJ. Pharmacokinetic studies in pregnancy. *Semin Perinatol.* 2020;44:151–227.

and the total plasma protein concentration decreases from 7.8 to 7.0 g/dL.[170] Maternal colloid osmotic pressure decreases by approximately 5 mm Hg during pregnancy.[21,171,172] The plasma cholinesterase activity decreases by approximately 25% during the first trimester and remains at that level until the end of pregnancy.[173]

Coagulation

Pregnancy is associated with enhanced platelet turnover, clotting, and fibrinolysis (Box 2.2). Thus, pregnancy represents a state of accelerated but compensated intravascular coagulation.

Increases in platelet factor 4 and beta-thromboglobulin signal elevated platelet activation, and the progressive increase in platelet distribution width and platelet volume are consistent with greater platelet consumption during pregnancy.[174–176] Platelet aggregation in response to collagen, epinephrine (adrenaline), adenosine diphosphate, and arachidonic acid is increased.[177] Some investigators have noted a decrease in platelet count,[176,178] whereas others have noted no change,[174,175] suggesting that increased platelet production compensates for greater activation. The platelet count usually decreases during the third trimester, with an estimated 8% of pregnant women having a platelet count < 150,000/mm^3 and 0.9% of pregnant women having a platelet count < 100,000/mm^3.[175,179] The most common causes of thrombocytopenia are **gestational thrombocytopenia**, hypertensive disorders of pregnancy, and idiopathic thrombocytopenia. The decrease in platelet count in the third trimester is caused by increased destruction and hemodilution.[180] Gestational thrombocytopenia is likely an exaggerated normal response.

The concentrations of most coagulation factors, including fibrinogen (factor I), proconvertin (factor VII), antihemophilic factor (factor VIII), Christmas factor (factor IX), Stuart-Prower factor (factor X), and Hageman factor (factor XII), increase during pregnancy. The increase in factor VIII is generally more marked in the third trimester. The concentrations of some factors increase by more than 100% (factors VII, VIII, IX, and fibrinogen).[180–183] Prothrombin (factor II) and serum calcium (factor IV) concentrations do not change, whereas the concentrations of thromboplastin antecedent (factor XI) and fibrin-stabilizing factor (factor XIII)

BOX 2.2 Changes in Coagulation and Fibrinolytic Parameters at Term Gestation[a]

Increased Factor Concentrations
- Factor I (fibrinogen)
- Factor VII (proconvertin)
- Factor VIII (antihemophilic factor)
- Factor IX (Christmas factor)
- Factor X (Stuart-Prower factor)
- Factor XII (Hageman factor)
- Von Willebrand Factor

Unchanged Factor Concentrations
- Factor II (prothrombin)
- Factor IV (ionized calcium)
- Factor V (proaccelerin)

Decreased Factor Concentrations
- Factor XI (thromboplastin antecedent)
- Factor XIII (fibrin-stabilizing factor)

Other Parameters
- Prothrombin time: shortened 20%
- Partial thromboplastin time: shortened 20%
- Thromboelastography: hypercoagulable
- Fibrinopeptide A: increased
- Antithrombin III: decreased
- Platelet count: no change or decreased
- Fibrin degradation products: increased
- Plasminogen: increased
- Plasminogen activator inhibitor-II: increased
- Protein C: unchanged
- Protein S: decreased

[a]Relative to nonpregnant state.

decrease.[182–184] Proaccelerin (factor V) levels are thought to be stable during pregnancy, although some sources suggest a slight increase. An increase in most factor concentrations, shortening of the prothrombin time and activated partial thromboplastin time,[181] an increase in fibrinopeptide A concentration, and a decrease in antithrombin III concentration suggest activation of the clotting system.[185] Protein S activity decreases steadily during pregnancy, reaching the lowest values at delivery.[186]

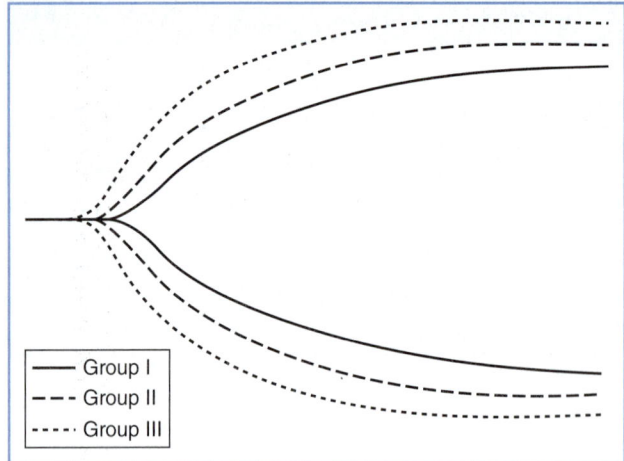

Fig. 2.8 Comparative thromboelastographs in nonpregnant (group I), nonlaboring term pregnant (group II), and laboring (group III) women. From Steer PL, Krantz HB. Thromboelastrography and sonoclot analysis in the healthy parturient. *J Clin Anesth*. 1993;5:419–424.

Thromboelastrography (TEG) demonstrates evidence of hypercoagulability in pregnancy. These changes (decrease in R and K values, increase in the α angle and maximum amplitude [MA], and decrease in measures of lysis) are observed as early as 10 to 12 weeks' gestation and are even greater during labor (Fig. 2.8).[187–189] Compared with samples taken during labor, TEG has demonstrated increased lysis in the postpartum period, possibly caused by the loss of placental expression of plasminogen activator inhibitor-2.[190] *In vitro*, exogenous oxytocin decreases R and K values, while increasing the α angle.[191] The *in vivo* effects of exogenous oxytocin are not known. Studies of **rotational thromboelastometry** during pregnancy also report reference values that show a positive correlation with increasing hypercoagulability and increasing gestational age.[192]

The greater concentration of fibrin degradation products signals increased fibrinolytic activity during gestation.[174] D-dimer values increase across gestation and remain higher than prepregnancy values in the postpartum period.[193,194] The marked elevation in the plasminogen concentration also is consistent with enhanced fibrinolysis.[195]

Hematology and Coagulation During the Puerperium

Blood loss during normal vaginal delivery and the early puerperium is approximately 600 mL,[196] compared with approximately 1000 mL during and within the first few hours of cesarean delivery.[196] The hematocrit in the immediate postpartum period is lower after cesarean delivery than after vaginal delivery because of the greater blood loss during cesarean delivery.[196] Regardless of the mode of delivery, the normal physiologic changes of pregnancy allow the healthy parturient to compensate for this blood loss. However, blood loss after either vaginal or cesarean delivery is often underestimated, and the discrepancy between actual and estimated blood loss is greater with increasing blood loss (see Chapter 37).[197]

Blood volume decreases to 125% of the prepregnancy level during the first postpartum week,[196] followed by a more gradual decline to 110% of the prepregnancy level at 6 to 9 weeks postpartum (see Fig. 2.6). The hemoglobin concentration and hematocrit decrease during the first 3 days postpartum, increase gradually during the next 3 days (because of a reduction in plasma volume), and continue to increase to prepregnancy measurements by 3 weeks postpartum.[198]

Albumin and total protein concentrations and colloid osmotic pressure decline after delivery and gradually return to prepregnancy levels by 6 weeks postpartum.[171] Plasma cholinesterase activity decreases below the predelivery level by the first postpartum day and remains at that decreased level during the next week.[173] Globulin concentrations are elevated throughout the first postpartum week.[169]

Beginning with delivery and during the first postpartum day, there is a rapid decrease in the platelet count and in the concentrations of fibrinogen, factor VIII, and plasminogen, and an increase in antifibrinolytic activity.[199] Clotting times remain shortened during the first postpartum day,[200] and viscoelastic testing remains consistent with a hypercoagulable state, although whether systemic fibrinolysis occurs is an area of active research.[190,191] During the first 3 to 5 days postpartum, increases are noted in the fibrinogen concentration and platelet count, changes that may account for the greater incidence of thrombotic complications during the puerperium.[200] The coagulation profile returns to the nonpregnant state by 2 to 3 weeks postpartum.[192,199]

THE IMMUNE SYSTEM

The blood leukocyte count increases progressively during pregnancy from the prepregnancy level, although there is a wide variation of normal values ranging from 3500 to 9000/mm³ prepregnancy to 5900 to 16,900/mm³ at term.[178] This change reflects an increase in the number of polymorphonuclear cells, with the appearance of immature granulocytic forms (myelocytes and metamyelocytes) in most pregnant women. The proportion of immature forms decreases during the last 2 months of pregnancy. The lymphocyte, eosinophil, and basophil counts decrease, whereas the monocyte count does not change. The leukocyte count increases to approximately 13,000/mm³ during labor and increases further to an average of 15,000/mm³ on the first postpartum day.[198] By the sixth postpartum day, the leukocyte count decreases to an average of 9250/mm³, although the count is still above normal at 6 weeks postpartum.

Despite an increased concentration, neutrophil function is impaired during pregnancy, as evidenced by depressed neutrophil chemotaxis and adherence.[201] This impairment may account for the greater incidence of infection during pregnancy and improved symptoms in some pregnant women with autoimmune diseases (e.g., **rheumatoid arthritis**). Levels of immunoglobulins A, G, and M are unchanged during gestation, but humoral antibody titers to certain viruses (e.g., **herpes simplex, measles, influenza type A**) are decreased.[202]

During pregnancy, the uterine mucosa is characterized by a large number of maternal immune cells found in close contact with the trophoblast. The fetal expression of paternal antigens requires adaptations in the maternal immune system so that the fetus is not perceived by the mother as "foreign."[203,204] This "immune tolerance" occurs because of a lack of fetal antigen expression, because of separation of the mother from the fetus, or from a functional suppression of the maternal lymphocytes.[205] During the first trimester of pregnancy, T lymphocytes express granulysin, a novel cytolytic protein that provides a protective role at the maternal-fetal interface.[206] Human T cells may be classified into T-helper cell types 1 and 2 (Th1 and Th2) on the basis of their cytokine production. Successful pregnancy is associated with a predominant Th2 state and a rise in an antiinflammatory cytokine profile. Th1 cytokines are detrimental to pregnancy.[207] These cells also produce natural antimicrobial agents within the uterus, which are important for prevention of uterine infection during pregnancy.[208] Maternal immunoglobulin E (IgE) production increases with pregnancy, and women with a history of pregnancy have higher baseline IgE and experience a slower decline in IgE levels as they age.[209]

NONPLACENTAL ENDOCRINOLOGY

Thyroid Function

The thyroid gland enlarges by 50% to 70% during pregnancy because of follicular hyperplasia and greater vascularity. The estrogen-induced increase in thyroid-binding globulin results in a 50% increase in total triiodothyronine (T_3) and thyroxine (T_4) concentrations during the first trimester, which are maintained until term.[210] The concentrations of free T_3 and T_4 do not change. The concentration of thyroid-stimulating hormone decreases during the first trimester but returns to the nonpregnant level shortly thereafter and undergoes no further change during the remainder of pregnancy. The fetal thyroid gland cannot produce thyroid hormone until the end of the first trimester and relies solely on maternal T_4 production during this critical time of development and organogenesis.

Approximately 4% to 7% of women of childbearing age are either hypothyroid or at risk for hypothyroidism during pregnancy.[211] Only 20% to 30% of affected women demonstrate symptoms of hypothyroidism, likely because some symptoms of hypothyroidism mimic features of pregnancy (e.g., fatigue).[212] In a large study of 502,036 pregnant women, 15% of tested women had **gestational hypothyroidism**, with 33% of these women demonstrating symptoms.[213] Based on these results, many physicians advocate universal screening, which appears to be cost effective, given the risk for decreased intelligence in the offspring, miscarriage, and postpartum bleeding if hypothyroidism is left untreated.[214]

Glucose Metabolism

Mean blood glucose concentration remains within the normal range during pregnancy, although the concentration may be lower in some women during the third trimester compared with nonpregnant individuals.[215] This finding is explained by the greater glucose demand of the fetus and the placenta. The relative hypoglycemic state results in fasting hypoinsulinemia. Pregnant women also exhibit exaggerated starvation ketosis.

Pregnant women are relatively insulin resistant because of hormones such as placental lactogen secreted by the placenta.[216] The blood glucose levels after a carbohydrate load are greater in pregnant women than in nonpregnant women, despite a hyperinsulinemic response. These changes resolve within 24 hours of delivery.

Adrenal Cortical Function

The concentration of corticosteroid-binding globulin (CBG) doubles during gestation as a result of an estrogen-induced enhancement of hepatic synthesis.[217] The elevated CBG value results in a 100% increase in the plasma cortisol concentration at the end of the first trimester and a 200% increase at term. The concentration of unbound, metabolically active cortisol at the end of the third trimester is 2.5 times the nonpregnant level. The increase in free cortisol results from greater production and reduced clearance. An increase in CBG concentration and a decrease in the serum albumin level affect the protein binding of corticosteroids. CBG binding capacity usually saturates at low concentrations of glucocorticoids. Clearance of betamethasone is greater during pregnancy, possibly because the drug is metabolized by placental enzymes.[218]

THE MUSCULOSKELETAL SYSTEM

Back pain during pregnancy is common and has a multifactorial etiology (see Chapter 46). One theory is that the enlarging uterus results in exaggerated lumbar lordosis, placing mechanical strain on the lower back. The hormonal changes of pregnancy may also play a role. Relaxin, a polypeptide hormone of the insulin-like growth factor family, is associated with remodeling of collagen fibers and pelvic connective tissue, permitting the aforementioned lordosis. The primary source of circulating relaxin is the corpus luteum; the placenta is a secondary source. Serum relaxin level in early pregnancy is positively correlated with the presence of back pain.[219] During pregnancy, gait also changes and there is an increase in anterior tilt of the pelvis to maintain body stability,[220] which may cause further stress on the vertebral column, leading to increased pain.

The enhancement of the lumbar lordosis during pregnancy alters the center of gravity over the lower extremities (Fig. 2.9) and may lead to other mechanical problems. Exaggerated lumbar lordosis tends to stretch the lateral femoral cutaneous nerve, which combined with compression under the inguinal ligament can result in **meralgia paresthetica**, with paresthesia or sensory loss over the anterolateral thigh. Anterior flexion of the neck and slumping of the shoulders usually accompany the enhanced lordosis, sometimes leading to a brachial plexus neuropathy.

Mobility of the sacroiliac, sacrococcygeal, and pubic joints increases during pregnancy in preparation for passage of the fetus. A widening of the pubic symphysis is evident by

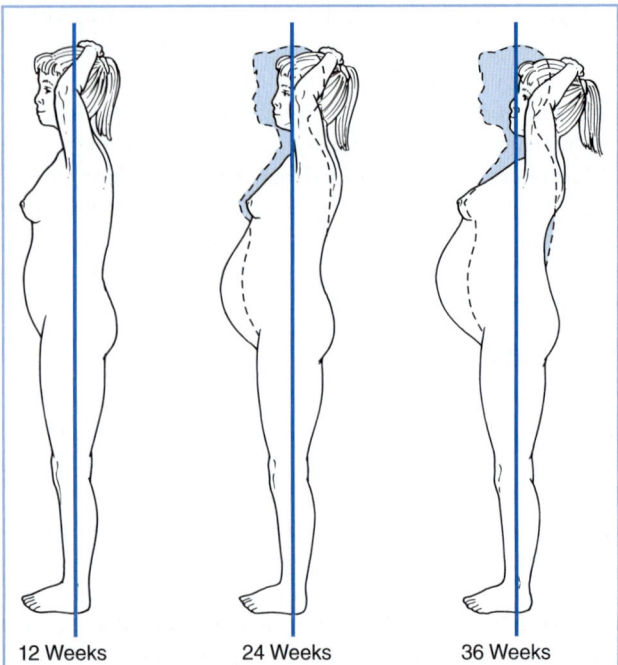

12 Weeks   24 Weeks   36 Weeks

Fig. 2.9 Changes in Posture During Pregnancy. The first and the subsequent dotted-line figures represent a woman's posture before growth of the uterus and its contents have affected the center of gravity. The second and third solid figures show that as the uterus enlarges and the abdomen protrudes, the lumbar lordosis is enhanced and the shoulders slump and move posteriorly. Modified from Beck AC, Rosenthal AH. *Obstetrical Practice.* Williams & Wilkins; 1955:146.

30 weeks' gestation. These changes are attributable to relaxin and the biomechanical strain of pregnancy on the ligaments.[221] Changes in posture and gait can lead to risk for falls. Relaxin may also contribute to the greater incidence of carpal tunnel syndrome and other neuropathies during pregnancy by changing the nature of the connective tissue so that more fluid is absorbed[222] and overall risk increases because of weight gain and edema.

The human fetus requires approximately 30 g of calcium for skeletal development by the time of term delivery.[223] Although intestinal absorption of calcium by the mother increases from as early as 12 weeks' gestation to meet this increased demand, it is insufficient to meet fetal demand and thus the maternal skeleton undergoes calcium resorption.[224] This does not cause long-term changes in skeletal calcium content or strength, and serum calcium levels remain stable during pregnancy. Pregnant women with twin gestation have a much higher calcium requirement. Compared with singleton pregnancies, there is a larger increase in maternal bone resorption in twin gestation.[225]

THE NERVOUS SYSTEM

Sleep

Sleep disturbances from mechanical and hormonal factors occur commonly during pregnancy. Latency and duration of rapid eye movement (REM) sleep are influenced by changes in progesterone and estrogen concentrations. Pregnant women have more complaints of insomnia and daytime sleepiness. The American Academy of Sleep Medicine defined **pregnancy-associated sleep disorder** as the occurrence of insomnia or excessive sleepiness that develops in the course of pregnancy.[226] In a cohort study of 189 healthy nulliparous women, Facco et al. reported that sleep duration was shorter in the third trimester (mean 7.0 [SD 1.2] hours) compared with the baseline period between 6 and 20 weeks' gestation (7.4 [1.2] hours).[227]

Sleep characteristics change as pregnancy progresses.[228] Early pregnancy is characterized by increased total sleep time and decreased stage 3 and 4 non-REM sleep, whereas late pregnancy is characterized by decreased total sleep time, increased waking after sleep onset, and decreased REM sleep.[228] Sleep may be poor for up to 3 months postpartum.[229] Upper airway changes lead to increased airflow resistance and snoring. Although only 4% of nonpregnant women snore, as many as 23% of pregnant women snore by the third trimester. Considerations for screening, diagnosing, and treating sleep apnea during pregnancy were described in a 2023 consensus guideline.[230]

Pregnancy is associated with **transient restless legs syndrome**, a disorder in which the patient experiences the need to move her legs. The incidence ranges from 15% in the first trimester to 23% in the third trimester.[231]

Central Nervous System

Cerebral blood flow increases in pregnancy. Nevo et al.[232] measured cerebral blood flow in 210 women at different gestational ages and found that it increased from 44.4 mL/min/100 g during the first trimester to 51.8 mL/min/100 g during the third trimester (Fig. 2.10). The increase was secondary to a decrease in cerebrovascular resistance and an increase in internal carotid artery diameter. Other changes in the brain that occur during pregnancy include (1) an increase in permeability of the blood-brain barrier caused by decreased cerebrovascular resistance with an increase in hydrostatic pressure and (2) an increase in capillary density in the posterior cerebral cortex.[233]

Women may experience an elevation in the threshold to pain and discomfort near the end of pregnancy and during labor, though this varies based on factors such as coping capacity.[234] The mechanism, although unclear, may be related to the effects of progesterone and endorphins. Elevated concentrations of endorphins and enkephalins are found in the plasma and CSF of parturients,[235] and opioid antagonists abolish pregnancy-induced analgesia to visceral stimulation in experimental animals.[236]

Vertebral Column

Anatomic and mechanical changes occur to the vertebral column during pregnancy. The apex of the thoracic curve shifts cephalad from T8 to T6–T7.[237] The volume of epidural fat and the epidural venous plexus enlarge and spinal CSF volume is reduced.[50]

In the lateral position, lumbar epidural pressure is positive in term pregnant women but negative in more than 90%

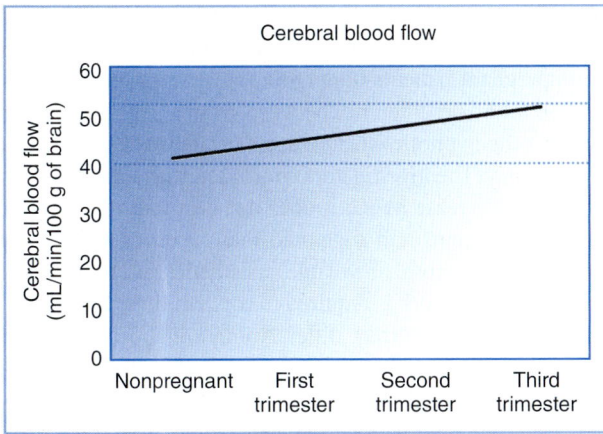

Fig. 2.10 Cerebral Blood Flow During Pregnancy. Cerebral blood flow increases as pregnancy progresses and is attributable to vasodilation from the hormonal changes of pregnancy. This increase in cerebral blood flow explains the increased risk for complications in patients with intracranial pathology as pregnancy progresses. Data from Nevo O, Soustiel JF, Thaler I. Maternal cerebral blood flow during normal pregnancy: a cross-sectional study. Am J Obstet Gynecol. 2010;203:475.e1–e6.

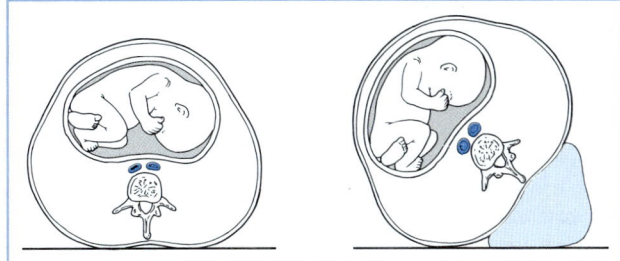

Fig. 2.11 Compression of the aorta and inferior vena cava in the supine (left) and lateral tilt (right) positions. Redrawn from Camann WR, Ostheimer GW. Physiologic adaptations during pregnancy. Int Anesthesiol Clin. 1990;28:2–10.

of nonpregnant women.[238] Turning a parturient from the lateral to the supine position increases the epidural pressure. Epidural pressure also increases during labor because of increased diversion of venous blood through the vertebral plexus secondary to either enhanced compression of the inferior vena cava in the supine position or greater intraabdominal pressure during pain and pushing. The epidural pressure returns to the nonpregnant level by 6 to 12 hours postpartum.

Despite compression of the dural sac by the epidural veins, the CSF pressure in pregnant women is the same as in nonpregnant women.[239] Uterine contractions and pushing during labor result in an increase in CSF pressure that is secondary to acute increases in epidural vein distention.

Sympathetic Nervous System

Dependence on the sympathetic nervous system for maintenance of hemodynamic stability increases progressively throughout pregnancy and reaches a peak at term.[240–242] The dependence on the sympathetic nervous system returns to that of the nonpregnant state by 36 to 48 hours postpartum.

ANESTHETIC IMPLICATIONS

Positioning

Aortocaval compression, decreased blood pressure and cardiac output, and impairment of uteroplacental blood flow can occur when a pregnant woman is placed in the supine position. This may compromise fetal well-being and neonatal outcome during labor or cesarean delivery.[243–245] Lee et al.[246] reported that when baseline maternal blood pressure was maintained with intravenous fluid and vasopressor administration during spinal anesthesia for cesarean delivery there was no difference in umbilical artery base excess or pH in patients who were supine or tilted 15 degrees. Additionally,

cardiac output was found to be not significantly different pre- and postspinal anesthesia when a prophylactic phenylephrine infusion was used.[247] It is suggested that if maternal blood pressure cannot be maintained at baseline, the supine position should be avoided after 20 weeks' gestation, and the uterus should be tilted more than 15 degrees (Fig. 2.11).[51,246]

Blood Replacement

At delivery, maternal vascular capacitance is reduced by the volume of the intervillous space (at least 500 mL). Therefore, during vaginal or cesarean delivery, this volume of blood does not need to be replaced and should not be considered in the estimation of blood loss for replacing red blood cells. Hemoconcentration occurs as maternal blood volume declines from 94 mL/kg at term to 76 mL/kg during the immediate postpartum period; however, with mobilization of edema fluid at postpartum day 1 to 2, the hematocrit may decline. This should be considered in the decision of whether a parturient should receive crystalloid, colloid, or blood for volume replacement.[159]

General Anesthesia

Airway Management, Oxygenation, and Ventilation

Changes in the maternal airway and respiratory physiology mandate modification of airway management during pregnancy (Box 2.3; see Chapter 29). The proportion of pregnant women with a Mallampati IV classification increases by 34% between 12 and 38 weeks' gestation.[248] Vascular engorgement of the airway results in edema of the oral and nasal pharynx, larynx, and trachea,[249] which may lead to difficult tracheal intubation and difficult mask ventilation. Airway edema may be exacerbated in patients with upper respiratory tract infection or preeclampsia and in those who have been pushing for a long time during the second stage of labor.

Pregnant women become hypoxemic more rapidly than nonpregnant women during episodes of apnea because FRC is reduced, oxygen consumption is increased, and FRC is less than closing capacity in up to 50% of supine individuals. During apnea accompanying rapid-sequence induction of general anesthesia, Pao_2 decreases twice as rapidly (139 versus 58 mm Hg/min [18.5 versus 7.7 kPa/min]) in pregnant versus nonpregnant women.[250] Denitrogenation (preoxygenation) is achieved faster in pregnant versus nonpregnant

BOX 2.3   Considerations for General Anesthesia During Pregnancy

Drugs
- Propofol
  - Induction dose decreased
  - Elimination half-life unaltered
- Volatile anesthetic agents
  - Minimum alveolar concentration decreased, but unclear whether hypnotic dose requirement differs from that in nonpregnant women
  - Speed of inhalation induction increased
- Succinylcholine (suxamethonium)
  - Duration of blockade unaltered
- Rocuronium
  - Increased sensitivity
- Chronotropic agents and vasopressors
  - Decreased sensitivity

Tracheal Intubation
- Increased rate of decline of Pao_2 during apnea
- Smaller endotracheal tube required (6.5 or 7.0 mm)
- Increased risk for difficult or failed mask ventilation
- Increased risk for failed intubation with traditional laryngoscopy
- Increased risk for bleeding with nasal instrumentation

women because of elevated minute ventilation and decreased FRC. However, after complete denitrogenation via inhalation of 100% oxygen, nonobese parturients tolerate only 2 to 3 minutes of apnea, versus 9 minutes in nonpregnant patients, before oxygen saturation decreases to less than 90%.

Ventilation during general anesthesia should be adjusted to maintain $Paco_2$ at approximately 30 mm Hg (4 kPa). This can be achieved with minute ventilation of 121 mL/kg per minute; in comparison, 77 mL/kg per minute is required to maintain a comparable $Paco_2$ in nonpregnant women.[251] Decreased plasma bicarbonate concentration reduces buffering capacity in pregnancy. Allowing the $Paco_2$ to increase to the normal level for nonpregnant women results in respiratory acidosis.

Intravenous and Inhalation Anesthetics

The **propofol** requirement decreases 10% during the first trimester[252]; this decrease does not correlate with progesterone levels. The elimination half-life of propofol is unaffected by pregnancy, though clearance may be higher.[253]

The rate of rise of alveolar to inspired anesthetic concentration ratio (F_A/F_I) of **volatile anesthetics**, and thus the speed of induction, is increased during pregnancy because of greater minute ventilation and reduced FRC, despite higher cardiac output.

The minimum alveolar concentration (MAC) for volatile anesthetics is up to 40% lower in pregnancy.[254–256] Although MAC is a spinal nociceptive reflex that involves both sensory and motor components,[257] practitioners have interpreted this decrease in MAC as indicating that pregnant patients have a decreased requirement for inhaled anesthetics. However, this interpretation has been questioned. Ueyama et al.[258] compared

bispectral index (BIS) values in 15 patients undergoing cesarean delivery with sevoflurane general anesthesia with the values in 15 nonpregnant patients undergoing elective gynecologic surgery and found no difference between groups. This finding suggests that the hypnotic effect of sevoflurane was not enhanced by pregnancy. The investigators concluded that although pregnancy may decrease MAC, it does not decrease volatile anesthetic requirements and suggested that parturients should be given the same dose of volatile anesthetics as nonpregnant patients. Further work is required to confirm these findings.

Laboring women may differ from nonlaboring women. Yoo et al.[259] observed lower BIS values with a standard sevoflurane-nitrous oxide anesthetic in women with prior labor compared with nonlaboring parturients. Similarly, Erden et al.[260] observed lower sevoflurane requirements to reach a BIS target value of 40 to 55 in laboring compared with nonlaboring parturients undergoing cesarean delivery.

Muscle Relaxants

Pseudocholinesterase activity is decreased by 24% before delivery and by 33% on the third postpartum day.[261] It returns to normal 2 to 6 weeks postpartum. The reduced activity does not usually result in clinically relevant prolongation of paralysis after a single dose of **succinylcholine (suxamethonium)**. Twitch height recovery after administration of succinylcholine is similar between pregnant and nonpregnant women, and recovery may even be faster because the larger volume of distribution results in a lower initial drug concentration and a shorter time before the threshold for recovery is attained. Pregnant women may be less sensitive than nonpregnant women to comparable plasma concentrations of succinylcholine, a feature that also may contribute to more rapid recovery during pregnancy.

Pregnant and postpartum women exhibit enhanced sensitivity to the aminosteroid muscle relaxants **vecuronium** and **rocuronium**.[262,263] The greater sensitivity to vecuronium is not explained by altered pharmacokinetics because the drug exhibits increased clearance and a shortened elimination half-life in pregnant women.[264] The mean onset time and clinical duration of **cisatracurium** are significantly shorter in women immediately after delivery than in nonpregnant women.[265]

Chronotropic Agents and Vasopressors

Pregnancy reduces the chronotropic response to **isoproterenol (isoprenaline)** and **epinephrine** because of downregulation of beta-adrenergic receptors.[266] These agents are less-sensitive markers of intravascular injection during administration of an epidural test dose in pregnant patients than in nonpregnant patients. Because of downregulation of adrenergic receptors, treatment of hypotension requires higher doses of vasopressors such as **phenylephrine** in pregnant women than in nonpregnant women.

Pharmacologic Changes During Pregnancy

The physiologic changes of pregnancy have important effects on the pharmacodynamics and pharmacokinetics of drugs administered during pregnancy (see Chapter 16). Pregnancy is associated with important changes to drug absorption, distribution, metabolism, and excretion (see Chapter 16). Pharmacogenomic variation during pregnancy affects the response to many common medications including opioids (e.g., codeine, hydromorphone, tramadol), antiemetics (e.g., ondansetron, metoclopramide), antihypertensives (e.g., metoprolol, labetalol, nifedipine), and antidepressants (e.g., amitriptyline). Some medications used in parturients may impact uteroplacental blood flow and others have no apparent effect provided maternal hemodynamics are maintained, likely related to the lack of autoregulation of uterine perfusion (see Chapter 3).

Neuraxial Analgesia and Anesthesia

Technical Considerations and Positioning

Increased lumbar lordosis during pregnancy may reduce the vertebral interspinous gap and change the lumbar angulation of spinous processes, thus creating technical difficulty in administering neuraxial anesthesia (Box 2.4 and Fig. 2.12; see Chapter 12). Widening of the pelvis results in a head-down tilt when a pregnant woman is in the lateral position (Fig. 2.13). This may increase the rostral spread of hyperbaric local anesthetics when injected intrathecally with patients in the lateral position. The flow of CSF from a spinal needle is unchanged throughout gestation because pregnancy does not alter CSF pressure.[239] However, flow rate may increase during a uterine contraction because of increased CSF pressure.

Local Anesthetic Dose Requirement

Pregnant patients show decreased local anesthetic dose requirement in the first trimester. This change occurs well before significant mechanical changes have occurred in the vertebral canal,[267] suggesting that there are pregnancy-induced alterations in nerve tissue sensitivity, either directly or indirectly from changes in hormone concentrations.[268]

Pregnant women exhibit a more rapid onset and a longer duration of spinal anesthesia than nonpregnant women who receive the same dose of local anesthetic. These results are consistent with enhanced neural sensitivity to local anesthetics; pregnancy-associated elevation in CSF pH may contribute to these effects.[269–271] The dose of hyperbaric local anesthetic required in term pregnant women is 25% lower than that in nonpregnant women.[272,273] This is attributed to the following factors: (1) reduction of spinal CSF volume, which accompanies distention of the vertebral venous plexus[50]; (2) enhanced

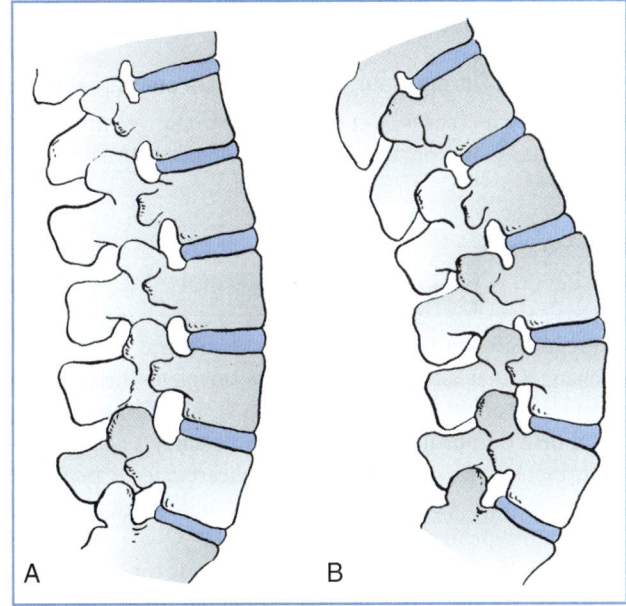

Fig. 2.12 Effects of Pregnancy on the Lumbar Spine. (A) Nonpregnant. (B) Pregnant. There is a marked increase in lumbar lordosis and a narrowing of the interspinous spaces during pregnancy. Modified from Bonica JJ. *Principles and Practice of Obstetric Analgesia and Anesthesia.* Vol. 1. FA Davis; 1967:35.

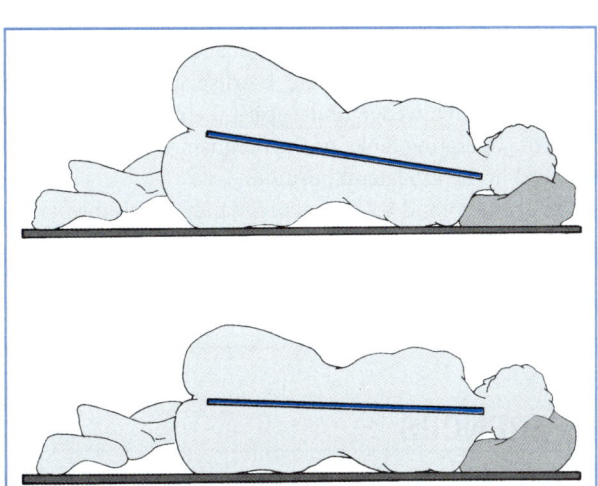

Fig. 2.13 Pelvic Widening and Resultant Head-Down Tilt in the Lateral Position During Pregnancy. *Upper panel*, Pregnant; *lower panel*, nonpregnant. Modified from Camann WR, Ostheimer GW. Physiological adaptations during pregnancy. *Int Anesthesiol Clin.* 1990;28:2–10.

neural sensitivity to local anesthetics; (3) increased rostral spread when injections are made with the patient in the lateral position; (4) inward displacement of intervertebral foraminal soft tissue, resulting from increased abdominal pressure[274]; and (5) a higher level of the apex of the thoracic kyphosis (the lowest point of the thoracic spinal canal in the supine position) during late pregnancy (see Fig. 12.4).[275] Spinal dose requirement changes rapidly in the postpartum period, with segmental dose requirement returning to that of nonpregnant women within 24 to 48 hours[276] as spinal CSF volume expands with the relief of vena caval compression. In contrast to spinal anesthesia, pregnancy appears to have less effect on the spread of epidural anesthesia.[277,278]

Hypotension During Neuraxial Analgesia and Anesthesia

Pregnancy increases dependence on the sympathetic nervous system for the maintenance of venous return

and SVR.[241] This, together with the effects of aortocaval compression, means that pregnant patients are particularly prone to hypotension and hemodynamic instability from the sympathetic block induced by neuraxial anesthesia. Management of hypotension is discussed in Chapter 26.

Effects of Neuraxial Anesthesia on Respiratory Function

FRC diminishes during neuraxial anesthesia, resulting in an increase in respiratory dead space and ventilation-perfusion mismatch. Abdominal muscles are important for forced expiration and coughing, and paralysis of these muscles during neuraxial anesthesia decreases PEF rate, maximum expiratory pressure, and the ability to increase intraabdominal and intrathoracic pressures during coughing.[279–281]

KEY POINTS

- Pregnancy results in various anatomic and physiologic changes that allow the mother to adapt to the growing fetus and allow the fetus to develop.
- Cardiac output increases during pregnancy as a result of an increase in stroke volume and heart rate. A pregnant woman with cardiovascular disease may not be able to meet this greater demand.
- Pregnant women have greater sympathetic tone than nonpregnant women.
- Beginning at mid-pregnancy, assumption of the supine position may result in compression of the inferior vena cava and aorta by the gravid uterus, which may result in decreases in both cardiac output and uteroplacental perfusion. Severe hypotension and bradycardia in the supine position is called the *supine hypotension syndrome.*
- Pregnant women should not lie supine after 20 weeks' gestation without aggressive maintenance of baseline blood pressure. The uterus should be displaced to the left by placement of a wedge underneath the right hip or by tilting the operating table, or the pregnant women should be placed in the full lateral position.
- The greater blood volume of pregnancy allows the parturient to tolerate the blood loss of delivery, within limits, with minimal hemodynamic perturbation. Maternal vascular capacitance is reduced at the time of delivery.

- Oxygen demand and delivery are greater during pregnancy and further increase during labor and delivery.
- Minute ventilation increases, whereas FRC decreases during pregnancy. It is not uncommon for the pregnant women to experience dyspnea.
- Pregnancy is a state of partially compensated respiratory alkalosis.
- Gastric volume, emptying, and pH are unaltered during pregnancy, but lower esophageal sphincter tone may be reduced with increased risk for gastroesophageal reflux.
- Pregnancy and the immediate postpartum period are considered hypercoagulable states.
- Mechanical changes in the vertebral column influence neuraxial analgesia and anesthesia.
- MAC values for the volatile anesthetics are decreased during pregnancy. However, it is unclear whether the hypnotic dose requirement is altered during pregnancy.
- Pregnant women have a rapid decrease in Pao_2 during periods of apnea.
- Pregnant women are at increased risk for failed tracheal intubation.
- Pregnant women are less responsive to vasopressors than nonpregnant women.

REFERENCES

1. Most J, Dervis S, Haman F, et al. Energy intake requirements in pregnancy. *Nutrients.* 2019;11:1812.
2. Institute of Medicine (U.S.) Committee to Reexamine IOM Pregnancy Weight Guidelines, Rasmussen KM, Yaktine AL. *Weight Gain During Pregnancy: Reexamining the Guidelines.* National Academies Press; 2009.
3. Amorim AR, Rossner S, Neovius M, et al. Does excess pregnancy weight gain constitute a major risk for increasing long-term BMI? *Obesity (Silver Spring).* 2007;15:1278–1286.
4. Eghbali M, Wang Y, Toro L, Stefani E. Heart hypertrophy during pregnancy: a better functioning heart? *Trends Cardiovasc Med.* 2006;16:285–291.
5. Cutforth R, MacDonald CB. Heart sounds and murmurs in pregnancy. *Am Heart J.* 1966;71:741–747.

6. Northcote RJ, Knight PV, Ballantyne D. Systolic murmurs in pregnancy: value of echocardiographic assessment. *Clin Cardiol.* 1985;8:327–328.

7. Holmes S, Kirkpatrick ID, Zelop CM, Jassal DS. MRI evaluation of maternal cardiac displacement in pregnancy: implications for cardiopulmonary resuscitation. *Am J Obstet Gynecol.* 2015;213:401.e1–e5.

8. Delgado C, Dawson K, Schwaegler B, et al. Hand placement during chest compressions in parturients: a pilot study to identify the location of the left ventricle using transthoracic echocardiography. *Int J Obstet Anesth.* 2020;43:31–35.

9. Schannwell CM, Zimmermann T, Schneppenheim M, et al. Left ventricular hypertrophy and diastolic dysfunction in healthy pregnant women. *Cardiology.* 2002;97:73–78.

10. Robson SC, Hunter S, Boys RJ, Dunlop W. Serial study of factors influencing changes in cardiac output during human pregnancy. *Am J Physiol.* 1989;256:H1060–H1065.

11. Spatling L, Fallenstein F, Huch A, et al. The variability of cardiopulmonary adaptation to pregnancy at rest and during exercise. *Br J Obstet Gynaecol.* 1992;99:1–40.

12. Iacobaeus C, Andolf E, Thorsell M, et al. Cardiac function, myocardial mechano-energetic efficiency, and ventricular-arterial coupling in normal pregnancy. *J Hypertens.* 2018;36:857–866.

13. Campos O, Andrade JL, Bocanegra J, et al. Physiologic multivalvular regurgitation during pregnancy: a longitudinal Doppler echocardiographic study. *Int J Cardiol.* 1993;40:265–272.

14. Carruth JE, Mivis SB, Brogan DR, Wenger NK. The electrocardiogram in normal pregnancy. *Am Heart J.* 1981;102:1075–1078.

15. Oram S, Holt M. Innocent depression of the S-T segment and flattening of the T-wave during pregnancy. *J Obstet Gynaecol Br Emp.* 1961;68:765–770.

16. Robson SC, Hunter S, Moore M, Dunlop W. Haemodynamic changes during the puerperium: a Doppler and M-mode echocardiographic study. *Br J Obstet Gynaecol.* 1987;94:1028–1039.

17. Petersen JW, Liu J, Chi YY, Lingis M, Williams RS, Rhoton-Vlasak A, Segal MS, Conrad KP, et al. Comparison of multiple non-invasive methods of measuring cardiac output during pregnancy reveals marked heterogeneity in the magnitude of cardiac output change between women. *Physiol Rep.* 2017;5:e13223.

18. Osman MW, Leone F, Nath M, et al. Diurnal variation and repeatability of arterial stiffness and cardiac output measurements in the third trimester of uncomplicated pregnancy. *J Hypertens.* 2017;35:2436–2442.

19. Capeless EL, Clapp JF. Cardiovascular changes in early phase of pregnancy. *Am J Obstet Gynecol.* 1989;161:1449–1453.

20. Laird-Meeter K, van de Ley G, Bom TH, et al. Cardiocirculatory adjustments during pregnancy – an echocardiographic study. *Clin Cardiol.* 1979;2:328–332.

21. Clark SL, Cotton DB, Lee W, et al. Central hemodynamic assessment of normal term pregnancy. *Am J Obstet Gynecol.* 1989;161:1439–1442.

22. Melchiorre K, Sharma R, Khalil A, Thilaganathan B. Maternal cardiovascular function in normal pregnancy: evidence of maladaptation to chronic volume overload. *Hypertension.* 2016;67:754–762.

23. Rubler S, Damani PM, Pinto ER. Cardiac size and performance during pregnancy estimated with echocardiography. *Am J Cardiol.* 1977;40:534–540.

24. Fok WY, Chan LY, Wong JT, et al. Left ventricular diastolic function during normal pregnancy: assessment by spectral tissue Doppler imaging. *Ultrasound Obstet Gynecol.* 2006;28:789–793.

25. Thaler I, Manor D, Itskovitz J, et al. Changes in uterine blood flow during human pregnancy. *Am J Obstet Gynecol.* 1990;162:121–125.

26. Rekonen A, Luotola H, Pitkänen M, et al. Measurement of intervillous and myometrial blood flow by an intravenous ^{133}Xe method. *Br J Obstet Gynaecol.* 1976;83:723–728.

27. Palmer SK, Zamudio S, Coffin C, et al. Quantitative estimation of human uterine artery blood flow and pelvic blood flow redistribution in pregnancy. *Obstet Gynecol.* 1992;80:1000–1006.

28. Flo K, Wilsgaard T, Vårtun A, Acharya G. A longitudinal study of the relationship between maternal cardiac output measured by impedance cardiography and uterine artery blood flow in the second half of pregnancy. *BJOG.* 2010;117:837–844.

29. Katz M, Sokal MM. Skin perfusion in pregnancy. *Am J Obstet Gynecol.* 1980;137:30–33.

30. Dunlop W. Serial changes in renal haemodynamics during normal human pregnancy. *Br J Obstet Gynaecol.* 1981;88:1–9.

31. U.S. Department of Health and Human Services. *Physical Activity Guidelines for Americans.* 2nd ed. U.S. Department of Health and Human Services; 2018.

32. American College of Obstetricians and Gynecologists. Committee Opinion No. 804: Physical activity and exercise during pregnancy and the postpartum period (reaffirmed 2023). *Obstet Gynecol.* 2020;135:e178–e188.

33. Gaston A, Cramp A. Exercise during pregnancy: a review of patterns and determinants. *J Sci Med Sport.* 2011;14:299–305.

34. Nascimento SL, Surita FG, Parpinelli MA, et al. The effect of an antenatal physical exercise programme on maternal/perinatal outcomes and quality of life in overweight and obese pregnant women: a randomised clinical trial. *BJOG.* 2011;118:1455–1463.

35. Szymanski LM, Satin AJ. Exercise during pregnancy: fetal responses to current public health guidelines. *Obstet Gynecol.* 2012;119:603–610.

36. Pernoll ML, Metcalfe J, Schlenker TL, et al. Oxygen consumption at rest and during exercise in pregnancy. *Respir Physiol.* 1975;25:285–293.

37. Ueland K, Novy MJ, Metcalfe J. Cardiorespiratory responses to pregnancy and exercise in normal women and patients with heart disease. *Am J Obstet Gynecol.* 1973;115:4–10.

38. Wolfe LA, Walker RM, Bonen A, McGrath MJ. Effects of pregnancy and chronic exercise on respiratory responses to graded exercise. *J Appl Physiol.* 1994;76:1928–1936.

39. Wilson M, Morganti AA, Zervoudakis I, et al. Blood pressure, the renin-aldosterone system and sex steroids throughout normal pregnancy. *Am J Med.* 1980;68:97–104.

40. Christianson RE. Studies on blood pressure during pregnancy. I. Influence of parity and age. *Am J Obstet Gynecol.* 1976;125:509–513.

41. de Haas S, Mulder E, Schartmann N, et al. Blood pressure adjustments throughout healthy and hypertensive pregnancy: a systematic review and meta-analysis. *Pregnancy Hypertens.* 2022;27:51–58.

42. Mikolajczyk RT, Zhang J, Ford J, Grewal J. Effects of interpregnancy interval on blood pressure in consecutive pregnancies. *Am J Epidemiol.* 2008;168:422–426.

43. Iwasaki R, Ohkuchi A, Furuta I, et al. Relationship between blood pressure level in early pregnancy and subsequent changes in blood pressure during pregnancy. *Acta Obstet Gynecol Scand*. 2002;81:918–925.

44. Gunderson EP, Chiang V, Lewis CE, et al. Long-term blood pressure changes measured from before to after pregnancy relative to nonparous women. *Obstet Gynecol*. 2008;112:1294–1302.

45. Kuate Defo A, Daskalopoulou SS. Alterations in vessel hemodynamics across uncomplicated pregnancy. *Am J Hypertens*. 2023;36:183–191.

46. Vinayagam D, Thilaganathan B, Stirrup O, et al. Maternal hemodynamics in normal pregnancy: reference ranges and role of maternal characteristics. *Ultrasound Obstet Gynecol*. 2018;51:665–671.

47. Kerr MG, Scott DB, Samuel E. Studies of the inferior vena cava in late pregnancy. *Br Med J*. 1964;1:522.4–533.

48. Kerr MG. The mechanical effects of the gravid uterus in late pregnancy. *J Obstet Gynaecol Br Commonw*. 1965;72:513–529.

49. Chun R, Baghirzada L, Tiruta C, Kirkpatrick AW. Measurement of intra-abdominal pressure in term pregnancy: a pilot study. *Int J Obstet Anesth*. 2012;21:135–139.

50. Hirabayashi Y, Shimizu R, Fukuda H, et al. Soft tissue anatomy within the vertebral canal in pregnant women. *Br J Anaesth*. 1996;77:153–156.

51. Higuchi H, Takagi S, Zhang K, et al. Effect of lateral tilt angle on the volume of the abdominal aorta and inferior vena cava in pregnant and nonpregnant women determined by magnetic resonance imaging. *Anesthesiology*. 2015;122:286–293.

52. Bieniarz J, Yoshida T, Romero-Salinas G, et al. Aortocaval compression by the uterus in late human pregnancy. IV. Circulatory homeostasis by preferential perfusion of the placenta. *Am J Obstet Gynecol*. 1969;103:19–31.

53. Lees MM, Scott DB, Kerr MG, Taylor SH. The circulatory effects of recumbent postural change in late pregnancy. *Clin Sci*. 1967;32:453–465.

54. McLennan CE. Antecubital and femoral venous pressure in normal and toxemic pregnancy. *Am J Obstet Gynecol*. 1943;45:568–591.

55. Fujita N, Higuchi H, Sakuma S, et al. Effect of right-lateral versus left-lateral tilt position on compression of the inferior vena cava in pregnant women determined by magnetic resonance imaging. *Anesth Analg*. 2019;128:1217–1222.

56. Eckstein KL, Marx GF. Aortocaval compression and uterine displacement. *Anesthesiology*. 1974;40:92–96.

57. Kinsella SM, Whitwam JG, Spencer JA. Aortic compression by the uterus: identification with the finapres digital arterial pressure instrument. *Br J Obstet Gynaecol*. 1990;97:700–705.

58. Abitbol MM. Aortic compression by pregnant uterus. *N Y State J Med*. 1976;76:1470–1475.

59. Kuo CD, Chen GY, Yang MJ, Tsai YS. The effect of position on autonomic nervous activity in late pregnancy. *Anaesthesia*. 1997;52:1161–1165.

60. Milsom I, Forssman L. Factors influencing aortocaval compression in late pregnancy. *Am J Obstet Gynecol*. 1984;148:764–771.

61. Clark SL, Cotton DB, Pivarnik JM, et al. Position change and central hemodynamic profile during normal third-trimester pregnancy and post partum. *Am J Obstet Gynecol*. 1991;164:883–887.

62. Drummond GB, Scott SE, Lees MM, Scott DB. Effects of posture on limb blood flow in late pregnancy. *Br Med J*. 1974;2:587–588.

63. Kinsella SM, Lohmann G. Supine hypotensive syndrome. *Obstet Gynecol*. 1994;83:774–788.

64. Armstrong S, Fernando R, Columb M, Jones T. Cardiac index in term pregnant women in the sitting, lateral, and supine positions: an observational, crossover study. *Anesth Analg*. 2011;113:318–322.

65. Howard BK, Goodson JH, Mengert WF. Supine hypotensive syndrome in late pegnancy. *Obstet Gynecol*. 1953;1:371–377.

66. Robson SC, Dunlop W, Boys RJ, Hunter S. Cardiac output during labour. *Br Med J (Clin Res Ed)*. 1987;295:1169–1172.

67. Ueland K, Hansen JM. Maternal cardiovascular dynamics. 3. Labor and delivery under local and caudal analgesia. *Am J Obstet Gynecol*. 1969;103:8–18.

68. Kjeldsen J. Hemodynamic investigations during labour and delivery. *Acta Obstet Gynecol Scand Suppl*. 1979;89:1–252.

69. Adams JQ, Alexander AM Jr. Alterations in cardiovascular physiology during labor. *Obstet Gynecol*. 1958;12:542–549.

70. Hendricks CH. The hemodynamics of a uterine contraction. *Am J Obstet Gynecol*. 1958;76:969–982.

71. Lee W, Rokey R, Miller J, Cotton DB. Maternal hemodynamic effects of uterine contractions by M-mode and pulsed-Doppler echocardiography. *Am J Obstet Gynecol*. 1989;161:974–977.

72. Goldsmith LT, Weiss G, Steinetz BG. Relaxin and its role in pregnancy. *Endocrinol Metab Clin North Am*. 1995;24:171–186.

73. Contreras G, Gutiérrez M, Beroíza T, et al. Ventilatory drive and respiratory muscle function in pregnancy. *Am Rev Respir Dis*. 1991;144:837–841.

74. LoMauro A, Aliverti A, Frykholm P, et al. Adaptation of lung, chest wall, and respiratory muscles during pregnancy: preparing for birth. *J Appl Physiol (1985)*. 2019;127:1640–1650.

75. Leontic EA. Respiratory disease in pregnancy. *Med Clin North Am*. 1977;61:111–128.

76. Wise RA, Polito AJ, Krishnan V. Respiratory physiologic changes in pregnancy. *Immunol Allergy Clin North Am*. 2006;26:1–12.

77. Grenville-Mathers R, Trenchard HJ. The diaphragm in the puerperium. *J Obstet Gynaecol Br Emp*. 1953;60:825–833.

78. Nørregaard O, Schultz P, Ostergaard A, Dahl R. Lung function and postural changes during pregnancy. *Respir Med*. 1989;83:467–470.

79. Russell IF, Chambers WA. Closing volume in normal pregnancy. *Br J Anaesth*. 1981;53:1043–1047.

80. Lemos A, de Souza AI, Figueiroa JN, et al. Respiratory muscle strength in pregnancy. *Respir Med*. 2010;104:1638–1644.

81. Harirah HM, Donia SE, Nasrallah FK, et al. Effect of gestational age and position on peak expiratory flow rate: a longitudinal study. *Obstet Gynecol*. 2005;105:372–376.

82. Grindheim G, Toska K, Estensen M-E, Rosseland LA. Changes in pulmonary function during pregnancy: a longitudinal cohort study. *BJOG*. 2012;119:94–101.

83. Hegewald MJ, Crapo RO. Respiratory physiology in pregnancy. *Clin Chest Med*. 2011;32:1–13.

84. Baldwin GR, Moorthi DS, Whelton JA, MacDonnell KF. New lung functions and pregnancy. *Am J Obstet Gynecol*. 1977;127:235–239.

85. Alaily AB. Carrol KB. Pulmonary ventilation in pregnancy. *Br J Obstet Gynaecol*. 1978;85:518–524.

86. Gee JB, Packer BS, Millen JE, Robin ED. Pulmonary mechanics during pregnancy. *J Clin Invest.* 1967;46:945–952.

87. Hignett R, Fernando R, McGlennan A, et al. A randomized crossover study to determine the effect of a 30 degrees head-up versus a supine position on the functional residual capacity of term parturients. *Anesth Analg.* 2011;113:1098–1102.

88. Bobrowski RA. Pulmonary physiology in pregnancy. *Clin Obstet Gynecol.* 2010;53:285–300.

89. Zwillich CW, Natalino MR, Sutton FD, Weil JV. Effects of progesterone on chemosensitivity in normal men. *J Lab Clin Med.* 1978;92:262–269.

90. Jensen D, Webb KA, Davies GA, O'Donnell DE. Mechanisms of activity-related breathlessness in healthy human pregnancy. *Eur J Appl Physiol.* 2009;106:253–265.

91. Jensen D, Duffin J, Lam YM, et al. Physiological mechanisms of hyperventilation during human pregnancy. *Respir Physiol Neurobiol.* 2008;161:76–86.

92. McAuley SE, Jensen D, McGrath MJ, Wolfe LA. Effects of human pregnancy and aerobic conditioning on alveolar gas exchange during exercise. *Can J Physiol Pharmacol.* 2005;83:625–633.

93. Moore LG, McCullough RE, Weil JV. Increased HVR in pregnancy: relationship to hormonal and metabolic changes. *J Appl Physiol.* 1987;62:158–163.

94. Templeton A, Kelman GR. Maternal blood-gases, (PAO_2-PaO_2), physiological shunt and V_D/V_T in normal pregnancy. *Br J Anaesth.* 1976;48:1001–1004.

95. Bader RA, Bader ME, Rose DF, Braunwald E. Hemodynamics at rest and during exercise in normal pregnancy as studies by cardiac catheterization. *J Clin Invest.* 1955;34:1524–1536.

96. Sady MA, Haydon BB, Sady SP, et al. Cardiovascular response to maximal cycle exercise during pregnancy and at two and seven months post partum. *Am J Obstet Gynecol.* 1990;162:1181–1185.

97. Shankar KB, Moseley H, Vemula V, et al. Arterial to end-tidal carbon dioxide tension difference during anaesthesia in early pregnancy. *Can J Anaesth.* 1989;36:124–127.

98. Shankar KB, Moseley H, Kumar Y, Vemula V. Arterial to end tidal carbon dioxide tension difference during caesarean section anaesthesia. *Anaesthesia.* 1986;41:698–702.

99. Shankar KB, Moseley H, Kumar Y, et al. Arterial to end-tidal carbon dioxide tension difference during anaesthesia for tubal ligation. *Anaesthesia.* 1987;42:482–486.

100. Dayal P, Murata Y, Takamura H. Antepartum and postpartum acid-base changes in maternal blood in normal and complicated pregnancies. *J Obstet Gynaecol Br Commonw.* 1972;79:612–624.

101. Seeds AE, Battaglia FC, Hellegers AE. Effects of pregnancy on the pH, PCO_2, and bicarbonate concentrations of peripheral venous blood. *Am J Obstet Gynecol.* 1964;88:1086–1089.

102. Lim VS, Katz AI, Lindheimer MD. Acid-base regulation in pregnancy. *Am J Physiol.* 1976;231:1764–1769.

103. Hägerdal M, Morgan CW, Sumner AE, Gutsche BB. Minute ventilation and oxygen consumption during labor with epidural analgesia. *Anesthesiology.* 1983;59:425–427.

104. Pearson JF, Davies P. The effect on continuous lumbar epidural analgesia on maternal acid-base balance and arterial lactate concentration during the second stage of labour. *J Obstet Gynaecol Br Commonw.* 1973;80:225–229.

105. Jouppila R, Hollmén A. The effect of segmental epidural analgesia on maternal and foetal acid-base balance, lactate, serum potassium and creatine phosphokinase during labour. *Acta Anaesthesiol Scand.* 1976;20:259–268.

106. Thalme B, Raabe N, Belfrage P. Lumbar epidural analgesia in labour. II. Effects on glucose, lactate, sodium, chloride, total protein, haematocrit and haemoglobin in maternal, fetal and neonatal blood. *Acta Obstet Gynecol Scand.* 1974;53:113–119.

107. Pearson JF, Davies P. The effect of continuous lumbar epidural analgesia on the acid-base status of maternal arterial blood during the first stage of labour. *J Obstet Gynaecol Br Commonw.* 1973;80:218–224.

108. Van de Putte P, Vernieuwe L, Perlas A. Term pregnant patients have similar gastric volume to non-pregnant females: a single-centre cohort study. *Br J Anaesth.* 2019;122:79–85.

109. Van Thiel DH, Gavaler JS, Stremple J. Lower esophageal sphincter pressure in women using sequential oral contraceptives. *Gastroenterology.* 1976;71:232–234.

110. Richter JE. Review article: the management of heartburn in pregnancy. *Aliment Pharmacol Ther.* 2005;22:749–757.

111. Fisher RS, Roberts GS, Grabowski CJ, Cohen S. Altered lower esophageal sphincter function during early pregnancy. *Gastroenterology.* 1978;74:1233–1237.

112. Marrero JM, Goggin PM, de Caestecker JS, et al. Determinants of pregnancy heartburn. *Br J Obstet Gynaecol.* 1992;99:731–734.

113. Wong CA, Loffredi M, Ganchiff JN, et al. Gastric emptying of water in term pregnancy. *Anesthesiology.* 2002;96:1395–1400.

114. La Salvia LA, Steffen EA. Delayed gastric emptying time in labor. *Am J Obstet Gynecol.* 1950;59:1075–1081.

115. Davison JS, Davison MC, Hay DM. Gastric emptying time in late pregnancy and labour. *J Obstet Gynaecol Br Commonw.* 1970;77:37–41.

116. O'Sullivan GM, Sutton AJ, Thompson SA, et al. Noninvasive measurement of gastric emptying in obstetric patients. *Anesth Analg.* 1987;66:505–511.

117. Sandhar BK, Elliott RH, Windram I, Rowbotham DJ. Peripartum changes in gastric emptying. *Anaesthesia.* 1992;47:196–198.

118. Wong CA, McCarthy RJ, Fitzgerald PC, et al. Gastric emptying of water in obese pregnant women at term. *Anesth Analg.* 2007;105:751–755.

119. Irwin R, Gyawali I, Kennedy B, et al. An ultrasound assessment of gastric emptying following tea with milk in pregnancy: a randomised controlled trial. *Eur J Anaesthesiol.* 2020;37:303–308.

120. Chiloiro M, Darconza G, Piccioli E, et al. Gastric emptying and orocecal transit time in pregnancy. *J Gastroenterol.* 2001;36:538–543.

121. Derbyshire EJ, Davies J, Detmar P. Changes in bowel function: pregnancy and the puerperium. *Dig Dis Sci.* 2007;52:324–328.

122. Parry E, Shields R, Turnbull AC. Transit time in the small intestine in pregnancy. *J Obstet Gynaecol Br Commonw.* 1970;77:900–901.

123. Murray FA, Erskine JP, Fielding J. Gastric secretion in pregnancy. *J Obstet Gynaecol Br Emp.* 1957;64:373–381.

124. Van Thiel DH, Gavaler JS, Joshi SN, et al. Heartburn of pregnancy. *Gastroenterology.* 1977;72:666–668.

125. Hong JY, Park JW, Oh JI. Comparison of preoperative gastric contents and serum gastrin concentrations in pregnant and nonpregnant women. *J Clin Anesth.* 2005;17:451–455.

126. Wyner J, Cohen SE. Gastric volume in early pregnancy: effect of metoclopramide. *Anesthesiology.* 1982;57:209–212.

127. Miller F. Nausea and vomiting in pregnancy: the problem of perception – is it really a disease? *Am J Obstet Gynecol.* 2002;186:S182–S183.

128. Gill SK, Maltepe C, Koren G. The effect of heartburn and acid reflux on the severity of nausea and vomiting of pregnancy. *Can J Gastroenterol.* 2009;23:270–272.

129. Carp H, Jayaram A, Stoll M. Ultrasound examination of the stomach contents of parturients. *Anesth Analg.* 1992;74:683–687.

130. Murphy DF, Nally B, Gardiner J, Unwin A. Effect of metoclopramide on gastric emptying before elective and emergency caesarean section. *Br J Anaesth.* 1984;56:1113–1116.

131. Roberts RB, Shirley MA. Reducing the risk of acid aspiration during cesarean section. *Anesth Analg.* 1974;53:859–868.

132. Kubli M, Scrutton MJ, Seed PT, O'Sullivan G. An evaluation of isotonic "sport drinks" during labor. *Anesth Analg.* 2002;94:404–408.

133. Lahiri SK, Thomas TA, Hodgson RM. Single-dose antacid therapy for the prevention of Mendelson's syndrome. *Br J Anaesth.* 1973;45:1143–1146.

134. Gin T, Cho AM, Lew JK, et al. Gastric emptying in the postpartum period. *Anaesth Intensive Care.* 1991;19:521–524.

135. James CF, Gibbs CP, Banner T. Postpartum perioperative risk of aspiration pneumonia. *Anesthesiology.* 1984;61:756–759.

136. Blouw R, Scatliff J, Craig DB, Palahniuk RJ. Gastric volume and pH in postpartum patients. *Anesthesiology.* 1976;45:456–457.

137. Lam KK, So HY, Gin T. Gastric pH and volume after oral fluids in the postpartum patient. *Can J Anaesth.* 1993;40:218–221.

138. Romalis G, Claman AD. Serum enzymes in pregnancy. *Am J Obstet Gynecol.* 1962;84:1104–1110.

139. Combes B, Shibata H, Adams R, et al. Alterations in sulfobromophthalein sodium-removal mechanisms from blood during normal pregnancy. *J Clin Invest.* 1963;42:1431–1442.

140. Blum A, Tatour I, Monir M, et al. Gallstones in pregnancy and their complications: postpartum acute pancreatitis and acute peritonitis. *Eur J Intern Med.* 2005;16:473–476.

141. Mendez-Sanchez N, Chavez-Tapia NC, Uribe M. Pregnancy and gallbladder disease. *Ann Hepatol.* 2006;5:227–230.

142. Ryan JP, Pellecchia D. Effect of progesterone pretreatment on guinea pig gallbladder motility in vitro. *Gastroenterology.* 1982;83:81–83.

143. Kern F Jr, Everson GT, DeMark B, et al. Biliary lipids, bile acids, and gallbladder function in the human female: effects of contraceptive steroids. *J Lab Clin Med.* 1982;99:798–805.

144. Jeyabalan A, Lain KY. Anatomic and functional changes of the upper urinary tract during pregnancy. *Urol Clin North Am.* 2007;34:1–6.

145. Rasmussen PE, Nielsen FR. Hydronephrosis during pregnancy: a literature survey. *Eur J Obstet Gynecol Reprod Biol.* 1988;27:249–259.

146. Davison JM, Hytten FE. Glomerular filtration during and after pregnancy. *J Obstet Gynaecol Br Commonw.* 1974;81:588–595.

147. Conrad KP. Maternal vasodilation in pregnancy: the emerging role of relaxin. *Am J Physiol Regul Integr Comp Physiol.* 2011;301:R267–R275.

148. Okada Y, Best SA, Jarvis SS, et al. Asian women have attenuated sympathetic activation but enhanced renal-adrenal responses during pregnancy compared to caucasian women. *J Physiol.* 2015;593:1159–1168.

149. Sims EA, Krantz KE. Serial studies of renal function during pregnancy and the puerperium in normal women. *J Clin Invest.* 1958;37:1764–1774.

150. Lind T, Godfrey KA, Otun H, Philips PR. Changes in serum uric acid concentrations during normal pregnancy. *Br J Obstet Gynaecol.* 1984;91:128–132.

151. Airoldi J, Weinstein L. Clinical significance of proteinuria in pregnancy. *Obstet Gynecol Surv.* 2007;62:117–124.

152. Higby K, Suiter CR, Phelps JY, et al. Normal values of urinary albumin and total protein excretion during pregnancy. *Am J Obstet Gynecol.* 1994;171:984–989.

153. Fishel Bartal M, Lindheimer MD, Sibai BM. Proteinuria during pregnancy: definition, pathophysiology, methodology, and clinical significance. *Am J Obstet Gynecol.* 2022;226:S819–S834.

154. American College of Obstetricians and Gynecologists Task Force on Hypertension in Pregnancy. Hypertension in pregnancy: report of the American College of Obstetricians and Gynecologists' Task Force on Hypertension in Pregnancy. *Obstet Gynecol.* 2013;122:1122–1131.

155. Baba Y, Ohkuchi A, Usui R, et al. Urinary protein-to-creatinine ratio indicative of significant proteinuria in normotensive pregnant women. *J Obstet Gynaecol Res.* 2016;42:784–788.

156. Smith NA, Lyons JG, McElrath TF. Protein:creatinine ratio in uncomplicated twin pregnancy. *Am J Obstet Gynecol.* 2010;203:381.e1–e4.

157. Davison JM, Hytten FE. The effect of pregnancy on the renal handling of glucose. *Br J Obstet Gynaecol.* 1975;82:374–381.

158. Aguree S, Gernand AD. Plasma volume expansion across healthy pregnancy: a systematic review and meta-analysis of longitudinal studies. *BMC Pregnancy Childbirth.* 2019;19:508.

159. Lund CJ, Donovan JC. Blood volume during pregnancy. Significance of plasma and red cell volumes. *Am J Obstet Gynecol.* 1967;98:394–403.

160. Taylor DJ, Lind T. Red cell mass during and after normal pregnancy. *Br J Obstet Gynaecol.* 1979;86:364–370.

161. Pritchard JA. Changes in the blood volume during pregnancy and delivery. *Anesthesiology.* 1965;26:393–399.

162. Cotes PM, Canning CE, Lind T. Changes in serum immunoreactive erythropoietin during the menstrual cycle and normal pregnancy. *Br J Obstet Gynaecol.* 1983;90:304–311.

163. Abbassi-Ghanavati M, Greer LG, Cunningham FG. Pregnancy and laboratory studies: a reference table for clinicians. *Obstet Gynecol.* 2009;114:1326–1331.

164. James AH. Iron deficiency anemia in pregnancy. *Obstet Gynecol.* 2021;138:663–674.

165. Hayashi Y, Ueyama H, Mashimo T, et al. Circulating mature adrenomedullin is related to blood volume in full-term pregnancy. *Anesth Analg.* 2005;101:1816–1820.

166. Hytten FE, Paintin DB. Increase in plasma volume during normal pregnancy. *J Obstet Gynaecol Br Emp.* 1963;70:402–407.

167. Duvekot JJ, Cheriex EC, Pieters FA, et al. Early pregnancy changes in hemodynamics and volume homeostasis are consecutive adjustments triggered by a primary fall in systemic vascular tone. *Am J Obstet Gynecol.* 1993;169:1382–1392.

168. Kennedy H, Haynes SL, Shelton CL. Maternal body weight and estimated circulating blood volume: a review and practical nonlinear approach. *Br J Anaesth.* 2022;129:716–725.

169. Coryell MN, Beach EF, Robinson AR, et al. Metabolism of women during the reproductive cycle. XVII. Changes in electrophoretic patterns of plasma proteins throughout the cycle and following delivery. *J Clin Invest.* 1950;29:1559–1567.

170. Mendenhall HW. Serum protein concentrations in pregnancy. I. Concentrations in maternal serum. *Am J Obstet Gynecol.* 1970;106:388–399.

171. Robertson EG, Cheyne GA. Plasma biochemistry in relation to oedema of pregnancy. *J Obstet Gynaecol Br Commonw.* 1972;79:769–776.

172. Wu PY, Udani V, Chan L, et al. Colloid osmotic pressure: variations in normal pregnancy. *J Perinat Med.* 1983;11:193–199.

173. Evans RT, Wroe JM. Plasma cholinesterase changes during pregnancy. Their interpretation as a cause of suxamethonium-induced apnoea. *Anaesthesia.* 1980;35:651–654.

174. Gerbasi FR, Bottoms S, Farag A, Mammen E. Increased intravascular coagulation associated with pregnancy. *Obstet Gynecol.* 1990;75:385–389.

175. Tygart SG, McRoyan DK, Spinnato JA, et al. Longitudinal study of platelet indices during normal pregnancy. *Am J Obstet Gynecol.* 1986;154:883–887.

176. Fay RA, Hughes AO, Farron NT. Platelets in pregnancy: hyperdestruction in pregnancy. *Obstet Gynecol.* 1983;61:238–240.

177. Norris LA, Sheppard BL, Bonnar J. Increased whole blood platelet aggregation in normal pregnancy can be prevented in vitro by aspirin and dazmegrel (UK38485). *Br J Obstet Gynaecol.* 1992;99:253–257.

178. Pitkin RM, Witte DL. Platelet and leukocyte counts in pregnancy. *JAMA.* 1979;242:2696–2698.

179. Kadir lRA, McLintock C. Thrombocytopenia and disorders of platelet function in pregnancy. *Semin Thromb Hemost.* 2011;37:640–652.

180. Thornton P, Douglas J. Coagulation in pregnancy. *Best Pract Res Clin Obstet Gynaecol.* 2010;24:339–352.

181. Talbert LM, Langdell RD. Normal values of certain factors in the blood clotting mechanism in pregnancy. *Am J Obstet Gynecol.* 1964;90:44–50.

182. Kasper CK, Hoag MS, Aggeler PM, Stone S. Blood clotting factors in pregnancy: factor 8 concentrations in normal and AHF-deficient women. *Obstet Gynecol.* 1964;24:242–247.

183. Stirling Y, Woolf L, North WR, et al. Haemostasis in normal pregnancy. *Thromb Haemost.* 1984;52:176–182.

184. Coopland A, Alkjaersig N, Fletcher AP. Reduction in plasma factor 13 (fibrin stabilizing factor) concentration during pregnancy. *J Lab Clin Med.* 1969;73:144–153.

185. Liu J, Yuan E, Lee L. Gestational age-specific reference intervals for routine haemostatic assays during normal pregnancy. *Clin Chim Acta.* 2012;413:258–261.

186. Szecsi PB, Jørgensen M, Klajnbard A, et al. Haemostatic reference intervals in pregnancy. *Thromb Haemost.* 2010;103:718–727.

187. Sharma SK, Philip J, Wiley J. Thromboelastographic changes in healthy parturients and postpartum women. *Anesth Analg.* 1997;85:94–98.

188. Steer PL, Krantz HB. Thromboelastography and sonoclot analysis in the healthy parturient. *J Clin Anesth.* 1993;5:419–424.

189. Karlsson O, Sporrong T, Hillarp A, et al. Prospective longitudinal study of thromboelastography and standard hemostatic laboratory tests in healthy women during normal pregnancy. *Anesth Analg.* 2012;115:890–898.

190. Shreeve NE, Barry JA, Deutsch LR, et al. Changes in thromboelastography parameters in pregnancy, labor, and the immediate postpartum period. *Int J Gynaecol Obstet.* 2016;134:290–293.

191. Butwick A, Harter S. An in vitro investigation of the coagulation effects of exogenous oxytocin using thromboelastography in healthy parturients. *Anesth Analg.* 2011;113:323–326.

192. Amgalan A, Allen T, Othman M, Ahmadzia HK. Systematic review of viscoelastic testing (TEG/ROTEM) in obstetrics and recommendations from the women's SSC of the ISTH. *J Thromb Haemost.* 2020;18:1813–1838.

193. Gong JM, Shen Y, He YX. Reference intervals of routine coagulation assays during the pregnancy and puerperium period. *J Clin Lab Anal.* 2016;30:912–917.

194. Cui C, Yang S, Zhang J, et al. Trimester-specific coagulation and anticoagulation reference intervals for healthy pregnancy. *Thromb Res.* 2017;156:82–86.

195. Hellgren M. Hemostasis during normal pregnancy and puerperium. *Semin Thromb Hemost.* 2003;29:125–130.

196. Ueland K. Maternal cardiovascular dynamics. VII. Intrapartum blood volume changes. *Am J Obstet Gynecol.* 1976;126:671–677.

197. Toledo P, McCarthy RJ, Hewlett BJ, et al. The accuracy of blood loss estimation after simulated vaginal delivery. *Anesth Analg.* 2007;105:1736–1740.

198. Taylor DJ, Phillips P, Lind T. Puerperal haematological indices. *Br J Obstet Gynaecol.* 1981;88:601–606.

199. Ygge J. Changes in blood coagulation and fibrinolysis during the puerperium. *Am J Obstet Gynecol.* 1969;104:2–12.

200. Bonnar J, McNicol GP, Douglas AS. Coagulation and fibrinolytic mechanisms during and after normal childbirth. *Br Med J.* 1970;2:200–203.

201. Krause PJ, Ingardia CJ, Pontius LT, et al. Host defense during pregnancy: neutrophil chemotaxis and adherence. *Am J Obstet Gynecol.* 1987;157:274–280.

202. Baboonian C, Griffiths P. Is pregnancy immunosuppressive? Humoral immunity against viruses. *Br J Obstet Gynaecol.* 1983;90:1168–1175.

203. Piccinni MP. Role of T-cell cytokines in decidua and in cumulus oophorus during pregnancy. *Gynecol Obstet Invest.* 2007;64:144–148.

204. Munoz-Suano A, Hamilton AB, Betz AG. Gimme shelter: the immune system during pregnancy. *Immunol Rev.* 2011;241:20–38.

205. Chen SJ, Liu YL, Sytwu HK. Immunologic regulation in pregnancy: from mechanism to therapeutic strategy for immunomodulation. *Clin Dev Immunol.* 2012;2012: 258391.

206. Vujaklija DV, Gulic T, Sucic S, et al. First trimester pregnancy decidual natural killer cells contain and spontaneously release high quantities of granulysin. *Am J Reprod Immunol.* 2011;66:363–372.

207. Abu-Raya B, Michalski C, Sadarangani M, Lavoie PM. Maternal immunological adaptation during normal pregnancy. *Front Immunol.* 2020;11:575197.

208. King AE, Kelly RW, Sallenave JM, et al. Innate immune defences in the human uterus during pregnancy. *Placenta.* 2007;28:1099–1106.

209. Rivara AC, Miller EM. Pregnancy and immune stimulation: re-imagining the fetus as parasite to understand age-related immune system changes in us women. *Am J Hum Biol.* 2017;29:e23041.

210. Harada A, Hershman JM, Reed AW, et al. Comparison of thyroid stimulators and thyroid hormone concentrations in the sera of pregnant women. *J Clin Endocrinol Metab.* 1979;48:793–797.

211. Dichtel LE, Alexander EK. Preventing and treating maternal hypothyroidism during pregnancy. *Curr Opin Endocrinol Diabetes Obes.* 2011;18:389–394.

212. Negro R, Schwartz A, Gismondi R, et al. Universal screening versus case finding for detection and treatment of thyroid hormonal dysfunction during pregnancy. *J Clin Endocrinol Metab*. 2010;95:1699–1707.

213. Blatt AJ, Nakamoto JM, Kaufman HW. National status of testing for hypothyroidism during pregnancy and postpartum. *J Clin Endocrinol Metab*. 2012;97:777–784.

214. Wang S, Teng WP, Li JX, et al. Effects of maternal subclinical hypothyroidism on obstetrical outcomes during early pregnancy. *J Endocrinol Invest*. 2012;35:322–325.

215. Felig P, Lynch V. Starvation in human pregnancy: hypoglycemia, hypoinsulinemia, and hyperketonemia. *Science*. 1970;170:990–992.

216. Fisher PM, Sutherland HW, Bewsher PD. The insulin response to glucose infusion in normal human pregnancy. *Diabetologia*. 1980;19:15–20.

217. Rosenthal HE, Slaunwhite WR Jr, Sandberg AA. Transcortin: a corticosteroid-binding protein of plasma. X. Cortisol and progesterone interplay and unbound levels of these steroids in pregnancy. *J Clin Endocrinol Metab*. 1969;29:352–367.

218. Pacheco LD, Ghulmiyyah LM, Snodgrass WR, Hankins GD. Pharmacokinetics of corticosteroids during pregnancy. *Am J Perinatol*. 2007;24:79–82.

219. Kristiansson P, Nilsson-Wikmar L, von Schoultz B, et al. Back pain in in-vitro fertilized and spontaneous pregnancies. *Hum Reprod*. 1998;13:3233–3238.

220. Branco MA, Santos-Rocha R, Vieira F, et al. Three-dimensional kinematic adaptations of gait throughout pregnancy and post-partum. *Acta Bioeng Biomech*. 2016;18:153–162.

221. Berg G, Hammar M, Möller-Nielsen J, et al. Low back pain during pregnancy. *Obstet Gynecol*. 1988;71:71–75.

222. Wilkinson M. The carpal-tunnel syndrome in pregnancy. *Lancet*. 1960;275:453–454.

223. Kovacs CS. Calcium and bone metabolism disorders during pregnancy and lactation. *Endocrinol Metab Clin North Am*. 2011;40:795–826.

224. Naylor KE, Iqbal P, Fledelius C, et al. The effect of pregnancy on bone density and bone turnover. *J Bone Miner Res*. 2000;15:129–137.

225. Nakayama S, Yasui T, Suto M, et al. Differences in bone metabolism between singleton pregnancy and twin pregnancy. *Bone*. 2011;49:513–519.

226. American Academy of Sleep Medicine. *International Classification of Sleep Disorders Revised: Diagnostic and Coding Manual*. American Academy of Sleep Medicine; 2000

227. Facco FL, Kramer J, Ho KH, et al. Sleep disturbances in pregnancy. *Obstet Gynecol*. 2010;115:77–83.

228. Santiago JR, Nolledo MS, Kinzler W, Santiago TV. Sleep and sleep disorders in pregnancy. *Ann Intern Med*. 2001;134:396–408.

229. Schweiger MS. Sleep disturbance in pregnancy. A subjective survey. *Am J Obstet Gynecol*. 1972;114:879–882.

230. Dominguez JE, Cantrell S, Habib AS, et al. Society of Anesthesia and Sleep Medicine and the Society for Obstetric Anesthesia and Perinatology consensus guideline on the screening, diagnosis, and treatment of obstructive sleep apnea in pregnancy. *Obstet Gynecol*. 2023;142:403–423.

231. Manconi M, Govoni V, De Vito A, et al. Pregnancy as a risk factor for restless legs syndrome. *Sleep Med*. 2004;5:305–308.

232. Nevo O, Soustiel JF, Thaler I. Maternal cerebral blood flow during normal pregnancy: a cross-sectional study. *Am J Obstet Gynecol*. 2010;203:475.e1–e6.

233. Cipolla MJ, Sweet JG, Chan SL. Cerebral vascular adaptation to pregnancy and its role in the neurological complications of eclampsia. *J Appl Physiol*. 2011;110:329–339.

234. Cogan R, Spinnato JA. Pain and discomfort thresholds in late pregnancy. *Pain*. 1986;27:63–68.

235. Abboud TK, Sarkis F, Hung TT, et al. Effects of epidural anesthesia during labor on maternal plasma beta-endorphin levels. *Anesthesiology*. 1983;59:1–5.

236. Iwasaki H, Collins JG, Saito Y, Kerman-Hinds A. Naloxone-sensitive, pregnancy-induced changes in behavioral responses to colorectal distention: pregnancy-induced analgesia to visceral stimulation. *Anesthesiology*. 1991;74:927–933.

237. Hirabayashi Y, Shimizu R, Fukuda H, et al. Anatomical configuration of the spinal column in the supine position. II. Comparison of pregnant and non-pregnant women. *Br J Anaesth*. 1995;75:6–8.

238. Messih MN. Epidural space pressures during pregnancy. *Anaesthesia*. 1981;36:775–782.

239. Marx GF, Zemaitis MT, Orkin LR. Cerebrospinal fluid pressures during labor and obstetrical anesthesia. *Anesthesiology*. 1961;22:348–354.

240. Assali NS, Prystowsky H. Studies on autonomic blockade. I. Comparison between the effects of tetraethylammonium chloride (TEAC) and high selective spinal anesthesia on blood pressure of normal and toxemic pregnancy. *J Clin Invest*. 1950;29:1354–1366.

241. Tabsh K, Rudelstorfer R, Nuwayhid B, Assali NS. Circulatory responses to hypovolemia in the pregnant and nonpregnant sheep after pharmacologic sympathectomy. *Am J Obstet Gynecol*. 1986;154:411–419.

242. Goodlin RC. Venous reactivity and pregnancy abnormalities. *Acta Obstet Gynecol Scand*. 1986;65:345–348.

243. Abitbol MM. Supine position in labor and associated fetal heart rate changes. *Obstet Gynecol*. 1985;65:481–486.

244. Huch A, Huch R, Schneider H, Rooth G. Continuous transcutaneous monitoring of fetal oxygen tension during labour. *Br J Obstet Gynaecol*. 1977;84:1–39.

245. Crawford JS, Burton M, Davies P. Time and lateral tilt at caesarean section. *Br J Anaesth*. 1972;44:477–484.

246. Lee AJ, Landau R, Mattingly JL, et al. Left lateral table tilt for elective cesarean delivery under spinal anesthesia has no effect on neonatal acid-base status: a randomized controlled trial. *Anesthesiology*. 2017;127:241–249.

247. Michelsen TM, Tronstad C, Rosseland LA. Blood pressure and cardiac output during caesarean delivery under spinal anaesthesia: a prospective cohort study. *BMJ Open*. 2021;11:e046102.

248. Pilkington S, Carli F, Dakin MJ, et al. Increase in Mallampati score during pregnancy. *Br J Anaesth*. 1995;74:638–642.

249. Dobb G. Laryngeal oedema complicating obstetric anaesthesia. *Anaesthesia*. 1978;33:839–840.

250. Archer GW Jr, Marx GF. Arterial oxygen tension during apnoea in parturient women. *Br J Anaesth*. 1974;46:358–360.

251. Rampton AJ, Mallaiah S, Garrett CP. Increased ventilation requirements during obstetric general anaesthesia. *Br J Anaesth*. 1988;61:730–737.

252. Mongardon N, Servin F, Perrin M, et al. Predicted propofol effect-site concentration for induction and emergence of anesthesia during early pregnancy. *Anesth Analg*. 2009;109:90–95.

253. Gin T, Gregory MA, Chan K, et al. Pharmacokinetics of propofol in women undergoing elective caesarean section. *Br J Anaesth*. 1990;64:148–153.

254. Palahniuk RJ, Shnider SM, Eger EI 2nd. Pregnancy decreases the requirement for inhaled anesthetic agents. *Anesthesiology*. 1974;41:82–83.

255. Abboud TK, Zhu J, Richardson M, et al. Desflurane: a new volatile anesthetic for cesarean section. Maternal and neonatal effects. *Acta Anaesthesiol Scand*. 1995;39:723–726.

256. Preckel B, Bolten J. Pharmacology of modern volatile anaesthetics. *Best Pract Res Clin Anaesthesiol*. 2005;19:331–348.

257. Jinks SL, Martin JT, Carstens E, et al. Peri-MAC depression of a nociceptive withdrawal reflex is accompanied by reduced dorsal horn activity with halothane but not isoflurane. *Anesthesiology*. 2003;98:1128–1138.

258. Ueyama H, Hagihira S, Takashina M, et al. Pregnancy does not enhance volatile anesthetic sensitivity on the brain: an electroencephalographic analysis study. *Anesthesiology*. 2010;113:577–584.

259. Yoo KY, Jeong CW, Kang MW, et al. Bispectral index values during sevoflurane-nitrous oxide general anesthesia in women undergoing cesarean delivery: a comparison between women with and without prior labor. *Anesth Analg*. 2008;106:1827–1832.

260. Erden V, Erkalp K, Yangin Z, et al. The effect of labor on sevoflurane requirements during cesarean delivery. *Int J Obstet Anesth*. 2011;20:17–21.

261. Shnider SM. Serum cholinesterase activity during pregnancy, labor and the puerperium. *Anesthesiology*. 1965;26:335–339.

262. Baraka A, Jabbour S, Tabboush Z, et al. Onset of vecuronium neuromuscular block is more rapid in patients undergoing caesarean section. *Can J Anaesth*. 1992;39:135–138.

263. Pühringer FK, Sparr HJ, Mitterschiffthaler G, et al. Extended duration of action of rocuronium in postpartum patients. *Anesth Analg*. 1997;84:352–354.

264. Dailey PA, Fisher DM, Shnider SM, et al. Pharmacokinetics, placental transfer, and neonatal effects of vecuronium and pancuronium administered during cesarean section. *Anesthesiology*. 1984;60:569–574.

265. Pan PH, Moore C. Comparison of cisatracurium-induced neuromuscular blockade between immediate postpartum and nonpregnant patients. *J Clin Anesth*. 2001;13:112–117.

266. DeSimone CA, Leighton BL, Norris MC, et al. The chronotropic effect of isoproterenol is reduced in term pregnant women. *Anesthesiology*. 1988;69:626–628.

267. Fagraeus L, Urban BJ, Bromage PR. Spread of epidural analgesia in early pregnancy. *Anesthesiology*. 1983;58:184–187.

268. Datta S, Lambert DH, Gregus J, et al. Differential sensitivities of mammalian nerve fibers during pregnancy. *Anesth Analg*. 1983;62:1070–1072.

269. Popitz-Bergez FA, Leeson S, Thalhammer JG, Strichartz GR. Intraneural lidocaine uptake compared with analgesic differences between pregnant and nonpregnant rats. *Reg Anesth*. 1997;22:363–371.

270. Flanagan HL, Datta S, Lambert DH, et al. Effect of pregnancy on bupivacaine-induced conduction blockade in the isolated rabbit vagus nerve. *Anesth Analg*. 1987;66:123–126.

271. Hirabayashi Y, Shimizu R, Saitoh K, et al. Acid-base state of cerebrospinal fluid during pregnancy and its effect on spread of spinal anaesthesia. *Br J Anaesth*. 1996;77:352–355.

272. Barclay DL, Renegar OJ, Nelson EW Jr. The influence of inferior vena cava compression on the level of spinal anesthesia. *Am J Obstet Gynecol*. 1968;101:792–800.

273. Hirabayashi Y, Shimizu R, Saitoh K, Fukuda H. Spread of subarachnoid hyperbaric amethocaine in pregnant women. *Br J Anaesth*. 1995;74:384–386.

274. Hogan QH, Prost R, Kulier A, et al. Magnetic resonance imaging of cerebrospinal fluid volume and the influence of body habitus and abdominal pressure. *Anesthesiology*. 1996;84:1341–1349.

275. Hirabayashi Y, Shimizu R, Fukuda H, et al. Anatomical configuration of the spinal column in the supine position. II. Comparison of pregnant and non-pregnant women. *Br J Anaesth*. 1995;75:6–8.

276. Abouleish EI. Postpartum tubal ligation requires more bupivacaine for spinal anesthesia than does cesarean section. *Anesth Analg*. 1986;65:897–900.

277. Grundy EM, Zamora AM, Winnie AP. Comparison of spread of epidural anesthesia in pregnant and nonpregnant women. *Anesth Analg*. 1978;57:544–546.

278. Kalas DB, Senfield RM, Hehre FW. Continuous lumbar peridural anesthesia in obstetrics. IV. Comparison of the number of segments blocked in pregnant and nonpregnant subjects. *Anesth Analg*. 1966;45:848–851.

279. Moir DD. Ventilatory function during epidural analgesia. *Br J Anaesth*. 1963;35:3–7.

280. Egbert LD, Tamersoy K, Deas TC. Pulmonary function during spinal anesthesia: the mechanism of cough depression. *Anesthesiology*. 1961;22:882–885.

281. von Ungern-Sternberg BS, Regli A, Bucher E, et al. The effect of epidural analgesia in labour on maternal respiratory function. *Anaesthesia*. 2004;59:350–353.

3

Uteroplacental Blood Flow

Joshua I. Rosenbloom, MD, MPH, FACOG, D. Michael Nelson, MD, PhD, and Yehuda Ginosar, BSc, MBBS

CHAPTER OUTLINE

BASIC PRINCIPLES OF HUMAN UTEROPLACENTAL BLOOD FLOW

The uteroplacental circulation provides nutrient and oxygen delivery and removal of waste products for the developing fetus. Understanding the regulation of uteroplacental circulation is an important foundation for the management of obstetric diseases and for the safe provision of obstetric anesthesia. The uteroplacental circulation can be affected by maternal disease, medications, parturition, and anesthesia. Abnormalities in uteroplacental circulation are implicated in the "Great Obstetric Syndromes" of preeclampsia, preterm birth, and intrauterine growth restriction.[1] Much of the available knowledge on the uteroplacental circulation comes from animal studies, which limits applicability to clinical care. Recently, computational modeling has provided new insights into the uteroplacental circulation.[2] Despite advances in our understanding, additional research is needed on the mechanisms underlying the establishment and regulation of uteroplacental blood flow, the effect of pharmacologic agents for improving pathologic conditions related to blood flow, and how alterations in uteroplacental blood flow affect pregnancy outcomes.

The physiology and pathophysiology of uteroplacental blood flow have been studied extensively in animals, especially sheep and rodents. However, major differences in placental organization, structure, and function exist among species. Therefore, caution must be exercised when extrapolating animal studies to clinical practice.

Some of the differences between animal and humans include:

1. **Degree of Separation of Maternal and Fetal Blood**

   The human placenta is **hemochorial**, with maternal blood in direct contact with fetal chorionic villi, while the sheep placenta is epitheliochorial, where maternal blood is separated from fetal chorionic tissue by maternal vascular endothelium and uterine epithelium.

2. **Organization of Units of Maternal-Fetal Exchange**

   The human placenta is **discoid**. The cotyledon is the basic unit of maternal-fetal placental exchange, consisting of a branching stem chorionic villus from the fetal side that traverses intervillous space to establish an anchoring villus in the decidua basalis of the maternal uterus. Within the chorioallantoic placenta, 15 to 25 cotyledons develop, which are tightly packed, separated by septa and sandwiched between the chorionic and basal plates of the placental disc.

By contrast, the sheep has a polycotyledonal placenta, where cotyledons are discrete and widely separated throughout the placenta.

3. **Depth of Trophoblast Remodeling of Uterine Vasculature in Pregnancy**

Normal human pregnancy is characterized by extensive **remodeling of uterine spiral arteries** by invading trophoblasts; this converts the high-resistance, low-flow, nonpregnant spiral arteries into low-resistance, high-flow spiral arteries. Trophoblast invasion occurs throughout the full depth of the decidua and into the inner third of the myometrium, which contrasts with limited invasion in rodents. Although rodents and humans both have hemochorial discoid placentas, the differences in the extent of trophoblast invasion and vascular remodeling make extrapolation between the two species problematic. For example, phenylephrine causes uterine artery vasoconstriction and impaired uteroplacental perfusion in rodents[3] and sheep[4,5] but not in human pregnancy. Indeed, failure to appreciate interspecies differences previously led to ephedrine long being considered the vasopressor of choice in obstetric anesthesia.

ANATOMY

The blood supply to the uterus is derived mainly from the uterine arteries (Fig. 3.1) with a smaller, variable contribution from the ovarian arteries. The uterine artery arises bilaterally from the anterior division of the internal iliac (hypogastric) artery, whereas the ovarian artery arises from the anterolateral abdominal aorta below the renal arteries. Vessel diameter and blood flow are greater in the uterine artery on the ipsilateral side of the placenta, compared with the contralateral artery.[6] Anastomoses are formed with the contralateral uterine artery, the vaginal arteries, and the ovarian arteries. The uterine arteries pass medially to the side of the uterus, where they supply branches to the cervix and vagina and ascend between the two layers of the broad ligament, yielding arcuate arteries that supply the body of the uterus to the junction with the fallopian tubes.

The arcuate arteries give rise to small branches that supply the outer myometrium and large-diameter radial arteries that penetrate deeply into the myometrium to reach the endometrium as approximately 200 convoluted spiral arteries.[7] The radial arteries also give rise to the basal arteries, which are subjacent to the endometrium but do not reach the luminal surface.[8] In early gestation, trophoblastic invasion into the lumens of the spiral arteries results in loss of vessel smooth muscle and contractile ability, producing vasodilation, decreased resistance, and increased blood flow. Abnormal or inadequate trophoblastic invasion is a hallmark of the histopathology of the uteroplacental circulation in preeclampsia (see Chapter 35).

Oxygenated maternal blood enters the intervillous space from the terminal openings of the spiral arteries that emanate from the basal plate, or decidua basalis, which is the junction of the chorioallantoic placenta with endometrium

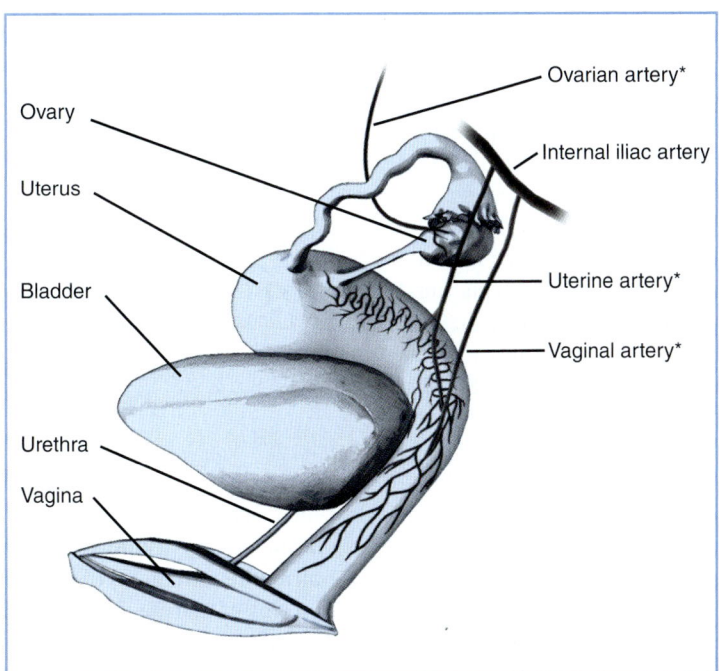

Fig. 3.1 Arterial Supply to the Female Reproductive Tract. *The female reproductive tract, particularly the uterus, has a rich network of collateral blood flow from both ipsilateral and contralateral vessels. Variations in the origin of arterial vessels and the presence of anastomoses (i.e., between left and right uterine arteries, or uterine to ovarian arteries) are common. During maternal hemorrhage, this network can thwart attempts to obtain hemostasis through vessel ligation or embolization. Illustration by Naveen Nathan, M.D., NorthShore University HealthSystem, University of Chicago Pritzker School of Medicine, Evanston, IL.

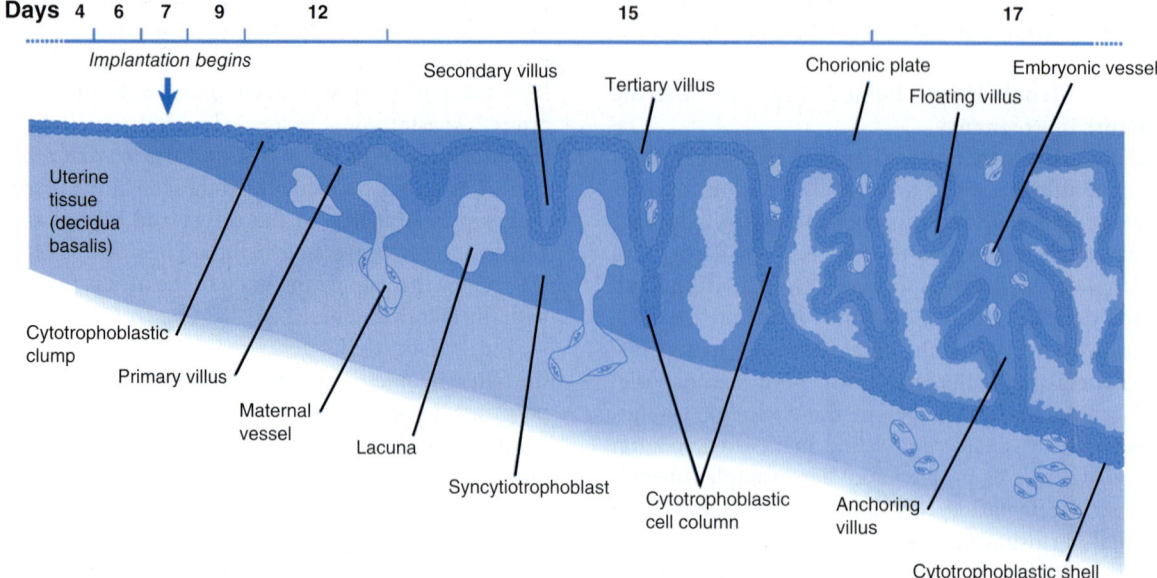

Fig. 3.2. Stages in the Formation of a Chorionic Villus. From Carlson, BM. *Human Embryology and Developmental Biology.* 7th ed. Elsevier; 2024.

of pregnancy, or decidua (Fig. 3.2). The branching chorio-allantoic villi occupy the intervillous space of the placenta, with maternal blood bathing the villous surfaces. These villi are covered by a trophoblast bilayer: an outer, terminally differentiated, multinucleated mass called syncytiotrophoblast, and a subjacent, proliferative, mononucleated stem cell population called cytotrophoblast. The syncytiotrophoblast is the primary site for exchange of oxygen, nutrients, and wastes between maternal and fetal blood. Maternal blood passively exits the intervillous space through multiple collecting veins in the decidua basalis that empty into uterine veins that drain via the internal iliac veins and also via the ovarian veins into the inferior vena cava on the right, and into the renal vein on the left.

Up to 90% of uterine blood perfuses the chorioallantoic placenta at term, with the remainder supplying the myometrium and nonplacental endometrium. Notably, the placental and nonplacental vasculatures are anatomically and functionally distinct. Moreover, regulation of perfusion through these vascular beds differs, which highlights the importance of distinguishing studies that measure total uteroplacental blood flow versus placental blood flow.

CHANGES DURING PREGNANCY

Uterine blood flow increases markedly during pregnancy, from less than 100 mL/min before pregnancy to 700 to 900 mL/min at term, depending on the method of measurement (Fig. 3.3). Uterine blood flow at term represents a greater proportion of cardiac output than in early pregnancy (12% versus 3.5%).[9] Sheep studies indicate that increases in uterine blood flow can be divided into three phases.[10] An initial phase likely controlled by ovarian secretion of estrogen and progesterone occurs before and during implantation and early placentation. A second phase results from the growth and

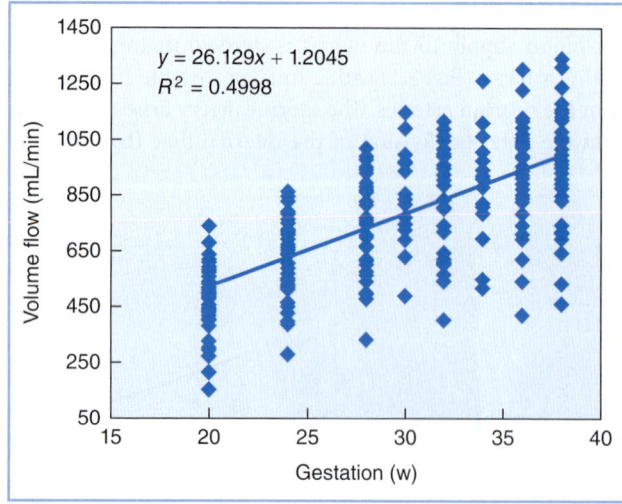

Fig. 3.3 Changes in Uterine Artery Blood Flow With Gestation. From Konje JC, Kaufmann P, Bell SC, Taylor DJ. A longitudinal study of quantitative uterine blood flow with the use of color power angiography in appropriate for gestational age pregnancies. *Am J Obstet Gynecol.* 2001;185:608–613.

remodeling of the uteroplacental vasculature to support placental development. The third phase results from progressive uterine artery vasodilation to meet the markedly increased nutrient requirements of the rapidly growing fetus. Expressed in terms of uterine weight, uterine flow per gram of tissue is particularly high in early gestation, and this ratio decreases as pregnancy progresses.[10] In comparison, umbilical blood flow, as a function of fetal weight, is relatively constant during pregnancy at 110 to 120 mL/min/kg,[11] although some studies showed a decrease in umbilical venous blood flow per kilogram fetal weight throughout gestation.[12] Uterine blood flow is higher in twin than in singleton pregnancy, but the flow per unit of estimated fetal weight is similar.[13]

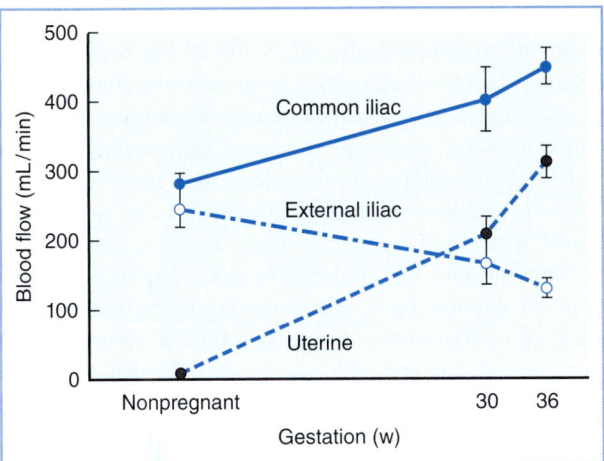

Fig. 3.4 Redistribution of Blood Flow in Pelvic Blood Vessels During Pregnancy Determined Unilaterally By Doppler Ultrasonography. Blood flow increased in the common iliac and uterine arteries but decreased in the external iliac artery, indicating that redistribution of flow favors uterine perfusion. Data are mean ± SEM. Modified from Palmer SK, Zamudio S, Coffin C, et al. Quantitative estimation of human uterine artery blood flow and pelvic blood flow redistribution in pregnancy. *Obstet Gynecol.* 1992;80:1000–1006.

Distribution of Blood Flow

The increase in uterine blood flow results from increases in uterine artery diameter and flow velocity.[14] The uterine artery diameter doubles from early pregnancy until week 21, is static until week 30, and then increases until at least week 36.[14] The mean flow velocity in the uterine artery increases eightfold over the course of gestation.[14] This increase in uterine and common iliac artery blood flow is associated with a decrease in external iliac artery flow, redistributing blood to the uterus (Fig. 3.4).[14]

Autoregulation

Vasoconstriction or vasodilation in response to changes in systemic arterial pressure maintains steady transcapillary fluid exchange.[15] In sheep, the nonpregnant uterine circulation and the nonplacental uterine circulation in pregnancy exhibit autoregulation, but autoregulation is limited in the uteroplacental circulation.[16,17] This occurs because the uteroplacental circulation is a dilated, low-resistance system with largely pressure-dependent perfusion, with limited ability to dilate or constrict. Importantly, the spiral arteries that supply the intervillous space lack the metaarterioles and precapillary sphincters that are essential for autoregulation.[15] However, studies are conflicting because of variation in the animal models and experimental conditions used; for example, uteroplacental autoregulation has been demonstrated in guinea pigs, rabbits, and sheep.[15,18] These discrepancies may be explained by the activity of the nonplacental uterine vasculature, which accounts for a small fraction of total uteroplacental blood flow but exhibits similar autoregulatory responses in pregnancy and nonpregnancy. In contrast, limited autoregulatory ability

exists in the placental circulation, which means that placental blood flow may diminish with reductions in maternal blood pressure (e.g., during hemorrhage or neuraxial anesthesia).

Changes During Parturition

Labor causes marked changes in uteroplacental perfusion. Uterine contractions decrease perfusion inversely proportional to the strength of the contraction and the increase in intrauterine pressure.[19] The uterine blood flow is limited when the intrauterine pressure exceeds 30 mm Hg, end-diastolic flow in the uterine artery ceases when the intrauterine pressure exceeds 35 mm Hg, and blood flow totally ceases when intrauterine pressure exceeds 60 mm Hg.[20] The strength of a normal uterine contraction in labor is 40 to 100 mm Hg. During uterine relaxation, there is a period of increased perfusion above baseline. The decrease in perfusion during a contraction causes autotransfusion into the central circulation of 300 to 500 mL, increasing the maternal stroke volume and cardiac output through increased cardiac preload.[21] This phenomenon can be significant for patients with maternal cardiac disease, who may poorly tolerate the autotransfusion associated with each contraction.

Hemodynamics

Uterine blood flow like other organs is determined by perfusion pressure and vascular resistance:

$$\text{Uterine blood flow} = \frac{\text{Uterine perfusion pressure}}{\text{Uterine vascular resistance}}$$
$$= \frac{\text{Mean uterine arterial pressure} - \text{Mean uterine venous pressure}}{\text{Uterine vascular resistance}} \quad (3.1)$$

There are several ways that uteroplacental blood flow may decrease (Box 3.1).

Decreased uterine arterial pressure may occur with: (1) hypovolemic or obstructive shock with reduced cardiac preload; (2) cardiogenic shock with reduced myocardial contractility; (3) distributive shock with reduced cardiac afterload (e.g., anaphylaxis, neurogenic shock, neuraxial anesthesia–induced sympatholysis); and (4) major cardiac arrhythmias.

Supine positioning with aortocaval compression may decrease uterine arterial pressure by reducing cardiac preload, mainly via impaired venous return from vena caval compression. Aortocaval compression also directly increases uterine venous pressure, further reducing uterine perfusion pressure. The Valsalva maneuver (while pushing during the second stage of labor) also increases uterine venous pressure.

As the uterus is a hollow muscular viscus, with the uterine artery on the outside and the placenta and fetus on the inside, uterine vascular resistance greatly increases during uterine contractions, leading to diminished or abolished uteroplacental perfusion. This is particularly relevant during long or obstructed labor and excessive oxytocin administration resulting in tachysystole or uterine tetany. Uterine vascular resistance also increases in response to endogenous vasoconstrictors released in response to stress, dehydration or hypovolemia, and exogenous vasoconstrictors (e.g., phenylephrine, norepinephrine [noradrenaline], ephedrine, or epinephrine [adrenaline]) administered during labor or cesarean delivery.

The hemodynamics of uteroplacental blood flow are uniquely associated with the coiled uterine spiral arteries, which in humans extend from the distal ends of the radial arteries in the myometrium into the decidua, terminating at the intervillous space (Fig. 3.5). The spiral geometry of these vessels provides a reserve of high resistance to flow when the requirement for uteroplacental blood supply is low,[22] and the ability to purge this reserve in pregnancy when the requirement for uteroplacental blood supply is high.[23]

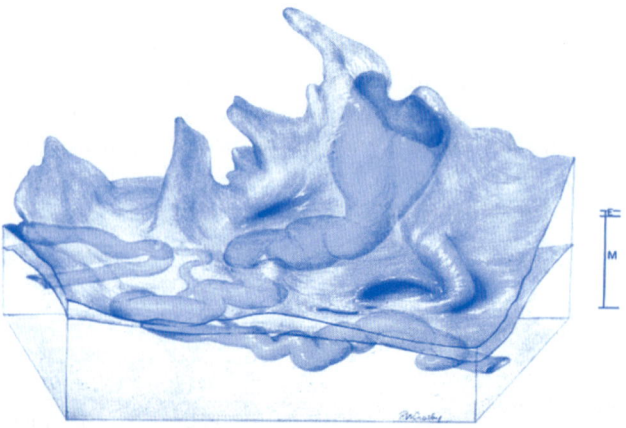

Fig. 3.5 Uterine Spiral Artery. Reconstructed serial sections of a spiral artery of a term human placenta passing through myometrium (M), endometrium (E), and the basal plate to the intervillous space. The widest arterial dimension was 2.4 mm. From Burton GJ, Woods AW, Jauniaux E, Kingdom JC. Rheological and physiological consequences of conversion of the maternal spiral arteries for uteroplacental blood flow during human pregnancy. *Placenta.* 2009;30:473–482.

The nonpregnant spiral artery has low flow and high resistance, with muscular walls under sympathetic neurovascular control. During normal human pregnancy, the uteroplacental circulation undergoes marked geometric and hemodynamic transformations from the influence of invading trophoblasts.[24,25] Spiral arteries are remodeled to become vessels with high flow and low resistance, no longer under sympathetic control, with distal segments transformed into inverted funnels opening into the intervillous space. The degree of spiral artery remodeling is quite nuanced. Using mathematical modeling of flow and resistance for the full range of spiral artery remodeling (Fig. 3.6), Zamir et al.[23] calculated that a conversion fraction, defined as the depth of remodeled vessel/total depth of tissue traversed by the spiral artery, of more than 80% was required to provide the uteroplacental perfusion needed for normal pregnancy. This mathematical and rheological approach complements pathologic observations that the depth of trophoblast invasion correlates with the adequacy or inadequacy of uteroplacental blood flow; failure of adequate remodeling in the first trimester has been associated with preeclampsia with severe features, fetal growth restriction (FGR), and prematurity.[1]

Mechanisms of Vascular Remodeling and Regulation

The increase in uteroplacental blood flow occurs primarily from a substantial decrease in uterine vascular resistance (Fig. 3.7) together with an increase in cardiac output and intravascular volume.[26] Although the mechanisms are incompletely understood, three main factors contribute to the decrease in vascular resistance: (1) vascular remodeling, (2) changes in vascular reactivity, and (3) the development of the widely dilated spiral arteries.[26]

Vascular remodeling of uterine arteries during pregnancy includes lengthening and straightening of coiled vessels[9] and vessel dilation. There is no change in the diameter of the common iliac or external iliac arteries, but the uterine artery diameter doubles by 21 weeks' gestation, and by 40 weeks, there is an eightfold increase in mean flow velocity.[14] The arcuate and radial arteries also dilate by 22% to 220%, depending on the species studied[26]; in rats and mice this is associated with an increase in distensibility and a decrease in elastin content.[27,28] Processes contributing to vascular remodeling include placentation with endovascular trophoblast invasion, increased shear stress, venoarterial exchange, and humoral factors.[26] A decrease in blood viscosity during pregnancy also has a minor effect on reducing uterine vascular resistance.[29]

A change in vascular reactivity during pregnancy is mediated by endothelial and vascular smooth muscle levels with an overall tendency for reduced tone, limited vasoconstriction, and increased vasodilation.[26] The growth of the placenta creates a low-resistance vascular pathway by the significant reduction of the intramyometrial microcirculation and the creation of an intervillous space.

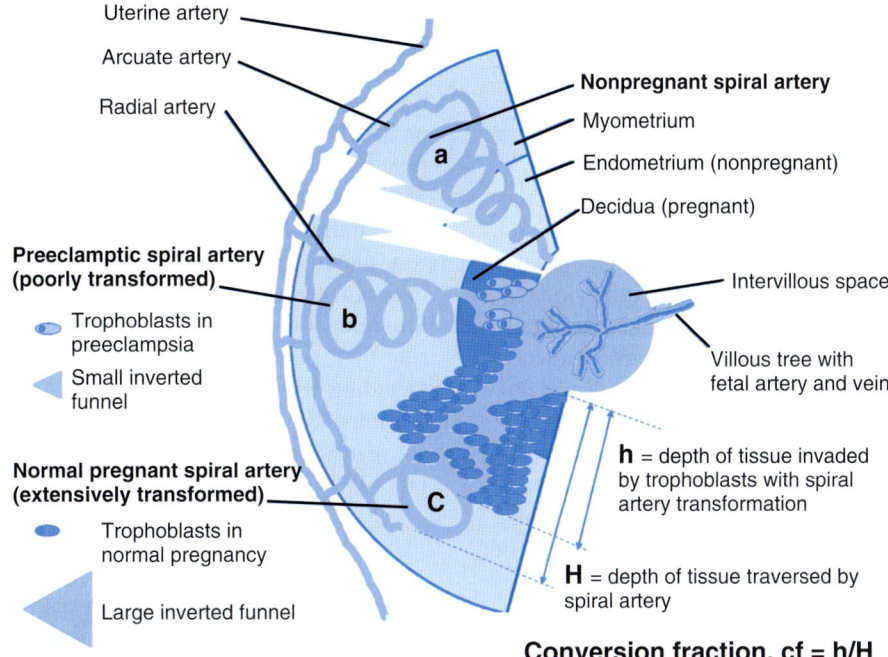

Conversion fraction, cf = h/H

Fig. 3.6 Spiral artery transformations in the decidua and myometrium of three physiologic scenarios: **(a) non-pregnancy,** indicated by presence of stroma and uterine epithelium, but absence of decidual layer; **(b) pregnancy with preeclampsia** with trophoblasts (beige) invading only the superficial decidua, causing minimal spiral artery transformation, and a small inverted funnel; **(c) normal pregnancy** with trophoblasts (green) invading through the decidua and the superficial myometrium, causing maximal spiral artery transformation, and a large inverted funnel. Spiral arteries during pregnancy (**b** and **c**) provide maternal blood to the intervillous space for gas exchange with the fetal artery and vein within the placental villi. The ratio of the depth of tissue of trophoblast-mediated spiral artery remodeling (h) to the total depth of the tissue through which the spiral artery traverses (H) is the conversion fraction (cf). From Zamir M, Nelson DM, Ginosar Y. Hemodynamic consequences of incomplete uterine spiral artery transformation in human pregnancy, with implications for placental dysfunction and preeclampsia. *J Appl Physiol (1985)*. 2021;130:457–465.

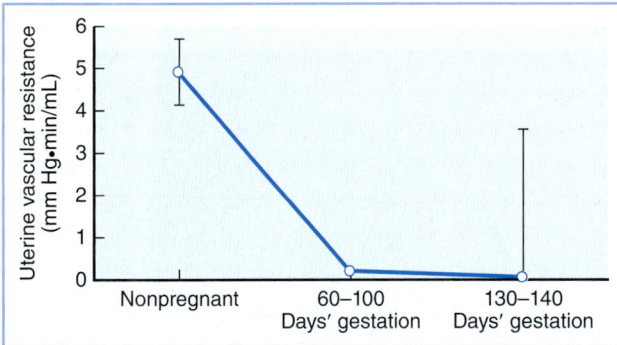

Fig. 3.7 Changes in Uterine Vascular Resistance With Gestation. Data are mean ± SE. Modified from Rosenfeld CR. Distribution of cardiac output in ovine pregnancy. *Am J Physiol.* 1977;232:H231–H235.

Effect of Endogenous Steroid Hormones

The endogenous steroid hormones are fundamental in short- and long-term uterine vascular changes during pregnancy, with estrogen as the primary driver of angiogenesis and vasodilation.[30,31] Plasma concentration of estrogen, initially derived from the ovaries and later predominantly from the placenta, rises concomitantly with the increase in uterine blood flow during pregnancy. Angiogenic and vasodilatory effects of estrogen are mediated via estrogen receptors ER-α and ER-β.[30] Most of these receptors are located in the nucleus and mediate genomic effects by regulating the transcription of genes that are responsible for the longer-term uterine angiogenic responses. There are also membrane receptors that mediate nongenomic effects by upregulating endothelial production of nitric oxide through the activation of endothelial nitric oxide synthase (eNOS) and the augmentation of eNOS protein expression.[32] Progesterone modulates the effect of estrogen on uterine blood flow by downregulating the expression of estrogen receptors; however, the exact effects of progesterone on uterine blood flow remain incompletely understood.[31,33]

Cortisol, the plasma level of which doubles during pregnancy, has both systemic and local effects on uterine blood flow. Systemically, cortisol contributes to regulation of uterine blood flow by increasing plasma volume. Although cortisol decreases eNOS protein expression and nitric oxide release, it potentiates the response to vasoconstrictor agents, including angiotensin II, vasopressin, and norepinephrine. Attenuation of these effects occurs during pregnancy.[31]

MEASUREMENT OF UTEROPLACENTAL BLOOD FLOW

Techniques used to measure uteroplacental blood flow in animals and humans have varied according to the experimental question, available technology, and ethical considerations. All methods have inherent potential for error. Many early studies measured flow in only one uterine artery, which may not reflect total flow, depending on the location of the placenta. Although placental perfusion is of greatest clinical interest, it is not always differentiated from total uterine blood flow, and the two uterine artery circulations vary independently. However, usually the measurement of intervillous blood flow provides a reasonable surrogate of placental blood flow.

The most common method of clinically assessing uterine artery flow is Doppler ultrasonography.[34] The uterine artery can be identified transabdominally or transvaginally; color flow aids vessel identification. Blood flow can be quantified by measuring the mean flow velocity and vessel cross-sectional area. Flow velocity measured by Doppler ultrasonography is angle-dependent and can be difficult to obtain correctly. An estimation of the volume of blood flow (Q) can be made by multiplying mean velocity (V) and vessel cross-sectional area (A), which is estimated with two-dimensional (B-mode) ultrasonography, that is, $Q = V \times A$. Measurement of absolute flow using this technique is difficult and prone to error, from inaccuracies in the measurement of vessel cross-sectional area (e.g., as arteries pulsate during the cardiac cycle) and velocity. Therefore, for diagnostic purposes, indices related to vascular impedance are derived from the flow velocity waveform that is independent of the angle of insonation. These rely on the uterine vascular bed normally having low resistance, with flow continuing during diastole. If distal resistance is increased, diastolic velocity decreases relative to systolic velocity, resulting in a waveform showing greater pulsatility. Commonly derived indices include the following:

$$\text{Systolic/diastolic (S/D) ratio} = \frac{\text{Systolic (max) velocity}}{\text{Diastolic (min) velocity}} \quad (3.2)$$

Pulatility index (PI)

$$= \frac{\text{Systolic (max) velocity} - \text{diastolic (min) velocity}}{\text{Mean velocity}} \quad (3.3)$$

Resistance index (RI)

$$= \frac{\text{Systolic (max) velocity} - \text{Diastolic (min) velocity}}{\text{Systolic (max) velocity}} \quad (3.4)$$

In early pregnancy, uterine artery flow is very pulsatile with high systolic flow and low diastolic flow. As gestation progresses, resistance gradually decreases. Abnormal patterns, including persistence of high resistance, diastolic notching, and the absence of end-diastolic flow or reversal of diastolic flow, are predictive of the development of abnormalities such as preeclampsia or FGR (Fig. 3.8). Doppler velocimetry is also applied to the umbilical vessels for antepartum fetal assessment (see Chapter 6). Other methods of evaluation include the use of two-dimensional and three-dimensional Doppler, power Doppler, contrast-enhanced ultrasonography, and functional magnetic resonance imaging (MRI). Blood oxygen level–dependent functional MRI (BOLD MRI), which does not require administration of contrast media, has been used to evaluate placental and fetal perfusion following hypoxia in pregnant sheep[35,36] and hyperoxia in pregnant humans.[37,38] Emerging functional MRI assessments of placental perfusion by the exchange of magnetically labeled water protons, including arterial spin labeling[39,40] and intravoxel incoherent motion (IVIM) echo planar imaging (EPI),[41] offer the benefit of avoiding radiation but suffer from low signal-to-noise ratios and long scan times.

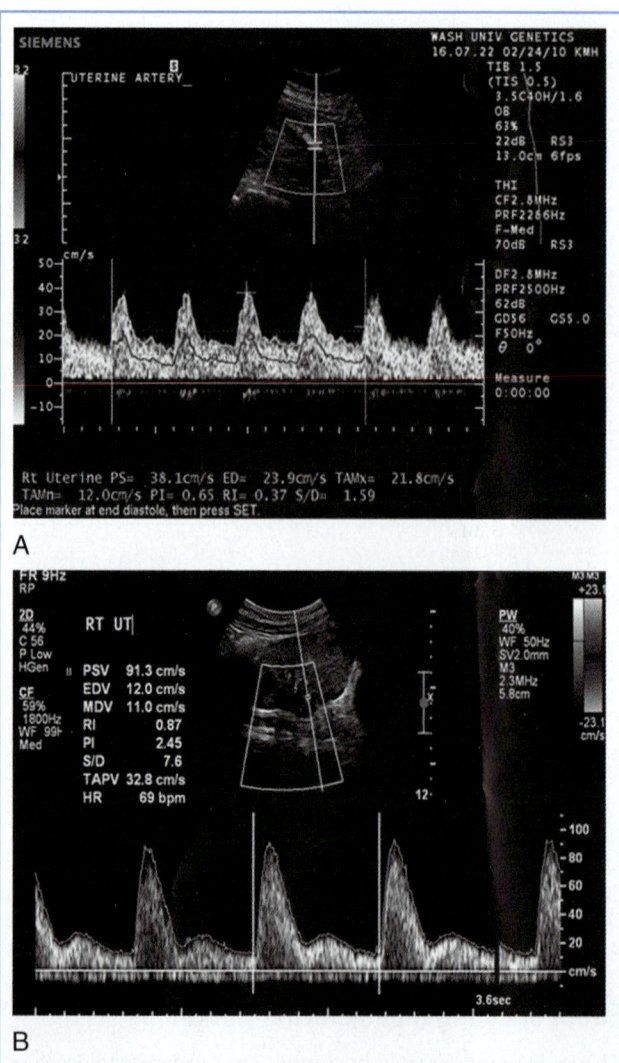

Fig. 3.8 Normal (A) and Abnormal (B) Uterine Artery Doppler Waveforms. The normal waveform has no notching and normal pulsatility. The abnormal waveform shows notching and increased pulsatility. From Tuuli M, Odibo AO. The role of serum markers and uterine artery Doppler in identifying at-risk pregnancies. *Clin Perinatol.* 2001;38:1–19.

CLINICAL ASSOCIATIONS

The "Great Obstetric Syndromes"

Preeclampsia

Of many competing theories of the underlying pathophysiology of preeclampsia (see Chapter 35), one implicates an imbalance of angiogenic and antiangiogenic factors. An increase in serum levels of soluble fms-like tyrosine kinase receptor-1 (sFlt-1), which is an antagonist of vascular endothelial growth factor and placental growth factor (PlGF), reduces angiogenesis.[42] Moreover, there is deficient remodeling of the uterine spiral arteries.[43] In normal pregnancy, the uterine spiral artery remodeling enhances vasodilation and decreases uterine vascular resistance.[43] However, in pregnancies complicated by preeclampsia, there is insufficient or shallow trophoblast invasion of the myometrial spiral arteries. This failure of spiral artery remodeling predisposes to hypoperfusion and chronic hypoxia.[43] Alternatively, flow volume in the placenta may be unaffected, but the pathologic spiral artery remodeling may lead to pulsatile, higher pressure flow within the placenta that is thought to cause damage to villi that mediate maternal-fetal transfer. In normal remodeling of spiral arteries, there is a loss of smooth muscle cells from the arterial walls; however, in the presence of insufficient remodeling, the vasoreactive muscle cells are not obliterated and contribute to increased vascular tone and contractility.[43] The abnormal flow thus contributes to ischemia-reperfusion injury and oxidative stress.

Clinically, the ratio of sFlt-1 to PlGF is used by some to predict the onset of preeclampsia in patients with clinical risk factors.[44] Additionally, the uterine artery Doppler pulsatility index (PI) is elevated in early pregnancy in patients who will subsequently develop preeclampsia.[45] Abnormal uterine artery Doppler PI is associated with abnormal spiral artery remodeling and thus is a surrogate for placental vascular insufficiency.[46] The administration of low doses of aspirin to patients at high risk of preeclampsia, based on early screening with uterine artery Doppler PI and biomarkers such as pregnancy-associated plasma protein A and PlGF, reduces the development of preterm preeclampsia.[47]

Fetal Growth Restriction

Etiologies for FGR include genetic, constitutional, infectious, maternal, and placental origins. Abnormal placental architecture is common, especially vascular abnormalities in villi, basal plate, or both.[48] Placental hypoperfusion yields relative hypoxia and increased vascular resistance. Cases of severe, early gestational onset of FGR commonly exhibit placental pathology with features of abnormal uteroplacental perfusion and defective extravillous trophoblast invasion.[46] There is a direct correlation between abnormal uterine artery Doppler measurements and defective spiral artery remodeling.[46] Importantly, FGR with abnormal uterine artery Doppler measurements is associated with lesions of the fetal stem arteries.[46] High resistance in the placenta evolves into deterioration of the Doppler pattern in the umbilical arteries. Normally, there is high flow in the umbilical arteries during diastole. With increased placental vascular resistance, there is diminished end-diastolic flow, resulting in an elevated umbilical artery PI. As resistance builds, there is absent, and ultimately reversal of, end-diastolic flow. The latter is a poor prognostic factor that increases the risk for intrauterine fetal demise and requires iatrogenic delivery as early as 30 weeks' gestation, depending on the clinical scenario.[49]

Preterm Delivery

Abnormalities in uteroplacental blood flow may contribute to the pathophysiology of spontaneous preterm birth. There is a higher risk of abnormal placentation, including abnormal transformation of the spiral arteries, in patients with spontaneous preterm birth.[50,51] The uterine artery Doppler pattern may be abnormal in patients who eventually will deliver preterm.[52] Further work is needed to understand the pathways underlying the abnormal uteroplacental blood flow seen in patients with preterm labor and delivery. Collectively, a common pathway underlying the "Great Obstetric Syndromes" implicates abnormal spiral artery remodeling and consequent abnormal uteroplacental perfusion.[1]

Effects of Labor and Disorders of Labor

Uterine Contractions

The placenta and fetus are located inside a hollow viscus with a muscular wall. Uterine contraction strength, timing, pulsatile nature, and uterine diastolic filling time during active labor markedly affect placental perfusion.

There are similarities between coronary artery blood flow to the subendocardial region of the contracting heart and uterine artery blood flow to the placenta (Fig. 3.9). In both cases, the arterial blood supply comes from the outer surface of a hollow organ and must cross a contracting muscular wall to perfuse a target on the inside of the wall (e.g., the subendocardium in the heart and the intervillous space of the placenta within the uterus). Importantly, perfusion is either completely occluded, as in the heart, or greatly reduced, as in the uteroplacental circulation, during the muscular contraction of systole. Flow only resumes during the muscular relaxation of diastole.

In active labor, a typical uterine contraction (systole) lasts from 40 to 60 seconds, and uterine relaxation (diastole) is typically 2 to 5 minutes in duration. Most fetuses tolerate the periodic cessation in placental perfusion during contraction; however, fetuses with underlying placental insufficiency may not tolerate labor. Excessive uterine contractions may be associated with oxytocin administration and may cause tachysystole with more than 5 contractions in 10 minutes or uterine tetany with a sustained contraction. There is a substantial reduction in uterine diastolic filling time with each condition. Even normal fetuses, with normal baseline placental function and perfusion, may suffer hypoxia from acute hypoperfusion. The risk of prolonged uterine contractions with short uteroplacental diastolic filling time is increased in cases of obstructed labor. A consequence of placental hypoperfusion with resulting hypoxia is fetal autonomic stimulation,

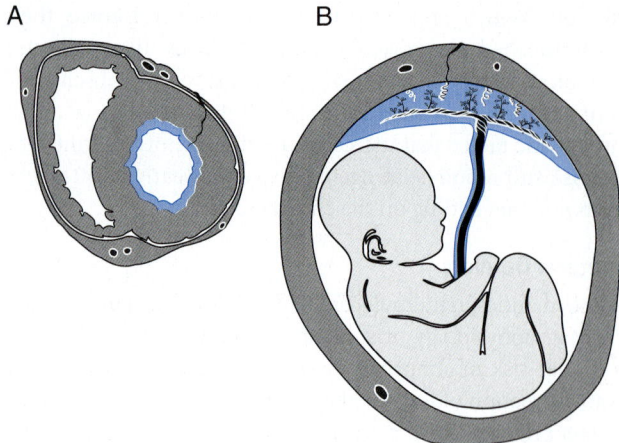

Fig. 3.9 The impact of uterine contractions on placental perfusion is comparable to that of myocardial contractions on subendocardial perfusion. *Blue areas* show "tissue at risk." Blood supply is indicated in *black*. (A) Subendocardial perfusion does not occur during cardiac systole, and during diastole, it is threatened when the filling time is short (tachycardia), arterial pressure is reduced (hypotension), or myocardial failure is present (elevated left ventricular end-diastolic pressure); an ischemic myocardium may be intolerant to moderately increased demand. (B) Placental perfusion is reduced during uterine systole (contraction), and during diastole it is threatened when filling time is short (tachysystole), arterial pressure is reduced (hypotension), or intrauterine pressure is elevated (obstructed labor); a fetus with chronic placental insufficiency may be intolerant to even normal labor. Illustration by Naveen Nathan, M.D., NorthShore University HealthSystem, University of Chicago Pritzker School of Medicine, Evanston, IL.

which may result in fetal heart rate (FHR) decelerations or fetal bradycardia during or shortly after uterine contractions. Intrauterine resuscitative measures include reducing uterine tone, either by stopping oxytocin infusion and/or administering tocolytic medication (see Chapter 8).

Umbilical Cord Prolapse

Prolapse of the umbilical cord in labor may cause fetal hypoxia via cord occlusion and vasospasm and is an obstetric emergency requiring expedited delivery (see Chapter 8).

Antepartum Hemorrhage

Antepartum hemorrhage has many causes and may compromise blood flow and oxygen delivery to the fetus (see Chapter 37).

Dystocia and Oxytocin Augmentation

Uterine tachysystole caused by oxytocin labor augmentation may acutely reduce placental perfusion. Evidence from monkeys, dogs, rabbits, and humans suggests that oxytocin-induced contractions cause a greater reduction in placental blood flow than spontaneous contractions.[53] Recovery of blood flow after uterine relaxation is slower in augmented versus spontaneous contractions.

Poor Placentation and Fetal Intolerance to Labor

Placental dysfunction, manifesting as FGR or preeclampsia, is associated with an increased risk of fetal intolerance to labor. A chronically hypoxic fetus poorly tolerates the superimposed hypoxia caused by uterine contractions, predisposing to fetal

hypoxia and acidosis.[54] The fetus may manifest an abnormal FHR tracing, which is associated with a loss of end-diastolic flow in the umbilical artery.[55]

Fetal Consequences of Inadequate Uteroplacental Blood Flow

Inadequate uteroplacental blood flow, whether acute and prolonged or chronic and persistent, can result in fetal acidosis, asphyxia, hypoxic-ischemic encephalopathy, and fetal death. The FHR tracing may show decelerations, loss of normal variability, bradycardia, or a combination of these abnormalities. The risk for fetal acidosis increases with the increasing deceleration area from baseline FHR, regardless of the shape of the decelerations.[56] There are three gradations in the hypoxic process: hypoxemia, hypoxia, and asphyxia.[54] Of interest, studies in monkeys have shown that hypoxic-ischemic encephalopathy evolves if cord occlusion persists for 15 to 18 minutes.[57] Notably, normal outcomes in human fetuses have been reported after even 25 minutes of acute bradycardia, while some neonates had neurologic findings after as little as 10 minutes of acute bradycardia.[57]

A common misconception is that most cases of **cerebral palsy** result from inadequate intrapartum uteroplacental blood flow. In actuality, 90% of cerebral palsy cases cannot be linked to intrapartum hypoxia (see Chapter 10).

Chronic Fetal Hypoperfusion and Diseases Presenting in Adult Life

Chronic placental hypoperfusion can affect the future health of both the mother and child. For example, evidence suggests that women with preeclampsia have a higher risk for developing cardiovascular disease[58,59] and possibly breast or ovarian cancer in later life.[60] Furthermore, the fetus has a higher lifetime risk of death from cardiovascular disease,[61,62] metabolic syndrome,[63] type 2 diabetes, and breast cancer.[62] The concept of developmental origins of health and disease[62] holds that an adverse intrauterine environment (e.g., impaired placental perfusion or dysfunction) can induce altered fetal and/or maternal phenotypes[64,65] via placental epigenetic and nutrient transport abnormalities.[66]

EFFECTS OF ANESTHESIA AND ANALGESIA ON UTEROPLACENTAL BLOOD FLOW

Anesthesia and analgesia can have *direct* and *indirect effects* on the fetus. General anesthesia may exert a direct effect (resulting in transient neonatal respiratory depression), whereas neuraxial analgesia and anesthesia exert predominantly indirect effects, of which the most important is alteration of uteroplacental blood flow. Nonanesthesia interventions that may impact the fetus via changes in uteroplacental blood flow include maternal supine posture, supplemental oxygen, and a prolonged uterine incision–delivery interval (see Chapter 26).

General Anesthesia
Direct Effects of General Anesthetic Drugs

Available data suggest that commonly used induction agents have minimal or no direct adverse effect on uteroplacental blood flow. Allen et al.[67] found that **thiopental (thiopentone)** inhibited the response of human myometrial arteries to contractile agents *in vitro* but had no effect on relaxation induced by prostacyclin. Alon et al.[68] reported that uterine blood flow did not change significantly during induction and maintenance of **propofol** anesthesia in pregnant sheep. Craft et al.[69] reported that uterine tone increased but uterine blood flow remained constant after an intravenous bolus of **ketamine** in pregnant sheep. Similarly, Strümper et al.[70] reported that neither racemic nor S+-ketamine affected uterine perfusion in pregnant sheep. Few data are available on the direct effects of **etomidate** on uteroplacental blood flow. Collectively, these data show relative safety, yet caution is warranted as many of the studies were conducted in sheep.

Indirect Effects of General Anesthetic Agents

During intravenous induction, uteroplacental perfusion may be affected by indirect mechanisms, such as the sympathetic response to laryngoscopy and tracheal intubation. Jouppila et al.[71] reported that intervillous blood flow decreased by 22% to 50% during the induction of anesthesia with **thiopental** 4 mg/kg, **succinylcholine** 1 mg/kg, and tracheal intubation. Gin et al.[72] compared **thiopental** 4 mg/kg and **propofol** 2 mg/kg in patients undergoing elective cesarean delivery and found that venous plasma concentrations of epinephrine and norepinephrine increased after tracheal intubation in both groups, but the maximum norepinephrine concentration was lower in the propofol group. No differences in neonatal outcomes were observed. Levinson et al.[73] found that intravenous **ketamine** increased blood pressure with a concomitant rise in uterine blood flow in pregnant sheep. The addition of a rapid-acting opioid (e.g., **alfentanil**, **remifentanil**) may minimize the increase in circulating catecholamines.[74,75]

Studies in pregnant sheep have shown that usual clinical doses (i.e., 0.5 to 1.5 minimum alveolar concentration [MAC]) of volatile anesthetic agents, including **isoflurane**, **desflurane**, and **sevoflurane**) have little or no effect on uterine blood flow, although deeper planes of anesthesia are associated with reductions in maternal cardiac output, blood pressure, and uterine blood flow.[76] Nonetheless, high concentrations (approximately 2 MAC) of inhalational anesthetic agents have been used during *ex utero* intrapartum treatment procedures without evidence of impaired fetal gas exchange.[77] A dose-dependent reduction in uterine tone caused by inhalational anesthetic agents would be expected to increase uterine blood flow in clinical circumstances in which tone is increased (e.g., hyperstimulation with oxytocin, cocaine overdose, placental abruption). Overall, there is little reason to choose a particular inhalational agent on the basis of uterine blood flow effects.

Vasoactive drugs have little direct effect on spiral artery tone owing to the trophoblast remodeling of the vessel walls in normal pregnancy. However, placental blood flow depends on maternal cardiac output,[78] which is reduced by most anesthetic drugs, with the exceptions of **ketamine** and **etomidate**. The impact of anesthetic drugs may be augmented in the presence of maternal dehydration, obstetric hemorrhage, or conversion to general anesthesia from neuraxial anesthesia.

The unresponsiveness of remodeled spiral arteries allows the use of vasoactive drugs to enhance maternal cardiac output without influencing placental blood flow directly, with some drugs shunting blood toward the uteroplacental circulation, as competing vascular beds vasoconstrict.[79]

Effects of Ventilation

Conflicting experimental data exist in animals regarding the effects of maternal hypercapnia on uteroplacental blood flow, ranging from hypoperfusion[80] or no change in pregnant sheep[81] to hyperperfusion in pregnant pigs.[82] BOLD MRI functional studies in pregnant rats showed that maternal exposure to 5% inspired CO_2 and 20% F_{IO_2} elicited an 80% reduction in placental perfusion.[83] With fetal asphyxia, functional MRI and Doppler ultrasound studies have demonstrated an increased perfusion index and fetal bradycardia in pregnant rats.[83] Hypercapnia induced direct vasodilation in the cerebral circulation in pregnant rats, with the predominant hemodynamic effect due to an increase in sympathetic tone and levels of circulating catecholamines, epinephrine and norepinephrine.[84]

The effect of hypocapnia on uteroplacental blood flow is controversial. Some investigators have noted that hyperventilation with hypocapnia causes fetal hypoxia and metabolic acidosis in animals,[85] whereas others have found no effect.[86] Levinson et al.[87] observed that positive pressure ventilation decreased uterine blood flow in pregnant sheep; however, because the addition of inhaled carbon dioxide did not improve uterine blood flow, the reduction in blood flow was attributed to the effects of mechanical hyperventilation.

Positive pressure ventilation can reduce venous return and cardiac output, particularly at high ventilatory pressures and in the presence of high levels of positive end-expiratory pressure. In pregnancy, this may be more marked for several reasons: (1) ventilation potentiates the hemodynamic compromise resulting from aortocaval compression, particularly in the hypovolemic parturient; and (2) respiratory compliance is reduced owing to raised intraabdominal pressure from the gravid uterus.

Neuraxial Anesthesia and Analgesia
Direct Effects of Neuraxial Anesthesia and Analgesia

Studies using Doppler ultrasound measurements, among other techniques, have shown that epidural and spinal analgesia do not normally have a significant direct affect on uteroplacental blood flow or fetal oxygenation.

Indirect Effects of Neuraxial Anesthesia and Analgesia

Uteroplacental blood flow may decrease after neuraxial anesthesia because of (1) maternal hypotension, (2) effects of vasopressors, or (3) decreased uteroplacental blood flow from anesthesia-related increases in uterine tone.

Maternal hypotension and vasopressors. Neuraxial anesthesia causes dose-dependent sympathectomy and vasodilation. In the absence of hypotension or reduced cardiac output, the effect on uteroplacental blood flow is minimal.[88]

However, the extensive neural blockade required for cesarean delivery may cause marked hypotension, which may be exacerbated by aortocaval compression and hypovolemia (see Chapter 26).

Limited data are available assessing vasopressors in the presence of fetal compromise or placental insufficiency. Erkinaro et al.[4] developed a sheep model to compare the effects of **phenylephrine** and **ephedrine** after a period of experimental fetal hypoxia. Hypotension was induced by epidural anesthesia and then corrected with either phenylephrine or ephedrine. In an initial study, ephedrine was associated with better restoration of uterine artery blood flow, but with no differences in fetal acid-base measurements or lactate concentration.[4] However, in a second study in which the placenta was embolized with microspheres to model placental insufficiency, phenylephrine and ephedrine had similar effects on uterine blood flow, fetal pH, and base excess, as found in the initial study, but fetal lactate concentration was greater in the phenylephrine group.[89] Although the investigators speculated that this might reflect impaired fetal clearance of lactate, the placental embolization may have narrowed the margin of safety for uteroplacental blood flow and increased fetal lactate production in the phenylephrine group.

In two studies, women with preeclampsia undergoing cesarean delivery with spinal anesthesia were randomized to receive phenylephrine or ephedrine for the prevention[90] or treatment[91] of spinal anesthesia–induced hypotension. Neither study identified differences between the two drugs in the acid-base status of the neonates, suggesting that either drug is appropriate for use in women with preeclampsia with potentially compromised uteroplacental circulation.

Ephedrine and phenylephrine both continue to be used clinically for maintaining maternal blood pressure during the administration of neuraxial anesthesia (see Chapter 26). Although most early experimental data in animals suggested that uteroplacental perfusion is better maintained with ephedrine than with alpha-adrenergic agonists, the applicability of those results to human pregnancy is unclear. Further, placental transfer of ephedrine may increase fetal myocardial oxygen consumption, increase fetal basal metabolic rate, and cause mild fetal metabolic acidosis, although the clinical significance of this is unclear.

Pregnancy is associated with a reduced response to endogenous and exogenous vasoconstrictors, including angiotensin II, endothelin, thromboxane, epinephrine, norepinephrine, phenylephrine, serotonin, and arginine vasopressin.[92–94] The relative refractoriness of the systemic and uterine circulations varies for different agents.

Concentrations of angiotensin II in maternal blood are increased twofold to threefold[95]; however, the vasopressor response to angiotensin II is attenuated.[96] This refractoriness is diminished in patients in whom preeclampsia develops.[96] The uterine circulation is less responsive to angiotensin II than the systemic circulation. Thus, the infusion of physiologic doses of angiotensin II has minimal effects on uteroplacental blood flow, while increasing systemic blood pressure.[97]

The difference in sensitivity of the uterine and systemic circulations to angiotensin II is an important physiologic adaptation during pregnancy. This response contributes to the redistribution of cardiac output, the increase in uterine blood flow, and possibly the maintenance of uterine blood flow during normal fluctuations in blood pressure.[98]

Sensitivity to vasoconstrictors, such as **epinephrine**, **norepinephrine**, and **phenylephrine**, is attenuated during pregnancy.[99] Larger doses of vasoconstrictors are typically required to maintain blood pressure during spinal anesthesia for cesarean delivery.[100] In contrast to the responses to angiotensin II, the uterine circulation is more responsive to the above agents compared with the response of the systemic circulation.[99] Importantly, during hemorrhage or other major stressors that result in large catecholamine release, uteroplacental perfusion is unlikely to be preferentially preserved above essential maternal perfusion.[101]

The mechanism underlying the difference in vascular sensitivity between the uterine and systemic circulations is unclear, but the distribution of receptor subtypes is believed to be important.[102] For example, there are two distinct subtypes of angiotensin II receptors: AT1R and AT2R. In most tissues, including systemic vascular smooth muscle, AT1R receptors are predominant and mediate vasoconstriction. However, AT2R receptors, which do not mediate smooth muscle contraction, account for 75% to 90% of angiotensin II binding in uterine artery and myometrium.[103,104]

Effects of anesthesia-related increases in uterine tone. Catecholamine levels increase during labor.[105] Epinephrine antagonizes the uterotonic effect of endogenous and exogenous oxytocin via direct tocolytic effects. Effective pain relief from neuraxial analgesia decreases circulating catecholamine levels,[105] which may result in stronger, more frequent, or sustained contractions; this may reduce uteroplacental blood flow and predispose to fetal bradycardia (see Chapter 24).[106]

Beneficial Effects of Neuraxial Analgesia and Anesthesia

Neuraxial analgesia has been used to improve fetal well-being in preeclampsia and FGR. With preeclampsia, the trophoblast invasion of the uterine decidua is impaired, causing spiral arteries to retain their nonpregnant smooth muscle, which makes them susceptible to vasoconstriction. Clinical studies have observed that sympathetic deafferentation induced by neuraxial anesthesia improved uteroplacental blood flow in women with preeclampsia.[107–110] In patients with preeclampsia and FGR, epidural **ropivacaine** caused a dose-dependent improvement in uterine artery blood flow, which was reversed by saline placebo.[111] Women with preeclampsia remote from term, who were treated with continuous antepartum epidural analgesia therapy, had longer enrollment-delivery intervals, some evidence of increased fetal growth, and reduced severity of preeclampsia, with less hypertension and a higher platelet count.[111,112] Although these studies were small,[111,112] nonrandomized,[111,112] and unblinded[111,112] or partially blinded,[113] the observed benefit of epidural analgesia is likely more than a consequence of vasodilation. Whereas systemic vasodilators (e.g., **nifedipine**) do not reliably improve placental blood flow,[114] probably because of simultaneous vasodilation of the uteroplacental vessels and competing vascular beds, neuraxial analgesia and anesthesia induce *segmental* vasodilation, reflex vasoconstriction in unanesthetized regions,[115,116] and redistribution of cardiac output toward vascular beds with sympathetic blockade, including the uteroplacental circulation.

Neuraxial Anesthesia for Cesarean Delivery

Elective cesarean delivery. With appropriate management of hemodynamic changes, neuraxial anesthesia has minimal impact on placental perfusion and fetal oxygenation during elective cesarean delivery. However, severe hypotension may decrease uteroplacental blood flow via reduction in perfusion pressure,[17] reflex release of endogenous vasoconstrictors, diversion of blood to the lower limbs,[117] and response to vasopressors.[5] The rapid and extensive sympathetic blockade during spinal anesthesia, and some methods used to treat hypotension, may account for the observation that umbilical arterial blood pH is lower with spinal anesthesia than with epidural or general anesthesia for cesarean delivery.[118]

Studies of the effect of bolus intravenous fluid administration have had mixed results. Most Doppler studies have shown that fluid preload before the initiation of neuraxial analgesia does not change vascular resistance indices,[119] although a decrease has been reported.[120]

Emergency cesarean delivery. For emergency cesarean delivery, in situations involving alteration in uterine activity, hemorrhage, or preeclampsia, the effects of epidural and spinal anesthesia on uteroplacental blood flow are of particular concern. Studies have reported conflicting results. In the setting of severe maternal hypotension, compromised uterine perfusion, or prior or partial anesthesia administration, neuraxial techniques may result in decreased uteroplacental blood flow; prompt interventions, such as administration of fluids, vasopressors, or blood, can help mitigate these effects.

EFFECTS OF NONANESTHETIC AGENTS

Alpha- and Beta-Adrenergic Receptor Antagonists

In patients with chronic or gestational hypertension, the effects of antihypertensive drugs on uteroplacental perfusion depend on the interaction of their effects on uterine vascular resistance and systemic blood pressure. Although studies of the response of uteroplacental blood flow to **labetalol** have had varying results in different animal species, showing an increase,[113] a decrease,[121] and no change,[122] studies in humans have generally demonstrated no significant change.[123,124] Studies of **methyldopa** in patients with preeclampsia have found either a reduction[125] or no change[126] in indices of uterine and placental vascular resistance. A multicenter trial showed that treating chronic hypertension with a blood pressure goal of less than 140/90 mm Hg was associated with improved maternal outcomes and no increased risk for small-for-gestational-age neonates.[127] This suggests that antihypertensive agents can effectively reduce maternal blood pressure with minimal impact on placental perfusion.

Calcium Channel Blockers

Most studies of **nifedipine** have shown no change in uteroplacental blood flow and no change or a decrease in uterine vascular resistance without evidence of fetal compromise.[114,128] A transient decrease of middle cerebral artery Doppler peak systolic velocity or PI has been observed with prolonged use of nifedipine, but the clinical significance is unclear.[128–130] **Verapamil** 0.2 mg/kg was shown to decrease maternal blood pressure and uterine blood flow in pregnant sheep,[131] although human data are lacking.

Nitroglycerin and Other Direct Vasodilators

Multiple studies have examined the effect of **nitroglycerin** on uteroplacental blood flow in patients with preeclampsia. In women with abnormal uterine artery blood flow at 24 to 26 weeks' gestation, an intravenous nitroglycerin infusion decreased uterine vascular resistance indices.[132] Similar responses have been observed with transdermal nitroglycerin administered for 3 days to patients with preeclampsia and FGR.[133] These responses are more pronounced in patients with preeclampsia compared with those in preterm labor without preeclampsia.[134] Moreover, an infusion of nitroglycerin in women with preeclampsia with severe features did not change the uterine artery PI.[134,135] Together, these findings suggest that when used as an acute tocolytic, nitroglycerin is unlikely to significantly affect uteroplacental blood flow despite having an effect on maternal blood pressure.

In animal models of pharmacologically induced hypertension, **hydralazine** reduced maternal blood pressure but increased uteroplacental blood flow, reflecting a decrease in uterine vascular resistance.[136,137] In humans, hydralazine treatment does not affect uterine or umbilical artery waveforms.[138]

Alpha-Adrenergic Receptor Agonists

Wallis et al.[139] found that the epidural injection of 2-chloroprocaine 1.5% with **epinephrine** (10 µg/mL) produced a small, brief reduction in uterine blood flow in pregnant sheep, whereas Alahuhta et al.[88] reported that epidural bupivacaine with epinephrine had no effect on intervillous blood flow in women undergoing cesarean delivery. Epinephrine added to epidural local anesthetics did not reduce uteroplacental blood flow in healthy women during labor.[140] However, one study observed that the addition of epinephrine (85 to 100 µg) to epidural bupivacaine increased Doppler indices of uteroplacental vascular resistance in hypertensive parturients with chronic fetal asphyxia.[107] Therefore, some anesthesia providers avoid epinephrine-containing local anesthetics in women with preeclampsia. Commonly, epinephrine (10 to 15 µg) is included in the epidural test dose. Marcus et al.[141] reported that repeated epidural injections of epinephrine (10 to 15 μg) did not decrease uterine blood flow in pregnant sheep; however, the same dose injected intravenously reduced uterine blood flow, with a maximum decrease of 43% observed at 1 minute.

Intravenous, but not epidural, administration of the α^2-adrenergic receptor agonist clonidine decreased uterine blood flow in gravid ewes.[142]

Umbilical arterial blood pH and base excess have been observed to be higher with the use of alpha-adrenergic receptor agonists compared with **ephedrine** for maintaining maternal blood pressure during spinal anesthesia for cesarean delivery.[143-145] A comparison of different infusion regimens of **phenylephrine**, titrated to maintain maternal systolic blood pressure near baseline, observed no depression of fetal pH and base excess despite very large total doses (up to 2500 μg) before delivery.[100] In contrast, large doses of ephedrine administered to maintain blood pressure during spinal anesthesia for cesarean delivery depressed umbilical arterial blood pH and base excess in a dose-dependent manner.[146] An explanation for the discrepancy between experimental and clinical data is complex and incompletely understood. Animal studies are not always appropriate models for clinical situations. Under clinical conditions, Doppler studies have shown some evidence that uterine vascular resistance is increased by alpha-adrenergic receptor agonists,[147] but this finding has not been consistent.[148] Although alpha-adrenergic receptor agonists increase uterine vascular resistance more than systemic vascular resistance, the observed difference in outcomes may primarily be a result of a differential effect in the myometrium, with relative sparing of the vessels that perfuse the placenta.[149] In addition, uteroplacental blood flow in humans has a margin of safety that allows modest decreases in uterine blood flow (e.g., caused by appropriate doses of alpha-adrenergic receptor agonists) to occur without compromising oxygen transfer.[150]

Finally, the propensity of ephedrine to worsen fetal acid-base status may be more related to direct beta-adrenergic receptor–mediated fetal metabolic effects.[150] Compared with phenylephrine, ephedrine crosses the placenta to a greater extent and is associated with higher fetal levels of lactate, glucose, epinephrine, and norepinephrine.[150] Thus, when considering the choice of vasopressor for clinical use, the anesthesia provider should consider the sum total effect on fetal oxygen supply and demand rather than the isolated effects on uteroplacental blood flow. In this respect, clinical studies do not favor the preferential use of ephedrine. Overall, studies comparing ephedrine and other vasopressors in humans have not demonstrated differences in neonatal clinical outcomes.

Other Inotropes

Inotropic drugs are rarely indicated in obstetric patients. On the basis of studies of normal pregnant sheep, **milrinone** and **amrinone** may increase uterine blood flow, whereas **dopamine** and **epinephrine** diminish flow.[151,152] During maternal resuscitation, the choice of inotropes should be based on the efficacy in the mother rather than the effects on uterine blood flow; restoration of spontaneous circulation and adequate uterine perfusion pressure is the priority (see Chapter 53).

Atrial and brain natriuretic peptides attenuate the response to **angiotensin II**, and intravenous infusion of atrial natriuretic peptide reduces blood pressure while increasing uterine blood flow in women with preeclampsia.[153] Protein kinase C activity is decreased in uterine but not systemic arteries of pregnant sheep and predisposes to vasodilation and an increase in uterine blood flow; this may have a regulatory effect on local ovarian and placental estrogen production.[154] Studies in rats have shown a decrease in endogenous endothelin-dependent vasoconstrictor tone in uteroplacental vessels, which may contribute to the increase in placental blood flow in late gestation.[155] Uterine vascular resistance in early pregnancy is increased by **relaxin**, which modulates the effects of estrogen and progesterone.[156] Placental protein 13 is a potent vasodilator of both uterine and systemic blood vessels *in vitro* and may contribute to the vasodilation that occurs during human pregnancy. The use of vasopressin to prevent spinal anesthesia–induced hypotension has been reported in patients with pulmonary hypertension.[157]

Prostaglandin Inhibitors

The greater synthesis and higher circulating concentrations of endothelial-derived vasodilators during pregnancy are believed to modulate systemic and uterine vascular responses to angiotensin II and other vasoconstrictors.[158] Uterine vascular production of prostacyclin is greater than systemic vascular production, which probably contributes to the maintenance of uteroplacental blood flow in opposition to the effects of circulating vasoconstrictors.[159] An enhanced response to angiotensin II during pregnancy has been demonstrated with the systemic and local infusion of **indomethacin**, which blocks prostacyclin production.[159] However, inhibition of prostaglandin synthesis by an infusion of indomethacin induces only a transient decrease in uteroplacental blood flow, indicating that uteroplacental blood flow is not solely dependent on the continued production of prostacyclin.[158] In the pregnant rabbit, indomethacin infusion causes a decrease in placental but not myometrial blood flow.[160] In contrast, in the dog, indomethacin resulted in an increase in placental blood flow.[161] In humans there was no change in the uterine artery Doppler pattern[162] or umbilical artery Doppler pattern[163] in patients undergoing indomethacin treatment.

Steroids

Steroid hormones regulate uteroplacental blood flow. **Betamethasone**, which may be administered to enhance fetal lung maturity, decreased umbilical artery PI and improved waveform from reversed to absent or even positive diastolic flow.[164–166] However, these effects are transient, and there was no effect on the uterine artery waveform. Notably, lack of improvement in fetal Doppler waveforms after betamethasone administration was associated with poor prognosis in cases of FGR.[167]

Magnesium Sulfate

Magnesium increases uterine blood flow in normotensive and hypertensive pregnant sheep.[168,169] Although hypermagnesemia was found to exacerbate maternal hypotension during epidural anesthesia in pregnant sheep, no reduction in uterine blood flow was observed.[168] In women in preterm labor[170] and in women with preeclampsia with severe features,[171] magnesium sulfate caused a modest decrease in Doppler indices of uterine vascular resistance. Overall, magnesium does not cause a clinically significant change in uteroplacental perfusion.

Oxygen Therapy

Although traditionally used as a therapy for intrauterine resuscitation, recent studies have shown that supplemental oxygen does not improve umbilical artery pH or neonatal outcomes.[167] Furthermore, supplemental oxygen administration when maternal oxygen saturation is normal does not increase umbilical artery Pao_2, and may even decrease it and placental blood flow (Fig. 3.10). Prolonged oxygen administration may impair placental transfer of oxygen.[172] The American College of Obstetricians and Gynecologists no longer recommends the routine use of oxygen supplementation for fetal intrauterine resuscitation in women with normal oxygen saturation,[173] although controversy remains.[174]

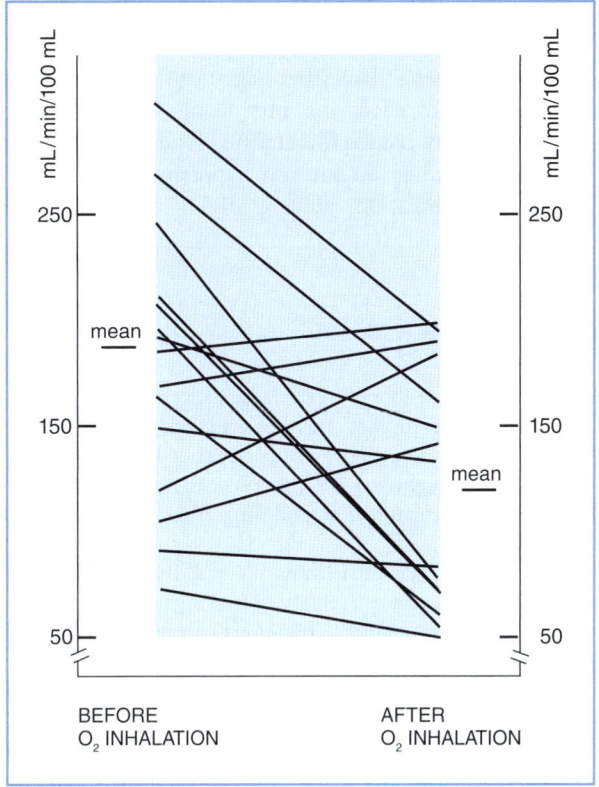

Fig. 3.10 Intervillous blood flow measured using a [133]Xenon method before and after inhalation of oxygen 5 L/min in 22 women with a pregnancy complication between 34 and 40 weeks' gestation. Data are shown for individual patients. Mean blood flow decreased significantly after inhalation of oxygen 5 L/min. Redrawn from Jouppila P, Kirkinen P, Koivula A, Jouppila R. The influence of maternal oxygen inhalation on human placental and umbilical venous blood flow. *Eur J Obstet Gynecol Reprod Biol.* 1983;16:151–156.

KEY POINTS

- Growth and development of the uteroplacental vasculature and progressive vasodilation allow uteroplacental blood flow to increase during pregnancy. Uteroplacental blood flow constitutes approximately 12% of maternal cardiac output at term.
- Many factors modulate the maintenance and regulation of uteroplacental blood flow, including altered responses to vasoconstrictors, increases in endothelium-derived vasodilators, and the effects of steroid hormones and shear stress.
- The uteroplacental circulation is a dilated, low-resistance vascular bed with limited ability for autoregulation. Flow may be reduced by a decrease in uterine arterial pressure, an increase in uterine venous pressure, or an increase in uterine vascular resistance.
- The uteroplacental circulation is composed of placental and nonplacental circulations that are anatomically and functionally dissimilar.
- Acute or chronic reductions in uteroplacental blood flow may threaten fetal viability and predispose to disorders such as preeclampsia and fetal growth restriction. In

situations of an acute reduction in uteroplacental perfusion, there is a limited margin of safety; exceeding this limit may decrease fetal oxygen uptake with resultant metabolic acidosis.
- Animal studies are the principal source of uteroplacental blood flow data; thus, clinicians should carefully consider interspecies differences and study methodology when extrapolating experimental findings to clinical practice.
- Doppler ultrasonography is the method most commonly used clinically to assess uteroplacental blood flow in humans. Abnormal waveforms and indices of resistance may be predictive of complications such as preeclampsia, fetal growth restriction, and preterm labor.
- Neuraxial anesthesia can increase uterine blood flow by reducing pain and stress or it can decrease uterine blood flow by causing hypotension.
- Although animal studies show that ephedrine protects uteroplacental blood flow better than alpha-adrenergic receptor agonists such as phenylephrine, umbilical arterial blood pH and base excess are lower after the administration of ephedrine. This effect may be related to a greater

propensity of ephedrine to cross the placenta and exert direct metabolic effects on the fetus.

- The doses of general anesthetic agents used clinically have minimal direct effects on uterine blood flow. General anesthesia may reduce the uterine blood flow by causing decreased cardiac output and hypotension. Conversely, noxious stimulation during light anesthesia may precipitate the release of catecholamines, which may result in decreased uterine blood flow.

- For cardiovascular emergencies in pregnant women, the choice of inotropic drug should depend primarily on the efficacy of the drugs to optimize the maternal condition, rather than on minor differences in uterine blood flow. Standard resuscitation drugs should be used in an emergency.

REFERENCES

1. Brosens I, Pijnenborg R, Vercruysse L, Romero R. The "Great Obstetrical Syndromes" are associated with disorders of deep placentation. *Am J Obstet Gynecol.* 2011;204:193–201.
2. Chappell J, Aughwane R, Clark AR, et al. A review of feto-placental vasculature flow modelling. *Placenta.* 2023;142:56–63.
3. Shapiro J, Ginosar Y, Gielchinsky Y, et al. BOLD-MRI demonstrates acute placental and fetal organ hypoperfusion with fetal brain sparing in response to phenylephrine but not ephedrine. *Placenta.* 2020;90:52–57.
4. Erkinaro T, Mäkikallio K, Kavasmaa T, et al. Effects of ephedrine and phenylephrine on uterine and placental circulations and fetal outcome following fetal hypoxaemia and epidural-induced hypotension in a sheep model. *Br J Anaesth.* 2004;93:825–832.
5. Ralston DH, Shnider SM, DeLorimier AA. Effects of equipotent ephedrine, metaraminol, mephentermine, and methoxamine on uterine blood flow in the pregnant ewe. *Anesthesiology.* 1974;40:354–370.
6. Konje JC, Kaufmann P, Bell SC, Taylor DJ. A longitudinal study of quantitative uterine blood flow with the use of color power angiography in appropriate for gestational age pregnancies. *Am J Obstet Gynecol.* 2001;185:608–613.
7. Browne VA, Julian CG, Toledo-Jaldin L, et al. Uterine artery blood flow, fetal hypoxia and fetal growth. *Philos Trans R Soc Lond B Biol Sci.* 2015;370:20140068.
8. Degner K, Magness RR, Shah DM. Establishment of the human uteroplacental circulation: a historical perspective. *Reprod Sci.* 2017;24:753–761.
9. Thaler I, Manor D, Itskovitz J, et al. Changes in uterine blood flow during human pregnancy. *Am J Obstet Gynecol.* 1990;162:121–125.
10. Rosenfeld CR, Morriss FH Jr, Makowski EL, et al. Circulatory changes in the reproductive tissues of ewes during pregnancy. *Gynecol Invest.* 1974;5:252–268.
11. Gill RW, Kossoff G, Warren PS, Garrett WJ. Umbilical venous flow in normal and complicated pregnancy. *Ultrasound Med Biol.* 1984;10:349–363.
12. Boito S, Struijk PC, Ursem NT, et al. Umbilical venous volume flow in the normally developing and growth-restricted human fetus. *Ultrasound Obstet Gynecol.* 2002;19:344–349.
13. Rigano S, Boito S, Maspero E, et al. OP15.01: absolute uterine artery blood flow volume is increased in twin human pregnancies compared to singletons. *Ultrasound Obstet Gynecol.* 2007;30:506.
14. Palmer SK, Zamudio S, Coffin C, et al. Quantitative estimation of human uterine artery blood flow and pelvic blood flow redistribution in pregnancy. *Obstet Gynecol.* 1992;80:1000–1006.
15. Verkeste CM, Saxena PR, Peeters LL. Lack of positive correlation between placental blood flow and mean arterial pressure in the non-anaesthetised guinea pig near term; an indication for autoregulation? *Eur J Obstet Gynecol Reprod Biol.* 1995;61:161–165.
16. Greiss FC Jr, Anderson SG. Pressure-flow relationship in the nonpregnant uterine vascular bed. *Am J Obstet Gynecol.* 1974;118:763–772.
17. Greiss FC Jr. Pressure-flow relationship in the gravid uterine vascular bed. *Am J Obstet Gynecol.* 1966;96:41–47.
18. Venuto RC, Cox JW, Stein JH, Ferris TF. The effect of changes in perfusion pressure on uteroplacental blood flow in the pregnant rabbit. *J Clin Invest.* 1976;57:938–944.
19. Assali NS, Dasgupta K, Kolin A, Holms L. Measurement of uterine blood flow and uterine metabolism. V. Changes during spontaneous and induced labor in unanesthetized pregnant sheep and dogs. *Am J Physiol.* 1958;195:614–620.
20. Li H, Gudmundsson S, Olofsson P. Uterine artery blood flow velocity waveforms during uterine contractions. *Ultrasound Obstet Gynecol.* 2003;22:578–585.
21. Lee W, Rokey R, Miller J, Cotton DB. Maternal hemodynamic effects of uterine contractions by M-mode and pulsed-Doppler echocardiography. *Am J Obstet Gynecol.* 1989;161:974–977.
22. Zamir M, Nelson DM, Ginosar Y. Geometric and hemodynamic characterization of uterine spiral arteries: the concept of resistance reserve. *Placenta.* 2018;68:59–64.
23. Zamir M, Nelson DM, Ginosar Y. Hemodynamic consequences of incomplete uterine spiral artery transformation in human pregnancy, with implications for placental dysfunction and preeclampsia. *J Appl Physiol (1985).* 2021;130:457–465.
24. Burton GJ, Woods AW, Jauniaux E, Kingdom JC. Rheological and physiological consequences of conversion of the maternal spiral arteries for uteroplacental blood flow during human pregnancy. *Placenta.* 2009;30:473–482.
25. Varberg KM, Dominguez EM, Koseva B, et al. Extravillous trophoblast cell lineage development is associated with active remodeling of the chromatin landscape. *Nat Commun.* 2023;14:4826.
26. Osol G, Mandala M. Maternal uterine vascular remodeling during pregnancy. *Physiology (Bethesda).* 2009;24:58–71.
27. Page KL, Celia G, Leddy G, et al. Structural remodeling of rat uterine veins in pregnancy. *Am J Obstet Gynecol.* 2002;187:1647–1652.
28. Forbes TR, Taku E. Vein size in intact and hysterectomized mice during the estrous cycle and pregnancy. *Anat Rec.* 1975;182:61–65.
29. Oosterhof H, Wichers G, Fidler V, Aarnoudse JG. Blood viscosity and uterine artery flow velocity waveforms in pregnancy: a longitudinal study. *Placenta.* 1993;14:555–561.

30. Rusidzé M, Gargaros A, Fébrissy C, et al. Estrogen actions in placental vascular morphogenesis and spiral artery remodeling: a comparative view between humans and mice. *Cells.* 2023;12:620.

31. Chang K, Lubo Z. Review article: steroid hormones and uterine vascular adaptation to pregnancy. *Reprod Sci.* 2008;15:336–348.

32. Pastore MB, Jobe SO, Ramadoss J, Magness RR. Estrogen receptor-α and estrogen receptor-β in the uterine vascular endothelium during pregnancy: functional implications for regulating uterine blood flow. *Semin Reprod Med.* 2012;30:46–61.

33. Chen JZ, Sheehan PM, Brennecke SP, Keogh RJ. Vessel remodelling, pregnancy hormones and extravillous trophoblast function. *Mol Cell Endocrinol.* 2012;349:138–144.

34. Urban G, Vergani P, Ghidini A, et al. State of the art: non-invasive ultrasound assessment of the uteroplacental circulation. *Semin Perinatol.* 2007;31:232–239.

35. Wedegärtner U, Kooijman H, Andreas T, et al. T2 and T2* measurements of fetal brain oxygenation during hypoxia with MRI at 3T: correlation with fetal arterial blood oxygen saturation. *Eur Radiol.* 2010;20:121–127.

36. Wedegärtner U, Tchirikov M, Schäfer S, et al. Functional MR imaging: comparison of BOLD signal intensity changes in fetal organs with fetal and maternal oxyhemoglobin saturation during hypoxia in sheep. *Radiology.* 2006;238:872–880.

37. Huen I, Morris DM, Wright C, et al. R_1 and R_2* changes in the human placenta in response to maternal oxygen challenge. *Magn Reson Med.* 2013;70:1427–1433.

38. Sørensen A, Peters D, Fründ E, et al. Changes in human placental oxygenation during maternal hyperoxia estimated by blood oxygen level-dependent magnetic resonance imaging (BOLD MRI). *Ultrasound Obstet Gynecol.* 2013;42:310–314.

39. Taso M, Aramendía-Vidaurreta V, Englund EK, et al. Update on state-of-the-art for arterial spin labeling (ASL) human perfusion imaging outside of the brain. *Magn Reson Med.* 2023;89:1754–1776.

40. Liu D, Shao X, Danyalov A, et al. Human placenta blood flow during early gestation with pseudocontinuous arterial spin labeling MRI. *J Magn Reson Imaging.* 2020;51:1247–1257.

41. Deng J, Zhang A, Zhao M, et al. Placental perfusion using intravoxel incoherent motion MRI combined with Doppler findings in differentiating between very low birth weight infants and small for gestational age infants. *Placenta.* 2023;135:16–24.

42. Stepan H, Herraiz I, Schlembach D, et al. Implementation of the sFlt-1/PlGF ratio for prediction and diagnosis of pre-eclampsia in singleton pregnancy: implications for clinical practice. *Ultrasound Obstet Gynecol.* 2015;45:241–246.

43. Staff AC, Fjeldstad HE, Fosheim IK, et al. Failure of physiological transformation and spiral artery atherosis: their roles in preeclampsia. *Am J Obstet Gynecol.* 2022;226:S895–S906.

44. Zeisler H, Llurba E, Chantraine F, et al. Predictive value of the sFlt-1:PlGF ratio in women with suspected preeclampsia. *N Engl J Med.* 2016;374:13–22.

45. Plasencia W, Maiz N, Bonino S, et al. Uterine artery Doppler at 11 + 0 to 13 + 6 weeks in the prediction of pre-eclampsia. *Ultrasound Obstet Gynecol.* 2007;30:742–749.

46. Mifsud W, Sebire NJ. Placental pathology in early-onset and late-onset fetal growth restriction. *Fetal Diagn Ther.* 2014;36:117–128.

47. Rolnik DL, Wright D, Poon LC, et al. Aspirin versus placebo in pregnancies at high risk for preterm preeclampsia. *New Engl J Med.* 2017;377:613–622.

48. Morley LC, Debant M, Walker JJ, et al. Placental blood flow sensing and regulation in fetal growth restriction. *Placenta.* 2021;113:23–28.

49. Baschat AA, Gembruch U, Harman CR. The sequence of changes in Doppler and biophysical parameters as severe fetal growth restriction worsens. *Ultrasound Obstet Gynecol.* 2001;18:571–577.

50. Brosens I, Puttemans P, Benagiano G. Placental bed research: I. The placental bed: from spiral arteries remodeling to the great obstetrical syndromes. *Am J Obstet Gynecol.* 2019;221:437–456.

51. Kim YM, Bujold E, Chaiworapongsa T, et al. Failure of physiologic transformation of the spiral arteries in patients with preterm labor and intact membranes. *Am J Obstet Gynecol.* 2003;189:1063–1069.

52. Misra VK, Hobel CJ, Sing CF. Placental blood flow and the risk of preterm delivery. *Placenta.* 2009;30:619–624.

53. Sato M, Noguchi J, Mashima M, et al. 3D power Doppler ultrasound assessment of placental perfusion during uterine contraction in labor. *Placenta.* 2016;45:32–36.

54. Olofsson P. Umbilical cord pH, blood gases, and lactate at birth: normal values, interpretation, and clinical utility. *Am J Obstet Gynecol.* 2023;228:S1222–S1240.

55. Weiss E, Hitschold T, Berle P. Umbilical artery blood flow velocity waveforms during variable deceleration of the fetal heart rate. *Am J Obstet Gynecol.* 1991;164:534–540.

56. Cahill AG, Tuuli MG, Stout MJ, et al. A prospective cohort study of fetal heart rate monitoring: deceleration area is predictive of fetal acidemia. *Am J Obstet Gynecol.* 2018;218:523.e1–e12.

57. Baxter P. Markers of perinatal hypoxia–ischaemia and neurological injury: assessing the impact of insult duration. *Dev Med Child Neurol.* 2020;62:563–568.

58. Ray JG, Vermeulen MJ, Schull MJ, Redelmeier DA. Cardiovascular health after maternal placental syndromes (CHAMPS): population-based retrospective cohort study. *Lancet.* 2005;366:1797–1803.

59. Bellamy L, Casas JP, Hingorani AD, Williams DJ. Pre-eclampsia and risk of cardiovascular disease and cancer in later life: systematic review and meta-analysis. *BMJ.* 2007;335:974.

60. Calderon-Margalit R, Friedlander Y, Yanetz R, et al. Preeclampsia and subsequent risk of cancer: update from the Jerusalem Perinatal Study. *Am J Obstet Gynecol.* 2009;200:63.e1–e5.

61. Osmond C, Barker DJ, Winter PD, et al. Early growth and death from cardiovascular disease in women. *BMJ.* 1993;307:1519–1524.

62. Barker DJP. Sir Richard Doll Lecture. Developmental origins of chronic disease. *Public Health.* 2012;126:185–189.

63. McMillen IC, Robinson JS. Developmental origins of the metabolic syndrome: prediction, plasticity, and programming. *Physiol Rev.* 2005;85:571–633.

64. Thornburg KL, O'Tierney PF, Louey S. Review: the placenta is a programming agent for cardiovascular disease. *Placenta.* 2010;31(suppl):S54–S59.

65. Lau C, Rogers JM, Desai M, Ross MG. Fetal programming of adult disease: implications for prenatal care. *Obstet Gynecol.* 2011;117:978–985.

66. Burton GJ, Fowden AL, Thornburg KL. Placental origins of chronic disease. *Physiol Rev.* 2016;96:1509–1565.

67. Allen J, Svane D, Petersen LK, et al. Effects of thiopentone and chlormethiazole on human myometrial arteries from term pregnant women. *Br J Anaesth.* 1992;68:256–260.

68. Alon E, Ball RH, Gillie MH, et al. Effects of propofol and thiopental on maternal and fetal cardiovascular and acid-base variables in the pregnant ewe. *Anesthesiology.* 1993;78:562–576.

69. Craft JB Jr, Coaldrake LA, Yonekura ML, et al. Ketamine, catecholamines, and uterine tone in pregnant ewes. *Am J Obstet Gynecol.* 1983;146:429–434.

70. Strümper D, Gogarten W, Durieux ME, et al. The effects of S+-ketamine and racemic ketamine on uterine blood flow in chronically instrumented pregnant sheep. *Anesth Analg.* 2004;98:497–502.

71. Jouppila P, Kuikka J, Jouppila R, Hollmén A. Effect of induction of general anesthesia for cesarean section on intervillous blood flow. *Acta Obstet Gynecol Scand.* 1979;58:249–253.

72. Gin T, O'Meara ME, Kan AF, et al. Plasma catecholamines and neonatal condition after induction of anaesthesia with propofol or thiopentone at caesarean section. *Br J Anaesth.* 1993;70:311–316.

73. Levinson G, Shnider SM, Gildea JE, DeLorimier AA. Maternal and foetal cardiovascular and acid-base changes during ketamine anaesthesia in pregnant ewes. *Br J Anaesth.* 1973;45:1111–1115.

74. Gin T, Ngan-Kee WD, Siu YK, et al. Alfentanil given immediately before the induction of anesthesia for elective cesarean delivery. *Anesth Analg.* 2000;90:1167–1172.

75. Ngan Kee WD, Khaw KS, Ma KC, et al. Maternal and neonatal effects of remifentanil at induction of general anesthesia for cesarean delivery: a randomized, double-blind, controlled trial. *Anesthesiology.* 2006;104:14–20.

76. Palahniuk RJ, Shnider SM. Maternal and fetal cardiovascular and acid-base changes during halothane and isoflurane anesthesia in the pregnant ewe. *Anesthesiology.* 1974;41:462–472.

77. Dahlgren G, Törnberg DC, Pregner K, Irestedt L. Four cases of the ex utero intrapartum treatment (EXIT) procedure: anesthetic implications. *Int J Obstet Anesth.* 2004;13:178–182.

78. Harris LK, Aplin JD. Vascular remodeling and extracellular matrix breakdown in the uterine spiral arteries during pregnancy. *Reprod Sci.* 2007;14:28–34.

79. Riley ET. Editorial I: Spinal anaesthesia for caesarean delivery: keep the pressure up and don't spare the vasoconstrictors. *Br J Anaesth.* 2004;92:459–461.

80. Walker AM, Oakes GK, Ehrenkranz R, et al. Effects of hypercapnia on uterine and umbilical circulations in conscious pregnant sheep. *J Appl Physiol.* 1976;41:727–733.

81. Faucher DJ, Laptook AR, Porter JC, Rosenfeld CR. Effects of acute hypercapnia on maternal and fetal vasopressin and catecholamine release. *Pediatr Res.* 1991;30:368–374.

82. Hanka R, Lawn L, Mills IH, et al. The effects of maternal hypercapnia on foetal oxygenation and uterine blood flow in the pig. *J Physiol.* 1975;247:447–460.

83. Ginosar Y, Gielchinsky Y, Nachmansson N, et al. BOLD-MRI demonstrates acute placental and fetal organ hypoperfusion

with fetal brain sparing during hypercapnia. *Placenta.* 2018;63:53–60.

84. Lioy F, Blinkhorn MT, Garneau C. Regional hemodynamic effects of changes in $PaCO_2$ in the vagotomized, sino-aortic de-afferented rat. *J Auton Nerv Syst.* 1985;12:301–313.

85. Motoyama EK, Rivard G, Acheson F, Cook CD. Adverse effect of maternal hyperventilation on the foetus. *Lancet.* 1966;1:286–288.

86. Lumley J, Renou P, Newman W, Wood C. Hyperventilation in obstetrics. *Am J Obstet Gynecol.* 1969;103:847–855.

87. Levinson G, Shnider SM, DeLorimier AA, Steffenson JL. Effects of maternal hyperventilation on uterine blood flow and fetal oxygenation and acid-base status. *Anesthesiology.* 1974;40:340–347.

88. Alahuhta S, Räsänen J, Jouppila R, et al. Uteroplacental and fetal haemodynamics during extradural anaesthesia for caesarean section. *Br J Anaesth.* 1991;66:319–323.

89. Erkinaro T, Kavasmaa T, Päkkilä M, et al. Ephedrine and phenylephrine for the treatment of maternal hypotension in a chronic sheep model of increased placental vascular resistance. *Br J Anaesth.* 2006;96:231–237.

90. Higgins N, Fitzgerald PC, van Dyk D, et al. The effect of prophylactic phenylephrine and ephedrine infusions on umbilical artery blood pH in women with preeclampsia undergoing cesarean delivery with spinal anesthesia: a randomized, double-blind trial. *Anesth Analg.* 2018;126:1999–2006.

91. Dyer RA, Emmanuel A, Adams SC, et al. A randomised comparison of bolus phenylephrine and ephedrine for the management of spinal hypotension in patients with severe preeclampsia and fetal compromise. *Int J Obstet Anesth.* 2018;33:23–31.

92. Weiner CP, Martinez E, Chestnut DH, Ghodsi A. Effect of pregnancy on uterine and carotid artery response to norepinephrine, epinephrine, and phenylephrine in vessels with documented functional endothelium. *Am J Obstet Gynecol.* 1989;161:1605–1610.

93. Weiner CP, Thompson LP, Liu KZ, Herrig JE. Endothelium-derived relaxing factor and indomethacin-sensitive contracting factor alter arterial contractile responses to thromboxane during pregnancy. *Am J Obstet Gynecol.* 1992;166:1171–1178.

94. Yang D, Clark KE. Effect of endothelin-1 on the uterine vasculature of the pregnant and estrogen-treated nonpregnant sheep. *Am J Obstet Gynecol.* 1992;167:1642–1650.

95. Wier RJ, Brown JJ, Fraser R, et al. Relationship between plasma renin, renin-substrate, angiotensin II, aldosterone and electrolytes in normal pregnancy. *J Clin Endocrinol Metab.* 1975;40:108–115.

96. Chesley LC, Talledo E, Bohler CS, Zuspan FP. Vascular reactivity to angiotensin II and norepinephrine in pregnant women. *Am J Obstet Gynecol.* 1965;91:837–842.

97. Rosenfeld CR, Naden RP. Uterine and nonuterine vascular responses to angiotensin II in ovine pregnancy. *Am J Physiol.* 1989;257:H17–H24.

98. Rosenfeld CR. Consideration of the uteroplacental circulation in intrauterine growth. *Semin Perinatol.* 1984;8:42–51.

99. Magness RR, Rosenfeld CR. Systemic and uterine responses to alpha-adrenergic stimulation in pregnant and nonpregnant ewes. *Am J Obstet Gynecol.* 1986;155:897–904.

100. Ngan Kee WD, Khaw KS, Ng FF. Comparison of phenylephrine infusion regimens for maintaining maternal

blood pressure during spinal anaesthesia for caesarean section. *Br J Anaesth*. 2004;92:469–474.

101. Bruce NW. Effects of acute maternal hemorrhage on uterineblood flow in the pregnant rat. *J Appl Physiol*. 1973;35:564–569.

102. Rosenfeld CR, DeSpain K, Word RA, Liu XT. Differential sensitivity to angiotensin II and norepinephrine in human uterine arteries. *J Clin Endocrinol Metab*. 2012;97:138–147.

103. Rosenfeld CR. Mechanisms regulating angiotensin II responsiveness by the uteroplacental circulation. *Am J Physiol Regul Integr Comp Physiol*. 2001;281:R1025–R1040.

104. Cox BE, Rosenfeld CR, Kalinyak JE, et al. Tissue specific expression of vascular smooth muscle angiotensin II receptor subtypes during ovine pregnancy. *Am J Physiol*. 1996;271:H212–H221.

105. Shnider SM, Abboud TK, Artal R, et al. Maternal catecholamines decrease during labor after lumbar epidural anesthesia. *Am J Obstet Gynecol*. 1983;147:13–15.

106. Friedlander JD, Fox HE, Cain CF, et al. Fetal bradycardia and uterine hyperactivity following subarachnoid administration of fentanyl during labor. *Reg Anesth*. 1997;22:378–381.

107. Alahuhta S, Räsänen J, Jouppila P, et al. Uteroplacental and fetal circulation during extradural bupivacaine-adrenaline and bupivacaine for caesarean section in hypertensive pregnancies with chronic fetal asphyxia. *Br J Anaesth*. 1993;71:348–353.

108. Jouppila P, Jouppila R, Hollmén A, Koivula A. Lumbar epidural analgesia to improve intervillous blood flow duringlabor in severe preeclampsia. *Obstet Gynecol*. 1982;59:158–161.

109. Mires GJ, Dempster J, Patel NB, Taylor DJ. Epidural analgesia and its effect on umbilical artery flow velocity waveform patterns in uncomplicated labour and labour complicated by pregnancy-induced hypertension. *Eur J Obstet Gynecol Reprod Biol*. 1990;36:35–41.

110. Ramos-Santos E, Devoe LD, Wakefield ML, et al. The effects of epidural anesthesia on the Doppler velocimetry ofumbilical and uterine arteries in normal and hypertensive patients during active term labor. *Obstet Gynecol*. 1991;77:20–26.

111. Ginosar Y, Nadjari M, Hoffman A, et al. Antepartum continuous epidural ropivacaine therapy reduces uterine artery vascular resistance in pre-eclampsia: a randomized, dose-ranging, placebo-controlled study. *Br J Anaesth*. 2009;102:369–378.

112. Kanayama N, Belayet HM, Khatun S, et al. A new treatment of severe pre-eclampsia by long-term epidural anaesthesia. *J Hum Hypertens*. 1999;13:167–171.

113. Eisenach JC, Mandell G, Dewan DM. Maternal and fetal effects of labetalol in pregnant ewes. *Anesthesiology*. 1991;74:292–297.

114. Moretti MM, Fairlie FM, Akl S, et al. The effect of nifedipine therapy on fetal and placental Doppler waveforms in preeclampsia remote from term. *Am J Obstet Gynecol*. 1990;163:1844–1848.

115. Matsukawa T, Sessler DI, Christensen R, et al. Heat flow and distribution during epidural anesthesia. *Anesthesiology*. 1995;83:961–967.

116. Ginosar Y, Weiniger CF, Kurz V, et al. Sympathectomy-mediated vasodilatation: a randomized concentration rangingstudy of epidural bupivacaine. *Can J Anaesth*. 2009;56:213–221.

117. Baumann H, Alon E, Atanassoff P, et al. Effect of epidural anesthesia for cesarean delivery on maternal femoral arterial and venous, uteroplacental, and umbilical blood flow velocities and waveforms. *Obstet Gynecol*. 1990;75:194–198.

118. Reynolds F, Seed PT. Anaesthesia for caesarean section and neonatal acid-base status: a meta-analysis. *Anaesthesia*. 2005;60:636–653.

119. Gogarten W, Struemper D, Gramke HF, et al. Assessment of volume preload on uteroplacental blood flow during epidural anaesthesia for caesarean section. *Eur J Anaesthesiol*. 2005;22:359–362.

120. Giles WB, Lah FX, Trudinger BJ. The effect of epidural anaesthesia for caesarean section on maternal uterine and fetal umbilical artery blood flow velocity waveforms. *BJOG*. 1987;94:55–59.

121. Morgan MA, Silavin SL, Dormer KJ, et al. Effects of labetalol on uterine blood flow and cardiovascular hemodynamics in the hypertensive gravid baboon. *Am J Obstet Gynecol*. 1993;168:1574–1579.

122. Ahokas RA, Mabie WC, Sibai BM, Anderson GD. Labetalol does not decrease placental perfusion in the hypertensive term-pregnant rat. *Am J Obstet Gynecol*. 1989;160:480–484.

123. Nylund L, Lunell NO, Lewander R, et al. Labetalol for the treatment of hypertension in pregnancy. Pharmacokinetics and effects on the uteroplacental blood flow. *Acta Obstet Gynecol Scand Suppl*. 1984;118:71–73.

124. Lunell NO, Nylund L, Lewander R, Sarby B. Acute effect of an antihypertensive drug, labetalol, on uteroplacental blood flow. *BJOG*. 1982;89:640–644.

125. Günenç O, Ciçek N, Görkemli H, et al. The effect of methyldopa treatment on uterine, umblical and fetal middle cerebral artery blood flows in preeclamptic patients. *Arch Gynecol Obstet*. 2002;266:141–144.

126. Montan S, Anandakumar C, Arulkumaran S, et al. Effects of methyldopa on uteroplacental and fetal hemodynamics in pregnancy-induced hypertension. *Am J Obstet Gynecol*. 1993;168:152–156.

127. Tita AT, Szychowski JM, Boggess K, et al. Treatment for mild chronic hypertension during pregnancy. *N Engl J Med*. 2022;386:1781–1792.

128. Guclu S, Gol M, Saygili U, et al. Nifedipine therapy for preterm labor: effects on placental, fetal cerebral and atrioventricular Doppler parameters in the first 48 hours. *Ultrasound Obstet Gynecol*. 2006;27:403–408.

129. Guclu S, Saygili U, Dogan E, et al. The short-term effect of nifedipine tocolysis on placental, fetal cerebral and atrioventricular Doppler waveforms. *Ultrasound Obstet Gynecol*. 2004;24:761–765.

130. Lima MM, Souza AS, Diniz C, et al. Doppler velocimetry of the uterine, umbilical and fetal middle cerebral arteries in pregnant women undergoing tocolysis with oral nifedipine. *Ultrasound Obstet Gynecol*. 2009;34:311–315.

131. Murad SH, Tabsh KM, Shilyanski G, et al. Effects of verapamil on uterine blood flow and maternal cardiovascular function in the awake pregnant ewe. *Anesth Analg*. 1985;64:7–10.

132. Ramsay B, De Belder A, Campbell S, et al. A nitric oxide donor improves uterine artery diastolic blood flow in normal early pregnancy and in women at high risk of pre-eclampsia. *Eur J Clin Invest*. 1994;24:76–78.

133. Cacciatore B, Halmesmäki E, Kaaja R, et al. Effects of transdermal nitroglycerin on impedance to flow in the uterine, umbilical, and fetal middle cerebral arteries in

pregnancies complicated by preeclampsia and intrauterine growth retardation. *Am J Obstet Gynecol.* 1998;179: 140–145.

134. Luzi G, Caserta G, Iammarino G, et al. Nitric oxide donors in pregnancy: fetomaternal hemodynamic effects induced in mild pre-eclampsia and threatened preterm labor. *Ultrasound Obstet Gynecol.* 1999;14:101–109.

135. Grunewald C, Kublickas M, Carlström K, et al. Effects of nitroglycerin on the uterine and umbilical circulation in severe preeclampsia. *Obstet Gynecol.* 1995;86:600–604.

136. Pedron SL, Reid DL, Barnard JM, et al. Differential effects of intravenous hydralazine on myoendometrial and placental blood flow in hypertensive pregnant ewes. *Am J Obstet Gynecol.* 1992;167:1672–1678.

137. Ring G, Krames E, Shnider SM, et al. Comparison of nitroprusside and hydralazine in hypertensive pregnant ewes. *Obstet Gynecol.* 1977;50:598–602.

138. Gudmundsson S, Gennser G, Marsal K. Effects of hydralazine on placental and renal circulation in pre-eclampsia. *Acta Obstet Gynecol Scand.* 1995;74:415–418.

139. Wallis KL, Shnider SM, Hicks JS, Spivey HT. Epidural anesthesia in the normotensive pregnant ewe: effects on uterine blood flow and fetal acid-base status. *Anesthesiology.* 1976;44:481–487.

140. Albright GA, Jouppila R, Hollmén AI, et al. Epinephrine does not alter human intervillous blood flow during epidural anesthesia. *Anesthesiology.* 1981;54:131–135.

141. Marcus MA, Gogarten W, Vertommen JD, et al. Haemodynamic effects of repeated epidural test-doses of adrenaline in the chronic maternal-fetal sheep preparation. *Eur J Anaesthesiol.* 1998;15:320–323.

142. Eisenach JC, Castro MI, Dewan DM, et al. Intravenous clonidine hydrochloride toxicity in pregnant ewes. *Am J Obstet Gynecol.* 1989;160:471–476.

143. Lee A, Ngan Kee WD, Gin T. A quantitative, systematic review of randomized controlled trials of ephedrine versus phenylephrine for the management of hypotension during spinal anesthesia for cesarean delivery. *Anesth Analg.* 2002;94:920–926.

144. Singh PM, Singh NP, Reschke M, et al. Vasopressor drugs for the prevention and treatment of hypotension during neuraxial anaesthesia for caesarean delivery: a Bayesian network meta-analysis of fetal and maternal outcomes. *Br J Anaesth.* 2020;124:e95–e107.

145. Heesen M, Rijs K, Hilber N, et al. Ephedrine versus phenylephrine as a vasopressor for spinal anaesthesia-induced hypotension in parturients undergoing high-risk caesarean section: meta-analysis, meta-regression and trial sequential analysis. *Int J Obstet Anesth.* 2019;37:16–28.

146. Ngan Kee WD, Khaw KS, Lee BB, et al. A dose-response study of prophylactic intravenous ephedrine for the prevention of hypotension during spinal anesthesia for cesarean delivery. *Anesth Analg.* 2000;90:1390–1395.

147. Alahuhta S, Räsänen J, Jouppila P, et al. Ephedrine and phenylephrine for avoiding maternal hypotension due to spinal anaesthesia for caesarean section. Effects on uteroplacental and fetal haemodynamics. *Int J Obstet Anesth.* 1992;1:129–134.

148. Ngan Kee WD, Lau TK, Khaw KS, Lee BB. Comparison of metaraminol and ephedrine infusions for maintaining arterial pressure during spinal anesthesia for elective cesarean section. *Anesthesiology.* 2001;95:307–313.

149. Greiss FC Jr. Differential reactivity of the myoendometrial and placental vasculatures: adrenergic responses. *Am J Obstet Gynecol.* 1972;112:20–30.

150. Ngan Kee WD, Khaw KS, Tan PE, et al. Placental transfer and fetal metabolic effects of phenylephrine and ephedrine during spinal anesthesia for cesarean delivery. *Anesthesiology.* 2009;111:506–512.

151. Fishburne JI Jr, Dormer KJ, Payne GG, et al. Effects of amrinone and dopamine on uterine blood flow and vascular responses in the gravid baboon. *Am J Obstet Gynecol.* 1988;158:829–837.

152. Santos AC, Baumann AL, Wlody D, et al. The maternal and fetal effects of milrinone and dopamine in normotensive pregnant ewes. *Am J Obstet Gynecol.* 1992;166:257–262.

153. Grunewald C, Nisell H, Jansson T, et al. Possible improvement in uteroplacental blood flow during atrial natriuretic peptide infusion in preeclampsia. *Obstet Gynecol.* 1994;84:235–239.

154. Magness RR, Rosenfeld CR, Carr BR. Protein kinase C in uterine and systemic arteries during ovarian cycle and pregnancy. *Am J Physiol.* 1991;260:E464–E470.

155. Ajne G, Nisell H, Wolff K, Jansson T. The role of endogenous endothelin in the regulation of uteroplacental and renal blood flow during pregnancy in conscious rats. *Placenta.* 2003;24:813–818.

156. Jauniaux E, Johnson MR, Jurkovic D, et al. The role of relaxin in the development of the uteroplacental circulation in early pregnancy. *Obstet Gynecol.* 1994;84:338–342.

157. Braun EB, Palin CA, Hogue CW. Vasopressin during spinal anesthesia in a patient with primary pulmonary hypertension treated with intravenous epoprostenol. *Anesth Analg.* 2004;99:36–37.

158. Magness RR, Mitchell MD, Rosenfeld CR. Uteroplacental production of eicosanoids in ovine pregnancy. *Prostaglandins.* 1990;39:75–88.

159. Magness RR, Rosenfeld CR, Hassan A, Shaul PW. Endothelial vasodilator production by uterine and systemic arteries. I. Effects of ANG II on PGI2 and NO in pregnancy. *Am J Physiol.* 1996;270:H1914–H1923.

160. Katz M, Creasy RK. Uterine blood flow distribution after indomethacin infusion in the pregnant rabbit. *Am J Obstet Gynecol.* 1981;140:430–434.

161. Gerber JG, Branch RA, Hubbard WC, Nies AS. Indomethacin is a placental vasodilator in the dog. The effect of prostaglandin inhibition. *J Clin Invest.* 1978;62:14–19.

162. Mari G, Kirshon B, Wasserstrum N, et al. Uterine blood flow velocity waveforms in pregnant women during indomethacin therapy. *Obstet Gynecol.* 1990;76:33–36.

163. Moise KJ, Mari G, Kirshon B, et al. The effect of indomethacin on the pulsatility index of the umbilical artery in human fetuses. *Am J Obstet Gynecol.* 1990;162:199–202.

164. Thuring A, Malcus P, Maršál K. Effect of maternal betamethasone on fetal and uteroplacental blood flow velocity waveforms. *Ultrasound Obstet Gynecol.* 2011;37:668–672.

165. Edwards A, Baker LS, Wallace EM. Changes in fetoplacental vessel flow velocity waveforms following maternal administration of betamethasone. *Ultrasound Obstet Gynecol.* 2002;20:240–244.

166. Ekin A, Gezer C, Solmaz U, et al. Effect of antenatal betamethasone administration on Doppler velocimetry of fetal and uteroplacental vessels: a prospective study. *J Perinat Med.* 2016;44:243–248.

167. Raghuraman N, Temming LA, Doering MM, et al. Maternal oxygen supplementation compared with room air for intrauterine resuscitation: a systematic review and meta-analysis. *JAMA Pediatr.* 2021;175:368–376.

168. Vincent RD Jr, Chestnut DH, Sipes SL, et al. Magnesium sulfate decreases maternal blood pressure but not uterine blood flow during epidural anesthesia in gravid ewes. *Anesthesiology.* 1991;74:77–82.

169. Dandavino A, Woods JR Jr, Murayama K, et al. Circulatory effects of magnesium sulfate in normotensive and renal hypertensive pregnant sheep. *Am J Obstet Gynecol.* 1977;127:769–774.

170. Keeley MM, Wade RV, Laurent SL, Hamann VD. Alterations in maternal-fetal Doppler flow velocity waveforms in preterm labor patients undergoing magnesium sulfate tocolysis. *Obstet Gynecol.* 1993;81:191–194.

171. Souza AS, Amorim MM, Coutinho IC, et al. Effect of the loading dose of magnesium sulfate (MgSO4) on the parameters of Doppler flow velocity in the uterine, umbilical and middle cerebral arteries in severe preeclampsia. *Hypertens Pregnancy.* 2010;29:123–134.

172. Watkins VY, Martin S, Macones GA, et al. The duration of intrapartum supplemental oxygen administration and umbilical cord oxygen content. *Am J Obstet Gynecol.* 2020;223:440.e1–e7.

173. American College of Obstetricians and Gynecologists. Practice Advisory: Oxygen supplementation in the setting of category II or III fetal heart tracings. https://www.acog.org/clinical/clinical-guidance/practice-advisory/articles/2022/01/oxygen-supplementation-in-the-setting-of-category-ii-or-iii-fetal-heart-tracings. Accessed June 11, 2025.

174. Burd J, Raghuraman N. Intrapartum oxygen for fetal resuscitation: state of the science. *Curr Obstet Gynecol Rep.* 2023;2:173–177.

4

The Placenta: Anatomy, Physiology, Transfer of Drugs, and Pathology

Mai He, MD, PhD, D. Michael Nelson, MD, PhD, and Sara Eyal, PhD

PLACENTAL PATHOLOGY

The human chorioallantoic placenta is at the maternal-fetal interface during pregnancy and is positioned to receive all drugs provided by the obstetric anesthesia provider in the course of supporting pregnant women. No longer considered a passive conduit for bilateral exchange, the placenta is a dynamic organ that performs critical functions in the immunologic, metabolic, nutritional, and hormonal maintenance of pregnancy. Placental dysfunction results in maladies with short- and long-term effects on both the mother and the fetus during pregnancy, into adulthood, and even into subsequent generations.[1,2] This chapter describes the anatomy, pathology, physiology, and pharmacology of the placenta, with attention to key aspects of importance to the obstetric anesthesia provider.

ANATOMY

Embryology

The fertilized egg, or zygote, undergoes cell divisions in the first week after conception, yielding a morula and then a blastocyst that implants interstitially within the endometrium of pregnancy, the decidua, about 9 days after conception. Importantly, the placenta and the conceptus develop within a $PO_2 < 15$ mm Hg (2.0 kPa) during the first 8 to 10 weeks, receiving nutrition from extracellular secretions of the endometrium and uterine glands called histiotroph.[3] During this early development, a developed blood circulation system does not exist, and premature oxygenation at the implantation site causes greater oxidative stress with placental maldevelopment ensuing in some pregnancies. From 10 to 12 weeks' gestation, perfusion of maternal blood into the intervillous space evolves to bathe the villous tree, allowing the maternal and fetal circulations to develop in close apposition, but without substantial interchange of maternal and fetal blood. This allows the physiologic transfer of gases, nutrients, and waste from 10 weeks' gestation until term in normal pregnancy.

A composite organ composed of uterine tissues (maternal contribution) and extraembryonic membranes (i.e., amnion, alloantois, chorion, and yolk sac; embryonic contribution), the human chorioallantoic placenta performs most of the functions of the newborn lungs, liver, intestines, kidneys, and endocrine glands.[4] As a consequence, although often simplistically referred to as affecting villous development and exchange or maternal-fetal circulation, placental maldevelopment and pathology can have significant implications. Maternal maladies that commonly affect the placenta are infection and inflammatory disorders.

Between 10 and 12 weeks' gestation, the branching villi contain fetal vessels enmeshed within a connective tissue core and delimited by a basement membrane on which rests a trophoblast bilayer: cytotrophoblasts, which form a continuous epithelium supporting syncytiotrophoblasts, which are a linear mass of nuclei.[4] The nuclei are bathed in maternal blood derived from openings in decidual spiral arterioles that perfuse the intervillous space. The branching villous tree increases surface area for exchange, and anchoring villi adhere the placenta to the uterine wall.[4]

Placental development is regulated by a complex interplay of genetic and environmental factors. Some key genes involved in the regulation of placental development include **Hox genes**, **IGFs** (insulin-like growth factors), **VEGF** (vascular endothelial growth factor), **HOXA10**, **FGFs** (fibroblast growth factors), and **HIFs** (hypoxia-inducible factors).[5] Epigenetic regulation changes gene expression without altering DNA sequences, and includes DNA methylation, histone modifications, noncoding

RNA, and environmental factors such as maternal diet, exposure to toxins, and stress. Emerging evidence supports the hypothesis of the developmental origins of health and disease, which states that individual developmental programming occurs via fine-tuning of fetal genetic and epigenetic traits *in utero* in response to a variety of stressors during pregnancy.[6] Indeed, the etiology of fetal growth restriction is multifactorial, encompassing fetal, maternal, and placental factors, with maladaptation of the placenta being the most common cause. Such placental dysfunction results in long-term, variable, adverse effects on both the offspring and the mother.

Anatomy, Vascular Architecture, and Histology

The human placenta is a disc-like structure attached to the maternal endometrium at the basal plate on one side with the opposite side having a fetal-facing surface, or chorionic plate, where the umbilical cord connects the fetus to the placenta (Fig. 4.1A). The basal plate of the delivered placenta exhibits indentations in the tissue demarcating cotyledons. Larger fetal chorionic vessels progressively branch into primary and secondary stem villi with smaller venules and arteries to create the fetal circulation. The maternal surface or basal plate serves as the insertion site of the anchoring villi within the decidua. Composed of connective tissue and blood vessels from the uterine wall and the umbilical cord, the chorionic

plate is covered by a single layer of amnion cells, or amniotic membrane, which secretes amniotic fluid. Amniotic fluid serves as a cushion for the fetus and as a means for exchange between the mother and fetus (see Fig. 4.1B).

Important features of placental anatomy are summarized in Box 4.1.

BOX 4.1   Pearls for Placental Anatomy

- **Chorionic plate:** The fetal side of the placenta rich in blood vessels that forms the umbilical cord.
- **Decidua basalis:** The maternal side of the placenta attached at the decidua, or endometrium, with decidual cells, which are modified endometrial cells, and remodeled spiral arterioles.
- **Intervillous space:** The area between the chorionic plate and decidua basalis where maternal blood circulates and exchange of nutrients, oxygen, and waste products occurs.
- **Chorionic villi:** Treelike projections on the chorionic plate that increase the surface area for exchange.
- **Trophoblastic shell:** The outer layer of the chorionic villi, adjacent to the decidua and consisting of both syncytiotrophoblast and cytotrophoblasts.
- **Umbilical cord:** Connects the fetus to the placenta, composed of two arteries and one vein.

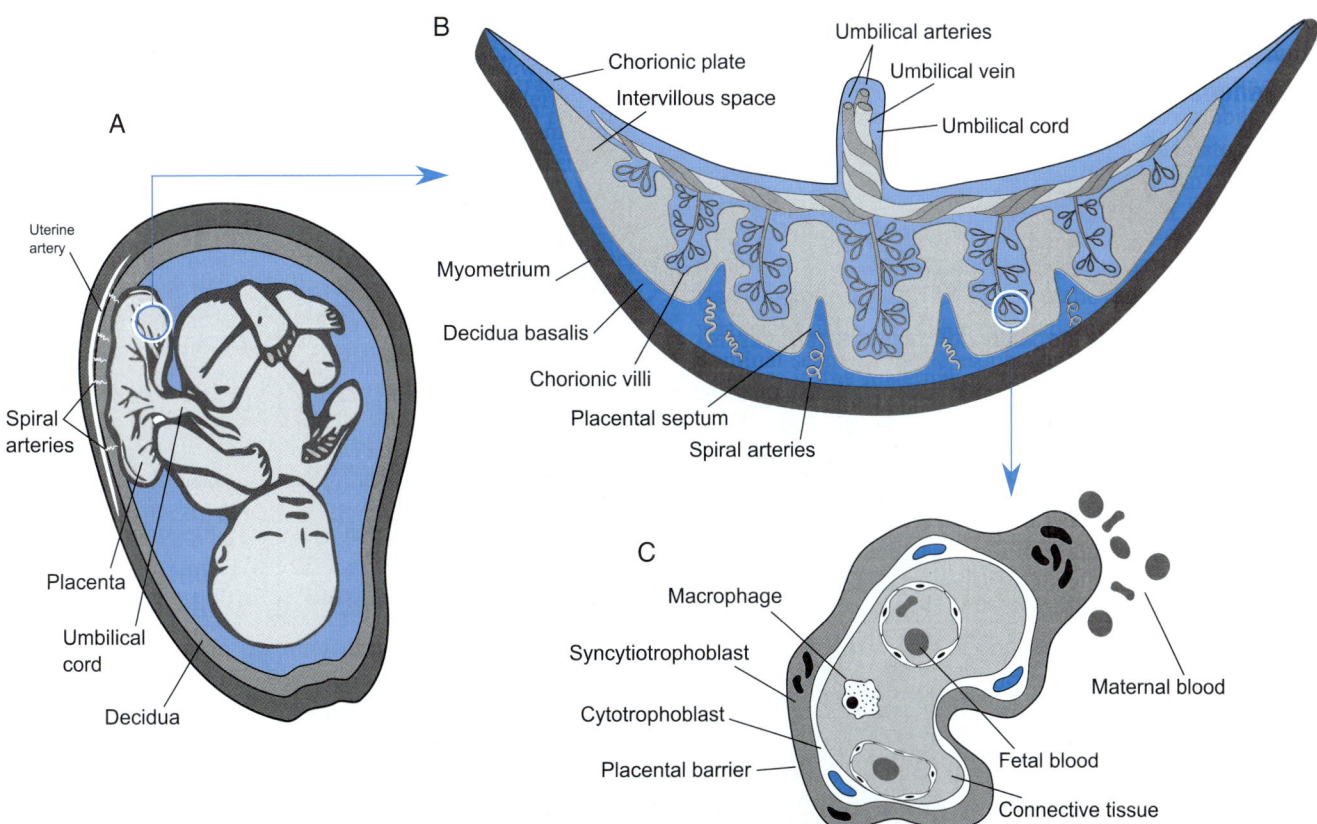

Fig. 4.1 Schematic Depiction of Anatomical Structures of the Human Placenta. (A) The placenta is an important organ for maternal-fetal physiologic exchange and attaches to the uterine wall. (B) Anatomical structure and composition of the human placenta. The umbilical vein transports oxygen and nutrient-rich blood from the placenta to fetus, while two umbilical arteries carry waste products from the fetus to the placenta. The intervillous space is filled with maternal blood, which enters through remodeled spiral arteries. (C) The major cell types and the placental barrier, consisting of syncytiotrophoblasts, cytotrophoblasts, and fetal endothelial cells. From Zhang B, Liang R, Zheng M, et al. Surface-functionalized nanoparticles as efficient tools in targeted therapy of pregnancy complications. *Int J Mol Sci.* 2019;20:3642.

Maternal Circulation

Under the initial hormonal influences of the corpus luteum, the uterine spiral arteries elongate and coil. Erosion of the decidua induces lateral looping of the already convoluted spiral arteries.[7] In late pregnancy, approximately 200 spiral arteries can supply approximately 600 mL/min of blood flow directly to the fetus through the placenta.[7] The vasodilation required to accommodate the increased flow is accomplished through wall replacement by cytotrophoblasts, which incorporate into the arterial wall and replace the elastic and muscular components with an extracellular matrix called the fibrinoid. Tightly coiled spiral arteries are thus transformed into distensible, thin-walled vessels that allow continuous blood supply in the placenta; vessel diameter increases up to 10-fold, while blood velocity and blood pressure decrease.[7] This physiologic conversion is a feature of all normal pregnancies. By contrast, if high blood velocity via nondilated spiral arteries persists, damage to the endothelium and endovascular trophoblast occurs, resulting in relative ischemia and the development of preeclampsia and fetal growth restriction.[8]

The intervillous space is a cavernous expanse that develops from the fusion of the trophoblastic lacunae and the erosion of the decidua by the expanding blastocyst. Folds in the basal plate form septae that divide the space into 13 to 30 anatomic compartments or lobules. Each lobule contains numerous villous trees, which are also known as **cotyledons** or **placentomes**. The intervillous space of the mature placenta can accommodate 350 mL of maternal blood.

Maternal arterial blood leaves the funnel-shaped spiral arteries and enters the intervillous space. The blood moves into the low-resistance area, where villi are loosely arranged within the intercotyledonary space before entering a region of densely packed intermediate and terminal villi where placental exchange predominates (Fig. 4.2).[9] Maternal venous blood collects between neighboring villous trees in an area called the perilobular zone. Collecting veins penetrate the maternal basal plate at the periphery of the villous trees to drain perilobular blood from the intervillous space.

Fetal Circulation

Two coiled umbilical arteries deliver fetal blood to the placenta and subsequently divide into chorionic arteries traversing the chorionic plate to supply the 50 villous trees located among placental lobules. At the base of each villous tree within the chorionic plate, the chorionic arteries are the main villous stem or truncal arteries as first-order vessels, which in turn branch into four to eight cotyledonary arteries as second-order vessels; as they pass toward the maternal basal plate, they further subdivide into ramulus chorii as third-order vessels and finally, terminal arterioles. The terminal arterioles lead through a neck region into a bulbous enlargement, where they form two to four narrow capillary loops. Here the large endothelial surface area and the near-absence

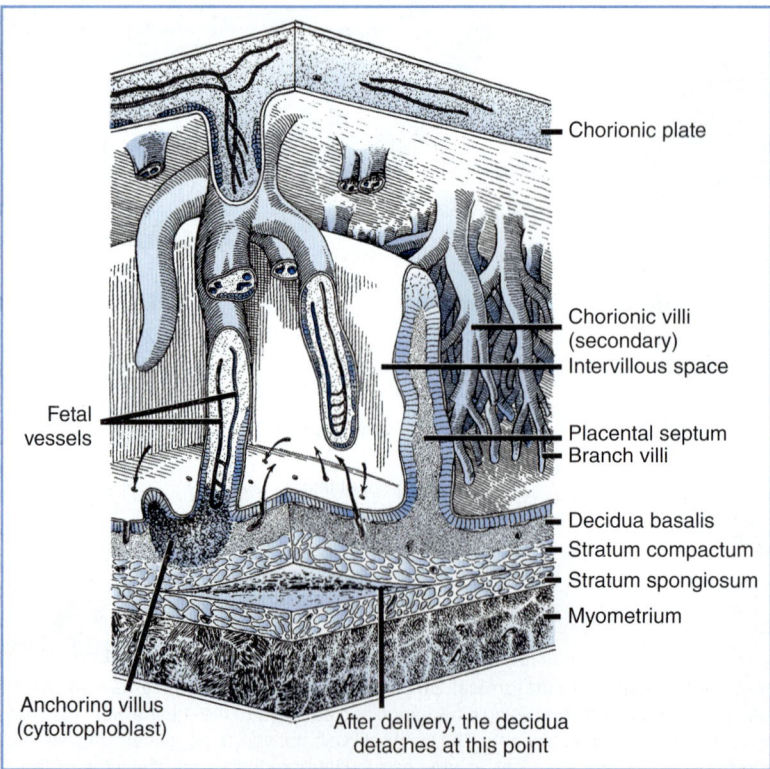

Fig. 4.2 **The Relationship Between the Villous Tree and Maternal Blood Flow.** *Arrows* indicate the maternal blood flow from the spiral arteries into the intervillous space and out through the spiral veins. Modified from Tuchmann-Duplessis H, David G, Haegel P. *Illustrated Human Embryology. Volume 1. Embryogenesis.* Springer Verlag; 1972:73.

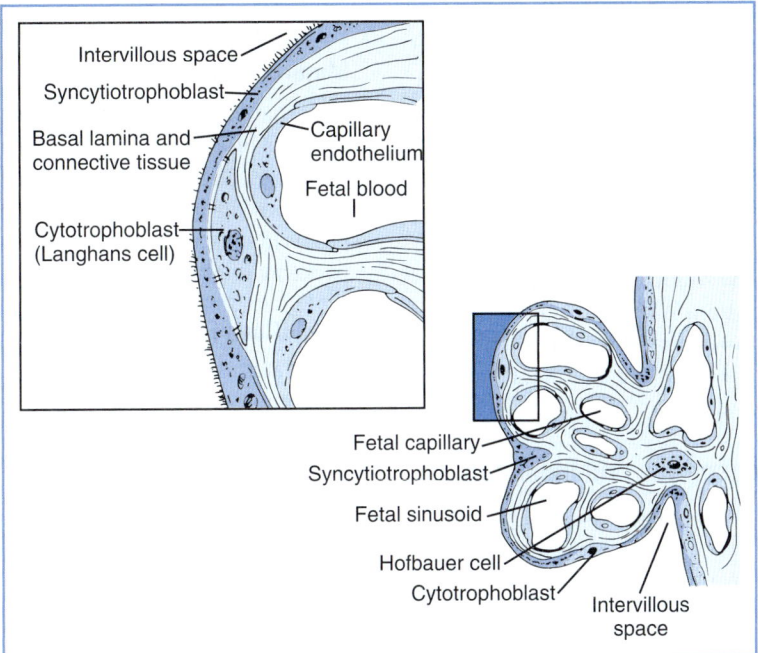

Fig. 4.3 Structure and Cellular Components of Terminal Villi. Right, Cellular morphology of two terminal villi. Left, higher magnification of the boxed region exhibiting the placental barrier between fetal and maternal blood. Modified from Kaufmann P. Basic morphology of the fetal and maternal circuits in the human placenta. *Contrib Gynecol Obstet.* 1985;13:5–17.

of connective tissue allow optimal maternal-fetal exchange (Fig. 4.3).[10]

The venous end of the capillary loops narrows and returns through the neck region to the collecting venules, which coalesce to form the larger veins in the stem of the villous trees as they perforate the chorionic plate to become chorionic veins. The venous tributaries combine to empty into the one umbilical vein that delivers oxygenated blood back to the fetus.

Chorionic Villi

The main component of the placental parenchyma is the chorionic villus. By the end of pregnancy, five types of villi comprise the placenta (see below). From the mesenchymal villi and immature intermediate villi, about 3 to 5 mature intermediate villi grow from the stem villous, and 10 to 12 branches of the terminal villi grow from the mature intermediate villi. These villi help communication between the chorionic plate and decidua. Most of the villi float freely in the intervillous space maternal blood while anchoring villi attach to the decidua for structural stability of the placenta.

Mesenchymal villi play a significant role early in the first trimester as the most primitive type of villi. The villi are mostly filled with mesenchymal cells that will later differentiate into myofibroblasts, fibroblasts, smooth muscle cells, endothelial cells, blood cells, and macrophages (see Fig. 4.1C).

Immature intermediate villi are prevalent in the mid-first trimester. These reticular structures contain fluid as well as macrophages called **Hofbauer cells**. Small arterioles and venules develop within the stroma.

Stem villi appear condensed with collagen fibers during the mid-first trimester. Additionally, there are fibroblasts and macrophages as well as muscularized arteries and veins, which define this type of villi.

Mature intermediate villi in mid-gestation are bundles of connective tissue with numerous peripheral capillaries, as well as some small terminal arterioles and collecting venules.

Terminal villi mainly evolve late in the second trimester through the third trimester. These villi have no stroma and predominantly contain sinusoidal capillaries.

Maternal-Fetal Interface

Villous maturation develops to reduce the distance between the maternal blood and fetal vessels to enhance maternal-fetal exchanges. The primary site of maternal-fetal exchange is the villous surface, especially at **vascular syncytial membranes** (**VSMs**; see Fig. 4.3), which are thinner areas of the placental villous membrane where the maternal and fetal circulations are separated by as little as 1 to 2 μm.[11] Increased VSM thickness, as witnessed in mothers with diabetes, predisposes to fetal hypoxia.

PHYSIOLOGY

The placenta exchanges molecules, including oxygen, nutrients, hormones, and waste, between the maternal and fetal circulations by passive diffusion and active transport. Moreover, the placenta performs a number of functions that are later assumed by the lungs, liver, gut, kidneys and endocrine glands, including secretion of immunologic factors for fetal protection, and hormones that influence both maternal and fetal metabolism.[4]

Maternal Recognition of Pregnancy

Human chorionic gonadotropin (hCG) is synthesized and released from the syncytiotrophoblast to stimulate luteal progesterone production needed to sustain pregnancy until 8 weeks' gestation, when the villous trophoblast assumes ongoing progesterone production. Without hCG production, progesterone from the corpus luteum diminishes and menstruation occurs with detachment of the endometrium containing the implanted blastocyst.[12]

Fetal Protection From Infectious and Immunologic Attack

The placenta tolerates the foreign antigens presented by the fetus and at the same time provides defense against numerous infections. The fetus inherits both maternal and paternal antigens and thus is an allograft that enjoys immune privileges that minimize the risk of rejection by the maternal immune system. The mechanisms of maternal tolerance to foreign fetal antigens are poorly understood. Potential mediator mechanisms include the modulation of leukocytes penetrating the maternal-fetal interface, functional alteration of leukocytes through decidual intercellular communication, human leukocyte antigen G expression, unique decidual natural killer cell (dNK) differentiation and recruitment to the implantation site, and apoptosis, among many others.[13,14]

The placenta also protects against microbial infection. Hofbauer cells in the stroma of the chorionic villi and the syncytial nature of the syncytiotrophoblast layer play critical roles in this protection of the fetus. Importantly, many leukocytes are located in the decidua of the implantation site to support a successful pregnancy, including dNK cells, decidual macrophages, and regulatory T (Treg) cells. Moreover, the placenta secretes antiviral molecules that limit viral infections and actively transport antibodies that protect the fetus via the expression of immunoglobulin G receptors on the surface of the syncytiotrophoblastic layer.[15,16]

Hormonal Function

Sophisticated transfer of substrate cholesterol and intermediate compounds in the maternal-fetal-placental unit allows placental enzymes to convert steroid precursors into estrogen and progesterone. This steroidogenic function of the placenta begins 35 to 47 days after ovulation, and the placental production of estrogen and progesterone ultimately exceeds that of the corpus luteum.[17] The placenta also produces and stores a wide array of enzymes, binding proteins, and polypeptide hormones. For example, the placenta produces not only hCG but also **human placental lactogen**, a growth hormone also known as human chorionic somatomammotropin, and factors that control hypothalamic function.[17] Production of protein and steroid hormones allows the placenta to influence and control the fetal environment.[18]

Regulation of Placental Blood Flow

Maternal Blood Flow

Maternal blood enters the intervillous cotyledon space at a pressure of 70 to 80 mm Hg in areas of the intervillous space that have relatively few villi. The pressure rapidly diminishes to 10 mm Hg and the velocity of blood flow decreases as blood passes into an area of higher resistance, created by the densely packed villi of the placentome.[19]

Fetal Blood Flow

The maternoplacental circulation relies on anatomical modifications of spiral arterioles to increase flow, while the increase in fetoplacental blood flow is primarily caused by vascular growth. Fetal perfusion of the placenta is not autoregulated and the placental vasculature is not innervated by the sympathetic nervous system. However, the fetus can modulate fetoplacental perfusion via (1) adrenomedullin release by the fetal adrenal glands, which maintains vascular tone; (2) net efflux and influx of water regulated by fetal blood pressure; and (3) local autoregulatory effects mediated by the paracrine vasodilators **nitric oxide** and **acetylcholine**.[20,21] Fetal blood pressure changes cause net influx and efflux of water across the placenta to affect fetal intravascular volume and perfusion. Maternal hyperglycemia and hypoxemia can alter regional fetal blood flow.[22] Endothelium-derived relaxing factors, especially **prostacyclin** and nitric oxide, are important in the control of the fetoplacental circulation.[23,24] Hypoxia-induced fetoplacental vasoconstriction is mediated by a reduction in the basal release of nitric oxide.[25] This vasoconstrictor activity is functionally similar to that found with hypoxic pulmonary vasoconstriction in the lung and allows optimal fetal oxygenation through redistribution of fetal blood flow to better-perfused lobules.[26] The placental vasculature constricts in response to graded hypoxia and may be more dependent on angiotensin II than catecholamines.[27]

Barrier Function

The fetus is sequestered in a unique microenvironment, generally independent of maternal sex or stress hormones and most environmental pollutants. This allows unimpaired development of the neuroendocrine and gonadal systems. The VSM of terminal villi is the thinnest and strictest physical barrier between fetal and maternal blood, consisting of endothelial cells of villous fetal capillaries, basement membranes of endothelium and trophoblast, and the villous trophoblast bilayer (see Fig. 4.3). However, the placenta is an incomplete barrier that permits bidirectional transfer of many substances. The transfer rate depends on the permeability of the substances across the VSM and the mechanisms (e.g., transporters) that restrict molecular movement; the syncytiotrophoblast expresses abundant transporters that are frequently the rate-limiting step for molecules crossing the placenta. Indeed, many substances undergo specific or nonspecific binding, metabolism, or sequestration within the placental tissues, thereby minimizing fetal exposure and accumulation; other substances are altered by the vast array of inducible and constitutive cytochrome P450 isoenzymes and transporters. Villous branching increases and villous diameters decrease, influencing the rate of diffusion.[19]

Transfer Functions/Transport Mechanisms

The placenta facilitates the transfer of oxygen from the mother to the fetus and the removal of carbon dioxide from the fetus to the mother. The placenta also acts as a filter, removing waste products from the fetus and excreting them into the maternal bloodstream for elimination. While the placenta acts somewhat as a barrier between the mother's bloodstream and the fetus, most drugs and chemicals can cross this barrier at variable concentrations to reach the fetus.[28]

Maternal and fetal blood can exchange cellular components by active adhesion and transmigration or as a result of disruption of the trophoblastic layer.[29] Fetal cells may be pluripotent and their DNA can be found in maternal organs for decades. These microchimeric fetal cells may contribute to maternal immunomodulation, development or worsening of autoimmune diseases (e.g., **thyroiditis**, **lupus**, **scleroderma**, and **asthma**), and healing of wounds, including neuronal tissue.[30]

The placenta releases extracellular vesicles of various sizes and functions. Macrovesicles from the syncytiotrophoblast (20 to 500 μm) carry fetal protein, RNA, and other substances; microvesicles from membranes of stressed or apoptotic cells (0.1 to 1 μm) and exosomes (20 to 100 nm) contribute to fetal-maternal communication.[31] Placental exosomes, nanovesicles 30 to 100 nm in size found in maternal circulation that contain proteins and transcription-related materials, exert a maternal immunosuppressive effect. Placental microparticles, which are vesicular products of syncytiotrophoblast larger than 100 nm, also contain RNA and DNA fragments and affect fetal and maternal apoptosis, angiogenesis, and inflammation. Syncytial nuclei from the placental villous tree also enter the maternal circulation, reside in maternal lungs, participate in maternal-fetal signaling, and assist in the delivery of retroviral proteins for immunomodulation.[32] Of interest, an excess of microparticles has been observed in early-onset preeclampsia.[33]

Substances are transferred across the placenta by several mechanisms via paracellular and transcellular pathways. Transcellular transport is the only route available for active transport, which involves carrier-mediated transport, endocytosis, and exocytosis (Fig. 4.4).[34]

Paracellular Transport

Paracellular transport refers to transport that occurs between cells and involves solute passage through intercellular shunt pathways described as placental channels. As the syncytiotrophoblast presents a contiguous surface membrane without lateral cell borders, the etiology of the paracellular route for passive diffusive transport is debated. Brownbill et al.[35] reported that channels proposed to be passage pathways within the syncytiotrophoblast were not apparent morphologically, but denudations of the surfacing trophoblast, some secondary to apoptosis, provided a functional passage available for diffusive transport. Placental channels allow nanoparticles smaller than 50 nm to cross the placenta via paracellular transport, based on the diffusion coefficient in water. Enhanced passage of substances was observed when placental structure and function were damaged by inflammation. Paracellular transport appears to be exclusively passive and downhill, occurring by diffusion or convection, and is driven by existing transepithelial gradients. For example, the paracellular route is the major urate transport pathway across the blood-placental barrier.[36]

Transcellular Transport

Transcellular transport occurs through cells, routed sequentially through membranes and the intervening cytoplasm. It occurs through the lipid membrane (e.g., lipophilic molecules and water) or within protein channels that traverse the lipid bilayer (e.g., charged substances such as ions).[37] There are two main ways that water can cross cell membranes: (1) simple diffusion through the lipid bilayer or transit through water-selective channels and (2) facilitated diffusion. The passive transfer of solutes across a membrane depends on (1) concentration and electrochemical differences across the membrane, which drive diffusion; (2) molecular weight; (3) lipid solubility; (4) degree of ionization; and (5) membrane surface area and thickness. Passive diffusion is a key mechanism for the transplacental transfer of lipophilic drugs with a molecular weight < 600 Daltons.[38]

Carrier-Mediated Transport

Carriers can mediate the transport of relatively lipid-insoluble molecules down their concentration gradient. Specifically, this mode of transfer exhibits (1) competitive and noncompetitive inhibition, (2) stereospecificity, (3) temperature influences, and (4) saturation kinetics. The latter characteristic is derived from the limited amount of membranous carrier protein complexes and the extent of interaction between the carrier and the substance undergoing transport. At high solute concentrations, a maximum rate of transfer is reached; thereafter, further increases in the concentration gradient do not affect the rate of transfer.[37]

Carriers can facilitate the membrane transfer of substrates down concentration gradients (facilitated diffusion) or against them (active transport). Examples of facilitated diffusion and active transport are the transplacental transfer of **glucose** and removal of **doxorubicin** from the placenta to maternal blood, respectively.

Placental carrier proteins can be generally divided into two major transporter superfamilies: **ABC (adenosine triphosphate binding cassette)** and **SLC (solute carrier)** transporters. Under most circumstances, SLC transporters mediate facilitated diffusion, whereas ABC transporters are involved in active transport. However, exceptions to this classification have been demonstrated.

Transporters of the Solute Carrier Superfamily

Placental SLCs mediate the transfer of hormones, nutrients, medications, and other exogenous compounds into and out of trophoblast cells and across the fetal capillaries. Examples

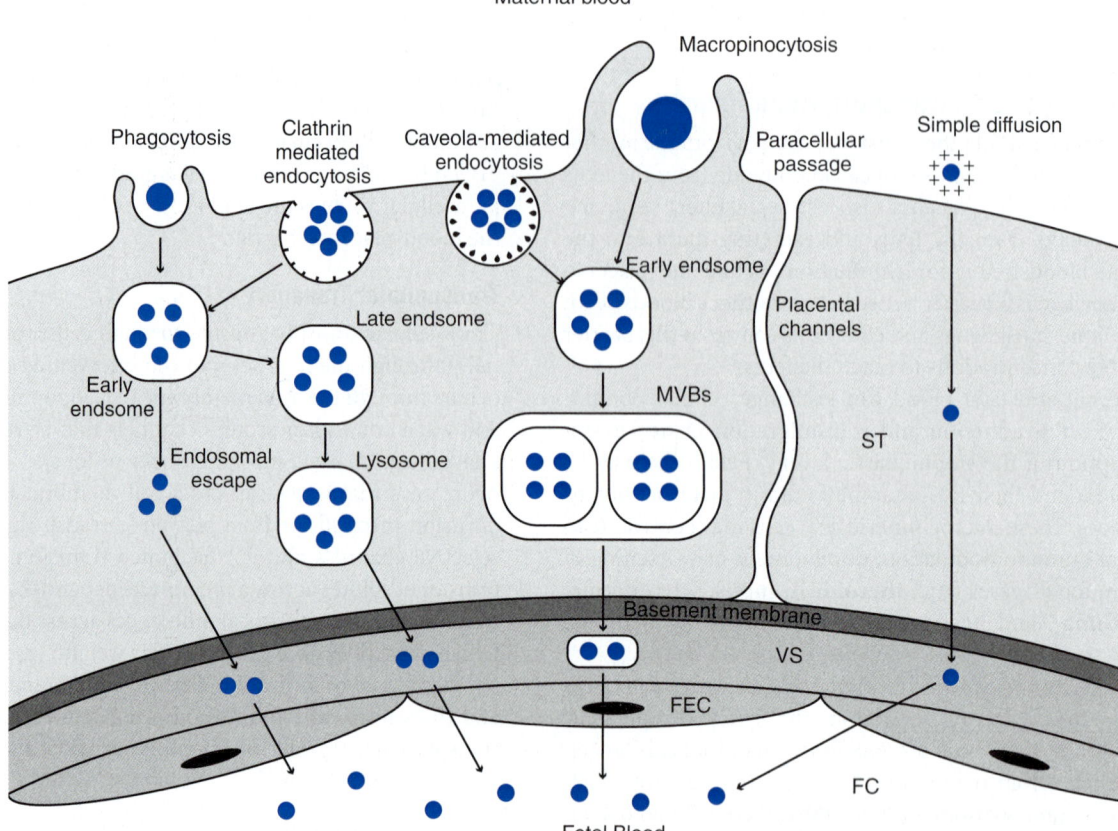

Fig. 4.4 Scheme Showing the Nanoparticle Transplacental Transport Mechanisms. Nanoparticles cross the placental barrier by paracellular passage and transcellular passage. The paracellular passage includes passive diffusion and carrier-mediated transport. Very small nanoparticles can penetrate syncytiotrophoblasts (*STs*) via placental channels and thereby enter the villous stroma (*VS*). Diffusion may then occur through the fetal endothelial cells (*FECs*) into the lumen of the fetal capillaries (*FCs*). The transcellular passage consists of endocytosis and exocytosis. Nanoparticles may be taken up by syncytiotrophoblasts via phagocytosis, clathrin-mediated endocytosis, caveolae-mediated endocytosis, and macropinocytosis, then they may be exocytosed through the endosomal escape pathway, lysosomal secretion, and multivesicular bodies (*MVBs*)–related secretion. After entering the VS, nanoparticles may cross the FEC by the same pathway and eventually enter into the fetal blood. Some cationic nanoparticles may be able to directly fuse the negatively charged trophoblast cell membrane and move toward the basal membrane by simple diffusion, thereby diffusing through the FECs into the fetal blood. From Zhang B, Liang R, Zheng M, et al. Surface-functionalized nanoparticles as efficient tools in targeted therapy of pregnancy complications. *Int J Mol Sci.* 2019;20:3642.

include organic anion transporting polypeptides, organic anion and cation transporters, monoamine transporters, and glucose and folate carriers. A nutrient or a drug may be transported across the placenta by several distinct transport mechanisms.

Cotransport

A special type of facilitated diffusion involves the uphill transport of a molecule linked to another substance traveling down its own concentration gradient. As such, the transfer is not directly driven by cellular energy expenditure. In most cases, sodium is the molecule that facilitates transport. For the membrane-bound carrier to transfer these molecules, both molecules must be bound to the carrier. This hybrid system is called secondary active transport or cotransport.[37] The transplacental transport of amino acids appears to occur principally through secondary active transport. Transporters

may be affected by disease states (e.g., **preeclampsia**) or signaling molecules (e.g., elevated steroid levels).[39]

Active Transport and Transporters

Active transport involves the movement of a substance across a cell membrane requiring energy from ATP hydrolysis. In general, active transport occurs against a concentration, electrical, or pressure gradient. Active transport also requires a protein membrane carrier that exhibits saturation kinetics and competitive inhibition. The best-known example of primary active ion transport is the translocation of sodium and potassium through the **sodium-potassium adenosine triphosphatase (Na+/K+ ATPase) pump**. Unlike most cell types, the placenta can self-generate creatinine, which assists in regeneration of ATP and meeting the high metabolic energy demands of the placenta.[40]

Placental active transport proteins for small molecules include the ABC transporters P-glycoprotein (P-gp), the breast cancer resistance protein (BCRP), and multidrug resistance proteins, as well as SLC transporters such as the sodium/multivitamin transporter and proteins involved in monoamine transport.[39] P-gp and BCRP are expressed on the microvillous surface membrane of the syncytiotrophoblast and play an important role in protecting the fetus from foreign and potentially teratogenic compounds. They additionally prevent compounds such as protease inhibitors from exerting therapeutic effects on the fetus.[41] Other P-gp substrates include all direct-acting oral anticoagulants (e.g., **dabigatran**), many immunosuppressive and chemotherapeutic agents, and some cardiovascular drugs (e.g., **verapamil**). Inhibition of these transporter proteins (e.g., P-gp inhibition by high-dose **cyclosporine**) can increase the fetal transfer of certain drugs.

Endocytosis and Exocytosis

Endocytosis of solutes by placental trophoblasts can involve pinocytosis and receptor-mediated endocytosis. **Pinocytosis** is an energy-requiring process in which the cell membrane invaginates around large macromolecules that exhibit negligible diffusion properties. Although the contents of pinocytotic vesicles are subject to intracellular digestion, studies have demonstrated that the vesicles can move across the cytoplasm and fuse with the membrane at the opposite pole, thereby potentially transferring certain molecules across the placenta. Receptor-mediated **endocytosis** is the selective internalization of extracellular ligands into cytoplasmic vesicles through their interactions with specific receptors. Examples of such receptors include the folate receptor (FR) alpha and the neonatal Fc receptors that bind IgG or IgG-based antibodies and transfer them from the maternal to the fetal circulation.[42]

Transfer of Respiratory Gases, Nutrients, and Monoamines

Oxygen. The placenta must provide approximately 8 mL O_2/min per kg fetal body weight for optimal fetal growth and development, while adults only require half this amount.[43] As the surrogate lung for the fetus, the placenta has only one-fifth the oxygen transfer efficiency of the adult lung.[44] The human lung has a surface area of 50 to 60 m^2 and a thickness of only 0.5 μm, which offers an abundant oxygen diffusion capacity. In comparison, the placenta has a markedly lower diffusion capacity because the total surface area is only 16 m^2 and the average tissue thickness is 3.5 μm. Furthermore, only 16% of uterine blood flow and 6% of umbilical blood flow are shunted through the placenta.[19]

Oxygen transfer across the placenta depends on the membrane surface area, membrane thickness, oxygen partial pressure gradient between maternal blood and fetal blood, oxygen affinity of maternal and fetal hemoglobin, and relative maternal and fetal blood flows. As physically dissolved oxygen diffuses across the villous membranes, bound oxygen is released by maternal hemoglobin in the intervillous space and diffuses across the villus to enter the fetal circulation and bind to fetal hemoglobin. Several factors affect the fetal blood PO_2 once equilibrium occurs in villous end capillaries. The equilibration of maternal and fetal PO_2 values suggests that a concurrent or parallel relationship exists between maternal and fetal blood within the area of exchange of the human placenta (Fig. 4.5).[19]

In humans, oxygen solubility is 10^{-4} M in plasma and 10^{-2} M in hemoglobin; thus, 99% of the oxygen content in blood is bound to hemoglobin. The maximum maternal arterial PO_2 is 425 mm Hg (56.7 kPa) with an FiO_2 of 100%, but the umbilical venous PO_2 is about 47 mm Hg (6.3 kPa), indicating a low oxygen diffusion capacity across the placenta.[45] The placenta receives less than 50% of the fetal cardiac output, and blood returning from the placenta admixes with the nonoxygenated blood in the fetal inferior vena cava, thus limiting fetal arterial PO_2.

The delivery of oxygen to the fetus is thus predominantly flow-limited, although some describe transfer as diffusion-limited because of the decreased ability of oxygen to cross the interhemal membrane. Maternal delivery of blood to the uterus is thus the predominant factor controlling fetal oxygen transfer. The relatively high fetal hemoglobin concentration of 17 mg/dL accounts for the large oxygen content and the net delivery of large quantities of oxygen to the fetus. Moreover, fetal hemoglobin has a higher oxygen affinity with a P50 (partial pressure when 50% saturated) of 18 mm Hg (2.4 kPa), compared with maternal hemoglobin that has a P50 of 27 mm Hg (3.6 kPa). This gradient produces a sink effect that enhances oxygen uptake by fetal red blood cells, keeping fetal Po_2 lower to promote the transfer of additional oxygen across the placenta. The **Bohr effect** also augments the transfer of oxygen from mother to fetus across the placenta. Specifically, fetal-maternal transfer of carbon dioxide makes maternal blood more acidic and fetal blood more alkalotic. These alterations of pH cause shifts in the maternal and fetal oxyhemoglobin dissociation curves, further enhancing the maternal oxygen transfer to the fetus in what is termed the **double Bohr effect**. Notably, this accounts for 2% to 8% of the transplacental transfer of oxygen.[46]

The placenta normally has a 50% reserve for changes in maternal or fetal blood flow by increasing venous extraction, a mechanism similar to that in adults. Based on umbilical venous-arterial differences, human fetal oxygen uptake at term is 0.25 mmol/kg per minute.[47] The metabolic activity of the placenta itself consumes up to 40% of the oxygen uptake. Placental oxygen consumption is stable, even with changes in maternal blood pressure and Po_2. Thirty percent of oxygen is for protein synthesis and another 30% for Na^+/K^+ ATPase activity. Of interest, the placental microanatomy changes in response to the chronic hypoxia found at high altitudes, with an increased capillary volume and decreased capillary thickness providing a doubling of the oxygen diffusion capacity.[48]

Carbon Dioxide. The transfer of CO_2 occurs through dissolved CO_2, carbonic acid (H_2CO_3), bicarbonate ion (HCO_3^-), carbonate ion (CO_3^{2-}), and carbaminohemoglobin. Equilibrium between CO_2 and HCO_3^- is maintained by a reaction catalyzed by carbonic anhydrase in red blood cells. The

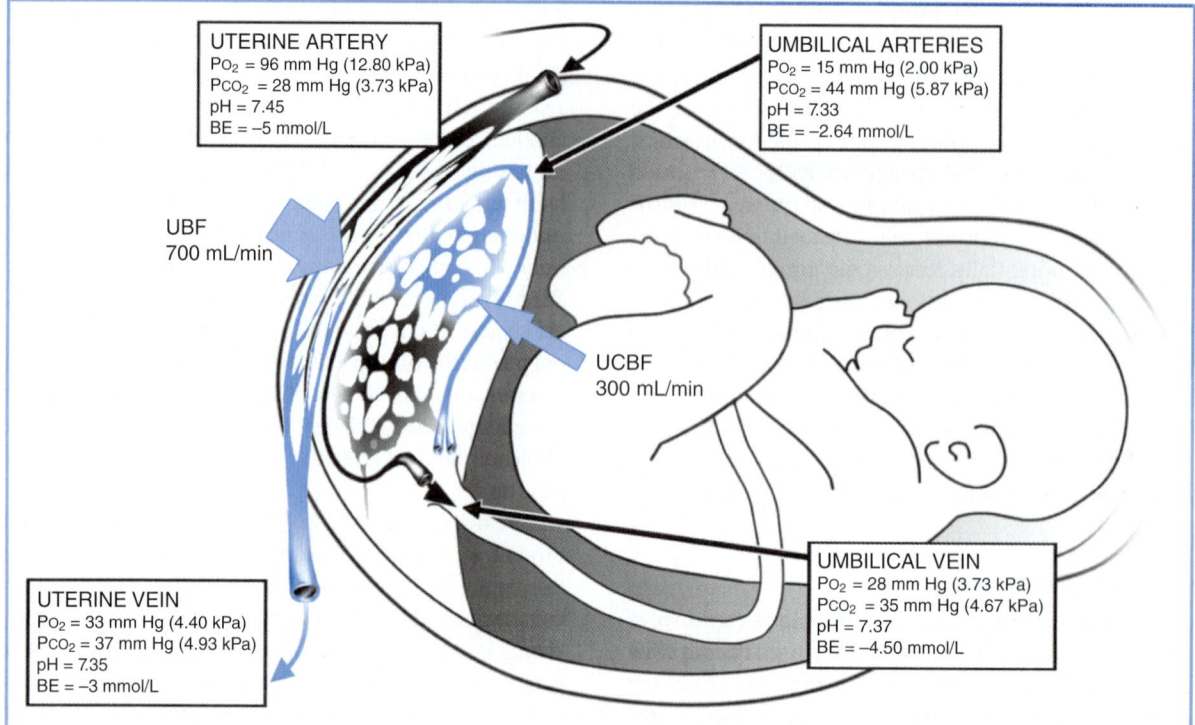

Fig. 4.5 The Concurrent Relationship Between the Maternal and Fetal Circulations Within the Placenta and the Manner in Which This Arrangement Affects Gas Transfer. These values were obtained from patients breathing room air during elective cesarean delivery. *BE*, Base excess; *PO₂*, partial pressure of oxygen; *PCO₂*, partial pressure of carbon dioxide; *UBF*, uterine blood flow; *UCBF*, umbilical cord blood flow. Blood gas data from Ramanathan S. *Obstetric Anesthesia*. Lea & Febiger; 1988:27. Illustration by Naveen Nathan, MD, NorthShore University Health System, University of Chicago Pritzker School of Medicine, Evanston, IL.

PCO_2 gradient between fetal blood (40 mm Hg [5.3 kPa]) and maternal blood (34 mm Hg [4.5 kPa]) drives fetal-maternal transfer. Carbon dioxide is 20 times more diffusible than oxygen, and the rapid movement of CO_2 from fetal capillary to maternal blood invokes a shift in the equilibrium of the carbonic anhydrase reaction, the **La Chatelier principle**, which produces more CO_2 for diffusion.[49] The transfer of CO_2 is augmented further by the **Haldane effect**, the production in the maternal blood of deoxyhemoglobin, which has a higher affinity for CO_2 than oxyhemoglobin. The resulting affinity may account for as much as 46% of the transplacental transfer of carbon dioxide.[42] Although a significant fetal-maternal concentration gradient exists for HCO_3^-, the charged nature of HCO_3^- impedes transfer, except as a source for CO_2 production through the carbonic anhydrase reaction.[50]

Glucose. Placental and fetal glucose demand is fulfilled by a stereospecific-facilitated diffusion system with glucose transporters, such as GLUT1 and GLUT3; the system is independent of insulin, a sodium gradient, or cellular energy.[51] Insulin does not cross the placenta; however, insulin receptors on the maternal side of the syncytiotrophoblast regulate nutrient transport through a signaling cascade involving the mammalian target of rapamycin complex (mTORC). Nutrient sensors for glucose, amino acids, oxygen, cytokines, growth factors, and energy levels stimulate mTORC1, a key sensing and signaling protein in the syncytiotrophoblast that regulates nutrient transport and growth.[52]

Amino Acids. Concentrations of amino acids are highest in the placenta, followed by umbilical venous blood and then maternal blood. The maternal-fetal transplacental transfer of amino acids is an active process that occurs principally through a linked translocation with sodium and facilitated diffusion. Examples of placental amino acid transporters include the L-type amino acid transporters LAT1 and LAT2, as well as sodium-coupled neutral amino acid transporters 1, 2, and 4.[53] Pregnancies with fetal growth restriction have reduced amino acid transport with an inability to increase transport despite higher maternal levels of essential amino acids than occur in healthy pregnancies.[54] Fetal growth restriction and hypoxia increase the breakdown of the amino acid tryptophan, which decreases production of serotonin as a vasodilator.[55]

Fatty Acids. Free fatty acids readily cross the human, but not ovine, placenta. The essential fatty acids, linoleic and alpha-linolenic acid, are transferred across the placenta with a peak of 7 g/day at term. The placental basal membrane has specific binding sites for very low–, medium-, and high-density lipoproteins. Lipase activity in the placenta converts triglycerides to nonessential fatty acids. The placenta does not elongate fatty acid chains, whereas the fetus does. Fatty acid transport occurs primarily by simple diffusion; however, the fatty acid–binding proteins FABPpm, FAT/CD36, and FATP facilitate transport. Nonessential fatty acids are albumin bound and may displace other protein-bound substances, including drugs.[56]

The placenta is a source of fatty acid synthase, which is responsible for straight chain fatty acid catabolism, and this pathway is regulated by ambient insulin levels. Dysregulation of placental fatty acid synthase may contribute to hypertension, insulin resistance, and fetal-placental growth abnormalities.[57]

Folate. Folates are B9 vitamins that are essential for fetal growth and development. Folate supplementation is recommended for women of reproductive age and during at least the first trimester of pregnancy, to reduce the risk of neural tube defects and adverse neurodevelopmental outcomes. Serum folate is almost entirely in the form of 5-methyltetrahydrofolate (5-MTHF). 5-MTHF and other folates are delivered across the placenta to the fetus by the coordinated activity of the reduced folate carrier, the proton-coupled folate transporter, and FRs α and β.[58]

Monoamines. Carriers that transfer monoamines across the placenta include the serotonin transporter, the norepinephrine transporter, the dopamine transporter, and the organic cation transporter 3.[59] In addition to endogenous monoamines, these carriers transfer to the fetus medications and drug of abuse, including amphetamines.[42] Monoamines can additionally accumulate and be metabolized within the placenta.[60] Inhibition of these transporters in the placenta (e.g., by some drugs of abuse) could lead to decreased placental blood flow, intrauterine growth restriction, and preterm delivery.

DRUG TRANSFER ACROSS THE PLACENTA

Drugs can be distributed to the fetus by the same mechanisms that transfer nutrients across the placenta (Fig. 4.6). All drugs that act on the brain cross the placenta because the placental molecular weight "sieve" is less strict than that of the blood-brain barrier (600 versus ~500 Da) and because the placenta contains a wider array of drug carriers.[61]

Transcellular diffusion is the major transfer mechanism for general anesthetic and sedative agents. The best examples of freely diffusible drugs are inhalation agents that yield in most cases equivalent maternal and fetal concentrations (Table 4.1).[42,62] Accordingly, the major factor determining the concentrations of such agents in fetal blood is their concentration in maternal blood.

Large molecules such as **heparins** and hydrophilic drugs are delivered to the fetus poorly. Yet many of these compounds, for example, **quaternary amine neuromuscular blocking agents**, are measurable in the fetal compartment, likely because of carrier-mediated uptake (see Table 4.1). Most drugs used in anesthesia are not good substrates for

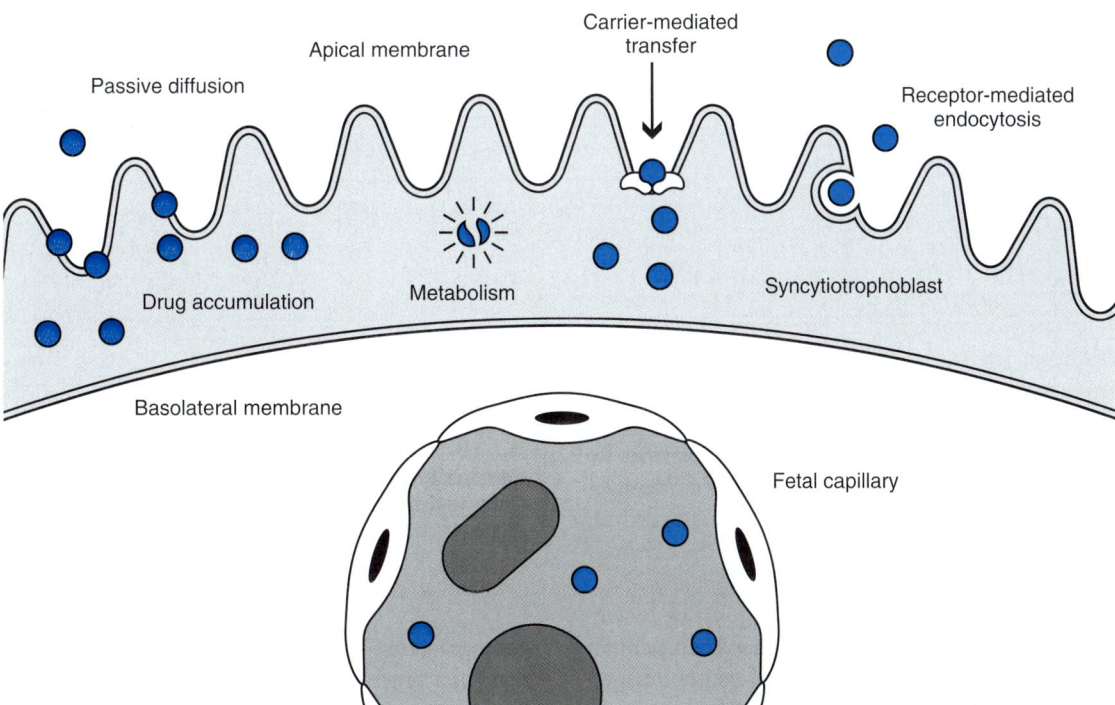

Fig. 4.6 Mechanisms of Drug Transfer Across the Syncytiotrophoblast. Drugs can cross the placenta by passive diffusion, carrier-mediated transfer (facilitated diffusion or active transport), or transcytosis. Within the syncytium, drugs can accumulate or undergo metabolism. Modified from Tetro N, Moushaev S, Rubinchik-Stern M, Eyal S. The placental barrier: the gate and the fate in drug distribution. *Pharm Res.* 2018;35:71.

TABLE 4.1   Examples of Transfer of Anesthetic Agents Across the Placenta

Drug	Cord:Maternal Partition[a]	Comments
Alfentanil[62,64]	0.29–0.35 (total) 0.97 (free)	
Atracurium	0.03–0.33	
Bupivacaine[62,64]	0.24–0.44 (total) 0.77–0.79 (free)	
Dantrolene	0.29–0.69	
Dexmedetomidine[71,72]	0.68 0.77	Cord:maternal ratio Cotyledon perfusion study
Diazepam	1–3	Transferred to the fetus from gestational week 6. At term, rapid distribution across the placenta, with distributional equilibrium 5–10 min after IV administration. Timing of administration with regard to uterine contractions can reduce fetal exposure
Etomidate	0.5	
Fentanyl[62,73]	0.23–0.73	Detectable in amniotic fluid before gestational week 12 but not later, and in fetal blood
Ketamine	0.61–1.03	
Lidocaine (Lignocaine)[62,64]	0.37–0.69 1.32	Given by IV infusion Ratio reported in an acidotic newborn following epidural anesthesia, and in nonacidotic newborns following local infiltration of the perineum
Magnesium sulfate	0.7–1	Prolonged retention in the newborn (days)
Meperidine (pethidine)	0.45–1.06	Detectable in cord blood 2 min after IV administration, in amniotic fluid 30 min after IM administration, and in the saliva of the newborns up to 48 h after IM administration
Methohexital[64,74]	~1 0.83	Rapid transfer A perfusion study; degree of transfer affected by protein binding
Midazolam	0.56–0.74	
Nalbuphine	0.37–1.24	
Nitrous oxide	~1	
Pancuronium[75,76]	0.1–0.4	
Propofol[62,64]	0.2–1.7	
Remifentanil	1–2	Shown to be metabolized by the fetus
Rocuronium	0.16	
Ropivacaine[62,64]	0.28–0.33 (total) 0.66–0.81 (free)	
Sulfentanil[64]	0.38–0.81	
Thiopental (thiopentone)[77,78]	0.43–1.08	
Vecuronium	0.11	

[a]Values are cord:maternal blood ratio of total drug concentration measured at term, and are based on data from Briggs GG, Freeman RK, Towers CV, Forinash AB. *Briggs Drugs in Pregnancy and Lactation: A Reference Guide to Fetal and Neonatal Risk*: Lippincott Williams & Wilkins; 2021, unless indicated otherwise.

efflux transporters, although they may interact with them to some extent.[63] Transcytosis is a major transplacental transfer pathway for **aminoglycosides**, **nanoparticle formulations**, and most **IgG-based therapeutic proteins**.[42]

The free (unbound to plasma proteins) drug concentrations in the maternal and the fetal circulations are usually comparable.[42] However, fetal-to-maternal ratios of the total drug concentrations in plasma can be affected by other factors, such as pH differences and different protein binding in the fetal and the maternal circulations. The fetal blood is slightly more acidic than maternal blood with a pH difference of 0.1, and weakly basic drugs such as **lidocaine** (lignocaine) can become "trapped" in the fetal compartment. The fetal:maternal ratio of α1-acid glycoprotein at term is 0.37, whereas that of albumin is 1.2. Based on these parameters, the fetal:maternal concentration ratio of a drug would be lower than unity if the placenta serves as an effective barrier for the drug (including transporter-mediated drug efflux), the drug is a weak acid, or it binds α1-acid glycoprotein.[42,64] The fetal:maternal ratio can be more than 1.0 for drugs that are weak bases, are transported to the fetus against a concentration gradient, or bind to albumin (at term) or to other fetal targets.[42,65,66]

Other factors that can affect the exposure of the fetus to medications include placental drug metabolism and drug accumulation. Drugs that undergo significant placental metabolism include structural analogues of endogenous compounds such as some **antiviral agents,** as well as **betamethasone, dexamethasone, buprenorphine,** and **methadone.** Placental accumulation has been demonstrated for **aminoglycosides, dexmedetomidine,** and recently also for **cannabinoids.**[42,62,67] Owing to drug accumulation, the placenta may serve as a depot compartment that could slowly release the drug to fetal blood over time.

The rate of transplacental transfer of readily diffusible drugs is largely influenced by the rate of placental blood flow. Flow plays a more minor rule in the placental kinetics of drugs that equilibrate over hours between the maternal and fetal compartments, such as **meperidine (pethidine)** and **cyclosporine.** The fetal accumulation of the latter may be higher upon repeated or continuous administration compared with a single, rapid intravenous bolus. Within the same pharmacologic class, some drugs may equilibrate between maternal and fetal blood more slowly than others.[42] For instance, the transplacental transfer of **midazolam** is slower compared with other benzodiazepines (e.g., **diazepam;** see Table 4.1).[62] Hydrophilic drugs such as **hexamethonium** may never reach distributional equilibrium because they are rapidly excreted by the fetus into the amniotic fluid.[42]

The physiologic parameters that determine the transfer of drugs across the placenta can change during the course of pregnancy. These include the surface area and the volume of the placenta, trophoblast thickness, placental blood flow, and transporter expression. For instance, P-gp expression in the syncytiotrophoblast is highest during the first trimester and lowest at term. In contrast, BCRP expression does not considerably change during pregnancy. Maternal pharmacokinetics can change as well with the gestational age.[42,65,66]

The placenta is not only a drug barrier but also a drug target. Even drugs that do not substantially cross the placenta can affect its function. Drugs, particularly **inhalation anesthetic agents,** can affect placental blood flow; others modulate the expression of placental transporters or receptors; and some directly inhibit placental carriers.[42] Placental drug transfer by diffusion, carriers, or other mechanisms may additionally be modified in the diseased placenta and during inflammation or systemic diseases that affect maternal pharmacokinetics.

Important features of placental pharmacology are summarized in Box 4.2.

BOX 4.2 Pearls for Placental Pharmacology

- All central nervous system drugs cross the placenta.
- Small lipophilic molecules are likely to have comparable free concentrations in maternal and fetal blood.
- Large or hydrophilic drugs can cross the placenta if they are substrates of placental carriers or receptors.
- Fetal exposure to drugs which slowly equilibrate between maternal and fetal blood can be reduced by minimizing the interval between drug administration and birth.
- Changes in fetal pH or fetal:maternal ratios of drug-binding proteins can affect the exposure of the fetus to some medications.
- Medications can affect the functions of the placenta, including the transfer of nutrients and other drugs.

PLACENTAL PATHOLOGY

There has been growing interest in the clinicopathologic correlation between placental abnormalities and adverse obstetric outcomes. In some cases, a skilled and systematic examination of the umbilical cord, fetal membranes, and placenta may provide insight into antepartum pathophysiology. Examination of the placenta often confirms a suspected clinical diagnosis (e.g., chorioamnionitis) and may shed light on conditions that have an immediate impact on offspring well-being or that may recur in subsequent pregnancies.

Placental structure is tightly associated with placental function, and structural placental changes cause placental dysfunction. Key structural components include those related to the maternal or fetal circulation or the maternal-fetal interface. Maldevelopment or injury of these components results in characteristic microscopic features and thus provides a system to classify placental pathology into maternal vascular malperfusion (MVM), fetal vascular malperfusion (FVM), acute inflammation and chronic inflammation, and others (Table 4.2).[68–70]

For example, maternal hypertensive disorders are associated with MVM, with small placentas and microscopic features related to superficial implantation and abnormal remodeling of decidual arterioles in the basal plate. This histopathology may be localized or global within the placental disc and may include infarction, accelerated villous maturation, distal villous hypoplasia, and decidual arteriopathy. Umbilical cord disorders can also produce FVM in the fetal circulation, including fetal vessel thrombosis, avascular villi, and villous stromal karyorrhexis. Multiple lesions may interact to affect downstream maternal or fetal organ function.

Commonly used ancillary tools in placental pathologic evaluation include special stains, such as iron stain for hemosiderin detection for chronic bleeding, Grocott methenamine silver stain for fungal microorganisms, and viral immunohistochemical (IHC) stains such as cytomegalovirus and parvovirus B19. IHC markers for placental tissue and cellular components include cytokeratins (CKs) as epithelial markers for amnion and trophoblast; vimentin for stromal cells; CD31, CD34, GLUT1, and factor VIII as endothelial markers; smooth muscle actin for smooth muscle; CD68 for Hofbauer cells; and the imprinting marker p57 to differentiate complete hydatidiform mole from partial hydatidiform mole and normal pregnancy.

TABLE 4.2   Common Placental Pathology, Suggested Definitions, and Potential Clinical Correlations

Pathology	Suggested Definition	Clinical Correlation
Maternal vascular malperfusion	The effects of inadequate spiral artery remodeling or spiral artery pathology, or high-velocity malperfusion	A spectrum of the "great obstetrical syndromes" that includes fetal growth restriction and preeclampsia; high-velocity malperfusion may be detrimental to placentation in early pregnancy and placental function in later pregnancy. Gross findings include placental hypoplasia, infarction, and retroplacental hemorrhage. Presents with bleeding during pregnancy and at delivery
Placental hypoplasia	Placental weight < 10th centile and/or a thin cord (< 10th centile or 8 mm diameter at term)	Often seen in the "great obstetrical syndromes"
Infarction	Any infarction seen in a preterm placenta and, at term, anything > 5% of nonperipheral infarction	Placental dysfunction and newborn brain lesions
Retroplacental hemorrhage	Grossly, there is blood accumulation on the maternal surface. Microscopically, blood accumulation beneath and dissecting the decidua and compression of the overlying intervillous space, with villous crowding, congestion, and/or intravillous hemorrhage with touching villi	Placental abruption
Distal villous hypoplasia	Paucity of villi in relation to the surrounding stem villi. The villi are thin, and syncytial knots are increased	Fetal growth restriction, placental dysfunction
Accelerated villous maturation	The presence of small or short hypermature villi for gestational period, usually accompanied by an increase in syncytial knots	Preeclampsia at early gestational age
Decidual arteriopathy (whether it is in the membrane roll or basal plate or both)	Including acute atherosis, fibrinoid necrosis with or without foam cells, mural hypertrophy, chronic perivasculitis, absence of spiral artery remodeling, arterial thrombosis, and persistence of intramural endovascular trophoblast in the third trimester	Preeclampsia, fetal growth restriction
Other Conditions That Also Affect Placental Intervillous Blood Flow		
Massive intervillous fibrin/ fibrinoid deposition		Maternal floor infarction, recurrent pregnancy loss[79]
Intervillous thrombi	Laminated red blood cells and fibrin present in the intervillous space	Transplacental bleeding
Fetal Vascular Malperfusion (Previously Known as "Fetal Thrombotic Vasculopathy") Likely Due to Obstruction of Fetal Blood Flow		
Fetal vascular malperfusion (can be seen in placentas from live-born individuals and in stillbirths)	Consisting of thrombosis, segmental avascular villi, and villous stromal-vascular karyorrhexis	Umbilical cord lesions, hypercoagulability, complications of fetal cardiac dysfunction, such as hypoxia
Thrombosis	A premortem process	Cord accidents
Avascular villi	Terminal villi showing total loss of villous capillaries and bland hyaline fibrosis of the villous stroma	Cord accidents

Continued

TABLE 4.2   Common Placental Pathology, Suggested Definitions, and Potential Clinical Correlations—cont'd

Pathology	Suggested Definition	Clinical Correlation
Villous stromal-vascular karyorrhexis (formerly known as hemorrhagic endovasculitis)	Terminal villi showing karyorrhexis of fetal cells (nucleated erythrocytes, leukocytes, endothelial cells, and/or stromal cells) with preservation of surrounding trophoblast	Cord accidents, intrauterine fetal demise
Stem vessel obliteration	Marked thickening of the vessel wall and resultant obliteration of the vascular lumen	Obstruction of fetal blood flow
Vascular ectasia	Vessels that are four times the luminal diameter of the surrounding corresponding vessel	Fetal hypoxia
Abnormal Villous Development		
Delayed villous maturation	A monotonous villous population with reduced numbers of vasculosyncytial membranes for the period of gestation, as well as a continuous cytotrophoblast layer and centrally placed capillaries	Often be seen in placentas from pregnancy complicated by maternal diabetes mellitus
Villous edema	Edematous villous stroma	Hydrops fetalis, parvovirus B19
Ascending Intrauterine Infection (Histologic Chorioamnionitis May Not Be Equivalent to Clinical Chorioamnionitis)		
Maternal inflammatory response	Acute subchorionitis, acute chorionitis, acute chorioamnionitis	Amniotic fluid infection
Fetal inflammatory response	Acute vasculitis of chorionic plate blood vessels, acute vasculitis of umbilical cord vessels, acute funisitis	Amniotic fluid infection, fetal/neonatal sepsis
Chronic Inflammation of Placenta[a]		
Chronic chorioamnionitis	Affects the chorioamniotic membranes	The most common lesion in late spontaneous preterm birth
Chronic villitis	When the inflammatory process affects the villous tree	
VUE	A destructive villous inflammatory lesion that is characterized by the infiltration of maternal T cells (CD8+ cytotoxic T cells) into chorionic villi	Has been reported in association with preterm and term fetal growth restriction, preeclampsia, fetal death, and preterm labor. Infants whose placentas have VUE are at risk for death and abnormal neurodevelopmental outcome at the age of 2 years
Chronic infectious villitis	Plasma cells often seen as a prominent inflammatory cells	Caused by specific infectious microorganisms (e.g., cytomegalovirus)
Chronic deciduitis	Involves the decidua basalis and consists of the presence of lymphocytes or plasma cells in the basal plate of the placenta	More common in pregnancies that result from egg donation and has been reported in a subset of patients with premature labor
Chronic histiocytic intervillositis	The intervillous infiltrate consists mostly of maternal mononuclear cells and fibrin depositions, which are both indicators for the severity of the intervillous infiltrate	Recurrent pregnancy loss
COVID placentitis[81,82]	Histologic manifestations have included variable degrees of histiocytic intervillositis, perivillous fibrin deposition, and syncytiotrophoblast necrosis	Experts recommended that placental infection be defined using techniques that allow virus detection and localization in placental tissue by one or more of the following methods: *in situ* hybridization with antisense probe (detects replication) or a sense probe (detects viral messenger RNA) or immunohistochemistry to detect viral nucleocapsid or spike proteins

TABLE 4.2   Common Placental Pathology, Suggested Definitions, and Potential Clinical Correlations—cont'd

Pathology	Suggested Definition	Clinical Correlation
Placental mesenchymal dysplasia[83]	A rare placental lesion characterized by stem villous cystic dilation and vesicle formation, placentomegaly, and vascular abnormalities	Can be associated with growth restriction, stillbirth, Beckwith-Wiedemann syndrome, and some chromosomal abnormalities, and needs to be distinguished from its main differential diagnosis, hydatidiform mole
Myometrial Invasion		
Placenta accreta spectrum[84,85]	Refers to the range of abnormally adhesive and penetrative placental tissue at a uterine scar. Divided into accreta, increta, and percreta based on degree of myometrial invasion	Incidence has increased and is now the leading indication for emergency peripartum hysterectomy in the setting of catastrophic hemorrhage from a nonseparating placenta
Other Significant Pathologies		
Amnion nodosum	Nodules of fetal skin, hair, and fat found on the amnion	Associated with severe, prolonged oligohydramnios, anhydramnios
Amnionic web and amniotic band syndrome	Amniotic membrane extending and spanning the angle made by the fetal surface from the base of the umbilical cord	Can be seen in congenital anomalies including amputation of fetal limbs
Villous capillary lesions	Chorangiosis, chorangioma, chorangiomatosis	Pregnancy complicated by maternal diabetes mellitus, high altitude, twin pregnancy, or hypoxia
Meconium staining	Passage of meconium *in utero*	Neonates are at risk for meconium aspiration

COVID, Coronavirus disease; *VUE*, villitis of unknown etiology.

[a]Chronic inflammatory lesions of the placenta are characterized by the infiltration of the organ by lymphocytes, plasma cells, and/or macrophages and may result from infections (viral, bacterial, parasitic) or be of immune origin (maternal antifetal rejection).[80]

Data from Khong TY, Mooney EE, Ariel I, et al. Sampling and definitions of placental lesions: Amsterdam Placental Workshop Group consensus statement. *Arch Pathol Lab Med.* 2016;140:698–713; Redline RW, Ravishankar S, Bagby CM, et al. Four major patterns of placental injury: a stepwise guide for understanding and implementing the 2016 Amsterdam consensus. *Mod Pathol.* 2021;34:1074–1092; Slack JC, Parra-Herran C. Life after Amsterdam: placental pathology consensus recommendations and beyond. *Surg Pathol Clin.* 2022;15:175–196, unless otherwise indicated.

KEY POINTS

- The placenta is a dynamic organ with a complex structure. It brings two circulations into close proximity for the exchange of blood gases, nutrients, and other substances (e.g., drugs).
- During pregnancy, anatomic adaptations result in near-maximal vasodilation of the uterine spiral arteries; this leads to a low-resistance pathway for the delivery of blood to the placenta. Consequently, adequate uteroplacental blood flow depends on the maintenance of a normal maternal perfusion pressure.
- Placental transfer involves all physiologic transport mechanisms that exist in other organ systems.
- Physical factors (e.g., molecular weight, lipid solubility, degree of ionization) affect the placental transfer of drugs and other substances. Maternal-fetal exchange is also affected by maternal and fetal blood flow, placental binding, placental metabolism, diffusion capacity, and plasma protein binding.
- Lipophilicity enhances the placental transfer and central nervous system uptake of general anesthetic agents. However, the placenta also absorbs highly lipophilic drugs, thereby creating a drug depot that limits initial drug transfer.
- Fetal acidemia can result in "ion trapping" of both local anesthetics and opioids.
- Vasoactive drugs cross the placenta and can affect fetal circulation and metabolism.
- Inflammation and infection may affect placental function and transport.
- Environmental factors influence epigenetic expression of genes, placental development, and fetal phenotypes.

REFERENCES

1. Muglia LJ, Benhalima K, Tong S, Ozanne S. Maternal factors during pregnancy influencing maternal, fetal, and childhood outcomes. *BMC Med*. 2022;20:418.

2. Azoulay L, Bouvattier C, Christin-Maitre S. Impact of intra-uterine life on future health. *Ann Endocrinol (Paris)*. 2022;83:54–58.

3. Burton GJ, Watson AL, Hempstock J, et al. Uterine glands provide histiotrophic nutrition for the human fetus during the first trimester of pregnancy. *J Clin Endocrinol Metab*. 2002;87:2954–2959.

4. Burton GJ, Fowden AL. The placenta: a multifaceted, transient organ. *Philos Trans R Soc Lond B Biol Sci*. 2015;370:20140066.

5. Hemberger M, Hanna CW, Dean W. Mechanisms of early placental development in mouse and humans. *Nat Rev Genet*. 2020;21:27–43.

6. Salmeri N, Carbone IF, Cavoretto PI, et al. Epigenetics beyond fetal growth restriction: a comprehensive overview. *Mol Diagn Ther*. 2022;26:607–626.

7. Ramsey EM, Donner MW. *Placental Vascular and Circulation: Anatomy, Physiology, Radiology, Clinical Aspects*. WB Saunders; 1980.

8. Roth CJ, Haeussner E, Ruebelmann T, et al. Dynamic modeling of uteroplacental blood flow in IUGR indicates vortices and elevated pressure in the intervillous space – a pilot study. *Sci Rep*. 2017;7:40771.

9. Freese UE. The fetal-maternal circulation of the placenta. I. Histomorphologic, plastoid injection, and x-ray cinematographic studies on human placentas. *Am J Obstet Gynecol*. 1966;94:354–360.

10. Kaufmann P. Basic morphology of the fetal and maternal circuits in the human placenta. *Contrib Gynecol Obstet*. 1985;13:5–17.

11. Sankar KD, Bhanu PS, Kiran S, et al. Vasculosyncytial membrane in relation to syncytial knots complicates the placenta in preeclampsia: a histomorphometrical study. *Anat Cell Biol*. 2012;45:86–91.

12. Theofanakis C, Drakakis P, Besharat A, Loutradis D. Human chorionic gonadotropin: the pregnancy hormone and more. *Int J Mol Sci*. 2017;18:1059.

13. Rackaityte E, Halkias J. Mechanisms of fetal T cell tolerance and immune regulation. *Front Immunol*. 2020;11:588.

14. Ander SE, Diamond MS, Coyne CB. Immune responses at the maternal-fetal interface. *Sci Immunol*. 2019;4:eaat6114.

15. Gude NM, Roberts CT, Kalionis B, King RG. Growth and function of the normal human placenta. *Thromb Res*. 2004;114:397–407.

16. Robbins JR, Bakardjiev AI. Pathogens and the placental fortress. *Curr Opin Microbiol*. 2012;15:36–43.

17. Penn AA. Endocrine and paracrine function of the human placenta. In: Polin RA, Abman SH, Rowitch DH, eds. *Fetal and Neonatal Physiology*. 5th ed. Elsevier; 2017:134–144.

18. Hill M, Pařízek A, Cibula D, et al. Steroid metabolome in fetal and maternal body fluids in human late pregnancy. *J Steroid Biochem Mol Biol*. 2010;122:114–132.

19. Faber JJ, Thornburg KL. *Placental Physiology: Structure and Function of Fetomaternal Exchange*. Raven Press; 1983.

20. Sastry BV. Human placental cholinergic system. *Biochem Pharmacol*. 1997;53:1577–1586.

21. Jerat S, DiMarzo L, Morrish DW, Kaufman S. Adrenomedullin-induced dilation of human placental arteries is modulated by an endothelium-derived constricting factor. *Regul Pept*. 2008;146:183–188.

22. Howard RB, Hosokawa T, Maguire MH. Hypoxia-induced fetoplacental vasoconstriction in perfused human placental cotyledons. *Am J Obstet Gynecol*. 1987;157:1261–1266.

23. Kuhn DC, Stuart MJ. Cyclooxygenase inhibition reduces placental transfer: reversal by carbacyclin. *Am J Obstet Gynecol*. 1987;157:194–198.

24. Myatt L, Brewer A, Brockman DE. The action of nitric oxide in the perfused human fetal-placental circulation. *Am J Obstet Gynecol*. 1991;164:687–692.

25. Coumans ABC, Garnier Y, Supçun S, et al. The role of nitric oxide on fetal cardiovascular control during normoxia and acute hypoxia in 0.75 gestation sheep. *J Soc Gynecol Investig*. 2003;10:275–282.

26. Ramasubramanian R, Johnson RF, Downing JW, et al. Hypoxemic fetoplacental vasoconstriction: a graduated response to reduced oxygen conditions in the human placenta. *Anesth Analg*. 2006;103:439–442.

27. Gao Q, Tang J, Li N, et al. A novel mechanism of angiotensin II-regulated placental vascular tone in the development of hypertension in preeclampsia. *Oncotarget*. 2017;8:30734–30741.

28. Audus KL. Controlling drug delivery across the placenta. *Eur J Pharm Sci*. 1999;8:161–165.

29. Dawe GS, Tan XW, Xiao ZC. Cell migration from baby to mother. *Cell Adh Migr*. 2007;1:19–27.

30. Clifton VL, Stark MJ, Osei-Kumah A, Hodyl NA. Review: The feto-placental unit, pregnancy pathology and impact on long term maternal health. *Placenta*. 2012;33(suppl):S37–S41.

31. Kohli S, Isermann B. Placental hemostasis and sterile inflammation: new insights into gestational vascular disease. *Thromb Res*. 2017;151(suppl 1):S30–S33.

32. Tong M, Chamley LW. Placental extracellular vesicles and feto-maternal communication. *Cold Spring Harb Perspect Med*. 2015;5:a023028.

33. Goswami D, Tannetta DS, Magee LA, et al. Excess syncytiotrophoblast microparticle shedding is a feature of early-onset pre-eclampsia, but not normotensive intrauterine growth restriction. *Placenta*. 2006;27:56–61.

34. Zhang B, Liang R, Zheng M, et al. Surface-functionalized nanoparticles as efficient tools in targeted therapy of pregnancy complications. *Int J Mol Sci*. 2019;20:3642.

35. Brownbill P, Edwards D, Jones C, et al. Mechanisms of alphafetoprotein transfer in the perfused human placental cotyledon from uncomplicated pregnancy. *J Clin Invest*. 1995;96:2220–2226.

36. Uehara I, Kimura T, Tanigaki S, et al. Paracellular route is the major urate transport pathway across the blood-placental barrier. *Physiol Rep*. 2014;2:e12013.

37. Hall JE. Transport of substances through a cell membrane. *Guyton and Hall Textbook of Medical Physiology*. 13th ed. Elsevier; 2015:47–59.

38. Pollex EK, Feig DS, Koren G. Oral hypoglycemic therapy: understanding the mechanisms of transplacental transfer. *J Matern Fetal Neonatal Med*. 2010;23:224–228.

39. Ghosh CMN. Drug permeation across the fetal maternal barrier. In: Janigro D, ed. *Mammalian Brain Development*. Humana Press; 2009:153–170.

40. Ellery SJ, Della Gatta PA, Bruce CR, et al. Creatine biosynthesis and transport by the term human placenta. *Placenta*. 2017;52:86–93.

41. Wang JS, Newport DJ, Stowe ZN, et al. The emerging importance of transporter proteins in the psychopharmacological treatment of the pregnant patient. *Drug Metab Rev*. 2007;39:723–746.

42. Tetro N, Moushaev S, Rubinchik-Stern M, Eyal S. The placental barrier: the gate and the fate in drug distribution. *Pharm Res*. 2018;35:71.

43. Longo L. Respiration in the fetal-placental unit. In: Cowett R, ed. *Principles of Perinatal-Neonatal Metabolism*. Springer-Verlag; 1991:304–315.

44. Dancis JSH. Physiology: transfer and barrier function. In: Gruenwald P, ed. *The Placenta and Its Maternal Supply Line: Effects of Insufficiency on the Fetus*. University Park Press; 1975:366.

45. Ramanathan S, Gandhi S, Arismendy J, et al. Oxygen transfer from mother to fetus during cesarean section under epidural anesthesia. *Anesth Analg*. 1982;61:576–581.

46. Hill EP, Power GG, Longo LD. A mathematical model of carbon dioxide transfer in the placenta and its interaction with oxygen. *Am J Physiol*. 1973;224:283–299.

47. Carter AM. Evolution of factors affecting placental oxygen transfer. *Placenta*. 2009;30(suppl A):S19–S25.

48. Reshetnikova OS, Burton GJ, Milovanov AP. Effects of hypobaric hypoxia on the fetoplacental unit: the morphometric diffusing capacity of the villous membrane at high altitude. *Am J Obstet Gynecol*. 1994;171:1560–1565.

49. Battaglia FC, Meschia G. Foetal and placental metabolisms: their interrelationship and impact upon maternal metabolism. *Proc Nutr Soc*. 1981;40:99–113.

50. Longo LD, Delivoria-Papadopoulos M, Forster RE 2nd. Placental CO_2 transfer after fetal carbonic anhydrase inhibition. *Am J Physiol*. 1974;226:703–710.

51. Novakovic B, Gordon L, Robinson WP, et al. Glucose as a fetal nutrient: dynamic regulation of several glucose transporter genes by DNA methylation in the human placenta across gestation. *J Nutr Biochem*. 2013;24:282–288.

52. Jansson T, Aye IL, Goberdhan DC. The emerging role of mTORC1 signaling in placental nutrient-sensing. *Placenta*. 2012;33(suppl 2):e23–e29.

53. McColl ER, Hurtarte M, Piquette-Miller M. Impact of inflammation and infection on the expression of amino acid transporters in the placenta: a minireview. *Drug Metab Dispos*. 2022;50:1251–1258.

54. Avagliano L, Garò C, Marconi AM. Placental amino acids transport in intrauterine growth restriction. *J Pregnancy*. 2012;2012:972562.

55. Murthi P, Wallace EM, Walker DW. Altered placental tryptophan metabolic pathway in human fetal growth restriction. *Placenta*. 2017;52:62–70.

56. Haggarty P. Fatty acid supply to the human fetus. *Annu Rev Nutr*. 2010;30:237–255.

57. Carreras-Badosa G, Prats-Puig A, Puig T, et al. Circulating fatty acid synthase in pregnant women: relationship to blood pressure, maternal metabolism and newborn parameters. *Sci Rep*. 2016;6:24167.

58. Zamek-Gliszczynski MJ, Sangha V, Shen H, et al. Transporters in drug development: International Transporter Consortium update on emerging transporters of clinical importance. *Clin Pharmacol Ther*. 2022;112:485–500.

59. Horackova H, Karahoda R, Vachalova V, et al. Functional characterization of dopamine and norepinephrine transport across the apical and basal plasma membranes of the human placental syncytiotrophoblast. *Sci Rep*. 2022;12:11603.

60. Ganapathy V. Drugs of abuse and human placenta. *Life Sci*. 2011;88:926–930.

61. Hamed R, Eyal AD, Berman E, Eyal S. In silico screening for clinical efficacy of antiseizure medications: not all central nervous system drugs are alike. *Epilepsia*. 2023;64:311–319.

62. Briggs GG, Freeman RK, Towers CV, Forinash AB. *Briggs Drugs in Pregnancy and Lactation: A Reference Guide to Fetal and Neonatal Risk*. 12th ed. Lippincott Williams & Wilkins; 2021.

63. Dagenais C, Graff CL, Pollack GM. Variable modulation of opioid brain uptake by P-glycoprotein in mice. *Biochem Pharmacol*. 2004;67:269–276.

64. Hutson JR, Garcia-Bournissen F, Davis A, Koren G. The human placental perfusion model: a systematic review and development of a model to predict in vivo transfer of therapeutic drugs. *Clin Pharmacol Ther*. 2011;90:67–76.

65. Jauniaux E, Gulbis B. In vivo investigation of placental transfer early in human pregnancy. *Eur J Obstet Gynecol Reprod Biol*. 2000;92:45–49.

66. Tsen LC, Tarshis J, Denson DD, et al. Measurements of maternal protein binding of bupivacaine throughout pregnancy. *Anesth Analg*. 1999;89:965–968.

67. Kumar A, Ieronimakis N, Unadkat J. Mechanisms of transplacental transfer of (-)-Δ 9-tetrahydrocannabinol (THC) in the human dual cotyledon, dual perfusion, placenta model. *FASEB J*. 2022;36. https://doi.org/10.1096/fasebj.2022.36.S1.0R546.

68. Khong TY, Mooney EE, Ariel I, et al. Sampling and definitions of placental lesions: Amsterdam Placental Workshop Group consensus statement. *Arch Pathol Lab Med*. 2016;140:698–713.

69. Redline RW, Ravishankar S, Bagby CM, et al. Four major patterns of placental injury: a stepwise guide for understanding and implementing the 2016 Amsterdam consensus. *Mod Pathol*. 2021;34:1074–1092.

70. Slack JC, Parra-Herran C. Life after Amsterdam: placental pathology consensus recommendations and beyond. *Surg Pathol Clin*. 2022;15:175–196.

71. Wang C, Liu S, Han C, et al. Effect and placental transfer of dexmedetomidine during caesarean section under epidural anaesthesia. *J Int Med Res*. 2017;45:964–972.

72. Ala-Kokko TI, Pienimaki P, Lampela E, et al. Transfer of clonidine and dexmedetomidine across the isolated perfused human placenta. *Acta Anaesthesiol Scand*. 1997;41:313–319.

73. Fleet JA, Belan I, Gordon AL, Cyna AM. Fentanyl concentration in maternal and umbilical cord plasma following intranasal or subcutaneous administration in labour. *Int J Obstet Anesth*. 2020;42:34–38.

74. Herman NL, Li AT, Van Decar TK, et al. Transfer of methohexital across the perfused human placenta. *J Clin Anesth*. 2000;12:25–30.

75. Booth PN, McLeod Watson MJ. K. Pancuronium and the placental barrier. *Anaesthesia*. 1977;32:320–323.

76. Duvaldestin P, Demetriou M, Henzel D, Desmonts JM. The placental transfer of pancuronium and its pharmacokinetics during caesarian section. *Acta Anaesthesiol Scand*. 1978;22:327–333.

77. Gaspari F, Marraro G, Penna GF, et al. Elimination kinetics of thiopentone in mothers and their newborn infants. *Eur J Clin Pharmacol*. 1985;28:321–325.

78. Morgan DJ, Blackman GL, Paull JD, Wolf LJ. Pharmacokinetics and plasma binding of thiopental. II: studies at cesarean section. *Anesthesiology*. 1981;54:474–480.

79. He M, Migliori A, Maari NS, Mehta ND. Follow-up and management of recurrent pregnancy losses due to massive perivillous fibrinoid deposition. *Obstet Med*. 2018;11:17–22.

80. Kim CJ, Romero R, Chaemsaithong P, Kim JS. Chronic inflammation of the placenta: definition, classification, pathogenesis, and clinical significance. *Am J Obstet Gynecol*. 2015;213:S53–S69.

81. Watkins JC, Torous VF, Roberts DJ. Defining severe acute respiratory syndrome coronavirus 2 (SARS-CoV-2) placentitis. *Arch Pathol Lab Med*. 2021;145:1341–1349.

82. Roberts DJ, Edlow AG, Romero RJ, et al. A standardized definition of placental infection by SARS-CoV-2, a consensus statement from the National Institutes of Health/Eunice Kennedy Shriver National Institute of Child Health and Human Development SARS-CoV-2 Placental Infection Workshop. *Am J Obstet Gynecol*. 2021;225:593.e1–e9.

83. Pawoo N, Heller DS. Placental mesenchymal dysplasia. *Arch Pathol Lab Med*. 2014;138:1247–1249.

84. Hecht JL, Baergen R, Ernst LM, et al. Classification and reporting guidelines for the pathology diagnosis of placenta accreta spectrum (PAS) disorders: recommendations from an expert panel. *Mod Pathol*. 2020;33:2382–2396.

85. Kapoor H, Hanaoka M, Dawkins A, Khurana A. Review of MRI imaging for placenta accreta spectrum: pathophysiologic insights, imaging signs, and recent developments. *Placenta*. 2021;104:31–39.

PART III

Fetal and Neonatal Assessment and Therapy

5

Fetal Physiology

Adrianne Rahde Bischoff, MD and Patrick J. McNamara, MB, BCH, BAO, MRCPCH, DCh, MSc, FASE

CHAPTER OUTLINE

FETAL ENVIRONMENT

Amniotic Fluid

The fetus is surrounded by amniotic fluid (*liquor amnii*), a complex fluid that changes as the pregnancy progresses. Amniotic fluid serves a number of vital roles, including the facilitation of fetal growth, the provision of a microgravity environment that cushions the fetus, and the generation of a defense mechanism against invading microbes.[1] The formation and maintenance of amniotic fluid is an intricate process that depends on fetal maturation, maternal hydration, hormonal status, and uteroplacental perfusion.

Amniotic fluid during early embryogenesis is principally derived from maternal plasma by the passage of water and solutes through aquaporin water channels expressed in the fetal-maternal membranes (amnion and chorion). The expression of aquaporins changes as gestation advances and with certain pathologic states, such as polyhydramnios.[2] Between 10 and 20 weeks' gestation, the volume of amniotic fluid increases in a predictable and linear manner from approximately 25 to 400 mL. During this period, the composition of amniotic fluid is similar to fetal extracellular fluid, owing to the absence of keratin in the fetal skin. Beyond 20 weeks' gestation, the volume of amniotic fluid is determined by the difference between production, from fetal urine and respiratory tract, and removal, through fetal swallowing.[3] The volume of amniotic fluid is also influenced by intramembranous (between amniotic fluid and fetal blood within the placenta) and transmembranous (between amniotic fluid and maternal blood within the uterus) pathways in both physiologic and pathophysiologic states.[4] Finally, the status of maternal hydration and the amount of decidual prolactin may alter the transfer of amniotic fluid through fetal and maternal tissues. Amniotic fluid volume plateaus at 800 to 1000 mL at around 28 weeks' gestation, after which it declines to approximately 400 mL at term.[3]

The *composition* of amniotic fluid undergoes more marked variation than its volume throughout gestation.[5] During the first trimester, amniotic fluid consists mostly of water and electrolytes and contains minimal protein. Keratinization of the fetal skin is complete by 25 weeks' gestation and decreases the permeability of fetal tissues to water and solutes. The impact of this process, coupled with the ability of the fetal kidneys to produce urine, results in increased amniotic fluid concentrations of urea and creatinine, decreased concentrations of sodium and chloride, and reduced osmolality. A variety of carbohydrates, proteins, lipids, electrolytes, enzymes, and hormones, which vary in concentration depending on the gestational age, are also present; some of these elements, particularly the amino acids taurine, glutamine, and arginine, serve a nutritive function for mitotic cells involved in trophoblastic growth and placental angiogenesis.[1] Many growth factors are found in amniotic fluid, many of which play an important role in fetal intestinal development.[1]

Antimicrobial defenses within the amniotic fluid are primarily composed of humoral mediators such as alpha-defensins, which are released from neutrophils, especially in the setting of preterm labor and/or chorioamnionitis. Other humoral mediators include lactoferrin, calprotectin, leukocyte protease inhibitor, and cathelicidin, which have significant activity against bacteria, viruses, and fungi.[6] Cellular mediators of the immune response are poorly characterized in amniotic fluid, and it remains unclear if the macrophages that are present serve a scavenging or an antimicrobial role. Neutrophils are usually absent from the amniotic fluid of a healthy fetus, and their presence typically signifies an inflammatory or infectious process.[1]

Biochemical and cellular analysis of amniotic fluid provides valuable information on chromosomal abnormalities, neural tube defects, prenatal infections, and most inborn errors of metabolism.[7,8] Several amniotic fluid-based indices, including the lecithin-sphingomyelin ratio, the phosphatidylglycerol level, lamellar body count, surfactant-to-albumin ratio, and electrical conductivity, can be used to assess fetal lung maturity.[9,10] Bilirubin levels can be determined by measuring the optical density of amniotic fluid, which assists in the monitoring of fetal hemolysis. Estimation of the amniotic fluid levels of S100-beta (a protein released from injured astrocytes) and cell-free fetal nucleic acids may serve as early screening tests for perinatal neurologic damage and fetal development, respectively.[11,12] Finally, amniotic fluid is a valuable reservoir for cell types of multiple lineages at different maturational ages; approximately 1% of these cells are pluripotent, thereby representing a novel source of stem cells.[13,14] Loss of amniotic fluid is one contributor to impaired lung development, and its most extreme form, pulmonary hypoplasia.

Oxygen Supply and Transport

The fetus has almost no oxygen reserve and depends on maternal sources of oxygen delivery via the placenta. Acute hypoxemia can have immediate, severe consequences, such as perinatal death, hypoxic-ischemic encephalopathy, and long-term consequences including cognitive impairment and cerebral palsy. Chronic reductions of oxygen supply may lead to fetal growth restriction (also known as intrauterine growth restriction) and may have long-term consequences for brain, heart, and kidney function through epigenetic changes. When tissue hypoxia occurs during critical periods of heart development, apoptosis of cardiomyocytes can result, potentially leading to a myocardium that is less resilient to ischemic insults in later life. In addition, chronic hypoxia can influence fetal development of brain and kidney function and metabolism, subsequently leading to problems in adulthood.[15,16]

Oxygenation of fetal tissues depends principally on the partial pressure of oxygen (Po_2) gradient between maternal and fetal blood, uteroplacental perfusion, and the different types of hemoglobin in maternal and fetal blood. The presence of fetal hemoglobin (hemoglobin F), with its higher concentration (approximately 18 g/dL) and greater affinity for oxygen than adult hemoglobin (see later discussion), results in a fetal arterial blood oxygen content that is similar to the adult, despite a lower oxygen tension and a similar rate of oxygen extraction.[17] The fetus grows and thrives in a hypoxemic

environment; specifically, the umbilical vein is the most oxygenated vessel in the fetal circulation and has a Po_2 of approximately 30 to 40 mm Hg (4.0 to 5.3 kPa). Tissue hypoxia, however, occurs when the demand for oxygen exceeds the available supply. In adult tissues, hypoxia typically occurs at $Po_2 < 20$ mm Hg (2.7 kPa; normal, approximately 40 mm Hg [5.3 kPa]). By contrast, in fetal tissues hypoxia occurs at $Po_2 < 17$ mm Hg (2.3 kPa; normal, approximately 20 to 25 mm Hg [2.7 to 3.3 kPa]). This implies that the environment for fetal development exhibits a smaller margin of safety before reaching a state of oxygen insufficiency and highlights the importance of maintaining adequate uteroplacental perfusion and fetal cardiac output to ensure fetal oxygen delivery.[18]

Placental oxygen concentration changes with gestation. In early pregnancy, the placental intervillous space is free of maternal blood cells, thereby requiring the embryo to rely on endometrial secretions and maternal plasma for its energy requirements.[19,20] During the first trimester the placenta has (1) a Po_2 of approximately 20 mm Hg (2.7 kPa); (2) only a few capillaries, which are located mainly in the center of the mesenchymal core; and (3) a trophoblastic layer that is twice the thickness of that in the second trimester.[21] Moreover, the fetal red blood cells are nucleated, and the exocoelomic cavity contains antioxidant molecules instead of an oxygen transport system. These anatomic and physiologic features, which limit the transfer of oxygen and the creation of free radicals, protect the highly sensitive embryo from the effects of oxidative stress and keep the embryonic cells in their pluripotent state.[22,23] At the end of the first trimester, an exponential increase in fetal growth creates a significant rise in the demand for oxygen and nutrients (Fig. 5.1). In response, cytotrophoblastic cells

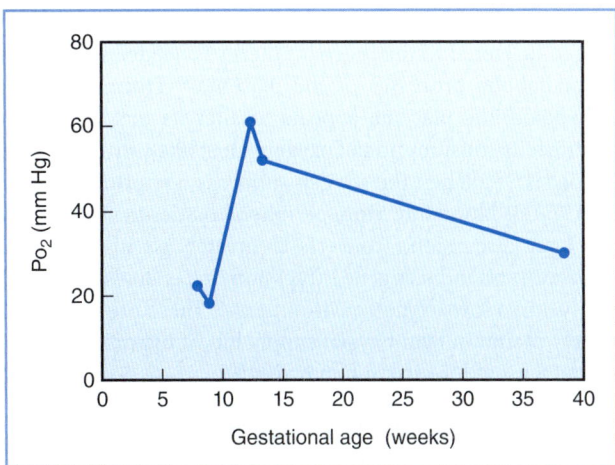

Fig. 5.1 The mean oxygen partial pressure (Po_2) throughout gestation in the human intervillous space. Data from Jauniaux E, Kiserud T, Ozturk O, et al. Amniotic gas values and acid-base status during acute maternal hyperoxemia and hypoxemia in the early fetal sheep. *Am J Obstet Gynecol.* 2000;182:661–665; Rodesch F, Simon P, Donner C, Jauniaux E. Oxygen measurements in endometrial and trophoblastic tissues during early pregnancy. *Obstet Gynecol.* 1992;80:283–285; and Schaaps JP, Tsatsaris V, Goffin F, et al. Shunting the intervillous space: new concepts in human uteroplacental vascularization. *Am J Obstet Gynecol.* 2005;192:323–332.

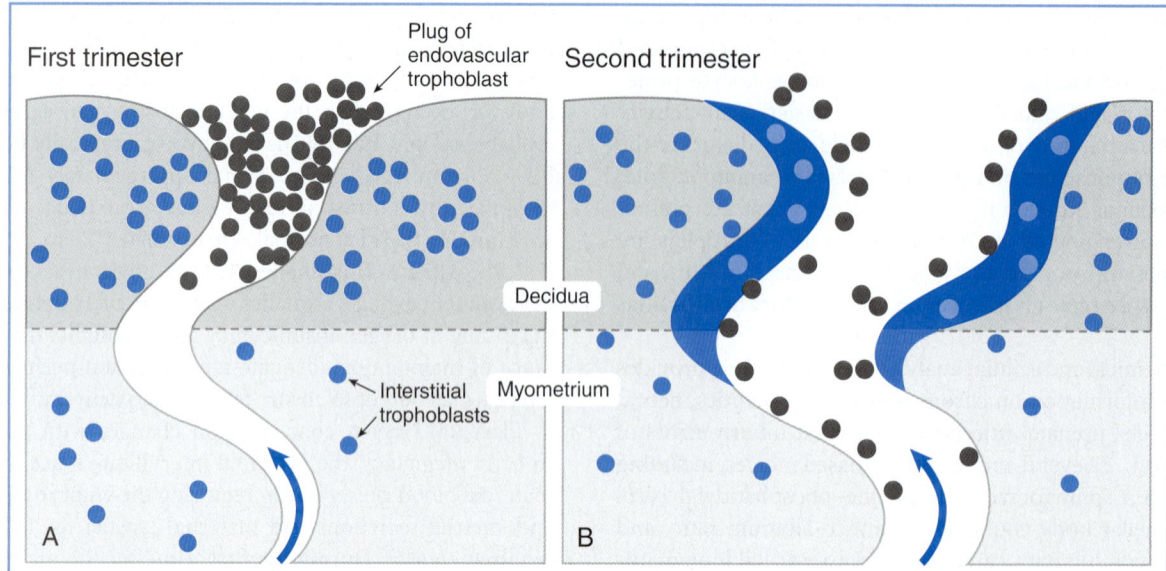

Fig. 5.2 Invasion and Remodeling of the Spiral Arteries by Endovascular and Interstitial Extravillous Trophoblasts. (A) In the first trimester, the terminal portion of the spiral artery is blocked by a plug of endovascular trophoblast. Early placental and embryonic development occurs in a state of low oxygen tension, and nutrition at this early stage is derived from secretions from maternal endometrial glands. (B) After 10 to 12 weeks' gestation, the endovascular trophoblast plug dissolves and the endovascular trophoblast migrates into the myometrium, replacing endothelial cells, which undergo apoptosis. Maternal blood is now able to enter the intervillous space, the oxygen tension increases to 60 mm Hg (8 kPa), and nutrition changes from histotrophic to hemotrophic. Modified from Pijnenborg R, Vercruysse L, Hanssens M. The uterine spiral arteries in human pregnancy: facts and controversies. *Placenta.* 2006;27:939–958.

interact with the smooth muscle of maternal spiral arteries, resulting in vessel dilation and the provision of oxygen-rich maternal blood flow to the placenta (Fig. 5.2).[24]

The placenta acts as both a conduit and consumer of oxygen. The placenta is metabolically active and performs important roles in carbohydrate and amino acid metabolism, protein synthesis, and substrate transport. Almost 40% of the oxygen delivered to the pregnant uterus is needed to support the metabolic processes of the placenta.[25] During periods of hypoxia, the placenta appears to alter its metabolism to diminish its consumption of oxygen, most likely by increasing glycolysis.[26,27] When the oxygen supply is compromised, the fetus shunts blood flow from peripheral tissues to vital organs (see later discussion), converts to greater use of anaerobic pathways, and induces gene expression that enables improved survival in a low-oxygen environment.[28] These processes can acutely maintain fetal oxygen supply but, if hypoxia is ongoing, fetal growth restriction may result.

Glucose and Lactate Metabolism

Glucose is the primary substrate for energy production in the fetus. Under normal conditions, gluconeogenesis is absent in mammalian fetuses and placental transfer is the only source of glucose.[29] Glucose uptake into the fetal tissues is regulated by glucose transporters whose expression varies in response to acute and chronic changes in fetal glucose concentration.[30] Fetal glucose concentration is linearly related to maternal concentration over a range of 3 to 5 mmol/L (54 to 90 mg/dL) (Fig. 5.3); studies in isolated placentas suggest that this

relationship continues up to a glucose concentration of 20 mmol/L (360 mg/dL).[31] The placenta uses the majority of glucose delivered to the uterus for oxidation, glycogen storage, and conversion to lactate, with the remainder being transferred to the umbilical venous blood by facilitated, carrier-mediated diffusion.

The umbilical cord blood glucose uptake is approximately 5 mg/kg/min at normal maternal arterial plasma glucose concentrations in sheep models.[32] It is estimated that lactate and amino acids provide approximately 25% each of the total fetal energy requirements.[33,34]

Lactate is produced even in well-oxygenated fetal lambs, with total lactate production being approximately 4 mg/kg/min.[35] Although the exact origin of fetal lactate is unclear, skeletal muscle and bone have been identified as sources of lactate production under resting conditions. Lactate production increases during episodes of acute hypoxemia, although this response may be blunted in fetuses previously exposed to oxidative stress.[36] Lactate consumption occurs in the fetal myocardium and liver.[37]

Amino Acid and Lipid Metabolism

The fetus uses amino acids for protein synthesis, growth, and oxidation. Most maternal-to-fetal amino acid transfer occurs against a concentration gradient and involves energy-dependent transfer mechanisms. Under conditions in which fetal aerobic metabolism is decreased, amino acid uptake by the placenta and fetus may be reduced because it involves an expenditure of energy. During maternal fasting, fetal amino

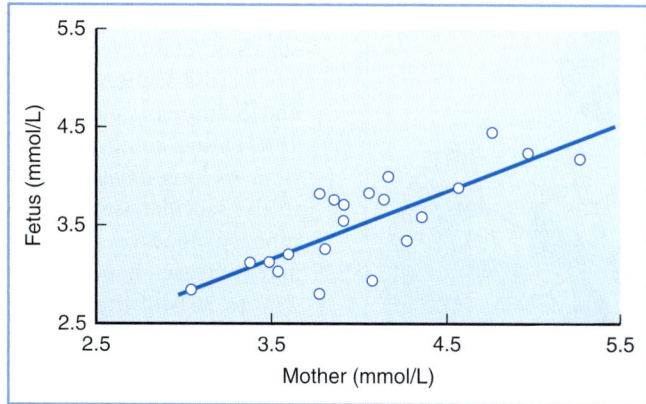

Fig. 5.3 The Linear Relationship Between Maternal and Fetal Blood Glucose Concentrations During the Third Trimester. Fetal blood was obtained by percutaneous umbilical cord blood sampling. From Kalhan SC. Metabolism of glucose and methods of investigation in the fetus and newborn. In: Polin RA, Fox WW, eds. *Fetal and Neonatal Physiology*. Vol I. WB Saunders; 1992:477–488.

acid uptake does not change; however, enhanced fetal proteolysis may occur, resulting in amino acid oxidation or gluconeogenesis.

Lipid products are transferred from the mother to the fetus. The fetus requires free fatty acids for growth, brain development, and the deposition of body fat for postnatal life. Fatty acids are transferred across the placenta by simple diffusion. Ketones are also transferred by simple diffusion, and in humans the maternal/fetal ketone ratio is approximately 2.0.[38] The fetus can use ketones as lipogenic substrates or as energy substrates in the brain, kidney, heart, liver, and placenta.[39] Beta-hydroxybutyrate (fatty acid) metabolism can occur in the placenta, brain, and liver during episodes of fetal hypoglycemia that result from maternal fasting.[39]

Thermoregulation

Intrauterine fetal temperature largely depends on maternal temperature. Owing to the high metabolic rate in the fetus, the net flow of heat is from the fetus to the mother. The fetus produces approximately twice as much weight-adjusted heat as the mother and maintains a temperature 0.5°C higher.[40,41] This maternal-fetal difference in temperature remains relatively constant and is referred to as the "heat clamp."[42]

The placental circulation is responsible for approximately 85% of the heat exchange between the mother and fetus. The remaining 15% is dissipated through the fetal skin and transferred through the amniotic fluid and the uterine wall to the maternal abdomen.[43] In animal models, fetal temperature may be rapidly affected by changes in umbilical blood flow.[44,45] In humans, fetal temperature increases during uterine contractions, which may be a result of intermittent obstruction of umbilical cord blood flow.[46] Whether this rise in fetal temperature contributes to acute hypoxic-ischemic brain damage in the setting of umbilical cord prolapse is unknown. However, relatively small increases in temperature increase the sensitivity of the fetal brain to hypoxic injury.[47]

Thermogenic mechanisms are not developed until the end of gestation and are largely inactive *in utero*. Newborns are at high risk for rapid heat loss due to amniotic fluid evaporation

and a sudden decrease in ambient temperature.[41] Because of their small muscle mass, neonates are incapable of significant heat production through shivering. Instead, nonshivering thermogenesis occurs in brown adipose tissue.

FETAL CARDIOVASCULAR SYSTEM

The cardiovascular system is one of the first functional organ systems in the developing fetus, evolving from its first appearance as a heart tube to its development as a four-chambered structure between 20 and 44 days' gestation. The valveless heart tube generates unidirectional flow beginning at approximately 21 days' gestation.

Circulatory Pattern

Fetal circulation differs significantly from the postnatal circulation. The fetal systemic circulation receives cardiac output from both the left and the right ventricle, with the ventricles working in *parallel*. In contrast, during postnatal life, the left and right circulations are separated, and the ventricles work in *series*. The fetal lungs are filled with fluid and do not participate in gas exchange. The pulmonary vascular resistance (PVR) is high.

Fetal blood flow is characterized by three anatomic shunts: the **ductus venosus**, the **foramen ovale**, and the **ductus arteriosus** (Fig. 5.4). Oxygenated blood travels from the placenta through the umbilical vein to the **ductus venosus**, which connects the umbilical vein with the inferior vena cava, thus bypassing the portal circulation and the liver. At mid-gestation, approximately 30% of the umbilical venous blood is shunted through the ductus venosus. From 30 to 40 weeks' gestation, this fraction decreases to approximately 20%, although a significant increase may occur in response to hypoxia.[48] Once in the right atrium, oxygenated blood preferentially flows through the **foramen ovale** and then to the left atrium and left ventricle, preferentially delivering well-oxygenated blood to the brain and the heart rather than the systemic circulation. Only a small amount of desaturated blood returns from the pulmonary veins and drains into the left atrium.

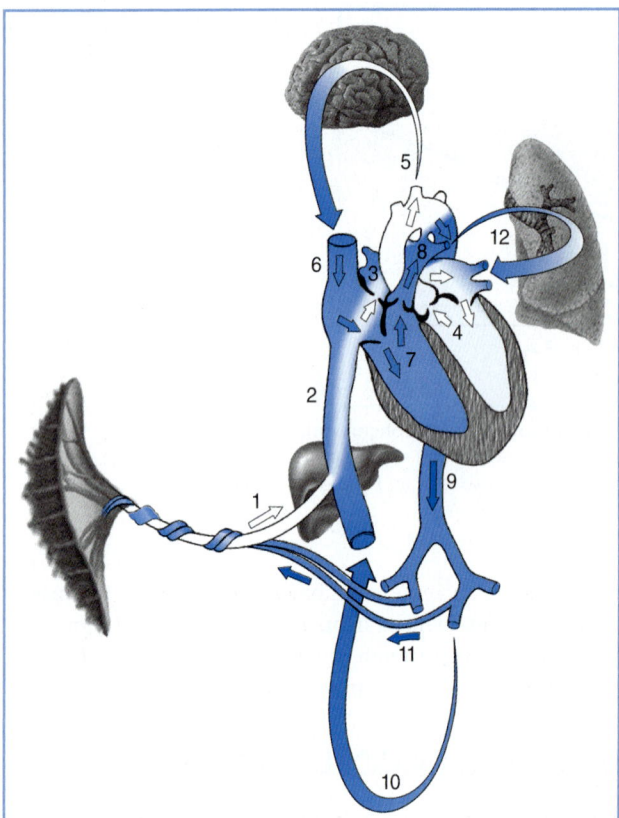

Fig. 5.4 The Fetal Circulation. Oxygenated blood leaves the placenta via the fetal umbilical vein *(1)*, enters the liver where flow divides between the portal sinus and the ductus venosus, and then empties into the inferior vena cava *(2)*. Inside the fetal heart, blood enters the right atrium, where most of the blood is directed through the foramen ovale *(3)* into the left atrium and ventricle *(4)*, and then enters the aorta. Blood is then sent to the brain *(5)* and myocardium, ensuring that these cells receive the highest oxygen content available. Deoxygenated blood returning from the lower extremities and the superior vena cava *(6)* is preferentially directed into the right ventricle *(7)* and pulmonary trunk. Most blood passes through the ductus arteriosus *(8)* into the descending aorta *(9)*, which in turn supplies the lower extremities *(10)* and the hypogastric arteries *(11)*. Blood returns to the placenta via the umbilical arteries for gas and nutrient exchange. A small amount of blood from the pulmonary trunk travels through the pulmonary arteries *(12)* to perfuse the lungs. *Arrows* in this figure depict the direction and oxygen content (*white* [oxygenated], *blue* [deoxygenated]) of the blood in circulation. Illustration by Naveen Nathan, MD, NorthShore University HealthSystem, University of Chicago Pritzker School of Medicine.

Deoxygenated blood from the head and upper extremities enters the right atrium through the superior vena cava and is preferentially directed into the right ventricle and the pulmonary artery. Because fetal PVR is higher than systemic vascular resistance (SVR), most of the pulmonary artery blood flow crosses the **ductus arteriosus** into the descending aorta, supplying the lower extremities and hypogastric arteries. Deoxygenated blood returns to the placenta via the umbilical arteries for gas and nutrient exchange.

PVR plays an important role in the fetal circulation. The small pulmonary arteries are compressed by fluid-filled alveoli; concomitantly, the lack of rhythmic distension

contributes to the mechanical impact on PVR. In the early stages of fetal development, PVR is elevated because of the small cross-sectional area and the lack of pulmonary vessels, and pulmonary blood flow comprises only approximately 13% of the combined cardiac output at 20 weeks' gestation. As lung development progresses from the canalicular to the saccular stage, there is a rapid proliferation of pulmonary blood vessels with a resultant relative drop in PVR and increase in pulmonary blood flow to approximately 25% to 30% of the combined cardiac output. Towards the third trimester, there is a secondary increase in PVR due to the response of pulmonary vasoconstrictor substances in response to oxygen.[17]

The relationship between PVR and pulmonary blood flow is inverse in late-gestation fetuses. PVR is the main determinant of the relative proportions of left ventricular filling that are driven by shunting of blood across the foramen ovale or by pulmonary venous return. Ultimately, this relationship is governed by the dynamic interplay between the different modulators of blood flow. For instance, fetal breathing increases pulmonary blood flow by up to fourfold owing to changes in capillary-interstitial transmural pressures, which in turns leads to a transient decrease in PVR. Pulmonary blood flow then increases and the shunt across the foramen ovale decreases.[49] This knowledge is particularly important to the understanding of maternal hypoxia and hyperoxia and the impact on delivery of oxygen to the fetal brain.

Several mechanisms protect the fetus from oxygen toxicity while still guaranteeing that oxygen delivery meets tissue demand. Although the fetal lungs do not participate in gas exchange, the pulmonary vasculature is reactive to oxygen and modulates blood flow to maintain oxygen delivery to the brain within a narrow range. Fetal sheep experiments of maternal hyperoxia demonstrated that significant increases in maternal arterial Po_2 are buffered by the placenta, resulting in an increase in umbilical vein Po_2 with little change in the fetal preductal circulation Po_2.[50]

Fetal oxygen delivery is regulated in the setting of maternal hypoxia by several mechanisms. Acutely, these include increased umbilical vein flow, dilation of the ductus venosus and the cerebral circulation, and decreased fetal oxygen content, which in turn increases PVR and decreases pulmonary blood flow. These changes, in turn, lead to a limited amount of desaturated blood returning to the left atrium from the pulmonary veins as well as preferential flow of blood coming from the umbilical vein through the foramen ovale and then to the ascending aorta.[17]

At birth, the fetus undergoes a significant and abrupt transition to a state of physiologic independence (see Chapter 9). Clamping of the umbilical cord results in a sudden increase in SVR and left ventricular afterload, and a reduction in right atrial preload. In addition, expansion of the lungs and increased alveolar oxygen tension result in decreased PVR. This allows for increased pulmonary blood flow, a decrease in right atrial pressure, and an increase in left atrial pressure, ultimately leading to the functional closure of both the foramen ovale and the ductus arteriosus.

Ductus Arteriosus

The ductus arteriosus, a vascular connection between the pulmonary artery and the proximal descending aorta, is responsible during fetal life for diverting deoxygenated blood away from the high-resistance pulmonary circuit into the systemic circulation. Of the total combined cardiac output, approximately 65% goes through the right ventricle and only 5% to 10% enters the fetal pulmonary circulation. The remainder is shunted through the ductus arteriosus to the descending aorta.[51,52] Prostaglandin E2 (PGE2) and prostacyclin I2 (PGI2) maintain the patency of the ductus arteriosus *in utero*. PGE2 is released from various fetal tissues and the placenta, with a higher circulating level in the fetus than the mother. Stimulation of PGE2 receptors results in an increased concentration of cyclic adenosine monophosphate, which, in turn, inhibits myosin light-chain kinase and results in ductus arteriosus relaxation.[53]

Following birth in term infants, the ductus arteriosus smooth muscle undergoes vasoconstriction, which leads to a functional closure of the lumen within the first couple of hours. This vasoconstriction is triggered primarily by the increase in oxygen tension through several mechanisms, as well as by increased lung catabolism of PGE2 and PGI2 with the removal of the placenta, and decreased ductus arteriosus expression of PGE2 receptors.[53–55] Reduction in endogenous nitric oxide production also contributes to postnatal ductus arteriosus closure.[56] Following smooth muscle vasoconstriction, ischemia-hypoxia of the muscle media of the ductus arteriosus occurs with an increase in vascular endothelial growth factor production. This is followed by vasa vasorum proliferation into the wall of the ductus arteriosus which, in combination with the attraction of mononuclear cells as well as platelet adhesion, ultimately leads to thrombotic sealing of the vasoconstricted ductus arteriosus, luminal remodeling, and anatomic occlusion.[57–60]

Blood Volume

Human fetal intravascular volume is approximately 110 mL/kg, which is a greater proportion than in postnatal life. Approximately 25% of this blood volume is contained within the placenta; the blood volume within the fetal body is estimated to be approximately 80 mL/kg.[61,62] Fetal intravascular volume is regulated through a complex interplay between the fetal heart, kidneys, and circulation and the placenta.[63] The fetus can adapt more quickly to changes in intravascular volume than the adult, owing to higher diffusion rates between the different fetal compartments.[64]

Transplacental transfer of water from mother to fetus depends on hydrostatic and osmotic pressures. The hydrostatic pressure is determined by the difference in pressures between the maternal intervillous space or capillaries and the fetal capillaries. The osmotic pressure is mainly determined by the presence of plasma proteins (i.e., colloid osmotic pressure). Transplacental water transfer is further regulated by angiotensin II. Adamson et al.[65,66] found that angiotensin II lowered the pressures in fetal placental exchange vessels, thereby promoting fluid transfer from the maternal to the fetal circulation.

The production of angiotensin II is under control of the renin-angiotensin-aldosterone system in the fetal kidneys. A reduction in fetal arterial pressure results in an increase in fetal plasma renin activity, which results in subsequent increases in angiotensin I and II. The resulting expansion of intravascular volume augments fetal cardiac output and arterial pressure.

Cardiac Development

During gestation, the fetal heart grows quickly and adapts to the continuously changing demands. The fetal myocardium grows primarily through hyperplasia, whereas after delivery, cardiac mass increases as a result of cell enlargement/hypertrophy.[67] This growth correlates with a prebirth transition from mononucleated cardiomyocytes to binucleated cardiomyocytes, which contribute to heart growth by hypertrophy. Interruption of the normal process of myocyte hyperplasia will lead to decreased myocardial endowment.

The number of cardiac myofibrils and the transition in the type of cardiac troponins that are present during prenatal development can alter fetal heart contractility.[68] The change from fetal to adult troponin is associated with decreased sensitivity of the contractile apparatus to calcium. A heightened calcium sensitivity is important in the early development of the fetal heart, when the sarcoplasmic reticulum is immature.[69] With advancing gestational age, ejection fraction declines, but cardiac output (per unit of fetal weight) does not change, owing to increasing ventricular volume. The fetal heart rate decreases over the course of gestation from 140 to 150 beats/min at 18 weeks' gestation to 120 to 140 beats/min at term.[70,71]

In utero developmental issues can have gestational and long-term heart consequences. Fetuses of mothers with diabetes mellitus were found to have signs of biventricular diastolic dysfunction, right ventricular systolic dysfunction, and septal hypertrophy in the third trimester, compared with control subjects.[72] Human growth-restricted fetuses have smaller, more spherical hearts, impaired systolic longitudinal function, and mild impairment in diastolic function, compared with matched non–growth-restricted fetuses; these alterations have been observed to persist when examined even 10 years later.[73]

Ventricular Responses to Changes in Preload and Afterload

The response of the fetal heart to changes in loading conditions differs from that of the adult heart. While the adult heart responds according to the Frank-Starling curve in a linear manner such that ventricular distention lengthens the diastolic fibers and results in augmented contractility, a number of studies have indicated that the fetal heart has a limited capacity to increase its stroke volume in response to an increase in preload (e.g., with intravenous fluid infusion).[74,75] Studies investigating the effects of afterload on fetal ventricular function have observed a significant decrease in right ventricular stroke volume in response to increases in arterial pressure.[74] The same phenomenon occurs in the left ventricle, although to a lesser degree. In a study of fetal lambs, in which gradual constriction of the descending aorta was applied, stroke volume was maintained until high mean arterial pressures were achieved, after which decreases were observed. This decrease in stroke volume in the presence of high mean arterial pressure may represent the exhaustion of "preload reserve," which will typically allow the maintenance of stroke volume in the setting of increased afterload.[76] All of these findings may be related to the immaturity of the myocardium with inherent diastolic dysfunction, which is partly due to paucity of contractile tissue, disorganized myofibrillar arrangement, and immature calcium handling.[77–79]

Cardiac Output and Distribution

In postnatal life, the right and left ventricles operate in series and their output is approximately equal; consequently, cardiac output is defined through measurements of output from either ventricle. However, in the fetus, the systemic circulation receives blood from both the left and right ventricle in parallel (i.e., the sum of the right and left ventricular outputs, except for a proportion of the right ventricular output that is delivered to the fetal lungs). At mid-gestation, the combined ventricular output (CVO) is approximately 210 mL/min, and it increases to approximately 1900 mL/min at 38 weeks' gestation (500 mL/min/kg).[75,80,81] During fetal life, the right ventricular volume is greater than the left ventricular volume during both systole and diastole, but stroke volume does not differ significantly between the two ventricles.[70]

Fetal cardiac output is sensitive to changes in fetal heart rate. As heart rate increases, cardiac output increases. As fetal heart rate decreases, fetal stroke volume increases only slightly, in part because of low fetal myocardial compliance. Although fetal bradycardia results in an extended diastolic filling time, the stiff fetal cardiac ventricles have limited ability to distend. Therefore, fetal bradycardia is associated with a marked drop in fetal cardiac output.

In both fetal and adult animals, approximately equal volumes of blood are delivered to oxygen-uptake organs (i.e., the placenta before delivery, the lungs after delivery) and the oxygen-consuming organs. Earlier studies investigating the organ distribution of CVO in the fetus were based on experiments on instrumented animals. However, significant interspecies differences exist. Recently, Abduljalil et al.[82] collated available published data and applied mathematical physiologically based pharmacokinetic modeling and simulation to estimate the distribution of CVO to different organs and tissues in the human fetus at different gestational ages (Table 5.1). This knowledge is important because fetal organ blood flow delivers not only nutrients but also chemicals and medications to which the pregnant woman may be exposed, intentionally or unintentionally. The distribution of the CVO to fetal organs changes in certain conditions and disease states (e.g., hypoxia, hypovolemia, preeclampsia, diabetes, fetal growth restriction).[82] For example, in human fetuses the brain receives approximately 14% to 18% of CVO,[82] but this fraction may be increased during circumstances of decreased placental perfusion, acidosis, or increased PCO_2.

TABLE 5.1 **Fetal Organ and Tissue Blood Flows as Percentages of Combined Ventricular Output at Different Gestational Ages Estimated From Physiologically Based Pharmacokinetic Modeling of Available Data**

	20 Weeks' Gestation	30 Weeks' Gestation	38 Weeks' Gestation
Brain	13.9	16.1	17.5
Lungs	22	22	22
Adipose	5	5	5
Bone	5	5	5
Skin	1	1	1
Muscle	6	6	6
Heart	3	3	3
Kidneys	7.8	6.6	5.6
Gut	2.1	2	2.7
Spleen	0.3	0.3	0.4
Pancreas	1	1	1
Hepatic artery	0.8	0.8	1
Placenta	24	19	16

Data from Abduljalil K, Pan X, Clayton R, et al. Fetal physiologically based pharmacokinetic models: systems information on fetal cardiac output and its distribution to different organs during development. *Clin Pharmacokinet.* 2021;60:741–757.

Regulation of Fetal Circulation

The autonomic nervous system is present early in gestation and plays a critical role in maintaining cardiovascular homeostasis. In the fetal chick heart, evidence of cholinergic innervation occurs as early as 3 days after fertilization (average incubation, 22 days). In the mammalian heart, inotropic and chronotropic responses to adrenergic agents have been measured as early as 4 to 5 weeks' gestation,[83] and the fetal myocardial pacemaker can be inhibited at this time by the cholinergic agonists carbamylcholine and acetylcholine.[84]

Most studies indicate that the parasympathetic system appears earlier than the sympathetic system (8 weeks' gestation versus 9 to 10 weeks' gestation),[83,85,86] becomes more dominant as pregnancy progresses, and is more functionally complete at birth (Fig. 5.5). As a result, the baseline fetal heart rate is slower at term than at 26 weeks' gestation.

Both parasympathetic and sympathetic systems undergo significant maturation during postnatal life, and full maturation of the vagal response is not observed until 1 to 2 months after delivery.[87,88] Similarly, although the contractile response of the fetal vasculature is less functional than the adult response, the fetal administration of an alpha-adrenergic receptor agonist can result in the redistribution of blood flow away from the kidneys, skin, and splanchnic organs and toward the heart, brain, placenta, and adrenal glands.[89] At birth, the autonomic nervous system mediates changes in heart rate and peripheral vascular resistance, and a redistribution of blood flow.[83]

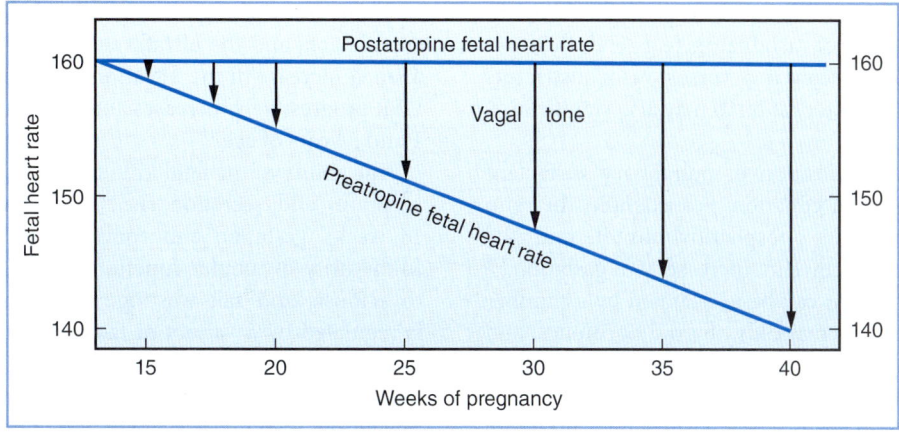

Fig. 5.5 The Growing Influence of the Parasympathetic Nervous System on Fetal Heart Rate as Gestation Progresses. This parasympathetic activity is reversible with administration of atropine. From Schifferli P, Caldeyro-Barcia R. Effects of atropine and beta-adrenergic drugs on the heart rate of the human fetus. In: Boréus LO, ed. *Fetal Pharmacology*. Raven Press; 1973:264.

Fetal cardiovascular function also adapts to varying metabolic and environmental conditions through regulation by the neurologic and endocrine systems. Most neuroregulation occurs in response to baroreceptor and chemoreceptor afferent input to the autonomic nervous system and through modulation of myocardial adrenergic receptor activity.

Arterial baroreceptor function has been demonstrated in several different fetal animal models. The predominant baroreceptors are located within the vessel walls of the aortic arch and at the bifurcations of the common carotid arteries. These receptors project signals to the vasomotor center in the medulla, from which autonomic responses emanate. The baroreceptors are functional early in fetal development and undergo continuous adaptation to the increases in blood pressure observed over time.[90] A sudden increase in fetal mean arterial pressure—as occurs with partial or complete occlusion of the umbilical arteries—results in cholinergic stimulation and subsequent fetal bradycardia.

Peripheral chemoreceptors are present within the vessel walls of the aortic arch and at the bifurcations of the common carotid arteries. In some animal species, peripheral chemoreceptors are transiently present in the adrenal glands but disappear after birth.[91] The fetal aortic chemoreceptors are responsive even to small changes in arterial oxygenation,[92,93] which contrasts with the less active fetal carotid chemoreceptors. Dawes et al.[94] concluded that the carotid chemoreceptors are important for postnatal respiratory control, whereas the aortic chemoreceptors are more involved in the control of cardiovascular responses and the regulation of oxygen delivery. Central chemoreceptors, located in the medulla oblongata, appear to play little if any role in fetal circulatory responses.

The neural control of the fetal circulation is far more dependent on chemoreceptor-mediated responses than in the adult circulation.[95] Acute fetal hypotension often stimulates a reflex response, which can include both bradycardia and vasoconstriction. Vasoconstriction is dependent on increases in both sympathetic autonomic activity and the rate of secretion of several vasoactive hormones, including arginine, vasopressin, renin, angiotensin, and aldosterone. Fetal bradycardia is most likely caused by activation of peripheral chemoreceptors.[95]

FETAL PULMONARY SYSTEM

The lungs begin as small, saccular outgrowths of the ventral foregut endoderm. Although sacculi with type I and II pneumocytes and ventilatory capacity are present during the last trimester, true alveoli develop at approximately 36 weeks' gestation. Most alveolar development occurs postnatally, within the first 6 to 18 months, when further maturation of the microvasculature and the air-blood barrier occurs.[96]

The pulmonary vasculature develops early in gestation, with continuity between its capillary plexus and the heart occurring as early as 34 days' gestation.[97,98] The size and number of pulmonary arteries and veins increases over time; however, vessel reactivity to local and hormonal influences is not detectable until after 20 weeks' gestation.[99,100] From 20 to 30 weeks' gestation, the growth in the size of the pulmonary vascular bed combined with a reduction in PVR results in greater pulmonary blood flow, from approximately 10% to 25% of the CVO. During this time, alterations in maternal oxygenation have no effect on the fetal pulmonary vasculature.[99,101] However, after 30 weeks' gestation, blood flow to the lungs decreases slightly owing to a significant increase in PVR, diminishing the fraction of CVO to approximately 20%.

After birth, with the onset of breathing, a significant reduction in PVR occurs and the pulmonary blood flow increases from 21% to 100% of cardiac output to enable gas exchange in the lungs.[102] A number of mechanical and molecular processes contribute to this perinatal pulmonary vasodilation. *In utero*, the fetal lungs are filled with fluid to maintain an appropriate level of expansion for normal pulmonary development.[103] The expulsion of lung liquid, particularly with a vaginal birth, likely decreases extraluminal pressure on the pulmonary vasculature and leads to a decrease in PVR.[104] Breathing movements, shear stress created by an abrupt surge in pulmonary blood flow, and the development of alveolar surface tension are other mechanical factors that can decrease PVR.[105] Finally, the relative predominance of vasodilators (e.g., endothelium-derived nitric oxide, prostacyclin) versus vasoconstrictors (e.g., platelet-activating factor) at birth may also significantly decrease PVR.[106,107]

The amount and composition of pulmonary surfactant changes over the course of gestation. For example, the ratio of phosphatidylglycerol to phosphatidylinositol, and the ratio of lecithin to sphingomyelin, increase with gestation.[108] Fetal surfactant production can be accelerated by a number of factors, including glucocorticoids, thyroid hormones, and autonomic neurotransmitters. A glucocorticoid surge in the last weeks of gestation is required for normal lung development.[109] In preterm birth, prior to this cortisol increase, there are low levels of surfactant with the subsequent development of infant respiratory distress syndrome (RDS). Consequently, the American College of Obstetricians and Gynecologists recommends a single course of corticosteroids for pregnant women between 24 and 34 weeks' gestation who are at risk for preterm delivery within 7 days.[110] In addition, there are recommendations to consider before and after these time intervals or for repeat dosing in select circumstances.

Antenatal corticosteroid treatment causes maturation of pulmonary epithelial cells, differentiation of type II cells, and activation of various components of surfactant (e.g., surfactant proteins and phospholipids); the treatment causes additional pulmonary alterations in the structural components, fluid metabolism, production of growth factors, and presence of antioxidant enzymes and adrenergic receptors. Maternal administration of glucocorticoids such as betamethasone or dexamethasone has been associated with a 35% to 40% reduction in RDS in preterm infants and a significant improvement in neonatal mortality.[111]

A relative disadvantage in respiratory morbidity and mortality of male infants born prematurely can be partially attributed to sex differences in surfactant production.[15,16] Higher levels of androgen and Müllerian-inhibiting substance in male fetuses adversely affect surfactant production, whereas estrogen promotes surfactant production in female fetuses.[16]

FETAL RENAL SYSTEM

Although fluid, electrolyte balance, and acid-base homeostasis are primarily regulated and maintained by the placenta, the fetal kidneys play an important role in fetal development through amniotic fluid production. Fetal glomeruli begin to develop at 8 to 9 weeks' gestation and start producing urine at 10 weeks' gestation, which contributes significantly to amniotic fluid production.[112,113] By 20 weeks' gestation, more than 90% of amniotic fluid is provided by the kidneys. Fetal oliguria and anuria can lead to lung hypoplasia and skeletal and tissue deformities (e.g., Potter sequence).[114] Glomerular filtration rate (GFR) increases over the course of gestation but remains low during fetal and early neonatal life. At birth, term newborns have a GFR of approximately 20 mL/min/1.73 m²,[115,116] which increases to approximately 50 mL/min/1.73 m² by 1 month of age.[116] This early increase in GFR is believed to result from a large increase in the glomerular capillary surface area and the ultrafiltration coefficient, together with a small increase in the filtration pressure.[117,118] Thereafter the GFR progressively increases and reaches adult levels between 1 and 2 years of age.[119]

The ability of the fetal kidneys to perform filtration, reabsorption, and secretion (i.e., tubular function) begins by 14 weeks' gestation and continues to develop postnatally. Immaturity of tubular function in preterm infants can lead to acidosis and salt wasting.[120,121] Renal function *in utero* is regulated by a variety of factors that control renal blood flow, glomerular filtration, and tubular function. The renin-angiotensin system is particularly important for normal fetal renal growth and development,[122] and maternal use of angiotensin-converting enzyme inhibitors or angiotensin receptor blockers is associated with renal agenesis and anomalies[123]; angiotensin II helps regulate blood pressure and the volume of fluid in the extravascular space.[124]

FETAL HEMATOLOGIC SYSTEM

Red blood cells, platelets, neutrophils, monocytes, and macrophages are all derived from a common progenitor cell.[125] In the developing embryo, hematopoiesis occurs at several anatomic sites in multiple waves. The first wave occurs in the yolk sac 30 days after conception and produces mostly primitive erythroid cells, but also macrophages and megakaryocytes.[126] The second wave also arises in the yolk sac but creates the same cells found in the adult human (i.e., erythroid, megakaryocyte, and several myeloid lineages). The third wave emerges from hematopoietic stem cells located within the major arteries of the embryo, yolk sac, and placenta. Hematopoietic stem cells migrate to the fetal liver and eventually seed the bone marrow, where they will reside for the remainder of life. The final wave of hematopoiesis produces all hematopoietic cell lineages, including B- and T-lymphocyte progenitor cells.[127,128]

Erythroid cells (red blood cells) are the first blood cells to develop. There are two developmentally and morphologically distinct erythroid lineages: primitive (embryonic) and definitive (adult). Cells of the primitive lineage support the transition from the rapidly growing embryo to fetus; primitive megaloblastic erythrocytes are much larger than definitive erythrocytes, express different globin genes, and differ in their oxygen-carrying capacity and response to low oxygen tension. By contrast, definitive erythrocytes are important during the transition from fetal to extrauterine life at birth. They are produced continuously from hematopoietic stem cells in the bone marrow and participate in a variety of normal physiologic processes throughout postnatal life.[125,129]

Fetal and adult human erythrocytes can be distinguished by their hemoglobin (hemoglobin F [HbF] and hemoglobin A [HbA]), respectively. The tetramer for HbF consists of two alpha (α) chains and two gamma (γ) chains ($\alpha_2\gamma_2$), whereas the tetramer for HbA includes two alpha (α) chains and two beta (β) chains ($\alpha_2\beta_2$). The gamma chain and the beta chain contain the same number of amino acids (146), but their sequences differ by a total of 39 amino acids.[130] The change

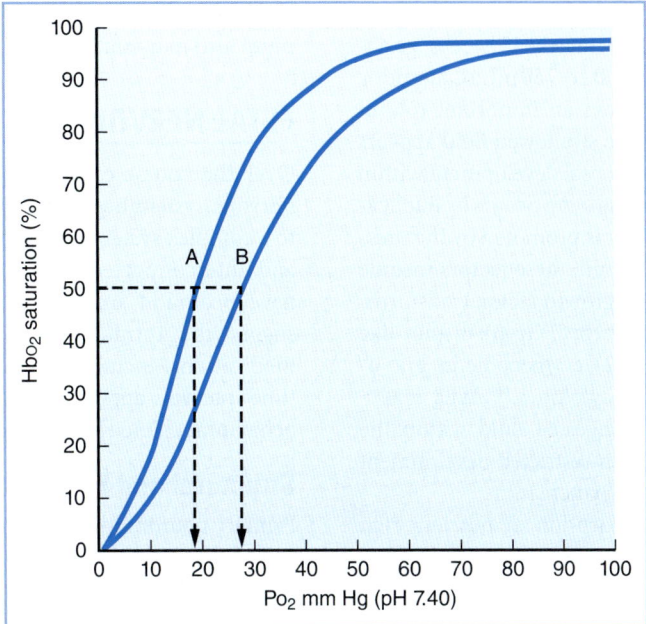

Fig. 5.6 Oxyhemoglobin Saturation Curves for Fetal (A) and Adult (B) Human Blood. The P_{50} is indicated by the *dashed vertical line*. Modified from Delivoria-Papadopoulos M, DiGiacomo JE. Oxygen transport. In: Polin RA, Fox WW, eds. *Fetal and Neonatal Physiology*. Vol 1. WB Saunders; 1992:807.

in expression from fetal to adult beta-globin genes begins at approximately 32 weeks' gestation and is completed after birth.[131]

HbF has a greater affinity for oxygen and a lower affinity for 2,3-diphosphoglycerate (DPG) and exhibits a leftward shift in the oxyhemoglobin dissociation curve compared with HbA (Fig. 5.6).[132] These differences result in greater arterial oxygen saturation in fetal versus maternal blood for any given arterial oxygen tension. This difference in oxygen affinity can be explained by a decreased interaction between the gamma chains of HbF and intraerythrocyte 2,3-DPG, the latter acting to lower oxygen affinity by binding and stabilizing the deoxygenated hemoglobin tetramer. As a consequence, 2,3-DPG decreases the oxygen affinity of HbF less than that of HbA.[133] Although fetuses and adults have similar intraerythrocyte 2,3-DPG concentrations, fetal blood exhibits a lower oxygen tension at which hemoglobin is 50% saturated (P_{50}). HbF levels begin to decrease toward the end of pregnancy, resulting in a corresponding increase in the P_{50}. At term, HbA accounts for approximately 25% of total hemoglobin, and the P_{50} is approximately 19 mm Hg (2.5 kPa).[134]

During the first few months of postnatal life, HbA levels increase, and 2,3-DPG concentration transiently increases above usual fetal and adult levels. Simultaneously, the affinity of neonatal blood for oxygen is equivalent to that of adult blood despite the persistence of 25% HbF.[132,134]

FETAL GASTROINTESTINAL SYSTEM

The gastrointestinal tract develops from the primitive digestive tube, which includes the foregut, midgut, and hindgut. The foregut receives its vascular supply from the celiac axis and gives origin to the oral cavity, pharynx, esophagus, stomach, and upper duodenum. The midgut, which receives its vascular supply from the superior mesenteric artery, develops into the distal duodenum, jejunum, ileum, cecum, appendix, and transverse colon. The hindgut receives its vascular supply from the inferior mesenteric artery, and it differentiates into the descending colon, the sigmoid colon, and the upper two-thirds of the rectum.[135] Intestinal villi appear by 7 weeks' gestation, and active absorption of glucose and amino acids occurs by 10 and 12 weeks' gestation, respectively.[136] Peristaltic waves and gastrointestinal motility are initiated by 8 weeks' gestation. Teniae, the three longitudinal ribbons of smooth muscle on the outside of the colon, appear by 12 weeks' gestation and contract to produce the haustra (bulges) in the colon.[137] In the small intestine, Auerbach and Meissner plexuses of parasympathetic nerves provide motor and secretomotor innervation, respectively; the two plexuses are present as early as 8 weeks' gestation.[136] Aggregations of lymphoid nodules (i.e., Peyer patches) develop by 20 weeks' gestation in the ileum.[138]

Although the fetal environment and neonatal gut were once believed to be sterile, *in utero* transmission of microbes from mother to infant likely occurs. Jiménez et al.[139] demonstrated that specific bacteria introduced to the gut of pregnant animals could be recovered in newborn meconium at the time of sterile cesarean delivery. Similarly in humans, Collado et al.[140] observed shared microbiota features in placental, amniotic fluid, and infant meconium samples obtained during elective cesarean delivery, suggesting *in utero* microbial gut colonization. The early-life microbiome is involved in immune system development, metabolic programming, neurodevelopment, and neonatal susceptibility to diseases.[141]

Swallowing

The fetus starts swallowing at approximately 15 weeks' gestation, and at term the fetus ingests 500 to 750 mL of amniotic fluid per day.[142] Fetal swallowing plays an important role in amniotic fluid homeostasis,[142] and the swallowed fluid appears to provide nutritional support for mucosal development within the gastrointestinal tract.[143] Intestinal growth occurs by duplication of intestinal crypts, a process that is promoted by the presence of trophic factors in amniotic fluid; these factors include epidermal growth factor, hepatocyte growth factor, transforming growth factor alpha (TGF-α) and beta (TGF-β), insulin-like growth factor-1 (IGF-1) and -2 (IGF-2), erythropoietin, granulocyte colony-stimulating factor, and cytokines.[144] Avila et al.[145] found that surgical obstruction of ingested fluid within the upper gastrointestinal tract resulted in restricted development of the gastrointestinal tract, liver, and pancreas.

The ingestion and intestinal absorption of nutrient-rich amniotic fluid also appear to play an important role in general fetal growth and development. In the fetal rabbit model, disorders of the upper gastrointestinal tract (e.g., esophageal obstruction, gastroschisis) lead to decreased intestinal nutrient absorption and decreased birth weight and crown-rump length.[146] Similar findings have been reported in human neonates with congenital esophageal atresia.[147]

Meconium

Meconium—which consists of water, intestinal secretions, squamous cells, lanugo hair, bile pigments, and blood—first appears in the fetal intestine between 10 and 12 weeks' gestation.[148] By 16 weeks' gestation, meconium moves into the colon.[149] Between 14 and 22 weeks' gestation, fetal colonic contents, as indicated by the presence of high levels of intestinal enzymes (e.g., disaccharidases, alkaline phosphatase), appear in the amniotic fluid.[150] After 22 weeks' gestation, a subsequent decline in the concentration of these gastrointestinal enzymes within the amniotic fluid is observed, which coincides with the development of anal sphincter tone.[150,151]

Meconium is continually cleared by fetal swallowing, leading to relatively clear amniotic fluid in most pregnancies. The presence of meconium-stained amniotic fluid may therefore represent either decreased clearance or increased passage of meconium, which is observed in the presence of fetomaternal stress factors such as hypoxia and infection, independent of fetal maturation.[148] Meconium-stained amniotic fluid occurs more frequently with advanced gestational age and is common in postterm pregnancies.[152]

Although many fetuses with meconium-stained amniotic fluid are born without adverse sequelae, meconium can have detrimental effects on fetal organs and the placenta. Meconium may cause umbilical cord vessel constriction, vessel necrosis, and the production of thrombi, which can lead to altered coagulation, cerebral palsy, and neonatal seizures.[153] In addition, meconium may reduce the antibacterial properties of amniotic fluid by altering zinc levels.[148] Fetal aspiration of meconium also may neutralize the action of surfactant, promote lung tissue inflammation through the activation of neutrophils, and possibly result in meconium aspiration syndrome (see Chapter 9). Finally, in the presence of perinatal hypoxia, meconium also may contribute to pulmonary hypertension.[148]

FETAL NERVOUS SYSTEM

Over the course of gestation, the human brain and central nervous system begin to develop from a few embryonic cells to a complex system in which billions of neurons are arranged and interconnected; small, seemingly minor changes may have profound implications. For example, animal studies suggest that intrauterine exposure to a variety of drugs and medications, including certain anesthetic agents, at specific time intervals appears to result in anatomic, functional, and behavioral changes following birth (see Chapter 10).

Structural and Functional Brain Development

Primary neuromodulation and neural tube formation occur by 4 weeks' gestation. By 8 weeks' gestation, the rostral end of the neural tube gives rise to the prosencephalon (forebrain), the mesencephalon (midbrain), and the rhombencephalon (hindbrain). These three segments further subdivide: the prosencephalon divides into the telencephalon and the diencephalon and the rhombencephalon divides into the metencephalon and myelencephalon. These five subdivisions establish the primary organization of the central nervous system.[154]

The human subplate, the developmental anlage of the cerebral cortex, develops between 13 and 15 postconceptional weeks as a temporary location for synapses with cortical and thalamic projections. The subplate layer disintegrates between 24 and 28 weeks' gestation. A significant increase in cortical development, organization, and synapse formation begins by 20 weeks' gestation and continues postnatally; during the third trimester alone, the cerebral cortex volume increases fourfold.[155,156]

The first fetal movements are witnessed near the end of the first trimester. These initial movements have simple patterns and originate from spontaneous discharges within the spine and brainstem. The fetal movements become more organized and complex as the pregnancy progresses, with higher brain centers modulating the activity of the brainstem and spine.

The exact onset of electrocortical activity is unknown, but electroencephalographic (EEG) activity can be recorded in preterm infants as early as 24 weeks' gestation. Fetal EEG activity differs from that in adults and is characterized by the presence of intermittent bursts of activity separated by periods of complete suppression. With maturation, these suppressed episodes become shorter and less frequent before completely disappearing in postnatal life. The early electrical activity within the nervous system controls several developmental processes, such as neuronal differentiation, migration, synaptogenesis, and formation of neuronal networks. For example, the initial spontaneous spinal and subcortical discharges are believed necessary for somatosensory development. As they elicit movements in the periphery, afferent signals establish topographic representation on the sensory cortex.[157–159]

Alterations in fetal brain and nervous system development can lead to major malformations.

Cerebral Metabolism

The immature brain, like the adult brain, relies mostly on oxidative metabolism to produce energy. Given the limited capacity for mitochondrial oxidative phosphorylation and the lower partial pressures of oxygen observed *in utero*, anaerobic glycolysis exhibits a greater role during this developmental period than after delivery.[160,161] In the presence of aerobic conditions, glucose is converted to pyruvic acid (glycolysis), which enters the Krebs cycle and the mitochondrial cytochrome system to create chemical energy.[162]

Although glucose represents the primary and predominant source of cerebral energy, the perinatal brain is uniquely capable of metabolizing other substrates, such as lactic acid and ketone bodies (e.g., β-hydroxybutyrate and acetoacetate). Lactic acid concentrations in the peripartum period are significantly elevated and may support over 50% of total cerebral oxidative metabolism in certain conditions such as hypoglycemia and hypoxia.[163,164] During hypoxic conditions, the fetal brain will also significantly decrease its energy consumption, as evidenced by fewer fetal movements and a slower EEG wave pattern.[165]

Cerebral Blood Flow

The development of the neural tube begins with formation of endothelium-lined vascular channels. By 10 weeks' gestation, an extensive network of leptomeningeal arteries covers the fetal brain, allowing vessels to sprout and penetrate the brain parenchyma. Subsequent vascular growth is most pronounced in rapidly developing areas of the brain.[160]

As described above, the fetal systemic circulation has unique features that ensure optimal oxygen delivery to the brain. The fetal circulatory system is much more sensitive to hypoxemia than that in the adult (Fig. 5.7).[166–168]

The redistribution of blood flow to the most actively developing regions of the fetal brain is at least partially the result of an adenosine-mediated mechanism. Adenosine, the breakdown product of adenosine triphosphate (ATP), accumulates during failure of ATP resynthesis and causes vasodilation of blood vessels and suppression of neuronal activity.[165] Other substances (e.g., nitric oxide, endogenous opioids, adrenomedullin) may also play a role in cerebral blood redistribution, but the exact mechanisms are incompletely understood.[169]

Nociception

Cutaneous sensory receptors are present in the human fetus at approximately 7 weeks' gestation, and a widespread network is established by 20 weeks' gestation. At term gestation, the density of cutaneous nociceptive receptors in the fetus is comparable to, and may even exceed, that of the adult. Although the development of sensory fiber-to-dorsal horn interneuron synapses has been reported to occur as early as 6 weeks' gestation,[170] differentiation of dorsal horn neurons begins at approximately 13 weeks' gestation; the laminar arrangement of dorsal horn neurons, replete with synaptic interconnections and neurotransmitter vesicles, is present in some regions of the spinal cord by 30 weeks' gestation.[171] At this time, the A-delta and C fibers make connections at the spinal cord level and with the surrounding dermatomes.

The neurons of the cerebral cortex develop by 20 weeks' gestation, and synaptogenesis of the thalamocortical connections is established between 20 and 24 weeks' gestation. Thalamocortical axons reach the somatosensory cortex at 24 to 26 weeks' gestation. Myelination of the pain pathways of the spinal cord and brainstem is completed during the second and third trimesters of gestation[172]; however, the process continues postnatally in other areas of the brain and in

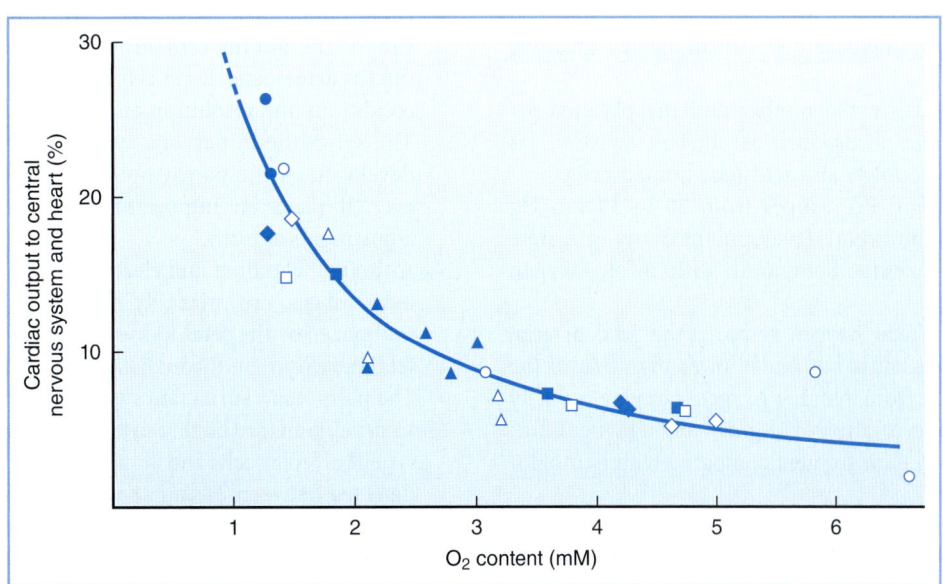

Fig. 5.7 The Redistribution of Cardiac Output to the Heart and Central Nervous System During Hypoxemia in Fetal Lambs. Each symbol represents a measurement from an individual fetal lamb. Modified from Sheldon RE, Peeters LLH, Jones MD Jr, et al. Redistribution of cardiac output and oxygen delivery in the hypoxic fetal lamb. *Am J Obstet Gynecol.* 1979;135:1071–1078.

peripheral nerve fibers. Although optimal pain processing requires myelination of pain pathways, cortical maturation, dendritic arborization, and thalamocortical fiber synaptogenesis, it is unclear when nociception, the capacity to feel pain, develops within the fetus. As early as 18 weeks' gestation, human fetuses demonstrate pituitary-adrenal, sympathoadrenal, and circulatory stress responses to noxious stimuli.[173–175] In studies of intrauterine blood transfusion in the human fetus, surgical needling of the intrahepatic vein (compared with needling of the insensate umbilical cord) is associated with evidence of a stress response, including increases in plasma beta-endorphin and cortisol levels and a diminution in the middle cerebral artery pulsatility index.[176] Administration of fentanyl 10 μg/kg blunts this stress response.[177]

The immaturity of thalamocortical connections before 25 weeks' gestation suggests that cortical processing of external input before 25 weeks' gestation is unlikely.[178] However, as early as 25 weeks' postmenstrual age, near-infrared spectroscopy has demonstrated cortical activity in response to noxious stimuli in preterm neonates.[179,180] Facial responses to painful stimuli (similar to those seen in adults) can be provoked in preterm neonates born and assessed as early as 25 weeks' gestation, which suggests the development of functional pathways from the spinal cord to the brain.[181,182] Nociceptive processing begins in the peripheral neurons, which relay signals through the spinothalamic tract, the thalamus, and ultimately the cerebral cortex, where conscious perception of pain occurs.[183] Current evidence suggests that fetal nociception at the level of the cortex occurs after the midpoint of pregnancy (i.e., between 24 and 30 weeks' gestation).

After birth, neonates appear to be more sensitive to pain, with lower pain thresholds, poor discriminative abilities, and a greater tendency to exhibit central sensitization in response to later noxious stimuli than adults. Early sensory experiences in the neonate can influence the development of nociceptive pathways.[184] Neonates and especially preterm infants who undergo numerous procedures in the neonatal intensive care unit and/or surgery have been observed to demonstrate altered pain perceptions later in life.[185] There is also evidence that early procedural pain is associated with thalamic development alterations in preterm neonates.[186] In the rodent model, tissue injury in early neonatal life results in an increased magnitude and duration of hyperalgesia after reinjury in later life, compared with those with no early-life pain experience.[184] Collectively, these observations have prompted some investigators to conclude that noxious events in neonates, when pain pathways are still undergoing a learning or "tuning process," may result in structural, functional, and behavioral alterations in adult pain processing. Some of these long-term consequences may be attenuated by preemptive analgesia.[187]

The foregoing neuroanatomic and neurochemical evidence, in addition to the well-characterized behavioral and physiologic responses to pain, indicate that both the fetus and newborn infant have nociceptive pathways capable of communicating nociceptive stimuli from the periphery to the cerebral cortex and regulating the response via efferent inhibitory pathways.

KEY POINTS

- Amniotic fluid serves several vital roles, including the facilitation of fetal and lung growth, the provision of a microgravity environment that cushions the fetus, and the generation of a defense mechanism against invading microbes.
- The fetus depends on the mother and the placenta for its basic metabolic needs, such as nutrient delivery, gas exchange, and electrolyte and acid-base homeostasis.
- Fetal arterial blood Po_2 ranges from 20 to 30 mm Hg (2.7 to 4.0 kPa), and fetal development exists in a state of relative hypoxemia compared with adult oxygen tension.
- Despite a lower fetal oxygen tension, the fetal arterial blood oxygen content is not much lower than that of the adult. This results from a higher oxygen-carrying capacity (hemoglobin concentration of 18 g/dL) and a higher affinity of hemoglobin F for oxygen, compared with hemoglobin A.
- The fetus produces approximately twice as much heat (on a weight-adjusted basis) and maintains a temperature 0.5 °C higher than the mother during the third trimester.
- The fetal circulation receives output from both the left and the right ventricle, with the ventricles working in parallel. Systemic blood flow consists of the sum of the right and left ventricular outputs, except for the small amount of blood delivered to the fetal lungs by the right ventricle.
- Fetal blood flow is characterized by three important shunts: the **ductus venosus**, the **foramen ovale**, and the **ductus arteriosus**. Birth is followed by changes in loading conditions and resolution of the fetal shunts.
- The sympathetic nervous system at birth is not as well developed as the parasympathetic nervous system; however, it plays an important role in the hemodynamic adjustments at birth.
- Although fetal fluid and electrolyte balance, and acid-base homeostasis, are primarily regulated and maintained by the placenta, the fetal kidneys play an important role in fetal development through amniotic fluid production.
- The pulmonary surfactant system is one of the last systems to develop before birth. Surfactant assembly occurs in the type II alveolar cells and components of surfactant are first detected between 24 and 28 weeks' gestation.
- Fetal hemoglobin has a greater oxygen affinity than adult hemoglobin, owing to a decreased interaction between hemoglobin F and 2,3-DPG. The P_{50} of fetal blood is significantly lower than that of adult blood.
- Fetal hypoxemia leads to a significant redistribution of cardiac output to the heart and the brain. This results

in both a global increase in cerebral blood flow and a redistribution of blood flow within the fetal brain.
- Fetal swallowing plays an important role in amniotic fluid homeostasis and the swallowed fluid appears to provide nutritional support for mucosal development within the gastrointestinal tract.

- The fetus has nociceptive pathways capable of communicating painful stimuli from the periphery to the cerebral cortex. Current evidence suggests that fetal nociception at the level of the cortex occurs after the midpoint of pregnancy (i.e., between 24 and 30 weeks' gestation).

REFERENCES

1. Underwood MA, Gilbert WM, Sherman MP. Amniotic fluid: not just fetal urine anymore. *J Perinatol.* 2005;25:341–348.
2. Prat C, Blanchon L, Borel V, et al. Ontogeny of aquaporins in human fetal membranes. *Biol Reprod.* 2012;86:48.
3. Brace RA, Wolf EJ. Normal amniotic fluid volume changes throughout pregnancy. *Am J Obstet Gynecol.* 1989;161:382–388.
4. Gilbert WM, Brace RA. Amniotic fluid volume and normal flows to and from the amniotic cavity. *Semin Perinatol.* 1993;17:150–157.
5. Gillibrand PN. Changes in the electrolytes, urea and osmolality of the amniotic fluid with advancing pregnancy. *J Obstet Gynaecol Br Commonw.* 1969;76:898–905.
6. Espinoza J, Chaiworapongsa T, Romero R, et al. Antimicrobial peptides in amniotic fluid: defensins, calprotectin and bacterial/permeability-increasing protein in patients with microbial invasion of the amniotic cavity, intra-amniotic inflammation, preterm labor and premature rupture of membranes. *J Matern Fetal Neonatal Med.* 2003;13:2–21.
7. Kramer K, Cohen HJ. Intrauterine fetal diagnosis for hematologic and other congenital disorders. *Clin Lab Med.* 1999;19:239–253.
8. Wilson RD. Amniocentesis and chorionic villus sampling. *Curr Opin Obstet Gynecol.* 2000;12:81–86.
9. Lewis PS, Lauria MR, Dzieczkowski J, et al. Amniotic fluid lamellar body count: cost-effective screening for fetal lung maturity. *Obstet Gynecol.* 1999;93:387–391.
10. Dubin SB. Assessment of fetal lung maturity. Practice parameter. *Am J Clin Pathol.* 1998;110:723–732.
11. Michetti F, Gazzolo D. S100B protein in biological fluids: a tool for perinatal medicine. *Clin Chem.* 2002;48:2097–2104.
12. Hui L, Bianchi DW. Cell-free fetal nucleic acids in amniotic fluid. *Hum Reprod Update.* 2011;17:362–371.
13. Klemmt PA, Vafaizadeh V, Groner B. The potential of amniotic fluid stem cells for cellular therapy and tissue engineering. *Expert Opin Biol Ther.* 2011;11:1297–1314.
14. Shaw SW, David AL, De Coppi P. Clinical applications of prenatal and postnatal therapy using stem cells retrieved from amniotic fluid. *Curr Opin Obstet Gynecol.* 2011;23:109–116.
15. Carter AM. Placental gas exchange and the oxygen supply to the fetus. *Compr Physiol.* 2015;5:1381–1403.
16. Fajersztajn L, Veras MM. Hypoxia: from placental development to fetal programming. *Birth Defects Res.* 2017;109:1377–1385.
17. Vali P, Lakshminrusimha S. The fetus can teach us: oxygen and the pulmonary vasculature. *Children (Basel).* 2017;4:67.
18. Rudolph A. *Congenital Diseases of the Heart: Clinical-Physiological Considerations.* 3rd ed. Wiley-Blackwell; 2009:1–24.
19. Burton GJ, Watson AL, Hempstock J, et al. Uterine glands provide histiotrophic nutrition for the human fetus during the first trimester of pregnancy. *J Clin Endocrinol Metab.* 2002;87:2954–2959.
20. Foidart JM, Hustin J, Dubois M, Schaaps JP. The human placenta becomes haemochorial at the 13th week of pregnancy. *Int J Dev Biol.* 1992;36:451–453.
21. Rodesch F, Simon P, Donner C, Jauniaux E. Oxygen measurements in endometrial and trophoblastic tissues during early pregnancy. *Obstet Gynecol.* 1992;80:283–285.
22. Schneider H. Oxygenation of the placental-fetal unit in humans. *Respir Physiol Neurobiol.* 2011;178:51–58.
23. Forristal CE, Wright KL, Hanley NA, et al. Hypoxia inducible factors regulate pluripotency and proliferation in human embryonic stem cells cultured at reduced oxygen tensions. *Reproduction.* 2010;139:85–97.
24. Jauniaux E, Watson A, Burton G. Evaluation of respiratory gases and acid-base gradients in human fetal fluids and uteroplacental tissue between 7 and 16 weeks' gestation. *Am J Obstet Gynecol.* 2001;184:998–1003.
25. Carter AM. Placental oxygen consumption. Part I: in vivo studies – a review. *Placenta.* 2000;21:S31–S37.
26. van Patot MC, Ebensperger G, Gassmann M, Llanos AJ. The hypoxic placenta. *High Alt Med Biol.* 2012;13:176–184.
27. Kay HH, Zhu S, Tsoi S. Hypoxia and lactate production in trophoblast cells. *Placenta.* 2007;28:854–860.
28. Patterson AJ, Zhang L. Hypoxia and fetal heart development. *Curr Mol Med.* 2010;10:653–666.
29. Kalhan SC, D'Angelo LJ, Savin SM, Adam PA. Glucose production in pregnant women at term gestation. Sources of glucose for human fetus. *J Clin Invest.* 1979;63:388–394.
30. Hay WW Jr. Placental-fetal glucose exchange and fetal glucose metabolism. *Trans Am Clin Climatol Assoc.* 2006;117:321–339.
31. Hauguel S, Desmaizieres V, Challier JC. Glucose uptake, utilization, and transfer by the human placenta as functions of maternal glucose concentration. *Pediatr Res.* 1986;20:269–273.
32. Hay WW Jr, Sparks JW, Wilkening RB, et al. Fetal glucose uptake and utilization as functions of maternal glucose concentration. *Am J Physiol.* 1984;246:E237–E242.
33. Gresham EL, James EJ, Raye JR, et al. Production and excretion of urea by the fetal lamb. *Pediatrics.* 1972;50:372–379.
34. Burd LI, Jones MD Jr, Simmons MA, et al. Placental production and foetal utilisation of lactate and pyruvate. *Nature.* 1975;254:710–711.
35. Battaglia FC, Meschia G. *An Introduction to Fetal Physiology.* Academic Press; 1986.
36. Gardner DS, Giussani DA, Fowden AL. Hindlimb glucose and lactate metabolism during umbilical cord compression and acute hypoxemia in the late-gestation ovine fetus. *Am J Physiol Regul Integr Comp Physiol.* 2003;284:R954–R964.
37. Sparks JW, Hay WW Jr, Bonds D, et al. Simultaneous measurements of lactate turnover rate and umbilical lactate uptake in the fetal lamb. *J Clin Invest.* 1982;70:179–192.

38. Palacin M, Lasuncion MA, Herrera E. Lactate production and absence of gluconeogenesis from placental transferred substrates in fetuses from fed and 48-H starved rats. *Pediatr Res.* 1987;22:6–10.

39. Shambaugh GE, Mrozak SC, Freinkel N. Fetal fuels. I. Utilization of ketones by isolated tissues at various stages of maturation and maternal nutrition during late gestation. *Metabolism.* 1977;26:623–635.

40. Power GG, Schroder H, Gilbert RD. Measurement of fetal heat production using differential calorimetry. *J Appl Physiol Respir Environ Exerc Physiol.* 1984;57:917–922.

41. Power GG, Blood AB. Perinatal thermal physiology. In: Polin RA, Fox MD, Abman SH, eds. *Fetal and Neonatal Physiology.* Saunders; 2011:615–624.

42. Asakura H. Fetal and neonatal thermoregulation. *J Nippon Med Sch.* 2004;71:360–370.

43. Gilbert RD, Schroder H, Kawamura T, et al. Heat transfer pathways between fetal lamb and ewe. *J Appl Physiol Respir Environ Exerc Physiol.* 1985;59:634–638.

44. Morishima HO, Yeh MN, Niemann WH, James LS. Temperature gradient between fetus and mother as an index for assessing intrauterine fetal condition. *Am J Obstet Gynecol.* 1977;129:443–448.

45. Kubonoya K, Yoneyama Y, Sawa R, et al. Brain temperature and metabolic responses during umbilical cord occlusion in fetal sheep. *Pflugers Arch.* 1998;436:667–672.

46. Rooth G, Huch A, Huch R, Peltonen R. Fetal-maternal temperature differences during labour. *Contrib Gynecol Obstet.* 1977;3:54–62.

47. Suzuki S, Murata T, Jiang L, Power GG. Hyperthermia prevents metabolic and cerebral flow responses to hypoxia in the fetal sheep. *J Soc Gynecol Investig.* 2000;7:45–50.

48. Kiserud T, Rasmussen S, Skulstad S. Blood flow and the degree of shunting through the ductus venosus in the human fetus. *Am J Obstet Gynecol.* 2000;182:147–153.

49. Prsa M, Sun L, van Amerom J, et al. Reference ranges of blood flow in the major vessels of the normal human fetal circulation at term by phase-contrast magnetic resonance imaging. *Circ Cardiovasc Imaging.* 2014;7:663–670.

50. Lakshminrusimha S, Saugstad OD. The fetal circulation, pathophysiology of hypoxemic respiratory failure and pulmonary hypertension in neonates, and the role of oxygen therapy. *J Perinatol.* 2016;36(suppl 2):S3–S11.

51. Teitel DF. Circulatory adjustments to postnatal life. *Semin Perinatol.* 1988;12:96–103.

52. Teitel DF, Iwamoto HS, Rudolph AM. Effects of birth-related events on central blood flow patterns. *Pediatr Res.* 1987;22:557–566.

53. Smith GC. The pharmacology of the ductus arteriosus. *Pharmacol Rev.* 1998;50:35–58.

54. Nakanishi T, Gu H, Hagiwara N, Momma K. Mechanisms of oxygen-induced contraction of ductus arteriosus isolated from the fetal rabbit. *Circ Res.* 1993;72:1218–1228.

55. Clyman RI. Mechanisms regulating the ductus arteriosus. *Biol Neonate.* 2006;89:330–335.

56. Seidner SR, Chen YQ, Oprysko PR, et al. Combined prostaglandin and nitric oxide inhibition produces anatomic remodeling and closure of the ductus arteriosus in the premature newborn baboon. *Pediatr Res.* 2001;50:365–373.

57. Clyman RI, Chan CY, Mauray F, et al. Permanent anatomic closure of the ductus arteriosus in newborn baboons: the roles of postnatal constriction, hypoxia, and gestation. *Pediatr Res.* 1999;45:19–29.

58. Levin M, McCurnin D, Seidner SR, et al. Postnatal constriction, ATP depletion, and cell death in the mature and immature ductus arteriosus. *Am J Physiol Regul Integr Comp Physiol.* 2006;290:R359–R364.

59. Waleh N, Seidner S, McCurnin D, et al. Anatomic closure of the premature patent ductus arteriosus: the role of CD14+/CD163+ mononuclear cells and VEGF in neointimal mound formation. *Pediatr Res.* 2011;70:332–338.

60. Echtler K, Stark K, Lorenz M, et al. Platelets contribute to postnatal occlusion of the ductus arteriosus. *Nat Med.* 2010;16:75–82.

61. Brace RA. Fetal blood volume responses to intravenous saline solution and dextran. *Am J Obstet Gynecol.* 1983;147:777–781.

62. Brace RA. Regulation of blood volume in utero. In: Hanson MA, Spencer JAD, Rodeck CH, eds. *Fetus and Neonate Physiology and Clinical Applications.* Cambridge University Press; 1993:75–99.

63. Faber JJ, Anderson DF. The placenta in the integrated physiology of fetal volume control. *Int J Dev Biol.* 2010;54:391–396.

64. Kiserud T. Physiology of the fetal circulation. *Semin Fetal Neonatal Med.* 2005;10:493–503.

65. Adamson SL, Morrow RJ, Bull SB, Langille BL. Vasomotor responses of the umbilical circulation in fetal sheep. *Am J Physiol.* 1989;256:R1056–R1062.

66. Adamson SL, Whiteley KJ, Langille BL. Pulsatile pressure-flow relations and pulse-wave propagation in the umbilical circulation of fetal sheep. *Circ Res.* 1992;70:761–772.

67. Kiserud T, Acharya G. The fetal circulation. *Prenat Diagn.* 2004;24:1049–1059.

68. Posterino GS, Dunn SL, Botting KJ, et al. Changes in cardiac troponins with gestational age explain changes in cardiac muscle contractility in the sheep fetus. *J Appl Physiol.* 2011;111:236–243.

69. Burrell JH, Boyn AM, Kumarasamy V, et al. Growth and maturation of cardiac myocytes in fetal sheep in the second half of gestation. *Anat Rec A Discov Mol Cell Evol Biol.* 2003;274:952–961.

70. Hamill N, Yeo L, Romero R, et al. Fetal cardiac ventricular volume, cardiac output, and ejection fraction determined with 4-dimensional ultrasound using spatiotemporal image correlation and virtual organ computer-aided analysis. *Am J Obstet Gynecol.* 2011;205:76.e1–e10.

71. Elmstedt N, Ferm-Widlund K, Lind B, et al. Fetal cardiac muscle contractility decreases with gestational age: a color-coded tissue velocity imaging study. *Cardiovasc Ultrasound.* 2012;10:19.

72. Miranda JO, Cerqueira RJ, Ramalho C, et al. Fetal cardiac function in maternal diabetes: a conventional and speckle-tracking echocardiographic study. *J Am Soc Echocardiogr.* 2018;31:333–341.

73. Sarvari SI, Rodriguez-Lopez M, Nuñez-Garcia M, et al. Persistence of cardiac remodeling in preadolescents with fetal growth restriction. *Circ Cardiovasc Imaging.* 2017;10:e005270.

74. Thornburg KL, Morton MJ. Filling and arterial pressures as determinants of RV stroke volume in the sheep fetus. *Am J Physiol.* 1983;244:H656–H663.

75. Gilbert RD. Control of fetal cardiac output during changes in blood volume. *Am J Physiol.* 1980;238:H80–H86.

76. Hawkins J, Van Hare GF, Schmidt KG, Rudolph AM. Effects of increasing afterload on left ventricular output in fetal lambs. *Circ Res.* 1989;65:127–134.

77. Friedman WF. The intrinsic physiologic properties of the developing heart. *Prog Cardiovasc Dis.* 1972;15:87–111.

78. Sheridan DJ, Cullen MJ, Tynan MJ. Qualitative and quantitative observations on ultrastructural changes during postnatal development in the cat myocardium. *J Mol Cell Cardiol.* 1979;11:1173–1181.

79. Smolich JJ. Ultrastructural and functional features of the developing mammalian heart: a brief overview. *Reprod Fertil Dev.* 1995;7:451–461.

80. Anderson DF, Bissonnette JM, Faber JJ, Thornburg KL. Central shunt flows and pressures in the mature fetal lamb. *Am J Physiol.* 1981;241:H60–H66.

81. Rudolph AM, Heymann MA. Circulatory changes during growth in the fetal lamb. *Circ Res.* 1970;26:289–299.

82. Abduljalil K, Pan X, Clayton R, et al. Fetal physiologically based pharmacokinetic models: systems information on fetal cardiac output and its distribution to different organs during development. *Clin Pharmacokinet.* 2021;60:741–757.

83. Papp JG. Autonomic responses and neurohumoral control in the human early antenatal heart. *Basic Res Cardiol.* 1988;83:2–9.

84. Long WA, Henry GW. Autonomic and central neuroregulation of fetal cardiovascular function. In: Polin RA, Fox WW, eds. *Fetal and Neonatal Physiology.* WB Saunders; 1992.

85. Smith RB. The development of the intrinsic innervation of the human heart between the 10 and 70 mm stages. *J Anat.* 1970;107:271–279.

86. Taylor IM, Smith RB. Cholinesterase activity in the human fetal heart between the 35- and 160-millimeter crown-rump length stages. *J Histochem Cytochem.* 1971;19:498–503.

87. Hata T, Matsuura H, Miyata M, et al. Autonomic modulation of sinus and atrioventricular nodes in premature low-birth-weight infants. *Pacing Clin Electrophysiol.* 2005;28:S288–S291.

88. Pickoff AS, Rios R, Stolfi A, Wang SN. Postnatal maturation of the response of the canine sinus node to critically timed, brief vagal stimulation. *Pediatr Res.* 1994;35:55–61.

89. Lorijn RH, Longo LD. Norepinephrine elevation in the fetal lamb: oxygen consumption and cardiac output. *Am J Physiol.* 1980;239:R115–R122.

90. Blanco CE, Dawes GS, Hanson MA, McCooke HB. Studies of carotid baroreceptor afferents in fetal and newborn lambs. In: Jones CT, Nathanielsz PW, eds. *The Physiological Development of the Fetus and Newborn.* Academic Press; 1985:596–598.

91. Long WA. Developmental pulmonary circulatory physiology. In: Long WA, ed. *Fetal and Neonatal Cardiology.* WB Saunders; 1990.

92. Boekkooi PF, Baan J Jr, Teitel D, Rudolph AM. Chemoreceptor responsiveness in fetal sheep. *Am J Physiol.* 1992;263:H162–H167.

93. Walker AM. Physiological control of the fetal cardiovascular system. In: Beard RW, Nathanielsz PW, eds. *Fetal Physiology and Medicine.* Marcel Dekker; 1984:287–316.

94. Dawes GS, Duncan SL, Lewis BV, et al. Cyanide stimulation of the systemic arterial chemoreceptors in foetal lambs. *J Physiol.* 1969;201:117–128.

95. Wood CE, Tong H. Central nervous system regulation of reflex responses to hypotension during fetal life. *Am J Physiol.* 1999;277:R1541–R1552.

96. Langston C, Kida K, Reed M, Thurlbeck WM. Human lung growth in late gestation and in the neonate. *Am Rev Respir Dis.* 1984;129:607–613.

97. Hall SM, Hislop AA, Haworth SG. Origin, differentiation, and maturation of human pulmonary veins. *Am J Respir Cell Mol Biol.* 2002;26:333–340.

98. Hall SM, Hislop AA, Pierce CM, Haworth SG. Prenatal origins of human intrapulmonary arteries: formation and smooth muscle maturation. *Am J Respir Cell Mol Biol.* 2000;23:194–203.

99. Rasanen J, Wood DC, Debbs RH, et al. Reactivity of the human fetal pulmonary circulation to maternal hyperoxygenation increases during the second half of pregnancy: a randomized study. *Circulation.* 1998:257–262.

100. Lewis AB, Heymann MA, Rudolph AM. Gestational changes in pulmonary vascular responses in fetal lambs in utero. *Circ Res.* 1976;39:536–541.

101. Rasanen J, Wood DC, Weiner S, et al. Role of the pulmonary circulation in the distribution of human fetal cardiac output during the second half of pregnancy. *Circulation.* 1996;94:1068–1073.

102. Gao Y, Cornfield DN, Stenmark KR, et al. Unique aspects of the developing lung circulation: structural development and regulation of vasomotor tone. *Pulm Circ.* 2016;6:407–425.

103. Hooper SB, Wallace MJ. Role of the physicochemical environment in lung development. *Clin Exp Pharmacol Physiol.* 2006;33:273–279.

104. Polglase GR, Wallace MJ, Morgan DL, Hooper SB. Increases in lung expansion alter pulmonary hemodynamics in fetal sheep. *J Appl Physiol.* 2006;101:273–282.

105. Gao Y, Raj JU. Regulation of the pulmonary circulation in the fetus and newborn. *Physiol Rev.* 2010;90:1291–1335.

106. Ibe BO, Hillyard RM, Raj JU. Heterogeneity in prostacyclin and thromboxane synthesis in ovine pulmonary vascular tree: effect of age and oxygen tension. *Exp Lung Res.* 1996;22:351–374.

107. Ibe BO, Portugal AM, Chaturvedi S, Raj JU. Oxygen-dependent PAF receptor binding and intracellular signaling in ovine fetal pulmonary vascular smooth muscle. *Am J Physiol Lung Cell Mol Physiol.* 2005;288:L879–L886.

108. Orgeig S, Morrison JL, Daniels CB. Prenatal development of the pulmonary surfactant system and the influence of hypoxia. *Respir Physiol Neurobiol.* 2011;178:129–145.

109. Lockwood CJ, Radunovic N, Nastic D, et al. Corticotropin-releasing hormone and related pituitary-adrenal axis hormones in fetal and maternal blood during the second half of pregnancy. *J Perinat Med.* 1996;24:243–251.

110. American College of Obstetrician and Gynecologists Committee on Obstetric Practice. Committee opinion No. 713: Antenatal corticosteroid therapy for fetal maturation (reaffirmed 2024). *Obstet Gynecol.* 2017;130:e102–e109.

111. Roberts D, Dalziel S. Antenatal corticosteroids for accelerating fetal lung maturation for women at risk of preterm birth. *Cochrane Database Syst Rev.* 2006;(3):CD004454.

112. Muller F, Dommergues M, Bussières L, et al. Development of human renal function: reference intervals for 10 biochemical markers in fetal urine. *Clin Chem.* 1996;42:1855–1860.

113. Moritz KM, Macris M, Talbo G, Wintour EM. Foetal fluid balance and hormone status following nephrectomy in the foetal sheep. *Clin Exp Pharmacol Physiol.* 1999;26:857–864.

114. Cuckow PM, Nyirady P, Winyard PJ. Normal and abnormal development of the urogenital tract. *Prenat Diagn.* 2001;21:908–916.

115. Vogtm BA, Dell KM. The kidney and the urinary tract. In: Martin RJ, Fanaroff AA, Walsh ML, eds. *Fanaroff and Martin's Neonatal Perinatal Medicine.* 11th ed. Elsevier; 2020:1871–1896.

116. Hunley TE, Kon V. Ichiwaka J. Glomerular circulation and function. In: Avner ED, Harmon WE, Niaudet P, Yoshiwaka N, eds. *Pediatric Nephrology.* 6th ed. Springer; 2009:31–64.

117. Turner AJ, Brown RD, Carlström M, et al. Mechanisms of neonatal increase in glomerular filtration rate. *Am J Physiol Regul Integr Comp Physiol*. 2008;295:R916–R921.

118. Guignard JP, Gouyon JB. Glomerular filtration rate in neonates. In: Polin RA, ed. *Nephrology and Fluid Electrolyte Physiology*. Saunders; 2008:1681–1704.

119. Hoseini R, Otukesh H, Rahimzadeh N, Hoseini S. Glomerular function in neonates. *Iran J Kidney Dis*. 2012;6:166–172.

120. Haycock GB, Aperia A. Salt and the newborn kidney. *Pediatr Nephrol*. 1991;5:65–70.

121. Baum M, Quigley R. Ontogeny of proximal tubule acidification. *Kidney Int*. 1995;48:1697–1704.

122. Gomez RA, Norwood VF. Developmental consequences of the renin-angiotensin system. *Am J Kidney Dis*. 1995;26:409–431.

123. Botelho Lourenço EL, Lima Ribeiro RC, Araújo VO, et al. Fetopathies associated with exposure to angiotensin converting enzyme inhibitor from *Tropaeolum majus* L. *Drug Chem Toxicol*. 2017;40:281–285.

124. Iwamoto HS, Rudolph AM. Effects of endogenous angiotensin II on the fetal circulation. *J Dev Physiol*. 1979;1:283–293.

125. Baron MH, Isern J, Fraser ST. The embryonic origins of erythropoiesis in mammals. *Blood*. 2012;119:4828–4837.

126. Laiosa MD, Tate ER. Fetal hematopoietic stem cells are the canaries in the coal mine that portend later life immune deficiency. *Endocrinology*. 2015;156:3458–3465.

127. Tavian M, Péault B. Embryonic development of the human hematopoietic system. *Int J Dev Biol*. 2005;49:243–250.

128. Dzierzak E, Speck NA. Of lineage and legacy: the development of mammalian hematopoietic stem cells. *Nat Immunol*. 2008;9:129–136.

129. Orkin SH, Zon LI. Hematopoiesis: an evolving paradigm for stem cell biology. *Cell*. 2008;132:631–644.

130. Perutz MF. The hemoglobin molecule. *Sci Am*. 1964;211:64–76.

131. Sankaran VG, Xu J, Orkin SH. Advances in the understanding of haemoglobin switching. *Br J Haematol*. 2010;149:181–194.

132. Delivoria-Papadopoulos M, McGowan JE. Oxygen transport and delivery. In: Polin RA, Fox WW, Abman SH, eds. *Fetal and Neonatal Physiology*. 4th ed. Elsevier Saunders; 2020:970–979.

133. Lorkin PA. Fetal and embryonic haemoglobins. *J Med Genet*. 1973;10:50–64.

134. Oski FA, Delivoria-Papadopoulos M. The red cell, 2,3-diphosphoglycerate, and tissue oxygen release. *J Pediatr*. 1970;77:941–956.

135. Ross AI. Organogenesis of the gastrointestinal tract. In: Polin R, Fox W, Abman S, eds. *Fetal and Neonatal Physiology*. 4th ed. Elsevier Saunders; 2011:1187–1197.

136. Grand RJ, Watkins JB, Torti FM. Development of the human gastrointestinal tract. A review. *Gastroenterology*. 1976;70:790–810.

137. Pace JL. The age of appearance of the haustra of the human colon. *J Anat*. 1971;109:75–80.

138. Cornes JS. Peyer's patches in the human gut. *Proc R Soc Med*. 1965;58:716.

139. Jiménez E, Marín ML, Martín R, et al. Is meconium from healthy newborns actually sterile? *Res Microbiol*. 2008;159:187–193.

140. Collado MC, Rautava S, Aakko J, et al. Human gut colonisation may be initiated in utero by distinct microbial communities in the placenta and amniotic fluid. *Sci Rep*. 2016;6:23129.

141. Walker RW, Clemente JC, Peter I, Loos RJF. The prenatal gut microbiome: are we colonized with bacteria in utero? *Pediatr Obes*. 2017;12:3–17.

142. Pritchard JA. Fetal swallowing and amniotic fluid volume. *Obstet Gynecol*. 1966;28:606–610.

143. Trahair JF, Harding R. Ultrastructural anomalies in the fetal small intestine indicate that fetal swallowing is important for normal development: an experimental study. *Virchows Arch A Pathol Anat Histopathol*. 1992;420:305–312.

144. Dasgupta S, Arya S, Choudhary S, Jain SK. Amniotic fluid: source of trophic factors for the developing intestine. *World J Gastrointest Pathophysiol*. 2016;7:38–47.

145. Avila CG, Harding R. The development of the gastrointestinal system in fetal sheep in the absence of ingested fluid. *J Pediatr Gastroenterol Nutr*. 1991;12:96–104.

146. Mulvihill SJ, Stone MM, Debas HT, Fonkalsrud EW. The role of amniotic fluid in fetal nutrition. *J Pediatr Surg*. 1985;20:668–672.

147. Jacobs DG, Wesson DE, Mago-Cao H, et al. Effect of esophageal ligation on the growth of fetal rabbits. *J Pediatr Gastroenterol Nutr*. 1989;8:245–251.

148. Ahanya SN, Lakshmanan J, Morgan BL, Ross MG. Meconium passage in utero: mechanisms, consequences, and management. *Obstet Gynecol Surv*. 2005;60:45–56.

149. Shwachman H, Antonowicz I. Studies on meconium. In: Lebenthal E, ed. *Textbook of Gastroenterology and Nutrition in Infancy*. Raven Press; 1981:81–93.

150. Potier M, Melancon SB, Dallaire L. Developmental patterns of intestinal disaccharidases in human amniotic fluid. *Am J Obstet Gynecol*. 1978;131:73–76.

151. Mulivor RA, Mennuti MT, Harris H. Origin of the alkaline phosphatases in amniotic fluid. *Am J Obstet Gynecol*. 1979;135:77–81.

152. Usher RH, Boyd ME, McLean FH, Kramer MS. Assessment of fetal risk in postdate pregnancies. *Am J Obstet Gynecol*. 1988;158:259–264.

153. Altshuler G, Arizawa M, Molnar-Nadasdy G. Meconium-induced umbilical cord vascular necrosis and ulceration: a potential link between the placenta and poor pregnancy outcome. *Obstet Gynecol*. 1992;79:760–766.

154. Stiles J, Jernigan TL. The basics of brain development. *Neuropsychol Rev*. 2010;20:327–348.

155. Kostović I. Structural and histochemical reorganization of the human prefrontal cortex during perinatal and postnatal life. *Prog Brain Res*. 1990;85:223–239.

156. Kostović I, Judas M. Transient patterns of cortical lamination during prenatal life: do they have implications for treatment? *Neurosci Biobehav Rev*. 2007;31:1157–1168.

157. Khazipov R, Sirota A, Leinekugel X, et al. Early motor activity drives spindle bursts in the developing somatosensory cortex. *Nature*. 2004;432:758–761.

158. Khazipov R, Luhmann HJ. Early patterns of electrical activity in the developing cerebral cortex of humans and rodents. *Trends Neurosci*. 2006;29:414–418.

159. Hellström-Westas L, Rosén I, Svenningsen NW. Cerebral function monitoring during the first week of life in extremely small low birthweight (ESLBW) infants. *Neuropediatrics*. 1991;22:27–32.

160. du Plessis AJ. Cerebral blood flow and metabolism in the developing fetus. *Clin Perinatol*. 2009;36:531–548.

161. Murthy MR, Rappoport DA. Biochemistry of the developing rat brain. II. Neonatal mitochondrial oxidations. *Biochim Biophys Acta*. 1963;74:51–59.

162. Vannucci S, Vannucci R. Perinatal brain metabolism. In: Polin R, Fox WA, Abman S, eds. *Fetal and Neonatal Physiology*. 4th ed. Elsevier; 2011.

163. Hernández MJ, Vannucci RC, Salcedo A, Brennan RW. Cerebral blood flow and metabolism during hypoglycemia in newborn dogs. *J Neurochem.* 1980;35:622–628.

164. Hellmann J, Vannucci RC, Nardis EE. Blood-brain barrier permeability to lactic acid in the newborn dog: lactate as a cerebral metabolic fuel. *Pediatr Res.* 1982;16:40–44.

165. Lutz PL. Mechanisms for anoxic survival in the vertebrate brain. *Annu Rev Physiol.* 1992;54:601–618.

166. Peeters LL, Sheldon RE, Jones MD Jr, et al. Blood flow to fetal organs as a function of arterial oxygen content. *Am J Obstet Gynecol.* 1979;135:637–646.

167. Jensen A, Roman C, Rudolph AM. Effects of reducing uterine blood flow on fetal blood flow distribution and oxygen delivery. *J Dev Physiol.* 1991;15:309–323.

168. Itskovitz J, LaGamma EF, Rudolph AM. Effects of cord compression on fetal blood flow distribution and O_2 delivery. *Am J Physiol.* 1987;252:H100–H109.

169. Pearce W. Hypoxic regulation of the fetal cerebral circulation. *J Appl Physiol.* 2006;100:731–738.

170. Okado N. Onset of synapse formation in the human spinal cord. *J Comp Neurol.* 1981;201:211–219.

171. Bijlani V, Rizvi TA, Wadhwa S. Development of spinal substrate for nociception in man. *NIDA Res Monogr.* 1988;87:167–179.

172. Gilles FJ, Shankle W, Dooling EC. Myelinated tracts: growth patterns. In: Gilles FJ, Leviton A, Dooling EC, eds. *The Developing Human Brain.* Wright & Co; 1983:117.

173. Giannakoulopoulos X, Teixeira J, Fisk N, Glover V. Human fetal and maternal noradrenaline responses to invasive procedures. *Pediatr Res.* 1999;45:494–499.

174. Gitau R, Fisk NM, Teixeira JM, et al. Fetal hypothalamic-pituitary-adrenal stress responses to invasive procedures are independent of maternal responses. *J Clin Endocrinol Metab.* 2001;86:104–109.

175. Teixeira J, Fogliani R, Giannakoulopoulos X, et al. Fetal haemodynamic stress response to invasive procedures. *Lancet.* 1996;347:624.

176. Giannakoulopoulos X, Sepulveda W, Kourtis P, et al. Fetal plasma cortisol and beta-endorphin response to intrauterine needling. *Lancet.* 1994;344:77–81.

177. Fisk NM, Gitau R, Teixeira JM, et al. Effect of direct fetal opioid analgesia on fetal hormonal and hemodynamic stress response to intrauterine needling. *Anesthesiology.* 2001;95:828–835.

178. Verriotis M, Chang P, Fitzgerald M, Fabrizi L. The development of the nociceptive brain. *Neuroscience.* 2016;338:207–219.

179. Slater R, Cantarella A, Gallella S, et al. Cortical pain responses in human infants. *J Neurosci.* 2006;26:3662–3666.

180. Bartocci M, Bergqvist LL, Lagercrantz H, Anand KJ. Pain activates cortical areas in the preterm newborn brain. *Pain.* 2006;122:109–117.

181. Whit Hall R, Anand KJS. Physiology of pain and stress in the newborn. *Neoreviews.* 2005;6:e61–e67.

182. Boyle EM, Freer Y, Wong CM, et al. Assessment of persistent pain or distress and adequacy of analgesia in preterm ventilated infants. *Pain.* 2006;124:87–91.

183. Fitzgerald M, Howard RF. The neurobiologic basis of pediatric pain. In: Schechter NL, Berde CB, Yaster M, eds. *Pain in Infants, Children and Adolescents.* 2nd ed. Lippincott Williams and Wilkins; 2003:19–42.

184. Beggs S, Currie G, Salter MW, et al. Priming of adult pain responses by neonatal pain experience: maintenance by central neuroimmune activity. *Brain.* 2012;135:404–417.

185. Derbyshire SW, Fitzgerald M. The painful consequences of neonatal nociceptive input. *Pain.* 2010;150:220–221.

186. Duerden EG, Grunau RE, Guo T, et al. Early procedural pain is associated with regionally-specific alterations in thalamic development in preterm neonates. *J Neurosci.* 2018;38:878–886.

187. Laprairie JL, Johns ME, Murphy AZ. Preemptive morphine analgesia attenuates the long-term consequences of neonatal inflammation in male and female rats. *Pediatr Res.* 2008;64:625–630.

6

Antepartum Fetal Assessment and Therapy

Anjali Kaimal, MD, MAS

Obstetric care involves antenatal assessment of the health of both the pregnant woman and the fetus. Routine fetal evaluations during pregnancy include the use of ultrasonography for determining gestational age or assessing fetal growth and well-being, chorionic villus or amniotic fluid sampling for genetic analysis, and fetal heart rate (FHR) monitoring during labor. In the setting of maternal, fetal, or obstetric complications, additional assessment methods can help guide management. This chapter reviews the available tests and interventions to assess and attempt to improve fetal well-being prior to delivery.

FETAL ASSESSMENT IN ROUTINE PREGNANCY CARE

Determination of Gestational Age

Gestational age at delivery is an important factor affecting neonatal outcome. Accurate knowledge of gestational age is essential for risk assessment and providing appropriate care and counseling. In women with regular 28-day menstrual cycles, the mean duration of a singleton pregnancy is 280 days (40 weeks) from the first day of the last normal menstrual period. *Term pregnancy* is defined as the period from 37 weeks' (259 days') to 42 weeks' (294 days') gestation, with neonatal outcomes varying widely across this period. For this reason, the designations of *early term* (37 0/7 to 38 6/7 weeks' gestation), *full term* (39 0/7 to 40 6/7 weeks' gestation), and *late term* (41 0/7 to 41 6/7 weeks' gestation) were adopted.[1] Delivery prior to 37 weeks is considered preterm, with anticipated complications varying based on the gestational age at delivery. Evaluation of fetal growth, efficient use of screening and diagnostic tests,

appropriate initiation of fetal surveillance, and optimal timing of delivery all depend on accurate dating of the pregnancy.

Recommendations for determining the gestational age and estimated due date (EDD) have been established by the American College of Obstetricians and Gynecologists (ACOG), the Society for Maternal-Fetal Medicine (SMFM), and the American Institute of Ultrasound in Medicine.[2] Assigning the EDD by the first day of the last menstrual period (LMP) is limited by inaccurate recall, irregular cycle lengths, and variations in ovulation timing. Ultrasonographic measurement of the embryo or fetus can improve the accuracy of the EDD, particularly when performed earlier in pregnancy. Gestational age determination is most accurate when ultrasonographic measurement of the fetus or embryo is performed in the first trimester (up to and including 13 6/7 weeks' gestation). For pregnancies achieved by assisted reproductive technology, the EDD should be assigned based on the age of the embryo and the date of transfer. When the LMP is recorded and the first accurate ultrasonographic examination is performed, the EDD should be determined, communicated to the patient, and documented in the medical record. Once established, the EDD should rarely be revised, as discrepancies between gestational age and fetal measurements may indicate an abnormality in fetal growth, such as macrosomia or fetal growth restriction (FGR).[3]

In the first trimester, before 14 0/7 weeks' gestation, the crown-rump length (CRL) measurement should be used to establish or confirm the gestational age; in the second and third trimesters, biometric measurements (i.e., biparietal diameter, head circumference, femur length, abdominal circumference) should be used. Assessment of gestational age in the third trimester (after 28 0/7 weeks' gestation) is the least accurate.[2]

Guidelines for revising the EDD are based on the initial ultrasonographic examination. Before 9 0/7 weeks' gestation, if the CRL and LMP dating differ by more than 5 days, the EDD should be revised using the CRL measurement. Ultrasonographic and LMP dating difference greater than 7 days (between 9 0/7 and 15 6/7 weeks' gestation), greater than 10 days (between 16 0/7 and 21 6/7 weeks' gestation), greater than 14 days (between 22 0/7 and 27 6/7 weeks' gestation), and greater than 21 days (at greater than 28 0/7 weeks' gestation) should be revised based on the ultrasonographic examination.[2] Pregnancies without ultrasonographic examination confirmation or revision of the EDD before 22 0/7 weeks' gestation should be considered suboptimally dated.[2,4] These pregnancies may benefit from a follow-up ultrasonographic examination 3 to 4 weeks later to confirm gestational age and assess interval growth.

Screening for Chromosomal Changes in Pregnancy

The ACOG and the SMFM guidance regarding screening for chromosomal abnormalities in pregnancy states[5]: "Testing for chromosomal abnormalities should be an informed patient choice based on provision of adequate and accurate information, the patient's clinical context, accessible health care resources, values, interests, and goals. All patients should be offered both screening and diagnostic tests, and all patients have the right to accept or decline testing after counseling." Historically, the detection of trisomy 21 (Down syndrome), the most common chromosomal abnormality in live-born infants, was a major focus due to the difficulty in ultrasonographic diagnosis. The availability of prenatal chromosomal microarray and whole exome sequencing of amniocentesis or chorionic villus samples has increased the options for obtaining prenatal genetic information. Such testing can provide reassurance or confirmation of screened or tested conditions, inform decisions regarding pregnancy continuation, and assist in pregnancy and/or delivery planning.

Screening for chromosomal changes can be performed by analysis of serum placental analytes specific to the first or second trimester, or by analysis of cell-free DNA, which is released into the maternal circulation by the placenta. The inclusion of an ultrasonographic nuchal translucency measurement with first or first and second trimester serum placental analyte assessment further improves detection rates. Cell-free DNA testing is the most sensitive and specific test for the common fetal aneuploidies (trisomy 13, 18, 21) and can be performed after 9 to 10 weeks' gestation. No single test performs optimally in all clinical situations, and all screening tests have the potential for false-positive or false-negative results. Pretest counseling should incorporate information regarding the conditions for which screening can be performed, the test characteristics, specific aspects of the patient's history that may impact risk of chromosomal changes, the ability to complete testing, and the interpretation of the test results. All serum screening modalities are less accurate in multiple gestations, and not all testing options are available, particularly for higher-order multiple gestations.

Prenatal Diagnosis of Fetal Chromosomal Abnormalities

Definitive prenatal fetal genetic information can be obtained by diagnostic testing via **chorionic villus sampling** (CVS) or **amniocentesis**.[6] A needle is inserted into the uterus under ultrasonographic guidance to obtain fetal cells from a placental sample (for CVS, performed at 10 to 13 weeks' gestation) or amniotic fluid (for amniocentesis, performed at 15 weeks' gestation and beyond). Risks common to all invasive procedures include bleeding, infection, isoimmunization, and pregnancy loss. Women who are Rh negative should receive $Rh_0(D)$ immune globulin before or after the procedure. Although risk for vertical transmission of viral infections (e.g., hepatitis B, hepatitis C, human immunodeficiency virus) with invasive procedures is low,[7,8] the patient should be made aware of these risks as part of a shared decision-making process. The risk of pregnancy loss associated with CVS is approximately 1 in 500, while the risk of pregnancy loss associated with amniocentesis is between 1 in 500 and 1 in 900.[6]

A unique CVS consideration involves the interpretation of the genetic test results. Because the fetus and placenta arise from the same cell, it is assumed that the genetic complements are identical, but this is not always the case. **Confined placental mosaicism** refers to the situation in which the karyotype of the chorionic villus is a mosaic (i.e., it contains two or more populations of cells with different karyotypes, usually one normal and one trisomic) but the karyotype of the fetus is normal. If mosaicism is detected on a CVS sample, it may be necessary to repeat the fetal karyotype with amniocentesis to provide additional information and to test for uniparental disomy, if indicated. Confined placental mosaicism can be associated with increased risk of growth restriction and warrants additional monitoring.[9]

Routine Ultrasonography

An ultrasonographic examination is recommended for all pregnant women,[3,10] given its ability to accurately determine gestational age, viability, fetal number, and placental location, and screen for fetal structural abnormalities in the second trimester. Significant variability exists in the sensitivity of routine ultrasonographic examinations for the detection of fetal anomalies; in a large review of 36 studies with over 900,000 fetuses, the detection rate for fetal anomalies ranged from 15% to 80%.[11] The detection rates for fetal malformations are improved when the examination is performed by an experienced operator at a tertiary center.[12] Central nervous system and urinary tract abnormalities are easier to detect than cardiac anomalies, and imaging of all abnormalities is more difficult in patients with high body mass index.[13]

The indications for first-trimester ultrasonography, which is performed before 14 0/7 weeks' gestation, are different from those for second- and third-trimester ultrasonography.[3] The first trimester is the ideal time to establish gestational age, fetal number (i.e., singleton versus multiple gestation), and chorionicity. First-trimester ultrasonography between 11.5 and 14 weeks' gestation can include assessment of the nuchal translucency, which, when thickened, is associated with an increased risk for aneuploidy and certain anomalies, such as cardiac, abdominal wall, and diaphragmatic defects.

Some aspects of fetal anatomy can be assessed in the first trimester, but ideally, a detailed fetal anatomic survey is performed at 18 to 22 weeks' gestation in all pregnant women to assess for fetal growth and anatomy. Placental location in relation to the cervix should also be documented at this time. If placenta previa is identified at 18 to 22 weeks' gestation, serial ultrasonographic examinations should follow placental location because only about 10% of placenta previas identified in the second trimester persist to term.[14,15] Other ultrasonographic elements that should be examined include the umbilical cord (i.e., number of vessels, placental and fetal insertion) and amniotic fluid volume. In pregnancies at high risk for fetal cardiac anomalies or preterm birth, fetal echocardiography and cervical length measurements, respectively, may be indicated. Certain fetal anomalies (e.g., achondroplasia, duodenal atresia) may only become evident later in pregnancy as the fetus develops.

Assessment of Fetal Well-Being

During routine or indicated visits throughout pregnancy, fetal well-being is assessed by confirming the FHR and fetal movements (quickening). Typically reported by 18 to 20 weeks' gestation by nulliparous women and by 16 to 18 weeks' gestation by parous women, the presence of **fetal movements** is correlated with fetal health. Decreased fetal movement, which is often observed with increasing gestational age, smoking, low amniotic fluid volume, anterior placentation, and antenatal corticosteroid therapy, is associated with adverse pregnancy events (e.g., umbilical cord compromise, placental abruption, stillbirth). For these reasons, a subjective decrease in perceived fetal movements in the third trimester should prompt an immediate investigation.

Evaluation of Fetal Growth

First described by Leopold and Sporlin in 1894,[16] a systematic physical examination of the gravid abdomen can determine the size, presentation, and lie of the fetus. Although the value of an abdominal examination is limited in the setting of a small fetus, maternal obesity, multiple pregnancy, uterine fibroids, or polyhydramnios, it is safe, well tolerated, and likely to add information to assist in antepartum management. The uterus can be palpated above the pelvic brim at approximately 12 weeks' gestation. Thereafter, fundal height should increase by approximately 1 cm per week, reaching the level of the umbilicus at 20 to 22 weeks' gestation (Fig. 6.1). Between 20 and 32 weeks' gestation, the fundal height (in centimeters) is approximately equal to the gestational age (in weeks) in healthy women of average weight with an appropriately growing fetus. However, a wide range of values exists for normal fundal height measurements, and maximal fundal height occurs at approximately 36 weeks' gestation, after which the lower uterine segment elongates and the fetus drops into the pelvis. For these reasons, fundal height measurements alone fail to identify growth restriction in more than 50% of fetuses.[17]

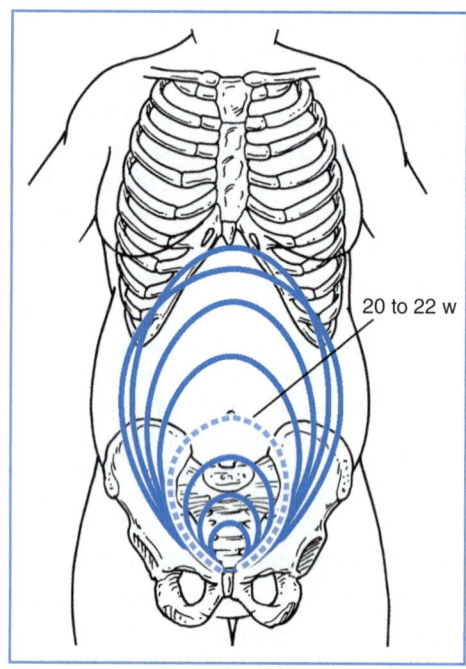

Fig. 6.1 Fundal height measurements in a singleton pregnancy with normal fetal growth.

If clinical findings suggest a fetal growth discrepancy between size and gestational age, ultrasonography is the modality of choice to evaluate alternative explanations, such as growth restriction, macrosomia, multifetal pregnancy, polyhydramnios, and uterine fibroids. FGR is associated with an increased risk of stillbirth as well as neonatal morbidity and mortality; once this diagnosis is made, management includes increasing antenatal surveillance and consideration for an earlier planned delivery.

Obstetric ultrasonography utilizes fetal measurements to estimate fetal weight; however, this approach has inherent limitations. First, regression equations used to create weight estimation formulas are derived primarily from cross-sectional data for infants delivered within an arbitrary period after the ultrasonographic examination. Second, growth curves for "normal" infants between 24 and 37 weeks' gestation rely on data collected from pregnancies delivered preterm, which may be complicated by some element of uteroplacental insufficiency, regardless of whether the delivery was spontaneous or indicated/iatrogenic. Third, ultrasonographic estimates of fetal weight are derived from mathematical formulas that use a combination of fetal measurements, most commonly the biparietal diameter, abdominal circumference, and femur length.[18] The abdominal circumference is the single most important measurement and is weighted more heavily in these formulas. Unfortunately, abdominal circumference is also the most difficult measurement to acquire, and small differences in the measured value result in large changes in the estimated fetal weight (EFW). A systematic review of ultrasonographic estimations of fetal weight found a significant margin of error, approximately 15%, across all studies.[19] Although the use of an intrauterine standard of EFW across gestation generally performed better than the use of a birthweight standard in predicting neonatal morbidity or mortality, neither significantly improved the accuracy of this detection.[20] Despite these limitations, ultrasonographic estimation of fetal weight with the use of an intrauterine growth standard remains the preferred approach for pregnancies at risk for growth restriction.[21]

Serial ultrasonographic evaluations of fetal weight are more useful than a single measurement in diagnosing abnormal fetal growth. The ideal interval for fetal growth evaluations is every 3 to 4 weeks; more frequent determinations may be misleading due to variations in the ultrasonographic measurements. However, in pregnancies complicated by growth restriction or fetal anomalies, evaluations can be performed as frequently as every 2 weeks. The use of customized fetal growth curves has not yet been shown to improve outcomes.[22]

Antepartum Fetal Testing

Antepartum fetal assessment is based on the theory that a change in fetal behavior can indicate a change in fetal status. With the goal of identifying the fetus at risk for preventable neurologic injury or death, antepartum fetal surveillance attempts to screen for neonatal hypoxemia and acidosis associated with infection, anemia, trauma, hypotension, or metabolic derangements. Testing cannot reliably predict or detect all causes of hypoxemia and acidosis, but those associated with progressive uteroplacental insufficiency are most likely to be identified. Antenatal fetal testing relies on the following assumptions: (1) progressive fetal asphyxia can lead to fetal death or permanent neurologic injury, (2) antenatal tests can discriminate between asphyxiated and nonasphyxiated fetuses, and (3) early detection of asphyxia with subsequent intervention can reduce the likelihood of an adverse perinatal outcome. Unfortunately, it is not clear whether these assumptions are reliable, and many adverse outcomes may not be anticipatable or preventable.

Despite these limitations, antepartum fetal testing, including the nonstress test (NST), biophysical profile (BPP), umbilical artery (UA) Doppler assessment, and contraction stress test (CST), are routinely used for high-risk pregnancies. While these tests can be used individually, given the wide variability in findings in normal and at-risk fetuses, a combination of testing modalities offers a more reliable assessment.[23]

Antepartum fetal tests should be interpreted in relation to the gestational age, presence or absence of congenital anomalies, and underlying clinical risk factors.[23] For example, a nonreassuring NST in a fetus with severe growth restriction at 32 weeks' gestation in the setting of heavy maternal vaginal bleeding has a much higher predictive value in identifying an adverse fetal outcome than an identical FHR tracing in a well-grown fetus at 40 weeks' gestation. The efficacy of antenatal fetal testing in preventing long-term neurologic injury has not been, nor will likely ever be, validated by prospective randomized clinical trials. Current recommendations rely predominantly on expert opinion and observational data.[24]

Nonstress Test

The fetal NST, also known as **fetal cardiotocography (CTG)**, investigates changes in the FHR pattern with time, reflecting the maturity of the autonomic nervous system; for this reason, it is less useful in the very preterm fetus (<28 weeks' gestation). The NST is noninvasive, simple to perform, inexpensive, and readily available in all obstetric units. Most obstetric care providers use the FHR interpretation criteria established in 1997, and updated in 2008, by the National Institute of Child Health and Human Development Research Planning Workshop (Table 6.1) (see Chapter 8).[25,26]

An NST is performed before the onset of labor via an externally placed Doppler ultrasound probe positioned on the maternal abdomen over the fetal heart. Sound waves emitted from the transducer are deflected by heart and heart valve movements. The shift in wave frequency is detected by a sensor and converted into a heart rate. The FHR is recorded for a period of 20 to 40 minutes during which the tracing is evaluated for the presence of periodic changes. Simultaneously, an external tocometer records myometrial tone, providing information about the timing and duration of contractions. The tocometer does not assess intrauterine pressure or the intensity of the contractions. A FHR tracing is designated *reactive* if there are two or more accelerations that peak (but do not necessarily remain) at least 15 bpm above the baseline for 15 seconds in a 20-minute period (Fig. 6.2).[25,26] In fetuses less than 32 weeks' gestation, FHR tracing is designated as reactive if there are two or more accelerations of at least 10 bpm above the baseline for 10 seconds. A reactive NST is regarded as evidence of fetal health.[27,28]

A nonreactive NST does not achieve sufficient accelerations within a 40-minute period; this finding does not necessarily indicate a compromised fetus, as most often it is secondary to a fetal sleep cycle.[29] The interpretation of a nonreactive NST must consider gestational age, the underlying clinical circumstance, and the results of previous NSTs. Only 65% of fetuses have a reactive NST by 28 weeks' gestation, whereas 95% do so by 32 weeks.[30,31] However, once a reactive NST has been documented, it should generally remain reactive throughout the remainder of the pregnancy. A nonreactive NST at term is associated with a poor perinatal outcome in only a minority of cases. It has a sensitivity of 57%, a positive predictive value of 13%, and a negative predictive value of 98% (assuming a prevalence of 4%) for a 5-minute Apgar score < 7. For permanent neurologic injury, a nonreactive NST at term has a 99.8% false-positive rate.[32]

Visual interpretation of the FHR tracing involves assessment of the following components: (1) baseline FHR, (2) baseline FHR variability, (3) presence of accelerations, (4) presence of periodic or episodic decelerations, and (5) changes of FHR pattern over time (see Table 6.1; see Fig. 8.4).[25,26] The patterns are categorized as **baseline**, **periodic** (i.e., associated with uterine contractions), or **episodic** (i.e., not associated with uterine contractions). Periodic changes are described as *abrupt* or *gradual* (defined as onset-to-nadir interval < 30 seconds or > 30 seconds, respectively).

TABLE 6.1	Interpretation of Antepartum Nonstress Test Results
Criterion	**Definition**
Baseline FHR	Defined as the approximate mean FHR during a 10-min segment and lasting at least 2 min. The normal FHR is defined as 110–160 bpm.
Baseline FHR variability	Described as fluctuations in baseline FHR ≥ 2 cycles/min. It is quantified visually as the amplitude of the peak to the trough in bpm. Variability is classified as follows: Absent: amplitude range undetectable Minimal: amplitude range detectable but less than or equal to 5 bpm Moderate: amplitude range 6–25 bpm Marked: amplitude range > 25 bpm The normal baseline FHR variability is defined as moderate variability.
Accelerations	Defined as an abrupt increase in FHR above baseline. At and after 32 weeks' gestation, an acceleration is defined as 15 bpm or more above baseline for 15 s or more but less than 2 min. Before 32 weeks' gestation, an acceleration is defined as 10 bpm or more above baseline for 10 s or more but less than 2 min. A **prolonged acceleration** is defined as an acceleration lasting 2 min or more but less than 10 min. If the duration is longer than 10 min, it is referred to as a "change in baseline" and not a prolonged acceleration.
Decelerations	Decelerations are not normal. However, some decelerations are a more serious sign of fetal compromise than others. The following three types of decelerations are recognized: **Early decelerations** are characterized by a gradual decrease and return to baseline FHR associated with a uterine contraction. The onset, nadir, and recovery of the deceleration are coincident with the beginning, peak, and ending of the uterine contraction. **Variable decelerations** are characterized by an abrupt decrease in the FHR to 15 bpm or more below the baseline and lasting for 15 s or more but less than 2 min. Abrupt is defined as less than 30 s from baseline to the nadir of the deceleration. When variable decelerations are associated with uterine activity, their onset, depth, and duration commonly vary with successive contractions. **Late decelerations** are characterized by a gradual decrease and return to baseline FHR associated with a uterine contraction. Importantly, the deceleration is delayed in timing, with the nadir of the deceleration occurring after the peak of the contraction. Onset, nadir, and recovery of the deceleration occur after the beginning, peak, and ending of the uterine contraction. A **prolonged deceleration** is defined as a deceleration lasting 2 min or more but less than 10 min. If the duration is longer than 10 min, it is referred to as a "change in baseline" and not a prolonged deceleration. **Recurrent decelerations** describe the presence of decelerations with more than 50% of uterine contractions in any 20-min period

FHR, Fetal heart rate.
Data from the National Institute of Child Health and Human Development Research Planning Workshop. Electronic fetal heart rate monitoring: research guidelines for interpretation. *Am J Obstet Gynecol.* 1997;177:1385–1390.

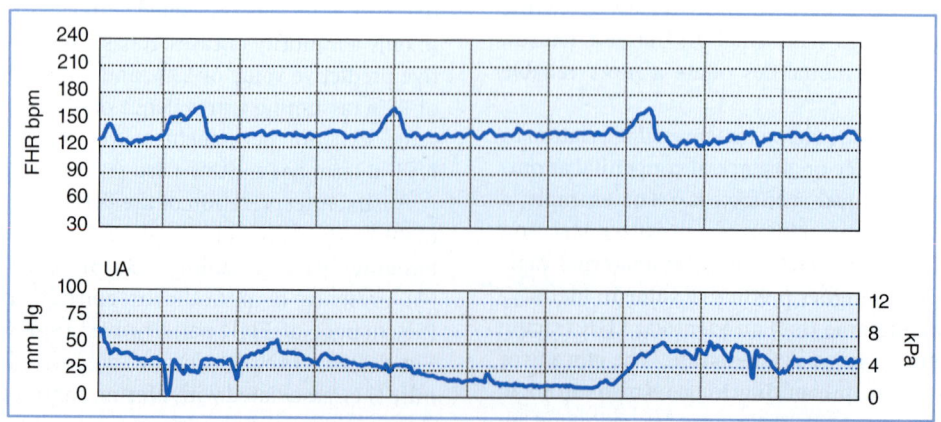

Fig. 6.2 A Normal (Reactive) Fetal Heart Rate (FHR) Tracing. The baseline FHR is normal (110–160 bpm), there is moderate variability (defined as 6 to 25 bpm from peak to trough), there are no decelerations, and there are two or more accelerations (defined as an increase in FHR of 15 bpm or more above baseline lasting at least 15 s) in a 20-min period.

A normal FHR tracing (Category 1) is defined as having a normal baseline rate (110 to 160 bpm), normal baseline variability (i.e., moderate variability, defined as 6 to 25 bpm from peak to trough), presence of accelerations, and absence of decelerations. FHR accelerations typically occur in response to fetal movement and usually indicate fetal health and adequate oxygenation (see Box 8.3).[25,26] **Abnormal FHR patterns** (Category 3) demonstrate absence of baseline variability combined with recurrent late or variable decelerations or substantial bradycardia. **Indeterminant FHR patterns** (Category 2) have characteristics between the two extremes of normal and abnormal tracings.[25,26]

Persistent fetal tachycardia (defined as an FHR > 160 bpm) may be associated with fetal hypoxia, maternal fever, chorioamnionitis (intrauterine infection), maternal administration of an anticholinergic or beta-adrenergic receptor agonist, fetal anemia, or tachyarrhythmia (Table 6.2). **Persistent fetal bradycardia** (FHR < 110 bpm) may be a result of congenital heart block, administration of a beta-adrenergic receptor antagonist, hypoglycemia, or hypothermia; it may also indicate fetal hypoxia.[25,26] Both tachyarrhythmias and bradyarrhythmias require immediate evaluation.

Baseline FHR variability, perhaps the most important component of the NST, is determined on a beat-to-beat basis by the competing influences of the sympathetic and parasympathetic nervous systems on the fetal sinoatrial node. The presence of FHR variability, characterized by fluctuations that are irregular in both amplitude and frequency,[25,26] indicates that the autonomic nervous system is functioning and that the fetus has normal acid-base status.

Variability is defined as absent, minimal, moderate, or marked. The older terms *short-term variability* and *long-term variability* are no longer used.[26] Normal (moderate) variability indicates the absence of cerebral hypoxia. In the setting of acute hypoxia, variability may be minimal or marked. Persistent or chronic hypoxia is typically associated with loss of variability. Reduced variability may be the result of maternal drug administration (see Table 6.2), fetal arrhythmia, or neurologic abnormality (e.g., anencephaly, structural abnormality, prior injury).[25,26]

Vibroacoustic Stimulation

Fetal vibroacoustic stimulation (VAS) refers to the response of the FHR to a vibroacoustic stimulus (82 to 95 dB) applied to the maternal abdomen for 1 to 2 seconds in the region of the fetal head. A FHR acceleration in response to VAS represents a positive result and is suggestive of fetal health. If VAS fails to produce an acceleration in the FHR, it may be repeated up to three times for progressively longer durations of up to 3 seconds.

As fetal sleep cycle is a common reason for a nonreactive NST, VAS can shorten the time needed to achieve a reactive NST and mitigate the need for further testing. In one study of low-risk women at term, VAS reduced the proportion of nonreactive NSTs over a 30-minute period from 14% to 9% and shortened the time needed to achieve a reactive NST by an average of 4.5 minutes.[33] VAS has no known adverse effect on fetal hearing, although data are limited.

TABLE 6.2 Drugs That Can Affect the Fetal Heart Rate Tracing

Effect on the Fetus	Drug
Fetal tachycardia	Atropine
	Epinephrine (adrenaline)
	Beta-adrenergic agonists (ritodrine, terbutaline)
Fetal bradycardia	Antithyroid medications (including propylthiouracil)
	Beta-adrenergic antagonists (e.g., propranolol)
	Intrathecal or epidural analgesia
	Methylergonovine (contraindicated before delivery)
	Oxytocin (if associated with excessive uterine activity)
Sinusoidal fetal heart rate pattern	Systemic opioid analgesia
Diminished variability	Atropine
	Anticonvulsants (but not phenytoin)
	Beta-adrenergic antagonists
	Antenatal corticosteroids (betamethasone, dexamethasone)
	Ethanol
	General anesthesia
	Hypnotics (including diazepam)
	Insulin (if associated with hypoglycemia)
	Magnesium sulfate
	Systemic opioid analgesia
	Promethazine

Biophysical Profile

The BPP combines an NST with an ultrasonographic scoring system performed over a 30-minute period. Each of the five components is awarded two points, for a total possible score of 10. Initially described for testing of postterm fetuses, the BPP has also been validated for use in term and preterm fetuses, but not during active labor.[34,35] The five variables described in the original BPP were (1) gross fetal body movements, (2) fetal tone (i.e., flexion and extension of limbs), (3) amniotic fluid volume, (4) fetal breathing movements, and (5) the NST (Table 6.3).[34] Outcomes for a BPP score of 8/10 are equivalent to those for a score of 10/10; thus, if all four ultrasonographic components are present, the NST is not required unless otherwise indicated.

The BPP's individual variables become apparent in the normal fetus in a predictable sequence; fetal tone appears at 7.5 to 8.5 weeks' gestation, fetal movement at 9 weeks, fetal breathing at 20 to 22 weeks, and FHR reactivity at 24 to 28 weeks.

TABLE 6.3 Characteristics of the Biophysical Profile

Biophysical Variable	Normal Score (Score = 2)	Abnormal Score (Score = 0)
Fetal breathing movements	At least one episode of FBM lasting at least 30 s	Absence of FBM altogether or no FBM episode ≥ 30 s Continuous breathing without cessation
Body or limb movements	At least three discrete body/limb movements in 30 min (episodes of active continuous movements should be regarded as a single movement)	Fewer than three episodes of body/limb movements over a 30-min period
Fetal tone	At least one episode of active extension with return to flexion of fetal limbs or trunk Opening and closing of hand or mouth	Slow extension with return to partial flexion Movement of limb in full extension Absence of fetal movements
Amniotic fluid evaluation	At least one pocket of AF ≥ 2 cm	No AF pockets or an AF pocket < 2 cm
Nonstress test	Moderate FHR variability Accelerations coupled with fetal movements	Minimal or no FHR variability Insufficient or absent accelerations Accelerations not coupled with fetal movement

AF, Amniotic fluid; *FBM,* fetal breathing movement; *FHR,* fetal heart rate.
Modified from Kaimal, AJ. Assessment of fetal health. In: Lockwood CJ, Copel JA, Dugoff L, et al., eds. *Creasy and Resnik's Maternal-Fetal Medicine: Principles and Practice.* 9th ed. Elsevier; 2023:560–573.e2.

In the setting of antepartum hypoxia, these characteristics typically disappear in the reverse order of their appearance (i.e., FHR reactivity is lost first, followed by fetal breathing, fetal movements, and finally fetal tone).[35] The amniotic fluid volume, which is composed almost entirely of fetal urine in the second and third trimesters, is not influenced by acute fetal hypoxia or acute central nervous system dysfunction. Rather, oligohydramnios (decreased amniotic fluid volume) in the latter half of pregnancy and in the absence of ruptured membranes is a reflection of chronic uteroplacental insufficiency and/or increased renal artery resistance leading to diminished urine output.[36] An adverse pregnancy outcome (including low Apgar scores and/or admission to the neonatal intensive care unit) is more common when oligohydramnios is present.[37,38] Periodic (i.e., weekly or twice weekly) screening for oligohydramnios in pregnancies at high risk for uteroplacental insufficiency (e.g., FGR) is important because amniotic fluid can become drastically reduced within 24 to 48 hours.[39]

Although each of the five components of the BPP are scored equally (two points if the variable is present or normal and 0 points if absent or abnormal), they are not equally predictive of adverse pregnancy outcome. For example, amniotic fluid volume is the variable that correlates most strongly with adverse pregnancy events. Clinical management in response to the BPP score is summarized in Table 6.4.[23] A score of 8 or 10 is regarded as reassuring; a score of 6 is considered equivocal, and a score of 4 or less is abnormal. A score of 0 or 2 suggests nonreassuring fetal status and should prompt evaluation for immediate delivery unless a reversible cause is identified.[23,35,40]

The *modified* BPP was developed to simplify and reduce the time necessary to complete an examination by focusing on the BPP components that are most predictive of outcome: (1) an NST, as an indicator of acute acid-base status; and (2) the amniotic fluid volume, as an index of uteroplacental function.[41,42] A *normal* modified BPP (reactive NST and a maximum vertical amniotic fluid pocket ≥ 2 cm) occurs in approximately 90% of examinations, and is as reliable as a full BPP in the prediction of fetal well-being. A full BPP is generally performed if an abnormal result is obtained and if the clinical situation and findings do not warrant an immediate intervention.

Contraction Stress Test

Also known as the oxytocin challenge test, the CST assesses the response of the FHR to uterine contractions induced by either intravenous oxytocin administration or nipple stimulation (which causes release of endogenous oxytocin from the maternal neurohypophysis). A minimum of three contractions for at least 40 seconds in a 10-minute period is required to interpret the test. A negative CST (no late or severe late decelerations with contractions) is reassuring and suggestive of a healthy, well-oxygenated fetus.

A positive CST (late or severe variable decelerations with at least 50% of the contractions) is suggestive of a fetus suffering from impaired maternal-to-fetal oxygen exchange during uterine contractions and is associated with adverse perinatal outcome in 35% to 40% of cases.[29] A CST is defined as *equivocal* if FHR decelerations occur in the presence of contractions that occur more frequently than every 2 minutes or last longer than 90 seconds, *equivocal-suspicious* if there are intermittent late decelerations or significant variable decelerations, and *unsatisfactory* if there are fewer than three contractions in 10 minutes or the FHR tracing is uninterpretable.[29] The combination of a positive CST and absence of FHR variability is especially ominous. It should be noted, however, that the false-positive rate of this test exceeds 50%.[27] If the CST is uninterpretable or equivocal, the test should be repeated in 24

TABLE 6.4 Recommended Management Based on Biophysical Profile

Score	Interpretation	Recommended Management
10/10 or 8/10 with normal AFV	Normal	No acute intervention; serial testing may be indicated by indication-specific protocols
8/10 with oligohydramnios	Chronic fetal compromise likely	Gestational age dependent: prove normal urinary tract, disprove undiagnosed rupture of membranes, consider antenatal corticosteroids if preterm
6/10 (normal AFV)	Equivocal test, fetal asphyxia not excluded	Repeat testing immediately: • If repeat score is 10/10, manage as 10 • For persistent 6/10, deliver if term • If preterm, repeat BPP within 24 h and deliver if less than 6/10
4/10	Acute fetal asphyxia likely (if oligohydramnios present, acute-on-chronic asphyxia likely)	Deliver by obstetrically appropriate method
2/10	Acute fetal asphyxia likely with chronic decompensation	Deliver for fetal indications (often requires cesarean delivery)
0/10	Severe, acute asphyxia virtually certain	Deliver immediately by cesarean if fetus is viable

AFV, Amniotic fluid volume; *BPP*, biophysical profile.
Modified from Kaimal, AJ. Assessment of fetal health. In: Lockwood CJ, Copel JA, Dugoff L, et al., eds. *Creasy and Resnik's Maternal-Fetal Medicine: Principles and Practice*. 9th ed. Elsevier; 2023:560–573.e2.

to 72 hours. Studies suggest that more than 80% of repeated tests are negative. The rate of antepartum intrauterine fetal demise within 1 week of a negative CST is 0.04%.[27]

Because this test is time-consuming, requires skilled nursing care, and necessitates an inpatient setting owing to the possibility of precipitating fetal compromise requiring emergency cesarean delivery, the CST is reserved for specific clinical indications. Moreover, there are contraindications to its use, including placenta previa, placental abruption, prior classical (high-vertical) cesarean delivery, and risk for preterm labor. Despite these limitations, the CST allows for indirect evaluation of fetal oxygenation during periods of uterine contractions and diminished uteroplacental perfusion and may therefore provide a better assessment of fetal well-being and fetal reserve than either the NST or the BPP (Table 6.5).[27,29,43]

Doppler Velocimetry

Doppler velocimetry can be used for the noninvasive measurement of fetal circulation, including blood flow in the UA, middle cerebral artery (MCA), and ductus venosus (DV). Doppler assessment of the UA is an evidence-based tool for the evaluation of pregnancies with FGR. Normally, UA resistance to blood flow from the fetus to the placenta falls progressively throughout pregnancy, reflecting an increase in the number of tertiary stem vessels. Factors that affect placental vascular resistance include gestational age, placental location, pregnancy complications (e.g., placental abruption, preeclampsia), and underlying maternal disease (e.g., chronic hypertension).[44]

Decreased diastolic flow with a resultant increase in the systolic-to-diastolic (S/D) ratio suggests an increase in placental vascular resistance.[45,46] Severely abnormal UA Doppler velocimetry (defined as absence of, or reversed diastolic

TABLE 6.5 False-Positive and False-Negative Rates for the Nonstress Test, Biophysical Profile, and Contraction Stress Test

Test	False-Negative Rate (per 1000 Live Births)[a]
Nonstress test	1.9
Biophysical profile	0.8
Contraction stress test	0.3

Data from References.[27, 40, 42]
[a]Data are presented as perinatal mortality rate within 1 w of a reactive nonstress test, a biophysical profile score of 8 or 10, or a negative contraction stress test after adjustments for congenital anomalies and known causes.

flow) is consistent with the obliteration of 50% to 70% of the terminal villi; this observation is most studied in the setting of FGR and is associated with poor perinatal outcomes (Fig. 6.3).[46–48] The SMFM published guidance regarding management of FGR in 2020; in the setting of reversed end-diastolic flow, delivery is recommended at 30 to 32 weeks' gestation, while for absent end-diastolic flow in the absence of other complications, delivery is recommended at 33 to 34 weeks' gestation.[22]

Preparation for delivery—including administration of corticosteroids for fetal lung maturity and transfer to a tertiary delivery center—should be considered when UA Doppler findings are abnormal in the setting of FGR, regardless of gestational age. However, in the presence of a normally grown fetus, it is unclear how to interpret such findings. For these reasons, UA Doppler velocimetry should not be performed routinely in pregnancies in the absence of growth restriction. UA Doppler velocimetry has not been shown to be useful in the evaluation of other types of high-risk pregnancies, including diabetic and postterm pregnancies, primarily because of a high false-positive rate.[49-53] Investigational indications include umbilical cord malformations, unexplained oligohydramnios, suspected or established preeclampsia, and, possibly, fetal cardiac anomalies.

MCA peak systolic velocity provides a noninvasive evaluation of fetal anemia, including moderate to severe cases resulting from isoimmunization.[54] When severe anemia

develops in a fetus, blood is preferentially shunted to the vital organs, such as the brain, which results in an increase in MCA peak systolic flow velocity.[54] This finding can help the maternal-fetal medicine specialist counsel affected patients about the need for cordocentesis and fetal blood transfusion. Doppler studies of other vessels (including the uterine artery, fetal aorta, DV, and fetal carotid arteries) have contributed to the knowledge of maternal-fetal physiology but as yet do not have evidence-based clinical applications.[22]

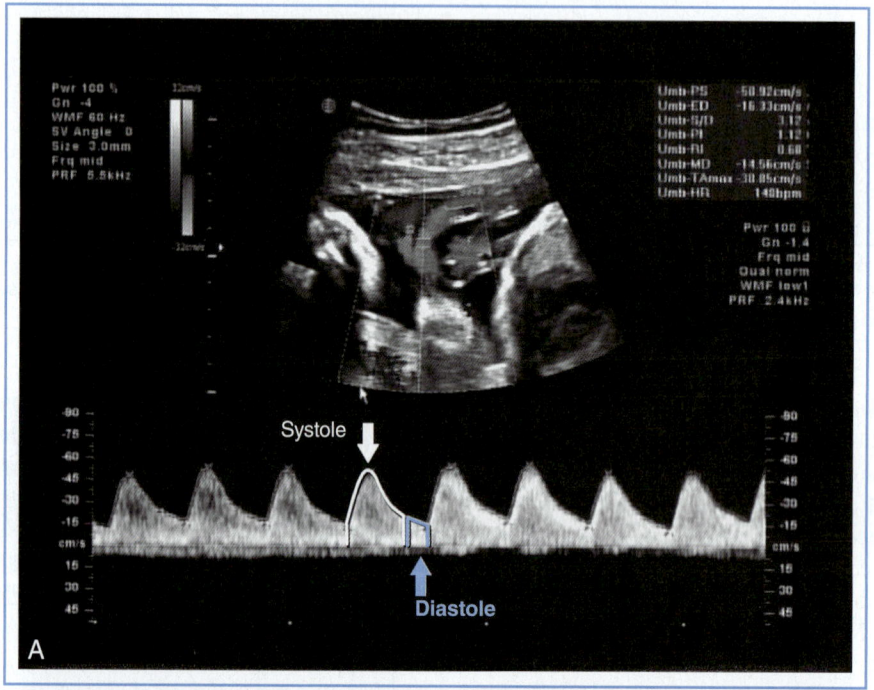

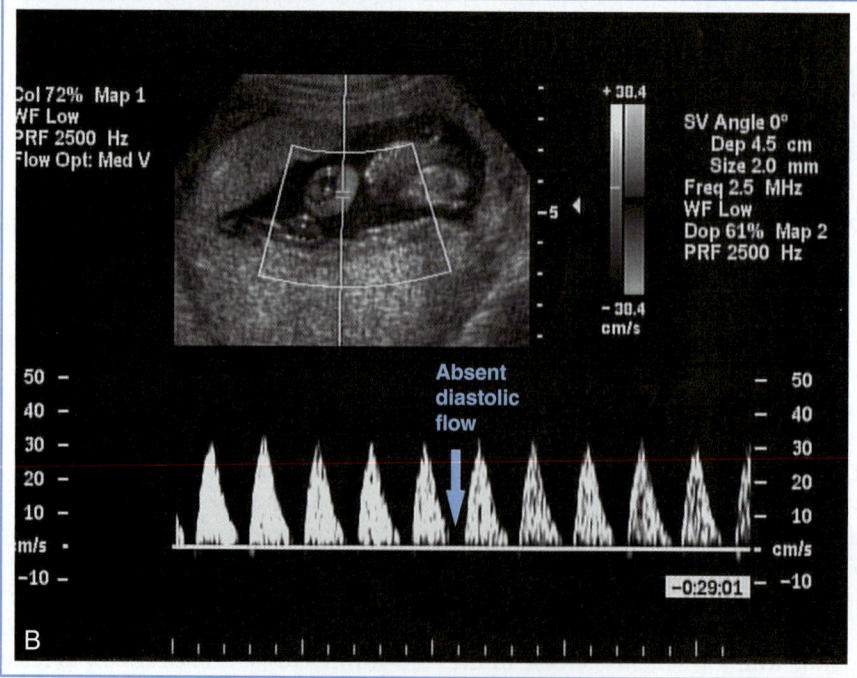

Fig. 6.3 **Umbilical Artery Doppler Velocimetry.** (A) Normal waveform in the umbilical artery as shown on Doppler velocimetry. Forward flow can be seen during both fetal systole and diastole. (B) Absent end-diastolic flow. Forward flow can be seen during systole, but there is no flow during diastole.

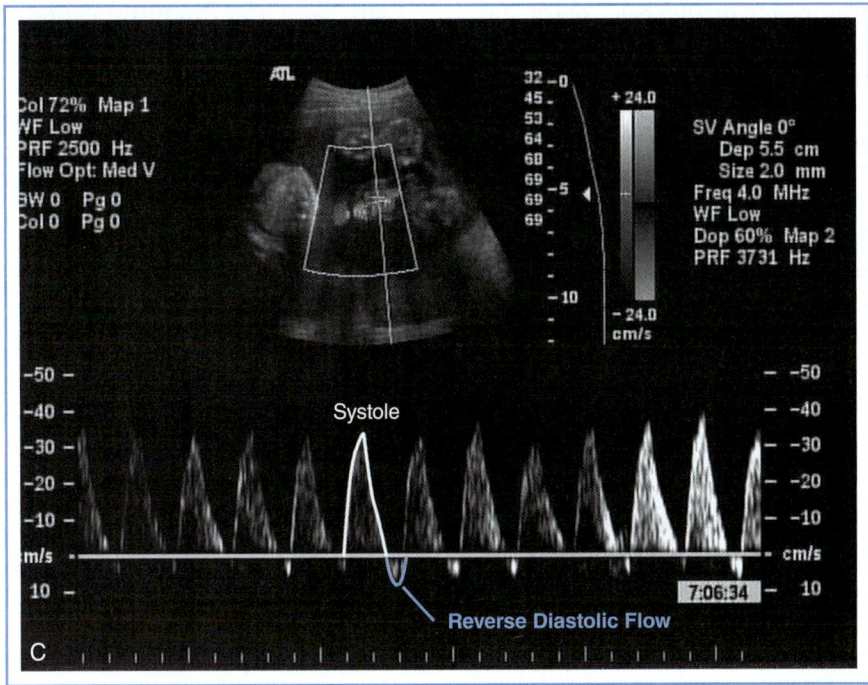

Fig. 6.3,cont'd (C) Reverse diastolic flow. Forward flow can be seen during systole, but there is reverse flow in the umbilical artery during diastole, which is suggestive of high resistance to blood flow in the placenta.

Multiple Modalities to Assess Fetal Well-Being

All standard tests to assess antepartum fetal well-being (i.e., NST, BPP, CST) are evaluated according to their ability to predict the absence of fetal death during the 1-week period after the test. The false-negative rate (defined as a reassuring test result with a subsequent bad outcome) for each of these tests are listed in Table 6.5.[27,29,40,42] The false-negative rates for all three tests are low. Because the NST has a high false-positive rate, some authorities consider it a screening test to identify fetuses requiring further assessment with either a BPP or a CST. No method of fetal assessment is perfect, and clinical judgment plays a large role in any management decision.

SELECTED SPECIAL CIRCUMSTANCES REQUIRING ADDITIONAL SURVEILLANCE AND COUNSELING

Fetal Growth Restriction

FGR is defined as an ultrasonographic EFW or an abdominal circumference less than the 10th percentile for the established gestational age.[22] FGR can result from a variety of maternal, fetal, and placental conditions and is associated with adverse perinatal outcomes, including intrauterine demise, neonatal morbidity, and neonatal mortality.[21] In addition, growth-restricted fetuses are at increased risk for adverse long-term health outcomes, including cardiovascular and endocrine disorders as well as neurologic impairment.[55]

Distinguishing the healthy, constitutionally small-for-gestational age fetus from the pathologically growth-restricted fetus is challenging. Fetuses with an EFW less than the 10th percentile are not necessarily pathologically growth restricted. Conversely, an EFW at or above the 10th percentile does not necessarily mean that an individual fetus has achieved its growth potential, and such a fetus may still be at risk for perinatal mortality and morbidity.[21]

Maternal disorders associated with FGR include any condition that can result in vascular disease or abnormal oxygenation, such as pregestational diabetes, hypertension, cardiac disease, autoimmune diseases, renal insufficiency, and malnutrition. Fetal conditions that may result in growth restriction include teratogen exposure (e.g., certain medications), intrauterine infection, aneuploidy (most often trisomy 13 and trisomy 18), and some structural malformations (e.g., abdominal wall defects, congenital heart disease). Placental pathology resulting in poor placental perfusion can lead to FGR. Umbilical cord abnormalities, such as velamentous or marginal cord insertion, have also been implicated in cases of FGR.[21] In more than half of cases of growth restriction, the etiology may be unclear even after a thorough investigation.[22]

FGR is associated with an increased risk for stillbirth.[21,22] When the EFW measures less than the 10th percentile, the risk for stillbirth is 1.5%, twice the risk for appropriately grown fetuses. The risk for stillbirth increases as the EFW decreases[56,57] and is further increased when FGR occurs in the context of oligohydramnios or abnormal diastolic blood flow in the UA.[58]

Early and accurate diagnosis of FGR, coupled with appropriate intervention, leads to an improvement in perinatal outcome. If FGR is suspected clinically by ultrasonography, a thorough evaluation of the mother and fetus is indicated. Referral to a maternal-fetal medicine specialist should be considered, particularly if growth restriction is severe, early onset, or associated with additional findings on ultrasonographic assessment (e.g., fetal anomalies, abnormal amniotic fluid volume). Every effort should be made to identify the cause of the FGR and to modify or eliminate contributing factors. Monitoring should include serial ultrasonographic examinations for growth and amniotic fluid volume, antenatal surveillance with UA velocimetry, and antepartum testing (NST or BPP). The timing of delivery should be based on 1) gestational age; 2) the underlying etiology, if known; 3) results of antepartum testing and interval growth scans; and 4) any additional risk factors for an adverse outcome, including maternal comorbidities.[21,22]

Fetal Macrosomia

Fetal macrosomia, historically defined as an absolute birth weight > 4000 or 4500 g regardless of gestational age,[59] should be differentiated from the term *large for gestational age*, which implies a birth weight at or greater than the 90th percentile for a given gestational age.

In general, the risk for labor abnormalities (e.g., cephalopelvic disproportion, dysfunctional labor), maternal morbidity (e.g., cesarean delivery, postpartum hemorrhage, significant vaginal lacerations), and newborn complications (e.g., 5-minute Apgar score < 4, birth injuries, assisted ventilation for longer than 30 minutes, neonatal intensive care unit admission) increases with birth weight between 4000 and 4499 g; newborn and maternal morbidity increases significantly with birth weight between 4500 and 4999 g; and perinatal mortality (e.g., stillbirth, neonatal mortality) increases with birth weight > 5000 g.[60] **Shoulder dystocia**, defined as a failure of delivery of the fetal shoulder(s) after initial attempts at downward traction during vaginal delivery, is among the most serious consequence of fetal macrosomia, and requires additional maneuvers to effect delivery.[61] The fetal injuries associated with shoulder dystocia include fracture of the clavicle and damage to the nerves of the brachial plexus, resulting in Erb-Duchenne paralysis (most of these resolve by 1 year of age). The overall prevalence of shoulder dystocia is 0.2% to 3.0% for all vaginal deliveries. In contrast, the risk for shoulder dystocia for neonates with birth weight ≥ 4500 g is 9% to 14%, and increases further in the setting of maternal diabetes to 20% to 50%.[62,63]

Fetal macrosomia can be determined clinically by abdominal palpation (e.g., Leopold maneuvers) or with ultrasonography. Although these two techniques appear to be equally accurate,[64] the ability to predict fetal macrosomia is poor, with a false-positive rate of 35% and a false-negative rate of 10%.[64,65] EFW measurements are less accurate in macrosomic fetuses than in normally grown fetuses, and factors such as low amniotic fluid volume, advancing gestational age, maternal obesity, and fetal position can compound these inaccuracies.

Despite the inaccuracy in the prediction of fetal macrosomia, an EFW should be documented by either clinical estimation or ultrasonography prior to delivery. Suspected fetal macrosomia is not an indication for induction of labor prior to 39 weeks' gestation because induction does not improve maternal or fetal outcomes and may increase the risk for cesarean delivery.[59] The ACOG recommends consideration of elective cesarean delivery when EFW exceeds 4500 g in women with diabetes mellitus, or when EBW exceeds 5000 g in women without diabetes mellitus.[59]

Late-Term and Postterm Pregnancy

Postterm pregnancy is defined as any pregnancy that continues to or beyond 42 weeks (294 days) from the first day of the last normal menstrual period or 14 days beyond the best obstetric estimate of the EDD, while a *late-term* pregnancy is defined as one between 41 0/7 and 41 6/7 weeks' gestation.[1] The prevalence of postterm pregnancy depends on the patient population (i.e., percentage of primigravidas, incidence of pregnancy complications, frequency of spontaneous preterm births) and the local practice patterns (e.g., use of ultrasonographic assessment of gestational age, cesarean delivery rates, use of labor induction). The incidence of postterm pregnancy in the United States has steadily decreased over time to 0.25% in 2021.[66] Compared with delivery at 40 weeks' gestation, postterm pregnancies pose significant risks to both the pregnant woman (higher risk for cesarean delivery, severe perineal injury, postpartum hemorrhage) and the fetus (stillbirth, fetal macrosomia, birth injury, meconium aspiration syndrome).[53] A 2020 systematic review of 34 randomized controlled trials including over 20,000 women concluded that induction of labor at term is associated with a decreased risk for perinatal death, stillbirth, neonatal intensive care unit admission, and cesarean delivery.[67] Additionally, the (ARRIVE trial (A Randomized Trial of Induction Versus Expectant Management) trial, published in 2018, found that induction of labor at 39 weeks' gestation in low-risk, nulliparous women resulted in a significantly decreased risk of cesarean delivery without an increased risk of neonatal adverse outcome.[68] For this reason, induction of labor after 42 0/7 weeks' and by 42 6/7 weeks' gestation is recommended, while induction of labor between 39 0/7 and 42 0/7 weeks' gestation can be considered.[53,69,70]

Late-term and postterm pregnancy is an indication for antenatal fetal surveillance,[24,53] although the efficacy of this approach has not been validated by prospective randomized trials. Options for evaluating fetal well-being include NST with or without amniotic fluid volume assessment, BPP, CST, or a combination of these modalities. The ACOG has recommended that antepartum fetal surveillance be initiated by 41 weeks' gestation and be performed once or twice weekly. Many experts advise twice-weekly testing with some evaluation of amniotic fluid volume at least weekly.

At term, evidence of fetal compromise (nonreassuring fetal test results) or **oligohydramnios** (i.e., low amniotic fluid volume) should prompt delivery.[53] Oligohydramnios, defined as amniotic fluid index ≤ 5 cm (sum of maximum vertical amniotic fluid pocket in each of the four quadrants) or a single deepest pocket measurement ≤ 2 cm, has been associated with an increased risk for fetal demise and is an indication for delivery at 36 0/7 to 37 6/7 weeks' gestation.[71] Recent studies concluded that the use of a deepest vertical pocket measurement ≤ 2 cm to diagnose oligohydramnios, rather than an amniotic fluid index ≤ 5 cm , was associated with a reduction of unnecessary interventions without an increase in adverse perinatal outcomes.[3,72,73] Adverse pregnancy outcomes (nonreassuring FHR tracing necessitating cesarean delivery, meconium aspiration syndrome, neonatal intensive care unit admission) are more common when oligohydramnios is present.[74] Screening of postterm patients for oligohydramnios is important because amniotic fluid can become dramatically reduced within 24 to 48 hours.[53]

ANTENATAL FETAL INTERVENTIONS

Continued assessment of the fetus throughout pregnancy is critical to optimizing pregnancy outcomes. In most cases, if fetal compromise is noted, the only intervention available is delivery. However, early delivery may also be associated with adverse outcomes, particularly at earlier gestational ages. Management should focus on developing a monitoring plan that collects data with the goal of optimizing the timing of delivery by balancing the risks of complications with ongoing pregnancy against the risks of preterm delivery. In certain situations, treatment may be available to improve neonatal outcome if preterm delivery is indicated or even to correct the underlying problem *in utero* (Table 6.6).[75] These interventions include noninvasive medical therapy (e.g., administration of

TABLE 6.6 Fetal Therapies	
Intervention	**Fetal Conditions**
Medication Therapy	
Antiarrhythmic agents	Fetal tachyarrhythmias
Stimulants	Fetal bradyarrhythmias
Corticosteroids	Prematurity, congenital adrenal hyperplasia
Ultrasound-Guided Procedures	
Amnioreduction	Polyhydramnios
Vesicocentesis	Lower urinary tract obstruction
Thoracentesis	Pleural effusion, macrocystic congenital pulmonary airway malformation
Pericardiocentesis	Pericardial effusion
Percutaneous umbilical blood sampling	Fetal anemia, genetic testing, direct fetal drug administration
Intrauterine transfusion	Fetal anemia, fetal thrombocytopenia
Thoracoamniotic shunt placement	Pleural effusion, macrocystic congenital pulmonary airway malformation
Vesicoamniotic shunt placement	Lower urinary tract obstruction
Interstitial laser coagulation	Twin reversed arterial perfusion sequence, bronchopulmonary sequestration, sacrococcygeal teratoma
Balloon valvuloplasty	Critical aortic stenosis
Selective Umbilical Cord Occlusion	
Radiofrequency ablation	Discordant twin anomalies
Bipolar umbilical cord coagulation	Twin-twin transfusion syndrome, twin anemia-polycythemia sequence, selective fetal growth restriction
Fetal Surgery	
Laser coagulation of placental anastomosis	Twin-twin transfusion syndrome, twin anemia-polycythemia sequence, selective fetal growth restriction
Ablation of posterior urethral valves	Lower urinary tract obstruction
Fetal biopsy	Definitive diagnosis
Ablation of feeding vessels	Chorangioma
Release of amniotic bands	Amniotic band sequence
Fetoscopic endoluminal tracheal occlusion	Congenital diaphragmatic hernia
Spina bifida closure	Myelomeningocele
Open maternal-fetal surgery	Myelomeningocele closure, lung lesion resection, sacrococcygeal teratoma debulking, mediastinal mass debulking
EXIT procedure	Cervical teratoma/lymphangioma, oral mass, severe micrognathia, congenital high airway obstruction syndrome, lung lesions, conjoined twin stabilization

EXIT, Ex utero intrapartum treatment.
Modified from Moldenhauer JS, Johnson A, Van Mieghem T. International Society for Prenatal Diagnosis 2022 DEBATE: there should be formal accreditation and ongoing quality assurance/review for units offering fetal therapy that includes public reporting of outcomes. *Prenat Diagn.* 2023;43:411–420.

corticosteroids to reduce the complications from preterm delivery) or invasive procedures (e.g., intrauterine transfusion, placement of a vesicoamniotic shunt, fetoscopic laser ablation of anastomotic vessels for twin-twin transfusion syndrome).[75] Some fetal interventions have been subjected to rigorous clinical trials and have been shown to be effective, whereas others remain investigational.

Antenatal Corticosteroids

The intervention that has had the greatest effect on perinatal outcome is antenatal maternal administration of corticosteroids prior to preterm delivery. *Respiratory distress syndrome* (RDS) refers to respiratory compromise presenting at or shortly after delivery because of a deficiency of pulmonary surfactant, an endogenous detergent that serves to decrease the surface tension within alveoli, thereby preventing alveolar collapse. Overall, neonatal RDS affects approximately 1% of live births, but not all infants are at equal risk. The pulmonary system is among the last of the fetal organ systems to become functionally mature. Thus, RDS is primarily, although not exclusively, a disease of preterm infants, with the incidence and severity highly dependent on gestational age. For example, RDS affects more than 80% of infants younger than 28 weeks' gestation and 10% infants born at 34 weeks' gestation.[76,77] RDS remains a major cause of perinatal morbidity and mortality in extremely preterm infants. In addition to gestational age, other factors influence the risk for RDS. For reasons that are not clear, African American race, female gender, preeclampsia, and intrauterine exposure to cigarette smoke have been associated with decreased risk for RDS.

In 1972, Liggins and Howie[78] demonstrated that the administration of a single course of two antenatal doses of a corticosteroid (betamethasone) reduced the incidence of RDS by 50%. A 2020 metaanalysis of 27 studies with more than 11,000 participants concluded that antenatal administration of corticosteroids to pregnant women at risk for preterm birth resulted in an improvement in overall neonatal survival and a reduction in RDS.[79] Maternally administered betamethasone and dexamethasone cross the placenta and induce cellular differentiation at the expense of growth. Type II pneumocytes in the lungs differentiate and begin making pulmonary surfactant, which accounts for the decrease in risk for RDS, and endothelial cells lining the vasculature undergo cellular maturation and stabilization, explaining the concomitant drop in the incidence of bleeding into the brain (intraventricular hemorrhage) and gastrointestinal tract (necrotizing enterocolitis).[80] Betamethasone and dexamethasone are the two corticosteroids used for this indication; prednisone, hydrocortisone, and other steroid preparations do not cross the placenta and therefore do not have a similar protective effect.

The National Institutes of Health and the ACOG have recommended that a single course of antenatal corticosteroids, either betamethasone (12 mg intramuscularly q24h × two doses) or dexamethasone (6 mg intramuscularly q12h × four doses), be given from 23 to 34 weeks' gestation to any pregnant women in whom delivery before 34 weeks' gestation is imminently anticipated.[81] More recently, the ACOG

has recommended a course of corticosteroids be considered for women with a singleton pregnancy between 34 0/7 and 36 6/7 weeks' gestation in whom the risk of preterm birth is high, who have not received a previous course of antenatal corticosteroids, and do not have any contraindications.[81]

Although the maximum benefit of antenatal corticosteroids is achieved 24 to 48 hours after the first injection, as little as 4 hours of treatment exerts some protective effect. This protective effect is at its peak for 7 days, after which further benefit is less clear. Multiple (three or more) courses of antenatal corticosteroids have been associated with FGR, smaller head circumference, and (in animals) abnormal myelination of the optic nerves; consequently, multiple courses are not recommended. A single repeat course of antenatal corticosteroids should be considered in women who are less than 34 0/7 weeks' gestation and at risk for preterm delivery within the next 7 days, at least 7 days after the prior dose.[81]

Fetal Surgery

Fetal surgery has been proposed in selected cases to prevent progressive organ damage or to restore normal anatomy and fetal development (see Chapter 7). Theoretically, the ideal circumstance for fetal surgery is a pregnancy in which the fetus has an isolated structural anatomic change that, if left untreated, will result in fetal or neonatal demise or significant, life-limiting effects that would be mitigated by *in utero* intervention. A detailed understanding of the natural history of the anatomic lesion is essential when one is considering whether to recommend surgery. Fetal surgery should not be attempted if the natural history of the disorder is unknown or if the chances of survival without *in utero* treatment are greater than the risks associated with the procedure. Most of the evidence for fetal interventions is observational.

Percutaneous umbilical cord blood sampling and transfusion of red blood cells to the fetus with **anemia** has been shown to improve survival in observational studies and is the recommended treatment approach, particularly between 18 and 35 weeks' gestation.[82]

In 2004, the results of a randomized control trial (the "Eurofoetus" trial) comparing endoscopic laser therapy to amnioreduction for twin--twin transfusion syndrome (TTTS) were published.[83] The trial was stopped early due to significant benefit in terms of survival of at least one twin to 28 days and 6 months, as well as improved neurologic outcome, with laser coagulation therapy. A 2020 metaanalysis including 2699 pregnancies undergoing laser coagulation therapy for TTTS reported survival rates of 50% to 70%, depending on stage.[84] A 2021 metaanalysis of 1499 TTTS survivors focused on risk factors for adverse neurodevelopmental outcome after laser therapy[85]; the overall incidence was 14%. The SMFM guidelines[86] recommend fetoscopic laser surgery as the standard treatment for stages II through stage IV TTTS presenting between 16 and 26 weeks' gestation.

Although pediatric benefit with open intrauterine fetal surgery for myelomeningocele repair has been observed, there are significant maternal risks, including the need for cesarean delivery with all future pregnancies (similar to that for women with a history of a classical cesarean delivery) as well as increased risk of uterine rupture.[87,88] Increasingly, fetal interventions are performed fetoscopically (rather than open); the minimally invasive approach is associated with a decreased risk of maternal complications.[89]

Before *in utero* surgery can be recommended, a thorough evaluation must be performed to (1) precisely characterize the defect, (2) exclude associated malformations, (3) perform a fetal genetic analysis, and (4) eliminate the possibility that the condition can be treated using less aggressive technologies. Detailed counseling about the risks and benefits of the proposed procedure is required prior to a shared decision-making process incorporating the patient's preferences and values. Such a discussion must include a detailed review of the risks to both the fetus and the mother, including preterm premature rupture of membranes, preterm labor and delivery, placental abruption, chorioamnionitis and sepsis, and maternal complications in the current pregnancy and future pregnancies.

KEY POINTS

- Accurate determination of gestational age is essential for the management of pregnancy complications and the effective use of antepartum fetal testing.
- Ultrasonography can be used to estimate gestational age, assess fetal growth, monitor amniotic fluid volume, and detect and characterize fetal anomalies.
- Appropriate fetal growth is strongly correlated with fetal health and can be assessed either clinically or with ultrasonography. Inappropriate fetal growth, particularly growth restriction, requires further evaluation.

- Pregnancies at increased risk for complications require additional fetal monitoring such as the nonstress test, biophysical profile, or contraction stress test. Serial, multimodal testing offers the most reliable information.
- The appropriate timing of delivery is a critical determinant of perinatal outcome. In general, delivery is indicated when the benefits of delivery to the fetus or mother outweigh the risks associated with continuing the pregnancy. Several variables should be considered in making such a decision, the most important of which are gestational age and fetal well-being.

REFERENCES

1. American College of Obstetricians and Gynecologists. Committee Opinion No. 579: Definition of term pregnancy (reaffirmed 2022). *Obstet Gynecol*. 2013;122:1139–1140.
2. American College of Obstetricians and Gynecologists. Committee Opinion No. 700: Methods for estimating the due date (reaffirmed 2022). *Obstet Gynecol*. 2017;129:e150–e154.
3. American College of Obstetricians and Gynecologists. American Institute of Ultrasound in Medicine Practice Bulletin No. 175: Ultrasound in pregnancy (reaffirmed 2022). *Obstet Gynecol*. 2016;128:e241–e256.
4. American College of Obstetricians and Gynecologists. Committee Opinion No. 688: Management of suboptimally dated pregnancies (reaffirmed 2024). *Obstet Gynecol*. 2017;129:e29–e32.
5. American College of Obstetricians and Gynecologists. Society for Maternal-Fetal Medicine Practice Bulletin No. 226: Screening for fetal chromosomal abnormalities (reaffirmed 2024). *Obstet Gynecol*. 2020;136:e48–e69.
6. American College of Obstetricians and Gynecologists. Practice Bulletin No. 162: Prenatal diagnostic testing for genetic disorders (reaffirmed 2024). *Obstet Gynecol*. 2016;127:e108–e122.
7. Du X, Zhang L, Liu Z, et al. Risk of mother-to-child transmission after amniocentesis in pregnant women with hepatitis B virus: a retrospective cohort study. *Am J Obstet Gynecol*. 2024;230:249.e1e8.
8. Floridia M, Masuelli G, Meloni A, et al. Amniocentesis and chorionic villus sampling in HIV-infected pregnant women: amulticentre case series. *BJOG*. 2017;124:1218–1223.
9. Spinillo SL, Farina A, Sotiriadis A, et al. Pregnancy outcome of confined placental mosaicism: meta-analysis of cohort studies. *Am J Obstet Gynecol*. 2022;227(5):714–727.e1. https://doi:10.1016/j.ajog.2022.07.034. Epub 2022 Aug 4. PMID: 35934121.

10. Salomon LJ, Alfirevic Z, Berghella V, et al. ISUOG Practice Guidelines (updated): performance of the routine mid-trimester fetal ultrasound scan. *Ultrasound Obstet Gynecol*. 2022;59:840–856.
11. Levi S. Ultrasound in prenatal diagnosis: polemics around routine ultrasound screening for second trimester fetal malformations. *Prenat Diagn*. 2002;22:285–295.
12. Grandjean H, Larroque D, Levi S. Sensitivity of routine ultrasound screening of pregnancies in the Eurofetus database. The Eurofetus Team. *Ann N Y Acad Sci*. 1998;847:118–124.
13. Dashe JS, McIntire DD, Twickler DM. Effect of maternal obesity on the ultrasound detection of anomalous fetuses. *Obstet Gynecol*. 2009;113:1001–1007.
14. Farladansky-Gershnabel S, Gluska H, Sharon-Weiner M, et al. Low lying placenta: natural course, clinical data, complications and a new model for early prediction of persistency. *J Matern Fetal Neonatal Med*. 2023;36:2204998.
15. Jansen C, Kleinrouweler CE, Kastelein AW, et al. Follow-up ultrasound in second-trimester low-positioned anterior and posterior placentae: prospective cohort study. *Ultrasound Obstet Gynecol*. 2020;56:725–731.
16. Leopold G, Sporlin L. Conduct of normal births through external examination alone. *Arch Gynaekol*. 1894;45:337.
17. Gardosi J, Francis A. Controlled trial of fundal height measurement plotted on customised antenatal growth charts. *Br J Obstet Gynaecol*. 1999;106:309–317.
18. Hadlock FP, Harrist RB, Carpenter RJ, et al. Sonographic estimation of fetal weight. The value of femur length in addition to head and abdomen measurements. *Radiology*. 1984;150:535–540.
19. Dudley NJ. A systematic review of the ultrasound estimation of fetal weight. *Ultrasound Obstet Gynecol*. 2005;25:80–89.

20. Blue NR, Mele L, Grobman WA, et al. Predictive performance of newborn small for gestational age by a United States intrauterine vs birthweight-derived standard for short-term neonatal morbidity and mortality. *Am J Obstet Gynecol MFM.* 2022;4:100599.

21. American College of Obstetricians and Gynecologists. Practice Bulletin No. 227: Fetal growth restriction. *Obstet Gynecol.* 2021;137:e16–e28.

22. Society for Maternal-Fetal Medicine Martins JG, Biggio JR, Abuhamad A. Society for Maternal-Fetal Medicine Consult Series #52: Diagnosis and management of fetal growth restriction (replaces Clinical Guideline Number 3, April 2012). *Am J Obstet Gynecol.* 2020;223:B2–B17.

23. Kaimal AJ. Assessment of fetal health. In: Lockwood CJ, Copel JA, Dugoff L, et al., eds. *Creasy and Resnick's Maternal-Fetal Medicine, Principles and Practice.* 9th ed. Elsevier; 2023:559–574.

24. American College of Obstetricians and Gynecologists. Committee Opinion No. 828: Indications for outpatient antenatal fetal surveillance (reaffirmed 2024). *Obstet Gynecol.* 2021;137:e177–e197.

25. National Institute of Child Health and Human Development Research Planning Workshop. Electronic fetal heart rate monitoring: research guidelines for interpretation. *Am J Obstet Gynecol.* 1997;177:1385–1390.

26. Macones GA, Hankins GD, Spong CY, et al. The 2008 National Institute of Child Health and Human Development workshop report on electronic fetal monitoring: update on definitions, interpretation, and research guidelines. *Obstet Gynecol.* 2008;112:661–666.

27. Freeman RK, Anderson G, Dorchester W. A prospective multi-institutional study of antepartum fetal heart rate monitoring. I. Risk of perinatal mortality and morbidity according to antepartum fetal heart rate test results. *Am J Obstet Gynecol.* 1982;143:771–777.

28. Boehm FH, Salyer S, Shah DM, Vaughn WK. Improved outcome of twice weekly nonstress testing. *Obstet Gynecol.* 1986;67:566–568.

29. American College of Obstetricians and Gynecologists. Practice Bulletin No. 229: Antepartum fetal surveillance (reaffirmed 2024). *Obstet Gynecol.* 2021;137:e116–e127.

30. Leveno KJ, Cunningham FG, Nelson S, et al. A prospective comparison of selective and universal electronic fetal monitoring in 34,995 pregnancies. *N Engl J Med.* 1986;315:615–619.

31. Smith CV, Phelan JP, Paul RH. A prospective analysis of the influence of gestational age on the baseline fetal heart rate and reactivity in a low-risk population. *Am J Obstet Gynecol.* 1985;153:780–782.

32. Nelson KB, Dambrosia JM, Ting TY, Grether JK. Uncertain value of electronic fetal monitoring in predicting cerebral palsy. *N Engl J Med.* 1996;334:613–618.

33. Smith CV, Phelan JP, Platt LD, et al. Fetal acoustic stimulation testing. II. A randomized clinical comparison with the nonstress test. . *Am J Obstet Gynecol.* 1986;155:131–134.

34. Manning FA. Dynamic ultrasound-based fetal assessment: thefetal biophysical profile score. *Clin Obstet Gynecol.* 1995;38:26–44.

35. Vintzileos AM, Campbell WA, Nochimson DJ, Weinbaum PJ. The use and misuse of the fetal biophysical profile. *Am J Obstet Gynecol.* 1987;156:527–533.

36. Oz AU, Holub B, Mendilcioglu I, et al. Renal artery Doppler investigation of the etiology of oligohydramnios in postterm pregnancy. *Obstet Gynecol.* 2002;100:715–718.

37. Tongsong T, Srisomboon J. Amniotic fluid volume as a predictor of fetal distress in postterm pregnancy. *Int J Gynaecol Obstet.* 1993;40:213–217.

38. Morris JM, Thompson K, Smithey J, et al. The usefulness of ultrasound assessment of amniotic fluid in predicting adverse outcome in prolonged pregnancy: a prospective blinded observational study. *BJOG.* 2003;110:989–994.

39. Clement D, Schifrin BS, Kates RB. Acute oligohydramnios in postdate pregnancy. *Am J Obstet Gynecol.* 1987;157:884–886.

40. Manning FA, Morrison I, Harman CR, et al. Fetal assessment based on fetal biophysical profile scoring: experience in 19,221 referred high-risk pregnancies. II. An analysis of false-negative fetal deaths. *Am J Obstet Gynecol.* 1987;157:880–884.

41. Nageotte MP, Towers CV, Asrat T, Freeman RK. Perinatal outcome with the modified biophysical profile. *Am J Obstet Gynecol.* 1994;170:1672–1676.

42. Miller DA, Rabello YA, Paul RH. The modified biophysical profile: antepartum testing in the 1990s. *Am J Obstet Gynecol.* 1996;174:812–817.

43. Manning FA, Morrison I, Lange IR, et al. Fetal assessment based on fetal biophysical profile scoring: experience in 12,620 referred high-risk pregnancies. I. Perinatal mortality byfrequency and etiology. *Am J Obstet Gynecol.* 1985;151:343–350.

44. Wenstrom KD, Weiner CP, Williamson RA. Diverse maternal and fetal pathology associated with absent diastolic flow in the umbilical artery of high-risk fetuses. *Obstet Gynecol.* 1991;77:374–378.

45. Giles WB, Trudinger BJ, Baird PJ. Fetal umbilical artery flow velocity waveforms and placental resistance: pathological correlation. *Br J Obstet Gynaecol.* 1985;92:31–38.

46. Nicolaides KH, Bilardo CM, Soothill PW, Campbell S. Absence of end diastolic frequencies in umbilical artery: a sign of fetal hypoxia and acidosis. *BMJ.* 1988;297:1026–1027.

47. Karsdorp VH, van Vugt JM, van Geijn HP, et al. Clinical significance of absent or reversed end diastolic velocity waveforms in umbilical artery. *Lancet.* 1994;344:1664–1668.

48. Zelop CM, Richardson DK, Heffner LJ. Outcomes of severely abnormal umbilical artery Doppler velocimetry in structurally normal singleton fetuses. *Obstet Gynecol.* 1996;87:434–438.

49. Farmakides G, Schulman H, Ducey J, et al. Uterine and umbilical artery Doppler velocimetry in postterm pregnancy. *J Reprod Med.* 1988;33:259–261.

50. Stokes HJ, Roberts RV, Newnham JP. Doppler flow velocity waveform analysis in postdate pregnancies. *Aust N Z J Obstet Gynaecol.* 1991;31:27–30.

51. Baschat AA. Doppler application in the delivery timing of the preterm growth-restricted fetus: another step in the right direction. *Ultrasound Obstet Gynecol.* 2004;23:111–118.

52. Landon MB, Gabbe SG, Bruner JP, Ludmir J. Doppler umbilical artery velocimetry in pregnancy complicated by insulin-dependent diabetes mellitus. *Obstet Gynecol.* 1989;73:961–965.

53. American College of Obstetricians and Gynecologists. Practice Bulletin No. 146: Management of late-term and postterm pregnancies (reaffirmed 2024). *Obstet Gynecol.* 2014;124:390–396.

54. Mari G, Adrignolo A, Abuhamad AZ, et al. Diagnosis of fetal anemia with Doppler ultrasound in the pregnancy complicated by maternal blood group immunization. *Ultrasound Obstet Gynecol.* 1995;5:400–405.

55. Fung C, Zinkhan E. Short- and long-term implications of small for gestational age. *Obstet Gynecol Clin North Am.* 2021;48:311–323.

56. Getahun D, Ananth CV, Kinzler WL. Risk factors for antepartum and intrapartum stillbirth: a population-based study. *Am J Obstet Gynecol.* 2007;196:499–507.

57. Papastefanou I, Ashoor G, Syngelaki A, et al. Relation of antepartum stillbirth to birthweight and gestational age: prospective cohort study. *BJOG.* 2024;131:200–206.

58. Vergani P, Roncaglia N, Locatelli A, et al. Antenatal predictors of neonatal outcome in fetal growth restriction with absent end-diastolic flow in the umbilical artery. *Am J Obstet Gynecol.* 2005;193:1213–1218.

59. American College of Obstetricians and Gynecologists. Practice Bulletin No. 216: Macrosomia (reaffirmed 2023). *Obstet Gynecol.* 2020;135:e18–e35.

60. Boulet SL, Alexander GR, Salihu HM, Pass M. Macrosomic births in the United States: determinants, outcomes, and proposed grades of risk. *Am J Obstet Gynecol.* 2003;188:1372–1378.

61. American College of Obstetricians and Gynecologists. Practice Bulletin No 178: Shoulder dystocia (reaffirmed 2024). *Obstet Gynecol.* 2017;129:e123–e133.

62. Nesbitt TS, Gilbert WM, Herrchen B. Shoulder dystocia and associated risk factors with macrosomic infants born in California. *Am J Obstet Gynecol.* 1998;179:476–480.

63. Gherman RB, Chauhan S, Ouzounian JG, et al. Shoulder dystocia: the unpreventable obstetric emergency with empiric management guidelines. *Am J Obstet Gynecol.* 2006;195:657–672.

64. Watson WJ, Soisson AP, Harlass FE. Estimated weight of the term fetus. Accuracy of ultrasound vs. clinical examination. *JReprod Med.* 1988;33:369–371.

65. Niswander KR, Capraro VJ, Van Coevering RJ. Estimation of birth weight by quantified external uterine measurements. *Obstet Gynecol.* 1970;36:294–298.

66. Osterman MJK, Hamilton BE, Martin JA, et al. Births: final data for 2021. *Natl Vital Stat Rep.* 2023;72:1–53.

67. Middleton P, Shepherd E, Morris J, et al. Induction of labour at or beyond 37 weeks' gestation. *Cochrane Database Syst Rev.* 2020;(7):CD004945.

68. Grobman WA, Rice MM, Reddy UM, et al. Labor induction versus expectant management in low-risk nulliparous women. *N Engl J Med.* 2018;379:513–523.

69. American College of Obstetricians and Gynecologists. Clinical practice update: management of full-term nulliparous individuals without a medical indication for delivery. *Obstet Gynecol.* 2025;145:e45–e50.

70. Society of Maternal-Fetal Publications Committee. SMFM statement on elective induction of labor in low-risk nulliparous women at term: the ARRIVE trial. *Am J Obstet Gynecol.* 2019;221:B2–B4.

71. American College of Obstetricians and Gynecologists. Committee Opinion No. 831: Medically indicated late-preterm and early-term deliveries. *Obstet Gynecol.* 2021;138:e35–e39.

72. Nabhan AF, Abdelmoula YA. Amniotic fluid index versus single deepest vertical pocket: a meta-analysis of randomized controlled trials. *Int J Gynaecol Obstet.* 2009;104:184–188.

73. Reddy UM, Abuhamad AZ, Levine D, et al. Fetal imaging: executive summary of a Joint Eunice Kennedy Shriver National Institute of Child Health and Human Development, Society for Maternal-Fetal Medicine, American Institute of Ultrasound in Medicine, American College of Obstetricians and Gynecologists, American College of Radiology, Society forPediatric Radiology, and Society of Radiologists in Ultrasound Fetal Imaging Workshop. *Am J Obstet Gynecol.* 2014;210:387–397.

74. Rabie N, Magann E, Steelman S, Ounpraseuth S. Oligohydramnios in complicated and uncomplicated pregnancy: a systematic review and meta-analysis. *Ultrasound Obstet Gynecol.* 2017;49:442–449.

75. Moldenhauer JS, Johnson A, Van Mieghem T. International Society for Prenatal Diagnosis 2022 DEBATE: there should be formal accreditation and ongoing quality assurance/review for units offering fetal therapy that includes public reporting of outcomes. *Prenat Diagn.* 2023;43:411–420.

76. Stoll BJ, Hansen NI, Bell EF, et al. Neonatal outcomes of extremely preterm infants from the NICHD Neonatal Research Network. *Pediatrics.* 2010;126:443–456.

77. Hibbard JU, Wilkins I, Sun L, et al. Respiratory morbidity in late preterm births. *JAMA.* 2010;304:419–425.

78. Liggins GC, Howie RN. A controlled trial of antepartum glucocorticoid treatment for prevention of the respiratory distress syndrome in premature infants. *Pediatrics.* 1972;50:515–525.

79. McGoldrick E, Stewart F, Parker R, Dalziel SR. Antenatal corticosteroids for accelerating fetal lung maturation for women at risk of preterm birth. *Cochrane Database Syst Rev.* 2020;(12):CD004454.

80. Leviton A, Kuban KC, Pagano M, et al. Antenatal corticosteroids appear to reduce the risk of postnatal germinal matrix hemorrhage in intubated low birth weight newborns. *Pediatrics.* 1993;91:1083–1088.

81. American College of Obstetricians and Gynecologists. Committee Opinion No. 713: Antenatal corticosteroid therapy for fetal maturation (reaffirmed 2024). *Obstet Gynecol.* 2017;130:e102–e109.

82. Society for Maternal-Fetal Medicine, et al.Mari G, Norton ME, et al. Society for Maternal-Fetal Medicine (SMFM) Clinical Guideline #8: The fetus at risk for anemia–diagnosis and management. *Am J Obstet Gynecol.* 2015;212:697–710.

83. Senat MV, Deprest J, Boulvain M, et al. Endoscopic laser surgery versus serial amnioreduction for severe twin-to-twin transfusion syndrome. *N Engl J Med.* 2004;351:136–144.

84. Di Mascio D, Khalil A, D'Amico A, et al. Outcome of twin-twin transfusion syndrome according to Quintero stage of disease: systematic review and meta-analysis. *Ultrasound Obstet Gynecol.* 2020;56:811–820.

85. Hessami K, Nassr AA, Sananès N, et al. Perinatal risk factors of neurodevelopmental impairment after fetoscopic laser photocoagulation for twin-twin transfusion syndrome: systematic review and meta-analysis. *Ultrasound Obstet Gynecol.* 2021;58:658–668.

86. Society for Maternal-Fetal Medicine (SMFM), Miller RS, Miller JL, et al. Society for Maternal-Fetal Medicine Consult Series #72: Twin-twin transfusion syndrome and twin anemia-polycythemia sequence. *Am J Obstet Gynecol.* 2024;231:B16–B37.

87. American College of Obstetricians and Gynecologists. Society for Maternal Fetal Medicine Committee Opinion No. 720: Maternal-fetal surgery for myelomeningocele (reaffirmed 2022). *Obstet Gynecol.* 2017;130:e164–e167.

88. Goodnight WH, Bahtiyar O, Bennett KA, et al. Subsequent pregnancy outcomes after open maternal-fetal surgery for myelomeningocele. *Am J Obstet Gynecol.* 2019;220:494.e1–e7.

89. Sacco A, Van der Veeken L, Bagshaw E, et al. Maternal complications following open and fetoscopic fetal surgery: a systematic review and meta-analysis. *Prenat Diagn.* 2019;39:251–268.

7

Anesthesia for Fetal Surgery and Other Intrauterine Procedures

Caitlin D. Sutton, MD and Mark D. Rollins, MD, PhD

Advances in prenatal diagnosis, imaging, and surgical equipment have all contributed to the development of fetal surgery. While most correctable malformations are best managed after delivery, antepartum recognition allows time for the coordination of appropriate prenatal and postnatal care; a minority of fetal abnormalities diagnosed *in utero* are amenable to intrauterine fetal surgery. Some defects, such as those that cause airway obstruction or irreversible end-organ damage, are particularly suitable for intrapartum intervention. This allows the benefit of intervention while the uteroplacental unit remains functional and often eliminates the urgency associated with undertaking the procedure in the postnatal period.

Guidelines for performing fetal surgery (Box 7.1) were originally developed more than 40 years ago but remain relevant today with only minimal modifications.[1] A consensus statement from the American Society of Anesthesiologists detailed anesthesia considerations for maternal-fetal interventions, highlighting that all fetal interventions should include multidisciplinary deliberation and planning.[2] A detailed preoperative evaluation should be completed to minimize risk to the pregnant patient. Potential maternal risks should be discussed as part of the consent process alongside the fetal benefits and risks, and clear expectations set for the patient's experience throughout the perioperative period. Guidelines from the American College of Obstetricians and Gynecologists and the American Academy of Pediatrics recommend that fetal treatment centers include a multidisciplinary comprehensive consent and counseling process, oversight of fetal research,

and participation in a data-sharing fetal intervention network.[3] Multidisciplinary guidance from the North American Fetal Therapy Network details expected fetal therapy center resources based on three levels of fetal care complexity.[4]

Fetal surgical interventions have historically been broadly categorized into three kinds of procedures: minimally invasive procedures, open surgical procedures, and intrapartum procedures. A summary of fetal conditions, therapy, and established interventions is detailed in Table 7.1, although newer conditions and indications are periodically emerging.

Minimally invasive procedures involving either fetoscopic or ultrasound-guided percutaneous procedures are typically performed near mid-gestation. They entail a lower risk for preterm labor and delivery than open procedures because they do not require a hysterotomy, yet the risk for preterm premature rupture of membranes (PROM) remains.[5]

Open surgical procedures involve both a maternal laparotomy and hysterotomy with use of pharmacologic agents to maintain uterine relaxation. These procedures are typically performed near mid-gestation and entail greater maternal and fetal risks compared with the minimally invasive techniques, including a significant risk for preterm PROM, preterm labor and delivery, uterine dehiscence, oligohydramnios, hemorrhage, pulmonary edema, and fetal mortality. In addition, after an open surgical procedure, a cesarean delivery is required for the pregnancy and all future deliveries owing to the location of the hysterotomy and the associated risks for uterine dehiscence or rupture.

BOX 7.1 Guidelines for Performing Fetal Procedures

1. Accurate diagnosis and staging is possible.
2. Other anomalies that would contraindicate fetal intervention are excluded.
3. Progression, severity, and prognosis of the condition are understood.
4. No effective postnatal therapy is currently available, and if not treated before birth, the anomaly would result in fetal death, irreversible organ damage, or other severe postnatal morbidity.
5. Intrauterine surgery has been proven feasible in animal models, with demonstrated reversal of the deleterious effects of the condition.
6. The maternal risk is acceptably low.
7. Interventions are performed in specialized multidisciplinary fetal treatment centers within strict protocols and approval of the local ethics committee, with informed consent obtained from the mother or parents.
8. There is access to high-level specialized medical care, including bioethical and psychosocial care and counseling.

Summarized from Harrison MR, Filly RA, Golbus MS, et al. Fetal treatment 1982. *N Engl J Med.* 1982;307:1651–1652; Sudhakaran N, Sothinathan U, Patel S. Best practice guidelines: fetal surgery. *Early Hum Dev.* 2012;88:15–19.

The *ex utero* intrapartum therapy (EXIT) procedure involves modification of a cesarean delivery to allow intrapartum fetal therapy while the fetus remains supported by placental gas exchange.[6,7] EXIT procedures are most often employed while (1) securing the airway by tracheal intubation, bronchoscopy, or tracheostomy in fetuses with congenital airway obstruction or neck mass; or (2) performing invasive fetal procedures required before delivery. The EXIT procedure enables the prevention of asphyxia in neonates in whom securing an airway after birth can be problematic. The procedure can also be used as a bridge to extracorporeal membrane oxygenation (ECMO) for a fetus with cardiopulmonary disease at risk for postnatal cardiac failure or failure of adequate pulmonary gas exchange.

As new surgical approaches have been developed, these three categories are no longer clearly defined. For example, fetal surgeries for neural tube defects (NTDs) can now be performed using various techniques, including laparotomy-assisted fetoscopic repair, "mini-laparotomy" fetoscopic repair, or even fully percutaneous fetoscopic repair. Additionally, fetal anomalies traditionally considered for EXIT procedures may be amenable to other approaches such as coordinated cesarean delivery with intervention immediately prior to or after delivery, with the goal of avoiding

TABLE 7.1 Fetal Conditions and Interventions

Fetal Condition	Therapy Rationale	Type	Intervention
Fetal anemia or thrombocytopenia	Prevention of heart failure and fetal hydrops	Ultrasound-guided	Intrauterine transfusion
Aortic stenosis or pulmonary atresia	Prevention of fetal hydrops, myocardial dysfunction, and hypoplastic left (or right) heart	Ultrasound-guided	Percutaneous fetal valvuloplasty
Hypoplastic left heart with intact atrial septum	Provision of a source of pulmonary blood flow, decreasing urgency of intervention at birth	Ultrasound-guided	Percutaneous fetal septoplasty
Obstructive uropathy	Bladder decompression with reduction in renal dysfunction, pulmonary hypoplasia, oligohydramnios, and limb malformation	Fetal ultrasound-guided and/or fetoscopy	Percutaneous vesicoamniotic shunting or fetoscopic laser ablation of urethral valves
Twin reversed arterial perfusion sequence	Prevention of high-output cardiac failure in the normal twin by stopping flow to the acardiac twin	Fetal ultrasound-guided and/or fetoscopy	Umbilical radiofrequency ablation or fetoscopic cord coagulation
Twin-to-twin transfusion syndrome	Reduction of twin-to-twin blood flow and prevention of cardiac failure	Fetoscopy	Fetoscopic laser photocoagulation of placental vessels and/or amnioreduction
Congenital diaphragmatic hernia	Prevention of pulmonary hypoplasia	Fetoscopy	Fetoscopic tracheal occlusion
Myelomeningocele	Reduction in hydrocephalus and hindbrain herniation with improved neurologic function and reduced spinal cord deficits	Open or fetoscopy	Closure of fetal defect *in utero*

(Continued)

TABLE 7.1	Fetal Conditions and Interventions—cont'd		
Fetal Condition	**Therapy Rationale**	**Type**	**Intervention**
Sacrococcygeal teratoma	Prevention of high-output cardiac failure, hydrops, and polyhydramnios	Fetal ultrasound-guided or open	Ablation of tumor vasculature or open fetal tumor debulking
Lung lesions	Reversal of pulmonary hypoplasia and cardiac failure (mid-gestation), prevention of respiratory and/or circulatory emergency at birth (peripartum)	Fetal image-guided, open, intrapartum or immediately postpartum	Thoracoamniotic shunting, open fetal lobectomy, EXIT allows for resection or chest decompression at time of delivery, PRESTO has second perioperative team immediately available
Fetal airway compromise	Secured airway and/or circulatory support to prevent respiratory compromise at birth	Open intrapartum	EXIT allows stabilization while on uteroplacental circulation

EXIT, Ex utero intrapartum therapy; *PRESTO,* procedure requiring a second team in the operating room.
Modified from Partridge EA, Flake AW. Maternal-fetal surgery for structural malformations. *Best Pract Res Clin Obstet Gynaecol.* 2012;26: 669–682; Hoagland MA, Chatterjee D. Anesthesia for fetal surgery. *Paediatr Anaesth.* 2017;27:346–357.

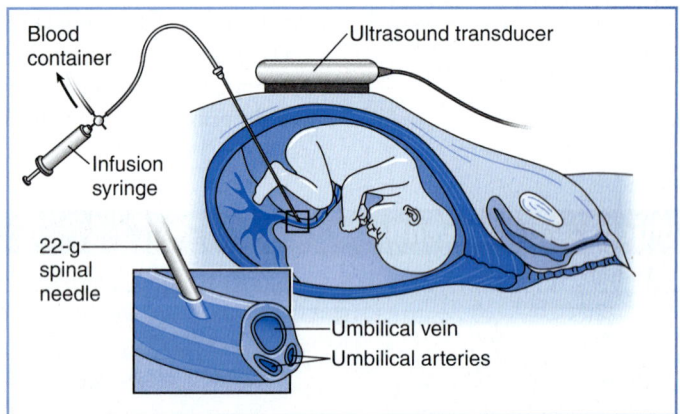

Fig. 7.1 Percutaneous Intrauterine Umbilical Cord Sampling and Transfusion. Illustration from University of California, San Francisco Fetal Treatment Center, San Francisco, CA.

potential maternal morbidity associated with an EXIT procedure. Procedures with intervention occurring immediately after delivery include many considerations similar to the EXIT procedure (e.g., the physiologic transition from fetal to neonatal circulation) and are referred to as a **procedure requiring a second team in the operating room** (**PRESTO**) or **cesarean section with immediate resection** (**CSIR,** pronounced like "scissor").[8,9]

INDICATIONS AND RATIONALE FOR FETAL SURGERY

Fetal Anemia and Intrauterine Transfusion

Fetal anemia can occur secondary to maternal alloimmunization, viral infections, homozygous thalassemia, maternal-fetal hemorrhage, and placental chorioangioma. The rate of fetal anemia secondary to rhesus D (RhD) sensitization has decreased to 1 in 500 pregnancies following the use of RhD immunoglobulin prophylaxis.[10] Serial Doppler studies of the middle cerebral artery (MCA) peak velocity are used to diagnose fetal anemia.[11,12] A sample of fetal umbilical cord blood just before starting the intrauterine transfusion (IUT) allows accurate assessment of fetal anemia.

IUTs are frequently performed using a 20- or 22-gauge needle with local anesthesia at the maternal needle insertion site. The needle is inserted percutaneously through the maternal abdomen and uterus under ultrasonographic guidance to access the umbilical vein (Fig. 7.1). The umbilical cord is often accessed near its placental insertion for stability, but a loop of umbilical cord or an intrahepatic portion of the umbilical vein can also be used. Before 18 weeks' gestation, intraperitoneal transfusion may be chosen for treatment of fetal anemia given that accessing the umbilical vein may not be possible.

The transfused volume of O-negative, cytomegalovirus (CMV)-negative, irradiated, leukocyte-depleted, packed red blood cells is determined based on the estimated fetal weight, gestational age, autologous hemoglobin, and hemoglobin of the sampled fetal blood.[13] Fetal hemoglobin level increases, then slowly decreases, so multiple IUTs are often required at 1- to 3-week intervals. Administration of a muscle relaxant to the fetus should be considered to decrease the chance of fetal movement dislodging the transfusion needle or shearing the cord vasculature.[14] The umbilical cord does not have pain receptors, but if the needle is advanced into the fetal abdomen for intraperitoneal access, fentanyl or another opioid should be administered to the fetus to blunt the stress response that results.[15] Providers should be prepared for a possible emergency cesarean delivery if the fetus is of viable age. The rate of fetal demise following IUT is approximately 3%.[12]

Obstructive Uropathy

Lower urinary tract obstruction (LUTO) occurs in approximately 1 in 4000 live births.[16] Congenital bilateral hydronephrosis results from fetal urethral obstruction at the bladder outlet, most commonly by either posterior urethral valves (PUVs, typically male fetuses) or urethral atresia. Other causes of fetal obstructive uropathy include obstruction at the ureteropelvic or vesicoureteric junction and a number of complex disorders in females (e.g., cloacal plate anomalies). LUTO may lead to progressive renal dysplasia and dysfunction, bladder distention, and oligohydramnios, and ultimately result in devastating developmental consequences, such as limb and facial deformities, pulmonary hypoplasia, and even neonatal death (Fig. 7.2).[17,18] Although postnatal correction relieves the obstruction, 25% to 30% of survivors develop end-stage kidney disease requiring dialysis by 5 years of age.[19] Early intrauterine intervention with placement of a **vesicoamniotic shunt (VAS)** allows drainage of urine from the fetal bladder into the amniotic cavity, and in animal models, improves dysplastic renal histology, restores normal urine flow and amniotic fluid volume, and results in improved lung growth and development.[20]

A VAS is a valveless, double-coiled catheter placed percutaneously with ultrasonographic guidance, with one coil in the urinary bladder and the other in the amniotic space. Common catheter-associated problems include: (1) difficult placement,

occlusion, and displacement; (2) fetal trauma, iatrogenic abdominal wall defects, and amnioperitoneal leaking; and (3) preterm PROM, preterm labor, and chorioamnionitis.[21] In a 2017 metaanalysis of primarily cohort studies, there was a perinatal survival improvement with VAS compared with conservative management (57.1% versus 38.8%, $P < .01$) but no difference in 2-year survival or postnatal renal function.[19]

Fetal cystoscopy is a more recent treatment in which a trocar-assisted fetoscope enters the fetal bladder under ultrasonographic guidance and allows direct visualization of the fetal urethra. Although not a viable treatment for urethral atresia, fetal cystoscopy facilitates diagnosis and treatment of LUTO caused by PUVs.[22] Once visualized, the PUVs are destroyed using guidewires and hydroablation or laser ablation. A two-center case-control study showed that both fetal cystoscopy and VAS improved the 6-month survival rate compared with no intervention in severe LUTO.[23]

A recent multicenter prospective clinical trial that examined the use of serial amnioinfusions (1 to 3 times each week) in fetuses with bilateral renal agenesis found that therapy mitigated lethal pulmonary hypoplasia, but was associated with higher preterm delivery and a low rate (35%) of survival to hospital discharge and long-term dialysis[24]; the survival rate was lower than anticipated in neonates born with renal failure (but not restricted to bilateral renal agenesis).[25] The trial was stopped early owing to concerns about neonatal morbidity and mortality despite demonstration of the intervention's efficacy.[24] Current evidence supports the use of fetal intervention for LUTO in selected fetuses in an effort to restore amniotic fluid volume, prevent pulmonary hypoplasia, and decrease perinatal mortality.[26]

Congenital Diaphragmatic Hernia

Congenital diaphragmatic hernia (CDH) occurs in approximately 1 in 2500 live-born infants and can cause significant morbidity and mortality from pulmonary hypoplasia and insufficiency. Survival rates have improved to greater than 70% over the past 25 years and are closely associated with the degree of pulmonary hypertension and respiratory

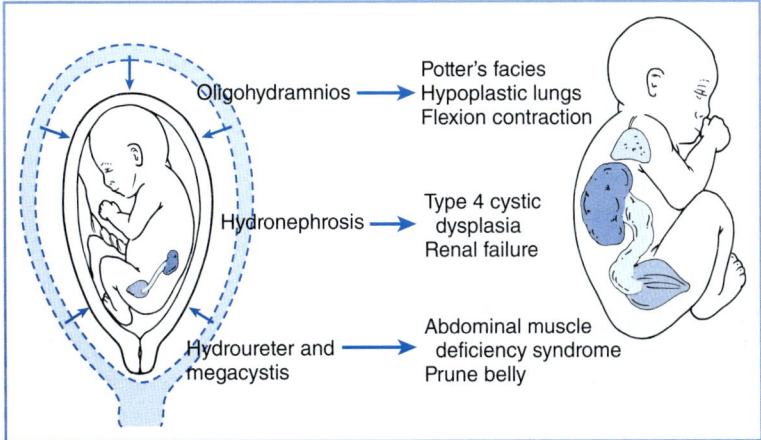

Fig. 7.2 Developmental Consequences of Fetal Urethral Obstruction. Obstructed fetal urinary flow results in hydronephrosis, hydroureter, megacystis, oligohydramnios, and pulmonary hypoplasia. Redrawn from Harrison MR, Filly RA, Parer JT, et al. Management of the fetus with a urinary tract malformation. *JAMA.* 1981;246:635–639.

insufficiency.[27,28] Significant morbidity occurs, despite optimal postnatal surgical management at tertiary care medical centers. Intrauterine intervention has the potential to decrease pulmonary hypoplasia and improve fetal lung development before delivery. Fetal lamb models of CDH demonstrated that parenchymal hypoplasia and associated pulmonary vascular changes could be reversed by correction *in utero*.[29] Primary open repairs of human CDH *in utero* have been undertaken with limited success.[30]

Tracheal occlusion impedes the normal egress of fetal lung fluid and results in expansion of the hypoplastic lung, thereby inducing lung growth, cellular maturation, and movement of the viscera out of the thorax in fetuses with CDH.[31] Once the trachea is occluded, fetal pulmonary fluid slowly accumulates and expands the lung, pushing the viscera out of the thorax. A small detachable balloon for endoluminal tracheal occlusion is placed in the trachea via percutaneous endoscopic endotracheal intubation and is left in place (Fig. 7.3).[32,33] Because of concern for tracheal damage by very early tracheal balloon placement,[34] the small detachable tracheal balloon is often placed via percutaneous endoscopic endotracheal intubation between 26 and 28 weeks' gestation and removed before birth by a second fetoscopic procedure near 34 weeks' gestation (if the fetus is still *in utero*).[35] This second procedure is performed to minimize the risk for preterm labor, avoid the need for the EXIT procedure, and possibly improve lung growth and minimize the reduction of type II alveolar cells associated with prolonged tracheal occlusion. If the balloon is still in place and delivery appears imminent, it must be removed or deflated prior to or at the time of delivery.

In 2021 two multicenter randomized Tracheal Occlusion To Accelerate Lung growth trials were published.[36,37] These trials compared postnatal CDH management with both late (30 to 32 weeks' gestation) fetoscopic endoluminal tracheal occlusion (FETO) intervention for moderate lung hypoplasia and earlier FETO intervention (27 to 30 weeks' gestation) for

severe lung hypoplasia. In both trials, the fetal tracheal balloon was removed in the 34th week of gestation. Compared with postnatal intervention, there was increased survival to discharge and to 6 months in fetuses with severe CDH treated *in utero* (40% versus 15%, $P = .009$).[36] The increased survival benefit was not statistically significant in the fetuses with moderate CDH that underwent *in utero* intervention compared with the postnatal group (survival to hospital discharge 63% vesus 50%, $P = .06$).[37] In both trials the fetal tracheal occlusion procedure resulted in higher rates of preterm PROM and preterm birth. Although promising, additional long-term follow-up in these patients is needed to better understand the efficacy of this intervention for CDH.[38]

Congenital Pulmonary Airway Malformation

Congenital pulmonary airway malformations (CPAMs) are pulmonary tumors with cystic and solid components usually isolated in a single lung. The incidence is approximately 1 in 25,000 pregnancies. Lesions are assessed by ultrasonography and can be classified as either macrocystic (≥ 5 mm diameter) or microcystic (< 5 mm diameter).[39] Lesions can regress, resulting in minimal associated morbidity, or progressively enlarge, often resulting in fetal hydrops (fetal heart failure). The size and growth of the lesions, rather than their specific type, are the primary determinants of overall prognosis. Small lesions detected *in utero* or in the neonate are treated after birth by surgical excision of the affected pulmonary lobe. Large lesions can cause mediastinal shift, hydrops, polyhydramnios, and pulmonary hypoplasia and can interfere with fetal or neonatal survival. In a retrospective single-institution review of 71 cases, the initial antenatal ultrasonographic ratio of CPAM volume-to-fetal head circumference (CPAM volume ratio [CVR]) was evaluated for hydrops formation and postnatal outcomes.[40] Fetuses with a CVR < 0.56 were noted to have no adverse postnatal outcomes, whereas a CVR > 0.56 had a positive predictive value for adverse postnatal outcomes of 33%. In addition, a CVR > 1.6 was associated with a greater risk for hydrops, and a CVR ≤ 1.6 with absence of a dominant cyst was associated with a less than 3% risk for hydrops.[41]

Depending on size, location, and other characteristics, CPAMs can be managed with either fetal intervention or postnatal resection.[42] Macrocystic lesions can be decompressed *in utero* by thoracocentesis or placement of shunt catheters between the cystic area and the amniotic cavity, resulting in sustained decompression and resolution of hydrops.[43] These *in utero* procedures are followed by postnatal surgery. However, not all lesions can be decompressed successfully with a shunt because the cysts are not always contiguous (i.e., in communication with each other) and can refill rapidly. In addition, thoracoamniotic shunts have associated risks, including malfunction, displacement, fetal hemorrhage, preterm PROM, preterm labor, and chorioamnionitis.[44] In a series of 68 fetuses with macrocystic CPAMs treated with thoracoamniotic shunts, the overall survival rate was 68% in hydropic and 88% in nonhydropic fetuses.[45] A 2023 single institution retrospective review of 31 fetuses that underwent thoracoamniotic shunts for congenital lung

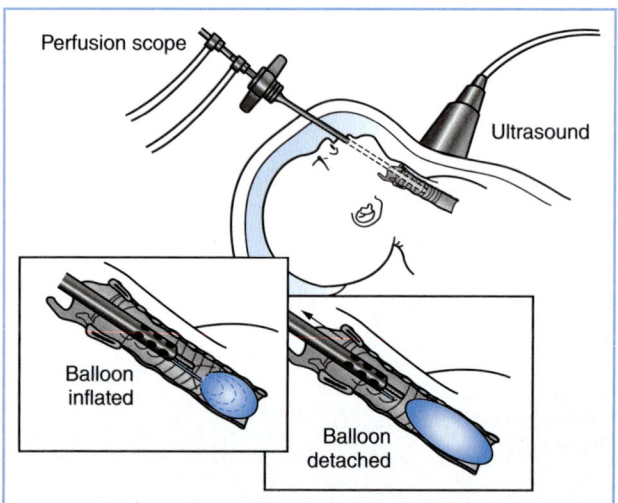

Fig. 7.3 **Fetal Tracheal Occlusion Using a Balloon.** From Harrison MR, Albanese CT, Hawgood SB, et al. Fetoscopic temporary tracheal occlusion by means of detachable balloon for congenital diaphragmatic hernia. *Am J Obstet Gynecol.* 2001;185:730–733.

Perfusion scope

Ultrasound

Balloon inflated

Balloon detached

malformations found long-term complications in 60% of the 15 surviving children (median age 11 years), including chest wall deformities and one phrenic nerve injury.[46] There was otherwise normal lung function without limitation in 14 of the 15 surviving children.

CPAMs inappropriate for drainage can be resected with open fetal surgery. Intrauterine pulmonary lobectomy for lesions associated with fetal hydrops has resulted in a 30-day postnatal survival rate of 50%, with tumor resection allowing for compensatory lung growth and resolution of hydrops.[47] Other less common options for fetal intervention include resection while on placental circulation (EXIT procedure), radiofrequency or laser ablation, and percutaneous ultrasound-guided sclerotherapy.[48] Maternal administration of **betamethasone** has been noted to improve fetal hydrops and overall outcome in selected fetuses with CPAM.[48–50]

Sacrococcygeal Teratoma

Sacrococcygeal teratoma (SCT) has an incidence of approximately 1 to 2 in 20,000 pregnancies and is associated with perinatal demise in 25% to 37% of cases.[51] Management requires serial ultrasonographic assessments, as some undergo rapid, substantial growth (e.g., volume 500 to 1000 cm[3])[52]; function as large arteriovenous (AV) fistulas; and result in high-output cardiac failure, hydrops fetalis, and placentomegaly. SCTs are staged using the **Altman criteria**,[53,54] which focus on their location. Stage I tumors are based entirely outside the pelvis and are suitable for intervention; by contrast, Stage IV tumors are completely within the pelvis and are not amenable to fetal resection. Tumor size is estimated based on a tumor volume-to-fetal weight ratio; large SCTs > 0.1 cm[3]/g (prior to 24 weeks' gestation) and those with rapid growth (>150 cm[3]/week) are associated with adverse outcomes, including tumor rupture and hemorrhage, as well as intrapartum dystocia.[53,55,56] Current surgical techniques do not allow complete resection of lesions that deeply invade the pelvis; however, in utero radiofrequency ablation, embolization, and thermocoagulation of the tumor or blood supply can reduce the tumor burden and resolve hydrops.[53,57] Large multicenter studies are needed to determine which therapies deliver the most definitive, optimal benefits (Fig. 7.4A).[53,58] During open fetal tumor resection (Fig. 7.4B), catheterization of a fetal limb or umbilical cord vein is required to allow fetal blood or fluid administration.

Some SCT cases are accompanied by "**maternal mirror**" or **Ballantyne syndrome**, a hyperdynamic state (i.e., hypertension, peripheral and pulmonary edema) in which the maternal physiology mimics the abnormal circulatory physiology of the hydropic fetus.[59,60] This syndrome is associated with a substantial increase in fetal mortality and maternal morbidity and requires aggressive management similar to that used for preeclampsia with severe features, a disease from which it must be distinguished. Platelet count, aspartate aminotransferase, alanine aminotransferase, and haptoglobin are typically unaffected in maternal mirror syndrome and may serve as diagnostic clues. Unfortunately, maternal mirror syndrome does not resolve quickly, even with rapid correction of the fetal pathophysiology, and severe life-threatening

maternal complications including pulmonary edema occur in about 20% of cases.[59,61]

Myelomeningocele

NTDs are characterized by a failure of neural tube fusion during development at the cranial level (**anencephaly**), spinal level (**spina bifida**), or both (**craniorachischisis**). There is wide heterogeneity in the birth prevalence of spina bifida, with rates of 3.4 to 3.7 per 10,000 births in most upper-middle-income and high-income countries versus rates that are 2- to 10-fold higher in world regions without folic acid fortification programs.[62,63] In contrast to anencephaly and craniorachischisis, spina bifida is not a lethal condition even in the most severe forms, such as **myeloschisis** or **myelomeningocele (MMC)**. In open MMCs, the spinous processes and overlying muscles and skin do not form normally, leading to exposure of the meninges and neural tissue. The exposed nerves can become inflamed and injured during the pregnancy from direct pressure as the fetus moves in utero and from amniotic fluid which becomes toxic to nerves in the third trimester (Fig. 7.5A).

The morbidity associated with spina bifida varies depending on the severity of the associated neuronal migrational abnormalities, known collectively as the **Chiari II malformation**, and the spinal level of the lesion. Patients can have paraparesis or paraplegia, neurogenic bowel and bladder, hydrocephalus, neuromuscular scoliosis, cranial nerve palsies, and neurocognitive deficits.[64]

Outcomes from prenatal repair of MMCs in animal models support a "two-hit" hypothesis in which the pathology is produced by both failure of the fetal neural tube to close, combined with prolonged exposure to the amniotic fluid.[65] The aim of fetal surgery is to reduce the damage that occurs in utero by creating a water-tight repair, thereby protecting the spinal cord and nerves from exposure to the amniotic fluid during the remaining gestation.

If the defect is not repaired in utero, surgical closure is generally performed within 72 hours after birth to prevent infection and preserve existing neurologic function. With postnatal NTD repair, hydrocephalus occurs in nearly all neonates with thoracic level lesions, approximately 85% of lumbar level lesions, and approximately 70% of sacral lesions.[66] Learning disabilities and cognitive defects are associated with the Chiari malformation, hydrocephalus, and damage to the white matter.[67] Despite treatment, permanent neurologic deficits such as central hypoventilation, vocal cord dysfunction, and oromotor and swallowing dysfunction can still occur in a minority (approximately 5%) of patients from underlying brainstem dysplasia associated with the Chiari II malformation. In addition, lifelong complications also include fecal incontinence (77%) and urinary incontinence with 54% requiring regular catheterization.[67] Orthopedic deformities such as clubbed feet, scoliosis, hip dislocation, and lower-extremity weakness are also common.[66]

Prenatal MMC repair is similar to a postnatal repair, but some modifications are necessary with fetal tissue. The first step in both procedures involves releasing the spinal cord from the skin by cutting the arachnoid membrane between

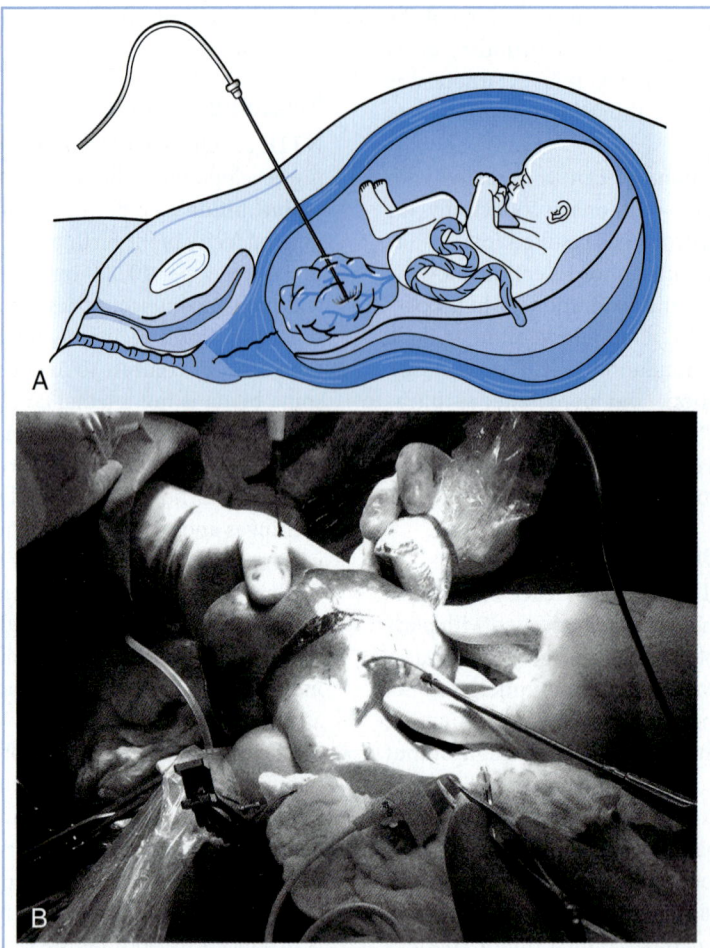

Fig. 7.4 *In Utero* Fetal Treatment of Sacrococcygeal Teratoma (SCT). (A) Radiofrequency ablation treatment of an SCT. (B) Open fetal surgery for *in utero* vascular ablation and tumor resection of SCT. Note pulse oximeter on fetal foot, placement of rectal temperature probe, and use of ultrasonography to monitor blood flow in SCT. (A) From Van Mieghem T, Al-Ibrahim A, Deprest J, et al. Minimally invasive therapy for fetal sacrococcygeal teratoma: case series and systematic review of the literature. *Ultrasound Obstet Gynecol.* 2014;43:611–619. (B) Illustration from author Mark Rollins during his affiliation with the UCSF Fetal Treatment Center, San Francisco, CA.

the placode and the junctional zone (Fig. 7.5B). Next, dura can be closed over the spinal cord but it is frequently very thin and fragile in a fetus and not water-tight; this layer can be augmented with myofascial flaps, followed by the closure of the skin.[68] Multiple surgical techniques exist to close the defect when there is not enough skin, including sewing in a patch, bipedicular advancement flaps, and rotational flaps.[69,70] The common goal of all these procedures is to achieve a water-tight closure to prevent exposure to amniotic fluid and further cerebrospinal fluid leakage (Fig. 7.5C).[71]

A randomized, prospective, multicenter clinical trial (the Management of Myelomeningocele Study [MOMS] trial) demonstrated that *in utero* repair improved motor function at 30 months of age and reduced the incidence of hydrocephalus.[72] Closure of the defect before 26 weeks' gestational age reverses hindbrain herniation.[73] The MOMS-II trial evaluated the original MOMS cohort at school age. The hydrocephalus benefit persisted and fetal patients who required a shunt were less likely to need a ventriculoperitoneal shunt revision (Table 7.2).

Open prenatal surgery portends the risk of uterine dehiscence. In 2019 the results from an international prospective observational registry of 77 subsequent pregnancies after open MMC repair demonstrated the risk of uterine rupture was 9.6%, with an additional risk of uterine dehiscence or thinning of 17.3%.[74] Other less invasive techniques, ranging from fully percutaneous to a "hybrid" laparotomy-assisted fetoscopic approach, have been developed with the aim of allowing a vaginal delivery and decreasing maternal and obstetric risks while producing equivalent neurosurgical results equivalent to the open method.[71,75,76] In 2021 the International Fetoscopic Myelomeningocele Repair Consortium reported the pregnancy and postnatal outcomes at 12 months in patients who underwent prenatal fetoscopic repair.[77] The average gestational age at delivery was 34 weeks, similar to that reported for open prenatal repairs, despite a higher rate of prelabor PROM (54.6% versus 32% to 46%). Neurologic outcomes at 12 months of life were similar.[78–80]

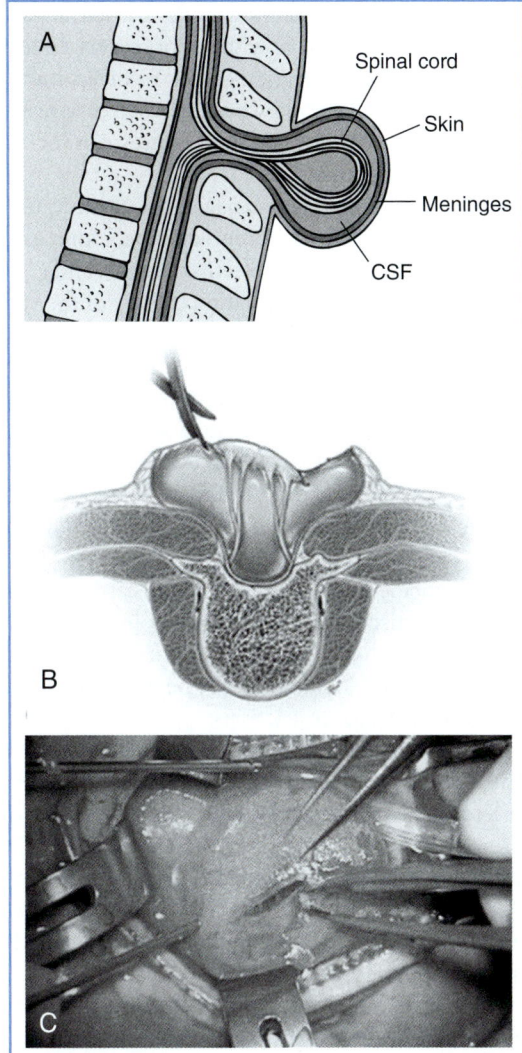

TABLE 7.2 Maternal and Fetal or Neonatal Complications for MOMS Trial Patients[a]

	Prenatal (n = 78)	Postnatal (n = 80)	P-Value
Maternal Outcomes			
Chorioamniotic membrane separation	20 (26%)	0	<.001
Pulmonary edema	5 (6%)	0	.03
Oligohydramnios	16 (21%)	3 (4%)	.001
Placental abruption	5 (6%)	0	.03
Spontaneous rupture of membranes	36 (46%)	6 (8%)	<.001
Spontaneous labor	30 (38%)	11 (14%)	<.001
Blood transfusion at delivery	7 (9%)	1 (1%)	.03
Hysterotomy site thin, or partial or complete dehiscence noted at delivery	27 (36%)	N/A	
Fetal Outcomes			
Fetal bradycardia during repair	8 (10%)	0	.003
Mean gestational age at birth (w)	34.1 ± 3.1	37.3 ± 1.1	<.001
Mean birth weight (g)	2383 ± 688	3039 ± 469	<.001
Respiratory distress syndrome	16 (21%)	5 (6%)	.008

Fig. 7.5 Myelomeningocele. (A) Spine with myelomeningocele. (B) Diagram demonstrating release of placode from arachnoid membrane. (C) Myelomeningocele repair during open *in utero* fetal surgery. Note the cystic membrane covering the deficit has been incised and meninges are visible inside the cystic cavity. The absorbable copolymer staples used during creation of the hysterotomy are visible along the uterine edges. *CSF,* Cerebrospinal fluid. (A) Modified from Kerr LM, Huether SE. Alterations of neurologic function in children. In: McCance KL, Huether SE, Brashers VL, Rote NS, eds. *Pathophysiology: The Biologic Basis for Disease in Adults and Children*, 7th ed. Elsevier; 2014:660–688. (B) Image created by Katherine Relyea, MS, CMI, and printed with permission from Baylor College of Medicine. (C) Illustration from author Mark Rollins during his affiliation with the UCSF Fetal Treatment Center, San Francisco, CA.

[a]The table lists only the maternal and fetal/neonatal complications that were significantly different (P < .05) between the prenatal and postnatal repair groups in the Management of Myelomeningocele Study (MOMS). Data for each group are shown as both an absolute number and as a percentage.
N/A, Not applicable.
Modified from Adzick NS, Thom EA, Spong CY, et al. A randomized trial of prenatal versus postnatal repair of myelomeningocele. *N Engl J Med.* 2011;364:993–1004.

Intraoperative anesthetic management typically consists of a combination of general endotracheal anesthesia administered to the mother and direct intramuscular (IM) opioid and muscle relaxant administered to the fetus.[81] To optimize operating conditions, significant uterine relaxation is required. In addition, intraoperative fetal monitoring is employed to detect early fetal compromise.

Complex Monochorionic Pregnancies

Up to one-third of twin pregnancies are monochorionic; these pregnancies are at risk for complications unique to monochorionic pregnancies, including twin-to-twin transfusion syndrome (TTTS), twin anemia-polycythemia sequence (TAPS), twin reverse arterial perfusion (TRAP), and conjoined twinning.

Twin-to-Twin Transfusion Syndrome

Some vascular anastomoses connect both fetal circulations in the shared placenta of almost all monochorionic twin pregnancies. In cases with a significant number of vascular anastomoses between the umbilical circulations, shared blood flow through the AV chorionic vessels can become unidirectional and imbalanced, resulting in TTTS.

Twin screening for TTTS starts by 16 weeks' gestation, with recognition typically occurring before 26 weeks' gestation.[82-84] TTTS typically complicates about 10% of monochorionic diamniotic pregnancies, or about 1 per 5000 births in general.[85] The twin serving as the recipient can develop polycythemia, polyuria, polyhydramnios, and hypertrophic cardiomyopathy; this twin is at risk for hydrops fetalis and fetal death. The twin serving as the donor is typically hypovolemic, growth restricted, and pressed against the endometrium in an oligohydramniotic sac (sometimes called the "stuck" twin). This twin is at risk for neonatal renal failure, tubular dysgenesis and dysfunction, and high cardiac output hydrops fetalis.

Typically, the diagnosis of TTTS requires the presence of (1) a monochorionic diamniotic pregnancy; (2) oligohydramnios, defined as a maximal vertical pocket (MVP) < 2 cm in one amniotic sac; and (3) polyhydramnios, defined as MVP > 8 cm in the other amniotic sac.[83] The most commonly used staging system describing the severity of TTTS was published by Quintero and is displayed in Table 7.3. Assessment of additional cardiac function parameters is predictive of outcome in the recipient twin.[86] Although the donor twin typically has normal cardiac function, the recipient twin can develop ventricular hypertrophy, atrioventricular valve regurgitation, ventricular diastolic and systolic dysfunction, and right ventricular outflow tract obstruction.

Fetuses with TTTS are at risk for neurologic injury with white matter lesions and long-term disability, preterm PROM, and preterm delivery. The incidence of preterm birth and neonatal morbidity increases as the stage/severity of TTTS increases, and when intervention is performed at an early gestational age (<18 weeks) or with a short cervix. In terms of mortality, if TTTS remains at Stage I or resolves, the overall survival rate is about 85%[85]; however, if TTTS progresses, the overall mortality rate of one or both fetuses can increase to greater than 80% if untreated.[87,88]

A variety of therapeutic management techniques have been used to treat TTTS: (1) amnioreduction, either as a one-time procedure or serially; (2) selective feticide; and (3) selective fetoscopic laser photocoagulation (SFLP) of the vascular anastomoses between the twins.

Amnioreduction can be performed any time after fusion of membranes (about 16 weeks' gestation) and is hypothesized to reduce the risk for preterm labor and improve placental blood flow. In a retrospective review, amnioreduction resulted in an overall birth survival rate of 78%, with 65% of recipient twins and 55% of donor twins alive at 1 month of age.[89]

Selective feticide is reserved for severe cases of TTTS or when there is a discordant fetal anomaly in one twin, with decreased overall chance of survival. In certain countries or regions, selective feticide may not be an option for some patients because of legal restrictions.

SFLP is routinely offered between 16 and 26 weeks' gestation. The US Food and Drug Administration (FDA) exemption for fetoscopic intervention on TTTS only applies for this time frame.[90] However, consensus from a recent Delphi study suggests that SFLP can be offered as early as 15 weeks and up to 28 weeks in selected cases.[91] The laser used for SFLP is typically inserted through a fetoscope to allow visualization of the vascular anastomoses to be ablated. The fetoscope enters the maternal abdomen and uterus in a placenta-free zone through a small percutaneously inserted cannula that allows passage into the recipient twin's amniotic sac (Fig. 7.6). The fetoscope placement is guided by ultrasonography and ideally positioned at 90 degrees to the placental vascular surface. Although typically positioned supine, in some situations the patient position may be dictated by the limited availability of a suitable entry point (e.g., predominantly anterior placenta). In rare instances where no such "window" can be identified, a laparoscopic-assisted technique requiring the placement of two trocars for pneumoperitoneum and manipulation of the uterus may be used.[92] After completion of the SFLP, an amnioreduction may be performed to decrease the risk for preterm labor.

The optimal management of Quintero Stage I TTTS is unknown; a recent systematic review and metaanalysis of Stage I TTTS demonstrated similar rates of survival with expectant management and laser therapy and slightly higher rates with amnioreduction (84.9%, 86.7%, and 92.2%, respectively, for survival of at least one twin; 67.9%, 69.7%, and 80.8%, respectively, for dual survival).[88,93] Approximately 30% of Quintero Stage I cases managed by amnioreduction or expectant management will ultimately progress to more severe stages.[94] Additional symptoms such as maternal discomfort with increasing polyhydramnios or cervical shortening may also prompt SFLP treatment. SFLP is the treatment

TABLE 7.3 Staging of Twin-to-Twin Transfusion Syndrome Severity

Stage	Parameter	Ultrasonographic Criteria
I	Amniotic fluid	MVP < 2 cm in donor twin amniotic sac and MVP > 8 cm in recipient twin amniotic sac
II	Fetal bladder	Inability to visualize the fetal bladder in the donor twin during 1 h of observation
III	Flow velocity change in UA, UV, or DV	Absent or reversed UA diastolic flow waveform Pulsatile UV flow waveform Reversed DV a-wave flow waveform
IV	Fetal hydrops	Presence of hydrops in either twin
V	Fetal demise	Absent fetal cardiac activity

DV, Ductus venosus; *MVP,* maximal vertical pocket; *UA,* umbilical artery; *UV,* umbilical vein.
Modified from Quintero RA, Morales WJ, Allen MH, et al. Staging of twin-to-twin transfusion syndrome. *J Perinatol.* 1999;19:550–555.

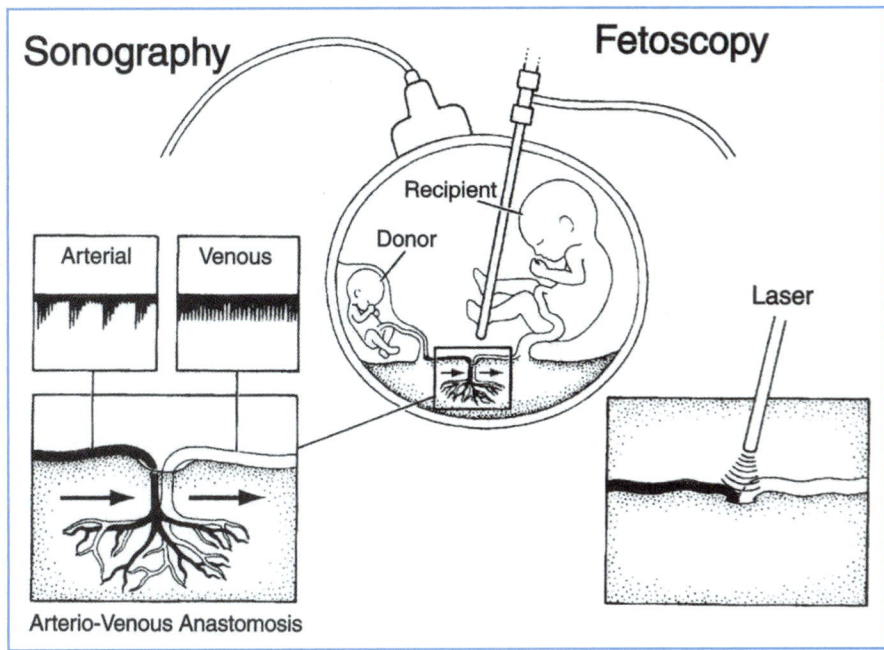

Fig. 7.6 *In utero* Fetoscopic Laser Ablation for Twin-to-Twin Transfusion Syndrome. Under ultrasound guidance, a fetoscope is inserted percutaneously into the recipient twin's amniotic sac. Using both ultrasonographic guidance and fetoscopic visualization, intertwin vessels are identified and ablated with the laser. From Graves CE, Harrison MR, Padilla BE. Minimally invasive fetal surgery. *Clin Perinatol*. 2017;44:729–751.

of choice for TTTS at Quintero Stages II to IV.[83,88] A 2004 randomized multicenter trial demonstrated the benefits of SFLP compared with amnioreduction for treatment of severe TTTS diagnosed between 15 and 26 weeks' gestation.[95] Rates of at least one twin survival were significantly higher in the laser treatment group. In addition, neurologic outcomes were better in the SFLP group. Survival of at least one twin is higher for earlier stages (86.9% for Stage I and 85% in Stage II), but remains moderately high even in higher stages (81.5% in Stage III and 82.8% in Stage IV), compared with Stage V (54.6%).[88]

The most common complications of SFLP are preterm PROM with subsequent preterm labor and delivery. Immediate perioperative concerns such as fetal bradycardia, inadvertent septostomy, bleeding from placental vessels, placental abruption, chorioamnionitis, and maternal pulmonary edema are rare. Maternal anesthesia is commonly managed with either neuraxial blockade or local anesthetic infiltration from skin to myometrium, with or without additional sedation.[2,96] In the rare case where a laparoscopy-assisted technique is performed, general anesthesia may be required.[92]

Twin Anemia-Polycythemia Sequence

TAPS is a type of chronic unbalanced sharing between fetuses that results in anemia in the donor twin and polycythemia in the recipient twin. In contrast to the large anastomoses that characterize TTTS, TAPS is believed to be related to the slow transfusion of blood from the donor to the recipient across tiny AV anastomoses. This leads to discordant hemoglobin concentrations, with one twin displaying chronic anemia while the other has polycythemia. The diagnosis is made postnatally based on the findings of a difference in hemoglobin

concentration > 8 g/dL between twins and either a reticulocyte count ratio > 1.7 or placental findings of small vascular anastomoses.[97]

Screening for TAPS during pregnancy is performed using MCA Doppler measurements, looking at both velocities and discordance between the twins, but there is neither consensus about the optimal approach to surveillance nor determination of diagnostic accuracy.[98] TAPS occurs spontaneously in up to 5% to 10% of monochorionic pregnancies, and can complicate up to 3% to 16% of TTTS cases after laser ablation.[98] The outcome of TAPS is highly variable.

Management options for TAPS include expectant management, early delivery, fetoscopic laser photocoagulation, or IUT for the anemic twin with or without partial exchange transfusion of the polycythemic twin.[99] The anesthetic management for these cases is similar to SFLP or IUT performed for other indications.

Twin Reversed Arterial Perfusion Sequence

In monochorionic twins, one twin can perfuse the other by retrograde blood flow though arterial-to-arterial anastomoses. TRAP sequence affects 1% of monozygotic twins, 1 in 35,000 pregnancies, and 1 in 30 triplet pregnancies. Inadequate perfusion of the recipient twin via only retrograde anastomotic flow results in the development of a set of nonviable anomalies that include acardia and acephalus. The acardiac twin is not viable, but its presence puts the entire pregnancy at risk during gestation. The viable ("pump") twin perfuses both itself and the acardiac twin and is at risk for high-output congestive heart failure, polyhydramnios, fetal growth restriction, preterm birth, and intrauterine fetal death if left untreated.

The goal of therapy is to stop the blood flow to the acardiac twin by targeting the acardiac twin's umbilical cord or intraabdominal vessels. This can be accomplished using various techniques such as intrafetal laser coagulation, bipolar cord coagulation, and radiofrequency ablation.[100] The procedures are typically guided by ultrasonography, and absence of flow to the nonviable acardiac twin is confirmed with Doppler imaging at the end of the procedure.

In the North American Fetal Therapy Network Registry, the reported overall pump-twin survival rate was 80.8% and the premature PROM rate was 17% after radiofrequency ablation, based on data from 98 patients from 22 institutions.[101] A metaanalysis and review of the literature noted the survival rate of the pump twin was also approximately 80% for most techniques.[102]

TRAP intervention procedures are typically performed with minimal sedation and either infiltration of local anesthesia at the ablation device insertion site or the administration of neuraxial anesthesia.

Congenital Heart Defects

Indications for catheter-based fetal cardiac interventions include (1) aortic valvuloplasty with the goal of preventing the development of hypoplastic left heart syndrome, (2) atrial septoplasty and stenting for hypoplastic left heart syndrome with an intact or highly restrictive atrial septum (HLHS-IAS), and (3) pulmonary valvuloplasty to prevent the need for single ventricle palliation for severe pulmonary stenosis and pulmonary atresia with intact ventricular septum (PS+PA/IVS). Fetal pericardiocentesis has also been employed to drain pericardial effusions.[103,104] Fetal intrapericardial teratomas have been successfully resected with *in utero* open fetal surgery or while on placental support during an EXIT procedure.[105,106]

For *in utero* aortic valvuloplasty, an angioplasty balloon is placed over a percutaneously inserted guide wire (Fig. 7.7), with technical success as high as 83%.[107] A 2023 systematic review and metaanalysis found that fetal aortic valvuloplasty was successfully performed in 84% of patients with conversion to biventricular circulation rate in 33% and a mortality rate of 20%.[108] The International Fetal Cardiac Intervention Registry (IFCIR) reported results of 108 patients from 15 centers over a 15-year period.[107] Fetal death occurred during the procedure in 8.3% of cases; another 8.3% of fetal patients died within 48 hours. Intraprocedure complications included fetal bradycardia, pericardial effusion, pleural effusion, balloon rupture, and death.[107]

The goals of atrial septoplasty (atrial perforation or balloon dilation) or stent placement for HLHS-IAS are to improve neonatal stability at delivery by creating an unobstructed atrial septum, and to reverse/reduce chronic changes to the pulmonary vascular bed, with the potential subsequent benefits of improving neonatal survival. The IFCIR reported[109] technical success in 77% of cases, with intraprocedure fetal death in 13% of cases. Survival to discharge after birth was poor at 35%, though when successful, fetal cardiac intervention was associated with neonatal stability at delivery and fewer cesarean deliveries.

Interventions are performed in PS+PA/IVS with the aim of improving growth of the tricuspid valve and right ventricle such that biventricular repair is possible and preventing or reversing hydrops in cases that have significant tricuspid regurgitation. The IFCIR has reported a technical success rate of 71%. Fetal complications occurred in over half of cases, including intraprocedure fetal death in 12% of cases and delayed fetal loss due to circular shunt from significant pulmonary insufficiency in an additional 3.4%. The most common other complications were pericardial effusion requiring

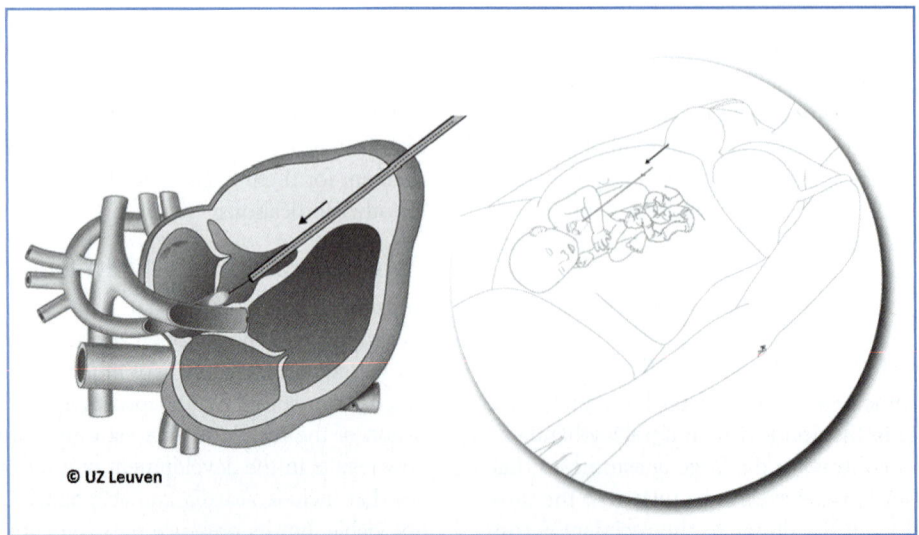

© UZ Leuven

Fig. 7.7 Percutaneous Fetal Aortic Valvuloplasty for Evolving Hypoplastic Left Heart Syndrome. The needle is inserted percutaneously through the maternal abdomen and uterus, then enters the apex of the fetal heart in alignment with the left ventricular outflow tract. A guidewire and a coronary dilation balloon catheter are advanced through the aortic valve, which is then dilated. From Van Mieghem T, Baud D, Devlieger R, et al. Minimally invasive fetal therapy. *Best Pract Res Clin Obstet Gynaecol.* 2012;26:711–725.

drainage in 48% and bradycardia requiring treatment in 36% of cases.[110]

Early descriptions of fetal cardiac intervention reported an approach involving a mini-laparotomy to facilitate fetal positioning; this was associated with improved technical success early in their experience, though all patients in this series underwent general anesthesia.[111] More recently, anesthetic management of these cases often involves the use of maternal neuraxial anesthesia. Fetal anesthesia is administered via ultrasound-guided direct IM injection of anesthetic drugs.

Maternal complications during fetal cardiac interventions are rare; however, anesthesia providers must be prepared for fetal resuscitation in these cases, which may involve drainage of pericardial effusions, administration of medications, or transabdominal fetal chest compressions.

SURGICAL BENEFITS AND RISKS

The primary goal of fetal interventions is to improve neonatal outcomes compared with postnatal interventions. In all cases, the direct, physiologic benefit of the intervention is to the fetus or fetuses, and these benefits must be weighed against the maternal, fetal, and obstetric risks from both clinical and ethical perspectives.

Serious maternal morbidity from intrauterine fetal surgery is relatively uncommon, but, by definition, the pregnant patient is having a procedure, with all its associated surgical and anesthetic risks, without direct physiologic benefit. Counseling and informed consent processes must take this unique situation into account. Maternal well-being must always be emphasized.

The fetal and obstetric risks of intrauterine surgery remain relatively high and include central nervous system injuries, membrane separation, PROM, placental abruption, preterm labor and delivery, significant blood loss, chorioamnionitis, postoperative amniotic fluid leaks with oligohydramnios, and fetal demise.[2,112] Preterm delivery accounts for significant morbidity and mortality. Chorioamniotic membrane separation can cause amniotic bands, umbilical cord strangulation, and fetal demise.[113] Improved techniques for sealing the membranes are being devised, including different surgical techniques for patching or membrane plication, sealants, and intra- or extraamniotic platelet or cryoprecipitate injections.[114–116]

The risks and benefits of each case must be weighed for patient- and situation-specific factors, with shared decision-making used when appropriate and feasible. Multidisciplinary evaluation and discussion can aid clinically and ethically sound decision-making for complex cases or those involving unique circumstances.

ANESTHETIC MANAGEMENT

Fundamental considerations for the anesthetic management of fetal surgery are similar to those for nonobstetric surgery during pregnancy (see Chapter 18). The safety of the mother is of paramount importance. Anesthesia providers should participate in preoperative assessment and exclude patients when their perioperative risk is unacceptably high relative to the potential fetal benefit. Early consultation allows time for optimizing perioperative concerns as well as setting appropriate expectations for the patient so that appropriately informed consent can be obtained. The specific surgical plan and requirements, including any intraoperative decision points that would warrant a change in approach, should be clear to the anesthesia provider to facilitate selecting an optimal anesthetic plan (Box 7.2).

Maternal analgesia and anesthesia can be provided by local infiltration, IV sedation, neuraxial anesthesia, general anesthesia, or a combination of these techniques. The choice of maternal anesthetic plan may be impacted by surgical, maternal, or fetal factors. For example, for a minimally invasive procedure, neuraxial anesthesia may be preferred over local anesthesia if maternal movement would be detrimental or if precise fetal positioning is critical, since success rates of external cephalic version have been shown to be higher when neuraxial anesthesia is used in term gestations.[117] Anesthetic management is also significantly impacted by the need for uterine relaxation. Complete uterine relaxation is typically necessary throughout open procedures, whereas fetoscopic cases require less tocolysis. The use of specific agents may impact certain aspects of maternal management (e.g., **magnesium sulfate** warrants judicious use of IV fluids and nondepolarizing muscle relaxants). Anesthesia providers caring for patients whose pregnancies are complicated by fetal anomalies must anticipate and identify impacts on maternal physiology, such as the development of mirror syndrome in the setting of fetal hydrops.

Fetal anesthesia can be administered via placental transfer of anesthetic agents administered to the mother, via direct fetal IV (peripheral fetal vein or umbilical vein), IM, or intracardiac administration of agents, or by a combination of these methods. It is important to note that administration of maternal anesthetic agents alone (e.g., volatile anesthetic agents) will not blunt a fetal stress response, and a plan for fetal analgesia is also required whenever a procedure will result in a noxious stimulus to the fetus. In general, a medication should be administered to the patient for whom its primary effect is intended, to optimize safety and efficacy while minimizing downsides to both the intended recipient as well as the "bystander." The operative team should be prepared for emergency situations such as maternal or fetal hemorrhage, need for intrauterine fetal resuscitation (e.g., fetal epinephrine [adrenaline] administration), and/or delivery and resuscitation of the neonate(s) when appropriate. In many fetal interventions, viability is impacted by the fetal anomaly in addition to the gestational age. All stakeholders, including the patient and clinical care team, should have a clear understanding of whether a cesarean delivery would be performed for fetal indications prior to arrival in the operating room.

Anesthesia for Minimally Invasive and Percutaneous Procedures

The anesthetic management for minimally invasive or percutaneous procedures should include plans for maternal analgesia

BOX 7.2   Questions to Aid Formulation of Anesthetic Plan

Procedure Related
- What category of procedure is planned?
  - Minimally invasive (ultrasound- or fiberoptic scope-guided)
  - Fetoscopic (percutaneous, mini-laparotomy, or laparotomy-assisted)
  - Open
  - EXIT
- What surgical steps are planned?
- Will a cesarean delivery be performed?
  - Planned
  - Only for maternal indications
  - For maternal or fetal indications
- What incisions are planned?
  - Location
  - Size
  - Number
- Will uterine irrigation be used?
- Will carbon dioxide insufflation be used?
  - Abdominal
  - Intrauterine
- Is intraoperative bleeding expected/possible?
  - Fetal
  - Maternal

Maternal Information
- Is maternal movement tolerated?
  - None (case requires maternal immobility during intervention)
  - Minimal (breathing or minor movement acceptable)
  - Yes
- To what extent will uterine relaxation be required during the procedure?
  - None
  - A portion of procedure
  - Throughout
- Are any specific uterotonics planned?

- Preoperative
- Intraoperative
- Postoperative
- What is the expected postoperative pain management plan?
  - Postoperative epidural analgesia
  - Postoperative fascial plane block
  - Postoperative systemic analgesics
- Is venous thromboembolism prophylaxis planned?
- What maternal medical concerns exist?
- Which teams should be contacted if emergency cesarean delivery is required in the postoperative period?

Fetal Information
- What is the gestational age?
- Is the fetus considered viable?
  - Intraoperative resuscitation plan
  - Plan for emergency delivery intraoperatively?
  - Plan for emergency delivery postoperatively?
  - Neonatal resuscitation plan?
- What is the estimated fetal weight?
- What is the placental location?
- Will fetal repositioning be necessary?
- Prior to neuraxial anesthesia or induction of anesthesia:
  - Document fetal heart rate
  - Fetal cardiac echocardiogram?
  - Fetal umbilical artery Doppler?
- What fetal monitoring is planned?
  - Intraoperatively
  - Postoperatively
- Will the fetus experience a noxious stimulus?
- Is fetal movement tolerated?
  - Yes
  - Decreased movement helpful but not required
  - No
- Is fetal hydrops present?
- What other fetal anomalies exist?

EXIT, *Ex utero* intrapartum therapy.

and anxiolysis as well as fetal anesthesia when appropriate. **Local anesthetic infiltration** of the maternal abdominal wall layers is sufficient to reduce maternal discomfort for many percutaneous procedures including amniocentesis, cordocentesis, intrauterine blood transfusion, needle aspiration of fetal cysts, shunt placement into the fetal bladder or thorax, or laser photocoagulation. **Neuraxial anesthesia** can also be used in these cases and may facilitate positioning, minimize maternal movement, and provide sensory coverage for multiple percutaneous instrumentation sites or a patient who has painful contractions. Supplemental **maternal anxiolysis** can be achieved through nonpharmacologic approaches and/or maternal administration of mild to moderate sedation.[118] Effective anxiolysis is of paramount importance, and the principles of trauma-informed care should be applied, such as frequent check-ins, respecting the patient's privacy, using a calm voice, maintaining focus on the patient, and avoiding unnecessary arm straps and oxygen masks.[119] **General anesthesia** is rarely necessary for minimally invasive procedures but may be required for certain maternal comorbidities or

the need for lateral or prone maternal positioning to optimize procedure success based on placental location and fetal position. Total intrauterine irrigation fluids to facilitate fetoscopic procedures should be closely monitored, as they can be absorbed into the maternal circulation and may increase the risk of pulmonary edema.[120]

Fetal movement may be hazardous for the fetus in certain cases. Placental transfer of maternally administered opioids and benzodiazepines can reduce, but not necessarily eliminate, fetal movement.[121] Reliable fetal immobility can be safely achieved with direct fetal IM or umbilical venous (UV) administration of **rocuronium** (e.g., 2.5 mg/kg IM, 1 mg/kg UV) or **vecuronium** (e.g., 0.2 mg/kg IM, 0.1 mg/kg UV) using ultrasonographic guidance. The onset of fetal paralysis occurs in 2 to 5 minutes, with an approximate duration of 1 to 2 hours.[122] The Society for Maternal-Fetal Medicine recommends considering the use of fetal paralytic agents for IUT procedures to decrease fetal movement.[14] For procedures that can cause noxious stimulation to the fetus, such as shunt catheter placement or cardiac septoplasty, an opioid (e.g., **fentanyl**

10 to 20 µg/kg) should also be administered to the fetus IM or UV to avoid a fetal stress response.[2,15] These seemingly high doses take into consideration the high volume of distribution related to the placental blood volume and have been shown to attenuate fetal stress response to noxious stimulus more effectively than lower doses.[15]

In case of emergency, the surgical team should be prepared to immediately administer appropriate fetal weight-based IM doses of resuscitative medications such as **atropine** (20 µg/kg) and **epinephrine** (1 to 10 µg/kg) and perform an emergency cesarean delivery if the fetus is viable. In specific cases (e.g., percutaneous fetal atrial septoplasty), other fetal resuscitative medications, such as **calcium**, **bicarbonate**, or **antiarrhythmics**, may be indicated.[123] The anesthesia provider should be prepared to provide maternal general anesthesia if required. The possible requirement for general anesthesia and a plan for fetal/neonatal resuscitation should be clearly discussed with the patient during the consent process.

Patients may receive preoperative **tocolytic agents** prior to these procedures. It can be helpful to incorporate the use of tocolytic agents into the preoperative "time out" or safety check, since some of these agents (e.g., **nifedipine**) may have hemodynamic effects and impact anesthetic management. Tocolysis typically is unnecessary after cordocentesis or IUT. For more invasive percutaneous procedures (e.g., shunt catheter placement, fetoscopic techniques), prophylactic perioperative tocolytic agents such as **indomethacin** or nifedipine may be administered to the mother.[124] **Acetaminophen (paracetamol)** and **oral opioids** are typically used for maternal postoperative analgesia.

Anesthesia for Open Fetal Surgery

When fetal surgery or an intrauterine procedure requires surgical access through a hysterotomy, general anesthesia is typically administered. Unique considerations for open fetal procedures include the need for profound uterine relaxation,

---

BOX 7.3 Perioperative Considerations for Open and Hybrid Fetal Surgery

Preoperative Considerations
- Complete maternal history and physical examination.
- Fetal workup to exclude other anomalies and imaging studies to determine fetal lesion, placental location, and estimated fetal weight. Consider fetal assessment (e.g., FHR, UA Doppler, fetal cardiac echocardiogram) immediately prior to induction.
- Maternal counseling by multidisciplinary team and preoperative team meeting
- Emergency delivery plan determined if needed based on gestational age
- Epidural catheter for postoperative analgesia placed and tested
- Prophylactic premedications for aspiration prophylaxis and tocolysis (e.g., indomethacin)
- Blood products available for potential maternal and fetal transfusion as appropriate
- Sequential compression devices on lower extremities for thrombosis prophylaxis
- Fetal resuscitation plan in place with drugs and fluid transferred to scrub nurse in unit doses
- Initiation of maternal warming (e.g., forced air warmer, fluid warmer)
- Completion of "time out" to ensure all appropriate staff, resources, and plans in place

Induction and Intraoperative Considerations
- Left uterine displacement and standard monitors
- Fetal assessment before induction
- Preoxygenation for 3 min before induction
- Rapid sequence induction and tracheal intubation
- Maternal $F_{IO_2} > 50\%$ and end-tidal CO_2 28–32 mm Hg (3.7–4.3 kPa)
- Ultrasonography to determine fetal and placental positioning
- Urinary catheter placed; additional large-bore IV access placed; possible arterial line (may be done preinduction)

- Prophylactic antibiotics
- Maternal blood pressure and heart rate maintained near pre-induction baseline (±10%) with intravenous phenylephrine, ephedrine, and/or glycopyrrolate
- Magnesium infusion for tocolysis initiated
- Appropriate uterine relaxation before hysterotomy performed
- High concentration of volatile anesthetic (2–3 MAC) or SIVA technique with IV remifentanil and propofol infusions combined with 1–1.5 MAC volatile anesthetic for open procedures
- Lower MAC requirements for hybrid procedures
- Intravenous nitroglycerin boluses or infusion if uterine relaxation not adequate
- Communication with fetal monitoring personnel
- Intramuscular administration of fetal opioid and neuromuscular blocking agent by surgeons
- Placement of fetal monitors as appropriate (e.g., intrauterine temperature and fetal pulse oximetry)
- Fetal IV access if significant fetal blood loss anticipated
- Fluid restriction to less than 2 L total to reduce risk for maternal pulmonary edema; consider colloid administration
- Maternal opioids as needed
- Epidural catheter activated for postoperative analgesia if appropriate
- Quantitative neuromuscular blockade monitoring recommended because of magnesium sulfate administration
- Tracheal extubation when patient is fully awake

Early Postoperative Considerations
- Postoperative debrief
- Continuation of tocolytic therapy
- Multimodal postoperative analgesia strategy (e.g., patient-controlled epidural analgesia, fascial plane blocks, scheduled acetaminophen; NSAIDs typically avoided)
- Uterine activity and fetal heart rate monitoring
- Ongoing fetal evaluation

CO_2, Carbon dioxide; *FHR*, fetal heart rate; F_{IO_2}, fraction of inspired oxygen; *IM*, intramuscular; *IV*, intravenous; *MAC*, minimum alveolar concentration; *SIVA*, supplemental intravenous anesthesia; *NSAIDs*, nonsteroidal antiinflammatory drugs; *UA*, umbilical artery.
Modified from Ferschl M, Ball R, Lee H, Rollins MD. Anesthesia for in utero repair of myelomeningocele. *Anesthesiology.* 2013,118:1211–1223.

intraoperative fetal monitoring, fetal anesthesia and analgesia, and postoperative maternal analgesia and uterine tocolysis (Box 7.3). In addition, significant maternal and fetal blood loss may occur, and the anesthesia providers must be prepared to provide maternal and fetal resuscitation.

Preoperatively, the mother receives agents for aspiration prophylaxis and uterine tocolysis (e.g., rectal/oral **indomethacin**), and an **epidural catheter** is placed for postoperative analgesia. The patient is positioned supine with left uterine displacement. A final assessment of the fetus and available personnel and resources is performed. Medications to provide fetal analgesia (e.g., **fentanyl** 10 to 20 μg/kg), immobility (e.g., **rocuronium** 2.5 mg/kg), and resuscitation (e.g., **atropine** 20 μg/kg, **epinephrine** 10 μg/kg) are prepared in separate, sterile, labeled syringes. Cross-matched blood should be available for maternal transfusion. In addition, O-negative, CMV-negative, irradiated, leukocyte-depleted, maternally cross-matched blood should be available for fetal transfusion.

Rapid-sequence induction of general anesthesia and tracheal intubation is performed. Fetal heart rate (FHR), umbilical cord blood flow, and fetal cardiac function are often monitored with ultrasonography during induction. Abnormalities in umbilical cord flow, flow across the ductus arteriosus, or fetal cardiac function may be an early sign of fetal compromise.[125] End-tidal carbon dioxide concentration should be maintained at baseline for pregnancy (28 to 32 mm Hg [3.7 to 4.3 kPa]). Initially, anesthesia is maintained with approximately 1 minimum alveolar concentration (MAC) of a volatile anesthetic agent or IV anesthetic agents while further preparations for surgery are undertaken, including (1) obtaining additional maternal vascular access/invasive monitoring, (2) prophylactic antibiotic administration, (3) urinary bladder catheterization, and (4) ultrasonographic assessment of fetal presentation and placental location. If invasive procedures are performed prior to anesthesia induction, consider pharmacologic anxiolysis and measures to minimize maternal pain and mental stress.[119] For open procedures with a high risk for significant fetal blood loss (e.g., resection of a fetal mass), a fetal IV catheter should be placed after hysterotomy, with all fluids administered to the fetus warmed. A maternal arterial catheter should be placed for maternal blood pressure monitoring if uterine tocolysis with a **nitroglycerin** infusion is planned or if maternal hemodynamic instability is anticipated. Total intraoperative maternal IV fluids are typically restricted (<2 L) to reduce the risk for postoperative pulmonary edema. Some fetal surgery centers administer colloid as a portion of the fluids to better maintain maternal blood pressure and/or choose to limit fluids even further. No clinical trials have proven a benefit of further fluid restriction in this setting.

A final surgical **time out** should occur before skin incision. A **phenylephrine** infusion with bolus doses of **ephedrine** and/or **glycopyrrolate** also can be administered to maintain maternal blood pressure and heart rate near baseline values. Maternal administration of a nondepolarizing muscle relaxant is usually not required, owing to the profound depth of anesthesia, but may be used to improve operative conditions.

A high concentration of a volatile anesthetic agent is typically administered to provide both maternal and fetal anesthesia as well as uterine relaxation. Adequate uterine relaxation may require greater than 2 MAC of a volatile anesthetic agent. Because high levels of volatile anesthetic agent are associated with fetal cardiac dysfunction and abnormal umbilical artery blood flow, some centers use **supplemental IV anesthesia** or other agents (e.g., **nitroglycerin**) to augment the uterine relaxation, allowing for a reduced concentration of the volatile anesthetic agent.[2,126,127] Administration of **magnesium sulfate** prior to hysterotomy may also reduce the dose of inhaled anesthetic agent required.[128] The uterus is assessed both visually and by palpation for contractions or increased tone. For circumstances in which volatile anesthetic agents or general anesthesia must be avoided (e.g., family history of malignant hyperthermia), neuraxial anesthesia can be administered and combined with an IV infusion of **nitroglycerin** to achieve uterine relaxation.[129] This technique does not improve fetal outcome and may be associated with more morbidity, as nitroglycerin administration during open fetal surgery has been associated with maternal pulmonary edema.[130]

Fetal well-being is periodically assessed with ultrasonography. In certain open cases, a sterile pulse oximetry probe may be attached to a fetal digit or limb. An opioid and a muscle relaxant are administered to the fetus IM, either before or after uterine incision with ultrasonographic guidance or direct vision, respectively. Some anesthesia providers also administer IM fetal **atropine** to prevent fetal bradycardia. Further studies are needed to determine the optimal anesthetic technique for ensuring maternal and fetal cardiovascular stability, optimal uteroplacental perfusion, and adequate fetal anesthesia to cause immobility and blockade of the fetal stress response.

The surgical team's approach to hemostasis, intrauterine fluid administration, and temperature management can have significant impact on both fetal and maternal well-being. The use of hemostatic surgical techniques on the uterus (i.e., cautery followed by full thickness sutures, compressive clamps along the tissue edge, or a stapling device) aim to minimize blood loss. During surgery, the exposed fetus and uterus are periodically bathed with warmed fluids to prevent desiccation and replace lost amniotic fluid. If an intrauterine infusion is used, it is important to minimize total irrigation fluid, as intrauterine irrigation fluid can be absorbed into the maternal circulation and may increase risk of pulmonary edema.[120] The intrauterine temperature is closely monitored to prevent fetal circulatory compromise associated with hypothermia.[131]

If magnesium sulfate has not already been administered, a loading dose is administered at initiation of uterine closure (4 to 6 g IV over 20 minutes), followed by an IV infusion of 1 to 2 g/h. As magnesium potentiates neuromuscular relaxation, close monitoring of twitch recovery is needed if a nondepolarizing muscle relaxant was administered, with **quantitative neuromuscular monitoring** recommended.[132] The volatile anesthetic agent can be decreased or discontinued after the magnesium sulfate bolus has been administered. Where available, **atosiban** can also be used in place of magnesium sulfate to maintain uterine relaxation during and after open fetal surgery.[133] Epidural analgesia can be initiated and maternal anesthesia is maintained with additional anesthetic drugs and opioids as appropriate.

Postoperative concerns include maternal and fetal pain, preterm PROM, preterm labor, infection, and a variety of potential fetal complications, including heart failure, intracranial hemorrhage, and demise.[2,112] Maternal analgesia can be maintained with an epidural infusion of a dilute solution of local anesthetic and opioid for several days. Effective analgesia may help prevent postoperative preterm labor.[134,135] Multimodal analgesia with **acetaminophen** and opioids can also be used to provide postoperative maternal analgesia. While a short course of **indomethacin** may be used for tocolysis (see later discussion), the use of **nonsteroidal antiinflammatory drugs** for analgesia is normally avoided to prevent constriction of the fetal ductus arteriosus. Epidural administration of a long-acting opioid (e.g., **morphine** 2 mg) can be considered just prior to epidural catheter removal.

Postoperative preterm labor is the "Achilles' heel" of fetal surgery.[112] Tocolysis after open fetal surgery is typically provided by an infusion of **magnesium sulfate**, although supplemental agents may include **indomethacin**, **nifedipine**, or **terbutaline**.[96] Not infrequently, two tocolytic agents are required to create uterine quiescence. Uterine activity and FHR are monitored closely during the first 2 to 3 postoperative days. The fetus is evaluated postoperatively by ultrasonography, and if indomethacin is used, periodic fetal echocardiography is performed to determine if premature closure of the ductus arteriosus has occurred. Unless preterm labor occurs, cesarean delivery is typically planned at 37 weeks' gestation to reduce the chance of labor onset and possible uterine rupture.

Anesthesia for Hybrid Procedures

The anesthetic approach for fetal surgeries performed using a "hybrid" approach depends on the technique used to access the intrauterine environment and the fetal procedure being performed. Generally, the anesthetic management is similar to that described for open procedures, with alterations to tocolysis, fetal monitoring, temperature management, and postoperative analgesia strategies.[81]

While preoperative tocolytic agents are typically administered as described for open procedures, the required degree of tocolysis is less. Volatile anesthetic agents are titrated to the minimum level necessary to prevent contractions; this approach decreases the amount of vasopressor support required for the mother and minimizes fetal myocardial depression associated with high MAC. During periods of direct uterine manipulation (e.g., port placement and removal), the volatile anesthetic agent may need to be increased (e.g., 1.2 to 1.4 MAC) to prevent contractions but can often be returned to prior levels (e.g., 0.8 to 1.0 MAC) during the fetal surgery when uterine manipulation is minimal.

Fetal blood is often prepared for hybrid procedures, but maternal blood loss is usually minimal and cross-matching maternal blood is not indicated except for rare situations (e.g., a positive maternal antibody screen). The carbon dioxide used for insufflation in these procedures is typically humidified and heated. Additional methods to ensure temperature homeostasis are available when the uterus is not open, such as the use of a plastic sheet placed over the uterus after port insertion to prevent the evaporative heat loss associated with an exteriorized uterus. As in open surgery, fetal well-being is periodically assessed with ultrasonography.

Postoperative analgesia is tailored to the specific surgical approach. Patients who undergo the less invasive approaches generally seem to have effective pain control with earlier (i.e., less than 24 hours postoperatively) transition from epidural to oral analgesia. Many centers use **fascial plane blocks** to facilitate this transition or in lieu of neuraxial analgesia.[136]

Anesthesia for the *Ex Utero* Intrapartum Treatment Procedure

Indications for an EXIT procedure may include **EXIT-to-airway** (e.g., cervical masses, severe craniofacial anomalies); **EXIT-to-resection** (e.g., thoracic masses, mediastinal masses, SCTs); and **EXIT-to-ECMO** (e.g., pulmonary insufficiency, cardiac anomaly).[137] Similar to open fetal surgery procedures, sustained uterine relaxation, maintenance of fetal perfusion, and delay of placental separation are necessary for a successful EXIT procedure. Preoperative concerns about uteroplacental insufficiency (e.g., FHR decelerations, fetal growth restriction, late-onset preeclampsia) should prompt discussion about the feasibility of an EXIT procedure. In all cases, a contingency plan should be in place should the placental support be abbreviated. Simulation or "run-throughs" in advance of the procedure help identify problems with equipment and staffing before they occur.

Anesthesia for EXIT procedures is typically performed with general anesthesia, with many considerations similar to those for open fetal surgery. Preparation for fetal monitoring, airway management, fetal/neonatal resuscitation, and postdelivery care should be completed before entering the operating room.[138] Fetal heart ultrasonography, a sterile pulse oximeter probe, and an end-tidal carbon dioxide indicator or gas analyzer are frequently used for fetal monitoring during the procedure. Unit doses of **atropine** (20 μg/kg) and **epinephrine** (10 μg/kg), as well as fetal analgesic and muscle relaxants agents (**fentanyl** 10 to 20 μg/kg and either **rocuronium** 2.5 mg/kg or **vecuronium** 0.2 mg/kg) are prepared and transferred in a sterile manner to the scrub nurse. Atropine (20 μg/kg) is sometimes administered to the fetus with the opioid and paralytic to reduce the risk of fetal bradycardia. A sterile ventilation bag with an air/oxygen source and manometer is available for the fetus, along with multiple endotracheal tube sizes and devices for fetal tracheal intubation, including rigid and flexible bronchoscopes, and equipment for creation of a surgical airway in the case of EXIT-to-airway.[139] Catheters for IV access as well as crystalloid and blood (O-negative, CMV-negative, leukocyte-depleted, irradiated, maternally cross-matched) should be available for fetal volume resuscitation if needed.

Preoperatively, a maternal epidural catheter may be placed, or intrathecal opioids may be administered, for postoperative analgesia. Maternal anesthetic considerations should include large-bore IV access, availability of uterotonic agents and cross-matched blood, and the ability to quickly obtain invasive maternal monitoring if not initially placed.

Techniques of maternal induction and tracheal intubation are similar to those typically used for cesarean delivery. Although techniques for maintenance of anesthesia vary among medical centers, administration of 1.5 to 3 MAC of a volatile anesthetic agent is often needed to achieve and maintain adequate uterine relaxation. Occasionally, **nitroglycerin** administered with a bolus dose (100 to 200 µg) or as an infusion may also be required to maintain appropriate uterine relaxation. Fetal anesthesia from the volatile anesthetic agent transferred across the placenta is typically supplemented by direct fetal IM administration of an opioid and muscle relaxant. The dosing of the fetal medications is dependent on the type of EXIT procedure (e.g., EXIT-to-airway, EXIT-to-resection). IM agents can be administered to the fetus either before uterine incision with ultrasonographic guidance or after uterine incision under direct visualization. Both cutting spinal and hypodermic needles should be available on the sterile field to allow for administration of fetal medications before or after hysterotomy as needed. Significant variability in serum fentanyl concentrations in umbilical cord blood has been documented during EXIT procedures,[140] and similar variability in onset of paralysis exists with muscle relaxants dependent on gestational age and likely the placental component of fetal blood volume.[122]

Following exposure of the uterus, the placental location and edges are determined by intraoperative ultrasonography. Similar to open fetal procedures, the uterine incision is extended using hemostatic surgical techniques (i.e., cautery followed by full thickness sutures, compressive clamps along the tissue edge, or a stapling device) to minimize blood loss. In the most common indication of EXIT-to-airway, the fetal head and shoulders are delivered in preparation for tracheal intubation. Warmed fluids are periodically irrigated over the fetus and into the uterine cavity and care is taken to avoid manipulation of the umbilical cord. The warmed crystalloid irrigation fluid helps maintain fetal euthermia and fetoplacental circulation while preventing decreased uterine volume, placental separation, and spasm of the cord vessels. The fetus is typically monitored with (1) a pulse oximeter probe placed on the fetal hand, (2) periodic cardiac ultrasonography, and/or (3) direct visualization. For more extensive procedures, such as fetal thoracotomy, or when there is fetal bradycardia suggestive of umbilical cord compression, the fetus can be delivered from the uterus and placed on the maternal chest and abdomen to facilitate the procedure.

The duration of the fetal procedure can range from a few minutes (e.g., bronchoscopy or intubation) to several hours (e.g., neck or thoracic mass resection, tracheostomy, or central intravascular cannulation). Although the majority of procedures require less than 1 hour, the anesthetic technique should be capable of providing maternal, fetal, and

uteroplacental stability over several hours.[141] Once surgery is completed and the trachea secured, fetal surfactant is administered if indicated. Fetal oxyhemoglobin saturation is typically 40% to 70% at this time,[142] but increases significantly to greater than 90% with ventilation of the fetal lungs.`

Upon umbilical cord clamping, the volatile anesthetic agent is reduced or eliminated to help achieve uterine tone and diminish the risk for postpartum hemorrhage. Typically a combination of an **opioid** and **propofol**, with or without **nitrous oxide**, is then used to maintain anesthesia. **Oxytocin** is administered, as well as other uterotonic agents if needed. Finally, **epidural analgesia** is used for postoperative pain control at most fetal centers and initiated prior to emergence from general anesthesia.[96]

If general anesthesia with a volatile anesthetic agent is contraindicated (e.g., history of malignant hyperthermia) an alternative technique for EXIT procedures involves the use of neuraxial anesthesia combined with IV infusions of **propofol**, **remifentanil**, and **nitroglycerin** to maintain uterine relaxation.[143] Without a volatile anesthetic agent, large doses of IV nitroglycerin (e.g., 10 to 20 µg/kg/min) are often required to achieve adequate uterine relaxation.[129] If large doses of nitroglycerin are to be administered for a prolonged period, an arterial catheter is recommended. Following prolonged EXIT procedures, the mother should be observed for evidence of pulmonary edema, which can be related to excessive IV fluids or absorption of uterine irrigation fluid, or administration of magnesium sulfate or nitroglycerin. Maternally administered IV **remifentanil** undergoes significant transfer across the placenta and can also serve as an adjuvant for fetal analgesia and immobility, though it should not be considered sufficient as a sole agent, as it will dissipate from the fetus rapidly following cord clamping.[121]

In an effort to decrease the risk of maternal morbidity associated with EXIT procedures, some centers are moving to coordinated deliveries with immediate neonatal intervention in an adjacent operating room, sometimes referred to as a **PRESTO** (procedure requiring a second team in the operating room) or **CSIR** (cesarean section with immediate resection).[9] This approach does not have the benefit of a controlled surgical intervention while the fetus is on placental bypass, but instead relies on preoperative coordination and immediate response of a multidisciplinary fetal operative team following delivery.

Fetal Response to Surgical Stimulation

Pain is a multidimensional, subjective, psychological construct that can exist in the absence of physical stimuli (e.g., phantom limb pain), and it includes emotional and affective components that require higher-level cortical processing.[144] As such, although pain is commonly associated with noxious physical stimuli, it is more than nociception or a simple reflex activity associated with a withdrawal response.[145] Attempts have been made to correlate pain with surgical stress; however, the stress response is mediated primarily in the spinal cord, brainstem, and/or basal ganglia, without involvement of the cortex.

In studies of intrauterine blood transfusion in the human fetus, surgical needling of the intrahepatic vein (in contrast to the insensate umbilical cord) is associated with evidence of a stress response, including increases in plasma beta-endorphin and cortisol concentrations and decreases in the MCA pulsatility index (determined by Doppler imaging).[146] These responses can be blunted by the fetal administration of fentanyl 10 µg/kg.[15] Human fetuses exhibit pituitary-adrenal, sympathoadrenal, and circulatory stress responses to noxious stimuli as early as 16 to 18 weeks' gestation.[135,147] Immature skin nociceptors likely begin to emerge at 10 weeks' gestation and are present by 17 weeks' gestation.[148] In internal organs, nociceptors develop slightly later. Peripheral nerve fibers that control movement grow into the spinal cord at about 8 weeks' gestation. When these fibers connect with nociceptors is unknown, but one human study suggests that nociceptive nerve fibers do not enter the spinal cord before about 19 weeks' gestation.[149] The cerebral cortex develops after the fetal spinal cord and brainstem. Thalamocortical connections to the somatosensory cortex are significantly developed at 24 to 30 weeks' gestation.[135,145]

The developing cerebral cortex consists of transient fetal zones where neuronal proliferation, cell migration, apoptosis, axonal outgrowth, and synaptogenesis occur according to a highly specific timetable. The cortical subplate is a temporary structure that serves as a waiting and organizing zone for various afferents destined for the cortex. It develops at about 13 weeks' gestation and recedes after 32 to 34 weeks' gestation.

Studies of fetal electroencephalograms (EEGs) at 24 weeks' gestation have demonstrated electrical activity only 2% of the time. At 30 weeks' gestation, EEGs begin showing patterns of wakefulness and sleep, but these are not concordant with fetal behavior. By 34 weeks' gestation, electrical activity is present 80% of the time, with more distinct wakefulness and sleep cycles similar to adult patterns.[150]

Two studies using near-infrared spectroscopy in preterm infants demonstrated differences in cerebral oxygenation over the somatosensory cortex with noxious and nonnoxious stimulation.[151,152] This appears to indicate that noxious information is at least transmitted to the infant cortex by 25 weeks' gestation. Similarly, preterm neonates also have demonstrated cortical evoked potentials after a heel lance.[153]

The exact onset of fetal *sentience*, the capacity to experience sensations such as pain, is unknown. Altogether, clinical observations of fetal and neonatal behavior, information about the development of mechanisms of pain perception, and studies of fetal and neonatal responses to noxious stimuli provide a compelling physiologic and philosophic rationale for the provision of adequate fetal anesthesia when a noxious stimulus is anticipated. Noxious stimulation during fetal life causes a stress response, which could have both short- and long-term adverse effects on the developing central nervous system. Although there is placental transfer of maternally administered volatile anesthetic agents, fetal opioid is required to blunt the fetal stress response. Administration of fetal analgesia has been the standard

practice worldwide since the inception of fetal surgery more than four decades ago,[154,155] and current guidelines recommend that opioid analgesia should be administered to the fetus during invasive fetal surgical procedures to attenuate autonomic responses that might be deleterious, avoid long-term consequences of nociception and physiologic stress on the fetus, and decrease fetal movement to optimize procedure outcome.[2,14]

Effects of Anesthesia on the Fetus

With maternal administration of general anesthesia, volatile anesthetics readily cross the placenta. The fetal level of volatile anesthetic agents depends on both the inspired maternal concentration as well as the duration of administration. Based on data from cesarean delivery, after 10 minutes of general anesthesia, fetal levels of both isoflurane and halothane reach approximately 70% of maternal levels.[156] Of interest, studies in sheep models have shown a lower fetal-to-maternal ratio of volatile anesthetic agents at 10 minutes, demonstrating that the fetal concentrations remain lower than maternal concentrations for significant periods of time (Fig. 7.8). High levels of maternal inhaled anesthetic agents (2 to 3 MAC) can affect fetal cardiac function and blood flow. A retrospective analysis of cardiac imaging from both open fetal cases and EXIT procedures noted severe left ventricular systolic dysfunction in the fetus with use of high concentrations of desflurane.[127] Echocardiographic findings from 100 open fetal MMC cases under desflurane anesthesia noted intraoperative ventricular dysfunction in 60% of cases, tricuspid regurgitation in 35%, and mitral valve regurgitation in 19%, with serious

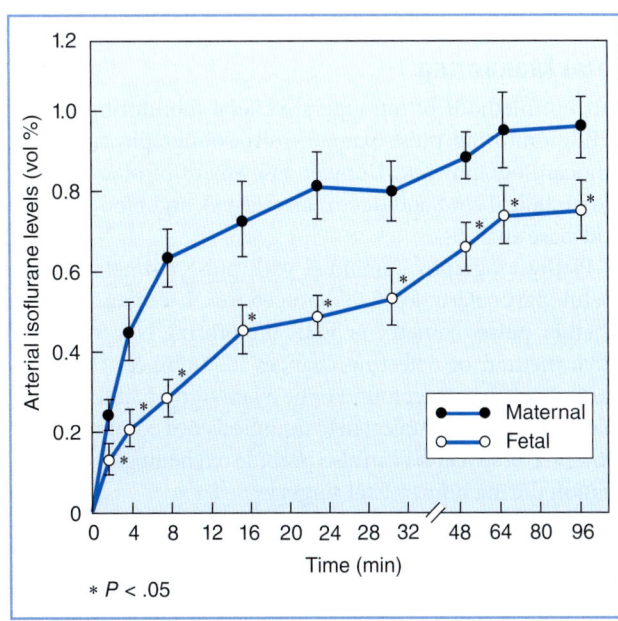

Fig. 7.8 Maternal and fetal arterial isoflurane concentrations in sheep during maternal administration of 2.0% isoflurane (mean ± SE). From Biehl DR, Yarnell R, Wade JG, Sitar D. The uptake of isoflurane by the foetal lamb in utero: effect on regional blood flow. *Can Anesth Soc J.* 1983;30:581–586.

cardiovascular events in 7% of cases.[157] In another review of open fetal surgery for MMC repair utilizing a volatile anesthetic agent (2 to 3 MAC), 34 of 37 fetuses developed intraoperative umbilical artery flow abnormalities.[158] Brief fetal exposure to deep maternal inhalation anesthesia (2 to 3 MAC) does not appear to result in significant fetal hypoxia, hypercarbia, or acidosis even after exposures of 2 hours if maternal arterial pressure is maintained.[159] However, others have noted acidosis after 45 minutes of fetal exposure to anesthesia.[160]

Questions regarding the relationship between anesthetic agents and neuronal apoptosis in the developing fetal brain exist (see Chapter 10). In 2003 an anesthetic regimen consisting of **midazolam**, **nitrous oxide**, and **isoflurane** was shown to alter neurons in the developing brain of 7-day-old rats and to cause long-term impairment of brain function.[161] Evidence for neuronal apoptosis in the developing brain after exposure to a wide range of anesthetic agents, such as **volatile anesthetic agents**, **propofol**, and **benzodiazepines**, has since been demonstrated in a variety of animal studies.[162] Although it remained unknown if anesthetic agents similarly affect human fetuses or neonates, in December 2016 the FDA issued a safety communication warning that "repeated or lengthy use of general anesthetic and sedation drugs during surgeries or procedures in children younger than 3 years or in pregnant women during their third trimester may affect the development of children's brains."[163] To date, high-quality human studies have found no differences in intelligence quotient or motor skills between children exposed to a single general anesthetic compared to those not exposed.[164,165] Currently no specific anesthetic agent (e.g., **volatile anesthetic agents**, **propofol**, **ketamine**, **benzodiazepines**) is known to be teratogenic or, alternatively, safer than another.[165]

Fetal Monitoring

Current methods of intraoperative fetal monitoring include FHR monitoring, pulse oximetry, ultrasonography (including echocardiography and Doppler assessment of blood flow in the umbilical cord and ductus arteriosus), and blood gas and acid-base analysis.

Plethysmography combined with pulse oximetry is very useful, particularly for EXIT procedures. It remains unclear whether pulse oximetry or FHR monitoring is a more sensitive method of detecting changes in umbilical cord flow. Bradycardia has been found to be a late sign of fetal compromise in fetal lambs subjected to umbilical cord compression.[166] However, bradycardia can also precede oxyhemoglobin desaturation during human fetal surgery.[167]

Ultrasonography is a crucial intraoperative fetal monitoring device. The FHR can be determined with visualization of the heart or with Doppler assessment of umbilical cord blood flow. Both absent and reversed umbilical artery diastolic flow are associated with increased perinatal morbidity and mortality in obstetric patients,[168] but the implications during fetal surgery remain unclear.[158] Abnormal ductus arteriosus flow patterns have been observed during open fetal surgery, but

the cause and implications remain unclear.[169] Fetal cardiac contractility and volume also can be assessed qualitatively by echocardiography. Unfortunately the sterile transducer often cannot be positioned continuously because its location interferes with surgery. When prolonged fetal bradycardia, oxyhemoglobin desaturation, and/or significant changes in fetal cardiac function and umbilical artery blood flow are noted, maneuvers should be done to improve uterine perfusion and relieve umbilical cord compression.[124] These maneuvers can include improving maternal blood pressure, cardiac output, and oxygenation through administration of vasoactive agents, fluids, and supplemental oxygen, as well as maximizing uterine relaxation. In severe cases requiring administration of fetal resuscitation drugs and/or fluids, fetal chest compressions (either transabdominal or *ex utero* depending on surgical approach) or emergent delivery may be necessary.

THE FUTURE OF FETAL THERAPY

Successful diagnosis and management of complex congenital anomalies and other fetal conditions amenable to prenatal intervention rely on well-organized, multidisciplinary, professional, and comprehensive fetal treatment programs to innovate new techniques, challenge dogma, and ensure ongoing success.

Although the rationale for prenatal fetal therapy seems straightforward, many issues remain problematic. Questions remain regarding the way fetal development is modulated by intrauterine intervention. Other questions revolve around maternal and fetal rights, safety, efficacy, long-term outcomes, cost-effectiveness, and societal resource allocation. Societal expectations and the availability of therapy must be balanced against the budgetary constraints in contemporary healthcare.

Fetal therapy must be evaluated carefully in properly conducted trials and undertaken only with great caution and informed maternal consent. Publication of outcomes in scientific journals and open communication with colleagues nationally and internationally facilitates the moral obligation of researchers to report all results to allow peer review of the merits and liabilities of fetal surgery. The principal concept of *primum non nocere* argues that it is unethical to undertake human trials until a procedure is appropriately tested in animals. Intervention should be undertaken only when there is a reasonable probability of long-term benefit and minimal maternal risk.

Through rapid innovation, the potential applications of fetal therapy are expanding. Recent advances in fetal therapy can be seen in use of *in utero* gene editing and stem cells,[170] fetal repair of gastroschisis,[171] and development of an artificial womb.[172] The advancement from innovation to research, and the subsequent transition to clinical care is complex and requires multidisciplinary and ethical oversight. It is critical to support these efforts in order to continue the progress of innovative fetal therapies.

KEY POINTS

- Most fetal malformations diagnosed *in utero* are not suitable for antenatal intervention. Fetal surgery is a reasonable option for anomalies that cause harm to the fetus before adequate organ development required for postnatal intervention (particularly lung maturity).
- Maternal safety is a primary consideration and must be weighed against potential long-term benefit to the fetus and neonate.
- Local or neuraxial anesthesia is normally suitable for percutaneous or minimally invasive procedures. Open or hybrid intrauterine procedures typically require administration of general anesthesia.
- Anesthetic considerations for intrauterine fetal surgery are similar to those for nonobstetric surgery in pregnant women. However, in addition to maintaining adequate maternal anesthesia and uteroplacental blood flow, fetal surgery typically requires (1) provision of anesthesia and analgesia for the fetus, (2) more intensive intraoperative fetal monitoring, and (3) intraoperative uterine relaxation.
- Randomized controlled trials have demonstrated improved outcomes with use of fetoscopic laser ablation to treat twin-to-twin transfusion syndrome and intrauterine open fetal repair to treat myelomeningocele.
- Preterm premature rupture of membranes and preterm labor after surgery are significant barriers to optimal outcomes with fetal surgery.
- There are many medical, social, ethical, and legal considerations regarding the efficacy and safety of intrauterine fetal surgery. Careful evaluation of fetal benefits and both fetal and maternal risks is fundamental to the decision as to when and whether fetal intervention is appropriate.

REFERENCES

1. Harrison MR, Filly RA, Golbus MS, et al. Fetal treatment 1982. *N Engl J Med*. 1982;307:1651–1652.
2. Chatterjee D, Arendt KW, Moldenhauer JS, et al. Anesthesia for maternal-fetal interventions: a consensus statement from the American Society of Anesthesiologists Committees on Obstetric and Pediatric Anesthesiology and the North American Fetal Therapy Network. *Anesth Analg*. 2021;132:1164–1173.
3. American College of Obstetricians and Gynecologists Committee on Ethics, American Academy of Pediatrics Committee on Bioethics. Committee Opinion No. 501: Maternal-fetal intervention and fetal care centers (reaffirmed in 2020). *Pediatrics*. 2011;128:e473–e478.
4. Baschat AA, Blackwell SB, Chatterjee D, et al. Care levels for fetal therapy centers. *Obstet Gynecol*. 2022;139:1027–1042.
5. Graves CE, Harrison MR, Padilla BE. Minimally invasive fetal surgery. *Clin Perinatol*. 2017;44:729–775.
6. Shieh HF, Wilson JM, Sheils CA, et al. Does the ex utero intrapartum treatment to extracorporeal membrane oxygenation procedure change morbidity outcomes for high-risk congenital diaphragmatic hernia survivors? *J Pediatr Surg*. 2017;52:22–25.
7. Joshi DSM, Antony K, Beninati M, Luks FI, Puricelli M, Lobeck IN. Indications, resource allocation, and outcomes associated with ex-utero intrapartum treatment procedures: a North American fetal therapy network survey. *Fetal Diagn Ther*. 2023;50:376–386.
8. Tran KM, Chatterjee D. New trends in fetal anesthesia. *Anesthesiol Clin*. 2020;38:605–619.
9. Creden SP, Portuondo J, Cheng LS, et al. Approach and technique for cesarean section to immediate resection for high-risk sacrococcygeal teratomas. *J Surg Res*. 2023;292: 38–43.
10. Practice Bulletin No. 181: Prevention of Rh D alloimmunization. *Obstet Gynecol*. 2017;130:e57–e70.
11. Oepkes D, Seaward PG, Vandenbussche FP, et al. Doppler ultrasonography versus amniocentesis to predict fetal anemia. *N Engl J Med*. 2006;355:156–164.

12. Prefumo F, Fichera A, Fratelli N, Sartori E. Fetal anemia: diagnosis and management. *Best Pract Res Clin Obstet Gynaecol*. 2019;58:2–14.
13. Crowe EP, Hasan R, Saifee NH, et al. How do we perform intrauterine transfusions? *Transfusion*. 2023;63:2214–2224.
14. Society for Maternal-Fetal Medicine, et al.Society of Family Planning, et al.Norton ME, et al. Society for Maternal-Fetal Medicine Consult Series #59: The use of analgesia and anesthesia for maternal-fetal procedures. *Contraception*. 2021;106:10–15.
15. Fisk NM, Gitau R, Teixeira JM, et al. Effect of direct fetal opioid analgesia on fetal hormonal and hemodynamic stress response to intrauterine needling. *Anesthesiology*. 2001;95:828–835.
16. Capone V, Persico N, Berrettini A, et al. Definition, diagnosis and management of fetal lower urinary tract obstruction: consensus of the ERKNet CAKUT-Obstructive Uropathy Work Group. *Nat Rev Urol*. 2022;19:295–303.
17. Harrison MR, Filly RA, Parer JT, et al. Management of the fetus with a urinary tract malformation. *JAMA*. 1981;246:635–639.
18. Farrugia MK, Kilby MD. Therapeutic intervention for fetal lower urinary tract obstruction: current evidence and future strategies. *J Pediatr Urol*. 2021;17:193–199.
19. Nassr AA, Shazly SAM, Abdelmagied AM, et al. Effectiveness of vesicoamniotic shunt in fetuses with congenital lower urinary tract obstruction: an updated systematic review and meta-analysis. *Ultrasound Obstet Gynecol*. 2017;49:696–703.
20. Glick PL, Harrison MR, Adzick NS, et al. Correction of congenital hydronephrosis in utero. IV: in utero decompression prevents renal dysplasia. *J Pediatr Surg*. 1984;19:649–657.
21. Smith-Harrison LI, Hougen HY, Timberlake MD, Corbett ST. Current applications of in utero intervention for lower urinary tract obstruction. *J Pediatr Urol*. 2015;11:341–347.
22. Farrugia MK. Fetal bladder outlet obstruction: embryopathology, in utero intervention and outcome. *JPediatr Urol*. 2016;12:296–303.
23. Ruano R, Sananes N, Sangi-Haghpeykar H, et al. Fetal intervention for severe lower urinary tract obstruction: amulticenter case-control study comparing fetal cystoscopy

with vesicoamniotic shunting. *Ultrasound Obstet Gynecol.* 2015;45:452–458.

24. Miller JL, Baschat AA, Rosner M, et al. Neonatal survival after serial amnioinfusions for bilateral renal agenesis: the Renal Anhydramnios Fetal Therapy Trial. *JAMA.* 2023;330:2096–2105.

25. Claes DJ, Richardson T, Harer MW, et al. Survival of neonates born with kidney failure during the initial hospitalization. *Pediatr Nephrol.* 2023;38:583–591.

26. Clayton DB, Brock JW. Current state of fetal intervention for lower urinary tract obstruction. *Curr Urol Rep.* 2018;19:12.

27. Burgos CM, Frenckner B, Luco M, et al. Right versus left congenital diaphragmatic hernia—what's the difference? *JPediatr Surg.* 2018;53:113–117.

28. de Buys Roessingh AS, Dinh-Xuan AT. Congenital diaphragmatic hernia: current status and review of the literature. *Eur J Pediatr.* 2018;53:393–406.

29. Harrison MR, Bressack MA, Churg AM, de Lorimier AA. Correction of congenital diaphragmatic hernia in utero. II. Simulated correction permits fetal lung growth with survival at birth. *Surgery.* 1980;88:260–268.

30. Harrison MR, Adzick NS, Flake AW, et al. Correction of congenital diaphragmatic hernia in utero. VI. Hard-earned lessons. *J Pediatr Surg.* 1993;28:1411–1417.

31. Russo FM, De Coppi P, Allegaert K, et al. Current and future antenatal management of isolated congenital diaphragmatic hernia. *Semin Fetal Neonatal Med.* 2017;22:383–390.

32. Deprest JA, Evrard VA, Van Ballaer PP, et al. Tracheoscopic endoluminal plugging using an inflatable device in the fetal lamb model. *Eur J Obstet Gynecol Reprod Biol.* 1998;81: 165–169.

33. Harrison MR, Albanese CT, Hawgood SB, et al. Fetoscopic temporary tracheal occlusion by means of detachable balloon for congenital diaphragmatic hernia. *Am J Obstet Gynecol.* 2001;185:730–733.

34. Jani J, Valencia C, Cannie M, et al. Tracheal diameter at birthin severe congenital diaphragmatic hernia treated by fetal endoscopic tracheal occlusion. *Prenat Diagn.* 2011;31:699–704.

35. Grivell RM, Andersen C, Dodd JM. Prenatal interventions for congenital diaphragmatic hernia for improving outcomes. *Cochrane Database Syst Rev.* 2015;(11):CD008925.

36. Deprest JA, Nicolaides KH, Benachi A, et al. Randomized trial of fetal surgery for severe left diaphragmatic hernia. *N Engl J Med.* 2021;385:107–118.

37. Deprest JA, Benachi A, Gratacos E, et al. Randomized trial of fetal surgery for moderate left diaphragmatic hernia. *N Engl J Med.* 2021;385:119–129.

38. Stolar CJH, Wilson JM, Losty PD, Flake AW. Fetal surgery for moderate and severe CDH—the TOTAL trials. *J Pediatr Surg.* 2022;57:552–553.

39. David M, Lamas-Pinheiro R, Henriques-Coelho T. Prenatal and postnatal management of congenital pulmonary airway malformation. *Neonatology.* 2016;110:101–115.

40. Yong PJ, Von Dadelszen P, Carpara D, et al. Prediction of pediatric outcome after prenatal diagnosis and expectant antenatal management of congenital cystic adenomatoid malformation. *Fetal Diagn Ther.* 2012;31:94–102.

41. Mann S, Wilson RD, Bebbington MW, et al. Antenatal diagnosis and management of congenital cystic adenomatoid malformation. *Semin Fetal Neonatal Med.* 2007;12:477–481.

42. Bose SK, Stratigis JD, Ahn N, et al. Prenatally diagnosed large lung lesions: timing of resection and perinatal outcomes. *JPediatr Surg.* 2023;58:2384–2390.

43. Wilson RD, Baxter JK, Johnson MP, et al. Thoracoamniotic shunts: fetal treatment of pleural effusions and congenital cystic adenomatoid malformations. *Fetal Diagn Ther.* 2004;19:413–420.

44. Gajewska-Knapik K, Impey L. Congenital lung lesions: prenatal diagnosis and intervention. *Semin Pediatr Surg.* 2015;24:156–159.

45. Cavoretto P, Molina F, Poggi S, et al. Prenatal diagnosis and outcome of echogenic fetal lung lesions. *Ultrasound Obstet Gynecol.* 2008;32:769–783.

46. Muntean A, Cazacu R, Ade-Ajayi N, et al. The long-term outcome following thoraco-amniotic shunting for congenital lung malformations. *J Pediatr Surg.* 2023;58:213–217.

47. Grethel EJ, Wagner AJ, Clifton MS, et al. Fetal intervention for mass lesions and hydrops improves outcome: a 15-year experience. *J Pediatr Surg.* 2007;42:117–123.

48. Baird R, Puligandla PS, Laberge JM. Congenital lung malformations: informing best practice. *Semin Pediatr Surg.* 2014;23:270–277.

49. Derderian SC, Coleman AM, Jeanty C, et al. Favorable outcomes in high-risk congenital pulmonary airway malformations treated with multiple courses of maternal betamethasone. *J Pediatr Surg.* 2015;50:515–518.

50. Kitagawa H, Pringle KC. Fetal surgery: a critical review. *Pediatr Surg Int.* 2017;33:421–433.

51. Van Mieghem T, Al-Ibrahim A, Deprest J, et al. Minimally invasive therapy for fetal sacrococcygeal teratoma: case series and systematic review of the literature. *Ultrasound Obstet Gynecol.* 2014;43:611–619.

52. Wilson RD, Hedrick H, Flake AW, et al. Sacrococcygeal teratomas: prenatal surveillance, growth and pregnancy outcome. *Fetal Diagn Ther.* 2009;25:15–20.

53. Peiró JL, Sbragia L, Scorletti F, et al. Management of fetal teratomas. *Pediatr Surg Int.* 2016;32:635–647.

54. Altman RP, Randolph JG, Lilly JR. Sacrococcygeal teratoma: American Academy of Pediatrics Surgical Section Survey-1973. *J Pediatr Surg.* 1974;9:389–398.

55. Coleman A, Shaaban A, Keswani S, Lim FY. Sacrococcygeal teratoma growth rate predicts adverse outcomes. *J Pediatr Surg.* 2014;49:985–989.

56. Gebb JS, Khalek N, Qamar H, et al. High tumor volume to fetal weight ratio is associated with worse fetal outcomes and increased maternal Rrsk in fetuses with sacrococcygeal teratoma. *Fetal Diagn Ther.* 2018;45:94–101.

57. Litwińska M, Litwińska E, Janiak K, et al. Percutaneous intratumor laser ablation for fetal sacrococcygeal teratoma. *Fetal Diagn Ther.* 2020;47:138–144.

58. Sananes N, Javadian P, Schwach Werneck Britto I, et al. Technical aspects and effectiveness of percutaneous fetal therapies for large sacrococcygeal teratomas: cohort study and literature review. *Ultrasound Obstet Gynecol.* 2016;47:712–719.

59. Braun T, Brauer M, Fuchs I, et al. Mirror syndrome: a systematic review of fetal associated conditions, maternal presentation and perinatal outcome. *Fetal Diagn Ther.* 2010;27:191–203.

60. Teles Abrao Trad A, Czeresnia R, Elrefaei A, et al. What do we know about the diagnosis and management of mirror syndrome? *J Matern Fetal Neonatal Med.* 2022;35:4022–4027.

61. Hirata G, Aoki S, Sakamaki K, et al. Clinical characteristics of mirror syndrome: a comparison of 10 cases of mirror syndrome with non-mirror syndrome fetal hydrops cases. *J Matern Fetal Neonatal Med*. 2016;29:2630–2634.

62. Atta CA, Fiest KM, Frolkis AD, et al. Global birth prevalence of spina bifida by folic acid fortification status: a systematic review and meta-analysis. *Am J Public Health*. 2016;106: e24–e34.

63. Kancherla V, Chadha M, Rowe L, et al. Reducing the burden of anemia and neural tube defects in low- and middle-income countries: an analysis to identify countries with an immediate potential to benefit from large-scale mandatory fortification of wheat flour and rice. *Nutrients*. 2021;13:244.

64. Lee SY, Papanna R, Farmer D, Tsao K. Fetal repair of neural tube defects. *Clin Perinatol*. 2022;49:835–848.

65. Yamashiro KJ, Farmer DL. Fetal myelomeningocele repair: a narrative review of the history, current controversies and future directions. *Transl Pediatr*. 2021;10:1497–1505.

66. Copp AJ, Adzick NS, Chitty LS, et al. Spina bifida. *Nat Rev DisPrimers*. 2015;1:15007.

67. Bowman RM, Lee JY, Yang J, et al. Myelomeningocele: the evolution of care over the last 50 years. *Childs Nerv Syst*. 2023;39:2829–2845.

68. Heuer GG, Moldenhauer JS, Scott Adzick N. Prenatal surgery for myelomeningocele: review of the literature and future directions. *Childs Nerv Syst*. 2017;33:1149–1155.

69. Mangels KJ, Tulipan N, Bruner JP, Nickolaus D. Use of bipedicular advancement flaps for intrauterine closure of myeloschisis. *Pediatr Neurosurg*. 2000;32:52–56.

70. Meuli M, Meuli-Simmen C, Mazzone L, et al. In utero plastic surgery in Zurich: successful use of distally pedicled random pattern transposition flaps for definitive skin closure during open fetal spina bifida repair. *Fetal Diagn Ther*. 2018;44: 173–178.

71. Belfort MA, Whitehead WE, Shamshirsaz AA, et al. Comparison of two fetoscopic open neural tube defect repair techniques: single- vs three-layer closure. *Ultrasound Obstet Gynecol*. 2020;56:532–540.

72. Adzick NS, Thom EA, Spong CY, et al. A randomized trial of prenatal versus postnatal repair of myelomeningocele. *N Engl J Med*. 2011;364:993–1004.

73. George E, MacPherson C, Pruthi S, et al. Long-term imaging follow-up from the Management of Myelomeningocele Study. *AJNR Am J Neuroradiol*. 2023;44:861–866.

74. Goodnight WH, Bahtiyar O, Bennett KA, et al. Subsequent pregnancy outcomes after open maternal-fetal surgery for myelomeningocele. *Am J Obstet Gynecol*. 2019;220:494–e7.

75. Chmait RH, Monson MA, Pham HQ, et al. Percutaneous/mini-laparotomy fetoscopic repair of open spina bifida: a novel surgical technique. *Am J Obstet Gynecol*. 2022;227:375–383.

76. Belfort MA, Whitehead WE, Shamshirsaz AA, et al. Fetoscopic open neural tube defect repair: development and refinement of a two-port, carbon dioxide insufflation technique. *Obstet Gynecol*. 2017;129:734–743.

77. Sanz Cortes M, Chmait RH, Lapa DA, et al. Experience of 300 cases of prenatal fetoscopic open spina bifida repair: report of the International Fetoscopic Neural Tube Defect Repair Consortium. *Am J Obstet Gynecol*. 2021;225:678–e11.

78. Moldenhauer JS, Adzick NS. Fetal surgery for myelomeningocele: after the management of myelomeningocele study (MOMS). *Semin Fetal Neonatal Med*. 2017;22:360–366.

79. Krispin E, Hessami K, Johnson RM, et al. Systematic classification and comparison of maternal and obstetrical complications following 2 different methods of fetal surgery for the repair of open neural tube defects. *Am J Obstet Gynecol*. 2023;229:53–e8.

80. Chmait RH, Monson MA, Chon AH. Advances in fetal surgical repair of open spina bifida. *Obstet Gynecol*. 2023;141:505–521.

81. Naus CA, Mann DG, Andropoulos DB, et al. "This is how we do it" Maternal and fetal anesthetic management for fetoscopic myelomeningocele repairs: the Texas Children's Fetal Center protocol. *Int J Obst Anesth*. 2025;61:104316. https://doi.org/10.1016/j.ijoa.2024.104316.

82. Benoit RM, Baschat AA. Twin-to-twin transfusion syndrome: prenatal diagnosis and treatment. *Am J Perinatol*. 2014;31:583–594.

83. Bamberg C, Hecher K. Twin-to-twin transfusion syndrome: controversies in the diagnosis and management. *Best Pract Res Clin Obstet Gynaecol*. 2022;84:143–154.

84. Khalil A, Rodgers M, Baschat A, et al. ISUOG Practice Guidelines: role of ultrasound in twin pregnancy. *Ultrasound Obstet Gynecol*. 2016;47:247–263.

85. Society for Maternal-Fetal Medicine Simpson LL. Twin-twin transfusion syndrome. *Am J Obstet Gynecol*. 2013;208:3–18.

86. Manning N, Archer N. Cardiac manifestations of twin-to-twin transfusion syndrome. *Twin Res Hum Genet*. 2016;19:246–254.

87. Roberts D, Neilson JP, Kilby MD, Gates S. Interventions for the treatment of twin-twin transfusion syndrome. *Cochrane Database Syst Rev*. 2014;(1):CD002073.

88. Di Mascio D, Khalil A, D'Amico A, et al. Outcome of twin-twin transfusion syndrome according to Quintero stage of disease: systematic review and meta-analysis. *Ultrasound Obstet Gynecol*. 2020;56:811–820.

89. Mari G, Roberts A, Detti L, et al. Perinatal morbidity and mortality rates in severe twin-twin transfusion syndrome: results of the International Amnioreduction Registry. *Am J Obstet Gynecol*. 2001;185:708–715.

90. Shanahan MA, Bebbington MW. Monochorionic twins: TTTS, TAPS, and selective fetal growth restriction. *Clin Obstet Gynecol*. 2023;66:825–840.

91. Krispin E, Javinani A, Odibo A, et al. Consensus protocols for management of early and late twin-twin transfusion syndrome: Delphi study. *Ultrasound Obstet Gynecol*. 2024;63:371–377.

92. Krispin E, Nassr AA, Espinoza J, et al. Outcomes of laparoscopy-assisted fetoscopic laser photocoagulation for twin-twin transfusion syndrome: an established alternative forinaccessible anterior placenta. *Prenat Diagn*. 2021;41: 1582–1588.

93. Nassr AA, Hessami K, Zargarzadeh N, et al. Fetoscopic laser photocoagulation versus expectant management for stage I twin-to-twin transfusion syndrome: a systematic review and meta-analysis. *Prenat Diagn*. 2023;43:1229–1238.

94. Khalil A, Cooper E, Townsend R, Thilaganathan B. Evolution of stage 1 twin-to-twin transfusion syndrome (TTTS): systematic review and meta-analysis. *Twin Res Hum Genet*. 2016;19:207–216.

95. Senat MV, Deprest J, Boulvain M, et al. Endoscopic laser surgery versus serial amnioreduction for severe twin-to-twin transfusion syndrome. *N Engl J Med*. 2004;351:136–144.

96. Wood CL, Zuk J, Rollins MD, et al. Anesthesia for maternal-fetal interventions: a survey of fetal therapy centers in the North American Fetal Therapy Network. *Fetal Diagn Ther.* 2021;48:361–371.

97. Slaghekke F, Kist WJ, Oepkes D, et al. Twin anemia-polycythemia sequence: diagnostic criteria, classification, perinatal management and outcome. *Fetal Diagn Ther.* 2010;27:181–190.

98. Mustafa HJ, Cermak R, Pedersen N, et al. Perinatal outcomes of pregnancies with twin-anemia polycythemia sequence complicating twin-to-twin transfusion syndrome using different twin-anemia polycythemia sequence diagnostic criteria. *Prenat Diagn.* 2022;42:985–993.

99. Baschat AA, Miller JL. Pathophysiology, diagnosis, and management of twin anemia polycythemia sequence in monochorionic multiple gestations. *Best Pract Res Clin Obstet Gynaecol.* 2022;84:115–126.

100. Brock CO, Johnson A. Twin reverse arterial perfusion: timing of intervention. *Best Pract Res Clin Obstet Gynaecol.* 2022;84:127–142.

101. Lee H, Bebbington M, Crombleholme TM. The North American Fetal Therapy Network Registry data on outcomes of radiofrequency ablation for twin-reversed arterial perfusion sequence. *Fetal Diagn Ther.* 2013;33:224–229.

102. Chaveeva P, Poon LC, Sotiriadis A, et al. Optimal method and timing of intrauterine intervention in twin reversed arterial perfusion sequence: case study and meta-analysis. *Fetal Diagn Ther.* 2014;35:267–279.

103. Junior EA, Tonni G, Martins WP. Outcomes of infants followed-up at least 12 months after fetal open and endoscopic surgery for meningomyelocele: a systematic review and meta-analysis. *J Evid Based Med.* 2016;9(3):125–135.

104. Garcia Rodriguez R, Rodriguez Guedes A, Garcia Delgado R, et al. Prenatal diagnosis of cardiac diverticulum with pericardial effusion in the first trimester of pregnancy with resolution after early pericardiocentesis. *Case Rep Obstet Gynecol.* 2015;2015:154690.

105. Rychik J, Khalek N, Gaynor JW, et al. Fetal intrapericardial teratoma: natural history and management including successful in utero surgery. *Am J Obstet Gynecol.* 2016;215:780–e7.

106. Nassr AA, Shazly SA, Morris SA, et al. Prenatal management of fetal intrapericardial teratoma: a systematic review. *Prenat Diagn.* 2017;37:849–863.

107. Patel ND, Nageotte S, Ing FF, et al. Procedural, pregnancy, and short-term outcomes after fetal aortic valvuloplasty. *Catheter Cardiovasc Interv.* 2020;96:626–632.

108. Mendel B, Kohar K, Amirah S, et al. The outcomes of fetal aortic valvuloplasty in critical aortic stenosis: a systematic review and meta-analysis. *Int J Cardiol.* 2023;382:106–111.

109. Jantzen DW, Moon-Grady AJ, Morris SA, et al. Hypoplastic left heart syndrome with intact or restrictive atrial septum: a report from the International Fetal Cardiac Intervention Registry. *Circulation.* 2017;136:1346–1349.

110. Hogan WJ, Grinenco S, Armstrong A, et al. Fetal cardiac intervention for pulmonary atresia with intact ventricular septum: International Fetal Cardiac Intervention Registry. *Fetal Diagn Ther.* 2020:1–9.

111. Wilkins-Haug LE, Tworetzky W, Benson CB, et al. Factors affecting technical success of fetal aortic valve dilation. *Ultrasound Obstet Gynecol.* 2006;28:47–52.

112. Al-Refai A, Ryan G, Van Mieghem T. Maternal risks of fetal therapy. *Curr Opin Obstet Gynecol.* 2017;29:80–84.

113. Sydorak RM, Hirose S, Sandberg PL, et al. Chorioamniotic membrane separation following fetal surgery. *J Perinatol.* 2002;22:407–410.

114. Chmait RH, Kontopoulos EV, Chon AH, et al. Amniopatch treatment of iatrogenic preterm premature rupture of membranes (iPPROM) after fetoscopic laser surgery for twin-twin transfusion syndrome. *J Matern Fetal Neonatal Med.* 2017;30:1349–1354.

115. Micheletti T, Eixarch E, Berdun S, et al. Ex-vivo mechanical sealing properties and toxicity of a bioadhesive patch as sealing system for fetal membrane iatrogenic defects. *Sci Rep.* 2020;10:18608.

116. Avilla-Royo E, Seehusen F, Devaud YR, et al. In vivo sealing of fetoscopy-induced fetal membrane defects by mussel glue. *Fetal Diagn Ther.* 2022;49:518–527.

117. Weiniger CF, Rabkin V. Neuraxial block and success of external cephalic version. *BJA Educ.* 2020;20:296–297.

118. American Society of Anesthesiologists Committee on Quality Management and Departmental Administration. Continuum of depth of sedation: definition of general anesthesia and levels of sedation/analgesia; 2019. https://www.asahq.org/standards-and-practice-parameters/statement-on-continuum-of-depth-of-sedation-definition-of-general-anesthesia-and-levels-of-sedation-analgesia. Accessed July 16, 2024.

119. Vogel TM, Coffin E. Trauma-informed care on labor and delivery. *Anesthesiol Clin.* 2021;39:779–791.

120. Katz SG, Somerville KP, Welsh A. Maternal pulmonary oedema during foetoscopic surgery. *Anaesth Intensive Care.* 2015;43:249–251.

121. Van de Velde M, Van Schoubroeck D, Lewi LE, et al. Remifentanil for fetal immobilization and maternal sedation during fetoscopic surgery: a randomized, double-blind comparison with diazepam. *Anesth Analg.* 2005;101:251–258.

122. Leveque C, Murat I, Toubas F, et al. Fetal neuromuscular blockade with vecuronium bromide: studies during intravascular intrauterine transfusion in isoimmunized pregnancies. *Anesthesiology.* 1992;76:642–644.

123. Donofrio MT, Moon-Grady AJ, Hornberger LK, et al. Diagnosis and treatment of fetal cardiac disease: a scientific statement from the American Heart Association. *Circulation.* 2014;129:2183–2242.

124. Hoagland MA, Chatterjee D. Anesthesia for fetal surgery. *Paediatr Anaesth.* 2017;27:346–357.

125. Cruz-Martínez R, Gámez-Varela A, Cruz-Lemini M, et al. Doppler changes in umbilical artery, middle cerebral artery, cerebroplacental ratio and ductus venosus during open fetal microneurosurgery for intrauterine open spina bifida repair. *Ultrasound Obstet Gynecol.* 2021;58:238–244.

126. Marsh BJ, Sinskey J, Whitlock EL, et al. Use of remifentanil for open in utero fetal myelomeningocele repair maintains uterine relaxation with reduced volatile anesthetic concentration. *Fetal Diagn Ther.* 2020;47:810–816.

127. Boat A, Mahmoud M, Michelfelder EC, et al. Supplementing desflurane with intravenous anesthesia reduces fetal cardiac dysfunction during open fetal surgery. *Paediatr Anaesth.* 2010;20:748–756.

128. Donepudi R, Huynh M, Moise KJ Jr, et al. Early administration of magnesium sulfate during open fetal myelomeningocele repair reduces the dose of inhalational anesthesia. *Fetal Diagn Ther.* 2019;45:192–196.

129. Rosen MA, Andreae MH, Cameron AG. Nitroglycerin for fetal surgery: fetoscopy and ex utero intrapartum treatment procedure with malignant hyperthermia precautions. *Anesth Analg.* 2003;96:698–700.

130. DiFederico EM, Burlingame JM, Kilpatrick SJ, et al. Pulmonary edema in obstetric patients is rapidly resolved except in the presence of infection or of nitroglycerin tocolysis after open fetal surgery. *Am J Obstet Gynecol.* 1998;179:925–933.

131. Aboud E, Neales K. The effect of maternal hypothermia on the fetal heart rate. *Int J Gynaecol Obstet.* 1999;66:163–164.

132. Thilen SR, Weigel WA, Todd MM, et al. 2023 American Society of Anesthesiologists Practice guidelines for monitoring and antagonism of neuromuscular blockade: a report by the American Society of Anesthesiologists Task Force on Neuromuscular Blockade. *Anesthesiology.* 2023;138:13–41.

133. Ochsenbein-Kölble N, Krähenmann F, Hüsler M, et al. Tocolysis for in utero surgery: atosiban performs distinctly better than magnesium sulfate. *Fetal Diagn Ther.* 2017;44:59–64.

134. Santolaya-Forgas J, Romero R, Mehendale R. The effect of continuous morphine administration on maternal plasma oxytocin concentration and uterine contractions after openfetal surgery. *J Matern Fetal Neonatal Med.* 2006;19:231–238.

135. Van de Velde M, De Buck F. Fetal and maternal analgesia/anesthesia for fetal procedures. *Fetal Diagn Ther.* 2012;31:201–209.

136. Patino M, Tran TD, Shittu T, et al. Enhanced recovery after surgery: benefits for the fetal surgery patient. *Fetal Diagn Ther.* 2021;48:392–399.

137. Bence CM, Wagner AJ. Ex utero intrapartum treatment (EXIT) procedures. *Semin Pediatr Surg.* 2019;28:150820.

138. Varela MF, Pinzon-Guzman C, Riddle S, et al. EXIT-to-airway: fundamentals, prenatal work-up, and technical aspects. *Semin Pediatr Surg.* 2021;30:151066.

139. Mosquera MS, Yuter S, Flake AW. Perinatal management of the anticipated difficult airway. *Semin Fetal Neonatal Med.* 2023;101485.

140. Tran KM, Maxwell LG, Cohen DE, et al. Quantification of serum fentanyl concentrations from umbilical cord blood during ex utero intrapartum therapy. *Anesth Analg.* 2012;114:1265–1267.

141. Hirose S, Farmer DL, Lee H, et al. The ex utero intrapartum treatment procedure: looking back at the EXIT. *J Pediatr Surg.* 2004;39:375–380.

142. Johnson N, Johnson VA, Fisher J, et al. Fetal monitoring with pulse oximetry. *Br J Obstet Gynaecol.* 1991;98:36–41.

143. Hofer IS, Mahoney B, Rebarber A, Beilin Y. An ex utero intrapartum treatment procedure in a patient with a family history of malignant hyperthermia. *Int J Obstet Anesth.* 2013;22:146–148.

144. Raja SN, Carr DB, Cohen M, et al. The revised International Association for the Study of Pain definition of pain: concepts, challenges, and compromises. *Pain.* 2020;161:1976–1982.

145. Lee SJ, Ralston HJ, Drey EA, et al. Fetal pain: a systematic multidisciplinary review of the evidence. *JAMA.* 2005;294:947–954.

146. Sekulic S, Gebauer-Bukurov K, Cvijanovic M, et al. Appearance of fetal pain could be associated with maturation of the mesodiencephalic structures. *J Pain Res.* 2016;9:1031–1038.

147. Brusseau R, Mizrahi-Arnaud A. Fetal anesthesia and pain management for intrauterine therapy. *Clin Perinatol.* 2013;40:429–442.

148. Terenghi G, Sundaresan M, Moscoso G, Polak JM. Neuropeptides and a neuronal marker in cutaneous innervation during human foetal development. *J Comp Neurol.* 1993;328:595–603.

149. Konstantinidou AD, Silos-Santiago I, Flaris N, Snider WD. Development of the primary afferent projection in human spinal cord. *J Comp Neurol.* 1995;354:11–12.

150. Bourel-Ponchel E, Gueden S, Hasaerts D, et al. Normal EEG during the neonatal period: maturational aspects from premature to full-term newborns. *Neurophysiol Clin.* 2021;51:61–88.

151. Bartocci M, Bergqvist LL, Lagercrantz H, Anand KJ. Pain activates cortical areas in the preterm newborn brain. *Pain.* 2006;122:109–117.

152. Slater R, Cantarella A, Gallella S, et al. Cortical pain responses in human infants. *J Neurosci.* 2006;26:3662–3666.

153. Slater R, Worley A, Fabrizi L, et al. Evoked potentials generated by noxious stimulation in the human infant brain. *Eur J Pain.* 2010;14:321–326.

154. Harrison MR, Golbus MS, Filly RA, et al. Fetal surgery for congenital hydronephrosis. *N Engl J Med.* 1982;306:591–593.

155. Harrison MR, Anderson J, Rosen MA, et al. Fetal surgery in the primate. I. Anesthetic, surgical, and tocolytic management to maximize fetal-neonatal survival. *J Pediatr Surg.* 1982;17:115–122.

156. Dwyer R, Fee JP, Moore J. Uptake of halothane and isoflurane by mother and baby during caesarean section. *Br J Anaesth.* 1995;74:379–383.

157. Rychik J, Cohen D, Tran KM, et al. The role of echocardiography in the intraoperative management of the fetus undergoing myelomeningocele repair. *Fetal Diagn Ther.* 2015;37:172–178.

158. Sinskey JL, Rollins MD, Whitlock E, et al. Incidence and management of umbilical artery flow abnormalities during open fetal surgery. *Fetal Diagn Ther.* 2018;43:274–283.

159. Hirose S, Sydorak RM, Tsao K, et al. Spectrum of intrapartum management strategies for giant fetal cervical teratoma. *JPediatr Surg.* 2003;38:446–450.

160. Gaiser RR, Kurth CD, Cohen D, Crombleholme T. The cesarean delivery of a twin gestation under 2 minimum alveolar anesthetic concentration isoflurane: one normal and one with a large neck mass. *Anesth Analg.* 1999;88:584–586.

161. Jevtovic-Todorovic V, Hartman RE, Izumi Y, et al. Early exposure to common anesthetic agents causes widespread neurodegeneration in the developing rat brain and persistent learning deficits. *J Neurosci.* 2003;23:876–882.

162. Bleeser T, Van Der Veeken L, Fieuws S, et al. Effects of general anaesthesia during pregnancy on neurocognitive development of the fetus: a systematic review and meta-analysis. *Br J Anaesth.* 2021;126:1128–1140.

163. Andropoulos DB, Greene MF. Anesthesia and developing brains—implications of the FDA warning. *N Engl J Med.* 2017;376:905–907.

164. Warner DO, Zaccariello MJ, Katusic SK, et al. Neuropsychological and behavioral outcomes after exposure of young children to procedures requiring general anesthesia. *Anesthesiology.* 2018;129:89–105.

165. McCann ME, De Graaff JC, Dorris L, et al. Neurodevelopmental outcome at 5 years of age after general

anaesthesia or awake-regional anaesthesia in infancy (GAS): an international, multicentre, randomised, controlled equivalence trial. *Lancet.* 2019;393:664–677.

166. Luks FI, Johnson BD, Papadakis K, et al. Predictive value of monitoring parameters in fetal surgery. *J Pediatr Surg.* 1998;33:1297–1301.

167. Izumi A, Minakami H, Sato I. Fetal heart rate decelerations precede a decrease in fetal oxygen content. *Gynecol Obstet Invest.* 1997;44:26–31.

168. Figueras F, Caradeux J, Crispi F, et al. Diagnosis and surveillance of late-onset fetal growth restriction. *Am J Obstet Gynecol.* 2018;218:S790–S802.e1.

169. Howley L, Wood C, Patel SS, et al. Flow patterns in the ductus arteriosus during open fetal myelomeningocele repair. *Prenat Diagn.* 2015;35:564–570.

170. Berkowitz CL, Luks VL, Puc M, Peranteau WH. Molecular and cellular in utero therapy. *Clin Perinatol.* 2022;49:811–820.

171. Joyeux L, Belfort MA, Coppi PD, et al. Complex gastroschisis: a new indication for fetal surgery? *Ultrasound Obstet Gynecol.* 2021;58:804–812.

172. Spencer BL, Mychaliska GB. Updates in neonatal extracorporeal membrane oxygenation and the artificial placenta. *Clin Perinatol.* 2022;49:873–891.

8

Intrapartum Fetal Assessment and Therapy

David B. Nelson, MD and Catherine Y. Spong, MD

CHAPTER OUTLINE

Assessment of fetal well-being during labor and at the time of delivery is paramount to ensure optimal health of the mother and infant. Since its introduction in the 1960s, fetal surveillance during labor has been predominantly managed with continuous monitoring of fetal heart rate (FHR). Yet, despite more than a half-century of widespread application, debate remains about the clinical application—and value—of electronic cardiotocography (CTG) as well as the mechanisms by which FHR patterns occur.[1] Understanding the interpretation of electronic FHR monitoring, its limitations, and the impact of the maternal condition is critical for intrapartum management as electronic FHR monitoring is the most common obstetric procedure.[2]

FETAL RISK DURING LABOR

Continuous electronic FHR monitoring during labor was introduced to identify fetal asphyxia, with the expectation that timely intervention would prevent cerebral palsy (CP).[3] A benefit attributed to electronic fetal monitoring is the near elimination of intrapartum fetal deaths, especially among preterm neonates.[4] Importantly, data supporting these observations are from epidemiologic studies, which provide associations but do not necessarily establish causation.[5,6] Additionally, widespread implementation of electronic fetal monitoring has been at the expense of increased operative interventions and a disappointing recognition that fetal neurologic injury and CP rates have remained essentially unchanged over decades (Fig. 8.1).[3,7]

Animal models have been used to study the hypothesis that intrapartum events can have long-term neurologic sequelae. Fetal monkeys subjected to hypoxia *in utero* suffer neurologic injuries similar to those seen in children who presumably suffered asphyxia *in utero*.[8–10] Complete asphyxia caused by total occlusion of the umbilical blood flow led to fetal arterial acidemia after approximately 8 minutes and neurologic injury following 10 minutes of occlusion.[11] Work with rodent, rabbit, piglet, and sheep models has shown similar patterns of damage.[12–16] Thus, fetal brain injury appears to be related to duration, frequency, and degree of cord occlusion.

In humans, a complex interplay of antepartum complications, suboptimal uterine perfusion, placental dysfunction, and intrapartum events can result in adverse neonatal outcome.[2] Various methods for the identification of high-risk pregnancies have been published.[17,18] High-risk pregnancies include, but are not limited to, pregnant individuals with (1) **medical complications** (e.g., hypertension, preeclampsia, diabetes mellitus, autoimmune disease, hemoglobinopathy); (2) **fetal complications** (e.g., fetal growth restriction, anomalies, preterm delivery, multiple gestation, hydrops fetalis); and (3) **intrapartum complications** (e.g., vaginal bleeding, maternal fever, meconium-stained amniotic fluid, oxytocin administration during labor). Owing to inadequate sensitivity, poor positive predictive values, and the inability to modify risk factor–related outcomes, the use of scoring systems has not been shown to improve pregnancy outcomes.[19–22] In a study of term pregnancies with fetal asphyxia, 63% had no known risk factors.[23]

Because of this, the magnitude of risk for intrapartum fetal neurologic injury is a matter of dispute with current data suggesting that it is unrealistic to expect detection of fetal asphyxia using FHR monitoring alone.[18] In 2014, the American College of Obstetricians and Gynecologists (ACOG) Task Force on Neonatal Encephalopathy developed criteria for intrapartum events that may be contributory to neurologic injury (Box 8.1). The Task Force concluded that 70% of fetal neurologic injuries result from events that occur before the onset of labor.[24] Only 4% of cases of neonatal encephalopathy result solely from intrapartum hypoxia, an incidence of approximately 1.5/1000.[23] The Task Force criteria

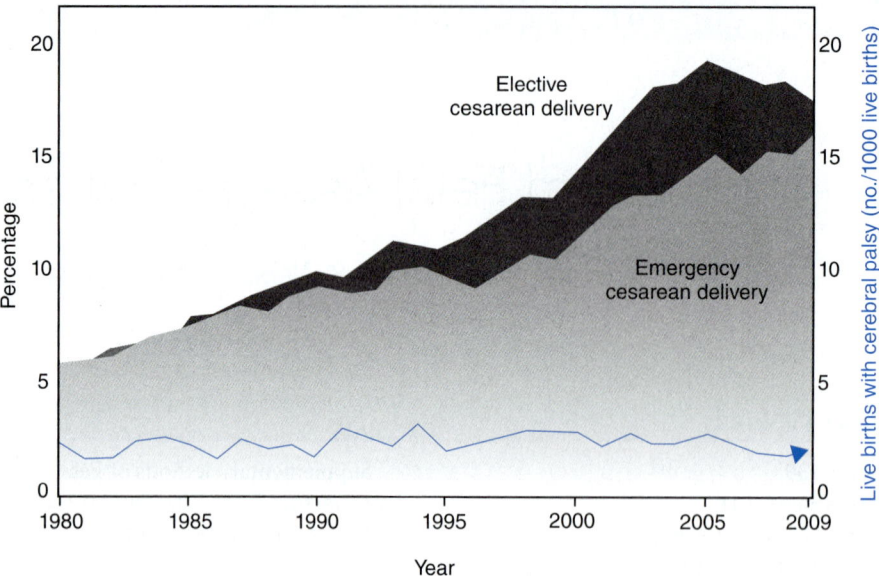

Fig 8.1 Percentage of Elective and Emergency Cesarean Deliveries and Live Births With Cerebral Palsy. The incidence of cerebral palsy has not changed despite a significant increase in the rate of cesarean delivery. Data from Nelson KB. Blair E. Prenatal factors in singletons with cerebral palsy born at or near term. *N Engl J Med.* 2015; 373:946–953.[3] Illustration by Naveen Nathan, MD, NorthShore University HealthSystem, University of Chicago Pritzker School of Medicine, Evanston, IL.

BOX 8.1 Neonatal Encephalopathy and Association With Peripartum Events

Definition of Neonatal Encephalopathy

Syndrome of disturbed neurologic function in the earliest days of life in an infant born at ≥35 weeks' gestation

Neonatal signs consistent with an acute peripartum or intrapartum event:

1. Apgar scores < 5 at 5 min and 10 min of life
2. Evidence of metabolic acidosis in umbilical cord arterial blood obtained at delivery (pH < 7.00, base deficit ≥ 12 mmol/L)
3. Neuroimaging evidence of acute brain injury seen on brain magnetic resonance imaging or magnetic resonance spectroscopy consistent with hypoxemia-ischemia
4. Presence of multisystem organ failure consistent with hypoxic-ischemic encephalopathy

Type and timing of contributing factors that are consistent with an acute peripartum or intrapartum event:

1. Sentinel hypoxic or ischemic event occurring immediately before or during labor and delivery (e.g., uterine rupture, abruption, amniotic fluid embolus)
2. Fetal heart rate monitor patterns consistent with an acute peripartum or intrapartum event
3. Type and timing of brain injury pattern based on imaging studies consistent with an etiology of an acute peripartum or intrapartum event
4. No evidence of other proximal or distal factors that could be contributing events

Developmental outcome is spastic quadriplegia or dyskinetic cerebral palsy.

Adapted from the American College of Obstetricians and Gynecologists. Executive summary: Neonatal encephalopathy and neurologic outcome, 2nd ed. Report of the American College of Obstetricians and Gynecologists' Task Force on Neonatal Encephalopathy. *Obstet Gynecol.* 2014;123:896–901.[24]

are consistent with clinical findings in a case series of neurologically impaired infants with intrapartum compromise.[25]

Thus, as defined by the ACOG Task Force, **neonatal encephalopathy** is a clinically defined syndrome of disturbed neurologic function in the earliest days of life in an infant born at or beyond 35 weeks' gestation, manifested by a subnormal level of consciousness, seizures, and often accompanied by difficulty with initiating and maintaining respiration and depression of tone and reflexes.[24] Hypoxic-ischemic encephalopathy (HIE) or birth asphyxia accounts for some, but not all, cases of neonatal encephalopathy. For example, case series of sentinel events (e.g., uterine rupture, umbilical cord prolapse, placental abruption, amniotic fluid embolus) during labor have been associated with HIE in surviving infants.[26]

With the current understanding of the pathophysiology of neonatal encephalopathy, and the contemporary technology used clinically, the extent to which obstetricians can prevent intrapartum injury remains unclear.[27–29] Given these uncertainties, efforts to understand placental physiology and pathophysiology are central to efforts to support the health of the pregnant woman and her fetus, both antepartum and intrapartum. The fetus depends on the placenta for the diffusion of nutrients and for respiratory gas exchange. Many factors affect placental transfer, including concentration gradients, villus surface area, placental permeability, and placental metabolism (see Chapter 4). Maternal hypertensive disease, congenital anomalies, and intrauterine infection are examples of conditions that may impair placental transfer.

One of the most important determinants of placental function is uterine blood flow.[30] A uterine contraction results in a transient decrease in uteroplacental blood flow. A placenta with borderline function before labor may be unable to support adequate gas exchange to prevent fetal asphyxia during labor. The healthy fetus may compensate for the effects of hypoxia during labor via (1) decreased oxygen consumption, (2) vasoconstriction of nonessential vascular beds, and (3) redistribution of blood flow to the vital organs (e.g., brain, heart, adrenal glands, placenta).[30-32] Humoral responses (e.g., release of epinephrine from the adrenal medulla) may enhance fetal cardiac function during hypoxia.[30] Prolonged or severe hypoxia overwhelms these compensatory mechanisms, resulting in fetal injury or death.

INTRAPARTUM FETAL ASSESSMENT

Electronic Fetal Heart Rate Monitoring

There is need for a sensitive yet specific method for the determination of fetal health during labor and delivery. Most contemporary methods include assessment of the FHR intermittently or continuously with Doppler ultrasonography. Alternatively, a fetal electrocardiography (ECG) electrode can be used. Experimental models have provided insight into FHR regulation. Both neuronal and humoral factors affect the intrinsic FHR. It has been proposed that parasympathetic outflow by means of the vagus nerve decreases the FHR, whereas sympathetic activity increases FHR and cardiac output.[33] Baroreceptors respond to increased blood pressure and chemoreceptors respond to decreased Pao_2 and increased $Paco_2$ to modulate the FHR through the autonomic nervous system. Cerebral cortical activity and hypothalamic activity affect the FHR through their effects on integrative centers in the medulla oblongata (Fig. 8.2).[34]

An electronic monitor simultaneously records the FHR and uterine contractions. Use of an electronic monitor allows determination of the **baseline rate** and **patterns** of the FHR and their relationship to uterine contractions. External or internal techniques allow continuous assessment of the FHR and uterine contractions (Fig. 8.3). Doppler ultrasonography detects the changes in fetal ventricular wall motion and blood flow in major vessels during each cardiac cycle. The monitor calculates the FHR by measuring the intervals between fetal myocardial contractions. Alternatively, an ECG lead attached to the fetal scalp enables the cardiotachometer to calculate the FHR by measuring each successive R-R interval.

The FHR tracing is typically superimposed over the uterine contraction pattern. Uterine contractions can be monitored externally with a tocodynamometer or internally with an intrauterine pressure catheter (IUPC). The tocodynamometer allows the determination of the approximate onset, duration, and offset of each uterine contraction. *Normal uterine activity* is defined as five or fewer contractions in 10 minutes, averaged over a 30-minute window.[2] *Tachysystole*, applied to either spontaneous or induced labor, is defined as more than five contractions in 10 minutes, averaged over 30 minutes, and should be categorized by the presence or absence of FHR decelerations.[2] The ACOG has recommended that the terms *hyperstimulation* and *hypercontractility* be abandoned.

An IUPC may be used to measure the relative strength, and the onset and offset, of each uterine contraction with

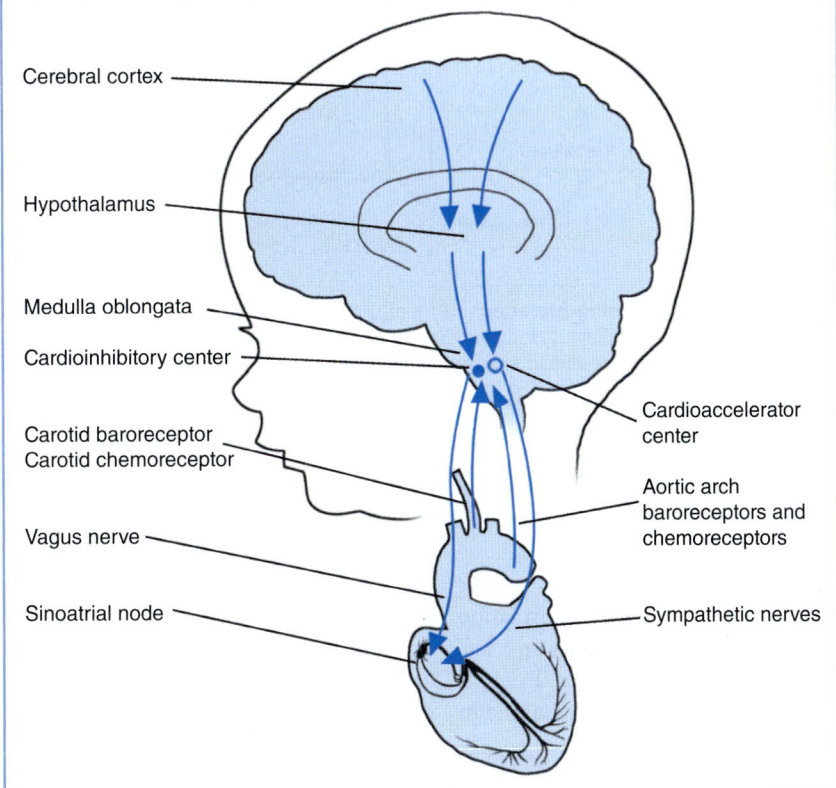

Fig 8.2 Regulation of Fetal Heart Rate. Illustration by Naveen Nathan, MD, NorthShore University HealthSystem, University of Chicago Pritzker School of Medicine, Evanston, IL.

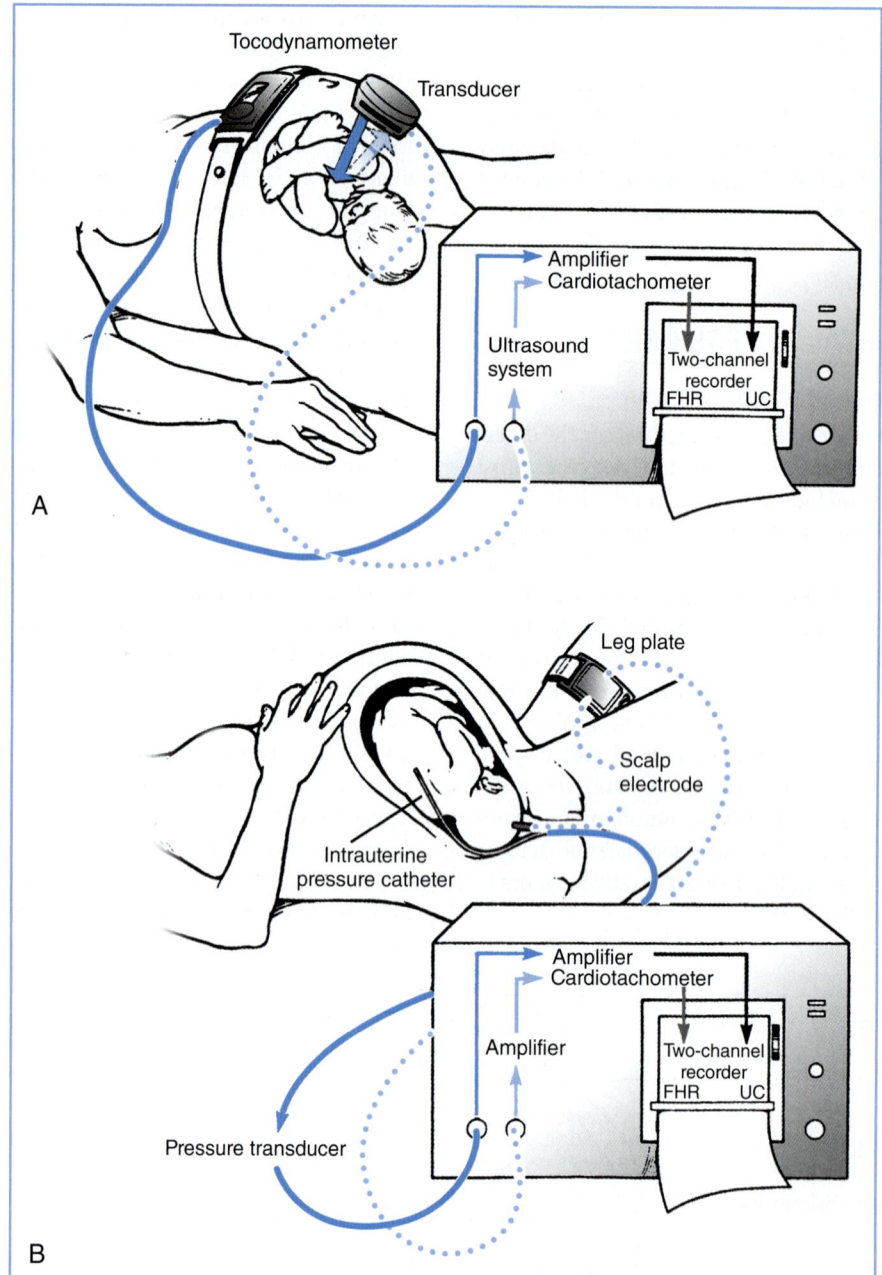

Fig 8.3 Electronic Fetal Monitoring Apparatus. (A) Instrumentation for external monitoring. Contractions are detected by the pressure-sensitive tocodynamometer, amplified, and then recorded. The fetal heart rate (FHR) is monitored with the Doppler ultrasound transducer, which emits and receives the reflected ultrasound signal that is then counted and recorded. (B) Techniques used for direct monitoring of FHR and uterine contractions (UCs). UCs are assessed with an intrauterine pressure catheter connected to a pressure transducer. This signal is then amplified and recorded. The fetal electrocardiogram is obtained by direct application of the scalp electrode, which is then attached to a leg plate on the mother's thigh. The signal is transmitted to the monitor, where it is amplified, counted by the cardiotachometer, and recorded. Illustration by Naveen Nathan, MD, NorthShore University HealthSystem, University of Chicago Pritzker School of Medicine, Evanston, IL.

greater precision than an external monitor. Such information may be used to distinguish among early, variable, and late FHR decelerations (see later). Additionally, the IUPC may be useful for obese parturients where the tocodynamometer lacks sensitivity.

The following features of the FHR pattern can be assessed: (1) **baseline** measurements, (2) **variability** (the extent to which the rate changes both instantaneously and over longer periods), (3) **accelerations**, and (4) **decelerations**, and their association with uterine contractions.

Baseline Fetal Heart Rate

A normal baseline FHR is defined as 110 to 160 beats per minute (bpm) and is determined by assessing the mean heart rate over a 10-minute period rounded to increments of 5 bpm.[2,35] In general, term fetuses have a lower baseline FHR than preterm fetuses because of greater parasympathetic nervous system activity. Laboratory studies suggest that bradycardia (caused by increased vagal activity) is the initial fetal response to acute hypoxemia. After prolonged hypoxemia, the fetus may experience tachycardia as a result of catecholamine secretion and sympathetic nervous system activity.[36] A baseline FHR < 110 bpm is termed *bradycardia* and a baseline FHR > 160 bpm is *tachycardia*.[2,35]

Fetal bradycardia may be caused by congenital heart block, fetal central nervous system (CNS) injury, or fetal hypoxia.[37–39] The most common cause of fetal tachycardia is maternal fever. Other causes include fetal cardiac arrhythmias and medications administered to the mother, such as beta-adrenergic receptor agonists (e.g., terbutaline for tocolysis). Epidural analgesia with local anesthetic agents (e.g., lidocaine, bupivacaine) can also lead to sympathetic blockade, maternal hypotension, transient uteroplacental insufficiency, and alterations in the FHR.[2] Parenteral opioids also may affect the FHR.[40] Lastly, FHR changes have been reported after an eclamptic seizure.[41] In a retrospective study of FHR tracings associated with eclampsia at Parkland Hospital, 79% of fetuses demonstrated prolonged bradycardia, and half of the fetuses developed fetal tachycardia after recovery from the episode of bradycardia.[41] The mean (± standard deviation) duration of bradycardia was 5.8 ± 3.0 minutes with a range of 2 to 15 minutes. FHR decelerations occurred, on average, 2.7 ± 1.6 minutes after the onset of the eclamptic seizure. Despite these periods of FHR decelerations associated with eclampsia, prioritization of maternal support and stabilization resulted in a favorable perinatal outcome without the need for immediate operative intervention in more than two-thirds of cases. Thus, an eclamptic seizure does not necessarily require immediate, emergent operative delivery for fetal indications.

Fetal Heart Rate Variability

FHR variability is the fluctuation in the baseline FHR that is irregular in amplitude and frequency.[2,35] Variability is usually quantified as the amplitude of peak-to-trough heart rate in beats per minute. Box 8.2 describes the variation of recorded findings. Baseline variability is defined as the irregular fluctuations in the baseline excluding accelerations and decelerations.[2,35] FHR variability increases over the course of gestation.[42] A representative FHR is shown in Fig. 8.4.

The presence of normal FHR variability reflects the presence of normal, intact pathways from and within the fetal cerebral cortex, midbrain, vagus nerve, and cardiac conduction system (see Fig. 8.2).[34] Variability is greatly influenced by the parasympathetic tone. Maternal administration of atropine, which readily crosses the placenta, can eliminate some variability. In humans, the sympathetic nervous system appears to have a lesser role in influencing variability.[34] Maternal administration of the beta-adrenergic receptor antagonist propranolol has little effect on FHR variability.[34]

During hypoxemia, fetal myocardial and cerebral blood flow increase to maintain oxygen delivery.[30,43,44] With severe

---

BOX 8.2 Definitions for Baseline Variability Based on Peak-to-Trough Amplitude

Baseline Variability
- Fluctuations in the baseline fetal heart rate that are irregular in amplitude and frequency
- Variability is visually quantitated as the amplitude of peak-to-trough in beats per minute
  - Absent: amplitude range undetectable
  - Minimal: amplitude rage detectable but 5 beats per minute or fewer
  - Moderate (normal): amplitude range 6–25 beats per minute
  - Marked: amplitude > 25 beats per minute

From American College of Obstetricians and Gynecologists. Practice Bulletin No. 106: Intrapartum fetal heart rate monitoring: nomenclature, interpretation, and general management principles (reaffirmed 2025). *Obstet Gynecol*. 2009;114:192–202.

---

hypoxemia, however, fetal blood flow cannot increase sufficiently to maintain oxygen delivery. The decompensation of cerebral blood flow and oxygen delivery results in a loss of FHR variability.[34] The absence of variability in an anencephalic fetus also suggests that the presence of FHR variability reflects the integrity of the CNS. In animal models, perfusion of the CNS with calcium results in depolarization of electroencephalographic activity, which abolishes FHR variability.

Clinically, the presence of normal FHR variability predicts early neonatal health, as defined by an Apgar score of greater than 7 at 5 minutes.[45] In a case series of monitored fetal deaths, no fetus had normal variability immediately before demise.[34] However, in a cohort of 500 deliveries, the presence or absence of variability was not associated with neonatal acidosis.[46] The differential diagnosis of decreased variability includes fetal hypoxia, fetal sleep state, fetal neurologic abnormality, and decreased CNS activity that results from exposure to drugs, such as opioids. Decreased FHR variability is observed following acute maternal meperidine administration and long-term administration of buprenorphine.[40,47] Magnesium sulfate, commonly used for fetal neuroprotection and eclampsia prevention, decreases FHR variability but without adverse neonatal effects.[48,49]

Accelerations

Accelerations are abrupt changes—onset-to-peak in 30 seconds—in the FHR from baseline.[2,35] Beyond 32 weeks' gestation, an acceleration is defined by a peak of at least 15 bpm above baseline and lasting at least 15 seconds. Before 32 weeks' gestation, a peak of 10 bpm above the baseline, lasting at least 10 seconds, is required. While an acceleration that extends for 2 minutes is considered prolonged, at 10 minutes it is considered a baseline change. During the antepartum period, the heart rate of the healthy fetus accelerates in response to fetal movement. Antepartum FHR accelerations signal fetal health, and their presence indicates a reactive nonstress test.

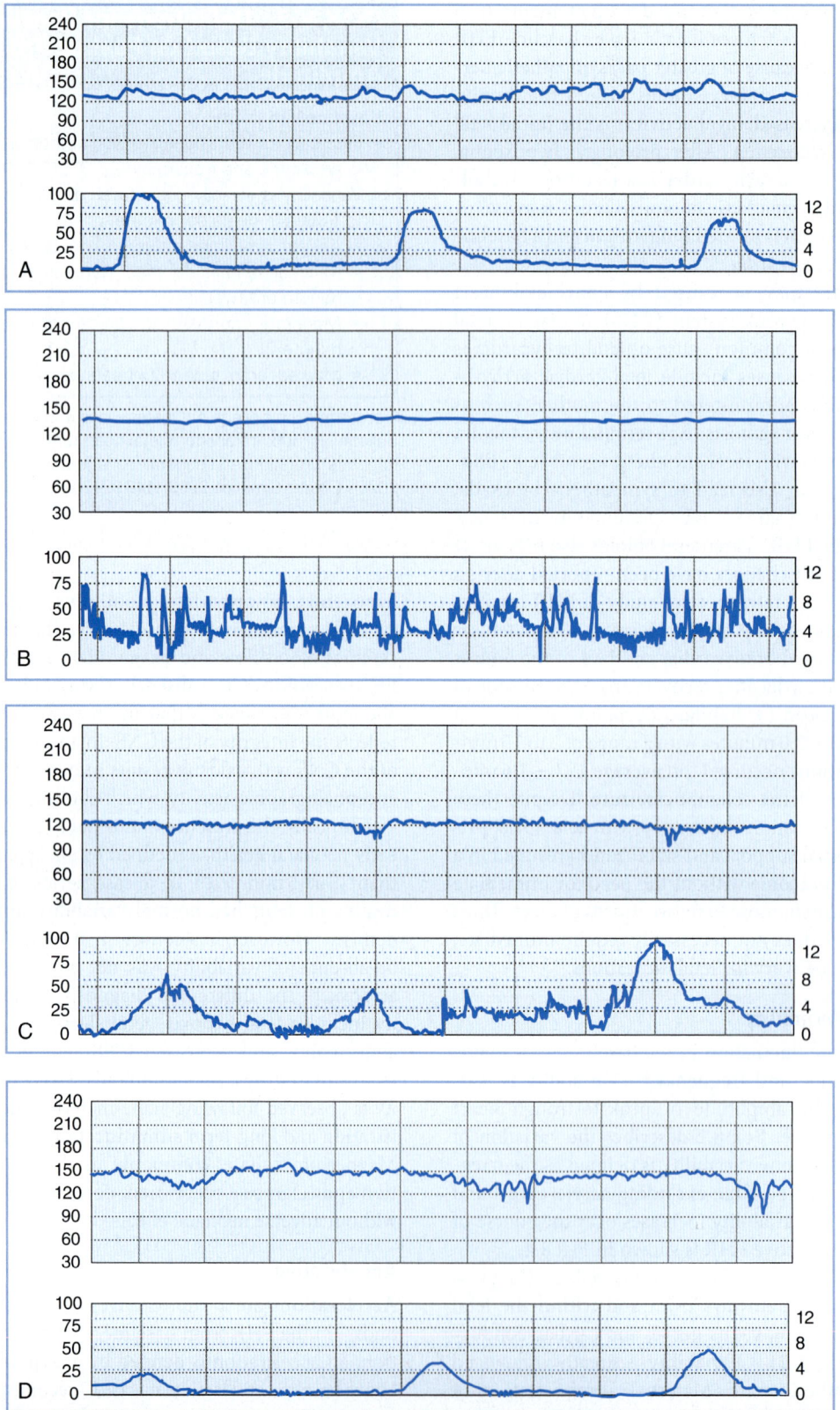

Fig 8.4 (A) Normal intrapartum fetal heart rate (FHR) tracing. The infant had Apgar scores of 8 and 8 at 1 and 5 min, respectively. (B) Absence of variability in an FHR tracing. Placental abruption was noted at cesarean delivery. The infant had an umbilical arterial blood pH of 6.75 and Apgar scores of 1 and 4, respectively. (C) Early FHR decelerations. After a normal spontaneous vaginal delivery, the infant had Apgar scores of 8 and 8, respectively. (D) Late FHR decelerations. The amniotic fluid surrounding this fetus was meconium stained. Despite the late FHR decelerations, the variability remained acceptable. The infant was delivered by cesarean delivery and had an umbilical venous blood pH of 7.30. Apgar scores were 9 and 9, respectively.

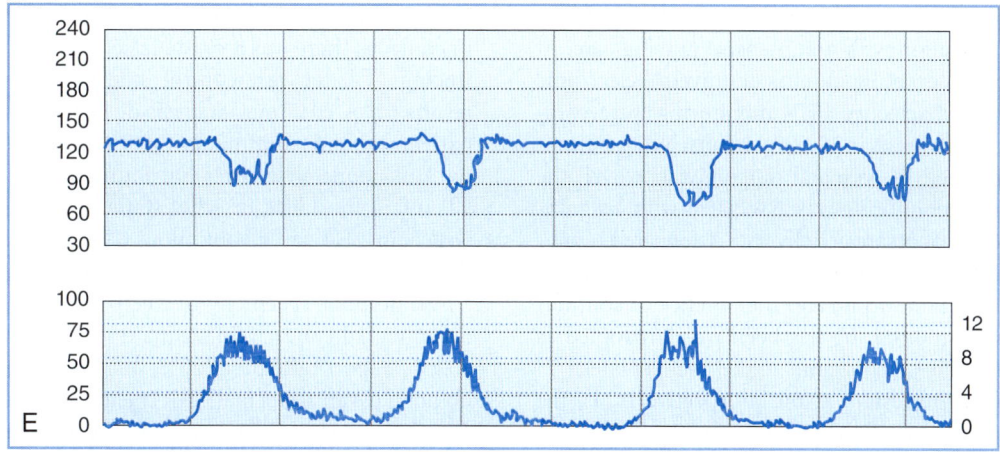

Fig 8.4, Con'd (E) Variable FHR decelerations. A tight nuchal cord was noted at low-forceps vaginal delivery. The infant had Apgar scores of 6 and 9, respectively. Numerical scales: *Left upper panel margin*, FHR in beats per minute; *left lower panel margin*, uterine pressure in mm Hg; *right lower panel margin*, uterine pressure in kilopascals (kPa).

Intrapartum accelerations most commonly preclude the existence of significant fetal metabolic acidosis. The absence of accelerations, however, does not necessarily suggest fetal compromise unless other nonreassuring findings are present.

Decelerations

Decelerations include early, late, or variable decelerations. **Early decelerations** occur simultaneously with uterine contractions. The onset and offset of each deceleration coincide with the onset and offset of the uterine contraction (see Fig. 8.4). In animal models, head compression can precipitate early decelerations.[36] In humans, early decelerations are believed to result from reflex vagal activity. Early decelerations are considered benign and not associated with fetal acidemia.

Late decelerations are delayed in timing with the nadir occurring after the peak of the contraction.[2,35] In most cases, the onset, nadir, and recovery of the deceleration occur after the beginning, peak, and ending of the contraction, respectively. Animal studies suggest that late decelerations represent a response to hypoxemia. The delayed onset of the deceleration reflects the time needed for the chemoreceptors to detect decreased oxygen tension and mediate the change in FHR by means of the vagus nerve.[36,50] Late decelerations may also result from decompensation of the myocardial circulation and myocardial failure. Clinical and animal studies suggest that late decelerations may be an overly sensitive indication of fetal asphyxia.[51] However, the combination of late decelerations and decreased or absent FHR variability is an ominous signal of fetal compromise.[52,53]

Variable decelerations vary in depth, shape, and duration. They often are abrupt in onset and offset. These are the most frequent decelerations identified during labor and are reported to occur in more than 80% of patients during the first stage of labor.[54] Variable decelerations result from baroreceptor- or chemoreceptor-mediated vagal activity or possible transient hypoxemia.[55,56] Experimental models and clinical studies suggest that umbilical cord occlusion, either partial

or complete, results in variable decelerations. During the second stage of labor, variable decelerations may result from compression of the fetal head. In this situation, dural stimulation leads to increased vagal discharge.[33] The healthy fetus can typically tolerate mild to moderate variable decelerations without decompensation. With prolonged, severe variable decelerations (<60 bpm) or persistent fetal bradycardia, it is difficult for the fetus to maintain cardiac output and umbilical blood flow.[33] Recurrent variable decelerations with minimal to moderate variability are indeterminant, whereas those with absent variability are deemed abnormal.[35]

Sinusoidal and **saltatory** patterns are two unusual FHR tracing patterns that may indicate fetal compromise. The sinusoidal FHR pattern is a regular, smooth, wavelike pattern that may signal fetal anemia.[57] Occasionally, maternal administration of an opioid, such as butorphanol, can lead to a sinusoidal FHR pattern. The saltatory pattern consists of excessive swings in variability (>25 bpm) and may signal the occurrence of acute fetal hypoxia; there is a weak association between this pattern and low Apgar scores.[58]

Limitations of Electronic Fetal Heart Rate Monitoring

Despite laboratory and early clinical data suggesting that FHR monitoring accurately reflects fetal health, controversy exists regarding the ability of this assessment tool to improve fetal and neonatal outcomes. It remains unclear why prospective studies have not confirmed greater benefit of the use of continuous electronic FHR monitoring during labor; the intensity of intrapartum assessment and care may play a role. In prospective trials, pregnant women were randomly assigned to receive intermittent FHR auscultation or continuous electronic FHR monitoring, but all patients were monitored by dedicated nursing staff who provided intensive intrapartum care. By contrast, the historical cohort studies compared patients who received continuous electronic FHR monitoring and intensive intrapartum care with patients who had intermittent FHR auscultation with nonintensive nursing care. At Parkland Hospital, alternating months of universal electronic FHR monitoring and selective FHR monitoring were compared over 3 years in more than 17,000 patients. No significant differences were noted in perinatal outcomes; however, the period of universal monitoring was associated with a significantly increased rate of cesarean delivery.[59] There are no published studies that have randomly assigned a group of patients to not receive FHR monitoring, and the practice of continuous electronic FHR monitoring has been widely adopted as standard practice in most labor units in the United States.

Consistent with the results of the prospective trials, the ACOG endorses the use of either intermittent auscultation or continuous electronic FHR monitoring during labor. In high-risk patients, the ACOG guidelines recommend that the obstetrician or nurse review the electronic FHR tracing every 15 minutes during the first stage of labor and every 5 minutes during the second stage.[2] For low-risk patients, the intervals may be lengthened to 30 minutes for the first stage and 15 minutes for the second stage.[2,60] The optimal interval for intermittent FHR monitoring has not been studied, but the intervals of 15 to 30 minutes in the active phase and every 5 minutes in the second stage have some indirect support.[7,61] Adherence to these standards for intermittent auscultation may be difficult to achieve in the clinical setting; in one study, this standard was met for only 3% of parturients.[62] A systematic review and metaanalysis compared intermittent use of handheld Doppler CTG to an obstetric stethoscope or fetoscope (nonelectronic device) and demonstrated no improvement in neonatal outcome but an increase in operative delivery.[63]

Several hypotheses to account for the apparent failure of intrapartum FHR monitoring to reduce the incidence of CP have been proposed and include the following:

- A large proportion of asphyxial damage begins before the onset of labor;
- Catastrophic, "sentinel" events (e.g., cord prolapse, placental abruption, uterine rupture) may not allow sufficient time for intervention before neurologic damage occurs;
- A larger proportion of very-low-birthweight infants survive and thus contribute to the number with CP;
- Infection is associated with abnormal FHR patterns and the subsequent development of CP, and it is unclear if early intervention offers any benefit in such cases;
- The amount of asphyxia required to cause permanent neurologic damage approximates the amount that causes fetal death, leaving a narrow window for intervention.[64] The number of children in whom CP develops from intrapartum asphyxia is probably small.[64]

Limitations of FHR monitoring include a poor positive predictive value in distinguishing between abnormal FHR tracings and abnormal outcomes. Because of this imprecision, the ACOG recommended that abnormal FHR tracings be described with the term *nonreassuring fetal status* rather than *fetal distress* or *birth asphyxia*.[24] In one population-based, case-control study of children with CP, FHR tracings were retrospectively reviewed. While a markedly higher incidence of

abnormal FHR tracings was found in children with CP than in controls, there was a 99.8% false-positive rate of abnormal tracings.[65] Later case-control studies have yielded similar results.[23,66] A 2017 metaanalysis of 13 trials, including 37,000 patients, found continuous CTG fetal monitoring reduced rates of neonatal seizures but found no clear differences in CP, infant mortality, or other standard measures of neonatal well-being. However, continuous CTG was associated with an increase in cesarean and operative vaginal births.[7]

While poor specificity of electronic fetal monitoring is a documented concern, inadequate sensitivity is also an issue. A 2017 report noted that 20% of fetuses born with acidemia do not have an abnormal FHR tracing even with expert retrospective evaluation.[29] A case-control study of infants with HIE showed that FHR monitoring the hour before delivery was poorly predictive of neurologic injury.[28] Further limitations of continuous FHR monitoring include: (1) poor intraobserver and interobserver agreement despite the use of trained observers, especially when FHR patterns are observed; (2) the required continual presence of a nurse or physician to assess the FHR tracing; (3) the inconvenience to the patient (e.g., confinement to bed and the application of monitor belts or a scalp electrode); and (4) the need to maintain the FHR tracings as legal documents.[68,69]

Despite little evidence for its efficacy, obstetricians rely on electronic FHR monitoring for the following three reasons: (1) professional obstetric organizations (e.g., ACOG) advise some form of monitoring during labor, (2) electronic FHR monitoring is logistically easier and less expensive than one-on-one nursing care during labor, and (3) individual (often anecdotal) experiences cause "many obstetricians [to] believe that in their own hands FHR monitoring is … efficacious."[70]

In 2008, the National Institute of Child Health and Human Development sponsored a workshop that resulted in the publication of updated definitions, interpretation, and research guidelines for intrapartum electronic FHR monitoring.[35] The published report proposed a three-tier system for the categorization of FHR patterns (Box 8.3).[35] The ACOG has adopted this system with suggested options for management.[2,60]

- **Category I (normal):** Strongly predictive of *normal* fetal acid-base status at the time of observation.
- **Category II (indeterminate):** Not predictive of *abnormal* fetal acid-base status, but without adequate evidence to classify as normal or abnormal.
- **Category III (abnormal):** Predictive of *abnormal* fetal acid-base status at the time of observation and thus requiring prompt evaluation (Box 8.4).[2,35]

In a large population review, at any one time, 78% of tracings were Category I, 22% of tracings were Category II, and 0.004% of the tracings were Category III.[71] Whereas only 0.2% of Category I tracings were associated with low Apgar scores and neonatal intensive care unit (NICU) admissions, this increased to 0.7% with Category II tracings, suggesting a greater association with increased short-term morbidity. A 2023 systematic review and metaanalysis evaluating the three-tier classification system concluded that the three-tiered interpretation system provides an approximate but

BOX 8.3 Three-Tiered Fetal Heart Rate (FHR) Interpretation System

Category I tracings include all of the following:
- Baseline rate: 110–160 beats per minute (bpm)
- Baseline FHR variability: moderate
- Accelerations: present or absent
- Late or variable decelerations: absent
- Early decelerations: present or absent

Category II tracings include:
- All tracings not categorized as Category I or Category III
- Baseline FHR
  - Bradycardia not accompanied by absent baseline variability
  - Tachycardia
- Baseline FHR variability
  - Minimal baseline variability
  - Absent baseline variability not accompanied by recurrent decelerations
  - Marked baseline variability
- Accelerations
  - Absence of induced accelerations after fetal stimulation
- Periodic or episodic decelerations
  - Recurrent variable decelerations accompanied by minimal or moderate variability
  - Prolonged deceleration ≥ 2 min but <10 min
  - Recurrent late decelerations with moderate baseline variability
  - Variable decelerations with other characteristics such as slow return to baseline, overshoots, or shoulders

Category III tracings include either:
- Absent baseline FHR variability and any of the following:
  - Recurrent late decelerations
  - Recurrent variable decelerations
  - Bradycardia
- Sinusoidal pattern

Modified from Macones GA, Hankins GD, Spong CY, et al. The 2008 National Institute of Child Health and Human Development workshop report on electronic fetal monitoring. *Obstet Gynecol.* 2008;112:661–666.[35]

BOX 8.4 Logistical Considerations in Preparation for Operative Delivery in the Setting of Category III Tracing

- Obtain informed consent (verbal or written as feasible)
- Assemble surgical team (surgeon, scrub technician, and anesthesia personnel)
- Assess patient transit time and location for operative delivery
- Ensure intravenous access
- Review status of laboratory tests (e.g., complete blood type and screen) and assess need for, and availability of, blood products
- Assess need for preoperative placement of indwelling Foley catheter
- Assemble personnel for neonatal resuscitation

From American College of Obstetricians and Gynecologists. Practice Bulletin No. 116: Management of intrapartum fetal heart rate tracings (reaffirmed 2025). *Obstet Gynecol.* 2010;116:1232–1240.[60]

imprecise measurement of neonatal prognosis.[72] Although the incidence of an Apgar score < 7 at 5 minutes and umbilical artery pH < 7.00 increased significantly with increasing FHR tracing category, approximately 98% of newborns with Category II tracings did not have adverse outcomes. Notably, of the 671 articles reviewed, only 3 publications met inclusion criteria.

Several other classification systems have been developed. For example, a five-tier FHR pattern interpretation system has been developed based on the Federal Homeland Security Classification of Risk in US airports (green = low risk, red = severe risk of acidemia, and/or evolution to a more serious pattern).[73] In a small retrospective study, the five-tier classification system performed better than the three-tier classification system in characterizing fetuses with acidemia who required subsequent admission to the NICU and respiratory support.[74] That said, this classification system is more complex, and in most US birthing facilities, the three-tier system is utilized as it is currently endorsed by national organizations.[2,35,60] Indeed, national organizations now have developed educational programs and clinical practicums for FHR monitoring using the three-tier system in obstetric practice.[75] Evidence for the impact of such training on neonatal and maternal outcomes is limited and requires further study.[76]

Methods for Improving the Efficacy of Electronic Fetal Heart Rate Monitoring

Several technologies have been employed to enhance the value of electronic FHR monitoring. To facilitate continual FHR assessment, many labor and delivery units transmit the tracings from the bedside to the nurses' station, referred to as "centralized" monitoring. Presumably, this practice facilitates a more rapid response to worrisome FHR tracings. Electronic archiving allows for the electronic storage and retrieval of FHR tracings and eliminates the need for long-term storage of the paper record. Storage, either using an electronic record or a paper FHR tracing, is necessary as a component of the medical record.[24] While commercially available programs with sound or light alerts have been developed, randomized controlled trials have not shown improvement over visual interpretation of tracings.[77–80] In fact, it is possible that intrapartum maternal overmonitoring can negatively impact care by generating alarm fatigue.[81] This has prompted some centers to explore risk-based alarm systems to reduce such fatigue.[82]

Supplemental Methods of Fetal Assessment

A normal electronic FHR monitor tracing is more than 99% accurate in predicting a 5-minute Apgar score > 7. Unfortunately, an abnormal FHR tracing has a false-positive rate > 99%.[2,60] Adding other fetal assessment tools may help identify the compromised fetus with greater specificity and allow appropriate intervention.

An older method used to confirm or exclude the presence of fetal acidosis when FHR monitoring suggests the presence of fetal compromise is **fetal scalp blood sampling** for pH or lactate. While supplementing FHR monitoring with fetal scalp blood pH assessment may decrease operative deliveries, there is no evidence to suggest improvement in fetal outcomes.[77,83,84] This technique is not currently performed at most birthing facilities in the United States. An alternative to fetal scalp blood sampling is **fetal scalp stimulation**.[85] The fetal scalp can be digitally stimulated during a vaginal examination or squeezed with an Allis clamp. The heart rate of a healthy, nonacidotic fetus accelerates in response to scalp stimulation; FHR acceleration is associated with a fetal pH > 7.20.[86,87] **Vibroacoustic stimulation** is the application of an artificial larynx to the maternal abdomen, which results in FHR acceleration in a healthy fetus and improves the specificity of FHR monitoring.[88] Used primarily in antepartum testing situations, there is less evidence for intrapartum use.[89] A metaanalysis of intrapartum stimulation tests (i.e., fetal scalp blood pH determination, Allis clamp scalp stimulation, vibroacoustic stimulation, digital fetal scalp stimulation) found the tests to be equivalent at predicting fetal acidemia, with digital fetal scalp stimulation having the greatest ease of use. However, all these tests are "less than perfect."[88]

Because FHR monitoring provides only an *indirect* measure of fetal oxygenation and acid-base status, alternative technologies such as **fetal pulse oximetry** and **ST waveform analysis of fetal ECG** have been evaluated to enhance assessment of fetal monitoring; neither improved neonatal outcome nor reduced cesarean births.[90] Recently, with the development of **artificial intelligence (AI)**, studies have suggested promise for AI and deep learning to enhance fetal surveillance.[91] In a retrospective study, concordance of intrapartum CTG between physicians and AI-based techniques was noted; however, AI-based monitoring resulted in a higher false-positive rate compared to clinical practice.[92]

The presence of **meconium-stained amniotic fluid** has long been associated with an increased risk for infant depression at birth. Moderate to thick meconium is associated with lower Apgar scores, lower umbilical arterial blood pH, an increased incidence of neonatal seizures, and higher rates of cesarean delivery and admission to an intensive care nursery.[93] Although approximately 4% to 22% of all deliveries are complicated by meconium-stained amniotic fluid, few of these infants experience neonatal depression. The odds ratio for complications increases with meconium, but most infants with neonatal complications have clear fluid.[93] Thus, meconium-stained fluid has a poor positive predictive value and poor sensitivity in predicting adverse neonatal outcomes.[93]

The physiology associated with the passage of meconium is incompletely understood. Ultrasonographic imaging suggests that the fetus regularly passes rectal contents into the amniotic fluid throughout gestation.[93] However, meconium-stained amniotic fluid is more common in pregnancies complicated by postterm or fetal growth restriction. Putative triggers for the passage of meconium include umbilical cord compression and hypoxia. The presence of meconium combined with an abnormal FHR tracing or another risk factor (e.g., fetal growth restriction) appears to be associated with an increased likelihood of neonatal depression.[93] Among newborns with meconium-stained amniotic fluid, approximately 3% to 12% develop significant neonatal respiratory compromise, termed **meconium aspiration syndrome**.[93] Antenatal risk factors for this syndrome include moderate or thick meconium (suggesting recent passage and lower amniotic fluid volume) and abnormal FHR tracings.[93] The lung injury likely originates from intrapartum fetal hypoxia.[93] Oropharyngeal suctioning at delivery has not proved beneficial (see Chapter 9).[94,95] Current recommendations state that newborns with meconium-stained amniotic fluid, regardless of vigor, should no longer receive routine suctioning; suctioning is reserved only for those with airway obstruction.[94,95]

INTRAPARTUM FETAL THERAPY FOR CATEGORIES II AND III FETAL HEART RATE PATTERNS

The identification of potential intrapartum fetal compromise with a Category II tracing should prompt a careful assessment of maternal, placental, and fetal factors. Attention to the etiology of fetal hypoxemia and the institution of appropriate treatments may mitigate fetal compromise. Clinical history, physical findings, laboratory findings, and fetal monitoring (e.g., FHR, ultrasonography) should be used in an attempt to identify the etiology.[96,97]

Correctable **maternal factors** that may contribute to fetal compromise include pathologic states that result in decreased oxygen delivery to the placenta. **Respiratory failure** caused by long-standing diseases (e.g., asthma) can be determined from history and physical findings, whereas additional laboratory measurements may be necessary to diagnose pneumonia, pulmonary edema, or viral infection (e.g., SARS-CoV-2 [COVID-19]) as an underlying cause. **Decreased oxygen delivery** to the placenta may result from acute (e.g., sepsis, hypotension) or chronic conditions. **Decreased uteroplacental perfusion** can result from reduced maternal cardiac output (e.g., cardiovascular disease) or chronic vascular disease (e.g., chronic hypertension, diabetes mellitus). Dehydration from prolonged labor is a more subtle cause of diminished uteroplacental perfusion.

Maternal hypotension related to neuraxial analgesia or aggressive antihypertensive therapy commonly results in FHR abnormalities, including fetal bradycardia. Appropriate therapy for treating maternal hypotension in this setting includes intravenous fluids and vasopressor administration. Immediately prior to delivery, neuraxial anesthesia-associated maternal hypotension has been associated both with fetal acidemia and hypoxia; thus, close attention to maternal blood pressure is vital prior to delivery.

Administration of **supplemental oxygen** was once thought to enhance fetal oxygenation, even in the previously normoxemic mother. However, this common practice, which is not supported by robust data, has been challenged. In 2021, a systematic review of 16 trials involving 2052 patients found an expected small increase in umbilical artery Pao_2, but no difference in umbilical artery pH, neonatal acidemia, admission to NICU, or any other meaningful clinical outcomes.[98] In a secondary analysis of a randomized trial, intrapartum oxygen supplementation, compared to room air, did not increase the rate of resolution of recurrent late and/or variable decelerations or high-risk Category II FHR tracings.[98] These findings prompted the ACOG to release a practice advisory in 2022 stating that routine use of oxygen supplementation in individuals with normal oxygen saturation is *not recommended* for fetal intrauterine resuscitation.[99]

Uterine tachysystole, which may result in decreased uteroplacental perfusion, is a known risk of the use of oxytocin or prostaglandin compounds for the induction of labor. Uterine contractions constrict the uterine spiral arteries, decreasing oxygen delivery to the placenta. A rare cause of fetal compromise is **uterine rupture**, which may result from uterine hyperstimulation, particularly in the setting of a uterine scar (e.g., prior cesarean delivery). **Placental abruption**, which may result in a partial or complete cessation of oxygen transfer to the fetus, can be associated with chronic or acute diseases. Long-standing vascular diseases, produced by chronic hypertension or smoking, and acute factors such as cocaine abuse and abdominal trauma, can precipitate a placental abruption.

The treatment of uteroplacental causes of fetal compromise includes correction of tachysystole by cessation of oxytocin infusion (Table 8.1). Oxytocin has a plasma half-life of 1 to 6 minutes, and consequently, it may take several minutes for the hypertonus to resolve. Alternatively, a tocolytic agent (e.g., terbutaline, nitroglycerin) may be administered.[96,97] Normal maternal circulation should be maintained by avoiding aortocaval compression with maternal position change, expanding intravascular volume, and administering a vasopressor (e.g., phenylephrine, ephedrine) if indicated.[100]

Obesity in pregnancy is a significant contributor to maternal and perinatal morbidity with a rising global prevalence among reproductive-aged women.[101] Application of monitors and interpretation of intrapartum FHR is often hindered because of increased soft tissue and abdominal mass. This may result in extensive time periods when the FHR cannot be monitored.[102] Internal monitoring with a fetal scalp electrode and IUPC—rather than external monitors—may be useful in such cases, but spontaneous or iatrogenic rupture of membranes and cervical dilation is required before applying these monitors.[101] As a consequence, in patients with obesity, the use of electrical uterine myography shows early promise and may eventually replace standard tocometry.[103]

Fetal factors may contribute to fetal hypoxemia and acidosis. **Umbilical cord prolapse** through the cervix causes cord compression and often results in sudden fetal bradycardia. In most circumstances, treatment of a prolapsed cord consists of manual elevation of the fetal head until emergency cesarean delivery can be accomplished. Only rarely should the umbilical cord be replaced back into the uterus and expectant care be attempted.[104] Reports from the developing world indicate that, in some cases, expeditious vaginal delivery may produce acceptable neonatal outcome.[105] Alternative methods to decompress a prolapsed umbilical cord include the use of the Trendelenburg position or an infusion of 500 to 700 mL of 0.9% saline into the maternal bladder until delivery can be expedited.[104,106,107]

More commonly, **umbilical cord compression** occurs within the uterus and manifests as variable FHR decelerations. Although there is limited evidence for improvements in short-term or long-term neonatal outcomes, **amnioinfusion** has been shown to decrease the recurrence of variable decelerations as well as the rate of cesarean delivery for "suspected fetal distress."[60,108] A 2012 systematic review and metaanalysis concluded that there was no advantage to *prophylactic* intrapartum amnioinfusion in patients with oligohydramnios compared with *therapeutic* amnioinfusion in patients with

TABLE 8.1	Intrauterine Resuscitation Measures for Category II or Category III Tracings	
Goal	**FHR Abnormality[a]**	**Potential Intervention(s)[b]**
Promote fetal oxygenation and improve uteroplacental blood flow	Recurrent late decelerations Prolonged decelerations or bradycardia Minimal or absent FHR variability	Initiate lateral positioning (either left or right) Administer intravenous fluid bolus Reduce uterine contraction frequency
Reduce uterine activity	Tachysystole with Category II or III tracing	Discontinue oxytocin or cervical ripening agents Consider administration of tocolytic medication (e.g., terbutaline)
Alleviate umbilical cord compression	Recurrent variable decelerations Prolonged decelerations or bradycardia	Initiate maternal repositioning Consider initiation of amnioinfusion If prolapsed umbilical cord is noted, elevate the presenting fetal part while preparations are underway for operative delivery

FHR, Fetal heart rate.

[a]Evaluation for the underlying suspected cause(s) is also an important step in management of abnormal FHR tracings.

[b]Depending on the suspected underlying cause(s) of FHR abnormality, combining multiple interventions simultaneously may be appropriate and potentially more effective than performing each intervention individually or serially.

From American College of Obstetricians and Gynecologists. Practice Bulletin No. 116: Management of intrapartum fetal heart rate tracings (reaffirmed 2025). *Obstet Gynecol.* 2010;116:1232–1240.[60]

both oligohydramnios and FHR abnormalities.[109] Initial studies suggested that in patients with thick, meconium-stained amniotic fluid, amnioinfusion might decrease the incidence of meconium aspiration syndrome and fetal acidosis. A meta-analysis, however, suggests no benefit of amnioinfusion in the setting of meconium unless decelerations resulting from oligohydramnios are present.[110]

Saline amnioinfusion requires a dilated cervix, ruptured membranes, and the placement of an IUPC. Equipment that allows simultaneous saline amnioinfusion and measurement of intrauterine pressure is preferred. Either normal saline or lactated Ringer's solution may be infused as a bolus or as a continuous infusion.[110] The ideal rate of infusion has not been determined, but a commonly used regimen consists of a bolus of as much as 800 mL (infused at a rate of 10–15 mL/min), followed by either a continuous infusion at a rate of 3 mL/min or repeated boluses of 250 mL, as needed.[110] The necessity of either an infusion pump or a fluid warmer has not been demonstrated.[110] Alleviation of abnormal FHR patterns generally requires 20 to 30 minutes.[110]

Although most studies suggest that amnioinfusion is safe for the mother and fetus, some complications have been reported. Overdistention of the uterus, a higher rate of maternal infection, and maternal respiratory distress, including cases of fatal amniotic fluid embolism, have occurred.[111,112] A causal relationship between amniotic fluid embolism and amnioinfusion has yet to be determined. Overdistention of the uterus may be controlled with proper documentation of fluid loss from the uterus during infusion, the provision of amnioinfusion by gravity instead of an infusion pump, and the use of ultrasonography to evaluate the intrauterine fluid volume.[110]

Maternal fever may increase fetal oxygen consumption. Obstetricians should treat maternal fever with acetaminophen, a cooling blanket, and antibiotics as indicated to maintain maternal and fetal euthermia. **Hyperglycemia** also increases fetal oxygen consumption, so administration of a large bolus of a glucose-containing solution is contraindicated.

Fetal cardiac failure results in inadequate umbilical blood flow and fetal hypoxemia and acidosis. **Fetal anemia** caused by maternal isoimmunization, fetal hemoglobinopathy, or fetal hemorrhage results in diminished fetal oxygen-carrying capacity. If intrapartum assessment suggests the presence of fetal compromise, and fetal therapy is unsuccessful in the presence of a Category III FHR tracing, the obstetrician should affect an expeditious delivery (see Box 8.4).[60]

KEY POINTS

- A normal FHR tracing accurately predicts fetal well-being. An abnormal tracing is not specific in the prediction of fetal compromise. Exceptions include the fetus with prolonged bradycardia or the fetus with late FHR decelerations and absence of variability; both suggest a high likelihood of fetal acidemia.
- Large, prospective, randomized studies have not confirmed that continuous electronic FHR monitoring confers substantial clinical benefit over intermittent FHR auscultation as performed by dedicated labor nurses.
- When a Category II FHR tracing occurs, fetal resuscitation *in utero* may be attempted with interventions that include maternal position change, treatment of uterine tachysystole, administration of an intravenous fluid bolus, and/or saline amnioinfusion.
- Routine use of maternal oxygen supplementation to parturients with normal oxygen saturation is not recommended for fetal intrauterine resuscitation.
- Maternal hypotension after initiation of neuraxial anesthesia has been associated both with fetal acidemia and hypoxia; therefore, close attention to maternal blood pressure is vital prior to delivery.

REFERENCES

1. Schifrin BS, Koos BJ, Cohen WR, Soliman M. Approaches to preventing intrapartum fetal injury. *Front Pediatr*. 2022;10:915344.
2. American College of Obstetricians and Gynecologists. ACOG Practice Bulletin No. 106: Intrapartum fetal heart rate monitoring: nomenclature, interpretation, and general management principles (reaffirmed 2025). *Obstet Gynecol*. 2009;114:192–202.
3. Nelson KB, Blair E. Prenatal factors in singletons with cerebral palsy born at or near term. *N Engl J Med*. 2015;373:946–953.
4. Vintzileos AM, Smulian JC. Timing intrapartum management based on the evolution and duration of fetal heart rate patterns. *J Matern Fetal Neonatal Med*. 2022;35:7936–7941.
5. Ananth CV, Chauhan SP, Chen HY, et al. Electronic fetal monitoring in the United States: temporal trends and adverse perinatal outcomes. *Obstet Gynecol*. 2013;121:927–933.
6. Resnik R. Electronic fetal monitoring: the debate goes on . . . and on . . . and on. *Obstet Gynecol*. 2013;121:917–918.
7. Alfirevic Z, Devane D, Gyte GM, Cuthbert A. Continuous cardiotocography (CTG) as a form of electronic fetal monitoring (EFM) for fetal assessment during labour. *Cochrane Database Syst Rev*. 2017;2:CD006066.
8. Jacobson Misbe EN, Richards TL, McPherson RJ, et al. Perinatal asphyxia in a nonhuman primate model. *Dev Neurosci*. 2011;33:210–221.
9. Brann AW Jr, Myers RE. Central nervous system findings in the newborn monkey following severe in utero partial asphyxia. *Neurology*. 1975;25:327–338.

10. Juul SE, Aylward E, Richards T, et al. Prenatal cord clamping in newborn *Macaca nemestrina*: a model of perinatal asphyxia. *Dev Neurosci*. 2007;29:311–320.

11. Myers RE. Two patterns of perinatal brain damage and their conditions of occurrence. *Am J Obstet Gynecol*. 1972;112:246–276.

12. Bernert G, Hoeger H, Mosgoeller W, et al. Neurodegeneration, neuronal loss, and neurotransmitter changes in the adult guinea pig with perinatal asphyxia. *Pediatr Res*. 2003;54:523–528.

13. Derrick M, Luo NL, Bregman JC, et al. Preterm fetal hypoxia-ischemia causes hypertonia and motor deficits in the neonatal rabbit: a model for human cerebral palsy? *J Neurosci*. 2004;24:24–34.

14. Drobyshevsky A, Derrick M, Luo K, et al. Near-term fetal hypoxia-ischemia in rabbits: MRI can predict muscle tone abnormalities and deep brain injury. *Stroke*. 2012;43:2757–2763.

15. Kellert BA, McPherson RJ, Juul SE. A comparison of high-dose recombinant erythropoietin treatment regimens in brain-injured neonatal rats. *Pediatr Res*. 2007;61:451–455.

16. Thoresen M, Satas S, Loberg EM, et al. Twenty-four hours of mild hypothermia in unsedated newborn pigs starting after a severe global hypoxic-ischemic insult is not neuroprotective. *Pediatr Res*. 2001;50:405–411.

17. Prior T, Mullins E, Bennett P, Kumar S. Prediction of fetal compromise in labor. *Obstet Gynecol*. 2014;123:1263–1271.

18. Locatelli A, Lambicchi L, Incerti M, et al. Is perinatal asphyxia predictable? *BMC Pregnancy Childbirth*. 2020;20:186.

19. Knox AJ, Sadler L, Pattison NS, et al. An obstetric scoring system: its development and application in obstetric management. *Obstet Gynecol*. 1993;81:195–199.

20. Kuru A, Sogukpinar N, Akman L, Kazandi M. The determination of high-risk pregnancy: the use of antenatal scoring system. *Clin Exp Obstet Gynecol*. 2013;40:381–383.

21. Devane D, Lalor JG, Daly S, et al. Cardiotocography versus intermittent auscultation of fetal heart on admission to labour ward for assessment of fetal wellbeing. *Cochrane Database Syst Rev*. 2017;(1):CD005122.

22. Bhartiya V, Sharma R, Kumar A, Srivastava H. Admission cardiotocography: a predictor of neonatal outcome. *J Obstet Gynaecol India*. 2016;66:321–329.

23. Low JA, Pickersgill H, Killen H, Derrick EJ. The prediction and prevention of intrapartum fetal asphyxia in term pregnancies. *Am J Obstet Gynecol*. 2001;184:724–730.

24. American College of Obstetricians and Gynecologists. Executive summary: Neonatal encephalopathy and neurologic outcome, second edition. Report of the American College of Obstetricians and Gynecologists' Task Force on Neonatal Encephalopathy. *Obstet Gynecol*. 2014;123:896–901.

25. Phelan JP, Korst LM, Martin GI. Application of criteria developed by the Task Force on Neonatal Encephalopathy and Cerebral Palsy to acutely asphyxiated neonates. *Obstet Gynecol*. 2011;118:824–830.

26. Nelson DB, Lucke AM, McIntire DD, et al. Obstetric antecedents to body-cooling treatment of the newborn infant. *Am J Obstet Gynecol*. 2014;211:155.e1–e6.

27. Maso G, Piccoli M, De Seta F, et al. Intrapartum fetal heart rate monitoring interpretation in labour: a critical appraisal. *Minerva Ginecol*. 2015;67:65–79.

28. Graham EM, Adami RR, McKenney SL, et al. Diagnostic accuracy of fetal heart rate monitoring in the identification of neonatal encephalopathy. *Obstet Gynecol*. 2014;124:507–513.

29. Clark SL, Hamilton EF, Garite TJ, et al. The limits of electronic fetal heart rate monitoring in the prevention of neonatal metabolic acidemia. *Am J Obstet Gynecol*. 2017;216:163.e1–e6.

30. Rainaldi MA, Perlman JM. Pathophysiology of birth asphyxia. *Clin Perinatol*. 2016;43:409–422.

31. Peeters LL, Sheldon RE, Jones MD Jr, et al. Blood flow to fetal organs as a function of arterial oxygen content. *Am J Obstet Gynecol*. 1979;135:637–646.

32. Cohn HE, Sacks EJ, Heymann MA, Rudolph AM. Cardiovascular responses to hypoxemia and acidemia in fetal lambs. *Am J Obstet Gynecol*. 1974;120:817–824.

33. Ball RH, Parer JT. The physiologic mechanisms of variable decelerations. *Am J Obstet Gynecol*. 1992;166:1683–1688.

34. Parer JT. *Handbook of Fetal Heart Rate Monitoring*, 2nd ed. W. B. Saunders Co; 1997.

35. Macones GA, Hankins GD, Spong CY, et al. The 2008 National Institute of Child Health and Human Development workshop report on electronic fetal monitoring: update on definitions, interpretation, and research guidelines. *Obstet Gynecol*. 2008;112:661–666.

36. Court DJ, Parer JT. *Experimental Studies of Fetal Asphyxia and Fetal Heart Rate Interpretation*. Perinatology Press; 1984:113–169.

37. Bravo-Valenzuela NJ, Rocha LA, Machado Nardozza LM, Junior EA. Fetal cardiac arrhythmias: current evidence. *Ann Pediatr Cardiol*. 2018;11:148–163.

38. Vintzileos AM, Smulian JC. Abnormal fetal heart rate patterns caused by pathophysiologic processes other than fetal acidemia. *Am J Obstet Gynecol*. 2023;228:S1144–S1157.

39. Lepercq J, Nghiem MA, Goffinet F. Fetal heart rate nadir during bradycardia and umbilical artery acidemia at birth. *Acta Obstet Gynecol Scand*. 2021;100:964–970.

40. Hill JB, Alexander JM, Sharma SK, et al. A comparison of the effects of epidural and meperidine analgesia during labor on fetal heart rate. *Obstet Gynecol*. 2003;102:333–337.

41. Ambia AM, Wells CE, Yule CS, et al. Fetal heart rate tracings associated with eclamptic seizures. *Am J Obstet Gynecol*. 2022;227:622.e1–e6.

42. Shuffrey LC, Myers MM, Odendaal HJ, et al. Fetal heart rate, heart rate variability, and heart rate/movement coupling in the Safe Passage Study. *J Perinatol*. 2019;39:608–618.

43. Jones M Jr, Sheldon RE, Peeters LL, et al. Fetal cerebral oxygen consumption at different levels of oxygenation. *J Appl Physiol Respir Environ Exerc Physiol*. 1977;43:1080–1084.

44. Fisher DJ, Heymann MA, Rudolph AM. Fetal myocardial oxygen and carbohydrate consumption during acutely induced hypoxemia. *Am J Physiol*. 1982;242:H657–H661.

45. Parer JT, King T, Flanders S, et al. Fetal acidemia and electronic fetal heart rate patterns: is there evidence of an association? *J Matern Fetal Neonatal Med*. 2006;19:289–294.

46. Cahill AG, Roehl KA, Odibo AO, Macones GA. Association and prediction of neonatal acidemia. *Am J Obstet Gynecol*. 2012;207:206.e1–e8.

47. Jansson LM, Velez M, McConnell K, et al. Maternal buprenorphine treatment and fetal neurobehavioral development. *Am J Obstet Gynecol*. 2017;216:529.e1–e8.

48. Verdurmen KMJ, Hulsenboom ADJ, van Laar J, Oei SG. Effect of tocolytic drugs on fetal heart rate variability: a systematic review. *J Matern Fetal Neonatal Med*. 2017;30:2387–2394.

49. Duffy CR, Odibo AO, Roehl KA, et al. Effect of magnesium sulfate on fetal heart rate patterns in the second stage of labor. *Obstet Gynecol*. 2012;119:1129–1136.

50. Westgate JA, Wibbens B, Bennet L, et al. The intrapartum deceleration in center stage: a physiologic approach to the interpretation of fetal heart rate changes in labor. *Am J Obstet Gynecol.* 2007;197:236.e1–e11.

51. Jia YJ, Chen X, Cui HY, et al. Physiological CTG interpretation: the significance of baseline fetal heart rate changes after the onset of decelerations and associated perinatal outcomes. *J Matern Fetal Neonatal Med.* 2021;34:2349–2354.

52. Williams KP, Galerneau F. Intrapartum fetal heart rate patterns in the prediction of neonatal acidemia. *Am J Obstet Gynecol.* 2003;188:820–823.

53. Sameshima H, Ikenoue T. Predictive value of late decelerations for fetal acidemia in unselective low-risk pregnancies. *Am J Perinatol.* 2005;22:19–23.

54. Melchior J, Bernard N. *Incidence and Pattern of Fetal Heart Rate Alterations During Labor,* 1st ed. Springer; 1985.

55. Sholapurkar SL. Categorization of fetal heart rate decelerations in American and European practice: importance and imperative of avoiding framing and confirmation biases. *J Clin Med Res.* 2015;7:672–680.

56. Lear CA, Galinsky R, Wassink G, et al. The myths and physiology surrounding intrapartum decelerations: the critical role of the peripheral chemoreflex. *J Physiol.* 2016;594:4711–4725.

57. Modanlou HD, Murata Y. Sinusoidal heart rate pattern: reappraisal of its definition and clinical significance. *J Obstet Gynaecol Res.* 2004;30:169–180.

58. Nunes I, Ayres-de-Campos D, Kwee A, Rosen KG. Prolonged saltatory fetal heart rate pattern leading to newborn metabolic acidosis. *Clin Exp Obstet Gynecol.* 2014;41:507–511.

59. Leveno KJ, Cunningham FG, Nelson S, et al. A prospective comparison of selective and universal electronic fetal monitoring in 34,995 pregnancies. *N Engl J Med.* 1986;315:615–619.

60. American College of Obstetricians and Gynecologists. Practice Bulletin No. 116: Management of intrapartum fetal heart rate tracings (reaffirmed 2025). *Obstet Gynecol.* 2010;116:1232–1240.

61. Lewis D, Downe S, FIGO Intrapartum Fetal Monitoring Expert Consensus Panel. FIGO consensus guidelines on intrapartum fetal monitoring: intermittent auscultation. *Int J Gynaecol Obstet.* 2015;131:9–12.

62. Morrison JC, Chez BF, Davis ID, et al. Intrapartum fetal heart rate assessment: monitoring by auscultation or electronic means. *Am J Obstet Gynecol.* 1993;168:63–66.

63. Martis R, Emilia O, Nurdiati DS, Brown J. Intermittent auscultation (IA) of fetal heart rate in labour for fetal well-being. *Cochrane Database Syst Rev.* 2017;(2):CD008680.

64. Freeman RK. Problems with intrapartum fetal heart rate monitoring interpretation and patient management. *Obstet Gynecol.* 2002;100:813–826.

65. Nelson KB, Dambrosia JM, Ting TY, Grether JK. Uncertain value of electronic fetal monitoring in predicting cerebral palsy. *N Engl J Med.* 1996;334:613–618.

66. Larma JD, Silva AM, Holcroft CJ, et al. Intrapartum electronic fetal heart rate monitoring and the identification of metabolic acidosis and hypoxic-ischemic encephalopathy. *Am J Obstet Gynecol.* 2007;197:301.e1–e8.

67. Blix E, Oian P. Interobserver agreements in assessing 549 labor admission tests after a standardized training program. *Acta Obstet Gynecol Scand.* 2005;84:1087–1092.

68. Figueras F, Albela S, Bonino S, et al. Visual analysis of antepartum fetal heart rate tracings: inter- and intra-observer agreement and impact of knowledge of neonatal outcome. *J Perinat Med.* 2005;33:241–245.

69. Palomaki O, Luukkaala T, Luoto R, Tuimala R. Intrapartum cardiotocography – the dilemma of interpretational variation. *J Perinat Med.* 2006;34:298–302.

70. Parer JT, King T. Fetal heart rate monitoring: is it salvageable? *Am J Obstet Gynecol.* 2000;182:982–987.

71. Jackson M, Holmgren CM, Esplin MS, et al. Frequency of fetal heart rate categories and short-term neonatal outcome. *Obstet Gynecol.* 2011;118:803–808.

72. Zullo F, Di Mascio D, Raghuraman N, et al. Three-tiered fetal heart rate interpretation system and adverse neonatal and maternal outcomes: a systematic review and meta-analysis. *Am J Obstet Gynecol.* 2023;229:377–387.

73. Parer JT, Ikeda T. A framework for standardized management of intrapartum fetal heart rate patterns. *Am J Obstet Gynecol.* 2007;197:26.e1–e6.

74. Coletta J, Murphy E, Rubeo Z, Gyamfi-Bannerman C. The 5-tier system of assessing fetal heart rate tracings is superior to the 3-tier system in identifying fetal acidemia. *Am J Obstet Gynecol.* 2012;206:226.e1–e5.

75. Association of Women's Health, Obstetric and Neonatal Nurses. Antepartum and intrapartum fetal heart rate monitoring: clinical competencies and education guide, 7th edition. *Nurs Womens Health.* 2022;26:e53–e61.

76. Kelly S, Redmond P, King S, et al. Training in the use of intrapartum electronic fetal monitoring with cardiotocography: systematic review and meta-analysis. *BJOG.* 2021;128:1408–1419.

77. Melamed N, Baschat A, Yinon Y, et al. FIGO (International Federation of Gynecology and Obstetrics) initiative on fetal growth: best practice advice for screening, diagnosis, and management of fetal growth restriction. *Int J Gynaecol Obstet.* 2021;152(Suppl 1):3–57.

78. Nunes I, Ayres-de-Campos D, Ugwumadu A, et al. Central fetal monitoring with and without computer analysis: a randomized controlled trial. *Obstet Gynecol.* 2017;129:83–90.

79. Devoe LD, Ross M, Wilde C, et al. United States multicenter clinical usage study of the STAN 21 electronic fetal monitoring system. *Am J Obstet Gynecol.* 2006;195:729–734.

80. Georgieva A, Redman CWG, Papageorghiou AT. Computerized data-driven interpretation of the intrapartum cardiotocogram: a cohort study. *Acta Obstet Gynecol Scand.* 2017;96:883–891.

81. Kern-Goldberger AR, Hamm RF, Raghuraman N, Srinivas SK. Reducing alarm fatigue in maternal monitoring on labor and delivery: a commentary on deimplementation in obstetrics. *Am J Perinatol.* 2023;40:1378–1382.

82. Kern-Goldberger AR, Nicholls EM, Plastino N, Srinivas SK. The impact of an intervention to improve intrapartum maternal vital sign monitoring and reduce alarm fatigue. *Am J Obstet Gynecol MFM.* 2023;5:100893.

83. Stal I, Wennerholm UB, Nordstrom L, et al. Fetal scalp blood sampling during second stage of labor – analyzing lactate or pH? A secondary analysis of a randomized controlled trial. *J Matern Fetal Neonatal Med.* 2022;35:1100–1107.

84. Wiberg-Itzel E, Lipponer C, Norman M, et al. Determination of pH or lactate in fetal scalp blood in management of intrapartum fetal distress: randomised controlled multicentre trial. *BMJ.* 2008;336:1284–1287.

85. Tahir Mahmood U, O'Gorman C, Marchocki Z, et al. Fetal scalp stimulation (FSS) versus fetal blood sampling (FBS) for women with abnormal fetal heart rate monitoring in labor: a prospective cohort study. *J Matern Fetal Neonatal Med.* 2018;31:1742–1747.

86. Clark SL, Gimovsky ML, Miller FC. The scalp stimulation test: a clinical alternative to fetal scalp blood sampling. *Am J Obstet Gynecol.* 1984;148:274–277.

87. Rathore AM, Ramji S, Devi CB, et al. Fetal scalp stimulation test: an adjunct to intermittent auscultation in non-reassuring fetal status during labor. *J Obstet Gynaecol Res.* 2011;37:819–824.

88. Skupski DW, Rosenberg CR, Eglinton GS. Intrapartum fetal stimulation tests: a meta-analysis. *Obstet Gynecol.* 2002;99:129–134.

89. East CE, Smyth RM, Leader LR, et al. Vibroacoustic stimulation for fetal assessment in labour in the presence of a nonreassuring fetal heart rate trace. *Cochrane Database Syst Rev.* 2013;(1): CD004664.

90. Belfort MA, Saade GR, Thom E, et al. A randomized trial of intrapartum fetal ECG ST-segment analysis. *N Engl J Med.* 2015;373:632–641.

91. Frasch MG, Strong SB, Nilosek D, et al. Detection of preventable fetal distress during labor from scanned cardiotocogram tracings using deep learning. *Front Pediatr.* 2021;9:736834.

92. Liu LC, Tsai YH, Chou YC, et al. Concordance analysis of intrapartum cardiotocography between physicians and artificial intelligence-based technique using modified one-dimensional fully convolutional networks. *J Chin Med Assoc.* 2021;84:158–164.

93. Vain NE, Batton DG. Meconium "aspiration" (or respiratory distress associated with meconium-stained amniotic fluid?). *Semin Fetal Neonatal Med.* 2017;22:214–219.

94. American College of Obstetricians and Gynecologists. Committee Opinion No 689: Delivery of a newborn with meconium-stained amniotic fluid (reaffirmed 2024). *Obstet Gynecol.* 2017;129:e33–e34.

95. Wyckoff MH, Aziz K, Escobedo MB, et al. Part 13: Neonatal resuscitation: 2015 American Heart Association guidelines update for cardiopulmonary resuscitation and emergency cardiovascular care. *Circulation.* 2015;132:S543–560.

96. Bullens LM, van Runnard Heimel PJ, van der Hout-van der Jagt MB, Oei SG. Interventions for intrauterine resuscitation in suspected fetal distress during term labor: a systematic review. *Obstet Gynecol Surv.* 2015;70:524–539.

97. Clark SL, Nageotte MP, Garite TJ, et al. Intrapartum management of category II fetal heart rate tracings: towards standardization of care. *Am J Obstet Gynecol.* 2013;209:89–97.

98. Raghuraman N, Temming LA, Doering MM, et al. Maternal oxygen supplementation compared with room air for intrauterine resuscitation: a systematic review and meta-analysis. *JAMA Pediatr.* 2021;175:368–376.

99. American College of Obstetricians and Gynecologists. Practice advisory: oxygen supplementation in the setting of category II or III fetal heart tracings (reaffirmed 2024). 2022. https://www.acog.org/clinical/clinical-guidance/practice-advisory/articles/2022/01/oxygen-supplementation-in-the-setting-of-category-ii-or-iii-fetal-heart-tracings. Accessed 21 May 2024.

100. Thurlow JA, Kinsella SM. Intrauterine resuscitation: active management of fetal distress. *Int J Obstet Anesth.* 2002;11:105–116.

101. Giouleka S, Tsakiridis I, Koutsouki G, et al. Obesity in pregnancy: a comprehensive review of influential guidelines. *Obstet Gynecol Surv.* 2023;78:50–68.

102. Brocato B, Lewis D, Mulekar M, Baker S. Obesity's impact on intrapartum electronic fetal monitoring. *J Matern Fetal Neonatal Med.* 2019;32:92–94.

103. Moni SS, Kirshenbaum R, Comfort L, et al. Noninvasive monitoring of uterine electrical activity among patients with obesity: a new external monitoring device. *Am J Obstet Gynecol MFM.* 2021;3:100375.

104. Lin MG. Umbilical cord prolapse. *Obstet Gynecol Surv.* 2006;61:269–277.

105. Enakpene CA, Omigbodun AO, Arowojolu AO. Perinatal mortality following umbilical cord prolapse. *Int J Gynaecol Obstet.* 2006;95:44–45.

106. Katz Z, Shoham Z, Lancet M, et al. Management of labor with umbilical cord prolapse: a 5-year study. *Obstet Gynecol.* 1988;72:278–281.

107. Bord I, Gemer O, Anteby EY, Shenhav S. The value of bladder filling in addition to manual elevation of presenting fetal part in cases of cord prolapse. *Arch Gynecol Obstet.* 2011;283: 989–991.

108. Hofmeyr GJ, Lawrie TA. Amnioinfusion for potential or suspected umbilical cord compression in labour. *Cochrane Database Syst Rev.* 2012;(1):CD000013.

109. Novikova N, Hofmeyr GJ, Essilfie-Appiah G. Prophylactic versus therapeutic amnioinfusion for oligohydramnios in labour. *Cochrane Database Syst Rev.* 2012;(9):CD000176.

110. Hofmeyr GJ, Xu H, Eke AC. Amnioinfusion for meconium-stained liquor in labour. *Cochrane Database Syst Rev.* 2014;(1): CD000014.

111. Dorairajan G, Soundararaghavan S. Maternal death after intrapartum saline amnioinfusion – report of two cases. *BJOG.* 2005;112:1331–1333.

112. Xu H, Hofmeyr J, Roy C, Fraser W. Intrapartum amnioinfusion for meconium-stained amniotic fluid: a systematic review of randomised controlled trials. *BJOG.* 2007;114:383–390.

9

Neonatal Assessment and Resuscitation

Susan W. Aucott, MD and Jamie D. Murphy, MD

The transition from intrauterine to extrauterine life represents the most important adjustment that a neonate will make. This transition occurs uneventfully after most deliveries and is dependent on the anatomic and physiologic condition of the infant, the ease or difficulty of the delivery, and the extrauterine environmental conditions. When the transition is unsuccessful, prompt assessment and supportive care must be initiated immediately.

At least one person skilled in neonatal resuscitation should be present at every delivery.[1,2] The resuscitation team may include personnel from the pediatric, anesthesiology, obstetric, respiratory therapy, and nursing services. The composition of the team varies among institutions, but there should be some form of 24-hour coverage in all hospitals that provide labor and delivery services.[1] A multidisciplinary team should participate in the process of ensuring that appropriate personnel and equipment are available for neonatal resuscitation.[1]

All personnel working in the delivery area should receive basic training in neonatal resuscitation to ensure prompt initiation of care before the arrival of the designated resuscitation team. The 2020 American Heart Association (AHA) Guidelines for Cardiopulmonary Resuscitation and Emergency Cardiovascular Care[2] reflect a review of scientific evidence by members of the American Academy of Pediatrics (AAP), the AHA, and the International Liaison Committee on Resuscitation. These guidelines have been incorporated into the Neonatal Resuscitation Program (NRP), which is the standardized training and certification program administered by the AAP. The NRP, originally sponsored by the AAP and

the AHA in 1987, is designed for use by all personnel who attend deliveries. To ensure the implementation of current guidelines for neonatal resuscitation, the AAP recommends that at least one NRP-certified practitioner attend every delivery.[1,3] The American Society of Anesthesiologists has emphasized that a single anesthesiologist should not be expected to assume responsibility for the concurrent care of both the mother and her child.[4] Rather, a second anesthesia provider or a qualified individual from another service should assume responsibility for the care of the neonate, except in an unforeseen emergency. Box 9.1 lists the qualifications of individuals delegated to perform neonatal resuscitation.

Although anesthesia providers are not usually the primary provider of neonatal resuscitation, they may be asked to assist in cases of difficult airway management or when the neonatal resuscitation team has not yet arrived. The anesthesia provider should be prepared to assist, provided that doing so does not compromise the care of the mother. Written hospital policies should identify the personnel responsible for neonatal resuscitation, and obstetric anesthesia providers should also maintain a high level of skill in neonatal resuscitation.

TRANSITION FROM INTRAUTERINE TO EXTRAUTERINE LIFE

Circulation

At birth, the circulatory system changes from a fetal circulation pattern, which is in parallel, through a transitional circulation, to an adult circulation pattern, which is in series (Fig. 9.1).[5] In the fetus, blood from the placenta travels through the umbilical vein and the ductus venosus to the inferior vena cava and the right side of the heart. The anatomic orientation of the inferior vena caval–right atrial junction favors shunting (i.e., streaming) of this well-oxygenated blood through the foramen ovale to the left side of the heart. The blood is then pumped through the ascending aorta, where branches that perfuse the upper part of the body (e.g., heart,

brain) exit proximal to the entrance of the ductus arteriosus.[6] Desaturated blood returns to the heart from the upper part of the body via the superior vena cava. The anatomic orientation of the superior vena caval–right atrial junction favors the streaming of blood into the right ventricle. Because fetal pulmonary vascular resistance is higher than systemic vascular resistance (SVR), approximately 90% of the right ventricular output passes through the ductus arteriosus and enters the aorta distal to the branches of the ascending aorta and aortic arch; therefore, blood that is less well-oxygenated perfuses the lower body, which has a lower oxygen consumption than the heart and brain. Deoxygenated blood from the fetus returns to the placental circulation via the umbilical arteries.

At the time of birth and during the subsequent period of circulatory transition, the amount of blood that shunts through the foramen ovale and ductus arteriosus diminishes, and flow becomes bidirectional. Clamping the umbilical cord (or exposing the umbilical cord to room air) results in increased SVR. Concurrently, expansion of the lungs and increased alveolar oxygen tension and pH result in decreased pulmonary vascular resistance and greater flow of pulmonary artery blood through the lungs.[7,8] Increased pulmonary artery blood flow results in improved oxygenation and higher left atrial pressure; the latter leads to a diminished shunt across the foramen ovale. Increased Po_2 and SVR and decreased pulmonary vascular resistance result in constriction of the

---

BOX 9.1 **Qualifications of Individuals Performing Neonatal Resuscitation**

- Ability to rapidly and accurately evaluate newborn condition
- Ability and authority to seek additional personnel and experts to assist with resuscitation
- Knowledge of risk factors predisposing to need for resuscitation
- Skills in airway management, chest compression, emergency administration of drugs and fluids, establishment of umbilical vein or intraosseous needle access, and maintenance of thermal stability

Modified from American Academy of Pediatrics, American College of Obstetricians and Gynecologists. Chapter 10: Care of the newborn. In: *Guidelines for Perinatal Care*. 8th ed. American Academy of Pediatrics; 2017:347–408.

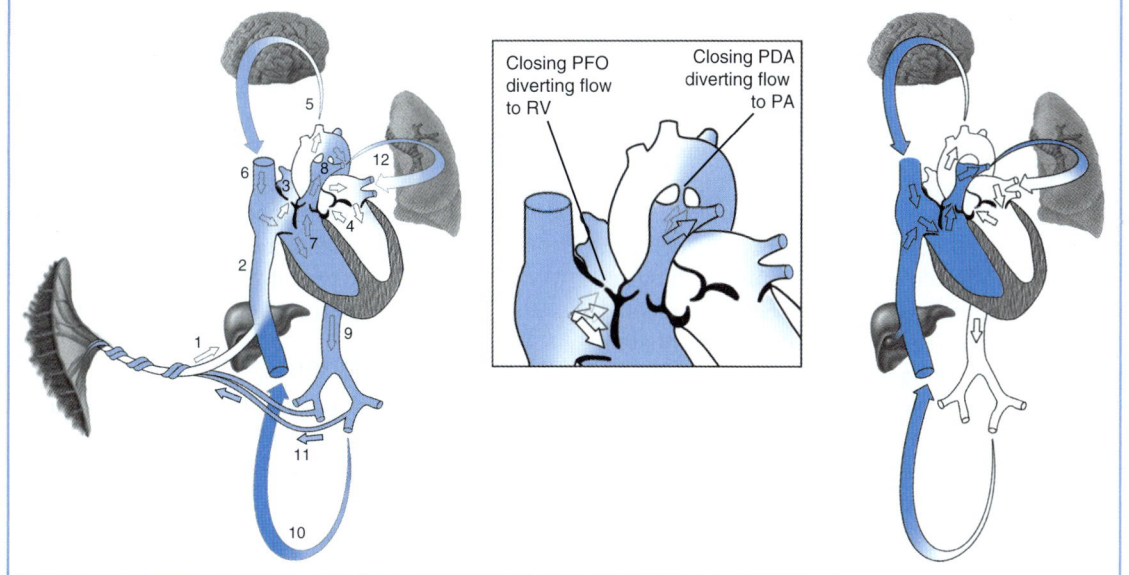

Fig. 9.1 Modification of Blood Flow Patterns From the Fetal *(Left)*, via the Transitional *(Center)*, to the Neonatal *(Right)* Circulation. In the fetal circulation, oxygenated blood *(white)* from the placenta travels through the umbilical vein *(1)* into the ductus venosus and the inferior vena cava *(2)*. The majority of oxygenated blood passes through the patent foramen ovale (PFO) from the right atrium to the left atrium *(3)* and ventricle *(4)*, and distributes this blood to the brain *(5)*. The deoxygenated blood *(blue)* from the brain and upper extremities enters the superior vena cava, mixing with a small portion of the oxygenated blood in the right atrium, before entering the right ventricle (RV, *7*). The mostly deoxygenated blood is transported into the pulmonary artery, where the majority is diverted through the patent ductus arteriosus (PDA, *8*) into the descending aorta *(9)*, thereby bypassing the lungs. Some blood enters the lower body *(10)*, but the majority returns to the placenta via the umbilical arteries *(11)*. A small amount of blood from the pulmonary artery enters the lungs *(12)*. During the transitional circulation, which occurs over a few days, the PFO closes, diverting blood from the right atrium to the right ventricle. Closure of the PDA diverts deoxygenated blood through the pulmonary arteries to the lungs. The neonatal circulation separates the oxygenated and deoxygenated blood flow pathways. Illustration by Naveen Nathan, MD, NorthShore University HealthSystem, University of Chicago Pritzker School of Medicine, Evanston, IL.

ductus arteriosus.[9,10] Together, these changes in vascular resistance result in functional closure of the foramen ovale and the ductus arteriosus. This process does not occur instantaneously, and arterial oxygen saturation (Sao_2) remains higher in the right upper extremity (which is preductal) than in the left upper extremity and the lower extremities until blood flow through the ductus arteriosus is minimal.[11] Differences in Sao_2 are usually minimal by 10 minutes and absent by 24 hours after birth. Provided there is no interference with the normal drop in pulmonary vascular resistance, both the foramen ovale and the ductus arteriosus close functionally as the infant transitions to an adult circulation.

Persistent pulmonary hypertension of the newborn (previously referred to as persistent fetal circulation) occurs when the pulmonary vascular resistance remains elevated after the time of birth. Factors that may exacerbate this problem include hypoxia, acidosis, hypovolemia, and hypothermia.[8,12] Maternal use of nonsteroidal antiinflammatory drugs may cause premature constriction of the ductus arteriosus in the fetus and thus predispose to persistent pulmonary hypertension of the newborn.[13]

Respiration

Fetal breathing movements have been observed *in utero* as early as 11 weeks' gestation. These movements increase with advancing gestational age but undergo a marked reduction within days of the onset of labor. They are stimulated by hypercapnia and maternal smoking and are inhibited by hypoxia and central nervous system (CNS) depressants (e.g., barbiturates). Under normal conditions, this fetal breathing activity results only in the movement of pulmonary dead space.[14]

The fetal lung contains a liquid composed of an ultrafiltrate of plasma, which is secreted by the lungs *in utero*[15]; the volume of this lung liquid is approximately 30 mL/kg. Partial reabsorption of this liquid occurs during labor and delivery, and approximately two-thirds is expelled from the lungs of the term neonate by the time of delivery.[16] Preterm infants and infants requiring cesarean delivery without labor may have a greater amount of residual lung liquid after delivery owing to a reduced catecholamine surge at delivery. This residual lung liquid leads to difficulty in the initiation and maintenance of normal breathing patterns and is the presumed cause of **transient tachypnea of the newborn (TTN)**.[17]

The first breath occurs approximately 9 seconds after delivery. Air enters the lungs as soon as the intrathoracic pressure begins to decrease. This air movement during the first breath is important because it establishes the neonate's functional residual capacity (Fig. 9.2).

Lung inflation is a major physiologic stimulus for the release of lung surfactant into the alveoli.[18] Surfactant, which is necessary for normal breathing, is present within the alveolar lining cells by 20 weeks' gestation[19] and within the lumen of the airways by 28 to 32 weeks' gestation. However, significant amounts of surfactant do not appear in terminal airways until 34 to 38 weeks' gestation unless its production has

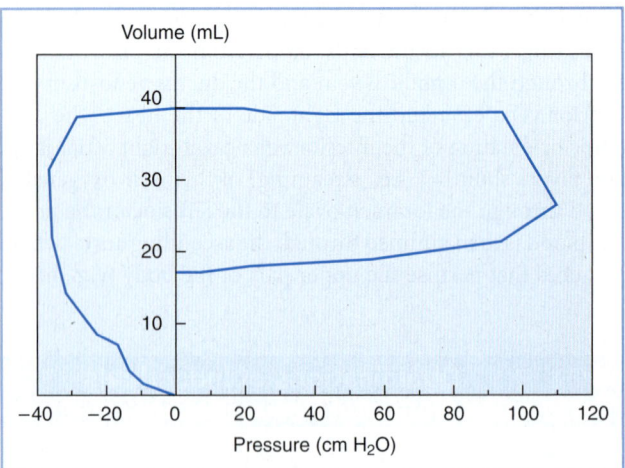

Fig. 9.2 Typical Pressure-Volume Loop of the Neonate's First Breath. The intrathoracic pressure decreases to −30 to −40 cm H_2O, drawing air into the lungs. The expiratory pressure is much greater than the inspiratory pressure. Modified from Milner AD, Vyas H. Lung expansion at birth. *J Pediatr.* 1982;101:879–886.

been stimulated by chronic stress or maternal corticosteroid administration.[20] Stress during labor and delivery can lead to the passage of meconium into the amniotic fluid and gasping efforts by the fetus, which may result in the aspiration of amniotic fluid into the lungs.[21]

Catecholamines

Transition to extrauterine life is associated with a catecholamine surge. In chronically catheterized sheep, catecholamine levels begin to rise a few hours before delivery and may be higher at the time of delivery than at any other time during life.[22] Catecholamines have an important role in the following areas: (1) the production and release of surfactant, (2) the transition to active sodium transport for absorption of lung fluid, (3) the mediation of preferential blood flow to vital organs during the period of stress that occurs during every delivery, and (4) thermoregulation of the neonate.

Thermal Regulation

Thermal stress challenges the neonate in the extrauterine environment. Neonates raise their metabolic rate and release norepinephrine in response to cold; this response facilitates the oxidation of brown fat, which contains numerous mitochondria. The oxidation results in **nonshivering thermogenesis**, the major mechanism for neonatal heat regulation.[23] This process may lead to significant oxygen consumption, especially if the neonate has not been dried and placed in an appropriate thermoneutral environment, for example, under a radiant warmer. Thermal stress is an even greater problem in infants with low fat stores, such as preterm infants or infants who are small for gestational age. An alternative method to eliminate heat loss from evaporation is to provide an occlusive wrap rather than drying the infant. For infants born at less than 28 weeks' gestation, the use of polythene wraps or bags is recommended to minimize heat loss.[24,25] For extreme preterm infants, increasing the ambient room temperature from 20°C to 23°C may minimize the risk for hypothermia.[26] The maintenance of a neutral thermal environment (i.e., 34°C to 35°C) is recommended.

In the neonate with a perinatal brain injury, however, mild hypothermia therapy through selective head or whole-body cooling is initiated in the first 6 hours of life and may be neuro-protective in the setting of hypoxia-ischemia.[27] Hyperthermia may worsen neurologic outcomes and should be avoided.[3,28] Hypothermia therapy, via selective head cooling or whole-body hypothermia, is usually continued for several days after initiation. Consequently, if an infant is delivered at a center where hypothermia therapy is unavailable, passive cooling can be initiated by turning the radiant warmer off while awaiting infant transfer.

Administration of neuraxial analgesia during labor is associated with an increase in maternal and fetal temperature, which might result in an increase in the frequency of neonatal sepsis evaluations (see Chapter 24).[29] However, a number of variables (e.g., preeclampsia/hypertension, gestational age, birth weight, meconium aspiration, respiratory distress at birth, hypothermia at birth, and group B beta-hemolytic streptococcal colonization of the maternal birth canal) have been observed to be strong predictors of neonatal sepsis evaluations, whereas maternal fever and epidural analgesia have not.[30] Confounding variables may influence the findings of these types of association studies; patients who choose either to receive or not receive neuraxial analgesia are inherently different. The incidence of actual neonatal sepsis is not different in term infants whose mothers either do or do not receive neuraxial analgesia.

In infants not requiring immediate resuscitation, providing skin-to-skin contact with the mother can allow for appropriate thermal regulation, enhance breastfeeding, and reduce maternal stress. This practice must be associated with close monitoring to prevent the infant from slipping off the mother and to detect **sudden unexpected postnatal collapse** (SUPC). Although rare, SUPC can be a fatal event in an otherwise healthy-appearing infant; prevention requires adequate personnel for observation, monitoring, and treatment.[31]

ANTEPARTUM AND INTRAPARTUM ASSESSMENT

Approximately 10% of neonates require some level of resuscitation.[3] The need for resuscitation can be predicted before labor and delivery with approximately 80% accuracy based on the presence of antepartum risk factors (Box 9.2).

Preterm delivery increases the likelihood that the neonate will require resuscitation. When a mother is admitted with either preterm labor or premature rupture of membranes, plans should be made for neonatal care in the event of delivery. The antenatal assessment of gestational age is based on the presumed date of the last menstrual period, the fundal height, and ultrasonographic measurements of the fetus. Unfortunately, it may be difficult to assess

---

BOX 9.2 Risk Factors Suggesting a Greater Need for Neonatal Resuscitation

Antepartum Risk Factors
- Maternal diabetes
- Hypertensive disorder of pregnancy
- Chronic hypertension
- Fetal anemia or isoimmunization
- Previous fetal or neonatal death
- Bleeding in second or third trimester
- Maternal infection
- Maternal cardiac, pulmonary, renal, thyroid, or neurologic disease
- Polyhydramnios
- Oligohydramnios
- Premature rupture of membranes
- Fetal hydrops
- Postterm gestation
- Multiple gestation
- Discrepancy between fetal size and dates (i.e., last menstrual period)
- Drug therapy (e.g., lithium carbonate, magnesium, adrenergic-blocking drugs)
- Maternal substance abuse
- Fetal malformation
- Diminished fetal activity
- No prenatal care
- Maternal age > 35 y

Intrapartum Risk Factors
- Emergency cesarean delivery
- Forceps or vacuum-assisted delivery
- Breech or other abnormal presentation
- Preterm labor
- Precipitous labor
- Chorioamnionitis
- Prolonged rupture of membranes (>18 h before delivery)
- Prolonged labor (>24 h)
- Macrosomia
- Category II or III fetal heart rate patterns
- Use of general anesthesia
- Uterine tachysystole with fetal heart rate changes
- Maternal administration of opioids within 4 h of delivery
- Meconium-stained amniotic fluid
- Prolapsed umbilical cord
- Placental abruption
- Placenta previa
- Significant intrapartum bleeding

Modified from *Textbook of Neonatal Resuscitation*. 8th ed. American Academy of Pediatrics and American Heart Association; 2021.

---

gestational age accurately because menstrual dates may be unknown or incorrect, the fundal height may be affected by abnormalities of fetal growth or amniotic fluid volume, and ultrasonographic assessment of fetal age is less precise after mid-pregnancy. The assessment of gestational age is most accurate in patients who receive prenatal care in early pregnancy; accurate knowledge of the gestational age enables the healthcare team to plan for the neonatal needs and to appropriately counsel the parents regarding neonatal morbidity and mortality. These plans and expectations must be formulated with caution and flexibility because the antenatal assessment may not accurately predict neonatal size, maturity, and/or condition at delivery.

A variety of **intrauterine insults** can impair the fetal transition to extrauterine life. For example, neonatal depression at birth can result from acute or chronic uteroplacental insufficiency or acute umbilical cord compression. Chronic uteroplacental insufficiency, regardless of its etiology, may result in fetal growth restriction. Fetal hemorrhage, viral or bacterial infection, meconium aspiration, and exposure to opioids or other CNS depressants also can result in neonatal depression. Although randomized trials have not confirmed that fetal heart rate (FHR) monitoring improves neonatal outcome, a nonreassuring FHR tracing is considered a predictor of the need for neonatal resuscitation (see Chapter 8).[32]

Infants with **congenital anomalies** (e.g., tracheoesophageal fistula, diaphragmatic hernia, CNS, and cardiac malformations) may need resuscitation and cardiorespiratory support. Ultrasonography allows for the antenatal diagnosis of many congenital anomalies and other fetal abnormalities (e.g., nonimmune hydrops). Obstetricians should communicate knowledge or suspicions regarding these entities to those who will provide care for the neonate in the delivery room to allow the resuscitation team to make specific resuscitation plans.

In the past, infants born by either elective or emergency cesarean delivery were considered more likely to require resuscitation than infants delivered vaginally. Evidence suggests that repeat cesarean deliveries and those performed for dystocia in patients without FHR abnormalities result in the delivery of infants at low risk for neonatal resuscitation, especially when the cesarean deliveries are performed with neuraxial anesthesia.[33–35] Infants delivered by elective repeat cesarean delivery are at higher risk for subsequent respiratory problems (e.g., TTN) than infants born vaginally. Infants born by cesarean delivery after a failed trial of labor are at a higher risk for neonatal sepsis than similar infants born vaginally.[36] Emergency cesarean delivery is a risk factor for the need for neonatal resuscitation.

NEONATAL ASSESSMENT

Apgar Score

Resuscitative efforts typically precede the performance of a thorough physical examination of the neonate. Because NRP instructions require simultaneous assessment and treatment, it is important that the neonatal assessment be both simple and sensitive. In 1953, Virginia Apgar, an anesthesiologist, described a simple method for neonatal assessment that could be performed while care was being delivered.[37] She suggested that this standardized and relatively objective scoring system would differentiate between infants who require resuscitation and those who need only routine care.[38]

The Apgar score is based on five parameters that are assessed at 1 and 5 minutes after birth. Further scoring at 5- or 10-minute intervals may be done if initial scores are low. The parameters are heart rate, respiratory effort, muscle tone, reflex irritability, and color. A score of 0, 1, or 2 is assigned for each of these five entities (Table 9.1). A total score of 8 to 10 is normal, a score of 4 to 7 indicates moderate impairment, and a score of 0 to 3 signals the need for immediate resuscitation. Dr. Apgar emphasized that this system does not replace a complete physical examination and serial observations of the neonate for several hours after birth.[39]

The Apgar score is widely used to assess neonates, although its value has been questioned. The scoring system may help predict mortality and neurologic morbidity in *populations* of infants, but Dr. Apgar cautioned against the use of the Apgar score to make these predictions in an *individual* infant. She noted that the risk for neonatal mortality was inversely proportional to the 1-minute score.[39] In addition, the 1-minute Apgar score was a better predictor of mortality within the first 2 days of life than within 2 to 28 days of life.

Several studies have challenged the notion that a low Apgar score signals perinatal asphyxia. In a prospective study of 1210 deliveries, Sykes et al.[40] noted a poor correlation between the Apgar score and the umbilical cord blood pH. Other studies, including those of low-birth-weight infants, have found that a low Apgar score is a poor predictor of neonatal acidosis, although a high score is reasonably specific for excluding the presence of severe acidosis.[41–47] By contrast,

TABLE 9.1	**Apgar Scoring System**			
		SCORE		
Parameter	**0**	**1**		**2**
Heart rate (bpm)	Absent	<100		>100
Respiratory effort	Absent	Irregular, slow, shallow, or gasping respirations		Robust, crying
Muscle tone	Absent, limp	Some flexion of extremities		Active movement
Reflex irritability (nasal catheter, oropharyngeal suctioning)	No response	Grimace		Active coughing and sneezing
Color	Cyanotic	Acrocyanotic (trunk pink, extremities blue)		Pink

the fetal biophysical profile has a good correlation with the acid-base status of the fetus and the neonate (see Chapter 6).[48] The biophysical profile includes the performance of a nonstress test and ultrasonographic assessment of fetal tone, fetal movement, fetal breathing movements, and amniotic fluid volume.

Additional studies have suggested that Apgar scores are poor predictors of long-term neurologic impairment.[49–51] The Apgar score is more likely to predict a poor neurologic outcome when the score remains 3 or less at 10, 15, and 20 minutes. However, when a child has cerebral palsy, low Apgar scores alone are not adequate evidence that perinatal hypoxia was responsible for the neurologic injury.[52]

The American College of Obstetricians and Gynecologists (ACOG) and AAP Task Force on Neonatal Encephalopathy recommend a comprehensive multidimensional assessment be performed of neonatal status and all potential contributing factors (maternal history, obstetric antecedents, intrapartum factors, placental pathology) to assess the likelihood that an acute peripartum or intrapartum event was sufficient to cause neonatal encephalopathy.[52] An Apgar score of less than 5 at 5 minutes and 10 minutes of age confers an increased risk of cerebral palsy, but most infants with low Apgar scores will not develop cerebral palsy.[52] If the 5-minute Apgar score is greater than or equal to 7, it is unlikely that peripartum hypoxia-ischemia caused the neonatal encephalopathy.[52]

In summary, the Apgar scoring system is used throughout the world; it is a convenient method for assessing the status of the neonate immediately after birth as well as the infant's response to resuscitation.[51] Low Apgar scores alone do not predict individual neonatal mortality or neurologic outcome; rather, Apgar scores can be low for a variety of reasons. Preterm delivery, congenital anomalies, neuromuscular diseases, antenatal drug exposure, manipulation at delivery, and subjectivity and error may influence the Apgar score.[51]

Umbilical Cord Blood Gas and pH Analysis

Umbilical cord blood gas and pH measurements reflect the fetal condition immediately before delivery and can be obtained routinely after delivery or measured only in cases of neonatal depression. These measurements may be a more objective indication of a neonate's condition than the Apgar score. However, because of the delay between obtaining the samples and reporting the results, decisions must be made based on clinical assessment until the results are available. The ACOG and AAP have recommended that cord blood gas measurements be obtained in cases for which fetal metabolic status is in question.[52]

The fetus produces carbonic acid (from oxidative metabolism) and lactic and beta-hydroxybutyric acids (primarily from anaerobic metabolism). Carbonic acid, which is often called *respiratory acid*, is cleared rapidly by the placenta as carbon dioxide when placental blood flow is normal. However, metabolic clearance of lactic and beta-hydroxybutyric acids requires hours; thus, these acids are called *metabolic* or *fixed*

acids. In the fetus, metabolic acidemia is more ominous than respiratory acidemia because the former reflects a significant amount of anaerobic metabolism.

The measured components of umbilical cord blood gas analysis are pH, Pco_2, Po_2, and bicarbonate (HCO_3^-). HCO_3^- is a major buffer in fetal blood. The measure of change in the buffering capacity of umbilical cord blood is reflected in the delta base, which is also known as the base excess or deficit; this value can be calculated from the pH, Pco_2, and HCO_3^-. Ideally, blood samples from both the umbilical artery and vein are collected. Umbilical artery blood gas measurements represent the fetal condition, whereas umbilical vein measurements reflect the maternal condition and uteroplacental gas exchange. Unfortunately, it may be difficult to obtain blood from the umbilical artery, especially when it is small, as it is in very low-birth-weight (VLBW) infants. Caution should be used in the interpretation of an isolated umbilical venous blood pH measurement, which can be normal despite the presence of arterial acidemia.

Proper blood sampling and handling are necessary. The measurements should be accurate, provided that (1) the umbilical cord is double-clamped immediately after delivery; (2) the samples are drawn within 20 minutes of delivery into a syringe containing the proper amount of heparin; and (3) the samples are analyzed within 20 minutes.[53,54] If the delay is longer than 20 minutes, the sample should be placed on ice. The base deficit and lactate values increase with longer delays and, thus, should be interpreted with caution.[52] The Po_2 measurement is more accurate if residual air bubbles are removed from the syringe.

Historically, a normal umbilical cord blood pH measurement was believed to be 7.2 or higher. However, investigators have challenged the validity of this number, given the lack of distinction between umbilical arterial and venous blood despite clear differences in their normal measurements.[55] There is no global consensus on the definition of acidemia.[56] One study noted that the median umbilical arterial blood pH in vigorous infants (those with 5-minute Apgar scores of ≥ 7) was 7.26, with a measurement of 7.10 representing the 2.5th percentile.[57] The statistical lower limit of umbilical artery pH is approximately 7.10 (mean minus two standard deviations).[56] A number of factors may also influence the umbilical arterial blood pH measurement. A fetus subjected to the stress of labor has a lower pH than one born by cesarean delivery without labor.[58] Offspring of nulliparous women tend to have a lower pH than offspring of parous women, a difference that is likely related to a difference in the duration of labor.[59] Other factors influencing fetal acid-base status include the maternal condition, temperature, gestational age, fetal body mass, and infection.[56] Delayed umbilical cord clamping is associated with lower pH and higher Pco_2, base deficit, and lactate because acidic metabolites, which have accumulated in peripheral tissue during labor, are washed into the central circulation as the infant begins to cry and move after delivery.[56]

Fetal arterial pH and Po_2 decrease and Pco_2 increases with gestational age, but base deficit values do not change.[52,56]

Preterm infants often have low Apgar scores despite the presence of normal umbilical cord blood gas and pH measurements; therefore, the assessment of umbilical cord blood may be especially helpful in the evaluation of preterm neonates whose low tone or poor respiratory effort may be related to gestational age alone.

Physicians should use strict definitions when interpreting umbilical cord blood gas and pH measurements. Terms such as *birth asphyxia* should be avoided in most cases.[52] *Acidemia* refers to an increase in the hydrogen ion concentration in the blood. *Acidosis* occurs when there is an increased hydrogen ion concentration in tissue. *Asphyxia* is a clinical situation that involves hypoxia (i.e., a decreased level of oxygen in tissue), damaging acidemia, and metabolic acidosis.

When acidemia is present, the type—respiratory, metabolic, or mixed—must be identified (Table 9.2).[60] Metabolic acidemia is more likely to be associated with acidosis than respiratory acidemia and is clinically more significant. Similarly, mixed acidemia with a high P_{CO_2}, an extremely low HCO_3^-, and a high base deficit is more ominous than a mixed acidemia with a high P_{CO_2} but only a slightly reduced HCO_3^- and a low base deficit. Mixed or metabolic acidemia (but not respiratory acidemia) is associated with an increased incidence of neonatal complications and death.[59]

In their study of 3506 term neonates, Goldaber et al.[61] noted that an umbilical arterial blood pH measurement < 7.00 was associated with a significantly higher incidence of neonatal death. All neonatal seizures in their study occurred in infants with an umbilical arterial blood pH < 7.05. By contrast, a short-term outcome study failed to show a good correlation between arterial blood pH and the subsequent health of an infant.[47] In the large study reported by Casey et al.,[62] umbilical arterial blood pH of ≤ 7.0 was a poorer predictor of the relative risk for neonatal death during the first 28 days of life than a 5-minute Apgar score of ≤ 3. However, 6264 infants were excluded from their study because umbilical arterial blood gas measurements could not be obtained and these infants had a higher incidence of neonatal death than those for whom blood gas measurements were obtained. In a separate review of 51,519 term deliveries, Yeh et al.[63] found an increased risk for adverse outcomes in infants with a pH < 7.10, with the lowest risk in infants with a pH between 7.26 and 7.30; however, 75% of infants with neurologic morbidity had a normal pH. Thus, it is important to remember that neonates may suffer multiorgan system damage, including neurologic injury, even in the absence of low pH and Apgar scores.

According to the ACOG/APP Task Force, an umbilical arterial blood pH < 7.0 and a base deficit ≥ 12 mmol/L at delivery are considered one part of the definition of an acute intrapartum hypoxic event sufficient to cause cerebral palsy.[52] The base deficit and bicarbonate (the metabolic component) values are the most significant factors associated with morbidity in neonates with an umbilical arterial blood pH < 7.0. Twenty-three percent of infants with an umbilical arterial base deficit of 12 to 16 mmol/L have moderate to severe

TABLE 9.2   Criteria Used to Define Types of Acidemia in Neonates With an Umbilical Arterial pH Measurement < 7.20

Classification	P_{CO_2}[a]	Base Deficit (mmol/L)
Respiratory	Elevated	<12
Metabolic	Normal	≥12
Mixed	Elevated	≥12

[a]Normal umbilical artery P_{CO_2} 45–55 mm Hg, normal umbilical vein P_{CO_2} 35–45 mm Hg.
Modified from Cahill AG. Intrapartum fetal evaluation. In: *Gabbe's Obstetrics: Normal and Problem Pregnancies*, 8th ed. Elsevier; 2021:267–294.

complications, which increases to 37% when the deficit is greater than 16 mmol/L.[52]

Abnormal FHR patterns and umbilical cord blood gas measurements are not consistently correlated with poor neonatal outcomes.[64] In a longitudinal study that evaluated outcomes at 6.5 years of age, Hafstrom et al.[65] found that infants with an umbilical arterial blood pH < 7.05 but a normal examination at birth had outcomes that did not differ from those for matched infants with a normal umbilical arterial blood pH.

As Virginia Apgar emphasized in 1962, the most important components of neonatal assessment are a careful physical examination and continued observation for several hours.[39] Additional information can be gained from the antenatal history, Apgar scores, and umbilical cord blood gas and pH measurements, provided that clinicians are aware of the proper methods of interpretation as well as the limitations of these methods of assessment.

Respiration and Circulation

There are some similarities between the initial assessment of the neonate and the initial assessment of an adult who requires resuscitation. In both situations, the physician should give immediate attention to the ABCs of resuscitation (i.e., airway, breathing, circulation).

The normal neonatal respiratory rate is between 30 and 60 breaths per minute. Breathing should begin by 30 seconds and be regular by 90 seconds of age. Failure of the neonate to breathe by 90 seconds of age represents either primary or secondary apnea. During *primary apnea*, but not secondary apnea, tactile stimulation can initiate breathing efforts. In addition, although heart rate may be low with both periods of apnea, a reduction in blood pressure occurs only during secondary apnea. Therefore, during evaluation of the apneic neonate, aggressive resuscitation must be initiated promptly if tactile stimulation does not result in the initiation of spontaneous breathing.

Assessment of the adequacy of respiratory function requires comprehensive observation for signs of neonatal respiratory distress. These signs include cyanosis, grunting,

TABLE 9.3	Targeted Preductal Spo_2 After Birth
Time After Birth (min)	**Spo_2 Target (%)**
1	60–65
2	65–70
3	70–75
4	75–80
5	80–85
10	85–95

From Aziz K, Lee HC, Escobedo MB, et al. Part 5: Neonatal resuscitation: 2020 American Heart Association guidelines for cardiopulmonary resuscitation and emergency cardiovascular care. *Circulation.* 2020;142(16_suppl_2):S524–S550.

flaring of the nares, retracting chest motions, and unequal breath sounds. The adequacy of respiratory function can also be assessed by the estimation of Sao_2. Pulse oximetry provides accurate estimates of Sao_2 during periods of stability but may overestimate values during rapid desaturation.[66] In addition, the Sao_2 (Spo_2) measurements may fluctuate in the delivery room as a result of the ongoing transition from the fetal to the neonatal circulation, and it may take more than 10 minutes to achieve a preductal Sao_2 > 95% in a healthy term infant. Targeted preductal Spo_2 values are shown in Table 9.3. Supplemental oxygen may be administered, titrated to achieve the normal range for healthy term infants after vaginal delivery.[3]

Pulse oximetry is recommended when resuscitation is anticipated, when positive pressure ventilation or supplemental oxygen is administered, or when central cyanosis persists beyond 5 to 10 minutes of life.[3] The pulse oximeter sensor should be applied to the neonate's right upper extremity, which receives preductal blood flow (see earlier discussion); because CNS blood flow is also preductal, right upper extremity Sao_2 measurements provide a more accurate assessment of CNS oxygenation.[11] Sensor placement can be difficult on skin that is wet and covered with vernix caseosa; therefore, it may be easier to place the sensor over the right radial artery, especially in preterm infants.[67]

Neonatal arterial blood sampling is technically difficult and thus rarely obtained in the delivery room. Cannulation of the umbilical artery is useful in infants who will require frequent blood sampling. This procedure often requires the use of microinstruments (especially in preterm and VLBW infants) and the ability to monitor the infant when obscured from view by surgical drapes; therefore, this procedure is usually performed in the neonatal intensive care unit (NICU).

The normal neonatal heart rate may be greater than 160 beats per minute (bpm) in the very early preterm neonate, but it should be within the range of 120 to 160 bpm by 28 weeks' gestational age. Clinical determination of the heart rate can be done by lightly grasping the base of the umbilical cord to feel the arterial pulsations or by listening to the apical heartbeat. These methods have been found to be less reliable than electrocardiography (ECG).[68] Additionally, several studies have found the ECG to be more accurate than pulse oximetry and is now recommended by the NRP for infants requiring resuscitation.[3]

Measurement of arterial blood pressure is not a priority during the initial assessment and resuscitation of the neonate.[3] However, observation for signs of abnormal circulatory function is considered essential. These signs include cyanosis, pallor, mottled coloring, prolonged capillary refill time, and weakness or absence of pulses in the extremities. One of the causes of abnormal circulatory function is hypovolemia, which should be anticipated in cases of bleeding from the umbilical cord or the fetal side of the placenta or whenever a neonate does not respond appropriately to resuscitation. The hypovolemic neonate may exhibit signs of abnormal circulatory function as well as tachycardia and tachypnea (neonatal hypovolemia usually does not accompany placental abruption, which may cause maternal bleeding, or other conditions associated with fetal asphyxia).

Neurologic Status

The initial neonatal neurologic assessment requires only simple observation. The neonate should demonstrate evidence of vigorous activity, including crying and active flexion of the extremities. Signs of possible neurologic abnormalities include apnea, seizures, hypotonia, and unresponsiveness. Neonates should be assessed for physical signs of hypoxic-ischemic encephalopathy. The modified Sarnat tool distinguishes three stages of encephalopathy based on physical signs and symptoms.[69] The stages of hypoxic-ischemic encephalopathy are associated with different outcomes: stage I, good; stage II, moderate; and stage III, poor.[69] Although detailed neurologic assessment, including head imaging, is performed after the neonate is transferred to the NICU, assessment of tone, baseline heart rate, respirations, and reflex activity is part of both the Apgar scoring system and the assessment for hypoxic-ischemic encephalopathy and is made initially in the delivery room.

Gestational Age

When assessing a very small neonate whose gestational age appears to be lower than that of viability, the evaluator must consider whether it is appropriate to initiate and maintain resuscitation efforts. The most accurate method of estimating gestational age combines consideration of the last menstrual period and early fetal ultrasound as well as physical and neurologic characteristics of the newborn. The neonatal gestational age is often assessed with the use of the scoring systems described initially by Dubowitz et al.[70] and subsequently modified by Ballard et al.,[71] using physical and neurologic criteria.

The Ballard score is most accurate when used to estimate gestational age at 30 to 42 hours, rather than during the first several minutes after birth, and is less accurate in very small preterm infants.[72,73]

Another commonly used criterion for the estimation of gestational age is birth weight. Normal values for birth weight are published and readily available. Although birth weight may help physicians estimate the gestational age of an otherwise healthy preterm infant, physicians cannot rely on birth weight to provide an accurate estimate of gestational age in an infant who suffered from fetal growth restriction or who is large for gestational age.

Because of the potential for inaccurate gestational age estimation in the delivery room, it is best not to use scoring systems to guide decisions regarding the initiation or continuation of neonatal resuscitation immediately after delivery. In most circumstances, the neonate's response to resuscitative efforts is the best indicator as to whether further intervention is warranted.

NEONATAL RESUSCITATION

The equipment and medications needed for neonatal resuscitation are listed in Box 9.3. Equipment, supplies, and medications should be checked regularly to ensure that all components are available and functional.[2]

Although previously published guidelines recommended suctioning of the mouth and nose after delivery of the head, current guidelines do *not* recommend routine intrapartum oropharyngeal and nasopharyngeal suctioning for infants born with either clear or meconium-stained amniotic fluid to avoid inducing bradycardia.[2,3]

Timing of cord clamping may vary by the gestational age and vigor of the infant. Current evidence supports a delay in cord clamping for more than 30 seconds after the delivery of term and late preterm infants (≥34 weeks' gestation) not requiring resuscitation.[2,74] In preterm infants, delayed cord clamping is associated with improved blood pressure and a lower incidence of intraventricular hemorrhage (IVH)[75]; no alterations in Apgar scores or need for delivery room resuscitation have been observed with this practice.[76] In nonvigorous term and late preterm infants, intact cord milking may be reasonable compared with early cord clamping (<30 seconds); however, cord milking is not recommended

---

BOX 9.3   Equipment and Drugs Needed for Neonatal Resuscitation

Suction Equipment
- Bulb syringe
- Mechanical suction and tubing
- Suction catheters: 5 F or 6 F, 8 F, and 10 F or 12 F
- 8-F feeding tube and 20-mL syringe
- Meconium aspiration device

Bag-and-Mask Equipment
- Neonatal resuscitation bag with a pressure-release valve or pressure manometer and valve to deliver positive end-expiratory pressure (the bag must be capable of delivering 90% to 100% oxygen) or a pressure-limiting T-piece resuscitator
- Face masks, term and preterm newborn sizes (masks with cushioned rim preferred)
- Supraglottic airway devices, term and preterm newborn sizes
- Air source with tubing
- Oxygen with flowmeter (flow rate up to 10 L/min) and tubing (including portable oxygen cylinders)
- Blender to mix air and oxygen to adjust oxygen delivery

Intubation Equipment
- Laryngoscope with straight blades: sizes 0 (preterm) and 1 (term)
- Extra bulbs and batteries for laryngoscope
- Tracheal tubes: 2.5, 3.0, 3.5, and 4.0 mm ID
- Stylet (optional)
- Scissors
- Tape or securing device for tracheal tube
- Alcohol sponges
- CO_2 detector (optional)
- Supraglottic airway (optional)

Medications
- Epinephrine 1:10,000 (0.1 mg/mL), 3- or 10-mL ampules
- Isotonic crystalloid (normal saline or lactated Ringer's solution) for volume expansion, 100 or 250 mL
- Sodium bicarbonate 4.2% (5 mEq/10 mL), 10-mL ampules
- Normal saline, 30 mL
- Dextrose 10%, 250 mL
- Normal saline "fish" or "bullet" (optional)
- Feeding tube: 5 F (optional)
- Umbilical vessel catheterization supplies:
  - Sterile gloves
  - Scalpel or scissors
  - Povidone-iodine solution
  - Umbilical tape
  - Umbilical catheters: 3.5 F, 5 F
  - Three-way stopcock
- Syringes: 1, 3, 5, 10, 20, and 50 mL
- Needles: 25-, 21-, and 18-gauge, or puncture device for needleless system

Miscellaneous
- Gloves and appropriate personal protection
- Radiant warmer or other heat source
- Firm, padded resuscitation surface
- Clock (timer optional)
- Warmed linens
- Stethoscope
- Tape: ½ or ¾ inch (1.25 or 1.9 cm)
- Cardiac monitor and electrodes and/or pulse oximeter with probe
- Oropharyngeal airways
- Polythene wrap or bags (for infants < 28 weeks' gestation)

ID, Internal diameter.
Modified from *Textbook of Neonatal Resuscitation*. 8th ed. American Academy of Pediatrics and American Heart Association; 2021.

for preterm infants less than 28 weeks' gestation age. Research is ongoing to determine the benefit of initiating resuscitation with an intact cord to promote improved venous return during initial breaths.[77,78]

Healthy, term neonates should be placed skin to skin with their mothers after an uneventful vaginal delivery.[2] After cesarean delivery, or after a vaginal delivery in which the need for resuscitation is anticipated, the neonate is transferred to the resuscitation area. The availability of sterile blankets allows the individual performing the delivery to remain sterile while transferring the infant; this issue is especially important during cesarean deliveries. The timing of delivery should be noted, assessment and appropriate resuscitative measures should be continued, and Apgar scores should be assigned at the appropriate intervals (Fig. 9.3).

Maintaining normal temperature during stabilization for nonasphyxiated infants is essential. The physician or nurse should place the infant beneath an overhead radiant warmer and promptly dry the skin of infants delivered at greater than 28 weeks' gestation. The infant who is delivered preterm at less than 28 weeks' gestation should be placed in a polythene bag or wrapping to prevent heat loss.[24,25] Additional methods to prevent hypothermia include increasing the room temperature, using a thermal mattress, and warm, humidified gases. Hypothermia can result in increased oxygen consumption and metabolic acidosis[79] and is associated with a significantly higher mortality rate among preterm infants.[3]

Selective cerebral hypothermia[80] or whole-body hypothermia[81,82] may protect against brain injury in the asphyxiated infant. The use of intentional hypothermia therapy requires an Neonatal Intensive Care Unit with defined protocols and multidisciplinary support. When assessing an infant for hypothermia therapy, the radiant warmer can be turned off to allow passive cooling. If the criteria for hypothermia therapy are not met on further assessment, the infant can be warmed slowly. Hyperthermia (>38.0°C) should be avoided in all infants.[2]

The neonate should be positioned in a way that allows the airway to remain open, with the head in the "sniffing" position (the neck flexed on the chest and the head extended on the neck, thereby aligning the oropharynx, pharynx, and hypopharynx). Suctioning of the mouth and nose with a bulb syringe may be necessary if secretions accumulate.

The neonate with a normal respiratory pattern, heart rate, and color requires no further intervention. Often the neonate has a normal respiratory pattern and heart rate but may not be pink. Acrocyanosis often persists for several minutes after delivery and does not require intervention. However, an evaluation for choanal atresia can be performed at this time with the gentle insertion of a small suction catheter through each nostril into the nasopharynx. Vigorous nasal suctioning should be avoided because it can cause trauma to the nasal mucosa and result in progressive edema and airway obstruction. The neonate is an obligate nasal breather; thus, choanal atresia is a potentially lethal anomaly that requires immediate attention. The classic clinical presentation for choanal atresia is an infant with cyanosis and respiratory distress at rest who becomes pink when crying. If this anomaly is present (as evidenced by failure of nasal passage of the catheter), the neonate should have an oral airway or endotracheal tube inserted and an evaluation performed for repair of the obstruction.

Tactile stimulation should be used if the neonate does not breathe immediately; this consists of gently rubbing the back and flicking the soles of the feet. Tactile stimulation does not trigger respiratory efforts during secondary apnea in the neonate. Therefore, if the neonate does not begin to breathe spontaneously after tactile stimulation, the evaluator should begin positive-pressure mask ventilation. If the neonate has an abnormally slow heart rate (i.e., <100 bpm), positive-pressure ventilation should be performed until the heart rate rises to the normal range. Overzealous tactile stimulation (e.g., slapping the back) is not useful; it provides no advantage over the more moderate methods and can cause traumatic injury. Infants with labored breathing, such as retractions or grunting, or persistent cyanosis may benefit from continuous positive airway pressure.

High concentrations of oxygen (as opposed to ambient air) can raise production of oxygen free radicals, which have been linked to hypoxia-reoxygenation injury.[83] Studies of term or near-term infants showed a significantly lower mortality rate with no evidence of harm when resuscitation was performed initially with room air rather than 100% oxygen.[84] The current guidelines for neonatal resuscitation for term infants recommend the initial use of room air for assisted ventilation.[2]

A 2018 metaanalysis[85] compared lower ($F_{IO_2} < 0.4$) versus higher ($F_{IO_2} \geq 0.4$) initial oxygen concentrations for the resuscitation of preterm infants. No difference in mortality or other outcomes was identified, although the quality of evidence was low. As a result, the current guidelines recommend resuscitation with 21% to 30% oxygen with titration as needed.[2] Sao_2 measurements of 85% to 92% are thought to be adequate and appropriate for neonates less than 35 weeks' gestation.

Positive-pressure ventilation must be performed correctly to ensure that it is effective and does not cause barotrauma. Current guidelines recommend the use of a T-piece resuscitator rather than a self-inflating bag to administer positive-pressive ventilation, particularly for preterm infants.[74] A self-inflating bag should be available as backup in the event of compressed gas failure. The face mask must be of appropriate size and shape to ensure a good seal around the nose and mouth. A variety of masks should be available to accommodate infants of all sizes and gestational ages. Use of a supraglottic airway (SGA), rather than a face mask, may be used to deliver positive-pressure ventilation for infants less than 34 weeks' gestation (see later).[74] For the infant with excessive occipital scalp edema (i.e., *caput succedaneum*), placing a small roll under the shoulders to alleviate hyperflexion of the neck may be helpful.

Neonatal Resuscitation Algorithm

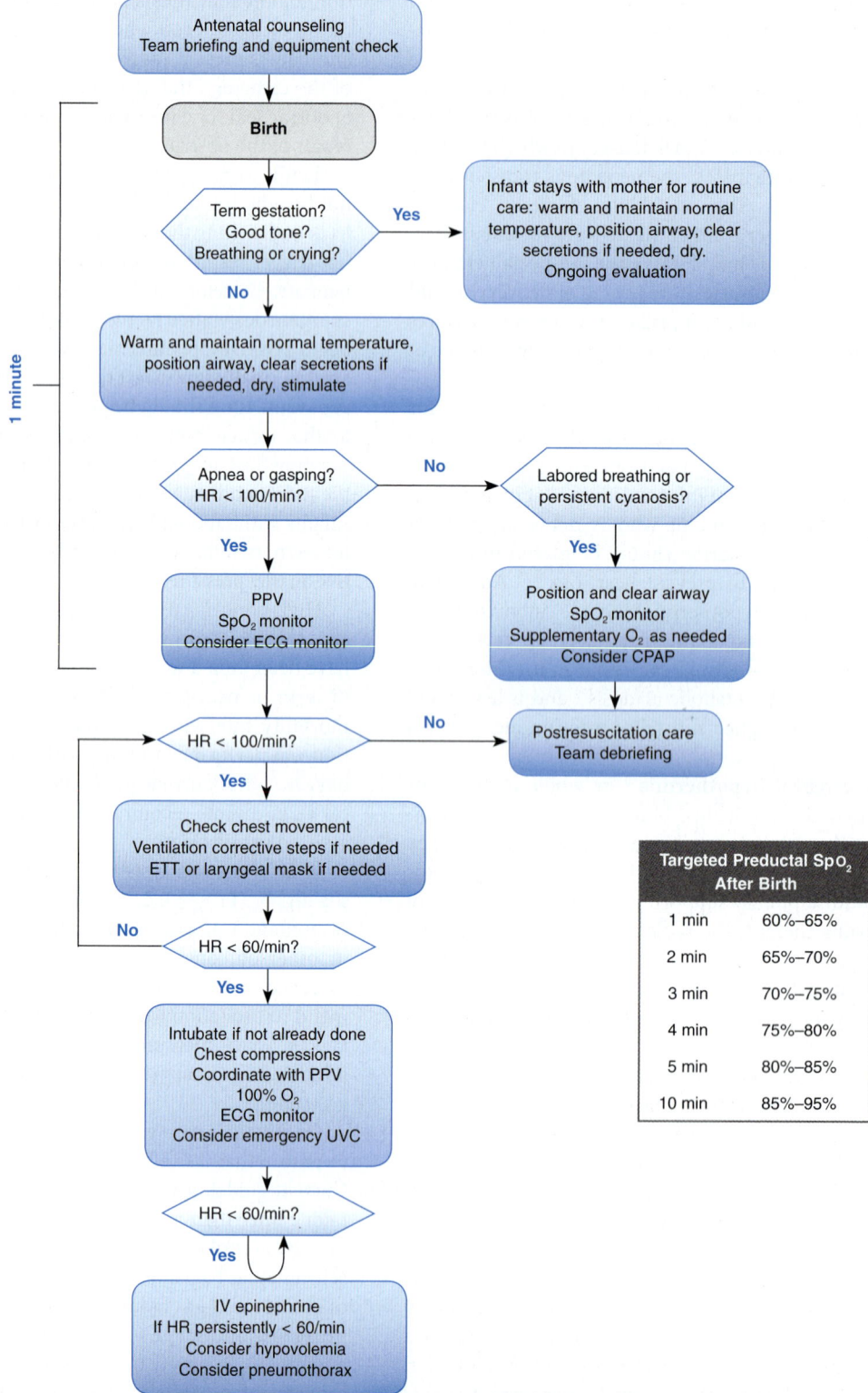

Targeted Preductal SpO₂ After Birth	
1 min	60%–65%
2 min	65%–70%
3 min	70%–75%
4 min	75%–80%
5 min	80%–85%
10 min	85%–95%

Fig. 9.3 **Algorithm for Resuscitation of the Newly Born Infant.** *CPAP,* Continuous positive airway pressure; *ECG,* electrocardiographic; *ETT,* endotracheal tube; *HR,* heart rate; *IV,* intravenous; *O₂,* oxygen; *SpO₂,* oxygen saturation; *UVC,* umbilical venous catheter. From Aziz K, Lee HC, Escobedo MB, et al. Part 5: Neonatal Resuscitation: 2020 American Heart Association Guidelines for Cardiopulmonary Resuscitation and Emergency Cardiovascular Care. *Circulation.* 2020;142:(16_suppl_2)S524–S550, with permission from the American Heart Association.

It has been suggested that during the first assisted breath, positive pressure at 30 cm H_2O in term infants should be maintained for 4 to 5 seconds at the end of inspiration to overcome the surface tension of the lungs and open the alveoli.[86] A 2015 review of the literature assessing the technique in human neonates found low-quality evidence of benefit for its use. The authors concluded that the safety and benefits of sustained inflation require further rigorous study.[3]

The neonatal response to a large, rapid inflation of the lungs is a sharp inspiration of its own (Head's paradoxical reflex).[87] Subsequent breaths should be delivered at a rate of 40 to 60 breaths per minute, with intermittent inspiratory pauses to prevent the development of atelectasis. The maximum pressure generated should range between 20 and 30 cm H_2O, with an inspiration-to-expiration ratio of approximately 1:1. In preterm infants, whose lungs may be more easily injured, initial inflation pressures of 20 to 25 cm H_2O may be adequate. If mask ventilation is needed for longer than 2 to 3 minutes, the stomach should be emptied with an orogastric catheter. Distention of the stomach with air can compromise respiratory function in the neonate. This maneuver should be performed with care because pharyngeal stimulation can result in bradycardia and apnea.[88]

The adequacy of respiratory resuscitation can be monitored from observation of its effect on heart rate; an increase in heart rate is the first consistently reliable sign of effective oxygenation. By contrast, changes in color occur slowly, are difficult to assess, and are a relatively poor index of successful resuscitation.

When the neonate's heart rate is higher than 100 bpm, positive-pressure ventilation can be stopped, and the infant can be reevaluated for spontaneous respiratory effort. Administration of naloxone is *not* recommended, even if opioid-induced respiratory depression is the suspected etiology. Naloxone can worsen the neurologic damage caused by asphyxia[89,90] and can precipitate acute neonatal opioid withdrawal, including seizure activity in cases of maternal opioid abuse. Assisted ventilation should be continued until resolution of the opioid effect rather than attempting to reverse it with naloxone.

If positive-pressure ventilation does not improve oxygenation (as reflected by an increase in heart rate), tracheal intubation is indicated. Tracheal intubation must be performed gently to avoid damage to the delicate neonatal neck and airway. The size of the neonate's head is large relative to that of its body; therefore, the neonate is in the optimal position when it lies supine. In most cases, it is not necessary to elevate or hyperextend the neonate's head during laryngoscopy.

The neonatal larynx is more anterior than that of the adult, and visualization often is easier when cricoid pressure is applied. The practitioner should hold the laryngoscope and apply cricoid pressure with the same hand. The thumb and first two fingers hold the base of the laryngoscope, the third finger rests on the mandible, and the fourth finger applies cricoid pressure. This technique promotes gentleness during airway manipulation. The distance from the gums to the larynx often is surprisingly short. A common mistake is to advance the laryngoscope blade too deeply—past the larynx and into the esophagus. When this error occurs, the larynx falls into view if the laryngoscope blade is withdrawn slowly.

The diameter of the endotracheal tube should be large enough to allow adequate ventilation and insertion of a suction catheter (if needed) but small enough to avoid causing trauma and subsequent subglottic stenosis. The ratio of internal diameter to gestational age should be less than 0.1 (e.g., 3.0 mm tube/35 weeks' gestation = 0.09).[91,92]

After tracheal intubation, positive-pressure ventilation should be resumed by means of an appropriate circuit (see earlier). Assessment of proper tube placement is accomplished by listening for breath sounds in both axillae. Exhaled CO_2 detection is the recommended method for confirming placement of the tube in the trachea.[3,93] False-negative results can occur in situations in which the infant is correctly intubated, with the tube in the trachea, but pulmonary blood flow is poor or absent. This may lead to unnecessary extubation in critically ill infants. The FiO_2 should be reduced as soon as possible, especially in the preterm neonate. The use of a pulse oximeter and an oxygen blender allows more targeted delivery of supplemental oxygen to the preterm infant immediately after birth. If the neonate is to remain intubated, a chest radiograph should be obtained to confirm the exact position of the endotracheal tube.

The skill and experience required for correct tracheal intubation and effective bag-and-mask ventilation may be lacking in providers who are inexperienced with neonatal resuscitation; as a consequence, SGAs have been evaluated as a potential alternative airway device for neonatal resuscitation.[94-96] The SGA is blindly inserted into the pharynx, and a cuff is inflated to provide a low-pressure seal around the larynx. When evaluated in term infants requiring resuscitation at delivery, use of the SGA was found to be highly successful and without complications.[94,95] The current neonatal resuscitation guidelines state that the SGA is an acceptable alternative means of establishing an airway in infants born at 34 weeks' gestation and later.[74]

One cause of unequal breath sounds and eventual circulatory collapse is a tension pneumothorax. Some physicians have recommended that providers of neonatal resuscitation be skilled in needle aspiration of a tension pneumothorax.[1] This maneuver is accomplished by placement of a 22- or 25-gauge needle in the second intercostal space in the midclavicular line (on the side where no breath or heart sounds are heard). Air will rush out of the needle hub, thereby reducing the tension pneumothorax.

In almost all resuscitations, the neonate responds to ventilatory support. Chest compressions are needed in only 0.03% of deliveries.[97] Chest compressions are indicated when the heart rate is less than 60 bpm despite adequate ventilation with supplemental oxygen for 30 seconds.[2]

The preferred method for providing chest compressions is with the thumbs of both hands and the hands encircling the chest.[2,3] Pressure is applied over the sternum just below an imaginary line drawn between the nipples; pressure applied over the lower part of the sternum or xiphoid can injure the abdomen. The sternum should be compressed to approximately one-third of the anteroposterior dimension of the chest, and the compression depth must be adequate to produce a palpable pulse.[3,98–100] The compression time should be slightly shorter than the release time, particularly in the very young infant.[101] Ventilation is compromised if the chest is compressed simultaneously with the administration of positive-pressure ventilation. The recommended ratio of compressions to breaths is 3:1.[3,102,103] This pattern is given at a rate of 120 events per minute, with 90 chest compressions and 30 breaths administered each minute. Respirations, heart rate, and color should be rechecked every 30 seconds. Compressions should be resumed until the heart rate is 60 bpm or higher. Positive-pressure ventilation with supplemental oxygen titrated to Sao_2 should be continued until the heart rate is higher than 100 bpm.

Medications are rarely required during neonatal resuscitation because most neonates who require resuscitative measures respond well to satisfactory oxygenation and ventilation alone.[2] However, a variety of pharmacologic agents should be available in the delivery room (see Box 9.3). **Epinephrine** (0.02 mg/kg or 0.2 mL/kg of a 1:10,000 solution) should be administered if the heart rate remains lower than 60 bpm after 30 seconds of adequate ventilation and chest compressions, with a 3 mL normal saline flush for all size infants.[3] Intravenous administration is the preferred route (via an umbilical venous line). While intravenous access is being established, intratracheal administration through an endotracheal tube may be considered; however, a larger dose of epinephrine (0.05 to 0.1 mg/kg) may be required. Administration of epinephrine is especially important if the heart rate is zero, and may require repeated dosing to be effective.[104] Epinephrine raises the heart rate (the major determinant of neonatal cardiac output) and restores coronary and cerebral blood flow (CBF).[105]

Sodium bicarbonate is not recommended during resuscitation. Because of its high osmolarity, this agent can cause hepatic injury at any gestational age and cerebral hemorrhage in the preterm infant[106,107]; it may also compromise myocardial and cerebral function.[108,109] It should be given only during prolonged resuscitation and when adequate ventilation and circulation have been established. Arterial blood gas measurements and serum chemistry determinations should guide the use of sodium bicarbonate, which generally occurs after stabilization.

Atropine is not recommended for use during neonatal resuscitation. Epinephrine is considered the drug of choice for the treatment of bradycardia.

Calcium administration is not recommended for neonatal resuscitation, unless it is given specifically to reverse the effect of magnesium, which may have crossed the placenta from the mother to the fetus. Evidence suggests that calcium administration causes cerebral calcification and decreases survival in stressed neonates.[110]

Volume expanders must be given strictly in recommended doses. A continuous infusion is dangerous in the neonate because it can easily result in the administration of an excessive fluid volume. Fluid overload can cause hepatic capsular rupture, brain swelling in the asphyxiated infant, or intracranial hemorrhage in the preterm infant. The recommended route of vascular access for neonates requiring access at the time of delivery is the umbilical vein.[2] The intraosseous route may be used if intravenous access is not feasible.

The cannulation of the umbilical vein involves insertion of a soft catheter into the cut end of the vein (Fig. 9.4). The catheter is advanced until blood return is noted, but no more than 2 cm past the abdominal surface. If ongoing vascular access is required during the neonate's hospital course, the soft umbilical catheter can be advanced through the ductus venosus into the inferior vena cava. Care must be taken to avoid leaving the tip in an intermediate location because of possible hepatic damage if a high-osmolarity substance is injected. Other complications of umbilical venous catheterization are hemorrhage and sepsis. The prolonged absence of vascular access in critically ill neonates can lead

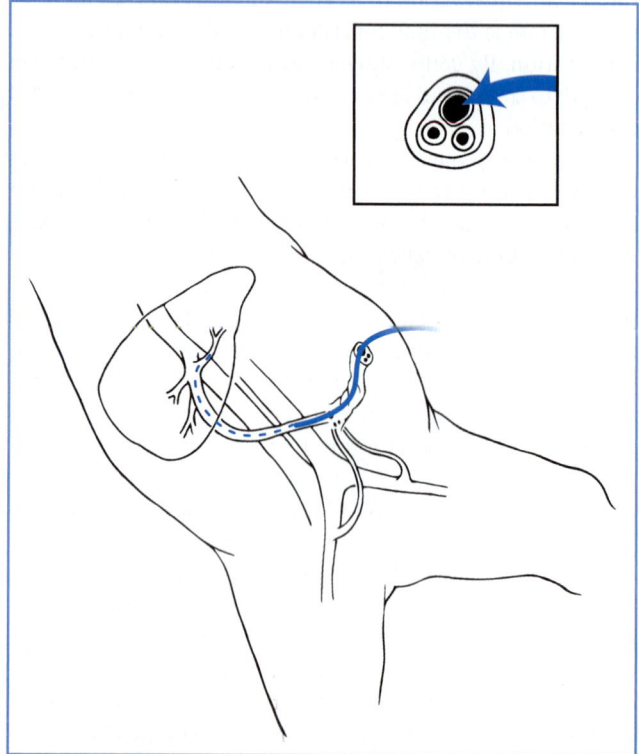

Fig. 9.4 Cannulation of the Umbilical Vein. A 3.5-F or 5-F umbilical catheter with a single end-hole and a radiopaque marker should be used. For emergency use, the catheter should be inserted into the vein of the umbilical stump until the tip of the catheter is just below the skin level but free flow of blood is present. If the catheter is inserted further, there is a risk for infusing solutions into the liver and possibly causing damage. Illustration by Naveen Nathan, MD, NorthShore University HealthSystem, University of Chicago Pritzker School of Medicine, Evanston, IL.

to hypoglycemia, which in association with hypoxia, can increase the risk for adverse neonatal outcomes.[111]

Intraosseous access is accomplished by insertion of a 20-gauge needle into the proximal tibia approximately 1 cm below the tibial tuberosity.[112] This technique may be easier to perform for practitioners who have little experience with intravenous or umbilical neonatal catheterization. Absorption from the neonatal bone marrow into the general circulation occurs almost immediately.[113,114] This rapid absorption results from the preponderance of red bone marrow over yellow bone marrow; yellow bone marrow is less vascular and is the dominant form of marrow after 5 years of age. Complications related to this technique are rare and include tibial fracture, which occurs more often in older children,[115] and osteomyelitis. The risk for infection is proportional to the duration of intraosseous infusion[116-118]; therefore, the needle should be removed after 1 to 2 hours and, if necessary, a more conventional route of access should be established.

Volume expanders should be considered when the infant demonstrates signs of shock, such as pale skin, poor perfusion, and weak pulse, or has not shown adequate response to other resuscitative measures. **Normal saline** is the preferred volume expander, given initially at 10 mL/kg over 5 to 10 minutes, with doses repeated as necessary after reassessment for ongoing hypovolemia.[2] Intravascular volume should be assessed through evaluation of heart rate, capillary refill time, and color. If significant blood loss is suspected, O-negative packed red blood cells may be used according to the same dosage regimen.[2] Red blood cells replete the oxygen-carrying capacity as well as the intravascular volume. O-negative blood should always be available for emergency use during neonatal resuscitation. Placental blood has been used for neonatal volume expansion, but this practice is discouraged in most institutions because of the risks for infection or transfusion of clotted blood. Albumin is not recommended.[2]

SPECIAL RESUSCITATION CIRCUMSTANCES

Meconium-Stained Amniotic Fluid

Meconium is present in the intestinal tract of the fetus after approximately 31 weeks' gestation. Meconium-stained amniotic fluid is present in 10% to 15% of all pregnancies; the incidence is higher in postterm pregnancies. Intrapartum passage of meconium may be associated with fetal stress and hypoxia.[119-121]

Meconium aspiration syndrome (MAS) is defined as respiratory distress in a neonate whose airway was exposed to meconium and whose chest radiograph exhibits characteristic findings, including pulmonary consolidation and atelectasis.[121] Treatment of MAS often involves the use of positive-pressure ventilation and is associated with a 5% to 20% incidence of pneumothorax from pulmonary air leaks.[122] It can be associated with persistent pulmonary hypertension

of the newborn. The use of extracorporeal membrane oxygenation (ECMO) and inhaled nitric oxide for the treatment of pulmonary hypertension associated with MAS has been shown to reduce mortality rates. In a US study published in 2009, the mortality in neonates admitted to the intensive care unit with MAS was 1.2%.[123]

In an attempt to reduce inhalation of meconium from the pharynx and thus prevent or reduce the severity of MAS, the practice of suctioning the mouth and pharynx after delivery of the head, and subsequent intubation to remove meconium from the trachea was a common practice. However, studies have documented that airway suctioning at birth does not prevent MAS and its associated mortality[2,121,124,125]; these studies indicated that MAS was primarily a result of intrauterine events such as asphyxia or sepsis. Hypoxia induces pathologic changes in the pulmonary vasculature, which results in pulmonary hypertension and respiratory distress after birth. The pulmonary damage is independent of meconium aspiration; therefore, it is not prevented by the suctioning of meconium. A prospective study designed to assess the efficacy of routine tracheal suctioning of meconium to prevent MAS indicated little or no benefit to this practice.[126] Current guidelines do not recommend routine intrapartum oropharyngeal and nasopharyngeal suctioning after delivery of the infant's head,[2,127] given that a large multicenter randomized trial showed no benefit to this practice in term-gestation infants.[128]

Amnioinfusion—the instillation of saline into the amniotic cavity—has been used successfully for reduction of cord compression in the presence of oligohydramnios during labor. It has also been proposed as a potential treatment to reduce the incidence of MAS in infants born to women with thick meconium staining of the amniotic fluid. A large multicenter randomized trial found no difference in rates of MAS or other neonatal disorders with the use of amnioinfusion.[129,130] Thus, the routine practice of amnioinfusion for meconium-stained fluid alone is not recommended.

Preterm Infant

The preterm neonate, especially the VLBW infant, is at higher risk for problems with multiple organ systems simply because of immaturity. During resuscitation, the physician should give special attention to the effect of prematurity on the lungs and the brain. Before maternal steroid use and the addition of surfactant and high-frequency ventilation to the therapeutic armamentarium of the neonatologist, neonatal respiratory distress syndrome caused by surfactant deficiency was the overwhelming obstacle to the attempted salvage of the very preterm infant.

Of the 1.5% of infants born before 28 weeks' gestation, mortality is impacted by gestational age, with a survival-to-discharge rate of 11% and 94% in infants born at 22 and 28 weeks, respectively.[131] However, 8.4% of these infants have moderate-to-severe cerebral palsy, and over 50% have moderate-to-severe neurodevelopmental impairment (see Chapter 10).

Markers for brain injury affecting preterm infants are IVH arising from the germinal matrix and periventricular leukomalacia. The brain injury may occur as a consequence of the IVH and its sequelae or as an associated finding. The incidence of IVH is directly related to gestational age; the lower the gestational age, the greater the risk for IVH.[132] Periventricular leukomalacia, which is the classic neuropathology associated with hypoxic-ischemic cerebral white matter injury in the preterm infant, commonly accompanies IVH.

The fragility of the immature subependymal germinal matrix predisposes the preterm infant to the development of IVH. The hemorrhage originates from the endothelial cell–lined vessels that course through the germinal matrix in free communication with the venous circulation (i.e., the capillary-venule junction). The hemorrhage can expand into the adjacent lateral ventricle. The pathogenesis of IVH is multifactorial; different combinations of factors are relevant in different patients.[132,133] The three major categories in the pathogenesis of IVH are intravascular, vascular, and extravascular. **Intravascular factors** include fluctuating CBF, which can result from respiratory disturbances in the ventilated preterm infant with neonatal respiratory distress syndrome,[134,135] increases in CBF,[136,137] increases in cerebral venous pressure,[138] decreases in CBF followed by reperfusion, and platelet and coagulation disturbances.[139] **Vascular factors** include the tenuousness of the capillary integrity of the germinal matrix and the vulnerability of the matrix capillaries to hypoxic-ischemic injury.[140] **Extravascular factors** include deficient vascular support, excessive fibrinolytic activity, and a possible postnatal decrease in extravascular tissue pressure.[141]

Of special interest in the discussion of antepartum and intrapartum care and neonatal resuscitation are the possible interventions that may prevent or lessen the severity of IVH. The best way to prevent germinal matrix IVH is to prevent preterm birth. Infection and inflammation are the most commonly identified causes of preterm birth at the lowest relevant gestational age.[142] Antenatal *treatment* of infections has not been proven to prevent preterm labor or premature rupture of membranes; however, *prevention* of infection, if possible, may be an important way to reduce the risk for IVH. Another intervention that lowers the incidence of IVH is the transportation of the preterm mother while the fetus is still *in utero* to a center that specializes in the care of high-risk neonates.[1]

Corticosteroids are currently the most beneficial antenatal pharmacologic intervention for the prevention of IVH. This effect was first noticed when obstetricians began giving betamethasone and dexamethasone to pregnant women to help accelerate fetal lung maturity. The mechanism behind this protection is thought to be improved neonatal cardiovascular stability, which results in less hypotension and less need for blood pressure treatment in these infants.[143] Antenatal betamethasone administration leads to lower placental vascular resistance and higher placental blood flow.[144] This improvement in placental blood flow may decrease impairment of the preterm infant's cerebral autoregulation. In addition, corticosteroids may stimulate the maturation of the germinal matrix. Recommendations regarding timing of corticosteroid administration have been published by the ACOG; corticosteroid administration is recommended for pregnant women between 24 0/7 weeks' and 33 6/7 weeks' gestation who are at risk for preterm delivery, while corticosteroid administration can be considered for at-risk pregnancies as early as 23 0/7 weeks' gestation.[145] A repeat course can be considered when there is risk for delivery within 7 days, and the woman is less than 34 0/7 weeks' gestation and the previous course of corticosteroids occurred more than 14 days previously (see Chapter 33).

Multiple studies have demonstrated a lower incidence of cerebral palsy in infants of mothers given **magnesium sulfate** for the treatment of preeclampsia or for tocolysis[146,147]; subsequent studies have observed a similar benefit when magnesium has been given specifically for fetal neuroprotection.[148–150] An ACOG Committee opinion[151] recommends the administration of magnesium sulfate to mothers in preterm labor. Maternal magnesium sulfate administration does not result in a decreased incidence of IVH, although the incidence of high-grade (grade III or IV) lesions may be reduced.[152] Although some investigators have suggested that antenatal exposure to magnesium sulfate results in a higher risk for adverse neonatal outcomes,[153] others have observed no association between umbilical cord blood magnesium concentration and the need for delivery room resuscitation when magnesium sulfate was administered for neuroprotection in anticipation of a preterm birth.[154]

Postnatal interventions that may prevent IVH include the avoidance of overly rapid infusion of volume expanders or hypertonic solutions such as sodium bicarbonate.[155] The establishment of adequate ventilation is the most beneficial immediate intervention that helps preserve cerebrovascular autoregulation in the preterm infant. The prevention of hypoxemia and hypercarbia is essential because they are both linked to pressure-passive cerebral circulation, which in turn leads to the development of IVH.[155]

Congenital Anomalies

Occasionally, neonatal resuscitation is complicated by congenital anomalies of the airway or diaphragm. These anomalies may manifest as respiratory distress, which resolves only when appropriate resuscitation techniques are used. For example, neonates are obligatory nose breathers. The diagnosis and management of choanal stenosis and atresia include placement of an oral airway or endotracheal tube until a definitive surgical procedure can be performed.

Other congenital anomalies that cause upper airway obstruction include (1) micrognathia, as in Pierre Robin sequence; (2) macroglossia, as in Beckwith-Wiedemann syndrome or glycogen storage disease type II; (3) laryngeal webs; (4) laryngeal atresia; (5) stenosis or paralysis at the level of the vocal cords; (6) subglottic stenosis; (7) subglottic webs; (8) tracheal agenesis; and (9) tracheal rings. Obstruction also can occur from tumors such as subglottic hemangiomas. The presence of a cleft palate may lead to difficulty with manual ventilation. In an infant with micrognathia or macroglossia, airway patency may be maintained if the neonate is kept in the prone position, which reduces posterior movement of the tongue into the pharynx. If macroglossia is extreme, use of an oral airway may be necessary to prevent complete obstruction of the pharynx by the tongue.

When respiratory distress and difficulty with bag-and-mask ventilation are encountered, laryngoscopy should be performed. The cause of the obstruction may be evident if it is supraglottic in location. Some supraglottic entities (e.g., laryngeal webs) may be treated successfully by passing an endotracheal tube through the obstruction and into the trachea. Subglottic lesions may require tracheostomy. The help of an otolaryngologist may be invaluable during resuscitation of a neonate with congenital airway obstruction. If there is antepartum evidence of such a condition (e.g., laryngeal stenosis), it is best to have an otolaryngologist present at the time of delivery. If obstruction is discovered after delivery, the resuscitator should not hesitate to call for surgical assistance.

Ex Utero Intrapartum Treatment Procedure

Fetal neck masses such as cervical teratoma and lymphangioma can lead to extrinsic airway compression. The resulting distortion of the airway can result in airway obstruction, and it may be difficult—if not impossible—to secure an airway in a timely fashion at delivery. These masses often are diagnosed before delivery because of the associated occurrence of polyhydramnios resulting from esophageal compression. In these rare cases, a multidisciplinary team should be assembled before delivery to assist in securing the airway at delivery. Liechty et al.[156] described a way of providing the time necessary to secure an airway, known as the *ex utero* intrapartum treatment (EXIT) procedure (see Chapter 7). During cesarean delivery, the obstetrician delivers the fetal head and shoulders but keeps the lower torso and umbilical cord intact within the uterus, thereby maintaining placental perfusion and oxygenation. The fetus can be given agents intramuscularly (e.g., fentanyl, muscle relaxant, atropine) to provide fetal analgesia and to prevent movement and breathing. The FHR and Sao$_2$ are monitored continuously via a pulse oximeter probe attached to the fetal hand. The pediatric surgeon can then perform direct laryngoscopy, rigid bronchoscopy, or tracheostomy if necessary. After establishment of the airway, the delivery of the infant is completed.

The EXIT procedure has been considered an option for fetuses with other congenital anomalies.[157] A common indication for the EXIT procedure is an intrinsic airway obstruction. Intrinsic airway obstruction of the larynx or upper trachea (e.g., laryngeal web, subglottic cyst, tracheal atresia) can lead to retention of bronchial secretions and subsequent pulmonary distention; this constellation of findings is often classified as **congenital high airway obstruction syndrome**. Use of the EXIT procedure resulted in the first long-term survival of a child with this syndrome.[158]

Indications for EXIT procedures continue to evolve and now include conditions such as severe congenital heart disease, in which the need for emergency ECMO at birth is anticipated. The EXIT procedure allows for the placement of arterial and venous cannulas before umbilical cord clamping, thereby avoiding an unstable period between the termination of placental perfusion and the institution of ECMO.[159] Other possible indications for the EXIT procedure include the resection of congenital cystic adenomatoid malformations and as a first step in separation procedures for conjoined twins with cardiovascular involvement.

Anesthetic considerations for the mother during an EXIT procedure include those relevant to general anesthesia for the mother undergoing cesarean delivery or other surgical procedures during pregnancy (see Chapters 7, 18, and 26). The anesthetic technique is dependent upon several variables including but not limited to the anticipated surgical approach, maternal medical history, and patient preferences, as well as minimizing the effect on fetal hemodynamics. Anesthetic management of EXIT procedures focuses on achieving maximal uterine muscle relaxation and maintaining uteroplacental perfusion and maternal hemodynamics while minimizing fetal cardiac dysfunction.[160]

Uterine relaxation is often achieved using volatile anesthetics, as well as adjuvant medications, including nitroglycerin, beta-adrenergic receptor agonists, and magnesium sulfate. Several volatile halogenated agents have been used for the EXIT procedure, including isoflurane, desflurane, and sevoflurane. To achieve maximal uterine muscle relaxation, high doses of a volatile agent may be required (up to 2 to 3 times the minimum alveolar concentration [MAC]). Prolonged neonatal exposure to volatile agents at the time of cesarean delivery can be associated with decreased 1-minute Apgar scores secondary to respiratory depression and hypotonia. In addition, fetal exposure to high-dose volatile anesthetic agents has been associated with fetal hypoxia and acidosis as well as fetal cardiac dysfunction, including ventricular dysfunction and bradycardia.[161] For this reason, combination techniques that lower volatile agent requirements are often employed to optimize relaxation while balancing fetal risk. In 2010, Boat et al. retrospectively examined the records of 39 patients undergoing EXIT procedures with high-dose desflurane (2 to 3 MAC) or supplemental intravenous anesthesia (SIVA) with propofol, remifentanil, and desflurane (1 to 1.5 MAC). The SIVA group achieved adequate uterine relaxation at lower MAC of desflurane (1 to 1.5 MAC) and had a lower incidence of fetal left ventricular dysfunction compared with the high-dose volatile agent group.[162]

In addition to volatile anesthetic agents, intravenous agents including nitroglycerin, magnesium sulfate, and beta-adrenergic receptor agonists have been utilized to optimize uterine relaxation. Nitroglycerin is the most common adjuvant as it allows for quick titration and is rapidly metabolized, facilitating rapid recovery of uterine tone after delivery of the neonate.[161] Additional benefits include rapid placental metabolism and minimal fetal hemodynamic changes, although careful titration is essential to avoid maternal hypotension and the accompanying uteroplacental perfusion. Intravenous boluses of 25- to 100-μg can be administered and titrated to effect, conferring uterine relaxation for up to 10 minutes.[163] Magnesium sulfate and beta-adrenergic receptor agonists, such as terbutaline, are much less frequently utilized during EXIT procedures because of their prolonged effects on uterine tone and adverse fetal side-effect profile. Neonates exposed to magnesium sulfate can present with hypotonia and lethargy upon delivery, while those exposed to beta-adrenergic receptor agonists can present with fetal tachycardia and metabolic derangements.[160]

Maintenance of uterine muscle relaxation is often complicated by vasodilation, which can lead to maternal hypotension, decreased uteroplacental blood flow, and decreased fetal cardiac output.[162] To maintain mean arterial pressure and ensure adequate uteroplacental perfusion, judicious vasopressor and intravenous fluid administration are required. Ephedrine and phenylephrine are the two most-used vasopressor agents in obstetric and fetal surgery. While both agents are considered safe for the mother and fetus, the efficacy of phenylephrine in the treatment of hypotension, and the higher umbilical artery blood pH and lower base excess compared with ephedrine, have resulted in phenylephrine being used as a first-line agent for the prevention and treatment of maternal hypotension.

Intraoperative monitoring, including continuous fetal pulse oximetry and heart rate monitoring, is critical throughout the EXIT procedure. Decreased baroreceptor activity and vasoconstrictive responses to hypovolemia make the fetus particularly susceptible to heat and evaporative fluid losses, as well as hypovolemia and hypoperfusion during exposure on the surgical field.[162] Effort should be made to maintain fetal temperature during the course of the procedure, including higher operating room temperatures and limiting exposure of fetal body parts not critical to the procedure to the outside environment. Blood for possible transfusion to the fetus should be immediately available at the time of the procedure and fetal hemoglobin and blood gases measured as indicated.

In a systematic review conducted by Kumar et al.,[164] neonatal mortality associated with EXIT procedures was reported as 10% (23 neonatal deaths/223 EXIT procedures) due to the inability to ventilate, oxygenate, or intubate ($n = 5$); pulmonary hypoplasia ($n = 11$); complex cardiac disease leading to heart failure and pulmonary hypertension ($n = 5$); and unexplained intraoperative bleeding ($n = 1$). The study reported no maternal or fetal complications due to the general or neuraxial anesthesia performed for the procedure.[164]

Other Congenital Anomalies

Esophageal atresia and **tracheoesophageal fistula** occur in 1 of 3000 births.[165] There are many variations of these anomalies, the most common being esophageal atresia with a distal tracheoesophageal fistula (80% to 90% of cases). Neonates with a tracheoesophageal fistula are at increased risk for the pulmonary aspiration of gastric contents through the fistula into the lung. Undiagnosed tracheoesophageal fistula should be suspected if bubbling secretions are observed during spontaneous or bag-and-mask ventilation. Once a tracheoesophageal fistula is suspected, bag-and-mask ventilation should be discontinued. Its use may contribute to overdistention of the gastrointestinal tract with air, possibly leading to difficulty in ventilation from impingement of the enlarged stomach on the diaphragm. A suction catheter should be placed in the esophageal pouch to facilitate the removal of oral secretions.

If mechanical ventilation is necessary, an endotracheal tube should be inserted with the tip distal to the entrance of the fistula. This positioning can be accomplished by performing an intentional right mainstem bronchial intubation followed by slowly withdrawing the tube until breath sounds are auscultated on the left; a lack of breath sounds over the stomach should then be confirmed. Percutaneous gastrostomy placement may be necessary during resuscitation to facilitate decompression of the gastrointestinal tract.

Congenital diaphragmatic hernia (CDH) occurs in approximately 2.3 in 10,000 live births.[166] The mortality rate from CDH is 30% to 60%.[167] In 80% to 90% of cases, the CDH occurs on the left side and is the result of herniation of the gut through the posterolateral defect of Bochdalek. During formation of the lung, herniation of the gut into the thoracic cavity results in hypoplasia of the lung tissue and pulmonary vasculature. This hypoplasia may be unilateral, but often it is bilateral because of the shift in mediastinal structures to the other side. CDH should be suspected when a neonate has respiratory difficulty and a scaphoid abdomen, resulting from the presence of abdominal contents in the thorax.

During resuscitation of the neonate with CDH, bag-and-mask ventilation is contraindicated because it results in further distention of the gut, with additional impingement on the lung. Tracheal intubation is recommended, followed by the placement of a nasogastric or orogastric tube to ensure decompression of the gastrointestinal tract. Ventilation should consist of low-positive-pressure breaths to decrease the risk for causing a pneumothorax on the side contralateral to the CDH. If a pneumothorax does occur, evacuation must occur promptly and is accomplished initially by placement of a 22-gauge needle into the second intercostal space in the midclavicular line and aspiration of air with an attached stopcock and syringe. Severe pulmonary hypertension often accompanies CDH. Maintenance of euthermia, normoxia, and adequate systemic blood pressure promotes pulmonary artery blood flow.

Whenever congenital anomalies of the respiratory tract are noted, the presence of other anomalies should be suspected. It is important to evaluate the neonate promptly for cardiac malformations, especially if appropriate resuscitative efforts are not successful. Echocardiography is used to evaluate cardiac structures and function.

ETHICAL CONSIDERATIONS

The current neonatal resuscitation guidelines address the ethical considerations of noninitiation or discontinuation of resuscitation in the delivery room.[2,3] Extremes of prematurity (<23 weeks' confirmed gestation) and severe congenital anomalies (e.g., anencephaly, confirmed trisomy 13 or 18) are examples of circumstances when noninitiation of resuscitation is considered appropriate. Because intrapartum confirmation of pertinent information may not be possible, it is recognized that initiation of resuscitation may occur and that its discontinuation may then be appropriate after further information has been obtained and discussion with family has occurred. In some cases, a trial of therapy may be appropriate, which does not always mandate continued support. In situations or conditions in which there is a high rate of survival and acceptable morbidity (i.e., ≥ 25 weeks' gestation and most congenital malformations), resuscitation is generally indicated. For those situations with a poor prognosis, including unlikely survival and potentially high morbidity (i.e., 22 to 24 weeks' gestation), the parents' desires regarding initiation of resuscitation should be supported (Table 9.4).[168]

Discontinuation of resuscitation of an infant with cardiopulmonary arrest may be appropriate if spontaneous circulation has not occurred in 20 minutes. After 10 minutes of asystole, survival itself and survival without severe disabilities are very unlikely.[2]

NEUROBEHAVIORAL TESTING

It is difficult to detect subtle neurobehavioral differences among neonates during the assignment of Apgar scores or the performance of the initial neurologic examination; therefore, investigators have developed and studied methods of documenting neonatal neurobehavioral status (Table 9.5). In the past, the neonate was considered incapable of exhibiting higher cortical function. However, investigators have noted that the term neonate is able to sense and respond to a variety of stimuli in a well-organized fashion.[169–171]

In 1973, Brazelton[172] described the Neonatal Behavioral Assessment Scale (NBAS) with the following four variables as key determinants of neonatal neurobehavior: (1) various prenatal influences (e.g., infection); (2) the maturity of the infant, especially its CNS; (3) the effects of analgesics and anesthetics administered to the mother before and during delivery; and (4) the effects of difficulties encountered during delivery (e.g., trauma). The NBAS was developed as a tool to detect neurobehavioral abnormalities that resulted from any of these four variables.

This scale consists of 47 individual tests with 27 evaluating behavior and 20 evaluating elicited or provoked responses. The 47 tests can be completed in approximately 45 minutes. The NBAS evaluates the ability of the neonate to perform complex motor behaviors, to alter the state of arousal, and to suppress meaningless stimuli. The goal is to provide an extensive evaluation of neonatal cortical function and to detect subtle differences among groups of infants. Habituation (i.e., the ability to suppress the response to meaningless, repetitive

TABLE 9.4 Interventions for Threatened and Imminent Periviable Birth

Intervention	WEEKS' GESTATION			
	22 0/7 to 22 6/7[a]	23 0/7 to 23 6/7	24 0/7 to 24 6/7	25 0/7 to 25 6/7
Cesarean delivery for fetal indication	Not recommended	Consider	Consider	Recommended
Neonatal assessment for resuscitation[b]	Consider	Consider	Recommended	Recommended
Antenatal corticosteroids	Not recommended	Consider	Recommended	Recommended
Tocolysis for preterm labor	Not recommended	Consider	Recommended	Recommended
Magnesium sulfate for neuroprotection	Not recommended	Consider	Recommended	Recommended
Antibiotics to prolong latency for premature rupture of membranes	Consider	Consider	Recommended	Recommended

[a]Administration of antibiotics to prolong latency may be considered between 20 0/7 and 21 6/7 weeks' gestation, but no other interventions are recommended.
[b]Factors in addition to gestational age may affect the chances of survival and should be considered in making the decision to initiate resuscitation or not.
Modified from American College of Obstetricians and Gynecologists and Society for Maternal-Fetal Medicine. Obstetric Care Consensus No. 6: Periviable birth (reaffirmed 2025). *Obstet Gynecol.* 2017;130:e187–e199.

TABLE 9.5 Neurobehavioral Tests for Neonates

Neurobehavioral Test	Items Tested	Focus	Uses
Brazelton (Neonatal Behavioral Assessment Scale)	45 individual tests taking 45 min	Early cortical function	Evaluates prenatal influences, effects of maturity, maternal medications, effects of difficult delivery
Scanlon (Early Neonatal Behavior Scale)	26 observations taking 6–10 min	Early cortical function	Evaluates effects of maternal medications
Amiel-Tison (Neurologic and Adaptive Capacity Score)	20 criteria taking 3–4 min	Motor tone	Differentiates drug-induced depression from depression related to asphyxia, trauma, or neurologic disease

stimuli) is considered an excellent indicator of normal early cortical function.[169]

In 1974, Scanlon et al.[173] described the Early Neonatal Behavioral Scale (ENNS), which consisted of tests that were easy to perform and score quantitatively during the neonatal period. The ENNS was developed primarily for the evaluation of the effects of maternal medications (e.g., analgesic and anesthetic agents) on neonatal neurobehavior. The ENNS consists of (1) 15 observations of muscle tone and power, reflexes (e.g., rooting, sucking, Moro), and response to stimuli (e.g., light, sound, pinprick); (2) 11 observations of the infant's state of wakefulness; (3) an assessment of the ability of the neonate to habituate to repetitive stimuli; and (4) an overall general assessment of neurobehavioral status. This test can be performed in 6 to 10 minutes.

In 1982, Amiel-Tison et al.[174] described the Neurologic and Adaptive Capacity Score (NACS) to differentiate neonatal depression secondary to maternally administered drugs from depression caused by asphyxia, birth trauma, or neurologic disease. Whereas the ENNS concentrates on the infant's habituation ability, the NACS emphasizes motor tone as a key indicator of drug-induced abnormal neurobehavior. The basis for this emphasis on neonatal motor tone is explained as follows: unilateral or upper body hypotonus may occur because of either birth trauma or anoxia, but global motor depression is more likely a result of anesthetic- or analgesic-induced depression. A total of 20 criteria are tested in the areas of adaptive capacity, passive tone (e.g., scarf sign), active tone (e.g., assessment of the flexor and extensor muscles of the neck), primary reflexes (e.g., Moro), and alertness. The total possible score is 40, and a score of 35 to 40 is considered normal. The NACS can be performed in 3 to 4 minutes.

Amiel-Tison et al.[174] examined interobserver reliability and assessed the correlation of results between the NACS and ENNS. The interobserver reliability was 93% for the NACS and 88% for the ENNS. Approximately 92% of infants with high scores on the ENNS scored equally well on the NACS. However, the reliability of the NACS has been questioned[175,176]; Halpern et al.[177] examined 200 healthy term infants with the NACS and found poor interobserver reliability. In contrast, in 2002, Amiel-Tison[178] reported her later experience with the NACS and documented good interobserver reliability.

Anesthesiologists have used neurobehavioral testing to document the effects of analgesic and anesthetic agents and techniques on neonatal neurobehavior. A number of studies have demonstrated transient, serum concentration–dependent depression of neonatal neurobehavior with the maternal administration of systemic agents (e.g., meperidine, diazepam).[179-181] However, in an NBAS examination that controlled for patient and labor and delivery characteristics, only decreased habituation was observed in neonates born to mothers who had received intravenous meperidine.[182] Similarly, maternal administration of intravenous fentanyl appears to minimally affect neonatal NACS examinations.[183]

As is the case with many studies of systemic agents, studies of epidural analgesia and anesthesia are often confounded by variables that are difficult to control, such as different patient populations, varied durations of labor, and multiple drug administrations. Scanlon et al.[173] introduced the ENNS in a study of the effect of maternal epidural anesthesia on neonatal neurobehavior. The researchers concluded that epidural anesthesia was associated with lower ENNS scores because of decreased muscle strength and tone. In this study, all patients who had received epidural anesthesia were considered part of one group, although 9 patients had received lidocaine and 19 had received mepivacaine. Further investigation showed that epidural lidocaine, even when administered in larger doses for cesarean delivery, does not affect ENNS scores.[184] The difference in ENNS scores between the epidural and non-epidural groups noted in the earlier study[173] was most likely related to the use of mepivacaine rather than lidocaine.[185] As was observed with lidocaine, epidurally administered bupivacaine, 2-chloroprocaine, and etidocaine—when given for cesarean delivery—do not affect ENNS scores.[184,186] Kuhnert et al.[187] assessed NBAS scores in a group of infants exposed to either epidural lidocaine or 2-chloroprocaine. Although the investigators observed subtle changes in neurobehavior in the group of infants whose mothers had received lidocaine, they concluded that other variables (e.g., mode of delivery) are more likely to affect performance on neurobehavioral testing.

Most, if not all, studies assessing neonatal behavioral scores after neuraxial or general anesthesia are observational. Baseline characteristics of women who chose neuraxial labor analgesia differ from those who use no or other forms of analgesia, and these differences are often not controlled for in observational studies. Similarly, baseline characteristics of women who receive neuraxial versus general anesthesia for cesarean delivery often differ. For example, Sepkoski et al.[188] compared NBAS scores between two groups of vaginally delivered infants. In one group, the mothers had received epidural bupivacaine, and in the other group, the mothers had received no anesthesia or analgesia. The infants in the epidural group showed less alertness, less orientation ability, and less motor function maturity than the infants in the control group. However, variables such as duration of labor, incidence of oxytocin administration, and incidence of operative delivery differed in the two groups. Earlier, Abboud et al.[189] performed ENNS examinations on vaginally delivered infants whose mothers had received epidural bupivacaine. In this study, epidural administration of bupivacaine did not affect the ENNS scores. The maternal doses of epidural bupivacaine and the maternal venous and umbilical cord blood bupivacaine concentrations were similar to those noted by Sepkoski et al.[188] Abboud et al.[189] also noted normal ENNS scores for infants whose mothers had received epidural lidocaine or 2-chloroprocaine.

Critics of the ENNS and NACS claim that the evaluations are unable to demonstrate subtle differences in neurobehavior that would be detected by the more comprehensive NBAS.[190] However, although some differences have been observed in NBAS performance among groups of infants exposed or not exposed to local anesthetics, confounding variables have prevented clear conclusions as to cause and effect.

Hodgkinson et al.[191] observed that the subarachnoid administration of tetracaine for cesarean delivery did not adversely affect ENNS performance. Other studies have indicated that NACS performance is not significantly affected by the maternal epidural administration of opioids[192–197] or epinephrine (in combination with a local anesthetic).[198–201]

The effects of general anesthetic agents on neonatal neurobehavior have been evaluated by the ENNS and NACS. In a prospective, randomized study, Abboud et al.[202] assessed NACS performance at 15 minutes, 2 hours, and 24 hours of age in infants whose mothers received general, epidural, or spinal anesthesia for cesarean delivery. Women who underwent general anesthesia received thiopental 4 mg/kg followed by enflurane 0.5% with nitrous oxide 50% in oxygen. Although the NACS was lower at both 15 minutes and 2 hours of age in the infants in the general anesthesia group than in the infants in the neuraxial anesthesia groups, no difference in NACS results was noted at 24 hours of age.

Hodgkinson et al.[191] used the ENNS to evaluate outcomes among three groups of infants, all of whom were delivered by elective cesarean delivery. One group of women received general anesthesia with thiopental 4 mg/kg followed by 50% nitrous oxide. A second group received general anesthesia with ketamine 1 mg/kg followed by 50% nitrous oxide. A third group received spinal anesthesia with tetracaine 6 to 8 mg. The ENNS evaluations were conducted at 4 to 8 hours of age and again at 24 hours. During the 4- to 8-hour examination, infants in the spinal anesthesia group scored significantly higher on multiple components of the ENNS than did infants in either of the general anesthesia groups. At 24 hours, infants in the spinal anesthesia group scored significantly higher than those in the thiopental group in alertness, total decrement score, and overall assessment. Similarly, infants in the spinal anesthesia group scored higher than those in the ketamine group in alertness and overall assessment. No significant differences existed between the scores of the thiopental group infants and the ketamine group infants.[191] Palahniuk et al.[203] observed similar results in a study that compared groups of infants whose mothers received either epidural anesthesia or general anesthesia for elective cesarean delivery. Infants whose mothers had received thiopental and nitrous oxide scored significantly lower in the alertness component of the ENNS than infants whose mothers had received epidural lidocaine with epinephrine.

Stefani et al.[204] observed that subanesthetic maternal doses of enflurane or nitrous oxide did not affect neonatal neurobehavior (as assessed by ENNS and NACS) at 15 minutes, 2 hours, and 24 hours of age. Abboud et al.[205] obtained similar results from NACS examinations of infants whose mothers had received subanesthetic doses of isoflurane.

The long-term effects of perinatal exposure to either general or neuraxial anesthesia at the time of cesarean delivery compared with vaginal delivery appear limited (see Chapter 10).

In a population-based birth cohort, Sprung et al.[206] found that children exposed to either general or neuraxial anesthesia during cesarean delivery were not more likely to develop learning disabilities than children who were delivered vaginally. Some controversy does exist, however, regarding the issue of repeated or lengthy use of general anesthesia, specifically in the third trimester of pregnancy. In 2017, the US Food and Drug Administration (FDA) issued a drug safety communication warning about the use of general anesthetics and sedation drugs in pregnant women and young children.[207] The statement reported that:

Published studies in pregnant animals and young animals have shown the use of general anesthetic and sedation drugs for more than 3 hours caused widespread loss of nerve cells in the brain. Studies in young animals suggest these changes result in long-term effects on the animals' behavior or learning. Studies have also been conducted in children, some of which support findings from previous animal studies, particularly after repeated or prolonged exposure to these drugs early in life. All the studies in children had limitations, and it is unclear whether any negative effects seen in children's learning or behavior were due to the drugs or to other factors, such as the underlying medical condition that led to the need for the surgery or procedure.

This statement focused on repeated or prolonged exposure, defined as greater than 3 hours, and was based primarily on animal studies with limited human data. Further research is needed to determine the true extent of neurologic impact in these cases. It is important to remember that the risks and benefits of exposure must be weighed with the indications for exposure. The ACOG, ASA, and FDA all agree that "anesthesia and sedation drugs are necessary for infants, children, and pregnant women who require surgery or other painful and stressful procedures, especially when they face life-threatening conditions requiring surgery that should not be delayed."[207] Patients should be appropriately counseled regarding the concerns or potential risk associated with prolonged exposure to anesthesia and sedative drugs, and decisions should be balanced with the benefits of such exposure.

In summary, subtle changes in neonatal neurobehavior may result from factors such as antepartum maternal drug exposure. Parent-infant bonding and the ability of the infant to breastfeed may be adversely affected by these neurobehavioral changes.[169] These transient effects may seem trivial to some observers but important to others. Regarding the long-term neurologic outcome of individual infants, performance during neurobehavioral assessment may aid the observer in the formulation of a prognosis. However, as demonstrated with Apgar scores, the prognostic value of an isolated test score is likely to be lower than the prognostic value of multiple factors considered together during the overall assessment of an individual infant.

KEY POINTS

- The anesthesia provider attending the mother should not be responsible for resuscitation of the neonate. However, all anesthesia providers should be prepared to assist during neonatal resuscitation when it is needed.
- Adverse conditions at birth (e.g., hypoxia, acidosis, profound hypovolemia, hypothermia) may impair the transition from intrauterine to extrauterine life. Impaired transition may manifest as persistent pulmonary hypertension of the newborn.
- The Apgar scoring system gives the practitioner a standard guide for assessing the need for neonatal resuscitation.
- No single factor should be considered prognostic of poor neurologic outcome. A combination of factors, including severe metabolic acidemia and Apgar scores of ≤ 3 beyond 5 minutes of life, are included among the criteria that suggest the occurrence of intrapartum hypoxia of sufficient severity to cause long-term neurologic impairment. However, not all infants who fulfill these criteria suffer permanent neurologic injury.
- Severe mixed or metabolic acidemia—but not respiratory acidemia alone—is associated with a higher incidence of neonatal complications and death.
- During evaluation of the apneic neonate, assisted ventilation should be initiated promptly if tactile stimulation does not result in the initiation of spontaneous breathing.
- Room air rather than 100% oxygen should be used for initial neonatal resuscitation in term infants, and 21% to 30% oxygen should be administered in preterm infants. If necessary, the administration and titration of supplemental oxygen should be guided by pulse oximetry.
- ECG monitoring of the heart rate rather than clinical assessment of the heart rate provides a more accurate evaluation of response to resuscitation.
- Meconium-exposed neonates do not require intrapartum or postpartum nasopharyngeal and oropharyngeal suctioning. Meconium-stained fluid may represent evidence of fetal compromise; thus, the infant may be more likely to require neonatal resuscitation.
- In most circumstances, decisions about the initiation or continuation of resuscitation in the delivery room should be based on the neonate's response to resuscitative efforts rather than an estimation of gestational age. Parental desires should be considered when the prognosis for infant survival is poor.

REFERENCES

1. American Academy of Pediatrics and American College of Obstetricians and Gynecologists. *Guidelines for Perinatal Care*. 8th ed.; 2017.
2. Aziz K, Lee HC, Escobedo MB, et al. Part 5: Neonatal resuscitation: 2020 American Heart Association guidelines for cardiopulmonary resuscitation and emergency cardiovascular care. *Circulation*. 2020;142:S524–S550.
3. Wyckoff MH, Aziz K, Escobedo MB, et al. Part 13: Neonatal resuscitation: 2015 American Heart Association guidelines update for cardiopulmonary resuscitation and emergency cardiovascular care. *Circulation*. 2015;132:S543–S560.
4. American Society of Anesthesiologists. *Statement on optimal goals for anesthesia care in obstetrics* 2021 https://www.asahq.org/standards-and-practice-parameters/statement-on-optimal-goals-for-anesthesia-care-in-obstetrics. Accessed 25 January 2024.
5. Rudolph AM, Heyman MA. Fetal and neonatal circulation and respiration. *Ann Rev Physiol*. 1974;36:187–207.
6. Rudolph AM. The changes in the circulation after birth. Their importance in congenital heart disease. *Circulation*. 1970;41:343–359.
7. Cassin S, Dawes GS, Mott JC, et al. The vascular resistance of the foetal and newly ventilated lung of the lamb. *J Physiol*. 1964;171:61–79.
8. Rudolph AM, Yuan S. Response of the pulmonary vasculature to hypoxia and H+ ion concentration changes. *J Clin Invest*. 1966;45:399–411.
9. Boreus LO, Malmfors T, McMurphy DM, Olson L. Demonstration of adrenergic receptor function and innervation in the ductus arteriosus of the human fetus. *Acta Physiol Scand*. 1969;77:316–321.
10. Assali NS, Morris JA, Smith RW, Manson WA. Studies on ductus arteriosus circulation. *Circ Res*. 1963;13:478–489.
11. Dimich I, Singh PP, Adell A, et al. Evaluation of oxygen saturation monitoring by pulse oximetry in neonates in the delivery system. *Can J Anaesth*. 1991;38:985–988.
12. Walsh-Sukys MC. Persistent pulmonary hypertension of the newborn. The black box revisited. *Clin Perinatol*. 1993;20:127–143.
13. Alano MA, Ngougmna E, Ostrea EM Jr, Konduri GG. Analysis of nonsteroidal antiinflammatory drugs in meconium and its relation to persistent pulmonary hypertension of the newborn. *Pediatrics*. 2001;107:519–523.
14. Adams FH, Moss AJ, Fagan L. The tracheal fluid in the fetal lamb. *Biol Neonat*. 1963;5:151–158.
15. Ross BB. Comparison of foetal pulmonary fluid with foetal plasma and amniotic fluid. *Nature*. 1963;199:1100.
16. Karlberg P. The adaptive changes in the immediate postnatal period, with particular reference to respiration. *J Pediatr*. 1960;56:585–604.
17. Alhassen Z, Vali P, Guglani L, et al. Recent advances in pathophysiology and management of transient tachypnea of newborn. *J Perinatol*. 2021;41:6–16.
18. Lawson EE, Birdwell RL, Huang PS, Taeusch HW Jr. Augmentation of pulmonary surfactant secretion by lung expansion at birth. *Pediatr Res*. 1979;13:611–614.
19. Platzker AC, Kitterman JA, Mescher EJ, et al. Surfactant in the lung and tracheal fluid of the fetal lamb and acceleration of its appearance by dexamethasone. *Pediatrics*. 1975;56:554–561.

20. Smrcek JM, Schwartau N, Kohl M, et al. Antenatal corticosteroid therapy in premature infants. *Arch Gynecol Obstet.* 2005;271:26–32.

21. Turbeville DF, McCaffree MA, Block MF, Krous HF. In utero distal pulmonary meconium aspiration. *South Med J.* 1979;72:535–536.

22. Hillman NH, Kallapur SG, Jobe AH. Physiology of transition from intrauterine to extrauterine life. *Clin Perinatol.* 2012;39:769–783.

23. Dahm LS, James LS. Newborn temperature and calculated heat loss in the delivery room. *Pediatrics.* 1972;49:504–513.

24. Cramer K, Wiebe N, Hartling L, et al. Heat loss prevention: a systematic review of occlusive skin wrap for premature neonates. *J Perinatol.* 2005;25:763–769.

25. Vohra S, Roberts RS, Zhang B, et al. Heat loss prevention (HeLP) in the delivery room: a randomized controlled trial of polyethylene occlusive skin wrapping in very preterm infants. *J Pediatr.* 2004;145:750–753.

26. Duryea EL, Nelson DB, Wyckoff MH, et al. The impact of ambient operating room temperature on neonatal and maternal hypothermia and associated morbidities: a randomized controlled trial. *Am J Obstet Gynecol.* 2016;214:505.e1–e7.

27. Jacobs SE, Berg M, Hunt R, et al. Cooling for newborns with hypoxic ischaemic encephalopathy. *Cochrane Database Syst Rev.* 2013;(1):CD003311.

28. Volpe JJ. Perinatal brain injury: from pathogenesis to neuro-protection. *Ment Retard Dev Disabil Res Rev.* 2001;7:56–64.

29. Sultan P, David AL, Fernando R, Ackland GL. Inflammation and epidural-related maternal fever: proposed mechanisms. *Anesth Analg.* 2016;122:1546–1553.

30. Kaul B, Vallejo M, Ramanathan S, Mandell G. Epidural labor analgesia and neonatal sepsis evaluation rate: a quality improvement study. *Anesth Analg.* 2001;93:986–990.

31. Feldman-Winter L, Goldsmith JP. Committee on Fetus and Newborn, Task Force on Sudden Infant Death Syndrome. Safe sleep and skin-to-skin care in the neonatal period for healthy term newborns. *Pediatrics.* 2016;138:e20161889

32. American Academy of Pediatrics and American Heart Association. *Textbook of Neonatal Resuscitation.* 8th ed. American Academy of Pediatrics; 2021.

33. Gordon A, McKechnie EJ, Jeffery H. Pediatric presence at cesarean section: justified or not? *Am J Obstet Gynecol.* 2005;193:599–605.

34. Atherton N, Parsons SJ, Mansfield P. Attendance of paediatricians at elective caesarean sections performed under regional anaesthesia: is it warranted? *J Paediatr Child Health.* 2006;42:332–336.

35. Algert CS, Bowen JR, Giles WB, et al. Regional block versus general anaesthesia for caesarean section and neonatal outcomes: a population-based study. *BMC Med.* 2009;7:20.

36. Hook B, Kiwi R, Amini SB, et al. Neonatal morbidity after elective repeat cesarean section and trial of labor. *Pediatrics.* 1997;100:348–353.

37. Apgar V. A proposal for a new method of evaluation of the newborn infant. *Curr Res Anesth Analg.* 1953;32:260–267.

38. Apgar V. The newborn (Apgar) scoring system. Reflections and advice. *Pediatr Clin North Am.* 1966;13:645–650.

39. Apgar V, James LS. Further observations on the newborn scoring system. *Am J Dis Child.* 1962;104:419–428.

40. Sykes GS, Molloy PM, Johnson P, et al. Do Apgar scores indicate asphyxia? *Lancet.* 1982;1:494–496.

41. Lauener PA, Calame A, Janecek P, et al. Systematic pH-measurements in the umbilical artery: causes and predictive value of neonatal acidosis. *J Perinat Med.* 1983;11:278–285.

42. Suidan JS, Young BK. Outcome of fetuses with lactic acidemia. *Am J Obstet Gynecol.* 1984;150:33–37.

43. Fields LM, Entman SS, Boehm FH. Correlation of the one-minute Apgar score and the pH value of umbilical arterial blood. *South Med J.* 1983;76:1477–1479.

44. Boehm FH, Fields LM, Entman SS, Vaughn WK. Correlation of the one-minute Apgar score and umbilical cord acid-base status. *South Med J.* 1986;79:429–431.

45. Page FO, Martin JN, Palmer SM, et al. Correlation of neonatal acid-base status with Apgar scores and fetal heart rate tracings. *Am J Obstet Gynecol.* 1986;154:1306–1311.

46. Luthy DA, Shy KK, Strickland D, et al. Status of infants at birth and risk for adverse neonatal events and long-term sequelae: a study in low birth weight infants. *Am J Obstet Gynecol.* 1987;157:676–679.

47. Josten BE, Johnson TR, Nelson JP. Umbilical cord blood pH and Apgar scores as an index of neonatal health. *Am J Obstet Gynecol.* 1987;157:843–848.

48. Vintzileosm AM, Gaffney SE, Salinger LM, et al. The relationships among the fetal biophysical profile, umbilical cord pH, and Apgar scores. *Am J Obstet Gynecol.* 1987;157:627–631.

49. Drage JS, Kennedy C, Berendes H, et al. The Apgar score as an index of infant morbidity. A report from the collaborative study of cerebral palsy. *Dev Med Child Neurol.* 1966;8:141–148.

50. Drage JS, Kennedy C, Schwarz BK. The Apgar score as an index of neonatal mortality. A report from the collaborative study of cerebral palsy. *Obstet Gynecol.* 1964;24:222–230.

51. American College of Obstetricians and Gynecologists and the American Academy of Pediatrics. The Apgar score. *Pediatrics.* 2015;136:819–822.

52. American College of Obstetrics and Gynecologists, American Academy of Pediatrics. *Neonatal Encephalopathy and Neurologic Outcome.* 2nd ed. American College of Obstetrics and Gynecologists; 2014.

53. White CR, Mok T, Doherty DA, et al. The effect of time, temperature and storage device on umbilical cord blood gas and lactate measurement: a randomized controlled trial. *J Matern Fetal Neonatal Med.* 2012;25:587–594.

54. Strickland DM, Gilstrap LC 3rd, Hauth JC, Widmer K. Umbilical cord pH and PCO2: effect of interval from delivery to determination. *Am J Obstet Gynecol.* 1984;148:191–194.

55. Miller JM Jr, Bernard M, Brown HL, et al. Umbilical cord blood gases for term healthy newborns. *Am J Perinatol.* 1990;7:157–159.

56. Olofsson P. Umbilical cord pH, blood gases, and lactate at birth: normal values, interpretation, and clinical utility. *Am J Obstet Gynecol.* 2023;228:S1222–S1240.

57. Helwig JT, Parer JT, Kilpatrick SJ, Laros RK Jr. Umbilical cord blood acid-base state: what is normal? *Am J Obstet Gynecol.* 1996;174:1807–1812.

58. Thorp JA, Sampson JE, Parisi VM, Creasy RK. Routine umbilical cord blood gas determinations? *Am J Obstet Gynecol.* 1989;161:600–605.

59. Vintzileos AM, Egan JF, Campbell WA, et al. Asphyxia at birth as determined by cord blood pH measurements in preterm and term gestations: correlations with neonatal outcome. *J Matern Fetal Med.* 1992;1:7–13.

60. Cahill AG. Intrapartum fetal evaluation. In: MB L, Galan H, Jauniaux E, et al., eds. *Gabbe's Obstetrics: Normal and Problem Pregnancies*. 8th ed. Elsevier; 2021:267–294.

61. Goldaber KG, Gilstrap LC 3rd, Leveno KJ, et al. Pathologic fetal acidemia. *Obstet Gynecol*. 1991;78:1103–1107.

62. Casey BM, McIntire DD, Leveno KJ. The continuing value of the Apgar score for the assessment of newborn infants. *N Engl J Med*. 2001;344:467–471.

63. Yeh P, Emary K, Impey L. The relationship between umbilical cord arterial pH and serious adverse neonatal outcome: analysis of 51,519 consecutive validated samples. *BJOG*. 2012;119:824–831.

64. Huddleston JF. Intrapartum fetal assessment. A review. *Clin Perinatol*. 1999;26:549–568.

65. Hafstrom M, Ehnberg S, Blad S, et al. Developmental outcome at 6.5 years after acidosis in term newborns: a population-based study. *Pediatrics*. 2012;129:e1501–e1507.

66. Jennis MS, Peabody JL. Pulse oximetry: an alternative method for the assessment of oxygenation in newborn infants. *Pediatrics*. 1987;79:524–528.

67. Kopotic RJ, Lindner W. Assessing high-risk infants in the delivery room with pulse oximetry. *Anesth Analg*. 2002;94:S31–S36.

68. Kamlin CO, O'Donnell CP, Everest NJ, et al. Accuracy of clinical assessment of infant heart rate in the delivery room. *Resuscitation*. 2006;71:319–321.

69. Sarnat HB, Sarnat MS. Neonatal encephalopathy following fetal distress. A clinical and electroencephalographic study. *Arch Neurol*. 1976;33:696–705.

70. Dubowitz LM, Dubowitz V, Goldberg C. Clinical assessment of gestational age in the newborn infant. *J Pediatr*. 1970; 77:1–10.

71. Ballard JL, Novak KK, Driver M. A simplified score for assessment of fetal maturation of newly born infants. *J Pediatr*. 1979;95:769–774.

72. Sanders M, Allen M, Alexander GR, et al. Gestational age assessment in preterm neonates weighing less than 1500 grams. *Pediatrics*. 1991;88:542–546.

73. Ballard JL, Khoury JC, Wedig K, et al. New Ballard score, expanded to include extremely premature infants. *J Pediatr*. 1991;119:417–423.

74. Yamada NK, Szyld E, Strand ML, et al. 2023 American Heart Association and American Academy of Pediatrics focused update on neonatal resuscitation: an update to the American Heart Association Guidelines for Cardiopulmonary Resuscitation and Emergency Cardiovascular Care. *Circulation*. 2024;149:e157–e166.

75. Rabe H, Reynolds G, Diaz-Rossello J. A systematic review and meta-analysis of a brief delay in clamping the umbilical cord of preterm infants. *Neonatology*. 2008;93:138–144.

76. Kaempf JW, Tomlinson MW, Kaempf AJ, et al. Delayed umbilical cord clamping in premature neonates. *Obstet Gynecol*. 2012;120:325–330.

77. Katheria A, Poeltler D, Durham J, et al. Neonatal resuscitation with an intact cord: a randomized clinical trial. *J Pediatr*. 2016;178:75–80.e3.

78. Katheria A, Lee HC, Knol R, et al. A review of different resuscitation platforms during delayed cord clamping. *J Perinatol*. 2021;41:1540–1548.

79. Schubring C. Temperature regulation in healthy and resuscitated newborns immediately after birth. *J Perinat Med*. 1986;14:27–33.

80. Gluckman PD, Wyatt JS, Azzopardi D, et al. Selective head cooling with mild systemic hypothermia after neonatal encephalopathy: multicentre randomised trial. *Lancet*. 2005;365:663–670.

81. Shankaran S, Laptook AR, Ehrenkranz RA, et al. Whole-body hypothermia for neonates with hypoxic-ischemic encephalopathy. *N Engl J Med*. 2005;353:1574–1584.

82. Papile LA. Systemic hypothermia – a "cool" therapy for neonatal hypoxic-ischemic encephalopathy. *N Engl J Med*. 2005;353:1619–1620.

83. Solberg R, Andresen JH, Escrig R, et al. Resuscitation of hypoxic newborn piglets with oxygen induces a dose-dependent increase in markers of oxidation. *Pediatr Res*. 2007;62:559–563.

84. Davis PG, Tan A, O'Donnell CP, Schulze A. Resuscitation of newborn infants with 100% oxygen or air: a systematic review and meta-analysis. *Lancet*. 2004;364:1329–1333.

85. Lui K, Jones LJ, Foster JP, et al. Lower versus higher oxygen concentrations titrated to target oxygen saturations during resuscitation of preterm infants at birth. *Cochrane Database Syst Rev*. 2018;(5):CD010239.

86. Vyas H, Milner AD, Hopkin IE, Boon AW. Physiologic responses to prolonged and slow-rise inflation in the resuscitation of the asphyxiated newborn infant. *J Pediatr*. 1981;99:635–639.

87. Thach BT, Taeusch HW Jr. Sighing in newborn human infants: role of inflation-augmenting reflex. *J Appl Physiol*. 1976;41:502–507.

88. Cordero L Jr, Hon EH. Neonatal bradycardia following nasopharyngeal stimulation. *J Pediatr*. 1971;78: 441–447.

89. Young RS, Hessert TR, Pritchard GA, Yagel SK. Naloxone exacerbates hypoxic-ischemic brain injury in the neonatal rat. *Am J Obstet Gynecol*. 1984;150:52–56.

90. Chernick V, Manfreda J, De Booy V, et al. Clinical trial of naloxone in birth asphyxia. *J Pediatr*. 1988;113:519–525.

91. Sherman JM, Lowitt S, Stephenson C, Ironson G. Factors influencing acquired subgottic stenosis in infants. *J Pediatr*. 1986;109:322–327.

92. Laing IA, Cowan DL, Ballantine GM, Hume R. Prevention of subglottic stenosis in neonatal ventilation. *Int J Pediatr Otorhinolaryngol*. 1986;11:61–66.

93. Ngan AY, Cheung PY, Hudson-Mason A, et al. Using exhaled CO2 to guide initial respiratory support at birth: a randomised controlled trial. *Arch Dis Child Fetal Neonatal Ed*. 2017;102:F525–F531.

94. Singh R, Mohan CVR, Taxak SMC. Controlled trial to evaluate the use of LMA for neonatal resuscitation. *J Anaesthesiol Clin Pharmacol*. 2005;21:303–306.

95. Trevisanuto D, Micaglio M, Pitton M, et al. Laryngeal mask airway: is the management of neonates requiring positive pressure ventilation at birth changing? *Resuscitation*. 2004;62:151–157.

96. Zanardo V, Weiner G, Micaglio M, et al. Delivery room resuscitation of near-term infants: role of the laryngeal mask airway. *Resuscitation*. 2010;81:327–330.

97. Jain L, Vidyasagar D. Cardiopulmonary resuscitation of newborns. Its application to transport medicine. *Pediatr Clin North Am*. 1993;40:287–302.

98. Orlowski JP. Optimum position for external cardiac compression in infants and young children. *Ann Emerg Med*. 1986;15:667–673.

99. Phillips GW, Zideman DA. Relation of infant heart to sternum: its significance in cardiopulmonary resuscitation. *Lancet.* 1986;1:1024–1025.

100. Finholt DA, Kettrick RG, Wagner HR, Swedlow DB. The heart is under the lower third of the sternum. Implications for external cardiac massage. *Am J Dis Child.* 1986;140: 646–649.

101. Dean JM, Koehler RC, Schleien CL, et al. Age-related effects of compression rate and duration in cardiopulmonary resuscitation. *J Appl Physiol.* 1990;68:554–560.

102. Fitzgerald KR, Babbs CF, Frissora HA, et al. Cardiac output during cardiopulmonary resuscitation at various compression rates and durations. *Am J Physiol.* 1981;241:H442–H448.

103. Babbs CF, Tacker WA, Paris RL, et al. CPR with simultaneous compression and ventilation at high airway pressure in 4 animal models. *Crit Care Med.* 1982;10:501–504.

104. Halling C, Sparks JE, Christie L, Wyckoff MH. Efficacy of intravenous and endotracheal epinephrine during neonatal cardiopulmonary resuscitation in the delivery room. *J Pediatr.* 2017;185:232–236.

105. Schleien CL, Dean JM, Koehler RC, et al. Effect of epinephrine on cerebral and myocardial perfusion in an infant animal preparation of cardiopulmonary resuscitation. *Circulation.* 1986;73:809–817.

106. Simmons MA, Adcock EW 3rd, Bard H, Battaglia FC. Hypernatremia and intracranial hemorrhage in neonates. *N Engl J Med.* 1974;291:6–10.

107. Papile LA, Burstein J, Burstein R, et al. Relationship of intravenous sodium bicarbonate infusions and cerebral intraventricular hemorrhage. *J Pediatr.* 1978;93:834–836.

108. Kette F, Weil MH, Gazmuri RJ. Buffer solutions may compromise cardiac resuscitation by reducing coronary perfusion presssure (erratum in JAMA 1991;266:3286). *JAMA.* 1991;266:2121–2126.

109. Kette F, Weil MH, von Planta M, et al. Buffer agents do not reverse intramyocardial acidosis during cardiac resuscitation. *Circulation.* 1990;81:1660–1666.

110. Changaris DG, Purohit DM, Balentine JD, et al. Brain calcification in severely stressed neonates receiving parenteral calcium. *J Pediatr.* 1984;104:941–946.

111. Tam EW, Haeusslein LA, Bonifacio SL, et al. Hypoglycemia is associated with increased risk for brain injury and adverse neurodevelopmental outcome in neonates at risk for encephalopathy. *J Pediatr.* 2012;161:88–93.

112. Fiser DH. Intraosseous infusion. *N Engl J Med.* 1990;322:1579–1581.

113. Hodge D 3rd, Delgado-Paredes C, Fleisher G. Intraosseous infusion flow rates in hypovolemic "pediatric" dogs. *Ann Emerg Med.* 1987;16:305–307.

114. Redmond AD, Plunkett PK. Intraosseous infusion. *Arch Emerg Med.* 1986;3:231–233.

115. La Fleche FR, Slepin MJ, Vargas J, Milzman DP. Iatrogenic bilateral tibial fractures after intraosseous infusion attempts in a 3-month-old infant. *Ann Emerg Med.* 1989;18:1099–1101.

116. Rosetti VA, Thompson BM, Miller J, et al. Intraosseous infusion: an alternative route of pediatric intravascular access. *Ann Emerg Med.* 1985;14:885–888.

117. Quilligan JJ Jr, Turkel H. Bone marrow infusion and its complications. *Am J Dis Child.* 1946;71:457–465.

118. Heinild S, Sondergaard T, Tudvad F. Bone marrow infusion in childhood experiences from a thousand infusions. *J Pediatr.* 1947;30:400–412.

119. Brown CA, Desmond MM, Lindley JE, Moore J. Meconium staining of the amniotic fluid; a marker of fetal hypoxia. *Obstet Gynecol.* 1957;9:91–103.

120. Matthews TG, Warshaw JB. Relevance of the gestational age distribution of meconium passage in utero. *Pediatrics.* 1979;64:30–31.

121. Osman A, Halling C, Crume M, et al. Meconium aspiration syndrome: a comprehensive review. *J Perinatol.* 2023;43: 1211–1221.

122. Wiswell TE, Tuggle JM, Turner BS. Meconium aspiration syndrome: have we made a difference? *Pediatrics.* 1990;85:715–721.

123. Singh BS, Clark RH, Powers RJ, Spitzer AR. Meconium aspiration syndrome remains a significant problem in the NICU: outcomes and treatment patterns in term neonates admitted for intensive care during a ten-year period. *J Perinatol.* 2009;29:497–503.

124. Davis RO, Philips JB 3rd, Harris BA Jr, et al. Fatal meconium aspiration syndrome occurring despite airway management considered appropriate. *Am J Obstet Gynecol.* 1985;151: 731–736.

125. Falciglia HS, Henderschott C, Potter P, Helmchen R. Does DeLee suction at the perineum prevent meconium aspiration syndrome? *Am J Obstet Gynecol.* 1992;167: 1243–1249.

126. Linder N, Aranda JV, Tsur M, et al. Need for endotracheal intubation and suction in meconium-stained neonates. *J Pediatr.* 1988;112:613–615.

127. American College of Obstetricians and Gynecologists. Committee Opinion No. 689: Delivery of a newborn with meconium-stained amniotic fluid (reaffirmed 2024). *Obstet Gynecol.* 2017;129:e33–e34.

128. Vain NE, Szyld EG, Prudent LM, et al. Oropharyngeal and nasopharyngeal suctioning of meconium-stained neonates before delivery of their shoulders: multicentre, randomised controlled trial. *Lancet.* 2004;364:597–602.

129. Fraser WD, Hofmeyr J, Lede R, et al. Amnioinfusion for the prevention of the meconium aspiration syndrome. *N Engl J Med.* 2005;353:909–917.

130. Ross MG. Meconium aspiration syndrome – more than intrapartum meconium. *N Engl J Med.* 2005;353:946–948.

131. Bell EF, Hintz SR, Hansen NI, et al. Mortality, in-hospital morbidity, care practices, and 2-year outcomes for extremely preterm infants in the US, 2013-2018. *JAMA.* 2022;327: 248–263.

132. Pande GS, Vagha JD. A review of the occurrence of intraventricular hemorrhage in preterm newborns and its future neurodevelopmental consequences. *Cureus.* 2023;15:e48968.

133. Tortorolo G, Luciano R, Papacci P, Tonelli T. Intraventricular hemorrhage: past, present and future, focusing on classification, pathogenesis and prevention. *Childs Nerv Syst.* 1999;15:652–661.

134. Perlman JM, McMenamin JB, Volpe JJ. Fluctuating cerebral blood-flow velocity in respiratory-distress syndrome. Relation to the development of intraventricular hemorrhage. *N Engl J Med.* 1983;309:204–209.

135. Perlman JM, Volpe JJ. Are venous circulatory abnormalities important in the pathogenesis of hemorrhagic and/or ischemic cerebral injury? *Pediatrics.* 1987;80:705–711.

136. Goddard J, Lewis RM, Armstrong DL, Zeller RS. Moderate, rapidly induced hypertension as a cause of intraventricular

hemorrhage in the newborn beagle model. *J Pediatr.* 1980;96:1057–1060.

137. Goldberg RN, Chung D, Goldman SL, Bancalari E. The association of rapid volume expansion and intraventricular hemorrhage in the preterm infant. *J Pediatr.* 1980;96:1060–1063.

138. Nakamura Y, Okudera T, Fukuda S, Hashimoto T. Germinal matrix hemorrhage of venous origin in preterm neonates. *Hum Pathol.* 1990;21:1059–1062.

139. Van de Bor M, Briet E, Van Bel F, Ruys JH. Hemostasis and periventricular-intraventricular hemorrhage of the newborn. *Am J Dis Child.* 1986;140:1131–1134.

140. Goldstein GW. Pathogenesis of brain edema and hemorrhage: role of the brain capillary. *Pediatrics.* 1979;64:357–360.

141. Gould SJ, Howard S. An immunohistochemical study of the germinal layer in the late gestation human fetal brain. *Neuropathol Appl Neurobiol.* 1987;13:421–437.

142. Goldenberg RL, Hauth JC, Andrews WW. Intrauterine infection and preterm delivery. *N Engl J Med.* 2000;342:1500–1507.

143. Moise AA, Wearden ME, Kozinetz CA, et al. Antenatal steroids are associated with less need for blood pressure support in extremely premature infants. *Pediatrics.* 1995;95:845–850.

144. Wallace EM, Baker LS. Effect of antenatal betamethasone administration on placental vascular resistance. *Lancet.* 1999;353:1404–1407.

145. American College of Obstetricians and Gynecologists. Committee Opinion No. 713: Antenatal corticosteroid therapy for fetal maturation (reaffirmed 2024). *Obstet Gynecol.* 2017;130:e102–e109.

146. Nelson KB, Grether JK. Can magnesium sulfate reduce the risk of cerebral palsy in very low birthweight infants? *Pediatrics.* 1995;95:263–269.

147. Paneth N, Jetton J, Pinto-Martin J, Susser M. Magnesium sulfate in labor and risk of neonatal brain lesions and cerebral palsy in low birth weight infants. The Neonatal Brain Hemorrhage Study Analysis Group. *Pediatrics.* 1997;99:e1.

148. Crowther CA, Hiller JE, Doyle LW, Haslam RR. Effect of magnesium sulfate given for neuroprotection before preterm birth: a randomized controlled trial. *JAMA.* 2003;290:2669–2676.

149. Marret S, Doyle LW, Crowther CA, Middleton P. Antenatal magnesium sulphate neuroprotection in the preterm infant. *Semin Fetal Neonatal Med.* 2007;12:311–317.

150. Rouse DJ, Hirtz DG, Thom E, et al. A randomized, controlled trial of magnesium sulfate for the prevention of cerebral palsy. *N Engl J Med.* 2008;359:895–905.

151. American College of Obstetricians and Gynecologists. Committee Opinion No. 455: Magnesium sulfate before anticipated preterm birth for neuroprotection (reaffirmed 2023). *Obstet Gynecol.* 2010;115:669–671.

152. Hirtz DG, Nelson K. Magnesium sulfate and cerebral palsy in premature infants. *Curr Opin Pediatr.* 1998;10:131–137.

153. Mittendorf R, Dambrosia J, Pryde PG, et al. Association between the use of antenatal magnesium sulfate in preterm labor and adverse health outcomes in infants. *Am J Obstet Gynecol.* 2002;186:1111–1118.

154. Johnson LH, Mapp DC, Rouse DJ, et al. Association of cord blood magnesium concentration and neonatal resuscitation. *J Pediatr.* 2012;160:573–577.e1.

155. Yanowitz TD. Cerebrovascular autoregulation among very low birth weight infants. *J Perinatol.* 2011;31:689–691.

156. Liechty KW, Crombleholme TM, Flake AW, et al. Intrapartum airway management for giant fetal neck masses: the EXIT (ex utero intrapartum treatment) procedure. *Am J Obstet Gynecol.* 1997;177:870–874.

157. Mosquera MS, Yuter S, Flake AW. Perinatal management of the anticipated difficult airway. *Semin Fetal Neonatal Med.* 2023;28:101485.

158. Crombleholme TM, Sylvester K, Flake AW, Adzick NS. Salvage of a fetus with congenital high airway obstruction syndrome by ex utero intrapartum treatment (EXIT) procedure. *Fetal Diagn Ther.* 2000;15:280–282.

159. Spiers A, Legendre G, Biquard F, et al. Ex utero intrapartum technique (EXIT): indications, procedure methods and materno-fetal complications – a literature review. *J Gynecol Obstet Hum Reprod.* 2022;51:102252.

160. Hoagland MA, Chatterjee D. Anesthesia for fetal surgery. *Paediatr Anaesth.* 2017;27:346–357.

161. Ngamprasertwong P, Vinks AA, Boat A. Update in fetal anesthesia for the ex utero intrapartum treatment (EXIT) procedure. *Int Anesthesiol Clin.* 2012;50:26–40.

162. Boat A, Mahmoud M, Michelfelder EC, et al. Supplementing desflurane with intravenous anesthesia reduces fetal cardiac dysfunction during open fetal surgery. *Paediatr Anaesth.* 2010;20:748–756.

163. Caponas G. Glyceryl trinitrate and acute uterine relaxation: a literature review. *Anaesth Intensive Care.* 2001;29:163–177.

164. Kumar K, Miron C, Singh SI. Maternal anesthesia for EXIT procedure: a systematic review of literature. *J Anaesthesiol Clin Pharmacol.* 2019;35:19–24.

165. Shaw-Smith C. Oesophageal atresia, tracheo-oesophageal fistula, and the VACTERL association: review of genetics and epidemiology. *J Med Genet.* 2006;43:545–554.

166. Paoletti M, Raffler G, Gaffi MS, et al. Prevalence and risk factors for congenital diaphragmatic hernia: a global view. *J Pediatr Surg.* 2020;55:2297–2307.

167. Doktor F, Antounians L, Miller J, et al. Seasonal variation of congenital diaphragmatic hernia: a review of the literature and database report from the United States and Canada. *Eur J Pediatr Surg.* 2023;33:11–16.

168. American College of Obstetricians and Gynecologists and Society for Maternal-Fetal Medicine. Obstetric Care Consensus No. 6: Periviable birth (reaffirmed 2025). *Obstet Gynecol.* 2017;130:e187–e199.

169. Brazelton TB, Scholl ML, Robey JS. Visual responses in the newborn. *Pediatrics.* 1966;37:284–290.

170. Ball W, Tronick E. Infant responses to impending collision: optical and real. *Science.* 1971;171:818–820.

171. Kearsley RB. The newborn's response to auditory stimulation: a demonstration of orienting and defensive behavior. *Child Dev.* 1973;44:582–590.

172. Brazelton TB. *Neonatal Behavior Assessment Scale.* Spastics International Medical Publications, William Heinemann Medical Books; 1973.

173. Scanlon JW, Brown WU Jr, Weiss JB, Alper MH. Neurobehavioral responses of newborn infants after maternal epidural anesthesia. *Anesthesiology.* 1974;40:121–128.

174. Amiel-Tison C, Barrier G, Shnider SM, et al. A new neurologic and adaptive capacity scoring system for evaluating obstetric medications in full-term newborns. *Anesthesiology.* 1982;56:340–350.

175. Brockhurst NJ, Littleford JA, Halpern SH. The neurologic and adaptive capacity score: a systematic review of its use in obstetric anesthesia research. *Anesthesiology.* 2000;92:237–246.

176. Camann W, Brazelton TB. Use and abuse of neonatal neurobehavioral testing. *Anesthesiology.* 2000;92:3–5.

177. Halpern SH, Littleford JA, Brockhurst NJ, et al. The neurologic and adaptive capacity score is not a reliable method of newborn evaluation. *Anesthesiology.* 2001;94:958–962.

178. Amiel-Tison C. Update of the Amiel-Tison neurologic assessment for the term neonate or at 40 weeks corrected age. *Pediatr Neurol.* 2002;27:196–212.

179. Brackbill Y, Kane J, Manniello RL, Abramson D. Obstetric meperidine usage and assessment of neonatal status. *Anesthesiology.* 1974;40:116–120.

180. Dailey PA, Baysinger CL, Levinson G, Shnider SM. Neurobehavioral testing of the newborn infant. Effects of obstetric anesthesia. *Clin Perinatol.* 1982;9:191–214.

181. Hodgkinson R, Bhatt M, Wang CN. Double-blind comparison of the neurobehaviour of neonates following the administration of different doses of meperidine to the mother. *Can Anaesth Soc J.* 1978;25:405–411.

182. Lieberman BA, Rosenblatt DB, Belsey E, et al. The effects of maternally administered pethidine or epidural bupivacaine on the fetus and newborn. *Br J Obstet Gynaecol.* 1979;86:598–606.

183. Rayburn WF, Smith CV, Leuschen MP, et al. Comparison of patient-controlled and nurse-administered analgesia using intravenous fentanyl during labor. *Anesthesiol Rev.* 1991;18:31–36.

184. Kileff ME, James FM 3rd, Dewan DM, Floyd HM. Neonatal neurobehavioral responses after epidural anesthesia for cesarean section using lidocaine and bupivacaine. *Anesth Analg.* 1984;63:413–417.

185. Brown WU, Bell GC, Lurie AO, et al. Newborn blood levels of lidocaine and mepivacaine in the first postnatal day following maternal epidural anesthesia. *Anesthesiology.* 1975;42:698–707.

186. Datta S, Corke BC, Alper MH, et al. Epidural anesthesia for cesarean section: a comparison of bupivacaine, chloroprocaine, and etidocaine. *Anesthesiology.* 1980;52:48–51.

187. Kuhnert BR, Harrison MJ, Linn PL, Kuhnert PM. Effects of maternal epidural anesthesia on neonatal behavior. *Anesth Analg.* 1984;63:301–308.

188. Sepkoski CM, Lester BM, Ostheimer GW, Brazelton TB. The effects of maternal epidural anesthesia on neonatal behavior during the first month. *Dev Med Child Neurol.* 1992;34:1072–1080.

189. Abboud TK, Khoo SS, Miller F, et al. Maternal, fetal, and neonatal responses after epidural anesthesia with bupivacaine, 2-chloroprocaine, or lidocaine. *Anesth Analg.* 1982;61:638–644.

190. Tronick E. A critique of the neonatal neurologic and adaptive capacity score (NACS). *Anesthesiology.* 1982;56:338–339.

191. Hodgkinson R, Bhatt M, Kim SS, et al. Neonatal neurobehavioral tests following cesarean section under general and spinal anesthesia. *Am J Obstet Gynecol.* 1978;132:670–674.

192. Hughes SC, Rosen MA, Shnider SM, et al. Maternal and neonatal effects of epidural morphine for labor and delivery. *Anesth Analg.* 1984;63:319–324.

193. Preston PG, Rosen MA, Hughes SC, et al. Epidural anesthesia with fentanyl and lidocaine for cesarean section: maternal effects and neonatal outcome. *Anesthesiology.* 1988;68:938–943.

194. Murakawa K, Abboud TK, Yanagi T, et al. Clinical experience of epidural fentanyl for labor pain. *J Anesth.* 1987;1:93–95.

195. Cohen SE, Tan S, Albright GA, Halpern J. Epidural fentanyl/bupivacaine mixtures for obstetric analgesia. *Anesthesiology.* 1987;67:403–407.

196. Abboud TK, Afrasiabi A, Zhu J, et al. Epidural morphine or butorphanol augments bupivacaine analgesia during labor. *Reg Anesth.* 1989;14:115–120.

197. Abboud TK, Zhu J, Afrasiabi A, et al. Epidural butorphanol augments lidocaine sensory anesthesia during labor. *Reg Anesth.* 1991;16:265–267.

198. Abboud TK, David S, Nagappala S, et al. Maternal, fetal, and neonatal effects of lidocaine with and without epinephrine for epidural anesthesia in obstetrics. *Anesth Analg.* 1984;63:973–979.

199. Abboud TK, Sheik-ol-Eslam A, Yanagi T, et al. Safety and efficacy of epinephrine added to bupivacaine for lumbar epidural analgesia in obstetrics. *Anesth Analg.* 1985;64:585–591.

200. Abboud TK, DerSarkissian L, Terrasi J, et al. Comparative maternal, fetal, and neonatal effects of chloroprocaine with and without epinephrine for epidural anesthesia in obstetrics. *Anesth Analg.* 1987;66:71–75.

201. Abboud TK, Afrasiabi A, Zhu J, et al. Bupivacaine/butorphanol/epinephrine for epidural anesthesia in obstetrics: maternal and neonatal effects. *Reg Anesth.* 1989;14:219–224.

202. Abboud TK, Nagappala S, Murakawa K, et al. Comparison of the effects of general and regional anesthesia for cesarean section on neonatal neurologic and adaptive capacity scores. *Anesth Analg.* 1985;64:996–1000.

203. Palahniuk RJ, Scatliff J, Biehl D, et al. Maternal and neonatal effects of methoxyflurane, nitrous oxide and lumbar epidural anaesthesia for caesarean section. *Can Anaesth Soc J.* 1977;24:586–596.

204. Stefani SJ, Hughes SC, Schnider SM, et al. Neonatal neurobehavioral effects of inhalation analgesia for vaginal delivery. *Anesthesiology.* 1982;56:351–355.

205. Abboud TK, Gangolly J, Mosaad P, Crowell D. Isoflurane in obstetrics. *Anesth Analg.* 1989;68:388–391.

206. Sprung J, Flick RP, Wilder RT, et al. Anesthesia for cesarean delivery and learning disabilities in a population-based birth cohort. *Anesthesiology.* 2009;111:302–310.

207. U.S. Food & Drug Administration. *FDA drug safety communication: FDA review results in new warnings about using general anesthetics and sedation drugs in young children and pregnant women.* 2016. www.fda.gov/Drugs/DrugSafety/ucm532356.htm. Accessed 24 January 2025.

10

Fetal and Neonatal Neurologic Injury

Tania F. Esakoff, MD, Sarah J. Kilpatrick, MD, PhD, and Arvind Palanisamy, MBBS, MD, FRCA

CHAPTER OUTLINE

The detection and diagnosis of fetal and neonatal brain injury have been advanced by improvements in functional imaging and the identification of potential biochemical markers. Evidence indicates that inflammatory mediators play an important role in the pathophysiology of fetal brain injury. Maternal administration of magnesium sulfate before anticipated early preterm birth reduces the risk for cerebral palsy in surviving infants. Induced hypothermia is beneficial for the treatment of neonatal hypoxic-ischemic encephalopathy. Rodent and nonhuman primate data suggest that fetal exposure to anesthetic agents may have harmful effects on neurogenesis and synapse formation in the developing brain. However, little progress has been made in reducing the incidence of neonatal brain injury and cerebral palsy.

FETAL BRAIN DEVELOPMENT

Generation of the various cell types that populate the developing brain, and their subsequent layering and organization, is a precisely regulated process encoded by genetic programs and modified by epigenetic influences.[1–4] Although such neurodevelopmental processes occur throughout the human life span, they are most robust and dynamic during the perinatal period.[5] Much of our understanding comes from studies in rodents and nonhuman primates.[6] Advances in neuroimaging have enabled studies of brain anatomy and neurobehavioral changes in the human fetus.

When pathways leading to orderly brain development are deconstructed, three major events appear critical to the establishment of functional synapses. **Neuronal proliferation**, **migration**, and **cellular differentiation** occur in a preordained fashion to establish early neural circuitry. These processes often overlap and occur at different rates in different brain regions. **Neurogenesis**, a term that encompasses both neuronal proliferation and subsequent survival, begins with neural stem/progenitor cells in neurogenic niches such as the subventricular zone and the subgranular zone of the dentate gyrus. These neural progenitor cells undergo mitosis to generate immature neurons that migrate in a radial fashion and laminate the cortex in an "inside-out" fashion.[7] Interneurons, which compose 10% to 15% of the total neuronal cells in the brain, originate from the ganglionic eminences in the developing brain.[8] These newly generated interneurons, which play an indispensable role in circuit inhibition, migrate in a tangential manner to populate distinct brain areas. Both forms of migration are guided by cell-intrinsic mechanisms and by structural scaffolds and humoral mediators such as **gamma-aminobutyric acid (GABA)** and **glutamate**.[9,10]

In humans, neurogenesis starts and peaks at 5 and 25 weeks' gestation, respectively, while neuronal migration is completed between 30 and 36 weeks' gestation.[11] Between 20 and 40 weeks' gestation, these processes are followed by the generation of an array of supporting glial cells, such as astrocytes and oligodendrocytes. Concurrently, synapse formation begins as early as the 10th week of gestation and continues to increase gradually at a rate of approximately 4% per week until the end of the second trimester. Subsequently, a robust and exponential increase in synapse formation (almost 40,000 synapses/min) occurs between 28 weeks' gestation and term.[12] These processes, together with the onset of myelination, result in a fivefold increase in brain volume and the appearance of morphologic features of the mature brain such as sulci and gyri. By 24 weeks' gestation, the fetus has all the neural machinery necessary to perceive pain[13]; this supports recommendations to provide fetal analgesia during fetal surgery from at least this point onward.[14]

Although the ontogeny of neurotransmitter systems is less well studied, animal and human data indicate that these systems appear very early in life, before the phase of active synaptogenesis.[11] The presence of these neuromodulatory substances before synapse formation supports the view that they serve a trophic role during early brain development, a role distinct from their predominant role of facilitating synaptic neurotransmission in the mature brain. Among these neurotransmitters, GABA remains the most widely studied (Fig. 10.1).[15] Although GABA has an inhibitory action in the mature brain, it serves an excitatory role during fetal brain development. The major mechanism for this role reversal is the differential expression of chloride ion transporters sodium potassium chloride cotransporter 1 (NKCC1) and potassium chloride cotransporter 2 (KCC2); these transporters increase the intracellular concentration of chloride in developing neurons.[16] On stimulation of **GABA receptors** that are expressed in neural progenitor cells and immature neurons, chloride ions are actively extruded, causing membrane depolarization rather than the hyperpolarization seen in mature neurons. This depolarizing effect of GABA decreases DNA synthesis and inhibits proliferation of neural progenitor cells,[17] causes concentration- and time-dependent effects on neuronal migration,[10] and plays a major role in activity-dependent synapse formation.[18]

The **N-methyl-d-aspartate (NMDA)-subtype glutamate receptors** originate later than the GABA receptors and remain functionally silent because of magnesium ion–induced channel blockade; thus, they play a limited role during early brain development. **Dopaminergic, cholinergic,** and **serotonergic** systems develop concomitantly and appear fully functional by the second trimester.[11] Pharmacologic interventions (e.g., **ethanol, antiseizure medications**) that act directly or indirectly on these powerful neuromodulator systems can induce long-lasting impairment of fetal brain development, mainly via impaired neurogenesis and/or altered neuronal migration.[19,20] Alteration of this excitation-inhibition balance is purportedly responsible for many childhood neurodevelopmental disorders.

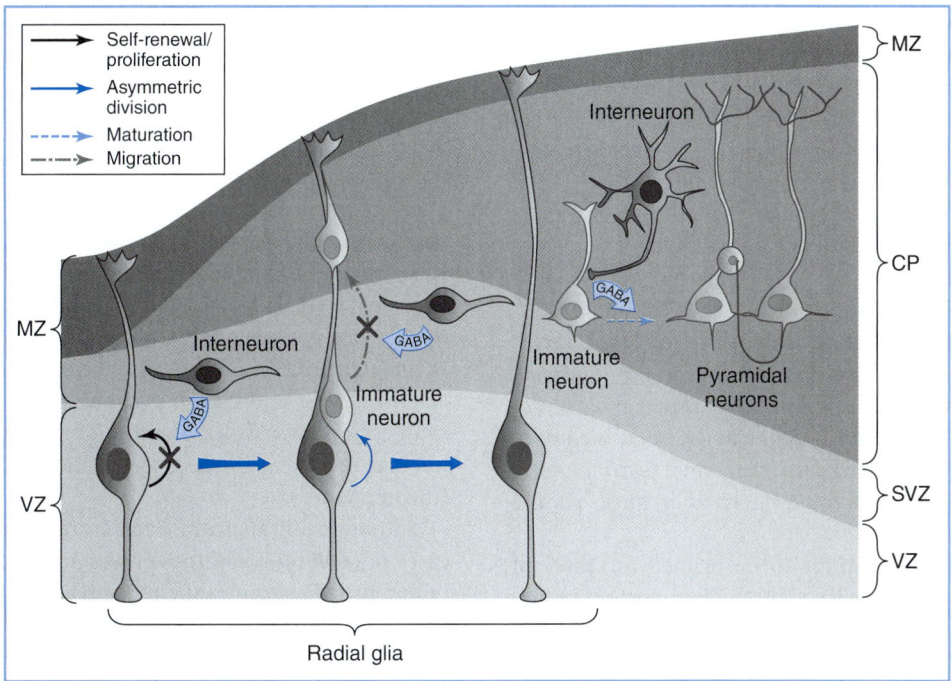

Fig. 10.1 The Role of Gamma-Aminobutyric Acid (GABA) in Regulating Embryonic Cortical Development. During corticogenesis, interneurons migrating in the subventricular zone can release GABA and activate GABAergic receptors on the radial glia, depolarizing these progenitors and decreasing their proliferation. Radial glia generate immature pyramidal neurons through asymmetric division, and the migration of these immature neurons along the radial fibers is decreased by GABA signaling. As young neurons assume their position in the cortex and begin to mature, GABA-mediated depolarization by the interneurons is required for the development of dendritic arbors and excitatory synaptic inputs from other pyramidal neurons. *CP,* Cortical plate; *MZ,* marginal zone; *VZ,* ventricular zone; *SVZ,* subventricular zone. From Wang DD, Kriegstein AR. Defining the role of GABA in cortical development. *J Physiol.* 2009;587:1873–1879.

Experimental studies have shown that the fetal **blood-brain barrier** is morphologically well developed and functionally competent at term,[21] although the exact time that blood-brain barrier competency is established in the human fetus is unknown.

CEREBRAL PALSY

History, Definition, and Significance

In 1861, John Little, an orthopedic surgeon, first described cerebral palsy in a report to the Obstetrical Society of London. Described as a neonatal neurologic disorder associated with difficult labor or birth trauma, the disorder was known as Little disease until William Osler coined the term *cerebral palsy* in 1888.[22] A precise definition and classification of cerebral palsy has proved elusive. In the foreword to the "Report on the Definition and Classification of Cerebral Palsy," published in 2007 in *Developmental Medicine and Child Neurology*, Peter Baxter[22] wrote, "This [supplement] illustrates the difficulties inherent in trying to agree what we mean by the terms we use and that a classification that suits one purpose, such as a diagnostic approach, may not always be ideal for others, such as therapy issues. Defining and classifying cerebral palsy is far from easy. We do need a consensus that can be used in all aspects of day-to-day care and for future research on cerebral palsy."

Today, **cerebral palsy** is defined as a nonprogressive disorder of the central nervous system (CNS) present since birth that includes some impairment of motor function or posture.[22] *Intellectual disability* (formerly known as *mental retardation*) may be present but is not an essential diagnostic criterion. Various forms of cerebral palsy differ in pathology, pathophysiology, and potential relationships with intrapartum events. Studies on cerebral palsy are difficult to interpret because of variations in duration of follow-up, birth weight classification, inclusion criteria for congenital abnormalities, and exclusion criteria for various causes of death. Terms such as *hypoxic-ischemic encephalopathy of the newborn*, *newborn asphyxia*, *birth asphyxia*, and *asphyxia neonatorum* are difficult to distinguish. Some authorities, including the American College of Obstetricians and Gynecologists (ACOG), have argued that the term *birth asphyxia* should be abandoned.[23]

Intrapartum events continue to be blamed for cases of cerebral palsy. It is widely believed that an intrapartum reduction in fetal oxygen delivery may cause cerebral palsy, and early primate studies demonstrated that perinatal asphyxia could cause brain injury.[24] Continuous electronic fetal heart rate (FHR) monitoring is believed to prompt delivery of at-risk fetuses and thus reduce asphyxial events, but despite a higher incidence of cesarean delivery, no reduction in the incidence of cerebral palsy has been observed since its widespread implementation during labor.[25,26] Further, among patients with new-onset late FHR decelerations, an estimated 99% of tracings would be false positive "if used as an indicator for subsequent development of cerebral palsy."[27]

Large randomized trials have not demonstrated better fetal and neonatal outcomes with continuous electronic FHR monitoring compared with intermittent FHR auscultation,[28,29] and there is little evidence that reassuring FHR tracings exclude the subsequent occurrence of cerebral palsy. A 1993 review of published FHR monitoring studies could not identify FHR patterns that were consistently associated with neurologic injuries and concluded, "We do not advocate the abandonment of the use of electronic fetal monitoring, but we do believe that it is yet to be proved to be of value in predicting or preventing neurologic morbidity."[30] A more focused application of FHR monitoring may ultimately be found useful. For example, fetal inflammatory changes, which can be associated with neurologic injury, may be associated with characteristic FHR findings.[31]

More recently, research has focused on whether expert, algorithm-assisted FHR interpretation may improve standard clinical care via earlier recognition of nonreassuring FHR tracings.[32] Although use of the algorithm identified more infants with acidemia (base deficit > 12 mol/L) than standard monitoring (46% versus 30%), less than 50% of the acidemic infants were identified.[32] Thus, the current application of electronic FHR monitoring provides incomplete data that should be evaluated in the clinical context.

Despite limitations in the use of intrapartum electronic FHR monitoring, it likely will continue to be used for the foreseeable future. In a review of medicolegal issues in FHR monitoring, Schifrin and Cohen[33] noted that despite its limitations, "Monitoring deserves credit for reducing intrapartum death, one of the original rationales for its development."

A 2008 workshop updated the definitions of various types of FHR tracings to simplify interpretation for providers.[34] A three-category system was developed. Category I FHR tracings provide reassuring evidence of fetal well-being and strongly predict *normal* fetal acid-base status at the time of observation. Category III tracings, the most ominous, predict *abnormal* fetal acid-base status at the time of observation and require prompt evaluation. Most FHR tracings are category II (indeterminate). Category II tracings are *not* predictive of *abnormal* fetal acid-base status, but do not provide sufficient evidence to be classified as either normal or abnormal; these tracings require continued surveillance and reevaluation (see Chapter 8).

Although intrapartum events are responsible for some cases of cerebral palsy, these cases are few.[35] After exclusion of infants with significant congenital anomalies, intrapartum events, including asphyxial insults, likely account for only 5% to 8% of all cases of cerebral palsy at all gestational ages,[36,37] and only 13% of infants born at 28 to 33 weeks' gestation.[38] It was estimated that only 16% of cerebral palsy cases may be preventable by placing a greater focus on earlier changes in FHR progression.[39] In 1999, the International Task Force on Cerebral Palsy published a consensus statement summarizing criteria that are necessary and suggestive of an intrapartum etiology for neurologic abnormalities (Box 10.1).[40] In 2010, a proposed evidence-based neonatal workup to confirm or refute allegations of intrapartum asphyxia was published.[41]

BOX 10.1 Criteria to Define an Acute Intrapartum Hypoxic Event as Sufficient to Cause Cerebral Palsy

Essential Criteria (All Four Must Be Met)

1. Evidence of metabolic acidosis in fetal umbilical cord arterial blood obtained at delivery (pH < 7 and base deficit ≥ 12 mmol/L)[a]
2. Early onset of severe or moderate neonatal encephalopathy in infants born at 34 or more weeks' gestation
3. Cerebral palsy of the spastic quadriplegic or dyskinetic type[b]
4. Exclusion of other identifiable etiologies, such as trauma, coagulation disorders, infectious conditions, and genetic disorders

Criteria That Collectively Suggest an Intrapartum Event—Within Close Proximity to Labor and Delivery (0–48 h)—but Are Nonspecific to Asphyxial Insults

1. A sentinel (signal) hypoxic event occurring immediately before or during labor
2. A sudden and sustained fetal bradycardia or the absence of fetal heart rate variability in the presence of persistent, late, or variable decelerations, usually after a hypoxic sentinel event when the pattern was previously normal
3. Apgar score ≤ beyond 5 min
4. Onset of multisystem involvement within 72 h of birth
5. Early imaging study showing evidence of acute nonfocal cerebral abnormality

[a]Buffer base is defined as the amount of buffer in blood available to combine with non-volatile acids. A buffer base of 34 mmol/L is equivalent to a whole blood base deficit of 12 mmol/L.

[b]Spastic quadriplegia and, less commonly, dyskinetic cerebral palsy are the only types of cerebral palsy associated with acute hypoxic intrapartum events. Spastic quadriplegia is not specific to intrapartum hypoxia. Hemiparetic cerebral palsy, hemiplegic cerebral palsy, spastic diplegia, and ataxia are unlikely to result from acute intrapartum hypoxia.

From Nelson KB, Grether JK. Potentially asphyxiating conditions and spastic cerebral palsy in infants of normal birth weight. *Am J Obstet Gynecol*. 1998;179:507–513.

BOX 10.2 Risk Factors for Neonatal Encephalopathy

Preconception Factors
- Increasing maternal age
- Mother unemployed, unskilled laborer, or stay-at-home
- No private health insurance
- Family history of seizures
- Family history of neurologic disorders
- Infertility treatment

Antepartum Factors
- Maternal thyroid disease
- Severe preeclampsia
- Bleeding in pregnancy
- Viral illness in pregnancy
- Postdates pregnancy
- Fetal growth restriction
- Placental abnormalities

Information compiled from Badawi N, Kurinczuk JJ, Keogh JM, et al. Antepartum risk factors for neonatal encephalopathy: the Western Australia case-control study. *BMJ*. 1998;317:1549–1553.

Epidemiology and Etiology

The varying forms of cerebral palsy suggest a multifactorial etiology. The Collaborative Perinatal Project was one of the largest studies of the antecedent factors associated with cerebral palsy.[42] This study evaluated the outcomes of 54,000 pregnancies among patients who delivered at 12 university hospitals between 1959 and 1966 and evaluated more than 400 variables in a univariate analysis[42]; identified potential risk factors were then subjected to a more rigorous multivariate analysis.[43] Maternal age, parity, socioeconomic status, smoking history, maternal diabetes, duration of labor, and use of anesthesia were not associated with cerebral palsy in the univariate analysis. The factors most strongly associated with cerebral palsy in the multivariate analysis were (1) maternal intellectual disability, (2) birth weight ≤ 2000 g, and (3) fetal malformations. Other factors associated with cerebral palsy included (1) breech presentation (but not vaginal breech delivery), (2) severe proteinuria (>5 g/24 h) during the second half of pregnancy, (3) third-trimester bleeding, and (4) gestational age ≤ 32 weeks. There was a slight association between cerebral palsy and fetal bradycardia, chorioamnionitis, and low placental weight. However, only 37% of the cases of cerebral palsy occurred in patients with one or more of these identified risk factors.

Rosen and Dickinson[44] reviewed studies from Europe, Australia, and the United States published between 1985 and 1990 and included data from 1959 to 1982. The incidence of cerebral palsy ranged from 1.8 to 4.9 (composite rate of 2.7) cases per 1000 live births. The incidence of certain conditions in infants with cerebral palsy was as follows: birth weight < 2500 g, 26%; diplegia, 34%; hemiplegia, 30%; quadriplegia, 20%; and extrapyramidal forms, 16%.

A large epidemiologic Australian study from 1998 noted an incidence of neonatal encephalopathy of 3.8 per 1000 term births and identified preconception and antepartum factors associated with neonatal encephalopathy (Box 10.2).[45] In a second study from 2011, the greatest risks for cerebral palsy included (1) preterm birth, (2) fetal growth restriction, (3) perinatal infection, and (4) multiple gestation.[46] Upper respiratory tract and gastrointestinal infections during pregnancy and operative vaginal delivery were not associated with cerebral palsy.[46] More recently, efforts to create a risk prediction model for cerebral palsy using both demographic and pregnancy factors have been attempted but are still in early stages of development in terms of application to patient care.[47] Evidence suggests that intrapartum factors alone are associated with neonatal encephalopathy in less than 5% of cases.[45,48] These data along with the recognition that most patients with identified risk factors do not have children with cerebral palsy, have led to a majority agreement that most cases of cerebral palsy cannot be predicted and that the identification of pregnancy-related conditions contributes minimally to the identification of individuals at risk for cerebral palsy.

In 2000, the ACOG and the American Academy of Pediatrics (AAP) convened the Neonatal Encephalopathy and Cerebral Palsy Task Force. The resulting landmark report,[49] released in 2003, was reviewed and endorsed by many groups. The Task Force extended the earlier international consensus statement regarding the requirements for establishing a causal relationship between intrapartum events and cerebral palsy (see Box 10.1).[40] The consensus statement led to several medicolegal conclusions[49]:

1. The only types of cerebral palsy associated with intrapartum hypoxia are spastic quadriplegia and, less commonly, dyskinesia.
2. Intellectual disability, learning disorders, and epilepsy should not be ascribed to birth asphyxia unless accompanied by spastic quadriplegia.
3. No statements about severity should be made before an affected child is 3 to 4 years of age, because mild cases may improve and dyskinesia may not be evident until then.
4. Intrapartum hypoxia sufficient to cause cerebral palsy is always accompanied by neonatal encephalopathy and seizures.

Phelan et al.[50] subsequently confirmed that fetuses who experienced a sudden and sustained deterioration of the FHR, and who subsequently were found to have cerebral palsy, demonstrated characteristics consistent with the ACOG/AAP Task Force criteria for intrapartum asphyxial injury.

Peripartum Asphyxia and Cerebral Palsy

Asphyxia may be defined as insufficient exchange of respiratory gases.[51] However, this definition does not include an index of severity or have any predictive value. Unfortunately, most studies have not used a uniform definition of *birth asphyxia*.[52]

In 1953 Virginia Apgar introduced a scoring system for identifying newborn infants in need of resuscitation and assessing the adequacy of subsequent resuscitation efforts.[53] Although the Apgar score has also been used to identify infants at risk for cerebral palsy, only a weak association has been found.[54] In the Collaborative Perinatal Project, only 1.7% of children with a 1-minute Apgar score ≤ 3 developed cerebral palsy.[55] Among infants who weighed more than 2500 g at delivery, the incidence of cerebral palsy was 4.7% if the 5-minute Apgar score was between 0 and 3 and 0.2% if the 5-minute Apgar score was greater than or equal to 7. Among infants who weighed less than 2500 g, the incidence of cerebral palsy was 6.7% and 0.8% with Apgar scores of 0 to 3 and greater than or equal to 7, respectively. Among all infants, a higher incidence of cerebral palsy was observed if the Apgar score remained less than or equal to 3 for more than 5 minutes. The incidence of early neonatal death increased among those infants with prolonged neonatal depression.

Most infants who subsequently manifest evidence of cerebral palsy have a normal 5-minute Apgar score. In the Collaborative Perinatal Project, only 15% of the infants in whom cerebral palsy later developed had a 5-minute Apgar score ≤ 3.[55] It should also be noted that preterm delivery is independently associated with a low Apgar score.

Although most cases of cerebral palsy are not attributable to intrapartum insults, intrapartum asphyxia does occur with serious consequences. However, the degree of asphyxia necessary to produce irreversible CNS injury is unclear. In some cases, an intrapartum insult that might have otherwise been innocuous might be superimposed on subclinical chronic fetal compromise and result in permanent injury.

Umbilical cord blood gas measurements are often used to diagnose suspected asphyxia. However, the definition of *normal* umbilical cord blood gas and pH measurements remains unclear.[51] In one study of 15,073 *vigorous* neonates (arbitrarily defined as having a 5-minute Apgar score ≥ 7) conducted between 1977 and 1993, the median umbilical arterial blood gas measurements (2.5th to 97.5th percentiles) were: pH 7.27 (7.10 to 7.38), P_{O_2} 17 (6 to 30) mm Hg [2.3 (0.8 to 6.9) kPa], P_{CO_2} 52 (35 to 74) mm Hg [6.9 (4.7 to 9.9) kPa], and base excess −4 (−11 to 1) mmol/L.[51] Only small differences in median pH and other measurements were present when infants were grouped according to gestational age. These data suggest that umbilical arterial blood pH in vigorous neonates can be as low as 7.10, and base excess may be as low as −11 mmol/L.

Although intrapartum events are most likely associated with a minority of cerebral palsy cases, clinical studies have attempted to define the associated extent and duration of perinatal asphyxia. Fee et al.[56] defined asphyxia as an umbilical arterial blood pH < 7.05 with a base deficit > 10 mmol/L; they concluded that this threshold was a poor predictor of adverse neurologic outcomes. Goodwin et al.[57] defined asphyxia as an umbilical arterial blood pH < 7.00; using this definition, hypoxic-ischemic encephalopathy and abnormal neurologic outcome were associated with acidemia. Goldaber et al.[58] also observed greater neonatal morbidity and mortality among term infants (birth weight > 2500 g) with an umbilical arterial blood pH < 7.00.

Low et al.[59,60] also studied complications of intrapartum asphyxia in term and preterm infants. They developed a complication score that expressed the magnitude of neonatal complications. Among term infants, the frequency and severity of newborn complications increased with the severity and duration of metabolic acidosis at birth. Importantly, respiratory acidosis at birth did not predict complications in newborns. Similar results were noted for preterm infants delivered between 32 and 36 weeks' gestation. In contrast, in infants delivered before 32 weeks' gestation, complications were similar in the control and asphyxia (defined as umbilical arterial blood buffer base < 30 mmol/L) groups. When this scoring system was used in term infants, the threshold for moderate or severe newborn complications was an umbilical arterial blood base deficit of 12 mmol/L.[60]

Relatively few studies have followed neurodevelopmental examinations for a sufficient duration to make meaningful conclusions about peripartum predictors of neurologic injury. Nagel et al.[61] performed such examinations in 30 children with umbilical arterial blood pH < 7.00 at delivery, 28 of whom survived the neonatal period. Evaluation at 1 to 3 years of age detected three children who had experienced an episode of hypertonia. Most of the children exhibited no major problems, with only one child displaying mild motor developmental delay. Another study examined neonatal complications (neonatal death, grade 3 or 4 intraventricular hemorrhage, gastrointestinal dysfunction, and neonatal seizures) in 35 newborns with umbilical arterial blood pH < 7.00 at delivery, three of whom died during the neonatal period.[62] Umbilical arterial blood base deficit ≥ 16 mmol/L and 5-minute Apgar score < 7 had 79% sensitivity and 81% specificity for predicting adverse neonatal outcomes.

Because metabolic acidosis may be a predictor of complications in newborns, the severity of intrapartum acidosis could be an important variable. Gull et al.[63] studied a small cohort of 27 patients with terminal bradycardia who were delivered vaginally. Not surprisingly, the umbilical arterial blood base deficit was greater in infants with end-stage bradycardia than in controls. The loss of short-term FHR variability for more than 4 minutes during terminal bradycardia correlated with the development of metabolic acidosis.

The relationship between umbilical arterial blood base excess values and the timing of hypoxic injury has been estimated in human and animal studies.[64] In a 2010 systematic review and metaanalysis, umbilical cord arterial blood pH < 7.00 was significantly associated with important, biologically plausible, adverse neonatal outcomes (i.e., neonatal mortality, hypoxic ischemic encephalopathy, intraventricular hemorrhage, periventricular leukomalacia, cerebral palsy).[65] Unfortunately, this relationship does not consider the role of previous or repetitive hypoxic episodes before the episode in question and therefore cannot accurately pinpoint the time of injury. Fortunately, the human fetus is quite robust, and episodes of intrauterine asphyxia usually yield a normal neonate. Blumenthal[66] concluded that there is a fine threshold between normality and death from asphyxia.

The increased presence of nucleated red blood cells in the umbilical circulation at delivery has been proposed as a marker of the occurrence and timing of intrauterine asphyxia.[67] However, data from these investigations demonstrated considerable variability and were influenced by birth weight and gestational age.[68] In 2014, the ACOG concluded that biomarkers predictive of long-term outcome after a hypoxic insult have not been identified, and that it is likely that a battery of such markers, in conjunction with clinical and imaging findings, rather than a single biomarker, would better predict outcome.[23]

Chorioamnionitis, Fever, and Cerebral Palsy

An association between cerebral palsy and chorioamnionitis has been demonstrated in preterm and term infants.[69,70] Intraamniotic infection and inflammation show direct evidence of causality between the intrauterine process and white matter injury.[71] Elevated maternal temperature is a sign of chorioamnionitis, but alone is insufficient for the diagnosis. Other signs include, but are not limited to, maternal and fetal tachycardia, foul-smelling amniotic fluid, uterine tenderness, and maternal leukocytosis. The diagnosis remains unproven until confirmed by placental culture or histologic examination.

The mechanism by which chorioamnionitis is associated with cerebral palsy is unclear; however, inflammatory cytokines may play a role (see discussion below).[72,73] A 2000 metaanalysis reported that both clinical and histologic chorioamnionitis were strongly associated with increased risk for cerebral palsy and periventricular leukomalacia in both preterm and term infants.[74] Similarly, in a 2010 metaanalysis, both histologic (pooled odds ratio [OR], 1.83; 95% confidence interval [CI], 1.17 to 2.89) and clinical chorioamnionitis (OR, 2.42; 95% CI, 1.52 to 3.84) were found to be significantly associated with cerebral palsy.[75] Preterm infants are particularly at risk, as up to 50% of cases of brain abnormalities in this population have been attributed to direct effect of moderate to severe acute histologic chorioamnionitis.[76]

Maternal temperature increases after administration of epidural labor analgesia in some women (see Chapter 24).[77] Although uncertain, the mechanism for this may be inflammatory. Epidural analgesia has been blamed for antibiotic administration to mothers with fever but no other evidence of chorioamnionitis, which may lead to unnecessary neonatal sepsis evaluations and antibiotic exposure.[78] Rather than treat all women with pyrexia for presumed chorioamnionitis, Mayer et al.[79] recommended that physicians make an effort to differentiate true chorioamnionitis from incidental maternal fever; they found that additional signs of chorioamnionitis were present in all cases in which the diagnosis was later confirmed by culture or pathologic examination. Neuraxial anesthesia is not a risk factor for cerebral palsy.[42]

PATHOPHYSIOLOGY OF FETAL ASPHYXIA

Intrauterine Hypoxemia and the Fetal Brain

The fetus is exclusively dependent on the placenta for oxygen and nutrients; thus, acute and chronic conditions that affect the placenta or the umbilical cord can deprive the fetus of these vital resources. Evidence from experimental animal models and humans suggests that both hypoxemic and inflammatory pathways interact and augment fetal brain damage.

The spectrum of neurologic injury in neonates depends on the duration and gestational age at hypoxemic-ischemic insult. Acute hypoxemia during the early- to mid-gestational period in sheep affects the predominant neurodevelopmental events such as neurogenesis and neuronal migration. Such hypoxemia causes the death of cerebellar Purkinje cells and hippocampal pyramidal neurons, and impaired neuronal migration.[80] In contrast, acute hypoxemia in late gestation appears to spare the hippocampus and cerebellum but causes neuronal death in the cerebral cortex and striatum.[81] Furthermore, acute perinatal anoxia causes long-term changes in dendritic arborization and synaptic connectivity.[82,83]

Experimental models of chronic hypoxemia, based on restriction of placental mass or blood flow, have demonstrated an array of completely different effects on the fetal brain. Chronic placental insufficiency relatively spares the fetal brain compared with other organ systems, although it results in reduced fetal brain weight. Overall, neurons appear to survive chronic and mild hypoxemia; even minor behavioral changes appear to resolve fully by adulthood in animal models. It is not known whether these effects are mediated by hypoxemia *per se*, or by other accompanying conditions such as chronic reduction of fetal nutrient supply or altered maternal-fetal endocrine status.

Dysregulation of neuronal calcium transport appears to be the initial pathway by which cerebral hypoxemia causes perinatal neuronal injury.[84] Hypoxia-induced changes in the NMDA receptor increase cellular permeability to calcium, triggering a variety of downstream effects, ultimately resulting in the generation of free radicals, peroxidation of lipid membranes, and nuclear fragmentation. It has long been recognized that developing oligodendroglia are highly vulnerable to excitotoxic injury in preterm infants.[85] Altered maturation or premature oligodendrocyte death can occur in areas of severe hypoxia-ischemia as a result of upregulation of inflammatory cytokines by activated microglia, elevated glutamate levels, or depleted levels of the antioxidant glutathione. It is highly likely that a combination of these mechanisms, modified by the nature and duration of insults and gestational age, determines the ultimate neurobehavioral phenotype.

Maternal Inflammation and Fetal Brain Injury

Although the development of the fetal brain is encoded by genetic programming, this is highly susceptible to environmentally induced epigenetic modifications and appears closely intertwined with maternal immune and endocrine systems. Experimental and epidemiologic studies reveal that maternal infection and inflammation early in pregnancy can cause an array of neurodevelopmental abnormalities in offspring such as schizophrenia and autism.[86-89] Among maternal infections, chorioamnionitis is the best characterized and investigated model of perinatal neuroinflammation. Human registry studies have confirmed an association between histological chorioamnionitis and cerebral palsy.[90] Although the exact contribution of maternal inflammation to perinatal brain injury is obscured because of the association of chorioamnionitis with preterm delivery and hypoxic-ischemic encephalopathy, inflammatory experimental models have revealed much information on cytokine induction, their transport across the placenta and amniotic fluid, and subsequent activation of the fetal immune system.

The mechanism by which maternal inflammation triggers a fetal immune response is likely multifactorial (Fig. 10.2). Despite the presence of circulating immune cells as early as 7 weeks' gestation in humans, antigen presentation is

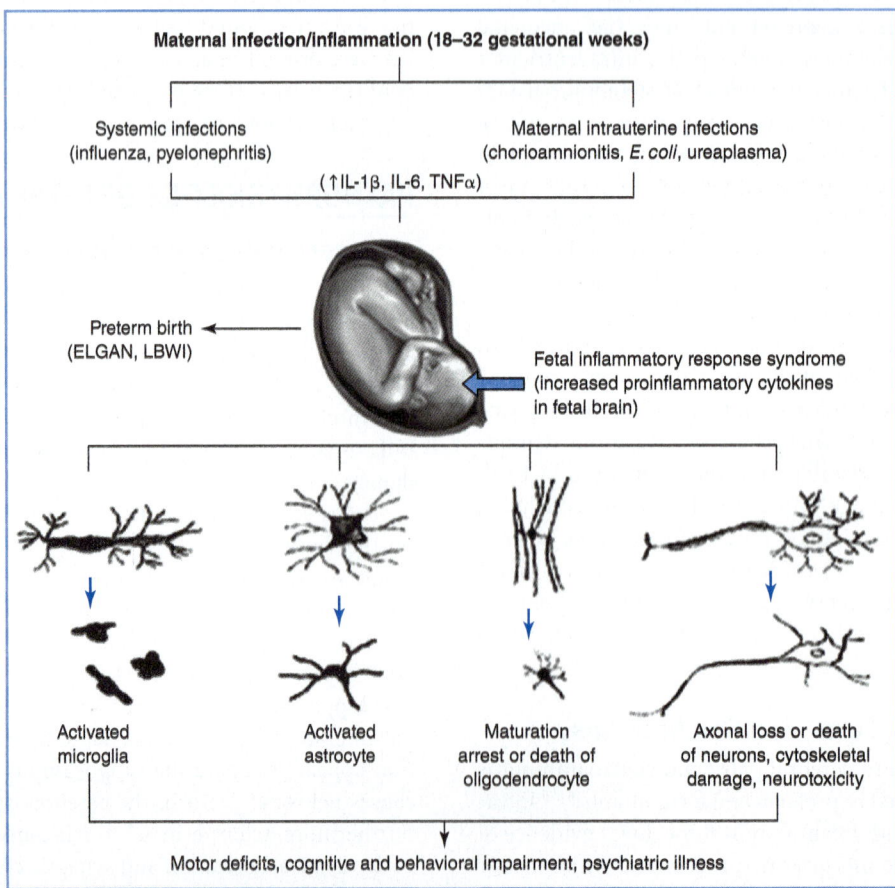

Fig. 10.2 Probable Mechanisms of Fetal Brain Injury With *In Utero* Exposure to Maternal Inflammation. *ELGAN*, Extremely low gestational age neonate; *IL*, interleukin; *LBWI*, low-birth-weight infant; *TNF*, tissue necrosis factor. From Burd I, Balakrishnan B, Kannan S. Models of fetal brain injury, intrauterine inflammation, and preterm birth. *Am J Reprod Immunol*. 2012;67:287–294.

suboptimal because of reduced expression of the major histocompatibility complex class II on antigen-presenting cells. Furthermore, the T cells are relatively immature. Therefore, maternally derived humoral mediators seem credible candidates to initiate and perpetuate an inflammatory cascade across the placenta. This idea has gained traction with the identification of maternal interleukin-6 (IL-6) in the fetal circulation as early as the second trimester, suggesting the possibility of transplacental transfer of proinflammatory cytokines.[91] Proinflammatory mediators such as IL-6 cause significant impairment of placental blood flow and fetal hypoxemia in animal models, dysregulate the barrier function of both the placenta and the immature fetal blood-brain barrier, trigger production of acute-phase proteins from the fetal liver, promote T-cell entry into the immature brain parenchyma, and disrupt the orderly patterning of the fetal cerebral cortex.[86,88,92–95] The role of inflammatory mediators in this phenomenon is reinforced by the direct correlation between plasma levels of IL-6 and the severity of functional deficits in offspring.[96,97] In addition to IL-6, cytokines such as IL-1β, IL-7, and IL-13 are upregulated in the fetal brain after a prenatal immune insult, which suggests collective activation of the innate fetal immune response.[98]

Both microglia (the major resident macrophages in the developing brain) and the complement system have been implicated as amplifiers of this immune response. During normal fetal development, microglia invade and colonize the fetal brain during the first and second trimesters[99] and are readily activated by proinflammatory mediators such as IL-1β. Activated microglial cells either cause a direct cytotoxic effect on oligodendrocytes and impair myelination or produce long-lasting alterations in neuronal-glial crosstalk, resulting in impaired synaptic function and subsequent neurodevelopmental disorders.[3,86,100]

At the cellular level, numerous mechanisms are involved in propagating the prenatal immune response. Intrauterine inflammation is linked to the metabolic demand of the fetal brain; in infants born before 30 weeks' gestation, chorioamnionitis was associated with increased total carotid artery blood flow (92 versus 63 mL/kg/min) and oxygen delivery (13.7 versus 10.1 mL/kg/min) compared with a control cohort without chorioamnionitis.[101] Whether the increase in oxygen delivery contributes to, or is a consequence of, fetal brain injury is unclear, but evidence suggests an enhanced susceptibility of the developing brain to oxidative stress.[102]

Collectively, robust experimental evidence suggests that prenatal inflammation alters fetal brain development at the molecular, cellular, and circuit levels. These findings are reinforced by epidemiologic studies that show a strong correlation between maternal infection/inflammation and neurodevelopmental disorders such as schizophrenia and autism.[87,103,104] Likewise, a study of placental histopathology of infants admitted to the neonatal intensive care unit (NICU) with hypoxic ischemic encephalopathy found that acute inflammation, including fetal inflammatory reaction, was higher in the moderate-severe hypoxic ischemic encephalopathy group than in the mild group.[105]

Animal Models of Fetal Asphyxia

Much of our knowledge of the fetal response to insufficient exchange of respiratory gases comes from animal models, which have limitations. Raju[106] reviewed the various animal models of fetal brain injury. At birth, sheep and guinea pig brains are much closer to maturity than the human brain. In this regard, rat pup and human brains are more similar to each other because they both undergo significant extrauterine development (Fig. 10.3).[107] Nonetheless, the importance of this distinction has been challenged. Previously, investigators relied mainly on morphologic milestones (e.g., the brain growth spurt) to compare species at different stages of development. A computerized method attempted to more accurately compare observations among 10 species (including humans) by evaluating the mathematical relationships of more than 100 developmental events and factors (e.g., evolutionary, genetic, neurochemical, neuroanatomic).[108] Although all events have not been cataloged for any one species, the iterative process allows information to be added to improve the theoretic model and is freely available online.[109] This method is not completely understood or accepted but may explain some of the variability in various models of developmental brain injury.

The chronically instrumented fetal lamb is similar in size to the human fetus, which facilitates placement of electrodes and vascular catheters in both the fetus and the mother. Investigators may obtain measurements while the mother (and fetus) remains anesthetized, or from awake animals that have recovered from surgery. Studies of animals with continuous instrumentation allow the assessment of fetal breathing movements, gross body movements, brain electrical activity (electroencephalogram), and blood gas and pH measurements. Blood concentrations of glucose, lactate, and various hormones can also be determined. Microdialysis techniques

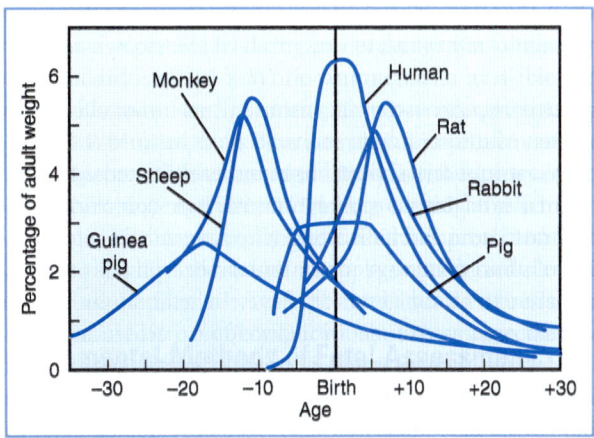

Fig. 10.3 Brain growth spurts of seven mammalian species expressed as first-order velocity curves of the increase in weight with age. The units of time for each species are as follows: guinea pig d); rhesus monkey (4 d); sheep (5 d); pig (w); human (mo); rabbit (2 d); rat (d). Rates are expressed as a percentage of adult weight for each unit of time. Modified from Dobbing J, Sands S. Comparative aspects of the brain growth spurt. *Early Hum Dev.* 1979;3:79–83.

have been used to evaluate neurotransmitter release within the fetal brain *in vivo*, in acute, exteriorized, and chronic preparations.[110,111] Other studies have measured fetal cerebral blood flow *in vivo* during episodes of hypoxemia[112] and during maternal infusion of ethanol.[113] These studies have enhanced understanding of the fetal brain response to pathophysiologic insults *in utero*, which ultimately may lead to improved diagnoses, treatment, and prevention of fetal brain injury.

Various methods have been used to produce fetal hypoxemia and acidemia in fetal lambs. Each method attempts to mimic one or more clinically relevant situation(s), including (1) decreased concentration of maternal inspired oxygen for several hours[114] or days[115]; (2) decreased uterine blood flow, which may be accomplished by placement of an adjustable clamp on the common iliac artery[116]; (3) decreased umbilical blood flow, either by total obstruction[117] or by means of a slow, progressive obstruction[118]; (4) selective uteroplacental embolization[119]; (5) maternal hemorrhage[120]; and (6) a combination of two insults, such as hypoxemia plus hypotension.[121]

Care must be exercised in the application of knowledge gained from hypoxia-ischemia studies conducted on nonfetal models (e.g., rat pups) to the problem of insufficient intrauterine gas exchange. The fetus and the fetal brain exist in a relatively hypoxemic environment. Despite preferential streaming of the most highly oxygenated blood to the brain and heart, the average Po_2 measured in the carotid artery of fetal lambs at term is approximately 22 mm Hg (2.9 kPa).[122] Further, unlike adult conditions in which global anoxia (i.e., cardiac arrest) or focal ischemia (i.e., stroke) is the clinical correlate, fetal asphyxia typically involves diminution, but not absence, of oxygen delivery, with variable degrees of respiratory or metabolic acidosis. A complete loss of cerebral blood flow rarely occurs, except as a terminal event. Of course, prolonged hypoxemia and decreased oxygen delivery can lead to acidemia and myocardial failure, followed by ischemia and rapid fetal demise. Fetal hypoxemia may result from the compromise of any or all of the steps involved in maternal-fetal oxygen transport (Box 10.3).[123] The impact of repeated hypoxic-ischemic insults, which may occur from various causes (e.g., repetitive umbilical cord occlusion, chronic abruption), should not be underestimated. Moreover, repeated brief insults may be harmful, as demonstrated in adult rats[124] and in fetal lambs.[125]

The neuropathology of intrauterine asphyxia depends, to some extent, on gestational age. In fetal lambs exposed to sustained hypoxemia with developing acidemia, immature fetuses demonstrated a predominantly periventricular injury, whereas mature fetuses had a primarily cortical injury, although there was some overlap (Fig. 10.4).[126] This finding is consistent with injury patterns in humans. Matsuda et al.[114] observed that the development of metabolic acidemia, reduced fetal breathing and body movements, and an altered sleep state were much less pronounced in midgestational fetal lambs subjected to hypoxemia than in fetal lambs at term.

BOX 10.3   Factors Decreasing Oxygen Transfer to the Fetus

Environmental Po_2
- High altitude

Maternal Cardiopulmonary Function
- Cyanotic heart disease

Oxygen Transport by Maternal Blood
- Anemia
- Cigarette smoking

Placental Blood Flow
- Hypertension
- Diabetes
- Placental abruption
- Uterine contractions

Placental Oxygen Transfer
- Placental abruption
- Placental infarcts

Umbilical Blood Flow and Fetal Circulation
- Occlusion
- Maternal heart disease

Oxygen Transport by Fetal Blood
- Anemia
- Hemorrhage

From Richardson B. The fetal brain: metabolic and circulatory responses to insufficient exchange of respiratory gases. *Clin Invest Med.* 1993;16:103–114.

Neuropathology of Fetal Asphyxia

The mechanism and timing of an asphyxial insult can affect the resulting fetal or neonatal pathology. Acute, complete asphyxia must be distinguished from incomplete, brief, or intermittent asphyxia or chronic hypoxemia. *Complete asphyxia* may occur in the setting of total placental abruption or umbilical cord occlusion (e.g., uterine rupture or umbilical cord prolapse), which if not treated rapidly leads to fetal demise. *Incomplete asphyxia* may occur whenever oxygen delivery to the fetus is inadequate to meet all of its needs (e.g., brief and/or repeated episodes of partial umbilical cord occlusion, placental embolization, or incomplete placental abruption). This latter category of asphyxia presumably contributes to the largest proportion of cases of cerebral palsy attributed to antepartum events. In these cases, the insult is not severe enough to lead to immediate fetal death but can profoundly affect fetal brain growth and development. Ongoing studies are attempting to determine whether there is a period *in utero* when the fetus is especially vulnerable to neurologic injury.

Using a primate model to perform seminal research on perinatal brain injury, Myers[24] identified two patterns of injury based on whether the fetus suffered complete or partial asphyxia. True complete asphyxia was demonstrated in fetal monkeys at term subjected to varying durations (0 to 25 minutes) of complete asphyxia. These fetuses were resuscitated

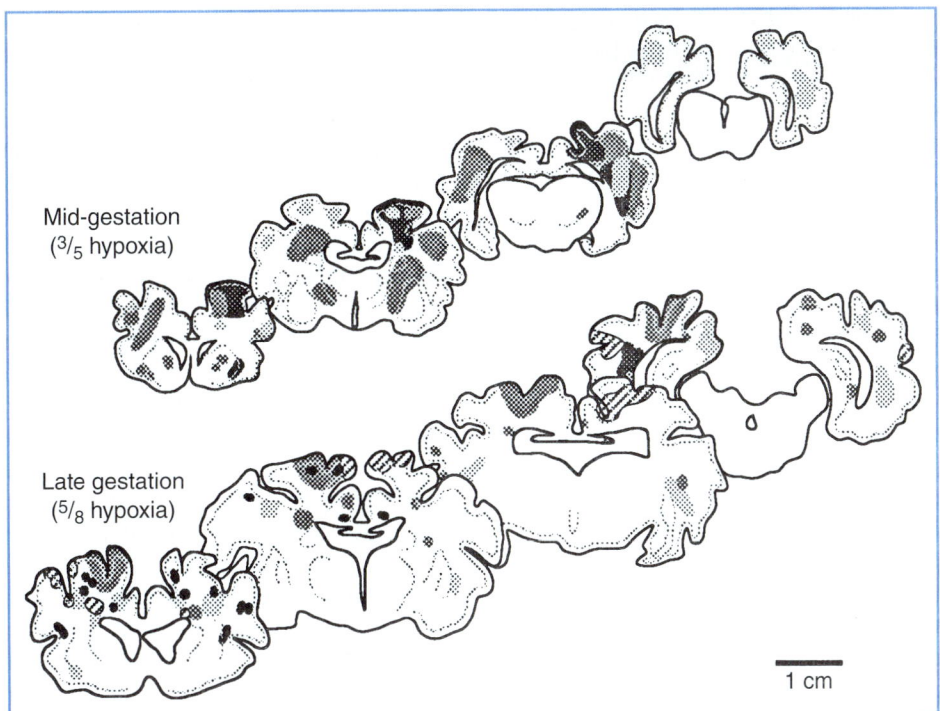

Mid-gestation
($^3/_5$ hypoxia)

Late gestation
($^5/_8$ hypoxia)

1 cm

Fig. 10.4 Composite diagram showing distribution of hypoxic injury in mid-gestational *(top)* and near-term *(bottom)* fetal lambs at 3 d after 8 h of arterial hypoxemia. Hypoxemia was produced by placing the pregnant ewe in a chamber with reduced ambient oxygen. Each *shading pattern* represents an individual animal. The severity of injury is not indicated in this diagram. From Penning DH, Grafe MR, Hammond R, et al. Neuropathology of the near-term and midgestation ovine fetal brain after sustained *in utero* hypoxemia. *Am J Obstet Gynecol.* 1994;170:1425–1432.

when possible, a procedure that often required the use of cardiac massage and epinephrine (adrenaline), and postmortem examinations revealed extensive pathology in brainstem areas. In humans, such a severe intrauterine insult would most likely be incompatible with extrauterine survival. If survival did occur, the infant would show obvious encephalopathy and multiorgan system dysfunction at birth. The second pattern (i.e., partial asphyxia) is more relevant to the discussion of human cerebral palsy. In studies of fetal monkeys subjected to partial asphyxia,[127] some animals demonstrated cortical necrosis, subcortical white matter damage, and basal ganglia damage. Although these two studies form the core of our knowledge of perinatal brain injury in primates, there were relatively few animals in each experimental group, and considerable variation in response occurred. Some animals suffered no injury, whereas others could not be resuscitated. Volpe[128] emphasized that the variation in neuropathology after intrauterine asphyxia depends on fetal gestational age and proposed a framework for these variations. He reported that the principal sites of injury in preterm fetuses are the white matter (especially periventricular white matter) and the basal ganglia, while older fetuses demonstrate injury primarily in the gray matter of the cortex and cerebellum. However, a 2023 study found that basal ganglia-thalamus injury accounted for three-fourths of cases of cerebral palsy in term or near-term infants.[38]

Cerebral white matter injury is a term that encompasses the full spectrum of periventricular leukomalacia. *Diffuse*

noncystic white matter injury is currently the predominant form of brain injury in children born prematurely.[129] The incidence of *cystic necrotic white matter injury* has declined markedly in the past several decades. The primary reason for white matter injury in preterm infants is the vulnerability of premyelinating oligodendrocytes to hypoxia-ischemia and inflammation.[129,130] Preterm infants have impaired cerebral blood flow autoregulation, particularly in vascular end zones and border zones.[131] Premyelinating oligodendrocytes are more susceptible to oxidative stress than mature cells because they lack antioxidant enzymes.[130]

Approximately one-third of preterm infants born between 24 and 32 weeks' gestation have evidence of diffuse white matter injury on magnetic resonance imaging (MRI).[132] These lesions cause disrupted white matter maturation and associated long-term neurodevelopmental consequences as these children grow.[129]

Fetal Adaptive Responses

The fetus has several adaptive responses for survival and growth in the relatively hypoxemic intrauterine environment; these adaptive changes to intrauterine hypoxemia vary between immature and mature fetuses. Fetal responses to asphyxia may be categorized as an alteration of fetal metabolism or maximization of fetal oxygen transport (Box 10.4).[123] Richardson[133] defined the *oxygen margin of safety* as the extent to which fractional oxygen extraction can increase and fetal arterial Po_2 can decrease before tissue oxygen supplies

Modified from Richardson B. The fetal brain: metabolic and circulatory responses to insufficient exchange of respiratory gases. *Clin Invest Med.* 1993;16:103–114.

BOX 10.4   Fetal Cerebral Responses to Asphyxia

Fetal Cerebral Metabolism
- Increased oxygen extraction
- Use of alternative energy sources
- Decreased growth
- Altered behavioral state

Fetal Cerebral O$_2$ Transport
- Redistribution of cerebral blood flow

are inadequate. Regardless of the etiology of decreased oxygen delivery to the fetus, fetal oxygen consumption is maintained by increasing oxygen extraction until oxygen delivery is approximately 50% of normal.[134] Lower levels of tissue oxygen tension result in progressive metabolic acidemia and a terminal decrease in oxygen consumption.[133]

Alterations in substrate use may affect the fetal response to insufficient exchange of respiratory gases. Unlike in adults, the fetal brain can use ketone bodies and lactate as alternative energy sources.[135] In gravid ewes, a reduction in uterine blood flow results in reduced fetal glucose consumption.[135] Current opinion holds that hyperglycemia should be avoided in adult humans at risk for ischemia.[136] Hyperglycemia may exacerbate metabolic acidosis by providing substrate for anaerobic metabolism, which increases lactic acid production. However, Vannucci and Mujsce,[137] citing experiments in neonatal rat pups, suggested that the immature brain may respond differently and that glucose administration may actually reduce hypoxic-ischemic brain injury. These investigators did not consider earlier work by Blomstrand et al.,[138] who studied the effects of hypoxia in the anesthetized, exteriorized fetal lamb and found that hyperglycemia accelerated the loss of somatosensory-evoked potentials, the onset of metabolic acidosis, and the reduction of cerebral oxygen consumption. Until these different observations are reconciled, the maintenance of normoglycemia *in utero* appears prudent.

During chronic hypoxemia, the fetus may also restrict the use of energy derived from oxidative metabolism to maintain essential cellular processes. This may lead to decreased somatic growth and fetal growth restriction. Using an ovine model of asphyxia, Hooper[139] detected decreased incorporation of tritiated [^{3}H]-thymidine (which reflects decreased DNA turnover and, presumably, decreased cell division) in fetal tissue. The decrease in incorporation of tritiated [^{3}H]-thymidine was not uniform in all tissues. The rates of DNA synthesis were maintained in most fetal tissues (including the fetal brain) but were greatly reduced in the lung, the skeletal muscle, and the thymus gland.

The fetus can conserve additional energy by decreasing breathing and gross body movements. Rurak and Gruber[140] demonstrated a 17% reduction in oxygen consumption in fetal lambs paralyzed by neuromuscular blockers. Perceptible fetal movements represent an index of fetal health. Many obstetric providers instruct their patients to count episodes of fetal activity for specified periods and to consult them if fetal movements are decreased or absent (see Chapter 6). Fetal hypoxemia results in decreases in both activity and rapid eye movement (REM) sleep in fetal lambs. REM sleep states are associated with an increased cerebral metabolic rate for oxygen (CMRo$_2$).[112] Thus, during periods of fetal stress, reductions in fetal body movements or REM sleep lead to a significant decline in fetal energy expenditure.

Oxygen deprivation typically results in a change in and/or redistribution of fetal cardiac output, the magnitude of which depends on the mechanism and severity of oxygen deprivation.[141] Sheldon et al.[142] demonstrated that fetal hypoxemia produced by decreasing maternal inspired oxygen concentration resulted in greater blood flow to the brain, myocardium, and adrenal glands. In fetal lambs, a brief (4-minute) complete arrest of uterine and ovarian blood flow resulted in a decrease in blood flow to all organs except the myocardium and adrenal glands.[143]

FETAL AND NEONATAL ASSESSMENT

Fetal Neurobehavioral Assessment

With advances in the understanding of prenatal brain development and imaging technology, there is considerable interest in monitoring and codifying fetal neurologic development and behavior to predict postnatal neurodevelopment.[144] The driving principle is that fetal behavioral patterns reflect complex interactions between the maternal environment and primitive neuronal network generators in the developing brain. It is widely agreed that most neurodevelopmental disorders have an intrauterine origin and that there is extensive neurobehavioral continuity from the fetal to the neonatal period.[145]

Although the assessment of high-risk pregnancies has included an analysis of certain aspects of fetal behavior, until recently there have been no unified scales for assessment of fetal neurobehavior. Current fetal neurobehavioral scales assess a variety of behaviors that can be categorized into the four main domains described by DiPietro[144]: (1) heart rate, (2) motor activity, (3) existing behavioral state, and (4) responsiveness to external stimuli. The Fetal Neurobehavioral Coding System (FENS) incorporates most elements of fetal behavior.[146] Using ultrasonography, FENS analysis can identify specific behaviors in fetuses with growth restriction; compared with normally developing fetuses, fetuses with growth restriction demonstrate a delayed appearance of behavioral states, longer behavioral state transitions, and disorganized behavioral patterns. These tests have been validated in other paradigms, including pregnancies that were complicated by maternal diabetes, substance abuse, and cigarette smoking.

A more comprehensive scale is the Kurjak Antenatal Neurodevelopmental Test, which includes an assessment of eight fetal parameters related to fetal behavior, general movements, and other physical signs (e.g., head circumference, presence or absence of overlapping cranial sutures, finger movements).[147] However, these fetal assessment studies are time-consuming and require specific training to codify behaviors. Moreover, because the brain structures driving such behaviors have not been clearly identified, it is difficult to understand the significance of any differences in behavior.

Fetal Neuroimaging Assessment

In vivo MRI provides details of the architecture of the developing brain beginning in the 18th gestational week and can quantify brain growth and structural abnormalities.[148] Other techniques, such as magnetic resonance (MR) tractography and functional fetal MRI, may enhance our understanding of normal brain development and thus facilitate identification of abnormal development. Until controlled trials demonstrate adequate sensitivity, specificity, and positive predictive power, these tests have limited clinical potential; any advantages will need to be balanced against possible detrimental effects of ultrasonography and MRI on fetal neuronal development and migration.[149]

Neonatal Radiologic Diagnosis of Cerebral Injury

MRI is useful for diagnosis of neonatal brain injury.[150] MRI can assist in the diagnosis of hypoxic-ischemic encephalopathy in newborn infants, provide three-dimensional evaluations to determine the volume of gray matter and the extent of white matter myelination (thus providing valuable insights into normal and abnormal brain development), and estimate the timing of the brain injury in patients with cerebral palsy.[150] Newer techniques, such as diffusion tensor imaging and MR spectroscopy, may offer advantages over conventional MRI when performed early (i.e., hours) after a hypoxic-ischemic insult. Diffusion tensor imaging detects the microscopic movement of water particles in brain tissue. MR spectroscopy analyzes the signal of protons attached to molecules such as glutamate, glutamine, and lactate, among others.[151] These methods detect acute chemical changes in brain tissue and may accurately predict motor outcome in preterm infants.[152] Injury patterns detected with these methods are present for several days and resolve over the next week, when the chronic injury becomes visible with conventional MRI. Identification of injuries with these techniques shortly after birth can support the hypothesis that injury occurred within days of delivery.[151] Thus, MR spectroscopy and diffusion tensor imaging are powerful new tools for timing the occurrence and understanding the pathophysiology of perinatal brain injury. Cerebral ultrasonography remains a useful technique in the early neurologic neonatal assessment, especially for the critically ill infant who might not be a candidate for transfer to an MRI facility.[153]

ANESTHESIA AND BRAIN INJURY

Anesthetic agents have profound effects on brain metabolism and synaptic transmission. These effects may be direct or indirect and protective or harmful.

Labor Analgesia and the Fetal Brain

Local anesthetic agents are given in lower concentrations for longer durations during labor analgesia than during surgery. Despite widespread use, there has been little attention to the neurodevelopmental consequences of antepartum and intrapartum fetal exposure to these drugs. Because neurodevelopmental events at term are quite different from those that occur during the second trimester, there is a need for experimental studies to investigate the effects of analgesic techniques and drugs administered during the third trimester of pregnancy.

Opioids

Among systemic opioids used for labor analgesia, meperidine (pethidine) remains the most widely studied. Although it is known that opioids cross the placenta and enter the fetal circulation,[154] the long-term effects of peripartum opioid exposure on the infant's neurodevelopmental trajectory are unclear. Only a few preclinical studies have addressed this question.[155,156] Endogenous opioid systems are active in the fetal brain; the presence of their cognate receptors at critical sites during this period suggests that these systems are intricately linked to early neurodevelopment.[157] Preclinical evidence suggests that opioid mechanisms play an important role in both early and adult neurogenesis by modulating neuronal progenitor proliferation and differentiation.[158,159] Of concern, fetal rat exposure to morphine during the entire second trimester alters offspring hippocampal development.[160] However, animal studies of opioid use in pregnancy should not be extrapolated to peripartum opioid use in humans because of differences in the gestational age and differences in drug dose and duration of administration. Only focused studies will reveal the true consequences of opioid administration for labor analgesia.

Neuraxial Techniques

Studies of neuraxial analgesia in labor usually focus on analgesic quality and obstetric and short-term neonatal outcomes. To date, no randomized trials have evaluated the long-term effects of neuraxial analgesia on brain development in offspring. Epidurally administered local anesthetics cross the placenta and enter the fetal circulation. Golub[161] randomized nonlaboring pregnant rhesus monkeys at term to receive epidural bupivacaine (total dose 1.2 mg/kg) or saline. No differences in specific cognitive deficits were identified between groups; however, exposed offspring demonstrated a prolonged increase in motor disturbance behaviors at 10 to 12 months of age, suggesting that perinatal interventions can alter postnatal behavioral ontogeny.

In humans, Flick et al.[162] examined the association between neuraxial labor analgesia and the incidence of childhood learning disabilities in a population-based birth cohort. The incidence of childhood learning disabilities was not associated with the use of neuraxial labor analgesia (adjusted hazard ratio, 1.05). In a prospective longitudinal study from China, neuraxial labor analgesia was not associated with delayed neurodevelopment in offspring at 2 years of age.[163] Finally, using administrative data from the Scottish National Health Service (2007 to 2016), Kearns et al.[164] reported that the use of epidural labor analgesia was associated with a reduced risk for developmental concerns in infants at 2 years of age (confounder-adjusted relative risk [RR], 0.96; 95% CI, 0.93 to 0.98), and specifically, fewer concerns regarding communication and fine motor skills.

Other studies have examined the relationship between neuraxial labor analgesia and autism spectrum disorders (ASDs). While some studies identified an association,[165] studies that used a sibling-matched design to control for genetic and environment factors that may contribute to ASD found no association.[166–168] Editorialists have concluded that accumulating data suggest that neuraxial labor analgesia does not cause ASD in offspring and that the observed association found in some studies is due to residual confounding.[169,170]

Inhalational Agents

The use of inhalational anesthetic agents during labor and delivery became popular after John Snow introduced the use of chloroform in the 1850s (see Chapter 1). Other agents, including nitrous oxide, trichloroethylene, cyclopropane, and methoxyflurane, were subsequently introduced and more recently the use of enflurane, isoflurane, desflurane, and sevoflurane has been described (see Chapter 23). Although halogenated inhalational anesthetic agents have been supplanted by neuraxial techniques for labor analgesia, nitrous oxide is still widely used, typically administered as 50% nitrous oxide in oxygen using a blender device (e.g., Nitronox in the United States) or premixed in a single cylinder (e.g., Entonox in the United Kingdom) (see Chapter 23).

Studies of the fetal and neonatal effects of inhalational anesthetic agents for labor analgesia generally have been of limited quality.[171] Available evidence suggests that they have minimal or no effect on Apgar and neurobehavioral scores immediately after delivery.[172,173] However, no study has evaluated long-term neurodevelopmental outcomes. This knowledge gap is critical because robust evidence suggests that early-life neural reprogramming, following pharmacologic and inflammatory insults, affects behavioral development later in life. Compelling animal evidence suggests that anesthetic agents administered during a critical period of brain development cause widespread neurodegeneration with subsequent learning, memory, and behavioral problems (see discussion below). Nitrous oxide, in particular, is now known to be a potent developmental neurotoxin in animal models, yet its effects (if any) on human neurodevelopment are unclear. Thus, although the pattern of nitrous oxide administration during labor is unlike its administration for surgical anesthesia, the administration of nitrous oxide for labor analgesia merits closer scrutiny.[174]

Maternal Anesthesia and the Fetal Brain

Many pregnant women continue to require general anesthesia for either pregnancy-related or nonobstetric surgical procedures. Commonly used anesthetic agents freely cross the placenta and reach the fetal brain, causing fetal sleep or sedation. Obstetric anesthesia research has focused primarily on the teratogenic effects of anesthetic agents administered during the first trimester (see Chapter 18) and the effects of anesthetic agents on neonatal behavior when administered during cesarean delivery. Historically, the second trimester was assumed to be a safe period for surgery and anesthesia, primarily because of a lack of targeted studies. However, extensive subsequent animal research has shown that anesthetic agents administered during the phase of synaptogenesis can induce a profound neurodegenerative response in the developing brain and cause functional impairment in offspring.[175,176] Human epidemiologic studies appear to support an association between early childhood exposure to anesthetic agents and subsequent functional impairment.[177,178] However, it is unclear whether these outcomes result from the underlying disease, surgery, or anesthesia, or a combination of these factors.

Because human synaptogenesis appears to begin during the third trimester, there is serious concern that intrauterine fetal exposure to anesthetic agents may result in similar functional impairment. Because there is no precise way to monitor human fetal brain development *in utero*, the potential long-term effects of maternal anesthesia on the fetal brain must be investigated in animal models. However, given the considerable differences in neural maturation among species (see Fig. 10.3 and Fig. 10.5), and the relative duration of anesthesia exposure in relation to the life span of the organism, these results should be interpreted with caution.[179]

The exact mechanisms by which anesthetic agents impair early brain development remain under investigation.[180] Anesthetic agent interactions with GABA and the NMDA-subtype of glutamate receptors decrease activity-dependent synapse formation and cause apoptotic neurodegeneration in multiple areas of the developing brain. These histopathologic changes have been well investigated, especially in the hippocampal formation, an area that is crucial for memory. Early exposure to anesthetic agents affects long-term potentiation in the hippocampus and affects spatial working memory in animal models.[175] These changes do not appear to be caused by direct cytotoxicity[181] but rather by a combination of effects on both neuronal and nonneuronal cells in the developing brain (Box 10.5).

Of specific concern are the effects of anesthetic agents on neurogenesis and synapse formation in the fetal brain. Human neural ontogeny suggests that the second trimester is a period of active fetal brain development, with neuroblast proliferation peaking between the 5th and 25th postmenstrual weeks. Because GABA and glutamate play a crucial role in these processes, there is concern that prolonged and nonphysiologic modulation of the fetal GABA and glutamatergic systems (e.g., during second-trimester maternal anesthesia) might affect neurogenesis, neuronal migration, and/or synapse formation.

In one of the first studies to simulate a clinically relevant scenario,[182] a single exposure to 1.4% isoflurane (1 MAC [minimum anesthetic concentration]) for 4 hours during the second trimester caused long-lasting impairment of

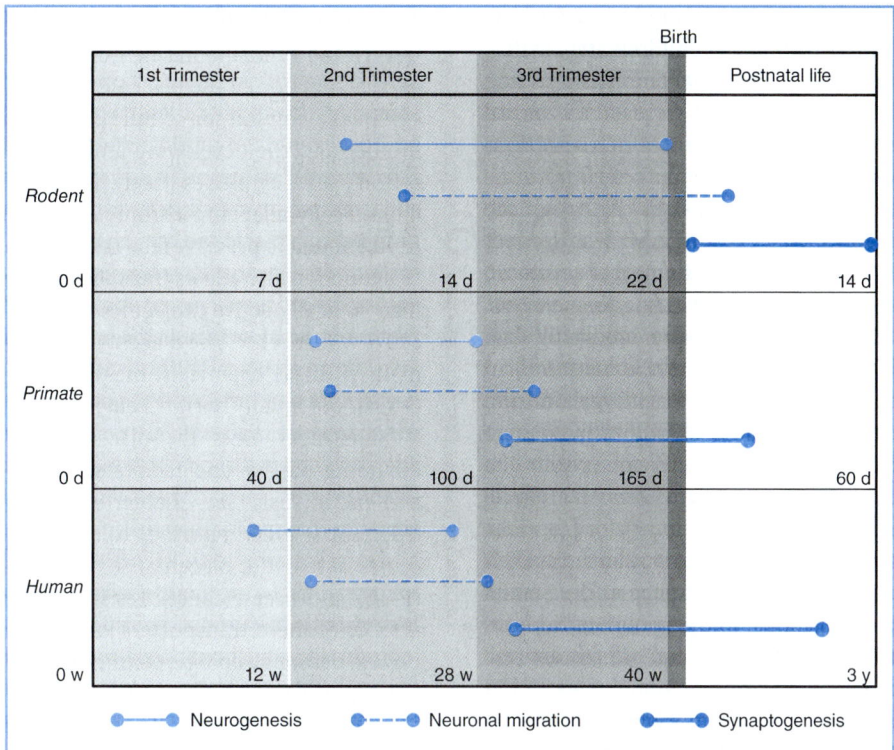

Fig. 10.5 Time Lines of Major Neurodevelopmental Events *In Utero* in Rodents, Nonhuman Primates, and Humans. Events are as marked in the figure legend (*d*, days; *w*, weeks; *y*, years). Synaptogenesis is predominantly a postnatal event in rodents, unlike that in primates and humans. From Palanisamy A. Maternal anesthesia and fetal neurodevelopment. *Int J Obstet Anesth.* 2012;21:152–162.

BOX 10.5 Salient Features of Developmental Anesthetic Neurotoxicity

- Apoptotic neuronal death during synaptogenesis
- Suppression of neurogenesis
- Morphologically abnormal synapse formation
- Altered dendritic spinogenesis
- Impairment of hippocampal long-term potentiation
- Deformation of neuronal and astroglial cytoskeletal protein
- Aberrant cell cycle reentry during neuronal mitosis
- Neuronal mitochondrial dysfunction
- Abnormal intraneuronal calcium homeostasis

From Palanisamy A. Maternal anesthesia and fetal neurodevelopment. *Int J Obstet Anesth.* 2012;21:152–162.

---

spatial working memory in rodent offspring. Although the exact mechanisms behind these behavioral disturbances are unclear, other studies suggest that mid-gestational exposure to isoflurane upregulates the proapoptotic protein caspase-12, decreases overall synapse numbers in the fetal hippocampus, and downregulates the plasticity-associated protein GAP-43.[183,184] Similar results have been reported in pregnant guinea pigs and macaques, suggesting that the fetal brain remains highly susceptible to maternal mid-trimester anesthesia.[185,186] Furthermore, isoflurane suppresses neurogenesis in rodents both *in vitro* and *in vivo*,[187,188] causing a depletion of the neural stem cell pool. At least *in vitro*, this phenomenon appears to be dose-dependent.[188] At present,

the impact of reduced neurogenesis on behavioral deficits and the effect of anesthetic agents on neuronal migration remain unknown.

Extension of these studies to the third trimester has yielded mixed results. In one rodent study, third-trimester maternal administration of 1.3% isoflurane for 6 hours had no effect on offspring neurodevelopment.[189] However, another dose-response study in term rodents found that maternal administration of 3% isoflurane, but not 1.3% isoflurane, for 1 hour caused fetal brain hippocampal neurodegeneration.[190] No neurodegenerative changes were observed after third-trimester exposure in guinea pigs.[185] Thus, in rodent models, it appears that the fetal brain is less vulnerable to the adverse effects of anesthetic agents during the third trimester. This could be caused by the stage of neurodevelopment, or more likely, by an increase in the levels of neuroprotective hormones such as estrogen, progesterone, neurosteroids, and oxytocin during the third trimester. Work from nonhuman primate models, however, shows that even a 5-hour exposure to either isoflurane (1% to 1.5%) or ketamine and propofol during the late second and early third trimester can cause a 2.5- to 5-fold increase in neuronal apoptosis in the fetal brain.[191–193]

Few studies have examined offspring neurodevelopmental effects after shorter-duration maternal anesthesia exposure. This knowledge gap is important because surgical anesthesia exposure in pregnant women is usually short. The relative safety of short exposures was supported by a population-based birth cohort study that sought to determine the incidence of learning disabilities in children after maternal administration of general or neuraxial anesthesia during cesarean or vaginal delivery.[194] Children exposed to general anesthesia during cesarean delivery were not more likely to develop learning disabilities compared with those born vaginally with no exposure to general anesthesia. Although the study was retrospective and used data from 1976 to 1982, it is reassuring that even the children whose mothers required emergency general anesthesia did not have a higher incidence of learning disability. In contrast, a human study using data from the US Medicaid database (1999 to 2013) identified an association between maternal exposure to anesthesia during nonobstetric surgery and disruptive or internalizing behavior disorder in offspring.[195] Again, it is difficult to separate the possible adverse effects of anesthetic agents from the effects of surgery and the underlying illness.[196]

Newer studies have explored the association between general anesthesia during the third trimester and ASDs in offspring, with inconclusive results. Using a propensity score-matched technique to adjust for underlying risk factors in a population-based data set derived from national registries in Taiwan, Chien et al.[197] reported that general anesthesia during cesarean delivery was associated with a 52% higher risk for developing autism than vaginal delivery. By contrast, a population-based sibling cohort study from Puerto Rico found no evidence for an association, although in this study both exposures during pregnancy and the first 2 years of life were included.[198] Further epidemiologic work is required to ascertain the effects of maternal anesthesia during nonobstetric surgery in the second trimester.

The wealth of anesthetic neurotoxicity studies prompted the US Food and Drug Administration (FDA) to issue an updated Drug Safety Communication in late 2016, warning that repeated or lengthy use of general anesthetic or sedative drugs during the third trimester of pregnancy or the first 3 years of life may have consequences for early brain development.[199] However, the results of recent prospective clinical trials suggest that short-duration exposure to anesthesia in children younger than 3 years of age does not have a detrimental effect on cognitive development.[200,201]

Fetal Neuroprotection

Throughout gestation, the fetus remains concealed, protected, and nourished by a combination of maternal anatomic and physiologic factors. For example, the amniotic fluid cushions the fetus against trauma, and the placenta serves as a conduit to ensure a continuous supply of nutrients. Despite these inbuilt protective mechanisms, the fetus remains vulnerable to maternal insults such as infection and fever, drugs, and acute changes in placental physiology. The developing CNS appears to be the organ system most susceptible to such insults. Understanding the developmental aspects of neuroprotective mechanisms will therefore enable generation of targeted neuroprotective therapies.

Role of the Placenta

One of the fundamental neuroprotective mechanisms is the barrier function of the placenta (see Chapter 4). The placenta serves as a conduit for chemical communication between the mother and the developing fetus; endocrine signals, growth factors, and cytokines freely traverse the placenta, which dynamically adapts to chronic changes in the maternal-fetal environment to preserve fetal growth and viability.[202] However, this function also allows transplacental transfer of many pharmacologically active molecules either by passive diffusion or active transport.[203] The placenta is capable of detoxification of many of these chemicals, making it the first line of defense against potentially harmful environmental agents.

Substances cross the placenta by several mechanisms, including passive and facilitated diffusion, active transport, and endocytosis (see Chapter 4). Molecules in the syncytiotrophoblast play important roles in active transport of molecules across the placenta, including phospho-glycoprotein (P-gp) and breast cancer resistance protein (BCRP).[203] The activity of these transporters varies with gestational age and certain pathophysiologic conditions (e.g., preeclampsia, intrauterine infection) and is influenced by the steroid hormones of pregnancy. Thus, it is possible that placental permeability to certain drugs depends on a complex interplay of several factors. In addition to this barrier function, the human placenta secretes large amounts of estrogen and progesterone, which enter the fetal circulation and serve as substrates for *de novo* neurosteroid synthesis in the fetal brain.[204] In particular, allopregnanolone has been shown to exert neuroprotective effects in the fetal brain (see discussion below).

Humoral Mechanisms

The intricate and symbiotic relationship between the fetus and maternal hormones throughout pregnancy has been extensively investigated. Much of our understanding comes from elaborate murine and primate research models in which changes in maternal levels of hormones closely parallel changes in the fetal plasma and/or brain. Throughout pregnancy, there is a gradual increase in many maternal hormones, such as progesterone, estradiol, and oxytocin.[205–207] At term or during labor, the levels of these hormones are 40- to 100-fold higher than in the nonpregnant state.

Many of these hormones freely cross the placenta and are transported to the fetal brain, where they profoundly influence neurodevelopment. For example, estradiol and progesterone influence neural stem cell proliferation, modulate apoptosis and synaptogenesis in a region-specific manner, alter subcellular signaling mechanisms, and promote dendritic growth and spinogenesis through specific receptor mechanisms.[205,206] Estradiol, in particular, prevents cell death in both neuronal and nonneuronal cell lines.

Maternal plasma oxytocin levels gradually increase during pregnancy and reach a peak during the second stage of labor. Oxytocin is particularly important because of its effects on GABAergic signaling in fetal neurons. Investigators showed that oxytocin transiently switched the action of GABA on immature rodent fetal neurons from *depolarizing* to *hyperpolarizing* at term gestation.[208] This finding raises the possibility that oxytocin protects the fetal brain during the stressful process of labor and delivery.[209]

NEUROPROTECTIVE THERAPIES

Magnesium Sulfate and Cerebral Palsy

There is historic controversy regarding the role of magnesium sulfate in preventing or possibly exacerbating fetal brain injury. Some controversy remains, but results of several large, randomized studies on the effect of antenatal maternal magnesium sulfate administration on offspring outcome has dramatically altered practice guidelines and clinical practice.[210-212] Although none of these studies demonstrated significant improvement in the primary outcome, all showed reduced cognitive morbidity, and none showed any increase in pediatric morbidity or mortality associated with magnesium sulfate use for neuroprotection.

In a placebo-controlled trial of women who were thought likely to deliver within 24 hours and before 30 weeks' gestation, Crowther et al.[210] reported a lower incidence of substantial gross motor dysfunction (3.4% versus 6.6%; RR, 0.51; 95% CI, 0.29 to 0.91) and combined death or substantial gross motor dysfunction (17% versus 22.7%; RR, 0.75; 95% CI, 0.59 to 0.96) in children whose mothers were randomized to receive antenatal magnesium sulfate treatment. In another large trial, which included women in preterm labor before 33 weeks' gestation, a significant reduction in death and/or gross motor dysfunction was again identified in the children whose mothers received magnesium sulfate (25.6% versus 30.8%; OR, 0.62; 95% CI, 0.41 to 0.99).[211] A reduction in death and/or motor or cognitive dysfunction (34.9% versus 40.5%; OR, 0.68; 95% CI, 0.47 to 0.99) was observed in the magnesium-exposed offspring at 2 years of age.[211] Finally, a randomized, controlled multicenter trial in the United States found that fetal exposure to magnesium sulfate within 24 hours of preterm delivery (between 24 and 32 completed weeks' gestational age) did not reduce the combined risk for moderate or severe cerebral palsy or death. However, fetal exposure to magnesium sulfate reduced the risk for moderate or severe cerebral palsy among survivors (1.9% versus 3.5%; RR, 0.55; 95% CI, 0.32 to 0.95) and was associated with a decreased overall rate of cerebral palsy (4.2% versus 7.3%; P = .004).[212]

Although the results are encouraging, it is difficult to compare trials owing to differences in inclusion criteria, study interventions/dosages, and outcomes. Nonetheless, it has been concluded from metaanalyses that fetal exposure to magnesium sulfate may reduce the risk for cerebral palsy without increasing the risk for neonatal death.[213,214]

In 2010, the ACOG and the Society for Maternal-Fetal Medicine (SMFM) released a joint opinion supporting antenatal maternal magnesium sulfate administration for fetal neuroprotection, stating that the available evidence suggests that magnesium sulfate administered before anticipated early preterm birth reduces the risk for cerebral palsy in surviving infants.[215] Physicians using magnesium sulfate for fetal neuroprotection should develop specific guidelines regarding inclusion criteria, treatment regimens, concurrent tocolysis, and monitoring. The ACOG and the SMFM have concluded that it is reasonable to use a protocol based on one of the large randomized trials[210-212]; magnesium sulfate should be offered to women at high risk for anticipated preterm delivery (<28 to 32 weeks' gestational age) within 24 hours. A loading dose of magnesium sulfate 4 to 6 g should be administered, followed by maintenance infusion of 1 to 2 g/h for 12 to 24 hours, at which point the risk for impending preterm delivery should be reassessed. If there is no longer a concern for impending delivery, the magnesium sulfate should be discontinued and restarted with active labor or when delivery is again thought to be imminent.

Hypothermia

Some investigators have described improved outcomes after the use of hypothermia in neonates at risk for hypoxic-ischemic encephalopathy. One group of investigators has described an experimental model of severe intrauterine hypoxia in preterm fetal sheep, in which asphyxia was produced by 25 minutes of complete umbilical cord occlusion.[216] Cerebral hypothermia (fetal extradural temperature reduced from 39°C to 29°C) decreased the loss of striatal neurons and oligodendroglia. This finding was associated with improved basal ganglia function after ischemia.

These and other experimental results prompted a randomized clinical trial of whole-body hypothermia for neonates with hypoxic-ischemic encephalopathy.[217] Eligible neonates were older than 36 weeks' gestational age, had moderate or severe encephalopathy, and were admitted to the NICU within 6 hours of birth. Body temperature was lowered to 33.5°C for 72 hours in neonates randomized to hypothermia treatment. Death or moderate to severe disability at 18 to 22 months of age occurred in 44% of 102 infants in the hypothermia group, compared with 62% of 106 infants in the control group (risk ratio, 0.72; 95% CI, 0.54 to 0.95; P = .01). Although encouraging, these results are at odds with those from another large multicenter randomized trial.[218] In an editorial attempting to reconcile these opposing results, several possible explanations were suggested.[219] Importantly, in the study that demonstrated no benefit, cooling began later and more time was required to achieve complete cooling because head (not total body) cooling was employed.[218] Moreover, the study that showed no benefit with hypothermia may have included infants who were so severely affected that no therapy would have been beneficial.[218] This highlights the importance of patient selection in these clinical trials.

In 2012, the whole-body hypothermia investigators published the results of follow-up evaluations of the original study subjects at 6 to 7 years of age. There was no difference in the combined primary outcome of death or an intelligence quotient (IQ) score < 70 (47% versus 62%, $P = .06$) between the hypothermia group and the control group.[220] The hypothermia group had a lower incidence of death or severe disability (41% versus 60%, $P = .03$), but there was no difference in moderate or severe disability (35% versus 38%, $P = .87$). Attention-executive dysfunction occurred in 4% of the hypothermia group versus 13% of the usual care group ($P = .19$), and visuospatial dysfunction occurred in 4% of the hypothermia group versus 3% of the usual care group ($P = .80$).[220] Thus, although there was no significant difference in the primary outcome, whole-body hypothermia decreased the incidence of death and did not increase the rate of a low IQ score or severe disability among survivors.

A 2013 metaanalysis of 11 randomized controlled trials of hypothermia therapy, which included 1505 term and late preterm infants, concluded that the benefits of cooling on survival and neurodevelopment outweigh the short-term adverse effects.[221] The authors advised that hypothermia should be instituted in term and late preterm infants with moderate-to-severe hypoxic-ischemic encephalopathy if identified before 6 hours of age. It remains unknown whether therapeutic hypothermia is beneficial in infants who have early-onset sepsis. A small study found similar outcomes in infants with proven sepsis and early-onset sepsis treated with hypothermia.[222] The authors suggested that therapeutic hypothermia should not be withheld from infants with early-onset sepsis. Further trials are necessary to identify appropriate cooling techniques and to refine patient selection.

Experimental Neuroprotection

Various other strategies for treating hypoxic-ischemic neonatal injuries, including administration of inflammatory mediator modulators, excitatory amino acid receptor agonists and antagonists, free radical scavengers, and platelet-activating factor antagonists have been suggested.[223,224] These emerging therapeutic strategies stem from basic neuroscience research on brain development and the pathophysiology of ischemic injury.

The role of white matter in the attenuation of hypoxic-ischemic brain damage (e.g., through uptake of excitatory amino acids or sequestration of potassium and hydrogen ions) is underappreciated,[225–227] and drugs that inhibit the release of excitatory amino acids or antagonize their receptors may be of benefit.[223] Multiple strategies may be necessary to inhibit the deleterious pathways initiated by brain ischemia and hypoxia.[228] A "brain cocktail," consisting of free radical scavengers, modifiers of nitric oxide activity, metabolic inhibitors, calcium and iron chelators, and drugs that affect the excitatory amino acid systems, may someday be administered to fetuses and neonates at risk for brain injury. Additional compounds that may inhibit CNS necrosis or apoptosis, either *in utero* or in the neonatal period, include agents that interrupt the inflammatory cascade, progesterone, and other steroids.

Erythropoietin (EPO) appears promising; EPO is known to have wide-ranging actions, including antiapoptotic, antioxidant, and antiinflammatory effects.[229] Indirectly, EPO may support angiogenesis and neovascularization.[229] In the first human clinical study, EPO administration in full-term neonates was associated with an almost 50% reduction in death and disability at 18 months when the hypoxic-ischemic injury was moderate but not severe.[230] A 2017 systematic review of studies in which EPO was administered to neonates born at greater than or equal to 35 weeks' gestation with perinatal asphyxia found that in six trials, EPO was administered alone, and in three trials it was administered with therapeutic hypothermia.[229] The authors concluded that long-term neurodevelopment outcomes are improved after EPO administration, and that EPO appears safe, without adverse effects.[229] However, the sample sizes were small in the included trials, and other study limitations precluded definitive conclusions.

Another agent with potential for fetal neuroprotection is **melatonin**, a highly effective antioxidant with reliable transplacental transfer and a wide therapeutic index. Administration of melatonin to fetal sheep compromised by experimental umbilical cord occlusion prevented oxidative stress, reduced lipid peroxidation, modulated microglial activation, and decreased the extent of brain damage.[231] The translational potential of other agents such as N-acetylcysteine, allopurinol, neurosteroids such as allopregnanolone, and anesthetic agents such as xenon, and creatine appears limited.

Further research has explored the role of umbilical cord blood cells in preventing brain injury. In a sheep model, umbilical cord blood cell administration at 12 hours after presumed hypoxia-ischemia reduced preterm white matter injury via antiinflammatory and antioxidant actions.[232]

Despite promising new therapies on the horizon, only a handful of currently used interventions are supported by evidence. A 2018 overview of Cochrane systematic reviews concluded that therapeutic hypothermia versus standard of care for newborns with hypoxic-ischemic encephalopathy can prevent cerebral palsy, and prophylactic methylxanthines (caffeine) versus placebo for tracheal extubation in preterm infants may reduce cerebral palsy risk. Early (<8 days of age) postnatal corticosteroids versus placebo or no treatment for chronic lung disease in preterm infants may increase cerebral palsy risk.[233]

The ability to accurately predict which fetuses are at risk for neurologic injury, and when, is currently rudimentary. The most vulnerable periods of fetal development are still unknown, and large studies are required to validate the use of noninvasive (e.g., advanced neuroimaging) fetal surveillance techniques.[234] Additional work has focused on identifying biomarkers of neurologic injury that could predict risk for cerebral palsy, thus identifying infants who would benefit from postdelivery interventions. The ability to identify these "at-risk" infants *in utero* or immediately after delivery is a necessary step in designing effective therapeutic regimens that interfere minimally with the normal trophic activities of the developing brain.

KEY POINTS

- Cerebral palsy is a nonprogressive disorder of the central nervous system that is present (but rarely obvious) at birth and involves some impairment of motor function or posture. Intellectual disability may or may not be present.
- The term *birth asphyxia* should be used sparingly, if at all, in medical records. More descriptive terms that describe the neonate's tone, color, respiratory effort, and metabolic status should be used when possible.
- The incidence of cerebral palsy is approximately 2 per 1000 live births and has not decreased despite the widespread use of intrapartum fetal heart rate monitoring and a higher cesarean delivery rate.
- The Apgar score is a poor predictor of cerebral palsy.
- Preterm delivery is a risk factor for cerebral palsy.
- Spastic quadriplegia and, less commonly, dyskinesia are the only types of cerebral palsy associated with acute intrapartum hypoxic events.
- Intrapartum hypoxia sufficient to cause cerebral palsy is always accompanied by neonatal encephalopathy and seizures.
- Fetal compensatory responses to hypoxemia *in utero* include (1) a redistribution of fetal cardiac output, with increased blood flow to the brain, myocardium, and adrenal glands; (2) decreased fetal energy consumption as a result of decreased fetal breathing and body movements; and (3) maintenance of essential cellular processes at the expense of fetal growth.
- Chorioamnionitis is associated with an increased risk for cerebral palsy. Epidural analgesia during labor is associated with an elevated maternal temperature (but not chorioamnionitis). Accurate diagnosis of chorioamnionitis may prevent unnecessary evaluations for sepsis in neonates of mothers with a rise in temperature during labor.
- No published data suggest that any given anesthetic drug or technique is more likely to protect fetal neurologic function (provided that the anesthetic technique is administered according to the recommended guidelines for good anesthesia practice).
- In animal models, exposure of the developing brain to anesthetic agents that interact with GABA and NMDA-type glutamate receptors induce a neurodegenerative response associated with subsequent functional impairment in adulthood. It remains to be determined whether exposure of human fetuses (via maternal anesthesia) and infants to these agents in clinically relevant doses leads to functional CNS impairment.

REFERENCES

1. Caviness VS Jr, Nowakowski RS, Bhide PG. Neocortical neurogenesis: morphogenetic gradients and beyond. *Trends Neurosci.* 2009;32:443–450.
2. Mitsuhashi T, Takahashi T. Genetic regulation of proliferation/differentiation characteristics of neural progenitor cells in the developing neocortex. *Brain Dev.* 2009;31:553–557.
3. Schafer DP, Lehrman EK, Kautzman AG, et al. Microglia sculpt postnatal neural circuits in an activity and complement-dependent manner. *Neuron.* 2012;74:691–705.
4. MacDonald JL, Roskams AJ. Epigenetic regulation of nervous system development by DNA methylation and histone deacetylation. *Prog Neurobiol.* 2009;88:170–183.
5. Amrein I, Isler K, Lipp HP. Comparing adult hippocampal neurogenesis in mammalian species and orders: influence of chronological age and life history stage. *Eur J Neurosci.* 2011;34:978–987.
6. Molnar Z, Clowry G. Cerebral cortical development in rodents and primates. *Prog Brain Res.* 2012;195:45–70.
7. Ayala R, Shu T, Tsai LH. Trekking across the brain: the journey of neuronal migration. *Cell.* 2007;128:29–43.
8. Pleasure SJ, Anderson S, Hevner R, et al. Cell migration from the ganglionic eminences is required for the development of hippocampal GABAergic interneurons. *Neuron.* 2000;28:727–740.
9. Belvindrah R, Lazarini F, Lledo PM. Postnatal neurogenesis: from neuroblast migration to neuronal integration. *Rev Neurosci.* 2009;20:331–346.
10. Heng JI, Moonen G, Nguyen L. Neurotransmitters regulate cell migration in the telencephalon. *Eur J Neurosci.* 2007;26:537–546.
11. de Graaf-Peters VB, Hadders-Algra M. Ontogeny of the human central nervous system: what is happening when? *Early Hum Dev.* 2006;82:257–266.
12. Levitt P. Structural and functional maturation of the developing primate brain. *J Pediatr.* 2003;143:S35–S45.
13. Lowery CL, Hardman MP, Manning N, et al. Neurodevelopmental changes of fetal pain. *Semin Perinatol.* 2007;31:275–282.
14. Ferschl M, Ball R, Lee H, Rollins MD. Anesthesia for in utero repair of myelomeningocele. *Anesthesiology.* 2013;118:1211–1223.
15. Wang DD, Kriegstein AR. Defining the role of GABA in cortical development. *J Physiol.* 2009;587:1873–1879.
16. Ben-Ari Y. Excitatory actions of GABA during development: the nature of the nurture. *Nat Rev Neurosci.* 2002;3:728–739.
17. LoTurco JJ, Owens DF, Heath MJ, et al. GABA and glutamate depolarize cortical progenitor cells and inhibit DNA synthesis. *Neuron.* 1995;15:1287–1298.
18. Ben-Ari Y, Gaiarsa JL, Tyzio R, Khazipov R. GABA: a pioneer transmitter that excites immature neurons and generates primitive oscillations. *Physiol Rev.* 2007;87:1215–1284.
19. Cuzon VC, Yeh PW, Yanagawa Y, et al. Ethanol consumption during early pregnancy alters the disposition of tangentially migrating GABAergic interneurons in the fetal cortex. *J Neurosci.* 2008;28:1854–1864.
20. Manent JB, Jorquera I, Mazzucchelli I, et al. Fetal exposure to GABA-acting antiepileptic drugs generates hippocampal and cortical dysplasias. *Epilepsia.* 2007;48:684–693.
21. Saunders NR, Liddelow SA, Dziegielewska KM. Barrier mechanisms in the developing brain. *Front Pharmacol.* 2012;3:46.
22. Baxter P. The definition and classification of cerebral palsy. *Dev Med Child Neurol.* 2007;49:1–44.

23. American College of Obstetricians and Gynecologists, American Academy of Pediatrics. *Neonatal Encephalopathy and Neurologic Outcome*. American College of Obstetricians and Gynecologists (reaffirmed 2019); 2014.

24. Myers RE. Two patterns of perinatal brain damage and their conditions of occurrence. *Am J Obstet Gynecol*. 1972;112:246–276.

25. Freeman R. Intrapartum fetal monitoring—a disappointing story. *N Engl J Med*. 1990;322:624–626.

26. Grant A, O'Brien N, Joy MT, et al. Cerebral palsy among children born during the Dublin randomised trial of intrapartum monitoring. *Lancet*. 1989;2:1233–1236.

27. Hankins GD, Erickson K, Zinberg S, Schulkin J. Neonatal encephalopathy and cerebral palsy: a knowledge survey of fellows of the American College of Obstetricians and Gynecologists. *Obstet Gynecol*. 2003;101:11–17.

28. Leveno KJ, Cunningham FG, Nelson S, et al. A prospective comparison of selective and universal electronic fetal monitoring in 34,995 pregnancies. *N Engl J Med*. 1986;315:615–619.

29. MacDonald D, Grant A, Sheridan-Pereira M, et al. The Dublin randomized controlled trial of intrapartum fetal heart rate monitoring. *Am J Obstet Gynecol*. 1985;152:524–539.

30. Rosen MG, Dickinson JC. The paradox of electronic fetal monitoring: more data may not enable us to predict or prevent infant neurologic morbidity. *Am J Obstet Gynecol*. 1993;168:745–751.

31. Freeman RK. Problems with intrapartum fetal heart rate monitoring interpretation and patient management. *Obstet Gynecol*. 2002;100:813–826.

32. Clark SL, Hamilton EF, Garite TJ, et al. The limits of electronic fetal heart rate monitoring in the prevention of neonatal metabolic acidemia. *Am J Obstet Gynecol*. 2017;216:163.e1–e6.

33. Schifrin BS, Cohen WR. Medical legal issues in fetal monitoring. *Clin Perinatol*. 2007;34:329–343.

34. Macones GA, Hankins GD, Spong CY, et al. The 2008 National Institute of Child Health and Human Development workshop report on electronic fetal monitoring: update on definitions, interpretation, and research guidelines. *Obstet Gynecol*. 2008;112:661–666.

35. Bakketeig LS. Only a minor part of cerebral palsy cases begin in labour. But still room for controversial childbirth issues in court. *BMJ*. 1999;319:1016–1017.

36. Blair E, Stanley FJ. Intrapartum asphyxia: a rare cause of cerebral palsy. *J Pediatr*. 1988;112:515–519.

37. Espinoza MI, Parer JT. Mechanisms of asphyxial brain damage, and possible pharmacologic interventions, in the fetus. *Am J Obstet Gynecol*. 1991;164:1582–1589.

38. Nakao M, Nanba Y, Okumura A, et al. Fetal heart rate evolution and brain imaging findings in preterm infants with severe cerebral palsy. *Am J Obstet Gynecol*. 2023;228:583.e1–e14.

39. Nakao M, Okumura A, Hasegawa J, et al. Fetal heart rate pattern in term or near-term cerebral palsy: a nationwide cohort study. *Am J Obstet Gynecol*. 2020;223:907.e1–e13.

40. MacLennan A. A template for defining a causal relation between acute intrapartum events and cerebral palsy: international consensus statement. *BMJ*. 1999;319:1054–1059.

41. Muraskas JK, Morrison JC. A proposed evidence-based neonatal work-up to confirm or refute allegations of intrapartum asphyxia. *Obstet Gynecol*. 2010;116:261–268.

42. Nelson KB, Ellenberg JH. Antecedents of cerebral palsy. I. Univariate analysis of risks. *Am J Dis Child*. 1985;139:1031–1038.

43. Nelson KB, Ellenberg JH. Antecedents of cerebral palsy. Multivariate analysis of risk. *N Engl J Med*. 1986;315:81–86.

44. Rosen MG, Dickinson JC. The incidence of cerebral palsy. *Am J Obstet Gynecol*. 1992;167:417–423.

45. Badawi N, Kurinczuk JJ, Keogh JM, et al. Intrapartum risk factors for newborn encephalopathy: the Western Australian case-control study. *BMJ*. 1998;317:1554–1558.

46. O'Callaghan ME, MacLennan AH, Gibson CS, et al. Epidemiologic associations with cerebral palsy. *Obstet Gynecol*. 2011;118:576–582.

47. Xiang S, Li L, Wang L, et al. A decision tree model of cerebral palsy based on risk factors. *J Matern Fetal Neonatal Med*. 2021;34:3922–3927.

48. American College of Obstetricians and Gynecologists. Executive summary: Neonatal encephalopathy and neurologic outcome, 2nd ed. Report of the American College of Obstetricians and Gynecologists' Task Force on Neonatal Encephalopathy. *Obstet Gynecol*. 2014;123:896–901.

49. American College of Obstetricians and Gynecologists, American Academy of Pediatrics. *Neonatal Encephalopathy and Cerebral Palsy: Defining the Pathogenesis and Pathophysiology*. American College of Obstetricians and Gynecologists; 2003.

50. Phelan JP, Korst LM, Martin GI. Application of criteria developed by the Task Force on Neonatal Encephalopathy and Cerebral Palsy to acutely asphyxiated neonates. *Obstet Gynecol*. 2011;118:824–830.

51. Helwig JT, Parer JT, Kilpatrick SJ, Laros RK Jr. Umbilical cord blood acid-base state: what is normal? *Am J Obstet Gynecol*. 1996;174:1807–1812.

52. Hull J, Dodd K. What is birth asphyxia? *Br J Obstet Gynaecol*. 1991;98:953–955.

53. Apgar V. A proposal for a new method of evaluation of the newborn infant. *Curr Res Anesth Analg*. 1953;32:260–267.

54. Marrin M, Paes BA. Birth asphyxia: does the Apgar score have diagnostic value? *Obstet Gynecol*. 1988;72:120–123.

55. Nelson KB, Ellenberg JH. Apgar scores as predictors of chronic neurologic disability. *Pediatrics*. 1981;68:36–44.

56. Fee SC, Malee K, Deddish R, et al. Severe acidosis and subsequent neurologic status. *Am J Obstet Gynecol*. 1990;162:802–806.

57. Goodwin TM, Belai I, Hernandez P, et al. Asphyxial complications in the term newborn with severe umbilical acidemia. *Am J Obstet Gynecol*. 1992;167:1506–1512.

58. Goldaber KG, Gilstrap LC 3rd, Leveno KJ, et al. Pathologic fetal acidemia. *Obstet Gynecol*. 1991;78:1103–1107.

59. Low JA, Lindsay BG, Derrick EJ. Threshold of metabolic acidosis associated with newborn complications. *Am J Obstet Gynecol*. 1997;177:1391–1394.

60. Low JA, Panagiotopoulos C, Derrick EJ. Newborn complications after intrapartum asphyxia with metabolic acidosis in the term fetus. *Am J Obstet Gynecol*. 1994;170:1081–1087.

61. Nagel HT, Vandenbussche FP, Oepkes D, et al. Follow-up of children born with an umbilical arterial blood pH < 7. *Am J Obstet Gynecol*. 1995;173:1758–1764.

62. Sehdev HM, Stamilio DM, Macones GA, et al. Predictive factors for neonatal morbidity in neonates with an umbilical

arterial cord pH less than 7.00. *Am J Obstet Gynecol.* 1997;177:1030–1034.

63. Gull I, Jaffa AJ, Oren M, et al. Acid accumulation during end-stage bradycardia in term fetuses: how long is too long? *Br J Obstet Gynaecol.* 1996;103:1096–1101.

64. Ross MG, Gala R. Use of umbilical artery base excess: algorithm for the timing of hypoxic injury. *Am J Obstet Gynecol.* 2002;187:1–9.

65. Malin GL, Morris RK, Khan KS. Strength of association between umbilical cord pH and perinatal and long term outcomes: systematic review and meta-analysis. *BMJ.* 2010;340:c1471.

66. Blumenthal I. Cerebral palsy—medicolegal aspects. *J R Soc Med.* 2001;94:624–627.

67. Phelan JP, Korst LM, Ahn MO, Martin GI. Neonatal nucleated red blood cell and lymphocyte counts in fetal brain injury. *Obstet Gynecol.* 1998;91:485–489.

68. Leikin E, Verma U, Klein S, Tejani N. Relationship between neonatal nucleated red blood cell counts and hypoxic-ischemic injury. *Obstet Gynecol.* 1996;87:439–443.

69. Murphy DJ, Johnson A. Placental infection and risk of cerebral palsy in very low birth weight infants. *J Pediatr.* 1996;129:776–778.

70. Grether JK, Nelson KB. Maternal infection and cerebral palsy in infants of normal birth weight. *JAMA.* 1997;278:207–211.

71. Stavsky M, Mor O, Mastrolia SA, et al. Cerebral palsy-trends in epidemiology and recent development in prenatal mechanisms of disease, treatment, and prevention. *Front Pediatr.* 2017;5:21.

72. Silverstein FS, Barks JD, Hagan P, et al. Cytokines and perinatal brain injury. *Neurochem Int.* 1997;30:375–383.

73. Dammann O, Leviton A. Maternal intrauterine infection, cytokines, and brain damage in the preterm newborn. *Pediatr Res.* 1997;42:1–8.

74. Wu YW, Colford JM Jr, Chorioamnionitis as a risk factor for cerebral palsy: a meta-analysis. *JAMA.* 2000;284:1417–1424.

75. Shatrov JG, Birch SC, Lam LT, et al. Chorioamnionitis and cerebral palsy: a meta-analysis. *Obstet Gynecol.* 2010;116:387–392.

76. Jain VG, Kline JE, He L, et al. Acute histologic chorioamnionitis independently and directly increases the risk for brain abnormalities seen on magnetic resonance imaging in very preterm infants. *Am J Obstet Gynecol.* 2022;227:623.e1–e13.

77. Patel S, Ciechanowicz S, Blumenfeld YJ, Sultan P. Epidural-related maternal fever: incidence, pathophysiology, outcomes, and management. *Am J Obstet Gynecol.* 2023;228(5S):S1283–S1304.e1.

78. Lieberman E Lang JM, Frigoletto F, Jr, et al. Epidural analgesia, intrapartum fever, and neonatal sepsis evaluation. *Pediatrics.* 1997;99:415–419.

79. Mayer DC, Chescheir NC, Spielman FJ. Increased intrapartum antibiotic administration associated with epidural analgesia in labor. *Am J Perinatol.* 1997;14:83–86.

80. Rees S, Breen S, Loeliger M, et al. Hypoxemia near mid-gestation has long-term effects on fetal brain development. *J Neuropathol Exp Neurol.* 1999;58:932–945.

81. Rees S, Inder T. Fetal and neonatal origins of altered brain development. *Early Hum Dev.* 2005;81:753–761.

82. Saraceno GE, Castilla R, Barreto GE, et al. Hippocampal dendritic spines modifications induced by perinatal asphyxia. *Neural Plast.* 2012;2012:873532.

83. Chen WF, Chang H, Wong CS, et al. Impaired expression of postsynaptic density proteins in the hippocampal CA1 region of rats following perinatal hypoxia. *Exp Neurol.* 2007;204:400–410.

84. McLean C, Ferriero D. Mechanisms of hypoxic-ischemic injury in the term infant. *Semin Perinatol.* 2004;28:425–432.

85. Back SA, Han BH, Luo NL, et al. Selective vulnerability of late oligodendrocyte progenitors to hypoxia-ischemia. *J Neurosci.* 2002;22:455–463.

86. Burd I, Balakrishnan B, Kannan S. Models of fetal brain injury, intrauterine inflammation, and preterm birth. *Am J Reprod Immunol.* 2012;67:287–294.

87. Hagberg H, Gressens P, Mallard C. Inflammation during fetal and neonatal life: implications for neurologic and neuropsychiatric disease in children and adults. *Ann Neurol.* 2012;71:444–457.

88. Boksa P. Effects of prenatal infection on brain development and behavior: a review of findings from animal models. *Brain Behav Immun.* 2010;24:881–897.

89. Patterson PH. Maternal infection and immune involvement in autism. *Trends Mol Med.* 2011;17:389–394.

90. Shevell A, Wintermark P, Benini R, et al. Chorioamnionitis and cerebral palsy: lessons from a patient registry. *Eur J Paediatr Neurol.* 2014;18:301–307.

91. Dahlgren J, Samuelsson AM, Jansson T, Holmäng A. Interleukin-6 in the maternal circulation reaches the rat fetus in mid-gestation. *Pediatr Res.* 2006;60:147–151.

92. Smith SE, Li J, Garbett K, et al. Maternal immune activation alters fetal brain development through interleukin-6. *J Neurosci.* 2007;27:10695–10702.

93. Deverman BE, Patterson PH. Cytokines and CNS development. *Neuron.* 2009;64:61–78.

94. Boles JL, Ross MG, Beloosesky R, et al. Placental-mediated increased cytokine response to lipopolysaccharides: a potential mechanism for enhanced inflammation susceptibility of the preterm fetus. *J Inflamm Res.* 2012;5:67–75.

95. Garay PA, Hsiao EY, Patterson PH, McAllister AK. Maternal immune activation causes age- and region-specific changes in brain cytokines in offspring throughout development. *Brain Behav Immun.* 2013;31:54–68.

96. Chiesa C, Pellegrini G, Panero A, et al. Umbilical cord interleukin-6 levels are elevated in term neonates with perinatal asphyxia. *Eur J Clin Invest.* 2003;33:352–358.

97. Samuelsson AM, Jennische E, Hansson HA, Holmäng A. Prenatal exposure to interleukin-6 results in inflammatory neurodegeneration in hippocampus with NMDA/GABA(A) dysregulation and impaired spatial learning. *Am J Physiol Regul Integr Comp Physiol.* 2006;290:R1345–R1356.

98. Arrode-Brusés G, Brusés JL. Maternal immune activation by poly I:C induces expression of cytokines IL-1beta and IL-13, chemokine MCP-1 and colony stimulating factor VEGF in fetal mouse brain. *J Neuroinflammation.* 2012;9:83.

99. Monier A, Evrard P, Gressens P, Verney C. Distribution and differentiation of microglia in the human encephalon during the first two trimesters of gestation. *J Comp Neurol.* 2006;499:565–582.

100. Paolicelli RC, Bolasco G, Pagani F, et al. Synaptic pruning by microglia is necessary for normal brain development. *Science.* 2011;333:1456–1458.

101. Stark MJ, Hodyl NA, Belegar VK, Andersen CC. Intrauterine inflammation, cerebral oxygen consumption and susceptibility to early brain injury in very preterm newborns. *Arch Dis Child Fetal Neonatal Ed.* 2016;101:F137–F142.

102. Perrone S, Tataranno LM, Stazzoni G, et al. Brain susceptibility to oxidative stress in the perinatal period. *J Matern Fetal Neonatal Med.* 2015;28(suppl 1): 2291–2295.

103. Brown AS, Derkits EJ. Prenatal infection and schizophrenia: a review of epidemiologic and translational studies. *Am J Psychiatry.* 2010;167:261–280.

104. Brown AS. Epidemiologic studies of exposure to prenatal infection and risk of schizophrenia and autism. *Dev Neurobiol.* 2012;72:1272–1276.

105. Espinoza ML, Brundler MA, Hasan SU, et al. Placental pathology as a marker of brain injury in infants with hypoxic ischemic encephalopathy. *Early Hum Dev.* 2022;174:105683.

106. Raju TN. Some animal models for the study of perinatal asphyxia. *Biol Neonate.* 1992;62:202–214.

107. Dobbing J, Sands J. Comparative aspects of the brain growth spurt. *Early Hum Dev.* 1979;3:79–83.

108. Clancy B, Finlay BL, Darlington RB, Anand KJ. Extrapolating brain development from experimental species to humans. *Neurotoxicology.* 2007;28:931–937.

109. Workman AD, Charvet CJ, Clancy B, et al. Modeling transformations of neurodevelopmental sequences across mammalian species. *J Neurosci.* 2013;33:7368–7383.

110. Penning DH, Chestnut DH, Dexter F, et al. Glutamate release from the ovine fetal brain during maternal hemorrhage. A study using chronic in utero cerebral microdialysis. *Anesthesiology.* 1995;82:521–530.

111. Reynolds JD, Penning DH, Dexter F, et al. Dose-dependent effects of acute in vivo ethanol exposure on extracellular glutamate concentration in the cerebral cortex of the near-term fetal sheep. *Alcohol Clin Exp Res.* 1995;19:1447–1453.

112. Richardson BS, Patrick JE, Abduljabbar H. Cerebral oxidative metabolism in the fetal lamb: relationship to electrocortical state. *Am J Obstet Gynecol.* 1985;153:426–431.

113. Richardson BS, Patrick JE, Bousquet J, et al. Cerebral metabolism in fetal lamb after maternal infusion of ethanol. *Am J Physiol.* 1985;249:R505–R509.

114. Matsuda Y, Patrick J, Carmichael L, et al. Effects of sustained hypoxemia on the sheep fetus at midgestation: endocrine, cardiovascular, and biophysical responses. *Am J Obstet Gynecol.* 1992;167:531–540.

115. Richardson BS, Carmichael L, Homan J, Patrick JE. Electrocortical activity, electroocular activity, and breathing movements in fetal sheep with prolonged and graded hypoxemia. *Am J Obstet Gynecol.* 1992;167:553–558.

116. Henderson JL, Reynolds JD, Dexter F, et al. Chronic hypoxemia causes extracellular glutamate concentration to increase in the cerebral cortex of the near-term fetal sheep. *Brain Res Dev Brain Res.* 1998;105:287–293.

117. Mallard EC, Gunn AJ, Williams CE, et al. Transient umbilical cord occlusion causes hippocampal damage in the fetal sheep. *Am J Obstet Gynecol.* 1992;167:1423–1430.

118. Clapp JF, Peress NS, Wesley M, Mann LI. Brain damage after intermittent partial cord occlusion in the chronically instrumented fetal lamb. *Am J Obstet Gynecol.* 1988;159: 504–509.

119. Clapp JF 3rd, Mann LI, Peress NS, Szeto HH. Neuropathology in the chronic fetal lamb preparation: structure-function correlates under different environmental conditions. *Am J Obstet Gynecol.* 1981;141:973–986.

120. Reynolds JD, Chestnut DH, Dexter F, et al. Magnesium sulfate adversely affects fetal lamb survival and blocks fetal cerebral blood flow response during maternal hemorrhage. *Anesth Analg.* 1996;83:493–499.

121. Hohimer AR, Chao CR, Bissonnette JM. The effect of combined hypoxemia and cephalic hypotension on fetal cerebral blood flow and metabolism. *J Cereb Blood Flow Metab.* 1991;11:99–105.

122. Robillard JE, Weitzman RE, Burmeister L, Smith FG Jr. Developmental aspects of the renal response to hypoxemia in the lamb fetus. *Circ Res.* 1981;48:128–138.

123. Richardson BS. The fetal brain: metabolic and circulatory responses to asphyxia. *Clin Invest Med.* 1993;16:103–114.

124. Lin B, Globus MY, Dietrich WD, et al. Differing neurochemical and morphological sequelae of global ischemia: comparison of single- and multiple-insult paradigms. *J Neurochem.* 1992;59:2213–2223.

125. Mallard EC, Williams CE, Gunn AJ, et al. Frequent episodes of brief ischemia sensitize the fetal sheep brain to neuronal loss and induce striatal injury. *Pediatr Res.* 1993;33:61–65.

126. Penning DH, Grafe MR, Hammond R, et al. Neuropathology of the near-term and midgestation ovine fetal brain after sustained in utero hypoxemia. *Am J Obstet Gynecol.* 1994;170: 1425–1432.

127. Brann AW Jr, Myers RE. Central nervous system findings in the newborn monkey following severe in utero partial asphyxia. *Neurology.* 1975;25:327–338.

128. Volpe JJ. Brain injury in the premature infant—current concepts of pathogenesis and prevention. *Biol Neonate.* 1992;62:231–242.

129. Back SA. Brain injury in the preterm infant: new horizons for pathogenesis and prevention. *Pediatr Neurol.* 2015;53: 185–192.

130. Lee YA. White matter injury of prematurity: its mechanisms and clinical features. *J Pathol Transl Med.* 2017;51: 449–455.

131. Alderliesten T, Lemmers PM, Smarius JJ, et al. Cerebral oxygenation, extraction, and autoregulation in very preterm infants who develop peri-intraventricular hemorrhage. *J Pediatr.* 2013;162:698–704.e2.

132. Miller SP, Ferriero DM, Leonard C, et al. Early brain injury in premature newborns detected with magnetic resonance imaging is associated with adverse early neurodevelopmental outcome. *J Pediatr.* 2005;147:609–616.

133. Richardson BS. Fetal adaptive responses to asphyxia. *Clin Perinatol.* 1989;16:595–611.

134. Edelstone DI. Fetal compensatory responses to reduced oxygen delivery. *Semin Perinatol.* 1984;8:184–191.

135. Gu W, Jones CT, Parer JT. Metabolic and cardiovascular effects on fetal sheep of sustained reduction of uterine blood flow. *J Physiol.* 1985;368:109–129.

136. Prakash A, Matta BF. Hyperglycaemia and neurological injury. *Curr Opin Anaesthesiol.* 2008;21:565–569.

137. Vannucci RC, Mujsce DJ. Effect of glucose on perinatal hypoxic-ischemic brain damage. *Biol Neonate.* 1992;62:215–224.

138. Blomstrand S, Hrbek A, Karlsson K, et al. Does glucose administration affect the cerebral response to fetal asphyxia? *Acta Obstet Gynecol Scand.* 1984;63:345–353.

139. Hooper SB, Bocking AD, White S, et al. DNA synthesis is reduced in selected fetal tissues during prolonged hypoxemia. *Am J Physiol.* 1991;261:R508–R514.

140. Rurak DW, Gruber NC. The effect of neuromuscular blockade on oxygen consumption and blood gases in the fetal lamb. *Am J Obstet Gynecol.* 1983;145:258–262.

141. Jensen A, Berger R. Fetal circulatory responses to oxygen lack. *J Dev Physiol.* 1991;16:181–207.

142. Sheldon RE, Peeters LL, Jones MD Jr, et al. Redistribution of cardiac output and oxygen delivery in the hypoxemic fetal lamb. *Am J Obstet Gynecol.* 1979;135:1071–1078.

143. Jensen A, Hohmann M, Künzel W. Dynamic changes in organ blood flow and oxygen consumption during acute asphyxia in fetal sheep. *J Dev Physiol.* 1987;9:543–559.

144. DiPietro JA. Neurobehavioral assessment before birth. *Ment Retard Dev Disabil Res Rev.* 2005;11:4–13.

145. Stanojevic M, Zaputovic S, Bosnjak AP. Continuity between fetal and neonatal neurobehavior. *Semin Fetal Neonatal Med.* 2012;17:324–329.

146. Salisbury AL, Fallone MD, Lester B. Neurobehavioral assessment from fetus to infant: the NICU Network Neurobehavioral Scale and the Fetal Neurobehavior Coding Scale. *Ment Retard Dev Disabil Res Rev.* 2005;11:14–20.

147. Honemeyer U, Talic A, Therwat A, et al. The clinical value of KANET in studying fetal neurobehavior in normal and at-risk pregnancies. *J Perinat Med.* 2013;41:187–197.

148. Prayer D, Kasprian G, Krampl E, et al. MRI of normal fetal brain development. *Eur J Radiol.* 2006;57:199–216.

149. Ang ES Jr, Gluncic V, Duque A, et al. Prenatal exposure to ultrasound waves impacts neuronal migration in mice. *Proc Natl Acad Sci U S A.* 2006;103:12903–12910.

150. Hinojosa-Rodríguez M, Harmony T, Carrillo-Prado C, et al. Clinical neuroimaging in the preterm infant: diagnosis and prognosis. *Neuroimage Clin.* 2017;16:355–368.

151. Panigrahy A, Blüml S. Advances in magnetic resonance neuroimaging techniques in the evaluation of neonatal encephalopathy. *Top Magn Reson Imaging.* 2007;18:3–29.

152. Nanba Y, Matsui K, Aida N, et al. Magnetic resonance imaging regional T1 abnormalities at term accurately predict motor outcome in preterm infants. *Pediatrics.* 2007;120:e10–e19.

153. Orman G, Benson JE, Kweldam CF, et al. Neonatal head ultrasonography today: a powerful imaging tool! *J Neuroimaging.* 2015;25:31–55.

154. Kuhnert BR, Kuhnert PM, Philipson EH, Syracuse CD. Disposition of meperidine and normeperidine following multiple doses during labor. II. Fetus and neonate. *Am J Obstet Gynecol.* 1985;151:410–415.

155. Golub MS, Donald JM. Effect of intrapartum meperidine on behavior of 3- to 12-month-old infant rhesus monkeys. *Biol Neonate.* 1995;67:140–148.

156. Golub MS, Eisele JH Jr, Donald JM. Obstetric analgesia and infant outcome in monkeys: infant development after intrapartum exposure to meperidine or alfentanil. *Am J Obstet Gynecol.* 1988;159:1280–1286.

157. Tripathi A, Khurshid N, Kumar P, Iyengar S. Expression of δ- and μ-opioid receptors in the ventricular and subventricular zones of the developing human neocortex. *Neurosci Res.* 2008;61:257–270.

158. Sargeant TJ, Day DJ, Miller JH, Steel RW. Acute in utero morphine exposure slows G2/M phase transition in radial glial and basal progenitor cells in the dorsal telencephalon of the E15.5 embryonic mouse. *Eur J Neurosci.* 2008;28:1060–1067.

159. Hauser KF, Houdi AA, Turbek CS, et al. Opioids intrinsically inhibit the genesis of mouse cerebellar granule neuron precursors in vitro: differential impact of μ and δ receptor activation on proliferation and neurite elongation. *Eur J Neurosci.* 2000;12:1281–1293.

160. Niu L, Cao B, Zhu H, et al. Impaired in vivo synaptic plasticity in dentate gyrus and spatial memory in juvenile rats induced by prenatal morphine exposure. *Hippocampus.* 2009;19:649–657.

161. Golub MS. Labor analgesia and infant brain development. *Pharmacol Biochem Behav.* 1996;55:619–628.

162. Flick RP, Lee K, Hofer RE, et al. Neuraxial labor analgesia for vaginal delivery and its effects on childhood learning disabilities. *Anesth Analg.* 2011;112:1424–1431.

163. Deng CM, Ding T, Liu ZH, et al. Impact of maternal neuraxial labor analgesia exposure on offspring's neurodevelopment: a longitudinal prospective cohort study with propensity score matching. *Front Public Health.* 2022;10:831538.

164. Kearns RJ, Shaw M, Gromski PS, et al. Association of epidural analgesia in women in labor with neonatal and childhood outcomes in a population cohort. *JAMA Netw Open.* 2021;4:e2131683.

165. Qiu C, Lin JC, Shi JM, et al. Association between epidural analgesia during labor and risk of autism spectrum disorders in offspring. *JAMA Pediatr.* 2020;174:1168–1175.

166. Hanley GE, Bickford C, Ip A, et al. Association of epidural analgesia during labor and delivery with autism spectrum disorder in offspring. *JAMA.* 2021;326:1178–1185.

167. Wall-Wieler E, Bateman BT, Hanlon-Dearman A, et al. Association of epidural labor analgesia with offspring risk of autism spectrum disorders. *JAMA Pediatr.* 2021;175:698–705.

168. Ren T, Zhang J, Yu Y, et al. Association of labour epidural analgesia with neurodevelopmental disorders in offspring: a Danish population-based cohort study. *Br J Anaesth.* 2022;128:513–521.

169. Wong CA, Stevens H. Labor epidural analgesia and autism spectrum disorder: is there an association? *JAMA.* 2021;326:1155–1157.

170. Butwick AJ, Abrams DA, Wong CA. Epidural labour analgesia and autism spectrum disorder: is the current evidence sufficient to dismiss an association? *Br J Anaesth.* 2022;128:393–398.

171. Likis FE, Andrews JC, Collins MR, et al. Nitrous oxide for the management of labor pain: a systematic review. *Anesth Analg.* 2014;118:153–167.

172. Reynolds F. The effects of maternal labour analgesia on the fetus. *Best Pract Res Clin Obstet Gynaecol.* 2010;24:289–302.

173. Stefani SJ, Hughes SC, Schnider SM, et al. Neonatal neurobehavioral effects of inhalation analgesia for vaginal delivery. *Anesthesiology.* 1982;56:351–355.

174. King TL, Wong CA. Nitrous oxide for labor pain: is it a laughing matter? *Anesth Analg.* 2014;118:12–14.

175. Jevtovic-Todorovic V, Hartman RE, Izumi Y, et al. Early exposure to common anesthetic agents causes widespread neurodegeneration in the developing rat brain and persistent learning deficits. *J Neurosci.* 2003;23:876–882.

176. Satomoto M, Satoh Y, Terui K, et al. Neonatal exposure to sevoflurane induces abnormal social behaviors and deficits in fear conditioning in mice. *Anesthesiology.* 2009;110:628–637.

177. Wilder RT, Flick RP, Sprung J, et al. Early exposure to anesthesia and learning disabilities in a population-based birth cohort. *Anesthesiology.* 2009;110:796–804.

178. Glatz P, Sandin RH, Pedersen NL, et al. Association of anesthesia and surgery during childhood with long-term academic performance. *JAMA Pediatr.* 2017;171:e163470.

179. McCann ME, Soriano SG. Does general anesthesia affect neurodevelopment in infants and children? *BMJ.* 2019;367:l6459.

180. Wang J, Liu Z. Research progress on molecular mechanisms of general anesthetic-induced neurotoxicity and cognitive impairment in the developing brain. *Front Neurol.* 2022;13:1065976.

181. Campbell LL, Tyson JA, Stackpole EE, et al. Assessment of general anaesthetic cytotoxicity in murine cortical neurones in dissociated culture. *Toxicology.* 2011;283:1–7.

182. Palanisamy A, Baxter MG, Keel PK, et al. Rats exposed to isoflurane in utero during early gestation are behaviorally abnormal as adults. *Anesthesiology.* 2011;114:521–528.

183. Kong F, Xu L, He D, et al. Effects of gestational isoflurane exposure on postnatal memory and learning in rats. *Eur J Pharmacol.* 2011;670:168–174.

184. Kong FJ, Tang YW, Lou AF, et al. Effects of isoflurane exposure during pregnancy on postnatal memory and learning in offspring rats. *Mol Biol Rep.* 2012;39:4849–4855.

185. Rizzi S, Carter LB, Ori C, Jevtovic-Todorovic V. Clinical anesthesia causes permanent damage to the fetal guinea pig brain. *Brain Pathol.* 2008;18:198–210.

186. Slikker W Jr, Zou X, Hotchkiss CE, et al. Ketamine-induced neuronal cell death in the perinatal rhesus monkey. *Toxicol Sci.* 2007;98:145–158.

187. Sall JW, Stratmann G, Leong J, et al. Isoflurane inhibits growth but does not cause cell death in hippocampal neural precursor cells grown in culture. *Anesthesiology.* 2009;110:826–833.

188. Culley DJ, Boyd JD, Palanisamy A, et al. Isoflurane decreases self-renewal capacity of rat cultured neural stem cells. *Anesthesiology.* 2011;115:754–763.

189. Li Y, Liang G, Wang S, et al. Effects of fetal exposure to isoflurane on postnatal memory and learning in rats. *Neuropharmacology.* 2007;53:942–950.

190. Wang S, Peretich K, Zhao Y, et al. Anesthesia-induced neurodegeneration in fetal rat brains. *Pediatr Res.* 2009;66:435–440.

191. Creeley CE, Dikranian KT, Dissen GA, et al. Isoflurane-induced apoptosis of neurons and oligodendrocytes in the fetal rhesus macaque brain. *Anesthesiology.* 2014;120:626–638.

192. Brambrink AM, Evers AS, Avidan MS, et al. Ketamine-induced neuroapoptosis in the fetal and neonatal rhesus macaque brain. *Anesthesiology.* 2012;116:372–384.

193. Creeley C, Dikranian K, Dissen G, et al. Propofol-induced apoptosis of neurones and oligodendrocytes in fetal and neonatal rhesus macaque brain. *Br J Anaesth.* 2013;110:i29–i38.

194. Sprung J, Flick RP, Wilder RT, et al. Anesthesia for cesarean delivery and learning disabilities in a population-based birth cohort. *Anesthesiology.* 2009;111:302–310.

195. Ing C, Silber JH, Lackraj D, et al. Behavioural disorders after prenatal exposure to anaesthesia for maternal surgery. *Br J Anaesth.* 2024;132:899–910.

196. Ende HB, Habib AS, Lim G, et al. Behavioural disorders after prenatal exposure to anaesthesia for maternal surgery: is it the anaesthesia or the surgery? *Br J Anaesth.* 2024;133:682–683.

197. Chien LN, Lin HC, Shao YH, et al. Risk of autism associated with general anesthesia during cesarean delivery: a population-based birth-cohort analysis. *J Autism Dev Disord.* 2015;45:932–942.

198. Creagh O, Torres H, Rivera K, et al. Previous exposure to anesthesia and autism spectrum disorder (ASD): a Puerto Rican population-based sibling cohort study. *Bol Asoc Med P R.* 2015;107:29–37.

199. United States Food and Drug Administration. FDA drug safety communication: FDA review results in new warnings about using general anesthetics and sedation drugs in young children and pregnant women; 2016. Available at: https://www.fda.gov/Drugs/DrugSafety/ucm532356.htm. Accessed November 12, 2024.

200. Davidson AJ, Disma N, de Graaff JC, et al. Neurodevelopmental outcome at 2 years of age after general anaesthesia and awake-regional anaesthesia in infancy (GAS): an international multicentre, randomised controlled trial. *Lancet.* 2016;387:239–250.

201. Sun LS, Li G, Miller TL, et al. Association between a single general anesthesia exposure before age 36 months and neurocognitive outcomes in later childhood. *JAMA.* 2016;315:2312–2320.

202. Petraglia F, Imperatore A, Challis JR. Neuroendocrine mechanisms in pregnancy and parturition. *Endocr Rev.* 2010;31:783–816.

203. Al-Enazy S, Ali S, Albekairi N, et al. Placental control of drug delivery. *Adv Drug Deliv Rev.* 2017;116:63–72.

204. Schubert K, Schade K. Placental steroid hormones. *J Steroid Biochem.* 1977;8:359–365.

205. Tsutsui K. Progesterone biosynthesis and action in the developing neuron. *Endocrinology.* 2008;149:2757–2761.

206. McCarthy MM. Estradiol and the developing brain. *Physiol Rev.* 2008;88:91–124.

207. de Geest K, Thiery M, Piron-Possuyt G, Vanden Driessche R. Plasma oxytocin in human pregnancy and parturition. *J Perinat Med.* 1985;13:3–13.

208. Tyzio R, Cossart R, Khalilov I, et al. Maternal oxytocin triggers a transient inhibitory switch in GABA signaling in the fetal brain during delivery. *Science.* 2006;314:1788–1792.

209. Khazipov R, Tyzio R, Ben-Ari Y. Effects of oxytocin on GABA signalling in the foetal brain during delivery. *Prog Brain Res.* 2008;170:243–257.

210. Crowther CA, Hiller JE, Doyle LW, Haslam RR. Effect of magnesium sulfate given for neuroprotection before preterm birth: a randomized controlled trial. *JAMA.* 2003;290:2669–2676.

211. Marret S, Marpeau L, Zupan-Simunek V, et al. Magnesium sulphate given before very-preterm birth to protect infant brain: the randomised controlled PREMAG trial. *BJOG.* 2007;114:310–318.

212. Rouse DJ, Hirtz DG, Thom E, et al. A randomized, controlled trial of magnesium sulfate for the prevention of cerebral palsy. *N Engl J Med.* 2008;359:895–905.

213. Crowther CA, Middleton PF, Voysey M, et al. Assessing the neuroprotective benefits for babies of antenatal magnesium sulphate: an individual participant data meta-analysis. *PLoS Med.* 2017;14:e1002398.

214. Shepherd ES, Goldsmith S, Doyle LW, et al. Magnesium sulphate for women at risk of preterm birth for neuroprotection of the fetus. *Cochrane Database Syst Rev.* 2024;(5):CD004661.

215. American College of Obstetricians and Gynecologists. Committee Opinion No. 455: Magnesium sulfate before anticipated preterm birth for neuroprotection (reaffirmed 2023). *Obstet Gynecol.* 2010;115:669–671.

216. George S, Scotter J, Dean JM, et al. Induced cerebral hypothermia reduces post-hypoxic loss of phenotypic striatal neurons in preterm fetal sheep. *Exp Neurol.* 2007;203:137–147.

217. Shankaran S, Laptook AR, Ehrenkranz RA, et al. Whole-body hypothermia for neonates with hypoxic-ischemic encephalopathy. *N Engl J Med.* 2005;353:1574–1584.

218. Gluckman PD, Wyatt JS, Azzopardi D, et al. Selective head cooling with mild systemic hypothermia after neonatal encephalopathy: multicentre randomised trial. *Lancet.* 2005;365:663–670.

219. Papile LA. Systemic hypothermia—a "cool" therapy for neonatal hypoxic-ischemic encephalopathy. *N Engl J Med.* 2005;353:1619–1620.

220. Shankaran S, Pappas A, McDonald SA, et al. Childhood outcomes after hypothermia for neonatal encephalopathy. *N Engl J Med.* 2012;366:2085–2092.

221. Jacobs SE, Berg M, Hunt R, et al. Cooling for newborns with hypoxic ischaemic encephalopathy. *Cochrane Database Syst Rev.* 2013;(1):CD003311.

222. Hakobyan M, Dijkman KP, Laroche S, et al. Outcome of infants with therapeutic hypothermia after perinatal asphyxia and early-onset sepsis. *Neonatology.* 2019;115:127–133.

223. Perlman JM. Intervention strategies for neonatal hypoxic-ischemic cerebral injury. *Clin Ther.* 2006;28:1353–1365.

224. Gao H, Jiang H. Current status and controversies in the treatment of neonatal hypoxic-ischemic encephalopathy: a review. *Medicine (Baltimore).* 2024;103:e38993.

225. Swanson RA. Astrocyte glutamate uptake during chemical hypoxia in vitro. *Neurosci Lett.* 1992;147:143–146.

226. Swanson RA, Choi DW. Glial glycogen stores affect neuronal survival during glucose deprivation in vitro. *J Cereb Blood Flow Metab.* 1993;13:162–169.

227. Ransom BR, Stys PK, Waxman SG. The pathophysiology of anoxic injury in central nervous system white matter. *Stroke.* 1990;21:III52–III57.

228. Volpe JJ. Brain injury in the premature infant—from pathogenesis to prevention. *Brain Dev.* 1997;19:519–534.

229. Garg B, Sharma D, Bansal A. Systematic review seeking erythropoietin role for neuroprotection in neonates with hypoxic ischemic encephalopathy: presently where do we stand. *J Matern Fetal Neonatal Med.* 2017:1–11.

230. Rees S, Harding R, Walker D. The biological basis of injury and neuroprotection in the fetal and neonatal brain. *Int J Dev Neurosci.* 2011;29:551–563.

231. Balduini W, Carloni S, Perrone S, et al. The use of melatonin in hypoxic-ischemic brain damage: an experimental study. *J Matern Fetal Neonatal Med.* 2012;25(suppl 1):119–124.

232. Li J, Yawno T, Sutherland AE, et al. Preterm umbilical cord blood derived mesenchymal stem/stromal cells protect preterm white matter brain development against hypoxia-ischemia. *Exp Neurol.* 2018;308:120–131.

233. Shepherd E, Salam RA, Middleton P, et al. Neonatal interventions for preventing cerebral palsy: an overview of Cochrane systematic reviews. *Cochrane Database Syst Rev.* 2018;(6):CD012409.

234. Parikh NA. Advanced neuroimaging and its role in predicting neurodevelopmental outcomes in very preterm infants. *Semin Perinatol.* 2016;40:530–541.

11

Quality, Patient Safety, and Medical Error

David J. Birnbach, MD, MPH and Klaus Kjaer, MD, MBA

CHAPTER OUTLINE

In 2000, the publication of the Institute of Medicine report *To Err Is Human: Building a Safer Health Care System* was a pivotal event for the healthcare system in the United States.[1] Prior to the publication of this report, many physicians and hospital administrators refused to acknowledge the frequent occurrence of preventable morbidity and the reality that our healthcare system was not adequately addressing the issue of patient safety. One estimate for annual error-induced mortality is greater than 250,000,[2] making medical errors the third-leading cause of death in the United States. Healthcare errors do not usually occur because of ill-trained medical personnel but rather are due to imperfect systems that trap both the patient and the healthcare provider. Regardless of the exact number, we now know that tens of thousands of patients die each year because of medical errors. Unfortunately, the labor and delivery suite is not immune to this phenomenon.

In the past several decades, numerous changes to medical care have been advocated with the goal of improving patient safety, including mandating minimum nurse-to-patient ratios,[3] reducing working hours of resident physicians,[4] use of care bundles,[5] and advancing the science of simulation training and teamwork.[6] As Pratt[7] eloquently stated, "Historically, medicine was simple, largely ineffective, and mostly safe (excluding perhaps trephination and bloodletting). Modern medicine is complex, highly effective, but dangerous." The field of patient safety attempts to reduce that danger.

Sadly, maternal mortality in the United States has risen over the last several decades, despite improvements in patient safety and healthcare—many of the deaths are judged preventable.[8] This is particularly troubling since this increase has occurred during a period (with the exception of COVID-19-related deaths) when global maternal death rates fell, thus making the United States an outlier for maternal mortality rates in the developed world.[9] Improved communication and collaboration among all stakeholders involved in perinatal health has been proposed as necessary to reverse this trend.[10] Although there have been significant developments to improve the safety of hospitalized patients, including scientific and policy approaches, human error continues to be a cause of morbidity and mortality. The numbers are staggering. A 2023 cross-sectional analysis of US-based observational data found that an estimated 795,000 Americans become permanently disabled or die annually across healthcare settings.[11]

Obstetric anesthesia practice has continued to evolve, but a study evaluating the epidemiology of anesthesia-related complications in obstetric units in a single state reported that the incidence of anesthesia-related complications during labor and delivery "remains a cause of concern, particularly in women undergoing cesarean delivery, living in rural areas, or having preexisting medical conditions."[12]

A 2023 report evaluating healthcare in the UK National Health Service considered what needed to be done to "close the gap between ambitious patient safety objectives and the reality of frontline practice."[13] The report outlined themes that lead to avoidable errors. These include failure to make the right diagnosis, delay in providing appropriate treatment, inadequate handoffs, and failure to listen to the concerns of the patients or their families. Of note, the report found that a failure to be honest when errors occur, poor-quality investigations, and inadequate learning responses all compounded the original errors. Although these statements were made generally about medical care in the National Health Service, they likely are pertinent to the practice of obstetrics and obstetric anesthesia globally.

In the recent past, strategies to reduce errors in obstetric care often focused on teamwork and team training, and that strategy continues to be a key to improving safety.[14] Improving interprofessional communication skills has been shown to reduce preventable adverse events.[15] However, consensus care bundles, such as the ones for prevention of venous thromboembolism,[16] obstetric hemorrhage,[17] and hypertension[18] are also vital for consistently preventing harm and improving parturient safety. Another imperative is to address racial disparities with a focus on patient safety (see Chapter 14). The Committee on Obstetric Anesthesia of the American Society of Anesthesiologists (ASA) has noted that significant disparities in maternal health exist in the peripartum period, most notably in maternal mortality, severe maternal morbidity, and in the use of neuraxial labor analgesia and general anesthesia for cesarean delivery.[19]

Adverse outcomes in the obstetric patient often involve issues related to lack of standardization, especially as relates to fetal heart rate (FHR) tracing interpretation, massive transfusion protocols, proper and early identification of patients at high-risk for adverse outcomes (especially for hemorrhage or failed tracheal intubation), and suboptimal communication among caregivers. Although the advent of new techniques and equipment has decreased the risk of failed intubation in the obstetric patient, lifesaving airway devices are not always used or even immediately available in all obstetric units and difficult intubation remains a concern. A large multicenter observational cohort study of more than 14,000 women receiving general anesthesia for cesarean delivery, using data from 2004 to 2019, reported that the risk of difficult intubation remains a very real and ongoing problem (1 in 49).[20] A 2017 UK review reported that anesthesiologists are not always prepared for a difficult airway and that videolaryngoscopy was less available in obstetric operating rooms than in other operating room suites.[21] A report from Japan confirmed that general anesthesia compared with neuraxial anesthesia for scheduled cesarean delivery is associated with greater odds for severe maternal morbidity, despite the availability of advanced airway equipment.[22] In addition, the increasing prevalence of chronic medical conditions in obstetric patients, such as heart disease, hypertension, morbid obesity, and diabetes, may be an important contributor to the high maternal morbidity and mortality rates in the United States.[23]

A 2022 ASA statement noted that anesthesiologists play a vital role in reducing maternal mortality and severe maternal morbidity.[24] The statement recommended ways in which anesthesiologists can contribute to these efforts at the local, regional, and national levels. Recommendations included: (1) a physician anesthesiologist should be an active member of each state's maternal mortality review committee, (2) antenatal anesthesiology consultations should be sought on high-risk patients, (3) physician anesthesiologists should be leaders in the implementation of the American College of Obstetricians and Gynecologists (ACOG) levels of maternal care,[25] and (4) regular institutional multidisciplinary simulation for maternal emergencies should include teaching or planning by a physician anesthesiologist and should include all team members who work on the obstetric unit, including the anesthesia providers.

Because of the high intensity and rapid changes that are common on the obstetric unit, a collaborative and respectful work environment is essential, but too often is not clearly present. A group of individuals working in the same environment who are not communicating with one another does not constitute a team.[26] This is especially true during crises such as maternal hemorrhage.[27] A team is a group of individuals who achieve a mutual goal through interdependent and adaptive actions. Characteristics of effective teams are listed in Table 11.1.

In addition, departmental silos can limit the ability to learn from our experiences. The reporting, trending, and sharing of suboptimal outcomes and near misses among all team members through a variety of approaches, including multidisciplinary rounds, are necessary to achieve a culture of safety. Joint efforts for review of suboptimal outcomes and near misses, including medical record reviews and joint meetings or morbidity and mortality presentations, should

TABLE 11.1 Characteristics of Effective Teams	
Knowledge/Skills/ Attitudes	**Characteristics of the Team**
Leadership	Roles are clear but not overly rigid. Team members believe leaders care about them.
Backup behavior	Members provide task assistance. Members provide feedback to each other.
Mutual performance monitoring	Members understand each other's roles.
Communication adaptability	Members communicate often and anticipate each other.
Mutual trust	Members trust each other and each other's intentions. Members' values are aligned.

Modified from Salas E, Sims DE, Klein C. Cooperation and teamwork at work. In: Spielberger CD, ed. *Encyclopedia of Applied Physiology*. Academic Press; 2004:499–505.

include the attendance and participation of anesthesia providers, obstetricians, neonatologists, midwives, and labor nurses. Discussions with patients and their families are also a part of optimal communication, shared decision-making, and necessary transparency (see Chapter 32).

Although there have been hundreds, if not thousands, of individual improvements that have contributed to safe anesthesia practices on the obstetric unit over the past half century, the ongoing occurrence of preventable harm suggests there is still much room for improvement.

PATIENT SAFETY AND MEDICAL ERRORS—BASICS AND DEFINITIONS

Medical error has been defined as a "failure of a planned action to be completed as intended, or the use of a wrong plan to achieve an aim."[1] Communication problems are consistently identified as a leading cause of medical errors in obstetrics, and perceptions are often misaligned.[28] The Joint Commission has reported that lack of effective communication, along with leadership and human factors, are often the primary causes of sentinel events (defined as a patient safety event that results in death, permanent harm, or severe temporary harm).[29]

Traditional assessments of medical error often blamed individuals and failed to address the broader issues that allowed the error to occur. New approaches are based on an understanding that humans, no matter how well trained and well meaning, will make errors and therefore the new approaches encourage creation of robust systems to minimize the likelihood of errors and their impact on patients when they occur. As James Reason said, "we can't change the human condition, but we can change the conditions under which humans work."[30] This paradigm change has borrowed heavily from other high-risk areas such as the aviation and nuclear power industries.[31]

In its simplest form, patient safety is freedom from accidental injury while receiving healthcare services. It includes the six dimensions of quality in healthcare, namely, safe, timely, effective, efficient, equitable, and patient centered.[32] However, the US Healthcare Research and Quality has expanded the definition of patient safety as follows: "Patient safety is a discipline in the health care sector that applies safety science methods toward the goal of achieving a trustworthy system of health care delivery. Patient safety is also an attribute of health care systems; it minimizes the incidence and impact of, and maximizes recovery from, adverse events."[33] This definition acknowledges that patient safety is an emerging discipline of building systems that produce highly reliable results with as few errors as possible. The discipline involves the quality of the delivered care as well as patient safety (see later).

There is currently widespread interest in changing our healthcare culture to build safer systems, including ensuring an appropriate physical work environment, developing redundancies in safety procedures, and the use of safety care bundles, especially as it relates to hemorrhage.[34] In addition,

---

> ## BOX 11.1 American College of Obstetricians and Gynecologists' Objectives for Patient Safety
>
> - Develop a commitment to encourage a culture of patient safety
> - Implement recommended safe medication practices
> - Reduce the likelihood of surgical errors
> - Improve communication with healthcare providers
> - Improve communication with patients
> - Establish a partnership with patients to improve safety
> - Make safety a priority in every aspect of practice

Summarized from American College of Obstetricians and Gynecologists' Committee on Patient Safety and Quality Improvement. Committee Opinion Number 447: Patient safety in obstetrics and gynecology (reaffirmed 2019). *Obstet Gynecol.* 2009;114:1424–1427.

---

it is essential to allow healthcare workers to report their mistakes, even those that do not cause harm to a patient, without fear of punishment, and to provide mechanisms for learning from errors. None of these steps will ultimately achieve the goal of a safe environment without the broad support of physicians, other healthcare workers, hospital administrators, and other key stakeholders. The ACOG Committee on Patient Safety[35] has highlighted objectives for the safe care of obstetric and gynecology patients (Box 11.1).

THE SWISS CHEESE MODEL

Patients are typically not injured by a single event resulting from the single act of a careless individual. More often, an underlying systems problem made the error possible, and numerous individual actions "fell through the cracks" of a system that allowed these actions to happen, ultimately resulting in harm to the patient. James Reason described the "Swiss cheese model" of error (Fig. 11.1), in which he explained how numerous contributing factors are responsible for the ultimate harm.[36] Reason developed this model to illustrate how analyses of major accidents and catastrophic systems failures tend to reveal multiple smaller failures that led up to the actual adverse event. In the model, each slice of cheese represents a safety barrier or precaution relevant to a particular hazard.

Fig. 11.2 illustrates the use of the Swiss cheese model to evaluate a near-miss event that occurred in a patient who almost underwent an unwanted surgical procedure. The events unfolded as follows:

1. A nulliparous woman in active labor at term arrived on the obstetric unit in severe pain. She did not speak English and was poorly understood by the unit's staff. Despite a policy requiring the use of a translator, no translator was used because the husband, who had some fluency in English, was helping to translate.
2. Because the patient was in such severe pain, both she and the nurse rushed through the initial intake interview. Based on hospital policy, in perceived compliance with patient privacy regulations, the husband was asked to leave the room during this interview.

3. There was another parturient on the unit with the same last name and similar-sounding first name. This was not that unusual for this hospital and although a policy existed for such an event, it was not followed. The white board used for team rounding used only patient initials,

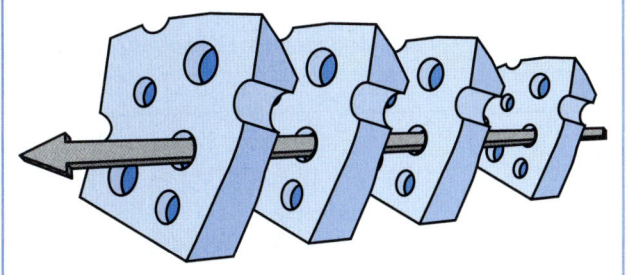

Fig. 11.1 James Swiss Cheese Model of Organizational Accidents. From Reason JT. *Human Error*. Cambridge University Press; 1990.

which prevented some of the staff from realizing that there were two patients with the same last name.

4. Shortly after admission the patient developed a category 3 FHR tracing. She was remote from delivery and was transported to the operating room for emergency cesarean delivery. The obstetric trainee who had just come on duty (and was not informed of the patient's name similarity at change-of-shift report) informed the labor nurse and anesthesiology trainee of the need for an emergency cesarean delivery. Mistaking the two patients, the procedure was booked for cesarean delivery plus bilateral tubal ligation. Unlike the other laboring patient with the same last name, this patient was nulliparous and did not wish to have a tubal ligation.

5. The procedure was temporarily delayed because of nursing shift change and the attending obstetrician urged the nurses to hurry. The obstetrician was known to have a "hot temper" and this exchange caused friction and breakdown of communication and teamwork.

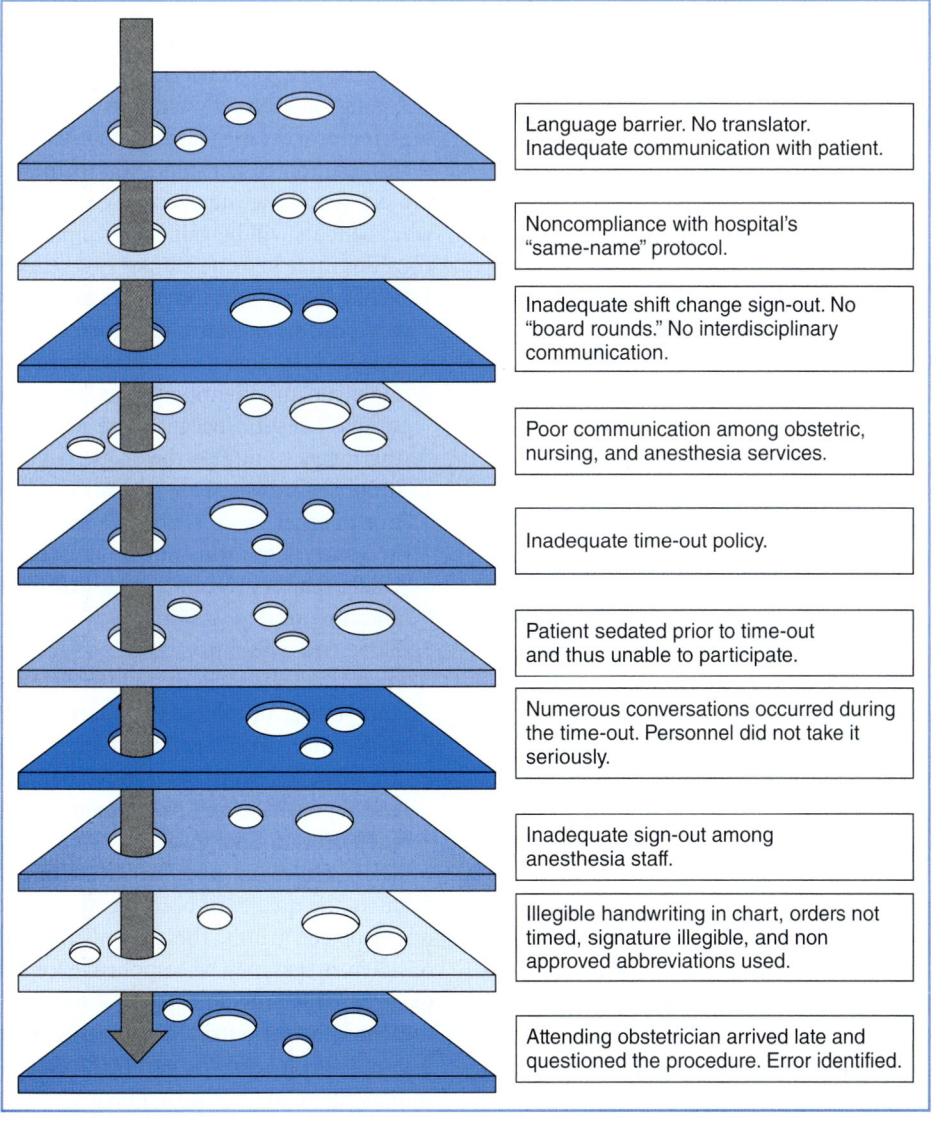

Language barrier. No translator. Inadequate communication with patient.

Noncompliance with hospital's "same-name" protocol.

Inadequate shift change sign-out. No "board rounds." No interdisciplinary communication.

Poor communication among obstetric, nursing, and anesthesia services.

Inadequate time-out policy.

Patient sedated prior to time-out and thus unable to participate.

Numerous conversations occurred during the time-out. Personnel did not take it seriously.

Inadequate sign-out among anesthesia staff.

Illegible handwriting in chart, orders not timed, signature illegible, and non approved abbreviations used.

Attending obstetrician arrived late and questioned the procedure. Error identified.

Fig. 11.2 "Swiss cheese" diagram of near-miss events illustrating how numerous layers/barriers to harm were breached and how these events almost resulted in permanent harm (permanent sterility) to the patient.

6. The patient arrived in the operating room and was extremely anxious and crying. Her husband was outside getting dressed for the operating room and no one in the room was able to communicate with her.

7. Because of the patient's severe anxiety and high risk for a panic attack, the anesthesiologist opted to administer intravenous fentanyl 50 µg prior to initiation of spinal anesthesia. The calming effect was greater than expected and the patient became very sedated.

8. A time-out was performed but was not performed correctly by the team as there were at least two additional conversations occurring at the same time as the time-out and the attending obstetrician was not present. The patient was similarly not involved with the time-out and would not have been able to participate even if not sedated due to the language barrier.

9. The attending obstetrician arrived prior to incision and on reviewing the medical record asked why a tubal ligation was planned for a nulliparous patient.

10. Immediate investigation revealed that the patient was misidentified and a major error was narrowly averted.

11. Because no harm befell the patient (near-miss event), there was no follow-up and no systems were put in place to prevent a similar occurrence in the future. Thus, there was failure to learn from the event. Multiple different actions could have identified the near-miss event earlier.

QUALITY ASSURANCE AND QUALITY IMPROVEMENT ON THE OBSTETRIC UNIT

Safety, and methods to improve safety, particularly by improving communication and developing a shared mental model, are critical to the care of the obstetric patient. However, quality of care, meaning not just avoiding error but achieving a set of desired health outcomes, is also essential. It is often stated that "if you can't measure it, you can't improve it." This premise is the foundation for building a system that supports both quality and patient safety.

While **quality assurance** (QA) is defined as the maintenance of a desired level of quality and a way to ensure that agreed-upon standards are met, **quality improvement** (QI) is the continuous process of creating systems to make things better. Both QA and QI are essential to building a robust quality program—putting the right processes in place and making sure they are executed reliably are both important drivers of achieving the best possible outcomes.[37]

Designing appropriate quality and safety activities is an important step towards achieving the goal of a safe obstetric unit and requires the identification of an area of unmet need. These areas of need may differ among hospitals. However, regardless of site, the area of need should ideally map to one of the six desirable outcomes of care systems—safe, timely, effective, efficient, equitable, and patient-centered care (Table 11.2).[38] Many opportunities exist for QI activities in every obstetric unit, no matter the type of hospital or unit. The key is to design the project so that there is agreement and acceptance from all

TABLE 11.2   Optimal Outcomes of Care Systems

Domain	Description
Safe	Avoiding harm from care meant to help patients
Effective	Providing care based on scientific data and consensus statements
Patient centered	Providing care that is respectful of and responsive to the individual patient
Timely	Reducing waits or harmful delays Offering alternatives if wait is lengthy Calling for backup when necessary
Efficient	Avoiding waste
Equitable	Providing care that does not vary in quality because of personal characteristics

Adapted from Fleisher LA. Quality anesthesia: medicine measures, patients decide. *Anesthesiology*. 2018;129:1063–1069.

stakeholders. One important method is soliciting feedback from key stakeholders, including patients, nurses, anesthesia providers, and obstetricians. QI projects are built on metrics, and these broadly fall into three categories—**structural metrics**, **process measures**, and **outcome measures**.

In addition to consideration of the business case for the project (i.e., how much money will the project cost versus what benefits will be gained), an optimal place to begin is to consider three key questions.

1. What do you (and your colleagues) want to improve? What need on the obstetric unit is strategically aligned with all stakeholders that is not currently being met?

2. How can the identified issue be improved? This is not a simple question because one needs to consider not only the metrics but also the scope, finances, and scale of the proposed project. Few projects can be completed in isolation of other processes on the unit. If other participants are necessary, how will they be identified and remunerated? Goals that are specific, measurable, assignable, realistic, and time related will improve success.

3. How will you know if a project was successful? This involves clearly identifying the deliverables of the project and setting up objective criteria for the success of each deliverable. To determine whether these criteria ultimately are met, relevant data must be collected, interpreted, and reported to key participants in the project within an agreed-upon time frame.

There are many possible indicators that can be used to evaluate the quality of both the obstetric and anesthetic care on the obstetric unit. These are often a key to identifying various factors that may be responsible for variability in the level of care that is provided. Some of these indicators can best be measured by an outside entity; this removes concerns with bias and reticence on the part of the unit's healthcare providers to participate in incident reporting. One example is the ASA Anesthesia Quality Institute, which has been a source of rich information for QI in the clinical practice of anesthesiology.[39]

The Society for Obstetric Anesthesia and Perinatology (SOAP) in the United States, the Obstetric Anesthetists' Association (OAA) in the United Kingdom, and similar professional societies in other countries issue position statements, consensus statements, and advisories that are helpful when reviewing the quality of delivered anesthesia care on a unit. The SOAP Center of Excellence (COE) designation recognizes excellent anesthesia care in individual obstetric units and sets a benchmark level of expected care with the goal of improving standards nationally.[40] In the United Kingdom, the OAA[38-41] undertook a collaborative Delphi project to identify key indicators to drive QI in obstetric anesthesia. They include (1) the percentage of unintentional dural punctures, (2) antenatal referral for anesthesia consultation in high-risk parturients, and (3) the percentage of neuraxial analgesia procedures that failed to provide adequate pain relief within 45 minutes of initiation. A follow-up survey of UK obstetric units found that most of the key indicator data are not routinely collected.[42]

The following are some examples of quality initiatives that can be undertaken to improve culture and safety in the obstetric suite using implementation science. **Implementation science**, at its core, aims to accelerate the adoption and integration of evidence-based practices into healthcare. Implementation of these initiatives is an opportunity to put into practice the evidence-based approaches published in the scientific literature. It reduces the variability that comes from the "I do it that way because I've always done it that way—regardless of the literature" attitude of many clinicians. Lane-Fall et al.[43] describe the goal of implementation science as making routine "the use of evidence-based practice, narrowing the gap between evidence and real-world practice."

Maternal Early Warning System

The Maternal Early Warning System is a list of abnormal parameters of blood pressure, respiratory rate, oxygen saturation, urine output, and mental status that indicate the need for urgent bedside evaluation.[44] Shields et al.[45] implemented a Maternal Early Warning Trigger Tool in pilot hospitals based on this framework and found that it was particularly well suited for detecting evolving sepsis and hypertensive disorders, had a good predictive value for patients who were ultimately admitted to the intensive care unit, and resulted in a significant improvement in maternal morbidity.

Opioid Prescribing After Cesarean Delivery

The opioid epidemic in the United States is a nationwide public health crisis.[46] Although opioid prescribing rates have declined in recent years, the increased availability and use of these highly addictive pain medications played an important role in the modern-day epidemic; this also includes the use of opioids in the postpartum patient (see Chapter 52). A population-based study using US data from 2003 to 2011 found that approximately 1 in 300 opioid-naive women become persistent opioid users following cesarean delivery.[47] A 2017 follow-up study showed that the amount of opioid prescribed after cesarean delivery exceeded the amount

actually used by a significant margin.[48] Subsequently, an implementation study demonstrated that a shared decision-making approach to opioid prescribing after cesarean delivery was associated with a 50% decrease in the amount of opioids prescribed postoperatively.[49]

Enhanced Recovery After Cesarean

Standardization is a way to reduce implicit bias in patient care, which has been identified as a contributor to disparities in maternal outcomes.[50] An example of standardization includes enhanced recovery after cesarean (ERAC) protocols.[51] The ERAC framework includes preoperative, intraoperative, and postoperative pathways (see Chapter 27). The intraoperative pathway recommendations focus on prevention of hypotension, maintenance of normothermia, optimal uterotonic administration, antibiotic prophylaxis, nausea/vomiting prophylaxis, multimodal analgesia, breastfeeding, fluid optimization, and delayed umbilical cord clamping.

Telemedicine

Implementing guidelines for improving maternal and fetal outcomes by leveraging telemedicine is an important opportunity. Potential benefits of telemedicine in obstetric anesthesia include cost savings, optimization of transfer decisions, improvement of resource allocation, better access, health provider education, greater patient satisfaction, increased range of care, and support of community-based care.[52]

Maternal Mental Health

Obstetric anesthesia care may influence maternal mental health. Anesthetic complications have been associated with postpartum posttraumatic stress disorder.[53] These complications include a negative delivery experience and pain during labor.[54] Plaat et al.[55] note that "a woman who experiences pain during caesarean section under neuraxial anesthesia is at risk of adverse psychological sequelae." Close attention to the diagnosis and management of pain during cesarean delivery is an important component of quality of obstetric anesthesia care.

Clinical Care Team Well-Being

Shanafelt et al.[56] have shown that healthcare provider burnout is associated with self-reported suboptimal patient care practices, including making medication errors, not discussing treatment options, and paying little attention to the personal impact of an illness on a patient. In 2009, Wallace et al.[57] proposed that physician wellness be used as a quality indicator, given its impact on both physician and patient outcomes. There are many drivers of clinical care team well-being,[58] and these drivers are important to address as part of a clinical quality and patient safety program. Training in high-performance teamwork is associated with significant improvement in supportive behavior among colleagues.[59]

CENTERS OF EXCELLENCE

The SOAP has developed a set of key recommendations for obtaining COE designation, with the aim of recognizing institutions and programs that demonstrate excellence in obstetric anesthesia care, setting a benchmark level of expected care to improve standards nationally, and providing a broad surrogate quality metric of institutions providing obstetric anesthesia care.[40] By defining a standard, the COE designation provides institutions with key performance indicators that can be measured and tracked over time. The COE recommendations, which include implementing the ASA and SOAP guidelines for obstetric care,[60] are listed in Box 11.2.

Similar to the SOAP Centers of Excellence, reviews of quality have been embraced by other specialties. The ACOG has developed a voluntary review of quality of care program that offers a confidential and unbiased site visit that includes obstetricians, perinatologists, labor nurses, midwives, and when requested or deemed necessary, anesthesiologists. The program has been assisting departments for more than 30 years. The 4-day visit includes medical record reviews and interviews with key stakeholders. Clinical issues include lack of adherence to guidelines and poor management decisions. Systems issues include evaluation of leadership, nursing staffing, and quality assessment process. In addition, obstetric as well as anesthesia policies and procedures are reviewed.

According to the ACOG, potential benefits of the program include the following:

- Identifying issues underlying adverse events
- Improving teamwork and trust

BOX 11.2   Society for Obstetric Anesthesia and Perinatology (SOAP) Centers of Excellence Recommendations[a]

1. Personnel and Staffing
   - Obstetric anesthesiologist leadership, specifically a board-certified physician anesthesiologist who has completed an Accreditation Council for Graduate Medical Education–accredited obstetric anesthesia fellowship and/or has equivalent expertise in obstetric anesthesia
   - In-house (24/7) coverage of obstetric patients, by at least one board-certified (or equivalent) physician anesthesiologist who is dedicated to covering the obstetric service without additional responsibilities for nonobstetric patients
   - Ability to mobilize (within a reasonable [30–60 min] time frame) additional anesthesia personnel in case of obstetric emergencies or high clinical volume beyond the capacity of in-house staff assigned to the obstetric service
2. Equipment, protocols, and policies
   - Availability of a massive transfusion protocol with O-negative blood and other blood products, and an emergency release system for available blood. Blood bank protocol needs to have been tested and be functional on the obstetric unit. Rapid-infuser device to assist with massive resuscitation readily available for use on the obstetric unit
   - Difficult airway cart (with laryngoscopes, endotracheal tubes, rescue airway devices [e.g., supraglottic airway device], videolaryngoscope, surgical airway equipment) immediately available on the obstetric unit. Suction and a means to deliver positive pressure ventilation immediately available in readily accessible locations where neuraxial analgesia/anesthesia and/or general anesthesia are administered. Lipid emulsion, appropriate supplies, and protocols that will allow a timely response to local anesthetic systemic toxicity
   - Multidisciplinary team–based approach with systems in place to ensure interprofessional communication and situational awareness on the obstetric unit. Daily multidisciplinary rounds or huddles to discuss management plans for women on the labor and delivery, antepartum, and postpartum units
   - Obstetric emergency response team with a policy that includes obstetric conditions and/or vital sign parameters that warrant activation, and means of notifying all members of the response team

   - An active multidisciplinary program with obstetric and anesthesia emergency simulation drills
   - Additional operating room (with nursing/technical/obstetric and anesthesia personnel) available at all times for emergency obstetric procedures (i.e., if all obstetric unit operating rooms are occupied)
3. Cesarean delivery management
   - A standardized clinical care pathway (e.g., enhanced recovery protocol) utilized by the institution and all obstetric anesthesia providers
   - Routine utilization of a pencil-point needle, 25 gauge or smaller for the provision of spinal anesthesia
   - Multimodal analgesia protocols and institutional efforts to minimize opioid use
   - Strategies to prevent maternal and fetal intraoperative hypothermia
   - Appropriate antibiotic prophylaxis to prevent surgical site infection
   - Spinal anesthesia-induced hypotension, nausea, and vomiting prophylaxis and treatment
4. Labor analgesia
   - Use of low-concentration local anesthetic solutions with neuraxial opioids for neuraxial labor analgesia
   - Combined spinal-epidural techniques available/offered in addition to standard labor epidural analgesia. Patient-controlled epidural analgesia and, ideally, programmed intermittent epidural boluses utilized for the provision of neuraxial labor analgesia
   - Routine utilization of flexible (flex-tipped/wire-reinforced) epidural catheters for labor epidural analgesia
   - Regular assessment of neuraxial labor analgesia effectiveness
5. Recommendations and guidelines implementation
   - At a minimum, evidence of implementation of the Practice Guidelines for Obstetric Anesthesia by the ASA Task Force on Obstetric Anesthesia and Society of Obstetric Anesthesia and Perinatology[60]
6. Quality assurance and patient follow-up

ASA, American Society of Anesthesiologists.
[a]SOAP Centers of Excellence. https://www.soap.org/centers-of-excellence_program. Accessed 13 July 2024.

- Enhancing the hospital's position for value-based payments
- Reducing the risk of malpractice claims

A review of their program has been published[61]; some of the anesthesia-related quality measures (when the group was accompanied by an anesthesiologist) included the following:

1. Preanesthetic airway examination is performed and documented.
2. Blood pressure is documented after administration of epidural analgesia, and corrected if hypotension occurs.
3. Unintentional dural puncture is clearly documented when it occurs.
4. Wait times for providing epidural analgesia are noted, and if long, alternative analgesia is offered.
5. Appropriate low-concentration local anesthetic solutions are used for epidural labor analgesia to minimize motor block.
6. A difficult airway cart is immediately available.
7. Procedure documentation is adequate.
8. Preoperative and postoperative notes are completed.
9. Appropriate medications are administered.
10. Estimated blood loss or quantitative blood loss is documented during hemorrhage.

These quality measures can be easily assessed by individuals in their own departments as part of a QI project.

An assessment of quality and safety indicators in anesthesia was summarized in a systematic review.[62] The authors identified 108 anesthetic clinical indicators; almost half were related to surgical or postoperative care. Most were process or outcome measures. They identified **descriptive, prescriptive,** **and proscriptive indicators**. Descriptive indicators were those that provided descriptive information. Prescriptive indicators were defined as those representing recommended or desired targets (e.g., preoperative antibiotic administration), and proscriptive indicators were defined as measures or actions that should not be performed (e.g., wrong medication).

LEVELS OF MATERNAL CARE

The ACOG and the Society for Maternal-Fetal Medicine proposed a system of regionalized levels of maternal care in 2015. The aim is to reduce maternal morbidity and mortality by establishing a structured system across geographic regions whereby risk-appropriate maternal care is provided by regional institutions with defined availability of personnel and resources.[25] Collaborative relationships between hospitals with differing levels of care allow women to give birth safely in their communities but facilitate transfer of care to a higher level of care when appropriate. The levels of care range from an accredited birthing center and Level I (basic care) to Level IV (regional perinatal healthcare centers).[25] The capability of each level includes the availability of specialized healthcare providers (obstetric providers, nursing services, and anesthesia providers (Table 11.3), as well as the ability to perform special services, including advanced imaging and intensive care. All facilities need to have the capability to triage, stabilize, and provide initial care while arranging transfer to a higher level of care, if necessary.

TABLE 11.3	Anesthesia Resources for Levels of Maternal Care	
Level	**Definition**	**Anesthesia Providers**
Accredited birth center	Care of low-risk women with uncomplicated pregnancy and anticipated uncomplicated birth	
Level I (basic care)	Care of low- to moderate-risk pregnancies	Anesthesia provider[a] available for labor analgesia and surgical anesthesia at all times
Level II (specialty care)	Level I care plus care of appropriate moderate- to high-risk antepartum, intrapartum, and postpartum conditions	Anesthesiologist readily available at all times
Level III (subspecialty care)	Level II plus care of more complex maternal conditions, obstetric complications, and fetal conditions	Board-certified anesthesiologist physically present at all times Director of obstetric anesthesia services is a board-certified anesthesiologist with fellowship training or experience in obstetric anesthesia
Level IV (regional perinatal health care centers)	Level III plus on-site medical and surgical care of the most complex conditions for critically ill pregnant women and fetuses throughout antepartum, intrapartum, and postpartum care	Board-certified anesthesiologist with obstetric anesthesiology fellowship training or experience in obstetric anesthesia physically present at all times

[a]Includes anesthesiologists, nurse anesthetists, or anesthesiologist assistants working with an anesthesiologist.
Summarized from American College of Obstetricians and Gynecologists, Society for Maternal-Fetal Medicine. Obstetric Care Consensus Number 9: Levels of maternal care (reaffirmed 2021). *Obstet Gynecol.* 2019;134:e41–e55.

SAFE LABOR ANALGESIA

Prior to the 1970s, a parturient desiring pain relief in labor was often given intravenous or intramuscular opioids, or combinations of medications such as scopolamine and opioids (so-called "twilight sleep"). Obstetricians often performed paracervical and pudendal blocks. Pulse oximetry and continuous FHR monitoring were not available; thus, maternal and fetal harm may not have been recognized. In the past four decades, anesthesiologists have played a key role in advancing safer alternatives for pain relief in labor, including improving the safety of neuraxial labor analgesia by transitioning to the use of low-concentration local anesthetics, adding neuraxial opioids, and innovating around the technology used to administer neuraxial drugs (see Chapter 24).

ADVANCES IN THE SAFETY OF SPINAL AND EPIDURAL TECHNIQUES FOR OPERATIVE DELIVERIES

The 1980s witnessed a dramatic increase in the use of neuraxial block for cesarean delivery. Since that time, many processes have been put in place to eliminate or reduce risks associated with neuraxial anesthesia, especially the risk of local anesthetic systemic toxicity (i.e., from an intravascular injection) or high- or total-spinal anesthesia (e.g., from an unintentional intrathecal injection) during the initiation of epidural anesthesia (see Chapter 12). Accidental injection of intravascular 0.75% bupivacaine intended for the epidural space was associated with numerous deaths. First reported by Albright in 1979, it ultimately resulted in the US Food and Drug Administration placing a black box warning recommending against the use of epidural 0.75% bupivacaine for obstetric anesthesia in 1983.[63] Further safety steps included the use of epidural test doses (see Chapter 12), incremental dosing, and perhaps most important, the availability of an intralipid antidote to treat local anesthesia systemic toxicity (LAST) (see Box 12.3 and Box 24.8).[64]

Similarly, advances in spinal anesthesia techniques have markedly improved safety. The use of hyperbaric spinal bupivacaine 0.75% greatly reduced the risk of total spinal anesthesia, and the use of agents with higher potential for adverse outcomes has decreased. For example, spinal tetracaine was associated with high spinal anesthesia, and epidural bupivacaine was associated with LAST. The use of pencil-point spinal needles has dramatically decreased the incidence of post-dural puncture headache after spinal anesthesia; the use of pencil-point spinal needles is now considered the standard of care.[65]

Improved Management of Hypotension Associated With Neuraxial Blockade

The incidence of severe hypotension associated with neuraxial blockade, while lower than in past decades, still occurs. The treatment of these hypotensive episodes has also changed dramatically over the past half century. Beginning in the 1970s, ephedrine became the predominant vasopressor used

for treatment of hypotension associated with neuraxial blockade in obstetrics. The origin of this preference for ephedrine was due to research published in the 1970s, primarily using a pregnant sheep model, wherein investigators found decreased uteroplacental perfusion when α-adrenergic receptor agonists were injected.[66] However, practice changed in the 1990s after human studies found that phenylephrine was safe, effective, and actually offered several advantages compared to ephedrine; one notable benefit was that phenylephrine was associated with less fetal acidemia than ephedrine.[67]

Guidelines and consensus statements have been very helpful to clinicians to guide management of hypotension during cesarean delivery (see Chapter 26). In 2018, Kinsella et al.[68] published an important international consensus statement for the management of vasopressors during cesarean delivery.

INCREASING THE SAFETY OF GENERAL ANESTHESIA IN OBSTETRICS

General anesthesia has long been considered a leading cause of anesthesia-related maternal mortality.[69] Studies evaluating fatalities associated with anesthesia for cesarean delivery have continued to identify general anesthesia as a risk factor.[69–71] Although the risk of failed tracheal intubation and aspiration associated with general anesthesia in the pregnant patient has likely decreased over the past several decades (see Chapter 28), general anesthesia still poses a greater risk than neuraxial anesthesia.[70] Overall, the risk of maternal mortality from anesthesia has dramatically decreased because of the greater use of neuraxial techniques and modern tools to facilitate improved difficult airway identification and management (see Chapter 29). These innovations include introducing routine use of pulse oximetry and capnography, as well as improved laryngoscopy tools such as videolaryngoscopy and the widespread use of supraglottic airway devices.

Preparation for an adverse anesthesia event, such as management of a difficult airway, is essential if the team is going to be able to effectively deal with the failed intubation. Simulation-based drills have become an essential tool in our fight against preventable morbidity and mortality associated with failed tracheal intubation, especially in light of the decreased general anesthesia experience that trainees are receiving on their obstetrics training rotations.[72] The development and dissemination of the ASA difficult airway algorithm[73] and the Obstetric Anaesthetists' Association and Difficult Airway Society guidelines[74] have undoubtedly reduced the incidence of maternal death associated with general anesthesia. These algorithms provide step-by-step directions on how to proceed in the event of a failed intubation, and simulation using these algorithms as cognitive aids improves preparedness for an emergency.

Team training has also likely had an impact in the reduction of morbidity and mortality associated with failed tracheal intubation and other obstetric emergencies. Team training is particularly useful for improving communication skills among multidisciplinary team members and developing nontechnical skills.[75] No longer is it enough for anesthesia providers to practice drills in a simulated environment alone. Ideally, groups of individuals, including anesthesia providers, obstetricians, labor nurses, and midwives are training together.[76] This multidisciplinary training is vital because backup assistance from other anesthesia providers is not always immediately available, and the anesthesia provider facing a failed tracheal intubation requires the help of others to manage oxygenation and ventilation safely without adverse effects on the mother and fetus.

TEAMS, IMPROVED EDUCATION, AND THE USE OF SIMULATION-BASED TEAM TRAINING

Healthcare in general, and care given to women in labor in particular, is a team activity. This is particularly true when the obstetrics team is faced with an emergency delivery on a busy obstetrics unit caring for high-risk parturients. Pronovost and Fleishlag[77] eloquently described the operating room environment as "among the most complex political, social, and cultural structures that exist, full of ritual, drama, hierarchy, and too often conflict." These authors concluded that poor teamwork contributes prominently to most adverse events, including those in the operating room. Salas et al.[78] have described teamwork as a complex yet elegant phenomenon. It can be defined as a "set of interrelated behaviors, actions, cognitions and attitudes that facilitate the required task work that must be completed."[78] Team behavior and coordination, particularly team information sharing, are critical for optimizing team performance.[79] Baker et al.[80] stated that to work together effectively, team members must possess specific knowledge, skills, and attitudes, including skill in monitoring each other's performance, knowledge of their own teammates' tasks, and a positive disposition toward working in a team. This description hardly coincides with an environment in which team members do not even know each other's names, a common occurrence in today's busy operating room environments.[81]

The Joint Commission recommended a risk reduction strategy for decreasing perinatal death or injury. This strategy includes the implementation of **team training** and mock emergency drills.[82] Box 11.3 highlights The Joint Commission goals.[83] Team training promotes the acquisition of adaptive behaviors, shared cognitions, and relevant attitudes. Salas et al.[84] described the making of a "dream team" through adaptive team performance. Fig. 11.3 illustrates the relationship between variables, emergent states, and multiple phases of team adaptation cycle.

Team training promotes the acquisition of adaptive behaviors, shared cognitions, and relevant attitudes. It is an instructional strategy that ideally combines practice-based delivery methods with realistic events, guided by teamwork competencies. Murray and Enarson[85] opined that "when a crisis complicates patient care, teamwork among health care professionals is frequently strained, resulting in more frequent as well as more serious failures in managing critical events." Obstetric anesthesia providers may be an integral

---

BOX 11.3 Key Joint Commission National Patient Safety Goals

- Improve the accuracy of patient identification
  - Use at least two patient identifiers when providing care
  - Before the start of any invasive procedure, conduct a "time-out" to confirm the correct patient, procedure, and site
- Improve the effectiveness of communication among caregivers
  - Read-back for verbal orders
  - Standardize list of abbreviations
  - Measure, assess, and if appropriate, take action to improve timeliness of reporting and the receipt of critical test results
  - Implement a standardized approach to hand-off communications
- Improve the safety of using medications
  - Standardize and limit the number of drug concentrations
  - Identify and review a list of look-alike/sound-alike drugs used by the organization
  - Label all medications
- Reduce the risk of healthcare-associated infections
  - Comply with US Centers for Disease Control hand-hygiene guidelines[a]
- Accurately and completely reconcile medication across the continuum of care
  - Implement a process for comparing the patient's current medications with those ordered for the patient
  - Communicate a complete list of the patient's medications to the next provider

[a]From US Centers for Disease Control. Clinical safety: hand hygiene for healthcare workers. February 24, 2024. https://www.cdc.gov/clean-hands/about/hand-hygiene-for-healthcare.html. Accessed 22 February 2025.
Modified from Grunebaum A. Error reduction and quality assurance in obstetrics. *Clin Perinatol.* 2007;34:489–502.

---

part of the miscommunication that occurs during crises. A systematic review of communication in the operating room demonstrated that anesthesia providers obtained low scores on communication.[86]

Although there was early skepticism, there is now wide consensus that team training improves patient safety and clinical outcomes.[87] It is not simply a matter of improved conditions compared to previous decades—team training has produced real benefits. The obstetric literature has highlighted a reduction in neonatal brachial plexus injury, maternal trauma related to forceps delivery, efficiency in performing timely cesarean delivery, and neonatal mortality, as well as improvements in the management of obstetric hemorrhage.[88,89] In addition, evidence suggests that medical simulation and team training allow recognition of potential areas of weakness in obstetric care. Maslovitz et al.[90] used simulation-based training to identify five recurrent mistakes in obstetric management committed by members of the managment team (Box 11.4). A 2022 systematic review and metaanalysis suggests a salutary effect of obstetric team training on obstetric outcomes but recommended that controlled trials targeted to identify the optimal methodology for effective team training are necessary going forward.[87]

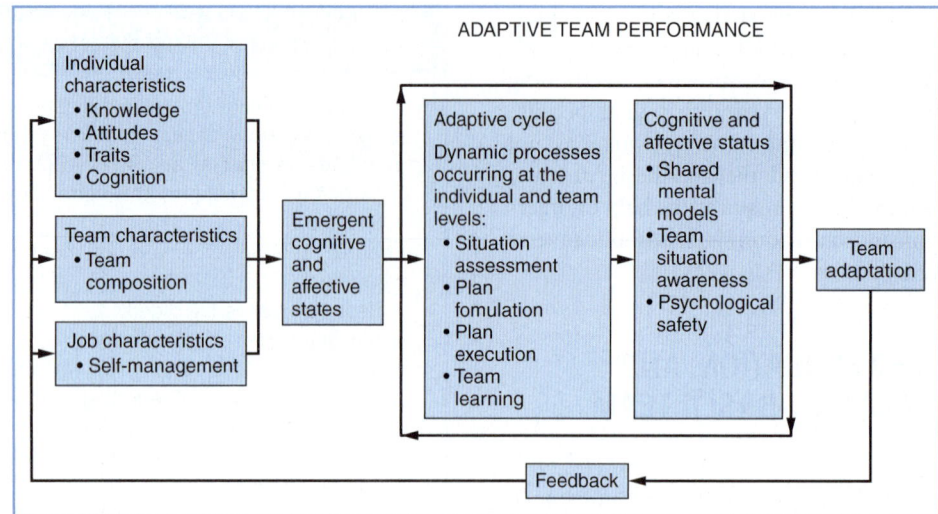

Fig. 11.3 Adaptive Team Performance. Modified from Salas E, Rosen MA, Burke CS, et al. The making of a dream team: when expert teams do best. In: Ericsson KA, Charness N, Hoffman RR, Feltovich RJ, eds. *The Cambridge Handbook of Expertise and Expert Performance*. Cambridge University Press; 2006:439–456.

BOX 11.4 Recurrent Mistakes in Peripartum Obstetric Care Observed in Simulation-Based Training

- Delay in recognition of postpartum hemorrhage
- Delay in transporting a bleeding patient to the operating room
- Unfamiliarity with prostaglandin administration to treat uterine atony
- Poor cardiopulmonary resuscitation techniques
- Inadequate documentation of shoulder dystocia
- Delayed administration of blood products to reverse disseminated intravascular coagulation

Adapted from Maslovitz S, Barkai G, Lessing JB, Ziv A, Many A. Recurrent obstetric management mistakes identified by simulation. *Obstet Gynecol.* 2007;109:1295–1300.

Simulation-based education, both *in situ* (performed in the actual clinical environment) as well as in a monitored and videotaped environment, has an important role in improving obstetric anesthesia safety. As the numbers of general anesthetics for cesarean delivery have decreased to low levels,[91] airway drills and learning to manage difficult airways and unanticipated failed tracheal intubations have moved from the clinical setting to one involving simulation-based training. These simulations and assessments may be a valuable educational tool for inexperienced trainees.[92] The effectiveness of this type of training has been demonstrated in several studies. For example, Goodwin et al.[93] showed significant improvement compared with baseline skills in the management of failed intubation after participation in simulated intubation drills. *In situ* simulation has also proven helpful in identifying and correcting institution-specific barriers that can delay emergency transport to the operating room.[94]

Drills are particularly effective when practiced in teams. Because anesthesiologists are pioneers in the field of patient safety,[14,95] they are particularly suited to help develop and implement safety strategies to minimize preventable harm on the obstetric suite. Obstetric drills that should involve anesthesia providers include obstetric crises such as hemorrhage, eclampsia, and shoulder dystocia as well as anesthetic crises such as failed tracheal intubation, intraoperative cardiac arrest, and malignant hyperthermia.

Another important safety area shown to be improved through simulation-based education is the accuracy of estimation of intraoperative blood loss during cesarean delivery. Toledo et al.[96] found that clinicians underestimated maternal blood loss by as much as 59% during simulated massive maternal hemorrhage, and the degree of error worsened as the blood loss volume increased. Following lectures on blood loss and simulation-based training, the average underestimation decreased to only 4%. Since postpartum hemorrhage is a leading cause of maternal morbidity and mortality, early recognition and mobilization of resources are essential.[97]

Training in perinatal emergencies with high-fidelity simulation has been shown to improve the speed with which anesthesia providers responded to those emergencies. Lipman et al.[98] used simulation-based assessment to evaluate optimal performance and identify gaps in cardiopulmonary resuscitation during simulated maternal cardiac arrest. The authors demonstrated numerous deficiencies in the performance of key advanced cardiac life support tasks, including correctly delivering chest compressions (56% correct), left uterine displacement (44% correct), switching chest compressors (33% correct), and appropriate defibrillation (6% correct). Box 11.5 highlights findings to facilitate effective collaboration in multidisciplinary team systems.[99]

Thomas et al.[100] have suggested that factors which influence the ability to work together may be categorized into provider characteristics (personal attributes, reputation, expertise), workplace factors (staffing, work environment, organization), and group influences (relationships, communication, existing

> ### BOX 11.5   Evidence-Based Practices for Improving Effective Collaboration in Multidisciplinary Team Systems
>
> - Team training targeting within-team skill development may improve team performance (but will not necessarily improve overall system performance).
> - Members of multidisciplinary team systems need to develop skills that facilitate effective processes within teams and between teams.
> - Coordination across teams through well-defined control mechanisms (e.g., norms, guidelines, charters, rules, meetings) supports more efficient and effective collaboration in complex environments.
> - Leadership processes can have significant positive effects on interteam coordination and multidisciplinary team performance.
> - Identifying patterns of leadership influence can help manage "who influences whom."

Modified from Shuffler ML, Carter DR. Teamwork situated in multiteam systems: key lessons learned and future opportunities. *Am Psychol.* 2018;73:390–406.

> ### BOX 11.6   Characteristics of High-Reliability Teams
>
> - Use closed-loop communication and other forms of information exchange to promote shared situational awareness.
> - Develop shared mental models that allow team members to monitor each others' performance and offer backup when needed.
> - Develop an organization that allows members to be assertive, to take advantage of functional expertise, and to seek input from other team members.
> - Seek and recognize complexities of team members' task environment and accordingly develop plans that promote adaptability.
> - Use semistructured feedback mechanisms such as team self-correction to manage and quickly learn from errors.
> - Assure psychological safety.

teamwork). These categories can be addressed, at least in part, by working together in teams in a simulated environment and evaluating teamwork and human performance.

Despite the inevitability of human error, some organizations that operate in complex environments can maintain an exceptionally safe workplace. These organizations have been termed **high-reliability organizations** (HROs). These organizations, which can include hospitals, have been defined as institutions in which individuals, working together in high-acuity situations facing great potential for error and disastrous consequences, consistently deliver care with positive results and minimal errors.[101] Specific leadership skills, including nonhierarchical leadership, transparent and continuous communication, deference to expertise, and ability to motivate, have been identified as vital.[102] Teams that exhibit behaviors that facilitate the characteristics and values held by these HROs are defined as high-reliability teams (Box 11.6).

Disruptive Behavior

Cultural factors may play a large role in team performance. These factors include attitudes, which may differ among nurses, obstetricians, and anesthesia providers as well as between resident and attending physicians, and motivation. Trust, while key to optimal teamwork, may be extremely problematic when there is disruptive behavior on the obstetric unit. Disruptive behavior includes angry outbursts, rudeness or verbal attacks, physical threats, intimidation, and sexual harassment. It can also include failure to comply with policies. The hostile environment that disruptive behaviors create makes it difficult for team members to advocate for the safe care of their patients.[103] Disruptive behavior often undermines patient safety and therefore cannot be tolerated in an organization that seeks safety and quality of care. Three to five percent of physicians exhibit disruptive behavior.

Studies have shown that as many as four "tense" communications occur between team members during each operating room procedure, with some of these events evolving into outright conflict.[104] In one survey of hospitals in California, Oregon, and Washington state in the United States, disruptive behavior was reported to occur on more than 60% of obstetric units.[105]

Institutions may face barriers in addressing disruptive behavior of individual healthcare providers. Leape and Fromson have called on the Federation of State Medical Boards, the American Board of Medical Specialties, and The Joint Commission to collaborate on developing better methods for expanding programs for responding to assessment and remediation of disruptive behavior.[104]

REDUCTION OF OPERATING ROOM–RELATED INFECTION

Healthcare-associated infection is found in approximately 10% of hospitalized patients, and the obstetric unit is no exception.[14] In fact, there are now multiple studies that have shown that some postoperative infections can be traced to contamination in the operating room.[106,107] Indeed, the anesthesia provider's inadequate hand hygiene in the period surrounding tracheal intubation may play a role in the transmission of infection.[108] Studies have now evaluated the anesthesia work area as a potential source of pathogen contamination.[109] Comprehensive infection control programs will increase patient safety related to infection and should include more frequent hand hygiene by anesthesia providers in and between operating rooms, improved environmental cleaning, vascular access care bundles, and greater infection surveillance.[109]

FUTURE TRENDS IN PATIENT SAFETY FOR OBSTETRIC CARE

The practice of obstetric anesthesia is now remarkably safe in the United States and other high-income countries. However, data suggest that the gains in safety that have occurred over the past half century in high-income countries have not been realized in low (see Chapter 15).[110] In addition, there continues to be great variability in the quality of anesthesia care provided in the United States despite the huge opportunities now available to facilitate delivery of more consistent quality of care. Unfortunately, not all obstetric units and individual anesthesia providers are meeting patient safety goals. Safety is a never-ending process and the need continues for further safety and quality research, expansion as well as dissemination of quality indicators, and use of consensus bundles and evidence-based practice, as well as outreach to low.

KEY POINTS

- Medical errors harm tens of thousands of patients each year.
- Gaps in communication among members of the healthcare team are often the primary cause of these errors.
- High-performance teamwork is essential to safe care of the pregnant patient.
- Structured high-performance team training can improve safety performance, especially in crisis situations.
- Factors that affect the ability of teams to work together include provider characteristics, workplace factors, and group influences.

- Goals of QI projects should be specific, measurable, attainable, relevant, and time bound.
- Identifying and tracking key performance indicators can drive performance in the quality of care delivered.
- The SOAP COE criteria are a key set of recommendations for achieving high-quality outcomes in obstetric anesthesia.

REFERENCES

1. Institute of Medicine (US) Committee on Quality of Health Care in America, Kohn LT, Corrigan JM, Donaldson MS. In: Kohn LT, Corrigan JM, Donaldson MS, eds. *To Err Is Human: Building a Safer Health System*. National Academies Press (US); 2000.
2. Makary MA, Daniel M. Medical error – the third leading cause of death in the US. *BMJ*. 2016;353:i2139.
3. Aiken LH, Clarke SP, Sloane DM, et al. Hospital nurse staffing and patient mortality, nurse burnout, and job dissatisfaction. *JAMA*. 2002;288:1987–1993.
4. Landrigan CP, Rothschild JM, Cronin JW, et al. Effect of reducing interns' work hours on serious medical errors in intensive care units. *N Engl J Med*. 2004;351:1838–1848.
5. Bernstein PS, Martin JN Jr, Barton JR, et al. National partnership for maternal safety: consensus bundle on severe hypertension during pregnancy and the postpartum period. *Anesth Analg*. 2017;125:540–547.
6. Greer JA, Lutgendorf MA, Ennen CS, et al. Obstetric simulation training and teamwork: immediate impact on knowledge, teamwork, and adherence to hemorrhage protocols. *Simul Healthc*. 2023;18:32–41.
7. Pratt SD. Focused review: simulation in obstetric anesthesia. *Anesth Analg*. 2012;114:186–190.
8. Ahn R, Gonzalez GP, Anderson B, et al. Initiatives to reduce maternal mortality and severe maternal morbidity in the United States: a narrative review. *Ann Intern Med*. 2020;173:S3–S10.
9. MacDorman MF, Declercq E, Cabral H, Morton C. Recent increases in the U.S. maternal mortality rate: disentangling trends from measurement issues. *Obstet Gynecol*. 2016;128:447–455.
10. Kilpatrick SJ. Next steps to reduce maternal morbidity and mortality in the USA. *Womens Health (Lond)*. 2015;11:193–199.
11. Newman-Toker DE, Nassery N, Schaffer AC, et al. Burden of serious harms from diagnostic error in the USA. *BMJ Qual Saf*. 2024;33:109–120.
12. Cheesman K, Brady JE, Flood P, Li G. Epidemiology of anesthesia-related complications in labor and delivery, New York State, 2002-2005. *Anesth Analg*. 2009;109:1174–1181.
13. Parliamentary and Health Service Ombudsman. *Broken Trust: Making Patient Safety More Than Just a Promise*. Parliamentary and Health Service Ombudsman; 2023. https://www.ombudsman.org.uk/publications/broken-trust-making-patient-safety-more-just-promise-0. Accessed 22 February 2025.
14. Birnbach DJ, Bateman BT. Obstetric anesthesia: leading the way in patient safety. *Obstet Gynecol Clin North Am*. 2019;46:329–337.
15. Hüner B, Derksen C, Schmiedhofer M, et al. Reducing preventable adverse events in obstetrics by improving interprofessional communication skills – results of an intervention study. *BMC Pregnancy Childbirth*. 2023;23:55.
16. D'Alton ME, Friedman AM, Smiley RM, et al. National partnership for maternal safety: consensus bundle on venous thromboembolism. *Anesth Analg*. 2016;123:942–949.
17. Fleischer A, Meirowitz N. Care bundles for management of obstetrical hemorrhage. *Semin Perinatol*. 2016;40:99–108.
18. Podovei M, Bateman BT. The consensus bundle on hypertension in pregnancy and the anesthesiologist: doing all the right things for all the patients all of the time. *Anesth Analg*. 2017;125:383–385.
19. American Society of Anesthesiologists Committe on Obstetric Anesthesia. *Statement on Reducing Maternal Peripartum Racial and Ethnic Disparities in Anesthesia Care*. American Society of Anesthesiologists; 2021. https://www.asahq.org/standards-and-practice-parameters/statement-on-reducing-maternal-peripartum-racial-and-ethnic-disparities-in-anesthesia-care. Accessed 22 February 2025.

20. Reale SC, Bauer ME, Klumpner TT, et al. Frequency and risk factors for difficult intubation in women undergoing general anesthesia for cesarean delivery: a multicenter retrospective cohort analysis. *Anesthesiology*. 2022;136:697–708.

21. Cook TM, Kelly FE. A national survey of videolaryngoscopy in the United Kingdom. *Br J Anaesth*. 2017;118:593–600.

22. Abe H, Sumitani M, Uchida K, et al. Association between mode of anaesthesia and severe maternal morbidity during admission for scheduled caesarean delivery: a nationwide population-based study in Japan, 2010-2013. *Br J Anaesth*. 2018;120:779–789.

23. Bateman BT, Mhyre JM, Hernandez-Diaz S, et al. Development of a comorbidity index for use in obstetric patients. *Obstet Gynecol*. 2013;122:957–965.

24. American Society of Anesthesiologists Committee on Obstetric Anesthesia. Statement on anesthesiologists' role in reducing maternal mortality and severe maternal morbidity. 2022. https://www.asahq.org/standards-and-practice-parameters/statement-on-anesthesiologists-role-in-reducing-maternal-mortality-and-severe-maternal-morbidity. Accessed 22 February 2025.

25. American College of Obstetricians and Gynecologists. Obstetric Care Consensus #9: Levels of maternal care (reaffirmed 2021). *Obstet Gynecol*. 2019;134:e41–e55.

26. Salas E, Reyes DL, McDaniel SH. The science of teamwork: progress, reflections, and the road ahead. *Am Psychol*. 2018;73:593–600.

27. Dulaney BM, Elkhateb R, Mhyre JM. Optimizing systems to manage postpartum hemorrhage. *Best Pract Res Clin Anaesthesiol*. 2022;36:349–357.

28. Rayburn WF, Jenkins C. Interprofessional Collaboration in Women's Health Care: collective competencies, interactive learning, and measurable improvement. *Obstet Gynecol Clin North Am*. 2021;48:1–10.

29. Guttman OT, Lazzara EH, Keebler JR, et al. Dissecting communication barriers in healthcare: a path to enhancing communication resiliency, reliability, and patient safety. *J Patient Saf*. 2021;17:e1465–e1471.

30. Reason J. Human error: models and management. *BMJ*. 2000;320:768–770.

31. Birnbach DJ, Rosen LF, Williams L, et al. A framework for patient safety: a defense nuclear industry-based high-reliability model. *Jt Comm J Qual Patient Saf*. 2013;39:233–240.

32. Institute of Medicine (US) Committee on Quality of Health Care in America. *Crossing the Quality Chasm: A New Health System for the 21st Century*. National Academies Press (US); 2001.

33. Emanuel L, Berwick D, Conway J, et al. What exactly is patient safety? In: Henriksen K, Battles JB, Keyes MA, Grady ML, eds. *Advances in Patient Safety: New Directions and Alternative Approaches (Vol 1: Assessment)*. Agency for Healthcare Research and Quality; 2008.

34. Escobar MF, Nassar AH, Theron G, et al. FIGO recommendations on the management of postpartum hemorrhage 2022. *Int J Gynaecol Obstet*. 2022;157(suppl 1):3–50.

35. American College of Obstetricians and Gynecologists Committee on Patient Safety and Quality Improvement. Opinion No. 447: Patient safety in obstetrics and gynecology (reaffirmed 2019). *Obstet Gynecol*. 2009;114:1424–1427.

36. Reason J. *Human Error*. Cambridge University Press; 1990.

37. Kjaer K. Quality assurance and quality improvement in the labor and delivery setting. *Anesthesiol Clin*. 2021;39:613–630.

38. Fleisher LA. Quality anesthesia: medicine measures, patients decide. *Anesthesiology*. 2018;129:1063–1069.

39. Liau A, Havidich JE, Onega T, Dutton RP. The National Anesthesia Clinical Outcomes Registry. *Anesth Analg*. 2015;121:1604–1610.

40. Carvalho B, Mhyre JM. Centers of Excellence for anesthesia care of obstetric patients. *Anesth Analg*. 2019;128:844–846.

41. Bamber JH, Lucas DN, Plaat F, et al. The identification of key indicators to drive quality improvement in obstetric anaesthesia: results of the Obstetric Anaesthetists' Association/National Perinatal Epidemiology Unit collaborative Delphi project. *Anaesthesia*. 2020;75:617–625.

42. Pritchard N, Lo Q, Wikner M, Bamber J. Collecting data for quality improvement in obstetric anaesthesia. *Int J Obstet Anesth*. 2019;39:142–143.

43. Lane-Fall MB, Cobb BT, Cené CW, Beidas RS. Implementation science in perioperative care. *Anesthesiol Clin*. 2018;36:1–15.

44. Mhyre JM, D'Oria R, Hameed AB, et al. The maternal early warning criteria: a proposal from the national partnership for maternal safety. *Obstet Gynecol*. 2014;124:782–786.

45. Shields LE, Wiesner S, Klein C, et al. Use of maternal early warning trigger tool reduces maternal morbidity. *Am J Obstet Gynecol*. 2016;214:527.e1–e6.

46. Lyden J, Binswanger IA. The United States opioid epidemic. *Semin Perinatol*. 2019;43:123–131.

47. Bateman BT, Franklin JM, Bykov K, et al. Persistent opioid use following cesarean delivery: patterns and predictors among opioid-naïve women. *Am J Obstet Gynecol*. 2016;215:353.e1–e18.

48. Bateman BT, Cole NM, Maeda A, et al. Patterns of opioid prescription and use after cesarean delivery. *Obstet Gynecol*. 2017;130:29–35.

49. Prabhu M, McQuaid-Hanson E, Hopp S, et al. A shared decision-making intervention to guide opioid prescribing after cesarean delivery. *Obstet Gynecol*. 2017;130:42–46.

50. White RS, Matthews KC, Tangel V, Abramovitz S. Enhanced recovery after surgery (ERAS) programs for cesarean delivery can potentially reduce healthcare and racial disparities. *J Natl Med Assoc*. 2019;111:464–465.

51. Bollag L, Lim G, Sultan P, et al. Society for Obstetric Anesthesia and Perinatology: consensus statement and recommendations for enhanced recovery after cesarean. *Anesth Analg*. 2021;132:1362–1377.

52. Duarte SS, Nguyen TT, Koch C, et al. Remote obstetric anesthesia: leveraging telemedicine to improve fetal and maternal outcomes. *Telemed J E Health*. 2020;26:967–972.

53. Vogel TM, Homitsky S. Antepartum and intrapartum risk factors and the impact of PTSD on mother and child. *BJA Educ*. 2020;20:89–95.

54. Dekel S, Stuebe C, Dishy G. Childbirth induced posttraumatic stress syndrome: a systematic review of prevalence and risk factors. *Front Psychol*. 2017;8:560.

55. Plaat F, Stanford SER, Lucas DN, et al. Prevention and management of intra-operative pain during caesarean section under neuraxial anaesthesia: a technical and interpersonal approach. *Anaesthesia*. 2022;77:588–597.

56. Shanafelt TD, Bradley KA, Wipf JE, Back AL. Burnout and self-reported patient care in an internal medicine residency program. *Ann Intern Med*. 2002;136:358–367.

57. Wallace JE, Lemaire JB, Ghali WA. Physician wellness: a missing quality indicator. *Lancet*. 2009;374:1714–1721.

58. Shanafelt TD, Noseworthy JH. Executive leadership and physician well-being: nine organizational strategies to promote engagement and reduce burnout. *Mayo Clin Proc*. 2017;92:129–146.

59. Weaver SJ, Rosen MA, Salas E, et al. Integrating the science of team training: guidelines for continuing education. *J Contin Educ Health Prof*. 2010;30:208–220.

60. American Society of Anesthesiologists and the Society for Obstetric Anesthesia and Perinatology. Practice guidelines for obstetric anesthesia: an updated report by the American Society of Anesthesiologists Task Force on Obstetric Anesthesia and the Society for Obstetric Anesthesia and Perinatology. *Anesthesiology*. 2016;124:270–300.

61. Lichtmacher A. Quality assessment tools: ACOG voluntary review of quality of care program, peer review reporting system. *Obstet Gynecol Clin North Am*. 2008;35:147–162.

62. Haller G, Stoelwinder J, Myles PS, McNeil J. Quality and safety indicators in anesthesia: a systematic review. *Anesthesiology*. 2009;110:1158–1175.

63. Larson CP Jr, Youssefzadeh K, Moon JS. The bupivacaine story: a tribute to George A. Albright, MD (1931-2020). *Anesth Analg*. 2022;135:1115–1119.

64. Macfarlane AJR, Gitman M, Bornstein KJ, et al. Updates in our understanding of local anaesthetic systemic toxicity: a narrative review. *Anaesthesia*. 2021;76(suppl 1):27–39.

65. Nath S, Koziarz A, Badhiwala JH, et al. Atraumatic versus conventional lumbar puncture needles: a systematic review and meta-analysis. *Lancet*. 2018;391:1197–1204.

66. Ralston DH, Shnider SM, DeLorimier AA. Effects of equipotent ephedrine, metaraminol, mephentermine, and methoxamine on uterine blood flow in the pregnant ewe. *Anesthesiology*. 1974;40:354–370.

67. Ngan Kee WD, Lee A, Khaw KS, et al. A randomized double-blinded comparison of phenylephrine and ephedrine infusion combinations to maintain blood pressure during spinal anesthesia for cesarean delivery: the effects on fetal acid-base status and hemodynamic control. *Anesth Analg*. 2008;107:1295–1302.

68. Kinsella SM, Carvalho B, Dyer RA, et al. International consensus statement on the management of hypotension with vasopressors during caesarean section under spinal anaesthesia. *Anaesthesia*. 2018;73:71–92.

69. Tsen LC, Pitner R, Camann WR. General anesthesia for cesarean section at a tertiary care hospital 1990-1995: indications and implications. *Int J Obstet Anesth*. 1998;7:147–152.

70. Hawkins JL, Chang J, Palmer SK, et al. Anesthesia-related maternal mortality in the United States: 1979-2002. *Obstet Gynecol*. 2011;117:69–74.

71. Guglielminotti J, Landau R, Li G. Adverse events and factors associated with potentially avoidable use of general anesthesia in cesarean deliveries. *Anesthesiology*. 2019;130:912–922.

72. Scavone BM, Toledo P, Higgins N, et al. A randomized controlled trial of the impact of simulation-based training on resident performance during a simulated obstetric anesthesia emergency. *Simul Healthc*. 2010;5:320–324.

73. Apfelbaum JL, Hagberg CA, Connis RT, et al. 2022 American Society of Anesthesiologists practice guidelines for management of the difficult airway. *Anesthesiology*. 2022;136:31–81.

74. Mushambi MC, Kinsella SM, Popat M, et al. Obstetric Anaesthetists' Association and Difficult Airway Society guidelines for the management of difficult and failed tracheal intubation in obstetrics. *Anaesthesia*. 2015;70:1286–1306.

75. Wu M, Tang J, Etherington C, et al. Interventions for improving teamwork in intrapartum care: a systematic review of randomised controlled trials. *BMJ Qual Saf*. 2020;29:77–85.

76. MacLennan K, Minehart RD, Vasco M, Eley VA. Simulation-based training in obstetric anesthesia: an update. *Int J Obstet Anesth*. 2023;54:103643.

77. Pronovost PJ, Freischlag JA. Improving teamwork to reduce surgical mortality. *JAMA*. 2010;304:1721–1722.

78. Salas E, Guthrie JWJ, Wilson-Donnelly KA, et al. Modeling team performance: the basic ingredients and research needs. In: Rouse WB, Boff KR, eds. *Organizational Simulation*. Wiley; 2005:185–228.

79. Kwon CS, Duzyj C. The impact of TeamSTEPPS training on obstetric team attitudes and outcomes on the labor and delivery unit of a regional perinatal center. *Am J Perinatol*. 2022;41(S01):e901–e910.

80. Baker DP, Day R, Salas E. Teamwork as an essential component of high-reliability organizations. *Health Serv Res*. 2006;41:1576–1598.

81. Birnbach DJ, Rosen LF, Fitzpatrick M, et al. Introductions during time-outs: do surgical team members know one another's names? *Jt Comm J Qual Patient Saf*. 2017;43:284–288.

82. Deering S, Johnston LC, Colacchio K. Multidisciplinary teamwork and communication training. *Semin Perinatol*. 2011;35:89–96.

83. Grunebaum A. Error reduction and quality assurance in obstetrics. *Clin Perinatol*. 2007;34:489–502.

84. Salas E, Rosen M, Burke C, et al. The making of a dream team: when expert teams do best. In: Ericsson K, Charness N, Feltovich P, Hoffman R, eds. *The Cambridge Handbook of Expertise and Expert Performance*. Cambridge University Press; 2006:439–456.

85. Murray D, Enarson C. Communication and teamwork: essential to learn but difficult to measure. *Anesthesiology*. 2007;106:895–896.

86. Weldon SM, Korkiakangas T, Bezemer J, Kneebone R. Communication in the operating theatre. *Br J Surg*. 2013;100:1677–1688.

87. Brogaard L, Glerup Lauridsen K, Lofgren B, et al. The effects of obstetric emergency team training on patient outcome: a systematic review and meta-analysis. *Acta Obstet Gynecol Scand*. 2022;101:25–36.

88. Marshall NE, Vanderhoeven J, Eden KB, et al. Impact of simulation and team training on postpartum hemorrhage management in non-academic centers. *J Matern Fetal Neonatal Med*. 2015;28:495–499.

89. Lutgendorf MA, Ennen CS, McGlynn A, et al. Interprofessional obstetric simulation training improves postpartum haemorrhage management and decreases maternal morbidity: a before-and-after study. *BJOG*. 2024;131:353–361.

90. Maslovitz S, Barkai G, Lessing JB, et al. Recurrent obstetric management mistakes identified by simulation. *Obstet Gynecol*. 2007;109:1295–1300.

91. Ring L, Landau R, Delgado C. The current role of general anesthesia for cesarean delivery. *Curr Anesthesiol Rep*. 2021;11:18–27.

92. Kiwalabye I, Cronjé L, Schoeman S, Sommerville T. A simulation-based study evaluating the preparedness of interns' post-anaesthesia rotation in managing a failed obstetric intubation scenario: is our training good enough? *S Afr Med J.* 2021;111:265–270.

93. Goodwin MW, French GW. Simulation as a training and assessment tool in the management of failed intubation in obstetrics. *Int J Obstet Anesth.* 2001;10:273–277.

94. Lipman SS, Carvalho B, Cohen SE, et al. Response times for emergency cesarean delivery: use of simulation drills to assess and improve obstetric team performance. *J Perinatol.* 2013;33:259–263.

95. Austin N, Goldhaber-Fiebert S, Daniels K, et al. Building comprehensive strategies for obstetric safety: simulation drills and communication. *Anesth Analg.* 2016;123:1181–1190.

96. Toledo P, McCarthy RJ, Burke CA, et al. The effect of live and web-based education on the accuracy of blood-loss estimation in simulated obstetric scenarios. *Am J Obstet Gynecol.* 2010;202:400.e1–e5.

97. Higgins N, Patel SK, Toledo P. Postpartum hemorrhage revisited: new challenges and solutions. *Curr Opin Anaesthesiol.* 2019;32:278–284.

98. Lipman SS, Daniels KI, Carvalho B, et al. Deficits in the provision of cardiopulmonary resuscitation during simulated obstetric crises. *Am J Obstet Gynecol.* 2010;203:179.e1–e5.

99. Shuffler ML, Carter DR. Teamwork situated in multiteam systems: key lessons learned and future opportunities. *Am Psychol.* 2018;73:390–406.

100. Thomas EJ, Sherwood GD, Mulhollem JL, et al. Working together in the neonatal intensive care unit: provider perspectives. *J Perinatol.* 2004;24:552–559.

101. Cochrane BS, Hagins M Jr, Picciano G, et al. High reliability in healthcare: creating the culture and mindset for patient safety. *Healthc Manage Forum.* 2017;30:61–68.

102. Logan-Athmer AL. The necessary leadership skillsets for the high-reliability organization framework adoption within acute healthcare organizations. *J Healthc Risk Manag.* 2022;42:31–36.

103. Wright C. The disruptive physician and impact on the culture of safety. *Curr Opin Anaesthesiol.* 2021;34:387–391.

104. Leape LL, Fromson JA. Problem doctors: is there a system-level solution? *Ann Intern Med.* 2006;144:107–115.

105. Veltman LL. Disruptive behavior in obstetrics: a hidden threat to patient safety. *Am J Obstet Gynecol.* 2007;196: 587.e1–e4.

106. Birnbach DJ, Rosen LF, Fitzpatrick M, et al. The use of a novel technology to study dynamics of pathogen transmission in the operating room. *Anesth Analg.* 2015;120:844–847.

107. Loftus RW, Koff MD, Birnbach DJ. The dynamics and implications of bacterial transmission events arising from the anesthesia work area. *Anesth Analg.* 2015;120:853–860.

108. Birnbach DJ, Rosen LF, Fitzpatrick M, et al. A new approach to pathogen containment in the operating room: sheathing the laryngoscope after intubation. *Anesth Analg.* 2015;121:1209–1214.

109. Munoz-Price LS, Bowdle A, Johnston BL, et al. Infection prevention in the operating room anesthesia work area. *Infect Control Hosp Epidemiol.* 2019;40:1–17.

110. Sobhy S, Zamora J, Dharmarajah K, et al. Anaesthesia-related maternal mortality in low-income and middle-income countries: a systematic review and meta-analysis. *Lancet Glob Health.* 2016;4:e320–e327.

PART IV

Foundations in Obstetric Anesthesia

12

Spinal and Epidural Analgesia and Anesthesia: Anatomy, Physiology, and Technique

Elizabeth M.S. Lange, MD and Naveen Nathan, MD

Successful administration and management of neuraxial anesthesia require a thorough understanding of neuroanatomy and the physiologic implications of commonly used neuraxial medications, as well as well-developed technical skills, and physiologic implications of commonly used neuraxial medications moderated by sound clinical judgment. The focus of this chapter is to characterize the anatomic and technical considerations for neuraxial anesthesia for obstetric anesthesia care. The reader is referred to Chapter 24 for a corresponding discussion of the physiologic and untoward effects of neuraxial analgesia in laboring women and to Chapter 26 for a discussion of neuraxial anesthesia for cesarean delivery.

ANATOMY

Neuraxial Anatomy
The Spinal Cord, Spinal Canal, and Meninges

The cephalad aspect of the spinal cord is continuous with the brainstem through the foramen magnum. The spinal cord terminates as the conus medullaris, most often at the level of the lower border of the first lumbar vertebral body. The conus medullaris is attached to the coccyx by means of a neural-fibrous band called the filum terminale, which is surrounded by the nerves of the lower lumbar and sacral roots, known as the cauda equina. Within the bony vertebral column are three membranes: the pia mater, the arachnoid mater, and the dura mater. The pia mater is a highly vascular membrane that closely

invests the spinal cord. The arachnoid mater is a delicate, nonvascular membrane closely adherent to the third and outermost layer, the dura. The subarachnoid space, located between the pia mater and arachnoid mater, contains (1) cerebrospinal fluid (CSF), (2) spinal nerves, (3) a trabecular network between the two membranes, (4) blood vessels that supply the spinal cord, and (5) lateral extensions of the pia mater—the dentate ligaments. The dura mater is a membrane, composed of collagen that encapsulates the spinal cord, the deeper meningeal layers, and the subarachnoid space. This layer forms a connective tissue sheath along the vertical axis of the central nervous system (CNS) that is contiguous with connective tissue covering the lateral extension of spinal nerve roots as they exit the intervertebral foramina. The interface between the dural and arachnoid layers has been described as a potential space capable of expansion after mechanical trauma. Unintentional injection of local anesthetic into this *subdural space* may explain some cases of failed spinal anesthesia. It may also explain the rare cases of high spinal anesthesia after the unintentional subdural injection of larger volumes of local anesthetic intended for *epidural* administration.[1] Although the spinal cord ends at the level of the bodies of L1 and L2 in most adults, the subarachnoid space and cauda equina continue to the S2 level (Fig. 12.1).

The Epidural Space

The epidural space is located external to the sac of the dura mater and contains loose connective tissue, adipose tissue, lymphatics, spinal nerve roots, and the internal vertebral

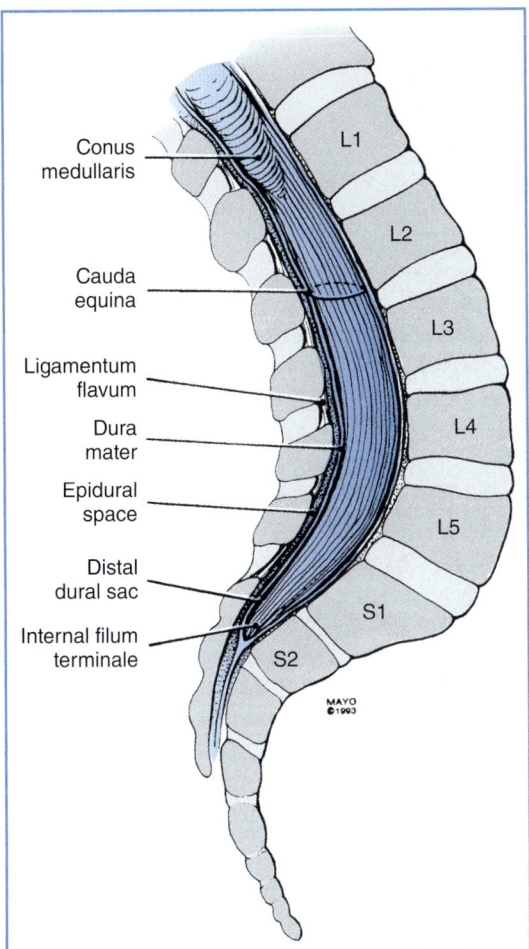

Fig. 12.1 Distal Neuraxial Anatomy. In pregnant women, the spinal cord usually ends at the lower border of the first lumbar vertebral body. The subarachnoid space continues to the second sacral vertebral level.

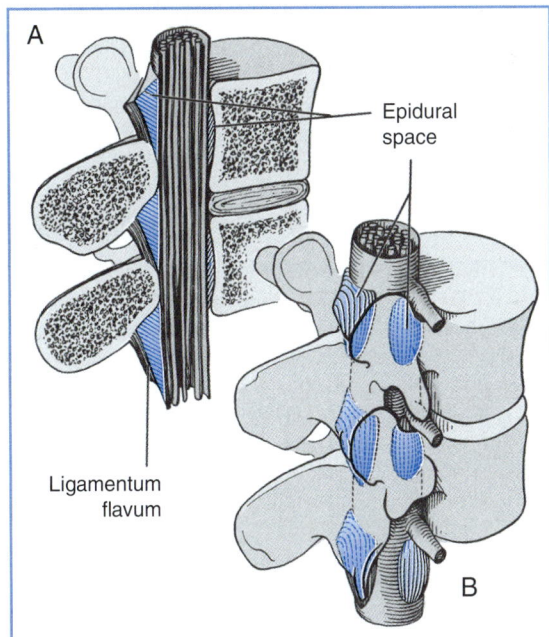

Fig. 12.2 (A) Sagittal section of the epidural space demonstrates that the contents of the epidural space depend on the level of the section. (B) Three-dimensional drawing of the epidural space shows the discontinuity of the epidural contents. However, this potential space can be dilated by the injection of fluid into the epidural space. Redrawn from Stevens RA. Neuraxial blocks. In: Brown DL, ed. *Regional Anesthesia and Analgesia*. Saunders; 1976:323.

venous plexus (Batson plexus) (Fig. 12.2). This space is bound by the posterior longitudinal ligament anteriorly, the ligamentum flavum and the periosteum of the lamina posteriorly, the pedicles of the vertebrae, and the intervertebral foramina with their contents laterally. The epidural space is closed at the foramen magnum, where the spinal dura attaches to the dura of the cranium and at the sacral hiatus by the sacrococcygeal ligament. Frequently, anatomic references will illustrate neuraxial anatomy by way of sagittal and/or transverse cross-section. This may result in the erroneous impression that the epidural space is a continuous columnar entity that envelops the dural sac at all points about its perimeter. Investigations using cryomicrotome sections and three-dimensional reconstruction of radiologic data verify that the epidural space is in fact discontinuous along the vertical and lateral axes of the spinal canal. It varies in anteroposterior thickness according to dermatomal distribution, being widest at the level of lumbar vertebrae and thinnest in the cervical region.[2] Epiduroscopy and epidurography at autopsy suggest the presence of a dorsal median connective tissue band in some individuals.[3] Anatomic dissection and computed tomographic epidurography have also suggested the presence of epidural space septa. This band

(or these septa) may provide an explanation for unilateral or incomplete epidural anesthesia.[4] However, an *in vivo* evaluation of 106 patients with epiduroscopy could not identify the presence of the dorsal median band, but did identify a fibrotic septa in some patients, suggesting that it may be a cadaveric artifact.[5]

The Vertebral Column and Ligaments

The ligamentum flavum lies posterior to the epidural space (Fig. 12.3). The lamina, the spinous processes of the vertebral bodies, and the interspinous ligaments lie posterior to the ligamentum flavum. Posterior to these structures is the supraspinous ligament (which extends from the external occipital protuberance to the coccyx), subcutaneous tissue, and skin. Historically, some have described the ligamentum flavum as a single ligament. In actuality, however, it is composed of two curvilinear ligaments that join in the middle and form an acute angle with a ventral opening.[6,7] Much like the epidural space, the ligamentum flavum is not uniform from skull to sacrum; indeed, it is not uniform even within a single intervertebral space. The thickness of the ligamentum flavum varies with vertebral level, body mass index (BMI), race, and age, as does the distance between the skin and epidural space.[8,9] In a mixed-race population of parturients with a BMI of approximately 25 kg/m² at the first prenatal visit, the mean (standard deviation [SD]) distance from the skin to the epidural space was 5.4 cm (1.1).[9] The distance was greater among black parturients and white parturients than among Asian parturients at any given BMI (Table 12.1).

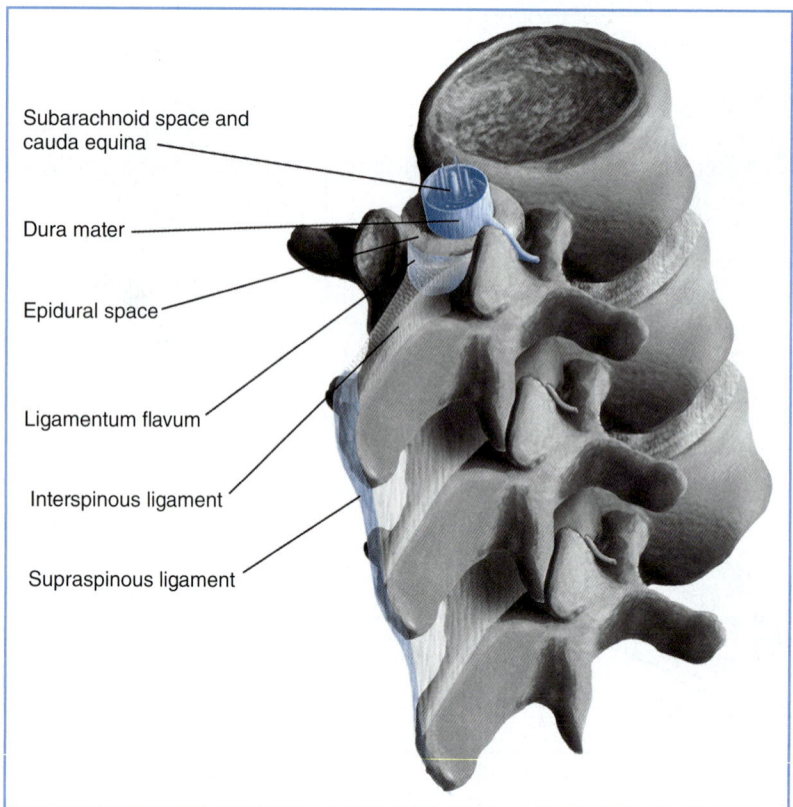

Subarachnoid space and cauda equina

Dura mater

Epidural space

Ligamentum flavum

Interspinous ligament

Supraspinous ligament

Fig. 12.3 Central Neuraxial Anatomy. Note the variable thickness of the ligamentum flavum, which is greatest in the midline and decreases laterally. Illustration by Naveen Nathan, MD, NorthShore University HealthSystem, University of Chicago Pritzker School of Medicine, Evanston, IL.

TABLE 12.1	Estimated Distance From the Skin to the Epidural Space			
	ESTIMATED DISTANCE (CM)			
BMI (kg/m²)	**White (n = 708)**	**Asian/British Asian (n = 24)**	**Black/British Black (n = 127)**	**Chinese (n = 126)**
20	4.7	4.5	5.0	4.4
25	5.3	5.1	5.7	4.7
30	6.0	5.7	6.5	5.1
35	6.6	6.2	7.2	5.4
40	7.2	6.8	8.0	5.7

Estimated distance from skin to lumbar epidural space after adjusting for body mass index (BMI) and race.
From Sharma V, Swinson AK, Hughes C, et al. Effect of ethnicity and body mass index on the distance from skin to lumbar epidural space in parturients. *Anaesthesia.* 2011;66:907–912.

Anatomic Changes of Pregnancy

The normal anatomic changes of pregnancy affect neuraxial anesthesia techniques. Uterine enlargement and vena caval compression result in engorgement of the epidural veins. Unintentional intravascular epidural catheter cannulation and injection of local anesthetic are more common in pregnant than in nonpregnant patients. In addition, vertebral foraminal veins are enlarged and may hinder local anesthetic access to nerve roots from the epidural space during administration of epidural anesthesia. The enlarged epidural veins and an increase in adipose tissue also may displace CSF from the thoracolumbar region of the subarachnoid space, as does the greater intraabdominal pressure of pregnancy; this displacement partly explains the lowered dose requirement for spinal anesthesia in pregnant women.[10] Subarachnoid dose

requirements are also affected by the lower specific gravity of CSF in pregnant patients than in nonpregnant patients.[11]

The hormonal changes of pregnancy affect the perivertebral ligamentous structures, including the ligamentum flavum. The ligamentum flavum may feel less dense and "softer" in pregnant women than in nonpregnant patients; thus sensing the passage of the epidural needle through the ligamentum flavum may be more challenging. It may also be more difficult for a pregnant patient to achieve flexion of the lumbar spine due to a progressive accentuation of lumbar lordosis. The relationship of surface anatomy to the vertebral column changes as pregnancy progresses. First, a pregnant woman's pelvis rotates on the long axis of the spinal column; thus the line joining the iliac crests (Tuffier's line) assumes a more cephalad relationship to the vertebral column (e.g., this imaginary line might cross the

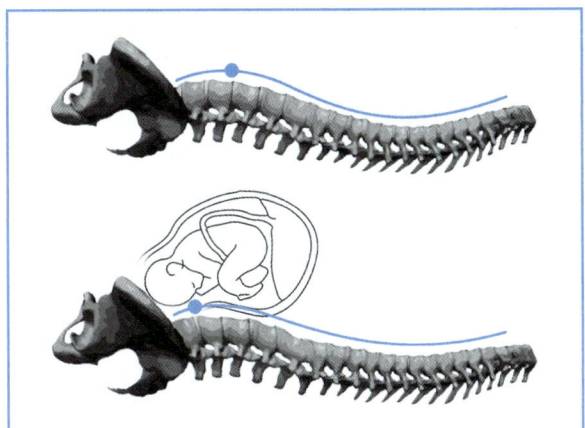

Fig. 12.4 The Curvature of the Spinal Column in the Nonpregnant *(Top)* and Pregnant Patient *(Bottom)*. The apex of the lumbar lordosis *(blue circle)* moves caudad in pregnancy. Additionally, the thoracic kyphosis is reduced and shifts cephalad. Illustration by Naveen Nathan, MD, NorthShore University HealthSystem, University of Chicago Pritzker School of Medicine, Evanston, IL.

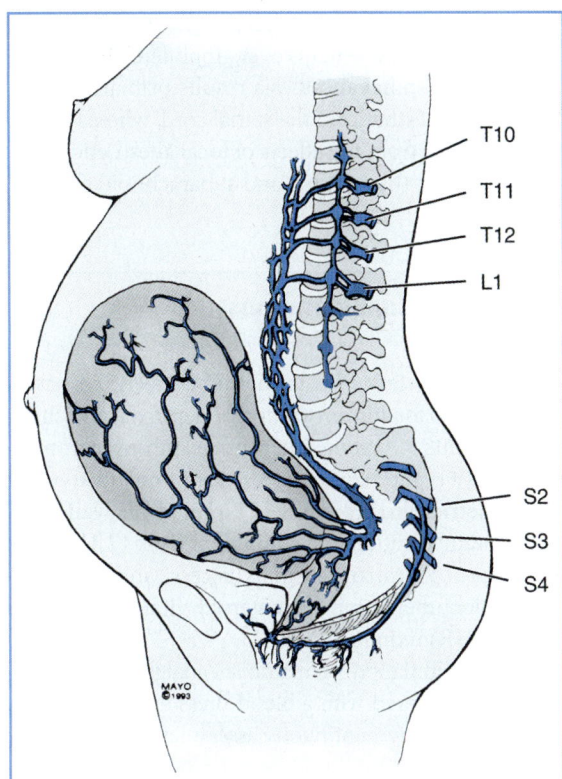

Fig. 12.5 Pain Pathways During Labor and Delivery. The afferent pain pathways from the cervix and uterus involve nerves that accompany sympathetic fibers and enter the neuraxis at T10 to L1. The pain pathways for the pelvic floor and perineum include the pudendal nerve fibers, which enter the neuraxis at S2 to S4.

vertebral column at the L3 to L4 interspace rather than the L4 to L5 interspace). Second, there is less space between adjacent lumbar spinous processes during pregnancy resulting in a narrower interspace. Third, magnetic resonance imaging has shown that the apex of the lumbar lordosis is shifted caudad during pregnancy, and the typical thoracic kyphosis in women is reduced during pregnancy.[12] These changes may influence the spread of subarachnoid anesthetic solutions in supine patients, leading to a higher sensory level in the pregnant patient (Fig. 12.4).[13] Finally, labor pain makes it more difficult for some women to assume and maintain an ideal position while the anesthesia provider performs neuraxial anesthesia.

PHYSIOLOGY

Obstetric Pain Pathways

Pain during the first stage of labor results primarily from changes in the lower uterine segment and cervix. Pain is transmitted by visceral afferent nerve fibers that accompany the sympathetic nerves and enter the spinal cord at the T10 to L1 segments. During the late first stage and second stage of labor, pain results from distention of the pelvic floor, vagina, and perineum. Pelvic pain is transmitted by somatic nerve fibers, which enter the spinal cord at the S2 to S4 segments (Fig. 12.5).

During cesarean delivery, additional nociceptive pathways are involved in the transmission of pain, and a T4 to T6 sensory level of anesthesia is required to provide adequate anesthesia, depending on the modality used to test the sensory level (i.e., touch, pinprick, or temperature).[14] Most cesarean deliveries are performed with a horizontal (e.g., Pfannenstiel) skin incision, which involves the infraumbilical T11 to T12 dermatomes. However, skin retraction, intraperitoneal manipulation, and diaphragmatic stimulation account for the higher dermatomal anesthesia requirement.

Physiology of Neural Blockade

Hormonal changes, anatomic changes, and decreases in CSF specific gravity likely are responsible for the lower local anesthetic dose requirements for spinal anesthesia in pregnant women. Local anesthetics produce conduction blockade primarily by blocking sodium channels in nerve membranes, thereby preventing the propagation of neural impulses. Differential blockade is manifested as differences in the extent of cephalad blockade of temperature discrimination and vasomotor tone, sensory loss to pinprick, sensory loss to touch, and motor function. Temperature discrimination and vasomotor tone are blocked to the greatest extent (i.e., most cephalad level) and motor function to the least extent. During spinal anesthesia, local anesthetics act directly on neural tissue in the subarachnoid space. Regression of anesthesia can be explained by the vascular uptake of local anesthetic from the subarachnoid space and spinal cord. Epidural anesthesia has a much smaller zone of differential motor-sensory-sympathetic blockade; this difference suggests that the mechanism of epidural anesthesia must involve more than simple diffusion across the dura. Nerve fiber size (i.e., smaller fibers are blocked more readily than larger fibers), myelination, and the length of nerve fiber exposed to local anesthetic are determinants of susceptibility to local anesthetic blockade and affect the extent of the differential zone of motor and sensory blockade.[15] With spinal anesthesia, the local anesthetic concentration required to block sufficient sodium channels to affect motor, sensory, and sympathetic function is less than that needed for the better-protected nerves found in the epidural space; thus a wider band of differential blockade occurs during spinal anesthesia than during epidural anesthesia.

The understanding of the mechanisms of spinal and epidural anesthesia likely remains oversimplified. Nonetheless, it seems clear that spinal anesthesia results primarily from the effects of local anesthetic on the spinal cord, whereas epidural anesthesia results from the effects of local anesthetic on nerve tissue within both the epidural and subarachnoid spaces.

TECHNIQUE

Preprocedural Considerations

Monitoring

The American Society of Anesthesiologists (ASA) has published guidelines for administration of neuraxial anesthesia in obstetric patients.[16] Among other things, these recommendations address (1) the required presence of qualified anesthesia and obstetric care providers, (2) immediate availability of resuscitation medication and equipment (Box 12.1), (3) mandatory preprocedural intravenous access, and (4) employment and documentation of maternal vital signs and fetal heart rate (FHR) monitoring.

During the initiation of neuraxial analgesia for labor, all patients are monitored with a blood pressure cuff and a pulse oximeter to facilitate continuous assessment of the maternal heart rate and oxygenation. Maternal blood pressure is measured every 1 to 2 minutes after the administration of the test and therapeutic doses of local anesthetic for approximately 15 to 20 minutes, or until the mother is hemodynamically stable. Subsequently (during maintenance of neuraxial analgesia), maternal blood pressure is measured every 15 to 30 minutes or more frequently if hypotension ensues. Continuous pulse oximetry during maintenance analgesia is used in selected patients (e.g., patients with obstructive sleep apnea or cardiovascular disease). Rarely, invasive hemodynamic monitoring is necessary. The sensory level of analgesia and the intensity of motor block

---

BOX 12.1 Suggested Resuscitation Equipment and Drugs That Should Be Available During Administration of Neuraxial Analgesia/Anesthesia

Drugs
- Hypnotic-amnestic agents (propofol, midazolam)
- Succinylcholine
- Ephedrine
- Epinephrine
- Phenylephrine
- Atropine
- Calcium chloride
- Sodium bicarbonate
- Naloxone

Equipment
- Oxygen source
- Suction source with tubing and catheters
- Self-inflating bag and mask for positive-pressure ventilation
- Face masks
- Oral airways
- Laryngoscope and assorted blades
- Endotracheal tubes with stylet
- Carbon dioxide detector

---

are assessed after the administration of the test and therapeutic doses of local anesthetic and at regular intervals thereafter.

The ASA Task Force on Obstetric Anesthesia[17] has made the following recommendation regarding FHR monitoring during the performance of neuraxial anesthesia procedures:

Fetal heart rate patterns should be monitored by a qualified individual before and after administration of neuraxial analgesia for labor. Continuous electronic recording of the fetal heart rate patterns may not be necessary in every clinical setting and may not be possible during placement of a neuraxial catheter.

The anesthesia provider cannot predict when hypotension will occur during the administration of neuraxial anesthesia. In addition, rapid onset of pain relief during the initiation of neuraxial labor analgesia is associated with nonreassuring FHR patterns (see Chapter 24).[18] Thus we believe that continuous electronic FHR monitoring should be performed both during (if possible) and after the administration of neuraxial analgesia in all laboring women. In some cases, the mother's position or maternal obesity precludes the use of an external Doppler device to monitor the FHR. In such cases, especially when there is concern regarding fetal well-being, it is helpful for the obstetric provider to place a fetal scalp electrode to monitor the FHR.

Contraindications, Informed Consent, Patient-Procedure Verification, and Partner's Presence

The American College of Obstetricians and Gynecologists states, "in the absence of a medical contraindication, maternal request is a sufficient medical indication for pain relief during labor and delivery," including neuraxial labor analgesia.[19] All patients should be informed of the risks, benefits of, and alternatives to neuraxial analgesia. The risk associated with neuraxial procedures relates to (1) the physical instrumentation of the spinal axis and (2) physiologic changes associated with medication administration via this anatomic route. Contraindications to needle or catheter placement include patient refusal or inability to cooperate, ongoing bleeding diathesis, infection either at the site of intended intervention or untreated systemic blood-borne illness, and increased intracranial pressure predisposing to cerebral herniation. Contraindications to injecting local anesthetics via the epidural or spinal route include severe hypovolemia and allergy to local anesthetics. It is unquestionable that patient refusal represents an absolute contraindication to an elective procedure. A thorough preoperative assessment of current fetal well-being, maternal volume status, intrapartum systemic opioid use, antibiotic administration for ongoing chorioamnionitis or other infectious process, and a brief reiteration of known maternal disease states, including allergies, will readily identify most of the major concerns that render neuraxial anesthesia potentially hazardous. The anesthesia provider should weigh the risks and benefits of neuraxial anesthesia for each patient.

Informed consent should include a frank discussion about anesthetic procedures and risks (see Chapter 32). Surveys of postpartum women have demonstrated that most parturients want to know the possible complications of epidural analgesia, even those that are rare.[20,21] It is best to relay this information before the onset of labor (e.g., during antenatal classes), or early in the intrapartum period, although doing so is not always feasible.[22] Some anesthesia providers fear that distressed, desperate, or sedated parturients may not understand the discussion of anesthetic procedures. A 2017 survey study of 206 postpartum women found no difference in recall of risks (discussed early after admission for labor) between women with and without pain at the time of the consent discussion.[23] The preanesthetic evaluation allows the physician to communicate a sense of concern and to demonstrate a commitment to the patient's care. Most laboring women understand the need for informed consent, and they appreciate the opportunity to participate in decisions about their care. Adequacy of consent can be demonstrated not only by documentation of information provided to the patient but also by the lack of patient objection to a procedure and the cooperation provided by the patient during the procedure. Before initiation of neuraxial anesthesia, a preprocedural verification process (i.e., "time-out") is performed in compliance with national patient safety recommendations. The participation of the patient, the anesthesia care provider, and a third party such as a member of the nursing staff may lead to the discovery of concerns that should be addressed before the initiation of neuraxial anesthesia.

Management of the pregnant patient occurs in a unique clinical care environment in which the presence of the patient's spouse or family members must be addressed. Most often, the dictates of local institutions will establish whether a partner's presence during administration of neuraxial labor analgesia is acceptable. Intuition may suggest that a partner who remains present during the placement of neuraxial analgesia may help alleviate the patient's ongoing anxiety regarding the procedure. Conversely, the partner may be so apprehensive or disruptive that the partner's presence becomes counterproductive to the care of the patient. Orbach-Zinger et al.[24] randomized 84 nulliparous women to either presence or absence of their partner during labor epidural catheter placement. Of interest, patient and partner anxiety, as measured by a validated anxiety questionnaire, was less when partners were absent during the procedure. Morell et al.[25] randomized 143 nulliparous patients to either presence or absence of a companion during labor epidural catheter placement. While anxiety scores were not different between groups, maternal satisfaction was improved with the presence of a companion during epidural catheter placement, and 89% of patients randomized to the group without a companion would have preferred to have a companion present during the procedure.

Patient Positioning

Pregnant women have an exaggerated lumbar lordosis, making it potentially more difficult for them to flex the lumbar spine. However, most pregnant patients have sufficient flexibility to facilitate the insertion of a needle into the epidural or subarachnoid space. Whether the block is initiated in the lateral or sitting position is a matter of provider and patient preference. Notable advantages of the lateral position include (1) orthostatic hypotension is less likely and (2) the position often facilitates continuous FHR monitoring during placement of the epidural catheter. Vincent and Chestnut[26] performed

a study in which they observed that neither the sitting nor the lateral position was consistently superior with regard to patient comfort. The sitting position is likely associated with a higher incidence of orthostatic hypotension and syncope. However, the sitting position is preferred—and may be required—in obese parturients, in whom identification of the midline is usually significantly easier in the sitting position.

One study demonstrated a greater reduction in maternal cardiac output with maximal lumbar flexion in the lateral decubitus position than in the sitting position during identification of the epidural space in laboring women.[27] The researchers speculated that maximal lumbar flexion in the lateral decubitus position results in concealed aortocaval compression. They recommended that "the tight fetal curl position be avoided," especially when the patient assumes the lateral decubitus position.

Aortocaval compression must be avoided to the extent possible (see Chapter 2). If maternal hydration is inadequate and if aortocaval compression is not avoided, the onset of anesthesia-induced sympathetic blockade may result in decreased venous return, cardiac output, and uteroplacental perfusion.

Maternal position during placement of the epidural catheter does not seem to affect the incidence of unintentional dural puncture. However, adoption of the lateral recumbent headdown position for epidural catheter placement may reduce the incidence of unintentional epidural venous puncture.[28]

When spinal or epidural anesthesia is performed with the patient in a lateral position, the patient's back should lie at, and parallel to, the edge of the bed, for at least two reasons. First, the edge is the firmest section of the mattress. If the patient lies away from the edge of the bed, the patient's weight will depress the mattress and the pelvis may rotate if the patient's knees extend past the far edge of the bed. Second, this position allows anesthesia providers to keep their elbows flexed, facilitating control of fine hand and wrist muscle movements. The plane of the entire back should be perpendicular to the mattress. When asked to flex the lower back, patients typically roll the top shoulder forward, an action that rotates the spine (which is undesirable) but does not flex the lower back.

Similarly, patients positioned sitting should have their feet supported by a stool with the backs of their knees against the edge of the bed, a maneuver that helps position the patient's back closer to the anesthesia provider. Alternatively, the cross-leg position may be a viable option in the sitting position. On preprocedural ultrasonography, the cross-leg position significantly increased the measured lengths of the posterior longitudinal ligament, ligamentum flavum, and interlaminar distance compared to standard positioning.[29] The shoulders should be relaxed symmetrically over the hips and buttocks. Beds in obstetric units often break at the foot, and the split in the mattress encourages the patient's seat to slope downhill if straddling the mattress split; this position will cause spine rotation and may make the procedure more difficult.

When spinal anesthesia is performed, the patient's position relative to the baricity of the anesthetic solution should be considered, because it influences the extent and latency of blockade as well as the incidence of hypotension. The incidence, timing, and extent of hypotension in the period immediately after initiation of the block depend on the type of block (i.e., spinal, epidural, or combined spinal-epidural [CSE]), drug characteristics (i.e., baricity, concentration, dose), patient position during the procedure, and patient position in the period following the procedure. For example, when spinal anesthesia is initiated with a hyperbaric solution for operative vaginal delivery, it often makes sense for the patient to be sitting to ensure the rapid onset of sacral anesthesia. Conversely, spinal anesthesia for cervical cerclage can be initiated with the patient in the steep lateral Trendelenburg position with a hypobaric anesthetic solution.

Posture has less influence on the spread of epidural anesthesia.[30,31] During epidural anesthesia, a unilateral block more likely results from the malposition of the catheter or an anatomic barrier within the epidural space than from patient position, particularly after a bolus injection. Norris and Dewan[30] observed that gravity did not augment the spread of anesthesia in patients receiving epidural anesthesia for cesarean delivery, and they concluded that posture does not need to be manipulated to ensure adequate bilateral epidural anesthesia. In at least two studies, it was noted that the use of the sitting position is not necessary for the development of good sacral anesthesia when large volumes of epidural local anesthetic are given for cesarean delivery.[30,31] However, Reid and Thorburn[31] observed that use of the sitting position appeared to delay the spread of anesthesia to the midthoracic dermatomes. In comparison with the bolus administration of epidural local anesthetic, the extent of blockade may be more gravity dependent when the anesthetic is administered as a continuous infusion over a prolonged period.

Some anesthesiologists contend that maternal position after epidural catheter placement affects the efficacy of epidural analgesia, but this is a matter of some dispute. Beilin et al.[32] observed that the placement of the laboring woman in the supine position with a 30-degree leftward tilt was associated with better epidural analgesia than maintenance of the left lateral decubitus position. In contrast, Preston et al.[33] observed no difference in analgesia and a significantly higher incidence of fetal bradycardia with the supine wedged position than with the full lateral position.

Aseptic Technique

An understanding of the importance of sterile technique and the gravity of infectious complications related to neuraxial anesthesia is crucial.[34,35] The incidence of epidural abscess and spinal meningitis is generally so low that many of the available recommendations are based on evidence from other domains of infection control (e.g., surgical wound site and central venous catheter–related infection).[36–38] Nonetheless, death and devastating neurologic compromise resulting from neuraxial infection can occur.

Infection of the epidural space tends to result in the formation of an abscess, most commonly formed by *Staphylococcus aureus* found in the epidermis of either the patient or the anesthesia provider. In contrast, meningitis associated with neuraxial procedures is most commonly caused by *Streptococcus viridans*. Viridans species of streptococcus may reside in the oronasopharyngeal tract of providers or patients or in the patient's vagina. Potential routes of infection include the (1)

epidural catheter track, (2) bloodstream, (3) equipment, and (4) injectate contamination. A more in-depth discussion of neuraxial infection is found in Chapter 31.

Guidelines describing aseptic technique for regional and neuraxial anesthetic procedures have been published by professional anesthesiology organizations and the US Centers for Disease Control and Prevention (CDC).[36,37,39] The following recommendations deserve emphasis:

1. Given that the oropharyngeal and skin flora of the anesthesia provider are implicated in many cases of neuraxial infection, the provider should don a surgical face mask and hat before initiation of spinal/epidural anesthesia. Microbial sampling in laminar-flow operating theaters has shown a 22-fold increase in bacterial counts when a face mask and hat are not worn.[40]
2. Washing hands with an alcohol-based antiseptic solution is recommended because this has been shown to be superior to antimicrobial soap. Jewelry (e.g., rings, watches) should be removed before and sterile gloves worn after hand cleansing.
3. The patient's skin should be decontaminated, preferably with a chlorhexidine-in-alcohol solution.[38] Evidence suggests that chlorhexidine has superior bactericidal and bacteriostatic efficacy compared with povidone-iodine.[41] If chlorhexidine is not available, then povidone-iodine with alcohol, rather than povidone-iodine alone, is preferred.[38] Of importance, the anesthesia provider is encouraged to exercise patience in allowing the antiseptic to dry, because a major mechanism of antisepsis is the desiccating action of alcohol.

Equipment and Placement of Needle/Catheter
Spinal Anesthesia

The first equipment decision involves determining whether to perform a single-shot or continuous spinal technique. Traditionally, a large-bore epidural needle and catheter are used for continuous spinal anesthesia because the US Food and Drug Administration (FDA) rescinded approval for the use of small-bore microcatheters in 1992. Therefore the risk for postdural puncture headache (PDPH) is significant. Continuous spinal analgesia or anesthesia using an "epidural" catheter sited in the subarachnoid space is useful after *unintentional* dural puncture with an epidural needle.

A 23-gauge, FDA-approved, spinal catheter is now available in the United States. The catheter is inserted using a "catheter-over-needle" technique. Initial observational study found that this catheter may have clinical utility[42]; however, a case series of five patients reported complications in all parturients, with three patients experiencing paresthesias and two PDPH.[43] Further study is required to determine the true incidence of complications and its utility for continuous spinal anesthesia in obstetric patients. Several commercial spinal catheters are available in Europe and have been used successfully in parturients, but at the current time, a single-shot technique is preferred for spinal anesthesia for most obstetric patients.

The primary equipment choice for spinal anesthesia concerns the type and size of the spinal needle. Cutting-bevel needles (e.g., Quincke) should be avoided because of the unacceptably high incidence of PDPH associated with their use. Instead, noncutting (pencil-point) needles (e.g., Whitacre,

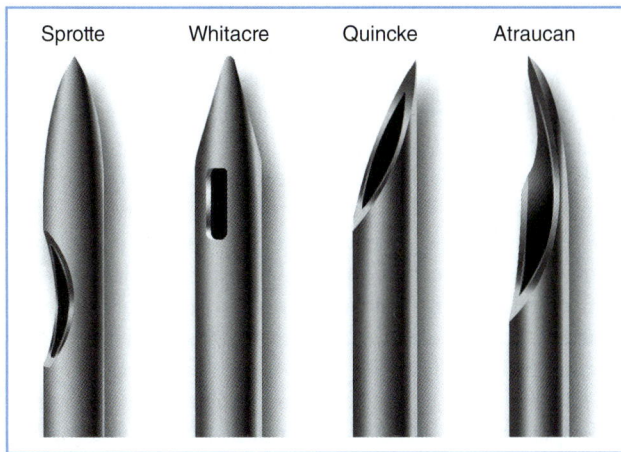

Fig. 12.6 Spinal Needle Assortment Often Used in Parturients. The Sprotte and Whitacre needles have cone-shaped bevels, whereas the Quincke and Atraucan needles have a cutting bevel. (Other sizes are available in some of these needle designs.)

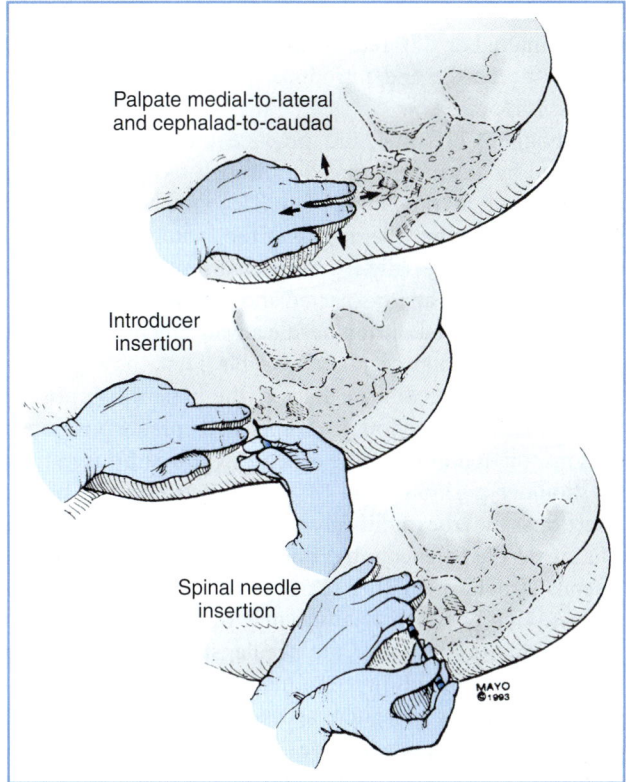

Fig. 12.7 The midline approach for spinal needle insertion requires accurate identification of a lumbar interspinous space. The palpating fingers are rolled in a medial-to-lateral and cephalad-to-caudad direction; an introducer is then inserted through the interspinous space almost perpendicular to the lumbar spinous process. Once the introducer is seated in the interspinous ligament, the spinal needle is inserted; the needle is stabilized in a tripod fashion during insertion (much like a dart being thrown).

Sprotte, Gertie Marx) should be used (Fig. 12.6). Pencil-point needles cause more trauma to the dura than occurs with cutting-bevel needles. This likely results in a more intense inflammatory response. Presumably, the inflammation results in more rapid closure of the dural defect.[44]

Needle size must also be determined. Larger needles offer a greater fidelity of tactile feedback as the anesthesia provider traverses tissue planes of variable impedance when performing spinal anesthesia. Furthermore, larger needles are more likely to withstand the high resistance encountered when contacting bone without bending or shearing. In general, the "ease-of-use" advantages associated with larger needles must be balanced against a lower incidence of PDPH with smaller needles. Most anesthesia providers use 25- or 27-gauge noncutting needles for routine spinal anesthesia in obstetric patients. The urgency of the procedure may also influence the choice of needle size. For example, a 25-gauge needle might be chosen for spinal anesthesia for an elective procedure, and a larger (e.g., 24-gauge or 22-gauge) needle might be chosen when the subarachnoid space must be entered quickly because of severe fetal compromise.

With a small-gauge needle (i.e., 24-gauge or smaller), use of an introducer needle is preferable. The introducer needle engages the interspinous ligament and more accurately guides the trajectory of the smaller spinal needle than is possible with use of a small-gauge spinal needle alone. The introducer needle also aids with skin puncture as it is often difficult to puncture the skin with noncutting needles.

Either the midline or the paramedian approach can be used to enter the subarachnoid space. The midline approach requires the patient to reduce her lumbar lordosis to allow access to the subarachnoid space between adjacent spinous processes in the lumbar region. Traditionally, the anesthesia provider identifies the interspinous space using a landmark technique, although there is growing use of preprocedural ultrasonography to identify the space (see later). The interspinous space may be identified with one (usually the thumb or index finger) or two fingers (usually the index and middle fingers) of the anesthesia provider's nondominant hand. The single finger "slides" along

the skin in the midline from cephalad to caudad until it "settles" into an interspinous space. The two fingers identify the interspinous space by palpating the caudad border of the more cephalad spine. The fingers identify the midline by rolling in a medial-to-lateral direction (Fig. 12.7).

Next, the anesthesia provider injects local anesthetic intradermally and subcutaneously. The introducer needle is inserted into the substance of the interspinous ligament. It is helpful if the introducer needle is embedded in the interspinous ligament; therefore obese patients may require a longer introducer needle. The introducer needle should lie in the sagittal midline plane. It is then grasped and steadied with the fingers of the nondominant hand while the dominant hand holds the spinal needle like a dart. The fifth finger may be used as a tripod against the patient's back to prevent patient movement from causing unintentional needle insertion to a level deeper than intended, and to "brake" the needle. As the needle passes through the ligamentum flavum and the dura, characteristic changes in resistance are noted. A "pop" is often perceived as the needle tip traverses the ligamentum flavum. A subsequent and more pronounced pop is perceived as the needle tip exits the dura-arachnoid. The stylet is removed, and CSF should appear in the needle hub. If CSF does not appear, the stylet is replaced, and the needle is advanced until another change in resistance or "pop" is appreciated and again checked for CSF flow. This process continues until either bone is encountered or CSF returns through the needle. If neither occurs, the needle and introducer are withdrawn, and the process is repeated.

Although with time and practice the tactile feedback produced by advancing a needle through tissues of variable resistance will become utterly familiar to the anesthesia provider, the novice may be unsure of the anatomic position of the needle tip, especially if unexpected resistance (i.e., contact with bone) or an unexpected and premature "pop sensation" is encountered during needle advancement. A stepwise problem-solving approach is reasonable. First, the anesthesia provider should reconfirm that (1) the patient has normal anatomy (i.e., not scoliotic), (2) she is acceptably positioned without rotation of the spine (often recognized by asymmetric shoulder position), and (3) the chosen point of needle insertion is the true midline plane. If these assertions are true, and the needle tip encounters bone, it is highly likely that the osseous structure is either the inferior or superior spinous process. One of two maneuvers may overcome this barrier. After slight withdrawal of the needle, simple angulation in a cephalad or caudad direction may redirect the needle trajectory sufficiently to achieve access to the central neuraxial canal. One must appreciate the "toughness" of the interspinous ligament. Even a 17-gauge epidural needle can be bent if the angle is changed without some prior retraction of the needle. Furthermore, if a spinal needle/introducer complex is used, care must be exercised that angulation of the spinal needle does not occur without first withdrawing the needle into the lumen of the introducer. Thereafter the entire spinal needle/introducer complex is angulated before the spinal

needle is readvanced. Angulation of the spinal needle without first withdrawing it into the introducer creates a fulcrum at the junction of the introducer tip where the spinal needle emerges and can potentially damage or even shear the delicate spinal needle (Fig. 12.8).

Alternatively, the introducer/needle complex may be withdrawn fully into subcutaneous tissue and either raised or lowered (cephalad or caudad) while still maintaining an angulation that is parallel to the original trajectory. Which approach is more effective may depend on the reason for the initial bone contact. If the patient has very narrow interspaces, then careful raising or lowering of the needle while maintaining a trajectory parallel to the floor may be appropriate. However, if the patient is overly flexed forward, it is possible that her lumbar spinous processes are projecting in a slightly upward angulation (relative to the perpendicular transverse plane). This may require that the needle be reangulated accordingly.

If bone is still encountered despite these considerations, it is likely that the needle tip is in fact *not* in the midline plane and is contacting the vertebral lamina. This may occur if the initial skin puncture is not in the midline, the needle tip deviates from the midline as it is advanced, or the patient's spine is rotated (either from poor positioning or scoliosis). Clues that the needle tip is not midline include (1) the patient complaining of lateralizing pain; (2) lack of CSF flow despite appropriate needle depth; and (3) the perception of "soft" or "mushy" tissue (paraspinous tissue) during needle advancement rather than the more "rigid" ligamentous tissue, or even a false "pop" as the needle tip exits the interspinous ligament laterally into paraspinous tissue. Much like the progressive modifications described earlier for correct alignment in the superioinferior

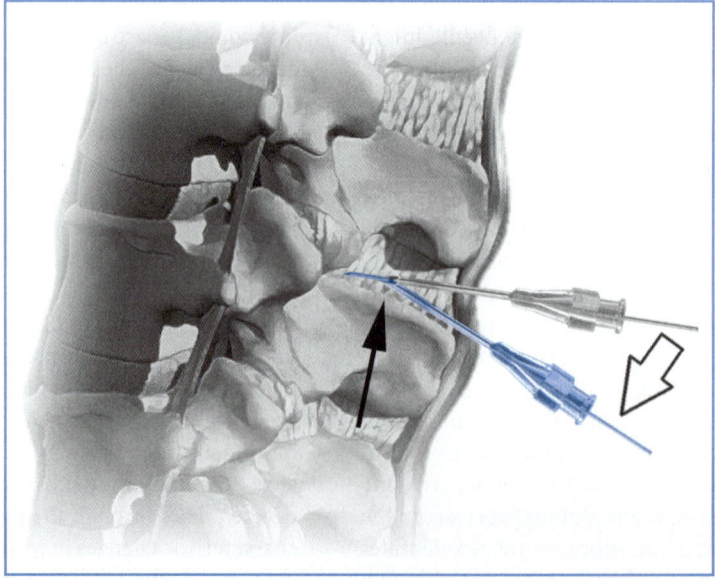

Fig. 12.8 Change of Needle Trajectory During Spinal Anesthesia. Note that if both the spinal needle and its introducer needle are manipulated without prior retraction of the spinal needle into the lumen of the introducer *(open arrow)*, a fulcrum is created *(dark arrow)* where the risk for bending or shearing the delicate spinal needle may occur. Illustration by Naveen Nathan, MD, NorthShore University HealthSystem, University of Chicago Pritzker School of Medicine, Evanston, IL.

plane, so too can these approaches be employed for redirecting in the lateral plane (Fig. 12.9). The novice is advised to make systematic changes in a stepwise fashion, rather than indiscriminately changing needle direction without first considering the anatomic problem.

Once CSF is freely dripping from the needle hub, the dorsum of the provider's nondominant hand steadies the spinal needle against the patient's back while the syringe with local anesthetic is attached to the needle. After aspirating to ensure the free flow of CSF, local anesthetic is injected at a rate of approximately 0.2 mL/s. After completion of the injection, some providers again aspirate approximately 0.2 mL of CSF

and reinject it into the subarachnoid space. This last step reconfirms the needle location and clears the needle of the remaining local anesthetic. The patient is then repositioned as appropriate.

For most patients, the midline approach is faster and less painful than the paramedian approach. The midline approach is also easier to teach than the paramedian approach because it requires mental projection of the anatomy in only two planes, whereas the paramedian approach requires appreciation of a third plane and estimation of the depth of the subarachnoid space from the skin (Fig. 12.10). Nevertheless, the paramedian approach is a useful technique that allows for

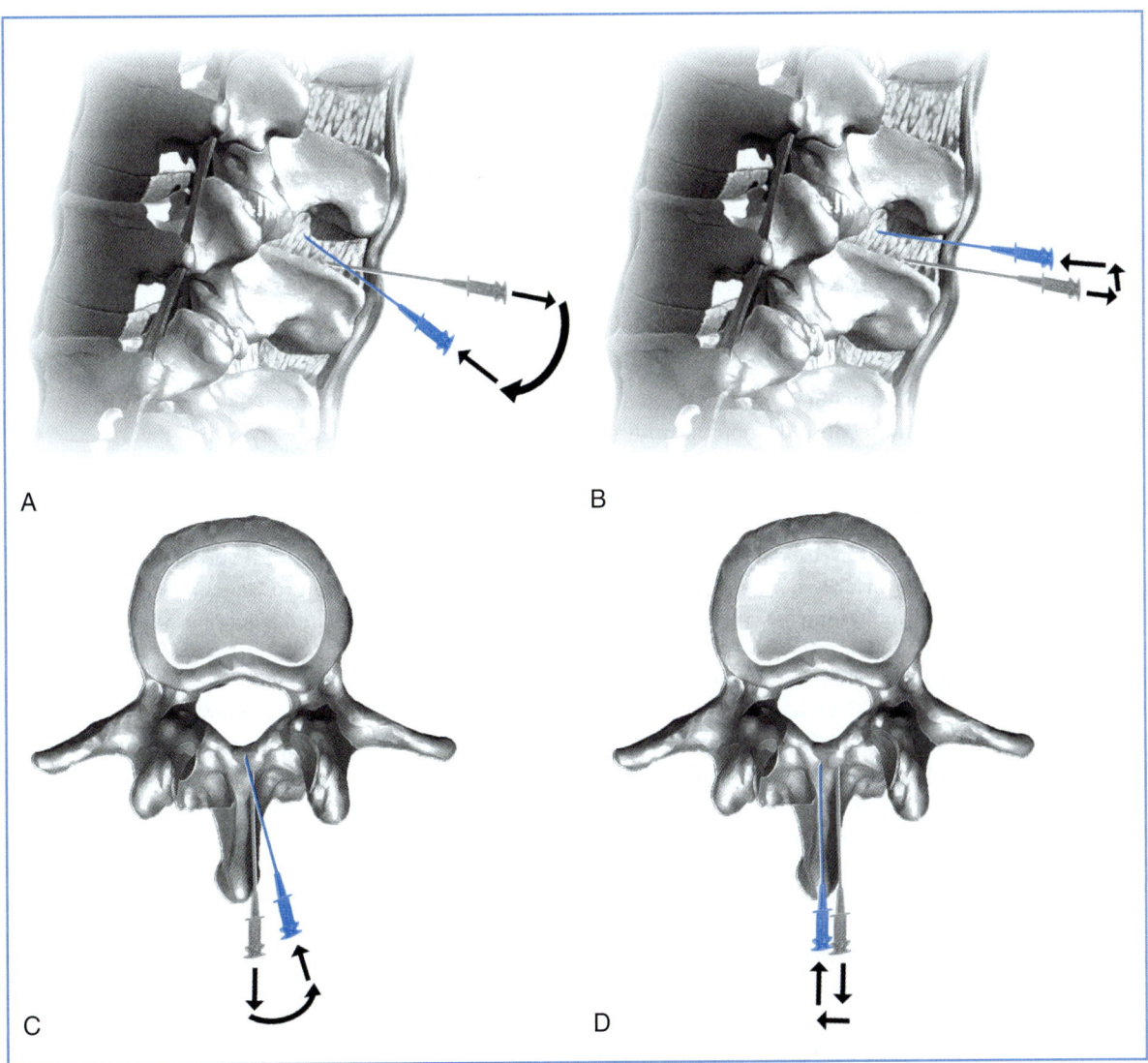

Fig. 12.9 Troubleshooting Contact With Bony Structures During Needle Placement. The *gray needle* represents the initial needle trajectory; the *blue needle* represents the adjusted needle trajectory. (A) Assuming correct midline needle placement, the needle can be retracted slightly and angulated to overcome a spinous process. (B) Alternatively, the needle may be "lifted" after slight retraction while keeping the original trajectory constant. (C) Assuming the needle is deviating from the midline plane and contacting lamina, an action similar to that in *A* may be executed. (D) Alternatively, a stepwise lateral shift similar in concept to that shown in *B* may correctly achieve midline alignment. Illustration by Naveen Nathan, MD, NorthShore University HealthSystem, University of Chicago Pritzker School of Medicine, Evanston, IL.

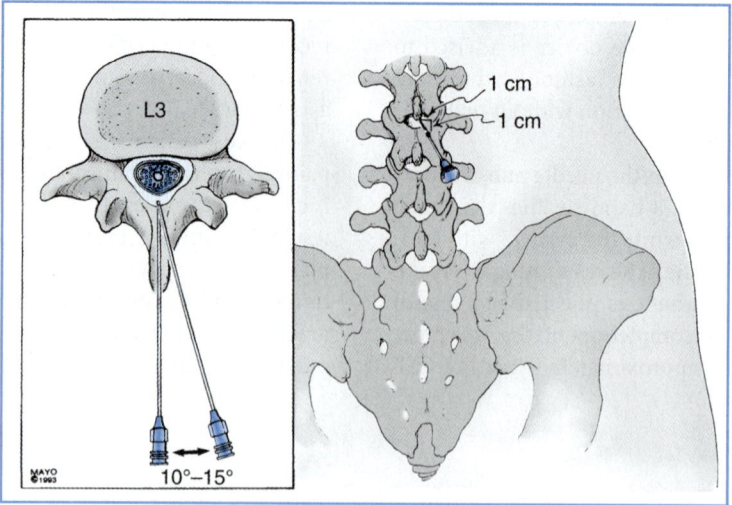

Fig. 12.10 Vertebral Anatomy of Midline and Paramedian Approaches for Spinal and Epidural Anesthesia. The midline approach requires anatomic projection in only two planes: sagittal and horizontal. The paramedian approach also requires consideration of the oblique plane. However, the paramedian approach requires less patient cooperation in reducing lumbar lordosis to allow for successful needle insertion. The paramedian needle insertion site is made 1 cm lateral and 1 cm caudad to the caudad edge of the more cephalad spinous process. The paramedian needle is inserted 10–15 degrees off the sagittal plane (inset).

the successful identification of the subarachnoid or epidural space in difficult cases. The paramedian approach does not require that the patient fully reduce her lumbar lordosis. This approach exploits the larger target that is available when the needle is inserted slightly off the midline.

A common error that is made with the paramedian approach is the insertion of the needle too far off the midline; the vertebral lamina then becomes a barrier to needle insertion. With the paramedian approach, the palpating fingers should again identify the caudad edge of the more cephalad spinous process. A skin wheal is raised 1 cm lateral and 1 cm caudad to this point; a longer needle is then used to infiltrate the deeper tissues in a cephalomedial plane. This step contrasts to the midline approach, in which the local anesthetic is not injected beyond the subcutaneous tissue. The spinal introducer is then inserted 10 to 15 degrees off the sagittal plane in a cephalomedial direction, and the spinal needle is advanced through the introducer needle toward the subarachnoid space. Another common error is to use an excessive cephalad angle with initial needle insertion. When the needle is inserted correctly and contacts bone, it is redirected slightly cephalad. If bone is again encountered, but at a deeper level, the slight stepwise increase in cephalad angulation is continued, and the needle is "walked" up and off the lamina. As with the midline approach, the characteristic feel of the ligamentum flavum and dura can be appreciated. The aim of the paramedian approach is to puncture the dura in the midline, even though the needle is inserted off the midline. Use of the paramedian approach requires insertion of a greater length of needle. Once CSF is obtained, the block is performed as it is with the midline approach.

During the performance of any nerve block technique, needle advancement should stop if the patient complains of pain. If pain is the result of inadequate soft tissue anesthesia, additional local anesthetic should be injected. Pain or paresthesias may also result from needle contact with central nerves or the spinal cord. Patient perception of paresthesias during the initiation of spinal anesthesia may indicate that the needle tip is in the subarachnoid space. The anesthesia provider should remove the stylet and check for CSF. If the paresthesia has resolved, the local anesthetic may be injected. If the paresthesia persists, however, the needle should be withdrawn and repositioned. In any case, the anesthesia provider should never inject the local anesthetic if the patient is complaining of paresthesias or lancinating pain, either of which may signal injection into a nerve or the spinal cord.

Epidural Anesthesia

Special equipment for epidural analgesia or anesthesia includes an epidural needle, an epidural catheter (for a continuous technique), and a loss-of-resistance syringe (for the loss-of-resistance technique to identify the epidural space). Single-shot epidural anesthesia is rarely used in obstetric practice because the major advantage of epidural over spinal anesthesia is the ability to provide continuous anesthesia or analgesia without puncturing the dura with a large needle. An epidural needle with a lateral opening (e.g., Hustead, Tuohy, Weiss) is most commonly used because it allows a catheter to be threaded through its orifice (Fig. 12.11).

Epidural anesthesia is typically initiated by injecting local anesthetic and adjuvants into the lumber epidural space. Although a caudal approach was used in the early era of neuraxial labor analgesia, it is now rarely used. Two methods are used to identify the epidural space during needle advancement: (1) hanging drop method and (2) loss-of-resistance method. Most anesthesia providers use the loss-of-resistance method (Fig. 12.12).

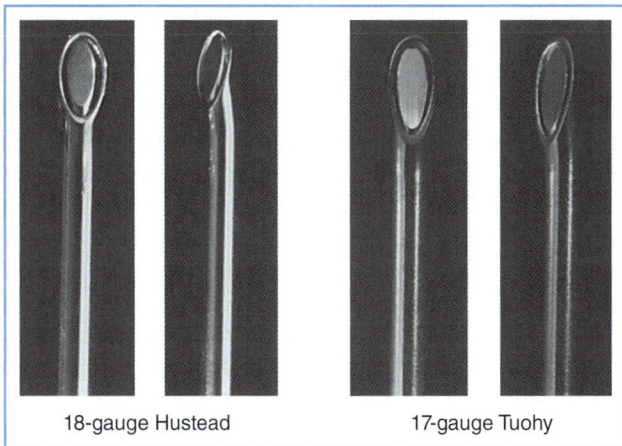

| 18-gauge Hustead | 17-gauge Tuohy |

Fig. 12.11 Epidural Needle Assortment Often Used in Parturients. Each needle is shown in an open-bevel view and an oblique orientation. The 18-gauge Hustead and 17-gauge Tuohy needles have lateral-facing openings, which direct epidural catheters to enter the epidural space more easily than if a single-shot Crawford needle design is used. (Other sizes and needle designs are available for obstetric epidural anesthesia.)

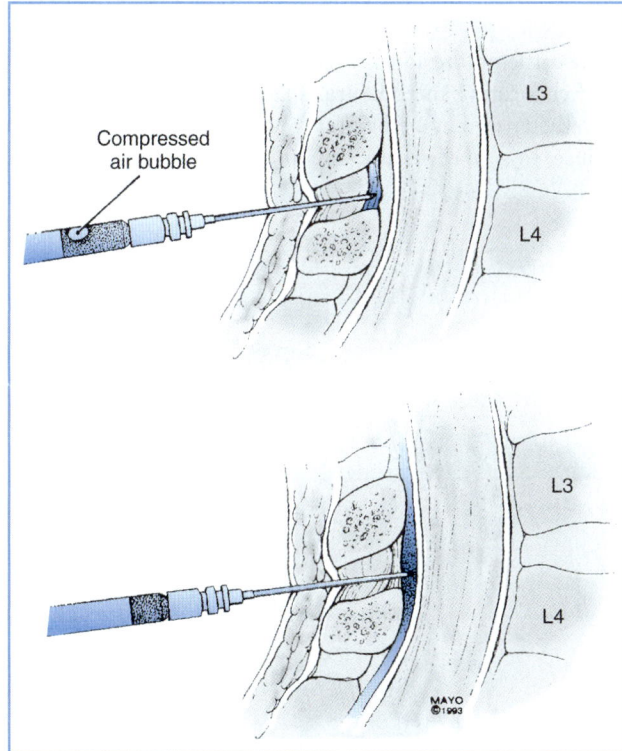

Fig. 12.12 Loss-of-Resistance Technique for Identifying the Epidural Space. The needle is first inserted into the interspinous ligament or ligamentum flavum, and a syringe containing an air bubble in saline is attached to the hub. After compression of the air bubble by pressure on the syringe-plunger, the needle is carefully advanced until a loss of resistance to syringe-plunger pressure is noted as the needle enters the epidural space.

The traditional loss-of-resistance syringe is a finely ground glass syringe with a Luer-lock connector. Plastic syringes are also available as are slip-tip syringes, and the choice is generally a matter of the anesthesia provider's preference. The

syringe is filled with 2 to 4 mL of saline, air, or saline with a small (0.25 to 0.5 mL) air bubble. There is some controversy regarding the use of air versus saline for detecting the point of loss of resistance.[45] Saline causes some syringe plungers to stick and may be confused with CSF during initiation of CSE anesthesia. Conversely, injection of air into the epidural space may contribute to patchy anesthesia[46] and unintentional pneumocephalus may increase the risk for headache.[47]

Results of investigations comparing air to saline for loss of resistance are conflicting. A 2014 metaanalysis that included 852 patients (most were obstetric patients) found no differences in inability to locate the epidural space, unintentional intravascular or intrathecal catheter placement, block failure, unblocked segments, or pain between the two mediums.[48] However, the confidence intervals of the relative risks were wide and the authors concluded that the evidence was of low quality. In a retrospective, single-institution study of loss of resistance to air versus saline by Segal and Arendt,[49] no significant differences in block success were found in 929 patients. The authors intentionally chose a retrospective approach to the question; they stated that because "it is impossible to mask the anesthesiologist to the medium used for loss-of-resistance, [they] hypothesized that randomized controlled trials might *overestimate* the difference between air and saline by forcing the operator to use a less-preferred technique in half of the subjects." Thus we recommend that anesthesia providers use the technique with which they are most comfortable. We use saline with a small bubble of air.

Regardless of the technique used, success depends on correct placement of the needle tip. The needle should be advanced sufficiently into the interspinous ligament before the syringe is attached or before the hanging drop of solution is placed into the needle hub. This approach has at least three advantages. First, it encourages the anesthesia provider to use proprioception while directing and advancing the needle. Second, it shortens the time required for successful identification of the epidural space. Third, it lowers the likelihood of a false-positive loss of resistance. Undoubtedly, this false-positive identification of the epidural space is responsible for many cases of unsuccessful epidural anesthesia; it is even possible to insert a catheter between the interspinous ligament and the ligamentum flavum.

During advancement of the needle-syringe assembly, the needle should be moved toward the epidural space by the provider's nondominant hand while the thumb of the dominant hand applies constant pressure on the syringe plunger, thereby compressing the small air bubble. Alternatively, the intermittent, oscillating technique is employed when using the loss-of-resistance to air technique. When the needle enters the epidural space, the pressure applied to the syringe plunger causes the saline solution or air to flow easily into the epidural space (see Fig. 12.12).

In most obstetric cases, the anesthesia provider inserts a catheter and uses an intermittent bolus or continuous infusion technique to maintain analgesia (see Chapter 24). Most practitioners insert the catheter before injecting local anesthetic to allow for the slow, incremental injection of local anesthetic/opioid solution and the more controlled development of epidural anesthesia. If the principal reason for using an epidural technique is the provision of continuous analgesia, it seems most practical to insert the catheter before injecting the therapeutic dose of local anesthetic so that correct catheter placement can be verified promptly.

Several types of single-use, disposable epidural catheters are available.[50] Catheters are made from plastic materials and differ as to the degree of "stiffness." Wire-embedded catheters are more flexible and are associated with a lower incidence of paresthesias and intravascular placement during catheter insertion.[28,51] The single-orifice catheter has one opening at its tip, whereas the multiorifice catheter has a closed "bullet" tip with three lateral orifices between 0.5 and 1.8 cm from the tip (Fig. 12.13).

The proposed advantage of single-orifice, open-end catheters is that the injection of drugs is restricted to a single anatomic site. In theory, this arrangement should facilitate the detection of intravenous or subarachnoid placement of the catheter. Likewise, a theoretical disadvantage of multiorifice, closed-end catheters is that local anesthetic may be injected into more than one anatomic site (e.g., both the epidural and subarachnoid spaces). A catheter initially placed in the epidural space can migrate into a vein or the subdural or subarachnoid space. Fortunately, this does not seem to be a common clinical problem. Regardless of the choice of catheter, aspiration should be performed before each dose of local anesthetic is injected.

An advantage of the multiorifice catheter over the single-orifice catheter is the consistent ability to aspirate fluid (either blood or CSF) when the catheter is in a vessel or the subarachnoid space.[52] Early studies suggested that multiorifice catheters may lead to more even distribution of local anesthetic and a lower incidence of "patchy" or unilateral anesthesia when the anesthetic is injected as a bolus.[53] With low infusion rates into the epidural space, such as those used with continuous epidural infusions, the solution exits only the most proximal hole,[54] and multiorifice catheters thus behave like single-orifice catheters. Use of higher infusion rates, such as those used with programmed intermittent epidural bolus (PIEB), will more consistently make use of all three orifices, depending on flow rate.[55] A randomized trial comparing single- and multiorifice wire-reinforced catheters found no differences in block initiation success, analgesia maintenance with a continuous epidural infusion, or complications.[56] In contrast, when labor analgesia was maintained with a PIEB technique, single-orifice catheters had improved analgesia and sacral coverage with fewer patient-controlled epidural analgesia boluses and less local anesthetic consumption compared with multiorifice catheters.[57] Additional studies are needed with the PIEB technique to fully delineate if single-orifice catheters are advantageous.

After locating the epidural space but prior to threading the catheter, it may be helpful to inject 5 to 10 mL of saline because this may reduce the incidence of epidural vein

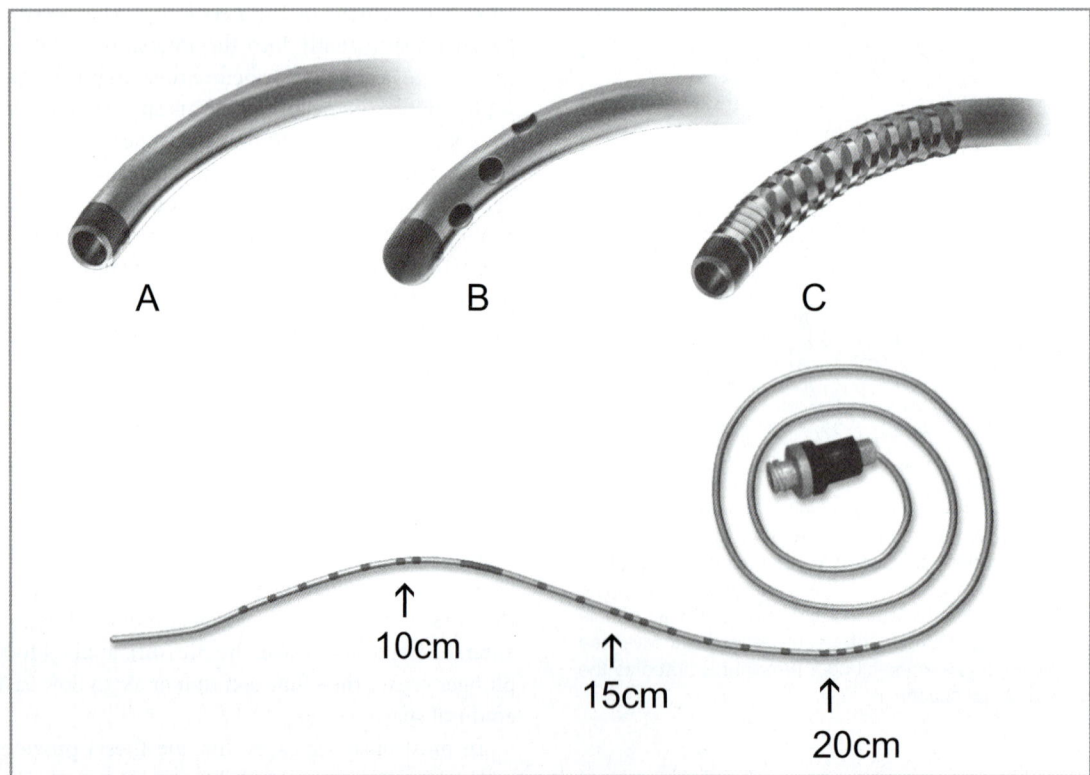

Fig. 12.13 Epidural Catheters. (A) Single-orifice catheter; (B) multiorifice catheter with bullet tip; (C) coiled wire reinforced catheter. *Bottom,* Epidural catheter with centimeter markings along distal end and Luer-lock connector at proximal end. Illustration by Naveen Nathan, MD, NorthShore University HealthSystem, University of Chicago Pritzker School of Medicine, Evanston, IL.

cannulation,[28] particularly when using stiffer epidural catheters. Six to eight centimeters of catheter are threaded into the epidural space before the epidural needle is removed. The catheter may then be pulled back until it is at the desired distance at the skin. Occasionally, the anesthesia provider will have difficulty advancing the catheter past the tip of the epidural needle. This difficulty may indicate that the epidural needle tip is not in the epidural space. However, if the provider is convinced that the needle is correctly placed, several maneuvers may facilitate catheter advancement. Having the patient take a deep breath often allows catheter advancement. Saline may be injected through the epidural needle if this has not been done. Although some providers rotate the epidural needle in an attempt to successfully advance the catheter, we do not recommend this maneuver because it may increase the risk for dural puncture. Instead, the epidural needle should be withdrawn 0.5 to 1 cm and again advanced into the epidural space. In a randomized trial comparing two different epidural kits from two different manufacturers with different epidural catheter and epidural needle types,[58] difficulty in threading the epidural catheter into the epidural space was significantly higher with one kit compared with the other. The authors suggested that variations in the morphologic features of the epidural needles and catheters, and their combination, may influence the success of siting the epidural catheter.

Many techniques are available for securing the epidural catheter at the skin entry site. A transparent, sterile adhesive dressing applied over the catheter after application of skin adhesive generally works well, and the periphery of the dressing can be reinforced with tape. The position of the epidural catheter may change significantly with patient movement from the sitting-flexed to the sitting-upright or lateral decubitus position.[59] Beilin et al.[60] found 5 cm was the optimal distance to thread a multiorifice catheter. Less than 5 cm led to catheter dislodgement and more than 5 cm led to a greater incidence of unilateral analgesia. D'Angelo et al.[61] found that the risk for catheter dislodgement was higher when single-orifice catheters were inserted 2 cm, but the risk for unilateral blockade was greater when catheters were inserted 6 to 8 cm. Therefore, if the catheter is to be used for a short period (e.g., during cesarean delivery), it should be left 2 to 4 cm into the epidural space. In contrast, if the catheter will be used for many hours (e.g., during labor), it should be left 4 to 6 cm into the space.[61] To minimize catheter movement at the skin, the patient should be positioned sitting upright or in the lateral position before the catheter is secured, especially if the patient is obese.[59] The epidural catheter should be labeled to decrease the risk of unintentional injection of a drug intended for intravascular injection.

The potential for the contamination of local anesthetic solutions has prompted the use of micropore filters during the administration of continuous epidural analgesia for labor. There is no evidence that filters decrease the rate of infection or of injection of undesirable foreign substances.[62] Additionally, filters may reduce the reliability of aspiration[63] and absorb local anesthetic solution, unless they are primed.[64]

We believe that micropore filters have little use in clinical obstetric anesthesia practice.

Combined Spinal-Epidural Anesthesia

CSE anesthesia combines the advantages and mitigates the disadvantages of single-shot spinal anesthesia and continuous epidural anesthesia (Box 12.2). Anesthesia is initiated with a subarachnoid injection of opioid with or without a local anesthetic and maintained via an epidural catheter. It is useful for both cesarean delivery anesthesia and labor analgesia. For cesarean delivery, the injection of the smaller dose of local anesthetic required for spinal (compared with epidural) anesthesia is inherently safer with regard to the possibility of unintentional intravascular injection. Additionally, the anesthesia provider can inject a local anesthetic dose that is lower than the ED_{95} (effective dose in 95% of cases) without fear of inadequate anesthesia. If surgical anesthesia is inadequate, the block can be "rescued" with epidural administration of local anesthetic. A randomized trial comparing 7, 8, and 9 mg of intrathecal bupivacaine administered as part of a CSE technique for cesarean delivery produced equivalent latencies to T4 sensory block with lower rates of maternal hypotension in the lowest-dose group.[65] The shorter duration of action seen in the low-dose (7 mg) group was easily addressed through the administration of local anesthetic via the indwelling epidural catheter. Compared with conventional epidural anesthesia for cesarean delivery, CSE anesthesia is associated with a more rapid onset of surgical anesthesia, less intraoperative pain and discomfort (because of a more dense block), better muscle relaxation, and less shivering and vomiting.[66]

The CSE technique is associated with a faster onset of labor analgesia, achieved with the subarachnoid injection of an

---

BOX 12.2 Advantages of Combined Spinal-Epidural Anesthetic Technique

Compared with epidural anesthesia
- Lower maternal, fetal, and neonatal plasma concentrations of anesthetic agents
- More rapid onset of analgesia and anesthesia
- Denser sensory blockade
- Complete early labor analgesia with opioid alone (no local anesthetic necessary)
- Lower failure rate for labor analgesia and conversion to surgical anesthesia

Compared with spinal anesthesia
- Technically easier in obese individuals: the epidural needle acts as an introducer for the spinal needle (it is easier to advance a rigid epidural needle)
- Ability to titrate anesthetic dose: start with low subarachnoid dose, and titrate to effect using epidural injection
- Results in less hypotension
- Ability to extend the extent of neuroblockade: spinal anesthesia for forceps delivery may be extended to epidural anesthesia for cesarean delivery after failed forceps delivery
- Continuous technique: ability to extend duration of anesthesia

opioid alone or an opioid combined with a small dose of local anesthetic. Studies differ as to whether CSE analgesia is associated with greater maternal satisfaction and fewer requests for supplemental analgesia. Goodman et al.[67] randomized 100 parous women in early labor to receive either CSE or conventional epidural analgesia. There were no differences in requests for supplemental analgesia, although pain scores were lower in the CSE group within the first 30 minutes. A single-institution randomized trial in 800 women found better first-stage analgesia and fewer requirements for treatment of breakthrough pain in women randomized to receive CSE compared with epidural analgesia.[68] A 2012 systematic review comparing CSE and epidural labor analgesia concluded that onset was faster with the CSE technique, but that there was no evidence for differences in maternal satisfaction, mode of delivery, ability to ambulate, or incidence of hypotension between the two techniques.[69] Several studies have found a lower incidence of failed epidural analgesia[70,71] as well as failed extension of epidural labor analgesia to cesarean delivery anesthesia[72] after the initiation of labor analgesia with a CSE technique. Presumably, verification of the correct placement of the spinal needle by visualization of CSF increases the likelihood that the tip of the epidural needle is correctly placed in the epidural space.

A purported disadvantage of the CSE technique is that correct placement of the epidural catheter in the epidural space cannot be verified until spinal analgesia or anesthesia wanes. Therefore it has been suggested that if a functioning epidural catheter is important to the safe care of the mother and fetus (e.g., in the setting of a suspected difficult airway or nonreassuring fetal status), an epidural rather than CSE technique is indicated. However, in a retrospective study that included 2395 neuraxial labor analgesia procedures, the CSE technique did not result in delayed recognition of epidural catheter failure, and the overall catheter failure rate was lower when the catheter was sited as part of CSE analgesia.[71] Therefore fear of unrecognized catheter malposition should not be a consideration when choosing a neuraxial technique.

There are several techniques for initiation of CSE anesthesia/analgesia. The most popular is the needle-through-needle technique, in which the epidural needle is sited in the epidural space and serves as an introducer for the spinal needle. The spinal needle passes through the epidural needle to puncture the dura. After injection of the subarachnoid dose, the spinal needle is removed, and the epidural catheter is threaded through the epidural needle. An alternative technique uses two skin punctures and two different interspaces: the spinal needle and epidural needle and catheter are introduced sequentially in two different interspaces.

The needle-through-needle technique requires a long spinal needle. Typically, a small (25-, 26-, or 27-gauge) noncutting needle is used to minimize the risk for PDPH. The tip of the spinal needle must protrude 12 to 17 mm beyond the tip of the epidural needle when the two needles are fully engaged (Fig. 12.14). Failure to puncture the dura and visualize CSF occurred in 25% of patients when the spinal needle protruded 9 mm, compared with no patients when the needle protruded

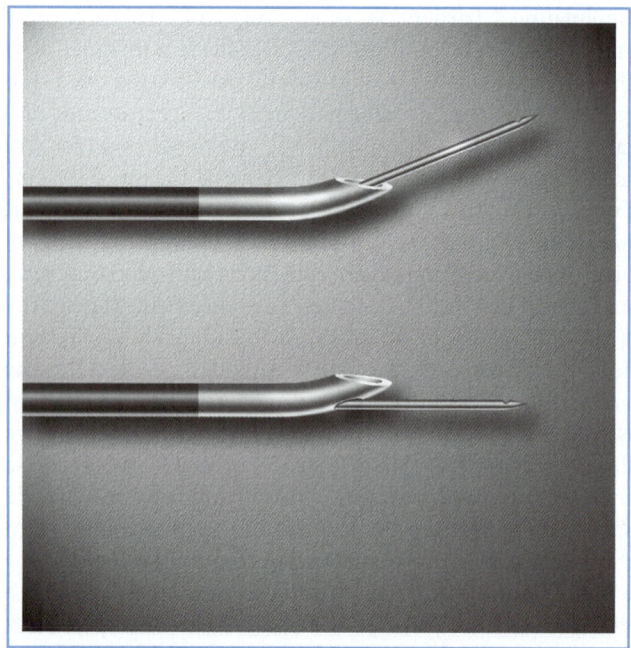

Fig. 12.14 Combined Spinal-Epidural Needle Configuration. *Top,* Spinal needle exits the epidural needle through the normal epidural needle bevel. Because the epidural needle bevel opening faces sideways, the spinal needle exits the epidural needle at a slight angle to the long axis of the epidural needle. *Bottom,* Spinal needle exits the epidural needle through a special orifice. The axes of the spinal and epidural needles are aligned. The spinal needle must protrude 12–17 mm from the tip of the epidural needle when the hubs are engaged, or the ability to puncture the dura with the spinal needle is compromised. Illustration by Naveen Nathan, MD, NorthShore University HealthSystem, University of Chicago Pritzker School of Medicine, Evanston, IL.

17 mm.[73] A 127-mm spinal needle is commonly used with a standard 9-cm epidural needle. However, because of differences in hub configurations among needles, the two hubs may not engage, and spinal needle protrusion may vary with specific needle combinations. Some manufacturers sell CSE needle "kits," in which the spinal needle is designed for a specific epidural needle. An additional small syringe (1 to 3 mL) is required for the spinal dose.

CSE anesthesia is initiated much like epidural anesthesia. The epidural needle is sited in the epidural space (Fig. 12.15). Before inserting the epidural catheter, the spinal needle is introduced through the epidural needle with the anesthesia provider's dominant hand, while the nondominant hand is anchored against the patient's back to serve as a brake for further advancement of the spinal needle. The provider usually perceives the tip of the spinal needle passing the tip of the epidural needle as a slight increase in resistance. Spinal needle advancement should stop immediately after the anesthesia provider perceives the dural puncture "pop." Dural puncture is verified by visualization of CSF after removal of the spinal needle stylet. The provider's nondominant hand is anchored on the patient's back, and the spinal and epidural needle hubs are grasped together between the thumb and index finger of this hand. The dominant hand attaches the spinal syringe. Aspiration of CSF before injection of the anesthetic solution is

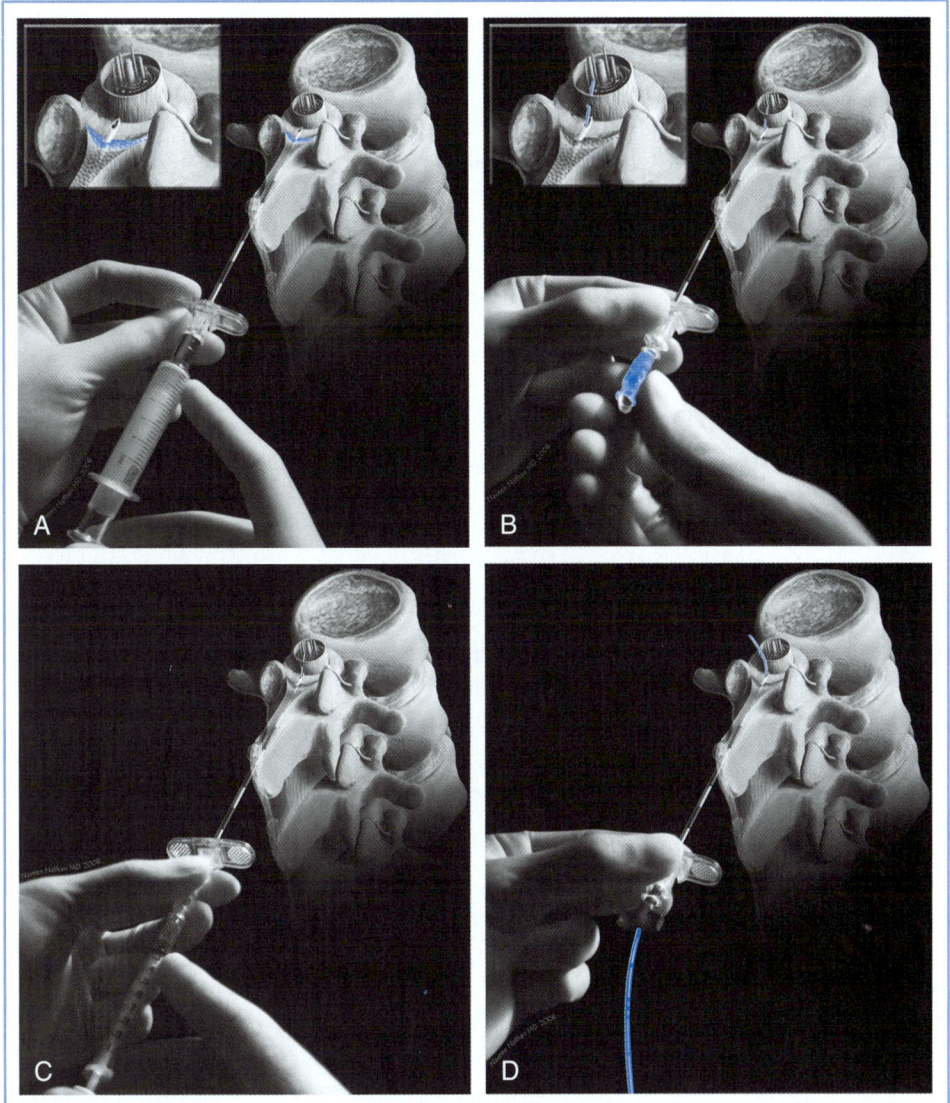

Fig. 12.15 Needle-Through-Needle Combined Spinal-Epidural Technique. (A) The epidural needle is sited in the epidural space. (B) The long spinal needle is passed through the epidural needle and punctures the dura mater. The operator's nondominant hand stabilizes the spinal and epidural needles, and the spinal needle stylet is withdrawn. Cerebrospinal fluid is seen spontaneously dripping from the spinal needle. (C) The syringe is attached to the spinal needle, and the intrathecal dose is injected. (D) The spinal needle is withdrawn, and the epidural catheter is threaded through the epidural needle into the epidural space. Illustration by Naveen Nathan, MD, NorthShore University HealthSystem, University of Chicago Pritzker School of Medicine, Evanston, IL.

not necessary.[74] After injection of the spinal dose and removal of the spinal syringe and needle as a unit, the epidural catheter is threaded in the usual fashion.

Failure to puncture the dura with the spinal needle, or to observe free-flowing CSF in the spinal needle, may occur in several circumstances (Fig. 12.16). The epidural needle tip may not be in the epidural space, or the needle tip may be correctly placed, but the spinal needle may fail to puncture the dura or may not reach the dura because of the depth of the posterior epidural space. Alternatively, the epidural needle may be angled away from the midline or in a sagittal plane off the midline, and the spinal needle may traverse the lateral epidural space without puncturing the dura. Although some clinicians elect to site the epidural catheter without observing

free flow of CSF in the spinal needle, this practice is associated with a higher catheter replacement rate (29%) than if free-flowing CSF is observed (4%).[74]

Dural Puncture Epidural Anesthesia

Dural puncture epidural (DPE) analgesia is another neuraxial technique that aims to exploit the advantages of CSE anesthesia while minimizing its shortcomings. It is procedurally identical to CSE anesthesia except for the omission of drug injection into the subarachnoid space. Presumably, excluding direct subarachnoid administration of opioid and local anesthetic at the time of dural puncture avoids the precipitous development of adverse effects such as hypotension and fetal bradycardia. However, the presence of the dural puncture

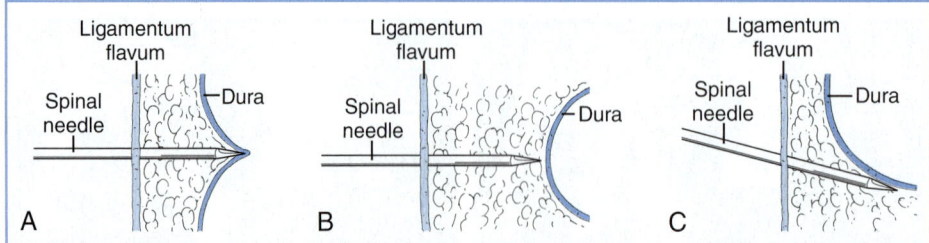

Fig. 12.16 Reasons for Failure of the Combined Spinal-Epidural Technique. (A) The spinal needle tents the dura but does not puncture it. (B) The spinal needle does not reach the dura. (C) The spinal needle passes to the side of the dural sac. Redrawn with permission from Riley ET, Hamilton CL, Ratner EF, Cohen SE. A comparison of the 24-gauge Sprotte and Gertie Marx spinal needles for combined spinal-epidural analgesia during labor. *Anesthesiology.* 2002;97:574.

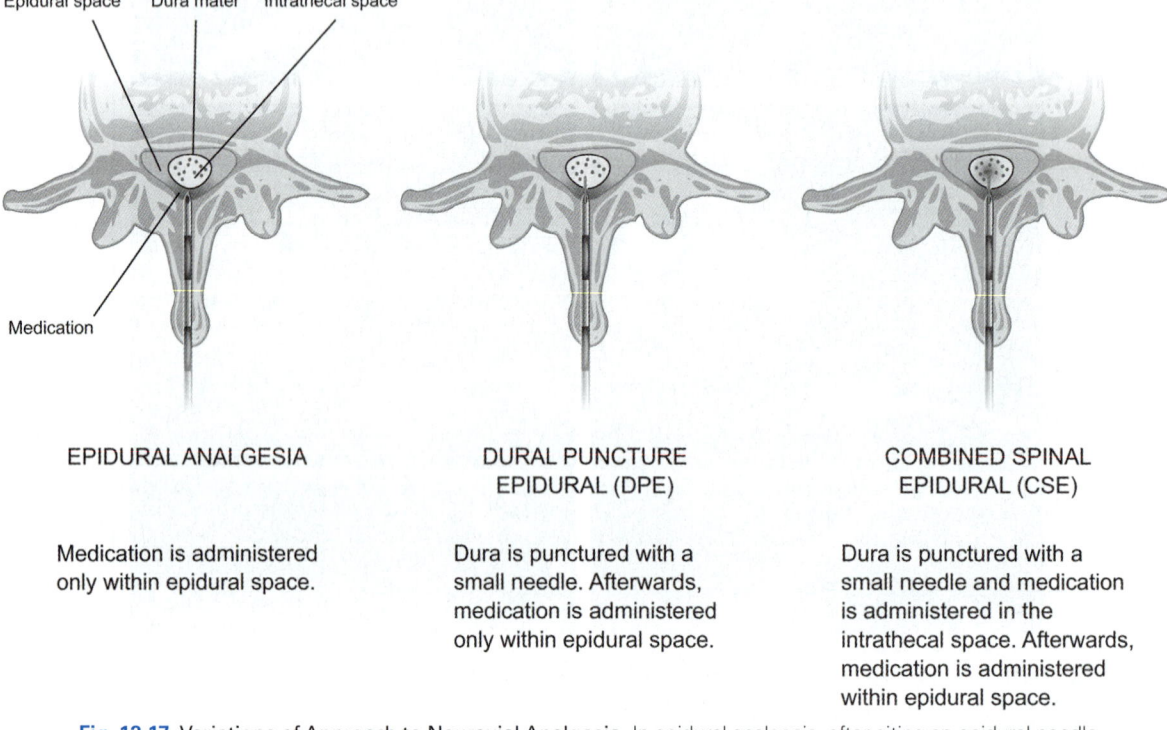

EPIDURAL ANALGESIA

Medication is administered only within epidural space.

DURAL PUNCTURE EPIDURAL (DPE)

Dura is punctured with a small needle. Afterwards, medication is administered only within epidural space.

COMBINED SPINAL EPIDURAL (CSE)

Dura is punctured with a small needle and medication is administered in the intrathecal space. Afterwards, medication is administered within epidural space.

Fig. 12.17 Variations of Approach to Neuraxial Analgesia. In epidural analgesia, after siting an epidural needle within the epidural space, a catheter is placed through which local anesthetic is administered. In DPE analgesia, a small hole is created in the dura by puncturing the dura using a spinal needle with a needle-through-needle technique prior to threading the epidural catheter. No medication is injected into the intrathecal space. Subsequent medication administered into the epidural space will have increased access to the cerebrospinal fluid due to the presence of a dural puncture. In CSE analgesia, a dose of local anesthetic and/or opioid is administered into the intrathecal space with a spinal needle inserted through the epidural needle using a needle-through-needle technique. Thereafter an epidural catheter is placed. Illustration byy Naveen Nathan, MD, NorthShore University HealthSystem, University of Chicago Pritzker School of Medicine, Evanston, IL.

allows for augmented transdural migration of epidurally injected drugs into the subarachnoid space. Hypothetically, this facilitates more reliable block of sacral dermatomes, which may be inadequately anesthetized with conventional epidural analgesia/anesthesia. The subarachnoid translocation of drugs may also act to compensate for an epidural catheter that would otherwise provide asymmetric block, leading to breakthrough pain and the requirement for manual top-up bolus injections of local anesthetic (Fig. 12.17).

Results of two early trials comparing traditional epidural to DPE analgesia were inconsistent.[75,76] Thomas et al.,[75] using

a 27-gauge spinal needle, found no differences in analgesia outcomes, including catheter manipulation and replacement rate, inadequate analgesia, unilateral block, sacral sparing, and the incidence of breakthrough pain. In contrast, Cappiello et al.,[76] using a 25-gauge spinal needle, found improved sacral analgesia, lower pain scores at 20 minutes, and a lower incidence of unilateral block in women randomized to receive DPE compared with epidural analgesia. A third trial compared epidural, CSE, and DPE analgesia.[77] Onset of analgesia (the primary outcome) was faster in the CSE group than in the epidural and DPE groups, but there was no difference between the epidural and DPE techniques. Compared with the traditional epidural technique, women randomized to receive DPE analgesia had a greater incidence of bilateral sacral block at 10 minutes and a lower incidence of asymmetric block at 30 minutes. Compared with CSE analgesia, women in the DPE group had a lower incidence of pruritus and hypotension. The combined incidence of uterine tachysystole and hypertonus was greater in the CSE compared with the epidural and DPE groups. Finally, a fourth trial comparing epidural to DPE analgesia found no difference in adequate analgesia at 10 minutes, but those in the DPE group had a shorter time to adequate analgesia (median time 8 versus 10 minutes).[78] There were no differences in complication rates, including maternal hypotension, nausea, and pruritus. Contreras et al.[79] compared analgesia characteristics in women randomized to DPE analgesia with a 25- or 27-gauge spinal needle. While onset of analgesia was slightly faster with the 25-gauge spinal needle, no differences were found in sacral block, motor block, and the number of top-up doses.

In larger retrospective studies, DPE analgesia has been associated with fewer catheter failures and replacements compared to the traditional epidural analgesia technique, with failure rates of 6.5% and 9.8%, respectively.[80] Thus DPE analgesia is frequently used clinically in high-risk obstetric populations such as complex cardiac patients and morbidly obese parturients. Tan et al.[81] conducted a double-blind randomized control trial comparing DPE analgesia with a 25-gauge spinal needle to traditional epidural analgesia in obese parturients. Although the study found no difference in a composite outcome (asymmetric block, epidural top-up doses, catheter adjustments/replacements, failure to extend analgesia to anesthesia for cesarean delivery), the range of BMI was wide and only 20% of the cohort had a BMI $\geq$ 50 kg/m², a group of patients in whom landmark identification of the interspinous space may be particularly challenging.[81]

Beyond quality of labor analgesia, there remains the question of whether differences exist between the DPE and epidural techniques when epidural labor analgesia is extended to epidural anesthesia for intrapartum cesarean delivery. Sharawi et al.[82] hypothesized that the time for extension of labor epidural analgesia to surgical anesthesia is faster in women who had epidural analgesia initiated with a DPE compared with a traditional epidural technique. Nonlaboring women undergoing scheduled cesarean delivery were randomized to receive "mock" labor analgesia initiated with a DPE or traditional epidural technique. Approximately 1 hour later, the block was extended with epidural 3% chloroprocaine, mimicking clinical care for laboring women who undergo urgent cesarean delivery. The investigators found that women in the DPE group had faster surgical extension (422 versus 655 seconds) and improved quality of anesthesia compared with the standard epidural technique.

A 2019 systematic review of randomized controlled studies compared DPE and traditional labor epidural analgesia (5 studies, 581 patients).[83] Although some studies found

advantages in speed of onset and pain scores in women randomized to receive DPE analgesia, results were not consistent. Further, the quality of the block was not different among groups. The authors attributed the lack of consistent results to differences in study design (e.g., differences in the gauge of the spinal needle chosen for the dural puncture, epidural loading solution, epidural loading volume, the time over which the loading dose was administered, and method used to maintain epidural analgesia). Further investigation is needed to better define the role of the DPE technique in the routine management of labor pain.

Ultrasonographic Guidance

The past two decades have witnessed an enormous increase in the use of ultrasound-guided regional anesthesia. Unlike the use of ultrasonography for vascular access and peripheral nerve block techniques, ultrasonography for neuraxial techniques is not used in real time. Most often, ultrasonography is a preprocedural tool used to aid the operator in the assessment of needle insertion site, needle angle, and estimated depth of the epidural space. A 2016 metaanalysis of randomized controlled trials and cohort studies comparing the traditional landmark technique to preprocedural ultrasonography as an adjunct to neuraxial procedures concluded that use of ultrasonography (1) results in more accurate identification of a given lumbar interspace, (2) allows accurate prediction of the depth of needle insertion to the epidural or intrathecal space, and (3) reduces technical difficulty (fewer attempts and needle redirections necessary for a successful procedure).[84] Evidence has not yet accumulated that preprocedural ultrasonography results in improved success of anesthesia and procedural safety (e.g., lower rate of complications such as unintentional dural puncture), although this could logically be assumed.

In the obstetric population, a host of randomized controlled trials have explored outcomes related to block placement and success comparing the traditional landmark-based technique versus the ultrasound-guided technique.[84] In many of these studies, an experienced ultrasonographer imaged the spine and marked the midline and interspaces on the skin, and a trainee performed the actual neuraxial procedure. In contrast, Arzola et al.[85] provided comprehensive neuraxial ultrasonography training to anesthesiology residents and fellows. Following training, low-risk women with easily palpable spinous processes requesting neuraxial labor analgesia were randomized to the use of preprocedural ultrasonography versus a traditional landmark technique; the trainee used the allocated technique to perform the procedure. There were no differences in epidural procedure time and number of attempted interspaces and needle passes between the two techniques. Total procedure time was longer in the ultrasonography group. An explanation for these findings is that expert ultrasonography skills are necessary to realize the advantages of the technique as an adjunct to neuraxial procedures. Another explanation is that ultrasonography offers no advantages in low-risk patients. Indeed, in a randomized controlled trial of CSE procedures for cesarean delivery performed by a single experienced anesthesiologist and ultrasonographer in women with palpable spinous processes, there were no differences in the first needle-pass success rate, number of needle passes, or patient satisfaction when women were randomized to an ultrasound-guided technique versus a traditional technique.[86] A 2021 metaanalysis evaluating obstetric patients in labor or presenting for cesarean delivery found preprocedural ultrasonography improved first-pass success without increasing time to perform the procedure. Further, the investigators found that ultrasonography decreased labor analgesia and anesthesia failure, intravascular canulation, postpartum back pain, and headache.[87] However, at the present time, an experienced anesthesiologist managing an uncomplicated pregnant patient is unlikely to benefit from the use of preprocedural ultrasonographic imaging.

There exist, however, unique clinical circumstances in which preprocedural imaging of neuraxial anatomy may be highly beneficial. Such may be the case in patients with morbid obesity; derangements of spinal anatomy resulting from scoliosis, spinal stenosis, or a history of spinal instrumentation; and in patients in whom identification of specific vertebral levels might be warranted (e.g., known preexisting disc herniation or nerve root compression at a specific interspace).[88] Creaney et al.[89] assessed the utility of preprocedural ultrasonography in pregnant patients with impalpable spinous processes presenting for spinal anesthesia for cesarean delivery. The mean BMI was approximately 40 kg/m². Although there was no difference in the total procedure time between groups, women in the ultrasonography group required fewer needle passes to locate the intrathecal space. Similarly, Park et al.[90] evaluated the use of preprocedural ultrasonography in patients with documented lumbar scoliosis and previous spinal surgery presenting for spinal anesthesia for orthopedic surgery. They found that patients in the ultrasonography group required fewer needle passes with higher first-pass success rate than the landmark technique.

Preprocedural ultrasonography is useful for estimating the distance from the skin to the epidural or intrathecal space.

In general, although studies have shown a high correlation between the ultrasonographic and actual measurement, ultrasonographic measurements underestimate the true distance from the skin to epidural space.[91,92] The factors that influence the small disparity between the predicted and actual distance include (1) differences between the angulation of the imaging beam versus the angulation of the needle; (2) differences between the degree of exerted pressure and skin compression of the ultrasound probe versus the needle; (3) current lack of fidelity in the ability of ultrasonography to discriminate between ligamentum flavum, epidural space, and dura mater; and (4) dependency of onscreen measurement tools (e.g., digital calipers) on operator skill and consistency. In a general obstetric population, the mean difference between the needle depth and ultrasonographic depth to the epidural space was 0.01 cm (95% confidence interval, −0.67 to 0.69 cm),[92] whereas in a second study by the same investigator group in which subjects were limited to obese parturients, the mean difference was 0.3 cm (95% confidence interval, −0.7 cm to 1.3 cm).[91]

A low-frequency (2- to 5-Hz) curvilinear probe allows visualization of neuraxial structures. Low-frequency waves are preferable owing to the requisite depth of penetration. The curvilinear array allows the capture of lateral structures such as the transverse processes. The ultrasound beam can be used to identify the spinous processes, and if these are not palpable, the interspinous spaces and the ligamentous structures. The ligamentum flavum-epidural space-dura mater will appear as a hyperechoic (white) complex, like bone, whereas the less dense subarachnoid space will appear hypoechoic (black).

Imaging is commonly performed in two planes: the longitudinal (sagittal) paramedian plane and the transverse plane. In the longitudinal paramedian plane, the probe is placed vertically over the sacral area, 2 to 3 cm lateral of the midline, and angled medially to focus on the neuraxial canal (Fig. 12.18). The sacrum is visualized as a hyperechoic line. As the probe is moved cephalad, a sawtooth pattern is visualized,

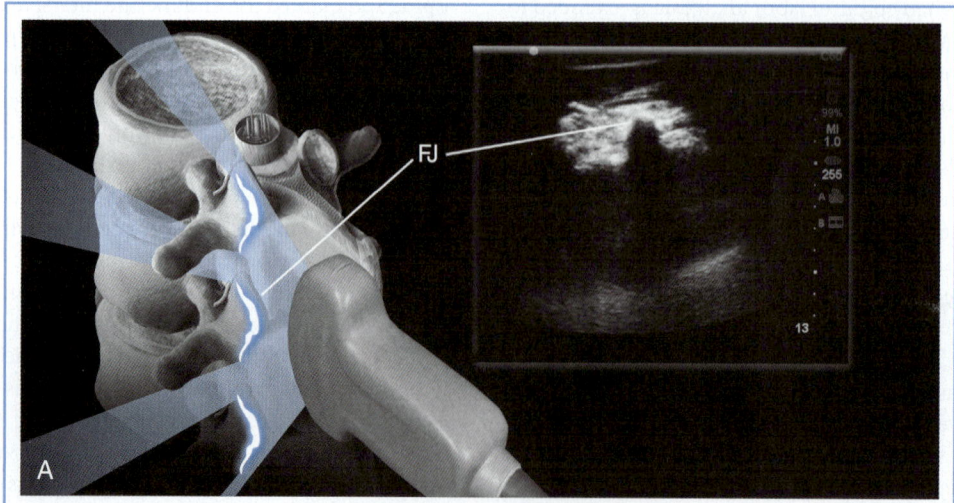

Fig. 12.18 Use of Ultrasonography. (A) Paramedian view: A so-called sawtooth pattern may be seen as the lamina and facet joints (*FJ*) are captured by this view, typically achieved 1 cm lateral to the midline sagittal plane.

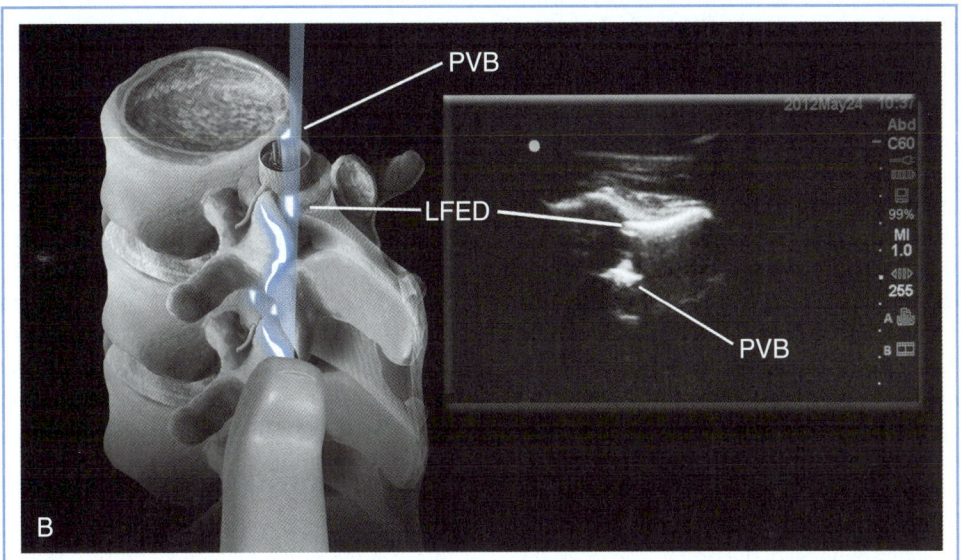

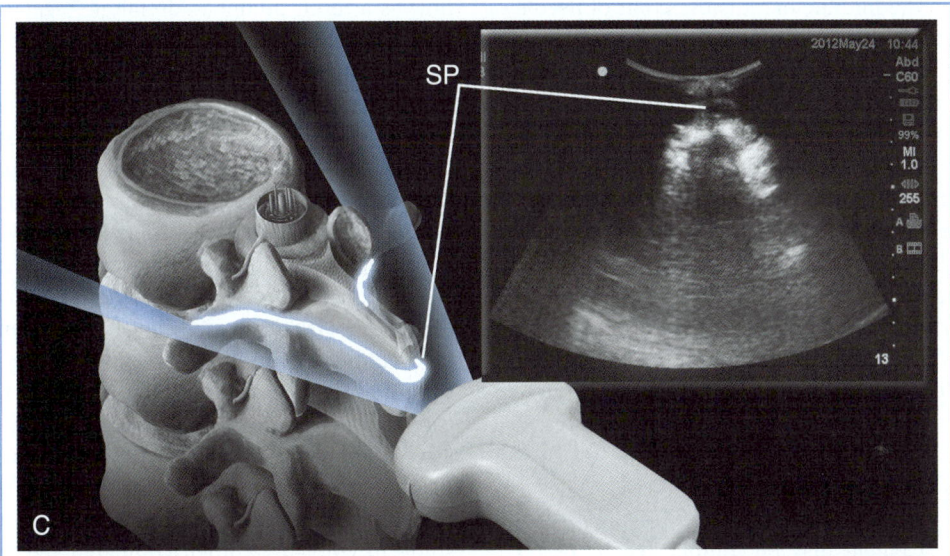

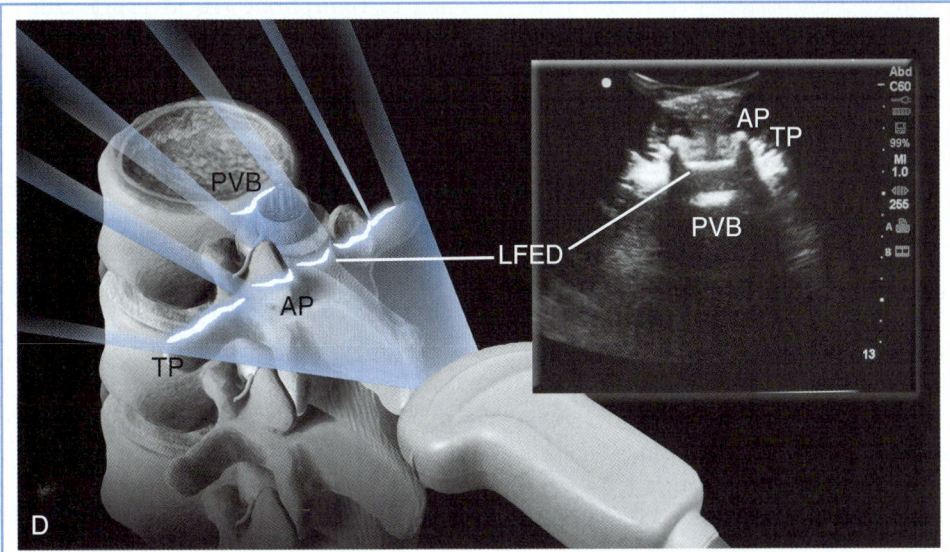

Fig. 12.18, cont'd (B) Paramedian view: By angulating the ultrasound probe, the ultrasound waves may escape through the interlaminar and transforaminal "windows" and capture the ligamentum flavum-epidural space-dura mater complex (*LFED*) as well as the posterior surface of the vertebral body (*PVB*). (C) Transverse spinous process view: A long, dark shadow is cast with little to no discernible anatomy beyond the osseous tip of the spinous process (*SP*). (D) Transverse interlaminar view: Ultrasound waves propagate through the interspinous ligament leading to signals partially reflected by the ligamentum LFED mater complex. The rays that continue to transmit through this complex encounter the posterior wall of the vertebral body (*PVB*). Articular processes (*APs*) and transverse processes (*TPs*) can be seen as well. Illustration by Naveen Nathan, MD, NorthShore University HealthSystem, University of Chicago Pritzker School of Medicine, Evanston, IL.

corresponding to the laminae of the vertebrae. The gaps between the teeth of the saw are the intervertebral spaces. The ultrasonographer can mark the chosen interspace on the skin as the probe is moved cephalad. Imaging in the transverse plane is used to identify the midline and assess the distance to the epidural space. The probe is positioned horizontally at the appropriate level and moved slightly cephalad and caudad to visualize the cephalad and caudad spinous processes. The midline is marked by centering the shadow cast by the spinous processes in the middle of the ultrasonographic image. The probe is then centered in the interspinous space and manipulated to achieve a clear view of the neuraxial canal structures. The midline of the ultrasonographic probe on both the left and right is marked on the skin, and these points are joined with a horizontal line after removal of the probe. The intersection of this line with the midline mark is the point of needle entry. The distance from the skin to the anterior aspect of the ligamentum flavum-dura mater complex is measured on the frozen image with ultrasonographic machine calipers.

There will likely be further study of novel software as technology advances to assist the less skilled ultrasonographer in performance of neuraxial procedures. One such example, is a proprietary software system that automatically identifies lumbar spine landmarks as the operator advances the ultrasound probe in a caudad to cephalad direction. In an early study, this system had 84% agreement with traditional lumbar ultrasonography compared to 70% with manual palpation.[93] Future technologic advances such as this may change the way preprocedural ultrasonography is used for performance of neuraxial procedures.

EPIDURAL TEST DOSE

Epidural catheter placement may be complicated by blood vessel or dural puncture with the needle or catheter. To prevent possible local anesthetic systemic toxicity (LAST) and high or total spinal anesthesia, the anesthesia provider must recognize the unintentional intravenous or subarachnoid placement of the needle or catheter. The purpose of the test dose is to allow early recognition of a malpositioned catheter. The ideal test dose must be readily available, safe, and effective. Its use should have a high sensitivity (i.e., low false-negative rate) and a high specificity (i.e., low false-positive rate). The intravascular and intrathecal test doses may be combined (a single injection to test for both intravascular and subarachnoid placement) or administered separately. A negative response to an epidural test dose does not guarantee the correct placement of the epidural catheter in the epidural space, nor does it guarantee that the catheter is not malpositioned in a blood vessel or the subarachnoid space. Rather, it decreases the likelihood that the catheter tip is in a blood vessel or the subarachnoid space.

Intravascular Test Dose

Intravascular placement of the epidural catheter may occur in as many as 7% to 8.5% of obstetric patients, although the rate may be lower with wire-embedded catheters.[28] Failure to recognize intravenous placement of the epidural catheter

and subsequent intravenous injection of a large dose of local anesthetic may lead to LAST, with CNS symptoms, seizures, cardiovascular collapse, and death.[94]

The most common intravascular test dose contains epinephrine 15 μg. In normal volunteers, intravenous injection of epinephrine 15 μg (3 mL of a 1:200,000 solution) reliably causes tachycardia.[95] An increase in heart rate of 20 beats per minute (bpm) within 45 seconds was 100% sensitive and specific for intravascular injection in patients who did not receive prior treatment with a beta-adrenergic receptor antagonist.[95] An increase in systolic blood pressure between 15 and 25 mm Hg was also observed.

Some anesthesiologists have expressed concerns about the use of an epinephrine-containing test dose in laboring women. Intravenous epinephrine may cause a decline in uterine blood flow as a result of alpha-adrenergic receptor–mediated constriction of the uterine arteries (Fig. 12.19).[96] However, this decrease in uterine blood flow is transient and comparable to the decrease that occurs during a uterine contraction. In healthy parturients, any transient effect of epinephrine on uterine blood flow likely represents a less severe insult than LAST. An epinephrine-containing test dose, however, may not be appropriate in parturients with severe hypertension, uteroplacental insufficiency, or cardiac pathology.

Concern has been expressed that the epinephrine-containing test dose lacks *specificity* in laboring women. The maternal tachycardic response to intravenous injection of epinephrine cannot always be distinguished from other causes of tachycardia (e.g., pain during a uterine contraction; Fig. 12.20).[97,98] Cartwright et al.[97] noted that 12% of laboring women had an increase in heart rate of at least 30 bpm after epidural injection of 3 mL of 0.5% bupivacaine without epinephrine. A study in laboring women compared the intravenous injection of epinephrine (10 to 15 μg) with that of saline; the sensitivity was 100%, the area under the receiver operator

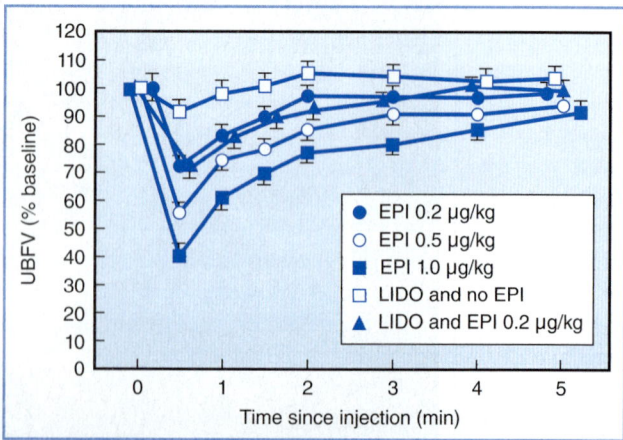

Fig. 12.19 The Effect of Intravenous Epinephrine (*EPI*), Lidocaine (*LIDO*), and Lidocaine With Epinephrine on Uterine Artery Blood Flow Velocity (*UBFV*) in the Pregnant Guinea Pig. The dose of lidocaine was 0.4 mg/kg. Values are presented as mean ± standard error of mean percentage of baseline. From Chestnut DH, Weiner CP, Martin JG, et al. Effect of intravenous epinephrine on uterine artery blood flow velocity in the pregnant guinea pig. *Anesthesiology.* 1986;65:633–636.

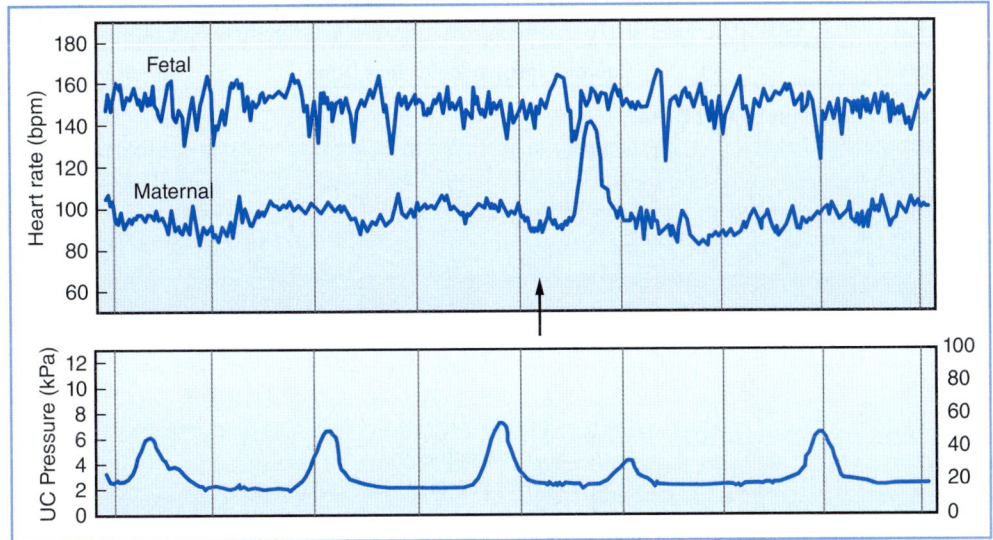

Fig. 12.20 Heart Rate of a Laboring Patient (Maternal Heart Rate [*MHR*]), Fetal Heart Rate, and Uterine Contractions (*UCs*) Are Shown. This tracing was obtained with the use of a fetal heart rate monitor with dual heart rate capacity. Note the variability of the MHR with uterine contractions. An intravenous injection of bupivacaine 12.5 mg and epinephrine 12.5 µg was administered *(arrow)*, mimicking a positive intravascular epidural test dose. Note the marked increase in MHR in response to intravenous injection. The maternal tachycardia had a duration of approximately 40 s. From Van Zundert AA, Vaes LE, De Wolf AM. ECG monitoring of mother and fetus during epidural anesthesia. *Anesthesiology.* 1987;66:584–585.

characteristic curve was 0.91 to 0.93, and the negative predictive value was 100%.[99] However, the positive predictive value was 55% to 73%. The results suggested that if a positive heart rate response to an epinephrine-containing test dose occurs in 20% of patients, 5% to 9% of epidural catheters would be identified incorrectly as intravascular and removed unnecessarily. Colonna-Romano and Nagaraj[100] concluded that the intravenous injection of an epinephrine-containing test dose results in "a sudden and fast acceleration in maternal heart rate within one minute." Thus careful assessment of the rate of increase in maternal heart rate may help distinguish a contraction-induced increase in heart rate from the effect of intravenously injected epinephrine, thereby improving the *specificity* of the epinephrine test. It is unclear whether such an assessment is clinically practical or will actually reduce the incidence of false-positive results.

Some anesthesiologists argue that the epinephrine-containing test dose lacks *sensitivity*. An increase in maternal heart rate of 25 bpm occurring within 2 minutes of drug injection and lasting at least 15 seconds was observed in only 5 of 10 laboring women who received intravenous epinephrine 15 µg.[101] Detection of intravenous epinephrine injection was improved when the authors retrospectively defined a positive maternal tachycardic response as a 10-bpm increase above the maximum maternal heart rate observed in the 2-minute period preceding the epinephrine injection. Others have confirmed that these revised criteria improve the sensitivity of the epinephrine-containing test dose in laboring women.[99] These findings stress the importance of tracking the chronotropic variability that occurs in laboring patients during neuraxial anesthesia procedures to reduce the risk for misinterpretation of the test dose.

The usefulness of an epinephrine-containing test dose also improves if additional information is obtained. For example, investigators administered intravenous bupivacaine 12.5 mg with epinephrine 12.5 µg or saline to laboring women.[102] They correctly identified the test solution in 39 of 40 women when they assessed maternal heart rate, blood pressure, uterine contractions, the timing of the injection, the presence of analgesia, and subjective signs and symptoms of intravascular injection (e.g., palpitations, lightheadedness, dizziness). The tachycardic response to intravenous epinephrine is not a reliable indicator of intravascular injection in patients who have received a beta-adrenergic receptor antagonist (e.g., labetalol).[103]

Other means of identifying intravascular placement of an epidural catheter have been proposed and may be clinically useful in specific patients (Table 12.2). Intravenous injection of 1 or 2 mL of air through a single-orifice catheter consistently produces changes in heart sounds as detected by the use of precordial Doppler ultrasonography.[104] (The external FHR monitor can be used for this purpose.) False-negative results may occur when small volumes of air are injected through a multiorifice epidural catheter; thus the air test is not a reliable test for intravascular injection when multiorifice epidural catheters are used.[105]

Local anesthetic–induced symptoms of subclinical CNS toxicity have also been evaluated as a means of recognizing unintentional intravenous injection. Colonna-Romano et al.[106] administered intravenous saline, lidocaine 100 mg, or 2-chloroprocaine 100 mg to laboring women. Observers blinded as to which substance was administered recorded the presence of CNS symptoms (i.e., dizziness, tinnitus, metallic or funny taste) after injection. Lidocaine 100 mg was a reliable

TABLE 12.2 Epidural Test Dose Regimens[a]

Test Dose Components	Positive Intravascular Test Dose	Positive Intrathecal Test Dose
Combined Intrathecal and Intravenous Test Dose:		
Lidocaine 1.5% with epinephrine 5 µg/mL (1:200,000): 3 mL	Increase in heart rate of 20 bpm within 1 min	Motor blockade at 3–5 min[b]
Bupivacaine 0.25% with epinephrine 5 µg/mL (1:200,000): 3 mL		
Intravenous Test Dose:		
Lidocaine 100 mg	Tinnitus, circumoral numbness, "dizziness"	
Bupivacaine 25 mg		
2-Chloroprocaine 100 mg		
Fentanyl 100 µg	Dizziness, drowsiness	
Air 1 mL	Change in Doppler heart sounds over right side of heart	
Intrathecal Test Dose:		
Lidocaine 40–60 mg		Motor blockade at 3–5 min[b]
Bupivacaine 7.5 mg		

[a]Test doses may be less sensitive in premedicated patients, patients treated with a beta-adrenergic receptor antagonist, pregnant patients, and anesthetized patients.
[b]Weakness in hip flexion.
Modified from Yilmaz M, Wong CA. Technique of neuraxial anesthesia. In: Wong CA, ed. *Spinal and Epidural Anesthesia.* McGraw-Hill; 2007:27–73.

marker of intravenous injection when the symptoms of tinnitus and metallic or funny taste were considered (sensitivity 100%; specificity 81%). 2-Chloroprocaine was less reliable (sensitivity 81% to 94%; specificity 69% to 81%). In a volunteer study, a dose of 1.5 mg/kg of 2-chloroprocaine was necessary to produce a probability of 90% that the subject would report symptoms of intravenous injection.[107]

Administration of fentanyl 100 µg has been described as a test for intravenous injection.[108] Dizziness was the most reliable symptom of intravenous fentanyl injection, with a sensitivity of 92% and a specificity of 92%.

Some situations reduce the reliability of subjective symptoms as a signal of intravenous injection of a drug. Tests that rely on the self-reporting of subjective symptoms require clear communication with the patient and thus are less useful when the anesthesia provider and patient speak different languages. Patient exhaustion and/or prior opioid administration also may affect the reliability of the test.

Lastly, the epidural catheter design and speed of injection may affect the reliability of the epidural test dose. An epinephrine-containing test dose should be injected rapidly; otherwise, rapid redistribution and metabolism of the drug decrease the actual dose administered to chronoreceptors. Multiorifice epidural catheters have three potential sites of exit for injected fluid or air, and the orifices may lie within two different body compartments. If injected too slowly, air or fluid preferentially exits the proximal orifice. The rate of injection used in clinical practice typically exceeds that required to ensure that fluid will exit all three orifices. In contrast, air must be injected at a much greater rate to ensure that it exits all three orifices; this rate is not practical for clinical use. The

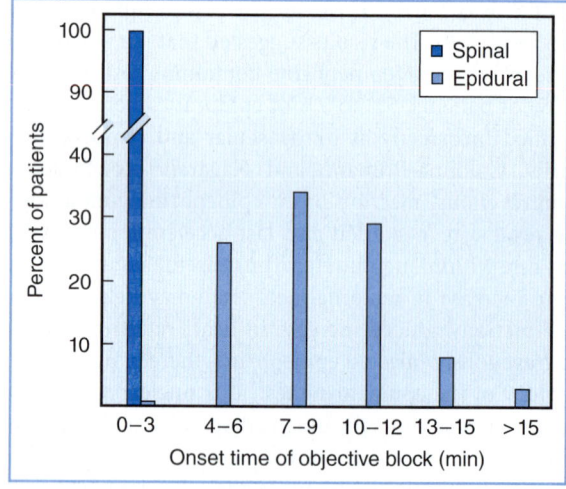

Fig. 12.21 Percentage of pregnant patients who demonstrated objective evidence of anesthesia (defined as the loss of sensation to pinprick) after epidural injection of 2–3 mL of 1.5% lidocaine with 1:200,000 epinephrine in 7.5% dextrose *(light teal bars)* (*n* = 250) or after intrathecal injection of 2 mL of 1.5% lidocaine with 1:200,000 epinephrine in 7.5% dextrose *(dark teal bar)* (*n* = 15). From Abraham RA, Harris AP, Maxwell LG, et al. The efficacy of 1.5% lidocaine with 7.5% dextrose and epinephrine as an epidural test dose for obstetrics. *Anesthesiology.* 1986;64:116–119.

distal orifice is both the most difficult to test and the one most likely to be positioned outside the epidural space.[109]

Intrathecal Test Dose

The intrathecal test dose should allow easy identification of subarachnoid (intrathecal) placement of the catheter without causing high or total spinal anesthesia and hemodynamic compromise. Bupivacaine (7.5 mg) and lidocaine (45 to 60 mg) are the local anesthetics most often used for an intrathecal test dose (Table 12.2; Fig. 12.21).[110,111] Ropivacaine 15 mg is *not* a useful intrathecal test dose agent because the slow onset of motor blockade precludes timely diagnosis of intrathecal injection.[112]

In a study of older, nonpregnant patients receiving continuous spinal anesthesia for surgery, Colonna-Romano et al.[111] used plain lidocaine 45 mg plus epinephrine 15 μg and assessed patient perception of lower-extremity warmth and heaviness, sensory loss to pinprick, and ability to perform a straight-leg raise. Patients usually perceived warmth in their legs within 1 minute of the intrathecal injection; however, impaired straight-leg raise 4 minutes after an intrathecal test dose injection was the only test that had a sensitivity of 100% for intrathecal injection. The application of these data to pregnant patients is unclear.

Richardson et al.[113] described the rapid onset (1 to 3 minutes) of high levels of spinal anesthesia with motor block and hypotension in five parturients who had received a test dose of plain lidocaine 45 mg plus epinephrine 15 μg. This solution is slightly hypobaric; thus the upright posture of these parturients during the injection may have contributed to the high sensory levels of anesthesia. The anesthesia provider must recognize the possible range of responses to the dose of local anesthetic used to assess the position of an epidural catheter and should perform a careful assessment of sensory, motor, and sympathetic function 3 to 5 minutes after administration of the test dose before concluding that the intrathecal test-dose result is negative. 2-Chloroprocaine is the only local anesthetic that can be used as a single, combined intravascular and intrathecal test dose in the nonpregnant patient; in most patients, 90 mg results in dense, but not total, spinal anesthesia after intrathecal injection and produces systemic signs of subclinical toxicity (tinnitus, funny taste) after intravascular injection.[114] The application to the pregnant woman is unclear.

The epidural injection of a local anesthetic-containing test dose augments *epidural* analgesia and should be considered in the calculation of the initial therapeutic dose of local anesthetic. Investigators have demonstrated that the test dose enhanced the density of epidural blockade and adversely affected the ability to ambulate.[115]

Ultimately, undetected intrathecal catheter insertion with negative aspiration of CSF is a rare event. With contemporary obstetric analgesic practice favoring a low-dose, low-concentration local anesthetic regimen in combination with an opioid, providers must weigh the risk of unwanted consequences of a positive traditional intrathecal test dose, including high spinal anesthesia, need for airway management, severe hypotension, and potential fetal compromise, with the risk of an unrecognized "untested" intrathecal catheter. Currently, there is lack of consensus on the need for a "traditional" epidural test dose. If a traditional test dose is not injected, the initial local anesthetic dose injected into the epidural catheter should not exceed the dose typically used as a test dose.[116] In an analysis of closed insurance claims between 2005 and 2015, 31% of claims filed for obstetric anesthesia care that resulted in maternal death or brain injury were due to high neuraxial block either at the time of epidural catheter placement or at the time of epidural dosing and likely attributable to an unrecognized intrathecal catheter.[117]

Techniques to Minimize Local Anesthetic Systemic Toxicity

No perfect test dose exists. Some anesthesia providers elect not to administer a test dose because it contributes to motor blockade.[115] In addition, aspiration of a *multiorifice* epidural catheter for blood has 98% sensitivity for detection of an intravascular location.[118] Unintentional intravascular injection of a small volume of solution containing a low concentration of local anesthetic is unlikely to result in serious morbidity. However, laboring women may need large doses of local anesthetic administered quickly (without incremental injection) for emergency operative delivery. The anesthesia provider must determine as soon as possible that the epidural catheter is correctly positioned within the epidural space. Even if no morbidity results, it is inconvenient for both the patient and the anesthesia provider to have to repeat the procedure and replace the catheter once the patient has been repositioned. Though the epinephrine-containing test dose provides an objective marker of intravascular injection that has stood the test of time, it is important to remember that pregnancy may lead to decreased sensitivity of beta-adrenergic receptor stimulation, and maternal heart rate may vary dramatically during labor. No matter whether a test dose is injected, drugs should be injected incrementally into the epidural space, because no test is 100% sensitive and catheters may migrate during use. Each incremental dose should be treated as a "test dose" (i.e., the dose should be small enough that it will not cause systemic toxicity if unintentionally injected intravascularly or total spinal anesthesia if injected intrathecally).

Steps to minimize the possibility of local anesthetic toxicity are summarized in Box 12.3. They include observation for passive return of CSF or blood (by lowering the proximal end of the epidural catheter below the insertion site),

---

> ### BOX 12.3   Steps to Decrease Risk for Unintentional Intravenous or Subarachnoid Injection of Local Anesthetic
>
> - Lower the proximal end of the catheter below the site of insertion. Observe for the passive return of blood or cerebrospinal fluid.
> - Aspirate before injecting each dose of local anesthetic.
> - Give the test dose between uterine contractions.
> - Use dilute solutions of local anesthetic during labor.
> - Do not inject more than 5 mL of local anesthetic as a single bolus.
> - Maintain verbal contact with the patient.
> - If little or no block is produced after the injection of an appropriate dose of local anesthetic, assume that the local anesthetic was injected intravenously and remove the catheter.

administration of the test dose between contractions, aspiration before each dose, incremental dose administration, maintaining verbal contact with the patient, and regular assessments throughout labor for an appropriate level and density of sensory and motor blockade (which indicates correct placement of the catheter in the epidural space).

CHOICE OF DRUGS[a]

The dose requirement of both epidural and spinal local anesthetics is decreased approximately 25% in pregnancy owing to anatomic and physiologic changes (see Chapter 2). These alterations begin to revert to the prepregnancy state within hours of delivery.

Spinal Anesthesia

Anesthesia providers may give spinal anesthesia for cerclage, nonobstetric surgery during pregnancy, operative vaginal delivery, cesarean delivery, removal of a retained placenta, postpartum tubal ligation, or labor analgesia. Cesarean delivery represents the most common indication for spinal anesthesia in pregnant women. Most anesthesia providers administer a hyperbaric solution of local anesthetic for spinal anesthesia in obstetric patients. Use of a hyperbaric solution compared with a plain solution without dextrose results in a faster onset of block and a higher maximum sensory level with a shorter duration of blockade.[119] The urgency and anticipated duration of surgery dictate the choice of local anesthetic agent. The most common choice in the United States is bupivacaine due to its long duration of action. Lidocaine is used less commonly. Ropivacaine and levobupivacaine may be used but are not approved for spinal administration in the United States, and levobupivacaine is not available in the United States. Preservative-free chloroprocaine is approved for spinal anesthesia and can be used for cesarean delivery,[120] but its duration of action is short, and therefore it may not be useful in all cases.[121]

Anesthesia providers often add an opioid to the local anesthetic to improve the quality of anesthesia, particularly with regard to visceral stimulation, and to provide postoperative analgesia.[122] The addition of an opioid to the local anesthetic decreases the incidence of intraoperative nausea and vomiting. The short-acting, lipid-soluble opioids (i.e., fentanyl, sufentanil) contribute to intraoperative anesthesia, and morphine or hydromorphone are often administered for postoperative analgesia.[123] Epinephrine may be added to prolong block duration and perhaps improve block density.[124] Clonidine may also prolong the duration of sensory blockade but is associated with sedation.[125] Dexmedetomidine may also prolong the duration of spinal anesthesia and reduce the incidence of shivering, but adequate studies of the safety of intrathecal dexmedetomidine are currently lacking.[126,127] (See Chapters 24, 26, and 27 for an in-depth discussion of adjuvants for neuraxial analgesia and anesthesia.)

Epidural Anesthesia

Local anesthetic agents available for epidural administration in obstetric patients include 2-chloroprocaine, lidocaine, mepivacaine, bupivacaine, and ropivacaine. Mepivacaine is used infrequently in obstetric anesthesia practice.

Bupivacaine remains a popular local anesthetic for analgesia during labor and vaginal delivery because of its differential sensory blockade, long duration of action, low frequency of tachyphylaxis, and low cost. Anesthesia providers infrequently administer bupivacaine for cesarean delivery because of the risk for cardiac toxicity and maternal mortality after unintentional intravascular injection of the drug (i.e., LAST).

Ropivacaine has gained popularity as an agent for epidural analgesia and anesthesia because it may result in less cardiac toxicity and greater differential sensory-motor blockade than bupivacaine.[128]

Levobupivacaine also has a more favorable safety profile than bupivacaine. Clinical trials have shown that ropivacaine and levobupivacaine have potency[129] and analgesic qualities similar to those of bupivacaine,[130,131] with the probable exception of less motor nerve block.[132]

Bupivacaine, ropivacaine, and levobupivacaine all have longer durations of action than lidocaine and are preferred over shorter-acting agents when a longer duration of anesthesia or analgesia is desirable. They are more commonly used for maintenance of epidural labor analgesia, whereas the shorter-acting agents are used for epidural surgical anesthesia. Despite some variation among reports, published clinical studies suggest no more than slight differences in onset, and no differences in quality or duration of neural blockade, among the three drugs. However, bupivacaine is more cardiotoxic than the other agents *in vitro* and probably after unintentional intravascular administration.[133] It would seem prudent to use ropivacaine or levobupivacaine rather than bupivacaine when a bolus dose of a concentrated solution is being given. When administered as a low-concentration infusion, improved safety has not been demonstrated with ropivacaine and levobupivacaine compared with bupivacaine.

The most popular choice of local anesthetic for epidural anesthesia for cesarean delivery is **2% lidocaine with epinephrine**. The addition of epinephrine (5 μg/mL) causes a modest prolongation of the block. The major advantage of epinephrine is that it improves the quality of epidural lidocaine anesthesia. Lam et al.[134] have shown that epidural labor analgesia can be extended to surgical anesthesia for cesarean delivery in 5.2 (1.5) minutes (mean [SD]) with the addition of bicarbonate and fentanyl to premixed 2% lidocaine with epinephrine.

Many anesthesia providers reserve **2-chloroprocaine** for cases in which rapid extension of epidural anesthesia for vaginal delivery or urgent cesarean delivery is necessary. The onset of surgical anesthesia was several minutes faster with 2-chloroprocaine compared with lidocaine with freshly mixed epinephrine and sodium bicarbonate in the setting of urgent cesarean delivery after epidural labor analgesia.[135] Therefore, when time is of the essence, 2-chloroprocaine is

---

[a]Chapter 13 contains a detailed discussion of anesthetic agents used for neuraxial anesthetic techniques.

the drug of choice. Typically, in an emergency, a large volume of concentrated local anesthetic solution is injected quickly. An additional advantage of 2-chloroprocaine in this situation is that it is rapidly metabolized by plasma esterases. Therefore the unintentional intravascular injection of a large volume of 2-chloroprocaine may be less likely to have serious adverse consequences.

As in spinal anesthesia, epidural opioids work synergistically with local anesthetics. Fentanyl 50 to 100 μg or sufentanil 5 to 10 μg is frequently added to an amide local anesthetic for both labor analgesia (allowing a lower dose of local anesthetic and less motor block) and cesarean delivery (resulting in a denser block with better blockade of visceral stimulation). **Sodium bicarbonate** may be added to lidocaine[136] and 2-chloroprocaine[137] (1 mEq/10 mL local anesthetic) to decrease latency.

COMPLICATIONS OF NEURAXIAL TECHNIQUES

Unintentional Dural Puncture

Unintentional dural puncture with an epidural needle occurs at a rate of approximately 1.5% in the obstetric population.[138] Approximately 52% of women will experience a PDPH after puncture with an epidural needle (see Chapter 30). Techniques to minimize the incidence of unintentional dural puncture include (1) identification of the ligamentum flavum during epidural needle advancement; (2) understanding the likely depth of the epidural space in an individual patient; (3) advancement of the needle between contractions, when unexpected patient movement is less likely; (4) adequate control of the needle-syringe assembly during advancement of the needle; and (5) clearing the needle of clotted blood or bone plugs. A study found the incidence of PDPH after unintentional dural puncture is less likely if the epidural needle bevel faced lateral rather than cephalad. However, an *in vitro* study using cadaver dura found that the fluid leakage rate through dural tears was not dependent on the orientation of the dura relative to the needle bevel.[139] We prefer to insert the epidural needle with the bevel oriented in a cephalad direction so that there is no need to rotate the needle bevel cephalad within the epidural space prior to placing the epidural catheter. Cephalad bevel orientation may also increase the likelihood of successful epidural anesthesia.[140]

The anesthesia provider has two options after unintentional dural puncture: site the epidural catheter within the subarachnoid space and use a continuous spinal anesthetic technique, or site the epidural catheter in a different interspace (i.e., starting afresh). Management may depend on the clinical setting. If advancement of an epidural needle results in dural trespass and the free flow of CSF is perceived in the barrel of the epidural syringe, the anesthesia provider should halt advancement of the epidural needle and either remove the epidural needle (if the plan is to resite the epidural catheter) or replace the stylet back into the lumen of the epidural needle to prevent further egress of CSF (if the plan is to administer intrathecal medication or perform a continuous spinal technique). Reinjection of CSF contained in the syringe should not be entertained because there is a high likelihood that air will concomitantly be introduced into the subarachnoid space and cause pneumocephalus. The risks and benefits of administering an intrathecal dose of anesthetic should be considered. Although intrathecal administration of local anesthetic through the epidural needle will result in rapid analgesia for an uncomfortable patient, the rapid efflux of CSF may render the injectate ineffective. Additionally, spinal analgesia may mask paresthesias during subsequent attempts at neuraxial anesthesia. Furthermore, spinal anesthesia may cause profound hypotension. If the patient is sitting, and likely to remain so for the next few minutes, the anesthesia provider may struggle to manage two problems instead of one (i.e., a challenging neuraxial procedure and maternal hypotension). However, rapid provision of analgesia may enable the patient to better assume an optimal position without moving when replacing the epidural needle. One option is to administer intrathecal opioid, thus providing analgesia without the risk for hypotension.

Evidence is conflicting as to whether the insertion of an epidural catheter through the dural puncture site decreases the incidence of PDPH.[141] Most studies are retrospective; a prospective study in which institutions were randomized to manage unintentional dural puncture with an intrathecal catheter or siting the epidural catheter in another interspace found no difference in the rate of PDPH or need for an epidural blood patch.[142] Continuous spinal anesthesia is an attractive option if identification of the epidural space has been difficult or if the anticipated duration of anesthesia or analgesia is relatively short (e.g., cesarean delivery, or vaginal delivery in parous women). The major disadvantage of an intrathecal catheter is the risk that it may be mistaken for an epidural catheter. Given that the local anesthetic dose required for epidural anesthesia is many times greater than that required for spinal anesthesia, unintentional administration of an epidural dose into the subarachnoid space will lead to total spinal anesthesia. Therefore, on a busy labor and delivery unit where multiple providers are providing anesthesia care, it may be safer to use an epidural catheter rather than an intrathecal catheter in women in whom the need for prolonged analgesia is anticipated.

Because of this concern the anesthesia provider may elect to initiate epidural anesthesia in another lumbar epidural interspace. However, even if the attempt results in a correctly placed catheter, the provider must be wary of an unexpectedly high level of anesthesia after the epidural administration of usual doses of local anesthetic. Leach and Smith[143] reported a patient who had an extensive block after unintentional dural puncture and subsequent epidural injection of bupivacaine. They presented radiologic evidence of the spread of local anesthetic from the epidural space to the subarachnoid space. The extent to which a dural tear affects the movement of substances from the epidural space to the subarachnoid space depends on the size of the hole, the lipophilicity of the drug (highly lipophilic drugs cross quickly regardless of the presence of a hole, whereas water-soluble drugs cross more quickly in the presence of a hole),[144] and whether the drug is administered into the epidural space as a bolus or an infusion. Rapid bolus administration of medications through an epidural catheter in a patient with a known dural puncture with a large-bore needle significantly increases the likelihood of high spinal anesthesia.

Unfortunately, there is no reliable method to decrease the risk for PDPH once dural puncture occurs. Studies regarding the utility of a prophylactic epidural blood patch (injection of autologous blood before removal of the epidural catheter and before onset of a headache) for the prevention of PDPH are conflicting,[145,146] but the only randomized and blinded trial found no difference in the incidence of headache in women who received a prophylactic blood patch compared with a sham patch.[146]

Occasionally, unintentional dural puncture is not recognized until the epidural catheter is threaded and CSF spontaneously appears at the proximal end of the catheter, or the catheter aspiration or intrathecal test dose is positive. Rarely, an epidural catheter that has been correctly sited in the epidural space may migrate into the subarachnoid space. The most significant clinical threat in this scenario is the continued use of a large-volume infusion of local anesthetic drug intended for epidural administration. An unrecognized spinal catheter was the cause of 24% of high neuraxial anesthetics reported to the Serious Complication Repository Project of the Society for Obstetric Anesthesia and Perinatology.[147] Thus, during prolonged epidural labor analgesia, the patient should be regularly monitored for evidence of high or dense neuraxial anesthesia.

Unintentional Intravascular or Subarachnoid Injection

The unintentional injection of large doses of local anesthetics into the subarachnoid space can lead to catastrophe. The rapid onset of high or total spinal anesthesia results in profound hypotension, loss of consciousness, and apnea secondary to hypoperfusion of the brain stem. Prompt treatment necessitates assisted ventilation, volume resuscitation, and pharmacologic support of blood pressure. Administration of chronotropic agents such as epinephrine may also be necessary if blockade of cardiac sympathetic drive results in bradycardia. The patient is at high risk for awareness in this setting, and the judicious use of an amnestic agent such as midazolam should be considered once cardiorespiratory stability has been restored.

Pregnant women are at higher risk for unintentional intravenous cannulation because of the engorgement of epidural veins. Intravascular injection of a local anesthetic may initially result in altered sensorium, tinnitus, and perioral numbness. Higher blood concentrations may result in seizures, and even-higher concentrations may cause dysrhythmias and cardiovascular collapse (see Chapter 13 and Box 24.8).

Inadequate Anesthesia

Pain during anesthesia represents a higher proportion of obstetric malpractice claims than of nonobstetric claims.[148,149] Active management of neuraxial labor analgesia and in-dwelling catheters is paramount to the care of obstetric patients.

The Society for Obstetric Anesthesia and Perinatology recommends regular assessment of neuraxial labor analgesia effectiveness as a key component for the Center of Excellence designation (see Chapter 11).[150] Regular assessment helps the timely identification of inadequate analgesia and epidural catheter malfunction. Ende et al.[151] implemented a rounding reminder within the electronic health record that not only decreased time between patient assessments but resulted in a significant decrease in the epidural catheter replacement rate from 14% preimplementation to 5% postimplementation.

During labor, inadequate epidural analgesia may result from the inadequate extent of sensory blockade, nonuniform blockade, or inadequate density of blockade. When called to evaluate breakthrough pain, the anesthesia provider should first evaluate the extent of bilateral sensory blockade in *both the cephalad and caudad directions* (see Box 24.7). Particularly if labor is progressing quickly, the extent of sacral blockade may not be adequate. In this case, epidural injection of a large volume of local anesthetic may improve sacral blockade. In contrast, if the extent of sensory blockade is adequate but the patient is still experiencing pain, the density of blockade may be insufficient. In this case, the provider should reestablish and maintain analgesia using a more concentrated solution of local anesthetic. Ende et al.[152] demonstrated that a standardized approach to evaluating breakthrough pain leads to earlier identification and replacement of nonfunctioning epidural catheters (Fig. 12.22).

Why do some obstetric epidural anesthetics fail over time? Collier[153] administered epidural radiocontrast agent in 25 parturients reporting unsatisfactory analgesia. The two major causes of inadequate block in this small study were transforaminal migration of the catheter tip and an obstructive barrier in the epidural space. Total block failure usually results from failure to identify the epidural space correctly or from malposition of the catheter tip outside the epidural space (e.g., in a neuroforamen). A unilateral block may occur despite the use of good technique. Unilateral blocks can often be prevented by limiting the length of catheter within the epidural space to 3 cm or less, but this may increase the risk for outward migration of the catheter over time. (Patients undergoing surgery remain still; by contrast, laboring women change position frequently.) Obese women seem to be at higher risk for outward migration of the catheter tip.[59]

Unilateral or patchy sensory blockade likely results from the nonuniform distribution of local anesthetic solution in the epidural space.[154] Whether catheter withdrawal in the setting of breakthrough pain is beneficial is not clear. Beilin et al.[155] compared catheter withdrawal followed by injection of local anesthetic with injection of local anesthetic without catheter withdrawal for the treatment of breakthrough pain. The ability to rescue analgesia was not different between the groups. Injection of a large volume of dilute local anesthetic solution (10 to 20 mL) into the epidural space usually corrects unilateral and patchy blockade, but if it does not, we recommend pulling the catheter back 1 to 2 cm and redosing. If analgesia cannot be rescued by pulling back the catheter and the second injection, strong consideration should be given to removing the catheter and replacing it at another interspace.

TOP UP REQUEST WORKFLOW

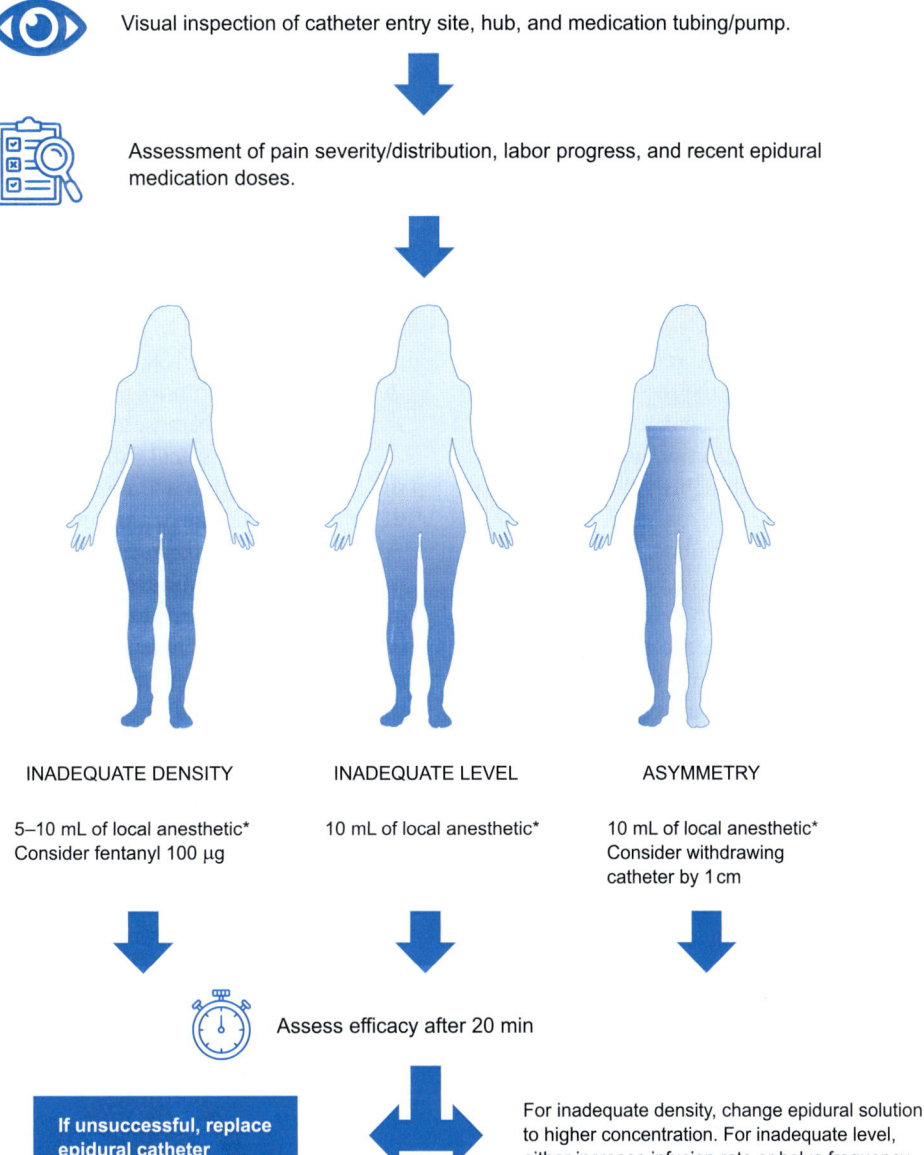

Visual inspection of catheter entry site, hub, and medication tubing/pump.

Assessment of pain severity/distribution, labor progress, and recent epidural medication doses.

INADEQUATE DENSITY	INADEQUATE LEVEL	ASYMMETRY
5–10 mL of local anesthetic* Consider fentanyl 100 µg	10 mL of local anesthetic*	10 mL of local anesthetic* Consider withdrawing catheter by 1 cm

Assess efficacy after 20 min

If unsuccessful, replace epidural catheter

For inadequate density, change epidural solution to higher concentration. For inadequate level, either increase infusion rate or bolus frequency.

* Ropivacaine 0.2% or Bupivacaine 0.125%

Fig. 12.22 Suggested Workflow Algorithm for Breakthrough Pain and Epidural Top-Up Requests During Labor. After confirming the integrity of the epidural infusion pump, tubing, catheter hub and insertion site, all patients should be assessed for the severity and distribution of their discomfort. Pain, despite a sufficient dermatomal level of analgesia, indicates a need for block of greater density (treated by increasing the concentration of the local anesthetic solution or adding adjuvants). An inadequate sensory level, however, requires increased volume of epidural solution. Lastly, an asymmetric block may be overcome with increased volume of epidural solution, with consideration for withdrawing the epidural catheter 1 cm. Failure to achieve satisfactory analgesia in any of these scenarios may necessitate replacement of the epidural catheter. Algorithm from Ende HB, Tran B, Thampy M, Bauchat JR, McCarthy RJ. Standardization of epidural top-ups for breakthrough labor pain results in a higher proportion of catheter replacements within 30 min of the first bolus dose. *Int J Obstet Anesth* 2021;47:103161. Illustration by Naveen Nathan, MD, NorthShore University HealthSystem, University of Chicago Pritzker School of Medicine, Evanston, IL.

The management of inadequate anesthesia is more problematic during cesarean delivery (see Chapter 26). Failure of spinal anesthesia may result from the maldistribution of local anesthetic within the subarachnoid space.[156] If inadequate spinal anesthesia is noted before incision, the anesthesia provider may augment the block with additional local anesthetic by either performing a second spinal anesthetic procedure or placing an epidural catheter, or both. However, care must be taken if performing a second spinal anesthetic procedure. In the ASA Closed-Claims Project database, Drasner and Rigler[157] identified three cases of cauda equina syndrome complicating spinal anesthesia. In two cases, "failed spinal" anesthesia had occurred, followed by a repeat injection of local anesthetic. The researchers recommended that anesthesia providers determine the presence of anesthesia in the sacral dermatomes before administering additional local anesthetic into the subarachnoid space. Additionally, they stated that if CSF was aspirated during the original procedure, it should be assumed that local anesthetic was delivered into the subarachnoid space, and the total dose of local anesthetic be limited to the maximum dose a clinician would consider reasonable to administer in a single injection.[157] If partial blockade is present (even if it is limited to the sacral dermatomes), the second dose should be reduced accordingly. It may also be advisable to perform the second procedure at a different interspace or make other changes to the original procedure (e.g., alter the patient's position, use a local anesthetic with different baricity, or straighten the lumbosacral curvature). Much of this complexity in decision making may be addressed by using an epidural technique as an alternative to repeat spinal anesthesia.

If the patient complains of pain after incision, the anesthesia provider must decide between the administration of inhalation or intravenous analgesia, and the administration of general anesthesia. Supplemental analgesia may be provided by administering 60% nitrous oxide in oxygen, small incremental boluses of ketamine (0.1 to 0.25 mg/kg), or small boluses of intravenous opioid. Infiltration of the surgical wound with local anesthetic is sometimes helpful, especially when spinal anesthesia regresses near the end of an unexpectedly long operation. Additionally, intraperitoneal chloroprocaine administration after infant delivery may aid in adjuvant anesthesia.[158] The anesthesia provider must ensure that the patient remains sufficiently alert to protect her airway. In most cases, severe pain unrelieved by modest doses of analgesic drug requires rapid-sequence induction of general anesthesia followed by tracheal intubation.

Risk factors for failed conversion of epidural labor analgesia to epidural anesthesia for intrapartum cesarean delivery include an increasing number of clinician-administered boluses during labor (requirement for top-up doses), greater urgency of cesarean delivery, and provision of anesthesia care by a nonobstetric anesthesiologist.[159] In some cases, inadequate epidural anesthesia results from failure to give a sufficient dose of local anesthetic or failure to wait a sufficient time after its administration. For example, after the epidural administration of 2% lidocaine with epinephrine, approximately 10 to 20 minutes must pass to achieve an adequate level of anesthesia, and additional local anesthetic may be needed to achieve an adequate density of blockade. In urgent cases or in cases with a "missed" segment, local infiltration with a local anesthetic often results in satisfactory anesthesia. Sometimes it is difficult to separate the beneficial effect of the local infiltration from the beneficial effect of waiting for the obstetrician to obtain, prepare, and inject the local anesthetic solution. If conversion to epidural anesthesia fails and is recognized prior to the start of the procedure, another epidural catheter can be placed or spinal anesthesia can be initiated. If spinal anesthesia is chosen the anesthesia provider should exercise caution because of a greater incidence of high spinal anesthesia in the setting of failed epidural anesthesia.[147,160] Presumably, the large volume of local anesthetic within, or near, the epidural space results in decreased lumbar CSF volume, which predisposes to high spinal anesthesia. It may be advisable to reduce the dose of intrathecal local anesthetic, particularly in the presence of partial epidural blockade.

Equipment Problems

The frequency of major equipment malfunction is very low during the administration of neuraxial anesthesia. Most anesthesia providers in the United States use disposable needles. If a needle should break, the portion of the needle that remains in the patient should be removed because it may migrate and cause injury.

An epidural or spinal catheter may shear and break off if the catheter is withdrawn through a needle; thus an epidural or spinal catheter should never be withdrawn in this manner. Rather, if the catheter must be withdrawn, the needle and catheter should be withdrawn as a unit. It is also possible to break a catheter during attempts at removing it, although this is rare. If resistance to catheter removal is encountered, the patient should assume a position that reduces lumbar lordosis, thereby lessening the kinking of the catheter between perivertebral structures. If position change is not successful, the catheter should be taped under tension to the patient's back and left undisturbed for several hours. The catheter usually works its way out and is then easy to remove. Once the catheter has been removed successfully, it should be examined to ensure that it has been removed completely. Complete removal of the catheter should be documented in the medical record.

Rarely, catheters do break on removal. We favor aggressive attempts to remove broken catheters located in the subarachnoid space to prevent the formation of dural adhesions.[161] However, it may be unnecessary to remove broken catheters located in the epidural space or in the ligaments as long as there is no catheter breaching the skin that may serve as a portal for infection. Rather, in these circumstances, the patient can be informed of the complication and observed over time. The incidence of catheter migration or other delayed sequelae appears to be low. Imaging (radiography, computed tomography, magnetic resonance) may help identify the precise location of a broken catheter.

During use, an epidural catheter occasionally becomes disconnected from the catheter connector. Options include replacing the epidural catheter or reconnecting the connector to the catheter. Langevin et al.[162] used an *in vitro* model to investigate whether microbial contamination precludes reconnection. They found that an area of the interior of the catheter distal to the disconnection may remain sterile for up to 8 hours if the fluid column within the catheter remains static (i.e., if "fluid does not move within the catheter when it is raised above the level of the patient").[162] Therefore they concluded that it *may* be safe to decontaminate the exterior of the catheter, cut the catheter with a sterile instrument, and reconnect it to a new sterile connector.

TEACHING NEURAXIAL ANESTHESIA PROCEDURES

Teaching mastery of neuraxial anesthesia is an important skill of academic anesthesiologists. A logical approach to learning neuraxial procedures might begin with self-study aimed at mastering the spatial geometry of the central neuraxis, via written or online material, spine models, sonoanatomy, or combinations of these. This may be followed by procedural practice on a simulator, followed by procedures performed on patients with close supervision of an experienced teacher. Beyond technical skills, the safe practice of neuraxial anesthesia requires knowledge of the pharmacologic and physiologic aspects of neuraxial procedures.

The importance of applying a consistent and thoughtful methodology when teaching procedural skills cannot be understated. Unlike videolaryngoscopy, which allows the observer real-time assessment of a trainee's mechanical technique, no such analogous technology facilitates guidance during neuraxial anesthesia procedures. Spinal and epidural anesthesia remain essentially "blind" procedures. E-learning tools such as computer-enhanced visual learning modules for neuraxial procedures have been shown to decrease mean procedure time and improve scores on procedural checklists.[163] The past decade has seen the development of high-fidelity simulators for teaching neuraxial techniques.[164] Use of low-technology simulators, such a vegetables and fruits, has also been described and may also be effective.[165]

Offering meaningful feedback is highly conducive to shaping procedural habits. An effective debriefing session results from a systematic approach to observation and analysis of clinical skill. One example is described by Chuan et al.[166] Their comprehensive checklist identifies 25 executable actions for regional anesthesia block procedures that are amenable to observation and assessment.

Mastery of technical skills requires practice. Kopacz et al.[167] determined that a 90% success rate is not attained and maintained until first-year anesthesiology residents perform approximately 45 spinal and 60 epidural procedures.

KEY POINTS

- Physiologic changes of pregnancy alter neuraxial anatomy; alterations include accentuation of lumbar lordosis, a "softer" ligamentum flavum, and decreased space in the spinal canal caused by vascular engorgement of epidural veins and increased adipose tissue.
- Physiologic changes of pregnancy cause a more pronounced response to neuraxial anesthesia–induced sympathetic blockade than is seen in nonpregnant patients. These include higher baseline sympathetic tone and aortocaval compression.
- Pregnant women, particularly those with neuraxial blockade, should not be cared for in the supine position but rather in lateral tilt or in the full lateral position.
- Correct patient positioning, equipment, and technique are important to the success and safety of neuraxial techniques.
- The midline approach is faster and less painful than the paramedian approach to the epidural or subarachnoid space. However, the paramedian approach may allow for the successful identification of the subarachnoid or epidural space in difficult cases.

- Use of a noncutting (pencil-point) needle for spinal anesthesia reduces the incidence of postdural puncture headache.
- Combined spinal-epidural anesthesia has the advantages of both spinal anesthesia and epidural anesthesia.
- The dural puncture epidural technique may provide many of the advantages of both the epidural and the combined-spinal epidural techniques, but further investigation is needed to better define the role of the technique in the routine management of labor pain.
- Approximately 20% to 30% less local anesthetic is required for epidural and spinal anesthesia in pregnant patients than in nonpregnant patients.
- Multiple techniques (e.g., test dose, aspiration, incremental dose injection) should be used to reduce the incidence and risk for unintentional subarachnoid or intravascular injection because not one technique will completely exclude all cases of malpositioned needles or catheters.

REFERENCES

1. Agarwal D, Mohta M, Tyagi A, Sethi AK. Subdural block and the anaesthetist. *Anaesth Intensive Care*. 2010;38:20–26.
2. Hogan QH. Epidural anatomy examined by cryomicrotome section. Influence of age, vertebral level, and disease. *Reg Anesth*. 1996;21:395–406.
3. Blomberg R. The dorsomedian connective tissue band in the lumbar epidural space of humans: an anatomical study using epiduroscopy in autopsy cases. *Anesth Analg*. 1986;65:747–752.
4. Savolaine ER, Pandya JB, Greenblatt SH, Conover SR. Anatomy of the human lumbar epidural space: new insights using CT-epidurography. *Anesthesiology*. 1988;68:217–220.
5. Marchesini M, Schiappa E, Raffaeli W. The dorsomedian ligamentous strand: an evaluation in vivo with epiduroscopy. *Med Sci (Basel)*. 2022;10
6. Hogan QH. Lumbar epidural anatomy. A new look by cryomicrotome section. *Anesthesiology*. 1991;75:767–775.
7. Zarzur E. Anatomic studies of the human ligamentum flavum. *Anesth Analg*. 1984;63:499–502.

8. Altinkaya N, Yildirim T, Demir S, et al. Factors associated with the thickness of the ligamentum flavum: is ligamentum flavum thickening due to hypertrophy or buckling? *Spine*. 2011;36:E1093–E1097.

9. Sharma V, Swinson AK, Hughes C, et al. Effect of ethnicity and body mass index on the distance from skin to lumbar epidural space in parturients. *Anaesthesia*. 2011;66:907–912.

10. Hogan QH, Prost R, Kulier A, et al. Magnetic resonance imaging of cerebrospinal fluid volume and the influence of body habitus and abdominal pressure. *Anesthesiology*. 1996;84:1341–1349.

11. Richardson MG, Wissler RN. Density of lumbar cerebrospinal fluid in pregnant and nonpregnant humans. *Anesthesiology*. 1996;85:326–330.

12. Hirabayashi Y, Shimizu R, Fukuda H, et al. Anatomical configuration of the spinal column in the supine position. II. Comparison of pregnant and non-pregnant women. *Br J Anaesth*. 1995;75:6–8.

13. Fassoulaki A, Gatzou V, Petropoulos G, Siafaka I. Spread of subarachnoid block, intraoperative local anaesthetic requirements and postoperative analgesic requirements in Caesarean section and total abdominal hysterectomy. *Br J Anaesth*. 2004;93:678–682.

14. Russell IF. A comparison of cold, pinprick and touch for assessing the level of spinal block at caesarean section. *Int J Obstet Anesth*. 2004;13:146–152.

15. Fink BR. Mechanisms of differential axial blockade in epidural and subarachnoid anesthesia. *Anesthesiology*. 1989;70:851–858.

16. American Society of Anesthesiologists Committee on Obstetric Anesthesia. Statement on neuraxial analgesia or anesthesia in obstetrics; 2021. https://www.asahq.org/standards-and-practice-parameters/statement-on-neuraxial-anesthesia-in-obstetrics. Accessed 14 January 2024.

17. American Society of Anesthesiologists. Practice guidelines for obstetric anesthesia: an updated report by the American Society of Anesthesiologists Task Force on Obstetric Anesthesia and the Society for Obstetric Anesthesia and Perinatology. *Anesthesiology*. 2016;124:270–300.

18. Abrao KC, Francisco RP, Miyadahira S, et al. Elevation of uterine basal tone and fetal heart rate abnormalities after labor analgesia: a randomized controlled trial. *Obstet Gynecol*. 2009;113:41–47.

19. American College of Obstetricians and Gynecologists. Practice Bulletin No. 209: Obstetric analgesia and anesthesia (reaffirmed 2024). *Obstet Gynecol*. 2019;133:e208–e225.

20. Jackson A, Henry R, Avery N, et al. Informed consent for labour epidurals: what labouring women want to know. *Can J Anaesth*. 2000;47:1068–1073.

21. Bethune L, Harper N, Lucas DN, et al. Complications of obstetric regional analgesia: how much information is enough? *Int J Obstet Anesth*. 2004;13:30–34.

22. Frohlich S, Tan T, Walsh A, Carey M. Epidural analgesia for labour: maternal knowledge, preferences and informed consent. *Ir Med J*. 2011;104:300–302.

23. Burkle CM, Olsen DA, Sviggum HP, Jacob AK. Parturient recall of neuraxial analgesia risks: impact of labor pain vs no labor pain. *J Clin Anesth*. 2017;36:158–163.

24. Orbach-Zinger S, Ginosar Y, Sverdlik J, et al. Partner's presence during initiation of epidural labor analgesia does not decrease maternal stress: a prospective randomized controlled trial. *Anesth Analg*. 2012;114:654–660.

25. Morell E, Peralta FM, Higgins N, et al. Effect of companion presence on maternal satisfaction during neuraxial catheter placement for labor analgesia: a randomized clinical trial. *Int J Obstet Anesth*. 2019;38:66–74.

26. Vincent RD, Chestnut DH. Which position is more comfortable for the parturient during identification of the epidural space? *Int J Obstet Anesth*. 1991;1:9–11.

27. Andrews PJ, Ackerman 3rd WE, Juneja MM. Aortocaval compression in the sitting and lateral decubitus positions during extradural catheter placement in the parturient. *Can J Anaesth*. 1993;40:320–324.

28. Mhyre JM, Greenfield ML, Tsen LC, Polley LS. A systematic review of randomized controlled trials that evaluate strategies to avoid epidural vein cannulation during obstetric epidural catheter placement. *Anesth Analg*. 2009;108:1232–1242.

29. Sharma M, Qasem F, Sebbag I, et al. The crossed-leg position increases the dimensions within the acoustic target window for neuraxial needle placement in term pregnancy: a prospective observational study. *Int J Obstet Anesth*. 2020;44:106–111.

30. Norris MC, Dewan DM. Effect of gravity on the spread of extradural anaesthesia for caesarean section. *Br J Anaesth*. 1987;59:338–341.

31. Reid JA, Thorburn J. Extradural bupivacaine or lignocaine anaesthesia for elective caesarean section: the role of maternal posture. *Br J Anaesth*. 1988;61:149–153.

32. Beilin Y, Abramovitz SE, Zahn J, et al. Improved epidural analgesia in the parturient in the 30 degree tilt position. *Can J Anaesth*. 2000;47:1176–1181.

33. Preston R, Crosby ET, Kotarba D, et al. Maternal positioning affects fetal heart rate changes after epidural analgesia for labour. *Can J Anaesth*. 1993;40:1136–1141.

34. US Centers for Disease Control and Prevention. Bacterial meningitis after intrapartum spinal anesthesia—New York and Ohio, 2008-2009. *MMWR Morb Mortal Wkly Rep*. 2010;59:65–69.

35. Baer ET. Post-dural puncture bacterial meningitis. *Anesthesiology*. 2006;105:381–393.

36. Siegel J, Rhinehart E, Jackson M, et al. 2007 Guideline for isolation precautions: preventing transmission of infectious agents in health care settings. https://www.cdc.gov/infection-control/hcp/isolation-precautions/?CDC_AAref_Val=https://www.cdc.gov/infectioncontrol/guidelines/isolation/. Accessed April 23, 2025.

37. American Society of Anesthesiologists and the American Society of Regional Anesthesia and Pain Medicine. Practice advisory for the prevention, diagnosis, and management of infectious complications associated with neuraxial techniques. *Anesthesiology*. 2017;126:585–601.

38. O'Grady NP, Alexander M, Burns LA, et al. Guidelines for the prevention of intravascular catheter-related infections. *Am J Infect Control*. 2011;39:S1–S34.

39. Association of Anaesthetists of Great Britain and Ireland. Infection control in anaesthesia. *Anaesthesia*. 2008;63:1027–1036.

40. Hubble MJ, Weale AE, Perez JV, et al. Clothing in laminar-flow operating theatres. *J Hosp Infect*. 1996;32:1–7.

41. Lai NM, Lai NA, O'Riordan E, et al. Skin antisepsis for reducing central venous catheter-related infections. *Cochrane Database Syst Rev*. 2016;(7):CD010140.

42. Tao W, Grant EN, Craig MG, et al. Continuous spinal analgesia for labor and delivery: an observational study with a 23-gauge spinal catheter. *Anesth Analg*. 2015;121:1290–1294.

43. McKenzie CP, Carvalho B, Riley ET. The Wiley spinal catheter-over-needle system for continuous apinal anesthesia: a case series of 5 cesarean deliveries complicated by paresthesias and headaches. *Reg Anesth Pain Med*. 2016;41:405–410.

44. Reina MA, de Leon-Casasola OA, Lopez A, et al. An in vitro study of dural lesions produced by 25-gauge Quincke and Whitacre needles evaluated by scanning electron microscopy. *Reg Anesth Pain Med*. 2000;25:393–402.

45. Shenouda PE, Cunningham BJ. Assessing the superiority of saline versus air for use in the epidural loss of resistance technique: a literature review. *Reg Anesth Pain Med*. 2003;28:48–53.

46. Beilin Y, Arnold I, Telfeyan C, et al. Quality of analgesia when air versus saline is used for identification of the epidural space in the parturient. *Reg Anesth Pain Med*. 2000;25:596–599.

47. Aida S, Taga K, Yamakura T, et al. Headache after attempted epidural block: the role of intrathecal air. *Anesthesiology*. 1998;88:76–81.

48. Antibas PL, do Nascimento Junior P, Braz LG, et al. Air versus saline in the loss of resistance technique for identification of the epidural space. *Cochrane Database Syst Rev*. 2014;(7):CD008938.

49. Segal S, Arendt KW. A retrospective effectiveness study of loss of resistance to air or saline for identification of the epidural space. *Anesth Analg*. 2010;110:558–563.

50. Toledano RD, Tsen LC. Epidural catheter design: history, innovations, and clinical implications. *Anesthesiology*. 2014;121:9–17.

51. Banwell BR, Morley-Forster P, Krause R. Decreased incidence of complications in parturients with the arrow (FlexTip Plus) epidural catheter. *Can J Anaesth*. 1998;45:370–372.

52. Norris MC, Fogel ST, Dalman H, et al. Labor epidural analgesia without an intravascular "test dose". *Anesthesiology*. 1998;88:1495–1501.

53. D'Angelo R, Foss ML, Livesay CH. A comparison of multiport and uniport epidural catheters in laboring patients. *Anesth Analg*. 1997;84:1276–1279.

54. Fegley AJ, Lerman J, Wissler R. Epidural multiorifice catheters function as single-orifice catheters: an in vitro study. *Anesth Analg*. 2008;107:1079–1081.

55. Du W, Song Y, Zhao Q, et al. The effect of open-end versus closed-end epidural catheter design on injection pressure and dye diffusion under various programmed intermittent epidural delivery rates: an in vitro study. *Int J Obstet Anesth*. 2022;51:103252.

56. Spiegel JE, Vasudevan A, Li Y, Hess PE. A randomized prospective study comparing two flexible epidural catheters for labour analgesia. *Br J Anaesth*. 2009;103:400–405.

57. Yi J, Li Y, Yuan Y, et al. Comparison of labor analgesia efficacy between single-orifice and multiorifice wire-reinforced catheters during programmed intermittent epidural boluses: a randomized controlled clinical trial. *Reg Anesth Pain Med*. 2023;48:61–66.

58. Pancaro C, Purtell J, LaBuda D, et al. Difficulty in advancing flexible epidural catheters when establishing labor analgesia: an observational open-label randomized trial. *Anesth Analg*. 2021;133:151–159.

59. Hamilton CL, Riley ET, Cohen SE. Changes in the position of epidural catheters associated with patient movement. *Anesthesiology*. 1997;86:778–784.

60. Beilin Y, Bernstein HH, Zucker-Pinchoff B. The optimal distance that a multiorifice epidural catheter should be threaded into the epidural space. *Anesth Analg*. 1995;81:301–304.

61. D'Angelo R, Berkebile BL, Gerancher JC. Prospective examination of epidural catheter insertion. *Anesthesiology*. 1996;84:88–93.

62. Tyagi A, Kumar R, Bhattacharya A, Sethi AK. Filters in anaesthesia and intensive care. *Anaesth Intensive Care*. 2003;31:418–433.

63. Charlton GA, Lawes EG. The effect of micropore filters on the aspiration test in epidural analgesia. *Anaesthesia*. 1991;46:573–575.

64. Westphal M, Hohage H, Buerkle H, et al. Adsorption of sufentanil to epidural filters and catheters. *Eur J Anaesthesiol*. 2003;20:124–126.

65. Leo S, Sng BL, Lim Y, Sia AT. A randomized comparison of low doses of hyperbaric bupivacaine in combined spinal-epidural anesthesia for cesarean delivery. *Anesth Analg*. 2009;109:1600–1605.

66. Choi DH, Kim JA, Chung IS. Comparison of combined spinal epidural anesthesia and epidural anesthesia for cesarean section. *Acta Anaesthesiol Scand*. 2000;44:214–219.

67. Goodman SR, Smiley RM, Negron MA, et al. A randomized trial of breakthrough pain during combined spinal-epidural versus epidural labor analgesia in parous women. *Anesth Analg*. 2009;108:246–251.

68. Gambling D, Berkowitz J, Farrell TR, et al. A randomized controlled comparison of epidural analgesia and combined spinal-epidural analgesia in a private practice setting: pain scores during first and second stages of labor and at delivery. *Anesth Analg*. 2013;116:636–643.

69. Simmons SW, Taghizadeh N, Dennis AT, et al. Combined spinal-epidural versus epidural analgesia in labour. *Cochrane Database Syst Rev*. 2012;(10):CD003401.

70. Pan PH, Bogard TD, Owen MD. Incidence and characteristics of failures in obstetric neuraxial analgesia and anesthesia: a retrospective analysis of 19,259 deliveries. *Int J Obstet Anesth*. 2004;13:227–233.

71. Booth JM, Pan JC, Ross VH, et al. Combined spinal epidural technique for labor analgesia does not delay recognition of epidural catheter failures: a single-center retrospective cohort survival analysis. *Anesthesiology*. 2016;125:516–524.

72. Lee S, Lew E, Lim Y, Sia AT. Failure of augmentation of labor epidural analgesia for intrapartum cesarean delivery: a retrospective review. *Anesth Analg*. 2009;108:252–254.

73. Riley ET, Hamilton CL, Ratner EF, Cohen SE. A comparison of the 24-gauge Sprotte and Gertie Marx spinal needles for combined spinal-epidural analgesia during labor. *Anesthesiology*. 2002;97:574–577.

74. Grondin LS, Nelson K, Ross V, et al. Success of spinal and epidural labor analgesia: comparison of loss of resistance technique using air versus saline in combined spinal-epidural labor analgesia technique. *Anesthesiology*. 2009;111:165–172.

75. Thomas JA, Pan PH, Harris LC, et al. Dural puncture with a 27-gauge Whitacre needle as part of a combined spinal-epidural technique does not improve labor epidural catheter function. *Anesthesiology*. 2005;103:1046–1051.

76. Cappiello E, O'Rourke N, Segal S, Tsen LC. A randomized trial of dural puncture epidural technique compared with the standard epidural technique for labor analgesia. *Anesth Analg*. 2008;107:1646–1651.

77. Chau A, Bibbo C, Huang CC, et al. Dural puncture epidural technique improves labor analgesia quality with fewer side effects compared with epidural and combined spinal epidural techniques: a randomized clinical trial. *Anesth Analg*. 2017;124:560–569.

78. Wilson SH, Wolf BJ, Bingham KN, et al. Labor analgesia onset with dural puncture epidural versus traditional epidural using a 26-gauge Whitacre needle and 0.125% bupivacaine bolus: a randomized clinical trial. *Anesth Analg*. 2018;126:545–551.

79. Contreras F, Morales J, Bravo D, et al. Dural puncture epidural analgesia for labor: a randomized comparison between 25-gauge and 27-gauge pencil point spinal needles. *Reg Anesth Pain Med*. 2019;44:750–753.

80. Berger AA, Jordan J, Li Y, et al. Epidural catheter replacement rates with dural puncture epidural labor analgesia compared with epidural analgesia without dural puncture: a retrospective cohort study. *Int J Obstet Anesth*. 2022;52:103590.

81. Tan HS, Reed SE, Mehdiratta JE, et al. Quality of labor analgesia with dural puncture epidural versus standard epidural technique in obese parturients: a double-blind randomized controlled study. *Anesthesiology*. 2022;136:678–687.

82. Sharawi N, Williams M, Athar W, et al. Effect of dural-puncture epidural vs standard epidural for epidural extension on onset time of surgical anesthesia in elective cesarean delivery: a randomized clinical trial. *JAMA Netw Open*. 2023;6:e2326710.

83. Heesen M, Rijs K, Rossaint R, Klimek M. Dural puncture epidural versus conventional epidural block for labor analgesia: a systematic review of randomized controlled trials. *Int J Obstet Anesth*. 2019;40:24–31.

84. Perlas A, Chaparro LE, Chin KJ. Lumbar neuraxial ultrasound for spinal and epidural anesthesia: a systematic review and meta-analysis. *Reg Anesth Pain Med*. 2016;41:251–260.

85. Arzola C, Mikhael R, Margarido C, Carvalho JC. Spinal ultrasound versus palpation for epidural catheter insertion in labour: a randomised controlled trial. *Eur J Anaesthesiol*. 2015;32:499–505.

86. Tawfik MM, Atallah MM, Elkharboutly WS, et al. Does preprocedural ultrasound increase the first-pass success rate of epidural catheterization before cesarean delivery? A randomized controlled trial. *Anesth Analg*. 2017;124:851–856.

87. Young B, Onwochei D, Desai N. Conventional landmark palpation vs. preprocedural ultrasound for neuraxial analgesia and anaesthesia in obstetrics—a systematic review and meta-analysis with trial sequential analyses. *Anaesthesia*. 2021;76:818–831.

88. Chin KJ, Perlas A, Chan V, et al. Ultrasound imaging facilitates spinal anesthesia in adults with difficult surface anatomic landmarks. *Anesthesiology*. 2011;115:94–101.

89. Creaney M, Mullane D, Casby C, Tan T. Ultrasound to identify the lumbar space in women with impalpable bony landmarks presenting for elective caesarean delivery under spinal anaesthesia: a randomised trial. *Int J Obstet Anesth*. 2016;28:12–16.

90. Park SK, Bae J, Yoo S, et al. Ultrasound-assisted versus landmark-guided spinal anesthesia in patients with abnormal spinal anatomy: a randomized controlled trial. *Anesth Analg*. 2020;130:787–795.

91. Balki M, Lee Y, Halpern S, Carvalho JC. Ultrasound imaging of the lumbar spine in the transverse plane: the correlation between estimated and actual depth to the epidural space in obese parturients. *Anesth Analg*. 2009;108:1876–1881.

92. Arzola C, Davies S, Rofaeel A, Carvalho JC. Ultrasound using the transverse approach to the lumbar spine provides reliable landmarks for labor epidurals. *Anesth Analg*. 2007;104:1188–1192.

93. Hetherington J, Brohan J, Rohling R, et al. A novel ultrasound software system for lumbar level identification in obstetric patients. *Can J Anaesth*. 2022;69:1211–1219.

94. Albright GA. Cardiac arrest following regional anesthesia with etidocaine or bupivacaine. *Anesthesiology*. 1979;51:285–287.

95. Guinard JP, Mulroy MF, Carpenter RL, Knopes KD. Test doses: optimal epinephrine content with and without acute beta-adrenergic blockade. *Anesthesiology*. 1990;73:386–392.

96. Chestnut DH, Weiner CP, Martin JG, et al. Effect of intravenous epinephrine on uterine artery blood flow velocity in the pregnant guinea pig. *Anesthesiology*. 1986;65:633–636.

97. Cartwright PD, McCarroll SM, Antzaka C. Maternal heart rate changes with a plain epidural test dose. *Anesthesiology*. 1986;65:226–228.

98. Chestnut DH, Owen CL, Brown CK, et al. Does labor affect the variability of maternal heart rate during induction of epidural anesthesia? *Anesthesiology*. 1988;68:622–625.

99. Colonna-Romano P, Lingaraju N, Godfrey SD, Braitman LE. Epidural test dose and intravascular injection in obstetrics: sensitivity, specificity, and lowest effective dose. *Anesth Analg*. 1992;75:372–376.

100. Colonna-Romano P, Nagaraj L. Tests to evaluate intravenous placement of epidural catheters in laboring women: a prospective clinical study. *Anesth Analg*. 1998;86:985–988.

101. Leighton BL, Norris MC, Sosis M, et al. Limitations of epinephrine as a marker of intravascular injection in laboring women. *Anesthesiology*. 1987;66:688–691.

102. Gieraerts R, Van Zundert A, De Wolf A, Vaes L. Ten ml bupivacaine 0.125% with 12.5 micrograms epinephrine is a reliable epidural test dose to detect inadvertent intravascular injection in obstetric patients. A double-blind study. *Acta Anaesthesiol Scand*. 1992;36:656–659.

103. Guinard JP, Mulroy MF, Carpenter RL, Knopes KD. Test doses: optimal epinephrine content with and without acute beta-adrenergic blockade. *Anesthesiology*. 1990;73:386–392.

104. Leighton BL, Norris MC, DeSimone CA, et al. The air test as a clinically useful indicator of intravenously placed epidural catheters. *Anesthesiology*. 1990;73:610–613.

105. Leighton BL, Topkis WG, Gross JB, et al. Multiport epidural catheters: does the air test work? *Anesthesiology*. 2000;92:1617–1620.

106. Colonna-Romano P, Lingaraju N, Braitman LE. Epidural test dose: lidocaine 100 mg, not chloroprocaine, is a symptomatic marker of i.v. injection in labouring parturients. *Can J Anaesth*. 1993;40:714–717.

107. Rathmell JP, Viscomi CM, Ashikaga T. Detection of intravascular epidural catheters using 2-chloroprocaine. Influence of local anesthetic dose and nalbuphine premedication. *Reg Anesth*. 1997;22:113–118.

108. Yoshii WY, Miller M, Rottman RL, et al. Fentanyl for epidural intravascular test dose in obstetrics. *Reg Anesth*. 1993;18:296–299.

109. Power I, Thorburn J. Differential flow from multihole epidural catheters. *Anaesthesia*. 1988;43:876–878.

110. Abraham RA, Harris AP, Maxwell LG, Kaplow S. The efficacy of 1.5% lidocaine with 7.5% dextrose and epinephrine as an epidural test dose for obstetrics. *Anesthesiology*. 1986;64:116–119.

111. Colonna-Romano P, Padolina R, Lingaraju N, Braitman LE. Diagnostic accuracy of an intrathecal test dose in epidural analgesia. *Can J Anaesth*. 1994;41:572–574.

112. Ngan Kee WD, Khaw KS, Lee BB, et al. The limitations of ropivacaine with epinephrine as an epidural test dose in parturients. *Anesth Analg*. 2001;92:1529–1531.

113. Richardson MG, Lee AC, Wissler RN. High spinal anesthesia after epidural test dose administration in five obstetric patients. *Reg Anesth.* 1996;21:119–123.

114. Mulroy MF, Neal JM, Mackey DC, Harrington BE. 2-Chloroprocaine and bupivacaine are unreliable indicators of intravascular injection in the premedicated patient. *Reg Anesth Pain Med.* 1998;23:9–13.

115. Cohen SE, Yeh JY, Riley ET, Vogel TM. Walking with labor epidural analgesia: the impact of bupivacaine concentration and a lidocaine-epinephrine test dose. *Anesthesiology.* 2000;92:387–392.

116. Massoth C, Wenk M. Epidural test dose in obstetric patients: should we still use it? *Curr Opin Anaesthesiol.* 2019;32:263–267.

117. Kovacheva VP, Brovman EY, Greenberg P, et al. A contemporary analysis of medicolegal issues in obstetric anesthesia between 2005 and 2015. *Anesth Analg.* 2019;128:1199–1207.

118. Norris MC, Ferrenbach D, Dalman H, et al. Does epinephrine improve the diagnostic accuracy of aspiration during labor epidural analgesia? *Anesth Analg.* 1999;88:1073–1076.

119. Khaw KS, Ngan Kee WD, Wong M, et al. Spinal ropivacaine for cesarean delivery: a comparison of hyperbaric and plain solutions. *Anesth Analg.* 2002;94:680–685.

120. Maes S, Laubach M, Poelaert J. Randomised controlled trial of spinal anaesthesia with bupivacaine or 2-chloroprocaine during caesarean section. *Acta Anaesthesiol Scand.* 2016;60:642–649.

121. Kim DH, Kahn R, Lee A, et al. Chloroprocaine provides safe, effective, short-acting spinal anesthesia ideal for ambulatory surgeries: a retrospective review. *HSS J.* 2020;16:280–284.

122. Dahlgren G, Hultstrand C, Jakobsson J, et al. Intrathecal sufentanil, fentanyl, or placebo added to bupivacaine for cesarean section. *Anesth Analg.* 1997;85:1288–1293.

123. Sharpe EE, Molitor RJ, Arendt KW, et al. Intrathecal morphine versus intrathecal hydromorphone for analgesia after cesarean delivery: a randomized clinical trial. *Anesthesiology.* 2020;132:1382–1391.

124. Katz D, Hamburger J, Gutman D, et al. The effect of adding subarachnoid epinephrine to hyperbaric bupivacaine and morphine for repeat cesarean delivery: a double-blind prospective randomized control trial. *Anesth Analg.* 2018;127:171–178.

125. Crespo S, Dangelser G, Haller G. Intrathecal clonidine as an adjuvant for neuraxial anaesthesia during caesarean delivery: a systematic review and meta-analysis of randomised trials. *Int J Obstet Anesth.* 2017;32:64–76.

126. Li XX, Li YM, Lv XL, et al. The efficacy and safety of intrathecal dexmedetomidine for parturients undergoing cesarean section: a double-blind randomized controlled trial. *BMC Anesthesiol.* 2020;20:190.

127. Yousef AA, Salem HA, Moustafa MZ. Effect of mini-dose epidural dexmedetomidine in elective cesarean section using combined spinal-epidural anesthesia: a randomized double-blinded controlled study. *J Anesth.* 2015;29:708–714.

128. Lyons G, Reynolds F. Toxicity and safety of epidural local anaesthetics. *Int J Obstet Anesth.* 2001;10:259–262.

129. Lyons G, Columb M, Wilson RC, Johnson RV. Epidural pain relief in labour: potencies of levobupivacaine and racemic bupivacaine. *Br J Anaesth.* 1998;81:899–901.

130. Beilin Y, Guinn NR, Bernstein HH, et al. Local anesthetics and mode of delivery: bupivacaine versus ropivacaine versus levobupivacaine. *Anesth Analg.* 2007;105:756–763.

131. Camorcia M, Capogna G. Epidural levobupivacaine, ropivacaine and bupivacaine in combination with sufentanil in early labour: a randomized trial. *Eur J Anaesthesiol.* 2003;20:636–639.

132. Lacassie HJ, Habib AS, Lacassie HP, Columb MO. Motor blocking minimum local anesthetic concentrations of bupivacaine, levobupivacaine, and ropivacaine in labor. *Reg Anesth Pain Med.* 2007;32:323–329.

133. Finucane BT. Ropivacaine cardiac toxicity–not as troublesome as bupivacaine. *Can J Anaesth.* 2005;52:449–453.

134. Lam DT, Ngan Kee WD, Khaw KS. Extension of epidural blockade in labour for emergency Caesarean section using 2% lidocaine with epinephrine and fentanyl, with or without alkalinisation. *Anaesthesia.* 2001;56:790–794.

135. Gaiser RR, Cheek TG, Gutsche BB. Epidural lidocaine versus 2-chloroprocaine for fetal distress requiring urgent cesarean section. *Int J Obstet Anesth.* 1994;3:208–210.

136. DiFazio CA, Carron H, Grosslight KR, et al. Comparison of pH-adjusted lidocaine solutions for epidural anesthesia. *Anesth Analg.* 1986;65:760–764.

137. Ackerman WE, Juneja MM, Denson DD, et al. The effect of pH and PCO2 on epidural analgesia with 2% 2-chloroprocaine. *Anesth Analg.* 1989;68:593–598.

138. Choi PT, Galinski SE, Takeuchi L, et al. PDPH is a common complication of neuraxial blockade in parturients: a meta-analysis of obstetrical studies. *Can J Anaesth.* 2003;50:460–469.

139. Angle PJ, Kronberg JE, Thompson DE, et al. Dural tissue trauma and cerebrospinal fluid leak after epidural needle puncture: effect of needle design, angle, and bevel orientation. *Anesthesiology.* 2003;99:1376–1382.

140. Huffnagle SL, Norris MC, Arkoosh VA, et al. The influence of epidural needle bevel orientation on spread of sensory blockade in the laboring parturient. *Anesth Analg.* 1998;87:326–330.

141. Heesen M, Hilber N, Rijs K, et al. Intrathecal catheterisation after observed accidental dural puncture in labouring women: update of a meta-analysis and a trial-sequential analysis. *Int J Obstet Anesth.* 2020;41:71–82.

142. Russell IF. A prospective controlled study of continuous spinal analgesia versus repeat epidural analgesia after accidental dural puncture in labour. *Int J Obstet Anesth.* 2012;21:7–16.

143. Leach A, Smith GB. Subarachnoid spread of epidural local anaesthetic following dural puncture. *Anaesthesia.* 1988;43:671–674.

144. Bernards CM, Kopacz DJ, Michel MZ. Effect of needle puncture on morphine and lidocaine flux through the spinal meninges of the monkey in vitro. Implications for combined spinal-epidural anesthesia. *Anesthesiology.* 1994;80:853–858.

145. Stein MH, Cohen S, Mohiuddin MA, et al. Prophylactic vs therapeutic blood patch for obstetric patients with accidental dural puncture—a randomised controlled trial. *Anaesthesia.* 2014;69:320–326.

146. Scavone BM, Wong CA, Sullivan JT, et al. Efficacy of a prophylactic epidural blood patch in preventing post dural puncture headache in parturients after inadvertent dural puncture. *Anesthesiology.* 2004;101:1422–1427.

147. D'Angelo R, Smiley RM, Riley ET, Segal S. Serious complications related to obstetric anesthesia: the serious complication repository project of the Society for Obstetric Anesthesia and Perinatology. *Anesthesiology.* 2014;120:1505–1512.

148. Szypula K, Ashpole KJ, Bogod D, et al. Litigation related to regional anaesthesia: an analysis of claims against the NHS in England 1995-2007. *Anaesthesia*. 2010;65:443–452.

149. Davies JM, Posner KL, Lee LA, et al. Liability associated with obstetric anesthesia: a closed claims analysis. *Anesthesiology*. 2009;110:131–139.

150. Carvalho B, Mhyre JM. Centers of Excellence for anesthesia care of obstetric patients. *Anesth Analg*. 2019;128:844–846.

151. Ende HB, French B, Shi Y, et al. Implementation of an epidural rounding reminder in the electronic medical record improves performance of standardized patient assessments during labor. *Appl Clin Inform*. 2023;14:238–244.

152. Ende HB, Tran B, Thampy M, et al. Standardization of epidural top-ups for breakthrough labor pain results in a higher proportion of catheter replacements within 30 min of the first bolus dose. *Int J Obstet Anesth*. 2021;47:103161.

153. Collier CB. Why obstetric epidurals fail: a study of epidurograms. *Int J Obstet Anesth*. 1996;5:19–31.

154. Hogan Q. Distribution of solution in the epidural space: examination by cryomicrotome section. *Reg Anesth Pain Med*. 2002;27:150–156.

155. Beilin Y, Zahn J, Bernstein HH, et al. Treatment of incomplete analgesia after placement of an epidural catheter and administration of local anesthetic for women in labor. *Anesthesiology*. 1998;88:1502–1506.

156. Fettes PD, Jansson JR, Wildsmith JA. Failed spinal anaesthesia: mechanisms, management, and prevention. *Br J Anaesth*. 2009;102:739–748.

157. Drasner K, Rigler ML. Repeat injection after a "failed spinal": at times, a potentially unsafe practice. *Anesthesiology*. 1991;75:713–714.

158. Togioka BM, Zarnegarnia Y, Bleyle LA, et al. Pharmacokinetics and tolerability of intraperitoneal chloroprocaine after fetal extraction in women undergoing cesarean delivery. *Anesth Analg*. 2022;135:777–786.

159. Bauer ME, Kountanis JA, Tsen LC, et al. Risk factors for failed conversion of labor epidural analgesia to cesarean delivery anesthesia: a systematic review and meta-analysis of observational trials. *Int J Obstet Anesth*. 2012;21:294–309.

160. Furst SR, Reisner LS. Risk of high spinal anesthesia following failed epidural block for cesarean delivery. *J Clin Anesth*. 1995;7:71–74.

161. Gompels B, Rusby T, Slater N. Fractured epidural catheter with retained fragment in the epidural space—a case study and proposed management algorithm. *BJA Open*. 2022;4:100095.

162. Langevin PB, Gravenstein N, Langevin SO, Gulig PA. Epidural catheter reconnection. Safe and unsafe practice. *Anesthesiology*. 1996;85:883–888.

163. Nixon HC, Stariha J, Farrer J, et al. Resident competency and proficiency in combined spinal-epidural catheter placement is improved using a computer-enhanced visual learning program: a randomized controlled trial. *Anesth Analg*. 2019;128:999–1004.

164. Vaughan N, Dubey VN, Wee MY, Isaacs R. A review of epidural simulators: where are we today? *Med Eng Phys*. 2013;35:1235–1250.

165. Raj D, Williamson RM, Young D, Russell D. A simple epidural simulator: a blinded study assessing the 'feel' of loss of resistance in four fruits. *Eur J Anaesthesiol*. 2013;30:405–408.

166. Chuan A, Graham PL, Wong DM, et al. Design and validation of the regional anaesthesia procedural skills assessment tool. *Anaesthesia*. 2015;70:1401–1411.

167. Kopacz DJ, Neal JM, Pollock JE. The regional anesthesia "learning curve". What is the minimum number of epidural and spinal blocks to reach consistency? *Reg Anesth*. 1996;21:182–190.

13

Local Anesthetics and Opioids

Ban Leong Sng, MBBS and Hon Sen Tan, MD, MMed, MHSc

CHAPTER OUTLINE

Local anesthetics and opioids are often used for pain relief in obstetric practice. Local anesthetics may be used for infiltration anesthesia or neuraxial block, whereas opioids are administered both systemically and neuraxially. The physiologic changes that occur during pregnancy may affect the pharmacology of both local anesthetics and opioids and may result in clinical effects on the mother and fetus.

LOCAL ANESTHETICS

Molecular Structure

All local anesthetics except cocaine contain an unsaturated carbon ring (aromatic portion), a tertiary amine, and an intermediate alkyl chain (Fig. 13.1). The intermediate alkyl chain is connected to the aromatic portion by either an ester or amide linkage and is the basis for the classification of local anesthetics as **amino-esters**, which are hydrolyzed by pseudocholinesterase, and **amino-amides**, which undergo hepatic microsomal metabolism (Table 13.1). The aromatic ring is a derivative of benzoic acid in amino-ester local anesthetics, while amino-amides contain an aniline homolog aromatic ring. The tertiary-amine confers properties of weak bases to local anesthetics by acting as a proton acceptor, and also increases water solubility when in its quaternary (i.e., "protonated") form. The Henderson-Hasselbalch equation predicts the relative proportions of local anesthetic that exist in the ionized (water-soluble) and un-ionized (water-insoluble) form. The lower the pK_a (acid dissociation constant) relative to physiologic pH, the greater the proportion of drug that exists in the un-ionized form. As the rate of diffusion across cell membranes is related to the proportion of un-ionized drug, local anesthetics with low pK_a have a faster onset of action than those with higher pK_a.

Clinical formulations of local anesthetics are prepared as hydrochloride salts to increase their solubility in water. These formulations are usually acidic (i.e., pH of 4 to 6) to enhance formation of the water-soluble quaternary tertiary-amine and to prevent oxidation of epinephrine, if present.

Enantiomers

With the exception of lidocaine, amino-amide local anesthetics are **enantiomeric compounds**, which exist as two or more compounds with the same molecular formula but are nonsuperimposable mirror images of each other. In the case of amino-amide local anesthetics, the single asymmetric carbon adjacent to the amino group results in two isomeric forms that are mirror images of each other. Enantiomers are classified by two naming conventions. The R/S system classifies enantiomers by their molecular geometry according to the Cahn-Ingold-Prelog priority rules. Alternatively, enantiomers can be classified based on their optical rotation properties, the direction in which the enantiomers rotate plane-polarized light. Enantiomers that rotate plane-polarized light clockwise are denoted as (+) or dextrorotatory, while those that rotate plane-polarized light anticlockwise are denoted (−) or levorotatory. This distinction is important because individual isomers of the same drug may have different biologic effects.

As a rule, the levorotatory isomer of a drug has greater vasoconstrictor activity and a longer duration of action, but less potential for systemic toxicity than the dextrorotatory form.[1]

In the past, local anesthetics contained a racemic (50:50) mixture of both dextrorotatory and levorotatory forms of the drug. However, with improved techniques of selective extraction, two commercially available single-isomer formulations of local anesthetic, ropivacaine and levobupivacaine, are now available. **Levobupivacaine** is the levorotatory isomer of bupivacaine; it is currently not marketed in the United States. **Ropivacaine** is a homolog of bupivacaine that is formulated as a single levorotatory isomer rather than as a racemic mixture.

The reduction in systemic toxicity observed with administration of the levorotatory isomers may be both drug and concentration dependent. For example, one study in isolated guinea pig hearts noted that bupivacaine isomers lengthened atrioventricular conduction time more than ropivacaine isomers did. In contrast to other measured variables, "atrioventricular conduction time showed evident stereoselectivity"

for bupivacaine at the lowest concentration studied (0.5 µM) but only at much higher concentrations for ropivacaine (>30 µM).[2]

Mechanism of Action

Local anesthetics act by inhibiting action potentials in excitable tissues, thereby blocking the transmission of pain impulses. At rest, the interior of a nerve cell is negatively charged in relation to its exterior. This resting potential of 60 to 90 mV exists because the concentration of positively charged sodium ions in the extracellular space greatly exceeds that in the intracellular space, while negatively charged ions such as proteins remain within the cell. The converse is true for potassium, with the intracellular concentration far exceeding that of the extracellular space. Excitation results in the opening of sodium membrane channels, which allows sodium ions to flow freely down their concentration gradient into the cell interior. Thus, the electrical potential within the nerve cell becomes less negative until, at the critical threshold of −55 mV, an action potential is generated by opening of voltage-gated sodium channels, permitting rapid influx of sodium into the cell. This depolarization initiates the same sequence of events in adjacent membrane segments, thus propagating the action potential downstream. Thereafter, sodium channels close and the membrane once again becomes impermeable to the influx of sodium. The negative resting membrane potential is reestablished as sodium-potassium pumps remove sodium from the cell by active transport, while increasing potassium levels within the resting cell.

Interference with sodium-ion conductance appears to be the mechanism by which local anesthetics reversibly inhibit the propagation of the action potential (Fig. 13.2).[3] Lipophilic (un-ionized) local anesthetic molecules cross the neuronal cell membrane and an equilibrium of ionized and un-ionized molecules is established intracellularly, dependent on the intracellular pH and pK$_a$ of the local anesthetic. Next, ionized molecules reversibly bind to voltage-gated sodium channels and inhibit their opening, thereby suppressing the generation of action potentials.

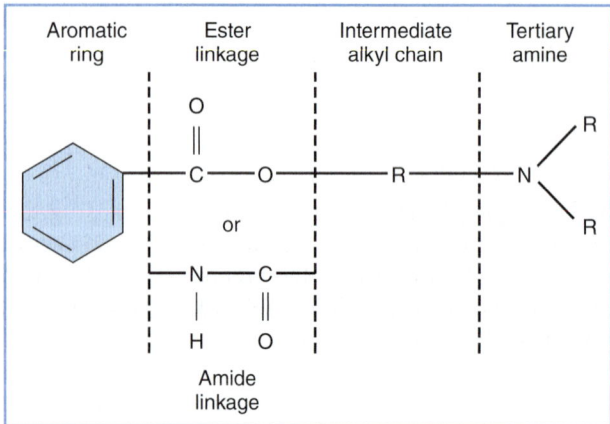

Fig. 13.1 Structure of the Molecule of a Local Anesthetic. *R*, Alkyl group. Modified from Santos AC, Pedersen H. Local anesthetics in obstetrics. In: Petrie RH, ed. *Perinatal Pharmacology*. Blackwell Scientific; 1989:373.

TABLE 13.1	**Physicochemical Characteristics and Fetal-to-Maternal (F/M) Blood Concentration Ratios at Delivery for Commonly Used Local Anesthetic Agents**				
	Molecular Weight (Base) (Da)	pK$_a$	Lipid Solubility[a]	% Protein Bound	F/M Ratio
Esters					
2-Chloroprocaine	271	8.9	0.14	—	—
Tetracaine	264	8.6	4.1	—	—
Amides					
Lidocaine	234	7.9	2.9	64	0.5–0.7
Bupivacaine (and levobupivacaine)	288	8.2	28	96	0.2–0.4
Ropivacaine	274	8.0	3	90–95	0.2

[a]*N*-heptane/pH = 7.4 buffer.
Modified from Santos AC, Pedersen H. Local anesthetics in obstetrics. In: Petrie RH, ed. *Perinatal Pharmacology*. Blackwell Scientific; 1989:375.

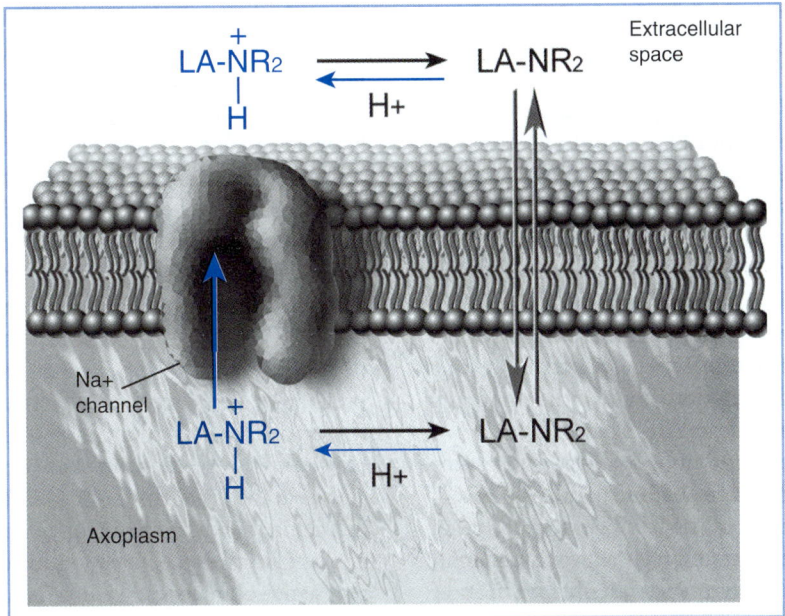

Fig. 13.2 Local Anesthetic Access to the Sodium Channel. The uncharged molecule (LA-NR$_2$) diffuses most easily across the lipid membrane and interacts with the sodium channel at an intramembranous site. The charged molecule (LA-NR$_2$H+) gains access to a specific receptor on the sodium channel in the intracellular space. Illustration by Naveen Nathan, MD, NorthShore University HealthSystem, University of Chicago Pritzker School of Medicine, Evanston, IL.

Pharmacodynamics

Pregnant women typically require smaller doses of local anesthetic than nonpregnant women for neuraxial blockade. This effect may be evident as early as the second trimester[4,5] and has been attributed to enhanced spread of local anesthetic caused by epidural venous engorgement. However, mechanical effects alone do not account for the observation that the spread of spinal and epidural analgesia in early pregnancy is similar to that in pregnant women at term.[4–6] Pregnancy may also enhance neuronal sensitivity to local anesthetics. For example, median nerve susceptibility to lidocaine was shown to increase during pregnancy.[7] Furthermore, in vitro studies demonstrated that the onset of neural blockade was faster, and lower concentrations of bupivacaine were required to block vagal fibers in pregnant compared to nonpregnant rabbits.[8]

Hormonal and biochemical changes may be responsible for the greater susceptibility to neural blockade during pregnancy. It has been speculated that these hormonal effects may be caused by progesterone or its metabolites since an enhanced effect of bupivacaine in isolated vagus fibers from nonpregnant, ovariectomized rabbits only occurred after long-term (4 days) but not short-term exposure to progesterone.[9] Moreover, the pH of cerebrospinal fluid (CSF) of pregnant women is higher, and the bicarbonate and total carbon dioxide content are lower, compared with age-matched nonpregnant controls; this may increase the proportion of local anesthetic that exists in the un-ionized form and facilitate diffusion of the drug across nerve membranes.[6]

Pharmacokinetics

Pregnancy is associated with progressive physiologic adaptations that may influence drug disposition (see Chapter 2).

However, it is difficult to predict with certainty the effects of pregnancy on the pharmacokinetics of an individual drug.

2-Chloroprocaine

2-Chloroprocaine is hydrolyzed rapidly by plasma pseudocholinesterase to chloroaminobenzoic acid and water. Although pregnancy is associated with a 30% to 40% decrease in pseudocholinesterase activity, the half-life of 2-chloroprocaine in maternal plasma in vitro is 11 to 21 seconds. After epidural injection, the half-life of 2-chloroprocaine in the mother ranges from 1.5 to 6.4 minutes.[10] The longer half-life after epidural administration results from continued absorption of the drug from the injection site. Administration of 2-chloroprocaine to patients with low pseudocholinesterase activity may result in prolonged local anesthetic effect and a greater potential for systemic toxicity.[11]

Lidocaine

The volume of the central compartment and the volume of distribution of lidocaine are greater in pregnant than in nonpregnant ewes.[12,13] Bloedow et al.[13] observed that the total body clearance of lidocaine was similar in the two groups of animals but the elimination half-life of lidocaine, which depends on the balance between volume of distribution and clearance, was longer in pregnant ewes.[13] In contrast, Santos et al.[12] concluded that the elimination half-life of lidocaine was similar in the two groups of sheep because the total body clearance of the drug was greater in pregnant than in nonpregnant animals. This discrepancy could result from differences in the complexity of the surgical preparation and the allowed recovery period. In pregnant women, the elimination half-life of lidocaine after epidural injection is approximately 114 minutes.[14]

Lidocaine is metabolized into two active compounds: monoethylglycinexylidide (MEGX) and glycinexylidide (GX). MEGX can be detected in maternal plasma within 10 to 20 minutes after neuraxial injection of lidocaine, whereas GX can be detected within 1 hour of epidural injection but rarely after subarachnoid injection.[15,16] Urinary excretion of unchanged lidocaine is negligible in sheep (i.e., less than 2% of the administered dose) and is not affected by pregnancy.[12]

The physiologic changes that occur during pregnancy are progressive. However, little information is available about the pharmacokinetics of local anesthetics before term. In one study, total clearance of lidocaine was similar at 119 and 138 days' gestation in gravid ewes (term is 148 days).[17]

Lidocaine is predominantly bound to alpha$_1$-acid glycoprotein (AAG) in plasma.[18] Given that pregnancy leads to a decreased concentration of AAG; the free plasma fraction of lidocaine tends to be higher in term pregnant women than in nonpregnant controls.[18] This increase in the free fraction of lidocaine occurs early in gestation and is progressive.[19]

Bupivacaine

At least two studies compared the pharmacokinetics of bupivacaine after epidural administration in pregnant and non-pregnant women.[20,21] The absorption rate, area under the concentration-time curve, and elimination half-life (12 to 13 hours) were similar in the two groups. The elimination half-life of bupivacaine after epidural administration is much longer than that after intravenous injection, largely because the drug is continuously absorbed over time from the epidural space.

In contrast to lidocaine,[12,13] the volume of distribution of bupivacaine is lower in pregnant than in nonpregnant sheep after intravenous injection.[21] The differences in gestational effects on the volume of distribution of the two local anesthetics may result from the greater binding of bupivacaine to plasma proteins during gestation (whereas the converse occurs with lidocaine).[21] In one study, urinary excretion of unchanged bupivacaine was not affected by pregnancy and was less than 1% of the administered dose.[20] Nonetheless, low concentrations of bupivacaine may be detected in the urine of pregnant women for as long as 3 days after delivery.[22]

Bupivacaine undergoes dealkylation in the liver to 2,6-pipecolyxylidide (PPX). After epidural injection of bupivacaine for cesarean delivery, PPX was detected in maternal plasma within 5 minutes and remained detectable for as long as 24 hours.[22] With the lower doses required for labor analgesia, PPX was found only if the block was maintained with multiple reinjections during a period that exceeded 4 hours.[23]

Pregnancy may affect metabolism of bupivacaine.[20] For example, pregnant women have higher serum PPX concentrations, but the unconjugated 4-hydroxy metabolite is not produced in significant amounts. The reason for this finding is unclear but may be related to effects of hormonal changes on hepatic enzyme systems. Both progesterone and estradiol are competitive inhibitors of microsomal oxidases, whereas reductive enzymes are induced by progesterone.[21]

Bupivacaine is bound extensively to AAG and albumin.[24] This protein binding is reduced during late pregnancy in humans.[25]

Long-acting pipechol amide local anesthetics, such as bupivacaine, are beneficial for neuraxial labor analgesia because they produce a relative motor-sparing block compared with other local anesthetics. The effective dose in 50% of cases (ED$_{50}$) for motor block after intrathecally administered bupivacaine was lower in pregnant than in nonpregnant women (3.96 and 4.14 mg, respectively).[26]

Ropivacaine

Pregnant sheep have a smaller volume of distribution and a slower clearance of ropivacaine than nonpregnant animals.[21] However, the relationship between volume of distribution and clearance is such that the elimination half-life is similar in pregnant and nonpregnant animals.

After intravenous injection in laboratory animals or non-pregnant volunteers, the elimination half-life of ropivacaine is shorter than that of bupivacaine.[21,27] The shorter elimination half-life of ropivacaine has been attributed to a faster clearance and a shorter mean residence time than that of bupivacaine.[21]

Peak plasma concentration (C$_{max}$) of 0.5% ropivacaine and 0.5% bupivacaine after epidural administration for cesarean delivery are similar (1.3 and 1.1 µg/mL, respectively).[28] The mean (± standard deviation [SD]) elimination half-life of ropivacaine is 5.2 ± 0.6 hours, which is shorter than that for bupivacaine (10.9 ± 1.1 hours). No difference in clearance between the two drugs has been noted.

Like bupivacaine, ropivacaine is metabolized by hepatic microsomal cytochrome P450. The major metabolite is PPX, and minor metabolites are 3'- and 4'-hydroxy-ropivacaine.[29]

Ropivacaine is highly bound (approximately 92%) to plasma proteins but less so than bupivacaine (96%).[30] Indeed, at plasma concentrations occurring during epidural anesthesia for cesarean delivery, the free fraction of ropivacaine is almost twice that of bupivacaine.[28] In pregnant women undergoing epidural analgesia, the free fraction of ropivacaine decreases as the concentration of AAG increases, up to the point at which the receptors are saturated.[31] However, there is little correlation between the free fraction and umbilical cord blood levels of ropivacaine at delivery.[31]

Extended-Release Local Anesthetics

The increasing demand for opioid-sparing analgesic techniques and rapid functional recovery have spurred development of extended-release local anesthetics aimed at providing sustained postoperative analgesia. Examples include Exparel (Pacira Pharmaceuticals, United States) and Zynrelef (HTX-011, Heron Therapeutics, United States).

Exparel consists of a preservative-free aqueous suspension of bupivacaine encapsulated within multivesicular liposomes (DepoFoam) at a nominal concentration of 13.3 mg/mL (liposomal bupivacaine). It is approved by the US Food and Drug Administration (FDA) for single-dose interscalene brachial plexus and sciatic nerve blocks, adductor canal blocks, and local infiltration.[32] The maximum recommended dose of liposomal bupivacaine for local infiltration is 266 mg (20 mL). Plasma levels of liposomal bupivacaine follow a bimodal distribution. The first plasma peak occurs within an hour after drug infiltration followed by a second peak approximately 12 to 36 hours later, although the rate of systemic absorption depends on multiple factors, including drug dose and vascularity of the administration site.[32,33] After bupivacaine is released from the liposomes and absorbed within the systemic circulation, its distribution and elimination are expected to mimic standard bupivacaine formulations.[32] Mixture of liposomal bupivacaine with water, hypotonic agents, or other local anesthetics is not recommended as these can disrupt the liposomal particles, resulting in rapid bupivacaine release.

Despite the prolonged sustained release of bupivacaine, the clinical superiority of liposomal bupivacaine over standard bupivacaine for postcesarean delivery analgesia is unclear (see Chapter 27). A systematic review comparing liposomal bupivacaine with standard bupivacaine for a heterogeneous mix of surgeries, including abdominal and orthopedic surgery, with the local anesthetic administered by varying routes including local infiltration, reported that liposomal bupivacaine was associated with statistically significantly lower mean pain score difference (−0.37 on numerical rating scale 0 to 10; 95% confidence interval [CI], −0.56 to −0.19) and opioid consumption reported in intravenous morphine equivalents ratio of means (0.85; 95% CI, 0.82 to 0.89) at 24 hours.[34] However, at 72 hours no significant reduction in mean pain score (−0.25; 95% CI, −0.71 to 0.20) was detected, although the ratio of morphine equivalents was significantly lower in patients who received liposomal bupivacaine (0.85; 95% CI, 0.77 to 0.95) than standard bupivacaine. The clinical relevance of these differences was questioned by the authors.[34]

Randomized trials suggest that transversus abdominis plane (TAP) block with liposomal bupivacaine may improve postcesarean delivery analgesia.[35,36] A multicenter randomized trial comparing TAP blocks with liposomal bupivacaine 266 mg plus bupivacaine 50 mg versus bupivacaine 50 mg alone after elective cesarean delivery under spinal anesthesia with intrathecal morphine 0.15 mg reported that the former regimen significantly reduced opioid consumption through 72 hours.[35] A second randomized trial comparing TAP block with liposomal bupivacaine 266 mg, intrathecal morphine 0.05 mg plus TAP block with liposomal bupivacaine 266 mg, and intrathecal morphine 0.15 mg alone reported that TAP block with liposomal bupivacaine resulted in noninferior opioid consumption through 72 hours and a lower incidence of adverse events compared to TAP block plus intrathecal morphine or intrathecal morphine alone.[36] Additional studies are warranted to determine the optimal dose of liposomal bupivacaine and whether there is a true benefit if the patient also receives intrathecal morphine.

Bupivacaine transfer into breast milk following TAP block with bupivacaine 52 mg plus liposomal bupivacaine 266 mg resulted in relative neonatal doses of less than 1% (<10% is considered to be acceptable by the FDA).[37]

Zynrelef is a formulation of slow-release bupivacaine combined with meloxicam, a nonsteroidal antiinflammatory drug (NSAID), encapsulated within a biodegradable polymer (Biochronomer). Slow-release bupivacaine-meloxicam is FDA-approved in adults for soft tissue or periarticular administration after bunionectomy, open inguinal herniorrhaphy, and total knee arthroplasty.[38] The pharmacokinetics, safety, and efficacy of slow-release bupivacaine-meloxicam for postcesarean delivery analgesia are still being investigated.

Effects of Preeclampsia

Pathophysiologic changes associated with preeclampsia (e.g., reduced hepatic blood flow, abnormal liver function, decreased intravascular volume) may also affect maternal blood concentrations of local anesthetics (see Chapter 35). For example, Ramanathan et al.[39] found that total body clearance of lidocaine after epidural injection was significantly lower in women with preeclampsia than in normotensive women; however, the elimination half-life of lidocaine was similar in the two groups. Nonetheless, decreased clearance may result in greater drug accumulation with repeated injections of lidocaine in women with preeclampsia. In contrast, long-acting amides have a relatively low hepatic extraction and changes in liver blood flow with preeclampsia may have less effect on the metabolic clearance.

Effect of Gestational Diabetes Mellitus

Gestational diabetes mellitus may have profound transient effects on the microcirculation. The placental transfer of lidocaine was unchanged for women at term with diabetes who received epidural lidocaine 200 mg, but the transfer of its metabolite, MEGX, was increased.[40] A weakness of the methodology was that umbilical artery/vein ratios were used to estimate placental transfer (see later).

Effect of Diurnal Variation

Pain may exhibit temporal variation in intensity because of diurnal neuroendocrine or external factors. In one study, the duration of action of epidural bupivacaine was approximately 25% longer when it was administered between 7:00 a.m. and 7:00 p.m. than between 7:00 p.m. and 7:00 a.m.[41] In contrast, another study found no diurnal variation with intrathecal bupivacaine administered for labor analgesia.[42] The authors suggested the diurnal variation may also be explained by external influences such as shift changes for nurses and anesthesiologists.[42]

Effect of Injectate Temperature

Latency of local anesthetic may be affected by temperature. For instance, onset of labor analgesia is faster when a solution of epidural bupivacaine 0.125% with fentanyl 2 µg/mL is injected at 37°C compared with 20°C.[43]

Toxicity

Systemic absorption or intravascular injection of a local anesthetic may result in **local anesthetic systemic toxicity**

(LAST). Toxicity most often involves the central nervous system (CNS), but cardiovascular toxicity also may occur. Less common are tissue toxicity and hypersensitivity reactions.

Central Nervous System Toxicity

The majority of LAST cases first present with CNS signs and symptoms.[44] Generally, the severity of CNS effects is proportional to the blood concentration of local anesthetic.[45] This relationship is well described for lidocaine (Fig. 13.3) and is classically described as a two-stage process of CNS excitation followed by depression.[46] Initially, the patient presents with prodromal symptoms such as numbness of the tongue, tinnitus, lightheadedness, or perioral numbness.[44] At high plasma concentrations, seizures occur because of a selective blockade of central inhibitory neurons that leads to increased CNS excitation.[47] At still higher concentrations, generalized CNS depression or coma may result from reversible blockade of both inhibitory and excitatory neuronal pathways. Finally, depression of the brainstem and cardiorespiratory centers may occur. However, it is important to note that LAST may not always present in this classical fashion when prodromal symptoms precede seizures, CNS depression, and cardiovascular toxicity. Instead, many cases of LAST first present with seizures or features of combined CNS and cardiovascular toxicity.[44] Hence, providers should remain vigilant for atypical manifestations, and any abnormal neurologic or cardiovascular signs and symptoms following local anesthetic administration should raise suspicion of LAST.

The relative CNS toxicity of a local anesthetic correlates with its potency. For lidocaine and bupivacaine, the ratio of the mean cumulative doses that cause seizures in dogs and human volunteers is approximately 4:1, which is similar to their relative anesthetic potencies.[48] Local anesthetics may be ranked in order of decreasing CNS toxicity as follows: bupivacaine, ropivacaine, levobupivacaine, lidocaine, and 2-chloroprocaine.[49]

Other factors (e.g., the speed of injection) may affect CNS toxicity,[50] and metabolic factors may also affect the seizure threshold. For example, in cats, an increase in $PaCO_2$ or a decrease in pH results in a reduction in the seizure-dose threshold for local anesthetics. Respiratory acidosis may result in delivery of more drug to the brain; alternatively, respiratory acidosis may result in "ion trapping" of the local anesthetic and/or an increase in the unbound fraction of drug available for pharmacologic effect.[51,52]

Cardiovascular Toxicity

Cardiovascular toxicity classically occurs in three phases. The first phase includes hypertension and tachycardia, followed by myocardial depression and hypotension. The terminal phase typically involves vasodilation, severe hypotension, and arrhythmias, including conduction blocks, tachyarrhythmias, and asystole.[46]

The cardiovascular system is typically much more resistant than the CNS to the toxic effects of local anesthetics. Severe, direct cardiovascular depression is rare, especially in association with the use of lidocaine. Prompt administration of oxygen and, if necessary, initiation of ventilatory and circulatory support usually prevent cardiac arrest after unintentional intravenous injection of lidocaine,[53] with progressive depression of myocardial function and profound vasodilation occurring only at extremely high plasma concentrations.[53] In contrast, the more potent amide local anesthetics (i.e., bupivacaine) have a narrower margin of safety, expressed as the ratio between the dose (or plasma concentration) required to produce cardiovascular collapse (CC) and the dose (or plasma concentration) required to produce seizures, termed the CC/CNS ratio.[53]

Specific Local Anesthetic Drugs and Systemic Toxicity

In general, agents with higher CC/CNS ratio have a greater margin of safety as earlier presentation of CNS features may facilitate diagnosis and treatment of LAST before cardiovascular collapse occurs. For instance, the greater cardiotoxicity of bupivacaine compared to lidocaine is reflected in CC/CNS ratios of 2 versus 7, respectively.[46]

A partial explanation for this discrepancy in cardiotoxicity may lie in the fact that supraconvulsant doses of bupivacaine (but not of lidocaine) precipitate lethal ventricular arrhythmias.[54,55] These arrhythmias may be caused by exaggerated electrophysiologic effects (e.g., depression of ventricular conduction) out of proportion to bupivacaine's anesthetic potency.[56] Two theories have been proposed to explain why malignant ventricular arrhythmias occur with bupivacaine but not with lidocaine. Both bupivacaine and lidocaine rapidly block cardiac sodium channels during systole, but bupivacaine dissociates from these channels during diastole at a much slower rate than lidocaine.[56] Thus, at physiologic heart rates, the diastolic period is of sufficient duration for lidocaine to dissociate from sodium channels,

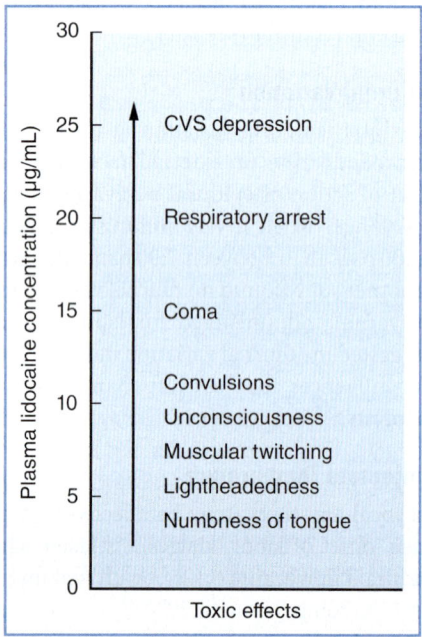

Fig. 13.3 Signs and Symptoms of Systemic Toxicity With Increasing Lidocaine Concentrations. *CVS,* Cardiovascular system. Modified from Carpenter RL, Mackey DC. Local anesthetics. In: Barash PG, Cullen BF, Stoelting RK, eds. *Clinical Anesthesia.* Lippincott; 1992:527.

whereas a bupivacaine block becomes intensified. This difference makes bupivacaine much more potent than lidocaine in depressing conduction and inducing reentrant-type ventricular arrhythmias. Alternatively, other investigators have suggested that high concentrations of local anesthetic in the brainstem may lead to systemic hypotension, bradycardia, and ventricular arrhythmias.[57] These effects occur more commonly with bupivacaine because of its high lipid solubility, which facilitates transfer across the blood-brain barrier. An echocardiographic study in anesthetized dogs suggested that bolus injection of bupivacaine results in systolic dysfunction, especially involving the right ventricle, which precedes the occurrence of arrhythmias.[58]

Systemic Toxicity of Ropivacaine and Levobupivacaine

In vitro, ropivacaine is intermediate between bupivacaine and lidocaine in its depressant effect on cardiac excitation and conduction as well as in its potential to induce reentrant-type ventricular arrhythmias.[30,59] In dogs, the margin of safety between convulsive or lethal doses and plasma concentrations of drug is greater for ropivacaine than for bupivacaine but less than that for lidocaine.[59] The arrhythmogenicity of ropivacaine in pigs also is intermediate between that of lidocaine and bupivacaine.[60] In sheep, the ratio of fatal doses of bupivacaine, ropivacaine, and lidocaine is 1:2:9.[61] Ropivacaine was found to cause fewer CNS symptoms and was 25% less toxic than bupivacaine (as defined by the doses and plasma concentrations that were tolerated) when administered to healthy male volunteers.[62]

However, studies comparing the systemic toxicity of ropivacaine and bupivacaine have used equal doses of each, and, therefore, cannot resolve the controversy as to whether ropivacaine truly is less cardiotoxic or merely less potent than bupivacaine. This issue is of concern only if larger doses of ropivacaine than bupivacaine are required to produce comparable regional block density. Indeed, several studies in laboring women suggest that epidural ropivacaine is 25% to 40% less potent than bupivacaine.[63–65] Thus, the need for a larger dose of ropivacaine may negate the expected benefits of its wider margin of safety. Long-acting amide local anesthetics—even the newer drugs—are very potent and may cause cardiac arrest with an unintentional intravascular injection or relative overdose. Indeed, cardiac arrest has been reported with the use of ropivacaine,[66,67] including one in a woman undergoing a cesarean delivery with epidural anesthesia.[68] However, in contrast to bupivacaine,[69] resuscitation from a cardiac arrest induced by ropivacaine may be successful more often than not.[66–68]

Evidence suggests that levobupivacaine causes fewer arrhythmias than the racemic drug. Levobupivacaine caused less inhibition of inactivated sodium channels than either the dextrorotatory or racemic drug.[70] In comparison with dextrorotatory and racemic bupivacaine, levobupivacaine resulted in less QRS widening and a lower frequency of malignant ventricular arrhythmias in isolated, perfused rabbit hearts.[71] Similarly, levobupivacaine produced less second-degree heart block and atrioventricular conduction delay than the other two forms of the drug in isolated perfused guinea pig hearts.[2]

In laboratory animals, the systemic toxicity of levobupivacaine is intermediate between that of bupivacaine and ropivacaine.[72] Potency ratio data for epidural bupivacaine, ropivacaine, and levobupivacaine in laboring women are inconsistent, but studies suggest that levobupivacaine is equipotent or slightly less potent than bupivacaine (see Chapter 24).[73,74] Altogether, published data and clinical experience suggest that the benefit of a lower risk for systemic toxicity with levobupivacaine is not obtained at the expense of efficacy. Like ropivacaine, levobupivacaine may cause cardiac arrest but is associated with a better response to resuscitation than racemic bupivacaine.[75]

Effects of Pregnancy on Systemic Toxicity

Central nervous system toxicity. Pregnancy-related hormones, such as estradiol and progesterone, have a neuroprotective effect in laboratory animals.[76] It is unclear whether pregnancy lowers the seizure threshold for amide local anesthetic agents. In one study, seizures occurred at lower doses of bupivacaine, levobupivacaine, and ropivacaine in pregnant than in nonpregnant ewes.[72] However, the difference was small (10% to 15%) and probably of negligible clinical significance. In studies in sheep and rats, pregnancy did not reduce the doses required to cause seizures after intravenous administration of mepivacaine, bupivacaine, or lidocaine.[55] Magnesium sulfate, which is frequently used in obstetric practice, does not affect the seizure-dose threshold of lidocaine.[77]

Cardiovascular toxicity. In 1979, Albright[69] alerted anesthesiologists to several cases of sudden and immediate cardiovascular collapse after unintentional intravascular injection of bupivacaine and etidocaine in pregnant women. Most of these cases were fatal, and subsequent controversy centered on whether resuscitation was instituted promptly and effectively or whether the cardiovascular collapse and inability to resuscitate were unique to bupivacaine. Nonetheless, the FDA restricted the use of the highest concentration (0.75%) of bupivacaine in pregnant women.

Several physiologic changes that occur during pregnancy place the parturient at higher risk for refractory cardiac arrest than the nonpregnant patient. First, reduced functional residual capacity and a higher metabolic rate hasten the onset of hypoxemia during periods of hypoventilation or apnea. Second, aortocaval compression decreases the efficacy of closed-chest cardiac massage in the supine position.[78] Third, a large bolus of drug injected into an epidural vein might reach the heart rapidly through a dilated azygous system. However, none of these factors adequately explains why cardiac arrest and difficult resuscitation are rare in parturients intoxicated with lidocaine or mepivacaine.[69,79]

Results of laboratory studies of the effects of pregnancy on bupivacaine cardiotoxicity are contradictory. Pregnancy-related hormones enhance the cardiotoxicity and arrhythmogenicity of bupivacaine *in vitro*.[80,81] For example, the magnitude and severity of bupivacaine-induced electrophysiologic changes are greater in myocardium obtained from nonpregnant rabbits treated with progesterone or beta-estradiol than in myocardium from untreated controls.[80,81] The electrophysiologic effects of lidocaine are less pronounced than those of bupivacaine, even in hormonally treated animals. Studies conducted *in vivo* have been less conclusive. In earlier investigations, significantly lower doses and plasma concentrations of bupivacaine, but not of mepivacaine or lidocaine, were required to produce circulatory collapse in pregnant than in nonpregnant sheep.[54,55] However, a study involving a larger number of sheep and more rigorous methods (e.g., randomization, blinding) failed to confirm that pregnancy enhances the cardiotoxicity of bupivacaine.[72] Progesterone does not increase myocardial sensitivity to ropivacaine.[82] Likewise, pregnancy does not enhance the systemic toxicity of ropivacaine or levobupivacaine in sheep.[72]

Extrapolation of results of animal studies to obstetric anesthesia practice is difficult, for several reasons. First, in the aforementioned sheep studies, the drug was administered by constant-rate intravenous infusion. In contrast, in pregnant women intoxicated with bupivacaine, cardiac arrest occurred after unintended intravascular injection of a large bolus of drug. Second, a potential for bias existed in the animal studies because randomization and blinding were not used in all studies and some relied on historical controls.[54,55] Third, it is unclear whether resuscitation in the reported clinical cases was accompanied by prompt and effective relief of aortocaval compression.[1,78]

Nonetheless, bupivacaine remains a popular local anesthetic for obstetric anesthesia. In current practice, heightened vigilance, use of an appropriate test dose, and fractionation of the therapeutic dose have made epidural anesthesia a safe technique for use in obstetric patients (see Chapter 12). Although LAST has been recognized for decades as an important potential cause of maternal mortality,[83] Hawkins et al.[84] noted that the number of maternal deaths resulting from LAST decreased after 1984, the year that the FDA withdrew approval for the epidural administration of 0.75% bupivacaine in obstetric patients. However, adherence to the aforementioned clinical precautions—rather than the proscription against the epidural administration of 0.75% bupivacaine (see Box 12.3)—is likely to be responsible for the lower number of maternal deaths caused by LAST. Anesthesia providers should be aware that intravenous injection of 0.25% and 0.5% bupivacaine can also cause LAST.

The availability of single levorotatory isomers of a local anesthetic may be advantageous because these drugs have a greater margin of safety than bupivacaine, with similar blocking properties, although at a higher cost. From the standpoint of systemic toxicity, the use of these isoforms may be more beneficial in parturients undergoing cesarean delivery, who require higher doses than administered for analgesia during labor. Nonetheless, a greater margin of safety with these new drugs should not be a substitute for proper technique.

Effects of Medical Comorbidity on Systemic Toxicity

Patients with cardiac disease may be at increased risk of LAST. In particular, those with preexisting conduction disorders may be susceptible to cardiovascular toxicity, while patients with cardiac dysfunction may be predisposed to local anesthetic–induced myocardial depression and arrhythmias.[46] Careful dosing and the use of less cardiotoxic agents may be considered.

In contrast, severe renal disease is typically associated with hyperdynamic circulation and reduced local anesthetic clearance, but increased AAG concentration. Hence, free plasma concentration of local anesthetics is largely unchanged and dose reduction is usually not required unless metabolic acidosis is present.[85]

Hepatic disease may reduce the clearance of local anesthetics, but this effect is mitigated by a larger volume of distribution and maintenance of AAG concentration. Dose adjustment may be considered in patients receiving multiple local anesthetic boluses or continuous infusion, and in those with cardiac and renal comorbidities.[85]

Effects of Block Type on Systemic Toxicity

Available evidence suggest that the risk of LAST varies with the type of block, with infiltration techniques and epidural blocks most commonly implicated.[44,86] This may be attributed to the dose of local anesthetic administered and site vascularity. For instance, fascial plane blocks such as the TAP block involve large volumes of local anesthetic administered into the intermuscular plane in contact with highly vascularized muscle tissue. It was reported that bilateral ultrasound-guided TAP blocks with bupivacaine following cesarean delivery may result in toxic plasma bupivacaine concentrations.[87]

Continuous local anesthetic infusion via a nerve catheter has also been associated with increased risk of LAST. Following nonobstetric abdominal surgery, bilateral TAP blocks with ropivacaine 100 mg per side and 10 mL/h infusion of 0.2% ropivacaine resulted in some patients exceeding toxic total plasma concentration thresholds, although unbound ropivacaine concentrations were much lower, possibly due to perioperative increase in AAG levels.[88]

Treatment of Systemic Toxicity

Meticulous attention to good technique and adherence to guidelines for maximum recommended dose are critical. (The use of a test dose to identify misplaced epidural catheters is discussed in Chapter 12.) Incremental injection of the therapeutic dose, use of the lowest effective dose, careful observation of the patient, and monitoring of vital signs may facilitate early detection and treatment of an impending reaction. In 2020, the American Society of Regional Anesthesia and Pain Medicine updated their checklist for managing LAST (see Chapter 24).[89]

Tissue Toxicity

Neurologic complications of neuraxial anesthesia are rare and result mostly from direct neural trauma, infection, injection of toxic doses of local anesthetic, or the injection of the wrong drug.

Several cases of prolonged or permanent sensory and motor deficits after subarachnoid injection of a large dose of 2-chloroprocaine intended for epidural block have been described.[90] Studies comparing the neurotoxicity of 2-chloroprocaine with that of other local anesthetics have yielded conflicting results, most likely related to the use of different methodologies and different species.[91,92] It has been suggested that neurotoxicity was caused by sodium metabisulfite, an antioxidant present in the commercial formulation used in the reported cases and a low pH (2.7 to 4.0) of the formulation.[91] In CSF rendered more acidic by 2-chloroprocaine, metabisulfite generates sulfur dioxide, which is lipid soluble and can diffuse into the nerve cells.[93] Intracellular hydration of sulfur dioxide generates sulfurous acid, which may cause profound intracellular acidosis and irreversible damage. In contrast, others have suggested that 2-chloroprocaine itself, and not metabisulfite, was the cause of neurologic deficits.[93]

Subsequently, the manufacturer released another preparation of 2-chloroprocaine, which was free of bisulfite but contained ethylenediaminetetraacetic acid (EDTA). This was followed by several reports of severe, incapacitating paralumbar pain and spasm associated with epidural injection of large volumes of the drug,[94] likely resulting from chelation of calcium by disodium EDTA and tetany of the affected muscles caused by local hypocalcemia. The current preparations of 2-chloroprocaine that are marketed for *epidural* and *spinal* administration do not contain EDTA or other preservatives. 2-Chloroprocaine intended for epidural administration is packaged in colored vials to reduce oxidation.

Lidocaine has been used for spinal anesthesia for more than 50 years, in thousands upon thousands of patients, with apparent safety. However, **cauda equina syndrome**, sacral nerve root deficits, or transient neurologic toxicity can occur after subarachnoid injection of lidocaine.[95,96] Neurotoxicity of local anesthetics is concentration dependent[97] and is not unique to lidocaine.[98,99] Some investigators have speculated that slow injection of local anesthetic through a spinal microcatheter results in maldistribution and pooling of high concentrations of hyperbaric lidocaine in the cauda equina area, resulting in increased risk for neurotoxicity and cauda equina syndrome.[95,96]

Milder manifestations of neurotoxicity also may occur. As early as 1954, mild, transient neurologic symptoms were reported after spinal anesthesia with lidocaine.[100] **Transient neurologic symptoms** (TNS) (dysesthesia or low back pain radiating to the buttocks, thighs, and calves) have been observed in surgical patients even after conventional (i.e., single-shot) spinal anesthesia with hyperbaric 5% lidocaine (see Chapter 31).[96] In 1994, in response to concerns that intrathecal injection of hyperbaric 5% lidocaine might be associated with TNS, the FDA Advisory Committee on Anesthetic Drugs recommended that the injected drug concentration be reduced by dilution with an equal volume of either preservative-free saline or CSF. However, Pollock et al.[101] reported that there was no difference in the incidence of TNS when spinal lidocaine 50 mg was diluted to 2%, 1%, or 0.5% solutions before administration and that the overall incidence of TNS did not differ from that of historic controls given 5% lidocaine.

Of interest, the exposure of frog sciatic nerve to lidocaine results in a progressive, irreversible loss of impulse activity beginning at a concentration of 1%.[97] The investigators of this study noted that "the range of lidocaine that produces such changes in mammalian nerve awaits determination."[97]

Generally, if pencil-point, side-hole spinal needles are used, it is recommended that the injection port should be directed cephalad. However, an epidemiologic survey did not implicate dose and needle-bevel direction as factors that affect the risk for TNS.[102] A metaanalysis of randomized controlled trials comparing spinal lidocaine with other local anesthetics found that the relative risk (RR) for development of TNS was lower with bupivacaine, levobupivacaine, prilocaine, and procaine than lidocaine (RR ranging from 0.10 to 0.23), but similar to mepivacaine and 2-chloroprocaine.[103] It has not been conclusively proven that TNS are manifestations of neurotoxicity.

Pregnancy may be associated with a reduced risk for TNS. Studies suggest that the incidence of TNS after spinal anesthesia with lidocaine or bupivacaine is equally low (<3%) in women having cesarean delivery and those undergoing postpartum tubal ligation.[104,105]

Allergic Reactions

True Ig-E-mediated immediate hypersensitivity reactions to a local anesthetic are rare and account for less than 1% of adverse reactions to local anesthetics.[106] Further, anaphylactic and anaphylactoid reactions may be the result of additives such as methylparaben and metabisulfite.[106] In a study of 164 patients referred to an allergy clinic for suspected local anesthetic allergy, none was found to be allergic.[107] Adverse reactions (e.g., CNS and cardiovascular symptoms) may mimic hypersensitivity but not actually be Ig-E-mediated reactions. The potential range of allergic manifestations is listed in Box 13.1.

Obstetricians should refer women with alleged allergy to an anesthesiologist for appropriate evaluation well before the

---

BOX 13.1   Non–IgE-Mediated Reactions to Local Anesthetics

- Psychomotor responses
  - Vasovagal episode
  - Hyperventilation or panic attack
- Endogenous sympathetic stimulation
- Responses to procedural trauma
- Delayed hypersensitivity reaction
- Non–IgE-mediated reaction to another agent
  - Epinephrine
  - Metabisulfite and other additives
- IgE-mediated reaction to another agent
  - Additives and preservatives
  - Latex
  - Antibiotic

Modified from Bhole MV, Manson AL, Seneviratne SL, Misbah SA. IgE-mediated allergy to local anaesthetics: separating fact from perception: a UK perspective. *Br J Anaesth*. 2012;108:903–911.

expected date of delivery. In many cases, a carefully obtained history excludes true hypersensitivity. If immediate hypersensitivity is suspected, patients should be referred to an allergist for further evaluation. Skin tested and graded challenge may be indicated.[106] Delayed reading of skin testing and patch testing may be considered if a delayed hypersensitivity reaction is suspected.[106] A second goal of allergy testing is to identify a safe alternative local anesthetic.

If the patient's history suggests a low risk of local anesthetic allergy, a single-dose local anesthetic challenge can be considered, particularly with an alternative class of local anesthetic (amides and esters).[106]

Management of an allergic reaction. Pharmacologic therapy of a severe allergic reaction involves (1) inhibition of mediator synthesis and release, (2) reversal of the effects of these mediators on target organs, and (3) prevention of the recruitment of other inflammatory processes. In general, catecholamines, especially epinephrine, but also phosphodiesterase inhibitors, antihistamines, and corticosteroids, have been used for this purpose. The Australian and New Zealand College of Anaesthetists with the Australian and New Zealand Anaesthetic Allergy Group have developed evidence-based guidelines for the management of perioperative anaphylaxis (Box 13.2).[108] Higher doses of catecholamines may be required in a patient who has a sympathetic blockade. Once the patient is stable, a serum tryptase level should be obtained; an elevated level is suggestive of anaphylaxis.

Effects on the Uterus and Placenta

Uterine Blood Flow

The association of paracervical block with fetal bradycardia has been attributed to the high concentration of local anesthetic deposited in the vicinity of the uterine arteries (see Chapter 23). Human uterine artery segments obtained at the time of cesarean hysterectomy constrict when exposed to high concentrations of lidocaine[109] or bupivacaine.[110]

These findings also have been confirmed in laboratory animals. Fishburne et al.[111] observed a dose-related decrease in uterine blood flow during uterine arterial infusion of 2-chloroprocaine, lidocaine, or bupivacaine in gravid ewes. However, when plasma local anesthetic concentrations mimic those that occur in ordinary clinical practice, local anesthetics have no adverse effect on uterine blood flow.[112–114]

Pregnancy itself may enhance uterine vascular reactivity to local anesthetic agents. Isolated human uterine artery segments obtained from term parturients constrict at a lower lidocaine concentration than uterine artery segments from nonpregnant patients.[109,115] Uterine artery sensitivity to local anesthetics increases as early as the second trimester of pregnancy and may be related to an increase in estrogen.[109,111] However, these studies were performed before the recognition of the importance of intact vascular endothelium in the *in vitro* assessment of vascular tone. The exact mechanism by which high concentrations of local anesthetics cause uterine artery vasoconstriction (while causing dilation in other vascular beds) is unclear. Clinical experience with the use of local anesthetics supports the view that clinical concentrations of

these drugs do not adversely affect the uterine vasculature (see Chapter 3).[116,117]

All local anesthetics can reduce uterine blood flow at plasma concentrations that greatly exceed those occurring during the routine practice of obstetric anesthesia.[111] There has been an added concern that the levorotatory isomers of local anesthetics, which produce vasoconstriction at clinical

---

BOX 13.2   Management of Anaphylaxis

Immediate management
- If cardiac arrest, follow ACLS guidelines (see Chapter 53 and Box 53.5).
- Discontinue or remove all triggers (e.g., chlorhexidine, synthetic colloids, latex).
  - Stop procedure; use minimal volatile anesthetic agents.
- Call for help.
- Maintain airway: Fio_2 1.0, consider need for tracheal intubation.
- Rapid large-volume fluid administration
  - Crystalloid bolus: 2 L, repeat as needed
  - Large-bore IV access
  - Elevate legs
- IV epinephrine bolus, repeat every 1–2 min as needed
  - Mild hypotension: 5–10 µg
  - Moderate hypotension: 20 µg
  - Life-threatening hypotension: 100–200 µg
  - Epinephrine infusion: 3–40 µg/min (0.05–0.5 µg/kg/min)

Refractory management
- Consider requesting more help.
- Consider cesarean delivery if still pregnant (deliver within 5 min of cardiovascular collapse).
- Make sure triggers have been removed.
- Monitoring: consider arterial line, transthoracic or transesophageal echocardiography.
- Resistant hypotension
  - Norepinephrine infusion: 3–40 µg/min (0.05–0.5 µg/kg/min)
  - Vasopressin bolus 1–2 U, then infusion 2 U/h
  - Glucagon: 1–2 mg IV every 5 min until a response
- Resistant bronchospasm
  - Continue epinephrine infusion.
  - Salbutamol metered dose inhaler 12 puffs (1200 µg)
  - Magnesium 2 g over 20 min
  - Consider volatile anesthetic agent or ketamine.
- Consider other diagnoses.

Postcrisis management
- Consider glucocorticoids: dexamethasone 0.1–0.4 mg/kg or hydrocortisone 2–4 mg/kg.
- Consider oral antihistamines.
- Consider canceling surgical procedure, ICU monitoring.
- Investigations: draw blood for tryptase level.
- Documentation in medical record, letter for patient, referral for allergy assessment

ACLS, Advanced cardiac life support; *IV*, intravenous.
Modified from Kolawole H, Marshall SD, Crilly H, et al. Australian and New Zealand Anaesthetic Allergy Group/Australian and New Zealand College of Anaesthetists perioperative anaphylaxis management guidelines. *Anaesth Intensive Care.* 2017;45:151–158.

doses,[118] may reduce uteroplacental perfusion and adversely affect fetal well-being. It is reassuring to note that ropivacaine, even at plasma concentrations that are almost two times greater than would be expected to occur during clinical use, does not reduce uterine blood flow or affect fetal heart rate (FHR), blood pressure, or acid-base measurements in pregnant sheep.[112] In humans, Doppler velocimetry studies have shown that ropivacaine has little effect on the uteroplacental or fetal circulation when it is administered to provide epidural anesthesia for cesarean delivery.[116] Similarly, clinically relevant plasma concentrations of levobupivacaine had no adverse effect on uterine blood flow.[112]

Umbilical Blood Flow

Fetal well-being also depends on the adequacy of perfusion of the placenta. The regulatory mechanisms that control flow through the umbilical vessels are poorly understood. Lidocaine does not affect spiral strips obtained from human umbilical artery segments at concentrations up to 5 μg/mL, but it produces relaxation in concentrations from 30 to 900 μg/mL.[119] Bupivacaine also does not constrict umbilical artery segments at clinically relevant concentrations of 0.3 and 1 μg/mL.[119] At higher concentrations, the effect of bupivacaine appears to be biphasic. Constriction occurs at concentrations of 5 to 25 μg/mL, and relaxation occurs at concentrations > 125 μg/mL.[119,120] Hypercarbia but not hypoxemia lessens the contractile response of umbilical vessels to bupivacaine *in vitro*.[121]

Decreases in umbilical blood flow of as much as 43% accompany intravenous administration of lidocaine 4 mg/kg in pregnant sheep.[122] However, plasma concentrations of the drug were higher than would be expected with clinical use, and all ewes exhibited signs of CNS toxicity, which may reduce umbilical blood flow itself.

Advances in noninvasive Doppler imaging have facilitated clinical assessment of umbilical cord blood flow velocity. The ratio of the systolic (S) peak to the diastolic (D) trough of the umbilical artery waveform is used as a measure of vascular resistance. The S/D ratio in the umbilical artery decreases during normal pregnancy, and high ratios usually are associated with fetal compromise (see Chapter 6). Local anesthetics administered for epidural anesthesia do not adversely affect the umbilical artery S/D ratio.[123,124] In fact, labor epidural analgesia with 1.5% lidocaine or 2% 2-chloroprocaine resulted in a decrease in the S/D ratio.[123,124] This favorable change may have resulted from pain relief. Other investigators have noted no appreciable change or a slight decrease in the S/D ratio after the epidural administration of amide local anesthetics for elective cesarean delivery.[116,117,125]

Uterine Tone and Contractility

Changes in uterine tone and contractility may affect uteroplacental perfusion. Local anesthetics exert direct effects on uterine smooth muscle. One study reported that exposure to high concentrations of local anesthetic *in vitro* led to contraction of human myometrial segments obtained at the time of cesarean delivery.[126] These findings have been corroborated

in laboratory animals.[127] Further, Belitzky et al.[128] observed that direct intramyometrial injection of 1% procaine resulted in uterine tachysystole and fetal compromise in pregnant women. In all of these reports, the myometrium was exposed to higher-than-normal concentrations of the drug. In other studies, intravenous infusion of lidocaine or bupivacaine that resulted in clinically relevant plasma concentrations did not affect uterine tone or uterine activity in pregnant ewes.[112,114] In a study using electrohysterogram monitoring, levobupivacaine caused less uterine muscle relaxation after intramyometrial injection in rats than did bupivacaine.[129]

2-Chloroprocaine and Morphine Interaction

Question exists as to whether epidural 2-chloroprocaine affects the efficacy of other drugs administered in the neuraxis. Previous administration of 2-chloroprocaine was observed to reduce the quality and duration of analgesia produced by subsequent epidural injection of morphine or fentanyl.[130,131] Several hypotheses have been proposed for this observation. Current evidence suggests that the most likely explanation is a "window" phenomenon whereby rapid regression of 2-chloroprocaine anesthesia occurs before the onset of epidural morphine analgesia. In a randomized noninferiority study, Lee et al.[132] found no difference in postoperative morphine equivalents for cesarean delivery when epidural morphine 3 mg was administered following epidural anesthesia with lidocaine compared with 2-chloroprocaine. After the initial dosing with either lidocaine with epinephrine or chloroprocaine, patients in both groups received additional boluses of epidural lidocaine with 1:200,000 epinephrine 30 minutes later to prevent 2-chloroprocaine anesthesia from waning before the onset of epidural morphine analgesia. Pain scores were also not different between the groups.

In another study in cesarean delivery patients,[133] combined spinal-epidural anesthesia was induced with spinal bupivacaine and fentanyl. Thirty minutes later, patients were randomized to receive epidural morphine 3 mg with or without 3% 2-chloroprocaine (150 mg). There were no differences between groups in time to first request for supplemental analgesia, pain scores, or need for supplemental analgesics. These results support the theory that the perceived antagonism of epidural morphine by 2-chloroprocaine is due to the rapid regression of 2-chloroprocaine anesthesia prior to onset of epidural morphine analgesia. Administering additional long-acting local anesthetics (e.g., lidocaine, bupivacaine) to fill this pharmacokinetic window until the onset of neuraxial morphine analgesia is indicated if epidural morphine is administered after epidural 2-chloroprocaine.

Potency of Bupivacaine, Ropivacaine, and Levobupivacaine

The levorotatory compounds ropivacaine and levobupivacaine were developed because of the concerns about the safety of high doses of bupivacaine. Many studies have addressed the question of relative potency among the three drugs. Ropivacaine is approximately 10 times less lipid soluble (N-heptane/buffer) than bupivacaine, a difference that is important for two reasons.[134] First, ropivacaine may penetrate more slowly into the large, heavily myelinated motor neurons, resulting in less motor block than occurs with bupivacaine. Second, the issue raises questions as to whether ropivacaine is equipotent to bupivacaine. Indeed, a higher dose of ropivacaine is required to produce a sensory and motor block comparable with that produced by bupivacaine after spinal injection.[135,136] Similarly, the EC_{50} (the local anesthetic concentration at which 50% of women have pain relief, also known as the minimum local anesthetic concentration) of epidural ropivacaine is almost twice as great as that of epidural bupivacaine in laboring women.[63]

Studies of the EC_{50} of epidural levobupivacaine are conflicting; one study found that levobupivacaine was essentially equipotent to bupivacaine,[73] whereas others suggested that ropivacaine and levobupivacaine have similar potency.[137,138] Spinal levobupivacaine may have a greater motor-sparing effect than bupivacaine when given for initiating labor analgesia.[139] Critics of the use of EC_{50} data to compare potency argue that it provides no information on the shape and slope of the dose-effect relationship, which can vary with drug concentration, and further, that it provides no information on the effective clinical dose (ED_{95} [effective dose in 95% of cases]).[140]

In obstetric anesthesia practice, the clinical effects of epidural levobupivacaine and ropivacaine are indistinguishable from those of epidural bupivacaine for labor analgesia.[141] The choice of bupivacaine, levobupivacaine, or ropivacaine does not affect the method of delivery or neonatal condition.[141] For cesarean delivery, epidural levobupivacaine 0.5% is virtually identical to epidural bupivacaine 0.5%.[142] The levorotatory isomers (ropivacaine and levobupivacaine) may provide a greater margin of safety when large volumes of a concentrated solution of local anesthetic are required (e.g., epidural anesthesia for cesarean delivery). However, there may be little advantage to using levobupivacaine or ropivacaine when dilute solutions are used for epidural labor analgesia or when a small dose is used for spinal anesthesia.

Placental Transfer

Most drugs, including local anesthetics, cross the placenta. The factors that influence the placental transfer of a drug include (1) the physicochemical characteristics of the drug, (2) the concentration of free drug in the maternal blood, (3) the permeability of the placenta, and (4) the hemodynamic events occurring within the fetal-maternal unit (see Chapter 4).

Local anesthetics cross placental membranes by a process of simple (i.e., passive) diffusion. The rate of transfer of a particular drug is described by the Fick equation, as follows:

$$\frac{Q}{t} = \frac{K \times A\,(C_m - C_f)}{D}$$

where Q/t is the rate of diffusion, K is the diffusion constant for the drug, A is the surface area available for transfer, C_m is the free drug concentration in the maternal blood,

C_f is the free drug concentration in the fetal blood, and D is the thickness of the trophoblastic epithelium. In general, K is affected by molecular size, lipid solubility, and degree of ionization.

Molecular Size

Compounds with a molecular weight of less than 500 Da cross the placenta easily, whereas drugs such as digoxin, which have a molecular weight > 500 Da, have a slower rate of diffusion. Molecular weights of local anesthetics range from 234 to 288 Da (see Table 13.1). These small differences in molecular weight should not affect the rate of placental transfer because the diffusion constant (K) is inversely proportional to the square root of the molecular weight.[143]

Ionization and Lipid Solubility

Local anesthetics are weak bases; they have a relatively low degree of ionization and considerable lipid solubility at physiologic pH. The basic un-ionized local anesthetic molecule is more lipid soluble than the ionized moiety and determines placental transfer in a protein-free perfusate.[144]

The relationship between pH and pK_a may affect drug accumulation in the fetus. For the amide local anesthetics, pK_a values are close enough to physiologic pH that changes in fetal pH may alter the balance between ionized and un-ionized drug. In the acidotic fetus, a greater proportion of drug in the ionized form results in a larger total amount of local anesthetic in fetal plasma, because of "ion trapping" (Fig. 13.4).[145–147] Elimination of lidocaine from fetal blood is slower in the asphyxiated fetus than in the nonasphyxiated fetus.[122] Accumulation of lidocaine may be greater in fetal tissues, where the pH is even lower than that in fetal blood.[147]

Protein Binding

Perhaps most confusing and least understood are the effects of protein binding on placental transfer. Amide local anesthetics are bound to AAG and to a lesser extent to albumin.[18] The extent of protein binding varies among the local anesthetic agents (see Table 13.1). For a given local anesthetic, the proportion of free drug increases as blood concentration increases because of the saturation of binding sites. Binding of local anesthetics in the fetal plasma is approximately half that in the mother.[148,149]

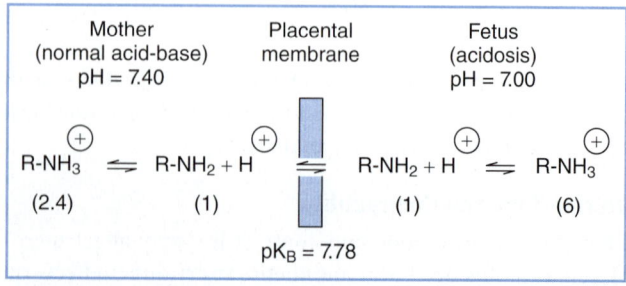

Fig. 13.4 "Ion Trapping" of a Local Anesthetic. The *numbers in parentheses* represent relative numbers of molecules. From the American College of Obstetricians and Gynecologists. *Obstet Gynecol.* 1976;48:29.

The fetal-to-maternal (F/M) blood concentration ratios of amide local anesthetic agents are listed in Table 13.1. The lower F/M blood concentration ratios of highly protein-bound drugs (e.g., bupivacaine) have been attributed to their more restricted placental transfer compared with less protein-bound drugs (e.g., lidocaine). Indeed, the rate of bupivacaine transfer across rabbit placenta perfused *in situ* is lower than that of lidocaine transfer.[150,151] Some investigators have suggested that protein binding in the maternal plasma should not affect the diffusion of drugs across the placenta because the dissociation from plasma proteins is essentially instantaneous.[143,152] In subsequent studies, the relatively low umbilical vein-to-maternal vein blood concentration ratio for bupivacaine has been attributed to differences in protein binding between maternal plasma and fetal plasma (Fig. 13.5).[148,149,153,154] Let us assume that the total concentration of lidocaine or bupivacaine in the maternal plasma is 2 mg/L. Lidocaine and bupivacaine are approximately 50% and 90% bound to maternal plasma proteins, respectively. Thus, the free concentrations of drug available for placental transfer are 1.0 and 0.2 mg/L, respectively. At equilibrium, the concentration of free drug is equal on the two sides of the placenta. In the fetus, however, lidocaine and bupivacaine are approximately 25% and 50% bound to fetal plasma proteins, respectively. Thus, the total lidocaine concentration in fetal plasma is 1.33 mg/L, resulting in an F/M ratio of 0.67; for bupivacaine, the corresponding values are 0.4 mg/L and 0.2, respectively.

In fact, accumulation of bupivacaine occurs in human fetuses whose mothers received the drug for epidural anesthesia.[22] After delivery, measurable plasma and urine concentrations persisted for as long as 3 days.[22] *In vitro* studies using a perfused human placental model have found that the placental transfer of ropivacaine is similar to that of bupivacaine.[155] Tissue concentrations of ropivacaine in fetal heart,

brain, liver, lung, kidneys, and adrenal glands were similar to those of bupivacaine.[112] Datta et al.[28] noted that the free fraction of ropivacaine at delivery was approximately twice that of bupivacaine in neonates whose mothers received the drug for epidural anesthesia during labor or cesarean delivery.

Maternal Blood Concentration of Drug

The maternal blood concentration of local anesthetic is determined by (1) the dose, (2) the site of administration, (3) metabolism and excretion, and (4) the effects of adjuvants such as epinephrine. For a given local anesthetic, the maternal blood concentration determines fetal drug exposure and is the only variable of the Fick equation that may be influenced by the clinician.

Dose. In general, higher doses result in higher maternal and fetal blood concentrations. For example, Kuhnert et al.[16] found that doubling the mean dose of epidural lidocaine from 300 to 595 mg almost doubled the concentration in umbilical cord blood. The elimination half-life of amide local anesthetics is relatively long; thus, repeated epidural injection or continuous infusion of the drug may lead to accumulation in the maternal plasma. This does not apply to 2-chloroprocaine, however, which is rapidly hydrolyzed by pseudocholinesterase.[10]

Site of administration. The rates of absorption and peak plasma concentrations depend on the vascularity at the site of administration. The peak plasma concentration of lidocaine is achieved within 9 to 10 minutes after paracervical block.[156] In contrast, absorption from the lumbar epidural space, which is less vascular, occurs at a slower rate; the peak plasma concentration is not achieved until 25 to 40 minutes after administration.[16] Injection of local anesthetic into the caudal rather than the lumbar epidural space may result in higher blood levels because of the need for a higher drug volume to provide

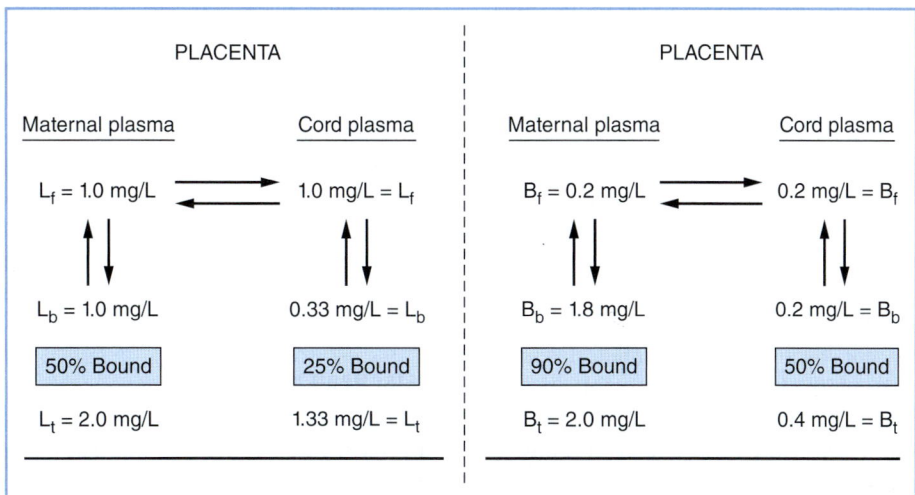

Fig. 13.5 Demonstration of how distribution of local anesthetics across the placenta may be predicted from differences in drug protein binding in maternal and fetal plasma. *Left,* lidocaine *(L); f, b, t,* free, bound, and total drug concentrations, respectively. *Right,* bupivacaine *(B).* Lidocaine umbilical cord-to-maternal plasma ratio (F/M) = 0.67; bupivacaine F/M = 0.20. From Mather LE, Tucker GT. Properties, absorption, and disposition of local anesthetic agents. In: Cousins MJ, Carr DB, Horlocker TT, Bridenbaugh PO, eds. *Neural Blockade in Clinical Anesthesia and Management of Pain.* 4th ed. Lippincott Williams & Wilkins; 2009:85.

comparable anesthesia to that provided by lumbar epidural injection.[157]

In the past, it was thought that subarachnoid administration of a local anesthetic resulted in less systemic absorption than epidural administration. However, peak blood concentrations of lidocaine have been reported to be similar after subarachnoid and epidural administration.[158] In another study, subarachnoid administration of lidocaine 75 mg for cesarean delivery resulted in low but measurable fetal plasma concentrations of the drug.[15]

Placenta. Maturation of the placenta may affect the rate of drug transfer. In pregnant mice, diazepam and its metabolites cross the placenta more rapidly in late pregnancy.[159] Uptake and metabolism of drugs by the placenta would be expected to reduce transfer to the fetus. However, placental drug uptake of local anesthetics is limited, and it is unlikely that this organ metabolizes the amide local anesthetic agents.[160] The same may not be true for the ester local anesthetics. For example, cocaine is biotransformed when it is incubated with human placental microsomal fraction, presumably because of cholinesterase activity within the placenta.[161] Placental metabolism of paraaminobenzoic acid also has been demonstrated.[162]

Teratogenicity

Local anesthetics are generally not considered teratogenic (see Chapter 17).

Fetal and Neonatal Effects

Pharmacokinetics

Local anesthetics, once transferred across the placenta, are distributed in the fetus. Factors that influence fetal tissue uptake of the drug include (1) fetal plasma protein binding, (2) lipid solubility, (3) the degree of ionization of the drug, and (4) hemodynamic changes that affect the distribution of fetal cardiac output. Fetal plasma protein-binding capacity of local anesthetics is approximately 50% that of maternal plasma; thus, there is greater availability of free drug in the fetus than in the mother.[148,149,163–165] Studies have examined the distribution of lidocaine in fetal tissues after an intravenous injection of the drug to animals.[17,166] The higher concentration of lidocaine in the liver, myocardium, and brain (compared with other fetal tissues) reflects rapid distribution of the drug to highly perfused tissues. Only the fetal liver had lidocaine concentrations that exceeded those in the mother. This finding is not surprising, given the high lipid content of the fetal liver and the fact that it receives most of the blood returning from the placenta by means of the umbilical vein.[166] Fetal asphyxia results in adaptations that increase blood flow to vital organs (e.g., brain, heart, adrenal glands).[167] The concentration of lidocaine in these organs is higher in asphyxiated fetuses than in healthy fetuses.[147,167]

Any drug that reaches the fetus undergoes metabolism and excretion. The term newborn has the hepatic enzymes necessary to metabolize local anesthetics.[15,16,168–170] Nonetheless, the elimination half-life of these drugs is longer in the neonate than in the adult.[169,170] The use of mepivacaine in obstetric epidural analgesia fell into disfavor after a report indicating

that the elimination half-life of the drug in the neonate was approximately 9 hours, or three times as long as the neonatal half-life for lidocaine.[171] It is ironic that the neonatal elimination half-life for bupivacaine may be as long as 14 hours.[172]

Morishima et al.[170] compared the pharmacokinetics of lidocaine among adult ewes and fetal and neonatal lambs. The metabolic (hepatic) clearance in the lambs was similar to that in adults, but renal clearance was greater in neonates. Nonetheless, the elimination half-life was prolonged in the lambs. This latter finding has been attributed to a greater volume of distribution in the neonatal lamb. Thus, at any given time, a smaller fraction of lidocaine accumulated in the body is available for clearance by hepatic metabolism. The greater renal clearance noted in neonates is a result of decreased protein binding, which increases the proportion of drug available for excretion.

The elimination half-life of local anesthetics in the fetus is similar to that in the adult because, unlike the newborn, the fetus can excrete drug across the placenta back to the mother.[149,170] With bupivacaine, this transfer may occur even though the total plasma drug concentration in the mother may exceed that in the fetus.[148]

Systemic Toxicity

In general, the neonate is more sensitive than the adult to the depressant effects of drugs. However, the seizure threshold for local anesthetics in the neonate appears to be similar to that in the adult. Morishima et al.[173] compared the relative CNS toxicity and cardiovascular toxicity of lidocaine in adult ewes and fetal and neonatal lambs. Greater doses (when calculated on a milligram-per-kilogram basis) were required to elicit toxic manifestations in the fetus and neonatal lamb than in the adult. However, the plasma concentrations of the drug associated with toxic manifestations were similar in the three groups of animals. The greater dose tolerated by fetuses than by neonates and adults was attributed to placental clearance of drug back to the mother and better maintenance of blood gas tensions during seizures. In the neonate, a large volume of distribution is most likely responsible for the high doses of local anesthetic required for fetal toxicity.

Studies of bupivacaine cardiotoxicity are inconsistent. *In vitro*, the sinoatrial node of neonatal guinea pigs was found to be more sensitive than that of adults to the cardiodepressant effect of bupivacaine.[174] In contrast, 2-day-old piglets demonstrated greater resistance than older animals to the arrhythmogenic and CNS effects of bupivacaine.[175]

Fetal Heart Rate

Changes in FHR after administration of local anesthetics are most often related to indirect effects such as maternal hypotension and uterine tachysystole (see Chapter 24). Local anesthetics probably have little direct effect on FHR, except perhaps after paracervical block. Rather, labor itself may be the single most important factor that alters FHR patterns.[176] Transient changes in FHR variability and an increase in the incidence of periodic decelerations have been observed during neuraxial analgesia in laboring women.[177,178] In contrast, in the absence of labor, FHR patterns are not affected even by the larger doses of local anesthetics required during epidural anesthesia for cesarean delivery.[176] The FHR changes noted in laboring women were transient and did not affect the condition of the newborns.[177,178] Further, Becker et al.[179] found no significant difference in the number or type of fetal electrocardiographic ST-segment changes (ST-waveform analysis events) in women with a high-risk singleton gestation who received epidural analgesia for labor compared with a control group of women who did not receive epidural analgesia.

Neurobehavioral Tests

Many neurobehavioral tests have been developed to detect subtle changes in organized behavior in the newborn. However, these tests are not reliable because they are subjective and lack specificity.[180] Other perinatal factors appear to have a more important effect on neonatal test performance than the choice of local anesthetic.[181]

Preterm Fetus and Newborn

It has become axiomatic that the preterm infant is more vulnerable than the term infant to the effects of analgesic and anesthetic drugs. Causes of enhanced drug sensitivity in the preterm newborn that have been postulated are as follows: (1) less protein is available for drug binding, (2) higher levels of bilirubin are present and may compete with the drug for protein binding, (3) greater access of the drug to the CNS occurs because of a poorly developed blood-brain barrier, (4) the preterm infant has greater total body water and less fat content, and (5) the preterm infant has a diminished ability to metabolize and excrete drugs. Unfortunately, few systematic studies have determined the maternal and fetal pharmacokinetics and pharmacodynamics of drugs throughout gestation; nevertheless, these deficiencies of the preterm infant may not be as serious as we have been led to believe. Although the plasma albumin and AAG concentrations are lower in the preterm fetus, these factors primarily affect drugs that are highly bound to these proteins. Most local anesthetics, however, exhibit only low to moderate degrees of binding in fetal plasma.[148,149]

The placenta efficiently eliminates fetal bilirubin. Thus, the hyperbilirubinemia of prematurity normally occurs in the postpartum period. Bupivacaine has been implicated as a possible cause of neonatal jaundice.[182] High affinity of the drug for fetal erythrocyte membranes may lead to a decrease in filterability and deformability, which may render red blood cells more prone to hemolysis.[182] However, increased bilirubin production has not been demonstrated in newborns whose mothers received bupivacaine for epidural anesthesia during labor and cesarean delivery.[183,184]

Greater total body water in the preterm fetus results in a larger volume of distribution for drugs. Thus, to achieve equal blood concentrations, the immature fetus must receive a greater amount of drug transplacentally than the mature fetus.

The diminished ability to metabolize or excrete drugs associated with prematurity is certainly not a universal

phenomenon. One study of the pharmacokinetics of lidocaine in preterm newborns noted that plasma clearance was similar to that in adults.[169]

During anesthesia for preterm labor, concerns about drug effects on the newborn are far less important than the prevention of asphyxia and trauma to the fetus. Indeed, healthy preterm fetal lambs tolerated clinically relevant plasma concentrations of lidocaine (e.g., approximately 1.5 μg/mL) as well as mature lambs.[17,185]

Fetal Asphyxia

Circulatory adaptations important for fetal survival during asphyxia result in increased blood flow and oxygen delivery to vital organs (e.g., heart, brain, adrenal glands).[167] Little information exists about the effects of local anesthetics on these fetal responses. Adaptation to asphyxia was unaffected in mature fetal lambs exposed to lidocaine.[167] In contrast, lidocaine adversely affected asphyxiated preterm fetal lambs, which experienced a further deterioration of acid-base status and a reduction in cardiac output and blood flow to the brain and heart (Fig. 13.6).[186] Similarly, in asphyxiated preterm fetal lambs, exposure to bupivacaine reduced blood flow to vital organs; however, FHR, blood pressure, and acid-base measurements did not change.[187]

After performing an *in vitro* study using perfused human placentas, Johnson et al.[188] suggested that bupivacaine might be preferable to lidocaine in the presence of fetal acidosis because the greater maternal protein binding of bupivacaine may limit its placental transfer. However, this methodology

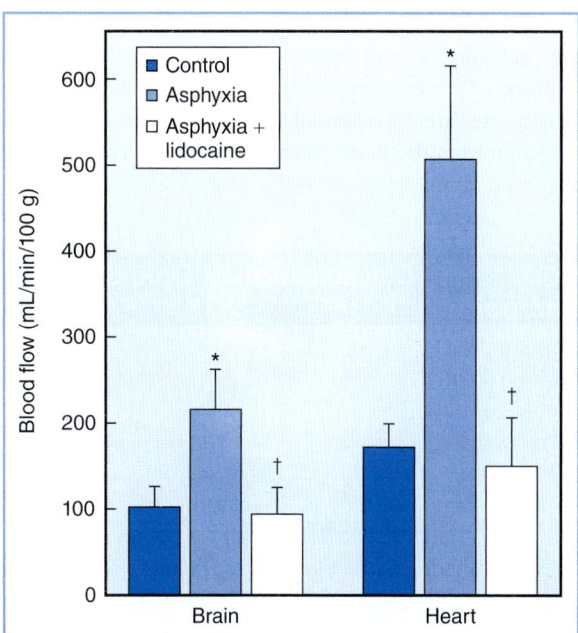

Fig. 13.6 Blood flow to the brain and heart in the preterm fetal lamb before and during asphyxia and during exposure to lidocaine while asphyxiated (mean ± SEM). *Significantly different from control. †Significantly different from asphyxia. Modified from Morishima HO, Pedersen H, Santos AC, et al. Adverse effects of maternally administered lidocaine on the asphyxiated preterm fetal lamb. *Anesthesiology.* 1989;71:110–115.

does not consider the potential for greater fetal tissue uptake of bupivacaine (than of lidocaine) because it is more lipid soluble and more protein bound than lidocaine.

In 1997, Santos et al.[187] reported that the effects of bupivacaine appeared less severe than those of lidocaine in asphyxiated preterm fetal lambs. However, the lidocaine data were generated in a separate experiment reported in 1989.[186] There are inherent limitations in a historical comparison of two studies performed 8 years apart. Further, it is unclear whether these findings are applicable to humans because both lidocaine and bupivacaine have enjoyed a long history of safe use in obstetric anesthesia practice; prospective clinical studies are required before one drug can be recommended over the other in the setting of fetal asphyxia.

OPIOIDS

Neuraxial opioid administration is unique in that it produces analgesia without loss of sensation or proprioception. Opioids are often coadministered with local anesthetic agents during intrapartum administration of neuraxial analgesia and anesthesia.

The term *opioid* refers to a series of compounds that are related to opium. These compounds may be classified as follows: (1) naturally occurring (e.g., morphine), (2) semisynthetic compounds (e.g., dihydromorphone), and (3) synthetic compounds (e.g., fentanyl) (Box 13.3). The only three naturally occurring opioids of clinical significance are morphine, codeine, and papaverine. These substances can be obtained from the poppy plant known botanically as *Papaver somniferum*. Development of synthetic drugs with morphine-like properties has led to development of the broad term *opioid*. These substances bind to several subpopulations of opioid receptors with resulting morphine-like effects. More than 40 years ago, identification of a dense concentration of opioid receptors in the dorsal horn of the spinal cord led to the use of neuraxial opioids as important adjuncts in obstetric anesthesia.

Opioid Receptors

Three broad opioid receptor systems have been identified: μ (mu: MOR), δ (delta: DOR), and κ (kappa: KOR) receptors.[189] Although there is a fourth receptor system,[190] the opiate receptor–like protein (ORL₁ or NOP), its role in pain modulation is not well characterized.[189] Each opioid receptor is encoded by a different gene and mediates different physiologic effects (Table 13.2). Although all these receptors may be involved with pain processing, the μ or κ receptors have the most important clinical pharmacologic effects.

Common pharmacologic effects (e.g., analgesia, respiratory depression) of morphine are mediated by μ-opioid receptors. Widely distributed throughout the brain and spinal cord, the μ, δ, and κ receptors are also present in a wide variety of peripheral tissues, including vascular, cardiac, airway/lung, and the gut. Opioids also act at several receptor sites with different affinities. Morphine has the greatest affinity for μ receptors and has less affinity for δ and κ receptors. However, morphine also has effects at δ and κ receptors when higher doses are administered. Responsible for analgesic, sedative, dysphoric, and diuretic effects,[189] δ and κ receptors are located both within the CNS and peripherally.[191] Peripheral κ agonists have been shown to modulate visceral pain, particularly in conditions that involve inflammation.[191]

The δ receptor is responsible for mediating some of the analgesic effects of the endogenous opioids (e.g., enkephalins, prodynorphan, proopiomelanocortin, proorphanin, endomorphins) in the spinal cord.[192] Few of the opioids have effects at the δ receptor in clinically relevant doses, but if a δ receptor agonist drug is administered in high doses (e.g., for treatment of pain in an opioid-tolerant patient), the drug may be less μ-receptor selective and produce δ-receptor effects.

BOX 13.3 Classification of Opioid Compounds

Naturally Occurring Compounds
- Morphine
- Codeine
- Papaverine
- Thebaine

Semisynthetic Compounds
- Heroin (diamorphine)
- Dihydromorphone
- Thebaine derivatives (e.g., etorphine, buprenorphine)

Synthetic Compounds
- Morphinan series (e.g., levorphanol, butorphanol)
- Diphenylpropylamine series (e.g., methadone)
- Benzomorphan series (e.g., pentazocine)
- Phenylpiperidine series (e.g., meperidine, fentanyl, sufentanil, alfentanil, remifentanil)

TABLE 13.2 Subtypes of Opioid Receptors

Receptor Type	Physiologic Response	Receptor Agonist
Mu (μ)	Analgesia Miosis Bradycardia Sedation Respiratory depression Decreased gastrointestinal transit	Morphine Fentanyl Sufentanil Meperidine
Kappa (κ)	Analgesia Sedation Respiratory depression Diuresis Psychotomimesis	Buprenorphine Pentazocine
Delta (δ)	Analgesia	Prodynorphin Endomorphins Enkephalins

Since their discovery, opioid receptors and their signaling continue to be an area of great research interest with potential development of better opioid analgesics with less risk for tolerance and addiction.

Molecular Structure

Naturally occurring opioids of significance can be divided into two distinct chemical classes, phenanthrenes (e.g., morphine) and benzylisoquinolines (e.g., papaverine, codeine; Fig. 13.7). The phenanthrenes are five-ring structures, and the benzylisoquinolines are three-ring structures. The semisynthetic opioids are morphine derivatives that have undergone relatively simple modifications of the morphine molecule. However, these modifications can produce profound alterations in the pharmacologic activity of the opioid. For example, substitution of an ester for the hydroxyl group on carbon 6 of morphine results in hydromorphone (Fig. 13.8). Synthetic opioids can be classified into the following four groups: (1) morphinan derivatives (e.g., levorphanol), (2) diphenyl or methadone derivatives (e.g., methadone, D-propoxyphene), (3) benzomorphan derivatives (phenazocine, pentazocine), and (4) phenylpiperidines (e.g., meperidine, fentanyl, alfentanil, sufentanil, remifentanil).

Morphine is the prototypical opioid with a five-ring structure that conforms to a *T* shape.[193] Three of the rings lie in one plane and the other two rings are perpendicular to the plane (Fig. 13.9). Although the analgesic activity of the opioid depends on its stereochemical structure,[194] the levorotatory isomer is usually the only isomer capable of producing analgesia. Morphine demonstrates several other characteristics that are common to other opioids: (1) a tertiary, positively charged basic nitrogen; (2) a quaternary carbon that is separated from the basic nitrogen by an ethane chain and attached to a phenyl group; (3) a phenolic hydroxyl group (morphine derivatives) or a ketone group (meperidine); and (4) the presence of an aromatic ring.[193]

A phenylpiperidine structure (i.e., an aromatic ring attached to a six-member ring containing five carbons and one nitrogen) is also part of the morphine molecule and is present in some other opioids (e.g., fentanyl; Fig. 13.10).[193] Phenylalanine and tyrosine moieties are structural elements that are important to all opioids, including endogenous neurotransmitters and modulators.[195,196]

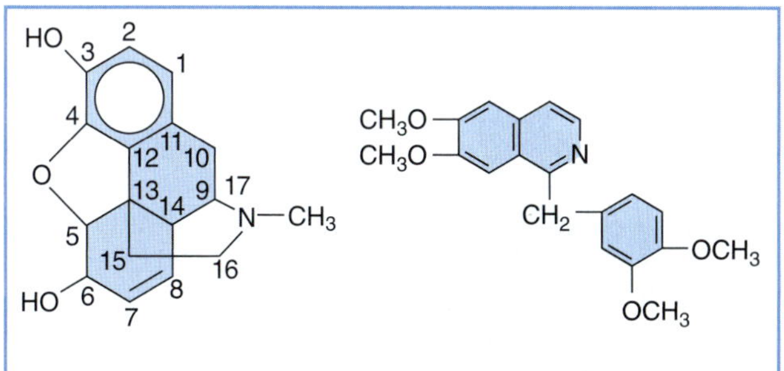

Mechanism of Action

Since the first clinical description of neuraxial opioid administration to treat cancer pain in 1979,[197] neuraxial opioid administration has become a mainstay in obstetric anesthesia practice. Clinical and laboratory research has focused on the mechanisms of synaptic transmission as well as the study of opioids and neurotransmitters that modulate this transmission.

Pain perception involves a complex series of nociceptive transmissions that begin with stimulation of sensory nerves in the periphery, resulting in generation of action potentials within the spinal cord and synaptic transmission to other supraspinal sites. Intraspinal administration of an opioid exploits the pharmacology of pain-modulating and pain-relieving systems that exist within the spinal cord (see Fig. 21.9). In early studies, Yaksh[198] demonstrated that morphine could produce selective suppression of nociceptive processing without affecting motor function, sympathetic tone, or proprioception when it was administered to the superficial layers of the dorsal horn of the spinal cord. However, when small amounts of opioid were administered to the cortex, the effects on nociceptive processing were negligible. Collectively, this work demonstrated that small doses of opioid can be selectively administered to a receptor site

Fig. 13.7 Naturally occurring opioids: phenanthrenes (e.g., morphine) and benzylisoquinolines (e.g., papaverine).

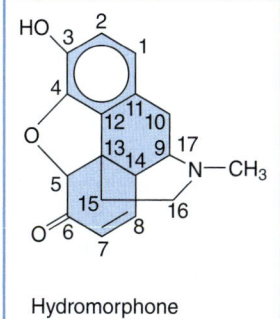

Fig. 13.8 Semisynthetic Opioids are Morphine Derivatives. For example, substitution of an ester for the hydroxyl group on carbon 6 of morphine results in hydromorphone.

Hydromorphone

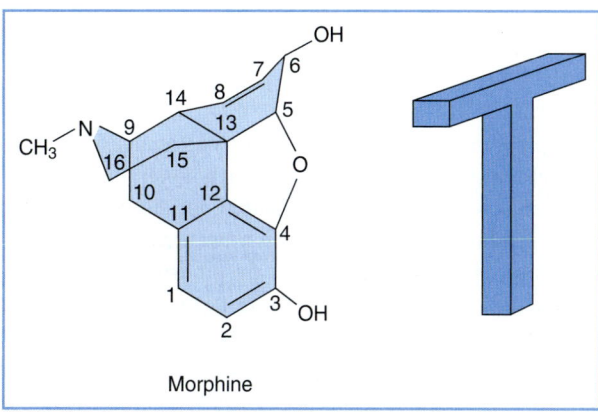

Morphine

Fig. 13.9 The *T*-Shaped Molecule of Morphine.

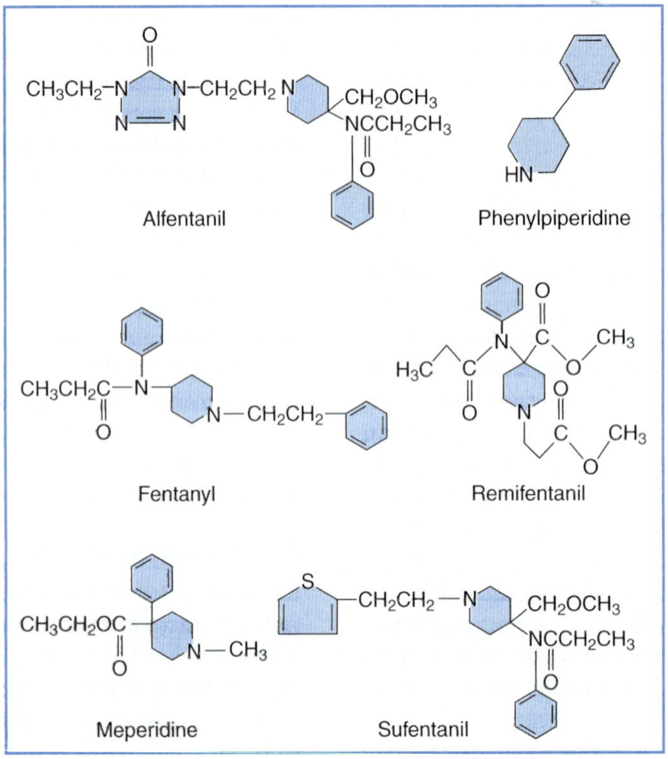

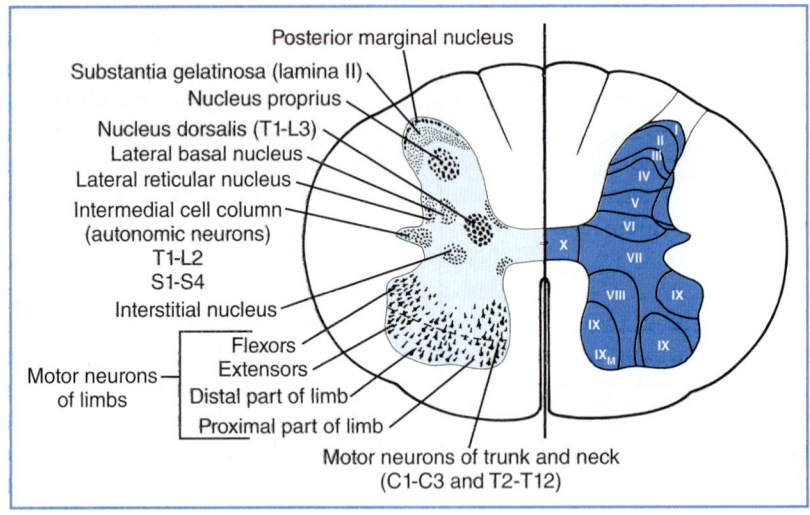

Fig. 13.10 Chemical structures of phenylpiperidine, meperidine, and the 4-anilinopiperidine derivatives fentanyl, sufentanil, alfentanil, and remifentanil.

Fig. 13.11 Architecture of the spinal cord, showing the gray matter nuclei (left) and Rexed laminae (right). From Ross BK, Hughes SC. Epidural and spinal narcotic analgesia. *Clin Obstet Gynecol.* 1987;30:552–565.

(i.e., spinal cord) and produce profound analgesia. In contrast, systemic administration of a much larger dose of opioid results in activation of multiple central and peripheral receptors to produce analgesia, but with unwanted side effects.

All opioids produce analgesia by binding to G protein–coupled opioid receptors. Activation of opioid receptors subsequently inhibits both adenylate cyclase and voltage-gated calcium channels. Inhibition of these calcium channels inhibits the release of excitatory afferent neurotransmitters, including glutamate, substance P, and other tachykinins.[189,199]

The result is inhibition of ascending nociceptive stimuli from the dorsal horn of the spinal cord.

Opioid receptors are nonuniformly distributed throughout the CNS. Although parenterally administered opioids most likely have both direct spinal and supraspinal effects, neuraxially administered opioids block the transmission of pain-related information by binding at presynaptic and postsynaptic receptor sites in the dorsal horn of the spinal cord (i.e., Rexed laminae I, II, V; Fig. 13.11). However, the rate and extent of neuraxial analgesia depend largely on the specific drug's physicochemical properties and ability to reach the opioid receptors in the spinal cord.

Pharmacokinetics and Pharmacodynamics

Many of the pharmacologic differences observed among neuraxially administered opioids depend on an opioid's ability to reach opioid receptors. An opioid's physicochemical properties, especially lipophilicity or hydrophilicity, largely determine the bioavailability of opioids administered within the neuraxis, as well as the drug's ability to produce CNS-mediated analgesia.

Before G protein-receptor activation can occur, the opioid must undergo a series of complex processes. Although several mechanisms have been proposed to explain the movement of opioids from the epidural space to the spinal cord, studies demonstrate that the only relevant mechanism is diffusion through the spinal meninges.[200,201] The opioid must traverse the dura and arachnoid membranes, diffuse through the CSF, and cross the pia membrane to reach the spinal cord (Fig. 13.12). Once the drug reaches the surface of the spinal cord, it must diffuse through the white matter and then the gray matter to reach the site of action, the dorsal horn.[202] The rate and extent of opioid transfer to receptors largely depend on a drug's physicochemical properties, particularly lipid solubility, because competing processes (e.g., uptake into the epidural fat or systemic circulation) limit the agent's diffusion to opioid receptors. Greater lipid solubility of a drug results in more rapid onset of analgesia. For example, fentanyl is a highly lipid-soluble opioid (i.e., 1000 times more lipid soluble than morphine); therefore, it has a more rapid onset of action than morphine (Table 13.3).

Latency, potency, and duration are also affected by other physicochemical properties, including molecular weight, pK_a, and protein binding. For example, the lower the pK_a, the greater the percentage of opioid existing in uncharged form (i.e., the anionic base) at a pH of 7.4. In the uncharged form, opioids penetrate the dura mater and dorsal horn more easily, resulting in a more rapid onset of analgesia.

The boundaries of the epidural space are the vertebral bodies, ligaments, and spinal meninges. Fat and the epidural venous plexus account for a large volume of the epidural space. The spinal meninges consist of the dura, arachnoid, and pia mater. Of these membranes, the arachnoid is the primary barrier for drug transfer from the epidural space to the spinal cord.[203] The arachnoid mater has multiple layers of overlapping cells that represent both a hydrophilic domain (consisting of extracellular and intracellular fluid) and a hydrophobic domain (the cell membranes).[201] For an opioid to navigate the arachnoid, it must diffuse through both domains before entering the CSF. Therefore, drugs of intermediate hydrophobicity move most readily across the arachnoid. Other physical characteristics of drugs (e.g., molecular weight) do not appear to play an important role in determining redistribution from the epidural space to the subarachnoid space.[201]

The efficacy of a drug also depends on its physicochemical properties, particularly lipid solubility. For example, the amount of drug that is sequestered in the epidural fat is entirely dependent on the drug's octanol-to-buffer distribution coefficient.[204] Consequently, lipophilic drugs (e.g., fentanyl) with a high octanol-to-buffer coefficient may never reach the arachnoid membrane and may partition in epidural fat. This lack of drug transfer across the meninges results in poor CSF bioavailability. Bernards et al.[204] used a porcine model to evaluate the movement of opioids from the epidural to the subarachnoid space. Alfentanil, fentanyl, and sufentanil were administered by bolus injection into the epidural

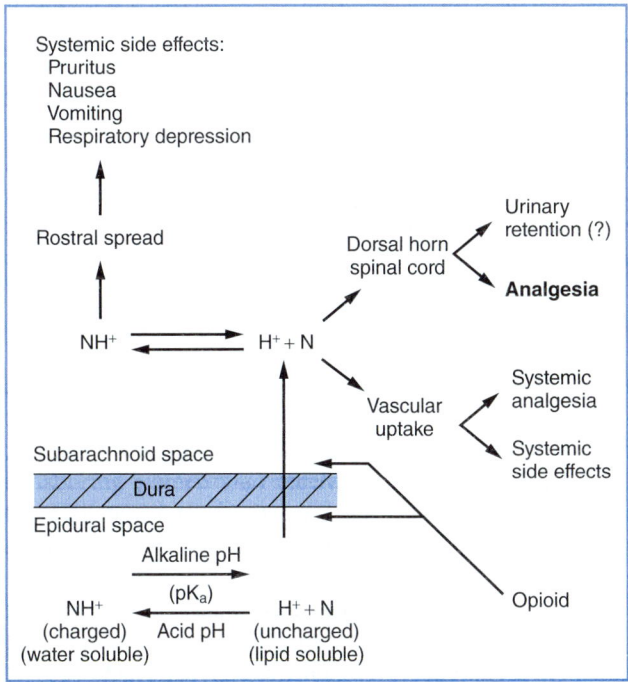

Fig. 13.12 Epidural opioids traverse the dura and arachnoid membranes, diffuse through cerebrospinal fluid, and cross the pia membrane before reaching the spinal cord. Several factors, including physicochemical properties (e.g., pK_a), affect the distribution of opioids within the neuraxis. From Ross BK, Hughes SC. Epidural and spinal narcotic analgesia. *Clin Obstet Gynecol.* 1987;30:552–565.

TABLE 13.3 Physicochemical Properties of Opioids Used for Neuraxial Analgesia

Opioid	Lipid Solubility[a]	pK_a	Protein Binding (%)
Morphine	0.70	7.9	35
Hydromorphone	1.28	8.1	19
Meperidine	39	8.5	70
Diamorphine	280	7.8	40
Fentanyl	717	8.4	84
Sufentanil	2842	8.0	93

[a]Octanol-water partition coefficient.
Data from Roy SD, Flynn GL. Solubility and related physicochemical properties of narcotic analgesics. *Pharm Res.* 1988;5:580–586; McLeod GA, Munishankar B, Columb MO. Is the clinical efficacy of epidural diamorphine concentration-dependent when used as analgesia for labour? *Br J Anaesth.* 2005;94:229–233.

space and opioid concentrations were continuously sampled and measured over time in the epidural and subarachnoid spaces and in the systemic venous and epidural plasma, using microdialysis techniques. They found a strong linear relationship between lipid solubility and mean residence time, indicating that more lipid-soluble opioids spend a longer time in the epidural space. Consequently these drugs partition themselves into the epidural fat with ongoing slow release back into the epidural space. Because of their long residence time in the epidural space, lipid-soluble drugs are found in lower concentrations in the CSF (i.e., decreased bioavailability to opioid receptors in the dorsal horn).

Several human studies have evaluated whether epidurally administered fentanyl produces analgesia by a selective spinal mechanism or by systemic absorption and redistribution. Results of studies of lipophilic opioids (administered by epidural infusion) have suggested that low concentrations of lipophilic opioids are subject to rapid vascular uptake from the epidural space or sequestration in epidural fat, thereby limiting access to the spinal cord.[205,206] However, the results of other studies have suggested a spinal effect when lipophilic opioids are administered by epidural bolus injection[207] or by epidural infusion of short duration.[208] Ginosar et al.[209] compared the analgesic effects of epidural bolus injection and epidural infusion of fentanyl in human volunteers. Study results suggested that epidural fentanyl infusion produced analgesia by uptake into the systemic circulation with redistribution to brain and peripheral opioid receptors. However, epidural bolus administration of fentanyl produced analgesia by selective spinal mechanisms.[209] These results were consistent with previous reports that an epidural fentanyl bolus results in a larger amount of fentanyl in the epidural space than occurs at any time during an epidural infusion of clinically relevant doses, leading to the greater availability of drug to activate opioid receptors in the dorsal horn of the spinal cord.

Although hydrophilic drugs (e.g., morphine) are subject to less systemic and epidural fat uptake than lipophilic drugs, the transfer of the former into the CSF is an inefficient process because they have difficulty in crossing the lipid bilayer of the arachnoid. However, despite these inefficiencies, morphine content in the spinal cord is significantly greater than lipophilic drug (e.g., fentanyl) content,[210] and morphine has much greater bioavailability in the spinal cord than do fentanyl and sufentanil.[204,210] Thus, although morphine clearly produces analgesia via a spinal mechanism, the extent of spinal analgesia produced by the neuraxial administration of fentanyl and sufentanil is less clear.

After a drug reaches the subarachnoid space, either by diffusion across the meninges or by direct injection into the CSF, its effects depend on its lipid solubility. All opioids produce at least some analgesia by spinal-specific mechanisms. Movement of these drugs within the CSF depends on their physicochemical properties. Drugs can diffuse within the CSF in either a cephalad or a caudad direction. Both morphine and fentanyl have been shown to move rapidly within the CSF.[211] Lipophilic drugs can also return to the epidural space by traversing previously mentioned structures.

Ummenhofer et al.[210] used a porcine model to investigate intrathecal administration of opioids. These investigators found that lipophilic opioids have a very large volume of distribution compared with hydrophilic drugs; the volume of distribution of sufentanil was 40 times greater than that of morphine. This is caused by sufentanil's extreme lipid solubility, with the drug rapidly leaving the CSF and entering the epidural fat, from where it is absorbed systemically.[212]

Neuraxial hydromorphone has been investigated as an alternative agent to morphine for postoperative cesarean analgesia. The estimated effective intrathecal morphine: hydromorphone dose ratio is 2:1.[213] Because morphine is more hydrophilic than hydromorphone, a shorter duration of analgesia can be expected with hydromorphone. Clinically, this may not be the case. In a prospective randomized study, Sharpe et al.[214] did not find a difference in pain scores during the first 24 hours when equipotent doses of intrathecal morphine (150 μg) or hydromorphone (75 μg) were administered for postoperative cesarean delivery pain. Although the time to first opioid request was shorter in the hydromorphone group (5.4 versus 12.1 hours), the study was underpowered to determine statistical significance. The adverse effect profiles of the two drugs were similar.

Extended-release epidural morphine (EREM) was developed to prolong the duration of a single epidural injection of morphine or obviate the need for a continuous infusion or multiple bolus doses. Multivesicular liposomal preparations gradually release morphine so that a larger epidural dose can be administered, providing analgesia for up to 48 hours (see Chapter 27). Studies that compared EREM 10 to 15 mg with conventional epidural morphine for provision of analgesia after cesarean delivery determined that EREM provided superior and prolonged analgesia without increasing the incidence of adverse effects (e.g., nausea, pruritus, sedation, respiratory depression).[215,216] This morphine formulation is not currently available in the United States.

In summary, the onset and duration of analgesia as well as adverse effects produced by neuraxial opioid administration depend on the specific type of opioid receptor that is activated as well as the dose, lipid solubility, and rate of movement and clearance of the opioid in the CSF.

Pharmacogenetics

Pain associated with labor and delivery is influenced by a multitude of physiologic, psychosocial, and environmental factors (see Chapter 21). Among these factors, genetic variations may also influence analgesic efficacy and related adverse effects. These pharmacogenetic factors have been extensively studied in relation to opioid analgesia, albeit with inconsistent results.[217] Nonetheless, studies on animals and human twins have estimated that 30% to 76% of interindividual variability in opioid requirement is attributable to genetic factors.[218]

Pharmacogenetic factors exert their effects in three ways: they can influence (1) the pharmacokinetics of opioids (how the drug is absorbed, distributed, metabolized, or eliminated), (2) opioid pharmacodynamics (the ability of opioids to act on their receptors and their downstream effects), and (3) the patient's pain perception (the complex interplay between nociceptive and antinociceptive mechanisms). In turn, these effects manifest clinically as interindividual variations in the dose required for analgesia and the incidence of opioid-related adverse effects.[219]

Of the pharmacokinetic processes, opioid metabolism plays a major role in determining plasma concentrations of the parent drug and active or inactive metabolites. Opioids (except remifentanil) are metabolized by hepatic cytochrome P450 enzymes, and single-nucleotide polymorphisms (SNPs) in the genes encoding these enzymes are associated with interindividual variations in the plasma concentrations of the parent drug and its metabolites.[219] For example, codeine is metabolized by CYP2D6 to its active moiety, morphine. Patients possessing SNPs that resulted in increased CYP2D6 activity were found to have high plasma concentrations of morphine after codeine administration and were at increased risk of codeine-related adverse effects. Conversely, patients with reduced CYP2D6 activity experience inadequate analgesia due to inadequate conversion of codeine to the active drug, morphine.[220] Similarly, SNPs in genes encoding enzymes involved in morphine (UGT2B7), tramadol (CYP2D6), and fentanyl or sufentanil (CYP3A4) metabolism may affect the plasma concentrations of the parent drug and metabolites, in turn altering their respective dose-response relationships.

Opioids exert their clinical effects through activation of G protein–coupled opioid receptors and their downstream signaling pathways. Additionally, opioids are substrates for P-glycoprotein (P-gp) drug transporter molecules, which influence the opioid available for binding to opioid receptors and, therefore, determine its pharmacodynamic activity. SNPs in the genes encoding opioid receptors and P-gp have been associated with variations in opioid efficacy.

In obstetric patients, the μ-opioid receptor gene *(OPRM1)* has been most widely studied, particularly polymorphism at position 118. At this position, guanine is substituted for adenosine in some individuals (A118G). The allelic frequency of this variant is population dependent; it is more common in Asians and less frequent in White and Black individuals.[217] In an early investigation of the role of the A118G variant in neuraxial opioid analgesia, Landau et al.[221] used both up-down sequential allocation and random allocation methods to estimate the ED_{50} of intrathecal fentanyl administered as part of combined spinal-epidural labor analgesia in nulliparous women who were A118 homozygotes or G118 hetero/homozygotes. The ED_{50} of intrathecal fentanyl was 1.5- to 2-fold higher in women with the wild-type allele (A118) compared with the minor allele (A118G).[221] However, when Wong et al.[222] evaluated the duration of intrathecal fentanyl analgesia (25 μg) in women who were classified into the same genetic groups, there were no differences between the groups in the duration of analgesia or treatment of breakthrough pain. A possible explanation was the high dose of intrathecal fentanyl.[222] Camorcia et al.[223] examined the effect of the A118G variant on the ED_{50} of epidural sufentanil in nulliparous women. Similar to the findings of Landau et al.,[221] the

estimated ED_{50} was significantly lower in women with the variant allele compared with women without the variant. Landau et al.[224] also evaluated the possible effects of common *OPRM1* SNPs on the analgesic efficacy of intravenous fentanyl labor analgesia; however, no differences were detected. The authors concluded that the study was likely underpowered to detect a difference between groups and, if differences exist, the impact on response to opioid labor analgesia is likely to be modest.

The potential role of the A118 genetic variant in influencing opioid analgesic requirements after cesarean delivery has been investigated in several studies. Wong et al.,[222] in a mixed race/ethnicity population, found no difference in duration of intrathecal morphine analgesia or need for supplemental analgesia in women carrying the variant allele. In contrast, Sia et al.[225] reported that Asian women with the variant allele had an *increased* incidence of breakthrough pain (as assessed by patient-controlled intravenous morphine requirements) after intrathecal administration of morphine compared with women without the variant allele. In a second study, the variant allele was found to independently predict increased postoperative morphine use in women undergoing cesarean delivery.[226]

The results of these studies are difficult to reconcile.[217,227] Although genetic components may influence patients' responses to nociceptive stimuli, current evidence suggests that genetic polymorphism in *OPRM1* plays a minor role, if any, in opioid pain management.[227,228] A metaanalysis examining the A118 genetic variant of *OPRM1* failed to identify a strong association between this variant allele and the response to opioids in different clinical settings.[228]

Finally, pain perception involves a complex interplay between intrinsic nociceptive and antinociceptive pathways, each step of which involves multiple molecular mechanisms that are subject to the influences of genetic variation. For example, catechol-*O*-methyltransferase (COMT) is an enzyme responsible for the methyl conjugation and metabolism of endogenous catecholamines such as adrenaline, noradrenaline, and dopamine. Studies of COMT variant (methionine is substituted for valine at position 15) demonstrated that the resultant decrease in COMT activity was associated with increased pain sensitivity, likely due to increased activation of peripheral $beta_2$- and $beta_3$-adrenergic receptors.[219,229] Finally, other factors besides genetics may influence pain and opioid response including (1) type of pain (visceral versus somatic), (2) type of opioid (hydrophilic versus hydrophobic), (3) route of administration, and (4) differences in metabolic pathways.

Toxicity

Any agent that is injected into the epidural or subarachnoid space should be administered with caution, owing to the potential for neurotoxicity and permanent neurologic damage. In general, the epidural space is more forgiving than the subarachnoid space (see Chapter 31). In many cases, clinicians have injected medications into the neuraxis that have not been well tested in animal models. Yaksh and Collins[230] have urged careful administration of neuraxial drugs, stating that "studies in animals should precede human use of spinally administered drugs."

The most commonly administered neuraxial opioids in obstetric patients are preservative-free formulations of morphine, fentanyl, and sufentanil. Preservative-free morphine is commercially available for both epidural and intrathecal administration. In the animal model, clinically relevant doses of preservative-free intrathecal morphine (<5 mg) were administered for 28 days via an indwelling subarachnoid catheter. Spinal cord blood flow and histopathology were unaffected.[231,232] To further evaluate preservative-free morphine for potential neurotoxicity, Yaksh et al.[233] studied the effects of continuous infusions of high-dose intrathecal morphine (1.5 to 12 mg/day for 28 days) in dogs. At higher doses (9 to 12 mg), the animals demonstrated allodynia soon after beginning the infusion, and at 12 mg, an inflammatory process developed and caused local tissue compression. In humans, long-term neuraxial opioid administration (up to 480 mg of epidural morphine over 124 days or 60 mg intrathecal morphine over 47 days) in patients with cancer pain resulted in no evidence of physiologic or neurologic adverse effects.[234]

Fentanyl is also available in a preservative-free formulation. Despite its widespread clinical use, few studies have assessed the histologic, physiologic, or clinical evidence of neurotoxicity with spinally administered fentanyl. One *in vitro* study evaluated the effects of fentanyl administration on nerve conduction.[235] Histopathologic studies of isolated rabbit vagus nerve axons did not show localized nerve damage after nerves were bathed in an isotonic solution of fentanyl. When axons were bathed in a hypotonic solution of fentanyl, permanent conduction deficits were noted. However, in clinical practice, large doses of fentanyl would be required to create a hypotonic intrathecal environment.

Although no formal neurotoxicology studies have evaluated sufentanil administration in humans, there are no clinical reports of neurotoxicity despite its widespread use. In one study, sufentanil was administered to cats through an indwelling intrathecal catheter over 5 days.[231] Sabbe et al.[236] administered clinically relevant doses of intrathecal sufentanil to dogs over several weeks and reported no histopathologic changes. In a sheep model, Rawal et al.[237] demonstrated dose-dependent spinal cord histopathologic changes after intrathecal administration of sufentanil (50 to 100 µg) every 6 hours for 72 hours. These doses are much larger than those used in clinical practice. It is possible that these findings reflect an artifact of experimental design (e.g., the frequent administration of a large-volume, hypotonic preparation).

Despite the paucity of data about possible neurotoxicity, both fentanyl and sufentanil are widely used in clinical practice. Although these drugs are not approved by the FDA for neuraxial use,[238] there are no published reports of neurologic deficits after epidural or intrathecal administration of either agent in humans. In general, anesthesia providers should exercise extreme caution before injecting any untested agent

TABLE 13.4   Incidence of Adverse Side Effects After Intrathecal Injection of 0.5 or 1.0 mg of Morphine

	INCIDENCE (%)		
Side Effect	Morphine 0.5 mg (*n* = 12)	Morphine 1 mg (*n* = 18)	Overall (*n* = 30)
Pruritus	58	94	80
Nausea/ vomiting	50	56	53
Urinary retention	42	44	43
Drowsiness	33	50	43
Respiratory depression	0	6	3

Modified from Abboud TK, Shnider SM, Dailey PA, et al. Intrathecal administration of hyperbaric morphine for the relief of pain in labour. *Br J Anaesth*. 1984;56:1351–1360.

into the spinal or epidural space to prevent irritation or damage to neural structures.

Adverse Effects

Neuraxial opioid administration is associated with beneficial effects as well as potential complications and side effects. Intrathecal administration of clinically relevant doses of morphine is associated with a high incidence of side effects, including somnolence, nausea and vomiting, pruritus, urinary retention, and respiratory depression (Table 13.4). However, epidural and intrathecal injection of more lipid-soluble opioids have fewer side effects.

Sensory Changes

An early study evaluating intrathecal sufentanil in laboring women reported sensory changes and hypotension, although no local anesthetics were administered.[239] Other investigators have reported high cervical sensory blockade associated with mental status changes, dysphagia, dyspnea, and automatisms after intrathecal sufentanil or fentanyl injection.[240,241] These symptoms are likely to be related to a dose-dependent opioid effect rather than neuraxial blockade–induced sympathectomy.[242] Further, these changes do not predict the quality or duration of analgesia or degree of hemodynamic change.[242] These sensory changes can be clinically significant, especially when they extend to the cervical dermatomes. Patients may feel that they cannot breathe or swallow, an effect that can be distressing. Fortunately, neither intrathecal sufentanil nor fentanyl affects the efferent limb of the nervous system, and motor function is not impaired. Patients should be reassured that their respiratory efforts are not impaired and that these symptoms will subside in 30 to 60 minutes. One report described the use of naloxone to treat the sensory changes associated with intrathecal sufentanil.[240]

Hypotension

Decreased blood pressure was reported in early studies that evaluated intrathecal opioid administration.[239,242] Although hypotension occurs in 5% to 10% of parturients who receive intrathecal opioids,[239,242] the incidence is higher when a local anesthetic or clonidine is added to the opioid. Early reports suggested that hypotension was caused by a sympathectomy, but later work suggests that hypotension results from pain relief[242] and decreased maternal levels of catecholamines, especially epinephrine.[243] Wang et al.[244] demonstrated that intrathecal opioids block the afferent information from A-delta and C-fibers to the spinal cord but that efferent nerve impulses (e.g., sympathetic efferents) are not directly blocked.

Other Adverse Effects of Opioids

Epidural and subarachnoid opioids are associated with other adverse effects, including nausea, vomiting, pruritus, respiratory depression, urinary retention, delayed gastric emptying, and recrudescence of herpes simplex virus infection. These topics are reviewed in Chapters 24, 26, and 27. Placental transfer and fetal and neonatal effects of opioids are discussed in Chapter 23.

Biased-Ligand Opioid Agonists

Biased-based opioid agonists are a class of opioid receptor agonists that selectively activate signaling pathways while avoiding or minimizing others. Recent evidence suggests that μ-receptor agonism activates the β-arrestin signaling pathway, in addition to G-protein signaling. The β-arrestin pathway is implicated in several opioid-related adverse effects, including respiratory depression, constipation, and tolerance.[245,246]

This suggests that preferential activation of G-protein signaling while minimizing β-arrestin activity may broaden the therapeutic window of opioids by reducing the risk of adverse effects. Oliceridine (previously TRV130) is the first of this new class of "biased-ligand" opioid agonists and has received FDA approval for the treatment of acute pain severe enough to require intravenous opioid analgesia.[247,248] At present, oliceridine is not approved for use during pregnancy or for neuraxial administration.

The structure of oliceridine is distinct from morphine and synthetic derivatives such as fentanyl, conferring exceptional selectivity for μ-opioid receptor activation while inducing only 14% of β-arrestin-2 activity compared to morphine.[247] Clinical trials of patients who underwent abdominoplasty and bunionectomy reported comparable or greater analgesic efficacy of oliceridine compared to morphine.[249–252] Initial studies also suggested that oliceridine is associated with lower risk of respiratory depression and gastrointestinal complications compared with morphine[247,253]; however, subsequent clinical trials were designed primarily to evaluate analgesic efficacy instead of safety outcomes. Given this important limitation, clinical studies either demonstrated reduced respiratory depression with oliceridine compared to morphine,[249,250,254,255] or no significant difference between the two drugs.[251] Clinical trial data for the incidence of gastrointestinal complications are limited, with two studies reporting a reduced incidence of nausea and vomiting, although no statistical analyses were performed.[250,251] Similarly, the safety of oliceridine in terms of cardiac arrhythmias and abuse potential is unclear, given the limited data available.[256] Research in the field is ongoing and may increase our opioid analgesia options in the future.

KEY POINTS

- Pregnancy enhances the effect of local anesthetic agents.
- Appropriate administration of epidural anesthesia does not adversely affect uterine tone or uterine or umbilical blood flow.
- Bupivacaine has greater cardiotoxicity than lidocaine because of its greater electrophysiologic effects, which predispose to ventricular arrhythmias.
- Amide local anesthetics formulated as the single S- (levorotatory) enantiomer, such as ropivacaine and levobupivacaine, have a lower potential for cardiotoxicity than racemic bupivacaine.
- Most local anesthetic toxicity cases first present with CNS signs and symptoms.
- The administration of lipid emulsion should be considered if serious local anesthetic systemic toxicity is suspected.
- Fetal acidosis results in accumulation of amide local anesthetic in the fetus.
- Local anesthetics, as used clinically, are not teratogenic.

- The elimination half-life of amide local anesthetics is longer in the newborn than in the adult because the former has a greater volume of distribution.
- The fetus and newborn seem to be no more vulnerable to the toxic effects of local anesthetics than the adult.
- Neuraxial opioid administration produces analgesia without loss of sensation or proprioception.
- The combination of a neuraxial local anesthetic and an opioid increases block density and allows for administration of a lower total dose of local anesthetic and a lower incidence of side effects.
- Spinal bioavailability of the hydrophilic drugs (e.g., morphine, hydromorphone) is greater than that of hydrophobic (lipophilic) opioids (e.g., fentanyl, sufentanil).
- Biased-ligand opioid agonists are a new class of opioids that selectively activate specific pathways that may increase efficacy and minimize adverse effects.

REFERENCES

1. Aberg G. Toxicological and local anaesthetic effects of optically active isomers of two local anaesthetic compounds. *Acta Pharmacol Toxicol (Copenh)*. 1972;31:273–286.
2. Graf BM, Abraham I, Eberbach N, et al. Differences in cardiotoxicity of bupivacaine and ropivacaine are the result of physicochemical and stereoselective properties. *Anesthesiology*. 2002;96:1427–1434.
3. Strichartz GR. The inhibition of sodium currents in myelinated nerve by quaternary derivatives of lidocaine. *J Gen Physiol*. 1973;62:37–57.
4. Bromage PR. Continuous lumbar epidural analgesia for obstetrics. *Can Med Assoc J*. 1961;85:1136–1140.
5. Lee GY, Kim CH, Chung RK, et al. Spread of subarachnoid sensory block with hyperbaric bupivacaine in second trimester of pregnancy. *J Clin Anesth*. 2009;21:482–485.
6. Fagraeus L, Urban BJ, Bromage PR. Spread of epidural analgesia in early pregnancy. *Anesthesiology*. 1983;58:184–187.
7. Butterworth JF, Walker FO, Lysak SZ. Pregnancy increases median nerve susceptibility to lidocaine. *Anesthesiology*. 1990;72:962–965.
8. Datta S, Lambert DH, Gregus J, et al. Differential sensitivities of mammalian nerve fibers during pregnancy. *Anesth Analg*. 1983;62:1070–1072.
9. Bader AM, Datta S, Moller RA, Covino BG. Acute progesterone treatment has no effect on bupivacaine-induced conduction blockade in the isolated rabbit vagus nerve. *Anesth Analg*. 1990;71:545–548.
10. Kuhnert BR, Kuhnert PM, Philipson EH, et al. The half-life of 2-chloroprocaine. *Anesth Analg*. 1986;65:273–278.
11. Monedero P, Hess P. High epidural block with chloroprocaine in a parturient with low pseudocholinesterase activity. *Can J Anaesth*. 2001;48:318–319.
12. Santos AC, Pedersen H, Morishima HO, et al. Pharmacokinetics of lidocaine in nonpregnant and pregnant ewes. *Anesth Analg*. 1988;67:1154–1158.
13. Bloedow DC, Ralston DH, Hargrove JC. Lidocaine pharmacokinetics in pregnant and nonpregnant sheep. *JPharm Sci*. 1980;69:32–37.
14. Downing JW, Johnson HV, Gonzalez HF, et al. The pharmacokinetics of epidural lidocaine and bupivacaine during cesarean section. *Anesth Analg*. 1997;84:527–532.
15. Kuhnert BR, Philipson EH, Pimental R, et al. Lidocaine disposition in mother, fetus, and neonate after spinal anesthesia. *Anesth Analg*. 1986;65:139–144.
16. Kuhnert BR, Knapp DR, Kuhnert PM, Prochaska AL. Maternal, fetal, and neonatal metabolism of lidocaine. *Clin Pharmacol Ther*. 1979;26:213–220.
17. Pedersen H, Santos AC, Morishima HO, et al. Does gestational age affect the pharmacokinetics and pharmacodynamics of lidocaine in mother and fetus? *Anesthesiology*. 1988;68:367–372.
18. Wood M, Wood AJ. Changes in plasma drug binding and alpha 1-acid glycoprotein in mother and newborn infant. *Clin Pharmacol Ther*. 1981;29:522–526.
19. Fragneto RY, Bader AM, Rosinia F, et al. Measurements of protein binding of lidocaine throughout pregnancy. *Anesth Analg*. 1994;79:295–297.
20. Pihlajamaki K, Kanto J, Lindberg R, et al. Extradural administration of bupivacaine: pharmacokinetics and metabolism in pregnant and non-pregnant women. *Br J Anaesth*. 1990;64:556–562.
21. Santos AC, Arthur GR, Lehning EJ, Finster M. Comparative pharmacokinetics of ropivacaine and bupivacaine in nonpregnant and pregnant ewes. *Anesth Analg*. 1997;85:87–93.
22. Kuhnert PM, Kuhnert BR, Stitts JM, Gross TL. The use of a selected ion monitoring technique to study the disposition ofbupivacaine in mother, fetus, and neonate following epidural anesthesia for cesarean section. *Anesthesiology*. 1981;55:611–617.
23. Reynolds F, Taylor G. Maternal and neonatal blood concentrations of bupivacaine: a comparison with lignocaine during continuous extradural analgesia. *Anaesthesia*. 1970;25:14–23.
24. Mather LE, Thomas J. Bupivacaine binding to plasma protein fractions. *J Pharm Pharmacol*. 1978;30:653–654.
25. Wulf H, Munstedt P, Maier C. Plasma protein binding of bupivacaine in pregnant women at term. *Acta Anaesthesiol Scand*. 1991;35:129–133.
26. Zhan Q, Huang S, Geng G, Xie Y. Comparison of relative potency of intrathecal bupivacaine for motor block in pregnant versus non-pregnant women. *Int J Obstet Anesth*. 2011;20:219–223.
27. Arthur GR, Feldman HS, Covino BG. Comparative pharmacokinetics of bupivacaine and ropivacaine, a new amide local anesthetic. *Anesth Analg*. 1988;67:1053–1058.
28. Datta S, Camann W, Bader A, VanderBurgh L. Clinical effects and maternal and fetal plasma concentrations of epidural ropivacaine versus bupivacaine for cesarean section. *Anesthesiology*. 1995;82:1346–1352.
29. Oda Y, Furuichi K, Tanaka K, et al. Metabolism of a new local anesthetic, ropivacaine, by human hepatic cytochrome P450. *Anesthesiology*. 1995;82:214–220.
30. Moller R, Covino BG. Cardiac electrophysiologic properties of bupivacaine and lidocaine compared with those of ropivacaine, a new amide local anesthetic. *Anesthesiology*. 1990;72:322–329.
31. Porter JM, Kelleher N, Flynn R, Shorten GD. Epidural ropivacaine hydrochloride during labour: protein binding, placental transfer and neonatal outcome. *Anaesthesia*. 2001;56:418–423.
32. US Food and Drug Administration. Highlights of Prescribing Information: Exparel; 2023. https://www.accessdata.fda.gov/drugsatfda_docs/label/2023/022496s044lbl.pdf. Accessed 13 July 2024
33. Hu D, Onel E, Singla N, et al. Pharmacokinetic profile of liposome bupivacaine injection following a single administration at the surgical site. *Clin Drug Investig*. 2013;33:109–115.
34. Dinges H-C, Wiesmann T, Otremba B, et al. The analgesic efficacy of liposomal bupivacaine compared with bupivacaine hydrochloride for the prevention of postoperative pain: a systematic review and meta-analysis with trial sequential analysis. *Reg Anesth Pain Med*. 2021;46:490–498.
35. Nedeljkovic SS, Kett A, Vallejo MC, et al. Transversus abdominis plane block with liposomal bupivacaine for pain after cesarean delivery in a multicenter, randomized, double-blind, controlled trial. *Anesth Analg*. 2020;131:1830.
36. Habib AS, Nedeljkovic SS, Horn J-L, et al. Randomized trial of transversus abdominis plane block with liposomal

bupivacaine after cesarean delivery with or without intrathecal morphine. *J Clin Anesth*. 2021;75:110527.

37. Mustafa HJ, Wong HL, Al-Kofahi M, et al. Bupivacaine pharmacokinetics and breast milk excretion of liposomal bupivacaine administered after cesarean birth. *Obstet Gynecol*. 2020;136:70.

38. US Food and Drug Administration. Highlights of Prescribing Information: Zynrelef; 2021. https://www.accessdata.fda.gov/drugsatfda_docs/label/2021/211988s000lbl.pdf. Accessed 13 July 2024

39. Ramanathan J, Bottorff M, Jeter JN, et al. The pharmacokinetics and maternal and neonatal effects of epidural lidocaine in preeclampsia. *Anesth Analg*. 1986;65:120–126.

40. Dantes Moises EC, de Barros Duarte L, Carvalho Cavalli R, et al. Transplacental distribution of lidocaine and its metabolite in peridural anesthesia administered to patients with gestational diabetes mellitus. *Reprod Sci*. 2015;22:791–797.

41. Debon R, Chassard D, Duflo F, et al. Chronobiology of epidural ropivacaine: variations in the duration of action related to the hour of administration. *Anesthesiology*. 2002;96:542–545.

42. Shafer SL, Lemmer B, Boselli E, et al. Pitfalls in chronobiology: a suggested analysis using intrathecal bupivacaine analgesia as an example. *Anesth Analg*. 2010;111:980–985.

43. Sviggum HP, Yacoubian S, Liu X, Tsen LC. The effect of bupivacaine with fentanyl temperature on initiation and maintenance of labor epidural analgesia: a randomized controlled study. *Int J Obstet Anesth*. 2015;24:15–21.

44. Gitman M, Barrington MJ. Local anesthetic systemic toxicity: a review of recent case reports and registries. *Reg Anesth Pain Med*. 2018;43:124–130.

45. Di Gregorio G, Neal JM, Rosenquist RW, Weinberg GL. Clinical presentation of local anesthetic systemic toxicity: a review of published cases, 1979 to 2009. *Reg Anesth Pain Med*. 2010;35:181–187.

46. Christie LE, Picard J, Weinberg GL. Local anaesthetic systemic toxicity. *BJA Educ*. 2015;15:136–142.

47. De Jong RH, Robles R, Corbin RW. Central actions of lidocaine–synaptic transmission. *Anesthesiology*. 1969;30:19–23.

48. Liu PL, Feldman HS, Giasi R, et al. Comparative CNS toxicity of lidocaine, etidocaine, bupivacaine, and tetracaine in awake dogs following rapid intravenous administration. *Anesth Analg*. 1983;62:375–379.

49. Covino BG, Vassallo HG. *Local Anesthetics: Mechanisms of Action and Clinical Use*. Grune & Stratton; 1976:126.

50. Scott DB. Evaluation of the toxicity of local anaesthetic agents in man. *Br J Anaesth*. 1975;47:56–61.

51. Englesson S, Grevsten S. The influence of acid-base changes on central nervous system toxicity of local anaesthetic agents. II. *Acta Anaesthesiol Scand*. 1974;18:88–103.

52. Burney RG, DiFazio CA, Foster JA. Effects of pH on protein binding of lidocaine. *Anesth Analg*. 1978;57:478–480.

53. de Jong RH, Ronfeld RA, DeRosa RA. Cardiovascular effects of convulsant and supraconvulsant doses of amide local anesthetics. *Anesth Analg*. 1982;61:3–9.

54. Santos AC, Pedersen H, Harmon TW, et al. Does pregnancy alter the systemic toxicity of local anesthetics? *Anesthesiology*. 1989;70:991–995.

55. Morishima HO, Pedersen H, Finster M, et al. Bupivacaine toxicity in pregnant and nonpregnant ewes. *Anesthesiology*. 1985;63:134–139.

56. Clarkson CW, Hondeghem LM. Mechanism for bupivacaine depression of cardiac conduction: fast block of sodium channels during the action potential with slow recovery from block during diastole. *Anesthesiology*. 1985;62:396–405.

57. Thomas RD, Behbehani MM, Coyle DE, Denson DD. Cardiovascular toxicity of local anesthetics: an alternative hypothesis. *Anesth Analg*. 1986;65:444–450.

58. Coyle DE, Porembka DT, Sehlhorst CS, et al. Echocardiographic evaluation of bupivacaine cardiotoxicity. *Anesth Analg*. 1994;79:335–339.

59. Feldman HS, Arthur GR, Covino BG. Comparative systemic toxicity of convulsant and supraconvulsant doses of intravenous ropivacaine, bupivacaine, and lidocaine in the conscious dog. *Anesth Analg*. 1989;69:794–801.

60. Reiz S, Haggmark S, Johansson G, Nath S. Cardiotoxicity of ropivacaine—a new amide local anaesthetic agent. *Acta Anaesthesiol Scand*. 1989;33:93–98.

61. Nancarrow C, Rutten AJ, Runciman WB, et al. Myocardial and cerebral drug concentrations and the mechanisms of death after fatal intravenous doses of lidocaine, bupivacaine, and ropivacaine in the sheep. *Anesth Analg*. 1989;69:276–283.

62. Scott DB, Lee A, Fagan D, et al. Acute toxicity of ropivacaine compared with that of bupivacaine. *Anesth Analg*. 1989;69:563–569.

63. Polley LS, Columb MO, Naughton NN, et al. Relative analgesic potencies of ropivacaine and bupivacaine for epidural analgesia in labor: implications for therapeutic indexes. *Anesthesiology*. 1999;90:944–950.

64. Capogna G, Celleno D, Fusco P, et al. Relative potencies of bupivacaine and ropivacaine for analgesia in labour. *Br J Anaesth*. 1999;82:371–373.

65. Ngan Kee WD, Ng FF, Khaw KS, et al. Determination and comparison of graded dose-response curves for epidural bupivacaine and ropivacaine for analgesia in laboring nulliparous women. *Anesthesiology*. 2010;113:445–453.

66. Chazalon P, Tourtier JP, Villevielle T, et al. Ropivacaine-induced cardiac arrest after peripheral nerve block: successful resuscitation. *Anesthesiology*. 2003;99:1449–1451.

67. Huet O, Eyrolle LJ, Mazoit JX, Ozier YM. Cardiac arrest after injection of ropivacaine for posterior lumbar plexus blockade. *Anesthesiology*. 2003;99:1451–1453.

68. Yoshida M, Matsuda H, Fukuda I, Furuya K. Sudden cardiac arrest during cesarean section due to epidural anaesthesia using ropivacaine: a case report. *Arch Gynecol Obstet*. 2008;277:91–94.

69. Albright GA. Cardiac arrest following regional anesthesia with etidocaine or bupivacaine. *Anesthesiology*. 1979;51:285–287.

70. Valenzuela C, Snyders DJ, Bennett PB, et al. Stereoselective block of cardiac sodium channels by bupivacaine in guinea pig ventricular myocytes. *Circulation*. 1995;92:3014–3024.

71. Mazoit JX, Boico O, Samii K. Myocardial uptake of bupivacaine: II. Pharmacokinetics and pharmacodynamics ofbupivacaine enantiomers in the isolated perfused rabbit heart. *Anesth Analg*. 1993;77:477–482.

72. Santos AC, DeArmas PI. Systemic toxicity of levobupivacaine, bupivacaine, and ropivacaine during continuous intravenous infusion to nonpregnant and pregnant ewes. *Anesthesiology*. 2001;95:1256–1264.

73. Lyons G, Columb M, Wilson RC, Johnson RV. Epidural pain relief in labour: potencies of levobupivacaine and racemic bupivacaine. *Br J Anaesth*. 1998;81:899–901.

74. Lacassie HJ, Habib AS, Lacassie HP, Columb MO. Motor blocking minimum local anesthetic concentrations of bupivacaine, levobupivacaine, and ropivacaine in labor. *Reg Anesth Pain Med*. 2007;32:323–329.

75. Foxall G, McCahon R, Lamb J, et al. Levobupivacaine-induced seizures and cardiovascular collapse treated with Intralipid. *Anaesthesia*. 2007;62:516–518.

76. Bourque M, Morissette M, Al Sweidi S, et al. Neuroprotective effect of progesterone in MPTP-treated male mice. *Neuroendocrinology*. 2016;103:300–314.

77. Kim YJ, McFarlane C, Warner DS, et al. The effects of plasma and brain magnesium concentrations on lidocaine-induced seizures in the rat. *Anesth Analg*. 1996;83:1223–1228.

78. Kasten GW, Martin ST. Resuscitation from bupivacaine-induced cardiovascular toxicity during partial inferior vena cava occlusion. *Anesth Analg*. 1986;65:341–344.

79. Marx GF. Cardiotoxicity of local anesthetics–the plot thickens. *Anesthesiology*. 1984;60:3–5.

80. Moller RA, Datta S, Fox J, et al. Effects of progesterone on the cardiac electrophysiologic action of bupivacaine and lidocaine. *Anesthesiology*. 1992;76:604–608.

81. Moller RA, Datta S, Strichartz GR. Beta-estradiol acutely potentiates the depression of cardiac excitability by lidocaine and bupivacaine. *J Cardiovasc Pharmacol*. 1999;34:718–727.

82. Moller RA, Covino BG. Effect of progesterone on the cardiac electrophysiologic alterations produced by ropivacaine and bupivacaine. *Anesthesiology*. 1992;77:735–741.

83. Bern S, Weinberg G. Local anesthetic toxicity and lipid resuscitation in pregnancy. *Curr Opin Anaesthesiol*. 2011;24:262–267.

84. Hawkins JL, Chang J, Palmer SK, et al. Anesthesia-related maternal mortality in the United States: 1979–2002. *Obstet Gynecol*. 2011;117:69–74.

85. Pere P, Ekstrand A, Salonen M, et al. Pharmacokinetics of ropivacaine in patients with chronic renal failure. *Br J Anaesth*. 2011;106:512–521.

86. Vasques F, Behr AU, Weinberg G, et al. A review of local anesthetic systemic toxicity cases since publication of the American Society of Regional Anesthesia Recommendations: to whom it may concern. *Reg Anesth Pain Med*. 2015;40:698–705.

87. Trabelsi B, Charfi R, Bennasr L, et al. Pharmacokinetics of bupivacaine after bilateral ultrasound-guided transversus abdominis plane block following cesarean delivery under spinal anesthesia. *Int J Obstet Anesth*. 2017;32:17–20.

88. Kumar SK, Rao V, Morris RG, et al. Ropivacaine (total and unbound) and AGP concentrations after transversus abdominis plane block for analgesia after abdominal surgery. *Ther Drug Monit*. 2014;36:759–764.

89. Neal JM, Neal EJ, Weinberg GL. American Society of Regional Anesthesia and Pain Medicine local anesthetic systemic toxicity checklist: 2020 version. *Reg Anesth Pain Med*. 2021;46:81–82.

90. Covino BG, Marx GF, Finster M, Zsigmond EK. Prolonged sensory/motor deficits following inadvertent spinal anesthesia. *Anesth Analg*. 1980;59:399–400.

91. Ready LB, Plumer MH, Haschke RH, et al. Neurotoxicity of intrathecal local anesthetics in rabbits. *Anesthesiology*. 1985;63:364–370.

92. Barsa J, Batra M, Fink BR, Sumi SM. A comparative in vivo study of local neurotoxicity of lidocaine, bupivacaine, 2-chloroprocaine, and a mixture of 2-chloroprocaine and bupivacaine. *Anesth Analg*. 1982;61:961–967.

93. Gissen AJ, Datta S, Lambert D. The chloroprocaine controversy: II. Is chloroprocaine neurotoxic? *Reg Anesth PainMed*. 1984;9:135–145.

94. Fibuch EE, Opper SE. Back pain following epidurally administered Nesacaine-MPF. *Anesth Analg*. 1989;69:113–115.

95. Rigler ML, Drasner K, Krejcie TC, et al. Cauda equina syndrome after continuous spinal anesthesia. *Anesth Analg*. 1991;72:275–281.

96. Schneider M, Ettlin T, Kaufmann M, et al. Transient neurologic toxicity after hyperbaric subarachnoid anesthesia with 5% lidocaine. *Anesth Analg*. 1993;76:1154–1157.

97. Bainton CR, Strichartz GR. Concentration dependence of lidocaine-induced irreversible conduction loss in frog nerve. *Anesthesiology*. 1994;81:657–667.

98. Lambert LA, Lambert DH, Strichartz GR. Irreversible conduction block in isolated nerve by high concentrations of local anesthetics. *Anesthesiology*. 1994;80:1082–1093.

99. Li DF, Bahar M, Cole G, Rosen M. Neurological toxicity of the subarachnoid infusion of bupivacaine, lignocaine or 2-chloroprocaine in the rat. *Br J Anaesth*. 1985;57:424–429.

100. Dripps RD, Vandam LD. Long-term follow-up of patients who received 10,098 spinal anesthetics: failure to discover major neurological sequelae. *J Am Med Assoc*. 1954;156:1486–1491.

101. Pollock JE, Liu SS, Neal JM, Stephenson CA. Dilution of spinal lidocaine does not alter the incidence of transient neurologic symptoms. *Anesthesiology*. 1999;90:445–450.

102. Freedman JM, Li DK, Drasner K, et al. Transient neurologic symptoms after spinal anesthesia: an epidemiologic study of 1,863 patients. *Anesthesiology*. 1998;89:633–641.

103. Forget P, Borovac JA, Thackeray EM, Pace NL. Transient neurological symptoms (TNS) following spinal anaesthesia with lidocaine versus other local anaesthetics in adult surgical patients: a network meta-analysis. *Cochrane Database Syst Rev*. 2019;(12):CD003006.

104. Aouad MT, Siddik SS, Jalbout MI, Baraka AS. Does pregnancy protect against intrathecal lidocaine-induced transient neurologic symptoms? *Anesth Analg*. 2001;92:401–404.

105. Philip J, Sharma SK, Gottumukkala VN, et al. Transient neurologic symptoms after spinal anesthesia with lidocaine in obstetric patients. *Anesth Analg*. 2001;92:405–409.

106. Jiang S, Tang M. Allergy to local anesthetics is a rarity: review of diagnostics and strategies for clinical management. *Clin Rev Allergy Immunol*. 2023;64:193–205.

107. Kvisselgaard AD, Mosbech HF, Fransson S, Garvey LH. Risk of immediate-type allergy to local anesthetics is overestimated-results from 5 years of provocation testing in a Danish allergy clinic. *J Allergy Clin Immunol Pract*. 2018;6:1217–1223.

108. Kolawole H, Marshall SD, Crilly H, et al. Australian and New Zealand Anaesthetic Allergy Group/Australian and New Zealand College of Anaesthetists perioperative anaphylaxis management guidelines. *Anaesth Intensive Care*. 2017;45:151–158.

109. Cibils LA. Response of human uterine arteries to local anesthetics. *Am J Obstet Gynecol*. 1976;126:202–210.

110. Noren H, Lindblom B, Kallfelt B. Effects of bupivacaine and calcium antagonists on human uterine arteries in pregnant and non-pregnant women. *Acta Anaesthesiol Scand*. 1991;35:488–491.

111. Fishburne JI FC Jr, Greiss JI FC Jr, Hopkinson R, Rhyne AL. Responses of the gravid uterine vasculature to arterial levels of local anesthetic agents. *Am J Obstet Gynecol.* 1979;133: 753–761.

112. Santos AC, Karpel B, Noble G. The placental transfer and fetal effects of levobupivacaine, racemic bupivacaine, and ropivacaine. *Anesthesiology.* 1999;90:1698–1703.

113. Chestnut DH, Weiner CP, Herrig JE. The effect of intravenously administered 2-chloroprocaine upon uterine artery blood flow velocity in gravid guinea pigs. *Anesthesiology.* 1989;70:305–308.

114. Biehl D, Shnider SM, Levinson G, Callender K. The direct effects of circulating lidocaine on uterine blood flow and foetal well-being in the pregnant ewe. *Can Anaesth Soc J.* 1977;24:445–451.

115. Gintautas J, Kraynack B, Havasi G, et al. Responses of isolated uterine arteries to local anesthetic agents. *Proc West Pharmacol Soc.* 1981;24:191–192.

116. Alahuhta S, Rasanen J, Jouppila P, et al. The effects of epidural ropivacaine and bupivacaine for cesarean section on uteroplacental and fetal circulation. *Anesthesiology.* 1995;83:23–32.

117. Giles WB, Lah FX, Trudinger BJ. The effect of epidural anaesthesia for caesarean section on maternal uterine and fetal umbilical artery blood flow velocity waveforms. *Br J Obstet Gynaecol.* 1987;94:55–59.

118. Kopacz DJ, Carpenter RL, Mackey DC. Effect of ropivacaine on cutaneous capillary blood flow in pigs. *Anesthesiology.* 1989;71:69–74.

119. Tuvemo T. Willdeck-Lund G. Smooth muscle effects of lidocaine, prilocaine, bupivacaine and etidocaine on the human umbilical artery. *Acta Anaesthesiol Scand.* 1982;26:104–107.

120. Noren H, Kallfelt B, Lindblom B. Influence of bupivacaine and morphine on human umbilical arteries and veins in vitro. *Acta Obstet Gynecol Scand.* 1990;69:87–91.

121. Halevy S, Rossner KL, Liu-Barnett M, et al. The response of umbilical vessels, with and without vascular endothelium, to local anesthesia in low PO2 and hypercarbia. *Reg Anesth.* 1995;20:316–322.

122. Morishima HO, Heymann MA, Rudolph AM, et al. Transfer of lidocaine across the sheep placenta to the fetus. Hemodynamic and acid-base responses of the fetal lamb. *Am J Obstet Gynecol.* 1975;122:581–588.

123. Marx GF, Elstein ID, Schuss M, et al. Effects of epidural block with lignocaine and lignocaine-adrenaline on umbilical artery velocity wave ratios. *Br J Obstet Gynaecol.* 1990;97: 517–520.

124. Marx GF, Patel S, Berman JA, et al. Umbilical blood flow velocity waveforms in different maternal positions and with epidural analgesia. *Obstet Gynecol.* 1986;68: 61–64.

125. Lindblad A, Marsal K, Vernersson E, Renck H. Fetal circulation during epidural analgesia for caesarean section. *Br Med J (Clin Res Ed).* 1984;288:1329–1330.

126. McGaughey HSJ, Corey EL, Eastwood D, Thorton WNJ. Effect of synthetic anesthetics on the spontaneous motility of human uterine muscle in vitro. *Obstet Gynecol.* 1962;19: 233–240.

127. Morishima HO, Covino BG, Yeh MN, et al. Bradycardia in the fetal baboon following paracervical block anesthesia. *Am J Obstet Gynecol.* 1981;140:775–780.

128. Belitzky R, Delard LG, Novick LM. Oxytocic effect of intramyometrial injection of procaine in a pregnant woman. *Am J Obstet Gynecol.* 1970;107:973–975.

129. Kaynak G, Iskender A, Albayrak M, et al. In vivo comparison of the effects of bupivacaine and levobupivacaine on the pregnant rat myometrium using electrohysterogram. *Gynecol Obstet Invest.* 2012;73:43–47.

130. Camann WR, Hartigan PM, Gilbertson LI, et al. Chloroprocaine antagonism of epidural opioid analgesia: a receptor-specific phenomenon? *Anesthesiology.* 1990;73:860–863.

131. Grice SC, Eisenach JC, Dewan DM. Labor analgesia with epidural bupivacaine plus fentanyl: enhancement with epinephrine and inhibition with 2-chloroprocaine. *Anesthesiology.* 1990;72:623–628.

132. Lee LO, Ramirez-Chapman AL, White DL, et al. Postcesarean analgesia with epidural morphine after epidural 2-chloroprocaine: a randomized noninferiority trial. *Anesth Analg.* 2023;136:86–93.

133. Hess PE, Snowman CE, Hahn CJ, et al. Chloroprocaine may not affect epidural morphine for postcesarean delivery analgesia. *J Clin Anesth.* 2006;18:29–33.

134. McClure JH. Ropivacaine. *Br J Anaesth.* 1996;76:300–307.

135. van Kleef JW, Veering BT, Burm AG. Spinal anesthesia with ropivacaine: a double-blind study on the efficacy and safety of 0.5% and 0.75% solutions in patients undergoing minor lower limb surgery. *Anesth Analg.* 1994;78:1125–1130.

136. Coppejans HC, Vercauteren MP. Low-dose combined spinal-epidural anesthesia for cesarean delivery: a comparison of three plain local anesthetics. *Acta Anaesthesiol Belg.* 2006;57:39–43.

137. Polley LS, Columb MO, Naughton NN, et al. Relative analgesic potencies of levobupivacaine and ropivacaine for epidural analgesia in labor. *Anesthesiology.* 2003;99: 1354–1358.

138. Benhamou D, Ghosh C, Mercier FJ. A randomized sequential allocation study to determine the minimum effective analgesic concentration of levobupivacaine and ropivacaine in patients receiving epidural analgesia for labor. *Anesthesiology.* 2003;99:1383–1386.

139. Vercauteren MP, Hans G, De Decker K, Adriaensen HA. Levobupivacaine combined with sufentanil and epinephrine for intrathecal labor analgesia: a comparison with racemic bupivacaine. *Anesth Analg.* 2001;93:996–1000.

140. D'Angelo R, James RL. Is ropivacaine less potent than bupivacaine? *Anesthesiology.* 1999;90:941–943.

141. Beilin Y, Guinn NR, Bernstein HH, et al. Local anesthetics and mode of delivery: bupivacaine versus ropivacaine versus levobupivacaine. *Anesth Analg.* 2007;105: 756–763.

142. Bader AM, Tsen LC, Camann WR, et al. Clinical effects and maternal and fetal plasma concentrations of 0.5% epidural levobupivacaine versus bupivacaine for cesarean delivery. *Anesthesiology.* 1999;90:1596–1601.

143. Mather L, Tucker G. Properties, absorption, and disposition of local anesthetic agents. In: Cousins MJ, Carr DB, Horlocker TT, Bridenbaugh PO, eds. *Neural Blockade in Clinical Anesthesia and Management of Pain.* 4th ed. Lippincott-Raven; 2009:48–95.

144. Ueki R, Tatara T, Kariya N, et al. Comparison of placental transfer of local anesthetics in perfusates with different pH values in a human cotyledon model. *J Anesth.* 2009;23: 526–529.

145. Biehl D, Shnider SM, Levinson G, Callender K. Placental transfer of lidocaine: effects of fetal acidosis. *Anesthesiology*. 1978;48:409–412.

146. Brown WU Jr, Bell GC, Alper MH. Acidosis, local anesthetics, and the newborn. *Obstet Gynecol*. 1976;48:27–30.

147. Morishima HO, Covino BG. Toxicity and distribution of lidocaine in nonasphyxiated and asphyxiated baboon fetuses. *Anesthesiology*. 1981;54:182–186.

148. Kennedy RL, Miller RP, Bell JU, et al. Uptake and distributionof bupivacaine in fetal lambs. *Anesthesiology*. 1986;65:247–253.

149. Kennedy RL, Bell JU, Miller RP, et al. Uptake and distribution of lidocaine in fetal lambs. *Anesthesiology*. 1990;72:483–489.

150. Hamshaw-Thomas A, Reynolds F. Placental transfer of bupivacaine, pethidine and lignocaine in the rabbit. Effect of umbilical flow rate and protein content. *Br J Obstet Gynaecol*. 1985;92:706–713.

151. Hamshaw-Thomas A, Rogerson N, Reynolds F. Transfer of bupivacaine, lignocaine and pethidine across the rabbit placenta: influence of maternal protein binding and fetal flow. *Placenta*. 1984;5:61–70.

152. Vella LM, Knott C, Reynolds F. Transfer of fentanyl across the rabbit placenta. Effect of umbilical flow and concurrent drug administration. *Br J Anaesth*. 1986;58:49–54.

153. Petersen MC, Moore RG, Nation RL, McMeniman W. Relationship between the transplacental gradients of bupivacaine and alpha 1-acid glycoprotein. *Br J Clin Pharmacol*. 1981;12:859–862.

154. Thomas J, Long G, Moore G, Morgan D. Plasma protein binding and placental transfer of bupivacaine. *Clin Pharmacol Ther*. 1976;19:426–434.

155. Johnson RF, Cahana A, Olenick M, et al. A comparison of the placental transfer of ropivacaine versus bupivacaine. *Anesth Analg*. 1999;89:703–708.

156. Petrie RH, Paul WL, Miller FC, et al. Placental transfer of lidocaine following paracervical block. *Am J Obstet Gynecol*. 1974;120:791–801.

157. Mazze RI, Dunbar RW. Plasma lidocaine concentrations after caudal, lumbar epidural, axillary block, and intravenous regional anesthesia. *Anesthesiology*. 1966;27:574–579.

158. Giasi RM, D'Agostino E, Covino BG. Absorption of lidocaine following subarachnoid and epidural administration. *Anesth Analg*. 1979;58:360–363.

159. Idanpaan-Heikkila JE, Taska RJ, Allen HA, Schoolar JC. Placental transfer of diazepam-14 C in mice, hamsters and monkeys. *J Pharmacol Exp Ther*. 1971;176:752–757.

160. Shnider SM, Way EL. The kinetics of transfer of lidocaine (Xylocaine) across the human placenta. *Anesthesiology*. 1968;29:944–950.

161. Roe DA, Little BB, Bawdon RE, Gilstrap LC 3rd. Metabolism of cocaine by human placentas: implications for fetal exposure. *Am J Obstet Gynecol*. 1990;163:715–718.

162. Van Petten GR, Hirsch GH, Cherrington AD. Drug-metabolizing activity of the human placenta. *Can J Biochem*. 1968;46:1057–1061.

163. Fletcher S, Carson R, Reynolds F, et al. Plasma total and free concentrations of bupivacaine and lignocaine in mother and fetus following epidural administration, singly or together. *IntJ Obstet Anesth*. 1992;1:135–140.

164. Tucker GT, Boyes RN, Bridenbaugh PO, Moore DC. Binding of anilide-type local anesthetics in human plasma. II. Implications in vivo, with special reference to transplacental distribution. *Anesthesiology*. 1970;33:304–314.

165. Ehrnebo M, Agurell S, Jalling B, Boreus LO. Age differences in drug binding by plasma proteins: studies on human foetuses, neonates and adults. *Eur J Clin Pharmacol*. 1971;3:189–193.

166. Finster M, Morishima HO, Boyes RN, Covino BG. The placental transfer of lidocaine and its uptake by fetal tissues. *Anesthesiology*. 1972;36:159–163.

167. Morishima HO, Santos AC, Pedersen H, et al. Effect of lidocaine on the asphyxial responses in the mature fetal lamb. *Anesthesiology*. 1987;66:502–507.

168. Blankenbaker WL, DiFazio CA, Berry FA Jr. Lidocaine and its metabolites in the newborn. *Anesthesiology*. 1975;42:325–330.

169. Mihaly GW, Moore RG, Thomas J, et al. The pharmacokinetics and metabolism of the anilide local anaesthetics in neonates. I. Lignocaine. *Eur J Clin Pharmacol*. 1978;13:143–152.

170. Morishima HO, Finster M, Pedersen H, et al. Pharmacokinetics of lidocaine in fetal and neonatal lambs and adult sheep. *Anesthesiology*. 1979;50:431–436.

171. Brown WU, Bell GC, Lurie AO, et al. Newborn blood levels of lidocaine and mepivacaine in the first postnatal day followingmaternal epidural anesthesia. *Anesthesiology*. 1975;42:698–707.

172. Lieberman BA, Rosenblatt DB, Belsey E, et al. The effects of maternally administered pethidine or epidural bupivacaine onthe fetus and newborn. *Br J Obstet Gynaecol*. 1979;86:598–606.

173. Morishima HO, Pedersen H, Finster M, et al. Toxicity of lidocaine in adult, newborn, and fetal sheep. *Anesthesiology*. 1981;55:57–61.

174. Bosnjak ZJ, Stowe DF, Kampine JP. Comparison of lidocaine and bupivacaine depression of sinoatrial nodal activity during hypoxia and acidosis in adult and neonatal guinea pigs. *Anesth Analg*. 1986;65:911–917.

175. Badgwell JM, Heavner JE, Kytta J. Bupivacaine toxicity in young pigs is age-dependent and is affected by volatile anesthetics. *Anesthesiology*. 1990;73:297–303.

176. Loftus JR, Holbrook RH, Cohen SE. Fetal heart rate after epidural lidocaine and bupivacaine for elective cesarean section. *Anesthesiology*. 1991;75:406–412.

177. Hehre FW, Hook R, Hon EH. Continuous lumbar peridural anesthesia in obstetrics. VI. The fetal effects of transplacental passage of local anesthetic agents. *Anesth Analg*. 1969;48:909–913.

178. Abboud TK, Afrasiabi A, Sarkis F, et al. Continuous infusion epidural analgesia in parturients receiving bupivacaine, chloroprocaine, or lidocaine—maternal, fetal, and neonatal effects. *Anesth Analg*. 1984;63:421–428.

179. Becker JH, Schaap TP, Westerhuis ME, et al. Intrapartum epidural analgesia and ST analysis of the fetal electrocardiogram. *Acta Obstet Gynecol Scand*. 2011;90:1364–1370.

180. Halpern SH, Littleford JA, Brockhurst NJ, et al. The neurologic and adaptive capacity score is not a reliable method of newborn evaluation. *Anesthesiology*. 2001;94:958–962.

181. Kuhnert BR, Harrison MJ, Linn PL, Kuhnert PM. Effects of maternal epidural anesthesia on neonatal behavior. *Anesth Analg*. 1984;63:301–308.

182. Clark DA, Landaw SA. Bupivacaine alters red blood cell properties: a possible explanation for neonatal jaundice

associated with maternal anesthesia. *Pediatr Res*. 1985;19:
341–343.

183. Gale R, Ferguson JE 2nd, Stevenson DK. Effect of epidural
analgesia with bupivacaine hydrochloride on neonatal
bilirubin production. *Obstet Gynecol*. 1987;70:692–695.

184. Alkan S, Tiras U, Dallar Y, Sunay D. Effect of anaesthetic
agents administered to the mothers on transcutaneous
bilirubin levels in the neonates. *Acta Paediatr*. 2010;99:
993–996.

185. Smedstad KG, Morison DH, Harris WH, Pascoe P. Placental
transfer of local anaesthetics in the premature sheep fetus. *Int
J Obstet Anesth*. 1993;2:34–38.

186. Morishima HO, Pedersen H, Santos AC, et al. Adverse effects
of maternally administered lidocaine on the asphyxiated
preterm fetal lamb. *Anesthesiology*. 1989;71:110–115.

187. Santos AC, Yun EM, Bobby PD, et al. The effects of
bupivacaine, L-nitro-L-arginine-methyl ester, and
phenylephrine on cardiovascular adaptations to asphyxia in
the preterm fetal lamb. *Anesth Analg*. 1997;85:1299–1306.

188. Johnson RF, Herman NL, Johnson HV, et al. Effects of fetal
pH on local anesthetic transfer across the human placenta.
Anesthesiology. 1996;85:608–615.

189. Yaksh T, Wallace M. Opioids, analgesia, and pain
management. In: Brunton L, Hilal-Dandan R, Knollman
BC, eds. *Goodman and Gilman's The Pharmacologic Basis of
Therapeutics*. 13th ed. McGraw-Hill Education; 2018:355-386.

190. Meunier JC, Mollereau C, Toll L, et al. Isolation and structure
of the endogenous agonist of opioid receptor-like ORL1
receptor. *Nature*. 1995;377:532–535.

191. Riviere PJ. Peripheral kappa-opioid agonists for visceral pain.
Br J Pharmacol. 2004;141:1331–1334.

192. Waldhoer M, Bartlett SE, Whistler JL. Opioid receptors. *Annu
Rev Biochem*. 2004;73:953–990.

193. Thorpe DH. Opiate structure and activity—a guide to
understanding the receptor. *Anesth Analg*. 1984;63:143–151.

194. Beckett AH. Analgesics and their antagonists: some steric and
chemical considerations. I. The dissociation constants of some
tertiary amines and synthetic analgesics, the conformations
of methadone-type compounds. *J Pharm Pharmacol*.
1956;8:848–859.

195. Portoghese PS, Alreja BD, Larson DL. Allylprodine analogues
as receptor probes. Evidence that phenolic and nonphenolic
ligands interact with different subsites on identical opioid
receptors. *J Med Chem*. 1981;24:782–787.

196. Gorin FA, Balasubramanian TM, Cicero TJ, et al. Novel
analogues of enkephalin: identification of functional groups
required for biological activity. *J Med Chem*. 1980;23:
1113–1122.

197. Wang JK, Nauss LA, Thomas JE. Pain relief by intrathecally
applied morphine in man. *Anesthesiology*. 1979;50:149–151.

198. Yaksh TL. Spinal opiate analgesia: characteristics and
principles of action. *Pain*. 1981;11:293–346.

199. Al-Hasani R, Bruchas MR. Molecular mechanisms of opioid
receptor-dependent signaling and behavior. *Anesthesiology*.
2011;115:1363–1381.

200. Bernards CM, Hill HF. The spinal nerve root sleeve is not a
preferred route for redistribution of drugs from the epidural
space to the spinal cord. *Anesthesiology*. 1991;75:827–832.

201. Bernards CM, Hill HF. Physical and chemical properties of
drug molecules governing their diffusion through the spinal
meninges. *Anesthesiology*. 1992;77:750–756.

202. Bernards CM. Understanding the physiology and
pharmacology of epidural and intrathecal opioids. *Best Pract
Res Clin Anaesthesiol*. 2002;16:489–505.

203. Bernards CM, Hill HF. Morphine and alfentanil permeability
through the spinal dura, arachnoid, and pia mater of dogs and
monkeys. *Anesthesiology*. 1990;73:1214–1219.

204. Bernards CM, Shen DD, Sterling ES, et al. Epidural,
cerebrospinal fluid, and plasma pharmacokinetics of epidural
opioids (part 1): differences among opioids. *Anesthesiology*.
2003;99:455–465.

205. Coda BA, Brown MC, Schaffer RL, et al. A pharmacokinetic
approach to resolving spinal and systemic contributions
to epidural alfentanil analgesia and side-effects. *Pain*.
1995;62:329–337.

206. Miguel R, Barlow I, Morrell M, et al. A prospective,
randomized, double-blind comparison of epidural and
intravenous sufentanil infusions. *Anesthesiology*. 1994;81:
346–352.

207. Liu SS, Gerancher JC, Bainton BG, et al. The effects
of electrical stimulation at different frequencies on
perception and pain in human volunteers: epidural versus
intravenous administration of fentanyl. *Anesth Analg*.
1996;82:98–102.

208. D'Angelo R, Gerancher JC, Eisenach JC, Raphael BL. Epidural
fentanyl produces labor analgesia by a spinal mechanism.
Anesthesiology. 1998;88:1519–1523.

209. Ginosar Y, Riley ET, Angst MS. The site of action of epidural
fentanyl in humans: the difference between infusion and bolus
administration. *Anesth Analg*. 2003;97:1428–1438.

210. Ummenhofer WC, Arends RH, Shen DD, Bernards CM.
Comparative spinal distribution and clearance kinetics of
intrathecally administered morphine, fentanyl, alfentanil, and
sufentanil. *Anesthesiology*. 2000;92:739–753.

211. Eisenach JC, Hood DD, Curry R, Shafer SL. Cephalad
movement of morphine and fentanyl in humans after
intrathecal injection. *Anesthesiology*. 2003;99:166–173.

212. Lu JK, Schafer PG, Gardner TL, et al. The dose-response
pharmacology of intrathecal sufentanil in female volunteers.
Anesth Analg. 1997;85:372–379.

213. Sviggum HP, Arendt KW, Jacob AK, et al. Intrathecal
hydromorphone and morphine for postcesarean delivery
analgesia: determination of the ED90 using a sequential
allocation biased-coin method. *Anesth Analg*. 2016;123:
690–697.

214. Sharpe EE, Molitor RJ, Arendt KW, et al. Intrathecal
morphine versus intrathecal hydromorphone for analgesia
after cesarean delivery: a randomized clinical trial.
Anesthesiology. 2020;132:1382–1391.

215. Carvalho B, Riley E, Cohen SE, et al. Single-dose,
sustained-release epidural morphine in the management of
postoperative pain after elective cesarean delivery: results of
a multicenter randomized controlled study. *Anesth Analg*.
2005;100:1150–1158.

216. Carvalho B, Roland LM, Chu LF, et al. Single-dose,
extended-release epidural morphine (DepoDur) compared
to conventional epidural morphine for post-cesarean pain.
Anesth Analg. 2007;105:176–183.

217. Landau R, Smiley R. Pharmacogenetics in obstetric
anesthesia. *Best Pract Res Clin Anaesthesiol*. 2017;31:23–34.

218. Young EE, Lariviere WR, Belfer I. Genetic basis of pain
variability: recent advances. *J Med Genet*. 2012;49:1–9.

219. Kumar S, Kundra P, Ramsamy K, Surendiran A. Pharmacogenetics of opioids: a narrative review. *Anaesthesia.* 2019;74:1456–1470.

220. Crews KR, Gaedigk A, Dunnenberger HM, et al. Clinical Pharmacogenetics Implementation Consortium guidelines for cytochrome P450 2D6 genotype and codeine therapy: 2014 update. *Clin Pharmacol Ther.* 2014;95:376–382.

221. Landau R, Kern C, Columb MO, et al. Genetic variability of the mu-opioid receptor influences intrathecal fentanyl analgesia requirements in laboring women. *Pain.* 2008;139: 5–14.

222. Wong CA, McCarthy RJ, Blouin J, Landau R. Observational study of the effect of mu-opioid receptor genetic polymorphism on intrathecal opioid labor analgesia and post-cesarean delivery analgesia. *Int J Obstet Anesth.* 2010;19: 246–253.

223. Camorcia M, Capogna G, Stirparo S, et al. Effect of mu-opioid receptor A118G polymorphism on the ED50 of epidural sufentanil for labor analgesia. *Int J Obstet Anesth.* 2012;21: 40–44.

224. Landau R, Liu SK, Blouin JL, Carvalho B. The effect of OPRM1 and COMT genotypes on the analgesic response to intravenous fentanyl labor analgesia. *Anesth Analg.* 2013;116:386–391.

225. Sia AT, Lim Y, Lim EC, et al. A118G single nucleotide polymorphism of human mu-opioid receptor gene influences pain perception and patient-controlled intravenous morphine consumption after intrathecal morphine for postcesarean analgesia. *Anesthesiology.* 2008;109:520–526.

226. Tan EC, Lim EC, Teo YY, et al. Ethnicity and OPRM variant independently predict pain perception and patient-controlled analgesia usage for post-operative pain. *Mol Pain.* 2009;5:32.

227. Wong CA. The promise of pharmacogenetics in labor analgesia…tantalizing, but not there yet. *Int J Obstet Anesth.* 2012;21:105–108.

228. Walter C, Lotsch J. Meta-analysis of the relevance of the OPRM1 118A>G genetic variant for pain treatment. *Pain.* 2009;146:270–275.

229. Crews KR, Monte AA, Huddart R, et al. Clinical pharmacogenetics implementation consortium guideline for CYP2D6, OPRM1, and COMT genotypes and select opioid therapy. *Clin Pharmacol Ther.* 2021;110:888–896.

230. Yaksh TL, Collins JG. Studies in animals should precede human use of spinally administered drugs. *Anesthesiology.* 1989;70:4–6.

231. Yaksh TL, Noueihed RY, Durant PA. Studies of the pharmacology and pathology of intrathecally administered 4-anilinopiperidine analogues and morphine in the rat and cat. *Anesthesiology.* 1986;64:54–66.

232. Matsumiya N, Dohi S. Effects of intravenous or subarachnoid morphine on cerebral and spinal cord hemodynamics and antagonism with naloxone in dogs. *Anesthesiology.* 1983;59:175–181.

233. Yaksh TL, Horais KA, Tozier NA, et al. Chronically infused intrathecal morphine in dogs. *Anesthesiology.* 2003;99:174–187.

234. Arner S, Rawal N, Gustafsson LL. Clinical experience of long-term treatment with epidural and intrathecal opioids—a nationwide survey. *Acta Anaesthesiol Scand.* 1988;32:253–259.

235. Power I, Brown DT, Wildsmith JA. The effect of fentanyl, meperidine and diamorphine on nerve conduction in vitro. *Reg Anesth.* 1991;16:204–208.

236. Sabbe MB, Grafe MR, Mjanger E, et al. Spinal delivery of sufentanil, alfentanil, and morphine in dogs. Physiologic and toxicologic investigations. *Anesthesiology.* 1994;81:899–920.

237. Rawal N, Nuutinen L, Raj PP, et al. Behavioral and histopathologic effects following intrathecal administration of butorphanol, sufentanil, and nalbuphine in sheep. *Anesthesiology.* 1991;75:1025–1034.

238. Bottros MM, Christo PJ. Current perspectives on intrathecal drug delivery. *J Pain Res.* 2014;7:615–626.

239. Cohen SE, Cherry CM, Holbrook RH Jr, et al. Intrathecal sufentanil for labor analgesia—sensory changes, side effects, and fetal heart rate changes. *Anesth Analg.* 1993;77: 1155–1160.

240. Scavone BM. Altered level of consciousness after combined spinal-epidural labor analgesia with intrathecal fentanyl and bupivacaine. *Anesthesiology.* 2002;96:1021–1022.

241. Fragneto RY, Fisher A. Mental status change and aphasia after labor analgesia with intrathecal sufentanil/bupivacaine. *Anesth Analg.* 2000;90:1175–1176.

242. Riley ET, Ratner EF, Cohen SE. Intrathecal sufentanil for labor analgesia: do sensory changes predict better analgesia and greater hypotension? *Anesth Analg.* 1997;84:346–351.

243. Cascio M, Pygon B, Bernett C, Ramanathan S. Labour analgesia with intrathecal fentanyl decreases maternal stress. *Can J Anaesth.* 1997;44:605–609.

244. Wang C, Chakrabarti MK, Whitwam JG. Specific enhancement by fentanyl of the effects of intrathecal bupivacaine on nociceptive afferent but not on sympathetic efferent pathways in dogs. *Anesthesiology.* 1993;79:766–773.

245. Ehrlich AT, Kieffer BL, Darcq E. Current strategies toward safer mu opioid receptor drugs for pain management. *Expert Opin Ther Targets.* 2019;23:315–326.

246. Raehal KM, Walker JK, Bohn LM. Morphine side effects in beta-arrestin 2 knockout mice. *J Pharmacol Exp Ther.* 2005;314:1195–1201.

247. DeWire SM, Yamashita DS, Rominger DH, et al. A G protein-biased ligand at the mu-opioid receptor is potently analgesic with reduced gastrointestinal and respiratory dysfunction compared with morphine. *J Pharmacol Exp Ther.* 2013;344:708–717.

248. US Food and Drug Administration. Highlights of Prescribing Information: Olinvyk; 2020. https://www.accessdata.fda.gov/drugsatfda_docs/label/2021/210730s001lbl.pdf. Accessed 5 August 2023.

249. Singla N, Minkowitz HS, Soergel DG, et al. A randomized, Phase IIb study investigating oliceridine (TRV130), a novel micro-receptor G-protein pathway selective (mu-GPS) modulator, for the management of moderate to severe acute pain following abdominoplasty. *J Pain Res.* 2017;10:2413–2424.

250. Singla NK, Skobieranda F, Soergel DG, et al. APOLLO-2: arandomized, placebo and active-controlled phase III study investigating oliceridine (TRV130), a G protein-biased ligand at the mu-opioid receptor, for management of moderate to severe acute pain following abdominoplasty. *Pain Pract.* 2019;19:715–731.

251. Viscusi ER, Skobieranda F, Soergel DG, et al. APOLLO-1: arandomized placebo and active-controlled phase III study investigating oliceridine (TRV130), a G protein-biased ligand at the micro-opioid receptor, for management of moderate-to-severe acute pain following bunionectomy. *J Pain Res*. 2019;12:927–943.

252. Viscusi ER, Webster L, Kuss M, et al. A randomized, phase 2 study investigating TRV130, a biased ligand of the mu-opioid receptor, for the intravenous treatment of acute pain. *Pain*. 2016;157:264–272.

253. Soergel DG, Subach RA, Burnham N, et al. Biased agonism of the mu-opioid receptor by TRV130 increases analgesia and reduces on-target adverse effects versus morphine: a randomized, double-blind, placebo-controlled, crossover study in healthy volunteers. *Pain*. 2014;155:1829–1835.

254. Ayad S, Demitrack MA, Burt DA, et al. Evaluating the incidence of opioid-induced respiratory depression associated with oliceridine and morphine as measured by the frequency and average cumulative duration of dosing interruption in patients treated for acute postoperative pain. *Clin Drug Investig*. 2020;40:755–764.

255. Dahan A, van Dam CJ, Niesters M, et al. Benefit and risk evaluation of biased mu-receptor agonist oliceridine versus morphine. *Anesthesiology*. 2020;133:559–568.

256. Tan HS, Habib AS. Safety evaluation of oliceridine for the management of postoperative moderate-to-severe acute pain. *Expert Opinion on Drug Safety*. 2021;20:1291–1298.

14

Racial and Ethnic Disparities in Obstetric Anesthesia Care

Paloma Toledo, MD, MPH, FASA

Racial and ethnic disparities are prevalent in healthcare,[1] and despite decades of public health initiatives to reduce and eliminate disparities, striking disparities persist. Disparities in health are a global concern. Disparities affect many vulnerable populations, including not only racial and ethnic minorities but also immigrants, asylum seekers, and nonnative speakers, as well as residents of rural communities.[2–6] Monitoring the trends in disparities is important for the creation of policies and programs targeted at reducing inequities.[2] While many examples of disparities exist in obstetric and obstetric anesthesia care, the disparities in maternal morbidity and mortality are among the most striking. Anesthesiologists and obstetricians have embraced achieving health equity as a goal. In this chapter, we will review the definitions of disparities, explore the underlying contributors to racial and ethnic disparities, and discuss approaches to achieve improvement in healthcare disparities, primarily in the United States.

DEFINITIONS

Race, in the historical context, was used to describe ancestry and people with shared physical traits. **Ethnicity** is also related to a shared ancestry, but denotes a shared culture (e.g., language, traditions, values). Race and ethnicity are social constructs; yet, to understand disparities within groups and develop targeted interventions, patients must be grouped by race and ethnicity. It is important to understand that misuse of race as a biologic construct may cause harm, and may actually magnify disparities.[7] **Genetic determinism** is the belief that genes determine all phenotypic differences between the socially defined races, and that differences in allelic frequency drive disparities.[8] However, in the United States, and worldwide, there is significant admixture among racial groups;

genetic variability within racial groups is greater than variability between groups.[9,10] Therefore, self-identified race may serve as a proxy for exposures, but is not a reliable proxy for genetic differences.

The US Office of Management and Budget "Race and Ethnic Standards for Federal Statistics and Administrative Reporting" classifies people into racial groups to facilitate comparing federal data. In 1997, the race categories were updated[11]; in this chapter, the following racial and ethnic categories are used: American Indian and Alaska Native, Asian, Black or African American, Native Hawaiian or Other Pacific Islander, White, and Hispanic. Nearly 3.6 million children were born in the United States in 2023,[12] and more than 30% of the US population self-identifies as a racial or ethnic minority.[13]

Multiple definitions for disparities exist, but the US Agency for Healthcare Research and Quality, which produces the annual *National Disparities Report*, defines **disparity** as a difference between two groups, where the absolute difference is statistically significant, and the relative difference is at least 10% worse for the nonreferent group.[1] The National Institute on Minority Health and Health Disparities (NIMHD) defines a health disparity as a health difference that adversely affects disadvantaged populations.[14] Currently designated health disparity populations include racial and ethnic minority groups, populations of less privileged socioeconomic status, underserved rural populations, sexual and gender minority groups, and people with disabilities.[14]

The root causes of disparities are complex; in healthcare, one conceptual model organizes the causes of disparities into patient factors, provider factors, and healthcare systems factors, which all interact with each other (Fig. 14.1).[15] Clinical care alone accounts for a small proportion of health

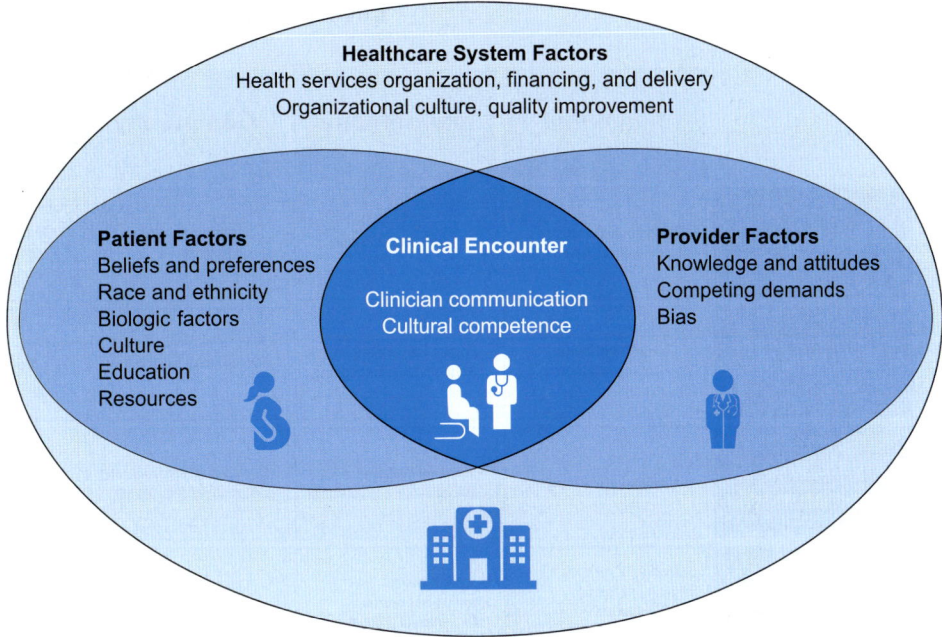

Fig. 14.1 Origins of Healthcare Disparities. Adapted from Kilbourne AM, Switzer G, Hyman K, et al. Advancing health disparities research within the health care system: a conceptual framework. *Am J Public Health.* 2006;96:2113–2121.

outcomes, whereas the social determinants of health account for as much as 50%.[16] The **social determinants of health** are defined by the World Health Organization as the nonmedical factors that influence health outcomes.[17] These factors include income, education, employment, housing, transportation, food insecurity, social inclusion, and nondiscrimination, as well as access to health services.[17] The NIMHD Minority Health and Health Disparities Research Framework incorporates the domains that influence health (e.g., biologic, behavioral, built environment, sociocultural environment, healthcare systems) and the levels of influence within those domains (e.g., individual, interpersonal, community, societal) in a matrix which expands on previous models to reflect the intersectionality of factors on both individual and population health (Fig. 14.2).[18]

DISPARITIES IN PRENATAL CARE AND OBSTETRIC DISEASE

Prenatal care, when established early and delivered with adequate quality, has been shown to improve pregnancy-related outcomes.[19] In 2022, the rates of late (defined as initiation of care in the third trimester) or no prenatal care were higher for Black, Hispanic, American Indian and Alaskan Native, and Native Hawaiian and Pacific Islander women compared to non-Hispanic White women (10.0%, 9.1%, 12.6%, 22.4%, versus 4.7%, respectively).[20] The barriers to access to prenatal care are likely multifactorial, but lack of appointment availability and long wait times disproportionately affect minority women compared to non-Hispanic White women using the same clinics.[21] Past experiences of racism may also pose a barrier to women initiating prenatal care. In one study, Black

and Hispanic women were three times more likely to report having experienced discrimination due to race, language, or culture than non-Hispanic White women.[22] Many of the conditions associated with severe maternal morbidity and mortality, such as obesity, hypertensive disorders of pregnancy, diabetes mellitus, and other chronic illnesses are more prevalent among minority women; therefore, increasing the access to prenatal care for medical optimization may improve health outcomes.[23–32] Studies have shown that public health department prenatal care programming is associated with improved Black maternal mortality rates.[33]

DISPARITIES IN NEURAXIAL LABOR ANALGESIA AND ANESTHESIA

Neuraxial labor analgesia, such as epidural analgesia or combined spinal-epidural analgesia, is the most effective treatment for the pain associated with childbirth.[34] Both the American College of Obstetricians and Gynecologists and the American Society of Anesthesiologists have promoted the use of neuraxial analgesia due to its efficacy and minimal effects on the neonate.[35] Yet, despite 73% of delivering women using neuraxial labor analgesia for pain control in the United States, Black and Hispanic women are less likely to use this modality of pain control in labor compared to non-Hispanic White women (adjusted odds ratio [aOR], 0.86 and 0.75, respectively).[36]

Studies documenting racial and ethnic disparities in use of neuraxial labor analgesia date back at least 20 years. In 2004, using the Georgia Medical Claims database, Rust et al.[37] compared neuraxial labor analgesia use by race and ethnicity. Fifty-three percent of the 29,833 women in the cohort used

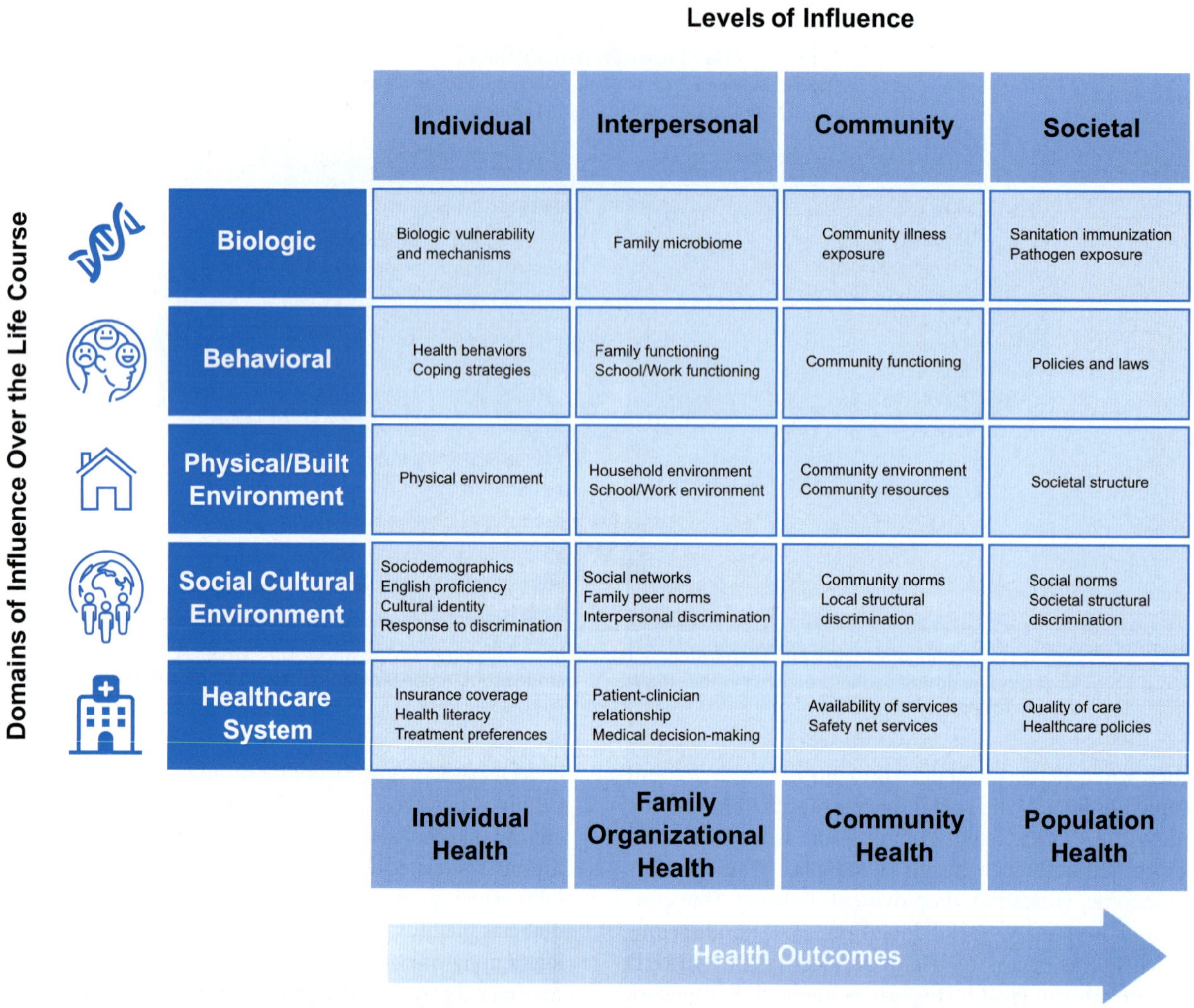

Levels of Influence

Domains of Influence Over the Life Course		Individual	Interpersonal	Community	Societal
	Biologic	Biologic vulnerability and mechanisms	Family microbiome	Community illness exposure	Sanitation immunization Pathogen exposure
	Behavioral	Health behaviors Coping strategies	Family functioning School/Work functioning	Community functioning	Policies and laws
	Physical/Built Environment	Physical environment	Household environment School/Work environment	Community environment Community resources	Societal structure
	Social Cultural Environment	Sociodemographics English proficiency Cultural identity Response to discrimination	Social networks Family peer norms Interpersonal discrimination	Community norms Local structural discrimination	Social norms Societal structural discrimination
	Healthcare System	Insurance coverage Health literacy Treatment preferences	Patient-clinician relationship Medical decision-making	Availability of services Safety net services	Quality of care Healthcare policies
		Individual Health	**Family Organizational Health**	**Community Health**	**Population Health**

Health Outcomes →

Fig. 14.2 National Institute on Minority Health and Health Disparities Research Framework. Adapted from National Institute on Minority Health and Health Disparities. NIMHD research framework. Available at: https://www.nimhd.nih.gov/about/overview/research-framework/nimhd-framework.html. Accessed 19 January 2025.

neuraxial analgesia, but differences existed by race and ethnicity. While 60% of non-Hispanic White women used neuraxial labor analgesia, only 50% of Black women and 35% of Hispanic women used it.[37] These disparities persisted even after controlling for patient age, metropolitan status, and the availability of anesthesiologists in the area. More contemporary studies have also documented racial and ethnic differences in the use of neuraxial analgesia for labor pain.[36,38–40] Differences in use may be driven by the anticipated desire for neuraxial labor analgesia. In one study, women who were Hispanic and non-Hispanic Black were less likely to anticipate neuraxial labor analgesia use than non-Hispanic White women (51%, 61%, and 83%, respectively, $P < .001$) at the time of admission to the hospital for childbirth.[38] Anticipated and actual use of neuraxial labor analgesia among Spanish-speaking Hispanic women were lower than among Hispanic women who speak English as their primary language.[39] Even after adjusting for age, marital status, income, obstetric provider type (obstetrician/midwife), and labor type, Spanish-speaking women were significantly less likely to anticipate

(aOR, 0.70; 97.5% confidence interval [CI], 0.53 to 0.92) and use (aOR, 0.88; 97.5% CI, 0.78 to 0.99) neuraxial labor analgesia compared to English-speaking Hispanic women.[39]

Knowledge and familiarity with neuraxial labor analgesia may differ by race and ethnicity. Misconceptions and fears have been shown to be important drivers in a patient's decision-making. In one survey, the rationale for avoiding neuraxial analgesia included fears of paralysis due to the procedure (76%), concerns about chronic back pain after the procedure (54%), and advice from friends and family against the use of neuraxial labor analgesia (36%).[41] After analgesic counseling, the anticipated use rate increased from a baseline of 14% to 38%.[41] In a randomized controlled trial,[40] 200 patients were randomized to a formalized language-concordant education program regarding labor neuraxial analgesia (consisting of a video, informational pamphlet, and in-person counseling) versus standard care. The Hispanic women who participated in the education program had an increased likelihood of using neuraxial labor analgesia compared with those who received standard care (risk ratio, 1.33; 95% CI, 1.02 to 1.74).

A patient's obstetric provider, and her provider's preferences, may also contribute to differences in the rates of neuraxial labor analgesia use as the provider may discuss analgesic options with the patient in the antepartum period. The rate of neuraxial anesthesia use is lower among patients who deliver with nonobstetricians (e.g., midwives).[42] While midwives historically cared for a smaller proportion of non-Hispanic White women than obstetricians,[43] a study published in 2014 indicated there were no longer significant differences in maternal race or ethnicity between patients cared for by the two types of providers.[44]

Racism may also contribute to disparities in neuraxial labor analgesia use. Several types of racism exist, including interpersonal, institutional, and structural. **Institutional and structural racism** are forms of racism that are embedded in systems, codified through laws or unwritten policies and established beliefs, which perpetuate unfair treatment to minority populations.[45,46] Structural racism has been identified as one of the key drivers of the social determinants of health for marginalized populations (Fig. 14.3).[46] A commonly cited example is redlining, a now outlawed practice, in which the government sanctioned certain geographical areas as Black neighborhoods, and deemed these areas hazardous for monetary lending by banks. This practice led to generational economic disadvantage.[47]

A cross-sectional study used 2017 US natality data to evaluate the association between structural racism and neuraxial analgesia use.[48] Structural racism was operationalized as an index of three Black-White inequity ratios (ratios for lower education, unemployment, and incarceration in jails) measured in the county of the delivery hospital. The index was stratified into terciles, with the third tercile corresponding to the highest level of structural racism. For Black women, after adjustment for sociodemographic and clinical characteristics, the adjusted odds of neuraxial labor analgesia use for women in the third tercile compared to the first tercile was reduced by 28.3% (95% CI, 26.9% to 29.6%).[48] For White women, this difference was 15.6% (95% CI, 14.7% to 16.5%). Given these differential effects observed in population-level data with multivariable risk adjustment, clinicians working in communities with substantial structural racism may not perceive any differences in the use of neuraxial analgesia.

Disparities in the use of neuraxial labor analgesia may impact disparities in the use of general anesthesia for cesarean delivery. While both neuraxial and general anesthesia are safe for cesarean delivery anesthesia, neuraxial anesthesia is preferred due to the numerous maternal and fetal benefits (see Chapter 26).[49,50] In two studies using data from the Maternal-Fetal Medicine Units Network cesarean delivery registry, non-Hispanic Black and Hispanic patients had the highest odds of undergoing general anesthesia for cesarean delivery compared with non-Hispanic White patients.[51,52] It is possible that the differential use of epidural labor analgesia among minority women contributed to the increased use of general anesthesia for cesarean delivery. In a retrospective analysis of 35,117 cesarean deliveries performed at a single academic institution between 2007 and 2018, 1147 cases (3.3%) were performed under general anesthesia.[53] The rates of general anesthesia were 5.0% for Black patients, 3.7% for Hispanic patients, 2.6% for Asian patients, and 2.8% for

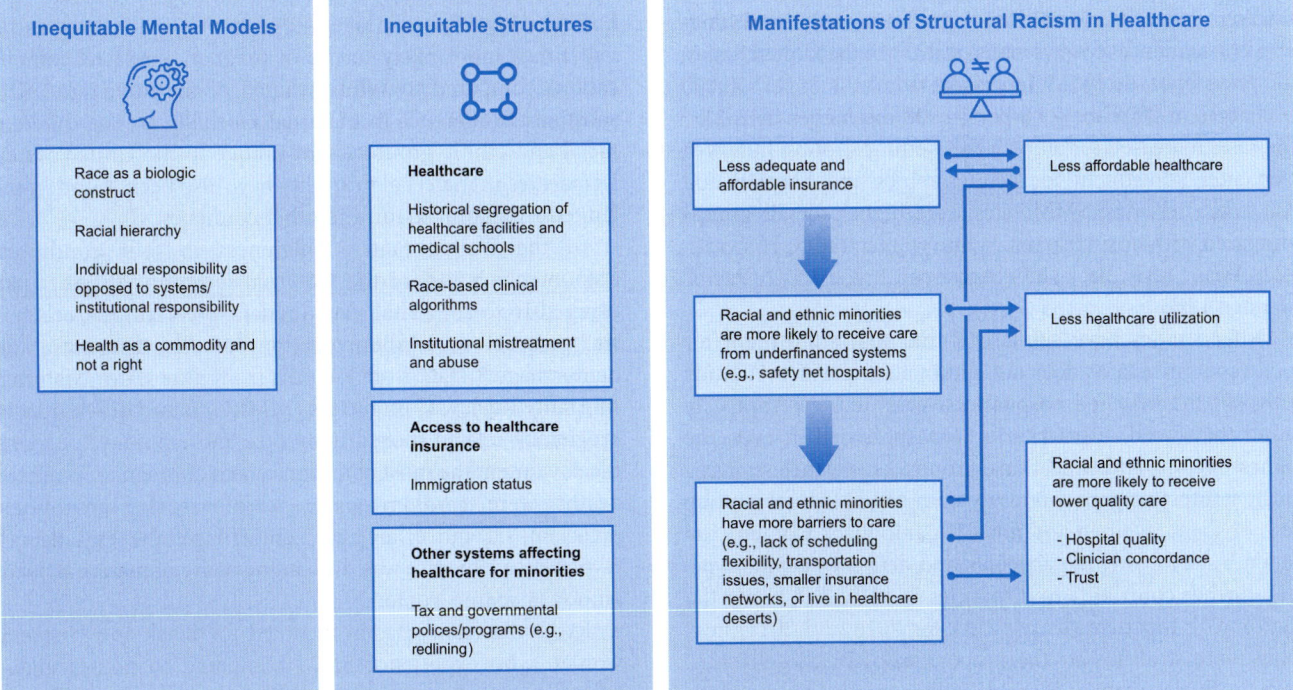

Fig. 14.3 Conceptual Map of Structural Racism in Healthcare. Adapted from Furtado K, Verdeflor A, Waidmann T. A conceptual map of structural racism in health care; 2023. https://Owww.urban.org/sites/default/files/2023-10/A%20Conceptual%20Map%20of%20Structural%20Racism%20in%20Health%20Care.pdf. Accessed 19 January 2025.

non-Hispanic White patients ($P < .001$). Among the patients who were in labor at the time of their cesarean delivery, 82.0% had neuraxial labor analgesia *in situ*. There were no racial or ethnic differences in the rates of general anesthesia use among those who had an epidural catheter *in situ* ($P = .16$).[53] These findings suggest that the extension of epidural *analgesia* to epidural surgical *anesthesia* may be one strategy for mitigating disparities in avoidable use of general anesthesia.[54]

Disparities in postpartum pain management have also been reported. In a retrospective cohort study of 1701 cesarean deliveries, severe pain after delivery (pain score $\geq 7/10$) was more common among women identifying as Black (28%) or Hispanic (22%) compared to those who identified as non-Hispanic White (20%) or Asian (15%).[55] Black and Hispanic women also had fewer pain assessments and received less opioid pain medication than non-Hispanic White women in the first 24 hours after delivery.[55] Other studies have shown that Black and Hispanic women have greater odds of a pain score $> 5/10$, but receive less inpatient pain medication (fewer morphine equivalents) than non-Hispanic White women, as well as fewer prescriptions for discharge opioid prescriptions.[56]

DISPARITIES IN SEVERE MATERNAL MORBIDITY

Multiple definitions for **severe maternal morbidity** (SMM) exist.[57] The US Centers for Disease Control and Prevention (CDC) define SMM as a composite of 21 indicators that can be extracted from administrative data.[58] The American College of Obstetrics and Gynecology and the Society for Maternal-Fetal Medicine define SMM as unintended outcomes in the birthing process that may have significant short- and long-term consequences to a woman's heath.[59] In the United States, the prevalence of SMM increased from 146.8 per 10,000 discharges in 2008 to 179.8 per 10,000 discharges in 2021.[60] The rates increased for all racial and ethnic groups; however, even after adjustment for demographics and hospital and visit characteristics, SMM rates were higher for all groups compared with non-Hispanic White women (aOR: Hispanic, 1.22; Asian, 1.33; Black, 1.39; American Indian, 1.41; Pacific Islander, 1.53).[60]

Other studies have similarly found that adjustment for socioeconomic status does not eliminate disparities. A study with 588,232 matched hospital deliveries in New York City found that racial disparities in SMM persisted in even the highest income and educational groups[61]; nevertheless, living in the poorest neighborhoods exacerbated SMM risk among both Hispanic women and non-Hispanic Black women. The patient's site of care, in particular, and delivery hospital type, may further contribute to disparities in SMM.[62–64] Using the Nationwide Inpatient Sample data for 2010 and 2011, hospitals were stratified by the proportion of Black deliveries. Seventy-four percent of Black deliveries occurred in medium and high Black-serving hospitals, and these hospitals had a higher rate of SMM than low Black-serving hospitals (18.8 versus 13.3 per 1000 deliveries).[62] Black women who delivered at high Black-serving hospitals had the highest rates of SMM (20.5 per 1000 deliveries).[62] The clustering of minoritized and under- and uninsured people in low-quality health systems is an example of structural racism.[46]

Disparities occur in many SMM conditions. Hemorrhage is a major contributor to SMM, and the incidence of postpartum hemorrhage (PPH) has been increasing (see Chapter 37).[65–68] The majority of hemorrhages are secondary to uterine atony,[65] and Hispanic ethnicity has been shown to be an independent risk factor for uterine atony requiring pharmacologic treatment.[69] Black women are 53% more likely to receive a blood transfusion than non-Hispanic White women.[70] Whether hemorrhage disparities are related to minority women experiencing more atony, having more underlying anemia, or a combination of other factors is not completely understood.

Black women are at higher risk for developing peripartum cardiomyopathy, are more likely to have severe disease at the time of diagnosis, and have worse recovery than non-Hispanic White women.[71–73]

DISPARITIES IN MATERNAL MORTALITY

Maternal mortality is discussed in detail in Chapter 39. Historically, in the United States, Black women are three to four times more likely to suffer peripartum death than non-Hispanic White women,[74–76] and disparities exist for American Indian and Alaska Native women as well.[77] Using data from the National Vital Statistics for 2021, the maternal mortality rate for non-Hispanic Black women was 2.6 times the rate for non-Hispanic White women.[77] Maternal mortality risk increases with increasing age among all racial groups; however, Black women over 40 years of age are three and a half times more likely to die of pregnancy-related complications compared to White women of the same age.[19] The substantial difference in maternal mortality among different racial and ethnic groups is not unique to the United States. Disparities in maternal mortality have also been found in the United Kingdom, Spain, and other countries.[4,78]

In the United States, differences in four conditions accounted for 59% of the maternal mortality disparity gap using 2016 to 2017 vital statistics data: preeclampsia/eclampsia, postpartum cardiomyopathy, embolic disorders, and hemorrhage.[79] Data from a report from nine states' Maternal Mortality Review Committees (MMRC) found differences in pregnancy-related mortality by race and ethnicity.[80] Among Black women, the most common causes of pregnancy-related deaths were cardiomyopathy, cardiovascular conditions, preeclampsia and eclampsia, hemorrhage, and embolism.[80] Hypertensive disease was the leading cause of maternal death among Hispanic women.[81]

Excess mortality has been noted for Black and Hispanic women who experience SMM compared to non-Hispanic White women. Among women with hypertensive disorders of pregnancy, Black women are 10 times more likely to die than non-Hispanic White women, and Hispanic women are eight times more likely to die than non-Hispanic White women.[82]

Disparities persist even after adjusting for confounders (e.g., age, marital status, and residence).[82] Similarly, other studies have found that Black women who experience preeclampsia, eclampsia, abruption, placenta previa, and PPH have a higher case fatality rate than non-Hispanic White women.[83]

Maternal geography, or site of care, may also contribute to disparities. States with a greater proportion of Black women in the population have higher rates of pregnancy-related deaths while states with fewer Black women have lower rates of pregnancy-related deaths.[84] It has been posited that population-based disparities may be a result of poverty, immigration, or rural location,[85] but Black women in Georgia are more likely to die in metropolitan, nonrural locations than rural locations.[86] Adjustment for access to care does not eliminate disparities. A study of pregnancy-associated deaths in the state of Louisiana from 2016 to 2017 found increased maternal mortality for women residing in maternity care deserts; however, even after adjustment for geographic access, the racial and ethnic disparities persisted.[87]

STRATEGIES FOR ADDRESSING DISPARITIES

Given that healthcare disparities are multifactorial, interventions at multiple levels will be required to reduce or eliminate them. In 2018, the National Partnership for Maternal Safety within the Council for Patient Safety in Women's Healthcare developed the *Reduction of Peripartum Racial and Ethnic Disparities Bundle*.[88] The bundle's recommendations were organized into four Rs (Readiness, Recognition and Prevention, Response, and Reporting and Systems Learnings), which are used in the other maternal safety bundles. The recommendations were organized into five themes: (1) measurement of disparities, (2) recognition of disparities at the personal and systems levels, (3) awareness of the magnitude of disparities, (4) communication barriers, and (5) differences in the structure of care. In 2021, the American Society of Anesthesiologists Committee on Obstetric Anesthesia released a *Statement on Reducing Maternal Peripartum Racial and Ethnic Disparities in Anesthesia Care*.[89] Actionable strategies for anesthesiologists are summarized in Box 14.1.

Measurement of Disparities

To measure baseline data and changes in patient outcomes, it is imperative that systems be implemented to accurately document patients' self-identified race and ethnicity. This will allow for the development of disparity dashboards, which have been recommended in the *Reduction of Peripartum Racial and Ethnic Disparities* bundle.[88] Staff assignment of the patient's race, or the use of surname to assign race and ethnicity, have been proven inaccurate.[92,93] The American Health Association's Health Research and Educational Trust developed a web-based tool to assist hospitals, health systems, and clinics with resources for systematically collecting race, ethnicity, and primary language data from patients.[94]

BOX 14.1   Recommendations for Anesthesia Providers for Reducing Peripartum Disparities

Ensure accurate documentation of race, ethnicity, and primary spoken language.

- Ensure that registration staff are trained on how to ask demographic questions to ensure patients understand why these data are being collected.
- Know how to access interpreter services.[a]

Race/ethnicity and primary spoken language data should be available in the electronic health record and used to create disparities dashboards.

- Define important process and outcome metrics (e.g., neuraxial analgesia use, unintentional dural puncture rate, general anesthesia rate) and stratify these data by race, ethnicity, and primary spoken language.
- Make stratified outcome metrics available to staff and leadership.

Recommendations specific to anesthesia providers

- Receive education on racial and ethnic disparities in anesthesia care and their root causes.
- Employ best practices for shared decision-making when discussing procedures (e.g., neuraxial labor analgesia).
- Work with other peripartum providers to identify women at risk for complications, engage in multidisciplinary peripartum planning, and develop and implement protocols and evidence-based safety bundles such as those from the American College of Obstetricians and Gynecologists Council on Patient Safety bundles.[90]
- Consider implementing the SOAP Enhanced Recovery after Cesarean recommendations[91]; implementation may minimize variation in care and reduce disparities.
- Anesthesia providers should engage in quality improvement initiatives that target reducing racial and ethnic disparities.

Engage in initiatives to support workforce diversity both within the anesthesia department, as well as within the institution.

- Encourage engagement in pipeline programs and mentorship of diverse learners across the pipeline.
- Evaluate culture of equity.
- Implement strategies, such as holistic interviewing.

SOAP, Society for Obstetric Anesthesia and Perinatology.
[a]Interpreter services should be utilized unless providers with second-language skills are proficient in the use of that language.
Recommendations adapted from American Society of Anesthesiologists Committee on Obstetric Anesthesia. Statement on Reducing Maternal Peripartum Racial and Ethnic Disparities in Anesthesia Care; 2021. https://www.asahq.org/standards-and-practice-parameters/statement-on-reducing-maternal-peripartum-racial-and-ethnic-disparities-in-anesthesia-care. Accessed 19 January 2025.

It is also important that clinicians are cognizant of patient's preferred primary spoken language, as communication barriers may contribute to healthcare disparities. At the national level, several measures are in place to ensure linguistic support to patients with limited English proficiency. The *National Culturally and Linguistically Appropriate Services (CLAS) Standards in Health and Health Care* state that an interpreter must be available to patients at no cost.[95] Title VI of the Equal Employment Opportunity Program prohibits national origin discrimination affecting persons with limited English proficiency.[96] Clinicians should be aware of how to access interpreter services at their institution and refrain from utilizing second-language skills to counsel patients if they are not proficient in the use of that language.[88]

Recognition of Disparities at the Personal and Systems Levels

Anesthesiologists should receive education about racial and ethnic disparities and actions that can be taken to reduce disparities. Ideally, this education can be delivered to anesthesiologists, obstetricians, and nursing staff, as addressing disparities will take multidisciplinary coordination. Protocols, such as enhanced recovery protocols and patient safety bundles should be implemented where possible, as these may help reduce variations in care, decrease implicit bias, and reduce disparities.[88,90,91,97–99]

Differential treatment for minoritized populations can exacerbate disparities. **Bias** can affect a clinician's perceptions and decisions and can impact patient-provider communication, treatment decisions, and ultimately, health outcomes.[100] Bias can be *explicit*, meaning that the individual is aware of the preference, or *implicit*, meaning that the individual's beliefs are not apparent to them, and differ from their explicit beliefs.[101] The Implicit Association Test (IAT) is the most common tool to measure implicit bias, and tests are available for multiple areas (e.g., race, gender, age).[102] In a retrospective study that evaluated the implicit and explicit preferences of 404,277 people who had taken the IAT, 2535 identified as physicians.[103] Similar to the nonphysician sample, physicians showed an implicit preference for White Americans relative to Black Americans. In a review of 15 studies that assessed implicit bias in healthcare, most adverse outcomes were related to patient-provider interactions, underscoring the need for providers to be aware of their own implicit biases and how it may influence cross-cultural communication.[104] Several states, including California, Delaware, Illinois, Maryland, and Michigan, have passed laws requiring implicit bias training for maternal healthcare providers.

At the institutional level, it is important to have a mechanism for patients, families, and staff to report inequitable care, episodes of disrespect, and miscommunication. If such an episode is reported, there should be a timely and tailored response.[88] Creating a culture where justice, equity, diversity, and inclusion are prioritized and valued is one strategy that leaders may use to promote institutional diversity.[105]

Initiatives to Identify and Reduce Racial and Ethnic Disparities

Perinatal providers should define the important process and outcome metrics that should be tracked in disparities dashboards.[88] These data, stratified by race, ethnicity, and primary spoken language (if applicable), should be disseminated regularly to the staff and leadership. Furthermore, when conducting reviews of SMM, mortality, and other clinically important metrics, the role of race, ethnicity, language, literacy, and other social determinants of health, including racism at the interpersonal and system level, should be evaluated.

One hospital system in Pennsylvania implemented disparities dashboards, regular reporting of a composite SMM metric by race and ethnicity, implicit bias training, and standardization of best practices, and was able to demonstrate a decreased risk of SMM over time for Black patients (aOR for SMM for 2021 versus 2019, 0.73; 95% CI, 0.62 to 0.86).[106] On a national level, state MMRCs use the Maternal Mortality Review Information Application (MMRIA) form to standardize data abstraction.[107] In 2022, a multidisciplinary working group of experts in maternal health, the CDC Division of Reproductive Health, and the CDC Foundation developed definitions of racism and discrimination that were added to the MMRIA form.[108] Structural racism, interpersonal racism, and discrimination were added as contributing factors for pregnancy-related deaths (Box 14.2).[108–111] By identifying these as contributing causes, MMRC recommendations may better target interventions to prevent future deaths.

Institutions should develop quality improvement projects that target disparities; yet, it is important to note that interventions may improve quality for all groups, or may disproportionately improve or worsen the care for the group experiencing the disparity.[112] Engaging patients and community partners as the intervention is developed is one strategy for ensuring the intervention is acceptable to patients, promotes the desired change, and increases sustainablility.[113]

The National Network of Perinatal Quality Collaboratives promotes data-driven quality improvement initiatives to improve patient outcomes.[114] At the state level, several perinatal quality collaboratives have engaged in birth equity initiatives, including the collaboratives in Illinois, Louisiana, and Massachusetts.[115–117] In Louisiana, this work resulted in improvement in the Black-White disparity ratio for PPH, from 2.1 at baseline to 1.3 after the intervention.[116] The rate of improvement was greater for Black women (50% improvement) than for non-Hispanic White women (15.7% improvement).[116]

Communication Barriers

Empowering **patient-centered care** is essential and should focus on individual patient's preferences and needs.[118] Communication between the patient and the provider is an important component of patient-centered care (see Chapter 32).[119,120] Patient-centered communication improves patient recall, satisfaction, and health outcomes,[121–123] and breakdowns in patient-provider communication may contribute to racial and ethnic disparities in healthcare.[111]

BOX 14.2 Definitions for Structural Racism, Interpersonal Racism, and Discrimination

Type of Racism	Definition
Structural racism	The systems of power based on historical injustices and contemporary social factors that systematically disadvantage people of color and advantage White people through inequities in housing, education, employment, earnings, benefits, monetary credit, media, healthcare, and criminal justice, among others
Interpersonal racism	Discriminatory interactions between individuals based on differential assumptions about the abilities, motives, and intentions of others, resulting in differential actions toward others based on their race. Racism can be conscious as well as unconscious, and it includes acts of commission and omission. It manifests as lack of respect, suspicion, devaluation, scapegoating, and dehumanization of others.
Discrimination	Treating someone less or more favorably based on the group, class, or category to which they belong, resulting from biases, prejudices, and stereotyping. Discrimination can manifest as differences in healthcare, clinical communication, and shared decision-making.

Definitions adapted from Bailey ZD, Krieger N, Agenor M, et al. Structural racism and health inequities in the USA: evidence and interventions. *Lancet*. 2017;389:1453–1463; Jones CP. Levels of racism: a theoretic framework and a gardener's tale. *Am J Public Health*. 2000;90:1212–1215; and Institute of Medicine, Smedley BD, Stith AY, Nelson, AR eds. *Unequal Treatment: Confronting Racial and Ethnic Disparities in Health Care*; 2003. https://www.ncbi.nlm.nih.gov/books/NBK220358/. Accessed 19 January 2025.

Medical discussions can be challenging when there are a variety of options to consider, and patients may not have enough understanding to make an informed decision,[124–126] particularly when challenged with low health literacy. Patients with low literacy are less likely to seek preventative care, understand medical instructions, and have higher mortality rates compared to patients with high literacy. Higher rates of low-health literacy exist among people who self-identify as racial and ethnic minorities compared to non-Hispanic White patients.[127]

The use of **shared decision-making** (see Chapter 32) is one strategy that can be used to reduce disparities. Briefly, shared decision-making is a process by which the clinician shares relevant risks and benefits on treatments, as well as their alternatives, and engages the patient (and potentially her partner or family) in a discussion about personal information and beliefs that would make a treatment more or less desirable.[128–130] **Shared decision-making tools** should be tailored so that cultural concerns (e.g., back pain and paralysis

regarding neuraxial labor analgesia[40,41,131]) are integrated into the tool.[132] The benefits of using decision aids have been demonstrated across populations, including the portion of the population with the lowest health literacy.[133–135] It is unknown to what extent shared decision-making has been integrated into obstetric anesthesia practice, but one study that assessed audio recordings of patient counseling about anesthetic options in an outpatient preoperative clinic found objective shared decision-making scores were low.[136]

Another area for improvement in healthcare disparities is diversity within the healthcare workforce.[111,137] **Underrepresented minorities in medicine** (URiM) are defined as racial or ethnic groups that have been historically underrepresented in medicine relative to their numbers in the general population.[138] Within the specialty of anesthesiology, the anesthesiologist physician workforce is neither reflective of the general patient population in the United States, nor of the general demographics of practicing physicians in all medical fields.[139] There are many ways in which increased workforce diversity reduces disparities. URiM physicians are more likely to work in underserved communities. Concordance between patients and their providers has been associated with improved patient-provider communication, patient satisfaction, and trust.[111,137,140,141] Furthermore, racial and ethnic concordance between patients and their physicians is associated with better patient experience measured using patient satisfaction survey scores.[142]

One secondary analysis of a cohort of women undergoing cesarean delivery under neuraxial anesthesia evaluated the association between racial and ethnic concordance and patient satisfaction.[143] Concordance between the patient and anesthesia team members was categorized as full concordance, partial concordance, discordance, and missing. Full concordance occurred in 4.5% of cases, partial concordance in 29.0%, discordance in 43.4%, and was missing in 23.1%. Satisfaction ratings did not differ among the concordance categories (88.9% for full concordance, 71.8% for partial concordance, 81.1% for discordance, and 78.5% for missing, $P = .02$).[143] While this study is likely underpowered, given the small number of patient-anesthesia team pairings with full concordance, the results underscore the view that, while racial concordance may be preferred, other attributes of the patient-provider relationship (e.g., respect, competence, trust) are also valued and inform patient assessment of their healthcare interactions.[144]

While a full discussion of strategies to increase the diversity of the physician workforce is outside the scope of this chapter, strategies such as holistic interviewing, engagement in pipeline programs, and an evaluation of the culture of equity within a department are actionable steps that may increase provider diversity.[145–148] Creation of community is important as diversity thrives in departments where there is a culture of inclusion.[145]

Differences in the Structure of Care

The structure of care in the peripartum period may be fractured for women from minoritized communities because they may receive their antepartum care in clinics where the obstetric providers do not have privileges at the hospital where the delivery will occur.[88] Healthcare coverage is also fragmented because some pregnant women gain insurance coverage during pregnancy only to lose it when they are no longer pregnant. Medicaid, the US government-sponsored health insurance program for low-income individuals, insures women with incomes up to 138% of the poverty level, yet disparities in Medicaid coverage exist.[149]

Historically, Medicaid only provided insurance coverage for 60 days after delivery. However, the majority of maternal deaths occur postpartum; thus, expanding Medicaid coverage to 1 year after delivery ensures that vulnerable patients do not lose access to postpartum healthcare. The American Rescue Plan Act of 2021 provided states with the option of extending postpartum Medicaid coverage from 60 days to 12 months. This option was made permanent under the Consolidated Appropriations Act of 2023. As of August 2024, all states except Arkansas have expanded postpartum Medicaid coverage to 1 year. Arkansas has expanded coverage for parents or other caretaker relatives who care for minor children. A cross-sectional study that utilized the Underlying Cause of Death 2006 to 2017 data files from the National Center for Health Statistics compared maternal death rates in states with and without Medicaid expansion.[150] There were 7 fewer deaths per 100,000 live births in Medicaid expansion states ($P = .002$).

KEY POINTS

- Healthcare disparities are a global issue and affect many vulnerable populations, including women who belong to racial and ethnic minority groups, immigrants, non-native speakers, asylum seekers, and residents of rural communities.
- Social determinants of health are the nonmedical factors that influence health outcomes, including income, education, employment, housing, transportation, food security, social inclusion, and nondiscrimination, as well as access to health services. These factors play an important role in health outcomes.
- Racial and ethnic disparities exist for the use of neuraxial labor analgesia and for neuraxial versus general anesthesia for cesarean deliveries. For women who are in labor, the extension of epidural analgesia to epidural anesthesia may be one strategy to mitigate disparities in avoidable use of general anesthesia for cesarean delivery.
- Racial and ethnic disparities in maternal mortality have been documented in the United States and worldwide. In the United States, the rate of maternal mortality has been three to four times higher for Black women compared to non-Hispanic White women.
- Multiple strategies have been suggested for reducing racial and ethnic disparities, including accurate measurement of race, ethnicity, and primary spoken language; use of dashboards to track disparities in outcome metrics; provider education about disparities and their root causes; reducing provider-patient communication barriers by shared decision-making; and engagement in programs to reduce workforce racial and ethnic disparities and increase workforce diversity.
- Protocols such as enhanced recovery protocols and patient safety bundles should be implemented when possible, as these may help reduce variations in care, decrease implicit bias, and reduce disparities.

REFERENCES

1. Agency for Healthcare Research and Quality. 2023 National healthcare quality and disparities report; 2023. https://www.ahrq.gov/research/findings/nhqrdr/nhqdr23/index.html. Accessed January 13, 2025.
2. Tangcharoensathien V, Lekagul A, Teo YY. Global health inequities: more challenges, some solutions. *Bull World Health Organ.* 2024;102:8686A.
3. Saucedo M, Deneux-Tharaux C, Bouvier-Colle MH. Understanding regional differences in maternal mortality: anational case-control study in France. *BJOG.* 2012;119:573–581.
4. Garcia-Tizon Larroca S, Arevalo-Serrano J, Ruiz Minaya M, et al. Maternal mortality trends in Spain during the 2000-2018 period: the role of maternal origin. *BMC Public Health.* 2022;22:337.
5. Eslier M, Azria E, Chatzistergiou K, et al. Association between migration and severe maternal outcomes in high-income countries: systematic review and meta-analysis. *PLoS Med.* 2023;20:e1004257.
6. Harrington KA, Cameron NA, Culler K, et al. Rural-urban disparities in adverse maternal outcomes in the United States, 2016–2019. *Am J Public Health.* 2023;113:224–227.
7. Vyas DA, Eisenstein LG, Jones DS. Hidden in plain sight - reconsidering the use of race correction in clinical algorithms. *N Engl J Med.* 2020;383:874–882.
8. Graves JL Jr, Goodman AH.*Why do races differ in disease incidence?. Racism, Not Race: Answers to Frequently Asked Questions.* Columbia University Press; 2022:94–98.
9. Lewontin RC. The apportionment of human diversity. *Evol Biol.* 1972;6:391–398.
10. Nei M, Roychoudhury AK. Gene differences between Caucasian, Negro, and Japanese populations. *Science.* 1972;177:434–436.
11. CDC National Center for Health Statistics. Race; 2024. https://www.cdc.gov/nchs/hus/sources-definitions/race.html. Accessed January 13, 2025.
12. US Centers for Disease Control, Martin, JA, Hamilton BE, Osterman MJK, Births in the United States, 2023; 2024. https://stacks.cdc.gov/view/cdc/158789. Accessed January 2025.
13. United States Census Bureau. Quick facts from the U.S. Census Bureau [updated October 15, 2024]; 2024. https://www.census.gov/quickfacts/. Accessed January 13, 2025.
14. National Institute on Minority Health and Health Disparities. Minority health and health disparities: Definitions and parameters; 2024. https://www.nimhd.nih.gov/

about/strategic-plan/nih-strategic-plan-definitions-and-parameters.html. Accessed January 13, 2025.

15. Kilbourne AM, Switzer G, Hyman K, et al. Advancing health disparities research within the health care system: aconceptual framework. *Am J Public Health.* 2006;96:2113–2121.

16. Hood CM, Gennuso KP, Swain GR, Catlin BB. County health rankings: relationships between determinant factors and health outcomes. *Am J Prev Med.* 2016;50:129–135.

17. World Health Organization. Social determinants of health. https://www.who.int/health-topics/social-determinants-of-health#tab=tab_1. Accessed January 13, 2025.

18. National Institute on Minority Health and Health Disparities. NIMHD research framework details; 2024. https://www.nimhd.nih.gov/about/overview/research-framework/nimhd-framework.html. Accessed January 13, 2025.

19. Creanga AA, Berg CJ, Syverson C, et al. Pregnancy-related mortality in the United States, 2006–2010. *Obstet Gynecol.* 2015;125:5–12.

20. Osterman MJK, Hamilton BE, Martin JA, et al. Births: final data for 2022. *Natl Vital Stat Rep.* 2024;73:1–56.

21. Beckmann CA, Buford TA, Witt JB. Perceived barriers to prenatal care services. *MCN Am J Matern Child Nurs.* 2000;25:43–46.

22. Attanasio L, Kozhimannil KB. Patient-reported communication quality and perceived discrimination in maternity care. *Med Care.* 2015;53:863–871.

23. Nguyen BT, Cheng YW, Snowden JM, et al. The effect of race/ethnicity on adverse perinatal outcomes among patients with gestational diabetes mellitus. *Am J Obstet Gynecol.* 2012;207:322.e1–e6.

24. Larsen WI, Strong JE, Farley JH. Risk factors for late postpartum preeclampsia. *J Reprod Med.* 2012;57:35–38.

25. Ramos GA, Caughey AB. The interrelationship between ethnicity and obesity on obstetric outcomes. *Am J Obstet Gynecol.* 2005;193:1089–1093.

26. Flegal KM, Carroll MD, Ogden CL, Curtin LR. Prevalence and trends in obesity among US adults, 1999–2008. *JAMA.* 2010;303:235–241.

27. Kominiarek MA, Vanveldhuisen P, Hibbard J, et al. The maternal body mass index: a strong association with delivery route. *Am J Obstet Gynecol.* 2010;203:264.e1–e7.

28. Vricella LK, Louis JM, Mercer BM, Bolden N. Anesthesia complications during scheduled cesarean delivery for morbidly obese women. *Am J Obstet Gynecol.* 2010;203:276.e1–e5.

29. HAPO Study Cooperative Research Group. Hyperglycaemia and Adverse Pregnancy Outcome (HAPO) study: associations with maternal body mass index. *BJOG.* 2010;117:575–584.

30. Makgoba M, Savvidou MD, Steer PJ. The effect of maternal characteristics and gestational diabetes on birthweight. *BJOG.* 2012;119:1091–1097.

31. Casey BM, Lucas MJ, McIntire DD, Leveno KJ. Pregnancy outcomes in women with gestational diabetes compared with the general obstetric population. *Obstet Gynecol.* 1997;90:869–873.

32. Gong J, Savitz DA, Stein CR, Engel SM. Maternal ethnicity and pre-eclampsia in New York City, 1995–2003. *Paediatr Perinat Epidemiol.* 2012;26:45–52.

33. Bekemeier B, Grembowski D, Yang YR, Herting JR. Local public health delivery of maternal child health services: are specific activities associated with reductions in Black-White mortality disparities? *Matern Child Health J.* 2012;16:615–623.

34. Anim-Somuah M, Smyth RM, Cyna AM, Cuthbert A. Epidural versus non-epidural or no analgesia for pain management in labour. *Cochrane Database Syst Rev.* 2018;(5):CD000331.

35. American College of Obstetricians and Gynecologists. Practice Bulletin No. 209: Obstetric analgesia and anesthesia (reaffirmed 2024). *Obstet Gynecol.* 2019;133:e208–e225.

36. Butwick AJ, Bentley J, Wong CA, et al. United States state-level variation in the use of neuraxial analgesia during labor for pregnant women. *JAMA Netw Open.* 2018;1:e186567.

37. Rust G, Nembhard WN, Nichols M, et al. Racial and ethnic disparities in the provision of epidural analgesia to Georgia Medicaid beneficiaries during labor and delivery. *Am J Obstet Gynecol.* 2004;191:456–462.

38. Toledo P, Sun J, Grobman WA, et al. Racial and ethnic disparities in neuraxial labor analgesia. *Anesth Analg.* 2012;114:172–178.

39. Toledo P, Eosakul ST, Grobman WA, et al. Primary spoken language and neuraxial labor analgesia use among Hispanic Medicaid recipients. *Anesth Analg.* 2016;122:204–209.

40. Togioka BM, Seligman KM, Werntz MK, et al. Education program regarding labor epidurals increases utilization by Hispanic Medicaid beneficiaries: a randomized controlled trial. *Anesthesiology.* 2019;131:840–849.

41. Orejuela FJ, Garcia T, Green C, et al. Exploring factors influencing patient request for epidural analgesia on admission to labor and delivery in a predominantly Latino population. *J Immigr Minor Health.* 2012;14:287–291.

42. Hueston WJ, McClaflin RR, Mansfield CJ, Rudy M. Factors associated with the use of intrapartum epidural analgesia. *Obstet Gynecol.* 1994;84:579–582.

43. Parker JD. Ethnic differences in midwife-attended US births. *Am J Public Health.* 1994;84:1139–1141.

44. Thornton P. Characteristics of spontaneous births attended by midwives and physicians in US hospitals in 2014. *J Midwifery Womens Health.* 2017;62:531–537.

45. Braveman PA, Arkin E, Proctor D, et al. Systemic and structural racism: definitions, examples, health damages, and approaches to dismantling. *Health Aff (Millwood).* 2022;41:171–178.

46. Furtado K, Verdeflor A, Waidmann T. A conceptual map of structural racism in health care; 2023. https://www.urban.org/sites/default/files/2023-10/A%20Conceptual%20Map%20of%20Structural%20Racism%20in%20Health%20Care.pdf. Accessed December 30, 2024.

47. Aaronson D, Hartley D, Mazumder B, Federal Reserve Bank of Chicago. The effects of the 1930s HOLC "redlining" maps. Working Papers, No. 2017-12 (revised August 2020); 2017. https://www.chicagofed.org/publications/working-papers/2017/wp2017-12. Accessed January 23, 2025.

48. Guglielminotti J, Lee A, Landau R, et al. Structural racism and use of labor neuraxial analgesia among non-Hispanic Black birthing people. *Obstet Gynecol.* 2024;143:571–581.

49. American Society of Anesthesiologists. Practice guidelines for obstetric anesthesia: an updated report by the American Society of Anesthesiologists Task Force on Obstetric Anesthesia and the Society for Obstetric Anesthesia and Perinatology. *Anesthesiology.* 2016;124:270–300.

50. Afolabi BB, Lesi FE. Regional versus general anaesthesia for caesarean section. *Cochrane Database Syst Rev.* 2012;(10):CD004350.

51. Butwick AJ, El-Sayed YY, Blumenfeld YJ, et al. Mode of anaesthesia for preterm Caesarean delivery: secondary analysis from the Maternal-Fetal Medicine Units Network Caesarean Registry. *Br J Anaesth.* 2015;115:267–274.

52. Butwick AJ, Blumenfeld YJ, Brookfield KF, et al. Racial and ethnic disparities in mode of anesthesia for cesarean delivery. *Anesth Analg.* 2016;122:472–479.

53. Thomas CL, Lange EMS, Banayan JM, et al. Racial and ethnic disparities in receipt of general anesthesia for cesarean delivery. *JAMA Netw Open.* 2024;7:e2350825.

54. Guglielminotti J, Landau R, Li G. Adverse events and factors associated with potentially avoidable use of general anesthesia in cesarean deliveries. *Anesthesiology.* 2019;130:912–922.

55. Johnson JD, Asiodu IV, McKenzie CP, et al. Racial and ethnic inequities in postpartum pain evaluation and management. *Obstet Gynecol.* 2019;134:1155–1162.

56. Badreldin N, Grobman WA, Yee LM. Racial disparities in postpartum pain management. *Obstet Gynecol.* 2019;134:1147–1153.

57. Snowden JM, Lyndon A, Kan P, et al. Severe maternal morbidity: a comparison of definitions and data sources. *Am J Epidemiol.* 2021;190:1890–1897.

58. Centers for Disease Control and Prevention. Identifying severe maternal morbidity (SMM) [updated May 15, 2024]; 2024. https://www.cdc.gov/maternal-infant-health/php/severe-maternal-morbidity/icd.html. Accessed January 19, 2025.

59. American College of Obstetricians and Gynecologists, Society for Maternal-Fetal Medicine, Kilpatrick SK, Ecker JL. Severe maternal morbidity: screening and review. *Am J Obstet Gynecol.* 2016;215:B17–B22.

60. Fink DA, Kilday D, Cao Z, et al. Trends in maternal mortality and severe maternal morbidity during delivery-related hospitalizations in the United States, 2008 to 2021. *JAMA Netw Open.* 2023;6:e2317641.

61. Howland RE, Angley M, Won SH, et al. Determinants of severe maternal morbidity and its racial/ethnic disparities in New York City, 2008-2012. *Matern Child Health J.* 2019;23:346–355.

62. Howell EA, Egorova N, Balbierz A, et al. Black-white differences in severe maternal morbidity and site of care. *Am J Obstet Gynecol.* 2016;214:122.e1–e7.

63. Garg B, Hersh A, Caughey AB, Pilliod RA. Severe maternal morbidity and Black-white differences in Washington State. *J Matern Fetal Neonatal Med.* 2022;35:5949–5956.

64. Mujahid MS, Kan P, Leonard SA, et al. Birth hospital and racial and ethnic differences in severe maternal morbidity in the state of California. *Am J Obstet Gynecol.* 2021;224:219.e1–e15.

65. Bateman BT, Berman MF, Riley LE, Leffert LR. The epidemiology of postpartum hemorrhage in a large, nationwide sample of deliveries. *Anesth Analg.* 2010;110:1368–1373.

66. Callaghan WM, Kuklina EV, Berg CJ. Trends in postpartum hemorrhage: United States, 1994-2006. *Am J Obstet Gynecol.* 2010;202:353.e1–e6.

67. Knight M, Callaghan WM, Berg C, et al. Trends in postpartum hemorrhage in high resource countries: a review and recommendations from the International Postpartum Hemorrhage Collaborative Group. *BMC Pregnancy Childbirth.* 2009;9:55.

68. Joseph KS, Rouleau J, Kramer MS, et al. Investigation of an increase in postpartum haemorrhage in Canada. *BJOG.* 2007;114:751–759.

69. Wetta LA, Szychowski JM, Seals S, et al. Risk factors for uterine atony/postpartum hemorrhage requiring treatment after vaginal delivery. *Am J Obstet Gynecol.* 2013;209:51.e1–e6.

70. Tangel VE, Matthews KC, Abramovitz SE, White RS. Racial and ethnic disparities in severe maternal morbidity and anesthetic techniques for obstetric deliveries: a multi-state analysis, 2007-2014. *J Clin Anesth.* 2020;65:109821.

71. Gentry MB, Dias JK, Luis A, et al. African-American women have a higher risk for developing peripartum cardiomyopathy. *J Am Coll Cardiol.* 2010;55:654–659.

72. Amos AM, Jaber WA, Russell SD. Improved outcomes in peripartum cardiomyopathy with contemporary. *Am Heart J.* 2006;152:509–513.

73. Kao DP, Hsich E, Lindenfeld J. Characteristics, adverse events, and racial differences among delivering mothers withperipartum cardiomyopathy. *JACC Heart Fail.* 2013;1:409–416.

74. Berg CJ, Callaghan WM, Syverson C, Henderson Z. Pregnancy-related mortality in the United States, 1998 to 2005. *Obstet Gynecol.* 2010;116:1302–1309.

75. Chang J, Elam-Evans LD, Berg CJ, et al. Pregnancy-related mortality surveillance—United States, 1991–1999. *MMWR Surveill Summ.* 2003;52:1–8.

76. Hoyert DL. National Center for Health Statistics: Maternal mortality rates in the United States, 2021. NCHS Health E-Stats; 2023. https://www.cdc.gov/nchs/data/hestat/maternal-mortality/2021/maternal-mortality-rates-2021.htm. Accessed November 15, 2024.

77. Fleszar LG, Bryant AS, Johnson CO, et al. Trends in state-level maternal mortality by racial and ethnic group in the United States. *JAMA.* 2023;330:52–61.

78. Small MJ, Allen TK, Brown HL. Global disparities in maternal morbidity and mortality. *Semin Perinatol.* 2017;41:318–322.

79. MacDorman MF, Thoma M, Declcerq E, Howell EA. Racial and ethnic disparities in maternal mortality in the United States using enhanced vital records, 2016-2017. *Am J Public Health.* 2021;111:1673–1681.

80. US Centers for Disease Control and Prevention. Report from nine maternal mortality review committees; 2018. https://stacks.cdc.gov/view/cdc/51660. Accessed January 19, 2025.

81. Hopkins FW, MacKay AP, Koonin LM, et al. Pregnancy-related mortality in Hispanic women in the United States. *Obstet Gynecol.* 1999;94:747–752.

82. Rosenberg D, Geller SE, Studee L, Cox SM. Disparities in mortality among high risk pregnant women in Illinois: a population based study. *Ann Epidemiol.* 2006;16:26–32.

83. Tucker MJ, Berg CJ, Callaghan WM, Hsia J. The Black-White disparity in pregnancy-related mortality from 5 conditions: differences in prevalence and case-fatality rates. *Am J Public Health.* 2007;97:247–251.

84. Moaddab A, Dildy GA, Brown HL, et al. Health care disparity and state-specific pregnancy-related mortality in the United States, 2005-2014. *Obstet Gynecol.* 2016;128:869–875.

85. MacKay AP, Berg CJ, Liu X, et al. Changes in pregnancy mortality ascertainment: United States, 1999-2005. *Obstet Gynecol.* 2011;118:104–110.

86. Platner M, Loucks TL, Lindsay MK, Ellis JE. Pregnancy-associated deaths in rural, nonrural, and metropolitan areas of Georgia. *Obstet Gynecol.* 2016;128:113–120.

87. Wallace M, Dyer L, Felker-Kantor E, et al. Maternity care deserts and pregnancy-associated mortality in Louisiana. *Womens Health Issues.* 2021;31:122–129.

88. Howell EA, Brown H, Brumley J, et al. Reduction of peripartum racial and ethnic disparities: a conceptual framework and maternal safety consensus bundle. *Obstet Gynecol.* 2018;131:770–782.

89. American Society of Anesthesiologists Committee on Obstetric Anesthesia. Statement on reducing maternal peripartum racial and ethnic disparities in anesthesia care; 2021. https://www.asahq.org/standards-and-practice-parameters/statement-on-reducing-maternal-peripartum-racial-and-ethnic-disparities-in-anesthesia-care. Accessed January 13, 2025.

90. Main EK, Goffman D, Scavone BM, et al. National partnership for maternal safety: consensus bundle on obstetric hemorrhage. *Anesth Analg.* 2015;121:142–148.

91. Bollag L, Lim G, Sultan P, et al. Society for Obstetric Anesthesia and Perinatology: consensus statement and recommendations for enhanced recovery after cesarean. *Anesth Analg.* 2021;132:1362–1377.

92. Boehmer U, Kressin NR, Berlowitz DR, et al. Self-reported vs administrative race/ethnicity data and study results. *Am J Public Health.* 2002;92:1471–1472.

93. Institute of Medicine, Ulmer C, McFadden B, Nerenz DR. *Race, Ethnicity, and Language Data: Standardization for Health Care Quality Improvement.* National Academies Press; 2009. https://pubmed.ncbi.nlm.nih.gov/25032349/. Accessed January 19, 2025.

94. Hasnain-Wynia R, Pierce D, Haque A, et al. *American Hospital Association: health research and educational trust disparities toolkit.* 2007. https://www.aha.org/ahahret-guides/2012-01-01-hret-disparities-toolkit. Accessed January 13, 2025.

95. U.S. Department of Health and Human Services. National culturally and linguistically appropriate services standards in health and health care; 2024. https://www.thinkculturalhealth.hhs.gov/Content/clas.asp. Accessed January 13, 2025.

96. Equal Employment Opportunity Program. Title VI, prohibition against national origin discrimination affecting limited English proficient persons. *Fed Regist.* 2004;69(7):1763–1768. National Archives. https://www.archives.gov/eeo/laws/title-vi.html. Accessed January 13, 2025.

97. Patel K, Zakowski M. Enhanced recovery after cesarean: current and emerging trends. *Curr Anesthesiol Rep.* 2021;11:136–144.

98. D'Alton ME, Friedman AM, Smiley RM, et al. National partnership for maternal safety: consensus bundle on venous thromboembolism. *Obstet Gynecol.* 2016;128:688–698.

99. Bernstein PS, Martin JN Jr, Barton JR, et al. National Partnership for Maternal Safety: consensus bundle on severe hypertension during pregnancy and the postpartum period. *Anesth Analg.* 2017;125:540–547.

100. Green AR, Carney DR, Pallin DJ, et al. Implicit bias among physicians and its prediction of thrombolysis decisions for black and white patients. *J Gen Intern Med.* 2007;22:1231–1238.

101. Greenwald AG, McGhee DE, Schwartz JL. Measuring individual differences in implicit cognition: the implicit association test. *J Pers Soc Psychol.* 1998;74:1464–1480.

102. Greenwald AG, Poehlman TA, Uhlmann EL, Banaji MR. Understanding and using the Implicit Association Test: III. Meta-analysis of predictive validity. *J Pers Soc Psychol.* 2009;97:17–41.

103. Sabin J, Nosek BA, Greenwald A, Rivara FP. Physicians' implicit and explicit attitudes about race by MD race, ethnicity, and gender. *J Health Care Poor Underserved.* 2009;20:896–913.

104. Hall WJ, Chapman MV, Lee KM, et al. Implicit racial/ethnic bias among health care professionals and its influence on health care outcomes: a systematic review. *Am J Public Health.* 2015;105:e60–e76.

105. Lee TH, Volpp KG, Cheung VG, Dzau VJ. Diversity and inclusiveness in health care leadership: three key steps. *NEJM Catalyst.* 2021;2:e1–e9.

106. Kern-Goldberger AR, Hirshberg A, James A, et al. Trends in severe maternal morbidity following an institutional team goal strategy for disparity reduction. *Am J Obstet Gynecol MFM.* 2024;6:101529.

107. Centers for Disease Control and Prevention. Maternal mortality review committees guides and tools; 2024. https://www.cdc.gov/maternal-mortality/php/mmrc/guides-tools.html. Accessed January 19, 2025.

108. Hardeman RR, Kheyfets A, Mantha AB, et al. Developing tools to report racism in maternal health for the CDC Maternal Mortality Review Information Application (MMRIA): findings from the MMRIA Racism & Discrimination Working Group. *Matern Child Health J.* 2022;26:661–669.

109. Bailey ZD, Krieger N, Agenor M, et al. Structural racism and health inequities in the USA: evidence and interventions. *Lancet.* 2017;389:1453–1463.

110. Jones CP. Levels of racism: a theoretic framework and a gardener's tale. *Am J Public Health.* 2000;90:1212–1215.

111. Institute of Medicine, Smedley BD, Stith A, Nelson A. *Unequal Treatment: Confronting Racial and Ethnic Disparities in Health Care.* National Academy Press; 2003. https://www.ncbi.nlm.nih.gov/books/NBK220358/. Accessed January 19, 2025.

112. Lion KC, Faro EZ, Coker TR. All quality improvement is health equity work: designing improvement to reduce disparities. *Pediatrics.* 2022;149.

113. Morain SR. Engaging community members to irradicate health disparities. *Am J Public Health.* 2020;110:143–144.

114. National Network of Perinatal Quality Collaboratives. https://nnpqc.org/. Accessed January 19, 2025.

115. Sullivan K, Belfort MB, Melvin P, et al. Leveraging the Massachusetts perinatal quality collaborative to address the COVID-19 pandemic among diverse populations. *J Perinatol.* 2021;41:2674–2683.

116. Louisiana Perinatal Quality Collaborative. 2023 annual report; 2023. https://lapqc.org/wp-content/uploads/LaPQC2023Report.pdf. Accessed January 13, 2025.

117. Illinois Perinatal Quality Collaborative. Birth equity—BE. Illinois Perinatal Quality Collaborative. https://ilpqc.org/birthequity/. Accessed January 13, 2025.

118. Institute of Medicine Committee on Health Care in America. *Crossing the Quality Chasm: A New Health System for the 21st Century.* National Academy Press; 2001. https://nap.nationalacademies.org/catalog/10027/crossing-the-quality-chasm-a-new-health-system-for-the. Accessed January 19, 2025.

119. Divi C, Koss RG, Schmaltz SP, Loeb JM. Language proficiency and adverse events in US hospitals: a pilot study. *Int J Qual Health Care.* 2007;19:60–67.

120. Bartlett G, Blais R, Tamblyn R, et al. Impact of patient communication problems on the risk of preventable adverse events in acute care settings. *CMAJ*. 2008;178:1555–1562.

121. Stewart MA. Effective physician-patient communication and health outcomes: a review. *CMAJ*. 1995;152:1423–1433.

122. Roter DL, Stewart M, Putnam SM, et al. Communication patterns of primary care physicians. *JAMA*. 1997;277:350–356.

123. Kohr MA, Parrish JM, Neef NA, et al. Communication skills training for parents: experimental and social validation. *J Appl Behav Anal*. 1988;21:21–30.

124. Zikmund-Fisher BJ, Couper MP, Singer E, et al. The DECISIONS study: a nationwide survey of United States adults regarding 9 common medical decisions. *Med Decis Making*. 2010;30:20S–34S.

125. Fagerlin A, Sepucha KR, Couper MP, et al. Patients' knowledge about 9 common health conditions: the DECISIONS survey. *Med Decis Making*. 2010;30:35S–52S.

126. Sepucha KR, Fagerlin A, Couper MP, et al. How does feeling informed relate to being informed? The DECISIONS survey. *Med Decis Making*. 2010;30:77S–84S.

127. National Center for Education Statistics. *The Health Literacy of America's Adults: Results from the 2003*. National Assessment of Adult Literacy; 2006. https://nces.ed.gov/pubsearch/pubsinfo.asp?pubid=2006483. Accessed January 19, 2025.

128. King JS, Moulton BW. Rethinking informed consent: the case for shared medical decision-making. *Am J Law Med*. 2006;32:429–501.

129. Kaplan RM. Shared medical decision making. A new tool for preventive medicine. *Am J Prev Med*. 2004;26:81–83.

130. King JS, Eckman MH, Moulton BW. The potential of shared decision making to reduce health disparities. *J Law Med Ethics*. 2011;39(suppl 1):30–33.

131. Toledo P, Sun J, Peralta F, et al. A qualitative analysis of parturients' perspectives on neuraxial labor analgesia. *Int J Obstet Anesth*. 2013;22:119–123.

132. Nathan AG, Marshall IM, Cooper JM, Huang ES. Use of decision aids with minority patients: a systematic review. *J Gen Intern Med*. 2016;31:663–676.

133. Volandes AE, Paasche-Orlow MK, Barry MJ, et al. Video decision support tool for advance care planning in dementia: randomised controlled trial. *BMJ*. 2009;338:b2159.

134. Meade CD, McKinney WP, Barnas GP. Educating patients with limited literacy skills: the effectiveness of printed and videotaped materials about colon cancer. *Am J Public Health*. 1994;84:119–121.

135. Davis TC, Berkel HJ, Arnold CL, et al. Intervention to increase mammography utilization in a public hospital. *J Gen Intern Med*. 1998;13:230–233.

136. Stubenrouch FE, Mus EMK, Lut JW, et al. The current level of shared decision-making in anesthesiology: an exploratory study. *BMC Anesthesiol*. 2017;17:95.

137. Cooper-Patrick L, Gallo JJ, Gonzales JJ, et al. Race, gender, and partnership in the patient-physician relationship. *JAMA*. 1999;282:583–589.

138. American Association of Medical Colleges. Underrepresented in medicine definition; 2019. https://www.aamc.org/what-we-do/equity-diversity-inclusion/underrepresented-in-medicine. Accessed January 13, 2025.

139. Toledo P, Duce L, Adams J, et al. Diversity in the American Society of Anesthesiologists leadership. *Anesth Analg*. 2017;124:1611–1616.

140. Saha S, Komaromy M, Koepsell TD, Bindman AB. Patient-physician racial concordance and the perceived quality and use of health care. *Arch Intern Med*. 1999;159:997–1004.

141. Shen MJ, Peterson EB, Costas-Muniz R, et al. The effects of race and racial concordance on patient-physician communication: a systematic review of the literature. *J Racial Ethn Health Disparities*. 2018;5:117–140.

142. Takeshita J, Wang S, Loren AW, et al. Association of racial/ethnic and gender concordance between patients and physicians with patient experience ratings. *JAMA Netw Open*. 2020;3:e2024583.

143. Sanchez J, Prabhu R, Guglielminotti J, Landau R. Racial and ethnic concordance between the patient and anesthesia team and patients' satisfaction with pain management during cesarean delivery. *Anesth Analg*. 2024;139:921–930.

144. Bogdan-Lovis E, Zhuang J, Goldbort J, et al. Do Black birthing persons prefer a Black health care provider during birth? Race concordance in birth. *Birth*. 2023;50:310–318.

145. Nwokolo OO, Coombs AAT, Eltzschig HK, Butterworth JF. Diversity and inclusion in anesthesiology. *Anesth Analg*. 2022;134:1166–1174.

146. Estime SR, Lee HH, Jimenez N, et al. Diversity, equity, and inclusion in anesthesiology. *Int Anesthesiol Clin*. 2021;59:81–85.

147. Toledo P, Wright CC, Vetter TR. Diversity, equity, and inclusion: more than words. *Anesth Analg*. 2023;137:722–723.

148. Mhyre JM, Jackson J, Lucero J, Goree J. Workforce solutions to address health disparities. *Curr Opin Anaesthesiol*. 2022;35:317–325.

149. Daw JR, Kolenic GE, Dalton VK, et al. Racial and ethnic disparities in perinatal insurance coverage. *Obstet Gynecol*. 2020;135:917–924.

150. Eliason EL. Adoption of Medicaid expansion is associated with lower maternal mortality. *Womens Health Issues*. 2020;30:147–152.

15

Obstetric Anesthesia in Low- and Middle-Income Countries

Medge D. Owen, MD and K. A. Kelly McQueen, MD, MPH, FASA

While there are many barriers to providing safe and equitable obstetric care in low- and middle-income countries (LMICs), the primary challenges in the 21st century relate to a lack of access to surgery and safe anesthesia care for the parturient. Many improvements made during the World Health Organization's (WHO) Millennium Development Goals campaign, including a goal to reduce maternal mortality, have succeeded in improving maternal outcomes. Measures have included increased contraception use, antiretroviral treatment for women with human immunodeficiency virus (HIV) infection, improved maternal education, higher family income levels, and a decrease in the global fertility rate.[1,2] Simply stated, fewer pregnancies lead to fewer maternal deaths. As a result of these efforts, the global maternal mortality ratio (MMR) declined from 339 to 223 deaths per 100,000 live births during the period 2000 to 2020, representing an annual reduction of 2.1% per year.[3] During this period, gradual improvements in MMR in sub-Saharan Africa occurred; however, this region of the world continues to report the highest rates of maternal mortality (see Chapter 39). Poor outcomes are the result of multifactorial health systems deficiencies, including lack of access to care and poor quality of care. Prior to 2015, limited focus on surgery and safe anesthesia care as a global public health priority[4] further contributed to stagnation in maternal mortality reduction in many LMICs. The World Bank definition of LMIC is shown in Table 15.1,[5] and the distribution of countries that fall into each category by region of the world is shown in Fig. 15.1.[6]

THE BURDEN OF DISEASE AND GLOBAL ANESTHESIA CRISIS

The Global Burden of Disease work, commissioned by the World Bank in 1990, measures the causes and trends of death and disability worldwide.[7] This important work has influenced public health policy, leading to more targeted global and national support to address various diseases in LMICs. The burden of both communicable and noncommunicable disease (NCD) in LMICs is highlighted in the World Bank's 2015 publication, *Disease Control Priorities*.[8] Surgery, as an intervention, along with safe anesthesia, impacts both communicable and NCDs such as trauma, cardiovascular disease, cancer, and maternal morbidity and mortality.

Historically, the lack of focus on surgery and safe anesthesia in LMICs by health ministries, the WHO, and other international organizations has limited investment in the infrastructure and workforce necessary for surgery and anesthesia. As disease in LMICs has shifted from communicable to NCDs during the last 30 years, and as populations live longer, individuals have developed more chronic diseases such as cardiovascular disease and cancer, many of which require surgery. Apart from the COVID-19 pandemic, the communicable disease burden has been markedly reduced; however, comparable improvements in the maternal burden of disease have not been made. Maternal morbidity and mortality remain unacceptably high in LMICs, and this reality is directly related to the lack of emergency and essential surgery and safe anesthesia.

Many factors contribute to the lack of timely access to surgery and safe anesthesia in LMICs, but none are more critical than the lack of adequate workforce, including physicians, nonphysician providers, and nurses.[9,10] In most of the 32 lowest-income countries, and especially in sub-Saharan Africa, the number of anesthesiologists is less than 1 per million population, and these physicians are often clustered in the largest cities at regional medical centers.[10] Fortunately, the training of nonphysician providers has been successful, and has allowed some growth toward the goal of more timely access to surgery and safe anesthesia, including cesarean delivery and surgical treatment of postpartum hemorrhage.[11] Improving the anesthesia workforce in LMICs, and thereby increasing access to timely surgery and patient safety, must be a goal for improving maternal peripartum care and related outcomes.

TABLE 15.1   Definition of Low- and Middle-Income Countries

World Bank Atlas Designation	Gross National Income per Capita
Low income	≤$1085
Lower middle income	$1086–$4255
Upper middle income	$4256–$13,205
High income	≥$13,205

The World Bank Atlas Method is used to calculate the 2023 income definitions based on Gross National Income/Gross National Project in 2021.
From Hamadeh N, Van Rompaey C, Metreau E, Eapen, SG. New World Bank country classification by income level: 2022-2023. https://blogs.worldbank.org/opendata/new-world-bank-country-classifications-income-level-2022-2023. Accessed 14 December 2024.

BARRIERS TO SURGERY AND ANESTHESIA IN LOW- AND MIDDLE-INCOME COUNTRIES

Paul Farmer, a renowned advocate for surgery and safe anesthesia in LMICs, summarized the barriers to providing safe surgery and anesthesia with 4 "S's," the need for space, staff, stuff, and systems.[12] These categories aptly summarize the challenge for providing safe obstetric anesthesia and peripartum care. Considering each of these barriers will facilitate understanding the current state in LMICs and address an approach to the solutions necessary for improving the care of mothers and their babies.

World Bank income classifications

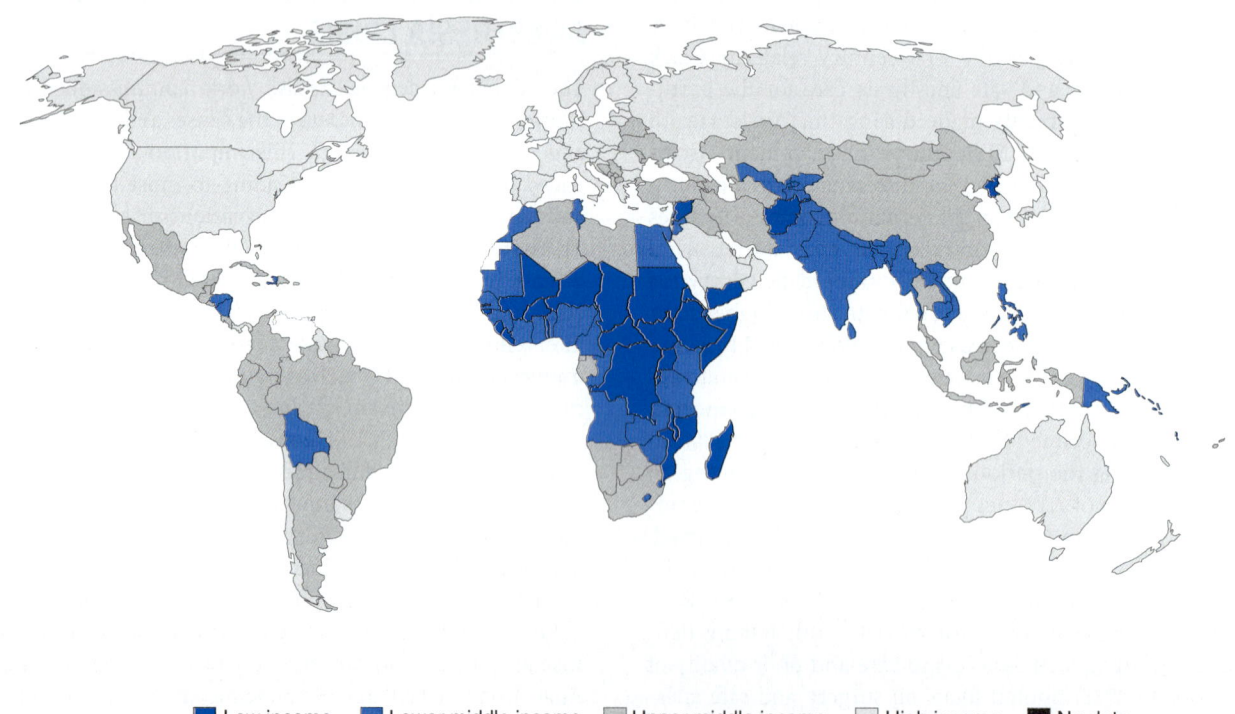

■ Low income   ■ Lower-middle income   ■ Upper-middle income   □ High income   ■ No data

Fig. 15.1 World Bank Country Classification by Gross National Income Level, 2023. Countries are divided into four categories based on gross national income per capita. Published open-access from Data Page: World Bank income groups, part of Roser M, Arriagag P, Hasell J, Ritchie H, Ortiz-Ospina E. Economic growth; 2023. Data adapted from World Bank. https://ourworldindata.org/grapher/world-bank-income-groups. Accessed 14 December 2024.

Infrastructure: Space

The infrastructural needs for surgical care and safe anesthesia have been surveyed and categorized as essential since early in the advocacy efforts for safe surgery within the global health agenda.[13-18] Essential to surgical systems, infrastructure includes everything from the bricks and mortar of operating rooms, to scalpels and cautery, and anesthesia machines and monitoring devices. Additionally, the infrastructure must be accessible to the population in need. For essential surgery, which is considered basic surgery without a high degree of specialization, the ideal access cadence is within 2 hours. The "Essential Surgery" section of the World Bank *Disease Control Priorities*, 3rd edition (DCP3), recommends that 44 cost-effective surgical procedures should be accessible within 2 hours of seeking care,[8] including cesarean delivery, dilation and curettage, and surgical treatment for hemorrhage. Beyond the infrastructure to provide surgery, it is essential to have the ability to monitor high-risk mothers to improve decision-making about when to intervene with surgical delivery. Additionally, oxygen and blood product availability must be considered.

Workforce: Staff

Many LMICs have too few practicing physicians to serve the populations in need. The availability of cesarean delivery in LMICs is an essential feature of obstetric care, but availability is often limited by lack of anesthesia and obstetric or surgical providers.[19,20] Many factors contribute to physician shortages, including poor access to medical education and residency training, and the exodus of LMIC physicians to higher-income countries (HICs), so-called brain drain. Specialty trained physicians are limited in most LMICs, and this is especially true for anesthesiologists in the lowest-income countries. The shortage of anesthesiologists and nonphysician anesthesia providers (NPAPs) has impacted surgical and obstetric care in many LMICs, but most notably in sub-Saharan Africa, where the crisis in anesthesia provision is most significant and the burden of surgical disease is the greatest (Table 15.2).

Until recently, little was known about the numbers of practicing anesthesiologists and NPAPs in LMICs, apart from reports by anesthesia and surgical missionaries noting that limitations in anesthesia care negatively impacted safety during surgery. Documentation of the number of anesthesia and surgical providers in LMICs began by a small group of interested researchers, and this eventually became a priority for the World Federation of Societies of Anesthesiologists (WFSA) and the WHO. Nicholas M. Greene advocated for training of NPAPs in sub-Saharan Africa after working in the harsh conditions of East Africa in the 1980s, where surgical access and safety were limited by the few trained anesthesia providers. Dr. Greene lobbied the American Society of Anesthesiologists (ASA) for many years before convincing the prestigious society to support the Overseas Teaching Program (OTP), whose initial aim in 1990 was to train nonphysicians to safely conduct anesthesia. The OTP continues today as the ASA Global Humanitarian Outreach Committee, which remains committed to the education and training of anesthesiologists and NPAPs in sub-Saharan Africa.

Anesthesia workforce surveys have been conducted since the late 2000s and are ongoing.[9,10] The WFSA Global Workforce Survey, the most comprehensive to date, has informed the global community and influenced planning for the education and training of physicians and NPAPs alike (Table 15.3 and Fig. 15.2).[21] The anesthesiology workforce crisis in LMICs was clearly illuminated in 2015 when several

TABLE 15.2 **Availability of Anesthesia Providers and Infrastructure Necessary for Cesarean Delivery in 26 Low- and Middle-Income Countries, 2009–13**

	Total (n = 719)	Facilities Performing Cesarean Delivery (N = 531)	Facilities Referring Cesarean Delivery (n = 67)
Personnel			
Anesthesiologist	172 (23.9%)	145 (27.3%)	4 (6.0%)[a]
General doctor providing anesthesia	66 (9.2%)	62 (11.7%)	0[b]
Nurse or NPAP	229 (31.8%)	202 (38.0%)	6 (9.0%)[a]
None present	389 (54.1%)	2 (0.4%)	57 (85.1%)[a]
Infrastructure			
Oxygen	525 (73.0%)	417 (78.5%)	21 (38.8%)[a]
Anesthesia machine	415 (57.7%)	350 (65.9%)	18 (33.3%)[a]
Blood bank	228 (31.7%)	199 (37.5%)	4 (7.4%)[a]

NPAP, Nonphysician anesthesia provider.
[a]$P < .001$, facilities performing cesarean delivery compared with facilities referring cesarean deliveries.
[b]$P < .003$, facilities performing cesarean delivery compared with facilities referring cesarean deliveries.
Data are based on a secondary analysis of facility-based survey data collected between 2009 and 2013 using the World Health Organization Situational Analysis Tool to Assess Emergency and Essential Surgical Care; Data from Olugunde R, Vogel JP, Cherian MN, et al. Assessment of cesarean delivery availability in 26 low- and middle-income countries: a cross-sectional study. *Am J Obstet Gynecol.* 2014;211:504.e1–e12.

TABLE 15.3 Density of Anesthesia Providers by World Bank 2021 Income Group and WHO Region, 2021–23

	PAP Number	PAP Density[a]	NPAP Number	NPAP Density[a]
Income Group				
High	194,106	16.1	94,065	7.8
Upper middle	215,808	7.5	53,369	1.9
Lower middle	87,229	3.0	13,231	0.5
Low	1637	0.3	10,288	1.7
WHO Region				
African	5949	0.6	15,422	1.4
Eastern Mediterranean	26,306	3.7	14,865	2.1
European	167,174	20.9	40,363	5.0
Americas	113,320	11.1	57,666	5.7
Southeast Asia	70,020	3.4	9049	0.4
Western Pacific	116,011	6.0	33,588	1.7

NPAP, Nonphysician anesthesia provider; *PAP*, physician anesthesia provider; *WHO*, World Health Organization.
[a]Provider density is reported as the number of providers per 100,000 population.
Adapted from Law TJ, Lipnick MS, Morriss W, et al. The Global Anesthesia Workforce Survey: updates and trends in the anesthesia workforce. *Anesth Analg.* 2024;139:15–24.

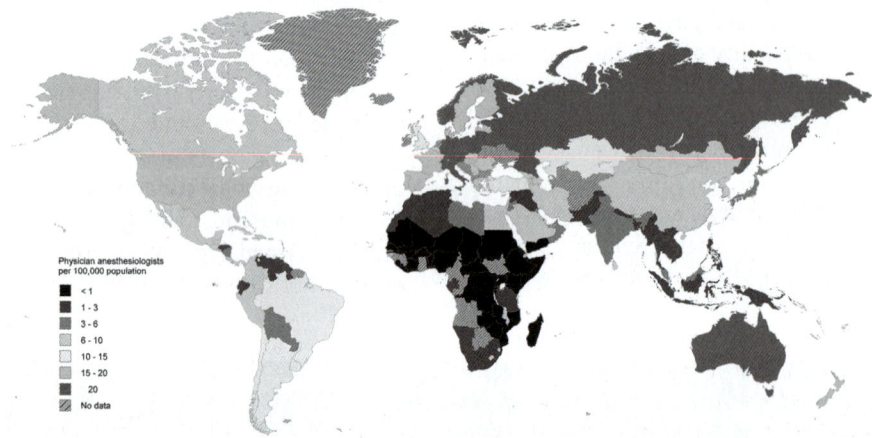

Fig. 15.2 Global distribution of physician anesthesia providers per 100,000 population (physician anesthesia provider density) by country. From Law TJ, Lipnick MS, Morriss W, et al. The Global Anesthesia Workforce Survey: updates and trends in the anesthesia workforce. *Anesth Analg.* 2024;139:15–24.

important bodies of work were published, namely the DCP3 *Essential Surgery* volume,[8] the Lancet Commission on Global Surgery (LCOGS),[11] and the World Health Assembly resolution on strengthening emergency and essential surgical care and anesthesia.[22] These reports underscored the anesthesia workforce crisis as the rate-limiting step for surgical access and patient safety and called for a commitment to workforce development to achieve safe anesthesia. It will take decades to train an adequate workforce of anesthesiologists to meet the needs of LMICs, but improving access and patient safety for patients in LMICs is an urgent need.

Fortunately, in many LMICs, there is a commitment to training nonphysician providers, including NPAPs.[19,20] Both task shifting and task sharing have been successfully applied to maternal and reproductive health in LMICs.[23] **Task shifting** is the deliberate shifting of a task or tasks that are specifically described and defined. The shift in responsibility frees up more highly trained individuals to provide more complex care. **Task sharing** involves a team of providers working together to deliver a procedure or service that they may not have delivered previously as individuals. Endorsed by the WHO, these strategies maximize health worker capacity and optimize performance in low-resource settings. Both task shifting and sharing are historically common in LMICs, where fully trained providers are scarce. The shifting or sharing may be an informal process that occurs out of necessity; however, a formal process that involves training, certification, and support offers better and safer options.

The delivery of peripartum care through task shifting is a sustainable option in LMICs. Examples include the shifting of responsibility from an obstetrician to a midwife, or from a midwife to a skilled birth attendant, freeing up the obstetrician or surgeon to provide cesarean delivery when needed. Similarly, anesthesia care delivery by a nurse anesthetist, general physician, or anesthesia technician allows critical surgery to continue in the absence of an anesthesiologist. Both examples are common in many LMICs. Task sharing is less common because of the shortage of anesthesiologists, especially in LMICs, thus limiting the availability of teams functioning together to provide anesthesia care.

Monitors, Medicines, and Other Stuff

Consistent with many operating spaces in LMICs, the labor and delivery areas and operating rooms for cesarean delivery frequently lack safety monitoring equipment, essential medicines, and access to blood products. A cross-sectional survey was conducted among 86 anesthesia providers working in national referral hospitals in five countries in East Africa (Uganda, Kenya, Tanzania, Rwanda, Burundi) to assess the ability to provide safe obstetric anesthesia.[24] None of the respondents worked in a facility that met all the requirements listed in the WFSA guidelines for safe anesthesia care. Although drugs for general and spinal anesthesia were generally present, the availability of safety monitors and airway supplies was limited. Even pulse oximetry and oxygen are not ubiquitous in LMICs. While governments may emphasize the need for basic safety monitoring, it may take years for every operating room and high acuity unit to be suitably equipped, as shown in a separate survey of cesarean delivery infrastructure in 26 LMICs (see Table 15.2).[20] International initiatives such as Lifebox (www.lifebox.org) are committed to providing durable, inexpensive, portable pulse oximeters with education to LMICs. Importantly, blood banks are also lacking in LMICs. For the care of women with peripartum or postpartum hemorrhage, the lack of access to transfusable blood is often catastrophic.

Consistent access to essential medicines is also a barrier to the anesthesia and obstetric care of women in the peripartum period. Essential medicines for the peripartum period include antibiotics, antihypertensive and antiemetic medications, general and local anesthetic agents, magnesium sulfate, and tocolytic agents. The WHO endorses an updated list of essential medicines every 2 years, but these medicines may not readily be available in every setting, and an absence of any of the essential medicines, including oxygen, can compromise the care of vulnerable patients, including the care of the mother and baby.[25] The WHO Essential Medicine List represents guidance to ministries of health and health systems, but these medications are not mandated. Similarly, there is no international governing body that requires ministries of health or local health systems to invest to ensure the availability of equipment, monitoring capability, basic surgical supplies, blood products, and essential medicines.

Systems

The fourth "S" in Farmer's guidance for successful healthcare delivery is "systems." The role of the system is often overlooked by many physicians from HICs who are committed to global health. Farmer noted that while space, staff, and stuff are essential for the delivery of healthcare, it is the system—operational processes, referral services, and medical records—that reorients the resources to provide quality medical care.[12] This need to focus on the system was proven true for addressing the HIV/AIDS epidemic; it is also true for the delivery of surgery and safe anesthesia, and especially true when addressing access to cesarean delivery and other life-saving obstetric procedures.

The evaluation of national surgical systems became a priority after the significant reports published in 2015,[8,26] and the unanimous commitment to emergency and essential surgery at the World Health Assembly.[22] The WHO and the Harvard Medical School Program in Global Surgery and Social Change (PGSSC) partnered[26] to create guidance for a process that would empower countries to perform their own evaluations, followed by the design of processes and systems to address the common barriers to safe surgical, obstetric, and anesthesia care. The National Surgery, Obstetric and Anesthesia Plans (NSOAPs) address infrastructure, workforce, and reusable and disposable resources for the care of surgical and obstetric patients.[11,26] The healthcare system is central to the ultimate success of the NSOAP process, and implementing the process has the potential to result in significant expansion of surgical, obstetric, and anesthesia care in LMICs (see later discussion).

CESAREAN DELIVERY IN LOW- AND MIDDLE-INCOME COUNTRIES

The timely access to cesarean delivery and other essential obstetric procedures is a significant barrier to improving maternal and fetal mortality in LMICs. Cesarean delivery is a common surgical procedure worldwide and is one of the most frequently performed surgeries in sub-Saharan Africa. In HICs, cesarean delivery rates are often considered excessively high and may approach 30% to 40% of births, but in sub-Saharan Africa, the cesarean delivery rate is often too low. In some countries and settings, it is as low as 1% of all births. The WHO recommends a 10% to 15% target cesarean delivery rate at the population level; cesarean delivery rates lower than this indicate inadequate access to emergency care, and rates exceeding this do not correlate with improved maternal or newborn outcomes.[27,28] The indications for cesarean delivery are universal.

Cesarean delivery rates are increasing worldwide, and this will inevitably increase the demand for anesthesia providers. A report on global cesarean delivery trends that included data from 169 countries representing 98.4% of the world's births estimated that 29.7 million cesarean births (cesarean birth rate, 21.1%; 95% confidence interval [CI], 19.9 to 22.4) occurred in 2015, almost double the 16.0 million (12.1%; 95% CI, 1.9 to 13.3) reported in 2000.[29] The increase has been attributed to a rise in facility-based births as well as an increase in cesarean deliveries conducted within facilities.[27] Wide variations in surgical delivery rates, however, are reported across LMICs. Even among LMICs, cesarean delivery rates vary widely. In Latin America and the Caribbean, the cesarean delivery rate is 10 times higher (44.3%) than it is in West and Central Africa (4.1%).[29] In 2015, the Dominican Republic had the highest national cesarean delivery rate (58.1%) and South Sudan the lowest (0.6%). In general, cesarean delivery rates are higher among wealthy and educated women, in urban areas, and in private hospitals, particularly in Brazil and China.[29–31]

Surgical delivery is considered a life-saving procedure; however, cesarean delivery may also be driven by nonmedical indications (maternal or obstetric provider choice), which may lead to unnecessary complications in current or subsequent pregnancies.[27,29] Reasons women may request cesarean delivery without a medical indication include fear of labor pain, pelvic floor damage, urinary incontinence, or reduced quality of sexual life, or superstitious beliefs.[32,33] Women who prefer cesarean delivery may perceive it to be safer, contrary to scientific evidence.[31,34,35] Obstetricians may be inclined to choose cesarean delivery due to convenience, financial incentives, or fear of litigation.[31–34] Cesarean delivery overuse should be monitored in LMICs, as it is associated with greater short- and long-term maternal mortality and morbidity compared with vaginal birth and leads to future risks for abnormal placentation such as placenta previa and placenta accreta.[32,36]

It is essential to evaluate the causes and variations of maternal and perinatal mortality associated with cesarean delivery across the LMIC spectrum. A 2019 meta-analysis of 116 studies in LMICs evaluated data from 2,933,457 cesarean deliveries and 6982 maternal deaths.[28] The risk of maternal death during cesarean delivery was higher in low-income than in middle-income countries ($P = .012$) and in teaching and tertiary hospitals than in other settings ($P = .014$). For every 1000 women undergoing cesarean delivery in LMICs, nearly 8 died (7.6; 95% CI, 6.6 to 8.6). This risk stands in stark contrast to eight maternal deaths per 100,000 cesarean deliveries in HICs such as the United Kingdom.[37] Women from sub-Saharan Africa had the highest risk of death (10.9 per 1000; 95% CI, 9.5 to 12.5) compared to other regions, although there were relatively few studies from Eastern Europe, Central Asia, and the Middle East. In addition, women undergoing emergency cesarean delivery in LMICs were twice as likely to die as those delivering by elective cesarean delivery. A third of all maternal deaths following cesarean delivery were attributed to postpartum hemorrhage (32%; 95% CI, 27% to 37%).[28] The risk of death associated with cesarean delivery has not substantially decreased over the past several decades and remains highest in countries with the lowest cesarean delivery rates.[28] It is clear that women having cesarean delivery in LMICs have disproportionately greater risks of death than do women in HICs.

To further investigate cesarean delivery outcomes in Africa, a prospective observational study was conducted in 183 hospitals across 22 countries in 2016.[36] Both elective and nonelective cesarean deliveries were included and followed for 7 days. Of 3684 patients, there were 20 maternal deaths (0.5%; 95% CI, 0.3% to 0.8%) and 633 complications (17.4%; 95% CI, 16.2% to 18.6%). Hemorrhage accounted for nearly 70% of the complications and 25% of the maternal deaths. Maternal mortality was independently associated with placenta previa, placental abruption, ruptured uterus, antepartum hemorrhage (odds ratio [OR], 4.47; 95% CI, 1.46 to 13.65), perioperative severe obstetric hemorrhage (OR, 5.87; 95% CI, 1.99 to 17.34), and anesthesia complications (OR, 11.47; 95% CI, 1.20 to 109.20). Maternal mortality related to cesarean delivery in Africa was 50 times higher than that in HICs and was influenced by peripartum hemorrhage and anesthesia complications.

The South African National Committee for Confidential Enquiry into Maternal Deaths (NCCEMD), initiated in 1998, is the most comprehensive audit of maternal outcomes in Africa. The 2011 to 2013 report found that the risk of death was nearly three times higher for women undergoing cesarean delivery than vaginal delivery.[38] In addition, the case fatality rate for death due to anesthesia complications was 0.02 per 10,000 for vaginal deliveries compared with 1.2 per 10,000 for cesarean deliveries, a sixfold difference. Furthermore, death from cesarean delivery was more likely in regions with the lowest cesarean delivery rates.

Type of Anesthesia for Cesarean Delivery

Anesthesia disproportionately contributes to maternal mortality in LMIC, primarily during cesarean delivery; therefore it is important to understand the attribution to death by the type of anesthetic. In a 2016 systematic review and meta-analysis of 140 studies from LMICs, investigators observed that complications from anesthesia related to cesarean delivery contributed to 13.8% (95% CI, 9.0 to 20.7) of all maternal deaths occurring during or after cesarean delivery.[39] The administration of general anesthesia tripled the odds of maternal death, with case fatality rates of 5.9 per 1000 and 1.2 per 1000 for general and neuraxial anesthesia, respectively.[39] General anesthesia also doubled the risk of perinatal death.

In a subset of studies, contributing factors were reported in 124 maternal deaths: over half of the deaths were attributed to airway complication and/or pulmonary aspiration; nearly one-third were related to staff incompetency, poor preoperative assessment, limited intraoperative monitoring, and equipment failure; and one-tenth were due to high spinal anesthesia or a drug-related event. The risk of death associated with anesthesia was higher in rural than in urban settings, and in low-income and lower-middle income than in upper-middle income countries.[39]

Many of the studies in the 2016 meta-analysis[39] were based in sub-Saharan Africa and may not reflect the full spectrum of anesthetic complications in LMICs. A secondary analysis of two large WHO surveys[40] (data from 2004 to 2005[41] and 2010 to 2011[42]) assessed associations between anesthetic technique and pregnancy outcomes for 129,742 cesarean deliveries in LMICs. For each of the WHO surveys, well-trained research assistants used pretested, standardized data collection forms to obtain data across various LMICs in Africa, Asia, Latin America, and the Middle East. The World Health Organization Global Survey (WHOGS) on Maternal and Perinatal Health[42] included 370 health facilities in 24 countries, and the World Health Organization Multicountry Survey (WHOMCS) on Maternal and Newborn Health[41] included 359 health facilities in 29 countries.[40] In each country, the capital city and two randomly selected provinces were sampled to identify seven facilities with over 1000 annual deliveries and the capacity to perform cesarean delivery. Spinal anesthesia was the most common anesthetic technique in both databases, accounting for 48.9% in the WHOGS and 57.1% in the WHOMCS.[40] Compared with general anesthesia, intended neuraxial anesthesia was associated with lower odds

of maternal death, maternal near-miss events, severe maternal outcome, and intensive care unit admission (Fig. 15.3).

In a 6-year retrospective review, Médecins Sans Frontières (MSF, also known as Doctors Without Borders) found that in over 75,000 surgeries conducted in low-resource settings, cesarean delivery was the most commonly performed surgery (35%), and spinal anesthesia was the most frequently administered type of anesthesia (46%).[43] The authors similarly reported a significantly lower odds of death associated with spinal than with general anesthesia with tracheal intubation (adjusted OR, 0.10; 95% CI, 0.05 to 0.18).

Although studies in low-resource settings have demonstrated better maternal outcomes when cesarean delivery is conducted with spinal anesthesia, neuraxial techniques are

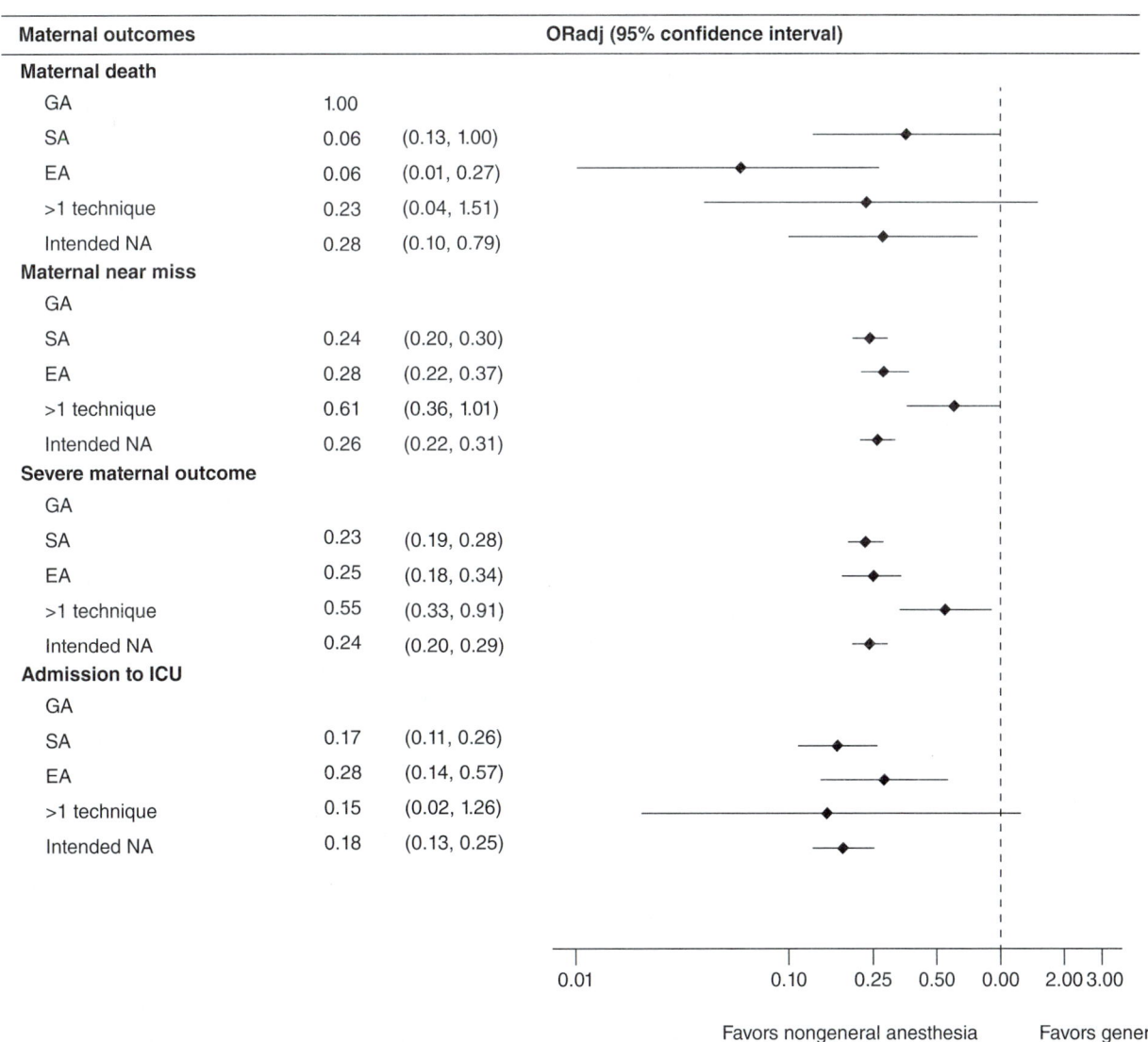

Fig. 15.3 Forest plot of the pooled estimates of maternal outcomes from WHO Global Survey (2004–08) and WHO Multicountry Survey (2010–11) data sets. Adjusted odds ratios (ORadj) are relative to the odds of outcomes for general anesthesia. Intended NA included data of women undergoing SA and EA and those who received more than one type of anesthesia. Admission to ICU is neonatal ICU admission. *EA*, Epidural anesthesia; *GA*, general anesthesia; *ICU*, neonatal intensive care unit; *NA*, neuraxial anesthesia; *SA*, spinal anesthesia. From Lumbiganon P, Moe H, Kamsa-Ard S, et al. Outcomes associated with anaesthetic techniques for caesarean section in low- and middle-income countries: a secondary analysis of WHO surveys. *Sci Rep.* 2020;10:10176.

not without risks. The 2008 to 2010 NCCEMD audit found that deaths due to spinal anesthesia had steadily increased over the preceding decade, accounting for more than half of the maternal deaths attributed to anesthesia.[44] The most recent NCCEMD audit (2017 to 2019) reported that over one-third of the 921 maternal deaths in women who received anesthesia were conducted using spinal anesthesia.[45] The author speculated that this finding is likely related to the increasing cesarean delivery rate across South Africa, the promotion of spinal anesthesia as a "safer" anesthesia technique, administration by physicians not fully trained or competent to manage complications of spinal anesthesia (such as hypotension, reflex bradycardia, and hemodynamic collapse), and use of spinal anesthesia for inappropriate conditions because it was the only form of anesthesia that the provider felt competent to provide.[44,46] There have been additional reports of substandard care and mortality in situations where a physician administered spinal anesthesia and then left the patient in the care of an unqualified person while the physician performed or assisted in the surgery or conducted neonatal resuscitation.[44,47] Sadly, maternal mortality from this practice has been reported in a country as advanced as Japan, where obstetricians often conduct both anesthesia and surgery on the same patient.[48]

The decision to use neuraxial or general anesthesia may be influenced by the severity of the indication for cesarean delivery. This may confound the observed association between mode of anesthesia and pregnancy outcome. Large database studies have not controlled for indication or patient comorbidities when comparing outcomes associated with neuraxial and general anesthesia, but audits have identified preventable morbidity and mortality. Whether general or spinal anesthesia is administered for cesarean delivery in low-resource settings, maternal morbidity and mortality related to substandard anesthesia practices are likely underreported.

Intravenous Ketamine Anesthesia

Intravenous ketamine administered as the sole anesthetic agent for cesarean delivery by minimally trained, unsupervised anesthesia officers has been described. Little data exist on the safety and outcomes of this technique. In Kenya, no maternal deaths were reported in a prospective case series of 401 emergency cesarean deliveries conducted with the use of intravenous ketamine without tracheal intubation by 54 trained, nonanesthesia providers.[49] A survey conducted in Sierra Leone found that intravenous ketamine without tracheal intubation was the second most common anesthetic technique administered for cesarean delivery, with spinal anesthesia the most common.[50] Similar findings have been reported in Zimbabwe.[51]

Deaths Attributable to Accidental Spinal Injection of Tranexamic Acid

An alarming increase in maternal deaths has been attributed to the accidental intrathecal administration of tranexamic acid (TXA). TXA is recommended for the treatment of postpartum hemorrhage and has quickly become a mainstay of care worldwide.[52] It is heat-stable and inexpensive; if stored in the operating room alongside local anesthetic solutions, similarly appearing glass ampules or vials can lead to drug administration errors. Intrathecal TXA is a potent neurotoxin, presenting with severe back and leg pain, refractory seizures, hypertension, tachycardia, and hemodynamic instability. There have been numerous case reports of accidental spinal TXA injection; death has resulted in approximately 50% of cases.[53] Accordingly, the WHO has issued a safety alert warning about this alarming trend.[54]

NEURAXIAL LABOR ANALGESIA IN LOW- AND MIDDLE-INCOME COUNTRIES

Anesthesia providers in many LMICs rarely care for obstetric patients outside the operating room, making it difficult to conduct neuraxial labor analgesia. The reasons for this are multifactorial and include insufficient anesthesia workforce; limited training and experience in obstetric anesthesia; fear of performing neuraxial anesthesia techniques in pregnant patients based on possible unforeseen complications; resistance from obstetricians and family members; lack of local anesthetic agents, other medications, and supplies (epidural catheters, infusion pumps, pencil-point spinal needles); lack of service coordination and appropriate staffing models to cover night shifts; and cost.[55–61] In some countries, patients must bear the cost of their own epidural kits and supplies.[59] Labor pain is generally perceived as "normal" and treatment of pain is not a priority. However, the need for anesthesia support on the labor ward is important, not only for providing pain relief, but also for enhancing multidisciplinary care and improving maternal and neonatal resuscitation, airway management, intensive care, and preoperative assessment.[56,60,62] Surveys suggest that women in low-income countries desire labor pain relief; however, many are unaware of the options or availability.[34,63,64] The literature is scant on the use of neuraxial labor analgesia in many LMICs.

Epidural Labor Analgesia
Eastern Europe

Even in relatively well-resourced middle-income countries with adequate numbers of anesthesia providers, the provision of neuraxial labor analgesia is limited.[55,59,61,65] Collaborations between nongovernmental organizations (NGO) and host institutions in LMICs have demonstrated some effectiveness in increasing the availability of neuraxial labor analgesia; however, use of these techniques remains limited. The NGO, Kybele, Inc., has worked in collaboration with several Eastern European countries and countries of the former Soviet Union to promote neuraxial anesthesia and analgesia use for cesarean and vaginal delivery with favorable results. In Croatia, a single 10-day training intervention in eight hospitals increased the average annual use of epidural labor analgesia from 1.2% to 2.3% across all sites for the year preceding and following the program.[65] In Serbia, a neighboring country with similar healthcare demographics, a training intervention conducted from 2012 to 2015 in a single regional hospital with 6500 annual births resulted in an increase of neuraxial labor analgesia from 1.2% in 2011 (baseline) to

10.5% in 2015.[55] Staffing constraints were cited as a barrier to the provision of neuraxial labor analgesia. All anesthesia staff members were available during the 8-hour workday, but only one anesthesiologist provided call coverage beginning midafternoon. This staffing model limited personnel available to perform labor analgesia at night, because the on-call person was also responsible for anesthesia for cesarean delivery. In addition, some obstetricians were resistant to change and did not support the distribution of patient informational brochures on analgesia and anesthesia options for vaginal and cesarean delivery. In the former Soviet county of Georgia, five hospitals were selected for participation in a multiyear project integrating clinical education, protocol development, quality improvement, and supply chain logistics.[59] Prior to 2007, 10% lidocaine was the only local anesthetic agent available and the antiquated technique of caudal labor analgesia was practiced. The program sought approval from the Health Ministry to bring bupivacaine, vasopressors, and supplies into the country for teaching demonstrations. Through continued engagement and early positive results, the Health Ministry approved the addition of bupivacaine to the national formulary. Additionally, the First Lady of Georgia became a strong advocate and proponent for more modern childbirth practices. The epidural kit supply chain improved and costs decreased, making labor analgesia more affordable. Consequently, the use of epidural labor analgesia increased from 20% in 2005 to over 40% in 2008 in participating hospitals, accounting for one-third of all deliveries in the capital city.

Kybele conducted six visits to neighboring Armenia between 2006 and 2015 to observe healthcare practices and to establish higher standards of obstetric anesthesia care.[61] Spinal anesthesia for cesarean delivery increased markedly across the country, but the use of epidural labor analgesia remained limited. Although epidural analgesia initially increased in seven hospitals from 2006 to 2012, by 2015, the use declined to less than 5% in all but two hospitals where labor epidural analgesia was sustained or increased. Epidural labor analgesia was not utilized outside the capital city, as there was typically only one anesthesiologist practicing in each hospital.

China. In China, the NGO, No Pain Labor & Delivery – Global Health Initiative, as well as recent governmental policies, have resulted in tremendous strides in promoting administration of neuraxial labor analgesia. A 2007 study reported that the estimated rate of neuraxial labor analgesia use in China was less than 1%.[66] Concomitantly, China also had one of the highest cesarean delivery rates in the world, which had grown to approximately half of the 16.4 million annual deliveries by 2010.[31] In essence, operative deliveries had become an accepted norm. The increase in the cesarean delivery rate occurred during the era of the one-child national policy and was driven by factors that included fear of malpractice litigation, cultural and superstitious beliefs, and fear of labor pain due to the limited availability of neuraxial labor analgesia.[33] These factors were compounded by a shortage of anesthesiologists and limited training in epidural labor analgesia, and wide disparity in care practices across urban and rural parts of the country.[67] In 2016, a national two-child policy was adopted, raising new concerns regarding advanced maternal age at childbirth

and risks associated with prior uterine surgery.[67] In an effort to decrease cesarean delivery rates and improve women's health, concerted efforts have been made to improve the provision of labor analgesia. The No Pain Labor & Delivery – Global Health Initiative began in 2008 with the goal of increasing the epidural labor analgesia rate by 10% by establishing 10 obstetric anesthesia-training centers over a 10-year period.[68] The program used annual 1-week visits by international expert clinicians with didactic and bedside education, daily debriefing and conferences, patient education books and social media education, and professional forums and the *Journal of No Pain Labor & Delivery – Global Health Initiative*. By 2020, 109 Chinese hospitals had been visited by over 1000 volunteer healthcare professionals from around the world. Four large-impact studies with approximately 74,465 parturients have confirmed that the implementation of 24-hour epidural pain relief services correlated with lower cesarean delivery rates in three hospital settings (a municipal maternity hospital, two academic institutions, and a rural hospital).[58,69–71]

In addition to the NGO collaboration, the National Health Commission in China issued two policies in 2018 to promote neuraxial labor analgesia.[72] The national policies aimed to improve neuraxial labor analgesia technical skills, promote a more scientific rationale for selecting the delivery mode, raise awareness regarding labor analgesia for hospital personnel, strengthen health education for pregnant women and their families, and make full use of training demonstrations in pilot hospitals. Accordingly, 913 pilot hospitals were selected for implementation.[73]

A study was undertaken to assess changes in the rates of neuraxial labor analgesia with data from China's National Maternal Near Miss Surveillance System.[74] Data were reviewed for 438 hospitals in 326 urban districts and rural counties in 30 provinces across China. Over the study period (2012 to 2019), 620,851 parturients received neuraxial labor analgesia from a population of 6,023,046 women who delivered vaginally. The estimated national neuraxial labor analgesia rate increased from 8.4% in 2012 to 16.7% in 2019.[74] Most provinces experienced a rapid rise in neuraxial labor analgesia use during this period, which was accelerated after 2018 with the introduction of the national pilot policy (Fig. 15.4).

The studies also evaluated the association between labor neuraxial analgesia and adverse maternal and perinatal outcomes in China.[58,69–71,74] There were no differences between women with and without neuraxial labor analgesia in the incidence of uterine atony, retained placenta, intrapartum fetal demise, and 1- and 5-minute Apgar scores < 7. However, women with neuraxial labor analgesia had higher incidences of genital tract trauma (adjusted relative risk [aRR], 1.53; 95% CI, 1.04 to 2.26) and maternal near miss (aRR, 1.35; 95% CI, 1.08 to 1.69) in nonpilot hospitals; these hospitals may have lacked sufficient equipment and personnel.[74]

India

In India, a diverse country with approximately 25 million annual births, epidural labor analgesia is infrequently used

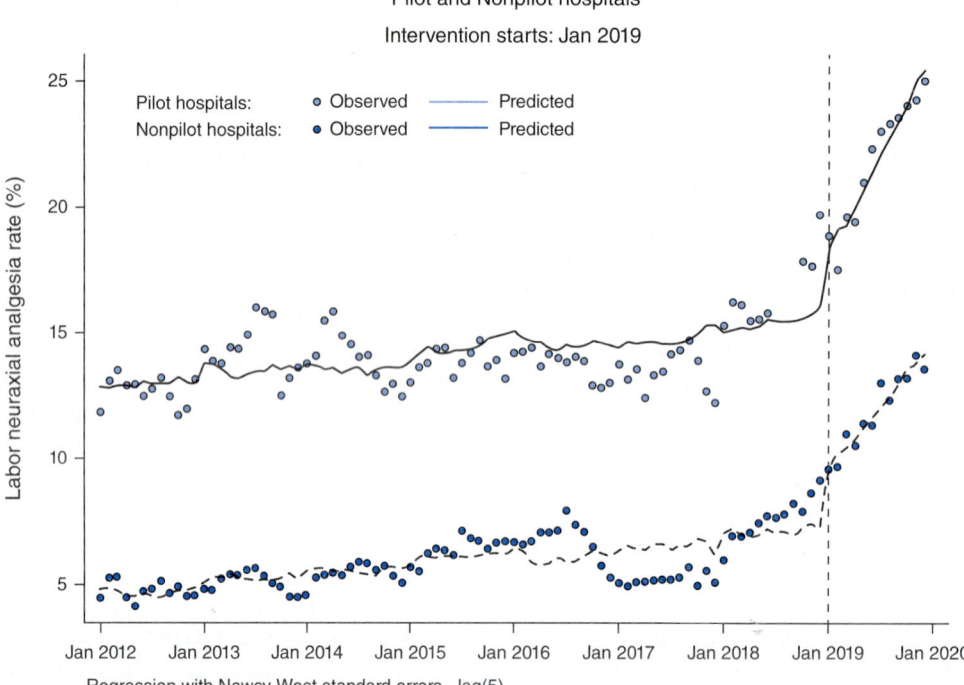

Fig. 15.4 Multiple-group interrupted time series analysis (ITSA) for comparisons on national monthly changes of labor neuraxial analgesia rates after initiation of the national policy promoting neuraxial labor analgesia in China (January 2019, *dotted line*). Promotion of neuraxial labor analgesia was officially implemented in 913 hospitals in China (primarily level-3 hospitals). The uptake of neuraxial labor analgesia increased in both pilot *(light dots)* and nonpilot (primarily level-2 hospitals) *(dark dots)*. The ITSA was adjusted for time-varying covariates, including proportion of maternal age ≥ 35 years old, women with college education or above, number of antenatal visits ≥ 7, and women with antepartum complications or medical diseases. From Mu Y, Wang X, Wang Y, et al. The trends and associated adverse maternal and perinatal outcomes of labour neuraxial analgesia among vaginal deliveries in China between 2012 and 2019: real-world observational evidence. *BMC Med.* 2021;19:74.

outside of private hospital settings. A recent survey conducted among 1351 anesthesiologists found that the highest rate of labor analgesia was in private (32.4%) and corporate hospitals (31.2%), followed by private medical colleges (21.1%), government medical colleges (12.4%), and government hospitals (3.0%).[75] These results suggest that labor analgesia is more consistently available for upper- and middle-income parturients, but much less available for the majority of women from rural and lower-income backgrounds who deliver in government hospitals. Labor analgesia was primarily conducted by anesthesiologists (71.3%), followed by both anesthesiologists and obstetricians (27.3%), and least commonly by obstetricians (1.4%). Epidural analgesia with intermittent bolus injection was employed most frequently (43.5%), followed by continuous infusion with intermittent boluses (37.9%). Other techniques included single-shot spinal analgesia, combined spinal-epidural analgesia, and patient-controlled epidural analgesia techniques. Bupivacaine (64.1%) and fentanyl (83.3%) were the most common epidural medications. India promotes up-to-date refresher training at the annual meeting of the Association of Obstetric Anaesthesiologists of India, established in 1983.

In Bhutan, a 4-year retrospective study found that of 15,119 patients, only 3.5% of women received either combined-spinal epidural, epidural, or single-shot spinal analgesia during

labor. Anesthesia staffing constraints and cultural beliefs were thought to limit the use of neuraxial labor analgesia.[76]

Latin America

Latin America represents a diverse group of countries with large gaps in research, knowledge, and health services related to obstetric anesthesia care.[48] Studies reflecting neuraxial labor analgesia use in various Latin America countries are limited. The WHO Multicountry Survey on Maternal and Newborn Health (WHOMCS) assessed labor analgesia practices in 29 countries across Latin America, Asia, the Middle East, and Africa, using data collected on 221,345 vaginal deliveries in 359 healthcare facilities in 2010 to 2011.[77] Pharmacologic analgesia interventions, including systemic analgesia (opioid or inhalational), neuraxial analgesia (epidural or spinal), or no pharmacologic intervention were compared by country and the Human Development Index (HDI), a composite measure of lifespan, education, and gross national income per capita. The use of epidural labor analgesia was higher among Latin American countries compared with Middle Eastern and sub-Saharan Africa countries, and in countries with a higher HDI (Table 15.4).[77] This study also found that neuraxial labor analgesia use was greater in nulliparous women, in women with higher education levels, and in women with previous cesarean delivery.[77]

TABLE 15.4 Use of Analgesia for Vaginal Birth in 29 Countries According to WHO Human Development Index and Regions, 2010–11

HDI and Country	LABOR ANALGESIA (%)		
	No Analgesia	Epidural Analgesia	Spinal Analgesia
Very High HDI			
Argentina	83	16	1
Japan	86	14	0.4
Qatar	82	18	0.4
High HDI			
Brazil	82	14	4
Ecuador	91	2	6
Lebanon	66	34	0.9
Mexico	71	29	0.1
Peru	98	2	0
Sri Lanka	99	1	0.2
Medium HDI			
Cambodia	99.6	0.1	0.3
China	94	5.6	0.1
India	99.8	0	0.1
Jordan	99	1	0
Mongolia	97	0	3
Nicaragua	99.6	0.2	0.1
OPT	94	6	0
Paraguay	89	8	3
Philippines	99.5	0.3	0.2
Thailand	99.7	0	0.3
Vietnam	86	13	1
Low HDI			
Afghanistan	99.9	0	0.1
Angola	99.9	0	0.1
DR Congo	99.7	0.2	0.1
Kenya	99.8	0.2	0
Nepal	99.4	0	0.6
Niger	100	0	0
Nigeria	100	0	0
Pakistan	98.3	0.1	1
Uganda	99.8	0	0.2

DR, Democratic Republic; *HDI*, Human Development Index; *OPT*, occupied Palestinian territories.
Data from Souza MA, Cecatti JG, Guida JP, et al. Analgesia for vaginal birth: secondary analysis from the WHO Multicountry Survey on Maternal and Newborn Health. *Int J Gynaecol Obstet.* 2021;152:401–408.

Educational strategies using simulation-based courses have been initiated by Confederación Latinoamericana de Sociedades de Anestesiología and the WFSA to improve obstetric anesthesia practices, and team training has been used to facilitate the management of obstetric emergencies.[48]

Middle East

The Middle Eastern region of the world similarly lacks studies on the use of neuraxial labor analgesia. The WHOMCS database reflects labor analgesia practices within some hospitals located in Qatar, Lebanon, Jordan, Palestine, Afghanistan, and Pakistan (see Table 15.4).[77] A 2019 3-month retrospective review of labor analgesia practices in Saudi Arabia was conducted in a tertiary referral hospital.[78] Intramuscular meperidine was used most frequently (35%). Epidural analgesia was administered to 32% of women, and spinal analgesia/intrathecal morphine and nitrous oxide were used in fewer than 1% of women. Approximately one-third of women received no form of analgesia. The authors stated that the study results may not reflect practice patterns across the country and that multicenter studies are needed to determine broader practices and care standards in Saudi Arabia.[78]

Sub-Saharan Africa

Neuraxial epidural analgesia use is extremely limited in sub-Saharan Africa (see Table 15.4).[79] A 2012 audit performed in an urban South African teaching hospital with over 7000 annual births found that only 2.2% of laboring patients had received epidural analgesia.[60] The primary reason was the posting of a single anesthesia provider who was simultaneously responsible for emergency surgery and labor analgesia. An epidural service was initiated in June 2014, whereby one anesthesia trainee was assigned to the labor ward during daytime hours, along with a staff nurse trained to manage epidural top-up doses and infusion adjustments. Following initiation, a 19-month audit was conducted from July 2014 to December 2015; 5.2% of women received epidural labor analgesia during this period. The authors surmised that the small number of patients who requested labor analgesia likely reflects a lack of patient knowledge about labor analgesia options. Overall use of epidural analgesia, however, remained low due to human resource allocation, nursing staff training, and patient education.

Spinal Labor Analgesia

In contrast to epidural analgesia, single-shot spinal analgesia may be a viable option for providing pain relief for labor in low-resource settings. It is simple to perform compared to an epidural technique, and it avoids the risk of unintentional dural puncture with a large-bore epidural needle and the associated risk of postdural puncture headache. The use of single-shot spinal analgesia minimizes the risk of local anesthetic systemic toxicity and high spinal anesthesia. It also requires less equipment (catheters, low-resistance syringes, infusion devices), all of which are generally unavailable in low-resource settings. Spinal analgesia has risks that must be discussed with the patient and anticipated; however, spinal labor analgesia services can be established with the development of simple protocols, staff education, and a few basic medications. Resuscitative agents (e.g., vasopressors) and equipment (e.g., self-inflating bag, face masks, endotracheal tubes) must be readily available. In labor and delivery suites that require parturients to walk to a separate delivery room, motor weakness from residual spinal analgesia must be considered.

Single-shot spinal labor analgesia is commonly utilized in some HICs, such as Finland, where studies have shown patient satisfaction and effectiveness.[80,81] In a study of 209 parturients, single-shot spinal labor analgesia with bupivacaine 2.5 mg and fentanyl 25 μg* provided pain relief for 101 ± 34 minutes (mean ± standard deviation [SD]) and 81% of women stated that they would request the same regimen again.[81] Single-shot spinal analgesia was also shown to be superior to paracervical block.[80] In a 2016 meta-analysis of five randomized, placebo-controlled trials, including 286 patients from HICs, the addition of intrathecal morphine (50 to 250 μg) extended the duration of the bupivacaine-fentanyl or sufentanil mixture by an average of 60 minutes.[82] A 2023 1-year retrospective review of 535 patients found that single-shot spinal labor analgesia was efficacious for most parturients; however, inadequate duration of analgesia was more frequent in nulliparous parturients and in parous women when analgesia was initiated early in labor.[83] The authors recommended this technique for use in resource-limited settings where other options for pain relief are unavailable.

Table 15.5 summarizes studies from LMICs utilizing single-shot spinal labor analgesia.[84-95] Many studies utilized spinal bupivacaine alone or in combination with fentanyl. A study from Nigeria found that the mean (± SD) duration of bupivacaine analgesia was shorter (62 ± 6 minutes) than bupivacaine combined with fentanyl (129 ± 22 minutes).[87] More patients receiving bupivacaine alone (52%) required a second spinal dose compared with those receiving bupivacaine with fentanyl (18%). The duration of labor and newborn outcomes were similar. Pruritus was more common with fentanyl administration (22% versus 0%); however, satisfaction was higher in the group that received fentanyl.

In a small study from Ghana describing the initiation of a labor analgesia service, 46 women received spinal bupivacaine; 6 (13%) required a second dose.[88] Protocol deviations were noted in 26 (57%) patients who received higher than the

recommended dose of bupivacaine 2.5 mg (range 3 to 6 mg), likely administered with the intent to extend the duration of pain relief. Opioid availability was limited; only four patients received bupivacaine combined with opioid (fentanyl 25 μg or meperidine 10 mg). Motor block was minimal and patients ambulated to an adjacent delivery room. Unfortunately, efforts to sustain the analgesia service were hampered by prolonged staff shortages and attrition.

A study from Turkey utilized bupivacaine 2.5 mg alone or in combination with fentanyl 15 or 25 μg in 105 patients.[90] The overall duration of analgesia was difficult to ascertain from the report; however, 21% of parturients in the bupivacaine-alone group required intravenous opioid supplementation compared with 9% in the fentanyl 15 μg group and 11% in the fentanyl 25 μg group. Pruritus was the most commonly reported side effect in all groups (9% to 11%) and Apgar scores were similar.

Several studies have compared single-shot spinal labor analgesia to an intermittent-bolus epidural technique. In a study of 80 multiparous women in Egypt, parturients were allocated to receive intrathecal hyperbaric bupivacaine 3.75 mg with fentanyl 25 μg or epidural bupivacaine 0.125% with 50 μg fentanyl (8 to 10 mL).[93] The block onset was slower (9 versus 5 minutes) in the epidural group but the mean (± SD) duration was longer (163 ± 17 versus 120 ± 3 minutes). Breakthrough pain in 25% of patients in the spinal group was treated with intravenous ketamine and perineal local infiltration, while in the epidural analgesia group it was treated with epidural top-up doses of bupivacaine 0.125% (30% of parturients in the epidural group). The spinal group had a shorter duration of labor, but pain scores, side effects, and satisfaction were similar between groups. The authors concluded that single-dose spinal analgesia is an effective alternative to epidural analgesia.

In an Iranian study, women were randomized to receive intrathecal bupivacaine 2.5 mg with fentanyl 50 μg or epidural bupivacaine 0.125% with fentanyl 50 μg (16 mL).[95] Breakthrough pain was treated with intramuscular meperidine in the spinal group and an epidural top-up dose in the epidural group. Initial pain scores were lower, and satisfaction was higher in the spinal group, although 13% of women in the spinal group reported pruritus. The authors found a longer mean (± SD) duration of analgesia in the spinal group (225 ± 19 versus 159 ± 37 minutes) and fewer women in the spinal group required supplemental analgesia (4% versus 28%). Labor duration and mode of delivery were similar. The authors recommended single-dose spinal analgesia as a simple and fast technique with high maternal satisfaction.

The addition of **spinal morphine** has been shown to extend the duration of spinal bupivacaine-fentanyl analgesia when used in laboring women in LMICs. In Kenya, the duration of analgesia was approximately 2 hours in women who received spinal bupivacaine-fentanyl compared with nearly 3 hours in women who received bupivacaine-fentanyl with intrathecal morphine.[86] The incidence of breakthrough pain was lower and satisfaction was greater in the women who received morphine. The incidence of adverse effects was higher in the women who received morphine, although the absolute incidence was low

---

* The Institute of Safe Medicine Practices (ISMP) has recommended that healthcare providers never use μg as an abbreviation for micrograms, but rather they should use mcg (https://www.ismp.org/sites/default/files/attachments/2017-11/Error%20Prone%20Abbreviations%202015.pdf, Accessed 11 August 2024). The use of the symbol μg is frequently misinterpreted and involved in harmful medication errors. The abbreviation may be mistaken for mg (milligrams), which would result in a 1000-fold overdose. The symbol μg should never be used when communicating medical information, including pharmacy and prescriber computer order entry screens, computer-generated labels, labels for drug storage bins, and medication administration records. However, most scholarly publications have continued to use the abbreviation μg. The editors have chosen to retain the use of the abbreviation μg throughout this text. However, the editors recommend the use of the abbreviation mcg in clinical practice.

(nausea [8% versus 4%], pruritus [15% versus 6%], shivering [6% versus 2%], hypotension [10% versus 4%]).

In another study from Ghana, spinal bupivacaine 2.5 mg, fentanyl 25 μg, and morphine 200 μg were administered to 332 patients; 28 (8%) required a second dose.[89] The primary outcome was ability to ambulate; no motor impairment was observed in 88% of parturients, and mild weakness occurred in 12%, allowing most women to walk to the delivery room. Pruritus occurred in 31% of parturients and nausea occurred in 27%; 14.5% of women received naloxone treatment. Fetal bradycardia occurred in 4% of women following the initiation of spinal analgesia.

A study from India compared intrathecal bupivacaine-fentanyl-morphine to the standard institutional systemic analgesia regimens consisting of intravenous and intramuscular pentazocine, diazepam, and tramadol.[92] If the visual analog scale (VAS) (0 to 10) pain score exceeded 5, intravenous ketamine was provided to supplement analgesia. Labor duration, mode of delivery, and Apgar scores were similar, but the pain scores were markedly lower in the spinal analgesia group (Fig. 15.5). The mean (± SD) duration of analgesia in the spinal group was 249 ± 24 minutes, similar to the reported length of labor (245 ± 20 minutes). Only two (5%) patients in the spinal group required rescue analgesia. Ninety-eight percent

TABLE 15.5	Studies in Low- and Middle-Income Countries Utilizing Single-Shot Spinal Labor Analgesia				
Author	**Country**	**n**	**Spinal Agents**		**Outcomes**
Krzysztof KM and Chandra S (2008)[84]	Indonesia	62	Bupivacaine 2.5 mg + morphine 0.25 mg + clonidine 45 μg		VAS pain score, analgesia duration, patient satisfaction, side effects
Fyneface-Ogan S, et al. (2012)[85]	Nigeria	90	Bupivacaine 2.5 mg versus bupivacaine 2.5 mg + fentanyl (dose not stated) versus bupivacaine 2.5 mg + dexmedetomidine 2.5 μg		Sensory and motor block, VPS pain score, analgesia duration, Apgar scores, umbilical venous pH, side effects
Tshibuyi PN, et al. (2013)[86]	Kenya	96	Bupivacaine 2.5 mg + fentanyl 25 μg versus bupivacaine 2.5 mg + fentanyl 25 μg + morphine 150 μg		Sensory and motor block, VAS pain score, analgesia duration, Apgar scores, patient satisfaction, side effects
Otokwala JG, et al. (2013)[87]	Nigeria	107	Bupivacaine 2.5 mg versus bupivacaine 2.5 mg + fentanyl 25 μg		Sensory and motor block, NPS pain score, analgesia duration, labor duration, Apgar score, umbilical artery pH
Olufolabi AJ, et al. (2015)[88]	Ghana	46	Bupivacaine 2.5 mg + fentanyl 25 μg or meperidine 10 mg, when available		VPS pain score, motor block, side effects
Anabah T, et al. (2015)[89]	Ghana	332	Bupivacaine 2.5 mg + fentanyl 25 μg + morphine 200 μg		VPS pain score, motor block, side effects
Bilge A, et al. (2017)[90]	Turkey	105	Bupivacaine 2.5 mg versus bupivacaine 2.5 mg + fentanyl 15 μg versus bupivacaine 2.5 mg + fentanyl 25 μg		VAS pain score, analgesia duration, Apgar scores, side effects
Khaled GM and Sabry AI (2020)[91]	Egypt	140	Bupivacaine 2.5 mg + dexamethasone 4 mg alone or combined with fentanyl 25 μg, morphine 100 μg, or dexmedetomidine 5 μg		VAS pain score, analgesia duration, sensory and motor block, Apgar scores, umbilical pH, side effects
Chauhan G, et al. (2020)[92]	India	100	Bupivacaine 2.5 mg + fentanyl 25 μg + morphine 250 μg versus IV/IM standard care		VAS pain score, analgesia duration, motor block, Apgar scores
Awad AA, et al. (2021)[93]	Egypt	80	Spinal bupivacaine 3.75 mg + fentanyl 25 μg versus epidural 0.125% bupivacaine 8–10 mL, fentanyl 50 μg		VAS pain score, sensory block onset time, motor block, analgesia duration, labor duration, patient satisfaction, side effects
Rathod S, et al. (2021)[94]	India	120	Bupivacaine 2.5 mg + fentanyl 25 μg + morphine 250 μg versus bupivacaine 2.5 mg + fentanyl 25 μg + dexmedetomidine 5 μg		Analgesia duration, labor duration, mode of delivery, Apgar scores, patient satisfaction
Rahmati J, et al. (2021)[95]	Iran	128	Spinal bupivacaine 2.5 mg + fentanyl 50 μg versus epidural 0.125% bupivacaine 16 mL + fentanyl 50 μg		VAS pain score, analgesia duration, labor duration, mode of delivery, patient satisfaction

IM, Intramuscular; IV, intravenous; NPS, numeric pain scale; VAS, visual analog scale (0–10 cm); VPS, verbal pain scale (0–10).

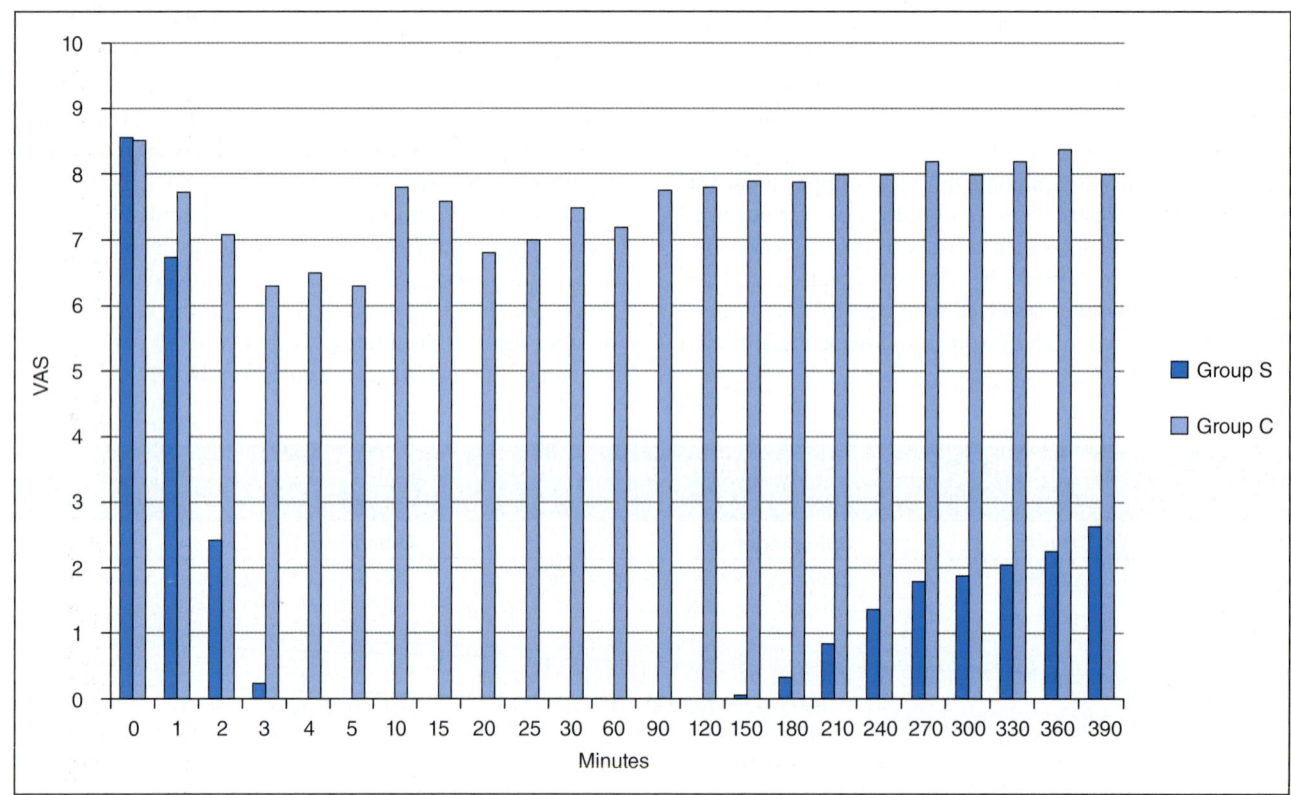

Fig. 15.5 Comparison of visual analog scale (VAS) pain scores (0 to 10) in 50 patients receiving intrathecal bupivacaine-fentanyl-morphine (Group S) and in 50 patients receiving the intravenous-intramuscular institutional standard of care (Group C). From Chauhan G, Samyal P, Pathania AA. Single-dose intrathecal analgesia: a safe and effective method of labor analgesia for parturients in low resource areas. *Ain-Shams J Anesthesiol.* 2020;12:23.

of parturients in the spinal group had a moderate to severe (Grade 2 to 3) motor block within 5 minutes of the intrathecal injection; however, this resolved within 30 minutes.

Other adjuvants, such as **spinal clonidine** and **dexmedetomidine**, have been evaluated.† A study in Indonesia reported a benefit from a combination of intrathecal bupivacaine 2.5 mg, morphine 250 μg, and clonidine 45 μg, although the duration of pain relief was unclear.[84] The mean VAS pain scores were never less than 3, the usual threshold for defining adequate analgesia, but remained less than 4 for at least 4 hours following injection. Adverse effects were reported in fewer than 10% of parturients and approximately 80% of women reported that they were "very satisfied" and would utilize spinal analgesia in the future.

In a Nigerian study, the addition of intrathecal dexmedetomidine 2.5 μg to bupivacaine extended mean (± SD) analgesia duration (defined as regression of S1 dermatome analgesia)

to 269 ± 16 minutes (bupivacaine only, 108 ± 22 minutes; bupivacaine-fentanyl, 123 ± 10 minutes).[85] Additional pain medication for episiotomy repair was required less frequently in the dexmedetomidine group (13%) than in the bupivacaine alone group (43%) and bupivacaine-fentanyl group (27%). Motor block and side effects were minimal.

A study from India prospectively evaluated intrathecal bupivacaine-fentanyl combined with either morphine 250 μg or dexmedetomidine 5 μg.[94] The mean (± SD) duration of analgesia was similar for both groups (morphine, 254 ± 13 minutes; dexmedetomidine, 254 ± 13 minutes). Maternal side effects were not reported; however, Apgar scores were similar. Finally, a study from Egypt randomized 140 multiparous women to receive either intrathecal bupivacaine 2.5 mg combined with dexamethasone 4 mg (control group), or the same drugs combined with either dexmedetomidine 5 μg, fentanyl 25 μg, or morphine 100 μg.[91] The mean (± SD) duration of analgesia was longest with the addition of dexmedetomidine (200 ± 25 minutes), followed by morphine (184 ± 18 minutes) and fentanyl (171 ± 14 minutes) compared to the control group (140 ± 4 minutes). The need for rescue analgesia was 26% in the bupivacaine-dexamethasone control group and 9% in the bupivacaine-dexamethasone-fentanyl group. More nausea, vomiting, and pruritus were reported in women receiving opioids, whereas sedation was associated with dexmedetomidine use. (Editor's note: Spinal

---

† The US Food and Drug Administration (FDA) package insert for Duraclon (epidural clonidine formulation) warns against the use of epidural clonidine in obstetric patients because of the risk of hypotension and bradycardia (see Chapter 24). Clonidine is not approved for spinal use; therefore, spinal administration is off label. Dexmedetomidine is not approved for epidural or spinal administration for any indication by the US FDA, and its use for epidural and spinal analgesia and anesthesia is off label.

dexamethasone has not been rigorously studied and combining multiple medications likely increases the risk of drug error and contamination.)

These studies demonstrate that single-shot spinal labor analgesia is effective and generally well tolerated across numerous LMIC settings. Although the duration of analgesia is prolonged when morphine or dexmedetomidine was combined with bupivacaine and fentanyl, it is unclear whether preservative-free morphine was used. Furthermore, the appropriate safety studies for spinal clonidine and dexmedetomidine must be conducted before the routine spinal use of these medications can be recommended.

EMERGING SOLUTIONS

The increasing global burden of cesarean delivery will require an expanded anesthesia workforce. It is imperative to grow the number of anesthesia providers and to improve the quality of anesthesia training to ensure the provision of safe care. Furthermore, the provision of pain relief is considered a basic human right and represents an index of healthcare quality and compassion. Healthcare professionals and government agencies must work to understand and address the multifactorial barriers that prevent women in LMICs from receiving pain relief when they desire it during labor. Moreover, providing analgesia during labor promotes multidisciplinary patient care. Anesthesia providers bring a unique set of skills to the care of high-risk obstetric patients, both in the labor ward and the operating room, that is well recognized in high-resource countries. Barriers that prevent the broader roles for involvement of anesthesia providers in maternal and neonatal care in LMICs should be addressed. This section highlights emerging solutions to address these challenges.

National Surgery, Obstetric, and Anesthesia Plans
Improving Infrastructure and Workforce

Founded in 1948, the WHO serves as the United Nations' health agency to promote global health and well-being. Each year, delegates from almost 200 member states meet in the **World Health Assembly** to define WHO priorities and policies. In 2015, member state delegates unanimously approved the **World Health Assembly Resolution on Emergency and Essential Surgical Care and Safe Anesthesia** to prioritize access to surgery, obstetric care, and safe anesthesia care.[22] Led by the WHO and the PGSSC within the Harvard Medical School, the NSOAP established a framework for countries to assess their infrastructure, workforce, and barriers to surgical care and safe anesthesia care.[96]

The NSOAP development process is iterative and time consuming and involves many steps because of the complexity and variability of surgical systems across the LMIC landscape. In 2018, the **Surgical Care System Strengthening: Developing National Surgery, Obstetric and Anesthesia Plans** was published as a guide to assist in the process of NSOAP creation.[26] A template for the NSOAP process was published in 2015 (Box 15.1).[26,97] Development of an NSOAP involves eight key steps:

> ### BOX 15.1 National Surgical Plan Components and Framework
>
> Infrastructure Components
> - Surgical facilities
> - Facility readiness
> - Blood product supply
> - Access and referral systems
>
> Workforce Components
> - Surgical, anesthesia, and obstetric providers
> - Allied health providers
>
> Service Delivery Components
> - Surgical volume
> - System coordination
> - Quality and safety
>
> Financing Components
> - Health financing and accounting
> - Budget allocation
>
> Information Management Components
> - Information systems
> - Research agenda

Summarized from Meara JG, Leather AJ, Hagander L, et al. Global Surgery 2030: evidence and solutions for achieving health, welfare, and economic development. *Lancet.* 2015:386:569–624.

(1) ministry support and ownership, (2) situation analysis and baseline assessments, (3) stakeholder engagement and priority setting, (4) drafting and validation, (5) monitoring and evaluation, (6) costing, (7) governance, and (8) implementation. Drafting an NSOAP involves defining the current gaps in care, synthesizing and prioritizing solutions, and providing an implementation and monitoring plan with a projected cost for the six domains of a surgical system: (1) infrastructure, (2) service delivery, (3) workforce, (4) information management, (5) finance, and (6) governance.[96] Progress in NSOAP development was hampered during the COVID-19 pandemic, but NSOAP implementation plans are currently being reinitiated. The recommended indicators are the same indicators recommended by the LCOGS, including access to timely essential surgery, specialist workforce density, surgical volume, perioperative mortality rate (POMR), and protection against impoverishing and catastrophic expenditure.[97] Zambia was the first country in sub-Saharan Africa to complete an NSOAP and other countries have followed, including Ethiopia, Rwanda, Tanzania, and Nigeria.[98–102]

Through the process of NSOAP development, countries are better understanding their anesthesiology workforce limitations and what is needed to meet the goals of timely and safe access to surgery. This information is intimately related to the provision of maternal care during childbirth, especially when a cesarean delivery or surgical treatment of hemorrhage is required. Countries that have completed NSOAPs are making efforts to train anesthesiologists and other nonphysician provider groups; however, it will take decades to increase the provider base to the capacity needed for access to safe surgery.

The NSOAP process has limitations and does not cover all aspects of a highly functional healthcare system; therefore, in the years following the LCOGS, additional metrics have been proposed. Access alone is not an adequate metric as systems begin to expand. Quality metrics are an obvious next step, since access to high-quality surgery, obstetric care, and safe anesthesia care is the ultimate goal.

Quality improvement is a systems process that is vitally important within sophisticated healthcare systems; however, the only clinical metric included in the NSOAP framework was POMR. Mortality reduction is vital, but the need for quality in surgery, obstetric care, and anesthesia care goes well beyond mortality. In 2018, the WHO produced a list of 100 Important Health Indicators, which included POMR and other important quality metrics such as the surgical site infection (SSI) and the MMR.[103] Kruk et al.[104] summarized the importance of quality programs in LMICs to improve surgical, obstetric, and anesthesia care.[104]

Education and Training

Until the provider base expands, efforts are underway to provide further training and credentialing to those providers who are "trained on the job" to perform anesthesia care as a subset of their current responsibilities. When anesthesia providers function without adequate training or access to safety monitoring, usually under the direction of a surgeon, higher-than-expected perioperative mortality in otherwise healthy young patients and children ensues.[105] Thus, there is a tremendous need to accelerate training of both physician and NPAPs in LMICs to increase the number of providers and to improve the quality of anesthesia care (Fig. 15.6).

A high degree of variation exists in the duration and quality of anesthesia training worldwide, including variation in curricula, limited exposure to subspecialty content, and lack of continuing educational opportunities. In Africa, most of the anesthesia care is provided by NPAPs comprised of nurse anesthetists or anesthesia technicians with 6 months to 3 years of training following high school or nursing school.[106] A 2016 to 2018 survey of anesthesia provider training and practice in Africa[107] revealed the degree of variation in NPAP training despite similar scope of practice. The authors suggested that this may be attributed to varied needs and resources in different settings, or a lack of consensus on training requirements (Table 15.6).

Training of both anesthesiologists and NPAPs is critically important to the future of global safe surgery. Ultimately, NSOAPs should address educational standardization and credentialing. However, the development of new anesthesia training programs is a significant undertaking requiring strong local leadership; international collaboration and funding support may benefit these programs.[108–110]

Anesthesiology Training Support Through International Societies

The WHO supports anesthesiology training through guidance to ministries of health and through partnerships with organizations that support the WHO vision. For example, the

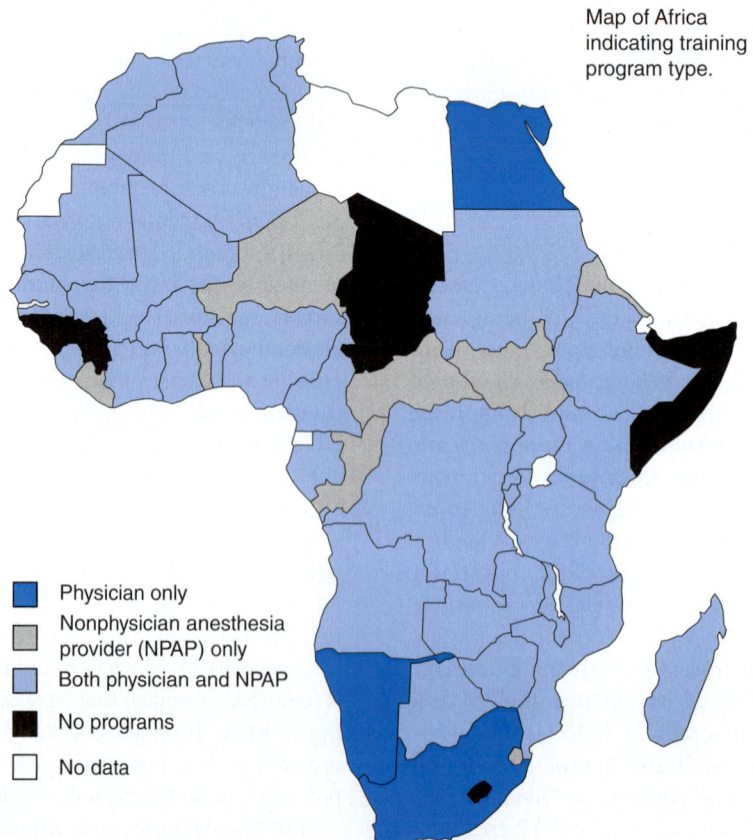

Map of Africa indicating training program type.

- ■ (blue) Physician only
- ■ (gray) Nonphysician anesthesia provider (NPAP) only
- ■ (light blue) Both physician and NPAP
- ■ (black) No programs
- □ (white) No data

Fig. 15.6 Map of Anesthesia Training Programs in Africa. The survey was conducted in 2016–17. *NPAP,* Nonphysician anesthesia provider. From Law TJ, Bulamba F, Ochieng JP, et al. Anesthesia provider training and practice models: a survey of Africa. *Anesth Analg.* 2019;129:839–846.

TABLE 15.6 Nonphysician Anesthesia Provider Training Programs in Africa, 2016–17

Questions[a]	
Is there a standardized examination?	33%
Is there a national professional society?	81%
Is there a practice guideline setting body?	33%
Does the program depend on foreign faculty?	28%
Program Characteristics[a]	
The majority of the curriculum is taught by physicians	48%
The majority of clinical supervision is done by physicians	23%
Teaching Modalities[b]	
Lectures in classroom	100%
In-theater supervision/instruction	100%
Workplace assessments	68%
Skills workshops in a classroom	55%
Simulation scenarios on mannequins	41%
Online materials	16%
Subspecialty Teaching[a]	
Obstetric anesthesia	100%
Pediatric anesthesia	95%
Regional anesthesia	83%
Trauma management	78%
Critical care	77%
Neuroanesthesia	66%

The data are from 70 respondents from 51 African countries surveyed 2016–17.
[a]Percent "yes" responses.
[b]Percent of respondents using the teaching modality.
Modified from Law TJ, Bulamba F, Ochieng JP, et al. Anesthesia provider training and practice models: a survey of Africa. *Anesth Analg.* 2019;129:839–846.

WHO partnered with PGSSC to create the NSOAP template and with the WFSA to endorse the 2018 Guidelines for Safe Anesthesia.[111] These guidelines provide direction to anesthesia professionals, their professional societies, and governments for improving and maintaining the quality and safety of anesthesia care. Work is being done by the WFSA, the ASA, and the Canadian Anesthesiologists' Society International Education Foundation to support anesthesiologist professional development. For example, the WFSA has initiated a subspecialty fellowship program[112] to support anesthesiologists from LMICs by providing financial assistance to successful applicants. Fellowships are either available or under development for pediatric, intensive care, regional, cardiac, neurosurgery, pain, and obstetric anesthesia subspecialties.[112] The ASA's Global Humanitarian Outreach Committee, previously called the OTP, has been supplementing local education for physician and nonphysician providers in sub-Saharan Africa since 1991. The program has served Zaire (prior to its transition to the Democratic Republic of Congo), Ghana, Tanzania, and Rwanda.

The College of Anaesthesiologists for East, Central, and Southern Africa, established in 2014, aims to provide structure in physician anesthesiology residency training in 10 sub-Saharan countries (Burundi, Ethiopia, Kenya, Malawi, Mozambique, Rwanda, Tanzania, Uganda, Zambia, and Zimbabwe). However, it faces real challenges because of too few specialist physician anesthesia members, thus restricting review and implementation of educational curricula in members' respective countries.[109]

The International Federation of Nurse Anesthetists (IFNA)[113] has numerous resources to guide nurse anesthesia program development. The IFNA has established a model curriculum for an 18- to 24-month certificate (nondegree) program, as well as a system for program recognition and accreditation. In addition, the IFNA website[113] contains a wealth of teaching material, practice standards, and guidelines available for download.

Obstetric Anesthesia Education and Training

Multiple levels of interventions are underway to help bridge the educational gap in obstetric anesthesia knowledge and skills in LMICs, although resources and research are still required to translate and promulgate best practices.[106] Some countries have developed short courses for nonanesthesiology physician providers. In India, a country contributing to nearly 20% of the global maternal mortality burden, a Life Saving Anesthetic Skills program was initiated to train medical officers not specialized in anesthesiology. The 18-week certification course teaches trainees how to perform spinal or general anesthesia for cesarean delivery in healthy parturients.[114] The program, which began in 2003, has been widely implemented across India. In South Africa, an Essential Steps in the Management of Obstetric Emergencies (ESMOE) course has been promoted for new medical officers. The course consists of 13 modules, one of which addresses obstetric anesthesia, as well as a hybrid learning model of *outreach*, whereby an anesthesiologist from a regional hospital visits a district hospital on a monthly basis for hands-on teaching, and *in-reach*, bringing general practitioners from district hospitals to referral hospitals for limited periods for exposure to high-acuity levels of care.[115] Careful evaluation and monitoring of such programs is important because inadequate training can lead to increased mortality, thus defeating the primary purpose.[116]

A well-established, short subspecialty course, Safer Anaesthesia from Education–Obstetrics (SAFE-OB), is a 3-day offering developed in 2010 by the Association of Anaesthetists of Great Britain and Ireland in conjunction with the WFSA. Following the first course in Uganda in 2011, SAFE-OB has been introduced in 47 countries to nearly 1200 trainers and 4000 anesthesia providers (as of January 2023).[117] SAFE-OB targets both physician and NPAPs with content relevant to maternal and neonatal morbidity and mortality (Box 15.2).[106,108] The training methodology involves didactic

> ### BOX 15.2   Key Educational Components of the Safer Anaesthesia From Education–Obstetrics (SAFE-OB) Course
>
> Preoperative preparation
> Airway management
> Obstetric general anesthesia
> Spinal anesthesia and complications
> Pregnancy physiology and critical care
> Maternal and newborn resuscitation
> Preeclampsia and eclampsia
> Obstetric hemorrhage
> Teamwork and communication
> WHO Surgical Safety Checklist

WHO, World Health Organization.
Summarized from Evans FM, Duarte JC, Haylock C, Morriss W. Are short subspecialty courses the education answer?. *Anesth Analg.* 2018;126:1305–1311; and Livingston P, Evans F, Nsereko E, et al. Safer obstetric anesthesia through education and mentorship: a model for knowledge translation in Rwanda. *Can J Anaesth.* 2014;61:1028–1039.

lectures, small-group discussions, skills stations, simulation, and self-reflection, adaptable to the local environment. Participants complete pre- and postcourse knowledge and structured skills-based assessments. Following training, participants are encouraged to utilize peer support and case-based journaling to contemplate care improvements. Another goal is to identify and equip local anesthesia providers who are capable of training others within their institutions, thus promoting local ownership and expanding the program's reach.

Several reports summarize outcomes following the introduction of SAFE-OB training outcomes in Africa. In Rwanda, course contents were contextualized before, during, and following training using knowledge-to-action cycles to promote knowledge uptake into clinical practice.[108] The evaluation of participant-maintained log books and semistructured interviews conducted 6 months following training suggested that there were improvements in preoperative assessment, preparation for anesthesia, systematic management of emergencies, use of left uterine displacement, and confidence in speaking up on the patient's behalf. In the Democratic Republic of Congo and Madagascar, participation in the SAFE-OB course resulted in knowledge and skill improvements, as well as self-reported changes in individual practice and organizational culture that were sustained over 12 to 18 months.[118] Perceived barriers to implementation included resistance from untrained peers, lack of senior clinical and administrative support, and resource limitations.

Similar results were reported in Ethiopia, utilizing a parallel study design, whereby trainees maintained knowledge and skills, and reported improved self-confidence and better communication within surgical teams when reassessed and interviewed 3 to 11 months following SAFE-OB training.[119] The study authors highlighted the limitations of interview-based reporting, including the possibility of biased participant

responses due to the desire to please the interviewer or fear of consequences. Direct observations of clinical care practices of the participants and team members would better ensure validity of the findings.[119]

In Kenya, the standard training format was enhanced by facility-based site visits 3 to 6 months following training to conduct semistructured interviews and to observe clinical practice.[120] Observations of clinical care were completed for 84 of 103 participants (81%). From 253 behaviors recorded, 145 (57%) were positive, which included preoperative preparation, sterile technique for spinal anesthesia, teamwork, communication, and advocacy. The most frequently occurring negative behaviors included failure to perform the WHO surgical safety checklist, failure to check the sensory level of spinal anesthesia, inadequate patient monitoring, and unsafe handling of blood products. These gaps identified areas where additional mentoring and reinforcement are needed. The authors conceded that baseline observations and additional research are required to attribute positive findings to the training.

Nongovernmental Organizations Supporting Obstetric Anesthesia Development

Health Volunteers Overseas

Health Volunteers Overseas (HVO)[121] is a US-based NGO founded in 1986 that aims to improve the quality and availability of healthcare in LMICs through teaching, training, and professional mentorship of the local health workforce. HVO deploys a short-term, highly skilled volunteer model to achieve its mission. HVO has sites specific for anesthesia education across Asia and Africa.

Médecins Sans Frontières

MSF (also known as Doctors Without Borders)[122] is an international organization that addresses surgical, medical, and obstetric care in LMICs, including those impacted by armed conflict, epidemics, natural disasters, and in locations otherwise devoid of healthcare resources. Surgeons, obstetricians, anesthesiologists, and nurse anesthetists are recruited as part of surgical teams that operate with standardized protocols, including essential equipment and medications. MSF provides patient care as well as training of local workers to build capacity and sustainability. Keeping the delivery of anesthesia care simple in low-resource settings is essential to facilitate efficacy, safety, and sustainability of its surgical missions. MSF won the Nobel Peace Prize in 1999 as a testament to the organization's commitment to addressing healthcare challenges within communities in crisis.

Kybele, Inc.

Kybele, Inc.[123] is an NGO founded in 2001 to promote safe childbirth worldwide through innovative healthcare partnerships. Kybele works with government and/or local hospital leaders to develop country-specific programs designed to improve national healthcare standards. Challenges and solutions are jointly identified at the local level in countries with sufficient infrastructure to sustain progress after training. Kybele typically conducts 1- to 2-week onsite training programs at regular intervals in a host country over several years. This builds relationships and trust with local hosts and encourages long-term progress and sustainability. It is vitally important to observe medical practices within host hospitals across the continuum of care to better understand gaps that may exist between theoretical knowledge, clinical practice, and standardized care processes.

Kybele strives to recruit practitioners across nationalities and disciplines. By 2024, over 388 healthcare providers representing 113 institutions have served as faculty. Gaining perspectives from multinational volunteers stimulate the vetting of diverse approaches and viewpoints that enhance creative solutions to healthcare challenges. Volunteer teams are comprised of obstetric anesthesiologists, obstetricians, neonatologists, nurses, midwives, and implementation scientists, among others. These faculty have collectively made over 1113 onsite visits; 42% have returned at least once. Training programs have focused on spinal, epidural, and general anesthesia; obstetric ultrasonography; neonatal resuscitation; laparoscopic surgery techniques; and postoperative pain management. Kybele reinforces these skills with operational capacity building such as leadership development, quality improvement, clinical guideline development, advocacy, monitoring, and evaluation.

Academic Partnerships

Academic partnerships in global health have offered bilateral opportunities for academic institutions in HICs and their counterparts in LMICs for many years. Academic partnerships specific to anesthesia and surgery collaboration in LMICs have been consistently expanding, particularly since 2015, with formal relationships providing education and training, including distance learning and research support. Within the United States alone, the number of academic programs supporting global surgery and anesthesia development has steadily increased, and interest among faculty, residents, fellows, and students continues to grow.

The literature tracking global health partnerships suggests that little is known about the effectiveness and sustainability of these partnerships.[124] As such, there is the need to establish guiding principles for global health engagements and partnerships, so that partnerships are equitable and mutually beneficial.[125] There is concern that some HIC global health enterprises may cause more harm than good by undermining local health systems, operating without appropriate licenses, capitalizing on research opportunities, and promoting the "global health experience" for the benefit of the HIC.[125] To this end, the Advocacy for Global Health Partnerships was established as a multisectoral coalition to lay out principles to guide ethical global health practices, referred to as the **Brocher Declaration** (Box 15.3).[125] Documenting the impact of appropriately balanced, long-term partnerships on increasing the number of trained anesthesia providers and improving patient safety and outcomes in LMICs are important to facilitate understanding the value of such

---

BOX 15.3   Six Principles of the Brocher Declaration

Mutual partnership with bidirectional input and learning
- Emphasize mutual partnership and bidirectionality—both parties have input and learn from one another.
- Recognize expertise and experience of host country health professionals.
- Establish equality, trust, and partnership as the foundations of all activities.

Empowered host country and community to define needs and activities
- Create programs based on the host country and community's priorities.
- Define activities so that external actors do not divert funds and efforts from real needs of the community.
- Align with national planning frameworks and WHO/SDG priorities.

Sustainable programs and capacity building
- Commit to long-term healthcare development and sustainability.
- Aim to strengthen health systems rather than providing unsustainable alternatives.
- Emphasize and utilize existing health systems.

Compliance with applicable laws, ethical standards, and code of conduct
- Comply with existing legal and regulatory frameworks in the host and originating countries and with local regulations for professional practice and drug distribution.
- Consider ethical principles including social justice, social contract, and utilitarian principles.
- Abide by common quality principles.

Humility, cultural sensitivity, and respect for all involved
- Respect the culture, history, strengths, expertise, and knowledge of host communities.
- Recognize the limitations of visitors' cursory understanding as nonmembers of the community and that they are subject to the constraints and biases of their own cultural backgrounds.
- Transform the current narrative of privileged volunteers gaining social capital with lower regard for the perspectives of the host communities to one of solidarity and respect.

Accountability for actions
- Evaluate programs appropriately so that negative outcomes and unintended consequences are reduced.
- Place special emphasis on the concerns of environmental impact due to the travel and activities involved.
- Ensure accountability to local authorities.

SDG, Sustainable Development Goals; *WHO,* World Health Organization.
From Prasad S, Aldrink M, Compton B, et al. Global health partnerships and the Brocher Declaration: principles for ethical short-term engagements in global health. *Ann Glob Health.* 2022;88:31.

---

partnerships. Since the need to support education, training, and research development in LMICs is so great, it is difficult to imagine that capacity can be built without external support, but ethical considerations must guide the engagement.

Improving Quality

Guidelines, Checklists, and Protocols

Practice guidelines are systematically assembled recommendations to guide clinicians in providing safe patient care based on the highest level of evidence and research findings. The guidelines are constructed through literature analysis and by expert opinion, and are modified as knowledge, technology, and practices evolve. Practice guidelines developed by and for HICs are common, but these should not be applied in LMIC settings without significant modification. Optimally, local practitioners in LMICs should lead their own guideline adaptation or development, considering the local culture, clinical needs, and available resources.[61] Practice guidelines specific to obstetric anesthesia are generally lacking in LMICs; however, anesthesiologists in several countries have recently completed national guideline development with partnership support.[31,61] In addition, three recent international consensus guidelines have been published with specific recommendations for variable resource countries for treatment of spinal hypotension,[126] use of uterotonic agents,[127] and management of intraoperative breakthrough pain during cesarean delivery with neuraxial anesthesia.[128]

The use of checklists has been shown to decrease complications and improve patient outcomes across diverse populations.[129–132] The most rigorously investigated checklist, the WHO Surgical Safety Checklist[133] (Fig. 15.7), has been implemented globally since 2009. It has been adapted for use in both HICs and LMICs and promoted by organizations invested in patient safety, including Lifebox and the WFSA. The WHO also has a childbirth checklist[134]; use of the checklist in LMICs is likely to improve patient safety both on the labor ward and in the operating room for cesarean delivery. For example, in East Africa, a context-relevant Safe Anesthesia Cesarean Delivery Checklist was developed and tested with the goal of improving adherence to best practice guidelines in the management of both elective and emergent cesarean delivery in sub-Saharan Africa.[135] Systematic observations of care revealed that essential safety steps were often skipped during emergencies involving hemorrhage, preeclampsia, and fetal compromise. Use of the cesarean delivery checklist during simulation exercises of peripartum hemorrhage and preeclampsia showed significant improvements in the completed steps.[135]

In addition to guidelines and checklists, most clinical protocols relevant to obstetric anesthesia have evolved from research conducted in high-resource settings. While pharmacologic and physiologic effects are similar across settings, protocol adaptations should be tested and validated in the clinical environments within which they will be used.[136] An example is the use of prophylactic vasopressors to prevent hypotension

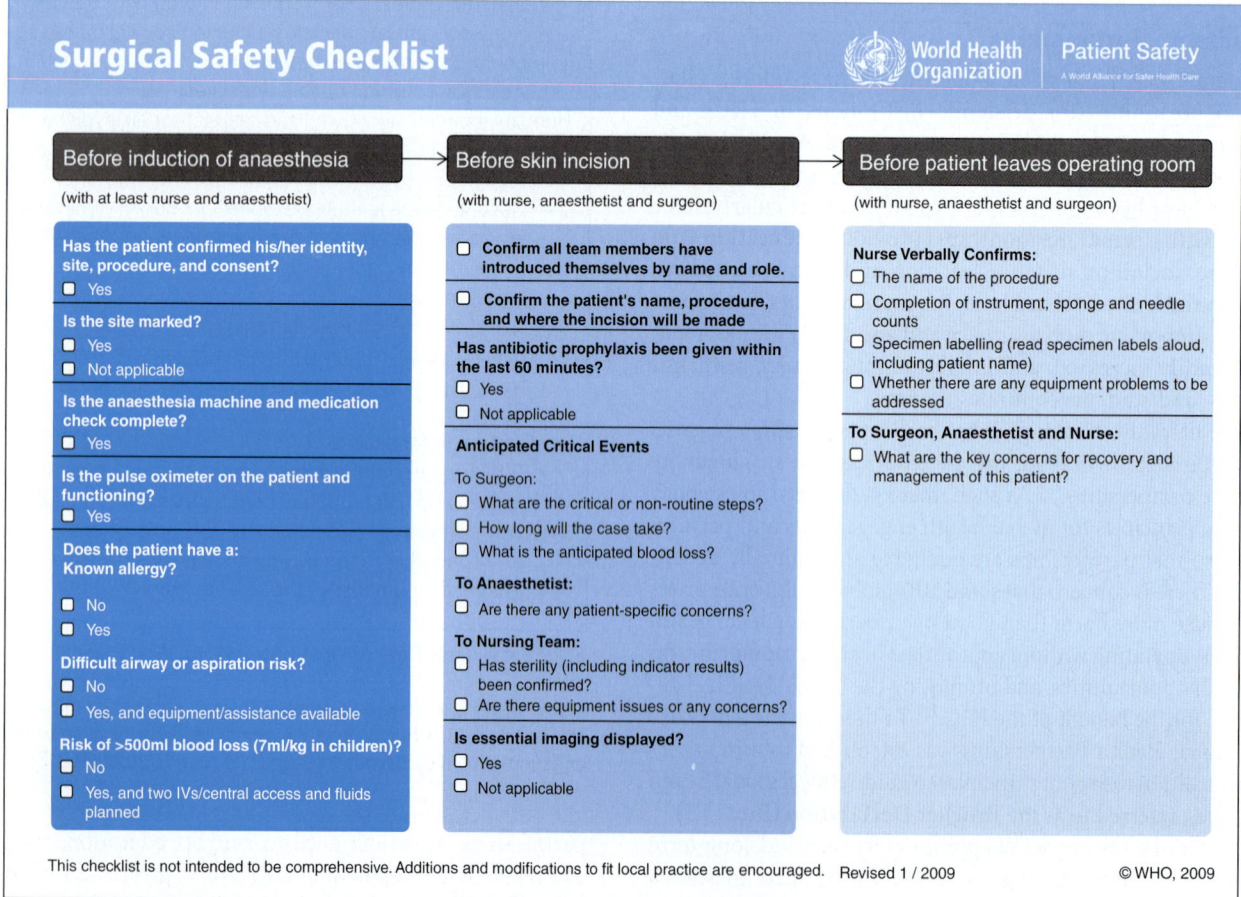

Fig. 15.7 World Health Organization Surgical Safety Checklist, Revised in 2009. Available from World Health Organization. WHO Surgical Safety Checklist. https://www.who.int/teams/integrated-health-services/patient-safety/research/safe-surgery/tool-and-resources. Accessed 14 December 2024.

after the initiation of spinal anesthesia. Historically, vasopressors were administered to treat hypotension once it occurred; however, newer consensus guidelines recommend the administration of prophylactic vasopressors (e.g., phenylephrine) (see Chapter 26).[126] Few low-resource countries use prophylactic phenylephrine infusions due to provider inexperience and/or infusion pump unavailability, yet in these settings, spinal hypotension may have the greatest negative impact.[137,138] However, meaningful guideline adaptations are being developed. In a 2017 study from South Africa,[137] women scheduled for cesarean delivery with spinal anesthesia were randomized to receive standard boluses of phenylephrine 50 to 100 µg or ephedrine 5 to 10 mg for the treatment of hypotension (n = 253), or a fixed rate, low-dose phenylephrine infusion 25 µg/min (n = 253) with vasopressor bolus treatment as needed. Hypotension was significantly less common in the prophylactic phenylephrine infusion group (47% versus 62%, $P = .001$). The authors concluded that given the inexperience of junior anesthetists in titrating infusions, a fixed, low-rate infusion of phenylephrine, supplemented with rescue bolus doses, allowed current treatment recommendations to be adapted for safety and simplicity in a low-resource setting.

In a prospective observational study at the same institution (n = 300),[139] the effectiveness and safety of administering a prophylactic phenylephrine infusion without an infusion pump were tested. Spinal anesthesia–induced hypotension was managed with one of two alternating protocols. The treatment group received an infusion of phenylephrine prepared by adding 500 µg to 1 L of crystalloid solution and administered by gravity flow through an 18-gauge intravenous cannula over 10 to 20 minutes (approximating a phenylephrine infusion at 25 to 50 µg/min). Women in the control group received the crystalloid solution without phenylephrine. In both groups, hypotension was treated with a bolus dose of phenylephrine, as needed. The incidence of hypotension was less in the phenylephrine group than in the control group (37% versus 51%, $P = .001$). There were four instances of bradycardia in each group (without the need for treatment with atropine) and six instances of systolic hypertension (>20% of baseline) in the phenylephrine group; the infusion was temporarily stopped per protocol, without further adverse sequelae. These studies have shown that equipment-dependent protocols developed in HICs can be modified into simple, pragmatic guidelines for use in low-resource environments.

Adaptations have also been made in the use of local anesthetic solutions for neuraxial anesthesia for cesarean delivery. For example, in North America, 0.75% hyperbaric bupivacaine with preservative-free morphine is often utilized to provide spinal anesthesia for cesarean delivery (see Chapter 26). Throughout Europe and Africa, 0.5% hyperbaric bupivacaine is the formulation most widely available. The South African ESMOE guidelines recommend the use of 9 mg (1.8 mL) 0.5% hyperbaric bupivacaine with fentanyl 10 µg (0.2 mL) for routine neuraxial anesthesia for cesarean delivery.[46] Furthermore, traditional steps for rapid-sequence induction of general anesthesia may need to be modified in low-resource settings, given the limited availability of video laryngoscopy.[115] These steps include apneic insufflation by face mask before tracheal intubation, low-pressure mask ventilation during induction if there is a risk of hypoxemia or difficult intubation, and early use of supraglottic airway devices for failed intubation. Although challenges exist in verifying outcome improvements after the introduction of protocols and recommendations in low-resource settings, in locations where morbidity and mortality rates are high, even minor improvements in anesthesia care standards can have substantial impact.

Quality Improvement and Implementation Science

Evidence suggests that guideline development, policy reform, and training interventions *alone* are insufficient to achieve sustainable best practices for mortality reduction. Focused training interventions are often narrowly focused and target specific knowledge and skills gaps, but do not address broader operational and leadership challenges that plague resource-restricted health systems. It has become increasingly clear that deaths in LMICs are now more likely to result from poor quality care than from poor access to care.[104]

In Tanzania, for example, in-service training was conducted for the management of postpartum hemorrhage. However, healthcare workers reported low facility readiness to provide appropriate care, despite the training.[140] They described deficiencies in essential supplies, blood product availability, communication, and leadership that impaired patient management and timely referrals. Rowe et al.[141] compared the effectiveness of various training strategies used to improve healthcare provider performance in LMICs in a systematic review of 337 studies. They found that standalone training was less effective than training combined with other interventions, such as infrastructure support, mentoring supervision, or group-based, quality improvement activities. In Ghana, a continuous quality improvement approach was used in addition to training and mentoring to strengthen capacity at a high-volume referral hospital.[142] Ninety-seven improvement activities were designed to enhance personnel, systems management, and communication across disciplines. After 5 years, 68% of the interventions were implemented. Maternal mortality decreased by 22.4%, despite a 50% increase in deliveries, lending support to an approach that incorporates a comprehensive strengthening systems and quality improvement.

In 2019, the WHO Global Ministerial Patient Safety Summit urged the use of *implementation science* principles to strengthen global patient safety efforts.[143] Implementation science can help determine what works, how it works, and how to best support and integrate the scale-up of healthcare interventions at regional and national levels. In 2022, White et al.[144] reviewed 45,128 articles from 47 LMICs to assess which implementation strategies were utilized in perioperative quality improvement interventions. They found that while many studies reported on the implementation of quality improvement initiatives in single centers, only 31 studies reported scaling-up strategies to multiple sites. The most implemented scale-up intervention was the WHO Surgical Safety Checklist, followed by SSI prevention. Three studies reported on neuraxial analgesia access and safety.[31,59,61] The studies were individually analyzed and compared to well-known implementation frameworks to look for similarities in approach and effectiveness. All studies utilized most components of the Yamey[145] and Barker[146] implementation frameworks, yet neither framework was directly referenced. This suggests that while many aspects of implementation may be intuitive to clinicians, the frameworks themselves are less well known. Because the literature on scale-up interventions in LMICs is sparse, White et al.[144] recommended a wider use of theoretical frameworks to guide the implementation process in consideration of which organizational and behavioral factors may help or hinder success of a scale-up effort, both in high- or low-resource settings. Additionally, for widespread implementation of clinician-driven quality improvement efforts, a larger multidisciplinary team should include implementation scientists with expertise in change management, quality improvement, behavior, and organizational change.[144] Failure to adequately implement improvement solutions within healthcare systems will mean that quality care will be unobtainable to those most in need.

KEY POINTS

- The care of mothers and newborns in low- and middle-income countries (LMICs) remains challenging due to many barriers, especially the lack of access to safe surgery and anesthesia.
- The National Surgery, Obstetric and Anesthesia Plans process holds promise for LMICs and may guide local implementation of steps to improve the access to surgical, obstetric, and anesthesia care.
- A practical commitment to the national anesthesia workforce is essential to the future of obstetric care and patient safety in LMICs.
- Labor analgesia in LMICs is not yet prioritized because of limitations in the workforce, essential medicines, and supplies.
- In most situations, neuraxial anesthesia (usually spinal) is preferred for a cesarean delivery; the safe conduct of neuraxial anesthesia should be reinforced in LMICs.

- Commitment to safe anesthesia and surgical access is required by ministries of health and local health systems; national medical schools must support anesthesia training and local hospitals must commit to anesthesiology residency training.
- An improvement in infrastructure, inclusive of supplies, equipment, safety monitors, and essential medicines, is required for safe obstetric anesthesia care.
- Even with increased commitment to anesthesia, obstetric, and surgical care in LMICs, the growth of quality healthcare will be slow and challenging.
- Quality initiatives are important to local and national evaluation of existing and new programs in LMICs.
- Implementation science methodology should be utilized to scale up key interventions to improve evidence-based maternal and newborn care in LMICs.

REFERENCES

1. Engmann CM, Khan S, Moyer CA, et al. Transformative innovations in reproductive, maternal, newborn, and child health over the next 20 years. *PLoS Med.* 2016;13:e1001969.
2. United Nations. The Millennium Development Goals Report; 2015. https://www.un.org/millenniumgoals/2015_MDG_Report/pdf/MDG%202015%20rev%20(July%201).pdf. Accessed 29 November 2024.
3. World Health Organization. Trends in maternal mortality 2000 to 2020: Estimates by WHO, UNICEF, UNFPA, World Bank Group and UNDESA/Population Division; 2023. https://iris.who.int/bitstream/handle/10665/366225/9789240068759-eng.pdf?sequence=1. Accessed 2 December 2024.
4. Truche P, Shoman H, Reddy CL, et al. Globalization of national surgical, obstetric and anesthesia plans: the critical link between health policy and action in global surgery. *Glob Health.* 2020;16:1.
5. Hamadeh N, Van Rompaey C, Metreau E, Eapen SG. *New World Bank Country Classification by Income Level: 2022-2023.* World Bank Blogs; 2022. https://blogs.worldbank.org/en/opendata/new-world-bank-country-classifications-income-level-2022-2023. Accessed 14 December 2024.
6. World Bank. World Bank income groups, 2023; 2024. https://ourworldindata.org/grapher/world-bank-income-groups. Accessed 14 December 2024.
7. Institute for Health Metrics and Evaluation. Global burden of disease. https://www.healthdata.org/research-analysis/gbd. Accessed 2 December 2024.
8. Debas HT, Donkor P, Gawande A, et al. Essential Surgery: Disease Control Priorities, vol. 1. 3rd ed. The World Bank; 2015. https://hdl.handle.net/10986/21568. Accessed 2 December 2024.
9. Dubowitz G, Detlefs S, McQueen KA. Global anesthesia workforce crisis: a preliminary survey revealing shortages contributing to undesirable outcomes and unsafe practices. *World J Surg.* 2010;34:438–444.
10. Kempthorne P, Morriss WW, Mellin-Olsen J, Gore-Booth J. The WFSA Global Anesthesia Workforce Survey. *Anesth Analg.* 2017;125:981–990.
11. Meara JG, Leather AJ, Hagander L, et al. Global Surgery 2030:evidence and solutions for achieving health, welfare, and economic development. *Lancet.* 2015;386: 569–624.
12. Farmer PE, Kim JY. Surgery and global health: a view from beyond the OR. *World J Surg.* 2008;32:533–536.

13. Knowlton LM, Chackungal S, Dahn B, et al. Liberian surgical and anesthesia infrastructure: a survey of county hospitals. *World J Surg.* 2013;37:721–729.
14. Kushner AL, Cherian MN, Noel L, et al. Addressing the Millennium Development Goals from a surgical perspective: essential surgery and anesthesia in 8 low- and middle-income countries. *Arch Surg.* 2010;145:154–159.
15. Notrica MR, Evans FM, Knowlton LM, McQueen KA. Rwandan surgical and anesthesia infrastructure: a survey of district hospitals. *World J Surg.* 2011;35:1770–1780.
16. Ologunde R, Maruthappu M, Shanmugarajah K, Shalhoub J. Surgical care in low and middle-income countries: burden and barriers. *Int J Surg.* 2014;12:858–863.
17. Solis C, Leon P, Sanchez N, et al. Nicaraguan surgical and anesthesia infrastructure: survey of Ministry of Health hospitals. *World J Surg.* 2013;37:2109–2121.
18. Vansell HJ, Schlesinger JJ, Harvey A, et al. Anaesthesia, surgery, obstetrics, and emergency care in Guyana. *J Epidemiol Glob Health.* 2015;5:75–83.
19. Kyei-Nimakoh M, Carolan-Olah M, McCann TV. Access barriers to obstetric care at health facilities in sub-Saharan Africa—a systematic review. *Syst Rev.* 2017;6:110.
20. Ologunde R, Vogel JP, Cherian MN, et al. Assessment of cesarean delivery availability in 26 low- and middle-income countries: a cross-sectional study. *Am J Obstet Gynecol.* 2014;211:504.e1–e12.
21. Law TJ, Lipnick MS, Morriss W, et al. The Global Anesthesia Workforce Survey: updates and trends in the anesthesia workforce. *Anesth Analg.* 2024;139:15–24.
22. World Health Organization 68th World Health Assembly. WHA68.15: Strengthening emergency and essential surgical care and anaesthesia as a component of universal health coverage; 2015. https://apps.who.int/gb/ebwha/pdf_files/wha68/a68_r15-en.pdf. Accessed 2 December 2024.
23. Dawson AJ, Buchan J, Duffield C, et al. Task shifting and sharing in maternal and reproductive health in low-income countries: a narrative synthesis of current evidence. *Health Policy Plan.* 2014;29:396–408.
24. Epiu I, Tindimwebwa JV, Mijumbi C, et al. Challenges of anesthesia in low- and middle-income countries: a cross-sectional survey of access to safe obstetric anesthesia in East Africa. *Anesth Analg.* 2017;124:290–299.
25. World Health Organization. World Health Organization Model List of Essential Medicines—23rd List, 2023; 2023. https://www.who.int/publications/i/item/WHO-MHP-HPS-EML-2023.02. Accessed 7 December 2024.
26. World Health Organization. Surgical care systems strengthening: Developing national surgical, obstetric and anaesthesia plans; 2017. https://iris.who.int/handle/10665/255566. Accessed 14 December 2024.
27. Boerma T, Ronsmans C, Melesse DY, et al. Global epidemiology of use of and disparities in caesarean sections. *Lancet.* 2018;392:1341–1348.
28. Sobhy S, Arroyo-Manzano D, Murugesu N, et al. Maternal and perinatal mortality and complications associated with caesarean section in low-income and middle-income countries: a systematic review and meta-analysis. *Lancet.* 2019;393:1973–1982.
29. Betran AP, Torloni MR, Zhang JJ, et al. WHO statement on caesarean section rates. *BJOG.* 2016;123:667–670.
30. Harrison MS, Goldenberg RL. Cesarean section in sub-Saharan Africa. *Matern Health Neonatol Perinatol.* 2016;2:6.
31. Hu LQ, Flood P, Li Y, et al. No Pain Labor & Delivery: a global health initiative's impact on clinical outcomes in China. *Anesth Analg.* 2016;122:1931–1938.
32. Betran AP, Temmerman M, Kingdon C, et al. Interventions to reduce unnecessary caesarean sections in healthy women and babies. *Lancet.* 2018;392:1358–1368.
33. Zhao P, Cai Z, Huang A, et al. Why is the labor epidural rate low and cesarean delivery rate high? A survey of Chinese perinatal care providers. *PLoS One.* 2021;16:e0251345.
34. Hug I, Chattopadhyay C, Mitra GR, et al. Maternal expectations and birth-related experiences: a survey of pregnant women of mixed parity from Calcutta, India. *Int J Obstet Anesth.* 2008;17:112–117.
35. Molina G, Weiser TG, Lipsitz SR, et al. Relationship between cesarean delivery rate and maternal and neonatal mortality. *JAMA.* 2015;314:2263–2270.
36. Bishop D, Dyer RA, Maswime S, et al. Maternal and neonatal outcomes after caesarean delivery in the African Surgical Outcomes Study: a 7-day prospective observational cohort study. *Lancet Glob Health.* 2019;7:e513–e522.
37. Royal College of Obstetricians & Gynaecologists. Consent Advice #14: Planned caesarean birth; 2022. https://www.rcog.org.uk/media/33cnfvs0/planned-caesarean-birth-consent-advice-no-14.pdf. Accessed 2 December 2024.
38. Gebhardt GS, Fawcus S, Moodley J, Farina Z. Maternal death and caesarean section in South Africa: results from the 2011-2013 Saving Mothers Report of the National Committee for Confidential Enquiries into Maternal Deaths. *S Afr Med J.* 2015;105:287–291.
39. Sobhy S, Zamora J, Dharmarajah K, et al. Anaesthesia-related maternal mortality in low-income and middle-income countries: a systematic review and meta-analysis. *Lancet Glob Health.* 2016;4:e320–e327.
40. Lumbiganon P, Moe H, Kamsa-Ard S, et al. Outcomes associated with anaesthetic techniques for caesarean section in low- and middle-income countries: a secondary analysis of WHO surveys. *Sci Rep.* 2020;10:10176.
41. Shah A, Faundes A, Machoki M, et al. Methodological considerations in implementing the WHO Global Survey for Monitoring Maternal and Perinatal Health. *Bull World Health Organ.* 2008;86:126–131.
42. Souza JP, Gülmezoglu AM, Carroli G, et al. The World Health Organization multicountry survey on maternal and newborn health: study protocol. *BMC Health Serv Res.* 2011;11:286.
43. Ariyo P, Trelles M, Helmand R, et al. Providing anesthesia care in resource-limited settings: a 6-year analysis of anesthesia services provided at Medecins Sans Frontieres Facilities. *Anesthesiology.* 2016;124:561–569.
44. Farina Z, Rout C. 'But it's just a spinal': combating increasing rates of maternal death related to spinal anaesthesia. *S Afr Med J.* 2012;103:81–82.
45. Lundgren AC. Trends in maternal deaths associated with anaesthesia in the triennium 2017–2019. *Obstet Gynaecol Forum.* 2020;30:48–49.
46. Bishop DG, Le Roux S. Troubleshooting obstetric spinal anaesthesia at district hospital level. *S Afr Fam Pract.* 2022;64:a5529.
47. Theron A, Rout CC. "Safe anaesthesia" for the South African rural obstetric patient in KwaZulu-Natal. *S Afr J Anaesth Analg.* 2014;20:233–237.
48. Bishop DG, Fernandes NL, Dyer RA, et al. Global issues in obstetric anaesthesia: perspectives from South Africa, Japan,

China, Latin America and North America. *Int J Obstet Anesth.* 2023;54:103648.

49. Burke TF, Mantena S, Opondo K, et al. A ketamine package for use in emergency cesarean delivery when no anesthetist is available: an analysis of 401 consecutive operations. *Int J Gynaecol Obstet.* 2022;158:377–384.

50. Lonnee HA, Taule K, Knoph Sandvand J, et al. A survey of anaesthesia practices at all hospitals performing caesarean sections in Sierra Leone. *Acta Anaesthesiol Scand.* 2021;65:404–419.

51. Lonnee HA, Madzimbamuto F, Erlandsen ORM, et al. Anesthesia for cesarean delivery: a cross-sectional survey of provincial, district, and mission hospitals in Zimbabwe. *Anesth Analg.* 2018;126:2056–2064.

52. World Health Organization. WHO recommendation on tranexamic acid for the treatment of postpartum haemorrhage; 2017. https://iris.who.int/bitstream/hand le/10665/259374/9789241550154-eng.pdf?sequence=1. Accessed 7 December 2024.

53. Patel S, Robertson B, McConachie I. Catastrophic drug errors involving tranexamic acid administered during spinal anaesthesia. *Anaesthesia.* 2019;74:904–914.

54. World Health Organization. Risk of medication errors with tranexamic acid injection resulting in inadvertent intrathecal injection; 2022. https://www.who.int/news/item/16-03-2022-risk-of-medication-errors-with-tranexamic-acid-injection-resulting-in-inadvertent-intrathecal-injection. Accessed 14 December 2024.

55. Baysinger CL, Pujic B, Velickovic I, et al. Increasing regional anesthesia use in a Serbian teaching hospital through an international collaboration. *Front Public Health.* 2017;5:134.

56. Engmann C, Olufolabi A, Srofenyoh E, Owen M. Multidisciplinary team partnerships to improve maternal and neonatal outcomes: the Kybele experience. *Int Anesthesiol Clin.* 2010;48:109–122.

57. Hodnett ED, Gates S, Hofmeyr GJ, Sakala C. Continuous support for women during childbirth. *Cochrane Database Syst Rev.* 2012;(10):CD003766.

58. Hu LQ, Zhang J, Wong CA, et al. Impact of the introduction of neuraxial labor analgesia on mode of delivery at an urban maternity hospital in China. *Int J Gynaecol Obstet.* 2015;129:17–21.

59. Ninidze N, Bodin S, Ivester T, et al. Advancing obstetric anesthesia practices in Georgia through clinical education and quality improvement methodologies. *Int J Gynaecol Obstet.* 2013;120:296–300.

60. van Zyl SF, Burke JL. Increasing the labour epidural rate in a state hospital in South Africa: challenges and opportunities. *SAfr J Anaesth Analg.* 2017;23:156–161.

61. Yuill G, Amroyan A, Millar S, et al. Establishing obstetric anesthesiology practice guidelines in the Republic of Armenia: a global health collaboration. *Anesthesiology.* 2017;127:220–226.

62. Dyer RA, Reed AR, James MF. Obstetric anaesthesia in low-resource settings. *Best Pract Res Clin Obstet Gynaecol.* 2010;24:401–412.

63. Kuti O, Faponle AF. Perception of labour pain among the Yoruba ethnic group in Nigeria. *J Obstet Gynaecol.* 2006;26:332–334.

64. Shaaban OM, Abbas AM, Mohamed RA, Hafiz H. Lack of pain relief during labor is blamable for the increase in the women demands towards cesarean delivery: a cross-sectional study. *Facts Views Vis ObGyn.* 2017;9:175–180.

65. Kopic D, Sedensky M, Owen M. The impact of a teaching program on obstetric anesthesia practices in Croatia. *Int J Obstet Anesth.* 2009;18:4–9.

66. Fan ZT, Gao XL, Yang HX. Popularizing labor analgesia in China. *Int J Gynaecol Obstet.* 2007;98:205–207.

67. Wu J, Yao SL. Obstetric anesthesia in China: associated challenges and long-term goals. *Chin Med J (Engl).* 2020;133:505–508.

68. ApgarCARE® International. No Pain Labor & Delivery – Global Health Initiative. www.nopainld.org. Accessed 14 December 2024.

69. Wang Q, Zheng SX, Ni YF, et al. The effect of labor epidural analgesia on maternal-fetal outcomes: a retrospective cohort study. *Arch Gynecol Obstet.* 2018;298:89–96.

70. Zhao Y, Gao Y, Sun G, et al. The effect of initiating neuraxial analgesia service on the rate of cesarean delivery in Hubei, China: a 16-month retrospective study. *BMC Pregnancy Childbirth.* 2020;20:613.

71. Drzymalski DM, Guo JC, Qi XQ, et al. The effect of the No Pain Labor & Delivery-Global Health Initiative on cesarean delivery and neonatal outcomes in China: an interrupted time-series analysis. *Anesth Analg.* 2021;132:698–706.

72. National Health Commission of the People's Republic of China. Opinions on strengthening and improving anaesthesia medical service [Chinese]; 2018. http://www.nhc.gov.cn/ yzygj/s3594q/201808/4479a1dbac7f43dcba54e6dce873a533. shtml. Accessed 7 December 2024.

73. National Health Commission of the People's Republic of China. Notice on carrying out the pilot work of labour analgesia; 2018. http://www.nhc.gov.cn/yzygj/pqt/201811/ e3d00e4a41f445fe89d100e6ee67c0a8.shtml. Accessed 7 December 2024.

74. Mu Y, Wang X, Wang Y, et al. The trends and associated adverse maternal and perinatal outcomes of labour neuraxial analgesia among vaginal deliveries in China between 2012 and 2019: a real-world observational evidence. *BMC Med.* 2021;19:74.

75. Narayanappa A, Gurulingaswamy S, Prabhakaraiah U, et al. Practice of labor analgesia among anesthesiologists across India: cross-sectional study. *Anesth Essays Res.* 2018;12:651–656.

76. Yoezer T, Gyeltshen D, Tshering J. Childbirth in Bhutan: a study on the use of neuraxial analgesia for labor pain. *Public Health Chall.* 2023;2:e73.

77. Souza MA, Cecatti JG, Guida JP, et al. Analgesia for vaginal birth: secondary analysis from the WHO Multicountry Survey on Maternal and Newborn Health. *Int J Gynaecol Obstet.* 2021;152:401–408.

78. Alshabibi M, Madkhali AM, Alkinani AA, et al. The trends ofobstetric anesthesia practice: in a tertiary care center in theKingdom of Saudi Arabia. *Saudi J Anaesth.* 2021;15: 383–386.

79. Wagstaff DT, Bulamba F, Fernando R. Obstetric anaesthesia over the next 10 years: Africa and Middle East. *Int J Obstet Anesth.* 2023;55:103877.

80. Junttila EK, Karjalainen PK, Ohtonen PP, et al. A comparison of paracervical block with single-shot spinal for labour analgesia in multiparous women: a randomised controlled trial. *Int J Obstet Anesth.* 2009;18:15–21.

81. Viitanen H, Viitanen M, Heikkilä M. Single-shot spinal block for labour analgesia in multiparous parturients. *Acta Anaesthesiol Scand*. 2005;49:1023–1029.

82. Al-Kazwini H, Sandven I, Dahl V, Rosseland LA. Prolonging the duration of single-shot intrathecal labour analgesia with morphine: a systematic review. *Scand J Pain*. 2016;13:36–42.

83. Kähkönen K, Väänänen A. Labour analgesia by single shot spinal for any parturient?—a retrospective one-year single centre audit. *Acta Anaesthesiol Scand*. 2023;67:1079–1084.

84. Kuczkowski KM, Chandra S. Maternal satisfaction with single-dose spinal analgesia for labor pain in Indonesia: a landmark study. *J Anesth*. 2008;22:55–58.

85. Fyneface-Ogan S, Gogo Job O, Enyindah CE. Comparative effects of single shot intrathecal bupivacaine with dexmedetomidine and bupivacaine with fentanyl on labor outcome. *ISRN Anesthesiol*. 2012;2012:816984.

86. Tshibuyl PN, Olang PO, Ogutu O, Chokwe TM. A comparative study on the efficacy of two regimens of single-shot spinal block for pain relief in women presenting in established labour. *East Afr Med J*. 2013;90:12–18.

87. Otokwala JG, Fyneface-Ogan S, Mato CN. Comparative effects of single shot low dose spinal bupivacaine only and bupivacaine with fentanyl on labour outcome. *Niger J Med*. 2013;22:279–285.

88. Olufolabi AJ, Atito-Narh E, Eshun M, et al. Teaching neuraxial anesthesia techniques for obstetric care in a Ghanaian referral hospital: achievements and obstacles. *Anesth Analg*. 2015;120:1317–1322.

89. Anabah T, Olufolabi A, Boyd J, George R. Low-dose spinal anaesthesia provides effective labour analgesia and does not limit ambulation. *S Afr J Anaesth Analg*. 2015;21:19–22.

90. Bilge A, Muge A, Ahmet G, et al. Comparison of different bupivacaine and fentanyl combinations when used with a single shut spinal block for labor analgesia. *J Anesth Clin Res*. 2017;8.

91. Khaled GM, Sabry AI. Outcomes of intrathecal analgesia in multiparous women undergoing normal vaginal delivery: arandomised controlled trial. *Indian J Anaesth*. 2020;64:109–117.

92. Chauhan G, Samyal P, Pathania AA. Single-dose intrathecal analgesia: a safe and effective method of labor analgesia for parturients in low resource areas. *Ain-Shams J Anesthesiol*. 2020;12:23.

93. Awad AA, Eldesoky GA, Alkafrawy MA. Effect of epidural bupivacaine versus intrathecal single dose in analgesia during normal vaginal labor of multiparous women. *Med J Cairo Univ*. 2021;89:431–438.

94. Rathod S, Syal GG, Sood R, Syal K. Intrathecal labor analgesia using dexmedetomidine: a viable alternative to epidural analgesia. *J South Asian Fed Obstet Gynaecol*. 2021;13:279–282.

95. Rahmati J, Shahriari M, Shahriari A, et al. Effectiveness of spinal analgesia for labor pain compared with epidural analgesia. *Anesth Pain Med*. 2021;11:e113350.

96. Sonderman KA, Citron I, Meara JG. National surgical, obstetric, and anesthesia planning in the context of global surgery: the way forward. *JAMA Surg*. 2018;153:959–960.

97. The Lancet. The Lancet Commission on Global Surgery; 2015. https://www.thelancet.com/commissions/global-surgery. Accessed 7 December 2024.

98. Citron I, Jumbam D, Dahm J, et al. Towards equitable surgical systems: development and outcomes of a national surgical,

obstetric and anaesthesia plan in Tanzania. *BMJ Glob Health*. 2019;4:e001282.

99. Sutherland TN, Rusats EL, Mutangana A, Banguti P. Formulation of a national surgical plan in Rwanda: a model for integration of physician and non-physician anaesthetists. *Br J Anaesth*. 2017;119:1232–1233.

100. Seyi-Olajide JO, Anderson JE, Williams OM, et al. National surgical, obstetric, anaesthesia and nursing plan, Nigeria. *Bull World Health Organ*. 2021;99:883–891.

101. Peters AW, Roa L, Rwamasirabo E, et al. National surgical, obstetric, and anesthesia plans supporting the vision of universal health coverage. *Glob Health Sci Pract*. 2020;8:1–9.

102. Peck GL, Hanna JS. The National Surgical, Obstetric, and Anesthesia Plan (NSOAP): recognition and definition of an empirically evolving global surgery systems science comment on "Global Surgery - Informing National Strategies for Scaling Up Surgery in Sub-Saharan Africa". *Int J Health Policy Manag*. 2018;7:1151–1154.

103. World Health Organization. 2018 Global Reference List of 100 Core Health Indicators (plus health-related SDGs); 2018. https://iris.who.int/handle/10665/259951. Accessed 8 December 2024.

104. Kruk ME, Gage AD, Arsenault C, et al. High-quality health systems in the Sustainable Development Goals era: time for a revolution. *Lancet Glob Health*. 2018;6:e1196–e1252.

105. Steffner KR, McQueen KA, Gelb AW. Patient safety challenges in low-income and middle-income countries. *Curr Opin Anaesthesiol*. 2014;27:623–629.

106. Evans FM, Duarte JC, Haylock Loor C, Morriss W. Are short subspecialty courses the educational answer? *Anesth Analg*. 2018;126:1305–1311.

107. Law TJ, Bulamba F, Ochieng JP, et al. Anesthesia provider training and practice models: a survey of Africa. *Anesth Analg*. 2019;129:839–846.

108. Livingston P, Evans F, Nsereko E, et al. Safer obstetric anesthesia through education and mentorship: a model for knowledge translation in Rwanda. *Can J Anaesth*. 2014;61:1028–1039.

109. Morriss WW, Milenovic MS, Evans FM. Education: the heart of the matter. *Anesth Analg*. 2018;126:1298–1304.

110. Potisek MG, Hatch DM, Atito-Narh E, et al. Where are they now? Evolution of a nurse anesthesia training school in Ghana and a survey of graduates. *Front Public Health*. 2017;5:78.

111. Gelb AW, Morriss WW, Johnson W, et al. World Health Organization-World Federation of Societies of Anaesthesiologists (WHO-WFSA) International Standards for a Safe Practice of Anesthesia. *Anesth Analg*. 2018;126:2047–2055.

112. World Federation of Societies of Anaesthesiologists. WFSA fellowship progamme. https://wfsahq.org/our-work/education-training/fellowship-programme/. Accessed 14 December 2024.

113. International Federation of Nurse Anesthetists. International Federation of Nurse Anesthetists International Federation of Nurse Anesthetists. https://ifna.site/. Accessed 14 December 2024.

114. Mavalankar D, Callahan K, Sriram V, et al. Where there is no anesthetist—increasing capacity for emergency obstetric care in rural India: an evaluation of a pilot program to train general doctors. *Int J Gynaecol Obstet*. 2009;107:283–288.

115. Bishop D, van Dyk D, Dyer RA. Safe obstetric anaesthesia in low- and middle-income countries—a perspective from Africa. *BJA Educ.* 2023;23:432–439.

116. Temlett L, Bishop DG, Moran N. Safe caesarean sections in South Africa: is internship training sufficient? *S Afr J Obstet Gynaecol.* 2022;28:4–9.

117. Fernandes NL, Lilaonitkul M, Subedi A, Owen MD. Global obstetric anaesthesia: bridging the gap in maternal health care inequities through partnership in education. *Int J Obstet Anesth.* 2023;55:103646.

118. White MC, Rakotoarisoa T, Cox NH, et al. A mixed-method design evaluation of the SAFE obstetric anaesthesia course at 4 and 12-18 months after training in the Republic of Congo and Madagascar. *Anesth Analg.* 2019;129:1707–1714.

119. Moore JN, Morriss WW, Asfaw G, et al. The impact of the Safer Anaesthesia from Education (SAFE) Obstetric Anaesthesia training course in Ethiopia: a mixed methods longitudinal cohort study. *Anaesth Intensive Care.* 2020;48:297–305.

120. Lilaonitkul M, Mishra S, Pritchard N, et al. Mixed methods analysis of factors influencing change in clinical behaviours of non-physician anaesthetists in Kenya following obstetric anaesthesia training. *Anaesthesia.* 2020;75:1331–1339.

121. Health Volunteers Overseas. Health Volunteers Overseas: Transforming lives through education. https://hvousa.org/. Accessed 14 December 2024.

122. Médecins Sans Frontières. Doctors Without Borders/Médecins Sans Frontières (MSF). www.doctorswithoutborders.org. Accessed 14 December 2024.

123. Kybele Incorporated™. Kybele: For safe childbirth worldwide. https://kybeleworldwide.org/. Accessed 14 December 2024.

124. Schriger SH, Binagwaho A, Keetile M, et al. Hierarchy of qualities in global health partnerships: a path towards equity and sustainability. *BMJ Glob Health.* 2021;6:e007132.

125. Prasad S, Aldrink M, Compton B, et al. Global health partnerships and the brocher declaration: principles for ethical short-term engagements in global health. *Ann Glob Health.* 2022;88:31.

126. Kinsella SM, Carvalho B, Dyer RA, et al. International consensus statement on the management of hypotension with vasopressors during caesarean section under spinal anaesthesia. *Anaesthesia.* 2018;73:71–92.

127. Heesen M, Carvalho B, Carvalho JCA, et al. International consensus statement on the use of uterotonic agents during caesarean section. *Anaesthesia.* 2019;74:1305–1319.

128. Plaat F, Stanford SER, Lucas DN, et al. Prevention and management of intra-operative pain during caesarean section under neuraxial anaesthesia: a technical and interpersonal approach. *Anaesthesia.* 2022;77:588–597.

129. Cadman V. Use of the WHO surgical safety checklist in low and middle income countries: a review of the literature. *JPerioper Pract.* 2018;28:334–338.

130. Hullfish KL, Miller T, Pastore LM, et al. A checklist for timeout on labor and delivery: a pilot study to improve communication and safety. *J Reprod Med.* 2014;59:579–584.

131. Vivekanantham S, Ravindran RP, Shanmugarajah K, et al. Surgical safety checklists in developing countries. *Int J Surg.* 2014;12:2–6.

132. White MC, Peven K, Clancy O, et al. Implementation strategies and the uptake of the World Health Organization surgical safety checklist in low and middle income countries: a systematic review and meta-analysis. *Ann Surg.* 2021;273:e196–e205.

133. World Health Organization. WHO Surgical Safety Checklist. https://www.who.int/teams/integrated-health-services/patient-safety/research/safe-surgery/tool-and-resources. Accessed 14 December 2024.

134. World Health Organization. WHO Safe Childbirth Checklist; 2015. https://iris.who.int/rest/bitstreams/886314/retrieve. Accessed 14 December 2024.

135. Alexander LA, Newton MW, McEvoy KG, et al. Development and pilot testing of a context-relevant safe anesthesia checklist for cesarean delivery in East Africa. *Anesth Analg.* 2019;128:993–998.

136. Zwane SF, Bishop DG, Rodseth RN. Hypotension during spinal anaesthesia for Caesarean section in a resource-limited setting: towards a consensus definition. *S Afr J Anaesth Analg.* 2019;25:1–5.

137. Bishop DG, Cairns C, Grobbelaar M, Rodseth RN. Prophylactic phenylephrine infusions to reduce severe spinal anesthesia hypotension during cesarean delivery in a resource-constrained environment. *Anesth Analg.* 2017;125:904–906.

138. van Dyk D, Dyer RA, Bishop DG. Spinal hypotension in obstetrics: context-sensitive prevention and management. *Best Pract Res Clin Anaesthesiol.* 2022;36:69–82.

139. Buthelezi AS, Bishop DG, Rodseth RN, Dyer RA. Prophylactic phenylephrine and fluid co-administration to reduce spinal hypotension during elective caesarean section in a resource-limited setting: a prospective alternating intervention study. *Anaesthesia.* 2020;75:487–492.

140. Alwy Al-Beity F, Pembe AB, Kwezi HA, et al. "We do what we can do to save a woman" health workers' perceptions of health facility readiness for management of postpartum haemorrhage. *Glob Health Action.* 2020;13:1707403.

141. Rowe AK, Rowe SY, Peters DH, et al. Effectiveness of strategies to improve health-care provider practices in low-income and middle-income countries: a systematic review. *Lancet Glob Health.* 2018;6:e1163–e1175.

142. Srofenyoh EK, Kassebaum NJ, Goodman DM, et al. Measuring the impact of a quality improvement collaboration to decrease maternal mortality in a Ghanaian regional hospital. *Int J Gynaecol Obstet.* 2016;134:181–185.

143. World Health Organization. Jeddah Declaration on Patient Safety to shape safer systems for future generations; 2019. https://www.who.int/news/item/04-03-2019-jeddah-declaration-on-patient-safety-to-shape-safer-systems-for-future-generations. Accessed 14 December 2024.

144. White MC, Ahuja S, Peven K, et al. Scaling up of safety and quality improvement interventions in perioperative care: a systematic scoping review of implementation strategies and effectiveness. *BMJ Glob Health.* 2022;7:e010649.

145. Yamey G. Scaling up global health interventions: a proposed framework for success. *PLoS Med.* 2011;8:e1001049.

146. Barker PM, Reid A, Schall MW. A framework for scaling up health interventions: lessons from large-scale improvement initiatives in Africa. *Implement Sci.* 2016;11:12.

PART V

Anesthesia Before and During Pregnancy

16

Pharmacology During Pregnancy and Lactation

Catherine S. Stika, MD, Emily A. Pinheiro, PhD, and Rupsa C. Boelig, MD, MS

CHAPTER OUTLINE

Because pregnant women become sick, and women with chronic medical problems become pregnant, care provided to pregnant women involves the administration of medications. In a prospective, longitudinal study of 9139 nulliparous pregnant women recruited in 2010 to 2013 at eight geographically diverse centers in the United States, 73.4% reported the use of at least one medication during pregnancy, excluding vitamins, supplements, and vaccines; 55.1% took medication in the first trimester.[1] These results are very similar to another cross-sectional, multinational, web-based study[2] which surveyed 9459 pregnant women in 2011 to 2012 and found 81.2% of respondents reported use of at least one prescribed or over-the-counter medication during pregnancy. The percentage was even higher for participants in Canada and the United States; 84.8% reported any medication use during pregnancy, with 75.6% taking drugs for a short-term illness and 64.2% reporting use of over-the-counter medications.

Once pregnant women are admitted to the hospital for birth, the number of drugs they are prescribed explodes. Parturients admitted for uncomplicated, term vaginal deliveries typically are prescribed multiple medications, including vitamins, oxytocics and other uterotonics, prophylactic and therapeutic antibiotics, analgesics including acetaminophen (paracetamol) prior to birth, opioids during labor, nonsteroidal antiinflammatory drugs (NSAIDs) postpartum, local anesthetics, antiemetics, antacids, histamine$_2$-receptor antagonists, anticoagulants, sedatives, antihistamines, stool softeners, antiflatulents, bowel stimulants, and topical perineal anesthetics.

Drugs may be prescribed to the pregnant patient to treat a maternal condition with incidental fetal transfer or to treat a fetal problem (e.g., supraventricular tachycardia) with maternal exposure. Historically, most publications addressing drug use during pregnancy have focused on fetal safety. While remaining cognizant of fetal safety, it is also important to consider maternal efficacy and safety. Because pregnant women are physiologically and pharmacologically different than nonpregnant women, it cannot be assumed that dosing strategies developed for nonpregnant, healthy adults will achieve comparable results when used during pregnancy.

The anesthesia provider administers numerous medications during the peripartum period and at other times during gestation, and postpartum if surgery or intensive care is required. Because optimal pain management requires an understanding of the pharmacologic environment, which may be influenced by pregnancy as well as drugs prescribed by other healthcare providers, it is important that all individuals who care for obstetric patients appreciate the profound effects of pregnancy on drug disposition and efficacy.

This chapter focuses on the changes in pharmacokinetics (PK) during pregnancy that affect drug disposition, using familiar medications for illustration. The unique pharmacodynamic (PD) change in pain thresholds that occurs during pregnancy will be discussed. Basic principles of teratology and fetal drug exposure, changes in the Pregnancy and Lactation Labeling Rule of the US Food and Drug Administration (FDA), and drug transfer during lactation will also be discussed.

PHARMACOKINETIC CHANGES DURING PREGNANCY

The changes during pregnancy that affect drug absorption, distribution, metabolism, and elimination can be divided into two broad categories: (1) normal obstetric physiology and (2) changes in hepatic metabolism. Although studies investigating the profound physiologic changes that occur during pregnancy were initially published in the earlier half of the 20th century, the first PK study describing the failure of a standard drug dose to achieve therapeutic concentrations during pregnancy was not published until 1977.[3] Since then, especially since the turn of the millennium with expansion of FDA and US National Institutes of Health support, the understanding of pregnancy as a special pharmacologic condition has advanced significantly. Although these pharmacologic changes are often described in the context of pregnant versus nonpregnant states, the pregnant state is not uniform; individual changes in maternal physiology and hepatic metabolism evolve with different trajectories across gestational ages. As a result, pregnant women in the third trimester handle drugs differently than in the second or first trimesters.

Hormonal Changes During Pregnancy

Reproductive hormones play important roles from ovulation and implantation, through gestation, and ultimately lactation. Although our understanding is evolving and incomplete, the same hormones that modulate obstetric physiology also play critical roles in changing the PK environment during pregnancy. After ovulation and implantation, the corpus luteum continues to be the primary source of increased estrogen and progesterone production. Circulating human chorionic gonadotropin (hCG) from the nascent trophoblast quickly replaces pituitary gonadotropins in support of ovarian steroidogenesis. Between gestation weeks 7 and 10, the site of hormonal production shifts from the corpus luteum to the placental syncytiotrophoblast (the luteal-placental shift). Plasma progesterone concentration increases from 1 to 2 ng/mL just before ovulation to a midluteal concentration of 10 to 35 ng/mL.[4–6] After implantation, the corpus luteum maintains production of progesterone until the placenta ramps up its synthetic machine and concentrations progressively rise to a peak of 100 to 200 ng/mL at term, a 10- to 20-fold increase compared with periovulation.[4]

Concentrations of the three maternal estrogens, estradiol (E2), estrone (E1), and estriol (E3), also progressively and dramatically increase during pregnancy.[7] Estradiol, the most potent of the three, increases approximately 500-fold, from a mean mid-follicular concentration of 50 pg/mL to approximately 25,000 pg/mL at term.[7,8] During the same time period, estriol increases 1000-fold.[9]

Plasma cortisol concentration also progressively increases during pregnancy from a prepregnancy low of 0 to 25 μg/dL, to 7 to 19 μg/dL in the first trimester, 10 to 42 μg/dL in the second trimester, and 12 to 50 μg/dL in the third trimester.[10] During pregnancy, the usual negative feedback relationship between corticotrophin-releasing hormone (CRH) and cortisol is attenuated.[11] Low cortisol concentrations typically trigger increases in hypothalamic CRH, which causes the anterior pituitary gland to secrete adrenocorticotrophic hormone (ACTH), which then stimulates the adrenal cortex to produce cortisol; as cortisol concentration rises, CRH and ACTH concentrations decrease. Paradoxically, during pregnancy, concentrations of CRH, ACTH, and cortisol are elevated above nonpregnant baseline values; the latter two increase approximately fourfold.[12] The source of the increased stimulation is the pregnancy itself; CRH is produced by the placental syncytiotrophoblast, fetal membranes, and the decidua.[13] Among multiple modulators, glucocorticoids increase placental CRH

with a *positive* feedback relationship.[14,15] Because the syncytiotrophoblast directly faces maternal vessels, placental CRH secreted into maternal vessels is responsible for most of the circulating maternal CRH. Maternal CRH progressively increases during gestation, until about 35 weeks, when it rapidly rises until labor onset, reaching concentrations 1000 to 10,000 times greater than nonpregnancy levels.[16] Desensitization of the pituitary gland to these extremely high CRH levels prevents pathologic elevations of ACTH and cortisol.[16] Placental CRH is thought to play a crucial role in regulation of both fetal maturation and the timing of delivery.[17] After delivery of the placenta, maternal hypothalamic CRH secretion, which had been suppressed by circulating cortisol concentrations, returns to normal function within 12 weeks.[11]

Impact of Obstetric Physiology on Pharmacokinetics

Increases in Blood Volume and Total Body Water

Blood volume increases substantially during pregnancy, starting from 6 to 8 weeks' gestation (see Chapter 2). Extracellular fluid and total body water also increase proportionally to patient weight.[18] In women in the third trimester of singleton pregnancy weighing 70 to 80 kg, the extracellular fluid space is approximately 0.255 L/kg compared with approximately 0.156 L/kg in nonpregnant women of similar weight.[19] The expansion of plasma volume and total body water increases the **volume of distribution (Vd)** of hydrophilic medications and reduces the concentration-to-dose ratio (C/D) of their *initial doses*. Vd is the theoretical volume that would be necessary to contain the administered dose at the measured plasma concentration:

$$Vd = dose/concentration.$$

Relevant drug examples.

Enoxaparin has a Vd that is essentially plasma volume. The maximum antifactor Xa activity after a 40-mg subcutaneous (SC) dose of enoxaparin is significantly lower in the first and third trimesters (mean 0.46 and 0.40 IU/mL, respectively) compared with 6 to 8 weeks postpartum (0.57 IU/mL).[20]

Ampicillin is hydrophilic and only 15% to 25% protein-bound; it readily distributes to approximately total body water. The maximum plasma ampicillin concentration (C_{max}) following a 500-mg oral dose was 41% lower during pregnancy compared with values attained when the same dose was given to the same women postpartum (mean 2.2 versus 3.7 μg/mL).[3]

Furosemide (frusemide) PK was studied in hypertensive women at term following an oral dose of 40 mg. Its **apparent volume of distribution (Vd/F)** was almost six times greater and C_{max} was 73% lower compared with values obtained from historic, nonpregnant subjects.[21] Given that furosemide is approximately 96% protein-bound to albumin in nonpregnant individuals, it was concluded that these findings were the result of both an increased free drug fraction due to lower albumin concentration and the marked increase of approximately 8 L in total body water that occurs in term pregnancy.

Because body fat has an extensive capacity to absorb lipophilic drugs, the Vd for these drugs greatly exceeds the actual volume of body fat. Although pregnant women gain body fat, the impact on Vd of lipophilic medications is insignificant because this change only minimally increases the already large Vd.

Decreased Protein Binding

Plasma protein concentrations decrease during pregnancy. **Albumin**, the most abundant of the plasma proteins, binds acidic and neutral compounds. Its concentration decreases from 4.2 g/dL in nonpregnancy to 3.6 g/dL by the midtrimester of pregnancy.[22] Another plasma protein, **alpha-1 acid glycoprotein (AGP)**, binds basic and some neutral drugs. Although earlier studies reported that AGP concentrations do not change during pregnancy,[23] more recent evidence has demonstrated a concentration reduction of almost 50% during the third trimester of pregnancy.[22,24,25] Lower plasma protein concentrations result in a greater free fraction of protein-bound drugs, resulting in greater drug effect, movement into other spaces, and availability for metabolism and/or clearance. Monitoring of free drug is often recommended during pregnancy for highly protein-bound medications that have a narrow therapeutic range (little difference between the minimal therapeutic and toxic concentrations) such as **digoxin**, **phenytoin**, and **free T4 (thyroxine)**.

Relevant drug examples.

Bupivacaine was shown to have a free fraction that was 52% higher in term laboring women than in nonpregnant women (median 8.2% versus 5.4%).[26]

Lidocaine (lignocaine) was shown to have a free fraction that was higher in term pregnant women than in nonpregnant women (mean 47.7% versus 32.0%).[24]

Midazolam was shown to have a free fraction that was 21% greater after oral administration at 28 to 32 weeks' gestation than after administration to the same women at 6 to 10 weeks postpartum (mean 0.71% versus 0.61%).[27]

Digoxin was shown to have a free fraction that was 5.8% greater after administration at 28 to 32 weeks' gestation than after administration to the same women at 6 to 10 weeks postpartum (mean 67% versus 63%).[27]

Increase in Cardiac Output

Cardiac output increases, with increases in both stroke volume and heart rate, and systemic vascular resistance decreases during pregnancy (see Chapter 2). These changes directly affect other processes that impact PK during pregnancy. Of primary importance, glomerular filtration rate (GFR) increases in parallel with cardiac output, which contributes to the enhanced renal clearance of some drugs.

Changes in Regional Blood Flow

The increased cardiac output during pregnancy is differentially distributed within the body. The placenta functions as a low-pressure, arteriovenous shunt and consumes 20% to 25% of cardiac output at term.[28] Renal blood flow increases to 30% to 40% above the prepregnancy baseline during the first and second trimesters, and then decreases to 10% above baseline in the third trimester.[29] Skin blood flow increases to dissipate heat generated by fetal metabolism[30]; blood flow to the developing breasts also

increases.[31] Arterial blood flow to the liver is unchanged but represents a lower percentage of cardiac output; however, beginning at 28 weeks' gestation, portal venous blood flow increases from 150% to 160% of nonpregnant levels.[32] The enhanced portal blood flow increases first-pass hepatic clearance of drugs with a high extraction ratio. Because of these hemodynamic changes, less cardiac output is available for skeletal muscle and other vascular beds, resulting in unpredictable and/or delayed absorption of medications administered intramuscularly.

Renal Clearance

Renal elimination comprises three components: (1) renal perfusion, (2) glomerular filtration, and (3) reabsorption and secretion within the nephric tubules. All three processes change with pregnancy (see Chapter 2). Stimulated by relaxin and nitric oxide, the increase in renal perfusion is detectable as early as 6 weeks' gestation,[29] and by 16 weeks' gestation it is 75% greater than the prepregnancy baseline. After this peak, it decreases during the late second to the early third trimester from 10% to 40% above baseline.[29,33,34] Although inulin clearance is the most accurate reflection of GFR, because of convenience, **creatinine clearance (CrCl)**, which includes a component of tubular secretion, has been used more commonly as an estimate of GFR during pregnancy.[29,35] CrCl begins to increase by the late luteal phase (20% greater than week 1 of the menstrual cycle), and is 45% above the follicular phase baseline by 9 weeks' gestation.[36] It peaks at approximately 50% above baseline in the late second to early third trimester before slightly decreasing closer to term. CrCl begins to decrease during the second postpartum week, with a return to normal values by 6 to 8 weeks after delivery.[29,37]

Renal Transporters and Renal Secretion and Reabsorption

Glomerular filtration of many drugs is supplemented by the net effects of tubular reabsorption and secretion. Straddling membrane surfaces, drug transporters control movement of drugs and other compounds into and out of cells. In the kidney, specific transporters are found on tubular cell membranes facing either the afferent blood vessels or urine where they facilitate movement of compounds either from the blood across the tubular cell and into urine (secretion) or from the urine back into the blood (reabsorption) (Fig. 16.1A). Pregnancy increases the activity of some of these transporters, which in general, increases renal clearance of their substrates.

Relevant drug examples.

Amoxicillin is primarily excreted unchanged through a combination of renal filtration plus the net effect of two opposing movements within the tubules: secretion into urine via the **organic anion transporter 1 (OAT1)** and **OAT3** and reabsorption out of the urine by the **peptide transporter 1 (PEPT1)**. Because of changes in both GFR and secretion, renal clearance of amoxicillin is increased by 50% in the second and third trimesters compared with the nonpregnant baseline.[38] Net amoxicillin secretion increases during pregnancy because of upregulation of OAT1 and OAT3 (secretion) and progesterone-induced downregulation of PEPT1 (reabsorption) (Fig. 16.1B).[38,39] Because of lower amoxicillin

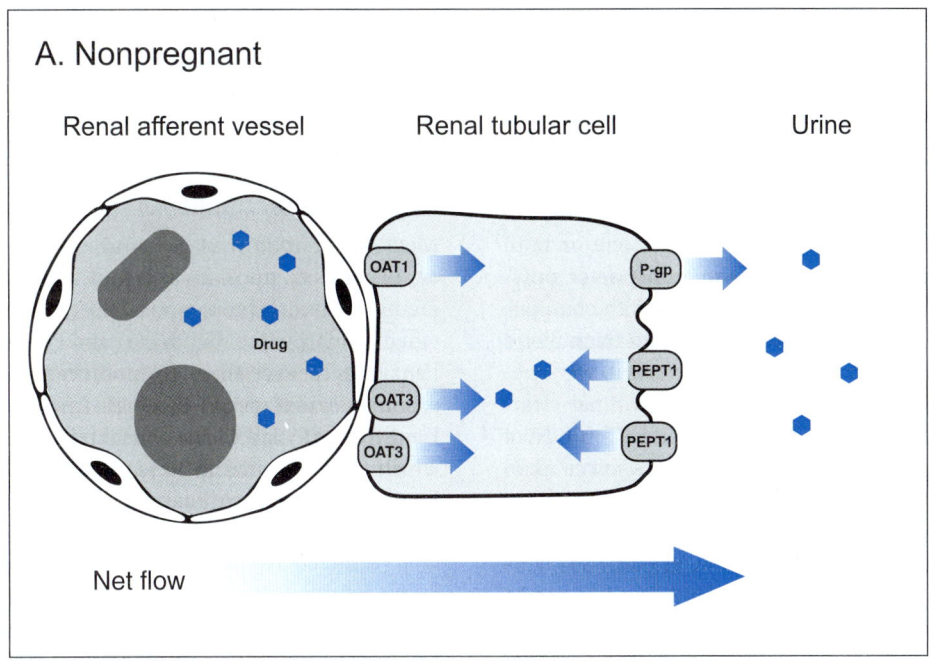

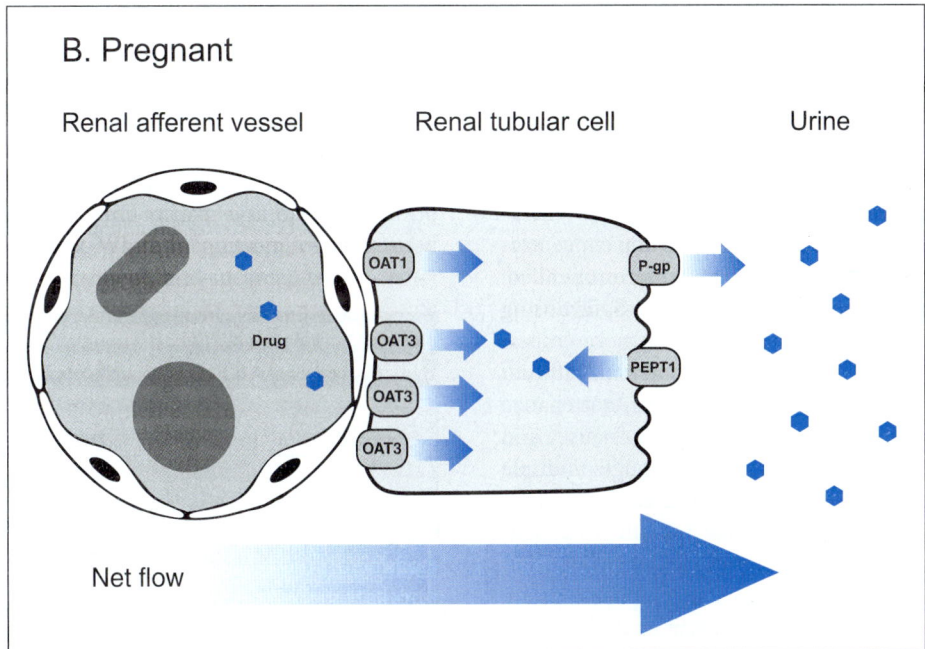

Fig. 16.1. Amoxicillin Excretion and Changes in Selected Renal Transporters in the Nonpregnant (A) and Pregnant (B) Patient. Transcription of OAT1 and OAT3, which move drug from afferent renal vessels into tubular cells, increases during pregnancy, and PEPT1, which removes drug from the urine is downregulated. This results in a net increase in renal secretion of amoxicillin during pregnancy compared to postpartum. *OAT1*, Organic anion transporter 1; *OAT3*, organic anion transporter 3; *PEPT1*, peptide transporter 1; *P-gp*, P-glycoprotein. Illustration by Naveen Nathan, MD, NorthShore University HealthSystem, University of Chicago Pritzker School of Medicine, Evanston, IL.

C_{max} secondary to the increase in its Vd, coupled with potential subtherapeutic concentrations at the end of the dosing interval from increased renal clearance, pregnant women may require larger and more frequent ampicillin dosing.

Metformin is eliminated unchanged by the kidneys with the assistance of another transporter, **organic cation transporter 2 (OCT2)**. Renal clearance of metformin is increased by 49% in the second trimester and by 29% in the third trimester compared with postpartum. Renal secretion of

metformin is also increased by 45% and 38%, in mid- and late-pregnancy, respectively, compared with postpartum.[40]

Digoxin is a well-known **probe substrate** (probe drugs have a metabolic pathway that is uniquely catalyzed by one enzyme[41]) for a third transporter, **P-glycoprotein (P-gp)**, whose activity is also enhanced during pregnancy.[42] With its long list of substrates, the efflux transporter, P-gp, plays a protective role, controlling drug movement out of cells in many tissues, including the intestines, liver, kidney, blood-brain barrier, and, importantly, the placenta.[43] Located on the apical, urine-facing surface of renal tubular cells, P-gp moves digoxin into the urine against its concentration gradient.[44] During the third trimester, the renal clearance of unbound digoxin was 52% higher and unbound digoxin renal secretion was 107% higher compared with postpartum.[27] The authors of this PK study hypothesized that this increase in digoxin secretion resulted from upregulation of either one or both transporters, P-gp and/or **organic anion transporter polypeptide**, another digoxin transporter located on the basolateral surface of the tubules, which moves digoxin from blood into the renal cell.[27]

Magnesium and **lithium** are cations whose renal clearances are enhanced during pregnancy.[45,46] In a PK study of magnesium therapy, magnesium clearance was lower (3.98 versus 5.88 L/h) and the steady-state concentration of magnesium was higher (7.2 versus 5.1 mg/dL) in women with preeclampsia than in women without preeclampsia who were receiving magnesium for fetal neuroprotection.[45] Women with greater maternal weight had lower serum magnesium concentrations immediately after the magnesium loading dose.[45]

Lithium clearance closely parallels CrCl. In pregnant women receiving lithium, its concentration rapidly falls during the first trimester, remains relatively stable during the second trimester—albeit significantly lower than nonpregnant values—and then either remains low or variably normalizes during the third trimester.[46–48] Because of its narrow therapeutic window, frequent monitoring of lithium concentrations with appropriate dose adjustment is recommended, especially during the first and third trimesters. Split dosing regimens (twice or three times daily) provide more consistent concentrations throughout the dosing interval. Lithium concentrations can vary in obstetric conditions that change either maternal hydration or renal clearance (e.g., nausea and vomiting, gastroenteritis, preeclampsia). Although multiple authors and societies have recommended decreasing or stopping lithium administration during labor,[49,50] some investigators have shown that lithium concentrations during labor do not significantly change, and that neonatal complications are not associated with lithium concentrations at birth.[51]

Levetiracetam, an anticonvulsant, is not appreciably protein-bound and is eliminated primarily by renal excretion with approximately 30% of the dose metabolized by nonhepatic enzymatic hydrolysis.[52] Large studies have shown that levetiracetam clearance is either the same in all three trimesters at approximately 43% above baseline,[53] or that it peaks in the second trimester and decreases slightly during the third trimester, at 1.22 and 1.15 times the baseline clearance, respectively.[54] In 2023, physiologically based PK modeling predicted that the steady-state area under the concentration-time curve (AUC) for levetiracetam decreased to 83%, 62%, and 67% of baseline values in the first, second, and third trimesters, respectively, and the recommended dose of levetiracetam should be 1.2, 1.6, and 1.5 times the baseline dose to maintain therapeutic concentrations in the first, second, and third trimesters, respectively.[55] Some authors have recommended

therapeutic dose monitoring starting in the first trimester with appropriate dose escalation to prevent seizures from subtherapeutic concentrations. Although C/D ratios do not return to prepregnancy baselines until 4 weeks postpartum, they begin increasing within 3 to 5 days after delivery.[56]

Hepatic Metabolism

Metabolic enzymes evolved to control concentrations of endogenous compounds and to detoxify dangerous environmental chemicals (xenobiotics). Hepatic metabolism is subdivided primarily into the **Phase I** and **Phase II enzymes**. Phase I enzymes catalyze chemical modifications of compounds, for example, oxidation or hydrolysis. The most important Phase I enzymes are the 12 **cytochrome P450 (CYP)** families, of which families 1, 2, and 3 are involved in drug metabolism.[57] Phase II enzymes facilitate simple biotransformation by adding readily available compounds (glucuronic acid, glutathione, amino acids, methyl, acetyl, and sulfate groups) to make molecules more hydrophilic and able to be renally excreted. Both Phase I and Phase II enzymes are affected by pregnancy, which can result in changes in drug concentrations, and consequently efficacy and/or toxicity (Table 16.1).

Phase I Drug-Metabolizing Enzymes and Pregnancy

CYP3A4/5. The CYP3A subfamily (CYP3A4, CYP3A5, and fetal/neonatal CYP3A7) is the most abundant of the cytochrome enzymes in humans and contributes to the metabolism of many endogenous compounds and 30% to 50% of drugs used today.[57] Induction of CYP3A4 by **enzyme-inducing**

TABLE 16.1. Changes in Drug-Metabolizing Enzymes[a] During Pregnancy

Enzyme	Increases	Decreases	No Known Change
CYP1A2		✓	
CYP2A6	✓		
CYP2B6			✓?
CYP2C9	✓		
CYP2C19		✓	
CYP2D6	✓		
CYP2E1	✓		
CYP3A4/5	✓		
UGT1A1	✓		
UGT1A4	✓		
UGT1A9	✓?		
UGT2B7	✓?		
NAT-2			✓?
SULT			✓?

[a]Results reflect functional phenotypes only.
CYP, Cytochrome P450; *NAT-2*: N-acetyltransferase-2;
SULT: sulfotransferases; *UGT,* uridine 5'-diphosphate glucuronosyltransferase.
? Data are inconclusive or inconsistent.

drugs (EIDs), such as **rifampin** and **carbamazepine**, occurs through stimulation of the xenobiotic sensing system, a mechanism that ramps up the metabolism when exposed to potentially toxic environmental chemicals.[58] EIDs bind to the nuclear receptors pregnane X receptor (PXR) and/or constitutive androstane receptor (CAR), both of which evolved from a primitive estrogen receptor. This complex then binds to the hormone-responsive element within DNA and upregulates transcription of the target gene(s) and subsequent production of their proteins, including CYP3A4/5.[59] Although numerous compounds can stimulate PXR/CAR, studies using cultured hepatocytes have suggested that the primary stimulus for induction of CYP3A4 during pregnancy is increased cortisol.[60]

For many, drugs metabolized by CYP3A, CYP3A4 and CYP3A5 work together, with increased clearance in individuals who have both CYP3A4 and a functional CYP3A5 phenotype. However, there are marked ethnic differences in the distribution of the major inactive CYP3A5*3 allele, which is present in 92% to 94% of Europeans, 71% to 75% of East Asians, 55% to 65% of South Asians, 60% to 66% of people with Hispanic ethnicity, but only 29% to 35% of people of African descent.[61] As a result, 65% to 71% of African Americans with functional CYP3A5 metabolize CYP3A4/5 drugs faster than other racial and ethnic groups. The impact of enhanced CYP3A5 metabolism is exemplified by **tacrolimus**; dosing guidelines recommend increased dosing for African American transplant recipients.[62] The impact of enhanced CYP3A5 metabolism on drugs used in obstetrics has not been well studied; however, investigators have reported that concentrations of the antimalarial drug **lumefantrine** are lower in pregnant women with the CYP3A5*1/*1 genotype, placing them at increased risk for treatment failure.[63] Similarly, in a study of **nifedipine** for tocolysis, high CYP3A5 expressors had lower average plasma nifedipine concentration and greater nifedipine clearance than those with inactive CYP3A5.[64]

Reflecting the importance CYP3A plays in the metabolism of many drugs used in obstetric care, numerous studies in pregnant women have confirmed enhanced clearance and reduced maximum concentrations of these medications. CYP3A activity has been shown to be induced by the end of the first trimester and it remains consistently elevated throughout pregnancy; however, it is not known how early it begins to increase in the first trimester or how quickly it normalizes postpartum.

Relevant drug examples.

Midazolam hydroxylation is a probe for CYP3A4/5 activity. After an oral dose of 2-mg midazolam, the apparent oral clearance of midazolam in the third trimester was 108% greater than postpartum.[27]

Dextromethorphan (a cough suppressant) *N*-demethylation is another probe for CYP3A activity. In a "cocktail" of two probe drugs, **dextromethorphan** and **caffeine**, Tracy et al.[65] showed that CYP3A activity had already increased by the early second trimester and remained elevated throughout pregnancy, at 35% to 38% above postpartum values.

Cholesterol is another probe for CYP3A activity. The metabolic ratio of 4β-hydroxycholesterol to cholesterol (4βOHC/C) was 26% greater in the third trimester of pregnancy compared with postpartum or nonpregnant controls as a result of increased CYP3A enzyme activity.[66] The 4βOHC/C metabolic ratios were similar in the late first trimester, and in the second and third trimesters, all approximately 50% greater than the ratios in nonpregnant women.[67]

Cortisol conversion to hydroxycortisol by CYP3A is enhanced during pregnancy as evidenced by the finding that the ratio of urinary 6-hydroxycortisol to 17-hydroxycorticosteroid (6-OHF/17-OHCS) was 4.9 times greater 1 week before delivery compared with 3 months after delivery.[68]

Betamethasone clearance by CYP3A4/5 increased 1.2- to 1.6-fold during the second and third trimesters of pregnancy compared with nonpregnancy.[69]

Nifedipine PK during pregnancy has been explored in two studies. Compared with historic, nonpregnant controls, nifedipine clearance was fourfold greater during the third trimester.[70] A similar fourfold increase in nifedipine clearance was observed in pregnant women treated for preterm labor as well as additional enhanced clearance in women with one or two active CYP3A5*1 alleles.[64]

Fentanyl is metabolized by CYP3A4 to its primary inactive metabolite norfentanyl.[71] Table 16.2 lists the drug-metabolizing enzymes involved with each of the opioid medications. The mean urinary metabolic ratio of norfentanyl/fentanyl (NF/F) in 420 pregnant women was approximately threefold larger than the ratio in nonpregnant individuals (44.6 versus 14.8, respectively)[72]; these authors also noted the wide range of values for NF/F in both groups, especially among the samples from pregnant subjects. In a PK study of intranasal fentanyl for labor analgesia, the median plasma fentanyl concentration 15 minutes after the first 50-μg dose was 0.21 ng/mL, which was approximately one-third less than the concentrations observed in nonpregnant subjects receiving fentanyl for dental surgery. An analgesic concentration of fentanyl (0.5 mg/mL) was reached in only 10 of 15 pregnant subjects.[73]

Oxycodone is metabolized approximately 45% by CYP3A4 to the inactive metabolite noroxycodone, and 19% by CYP2D6 to the active metabolite, oxymorphone.[74,75] Both the parent drug and its two metabolites also undergo glucuronidation by uridine 5′-diphosphate glucuronosyltransferase (UGT) 2B7 and UGT2B4 prior to renal excretion.[75] In a PK study of pregnant women receiving intravenous oxycodone for analgesia during the first stage of labor, the Vd was smaller, clearance was greater, and the elimination half-life of oxycodone was shorter (2.6 versus 3.8 hours) compared with nonpregnant volunteers.[76]

Tacrolimus is primarily metabolized by CYP3A4/5. Clearance of tacrolimus was shown to be 39% greater in the third trimester compared with postpartum.[77]

Lumefantrine, an antimalarial drug, is extensively metabolized by CYP3A4. In pregnant women, day 7 mean lumefantrine concentrations were significantly lower than in nonpregnant women (geometric mean ratio 1.40), increasing the risk for subtherapeutic concentrations and treatment failure.[63]

Protease inhibitors are primarily metabolized by CYP3A4. Because maintaining therapeutic concentrations is critical in

TABLE 16.2. Drug-Metabolizing Enzymes Involved in Opioid Metabolism

Opioid	Active Drug[a]	CYP3A	CYP2D6	CYP2B6	CYP2C19	Other CYPs	UGTs	Other Enzymes
Alfentanil		✓						
Buprenorphine		✓				CYP2C8	UGT2B7, UGT1A1, UGT1A3	
Butorphanol								Probably hepatic; enzymes not identified
Codeine[a]	Morphine and Morphine-6-glucuronide	✓	✓				UGT2B7, UGT2B4	
Fentanyl		✓						
Hydrocodone[a]	Hydromorphone and Dihydrocodone	✓	✓ (minor)					
Hydromorphone		✓					UGT2B7	SULT1A3
Meperidine (Pethidine)		✓		✓	✓	(minor: 2C8, 2D6, 2C9)	UGT2B4, UGT2B7	
Methadone		✓		✓	✓	(minor:2C8)	UGT2B7	
Morphine		✓ (minor)					UGT2B7	SULTs (minor: UGT1A1, UGT1A3, UGT1A8, UGT1A9, UGT1A10, UGT2B4, UGT2B15, UGT2B17)
Nalbuphine								Probably hepatic; enzymes not identified
Oxycodone		✓	✓				UGT2B4, UGT2B7	
Oxymorphone		✓	✓				UGT2B7	
Remifentanil								Hydrolysis by nonspecific blood and tissue esterases
Sufentanil		✓						
R,R-Tramadol/S,S-Tramadol[b]	O-Desmethyltramadol (M1)	✓	✓	✓			UGT2B7, UGT1A8	

[a]Administered drug is an inactive prodrug that is converted to the active drug; enzymes in the table are involved in conversion of the prodrug to the active drug or conjugating the prodrug.
[b]Tramadol is a racemic mixture of S/S and R/R enantiomers; M1 has greater mu-opioid activity (R,R-M1 > S,S-M1) than the parent tramadol. Although CYP enzymes metabolize both enantiomers, CYP2D6 preferentially metabolizes S,S-tramadol to the M1 metabolite, and CYP3A4 and CYP2B6 preferentially metabolize R,R-tramadol to N-desmethyltramadol (M2).
CYP, Cytochrome P450; NAT-2, N-acetyltransferase-2; SULT, sulfotransferase; UGT, uridine 5'-diphosphate glucuronosyltransferase.

the treatment of human immunodeficiency virus (HIV) disease, antiretroviral therapies have been better studied than any other class of drugs during pregnancy. Compared with postpartum values, the AUC of **darunavir** during the second and third trimesters is 38% to 39% smaller with once daily dosing and 26% smaller with twice daily dosing.[78] The AUC of **indinavir** was decreased by 68% at 30 to 32 weeks' gestation compared with values from the same women postpartum.[79] The geometric mean ratio of third trimester and postpartum **lopinavir** AUC (when administered as lopinavir/ritonavir) was 0.72, and 82% of the pregnant women did not meet target lopinavir AUC.[80] Because **atazanavir** AUC and trough concentration (C_{min}) are reduced by 6% to 47% during pregnancy, even when coadministered with the pharmacoenhancer, ritonavir,[81,82] some experts have recommended that the higher dose (atazanavir 400 mg/ritonavir 100 mg once daily) be used during pregnancy.[81,83]

Carbamazepine, an anticonvulsant, is converted to its 10,11-epoxide metabolite primarily by CYP3A4 with a minor contribution by CYP2C8. Carbamazepine is a well-known EID, stimulating its own metabolism through upregulation of transcription of CYP3A4 via the xenobiotic sensors, PXR and CAR. However, compared with nonpregnant baselines, no significant change in carbamazepine clearance was reported to occur during pregnancy.[84]

Methadone is N-demethylated mainly by CYP2B6 and CYP3A4, although there is some stereo-specificity among the minor enzymes involved in metabolism of its S- and R-enantiomers.[85] Methadone clearance increases during pregnancy, presumably because of increased CYP3A4 activity, necessitating dose escalation to maintain therapeutic plasma concentrations.[86–89]

Buprenorphine is metabolized by either (1) N-dealkylation to norbuprenorphine by CYP3A4 with some contribution by CYP2C8,[90] followed by glucuronidation by UGT1A1 and UGT1A3,[91] or (2) direct glucuronidation by UGT1A1, UGT1A3, and UGT2B7.[91] Metabolism via both pathways is increased during pregnancy.[91] Because plasma concentrations decreased below the theoretical level required to prevent withdrawal symptoms with the standard 12-hourly dosing in 50% to 80% of pregnant women, changing to a three to four times daily dosing schedule may be helpful to sustain therapeutic buprenorphine concentrations and improve adherence.[92]

Ketamine is converted to norketamine by both CYP3A4 and CYP2B6, with some studies supporting CYP2B6 as the dominant enzyme and others showing a primary role for CYP3A4.[93–95] Although there are no published PK studies of ketamine during pregnancy, given the involvement of CYP3A4, ketamine metabolism is most likely enhanced. Additional support for this hypothesis comes from PK studies of ketamine in women taking combined estrogen and progestin contraceptives, which showed that ketamine clearance was increased by 20% compared with men.[96]

CYP2D6. After CYP3A, CYP2D6 is the next most important CYP enzyme, contributing to the metabolism of about 20% of medications.[57] CYP2D6 has pharmacogenetic variants that are associated with estimated 1000-fold differences in activity: phenotypic **extensive metabolizers (EMs)** have two normally active alleles, **poor metabolizers (PMs)** have two loss-of-function alleles, **intermediate metabolizers (IMs)** have one active and one loss-of-function allele, and **ultrarapid metabolizers (UMs)** have multiple copies of an otherwise normally active allele. Allelic distribution varies by ethnicity; CYP2D6 PMs are most prevalent among the White population (7% to 10%), followed by African (1.9% to 7.3%), Hispanic ethnicity (2.2% to 6.6%), and Asian (0% to 1.2%). In contrast, UMs are more common in Arabian, East African, and Mediterranean populations (8.7% to 29%), but relatively infrequent among people of European descent (0.8% to 1.3%).[97]

Typically, CYP2D6 activity is not induced by PXR/CAR and the xenobiotic sensing system; the usual EIDs, **rifampin** and **carbamazepine**, do not change CYP2D6 activity. However, during pregnancy, studies examining CYP2D6 substrates have shown enhanced metabolism.[65,98–102] The exact mechanism by which this occurs is not known. Unlike CYP3A activity during pregnancy, which stays consistently elevated from the first trimester through delivery, CYP2D6 activity progressively increases by 25% in the late first/early second trimester to 48% in the late third trimester.[65] However, the increased activity is observed only in the EMs and UMs, with less change seen in the IMs, and no change in the PMs.[101,102] CYP2D6 activity is enhanced to such a degree during pregnancy that **clonidine**, which is primarily renally cleared, appears to switch to CYP2D6 metabolism as its primary elimination mechanism during pregnancy.[98,103]

Relevant drug examples.

Oral **metoprolol** was shown to have an apparent clearance 2 to 13 times greater in the third trimester compared with postpartum, and plasma concentrations during the third trimester were 12% to 55% of those after delivery.[99] In another study, the apparent clearance after oral administration in CYP2D6 EMs was 1.8-fold higher in mid-pregnancy and threefold higher in late pregnancy compared with postpartum. Metoprolol clearance in the CYP2D6 IMs progressively increased during pregnancy but was consistently lower than in the EMs.[100]

Dextromethorphan is O-demethylated by CYP2D6 to dextrorphan. By comparing dextromethorphan/dextrorphan metabolic ratios, CYP2D6 activity was shown to be 26% greater at 14 to 18 weeks', 35% greater at 24 to 28 weeks', and 48% greater at 36 to 40 weeks' gestation compared with postpartum.[65] When stratified by CYP2D6 phenotype, metabolism of dextromethorphan during pregnancy was increased in CYP2D6 EMs and IMs but decreased in PMs, compared with postpartum.[102]

Clonidine was shown to have apparent oral clearance that was twofold greater in the second and third trimesters compared with historic, nonpregnant controls (440 versus 245 mL/min) without significant change in renal clearance.[98]

Paroxetine concentrations in women taking the drug during pregnancy were found to progressively decrease in CYP2D6 EMs, while concentrations in IMs and PMs did not change or increased, respectively.[101]

CYP1A2. The CYP1 family of enzymes comprises three enzymes: CYP1A1, CYP1A2, and CYP1B1. CYP1A2 is found only in the liver and the other two only in extrahepatic tissues. CYP1A2 contributes to the metabolism of approximately 10% of medications, including **caffeine, theophylline, tricyclic antidepressants, acetaminophen** (minor), and **estrogens**.[104] Among the compounds that inhibit CYP1A2, **estradiol** downregulates its transcription and decreases its activity.[105–107] **Caffeine** metabolism is remarkably complex, but more than 95% is by CYP1A2.[108] Using caffeine metabolism as a probe for CYP1A2, compared with postpartum, CYP1A2 activity was shown to progressively decrease during pregnancy with reductions of 32.8% at 14 to 18 weeks', 48.1% at 24 to 28 weeks', and 65.2% at 36 to 40 weeks' gestation.[65]

CYP2A6. CYP2A6 is involved with the metabolism of approximately 3% of commonly used medications.[57] It is the primary enzyme responsible for the oxidation of **nicotine** and **cotinine**. CYP2A6 is highly polymorphic with approximately 40 allelic variations that differ in their level of activity.[109] Estrogen induces activity of CYP2A6 through the estrogen receptor (ERα), which acts as a transcription factor when bound to a promoter element associated with the CYP2A6 gene.[110] Nicotine C-oxidation via CYP2A6 was shown to be higher in early and late pregnancy (1.07-fold and 1.11-fold, respectively) compared with postpartum, as determined by analyzing urine samples from pregnant smokers.[111] In addition, nicotine N-glucuronidation by UGT2B10 was increased during early and late pregnancy (1.33-fold and 1.67-fold, respectively) compared with postpartum.[111]

CYP2B6. The status of CYP2B6 activity during pregnancy is unclear. Although estradiol induces transcription of CYP2B6 RNA in cultured hepatocytes,[112] studies of medications metabolized by CYP2B6 during pregnancy are either less definitive or show no significant changes. Assessing specific CYP2B6 activity is often problematic because CYP2B6 contributes to the metabolism of approximately 25% to 30% of the drugs metabolized by CYP3A4, and few drugs are uniquely metabolized by CYP2B6.[113]

Relevant drug examples.

Efavirenz, an antiretroviral medication, is a probe drug for CYP2B6. Its PK parameters were either not significantly different during pregnancy compared with postpartum or insufficiently different to warrant a dosing adjustment.[114,115]

Bupropion, a smoking cessation drug, is metabolized by CYP2B6 to hydroxybupropion. The metabolic ratio of hydroxybupropion to bupropion (OHBUP/BUP) has been used as a CYP2B6 probe. Compared with postpartum, no significant changes were observed in the OHBUP/BUP ratio or OHBUP concentrations in mid- or late pregnancy.[116] These findings were confirmed in a subsequent study; steady-state plasma concentrations and clearances of the bupropion enantiomers and metabolites were not different during pregnancy and the distant postpartum period.[117]

Methadone C/D ratios, conversely, decrease and clearance increases during pregnancy[88]; however, it is not known whether these changes occur because of the increased activity of CYP3A4 or CYP2B6, because both metabolize methadone.

CYP2C9. **Estradiol** increases CYP2C9 activity in cultured hepatocytes by unknown mechanisms that do not involve increased mRNA transcription.[118] This observation has been confirmed by PK studies during pregnancy with drugs metabolized by CYP2C9.

Relevant drug examples.

Indomethacin's apparent oral clearance in the second trimester was greater (14.5 versus 6.5 to 9.8 L/h) and the mean plasma concentration after a 25-mg oral dose was 37% lower compared with historic controls.[119]

Glyburide clearance in pregnant women with type 2 diabetes mellitus was twofold higher during the third trimester compared with nonpregnant women.[120] Using modeling simulations, the authors of this study predicted that, compared with the usual twice daily dose of 1.25 to 10 mg, glyburide would have to be increased during pregnancy to as much as 23.75 mg twice daily for optimal glucose control.

CYP2C19. Similar to CYP2D6, CYP2C19 has common phenotypes with dramatically different activity: poor (two loss-of-function or no-function alleles), intermediate (one loss-of-function and one normal-function or gain-of-function allele), extensive (two normal-function alleles), rapid (one normal-function and one gain-of-function allele), and UMs (two gain-of-function alleles).[121] Hepatocyte studies confirm downregulation of CYP2C19 expression by estrogens.[122]

Relevant drug examples.

Proguanil conversion to the active antimalarial drug cycloguanil is decreased by approximately 60% during the third trimester of pregnancy in CYP2C19 EMs. This conversion was also decreased in women taking estrogen-containing contraceptives. Pregnancy did not affect the metabolic activity of CYP2C19 PMs.[123] These authors recommended an increase in proguanil dosing during pregnancy.[124]

Esomeprazole (S-omeprazole) is primarily metabolized by CYP2C19 to a desmethyl metabolite and a 5-hydroxy metabolite, while a smaller amount is metabolized by CYP3A4 to 3-hydroxyomeprazole.[125,126] After a single dose, esomeprazole clearance was 42.2% lower in pregnant versus nonpregnant patients.[127]

CYP2E1. CYP2E1 is an unusual CYP enzyme; it is not activated by nuclear receptors but rather induced by **human placental lactogen (hPL)** through the phosphoinositol 3-kinase pathway.[128] Because of the enzyme's preference for small molecules, CYP2E1 is not involved in the metabolism of many drugs. During pregnancy, hPL increases 10-fold.

Relevant drug examples.

Ethanol is a substrate for CYP2E1 (ethanol oxidation) as well as both an inducer and inhibitor.

Acetaminophen metabolism by CYP2E1 is responsible for hepatotoxicity.[129]

Halothane, isoflurane, sevoflurane, enflurane, and **desflurane** are metabolized predominantly by CYP2E1.[130–132] However, with the exception of sevoflurane, of which 5% to 8% is metabolized, metabolism of the newer halogenated anesthetic agents is minimal.[133] Less than 2% of isoflurane can be recovered in the urine as metabolites and an even smaller amount of desflurane (<0.02%) is metabolized.[133] The impact of increased CYP2E1 activity during pregnancy on sevoflurane metabolism has not been studied.

Caffeine is primarily (70% to 80%) metabolized via 3-*N* demethylation to paraxanthine by CYP1A2. Only 7% to 8% is converted to theobromine by CYP1A2 and CYP2E1 (1-N demethylation) and another 7% to 8% is metabolized to theophylline by CYP2C8/9, CYP3A4, and possibly CYP2E1 and CYP1A2 (7-N demethylation). Of the remainder, approximately 15% is C-8 hydroxylated by CYP1A2, CYP3A4, CYP2C8/9, and CYP2E1.[134] However, in a PK study in pregnant women, the dominant metabolite was theobromine rather than paraxanthine, reflecting suppression of CYP1A2 and induction of CYP2E1 during pregnancy.[135] CYP2E1 activity and theobromine concentration were shown to be increased in pregnant women by consumption of charbroiled meat (a known inducer of CYP2E1 activity) and by acetaminophen use (twofold and fivefold increases, respectively).[135]

Phase II Drug-Metabolizing Enzymes and Pregnancy

Uridine 5′-diphosphate glucuronosyltransferases.
Mammalian UGTs are divided into two families: UGT1 and UGT2. In humans, the UGT1A gene cluster is located on chromosome 2q37 and contains nine functional isoforms: UGT1A1, and UGT1A3 through UGT10, plus four defunct pseudogenes. UGT2A (three isoforms) and UGT2B (seven isoforms) subfamilies are located on chromosome 4q13. UGT enzymes are primarily produced within the liver and gastrointestinal tract, but they also play significant roles in the kidney and can be found in the pancreas, trachea, lung, heart, bone marrow, spleen, thymus, adrenal gland, thyroid, ovary, uterus, cervix, placenta, breast, testis, prostate, adipose, skeletal muscle, brain, nasal mucosa, and bladder.[136] Expression of UGTs and their activities vary significantly among individuals and is influenced by multiple transcription factors, many of which are either enzyme- or family-specific (e.g., inducing UGT1A but not UGT2B). Each enzyme also has numerous pharmacogenetic variants with variable degrees of function. Some drugs are uniquely conjugated by one of the UGT enzymes; many compounds are substrates of multiple UGTs.[137]

UGT1A1.
UGT1A1 metabolizes **labetalol** and **bilirubin** as well as several of the antiretroviral integrase inhibitors, **bictegravir**, **dolutegravir**, and **raltegravir**. It contributes to the metabolism of **acetaminophen**, many **NSAIDs**, and **statins**, as well as **morphine** and **buprenorphine**.[136] In hepatocyte studies, progesterone is one of several factors that increase transcription of UGT1A1.[136,138] During pregnancy, UGT1A1 activity progressively increases across gestational age.[139]

Relevant drug examples.
Oral **labetalol**, taken by pregnant women for chronic hypertension, was shown to have apparent clearance that was 1.4-fold greater in the late first trimester and 1.6-fold greater at term compared with postpartum.[139] In an earlier study, the elimination half-life of labetalol in the third trimester was shorter than in nonpregnant controls (1.7 versus 6 to 8 hours).[140] Authors of both studies[139,140] advised that the dosing interval for labetalol may need to be shortened during pregnancy to maintain hypertensive control.

UGT1A4.
Of all the metabolic enzyme processes studied during pregnancy, none changes as dramatically as UGT1A4

glucuronidation. UGT1A4 is either the primary or contributing enzyme for approximately two dozen medications, including **lamotrigine**, **valproic acid**, **midazolam**, multiple **antipsychotics**, **cyclobenzaprine**, **amitriptyline**, **phenytoin**, and **ethinyl estradiol**. Using hepatocyte cultures, estrogen has been shown to upregulate UGT1A4 transcription.[141]

Relevant drug examples.
Lamotrigine, an anticonvulsant and mood-stabilizing drug, is primarily metabolized by UGT1A4.[142] When lamotrigine was administered to women taking oral contraceptives, its clearance did not change in women taking progestin-only pills, while it increased, and breakthrough seizures occurred, in women taking combination estrogen and progestin contraceptives.[143] Subsequent investigations have shown that enhanced lamotrigine clearance begins from as early as 5 weeks' gestation and progressively increases until it peaks in the third trimester at 248% to 330% above baseline.[144-146] However, not all pregnant women exhibit the same marked increase in glucuronidation. In a PK study of women receiving lamotrigine who were pregnant or planning pregnancy, Polepally et al.[147] identified two subpopulations: in 77% of 64 pregnancies, third trimester oral lamotrigine clearance increased 219% above baseline, where as in 23%, it rose by only 21%. Factors that differentiate these populations have not been identified. Many authors recommend monthly drug monitoring with serial dose increases to maintain stable therapeutic lamotrigine concentrations during pregnancy.[144] Because clearance of lamotrigine falls rapidly after delivery and returns to nonpregnant levels by 3 weeks postpartum, dose tapering should begin within the first week after delivery to prevent possible lamotrigine toxicity.[144]

Dexmedetomidine is hepatically metabolized to inactive metabolites by two pathways: (1) direct glucuronidation by UGT1A4 and UGT2B10 and (2) hydroxylation of a smaller fraction by CYP2A6.[148] Although induction mechanisms for UGT2B10 are currently unknown,[136] UGT1A4 and CYP2A6 are both upregulated by estrogen. No studies exploring the maternal PK of dexmedetomidine have been performed.

UGT2B7.
UGT2B7 contributes to the glucuronidation of approximately 35% of commonly used medications. Important substrates include (1) the opioid drugs **morphine**, **codeine**, **buprenorphine**, and **naloxone**; (2) other drugs, including **zidovudine**, **efavirenz**, **haloperidol**, **ethanol**, **lorazepam**, **NSAIDs**, and **chloramphenicol**; (3) the endogenous compounds **bile acids**, **fatty acids**, and **retinoic acids**; and (4) multiple steroid hormones, including **estrogens**, **catecholestrogens**, **androgens**, **glucocorticoids**, and **mineralocorticoids**.[136] UGT2B7 is widely distributed throughout the body: in the liver, small intestine, kidney, breast, lung, placenta, adipose, skin, pancreas, bladder, uterus, brain, and adrenal.[136] Regulation of UGT2B7 transcription involves a system unrelated to the xenobiotic nuclear receptors that induce some of the CYP and UGT1A genes. Instead, UGT2B7 is regulated by the transcription factors, hepatocyte nuclear factor 1α (HNF1α) and HNF4α with contributions from caudal-related homeobox transcription factor 2 (CDX-2).[136] Classic hormonal changes during pregnancy do not appear to influence this regulatory system.[138,149,150]

Relevant drug examples.

Zidovudine is metabolized (60% to 70%) to its inactive metabolite 5′-glucuronyl zidovudine exclusively by UGT2B7, making it an ideal probe for UGT2B7 activity.[151] In multiple PK studies performed in pregnant women, zidovudine total body clearance, maximum concentration, and elimination half-life were not significantly different from the same parameters in nonpregnant adults.[149,150]

Morphine is metabolized predominantly by UGT2B7. In nonpregnant adults, approximately 60% is glucuronidated to inactive morphine-3-glucuronide (M3G), while 5% to 10% is glucuronidated to the active metabolite, morphine-6-glucuronide (M6G).[151–153] A third pathway, catalyzed primarily by CYP3A4 and CYP2C8, is *N*-demethylation to normorphine.[152] UGT2B7 is the dominant enzyme facilitating both glucuronidation pathways[151]; however, *in vitro* studies have shown that other UGTs can participate, including UGT2B4, UGT2B15, UGT2B17, UGT1A1, UGT1A3, UGT1A9, and UGT1A10 in the formation of M3G, and UGT2B4, UGT1A1, UGT1A3, and UGT1A8 to produce M6G.[152,154,155] In a PK study of morphine used for labor analgesia, its elimination half-life was approximately 49% shorter, plasma clearance was 70% greater, and the metabolic ratio of M3G/morphine at 10 minutes was 88% greater in pregnant women compared with nonpregnant subjects.[156] Given that UGT2B7 has been shown not to change during pregnancy, one potential explanation for the increased metabolism is that minor UGT enzymes, which are known to increase their activity during pregnancy, assume greater responsibility for morphine metabolism.

UGT1A6. In addition to metabolizing the endogenous hormone **serotonin**, UGT1A6 conjugates **acetaminophen** and **aspirin**.[136] Although UGT1A6 may weakly respond to PXR/CAR induction, its primary transcription control appears to be exerted through the aryl hydrocarbon receptor (AhR), which influences transcription similar to PXR/CAR.[136]

UGT1A9. UGT1A9 conjugates a variety of compounds, including **ethanol**, **nicotine**, **NSAIDs**, **propranolol**, **hydroxywarfarin**, **furosemide**, **acetaminophen**, and **cannabinol**.[136] Transcriptional regulation of UGT1A9 appears to involve similar mechanisms as UGT2B7: HNF1α and HNF4α with CDX-2.

Relevant drug examples.

Propofol and its hydroxy metabolite (created by CYP2C9 and CYP2B6) are exclusively conjugated by UGT1A9. In a study of women who received propofol anesthesia for first-trimester termination of pregnancy, specific UGT1A9 pharmacogenetic variants shortened the duration of effective analgesia and sedation.[157] Propofol clearance was shown to be 30% faster in women having cesarean delivery compared with women undergoing laparoscopic sterilization.[158] In the latter study, the authors did not analyze metabolites, so it is unknown which pathway (UGT1A9 and/or CYP2C9/2B6) drove the increase in propofol clearance.

Furosemide elimination in nonpregnant individuals is 40% to 70% by unchanged drug excretion in urine and 20% to 30% by metabolism within the kidney and liver by UGT1A9 and UGT1A1.[159,160] In hypertensive women at term, the median apparent oral clearance was two- to threefold higher (25.3 L/h) compared with historical data from nonpregnant individuals (8.3 to 15.7 L/h) after administration of 40 mg.[21] Of interest, glucuronidation played a more dominant role in furosemide elimination in pregnant patients, contributing to 90% of total clearance (22.7 L/h), compared with 60% (3.7 to 10.6 L/h) in the nonpregnant controls.[21] It is unknown whether UGT1A9 contributes to the increase in glucuronidation or if it is solely by UGT1A1.

Acetaminophen (paracetamol) is metabolized through three different pathways. In nonpregnant adults, approximately 47% to 62% is converted to an inactive glucuronide (by UGT1A6 and UGT1A9 with minor contribution from UGT1A1 and UGT2B15), and 30% to 44% is sulfate conjugated. Eight to 10% is oxidized to the reactive metabolite, *N*-acetyl-*p*-benzoquinone-imine (NAPQI), primarily by CYP2E1, with minor contribution from CYP3A4, CYP1A2, CYP2D6, and CYP2A6. NAPQI is rapidly conjugated by hepatic glutathione, thereby preventing hepatic toxicity at therapeutic dosing. Less than 5% is excreted in the urine as unchanged drug.[161]

When acetaminophen was given intravenously to women after cesarean delivery (2-g loading dose followed by 1 g 6-hourly maintenance doses), total clearance was almost twice as high (21.1 versus 11.7 L/h) compared with a subset of the same patients who received a 2-g loading dose 10 to 15 weeks postpartum.[161] Further analysis revealed that the increase in clearance was due to enhanced glucuronidation (11.6 versus 4.76 L/h), increased oxidation (4.95 versus 2.77 L/h), and increased urinary excretion of unchanged drug (1.15 versus 0.75 L/h). In contrast, sulfate conjugation was unchanged. Increased acetaminophen clearance during pregnancy has been confirmed in other studies.[162,163] Although increasing the acetaminophen dose may counter the impact of this increased clearance, caution was advised because a higher dose would also increase production of NAPQI and the risk of hepatoxicity.[161] Increased acetaminophen clearance also occurs in women taking oral combination hormonal contraceptives. Compared with controls, plasma acetaminophen clearance was approximately 64% higher (470 versus 287 mL/min) and the elimination half-life was lower (1.67 versus 2.40 hours).[164] Hormonal contraception also increased glucuronidation without change in sulfation. It is not known which of the reproductive hormones is responsible for the induction of glucuronidation and which of the UGT enzymes is/are induced.

UGT2B15. UGT2B15 is widely expressed throughout the body, including in reproductive organs, and is involved in the metabolism of endogenous steroids and a number of drugs, including **acetaminophen**, **oxazepam**, and **lorazepam**.[136] Control of its transcription is complex but studies have identified the presence of an estrogen receptor binding site with estradiol upregulation.[136]

Relevant drug examples.

Lorazepam is administered as a racemic mixture of which only the *S*-enantiomer is biologically active. Both enantiomers are metabolized by the same enzymes (predominantly UGT2B15, plus UGT2B4 and UGT2B7) as well as stereo-specific enzymes (*R*-lorazepam is also metabolized by

UGT1A7 and UGT1A10).[165] In a PK study of oral lorazepam (2 mg) in laboring women, the apparent Vd was increased (mean 178.8 L) compared with historic controls (93 to 116 L), owing to decreased protein binding and increased total body water.[166] Apparent clearance after oral lorazepam administration was approximately twofold higher (mean 2.61 mL/min kg) compared with historic controls (0.84 to 1.8 mL/min kg) and the mean elimination half-life was lower (10 hours) compared with 16 hours in historic controls.[166]

Other Phase II enzymes. In an early study, *N*-acetyltransferase-2 (NAT-2) activity was shown to be significantly decreased during pregnancy using caffeine metabolism (a secondary pathway).[167] However, subsequent studies have reported different results. Also using caffeine, the activity of NAT-2 in pregnant women (all fast acetylators), decreased by only 13% and only during early pregnancy; NAT-2 activity returned to nonpregnant levels during mid- and late pregnancy.[168] The absence of significant change in NAT-2 activity between pregnant and nonpregnant individuals was confirmed using hydralazine. Although there was a clear difference between fast and slow acetylators, and the study did not explore the first trimester, the authors demonstrated that hydralazine PK during the second and third trimesters of pregnancy was reasonably comparable with that of nonpregnant subjects in prior studies.[169] Although activity of SULT2A1, one of the most important of the sulfotransferase (SULT) enzymes, is upregulated by estradiol in cultured hepatocytes,[170] sulfation of acetaminophen during pregnancy does not appear to change.[161] Very little is known about the activity of other Phase II enzymes during pregnancy.

Medications Metabolized by Enzymes Affected Variably During Pregnancy

Meperidine (pethidine) transformation to its active metabolite, normeperidine (norpethidine), is catalyzed by CYP2B6, CYP3A4, and CYP2C19. *In vitro* hepatocyte studies have shown that CYP2B6, CYP3A4, and CYP2C19 account for 57%, 28%, and 15%, respectively, of the total intrinsic clearance of meperidine.[171] In a PK study of meperidine administered to pregnant women in labor, no differences were observed in metabolism or clearance of meperidine, compared with nonpregnant controls in the early follicular phase (low estradiol/no progesterone).[172] One possible explanation for these findings is that the *decrease* in CYP2C19 activity counters the *increase* in CYP3A4 activity. Based on current knowledge, CYP2B6 does not change, resulting in no significant net change in meperidine metabolism.

Sertraline is metabolized to its desmethyl metabolite by CYP2C19 and CYP3A4, with minor contributions by CYP2C9, CYP2B6, and CYP2D6.[173,174] Studies have shown that the CYP2C19 phenotype impacts sertraline metabolism and dosing requirements in nonpregnant patients; lacking one of the primary enzymes that metabolize sertraline, CYP2C19 PMs have higher sertraline C/D ratios and often require lower starting doses.[175,176] In a PK study of sertraline across pregnancy and postpartum, the mean pregnant and postpartum C/D ratios in women with functional CYP2C19

activity (EMs/UMs/rapid metabolizers) were not significantly different because the *increase* in CYP3A4 metabolism was countered by the *decrease* in CYP2C19 activity.[177] However, a significant difference was observed in CYP2C19 PMs/IMs; with primarily CYP3A4 to metabolize sertraline, their mean C/D ratios during pregnancy were approximately 50% lower than postpartum, potentially placing them at risk of inadequate therapy during pregnancy.[177]

PHARMACODYNAMIC CHANGES DURING PREGNANCY: IMPACT ON ANESTHETIC AND ANALGESIC DRUGS

Distinct from PK, which focuses on the processes that affect drug concentration, **PD** relates to the interaction of the drug with its environment, its receptor or enzyme binding site, and ultimately its impact on downstream biochemical and physiologic effects. Although the complex physiologic changes that occur during pregnancy affect the PD environment of many of the medications we use, this discussion will focus on the perception of pain in the pregnant woman and its impact on drugs used for anesthesia and analgesia.

Endogenous opioids, acting through their respective receptors, modulate pain and influence other functions by inhibiting voltage-gated calcium channels and/or by opening potassium channels, both of which inhibit neuronal excitability.[178] Opioid receptors are located within the brain, spinal cord, peripheral neurons, gastrointestinal tract, heart, immune cells, and other tissues, including extensively within the placenta.[178–180] Early research dating back to the 1980s has identified both kappa-[181] (most prevalent) and mu-opioid receptors[182] within the placenta, as well as all three endogenous opioid families: **β-endorphin**, **enkephalins** (both methionine and leucine), and **dynorphins**, with dynorphin 1 to 8 being the major form in the human chorionic villi.[183] One of the endogenous opioids, β-endorphin, is derived from proopiomelanocortin (POMC), a protein that is cleaved into four different peptides: ACTH, α-melanocyte-stimulating hormone, β-lipotropin, and β-endorphin.[11] The placenta synthesizes significant amounts of CRH, which induces placental production of POMC and β-endorphin.[184] Although placental opioids are known to increase nitric oxide locally,[182] stimulate release of hCG[185] and hPL,[186] and suppress interleukin-8 (IL-8) production (which could otherwise initiate preterm labor),[187] the full extent of the role of placental opioids remains elusive.

Beyond the placenta, endogenous opioids contribute to the support of pregnancy through the regulation of several neuroendocrine systems which optimize fetal growth, protect the fetus from maternal stress, inhibit preterm labor throughout gestation, and facilitate parturition and subsequent lactation.[188] Endogenous opioids inhibit posterior pituitary secretion of oxytocin, thus expanding oxytocin storage during pregnancy until just before labor onset.[188] They inhibit dopamine secretion into the hypothalamic-hypophyseal portal blood system, thereby promoting prolactin surges both in early pregnancy and during lactation.[188] Endogenous opioids also contribute to attenuation of the hypothalamic-pituitary-adrenal axis response to psychologic and physical stressors during pregnancy, including increasing the threshold for perception of pain.[188]

The physiologic changes that occur during human pregnancy and parturition create opioid-mediated maternal analgesia that operates through the spinal cord dynorphin/kappa-opioid system.[189] Evidence to support the role of endogenous opioids in pregnancy-induced analgesia can be found in experiments with other mammals. Maternal pain thresholds were evaluated across pregnancy and postpartum in pregnant rats by measuring the intensity of an electric shock that elicited reflexive jumping. Pain thresholds gradually rose during the second half of gestation and then rapidly increased 1 to 2 days before parturition. This increased pain threshold was abolished by exposure to the opioid antagonist naltrexone.[190] Administration of estradiol and progesterone in concentrations that simulate pregnancy to nonpregnant, ovariectomized rats produced elevated pain thresholds similar to that observed during actual pregnancy.[189] These changes were blocked by naltrexone. Administration of estrogen and progesterone separately or sequentially failed to produce the increased pain thresholds.[189] In response to mild thermal stimulation, pregnant pigs exhibited increased pain thresholds so profound that just before labor the majority of the sows failed to respond at all.[191] Administration of naloxone to half of the sows during labor reversed this tolerance.

Similar results have been reported in human pregnancies, although the findings have not been as consistent as those in animals. Compared with nonpregnant controls, heat pain thresholds progressively increased in both the forearm and T10 dermatome in pregnant women when tested during the early and late third trimester and early labor. The contact heat-evoked potentials were significantly lower at 40 weeks' compared with 32 weeks' gestation, supporting a general inhibitory mechanism during pregnancy that increases at term.[192] Other investigators reported that heat pain tolerance was higher before delivery and 1 to 2 days postdelivery in pregnant women than in nonpregnant conrols.[193] In contrast, a subsequent study by the same authors observed no change in pain evaluations (conditioned pain modulation, mechanical temporal stimulation and temperature pain scores) in the first, second, and third trimesters compared with 6 to 12 weeks postpartum.[194]

This reduced capacity to feel pain is one mechanism that underlies the changes in dosing requirement observed in pregnant women for both anesthetic and analgesic medications; minimal alveolar concentration (MAC) values for volatile anesthetic agents during pregnancy are reduced. MAC values for **isoflurane**, **halothane**, and **methoxyflurane** in anesthetized pregnant ewes were reduced by 25% to 40% compared with nonpregnant ewes.[195] Similarly, MAC values for halothane in pregnant rats were decreased by 19% during midgestation and by 16% at term, and returned to control values by 5 days postpartum.[196]

The MAC values for volatile anesthetic agents during pregnancy were first evaluated in women undergoing early pregnancy termination (8 to 12 weeks).[197] Using transcutaneous electrical stimulation to elicit pain, isoflurane MAC was decreased by 28% compared with nonpregnant controls. In a subsequent study in a similar population, MAC for enflurane was decreased by 30% and halothane by 27% compared with MAC values in nonpregnant women undergoing laparoscopy.[198] The authors then evaluated MAC for isoflurane at 28 to 126 hours after delivery in women undergoing tubal ligation.[199] The 30% reduction in MAC persisted for 24 to 36 hours after delivery and then gradually returned to normal values by 72 hours after delivery. Other investigators performed a similar study with isoflurane in women undergoing postpartum tubal ligation and confirmed the findings[200]; MAC for isoflurane was reduced by 28% within the first 12 hours after delivery and returned to normal values by 25 hours.

Some authors have hypothesized that increased progesterone is responsible for the observed changes in the MAC values for volatile anesthetic agents. The addition of progesterone reduced the MAC for halothane in rabbits,[201] and lower concentrations of **sevoflurane** were needed to maintain a constant bispectral index in women during the luteal phase of the menstrual cycle when ovarian progesterone is elevated compared with the follicular phase when progesterone concentrations are negligible.[202] However, studies in human pregnancy and postpartum have inconsistently correlated changes in MAC to progesterone concentrations.[200,203]

Local anesthetics employed for nerve blocks have faster onset and longer duration during pregnancy. The time to onset of a conduction block of the vagus nerve with **bupivacaine** was faster in both an *in vitro* sheath nerve preparation[204] and live animal studies[205] in pregnant compared with nonpregnant rabbits. **Lidocaine** blockade of the sciatic nerve was achieved at the same time in pregnant versus nonpregnant rats, but it lasted 48% longer in the pregnant rats and the lidocaine concentration at return of deep pain sensation was 43% lower in the pregnant animals.[206] The same phenomenon was observed in humans; median nerve block at the wrist with lidocaine inhibited sensory nerve action potentials to a greater extent in pregnant woman compared with nonpregnant subjects.[207]

Dosing for neuraxial anesthesia during pregnancy is also affected by anatomic factors; pregnant women have increased epidural blood volume, especially in the supine position, which decreases the capacity of the epidural space and volume of lumbar cerebral spinal fluid (see Chapter 2). By itself, this increases the spread of local anesthetic within the subarachnoid space.[208–210] In a study of motor block with intrathecal plain **bupivacaine** in pregnant and nonpregnant women undergoing cesarean delivery or elective gynecologic surgery, the ED_{50} (median effective dose) was 3.96 mg for pregnant women versus 4.51 mg for nonpregnant women.[211] In a similar study, the ED_{50} for motor block with intrathecal bupivacaine was 3.4 mg for pregnant women versus 5.2 mg for nonpregnant women.[212]

GENERAL PRINCIPLES OF TERATOLOGY AND DRUG USE DURING PREGNANCY

Safe use of drugs during pregnancy includes consideration of not only maternal safety but also potential fetal impact. A fetal effect of particular concern is teratogenesis. A broad definition of a teratogen is a substance that has an adverse effect on the developing fetus by altering the growth, structure, or function of the developing embryo. The principles of teratology as outlined by Wilson[213] are shown in Box 16.1. Potential fetal risks from intrauterine exposure to anesthetic drugs are summarized in Table 16.3. Structural and behavioral teratology of anesthetic agents are discussed in Chapters 10 and 18. Data for nonanesthetic drugs are shown in Appendix 16.1 (online only).

Specific Highly Teratogenic Drugs

Some drugs are so highly teratogenic that two simultaneous forms of reliable contraception are recommended or required during treatment of either partner, sometimes to be continued for months or years after stopping the drug. Examples include: (1) **thalidomide** (and analogs), which is still used to treat erythema nodosum leprosum and multiple myeloma (fetal effect: severe malformations of the limbs [phocomelia], axial skeleton, head, face, eyes, ears, tongue, teeth, gastrointestinal tract, central nervous system, cardiovascular system, and respiratory systems)[236]; (2) the antiviral **ribavirin**, which is used for hepatitis C and viral hemorrhagic fevers (fetal effect: severe malformations and embryolethality at doses below recommended human doses reported in animal data)[214]; (3) **isotretinoin**, which is used for cystic acne (fetal effect: profound, extensive abnormalities of the central nervous, craniofacial and cardiovascular systems)[237]; and (4) **acitretin**, another retinoid that is used for severe psoriasis and is sequestered in fat tissue for at least 3 years.[214] In Europe, use of **valproate** requires a pregnancy prevention program (fetal effect: cardiovascular, craniofacial, genitourinary, and musculoskeletal malformations plus cognitive developmental delay).[238]

Drug Labeling for Pregnancy and Lactation

In 2014, the FDA published the **Pregnancy and Lactation Labeling Rule (PLLR)**.[239] This rule supplanted the previously used letter (ABCDX) categories, which were oversimplified and of limited utility in risk-benefit decision making. The PLLR was implemented on June 30, 2015, and applies to all prescription drugs approved on or after June 30, 2001. The label must be updated whenever new information is available and thus should serve as a reliable source of up-to-date information in a standardized format. The PLLR requires narrative descriptions of available data in three categories under the "Use in Specific Populations" section: (1) Pregnancy, (2) Lactation, and (3) Females and Males of Reproductive Potential (Box 16.2).

The PLLR guidelines are designed to overcome several limitations of the former letter-based categories, but many prescribers remain unfamiliar with the updated labeling guidelines. A 2018 survey of members of the American Academy of Allergy, Asthma, and Immunology found that less than half of respondents were aware of the updated labeling guidelines and 95% of respondents continued to use the former letter categories to make decisions.[240] Fifty-six percent of respondents indicated that the PLLR narrative format was unhelpful compared with the letter-based categories. The utility of the PLLR narrative is inherently confined by the amount of pregnancy and lactation data available for a particular

---

BOX 16.1 Principles of Teratology[a]

1. A teratogen produces a specific abnormality or constellation of abnormalities.
   Example: Fetal warfarin syndrome consists of facial and skeletal anomalies.[b]
2. There is a dose-effect relationship with progressively higher doses leading to more severe findings.
   Example: More frequent malformations are associated with doses of warfarin > 5 mg/d.[c]
3. A teratogen must reach the fetus in a sufficient amount to cause this effect.
   Example: Drugs that do not cross the placenta (e.g., heparin) cannot be teratogenic; drugs that have very limited fetal exposure because of either placental export or fetal metabolism are unlikely to be teratogenic.
4. Teratogen exposure must happen at a stage in fetal development to cause that effect.
   Example: Development of most organs and structures (organogenesis) occurs very early during pregnancy (beginning at approximately 2 weeks' gestation) and is largely complete by approximately 12 weeks' gestation. Neurodevelopment occurs throughout gestation and neonatal life (Fig. 16.2). Exposure to a specific drug at less than 4 weeks' gestation may cause miscarriage, at 2–8 weeks' gestation may cause major congenital heart defects, and at greater than 12 weeks' gestation may have no adverse structural impact at all. A drug that is teratogenic and causes neural tube development anomalies may have no effect when introduced in the second trimester because the neural tube is formed by this time. In contrast, drugs that could potentially impact neurodevelopment such as psychoactive agents have risk of teratogenicity throughout gestation.
5. Susceptibility to teratogenesis depends on the genotype of both mother and fetus.
   Example: Severity of fetal hydantoin syndrome depends on genotype-related alterations in activity of epoxide hydrolase.[d]

[a]Wilson JG. Experimental studies on congenital malformations. *J Chronic Dis*. 1959;10:111–130.
[b]Warkany J. Warfarin embryopathy. *Teratology*. 1976;14:205–209.
[c]Vitale N, De Feo M, De Santo LS, et al. Dose-dependent fetal complications of warfarin in pregnant women with mechanical heart valves. *J Am Coll Cardiol*. 1999;33:1637–1641.
[d]Buehler BA, Delimont D, van Waes M, Finnell RH. Prenatal prediction of risk of the fetal hydantoin syndrome. *N Engl J Med*. 1990;322:1567–1572.

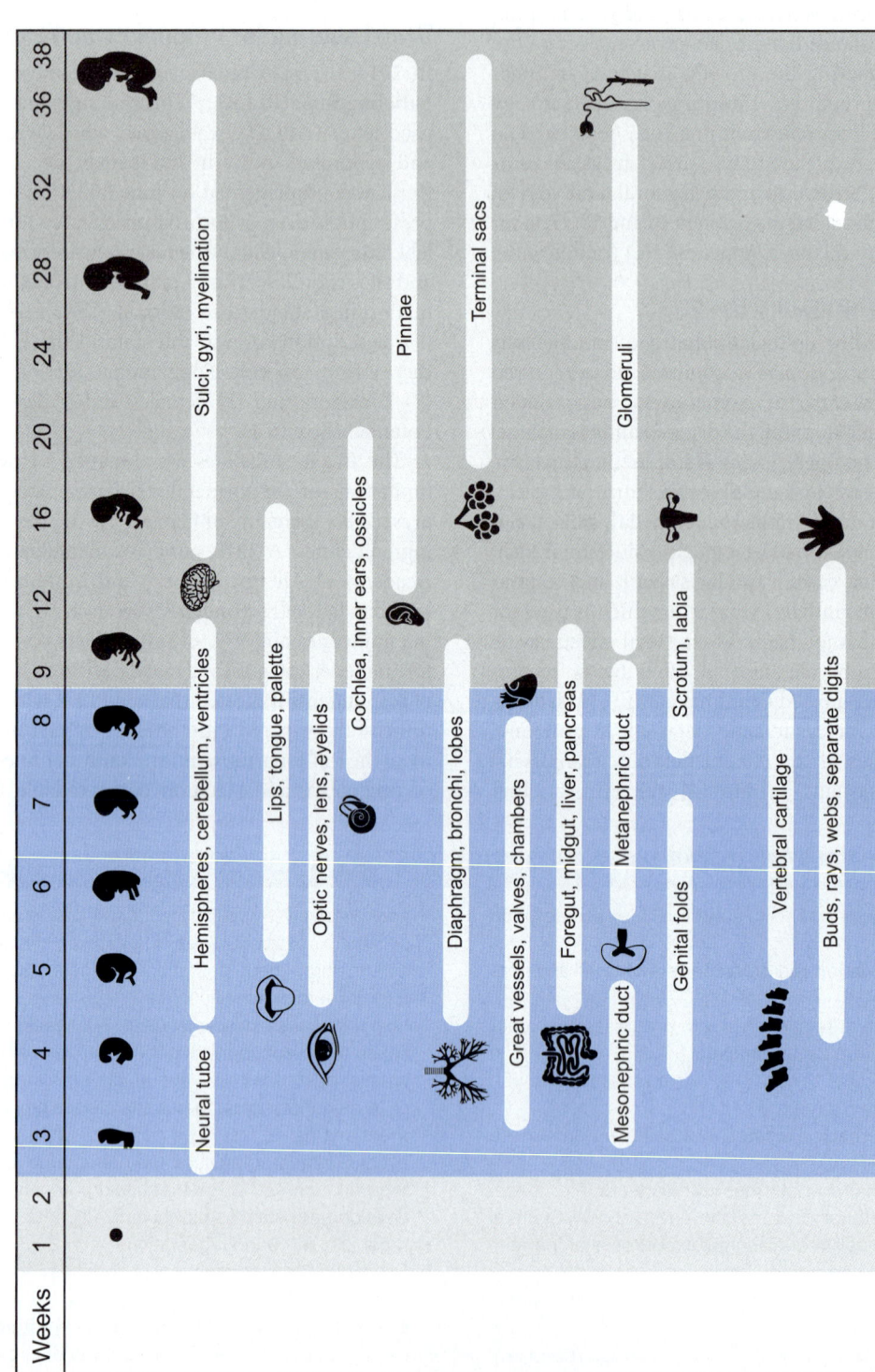

Fig. 16.2. Embryo-fetal development according to gestational age determined by the first day of the last menses. Times are approximate. Illustration by Naveen Nathan, MD, NorthShore University HealthSystem, University of Chicago Pritzker School of Medicine, Evanston, IL.

TABLE 16.3.   Potential Fetal Risks From Intrauterine Exposure to Anesthetic Drugs

Drug	Class	Comments/Potential Risks
General Anesthetic Drugs[a,b]		
Desflurane[214,215]	Inhalational halogenated anesthetic	No reports of potential teratogenicity from exposure early in human pregnancy. Not teratogenic in animals. Can cause neonatal depression, which may last up to 24 h. Dose-related relaxation of gravid uterine muscle reversible with oxytocin.
Isoflurane[214,216]	Inhalational halogenated anesthetic	No reports of potential teratogenicity from exposure early in human pregnancy. Not teratogenic in animals. Can cause neonatal depression, which may last up to 24 h. Dose-related relaxation of gravid uterine muscle reversible with oxytocin.
Sevoflurane[214,215]	Inhalational halogenated anesthetic	No reports of potential teratogenicity from exposure early in human pregnancy. Teratogenic in mice (cleft palate). Can cause neonatal depression, which may last up to 24 h. Dose-related relaxation of gravid uterine muscle reversible with oxytocin.
Ketamine[214,217,218]	General anesthetic, nonbarbiturate, phencyclidine derivative (NMDA receptor antagonist)	For isolated use for anesthesia indications, excluding chronic use for treatment of depression: no reports of malformations from exposure in humans or animals; however, no first trimester reports. Rapidly crosses the placenta. Maternal (hypertension) and neonatal (neonatal depression, increased skeletal muscle tone) adverse effects were observed with higher doses (1.5–2.2 mg/kg) in earlier studies and are less common with lower doses (0.2–0.5 mg/kg). Neonatal depression lower or absent with induction to delivery time < 10 min.
Nitrous oxide (N_2O)[214,219-225]	General anesthetic, sedative, analgesic, inorganic gas	Animal studies have suggested that exposure increases risks of dose-related fetal loss, growth restriction, skeletal malformations, major anomalies, and lower male-to-female sex ratios of surviving fetuses. However, with few exceptions, these studies were performed with exposures much higher and much longer than typical surgical exposures. 1970s and early 1980s studies of personnel in dental offices using N_2O sedation and hospital ORs prior to universal installation of anesthetic gas scavenging implicated occupational exposure in increased risk of spontaneous abortion with a dose-response association with duration of exposure versus unexposed subjects. In 1985, combined data showed RR 1.3 (95% CI, 1.2 to 1.4) for spontaneous abortion in pregnant physicians and nurses working in ORs. Although the OR environment contains other anesthetic agents, studies were performed in N_2O-only environments. Exposure is shorter for individual operations. In The Collaborative Perinatal Project, 76 of 50,282 monitored pregnancies were exposed to N_2O during first trimester surgery and there was no evidence of association with observed defects. The concomitant use of N_2O and ketamine (both NMDA receptor antagonists) without addition of a GABA agonist (e.g., halothane, isoflurane, propofol, benzodiazepines) was shown in animals to potentiate neurotoxicity of N_2O, especially in immature brains. When children aged 5–13 y born to mothers exposed to waste anesthetic gases during pregnancy were compared with unexposed controls, developmental milestones were similar, but exposed children had significantly lower gross motor ability and evidence of inattention/hyperactivity, and level of exposure negatively correlated with fine motor ability and IQ performance; it was concluded that occupational exposure to waste anesthetic gases during pregnancy might be a risk factor for minor neurologic deficits in the offspring. N_2O used for labor analgesia does not affect uterine activity, and does not adversely affect neonatal neurobehavior at 15 min, 2 h, or 24 h of age compared with unexposed neonates.
Propofol[214,226,227]	General anesthetic and hypnotic	Most reports have shown no difference in Apgar scores or time to sustained spontaneous respiration in infants exposed to propofol versus other general anesthetics, and no correlation has been found between Apgar scores and umbilical blood concentration of propofol. However, one study reported lower Apgar scores in infants exposed to propofol compared with infants born by spontaneous vaginal delivery.
Local Anesthetic Drugs		
2-Chloroprocaine[228]	Amino-ester local anesthetic	Rapid hydrolysis by esterases minimizes fetal exposure. No detectable parent drug in umbilical vein after perineal infiltration for episiotomy.
Bupivacaine[229]	Amino-amide local anesthetic	Lowest fetal/maternal total concentration ratio among amide-type agents owing to extensive binding to maternal alpha-1-acid glycoprotein. As a weak base, it may accumulate in the fetus in the setting of fetal acidosis.

(Continued)

TABLE 16.3. Potential Fetal Risks From Intrauterine Exposure to Anesthetic Drugs—cont'd

Drug	Class	Comments/Potential Risks
Lidocaine (lignocaine)[230–233]	Amino-amide local anesthetic	Crosses the placenta but no reported harm from exposure in the first 4 mo of pregnancy. Most studies during delivery have suggested no adverse fetal effects. One report of infant hypotonia and tonic seizures 1 h after birth and toxic levels of lidocaine following maternal perineal nerve block.
Ropivacaine[229,234]	Amino-amide local anesthetic	Increased free drug concentrations compared with bupivacaine owing to lower lipid solubility and protein binding; however, adverse fetal effects not reported. As a weak base, it may accumulate in the fetus in the setting of fetal acidosis.

[a]FDA Drug Safety Communication (December 16, 2016): FDA review resulted in new warnings about using general anesthetics and sedation drugs in young children and pregnant women. "The U.S. FDA is warning that repeated or lengthy use of general anesthetic and sedation drugs during surgeries or procedures in children younger than 3 years or in pregnant women during their third trimester may affect the development of children's brains. Consistent with animal studies, recent human studies suggest that a single, relatively short exposure to general anesthetic and sedation drugs in infants or toddlers is unlikely to have negative effects on behavior or learning…health care professionals should balance the benefits of appropriate anesthesia in young children and pregnant women against the potential risks, especially for procedures that may last longer than 3 hours or if multiple procedures are required in children under 3 years…This list includes anesthetic and sedation drugs that block NMDA receptors and/or potentiate GABA activity."[235] (See Chapter 10.)

[b]Because of adverse safety profiles, enflurane and halothane are not in common use in the United States and therefore are not included.

CI, Confidence interval; *FDA,* US Food and Drug Administration; *GABA,* gamma-amino-butyric acid; *IQ,* intelligence quotient; *NMDA,* N-methyl-D-aspartate; *OR,* operating room; *RR,* risk ratio.

BOX 16.2 Food and Drug Administration Pregnancy and Lactation Labeling Rule

Pregnancy Section

1. *Pregnancy Exposure Registry:* This section is only required if a scientifically acceptable registry exists that includes the labeled drug. It lists contact information to enroll in the registry or obtain additional information.
2. *Risk Summary:* This section describes the risk of adverse developmental outcomes based on all relevant human, animal, and pharmacologic data. Adverse developmental outcomes include structural abnormalities, embryo-fetal and/or infant mortality, functional impairment, and alterations to growth. Information on the background risk of major birth defects and miscarriage should be included for systemically absorbed medications.
3. *Clinical Considerations:* This section provides information to aid healthcare providers in prescribing and provision of risk-benefit counseling. Where information is available, this section includes five subheadings: (1) disease-associated maternal and/or embryo/fetal risk, (2) dose adjustments during pregnancy and the postpartum period, (3) maternal adverse reactions, (4) fetal/neonatal adverse reactions, and (5) labor or delivery.

4. *Data:* This section describes the data that provided the scientific basis for the information presented in the "Risk Summary" and "Clinical Considerations" sections.

Lactation Section

1. *Risk Summary:* This section summarizes information on the presence of a drug and/or its active metabolite(s) in human milk, the effect of the drug/metabolite(s) on the breastfed child, and the effect of the drug/metabolite(s) on milk production.
2. *Clinical Considerations:* This section includes information on methods to minimize exposure of the breastfed child and available interventions for monitoring and mitigating adverse drug reactions in the breastfed child.
3. *Data:* This section describes the data that provided the scientific basis for the information presented in the "Risk Summary" and "Clinical Considerations" sections.

Females and Males of Reproductive Potential Section

Pregnancy Testing, Contraception, and Infertility: These sections address whether pregnancy testing or contraception is recommended or required before, during, or after drug therapy and available data regarding adverse effects on fertility.

Modified from Food and Drug Administration. Content and format of labeling for human prescription drug and biological products: requirements for pregnancy and lactation labeling. *Fed Regist.* 2014;79:72064–72103.

---

drug. An analysis of new drugs approved between 2010 and 2019 found that only 10.7% and 2.8% had available human data for pregnancy and lactation, respectively. Nearly half of medications evaluated had no animal or human lactation data.[241] It will be imperative to continue to evaluate awareness and perceived utility of the PLLR system as the number of medications that are PLLR-compliant and the amount of available human data increase.

Drug Use During Lactation

Studies estimate that 66% to 84% of breastfeeding women use medication(s) during lactation.[242,243] Nursing parents are understandably concerned about the transfer of drugs and chemicals to breast milk. Accurate advice is important to prevent unnecessary cessation of breastfeeding or discontinuation of appropriate drug treatment. Unfortunately, nearly half of all medications have no data on use during lactation, and less than 5% have available human data.[241,244] The most comprehensive up-to-date information for individual agents can be found in the **Drugs and Lactation Database (LactMed) of the National Library of Medicine's Toxicology Data Network (TOXNET).**[245] Potential infant risks from anesthetic drugs in lactating mothers are summarized in Table 16.4. Data for nonanesthetic drugs are shown in Appendix 16.2 (online only).

TABLE 16.4 Potential Infant Risks From Anesthetic Drugs in Lactating Mothers

Drug	Class	Neonatal Exposure M/P, RID (%)	Lactation Recommendation	Comments/Potential Risks
General Anesthetic Drugs[a]				
Because a combination of anesthetic agents is normally used, the interval postprocedure for which the lactating mother should abstain (pump and dump) before resuming breastfeeding should be based on the most problematic medication. Breastfeeding immediately prior to anesthesia may decrease anesthetic requirements.[246]				
Desflurane[214,247]	Inhalational halogenated anesthetic	n/a	Compatible with breastfeeding	No published data on desflurane during lactation. Probably excreted into breast milk; however, because plasma half-life is very short and oral absorption is poor, minimal infant exposure is expected. Breast milk concentrations should be lower than with other halogenated agents because of low blood and tissue solubility and rapid washout. No waiting period or discarding of milk is required.
Isoflurane[248]	Inhalational halogenated anesthetic	n/a	Compatible with breastfeeding	No published data on isoflurane during lactation. Probably excreted into breast milk; however, because plasma half-life is short and oral absorption is poor, minimal infant exposure is expected. No waiting period or discarding of milk is required.
Sevoflurane[249]	Inhalational halogenated anesthetic	n/a	Compatible with breastfeeding	No published data on sevoflurane during lactation. Sevoflurane is probably excreted into breast milk; however, because the plasma half-life is short and the drug is poorly orally absorbed, the infant exposure is expected to be minimal. No waiting period or discarding of milk is required.
Nitrous oxide[214,250]	General anesthetic, sedative, analgesia, inorganic gas	n/a	Compatible with breastfeeding	No data. Because the plasma half-life of nitrous oxide is less than 3 min, extensive passage into milk is not expected and the infant is not expected to absorb it.
Ketamine[214,251]	General anesthetic nonbarbiturate, phencyclidine derivative	RID: 0.65% after 0.5 mg/kg 0.77% after 1 mg/kg Variable dosages: 0.34%–0.57%	Compatible with breastfeeding Consider an 11-h postdose abstention period (pump and dump)	Excreted with active metabolite, norketamine, into milk in very low concentrations. Oral bioavailability is low for both, so expected to pose little risk to breastfed infants. Elimination half-life approximately 2.17 h. Some authors have recommended an 11-h postdose abstention period (pump and dump), after which the drug should be undetectable in maternal plasma. Monitor infant for sedation and poor feeding.
Propofol[214,252]	General anesthetic and hypnotic	RID: 0.2%	Compatible with breastfeeding	Amounts of propofol in breast milk are small and not expected to be absorbed by the infant. Discarding milk or deferring breastfeeding based on propofol exposure is not required. A green discoloration of breast milk following propofol use has been reported by some authors.

(Continued)

TABLE 16.4.	**Potential Infant Risks From Anesthetic Drugs in Lactating Mothers—cont'd**			
Drug	Class	Neonatal Exposure M/P, RID (%)	Lactation Recommendation	Comments/Potential Risks
Local Anesthetic Drugs				
Bupivacaine[253–255]	Amino-amide local anesthetic	M/P: 0.34–0.37 RID: <1%	Compatible with breastfeeding	Among breastfed infants of mothers who received bupivacaine during delivery, 2/42 had transient tachypnea of unknown origin but none required readmission.
2-Chloroprocaine[256]	Amino-ester local anesthetic	n/a	Probably compatible; however, because of the absence of data, an alternative drug may be preferred	There are no published data on the use of 2-chloroprocaine during breastfeeding. Based on known low excretion of other local anesthetics into breastmilk and the extremely short half-life of 2-chloroprocaine, it is unlikely to adversely affect the breastfed infant.
Lidocaine[255]	Amino-amide local anesthetic	M/P: 1.07	Compatible with breastfeeding	No adverse effects reported
Ropivacaine[257]	Amino-amide local anesthetic	M/P: 0.23–0.25	Compatible with breastfeeding	No adverse effects reported

[a]Because of adverse safety profiles, enflurane and halothane are not in common use in the United States and therefore are not included.
M/P, Ratio of drug concentration in milk/drug concentration in maternal plasma; *n/a*, not available; *RID*, relative infant dose (%) = infant dose (mg/kg/d)/maternal dose (mg/kg/d) × 100.

Infant exposure to maternal medication can be minimized simply by breastfeeding just prior to drug administration. For medications that were also taken during pregnancy, it is important to note that medication exposure through breast milk will almost always be much lower than fetal exposure *in utero*. Thus, it is generally appropriate to continue medications that were used during pregnancy while breastfeeding. Few medications are truly contraindicated during lactation. These include **antineoplastics**, **ergot alkaloids**, some **anticonvulsants**, **gold**, **iodine**, **radiopharmaceuticals**, and **recreational drugs**.[258]

Maternal drugs may also affect lactation, and some are used therapeutically for this purpose. **Galactagogues** are medications or herbal therapies intended to increase milk production. However, the quality and quantity of available data on galactagogue efficacy are low.[259] A systematic review and metaanalysis of two commonly used off-label galactagogues, **domperidone** and **metoclopramide**, found a significant increase in milk supply among mothers of preterm infants with low supply with domperidone but not metoclopramide.[260] Domperidone is not approved for the purpose of increasing milk production in the United States because of safety concerns, including arrhythmias, cardiac arrest, and sudden death. The effect of herbal compounds such as **fenugreek** on milk production in well-controlled trials is mixed, though a network metaanalysis of multiple studies found a significant effect of fenugreek compared with controls.[261]

Drugs that increase the secretion of prolactin could theoretically stimulate milk production, though a direct relationship between prolactin levels and milk volume has not been established.[262] Drugs associated with increased prolactin levels include dopamine antagonists such as **phenothiazines** and **haloperidol**, and antipsychotics such as **sulpiride** and **risperidone**.[263] Drugs that may decrease milk production include **first-generation anticholinergics**, **high-dose estrogen**, and dopamine agonists such as **bromocriptine** and **cabergoline**.[264]

Transfer of Drugs to Breast Milk

Transfer of drugs between plasma and breast milk largely occurs via passive diffusion and is bidirectional. During colostrum production in the first 3 to 4 days postpartum, the mammary epithelium allows passage of large molecules and cells. Although this suggests a higher potential for drug transfer in early breastfeeding, minimal milk intake during this early period is likely to limit infant exposure. Over the first week postpartum, mammary epithelial cells establish tight junctions that limit transfer of large molecules. Most drugs move between blood and breast milk via passive diffusion down the concentration gradient formed by the nonionized, unbound drug on either side of the semipermeable lipid barrier. Large molecules such as **monoclonal antibodies** and **heparins** typically cannot diffuse into breast milk, although inflammatory conditions such as mastitis can disrupt the epithelial barrier and allow for increased paracellular drug transfer into breast milk.[265,266]

Additional properties beyond molecular weight that affect the concentration in breast milk include lipid solubility, protein binding, and degree of ionization. Highly lipid-soluble drugs pass more readily into breast milk. Fat is the most variable macronutrient in breast milk, and higher concentrations will favor higher concentrations of lipid-soluble drugs. Fat content is higher in hindmilk compared with foremilk, during the day compared with early morning and at night, and earlier in the postpartum period.[267]

Ionization status also affects drug concentrations in breast milk. Breast milk is more acidic than plasma, which allows ionized weak bases to concentrate in breast milk while ionized weak acids concentrate in plasma. For example, breast milk concentrations of **codeine**, a weak base, are 1.5 times higher than plasma concentrations. Other weak bases that may disproportionately concentrate in breast milk include **amphetamines** and **benzodiazepines**. The degree to which this phenomenon occurs is influenced by breast milk pH, which can vary from 6.7 to 7.4.[265,268]

Protein binding also affects the transfer of drugs into breast milk. Protein concentrations are significantly higher in plasma than breast milk (75 versus 8 to 9 g/L), and the majority of proteins in breast milk have low affinity for drug binding.[266] Consequently, highly protein-bound drugs tend to be retained in the plasma. Drugs that are more than 85% protein bound do not typically result in infant exposure. Exceptions have been noted for drugs that were also administered during pregnancy or during delivery as well as for those given at high doses in the first week postpartum.[269]

Although most drugs move by passive diffusion, a small number undergo active transport. The sodium iodide transporter and the breast cancer resistance protein actively transport substrates into breast milk. This leads to an increased concentration of transporter substrates in breast milk, including **iodide, acyclovir, cimetidine, methotrexate, and nitrofurantoin**.[270-272]

Approximations of infant exposure are often quantified as the **relative infant dose (RID)**:

$$\text{RID (\%)} = \frac{\text{Infant Dose (mg/kg/day)}}{\text{Maternal Dose (mg/kg/day)}} \times 100$$

The infant dose for the RID can be determined from the maternal plasma concentration ($C_{maternal}$), the ratio between milk and plasma concentrations (M/P), and the volume of milk ingested (V_{milk}), which is estimated to be 150 mL/kg/day if the specific value is unknown.

$$\text{Infant dose} = C_{maternal} \times M/P \times V_{milk}$$

A World Health Organization Working Group proposed that drugs with an RID > 10% of the lowest maternal or infant weight-adjusted dose may not be safe in breastfeeding and drugs with an RID > 25% should be avoided.[266] Others have proposed a more conservative 5% threshold. Importantly, the RID does not account for infant age, pharmacogenomic factors, active metabolites, or variable toxicity among drugs.[265]

Infant age modifies risk owing to both changes in volume of milk consumption and maturation of infant metabolic and excretory pathways. These differences can result in prolonged drug half-lives in neonates. Among reported adverse events in breastfed infants, approximately two-thirds occurred in the first month postpartum and three-quarters within the first 2 months.[273]

Maternal and infant pharmacogenomics can also affect toxicity. For example, the prodrug, **codeine**, and its active metabolite, **morphine**, are generally found at clinically insignificant concentrations in breast milk, and a large, population-based cohort study found no association between adverse infant outcomes and maternal codeine use.[274] However, a report of infant death secondary to maternal codeine use highlights the potential impact of pharmacogenomic variants.[275] The mother in this case was determined to be a CYP2D6 UM, resulting in much more rapid conversion of codeine to morphine. While this case represents an extremely rare event, it underscores the potential for pharmacogenomic variants to significantly modify infant exposures in breastfeeding.

KEY POINTS

- Approximately two-thirds of pregnant women in North America report the use of over-the-counter medications.
- Much of the care provided to pregnant patients involves the use of medications.
- Drugs administered to the pregnant patient may be prescribed to treat a maternal condition with incidental fetal transfer, or they may be prescribed to treat a fetal problem with maternal exposure.
- Because of the physiologic, pharmacokinetic, and pharmacodynamic changes that occur during gestation, pregnancy is considered the fifth special pharmacologic population (in addition to people with hepatic disease, people with renal disease, children, and geriatric adults).
- Dosing strategies developed for healthy nonpregnant adults may not achieve comparable results when prescribed for pregnant patients.
- Concentrations of reproductive hormones as well as cortisol dramatically increase during pregnancy.
- The expansion of plasma volume and total body water increases the volume of distribution of hydrophilic medications and reduces the concentration-to-dose ratio of their initial doses.
- The plasma proteins albumin and alpha-1 acid glycoprotein have lower concentrations during pregnancy; this results in protein-bound drugs having a greater free fraction for (1) drug effect, (2) movement of drug into nonplasma spaces (tissue concentrations are increased), and (3) drug availability for metabolism and/or clearance. Monitoring of free drug is often recommended during pregnancy for drugs that are highly protein-bound and have a narrow therapeutic range.
- Increased cardiac output during pregnancy leads to increased glomerular filtration, which, coupled with changes in activity of renal drug transporters, increases the renal clearance of many drugs.
- The activities of drug-metabolizing enzymes are variably affected during pregnancy; activities may increase or decrease, and a few do not change, compared with the nonpregnant state.

- An increase in endogenous opioids promotes maintenance of the pregnant state and enhances fetal health via multiple pathways.
- Endogenous opioids increase pain threshold during pregnancy; this contributes to a reduction in the MAC values of volatile anesthetic agents and faster onset and longer duration of local anesthetics employed for nerve blocks in pregnant patients.
- Teratogens are substances that adversely affect the developing fetus by altering its growth, structure, or function.
- A teratogen produces a specific abnormality or constellation of abnormalities with a dose-effect relationship.
- Teratogen exposure must occur at a specific stage of gestation to have an effect.

- Susceptibility to teratogenesis is affected by the genotype of both mother and fetus.
- The 2014 FDA Pregnancy and Lactation Labeling Rule supplanted the previous letter system and provides detailed information regarding pregnancy, lactation, and reproductive effects of drugs.
- Most drug transfer to breast milk occurs via passive diffusion and is bidirectional. Drug transport is affected by molecular size, lipid solubility, protein binding, and degree of ionization.
- The NICHD Drugs and Lactation Database (LactMed) (https://www.ncbi.nlm.nih.gov/books/NBK501922/) provides the most comprehensive and up-to-date information for the use of specific medications during breastfeeding.

REFERENCES

1. Haas DM, Marsh DJ, Dang DT, et al. Prescription and other medication use in pregnancy. *Obstet Gynecol*. 2018;131: 789–798.
2. Lupattelli A, Spigset O, Twigg MJ, et al. Medication use in pregnancy: a cross-sectional, multinational web-based study. *BMJ Open*. 2014;4:e004365.
3. Philipson A. Pharmacokinetics of ampicillin during pregnancy. *J Infect Dis*. 1977;136:370–376.
4. Tulchinsky D, Hobel CJ. Plasma human chorionic gonadotropin, estrone, estradiol, estriol, progesterone, and 17 alpha-hydroxyprogesterone in human pregnancy. 3. Early normal pregnancy. *Am J Obstet Gynecol*. 1973;117:884–893.
5. Mishell DR Jr, Thorneycroft IH, Nagata Y, et al. Serum gonadotropin and steroid patterns in early human gestation. *Am J Obstet Gynecol*. 1973;117:631–642.
6. Taylor HS, Pal L, Seli E. *The Endocrinology of Pregnancy*. 9th ed. Wolters Kluwer; 2020:196–252.
7. Soldin OP, Guo T, Weiderpass E, et al. Steroid hormone levels in pregnancy and 1 year postpartum using isotope dilution tandem mass spectrometry. *Fertil Steril*. 2005;84:701–710.
8. Buster JE, Abraham GE. The applications of steroid hormone radioimmunoassays to clinical obstetrics. *Obstet Gynecol*. 1975;46:489–499.
9. Buster JE, Sakakini J Jr, Killam AP, Scragg WH. Serum unconjugated estriol levels in the third trimester and their relationship to gestational age. *Am J Obstet Gynecol*. 1976;125:672–676.
10. Abbassi-Ghanavati M, Greer LG, Cunningham FG. Pregnancy and laboratory studies: a reference table for clinicians. *Obstet Gynecol*. 2009;114:1326–1331.
11. Mastorakos G, Ilias I. Maternal and fetal hypothalamic-pituitary-adrenal axes during pregnancy and postpartum. *Ann N Y Acad Sci*. 2003;997:136–149.
12. Carr BR, Parker CR Jr, Madden JD, et al. Maternal plasma adrenocorticotropin and cortisol relationships throughout human pregnancy. *Am J Obstet Gynecol*. 1981;139:416–422.
13. Petraglia F, Florio P, Nappi C, Genazzani AR. Peptide signaling in human placenta and membranes: autocrine, paracrine, and endocrine mechanisms. *Endocr Rev*. 1996;17:156–186.
14. Jones SA, Brooks AN, Challis JR. Steroids modulate corticotropin-releasing hormone production in human fetal membranes and placenta. *J Clin Endocrinol Metab*. 1989;68:825–830.
15. Robinson BG, Emanuel RL, Frim DM, Majzoub JA. Glucocorticoid stimulates expression of corticotropin-releasing hormone gene in human placenta. *Proc Natl Acad Sci U S A*. 1988;85:5244–5248.
16. Thomson M. The physiological roles of placental corticotropin releasing hormone in pregnancy and childbirth. *J Physiol Biochem*. 2013;69:559–573.
17. Smith R, Nicholson RC. Corticotrophin releasing hormone and the timing of birth. *Front Biosci*. 2007;12:912–918.
18. Petersen VP. Body composition and fluid compartments in normal, obese and underweight human subjects. *Acta Med Scand*. 1957;158:103–111.
19. Frederiksen MC, Ruo TI, Chow MJ, Atkinson AJ Jr. Theophylline pharmacokinetics in pregnancy. *Clin Pharmacol Ther*. 1986;40:321–328.
20. Casele HL, Laifer SA, Woelkers DA, Venkataramanan R. Changes in the pharmacokinetics of the low-molecular-weight heparin enoxaparin sodium during pregnancy. *Am J Obstet Gynecol*. 1999;181:1113–1117.
21. Gonçalves PVB, Moreira FL, Benzi JRL, et al. A pilot study of the maternal-fetal pharmacokinetics of furosemide in plasma, urine, and amniotic fluid of hypertensive parturient women under cesarean section. *J Clin Pharmacol*. 2020;60:1655–1661.
22. Mendenhall HW. Serum protein concentrations in pregnancy. I. Concentrations in maternal serum. *Am J Obstet Gynecol*. 1970;106:388–399.
23. Chu CY, Singla VP, Wang HP, et al. Plasma alpha 1-acid glycoprotein levels in pregnancy. *Clin Chim Acta*. 1981;112:235–240.
24. Wood M, Wood AJ. Changes in plasma drug binding and alpha 1-acid glycoprotein in mother and newborn infant. *Clin Pharmacol Ther*. 1981;29:522–526.
25. Bardy AH, Hiilesmaa VK, Teramo K, Neuvonen PJ. Protein binding of antiepileptic drugs during pregnancy, labor, and puerperium. *Ther Drug Monit*. 1990;12:40–46.
26. Wulf H, Münstedt P, Maier C. Plasma protein binding of bupivacaine in pregnant women at term. *Acta Anaesthesiol Scand*. 1991;35:129–133.

27. Hebert MF, Easterling TR, Kirby B, et al. Effects of pregnancy on CYP3A and P-glycoprotein activities as measured by disposition of midazolam and digoxin: a University of Washington specialized center of research study. *Clin Pharmacol Ther.* 2008;84:248–253.

28. Metcalfe J, Romney SL, Ramsey LH, et al. Estimation of uterine blood flow in normal human pregnancy at term. *J Clin Invest.* 1955;34:1632–1638.

29. Odutayo A, Hladunewich M. Obstetric nephrology: renal hemodynamic and metabolic physiology in normal pregnancy. *Clin J Am Soc Nephrol.* 2012;7:2073–2080.

30. Ginsburg J, Duncan SL. Peripheral blood flow in normal pregnancy. *Cardiovasc Res.* 1967;1:132–137.

31. Thoresen M, Wesche J. Doppler measurements of changes in human mammary and uterine blood flow during pregnancy and lactation. *Acta Obstet Gynecol Scand.* 1988;67:741–745.

32. Nakai A, Sekiya I, Oya A, et al. Assessment of the hepatic arterial and portal venous blood flows during pregnancy with Doppler ultrasonography. *Arch Gynecol Obstet.* 2002;266:25–29.

33. Davison JM, Dunlop W. Renal hemodynamics and tubular function normal human pregnancy. *Kidney Int.* 1980;18:152–161.

34. Dunlop W. Renal physiology in pregnancy. *Postgrad Med J.* 1979;55:329–332.

35. Dodge WF, Travis LB, Daeschner CW. Comparison of endogenous creatinine clearance with inulin clearance. *Am J Dis Child.* 1967;113:683–692.

36. Davison JM, Noble MC. Serial changes in 24 hour creatinine clearance during normal menstrual cycles and the first trimester of pregnancy. *Br J Obstet Gynaecol.* 1981;88:10–17.

37. Cheung KL, Lafayette RA. Renal physiology of pregnancy. *Adv Chronic Kidney Dis.* 2013;20:209–214.

38. Andrew MA, Easterling TR, Carr DB, et al. Amoxicillin pharmacokinetics in pregnant women: modeling and simulations of dosage strategies. *Clin Pharmacol Ther.* 2007;81:547–556.

39. Peng J, Ladumor MK, Unadkat JD. Prediction of pregnancy-induced changes in secretory and total renal clearance of drugs transported by organic anion transporters. *Drug Metab Dispos.* 2021;49:929–937.

40. Eyal S, Easterling TR, Carr D, et al. Pharmacokinetics of metformin during pregnancy. *Drug Metab Dispos.* 2010;38:833–840.

41. Fuhr U, Hsin CH, Li X, et al. Assessment of pharmacokinetic drug-drug interactions in humans: in vivo probe substrates for drug metabolism and drug transport revisited. *Annu Rev Pharmacol Toxicol.* 2019;59:507–536.

42. Greiner B, Eichelbaum M, Fritz P, et al. The role of intestinal P-glycoprotein in the interaction of digoxin and rifampin. *J Clin Invest.* 1999;104:147–153.

43. Ahmed Juvale II, Abdul Hamid AA, Abd Halim KB, Che Has AT. P-glycoprotein: new insights into structure, physiological function, regulation and alterations in disease. *Heliyon.* 2022;8:e09777.

44. Ivanyuk A, Livio F, Biollaz J, Buclin T. Renal drug transporters and drug interactions. *Clin Pharmacokinet.* 2017;56:825–892.

45. Brookfield KF, Su F, Elkomy MH, et al. Pharmacokinetics and placental transfer of magnesium sulfate in pregnant women. *Am J Obstet Gynecol.* 2016;214:737.

46. Clark CT, Newmark RL, Wisner KL, et al. Lithium pharmacokinetics in the perinatal patient with bipolar disorder. *J Clin Pharmacol.* 2022;62:1385–1392.

47. Wesseloo R, Liu X, Clark CT, et al. Risk of postpartum episodes in women with bipolar disorder after lamotrigine or lithium use during pregnancy: a population-based cohort study. *J Affect Disord.* 2017;218:394–397.

48. Westin AA, Brekke M, Molden E, et al. Changes in drug disposition of lithium during pregnancy: a retrospective observational study of patient data from two routine therapeutic drug monitoring services in Norway. *BMJ Open.* 2017;7:e015738.

49. American Psychiatric Association. Practice guideline for the treatment of patients with bipolar disorder (revision). *Am J Psychiatry.* 2002;159:1–50.

50. Malhi GS, Bassett D, Boyce P, et al. Royal Australian and New Zealand College of Psychiatrists clinical practice guidelines for mood disorders. *Aust N Z J Psychiatry.* 2015;49:1087–1206.

51. Molenaar NM, Poels EMP, Robakis T, et al. Management of lithium dosing around delivery: an observational study. *Bipolar Disord.* 2021;23:49–54.

52. De Smedt T, Raedt R, Vonck K, Boon P. Levetiracetam: part II, the clinical profile of a novel anticonvulsant drug. *CNS Drug Rev.* 2007;13:57–78.

53. Berlin M, Barchel D, Gandelman-Marton R, etal. Therapeutic levetiracetam monitoring during pregnancy: "mind the gap". *Ther Adv Chronic Dis.* 2019;10:2040622319851652.

54. Li Y, Wang ML, Guo Y, et al. Population pharmacokinetics and dosing regimen optimization of levetiracetam in epilepsy during pregnancy. *Br J Clin Pharmacol.* 2023;89:1152–1161.

55. Chen J, You X, Wu W, et al. Application of PBPK modeling in predicting maternal and fetal pharmacokinetics of levetiracetam during pregnancy. *Eur J Pharm Sci.* 2023;181:106349.

56. Westin AA, Reimers A, Helde G, et al. Serum concentration/dose ratio of levetiracetam before, during and after pregnancy. *Seizure.* 2008;17:192–198.

57. Zhao M, Ma J, Li M, et al. Cytochrome P450 enzymes and drug metabolism in humans. *Int J Mol Sci.* 2021;22:12808.

58. Tolson AH, Wang H. Regulation of drug-metabolizing enzymes by xenobiotic receptors: PXR and CAR. *Adv Drug Deliv Rev.* 2010;62:1238–1249.

59. Mackowiak B, Wang H. Mechanisms of xenobiotic receptor activation: direct vs. indirect. *Biochim Biophys Acta.* 2016;1859:1130–1140.

60. Sachar M, Kelly EJ, Unadkat JD. Mechanisms of CYP3A induction during pregnancy: studies in HepaRG cells. *AAPS J.* 2019;21:45.

61. Xie HG, Wood AJ, Kim RB, et al. Genetic variability in CYP3A5 and its possible consequences. *Pharmacogenomics.* 2004;5:243–272.

62. Lamba J, Hebert JM, Schuetz EG, et al. PharmGKB summary: very important pharmacogene information for CYP3A5. *Pharmacogenet Genomics.* 2012;22:555–558.

63. Mutagonda RF, Minzi OMS, Massawe SN, et al. Pregnancy and CYP3A5 genotype affect day 7 plasma lumefantrine concentrations. *Drug Metab Dispos.* 2019;47:1415–1424.

64. Haas DM, Quinney SK, Clay JM, et al. Nifedipine pharmacokinetics are influenced by CYP3A5 genotype when used as a preterm labor tocolytic. *Am J Perinatol.* 2013;30:275–281.

65. Tracy TS, Venkataramanan R, Glover DD, et al. Temporal changes in drug metabolism (CYP1A2, CYP2D6 and CYP3A activity) during pregnancy. *Am J Obstet Gynecol.* 2005;192:633–639.

66. Nylén H, Sergel S, Forsberg L, et al. Cytochrome P450 3A activity in mothers and their neonates as determined by plasma 4β-hydroxycholesterol. *Eur J Clin Pharmacol.* 2011;67:715–722.

67. Kim AH, Kim B, Rhee SJ, et al. Assessment of induced CYP3A activity in pregnant women using 4β-hydroxycholesterol: cholesterol ratio as an appropriate metabolic marker. *Drug Metab Pharmacokinet.* 2018;33:173–178.

68. Ohkita C, Goto M. Increased 6-hydroxycortisol excretion in pregnant women: implication of drug-metabolizing enzyme induction. *DICP.* 1990;24:814–816.

69. Della Torre M, Hibbard JU, Jeong H, Fischer JH. Betamethasone in pregnancy: influence of maternal body weight and multiple gestation on pharmacokinetics. *Am J Obstet Gynecol.* 2010;203:254.e1e12.

70. Prevost RR, Akl SA, Whybrew WD, Sibai BM. Oral nifedipine pharmacokinetics in pregnancy-induced hypertension. *Pharmacotherapy.* 1992;12:174–177.

71. Labroo RB, Paine MF, Thummel KE, Kharasch ED. Fentanyl metabolism by human hepatic and intestinal cytochrome P450 3A4: implications for interindividual variability in disposition, efficacy, and drug interactions. *Drug Metab Dispos.* 1997;25:1072–1080.

72. Wanar A, Saia K, Field TA. Accelerated fentanyl metabolism during pregnancy and impact on prenatal drug testing. *Matern Child Health J.* 2023;27:1944–1948.

73. Kokki M, Heikkinen AT, Raatikainen K, et al. Pharmacokinetics of intranasal fentanyl in parturient. *Br J Anaesth.* 2015;115:635–636.

74. Lalovic B, Phillips B, Risler LL, et al. Quantitative contribution of CYP2D6 and CYP3A to oxycodone metabolism in human liver and intestinal microsomes. *Drug Metab Dispos.* 2004;32:447–454.

75. Romand S, Spaggiari D, Marsousi N, et al. Characterization of oxycodone in vitro metabolism by human cytochromes P450 and UDP-glucuronosyltransferases. *J Pharm Biomed Anal.* 2017;144:129–137.

76. Kokki M, Franco MG, Raatikainen K, et al. Intravenous oxycodone for pain relief in the first stage of labour—maternal pharmacokinetics and neonatal exposure. *Basic Clin Pharmacol Toxicol.* 2012;111:182–188.

77. Zheng S, Easterling TR, Umans JG, et al. Pharmacokinetics of tacrolimus during pregnancy. *Ther Drug Monit.* 2012;34:660–670.

78. Stek A, Best BM, Wang J, et al. Pharmacokinetics of once versus twice daily darunavir in pregnant HIV-infected women. *J Acquir Immune Defic Syndr.* 2015;70:33–41.

79. Unadkat JD, Wara DW, Hughes MD, et al. Pharmacokinetics and safety of indinavir in human immunodeficiency virus-infected pregnant women. *Antimicrob Agents Chemother.* 2007;51:783–786.

80. Stek AM, Mirochnick M, Capparelli E, et al. Reduced lopinavir exposure during pregnancy. *AIDS.* 2006;20:1931–1939.

81. Conradie F, Zorrilla C, Josipovic D, et al. Safety and exposure of once-daily ritonavir-boosted atazanavir in HIV-infected pregnant women. *HIV Med.* 2011;12:570–579.

82. Mirochnick M, Best BM, Stek AM, et al. Atazanavir pharmacokinetics with and without tenofovir during pregnancy. *J Acquir Immune Defic Syndr.* 2011;56:412–419.

83. Kreitchmann R, Best BM, Wang J, et al. Pharmacokinetics of an increased atazanavir dose with and without tenofovir during the third trimester of pregnancy. *J Acquir Immune Defic Syndr.* 2013;63:59–66.

84. Johnson EL, Stowe ZN, Ritchie JC, et al. Carbamazepine clearance and seizure stability during pregnancy. *Epilepsy Behav.* 2014;33:49–53.

85. Chang Y, Fang WB, Lin SN, Moody DE. Stereo-selective metabolism of methadone by human liver microsomes and cDNA-expressed cytochrome P450s: a reconciliation. *Basic Clin Pharmacol Toxicol.* 2011;108:55–62.

86. Pond SM, Kreek MJ, Tong TG, et al. Altered methadone pharmacokinetics in methadone-maintained pregnant women. *J Pharmacol Exp Ther.* 1985;233:1–6.

87. Wolff K, Boys A, Rostami-Hodjegan A, et al. Changes to methadone clearance during pregnancy. *Eur J Clin Pharmacol.* 2005;61:763–768.

88. Bogen DL, Perel JM, Helsel JC, et al. Pharmacologic evidence to support clinical decision making for peripartum methadone treatment. *Psychopharmacology (Berl).* 2013;225:441–451.

89. McCarthy JJ, Vasti EJ, Leamon MH, et al. The use of serum methadone/metabolite ratios to monitor changing perinatal pharmacokinetics. *J Addict Med.* 2018;12:241–246.

90. Kobayashi K, Yamamoto T, Chiba K, et al. Human buprenorphine N-dealkylation is catalyzed by cytochrome P450 3A4. *Drug Metab Dispos.* 1998;26:818–821.

91. Zhang H, Bastian JR, Zhao W, et al. Pregnancy alters CYP- and UGT-mediated metabolism of buprenorphine. *Ther Drug Monit.* 2020;42:264–270.

92. Caritis SN, Bastian JR, Zhang H, et al. An evidence-based recommendation to increase the dosing frequency of buprenorphine during pregnancy. *Am J Obstet Gynecol.* 2017;217:459.e1e6.

93. Yanagihara Y, Kariya S, Ohtani M, et al. Involvement of CYP2B6 in n-demethylation of ketamine in human liver microsomes. *Drug Metab Dispos.* 2001;29:887–890.

94. Hijazi Y, Boulieu R. Contribution of CYP3A4, CYP2B6, and CYP2C9 isoforms to N-demethylation of ketamine in human liver microsomes. *Drug Metab Dispos.* 2002;30:853–858.

95. Desta Z, Moaddel R, Ogburn ET, et al. Stereoselective and regiospecific hydroxylation of ketamine and norketamine. *Xenobiotica.* 2012;42:1076–1087.

96. Sigtermans M, Dahan A, Mooren R, et al. S(+)-ketamine effect on experimental pain and cardiac output: a population pharmacokinetic-pharmacodynamic modeling study in healthy volunteers. *Anesthesiology.* 2009;111:892–903.

97. Bernard S, Neville KA, Nguyen AT, Flockhart DA. Interethnic differences in genetic polymorphisms of CYP2D6 in the U.S. population: clinical implications. *Oncologist.* 2006;11:126–135.

98. Buchanan ML, Easterling TR, Carr DB, et al. Clonidine pharmacokinetics in pregnancy. *Drug Metab Dispos.* 2009;37:702–705.

99. Högstedt S, Rane A. Plasma concentration-effect relationship of metoprolol during and after pregnancy. *Eur J Clin Pharmacol.* 1993;44:243–246.

100. Ryu RJ, Eyal S, Easterling TR, et al. Pharmacokinetics of metoprolol during pregnancy and lactation. *J Clin Pharmacol.* 2016;56:581–589.

101. Ververs FF, Voorbij HA, Zwarts P, et al. Effect of cytochrome P4502D6 genotype on maternal paroxetine plasma concentrations during pregnancy. *Clin Pharmacokinet.* 2009;48:677–683.

102. Wadelius M, Darj E, Frenne G, Rane A. Induction of CYP2D6 in pregnancy. *Clin Pharmacol Ther.* 1997;62:400–407.

103. Claessens AJ, Risler LJ, Eyal S, et al. CYP2D6 mediates 4-hydroxylation of clonidine in vitro: implication for pregnancy-induced changes in clonidine clearance. *Drug Metab Dispos.* 2010;38:1393–1396.

104. Kwon YJ, Shin S, Chun YJ. Biological roles of cytochrome P450 1A1, 1A2, and 1B1 enzymes. *Arch Pharm Res.* 2021;44:63–83.

105. Pollock BG, Wylie M, Stack JA, et al. Inhibition of caffeine metabolism by estrogen replacement therapy in postmenopausal women. *J Clin Pharmacol.* 1999;39: 936–940.

106. Walker AA, Dickmann L, Isoherranen N. Pregnancy decreases rat CYP1A2 activity and expression. *Drug Metab Dispos.* 2011;39:4–7.

107. Shelepova T, Nafziger AN, Victory J, et al. Effect of a triphasic oral contraceptive on drug-metabolizing enzyme activity as measured by the validated Cooperstown 5+1 cocktail. *J Clin Pharmacol.* 2005;45:1413–1421.

108. Kalow W, Tang BK. The use of caffeine for enzyme assays: a critical appraisal. *Clin Pharmacol Ther.* 1993;53:503–514.

109. Raunio H, Rahnasto-Rilla M. CYP2A6: genetics, structure, regulation, and function. *Drug Metabol Drug Interact.* 2012;27:73–88.

110. Higashi E, Fukami T, Itoh M, et al. Human CYP2A6 is induced by estrogen via estrogen receptor. *Drug Metab Dispos.* 2007;35:1935–1941.

111. Taghavi T, Arger CA, Heil SH, et al. Longitudinal influence of pregnancy on nicotine metabolic pathways. *J Pharmacol Exp Ther.* 2018;364:238–245.

112. Koh KH, Jurkovic S, Yang K, et al. Estradiol induces cytochrome P450 2B6 expression at high concentrations: implication in estrogen-mediated gene regulation in pregnancy. *Biochem Pharmacol.* 2012;84:93–103.

113. Walsky RL, Astuccio AV, Obach RS. Evaluation of 227 drugs for in vitro inhibition of cytochrome P450 2B6. *J Clin Pharmacol.* 2006;46:1426–1438.

114. Cressey TR, Stek A, Capparelli E, et al. Efavirenz pharmacokinetics during the third trimester of pregnancy and postpartum. *J Acquir Immune Defic Syndr.* 2012;59: 245–252.

115. Kreitchmann R, Schalkwijk S, Best B, et al. Efavirenz pharmacokinetics during pregnancy and infant washout. *Antivir Ther.* 2019;24:95–103.

116. Fokina VM, Xu M, Rytting E, et al. Pharmacokinetics of bupropion and Its pharmacologically active metabolites in pregnancy. *Drug Metab Dispos.* 2016;44:1832–1838.

117. Fay EE, Czuba LC, Sager JE, et al. Pregnancy has no clinically significant effect on the pharmacokinetics of bupropion or its metabolites. *Ther Drug Monit.* 2021;43:780–788.

118. Choi SY, Koh KH, Jeong H. Isoform-specific regulation of cytochromes P450 expression by estradiol and progesterone. *Drug Metab Dispos.* 2013;41:263–269.

119. Rytting E, Nanovskaya TN, Wang X, et al. Pharmacokinetics of indomethacin in pregnancy. *Clin Pharmacokinet.* 2014;53:545–551.

120. Hebert MF, Ma X, Naraharisetti SB, et al. Are we optimizing gestational diabetes treatment with glyburide? The pharmacologic basis for better clinical practice. *Clin Pharmacol Ther.* 2009;85:607–614.

121. Tornio A, Backman JT. Cytochrome P450 in pharmacogenetics: an update. *Adv Pharmacol.* 2018;83:3–32.

122. Mwinyi J, Cavaco I, Pedersen RS, et al. Regulation of CYP2C19 expression by estrogen receptor alpha: implications for estrogen-dependent inhibition of drug metabolism. *Mol Pharmacol.* 2010;78:886–894.

123. McGready R, Stepniewska K, Seaton E, et al. Pregnancy and use of oral contraceptives reduces the biotransformation of proguanil to cycloguanil. *Eur J Clin Pharmacol.* 2003;59: 553–557.

124. McGready R, Stepniewska K, Edstein MD, et al. The pharmacokinetics of atovaquone and proguanil in pregnant women with acute falciparum malaria. *Eur J Clin Pharmacol.* 2003;59:545–552.

125. Andersson T, Hassan-Alin M, Hasselgren G, et al. Pharmacokinetic studies with esomeprazole, the (S)-isomer of omeprazole. *Clin Pharmacokinet.* 2001;40:411–426.

126. Li XQ, Weidolf L, Simonsson R, Andersson TB. Enantiomer/enantiomer interactions between the S- and R- isomers of omeprazole in human cytochrome P450 enzymes: major role of CYP2C19 and CYP3A4. *J Pharmacol Exp Ther.* 2005;315:777–787.

127. Gebreyesus MS, Decloedt EH, Cluver CA, et al. Population pharmacokinetics of esomeprazole in patients with preterm preeclampsia. *Br J Clin Pharmacol.* 2022;88:4639–4645.

128. Lee JK, Chung HJ, Fischer L, et al. Human placental lactogen induces CYP2E1 expression via PI 3-kinase pathway in female human hepatocytes. *Drug Metab Dispos.* 2014;42:492–499.

129. Guengerich FP. Cytochrome P450 2E1 and its roles in disease. *Chem Biol Interact.* 2020;322:109056.

130. Kharasch ED, Thummel KE. Identification of cytochrome P450 2E1 as the predominant enzyme catalyzing human liver microsomal defluorination of sevoflurane, isoflurane, and methoxyflurane. *Anesthesiology.* 1993;79:795–807.

131. Kharasch ED, Thummel KE, Mautz D, Bosse S. Clinical enflurane metabolism by cytochrome P450 2E1. *Clin Pharmacol Ther.* 1994;55:434–440.

132. Restrepo JG, Garcia-Martin E, Martinez C, Agundez JA. Polymorphic drug metabolism in anaesthesia. *Curr Drug Metab.* 2009;10:236–246.

133. Preckel B, Bolten J. Pharmacology of modern volatile anaesthetics. *Best Pract Res Clin Anaesthesiol.* 2005;19:331–348.

134. Kot M, Daniel WA. The relative contribution of human cytochrome P450 isoforms to the four caffeine oxidation pathways: an in vitro comparative study with cDNA-expressed P450s including CYP2C isoforms. *Biochem Pharmacol.* 2008;76:543–551.

135. Alcorta-García MR, López-Villaseñor CN, Sánchez-Ferrer G, et al. Modulation of CYP2E1 metabolic activity in a cohort of confirmed caffeine ingesting pregnant women with preterm offspring. *Mol Cell Pediatr.* 2020;7:4.

136. Hu DG, Meech R, McKinnon RA, Mackenzie PI. Transcriptional regulation of human UDP-glucuronosyltransferase genes. *Drug Metab Rev.* 2014;46:421–458.

137. Oda S, Fukami T, Yokoi T, Nakajima M. A comprehensive review of UDP-glucuronosyltransferase and esterases for drug development. *Drug Metab Pharmacokinet*. 2015;30:30–51.

138. Jeong H, Choi S, Song JW, et al. Regulation of UDP-glucuronosyltransferase (UGT) 1A1 by progesterone and its impact on labetalol elimination. *Xenobiotica*. 2008;38:62–75.

139. Fischer JH, Sarto GE, Hardman J, et al. Influence of gestational age and body weight on the pharmacokinetics of labetalol in pregnancy. *Clin Pharmacokinet*. 2014;53:373–383.

140. Rogers RC, Sibai BM, Whybrew WD. Labetalol pharmacokinetics in pregnancy-induced hypertension. *Am J Obstet Gynecol*. 1990;162:362–366.

141. Chen H, Yang K, Choi S, et al. Up-regulation of UDP-glucuronosyltransferase (UGT) 1A4 by 17β-estradiol: a potential mechanism of increased lamotrigine elimination in pregnancy. *Drug Metab Dispos*. 2009;37:1841–1847.

142. Tomson T, Ohman I, Vitols S. Lamotrigine in pregnancy and lactation: a case report. *Epilepsia*. 1997;38:1039–1041.

143. Reimers A, Helde G, Brodtkorb E. Ethinyl estradiol, not progestogens, reduces lamotrigine serum concentrations. *Epilepsia*. 2005;46:1414–1417.

144. Fotopoulou C, Kretz R, Bauer S, et al. Prospectively assessed changes in lamotrigine-concentration in women with epilepsy during pregnancy, lactation and the neonatal period. *Epilepsy Res*. 2009;85:60–64.

145. Karanam A, Pennell PB, French JA, et al. Lamotrigine clearance increases by 5 weeks gestational age: relationship to estradiol concentrations and gestational age. *Ann Neurol*. 2018;84:556–563.

146. Ohman I, Beck O, Vitols S, Tomson T. Plasma concentrations of lamotrigine and its 2-N-glucuronide metabolite during pregnancy in women with epilepsy. *Epilepsia*. 2008;49:1075–1080.

147. Polepally AR, Pennell PB, Brundage RC, et al. Model-based lamotrigine clearance changes during pregnancy: clinical implication. *Ann Clin Transl Neurol*. 2014;1:99–106.

148. Weerink MAS, Struys M, Hannivoort LN, et al. Clinical pharmacokinetics and pharmacodynamics of dexmedetomidine. *Clin Pharmacokinet*. 2017;56:893–913.

149. Watts DH, Brown ZA, Tartaglione T, et al. Pharmacokinetic disposition of zidovudine during pregnancy. *J Infect Dis*. 1991;163:226–232.

150. O'Sullivan MJ, Boyer PJ, Scott GB, et al. The pharmacokinetics and safety of zidovudine in the third trimester of pregnancy for women infected with human immunodeficiency virus and their infants: phase I acquired immunodeficiency syndrome clinical trials group study (protocol 082). Zidovudine Collaborative Working Group. *Am J Obstet Gynecol*. 1993;168:1510–1516.

151. Court MH, Krishnaswamy S, Hao Q, et al. Evaluation of 3'-azido-3'-deoxythymidine, morphine, and codeine as probe substrates for UDP-glucuronosyltransferase 2B7 (UGT2B7) in human liver microsomes: specificity and influence of the UGT2B7*2 polymorphism. *Drug Metab Dispos*. 2003;31:1125–1133.

152. Thorn CF, Klein TE, Altman RB. Codeine and morphine pathway, pharmacokinetics. PharmGKB; 2022. https://www.pharmgkb.org/pathway/PA146123006. Accessed July 14, 2024.

153. van Dorp EL, Romberg R, Sarton E, et al. Morphine-6-glucuronide: morphine's successor for postoperative pain relief? *Anesth Analg*. 2006;102:1789–1797.

154. Ohno S, Kawana K, Nakajin S. Contribution of UDP-glucuronosyltransferase 1A1 and 1A8 to morphine-6-glucuronidation and its kinetic properties. *Drug Metab Dispos*. 2008;36:688–694.

155. Stone AN, Mackenzie PI, Galetin A, et al. Isoform selectivity and kinetics of morphine 3- and 6-glucuronidation by human UDP-glucuronosyltransferases: evidence for atypical glucuronidation kinetics by UGT2B7. *Drug Metab Dispos*. 2003;31:1086–1089.

156. Gerdin E, Salmonson T, Lindberg B, Rane A. Maternal kinetics of morphine during labour. *J Perinat Med*. 1990;18:479–487.

157. Wang YB, Zhang RZ, Huang SH, et al. Relationship between UGT1A9 gene polymorphisms, efficacy, and safety of propofol in induced abortions amongst Chinese population: a population-based study. *Biosci Rep*. 2017;37:BSR20170722.

158. Gin T, Gregory MA, Chan K, et al. Pharmacokinetics of propofol in women undergoing elective caesarean section. *Br J Anaesth*. 1990;64:148–153.

159. Kerdpin O, Knights KM, Elliot DJ, Miners JO. In vitro characterisation of human renal and hepatic frusemide glucuronidation and identification of the UDP-glucuronosyltransferase enzymes involved in this pathway. *Biochem Pharmacol*. 2008;76:249–257.

160. Ellison DH. Clinical pharmacology in diuretic use. *Clin J Am Soc Nephrol*. 2019;14:1248–1257.

161. Kulo A, Peeters MY, Allegaert K, et al. Pharmacokinetics of paracetamol and its metabolites in women at delivery and post-partum. *Br J Clin Pharmacol*. 2013;75:850–860.

162. Allegaert K, Peeters MY, Beleyn B, et al. Paracetamol pharmacokinetics and metabolism in young women. *BMC Anesthesiol*. 2015;15:163.

163. Kulo A, van de Velde M, de Hoon J, et al. Pharmacokinetics of a loading dose of intravenous paracetamol post caesarean delivery. *Int J Obstet Anesth*. 2012;21:125–128.

164. Mitchell MC, Hanew T, Meredith CG, Schenker S. Effects of oral contraceptive steroids on acetaminophen metabolism and elimination. *Clin Pharmacol Ther*. 1983;34:48–53.

165. Uchaipichat V, Suthisisang C, Miners JO. The glucuronidation of R- and S-lorazepam: human liver microsomal kinetics, UDP-glucuronosyltransferase enzyme selectivity, and inhibition by drugs. *Drug Metab Dispos*. 2013;41:1273–1284.

166. Papini O, da Cunha SP, da Silva Mathes Ado C, et al. Kinetic disposition of lorazepam with focus on the glucuronidation capacity, transplacental transfer in parturients and racemization in biological samples. *J Pharm Biomed Anal*. 2006;40:397–403.

167. Bologa M, Tang B, Klein J, et al. Pregnancy-induced changes in drug metabolism in epileptic women. *J Pharmacol Exp Ther*. 1991;257:735–740.

168. Tsutsumi K, Kotegawa T, Matsuki S, et al. The effect of pregnancy on cytochrome P4501A2, xanthine oxidase, and N-acetyltransferase activities in humans. *Clin Pharmacol Ther*. 2001;70:121–125.

169. Han LW, Ryu RJ, Cusumano M, et al. Effect of N-acetyltransferase 2 genotype on the pharmacokinetics of hydralazine during pregnancy. *J Clin Pharmacol*. 2019;59:1678–1689.

170. Li W, Ning M, Koh KH, et al. 17β-Estradiol induces sulfotransferase 2A1 expression through estrogen receptor α. *Drug Metab Dispos*. 2014;42:796–802.

171. Ramírez J, Innocenti F, Schuetz EG, et al. CYP2B6, CYP3A4, and CYP2C19 are responsible for the in vitro N-demethylation of meperidine in human liver microsomes. *Drug Metab Dispos*. 2004;32:930–936.

172. Kuhnert BR, Kuhnert PM, Prochaska AL, Sokol RJ. Meperidine disposition in mother, neonate, and nonpregnant females. *Clin Pharmacol Ther*. 1980;27:486–491.

173. Greenblatt DJ, von Moltke LL, Harmatz JS, Shader RI. Human cytochromes mediating sertraline biotransformation: seeking attribution. *J Clin Psychopharmacol*. 1999;19:489–493.

174. Kobayashi K, Ishizuka T, Shimada N, et al. Sertraline N-demethylation is catalyzed by multiple isoforms of human cytochrome P-450 in vitro. *Drug Metab Dispos*. 1999;27:763–766.

175. Rudberg I, Hermann M, Refsum H, Molden E. Serum concentrations of sertraline and N-desmethyl sertraline in relation to CYP2C19 genotype in psychiatric patients. *Eur J Clin Pharmacol*. 2008;64:1181–1188.

176. Wang JH, Liu ZQ, Wang W, et al. Pharmacokinetics of sertraline in relation to genetic polymorphism of CYP2C19. *Clin Pharmacol Ther*. 2001;70:42–47.

177. Stika CS, Wisner KL, George AL Jr, et al. Changes in sertraline plasma concentrations across pregnancy and postpartum. *Clin Pharmacol Ther*. 2022;112:1280–1290.

178. Waldhoer M, Bartlett SE, Whistler JL. Opioid receptors. *Annu Rev Biochem*. 2004;73:953–990.

179. Pathan H, Williams J. Basic opioid pharmacology: an update. *Br J Pain*. 2012;6:11–16.

180. Rosenfeld CS. The placenta as a target of opioid drugs. *Biol Reprod*. 2022;106:676–686.

181. Mansson E, Bare L, Yang D. Isolation of a human kappa opioid receptor cDNA from placenta. *Biochem Biophys Res Commun*. 1994;202:1431–1437.

182. Mantione KJ, Angert RM, Cadet P, et al. Identification of a micro opiate receptor signaling mechanism in human placenta. *Med Sci Monit*. 2010;16:BR347–BR352.

183. Ahmed MS, Cemerikic B, Agbas A. Properties and functions of human placental opioid system. *Life Sci*. 1992;50:83–97.

184. Zoumakis E, Margioris AN, Makrigiannakis A, et al. Human endometrium as a neuroendocrine tissue: expression, regulation and biological roles of endometrial corticotropin-releasing hormone (CRH) and opioid peptides. *J Endocrinol Invest*. 1997;20:158–167.

185. Cemerikic B, Cheng J, Agbas A, Ahmed MS. Opioids regulate the release of human chorionic gonadotropin hormone from trophoblast tissue. *Life Sci*. 1991;49:813–824.

186. Petit A, Gallo-Payet N, Lehoux JG, et al. Adenosine 3':5'-cyclic monophosphate (cAMP) is not the mediator of kappa opiate effect on human placental lactogen release. *Life Sci*. 1991;49:465–472.

187. Nandhra TS, Carson RJ. β-endorphin inhibits the production of interleukin-8 by human chorio-decidual cells in culture. *Mol Hum Reprod*. 2000;6:555–560.

188. Brunton PJ. Endogenous opioid signalling in the brain during pregnancy and lactation. *Cell Tissue Res*. 2019;375:69–83.

189. Dawson-Basoa MB, Gintzler AR. 17-β-estradiol and progesterone modulate an intrinsic opioid analgesic system. *Brain Res*. 1993;601:241–245.

190. Gintzler AR. Endorphin-mediated increases in pain threshold during pregnancy. *Science*. 1980;210:193–195.

191. Jarvis S, McLean KA, Chirnside J, et al. Opioid-mediated changes in nociceptive threshold during pregnancy and parturition in the sow. *Pain*. 1997;72:153–159.

192. Draisci G, Catarci S, Vollono C, et al. Pregnancy-induced analgesia: a combined psychophysical and neurophysiological study. *Eur J Pain*. 2012;16:1389–1397.

193. Carvalho B, Angst MS, Fuller AJ, et al. Experimental heat pain for detecting pregnancy-induced analgesia in humans. *Anesth Analg*. 2006;103:1283–1287.

194. Carvalho B, Granot M, Sultan P, et al. A longitudinal study to evaluate pregnancy-induced endogenous analgesia and pain modulation. *Reg Anesth Pain Med*. 2016;41:175–180.

195. Palahniuk RJ, Shnider SM, Eger EI 2nd. Pregnancy decreases the requirement for inhaled anesthetic agents. *Anesthesiology*. 1974;41:82–83.

196. Strout CD, Nahrwold ML. Halothane requirement during pregnancy and lactation in rats. *Anesthesiology*. 1981;55:322–323.

197. Gin T, Chan MT. Decreased minimum alveolar concentration of isoflurane in pregnant humans. *Anesthesiology*. 1994;81:829–832.

198. Chan MT, Mainland P, Gin T. Minimum alveolar concentration of halothane and enflurane are decreased in early pregnancy. *Anesthesiology*. 1996;85:782–786.

199. Chan MT, Gin T. Postpartum changes in the minimum alveolar concentration of isoflurane. *Anesthesiology*. 1995;82:1360–1363.

200. Zhou HH, Norman P, DeLima LG, et al. The minimum alveolar concentration of isoflurane in patients undergoing bilateral tubal ligation in the postpartum period. *Anesthesiology*. 1995;82:1364–1368.

201. Datta S, Migliozzi RP, Flanagan HL, Krieger NR. Chronically administered progesterone decreases halothane requirements in rabbits. *Anesth Analg*. 1989;68:46–50.

202. Erden V, Yangn Z, Erkalp K, et al. Increased progesterone production during the luteal phase of menstruation may decrease anesthetic requirement. *Anesth Analg*. 2005;101:1007–1011.

203. Lee J, Lee J, Ko S. The relationship between serum progesterone concentration and anesthetic and analgesic requirements: a prospective observational study of parturients undergoing cesarean delivery. *Anesth Analg*. 2014;119:901–905.

204. Datta S, Lambert DH, Gregus J, et al. Differential sensitivities of mammalian nerve fibers during pregnancy. *Anesth Analg*. 1983;62:1070–1072.

205. Flanagan HL, Datta S, Lambert DH, et al. Effect of pregnancy on bupivacaine-induced conduction blockade in the isolated rabbit vagus nerve. *Anesth Analg*. 1987;66:123–126.

206. Popitz-Bergez FA, Leeson S, Thalhammer JG, Strichartz GR. Intraneural lidocaine uptake compared with analgesic differences between pregnant and nonpregnant rats. *Reg Anesth*. 1997;22:363–371.

207. Butterworth JF, 4th Walker FO, Lysak SZ. Pregnancy increases median nerve susceptibility to lidocaine. *Anesthesiology*. 1990;72:962–965.

208. Hirabayashi Y, Shimizu R, Fukuda H, et al. Soft tissue anatomy within the vertebral canal in pregnant women. *Br J Anaesth*. 1996;77:153–156.

209. Hirabayashi Y, Shimizu R, Fukuda H, et al. Effects of the pregnant uterus on the extradural venous plexus in the supine

and lateral positions, as determined by magnetic resonance imaging. *Br J Anaesth.* 1997;78:317–319.

210. Onuki E, Higuchi H, Takagi S, et al. Gestation-related reduction in lumbar cerebrospinal fluid volume and dural sac surface area. *Anesth Analg.* 2010;110:148–153.

211. Zhan Q, Huang S, Geng G, Xie Y. Comparison of relative potency of intrathecal bupivacaine for motor block in pregnant versus nonpregnant women. *Int J Obstet Anesth.* 2011;20:219–223.

212. Camorcia M, Capogna G, Columb MO. Effect of sex and pregnancy on the potency of intrathecal bupivacaine: determination of ED_{50} for motor block with the up-down sequential allocation method. *Eur J Anaesthesiol.* 2011;28:240–244.

213. Wilson JG. Experimental studies on congenital malformations. *J Chronic Dis.* 1959;10:111–130.

214. Briggs GG, Freeman RK, Towers CV, Forinash AB. *Brigg's Drugs in Pregnancy and Lactation: A Reference Guide to Fetal and Neonatal Risk.* 12th ed. Lippincott Williams & Wilkins; 2021.

215. Yildiz K, Dogru K, Dalgic H, et al. Inhibitory effects of desflurane and sevoflurane on oxytocin-induced contractions of isolated pregnant human myometrium. *Acta Anaesthesiol Scand.* 2005;49:1355–1359.

216. Munson ES, Embro WJ. Enflurane, isoflurane, and halothane and isolated human uterine muscle. *Anesthesiology.* 1977;46:11–14.

217. Nishijima M. Ketamine in obstetric anesthesia: special reference to placental transfer and its concentration in blood plasma. *Acta Obstet Gynaecol Jpn.* 1972;19:80–93.

218. Baraka A, Louis F, Dalleh R. Maternal awareness and neonatal outcome after ketamine induction of anaesthesia for Caesarean section. *Can J Anaesth.* 1990;37:641–644.

219. Buring JE, Hennekens CH, Mayrent SL, et al. Health experiences of operating room personnel. *Anesthesiology.* 1985;62:325–330.

220. Heinonen OPSD, Shapiro S. *Birth Defects and Drugs in Pregnancy.* Publishing Sciences Group; 1977.

221. Jevtovic-Todorovic V, Benshoff N, Olney JW. Ketamine potentiates cerebrocortical damage induced by the common anaesthetic agent nitrous oxide in adult rats. *Br J Pharmacol.* 2000;130:1692–1698.

222. Ratzon NZ, Ornoy A, Pardo A, et al. Developmental evaluation of children born to mothers occupationally exposed to waste anesthetic gases. *Birth Defects Res A Clin Mol Teratol.* 2004;70:476–482.

223. Olney JW, Farber NB, Wozniak DF, et al. Environmental agents that have the potential to trigger massive apoptotic neurodegeneration in the developing brain. *Environ Health Perspect.* 2000;108(suppl 3):383–388.

224. Stefani SJ, Hughes SC, Schnider SM, et al. Neonatal neurobehavioral effects of inhalation analgesia for vaginal delivery. *Anesthesiology.* 1982;56:351–355.

225. Baxi LV, Petrie RH. Pharmacologic effects on labor: effects of drugs on dystocia, labor, and uterine activity. *Clin Obstet Gynecol.* 1987;30:19–32.

226. Gin T, Gregory MA, Chan K, Oh TE. Maternal and fetal levels of propofol at caesarean section. *Anaesth Intensive Care.* 1990;18:180–184.

227. Celleno D, Capogna G, Tomassetti M, et al. Neurobehavioural effects of propofol on the neonate following elective caesarean section. *Br J Anaesth.* 1989;62:649–654.

228. Philipson EH, Kuhnert BR, Syracuse CD. 2-Chloroprocaine for local perineal infiltration. *Am J Obstet Gynecol.* 1987;157:1275–1278.

229. Nau H. Clinical pharmacokinetics in pregnancy and perinatology. I. Placental transfer and fetal side effects of local anaesthetic agents. *Dev Pharmacol Ther.* 1985;8:149–181.

230. Abboud TK, Sarkis F, Blikian A, et al. Lack of adverse neonatal neurobehavioral effects of lidocaine. *Anesth Analg.* 1983;62:473–475.

231. Demeulemeester V, Van Hautem H, Cools F, Lefevere J. Transplacental lidocaine intoxication. *J Neonatal Perinatal Med.* 2018;11:439–441.

232. Abboud TK, Afrasiabi A, Sarkis F, et al. Continuous infusion epidural analgesia in parturients receiving bupivacaine, chloroprocaine, or lidocaine—maternal, fetal, and neonatal effects. *Anesth Analg.* 1984;63:421–428.

233. Li JN, Nijhawan RI, Srivastava D. Cutaneous surgery in patients who are pregnant or breastfeeding. *Dermatol Clin.* 2019;37:307–317.

234. McCrae AF, Westerling P, McClure JH. Pharmacokinetic and clinical study of ropivacaine and bupivacaine in women receiving extradural analgesia in labour. *Br J Anaesth.* 1997;79:558–562.

235. FDA Drug Safety Communication: FDA review results in new warnings about using general anesthetics and sedation drugs in young children and pregnant women US Food & Drug Administration; 2016. https://www.fda.gov/drugs/drug-safety-and-availability/fda-drug-safety-communication-fda-review-results-new-warnings-about-using-general-anesthetics-and. Accessed July 14, 2024.

236. Newman CG. The thalidomide syndrome: risks of exposure and spectrum of malformations. *Clin Perinatol.* 1986;13:555–573.

237. Lammer EJ, Chen DT, Hoar RM, et al. Retinoic acid embryopathy. *N Engl J Med.* 1985;313:837–841.

238. Angus-Leppan H, Liu RSN. Weighing the risks of valproate in women who could become pregnant. *BMJ.* 2018;361:k1596.

239. Food and Drug Administration. Content and format of labeling for human prescription drug and biological products: requirements for pregnancy and lactation labeling. *Fed Regist.* 2014;79:72064–72103.

240. Namazy J, Chambers C, Sahin L, et al. Clinicians' perspective of the new pregnancy and lactation labeling rule (PLLR): results from an AAAAI/FDA survey. *J Allergy Clin Immunol Pract.* 2020;8:1947–1952.

241. Byrne JJ, Saucedo AM, Spong CY. Evaluation of drug labels following the 2015 pregnancy and lactation labeling rule. *JAMA Netw Open.* 2020;3:e2015094.

242. de Waard M, Blomjous BS, Hol MLF, et al. Medication use during pregnancy and lactation in a Dutch population. *J Hum Lact.* 2019;35:154–164.

243. McClatchey AK, Shield A, Cheong LH, et al. Why does the need for medication become a barrier to breastfeeding? A narrative review. *Women Birth.* 2018;31:362–366.

244. Mazer-Amirshahi M, Samiee-Zafarghandy S, Gray G, van den Anker JN. Trends in pregnancy labeling and data quality for US-approved pharmaceuticals. *Am J Obstet Gynecol.* 2014;211:690.e1–e11.

245. National Library of Medicine Lactation Database (LactMed). Drugs and Lactation Database (LactMed). https://www.ncbi.nlm.nih.gov/books/NBK501922/#IX-D. Accessed July 14, 2024.

246. Bhaskara B, Dayananda VP, Kannan S, et al. Effect of breastfeeding on haemodynamics and consumption of propofol and sevoflurane: a state entropy guided comparative study. *Indian J Anaesth.* 2016;60:180–186.

247. National Library of Medicine Lactation Database (LactMed). Desflurane; 2020. https://www.ncbi.nlm.nih.gov/books/NBK501500/. Accessed July 14, 2024.

248. National Library of Medicine Lactation Database (LactMed). Isoflurane; 2020. https://www.ncbi.nlm.nih.gov/books/NBK501499/. Accessed July 14, 2024.

249. National Library of Medicine Lactation Database (LactMed). Sevoflurane; 2020. https://www.ncbi.nlm.nih.gov/books/NBK501504/. Accessed July 14, 2024.

250. National Library of Medicine Lactation Database (LactMed). Nitrous Oxide; 2023. https://www.ncbi.nlm.nih.gov/books/NBK501501/. Accessed July 14, 2024.

251. National Library of Medicine Lactation Database (LactMed). Ketamine; 2023. https://www.ncbi.nlm.nih.gov/books/NBK500566/. Accessed July 14, 2024.

252. National Library of Medicine Lactation Database (LactMed). Propofol; 2021. https://www.ncbi.nlm.nih.gov/books/NBK501298/. Accessed July 14, 2024.

253. Mustafa HJ, Wong HL, Al-Kofahi M, et al. Bupivacaine pharmacokinetics and breast milk excretion of liposomal bupivacaine administered after cesarean birth. *Obstet Gynecol.* 2020;136:70–76.

254. Bolat E, Bestas A, Bayar MK, et al. Evaluation of levobupivacaine passage to breast milk following epidural anesthesia for cesarean delivery. *Int J Obstet Anesth.* 2014;23:217–221.

255. Ortega D, Viviand X, Lorec AM, et al. Excretion of lidocaine and bupivacaine in breast milk following epidural anesthesia for cesarean delivery. *Acta Anaesthesiol Scand.* 1999;43:394–397.

256. National Library of Medicine Lactation Database (LactMed). Chloroprocaine; 2018. https://www.ncbi.nlm.nih.gov/books/NBK501609/. Accessed July 14, 2024.

257. Matsota PK, Markantonis SL, Fousteri MZ, et al. Excretion of ropivacaine in breast milk during patient-controlled epidural analgesia after cesarean delivery. *Reg Anesth Pain Med.* 2009;34:126–129.

258. Moretti ME, Lee A, Ito S. Which drugs are contraindicated during breastfeeding? Practice guidelines. *Can Fam Physician.* 2000;46:1753–1757.

259. Foong SC, Tan ML, Foong WC, et al. Oral galactagogues (natural therapies or drugs) for increasing breast milk production in mothers of non-hospitalised term infants. *Cochrane Database Syst Rev.* 2020;(5):CD011505.

260. Shen Q, Khan KS, Du MC, et al. Efficacy and safety of domperidone and metoclopramide in breastfeeding: a systematic review and meta-analysis. *Breastfeed Med.* 2021;16:516–529.

261. Khan TM, Wu DB, Dolzhenko AV. Effectiveness of fenugreek as a galactagogue: a network meta-analysis. *Phytother Res.* 2018;32:402–412.

262. Anderson PO, Valdes V. A critical review of pharmaceutical galactagogues. *Breastfeed Med.* 2007;2:229–242.

263. La Torre D, Falorni A. Pharmacological causes of hyperprolactinemia. *Ther Clin Risk Manag.* 2007;3:929–951.

264. Anderson PO. Drugs that suppress lactation, part 2. *Breastfeed Med.* 2017;12:199–201.

265. Anderson PO, Sauberan JB. Modeling drug passage into human milk. *Clin Pharmacol Ther.* 2016;100:42–52.

266. Anderson PO. Drugs in lactation. *Pharm Res.* 2018;35:45.

267. Ballard O, Morrow AL. Human milk composition: nutrients and bioactive factors. *Pediatr Clin North Am.* 2013;60:49–74.

268. Ansell C, Moore A, Barrie H. Electrolyte pH changes in human milk. *Pediatr Res.* 1977;11:1177–1179.

269. Anderson GD. Using pharmacokinetics to predict the effects of pregnancy and maternal-infant transfer of drugs during lactation. *Expert Opin Drug Metab Toxicol.* 2006;2:947–960.

270. Oo CY, Kuhn RJ, Desai N, McNamara PJ. Active transport of cimetidine into human milk. *Clin Pharmacol Ther.* 1995;58:548–555.

271. Darrouzet E, Lindenthal S, Marcellin D, et al. The sodium/iodide symporter: state of the art of its molecular characterization. *Biochim Biophys Acta.* 2014;1838:244–253.

272. Ito N, Ito K, Ikebuchi Y, et al. Prediction of drug transfer into milk considering breast cancer resistance protein (BCRP)-mediated transport. *Pharm Res.* 2015;32:2527–2537.

273. Anderson PO, Pochop SL, Manoguerra AS. Adverse drug reactions in breastfed infants: less than imagined. *Clin Pediatr (Phila).* 2003;42:325–340.

274. Juurlink DN, Gomes T, Guttmann A, et al. Postpartum maternal codeine therapy and the risk of adverse neonatal outcomes: a retrospective cohort study. *Clin Toxicol (Phila).* 2012;50:390–395.

275. Koren G, Cairns J, Chitayat D, et al. Pharmacogenetics of morphine poisoning in a breastfed neonate of a codeine-prescribed mother. *Lancet.* 2006;368:704.

17

Problems of Early Pregnancy

Emily E. Sharpe, MD and Margaret E. Long, MD

Obstetric disease of early pregnancy may result in significant maternal morbidity and even mortality. Safe care of patients with obstetric disease involves a thorough understanding of the physiologic changes of early pregnancy as well as the specific issues associated with each pathologic condition. Many of these profound physiologic changes occur in the first trimester (see Chapter 2).

ASSISTED REPRODUCTION

Assisted Reproductive Technology Procedures

Fertility treatments that involve handling of eggs or embryos are referred to as assisted reproductive technology (ART) procedures. These procedures address etiologies related to oocyte, sperm, uterus, a combination of factors, or unknown factors. While ART is commonly utilized for primary and secondary infertility, other indications include fertility preservation prior to cytotoxic therapy, delayed childbearing, genetic disorders or sex screening (preimplantation genetic diagnosis), and childbearing for same-sex couples or individuals without partners.

Ovarian Stimulation

While natural cycles usually generate one oocyte, ovarian stimulation utilizes follicle-stimulating hormone, human menopausal gonadotropin, or both to develop multiple ovarian follicles in one cycle to increase the number available for retrieval. Hormonal regimens typically include a gonadotropin-releasing hormone (GnRH) analog to prevent the pituitary from inducing premature ovulation.[1] When mature follicles are confirmed by ultrasonographic and estradiol monitoring, human chorionic gonadotropin (hCG) (or GnRH agonists in some circumstances) is later added to initiate the ovulation cascade in preparation for oocyte retrieval. Cycles may be canceled, most commonly because of poor ovarian response, but occasionally because of hyperstimulation. All visible ovarian follicles are aspirated 34 to 36 hours after hCG administration (see later discussion), with each follicle usually containing a single oocyte.[1]

After oocyte retrieval, luteal phase support with transvaginal or intramuscular progesterone is used until the first positive pregnancy test or completion of the first trimester.

Oocyte Retrieval

Oocyte retrievals are typically performed transvaginally with ultrasonographic guidance (Fig. 17.1).[2] Laparoscopic oocyte retrieval may be required if transvaginal access to the ovaries is not possible. The 34- to 36-hour timing of oocyte retrieval after hCG administration is necessary to prevent oocyte loss through ovulation.[1] A vaginal ultrasound probe is used to guide the needle into a follicle so the fluid and oocyte can

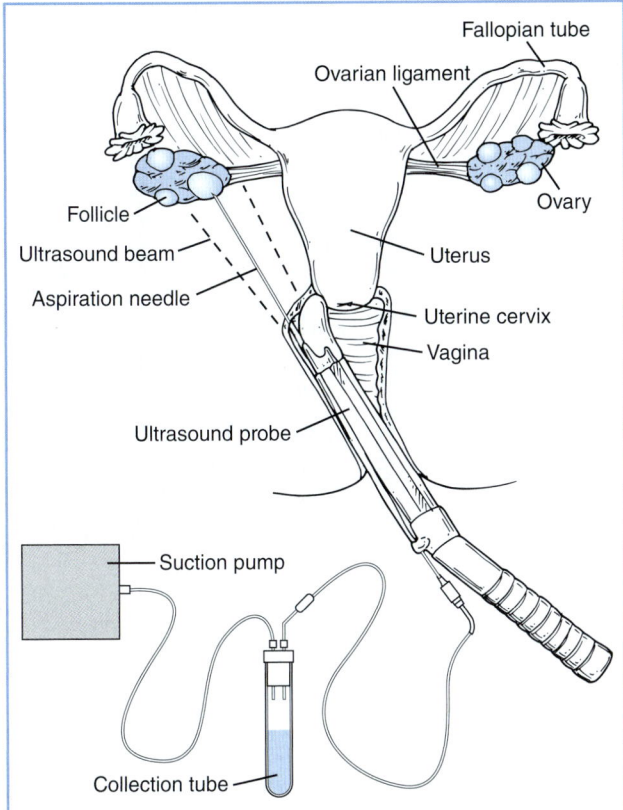

Fig. 17.1 Transvaginal Ultrasound-Guided Oocyte Retrieval. The ultrasonographic probe is placed in the vagina and advanced into the posterior fornix. The needle, previously inserted through the needle guide, is advanced through the vaginal wall and ovarian capsule. Redrawn from Steinbrook R. Egg donation and human embryonic stem-cell research. *N Engl J Med.* 2006;354:324–326. Copyright © 2006 Massachusetts Medical Society. All rights reserved.

be aspirated for subsequent *in vitro* care, fertilization, and embryo management. Some may choose to cryopreserve oocytes for later fertilization and pregnancy, especially in the absence of a partner.

In Vitro Fertilization

Although the term *in vitro fertilization* (IVF) is often used synonymously with ART, technically it applies only to the process of oocyte fertilization with spermatozoa in culture media. IVF provides the opportunity to manage male factor infertility by increasing the concentration of sperm, performing intracytoplasmic sperm injection, or using sperm collected from the testis or epididymis. Embryo selection based on probable implantation success, assisted hatching, preimplantation genetic testing for aneuploidy or certain inherited disorders, and cryopreservation of embryos are other opportunities provided by IVF in addition to management of ovulation and tubal disorders.[1]

Embryo Transfer

One or more embryos resulting from a current IVF cycle or thawed cryopreserved embryos from a prior IVF cycle are transferred via a catheter into the uterine cavity. A single embryo is often transferred to reduce the risk for multiple gestation and associated complications.[3] Other forms of transfer are less common, require at least one normal fallopian tube, and occur via laparoscopy as zygote intrafallopian transfer (ZIFT) or gamete intrafallopian transfer (GIFT).[1]

Ovarian Tissue Cryopreservation

Ovarian tissue cryopreservation is an option for fertility preservation for individuals who cannot have ovarian stimulation.[4] Prepubescent girls and women who require immediate cytotoxic therapy can have laparoscopy for removal of the outer portion of the ovary where most of the oocytes are located. This tissue is then frozen until it can be reimplanted.

Success of Assisted Reproductive Technology

The Society for Assisted Reproductive Technology and the American Society for Reproductive Medicine collaborate with the US Centers for Disease Control and Prevention (CDC) to maintain a data registry and analyze the results of all ART cycles initiated during each calendar year in the United States.[5]

Diminished ovarian reserve due to age or other factors has the largest impact on IVF success. Recently published data indicate that the percentage of intended egg retrievals that resulted in live births was 51.1% for recipients less than 35 years of age and 7.6% for recipients greater than 40 years of age. For those with diminished ovarian reserve, live births occurred in 30.4% for recipients less than 35 years of age and 6.2% for recipients greater than 40 years of age.[5] For the latter individuals, live birth rates increase with use of donor eggs or embryos.

Obstetric Complications

Rarely, ovarian stimulation with gonadotropins can lead to **ovarian hyperstimulation syndrome (OHSS)** in which multiple follicles cause ovarian enlargement and third space sequestration of fluids occurs.[6] Patient characteristics and response to ovarian stimulation can help predict those at highest risk. Mild OHSS can cause self-limited symptoms including nausea and vomiting, diarrhea, abdominal pain, and dyspnea. In 1% to 5% of cycles, moderate to severe OHSS develops with ascites, hemoconcentration, and leukocytosis. With severe or critical OHSS, patients have more severe intravascular volume depletion and may have renal impairment, electrolyte abnormalities, hydrothorax, pleural or pericardial effusions, and thrombosis among other potentially life-threatening complications. Treatment for OHSS involves supportive care and fluid replacement along with prophylactic anticoagulation.[6]

Anesthetic implications of OHSS include increased free drug concentrations. Rarely, an emergency laparoscopy or laparotomy is required for ovarian torsion. Abdominal paracentesis and thoracentesis may be necessary before the induction of general anesthesia in patients with respiratory compromise caused by massive ascites or pleural effusions.

Multiple-gestation pregnancies have decreased with use of cryopreservation and increased use of single embryo transfers. Triplet and other higher-order multiple births occur in less than 0.1% of embryo transfer cycles. Singleton births occurred after 34.5%, and twin births after 2.3%, of embryo transfer cycles in 2020.[5]

Ectopic pregnancy occurs more frequently after ART or ovulation induction.[3] Rates of ectopic pregnancy after ART have decreased, possibly because of the practice of transferring fewer embryos. Rates of **heterotopic pregnancy**, a simultaneous intrauterine and ectopic pregnancy, are elevated after ART, especially if more than one embryo is transferred.

Preterm and low-birth-weight infants are more common with ART singleton pregnancies than with naturally conceived pregnancies after controlling for maternal age and parity.[3] Rather than being the cause of this morbidity, ART may well be a marker for underlying conditions that cause the morbidity.[7] In addition, ART pregnancies are at higher risk for **placenta previa** (relative risk [RR], 6.02; 95% confidence interval [CI], 2.79 to 13.01).[3]

Effects of Anesthesia on Reproduction

General Considerations

In 1987 Boyers et al.[8] reported that oocytes recovered by laparoscopic techniques in patients who had received general anesthesia (isoflurane or enflurane with a 50% nitrous oxide-oxygen mixture) were less likely to be fertilized if the procedure was prolonged. Specifically, fertilization rates for the first- and last-recovered oocytes were 69% and 54%, respectively, when the difference in exposure time exceeded 5 minutes. The investigators implicated either (1) the acidification of follicular fluid by intraperitoneal carbon dioxide or (2) the effects of anesthesia.

The potential association between anesthetic techniques and agents and outcomes of ART procedures must be interpreted with caution. Studies have differed in retrieval method,[9] and the anesthetic agents administered may not have been disclosed.[10] In addition, conclusions based on animal data may not be fully applicable to humans owing to interspecies and assay method differences.[11]

Assessment of specific anesthetic drugs must also be interpreted in context; relevant factors include (1) the method of administration, (2) dose of anesthetic agents, (3) combination with other drugs, (4) timing of administration, and (5) duration of exposure. Anesthetic agents may affect unfertilized oocytes and fertilized embryos differently. Finally, there may be greater free concentrations of some agents (e.g., bupivacaine) during ART stimulation because of a decrease in plasma protein binding capacity associated with hormonal manipulation.[12]

Local Anesthetic Agents

In animal models, the effect of local anesthetic agents on reproductive physiology appears to be related to the agent, timing, and dose of exposure. Using mouse oocytes incubated with known concentrations of **lidocaine**, **bupivacaine**, or **2-chloroprocaine**, Schnell et al.[13] demonstrated that lidocaine and 2-chloroprocaine adversely affected both fertilization and embryo development at a concentration of 1.0 μg/mL (Figs. 17.2 and 17.3). In contrast, bupivacaine produced adverse

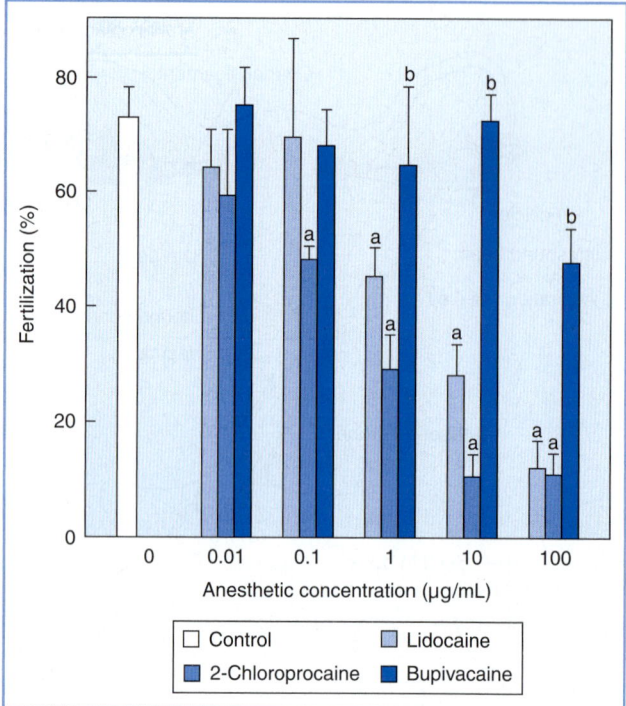

Fig. 17.2 Fertilization of mouse oocytes at 48 h (mean ± SD) for each anesthetic exposure group. *a*, *P* < .05 (anesthetics compared with control); *b*, *P* < .05 (lidocaine and 2-chloroprocaine compared with bupivacaine). Modified from Schnell VL, Sacco AG, Savoy-Moore RT, et al. Effects of oocyte exposure to local anesthetics on in vitro fertilization and embryo development in the mouse. *Reprod Toxicol.* 1992;6:323–327, with permission from Elsevier Science.

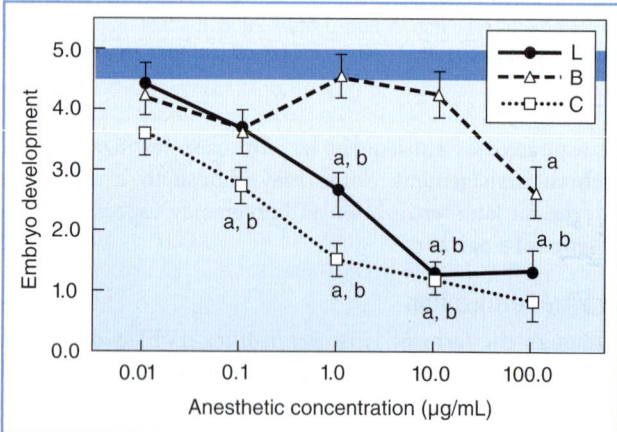

Fig. 17.3 Embryo Development Scores (Mean ± SD) at 72 h as a Function of Anesthetic Concentration. *Shaded area* represents embryo development score (4.75 ± 0.28) for the control mouse embryos. *a*, *P* < .01 (lidocaine [L], bupivacaine [B], and 2-chloroprocaine [C] compared with control); *b*, *P* < .01 (bupivacaine compared with lidocaine and 2-chloroprocaine). Modified from Schnell VL, Sacco AG, Savoy-Moore RT, et al. Effects of oocyte exposure to local anesthetics on in vitro fertilization and embryo development in the mouse. *Reprod Toxicol.* 1992;6:323–327.

effects only at the highest concentration studied (100 μg/mL). Similarly, Del Valle and Orihuela[14] demonstrated that 24% of mouse embryos exposed to lidocaine 10 μg/mL showed evidence of degeneration, compared with none in a control group.

However, these *in vitro* findings may have limited clinical relevance, given the lower anesthetic concentrations administered in clinical practice and the washing and screening procedures oocytes undergo before fertilization and transfer.

Human trial data appear to indicate minimal oocyte and embryo alterations with local anesthetics used during oocyte retrieval procedures. Wikland et al.[15] reported that the incidence of oocyte fertilization and clinical pregnancy was not reduced among women who received a modified paracervical block with lidocaine for transvaginal oocyte retrieval.

Opioids and Benzodiazepines

Fentanyl, **alfentanil**, **remifentanil**, and **meperidine (pethidine)** do not appear to interfere with either fertilization or preimplantation embryo development in animal and human trials.[16,17] When given during oocyte retrieval, fentanyl and alfentanil were detected in extremely low (or undetectable) concentrations in follicular fluid.

Midazolam administered systemically in preovulatory mice did not impair fertilization or embryo development *in vivo* or *in vitro*, even when given in doses up to 500 times greater than those used clinically.[18] In humans, when used in small bolus or infusion doses for anxiolysis and sedation for ART, midazolam was not detected in follicular fluid and does not appear to be teratogenic.[19,20]

Intravenous Anesthetic Agents

Most animal and human trials suggest that **propofol** has minimal to no detrimental effects on fertilization and early embryo development,[21-25] despite accumulating in a dose- and duration-dependent manner within the follicular fluid.[26-28] Hamster oocytes exposed to very high concentrations of propofol (20 µg/mL) demonstrated no DNA damage when evaluated by sister chromatid exchange assays, a sensitive index of genotoxic effects.[29] A smaller incidence of ongoing pregnancies was observed among women given propofol-nitrous oxide anesthesia for ZIFT procedures compared with thiopental-nitrous oxide-isoflurane anesthesia.[30] Further investigation is necessary to further elucidate the full effects of propofol on various reproductive outcomes.

Ketamine (0.75 mg/kg), administered with **midazolam** (0.06 mg/kg), has been reported to be an acceptable alternative to general anesthesia with isoflurane for oocyte retrieval.[31] No differences in reproductive outcomes were observed; however, the study was not powered to adequately assess this result.

Nitrous Oxide

Nitrous oxide reduces methionine synthetase activity, nonmethylated folate derivatives, and DNA synthesis in animals and humans.[32,33] Nitrous oxide also impairs the function of mitotic spindles in cell cultures.[34] Although Warren et al.[35] reported that two-cell mouse embryos exposed to nitrous oxide within 4 hours of the expected onset of cleavage were less likely to develop to the blastocyst stage (Fig. 17.4), this difference had resolved by later stages of embryo development.

Clinical studies of anesthesia for laparoscopic ART procedures support the administration of nitrous oxide.[22,30,36] In

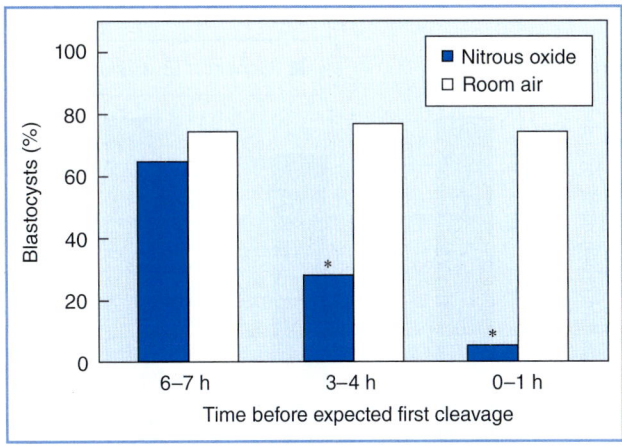

Fig. 17.4 Developmental outcome of two-cell mouse embryos exposed to 60% nitrous oxide/40% oxygen for 30 min *in vitro*. Administration of nitrous oxide within 4 h of anticipated cleavage decreased the percentage of embryos reaching the blastocyst stage. *$P < .05$ compared with the room air (i.e., control) group. Modified from Warren JR, Shaw B, Steinkampf MP. Effects of nitrous oxide on preimplantation mouse embryo cleavage and development. *Biol Reprod.* 1990;43:158–161.

a multicenter study, Beilin et al.[22] observed a delivery rate of 35% among women given nitrous oxide compared with 30% among women who did not receive nitrous oxide.

Volatile Halogenated Agents

Volatile halogenated anesthetic agents have been observed to depress DNA synthesis and mitosis in cell cultures.[37,38] Sturrock and Nunn[37] noted that volatile halogenated agents prevent cytoplasmic cleavage during mitosis, leading to a greater number of abnormal mitotic figures (e.g., tripolar and tetrapolar nuclear phases). **Isoflurane** adversely affects embryo development *in vitro*. Warren et al.[39] reported that two-cell mouse embryos exposed to 3% (but not 1.5%) isoflurane for 1 hour were less likely to develop to the blastocyst stage (Fig. 17.5), but only when isoflurane was given within 4 hours of the predicted onset of cleavage.

Volatile halogenated agents have been compared in clinical studies. In a retrospective sequential study design, Wilhelm et al.[16] noted lower pregnancy rates in patients undergoing oocyte retrieval with general anesthesia (isoflurane or propofol in combination with 60% nitrous oxide in oxygen) than in subsequent patients who received analgesia with a remifentanil-based technique. However, it is possible physician-related factors may have improved the outcomes in the later sedation analgesia phase of the study.[16] Another retrospective study by Piroli et al.[40] comparing four anesthetic methodologies (**topical local anesthetic**, **propofol**, **thiopental**, and **sevoflurane**) found similar outcomes in fertilization rate and embryo development but a decrease in the number of quality embryos in the sevoflurane group.

Although these data suggest that specific volatile halogenated agents may affect ART outcomes, the mechanisms remain incompletely evaluated. Caution is advised in the selection of newer agents, such as **sevoflurane** and **desflurane**, until further work has been done.

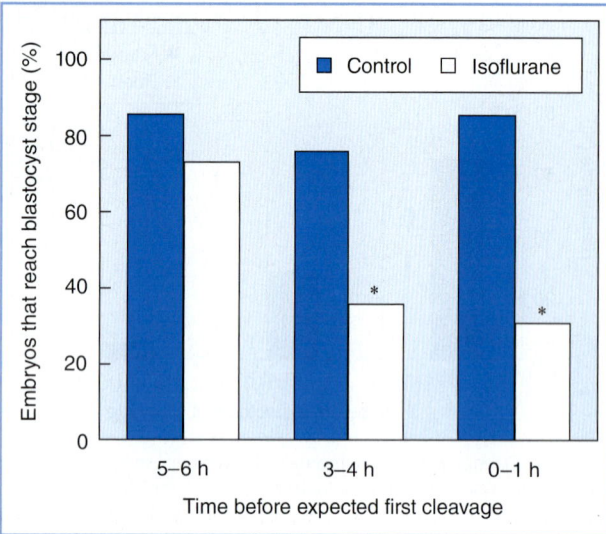

Fig. 17.5 Developmental outcome of two-cell mouse embryos exposed *in vitro* to 3% isoflurane for 30 min at various times in relation to expected onset of the first cleavage *in vitro*. *P < .01. Modified from Warren JR, Shaw B, Steinkampf MP. Inhibition of pre-implantation mouse embryo development by isoflurane. *Am J Obstet Gynecol.* 1992;166:693–698.

Antiemetic Agents

At least one study noted that **droperidol** and **metoclopramide** rapidly induce hyperprolactinemia with subsequent impairment of ovarian follicle maturation and corpus luteum function.[41] Moreover, Forman et al.[42] demonstrated that low plasma prolactin concentrations during ART procedures were associated with a higher incidence of pregnancy. In contrast, when a single dose of intravenous metoclopramide 10 mg was given the day preceding oocyte retrieval, a prolactin level increase of greater than 200% yielded larger follicles, more mature oocytes, and improved IVF success rates.[43] The effects of other antiemetic agents, such as **ondansetron**, have not been studied.

Anesthetic Management

Although most patients undergoing ART procedures are young and otherwise healthy, the use of ART procedures in patients with a growing spectrum of pathologic processes, such as morbid obesity, cancer (with oocyte retrieval performed before chemotherapy or radiation therapy), and severe cardiac, pulmonary, or renal morbidities (with oocyte retrieval performed for embryo transfer in surrogate gestational carriers), requires careful assessment of individual patients.

All patients should follow the American Society of Anesthesiologists fasting guidelines.[44] In the event that a patient does not adhere to fasting guidelines, the decision to delay or cancel the procedure should be made after careful analysis of the potential risks and benefits. If the window for maximal oocyte retrieval (34 to 36 hours after hCG administration) is missed, ovulation with loss of oocytes can occur, invalidating the considerable effort and expense incurred to

that point. Moreover, if oocyte retrieval is not performed, the patient is at increased risk for OHSS, with its potential for significant morbidity. In contrast, the risk for pulmonary aspiration of gastric contents may be low, particularly when spinal anesthesia is administered.

The ideal anesthetic technique provides effective pain relief with minimal postoperative nausea, sedation, pain, and psychomotor impairment.

Ultrasound-Guided Transvaginal Oocyte Retrieval

Although transvaginal oocyte retrievals can be performed under **paracervical**, **spinal**, **epidural**, and **general anesthetic** techniques, **conscious or deep sedation analgesia** (often administered as a component of **monitored anesthesia care**) is the most commonly used technique.[45,46] Although usually adequate for surgical analgesia, deep sedation analgesia may need to progress to loss of consciousness (i.e., general anesthesia) to prevent patient movement at critical points in the procedure.[47] A Cochrane systematic review of 24 randomized controlled trials with 3160 women found no anesthetic modality was superior to another, and evidence was insufficient to show any influence on pregnancy rates.[48]

Because paracervical anesthesia incompletely blocks sensation from the vaginal and ovarian pain fibers, additional analgesia is required.[49] Epidural and spinal techniques provide excellent anesthesia with minimal oocyte exposure to anesthetic agents.

General anesthesia can be provided by **total intravenous anesthesia** using **propofol** (titrated) and an opioid (e.g., **fentanyl** 50 to 100 μg). Most patients can be managed with spontaneous ventilation using a mask or supraglottic airway (SGA), but individuals with significant risk factors for aspiration should undergo tracheal intubation with a cuffed endotracheal tube. Maintenance of anesthesia with a volatile halogenated agent has been used successfully; however, greater rates of nausea and emesis and more unplanned admissions have been observed with this technique than with a propofol, alfentanil, and air-oxygen mixture.[50]

Embryo Transfer

Described as relatively painless, transcervical embryo transfer procedures are most commonly performed without analgesia or anesthesia; however, on rare occasions, intravenous sedation analgesia or regional or general anesthesia may be requested. In contrast, transabdominal gamete or embryo transfer procedures (i.e., GIFT, ZIFT) are usually performed via laparoscopy under local, neuraxial, or general anesthesia.

Pneumoperitoneum and the Trendelenburg Position

Carbon dioxide is usually used to establish pneumoperitoneum. GIFT and ZIFT procedures are often performed with the patient in the Trendelenburg position to facilitate visualization of the fallopian tubes and other pelvic structures. Hemodynamic effects of moderate pneumoperitoneum (<20 mm Hg) in a patient in the Trendelenburg position include increased mean arterial and central venous pressures, increased systemic vascular resistance, and decreased stroke volume and cardiac output.[51] Heart rate usually does not change, but in some patients pneumoperitoneum may elicit sinus bradycardia, heart block, or even cardiac arrest. Finally, pneumoperitoneum aggravates the respiratory effects of the Trendelenburg position (e.g., reduced chest wall compliance, increased venous admixture). Overall, most healthy patients easily tolerate the cardiovascular and pulmonary effects of intraabdominal pressures < 20 mm Hg.

Laparoscopic-Assisted Reproductive Technology

The anesthetic plan for intrafallopian transfer procedures is typically dictated by the method (i.e., transabdominal or transvaginal) of oocyte retrieval. Many ART programs harvest oocytes transabdominally during pelvic laparoscopy; the principal advantage is that the patient is positioned and anesthetized once for both the retrieval and transfer portions of the procedure. The major disadvantage of this technique is that oocytes are exposed to both carbon dioxide pneumoperitoneum and anesthetic agents. Induction is usually performed with intravenous **propofol**, **lidocaine**, **fentanyl**, and either **succinylcholine (suxamethonium)** or **rocuronium**. Subsequently, anesthesia is maintained with a **propofol infusion** or a volatile halogenated agent in oxygen and air, with or without a short-acting muscle relaxant.

Alternatively, oocytes can be retrieved transvaginally and transferred—as oocytes or embryos—laparoscopically. This technique is most commonly used with ZIFT procedures, whereby oocyte retrieval and IVF occur on the preceding day.

Some patients prefer **spinal** or **epidural anesthesia** for GIFT procedures. Healthy, nonobese patients have been reported to successfully undergo laparoscopic surgery in the Trendelenburg position with high thoracic (i.e., T2 to T4) spinal or epidural anesthesia.[52–55] Limiting intraperitoneal pressure to less than 10 mm Hg may facilitate the use of neuraxial anesthesia for these procedures. Obese women are not ideal candidates for neuraxial anesthesia for laparoscopic surgery.

Postoperative Management

The incidence of anesthetic or surgical complications requiring hospital admission after ART procedures is low.[1,56] The most common indications for hospitalization are hemoperitoneum and syncope after oocyte retrieval, and nausea, vomiting, and bowel injury after laparoscopic procedures. Abdominal pain and uterine cramping occur commonly after oocyte retrieval. Incisional pain and referred shoulder pain because of diaphragmatic irritation can also occur after laparoscopic ART procedures. Postprocedural discomfort is related primarily to the number of follicles retrieved (rather than the hormonal alterations induced by the stimulation cycle) and can be effectively managed with the use of a heating pad and small doses of intravenous fentanyl (25 to 50 μg) or oral analgesics such as acetaminophen (paracetamol) 500 to 1000 mg.[48,57]

Nausea and emesis can also occur; however, exposure to droperidol and metoclopramide should be limited as they have been shown to induce hyperprolactinemia with subsequent impairment of ovarian follicle maturation and corpus luteum function.[41] Treatment with nondopaminergic agents can be considered. Before discharge, patients should be able to drink and retain liquids, ambulate, and void. Patients undergoing anesthesia for an ART procedure should be contacted 24 hours after the procedure to allow assessment of recovery and potential complications.

ECTOPIC PREGNANCY

Ectopic pregnancy occurs when a fertilized ovum implants outside the endometrial lining of the uterus. Death, infertility, and recurrent ectopic pregnancy are possible sequelae. Since ectopic pregnancy rates are not currently tracked in the United States, only estimates from older data are available. Based on emergency department data from 2006 to 2013, the ratio of ectopic pregnancy to live births was 12.3 per 1000, with the ratio increasing during this time.[58]

Hemorrhage from ruptured ectopic pregnancy is the leading cause of pregnancy-related maternal death during the first trimester and accounted for 2.7% of all pregnancy-related maternal deaths in the United States from 2011 to 2013.[59] While many who have had an ectopic pregnancy subsequently suffer from infertility or another ectopic pregnancy, over half will have a subsequent live birth.[60]

The number of deaths from ectopic pregnancy has decreased in the United States since the 1980s. The ectopic pregnancy mortality ratio decreased from 1.15 deaths per 100,000 live births from 1980 to 1984 to 0.6 deaths per 100,000 live births in 2018.[61,62] The CDC attributed this decline in ectopic pregnancy mortality to improvements in pregnancy testing, pelvic ultrasonography, and improved therapeutic modalities, including laparoscopic surgery and medical management.[63] Delays in seeking healthcare are associated with death from ectopic pregnancy. Young patients, racial minorities, and those with poor socioeconomic status are disproportionately represented among deaths from ectopic pregnancy.[64] In the United Kingdom, ectopic pregnancy was the most frequent cause of maternal death in early pregnancy between 2018 and 2020.[64]

Factors that alter the risk for ectopic pregnancy include: (1) previous ectopic pregnancy (10% recurrence risk); (2) treatment for infertility (e.g., IVF, ovulation induction); (3) prior pelvic infection (e.g., pelvic inflammatory disease, ruptured appendix); (4) prior pelvic or fallopian tube surgery (e.g., tubal ligation, endometriosis surgery); and (5) advanced maternal age.[65] However, half of patients with an ectopic pregnancy have no identifiable risk factors. Intrauterine device (IUD) use is associated with a lower risk for ectopic pregnancy than that of the general population, but in the rare event that a pregnancy does occur, the ectopic pregnancy potential is up to 53%.[65]

The fertilized ovum can implant in a variety of locations other than the uterine cavity (Fig. 17.6). Most ectopic pregnancies (>90%) are **tubal**, but they can also implant in the **ovary**, **cervix**, **abdomen**, and **cesarean scar**. Delay in diagnosis and treatment increases morbidity and mortality.[65]

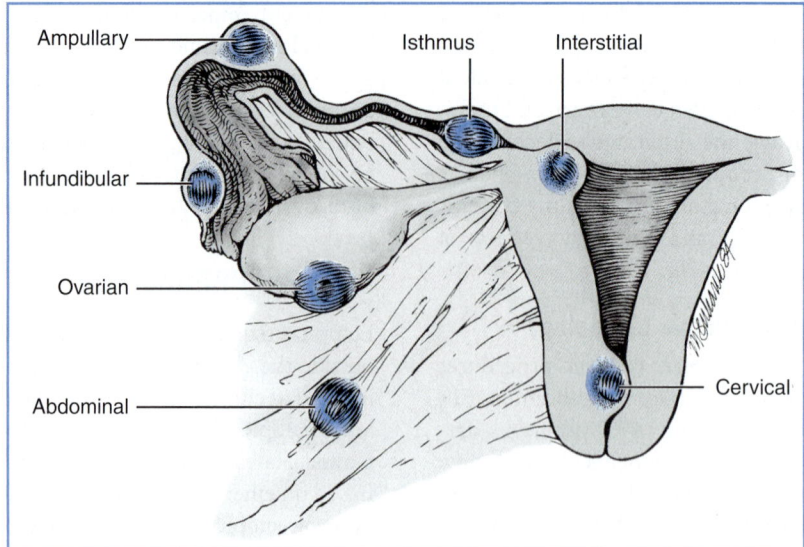

Fig. 17.6 Potential Locations of Ectopic Pregnancies. The majority occur in the ampullary portion of the fallopian tube. Modified from DeCherney AH, Seifer DB. Ectopic pregnancy. In: Gabbe SG, Niebyl JR, Simpson JL, eds. *Obstetrics: Normal and Problem Pregnancies*, 2nd ed. Churchill Livingstone; 1991:811.

In patients who have infertility, undergo ovulation induction, or undergo ART procedures, ectopic pregnancies are more common. ART, especially IVF with ovulation induction and transfer of multiple embryos, is associated with heterotopic pregnancy. The risk for heterotopic pregnancy in the general population is 3 to 25 per 100,000 pregnancies, while the risk after IVF may be as high as 1000 per 100,000 pregnancies.[65]

Clinical Presentation

The clinical presentation of the patient with an ectopic pregnancy depends on the gestational age, site of implantation, and extent of hemorrhage. **Abdominal pain** or **vaginal bleeding** in a reproductive age female requires evaluation for pregnancy. Before rupture, the signs and symptoms of ectopic pregnancy may be absent or subtle. Patients with hemorrhage (with or without tubal rupture) may experience dizziness or syncope, may have the urge to defecate because of the effect of blood in the cul-de-sac, and may have shoulder pain from diaphragmatic irritation by intraabdominal blood. As with many young, healthy patients, compensation for blood loss can occur with minimal symptoms initially, followed by rapid decompensation.

Diagnosis

Ectopic pregnancy should be excluded in any patient who has pelvic pain or vaginal bleeding and a positive pregnancy test. In a woman of reproductive age, the symptoms of ectopic pregnancy must be differentiated from early pregnancy loss (EPL), normal intrauterine pregnancy, abortion complications, and nonpregnancy-related causes of pelvic pain or vaginal bleeding.[65]

Pregnancy of unknown location (PUL) is present when a hCG test is positive and presumed due to pregnancy but the site of implantation is undetermined.[65] Transvaginal

ultrasonography can reliably confirm the presence of an intrauterine pregnancy. An intrauterine gestational sac with a yolk sac, embryo, or both is the earliest confirmation of an intrauterine pregnancy and should be visualized by 6 weeks' gestation. A gestational sac in the adnexa with a yolk sac, fetus, or both confirms the diagnosis of ectopic pregnancy; however, an ectopic pregnancy is often difficult to visualize. Findings suggesting ectopic pregnancy include ultrasonographic visualization of an adnexal mass and free fluid in the cul-de-sac in the absence of an intrauterine pregnancy.[65]

While early diagnosis of ectopic pregnancy is challenging, prompt identification and treatment decreases morbidity and mortality. If concern exists for ectopic pregnancy with a PUL, serial hCG measurements spaced 48 hours apart combined with periodic ultrasonographic evaluation can help clarify the viability of the pregnancy regardless of location.[65] The serum hCG criteria for a viable pregnancy have evolved and become more conservative in several ways. The rate of rise in hCG has been found to vary with the initial hCG value. Additionally, the discriminatory level, the level of hCG at which an intrauterine pregnancy should be visible with ultrasonography, has been raised. The level of hCG does not predict the risk for ectopic pregnancy rupture. Decreasing or plateauing hCG levels typically indicate a nonviable pregnancy.[65]

Uterine aspiration or curettage can be performed when a PUL has been found nonviable or is undesired. Identification of chorionic villi confirms an intrauterine pregnancy. Absence of villi signals either an early intrauterine pregnancy loss or an ectopic pregnancy. Follow-up hCG monitoring is required in this instance until the hCG level is negative, as ectopic pregnancies can still rupture with falling hCG levels.[65]

Obstetric Management

Management options for ectopic pregnancy include expectant, medical, and surgical. Management choice depends on the characteristics of the ectopic pregnancy, access to follow-up care, and patient preferences and fertility desires.[65] Patients with ectopic pregnancies who are Rh-negative should receive Rho(D) immune globulin.[66]

Expectant management has been studied in patients with hCG levels plateauing at less than 1500 mIU/mL who are hemodynamically stable with an identified ectopic pregnancy or PUL. While outcomes compared favorably to single-dose methotrexate therapy, some do not feel that the risk-benefit balance favors expectant management.[67,68] For patients with an initial hCG of less than 200 mIU/mL, the success rate is 88%.[65] Evidence of failed expectant management includes pain, inadequate decrease in hCG levels, or hemoperitoneum due to tubal rupture.

Medical management with methotrexate has become a common management strategy for ectopic pregnancies. Candidates for this therapy cannot have a ruptured ectopic pregnancy or any medical contraindications to methotrexate therapy (e.g., lactation, immunodeficiency, or moderate to severe hematologic, hepatic, renal, pulmonary, or peptic ulcer disease) and must be willing and able to participate in posttreatment monitoring.[65] Relative contraindications are summarized in Box 17.1.[65] Methotrexate regimens to manage ectopic pregnancy utilize one or more intramuscular injections in addition to symptom and hCG monitoring to identify those who require additional methotrexate or surgical management. Success rates vary from 70% to 95% and vary with initial hCG level and regimen used. Side effects of methotrexate are summarized in Box 17.1. An optimal management regimen has not been identified with an ideal balance of efficacy and few side effects, but one- and two-dose regimens are most common. Compared with surgical management, medical management of ectopic pregnancy results in no difference in overall tubal preservation, tubal patency, risk for repeat ectopic pregnancy, or success of future pregnancies.

Surgical management is indicated for hemodynamic instability or evidence of intraperitoneal bleeding or pain from rupture. Other indications for surgical management include absolute or relative contraindications to methotrexate therapy, failure of medical therapy, and patient preference. Except when large-volume intraperitoneal bleeding is anticipated, laparoscopic surgery is typically performed. Partial or complete salpingectomy removes the ectopic pregnancy and fallopian tube, whereas a salpingostomy opens the tube to remove only the ectopic pregnancy. Choice of technique depends on the patient's reproductive plans, degree of tubal damage, and condition of the contralateral tube. Salpingostomy has a higher subsequent intrauterine pregnancy rate but also an increased risk for recurrent ectopic pregnancy. Poor visualization at laparoscopy due to hemorrhage may require conversion to laparotomy.[65] To aid hemostasis during laparoscopic removal of the ectopic pregnancy, some surgeons inject dilute vasopressin into the surface of the fallopian tube. This agent causes marked blanching of the tube and results in a relatively bloodless surgical field. If the vasopressin is mixed incorrectly or accidentally injected intravenously, a marked increase in maternal blood pressure may occur.

Interstitial pregnancy occurs in 2% of ectopic pregnancies. Interstitial pregnancy results from implantation in the interstitial portion of the tube, where it traverses the myometrium.[69] This may go unrecognized and may manifest as uterine wall rupture, massive hemorrhage, and shock, resulting in a 2% to 5% mortality rate.[70] IVF, ipsilateral salpingectomy, uterine anomalies, and prior ectopic pregnancy are risk factors.[69] Salpingectomy has become a more common method of tubal sterilization in recent years. If diagnosed prior to rupture, interstitial ectopic pregnancy may be managed with systemic or local methotrexate therapy or selective arterial embolization. At a low initial hCG level with subsequent decline, expectant management may be considered. Surgical resection of an interstitial ectopic pregnancy via cornuotomy may be chosen initially or after failure of medical management, whereas a cornual wedge resection or hysterectomy may be required because of hemorrhage. Cornual wedge resection has a risk for uterine rupture with a future pregnancy.[69]

Cervical pregnancy occurs in 0.4% of ectopic pregnancies. Cervical pregnancy can result in massive, relatively painless hemorrhage because of the inability of the cervix to contract. Differentiating a cervical ectopic pregnancy from an evolving EPL can be challenging. Risk factors include prior dilation and curettage (D & C), prior cesarean delivery, or IVF for the current pregnancy. Owing to its rarity, standardized treatments have not been identified but may include uterine artery embolization (UAE), vaginal or laparoscopic ligation of the cervical branch of the uterine artery, hysteroscopic excision, local or systemic methotrexate, balloon tamponade, partial or

---

BOX 17.1 Contraindications and Relative Contraindications to Methotrexate for Ectopic Pregnancy Management and Side Effects

Contraindications
- Ruptured ectopic pregnancy
- Heterotopic pregnancy with desired, viable intrauterine pregnancy
- Lactation
- Immunodeficiency
- Moderate to severe hematologic, hepatic, renal, pulmonary, or peptic ulcer disease
- Inability to participate in posttreatment monitoring

Relative Contraindications
- Ectopic pregnancy more than 4 cm in diameter
- Embryonic cardiac activity visualized on transvaginal ultrasonography
- Initial serum hCG level > 5000 mIU/mL
- Refusal to accept blood products

Side Effects of Methotrexate (Vary With Total Dose)
- Abdominal pain, often 2–3 d after administration
- Vomiting
- Stomatitis
- Neutropenia
- Pneumonitis

complete cervical excision, hysterectomy, or combinations of the above.[69]

Ovarian ectopic pregnancy occurs in 1% to 3% of ectopic pregnancies. It is more common after ART and results when the gestation implants within the ovary.[69] Diagnosis of ovarian ectopic pregnancy is difficult using ultrasonography, and patients often present with intraperitoneal bleeding. Localization of the ectopic pregnancy may occur intraoperatively or on histologic examination. Treatment options include oophorectomy, ovarian wedge resection, or limited removal of the pregnancy only.

Cesarean scar ectopic pregnancy (CSEP) occurs in 4% to 6% of ectopic pregnancies. CSEP occurs in 1 in 500 to 560 pregnant patients with a prior low transverse cesarean delivery. In these cases a gestational sac implants in a uterine scar defect (niche or isthmocele) from a prior cesarean delivery.[69] Pain, bleeding, or no symptoms may precede ultrasonographic diagnosis, though the presenting symptom may be hemorrhagic shock.[71] Two types of CSEP occur. **Type I CSEP** develops with viable pregnancy growth into the uterine cavity, and **type II CSEP** develops with nonviable pregnancy growth toward the myometrium and bladder. The risk for uterine rupture and hemorrhage, possibly requiring hysterectomy, necessitates prompt identification and management of type II CSEP.[69] Type I CSEP can lead to **placenta accreta spectrum disorder** with risk for severe hemorrhage later in pregnancy or at delivery. For those with EPL and manageable bleeding, expectant management is an option but can be associated with development of a uterine arteriovenous malformation.[69,71] Expectant management of a viable pregnancy is not recommended by the Society for Maternal-Fetal Medicine (SMFM) because of the high risk for potentially life-threatening morbidity.[71] In the absence of definitive management options, various interventions may be used depending on presentation and the patient's desire for fertility. Surgical resection transvaginally or laparoscopically or ultrasound-guided uterine aspiration are operative interventions recommended by the SMFM, and hysterectomy may be considered.[71] Local injection of methotrexate into the gestation may be used with or without another intervention. Potassium chloride injection may be considered for a heterotopic gestation. UAE and balloon catheters have also been utilized.

Abdominal pregnancy, which occurs in 1% of ectopic pregnancies, results from implantation in the peritoneal cavity, not including the fallopian tubes, ovaries, broad ligament, or cervix. Risk factors are thought to be similar to those for other ectopic pregnancies. Maternal mortality is about nine times higher than with other ectopic pregnancies, and fetal mortality may be 45% to 90%.[69] Possibly because of minimal or vague symptoms, abdominal ectopic pregnancies are often diagnosed later in gestation than other ectopic pregnancies. Given the challenges in clinical and ultrasonographic identification of abdominal ectopic pregnancies, most cases are not diagnosed preoperatively. Magnetic resonance imaging may aid in diagnosis and identification of the placental implantation site. While laparoscopic surgery may be sufficient for first-trimester cases, laparotomy is typically undertaken for later gestations. The risk for hemorrhage depends on the site

of placental implantation and is lower with attachment to the uterine serosa and higher with attachment to the spleen, liver, iliac vessels, or omentum. Multiple factors impact the decision to remove the placenta or leave it *in situ*, as both options can result in mortality. The risk for immediate torrential hemorrhage with placental removal is balanced against future complications, which may include secondary hemorrhage, sepsis, preeclampsia, and coagulopathy. In specific circumstances, after careful evaluation and maternal counseling, expectant management has occurred with tertiary center monitoring and availability of a multidisciplinary team.[69]

Heterotopic pregnancy is rare in spontaneous pregnancies, but occurs in up to 1% of IVF pregnancies. Diagnosis can be challenging and relies on symptoms and ultrasonography, with a high index of suspicion required after IVF. Management is typically surgical as systemic methotrexate is contraindicated in the presence of a desired, viable intrauterine pregnancy.[65]

Anesthetic Management

Patients with an unruptured tubal pregnancy typically have normal intravascular volume, minimal bleeding before and during surgery, and low anesthetic and surgical risk. Anesthetic considerations for laparoscopy or laparotomy are summarized in Box 17.2. Although most patients may prefer general anesthesia, neuraxial anesthesia with an upper sensory level of at least T4 may be an alternative in selected patients. Shoulder pain from diaphragmatic irritation may occur and can be treated with intravenous analgesics (e.g., fentanyl 1 to 2 μg/kg).

A ruptured ectopic pregnancy may be associated with significant preoperative blood loss, but estimation of the extent of blood loss is difficult because healthy patients may maintain a normal blood pressure despite a markedly reduced circulating blood volume. General anesthesia, with preparation for hemorrhage, is preferred if significant bleeding has occurred (e.g., ruptured tubal pregnancy) or is likely to occur (e.g., cervical, interstitial, cornual, cesarean scar, or abdominal ectopic pregnancy, or early placenta accreta). Intraoperative autologous blood transfusion can be used, and it may be useful especially in developing countries, where blood bank supplies may be limited and women typically present late with significant hemoperitoneum and/or hypovolemic shock.[72] The desire to preserve fertility often results in greater blood loss as tissue and organ preservation are attempted. Studies that evaluated obstetric-related intensive care unit admissions found that approximately 9% to 10% of admissions were related to complications from ectopic pregnancies or abortion.[73,74]

EARLY PREGNANCY LOSS, ABORTION, AND MID-TRIMESTER PREGNANCY LOSS

Changing terminology now refers to spontaneous, incomplete, and missed abortions as **early pregnancy loss (EPL)**.[75] EPL is defined as a nonviable intrauterine gestation prior to 13 weeks' gestation, which is identified by the presence of a gestational sac that is empty or contains an embryo or fetus without cardiac activity. The term *abortion* is now limited to

BOX 17.2 Suggested Anesthetic Techniques for Laparoscopy or Laparotomy for Patients With Ectopic Pregnancy

General Considerations

- Blood typing and antibody screening
- Aspiration prophylaxis if patient not appropriately fasted
- Routine noninvasive monitors
- Large-bore peripheral intravenous catheter
- Urinary catheter
- If major bleeding has occurred or is expected to occur (e.g., ruptured tubal, interstitial, cervical, uterine scar, or abdominal ectopic pregnancy):
  - Two or more large-bore intravenous catheters
  - Typing and cross-matching of blood
  - Consideration of invasive hemodynamic monitoring (e.g., arterial catheter, central venous catheter)
  - Consideration of intraoperative cell salvage
- Although general anesthesia is usually preferred, neuraxial (spinal or epidural) anesthesia may be considered for hemodynamically stable patients with a low likelihood of significant hemorrhage (i.e., unruptured tubal pregnancy):
  - Intravenous fluids, vasopressors, supplemental oxygen, and minimal sedation given as clinically indicated

General Anesthesia

- Rapid-sequence induction with cricoid pressure if the patient is not appropriately fasted
- Induction: propofol (ketamine or etomidate should be considered if patient is hemodynamically unstable)
- Muscle relaxant
- Tracheal intubation
- Maintenance: volatile or intravenous anesthetic agents
- Placement of an oral gastric tube, performance of suctioning, and removal of the tube
- Reversal of neuromuscular blockade and extubation when the patient is awake and responds to verbal commands

Spinal Anesthesia

- Single injection with a small-gauge pencil-tip spinal needle: hyperbaric bupivacaine 12–15 mg with fentanyl 10–25 µg to achieve T4 sensory blockade

Epidural Anesthesia

- Placement of mid-lumbar epidural catheter
- Lidocaine 2% with epinephrine 5 µg/mL (1:200,000), approximately 20 mL, and fentanyl 100 µg, injected incrementally, to achieve T4 sensory blockade

medical or surgical procedures to terminate a pregnancy that does not result in a live birth, which may be performed electively or for medical reasons.[76]

EPL occurs in 10% to 15% of clinically recognized pregnancies overall, with the frequency varying with age: 9% to 17% at ages 20 to 30 years, 40% at age 35 years, 40% at age 40 years, and 80% at age 45 years.[75,77] When subclinical pregnancies are also considered, the incidence of spontaneous pregnancy loss may be as high as 60%.[78] Although most spontaneous pregnancy losses manifest clinically at 8 to 14 weeks' gestation, ultrasonography suggests that fetal demise usually occurs before 8 weeks' gestation.

Recurrent pregnancy loss refers to the spontaneous loss of two or more pregnancies confirmed by ultrasonography or histopathology.[79] Two consecutive EPLs are thought to occur in less than 5% of pregnant women and three or more in about 1%.[79] Identifiable etiologies include cytogenetic abnormalities, antiphospholipid antibody syndrome, anatomic abnormalities, and hormonal or metabolic abnormalities; however, an etiology usually is not identified. A Canadian study noted that high/very high healthcare use in the prior 2 years—a measure of baseline maternal morbidity—was associated with a twofold increase in the risk for a first EPL loss compared with a live birth. Other risk factors were use of infertility drugs, living in a disadvantaged neighborhood, and prior suicide attempt.[80] Most couples with recurrent pregnancy loss are able to conceive again and have a live birth.

A total of 620,327 legal abortions were reported in the United States in 2020, a rate of 11.2 abortions per 1000 women and a ratio of 198 abortions per 1000 live births.[76] The total number of abortions and rate of abortions (number of abortions per 1000 women) in the United States are at historic lows since surveillance began by the CDC in 1969.[76] In 2020, 51% were early medical abortions at less than or equal to 9 weeks' gestation, 40% were surgical abortions at less than or equal to 13 weeks' gestation, 6.7% were surgical abortions at greater than 13 weeks' gestation, and 2.4% were medical abortion at greater than 9 weeks' gestation.[76] Abortion is safer for the mother than carrying a pregnancy to term; the case fatality rate from 2013 to 2019 has decreased to 0.43 deaths per 100,000 reported legal abortions,[76] compared with 17.4 per 100,000 live births.[81] Unsafe abortions do not utilize medically recommended methods, are performed by individuals without necessary skills, occur outside appropriate pregnancy durations, take place in substandard environments, or a combination of these.[82] A global study estimated that the proportion of unsafe abortions was higher in countries with restrictive abortion laws compared with those with less restrictive laws.[82]

Judicial and legislative changes have decreased access to legal abortion in the United States. As of June 2023, 41% of women in the United States do not have access to an abortion clinic within a 30-minute drive, and 23% do not have access within a 90-minute drive.[83] Worldwide, in high-income countries, the rates of unintended pregnancy and abortion were lower in 2015 to 2019 if abortion was not restricted. Abortion restrictions in high-income countries increased rather than reduced abortion rates.[84] With restrictions limiting access to legal abortion in the United States, monitoring is required to determine whether complications from unsafe abortions may increase.

About 7% of women in the United States attempt self-managed abortion (SMA) at some point in their lifetime.[85] SMAs occur outside of formal healthcare and may include self-sourcing of medical abortion drugs, use of herbal or toxic substances, and physical methods. People of color, those with lower income, or people living in states with more legal restrictions on abortion appear to have higher rates of SMA.[86]

Mid-trimester pregnancy loss is variably defined as occurring between 13 and 20 weeks', and up to 24 weeks', gestation. The estimated incidence is 2% to 3% of diagnosed pregnancies.[87] Etiologies include placental or cervical insufficiency, fetal anomalies, antiphospholipid antibody syndrome, infection, and previable rupture of membranes; however, 50% to 60% of cases have no identified etiology.[87]

Second-trimester abortions comprise a small fraction of total abortions performed in the United States. In 2021, 93.5% of abortions were performed at less than or equal to 13 weeks' gestation, 5.7% of abortions were performed at 14 to 20 weeks' gestation, and 0.9% were performed at greater than or equal to 21 weeks' gestation.[76,88] Indications for pregnancy terminations in the second trimester include major fetal anatomic or genetic anomalies, previable premature rupture of membranes, preeclampsia, and maternal morbidity. Delays in first-trimester abortion access (e.g., diagnostic delays, financial hurdles, referral difficulties, travel requirements, delayed provider identification) also result in second-trimester abortions. Lower socioeconomic status and multiple disruptive life events are associated with higher risk for second-trimester abortion.[88] Abortion restrictions have been directed more toward second trimester procedures. A maternal morbidity rate of 57% and a 96% perinatal death rate occurred with legally mandated expectant management of previable premature rupture of membranes, compared with a 33% maternal morbidity rate when immediate pregnancy interruption was available and performed.[89]

Clinical Presentation

The clinical presentation and management of spontaneous EPL vary. Bleeding may be accompanied by cramping or backache. While historically recommended, alteration of daily activities (e.g., reduced activity or bedrest) does not impact outcome. Approximately 25% of pregnancies are complicated by first trimester bleeding; approximately half of affected women progress to a spontaneous pregnancy loss, with the percentage increasing to about 80% if both cramping and bleeding are present.[90]

Ultrasonographic and hCG criteria for diagnosing EPL have become more conservative based on observational data and a desire to avoid intervention in pregnancies that are viable and desired. Follow-up ultrasonography is indicated when the ultrasonographic diagnostic criteria are not definitively confirmed initially. Once an intrauterine site of pregnancy is confirmed by ultrasonography, hCG testing is no longer helpful in determining viability.

Fetal death in the second trimester, up to 20 to 24 weeks' gestation, is a **mid-trimester pregnancy loss** and is more likely to require medical intervention. Presenting signs and symptoms may include decreased fetal movement, vaginal bleeding, pain, and/or rupture of membranes, or no symptoms may occur.[87] Very rarely, coagulation defects, such as disseminated intravascular coagulation, may complicate mid-trimester loss in patients who have longer retention of fetal tissue and/or those who suffer the pregnancy loss at a more advanced gestational age.

Obstetric Management

First-trimester pregnancy losses can be managed expectantly, medically, or surgically. Factors such as gestational age, patient preference, treatment availability, and cost can all

impact management, but the long-term outcome is similar. A woman who is asymptomatic or minimally symptomatic may utilize any management option. Active vaginal bleeding (especially if heavy) typically requires surgical intervention to prevent excessive blood loss and potential shock. Medical disorders that would increase the patient's risk for bleeding or decrease maternal tolerance of blood loss or current infection are also indications for surgical management.

Conservative management incurs the least initial medical intervention and cost, but the highest chance of serious complications, including need for unplanned or emergency surgery. While most pregnancy losses occur in the early first trimester, spontaneous expulsion of tissue may not occur until the late first trimester. With expectant management, 64% of women will have complete passage of products of conception but some will require surgical intervention for bleeding. Conservative management has higher likelihood of success in early gestations.[77]

Medical management provides more control over timing of tissue expulsion without a procedure. Combination treatment of EPL with **misoprostol** and **mifepristone** results in a higher expulsion completion rate of 90.9% and a lower risk for surgical intervention than misoprostol alone, which has a 78% to 83% expulsion completion rate.[77,91] The potential for an ongoing viable pregnancy after medical abortion with misoprostol alone is about 6% but decreases with increasing number of doses.[91] When a combination of mifepristone and misoprostol is available, it is more effective in managing both EPL and medical abortions than misoprostol alone. Combination regimens involve oral administration of mifepristone and then misoprostol (buccal [FDA-approved], vaginal or sublingual) 24 to 48 hours later. Misoprostol-only regimens use 800-μg doses via buccal, vaginal, or sublingual routes, with the number of doses depending on clinical circumstances.[75,91] The likelihood of medical management success for EPL and abortion is greater with earlier gestations.[75,91]

For second-trimester (13 to 24 weeks' gestation) pregnancy loss or termination, management techniques are similar, although lower doses of medication and shorter time to completion are seen with pregnancy loss. Medical management options include mifepristone with misoprostol, misoprostol alone, high-dose intravenous oxytocin, or vaginal prostaglandin E_2.[92] Combining mifepristone and misoprostol optimizes efficacy and efficiency, with 95% completion within 24 hours compared with 80% to 85% completion with misoprostol alone.[92] While two or more prior cesarean deliveries increase the risk for uterine rupture, possibly to 2.5%, this is not considered a contraindication, especially when the alternative is hysterotomy.[93] Other methods are less commonly used. Use of a transcervical balloon catheter in combination with misoprostol alone has shortened time to completion but osmotic dilators have not.[93] Evidence regarding use of cervical preparation prior to mifepristone in combination with misoprostol is lacking.[93] Misoprostol, 15-methyl-prostaglandin $F2_\alpha$ (carboprost), or a procedural uterine evacuation may be required for retained placental tissue, though the ideal timing of intervention in the absence of hemorrhage is unclear. Compared with dilation and evacuation (D & E), medical induction at 13 to 24 weeks' gestation was less successful and had higher morbidity with an adjusted RR of 8.5 (95% CI, 3.7 to 19.8).[94]

The cervix can be prepared for a procedure to empty the uterus with vaginal misoprostol or intracervical laminaria, but this is not often required in first-trimester procedures. Procedures to empty the uterus include suction aspiration with a manual or electric vacuum, D & C, and D & E. Procedures currently described as "D & C" in practice may or may not include mechanical cervical dilation prior to suction aspiration with or without subsequent sharp curettage. D & E is the procedural method used to empty the uterus from 13 to 24 weeks' gestation due to ossified fetal bones that are present beginning at 13 to 15 weeks' gestation; this involves greater cervical dilation followed by evacuation of the uterus with suction and the aid of surgical forceps. Oxytocin and/or an ergot alkaloid (e.g., methylergonovine) increases uterine tone and may be administered intraoperatively and/or postoperatively to decrease the amount of uterine bleeding. To prevent massive maternal blood loss during a medically induced vaginal delivery, D & E is the procedure of choice for mid-trimester pregnancy loss up to 24 weeks with placenta previa or active bleeding. In the presence of infection, D & E may be delayed until after antibiotics have been administered.[92] Rho(D) immune globulin prophylaxis is widely recommended in the United States for pregnancies ending after 10 weeks' gestation. With conservative, medical or aspiration management of pregnancies at less than or equal to 12 0/7 weeks' gestation, Rho(D) immune globulin prophylaxis is no longer routinely recommended but may occur with shared decision making.[66,95,96]

An IUD may be placed immediately after a procedure for a first- or second-trimester pregnancy loss or abortion in the absence of sepsis. In cases of medical management, confirmation of completion including placental delivery must occur prior to IUD placement.[97]

Obstetric Complications

Complications of conservative management of EPL, medical management of EPL and abortion, and medical SMA are similar. Care may be sought because of pain, bleeding, and other symptoms that may or may not require intervention. Providers should only request information necessary to provide care.[97]

Complications of procedural management of EPL, abortion, mid-trimester pregnancy loss, and self-managed procedural abortion include cervical laceration, uterine perforation, hemorrhage, retained products of conception, infection, and sepsis. The risk for these complications is increased in pregnancies that have progressed beyond the first trimester, but the risk is still less than delivery later in pregnancy. Complications are higher if procedures occurred in unsafe environments.[75,88,94,98] Infection after EPL or abortion occurs in 0.9% to 2% of patients, with no clear variation based on indication or method of management except for unsafe procedures. The American College of Obstetricians and Gynecologists recommends administration of antimicrobial prophylaxis (e.g., a single dose of doxycycline 200 mg 1 hour before the procedure) for women undergoing uterine evacuation for induced abortion; this regimen has been shown to reduce infection risk by 41%.[75,99] Because the risk of infection after suction curettage for missed EPL should be similar to that after induced abortion, despite a lack of data, antibiotic prophylaxis should also be considered for these patients.[75,99] The benefit of antibiotic prophylaxis for the medical management of EPL and medical abortion is unknown, and the routine use of prophylactic antibiotics is not recommended in these circumstances.[95]

Infection may present as increasing abdominal pain, tachycardia, fever, uterine tenderness, or feeling unwell 24 hours or more after the onset of vaginal bleeding or a procedure. Use of multiple doses of misoprostol can cause temperature elevation in 5% to 10% of patients, potentially complicating identification of infection, although temperature should normalize within 2 hours after the medication is discontinued.[93] For those presenting with symptoms of infection, evaluation for retained products of conception is warranted. Uterine perforation should be considered after procedural management, especially if the procedure was unsafe. Prompt administration of broad-spectrum intravenous antibiotics is indicated. If infection leads to organ dysfunction and sepsis, fluid resuscitation and other support may be required. Toxic shock from *Clostridium* species can occur and presents with flulike symptoms that can progress rapidly to refractory hypotension and death. Hemoconcentration and marked leukocytosis are often present with *Clostridium* toxic shock.[75,88,94,95]

The risk for uterine perforation during D & C in a recently delivered patient may be as high as 5%.[100] Predisposing factors may include retroverted uterus, infection, later gestational age, and nulliparity. Midline perforation of the fundus with a blunt instrument may be managed with close observation. Use of a sharp instrument poses a greater risk for injury requiring further evaluation and management. Bleeding from vascular damage may be intraabdominal, retroperitoneal, or in the broad ligament. Bowel injury can also be difficult to identify. Laparoscopy, cystoscopy, or other evaluation may be required to evaluate and repair injury. Lower genital tract or bowel injury should be excluded, and the uterus should be promptly evaluated for the presence of retained tissue.

Preexisting anemia, infection, retained products of conception, cervical laceration, uterine perforation, and choice of medical or surgical management may affect decisions regarding transfusion after a first- or mid-trimester pregnancy loss or abortion.[75,92,94,95] Medical management is associated with higher transfusion rate (0.1%) compared with procedural management (0.01%) of first-trimester abortion.[95] Mid-trimester procedural and medical management have similar transfusion rates.[92] Medical management of a mid-trimester abortion may be associated with hemorrhage in 2% to 20% of cases, with rare need for transfusion.[93] The presence of placenta accreta spectrum markedly increases this risk.

Rho(D) immune globulin should be administered to prevent Rh alloimmunization when indicated. Rho(D) immune globulin administration for first trimester bleeding less than 12 weeks' gestation without pregnancy loss is optional based on immune globulin availability and patient and provider preference. In Rh-negative women who have a pregnancy loss, the risk for alloimmunization is 1.5% to 2% with a spontaneous loss and 4% to 5% after a D & C procedure. While Rho(D) immune globulin is considered in Rh-negative patients after a spontaneous loss, it is indicated at any gestation after a D & C for an early pregnancy loss, a medication managed or surgical termination of pregnancy greater than 12 0/7 weeks' gestation, or treatment of ectopic pregnancy with medication or surgery.[66]

Anesthetic Management

Several anesthetic techniques are appropriate for D & C and D & E procedures (Box 17.3). The choice depends on several factors (e.g., whether the cervix is dilated; the gestational age and ossification of the fetus; the presence of significant blood loss, sepsis, or a full stomach; and the emotional state and preference of the patient). Dilation of the cervix is relatively painful, whereas suction and curettage are less painful. If the cervix is dilated and the products of conception can be curettaged and suctioned, local anesthesia only (paracervical block), or sedation with or without a paracervical block, may suffice.[101] The World Health Organization (WHO) recommends routine availability of pain medication regardless of gestational age.[93] If the cervix is not dilated, paracervical block and sedation, spinal or epidural anesthesia (with sensory blockade from T10 to S4), or general anesthesia should be used. Indications for general anesthesia may include high risk for hemorrhage; active vomiting; full stomach; or a gestational age ≥ 15 weeks, which requires a greater degree of cervical dilation for a D & E procedure. Selected patients may benefit from premedication with a short-acting benzodiazepine (e.g., **midazolam**). The SMFM has stated that the fetus does not perceive pain until 24 to 25 weeks' gestation, and does not recommend the administration of fetal analgesia during pregnancy termination.[102]

Monitored anesthesia care or deep sedation ensures patient comfort, avoids airway instrumentation, and incurs both shorter operating room time and shorter recovery time.[103] In a retrospective, cohort study of 5579 patients receiving moderate or deep sedation without tracheal

---

BOX 17.3   Suggested Anesthetic Techniques for Dilation and Uterine Suction Curettage (D & C) or Evacuation (D & E) for Early Pregnancy Loss or Induced Abortion

General Considerations

- A paracervical block alone or with moderate sedation may be used for D & C. Patients may have significant discomfort and anxiety
- Blood typing and antibody screening or typing and cross-matching in patients with a large blood loss or those with advanced gestation
- Aspiration prophylaxis if patient is not appropriately fasted
- Routine noninvasive monitors
- One peripheral intravenous catheter
- Administration of a short-acting benzodiazepine (e.g., midazolam) may be indicated for patients who prefer anxiolysis, sedation, and/or amnesia
- Ketorolac and acetaminophen may reduce postoperative pain
- Monitored anesthesia care (moderate or deep sedation, natural airway) is an option in healthy, stable patients who have appropriately fasted. A paracervical block can facilitate this anesthetic
- Neuraxial (spinal or epidural) anesthesia is an option for hemodynamically stable patients without sepsis
- General anesthesia may be most appropriate for patients at high risk for hemorrhage, active vomiting, or a full stomach, or for patients requiring a D & E procedure (e.g., gestation > 15 w with large fetal size and fetal ossification)
- Intravenous fluids, vasopressors, supplemental oxygen, and sedation given as clinically indicated
- Uterotonics should be available, such as oxytocin, methylergonovine, carboprost, or misoprostol
- In patients with significant blood loss: observe the patient in the operating room for evidence of hypotension for at least 5 min after the legs have been lowered from the lithotomy to the supine position

Monitored Anesthesia Care (Moderate or Deep Sedation)

- Well tolerated when the cervix is dilated and gestational age is first trimester

- Paracervical block
- Intravenous analgesia with fentanyl, alfentanil, or remifentanil and sedation with propofol. May add midazolam as needed for anxiolysis

Spinal Anesthesia

- Sensory blockade from T10 to S4
- Single injection with a small-gauge spinal needle
- Hyperbaric bupivacaine 7.5–10 mg, 2-chloroprocaine 40–50 mg, mepivacaine 45–70 mg, or lidocaine 40 mg, with fentanyl 10–20 µg

Epidural Anesthesia

- Placement of mid-lumbar epidural catheter
- Lidocaine 2% with epinephrine 5 µg/mL (12–15 mL) and fentanyl 50–100 µg, injected incrementally, to achieve sensory blockade from T10 to S4

General Anesthesia

- Rapid-sequence induction with cricoid pressure if the patient is not appropriately fasted
- Induction: propofol or thiopental (ketamine or etomidate in cases of severe hemorrhage and hemodynamic instability)
- Mask anesthesia or supraglottic airway during early pregnancy if patient is appropriately fasted and hemodynamically stable; otherwise, tracheal intubation with a muscle relaxant
- Maintenance: intravenous anesthetic agents (propofol infusion) and short duration opioid (e.g., fentanyl or alfentanil). Nitrous oxide or volatile anesthetic (<0.5 MAC) may be added
- High concentration (>0.5 MAC) of a volatile anesthetic agent should be avoided if there is significant bleeding or evidence of uterine atony
- Insertion and removal of an oral gastric tube (if trachea is intubated) to evacuate the stomach
- Tracheal extubation when the patient is awake and responds to verbal commands

MAC, Minimum alveolar concentration.

intubation (administered by registered nurses and certified registered nurse anesthetists) at a free-standing abortion center, there were no perioperative pulmonary complications or anesthesia-related adverse events.[104] In a retrospective study of 4481 second-trimester D & E procedures, 2523 patients (56%) received deep sedation without tracheal intubation (administered by an anesthesiologist).[105] Of these cases, there were seven cases of anesthesia-related complications, with two cases of pulmonary aspiration (0.08%; 95% CI, 0.01% to 0.29%), four cases of upper airway obstruction (0.16%; 95% CI, 0.04% to 0.41%), and one case of lingual nerve injury (0.04%; 95% CI, 0.001% to 0.22%).[105] Intravenous sedation without tracheal intubation for first- and second-trimester abortions may be considered.

Neuraxial anesthesia should be considered in response to patient preference, in patients with a difficult airway, or severe cardiovascular or pulmonary disease.[103] Sensory blockade from T10 to S4 is necessary for the procedure. There are few data regarding optimal neuraxial anesthesia management for D & C and D & E procedures; however, data from other types of procedures can guide management. A **hyperbaric bupivacaine** single injection of intrathecal **hyperbaric bupivacaine** (7.5 to 10 mg) and **fentanyl** (10 to 20 µg) is sufficient. However, compared with intrathecal bupivacaine, intrathecal **mepivacaine** 2% and intrathecal **2-chloroprocaine** 3% have an earlier return to motor function, which facilitates discharge.[106,107]

Typically, the cervix is already dilated in patients who have had significant preoperative bleeding. Rarely does a patient with a closed cervix have significant, visible bleeding. In the presence of significant bleeding, intravascular volume should be restored first. A paracervical block and sedation may then be adequate. Substantial hemorrhage represents a relative contraindication to the use of spinal or epidural anesthesia.

General anesthesia may be induced with **propofol**, although **ketamine** or **etomidate** may be preferred in patients with significant bleeding and hemodynamic instability. Large doses (1.5 to 2.0 mg/kg) of ketamine may increase uterine tone.[108]

Drugs administered for general anesthesia may influence blood loss during the procedure. Volatile anesthetic agents cause dose-dependent relaxation of uterine smooth muscle[109] and have been associated with increased uterine bleeding.[110] A systematic review found bleeding was higher in patients randomized to receive a volatile anesthetic agent compared with propofol, with a mean difference of 164 (95% CI, 44 to 286) mL.[110]

For D & E procedures, general anesthesia is commonly maintained with oxygen, a propofol infusion, and an opioid. **Nitrous oxide** or a low concentration (<0.5 minimum alveolar concentration [MAC]) of a volatile anesthetic agent may be added. The volatile anesthetic agent should be avoided or discontinued if there is any evidence of uterine atony. In most cases, **oxytocin** is administered intravenously to increase uterine tone and decrease blood loss. Oxytocin is typically administered via an infusion pump with or without a 1 to 3 IU bolus. Oxytocin receptor expression increases with gestation. Therefore, uterine atony in early pregnancy may best be treated with **misoprostol**, **carboprost**, or **methylergonovine**.

The D & C or D & E procedure is performed with the patient in the lithotomy position. After the procedure is completed and the patient's legs are lowered, hypotension may develop in patients who have lost a substantial amount of blood, especially if neuraxial anesthesia has been used.

CERVICAL INSUFFICIENCY OR INCOMPETENCE

Cervical insufficiency is the inability of the cervix to hold a pregnancy in the uterus through the second trimester in the absence of labor. The definition and diagnostic criteria for cervical insufficiency have changed over time because of difficulty in separating it from other processes that lead to preterm delivery. Cervical insufficiency is a clinical diagnosis. Vaginal bleeding, rupture of membranes, and labor may result from cervical insufficiency, but to meet the diagnostic criteria these cannot be antecedent events. The etiology of cervical insufficiency remains unclear, and acquired factors such as obstetric cervical laceration, treatment of cervical intraepithelial lesions, or mechanical dilation for a gynecologic procedure may contribute to an increased risk. Congenital factors may include collagen disorders, Müllerian disorders, and biologic variation.[111]

Diagnosis

Symptoms of cervical insufficiency include altered vaginal discharge, lower abdominal or back pressure or discomfort, vaginal fullness, and urinary frequency. The diagnosis is definitive if delivery occurs in the second trimester before 24 weeks' gestation in the absence of bleeding, infection, or labor as the initial symptom. Cervical dilation or prolapse of membranes through the cervix in the absence of other findings or symptoms provides sufficient certainty of cervical insufficiency. A short cervix on ultrasonographic measurement is associated with preterm birth but is not sufficient to diagnose cervical insufficiency. As success of cerclage is less when the cervix is dilated or membranes are prolapsed, various means of screening asymptomatic women have been proposed, but no satisfactory test has been identified.[111]

Obstetric Management

Cervical cerclage may be placed based on prior obstetric history, current symptoms and findings, or both. For women with two or more second trimester losses that suggest cervical insufficiency, a history-indicated cerclage may be placed at 12 to 14 weeks' gestation. Alterations in maternal activity have not proven effective. Cervical pessaries may be helpful in a subset of high-risk individuals. A rescue or emergency cerclage is placed in the setting of symptoms such as pelvic pressure, cramping, or altered vaginal discharge and evidence of cervical insufficiency before 25 weeks' gestation. A dilated or short cervix found on visual or digital examination or a short cervix on transvaginal ultrasonography provide evidence of cervical insufficiency. Rescue or emergency cerclage carries greater risk for complications and a lower success rate. Some women will be found to have a short cervix during routine screening anatomy ultrasonography, while others with risk factors may have serial ultrasonographic examinations to detect development of a short cervix. With a history of prior preterm birth at less than 34 weeks' gestation along with a short cervix (<2.5 cm) noted on ultrasonography before 24 weeks' gestation, cerclage placement is associated with improved outcome.[112] In these women, an estimated 20 cerclages are needed to prevent one perinatal death, and more than 6500 infants per year could be saved in the United States by this management.[113] In contrast, cerclage placement appears to worsen the outcome in women with a multifetal gestation regardless of cervical length.

Transvaginal cerclages are most common and include the modified **Shirodkar cerclage** and **McDonald cerclage**. A nonabsorbable ligature (e.g., polyester, large-gauge polypropylene, or polyester suture) is placed around the cervix at or near the level of the internal cervical os. In the more invasive modified Shirodkar procedure, the cervical mucosa is incised anteriorly and posteriorly with dissection of the bladder and rectum off the cervix. The ligature is placed submucosally and then tied, and the mucosal incisions are closed. The cervical mucosa is left intact with the McDonald cerclage; a purse-string ligature is placed around the cervix and then tied (Fig. 17.7). These two procedures result in comparable rates of fetal survival in patients with no history of a previous cerclage.[111,114] The cerclage is removed at 36 to 37 weeks' gestation, or earlier if there is rupture of membranes, signs of labor, or infection. McDonald cerclage may be removed in a clinic setting but Shirodkar cerclage may require tissue dissection for removal.[111]

Transvaginal cerclage can be performed in most patients with an incompetent cervix. However, if no substantial cervical tissue is present (e.g., severe cervical laceration, shortening, or scarring) or if spontaneous delivery occurred prior to 28 weeks' gestation with a previous transvaginal cerclage, a **transabdominal cerclage** may be performed. Compared with repeat transvaginal cerclage in those who delivered prior to

33 to 34 weeks' gestation with a cerclage in place, transabdominal cerclage either before or during pregnancy was associated with reduced risk for recurrent preterm birth. Most patients with transabdominal cerclage undergo cesarean delivery. The cerclage may be placed via open, laparoscopic, or robotic surgery depending on clinical situation and available resources. The transabdominal cerclage can remain *in situ* if further pregnancies are desired, or it can be removed at the time of cesarean delivery.[115]

Contraindications to cerclage procedures include preterm labor, vaginal bleeding, fetal anomalies, fetal death, rupture of membranes, placental abruption, and evidence of intrauterine infection. Some obstetric providers obtain specimens for culture of the amniotic fluid and/or cervix before placement of a cerclage. Although the efficacy of perioperative antibiotics and/or tocolytic drugs has not been confirmed, some obstetric providers may choose to use them.[111]

The greatest risk during the performance of emergency cerclage is **rupture of the membranes**. Several techniques have been described to facilitate replacement of the bulging fetal membranes into the uterus. Uterine relaxation is essential, which can be facilitated by administration of a volatile anesthetic agent. Alternatively, a uterine relaxant like nitroglycerin may be administered. The steep Trendelenburg position allows for gravity assistance.

To assist in reduction of herniated membranes, some obstetric providers fill the urinary bladder with sterile saline. Insertion of a 16-mm Foley catheter into the cervical canal with subsequent inflation of the balloon with 30 to 60 mL of saline has also been described.[116] The balloon is deflated and the catheter is removed at the end of the procedure.

The risk for complications with cervical cerclage varies widely with the clinical situation and technique. Immediate complications include rupture of the fetal membranes, hemorrhage, and preterm labor. Transabdominal cerclage placement incurs risk for bowel, bladder, and vascular injury.[115] Delayed complications of all cerclages include infection,

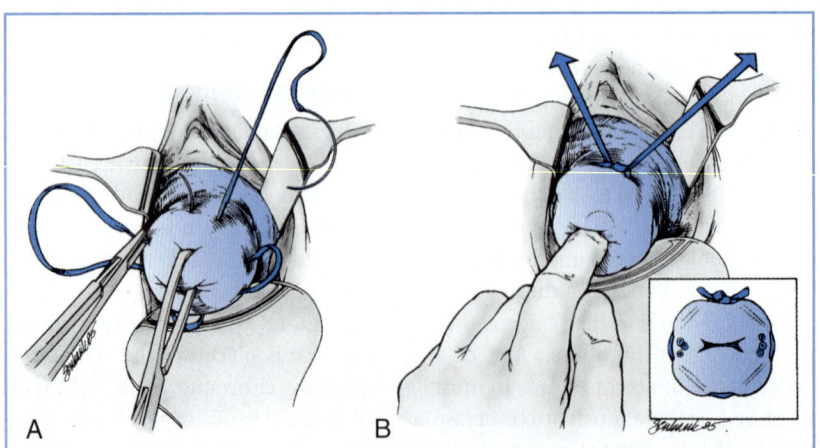

Fig. 17.7 Placement of Sutures for McDonald Cervical Cerclage. (A) A double-headed polyester fiber (Mersilene) band with four "bites" is placed in the cervix, avoiding the vessels. (B) The suture is placed high up on the cervix, close to the cervical-vaginal junction, approximately at the level of the internal os. Modified from Iams JD. Preterm birth. In: Gabbe SG, Niebyl JR, Simpson JL, eds. *Obstetrics: Normal and Problem Pregnancies*, 4th ed. Churchill Livingstone; 2002:803.

suture displacement, cervical stenosis secondary to scarring, and cervical lacerations and uterine rupture if labor proceeds with the cerclage in place. Rarely, sepsis may result in death.[111]

Anesthetic Management

Transvaginal cervical cerclage is usually performed under spinal, epidural, or general anesthesia (Box 17.4). The degree of cervical dilation may influence the choice of anesthesia. If the cervix is not dilated, spinal, epidural, or general anesthesia may be administered. Neuraxial anesthesia is commonly used and provides dense sensory blockade, maintenance

of airway reflexes, and reduced sedation, while limiting fetal exposure to anesthetic agents and reducing postoperative nausea and vomiting. Sensory blockade from sacral dermatomes to T10 is necessary, because both the cervix (L1 to T10) and vagina and perineum (S2 to S4) require anesthesia. **Bupivacaine** is commonly used for spinal anesthesia but its prolonged duration of action may be associated with delayed discharge from the hospital. **2-Chloroprocaine** has a shorter duration of action than bupivacaine; a prospective, dose-finding study estimated that the effective dose for 90% of patients (ED_{90}) of intrathecal 2-chloroprocaine combined with fentanyl 10 µg for elective cervical cerclage placement was 49.5 mg (95% CI, 45.0 to 50.1).[117] A comparison of intrathecal 50-mg 2-chloroprocaine 3% with 9-mg hyperbaric bupivacaine 0.75%, both with fentanyl 15 µg, found no difference in time to motor block resolution (109 versus 112 minutes, respectively; $P = .66$). However, time to sensory block resolution (143 versus 198 minutes; $P = .002$) and time to recovery room discharge (76 minutes shorter; $P < .0005$) were significantly shorter in patients who received 2-chloroprocaine than in patients who received bupivacaine.[106] There is no consensus on the ideal local anesthetic for cervical cerclage placement procedures, and intrathecal **lidocaine** and **mepivacaine** can also be considered. Administration of neuraxial anesthesia obviates the need for tracheal intubation and the possibility of coughing on the endotracheal tube. Although some physicians worry that the acute dorsiflexion needed during initiation of the neuraxial blockade may raise intrauterine pressure, many prefer the avoidance of general anesthesia during pregnancy whenever possible.

If the cervix is dilated—especially if the fetal membranes are bulging—the choice of anesthesia is less straightforward. The advantages and disadvantages of each anesthetic technique must be weighed carefully. It is important to produce adequate analgesia for the mother and to prevent an increase in intraabdominal and intrauterine pressure that may lead to further bulging and possible rupture of the fetal membranes.

General anesthesia may be preferred in the patient with a dilated cervix and bulging fetal membranes. Administration of a volatile anesthetic agent relaxes uterine smooth muscle and results in a decrease in intrauterine pressure. A decrease in intrauterine pressure facilitates replacement of the bulging membranes and placement of the cerclage. On occasion, amniocentesis may be performed before or during a cerclage procedure to decrease intrauterine pressure and facilitate reduction of the fetal membranes. During induction and maintenance of general anesthesia, it is important to avoid endotracheal tube–induced coughing, which might raise intrauterine pressure. In addition, vomiting significantly raises intrauterine pressure.

Few clinical studies have compared obstetric outcomes after administration of neuraxial anesthesia and general anesthesia for cerclage. One retrospective study observed no difference in fetal outcome after administration of either general anesthesia (375 cases) or epidural anesthesia (114 cases).[118]

Another study found no significant difference in plasma oxytocin levels or postoperative uterine activity between women who received either spinal or general anesthesia for a Shirodkar cerclage.[119] A more recent prospective case-control study compared outcomes after general anesthesia (141 cases) and spinal anesthesia (156 cases) for emergency cervical cerclage placement and found no significant differences in preterm delivery, miscarriage rate, or maternal and neonatal outcomes.[120]

In theory, it is possible that replacement of bulging membranes and closure of the cervix may raise intrauterine pressure with a subsequent reduction in placental blood flow. In this case, it would be reasonable to give a tocolytic agent to help reduce intrauterine pressure.

Removal of a McDonald cerclage often does not require anesthesia. Anesthesia (e.g., paracervical block, spinal anesthesia, epidural anesthesia) is usually necessary for removal of a Shirodkar cerclage. If the Shirodkar cerclage is epithelialized, some obstetric providers elect to leave it intact and perform an elective cesarean delivery.

Labor often begins within a few hours or days after suture removal. If an epidural catheter was placed for cerclage removal, the epidural anesthetic can be allowed to regress while the patient is observed for evidence of cervical dilation and the onset of labor. When labor begins, epidural labor analgesia can be initiated by injection of drugs through the *in situ* catheter.

GESTATIONAL TROPHOBLASTIC DISEASE

In a normal pregnancy, trophoblastic tissue forms the placenta. Abnormal trophoblastic development after abnormal fertilization results in **gestational trophoblastic disease (GTD)**. Benign varieties include complete and partial **hydatidiform moles** and placental site nodules. Atypical placental site nodules have malignant potential. Malignant varieties, known as **gestational trophoblastic neoplasia (GTN)**, include **invasive mole**, **choriocarcinoma**, **placental site trophoblastic tumor**, and **epithelioid trophoblastic tumor**.[121]

Risk factors for hydatidiform mole include history of a hydatidiform mole (more so if a complete mole) and, more impactfully, extremes of reproductive age (less than 15 years and greater than 45 years). Brazil and parts of Asia including India have higher incidences of molar pregnancy (around 2 to 6 per 100,000 pregnancies) than Europe and North America (1 to 2 per 100,000 pregnancies). Choriocarcinoma is less common in Europe and North America (3 per 100,000 deliveries) than in Southeast Asia (about 23 per 100,000 deliveries). Placental site trophoblastic tumor at 1 per 100,000 deliveries and epithelioid trophoblastic tumor at 0.1 per 100,000 deliveries are rarer forms of malignant GTD.[121]

Produced by the cytotrophoblast and syncytiotrophoblast, hCG serves as a perfect tumor marker aiding in diagnosis, monitoring of therapy, and detection of recurrent disease. Metastatic disease does not preclude cure with GTN.[121]

Categorization and Etiology

Complete and Partial Hydatidiform Mole

The two types of hydatidiform moles vary in karyotype and histology. A complete mole lacks maternal DNA and is diploid with a 46XX or 46XY karyotype from duplication of chromosomes from a single sperm (80%) or fertilization by two sperms (20%). A fetus does not develop but hydropic villi do and may be accompanied by theca lutein ovarian cysts. In contrast, partial moles are typically triploid after fertilization of an ovum with haploid maternal DNA by two sperms. A nonviable fetus is present and cystic changes occur in the placenta. Preevacuation, it may be diagnosed as an EPL. Flow cytometry may be used on products of conception to differentiate between these two conditions. Early hCG testing and ultrasonography have led to diagnosis earlier in pregnancy and a reduced occurrence of preeclampsia, hyperthyroidism, and respiratory failure. Hyperemesis, anemia, and uterine enlargement are other presenting symptoms that have decreased with earlier diagnosis.[121]

Gestational Trophoblastic Neoplasia and Atypical Placental Site Nodule

GTN can occur after a molar pregnancy (50%), a term or preterm pregnancy (25%), or an ectopic pregnancy or EPL (25%).[121] Abnormal uterine bleeding postpartum may be the presenting symptom, but sequelae of bleeding from metastatic sites in the lung, liver, spleen, brain, spine, and intestine may also occur.[122] The antecedent pregnancy may be unrecognized.

Atypical placental site nodules coexist with or develop into placental site trophoblastic tumor or epithelioid trophoblastic tumor in 10% to 15% of cases. These three forms variably produce hCG and develop primarily in the placental bed (atypical placental site nodules and placental site trophoblastic tumor) or cervix or lower uterine segment (epithelioid trophoblastic tumor).[122]

Medical Complications

Earlier diagnosis has decreased the risk for complications at presentation and during uterine evacuation. In the absence of early hCG testing and ultrasonography, vaginal bleeding, sometimes with passage of villi, may be the presenting symptom.[122] Complications can occur in 25% of those with a 14 to 16 weeks' gestational size uterus or larger.[123] Nausea and vomiting of pregnancy are common and may be severe.[121] Preoperative anemia may develop secondary to vaginal or concealed bleeding. The homology of hCG and thyroid-stimulating hormone (TSH) can lead to hyperthyroidism at very high hCG levels. This in turn increases the risk for thyroid storm. Uterine enlargement greater than 16 weeks' gestational size is associated with a greater risk for intraoperative complications including hemorrhage, uterine perforation, and respiratory distress.[122] Trophoblastic embolization, hyperthyroidism, preeclampsia, anemia, and iatrogenic fluid overload may contribute to a risk for acute respiratory distress syndrome.[123] Theca lutein cysts develop more commonly with complete moles and result from hCG stimulation of the ovary. Surgical intervention for torsion or rupture is rarely required.[123] The occurrence of first-trimester preeclampsia (new-onset hypertension and proteinuria) is extremely rare in the absence of GTD. Emptying the uterus of GTD and antihypertensive therapies are the cornerstones of primary management.

Obstetric Management
Complete and Partial Hydatidiform Moles

Management is primarily with suction D & C, although if fertility preservation is not desired, a hysterectomy can be performed per patient preference (80% reduction in GTN). Preoperatively, assessment of complete blood count and serum creatinine, and performance of type and screen or cross-match are appropriate given the risk for hemorrhage. Uterotonic medications such as an oxytocin infusion may be administered during the procedure. Medical evacuation of the uterus is contraindicated because of the risk for hemorrhage and higher rates of GTN. Rho(D) immune globulin is indicated for Rh-negative patients. Hemorrhage and pulmonary compromise are potential intraoperative complications. After D & C or hysterectomy, hCG monitoring is initiated to detect postmolar GTN development, which occurs in about 20% of complete moles and 4% of partial moles. Multiple guidelines exist recommending hCG monitoring strategies. Normalization of hCG level within 56 days of uterine evacuation or hysterectomy is associated with a 0.02% to 0.03% risk for postmolar GTN, so duration of monitoring may be shorter than previously recommended.[121] Patients at highest risk for postmolar GTN development after molar pregnancy include those with an initial hCG over 100,000 mIU/mL, age older than 40 years, presence of theca lutein cyst, and uterine size greater than dates.[121] The risk for postmolar GTN increases with age and may reach 60% after uterine evacuation in those older than 50 years regardless of hCG level. The combination of hCG over 175,000 mIU/mL and age older than 40 years increases postmolar GTN risk after uterine evacuation to 85%.[121]

Specific care of GTN is beyond the scope of this chapter. GTN often presents with bleeding sequelae and metastatic forms can appear in any organ, but most frequently the lung, brain, or liver.[121,122]

While postmolar GTN can be diagnosed by histology, it may also be diagnosed based on a plateaued hCG level, a rising hCG level, or clinical or radiologic evidence of metastatic disease. Biopsy of highly vascular metastatic disease can result in profuse bleeding. The Féderation Internationale de Gynécolgie et d'Obstétrique (FIGO) anatomic stage and WHO risk scores predict disease progression and response to single agent chemotherapy. Low-risk GTN, as determined by FIGO stage and score, has an almost 100% complete remission rate overall. Disease with higher FIGO stage and score can have drug resistance and is managed with multiagent chemotherapy.[121] Induction chemotherapy may be given initially to ultra-high-risk patients to reduce early death from sudden tumor collapse.[122]

Anesthetic Management

Preoperative assessment of the patient with a molar pregnancy consists of evaluation for specific complications of molar pregnancy, including hyperemesis gravidarum, gestational hypertension and preeclampsia, anemia, and thyrotoxicosis. The main anesthetic considerations include the potential for rapid and significant blood loss and the risk for cardiopulmonary distress with uterine evacuation. The anesthesia provider should establish adequate intravenous access, and blood products should be immediately available. Invasive arterial pressure and/or central venous pressure monitoring may be indicated in the patient with hypoxemia, severe anemia, hemorrhage, severe gestational hypertension or preeclampsia, hyperthyroidism, or a uterus greater than 16 weeks' gestation size.

Although neuraxial anesthesia has been described, general anesthesia is often preferred because of the potential for rapid, substantial blood loss and cardiopulmonary distress during evacuation of the uterus (Box 17.5). For patients with acute hemorrhage and hypovolemia, induction with **propofol** may cause marked hypotension. In hyperthyroid patients, **ketamine** may result in marked tachycardia.[124] **Etomidate** may be considered for patients with preoperative bleeding and preoperative evidence of hyperthyroidism. Anesthesia can be maintained using either an inhalational or intravenous technique, although it may be necessary to avoid volatile anesthetic agents in some patients to optimize uterine contractility.[125] Care should be exercised with the use of a propofol infusion in hemodynamically unstable patients.

An intravenous **oxytocin** infusion (6 to 15 IU/h) should begin either before or during uterine evacuation.[123] Oxytocin helps the uterus contract, facilitating safe curettage and reducing blood loss. Some obstetric providers have speculated

---

BOX 17.5 Suggested Anesthetic Technique for Patients With Gestational Trophoblastic Disease

Preoperative Evaluation
- Evaluation for complications of molar pregnancy
- Baseline arterial blood gas measurements

General Anesthesia
- Routine noninvasive monitors
- Consider invasive hemodynamic monitoring in patients with hypoxemia, gestational hypertension or preeclampsia, severe anemia, hyperthyroidism, or a uterine size > 16 w
- Two large-gauge peripheral intravenous catheters
- Immediate availability of blood
- Induction: etomidate if evidence of hemorrhage or hemodynamic instability
- Tracheal intubation with a muscle relaxant
- Maintenance: inhalation or intravenous technique; avoid volatile agents if optimization of uterine contractility is required, and exercise caution with the use of a propofol infusion in hemodynamically unstable patients
- Oxytocin infusion (6–15 IU/h) after cervical dilation or after partial uterine evacuation

that oxytocin may decrease trophoblastic embolization by constricting the uterine veins.[123] Postoperatively, the patient should be monitored closely for any evidence of uterine hemorrhage or cardiopulmonary distress.

NAUSEA AND VOMITING OF PREGNANCY AND HYPEREMESIS GRAVIDARUM

As many as 50% to 80% of women experience nausea and 50% experience vomiting or retching during pregnancy. This can result in impaired quality of life, missed work, and use of medical resources. Delay in management can result in more refractory symptoms and subsequently increased risk for complications and hospitalization. Although it has been referred to as *morning sickness*, symptoms can occur at any time of day. Symptoms typically improve or resolve by the end of the first trimester.[126]

On rare occasions (0.3% to 3% of pregnancies), women experience a persistent and severe form of nausea and vomiting called **hyperemesis gravidarum**.[126] Evidence of acute starvation (marked ketonuria) and loss of 5% of prepregnant weight are potential but not universally accepted diagnostic criteria. Tests of electrolytes, liver function, and thyroid function may be mildly abnormal. In early pregnancy, hyperemesis gravidarum is the most common reason for hospital admission.[126]

Risk factors for hyperemesis gravidarum include multiple gestation, GTD, thyrotoxicosis, history of motion sickness, migraine headaches, and personal or family history of hyperemesis.[126] Diagnosis is by exclusion, and if symptoms begin after 9 weeks' gestation, many other underlying diseases should be ruled out. The presence of symptoms prior to pregnancy or findings such as fever, more than mild abdominal tenderness, or other localizing signs may suggest alternative diagnoses including gastrointestinal diseases (e.g., gastroenteritis, peptic ulcer disease, gastroparesis, hepatitis, cholecystitis, pancreatitis, gastroparesis, partial bowel obstruction, appendicitis), genitourinary diseases (e.g., pyelonephritis, uremia, ovarian torsion, kidney stones, fibroid degeneration), metabolic disorders (e.g., diabetic ketoacidosis, hyperthyroidism, hyperparathyroidism, Addison disease), neurologic disorders (e.g., pseudotumor cerebri, migraine headaches,

central nervous system tumors), psychiatric disorders, acute fatty liver of pregnancy, drug toxicity, cannabis use, and preeclampsia, among others. Gastroesophageal reflux disease may exacerbate vomiting throughout pregnancy. Markedly abnormal laboratory values suggest an etiology other than hyperemesis gravidarum.

Serious maternal complications may include Wernicke encephalopathy (deficiency of vitamin B1), acute tubular necrosis, esophageal rupture, and pneumothorax and splenic avulsion.[126]

Timely management of nausea and vomiting of pregnancy is thought to reduce progression to hyperemesis gravidarum. In addition to lifestyle interventions, early initiation of vitamin B6 and doxylamine, potentially prior to symptoms in those with a prior history of hyperemesis gravidarum, is recommended because of long-term evidence of safety and efficacy. Escalating therapy involves layering of additional therapies if needed. The potential exists for extrapyramidal effects, neuroleptic malignant syndrome, and QT interval prolongation depending on medication combinations used. Dehydration is managed with intravenous rehydration and correction of electrolyte abnormalities. Antithyroid medications are not indicated for suppressed TSH and elevated free T4 (thyroxine) in early pregnancy (gestational thyrotoxicosis). Interventions of last resort include corticosteroids, parenteral nutrition, and a peripherally inserted central venous catheter.[126]

CORPUS LUTEUM CYSTS

The corpus luteum provides hormonal pregnancy support with progesterone production until the placenta is established. Symptomatic corpus luteum cysts occasionally occur during early pregnancy but typically resolve over several weeks. Larger cysts may result in ovarian torsion, which can require surgical intervention. Otherwise, mild bleeding from a corpus luteum can progress into hemorrhage, more commonly in those with bleeding disorders or receiving pharmacologic anticoagulation. Supportive care for hemorrhage and improvement in clotting function may be sufficient, although ovarian cystectomy or oophorectomy may be required to control bleeding.[127] If the cyst is removed, supplemental progesterone is administered until 10 to 12 weeks' gestation.

KEY POINTS

- Assisted reproductive technology (ART) includes techniques that are being applied to an increasingly diverse population of patients with a wide range of comorbidities.
- ART procedures usually involve a regimen of hormonal stimulation and oocyte retrieval followed by *in vitro* fertilization with either fresh embryo transfer or embryo cryopreservation for later transfer into the uterus transcervically.
- Hormonal stimulation results in multiple oocytes for retrieval. On occasion, ovarian hyperstimulation syndrome can occur, with severe cases being associated with

- ascites, pleural effusion, hemoconcentration, oliguria, and thromboembolic events.
- Sedation analgesia, neuraxial anesthesia, and general anesthesia have all been used successfully to anesthetize women for ART procedures. Deep sedation may have to progress to loss of consciousness (i.e., general anesthesia) to prevent patient movement at critical times during the procedure.
- Laboratory studies have suggested that local anesthetics, nitrous oxide, and volatile halogenated anesthetic agents interfere with some aspects of reproductive physiology

in vitro. However, few clinical data have shown that brief administration of any contemporary anesthetic agent for an ART procedure adversely affects live-birth rates.

- General anesthesia may be administered by mask or supraglottic airway (SGA) for selected extraabdominal procedures during the first 18 to 20 weeks of pregnancy, provided that the patient is appropriately fasted and there is no difficulty with mask ventilation. Some anesthesia providers prefer to limit the use of mask anesthesia or the SGA to the first 12 to 14 weeks of pregnancy.
- Most ectopic pregnancies are located in one of the fallopian tubes. Ruptured tubal pregnancies, as well as interstitial, cervical, cesarean scar, and abdominal ectopic pregnancies, as well as mid-trimester pregnancies with placenta accreta spectrum, may result in substantial hemorrhage.
- The most painful part of a dilation and uterine evacuation procedure is the dilation of the cervix. If the cervix is already dilated and the fetal size is first trimester, sedation (with or without paracervical block) often suffices. If the cervix is closed, either a paracervical block with sedation or neuraxial or general anesthesia may be necessary. If the fetal size is advanced (>13 to 15 weeks' gestation), many anesthesia providers prefer general anesthesia because of the greater surgical stimulation and risk for bleeding complications.
- Neuraxial anesthesia is an excellent choice for prophylactic cervical cerclage. In a patient who requires emergency cervical cerclage, it is important to prevent a marked increase in intraabdominal and intrauterine pressures, which might cause rupture of bulging fetal membranes.
- The patient with a molar pregnancy may have hyperemesis gravidarum, gestational hypertension, severe anemia, and/or hyperthyroidism. These complications are more common in patients with excessive uterine size.
- Rapid and profound blood loss is possible with uterine evacuation of a molar pregnancy, and acute cardiopulmonary distress can develop after uterine evacuation.

REFERENCES

1. The American Society for Reproductive Medicine. Assisted reproductive technology: a guide for patients revised 2018. https://www.reproductivefacts.org/news-and-publications/fact-sheets-and-infographics/assisted-reproductive-technologies-booklet/?_t_tags=siteid:db69d13f-2074-446c-b7f0-d15628807d0c,language:en&_t_hit.id=ASRM_Models_Pages_ContentPage/_23a74fae-ee79-415c-bd20-386cc14b0a16_en&_t_hit.pos=9. Accessed January 2024.
2. Wikland M, Enk L, Hammarberg K, Nilsson L. Use of a vaginal transducer for oocyte retrieval in an IVF/ET program. *J Clin Ultrasound*. 1987;15:245–251.
3. Grady R, Alavi N, Vale R, et al. Elective single embryo transfer and perinatal outcomes: a systematic review and meta-analysis. *Fertil Steril*. 2012;97:324–331.
4. American Society for Reproductive Medicine. Female cancer, cryopreservation, and fertility; 2014. https://www.reproductivefacts.org/globalassets/_rf/news-and-publications/bookletsfact-sheets/english-pdf/female_cancer_cryopreservation_and_fertility_factsheet.pdf. Accessed January 2024.
5. US Centers for Disease Control and Prevention. ART Success Rates. https://www.cdc.gov/art/artdata/. Accessed January 2024.
6. Practice Committee of the American Society for Reproductive Medicine. Prevention and treatment of moderate and severe ovarian hyperstimulation syndrome: a guideline. *Fertil Steril*. 2016;106:1634–1647.
7. Sunderam S, Kissin DM, Zhang Y, et al. Assisted reproductive technology surveillance—United States, 2018. *MMWR Surveill Summ*. 2022;71:1–19.
8. Boyers SP, Lavy G, Russell JB, DeCherney AH. A paired analysis of in vitro fertilization and cleavage rates of first-versus last-recovered preovulatory human oocytes exposed to varying intervals of 100% CO_2 pneumoperitoneum and general anesthesia. *Fertil Steril*. 1987;48:969–974.
9. Lefebvre G, Vauthier D, Seebacher J, et al. In vitro fertilization: a comparative study of cleavage rates under epidural and general anesthesia-interest for gamete intrafallopian transfer. *J In Vitro Fert Embryo Transf*. 1988;5:305–306.
10. Lewin A, Margalioth EJ, Rabinowitz R, Schenker JG. Comparative study of ultrasonically guided percutaneous aspiration with local anesthesia and laparoscopic aspiration of follicles in an in vitro fertilization program. *Am J Obstet Gynecol*. 1985;151:621–625.
11. Davidson A, Vermesh M, Lobo RA, Paulson RJ. Mouse embryo culture as quality control for human in vitro fertilization: the one-cell versus the two-cell model. *Fertil Steril*. 1988;49:516–521.
12. Tsen LC, Arthur GR, Datta S, et al. Estrogen-induced changes in protein binding of bupivacaine during in vitro fertilization. *Anesthesiology*. 1997;87:879–883.
13. Schnell VL, Sacco AG, Savoy-Moore RT, et al. Effects of oocyte exposure to local anesthetics on in vitro fertilization and embryo development in the mouse. *Reprod Toxicol*. 1992;6:323–327.
14. Del Valle LJ, Orihuela PA. Cleavage and development in cultured preimplantation mouse embryos exposed to lidocaine. *Reprod Toxicol*. 1996;10:491–496.
15. Wikland M, Evers H, Jakobsson AH, et al. The concentration of lidocaine in follicular fluid when used for paracervical block in a human IVF-ET programme. *Hum Reprod*. 1990;5:920–923.
16. Wilhelm W, Hammadeh ME, White PF, et al. General anesthesia versus monitored anesthesia care with remifentanil for assisted reproductive technologies: effect on pregnancy rate. *J Clin Anesth*. 2002;14:1–5.
17. Matsota P, Sidiropoulou T, Batistaki C, et al. Analgesia with remifentanil versus anesthesia with propofol-alfentanil for transvaginal oocyte retrieval: a randomized trial on their impact on in vitro fertilization outcome. *Middle East J Anaesthesiol*. 2012;21:685–692.
18. Swanson RJ, Leavitt MG. Fertilization and mouse embryo development in the presence of midazolam. *Anesth Analg*. 1992;75:549–554.
19. Chopineau J, Bazin JE, Terrisse MP, et al. Assay for midazolam in liquor folliculi during in vitro fertilization under anesthesia. *Clin Pharm*. 1993;12:770–773.
20. Casati A, Valentini G, Zangrillo A, et al. Anaesthesia for ultrasound guided oocyte retrieval: midazolam/remifentanil

versus propofol/fentanyl regimens. *Eur J Anaesthesiol.* 1999;16:773–778.

21. Rosenblatt MA, Bradford CN, Bodian CA, Grunfeld L. The effect of a propofol-based sedation technique on cumulative embryo scores, clinical pregnancy rates, and implantation rates in patients undergoing embryo transfers with donor oocytes. *J Clin Anesth.* 1997;9:614–617.

22. Beilin Y, Bodian CA, Mukherjee T, et al. The use of propofol, nitrous oxide, or isoflurane does not affect the reproductive success rate following gamete intrafallopian transfer (GIFT). *Anesthesiology.* 1999;90:36–41.

23. Pierce ET, Smalky M, Alper MM, et al. Comparison of pregnancy rates following gamete intrafallopian transfer (GIFT) under general anesthesia with thiopental sodium or propofol. *J Clin Anesth.* 1992;4:394–398.

24. Christiaens F, Janssenswillen C, Van Steirteghem AC, et al. Comparison of assisted reproductive technology performance after oocyte retrieval under general anaesthesia (propofol) versus paracervical local anaesthetic block: a case-controlled study. *Hum Reprod.* 1998;13:2456–2460.

25. Hein HA, Putman JM. Is propofol a proper proposition for reproductive procedures? *J Clin Anesth.* 1997;9:611–613.

26. Christiaens F, Janssenswillen C, Verborgh C, et al. Propofol concentrations in follicular fluid during general anaesthesia for transvaginal oocyte retrieval. *Hum Reprod.* 1999;14:345–348.

27. Ben-Shlomo I, Moskovich R, Golan J, et al. The effect of propofol anaesthesia on oocyte fertilization and early embryo quality. *Hum Reprod.* 2000;15:2197–2199.

28. Imoedemhe DA, Sigue AB, Abdul Ghani I, et al. An evaluation of the effect of the anesthetic agent profofol (Diprivan) on the outcome of human in vitro fertilization. *J Assist Reprod Genet.* 1992;9:488–491.

29. Tomioka S, Nakajo N. No genotoxic effect of propofol in Chinese hamster ovary cells: analysis by sister chromatid exchanges. *Acta Anaesthesiol Scand.* 2000;44:1261–1265.

30. Vincent RD, Syrop CH, Van Voorhis BJ, et al. An evaluation of the effect of anesthetic technique on reproductive success after laparoscopic pronuclear stage transfer: propofol/nitrous oxide versus isoflurane/nitrous oxide. *Anesthesiology.* 1995;82:352–358.

31. Ben-Shlomo I, Moskovich R, Katz Y, Shalev E. Midazolam/ketamine sedative combination compared with fentanyl/propofol/isoflurane anaesthesia for oocyte retrieval. *Hum Reprod.* 1999;14:1757–1759.

32. Koblin DD, Waskell L, Watson JE, et al. Nitrous oxide inactivates methionine synthetase in human liver. *Anesth Analg.* 1982;61:75–78.

33. Baden JM, Serra M, Mazze RI. Inhibition of fetal methionine synthase by nitrous oxide. *Br J Anaesth.* 1984;56:523–526.

34. Kieler J. The cytotoxic effect of nitrous oxide at different oxygen tensions. *Acta Pharmacol Toxicol (Copenh).* 1957;13:301–308.

35. Warren JR, Shaw B, Steinkampf MP. Effects of nitrous oxide on preimplantation mouse embryo cleavage and development. *Biol Reprod.* 1990;43:158–161.

36. Rosen MA, Roizen MF, Eger II E, et al. The effect of nitrous oxide on in vitro fertilization success rate. *Anesthesiology.* 1987;67:42–44.

37. Sturrock JE, Nunn JF. Mitosis in mammalian cells during exposure to anesthetics. *Anesthesiology.* 1975;43:21–33.

38. Nunn JF, Lovis JD, Kimball KL. Arrest of mitosis by halothane. *Br J Anaesth.* 1971;43:524–530.

39. Warren JR, Shaw B, Steinkampf MP. Inhibition of preimplantation mouse embryo development by isoflurane. *Am J Obstet Gynecol.* 1992;166:693–698.

40. Piroli A, Marci R, Marinangeli F, et al. Comparison of different anaesthetic methodologies for sedation during in vitro fertilization procedures: effects on patient physiology and oocyte competence. *Gynecol Endocrinol.* 2012;28:796–799.

41. Kauppila A, Leinonen P, Vihko R, Ylöstalo P. Metoclopramide-induced hyperprolactinemia impairs ovarian follicle maturation and corpus luteum function in women. *J Clin Endocrinol Metab.* 1982;54:955–960.

42. Forman R, Fishel SB, Edwards SR, Walters E. The influence of transient hyperprolactinemia on in vitro fertilization in humans. *J Clin Endocrinol Metab.* 1985;60:517–522.

43. Mendes MC, Ferriani RA, Sala MM, et al. Effect of transitory hyperprolactinemia on in vitro fertilization of human oocytes. *J Reprod Med.* 2001;46:444–450.

44. American Society of Anesthesiologists. Practice guidelines for preoperative fasting and the use of pharmacologic agents to reduce the risk of pulmonary aspiration: application to healthy patients undergoing elective procedures: an updated report by the American Society of Anesthesiologists Task force on Preoperative Fasting and the Use of Pharmacologic Agents to Reduce the Risk of Pulmonary Aspiration. *Anesthesiology.* 2017;126:376–393.

45. Thanikachalam P, Govindan DK. Pain management during ultrasound guided transvaginal oocyte retrieval—a narrative review. *J Hum Reprod Sci.* 2023;16:2–15.

46. Guasch E, Gómez R, Brogly N, Gilsanz F. Anesthesia and analgesia for transvaginal oocyte retrieval. Should we recommend or avoid any anesthetic drug or technique? *Curr Opin Anaesthesiol.* 2019;32:285–290.

47. Hong JY, Jee YS, Luthardt FW. Comparison of conscious sedation for oocyte retrieval between low-anxiety and high-anxiety patients. *J Clin Anesth.* 2005;17:549–553.

48. Kwan I, Wang R, Pearce E, Bhattacharya S. Pain relief for women undergoing oocyte retrieval for assisted reproduction. *Cochrane Database Syst Rev.* 2018;(5):CD004829.

49. Ng EHY, Tang OS, Chui DKC, Ho PC. Comparison of two different doses of lignocaine used in paracervical block during oocyte collection in an IVF programme. *Hum Reprod.* 2000;15:2148–2151.

50. Raftery S, Sherry E. Total intravenous anaesthesia with propofol and alfentanil protects against postoperative nausea and vomiting. *Can J Anaesth.* 1992;39:37–40.

51. McKenzie R, Wadhwa RK, Bedger RC. Noninvasive measurement of cardiac output during laparoscopy. *J Reprod Med.* 1980;24:247–250.

52. Silva PD, Kang SB, Sloane KA. Gamete intrafallopian transfer with spinal anesthesia. *Fertil Steril.* 1993;59:841–843.

53. Chung PH, Yeko TR, Mayer JC, et al. Gamete intrafallopian transfer. Comparison of epidural vs. general anesthesia. *J Reprod Med.* 1998;43:681–686.

54. Pusapati RN, Sivashanmugam T, Ravishankar M. Respiratory changes during spinal anaesthesia for gynaecological laparoscopic surgery. *J Anaesthesiol Clin Pharmacol.* 2010;26:475–479.

55. Ciofolo MJ, Clergue F, Seebacher J, et al. Ventilatory effects of laparoscopy under epidural anesthesia. *Anesth Analg.* 1990;70:357–361.

56. Stojnic J, Bila J, Tulic L, et al. Severe hemoperitoneum due to ovarian bleeding after transvaginal oocyte retrieval with surgical management: a retrospective analysis and comprehensive review of the literature. *Medicina (Kaunas)*. 2023;59:307.

57. Frederiksen Y, Mehlsen MY, Matthiesen SM, et al. Predictors of pain during oocyte retrieval. *J Psychosom Obstet Gynaecol*. 2017;38:21–29.

58. Mann LM, Kreisel K, Llata E, et al. Trends in ectopic pregnancy diagnoses in United States emergency departments, 2006-2013. *Matern Child Health J*. 2020;24:213–221.

59. Creanga AA, Syverson C, Seed K, Callaghan WM. Pregnancy-related mortality in the United States, 2011-2013. *Obstet Gynecol*. 2017;130:366–373.

60. Lund Kårhus L, Egerup P, Wessel Skovlund C, Lidegaard Ø. Long-term reproductive outcomes in women whose first pregnancy is ectopic: a national controlled follow-up study. *Hum Reprod*. 2013;28:241–246.

61. Hoyert DL, Miniño AM. Maternal mortality in the United States: changes in coding, publication, and data release, 2018. *Natl Vital Stat Rep*. 2020;69:1–18.

62. Creanga AA, Shapiro-Mendoza CK, Bish CL, et al. Trends in ectopic pregnancy mortality in the United States: 1980-2007. *Obstet Gynecol*. 2011;117:837–843.

63. US Centers for Disease Control and Prevention. Ectopic pregnancy mortality—Florida, 2009-2010. *MMWR Morb Mortal Wkly Rep*. 2012;61:106–109.

64. Knight M, Bunch K, Patel R, et al. *Saving Lives, Improving Mothers' Care Core Report—Lessons Learned to Inform Maternity Care From the UK and Ireland Confidential Enquiries Into Maternal Deaths and Morbidity 2018-20*. National Perinatal Epidemiology Unit, University of Oxford; 2022.

65. American College of Obstetricians and Gynecologists. Practice Bulletin No. 193: Tubal ectopic pregnancy (reaffirmed 2022). *Obstet Gynecol*. 2018;131:e91–e103.

66. American College of Obstetricians and Gynecologists. Practice Bulletin No. 181: Prevention of Rh D alloimmunization (reaffirmed 2024). *Obstet Gynecol*. 2017;130:e57–e70.

67. van Mello NM, Mol F, Verhoeve HR, et al. Methotrexate or expectant management in women with an ectopic pregnancy or pregnancy of unknown location and low serum hCG concentrations? A randomized comparison. *Hum Reprod*. 2013;28:60–67.

68. Jurkovic D, Memtsa M, Sawyer E, et al. Single-dose systemic methotrexate vs expectant management for treatment of tubal ectopic pregnancy: a placebo-controlled randomized trial. *Ultrasound Obstet Gynecol*. 2017;49:171–176.

69. Sokalska A, Rambhatla A, Dudley C, Bhagavath B. Nontubal ectopic pregnancies: overview of diagnosis and treatment. *Fertil Steril*. 2023;120:553–562.

70. Brincat M, Bryant-Smith A, Holland TK. The diagnosis and management of interstitial ectopic pregnancies: a review. *Gynecol Surg*. 2019;16. https://doi.org/10.1186/s10397-018-1054-4.

71. Society for Maternal-Fetal Medicine (SMFM), Miller R, Gyamfi-Bannerman C. Society for Maternal-Fetal Medicine Consult Series No. 63: Cesarean scar ectopic pregnancy. *Am J Obstet Gynecol*. 2022;227:B9–B20.

72. Selo-Ojeme DO, Feyi-Waboso PA. Salvage autotransfusion versus homologous blood transfusion for ruptured ectopic pregnancy. *Int J Gynaecol Obstet*. 2007;96:108–111.

73. Wanderer JP, Leffert LR, Mhyre JM, et al. Epidemiology of obstetric-related ICU admissions in Maryland: 1999-2008. *Crit Care Med*. 2013;41:1844–1852.

74. Aoyama K, Pinto R, Ray JG, et al. Variability in intensive care unit admission among pregnant and postpartum women in Canada: a nationwide population-based observational study. *Crit Care*. 2019;23:381.

75. American College of Obstetricians and Gynecologists. Practice Bulletin No. 200: Early pregnancy loss (reaffirmed 2025). *Obstet Gynecol*. 2018;132:e197–e207.

76. Kortsmit K, Nguyen AT, Mandel MG, et al. Abortion surveillance—United States, 2020. *MMWR Surveill Summ*. 2022;71:1–27.

77. Ghosh J, Papadopoulou A, Devall AJ, et al. Methods for managing miscarriage: a network meta-analysis. *Cochrane Database Syst Rev*. 2021;(6):CD012602.

78. Wilcox AJ, Weinberg CR, O'Connor JF, et al. Incidence of early loss of pregnancy. *N Engl J Med*. 1988;319:189–194.

79. The Practice Committee of the American Society for Reproductive Medicine. Evaluation and treatment of recurrent pregnancy loss: a committee opinion. *Fertil Steril*. 2012;98:1103–1111.

80. Strumpf E, Lang A, Austin N, et al. Prevalence and clinical, social, and healthcare predictors of miscarriage. *BMC Pregnancy Childbirth*. 2021;21:185.

81. Joseph KS, Boutin A, Lisonkova S, et al. Maternal mortality in the United States: recent trends, current status, and future considerations. *Obstet Gynecol*. 2021;137:763–771.

82. Ganatra B, Gerdts C, Rossier C, et al. Global, regional, and subregional classification of abortions by safety, 2010-14: estimates from a Bayesian hierarchical model. *Lancet*. 2017;390:2372–2381.

83. Alterio M, Von Davies R, Tobias M, et al. A geospatial analysis of abortion access in the United States after the reversal of Roe v Wade. *Obstet Gynecol*. 2023;142:1077–1085.

84. Bearak J, Popinchalk A, Ganatra B, et al. Unintended pregnancy and abortion by income, region, and the legal status of abortion: estimates from a comprehensive model for 1990-2019. *Lancet Glob Health*. 2020;8:e1152–e1161.

85. Ralph L, Foster DG, Raifman S, et al. Prevalence of self-managed abortion among women of reproductive age in the United States. *JAMA Netw Open*. 2020;3:e2029245.

86. Aiken ARA, Starling JE, Gomperts R. Factors associated with use of an online telemedicine service to access self-managed medical abortion in the US. *JAMA Netw Open*. 2021;4:e2111852.

87. McNamee KM, Dawood F, Farquharson RG. Mid-trimester pregnancy loss. *Obstet Gynecol Clin North Am*. 2014;41:87–102.

88. American College of Obstetricians and Gynecologists. Practice Bulletin No. 135: Second-trimester abortion (reaffirmed 2022). *Obstet Gynecol*. 2013;121:1394–1406.

89. Society for Maternal-Fetal Medicine. Clinical considerations for management of severe complications when abortion care is restricted; 2022. https://www.smfm.org/publications/450-clinical-considerations-for-management-of-severe-complications-when-abortion-care-is-restricted. Accessed January 2024.

90. Sapra KJ, Buck Louis GM, Sundaram R, et al. Signs and symptoms associated with early pregnancy loss: findings from a population-based preconception cohort. *Hum Reprod*. 2016;31:887–896.

91. Raymond EG, Mark A, Grossman D, et al. Medication abortion with misoprostol-only: a sample protocol. *Contraception*. 2023;121:109998.

92. Borgatta L, Kapp N. Labor induction abortion in the second trimester. *Contraception.* 2011;84:4–18.

93. Zwerling B, Edelman A, Jackson A, et al. Society of Family Planning Clinical Recommendation: medication abortion between 14 0/7 and 27 6/7 weeks of gestation: jointly developed with the Society for Maternal-Fetal Medicine. *Am J Obstet Gynecol.* 2023. https://doi.org/10.1016/j.ajog.2023.09.097.

94. American College of Obstetricians and Gynecologist and the Society for Maternal Fetal Medicine, Metz TD, Berry RS, et al. Obstetric Care Consensus No. 10: Management of stillbirth. *Am J Obstet Gynecol.* 2020;222:B2–B20.

95. American College of Obstetricians and Gynecologists. Practice Bulletin N. 225: Medication abortion up to 70 days of gestation (reaffirmed 2023). *Obstet Gynecol.* 2020; 136:e31–e47.

96. American College of Obstetricians and Gynecologists. Clinical Practice Update: Rh D immune globulin administration after abortion or pregnancy loss at less than 12 weeks' gestation. *ObstetGynecol.* 2024;144:e140–e143.

97. American College of Obstetricians and Gynecologists. Committee Opinion No. 833: Access to postabortion contraception (reaffirmed 2024). *Obstet Gynecol.* 2021;138:e91–e95.

98. American College of Obstetricians and Gynecologists. Committee Statement No. 13: Self-managed abortion. *Obstet Gynecol.* 2024;144:e152–e9.

99. American College of Obstetricians and Gynecologists. Practice Bulletin No. 195: Prevention of infection after gynecologic procedures (reaffirmed 2022). *Obstet Gynecol.* 2018;131:e172–e189.

100. Ben-Baruch G, Menczer J, Shalev J, et al. Uterine perforation during curettage: perforation rates and postperforation management. *Isr J Med Sci.* 1980;16:821–824.

101. Allen RH, Singh R. Society of Family Planning clinical guidelines pain control in surgical abortion part 1—local anesthesia and minimal sedation. *Contraception.* 2018;97: 471–477.

102. Norton ME, Cassidy A, Ralston SJ, et al. Society for Maternal-Fetal Medicine Consult Series No. 59: The use of analgesia and anesthesia for maternal-fetal procedures. *Am J Obstet Gynecol.* 2021;225:B2–B8.

103. Ozery E, Ansari J, Kaur S, et al. Anesthetic considerations for second-trimester surgical abortions. *Anesth Analg.* 2023;137:345–353.

104. Gokhale P, Lappen JR, Waters JH, Perriera LK. Intravenous sedation without intubation and the risk of anesthesia complications for obese and non-obese women undergoing surgical abortion: a retrospective cohort study. *Anesth Analg.* 2016;122:1957–1962.

105. Aksel S, Lang L, Steinauer JE, et al. Safety of deep sedation without intubation for second-trimester dilation and evacuation. *Obstet Gynecol.* 2018;132:171–178.

106. Lee A, Shatil B, Landau R, et al. Intrathecal 2-chloroprocaine 3% versus hyperbaric bupivacaine 0.75% for cervical cerclage: a double-blind randomized controlled trial. *Anesth Analg.* 2022;134:624–632.

107. Siddiqi A, Mahmoud Y, Secic M, et al. Mepivacaine versus bupivacaine spinal anesthesia for primary total joint arthroplasty: a systematic review and meta-analysis. *J Arthroplasty.* 2022;37:1396–1404.e5.

108. Oats JN, Vasey DP, Waldron BA. Effects of ketamine on the pregnant uterus. *Br J Anaesth.* 1979;51:1163–1166.

109. Munson ES, Embro WJ. Enflurane, isoflurane, and halothane and isolated human uterine muscle. *Anesthesiology.* 1977;46:11–14.

110. Lee HA, Kawakami H, Mihara T, et al. Impact of anesthetic agents on the amount of bleeding during dilatation and evacuation: a systematic review and meta-analysis. *PLoS One.* 2021;16:e0261494.

111. American College of Obstetricians and Gynecologists. Practice Bulletin No.142: Cerclage for the management of cervical insufficiency (reaffirmed 2024). *Obstet Gynecol.* 2014;123:372–379.

112. Owen J, Hankins G, Iams JD, et al. Multicenter randomized trial of cerclage for preterm birth prevention in high-risk women with shortened midtrimester cervical length. *Am J Obstet Gynecol.* 2009;201:375.e1–e8.

113. Berghella V, Rafael TJ, Szychowski JM, et al. Cerclage for short cervix on ultrasonography in women with singleton gestations and previous preterm birth: a meta-analysis. *Obstet Gynecol.* 2011;117:663–671.

114. Odibo AO, Berghella V, To MS, et al. Shirodkar versus McDonald cerclage for the prevention of preterm birth in women with short cervical length. *Am J Perinatol.* 2007;24:55–60.

115. Temming L, Mikhail E. Society for Maternal-Fetal Medicine Consult Series No. 65: Transabdominal cerclage. *Am J Obstet Gynecol.* 2023;228:B2–B10.

116. Rust OA, Roberts WE. Does cerclage prevent preterm birth? *Obstet Gynecol Clin North Am.* 2005;32:441–456.

117. Sharawi N, Tan HS, Taylor C, et al. ED 90 of intrathecal chloroprocaine with fentanyl for prophylactic cervical cerclage: a sequential allocation biased-coin design. *Anesth Analg.* 2022;134:834–842.

118. Crawford JS, Lewis M. Nitrous oxide in early human pregnancy. *Anaesthesia.* 1986;41:900–905.

119. Yoon HJ, Hong JY, Kim SM. The effect of anesthetic method for prophylactic cervical cerclage on plasma oxytocin: a randomized trial. *Int J Obstet Anesth.* 2008;17:26–30.

120. Wang Y, Ning X, Yu Y, et al. Comparison of outcomes following general anesthesia and spinal anesthesia during emergency cervical cerclage in singleton pregnant women in the second trimester at a single center. *Med Sci Monit.* 2022;28:e934771.

121. Horowitz NS, Eskander RN, Adelman MR, Burke W. Epidemiology, diagnosis, and treatment of gestational trophoblastic disease: a Society of Gynecologic Oncology evidenced-based review and recommendation. *Gynecol Oncol.* 2021;163:605–613.

122. Ngan HYS, Seckl MJ, Berkowitz RS, et al. Diagnosis and management of gestational trophoblastic disease: 2021 update. *Int J Gynaecol Obstet.* 2021;155(suppl 1):86–93.

123. Soper JT. Gestational trophoblastic disease: current evaluation and management. *Obstet Gynecol.* 2021;137:355–370.

124. Kaplan JA, Cooperman LH. Alarming reactions to ketamine in patients taking thyroid medication—treatment with propranolol. *Anesthesiology.* 1971;35:229–230.

125. Ackerman WI. Anesthetic considerations for complicated hydatidiform molar pregnancies. *Anesth Rev.* 1984;11:20–24.

126. American College of Obstetricians and Gynecologists. Practice Bulletin No. 189: Nausea and vomiting of pregnancy (reaffirmed 2024). *Obstet Gynecol.* 2018;131:e15–e30.

127. Hoffman R, Brenner B. Corpus luteum hemorrhage in womenwith bleeding disorders. *Womens Health (Lond).* 2009;5:91–95.

18

Nonobstetric Surgery During Pregnancy

Jeanette R. Bauchat, MD, MS and Marc Van de Velde, MD, PhD, EDRA, FESAIC

CHAPTER OUTLINE

BACKGROUND: EPIDEMIOLOGY OF PREGNANCY DURING NONOBSTETRIC SURGERY

It has been estimated that nonobstetric surgery is performed in 0.48% to 0.7% of pregnancies.[1–3] Based on total birth rates, this suggests that approximately 17,000 to 25,000 surgeries during pregnancy occur annually in the United States and in the European Union.[4] Pregnancy sometimes may be unrecognized at the time of surgery. Estimates of the incidence of positive pregnancy tests in women of childbearing age presenting for orthopedic and elective sterilization procedures have ranged from 0.002% to 2.6%.[5] Medical history alone may not be a reliable means of excluding pregnancy in women presenting for elective surgery; however, the practice of mandating pregnancy testing for every woman of childbearing age is controversial. A number of concerns have been raised; mandatory testing does not fully consider patient autonomy and likely disproportionately affects the most vulnerable patient populations, including minorities and women of lower socioeconomic status.[6] Moreover, the medicolegal and health implications of a false-positive or false-negative pregnancy test have not been fully explored; litigation has occurred as a result of failure to follow up on routine preoperative pregnancy tests and pregnancy loss following surgery.[7]

The American Society of Anesthesiologists (ASA) has stated: "Pregnancy testing may be offered to female patients of childbearing age and for whom the result would alter the patient's management. Informed consent or assent of the risks, benefits, and alternatives related to preoperative pregnancy testing should be obtained."[8] The UK National Institute for Health and Clinical Excellence has issued preoperative screening guidelines recommending the development of institutional protocols that include "… criteria for inquiry or consented testing, what information is provided to patients, how pregnancy status is recorded, and the procedures for the management of consent and disclosure, particularly for groups who may find discussion of pregnancy a sensitive issue."[9]

Surgery may be necessary during any stage of pregnancy. A retrospective review of pregnancies complicated by surgery in a single tertiary-referral hospital in Belgium found that 32%, 44%, and 24% of cases were in the first, second, and third trimesters, respectively.[1] Indications for pregnancy-related surgery include cervical incompetence, the presence of ovarian cysts, and conditions amenable to fetal surgery (see Chapter 7). Indications for nonpregnancy-related surgery include the presence of acute abdominal disease, malignancy, and trauma. The Hospital Episode Statistics database, which records all admissions to English National Health Service (NHS) hospitals indicated that of 6,486,280 pregnancies, 47,628 received nonobstetric surgery, with abdominal surgery the most commonly performed (35.3%).[2] The American College of Surgeons' National Surgical Quality Improvement Program (NSQIP) database demonstrated higher rates of emergency surgery (50.5% in 2764 pregnant women versus 13.2% in 516,705 nonpregnant women) with no difference in 30-day mortality.[3]

When caring for pregnant women undergoing nonobstetric surgery, anesthesia providers may need to modify standard anesthetic or enhanced recovery after surgery (ERAS) protocols to accommodate pregnancy-induced maternal physiologic changes and the presence of the fetus. The Global

Burden of Disease Maternal Mortality Collaborators[1,10] and other maternal mortality databases, such as the Confidential Enquiries into Maternal Deaths in the United Kingdom,[11] have demonstrated that mothers may die, even in early pregnancy, of hemorrhage, hypertensive disorders, thromboembolism, and sepsis. In developed countries, many maternal deaths are considered preventable; multidisciplinary care should ideally follow protocols and guidelines developed for specific scenarios, which can occur during or after nonobstetric surgical procedures.[11,12] Two studies retrospectively analyzed data from the NSQIP database for pregnant women undergoing surgery.[3,13] Reassuringly, the rate of major complications (e.g., infections, reoperation, wound complications, respiratory complications, venous thromboembolism, blood transfusion, maternal death) for antenatal nonobstetric surgery was approximately 7%, which was not different from the rate in nonpregnant women.[13]

MATERNAL PHYSIOLOGY: IMPLICATIONS DURING SURGERY

During pregnancy, profound changes in physiology result from increased concentrations of various hormones, mechanical effects of the gravid uterus, greater metabolic demand, and the hemodynamic consequences of the low-pressure placental circulation, all of which have anesthetic implications during a surgical procedure (see Chapter 2).

Respiratory System and Airway

Alveolar ventilation increases by 30% or more by mid-pregnancy. This increase results in chronic respiratory alkalosis with a $PaCO_2$ of 28 to 32 mm Hg (3.7 to 4.3 kPa), a slightly alkaline pH (approximately 7.44), and decreased levels of bicarbonate and buffer base. Although oxygen consumption and alveolar ventilation are increased, PaO_2 usually increases only slightly or remains within the normal range. Adjusting mechanical ventilation parameters to maintain the lower $PaCO_2$ of pregnancy, particularly during laparoscopic insufflation, is critical for a physiologically normal acid-base status. Functional residual capacity (FRC) diminishes by approximately 20% as the uterus expands, resulting in decreased oxygen reserve; other factors (e.g., morbid obesity; perioperative intraabdominal distention; placement of the patient in the supine, Trendelenburg, or lithotomy position; induction of anesthesia) may further decrease FRC, increase oxygen consumption, and diminish buffering capacity, resulting in the rapid development of hypoxemia and acidosis during periods of hypoventilation or apnea.

Weight gain during pregnancy and capillary engorgement of the respiratory tract mucosa lead to more frequent problems with mask ventilation and tracheal intubation (see Chapter 29). Difficult airway management and failed intubation (a leading cause of anesthesia-related maternal death) is as much a risk during early pregnancy with nonobstetric surgery as it is during cesarean delivery.[11] In 2015, the Obstetric Anaesthetists' Association and the Difficult Airway Society developed a difficult airway algorithm that was designed for the unique challenges of managing an obstetric patient, including considerations for fetal status and urgency of cesarean delivery; this algorithm is relevant to airway management for women with a viable fetus undergoing nonobstetric surgery (see Figs. 29.12–29.14).[14]

Cardiovascular System

During the second half of pregnancy, compression of the inferior vena cava by the gravid uterus reduces venous return and cardiac output; in 10% of pregnant women, these effects can precipitate significant vasovagal symptoms and signs, which are collectively known as the "supine hypotension syndrome of pregnancy."[15] During mid-pregnancy, patient movement from the supine to the left lateral position reduces vena caval compression, resulting in an increase in left ventricular ejection fraction (8%), end-diastolic volume (25%), and stroke volume.[16] By late pregnancy, the same patient movement results in even greater increases in these parameters; for example, cardiac output increases by up to 24%.[16] Although magnetic resonance imaging (MRI) studies of vena caval compression indicate virtually no compression with 30 degrees of left lateral tilt,[17] most surgeries cannot be performed in this position. Therefore, after 18 to 20 weeks' gestation, some degree of left lateral tilt should be applied, acknowledging that maternal or fetal hemodynamic instability may warrant a further increase in tilt, if necessary.

Hematologic System

Blood volume expansion begins as early as the first trimester and ultimately achieves a 30% to 45% increase by term gestation. The smaller increase in red blood cell than plasma volume results in dilutional anemia, allowing moderate blood loss to be well tolerated.[18] Hemoglobin levels that define anemia during pregnancy vary by gestational age: <11 g/dL in the first trimester, <10.5 g/dL in the second trimester, and <11 g/dL in the third trimester.[18] Pregnancy is associated with benign leukocytosis; thus, the white blood cell count is an unreliable indicator of infection. In general, pregnancy induces a hypercoagulable state, with increases in fibrinogen; factors VII, VIII, X, and XII; and fibrin degradation products.

Pregnancy is associated with enhancement of platelet turnover, clotting, and fibrinolysis; although a wide variation in the platelet count has been observed, functionally some pregnant women with thrombocytopenia may still be hypercoagulable. Pregnancy represents a state of accelerated but compensated intravascular coagulation. Given the high risk of mortality associated with thromboembolism, thromboprophylaxis management should be applied to pregnant surgical patients (see discussion below).[19,20]

Gastrointestinal System

Incompetence of the lower esophageal sphincter and distortion of gastric and pyloric anatomy during pregnancy increase the risk for gastroesophageal reflux, despite similar gastric emptying rates in pregnant and nonpregnant patients.[21] It is unclear at what gestational age the risk for aspiration becomes significant; gastroesophageal reflux starts early in the first trimester, and other mechanically induced factors become more relevant later in pregnancy. The feasibility of assessing gastric contents using ultrasonography has been investigated[22];

further study is needed to determine whether assessing gastric contents before the induction of anesthesia can be used to inform anesthetic management and reduce the risk for aspiration. It seems prudent to consider the pregnant patient as having a higher risk for aspiration from the beginning of the second trimester.[23]

Altered Responses to Anesthesia

A 30% to 40% decrease in the minimum alveolar concentration (MAC) of volatile anesthetic agents has been observed in pregnancy, correlating with higher serum progesterone levels.[24] Although **thiopental (thiopentone)** requirement begins to decrease in early pregnancy,[25] the effects of pregnancy on **propofol** requirement are conflicting and appear unrelated to progesterone levels.[25,26] The relatively high risk for intraoperative awareness (estimated risk 1 in 670 general anesthetics) observed in pregnant women during cesarean delivery is attributable, in part, to the need for rapid-sequence induction of general anesthesia, omission or reduction in analgesic (opioids) and anesthetic medications, and need for urgent surgery.[27,28] These circumstances may also be encountered during nonobstetric surgery in pregnancy, and depth of anesthesia monitoring should be considered.[27,28]

Plasma cholinesterase levels decrease by approximately 25% from early in pregnancy until the seventh postpartum day. However, prolonged neuromuscular blockade with **succinylcholine (suxamethonium)** is uncommon because the larger volume available for drug distribution offsets the impact of decreased drug hydrolysis.[29] The anesthesia provider should monitor all forms of neuromuscular blockade with a nerve stimulator to ensure adequate muscle relaxation as well as reversal before extubation of the trachea.

Decreased protein binding associated with lower albumin and alpha-glycoprotein concentrations during pregnancy may result in a larger fraction of unbound drug, with the potential for greater drug toxicity during pregnancy.[30] Pregnancy-associated changes in volume of distribution (caused by changes in body composition and/or plasma protein–binding capacity), metabolic activity, and hepatic or renal elimination (caused by changes in glomerular filtration rate and tubular transport processes) may contribute to changes in drug effects and metabolism, including the need for a higher initial loading dose of any given medication (see Chapter 16).[31] For example, in pregnant women, **cefazolin** clearance is approximately twice as high between 20 and 40 weeks' gestation, and **acetaminophen (paracetamol)** clearance is increased, compared with nonpregnant women.[31] Pregnant surgical patients may require drugs for which limited pharmacokinetic and pharmacodynamic information during pregnancy is available; judicious use of such agents is advisable.

Neuraxial anesthesia dosing may also be affected by pregnancy.[32] Increased intraabdominal pressure and vena caval compression can result in compression of the intrathecal sac, reduced capacity of the epidural space, and distention of the epidural venous plexus; these changes can increase the risk for intravascular injection of local anesthetics during epidural administration and the dermatomal spread of local anesthetics during administration of spinal and epidural anesthesia (see Chapter 12).

FETAL CONSIDERATIONS

Possible fetal risks of antenatal surgery include: (1) the effects of the disease process itself or related therapy; (2) the concern for teratogenicity associated with maternal physiologic derangements or nonpharmacologic and pharmacologic agent exposure during the perioperative period; and (3) early pregnancy loss or preterm labor and delivery, resulting in low birth weight (LBW) and other morbidities associated with prematurity.

Risks for Teratogenicity and Reproductive Hazards

Teratogenicity has been defined as any significant postnatal change in function or form in an offspring after prenatal treatment. Concern about the potential harmful effects of anesthetic agents stems from their known effects on mammalian cells, which include reversible decreases in cell motility, prolongation of DNA synthesis, and inhibition of cell division. Prospective clinical studies of the teratogenic effects of anesthetic agents are impractical owing to the large number of drug-exposed patients required; consequently, investigations have taken one of the following directions: (1) small animal studies of the reproductive effects of anesthetic agents, (2) epidemiologic surveys of operating room personnel routinely exposed to subanesthetic concentrations of inhalation agents, and (3) outcome studies in women who have undergone surgery while pregnant.

Principles of Teratogenicity

A number of important factors influence the teratogenic potential of a substance: species susceptibility, dose of the substance, duration and timing of exposure, and genetic predisposition.[33] A teratogen may cause malformations following the single administration of a high dose, or the long-term administration of a low dose; however, this does not mean that a single, short exposure of a "normal" dose (e.g., during a typical anesthetic) would incur risk. In addition, a small dose of a teratogen may cause an effect in susceptible early embryos, whereas a much larger dose in the fetus may prove harmless. Finally, the results of studies performed in small animals cannot necessarily be extrapolated to other species, especially humans. Although many drugs or agents have been listed in catalogues of teratogenic agents owing to their effects in animals, very few are proven human teratogens.[33]

Manifestations of teratogenicity include death, structural abnormality, growth restriction, and functional deficiency.[33] Structural abnormalities can lead to death if they are severe, although death may occur in the absence of congenital anomalies. Growth restriction is a manifestation of teratogenesis and may relate to multiple factors, including placental insufficiency and genetic and environmental factors. Functional deficiencies include behavioral and learning abnormalities, the study of which is called behavioral teratology (see below). The stage of gestation at which exposure occurs determines the target organs or tissues, the types of defects, and the severity of damage. Most structural abnormalities result from exposure during the period of organogenesis (days 31 to 71 after the first day of the last menstrual period). Fig. 18.1

shows the critical stages of development and the related susceptibility of different organs to teratogens. Functional deficiencies are usually associated with exposure during late pregnancy or even after birth because the human central nervous system (CNS) continues to mature until the second year of life.[34]

Consideration of the possible teratogenicity of anesthetic agents must be viewed against the naturally high occurrence of adverse pregnancy outcomes. Roberts and Lowe[35] estimated that as many as 80% of human conceptions are ultimately lost. The rates of spontaneous miscarriage from 5 to 20 weeks' gestation range from 11% to 22%.[36] The incidence of congenital anomalies among humans is approximately 3%, and of these, less than 1% are attributable to exposure to drugs and environmental toxins (Table 18.1). Several criteria are used to determine whether a drug is a human teratogen: (1) proven exposure to the drug at the critical time of development; (2) consistent findings in two or more high-quality epidemiologic studies; (3) careful delineation of the clinical cases, ideally with the identification of a specific defect or syndrome; and (4) an association that "makes biological sense."[33] Documentation of teratogenicity in experimental animals is important but not essential. The drugs or factors that are proven human teratogens do not include anesthetic agents (which are listed as "unlikely teratogens") or any drug routinely used during anesthesia (Fig. 18.2) (see Chapter 16).

Potential Teratogenicity of Nonpharmacologic Agents in the Perioperative Setting

Maternal Metabolic Derangements. Anesthesia and surgery can cause derangements of maternal physiology that may result in hypoxia, hypercapnia, stress, and abnormalities of

TABLE 18.1 Etiology of Human Developmental Defects

Causes of Developmental Defects in Humans	Percentage
Genetic transmission	15–20
Chromosomal abnormality	5
Maternal condition	4
Maternal infection	3
Maternal metabolic imbalance	1–2
Drugs/chemicals/radiation	<1
Unknown	65–70

Modified from Brent RL, Beckman DA. Environmental teratogens. *Bull N Y Acad Med.* 1990;66:123–163.

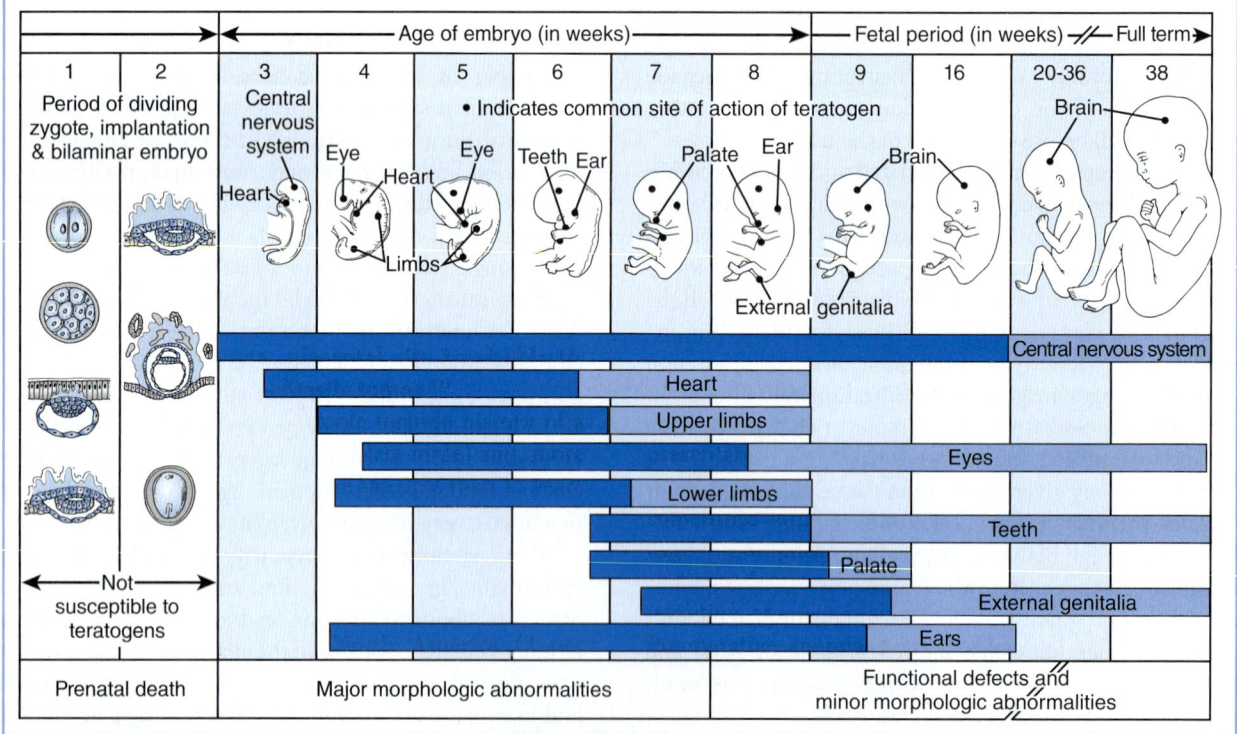

Fig. 18.1 Critical Periods in Human Development. During the first 2 w of development, the embryo typically is not susceptible to teratogens. During these predifferentiation stages, a substance either damages all or most cells of the embryo, resulting in its death, or damages only a few cells, allowing the embryo to recover without development of defects. The dark bars denote highly sensitive periods, whereas the light bars indicate periods of lesser sensitivity. The ages shown refer to the actual ages of the embryo and fetus. Clinical estimates of gestational age represent intervals beginning with the first day of the last menstrual period. Because fertilization typically occurs 2 w after the first day of the last menstrual period, the reader should add 14 d to the ages shown here to convert to the estimated gestational ages that are used clinically. Redrawn from Moore KL. *The Developing Human.* 4th ed. WB Saunders; 1993:156.

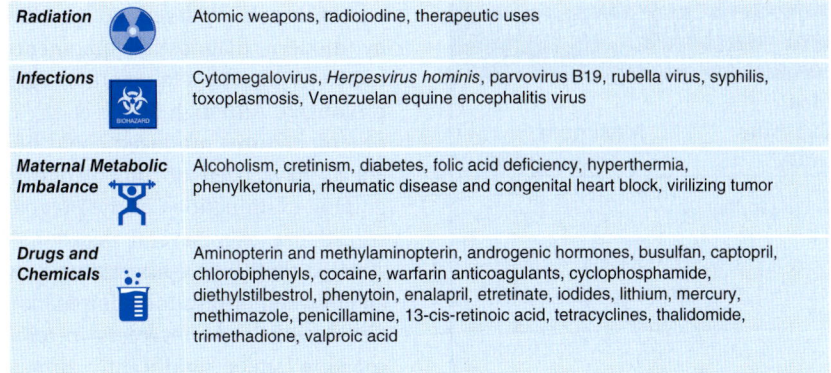

Radiation	Atomic weapons, radioiodine, therapeutic uses
Infections	Cytomegalovirus, *Herpesvirus hominis*, parvovirus B19, rubella virus, syphilis, toxoplasmosis, Venezuelan equine encephalitis virus
Maternal Metabolic Imbalance	Alcoholism, cretinism, diabetes, folic acid deficiency, hyperthermia, phenylketonuria, rheumatic disease and congenital heart block, virilizing tumor
Drugs and Chemicals	Aminopterin and methylaminopterin, androgenic hormones, busulfan, captopril, chlorobiphenyls, cocaine, warfarin anticoagulants, cyclophosphamide, diethylstilbestrol, phenytoin, enalapril, etretinate, iodides, lithium, mercury, methimazole, penicillamine, 13-cis-retinoic acid, tetracyclines, thalidomide, trimethadione, valproic acid

Fig. 18.2 Teratogenic Agents in Humans. Known teratogens in humans, including radiation, infection, maternal metabolic imbalances, and specific drugs and chemicals. Modified from Shepard TH, Lemire RJ. *Catalog of Teratogenic Agents.* 13th ed. Johns Hopkins University Press; 2010.

temperature and carbohydrate metabolism. These states can increase oxidative stress and be teratogenic or may enhance the teratogenicity of other agents.[37,38]

Severe **hypoglycemia** and prolonged **hypoxia** and **hypercarbia** have caused congenital anomalies in laboratory animals, but there is no evidence to support teratogenicity after brief episodes in humans. Prolonged exposure to **hyperglycemia** is a known teratogen causing cardiac, CNS, and skeletal abnormalities, but any organ system can be affected.[39] Anomalies are tightly linked with duration and degree of hyperglycemia, particularly in the first trimester,[39] but it is unlikely that a brief period of intraoperative hyperglycemia has any teratogenic effects. Although severe hypoxemia causes structural teratogenesis in animals and humans, the chronic hypoxemia experienced by mothers at high altitudes results in small-for-gestational-age infants but without an increase in congenital defects.[40] Maternal stress and anxiety have been associated with poor fetal neurocognitive development (behavioral teratogenicity).[41] Studies following obstetric outcomes in women in war zones have demonstrated that maternal emotional trauma and posttraumatic stress disorder may affect fetal growth[42] and increase the risk for miscarriage and hypertensive disorders of pregnancy,[43] but these studies may be confounded by the lack of infrastructure to meet basic prenatal healthcare needs. Hypothermia is not teratogenic, whereas hyperthermia is teratogenic in both animals and humans.[44] Congenital anomalies, especially involving the CNS, have repeatedly been associated with maternal fever during the first half of pregnancy. It must be remembered that fetal temperature is on average 0.5°C to 1°C higher than maternal temperature. Embryonic oxidative stress from reactive oxygen species has been implicated as one of the mechanisms involved in teratogenicity of many agents.[38]

Radiation Exposure During Diagnostic Examinations and Procedures.
Ionizing radiation is a human teratogen that can result in an increased, dose-related risk for malignant disease, genetic disease, congenital anomalies, and/or fetal death.[45] Radiation is expressed as grays (Gy) or milligrays (mGy) (1 Gy = 100 rad) and is evaluated as cumulative dose (i.e., background radiation and medical diagnostic radiation) throughout the entire pregnancy. No dose of radiation is

considered safe, but the type and severity of effects vary with the radiation exposure to the uterus and fetus and with the gestational age of the fetus (Table 18.2). Background radiation during gestation is 1.3 to 5.8 mGy.[46] There is no evidence that radiation exposure below 50 mGy is associated with a teratogenic effect in either humans or animals.[46] In contrast with the negligible risk for teratogenicity, observational studies suggest that there is a slightly higher risk for childhood cancer at radiation doses of 10 mGy or higher.[46] The relative risk for childhood malignancy after maternal abdominal radiation exposure has been estimated to be 2.28 (95% confidence interval [CI], 1.31 to 3.97).[46] The absorbed fetal dose for all conventional radiographic imaging inside or outside the abdomen and pelvis is negligible and is well below 50 mGy, with most falling under 5 mGy (Table 18.3). However, direct radiographic examination using computed tomography or fluoroscopy of the abdomen and pelvis may result in significant fetal radiation exposure, with doses that may approach 100 mGy. Interventional radiologic procedures (e.g., cerebral angiography, cerebral embolization, endoscopic retrograde cholangiopancreatography) are frequently complex and prolonged, particularly when surgery is not an option. These

TABLE 18.2 Radiation Exposure by Gestational Age and Outcomes

Radiation Dose (cGy)	Gestational Age	Fetal Effects
<5	All stages	No fetal effects
10	<8 w	Miscarriage
5–50	8–15 w	Growth restriction Mental retardation
5–50	16 w–birth	Increase childhood cancer (0.3%–6%)
>50	16 w–birth	Childhood cancer (>6%)
	>25 w	Death

Modified from Rimawi BH, Green V, Lindsay M. Fetal implications of diagnostic radiation exposure during pregnancy: evidence-based recommendations. *Clin Obstet Gynecol.* 2016;59:412–418.

TABLE 18.3   Fetal Radiation Exposure for Common Diagnostic Procedures

Procedure	Mean Exposure (mGy)	Maximum Exposure (mGy)
Conventional Radiographic Examination		
Abdomen	1.4	4.2
Chest	<0.01	<0.01
Intravenous urogram	1.7	10
Lumbar spine	1.7	10
Pelvis	1.1	4
Skull	<0.01	<0.01
Thoracic spine	<0.01	<0.01
Fluoroscopic Examination		
Barium meal (upper GI)	1.1	5.8
Barium enema	6.8	24
Computed Tomography		
Abdomen	8.0	49
Head	0.06	0.96
Chest	<0.005	<0.005
Lumbar spine	2.4	8.6
Pelvis	25	79

GI, Gastrointestinal.
From Valentin J. Pregnancy and medical radiation. ICRP Publication 84. Ann ICRP. 2000;30:1–43.

procedures, especially the abdominal interventions, expose the fetus to a significant radiation dose, sometimes more than 50 mGy; thus, professional societies have developed guidance for the use of these technologies during pregnancy.[47,48]

If the mother's condition necessitates diagnostic testing and radiation exposure, and no other acceptable imaging modality is available, testing should not be withheld if the benefits to the mother (and, by extension, the fetus) are judged to outweigh the risks. Delayed diagnosis of a critical condition may result in significant harm to the maternal/fetal dyad. The consultation with the radiologist should include discussion of the optimal diagnostic modality that adheres to the **ALARA principle** (as low as reasonably achievable) for radiation and minimizes the absorbed dose, through abdominal shielding, scan length reduction, and milliampere modulation. The avoidance or minimization of IV radiopaque iodinated contrast media, which crosses the placenta and theoretically can cause neonatal hypothyroidism, should be considered as well.[48]

Diagnostic ultrasonography during pregnancy has long been considered devoid of embryotoxic effects. In animals, ultrasound intensities up to $20\,W/cm^2$ have been found to be safe.[49,50] However, in rat models, when higher intensities ($>30\,W/cm^2$) have been used, or when repeated exposure has occurred during early pregnancy, postnatal neurobehavioral effects have been described.[50,51] Ultrasound waves produced by modern diagnostic equipment can induce significant increases in fetal temperature, especially when imaging is prolonged. Although Miller et al.[52] concluded that the range of temperatures produced could be teratogenic, no biologic effects have been documented from diagnostic ultrasonographic examinations in the pregnant patient, despite widespread use over several decades. Nonetheless, it must be stressed that these epidemiologic studies were conducted in an era when ultrasound equipment was less potent and associated with lower increases in temperature. Doppler interrogation emits significantly more acoustic intensity, and subsequently more heat, than pulse-echo imaging equipment. Therefore, ultrasonographic examinations should be used judiciously, keeping the exposure time and acoustic output to the lowest level possible.

Gadolinium-based MRI contrast agents readily cross the placenta, enter the fetal circulation, and are excreted by the fetal kidneys into the amniotic fluid, where they may be swallowed by the fetus or resorbed by the mother. Gadolinium can be detected in the brain, bone, and liver in mammalian models.[53] A large retrospective study designed to evaluate the effects of MRI exposure interrogated a Canadian universal healthcare database of all births after 20 weeks' gestation from 2003 to 2015.[54] The relative risk for stillbirth was higher (1.68) among those pregnancies in which the fetus was exposed to gadolinium-MRI in the first trimester ($n = 1737$) compared with no MRI ($n = 1{,}418{,}451$); no conclusion could be made for MRI with and without gadolinium because of small sample sizes.[54] Gadolinium can cause fetal bradycardia, late fetal heart rate (FHR) decelerations, and preterm labor.[55] Adequately performed studies on the effects of gadolinium in pregnancy have not yet been performed. The American College of Radiology and the American College of Obstetricians and Gynecologists (ACOG) recommend that IV gadolinium be avoided during pregnancy and used only if absolutely essential.[48,56]

Potential Teratogenicity of Pharmacologic Agents in the Perioperative Setting

Animal studies. Early rodent studies documented teratogenicity (CNS malformations, skeletal abnormalities, and growth restriction) after exposure to a variety of opioids; however, these conclusions have been challenged because opioids given in large bolus injections can cause respiratory depression and impaired feeding, which may be teratogenic. In a rat study designed to avoid such problems, Fujinaga and Mazze[57] maintained clinically relevant concentrations of **morphine** and failed to observe structural anomalies, although fetal growth restriction was present, and offspring mortality was increased. Using the same methodology, Fujinaga et al.[58,59] found **fentanyl, sufentanil,** and **alfentanil** completely devoid of teratogenic effects. Additional mouse studies have confirmed the absence of structural teratogenicity with opioids.[60]

Use of tranquilizers and anxiolytics in pregnancy has been investigated less rigorously than opioids. Animal studies have demonstrated structural or behavioral teratogenesis after exposure to some of the **barbiturate**, **phenothiazine**, and **tricyclic antidepressant** agents.[61,62] The reader is referred to standard teratology reference sources and package inserts for animal and human data related to specific drugs.[33]

Studies in rodents and nonhuman primates indicate that exposure of the immature brain to anesthetic agents such as **propofol**, **thiopental**, and **ketamine** (i.e., agents classified as N-methyl-d-aspartate [NMDA] antagonists and gamma-aminobutyric acid [GABA] agonists) are associated with brain cell apoptosis and functional learning deficits (see Chapter 10).[63,64] A metaanalysis by Bleeser et al.[34] demonstrated that anesthesia-induced neurotoxicity during pregnancy is a consistent finding in animal studies, with neurodegeneration increasing with longer duration, greater dosage, and higher frequency of agent exposure.[64,65]

However, recent animal and human evidence of exposure of the fetal brain to various anesthetic agents has been reassuring. Using a rabbit model, Van der Veeken et al.[66] injected anesthetic agents and neuromuscular blocking agents into the fetus and observed no brain modifications; the addition of fetal surgery yielded no neurodevelopmental effects.[67] In a similar rabbit model, 2 hours of maternal exposure to general anesthesia and laparotomy, with minimal organ and no fetal manipulation, resulted in slower offspring motor neurodevelopment, but the effect was almost undetectable by 7 weeks.[68] By contrast, no fetal neuronal injury or neurobehavioral impairments were observed in an ovine model with maternal exposure to anesthesia for 5 hours.[69] A rabbit study of maternal **sevoflurane** anesthesia for laparotomy produced neurodevelopmental effects, which were not prevented with the addition of xenon.[70]

Human studies. Teratogenesis has not been associated with any of the commonly used induction agents, including **barbiturates**, **ketamine**, and **benzodiazepines**, when administered in clinical doses during anesthesia.[33] In a bidirectional cohort study, Bleeser et al.[71] reported no neurodevelopmental changes in the fetus and neonate when exposed to anesthesia prenatally.

Studies of long-term sedative-hypnotic therapy have associated teratogenicity with some agents, but affirmative studies have been retrospective and have had methodologic flaws. In a prospective evaluation of children with birth defects, a higher risk for cleft lip was not found when mothers ingested **diazepam** during the first trimester.[72] The present consensus among teratologists is that diazepam is not a proven human teratogen.[33] Moreover, no evidence suggests that a single dose of a benzodiazepine (e.g., **midazolam**) is harmful to the fetus.

Obstetric complications of prenatal opioid exposure are well documented and include preterm birth, small for gestational age, LBW, reduced head circumference, and sudden infant death (see Chapters 42 and 52).[73] The evidence supporting structural teratogenicity of opioids in humans is of low quality, but in a systematic review of case-control and cohort studies, Lind et al.[73] found a positive association between **fetal opioid exposure** and congenital anomalies (e.g., cleft lip, cleft palate, atrial septal defect, clubfoot) in 17 of 30 studies. **Neonatal opioid withdrawal syndrome**[74]

and impaired cognition, psychomotor skills, and behavioral development have been observed in infants and children exposed to opioids *in utero*.[75,76] However, many studies did not correct for socioeconomic or environmental factors that might also influence neurobehavioral development.

Attempts should be made to reduce cumulative dose of opioid medications prescribed to pregnant women while ensuring adequate pain management. Analgesic and anesthetic techniques, such as regional, peripheral nerve, and field blocks, and surgical techniques, such as laparoscopy, that reduce the need for postoperative opioids should be used preferentially in pregnant women. Multimodal analgesia, including maximizing the use of nonopioid medications that are considered safe in pregnancy (e.g., **acetaminophen**), should be considered.

Local Anesthetics

No evidence supports morphologic or behavioral teratogenicity with **lidocaine (lignocaine)** administration in rats,[77] or with the clinical administration of local anesthetics, with the exception of **cocaine**. Maternal cocaine abuse is associated with adverse reproductive outcomes, including abnormal neonatal behavior and, in some reports, a higher incidence of congenital defects of the genitourinary, cardiac, facial, and gastrointestinal tracts.[78] The greatest risk to the fetus most likely results from the high incidence of placental abruption and preterm delivery associated with maternal cocaine use (see Chapter 52).

Muscle Relaxants and Muscle Relaxant Reversal Agents

Testing muscle relaxants for teratogenicity using standard *in vivo* animal study techniques is complicated by the requirement for very low drug doses or the need for mechanical ventilation (a complex undertaking in rodents). Fujinaga et al.[79] used a whole-embryo rat culture system to investigate the reproductive toxicity of high doses of **d-tubocurarine**, **pancuronium**, **atracurium**, and **vecuronium**. Although dose-dependent toxicity was manifested, these effects occurred only at concentrations 30-fold greater than those encountered in clinical practice. Given that fetal blood concentrations of muscle relaxants are only 10% to 20% of maternal concentrations, these drugs appear to have a wide margin of safety when administered to the mother during organogenesis.

Sugammadex, an agent that rapidly reverses paralysis by forming a complex with neuromuscular blocking agents, has not been robustly investigated in pregnant women.[80] In women undergoing cesarean delivery with general anesthesia and **rocuronium** for rapid-sequence induction, the dosing and response to sugammadex were similar to those in nonpregnant patients.[81] Known risks of sugammadex include anaphylaxis (0.3%), bradycardia, and cardiac arrest.[80] Because of binding properties to progestogen (synthetic progesterone), the theoretical risk of inducing preterm labor, and the paucity of evidence regarding lactation, in 2019 the Society for Obstetric Anesthesia and Perinatology (SOAP) recommended that sugammadex be avoided in early pregnancy and that it be avoided or used with caution in late or term pregnancy.[82]

However, this guidance has been questioned as a result of (1) an analysis of the chemical and pharmacokinetic profile differences from endogenous progesterone, (2) a growing number of case series indicating an absence of adverse effects, and (3) a risk/benefit assessment that considers the potential occurrence of residual neuromuscular blockade when **neostigmine/ glycopyrrolate** is used for reversal.[83] Although used for decades, neostigmine in high dosages has been noted to be teratogenic to vertebral column and beak formation in chicks.[84]

Inhalation Anesthetics

Animal Studies. Under certain conditions, the **volatile halogenated anesthetic agents** can produce teratogenic changes in chicks or small rodents. Long-term exposure to subanesthetic concentrations of **halothane** caused fetal growth restriction in rats but no increase in the incidence of congenital anomalies,[85] whereas **isoflurane** had no adverse effects.[86]

Significant reproductive effects have occurred with anesthetic concentrations of volatile anesthetic agents, including fetal skeletal abnormalities or death, following repeated or prolonged maternal exposure in rodents.[87,88] Teratogenicity in these studies was most likely caused by the physiologic changes (e.g., profound hypothermia, hypoventilation) associated with anesthesia rather than by the anesthetic agents themselves. Moreover, some strains of mice are especially likely to demonstrate anomalies, such as a cleft palate. Mazze et al.[89] exposed rats to 0.75 MAC of **halothane, isoflurane**, or **enflurane**, or 0.55 MAC of **nitrous oxide**, for 6 hours daily on 3 consecutive days at various stages of pregnancy. The animals remained conscious throughout the study, and normal feeding and sleep patterns were preserved. Under these conditions, no teratogenic effects were associated with any of the volatile agents. The only positive finding was a threefold increase in the rate of fetal resorption with nitrous oxide. No evidence has suggested reproductive toxicity with either **sevoflurane** or **desflurane** in clinical concentrations.

In contrast with the volatile halogenated agents, **nitrous oxide** is a weak teratogen in rodents under certain conditions, even when normal homeostasis is maintained. Rats continually exposed to 50% to 70% nitrous oxide for 2 to 6 days (starting on day 8 of gestation) had an increased incidence of congenital abnormalities.[89,90] To exclude the possibility that adverse effects were a consequence of the anesthetic state, Lane et al.[91] exposed rats to 70% nitrous oxide or to a similar concentration of **xenon** (a slightly more potent anesthetic devoid of biochemical effects) for 24 hours on day 9 of gestation; abnormalities occurred only in the nitrous oxide group. With the exception of one study in which extremely prolonged exposure to a low concentration of nitrous oxide had some minor effects,[92] at least 50% nitrous oxide has been required to consistently produce anomalies.[90] The threshold exposure time has not been rigorously determined, although exposure for at least 24 hours typically was necessary.

In vivo and embryo culture studies in rats have confirmed that nitrous oxide has several adverse reproductive effects, each of which results from exposure at a specific period of susceptibility.[93,94] Fetal resorptions occurred after exposure on days 8 and 11 of gestation, skeletal anomalies after exposure

on day 8 or 9, and visceral anomalies (including *situs inversus*) only when exposure occurred on day 8.[95]

Initially, teratogenicity associated with nitrous oxide was thought to result from its oxidation of vitamin B12, which interferes with its function as a coenzyme for methionine synthase.[96] Transmethylation from methyl-tetrahydrofolate to homocysteine, with subsequent production of tetrahydrofolate (THF) and methionine, is catalyzed by methionine synthase (Fig. 18.3). Thus, methionine synthase inhibition could cause a decrease in THF (with a resultant decrease in DNA synthesis) and lower methionine levels (with resultant impairment of methylation reactions). Nitrous oxide rapidly inactivates methionine synthase in both animals[97] and humans.[98] Prolonged human exposure to nitrous oxide leads to adverse neurologic and hematologic outcomes, the latter probably resulting from diminished DNA synthesis.[96]

Considerable evidence indicates that methionine synthase inhibition and a consequent lack of THF are not solely responsible for the teratogenic effects of nitrous oxide. Additional studies have implicated alpha-1 adrenergic receptor stimulation in the production of *situs inversus* by nitrous oxide.[99] Postulated mechanisms by which sympathetic stimulation might have adverse reproductive effects include a decrease in uterine blood flow and overstimulation of G protein–dependent membrane signal transduction pathways.[100] There is also evidence that nitrous oxide may cause neuronal apoptosis in rats, in part, as a result of oxidative stress.[101]

In summary, evidence suggests that the etiology of nitrous oxide teratogenicity in rats is complex and multifactorial. Determination of the relative roles of methionine deficiency and sympathetic stimulation or other mechanisms awaits further study. Although nitrous oxide is considered a weak teratogen in rats and mice, reproductive effects occur only after prolonged exposure to high concentrations that are unlikely to be encountered in humans during clinical anesthesia. Whether nitrous oxide administration is associated with neuronal apoptosis and learning impairments in humans remains to be determined.

Human Studies. Epidemiologic surveys dating to the early 1970s suggested that reproductive hazards (e.g., spontaneous abortion, congenital anomalies) were associated with **occupational exposure to waste anesthetic agents**, principally **nitrous oxide**, in the operating room and during dental

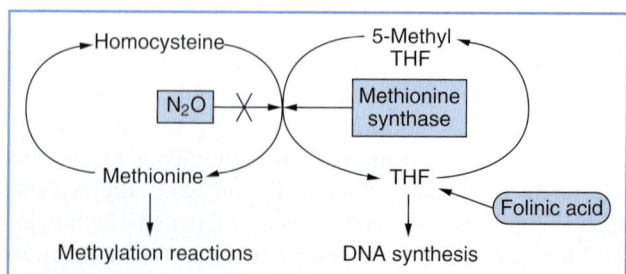

Fig. 18.3 Pathway of Methionine Synthase Inhibition by Nitrous Oxide (N$_2$O). Metabolic consequences include impaired DNA synthesis and methylation reactions. *THF*, Tetrahydrofolate. Illustration M. Fujinaga, Palo Alto, CA.

surgery. Critical reviews of these studies questioned their conclusions, noting that response bias, inappropriate control groups, lack of verification of medical data, and exposure to multiple environmental factors made definitive conclusions impossible.[102-104] By the late 1970s and 1980s, more rigorous studies had not confirmed an association between operating room work and exposure to anesthetic agents with higher reproductive risk.[105,106]

Dimich-Ward et al.[107] studied the risk for fetal anomalies in live and stillborn births in an offspring cohort study of registered nurses ($n = 22,611$) in the British Columbia Vital Statistics Registry (1986 to 2000). In nurses exposed to the operating room environment, an increased risk for congenital anomalies was associated with exposure to halogenated anesthetic agents (odds ratio [OR], 1.49) or nitrous oxide (OR, 1.42). The Nurse's Health Study-II ($n = 8461$), published in 2012, compared the risk for spontaneous abortion in nurses exposed to anesthetic gases (e.g., **nitrous oxide, halothane, enflurane, and isoflurane**) versus those who were not exposed, with correction for age, parity, shift work, and hours worked.[108] The odds for abortion were not different between groups. A major limitation of these studies[107,108] was the failure to correct for tobacco use or alcohol consumption; the relative risk for spontaneous abortion is increased with cigarette smoking (1.8), one or two alcoholic drinks per day (1.98), and more than three drinks per day (3.53).[109]

Using a questionnaire-based survey of 744 pregnancies in 2028 female veterinarians, Shirangi et al.[110] observed that the prevalence of preterm birth (before 37 weeks' gestation) was higher in those exposed to unscavenged anesthetic gases (7.3%) compared with the general Australian population (5.7%) during the same period. The identity of the specific anesthetic gas used was not requested; however, **halothane**, **nitrous oxide**, **enflurane**, and **methoxyflurane** were commonly used during the study period. A hazards model predicted a 2.5-fold increase in preterm delivery risk in women exposed to unscavenged gas for one or more hours per week compared with an unexposed group.[110]

It is possible that the higher waste levels of nitrous oxide encountered in dentists' offices compared with operating rooms pose a reproductive risk, but overall the epidemiologic data do not support an increased risk for congenital anomalies with long-term occupational exposure to nitrous oxide.[111,112] However, nitrous oxide is more potent than carbon dioxide in trapping heat in the ozone layer, with potential relevance to climate change.

Studies of Surgery Performed During Pregnancy

Studies from the 1960s to 1980s indicated that surgery during pregnancy increased the risk of spontaneous abortion, fetal mortality, preterm delivery, and LBW, but not congenital anomalies.[113-116]

In the largest study to date investigating anesthesia type and pregnancy outcomes, Mazze and Källén[117] linked data from three Swedish healthcare registries (the Medical Birth Registry, the Registry of Congenital Malformations, and the Hospital Discharge Registry) for the years 1973 to 1981.

Among the population of 720,000 pregnant women, 5405 (0.75%) had nonobstetric surgery, including 2252 who had procedures during the first trimester. Of the women who had surgery, 54% received general anesthesia, which included nitrous oxide in 97% of cases. The researchers found a higher incidence of LBW and very low birth rate infants in the surgical group, which resulted from both preterm delivery and fetal growth restriction, but no difference in the incidence of stillbirth or the overall incidence of congenital anomalies. Although the overall rate of anomalies among infants of women who had first-trimester operations was not higher, this group did have a higher-than-expected incidence of neural tube defects (6.0 observed versus 2.5 expected). Five of the six women whose infants had these defects were among the 572 women who had had surgery during gestational weeks 4 to 5, which is the period of neural tube formation; the researchers cautioned that this finding could have been a chance association.[117] However, if a true causal relationship exists between neural tube defects and anesthesia at this stage of gestation, it could represent an eightfold to ninefold increase in the risk for this anomaly (i.e., an absolute risk of almost 1%). A case-control study of infants born in Atlanta between 1968 and 1980 gathered information regarding first-trimester exposure to general anesthesia from the mothers of 694 infants with major CNS defects and 2984 control mothers.[118] A significant association was found between general anesthesia exposure and hydrocephalus in conjunction with another major defect (the strongest association was with hydrocephalus and eye defects). Two additional studies[119,120] from the 1980s focused on the risks associated with nitrous oxide anesthesia during early pregnancy; no increase in the incidence of spontaneous abortion or congenital abnormalities was identified. Limitations of these studies include their retrospective nature; a lack of information about the types of surgery, the anesthetic agents used, and the presence or absence of surgical complications; and the fact that they were conducted decades ago with older anesthetic and surgical techniques.[117,118]

A population-based, case-control study from the National Birth Defects Prevention Study (1997 to 2011), that involved 10 American states was designed to investigate risk factors for more than 30 major structural birth defects in pregnancies.[121] In the periconceptional period, the most common procedures utilizing general anesthesia were dental procedures (16.7%), cholecystectomy (9.5%), and cervical cerclage (9.5%, $n = 8$). As expected, acute abdominal conditions in the second and third trimester most commonly required general anesthesia, including appendectomy (12.1%), cholecystectomy (15.2%), and kidney stone/ureteral stent procedures (13.6%). No association was found between any of the 30 birth defects and general anesthesia exposure at any time point in the pregnancies between those exposed versus those not exposed to surgery in pregnancy.

A cohort study conducted from 2003 to 2012 of 19,926 pregnant women in the Nationwide Inpatient Sample, which accounts for 20% of patients discharged from US community hospitals, sought to analyze risk factors for adverse outcomes associated with appendectomy and cholecystectomy.[122] An adverse obstetric outcome occurred in 4.8% of women, the most common being preterm delivery (35.4%), preterm labor without preterm delivery (26.4%), and miscarriage (25.7%).[122] Preexisting obstetric risk factors were the largest contributors to adverse pregnancy outcomes, including cervical incompetence (adjusted OR, 24.3), prior preterm labor in pregnancy (adjusted OR, 18.3), and vaginitis/vulvovaginitis (adjusted OR, 5.2).[122] Other risk factors included non-Caucasian ethnicity, multiple gestation, open surgical technique, and increased disease severity (e.g., peritonitis, sepsis). Specific anesthetic techniques or agents could not be determined from the database.

A retrospective analysis of 6.5 million pregnancies in English NHS hospitals between 2002 and 2012 identified 47,628 pregnancies in which nonobstetric surgery occurred.[2] The risk of adverse birth outcomes was higher in pregnant women having surgery than in those who did not have surgery, with adjusted risk (AR, the additional difference in risk in mothers undergoing nonobstetric surgery) values calculated as 0.7% (95% CI, 0.4 to 0.9) for miscarriage, 0.4% (95% CI, 0.3 to 0.4) for stillbirth, 3.2% (95% CI, 2.9 to 3.4) for preterm delivery, 2.6% (95% CI, 2.5 to 2.9) for LBW, and 4.0% (95% CI, 3.6 to 4.5) for cesarean delivery.

In a retrospective review of hospital records from 2001 to 2016, Devroe et al.[1] compared 171 patients who had nonobstetric surgery during pregnancy with 684 nonexposed control patients matched for age, time of delivery, and parity. They found that in women who had surgery, delivery was earlier and more frequently preterm (25% versus 17%), and birth weight was lower (median 3.16 kg [95% CI, 3.06 to 3.26]) versus 3.27 kg (3.22 to 3.32). When surgery was conducted under general anesthesia, LBW was more frequent (22% versus 6%). Laparoscopic surgery did not increase the incidence of adverse pregnancy outcomes.

In summary, nonobstetric anesthesia and surgery are associated with a higher incidence of abortion, fetal growth restriction, and perinatal mortality, which can often be attributed to the procedure, the site of surgery (i.e., proximity to the uterus), and/or the underlying maternal or obstetric conditions. Evidence does not suggest that anesthesia during pregnancy, *per se*, results in an overall increase in congenital abnormalities, or that a relationship exists between the type of anesthesia provided and adverse pregnancy outcomes.

Behavioral Teratology

Some teratogens produce enduring behavioral abnormalities without any observable morphologic changes. The CNS may be especially sensitive to such influences during the period of major myelination, which in humans extends from the fourth intrauterine month to the second postnatal month (see Chapter 10).

Currently used general anesthetic agents act mainly by one of two principal mechanisms: (1) the potentiation of GABA$_A$ receptors (**benzodiazepines**, **halogenated volatile anesthetic agents**, and **barbiturates**) or (2) the antagonism of NMDA receptors (**nitrous oxide, ketamine**). Drugs that act by either of these mechanisms appear to induce widespread neuronal apoptosis in animal models. In a review of 65 animal studies on the influence of anesthetic agents on brain development, Bleeser et al.[34] found that all anesthetic agents tested were associated with impaired learning and memory and direct neuronal injury. Although most of these studies used very high drug doses and maintained hemodynamic parameters poorly, their data have been used to direct clinical studies and issue policy guidance.

In 2016, the US Food and Drug Administration issued a "Drug Safety Communication" warning that "…repeated or lengthy use of general anesthetic and sedation drugs during surgeries or procedures in children younger than 3 years or in pregnant women during their third trimester may affect the development of children's brains."[123] Because most repeated or lengthy procedures in pregnant women and in children younger than 3 years of age are urgent or necessary, and alternative anesthetic techniques are not feasible for many of these surgical procedures, the implications for anesthetic and surgical practice will primarily be to discuss the timing and the relative advantages and risks of different procedures.

Using validated postoperative neurodevelopmental testing in human children, the Pediatric Anesthesia and Neurodevelopment Assessment (PANDA) trial[124] and the General Anesthesia versus Spinal Anesthesia (GAS) trial[125] determined that a brief, single exposure to general anesthesia did not lead to poorer neurodevelopmental outcomes in children exposed to general anesthesia compared with control groups.[124,125] The international, multicenter GAS trial randomized infants (younger than 60 weeks' postmenstrual age, born at more than 26 weeks' gestation) who were undergoing inguinal herniorrhaphy to awake-regional ($n = 238$) or sevoflurane-based general anesthesia ($n = 294$). No difference was found in the secondary outcome, the composite cognitive score of the Bayley Scales of Infant and Toddler Development III, assessed at 2 years of age.[125] The result of the primary outcome, the 5-year full-scale intelligence quotient, indicated no difference between the group that received awake-regional ($n = 205$) and sevoflurane-based general anesthesia ($n = 242$).[126] The sibling-matched cohort design PANDA trial evaluated whether a single exposure to general anesthesia in healthy children younger than 3 years of age (determined retrospectively) was associated with a risk for impaired global cognitive function (IQ) or other neurocognitive functions and behaviors in children 8 to 15 years of age (assessed prospectively).[124] No differences were found in global cognitive function or neurodevelopmental outcomes in 105 sibling-matched pairs. Similarly, Bleeser et al.[71] performed a bidirectional cohort study with retrospective identification of children (2 to 18 years) who were prenatally exposed to anesthesia while their mothers underwent nonobstetric surgery during pregnancy. The neurodevelopmental outcomes of these children were compared, using parental questionnaires, with those from unexposed children to evaluate executive functioning, psychosocial problems, learning disorders, and diagnoses listed in the fifth edition of the *Diagnostic and Statistical Manual of Mental Disorders* (DSM-5). The study did not find evidence in the general population for an association between prenatal exposure to anesthesia and impaired neurodevelopmental outcomes.

Assessment of the impact of anesthetic agents should also consider influence of surgery, which can independently result in derangements in maternal physiology (e.g., hypoxia, stress, hypoglycemia) that can lead to apoptosis during the critical period of neuronal development.[127] Moreover, painful stimuli *per se* can cause also lead to long-term behavioral changes.[128]

Fetal Heart Rate Monitoring

Continuous FHR monitoring (using transabdominal Doppler ultrasonography) may be feasible beginning at 18 to 20 weeks' gestation, although technical problems may limit its use until after 22 weeks' gestation.[129] Transabdominal monitoring may not be possible during abdominal procedures or when the mother is very obese; the intraoperative use of transvaginal Doppler ultrasonography may be considered in selected cases.

The ACOG and ASA have jointly published guidelines for clinical management and fetal monitoring during nonobstetric surgery, which are summarized in Fig. 18.4.[130] In patients with a previable fetus, it is generally sufficient to ascertain the FHR by Doppler ultrasonography before and after the procedure. In patients with a viable fetus, at a minimum, simultaneous electronic FHR and contraction monitoring should be performed before and after the procedure to assess fetal well-being and the absence of contractions.[130] The ACOG/ASA guidelines state that "intraoperative electronic fetal monitoring may be appropriate when all of the following apply: (1) the fetus is viable; (2) it is physically possible to perform intraoperative electronic fetal monitoring; (3) a healthcare provider with obstetric surgery privileges is available; (4) when possible, the woman has provided informed consent that allows for emergency cesarean delivery for fetal indications; and (5) the nature of the planned surgery will allow the safe interruption or alteration of the procedure to provide access to perform emergency delivery."[130] However, a survey of members of the Association of Professors of Gynecology and Obstetrics indicated that only 43% routinely used intraoperative FHR monitoring.[131]

FHR variability, typically used as an indicator of fetal well-being, is present by 25 to 27 weeks' gestation. Most anesthetic agents and opioids reduce FHR variability. When uterine contractions are not monitored, FHR interpretation is very limited. Persistent, severe fetal bradycardia typically indicates true fetal compromise.

Intraoperative FHR monitoring requires the presence of a provider who can interpret the FHR tracing. In addition, a multidisciplinary plan should address how to proceed in the event of persistent, nonreassuring fetal status, including whether to interrupt ongoing surgery to perform an emergency cesarean delivery. Intraoperative FHR monitoring may allow for the optimization of the maternal condition if the fetus shows signs of compromise. An unexplained change in FHR baseline mandates the evaluation of maternal position, blood pressure, oxygenation, and acid-base status, and the inspection of the surgical site to ensure that neither surgeons nor retractors are impairing uteroplacental perfusion.

Fetal Effects of Anesthesia
Maintenance of Fetal Well-Being

The most serious fetal risk associated with maternal surgery during pregnancy is intrauterine asphyxia. Fetal oxygenation is critically dependent on the maintenance of normal maternal arterial oxygen tension, oxygen-carrying capacity, oxygen affinity, and uteroplacental perfusion.

Maternal and Fetal Oxygenation. Transient mild to moderate decreases in maternal PaO_2 are well tolerated by the fetus, primarily because fetal hemoglobin has a high affinity for oxygen. Severe maternal hypoxemia results in fetal hypoxia and, if persistent, may cause fetal death. Any complication that causes profound maternal hypoxemia (e.g., difficult tracheal intubation, esophageal intubation, pulmonary aspiration, total spinal anesthesia, local anesthetic systemic toxicity [LAST]) is a potential threat to the fetus.

Studies of isolated human placental vessels have suggested that hyperoxia may cause uteroplacental vasoconstriction, with potential impairment of fetal oxygen delivery[132,133]; however, this concern has proved to be unfounded. Studies in pregnant women have demonstrated better fetal oxygenation with increasing maternal PaO_2; however, fetal PaO_2 never exceeds 60 mm Hg (8.0 kPa), even when maternal PaO_2 increases to 600 mm Hg (80 kPa). This physiologic limitation exists, in part, because of the low diffusion capacity of oxygen in the placenta, as well as the admixture of blood returning

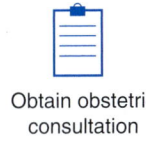

Obtain obstetric consultation

Delay elective, not emergency cases

Discuss timing of FHR monitoring

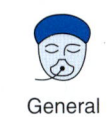

General anesthesia safe

Monitor/plan for preterm delivery

Thromboembolism prophylaxis

Fig. 18.4 Summary of Guidelines for Clinical Management of Nonobstetric Surgery During Pregnancy. *FHR,* Fetal heart rate. From American College of Obstetricians and Gynecologists. Committee Opinion No. 775: Nonobstetric surgery during pregnancy (reaffirmed 2021). *Obstet Gynecol.* 2019;133:e285–e286.

to the fetus from the placenta with deoxygenated blood from the fetal inferior vena cava (see Chapter 4). Thus, intrauterine retrolental fibroplasia and premature closure of the ductus arteriosus cannot result from high maternal PaO_2. McClaine et al.[134] observed that the maternal administration of general anesthesia for 4 hours in gravid ewes produced an initial—but not sustained—increase in fetal systemic oxygenation, but a sustained increase in cerebral oxygenation. The investigators hypothesized that the increase in fetal cerebral oxygenation resulted from greater cerebral perfusion, lower cerebral metabolic rate, or both. Histologic examination found no evidence of neurotoxicity.

Maternal Carbon Dioxide and Acid-Base Status. Maternal hypercapnia can cause fetal acidosis because fetal $PaCO_2$ correlates directly with maternal $PaCO_2$. Although mild fetal respiratory acidosis is of little consequence, severe acidosis can cause fetal myocardial depression and hypotension. Maternal hyperventilation with low maternal $PaCO_2$ and high pH can adversely affect fetal oxygenation by several mechanisms.[135–137] Respiratory or metabolic alkalosis can compromise maternal-fetal oxygen transfer by causing umbilical artery constriction[135] and by shifting the maternal oxyhemoglobin dissociation curve to the left.[136] In addition, hyperventilation, independent of changes in $PaCO_2$, may reduce uterine blood flow and cause fetal acidosis.[137] This decrease most likely is a consequence of mechanical ventilation, whereby increased intrathoracic pressure reduces venous return and cardiac output, which in turn decreases uteroplacental perfusion. Thus, hyperventilation should be avoided in the pregnant surgical patient. Rather, the $PaCO_2$ should be kept in the normal range for pregnancy.

Uteroplacental Perfusion. Maternal hypotension from any cause can jeopardize uteroplacental perfusion and cause fetal asphyxia (see Chapter 3). The most common causes of hypotension in the pregnant patient undergoing surgery include (1) deep levels of general anesthesia, (2) sympathectomy with high sensory levels of spinal or epidural blockade, (3) aortocaval compression, (4) hemorrhage, and (5) hypovolemia. In monkeys, prolonged hypotension (i.e., systolic blood pressure < 75 mm Hg) caused by deep halothane anesthesia resulted in fetal hypoxia, acidosis, and hypotension.[138] After as much as 5 hours of severe partial asphyxia *in utero* (pH < 7.00 for at least 1 hour), neonatal monkeys were depressed and experienced seizures. Postnatal survival was poor and pathologic brain changes included swelling, necrosis, and hemorrhage. The clinical course and neuropathologic findings in these animals resembled those in infants known to have suffered severe intrauterine asphyxia and who died within a few days of birth.

However, good fetal and neonatal outcomes have been reported following deliberate use of moderate degrees of hypotension, usually to facilitate performance of a neurosurgical procedure in otherwise healthy women[139]; maternal systolic blood pressures were maintained at 70 to 80 mm Hg, with transient periods as low as 50 mm Hg. These blood pressure parameters likely cannot be extrapolated to maternal conditions such as gestational hypertension, preeclampsia,

or other conditions that predispose to uteroplacental insufficiency. In surgical circumstances necessitating maternal hypotension, the risk to the fetus must be balanced against the risk for uncontrolled maternal bleeding or stroke.

The multiple factors that influence uteroplacental blood flow are discussed in detail in Chapter 3. Of relevance to the pregnant surgical patient are drugs that cause uterine artery vasoconstriction. Preoperative anxiety and light anesthesia increase circulating catecholamines, possibly impairing uterine blood flow.[140] Drugs that cause uterine tachysystole (e.g., **ketamine** in early pregnancy in doses more than 2 mg/kg,[141] toxic doses of local anesthetics[142]) may increase vascular resistance of the vessels perfusing the uterus and placenta, decreasing perfusion.

Although historically **ephedrine** was the preferred first-line agent for the treatment of hypotension during the administration of neuraxial anesthesia in obstetric patients, evidence now supports the use of an alpha-adrenergic receptor agonist such as **phenylephrine** as the drug of choice for this purpose (see Chapter 26).[143] Human studies in women receiving neuraxial anesthesia, including those that directly evaluated uterine vascular resistance by Doppler ultrasonography, have demonstrated no differences in uterine blood flow parameters when ephedrine or phenylephrine infusions were used to maintain baseline mean arterial pressure.[144] Moreover, a metaanalysis of randomized controlled trials comparing ephedrine with phenylephrine for the treatment of hypotension during spinal anesthesia for cesarean delivery concluded the following: (1) there was no difference between phenylephrine and ephedrine for the prevention and treatment of maternal hypotension, (2) maternal bradycardia was more likely to occur with phenylephrine than with ephedrine, (3) women treated with phenylephrine had neonates with higher umbilical arterial blood pH measurements than those given ephedrine, and (4) there was no difference between the two vasopressors in the incidence of true fetal acidosis (i.e., umbilical arterial blood pH < 7.20).[145]

Ngan Kee et al.[146] demonstrated that placental transfer was greater for ephedrine than phenylephrine, with less early metabolism and/or redistribution in the fetus. Fetal concentrations of lactate, glucose, and catecholamines were also higher with ephedrine than phenylephrine, thus supporting the hypothesis that the lower fetal pH observed with ephedrine is related to metabolic effects secondary to stimulation of fetal beta-adrenergic receptors. Recently, **norepinephrine (noradrenaline)** has been observed to successfully prevent and treat spinal anesthesia–induced maternal hypotension and appears as safe as other vasopressors.[147,148]

Effects of Inhalation Agents on the Fetus

Volatile halogenated anesthetic agents are a common component of general anesthesia; the depressant effect of these agents on uterine myometrial contractility may be beneficial for prevention of preterm labor. These agents transfer readily across the placenta and can affect the fetus directly (by depressing the fetal cardiovascular system or CNS) or indirectly (by causing maternal hypoxia or hypotension). Studies in gravid ewes have shown minimal fetal effects with maternal administration of moderate concentrations of volatile agents.[149] During the inhalation of 1.0 and 1.5 MAC **halothane** or **isoflurane**, uterine artery vasodilation compensated for small decreases in maternal blood pressure to maintain uterine perfusion; however, the inhalation of 2.0 MAC concentrations for prolonged periods induced marked reductions in maternal blood pressure and uteroplacental blood flow, which resulted in fetal hypoxia, diminished fetal cardiac output, and fetal acidosis.[150]

The effects of anesthesia on the healthy fetal lamb may be minimal, but the effects on a stressed fetal lamb remain unclear. In one study, the administration of 1% halothane to the mothers of asphyxiated fetal lambs caused severe fetal hypotension, acidosis, and decreases in cerebral blood flow and oxygen delivery.[150] In other studies, acidosis that was less severe in magnitude or duration was associated with the maintenance of fetal cardiac output and a preservation of the balance between oxygen supply and demand.[151,152] The protective compensatory mechanisms that exist during asphyxia may be abolished by high but not low concentrations of volatile agents.

In a study in pregnant rabbits, Bleeser et al.[153] evaluated 2 hours of **sevoflurane** anesthesia without vasopressors to restore normal blood pressure and compared it with 2 hours of sevoflurane exposure with restoration of blood pressure using **norepinephrine**; treatment of anesthesia-induced hypotension using norepinephrine did not affect neuron densities but was associated with impairment of several secondary fetal outcomes. Further studies are needed to investigate measurable and meaningful clinical outcomes, including threshold blood pressures in pregnant women undergoing general anesthesia.

The relevance of the above data to women undergoing surgery during pregnancy is unclear. Provided that maternal hypotension is prevented, FHR decelerations are not expected, but diminished FHR variability typically occurs as the fetus becomes anesthetized. If intraoperative FHR monitoring shows signs of fetal compromise, corrective maneuvers should be implemented (Box 18.1), including the consideration of conversion to IV anesthesia.

Effects of Systemic Agent on the Fetus

Opioids and induction agents decrease FHR variability, possibly to a greater extent than inhalation agents.[154,155] This finding most likely relates to an anesthetized fetus, but warrants vigilance for maternal hypotension or other abnormalities. Fetal respiratory depression is most relevant when cesarean delivery is performed at the same time as the surgical procedure. Even then, high-dose opioid anesthesia need not be avoided if indicated for maternal reasons (e.g., anesthesia for patients with cardiac disease), although the neonatologist should be informed so preparations can be made to support neonatal respiration. Some data indicate that **remifentanil** may result in less neonatal depression than longer-acting opioids.[156]

Maternal administration of **muscle relaxants** and **muscle relaxant reversal agents** typically is not problematic for the fetus. The rapid IV injection of an **anticholinesterase agent** could stimulate acetylcholine release and theoretically increase uterine tone and precipitate preterm labor.[157] Although this concern is unproven, slow administration of an anticholinesterase agent (after prior injection of an anticholinergic agent) is recommended. **Atropine** rapidly crosses the placenta and, when given in large doses, causes fetal tachycardia and loss of FHR variability.[158] Although neither atropine nor **glycopyrrolate** significantly affects FHR when standard clinical doses are administered,[159] glycopyrrolate is often recommended because it crosses the placenta less readily. Limited transplacental passage of **neostigmine** is expected, but mild fetal bradycardia was reported in one patient at 31 weeks' gestation when neostigmine was administered with glycopyrrolate during emergence from general anesthesia.[160] This problem did not occur during the administration of a second general anesthetic to the same patient 4 days later, when atropine was administered with neostigmine, presumably because atropine undergoes greater placental transfer than glycopyrrolate.

PRACTICAL CONSIDERATIONS

Timing of Surgery

The ACOG/ASA committee opinion on nonobstetric surgery during pregnancy states that elective surgery should not be performed during pregnancy and that necessary surgery should not be denied because of trimester considerations; however, should surgery be deemed necessary, the second trimester is preferred because of its association with the lowest risk for spontaneous abortion and preterm labor.[130]

Urgent operations are often indicated for abdominal emergencies, some malignancies, and neurosurgical and cardiac conditions. The management and timing of most acute surgical procedures should mimic that for nonpregnant patients. In the event of a serious maternal illness necessitating emergency surgery, the remote fetal risks associated with anesthesia and surgery are of secondary importance. The primary goal is to preserve the life of the mother. Successful neonatal outcomes in complex, high-risk procedures requiring

---

BOX 18.1 Maneuvers for Intrauterine Fetal Resuscitation During Nonobstetric Surgery

- Increase left uterine displacement
- Increase oxygen concentration
- Optimize blood pressure management via vasopressors and fluids
- Release surgical retraction, manipulation, or abdominal insufflation
- Ensure appropriate end-tidal CO_2 level of 28 to 32 mm Hg (3.7 to 4.3 kPa).
- Evaluate and correct acid-base status
- Check maternal hemoglobin
- Consider administration of uterine relaxation agents (e.g., nitroglycerin, terbutaline, increased concentration of volatile agent) if uterine hypertonus or tetany occurs

induced hypothermia, induced hypotension, and cardiopulmonary bypass have been reported.

The decision to perform simultaneous cesarean delivery with maternal surgery depends on several factors. Cesarean delivery may be performed immediately before the surgical procedure to either improve maternal physiologic parameters during the planned surgery or to avoid risks to a viable fetus associated with special patient positioning (e.g., the sitting or prone position), life-threatening airway pathologies, prolonged anesthesia, major intraoperative blood loss, maternal hyperventilation, deliberate hypotension, or cardiopulmonary bypass.

Prevention of Preterm Labor

Most epidemiologic studies of women who undergo nonobstetric surgery during pregnancy have reported a higher incidence of abortion, preterm labor, and preterm delivery. Whether the surgery, manipulation of the uterus, or the underlying condition is responsible is unclear. In a study of 778 women who underwent appendectomy during pregnancy, Mazze and Källén[161] found that 22% of women who underwent surgery between 24 and 36 weeks' gestation delivered in the week after surgery. In the women in whom pregnancy continued beyond 1 week after surgery, there was no further increase in the rate of preterm birth. Second-trimester procedures and operations that do not involve uterine manipulation carry the lowest risk for preterm labor.

Magnesium sulfate is commonly used in pregnancy as a tocolytic, anticonvulsant, or fetal neuroprotective agent. Antenatal magnesium sulfate has been shown to reduce the incidence and severity of cerebral palsy after very preterm birth (see Chapter 10).[162] Magnesium also has effects that are relevant to the delivery of anesthesia, including an increase in the rate of onset of neuromuscular blockade,[163] the reestablishment of neuromuscular blockade in patients recovering from a nondepolarizing muscle relaxant,[164] and a reduction in general anesthetic agent dose requirement.[165]

Although the volatile agents depress myometrial irritability and thus are theoretically advantageous for abdominal procedures, there is no evidence that any one anesthetic agent or technique positively or negatively influences the risk for preterm labor. Published data do not support the routine use of prophylactic tocolytic agents. Whether greater surveillance and early tocolytic therapy will reduce the risk for preterm delivery after surgery during pregnancy is not known. Monitoring for uterine contractions may be performed intraoperatively with an external tocodynamometer (if technically feasible) and for several days postoperatively, allowing tocolytic therapy to be instituted, if appropriate. Additional surveillance is necessary in patients who receive potent postoperative analgesics as they may be unaware of mild uterine contractions.

Emergency Abdominal Surgery

Acute abdominal disease occurs infrequently in pregnancy; the most common causes include appendicitis (1 in 500 to 1 in 2000 pregnancies), cholecystitis (1 in 1600 to 1 in 10,000 pregnancies), and bowel obstruction (1 in 1500 to 1 in 16,000 pregnancies).[166,167] Accurate diagnosis, especially of an acute abdominal crisis (e.g., appendicitis, cholecystitis), can be very difficult during pregnancy, and several conditions must be considered in the differential diagnosis (Table 18.4).[168] Nausea, vomiting, constipation, and abdominal distention are common symptoms of both normal pregnancy and acute abdominal disease. Abdominal tenderness may be indistinguishable from ligamentous or uterine contraction pain. The expanding uterus makes the physical examination of the abdomen difficult. Because the white blood cell count in normal pregnancy may reach $15,000/mm^3$ ($15 \times 10^9/L$), it must be markedly elevated to be diagnostically helpful. Additional delay may result from the reluctance to perform imaging studies involving radiation or contrast medium. However, using data from the NSQIP from 2005 to 2009, Silvestri et al.[169] found no difference in 30-day postoperative morbidity or mortality in 857 pregnant and 20,029 nonpregnant appendectomy cases and

TABLE 18.4	Nonobstetric Abdominal Crises in Pregnancy	
Medical Conditions	**Gynecologic Surgical Conditions**	**Nongynecologic Surgical Conditions**

• Abdominal crises caused by systemic disease
  • Sickle cell disease
  • Diabetic ketoacidosis
  • Porphyria
• Renal disease
  • Glomerulonephritis
  • Pyelonephritis
• Pulmonary disease
  • Basal pneumonia with pleurisy
• Cholecystitis and pancreatitis (early, uncomplicated)
• Myocardial infarction, pericarditis
• Substance use disorder (withdrawal symptoms)
	• Ovarian cyst/tumor
	  • Rupture
	  • Torsion
	  • Hemorrhage
	  • Infection
	• Torsion of a fallopian tube
	• Tubo-ovarian abscess
	• Uterine myoma
	  • Degeneration
	  • Infection
	• Ovarian torsion
		• Acute appendicitis
		• Acute cholecystitis and its complications
		• Acute pancreatitis and its complications
		• Intestinal obstruction
		• Trauma with visceral injury or hemorrhage
		• Vascular accidents (e.g., ruptured abdominal aneurysm)
		• Peptic ulcer

Modified from Fainstat T, Bhat N. Surgical resolution of nonobstetric abdominal crises complicating pregnancy. In: Baden JM, Brodsky JB, eds. *The Pregnant Surgical Patient*. Futura Publishing; 1985:154.

436 pregnant and 32,915 nonpregnant cholecystectomy cases. Moore et al.[3] used 2006 to 2011 data from the NSQIP to compare 2764 (0.5%) pregnant and 516,705 (99.5%) nonpregnant women undergoing general surgery. No difference in 30-day postoperative mortality or morbidity were noted between groups, but pregnant women tended to be younger, have fewer comorbidities than the general population, and were more likely to be undergoing emergency surgery. Similar findings in another NSQIP study of 2005 to 2012 data demonstrated that pregnant patients were more likely to have emergency surgery (52% versus 11%) and to be admitted as an inpatient (71% versus 54%) compared with their nonpregnant peers.[170] Although there is likely significant overlap in the data from these NSQIP studies, they indicated a 6% overall incidence of 30-day major postoperative complications that did not vary by pregnancy status.[169,170] Although it is reassuring that the risk to the mother is comparable to that in nonpregnant women undergoing similar surgical procedures, the severity of disease significantly affects fetal outcomes in pregnant women with acute abdominal disease.[122]

Laparoscopy

Laparoscopy is performed during pregnancy for both diagnostic and therapeutic indications with increasing frequency.[171-174] Concerns exist about the effects of laparoscopy on fetal well-being, especially the risks for (1) uterine or fetal trauma, (2) fetal acidosis from absorbed carbon dioxide, and (3) decreased maternal cardiac output and uteroplacental perfusion resulting from an iatrogenic increase in intraabdominal pressure. In some animal studies, maternal and fetal acidosis and tachycardia have occurred during intraabdominal insufflation, perhaps because maternal ventilation was guided by measurements of end-tidal rather than arterial carbon dioxide levels.[175] Uteroplacental perfusion decreased by 61% in one study in which gravid ewes were subjected to CO_2 pneumoperitoneum at a pressure of 20 mm Hg (although there were no adverse fetal consequences).[176] It is unclear whether the severity of acidosis and decrement in uteroplacental perfusion are related to insufflation pressure.[175]

Many practitioners believe, however, that the potential benefits of laparoscopic surgery compared with open abdominal surgery outweigh the risks. Potential benefits include (1) shorter hospitalization; (2) less postoperative pain; (3) decreased risk for thromboembolic and wound complications; and (4) faster return to normal activities, including earlier return of normal gastrointestinal function, less uterine irritability, and less fetal depression.[171] In a survey of laparoscopic surgeons, Reedy et al.[172] obtained data from 413 laparoscopic procedures performed during pregnancy and reviewed an additional 55 previously published cases. Among the procedures surveyed, 48% were cholecystectomies, 28% were adnexal operations, 16% were appendectomies, and 8% were diagnostic procedures. Thirty-two percent of operations were performed in the first trimester, 54% in the second, and 13% in the third. Several principally retrospective trials comparing open and laparoscopic interventions reported no maternal and fetal outcome differences.[173,174]

Human clinical studies and experience suggest that the fetal effects of the CO_2 pneumoperitoneum and increased intraabdominal pressure are limited. In one clinical study, there were no differences in the maternal pH, $PaCO_2$, or arterial–to–end-tidal CO_2 pressure gradients before, during, or after termination of the pneumoperitoneum during laparoscopy.[177] Steinbrook and Bhavani-Shankar[178] used thoracic electrical bioimpedance cardiography to measure changes in cardiac output in four pregnant women undergoing laparoscopic cholecystectomy. They observed hemodynamic changes similar to those that typically occur during laparoscopic surgery in nonpregnant patients (i.e., decrease in cardiac index with concurrent increases in mean arterial pressure and systemic vascular resistance). Reported clinical experiences with laparoscopy during pregnancy generally have been favorable with the rare occurrence of complications, such as intraoperative perforation of the uterus with the Veress needle.[172] Nonetheless, Amos et al.,[179] in a case series, reported fetal deaths following four of seven laparoscopic procedures. Some practitioners have suggested the use of gasless laparoscopic techniques to avoid the potential fetal effects of CO_2 pneumoperitoneum.[180,181]

Careful selection and conduct of surgical and anesthetic techniques can assist in avoiding complications associated with laparoscopic surgery during pregnancy. The surgeon should be experienced with the technique, and the anesthesia provider must be aware of the accompanying physiologic alterations, including the cardiorespiratory implications. The Society of American Gastrointestinal and Endoscopic Surgeons has published guidelines for the management of pregnant women undergoing laparoscopic procedures.[182] Selected recommendations that have strong evidence are depicted in Fig. 18.5. The guidelines emphasize that the indications for laparoscopic surgery in pregnant patients do not differ from those for nonpregnant patients and may be performed during any trimester of pregnancy. Recent European guidelines for the treatment of appendicitis during pregnancy have formally endorsed low-pressure pneumoperitoneum laparoscopy during pregnancy.[183]

Ultrasound for initial imaging

Limit imaging to 50–100 mGy

Laparoscopy safe in pregnancy

Carbon dioxide monitoring

Left uterine displacement during surgery

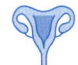
No prophylactic tocolysis unless already in preterm labor

Fig. 18.5 Selected recommendations for the use of laparoscopy during pregnancy from the Society of American Gastrointestinal and Endoscopic Surgeons. From Pearl JP, Price RR, Tonkin AE, et al. *Guidelines for the Use of Laparoscopy During Pregnancy.* 2017. https://www.sages.org/publications/guidelines/guidelines-for-diagnosis-treatment-and-use-of-laparoscopy-for-surgical-problems-during-pregnancy/. Accessed 28 August 2024.

General anesthesia is used in most laparoscopic procedures, although the use of epidural anesthesia has also been described.[172] The Trendelenburg position exacerbates decreases in FRC and increases in hypoxemia from airway closure. Hyperventilation, which may be necessary to maintain normal maternal $PaCO_2$, may reduce uteroplacental perfusion and affect fetal oxygenation. Hypotension may result from pneumoperitoneum, aortocaval compression, or use of the reverse Trendelenburg position, and a vasopressor may be needed to maintain maternal blood pressure.[184] As with open surgery, fetal well-being is best preserved by maintaining maternal oxygenation, acid-base status, and hemodynamic parameters within normal pregnancy limits. The FHR and uterine tone should be monitored before and after surgery (see discussion above).

Electroconvulsive Therapy

Serious psychiatric conditions occurring during pregnancy are associated with significant risks, including mortality (see Chapter 49).[185,186] For several of these conditions, electroconvulsive therapy (ECT) is a recommended therapeutic option. In pregnancy, ECT can be beneficial since it allows the avoidance of prolonged medication use (such as benzodiazepines and antidepressants); however, ECT has been associated with cases of placental abruption, vaginal bleeding, preterm labor, and FHR changes.[186] In 2018 recommendations for the use of ECT in pregnancy were published following an extensive literature review.[185] ECT appears safe during pregnancy but must be balanced against the potential risks of uterine contractions and preterm labor. There is no evidence of an association of ECT with congenital anomalies, either morphologic or behavioral, or later neurocognitive disturbances.

Anesthetic Management

Enhanced Recovery After Surgery

ERAS protocols are evidence-based practices in the perioperative period used worldwide that have demonstrated improved surgical outcomes while reducing complications and length of hospital stay.[187] Many institutions have implemented these protocols for pregnant patients undergoing obstetric and nonobstetric surgery.[188] However, anesthesia providers should reconsider or omit certain components, such as **nonsteroidal antiinflammatory drugs (NSAIDs)**, to avoid potentially harmful fetal exposure. The use of drugs with known and proven fetal safety is optimal.

Preoperative Management

Nonobstetric surgery in the pregnant patient should be performed in an institution where appropriate multidisciplinary personnel and care are readily available.[189] Appropriate blood management strategies should be considered.

Anemia in pregnancy occurs in approximately 21.6 per 1000 women in the United States.[190] When due to iron deficiency, anemia can be treated with IV administration of iron, which increases hemoglobin levels more rapidly (2 weeks) than with oral (>6 weeks) therapy.[191,192]

The Joint Opinion of ACOG and the ASA recommendations should be included in preoperative considerations[130] (see Fig. 18.4). An obstetric consultation, often with a maternal-fetal medicine specialist, will allow the patient to consider the risks/benefits of surgery, appreciate the signs/symptoms of preterm labor, and understand the fetal monitoring required. The preoperative history and physical examination should include a pregnancy history and assessment of gestational age. The anesthesia informed consent should include discussion of the risks and benefits of maternal and fetal anesthetic exposure. Pregnant women are at increased risk for acid aspiration after 18 to 20 weeks' gestation (see discussion above). Pharmacologic precautions against acid aspiration may include the preanesthetic administration of a **histamine H_2-receptor antagonist**, **metoclopramide**, and a clear nonparticulate antacid such as **sodium citrate**. Considerations for multimodal analgesia should include **acetaminophen (paracetamol)** and **regional anesthetic blockade**, if appropriate, but other medications such as **gabapentinoids** should likely be omitted given their minimal or unproven universal benefit.[193]

FHR monitoring is typically performed prior to and following the surgical procedure. Intraoperative FHR monitoring may be considered when technically feasible, depending on the ease of monitoring, the type and site of surgery, and gestational age (see discussion above).

Intraoperative Management

Choice of Anesthetic Technique. Maternal indications and consideration of the site and nature of the surgery should guide the choice of anesthesia. No study has found an association between improved fetal outcome and any specific anesthetic technique, except for a single retrospective medical record analysis in which the use of general anesthesia was associated with significantly lower birth weight despite similar gestational age at delivery.[194] However, when possible, local, regional (with the exception of paracervical block), or neuraxial anesthesia are preferred, in order to limit systemic drug exposure and minimize airway and respiratory complications. Appropriate measures should be used to minimize intraoperative hypotension, and anesthesia providers should be vigilant to the signs of high neuraxial blockade and LAST.

Prevention of Aortocaval Compression. Beginning at 18 to 20 weeks' gestation, the pregnant patient should be transported and positioned on her side, with the uterus displaced leftward, to minimize aortocaval compression.

Monitoring. Maternal monitoring should include noninvasive or invasive blood pressure measurement, electrocardiography, pulse oximetry, capnography, temperature monitoring, and a peripheral nerve stimulator. Because of the potential for altered sensitivity to and metabolism of anesthetic agents, there may be a higher risk of awareness, so use of a depth of anesthesia monitor is prudent. Avoidance of hypoxemia, hypotension, acidosis, and hyperventilation are critical; however, hyperventilation should be avoided. End-tidal CO_2 should be maintained in the normal range of 28 to 32 mm Hg (3.7 to 4.3 kPa) for pregnancy.

General Anesthesia Technique. A commonly used general anesthetic technique employs denitrogenation (preoxygenation), an opioid, rapid-sequence induction with a fast-acting induction agent (e.g., propofol) and muscle relaxant, and a moderate concentration of a volatile halogenated agent. Drugs with a history of safe use during pregnancy include thiopental, propofol, morphine, fentanyl, succinylcholine, and the nondepolarizing muscle relaxants. Scientific evidence does not support the avoidance of nitrous oxide during pregnancy, particularly after the sixth gestational week.[195]

Although rapid-sequence induction with the application of cricoid pressure has been a long-standing practice for the induction of general anesthesia, some experts have suggested that it is unnecessary in fasted pregnant women undergoing elective surgery and may make tracheal intubation more challenging (see Chapter 29).[196] It has been commonly accepted that general anesthesia mandates tracheal intubation from 18 to 20 weeks' gestation or if the stomach is full. However, two retrospective studies (combined *n* = 3700) reported the use of supraglottic airway devices with esophageal drains in pregnant women undergoing elective cesarean delivery with no reported cases of aspiration.[197,198] Women in these studies followed fasting guidelines and had normal body mass index, and the airway devices were placed using aspiration precautions (i.e., preoperative antacid administration, cricoid pressure, and rapid-sequence induction). Although these studies do not definitively demonstrate safety, these devices may be an alternative airway management technique for women for whom avoidance of tracheal intubation or neuromuscular paralysis is desirable (e.g., professional singer, patient with myotonic dystrophy). A systematic review of gastric ultrasonography in pregnant women indicated its reliability in assessing gastric volume, but an inability to predict aspiration risk or need for rapid-sequence induction.[199]

Postoperative Management

The FHR and uterine activity should be monitored during recovery from anesthesia. Adequate analgesia should be ensured with systemic or neuraxial opioids, acetaminophen, or neural blockade. NSAIDs should be avoided in pregnancy, especially in the first and third trimesters. Maternal safety organizations recommend mechanical compression devices for thromboembolism prophylaxis in all women undergoing cesarean delivery and pharmacologic prophylaxis in women with additional risk factors, including obesity, thrombophilia, prolonged immobility, and any condition that may increase the risk for venous thromboembolism.[19,20] Many of the principles recommended in these guidelines should be applied to pregnant patients undergoing nonobstetric surgery.

Maternal Cardiac Arrest and Resuscitation

Although standard **Basic Life Support** and **Advanced Cardiac Life Support** principles should apply, the anatomic and physiologic changes of pregnancy, and the presence of a fetus, require several specific modifications to resuscitation protocols (see Chapter 41 and Box 41.18). The neonatal resuscitation team should be part of the maternal cardiac arrest team, as the fetus will likely need immediate resuscitation upon delivery. The reversible causes of cardiac arrest during pregnancy are similar to those in nonpregnant patients; however, additional causes specific to pregnancy include amniotic fluid embolism, eclampsia, placental abruption, and hemorrhage.

KEY POINTS

- A significant number of women undergo anesthesia and surgery during pregnancy for procedures unrelated to delivery. Necessary maternal surgical intervention should not be delayed for fetal considerations.
- Maternal risks are associated with the anatomic and physiologic changes of pregnancy (e.g., difficult intubation, aspiration) and with the underlying maternal disease.
- Fetal risks associated with surgery include fetal death, preterm labor, growth restriction, and low birth weight. Fetal risks may be further altered by the anesthetic, the operation, or the underlying maternal disease.
- Clinical studies suggest that anesthesia and surgery during pregnancy do not increase the risk for congenital anomalies or neurodevelopmental compromise.
- No anesthetic agent is a proven teratogen in humans, although some anesthetic agents, specifically nitrous oxide, are teratogenic in animals under certain conditions.

- The use of fetal heart rate monitoring in the perioperative period requires a multidisciplinary discussion with the patient, obstetric provider, surgeon, anesthesia provider, and possibly the neonatologist.
- The anesthetic management of the pregnant surgical patient should focus on the avoidance of hypoxemia, hypotension, acidosis, and hyperventilation, and should include clinical monitors appropriate for the anesthetic and surgical interventions.
- Enhanced recovery after surgery protocols should be followed to for nonobstetric surgery in pregnancy, but some protocol components will require modification to reduce fetal exposure to select medications.

REFERENCES

1. Devroe S, Bleeser T, Van de Velde M, et al. Anesthesia for non-obstetric surgery during pregnancy in a tertiary referral center: a 16-year retrospective, matched case-control, cohort study. *Int J Obstet Anesth.* 2019;39:74–81.
2. Balinskaite V, Bottle A, Sodhi V, et al. The risk of adverse pregnancy outcomes following nonobstetric surgery during pregnancy: estimates from a retrospective cohort study of 6.5 million pregnancies. *Ann Surg.* 2017;266:260–266.
3. Moore HB, Juarez-Colunga E, Bronsert M, et al. Effect of pregnancy on adverse outcomes after general surgery. *JAMA Surg.* 2015;150:637–643.
4. Osterman MJK, Hamilton BE, Martin JA, et al. Births: final data for 2021. *Natl Vital Stat Rep.* 2023;72:1–53.
5. Kasliwal A, Farquharson RG. Pregnancy testing prior to sterilisation. *BJOG.* 2000;107:1407–1409.
6. Iseyemi A, Zhao Q, McNicholas C, Peipert JF. Socioeconomic status as a risk factor for unintended pregnancy in the contraceptive CHOICE project. *Obstet Gynecol.* 2017;130:609–615.
7. Lamont T, Coates T, Mathew D, et al. Checking for pregnancy before surgery: summary of a safety report from the National Patient Safety Agency. *BMJ.* 2010;341:c3402.
8. American Society of Anesthesiologists. Statement on pregnancy testing prior to anesthesia and surgery. https://www.asahq.org/standards-and-practice-parameters/statement-on-pregnancy-testing-prior-to-anesthesia-and-surgery. Accessed 21 March 2024.
9. National Institute for Health and Clinical Excellence. Guideline No. 45: Routine preoperative tests for elective surgery. Available at https://www.nice.org.uk/guidance/ng45. Accessed 21 March 2024.
10. Global Burden of Disease 2015 Maternal Mortality Collaborators. Global, regional, and national levels of maternal mortality, 1990-2015: a systematic analysis for the Global Burden of Disease Study 2015. *Lancet.* 2016;388:1775–1812.
11. Knight M, Bunch K, Patel R, et al. *Saving Lives, Improving Mothers' Care Core Report – Lessons Learned to Inform Maternity Care From the UK and Ireland Confidential Enquiries Into Maternal Deaths and Morbidity 2018-20.* National Perinatal Epidemiology Unit, University of Oxford; 2022.
12. Geller SE, Rosenberg D, Cox SM, et al. The continuum of maternal morbidity and mortality: factors associated with severity. *Am J Obstet Gynecol.* 2004;191:939–944.
13. Erekson EA, Brousseau EC, Dick-Biascoechea MA, et al. Maternal postoperative complications after nonobstetric antenatal surgery. *J Matern Fetal Neonatal Med.* 2012;25:2639–2644.
14. Mushambi MC, Kinsella SM, Popat M, et al. Obstetric Anaesthetists' Association and Difficult Airway Society guidelines for the management of difficult and failed tracheal intubation in obstetrics. *Anaesthesia.* 2015;70:1286–1306.
15. Kinsella SM, Lohmann G. Supine hypotensive syndrome. *Obstet Gynecol.* 1994;83:774–788.
16. Rossi A, Cornette J, Johnson MR, et al. Quantitative cardiovascular magnetic resonance in pregnant women: cross-sectional analysis of physiological parameters throughout pregnancy and the impact of the supine position. *J Cardiovasc Magn Reson.* 2011;13:31.
17. Higuchi H, Takagi S, Zhang K, et al. Effect of lateral tilt angle on the volume of the abdominal aorta and inferior vena cava in pregnant and nonpregnant women determined by magnetic resonance imaging. *Anesthesiology.* 2015;122:286–293.
18. American College of Obstetricians and Gynecologists. Practice Bulletin No. 233: Anemia in pregnancy (reaffirmed 2024). *Obstet Gynecol.* 2021;138:e55–e64.
19. D'Alton ME, Friedman AM, Smiley RM, et al. National Partnership for Maternal Safety: consensus bundle on venous thromboembolism. *Anesth Analg.* 2016;123:942–949.
20. Royal College of Obstetricians and Gynaecologists. Green-top Guideline No. 37a. Reducing the risk of venous thromboembolism during pregnancy and the puerperium. Available at https://www.rcog.org.uk/globalassets/documents/guidelines/gtg-37a.pdf. Accessed 27 August 2024.
21. Macfie AG, Magides AD, Richmond MN, Reilly CS. Gastric emptying in pregnancy. *Br J Anaesth.* 1991;67:54–57.
22. Arzola C, Perlas A, Siddiqui NT, et al. Gastric ultrasound in the third trimester of pregnancy: a randomised controlled trial to develop a predictive model of volume assessment. *Anaesthesia.* 2018;73:295–303.
23. Brock-Utne JG, Dow TG, Dimopoulos GE, et al. Gastric and lower oesophageal sphincter (LOS) pressures in early pregnancy. *Br J Anaesth.* 1981;53:381–384.
24. Gin T, Chan MT. Decreased minimum alveolar concentration of isoflurane in pregnant humans. *Anesthesiology.* 1994;81:829–832.
25. Higuchi H, Adachi Y, Arimura S, et al. Early pregnancy does not reduce the C_{50} of propofol for loss of consciousness. *Anesth Analg.* 2001;93:1565–1569.
26. Mongardon N, Servin F, Perrin M, et al. Predicted propofol effect-site concentration for induction and emergence of anesthesia during early pregnancy. *Anesth Analg.* 2009;109:90–95.
27. Robins K, Lyons G. Intraoperative awareness during general anesthesia for cesarean delivery. *Anesth Analg.* 2009;109:886–890.
28. Pandit JJ, Andrade J, Bogod DG, et al. 5th National Audit Project (NAP5) on accidental awareness during general anaesthesia: summary of main findings and risk factors. *Br J Anaesth.* 2014;113:549–559.
29. Leighton BL, Cheek TG, Gross JB, et al. Succinylcholine pharmacodynamics in peripartum patients. *Anesthesiology.* 1986;64:202–205.
30. Tsen LC, Tarshis J, Denson DD, et al. Measurements of maternal protein binding of bupivacaine throughout pregnancy. *Anesth Analg.* 1999;89:965–968.
31. Ansari J, Carvalho B, Shafer SL, Flood P. Pharmacokinetics and pharmacodynamics of drugs commonly used in pregnancy and parturition. *Anesth Analg.* 2016;122:786–804.
32. Finster M. Pediatric and obstetrical anesthesia. In: Stanley TH, Schafer PG, eds. *Developments in Critical Care Medicine and Anesthesiology.* Springer; 1995.
33. Schafer C, Peters P, Miller R. *Drugs During Lactation and Pregnancy: Treatment Options and Risk Assessments.* 3rd ed. Elsevier; 2015.
34. Bleeser T, Van Der Veeken L, Fieuws S, et al. Effects of general anaesthesia during pregnancy on neurocognitive development of the fetus: a systematic review and meta-analysis. *Br J Anaesth.* 2021;126:1128–1140.
35. Roberts C, Lowe C. Where have all the conceptions gone? *Lancet.* 1975;305:498–499.

36. Ammon Avalos L, Galindo C, Li DK. A systematic review to calculate background miscarriage rates using life table analysis. *Birth Defects Res A Clin Mol Teratol.* 2012;94:417–423.

37. Wells PG, McCallum GP, Lam KC, et al. Oxidative DNA damage and repair in teratogenesis and neurodevelopmental deficits. *Birth Defects Res C Embryo Today.* 2010;90:103–109.

38. Ornoy A. Embryonic oxidative stress as a mechanism of teratogenesis with special emphasis on diabetic embryopathy. *Reprod Toxicol.* 2007;24:31–41.

39. Gabbay-Benziv R, Reece EA, Wang F, Yang P. Birth defects in pregestational diabetes: defect range, glycemic threshold and pathogenesis. *World J Diabetes.* 2015;6:481–488.

40. Julian CG. High altitude during pregnancy. *Clin Chest Med.* 2011;32:21–31.

41. O'Connor TG, Monk C, Fitelson EM. Practitioner review: maternal mood in pregnancy and child development – implications for child psychology and psychiatry. *J Child Psychol Psychiatry.* 2014;55:99–111.

42. Koen N, Brittain K, Donald KA, et al. Psychological trauma and posttraumatic stress disorder: risk factors and associations with birth outcomes in the Drakenstein Child Health Study. *Eur J Psychotraumatol.* 2016;7:28720.

43. Punamaki RL, Diab SY, Isosavi S, et al. Maternal pre- and postnatal mental health and infant development in war conditions: the Gaza Infant Study. *Psychol Trauma.* 2018;10:144–153.

44. Dreier JW, Andersen AM, Berg-Beckhoff G. Systematic review and meta-analyses: fever in pregnancy and health impacts in the offspring. *Pediatrics.* 2014;133:e674–e688.

45. Rimawi BH, Green V, Lindsay M. Fetal implications of diagnostic radiation exposure during pregnancy: evidence-based recommendations. *Clin Obstet Gynecol.* 2016;59:412–418.

46. Lowe SA. Diagnostic radiography in pregnancy: risks and reality. *Aust N Z J Obstet Gynaecol.* 2004;44:191–196.

47. Dauer LT, Thornton RH, Miller DL, et al. Radiation management for interventions using fluoroscopic or computed tomographic guidance during pregnancy: a joint guideline of the Society of Interventional Radiology and the Cardiovascular and Interventional Radiological Society of Europe with endorsement by the Canadian Interventional Radiology Association. *J Vasc Interv Radiol.* 2012;23:19–32.

48. American College of Obstetricians and Gynecologists. Committee Opinion No. 723: Guidelines for diagnostic imaging during pregnancy and lactation (reaffirmed 2021). *Obstet Gynecol.* 2017;130:e210–e216.

49. Fisher JE Jr, Acuff-Smith KD, Schilling MA, et al. Teratologic evaluation of rats prenatally exposed to pulsed-wave ultrasound. *Teratology.* 1994;49:150–155.

50. Vorhees CV, Acuff-Smith KD, Schilling MA, et al. Behavioral teratologic effects of prenatal exposure to continuous-wave ultrasound in unanesthetized rats. *Teratology.* 1994;50:238–249.

51. Hande MP, Devi PU. Teratogenic effects of repeated exposures to X-rays and/or ultrasound in mice. *Neurotoxicol Teratol.* 1995;17:179–188.

52. Miller MW, Nyborg WL, Dewey WC, et al. Hyperthermic teratogenicity, thermal dose and diagnostic ultrasound during pregnancy: implications of new standards on tissue heating. *Int J Hyperthermia.* 2002;18:361–384.

53. Khairinisa MA, Takatsuru Y, Amano I, et al. The effect of perinatal gadolinium-based contrast agents on adult mice behavior. *Invest Radiol.* 2018;53:110–118.

54. Ray JG, Vermeulen MJ, Bharatha A, et al. Association between MRI exposure during pregnancy and fetal and childhood outcomes. *JAMA.* 2016;316:952–961.

55. Gatta G, Di Grezia G, Cuccurullo V, et al. MRI in pregnancy and precision medicine: a review from literature. *J Pers Med.* 2022;12:9.

56. Kanal E, Barkovich AJ, Bell C, et al. ACR guidance document on MR safe practices: 2013. *J Magn Reson Imaging.* 2013;37:501–530.

57. Fujinaga M, Mazze RI. Teratogenic and postnatal developmental studies of morphine in Sprague-Dawley rats. *Teratology.* 1988;38:401–410.

58. Fujinaga M, Stevenson JB, Mazze RI. Reproductive and teratogenic effects of fentanyl in Sprague-Dawley rats. *Teratology.* 1986;34:51–57.

59. Fujinaga M, Mazze RI, Jackson EC, Baden JM. Reproductive and teratogenic effects of sufentanil and alfentanil in Sprague-Dawley rats. *Anesth Analg.* 1988;67:166–169.

60. Martin LV, Jurand A. The absence of teratogenic effects of some analgesics used in anaesthesia. Additional evidence from a mouse model. *Anaesthesia.* 1992;47:473–476.

61. Finnell RH, Shields HE, Taylor SM, Chernoff GF. Strain differences in phenobarbital-induced teratogenesis in mice. *Teratology.* 1987;35:177–185.

62. Tonge SR. Permanent alterations in catecholamine concentrations in discrete areas of brain in the offspring of rats treated with methylamphetamine and chlorpromazine. *Br J Pharmacol.* 1973;47:425–427.

63. Vutskits L, Davidson A. Update on developmental anesthesia neurotoxicity. *Curr Opin Anaesthesiol.* 2017;30:337–342.

64. Bleeser T, Brenders A, Hubble TR, et al. Preclinical evidence for anaesthesia-induced neurotoxicity. *Best Pract Res Clin Anaesthesiol.* 2023;37:16–27.

65. Xiong M, Zhang L, Li J, et al. Propofol-induced neurotoxicity in the fetal animal brain and developments in modifying these effects – an updated review of propofol fetal exposure in laboratory animal studies. *Brain Sci.* 2016;6:11.

66. van der Veeken L, Inversetti A, Galgano A, et al. Fetally-injected drugs for immobilization and analgesia do not modify fetal brain development in a rabbit model. *Prenat Diagn.* 2021;41:1164–1170.

67. Van der Veeken L, Emam D, Bleeser T, et al. Fetal surgery has no additional effect to general anesthesia on brain development in neonatal rabbits. *Am J Obstet Gynecol MFM.* 2022;4:100513.

68. Van der Veeken L, Van der Merwe J, Devroe S, et al. Maternal surgery during pregnancy has a transient adverse effect on the developing fetal rabbit brain. *Am J Obstet Gynecol.* 2019;221:355.e1–e19.

69. Bleeser T, Basurto D, Russo F, et al. Effects of cumulative duration of repeated anaesthesia exposure on foetal brain development in the ovine model. *J Clin Anesth.* 2023;85:111050.

70. Devroe S, Van der Veeken L, Bleeser T, et al. The effect of xenon on fetal neurodevelopment following maternal sevoflurane anesthesia and laparotomy in rabbits. *Neurotoxicol Teratol.* 2021;87:106994.

71. Bleeser T, Devroe S, Lucas N, et al. Neurodevelopmental outcomes after prenatal exposure to anaesthesia for maternal surgery: a propensity-score weighted bidirectional cohort study. *Anaesthesia.* 2023;78:159–169.

72. Shiono PH, Mills JL. Oral clefts and diazepam use during pregnancy. *N Engl J Med.* 1984;311:919–920.

73. Lind JN, Interrante JD, Ailes EC, et al. Maternal use of opioids during pregnancy and congenital malformations: a systematic review. *Pediatrics*. 2017;139:e20164131.

74. Patrick SW, Davis MM, Lehman CU, Cooper WO. Increasing incidence and geographic distribution of neonatal abstinence syndrome: United States 2009 to 2012. *J Perinatol*. 2015;35:667.

75. Baldacchino A, Arbuckle K, Petrie DJ, McCowan C. Neurobehavioral consequences of chronic intrauterine opioid exposure in infants and preschool children: a systematic review and meta-analysis. *BMC Psychiatry*. 2014;14:104.

76. Baldacchino A, Arbuckle K, Petrie DJ, McCowan C. Erratum: Neurobehavioral consequences of chronic intrauterine opioid exposure in infants and preschool children: a systematic review and meta-analysis. *BMC Psychiatry*. 2015;15:134.

77. Fujinaga M, Mazze RI. Reproductive and teratogenic effects of lidocaine in Sprague-Dawley rats. *Anesthesiology*. 1986;65:626–632.

78. Briggs GG, Freeman RK, Towers CV, Forinash AB. *Drugs in Pregnancy and Lactation: A Reference Guide to Fetal and Neonatal Risk*. 12th ed. Lippincott Williams & Wilkins; 2021.

79. Fujinaga M, Baden JM, Mazze RI. Developmental toxicity of nondepolarizing muscle relaxants in cultured rat embryos. *Anesthesiology*. 1992;76:999–1003.

80. Sugammadex package insert: Highlights of prescribing information. 2015. https://www.accessdata.fda.gov/drugsatfda_docs/label/2015/022225lbl.pdf. Accessed 27 August 2024.

81. Pühringer FK, Kristen P, Rex C. Sugammadex reversal of rocuronium-induced neuromuscular block in Caesarean section patients: a series of seven cases. *Br J Anaesth*. 2010;105:657–660.

82. Ad Hoc task force: Willett, Butwick, Togioka, et al. Statement on Sugammadex During Pregnancy and Lactation. Society of Obstetric Anesthesia and Perinatology; 2019. https://www.soap.org/assets/docs/SOAP_Statement_Sugammadex_During_Pregnancy_Lactation_APPROVED.pdf. Accessed 27 August 2024.

83. Gaston IN, Lange EMS, Farrer JR, Toledo P. Sugammadex use for reversal in nonobstetric surgery during pregnancy: a reexamination of the evidence. *Anesth Analg*. 2023;136:1217–1219.

84. Landauer W. Cholinomimetic teratogens: studies with chicken embryos. *Teratology*. 1975;12:125–145.

85. Wharton RS, Mazze RI, Baden JM, et al. Fertility, reproduction and postnatal survival in mice chronically exposed to halothane. *Anesthesiology*. 1978;48:167–174.

86. Mazze RI. Fertility, reproduction, and postnatal survival in mice chronically exposed to isoflurane. *Anesthesiology*. 1985;63:663–667.

87. Mazze RI, Wilson AI, Rice SA, Baden JM. Fetal development in mice exposed to isoflurane. *Teratology*. 1985;32:339–345.

88. Basford AB, Fink BR. The teratogenicity of halothane in the rat. *Anesthesiology*. 1968;29:1167–1173.

89. Mazze RI, Fujinaga M, Rice SA, et al. Reproductive and teratogenic effects of nitrous oxide, halothane, isoflurane, and enflurane in Sprague-Dawley rats. *Anesthesiology*. 1986;64:339–344.

90. Mazze RI, Wilson AI, Rice SA, Baden JM. Reproduction and fetal development in rats exposed to nitrous oxide. *Teratology*. 1984;30:259–265.

91. Lane GA, Nahrwold ML, Tait AR, et al. Anesthetics as teratogens: nitrous oxide is fetotoxic, xenon is not. *Science*. 1980;210:899–901.

92. Vieira E, Cleaton-Jones P, Austin JC, et al. Effects of low concentrations of nitrous oxide on rat fetuses. *Anesth Analg*. 1980;59:175–177.

93. Fujinaga M, Baden JM, Mazze RI. Susceptible period of nitrous oxide teratogenicity in Sprague-Dawley rats. *Teratology*. 1989;40:439–444.

94. Fujinaga M, Baden JM. Critical period of rat development when sidedness of asymmetric body structures is determined. *Teratology*. 1991;44:453–462.

95. Baden JM, Fujinaga M. Effects of nitrous oxide on day 9 rat embryos grown in culture. *Br J Anaesth*. 1991;66:500–503.

96. Chanarin I. Cobalamins and nitrous oxide: a review. *J Clin Pathol*. 1980;33:909–916.

97. Koblin DD, Watson JE, Deady JE, et al. Inactivation of methionine synthetase by nitrous oxide in mice. *Anesthesiology*. 1981;54:318–324.

98. Koblin DD, Waskell L, Watson JE, et al. Nitrous oxide inactivates methionine synthetase in human liver. *Anesth Analg*. 1982;61:75–78.

99. Fujinaga M, Maze M, Hoffman BB, Baden JM. Activation of alpha-1 adrenergic receptors modulates the control of left/right sidedness in rat embryos. *Dev Biol*. 1992;150:419–421.

100. Fujinaga M, Baden JM, Suto A, et al. Preventive effects of phenoxybenzamine on nitrous oxide-induced reproductive toxicity in Sprague-Dawley rats. *Teratology*. 1991;43:151–157.

101. Jevtovic-Todorovic V, Hartman RE, Izumi Y, et al. Early exposure to common anesthetic agents causes widespread neurodegeneration in the developing rat brain and persistent learning deficits. *J Neurosci*. 2003;23:876–882.

102. Buring JE, Hennekens CH, Mayrent SL, et al. Health experiences of operating room personnel. *Anesthesiology*. 1985;62:325–330.

103. Tannenbaum TN, Goldberg RJ. Exposure to anesthetic gases and reproductive outcome. A review of the epidemiologic literature. *J Occup Med*. 1985;27:659–668.

104. Mazze RI, Lecky JH. The health of operating room personnel. *Anesthesiology*. 1985;62:226–228.

105. Ericson HA, Källén AJ. Hospitalization for miscarriage and delivery outcome among Swedish nurses working in operating rooms 1973-1978. *Anesth Analg*. 1985;64:981–988.

106. Spence AA. Environmental pollution by inhalation anaesthetics. *Br J Anaesth*. 1987;59:96–103.

107. Dimich-Ward H, Le Nhu D, Beking K, et al. Congenital anomalies in the offspring of nurses: association with area of employment during pregnancy. *Int J Occup Environ Health*. 2011;17:195–201.

108. Lawson CC, Rocheleau CM, Whelan EA, et al. Occupational exposures among nurses and risk of spontaneous abortion. *Am J Obstet Gynecol*. 2012;206:327.e1–e8.

109. Harlap S, Shiono PH. Alcohol, smoking, and incidence of spontaneous abortions in the first and second trimester. *Lancet*. 1980;2:173–176.

110. Shirangi A, Fritschi L, Holman CD. Associations of unscavenged anesthetic gases and long working hours with preterm delivery in female veterinarians. *Obstet Gynecol*. 2009;113:1008–1017.

111. Cohen EN, Gift HC, Brown BW, et al. Occupational disease in dentistry and chronic exposure to trace anesthetic gases. *J Am Dent Assoc*. 1980;101:21–31.

112. Rowland AS, Baird DD, Weinberg CR, et al. Reduced fertility among women employed as dental assistants exposed to high levels of nitrous oxide. *N Engl J Med*. 1992;327:993–997.

113. Smith BE. Fetal prognosis after anesthesia during gestation. *Anesth Analg.* 1963;42:521–526.

114. Shnider SM, Webster GM. Maternal and fetal hazards of surgery during pregnancy. *Am J Obstet Gynecol.* 1965;92:891–900.

115. Duncan PG, Pope WD, Cohen MM, Greer N. Fetal risk of anesthesia and surgery during pregnancy. *Anesthesiology.* 1986;64:790–794.

116. Brodsky JB, Cohen EN, Brown BW Jr, et al. Surgery during pregnancy and fetal outcome. *Am J Obstet Gynecol.* 1980;138:1165–1167.

117. Mazze RI, Källén B. Reproductive outcome after anesthesia and operation during pregnancy: a registry study of 5405 cases. *Am J Obstet Gynecol.* 1989;161:1178–1185.

118. Sylvester GC, Khoury MJ, Lu X, Erickson JD. First-trimester anesthesia exposure and the risk of central nervous system defects: a population-based case-control study. *Am J Public Health.* 1994;84:1757–1760.

119. Crawford JS, Lewis M. Nitrous oxide in early human pregnancy. *Anaesthesia.* 1986;41:900–905.

120. Aldridge LM, Tunstall ME. Nitrous oxide and the fetus. A review and the results of a retrospective study of 175 cases of anaesthesia for insertion of Shirodkar suture. *Br J Anaesth.* 1986;58:1348–1356.

121. Fisher SC, Siag K, Howley MM, et al. Maternal surgery and anesthesia during pregnancy and risk of birth defects in the National Birth Defects Prevention Study, 1997-2011. *Birth Defects Res.* 2020;112:162–174.

122. Sachs A, Guglielminotti J, Miller R, et al. Risk factors and risk stratification for adverse obstetrical outcomes after appendectomy or cholecystectomy during pregnancy. *JAMA Surg.* 2017;152:436–441.

123. U.S. Food and Drug Administration. FDA Drug Safety Communication: FDA review results in new warnings about using general anesthetics and sedation drugs in young children and pregnant women. Available at https://www.fda.gov/Drugs/DrugSafety/ucm532356.htm. Accessed 27 August 2024.

124. Sun LS, Li G, Miller TL, et al. Association between a single general anesthesia exposure before age 36 months and neurocognitive outcomes in later childhood. *JAMA.* 2016;315:2312–2320.

125. Davidson AJ, Disma N, de Graaff JC, et al. Neurodevelopmental outcome at 2 years of age after general anaesthesia and awake-regional anaesthesia in infancy (GAS): an international multicentre, randomised controlled trial. *Lancet.* 2016;387:239–250.

126. McCann ME, de Graaff JC, Dorris L, et al. Neurodevelopmental outcome at 5 years of age after general anaesthesia or awake-regional anaesthesia in infancy (GAS): an international, multicentre, randomised, controlled equivalence trial. *Lancet.* 2019;393:664–677.

127. Bhutta AT, Anand KJ. Vulnerability of the developing brain. Neuronal mechanisms. *Clin Perinatol.* 2002;29:357–372.

128. Ruda MA, Ling QD, Hohmann AG, et al. Altered nociceptive neuronal circuits after neonatal peripheral inflammation. *Science.* 2000;289:628–631.

129. Biehl DR. Foetal monitoring during surgery unrelated to pregnancy. *Can Anaesth Soc J.* 1985;32:455–459.

130. American College of Obstetricians and Gynecologists. Committee Opinion No. 775: Nonobstetric surgery during pregnancy (reaffirmed 2021). *Obstet Gynecol.* 2019;133:e285–e286.

131. Kilpatrick CC, Puig C, Chohan L, et al. Intraoperative fetal heart rate monitoring during nonobstetric surgery in pregnancy: a practice survey. *South Med J.* 2010;103:212–215.

132. Panigel M. Placental perfusion experiments. *Am J Obstet Gynecol.* 1962;84:1664–1683.

133. Khazin AF, Hon EH, Hehre FW. Effects of maternal hyperoxia on the fetus. I. Oxygen tension. *Am J Obstet Gynecol.* 1971;109:628–637.

134. McClaine RJ, Uemura K, de la Fuente SG, et al. General anesthesia improves fetal cerebral oxygenation without evidence of subsequent neuronal injury. *J Cereb Blood Flow Metab.* 2005;25:1060–1069.

135. Motoyama EK, Rivard G, Acheson F, Cook CD. The effect of changes in maternal pH and P-CO$_2$ on the P-O$_2$ of fetal lambs. *Anesthesiology.* 1967;28:891–903.

136. Kambam JR, Handte RE, Brown WU, Smith BE. Effect of normal and preeclamptic pregnancies on the oxyhemoglobin dissociation curve. *Anesthesiology.* 1986;65:426–427.

137. Levinson G, Shnider SM, DeLorimier AA, Steffenson JL. Effects of maternal hyperventilation on uterine blood flow and fetal oxygenation and acid-base status. *Anesthesiology.* 1974;40:340–347.

138. Brann AW Jr, Myers RE. Central nervous system findings in the newborn monkey following severe in utero partial asphyxia. *Neurology.* 1975;25:327–338.

139. Newman B, Lam AM. Induced hypotension for clipping of a cerebral aneurysm during pregnancy: a case report and brief review. *Anesth Analg.* 1986;65:675–678.

140. Shnider SM, Wright RG, Levinson G, et al. Uterine blood flow and plasma norepinephrine changes during maternal stress in the pregnant ewe. *Anesthesiology.* 1979;50:524–527.

141. Oats JN, Vasey DP, Waldron BA. Effects of ketamine on the pregnant uterus. *Br J Anaesth.* 1979;51:1163–1166.

142. Greiss FC Jr, Still JG, Anderson SG. Effects of local anesthetic agents on the uterine vasculatures and myometrium. *Am J Obstet Gynecol.* 1976;124:889–899.

143. Habib AS. A review of the impact of phenylephrine administration on maternal hemodynamics and maternal and neonatal outcomes in women undergoing cesarean delivery under spinal anesthesia. *Anesth Analg.* 2012;114:377–390.

144. Guo R, Xue Q, Qian Y, et al. The effects of ephedrine and phenylephrine on placental vascular resistance during cesarean section under epidural anesthesia. *Cell Biochem Biophys.* 2015;73:687–693.

145. Lee A, Ngan Kee WD, Gin T. A quantitative, systematic review of randomized controlled trials of ephedrine versus phenylephrine for the management of hypotension during spinal anesthesia for cesarean delivery. *Anesth Analg.* 2002;94:920–926.

146. Ngan Kee WD, Khaw KS, Tan PE, et al. Placental transfer and fetal metabolic effects of phenylephrine and ephedrine during spinal anesthesia for cesarean delivery. *Anesthesiology.* 2009;111:506–512.

147. Ngan Kee WD, Lee SW, Ng FF, et al. Randomized double-blinded comparison of norepinephrine and phenylephrine for maintenance of blood pressure during spinal anesthesia for cesarean delivery. *Anesthesiology.* 2015;122:736–745.

148. Liu P, He H, Zhang SS, et al. Comparative efficacy and safety of prophylactic norepinephrine and phenylephrine in spinal anesthesia for cesarean section: a systematic review and meta-analysis with trial sequential analysis. *Front Pharmacol.* 2022;13:1015325.

149. Palahniuk RJ, Shnider SM. Maternal and fetal cardiovascular and acid-base changes during halothane and isoflurane anesthesia in the pregnant ewe. *Anesthesiology*. 1974;41:462–472.

150. Palahniuk RJ, Doig GA, Johnson GN, Pash MP. Maternal halothane anesthesis reduces cerebral blood flow in the acidotic sheep fetus. *Anesth Analg*. 1980;59:35–39.

151. Baker BW, Hughes SC, Shnider SM, et al. Maternal anesthesia and the stressed fetus: effects of isoflurane on the asphyxiated fetal lamb. *Anesthesiology*. 1990;72:65–70.

152. Cheek DB, Hughes SC, Dailey PA, et al. Effect of halothane on regional cerebral blood flow and cerebral metabolic oxygen consumption in the fetal lamb in utero. *Anesthesiology*. 1987;67:361–366.

153. Bleeser T, Van Der Veeken L, Basurto D, et al. Neurodevelopmetal effects of maternal blood pressure management with noradrenaline during general anaesthesia for nonobstetric surgery in the pregnant rabbit model. *Eur J Anaesthesiol*. 2022;39:511–520.

154. Johnson ES, Colley PS. Effects of nitrous oxide and fentanyl anesthesia on fetal heart-rate variability intra- and postoperatively. *Anesthesiology*. 1980;52:429–430.

155. Liu PL, Warren TM, Ostheimer GW, et al. Foetal monitoring in parturients undergoing surgery unrelated to pregnancy. *Can Anaesth Soc J*. 1985;32:525–532.

156. Heesen M, Klöhr S, Hofmann T, et al. Maternal and foetal effects of remifentanil for general anaesthesia in parturients undergoing caesarean section: a systematic review and meta-analysis. *Acta Anaesthesiol Scand*. 2013;57:29–36.

157. McNall PG, Jafarnia MR. Management of myasthenia gravis in the obstetrical patient. *Am J Obstet Gynecol*. 1965;92:518–525.

158. Hellman LM, Johnson HL, Tolles WE, Jones EH. Some factors affecting the fetal heart rate. *Am J Obstet Gynecol*. 1961;82:1055–1063.

159. Abboud T, Raya J, Sadri S, et al. Fetal and maternal cardiovascular effects of atropine and glycopyrrolate. *Anesth Analg*. 1983;62:426–430.

160. Clark RB, Brown MA, Lattin DL. Neostigmine, atropine, and glycopyrrolate: does neostigmine cross the placenta? *Anesthesiology*. 1996;84:450–452.

161. Mazze RI, Källén B. Appendectomy during pregnancy: a Swedish registry study of 778 cases. *Obstet Gynecol*. 1991;77:835–840.

162. Doyle LW. Antenatal magnesium sulfate and neuroprotection. *Curr Opin Pediatr*. 2012;24:154–159.

163. Kim MH, Oh AY, Jeon YT, et al. A randomised controlled trial comparing rocuronium priming, magnesium pre-treatment and a combination of the two methods. *Anaesthesia*. 2012;67:748–754.

164. Hans GA, Bosenge B, Bonhomme VL, et al. Intravenous magnesium re-establishes neuromuscular block after spontaneous recovery from an intubating dose of rocuronium: a randomised controlled trial. *Eur J Anaesthesiol*. 2012;29:95–99.

165. Olgun B, Oğuz G, Kaya M, et al. The effects of magnesium sulphate on desflurane requirement, early recovery and postoperative analgesia in laparascopic cholecystectomy. *Magnes Res*. 2012;25:72–78.

166. Bouyou J, Gaujoux S, Marcellin L, et al. Abdominal emergencies during pregnancy. *J Visc Surg*. 2015;152:S105–S115.

167. Coleman MT, Trianfo VA, Rund DA. Nonobstetric emergencies in pregnancy: trauma and surgical conditions. *Am J Obstet Gynecol*. 1997;177:497–502.

168. Cherry SH. The pregnant patient: need for surgery unrelated to pregnancy. *Mt Sinai J Med*. 1991;58:81–84.

169. Silvestri MT, Pettker CM, Brousseau EC, et al. Morbidity of appendectomy and cholecystectomy in pregnant and nonpregnant women. *Obstet Gynecol*. 2011;118:1261–1270.

170. Abdelwahab M, Lynch CD, Schneider P, et al. Postoperative complications after non-obstetric surgery among pregnant patients in the National Surgical Quality Improvement Program, 2005-2012. *Am J Surg*. 2022;223:364–369.

171. Fatum M, Rojansky N. Laparoscopic surgery during pregnancy. *Obstet Gynecol Surv*. 2001;56:50–59.

172. Reedy MB, Galan HL, Richards WE, et al. Laparoscopy during pregnancy. A survey of laparoendoscopic surgeons. *J Reprod Med*. 1997;42:33–38.

173. Buser KB. Laparoscopic surgery in the pregnant patient: results and recommendations. *JSLS*. 2009;13:32–35.

174. Corneille MG, Gallup TM, Bening T, et al. The use of laparoscopic surgery in pregnancy: evaluation of safety and efficacy. *Am J Surg*. 2010;200:363–367.

175. Cruz AM, Southerland LC, Duke T, et al. Intraabdominal carbon dioxide insufflation in the pregnant ewe. Uterine blood flow, intraamniotic pressure, and cardiopulmonary effects. *Anesthesiology*. 1996;85:1395–1402.

176. Barnard JM, Chaffin D, Droste S, et al. Fetal response to carbon dioxide pneumoperitoneum in the pregnant ewe. *Obstet Gynecol*. 1995;85:669–674.

177. Bhavani-Shankar K, Steinbrook RA, Brooks DC, Datta S. Arterial to end-tidal carbon dioxide pressure difference during laparoscopic surgery in pregnancy. *Anesthesiology*. 2000;93:370–373.

178. Steinbrook RA, Bhavani-Shankar K. Hemodynamics during laparoscopic surgery in pregnancy. *Anesth Analg*. 2001;93:1570–1571.

179. Amos JD, Schorr SJ, Norman PF, et al. Laparoscopic surgery during pregnancy. *Am J Surg*. 1996;171:435–437.

180. Tanaka H, Futamura N, Takubo S, Toyoda N. Gasless laparoscopy under epidural anesthesia for adnexal cysts during pregnancy. *J Reprod Med*. 1999;44:929–932.

181. Melgrati L, Damiani A, Franzoni G, et al. Isobaric (gasless) laparoscopic myomectomy during pregnancy. *J Minim Invasive Gynecol*. 2005;12:379–381.

182. Pearl J.P., Price R.R., Tonkin A.E., et al. Guidelines for the Use of Laparoscopy During Pregnancy. 2017. https://www.sages.org/publications/guidelines/guidelines-for-diagnosis-treatment-and-use-of-laparoscopy-for-surgical-problems-during-pregnancy/. Accessed 27 August 2024.

183. Adamina M, Andreou A, Arezzo A, et al. EAES rapid guideline: systematic review, meta-analysis, GRADE assessment, and evidence-informed European recommendations on appendicitis in pregnancy. *Surg Endosc*. 2022;36:8699–8712.

184. Steinbrook RA, Brooks DC, Datta S. Laparoscopic cholecystectomy during pregnancy. Review of anesthetic management, surgical considerations. *Surg Endosc*. 1996;10:511–515.

185. Ward HB, Fromson JA, Cooper JJ, et al. Recommendations for the use of ECT in pregnancy: literature review and proposed clinical protocol. *Arch Womens Ment Health*. 2018;21:715–722.

186. Sinha P, Goyal P, Andrade C. A meta-review of the safety of electroconvulsive therapy in pregnancy. *J ECT*. 2017;33:81–88.

187. ERAS Society Guidelines. https://erassociety.org/guidelines/. Accessed 27 August 2024.

188. Bollag L, Lim G, Sultan P, et al. Society for Obstetric Anesthesia and Perinatology: consensus statement and recommendations for enhanced recovery after cesarean. *Anesth Analg.* 2021;132:1362–1377.

189. American College of Obstetricians and Gynecologists and American Society of Anesthesiologists. ACOG Committee Opinion No. 696: Nonobstetric surgery during pregnancy (interim update). *Obstet Gynecol.* 2017;129:777–778.

190. Adebisi OY, Strayhorn G. Anemia in pregnancy and race in the United States: blacks at risk. *Fam Med.* 2005;37:655–662.

191. Lewkowitz AK, Gupta A, Simon L, et al. Intravenous compared with oral iron for the treatment of iron-deficiency anemia in pregnancy: a systematic review and meta-analysis. *J Perinatol.* 2019;39:519–532.

192. Sultan P, Bampoe S, Shah R, et al. Oral vs intravenous iron therapy for postpartum anemia: a systematic review and meta-analysis. *Am J Obstet Gynecol.* 2019;221:19–29.e13.

193. Verret M, Lauzier F, Zarychanski R, et al. Perioperative use of gabapentinoids for the management of postoperative acute pain: a systematic review and meta-analysis. *Anesthesiology.* 2020;133:265–279.

194. Jenkins TM, Mackey SF, Benzoni EM, et al. Non-obstetric surgery during gestation: risk factors for lower birthweight. *Aust N Z J Obstet Gynaecol.* 2003;43:27–31.

195. Sanders RD, Weimann J, Maze M. Biologic effects of nitrous oxide: a mechanistic and toxicologic review. *Anesthesiology.* 2008;109:707–722.

196. de Souza DG, Doar LH, Mehta SH, Tiouririne M. Aspiration prophylaxis and rapid sequence induction for elective cesarean delivery: time to reassess old dogma? *Anesth Analg.* 2010;110:1503–1505.

197. Halaseh BK, Sukkar ZF, Hassan LH, et al. The use of ProSeal laryngeal mask airway in caesarean section – experience in 3000 cases. *Anaesth Intensive Care.* 2010;38:1023–1028.

198. Yao WY, Li SY, Sng BL, et al. The LMA Supreme in 700 parturients undergoing cesarean delivery: an observational study. *Can J Anaesth.* 2012;59:648–654.

199. Howle R, Sultan P, Shah R, et al. Gastric point-of-care ultrasound (PoCUS) during pregnancy and the postpartum period: a systematic review. *Int J Obstet Anesth.* 2020;44:24–32.

PART VI

Labor and Vaginal Delivery

19

Obstetric Management of Labor and Vaginal Delivery

Akila Subramaniam, MD, MPH and Alan T.N. Tita, MD, PhD

THE PROCESS OF LABOR AND DELIVERY

Labor, which is also called *parturition*, is the process by which sufficiently frequent and strong uterine contractions cause thinning (i.e., effacement) and dilation of the cervix, thereby permitting passage of the fetus from the uterus through the birth canal.

Onset of Labor

Timing

Fewer than 10% of pregnancies end on the expected date of delivery (EDD), although most births occur within 7 days of the EDD. In the United States, approximately 10% of births occur preterm (before 37 weeks' gestation) (see Chapter 33), and approximately 5% to 7% of pregnancies remain undelivered at 42 weeks' gestation (*postterm*). These rates are lower for carefully dated pregnancies.

Mechanism

The cause of the onset of labor in women—either term or preterm—remains unknown. In other mammalian species, a decrease in serum progesterone concentration in association with an increase in estrogen concentration is followed by increases in prostaglandin production, the number of myometrial oxytocin receptors, and myometrial gap junction formation. In sheep, the fetus apparently triggers parturition through a surge in fetal cortisol production. In women, progesterone concentrations do not decline before the onset of labor, and no surge in fetal cortisol secretion occurs. The laboring human uterus does manifest increases in prostaglandin production, oxytocin receptors, and myometrial gap junction formation.[1,2] Preterm and postterm deliveries both constitute important obstetric problems. Better understanding of the mechanism of the onset of human labor may lead to new approaches to preventing the preterm and postterm onset of parturition.

Stages of Labor

By convention, labor is divided into three stages. The first (cervical) stage begins with the maternal perception of regular, painful uterine contractions with documented cervical change and ends with the complete dilation of the cervix. The first stage of labor is divided into latent and active phases (see later). Complete cervical dilation (10 cm) is necessary to allow movement of the term fetus from the uterus into the vagina. Preterm fetuses require less than 10 cm of cervical dilation. The second (pelvic) stage of labor begins with the complete dilation of the cervix and ends with the birth of the infant. The third (placental) stage begins with the birth of the infant and ends with the delivery of the placenta. Some authorities identify a fourth stage of labor, corresponding to the first postpartum hour, during which postpartum hemorrhage is most likely to occur.

Components of Labor and Delivery

The events that occur during labor and vaginal delivery can be thought of as belonging to the three components of the process: (1) the **powers** (uterine contractions and, in the second stage, the addition of voluntary maternal expulsive efforts); (2) the **passageway** (the bony pelvis and the soft tissues contained therein); and (3) the **passenger** (the fetus). The interaction of these three components determines the success or failure of the process.

The Powers

The uterus, which is a smooth muscle organ, contracts throughout gestation with variable frequency. In some women, the uterus remains relatively quiescent until the abrupt onset of labor. In others, the uterus contracts several times per hour for days without causing pain or even a clear perception of uterine contractions. The parturient verifies the onset of labor when she perceives regular, uncomfortable uterine contractions.

During labor, the frequency, duration, and intensity of uterine contractions increase. During the latent phase of the first stage of labor, the contractions may occur every 5 to 7 minutes, last 30 to 40 seconds, and develop intrauterine pressures (intensity) of 20 to 30 mm Hg above basal tone (10 to 15 mm Hg). In the active phase, contractions typically occur every 2 to 3 minutes, last 50 to 70 seconds, and are 40 to 60 mm Hg in intensity. This higher intensity reflects a more widespread propagation of the contractions, with the recruitment of more myometrial cells.

Retraction accompanies contraction as the myometrial cells shorten. The walls of the upper, contractile portion of the uterus thicken. Cervical dilation and effacement reflect the traction placed on the cervix by the contracting uterus. The passive lower uterine segment enlarges and becomes thinner as cervical tissue is pulled over the fetal presenting part by traction from the upper portion of the uterus. At the end of the first stage of labor, there is complete cervical dilation. If there is no mechanical obstruction, additional uterine contractions force the fetus to descend through the birth canal. When this occurs, the parturient often perceives an urge to defecate, reflecting pressure on the rectum. The parturient's expulsive efforts add to the force of uterine contractions to hasten descent and shorten the second stage of labor.

The Passageway

The fetus is ideally of a size and conformation that there is no mechanical mismatch with the bony pelvis. The type and size of the pelvis constitute important predictors of the success of vaginal delivery. Rarely, an ovarian or uterine tumor (e.g., leiomyoma), cervical cancer, or a vaginal septum may impede passage of the fetus through the birth canal.

Four pelvic types have been described on the basis of the shape of the pelvic inlet (the plane bounded by the upper inner pubic symphysis, the linea terminalis of the iliac bones, and the sacral promontory) (Table 19.1).[3]

The most common pelvic type, the **gynecoid** pelvis, is particularly well suited to accommodate the flexed fetal head within the bony pelvis. The inlet is round or oval, with the transverse diameter only slightly greater than the anteroposterior diameter. The pelvic sidewalls are straight and do not converge, the ischial spines are not prominent, the sacrum is hollow, and the subpubic arch is wide. The absence of prominent ischial spines is an important feature because the distance between them—the transverse diameter of the midpelvis—is the narrowest pelvic dimension. The other pelvic types are thought to be less favorable for vaginal delivery.

Radiographic pelvimetry was historically thought to provide more information regarding pelvic dimensions and features than can be obtained by clinical pelvimetry alone. However, large metaanalyses have shown no utility in its use for clinical management because of its poor ability to predict a successful vaginal birth[4] and its association with an increased rate of cesarean delivery. Computed tomography and magnetic resonance imaging are associated with less or no ionizing radiation exposure, but data are limited on their utility for predicting a successful vaginal delivery.

In the absence of a history of pelvic fracture or rare musculoskeletal disease (e.g., a dwarfing condition), there are few circumstances in which the pelvic anatomy precludes a trial of labor. A pelvis with smaller-than-average dimensions may be adequate for a particular fetus if the head is well flexed, molding is sufficient (i.e., overlapping of the fetal unfused skull bones), and contractions are adequate (>200 Montevideo units).[5]

The Passenger

Fetal size and the relationship of the fetus to the maternal pelvis can affect labor progress. The **lie** of the fetus (the relationship of the long axis of the fetus to the long axis of the mother) can be transverse, oblique, or longitudinal. In the first two, vaginal delivery is impossible unless the fetus is very immature.

The **presentation** denotes that portion of the fetus overlying the pelvic inlet. The presentation may be cephalic, breech, or shoulder. Cephalic presentations are further subdivided into vertex, brow, or face presentations according to the degree of flexion of the neck. In more than 95% of labors at term, the presentation is cephalic and the fetal head is well flexed (i.e., vertex presentation).

TABLE 19.1 Features Determined by Clinical Pelvimetry as Related to Pelvic Type

Suboptimal Features	PELVIC TYPE			
	Gynecoid	Android	Anthropoid	Platypelloid
Promontory reached (diagonal conjugate ≤ 12 cm)	−	±	−	+
Sacrum flat/forward (versus curved)	−	+	−	+
Spines prominent (found by medical student)	−	+	+	−
Sacrosciatic notch narrow (≤2 fingerbreadths)	−	+	−	−
Subpubic arch narrow (acute angle)	−	+	+	−

+, Present; −, absent; ±, variable.

From Zlatnik FJ. Normal labor and delivery and its conduct. In: Scott JR, DiSaia PJ, Hammond CB, Spellacy WN, eds. *Danforth's Obstetrics and Gynecology*. 6th ed. JB Lippincott; 1990:161–188.

BOX 19.1   Positions of the Occiput in Labor, Listed in Order of Decreasing Frequency

- Left occiput transverse (LOT)
- Right occiput transverse (ROT)
- Left occiput anterior (LOA)
- Right occiput posterior (ROP)
- Right occiput anterior (ROA)
- Left occiput posterior (LOP)
- Occiput anterior (OA)
- Occiput posterior (OP)

BOX 19.2   The Cardinal Movements of Labor

- Engagement
- Descent
- Flexion
- Internal rotation
- Extension
- External rotation
- Expulsion

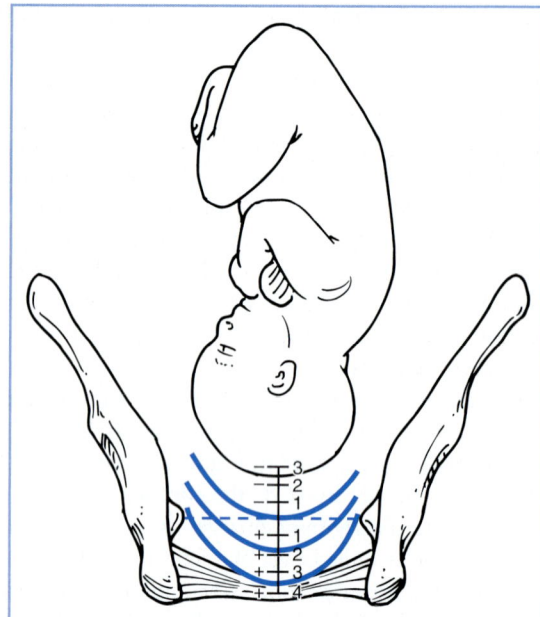

Fig. 19.1 Stations of the fetal head. Redrawn from Zlatnik FJ. Normal labor and delivery and its conduct. In: Scott JR, DiSaia PJ, Hammond CB, Spellacy WN, eds. *Danforth's Obstetrics and Gynecology.* 7th ed. JB Lippincott; 1994:116.

The **position** of the fetus denotes the relationship of a specific presenting fetal bony point to the maternal pelvis. In vertex presentations, that bony point is the *occiput*. During vaginal examination, palpation of the sagittal suture and fontanels permits determination of the fetal position. Positions of the occiput are listed in Box 19.1. Other markers for position are the sacrum for breech presentation, the mentum for face presentation, and the acromion for shoulder presentation. (See Chapter 34 for a discussion of nonvertex presentations.)

The Mechanism of Labor

The *mechanism of labor* refers to the changes in fetal conformation and position (cardinal movements) (Box 19.2) that occur during descent through the birth canal during the late first and the second stage of labor.

The first cardinal movement is **engagement**, which denotes passage of the biparietal diameter (BPD) (i.e., the widest transverse diameter of the fetal head) through the plane of the pelvic inlet. Obstetricians judge that engagement has occurred when the leading bony point of the fetal head is palpable at the level of the ischial spines. This is a reasonable proxy because the distance between the leading bony point and the BPD is typically less than the distance between the ischial spines and the plane of the pelvic inlet. If the leading bony point is at the level of the spines, the vertex is said to be at zero station. If the leading bony point is 1 cm above the level of the spines, the station is designated as –1. Similarly, +1, +2, and +3 indicate that the leading bony point is 1, 2, and 3 cm below the ischial spines, respectively (Fig. 19.1). At +5 station, delivery is imminent. *Station* refers to palpation of the leading bony point. Often, marked edema of the scalp

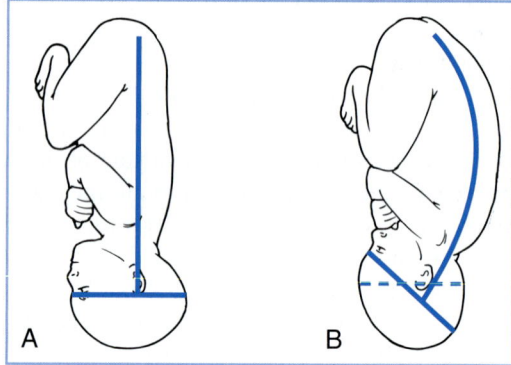

Fig. 19.2 (A) Relation of the head to the vertebral column before flexion. (B) Relation of the head to the vertebral column after flexion. Redrawn from Zlatnik FJ. Normal labor and delivery and its conduct. In: Scott JR, DiSaia PJ, Hammond CB, Spellacy WN, eds. *Danforth's Obstetrics and Gynecology.* 6th ed. JB Lippincott; 1990:174.

(i.e., caput succedaneum) occurs during labor. In such cases, the bony skull may be 2 to 3 cm higher than the scalp.

The second cardinal movement is **descent**, although descent occurs throughout the birth process. The third cardinal movement is **flexion**. A very small fetus can typically descend through the maternal pelvis without increased flexion. However, under the usual circumstances at term, the force from uterine contractions from above the fetus and resistance from below enhance flexion of the occiput (Fig. 19.2).

The fourth cardinal movement is **internal rotation**. The fetus meets the narrowest pelvic dimension, the transverse diameter between the ischial spines, at the level of the midpelvis. Because the BPD of the fetal head is slightly smaller than the suboccipitobregmatic diameter, the vertex typically negotiates the mid-pelvis with the sagittal suture in an antero-posterior direction. *Internal rotation* describes the change in the position of the vertex from occiput transverse or oblique to anteroposterior. The occiput tends to rotate to the roomiest part of the pelvis; thus, in gynecoid pelvises, the fetus is delivered in an occiput anterior position.

The next cardinal movement is **extension**, which occurs as the fetal head delivers (Fig. 19.3). Subsequently, the occiput rotates to the side (**external rotation**) as the shoulders pass through the mid-pelvis in an oblique diameter. The anterior shoulder moves under the pubic symphysis. With gentle downward traction, it passes from the birth canal, and **expulsion** of the remainder of the fetus occurs.

Abnormalities of the pelvis affect the mechanism of labor in specific ways. In an **anthropoid** pelvis, where the anteroposterior diameter of the pelvic inlet exceeds the transverse diameter, internal rotation to the occiput posterior position rather than the occiput anterior position often occurs. Delivery occurs with the occiput in the posterior position, or rotation to the occiput anterior position occurs just before delivery. In cases of persistent occiput posterior position, delivery occurs by flexion rather than extension of the fetal head (see Fig. 19.3).

In **platypelloid** pelvises, internal rotation may not take place. The widest diameter is the transverse diameter, and descent of the vertex may occur with the occiput in the transverse position; rotation to the occiput anterior position occurs only at delivery.

Clinical Course

Admission

When a patient enters the labor and delivery unit, the first question that must be asked is "why?" Did she come because of regular, painful uterine contractions; decreased fetal activity; vaginal bleeding; ruptured membranes (chorioamnion); or some other reason? If the presumptive diagnosis is labor, is the fetus at term?

The time of the onset of labor and the status of the membranes should be determined. Observation of the patient's demeanor coupled with the assessment of cervical effacement and dilation will signal whether the patient is in the latent or active phase of the first stage of labor. In patients with vaginal bleeding, manual examination of the cervix is deferred until after ultrasonography, unless placenta previa has been previously ruled out, to avoid exacerbation of bleeding. To decrease the risk of infection, cervical examination may also be deferred in patients with prelabor rupture of membranes.

Abdominal examination or ultrasonography is used to establish presentation and an estimate of fetal size. With most obstetric services, external electronic fetal heart rate (FHR) monitoring is used on admission to assess fetal condition. The baseline rate and variability and the presence or absence of accelerations and decelerations are of interest (see Chapter 8).

Subsequent Care

The maternal vital signs and FHR are recorded periodically. In some obstetric services, continuous electronic FHR monitoring is used universally; with other services, FHR is monitored via intermittent auscultation. In low-risk patients, it is acceptable to record the FHR every 30 minutes in the first part of the first stage of labor, every 15 minutes in the latter part of the first stage, and every 5 minutes in the second stage. During latent labor, the patient may ambulate or assume any position of comfort on the labor bed or in a chair. During active labor, some women choose to lie down. Evidence supports that ambulation should be recommended in the first stage of labor for women without neuraxial analgesia; for those with neuraxial analgesia, either ambulating or not is acceptable.[5] For women with low-risk pregnancies, choices concerning analgesia or anesthesia are made according to the patient's wishes. For some women with maternal, obstetric, or fetal comorbidities, clinicians may suggest neuraxial analgesia to decrease the maternal stress of labor or facilitate operative vaginal delivery (see Chapter 24).

During labor, those providing obstetric care must focus on the following two critical questions:
1. Is the fetus tolerating labor in a satisfactory fashion or is there evidence of fetal compromise (see Chapter 8)?
2. What is the progress of labor?

Labor Progress: The Labor Curve

One of the central tasks of those providing intrapartum care is to determine whether labor is progressing, and if not, to determine the significance of the delay and what the response should be. It is important to note that there is significant

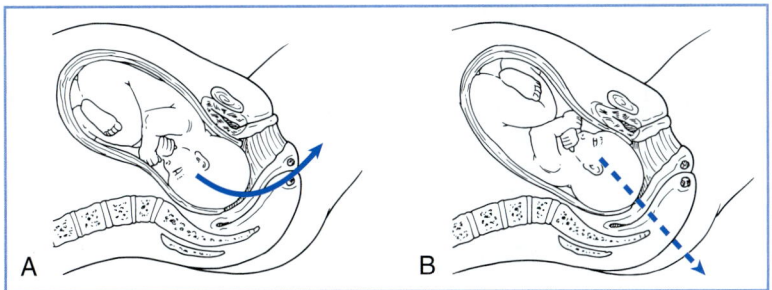

Fig. 19.3 Vertex Presentations. (A) Occiput anterior position. (B) Occiput posterior position. Redrawn from Zlatnik FJ. Normal labor and delivery and its conduct. In: Scott JR, DiSaia PJ, Hammond CB, Spellacy WN, eds. *Danforth's Obstetrics and Gynecology.* 6th ed. JB Lippincott; 1990:174.

variation in the "normal" progress of labor; different definitions are used globally depending on the population. Many methods of measuring the progress of labor have been proposed, but there is no widely accepted definition of the "normal" progress of labor.[6] A general overview of methods of labor progression assessment is detailed below.

A generation of obstetricians is indebted to Emanuel Friedman, whose landmark studies of labor provided a foundational framework for judging labor progress.[7] Friedman's approach was straightforward. He graphed cervical dilation on the *y*-axis and elapsed time on the *x*-axis for thousands of labors. He considered nulliparous and parous patients separately, delineated the difference between latent and active phase, and offered guidance for the statistical limits of normal.[7] Based on Friedman's labor curve, Peisner and Rosen[8] evaluated the progress of labor for 1060 nulliparous women and 639 parous women. After excluding women with protracted or arrested labor, these researchers noted that 60% of the women had reached the latent-active phase transition by 4 cm of cervical dilation and 89% did so by 5 cm.

Parity, referring to previous pregnancies of at least 20 weeks' gestation, is an important determinant of labor length. For example, a pregnant woman who is gravida 2, para 1 is pregnant for the second time, and her first pregnancy resulted in delivery after 20 weeks' gestation. Fourteen hours is the suggested limit of the latent phase in the *parous* woman. According to Friedman, in the active phase of the first stage of labor, a nulliparous woman's cervix should dilate at a rate of at least 1.2 cm per hour, and a parous woman's cervix should dilate at least 1.5 cm per hour. (The slopes of the dilation curves in Fig. 19.4 represent the lower limits of normal.) If a woman's cervix fails to dilate at the appropriate rate during the active phase of labor, she is said to have **primary dysfunctional labor**. Graphically, her cervical dilation "falls off the curve." If cervical dilation ceases during a 2-hour period in the active phase of labor, **secondary arrest of dilation** has occurred.

Studies published in 2002 and 2010 using data from a large database of women who gave birth in the United States reported slower rates of cervical dilation and engendered an ongoing transition toward the use of the Zhang "contemporary labor curve."[9,10] These newer data have been adopted into new labor management practice guidelines.[11] These labor curves reveal that cervical dilation is particularly slow prior to 6-cm cervical dilation and that the deceleration phase described by Friedman is usually absent. Therefore, 6 cm, rather than 4 cm, of cervical dilation more accurately reflects the start of the active phase in contemporary labor curves and should be used to define the active phase for labor management.[10,11] Furthermore, in the active phase, the absence of cervical change over at least 4 hours rather than 2 hours is a better definition of labor arrest. Estimates of contemporary rates of cervical dilation from 4 cm (when patients are often admitted to the maternity unit) by parity are shown in Table 19.2. Nulliparous women have a slower cumulative rate of cervical dilation overall. However, before 6 cm of dilation, the time intervals required to dilate 1 cm are similar between nulliparous and parous women. While these "contemporary labor curves" have been emphasized in new practice guidelines, it is important to note the ongoing need for prospective evaluation of these new criteria, as comparisons of labor managed using the Friedman and Zhang labor curves have yielded mixed results.[12,13] Furthermore, the routine use of a partogram (labor curve) to monitor labor progress (regardless of the labor curve utilized) is no longer recommended.[5]

TABLE 19.2 Rate of Spontaneous Cervical Dilation by Parity

Cervical Dilation	Nulliparous: Median Time (h) (95th Percentile)	Parous: Median Time (h) (95th Percentile)
First Stage		
4–5 cm	1.3 (6.4)	1.4 (7.1)
5–6 cm	0.8 (3.2)	0.8 (3.4)
6–7 cm	0.6 (2.2)	0.5 (1.8)
7–8 cm	0.5 (1.6)	0.4 (1.2)
8–9 cm	0.5 (1.4)	0.3 (1.0)
9–10 cm	0.5 (1.8)	0.3 (0.9)
Second Stage		
10 cm to delivery (epidural analgesia)	1.1 (3.6)	0.4 (2.0)
10 cm to delivery (no epidural analgesia)	0.6 (2.8)	0.2 (1.3)

Modified from Zhang J, Landy HJ, Branch DW, et al. for the Consortium on Safe Labor. Contemporary patterns of spontaneous labor with normal neonatal outcomes. *Obstet Gynecol.* 2010;116:1281–1287.

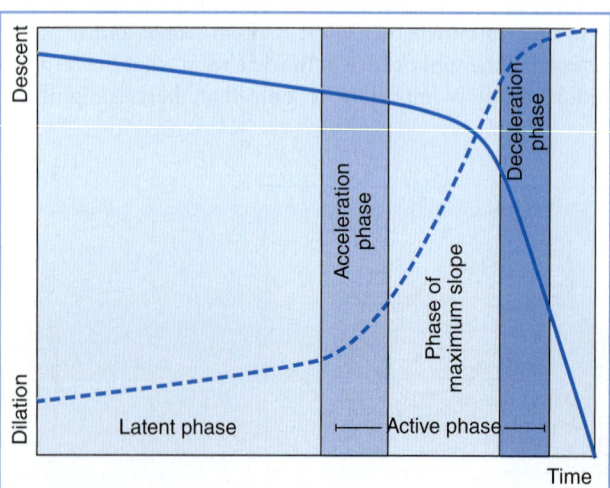

Fig. 19.4 The Friedman Curve. From Friedman EA. Patterns of labor as indicators of risk. *Clin Obstet Gynecol.* 1973;16:172–183.

TABLE 19.3   The Bishop Cervix Score[a]

Component	SCORE			
	0	1	2	3
Dilation (cm)	0	1–2	3–4	5+
Effacement (%)	0–30	40–50	60–70	80+
Station	–3	–2	–1/0	+1
Consistency	Firm	Medium	Soft	
Position	Posterior	Mid	Anterior	

[a]Modified Bishop Score: Effacement is replaced by cervical length: 0 points for >3 cm, 1 for >2 cm, 2 for >1 cm, 3 for >0 cm.
From Bishop EH. Pelvic scoring for elective induction. *Obstet Gynecol.* 1964;24:266–268.

Abnormalities of the latent phase and active phase differ in associated factors, apparent causes, and significance. A prolonged latent phase is more likely if labor begins with an unfavorable (long, closed, firm) cervix.[7] The Bishop score (Table 19.3) helps quantitate the favorability of the cervix; the higher the score, the shorter the labor and the less likelihood of labor failure.[14] This finding is not surprising, because a high Bishop score indicates that the cervix is ready to dilate with uterine contractions (i.e., the cervix will soon enter the active phase). By contrast, a low score suggests that many hours of uterine contractions may be needed to soften and efface the cervix.

Some women with a prolonged latent phase are not in true labor, but rather in "false labor" with Braxton-Hicks contractions; this diagnosis is made in retrospect. After hours of regular, painful contractions, uterine activity may cease without the occurrence of appreciable cervical dilation. Several hours or days later, the patient may reappear in true labor.

Studies published in 1993 and 2011[15,16] reported an increased risk for cesarean delivery, chorioamnionitis, endometritis, excessive blood loss, depressed Apgar scores, and need for neonatal resuscitation with a prolonged latent phase. Primary dysfunctional labor and arrest of dilation during the active phase may indicate cephalopelvic disproportion.[7,17,18] Whether using the historic Friedman or contemporary Zhang labor curve, it is clear that women who experience active-phase arrest of dilation are more likely to require cesarean delivery than women without arrest (regardless of definition) during the active phase.

In summary, the contemporary view of labor progress is that delays in the latent phase of the first stage of labor may be associated with fetopelvic disproportion or the need for cesarean delivery, but this is not universal, as some women may still achieve vaginal birth with prolonged labor without adverse outcomes.[19] Delays in the active phase predict fetopelvic disproportion, although not with precision. Given current obstetric practice and fetal monitoring techniques, it is unclear whether first-stage labor abnormalities are intrinsically associated with neonatal depression at delivery.[20,21]

First stage of labor. Intravenous **oxytocin** administration during the first stage of labor leads to shorter duration of labor and facilitates successful vaginal delivery.[17] Labor is shortened by approximately 2 hours without increasing the risk of cesarean delivery.[5] Commonly, oxytocin is administered concomitantly with amniotomy to further shorten the duration of the first stage of labor, especially in women with slow progression of labor. The risks associated with oxytocin stimulation are both maternal and fetal, but are uncommon.[5] If mechanical obstruction to delivery exists, greater uterine activity predisposes the patient to *uterine rupture*, a grave obstetric complication. Multiparity and prior uterine surgery are additional predisposing factors to uterine rupture. Oxytocin has an antidiuretic effect, and iatrogenic *water intoxication* accompanied by seizures and even coma and death have been reported. In these cases, however, oxytocin was administered over many hours (often days) in electrolyte-free solutions, with little attention paid to maternal urine output. Infusion of electrolyte-containing solutions and close attention to the parturient's fluid balance should prevent this complication. *Uterine tachysystole* with FHR decelerations is another risk of exogenous oxytocin infusion. The force generated during uterine contractions interrupts blood flow through the intervillous space; uterine contractions can be regarded as episodes of "fetal breath-holding." If the contractions are too frequent (i.e., at intervals < 2 minutes, defined as uterine tachysystole), there may be insufficient time for placental gas exchange during uterine diastole, the fetus may become hypoxemic, and fetal compromise may result. Continuous FHR and maternal contraction observation using tocometry permit a timely diagnosis of uterine tachysystole. Decreasing the oxytocin infusion rate, temporarily discontinuing the oxytocin, or, in some instances, administering a tocolytic (e.g., terbutaline, nitroglycerin) can promptly correct the problem.

Currently, in the United States, oxytocin for inducing or augmenting labor is given intravenously, typically by infusion pump. Continuous electronic FHR monitoring is used, and a physician or nurse monitors the FHR pattern.

The variability in protocols for oxytocin induction or augmentation of labor reflects confusion in the literature.[22–26] The goal is to increase uterine activity to efficiently and effectively promote cervical dilation without causing fetal compromise as a result of uterine tachysystole. However, the best way to do this is unclear. Recommended starting doses of oxytocin vary from 1 to 6 mU/min; additional drug is administered until a satisfactory labor pattern is achieved. Dosage increments typically vary from 1 to 6 mU at intervals of 15 to 40 minutes. High-dose oxytocin regimens involve the use of higher starting doses and incremental dose increases of 4 mU/min or greater. A systematic review of available trials suggests that the use of a higher-dose regimen for labor augmentation is associated with shortened labor and a decrease in the incidence of cesarean delivery and thus may be considered.[5,27,28]

The amnion contains the amniotic fluid and helps protect the uterine contents from the microbial flora of the vagina and provides mechanical protection for the fetus and umbilical cord during fetal growth and movement. In the absence of intervention, the membranes generally rupture at the onset of labor or near full cervical dilation. If the membranes are intact, the question arises as to whether they should be artificially ruptured during labor. If so, when? Because there is concern about infection once the membranes are ruptured, the performance of an amniotomy commits the mother to delivery. The traditional thought was that amniotomy should not be done early in the labor course. However, newer data, including metaanalyses, suggest that early amniotomy (i.e., amniotomy at cervical dilation < 4 cm or soon after mechanical cervical ripening with a balloon) decreases the time to complete dilation and vaginal delivery, especially in nulliparous women, without an increase in adverse perinatal outcomes.[29–31] While routine amniotomy in normally progressing spontaneous labor is not recommended, early amniotomy is routinely advised in the treatment of dysfunctional labor and for the prevention of dysfunctional labor.[5]

Second stage of labor. When the cervix has been completely retracted to form the lower uterine segment and is therefore not palpable on vaginal examination, full or complete dilation has been achieved, and the second stage of labor begins. Strong uterine contractions coupled with voluntary expulsive efforts by the parturient cause the fetal presenting part to descend through the pelvis, resulting in delivery. At complete cervical dilation, there is frequently an increase in bloody vaginal show, the parturient may vomit, and she may report rectal pressure. This sensation of needing to "bear down" encourages strong Valsalva maneuvers during uterine contractions. The duration of the second stage of labor is influenced by parity and the presence or absence of epidural analgesia.[11] In the Zhang et al. study (Consortium on Safe Labor),[9] the 95th percentile threshold for the duration of the second stage of labor was approximately 1 hour longer in parturients who received epidural analgesia compared with those who did not.

The contemporary obstetrician, although less concerned about the elapsed time during the second stage of labor than were obstetricians historically, continues to balance the risks of prematurely performing a cesarean delivery with the risks of adverse outcomes associated with a prolonged second stage. While studies have shown that a prolonged second-stage of labor is associated with an increase in maternal obstetric trauma, postpartum hemorrhage, infection, neonatal depression, and admission to the neonatal intensive care unit, particularly in the setting of difficult operative vaginal delivery, the contemporary view is that the second stage of labor does not need to be terminated at an arbitrary time provided that progress in descent continues and the FHR pattern is reassuring.[32,33] Allowing a longer second-stage duration is an acceptable practice to decrease the rate of unnecessary cesarean deliveries.[9,11]

If the parturient is allowed to choose her own position during labor and delivery, she often chooses not to stay in one place.[34] Without instruction from birth attendants, the parturient frequently chooses to walk or sit in a chair during latent labor. In the active phase of the first stage, however, she often returns to the labor bed. During the second stage of labor, some women assume the squatting position, whereas others, with their legs supported by the nurse and the father of the baby, assume a semisitting position. The goal is to achieve a position in which the parturient's Valsalva efforts are most effective. The patient should avoid the supine position without left uterine displacement, which results in aortocaval compression. Aortocaval compression seems to be less severe with the patient in the semisitting position, and it is avoided altogether with the patient in the lateral position.

An episiotomy is a perineal incision extending either directly posterior from 6 o'clock (midline) or in a 45-degree angle to either side (mediolateral). The former causes less discomfort, is more anatomic, and is easier to repair than the latter. The mediolateral episiotomy's advantage is that extension through the anal sphincter and rectal mucosa is less likely to occur, but its major disadvantage is that it may cause more bleeding or severe postpartum pain. In the past, as the fetal head distended the perineum shortly before delivery, an episiotomy was often performed to shorten labor and to protect against the subsequent development of uterine prolapse, cystocele, and rectocele.

The role of episiotomy in contemporary obstetrics is limited.[35] Tears involving the anal sphincter (third degree) and rectal mucosa (fourth degree) are actually more common after midline episiotomy than if episiotomy is not performed. In the absence of an episiotomy, however, anterior periurethral lacerations are common. These rarely cause immediate problems, but data on long-term outcomes are lacking. Given the recognized association between midline episiotomies and third- and fourth-degree tears, the association of these tears with long-term morbidity, and the failure to observe any benefits to routine episiotomy, more restrictive use of this incision is now recommended.[35,36] An episiotomy may still be indicated in some instances of operative vaginal delivery of a large infant with suspected fetal compromise, or to manage shoulder dystocia.[37]

The timing of initiation of maternal pushing efforts has been understudied. Pushing immediately upon full cervical dilation or allowing for spontaneous fetal descent (delayed pushing) have both been commonly used, but neither has been the "gold standard." A 2018 randomized trial in nulliparous patients with neuraxial analgesia compared immediate and delayed pushing; the timing of pushing effort did not affect the rate of vaginal delivery.[38] There were no differences in neonatal outcomes or perineal lacerations; however, immediate pushing was associated with decreased chorioamnionitis and postpartum hemorrhage. Current American College of Obstetricians and Gynecologists (ACOG) guidelines recommend pushing commence when complete cervical dilation is achieved (immediate pushing).[11]

Third stage of labor. The third stage of labor begins with the delivery of the infant and ends with the delivery of the placenta. The placenta typically separates from the uterine wall within a few contractions after delivery of the infant, and expulsion of the placenta follows a few minutes later.

When the placenta has separated from the uterine wall, gentle traction on the umbilical cord, coupled with suprapubic pressure to elevate the uterus, serves to facilitate delivery of the placenta and membranes. In the absence of excessive bleeding, the obstetrician waits for the signs of placental separation before attempting to deliver it. Exerting traction on the umbilical cord before the placenta has separated may result in complications. The umbilical cord may separate from the placenta, making extraction of the placenta more challenging. A much more serious complication is *uterine inversion*. In cases of fundal implantation of the placenta, excessive umbilical cord traction before the placenta has separated can turn the uterus inside out, resulting in severe hemorrhage (see Chapter 37).

If the placenta does not separate from the uterus in a timely fashion (prolonged third stage) or if significant bleeding occurs, manual removal of the placenta is indicated. Although some obstetricians advocate performing this procedure with sedation or systemic analgesia, neuraxial anesthesia, or general anesthesia if neuraxial anesthesia is not feasible, is typically warranted. The obstetrician's hand is passed into the uterine cavity, and the edge of the placenta is identified. The hand is used as a trowel to separate the placenta from the uterine wall. If the obstetrician cannot easily develop a plane between the placenta and the uterine wall, the diagnosis of *placenta accreta* should be considered. Placenta accreta typically results in severe hemorrhage, which frequently mandates emergency hysterectomy (see Chapter 37).

Classically, a duration of 30 minutes has been used to define a prolonged third stage; however, data from a study published in 2016 suggest that the incidence of postpartum hemorrhage is increased if the third stage of labor duration exceeds 20 minutes.[39] However, in the absence of significant bleeding, more time may be allowed for placental separation, particularly at earlier gestational ages when it may be difficult to access the uterus and the umbilical cord is too small to achieve traction without avulsion.

After delivery, and either before or after the placenta has been removed, uterotonic agents are administered to reduce bleeding. **Oxytocin** is universally recommended as a prophylactic agent to reduce postpartum bleeding and may be given intravenously in a dilute solution, or 10 units may be given intramuscularly (see Chapter 37).[40]

If the uterus does not respond to oxytocin, other uterotonic agents are typically administered. **Methylergonovine** (0.2 mg every 2 to 4 hours) has long been available for intramuscular administration. It contracts vascular smooth muscle and may cause hypertension. Methylergonovine should not be given intravenously except in cases of severe, life-threatening hemorrhage. In such cases, the physician should give the drug slowly and carefully monitor the maternal blood pressure.

15-Methylprostaglandin $F_{2\alpha}$ (carboprost) administered intramuscularly (0.25 mg every 15 to 90 minutes, maximum of 8 doses) has been demonstrated to be an effective uterotonic agent if other drugs, such as oxytocin, have failed.[41] 15-Methylprostaglandin $F_{2\alpha}$ may cause bronchospasm and its use is relatively contraindicated in patients with asthma.

Use of tranexamic acid (TXA) has been studied with mixed results (see Chapter 37). A large US trial of prophylactic TXA administration to women undergoing cesarean delivery found no benefit.[42] As such, TXA is only considered an adjunct agent (not a first-line agent) for bleeding control in the postpartum period.[40,42]

Most obstetricians in the United States do not use oxytocin or other uterotonic agents until the placenta has been delivered, whereas globally, obstetricians may administer these agents immediately after delivery of the infant or even with delivery of the anterior shoulder. The timing likely does not matter.[43] Immediately after the delivery of the placenta, if the obstetrician suspects an abnormality, the hand can be passed into the uterine cavity. Within several minutes, however, the cervix and birth canal contract. Subsequent uterine exploration typically requires the administration of anesthesia and/or a uterine relaxation agent (e.g., nitroglycerin).

Fourth stage of labor. Many obstetricians consider the first 60 minutes after delivery of the placenta to be the fourth stage of labor. Labor is completed, but this designation emphasizes that the patient must be watched carefully for postpartum bleeding. Postpartum hemorrhage is defined as estimated blood loss $\geq$ 1000 mL regardless of mode of delivery, or any blood loss with symptoms of hypovolemia within 24 hours after delivery. More than 80% of cases of postpartum hemorrhage result from uterine atony; less common causes are vaginal/cervical lacerations, thrombotic disorders, or abnormal placentation (retained placenta, placenta accreta).[40] If uterine atony is not identified during the first hour after delivery, it is unlikely to occur subsequently. The patient should be evaluated frequently to be certain that excessive bleeding is not occurring and that the uterus remains contracted. Considerable blood loss can occur in the presence of "normal" vital signs; a modest increment in additional blood loss can then be followed by profound shock. Uterine relaxation and excessive bleeding after delivery are initially treated with uterine massage and further uterotonic drug administration (see Chapter 37). Management options for persistent hemorrhage include uterine tamponade, uterine vacuum compression devices, surgery, and vascular embolization.

SPECIAL SITUATIONS

Prelabor Rupture of Membranes

Prelabor rupture of the membranes (PROM) is defined as a rupture of the fetal membranes (i.e., the chorioamnion) before the onset of labor. It may occur preterm (before 37 weeks' gestation) or at term.

Preterm Prelabor Rupture of Membranes

The most significant complication of preterm PROM is preterm birth.[44] Although the length of the *latent period* (the interval between membrane rupture and the onset of labor) is inversely related to gestational age, only one in five women with preterm PROM have latent periods exceeding 1 week. Indeed, PROM is the precipitating factor in nearly one-third of preterm deliveries. Chorioamnionitis is a risk factor for preterm PROM; both chorioamnionitis and prolapse of the umbilical cord are risks of PROM. If membrane rupture occurs during the second trimester and if the fetus experiences a long exposure to oligohydramnios, there is risk for pulmonary hypoplasia, perinatal death, neonatal sepsis, and orthopedic deformities.

Current management of preterm PROM is conservative. The diagnosis is confirmed by inspection, nitrazine, and fern testing, or rarely by ultrasound-guided instillation of dye into the amniotic fluid and observation of its passage vaginally (commercial testing kits are available with variable test characteristics).[45] Electronic FHR monitoring is used to identify variable FHR decelerations that signal umbilical cord compression. The mother is also evaluated for fever and uterine tenderness, which may indicate chorioamnionitis. If these are absent, the clinician awaits the onset of labor or the subsequent development of infection. The adjunctive use of maternally administered corticosteroids to enhance fetal pulmonary maturity, and antibiotics to prevent chorioamnionitis and delay the onset of labor, is indicated.[45–47] Current evidence does not support the use of tocolytic therapy to prolong pregnancy.[45,48] Delivery is recommended routinely at 34 weeks' gestation (a point beyond which the rate of severe neonatal morbidity and mortality is very low).[45] Recent studies have suggested some benefit for expectant management of preterm PROM between 34 and 37 weeks' gestation; however, in these cases, hospitalization and close observation are warranted.

Term Prelabor Rupture of Membranes

Approximately 8% of term pregnancies are complicated by PROM; the natural history is summarized in Table 19.4.[45,49,50] Although chorioamnionitis is more likely to occur preterm than at term with PROM, no clear relationship exists between the length of the latent period and chorioamnionitis in the preterm patient.[51] By contrast, chorioamnionitis at term is more likely if the latent period exceeds 24 hours. The relationship between prolonged latency and chorioamnionitis accounts for the usual practice in the United States of immediate oxytocin induction of labor for a woman with PROM at term if she is not already in active labor.[45,52] Expectant management for a short period of time may be offered to the patient.[45]

Chorioamnionitis

If chorioamnionitis develops, the fetus must be delivered. Intrapartum antibiotic administration improves the outcome for both the mother and infant.[53] Ampicillin and gentamicin are often chosen to combat group B streptococcus and

Escherichia coli, which are important neonatal pathogens. Because no relationship exists between the number of hours that chorioamnionitis has been present and perinatal outcome, chorioamnionitis alone is not an indication for cesarean delivery.[54–57] Antibiotics, oxytocin, and close observation of the mother and fetus are indicated.

Induction of Labor

Induction of labor is defined as a surgical or medical intervention that leads to uterine contractions that progressively dilate the cervix. Because elective and indicated inductions differ in terms of eligibility criteria, they are considered separately, even though the methods used are similar.

Factors associated with the success of induction (elective or indicated) of labor include (1) a parous patient, (2) a singleton vertex presentation, (3) a certain gestation of at least 39 weeks, (4) a favorable cervix, and (5) no contraindications to labor and vaginal delivery. The Bishop score (see Table 19.3) helps quantitate the favorability of the cervix.[14] Bishop observed that a score of 9 or greater was not associated with induction failure. With the modified Bishop score, cervical length replaces cervical effacement. When the components of the Bishop score are considered separately in terms of their effects on the latent phase, dilation is most critical. Cervical effacement (or length), fetal station, and consistency are each half as important, and cervical position has little effect.[58]

If the Bishop score is favorable, amniotomy or oxytocin administration suffices as a means of inducing labor; some obstetricians reserve oxytocin for the patient who is not experiencing uterine contractions 4 to 6 hours after amniotomy. Amniotomy can be performed early in the morning with anticipated delivery in the afternoon. Often, however, the cervix is not favorable, and induction is typically initiated with the application of cervical ripening agents (prostaglandin E analogues) or the use of a balloon catheter bulb for 12 hours[59] to mechanically dilate the cervix.[60]

Both mechanical and pharmacologic techniques are effective in improving the Bishop score; both improve rates of successful vaginal delivery with the most efficacy reported for mechanical balloons and oral misoprostol.[59,61] These measures can even be instituted the evening before the planned induction. One additional advantage for a balloon catheter is that the catheter can be placed in the outpatient setting in low-risk patients.

A commonly used pharmacologic method involves the topical application of prostaglandin E_2, either in the vagina or in the cervical canal. Prostaglandin E_2 has a local effect in the initiation of softening, effacement, and dilation of the cervix, and it also has an oxytocin-like effect on the myometrium. Women treated with prostaglandin E_2 commonly experience contractions and labor before amniotomy or oxytocin administration. The same is true for misoprostol, a prostaglandin E_1 analogue that is now widely used for cervical ripening and labor induction.[62] Prostaglandins should not be administered to induce labor in women with a prior cesarean delivery because their use is associated with an increased risk for

TABLE 19.4 **Natural History of Prelabor Rupture of the Membranes at Term**	
Variable	Value
Prevalence	8%
Delivery within 33 h of membrane rupture with expectant management	50%
Delivery between 97 and 104 h of membrane rupture after induction of labor	95%

Data from American College of Obstetricians and Gynecologists. Practice Bulletin No. 217: Prelabor rupture of membranes (reaffirmed 2023). *Obstet Gynecol.* 2020;135:e80–e97.

uterine rupture. Overall, mechanical dilation with a balloon catheter bulb or prostaglandin E$_1$ analogues are considered equally efficacious methods of cervical ripening.[59]

Elective Induction

The rationale for elective induction of labor is convenience, both for the patient and for the physician. Because it is elective, the delivery should be easily accomplished, and the risks should approach zero. Elective inductions have been criticized by some physicians because of the possibilities of induction failure and iatrogenic prematurity.[63] However, a 2016 randomized controlled study noted no increase in the risk for cesarean delivery or adverse perinatal outcomes in women older than 35 years of age undergoing elective induction of labor at 39 weeks' gestation.[64] A large, multicenter, randomized trial published in 2018 found that elective induction of labor in low-risk nulliparous women at 39 weeks' gestation did not result in a greater frequency of adverse perinatal outcomes than expectant management, and it resulted in a lower frequency of cesarean delivery.[65] Metaanalyses of observational studies have confirmed these findings.[66]

As a result of this large, multicenter trial,[65] elective induction of labor at 39 weeks' gestation is rapidly becoming the standard of care in the United States. To counteract the volume of elective inductions, alternative outpatient methods of induction are currently being evaluated in multicenter trials using a balloon catheter; early, small trials and metaanalyses show promising results, especially in nulliparous women.[67-69]

Indicated Induction

Induction of labor is performed when delivery is indicated for maternal or fetal reasons and both the mother and fetus can tolerate labor and vaginal delivery. An indicated induction of labor often arises in the setting of medical comorbidities (such as pregestational diabetes or hypertension) or an obstetric complication such as preeclampsia or fetal growth restriction (also known as *intrauterine growth restriction*). The physician is dealing with a complicated pregnancy when performing an indicated induction of labor; therefore, close maternal and fetal monitoring are indicated. When considering the critical question whether induction should be undertaken, the obstetrician must weigh the perinatal risks of continued intrauterine versus extrauterine existence and must also consider the potential adverse maternal consequences of induction of labor, including a higher risk for infection and/or cesarean delivery. Approaches to induction of labor for this group of patients mirror those described for elective induction of labor.

Operative Vaginal Delivery

Cesarean delivery is the most common surgical procedure worldwide, and global efforts to decrease the primary cesarean delivery rate have been initiated in the last decade. This safe operation is preferable to the continuation of labor in the setting of genuine fetal compromise or to the performance of a difficult and traumatic vaginal delivery. Unfortunately, however, more traditional obstetric interventions (e.g., labor,

additional labor, operative vaginal delivery) are often bypassed in favor of cesarean delivery, perhaps for medicolegal rather than for medical concerns. The appropriate use of operative vaginal delivery techniques requires an accurate assessment of the situation, technical skills, and an honest and humble physician. Unfortunately, rates of operative vaginal delivery continue to decrease across the United States. Those currently in obstetrics training perform far fewer operative vaginal deliveries than in previous years, endangering the future of this pivotal practice critical to avoiding unnecessary cesarean deliveries.[70]

Carefully selected and performed forceps- or vacuum-assisted delivery shortens the second stage of labor in cases of nonreassuring fetal status, maternal illness or exhaustion, and/or undue prolongation of labor with little or no progress. The station of the presenting vertex is critical to the safety of the procedure for mother and infant. The current ACOG classification permits a rational approach to operative vaginal delivery (Box 19.3).[71,72]

For any operative vaginal delivery, adequate anesthesia is required. Outlet operative deliveries are considered to be safe for both mother and fetus. The low station typically rules out cephalopelvic disproportion, and little traction is required. Outlet operative deliveries shorten the second stage by only a few minutes. Sustained fetal bradycardia is a common indication for outlet operative delivery. The higher the head, the more traction is required to achieve fetal descent. Rotation increases the likelihood of vaginal tears.[72] The obstetrician must avoid excessive traction and must be willing to abandon the attempt in favor of cesarean delivery if vaginal delivery does not proceed easily with notable descent with the first pulling action.

Mid-pelvic deliveries reflect a more complicated problem.[73,74] If the station is overestimated, the vertex may not be engaged. Midpelvic deliveries should be regarded as "trials." Few obstetricians are currently trained in mid-pelvic operative deliveries.

Although operative vaginal delivery was traditionally accomplished with obstetric forceps, use of a soft plastic cup vacuum extractor is now more common than the use of

---

BOX 19.3   Classification of Forceps Delivery

Outlet Forceps Delivery
- Scalp is visible.
- Skull has reached the pelvic floor, and the head is on the perineum.
- Sagittal suture is in the anteroposterior diameter or within 45 degrees (e.g., occiput anterior, left occiput anterior, right occiput posterior).

Low Forceps Delivery
- Station is +2 or greater.
- Hollow of the sacrum is filled.

Mid-Forceps Delivery
- Vertex is engaged, but the station is 0 or +1.

forceps.[75–78] Neither technique is uniformly better than the other. The vacuum extractor is easier to apply, especially if the obstetrician is uncertain of the position of the occiput, and it is most likely associated with less maternal trauma. A maximum of three pull attempts should be allowed with a vacuum device. Forceps—but not the vacuum extractor—permit the correction of deflection or slight abnormalities of position that may impede progress. The vacuum extractor is more likely to slip off; whether this feature enhances safety is unknown. Neonatal results are comparable, but intracranial and retinal hemorrhages, which are of unclear significance, are more likely with vacuum extraction. The risk of maternal trauma (e.g., vaginal lacerations) is greater with forceps deliveries.

Ideally, the obstetrician should be trained to use both forceps and vacuum techniques and should individualize their use. A 2017 study observed that mandating resident competency in the use of forceps before beginning training with vacuum extraction was associated with greater use of epidural analgesia, more forceps deliveries, fewer cases of postpartum hemorrhage, and no increase in perineal injury or neonatal morbidity.[79] However, recent data show decreases in rates of both vacuum and forceps use, with the preferred method of operative delivery being institution dependent as well as based on operator comfort level.

Persistent occiput-posterior positions often occur in anthropoid and android pelvises. In modern obstetrics, the infants in most of these cases are delivered with the occiput posterior. Extension of the episiotomy is a common complication in this circumstance; this argues for the consideration of a mediolateral episiotomy. Deep transverse arrest of the occiput was traditionally managed with rotation and delivery with Kielland forceps. Current trainees typically have little experience with this instrument, and they are more likely to proceed with a cesarean delivery in this circumstance.

Nonvertex Presentations

A persistent brow presentation or a transverse lie mandates cesarean delivery. Most face presentations and selected breech presentations can be safely delivered vaginally.[80] However, in response to a large, international, multicenter trial published in 2000, in which planned vaginal delivery was associated with worse perinatal outcomes than planned cesarean delivery,[81] the ACOG now recommends cesarean delivery for persistent singleton breech presentation at term as the preferred mode of delivery for most physicians, particularly in light of diminishing experience in vaginal breech deliveries.[82] In cases where shared decision-making has been performed, a term singleton vaginal breech delivery may be reasonable using hospital-specific protocols, detailed informed consent, and a trained provider.

Fetal Death

If fetal death has occurred, the obstetrician no longer has two patients, making maternal safety the only concern. Although placenta previa or absolute cephalopelvic disproportion may indicate cesarean delivery, the obstetrician is often more willing to choose a more complicated operative vaginal delivery than if the fetus were living.

Shoulder Dystocia

With vertex presentations, most mechanical difficulties are resolved with delivery of the head. Once the head is delivered, the remainder of the fetus follows easily. In as many as 3% of vaginal deliveries, this is not the case. After the (often large) head is delivered, it seems to be "sucked" back into the perineum (the turtle sign). With maternal pushing and gentle traction, nothing happens. In this case, the anterior shoulder is trapped above the pubic symphysis. This serious complication is called *shoulder dystocia*. If delivery is not accomplished soon, umbilical cord compression may result in asphyxia. Excessive traction on the fetal head may result in damage to the brachial plexus (e.g., Erb palsy), which may be permanent or temporary. During the manipulations undertaken to effect delivery, a fracture of the fetal clavicle or humerus may result.

Risk factors for shoulder dystocia are those that predict or reflect mechanical difficulty (Box 19.4).[37,83–85] Women with diabetes mellitus are predisposed to shoulder dystocia, not only because fetal macrosomia is more common but also because the fetus of a mother with diabetes has a shoulder circumference that is disproportionately large relative to the head circumference. Desultory labor may be a harbinger of mechanical mismatch, and operative vaginal delivery can exacerbate the situation. Although risk factors are known, it is important to recognize that shoulder dystocia cannot be accurately predicted or prevented.[37]

Appropriate management of shoulder dystocia begins with the recognition that there is sufficient time to deliver the infant safely. Neuraxial anesthesia is ideal. Episiotomy can be considered to allow space for the operator's hands to perform the shoulder dystocia maneuvers. The anterior shoulder is typically stuck behind the pubic symphysis. Although greater posterior room does not directly permit delivery, it does permit vaginal manipulations that may be necessary to effect delivery. Table 19.5 lists one plan of management for shoulder dystocia, but other choices are available.[37,83,86] Emergency drills and simulation training may improve proficiency in the management of shoulder dystocia.

If suprapubic pressure (directed toward the floor) coupled with gentle traction on the head is not efficacious, the mother's thighs are removed from their supports and are hyperflexed alongside her abdomen. This maneuver (i.e., the McRoberts maneuver) elevates the symphysis in

---

BOX 19.4 Risk Factors for Shoulder Dystocia

- Fetal macrosomia
- Maternal diabetes mellitus
- Delayed active phase of labor
- Prolonged second stage of labor
- Operative vaginal delivery

TABLE 19.5 Management of Shoulder Dystocia	
Maneuver	**Desired Result**
Suprapubic pressure	Anterior shoulder dislodged from above pubic symphysis
Hyperflexion of maternal thighs alongside abdomen (McRoberts maneuver)	Cephalad rotation of pubic symphysis
Intravaginal pressure on posterior shoulder	Anteroposterior position of shoulders transformed to oblique position
Delivery of posterior arm	Once accomplished, added room permits delivery
Cephalic replacement (Zavanelli maneuver)	Cesarean delivery

a cephalad direction and often frees the impacted shoulder and allows easy delivery. If the McRoberts maneuver is not successful, the 2017 ACOG guidelines recommend attempts to deliver the posterior arm as the next step.[37] Despite previous assumptions to the contrary, vaginal delivery of the head does not necessarily commit one to vaginal birth of the infant. Cephalic replacement (i.e., the Zavanelli maneuver) and cesarean delivery must be considered as a last resort. If all measures have failed, the position of the vertex is rotated back to the position prior to external rotation (usually occiput anterior), flexion is achieved, and the head is elevated, which may be facilitated by tocolysis (e.g., sublingual nitroglycerin 0.4 mg, intravenous nitroglycerin 100 µg, subcutaneous or intravenous terbutaline 0.25 mg, or general anesthesia with a volatile anesthetic agent). After the fetal head has been placed back into the vagina, prompt cesarean delivery is performed.[86]

KEY POINTS

- The outcome of labor reflects the interaction of three components: the powers, the passageway, and the passenger.
- Assuming that the fetus is tolerating labor satisfactorily, an important obstetric determination is whether the patient is in the latent or the active phase of the first stage of labor.
- Early amniotomy and intrapartum oxytocin administration shorten labor.
- Oxytocin is a valuable obstetric medication that increases vaginal delivery rates and shortens labor. Higher-dose regimens can be considered.
- Expectant management is the standard choice for the very preterm patient with prelabor rupture of membranes. Induction of labor is generally undertaken in patients exhibiting this condition at term.
- Elective induction of labor is an appropriate choice for all low-risk patients, regardless of cervical favorability; however, this should be an individualized decision between the patient and provider.
- The declining numbers of operative vaginal deliveries may reflect medicolegal concerns and challenges in obstetrical training, rather than new scientific information.

REFERENCES

1. Casey ML, MacDonald PC. Biomedical processes in the initiation of parturition: decidual activation. *Clin Obstet Gynecol*. 1988;31:533–552.
2. Garfield RE. Control of myometrial function in preterm versus term labor. *Clin Obstet Gynecol*. 1984;27:572–591.
3. Lund KJ, McManaman J. Normal labor, delivery, newborn care, and puerperium. In: Gibbs RS, Karlan BY, Haney AF, Nygaard IE, eds. *Danforth's Obstetrics and Gynecology*. 10th ed. Lippincott Williams & Wilkins; 2008:22–42.
4. Pattinson RC, Cuthbert A, Vannevel V. Pelvimetry for fetal cephalic presentations at or near term for deciding on mode of delivery. *Cochrane Database Syst Rev*. 2017;(3):CD000161.
5. Alhafez L, Berghella V. Evidence-based labor management: first stage of labor (part 3). *Am J Obstet Gynecol MFM*. 2020;2:100185.
6. Lundborg L, Aberg K, Sandstrom A, et al. First stage progression in women with spontaneous onset of labor: a large population-based cohort study. *PLoS One*. 2020;15:e0239724.
7. Friedman EA. *Labor: Clinical Evaluation and Management*. 2nd ed. Appleton-Century-Crofts; 1978.
8. Peisner DB, Rosen MG. Transition from latent to active labor. *Obstet Gynecol*. 1986;68:448–451.

9. Zhang J, Landy HJ, Branch DW, et al. For the consortium on safe labor. Contemporary patterns of spontaneous labor with normal neonatal outcomes. *Obstet Gynecol*. 2010;116:1281–1287.
10. Zhang J, Troendle J, Yancey M. Reassessing the labor curve in nulliparous women. *Am J Obstet Gynecol*. 2002;187:824–828.
11. American College of Obstetricians and Gynecologists. Clinical practice guideline No. 8: First and second stage labor management. *Obstet Gynecol*. 2024;143:144–162.
12. Limas MM, Shah SC, Turrentine MA. Cesarean delivery rate in nulliparous women in the second stage of labor when using Zhang compared with Friedman labor curves: a systematic review and meta-analysis. *Obstet Gynecol*. 2023;141:1089–1097.
13. Thuillier C, Roy S, Peyronnet V, et al. Impact of recommended changes in labor management for prevention of the primary cesarean delivery. *Am J Obstet Gynecol*. 2018;218:341.e1–e9.
14. Bishop EH. Pelvic scoring for elective induction. *Obstet Gynecol*. 1964;24:266–268.
15. Rouse DJ, Weiner SJ, Bloom SL, et al. for the Eunice Kennedy Shriver National Institute of Child Health and Human Development (NICHD) Maternal-Fetal Medicine Units Network (MFMU). Failed labor induction: toward an objective diagnosis. *Obstet Gynecol*. 2011;117:267–272.

16. Chelmow D, Kilpatrick SJ, Laros RK. Maternal and neonatal outcomes after prolonged latent phase. *Obstet Gynecol.* 1993;81:486–491.

17. Henry DE, Cheng YW, Shaffer BL, et al. Perinatal outcomes in the setting of active phase arrest of labor. *Obstet Gynecol.* 2008;112:1109–1115.

18. Bottoms SF, Hirsch VJ, Sokol RJ. Medical management of arrest disorders of labor: a current overview. *Am J Obstet Gynecol.* 1987;156:935–939.

19. Friedman EA. Patterns of labor as indicators of risk. *Clin Obstet Gynecol.* 1973;16:172–183.

20. Blankenship SA, Raghuraman N, Delhi A, et al. Associaion of abnormal first stage of labor duration and maternal and neonatal morbidity. *Am J Obstet Gynecol.* 2020;223:445.e1–e15.

21. Harper LM, Caughey AB, Roehl KA, et al. Defining an abnormal first stage of labor based on maternal and neonatal outcomes. *Am J Obstet Gynecol.* 2014;210:536.e1–e7.

22. O'Driscoll K, Meagher D. *Active Management of Labour: The Dublin Experience.* 2nd ed. Baillière Tindall; 1986.

23. Satin AJ, Leveno KJ, Sherman ML, et al. High versus low dose oxytocin for labor stimulation. *Obstet Gynecol.* 1992;80:111–116.

24. Xenakis EM, Langer O, Piper JM, et al. Low-dose versus high-dose oxytocin augmentation of labor: a randomized trial. *Am J Obstet Gynecol.* 1995;173:1874–1878.

25. Satin AJ, Hankins GDV, Yeomans ER. A prospective study of two dosing regimens of oxytocin for the induction of labor in patients with unfavorable cervices. *Am J Obstet Gynecol.* 1991;165:980–984.

26. Merrill DC, Zlatnik FJ. Randomized, double-masked comparison of oxytocin dosage in induction and augmentation of labor. *Obstet Gynecol.* 1999;94:455–463.

27. Kenyon S, Tokumasu H, Dowswell T, et al. High dose versus low dose oxytocin for augmentation of delayed labour. *Cochrane Database Syst Rev.* 2013;(7):CD007201.

28. Wei SQ, Luo ZC, Qi HP, et al. High-dose vs low-dose oxytocin for labor augmentation: a systematic review. *Am J Obstet Gynecol.* 2010;203:296–304.

29. Battarbee AN, Palatnik A, Peress DA, Grobman WA. Association of early amniotomy after Foley balloon catheter ripening and duration of nulliparous labor induction. *Obstet Gynecol.* 2016;128:592–597.

30. Macones GA, Cahill A, Stamilio DM, Odibo AO. The efficacy of early amniotomy in nulliparous labor induction: a randomized controlled trial. *Am J Obstet Gynecol.* 2012;207:403.e1–e5.

31. Kim SW, Nasioudis D, Levine LD. Role of early amniotomy with induced labor: a systematic review of literature and meta-analysis. *Am J Obstet Gynecol MFM.* 2019;1:100052.

32. Allen VM, Baskett TF, O'Connell CM, et al. Maternal and perinatal outcomes with increasing duration of the second stage of labor. *Obstet Gynecol.* 2009;113:1248–1258.

33. Rouse DJ, Weiner SJ, Bloom SL, et al. Second stage labor duration in nulliparous women: relationship to maternal and perinatal outcomes. Eunice Kennedy Shriver National Institute of Child Human Development Maternal-Fetal Medicine Units Network. *Am J Obstet Gynecol.* 2009;201:357.

34. Carlson JM, Diehl JA, Sachtleben-Murray M, et al. Maternal position during parturition in normal labor. *Obstet Gynecol.* 1986;68:443–447.

35. American College of Obstetricians and Gynecologists. Practice Bulletin No. 198: Prevention and management of obstetric lacerations at vaginal delivery (reaffirmed 2022). *Obstet Gynecol.* 2018;132:e87–e102.

36. Hartmann K, Viswanathan M, Palmieri R, et al. Outcomes of routine episiotomy: a systematic review. *JAMA.* 2005;293:2141–2148.

37. American College of Obstetricians and Gynecologists. Practice Bulletin No. 178: Shoulder dystocia (reaffirmed 2024). *Obstet Gynecol.* 2017;129:e123–e133.

38. Cahill AG, Srinivas SK, Tita ATN, et al. Effect of immediate vs delayed pushing on rates of spontaneous vaginal delivery among nulliparous women receiving neuraxial analgesia: a randomized clinical trial. *JAMA.* 2018;320:1444–1454.

39. Frolova AI, Sout MJ, Tuuli MG, et al. Duration of the third stage of labor and risk of postpartum hemorrhage. *Obstet Gynecol.* 2016;127:951–956.

40. American College of Obstetricians and Gynecologists. Practice Bulletin No. 183: Postpartum hemorrhage (reaffirmed 2024). *Obstet Gynecol.* 2017;130:e168–e186.

41. Hayashi RH, Castillo MS, Noah ML. Management of severe postpartum hemorrhage due to uterine atony using an analogue of prostaglandin F2 alpha. *Obstet Gynecol.* 1981;58:426–429.

42. Pacheco LD, Clifton RG, Saade GR, et al. Tranexamic acid to prevent obstetrical hemorrhage after cesarean delivery. *N Engl J Med.* 2023;388:1365–1375.

43. Jackson KW, Allbert JR, Schemmer GK, et al. A randomized controlled trial comparing oxytocin administration before and after placental delivery in the prevention of postpartum hemorrhage. *Am J Obstet Gynecol.* 2001;185:873–877.

44. Malee MP. Expectant and active management of preterm premature rupture of membranes. *Obstet Gynecol Clin North Am.* 1992;19:309–315.

45. American College of Obstetricians and Gynecologists. Practice Bulletin, Number 217: Prelabor rupture of membranes (reaffirmed 2023). *Obstet Gynecol.* 2020;135:e80–e97.

46. Mercer BM, Miodovnik M, Thurnau GR, et al. for the National Institute of Child Health and Human Development Maternal-Fetal Medicine Units Network. Antibiotic therapy for reduction of infant morbidity after preterm premature rupture of the membranes: a randomized controlled trial. *JAMA.* 1997;278:989–995.

47. American College of Obstetricians and Gynecologists. Practice Bulletin No. 199: Use of prophylactic antibiotics in labor and delivery (reaffirmed 2025). *Obstet Gynecol.* 2018;132:e103–e119.

48. Mercier BM. Is there a role for tocolytic therapy during conservative management of preterm premature rupture of membranes? *Clin Obstet Gynecol.* 2007;50:487–496.

49. American College of Obstetricians and Gynecologists. Practice Bulletin No. 172: Premature rupture of membranes. *Obstet Gynecol.* 2016;128:e165–e177.

50. Zlatnik FJ. Management of premature rupture of membranes at term. *Obstet Gynecol Clin North Am.* 1992;19:353–364.

51. Aziz N, Cheng YW, Caughey AB. Factors and outcomes associated with longer latency in preterm premature rupture of membranes. *J Matern Fetal Neonatal Med.* 2008;21:821–825.

52. Melamed N, Berghella V, Ananth CV, et al. Optimal timing of labor induction after prelabor rupture of membranes at term: a secondary analysis of the TERMPROM study. *Am J Obstet Gynecol.* 2023;228:326.e1–e13.

53. Gibbs RS, Dinsmoor MJ, Newton ER, Ramamurthy RS. A randomized trial of intrapartum versus immediate postpartum treatment of women with intra-amniotic infection. *Obstet Gynecol.* 1988;72:823–828.

54. American College of Obstetricians and Gynecologists. Committee Opinion No. 712: Intrapartum management of intraamniotic infection (reaffirmed 2022). *Obstet Gynecol.* 2017;130:e95–e101.

55. Gibbs RS, Castillo MS, Rodgers PJ. Management of acute chorioamnionitis. *Am J Obstet Gynecol.* 1980;136:709–713.

56. Hauth JC, Gilstrap LC, Hankins GDV, Connor KD. Term maternal and neonatal complications of acute chorioamnionitis. *Obstet Gynecol.* 1985;66:59–62.

57. Rouse DJ, Landon M, Leveno KJ, et al. The Maternal-Fetal Medicine Units cesarean registry: chorioamnionitis at term and its duration-relationship to outcomes. *Am J Obstet Gynecol.* 2004;191:211–216.

58. Friedman EA, Niswander KR, Bayonet-Rivera NP, Sachtleben MR. Relation of prelabor evaluation to inducibility and the course of labor. *Obstet Gynecol.* 1966;28:495–501.

59. Berghella V, Bellussi F, Schoen CN. Evidence-based labor management: induction of labor (part 2). *Am J Obstet Gynecol MFM.* 2020;2:100136.

60. American College of Obstetricians and Gynecologists. Practice Bulletin No. 107: Induction of labor (reaffirmed 2024). *Obstet Gynecol.* 2009;114:386–397.

61. Bernstein P. Prostaglandin E2 gel for cervical ripening and labour induction: a multicentre placebo-controlled trial. *Can Med Assoc J.* 1991;145:1249–1254.

62. Hofmeyr GJ, Gülmezoglu AM, Pileggi C. Vaginal misoprostol for cervical ripening and induction of labour. *Cochrane Database Syst Rev.* 2010;(10):CD000941.

63. Rayburn WF, Zhang J. Rising rates of labor induction: present concerns and future strategies. *Obstet Gynecol.* 2002;100:164–167.

64. Walker KF, Bugg GJ, Macpherson M, et al. Randomized trial of labor induction in women 35 years of age or older. *N Engl J Med.* 2016;374:813–822.

65. Grobman WA, Rice MM, Reddy UM, for the Eunice Kennedy Shriver National Institute of Child Health and Human Development Maternal-Fetal Medicine Units Network. Labor induction versus expectant management in low-risk nulliparous women. *N Engl J Med.* 2018;379:513–522.

66. Grobman WA, Caughey AB. Elective induction of labor at 39 weeks compared with expectant management: a meta-analysis of cohort studies. *Am J Obstet Gynecol.* 2019;221:304–310.

67. Ausbeck EB, Jauk VC, Xue Y, et al. Outpatient Foley catheter for induction of labor in nulliparous women: a randomized controlled trial. *Obstet Gynecol.* 2020;136:597–606.

68. Kuper SG, Jauk VC, George DM, et al. Outpatient Foley catheter for induction of labor in parous women: a randomized controlled trial. *Obstet Gynecol.* 2018;132:94–101.

69. Pierce-Williams R, Lesser H, Saccone G, et al. Outpatient cervical ripening with balloon catheters: a systematic review and meta-analysis. *Obstet Gynecol.* 2022;139:255–268.

70. Merriam AA, Ananth CV, Wright JD, et al. Trends in operative vaginal delivery, 2005-2013: a population-based study. *BJOG.* 2017;124:1365–1372.

71. American College of Obstetricians and Gynecologists. Practice Bulletin Number 219: Operative vaginal birth (reaffirmed 2025). *Obstet Gynecol.* 2020;135:e149–e159.

72. Yeomans ER. Operative vaginal delivery. *Obstet Gynecol.* 2010;115:645–653.

73. Bashore RA, Phillips WH, Brinkman CR. A comparison of the morbidity of midforceps and cesarean delivery. *Am J Obstet Gynecol.* 1990;162:1428–1434.

74. Robertson PA, Laros RK, Zhao RL. Neonatal and maternal outcome in low-pelvic and midpelvic operative deliveries. *Am J Obstet Gynecol.* 1990;162:1436–1442.

75. Berkus MD, Ramamurthy RS, O'Connor PS, et al. Cohort study of silastic obstetric vacuum cup deliveries. I. Safety of the instrument. *Obstet Gynecol.* 1985;66:503–509.

76. Dell DL, Sightler SE, Plauche WC. Soft cup vacuum extraction: a comparison of outlet delivery. *Obstet Gynecol.* 1985;66:624–628.

77. Broekhuizen FF, Washington JM, Johnson F, Hamilton PR. Vacuum extraction versus forceps delivery: indications and complications, 1979-1984. *Obstet Gynecol.* 1987;69:338–342.

78. Williams MC, Knuppel RA, O'Brien WF, et al. A randomized comparison of assisted vaginal delivery by obstetric forceps and polyethylene vacuum cup. *Obstet Gynecol.* 1991;78:789–794.

79. Skinner S, Davies-Tuck M, Wallace E, Hodges R. Perinatal and maternal outcomes after training residents in forceps before vacuum instrumental birth. *Obstet Gynecol.* 2017;130:151–158.

80. Weiner CP. Vaginal breech delivery in the 1990s. *Clin Obstet Gynecol.* 1992;35:559–569.

81. Hannah ME, Hannah WJ, Hewson SA, et al., for the Term Breech Trial Collaborative Group. Planned caesarean section versus planned vaginal birth for breech presentation at term: a randomized multicentre trial. *Lancet.* 2000;356:1375–1383.

82. American College of Obstetricians and Gynecologists. Committee Opinion No. 745: Mode of term singleton breech delivery (reaffirmed 2023). *Obstet Gynecol.* 2018;132:e60–e63.

83. O'Leary JA, Leonetti HB. Shoulder dystocia: prevention and treatment. *Am J Obstet Gynecol.* 1990;162:5–9.

84. Gross TL, Sokol RJ, Williams T, Thompson K. Shoulder dystocia: a fetal-physician risk. *Am J Obstet Gynecol.* 1987;156:1408–1414.

85. Langer O, Berkus MD, Huff RW, Samueloff A. Shoulder dystocia: should the fetus weighing 4000 grams be delivered by cesarean section? *Am J Obstet Gynecol.* 1991;165:831–837.

86. Sandberg EC. The Zavanelli maneuver: 12 years of recorded experience. *Obstet Gynecol.* 1999;93:312–317.

20

Trial of Labor and Vaginal Birth After Cesarean Delivery

Britany L. Raymond, MD and David H. Chestnut, MD

In 1916, Edward Cragin[1] stated, "Once a cesarean, always a cesarean." This edict has had a profound effect on obstetric practice. Cesarean delivery is now the most frequently performed major surgery in the United States, with rates increasing from 5.5% of all deliveries in 1970 to 32.1% in 2021 (Fig. 20.1).[2] This rapid acceleration is primarily driven by an increase in the number of primary cesarean deliveries and is influenced by the vaginal birth after cesarean (VBAC) rate.[3] The overall cesarean rate is likely to continue rising, as the majority of women who undergo a primary cesarean will elect for a repeat cesarean with subsequent deliveries.[2]

For many years, most US physicians ignored Cragin's subsequent statement, "Many exceptions occur."[1] In 1981, the National Institute of Child Health and Human Development Conference on Childbirth concluded that VBAC is an appropriate option for many women.[4] In 1991, Rosen et al.[5] modified Cragin's original dictum as follows: "Once a cesarean, a trial of labor should precede a second cesarean except in the most unusual circumstances." In 1988 and again in 1994, the American College of Obstetricians and Gynecologists (ACOG)[6] concluded:

> *The concept of routine repeat cesarean birth should be replaced by a specific decision process between the patient and the physician for a subsequent mode of delivery.... In the absence of a contraindication, a woman with one previous cesarean delivery with a lower uterine segment incision should be counseled and encouraged to undergo a trial of labor in her current pregnancy.*

In just a few short years following the ACOG's support, the VBAC rate rose to its highest ever at 28.3% in 1996, contributing to a significant reduction in the overall cesarean delivery rate across the country.[7] However, the safety of trial of labor after cesarean (TOLAC) came under scrutiny as cases of uterine rupture and complications were reported.[8,9] In response, the ACOG[10] cautioned that TOLACs should be limited to institutions with appropriate emergency equipment, and further stated that physicians should be *immediately* available, rather than *readily* available. Subsequently, the VBAC rates sharply declined to 9.2% in 2004 and have yet to fully recover[2,7] despite a 2010 National Institutes of Health (NIH) consensus development conference statement supporting TOLAC as a reasonable option for many pregnant women with one prior low transverse uterine incision.[11]

PRIMARY CESAREAN DELIVERY: CHOICE OF UTERINE INCISION

Obstetric practice in 1916 hardly resembled obstetric practice today. In 1916, only 1% to 2% of all infants were delivered by cesarean. Most cesarean deliveries were performed in patients with a contracted bony pelvis, and obstetricians uniformly performed a classic uterine incision (i.e., a long vertical incision in the upper portion of the uterus) (Fig. 20.2). In 1922, De Lee and Cornell[12] advocated the performance of a vertical incision in the lower uterine segment. Unfortunately, low-vertical

Temporal Trends of Cesarean Delivery and VBAC Rates in the United States

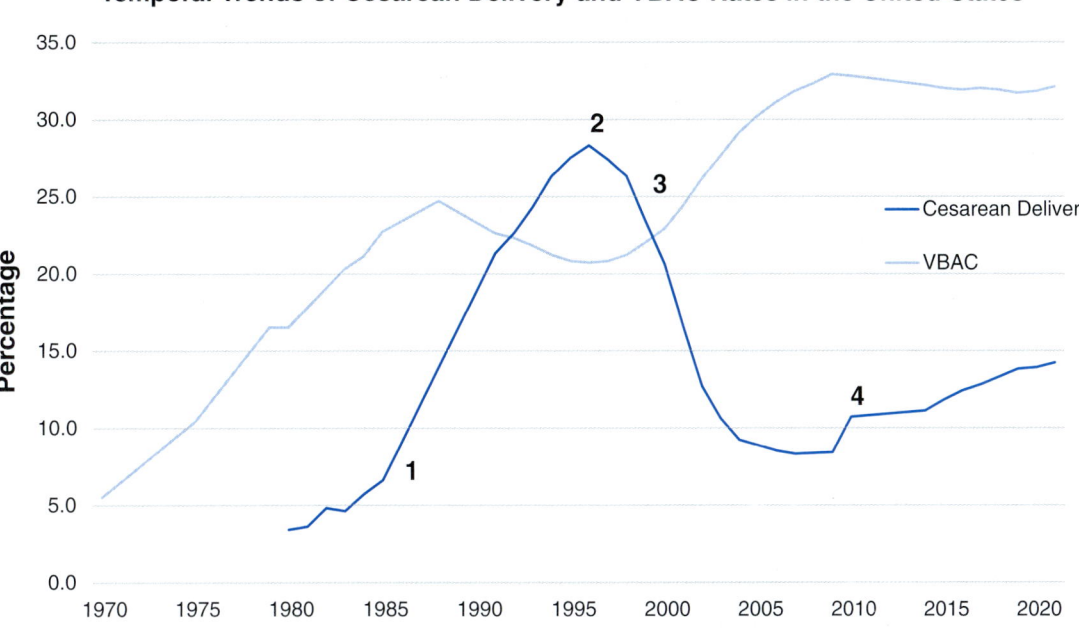

Fig. 20.1 Temporal trends of cesarean delivery and vaginal birth after cesarean (VBAC) rates in the context of the release of important publications and professional guidelines. 1 (1988): The American College of Obstetricians and Gynecologists (ACOG) news release encourages VBAC, noting a previous cesarean is not an indication for performing a repeat cesarean. 2 (1996): Publication of McMahon et al. landmark study in the *New England Journal of Medicine* describing adverse maternal and neonatal outcomes during attempted VBAC. 3 (1999): The ACOG updates its Practice Bulletin to recommend that emergency staff be "immediately available" at centers offering VBAC. 4 (2010): National Institutes of Health (NIH) Consensus Panel Statement released, "Vaginal birth after cesarean: new insights." Data are summarized from (1) Centers for Disease Control and Prevention (CDC). Rates of cesarean delivery–United States, 1993. *MMWR Morb Mortal Wkly Rep* 1995;44:303–307. (2) Osterman MJK, Hamilton BE, Martin JA, Driscoll AK, Valenzuela CP. *Births: Final Data for 2022.* National Vital Statistics National Center for Health Statistics Reports; 2024; https://doi.org/10.15620/cdc:145588. Accessed 14 March 2025. (3) Taffel SM, Placek PJ, Liss T. Trends in the United States cesarean section rate and reasons for the 1980-85 rise. *Am J Public Health.* 1987;77:955–5990.

incisions rarely are confined to the lower uterine segment. Such incisions often extend to the body of the uterus, which does not heal as well as the lower uterine segment. Kerr[13] later advocated the performance of a low-transverse uterine incision (see Fig. 20.2). A low-transverse uterine incision results in less blood loss and is easier to repair than a classic uterine incision.[14] Further, a low-transverse uterine incision is more likely to heal satisfactorily and to maintain its integrity during a subsequent pregnancy. Thus, obstetricians prefer to make a low-transverse uterine incision during most cesarean deliveries.

Obstetricians reserve the low-vertical incision for patients whose lower uterine segment does not have enough width to allow safe delivery. Preterm parturients may have a narrow lower uterine segment. In these patients, delivery through a transverse uterine incision may cause an extension of the incision into the vessels of the broad ligament. For example, a patient with preterm labor at 26 weeks' gestation may undergo cesarean delivery because of a breech presentation, and the obstetrician may perform a low-vertical incision to facilitate an atraumatic delivery of the fetal head.

Obstetricians rarely perform a classic uterine incision in modern obstetric practice, as it places the patient at high risk

for catastrophic uterine rupture during a subsequent pregnancy.[15] Such uterine rupture may occur before or during labor, and it often results in maternal and perinatal morbidity or mortality. An obstetrician may perform a classic uterine incision when the need for extensive intrauterine manipulation of the fetus (e.g., delivery of a fetus with a transverse lie) is anticipated. Some obstetricians prefer a classic uterine incision in patients with an anterior placenta previa. In such cases, the performance of a classic incision allows the obstetrician to avoid cutting through the placenta, which might result in significant hemorrhage. The obstetrician may perform a classic uterine incision in women with morbid obesity in whom it is difficult to expose the lower uterine segment, especially when the skin incision is supraumbilical.

ELIGIBILITY AND SELECTION CRITERIA

The ACOG[15] has concluded that "most women with one previous cesarean delivery with a low-transverse incision are candidates for and should be counseled about and offered TOLAC."

Most studies suggest a high likelihood of success with TOLAC, averaging around 68.4%.[16] Wu et al.[16] performed a

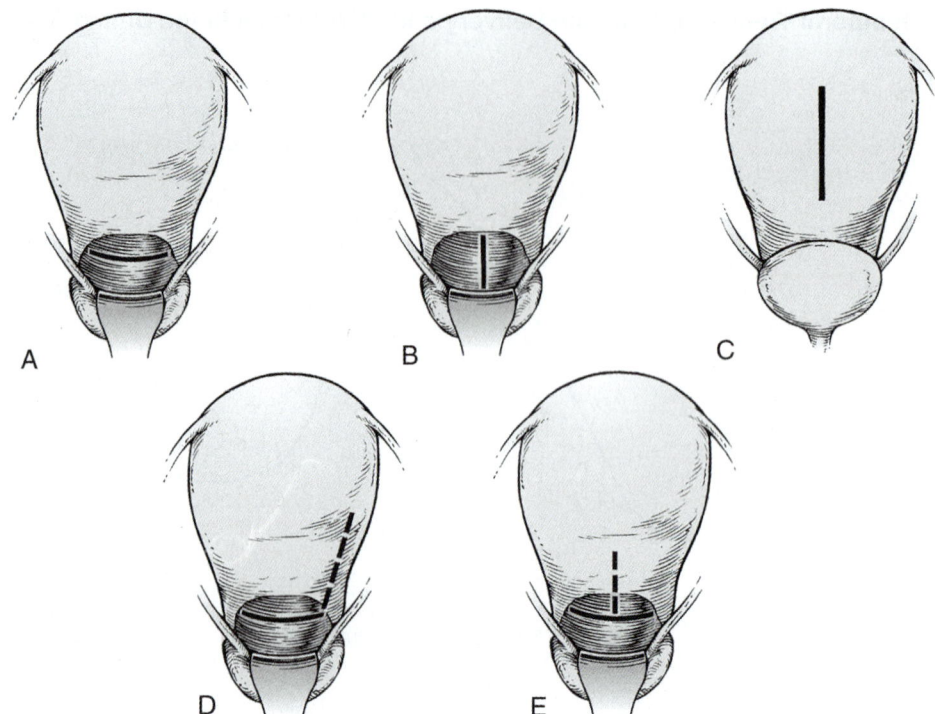

Fig. 20.2 Uterine Incisions for Cesarean Delivery. (A) Low-transverse incision. The bladder is retracted downward, and the incision is made in the lower uterine segment, curving gently upward. If the lower segment is poorly developed, the incision also can curve sharply upward at each end to avoid extending into the ascending branches of the uterine arteries. (B) Low-vertical incision. The incision is made vertically in the lower uterine segment after reflection of the bladder, with avoidance of extension into the bladder below. If more room is needed, the incision can be extended upward into the upper uterine segment. (C) Classic incision. The incision is entirely within the upper uterine segment and can be at the level shown or in the fundus. (D) J-shaped incision. If more room is needed when an initial transverse incision has been made, either end of the incision can be extended upward into the upper uterine segment and parallel to the ascending branch of the uterine artery. (E) T-shaped incision. More room can be obtained in a transverse incision by an upward midline extension into the upper uterine segment. From Berghella V, MacKeen AD, Jauniaux E. Cesarean delivery. In: Landon MB, Gatan HL, Jauniaux ERM, et al., eds. *Gabbe's Obstetrics: Normal and Problem Pregnancies.* 8th ed. Elsevier;2021:375–394.

BOX 20.1 Predictors of VBAC Success

- History of a previous VBAC
- High Bishop score upon admission
- Prior vaginal birth before cesarean
- Fetal malpresentation as the indication for previous cesarean
- White race

VBAC, Vaginal birth after cesarean.
Data from Wu Y, Kataria Y, Wang Z, et al. Factors associated with successful vaginal birth after a cesarean section: a systematic review and meta-analysis. *BMC Pregnancy Childbirth.* 2019;19:360.

---

metaanalysis of 94 studies to examine factors associated with successful VBAC. History of a previous VBAC was associated with the highest rate of success (Box 20.1). Other positively associated factors included a higher Bishop score upon admission (see Chapter 19) and a prior vaginal birth before cesarean. A history of dystocia or arrest of labor necessitating a previous cesarean was associated with the lowest adjusted odds of success. Other factors associated with decreased odds of success included diabetes mellitus, non-White race, fetal macrosomia, and dystocia or failure to progress as the indication for a prior cesarean.

Investigators have developed scoring systems for predicting the success or failure of TOLAC. Grobman et al.[17] developed a nomogram specifically for women undergoing TOLAC at term gestation with one previous low-transverse cesarean delivery, a singleton gestation, and a vertex fetal presentation. The original nomogram incorporated six variables that may be ascertained at the first prenatal visit; these variables included maternal age, body mass index, race and ethnicity, prior vaginal delivery, prior VBAC, and a recurring indication for cesarean delivery. This model was validated in multiple subsequent studies.[18-20] In 2021, recognizing that differences in outcome by race reflect systemic racism and social determinants of health, Grobman et al. reanalyzed the data without including race and ethnicity as independent variables.[21] An online version of the updated VBAC calculator tool is now available.[22] One calculator can be used in early pregnancy, and a second calculator that includes gestational age and details of the cervical examination can be used on admission for delivery.[22]

Previous Low-Vertical Incision

Some obstetricians allow a trial of labor after a previous low-vertical uterine incision provided that there is documentation that the uterine incision was confined to the lower uterine segment (low-vertical uterine incisions often extend above the lower uterine segment, especially when performed in preterm patients). Martin et al.[23] reviewed the obstetric literature to summarize outcomes among women who attempted VBAC after a previous low-vertical cesarean delivery. The authors were able to identify 10 studies reporting the complete outcomes for 372 patients. Although four (1%) uterine ruptures were described, only two ruptures involved the previous low-vertical incision; the other two ruptures occurred at uterine sites anatomically remote from the previous scar. Therefore, the authors concluded that a low-vertical incision that does not extend beyond the lower uterine segment should not be a contraindication to TOLAC in uncomplicated singleton pregnancies. The ACOG[15] concluded that there is no consistent evidence of an increased risk for uterine rupture in women with a previous low-vertical uterine incision and that obstetricians and patients may choose to undergo TOLAC in the presence of a documented prior low-vertical uterine incision.

Unknown Uterine Scar

For some patients, there is no documentation of the type of uterine incision performed during a previous cesarean delivery. Some obstetricians require documentation of the type of previous uterine incision before they allow a patient to attempt VBAC. Smith et al.[24] found that the incidence of uterine rupture did not differ in women with an unknown scar compared to those with a known low-transverse uterine incision. An explanation for this finding is that most patients with an unknown uterine scar have a low-transverse uterine incision scar from the previous cesarean delivery. Ultrasonography may help the obstetrician confirm the presence of a low-transverse uterine scar in the pregnant woman with an unknown uterine scar.[25] The ACOG[15] concluded that "women with one previous cesarean delivery with an unknown uterine scar type may be candidates for TOLAC, unless there is a high clinical suspicion of a previous classical uterine incision, such as cesarean delivery performed at an extremely preterm gestational age."

History of More Than One Cesarean Delivery

Results of studies that have assessed outcomes of TOLAC in women with a history of more than one cesarean delivery are inconsistent. One large multicenter study found no increased risk for uterine rupture (0.9% versus 0.7%) in women with more than one previous cesarean delivery compared to women with only one previous cesarean delivery.[26] A second large study observed that the risk for uterine rupture increased from 0.9% to 1.8% during TOLAC in women with two previous cesarean deliveries.[27] Both studies observed that TOLAC was associated with an increase in maternal morbidity in women with more than one previous cesarean delivery, although the absolute magnitude of the difference in morbidity was relatively small.[26,27] Data regarding the risk for TOLAC in women with more than two previous cesarean deliveries are limited.[28] The ACOG[15] concluded that it is reasonable to consider TOLAC for women with two previous low-transverse cesarean deliveries. The Royal College of Obstetricians and Gynaecologists (RCOG)[29] stated that "women who have had two or more prior lower segment caesarean deliveries may be offered VBAC after counseling by a senior obstetrician," while the Society of Obstetricians and Gynaecologists of Canada (SOGC) advises that "women with 2 prior Caesarean sections appear to have similar vaginal birth after Caesarean rates as those with 1 prior Caesarean section. Women should be informed of a higher risk of uterine rupture in trial of labor after Caesarean with more than 1 Caesarean section."[30] The VBAC prediction model developed for singleton gestation was found to be valid for predicting VBAC success in women with two prior cesarean deliveries.[31]

Twin Gestation

Some obstetricians believe that uterine overdistention, which occurs with twin gestation, increases the risk for uterine rupture in patients with a history of previous cesarean delivery. Studies consistently suggest otherwise but are limited by the small number of patients.[32,33] Cahill et al.[34] performed a retrospective cohort study of 25,005 obstetric patients with at least one previous cesarean delivery, which included 535 patients with a twin pregnancy. The investigators observed that women with a twin gestation were less likely to attempt VBAC, but were no more likely to have a failed VBAC or to experience major morbidity than women with a singleton gestation. Likewise, a report from the Maternal-Fetal Medicine Unit Cesarean Registry[35] included outcome measures for 186 women with a twin gestation who attempted VBAC; 120 (64.5%) delivered vaginally. Women who attempted TOLAC with twin gestation had no higher risk for transfusion, endometritis, intensive care unit admission, or uterine rupture than women who underwent elective repeat cesarean delivery. The investigators concluded that TOLAC in women with a twin gestation after previous cesarean delivery does not appear to be associated with a higher risk for maternal morbidity.[35]

In contrast, another large population study by Ford et al.[36] reported a statistically significant increase in uterine rupture rate associated with TOLAC compared with elective cesarean delivery for twin gestation. The authors reviewed outcomes of 6555 women with a twin gestation who delivered between 1993 and 2002. Among 1850 women who underwent TOLAC, 836 (45.2%) delivered vaginally. The rate of uterine rupture was higher in the TOLAC group compared to the elective cesarean delivery group (0.9% versus 0.1%), but the rate of wound complications was lower in the TOLAC group (0.6% versus 1.3%).

The ACOG[15] concluded that "women with one previous cesarean delivery with a low-transverse [uterine] incision, who are otherwise appropriate candidates for twin vaginal delivery, are considered candidates for TOLAC." While the SOGC guidelines[30] are aligned with the ACOG, the RCOG[29] takes a more conservative approach, stating that "there is uncertainty about the safety and efficacy of planned VBAC in pregnancies complicated by … twin gestation."

Suspected Macrosomia

The ACOG's stance on macrosomia (fetal weight > 4000 g) and TOLAC eligibility has shifted over the years. In 1994 the ACOG[6] concluded that macrosomia does not contraindicate TOLAC. However, in 1999, the ACOG[10] revised its recommendations to include suspected macrosomia on the list of TOLAC eligibility criteria that are controversial. While macrosomia is well established as a risk factor associated with reduced success rates of TOLAC,[16,37,38] studies examining the incidence of uterine rupture report conflicting results.[37,39,40] The 2019 ACOG guidelines[15] encourage providers to consider current fetal weight relative to past birth weights, but concluded that "suspected macrosomia alone should not preclude the possibility of TOLAC."

Gestation Beyond 40 Weeks

Studies have consistently demonstrated decreased rates of successful VBAC in women who undergo TOLAC after 40 weeks' gestation.[41-43] The largest study[42] assessing the incidence of uterine rupture in women with advanced gestation undergoing TOLAC did not report an elevated risk in this population. The ACOG[15] acknowledges that the likelihood of successful VBAC may be diminished in more advanced gestations, but a "gestational age greater than 40 weeks alone should not preclude TOLAC."

Breech Presentation and External Cephalic Version

Breech presentation itself does not increase the risk for uterine rupture. In contemporary practice, most obstetricians do not allow a trial of labor in *any* patient with a breech presentation. Thus, most patients with a breech presentation undergo elective cesarean delivery, with or without a history of previous cesarean delivery. The ACOG[15] concluded that external cephalic version is not contraindicated in women with breech presentation and a previous low-transverse uterine incision who are at low risk for adverse maternal and neonatal outcomes from external cephalic version and TOLAC.

Social Factors and Counseling

Some women reject TOLAC because they have experienced prolonged, painful labor during a previous pregnancy. They fear that they will again experience a prolonged, painful labor and ultimately need a repeat cesarean delivery. This fear is more common in women who have delivered in smaller hospitals without the availability of neuraxial analgesia during labor. Other women reject TOLAC because they prefer to schedule the date of elective repeat cesarean delivery, permitting prearrangement of responsibilities such as childcare. Kirk et al.[44] questioned 160 women regarding factors affecting their choice between TOLAC and elective repeat cesarean delivery. These investigators concluded that "social exigencies appeared to play a more important role than an assessment of the medical risks in making these decisions." Similarly,

Joseph et al.[45] observed that fear and inconvenience are the most common deterrents to attempted VBAC. Finally, some women reject TOLAC because of their concern about the adverse effects of labor and vaginal delivery on the maternal pelvic floor, with the risk for subsequent problems such as urinary and fecal incontinence.

A lack of appropriate education and counseling may also contribute to low TOLAC rates. Several survey studies have reported that TOLAC-eligible women are not adequately informed about the risks and benefits of TOLAC compared with elective repeat cesarean delivery.[46-48] Bernstein et al.[47] found that only 4% of eligible patients electing a repeat cesarean delivery knew that the success rate of TOLAC could be as high as 60% to 80%, and more than half were unaware that the recovery from a cesarean is longer than with vaginal delivery. Alarmingly, one study[46] found that 62% of TOLAC-eligible women had received counseling recommending a repeat elective cesarean delivery without mention of TOLAC, despite having at least three antenatal visits. The impact of patient education cannot be understated; Sindiani et al.[48] reported that the single independent factor that influenced a woman's choice of mode of delivery was whether the woman received counseling on the risks of TOLAC. Women counseled on the risks of TOLAC were four times more likely to elect a TOLAC than those not counseled. Interestingly, some studies have reported that women establish their initial preference for mode of delivery based on outside sources of information and opinion from friends and family; subsequent antenatal counseling by a medical professional had limited effect or influence on their final decision.[49,50] However, provider bias during counseling can have a significant impact, as patients are much more likely to select a mode of delivery if they perceive it to be a strong provider preference.[46,47,50]

Cox[50] discussed and emphasized the importance of shared decision-making when choosing the mode of delivery after a previous cesarean. Patient-centered decision aids[51,52] have been suggested as tools to assist providers and patients in this process, and perhaps improve education in effort to increase the TOLAC rate. However, the PROCEED[51] trial, a multicenter study of 1485 patients, failed to show that use of a decision support tool influenced the TOLAC rate compared with usual care (43.3% versus 46.2%). Regardless of how one approaches a shared decision-making conversation, it is important to include a discussion about a patient's family planning goals, as the risk for a placenta accreta spectrum and major hemorrhage in subsequent pregnancies increases with each cesarean delivery (see Chapter 37).[53] A patient who is planning to have several children should take this into consideration when deciding between TOLAC and repeat cesarean delivery. In 2019, the ACOG[15] emphasized: "After counseling, the ultimate decision to undergo TOLAC or a repeat cesarean delivery should be made by the patient in consultation with her obstetrician or obstetric care provider. The potential risks and benefits of both TOLAC and elective repeat cesarean delivery should be discussed. Documentation of counseling and the management plan should be included in the medical record."

In addition to patient preferences, the low frequency of TOLAC has resulted, in part, from physician preferences. One survey[54] of privately practicing obstetricians revealed the most common reasons for discontinuing TOLAC in their clinical practice included maternal-fetal safety concerns about uterine rupture and medicolegal consequences. Physicians who did not offer TOLAC to their patients were more likely to have been in practice less than 10 years, report previous experience with a morbid uterine rupture, and indicate prior involvement in medical malpractice litigation.

Economic Factors

In many cases, physician reimbursement is greater for elective repeat cesarean delivery than for VBAC, despite the fact that VBAC requires greater physician effort.[55] Stafford[55] reviewed the impact of nonclinical factors on the performance of repeat cesarean delivery in California. He observed that "proprietary hospitals, with the greatest incentive to maximize reimbursement, had the highest repeat cesarean [delivery] rates." Nonteaching hospitals and hospitals with low-volume obstetric services had lower VBAC rates than teaching hospitals and hospitals with high-volume obstetric services. Likewise, Hueston and Rudy[56] found that women who undergo elective repeat cesarean delivery are more likely to have private insurance than women who attempt VBAC. Stafford[55] concluded: "Because a cesarean [delivery] is nearly twice as costly as a vaginal birth, … the higher repeat cesarean [delivery] rates associated with proprietary hospitals, non-teaching hospitals, and low-volume hospitals contribute to increased health care expenditures." Furthermore, a 2017 systematic review by Rogers et al.[57] determined, "After a review of all the available evidence, we conclude that for women who are likely to have a successful vaginal delivery, routine elective repeat cesarean delivery may result in excess morbidity and cost from a population perspective."

From an individual patient perspective, evaluating the cost effectiveness between the two modes of delivery is complex and involves several factors, the most important of which is the likelihood of a successful VBAC. A failed TOLAC requiring a subsequent cesarean delivery may offset any financial benefit initially anticipated, particularly if the delivery becomes an emergency or results in serious maternal or neonatal morbidity. One analytic model examining marginal cost per quality-adjusted life years determined TOLAC to be more cost-effective than an elective repeat cesarean when the predicted VBAC success rate is greater than 47.2%.[58]

Medicolegal Factors

Uterine rupture is one of the most morbid complications of TOLAC. Unfortunately, there is inconsistency and confusion in reports of the incidence of asymptomatic uterine scar dehiscence as opposed to frank uterine rupture. **Uterine scar dehiscence** may be defined as a uterine wall defect that does not result in fetal compromise or maternal hemorrhage and that does not require emergency cesarean delivery or postpartum laparotomy. In contrast, **uterine rupture** may be accompanied by extrusion of the fetus or placenta and results in fetal compromise, maternal hemorrhage, or both, sufficient to require cesarean delivery or postpartum laparotomy.[59]

Obstetricians understandably fear that they will be found liable if an adverse event occurs during TOLAC. In one case, a jury awarded a verdict of $98.5 million because of a delayed diagnosis of uterine rupture.[60] Phelan[61] cited another court decision that he predicted would have a "chilling effect on the future of VBAC." In this case, the fetal heart rate (FHR) was normal until it abruptly decreased to 80 beats per minute at a cervical dilation of 9 cm. The interval between the onset of the FHR deceleration and emergency cesarean delivery was 27 minutes. At delivery, the fetal head was found in the left adnexa. The mother required transfusion, and the child suffered from developmental delay and cerebral palsy. The court found that the defendants were negligent in their failure to deliver the infant in a timely manner and to provide adequate informed consent. The court also concluded that "the ACOG 30-minute rule[62] represented the maximum period of elapse" and did not represent the minimum standard of care. As a result of this verdict, Phelan[61] proposed the use of a VBAC consent form that includes the following statement: "I understand that if my uterus ruptures during my VBAC, there may not be sufficient time to operate and to prevent the death of or permanent brain injury to my baby." Flamm[63] responded that "widespread implementation of this or similar consent forms essentially would mean the end of VBAC."

Greene[64] wrote a sobering editorial on the risks associated with attempted VBAC. Observing that the study performed by Lydon-Rochelle et al.[65] found that spontaneous labor following a cesarean delivery was associated with a tripling of the risk for uterine rupture (i.e., a uterine rupture rate of 5.2 per 1000 women who had spontaneous onset of labor versus 1.6 per 1000 women who underwent elective repeat cesarean delivery without labor), he stated that "there is no reason to believe that improvements in clinical care can substantially reduce the risks of uterine rupture and perinatal mortality." Greene[64] concluded his 2001 editorial as follows:

> After a thorough discussion of the risks and benefits of attempting a vaginal delivery after cesarean section, a patient might ask, "But doctor, what is the safest thing for my baby?" Given the findings of Lydon-Rochelle et al., my unequivocal answer: elective repeat cesarean section.

An analysis of obstetric closed claims cases determined that 80% of claims involving TOLAC could be avoided if TOLAC was offered only to women who present in spontaneous labor, follow a normal labor curve without augmentation, and maintain a favorable FHR tracing.[66] While adoption of this strategy may reduce litigation, its conservative nature would greatly restrict the number of candidates eligible for TOLAC.

Institutional Factors

Most studies of VBAC have been conducted in university or tertiary care hospitals with in-house obstetricians, anesthesia providers, and operating room staff. However, a 2007 study[67] evaluated outcomes for women who attempted VBAC in 17 diverse hospitals, including six university hospitals, five community hospitals with an obstetrics-gynecology residency program, and six community hospitals without an obstetrics-gynecology residency program. The incidence of uterine rupture with attempted VBAC was significantly higher in community hospitals than in university hospitals (1.2% versus 0.6%, respectively), but the rates of maternal blood transfusion and composite adverse maternal outcome were identical in community and university hospitals.[67] However, several studies have demonstrated worse neonatal outcomes when TOLAC is attempted in out-of-hospital birth settings, such as the home or at a birthing center.[68,69]

The ACOG and the Society for Maternal-Fetal Medicine have recommended that attempted VBAC should occur in a level I center or higher (see Table 11.3).[15] Furthermore, the ACOG,[15] RCOG,[29] and SOGC[30] specify that emergency equipment and personnel should be immediately available. Critics have suggested that these guidelines are too restrictive and ultimately limit women's access to TOLAC, particularly at smaller centers and in more rural areas.[70]

Professional Society Practice Guidelines

In 1999, the ACOG[10] issued guidelines stating that because uterine rupture may be catastrophic, TOLAC should be attempted in institutions equipped to respond to emergencies with physicians *immediately* available to provide emergency care. However, the ACOG[10] also noted that "the operational definition of 'immediately available' personnel and facilities remains the purview of each local institution." Likewise, the RCOG[29] has stated that planned VBAC should be conducted in a facility "with resources available for immediate caesarean delivery and advanced neonatal resuscitation."

The 2010 NIH consensus development panel[11] noted that approximately one-third of hospitals and one-half of obstetric physicians in the United States no longer offered TOLAC, largely because of fear of liability and litigation. The panel[11] expressed concern that practice guidelines have created barriers that prevent women from choosing TOLAC and that pregnant women should be given the opportunity to make informed decisions about the risks and benefits of TOLAC versus elective repeat cesarean delivery. The panel[11] also urged professional societies to reassess the requirement for immediate availability of surgical and anesthesia providers.

Subsequently, the ACOG[15] stated that restricting access was not the intention of their "immediately available" requirement. The ACOG[15] noted that "much of the data concerning the safety of TOLAC is from centers capable of performing a timely emergency cesarean delivery." Further, they stated that "although there is reason to think that more rapid availability of cesarean delivery may provide a small incremental benefit in safety, comparative data examining in detail the effect of alternate systems and response times are not available."

Holmgrem et al.[59] reviewed neonatal outcomes of 36 uterine ruptures occurring in 11,195 TOLAC cases from 2000 to 2009. The primary outcome was an Apgar score < 7 or umbilical artery pH < 7.0. The authors emphasized

that mere minutes count; the mean (standard deviation) decision-to-delivery times for neonates with and without adverse outcomes were 23.3 ($\pm$10.8) and 16.0 ($\pm$7.7) minutes, respectively ($P = .02$). In 2018, Al-Zirqi et al.[71] reviewed 41 years of population-based registry data to investigate the infant outcomes after uterine rupture. They concluded that decision-to-delivery time of less than 20 minutes limited the incidence of infant death. In comparison, a decision-to-delivery time > 30 minutes increased the odds of infant death over 16-fold. Birnbach et al.[72] reviewed the impact of anesthesia provider availability on the incidence of VBAC in the United States. They concluded that the "immediately available" requirement necessitates having an in-hospital anesthesia provider who is not performing another simultaneous anesthetic. Their economic analysis prompted a conclusion that "the minimum requirement to provide immediate anesthesia care for all deliveries would be to have all deliveries at facilities with greater than 1500 deliveries annually."

In 2019, the ACOG[15] modified their practice bulletin as follows:

> *Women attempting TOLAC should be cared for in a level I center or higher. Level I facilities must have the ability to begin emergency cesarean delivery within a time interval that best considers maternal and fetal risks and benefits with the provision of emergency care… The decision to offer and pursue TOLAC in a setting in which the option of emergency cesarean delivery is limited should be carefully considered by patients and their obstetricians or other obstetric care providers.*

Further, the ACOG[15] also encourages respect for patient autonomy, as follows:

> *Respect for patient autonomy also dictates that even if a center does not offer TOLAC, such a policy cannot be used to force women to have cesarean delivery or to deny care to women in labor who decline to have a repeat cesarean delivery.*

Similarly, the American Society of Anesthesiologists states, "The immediate availability of appropriate facilities and personnel (including obstetric anesthesia; nursing personnel; and a physician capable of monitoring labor and performing cesarean delivery, including an emergency cesarean delivery) is optimal. When resources for immediate cesarean delivery are not available … patients should be clearly informed of the potential increase in risk and the management alternatives."[73] Finally, the American Academy of Family Physicians practice guidelines state,[74] "Women at risk of uterine rupture or other complications who are still able to consider [TOLAC/VBAC] need to deliver at facilities that have the ability to effectively manage these complications. Information is lacking about how appropriate [TOLAC/VBAC] may be in different types of facilities … thus, there is little guidance about the settings in which to perform [TOLAC/VBAC] when looking at only the type or location of the facility, or the number of deliveries performed."

Contraindications

Contraindications to planned TOLAC include[15]:

- Previous classic or T-shaped incision or extensive transfundal uterine surgery
- Previous uterine rupture
- Medical or obstetric complication that precludes labor and vaginal delivery
- Inability to perform emergency cesarean delivery because of unavailable surgeon, anesthesia provider, or operating room staff (see earlier).

MATERNAL AND NEONATAL OUTCOMES

The highest risk for maternal morbidity and mortality is associated with unsuccessful TOLAC.[11] The ACOG[15] concluded that women with at least a 60% to 70% chance of successful VBAC have equal or less maternal morbidity when they undergo TOLAC than women who undergo elective repeat cesarean delivery. Conversely, the ACOG[15] also noted that women who have a lower than 60% probability of successful VBAC have a greater likelihood of morbidity than women who undergo elective repeat cesarean delivery. Thus, the ability to identify women with a high likelihood of successful VBAC would improve the safety of TOLAC.

Maternal Outcomes

In a 2004 systematic review of published studies of attempted VBAC, Guise et al.[75] observed no significant difference in the incidence of maternal death or hysterectomy between women who attempted a trial of labor and those who underwent repeat cesarean delivery. Uterine rupture was more common in the women who attempted a trial of labor, but the rates of asymptomatic uterine dehiscence did not differ.

Wen et al.[76] performed a retrospective cohort comparison of outcomes after TOLAC or elective repeat cesarean delivery in 308,755 Canadian women with a history of previous cesarean delivery. These investigators observed that the rates of uterine rupture (0.65%), transfusion (0.19%), and hysterectomy (0.10%) were significantly higher in the TOLAC group. However, the maternal in-hospital death rate was significantly lower in the TOLAC group (1.6 per 100,000) than in the elective cesarean delivery group (5.6 per 100,000). Similarly, Guise et al.[77] observed a lower maternal mortality rate in women who underwent TOLAC than in women who underwent elective repeat cesarean delivery (0.004% versus 0.013%, respectively).

Rossi and D'Addario[78] performed a metaanalysis of studies published from 2000 to 2007 that compared maternal morbidity in women who underwent TOLAC versus women who underwent elective repeat cesarean delivery. Successful VBAC occurred in 17,905 (73%) of 24,349 women who underwent TOLAC. Overall maternal morbidity did not differ between women who underwent TOLAC and women who underwent elective repeat cesarean delivery. Likewise, the incidence of blood transfusion and hysterectomy did not differ between the two groups. The incidence of uterine rupture was higher in the TOLAC group (1.3% versus 0.4%). Further, maternal morbidity, uterine rupture, blood transfusion, and hysterectomy were more common in women who had a *failed* TOLAC.

In 2010, the NIH convened a consensus panel[11] to review birth outcomes associated with TOLAC and elective repeat cesarean delivery in developed countries. The panel performed the most comprehensive review of its time, including 41 studies of maternal outcomes and 11 studies of neonatal outcomes. The panel determined the overall benefits of TOLAC "are directly related to having a [successful] VBAC as these women typically have the lowest morbidity." Likewise, the panel noted that the harms of TOLAC "are associated with an unsuccessful trial of labor resulting in cesarean delivery because these deliveries have the highest morbidity." However, the panel concluded that women who undergo TOLAC, regardless of the ultimate mode of delivery, are at decreased risk for maternal mortality compared with women who undergo elective repeat cesarean delivery. The panel also cited low-grade evidence of a shorter hospitalization overall for women attempting TOLAC compared with women undergoing elective repeat cesarean delivery.

In 2022, Fitzpatrick et al.[79] aimed to provide an updated review since the publication of the 2010 NIH consensus panel of the evidence regarding short- and long-term outcomes for women and their children following TOLAC versus elective repeat cesarean delivery. The authors also investigated additional outcomes that were not included in the 2010 review, such as maternal mental health and childhood health problems. The authors identified 47 eligible studies, including 2 randomized controlled trials, 44 cohort studies, and 1 case control study. Since the 2010 review, nine studies reported on maternal mortality. A total of four maternal deaths were reported, all of which occurred in the elective repeat cesarean group. Some 31 studies reported rates of uterine rupture, which varied from 0.00% to 4.8% in the TOLAC group and 0.00% to 2.9% in the elective repeat cesarean group. An increased risk of uterine rupture with TOLAC was reported in 16/31 studies. The risk of rupture was more apparent when labor was induced or augmented. The remaining 15/31 studies found no statistically significant difference between groups, or they reported no uterine ruptures in either group. However, the authors noted that most of these studies were small. Of studies reporting the incidence of hysterectomy, most (12/14) found there was no significant difference in risk between planned mode of delivery.

Outcomes for hemorrhage were more variable, with the authors noting a lack of consistency on the definition of hemorrhage among studies. Overall, the authors identified 18 publications reporting the risk of maternal hemorrhage since the 2010 NIH review. Half of the studies (9/18) found an increased risk of hemorrhage among the TOLAC cohorts (relative risk ranging from 1.25 to 9.90). Only two studies found a reduced risk of hemorrhage among TOLAC patients, and the remaining seven found no risk difference between groups. A comparison of infection rates was also challenging to perform, as the definition criteria for infection varied substantially among studies. However, the absolute risks of infection were nearly identical between groups (TOLAC, 0.02% to 15.7%; elective repeat cesarean, 0.00% to 15.7%). TOLAC was favored for reduced length of hospitalization (5/7 studies) and increased rates of breastfeeding (2/2 studies). Similar to the 2010 NIH panel review,[11] the authors were unable to identify any studies reporting the incidence of urinary or fecal incontinence. The investigators also explored the impact of mode of delivery on maternal mental health, which was not an outcome included in the 2010 review. Only two eligible studies were identified: one small RCT[80] reported no significant risk difference, while a large population cohort study[81] found TOLAC was associated with a 17% reduced risk of the mother being prescribed an antidepressant in the first year after delivery. Ultimately, the authors concluded, "Collectively, the evidence supports existing consensus that there are risks and benefits associated with both planned VBAC and [elective repeat cesarean], and therefore women without contraindications to VBAC should be given an informed choice about planned mode of birth after previous cesarean section."

Neonatal Outcomes

The 2010 NIH consensus development panel[11] concluded that the perinatal mortality rate (death between 20 weeks' gestation and 28 days of life) is increased with TOLAC compared with elective repeat cesarean delivery (130 deaths per 100,000 infants compared with 50 deaths per 100,000 infants, respectively). Likewise, the panel concluded that the neonatal mortality rate (death in the first 28 days of life) is also increased with TOLAC compared with elective repeat cesarean delivery (110 deaths per 100,000 infants versus 50 deaths per 100,000 infants, respectively).[11] The updated 2022 review by Fitzpatrick et al.[79] identified an additional five studies reporting on perinatal mortality. The three largest of these studies reported a fivefold to sevenfold increased risk of mortality for infants born after TOLAC. Twelve additional studies reported on neonatal mortality, most (9/12) failing to identify a significant risk difference between groups. The three remaining studies favored elective repeat cesarean delivery, reporting a 1.4-fold to 2-fold increased risk of mortality among neonates born after TOLAC.

However, elective cesarean delivery may result in some cases of iatrogenic neonatal respiratory sequelae, including respiratory distress syndrome and transient tachypnea of the newborn. Kamath et al.[82] observed that newborns born after elective repeat cesarean delivery had significantly higher rates of respiratory morbidity and neonatal intensive care unit admission—and a longer length of hospital stay—than infants whose mothers attempted VBAC. However, the 2010 NIH consensus development panel[11] concluded that there is insufficient evidence to determine whether substantial differences in respiratory outcomes occur in infants born via elective repeat cesarean delivery compared with infants born after TOLAC. Additional results from the study by Fitzpatrick et al.[79] challenge the respiratory benefits of TOLAC reported by Kamath et al.[82] Only one of three identified studies found a reduction in transient tachypnea of the newborn among neonates born after TOLAC. Furthermore, the authors identified a possible trend toward increased respiratory risk among

neonates born after TOLAC. Of eight additional publications reporting ventilatory support requirements, half found a small increased risk (1.1-fold to 1.2-fold) among neonates born after TOLAC. Two of three studies examining neonatal tracheal intubation reported a significantly increased risk (1.5-fold to 6-fold) in the TOLAC group.

The 2022 review[79] expanded upon the 2010 NIH panel work[11] by investigating outcomes related to childhood health. A population-based study was identified; it found no difference in various childhood medical conditions (e.g., asthma, cancer, type 1 diabetes mellitus) between modes of delivery up through 21 years of age.[83] The authors identified two population-based studies reporting on the incidence of learning disabilities; neither of them demonstrated a difference between planned TOLAC and planned cesarean delivery.[83,84] However, one study[83] reported an increased risk of learning disabilities among children born by cesarean after a failed TOLAC compared to successful VBAC (3.7% versus 2.3%; adjusted odds ratio, 1.64; 95% confidence interval [CI], 1.17 to 2.29).

OBSTETRIC MANAGEMENT

Intravenous Access and Availability of Blood

It seems prudent to recommend the early establishment of intravenous access in women who undergo TOLAC. Resources for transfusion of blood and blood products should be readily available.

Fetal Heart Rate Monitoring

The ACOG,[15] SOGC,[30] and RCOG[29] recommend continuous electronic FHR monitoring for the duration of a TOLAC, as FHR abnormalities can be a key indicator of uterine rupture.[85,86] Rodriguez et al.[87] reviewed 76 cases of uterine rupture at their hospital. A nonreassuring FHR pattern occurred in 59 of the 76 patients and was the most reliable sign of uterine rupture.

Intrauterine Pressure Monitoring

The intrauterine pressure catheter provides a quantitative measurement of uterine tone both during and between contractions. In the past, some obstetricians contended that an intrauterine pressure catheter should be used in all patients who undergo TOLAC, arguing that a loss of intrauterine pressure and cessation of labor will signal the occurrence of uterine rupture. In one study,[87] 39 patients had an intrauterine pressure catheter at the time of uterine rupture. None of these patients experienced an apparent decrease in resting uterine tone or cessation of labor, but four patients experienced an increase in baseline uterine tone. In these four patients, the increase in baseline uterine tone was associated with severe variable FHR decelerations that prompted immediate cesarean delivery. The authors concluded that the information obtained from the use of the intrauterine pressure catheter did not help obstetricians make the diagnosis of uterine rupture.[87] This conclusion was replicated by Devoe et al.[88] using a controlled model of uterine rupture. In 2019, the ACOG[15] concluded, "There are no data to suggest that intrauterine pressure catheters or fetal scalp electrodes are superior to external forms of continuous monitoring. In addition, there is evidence that the use of intrauterine pressure catheters does not help in the diagnosis of uterine rupture."

Use of Prostaglandins

The ACOG[15] has acknowledged that studies examining the relationship between prostaglandin use and uterine rupture during TOLAC offer mixed results. However, the ACOG[15] cited evidence from small studies that observed an increased risk for uterine rupture after the use of misoprostol (prostaglandin E_1) in women who attempted VBAC. Therefore, the ACOG[15] has concluded that "misoprostol should not be used for third trimester cervical ripening or labor induction in patients who have had a cesarean delivery or major uterine surgery." The RCOG[29] concluded that "induction of labor using mechanical methods (amniotomy or Foley catheter) is associated with a lower risk for scar rupture compared with induction using prostaglandins."

Induction and Augmentation of Labor

Induction of labor is less likely to result in a successful VBAC than spontaneous labor.[89–91] A 2019 metaanalysis[16] determined that the odds ratio for a successful VBAC following induction of labor was 0.58 (95% CI, 0.50 to 0.67) compared to spontaneous labor. Independent of induction, studies regarding augmentation of labor utilizing oxytocin have demonstrated conflicting results.[5,55,92,93] In a 1991 meta-analysis, Rosen et al.[5] noted that the use of oxytocin did not increase the risk for uterine scar dehiscence or rupture during TOLAC. In contrast, in one large retrospective study of more than 20,000 women, uterine rupture was nearly five times more common among women undergoing induction of labor with oxytocin than in those who had an elective repeat cesarean delivery.[65] Zelop et al.[92] observed a higher rate of uterine rupture in women undergoing oxytocin induction of labor for attempted VBAC than in similar women attempting VBAC with spontaneous labor. The ACOG[15] has concluded that "the varying outcomes of available studies and small absolute magnitude of the risk reported in those studies support that oxytocin augmentation may be used in patients undergoing TOLAC." While the RCOG[29] and SOGC[30] do not conclude oxytocin is contraindicated in TOLAC, both of these societies advise providers to counsel women about increased risk, with the RCOG specifying, "Women should be informed of the twofold to threefold increased risk of uterine rupture and around 1.5-fold increased risk of caesarean delivery in induced and/or augmented labor compared with spontaneous VBAC labor."

ANESTHETIC MANAGEMENT

In the past, some obstetricians contended that epidural analgesia might mask the pain of uterine scar separation or rupture and thereby delay the diagnosis of uterine scar dehiscence or rupture.[94,95] Plauché et al.[94] stated, "Regional anesthesia,

such as epidural anesthesia, blunts the patient's perception of symptoms and the physician's ability to elicit signs of early uterine rupture." Others have argued that the sympathectomy associated with epidural anesthesia might attenuate the maternal compensatory response to the hemorrhage, preventing the compensatory tachycardia and vasoconstriction that occur during hemorrhage. However, consensus[15] now exists that these concerns do not preclude administration of neuraxial analgesia during TOLAC, for several reasons.

First, maternal pain, uterine tenderness, and tachycardia have low sensitivity and specificity as diagnostic signs or symptoms of lower uterine segment scar dehiscence and rupture. Some uterine scars even separate painlessly, as obstetricians occasionally discover an asymptomatic lower uterine segment scar dehiscence at the time of elective repeat cesarean delivery. Nahum and Pham[96] performed a review of the literature to evaluate the prevalence of symptoms among patients with uterine rupture. Among 9 studies of 118 uterine ruptures, abdominal pain was reported in only 26% of patients. Overall, abdominal pain was the sixth most common finding behind prolonged FHR deceleration (80%), abnormal FHR pattern (54%), uterine tachysystole (40%), vaginal bleeding (37%), and shock (33%). Also, Case et al.[97] reported 20 patients with a history of previous cesarean delivery in whom the indication for urgent repeat cesarean delivery was severe hypogastric pain, tenderness, or both. At surgery, they confirmed the presence of scar dehiscence in only 1 of the 20 patients.

Second, there is insufficient evidence that abdominal pain, if it occurs, would be masked by epidural analgesia. In fact, epidural analgesia may allow for the acute pain of a uterine rupture to be more distinguishable and recognizable compared to that in laboring women without epidural analgesia. Johnson and Oriol[98] reviewed 14 studies of nearly 11,000 TOLAC patients, 1623 of whom received epidural analgesia. Of those who experienced uterine rupture, 5 of 14 patients (35%) with epidural analgesia reported abdominal pain, compared with 4 of 23 patients (17%) without epidural analgesia. Importantly, these investigators observed that epidural analgesia did not delay the diagnosis of uterine rupture. Eckstein et al.[99] suggested that the unexpected development of pain during previously successful epidural analgesia might be indicative of uterine rupture. A 2010 study[100] found evidence of "epidural dose escalation immediately before uterine rupture in women who attempted VBAC, when compared with women who did not have uterine rupture." The authors concluded that "clinical suspicion for uterine rupture should be high in women who require frequent epidural dosing during a VBAC trial."[100] Likewise, the RCOG[29] stated that "an increasing requirement for pain relief in labour should raise awareness of the possibility of an impending uterine rupture." Thus, epidural analgesia may improve the specificity of abdominal pain as a symptom of uterine scar separation or rupture.

Third, several published series have reported the successful use of epidural analgesia in women undergoing TOLAC.[98,101] There is little evidence that epidural analgesia either decreases the likelihood of vaginal delivery or adversely affects maternal or neonatal outcome in women who have uterine scar separation or rupture. Flamm et al.[102] reported a multicenter study of 1776 patients who attempted VBAC. Approximately 134 (74%) of 181 women who received epidural analgesia delivered vaginally, compared with 1180 (74%) of 1595 women who did not receive epidural analgesia. A 2017 retrospective study[101] from Israel reported a slightly higher rate of successful VBAC in women who received labor epidural analgesia than in women who did not (91.3% versus 88.2%), but women in the epidural group had a higher rate of operative vaginal delivery (11.7% versus 2.8%). A 2019 multicenter study[103] in China also found a significantly higher rate of vaginal delivery among TOLAC patients with epidural analgesia compared to those without (86% versus 70%). Although the rates of operative delivery were not different between the two patient groups, the occurrence of episiotomy was higher for women with epidural analgesia (43.4% versus 28.2%).

Fourth, in the past, some obstetricians favored the use of epidural analgesia because it facilitates postpartum uterine exploration to assess the integrity of the uterine scar. Meehan et al.[104] earlier supported routine postpartum palpation of the uterine scar. However, the same author[105] subsequently acknowledged that it is not necessary to repair all such defects. Many obstetricians manage asymptomatic uterine scar dehiscence with "expectant observation." Thus, they argue that routine palpation of the uterine scar is unnecessary after successful VBAC.[14]

Fifth, epidural analgesia facilitates rapid induction of safe surgical anesthesia should cesarean delivery or postpartum laparotomy be required.[106]

Finally, it is inhumane to deny effective analgesia to women who undergo TOLAC. Further, the ACOG[15] has concluded that adequate pain relief may encourage more women to choose TOLAC. Thus, the availability and use of neuraxial analgesia may decrease the incidence of unnecessary repeat cesarean delivery.

The ACOG[15] has stated that good and consistent scientific evidence supports a conclusion that epidural analgesia may be used during TOLAC. In our judgment, the availability of neuraxial analgesia is an essential component of a successful VBAC program.

KEY POINTS

- Cesarean delivery is the most commonly performed major operation in the United States.
- A trial of labor after cesarean (TOLAC) is successful in approximately 70% of women in whom a low-transverse uterine incision was made during a previous cesarean delivery.
- A previous vaginal delivery, specifically a previous vaginal birth after cesarean (VBAC), is the greatest predictor for successful VBAC. Maternal factors that lower the likelihood of successful VBAC include advancing age, obesity, hypertensive disorders, and diabetes. Labor induction and the indication for a previous cesarean should also be considered as factors that affect a TOLAC's success.
- The American College of Obstetricians and Gynecologists has recommended that resources for performing emergency cesarean delivery should be immediately available for women undergoing TOLAC. Other groups have argued that this guideline is too restrictive and has created barriers that prevent women from choosing TOLAC.
- Continuous electronic fetal heart rate monitoring represents the best means of detecting uterine rupture.
- Women are more likely to undergo TOLAC if they know that they will receive effective analgesia during labor.
- Epidural analgesia does not delay the diagnosis of uterine rupture or decrease the likelihood of successful VBAC.

REFERENCES

1. Cragin EB. Conservatism in obstetrics. *New York Med J.* 1916;104:1–3.
2. Osterman MJK, Hamilton BE, Martin JA, et al. Births: final data for 2021. *Natl Vital Stat Rep.* 2023;72:1–53.
3. Osterman M. Changes in primary and repeat cesarean delivery: United States, 2016–2021. Report No. 21. *Vital Statistics Rapid Release.* 2022;21. https://stacks.cdc.gov/view/cdc/117432. Accessed 15 March 2025.
4. U.S. Department of Health and Human Services, Public Health Service, National Institutes of Health. *Repeat cesarean birth. Cesarean Childbirth NIH Publication No 82-2067.* United States Government Printing Office; 1981.
5. Rosen MG, Dickinson JC, Westhoff CL. Vaginal birth after cesarean: a meta-analysis of morbidity and mortality. *Obstet Gynecol.* 1991;77:465–470.
6. American College of Obstetricians and Gynecologists Committee on Obstetric Practice. Committee Opinion No. 143: Vaginal delivery after a previous cesarean birth. *Int J Gynaecol Obstet.* 1994;48:127–129.
7. Menacker F, Declercq E, Macdorman MF. Cesarean delivery: background, trends, and epidemiology. *Semin Perinatol.* 2006;30:235–241.
8. McMahon MJ, Luther ER, Bowes WA, Olshan AF. Comparison of a trial of labor with an elective second cesarean section. *N Engl J Med.* 1996;335:689–695.
9. Yeh J, Wactawiski-Wende J, Shelton JA, Reschke J. Temporal trend in the rates of trial of labor in low-risk pregnancies and their impact on the rates and success of vaginal birth after cesarean delivery. *Am J Obstet Gynecol.* 2006;194:144–152.
10. American College of Obstetricians and Gynecologists. Practice Bulletin Number 5: Vaginal birth after previous cesarean delivery. *Int J Gynaecol Obstet.* 1999;66:197–204.

11. National Institutes of Health Consensus Development Conference Statement. Vaginal birth after cesarean: new insights. *Obstet Gynecol.* 2010;115:1279–1295.

12. De Lee JB, Cornell EL. Low cervical cesarean section (laparotrachelotomy). *JAMA.* 1922;79:109–112.

13. Kerr JMM. The technique of cesarean section, with special reference to the lower uterine segment incision. *Am J Obstet Gynecol.* 1926;12:729–734.

14. Berghella V, MacKeen AD, Jauniaux E. Cesarean delivery. In: Landon MB, Gatan HL, Jauniaux ERM, et al., eds. *Gabbe's Obstetrics: Normal and Problem Pregnancies.* 8th ed. Elsevier; 2021:375–394.

15. American College of Obstetricians and Gynecologists and Society for Maternal-Fetal Medicine. Practice Bulletin No. 205: Vaginal birth after cesarean delivery (reaffirmed 2024). *Obstet Gynecol.* 2019;133:e110–e127.

16. Wu Y, Kataria Y, Wang Z, et al. Factors associated with successful vaginal birth after a cesarean section: a systematic review and meta-analysis. *BMC Pregnancy Childbirth.* 2019;19:360.

17. Grobman WA, Lai Y, Landon MB, et al. Development of a nomogram for prediction of vaginal birth after cesarean delivery. *Obstet Gynecol.* 2007;109:806–812.

18. Chaillet N, Bujold E, Dube E, Grobman WA. Validation of a prediction model for vaginal birth after caesarean. *J Obstet Gynaecol Can.* 2013;35:119–124.

19. Costantine MM, Fox KA, Pacheco LD, et al. Does information available at delivery improve the accuracy of predicting vaginal birth after cesarean? Validation of the published models in an independent patient cohort. *Am J Perinatol.* 2011;28:293–298.

20. Costantine MM, Fox K, Byers BD, et al. Validation of the prediction model for success of vaginal birth after cesarean delivery. *Obstet Gynecol.* 2009;114:1029–1033.

21. Grobman WA, Sandoval G, Rice MM, et al. Prediction of vaginal birth after cesarean delivery in term gestations: a calculator without race and ethnicity. *Am J Obstet Gynecol.* 2021;225:664.e1–e7.

22. Maternal-Fetal Medicine Units Network. Vaginal birth after cesarean. https://mfmunetwork.bsc.gwu.edu/web/mfmunetwork/vaginal-birth-after-cesarean-calculator. Accessed 15 March 2025.

23. Martin JN Jr, Perry KG Jr, Roberts WE, Meydrech EF. The case for trial of labor in the patient with a prior low-segment vertical cesarean incision. *Am J Obstet Gynecol.* 1997;177:144–148.

24. Smith D, Stringer E, Vladutiu CJ, et al. Risk of uterine rupture among women attempting vaginal birth after cesarean with an unknown uterine scar. *Am J Obstet Gynecol.* 2015;213:80.e1–e5.

25. Lonky NM, Worthen N, Ross MG. Prediction of cesarean section scars with ultrasound imaging during pregnancy. *J Ultrasound Med.* 1989;8:15–19.

26. Landon MB, Spong CY, Thom E, et al. Risk of uterine rupture during a trial labor in women with multiple and single prior cesarean delivery. *Obstet Gynecol.* 2006;108:12–20.

27. Macones GA, Cahill A, Pare E, et al. Obstetric outcomes in women with two prior cesarean deliveries: is vaginal birth after cesarean delivery a viable option? *Am J Obstet Gynecol.* 2005;192:1223–1228.

28. Cahill AG, Tuuli M, Odibo AO, et al. Vaginal birth after caesarean for women with three or more prior caesareans: assessing safety and success. *BJOG.* 2010;117:422–427.

29. Royal College of Obstetricians and Gynaecologists. Birth after previous caesarean birth. Green-top Guideline No. 45., October, 2015. https://www.rcog.org.uk/globalassets/documents/guidelines/gtg_45.pdf. Accessed 15 March 2025.

30. Dy J, DeMeester S, Lipworth H, Barrett J. No. 382-Trial of labour after caesarean. *J Obstet Gynaecol Can.* 2019;41:992–1011.

31. Metz TD, Allshouse AA, Faucett AM, Grobman WA. Validation of a vaginal birth after cesarean delivery prediction model in women with two prior cesarean deliveries. *Obstet Gynecol.* 2015;125:948–952.

32. Myles T. Vaginal birth of twins after a previous cesarean section. *J Matern Fetal Med.* 2001;10:171–174.

33. Sansregret A, Bujold E, Gauthier RJ. Twin delivery after a previous caesarean: a twelve-year experience. *J Obstet Gynaecol Can.* 2003;25:294–298.

34. Cahill A, Stamilio DM, Pare E, et al. Vaginal birth after cesarean (VBAC) attempt in twin pregnancies: is it safe? *Am J Obstet Gynecol.* 2005;193:1050–1055.

35. Varner MW, Leindecker S, Spong CY, et al. The maternal-fetal medicine unit cesarean registry: trial of labor with a twin gestation. *Am J Obstet Gynecol.* 2005;193:135–140.

36. Ford AD, Bateman BT, Simpson LL. Vaginal birth after cesarean delivery in twin gestations: a large, nationwide sample of deliveries. *Am J Obstet Gynecol.* 2006;195:1138–1142.

37. Elkousy MA, Sammel M, Stevens E, et al. The effect of birth weight on vaginal birth after cesarean delivery success rates. *Am J Obstet Gynecol.* 2003;188:824–830.

38. Peaceman AM, Gersnoviez R, Landon MB, et al. The MFMU cesarean registry: impact of fetal size on trial of labor success for patients with previous cesarean for dystocia. *Am J Obstet Gynecol.* 2006;195:1127–1131.

39. Flamm BL, Goings JR. Vaginal birth after cesarean section: is suspected fetal macrosomia a contraindication? *Obstet Gynecol.* 1989;74:694–697.

40. Leung AS, Farmer RM, Leung EK, et al. Risk factors associated with uterine rupture during trial of labor after cesarean delivery: a case-control study. *Am J Obstet Gynecol.* 1993;168:1358–1363.

41. Zelop CM, Shipp TD, Cohen A, et al. Trial of labor after 40 weeks' gestation in women with prior cesarean. *Obstet Gynecol.* 2001;97:391–393.

42. Coassolo KM, Stamilio DM, Pare E, et al. Safety and efficacy of vaginal birth after cesarean attempts at or beyond 40 weeks of gestation. *Obstet Gynecol.* 2005;106:700–706.

43. Kiran TS, Chui YK, Bethel J, Bhal PS. Is gestational age an independent variable affecting uterine scare rupture rates? *Eur J Obstet Gynecol Reprod Biol.* 2006;126:68–71.

44. Kirk EP, Doyle KA, Leigh J, Garrard ML. Vaginal birth after cesarean or repeat cesarean section: medical risks or social realities. *Am J Obstet Gynecol.* 1990;162:1398–1405.

45. Joseph GF, Stedman CF, Robichaux AG. Vaginal birth after cesarean section: the impact of patient resistance to a trial of labor. *Am J Obstet Gynecol.* 1991;164:1441–1447.

46. Biraboneye SP, Ogutu O, van Roosmalen J, et al. Trial of labour or elective repeat caesarean delivery: are women making an informed decision at Kenyatta national hospital? *BMC Pregnancy Childbirth.* 2017;17:260.

47. Bernstein SN, Matalon-Grazi S, Rosenn BM. Trial of labor versus repeat cesarean: are patients making an informed decision? *Am J Obstet Gynecol.* 2012;207:e1–e6.

48. Sindiani A, Rawashdeh H, Obeidat N, et al. Factors that influenced pregnant women with one previous caesarean section regarding their mode of delivery. *Ann Med Surg (Lond).* 2020;55:124–130.

49. Kaimal AJ, Grobman WA, Bryant A, et al. The association of patient preferences and attitudes with trial of labor after cesarean. *J Perinatol.* 2019;39:1340–1348.

50. Cox KJ. Counseling women with a previous cesarean birth: toward a shared decision-making partnership. *J Midwifery Womens Health.* 2014;59:237–245.

51. Kuppermann M, Kaimal AJ, Blat C, et al. Effect of a patient-centered decision support tool on rates of trial of labor after previous cesarean delivery: the PROCEED randomized clinical trial. *JAMA.* 2020;323:2151–2159.

52. Shorten A, Shorten B, Keogh J, et al. Making choices for childbirth: a randomized controlled trial of a decision-aid for informed birth after cesarean. *Birth.* 2005;32:252–261.

53. Saleh AM, Dudenhausen JW, Ahmed B. Increased rates of cesarean sections and large families: a potentially dangerous combination. *J Perinat Med.* 2017;45:517–521.

54. Wells CE. Vaginal birth after cesarean delivery: views from the private practitioner. *Semin Perinatol.* 2010;34:345–350.

55. Stafford RS. The impact of nonclinical factors on repeat cesarean section. *JAMA.* 1991;265:59–63.

56. Hueston WJ, Rudy M. Factors predicting elective repeat cesarean delivery. *Obstet Gynecol.* 1994;83:741–744.

57. Rogers AJ, Rogers NG, Kilgore ML, et al. Economic evaluations comparing a trial of labor with an elective repeat cesarean delivery: a systematic review. *Value Health.* 2017;20:163–173.

58. Gilbert SA, Grobman WA, Landon MB, et al. Lifetime cost-effectiveness of trial of labor after cesarean in the United States. *Value Health.* 2013;16:953–964.

59. Holmgren C, Scott JR, Porter TF, et al. Uterine rupture with attempted vaginal birth after cesarean delivery: decision-to-delivery time and neonatal outcome. *Obstet Gynecol.* 2012;119:725–731.

60. Freeman G. $98.5 million verdict in missed uterine rupture. *Ob-Gyn Malpractice Prev.* 1996;3:41–48.

61. Phelan JP. VBAC: Time to reconsider? *OBG Management.* 1996:62–68.

62. American College of Obstetricians and Gynecologists Committee on Professional Standards. *Standards for Obstetric-gynecologic Services.* American College of Obstetricians and Gynecologists; 1982.

63. Flamm BL. Once a cesarean, always a controversy. *Obstet Gynecol.* 1997;90:312–315.

64. Greene MF. Vaginal delivery after cesarean section: is the risk acceptable? *N Engl J Med.* 2001;345:54–55.

65. Lydon-Rochelle M, Holt VL, Easterling TR, Martin DP. Risk of uterine rupture during labor among women with a prior cesarean delivery. *N Engl J Med.* 2001;345:3–8.

66. Clark SL, Belfort MA, Dildy GA, Meyers JA. Reducing obstetric litigation through alterations in practice patterns. *Obstet Gynecol.* 2008;112:1279–1283.

67. DeFranco EA, Rampersad R, Atkins KL, et al. Do vaginal birth after cesarean outcomes differ based on hospital setting? *Am J Obstet Gynecol.* 2007;197:400.e1–e6.

68. Cox KJ, Bovbjerg ML, Cheyney M, Leeman LM. Planned home VBAC in the United States, 2004-2009: outcomes, maternity care practices, and implications for shared decision making. *Birth.* 2015;42:299–308.

69. Tilden EL, Cheyney M, Guise JM, et al. Vaginal birth after cesarean: neonatal outcomes and United States birth setting. *Am J Obstet Gynecol.* 2017;216:403.e1–e8.

70. Leeman LM, King VJ. Increasing patient access to VBAC: new NIH and ACOG recommendations. *Am Fam Physician.* 2011;83:121–122, 127.

71. Al-Zirqi I, Daltveit AK, Vangen S. Infant outcome after complete uterine rupture. *Am J Obstet Gynecol.* 2018;219:109.e1–e9.

72. Birnbach DJ, Bucklin BA, Dexter F. Impact of anesthesiologists on the incidence of vaginal birth after cesarean in the United States: role of anesthesia availability, productivity, guidelines, and patient safety. *Semin Perinatol.* 2010;34:318–324.

73. American Society of Anesthesiologists Committee on Obstetrics and Anesthesia. Statement on optimal goals for anesthesia care in obstetrics. 2021. https://www.asahq.org/standards-and-practice-parameters/statement-on-optimal-goals-for-anesthesia-care-in-obstetrics. Accessed 7 January 2024.

74. Hauk L. Planning for labor and vaginal birth after cesarean delivery: guidelines from the AAFP. *Am Fam Physician.* 2015;91:197–198.

75. Guise JM, Berlin M, McDonagh M, et al. Safety of vaginal birth after cesarean: a systematic review. *Obstet Gynecol.* 2004;103:420–429.

76. Wen SW, Rusen ID, Walker M, et al. Comparison of maternal mortality and morbidity between trial of labor and elective cesarean section among women with previous cesarean delivery. *Am J Obstet Gynecol.* 2004;191:1263–1269.

77. Guise JM, Denman MA, Emeis C, et al. Vaginal birth after cesarean: new insights on maternal and neonatal outcomes. *Obstet Gynecol.* 2010;115:1267–1278.

78. Rossi AC, D'Addario V. Maternal morbidity following a trial of labor after cesarean section vs. elective repeat cesarean delivery: a systematic review with metaanalysis. *Am J Obstet Gynecol.* 2008;199:224–231.

79. Fitzpatrick KE, Quigley MA, Kurinczuk JJ. Planned mode of birth after previous cesarean section: a structured review of the evidence on the associated outcomes for women and their children in high-income setting. *Front Med (Lausanne).* 2022;9:920647

80. Law LW, Pang MW, Chung TK, et al. Randomised trial of assigned mode of delivery after a previous cesarean section – impact on maternal psychological dynamics. *J Matern Fetal Neonatal Med.* 2010;23:1106–1113.

81. Fitzpatrick KE, Quigley MA, Smith DJ, Kurinczuk JJ. Planned mode of birth after previous caesarean section and women's use of psychotropic medication in the first year postpartum: a population-based record linkage cohort study. *Psychol Med.* 2022;52:3210–3221.

82. Kamath BD, Todd JK, Glazner JE, et al. Neonatal outcomes after elective cesarean delivery. *Obstet Gynecol.* 2009;113:1231–1238.

83. Black M, Bhattacharya S, Philip S, et al. Planned repeat cesarean section at term and adverse childhood health outcomes: a record-linkage study. *PLoS Med.* 2016;13:e1001973.

84. Fitzpatrick KE, Kurinczuk JJ, Quigley MA. Planned mode of birth after previous caesarean section and special educational needs in childhood: a population-based record linkage cohort study. *BJOG.* 2021;128:2158–2168.

85. Sheiner E, Levy A, Ofir K, et al. Changes in fetal heart rate and uterine patterns associated with uterine rupture. *J Reprod Med.* 2004;49:373–378.

86. Ridgeway JJ, Weyrich DL, Benedetti TJ. Fetal heart rate changes associated with uterine rupture. *Obstet Gynecol.* 2004;103:506–512.

87. Rodriguez MH, Masaki DI, Phelan JP, Diaz FG. Uterine rupture: are intrauterine pressure catheters useful in the diagnosis? *Am J Obstet Gynecol.* 1989;161:666–669.

88. Devoe LD, Croom CS, Youssef AA, Murray C. The prediction of "controlled" uterine rupture by the use of intrauterine pressure catheters. *Obstet Gynecol.* 1992;80:626–629.

89. Landon MB, Leindecker S, Spong CY, et al. The MFMU cesarean registry. Factors affecting the success of trial of labor after previous cesarean delivery. *Am J Obstet Gynecol.* 2005;193:1016–1023.

90. Delaney T, Young DC. Spontaneous versus induced labor after a previous cesarean delivery. *Obstet Gynecol.* 2003;102:39–44.

91. Grinstead J, Grobman WA. Induction of labor after one prior cesarean: predictors of vaginal delivery. *Obstet Gynecol.* 2004;103:534–538.

92. Zelop CM, Shipp TD, Repke JT, et al. Uterine rupture during induced or augmented labor in gravid women with one prior cesarean delivery. *Am J Obstet Gynecol.* 1999;181:882–886.

93. Harper LM, Cahill AG, Boslaugh S, et al. Association of induction of labor and uterine rupture in women attempting vaginal birth after cesarean: a survival analysis. *Am J Obstet Gynecol.* 2012;206:51.e1–e5.

94. Plauché WC, Von Almen W, Muller R. Catastrophic uterine rupture. *Obstet Gynecol.* 1984;64:792–797.

95. Abraham R, Sadovsky E. Delay in the diagnosis of rupture of the uterus due to epidural anesthesia in labor. *Gynecol Obstet Invest.* 1992;33:239–240.

96. Nahum GG, Pham KQ. Uterine Rupture in Pregnancy. Medscape; 2018. https://reference.medscape.com/article/275854-overview#a5. Accessed 15 March 2025.

97. Case BD, Corcoran R, Jeffcoate N, Randle GH. Caesarean section and its place in modern obstetric practice. *J Obstet Gynaecol Br Commonw.* 1971;78:203–214.

98. Johnson C, Oriol N. The role of epidural anesthesia in trial of labor. *Reg Anesth.* 1990;15:304–308.

99. Eckstein KL, Oberlander SG, Marx GF. Uterine rupture during extradural blockade. *Can Anaesth Soc J.* 1973;20:566–568.

100. Cahill AG, Odibo AO, Allsworth JE, Macones GA. Frequent epidural dosing as a marker for impending uterine rupture in patients who attempt vaginal birth after cesarean delivery. *Am J Obstet Gynecol.* 2010;202:355.e1–e5.

101. Grisaru-Granovsky S, Bas-Lando M, Drukker L, et al. Epidural analgesia at trial of labor after cesarean (TOLAC): a significant adjunct to successful vaginal birth after cesarean (VBAC). *J Perinat Med.* 2018;46:261–269.

102. Flamm BL, Lim OW, Jones C, et al. Vaginal birth after cesarean section: results of a multicenter study. *Am J Obstet Gynecol.* 1988;158:1079–1084.

103. Sun J, Yan X, Yuan A, et al. Effect of epidural analgesia in trial of labor after cesarean on maternal and neonatal outcomes in China: a multicenter, prospective cohort study. *BMC Pregnancy Childbirth.* 2019;19:498.

104. Meehan FP, Moolgaoker AS, Stallworthy J. Vaginal delivery under caudal analgesia after caesarean section and other major uterine surgery. *Br Med J.* 1972;2:740–742.

105. Meehan FP, Burke G, Kehoe JT, Magani IM. True rupture/scar dehiscence in delivery following prior section. *Int J Gynecol Obstet.* 1990;31:249–255.

106. Bucklin BA. Vaginal birth after cesarean delivery. *Anesthesiology.* 2003;99:1444–1448.

The Pain of Childbirth and Its Effect on the Mother and the Fetus

Peter H. Pan, MD, MSEE and Jessica M. Meister Berger, MD, JD

CHAPTER OUTLINE

Pain is defined as "an unpleasant sensory and emotional experience associated with, or resembling that associated with, actual or potential tissue damage."[1] The gate control theory of pain, described in 1965 by Melzack and Wall,[2] revolutionized the understanding of the mechanisms responsible for pain and analgesia. Originally explained as the regulation of pain signals from the peripheral nerve to the spinal cord by the activity of other peripheral nerves, interneurons in the spinal cord, and central supraspinal centers (Fig. 21.1), the theory has been refined with the concept of a neuromatrix, a remarkably dynamic system capable of undergoing rapid change.[3] Neural circuits and intraneural mechanisms regulate sensitivity at peripheral afferents; along conducting axons of peripheral nerves; in the spinal cord, pons, medulla, and thalamus; and at cortical sites of pain transmission and projection. The experience of pain is a summation of these ascending and descending inputs. For example, application of capsaicin to the skin alters spinal gating mechanisms within 10 minutes, resulting in a light touch signal being interpreted as burning pain.[4]

Despite extensive research into mechanisms and treatments for chronic pain, comparatively little research on the neurophysiologic basis or therapies for labor pain has been performed. This discrepancy has led to vastly different approaches to the treatment of patients with chronic versus obstetric pain. A patient with chronic pain typically undergoes a sophisticated physical assessment of sensory function, is offered therapies from nearly a dozen different classes of analgesics, and can benefit from the enormous resources expended by the pharmaceutical industry to introduce agents that act on novel receptors or enzymes. By contrast, a laboring parturient receives no physical assessment of sensory function and is offered only a handful of systemic drugs that act primarily through the anatomic blockade of neural traffic. While there are pertinent differences between chronic pain and obstetric populations, most notably consideration of fetal effects, studies indicate that sex and gender influence multiple dimensions of pain; further, gender disparities in the treatment of pain are well documented. Female patients are more likely to have pain conditions, may be undertreated for pain, and have pain that is more readily dismissed.[4,5] Whether these disparities are reflected in the comparative dearth of research and treatment of labor pain is a worthwhile question.

The concept of pain as extending beyond a mere sensory and emotional experience has evolved with a multidimensional theory known as the biopsychosocial model of pain.[6] This model postulates that the experience and significance of pain is influenced by—and reciprocally influences—complex social, biological, and psychological constructs. The pain experience, then, is affected by an individual's biologic predisposition and innumerable social factors, and is modulated by the individual's coping mechanisms and other psychological responses. Unlike most forms of chronic pain, pain associated with labor and childbirth tends to occupy a unique significance in these dimensions.

In this chapter, the application of the biopsychosocial model of pain is explored, and the basis for current therapy (anatomy), the basis for future therapy (neurophysiology), and the effects of labor pain on the mother and the infant are reviewed.

BIOPSYCHOSOCIAL MODEL OF PAIN

The conceptualization of the pain experience and its complexity has evolved beyond mere biomechanics and now recognizes a robust multidimensional interplay between a person's unique social and cultural context, psychological condition, and biological comorbidities and predisposition.[6] These three dimensions not only inform the experience of pain but are simultaneously influenced by the occurrence of pain (Fig. 21.2). This reciprocal relationship, classically described in chronic pain, has been recognized in the obstetric population as well.[7,8] Treating obstetric pain requires clinical

recognition of and sensitivity to an individual's unique protective and adverse risk factors, as well as understanding the multidimensional lens through which the parturient experiences labor pain. Optimization of protective factors presents a future opportunity to enhance the treatment of obstetric pain and reduce the sequelae of severe labor pain. Throughout this chapter, the biopsychosocial model, and the notion of pain as a highly complex interplay, will be revisited as it applies to multiple aspects of labor pain. The biopsychosocial model has been criticized for lacking clear parameters for application; certainly, addressing the multiple dimensions and mitigating risk factors requires long-term, large-scale efforts[9] and is not pragmatic in the setting of labor. Saxbe[9] proposed that the primary utility of the biopsychosocial model in the treatment of labor pain is enhanced clinician awareness of, and sensitivity to, the highly complex dynamics that inform a patient's pain, and subsequent eradication of a simplistic notion of labor pain as a mere sensory experience to be pharmacologically muted. In understanding labor pain and childbirth through the biopsychosocial lens, the clinician invites an improved patient–physician therapeutic relationship, enhanced multidisciplinary teamwork, compassionate care, and improved patient outcomes.

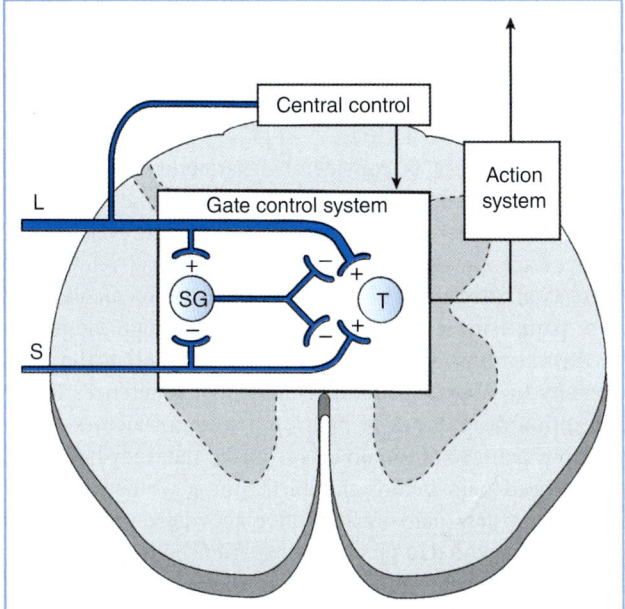

Fig. 21.1 Gate Control Theory of Pain. Activity in small-diameter afferents (S) stimulates transmission cells in the spinal cord (T), which send signals supraspinally and results in the perception of pain. Small-diameter afferents also inhibit cells in the spinal cord substantia gelatinosa (SG), the activity of which reduces excitatory input to T cells. Activity in large-diameter afferents (L) also stimulates T cells in a manner that is perceived as nonpainful and excites SG cells to "close the gate" and reduce small-diameter afferent activation of T cells. The gate mechanism is under regulation by central sites. From Melzack R, Wall PD. Pain mechanisms: a new theory. *Science.* 1965;150:971–975.

MEASUREMENT AND SEVERITY OF LABOR PAIN

The recognition and acceptance of chronic pain, which frequently lacks an obvious outward cause, contrasts with the recurrent denial of labor pain, which is accompanied by visible tissue injury. Dick-Read[10] suggested that labor is a natural process not considered painful by women in some indigenous cultures and should be handled with education and preparation rather than through pain medications. Aspects of this theory align with the biopsychosocial model of pain, in which biologic predisposition as well as family and cultural context

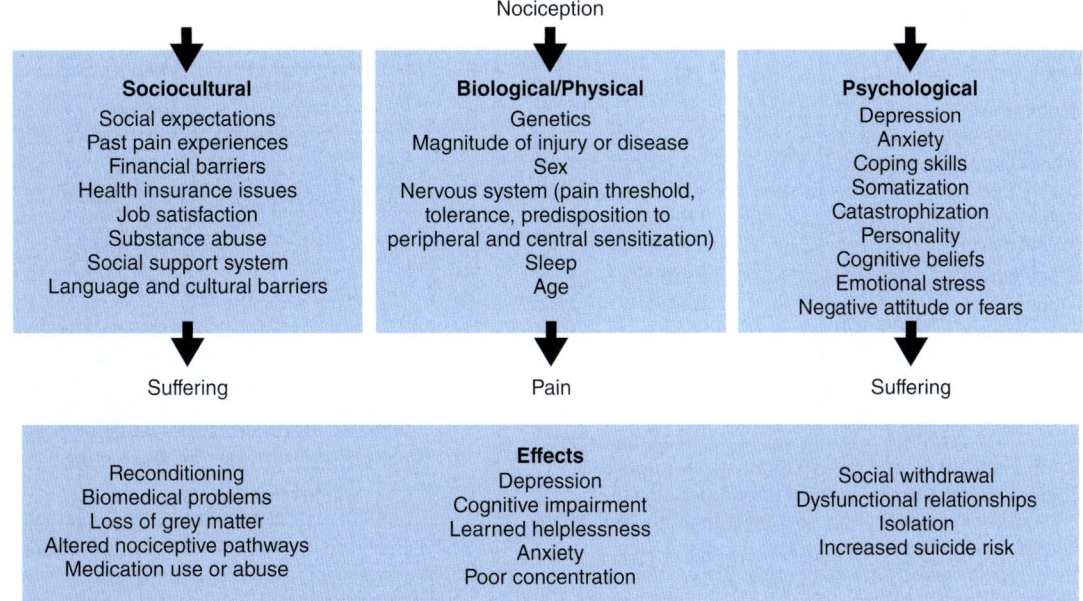

Fig. 21.2 The Biopsychosocial Model of Pain. Biological predisposition, psychological constructs, and social context mutually inform the experience of, and response to, pain. Modified from Cohen SP, Vase L, Hooten WM. Chronic pain: an update on burden, best practices, and new advances. *Lancet.* 2021;397:2082–2097.

are understood to influence the pain experience.[6] Lamaze[11] popularized psychoprophylaxis as a method of birth preparation. This method now forms the basis for prepared childbirth training in the developed world, highlighting the efficacy of optimizing coping mechanisms and psychological response to pain in the biopsychosocial model.

The severity of labor pain has been recognized previously. Melzack,[12] using a questionnaire developed to assess the intensity and emotional impact of pain, observed that nulliparous women with no prepared childbirth training rated labor pain to be as painful as a digit amputation without anesthesia (Fig. 21.3).[12] More than 30 years before Melzack's quantification of pain, Javert and Hardy[13,14] trained subjects to reproduce the intensity of labor pain with the sensation of noxious heat applied to the skin from a radiant heat source. In these experiments, several women achieved "ceiling pain"—resulting in second-degree burns to the skin—when they attempted to match the intensity of uterine contraction pain.[13] Individual women also reported a close positive correlation between cervical dilation and pain intensity. Analysis of the investigators' original data[13] indicates a high likelihood of severe pain as labor progresses, with a time course closely associated with cervical dilation (Fig. 21.4). Other investigators have noted that uterine pressure during contractions accounts for more than 90% of the variability in labor pain intensity.[15] These observations are consistent with the conclusion that cervical distention is the primary cause of pain during the first stage of labor.

To objectively measure pain in laboring women, Charier et al.[16] studied the physiologic fluctuations of the iris, which is dependent on the input from the sympathetic and parasympathetic systems. By measuring the variation coefficient of the pupillary diameter (VCPD) as a mathematical extraction of pupil size fluctuation in 40 laboring women, these researchers were able to demonstrate a stronger correlation ($r = 0.77$ versus $r = 0.42$) with numerical pain scores in labor during a uterine contraction than pupillary diameter alone.

However, there is considerable variability in the rated intensity of pain during labor. Nulliparous women rate labor pain as more severe than do parous women; however, the differences are small and of questionable clinical relevance.[17] There is a correlation between the intensity of menses and labor pain, especially back discomfort,[17] although the reason for this relationship is unknown. It is possible that the rated intensity of labor pain reflects individual differences in the perception of all types of pain. In a study of factors affecting labor pain, 10 of 97 subjects reported that they had never experienced pain before childbirth; these women reported significantly less pain during labor and delivery compared with women who had previously experienced pain.[18] In other studies, the variability of pain after cesarean delivery could be predicted with preoperative quantitative sensory testing, such as rating the intensity of pain with a standardized noxious thermal stimulus, psychological constructs, and their combinations.[19,20]

The mechanism by which people perceive different levels of pain from the same stimulus remains unclear. A study involving brain imaging and a fixed acute noxious heat stimulus showed a strong correlation between verbal pain assessment and the level of activation of various cortical brain regions,

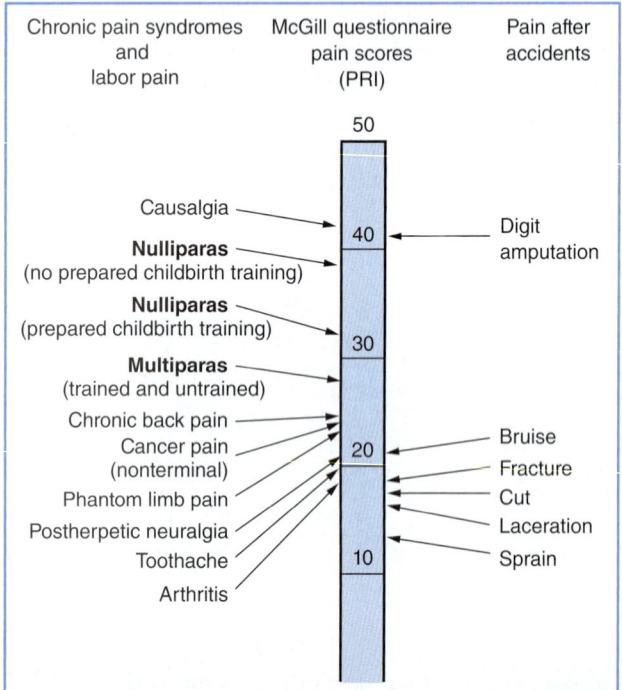

Fig. 21.3 A Comparison of Pain Scores Obtained Through the McGill Pain Questionnaire. Scores were collected from women in labor, patients in a general hospital clinic, and patients in the emergency department after accidents involving traumatic injury. Note the modest difference in pain scores between nulliparous women with and without prepared childbirth training. *PRI*, Pain rating index, which represents the sum of the rank values of all the words chosen from 20 sets of pain descriptors. Modified from Melzack R. The myth of painless childbirth (The John J. Bonica Lecture). *Pain.* 1984;19:321–337.

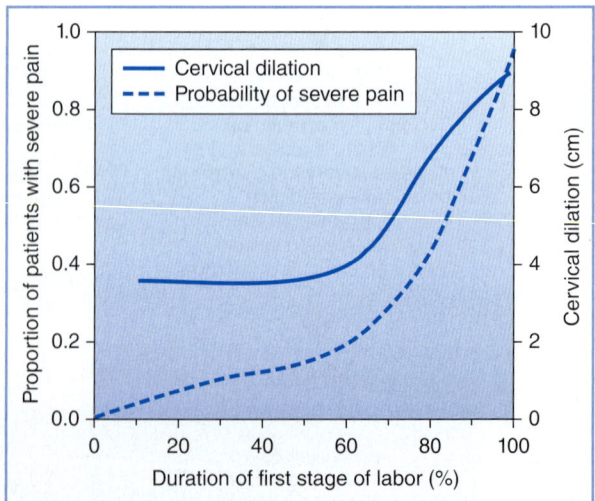

Fig. 21.4 Likelihood of Severe Pain During Labor. A significant minority of women (approximately one-third) have severe pain in early labor, and the proportion of women with severe pain increases to nearly 90% later in labor, in close relationship with cervical dilation. Data from Hardy JD, Javert CT. Studies on pain: measurements of pain intensity in childbirth. *J Clin Invest.* 1949;28:153–162.

especially the contralateral somatosensory cortex and anterior cingulate cortex.[21] The investigators also found that the degree of activation of the thalamus was essentially identical in all subjects, suggesting that differences in perceived pain resulted from modulation at suprathalamic levels rather than in the peripheral nerves or spinal cord. The situation in labor may be more complex. For example, a large genetic polymorphism regulates cytokine production and function as well as pregnancy outcome.[22] It is possible that interindividual differences in labor pain may partially reflect genetic differences in cytokine production or response.

In evaluating and studying labor pain and its treatment, most studies have assessed labor pain using a set of discrete pain scores. However, labor pain is a complex, subjective, multidimensional, and dynamically changing experience with both sensory and affective components that are influenced by many factors. Therefore, better identification of the covariates that affect labor progress and its associated pain is needed. Conell-Price et al.[23] developed and validated a dynamic model to account for labor progress in the assessment of labor pain. Subsequently, Debiec et al.[24] combined a biexponential model describing labor progress with a sigmoidal labor pain model to assess the influence of patient covariates on labor pain. Both studies used retrospective patient data to develop and test their models. In the former study,[23] the prediction error for the pain scores was large, but the purpose of the model was to identify and remove variability associated with labor progress so that other factors (e.g., genetic polymorphisms) could be quantitatively studied; the authors reported that cervical dilation accounted for only 16% to 20% of the variability in reported pain. In the latter study,[24] the covariate of ethnicity was found to have a statistically significant but clinically trivial effect on labor progress. The modeling described by these investigators provides a useful quantitative tool for future studies to identify and assess the effects of patient and/or environmental covariates on labor progress, labor pain, and therapeutic responses. Better understanding of underlying causes of interindividual variability in labor progress, labor pain, and therapeutic responses is likely to lead to more tailored therapy.

In summary, although significant variability exists in the rated intensity of pain during labor and delivery, the majority of women experience more than minimal pain. The close correlation between cervical dilation and the rated severity of pain implies the existence of a causal relationship and increases the likelihood that a parturient will request analgesia as labor progresses.

PERSONAL SIGNIFICANCE AND MEANING

Significant interpersonal variation exists in the experience of, and response to, pain.[25] The biopsychosocial model of pain permits a greater understanding of how different parturients undergoing a physiologically similar birth event can have vastly different pain experiences that can extend into chronic sequelae such as depression and posttraumatic stress disorder (PTSD). Recognition of an intensity-discriminatory

component and an emotional-cognitive component of labor pain has fostered current interventions heavily weighted toward the first component and assumes that labor pain is severe and is an appropriate context for pharmacologic treatment. Largely ignored are interventions addressing the emotional-cognitive component, including exploration into the considerable variation in coping strategies and the personal meaning of labor pain.[26] Williams and Craig[27] suggested that the definition of pain should include these often overlooked cognitive and social elements, and Whitburn et al.[28] suggested a further definitional extension to etiologies that do not include tissue damage. These alterations, which are reflected by the biopsychosocial model, would make the experience and study of pain more relevant to the labor experience.

Although many obstetric patients rate the pain of labor and delivery as being severe, the qualitative descriptors often reflect an emotional context. In a pioneering study of the quantification of pain, Bajaj et al.[29] compared pain descriptors among four groups of patients who were in labor, had experimental cervical dilation, were undergoing spontaneous abortion, or who had dysmenorrhea (Table 21.1). Women with dysmenorrhea used words that indicate suffering, such as "punishing" and "wretched," whereas those in labor did not. Some researchers have drawn parallels between the pain of labor with that derived from mountain climbing, which is associated with a sense of euphoria.[26] However, other have found no deeper or spiritual meaning, believing it to be similar to "normal" parts of human life that involved discomfort (e.g., trauma, severe dental disease, cancer). Elements related to pregnancy, such as whether it was desired or planned, or if substantive efforts were employed (e.g., assisted reproductive technologies, repeated pregnancy losses), may also influence labor pain and the likelihood of long-term sequelae, but remain largely unexplored.[8]

In summary, there are large interindividual differences in how parturients experience the personal significance or meaning of labor pain. These different perceptions can lead to a long-term sense of failure and guilt when pharmacologic pain relief is accepted or emotional trauma when it is withheld. The use of educational interventions and improved management of labor expectations may improve the birth experience by creating realistic pain expectations during labor and delivery.[30]

ANATOMIC BASIS OF LABOR PAIN

First Stage of Labor

Several lines of evidence suggest that the pain experienced during the first stage of labor is transduced by afferents with peripheral terminals in the cervix and lower uterine segment rather than the uterine body, as is often depicted (Fig. 21.5). Uterine body afferents fire in response to distention, but in the absence of inflammation, uterine body distention has no or minimal effect on the behavior of laboratory animals.[31,32] These observations suggest that uterine body afferents may be an important site of chronic inflammatory disease and

TABLE 21.1 **Word Descriptors From the McGill Pain Questionnaire Used to Describe Pain From the Uterus and Cervix**

Pain Descriptors	Balloon Distention of the Cervix[a]	Labor[b]	Abortion[c]	Dysmenorrhea[a]
	TYPE/SOURCE OF PAIN			
Sensory	Shooting, boring, sharp, hot, dull, taut	Throbbing, shooting, sharp, cramping, aching, taut	Cutting, cramping, tugging, pulling, aching	Pulsing, beating, shooting, pricking, boring, drilling, sharp, cutting, pinching, pressing, cramping, tugging, pulling, hot, stinging, dull, hurting, heavy, taut
Affective		Exhausting, tiring, frightening, grueling	Tiring	Tiring, sickening, punishing, wretched
Evaluative	Annoying		Intense	Annoying, intense
Miscellaneous	Drawing, squeezing	Tearing	Numb, squeezing	Piercing, drawing, squeezing, nagging

[a]Data from Bajaj P, Drewes AM, Gregersen H, et al. Controlled dilatation of the uterine cervix: an experimental visceral pain model. *Pain.* 2002;99:433–442.
[b]Data from Niven C, Gijsbers K. A study of labour pain using the McGill Pain Questionnaire. *Soc Sci Med.* 1984;19:1347–1351.
[c]Data from Wells N. Pain and distress during abortion. *Health Care Women Int.* 1991;12:293–302.

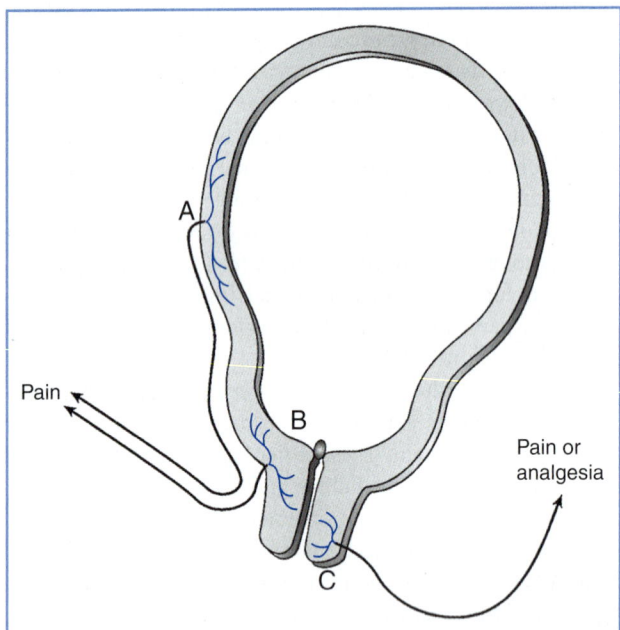

Fig. 21.5 Uterocervical Afferents Activated During the First Stage of Labor. Uterine body afferents (A) partially regress during pregnancy and may contribute to the pain of the first stage of labor. However, the major input is from afferents in the lower uterine segment and endocervix (B). By contrast, at least in animals, the activation of afferents that innervate the vaginal surface of the cervix (C) results in analgesia, not pain, and they enter the spinal cord in sacral areas rather than at the site of referred pain in labor.

chronic pelvic pain but are much less relevant to acute obstetric and uterine cervical pain. In addition, afferents to the uterine body regress during normal pregnancy, whereas those to the cervix and lower uterine segment do not.[33] This denervation of the myometrium may protect against preterm labor by limiting α_1-adrenergic receptor stimulation by locally released norepinephrine (noradrenaline). Javert and Hardy[13] reproduced the pain of uterine contractions in women during labor by manual distention of the cervix. Bonica and Chadwick[34] later confirmed that women undergoing cesarean delivery under a local anesthetic field block experience pain from cervical distention, which mimics that of labor pain, but do not experience pain from uterine distention.[35]

The uterine cervix has dual innervation; afferents innervating the endocervix and lower uterine segment have cell bodies in thoracolumbar dorsal root ganglia (DRG), whereas afferents innervating the vaginal surface of the cervix and upper vagina have cell bodies in sacral DRG.[36] These two innervations result in different sensory input and referral of pain. Pelvic afferents innervating the vaginal surface of the cervix are almost exclusively C fibers, with the majority containing the peptides substance P and calcitonin gene-related peptide (CGRP). These afferents express alpha and beta estrogen receptors and have an innervation pattern that is not affected by pregnancy.[34,37,38] Stimulation of the vaginal surface of the cervix in rats results in antinociception, lordosis, ovulation, and a hormonal state of pseudopregnancy, all of which are related to mating behaviors in this species.[39] In rats, these vaginal afferent terminals are activated only during delivery and not during labor, which suggests that they are not relevant to the pain of the first stage of labor.[40] By contrast, dilation of the endocervix in rats results in the activation of afferents entering the lower thoracic spinal cord and nociception rather than antinociception. These afferents, which are mostly or exclusively C fibers,[41] are activated during the first stage of labor, suggesting that they are relevant to pain during this period.

More than 90 years ago, experiments in dogs allowed Cleland[42] to identify T11–T12 as the segmental level of entry into the spinal cord of afferents that transmit the pain of the first stage of labor. Because dysmenorrhea could be treated through the destruction of the superior or inferior hypogastric plexus,[43] Cleland[42] reasoned that the sensory afferents and sympathetic efferents were likely intermingled; he subsequently demonstrated that the bilateral blockade of the lumbar paravertebral sympathetic chain could produce analgesia during the first stage of labor. First-stage labor pain is transmitted by afferents that have cell bodies in T10–L1 DRG and pass through the paracervical region, the hypogastric nerve and plexus, and the lumbar sympathetic chain.

Classical teaching states that pain-transmitting C and A-delta nerve fibers enter the spinal cord through the dorsal roots and terminate in a dense network of synapses in the ipsilateral superficial laminae (I and II) of the dorsal horn, with minimal rostrocaudal extension of fibers. Whereas this characterization is true for somatic afferents, visceral C fiber afferents enter the cord primarily—but not exclusively—through the dorsal roots and terminate in a loose network of synapses in the superficial and deep dorsal horn and the ventral horn. These afferents also cross to the contralateral dorsal horn, with extensive rostrocaudal extension of fibers. This anatomic distinction underlies the precise localization of somatic pain and the diffuse localization of visceral pain, which may cross the midline; it may also determine the potency or efficacy of drugs that must reach afferent terminals, such as intrathecal opioids.

Pain-transmitting neurons in the spinal cord dorsal horn send axons to the contralateral ventral spinothalamic tract (stimulating thalamic neurons) with further projections to the somatosensory cortex, where pain is perceived. These spinal neurons also send axons through the spinoreticular and spinomesencephalic tracts to provide signals to the areas of vigilance (locus coeruleus, reticular formation), cardiorespiratory regulation (nucleus tractus solitarius, caudal medulla), and reflex descending inhibition (periaqueductal gray, locus coeruleus and subcoeruleus, nucleus raphe magnus, rostral medial medulla, cerebellum). Thalamic activation from painful stimuli results in the activation not only of the somatosensory cortex but also areas of memory (prefrontal cortex), motor response (M1 motor cortex), and emotional response (insular cortex, anterior cingulate cortex). Supraspinal pain pathways activated by pain of the first stage of labor can be briefly described sequentially, starting with the ascending pathways projecting to the pons and the medulla, thereby activating centers of cardiorespiratory control and descending pathways as well as the thalamus, which in turn sends projections to the anterior cingulate, motor, somatosensory, and limbic regions.

The anatomic basis for pain of the first stage of labor implies that amelioration of pain requires blockade of peripheral afferents (by paracervical, paravertebral, lumbar sympathetic, or epidural [T10–L1 dermatome] block) or of spinal cord transmission (by intrathecal injection of local anesthetic and/or opioid) (Fig. 21.6). Given the widespread distribution of visceral synapses in the spinal cord, intrathecally administered drugs must have physicochemical properties that facilitate deep penetration into the spinal cord to effectively reach and block the terminals responsible for pain transmission.

In particular, the lipophilicity of opioids and the ionization state of local anesthetics affect the rate of uptake across cellular membranes, thereby influencing the onset and clinical efficacy of the drug when administered in the epidural or intrathecal space.

Second Stage of Labor

Pain during the second stage of labor is transmitted by the same afferents activated during the first stage of labor but with additional afferents that innervate the cervix (vaginal surface), vagina, and perineum. These additional afferents are somatic, coursing through the pudendal nerve DRG at S2 to S4. Thus, the pain specific to the second stage of labor is precisely localized to the vagina and perineum and reflects distention, ischemia, and frank injury, either by stretching to the point of disruption or by surgical incision. Studies in nonpregnant women indicate a minor analgesic effect of mechanical self-stimulation of the vaginal surface of the cervix[44]; this effect may result from the stimulation of C fibers, because in women with a high oral intake of capsaicin, the activity of such fibers is reduced.[45] The relevance of this minor effect in reducing the pain of the second stage of labor has not been examined; however, it does suggest that noxious input during labor may activate endogenous analgesia (see later discussion).

The anatomic basis for pain of the second stage of labor implies that analgesia for this stage can be obtained by augmenting the methods used to treat the pain of the first stage of labor with caudad extension of the epidural blockade from T10 to S4, or alternatively with a bilateral pudendal nerve block for sacral analgesia (see Fig. 21.6).

NEUROPHYSIOLOGIC BASIS

Peripheral Afferent Terminals

Visceral nociceptors, such as those that transduce the pain of the first stage of labor, are activated by stretching and distention. However, unlike somatic afferents, they are not activated by cutting. With each uterine contraction, pressure is transmitted to stretch the uterine cervix, leading to the activation of these visceral afferent nerve terminals. How mechanical distention results in the depolarization of the nerve terminal and the generation of an action potential is not entirely known, but the following mechanisms are likely:

1. Several ion channels respond to the distortion of the cell membrane. One of them, brain sodium channel-1 or acid-sensing ion channel-2 (ASIC-2), is exclusively expressed in sensory afferents and might directly depolarize the nerve terminal by opening its channel when the membrane is distorted (Fig. 21.7).[46]
2. Mechanical distortion may result in the acute release of a short-acting neurotransmitter that directly stimulates ion channel receptors on nerve terminals. Although this process has not yet been examined in the uterine cervix, studies have observed that stretching the bladder urothelium releases adenosine triphosphate, which directly stimulates

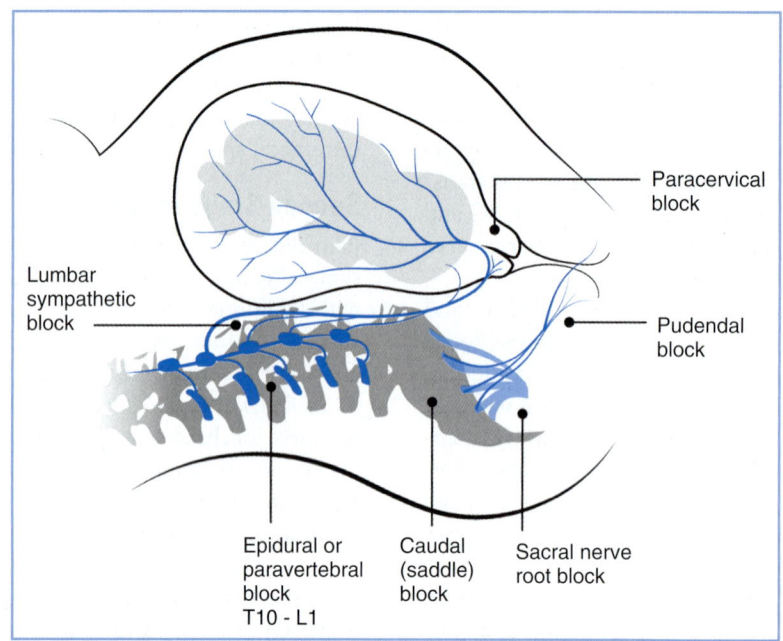

Fig. 21.6 Transmission and Blockade of Labor Pain. Labor pain has a visceral component (e.g., release of potassium, bradykinin, histamine, and serotonin) and a somatic component (e.g., mechanoreceptors). Noxious stimuli invoke nociceptive responses in the paracervical region and the pelvic and hypogastric plexus, as well as the lumbar sympathetic chain. Through the white rami communicantes of the T10, T11, T12, and L1 spinal nerves, nociceptive signals enter the dorsal horn of the spinal cord. Blockade at different levels along this path (sacral nerve root block of S2–S4, pudendal block, paracervical block, low caudal or true saddle block, lumbar sympathetic block, segmental epidural block of T10–L1, and paravertebral block T10–L1) can alleviate the visceral and somatic components of labor pain. Illustration by Naveen Nathan, MD, NorthShore University HealthSystem, University of Chicago Pritzker School of Medicine.

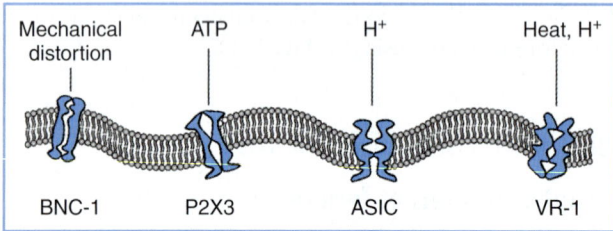

Fig. 21.7 Afferent nerve endings contain multiple excitatory ligand-gated ion channels, including those that respond to mechanical distortion: *BNC-1*, Brain sodium channel-1; *ATP*, adenosine triphosphate; *P2X3*, purinergic receptor; *H+*, hydrogen ion; *ASIC*, acid-sensing ion channel; *VR-1*, vanilloid receptor type 1.

a type of ligand-gated ion channel, P2X3, on sensory afferents in the bladder wall.[47] Because P2X3 receptors are widely expressed in C fibers,[48] this mechanism might be responsible for the pain resulting from the acute distention of the uterine cervix.

3. Local ischemia during contractions may result in gated or spontaneous activity of other ion channels. Some of these ion channels—the ASIC family—respond directly to the low pH that occurs during ischemia,[49] whereas other classes of ion channels may be activated to open spontaneously. For example, the vanilloid receptor type 1 (VR-1) is a receptor-gated ion channel that responds to noxious heat and capsaicin-like ligands.[50] VR-1 receptor-gated ion channels are not normally open in the absence of high temperature or capsaicin-like ligands; however, in the presence of

low pH, these channels open at room temperature. It is likely that VR-1 receptors are expressed on visceral afferent terminals, given that the application of capsaicin or heat to the distal esophagus in humans results in pain.[51] VR-1 receptors in the visceral afferent fibers implicated in the first stage of labor pain are presumed to demonstrate similar activation in response to the low pH produced by contraction-induced ischemia.[50]

Uterine cervical afferents (including the C fibers innervating the vaginal surface of the cervix) contain substance P, CGRP, and the enzyme nitric oxide synthase.[52] C fibers can be divided into two groups: (1) those that contain substance P and CGRP and respond to nerve growth factor through actions on tyrosine kinase A receptors, and (2) those that contain somatostatin and respond to glially derived growth factor through actions on a c-ret complex.[53] Other compounds commonly contained in C fiber terminals include glutamate, vasoactive intestinal peptide, and neuropeptide Y. The variable role of C fiber subtypes in the transmission of pain is also unclear. Given that somatostatin typically inhibits substance P release and pain transmission,[54,55] the net transmission of nociception at the spinal cord level may reflect a complex interaction between excitatory and inhibitory C fiber subtypes.

The numerous ion channels involved in the neurophysiology of pain during the first stage of labor may represent important new targets for local or systemic analgesic drug delivery. As an understanding of the classification, function, and relevance of different C fiber subtypes remains in its infancy, research involving these endocervical subtypes may ultimately benefit the treatment of labor pain.

Role of Sensitization

Nociceptors typically respond to high-threshold stimuli. Peripheral afferent terminals, which can change their properties in response to various conditions, can be directly stimulated by the low pH associated with inflammation and ischemia (Fig. 21.8); selective ligand-gated ion channels on these terminals can also be stimulated by the release of bradykinin.[56] In addition, peripheral inflammation can sensitize afferent terminals within minutes to hours, thereby altering their gene expression and leading to a large amplification of pain signaling.[57]

Peripheral inflammation is commonly associated with pain resulting from acute postoperative and chronic arthritic conditions, but it may also play an essential role in labor pain. Both the cervical ripening process and labor itself result from local synthesis and release of various inflammatory products including macrophages and leukocytes in the term cervix, inducible nitric oxide synthetase, and proinflammatory cytokines and metalloproteinases that degrade the cervical extracellular matrix.[58] The clinical utility of these inflammatory mediators includes agents (e.g., prostaglandin E$_2$ [PGE$_2$]) that prepare the cervix for labor induction and inhibitors (e.g., indomethacin) that slow preterm labor.

PGE$_2$ is an especially important sensitizing agent for uterine cervical afferents. In most species, the onset of labor is triggered by a sudden decline in circulating estrogen concentration. This decrease removes a tonic block on the expression of cyclooxygenase, leading to an increase in local production of prostaglandins, especially PGE$_2$.[59] PGE$_2$ is central to a variety of processes that allow ripening and dilation of the uterine cervix. During the 24 to 72 hours preceding the onset of labor, collagen in the cervix becomes disorganized owing to the activation of prostaglandin receptors and the activity of inflammatory cytokines (mostly interleukin-1-beta [IL-1β] and tumor necrosis factor-alpha [TNF-α]) and matrix metalloproteinases (especially types 2 and 9).[60,61] A series of studies in the rat paw have demonstrated that PGE$_2$ induces peripheral sensitization in a sex-independent manner by activation of protein kinase A[62] and nitric oxide synthase.[63]

Cytokines and growth factors are released into the uterine cervix immediately before and during labor. Cytokine IL-1β enhances cyclooxygenase activity and substance P release in the DRG and spinal cord.[64,65] TNF-α increases the spontaneous activity of afferent fibers[66] and enhances CGRP release and VR-1 receptor expression in DRG cells in culture.[67] Nerve growth factor also induces mechanical hypersensitivity.[68] These sensitizing substances (prostaglandins, cytokines, and growth factors) signal peripheral nerves in a manner that results in changes in DRG cell number, peptide expression and release, receptor and ion channel expression, and biophysical properties. For example, inflammatory mediators alter the expression of sodium (Na$^+$) channel subtypes,[69,70] thereby resulting in more rapid, repetitive firing capability[71] and spontaneous afferent activity.[72] Thus, sensitized peripheral afferents may fire at a lower stimulus threshold and more frequently, though the intensity and nature of the stimulus may be objectively unchanged.

Estrogen receptor signaling can dramatically affect the structure of the uterine cervix and possibly modulate pain responses. Long-term estrogen exposure sensitizes a subset of mechanosensitive afferents innervating the uterine cervix. The hypogastric afferents that innervate the uterine cervix are polymodal and contain high-threshold (HT) and low-threshold (LT) fibers. Long-term estrogen exposure increases the spontaneous activities of both HT and LT fibers, but only HT fibers show greater responses to uterine cervical distention.[73] Long-term estrogen exposure also increases the proportion of hypogastric afferents innervating the uterine cervix, which express transient receptor potential vanilloid type 1 (TRPV-1). Capsazepine, a TRPV-1 channel antagonist, reduces the hypogastric afferent responses to cervical distention in estrogen-treated animals but not in ovariectomized animals without estrogen replacement.[74,75] These data suggest that the TRPV-1 receptor is important for estrogen-induced sensitization and amplification of pain responses to uterine cervical distention and thus represents a potential new target for preventing or treating such pain.

Implications of peripheral sensitization of cervical afferents during labor include:

1. Braxton-Hicks contractions, prior to the onset of this inflammatory process, may be as powerful as labor contractions but with significantly less pain.
2. Pain may increase with the progress of labor as a result of sensitization.

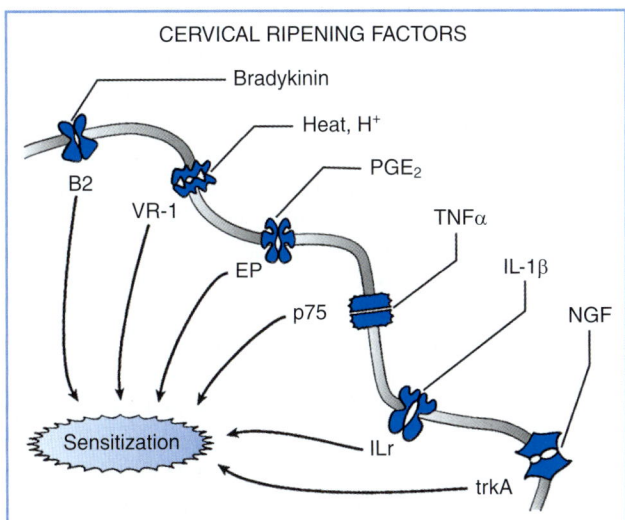

Fig. 21.8 Effects of Inflammation From Cervical Ripening on Afferent Terminals. A variety of factors, including bradykinin, heat and hydrogen ions, prostaglandins (including PGE$_2$), tumor necrosis factor-α (TNFα), interleukin-1 beta (IL-1β), and nerve growth factor (NGF), act on their cognate receptors to sensitize nerve endings and amplify the perception and severity of pain from nerve stimulation. *B2*, Bradykinin-2 receptor; *EP*, prostaglandin E receptor; *ILr*, interleukin-1 receptor; *p75*, p75 tumor necrosis factor-α receptor; *trkA*, tyrosine kinase A; *VR-1*, vanilloid receptor type 1.

3. Inflammatory mediators may provide new targets to treat labor pain.

Inhibitory Receptors

Given the multiplicity of direct excitatory and sensitizing mechanisms on peripheral terminals, more plausible peripheral targets are the endogenous inhibitory receptors expressed on the afferent terminals (Fig. 21.9). Although μ-opioid receptors have achieved the widest attention and are expressed in some afferents in the setting of inflammation,[76] the efficacy of local instillation of morphine has proved disappointing,[77] with the exception of an intraarticular injection.[78] Moreover, antinociception by μ-opioid receptor agonists to uterine cervical distention occurs in the central, but not peripheral, nervous system.[59]

κ-Opioid receptor agonists may effectively treat visceral pain owing to the presence of these receptors in visceral (but not somatic) afferents, at least in the gastrointestinal tract.[79] κ-Opioid receptor agonists can also produce antinociception in response to uterine cervical distention through actions in the peripheral nervous system.[40,80] Pharmaceutical firms are developing drugs of this class that are restricted to the periphery, have few central side effects,[81,82] and presumably express little potential for placental transfer; potentially, such agents could be useful for labor analgesia.

Estrogen and progesterone can alter the analgesic response to opioids. In most cases involving somatic stimulation, tonic estrogen treatment reduces the efficacy of μ-opioid but not κ-opioid receptor agonists.[83] Further, κ-opioid receptor agonists have greater analgesic efficacy in women than in men.[84] In animals, tonic estrogen exposure reduces the inhibitory responses to uterine cervical distention by morphine but not to the κ-opioid receptor agonist U-50488.[85] In contrast, the inhibitory action of *intrathecal* morphine against responses to uterine cervical distention is unaffected by tonic estrogen exposure,[86] which is consistent with the observation that

intrathecal opioids relieve the pain of the first (visceral), but not second (mostly somatic), stage of labor.

Implications of inhibitory receptors on afferent terminals are that κ- but not μ-opioid receptor agonists may produce pain relief through their actions in the periphery. Selective, peripherally restricted drugs are under development for the systemic treatment of visceral pain. In addition, estrogen-dependent inhibition of the supraspinal (but not the spinal) analgesic action of μ-opioid receptor agonists may underlie the limited analgesic effect produced by systemic opioids,[87] a finding that is in contrast to the efficacy of intrathecal opioids[88] in relieving the pain of the first stage of labor.

Peripheral Nerve Axons

The current approach to labor analgesia relies primarily on an understanding of the afferent axons and their level of entry into the spinal cord and on the central administration of local anesthetics to block afferent traffic conduction. Axons are considered conduits that allow for the propagation of action potentials by the transitory opening of sodium and other ion channels.

Although a number of voltage-gated sodium channel subtypes exist, most studies have focused on three specific subtypes that are expressed in sensory but not motor afferents.[89] Two of these, NaV1.8 and NaV1.9, are relatively resistant to blockade by tetrodotoxin (TTX-R); NaV1.9 is often referred to as "persistent," owing to its very slow inactivation kinetics.[90] Inflammation and injury to nerves decrease the TTX-R current density in afferent cell bodies.[91] Some investigators have suggested that NaV1.8 is selectively trafficked to the periphery after injury and inflammation[91] and that a reduction of its expression reduces hypersensitivity.[92] Other investigators, using sucrose gap measurements of compound action potentials, have demonstrated a shortened refractory period and a decrease in delayed depolarization after nerve injury[93,94] that are consistent with the greater expression of rapidly repriming tetrodotoxin-sensitive (TTX-S) channels and the decreased expression of kinetically slow TTX-R channels. To date, these studies have focused primarily on peripheral nerve injury models of chronic pain, and neither the subtypes nor their change during the cervical inflammation of labor has been studied. In one animal study, dexmedetomidine was shown to reduce NaV1.8 currents in DRG neurons and decrease excitability of small sensory neurons via increased activation threshold and decreased rate of firing.[95]

Selective subtype-specific sodium channel blockers could improve both the safety and efficacy of the treatment of labor pain, because such agents would potentially not interact with sodium channels in the brain, heart, or motor nerve fibers. Some investigators have observed that injection of the antidepressant amitriptyline, an agent known to block the NaV1.8 sodium channel, around the peripheral nerves provides a neural blockade two- to fivefold longer than that provided by injection of long-acting local anesthetics.[96,97]

Another subject of current research is the prolongation of selective antinociception without motor or sympathetic block via manipulation of the TRPV-1 receptor, a

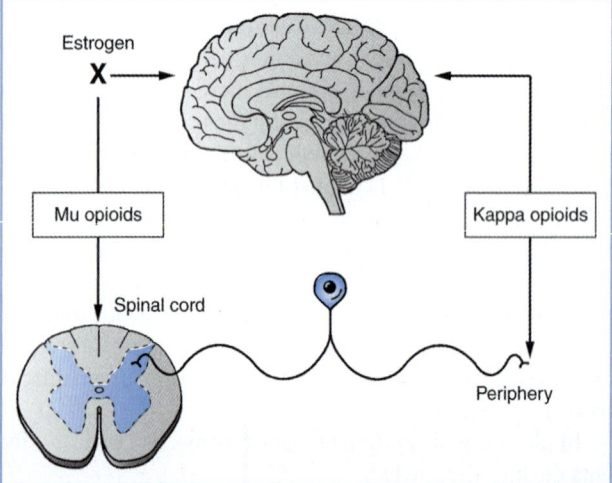

Fig. 21.9 κ-Opioid receptor agonists act primarily at visceral afferent terminals in the periphery and in the supraspinal central nervous system to provide analgesia during the first stage of labor, whereas μ-opioid receptor agonists act in the spinal cord and the supraspinal central nervous system. Estrogens block the effect of μ-opioid receptor agonists at supraspinal sites.

nonselective ligand-gated cation channel. TRPV-1 receptors are expressed in peripheral primary afferent neurons, nociceptive C and A-delta fibers, and the DRG, as well as the structures involving the endogenous antinociceptive descending pathway. TRPV-1 receptors can be activated by capsaicin, heat, and endovanilloids, leading to release of substance P and activation of inhibitory neurons in laminae I, III, and IV. Further, activation of the TRPV-1 receptors causes opening of the small TRPV-1 channels on the neurons and allows size-selective entry of coadministered charged molecules. Permanently charged local anesthetic, when applied alone, cannot cross the nerve membrane to exert its effect on sodium channels in small sensory neurons. When applied in the presence of capsaicin or other TRPV-1 agonists, the permanently charged local anesthetic becomes permeant to exert its local anesthetic effect. Binshtok et al.[98] reported the inhibition of nociceptors by TRPV-1-mediated entry of impermeant sodium channel blockers. However, stimulation of TRPV-1 receptors, such as with capsaicin alone, also results in the induction of receptor-mediated acute pain. Rodent studies indicate that the coapplication of lidocaine and its quaternary permanently charged derivative QX-314, which activate and enter TRPV-1 channels, respectively, produces a prolonged, predominantly nociceptor-selective block without the nocifensive behavior associated with capsaicin.[99] The issues of pain elicited with administration of TRPV-1 agonists such as capsaicin and, more importantly, the neurotoxicity of permanently charged Na[+] channel blockers remain to be overcome and require further research. Should future research prove the absence of toxicity, it is conceivable that amitriptyline or other agents that interact with Na[+] channel subtypes and/or TPRV-1 receptors could be considered for single-injection techniques to produce prolonged and selective analgesia for labor pain and postoperative pain relief.

Interactions among the numerous ion channels expressed on axons can alter neural conduction. An example is the transient refractory period caused by the membrane hyperpolarization following a short burst of nerve firing. This phenomenon results from activation of the Na[+]/K[+] exchange pump and dampens high-frequency nerve activity. The Na[+]/K[+] exchange pump activity, in turn, can be reduced by a hyperpolarization-induced current termed I_h. Drugs that block the I_h current enhance the hyperpolarization caused by the Na[+]/K[+] exchange pump and ultimately serve to reduce nerve traffic[100] and provide prolonged analgesia.[101] A second example is the desensitization of VR-1 receptors present on the axons of C fibers. The perineural injection of drugs that desensitize these receptors without first stimulating them avoids the induction of receptor-mediated acute pain and instead produces prolonged selective sensory analgesia without motor effects.[102] The mechanism by which VR-1 receptor desensitization alters the transmission of action potentials is under investigation.

Implications of the neurophysiology of axonal transmission of labor pain are that sodium channel subtype-selective agents, or those that affect other ion channels expressed on axons, may provide safer and more selective tools for regional analgesic techniques.

Spinal Cord

When action potentials invade the central terminals of C and A-delta fiber afferents in the spinal cord, voltage-gated calcium channels open. Increased intracellular calcium triggers a multistep process of neurotransmitter docking and fusion with the plasma membrane, which results in neurotransmitter release.[103] Inhibition of these calcium channels, such as by gabapentin, and the consequent neurotransmitter release, produces antinociception to visceral stimulation.[104]

A nociceptive stimulus can result in the release of multiple excitatory neurotransmitters, including amino acids (glutamate, aspartate) and peptides (especially substance P, CGRP, and neurokinin A) that interact with specific receptors on spinal cord neurons. Although the stimulation of neurokinin receptors is necessary for the perception of moderate to severe pain,[105] a complex and poorly understood interplay exists among these released neurotransmitters.

As described, neurotransmitter release at sensory afferent terminals is controlled by presynaptic receptors that act primarily by altering the flux of intracellular calcium when an action potential arrives. Some of these neurotransmitters are excitatory; for example, the action of acetylcholine on nicotinic acetylcholine receptors amplifies further neurotransmitter release.[106] Gamma-aminobutyric acid (GABA) is the key endogenous inhibitory neurotransmitter in the nervous system, and stimulation of GABA receptors significantly reduces the afferent terminal release of other neurotransmitters.[107] Multiple compounds produce analgesia by enhancing the release of GABA at afferent terminals in the spinal cord. The coexistence of excitatory and inhibitory systems can make the response to a neurotransmitter or an exogenously administered agent, such as a local anesthetic drug given intrathecally, difficult to predict. For example, acetylcholine can enhance or reduce the afferent terminal release of neurotransmitters by actions on nicotinic and muscarinic receptors, respectively.[108,109] The net effect of acetylcholine appears to be inhibitory, which is indicated by the analgesic effect of intrathecal administration of the cholinesterase inhibitor neostigmine.[110]

The primary mechanism of action of the neurotransmitter enkephalin, which is released by spinal cord interneurons, and of norepinephrine, which is released by axons descending from pontine centers, is the inhibition of neurotransmitter release from primary afferent terminals. These substances act on μ-opioid and α_2-adrenergic receptors, respectively,[111,112] and may produce some of the similar effects observed after the intrathecal administration of opioids and α_2-adrenergic agonists for the treatment of labor pain.

Amino acids and peptides released from sensory afferents stimulate a heterogeneous group of spinal cord neurons, including neurons that project to supraspinal structures, interneurons that modulate transmission at the afferent terminal itself (the "gate" of the control theory), and interneurons that stimulate motor and sympathetic nervous system reflexes. Large and sustained glutamate release from an intensely noxious stimulus can activate *N*-methyl-D-aspartate (NMDA) receptors, resulting in sustained depolarization and enhanced excitability of projection neurons (Fig. 21.10).[113] Although the intrathecal injection of NMDA receptor antagonists (e.g., ketamine) has been restricted because of neurotoxicity concerns,[114] systemic infusion of magnesium sulfate has been observed to produce postoperative analgesia.[115] Magnesium is an endogenous inhibitory modulator of NMDA receptors, and it is conceivable that magnesium sulfate administered systemically for obstetric indications may have a minor effect on labor pain.

Prolonged and intense nociceptive stimuli can produce sensitization and amplification of pain signaling at the spinal cord level that mirrors the peripheral sensitization resulting from inflammation. Some of these processes are a direct consequence of receptors (e.g., NMDA receptors) that are activated only with highly intense and prolonged stimulation or by the long-term release of neurotransmitters that simultaneously activate the glutamate and substance P receptors on the same cell. Others reflect the synthesis and release of classic "inflammatory" substances by the spinal cord glial cells in response to prolonged afferent stimulation from nitric oxide and prostaglandins, especially PGE_2. Some nonopioid analgesic drugs produce analgesia by actions exclusively (e.g., acetaminophen [paracetamol]) or primarily (e.g., aspirin) in the central nervous system, especially the spinal cord.[116]

Spinal sensitization processes represent a novel target for the treatment of labor pain. More than 90 years ago, Cleland[42] noted the presence of hypersensitivity to light touch on the skin of dermatomes T11 and T12 in laboring women, which likely represents the enhanced sensitivity of spinal cord neurons receiving both visceral input from the cervix and skin input at those levels.[117] When the visceral stimulation to these dermatomes was blocked by a paravertebral local anesthetic injection, Cleland[42] observed that the hypersensitivity was ablated; this observation is consistent with the later finding that ongoing C fiber input is required for hypersensitivity to occur.[118]

Uterine cervical distention results in a pattern of spinal cord neuronal activation similar to that witnessed during labor and delivery. In a study in rats reported by Tong et al.,[119] uterine cervical distention significantly increased c-fos immunoreactivity in the spinal cord from T12 to L2, with most of the c-fos expression occurring in the deep dorsal horn and central canal regions. Uterine cervical distention–evoked c-fos expression was prevented by prior infiltration of lidocaine into the cervix or by intrathecal administration of ketorolac (a cyclooxygenase [COX] inhibitor) in a dose-dependent manner.[119] Intrathecal administration of indomethacin (a nonspecific COX inhibitor) and the selective COX-2 inhibitor SC-58238 effectively ablated uterine cervical distention–induced electromyographic activity without altering the hemodynamic response,. By contrast, the selective COX-1 inhibitor SC-58360 was ineffective in ablating uterine cervical distention–induced electromyographic activity, as was ketorolac, an agent with higher affinity for COX-1 than COX-2.[120] Together, these data suggest that targeting COX-2 is necessary to treat the acute visceral pain often associated with brief infrequent contractions in late pregnancy; therefore, intrathecal ketorolac would be predicted to be ineffective. However, in the setting of sustained, frequent, and repetitive contractions for a prolonged period (as occurs during active labor), intrathecal ketorolac might be effective. The intrathecal injection of ketorolac has been introduced into experimental human trials[121] and warrants examination as a potential modality for selective treatment of labor pain.

The neurophysiologic basis for labor pain in the spinal cord implies that purely inhibitory mechanisms (e.g., opioid and α_2-adrenergic receptors) can be mimicked by the intrathecal injection of agonists to these receptors. However, the administration of other agents (e.g., acetylcholine) in this location has less predictable results. Central sensitization mechanisms in the spinal cord most certainly occur during labor, and future treatments may target these mechanisms.

Ascending and Descending Projections

Spinal cord neurons project to multiple brainstem sites as well as the thalamus. Descending systems, which are activated primarily by stimulation of the nucleus raphe magnus, the periaqueductal gray, and the locus coeruleus, modulate pain transmission as described in the gate control theory.[122] Activation of descending pathways results in the spinal release of endogenous ligands for serotonergic, opioid, and α_2-adrenergic receptor-mediated analgesia. Spillover of neurotransmitters into the cerebrospinal fluid has been used as a measure of activation of these systems. Studies measuring these substances in laboring women have shown no increase in enkephalin but an increase in norepinephrine.[123] These descending inhibitory systems can be activated by psychoprophylactic methods,[124] and agents that prolong or intensify the action of these ligands, such as enkephalinase inhibitors and monoamine reuptake inhibitors, might further enhance analgesia.[125]

Brainstem activation by the pain of labor leads to other reflexes, such as increases in sympathetic nervous system

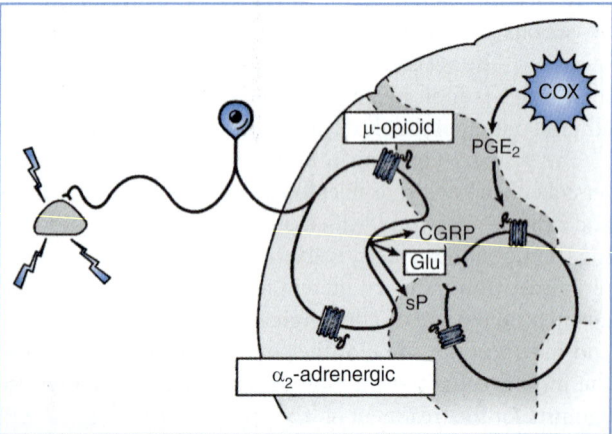

Fig. 21.10 Pain Transmission in the Spinal Cord. Excitatory transmission occurs directly by release of amino acids such as glutamate (Glu) and peptides (sP [substance P], CGRP [calcitonin gene–related peptide]) and indirectly via activation of enzymes such as cyclooxygenase (COX) in nearby glia, which synthesize prostaglandins, including prostaglandin E_2 (PGE_2). Inhibitory mechanisms are primarily presynaptic, with µ-opioid and α_2-adrenergic receptors being the most common (or at least the most studied).

activity and respiratory drive and, with prolonged activation, stimulation of descending pathways that amplify rather than reduce pain transmission at the spinal cord.[126,127] The circuitry and pharmacology of such pain-enhancing systems in the brainstem and their potential applications for treatment are under current investigation.

Our understanding of the areas of the brain activated during labor pain is limited, although studies of other types of experimental nociception in healthy volunteers indicate that visceral pain is considered more unpleasant than somatic pain. This difference reflects, in part, the greater activation of centers for negative emotions, including fear. Although distraction methods do not alter the thalamic activation from noxious stimulation, a reduction in cortical activation and the report of pain have been observed,[128] supporting a suprathalamic mechanism of psychoprophylaxis in the reduction of pain.

The neurophysiologic basis of labor pain and ascending projections suggests the activation of multiple supraspinal sites. Some of these sites stimulate potentially detrimental cardiorespiratory reflexes. Other sites, which send descending projections modulating transmission in the spinal cord, may be targeted for the provision of analgesia. In addition, suprathalamic modulation of pain signals appears to partially account for interindividual differences in pain perception and for the relative efficacy of psychoprophylaxis in reducing the intensity of reported pain.

EFFECT ON THE MOTHER

Obstetric Course

Several aspects of labor pain can affect the course of labor and delivery (Fig. 21.11). Pain enhances the activity of the sympathetic nervous system, leading to increased plasma concentrations of catecholamines, especially epinephrine (adrenaline). The provision of labor analgesia reduces the plasma concentration of epinephrine and its associated beta-adrenergic tocolytic effects on the myometrium. This process may underlie the observations by some investigators who have noted, either anecdotally or under controlled conditions, a shift from dysfunctional to normal labor patterns in some women when analgesia is achieved with paravertebral[42,44] or epidural[129] blocks or with systemic meperidine (pethidine) analgesia.[130] The abrupt reduction in plasma epinephrine concentration following the rapid onset of neuraxial analgesia may result in an acute reduction of beta-adrenergic tocolysis and a transient period of uterine hyperstimulation. In some cases, these changes may lead to transient fetal stress and fetal heart rate abnormalities.[131,132] Therefore, the presence of a dysfunctional labor pattern or fetal monitoring suggestive of fetal compromise are important considerations in the decision to institute neuraxial blockade. Some studies have found that prolonged fetal decelerations are more common following the combined spinal-epidural technique than conventional epidural or dural puncture epidural techniques,[133] while others have found minimal difference; regardless, fetal

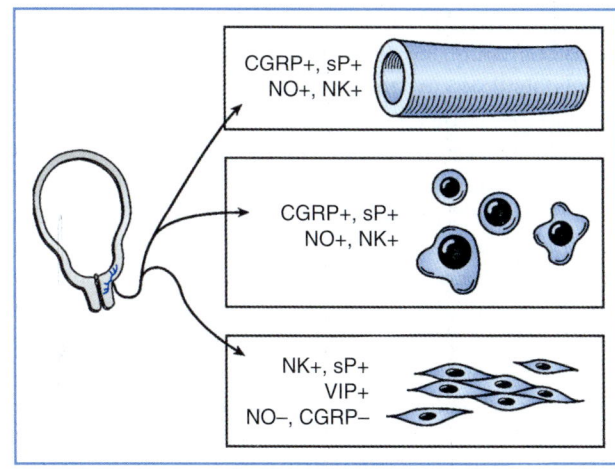

Fig. 21.11 Aspects of Pain That May Affect the Course of Labor. In addition to indirect effects (e.g., beta-adrenergic tocolysis from increased secretion of epinephrine, greater release of oxytocin via Ferguson reflex), depolarization of afferent terminals in the lower uterine segment and cervix can directly alter aspects of labor. Substances released by nerve terminals include those that increase local blood flow (CGRP [calcitonin gene–related peptide], sP [substance P], NO [nitric oxide], NK [neurokinin]), those that stimulate immune cell function, and those that stimulate (+) or inhibit (–) myometrial smooth muscle activity, including vasoactive intestinal peptide (VIP).

heart rate alterations can occur following any technique of neuraxial block and thus the maternal and fetal conditions should always be observed.[134]

Ferguson's reflex, a neuroendocrine response by which fetal distention of the cervix stimulates maternal oxytocin production and release, involves neural input from ascending spinal tracts (especially from sacral sensory input) to the midbrain. Although spontaneous labor and delivery occur in women with spinal cord injury, which disrupts this tract,[135] some investigators have argued that neuraxial analgesia can inhibit this reflex and prolong labor, especially the second stage. However, strong evidence for this does not exist. Some studies have noted a reduction in plasma oxytocin concentration with epidural local anesthetic[136] or intrathecal opioid[137] analgesia, whereas others have not noted such a reduction.[138]

Papka and Shew[33] suggested that afferent terminals in the lower uterine segment and cervix might have an important secretory (efferent) function in the regulation of labor. Afferent terminals contain many substances that stimulate (substance P, glutamate, vasoactive intestinal peptide) or inhibit (CGRP, nitric oxide) myometrial activity, and these substances can be released locally into the cervix and lower uterine segment when terminals are depolarized by contraction-related tissue distortion. In addition, depolarization of the afferent terminal can result in an action potential that, upon reaching a site of nerve branching, invades adjacent branches and travels distally to depolarize distant terminals of the same nerve. This axon reflex has long been recognized to occur in somatic nerves; owing to the more extensive arborizations believed to exist in visceral nerves, local stimulation should result in more widespread release of these transmitters. Therefore, it is tempting to speculate that these axon reflexes are more profoundly affected when local anesthetic is administered closer to the terminals associated with cervical dilation and labor (e.g., as occurs with paracervical and paravertebral blocks) than occurs when local anesthetic is administered farther away from the terminals (e.g., with epidural block). This speculation would imply that the net effect of afferent terminal-released substances inhibits rather than accelerates labor. A Cochrane review of studies comparing paracervical, uterosacral, and intracervical injection of local anesthetic versus placebo for pain with cervical dilation found that, compared with placebo, paracervical local anesthetic provided pain relief with cervical dilation; excluding placebo, the other techniques yielded comparatively equivocal results, which were thought to be inferior to neuraxial blockade for cervical dilation.[139]

In summary, neural stimulation through pain pathways leads to the release of substances that either increase (oxytocin) or inhibit (epinephrine) uterine activity and cervical dilation. Therefore, the effect of analgesia on the course of labor can vary between and within individuals. In addition, axon reflexes can result in the release of neurotransmitters from afferents into the lower uterine segment and cervix. It is hoped that future investigation will determine whether the proximity of local anesthetic deposition affects the response of cervical dilation and labor.

Cardiac, Respiratory, and Gastrointestinal Effects

Labor exerts stresses on the cardiovascular and respiratory systems. The elevated plasma catecholamine concentrations observed during labor pain can further increase maternal cardiac output and peripheral vascular resistance and decrease uteroplacental perfusion. Even transient stress is associated with dramatic increases in plasma concentration of norepinephrine and subsequent decreases in uterine blood flow (Fig. 21.12). Plasma epinephrine concentrations in women with painful labor are similar to those observed after an intravenous bolus of epinephrine 15 μg[140]; intravenous bolus injection of epinephrine 10 to 20 μg resulted in a significant (albeit transient) reduction in uterine blood flow in gravid ewes.[141] Effective neuraxial analgesia, provided by epidural local anesthetic[142] or intrathecal opioid administration,[143] significantly reduced (50%) maternal catecholamine concentrations. By contrast, neonatal plasma catecholamine concentrations do not appear to be altered by maternal neuraxial anesthetic techniques; this relative independence of neonatal catecholamine responses may be important for the neonatal adaptation to extrauterine life.[144]

The physiologic changes of pregnancy result in increased minute ventilation, with respiratory alkalosis, as a mechanism to meet the demands of increased oxygen requirements for the parturient and the fetus. The intermittent pain of uterine contractions also stimulates the respiratory system, leading to periods of intermittent hyperventilation. In the absence of supplemental oxygen administration, compensatory periods of hypoventilation between contractions result in transient episodes of maternal, and even fetal, hypoxemia (Fig. 21.13). Treatment of labor pain with epidural analgesia minimizes the increase in net minute ventilation and the accompanying

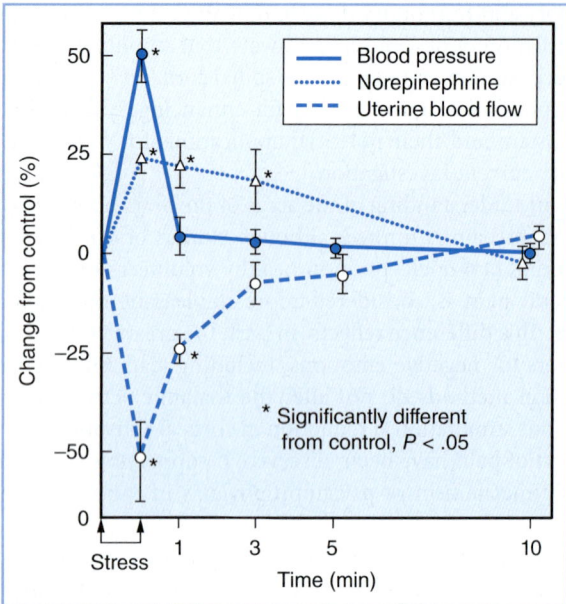

Fig. 21.12 Effect of a painful stimulus on the hind leg on maternal blood pressure, norepinephrine concentrations, and uterine blood flow in gravid ewes. The increase in blood pressure was transient, but plasma norepinephrine concentrations remained elevated for several minutes; the elevation is reflected in the slow return of uterine blood flow to normal. From Shnider SM, Wright RG, Levinson G, et al. Uterine blood flow and plasma norepinephrine changes during maternal stress in the pregnant ewe. *Anesthesiology.* 1979;50:524–527.

increase in oxygen consumption.[145] In general, the cardiovascular and respiratory system changes induced by labor pain are well tolerated by healthy parturients (with normal uteroplacental perfusion) and their fetuses. Some authors have concluded that these changes are of minimal relevance in uncomplicated labor.[27] However, in the presence of maternal or fetal disease or compromise, significant cardiopulmonary alterations may lead to maternal or fetal decompensation; effective analgesia may be especially important in such cases.

Labor pain, anxiety, and emotional stress increase gastrin release and inhibit the segmental and suprasegmental reflexes of gastrointestinal and urinary motility. This in turn results in an increase in gastric acidity and volume, and a delay in bladder emptying.[146] These changes are further aggravated by the recumbent position, opioids, and other depressant medications (e.g., barbiturates), putting laboring parturients at risk for pulmonary aspiration of gastric contents, especially during emergency induction of general anesthesia for cesarean delivery. There are no known studies examining the severity of labor pain with rate of gastric emptying, but in nonpregnant subjects even mild to moderate pain has been demonstrated to slow gastric motility and delay gastric emptying.[147] Thus, the physiologic impairment that occurs due to pregnancy may be further compounded by the presence of uncontrolled labor pain. Effective neuraxial labor analgesia has been found to facilitate gastric emptying in laboring patients compared with those without neuraxial blockade.[148]

In summary, pain-induced activation of the sympathetic nervous system during labor is associated with cardiovascular, respiratory, and gastrointestinal effects that may alter

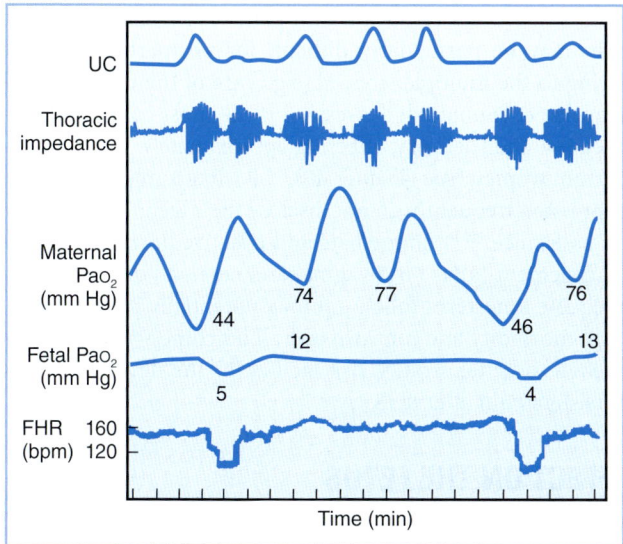

UC

Thoracic
impedance

Maternal
Pao₂
(mm Hg)

74   77

44   12   76

Fetal Pao₂
(mm Hg)

46   13

5   4

FHR   160
(bpm)   120

Time (min)

Fig. 21.13 Maternal and fetal hypoxemia during hypoventilation between uterine contractions (UC), which are associated with maternal hyperventilation. *FHR,* Fetal heart rate. From Bonica JJ. Labour pain. In Wall PD, Melzack R, eds. Textbook of Pain. Churchill Livingstone; 1984, as redrawn from Huch A, Huch R, Schneider H, Rooth GL. Continuous transcutaneous monitoring of fetal oxygen tension during labour. *Br J Obstet Gynaecol.* 1977;84(suppl):1–39.

maternal and fetal well-being. The provision of effective neuraxial analgesia may mitigate many of these cardiopulmonary effects.

Psychological Effects

The interindividual experience of labor pain is highly variable and is influenced by social, cultural, and psychological factors. The reciprocal interplay between labor pain and psychological conditions is similarly complex, and labor pain may predispose patients to a multitude of sequelae including PTSD and depression. For some, the pain of labor may contribute to birth trauma, predisposing as many as one of every three parturients to the development of PTSD.[149] Parturients who perceive the labor and delivery process as positive and nonthreatening may undergo pain without suffering,[26] and in laboring patients who did not perceive their pain as "suffering"[149] numerical pain scores were not predictive of the development of postpartum PTSD. These findings are consistent with the biopsychosocial model of pain, suggesting the cognitive interpretation of a pain experience influences an individual's psychological outcomes.

Although the acceptance of labor analgesia has a minor overall effect on maternal satisfaction with the labor and delivery process,[150] individual patients may ascribe significant personal meaning to their decision regarding analgesia. Billewicz-Driemel and Milne[151] reported that a small proportion (<5%) of women who requested and received epidural labor analgesia described a sense of deprivation from having missed the natural labor experience in its entirety; some of these women may subsequently seek psychiatric counseling.[152]

By contrast, unrelieved severe labor pain can have psychological and physical consequences, including depression and

negative thoughts about sexual relationships.[17] In a 5-year study in Sweden, 43 women requested elective cesarean delivery owing to a fear of labor and vaginal delivery.[153] The prevalence of tocophobia (fear of childbirth) is notable in some countries with high elective cesarean delivery rates, such as Brazil.[154] Frank psychotic reactions resembling PTSD can occur after childbirth, although the incidence is rare (<1%).[155]

Psychological consequences of labor pain are complex, and influenced by predisposing and protective factors, as well as the personal significance an individual attaches to the pain of labor and childbirth. Psychological harm can be experienced through the provision or withholding of labor analgesia, as well as the occurrence or perception of birth trauma, underscoring the tremendous variability in the meaning of labor pain for different women.

Pain After Delivery

Many women undergo delivery without negative sequelae, but some may experience significant persistent postpartum pain and even depression. Pain is the most frequent postpartum complaint.[8] Studies of acute and chronic postpartum pain have shown a 7% incidence of perineal pain at 8 weeks after vaginal delivery,[156] a 43% incidence of hyperalgesia at 48 hours, and a 23% incidence of residual pain at 6 months after cesarean delivery.[157] In a multicenter, prospective, longitudinal cohort study of 1288 parturients delivering either by cesarean or vaginal delivery, Eisenach et al.,[158] using regression analyses and propensity adjustment, reported a 10.9% prevalence of severe acute pain within 36 hours postpartum, whereas the prevalences of persistent pain and depression at 8 weeks postpartum were 9.8% and 11.2%, respectively. The severity of acute postpartum pain, but not the mode of delivery, was independently related to risk for persistent pain and depression at 8 weeks postpartum, both of which also resulted in negative effects on activities of daily living and on sleep. Women with severe acute postpartum pain had 2.5- and 3.0-fold increases in risk for persistent pain and depression, respectively, compared with those with mild acute postpartum pain. These findings suggest these morbidities may not be related to degrees of physical tissue trauma but rather may be related to an individual's pain response to that injury.

Although there is significant interindividual variability with regard to acute postpartum pain,[21] the severity of acute postoperative pain in nonobstetric surgical patients has been correlated with the occurrence of chronic pain.[159] Whether the presence and severity of labor pain or the presence and severity of acute postpartum pain after either vaginal or cesarean delivery predicts the occurrence of chronic pain is under investigation. Studies in animals suggest that acute intervention at the time of tissue injury reduces the likelihood of developing chronic pain,[160] indicating that the severity of acute pain may be an active participatory component in the pathophysiology of transitioning from acute to chronic pain.[158] In a prospective cohort study of 241 parturients undergoing vaginal delivery, Ding et al.[161] reported that the use of epidural labor analgesia was associated with a decreased risk for postpartum depression (odds ratio, 0.31; 95% confidence interval, 0.12 to 0.82;

$P = .018$). Attentive pain treatment and follow-up during the early postpartum period may potentially reduce long-term morbidities and improve overall outcomes.

The reported incidence of chronic pain after delivery varies widely because of differences in the definitions, the inclusion or exclusion of chronic pain, and the imprecision in separating acute from preexisting pain. Long-term follow-up of postpartum patients showed that the incidence of chronic pain (defined as new pain that began at the time of labor and delivery) at 6 months and 1 year was remarkably low at 3% and 0.1%, respectively, compared with nonobstetric surgeries with similar tissue injury.[162] In a sciatic nerve injury–induced neuropathic pain model in rats, the birthing plus nursing of pups in combination, but not individually, appeared protective against the development of surgical nerve injury–induced hypersensitivity to pain. This protection is likely mediated by spinal oxytocin because the protective effect is abolished by administration of spinal atosiban, an oxytocin antagonist.[163]

Most pain research examines pain scores at predefined time points in the postoperative or postpartum period but neglects the day-to-day experiences of pain recovery following surgery. Houle et al.[164] applied growth curve modeling to patients undergoing cesarean delivery or lower limb total joint arthroplasty by evaluating daily pain scores; a Bayesian change-point model, rather than the traditional log(time) model, was observed to be a better fit to the diminution of postoperative pain scores and suggested that "meaningful subpopulations of experience may exist" wherein patients do not recover in the same manner after the same surgery.

Further research is needed to better define protective and/or predictive factors in patients who are at risk for developing severe acute and/or chronic postpartum pain. Coupled status, higher education, and employment appear to be protective factors in studies of postpartum pain.[8] Persistent or chronic pain may be particularly difficult for postpartum patients owing to the multiple stresses (e.g., care of the neonate) and sequelae encountered; depression is the most common complication after delivery, affecting approximately 13% of postpartum women (see Chapter 49).[165] Postpartum patients with depression frequently do not disclose their feelings nor desire for assistance.[166,167] Immediate and effective postpartum pain management (after both vaginal and cesarean delivery) with adequate long-term follow-up may potentially prevent long-term morbidity and improve overall outcomes.[167] Research is needed to better stratify risk factors for the development of persistent pain after delivery.

EFFECT ON THE FETUS

The absence of direct neural connections from the mother to the fetus appears to limit the direct fetal effects of maternal labor pain. However, labor pain and processes can indirectly affect systems that determine uteroplacental perfusion. First, pain influences the release of oxytocin and epinephrine, which are important determinants of uterine contraction frequency and intensity. Abrupt changes in plasma catecholamines due to labor analgesia can influence uterine tone, as previously discussed, which may impact the fetus. Second, the effect of pain on the release of norepinephrine and epinephrine modulates uterine artery vasoconstriction. Third, the episodic hyperventilation and hypoventilation associated with painful contractions can result in maternal oxyhemoglobin desaturation and decreased fetal oxygen delivery. Although these effects are well tolerated in normal circumstances and are effectively blocked by analgesia, fetal well-being may be affected in situations of limited uteroplacental reserve.

SUMMARY

The personal significance and long-term impact of labor pain are highly complex and must be understood within the context of an individual's biological, psychological, and social framework. Anatomically, pain during the first stage of labor results from the stimulation of visceral afferents that innervate the lower uterine segment and cervix, intermingle with sympathetic efferents, and enter the spinal cord at the T10 to L1 segments. Pain during the second stage of labor results from the additional stimulation of somatic afferents that innervate the vagina and perineum, travel within the pudendal nerve, and enter the spinal cord at the S2 to S4 segments. These pain signals are processed in the spinal cord and are transmitted to brainstem, midbrain, and thalamic sites, the last with projections to the cortex, implicating the sensory-emotional experience of pain. Current obstetric anesthesia practice relies nearly exclusively on the blocking of pain transmission by deposition of local anesthetic, with or without adjuncts, along the afferent nerves from sites near the peripheral afferent terminals to sites near their central terminals.

The neurophysiology of visceral pain, especially in relation to labor pain, continues to be investigated, with considerable academic and pharmaceutical targeting of (1) the normal ionic transduction mechanisms and processes of sensitization in peripheral afferent terminals, (2) the mechanisms of inhibition available in the spinal cord and brainstem, and (3) the processes by which conscious distraction methods can be amplified and relieve pain. The biopsychosocial model of pain highlights the complex social, cultural, physical, and emotional contexts that mutually inform the experience of, and response to, pain. Labor pain is an intensely variable and personal experience, the meaning of which is shaped by a multitude of factors beyond the purview of the anesthesia provider. By endeavoring to understand these dynamics, to respect the individual patient's experience, and to honor patient autonomy and capacity despite often intense pain and rapidly evolving clinical scenarios, the anesthesia provider is best positioned to establish a strong therapeutic alliance and confer protective benefit against the evolution of labor pain to PTSD and chronic pain.

KEY POINTS

- The biopsychosocial model of pain highlights the complex biological, psychological, and sociological factors that summate to produce a person's experience of pain. Labor pain is often uniquely associated with personal, cultural, and existential significance.
- Labor pain exists and may be severe, with a close correlation between cervical dilation and pain during the first stage.
- The first stage of labor involves visceral pain from the lower uterine segment and endocervix, which results in hypersensitivity to convergent somatic dermatomes. This pain is most likely amplified over time because of the sensitization of peripheral and central pain-signaling pathways. The second stage of labor results in somatic pain from the vagina and perineum and is briefer than the first stage.
- Afferent terminals transduce a mechanical process into electrical signals, which are probably amplified by the release of prostaglandins, cytokines, and growth factors into the cervix as part of the normal disruption of collagen that allows the cervix to soften and dilate.
- Pain transmission in the spinal cord is not hardwired; it is remarkably and rapidly plastic, and it is altered by local neuronal activity that releases μ-opioid receptor agonists and descending pathways that release α_2-adrenergic and serotonergic receptor agonists.
- There are large individual differences in pain perception, which likely reflect differences at suprathalamic sites. The activation of suprathalamic sites is the primary mechanism of action for distraction methods of analgesia.
- Labor pain alters the obstetric course and the maternal cardiac and respiratory function in a complex manner that normally is well tolerated, can sometimes be detrimental to both mother and fetus, and is alleviated by analgesia.
- Physiologic changes of pregnancy and pain both decrease gastric emptying; gastric emptying is facilitated by effective neuraxial labor analgesia.
- The pain of labor does not affect a patient's ability to understand or to participate in informed consent discussions and medical decision-making. Patients in severe pain do not lose their autonomy because of pain, and pain does not constitute an implied or emergency exception to the medicolegal doctrine of informed consent.
- Labor pain carries meaning in distinction from most other causes of severe pain; the treatment of labor pain should be applied within this context.
- Acute postpartum pain after either vaginal or cesarean delivery deserves attention and treatment; the factors or mechanisms responsible for the development of persistent or chronic postpartum pain, depression, and PTSD are under investigation.

REFERENCES

1. Merskey H, Albe-Fessard DG, Bonica JJ, et al. Pain terms: a list with definitions and notes on usage. Recommended by the IASP Subcommittee on Taxonomy. *Pain.* 1979;6:249–252.
2. Melzack R, Wall PD. Pain mechanisms: a new theory. *Science.* 1965;150:971–979.
3. Melzack R. From the gate to the neuromatrix. *Pain.* 1999;82: S121–S126.
4. Simone DA, Baumann TK, LaMotte RH. Dose-dependent pain and mechanical hyperalgesia in humans after intradermal injection of capsaicin. *Pain.* 1989;38:99–107.
5. Fillingim RB, King CD, Ribeiro-Dasilva MC, et al. Sex, gender, and pain: a review of recent clinical and experimental findings. *J Pain.* 2009;10:447–485.
6. Cohen SP, Vase L, Hooten WM. Chronic pain: an update on burden, best practices, and new advances. *Lancet.* 2021;397: 2082–2097.
7. Duberstein ZT, Brunner J, Panisch LS, et al. The biopsychosocial model and perinatal health care: determinants of perinatal care in a community sample. *Front Psychiatry.* 2021;12:746803.
8. Badreldin N, Ditosto JD, Grobman WA, Yee LM. Maternal psychosocial factors associated with postpartum pain. *Am J Obstet Gynecol MFM.* 2023;5:100908.
9. Saxbe DE. Birth of a new perspective? A call for biopsychosocial research on childbirth. *Curr Dir Psychol Sci.* 2017;26:81–86.
10. Dick-Read G. *Childbirth Without fear: The Principles and Practice of Natural Childbirth.* 2nd ed. Harper & Brothers; 1953.
11. Lamaze F.*Qu'est-ce que l'accouchement sans douleur par la methode psychoprophylactique: ses principes, sa realisation, ses resultats.* Savoir et Connaitre; 1956.
12. Melzack R. The myth of painless childbirth (the John J. Bonica lecture). *Pain.* 1984;19:321–337.
13. Javert CT, Hardy JD. Influence of analgesic on pain intensity during labor; with a note on natural childbirth. *Anesthesiology.* 1951;12:189–215.
14. Hardy JD, Javert CT. Studies on pain: measurements of pain intensity in childbirth. *J Clin Invest.* 1949;28:153–162.
15. Algom D, Lubel S. Psychophysics in the field: perception and memory for labor pain. *Percept Psychophys.* 1994;55:133–141.
16. Charier DJ, Zantour D, Pichot V, et al. Assessing pain using the variation coefficient of pupillary diameter. *J Pain.* 2017;18:1346–1353.
17. Melzack R, Taenzer P, Feldman P, Kinch RA. Labour is still painful after prepared childbirth training. *Can Med Assoc J.* 1981;125:357–363.
18. Niven CA, Gijsbers KJ. Do low levels of labour pain reflect low sensitivity to noxious stimulation? *Soc Sci Med.* 1989;29: 585–588.
19. Granot M, Lowenstein L, Yarnitsky D, et al. Postcesarean section pain prediction by preoperative experimental pain assessment. *Anesthesiology.* 2003;98:1422–1426.
20. Pan PH, Coghill R, Houle TT, et al. Multifactorial preoperative predictors for postcesarean section pain and analgesic requirement. *Anesthesiology.* 2006;104:417–425.
21. Coghill RC, McHaffie JG, Yen YF. Neural correlates of interindividual differences in the subjective experience of pain. *Proc Natl Acad Sci U S A.* 2003;100:8538–8542.

22. Reid JG, Simpson NA, Walker RG, et al. The carriage of pro-inflammatory cytokine gene polymorphisms in recurrent pregnancy loss. *Am J Reprod Immunol.* 2001;45:35–40.

23. Conell-Price J, Evans JB, Hong D, et al. The development and validation of a dynamic model to account for the progress of labor in the assessment of pain. *Anesth Analg.* 2008;106:1509–1515.

24. Debiec J, Conell-Price J, Evansmith J, et al. Mathematical modeling of the pain and progress of the first stage of nulliparous labor. *Anesthesiology.* 2009;111:1093–1110.

25. Fillingim RB. Individual differences in pain: understanding the mosaic that makes pain personal. *Pain.* 2017;158(suppl 1):S11–S18.

26. Lowe NK. The nature of labor pain. *Am J Obstet Gynecol.* 2002;186:S16–S24.

27. Williams ACC, Craig KD. Updating the definition of pain. *Pain.* 2016;157:2420–2423.

28. Whitburn LY, Jones LE, Davey MA, Small R. Supporting the updated definition of pain. But what about labour pain? *Pain.* 2017;158:990–991.

29. Bajaj P, Drewes AM, Gregersen H, et al. Controlled dilatation of the uterine cervix-an experimental visceral pain model. *Pain.* 2002;99:433–442.

30. Shnol H, Paul N, Belfer I. Labor pain mechanisms. *Int Anesthesiol Clin.* 2014;52:1–17.

31. Robbins A, Sato Y, Hotta H, Berkley KJ. Responses of hypogastric nerve afferent fibers to uterine distension in estrous or metestrous rats. *Neurosci Lett.* 1990;110:82–85.

32. Bradshaw HB, Temple JL, Wood E, Berkley KJ. Estrous variations in behavioral responses to vaginal and uterine distention in the rat. *Pain.* 1999;82:187–197.

33. Papka R, Shew R. *Neural Input to the Uterus and Influence on Uterine Contractility.* CRC Press; 1993:375–399.

34. Papka RE, Storey-Workley M, Shughrue PJ, et al. Estrogen receptor-alpha and -beta immunoreactivity and mRNA in neurons of sensory and autonomic ganglia and spinal cord. *Cell Tissue Res.* 2001;304:193–214.

35. Bonica J, Chadwick H. *Labour Pain.* Churchill Livingstone; 1989:482–499.

36. Berkley KJ, Robbins A, Sato Y. Functional differences between afferent fibers in the hypogastric and pelvic nerves innervating female reproductive organs in the rat. *J Neurophysiol.* 1993;69:533–544.

37. Papka RE, Storey-Workley M. Estrogen receptor-alpha and -beta coexist in a subpopulation of sensory neurons of female rat dorsal root ganglia. *Neurosci Lett.* 2002;319:71–74.

38. Pokabla MJ, Dickerson IM, Papka RE. Calcitonin gene-related peptide-receptor component protein expression in the uterine cervix, lumbosacral spinal cord, and dorsal root ganglia. *Peptides.* 2002;23:507–514.

39. Komisaruk BR, Wallman J. Antinociceptive effects of vaginal stimulation in rats: neurophysiological and behavioral studies. *Brain Res.* 1977;137:85–107.

40. Papka RE, Hafemeister J, Puder BA, et al. Estrogen receptor-alpha and neural circuits to the spinal cord during pregnancy. *J Neurosci Res.* 2002;70:808–816.

41. Sandner-Kiesling A, Pan HL, Chen SR, et al. Effect of kappa opioid agonists on visceral nociception induced by uterine cervical distension in rats. *Pain.* 2002;96:13–22.

42. Cleland J. Paravertebral anaesthesia in obstetrics. *Surg Gynecol Obstet.* 1933;57:51–62.

43. Cotte G. Sur le traitement des dysmenorrhées rébelles par la sympathectomie hypogastrique périarterielle ou la section du nerf présacre. *Lyon Med.* 1925;LVI:153.

44. Whipple B, Komisaruk BR. Elevation of pain threshold by vaginal stimulation in women. *Pain.* 1985;21:357–367.

45. Whipple B, Martinez-Gomez M, Oliva-Zarate L, et al. Inverse relationship between intensity of vaginal self-stimulation-produced analgesia and level of chronic intake of a dietary source of capsaicin. *Physiol Behav.* 1989;46:247–252.

46. Lingueglia E, de Weille JR, Bassilana F, et al. A modulatory subunit of acid sensing ion channels in brain and dorsal root ganglion cells. *J Biol Chem.* 1997;272:29778–29783.

47. Cockayne DA, Hamilton SG, Zhu QM, et al. Urinary bladder hyporeflexia and reduced pain-related behaviour in P2X3-deficient mice. *Nature.* 2000;407:1011–1015.

48. Burnstock G. P2X receptors in sensory neurones. *Br J Anaesth.* 2000;84:476–488.

49. Waldmann R, Champigny G, Lingueglia E, et al. H(+)-gated cation channels. *Ann N Y Acad Sci.* 1999;868:67–76.

50. Drewes AM, Schipper KP, Dimcevski G, et al. Multimodal assessment of pain in the esophagus: a new experimental model. *Am J Physiol Gastrointest Liver Physiol.* 2002;283:G95–G103.

51. Julius D, Basbaum AI. Molecular mechanisms of nociception. *Nature.* 2001;413:203–210.

52. Papka RE, McNeill DL, Thompson D, Schmidt HH. Nitric oxide nerves in the uterus are parasympathetic, sensory, and contain neuropeptides. *Cell Tissue Res.* 1995;279:339–349.

53. Bennett DL, Michael GJ, Ramachandran N, et al. A distinct subgroup of small DRG cells express GDNF receptor components and GDNF is protective for these neurons after nerve injury. *J Neurosci.* 1998;18:3059–3072.

54. Kim SJ, Chung WH, Rhim H, et al. Postsynaptic action mechanism of somatostatin on the membrane excitability in spinal substantia gelatinosa neurons of juvenile rats. *Neuroscience.* 2002;114:1139–1148.

55. Carlton SM, Du J, Zhou S, Coggeshall RE. Tonic control of peripheral cutaneous nociceptors by somatostatin receptors. *J Neurosci.* 2001;21:4042–4049.

56. Linhart O, Obreja O, Kress M. The inflammatory mediators serotonin, prostaglandin E2 and bradykinin evoke calcium influx in rat sensory neurons. *Neuroscience.* 2003;118:69–74.

57. Woolf CJ, Costigan M. Transcriptional and posttranslational plasticity and the generation of inflammatory pain. *Proc Natl Acad Sci U S A.* 1999;96:7723–7730.

58. Yellon SM. Immunobiology of cervix ripening. *Front Immunol.* 2019;10:3156.

59. Sato T, Michizu H, Hashizume K, Ito A. Hormonal regulation of PGE2 and COX-2 production in rabbit uterine cervical fibroblasts. *J Appl Physiol.* 2001;90(1985):1227–1231.

60. Lyons CA, Beharry KD, Nishihara KC, et al. Regulation of matrix metalloproteinases (type IV collagenases) and their inhibitors in the virgin, timed pregnant, and postpartum rat uterus and cervix by prostaglandin E_2-cyclic adenosine monophosphate. *Am J Obstet Gynecol.* 2002;187:202–208.

61. Stygar D, Wang H, Vladic YS, et al. Increased level of matrix metalloproteinases 2 and 9 in the ripening process of the human cervix. *Biol Reprod.* 2002;67:889–894.

62. Aley KO, Levine JD. Role of protein kinase A in the maintenance of inflammatory pain. *J Neurosci.* 1999;19:2181–2186.

63. Aley KO, McCarter G, Levine JD. Nitric oxide signaling in pain and nociceptor sensitization in the rat. *J Neurosci*. 1998;18:7008–7014.

64. Samad TA, Moore KA, Sapirstein A, et al. Interleukin-1β-mediated induction of Cox-2 in the CNS contributes to inflammatory pain hypersensitivity. *Nature*. 2001;410:471–475.

65. Inoue A, Ikoma K, Morioka N, et al. Interleukin-1β induces substance P release from primary afferent neurons through the cyclooxygenase-2 system. *J Neurochem*. 1999;73:2206–2213.

66. Leem JG, Bove GM. Mid-axonal tumor necrosis factor-alpha induces ectopic activity in a subset of slowly conducting cutaneous and deep afferent neurons. *J Pain*. 2002;3:45–49.

67. Winston J, Toma H, Shenoy M, Pasricha PJ. Nerve growth factor regulates VR-1 mRNA levels in cultures of adult dorsal root ganglion neurons. *Pain*. 2001;89:181–186.

68. Rueff A, Dawson AJ, Mendell LM. Characteristics of nerve growth factor induced hyperalgesia in adult rats: dependence on enhanced bradykinin-1 receptor activity but not neurokinin-1 receptor activation. *Pain*. 1996;66:359–372.

69. Waxman SG, Kocsis JD, Black JA. Type III sodium channel mRNA is expressed in embryonic but not adult spinal sensory neurons, and is reexpressed following axotomy. *J Neurophysiol*. 1994;72:466–470.

70. Kim CH, Oh Y, Chung JM, Chung K. The changes in expression of three subtypes of TTX sensitive sodium channels in sensory neurons after spinal nerve ligation. *Brain Res Mol Brain Res*. 2001;95:153–161.

71. Black JA, Cummins TR, Plumpton C, et al. Upregulation of a silent sodium channel after peripheral, but not central, nerve injury in DRG neurons. *J Neurophysiol*. 1999;82:2776–2785.

72. Liu CN, Wall PD, Ben-Dor E, et al. Tactile allodynia in the absence of C-fiber activation: altered firing properties of DRG neurons following spinal nerve injury. *Pain*. 2000;85:503–521.

73. Liu B, Eisenach JC, Tong C. Chronic estrogen sensitizes a subset of mechanosensitive afferents innervating the uterine cervix. *J Neurophysiol*. 2005;93:2167–2173.

74. Yan T, Liu B, Du D, et al. Estrogen amplifies pain responses to uterine cervical distension in rats by altering transient receptor potential-1 function. *Anesth Analg*. 2007;104:1246–1250.

75. Tong C, Conklin D, Clyne BB, et al. Uterine cervical afferents in thoracolumbar dorsal root ganglia express transient receptor potential vanilloid type 1 channel and calcitonin gene-related peptide, but not P2X3 receptor and somatostatin. *Anesthesiology*. 2006;104:651–657.

76. Mousa SA, Zhang Q, Sitte N, et al. β-Endorphin-containing memory-cells and μ-opioid receptors undergo transport to peripheral inflamed tissue. *J Neuroimmunol*. 2001;115:71–78.

77. Picard PR, Tramèr MR, McQuay HJ, Moore RA. Analgesic efficacy of peripheral opioids (all except intra-articular): a qualitative systematic review of randomised controlled trials. *Pain*. 1997;72:309–318.

78. Kalso E, Tramèr MR, Carroll D, et al. Pain relief from intra-articular morphine after knee surgery: a qualitative systematic review. *Pain*. 1997;71:127–134.

79. Sengupta JN, Su X, Gebhart GF. Kappa, but not mu or delta, opioids attenuate responses to distention of afferent fibers innervating the rat colon. *Gastroenterology*. 1996;111:968–980.

80. Sandner-Kiesling A, Eisenach JC. Pharmacology of opioid inhibition to noxious uterine cervical distension. *Anesthesiology*. 2002;97:966–971.

81. Gebhart GF, Su X, Joshi S, et al. Peripheral opioid modulation of visceral pain. *Ann N Y Acad Sci*. 2000;909:41–50.

82. Binder W, Walker JS. Effect of the peripherally selective κ-opioid agonist, asimadoline, on adjuvant arthritis. *Br J Pharmacol*. 1998;124:647–654.

83. Cicero TJ, Nock B, O'Connor L, Meyer ER. Role of steroids in sex differences in morphine-induced analgesia: activational and organizational effects. *J Pharmacol Exp Ther*. 2002;300:695–701.

84. Gear RW, Miaskowski C, Gordon NC, et al. Kappa-opioids produce significantly greater analgesia in women than in men. *Nat Med*. 1996;2:1248–1250.

85. Sandner-Kiesling A, Eisenach JC. Estrogen reduces efficacy of μ- but not κ-opioid agonist inhibition in response to uterine cervical distension. *Anesthesiology*. 2002;96:375–379.

86. Shin SW, Eisenach JC. Intrathecal morphine reduces the visceromotor response to acute uterine cervical distension in an estrogen-independent manner. *Anesthesiology*. 2003;98:1467–1471.

87. Olofsson C, Ekblom A, Ekman-Ordeberg G, et al. Lack of analgesic effect of systemically administered morphine or pethidine on labour pain. *Br J Obstet Gynaecol*. 1996;103:968–972.

88. Leighton BL, DeSimone CA, Norris MC, Ben-David B. Intrathecal narcotics for labor revisited: the combination of fentanyl and morphine intrathecally provides rapid onset of profound, prolonged analgesia. *Anesth Analg*. 1989;69:122–125.

89. Goldin AL, Barchi RL, Caldwell JH, et al. Nomenclature of voltage-gated sodium channels. *Neuron*. 2000;28:365–368.

90. Renganathan M, Cummins TR, Waxman SG. Nitric oxide blocks fast, slow, and persistent Na+ channels in C-type DRG neurons by S-nitrosylation. *J Neurophysiol*. 2002;87:761–775.

91. Gold MS, Weinreich D, Kim CS, et al. Redistribution of Na(V)1.8 in uninjured axons enables neuropathic pain. *J Neurosci*. 2003;23:158–166.

92. Lai J, Gold MS, Kim CS, et al. Inhibition of neuropathic pain by decreased expression of the tetrodotoxin-resistant sodium channel, NaV1.8. *Pain*. 2002;95:143–152.

93. Nonaka T, Honmou O, Sakai J, et al. Excitability changes of dorsal root axons following nerve injury: implications for injury-induced changes in axonal Na(+) channels. *Brain Res*. 2000;859:280–285.

94. Sakai J, Honmou O, Kocsis JD, Hashi K. The delayed depolarization in rat cutaneous afferent axons is reduced following nerve transection and ligation, but not crush: implications for injury-induced axonal Na+ channel reorganization. *Muscle Nerve*. 1998;21:1040–1047.

95. Gu XY, Liu BL, Zang KK, et al. Dexmedetomidine inhibits Tetrodotoxin-resistant Nav1.8 sodium channel activity through Gi/o-dependent pathway in rat dorsal root ganglion neurons. *Mol Brain*. 2015;8:15.

96. Gerner P, Mujtaba M, Sinnott CJ, Wang GK. Amitriptyline versus bupivacaine in rat sciatic nerve blockade. *Anesthesiology*. 2001;94:661–667.

97. Gerner P, Mujtaba M, Khan M, et al. N-phenylethyl amitriptyline in rat sciatic nerve blockade. *Anesthesiology*. 2002;96:1435–1442.

98. Binshtok AM, Bean BP, Woolf CJ. Inhibition of nociceptors by TRPV1-mediated entry of impermeant sodium channel blockers. *Nature*. 2007;449:607–610.

99. Binshtok AM, Gerner P, Oh SB, et al. Coapplication of lidocaine and the permanently charged sodium channel blocker QX-314 produces a long-lasting nociceptive blockade in rodents. *Anesthesiology*. 2009;111:127–137.

100. Dalle C, Schneider M, Clergue F, et al. Inhibition of the I_h current in isolated peripheral nerve: a novel mode of peripheral antinociception? *Muscle Nerve*. 2001;24:254–261.

101. Chaplan SR, Guo HQ, Lee DH, et al. Neuronal hyperpolarization-activated pacemaker channels drive neuropathic pain. *J Neurosci*. 2003;23:1169–1178.

102. Kissin I, Bright CA, Bradley EL, Jr. Selective and long-lasting neural blockade with resiniferatoxin prevents inflammatory pain hypersensitivity. *Anesth Analg*. 2002;94:1253–1258.

103. Ludwig M, Sabatier N, Bull PM, et al. Intracellular calcium stores regulate activity-dependent neuropeptide release from dendrites. *Nature*. 2002;418:85–89.

104. Feng Y, Cui M, Willis WD. Gabapentin markedly reduces acetic acid-induced visceral nociception. *Anesthesiology*. 2003;98:729–733.

105. Cao YQ, Mantyh PW, Carlson EJ, et al. Primary afferent tachykinins are required to experience moderate to intense pain. *Nature*. 1998;392:390–394.

106. Khan IM, Marsala M, Printz MP, et al. Intrathecal nicotinic agonist-elicited release of excitatory amino acids as measured by in vivo spinal microdialysis in rats. *J Pharmacol Exp Ther*. 1996;278:97–106.

107. Riley RC, Trafton JA, Chi SI, Basbaum AI. Presynaptic regulation of spinal cord tachykinin signaling via GABA(B) but not GABA(A) receptor activation. *Neuroscience*. 2001;103:725–737.

108. Li DP, Chen SR, Pan YZ, et al. Role of presynaptic muscarinic and GABA(B) receptors in spinal glutamate release and cholinergic analgesia in rats. *J Physiol*. 2002;543:807–818.

109. Baba H, Kohno T, Okamoto M, et al. Muscarinic facilitation of GABA release in substantia gelatinosa of the rat spinal dorsal horn. *J Physiol*. 1998;508(Pt 1):83–93.

110. Lauretti GR, Hood DD, Eisenach JC, Pfeifer BL. A multi-center study of intrathecal neostigmine for analgesia following vaginal hysterectomy. *Anesthesiology*. 1998;89:913–918.

111. Lombard MC, Besson JM. Attempts to gauge the relative importance of pre- and postsynaptic effects of morphine on the transmission of noxious messages in the dorsal horn of the rat spinal cord. *Pain*. 1989;37:335–345.

112. Kuraishi Y, Hirota N, Sato Y, et al. Noradrenergic inhibition of the release of substance P from the primary afferents in the rabbit spinal dorsal horn. *Brain Res*. 1985;359:177–182.

113. Headley PM, Grillner S. Excitatory amino acids and synaptic transmission: the evidence for a physiological function. *Trends Pharmacol Sci*. 1990;11:205–211.

114. Karpinski N, Dunn J, Hansen L, Masliah E. Subpial vacuolar myelopathy after intrathecal ketamine: report of a case. *Pain*. 1997;73:103–105.

115. Wilder-Smith CH, Knopfli R, Wilder-Smith OH. Perioperative magnesium infusion and postoperative pain. *Acta Anaesthesiol Scand*. 1997;41:1023–1027.

116. Svensson CI, Yaksh TL. The spinal phospholipase-cyclooxygenase-prostanoid cascade in nociceptive processing. *Annu Rev Pharmacol Toxicol*. 2002;42:553–583.

117. Roza C, Laird JM, Cervero F. Spinal mechanisms underlying persistent pain and referred hyperalgesia in rats with an experimental ureteric stone. *J Neurophysiol*. 1998;79:1603–1612.

118. Ossipov MH, Lopez Y, Nichols ML, et al. The loss of antinociceptive efficacy of spinal morphine in rats with nerve ligation injury is prevented by reducing spinal afferent drive. *Neurosci Lett*. 1995;199:87–90.

119. Tong C, Ma W, Shin SW, et al. Uterine cervical distension induces cFos expression in deep dorsal horn neurons of the rat spinal cord. *Anesthesiology*. 2003;99:205–211.

120. Du D, Eisenach JC, Ririe DG, Tong C. The antinociceptive effects of spinal cyclooxygenase inhibitors on uterine cervical distension. *Brain Res*. 2004;1024:130–136.

121. Eisenach JC, Curry R, Hood DD, Yaksh TL. Phase I safety assessment of intrathecal ketorolac. *Pain*. 2002;99:599–604.

122. Basbaum AI, Fields HL. Endogenous pain control mechanisms: review and hypothesis. *Ann Neurol*. 1978;4:451–462.

123. Eisenach JC, Dobson CE, 2nd, Inturrisi CE, et al. Effect of pregnancy and pain on cerebrospinal fluid immunoreactive enkephalins and norepinephrine in healthy humans. *Pain*. 1990;43:149–154.

124. Benedetti F, Arduino C, Amanzio M. Somatotopic activation of opioid systems by target-directed expectations of analgesia. *J Neurosci*. 1999;19:3639–3648.

125. Millan M. *Somatotopic Activation of Opioid Systems by Target-Directed Expectations of Analgesia*. Springer-Verlag; 1997:385–446.

126. Zhuo M, Sengupta JN, Gebhart GF. Biphasic modulation of spinal visceral nociceptive transmission from the rostroventral medial medulla in the rat. *J Neurophysiol*. 2002;87:2225–2236.

127. Al-Chaer ED, Traub RJ. Biological basis of visceral pain: recent developments. *Pain*. 2002;96:221–225.

128. Jones AK, Kulkarni B, Derbyshire SW. Pain mechanisms and their disorders. *Br Med Bull*. 2003;65:83–93.

129. Moir DD, Willocks J. Management of incoordinate uterine action under continuous epidural analgesia. *Br Med J*. 1967;3:396–400.

130. Riffel HD, Nochimson DJ, Paul RH, Hon EH. Effects of meperidine and promethazine during labor. *Obstet Gynecol*. 1973;42:738–745.

131. Abrao KC, Francisco RPV, Miyadahira S, et al. Elevation of uterine basal tone and fetal heart rate abnormalities after labor analgesia: a randomized controlled trial. *Obstet Gynecol*. 2009;113:41–47.

132. Mardirosoff C, Dumont L, Boulvain M, Tramèr MR. Fetal bradycardia due to intrathecal opioids for labour analgesia: a systematic review. *BJOG*. 2002;109:274–281.

133. Okahara S, Inoue R, Katakura Y, et al. Comparison of the incidence of fetal prolonged deceleration after induction of labor analgesia between dural puncture epidural and combined spinal epidural technique: a pilot study. *BMC Pregnancy Childbirth*. 2023;23:182.

134. Patel NP, El-Wahab N, Fernando R, et al. Fetal effects of combined spinal-epidural vs epidural labour analgesia: a prospective, randomised double-blind study. *Anaesthesia*. 2014;69:458–467.

135. Hingson R, Hellman L. *Anatomic and physiologic considerations*. JB Lippincott; 1956:74.

136. Rahm VA, Hallgren A, Högberg H, et al. Plasma oxytocin levels in women during labor with or without epidural analgesia: a prospective study. *Acta Obstet Gynecol Scand*. 2002;81:1033–1039.

137. Stocche RM, Klamt JG, Antunes-Rodrigues J, et al. Effects of intrathecal sufentanil on plasma oxytocin and cortisol concentrations in women during the first stage of labor. *Reg Anesth Pain Med*. 2001;26:545–550.

138. Scull TJ, Hemmings GT, Carli F, et al. Epidural analgesia in early labour blocks the stress response but uterine contractions remain unchanged. *Can J Anaesth*. 1998;45:626–630.

139. Tangsiriwatthana T, Sangkomkamhang US, Lumbiganon P, Laopaiboon M. Paracervical local anaesthesia for cervical dilatation and uterine intervention. *Cochrane Database Syst Rev*. 2009:CD005056.

140. Leighton BL, Norris MC, Sosis M, et al. Limitations of epinephrine as a marker of intravascular injection in laboring women. *Anesthesiology*. 1987;66:688–691.

141. Hood DD, Dewan DM, James FM, 3rd. Maternal and fetal effects of epinephrine in gravid ewes. *Anesthesiology*. 1986;64:610–613.

142. Shnider SM, Abboud TK, Artal R, et al. Maternal catecholamines decrease during labor after lumbar epidural anesthesia. *Am J Obstet Gynecol*. 1983;147:13–15.

143. Cascio M, Pygon B, Bernett C, Ramanathan S. Labour analgesia with intrathecal fentanyl decreases maternal stress. *Can J Anaesth*. 1997;44:605–609.

144. Jouppila R, Puolakka J, Kauppila A, Vuori J. Maternal and umbilical cord plasma noradrenaline concentrations during labour with and without segmental extradural analgesia, and during caesarean section. *Br J Anaesth*. 1984;56:251–255.

145. Hagerdal M, Morgan CW, Sumner AE, Gutsche BB. Minute ventilation and oxygen consumption during labor with epidural analgesia. *Anesthesiology*. 1983;59:425–427.

146. Buchan AS, Sharwood-Smith GH. Physiological changes in pregnancy. In: Buchan AS, Sharwood-Smith GH, eds. *The Simpson Handbook of Obstetric Anaesthesia*. Albamedia on behalf of The Royal College of Surgeons of Edinburgh; 1999.

147. Hasuo H, Kusunoki H, Kanbara K, et al. Tolerable pain reduces gastric fundal accommodation and gastric motility in healthy subjects: a crossover ultrasonographic study. *Biopsychosoc Med*. 2017;11:4.

148. Bouvet L, Schulz T, Piana F, et al. Pregnancy and labor epidural effects on gastric emptying: a prospective comparative study. *Anesthesiology*. 2022;136:542–550.

149. Garthus-Niegel S, Knoph C, von Soest T, et al. The role of labor pain and overall birth experience in the development of posttraumatic stress symptoms: a longitudinal cohort study. *Birth*. 2014;41:108–115.

150. Hodnett ED. Pain and women's satisfaction with the experience of childbirth: a systematic review. *Am J Obstet Gynecol*. 2002;186:S160–S172.

151. Billewicz-Driemel AM, Milne MD. Long-term assessment of extradural analgesia for the relief of pain in labour. II: sense of "deprivation" after extradural analgesia in labour: relevant or not? *Br J Anaesth*. 1976;48:139–144.

152. Stewart DE. Psychiatric symptoms following attempted natural childbirth. *Can Med Assoc J*. 1982;127:713–716.

153. Ryding EL. Psychosocial indications for cesarean section. A retrospective study of 43 cases. *Acta Obstet Gynecol Scand*. 1991;70:47–49.

154. Imakawa CSO, Nadai MN, Reis M, et al. Is it necessary to evaluate fear of childbirth in pregnant women? A scoping review. *Rev Bras Ginecol Obstet*. 2022;44:692–700.

155. Ballard CG, Stanley AK, Brockington IF. Post-traumatic stress disorder (PTSD) after childbirth. *Br J Psychiatry*. 1995;166:525–528.

156. Macarthur AJ, Macarthur C. Incidence, severity, and determinants of perineal pain after vaginal delivery: a prospective cohort study. *Am J Obstet Gynecol*. 2004;191:1199–1204.

157. Lavand'homme PM, Roelants F, Waterloos H, De Kock MF. Postoperative analgesic effects of continuous wound infiltration with diclofenac after elective cesarean delivery. *Anesthesiology*. 2007;106:1220–1225.

158. Eisenach JC, Pan PH, Smiley R, et al. Severity of acute pain after childbirth, but not type of delivery, predicts persistent pain and postpartum depression. *Pain*. 2008;140:87–94.

159. Kehlet H, Jensen TS, Woolf CJ. Persistent postsurgical pain: risk factors and prevention. *Lancet*. 2006;367:1618–1625.

160. Hefferan MP, O'Rielly DD, Loomis CW. Inhibition of spinal prostaglandin synthesis early after L5/L6 nerve ligation prevents the development of prostaglandin-dependent and prostaglandin-independent allodynia in the rat. *Anesthesiology*. 2003;99:1180–1188.

161. Ding T, Wang DX, Qu Y, et al. Epidural labor analgesia is associated with a decreased risk of postpartum depression: a prospective cohort study. *Anesth Analg*. 2014;119:383–392.

162. Eisenach JC, Pan P, Smiley RM, et al. Resolution of pain after childbirth. *Anesthesiology*. 2013;118:143–151.

163. Gutierrez S, Liu B, Hayashida K, et al. Reversal of peripheral nerve injury-induced hypersensitivity in the postpartum period: role of spinal oxytocin. *Anesthesiology*. 2013;118:152–159.

164. Houle TT, Miller S, Lang JE, et al. Day-to-day experience in resolution of pain after surgery. *Pain*. 2017;158:2147–2154.

165. Wisner KL, Parry BL, Piontek CM. Clinical practice. Postpartum depression. *N Engl J Med*. 2002;347:194–199.

166. Brown S, Lumley J. Maternal health after childbirth: results of an Australian population based survey. *Br J Obstet Gynaecol*. 1998;105:156–161.

167. Lydon-Rochelle MT, Holt VL, Martin DP. Delivery method and self-reported postpartum general health status among primiparous women. *Paediatr Perinat Epidemiol*. 2001;15:232–240.

22

Childbirth Preparation and Nonpharmacologic Analgesia

Rebecca D. Minehart, MD, MSHPEd and Marie E. Minnich, MD, MMM, MBA, CPE

CHAPTER OUTLINE

At their core, the experiences of labor and birthing a child are intensely personal, intimate processes for many women, regardless of culture or background. While anesthesia providers may have a particular view of what is important to someone during childbirth, including pain management strategies, our goals should be to understand each woman's values and beliefs and to recommend therapies when appropriate, considering medical and obstetric considerations and personal wishes. Some parturients seek nonpharmacologic strategies to cope with the pain of labor; these strategies may be independent of, or complementary to, more traditional forms of labor pain relief such as neuraxial analgesia. Studies of nonpharmacologic approaches to pain management during labor compared with the usual care, such as neuraxial or intravenous pain relief, have found that some nonpharmacologic strategies, such as water immersion, acupuncture, and upright maternal positioning, are associated with reductions in various obstetric interventions (e.g., use of oxytocin).[1-3] While some evidence regarding nonpharmacologic approaches may appear less rigorous than that supporting pharmacologic-based forms of pain relief, many of these nonpharmacologic approaches are rooted in pain-based theories, including (1) the gate control theory (e.g., light massage, water immersion, ambulation, birthing balls); (2) diffuse noxious inhibitory control (e.g., sterile water injections, acupuncture, acupressure, transcutaneous electrical nerve stimulation [TENS]); and (3) central nervous system control (e.g., antenatal education, continuous support during labor, meditation, hypnosis, aromatherapy).[1] This chapter seeks to provide obstetric anesthesia providers with a comprehensive knowledge of nonpharmacologic labor strategies and how they may influence the labor pain experience and obstetric interventions. This lays the groundwork for informed discussion of pain relief options among patients, nurses, obstetricians, and anesthesia providers.

PAIN PERCEPTION

Anesthesia providers are indebted to Ronald Melzack and colleagues for their early studies of the pain of childbirth.[4] In 1975 Melzack described the use of the McGill Pain Questionnaire to investigate differences among pain modalities.[5] In a subsequent study, he and colleagues found that labor pain is one of the most intense types of pain among those studied, although the results were associated with factors such as a history of menstrual difficulties and lower socioeconomic status (higher scores).[4] In general, parous women had lower pain scores than nulliparous women, but the responses varied widely within the groups (Figs. 22.1 and 22.2). Early studies identified a modest decrease in the average pain score among nulliparous women who participated in childbirth preparation, but the training did not eliminate pain in these women.[4,6] More recent studies have focused on pregnant women's experiences of childbirth and have shown potential benefits from attending childbirth preparation training, including lowered anxiety assessments, shorter duration of the first stage of labor, lower epidural analgesia usage rates, lower rates of cesarean delivery, and enhanced labor satisfaction.[7-10] While this body of evidence is encouraging, higher-quality studies are needed.

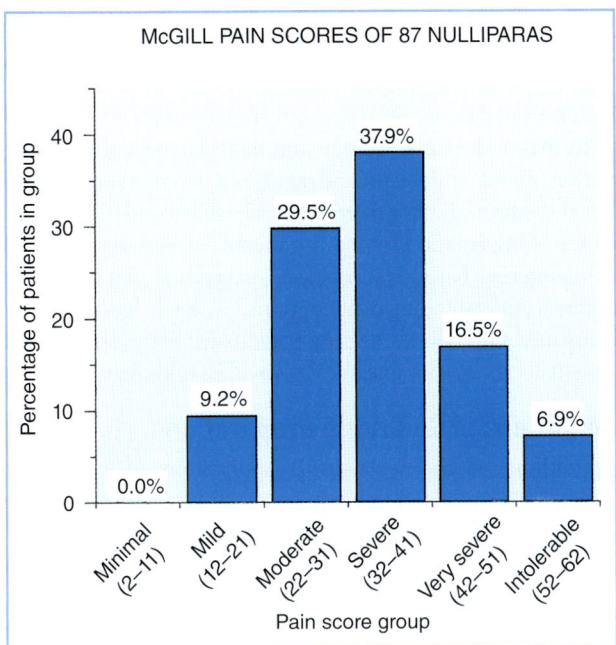

Fig. 22.1 The severity of pain during labor as assessed by the McGill Pain Questionnaire for 87 nulliparous women. Modified from Melzack R, Taezner P, Feldman P, Kinch RA. Labour is still painful after prepared childbirth training. *Can Med Assoc J.* 1981;125:357–363.

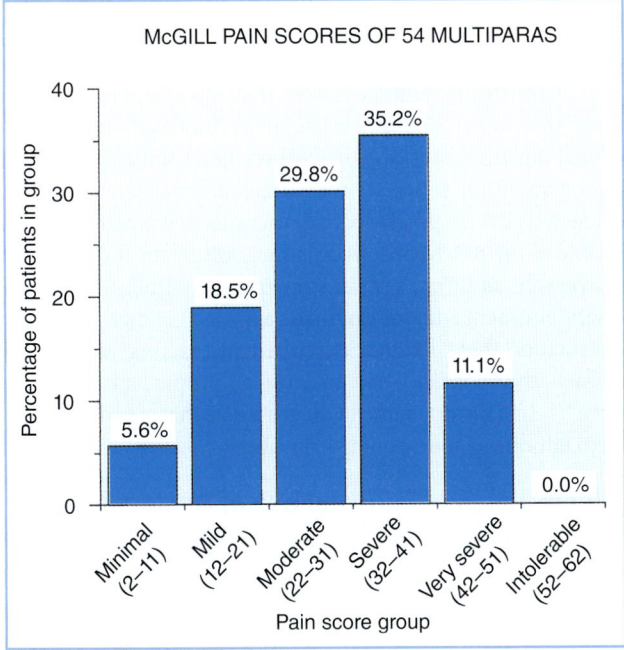

Fig. 22.2 The severity of pain during labor as assessed by the McGill Pain Questionnaire for 54 parous women. Modified from Melzack R, Taezner P, Feldman P, Kinch RA. Labour is still painful after prepared childbirth training. *Can Med Assoc J.* 1981;125:357–363.

HISTORY OF CHILDBIRTH PREPARATION AND INTERVENTION

As one traces the history of the evolution of childbirth analgesia, there is tension in the balance between the degree of medicalization, maternal participation, and pain management. Before the mid-19th century, childbirth occurred at home

in the company of family and friends, without medication or medical intervention. The specialty of obstetrics was developed to decrease maternal mortality. Interventions initially developed for the management of complications became accepted and practiced as routine obstetric care. Physicians first administered anesthesia for childbirth during this period (see Chapter 1); the 1848 meeting of the American Medical Association included reports of the use of ether and chloroform in approximately 2000 obstetric cases.[11] The combination of morphine and scopolamine (i.e., twilight sleep) gained popularity in the early 1910s, followed by great alarm with increasing reports of newborn apneic events.[12] Nonetheless, these techniques were widely used, and influential women advocated that they be made available to all parturients.[13] Together, these developments moved childbirth from the home and family unit to the hospital environment.[14] As this move occurred, women maintained their desire to be active participants during childbirth.

In his original publication entitled *Childbirth Without Fear*, Dick-Read[15] asserted his belief that childbirth was not inherently painful. He opined that the pain of childbirth results from a "fear-tension-pain syndrome." He believed—and taught—that antepartum instruction about muscle relaxation and elimination of fear would prevent labor pain. Some readers incorrectly concluded that he advocated a return to primitive obstetrics, but this was not the case. Review of his practice reveals that he used the available obstetric techniques—including analgesia, anesthesia, episiotomy, forceps, and abdominal delivery—as appropriate for the individual patient. However, he cautioned against the routine use of these procedures and encouraged active participation of mothers in the delivery of their infants. Unfortunately, he did not use the scientific method to validate his beliefs.

Although Dick-Read was the earliest proponent of so-called "natural" childbirth, it was Fernand Lamaze who introduced the Western world to "psychoprophylaxis."[16] His publications were based on techniques that he observed while traveling in Russia, often derived from the teachings of Velvovsky.[17] Again, no data were presented to link these treatments to outcomes. The "Lamaze method" became popular in the United States after Marjorie Karmel wrote about her childbirth experience under the care of Dr. Lamaze.[18] Within 1 year of the publication of her book, *Thank You, Dr. Lamaze: A Mother's Experiences in Painless Childbirth*, the American Society for Psychoprophylaxis in Obstetrics was born and organizations such as the International Childbirth Education Association and the La Leche League were formed.[19] These organizations actively encouraged a renewed emphasis on family-centered maternity care, and society was receptive. Women and their partners were ready to actively participate in childbirth and to have input in decisions about obstetric and anesthetic interventions. Childbirth preparation methods were taught and used extensively, despite a lack of scientific validation of their efficacy.

In 1975 Leboyer[20] described a modification of natural childbirth in his book *Birth Without Violence*. He advocated childbirth in a dark, quiet room; gentle massage of the newborn without routine suctioning; and a warm bath soon after birth. He opined that these maneuvers result in a less shocking first-separation experience and a healthier, happier infancy and childhood. Although there are few controlled studies of this method, published observations do not support his claim of superiority.[21,22]

Childbirth Education and Preparation

The major goals of childbirth education that were initially promoted by Dick-Read are taught with little modification in formal childbirth preparation classes today (Box 22.1). Most current classes credit Lamaze with the major components of childbirth preparation, even though Dick-Read was the first to promote patient education, relaxation training, breathing exercises, and paternal participation.[23] Some instructors and training manuals claim other benefits of childbirth preparation (Box 22.2),[24,25] although a 2015 review of the Bradley method and HypnoBirthing methods called for more rigorous study with transparent methods rather than self-reported outcomes.[26] A 2007 systematic review concluded that there is insufficient evidence to evaluate the efficacy of antenatal childbirth education on childbirth and parenting outcomes,[27] although a 2023 scoping review emphasized the need for more rigorous study.[3] Despite the lack of high-quality evidence and variability in teaching quality,[8] childbirth preparation classes are broadly available and often attended.

Socioeconomic disparities exist in childbirth education class attendance.[28,29] In addition, the effect of childbirth education on attitude and childbirth experience depends, in part, on the social class to which the mother belongs. Although investigators have found that childbirth classes have a positive effect on the attitudes of both parents of all social classes, this effect is more pronounced among "working-class"[30] and indigent women[31]; this latter finding probably reflects the greater availability and use of other educational materials by middle- and upper-class women. Childbirth classes often are the only—or at least the primary—source of information for working-class and indigent women. Attendance is also associated with improved

---

BOX 22.1   Goals of Childbirth Preparation

- Patient education about pregnancy, labor, and delivery
- Relaxation training
- Instruction in breathing techniques
- Participation of father/support person
- Early parental bonding

BOX 22.2   Purported Benefits of Childbirth Preparation

- Greater maternal control and cooperation
- Decreased maternal anxiety
- Reduced maternal pain
- Decreased maternal need for analgesia/anesthesia
- Shorter labor
- Diminished maternal morbidity
- Less fetal stress/distress
- Strengthened family relationships because of the shared birth experience

---

postpartum practices (e.g., safe newborn sleeping practices, breastfeeding).[8] Contemporary analyses suggest that privately insured women who attend childbirth education classes may benefit from a lower elective cesarean delivery rate.[8]

In the modern era, women and their partners obtain information about childbirth and analgesia from many sources. Social media and other internet sites have become the primary source of information for many patients.[32-34] However, variability in internet-based information quality may limit pregnant women's understanding of her options.[35] Knowledge of information sources and biases held by patients facilitates shared decision-making between anesthesia providers and their patients.

Limitations of Childbirth Preparation

Limitations of the widespread application of psychoprophylaxis and other childbirth preparation methods remain. Proponents assume that these techniques are easily used during labor and delivery; however, Copstick et al.[36] found that patients were able to use the coping techniques in the early first stage of labor but that the successful use of the coping skills became less and less common as labor progressed. By the onset of the second stage, less than one-third of mothers were able to use any of the breathing or postural techniques taught during their childbirth classes.[36] The method of preparation influences the pregnant woman's ability to use breathing and relaxation techniques. Bernardini et al.[37] observed that self-taught pregnant women are less likely to practice the techniques during the prenatal period or to use the techniques during labor.

Childbirth preparation classes may also set false expectations. If a woman does not relate to the "normal" delivery discussed during classes, she may experience a sense of failure or inferiority. Both Stewart[38] and Guzman Sanchez et al.[39] have discussed adverse psychological reactions in women who were unable to use psychoprophylaxis successfully during labor and delivery. In addition, several women have written about their disappointment with the dogmatic approach of their childbirth instructors; these women described instructors who rigidly defined the "correct" way to have a "proper" birth experience.[40,41] In contrast, some evidence exists that antenatal childbirth education courses may help ease the fear of childbirth.[42]

Effects on Labor Pain and Use of Analgesics

Little scientific evidence supports the efficacy of childbirth preparation in mitigating labor pain. Psychology, nursing, obstetric, anesthesia, and lay journals provide extensive discussions of childbirth preparation, but most articles describe anecdotal clinical experiences with an assumption that it offers benefits for the mother and child. Outcome studies often do not include a group of women who were randomly assigned to an untreated or a placebo-controlled group, and statistical analysis is often incomplete. Older studies have reported a *decreased* use of analgesic medications[43,44] or regional anesthesia,[43,44] shorter first stage of labor,[45] and a lower incidence of nonreassuring fetal status[46] and cesarean delivery,[46] whereas others reported *no change* in the use of analgesics,[45-49] duration of labor,[46-52] rate of operative vaginal[47-49] or cesarean delivery,[49-51] or incidence of nonreassuring fetal status.[45,48,52] A 2013 systematic review[53] found

TABLE 22.1 Effects of Childbirth Preparation Training

Study	Analgesic Use	Neuraxial Anesthesia	Duration of Labor	Cesarean Delivery Rate	Operative Delivery Rate	Fetal Distress	Oxytocin Use
Patton et al.[48]	NC	NC	NC	NC	NC	NC	↑
Hetherington[55]	↓	↓	—	—	↓	—	—
Zax et al.[50]	↓	↓	NC	—	—	—	—
Scott and Rose[52]	↓	↓	NC	NC	↓	NC	NC
Hughey et al.[46]	NC	↓	NC	↓	↓	↓	NC
Sturrock and Johnson[49]	NC	—	NC	NC	NC	—	—
Brewin and Bradley[47]	NC	NC	NC	NC	NC	—	—
Delke et al.[45]	NC	—	↓	—	—	NC	NC
Yohai et al.[7]	NC	NC	↓	NC	—	—	—
Vanderlaan et al.[8]	—	—	—	↓	—	—	—

NC, No change; ↑, increased; ↓, decreased; —, not studied/reported.

a paradoxical increase in labor epidural analgesia use and induction of labor among those who attended childbirth classes, although benefits included fewer admissions for false labor, decreased anxiety about childbirth, and enhanced partner engagement. A 2020 retrospective review of 197 low-risk, nulliparous women who self-selected to attend or not attend childbirth classes noted that the attendees were less likely to undergo induction of labor and had lower use of analgesic medications during labor.[54] There was no significant difference between groups in maternal satisfaction or perception of control. These diverse findings may reflect different patient populations, poor study design, or researcher bias. Table 22.1 summarizes several studies of childbirth preparation training and their association with labor outcome.

To elucidate the effect of the coping techniques taught in childbirth classes, several investigators have attempted to quantify changes in pain threshold, pain perception, anxiety levels, and physiologic responses to standardized stimuli by evaluating nonpregnant and nulliparous women in laboratory settings.[56–60] Studies varied in the stimulus applied, the coping techniques studied, and the parameters analyzed. Together, these studies suggest that *practicing* these techniques facilitates their efficacy and that newer cognitive techniques (e.g., systematic desensitization, sensory transformation) may be more effective than traditional Lamaze techniques of varied breathing patterns and relaxation. Further studies may help refine childbirth preparation to maximize the positive psychophysiologic effects.

NONPHARMACOLOGIC ANALGESIC TECHNIQUES

Nonpharmacologic analgesic techniques range from those that require minimal specialized equipment and training and are widely available to those that are offered only by institutions with the necessary equipment and trained personnel (Box 22.3). Most published studies assessing nonpharmacologic methods of labor analgesia are of poor quality.[61–64] Several comprehensive reviews of alternative therapies for pain management provide a foundation for discussion with

BOX 22.3 Nonpharmacologic Analgesic Techniques

Minimal Training/Equipment
- Emotional support
- Touch and massage
- Therapeutic use of heat and cold
- Hydrotherapy
- Vertical position

Specialized Training/Equipment
- Biofeedback
- Sterile water injection
- Transcutaneous electrical nerve stimulation
- Acupuncture
- Hypnosis
- Virtual reality

patients and obstetric providers[61–63]; however, clinical evidence is insufficient on techniques such as music therapy, aromatherapy, and chiropractic manipulation. These techniques may provide intangible benefits that pregnant women may consider to be an important part of their labor experience.

Continuous Labor Support

Continuous support during labor is essential to the process of a satisfying childbirth experience. Typically, the pregnant woman's partner, family member, and/or friend provide this support. Research has noted that partner participation is associated with decreased maternal anxiety and medication requirements.[65] Studies evaluating the benefits of emotional support provided by doulas or other unrelated individuals on the mode of delivery, feelings about the birth experience, use of labor analgesia, oxytocin augmentation, duration of labor, perineal trauma, breastfeeding outcomes, and Apgar scores, among other outcomes, suggest that the companionship of another woman who is not part of the medical establishment may reduce a parturient's anxiety more effectively than the companionship provided by her partner.[51,66] A patient's sense of isolation adversely affects her perception of labor. In one

TABLE 22.2　**Systematic Review: Continuous Labor Support Versus Usual Care**

Outcome	Number of Trials	Number of Subjects	Relative Risk[a]	95% Confidence Interval
Use of neuraxial analgesia	9	11,444	0.93	0.88 to 0.99
Use of any analgesia	15	12,433	0.90	0.84 to 0.96
Spontaneous vaginal delivery	21	14,369	1.08	1.04 to 1.12
Operative vaginal delivery	19	14,118	0.90	0.85 to 0.96
Cesarean delivery	24	15,347	0.75	0.64 to 0.88
Negative feelings about childbirth experience	11	11,133	0.69	0.59 to 0.79
Labor duration	13	5429	−0.69 h[b]	−1.04 to −0.34
Infant with a low 5-min Apgar score	14	12,615	0.62	0.46 to 0.85

[a]For women who received continuous support compared with no support.
[b]Weighted mean difference.
Data from Bohren MA, Hofmeyr GJ, Sakala C, et al. Continuous support for women during childbirth. *Cochrane Database Syst Rev.* 2017;(7): CD003766.[66]

study, women randomly assigned to receive intrapartum support from a friend or female relative who was chosen by the parturient and trained as a doula were more likely to have positive feelings about their delivery and had a higher rate of breastfeeding 6 to 8 weeks after delivery than women who were randomly assigned to receive usual care.[51]

A 2017 metaanalysis evaluated results from 26 studies that included 15,858 women who were randomly assigned to receive either continuous childbirth support or usual care (Table 22.2).[66] The pooled data suggest that women who receive one-on-one support during labor are less likely to use any type of analgesia and report negative feelings about the childbirth experience, and are more likely to have a spontaneous vaginal delivery, although evidence was generally of low quality.[66] The benefits were greater when the support person was present in a doula (trained labor companion) role. In addition, the mean duration of labor was slightly shorter (approximately 41 minutes) in the women who received continuous support during labor, and the likelihood of a low 5-minute Apgar score was less.

These results have important implications for obstetric care, although they may not be generalizable. Results from trials in North America do not appear as striking as those from Europe or Africa.[61] The aforementioned systematic review of continuous labor support concluded that the preponderance of evidence suggests that all parturients should have access to emotional support, whether it is provided by the partner, a family member, a labor companion (e.g., doula), or professional hospital staff.[66] Further studies should compare different models of continuous childbirth support and should include longer-term outcomes, including breastfeeding and postpartum depression.

Touch and Massage

Various touch and massage techniques are discussed with women and their support persons during childbirth preparation classes. These techniques include effleurage (e.g., long, light stroking of the back or abdomen), counterpressure to alleviate back discomfort, and reassuring pats.[61,67] While a 2018 systematic review found low-quality evidence that massage provided reduced self-reported pain intensity, other outcomes showed no difference based on very low-quality evidence.[68] Touch and

massage can provide a comfort that is generally appreciated by women during labor. These measures may be used by the pregnant woman, her support person, or the professional staff members providing intrapartum care. The techniques are easily discontinued. In some cases, touch and massage may reduce discomfort. More often, touch and massage transmit a sense of caring, which fosters a sense of security and well-being.

Therapeutic Use of Heat and Cold

Another simple technique for alleviating labor pain is the therapeutic use of temperature (hot or cold) applied to various regions of the body. Warm compresses may be placed on localized areas or a warm blanket may cover the entire body. Alternatively, ice packs may be placed on the low back or perineum to decrease pain perception. Studies of the therapeutic use of heat and cold during labor are of low quality.[68] The use of superficial heat and cold for comfort is widespread (if not completely understood), and it has no discernible risk to the mother or the fetus.[61] Cold and heat should not be applied to anesthetized skin as diminished awareness may increase the potential for damage to the skin.

Aromatherapy

Aromatherapy is the use of essential oils, which are fragrant, volatile organic compounds obtained by distillation of plant material. The oils are commonly combined with a carrier oil and massaged into the skin, inhaled, or mixed in a bath. Two metaanalyses showed pain-reducing benefits for labor with the use of aromatherapy.[69,70] Another metaanalysis investigating types of aromatherapy showed reduced pain in the first stage of labor with lavender oil, jasmine oil, rose oil, chamomile oil, boswellia oil, and bitter orange oil.[71] Given the widespread availability and relative affordability of aromatherapy diffusers and oils, they should be included in the childbirth experience if desired by the patient, barring any hypersensitivity to these compounds.

Hydrotherapy

Hydrotherapy may involve a simple shower or tub bath or may include the use of a whirlpool or large tub specially equipped for pregnant women. Purported benefits of hydrotherapy include decreased anxiety and pain and greater uterine contraction efficiency. Results of randomized, controlled trials comparing water baths with usual care are inconsistent; a 2018 systematic review found that of all purported benefits, only a small reduction in the use of neuraxial analgesia was observed.[72] A 2024 systematic review of randomized clinical trials found a modest decrease in pain but no decrease in the duration of the first stage of labor, and no significant impact on neonatal 5-minute Apgar scores.[73]

Laboring Position

Several investigators have studied the effects of various laboring body positions on pain perception and labor outcome. These positions are broadly categorized as *vertical* (e.g., sitting, standing, walking, squatting) or *horizontal* (e.g., supine, lateral). In many cases, studies of positional techniques have focused on those women who did not employ neuraxial analgesia techniques. A 2017 systematic review found the upright compared to the supine position in laboring women without epidural analgesia was associated with no difference in the rate of cesarean delivery or admission to the neonatal intensive care unit, but a slightly shorter duration of the second stage of labor (mean difference –6.2 minutes), reduced performance of episiotomy and operative vaginal delivery, and increased incidence of estimated blood loss > 500 mL.[74] A 2022 metaanalysis of studies evaluating the use of a birthing ball on labor pain scores for women without epidural labor analgesia found a significantly lower pain score (by 1.7 points on a 11-point scale) but no other differences in delivery outcomes.[75]

Ambulation in the presence of neuraxial analgesia does not appear to influence the outcome of labor.[76–78] In a prospective, randomized study, Bloom et al.[77] noted that walking did not shorten the duration of the first stage of labor or reduce the requirement for oxytocin augmentation, the use of analgesia, or the requirement for operative delivery. They concluded that "walking neither enhanced nor impaired active labor and was not harmful to the mothers or their infants."[77] In a 2013 metaanalysis comparing outcomes in women with epidural analgesia randomized to upright and ambulant positions or recumbent positions, there were no differences in any maternal or neonatal outcome, including mode of delivery.[76]

Several studies have assessed maternal position during the second stage of labor. In a review of evidence-based management of the second stage of labor, Gimovsky and Berghella[79] recommended that women without neuraxial analgesia assume upright positions during the second stage of labor. There is renewed interest in the squatting or modified squatting position, which provides greater comfort for some women during childbirth. It is unclear whether birthing cushions or stools confer any benefit to the mother or the newborn.

Other than the possibility of greater blood loss, upright positions during labor are not typically associated with harm to the mother or newborn and may aid maternal comfort.

Biofeedback

Biofeedback is a relaxation method that is used as an adjunct to the relaxation training taught in Lamaze and other childbirth education programs. Two biofeedback procedures may be applicable to the laboring woman: skin-conductance (autonomic) and electromyographic (voluntary muscle) relaxation. St James-Roberts et al.[80] demonstrated that electromyographic but not skin-conductance biofeedback techniques could be taught effectively in Lamaze classes, although they noted no difference in duration of the first stage of labor, use of epidural analgesia, incidence of operative delivery, or Apgar scores among electromyographic, skin-conductance, and control groups. In a small study, Duchene et al.[81] reported reduced pain perception during labor and delivery, and a lower rate of epidural analgesia use (40% versus 70% for the control group) with electromyographic biofeedback; there was no difference between groups in Apgar scores. A 2011 systematic review assessing the effectiveness of biofeedback found that most studies had a high risk for bias, and although some studies demonstrated reduced use of analgesic medications with biofeedback, there was insufficient evidence to conclude that biofeedback was efficacious.[82]

In summary, biofeedback training does not appear to confer substantial benefit beyond that of traditional relaxation training taught in childbirth education classes.

Sterile Water Injections

Intradermal or subcutaneous water injections are used to treat lower back pain, which is a common complaint during labor. The technique consists of injecting 0.05 to 0.1 mL of sterile water at four sites on the lower back (over each posterior superior iliac spine, and at 1 cm medial and 3 cm caudad to the posterior superior iliac spine on both sides of the back) (Fig. 22.3). The injections themselves are acutely painful for 20 to 30 seconds, but as the injection pain fades, so does lower back pain. As the afferent nerve fibers that innervate the uterus and cervix, as well as the nerve fibers that

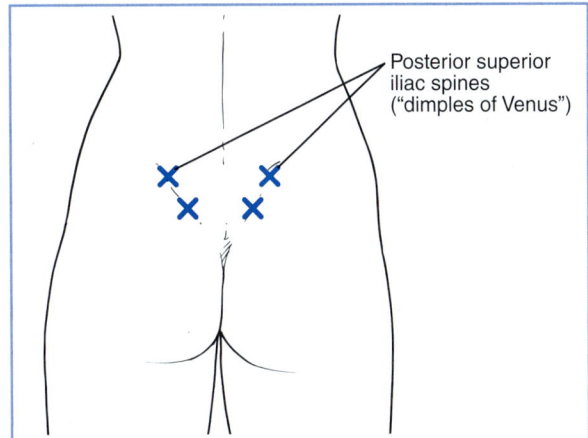

Fig. 22.3 Placement of Intradermal Water Blocks (x). Approximately 0.05 to 0.1 mL of sterile water is injected intradermally to form a small bleb over each posterior superior iliac spine and at 3 cm below and 1 cm medial to each spine on both sides of the back (i.e., for a total of four injections). The exact locations of the injections do not appear to be critical to the block success but can be placed at which points the laboring person feels the most discomfort. From Simkin P. Update on nonpharmacologic approaches to relieve labor pain and prevent suffering. *J Midwifery Womens Health*. 2004;49:489–504.

innervate the lower back, enter the spinal cord at the T10 to L1 spinal segments, a component of the pain may be referred pain. A 2012 systematic review assessing the effectiveness of intracutaneous or subcutaneous sterile water injections during labor concluded that there is little robust evidence that these injections effectively reduce back pain or labor pain.[83] A subsequent 2022 systematic review comparing intradermal and subdermal sterile water injections with a control group showed that both intradermal and subdermal injections may be superior to control in reducing labor pain after 10 minutes.[84] There were no adverse events or significant differences in cesarean delivery rates.

Transcutaneous Electrical Nerve Stimulation

TENS involves the transmission of low-voltage electrical current to the skin via surface electrodes. Advantages of TENS are that it is easy to use and discontinue, is noninvasive, and has no demonstrable harmful effects on the fetus. The disadvantage is the occasional interference with electronic fetal heart rate monitoring. Chao et al.[85] evaluated the use of TENS at specific acupuncture points and observed a reduction in pain perception. However, a 2011 systematic review of nine trials in more than 1000 women concluded that TENS did not reduce labor pain and did not reduce the use of additional analgesic agents.[86] There also was no effect on the duration of labor or the incidence of operative vaginal delivery. A 2020 metaanalysis found modest beneficial effects in reducing pain scores, although the authors noted very low quality of evidence and a high risk of bias.[87] Advocating widespread use of TENS does not seem warranted, although it may be offered to women if they desire to use it and it is available.

Acupuncture and Acupressure

Traditional Chinese medicine includes extensive use of acupuncture. Given that acupuncture can provide analgesia, there is interest in its use for intrapartum analgesia. Early observational reports described conflicting results as to the efficacy of intrapartum acupuncture and a lack of standardization of the acupuncture points to be stimulated.

A 2020 systematic review and metaanalysis of 28 acupuncture trials including 3960 women concluded that acupuncture may hold promise as a nonpharmacologic option for labor analgesia and may reduce the rates of epidural analgesia; however, the evidence was of low quality and larger studies are required for definitive conclusions.[88] All of the randomized, controlled acupuncture studies were performed outside the United States, in countries in which the use of neuraxial labor analgesia is less available or less utilized than in the United States. As acupuncture requires trained personnel, it is unlikely that either acupuncture or acupressure will gain widespread acceptance in the United States for intrapartum analgesia.

Hypnosis

The use of hypnosis for obstetric analgesia is not new.[89] Early proponents touted safety for the mother and the fetus, lower analgesic requirements, and shorter labor as the major advantages of intrapartum hypnosis. Whether hypnosis differs substantially from other childbirth preparation techniques is an unresolved controversy. Fee and Reilley[90] concluded that the breathing and relaxation exercises used in childbirth preparation do not represent a hypnotic trance as evidenced by the successful teaching of childbirth preparation exercises to women who are not susceptible to hypnosis. However, women susceptible to hypnosis may achieve a state much like a hypnotic trance when using the same exercises.

Instruction in the techniques of self-hypnosis typically occurs before the onset of labor and may entail visits to the hypnotist or involvement in a childbirth education program such as HypnoBirthing. Although proponents previously suggested that successful hypnosis training should begin early in the third trimester, Rock et al.[91] found that hypnosis could be introduced to untrained, nonvolunteer patients during labor. A 2016 metaanalysis included nine randomized controlled trials of hypnosis; in eight trials the intervention was antenatal hypnosis training, and in one trial the intervention occurred during labor.[92] Women in the hypnosis group were less likely to use pharmacologic analgesia, but the evidence was judged to be of very low quality.[92] There were no differences in any other outcomes, including coping with labor and rate of spontaneous vaginal birth. The authors concluded that further high-quality, large trials are needed.

In summary, limitations to the widespread use of hypnosis include (1) antepartum training sessions are required, (2) trained hypnotherapists must be available during labor, and (3) it offers no clear benefit.

New Techniques

Virtual reality is emerging as a possible tool for managing labor pain and anxiety, as it provides distraction.[93] A 2022 metaanalysis of 12 studies with 1095 participants suggested that virtual reality may reduce pain scores during labor, reduce anxiety, and improve satisfaction with delivery, without any positive or negative effects on the course of labor.[93] As technology and equipment evolves, this new technology may provide additional sources of comfort for those choosing to engage with it.[79]

IMPLICATIONS FOR ANESTHESIA PROVIDERS

Childbirth preparation classes and nonpharmacologic analgesic techniques do not achieve the same level of pain relief as neuraxial labor analgesia. Thus, some might question whether it is important for anesthesia providers to have knowledge of these techniques. As our contributions to the care of the obstetric patient and her family extend well beyond the administration of neuraxial analgesia, it is important for anesthesia providers to be knowledgeable about nonpharmacologic analgesic techniques. In addition, epidural analgesia/anesthesia does not eliminate the beneficial effects of other comfort measures, such as massage and continued emotional support from family and friends.

Although anesthesia providers usually have little involvement in prenatal education classes, our active participation in childbirth preparation may help patients receive more accurate information about the risks and benefits of analgesia/anesthesia for labor during vaginal and cesarean delivery. Well-informed patients are more likely to accept the obstetric and anesthetic interventions that may become necessary during labor. Women with medical or obstetric comorbidities that may increase anesthetic risk should be encouraged to discuss these problems with an anesthesia provider before the onset of labor, ideally in an antepartum consultation. A survey study confirmed that most women would prefer a prelabor visit with their anesthesiologist.[94]

Much has been written in professional and lay journals concerning the "proper" childbirth experience. Each patient's expectations of labor will influence her childbirth experience. There is a growing movement toward patient-centered maternity care (see Chapter 32), and a need for widespread adoption of practices that support inclusion of women's values and beliefs in the birthing process.[95] Major contributors to women's satisfaction during childbirth are related to the presence of a competent, humane provider during labor and delivery who provides medical interventions when necessary.[96] Our interactions with the patient, family, and obstetrician will influence perceptions of the childbirth experience.[96]

Ideally, "success" will be defined as a positive childbirth experience regardless of the mode of delivery, use of analgesia and anesthesia, or other arbitrary definitions.

Whenever possible, anesthesia providers should provide safe anesthetic care that is compatible with reasonable patient expectations. Future studies on the efficacy of childbirth education and nonpharmacologic analgesic techniques should evaluate the patient's overall experience and satisfaction in a scientifically robust manner.

KEY POINTS

- No nonpharmacologic technique consistently provides the quality of intrapartum pain relief that is provided by neuraxial analgesia.
- Childbirth preparation does not eliminate the pain of labor or substantially reduce the use of analgesia/anesthesia, but it is associated with a decrease in the maternal anxiety associated with labor.
- The preponderance of evidence recommends that all parturients have access to emotional support, whether it is provided by the partner, a family member, a labor companion (e.g., doula), or professional hospital staff.

- Biofeedback, transcutaneous electrical nerve stimulation, acupuncture, intradermal water injections, and hypnosis may provide mild analgesic benefits for some patients, but high-quality evidence is lacking.
- Newer techniques such as the use of virtual reality as an effective distraction from labor pain show some early promise, but further study is needed.
- Anesthesia providers should become active participants in childbirth education. They should facilitate honest discussion of the risks and benefits of a broad range of available analgesic/anesthetic and comfort techniques.

REFERENCES

1. Chaillet N, Belaid L, Crochetiere C, et al. Nonpharmacologic approaches for pain management during labor compared with usual care: a meta-analysis. *Birth*. 2014;41:122–137.
2. Alhafez L, Berghella V. Evidence-based labor management: first stage of labor (part 3). *Am J Obstet Gynecol MFM*. 2020;2:100185.
3. Zuarez-Easton S, Erez O, Zafran N, et al. Pharmacologic and nonpharmacologic options for pain relief during labor: an expert review. *Am J Obstet Gynecol*. 2023;228:S1246–S1259.
4. Melzack R, Taenzer P, Feldman P, Kinch RA. Labour is still painful after prepared childbirth training. *Can Med Assoc J*. 1981;125:357–363.
5. Melzack R. The McGill pain questionnaire: major properties and scoring methods. *Pain*. 1975;1:277–299.
6. Melzack R. The myth of painless childbirth (the John J. Bonica lecture). *Pain*. 1984;19:321–337.
7. Yohai D, Alharar D, Cohen R, et al. The effect of attending a prenatal childbirth preparedness course on labor duration and outcomes. *J Perinat Med*. 2018;46:47–52.
8. Vanderlaan J, Gatlin T, Shen J. Outcomes of childbirth education in PRAMS, phase 8. *Matern Child Health J*. 2023;27:82–91.
9. Chen I, Opiyo N, Tavender E, et al. Non-clinical interventions for reducing unnecessary caesarean section. *Cochrane Database Syst Rev*. 2018;(9):CD005528.
10. Levett KM, Dahlen HG, Smith CA, et al. Cost analysis of the CTLB Study, a multitherapy antenatal education programme to reduce routine interventions in labour. *BMJ Open*. 2018;8:e017333.
11. Speert H.*Obstetrics and Gynecology in America: A History*. Waverly Press; 1980.
12. Pitcock CD, Clark RB. From Fanny to Fernand: the development of consumerism in pain control during the birth process. *Am J Obstet Gynecol*. 1992;167:581–587.
13. Wertz RW, Wertz DC. *Lying-in: A History of Childbirth in America*. Free Press; 1977.
14. Devitt N. The transition from home to hospital birth in the United States, 1930-1960. *Birth Fam J*. 1977;4:47–58.
15. Dick-Read G. *Childbirth Without Fear: The Principles and Practice of Natural Childbirth*. Harper & Brothers; 1944.
16. Lamaze F. *Painless Childbirth, Psychoprophylactic Method*. Burke; 1958.
17. Velvovsky I, Platonov K, Ploticher V, Shugom E. *Painless Childbirth Through Psychoprophylaxis: Lectures for Obstetricians*. Foreign Languages Publishing House; 1960.

18. Karmel M. *Thank You, Dr. Lamaze: A Mother's Experiences in Painless Childbirth*. Lippincott; 1959.

19. Karmel M. *Thank You, Dr. Lamaze: A Mother's Experiences in Painless Childbirth*. 2nd ed. Harper & Row; 1981.

20. Leboyer F. *Birth Without Violence*. Knopf (distributed by Random House); 1975.

21. Nelson NM, Enkin MW, Saigal S, et al. A randomized clinical trial of the leboyer approach to childbirth. *N Engl J Med*. 1980;302:655–660.

22. Saigal S, Nelson NM, Bennett KJ, Enkin MW. Observations on the behavioral state of newborn infants during the first hour of life. A comparison of infants delivered by the leboyer and conventional methods. *Am J Obstet Gynecol*. 1981;139:715–719.

23. Beck NC, Geden EA, Brouder GT. Preparation for labor: a historical perspective. *Psychosom Med*. 1979;41:243–258.

24. Beck NC, Hall D. Natural childbirth. A review and analysis. *Obstet Gynecol*. 1978;52:371–379.

25. Lindell SG. Education for childbirth: a time for change. *J Obstet Gynecol Neonatal Nurs*. 1988;17:108–112.

26. Varner CA. Comparison of the bradley method and HypnoBirthing childbirth education classes. *J Perinat Educ*. 2015;24:128–136.

27. Gagnon AJ, Sandall J. Individual or group antenatal education for childbirth or parenthood, or both. *Cochrane Database Syst Rev*. 2007;(3):CD002869.

28. Lu MC, Prentice J, Yu SM, et al. Childbirth education classes: sociodemographic disparities in attendance and the association of attendance with breastfeeding initiation. *Matern Child Health J*. 2003;7:87–93.

29. Toledo P, Sun J, Grobman WA, et al. Racial and ethnic disparities in neuraxial labor analgesia. *Anesth Analg*. 2012;114:172–178.

30. Nelson MK. The effect of childbirth preparation on women of different social classes. *J Health Soc Behav*. 1982;23:339–352.

31. Zacharias JF. Childbirth education classes: effects on attitudes toward childbirth in high-risk indigent women. *JOGN Nurs*. 1981;10:265–267.

32. Declercq ER, Sakala C, Corry MP, et al. Major survey findings of listening to mothers (SM) III: new mothers speak out: report of national surveys of women's childbearing experiences conducted October-December 2012 and January-April 2013. *J Perinat Educ*. 2014;23:17–24.

33. Toledo P, Pumarino J, Grobman WA, et al. Patients' preferences for labor analgesic counseling: a qualitative analysis. *Birth*. 2017;44:345–351.

34. Heim MA, Makuch MY. Pregnant women's knowledge of non-pharmacological techniques for pain relief during childbirth. *Eur J Midwifery*. 2022;6:5.

35. D'Souza RS, D'Souza S, Sharpe EE. YouTube as a source of medical information about epidural analgesia for labor pain. *Int J Obstet Anesth*. 2021;45:133–137.

36. Copstick S, Hayes RW, Taylor KE, Morris NF. A test of a common assumption regarding the use of antenatal training during labour. *J Psychosom Res*. 1985;29:215–218.

37. Bernardini JY, Maloni JA, Stegman CE. Neuromuscular control of childbirth-prepared women during the first stage of labor. *JOGN Nurs*. 1983;12:105–111.

38. Stewart DE. Psychiatric symptoms following attempted natural childbirth. *Can Med Assoc J*. 1982;127:713–716.

39. Guzman Sanchez A, Segura Ortega L, Panduro Baron JG. Psychological reaction due to failure using the Lamaze method. *Int J Gynaecol Obstet*. 1985;23:343–346.

40. Tuteur A. Opinion: How the natural birth industry sets mothers up for guilt and shame. The Washington Post; 2016. https://www.washingtonpost.com/opinions/how-the-natural-birth-industry-sets-mothers-up-for-guilt-and-shame/2016/05/06/8720e956-1241-11e6-81b4-581a5c4c42df_story.html?utm_term=.a923c0b0808a. Accessed 31 July 2024.

41. Edwards K. Why are we still trying to talk women out of epidurals?: The Sydney Morning Herald; 2016. http://www.smh.com.au/lifestyle/life-and-relationships/parenting/why-are-we-still-trying-to-talk-women-out-of-epidurals-20160916-gri7a7.html. Accessed 31 July 2024.

42. Moghaddam Hosseini V, Nazarzadeh M, Jahanfar S. Interventions for reducing fear of childbirth: a systematic review and meta-analysis of clinical trials. *Women Birth*. 2018;31:254–262.

43. Ricchi A, La Corte S, Molinazzi MT, et al. Study of childbirth education classes and evaluation of their effectiveness. *Clin Ter*. 2020;170:e78–e86.

44. Leutenegger V, Grylka-Baeschlin S, Wieber F, et al. The effectiveness of skilled breathing and relaxation techniques during antenatal education on maternal and neonatal outcomes: a systematic review. *BMC Pregnancy Childbirth*. 2022;22:856.

45. Delke I, Minkoff H, Grunebaum A. Effect of Lamaze childbirth preparation on maternal plasma beta-endorphin immunoreactivity in active labor. *Am J Perinatol*. 1985;2:317–319.

46. Hughey MJ, McElin TW, Young T. Maternal and fetal outcome of Lamaze-prepared patients. *Obstet Gynecol*. 1978;51:643–647.

47. Brewin C, Bradley C. Perceived control and the experience of childbirth. *Br J Clin Psychol*. 1982;21:263–269.

48. Patton LL, English EC, Hambleton JD. Childbirth preparation and outcomes of labor and delivery in primiparous women. *J Fam Pract*. 1985;20:375–378.

49. Sturrock WA, Johnson JA. The relationship between childbirth education classes and obstetric outcome. *Birth*. 1990;17:82–85.

50. Zax M, Sameroff AJ, Farnum JE. Childbirth education, maternal attitudes, and delivery. *Am J Obstet Gynecol*. 1975;123:185–190.

51. Campbell D, Scott KD, Klaus MH, Falk M. Female relatives or friends trained as labor doulas: outcomes at 6 to 8 weeks postpartum. *Birth*. 2007;34:220–227.

52. Scott JR, Rose NB. Effect of psychoprophylaxis (Lamaze preparation) on labor and delivery in primiparas. *N Engl J Med*. 1976;294:1205–1207.

53. Ferguson S, Davis D, Browne J. Does antenatal education affect labour and birth? A structured review of the literature. *Women Birth*. 2013;26:e5–e8.

54. Mueller CG, Webb PJ, Morgan S. The efects of childbirth education on maternity outcomes and maternal satisfaction. *J Perinat Educ*. 2020;29:16–22.

55. Hetherington SE. A controlled study of the effect of prepared childbirth classes on obstetric outcomes. *Birth*. 1990;17:86–90.

56. Geden E, Beck NC, Brouder G, et al. Self-report and psychophysiological effects of Lamaze preparation: an analogue of labor pain. *Res Nurs Health*. 1985;8:155–165.

57. Geden EA, Beck NC, Anderson JS, et al. Effects of cognitive and pharmacologic strategies on analogued labor pain. *Nurs Res*. 1986;35:301–306.

58. Manderino MA, Bzdek VM. Effects of modeling and information on reactions to pain: a childbirth-preparation analogue. *Nurs Res*. 1984;33:9–14.

59. Worthington EL Jr, Martin GA. A laboratory analysis of response to pain after training three Lamaze techniques. *J Psychosom Res*. 1980;24:109–116.

60. Whipple B, Josimovich JB, Komisaruk BR. Sensory thresholds during the antepartum, intrapartum and postpartum periods. *Int J Nurs Stud*. 1990;27:213–221.

61. Simkin P, Bolding A. Update on nonpharmacologic approaches to relieve labor pain and prevent suffering. *J Midwifery Womens Health*. 2004;49:489–504.

62. Markley JC, Rollins MD. Non-neuraxial labor analgesia: options. *Clin Obstet Gynecol*. 2017;60:350–364.

63. Arendt KW, Tessmer-Tuck JA. Nonpharmacologic labor analgesia. *Clin Perinatol*. 2013;40:351–371.

64. Jones L, Othman M, Dowswell T, et al. Pain management for women in labour: an overview of systematic reviews. *Cochrane Database Syst Rev*. 2012;(3):CD009234.

65. Van Leugenhaege L, Degraeve J, Jacquemyn Y, et al. Factors associated with the intention of pregnant women to give birth with epidural analgesia: a cross-sectional study. *BMC Pregnancy Childbirth*. 2023;23:598.

66. Bohren MA, Hofmeyr GJ, Sakala C, et al. Continuous support for women during childbirth. *Cochrane Database Syst Rev*. 2017;(7):CD003766.

67. Smith CA, Levett KM, Collins CT, Jones L. Massage, reflexology and other manual methods for pain management in labour. *Cochrane Database Syst Rev*. 2012;(2):CD009290.

68. Smith CA, Levett KM, Collins CT, et al. Massage, reflexology and other manual methods for pain management in labour. *Cochrane Database Syst Rev*. 2018;(3):CD009290.

69. Chen SF, Wang CH, Chan PT, et al. Labour pain control by aromatherapy: a meta-analysis of randomised controlled trials. *Women Birth*. 2019;32:327–335.

70. Liao CC, Lan SH, Yen YY, et al. Aromatherapy intervention on anxiety and pain during first stage labour in nulliparous women: a systematic review and meta-analysis. *J Obstet Gynaecol*. 2021;41:21–31.

71. Kaya A, Yesildere Saglam H, Karadag E, Gursoy E. The effectiveness of aromatherapy in the management of labor pain: a meta-analysis. *Eur J Obstet Gynecol Reprod Biol X*. 2023;20:100255.

72. Cluett ER, Burns E, Cuthbert A. Immersion in water during labour and birth. *Cochrane Database Syst Rev*. 2018;(5):CD000111.

73. Mellado-García E, Díaz-Rodríguez L, Cortés-Martín J, et al. Hydrotherapy in pain management in pregnant women: a meta-analysis of randomized clinical trials. *J Clin Med*. 2024;13

74. Gupta JK, Sood A, Hofmeyr GJ, Vogel JP. Position in the second stage of labour for women without epidural anaesthesia. *Cochrane Database Syst Rev*. 2017;(5):CD002006.

75. Grenvik JM, Rosenthal E, Wey S, et al. Birthing ball for reducing labor pain: a systematic review and meta-analysis of randomized controlled trials. *J Matern Fetal Neonatal Med*. 2022;35:5184–5193.

76. Lawrence A, Lewis L, Hofmeyr GJ, Styles C. Maternal positions and mobility during first stage labour. *Cochrane Database Syst Rev*. 2013;(10):CD003934.

77. Bloom SL, McIntire DD, Kelly MA, et al. Lack of effect of walking on labor and delivery. *N Engl J Med*. 1998;339:76–79.

78. Nageotte MP, Larson D, Rumney PJ, et al. Epidural analgesia compared with combined spinal-epidural analgesia during labor in nulliparous women. *N Engl J Med*. 1997;337:1715–1719.

79. Gimovsky AC, Berghella V. Evidence-based labor management: second stage of labor (part 4). *Am J Obstet Gynecol MFM*. 2022;(4):100548.

80. St James-Roberts I, Chamberlain G, Haran FJ, Hutchinson CM. Use of electromyographic and skin-conductance biofeedback relaxation training of facilitate childbirth in primiparae. *J Psychosom Res*. 1982;26:455–462.

81. Duchene P. Effects of biofeedback on childbirth pain. *J Pain Symptom Manage*. 1989;4:117–123.

82. Barragan Loayza IM, Sola I, Juando Prats C. Biofeedback for pain management during labour. *Cochrane Database Syst Rev*. 2011;(6):CD006168.

83. Derry S, Straube S, Moore RA, et al. Intracutaneous or subcutaneous sterile water injection compared with blinded controls for pain management in labour. *Cochrane Database Syst Rev*. 2012;(1):CD009107.

84. Huang CY, Lo SF, Chou SH, Shih CL. Analgesic effects of sterile water injection in the management of low back pain during labor: a systematic review and meta-analysis. *Int J Gynaecol Obstet*. 2022;159:642–650.

85. Chao AS, Chao A, Wang TH, et al. Pain relief by applying transcutaneous electrical nerve stimulation (TENS) on acupuncture points during the first stage of labor: a randomized double-blind placebo-controlled trial. *Pain*. 2007;127:214–220.

86. Mello LF, Nobrega LF, Lemos A. Transcutaneous electrical stimulation for pain relief during labor: a systematic review and meta-analysis. *Rev Bras Fisioter*. 2011;15:175–184.

87. Thuvarakan K, Zimmermann H, Mikkelsen MK, Gazerani P. Transcutaneous electrical nerve stimulation as a pain-relieving approach in labor pain: a systematic review and meta-analysis of randomized controlled trials. *Neuromodulation*. 2020;23:732–746.

88. Smith CA, Collins CT, Levett KM, et al. Acupuncture or acupressure for pain management during labour. *Cochrane Database Syst Rev*. 2020;(2):CD009232.

89. August R. *Hypnosis in Childbirth*. McGraw Hill; 1961.

90. Fee AF, Reilley RR. Hypnosis in obstetrics: a review of techniques. *J Am Soc Psychosom Dent Med*. 1982;29:17–29.

91. Rock NL, Shipley TE, Campbell C. Hypnosis with untrained, nonvolunteer patients in labor. *Int J Clin Exp Hypn*. 1969;17:25–36.

92. Madden K, Middleton P, Cyna AM, et al. Hypnosis for pain management during labour and childbirth. *Cochrane Database Syst Rev*. 2016;(5):CD009356.

93. Xu N, Chen S, Liu Y, et al. The effects of virtual reality in maternal delivery: systematic review and meta-analysis. *JMIR Serious Games*. 2022;10:e36695.

94. Beilin Y, Rosenblatt MA, Bodian CA, et al. Information and concerns about obstetric anesthesia: a survey of 320 obstetric patients. *Int J Obstet Anesth*. 1996;5:145–151.

95. de Labrusse C, Ramelet AS, Humphrey T, Maclennan SJ. Patient-centered care in maternity services: a critical appraisal and synthesis of the literature. *Womens Health Issues*. 2016;26:100–109.

96. Behruzi R, Hatem M, Goulet L, et al. Understanding childbirth practices as an organizational cultural phenomenon: a conceptual framework. *BMC Pregnancy Childbirth*. 2013;13:205–214.

23

Systemic and Nonneuraxial Regional Labor Analgesia

Valerie Zaphiratos, MSc, MD, FRCPC and
Ronald B. George, MD, FRCPC

Systemic drugs have been used to decrease the pain of childbirth since 1847, when James Young Simpson used diethyl ether to anesthetize a parturient with a deformed pelvis. Since that time, the provision of labor analgesia has advanced significantly. The growth of labor analgesia owes its progress to the heightened awareness of the neonatal effects of sedating medications or general anesthesia administered during vaginal delivery and a greater desire of parturients to actively participate in their childbirth experience.

In the modern era, systemic drug administration provides less effective labor analgesia with greater side effects compared with neuraxial techniques (epidural, spinal, combined spinal-epidural, dural-puncture epidural). As a consequence, a significant and growing number of parturients receive neuraxial labor analgesia globally, particularly in North America (60% to 75% rate of use).[1,2]

However, the use of systemic analgesia remains the most common practice worldwide. Many parturients labor and deliver in an environment where safe neuraxial analgesia is not available. Some parturients decline neuraxial analgesia or choose to receive systemic analgesia. Finally, some parturients may have a medical condition that contraindicates a neuraxial procedure (e.g., coagulopathy) or presents technical challenges (e.g., severe scoliosis, the presence of spinal hardware).

PARENTERAL OPIOIDS

Opioids are the most widely used systemic medications for labor analgesia owing to their low cost, ease of use, and the lack of need for specialized equipment and personnel. These drugs act at opioid receptors (Table 23.1).[3] Although associated with a high frequency of maternal side effects (e.g., nausea, vomiting, delayed gastric emptying, dysphoria, drowsiness, hypoventilation) and the potential for adverse neonatal effects, opioid use has been augmented by the availability of patient-controlled delivery systems.

There is little scientific evidence to suggest that one opioid is superior to another, as analgesia and side effects are largely dose-dependent rather than drug-dependent; most often, drug selection is based on local policies and provider preferences (Table 23.2). As a result of their high lipid solubility and low molecular weight (<500 Da), all opioids readily cross the placenta by diffusion and are associated with the risk for neonatal respiratory depression and neurobehavioral changes. Opioids may also affect the fetus *in utero* and neonate, who are particularly susceptible to opioid-induced side effects for several reasons. The metabolism and elimination of these drugs are prolonged compared with adults, and the blood-brain barrier is less well developed, allowing for greater central effects. Opioids may result in decreased variability of the fetal heart rate (FHR), although this change usually does not reflect a worsening of fetal oxygenation or acid-base status. The likelihood of neonatal respiratory depression depends on the dose and timing of opioid administration, as well as the presence of active metabolites. In a multicenter randomized trial, Halpern et al.[4] demonstrated an increased need for active neonatal resuscitation in a group that received parenteral opioid via patient-controlled analgesia (PCA) compared with a group that received local anesthetic plus opioid via patient-controlled epidural analgesia (PCEA) (52% versus 31%).

TABLE 23.1 Opioid Receptor Type Classification

Classification	Effects
μ_1, μ_2, μ_3	Analgesia, miosis, euphoria, respiratory depression, bradycardia
κ	Analgesia, sedation, miosis
δ	Analgesia, respiratory depression
Nociception	Inhibition of opioid analgesia
ζ	Tissue growth, embryonic development

Intermittent Bolus Parenteral Opioids

Opioids may be given intermittently by subcutaneous (SC), intramuscular (IM), or intravenous (IV) injection. The route and timing of administration influence maternal uptake and placental transfer to the fetus. The SC and IM routes have the advantage of ease of administration but are painful. Absorption varies with the site of injection and depends on local and regional blood flow; consequently, the onset, quality, and duration of analgesia are highly variable. IV administration is generally preferred when available, as it offers several advantages: the onset of analgesia is fast, the timing and magnitude of the peak plasma concentration of the drug are predictable, and titration to desired effect is possible.

Morphine

First isolated in 1806 and named after *Morpheus*, the Greek god of dreams, morphine was used only briefly for labor analgesia because of associated neonatal depression. In the early 1900s, morphine reappeared in combination with **scopolamine** ("twilight sleep"), but its use would often result in maternal sedation and neonatal depression.

With a high affinity for μ-opioid receptors, morphine is a potent long-acting analgesic. Morphine is principally metabolized by conjugation in the liver, with up to 70% transformed into largely inactive morphine-3-glucuronide. The remainder is transformed into the active metabolite morphine-6-glucuronide, an opioid agonist that is 13 times more potent than morphine.[5] Both metabolites are excreted in the urine and have elimination half-lives of up to 4.5 hours in the presence of normal renal function. Morphine rapidly crosses the placenta, and a fetal-to-maternal blood concentration ratio of 0.96 is observed at 5 minutes. The elimination half-life of morphine is longer in neonates than in adults.

Morphine can be given every 4 hours IV (0.05 to 0.1 mg/kg) or IM (0.1 to 0.2 mg/kg), with a peak effect observed in 10 and 30 minutes, respectively. The duration of action when given IV or IM is 3 to 4 hours.[5] As an intrapartum opioid analgesic, morphine is infrequently used owing to its long half-life and maternal side effects such as respiratory depression and histamine release, which may result in rash and pruritus. Like many opioids, morphine is emetogenic and is associated with sedation and dysphoria with increasing doses.[5] Despite these limitations, IM morphine 10 to 15 mg is sometimes used in early labor, concomitantly with

an antiemetic (e.g., IM **dimenhydrinate** 25 mg), to provide analgesia with sedation.

Olofsson et al.[6] assessed the analgesic efficacy of IV morphine (0.05 mg/kg every third contraction, to a maximum dose of 0.2 mg/kg) and observed clinically insignificant reductions in labor pain intensity. The same investigators also compared IV morphine (up to 0.15 mg/kg) with IV **meperidine (pethidine)** (up to 1.5 mg/kg) and found that both groups had high pain scores despite high levels of maternal sedation.[7] A randomized controlled trial that compared morphine 2 mg with IV **acetaminophen (paracetamol)** 1000 mg for early labor analgesia observed no differences in visual analog scale (VAS) pain scores at baseline and at 15 and 60 minutes.[8] However, within 2 hours of administration, more patients receiving acetaminophen required rescue analgesia (52.9% versus 17.6%; $P < .01$).

Pregnancy alters the pharmacokinetics of morphine, with greater plasma clearance, shorter elimination half-life, and earlier peak metabolite levels. In theory, these characteristics should reduce fetal exposure. Possible neonatal respiratory depression has been attributed to an increased permeability of the neonatal brain. In a small study, Way et al.[9] observed that IV morphine given to newborns appeared to cause greater respiratory depression than an equipotent dose of meperidine when response to carbon dioxide was measured. However, no cases of neonatal depression after morphine administration during labor were observed in one study.[10]

Meperidine

In 1947 meperidine (pethidine) was the first synthetic opioid used for labor analgesia and quickly displaced morphine in the United Kingdom.[11] An agonist that binds to both μ- and κ-opioid receptors, meperidine is estimated to have 10% of the analgesic potency of morphine. The usual dose is 50 to 100 mg IM, which can be repeated every 4 hours. The onset of analgesia occurs in 10 to 15 minutes, but 45 minutes may be required to reach peak effect. The duration of action is typically 2 to 3 hours.

Meperidine is highly lipid soluble, readily crosses the placenta, and equilibrates between the maternal and fetal compartments within 6 minutes. Meperidine is metabolized in the liver to **normeperidine (norpethidine)**, a pharmacologically active metabolite that may cause prolonged neonatal side effects.[12] The action of meperidine, but not normeperidine, is reversed by naloxone; consequently, antagonism with naloxone may exacerbate normeperidine-induced seizures owing to suppression of the anticonvulsant effect of meperidine.

Historically, meperidine was given to decrease the length of the first stage of labor in cases of dystocia. However, Sosa et al.[13] reported that, compared with placebo, meperidine 100 mg given IV was associated with no differences in the duration of active labor or operative delivery rate, but greater requirement for oxytocin augmentation (relative risk [RR] 2.24, 95% confidence interval [CI], 1.13 to 4.43). Moreover, maternal administration of meperidine has been associated with increased umbilical cord arterial acidemia, altered neonatal behavior,[14] and lower Apgar scores and neonatal muscle

TABLE 23.2   Systemic Opioids for Labor Analgesia

Drug	Usual Dose (IV/IM)	Time to Peak Effect (IV/IM)	Duration of Action	Comments
Meperidine (Pethidine)	25–50 mg IV 50–100 mg IM	5–10 min IV 45 min IM	2–3 h	Maximal neonatal depression 3–5 h after dose Has an active metabolite with a long half-life
Morphine	2–5 mg IV 10–15 mg IM	10 min IV 30 min IM	3–4 h	Possibly more neonatal respiratory depression than with meperidine Has an active metabolite
Diamorphine	5–10 mg IV 5–10 mg IM	2–5 min IV 5–10 min IM	90 min	Morphine prodrug More euphoria, less nausea than with morphine
Fentanyl	25–50 µg IV	2–4 min IV	30–60 min	Usually administered as an infusion or by PCA Accumulates during an infusion Less neonatal depression than with meperidine
Nalbuphine	10–20 mg IV 10–20 mg IM/SC	2–3 min IV 15 min IM/SC	3–6 h	Opioid agonist/antagonist Ceiling effect on respiratory depression Lower neonatal neurobehavioral scores than with meperidine
Butorphanol	1–2 mg IV 1–2 mg IM	5–10 min IV 30–60 min IM	4–6 h	Opioid agonist/antagonist Ceiling effect on respiratory depression
Meptazinol	50–100 mg IM	30 min IM	2–3 h	Partial opioid agonist Less sedation and respiratory depression than with other opioids
Pentazocine	30–60 mg IV 30–60 mg IM	2–3 min IV 20 min IM	3–4 h	Opioid agonist/antagonist Psychomimetic effects possible
Tramadol	50–100 mg IV 50–100 mg IM	10 min IM	2–4 h	Mixed action Lower efficacy and more side effects compared with meperidine

IM, Intramuscular; *IV*, intravenous; *PCA*, patient-controlled analgesia; *SC*, subcutaneous.

tone. Maternal side effects include a high incidence of nausea, vomiting, and dysphoria.

Elbohoty et al.[15] reported that IV meperidine 50 mg produced labor analgesia that was comparable to that produced by IV acetaminophen 1000 mg but with a greater incidence of adverse effects (64% versus 0%). Zuarez-Easton et al.[16] reported that labor pain intensity, side effects, and maternal satisfaction did not differ after IV meperidine 50 mg or inhaled **nitrous oxide**. A review of 62 randomized controlled trials from 1972 to 2018 found that meperidine had similar or inferior analgesic efficacy compared with other analgesics for acute postoperative or labor pain and was associated with more sedation and respiratory depression.[17] Despite the availability of newer and more effective analgesics with fewer side effects, meperidine remains commonly administered for labor analgesia, most likely because of familiarity, ease of administration, availability, and low cost.

Diamorphine

Diamorphine (3,6-diacetylmorphine, heroin) is a synthetic derivative twice as potent as its parent morphine and used in some countries for labor analgesia.[11] As a prodrug,

diamorphine has no direct affinity for opioid receptors; however, when rapidly hydrolyzed by plasma esterases, the active metabolites provide faster analgesia onset with more euphoria and less nausea and vomiting than morphine.[5] These pharmacokinetic properties may predispose to maternal, as well as neonatal, respiratory depression owing to rapid placental transfer.

In a two-center double-blind randomized controlled trial that compared IM diamorphine 7.5 mg with IM meperidine 150 mg for labor analgesia in 484 parturients, Wee et al.[18] found that analgesia was modestly better but the mean length of labor was 82 (95% CI, 39 to 124) minutes longer with diamorphine. No differences in maternal sedation, nausea and vomiting, or primary neonatal outcomes were observed. In a single-center retrospective observational safety study, patients who chose PCA remifentanil, IM diamorphine, or epidural analgesia, experienced similar neonatal adverse events.[19]

Despite the risk of maternal and neonatal respiratory depression, diamorphine is still used for labor analgesia in some developed countries with low epidural analgesia rates, such as the United Kingdom, but it is seldom used in the United States or Canada.[19]

Nalbuphine

Nalbuphine is a mixed agonist-antagonist opioid analgesic with agonist activity at κ-opioid receptors, thereby producing analgesia, and partial agonist activity at μ-opioid receptors, thus resulting in less respiratory depression.[20] A partial agonist is a drug that has receptor affinity but produces a submaximal effect compared with a full agonist, even when given at very high doses.[5]

Nalbuphine can be administered by IM, IV, or SC injection, with a usual dose of 10 to 20 mg every 4 to 6 hours. The onset of analgesia occurs within 2 to 3 minutes of IV administration and within 15 minutes of IM or SC administration. The drug is metabolized in the liver to inactive compounds that are then secreted into bile and excreted in feces.[20]

Nalbuphine and morphine are of equal analgesic potency and result in sedation and respiratory depression at similar doses. However, because of its mixed receptor affinity, nalbuphine demonstrates a ceiling effect for respiratory depression at a dose of 0.5 mg/kg.[20] Nalbuphine causes less nausea, vomiting, and dysphoria than morphine.

Wilson et al.[21] performed a randomized, double-blind comparison of IM nalbuphine 20 mg and meperidine 100 mg for labor analgesia. Nalbuphine was associated with less nausea and vomiting but more maternal sedation. Analgesia was comparable between the groups. Neonatal neurobehavioral scores were lower in the nalbuphine group at 2 to 4 hours, but there was no difference between groups at 24 hours. The mean umbilical vein-to-maternal vein concentration ratio was higher with nalbuphine (0.78) than with meperidine (0.61). A subsequent study failed to demonstrate an analgesic advantage with either drug but again reported transient neonatal neurologic depression with nalbuphine.[22]

Nicolle et al.,[23] evaluating the transplacental transfer and neonatal pharmacokinetics of IM or IV nalbuphine in 28 laboring parturients, found a high umbilical vein-to-maternal vein concentration ratio of 0.74, which did not correlate with the administered dose. The estimated neonatal half-life was 4.1 hours, which is greater than the adult half-life and, more importantly, longer than the half-life of naloxone. There was a transient reduction in FHR variability in 54% of the fetuses, which was not associated with the plasma concentration of nalbuphine. Analgesia was rated as effective by only 54% of parturients.

Like morphine, nalbuphine is occasionally used for early labor analgesia; more commonly, its antagonistic properties are employed to treat pruritus from neuraxial or IV opioids.

Fentanyl

Fentanyl is a synthetic opioid that is highly lipid-soluble, protein-bound, and selective for the μ-opioid receptor, with an analgesic potency 100 times that of morphine. Its rapid onset (peak effect 2 to 4 minutes), short duration of action (30 to 60 minutes), and lack of active metabolites make it attractive for labor analgesia. Fentanyl is most commonly administered via PCA.

Small doses of fentanyl undergo rapid redistribution, but large or repeated doses may accumulate.[5] Importantly, clearance of fentanyl by elimination represents only 20% of that occurring by redistribution, resulting in a rapid increase in context-sensitive half-time when using an infusion over 2 hours of duration.[5] In contrast to morphine, fentanyl is metabolized to several inactive metabolites in the liver that are excreted in the urine. After 2 hours of infusion, it takes at least 50 minutes for plasma concentration to decrease by 50%.[5] Thus, to avoid neonatal effects, in many labor analgesia studies fentanyl was stopped before the second stage of labor.[24-26]

Fentanyl readily crosses the placenta; however, the average umbilical vein-to-maternal vein ratio remains low, most likely owing to a significant degree of maternal protein binding and drug redistribution. In a chronically instrumented sheep model, Craft et al.[27] detected fentanyl in fetal plasma as early as 1 minute after maternal administration; however, maternal plasma levels were approximately 2.5 times greater than fetal plasma levels.

Rayburn et al.[28] compared parturients receiving IV fentanyl (50 to 100 μg every hour at maternal request) with those who did not receive analgesia. All patients receiving fentanyl (mean dose 140 [range 50 to 600] μg) experienced brief analgesia (mean 45 minutes), sedation, and a transient reduction in FHR variability (mean 30 minutes). There were no differences between groups in neonatal Apgar scores, respiratory status, or Neurologic and Adaptive Capacity Scores (NACS). In a similar comparison of IV fentanyl (50 to 100 μg every hour) with an equianalgesic dose of meperidine (25 to 50 mg every 2 to 3 hours), Rayburn et al.[29] observed less sedation, vomiting, and neonatal naloxone administration with fentanyl, but no difference in NACS. The two groups experienced similarly high pain scores, suggesting that both drugs have poor analgesic efficacy at the studied doses.

Fentanyl boluses administered during labor are most often used as a bridge to neuraxial analgesia or opioid PCA but can also be used for analgesia throughout labor. When fentanyl is used throughout labor, naloxone should be readily available for administration to the mother or neonate, and oxygen saturation monitoring for the neonate should be considered.

Other Opioids

Compared with meperidine, **butorphanol**, **meptazinol**, and **pentazocine** provide similar or less analgesia, with greater cost or side effects. Butorphanol does not confer additional analgesic benefit compared with meperidine.[30] Meptazinol is costly, confers similar benefit to meperidine, is rarely used in the United Kingdom, and unavailable in the United States and Canada.[31] Pentazocine provides similar analgesia to meperidine, but psychomimetic effects such as dysphoria and hallucinations complicate its use.[32]

Tramadol, an atypical racemic mixture of two enantiomers, is a weak, synthetic drug that has affinity for all opioid receptors, but particularly the μ-opioid subtype. Administered orally, IM, or IV at a dose of 50 to 100 mg every 4 to 6 hours in adults, the analgesic potency of tramadol is equal to that of meperidine and one-fifth to one-tenth that of morphine. Tramadol and its active M1 metabolite *O*-desmethyltramadol readily cross the placenta, and an umbilical vein-to-maternal vein ratio of 0.94 has been observed at delivery.[33] In a comparison of IM tramadol 100 mg and meperidine 100 mg for labor analgesia, Keskin et al.[34] observed greater pain relief and a lower incidence of nausea and fatigue with meperidine. By contrast, Viegas et al.[35] conducted a randomized, double-blind trial to compare IM administration of tramadol 50 mg, tramadol 100 mg, and meperidine 75 mg. Tramadol and meperidine provided similar labor analgesia; however, a higher incidence of maternal and neonatal adverse effects was observed with meperidine.

Codeine seldom has been studied for labor analgesia and produces limited analgesic benefit. Tramadol and codeine are not widely available in parenteral formulation. In addition, the US Federal Drug Administration issued a strong warning against the use of codeine and tramadol for lactating women because of the risk of serious adverse reactions (sedation, hypopnea or apnea, breastfeeding difficulties, and death) in breastfed infants born to mothers who are CYP2D6 ultrametabolizers.[14,36]

Patient-Controlled Analgesia

First described in parturients with thrombocytopenia who were unable to receive neuraxial analgesia, the use of PCA has grown in availability and popularity.[37] Suggested advantages of PCA include: (1) superior pain relief with lower doses of drug, (2) less risk for maternal respiratory depression compared with bolus IV administration, (3) less placental transfer of drug, (4) less need for antiemetic agents, and (5) greater patient satisfaction.[38] For these reasons, PCA is a common method of labor analgesia when neuraxial analgesia is not available, contraindicated, or unsuccessful. The parturient can tailor the administration of analgesia according to individual needs; furthermore, with some regimens, the bolus dose can be titrated as labor progresses. The smaller, more frequent dosing of PCA may result in a more stable plasma drug concentration and thus a more consistent analgesic effect compared with that of intermittent bolus administration regimens.[38]

However, PCA for labor analgesia is not without limitations. Despite the frequency of dose administration, the coordination of peak opioid concentrations with uterine contractions can be difficult and may result in suboptimal analgesia. In addition, the relatively small doses of opioid may be less effective at controlling pain as labor progresses. A variety of drugs, doses, and regimens for PCA have been studied, including comparisons with and without a continuous IV infusion (Table 23.3). The safest and most effective opioids used for PCA for labor analgesia are **fentanyl** and **remifentanil**. Rarely administered by PCA for labor analgesia in parturients with a live fetus, **morphine**, **diamorphine**, and **meperidine** are options for those with intrauterine fetal demise.[37]

TABLE 23.3   Opioids Used for Intravenous Patient-Controlled Analgesia in Labor

Drug	Bolus Dose	Lockout Interval (min)
Fentanyl	10–25 μg	5–12
Remifentanil (bolus only)	0.2–0.5 μg/kg (low dose initially, then titrated to effect)	2–3
Remifentanil (background infusion with bolus dose)[a]	Infusion rate: 0.025–0.1 μg/kg/min Bolus dose: 0.25 μg/kg	2–3

[a]Background infusion of remifentanil used concomitantly with patient-controlled analgesia bolus is not recommended by the RemiPCA SAFE network.[39]

Fentanyl

The pharmacologic profile of fentanyl (e.g., rapid onset, high potency, short duration of action, absence of active metabolites) has resulted in its selection as one of the most commonly used opioids for PCA during labor and delivery since the early 1990s.

Rayburn et al.[40] compared fentanyl PCA (bolus 10 μg, lockout interval 12 minutes) with intermittent IV nurse-administered boluses (50 to 100 μg every hour, on demand). The degree of analgesia, adverse maternal effects, and neonatal outcomes (e.g., Apgar scores, naloxone requirement, neurobehavioral scores) were similar between the two groups. The two groups used a similar total amount of fentanyl, had comparable umbilical serum concentrations of fentanyl, and had incomplete analgesia during late labor.

Nikkola et al.[26] observed that fentanyl PCA (loading dose 50 μg, bolus 20 μg, lockout interval 5 minutes) provided a moderate reduction in labor pain in 50% of parturients; however, less overall pain relief was experienced compared with parturients who received epidural analgesia. The use of fentanyl was also associated with a higher incidence of maternal dizziness and sedation.

Morley-Forster and Weberpals[41] observed a 44% incidence of moderate neonatal depression (1-minute Apgar score < 6) in a retrospective review of 32 neonates whose mothers had received fentanyl PCA using various regimens during labor. A total of 9.4% of the neonates required naloxone; the total dose of fentanyl was higher in the mothers of neonates who required naloxone than in those who did not (mean 770 [SD 233] μg versus 298 [287] μg, respectively). By contrast, in a retrospective evaluation of fentanyl PCA (loading dose 50 μg, bolus 20 μg, lockout interval 5 minutes) compared with no analgesia during labor, Miyakoshi et al.[25] observed comparable Apgar scores, similar mean umbilical arterial blood pH measurements, and no requirement for naloxone in 258 neonates exposed to fentanyl PCA. Maternal pain scores with PCA fentanyl were decreased significantly from baseline for the first 3 hours after initiation, with 6.2% experiencing nausea, but none exhibiting maternal respiratory depression or excessive sedation.

Halpern et al.[4] randomized 242 laboring patients to receive either PCA fentanyl (loading dose 100 μg plus additional doses of 50 μg until adequate pain relief, bolus 25 to 50 μg, lockout interval 10 minutes) or epidural analgesia. There were no differences in rates of cesarean delivery or instrumentation, however, the PCA fentanyl group had greater use of antiemetics (17% versus 6.4%; $P = .01$); experienced more sedation (39% versus 5%; $P < .001$); and had more pain, lower maternal satisfaction, and more neonates requiring active resuscitation (52% versus 31%; $P = .001$) and naloxone (17% versus 3%; $P < .001$). Some 33% of the parturients in the PCA fentanyl group requested epidural analgesia.

Remifentanil

Remifentanil is an ultra-short-acting, synthetic anilinopiperidine derivative with selective activity at the μ-opioid receptor, and a small volume of distribution (0.39 L/kg). Functional brain magnetic resonance imaging revealed an onset time of 20 to 30 seconds, peak concentration within 80 to 90 seconds at the cortical loci, and a blood-brain equilibration time of 1.2 to 1.4 minutes.[42] Remifentanil undergoes rapid hydrolysis by nonspecific plasma and tissue esterases to inactive metabolites, independent of organ metabolism, resulting in a short elimination half-life of approximately 9.5 minutes. The context-sensitive half-time is 3.5 minutes, irrespective of the duration of infusion. The effective analgesic half-life is 6 minutes, thus allowing effective analgesia for consecutive uterine contractions. Plasma concentrations of remifentanil in pregnant patients are approximately half those found in nonpregnant patients.[43] This difference may be caused by the greater volume of distribution (increased blood volume and reduced protein binding), greater clearance (increased cardiac output and renal perfusion), and higher esterase activity during pregnancy.

Remifentanil is rapidly titratable, allowing for dose adjustments with labor progress or in response to side effects. Termination of a continuous remifentanil infusion results in a 50% recovery in minute ventilation within 5.4 minutes. Although remifentanil readily crosses the placenta, resulting in a fetal-to-maternal blood ratio of 0.88, the lower umbilical artery-to-vein concentration ratio of 0.29 demonstrates that the drug is extensively redistributed and/or metabolized by the fetus.[43] Kan et al.[43] also found no adverse neonatal effects after a remifentanil infusion during cesarean delivery.

With ultrarapid pharmacokinetics, remifentanil does not accumulate with time and can be used during the second stage of labor with less concern for neonatal side effects. However, the rapid onset and offset of remifentanil, with peak effect-site concentrations at 1 to 2 minutes, may not provide adequate or sustained analgesia for the desired or subsequent uterine contraction, respectively. Thus, the use of PCA remifentanil requires training of patients to appropriately time the bolus dose with contractions.

Efficacy and Optimal Regimen. Owing to its ultra-short action, delivery of remifentanil is limited to PCA bolus, a continuous infusion, or a combination of the two. Although a number of studies have compared remifentanil with other opioids using fixed, nontitratable PCA doses, Volmanen

et al.[44] attempted to determine the minimum effective dose of remifentanil for labor analgesia during the first stage of labor. Using an initial bolus dose of 0.2 μg/kg, and dose increases of 0.2 μg/kg (lockout interval 1 minute) over a 1-hour study period, the median effective bolus dose was observed to be 0.4 μg/kg (range 0.2 to 0.8 μg/kg). However, frequent episodes of maternal oxygen saturation < 94% (10 of 17 subjects), maternal sedation, and reduced FHR variability were observed.

Balki et al.[45] compared the effect of a fixed remifentanil bolus dose with a titratable background infusion versus a fixed background infusion with a titratable bolus dose. Both groups started with a remifentanil bolus dose of 0.25 μg/kg (lockout interval 2 minutes) and a background infusion rate of 0.025 μg/kg/min. If analgesia was inadequate, either the background infusion or bolus dose was increased in a stepwise manner to a maximum of 0.1 μg/kg/min or 1 μg/kg, respectively. The mean pain scores, satisfaction scores, and cumulative remifentanil doses were similar in the two groups; only one patient eventually requested epidural analgesia. The incidence of maternal side effects was higher in the escalating bolus dose group, including drowsiness (100% versus 30%) and frequency of oxygen saturation < 95% (60% versus 40%). There was no difference in the incidence of adverse neonatal effects. The investigators advocated the use of a titrated background infusion (range, 0.025 to 0.1 μg/kg/min) with a constant PCA bolus dose (0.25 μg/kg, lockout interval 2 minutes).[45]

D'Onofrio et al.[46] conducted an observational study of 205 parturients in whom a continuous infusion of remifentanil was titrated (initial to maximum dose range, 0.025 to 0.15 μg/kg/min) with a goal of achieving pain scores ≤ 4/10 during contractions. Adequate analgesia was achieved within 30 minutes but required a median remifentanil infusion dose of 0.075 μg/kg/min. The oxygen saturation remained greater than 95% in all patients without supplemental oxygen, and there were no reported neonatal side effects.

Together, these studies suggest that fixed-dose remifentanil PCA protocols are less effective than titratable regimens, with the potential for low doses resulting in poor analgesia, underdosing, and maternal dissatisfaction, and high doses resulting in adverse effects such as maternal sedation, respiratory depression, and oxygen desaturation. Evidence is conflicting as to whether the use of a background infusion confers additional benefits, particularly given the greater risk for maternal sedation and respiratory depression.[45,47]

Rehberg et al.[48] sought to improve labor analgesia and reduce side effects by altering the timing of the remifentanil PCA bolus. A handheld dynamometer was used to determine the peak effect of the next contraction; however, because of contraction variability, analgesia was not substantially improved. The analgesic benefit of remifentanil may be best optimized by instructing parturients to press the PCA button at the first perception of a contraction, given that the peak analgesic effect occurs within 1 to 3 minutes.[20]

Leong et al.[49] devised an automated closed interactive feedback system ("step-up–step-down" regimen) with the input of continuous monitoring devices (pulse oximeter and heart rate) to modulate drug delivery and improve labor analgesia and safety. The vital sign–controlled, patient-assisted IV analgesia prototype initially administered small boluses of remifentanil, with dosing alterations based on the presence or absence of patient demands over a predefined period. In the 29 parturients who used the device, despite all using supplemental oxygen, 52% experienced oxygen desaturation < 95% for more than 60 seconds, and 24% experienced a heart rate < 60 beats/min for more than 60 seconds. The median dose of remifentanil was 0.07 µg/kg/min, and the system automatically reduced dosages and temporarily halted remifentanil administration when desaturation and bradycardia thresholds were achieved. Additional analgesia, including nitrous oxide or an epidural technique, was required by 31% of parturients.

Side effects. Remifentanil can cause respiratory depression through reductions in the ventilatory rate and tidal volume. Although the safety profile of remifentanil PCA in labor has been specifically evaluated, the data are conflicting.[46,50] Volikas et al.[50] investigated the maternal and neonatal effects of remifentanil PCA (bolus dose 0.5 µg/kg, lockout interval 2 minutes) in 50 parturients. Effective analgesia was reported in 86% of study participants, and 44% experienced slight drowsiness (but were rousable to voice and maintained oxygen saturation > 93%). Mild itching and FHR changes occurred in the first 20 minutes of remifentanil PCA but did not require treatment. Umbilical cord blood gas measurements and neonatal Apgar scores and neurologic examinations were all within normal limits.

A survey of 61 Dutch hospitals reviewed 27 maternal and 2 neonatal serious adverse events related to remifentanil PCA.[51] The majority of maternal serious adverse events were oxygen desaturation (23 cases), followed by apnea (6 cases), bradycardia (4 cases), and 1 maternal cardiac arrest; the 2 neonatal adverse events were respiratory depression. In five cases of maternal apnea, a background infusion was used in addition to PCA boluses.

With the use of oxygen saturation and end-tidal CO_2 monitoring, Stocki et al.[52] reported a moderate number of apneic events (respiratory arrest greater than 20 seconds), low respiratory rates, and hypoxemic events in laboring parturients who received remifentanil PCA, compared with none in those who received epidural analgesia. These findings suggest that the analgesia onset from a bolus dose of remifentanil may occur after the cessation of uterine contractions (which have an average duration of 60 to 70 seconds). Although Thurlow et al.[53] encouraged parturients to activate a bolus dose at the very first detection of a contraction, or even between contractions, Volmanen et al.[54] indicated that the onset of electroencephalographic depression and subsequent onset of peak respiratory depression does not happen until approximately 2.5 minutes after bolus injection. Consequently, bolus administration can frequently miss the uterine contraction.

Weiniger et al.[55] evaluated candidate variables (i.e., respiratory rate, end-tidal CO_2, pulse oximetry, heart rate, and integrated pulmonary index) to serve as early warning apnea alerts (defined as any variable value below a prespecified threshold for 15 seconds). A total of 331 immediate early warning alerts and 62 episodes of apnea (defined as maximal CO_2 < 5 mm Hg for at least 30 consecutive seconds) occurred among 10 of 19 patients (56.2%) who received remifentanil PCA. Alerts for end-tidal CO_2, respiratory rate, and integrated pulmonary index detected most episodes of apnea, pulse oximetry alerts missed the majority of apneic episodes, and all variables had a low positive predictive rate, indicating the limitations of respiratory monitors for early warning apnea surveillance in this setting.

The use of remifentanil PCA during labor results in a variable range in the incidences of maternal sedation, dizziness, nausea, vomiting, and pruritus. The wide incidence of nausea (0% to 60%)[45,46] may reflect an opioid-induced increase in vagal activity, which can decrease mean arterial pressure and heart rate; however, this has not been reported in laboring patients receiving remifentanil PCA, perhaps reflecting the doses administered and/or the high maternal sympathetic activity during labor. Pruritus occurs in approximately 16% of parturients.[24] In 140 parturients randomly assigned to either remifentanil PCA or epidural analgesia, Douma et al.[56] observed fever (temperature > 38°C) in 10% of remifentanil PCA patients compared with 37% in epidural analgesia patients.

Opioid-induced loss of FHR variability, a potential indicator of fetal compromise, may create diagnostic confusion in a labor setting.[57] Comparison studies have reported a lower incidence of FHR abnormalities with remifentanil than with meperidine.[47] However, similar to other opioids, available data suggest that remifentanil might induce fetal and neonatal acidosis.

Many studies have suggested that continuous patient monitoring is required with remifentanil use during labor. Van de Velde and Carvalho[58] suggested that monitoring for respiratory depression should ideally evaluate respiratory rate and sedation (one-to-one nursing or midwifery care), determine the adequacy of ventilation (capnography, apnea monitor), and evaluate oxygenation (pulse oximetry). Routine use of supplemental oxygen may increase the duration of apnea and reduce the sensitivity of pulse oximetry for detecting hypoventilation. A method for assisting ventilation (e.g., a self-inflating ventilating bag) should be immediately available.

The RemiPCA SAFE Network (https://www.remipca.org/php/en/index.php), which currently over 40 international hospital centers, was established to create international standards and monitor maternal and neonatal outcomes associated with the use of remifentanil PCA for labor. Melber et al.[39] published findings from the self-reported RemiPCA network database from 2010 to 2015, which included 5740 pregnant patients; the most frequent maternal side effects were hypoxemia (Spo_2 < 94%) (27%), sedation (26%), nausea/vomiting (17%), and pruritus (3%). Although no parturients required assisted ventilation or cardiopulmonary resuscitation, neonatal oxygen supplementation was required in 7% of neonates, and cardiopulmonary resuscitation potentially related to remifentanil was required in 0.3% of neonates. Of interest, no complications were reported in centers that used remifentanil PCA at least 10 times per year, suggesting the value of familiarity with use.[59] To decrease maternal adverse events, three operational changes were adopted by the RemiPCA network in 2013: (1) use of a 4-hour minimum time interval between the administration of long-acting opioids and the initiation of remifentanil PCA, (2) reduction of the bolus dose maximum to 30 μg (ideal range 10 to 30 μg), and (3) use of a supplemental oxygen administration threshold of $Spo_2 < 94\%$.

To date, the studies of remifentanil administration for labor analgesia have included only healthy parturients with low-risk singleton pregnancies. Given the significant risk for maternal and neonatal sedation, respiratory depression, and oxygen desaturation with remifentanil PCA, the use of continuous pulse oximetry and continuous (or near continuous) one-to-one nursing care is critical for its safe use. An anesthesia provider should be notified if excess sedation, respiratory rate < 8 breaths/min, and/or oxygen saturation < 94%, despite supplemental oxygen, occurs.[60]

Comparison with other forms of labor analgesia. The efficacy of remifentanil PCA has been compared with that of other labor analgesic agents and regimens (Table 23.4).

TABLE 23.4 Trials Comparing Remifentanil Patient-Controlled Analgesia With Alternative Labor Analgesia With Analgesia as a Primary Outcome

Reference	Number of Subjects	Study Design	Groups; Drugs; Doses	Primary Data	Comments
Volikas and Male 2001[61]	17	Double-blinded, randomized	n = 8; Meperidine PCA 10-mg bolus, 5-min lockout n = 9; Remifentanil PCA 0.5-μg/kg bolus, 2-min lockout	VAPS hourly VAPS after delivery	Lower mean VAPS hourly with remifentanil (P = .0496) Lower mean VAPS after delivery with remifentanil (P = .03)
Thurlow et al. 2002[53]	36	Unblinded, randomized	n = 18; Meperidine 100 mg IM n = 18; Remifentanil PCA 20-μg bolus, 3-min lockout	VAPS at 1 h after analgesia Maximum VAPS at 2 h after analgesia	Lower VAPS with remifentanil at 1 h (48 mm versus 72 mm; P = .0004) Lower max VAPS with remifentanil during first 2 h (66.5 mm versus 82.5 mm; P = .009)
Blair et al. 2005[47]	39	Double-blinded, randomized	n = 19; Meperidine PCA 15-mg bolus, 10-min lockout n = 20; Remifentanil PCA 40-μg bolus, 2-min lockout	VAPS every 30 min VAPS "overall" at 2 h after delivery	Similar VAPS in labor and overall between groups (overall pain score 63.6 mm with remifentanil versus 68.6 mm with meperidine) (P = NS)
Evron et al. 2005[62]	88	Double-blinded, randomized	n = 45; Meperidine 75–200 mg IV n = 43; Remifentanil PCA increasing bolus dose in 5-μg increments (range 20–70 μg), 3-min lockout	VAPS at 1 h after analgesia VAPS at end of first stage of labor	Lower VAPS with remifentanil at 1 h (35.8 mm versus 58.8 mm, P < .001) Lower VAPS with remifentanil at end of first stage (32.6 mm versus 53.5 mm, P < .001)
Douma et al. 2010[24]	159	Double-blinded, randomized	n = 53; Meperidine PCA 49.5 mg load, 5-mg bolus, 10-min lockout n = 52; Remifentanil PCA 40-μg load, 40-μg bolus, 2-min lockout n = 54; Fentanyl PCA 50-μg load, 20-μg bolus, 5-min lockout	VAPS hourly	Greatest reduction in VAPS observed at 1 h in all three groups Greater reduction in VAPS at 1 h with remifentanil (3.2 cm), fentanyl (1.4 cm), and meperidine (0.8 cm) Similar VAPS among groups beyond first hour

(Continued)

TABLE 23.4 **Trials Comparing Remifentanil Patient-Controlled Analgesia With Alternative Labor Analgesia With Analgesia as a Primary Outcome—cont'd**

Reference	Number of Subjects	Study Design	Groups; Drugs; Doses	Primary Data	Comments
Ng et al. 2011[63]	68	Double-blind, randomized	n = 34; Meperidine 50 mg IM < 60 kg, 75 mg ≥ 60 kg n = 34; Remifentanil PCA 25-μg bolus < 60 kg, 30-μg bolus ≥ 60 kg, 3.75–4.5-min lockout	VAPS hourly	Lower mean VAPS with remifentanil (P = .001) Lowest VAPS with remifentanil at 2 h after analgesia (44% relative reduction from baseline)
Marwah et al. 2012[64]	98	Retrospective cohort	n = 47; Remifentanil PCA 0.25-μg/kg bolus, 2-min lockout and background infusion 0.025–0.05 μg/kg/min n = 51; Fentanyl PCA 20–50-μg bolus, 3–6-min lockout	Hourly verbal pain score scale 0–10	Mean pain score with remifentanil 4.1 (baseline 7.6) Mean pain score with fentanyl 4.9 (baseline 8.2)
Wilson et al. 2018[60]	401	Open-label multicenter randomized controlled trial	n = 201; Remifentanil PCA 40-μg bolus, 2-min lockout n = 199; Meperidine 100 mg IM q4h, maximum 400 mg/24 h	Request for epidural analgesia	41% requested epidural analgesia with meperidine versus 19% with remifentanil (RR, 0.48; 95% CI, 0.34 to 0.66; P < .0001)
Volmanen et al. 2005[65]	15	Double-blind, randomized, crossover	All participants had 20 min of 50% nitrous oxide or remifentanil PCA (0.4 μg/kg bolus, 1-min lockout) followed by 20-min washout period (no analgesia) then 20 min of the other analgesic. n = 9; Group 1 remifentanil then nitrous oxide n = 6; Group 2 nitrous oxide then remifentanil	Pain intensity difference (PID = mean pain score without analgesia minus mean pain score with analgesia)	Higher PID with remifentanil (1.5 versus 0.5, P = .01)
Volmanen et al. 2008[66]	45	Double-blind, randomized	n = 24; Remifentanil PCA 0.1–0.9-μg/kg bolus (0.1-μg/kg increments), 1-min lockout n = 21; Epidural 20 mL of levobupivacaine 0.625 mg/mL with fentanyl 2 μg/mL	Pain after each contraction (0–10)	Higher median pain scores with remifentanil (7.3 versus 5.2, P = .009)
Douma et al. 2011[67]	20	Randomized unblinded controlled	n = 10; Remifentanil PCA 40-μg load, 40-μg bolus, 2-min lockout n = 10; Epidural 0.2% ropivacaine 12.5-mL initial bolus, infusion 0.1% ropivacaine and sufentanil 0.5 μg/mL at 10 mL/h	VAPS hourly	Greater decrease in pain scores with epidural at all time intervals (n = 6 per group analyzed)
Stocki et al. 2014[52]	39	Randomized unblinded controlled noninferiority study	n = 19; Remifentanil PCA 20–60-μg bolus, 1–2-min lockout n = 20; PCEA 0.1% bupivacaine and fentanyl 2 μg/mL, 15-mL initial dose, 10-mL bolus, 20-min lockout, basal infusion 5 mL/h	Mean NRS pain scores assessed hourly	Mean NRS reduction at 30 min with remifentanil 4.5 versus 7.1 with PCEA, pain score at 30 min 3.7 with remifentanil versus 1.5 with PCEA

(Continued)

TABLE 23.4 Trials Comparing Remifentanil Patient-Controlled Analgesia With Alternative Labor Analgesia With Analgesia as a Primary Outcome—cont'd

Reference	Number of Subjects	Study Design	Groups; Drugs; Doses	Primary Data	Comments
Freeman et al. 2015[68]	1414	Multicenter randomized controlled equivalence trial	n = 447; Remifentanil PCA 20–40-µg bolus (initial 30-µg bolus), 3-min lockout n = 347; Epidural using various regimens: ropivacaine/sufentanil (37%), bupivacaine/sufentanil (46%), levobupivacaine/sufentanil (6%), and bupivacaine/fentanyl. No doses specified	Hourly satisfaction scores for pain relief	Area under the curve for satisfaction scores lower with remifentanil
Tveit et al. 2012[69]	37	Unblinded, randomized	n = 17; Remifentanil PCA 0.15–1.05-µg/kg bolus (0.15-µg/kg increments), 2-min lockout n = 20; Epidural ropivacaine 1 mg/mL with fentanyl 2 µg/mL. Loading dose 15 mL, then 10 mL/h infusion	VAPS every 15 min	Similar VAPS between groups at end of first stage and during second stage Similar maximum reduction in VAPS between groups

CI, Confidence interval; *IM*, intramuscular; *NRS*, numeric rating scale; *NS*, nonsignificant; *PCA*, patient-controlled analgesia; *PCEA*, patient-controlled epidural analgesia; *RR*, relative risk; *VAPS*, visual analog pain score.

Remifentanil versus fentanyl. Douma et al.[24] compared remifentanil PCA (loading dose 40 µg, bolus 40 µg, lockout interval 2 minutes), fentanyl PCA (loading dose 50 µg, bolus 20 µg, lockout interval 5 minutes), and meperidine PCA (loading dose 49.5 mg, bolus 5 mg, lockout interval 10 minutes) in 159 laboring patients. The decrease in pain scores was mild to moderate and similar in all groups, except after 1 hour of initiation, when the remifentanil group had better analgesia. Patients receiving meperidine had the highest crossover rate to epidural analgesia. Remifentanil PCA had greater sedation and pruritus than the other two groups. Compared with PCA meperidine, PCA remifentanil had more oxygen desaturation, but greater overall satisfaction. Neonatal outcomes were similar in all groups.

In a retrospective observation study, Marwah et al.[64] compared 98 laboring parturients who had received PCA fentanyl (bolus 25 to 50 µg, lockout interval 3 to 6 minutes) or PCA remifentanil (bolus 0.25 µg/kg, lockout interval 2 minutes, infusion 0.025 to 0.05 µg/kg/min). Decreases in pain scores were similar and moderate in both groups. Maternal sedation and desaturation were higher in the PCA remifentanil group, while the PCA fentanyl group had greater need for neonatal resuscitation (excluding confounders, 44% versus 8%; OR, 8.56; 95% CI, 2.17 to 33.77), and a greater percentage of neonates with 1-minute Apgar score < 7 (39% versus 18%; OR 2.83; 95% CI, 1.07 to 7.53). No neonate required naloxone and the umbilical cord gas measurements were similar between groups and within normal range.

Overall, remifentanil PCA offers similar or marginally better analgesia and satisfaction than fentanyl PCA, with significantly more maternal side effects of sedation, respiratory depression, and hypoxemia. Conversely, fentanyl PCA accumulates with repeated doses, especially after 2 hours duration,

and pharmacodynamically mimics an infusion. The advantage of such an accumulation diminishes the need to time the PCA bolus with contractions compared with remifentanil PCA. However, fentanyl accumulation has been shown to impact neonatal outcomes with an increased need for neonatal resuscitation and decreased Apgar scores at 1 minute. Thus, the choice of opioid PCA for each healthcare center should consider available labor resources for maternal monitoring and patient education, proximity of anesthesia providers to the labor and delivery ward, and in-house availability of specialized neonatal healthcare personnel, such as pediatricians.

Remifentanil versus meperidine. Thurlow et al.[53] conducted a randomized unblinded study in 36 patients that compared remifentanil PCA (bolus 20 µg, lockout interval 3 minutes) with IM meperidine 100 mg. The remifentanil group had lower pain scores (median maximum pain score 66/100 mm versus 82/100 mm, P = .009) within the first 2 hours of commencing analgesia. However, parturients in the remifentanil group also used nitrous oxide analgesia (56%) and experienced more sedation and episodes of oxygen saturation < 94%. No difference in Apgar scores was found.

Ng et al.[63] conducted a randomized, double-blind study in which 69 patients used a PCA device containing either remifentanil (PCA group) or 0.9% saline (meperidine group), and also received an IM injection of either saline (PCA group) or meperidine (meperidine group). The doses administered depended on patient weight; parturients < 60 or ≥ 60 kg were given a bolus dose of remifentanil of 25 or 30 µg, respectively. Similarly, the dose of meperidine was either 50 or 75 mg. The PCA lockout interval was 3.75 to 4.5 minutes with no background infusion. Maternal analgesia was greater (particularly in the first 2 hours after initiation), the median time to first rescue analgesic request was longer (8.0 versus 4.9 hours), and maternal satisfaction scores were higher in the remifentanil PCA group compared with the meperidine group. There was no difference between groups in maternal sedation, nausea, oxygen saturation, and neonatal outcomes.

Blair et al.[47] observed that the use of remifentanil PCA (bolus 40 μg, lockout interval 2 minutes) resulted in higher maternal satisfaction scores and modest analgesic benefit compared with meperidine PCA (bolus 15 mg, lockout interval 10 minutes).

In a systematic review of seven randomized controlled trials ($n = 349$), Leong et al.[70] evaluated the administration of remifentanil versus meperidine via a variety of drug delivery methods (e.g., PCA, continuous infusion, IM) for labor analgesia. The use of remifentanil reduced mean VAS pain scores by 25 mm more than meperidine in the first hour, and was associated with a conversion rate to epidural analgesia of less than 10%. Similarly, Schnabel et al.,[71] in a metaanalysis comparing PCA remifentanil, PCA meperidine, and epidural analgesia, reported that parturients who received remifentanil PCA had lower mean pain scores after 1 hour, a lower crossover rate to epidural analgesia, and higher satisfaction scores than those who received meperidine.

In the 2018 RESPITE study comparing IM meperidine with PCA remifentanil in 400 laboring parturients, 41% and 19% of parturients in the meperidine and remifentanil groups, respectively, requested epidural analgesia (RR 0.48; 95% CI, 0.34 to 0.66; $P < .0001$).[60] Parturients in the remifentanil group also had fewer operative vaginal deliveries, lower pain scores, and higher satisfaction compared with those in the meperidine group. A subsequent qualitative exploration study by the same authors interviewed 49 patients from the original RESPITE study.[72] Those who received PCA remifentanil reported feeling more effective analgesia, alert, and in control during their birth experience compared with the meperidine group. Side effects including nausea and cognitive effects were present in both groups. Overall, compared with meperidine, PCA remifentanil has been shown to provide better analgesia, less conversion to epidural analgesia, and higher maternal satisfaction.

Remifentanil versus nitrous oxide. Volmanen et al.[65] performed a double-blind crossover trial that compared remifentanil (bolus 0.4 μg/kg, lockout interval 1 minute) with 50% nitrous oxide during the first stage of labor. The 20 patients used both analgesics in a random order for 20 minutes, with an intervening washout period of 20 minutes. Pain relief (although modest), maternal sedation, and patient satisfaction were greater in the remifentanil group. No difference in the incidence of FHR changes was observed between the two groups.

Remifentanil versus epidural analgesia. A large metaanalysis found that PCA fentanyl and remifentanil provided inferior labor analgesia at 30, 60, 120, and 180 minutes, and greater sedation, nausea, and vomiting compared with various epidural techniques; the analgesia curves further diverged as labor progressed.[73] A Cochrane review concluded that PCA remifentanil compared with epidural analgesia was associated with less maternal satisfaction (seven trials) and

higher pain intensity (four trials) and no differences in delivery mode (nine trials) or assisted birth (eight trials).[74] Two additional metaanalyses concluded that PCA remifentanil provides inferior labor analgesia (mean difference in effect size 3.0 cm/10 cm [95% CI, 0.7 to 5.2] at 2 hours) and satisfaction compared with epidural analgesia.[71,75]

In a randomized, double-blind trial, Volmanen et al.[66] compared PCA remifentanil (mean effective bolus 0.5 [range 0.3 to 0.7] μg/kg, lockout interval 1 minute) with lumbar epidural analgesia (20-mL levobupivacaine 0.0625% with fentanyl 2 μg/mL). All patients received an epidural technique and PCA remifentanil or saline. Parturients receiving epidural analgesia had a more significant and rapid reduction in pain scores than those receiving remifentanil (10 versus 40 minutes to reach the individual effective dose), but median "pain relief" scores were similar between the two groups. The investigators postulated that high maternal satisfaction with PCA remifentanil may be the result of factors other than the degree of analgesia produced.

Stocki et al.[52] conducted an unblinded controlled noninferiority study in 39 healthy parturients randomized to receive PCA remifentanil (titrated from 20 to 60 μg, lockout interval 1 to 2 minutes), or PCEA (0.1% bupivacaine with 2 μg/mL fentanyl). Analgesia with remifentanil was inferior to the epidural technique at all time points, but maternal satisfaction was similar. All apnea events occurred in the patients receiving remifentanil, who also had lower mean respiratory rates and oxygen saturation. In a multicenter trial of 1414 parturients randomized to receive PCA remifentanil or epidural analgesia, Freeman et al.[68] found higher satisfaction and analgesia in parturients who received epidural analgesia.

Morphine

Morphine is rarely administered by PCA for labor analgesia except for parturients with intrauterine fetal demise.[37] The accumulation of the active metabolite morphine-6-glucuronide, which is a potent respiratory depressant, is a concern in parturients with a live fetus. No studies have compared the analgesic efficacy of morphine administered by PCA versus intermittent bolus administration during labor.

OPIOID ANTAGONISTS

Naloxone is a pure opioid antagonist at the μ-, κ-, and δ-opioid receptors, although it has the greatest affinity for the μ-opioid receptor.[5,20] It is the drug of choice to treat adverse opioid effects in both the mother and the newborn, and it may be given IV, SC, or IM. The onset of action after an IV dose (1 to 4 μg/kg) is 2 minutes, with duration of action 30 to 40 minutes; this duration may be less than that of the opioid whose action it antagonizes, and repeated doses or an infusion may be necessary. The administration of naloxone during labor or before delivery may reverse the quality of maternal analgesia and confer only a limited reduction in maternal side effects.

Naloxone was previously administered to neonates with diminished respiratory drive who had been exposed to maternal opioids prior to delivery.[76] Although a metaanalysis indicated that naloxone increased alveolar ventilation in the 6 hours after birth, there is insufficient evidence to determine the safety or efficacy of administering naloxone to neonates in this setting. Current guidelines recommend that all neonates with apnea or decreased respiratory drive be managed with appropriate respiratory support, regardless of prior *in utero* opioid exposure.[77] Naloxone should not be given to the neonate of a mother who is opioid-dependent or on methadone maintenance therapy, as this action may provoke withdrawal activity and seizures.

OPIOID ADJUNCTS AND SEDATIVES

Historically, although many drugs have been used as adjuncts to parenteral opioid analgesia, most are now infrequently used owing to their association with maternal sedation and neonatal depression and more safe and effective neuraxial and PCA opioid technique options.

Barbiturates are sedative agents with no analgesic effect. They are lipid soluble, rapidly cross the placenta, are detectable in fetal blood, and can result in neonatal depression, especially if combined with systemic opioid administration.

Phenothiazines (e.g., chlorpromazine, promethazine, propiomazine) are dopamine antagonists that have sedative, antiemetic, and antipsychotic properties. They rapidly cross the placenta and reduce FHR variability. Neurobehavioral outcomes after the maternal administration of these agents have not been studied carefully, but there is no evidence that they cause neonatal respiratory depression. Phenothiazines (particularly chlorpromazine) may cause hypotension from alpha-adrenergic receptor blockade, and they may produce unwanted extrapyramidal movements.[20] Parenterally administered promethazine (25 to 50 mg) has an onset of 15 minutes and a duration of action of up to 20 hours; it rapidly crosses the placenta, resulting in detectable fetal levels within 1 to 2 minutes of maternal IV administration.[20] Propiomazine is a mild respiratory depressant that may further depress maternal ventilation when coadministered with opioids. It has a faster onset and shorter duration of action than promethazine.

Metoclopramide is a procainamide derivative that can increase gastric motility and reduce nausea and vomiting. As an antagonist at central dopamine receptors, it can also cause drowsiness.[20] After meperidine administration for labor analgesia, Vella et al.[78] found metoclopramide as effective as promethazine for reducing the incidence of nausea and vomiting. Reduced pain scores and nitrous oxide use were observed in those who received metoclopramide compared with those who received promethazine or placebo; this may reflect either an antianalgesic effect of promethazine or a possible analgesic effect of metoclopramide.

Benzodiazepines (e.g., diazepam, lorazepam, midazolam) have been used for sedation in labor but are associated with significant side effects. **Diazepam** rapidly crosses the placenta and accumulates in the fetus at concentrations that may exceed maternal concentrations. The elimination half-life of the parent drug is 24 to 48 hours, but active metabolites may persist for up to 120 hours. Diazepam may cause maternal and neonatal respiratory depression, as well as neonatal hypotonia, impaired thermoregulation, and an abnormal stress response. These effects may be dose related. **Lorazepam** has a half-life of 12 hours and is metabolized to an inactive glucuronide. McAuley et al.[79] gave lorazepam 2 mg or placebo prior to the IM administration of meperidine 100 mg for labor analgesia. Analgesia was better in the lorazepam group, but lorazepam administration was associated with a nonsignificant increase in neonatal respiratory depression. Neonatal neurobehavioral scores were similar in the two groups. Amnesia was common with lorazepam.

Midazolam has a rapid onset of action and an elimination half-life of 1 to 4 hours.[20] It is metabolized in the liver to one major and several minor pharmacologically active compounds, which may persist in patients with critical illnesses accompanied by hepatic and/or renal impairment. Midazolam readily crosses the placenta and when used at high doses (e.g., induction of general anesthesia) can result in neonatal hypotonia. Midazolam causes potent anterograde amnesia, a characteristic that may be undesirable for the childbirth experience.

Ketamine is a phencyclidine derivative that acts as a noncompetitive antagonist at the *N*-methyl-D-aspartate (NMDA) receptor and, at high doses, as an agonist at μ-opioid receptors. Most commonly given by IV or IM injection, ketamine in small doses (0.2 to 0.5 mg/kg IV) can provide dissociative analgesia, whereas larger doses (1 to 2 mg/kg IV, 5 to 10 mg/kg IM) can be used to induce general anesthesia.

When given intravenously, ketamine has an onset within 30 seconds and a duration of action of 5 to 10 minutes; intramuscular administration has an onset of 2 to 8 minutes with a duration of 10 to 20 minutes.[20] Ketamine is hepatically metabolized to active metabolites, which are excreted in the urine.

Ketamine's sympathomimetic properties cause an increase in heart rate, systolic pressure, and cardiac output, which should be avoided in patients with preeclampsia or hypertension. Joselyn et al.[80] reported acceptable labor analgesia with an IV infusion of ketamine (bolus 0.1 mg/kg with an infusion of 0.2 mg/kg/h, titrated to effect). The average infusion rate was 0.17 mg/kg/h, yielding an average total dose of 57 mg (range 18 to 160 mg). No unpleasant hallucinations were experienced; however, with the initial dose, emesis and transient lightheadedness and nystagmus occurred. All neonates had a 5-minute Apgar score of 9 or 10.

Ketamine may also provide effective analgesia just before vaginal delivery in parturients without neuraxial anesthesia, or it may be used as an adjunctive agent in parturients with unsatisfactory neuraxial analgesia/anesthesia. Using incremental doses of IV ketamine (0.2 to 0.4 mg/kg, up to a maximum dose of 100 mg) immediately before delivery, Akamatsu et al.[81] reported that 78 of 80 parturients experienced complete analgesia with no adverse maternal or neonatal effects. The occurrence of amnesia and a dreamlike state was high, but only one woman found this unpleasant.

Administration of small doses of ketamine (10- to 20-mg doses, repeated at intervals of 2 to 5 minutes, while not exceeding a total dose of 1 mg/kg during a 30-minute period) is associated with a low incidence of hallucinations; however, amnesia is common. In these settings, the anesthesia provider must maintain continual verbal contact with the patient and must ensure that the patient remains sufficiently awake to maintain adequate ventilation and protect their airway.

Dexmedetomidine is a highly specific and selective alpha-2 adrenergic receptor agonist that has been increasingly used in obstetric anesthesia.[82] It produces dose-dependent sedation, anxiolysis, and analgesia, with minimal respiratory depression, and suppression of the stress response to surgery. After IV administration, dexmedetomidine exhibits a rapid distribution phase with a half-life of 6 minutes, a terminal elimination half-life of 2 hours,[83] and low maternal-to-fetal transfer.[84] In 20 parturients undergoing cesarean delivery under epidural anesthesia with dexmedetomidine sedation, the umbilical vein-to-maternal vein concentration ratio was 0.68.[85] Following cord clamping, administration of a dexmedetomidine infusion at 0.6 μg/kg/h led to negligible amounts in breastmilk.[86] In the nonobstetric population, preprocedural and procedural sedation is provided by a loading dose of 1 μg/kg over 10 to 20 minutes followed by an infusion at 0.2 to 0.7 μg/kg/h.[83] Doses of 10 to 30 μg alleviate shivering during cesarean delivery.[87]

Two case reports described the use of dexmedetomidine for intrapartum analgesia.[88,89] Dexmedetomidine provided successful labor analgesia in a patient with preeclampsia, with limited changes in maternal blood pressure, but pain scores of 2 to 3/10 for the 3 hours of the infusion[88]; although cesarean delivery under general anesthesia was necessary because of persistent late FHR decelerations, the neonate was lively with high Apgar scores. In the second case, a dexmedetomidine infusion significantly improved labor analgesia, with easily rousable sedation, when used as an adjunct to unsatisfactory PCA fentanyl in a parturient with spina bifida occulta and a tethered spinal cord reaching L5 to S1.[89] There were no maternal or fetal hemodynamic changes. The dexmedetomidine infusion was continued during cesarean delivery under general anesthesia and a healthy baby with normal Apgar scores was delivered. A randomized controlled trial of 60 women reported that when a dexmedetomidine infusion was added to remifentanil PCA, total remifentanil consumption was 53.3% lower and there were fewer instances of oxygen desaturation compared with remifentanil PCA alone.[90]

INHALATIONAL ANALGESIA

Although the use of inhalational analgesia for labor analgesia varies by country, only nitrous oxide has achieved wide clinical use.

Nitrous Oxide

Globally, nitrous oxide (N_2O) is the most common inhalational agent used for labor analgesia.[91] It was introduced in the late 1800s and further popularized when equipment for self-administration was introduced by Minnitt in England in 1934. Typically it is administered as 50% nitrous oxide in oxygen using a blender device (e.g., Nitronox in the United States and Canada) or premixed in a single cylinder (e.g., Entonox in the United Kingdom); when provided alone or in combination with other forms of analgesia, the incidence of its use during labor ranges from 1% (or less) in the United States to over 50% in many parts of Europe, Scandinavia, and the United Kingdom. The National Institute for Health and Care Excellence in the United Kingdom recommends that Entonox should be available in all birth settings.[92]

A tasteless and odorless gas that is nonirritating to the airway, nitrous oxide is a weak anesthetic agent with a minimum alveolar concentration (MAC) > 100% at 1 atmosphere. Although incompletely understood, the mechanism of action of nitrous oxide involves supraspinal NMDA receptor antagonism, the release of corticotropin-releasing factor, stimulation of opioid and noradrenergic supraspinal receptors, and the inhibition GABAergic supraspinal interneurons leading to disinhibition of spinal adrenergic and GABAergic neurons.[93,94] Because of its low blood/gas solubility, nitrous oxide has a very rapid onset and offset, reaches peak brain concentration within 60 seconds in laboring patients, and undergoes minimal metabolism.[95]

Nitrous oxide does not interfere with uterine activity, but it readily crosses the placenta, and a fetal-to-maternal concentration ratio of 0.8 occurs within 15 minutes; however, no apparent detrimental effects on FHR, Apgar scores, or umbilical cord blood gas measurements have been reported.[93] Even when used immediately prior to delivery, there is no evidence that nitrous oxide causes neonatal respiratory depression or altered neurobehavioral scores. The neonate rapidly eliminates nitrous oxide by respiration, resulting in a half-life of less than 3 minutes.[93]

A systematic review of 12 randomized controlled trials concluded that nitrous oxide is not a potent labor analgesic, with less effectiveness than epidural analgesia, but confers benefit and high levels of satisfaction for some.[96] Similarly, Zuarez-Easton et al.[16] demonstrated in a randomized trial that although meperidine and nitrous oxide had similar, but limited efficacy for providing labor analgesia, maternal satisfaction and desire for subsequent labor use was substantial with nitrous oxide. Richardson et al.[97] observed that patients who received nitrous oxide alone for labor and vaginal delivery were as likely to express satisfaction with their anesthesia care as patients who received neuraxial analgesia, despite being less likely to report excellent analgesia. Further, among all laboring patients who experienced poor analgesia effectiveness, those who used nitrous oxide alone were more likely to report high satisfaction than patients who received epidural analgesia alone (OR 2.5; 95% CI, 1.4 to 4.5; $P = .002$). The authors concluded that analgesia quality is not the only contributor to maternal satisfaction.

Although a low incidence of serious adverse events (3 per 10,000 administrations of 50% nitrous oxide in oxygen) has been reported, suitable equipment must be available to ensure safe administration. An apparatus that limits the concentration of nitrous oxide (e.g., a nitrous oxide/oxygen blender or a premixed 1:1 cylinder) is required and should be checked periodically for correct delivery concentration. Inhalation should occur through a mask or mouthpiece containing a one-way demand valve, which opens only when negative inspiratory pressure is applied, to limit gas delivery in a drowsy patient and pollution from unscavenged gases.[98]

Environmental pollution from unscavenged gases may be significant, and it remains unclear whether regular occupational exposure to subanesthetic concentrations of nitrous oxide results in significant health risks for healthcare workers. Overall, epidemiologic data do not suggest the presence of higher reproductive risks in healthcare workers exposed to nitrous oxide in the work environment (see Chapters 16 and 18). Established emission factors and lifecycle assessments were used to calculate carbon dioxide equivalents (CO_2e) related to drug manufacture, disposables packaging, administration pump electricity use, and unmetabolized gas emissions.[93] Inhalation of Entonox was associated with the highest carbon emissions at 237.33 kgCO_2e. Epidural analgesia and remifentanil PCA produce significantly less carbon emissions, with 1.2 kgCO_2e and 0.75 kgCO_2e, respectively. Coming practice recommendations will include environmental impact in the rationale for preference of neuraxial and intravenous analgesia techniques over nitrous oxide.[99]

Although nitrous oxide has limited effects on cardiovascular and ventilatory drive, it can depress ventilation through a reduction in tidal volume; this effect is partially compensated by an increase in respiratory rate. Hyperventilation with associated hypocapnia during uterine contractions, rather than diffusion hypoxemia, may be the cause of occasional oxygen desaturation.[100] It is unclear whether the incidence of intrapartum maternal hypoxemia differs among those who use nitrous oxide compared with those who receive no analgesia during labor. However, the risk for maternal hypoxemia with nitrous oxide may be more common with the concomitant administration of opioids or other sedatives; the entire obstetric care team should be aware of this possibility.

The most common maternal side effects of nitrous oxide are nausea and vomiting (occurring in up to 33% of parturients), drowsiness, dizziness, and the presence of paresthesias, which may be related to maternal hyperventilation during contractions.[93] In a systematic review of 29 studies by Likis et al.,[96] nausea was reported to occur at rates up to 45% and dizziness up to 23%.

Significant adverse effects on the neonate have not been reported. Umbilical cord blood gas measurements and neonatal Apgar scores when parturients used nitrous oxide were not different compared with those when parturients used other forms of labor pain relief or no analgesia.[96] However, neuroapoptosis in rodents exposed to large doses of nitrous oxide (and other anesthetic agents) at specific growth time points of the developing brain indicates the need for further clinical and research studies.[101]

Volatile Halogenated Agents

While several studies have examined the use of volatile anesthetic agents for labor analgesia, most required special breathing equipment, did not address the issue of unscavenged gases, and were unable to demonstrate a meaningful clinical application in modern labor analgesia. Moreover, all volatile halogenated agents cause dose-dependent relaxation of uterine smooth muscle; when uterine tone is desirable, volatile anesthetic concentrations > 0.5 MAC are not recommended.

Enflurane and Isoflurane

Abboud et al.[102] compared the analgesic effects of 0.25% to 1.25% enflurane with the administration of 30% to 60% nitrous oxide, both given in oxygen during the second stage of labor in 105 parturients. Satisfactory pain relief was reported in approximately 89% and 76% of parturients in the enflurane and nitrous oxide groups, respectively. There were no differences observed in maternal blood loss, Apgar scores, or umbilical cord blood gas measurements.

McLeod et al.[103] observed improved labor analgesia with the self-administration of 0.75% isoflurane in oxygen compared with Entonox. Subsequent studies observed satisfactory pain relief with minimal levels of drowsiness with various concentrations of an isoflurane-Entonox mixture. In 221 parturients in whom Entonox provided inadequate analgesia, Ross et al.[104] observed that 75% continued for more than 1 hour with a 0.25% isoflurane-Entonox premixture. No mother experienced significant sedation or loss of consciousness, and there was no adverse effect on Apgar scores, neonatal respiratory status, or maternal blood loss.

Desflurane

Because of its low blood-gas partition coefficient, desflurane has a rapid onset and offset; however, the notable airway irritation and amnesia (23%) make it a less attractive option for inhalation analgesia. Abboud et al.[105] compared inhalation of 1% to 4.5% desflurane versus 30% to 60% nitrous oxide, both in oxygen, and found similar analgesia scores and neonatal outcomes between groups.

Sevoflurane

With a short onset and offset of action, sevoflurane causes less airway irritation and has a less unpleasant odor than the other volatile agents. Toscano et al.[106] conducted a safety and feasibility pilot study of 50 parturients breathing 2% to 3% sevoflurane in an oxygen/air mixture via a compact anesthesia delivery system. Using an end-tidal sevoflurane goal of 1.2% to 1.4% (0.8 to 0.9 MAC during pregnancy) at the peak of uterine contractions, pain scores were lower with sevoflurane than without sevoflurane (mean 3.3 [SD 1.5] versus 8.7 [1.0], respectively, on a scale of 0 to 10). No episodes of desaturation, loss of consciousness, or adverse effects on FHR or neonatal Apgar scores were reported.

In an escalating dose study, Yeo et al.[107] determined that 0.8% sevoflurane was the optimal concentration for labor analgesia, beyond which an increased level of sedation with no additional analgesic benefit was observed. Ng et al.[108] randomized 48 primigravid parturients to receive either 0.8% sevoflurane (via an inhaler attached to wall gas supply) or Entonox. No significant difference in median pain scores or adverse effects were observed.

NONNEURAXIAL REGIONAL ANALGESIA

Alternative regional analgesic techniques for labor and vaginal delivery are less frequently used in centers with high rates of neuraxial analgesia use. Nonetheless, many parturients have contraindications, limited access to, or no desire for neuraxial analgesia.

Paracervical Block

During the first stage of labor, pain results primarily from dilation of the cervix and distention of the lower uterine segment and upper vagina. Although now used infrequently, obstetric providers can provide first-stage labor analgesia by performing a paracervical block to diminish transmission through the paracervical ganglion—also known as the *Frankenhäuser ganglion*—which lies immediately lateral and posterior to the cervicouterine junction.

Paracervical block does not adversely affect the progress of labor, the function of peripheral sensory or motor nerves, or the somatic sensory fibers from the lower vagina, vulva, and perineum. Satisfactory analgesia is achieved during the first stage of labor in 50% to 75% of parturients, with lower success in multiparous patients who may experience sudden and rapid descent of the fetal presenting part.[109] Junttila et al.[110] reported on 104 multiparous laboring women who were randomized to receive paracervical block using bupivacaine or single-shot spinal anesthesia using bupivacaine/sufentanil; women who received a paracervical block had a smaller decrease in pain scores, but 43% achieved a pain score ≤ 3/10 and 51% indicated willingness to receive this method of labor analgesia in a future pregnancy.

Technique

A paracervical block is performed with the patient in a modified lithotomy position with the uterus displaced leftward. A needle guide is used to define and limit the depth of the injection and to reduce the risk for vaginal or fetal injury. The needle and needle guide are introduced into the vaginal fornix with the left hand for the left side of the pelvis, and vice versa for the right side, at the 4-o'clock or the 8-o'clock positions (Fig. 23.1). The needle is advanced through the vaginal mucosa to a depth of 2 to 3 mm, with a total of 5 to 10 mL of local anesthetic, without epinephrine (adrenaline), injected on each side; as direct fetal part injection may inadvertently occur, the FHR should be observed for 5 to 10 minutes after each injection.[111]

Choice of Local Anesthetic

The paracervical block requires small volumes of a dilute solution of local anesthetic. There is no indication for more than 10 mL of local anesthetic on each side or the use of concentrated solutions such as 2% lidocaine (lignocaine), 0.5% bupivacaine, or 3% 2-chloroprocaine. Nieminenm and Puolakka[112] observed that a paracervical block with 10 mL of 0.125% bupivacaine versus 0.25% bupivacaine provided similar analgesia. Bupivacaine has greater cardiotoxicity than other local anesthetic agents, and some investigators have observed a higher incidence of fetal bradycardia or perinatal death with this agent used for paracervical blockade.[113]

The rapid enzymatic hydrolysis of 2-chloroprocaine yields the shortest intravascular half-life among clinically available local anesthetics, which may be advantageous if an

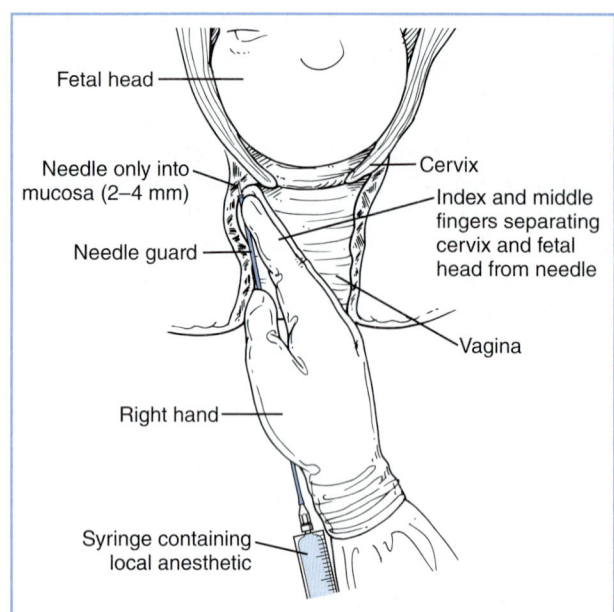

Fig. 23.1 Technique of Paracervical Block. Notice the position of the hand and fingers in relation to the cervix and fetal head. No undue pressure is applied at the vaginal fornix by the fingers or the needle guide, and the needle is inserted to a shallow depth. Redrawn from Abouleish E. *Pain Control in Obstetrics.* JB Lippincott; 1977:344.

BOX 23.1 Maternal Complications of Paracervical Block

- Vasovagal syncope
- Laceration of the vaginal mucosa
- Local anesthetic systemic toxicity
- Parametrial hematoma
- Postpartum neuropathy
- Paracervical, retropsoal, or subgluteal abscess

---

unintentional intravascular or fetal injection occurs. Philipson et al.[114] performed a paracervical block with 10 mL of 1% 2-chloroprocaine in 16 healthy parturients, and detected only trace concentrations of 2-chloroprocaine at delivery in 1 (6%) maternal and 4 (25%) umbilical cord venous blood samples.

Maternal Complications

Maternal complications of paracervical block are uncommon but potentially serious, including local anesthetic systemic toxicity, postpartum neuropathy, and infection (Box 23.1).[115,116]

Fetal Complications

Direct fetal scalp injection of 10 to 20 mL of local anesthetic during paracervical block can cause local anesthetic toxicity and fetal death[117]; fetal scalp injection appears more likely in the presence of an uncomfortable parturient with advanced (i.e., greater than 8 cm) cervical dilation.

The most common fetal complication after injection of local anesthetic is fetal bradycardia, which typically develops within 2 to 10 minutes and resolves within 5 to 10 minutes, but can persist for as long as 30 minutes. In a review of four randomized controlled trials published between 1975 and 2000, Rosen[118] reported that the incidence of postparacervical block fetal bradycardia was 15%. Volmanen et al.[119] reviewed four reasonably sized studies of paracervical block ($n > 200$), using a superficial injection technique with 0.125% or 0.25% bupivacaine. Among the 1361 patients in these studies, the incidence of fetal bradycardia was 2.2%, with most being transient and not requiring emergency cesarean delivery.[119]

The etiology of fetal bradycardia after paracervical block is unclear. Manipulation of the fetal head, uterus, or uterine blood vessels during performance of the block may cause reflex fetal bradycardia. Investigators have also speculated that the FHR changes result from rapid transplacental passage of local anesthetic into the fetal circulation, with subsequent effects on the fetal heart or FHR regulatory centers, or direct injection of local anesthetic into the fetal head or uterine blood vessels.[120-122] However, fetal bradycardia has not consistently occurred in documented cases of fetal local anesthetic toxicity. Freeman et al.[123] injected mepivacaine 300 mg directly into the scalp of two anencephalic fetuses. The QRS complex widened and the PR interval lengthened in the fetal electrocardiogram (ECG), and both fetuses died, but fetal bradycardia did not occur before fetal death. In contrast, the investigators observed no widening of the QRS complex or lengthening of the PR interval in normal fetuses demonstrating bradycardia after paracervical block. Rather, the fetal ECG changes were consistent with sinoatrial node suppression with a wandering atrial pacemaker. The investigators suggested that a mechanism other than direct fetal myocardial depression is responsible for fetal bradycardia after a paracervical block.

Myometrial injection of local anesthetic also may cause greater uterine activity. Following a paracervical block with either lidocaine or 2-chloroprocaine in pregnant baboons with normal and acidotic fetuses, Morishima et al.[124] observed a transient increase in uterine activity and a reduction in uterine blood flow in 73% of the mothers. Approximately 33% of the normal fetuses and all the acidotic fetuses had bradycardia after paracervical block. This suggests that a paracervical block should be avoided in the presence of fetal compromise.

Uterine and/or umbilical artery vasoconstriction. The deposition of local anesthetic in close proximity to the uterine arteries may alter perfusion.[125] Manninen et al.[126] observed that a paracervical injection of 10 mL of 0.25% bupivacaine led to an increase in the uterine artery pulsatility index—an estimate of uterine vascular resistance—in healthy nulliparous patients, suggesting that a paracervical block may result in uterine artery vasoconstriction.

In contrast, Puolakka et al.,[120] using a xenon isotope in 10 parturients, observed no decrease in mean intervillous blood flow before and after a paracervical block with 10 mL of 0.25% bupivacaine. Using Doppler ultrasonography in 12 healthy parturients, Räsänen and Jouppila[127] observed no significant change in either uterine or umbilical artery pulsatility index after a paracervical block with 10 mL of 0.25% bupivacaine.

Regardless of the etiology, the severity and duration of fetal bradycardia correlate with the incidence of fetal acidosis and subsequent neonatal depression.

Recommendations

A paracervical block may be an appropriate technique in circumstances in which neuraxial analgesia is contraindicated or unavailable. The following recommendations seem reasonable:

1. Perform a paracervical block only in healthy parturients at term who have no evidence of uteroplacental insufficiency or fetal compromise.
2. Continuously monitor the FHR and uterine activity before, during, and after performance of a paracervical block. Perform a paracervical block only in patients with a reassuring FHR tracing. An exception would be a patient whose fetus has an anomaly incompatible with life (e.g., anencephaly).
3. Do not perform a paracervical block when the cervix is dilated 8 cm or more.
4. Establish intravenous access before performing a paracervical block.
5. Maintain left uterine displacement during and after performance of the block.
6. Limit the depth of injection to approximately 3 mm.
7. Aspirate before each injection of local anesthetic.
8. Administer small volumes of a dilute solution of local anesthetic; 2-chloroprocaine is the agent of choice.
9. After injecting the local anesthetic on one side, wait 5 to 10 minutes and observe the FHR before injecting the local anesthetic on the other side.
10. Avoid the administration of epinephrine-containing local anesthetic solutions.
11. Monitor the mother's blood pressure and watch for signs of local anesthetic systemic toxicity. Maintain normal maternal blood pressure.
12. If fetal bradycardia should occur, try to achieve fetal resuscitation *in utero*. Discontinue oxytocin and ensure that the patient is on her left side. Perform operative delivery if the fetal bradycardia persists beyond 10 minutes.

Lumbar Sympathetic Block

Paravertebral lumbar sympathetic block interrupts the transmission of pain impulses from the cervix and lower uterine segment to provide analgesia for the first stage of labor. The lumbar sympathetic trunk is located anterolaterally from L1 to L4, with the densest portion of the ganglia being located at L2 and L3, which is where the block is commonly performed.[128] First-stage labor analgesia from a lumbar sympathetic block lasts an average of 4.5 hours, which is comparable to that provided by paracervical block but with less risk for fetal bradycardia[129]; both blocks require additional analgesia for delivery. Compared with epidural analgesia, a lumbar sympathetic block is technically more difficult and painful.

A lumbar sympathetic block may have a favorable effect on the progress of labor. Leighton et al.[130] randomized 36 nulliparous term laboring parturients to receive lumbar sympathetic block or epidural analgesia and found that women who received a lumbar sympathetic block had more rapid cervical dilation in the first 2 hours and a shorter second stage of labor.

Similar to neuraxial analgesia, coagulopathy is a contraindication to a lumbar sympathetic block, given the proximity of the neuraxis and the needle depth required.[128] A lumbar sympathetic block may be an alternative when a history of previous back surgery precludes the administration of epidural analgesia, or for women who desire first-stage analgesia without any motor block or loss of perineal sensation.

Maternal complications are uncommon and include hypotension,[130] local anesthetic systemic toxicity, total spinal anesthesia, retroperitoneal hematoma, Horner's syndrome,[131] and post–dural puncture headache.[132] Fetal complications are unlikely unless hypotension or increased uterine activity results in decreased uteroplacental perfusion.

During the past four decades, the lumbar sympathetic block has all but disappeared from obstetric anesthesia practice in North America for several reasons. Most anesthesia providers minimize motor block during epidural analgesia by giving dilute solutions of local anesthetic with an opioid. For those patients who especially want to retain full perineal sensation, anesthesia providers may use an opioid-only epidural or spinal technique. Thus, there are few patients for whom a lumbar sympathetic block holds unique advantages. Further, the procedure often is painful, and few obstetric anesthesia providers have acquired and maintained the required proficiency.

Paravertebral block

A paravertebral block is most commonly performed with ultrasonographic guidance to provide analgesia for video-assisted thoracoscopy and anesthesia and analgesia for breast surgery.[133,134] Anterolaterally the paravertebral space is bound by the parietal pleura, and by the costotransverse ligament posteriorly, and contains the intercostal nerve, the dorsal rami, the intercostal vessels, and the sympathetic chain. A paravertebral injection may remain localized to the space injected, or it may spread caudally and rostrally, to the intercostal space laterally, the epidural space medially, or with a combination of spread.[135]

Varying degrees of epidural spread have been shown in up to 70% of patients. Although needle placement differs from the lumbar sympathetic block, a common side effect of paravertebral block includes a sympathetic block. Contraindications include coagulopathy because of the proximity to the neuraxis and the needle depth required to perform the block. Complications include vascular puncture, hypotension, pleural puncture, and pneumothorax.[135]

Nair and Henry[136] described the use of a paravertebral block for labor analgesia. Initially, all four levels from T10 to L1 bilaterally were injected, then subsequently single-shot bilateral blocks at T11, or both T11 and T12 were used to provide effective analgesia for the first stage of labor with stable hemodynamics and a duration of 3 to 4 hours. A paravertebral block may be an alternative in selected patients when medical contraindications or resource constraints preclude the use of epidural analgesia.

Erector Spinae Plane Block

The erector spinae plane (ESP) block was first described for the treatment of neuropathic chest pain. Injected local anesthetic spreads to the paravertebral and epidural spaces in both cranial and caudal directions, thereby potentially producing both somatic and visceral analgesia in multiple segments.[137] Current evidence for ESP blocks in labor analgesia is limited to case reports. Vilchis Rentería et al.[138] reported four cases in which they administered ESP for labor analgesia. Using bilateral single-shot options and unilateral catheter techniques with large volumes of a concentrated solution of local anesthetic at the L4 transverse process, a modest decrease in pain scores was achieved. Yasar and Uysal reported the use of ESP block in three laboring patients who did not wish to have epidural analgesia. The blocks were performed under ultrasound guidance at the level of the T11 transverse process using bilateral injection of 10-mL bupivacaine 0.25%, followed by catheter insertion. Pain scores decreased in the first stage of labor for all patients, but analgesia was not effective in the second stage of labor.[139]

Quadratus Lumborum Block

A quadratus lumborum block (QLB) can provide the dermatomal coverage (T4 to L2) necessary for first-stage labor analgesia. There are three variations based on needle tip orientation during injection: anterior, lateral, and posterior. Unlike transversus abdominal plane (TAP) block, QLB provides somatic and visceral analgesia, likely because of spread to the paravertebral space.[140] In obstetric patients, QLB mostly has been described for postoperative analgesia when the use of long-acting neuraxial opioids is not possible. However, de Haan et al.[141] described the use of ultrasound-guided bilateral posterior QLB using bupivacaine 0.5% to provide labor analgesia in a patient with Hemophilia A who declined neuraxial analgesia. The patient had complete relief of contraction pain, although she reported postpartum that she had experienced perineal pain during the second stage of labor.

Pudendal Nerve Block

During the second stage of labor, pain results from distention of the lower vagina, vulva, and perineum. The pudendal nerve, which includes somatic nerve fibers from the anterior primary divisions of the second, third, and fourth sacral nerves, represents the primary source of sensory innervation to this area, as well as motor innervation to the perineal muscles and to the external anal sphincter.

The pudendal nerve block became popular for labor analgesia when Klink[142] and Kohl[143] described the anatomy and reported modified techniques in the 1950s. The objective is to block the pudendal nerve distal to its formation by the anterior divisions of S2 to S4 but proximal to its division into its terminal branches (i.e., dorsal nerve of the clitoris, perineal nerve, and inferior hemorrhoidal nerve). While able to provide satisfactory anesthesia for spontaneous vaginal delivery and perhaps for outlet-forceps delivery, the pudendal nerve block provides inadequate anesthesia for mid-forceps delivery, postpartum examination and repair of the upper vagina and cervix, and manual exploration of the uterine cavity.[144]

Efficacy and Timing

The efficacy of pudendal nerve block varies according to obstetric training and experience, with bilateral success rates of approximately 50% and 25% using the transvaginal and transperineal routes, respectively.[145]

The pudendal nerve block is typically provided upon patient request at the onset of the second stage of labor or immediately before delivery. There are few data about the effect of the timing of the pudendal nerve block on the duration of the second stage of labor. The pudendal nerve block has demonstrated less reliability for second-stage labor analgesia, greater efficacy for episiotomy and repair,[146] and, when performed with a nerve stimulator-guided deposition with ropivacaine, less discomfort or need for supplemental analgesia for the first 48 hours following a vaginal delivery and episiotomy repair.[147]

Technique

The transvaginal approach uses a needle guide (i.e., Iowa trumpet or Kobak needle guide) to prevent injury to the vagina and fetus. In contrast to the paracervical block technique, the needle must protrude 1.0 to 1.5 cm beyond the needle guide to allow adequate penetration for local anesthetic injection. The obstetric provider introduces the needle and needle guide into the vagina with the left hand for the left side of the pelvis and vice versa for the right side (Fig. 23.2). The needle is introduced through the vaginal mucosa and sacrospinous ligament, just medial and posterior to the ischial spine. As the pudendal artery lies near the pudendal nerve, aspiration must occur before and during injection of 7 to 10 mL of local anesthetic on each side. With the patient in the lateral decubitus position, a transcutaneous approach with a 5 to 2 MHz ultrasound probe can be used[148]; the probe is placed below the ischial spine, perpendicular to the skin oriented along the

line connecting the greater trochanter and the posterior superior iliac spine. The probe is then shifted in a parallel manner inferomedially; the pudendal nerve is located between the gluteus maximus and the levator ani muscles, medial to the obturator internus. The needle is advanced in a medial to lateral direction using an in-plane technique until within the immediate vicinity of the pudendal nerve.

Choice of Local Anesthetic

Rapid maternal absorption of the local anesthetic occurs after the performance of a pudendal nerve block; thus, concentrated solutions of local anesthetic should not be used.[149] Zador et al.[149] detected measurable concentrations of lidocaine in maternal venous and fetal scalp capillary blood samples within 5 minutes, and peak concentrations between 10 and 20 minutes of the injection of 20 mL of 1% lidocaine. Kuhnert et al.[150] reported that a pudendal nerve block versus epidural analgesia yielded similar neonatal urine concentrations of lidocaine and its metabolites.

A pudendal nerve block with 2-chloroprocaine may need to be repeated, given its short duration of action. Merkow et al.[151] evaluated neonatal neurobehavior in infants whose mothers received 30 mL of 0.5% bupivacaine, 1% mepivacaine, or 3% 2-chloroprocaine for a pudendal nerve block and perineal infiltration before delivery. Neonatal response to pinprick at 4 hours was better in the mepivacaine group; otherwise, there were no significant differences among groups in neurobehavioral scores at 4 and 24 hours after delivery.

The addition of epinephrine to the local anesthetic solution may minimally affect the quality of pudendal nerve block. In 151 patients randomized to receive pudendal nerve block with 20 mL of 1% mepivacaine either with or without epinephrine, Schierup et al.[152] observed that the addition of epinephrine slightly improved the duration, but not quality, of the anesthesia, and slightly reduced the maternal venous blood mepivacaine concentrations with no difference in umbilical cord blood concentrations.

Complications

Maternal complications of a pudendal nerve block are uncommon but may be serious (Box 23.2). Local anesthetic systemic toxicity may result from either direct intravascular injection or systemic absorption, particularly if repeated injections are administered. Vaginal, ischiorectal, and retroperitoneal hematomas, while typically small and without need to intervene operatively, may result from trauma to the pudendal artery.[153] Subgluteal and retropsoal abscesses are rare but can result in significant morbidity or mortality.[116,154]

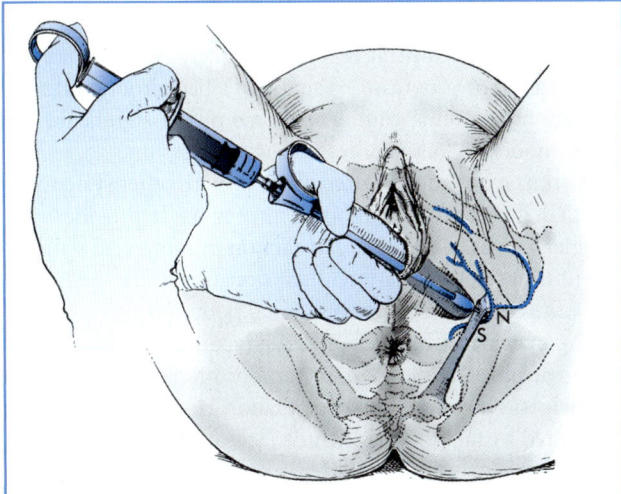

Fig. 23.2 Local Infiltration of the Pudendal Nerve. Transvaginal technique showing the needle extended beyond the needle guard and passing through the sacrospinous ligament *(S)* to reach the pudendal nerve *(N)*. From Cunningham FG, MacDonald PC, Gant NF, et al. *Williams Obstetrics*. 20th ed. Appleton & Lange; 1997:389.

> ### BOX 23.2 Maternal Complications of Pudendal Nerve Block
>
> - Laceration of the vaginal mucosa
> - Local anesthetic systemic toxicity
> - Vaginal, ischiorectal, or retroperitoneal hematoma
> - Retropsoal or subgluteal abscess

Fetal complications are rare and result primarily from fetal trauma and/or direct injection of local anesthetic. Pagès et al.[155] reported three cases of neonatal lidocaine intoxication following a maternal pudendal nerve block before delivery; all three infants had complete recovery.

Perineal Infiltration

Perineal infiltration is perhaps the most common local anesthetic technique used for vaginal delivery, and sometimes given simultaneously with a pudendal nerve block. With no large nerve fibers to be blocked, rapid onset of anesthesia is obtained with injection of local anesthetic into the posterior fourchette. However, perineal infiltration provides anesthesia only for episiotomy and repair. In a prospective randomized trial, perineal infiltration of saline-placebo provided postpartum analgesia that was equivalent to that provided by infiltration of either ropivacaine or lidocaine in parturients who underwent mediolateral episiotomy at vaginal delivery.[156]

Choice of Local Anesthetic

Philipson et al.[157] evaluated the pharmacokinetics of perineal infiltration of 1% or 2% lidocaine without epinephrine during the crowning phase of the second stage of labor in 15 healthy parturients. With a mean (SD) dose of lidocaine of 79 (3) mg, and mean drug-to-delivery interval of 7.8 (7.0) minutes, lidocaine was detected in maternal plasma as early as 1 minute after injection, with peak concentrations 3 to 15 minutes after injection. Despite the administration of small doses of lidocaine and short drug-to-delivery intervals, the rapid placental transfer resulted in a mean fetal-to-maternal lidocaine concentration ratio of 1.32, which was significantly higher than the reported ratio with paracervical block, pudendal nerve block, or epidural anesthesia for vaginal or cesarean delivery. Fetal tissue acidosis may increase the fetal-to-maternal lidocaine ratio.

In 17 parturients receiving perineal infiltration of 1% or 2% 2-chloroprocaine shortly before delivery, Philipson et al.[158] observed adequate anesthesia for simple episiotomy repair with a mean (SD) dose of 2-chloroprocaine of 81.8 (27.0) mg, and a mean drug-to-delivery interval of 6.7 (4.3) minutes. At delivery, 2-chloroprocaine was not detected in maternal or neonatal plasma and in only one umbilical cord venous blood sample; thus, the authors concluded that 2-chloroprocaine may be preferable to lidocaine for perineal infiltration. In contrast, the drug's metabolite, chloroaminobenzoic acid, was consistently detected in maternal plasma, umbilical cord venous plasma, and neonatal urine, with a fetal-to-maternal ratio of chloroaminobenzoic acid of 0.80; chloroaminobenzoic acid can inhibit the action of sulfonamides, but does not have other clinical implications.

Complications

The presence of a molded head in the occiput posterior position may predispose to unintentional direct injection of the fetal scalp. Newborn local anesthetic toxicity after administration of small doses (6 to 10 mL) of 1% to 2% lidocaine for maternal perineal infiltration has been reported.[159] In such cases, the infants were initially vigorous but required tracheal intubation 15 minutes after delivery. No lidocaine was detected in umbilical cord blood, but neonatal blood samples revealed concentrations of 14 µg/mL at 2 hours and 13.8 µg/mL at 6.5 hours.[160] Small scalp puncture wounds suggested that the lidocaine toxicity resulted from direct fetal scalp injection. Pignotti et al.[161] reported two cases of neonatal local anesthetic toxicity. In one case, lidocaine and prilocaine cream had been applied to the maternal perineum. In the second case, 10 mL of 2% mepivacaine had been injected into the perineum. Although both infants required tracheal intubation and mechanical ventilation, neurodevelopmental outcome was normal at 12 months of age.

KEY POINTS

- Systemic analgesia is commonly used around the world for labor analgesia.
- All opioid analgesic drugs rapidly cross the placenta and cause a transient reduction in fetal heart rate variability.
- Neonates whose mothers received systemic opioid analgesia are more likely to exhibit neonatal depression than those mothers who received no analgesia or epidural analgesia.
- The safest and most effective opioids used for patient-controlled analgesia (PCA) for labor analgesia are fentanyl and remifentanil.
- Remifentanil PCA offers similar or marginally better analgesia and satisfaction than fentanyl PCA, with significantly more maternal side effects of sedation, respiratory depression, and hypoxemia.
- The choice of opioid PCA for each healthcare center should consider resources available during labor for maternal monitoring and patient education, and availability of specialized neonatal personnel.

- The optimal remifentanil PCA regimen has not yet been determined, but titrated regimens likely confer an advantage as labor progresses. The use of a background infusion warrants extreme caution because of the significant risk for moderate to severe respiratory depression.
- Nitrous oxide may be used alone or with other systemic or inhaled agents. Inhalation of nitrous oxide provides variable analgesia, but high satisfaction in motivated patients. Future use of inhalational labor analgesia may be limited by the concern for environmental pollution.
- A paracervical block, lumbar sympathetic block, erector spinae block, and quadratus lumborum block may provide analgesia for the first stage of labor. However, their use is limited by factors that include lack of provider familiarity or experience, limited evidence of efficacy, and side effects.
- A pudendal nerve block may provide satisfactory anesthesia for spontaneous vaginal delivery and instrumental delivery but it provides inadequate anesthesia for manual exploration of the uterine cavity.

REFERENCES

1. Butwick AJ, Bentley J, Wong CA, et al. United States state-level variation in the use of neuraxial analgesia during labor for pregnant women. *JAMA Netw Open.* 2018;1:e186567.
2. Canadian Institute for Health Information (CIHI). Inpatient hospitalization, surgery, newborn, alternate level of care and childbirth satistics, 2017–2018; 2019. https://secure.cihi.ca/free_products/dad-hmdb-childbirth-quick-stats-2017-2018-snapshot-en-web.pdf. Accessed March 31, 2024.
3. Corbett AD, Henderson G, McKnight AT, Paterson SJ. 75 years of opioid research: the exciting but vain quest for the Holy Grail. *Br J Pharmacol.* 2006;147(suppl 1):S153–S162.
4. Halpern SH, Muir H, Breen TW, et al. A multicenter randomized controlled trial comparing patient-controlled epidural with intravenous analgesia for pain relief in labor. *Anesth Analg.* 2004;99:1532–1538.
5. Peck T, Hill S, Williams M. *Pharmacology for Anaesthesia and Intensive Care.* 3rd ed. Cambridge University Press; 2008.
6. Olofsson C, Ekblom A, Ekman-Ordeberg G, et al. Analgesic efficacy of intravenous morphine in labour pain: a reappraisal. *Int J Obstet Anesth.* 1996;5:176–180.
7. Olofsson C, Ekblom A, Ekman-Ordeberg G, et al. Lack of analgesic effect of systemically administered morphine or pethidine on labour pain. *Br J Obstet Gynaecol.* 1996;103:968–972.
8. Ankumah NE, Tsao M, Hutchinson M, et al. Intravenous acetaminophen versus morphine for analgesia in labor: a randomized trial. *Am J Perinatol.* 2017;34:38–43.
9. Way WL, Costley EC, Leongway E. Respiratory sensitivity of the newborn infant to meperidine and morphine. *Clin Pharmacol Ther.* 1965;6:454–461.
10. Gerdin E, Salmonson T, Lindberg B, Rane A. Maternal kinetics of morphine during labour. *J Perinat Med.* 1990;18:479–487.
11. Tuckey JP, Prout RE, Wee MY. Prescribing intramuscular opioids for labour analgesia in consultant-led maternity units: a survey of UK practice. *Int J Obstet Anesth.* 2008;17:3–8.
12. Reynolds F. Labour analgesia and the baby: good news is no news. *Int J Obstet Anesth.* 2011;20:38–50.
13. Sosa CG, Balaguer E, Alonso JG, et al. Meperidine for dystocia during the first stage of labor: a randomized controlled trial. *Am J Obstet Gynecol.* 2004;191:1212–1218.
14. Martin E, Vickers B, Landau R, Reece-Stremtan S. ABM Clinical Protocol #28, Peripartum analgesia and anesthesia for the breastfeeding mother. *Breastfeed Med.* 2018;13:164–171.
15. Elbohoty AE, Abd-Elrazek H, Abd-El-Gawad M, et al. Intravenous infusion of paracetamol versus intravenous pethidine as an intrapartum analgesic in the first stage of labor. *Int J Gynaecol Obstet.* 2012;118:7–10.
16. Zuarez-Easton S, Zafran N, Garmi G, et al. Meperidine compared with nitrous oxide for intrapartum pain relief in multiparous patients: a randomized controlled trial. *Obstet Gynecol.* 2023;141:4–10.
17. Ching Wong SS, Cheung CW. Analgesic efficacy and adverse effects of meperidine in managing postoperative or labor pain: a narrative review of randomized controlled trials. *Pain Physician.* 2020;23:175–201.
18. Wee MYK, Tuckey JP, Thomas PW, Burnard S. A comparison of intramuscular diamorphine and intramuscular pethidine for labour analgesia: a two-centre randomised blinded controlled trial. *BJOG.* 2014;121:447–454.
19. Murray H, Hodgkinson P, Hughes D. Remifentanil patient-controlled intravenous analgesia during labour: a retrospective observational study of 10 years' experience. *Int J Obstet Anesth.* 2019;39:29–34.
20. Sasada M, Smith S. *Drugs in Anaesthesia & Intensive Care.* 3rd ed. Oxford University Press; 2003.
21. Wilson CM, McClean E, Moore J, Dundee JW. A double-blind comparison of intramuscular pethidine and nalbuphine in labour. *Anaesthesia.* 1986;41:1207–1213.
22. Dan U, Rabinovici Y, Barkai G, et al. Intravenous pethidine and nalbuphine during labor: a prospective double-blind comparative study. *Gynecol Obstet Invest.* 1991;32:39–43.
23. Nicolle E, Devillier P, Delanoy B, et al. Therapeutic monitoring of nalbuphine: transplacental transfer and estimated pharmacokinetics in the neonate. *Eur J Clin Pharmacol.* 1996;49:485–489.
24. Douma M, Verwey R, Kam-Endtz C, et al. Obstetric analgesia: a comparison of patient-controlled meperidine, remifentanil, and fentanyl in labour. *Br J Anaesth.* 2010;104:209–215.
25. Miyakoshi K, Tanaka M, Morisaki H, et al. Perinatal outcomes: intravenous patient-controlled fentanyl versus no analgesia in labor. *J Obstet Gynaecol Res.* 2013;39:783–789.
26. Nikkola EM, Ekblad UU, Kero PO, et al. Intravenous fentanyl PCA during labour. *Can J Anaesth.* 1997;44:1248–1255.
27. Craft JB Jr, Coaldrake LA, Bolan JC, et al. Placental passage and uterine effects of fentanyl. *Anesth Analg.* 1983;62:894–898.
28. Rayburn W, Rathke A, Leuschen MP, et al. Fentanyl citrate analgesia during labor. *Am J Obstet Gynecol.* 1989;161:202–206.
29. Rayburn WF, Smith CV, Parriott JE, Woods RE. Randomized comparison of meperidine and fentanyl during labor. *Obstet Gynecol.* 1989;74:604–606.
30. Nelson KE, Eisenach JC. Intravenous butorphanol, meperidine, and their combination relieve pain and distress in women in labor. *Anesthesiology.* 2005;102:1008–1013.
31. Morrison CE, Dutton D, Howie H, Gilmour H. Pethidine compared with meptazinol during labour. A prospective randomised double-blind study in 1100 patients. *Anaesthesia.* 1987;42:7–14.
32. Mowat J, Garrey MM. Comparison of pentazocine and pethidine in labour. *Br Med J.* 1970;2:757–759.
33. Claahsen-van der Grinten HL, Verbruggen I, van den Berg PP, et al. Different pharmacokinetics of tramadol in mothers treated for labour pain and in their neonates. *Eur J Clin Pharmacol.* 2005;61:523–529.
34. Keskin HL, Keskin EA, Avsar AF, et al. Pethidine versus tramadol for pain relief during labor. *Int J Gynaecol Obstet.* 2003;82:11–16.
35. Viegas OA, Khaw B, Ratnam SS. Tramadol in labour pain in primiparous patients. A prospective comparative clinical trial. *Eur J Obstet Gynecol Reprod Biol.* 1993;49:131–135.
36. Jin J. Risks of codeine and tramadol in children. *JAMA.* 2017;318:1514.
37. Saravanakumar K, Garstang JS, Hasan K. Intravenous patient-controlled analgesia for labour: a survey of UK practice. *Int J Obstet Anesth.* 2007;16:221–225.
38. McIntosh DG, Rayburn WF. Patient-controlled analgesia inobstetrics and gynecology. *Obstet Gynecol.* 1991;78:1129–1135.
39. Melber AA, Jelting Y, Huber M, et al. Remifentanil patient-controlled analgesia in labour: six-year audit of outcome data

of the RemiPCA SAFE Network (2010-2015). *Int J Obstet Anesth.* 2019;39:12–21.

40. Rayburn WF, Smith CV, Leuschen MP, et al. Comparison of patient-controlled and nurse-administered analgesia using intravenous fentanyl during labor. *Anesthesiol Rev.* 1991;18:31–36.

41. Morley-Forster PK, Weberpals J. Neonatal effects of patient-controlled analgesia using fentanyl in labor. *Int J Obstet Anesth.* 1998;7:103–107.

42. Leppa M, Korvenoja A, Carlson S, et al. Acute opioid effects on human brain as revealed by functional magnetic resonance imaging. *Neuroimage.* 2006;31:661–669.

43. Kan RE, Hughes SC, Rosen MA, et al. Intravenous remifentanil: placental transfer, maternal and neonatal effects. *Anesthesiology.* 1998;88:1467–1474.

44. Volmanen P, Akural EI, Raudaskoski T, Alahuhta S. Remifentanil in obstetric analgesia: a dose-finding study. *Anesth Analg.* 2002;94:913–917.

45. Balki M, Kasodekar S, Dhumne S, et al. Remifentanil patient-controlled analgesia for labour: optimizing drug delivery regimens. *Can J Anaesth.* 2007;54:626–633.

46. D'Onofrio P, Novelli AM, Mecacci F, Scarselli G. The efficacy and safety of continuous intravenous administration of remifentanil for birth pain relief: an open study of 205 parturients. *Anesth Analg.* 2009;109:1922–1924.

47. Blair JM, Dobson GT, Hill DA, et al. Patient controlled analgesia for labour: a comparison of remifentanil with pethidine. *Anaesthesia.* 2005;60:22–27.

48. Rehberg B, Wickboldt N, Juillet C, Savoldelli G. Can remifentanil use in obstetrics be improved by optimal patient-controlled analgesia bolus timing? *Br J Anaesth.* 2015;114:281–289.

49. Leong WL, Sng BL, Zhang Q, et al. A case series of vital signs-controlled, patient-assisted intravenous analgesia (VPIA) using remifentanil for labour and delivery. *Anaesthesia.* 2017;72:845–852.

50. Volikas I, Butwick A, Wilkinson C, et al. Maternal and neonatal side-effects of remifentanil patient-controlled analgesia in labour. *Br J Anaesth.* 2005;95:504–509.

51. Logtenberg SLM, Vink ML, Godfried MB, et al. Serious adverse events attributed to remifentanil patient-controlled analgesia during labour in The Netherlands. *Int J Obstet Anesth.* 2019;39:22–28.

52. Stocki D, Matot I, Einav S, et al. A randomized controlled trial of efficacy and respiratory effects of patient-controlled intravenous remifentanil analgesia and patient controlled epidural analgesia in laboring women. *Anesth Analg.* 2014;118:589–597.

53. Thurlow JA, Laxton CH, Dick A, et al. Remifentanil by patient-controlled analgesia compared with intramuscular meperidine for pain relief in labour. *Br J Anaesth.* 2002;88:374–378.

54. Volmanen PVE, Akural EI, Raudaskoski T, et al. Timing of intravenous patient-controlled remifentanil bolus during early labour. *Acta Anaesthesiol Scand.* 2011;55:486–494.

55. Weiniger CF, Carvalho B, Stocki D, Einav S. Analysis of physiological respiratory variable alarm alerts among laboring women receiving remifentanil. *Anesth Analg.* 2017;124:1211–1288.

56. Douma MR, Stienstra R, Middeldorp JM, et al. Differences in maternal temperature during labour with remifentanil patient-controlled analgesia or epidural analgesia: a randomised controlled trial. *Int J Obstet Anesth.* 2015;24:313–322.

57. Van de Velde M, Van Schoubroeck D, Lewi LE, et al. Remifentanil for fetal immobilization and maternal sedation during fetoscopic surgery: a randomized, double blind comparison with diazepam. *Anesth Analg.* 2005;101:251–258.

58. Van de Velde M, Carvalho B. Remifentanil for labor analgesia: an evidence-based narrative review. *Int J Obstet Anesth.* 2016;25:66–74.

59. Karol D, Weiniger CF. Update on non-neuraxial labor analgesia. *Curr Anesthesiol Rep.* 2021;11:348–354.

60. Wilson MJA, MacArthur C, Hewitt CA, et al. Intravenous remifentanil patient-controlled analgesia versus intramuscular pethidine for pain relief in labour (RESPITE): an open-label, multicentre, randomised controlled trial. *Lancet.* 2018;392:662–672.

61. Volikas I, Male D. A comparison of pethidine and remifentanil patient-controlled analgesia in labour. *Int J Obstet Anesth.* 2001;10:86–90.

62. Evron S, Glezerman M, Sadan O, et al. Remifentanil: a novel systemic analgesic for labor pain. *Anesth Analg.* 2005;100:233–238.

63. Ng TK, Cheng BC, Chan WS, et al. A double-blind randomised comparison of intravenous patient-controlled remifentanil with intramuscular pethidine for labour analgesia. *Anaesthesia.* 2011;66:796–801.

64. Marwah R, Hassan S, Carvalho JC, Balki M. Remifentanil versus fentanyl for intravenous patient-controlled labor analgesia: an observational study. *Can J Anesth.* 2012;59:246–254.

65. Volmanen P, Akural E, Raudaskoski T, et al. Comparison of remifentanil and nitrous oxide in labour analgesia. *Acta Anaesthesiol Scand.* 2005;49:453–458.

66. Volmanen P, Sarvela J, Akural EI, et al. Intravenous remifentanil vs. epidural levobupivacaine with fentanyl for pain relief in early labour: a randomised, controlled, double-blinded study. *Acta Anaesthesiol Scand.* 2008;52:249–255.

67. Douma MR, Middeldorp JM, Verwey RA, et al. A randomised comparison of intravenous remifentanil patient-controlled analgesia with epidural ropivacaine/sufentanil during labour. *Int J Obstet Anesth.* 2011;20:118–123.

68. Freeman LM, Bloemenkamp KW, Franssen MT, et al. Patient controlled analgesia with remifentanil versus epidural analgesia in labour: randomised multicentre equivalence trial. *BMJ.* 2015;350:h846.

69. Tveit TO, Seiler S, Halvorsen A, Rosland JH. Labour analgesia: a randomised, controlled trial comparing intravenous remifentanil and epidural analgesia with ropivacaine and fentanyl. *Eur J Anaesthesiol.* 2012;29:129–136.

70. Leong WL, Sng BL, Sia AT. A comparison between remifentanil and meperidine for labor analgesia: a systematic review. *Anesth Analg.* 2011;113:818–825.

71. Schnabel A, Hahn N, Broscheit J, et al. Remifentanil for labour analgesia: a meta-analysis of randomised controlled trials. *Eur J Anaesthesiol.* 2012;29:177–185.

72. Moran VH, Thomson G, Cook J, et al. Qualitative exploration of women's experiences of intramuscular pethidine or remifentanil patient-controlled analgesia for labour pain. *BMJ Open.* 2019;9:e032203.

73. Wydall S, Zolger D, Owolabi A, et al. Comparison of different delivery modalities of epidural analgesia and intravenous analgesia in labour: a systematic review and network meta-analysis. *Can J Anaesth.* 2023;70:406–442.

74. Weibel S, Jelting Y, Afshari A, et al. Patient-controlled analgesia with remifentanil versus alternative parenteral methods for pain management in labour. *Cochrane Database Syst Rev*. 2017;(4):CD011989.

75. Liu ZQ, Chen XB, Li HB, et al. A comparison of remifentanil parturient-controlled intravenous analgesia with epidural analgesia: a meta-analysis of randomized controlled trials. *Anesth Analg*. 2014;118:598–603.

76. Moe-Byrne T, Brown JVE, McGuire W. Naloxone for opioid-exposed newborn infants. *Cochrane Database Syst Rev*. 2018;(10):CD003483.

77. Weiner G, Zaichkin J, eds. *Textbook of Neonatal Resuscitation. Lesson 10: Special Considerations*. 8th ed. American Academy of Pediatrics; 2021:243–263.

78. Vella L, Francis D, Houlton P, Reynolds F. Comparison of the antiemetics metoclopramide and promethazine in labour. *Br Med J (Clin Res Ed)*. 1985;290:1173–1175.

79. McAuley DM, O'Neill MP, Moore J, Dundee JW. Lorazepam premedication for labour. *Br J Obstet Gynaecol*. 1982;89:149–154.

80. Joselyn AS, Cherian VT, Joel S. Ketamine for labour analgesia. *Int J Obstet Anesth*. 2010;19:122–123.

81. Akamatsu TJ, Bonica JJ, Rehmet R, et al. Experiences with the use of ketamine for parturition. I. Primary anesthetic for vaginal delivery. *Anesth Analg*. 1974;53:284–287.

82. Sng BL, Dabas R, Sia AT. Intravenous dexmedetomidine use in obstetric anaesthesia: a weapon in our armoury? *Int J Obstet Anesth*. 2018;36:1–2.

83. Naaz S, Ozair E. Dexmedetomidine in current anaesthesia practice—a review. *J Clin Diagn Res*. 2014;8:GE01–GE04.

84. Ala-Kokko TI, Pienimäki P, Lampela E, et al. Transfer of clonidine and dexmedetomidine across the isolated perfused human placenta. *Acta Anaesthesiol Scand*. 1997;41:313–319.

85. Wang C, Liu S, Han C, et al. Effect and placental transfer of dexmedetomidine during caesarean section under epidural anaesthesia. *J Int Med Res*. 2017;45:964–972.

86. Yoshimura M, Kunisawa T, Suno M, et al. Intravenous dexmedetomidine for cesarean delivery and its concentration in colostrum. *Int J Obstet Anesth*. 2017;32:28–32.

87. Lamontagne C, Lesage S, Villeneuve E, et al. Intravenous dexmedetomidine for the treatment of shivering during Cesarean delivery under neuraxial anesthesia: a randomized-controlled trial. *Can J Anaesth*. 2019;66:762–771.

88. Abu-Halaweh SA, Al Oweidi AK, Abu-Malooh H, et al. Intravenous dexmedetomidine infusion for labour analgesia in patient with preeclampsia. *Eur J Anaesthesiol*. 2009;26:86–87.

89. Palanisamy A, Klickovich RJ, Ramsay M, et al. Intravenous dexmedetomidine as an adjunct for labor analgesia and cesarean delivery anesthesia in a parturient with a tethered spinal cord. *Int J Obstet Anesth*. 2009;18:258–261.

90. Abdalla W, Ammar MA, Tharwat AI. Combination of dexmedetomidine and remifentanil for labor analgesia: A double-blinded, randomized, controlled study. *Saudi J Anaesth*. 2015;9:433–438.

91. Rooks J. Nitrous oxide for pain in labor—why not in the United States? *Birth*. 2007;34:3–5.

92. National Institute for Health and Care Excellence. Intrapartum care; 2023. https://www.nice.org.uk/guidance/ng235. Accessed April 1, 2024.

93. Rosen MA. Nitrous oxide for relief of labor pain: a systematic review. *Am J Obstet Gynecol*. 2002;186:S110–S126.

94. Zafirova Z, Sheehan C, Hosseinian L. Update on nitrous oxide and its use in anesthesia practice. *Best Pract Res Clin Anaesthesiol*. 2018;32:113–123.

95. Waud BE, Waud DR. Calculated kinetics of distribution of nitrous oxide and methoxyflurane during intermittent administration during obstetrics. *Anesthesiology*. 1970;32:306–316.

96. Likis FE, Andrews JC, Collins MR, et al. Nitrous oxide for the management of labor pain: a systematic review. *Anesth Analg*. 2014;118:153–167.

97. Richardson MG, Lopez BM, Baysinger CL, et al. Nitrous oxide during labor: maternal satisfaction does not depend exclusively on analgesic effectiveness. *Anesth Analg*. 2017;124:548–553.

98. Pearson F, Sheridan N, Pierce JMT. Estimate of the total carbon footprint and component carbon sources of different modes of labour analgesia. *Anaesthesia*. 2022;77:486–488.

99. Kampman JM, Sperna Weiland NH. Anaesthesia and environment: impact of a green anaesthesia on economics. *Curr Opin Anaesthesiol*. 2023;36:188–195.

100. Einarsson S, Stenqvist O, Bengtsson A, et al. Gas kinetics during nitrous oxide analgesia for labour. *Anesthesia*. 1996;51:449–452.

101. Jevtovic-Todorovic V, Hartman RE, Izumi Y, et al. Early exposure to common anesthetic agents causes widespread neurodegeneration in the developing rat brain and persistent learning deficits. *J Neurosci*. 2003;23:876–882.

102. Abboud TK, Shnider SM, Wright RG, et al. Enflurane analgesia in obstetrics. *Anesth Analg*. 1981;60:133–137.

103. McLeod DD, Ramayya GP, Tunstall ME. Self-administered isoflurane in labour. A comparative study with Entonox. *Anaesthesia*. 1985;40:424–426.

104. Ross JA, Tunstall ME, Campbell DM, Lemon JS. The use of 0.25% isoflurane premixed in 50% nitrous oxide and oxygen for pain relief in labour. *Anaesthesia*. 1999;54:1166–1172.

105. Abboud TK, Swart F, Zhu J, et al. Desflurane analgesia for vaginal delivery. *Acta Anaesthesiol Scand*. 1995;39:259–261.

106. Toscano A, Pancaro C, Giovannoni S, et al. Sevoflurane analgesia in obstetrics: a pilot study. *Int J Obstet Anesth*. 2003;12:79–82.

107. Yeo ST, Holdcroft A, Yentis SM, Stewart A. Analgesia with sevoflurane during labour: I. Determination of the optimum concentration. *Br J Anaesth*. 2007;98:105–109.

108. Ng KWS, Chan Y, Shariffuddin II, et al. Abstract PR210: Sevonox study: a comparison of 0.8% sevoflurane & Entonox for labour analgesia. *Anesth Analg*. 2016;123(3S):271–272.

109. Palomäki O, Huhtala H, Kirkinen P. What determines the analgesic effect of paracervical block? *Acta Obstet Gynecol Scand*. 2005;84:962–966.

110. Junttila EK, Karjalainen PK, Ohtonen PP, et al. A comparison of paracervical block with single-shot spinal for labour analgesia in multiparous women: a randomised controlled trial. *Int J Obstet Anesth*. 2009;18:15–21.

111. King JC, Sherline DM. Paracervical and pudendal block. *Clin Obstet Gynecol*. 1981;24:587–595.

112. Nieminenm K, Puolakka J. Effective obstetric paracervical block with reduced dose of bupivacaine: a prospective randomized double-blind study comparing 25 mg (0.25%) and 12.5 mg (0.125%) of bupivacaine. *Acta Obstet Gynecol Scand*. 1997;76:50–54.

113. Teramo K. Effects of obstetrical paracervical blockade on the fetus. *Acta Obstet Gynecol Scand*. 1971;16:1–55.

114. Philipson EH, Kuhnert BR, Syracuse CB, et al. Intrapartum paracervical block anesthesia with 2-chloroprocaine. *Am J Obstet Gynecol*. 1983;146:16–22.

115. Gaylord TG, Pearson JW. Neuropathy following paracervical block in the obstetric patient. *Obstet Gynecol.* 1982;60: 521–525.

116. Svancarek W, Chirino O, Schaefer G, Blythe JG. Retropsoas and subgluteal abscesses following paracervical and pudendal anesthesia. *JAMA.* 1977;237:892–894.

117. Chase D, Brady JP. Ventricular tachycardia in a neonate with mepivacaine toxicity. *J Pediatr.* 1977;90:127–129.

118. Rosen MA. Paracervical block for labor analgesia: a brief historic review. *Am J Obstet Gynecol.* 2002;186:S127–S130.

119. Volmanen P, Palomäki O, Ahonen J. Alternatives to neuraxial analgesia for labor. *Curr Opin Anaesthesiol.* 2011;24:235–241.

120. Puolakka J, Jouppila R, Jouppila P, Puukka M. Maternal and fetal effects of low-dosage bupivacaine paracervical block. *J Perinat Med.* 1984;12:75–84.

121. Shnider SM, Asling JH, Margolis AJ, et al. High fetal blood levels of mepivacaine and fetal bradycardia. *N Engl J Med.* 1968;279:947–948.

122. Asling JH, Shnider SM, Margolis AJ, et al. Paracervical block anesthesia in obstetrics. II. Etiology of fetal bradycardia following paracervical block anesthesia. *Am J Obstet Gynecol.* 1970;107:626–634.

123. Freeman RK, Gutierrez NA, Ray ML, et al. Fetal cardiac response to paracervical block anesthesia. I. *Am J Obstet Gynecol.* 1972;113:583–591.

124. Morishima HO, Covino BG, Yeh MN, et al. Bradycardia in the fetal baboon following paracervical block anesthesia. *Am J Obstet Gynecol.* 1981;140:775–780.

125. Norén H, Lindblom B, Källfelt B. Effects of bupivacaine and calcium antagonists on human uterine arteries in pregnant and non-pregnant women. *Acta Anaesthesiol Scand.* 1991;35:488–491.

126. Manninen T, Aantaa R, Salonen M, et al. A comparison of the hemodynamic effects of paracervical block and epidural anesthesia for labor analgesia. *Acta Anaesthesiol Scand.* 2000;44:441–445.

127. Räsänen J, Jouppila P. Does a paracervical block with bupivacaine change vascular resistance in uterine and umbilical arteries? *J Perinat Med.* 1994;22:301–308.

128. Alexander CE, De Jesus O, Varacallo M. *Lumbar sympathetic block. StatPearls [Internet].* StatPearls Publishing; 2023.

129. Meguiar RV, Wheeler AS. Lumbar sympathetic block with bupivacaine: analgesia for labor. *Anesth Analg.* 1978;57: 486–490.

130. Leighton BL, Halpern SH, Wilson DB. Lumbar sympathetic blocks speed early and second stage induced labor in nulliparous women. *Anesthesiology.* 1999;90: 1039–1046.

131. Wills M, H, Korbon GA, Arasi R. Horner's syndrome resulting from a lumbar sympathetic block. *Anesthesiology.* 1988;68:613–614.

132. Artuso JD, Stevens RA, Lineberry PJ. Post dural puncture headache after lumbar sympathetic block: a report of two cases. *Reg Anesth.* 1991;16:288–291.

133. Clairoux A, Soucy-Proulx M, Pretto F, et al. Intrapandemic regional anesthesia as practice: a historical cohort study in patients undergoing breast cancer surgery. *Can J Anaesth.* 2022;69:485–493.

134. Sandeep B, Huang X, Li Y, et al. A comparison of regional anesthesia techniques in patients undergoing video-assisted thoracic surgery: a network meta-analysis. *Int J Surg.* 2022;105:106840.

135. Slinchenkova K, Lee K, Choudhury S, et al. A review of the paravertebral block: benefits and complications. *Curr Pain Headache Rep.* 2023;27:203–208.

136. Nair V, Henry R. Bilateral paravertebral block: a satisfactory alternative for labour analgesia. *Can J Anaesth.* 2001;48: 179–184.

137. Adhikary SD, Bernard S, Lopez H, Chin KJ. Erector spinae plane block versus retrolaminar block: a magnetic resonance imaging and anatomical study. *Reg Anesth Pain Med.* 2018;43:756–762.

138. Vilchis Rentería JS, Peng PWH, Forero M. The erector spinae plane block for obstetric analgesia: a case series of a novel technique. *Anaesth Rep.* 2020;8:e12083.

139. Yasar E, Uysal AI. Erector spinae plane blockade in the first stage of labour: a case series. *Braz J Anesthesiol.* 2022;72: 519–521.

140. Chin KJ, McDonnell JG, Carvalho B, et al. Essentials of our current understanding: abdominal wall blocks. *Reg Anesth Pain Med.* 2017;42:133–183.

141. de Haan JB, Tabba S, Lee LO, et al. Posterior quadratus lumborum block for labor analgesia: a case report. *A A Pract.* 2020;14:e01193.

142. Klink EW. Perineal nerve block: an anatomic and clinical study in the female. *Obstet Gynecol.* 1953;1:137–146.

143. Kohl GC. New method of pudendal nerve block. *Northwest Med.* 1954;53:1012–1013.

144. Hutchins CJ. Spinal analgesia for instrumental delivery: a comparison with pudendal nerve block. *Anaesthesia.* 1980;35:376–377.

145. Scudamore JH, Yates MJ. Pudendal block—a misnomer? *Lancet.* 1966;1:23–24.

146. Pace MC, Aurilio C, Bulletti C, et al. Subarachnoid analgesia in advanced labor: a comparison of subarachnoid analgesia and pudendal block in advanced labor. Analgesic quality and obstetric outcome. *Ann N Y Acad Sci.* 2004;1034: 356–363.

147. Aissaoui Y, Bruyère R, Mustapha H, et al. A randomized controlled trial of pudendal nerve block for pain relief after episiotomy. *Anesth Analg.* 2008;107:625–629.

148. Xu J, Zhou R, Su W, et al. Ultrasound-guided bilateral pudendal nerve blocks of nulliparous women with epidural labour analgesia in the second stage of labour: a randomised, double-blind, controlled trial. *BMJ Open.* 2020;10:e035887.

149. Zador G, Lindmark G, Nilsson BA. Pudendal block in normal vaginal deliveries: clinical efficacy, lidocaine concentrations in maternal and foetal blood, foetal and maternal acid-base values and influence on uterine activity. *Acta Obstet Gynecol Scand Suppl.* 1974;34:51–64.

150. Kuhnert BR, Knapp DR, Kuhnert PM, Prochaska AL. Maternal, fetal, and neonatal metabolism of lidocaine. *Clin Pharmacol Ther.* 1979;26:213–220.

151. Merkow AJ, McGuinness GA, Erenberg A, Kennedy RL. The neonatal neurobehavioral effects of bupivacaine, mepivacaine, and 2-chloroprocaine used for pudendal block. *Anesthesiology.* 1980;52:309–312.

152. Schierup L, Schmidt JF, Jensen AT, Rye BAO. Pudendal block in vaginal deliveries: mepivacaine with and without epinephrine. *Acta Obstet Gynecol Scand.* 1988;67: 195–197.

153. Kurzel RB, Au AH, Rooholamini SA. Retroperitoneal hematoma as a complication of pudendal block: diagnosis made by computed tomography. *West J Med.* 1996;164: 523–525.

154. Hibbard LT, Snyder EN, McVann RM. Subgluteal and retropsoal infection in obstetric practice. *Obstet Gynecol.* 1972;39:137–150.

155. Pagès H, de la Gastine B, Quedru-Aboane J, et al. Lidocaine intoxication in newborn following maternal pudendal anesthesia: report of three cases. *J Gynecol Obstet Biol Reprod (Paris).* 2008;37:415–418.

156. Schinkel N, Colbus L, Soltner C, et al. Perineal infiltration with lidocaine 1%, ropivacaine 0.75%, or placebo for episiotomy repair in parturients who received epidural labor analgesia: a double-blind randomized study. *Int J Obstet Anesth.* 2010;19:293–297.

157. Philipson EH, Kuhnert BR, Syracuse CD. Maternal, fetal, and neonatal lidocaine levels following local perineal infiltration. *Am J Obstet Gynecol.* 1984;149:403–407.

158. Philipson EH, Kuhnert BR, Syracuse CD. 2-Chloroprocaine for local perineal infiltration. *Am J Obstet Gynecol.* 1987;157:1275–1278.

159. Kim WY, Pomerance JJ, Miller AA. Lidocaine intoxication in a newborn following local anesthesia for episiotomy. *Pediatrics.* 1979;64:643–645.

160. De Praeter C, Vanhaesebrouck P, De Praeter N, Govaert P. Episiotomy and neonatal lidocaine intoxication (letter). *Eur J Pediatr.* 1991;150:685–686.

161. Pignotti MS, Indolfi G, Ciuti R, Donzelli G. Perinatal asphyxia and inadvertent neonatal intoxication from local anaesthetics given to the mother during labour. *BMJ.* 2005;330:34–35.

24

Epidural and Spinal Analgesia: Anesthesia for Labor and Vaginal Delivery

Cynthia A. Wong, MD

CHAPTER OUTLINE

Epidural analgesia and spinal analgesia are the most effective methods of intrapartum pain relief in contemporary clinical practice.[1] During the first stage of labor, pain results primarily from distention of the lower uterine segment and cervix. Painful impulses are transmitted via visceral afferent nerve fibers, which accompany sympathetic nerve fibers and enter the spinal cord at the 10th, 11th, and 12th thoracic and 1st lumbar spinal segments. As labor progresses and the fetus descends in the birth canal, distention of the vagina and perineum results in painful impulses that are transmitted via the pudendal nerve to the second, third, and fourth sacral spinal segments. Neuraxial analgesia is the only form of analgesia that provides complete pain relief for both stages of labor. During the first stage of labor, visceral pain impulses entering the spinal cord at T10 to L1 must be blocked. During the late first stage of labor and the second stage of labor, somatic impulses entering the spinal cord from S2 to S4 must also be blocked (see Chapter 21).

In a survey of 1000 consecutive women who chose a variety of analgesic techniques for labor and vaginal delivery (including nonpharmacologic methods, transcutaneous electrical nerve stimulation [TENS], intramuscular meperidine [pethidine], inhalation of nitrous oxide, epidural analgesia, and a combination of these techniques), pain relief and overall satisfaction with the birth experience were greater in patients who received epidural analgesia.[2] Similarly, randomized studies that have compared epidural analgesia with systemic opioids and/or inhalation analgesia (i.e., nitrous oxide) and other nonpharmacologic techniques (e.g., TENS, continuous support) have shown that pain scores are lower and patients are more satisfied with neuraxial analgesia.[3]

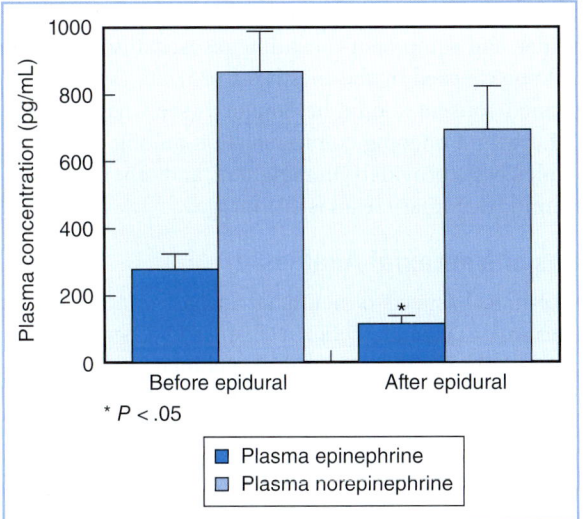

Fig. 24.1 Influence of Epidural Analgesia on Maternal Plasma Concentrations of Catecholamines During Labor. *$P < .05$ compared with before initiation of epidural analgesia. Modified from Shnider SM, Abboud TK, Artal R, et al. Maternal catecholamines decrease during labor after lumbar epidural anesthesia. *Am J Obstet Gynecol*. 1983;147:13–15.

The provision of analgesia for labor may result in other benefits. Effective neuraxial analgesia reduces maternal plasma concentrations of catecholamines (Fig. 24.1).[4] Decreased alpha- and beta-adrenergic receptor stimulation may result in better uteroplacental perfusion and more effective uterine activity.[5,6] Painful uterine contractions result in maternal hyperventilation, which in turn leads to maternal respiratory alkalosis, a leftward shift of the oxyhemoglobin dissociation curve, increased maternal hemoglobin affinity for oxygen, and reduced oxygen delivery to the fetus.[7] Hypocarbia also leads to hypoventilation between contractions, which may cause a decrease in maternal Pao_2. Effective epidural analgesia blunts this "hyperventilation-hypoventilation" cycle.[8] Additionally, one study showed that paternal anxiety levels were lower, and both paternal involvement in the childbirth process and paternal satisfaction were greater, in men whose partners received epidural analgesia than in those whose partners did not.[9] Finally, the presence of an epidural catheter and effective epidural *analgesia* facilitate the rapid initiation of epidural *anesthesia* for emergency intrapartum cesarean delivery. Neuraxial anesthesia for cesarean delivery is associated with greater overall maternal safety than emergency administration of general anesthesia (see Chapter 26).

Neuraxial analgesia is not used by all laboring women, although surveys of obstetric anesthesia practice in the United States have shown that its use has grown over the past four decades.[10] Data collected from the US Standard Certificate of Live Birth in 2015 indicated that 73% of laboring women who had a singleton gestation received neuraxial analgesia. The rate was higher among non-Hispanic White women than in women of other races/ethnicities, and it was also higher in larger maternal units than in smaller units.[10,11] In France in 2021, 85% of laboring women used neuraxial analgesia.[12]

In China, the use of neuraxial labor analgesia continues to grow.[13]

The availability of skilled anesthesia providers influences the neuraxial analgesia rate.[10] Other factors include the information and advice provided to pregnant women by obstetric providers, nurses, and childbirth education instructors. The personal and cultural expectations of a laboring woman,[14] as well as obstetric complications, also affect the childbirth experience and the use of neuraxial analgesia (see Chapters 14, 21, and 22).

Ideally, the anesthesia provider should tailor the analgesic technique to meet the individual parturient's needs. Factors that should be considered in formulating an analgesic plan for individual parturients include the parturient's preferences for analgesia, coexisting maternal disease, the airway examination, fetal status, spontaneous versus induced labor, stage of labor at the time of request for analgesia, and anticipated risk for operative delivery. The risks and benefits of the various neuraxial techniques should be assessed for each parturient. Good technique requires thoughtful preparation and meticulous attention to detail to ensure maternal and fetal safety.

The ideal labor analgesic technique is safe for both the mother and the infant, does not interfere with the progress of labor and delivery, and provides flexibility in response to changing conditions. In addition, the ideal technique provides consistent pain relief, minimizes undesirable side effects (e.g., motor block), and minimizes ongoing demands on the anesthesia provider's time. No single technique or anesthetic agent is ideal for all parturients. Guidelines promulgated by professional organizations address obstetric anesthesia care.[15-18] All obstetric anesthesia providers should review their country's respective guidelines. Specific neuraxial techniques for labor analgesia, including their advantages, disadvantages, side effects, and complications, are considered in this chapter.

PREPARATION FOR NEURAXIAL ANALGESIA

Indications and Contraindications

Neuraxial analgesia is indicated to treat the pain of labor. In its 2019 Practice Bulletin, *Obstetric Analgesia and Anesthesia*, the American College of Obstetricians and Gynecologists (ACOG) reaffirmed an earlier opinion jointly published by the American Society of Anesthesiologists (ASA) and ACOG, which stated that "in the absence of a medical contraindication, maternal request is a sufficient medical indication for pain relief during labor."[18] Furthermore, the ACOG[18] has stated that "decisions regarding analgesia should be closely coordinated among the obstetrician-gynecologist or other obstetric care provider, the anesthesiologist, the patient, and skilled support personnel." Neuraxial analgesia is an appropriate treatment for the pain of labor, including early labor (defined as regular uterine contractions that cause progressive effacement and dilation of the uterine cervix). Randomized controlled trials[19] have confirmed that initiation of neuraxial analgesia in early labor does not increase the risk for cesarean delivery (see later discussion).

Neuraxial analgesia may facilitate an atraumatic vaginal breech delivery, the vaginal delivery of twin infants, and vaginal delivery of a preterm infant (see Chapters 33 and 34). By providing effective pain relief, neuraxial analgesia facilitates blood pressure control in women with preeclampsia (see Chapter 35). Neuraxial analgesia also blunts the hemodynamic effects of uterine contractions (e.g., sudden increase in cardiac preload) and the associated pain response (tachycardia, increased systemic vascular resistance, hypertension, hyperventilation) in patients with other medical comorbidities (e.g., mitral stenosis, spinal cord injury, intracranial neurovascular disease, asthma; see Chapters 41, 47, and 51).

Box 24.1 lists the contraindications to administration of epidural or spinal analgesia. Some anesthesia providers have suggested that systemic maternal infection, preexisting neurologic disease, or severe stenotic heart lesions are relative contraindications to neuraxial analgesia. However, most cases of systemic infection (especially if properly treated), or neurologic or cardiac disease, do not contraindicate the administration of neuraxial analgesia (see Chapters 36, 41, and 47). It is controversial whether mild or isolated abnormalities in tests of blood coagulation preclude the use of neuraxial analgesia. The dose and timing of administration of drugs administered for thromboprophylaxis must also be considered (see Chapter 44). The anesthesia provider should consider the risks and benefits of neuraxial analgesia for each patient individually.

Thorough preparation for neuraxial labor analgesia involves several steps (Box 24.2). These include (1) a review of the parturient's obstetric history; (2) a focused preanesthetic evaluation that includes maternal obstetric, anesthetic, and health history; and (3) a brief physical examination (i.e., vital signs, airway, heart, lungs, and back).[15] Routine measurement of the platelet count and other laboratory measurements are not necessary, except in selected patients.[15] Similarly, routine intrapartum blood typing and screening or cross-matching is not necessary in healthy parturients, although consideration should be given to sending a blood sample to the blood bank (to facilitate the rapid availability of blood products in case of emergency need).[15] For parturients at increased risk for hemorrhage and for those with antenatal anemia (see Chapter 44), intrapartum typing and screening or cross-matching should be performed. Fetal well-being should be assessed by a skilled provider, and equipment (including resuscitation equipment) should be checked by the anesthesia provider (see Box 12.1). Informed consent should be obtained (see Chapters 12 and 32). Early and ongoing communication among the obstetric and anesthesia providers, nursing staff, and other members of the multidisciplinary team is encouraged.

Types of Neuraxial Analgesia

The technical aspects of neuraxial analgesic/anesthetic techniques are discussed in detail in Chapter 12. These techniques include continuous epidural, combined spinal-epidural (CSE), dural-puncture epidural (DPE), and occasionally, continuous or single-shot spinal analgesia or caudal analgesia. There are advantages and disadvantages to each technique (Table 24.1).

Epidural Analgesia

Continuous lumbar epidural analgesia has been the mainstay of neuraxial labor analgesia for decades. Placement of an epidural catheter allows analgesia to be maintained until after delivery. No dural puncture is required. The presence of a catheter and effective *analgesia* allow the conversion to epidural surgical *anesthesia* should intrapartum cesarean delivery be necessary. Injection of a local anesthetic in the lumbar epidural space allows both cephalad and caudad spread of the anesthetic solution.

Analgesia is initiated by bolus injection of drug(s) through the epidural needle, catheter, or both. Analgesia is maintained with intermittent bolus injections, a continuous epidural infusion (CEI), or a combination of these techniques, administered by the anesthesia provider, the patient, or an infusion

---

BOX 24.1 Contraindications to Epidural and Spinal Analgesia

- Patient refusal or inability to cooperate
- Increased intracranial pressure secondary to a mass lesion
- Skin or soft tissue infection at the site of needle placement
- Frank coagulopathy
- Recent pharmacologic anticoagulation[a]
- Uncorrected maternal hypovolemia (e.g., hemorrhage)
- Inadequate training in or experience with the technique
- Inadequate resources (e.g., staff, equipment) for monitoring and resuscitation

[a]Safety depends on specific drug and timing and dose of the most recent drug administration.

BOX 24.2 Checklist: Preparation for Neuraxial Labor Analgesia

1. Communicate (early) with the obstetric provider.
   - Review parturient's obstetric history.
2. Perform focused preanesthetic evaluation.
   - Review maternal obstetric, anesthetic, and health history.
   - Perform targeted physical examination (vital signs, airway, heart, lungs, back).
3. Review relevant laboratory measurements and imaging studies.
4. Consider need for blood typing and screening or cross-matching.
5. Formulate analgesia plan.
6. Obtain informed consent.
7. Perform equipment check:
   - Check routine equipment and drugs.
   - Check emergency resuscitation equipment.
8. Obtain peripheral intravenous access.
   - Confirm the free flow of a crystalloid solution.
9. Apply maternal monitors (blood pressure, heart rate, pulse oximetry).
10. Monitor fetal heart rate.
11. Perform a team time-out.

TABLE 24.1 Advantages and Disadvantages of Neuraxial Techniques in Labor

Neuraxial Technique	Advantages	Disadvantages
Continuous epidural	Continuous analgesia No dural puncture required Ability to extend analgesia to anesthesia for cesarean delivery	Slow onset of analgesia Larger drug doses required compared with spinal techniques Greater risk for maternal local anesthetic systemic toxicity Greater fetal drug exposure
Combined spinal-epidural	Continuous analgesia Low doses of local anesthetic and opioid Rapid onset of analgesia Rapid onset of sacral analgesia Ability to extend analgesia to anesthesia for cesarean delivery Complete analgesia with opioid alone Decreased incidence of failed epidural analgesia	Increased incidence of pruritus Possible higher risk for fetal bradycardia
Dural-puncture epidural	Continuous analgesia Possible earlier sacral analgesia than epidural analgesia Ability to extend analgesia to anesthesia for cesarean delivery	Intermediate onset of analgesia Larger drug doses required compared with spinal techniques Greater risk for maternal local anesthetic systemic toxicity Greater fetal drug exposure
Continuous spinal	Low doses of local anesthetic and opioid Rapid onset of analgesia Ability to extend analgesia to anesthesia for cesarean delivery	Large dural puncture increases risk for post–dural puncture headache Possibility of overdose and total spinal anesthesia if the spinal catheter is mistaken for an epidural catheter Careful titration to treat breakthrough pain may delay effective analgesia
Continuous caudal	Continuous analgesia Avoids need to access neuraxial canal through lumbar interspace in patients with previous lumbar spine surgery	Requires large volumes/doses of drugs May be technically more difficult than other neuraxial techniques Possible higher risk for infection than with other neuraxial techniques Risk for inadvertent fetal injection
Single-shot spinal	Technically simple Rapid onset of analgesia Immediate sacral analgesia Low drug doses	Limited duration of analgesia

pump. The catheter is removed after delivery when there is no further need for analgesia or anesthesia.

Combined Spinal-Epidural Analgesia

The CSE technique has become increasingly popular in the past 30 years. Onset of complete analgesia is significantly faster than with epidural techniques (2 to 5 minutes versus 10 to 15 minutes, respectively).[20] More women with spinal analgesia had effective analgesia at 10 minutes (relative risk [RR], 1.9; 95% confidence interval [CI], 1.5 to 2.5).[20] In particular, the onset of sacral analgesia is significantly slower after the initiation of lumbar epidural analgesia than spinal analgesia. It may take several hours of lumbar epidural infusion, or several bolus injections of local anesthetic into the lumbar epidural space, to achieve sacral analgesia. Rapid onset of sacral analgesia is advantageous in the parturient in whom analgesia is initiated late in the first stage of labor or in a parous parturient with rapid progress of labor. Spinal analgesia requires significantly lower drug doses to attain effective analgesia compared with epidural analgesia; therefore the risk for local anesthetic systemic toxicity (LAST) is decreased. In addition, there is less systemic absorption of spinal anesthetic agents into the maternal circulation, so maternal and fetal plasma drug concentrations are lower with spinal than with epidural analgesia.

An additional advantage of spinal analgesia is that complete analgesia for early labor can be accomplished with the intrathecal injection of a lipid-soluble opioid without the addition of a local anesthetic. Thus, motor blockade is avoided and the risk for hypotension is lower.[21] This method is ideal for patients who wish to ambulate or for those with preload-dependent cardiac conditions such as stenotic heart lesions. Finally, use of the CSE technique may lower the incidence of failure of epidural analgesia (e.g., a nonfunctioning epidural catheter).[22,23] The likelihood of an epidural catheter placed for labor analgesia failing to provide satisfactory anesthesia for a subsequent cesarean delivery was more than five times higher for catheters placed as part of an epidural technique than for catheters placed as part of a CSE technique.[23]

CSE analgesia has several possible undesirable side effects. Dural puncture is required for initiation, although use of small-gauge pencil-point needles does not appear to increase the risk for post–dural puncture headache.[20] The incidence of pruritus is higher with intrathecal opioid administration than with epidural opioid administration.[20] Another purported disadvantage of the CSE technique is that the correct placement of the epidural catheter in the epidural space cannot be verified until spinal analgesia or anesthesia wanes. However, in a retrospective study that included 2395 neuraxial labor analgesia procedures, the CSE technique did not result in delayed recognition of epidural catheter failure, and the overall catheter failure rate was lower when the catheter was placed as part of CSE analgesia.[22]

The most common CSE technique for labor analgesia is the needle-through-needle technique in a midlumbar interspinous space (see Chapter 12). Analgesia is maintained via the epidural catheter, as with traditional epidural analgesia.

Dural-Puncture Epidural Analgesia

DPE analgesia is a modification of the CSE technique in which a dural puncture is made with a small-gauge spinal needle, but no drug is injected into the subarachnoid space. In theory, the technique combines some benefits of CSE and epidural analgesia, while mitigating the adverse effects of each technique. Results of studies comparing DPE analgesia with epidural analgesia and CSE analgesia have been inconsistent.[24] In a 2022 metaanalysis comparing DPE and epidural analgesia (10 trials, $n = 1099$), onset of analgesia was faster in women randomized to receive DPE.[25] There were, however, no differences in secondary outcomes, including quality of block (unilateral block, sacral-sparing, incidence of breakthrough pain), mode of delivery, and incidence of fetal bradycardia or other adverse effects.[25] The study was underpowered for many of these outcomes. In a randomized comparison of epidural, CSE, and DPE techniques, DPE analgesia had longer latency, but a lower incidence of pruritus, hypotension, and uterine tachysystole compared with CSE analgesia.[26] When loss of resistance is unclear, insertion of a spinal needle to verify cerebrospinal fluid (CSF) may be a useful technique to confirm placement of the epidural needle tip in the epidural space. In the setting of intrapartum cesarean delivery, the time to onset of surgical epidural anesthesia may be faster when an epidural catheter sited using a DPE technique is topped up for surgical anesthesia compared with a catheter sited using a traditional epidural technique (no dural puncture).[27]

Continuous Spinal Analgesia

Continuous spinal analgesia is used occasionally for labor analgesia but is not practical for most parturients. Several spinal catheters are commercially available in the United States and Europe, but their use for continuous labor analgesia has not been well studied. Because the available catheters require dural puncture with a large-gauge needle, the technique may be associated with an unacceptably high incidence of post–dural puncture headache. However, continuous spinal analgesia is a management option in patients with unintentional dural puncture. When a patient has a spinal catheter, clear communication is essential to ensure that any anesthesia provider managing labor analgesia administers appropriate intrathecal local anesthetic and opioid doses. Intrathecal doses are much lower than doses intended for the epidural space, and if a typical epidural dose is administered intrathecally, high- or total-spinal anesthesia may result. In the event of inadequate spinal analgesia, careful titration is necessary; it may require additional time to distinguish between insufficient drug administration (while the catheter remains in the intrathecal space), catheter tip movement (withdrawal) into the epidural space, or complete catheter dislodgement. As long as catheter dislodgement is prevented during patient transport and positioning, effective continuous spinal analgesia can readily be converted to surgical anesthesia, if necessary.

Caudal Analgesia

Continuous caudal epidural analgesia is used infrequently in modern obstetric anesthesia practice. It is technically more difficult to place a caudal catheter than a lumbar epidural catheter. Large volumes of anesthetic solution are required to extend neuroblockade to the low thoracic spinal segments, resulting in higher maternal plasma concentrations of drug. There is a risk for needle/catheter misplacement and direct injection into the fetus if the needle is inadvertently directed lateral to the coccyx rather than into the sacral hiatus. However, this technique is useful for parturients in whom access to the lumbar spinal canal is not possible (e.g., because of a fused lumbar spine); ultrasonographic guidance may improve both safety and efficacy of the technique.[28]

Single-Shot Techniques

In general, single-shot techniques (spinal, lumbar epidural, or caudal) are less useful for most laboring women because of their limited duration of action; they are generally not used in high-resource settings. However, single-shot techniques may be useful in low-resource settings (see Chapter 15). A single-shot spinal procedure is simpler to perform than epidural- and catheter-based techniques and requires less equipment, often not available in low-resource settings. A spinal technique avoids the risk of unintentional dural puncture with a large-bore epidural needle, and the risks of local anesthetic toxicity and high spinal anesthesia are minimal.

In both high- and low-resource settings, a single-shot spinal technique may be indicated for parturients who require analgesia or anesthesia shortly before anticipated vaginal delivery or in settings in which continuous neuraxial analgesia is not possible.[29] Intrathecal morphine has been combined with bupivacaine and sufentanil or fentanyl in an attempt to prolong analgesia. A 2016 metaanalysis of five randomized-controlled trials comparing single-shot spinal labor analgesia (bupivacaine and sufentanil or fentanyl) with and without morphine concluded that additional adequately powered trials are necessary to determine the benefits and harms of the technique.[30]

Informed Consent

Informed consent is an important aspect of preparation for neuraxial labor analgesia (see Chapters 12 and 32). The preanesthetic evaluation and informed consent process allow the anesthesia provider to allay the parturient's concerns and to demonstrate a commitment to her care. Most laboring women understand the need for informed consent and appreciate the opportunity to participate in decisions about their care.

Equipment and Monitors

Resuscitation equipment, drugs, and supplies must be immediately available for the management of serious complications of neuraxial analgesia (e.g., hypotension, total spinal anesthesia, LAST) (see Box 12.1).[15] Emergency airway equipment should be checked before the administration of neuraxial analgesia.

During the initiation of neuraxial analgesia, the parturient's oxygen saturation should be measured continuously and the blood pressure should be assessed every 2 to 3 minutes for 15 to 20 minutes after the neuraxial anesthetic administration, or until the mother is hemodynamically stable (see Chapter 12). The fetal heart rate (FHR) should be monitored before and after the initiation of neuraxial analgesia; it may be difficult to monitor the FHR during the actual procedure.[15] During maintenance of neuraxial analgesia, maternal blood pressure should be measured every 15 to 30 minutes, or more frequently if hypotension ensues. The sensory level of analgesia and the intensity of motor block (Box 24.3) should be assessed after the administration of the test and therapeutic doses of local anesthetics. Subsequently, sensory level, motor block, and pain control should be assessed at regular intervals.

Before the initiation of neuraxial analgesia, ultrasonographic imaging of the back may be helpful, especially in parturients whose landmarks are difficult to palpate (see Chapter 12).

Intravenous Hydration

Placement of an intravenous catheter (preferably 18-gauge or larger) and correction of hypovolemia with intravenous hydration are necessary before the initiation of neuraxial analgesia to mitigate hypotension that can result from sympathetic blockade. Data from small studies are conflicting as to whether a fluid bolus administered immediately before the initiation of analgesia decreases the risk for nonreassuring FHR patterns.[31–35] The ASA Task Force on Obstetric Anesthesia is silent on intravenous fluid management,[15] although many anesthesia providers administer approximately 500 mL of lactated Ringer's solution (without dextrose) immediately before or during the initiation of analgesia. Severe hypotension is less likely with the contemporary practice of administering a dilute solution of local anesthetic for epidural analgesia or an intrathecal opioid for spinal analgesia.

Studies of intravenous hydration and spinal anesthesia for cesarean delivery suggest that there is no advantage to administering the fluid before the initiation of anesthesia (preload) compared with administering the fluid at the time of initiation of anesthesia (coload).[36] Fluid administration should be judicious in parturients at risk for pulmonary edema (e.g., women with preeclampsia with severe features, heart disease). Anesthesia and obstetric providers should avoid the bolus administration of dextrose-containing solutions in laboring women.

Maternal Positioning

Either the lateral decubitus or the sitting position can be used during initiation of neuraxial analgesia (see Chapter 12). Factors to consider when positioning the parturient for the procedure include patient comfort, avoidance of aortocaval compression, ability to monitor the FHR, provider comfort and experience, and optimal positioning of the spine and palpation of landmarks. Patient position relative to the baricity of the anesthetic solution should be considered during initiation of spinal analgesia/anesthesia. There is no evidence that patient position during an epidural catheter insertion and the initial bolus injection of anesthetic solution influences the extent of neuroblockade.[37] After completion of the procedure, parturients should be monitored for the first 15 to 30 minutes, usually in the lateral position to minimize aortocaval compression during the onset of neuraxial labor analgesia.[38] Patient position generally does not influence sensory block distribution if bolus maintenance techniques are used (see later discussion). However, if analgesia is maintained with a continuous infusion technique, sensory block may become more extensive or dense on the dependent side over time. Regular changes in maternal position are encouraged to avoid development of one-sided sensory blockade and compression injury.

INITIATION OF EPIDURAL ANALGESIA

A procedure for initiating epidural labor analgesia is outlined in Box 24.4. Commonly, after siting the epidural catheter in the epidural space, a test dose is administered to rule out intrathecal or intravascular placement of the epidural catheter. After a negative test dose, epidural analgesia is established with incremental injection of a local anesthetic, usually in combination with a lipid-soluble opioid. Maternal vital signs are monitored, and clinical analgesia is verified.

Epidural Test Dose

The purpose of the test dose is to help identify unintentional cannulation of a vein or the subarachnoid space. The test dose should contain a dose of local anesthetic and/or another

---

> **BOX 24.3 Assessment of Motor Block**
>
> - Complete: patient unable to move feet or knees
> - Almost complete: patient able to move feet only
> - Partial: patient just able to move knees
> - None: patient capable of full flexion of knees and feet

Modified from Bromage PR. *Epidural Analgesia*. WB Saunders; 1978:144.

BOX 24.4 Suggested Procedure for Initiation of Epidural Labor Analgesia

1. Complete preparation for neuraxial analgesia checklist (see Box 24.2).
2. Position the patient with the help of an assistant (lateral decubitus or sitting).
3. Initiate maternal blood pressure and pulse oximetry monitoring and fetal heart rate monitoring.
4. Initiate an intravenous fluid bolus (e.g., 500 mL of lactated Ringer's solution).
5. Site epidural catheter in epidural space using sterile technique.
6. Administer an epidural test dose (see Table 12.2).
7. If the test dose is negative, secure epidural catheter and position patient in the lateral position.
8. Administer 5 to 15 mL of epidural local anesthetic, in 5-mL increments (usually low concentration of local anesthetic combined with a lipid-soluble opioid [see Table 24.2]).
9. Monitor maternal blood pressure every 2 to 3 min for 15 to 20 min, or until the parturient is hemodynamically stable.
10. Assess the pain score and extent of sensory blockade (cephalad and caudad).
11. Initiate maintenance epidural analgesia (see Table 24.5).

---

marker sufficient to allow the recognition of intravenous or subarachnoid injection but not so large as to cause LAST or total spinal anesthesia. The most common *intravascular* test dose contains epinephrine (adrenaline) (see Chapter 12).

The use of the epinephrine test dose in obstetrics is not without detractors. Some anesthesia providers fear that intravenous injection of epinephrine may decrease uteroplacental perfusion and precipitate fetal compromise. However, there has been no report of adverse neonatal outcome after intravenous injection of an epinephrine-containing test dose. Another argument against routine use of a test dose is that aspiration of multiorifice catheters is 98% sensitive in identifying their intravascular location.[39] (The sensitivity of aspiration is significantly lower for single-orifice catheters.) The epinephrine test dose is less specific in laboring women because cyclic changes in the maternal heart rate complicate the interpretation of its effects.[40] For this reason, if used, the test dose should be given immediately after a uterine contraction so there is less confusion as to whether tachycardia is caused by pain or intravenous epinephrine. In some cases (e.g., hypertensive crisis, critical aortic stenosis), a test dose containing epinephrine is best avoided. Other methods of detecting intravascular injection[41] are discussed in Chapter 12.

The local anesthetic component of the test dose tests for unintended intrathecal catheter placement.[41] Because modern epidural labor analgesia involves the infusion of low-concentration local anesthetic solution, unintentional intravascular or intrathecal administration is not likely to result in cardiovascular collapse or total spinal anesthesia.

Proponents of using a test dose argue that it still has a role in obstetric anesthesia practice.[42] Large volumes of concentrated local anesthetic solution are still routinely administered for emergency cesarean delivery. Although not a safety issue, it is easier for the parturient and anesthesia provider to identify a misplaced catheter at the time of initial placement and to replace the catheter at that time rather than identify the misplaced catheter after the sterile field has been breached and the parturient repositioned. No matter whether a formal test dose is used or not, it is imperative for the anesthesia provider to take the time to look for evidence of unintentional intrathecal or intravascular injection of local anesthetic. Finally, every anesthesia provider should remember that no single test dose regimen can exclude every case of unintentional intravenous or subarachnoid injection. Box 12.3 summarizes steps that may be taken to decrease the risk for unintentional intravenous or subarachnoid injection of local anesthetic.

Choice of Drugs

The ideal analgesic drug for labor provides rapid onset of effective analgesia with minimal motor blockade, minimal risk for maternal toxicity, and has negligible effect on uterine activity and uteroplacental perfusion. It would undergo limited transplacental transfer and thus have minimal direct effect on the fetus. Finally, this ideal agent would have a long duration of action. Although this perfect analgesic drug does not exist, the combination of a local anesthetic with an opioid allows us to approach this goal.

Traditionally, local anesthetics were administered to block both the visceral pain of labor (lower uterine segment distention and cervical dilation) and the somatic pain (descent of the fetus in the birth canal). In 1976, investigators identified dense concentrations of opioid receptors in the dorsal horn of the spinal cord.[43] The application of small doses of an opioid to these receptor sites generates a specific and profound opioid response.[43] Intrathecal opioids effectively relieve the visceral pain of the early first stage of labor, although they must be combined with a local anesthetic to effectively relieve the somatic pain of the late first stage and the second stage of labor. The combination of a local anesthetic with a lipid-soluble opioid allows for the use of lower doses of each agent, thus minimizing undesirable side effects. For example, when used alone without an opioid, the local anesthetic dose required for effective epidural analgesia is associated with an unacceptably high incidence of motor blockade. Similarly, used alone, high doses of epidural opioid are required for satisfactory analgesia during early labor, and such doses are associated with significant systemic absorption and systemic side effects. The addition of an opioid to the local anesthetic also shortens latency,[44] an important aspect of labor analgesia, especially with the use of long-acting local anesthetics that usually also have long latency. Thus, contemporary epidural labor analgesia practice most often incorporates low doses of a long-acting local anesthetic combined with a lipid-soluble opioid.

Local Anesthetics

Bupivacaine. Historically, the amide local anesthetic bupivacaine has been the most commonly used agent for epidural labor analgesia. Bupivacaine is highly protein-bound, a feature that limits transplacental transfer. The umbilical vein–to–maternal vein concentration ratio is approximately 0.3.[45] With a single epidural bolus dose, the duration of analgesia is approximately 90 minutes. Epidural bupivacaine (e.g., 10 to 20 mL of a 0.0625% or 0.125% solution) combined with fentanyl or sufentanil is adequate to initiate labor analgesia in most parturients (Table 24.2).

The potency of local anesthetics for neuraxial labor analgesia is often assessed and compared by determining the dose (ED_{50}) or concentration (EC_{50}) of epidural solution that achieves effective analgesia in half of women. Early studies that used up-and-down methodology focused on the median effective concentration of local anesthetic solution when administered as a 20-mL epidural bolus, referred to as the minimum local anesthetic concentration (MLAC). MLAC is lower for women in early labor than in late labor,[46] and it is also lower when the local anesthetic is combined with a lipid-soluble opioid.[47] Subsequent work has expanded this concept to evaluate additional variables, such as drug dose, volume, and speed of injection, across a range of efficacies and clinical outcomes.[48]

It is important to consider the local anesthetic *dose* and *concentration* for initiation and maintenance of epidural analgesia. Christiaens et al.[49] randomly assigned parturients to receive epidural bupivacaine 20 mg diluted in 4, 10, or 20 mL (0.5%, 0.2%, and 0.1% solutions, respectively). Analgesia in the 10- and 20-mL groups was superior to that in the 4-mL group, and duration of analgesia was longest in the 20-mL group. Lyons et al.[50] compared the minimum local anesthetic volume and minimum local anesthetic dose for 0.125% and 0.25% bupivacaine for epidural labor analgesia. Bupivacaine 0.125% produced analgesia equivalent to that provided by bupivacaine 0.25%, with a 50% increase in required volume and a 25% reduction in dose (Table 24.3). Stated differently, a dose-sparing effect is achieved by administering a 0.125% solution of bupivacaine rather than a 0.25% solution. Together, these data suggest that epidural analgesia and safety are improved with the use of low concentration–high volume local anesthetic solutions.

Ropivacaine. Ropivacaine is an amide local anesthetic similar to bupivacaine in structure and pharmacodynamics (see Chapter 13). Ropivacaine is cleared more rapidly than bupivacaine after intravenous administration in both pregnant and nonpregnant sheep. Consequently, a larger dose of drug—but not a higher plasma concentration—is required to produce LAST.[51] These findings suggest that ropivacaine may have a greater margin of safety than bupivacaine if unintentional intravenous injection occurs in pregnant women.

TABLE 24.2 Drugs Used for Initiation of Epidural and Spinal Labor Analgesia

Drug	Epidural Analgesia[a]	Spinal Analgesia
Local Anesthetics[b]		
Bupivacaine	0.0625%–0.125%	1.25–2.5 mg
Ropivacaine	0.08%–0.2%	2.0–3.5 mg
Levobupivacaine	0.0625%–0.125%	2.0–3.5 mg
Lidocaine[c]	0.75%–1.0%	NA
Opioids[b]		
Fentanyl	50–100 μg	15–25 μg[d]
Sufentanil	5–10 μg	1.5–5 μg[d]
Morphine[c]	NA	125–250 μg[d]
Meperidine[c]	NA	10–20 mg

[a]The volume required to initiate epidural labor analgesia is 10–20 mL of local anesthetic solution.
[b]The local anesthetic dose/concentration and the fentanyl or sufentanil dose are reduced if the drugs are combined or if a local anesthetic-containing epidural test dose is administered before the initial therapeutic dose. The dose of opioid should be reduced, or the opioid omitted, if the parturient has recently received systemic opioid analgesia.
[c]Lidocaine, morphine, and meperidine are not commonly used for labor analgesia because of their short duration of action (lidocaine), long latency (morphine), and high incidence of nausea and vomiting (morphine and meperidine).
[d]Opioids may be administered without local anesthetics when spinal analgesia is induced in early labor. The incidence of pruritus and sedation is dose-dependent. The addition of spinal or epidural local anesthetic is necessary for women in advanced labor.
Note: The suggested doses are based on clinical studies, potency ratios, and clinical experience.
NA, Not applicable.

TABLE 24.3 Comparison of Epidural Bupivacaine 0.125% and 0.25%: Median Effective Volume and Dose

	Bupivacaine 0.125%[a]	Bupivacaine 0.25%[a]
Median Effective Volume[b]		
Up-down analysis (mL)	13.6 (12.4 to 14.8)	9.2 (6.9 to 11.5)
Probit analysis (mL)	13.5 (11.4 to 15.9)	8.6 (7.2 to 10.3)
Median Effective Dose[c]		
Up-down analysis (mg)	17.0 (15.5 to 18.5)	23.1 (17.2 to 28.9)
Probit analysis (mg)	16.8 (14.2 to 19.9)	21.5 (17.9 to 25.7)

[a]95% confidence intervals shown in parentheses, which were calculated using up-down sequential and probit analysis.
[b]Median effective volume at a fixed local anesthetic concentration.
[c]Median effective dose at a fixed local anesthetic concentration.
Modified from Lyons GR, Kocarev MG, Wilson RC, Columb MO. A comparison of minimum local anesthetic volumes and doses of epidural bupivacaine (0.125% w/v and 0.25% w/v) for analgesia in labor. *Anesth Analg.* 2007;104:412–415.

However, many early investigations assumed that ropivacaine and bupivacaine are equipotent; subsequent studies have demonstrated that ropivacaine is 25% to 40% less potent than bupivacaine.[52–54] In one study that characterized the full dose-response curves, the slope of the bupivacaine and ropivacaine curves were similar, suggesting that the nature of the drug-receptor interaction is not different between the two drugs.[54] When ropivacaine concentrations are adjusted for this difference in potency, there is a less clear advantage for ropivacaine in terms of the risk for systemic toxicity.[52] In reality, LAST is not usually a major concern with the contemporary administration of a dilute solution of local anesthetic for epidural labor analgesia.

Early clinical studies suggested that ropivacaine is associated with the desirable characteristic of less motor block than bupivacaine.[55,56] However, these studies also compared equal concentrations of ropivacaine and bupivacaine, and the observed lower degree of motor blockade may reflect the lesser potency of ropivacaine. A study of the relative motor-blocking potencies of epidural ropivacaine and bupivacaine showed that ropivacaine was less potent than bupivacaine in terms of motor blockade,[57] a finding that corresponded to the relative analgesic potencies of the two drugs.[52,53] The differences in potency of motor blockade may not be relevant with the use of low concentrations of local anesthetic. Several clinical studies[58–60] and a well-conducted metaanalysis of studies that compared epidural ropivacaine and bupivacaine[61] did not demonstrate an advantage for ropivacaine in terms of outcome of labor (see later discussion).[59–61]

There is no clear evidence of greater patient safety, lower risk for operative vaginal delivery, or other improved outcomes when ropivacaine is used to provide epidural labor analgesia.[60,62] A 2010 review concluded that there is no advantage to the routine use of ropivacaine compared with bupivacaine for labor analgesia.[62] In contrast, ropivacaine offers greater patient safety in settings in which high concentrations and greater volumes of drugs are administered (e.g., brachial plexus blockade or epidural anesthesia for cesarean delivery).[63]

Like bupivacaine, ropivacaine is often combined with fentanyl or sufentanil for labor analgesia. Ropivacaine concentrations used to initiate epidural analgesia range from 0.08% to 0.2% (see Table 24.2). Higher concentrations are used if the drug is administered without an opioid.

Levobupivacaine. Levobupivacaine is the levorotatory enantiomer of bupivacaine (which is a racemic mixture). It is not available in the United States. Both preclinical and clinical studies have suggested that, like ropivacaine, levobupivacaine has less potential for cardiotoxicity than bupivacaine when equal doses of the two drugs are compared.[64,65] One study found that levobupivacaine was essentially equipotent to bupivacaine with a potency ratio of 0.98; however, the 95% CI was wide (0.67 to 1.41).[66] Other studies have suggested that levobupivacaine and ropivacaine have similar potency.[67,68] In an MLAC study that compared the motor blocking potency of bupivacaine and levobupivacaine,[69] levobupivacaine was less potent than bupivacaine (potency ratio, 0.87; 95% CI, 0.77 to

0.98).[69] Beilin et al. compared epidural bupivacaine, ropivacaine, and levobupivacaine (0.0625% with fentanyl 2 μg/mL*) for labor analgesia and found no differences among groups in obstetric outcomes, although the incidence of motor blockade was lower in the ropivacaine and levobupivacaine groups. Therefore, although epidural bupivacaine is more potent than ropivacaine for both sensory and motor blockade during labor, and may be more potent than levobupivacaine, there do not appear to be any clinical advantages of one drug over the other two drugs for epidural labor analgesia.

Lidocaine. Lidocaine is an amide local anesthetic with a duration of action intermediate between those of bupivacaine and 2-chloroprocaine. During labor, the administration of a 0.75% to 1.0% solution of lidocaine typically provides satisfactory analgesia. However, lidocaine is not commonly used for initiation or maintenance of epidural labor analgesia (except for the epidural test dose), in part because of its shorter duration of action in comparison with bupivacaine, ropivacaine, and levobupivacaine. Lidocaine is less protein-bound than these other amide local anesthetics, and at delivery, the umbilical vein–to–maternal vein lidocaine concentration ratio is approximately twice that of bupivacaine.[70] Early studies discouraged the epidural administration of lidocaine in pregnant women because epidural lidocaine was associated with abnormal neonatal neurobehavioral findings.[71] Subsequently, larger, more carefully controlled studies have demonstrated that the epidural administration of lidocaine, bupivacaine, and 2-chloroprocaine has similar neonatal outcomes.[72,73] Although some investigators have observed subtle differences in neurobehavior between infants exposed to lidocaine and those exposed to other local anesthetics, these differences are within the inherent variability of the examinations and are not clinically significant. Other factors (e.g., mode of delivery) appear to be much more important determinants of neonatal condition.

2-Chloroprocaine. An ester local anesthetic, 2-chloroprocaine has a rapid onset of action. Epidural administration of 10 mL of 2% 2-chloroprocaine provides effective analgesia for approximately 40 minutes. The short duration of action limits its usefulness during labor. In obstetric practice, 2-chloroprocaine is most commonly used for extension of epidural labor analgesia for operative vaginal delivery (see later discussion) or emergency cesarean delivery (see Chapter 26).

---

*The Institute of Safe Medicine Practices has recommended that healthcare providers never use μg as an abbreviation for micrograms, but rather they should use mcg (https://www.ismp.org/sites/default/files/attachments/2017-11/Error%20Prone%20Abbreviations%202015.pdf, Accessed August 11, 2024). The use of the symbol μg is frequently misinterpreted and involved in harmful medication errors. The abbreviation may be mistaken for mg (milligrams), which would result in a 1000-fold overdose. The symbol μg should never be used when communicating medical information, including pharmacy and prescriber computer order entry screens, computer-generated labels, labels for drug storage bins, and medication administration records. However, most scholarly publications have continued to use the abbreviation μg. The editors have chosen to retain the use of the abbreviation μg throughout this text. However, the editors recommend the use of the abbreviation mcg in clinical practice.

Opioids

Lipid-soluble opioids: fentanyl and sufentanil. In contemporary practice, the lipid-soluble opioids play a central role alongside local anesthetics for the provision of neuraxial labor analgesia. The addition of lipid-soluble opioids to local anesthetics shortens latency and improves quality of analgesia. Permeability (of the dura-arachnoid) is not a rate-limiting factor; increasing the concentration gradient (by administration of a larger dose) facilitates faster entry into the spinal cord. The high lipid solubility of these agents also results in a shorter duration of action and greater systemic absorption than occurs with water-soluble drugs.

Some investigators have suggested that the improved analgesia results from a supraspinal action rather than a primary spinal action. However, several studies have refuted this, including studies of epidural opioid administration by bolus[74] and continuous infusion.[75] Vella et al.[74] observed that the initiation of epidural analgesia with 0.25% bupivacaine with *epidural* fentanyl 80 μg resulted in more rapid, complete, and prolonged analgesia than *intravenous* fentanyl 80 μg, even though plasma fentanyl concentrations were higher in the intravenous group. Similarly, D'Angelo et al.[75] demonstrated that a CEI but not an intravenous infusion of fentanyl reduced epidural bupivacaine requirements in laboring women. Polley et al.[76] determined that the MLAC of epidural bupivacaine administered as a 20-mL bolus in laboring women was reduced from 0.064% to 0.034% when epidural rather than intravenous fentanyl was coadministered with bupivacaine. Ginosar et al.[77] determined that the MLAC of bupivacaine administered by *CEI* during labor was lower by a factor of three when it was coadministered with an epidural (rather than intravenous) fentanyl infusion. Finally, in a volunteer study,[78] lumbar epidural *bolus* administration of fentanyl resulted in tolerance of experimental pain at a lumbar but not a cranial dermatome, whereas lumbar epidural fentanyl *infusion* resulted in pain tolerance at both dermatomes, suggesting vascular absorption and a systemic effect of the fentanyl. Thus, the site(s) of action of fentanyl after epidural administration may depend on dose and mode of administration.

Pain and analgesic requirements are highly variable and depend on several factors, including parity, stage of labor, presence of ruptured membranes, and oxytocin augmentation. One study reported that the ED_{50} of epidural sufentanil was higher in women undergoing prostaglandin induction of labor than in women with spontaneous labor.[79] Conell-Price et al.[80] developed a model of labor pain in nulliparous women and found that the use of oxytocin was associated with 48% more pain at the start of labor.

The high doses of epidural fentanyl or sufentanil required to provide complete labor analgesia (administered alone without local anesthetic) are associated with significant adverse effects. Capogna et al.[81] sought to determine the median effective analgesic dose (ED_{50}) of epidural fentanyl and sufentanil alone (no local anesthetic) for the initiation of epidural analgesia in nulliparous women with a cervical dilation between 2 and 4 cm. The ED_{50} of fentanyl was 124 μg (95% CI, 118 to 131 μg), and the ED_{50} of sufentanil was 21 μg (95% CI, 20 to

22 μg), with a potency ratio of 5.9:1. Pruritus and sedation were common; side effects precluded significant dose escalation to establish the ED_{95} or to manage analgesia for more advanced labor.

Lipophilic opioids and local anesthetics have dose-sparing effects when combined. Indeed, even the lidocaine epidural test dose appears to augment the efficacy of a lipophilic opioid bolus to establish analgesia. In a study comparing sufentanil alone, sufentanil with bupivacaine, and bupivacaine alone,[82] women randomly assigned to the sufentanil-alone (30 μg) group experienced satisfactory analgesia after the initial dose but not after subsequent doses. In this study, the initial dose was administered after an epidural test dose that contained lidocaine 60 mg. A second study compared the administration of epidural fentanyl or sufentanil immediately after a lidocaine 45-mg/epinephrine 15-μg test dose for the initiation of analgesia for women in early labor.[83] There were no differences in analgesic onset, quality, or duration between women randomly assigned to receive either fentanyl 100 μg or sufentanil 20 μg, with both groups experiencing effective pain relief that lasted, on average, more than 2 hours.[83] In a third study, when epidural fentanyl 100 μg was administered after a lidocaine and epinephrine test dose, the diluent volume (2 to 20 mL) did not affect the onset or duration of epidural labor analgesia, with analgesia lasting approximately 2 hours in all groups.[84] This finding differs from local anesthetic solutions, where higher volumes of more dilute solutions have dose-sparing effects (Table 24.3).

In clinical practice, either fentanyl or sufentanil is frequently combined with a low-concentration, long-acting amide local anesthetic to both initiate and maintain epidural labor analgesia. The addition of a lipid-soluble opioid to a local anesthetic for neuraxial labor analgesia decreases latency, prolongs the duration of analgesia, and improves the quality of analgesia.[85–87] For example, 86% of women rated their analgesia as excellent after epidural analgesia was initiated with bupivacaine combined with sufentanil, compared with 50% of those who received bupivacaine without sufentanil.[86] The percentage of women who experienced no or short periods of pain during the first stage of labor was 94% in women who received sufentanil and 76% in women who did not.[88] After initiation of analgesia with 0.125% bupivacaine with epinephrine 1.25 μg/mL, 43% of women randomly assigned to receive epidural fentanyl 100 μg rated their analgesia as excellent, compared with 6% in a control group that did not receive fentanyl.[87]

Epidural opioid administration allows the anesthesia provider to use a more dilute solution of local anesthetic to initiate epidural labor analgesia.[89] Epidural fentanyl and sufentanil decrease epidural bupivacaine requirement during labor in a dose-dependent fashion (Fig. 24.2).[47,90] The reduction in MLAC by the addition of fentanyl or sufentanil is observed with levobupivacaine,[91,92] ropivacaine,[92,93] and 2-chloroprocaine[94] as well as bupivacaine.

The dose-sparing effects of fentanyl and sufentanil are also evident when the drugs are combined with a low-concentration solution of bupivacaine used for the maintenance of analgesia

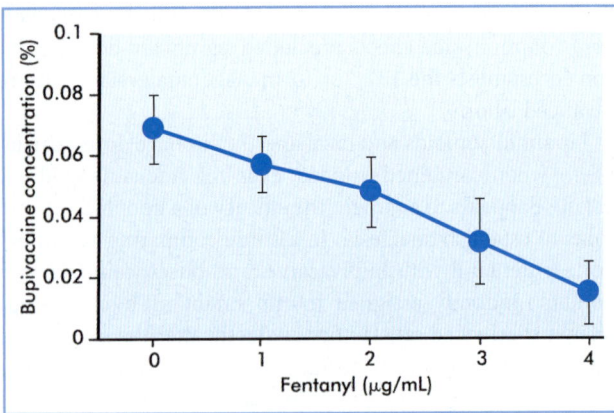

Fig. 24.2 The effect of epidural fentanyl on the minimum local anesthetic concentration (defined as the effective concentration in 50% of subjects [EC_{50}] for epidural bupivacaine analgesia during labor. Data are expressed as median concentrations with 95% confidence intervals. Data from Lyons G, Columb M, Hawthorne L, Dresner M. Extradural pain relief in labour: bupivacaine sparing by extradural fentanyl is dose dependent. *Br J Anaesth.* 1997;78:493–496.

throughout labor. For example, in women randomly assigned to receive bupivacaine/epinephrine with or without fentanyl 100 μg, the total bupivacaine dose was 55 or 110 mg, respectively.[87] The advantages of a lower total dose of local anesthetic include (1) decreased risk for LAST, (2) decreased risk for high- or total-spinal anesthesia, (3) decreased plasma concentrations of local anesthetic in the fetus and neonate, and (4) decreased intensity of motor blockade.

There are few rigorous *dose-response* studies of epidural fentanyl or sufentanil combined with bupivacaine for initiation of epidural labor analgesia. Herman et al.[95] randomly assigned 100 laboring women with a cervical dilation of 5 cm or less to receive 0.125% bupivacaine 10 mL, combined with fentanyl 0 to 100 μg (in 25-μg increments) or sufentanil 0 to 25 μg (in 5-μg increments), injected after a negative epidural test dose (bupivacaine 7.5 mg with epinephrine 15 μg). Using probit analysis, these researchers calculated the effective dose in 95% of subjects (ED_{95}) to be 50 μg for fentanyl and 8 μg for sufentanil; these figures equate to a sufentanil-to-fentanyl potency ratio of 6.3:1. Therefore, data suggest that the potency ratio of sufentanil to fentanyl administered into the epidural space is approximately 6:1, regardless of whether administered in the presence[95] or absence[81] of a local anesthetic solution.

The range of fentanyl and sufentanil doses used for the initiation of epidural labor analgesia is shown in Table 24.2. It is not clear whether higher doses of epidural lipophilic opioid (e.g., fentanyl 100 versus 50 μg) provide superior analgesia.[86,87,96,97] Data are inconsistent, but overall suggest that higher doses result in more pruritus and neonatal depression (see later discussion). Current evidence supports the administration of epidural opioid doses at the lower end of the dose range, which are frequently sufficient for nulliparous women, for women in early labor, or when the opioid is coadministered with a local anesthetic. Fortunately, with a catheter-based epidural technique, relatively conservative initial doses

may be augmented with additional local anesthetic and lipophilic opioid solution through the epidural catheter if satisfactory analgesia is not achieved with the initial bolus dose.

Other opioids. **Morphine** was one of the first opioids used for labor analgesia. However, the inconsistent analgesia, long latency (30 to 60 minutes), along with the introduction of lipid-soluble opioids and epidural infusion pumps into clinical practice, have made the use of epidural morphine for continuous labor analgesia largely obsolete.

Several groups of investigators have reported the use of epidural **hydromorphone** for labor analgesia.[98–100] The lipid solubility of hydromorphone lies between those of morphine and fentanyl, but is closer to that of morphine (see Table 13.3).[101] In a large prospective observational study, effective labor analgesia was obtained by initiating analgesia with 0.25% bupivacaine (20 to 25 mg) with epinephrine (40 to 50 μg), followed by hydromorphone 100 μg.[98] However, Mhyre[100] observed that effective labor analgesia could not be provided by 0.035% bupivacaine (7 mg) with hydromorphone 100 to 110 μg. In another trial, parturients were randomly assigned to receive either epidural hydromorphone 300 μg or saline-control immediately after the initiation of analgesia with lidocaine 45 mg, epinephrine 15 μg, and fentanyl 100 μg.[99] The duration of analgesia and side effects were similar in the two groups. At the current time, further investigation is required before hydromorphone can be recommended for epidural labor analgesia.

Meperidine may be used effectively alone (without a local anesthetic), in part because it possesses local anesthetic properties.[102] When given during labor, epidural meperidine 100 mg provides analgesia similar to that provided by 0.25% bupivacaine, with less motor blockade. However, this dose of epidural meperidine produces more sedation, nausea, and pruritus than epidural bupivacaine. Handley and Perkins[103] observed that the addition of meperidine 25 mg to 0.125%, 0.187%, or 0.25% bupivacaine (10 mL) provided adequate analgesia for the first stage of labor. Epidural administration of meperidine effectively prevents or treats the shivering that often occurs during labor.[104] Massad et al. randomly allocated women to receive 0.1% bupivacaine with either meperidine 1 mg/mL or fentanyl 2 μg/mL.[105] No differences were noted between groups in analgesic characteristics, except that women in the meperidine group had a higher incidence of nausea and vomiting. Currently there is no evidence that meperidine alone or in combination with bupivacaine has any advantages over a combination of a long-acting amide local anesthetic and a lipid-soluble opioid.

Several studies described the use of **alfentanil** with bupivacaine for labor analgesia.[106,107] Alfentanil has lower lipid solubility than both fentanyl and sufentanil. Only a few small studies have compared alfentanil with other opioids for labor analgesia.

Butorphanol is a lipid-soluble opioid agonist-antagonist with weak μ-receptor and strong κ-receptor activity. Because κ-opioid receptors appear to be involved in the modulation of visceral pain, κ-receptor agonists may be useful agents for the relief of labor pain, which has a significant visceral component (see Chapter 21).[108–110] Somnolence is the most prominent side effect of epidural butorphanol. The addition of butorphanol 1, 2, or 3 mg to 0.25% bupivacaine (25 mg) shortened latency and prolonged the duration of analgesia in comparison with epidural bupivacaine alone in one study.[109] The investigators concluded that the optimal dose of butorphanol was 2 mg. Of concern was the observation of a transient sinusoidal FHR pattern in the 3-mg group that was not unlike that seen after the intravenous administration of butorphanol.[110] However, there was no difference among groups in Apgar scores, umbilical cord blood gas and pH measurements, or neurobehavioral scores. Similarly, Abboud et al.[108] observed that the addition of butorphanol 1 or 2 mg to 0.25% bupivacaine resulted in better quality and longer duration of analgesia than the epidural administration of bupivacaine alone, without maternal or neonatal side effects. However, some anesthesia providers have noted that the epidural administration of butorphanol results in somnolence and occasional dysphoria, which are side effects of κ-receptor stimulation.

Diamorphine (heroin) is available for epidural analgesia in the United Kingdom. Using isobolographic analysis, McLeod et al.[111] concluded that the combination of diamorphine and levobupivacaine is additive when used for first-stage labor analgesia. Several studies from the United Kingdom have reported diamorphine doses between 250 and 500 µg/h (i.e., diamorphine 25 to 50 µg/mL combined with a low concentration of bupivacaine).[106,112] Whether diamorphine offers any advantages over fentanyl or sufentanil has not been studied. It is not available for clinical administration in the United States.

Adjuvants

Although the contemporary mainstay of epidural labor analgesia includes administration of a long-acting amide local anesthetic combined with a lipid-soluble opioid, other drugs may be added as adjuvants. Adjuvants may prolong the duration of analgesia or decrease the required anesthetic dose, thus reducing the risk for specific side effects.

Epinephrine. Some anesthesia providers add a low dose of epinephrine (1.25 to 5 µg/mL [1:800,000 to 1:200,000]) to the local anesthetic solution (Table 24.4). The addition of epinephrine shortens the latency and prolongs the duration of epidural bupivacaine analgesia.[113,114] The MLAC of bupivacaine with epinephrine (66 µg) was reported to be 29% lower than that of bupivacaine without epinephrine,[115] perhaps as a result of the stimulation of alpha-adrenergic receptors in the spinal cord.

The addition of epinephrine to the local anesthetic has a variable effect on the systemic uptake of the local anesthetic in obstetric patients.[116–118] The systemic absorption of epinephrine may increase maternal heart rate and transiently decrease uterine activity as a result of betaadrenergic receptor stimulation.[113,119,120] However, some studies have shown that the addition of epinephrine to bupivacaine, lidocaine, or levobupivacaine does not result in longer labor than the epidural administration of bupivacaine or lidocaine without epinephrine[119,121] or levobupivacaine-sufentanil without epinephrine.[122] Epidural administration of an epinephrine-containing local anesthetic solution does not adversely affect intervillous blood flow[123] or neonatal outcome.[114,116,122] One disadvantage of the use of epinephrine is that it increases the intensity of motor blockade.[121,122] The addition of epinephrine may improve the efficacy of epidural opioids,[124] but the enhanced effect is insufficient to make the use of epidural opioids (without local anesthetic) an attractive regimen for the duration of labor. Finally, the addition of a third drug to the local anesthetic/opioid solution may increase the risk for drug error and contamination. For these reasons, we do not routinely administer epinephrine-containing local anesthetic solutions during labor. However, other anesthesia providers have a different view, and some consider epinephrine a useful adjuvant, especially when added to a very dilute solution of local anesthetic with an opioid.

Clonidine. Analgesia is enhanced by the direct stimulation of alpha$_2$-adrenergic receptors and the inhibition of neurotransmitter release in the dorsal horn of the spinal cord (see Chapter 21). Evidence is accumulating that the interaction of clonidine with opioids is synergistic for producing analgesia.[125] Epidural administration of clonidine alone provides modest analgesia. Studies have evaluated the epidural administration of clonidine as an adjuvant to a local anesthetic alone,[126–129] to local anesthetic and opioid combinations,[130–134]

TABLE 24.4 Adjuncts to Neuraxial Labor Analgesia

| Adjunct Drug | EPIDURAL ANALGESIA | | SPINAL ANALGESIA |
	Initiation Bolus Dose[a]	Maintenance Infusion Dose[a]	Initiation Bolus Dose
Epinephrine	25–75 µg[b]	25–50 µg/h[b]	2.25–200 µg
Clonidine	75–100 µg	10–30 µg/h[c]	15–30 µg
Neostigmine	500–750 µg	25–75 µg/h[d]	NR
Morphine	NA	NA	100–250 µg (0.1–0.25 mg)

[a]Adjuncts are usually coadministered with a low-concentration local anesthetic solution (e.g., bupivacaine < 0.08%), often with a lipid-soluble opioid. There is extensive experience with epidural clonidine for labor analgesia in some European countries but less overall experience with epidural neostigmine.
[b]Usually administered in a 1:800,000 to 1:200,000 solution (1.25–5 µg/mL).
[c]Administered in a concentration of 0.75–1.5 µg/mL.
[d]Administered in a concentration of 4 µg/mL.
NA, Not applicable; *NR*, not recommended.

to fentanyl,[135] and to neostigmine (see later discussion).[136,137] Clonidine 60 µg, but not 30 µg, decreased the MLAC of ropivacaine by approximately two-thirds.[138] In another study,[128] clonidine 75 µg and sufentanil 5 µg both reduced the MLAC of ropivacaine by about two-thirds. Unlike epinephrine, clonidine does not increase the motor blockade that results from the epidural administration of a local anesthetic, but it does potentiate both the quality and duration of analgesia.[130–134] However, in a warning on the package insert, the manufacturer of Duraclon (the epidural clonidine formulation approved by the US Food and Drug Administration [FDA]) recommends against its use in obstetric patients because of the risk for hypotension[129–131,134,138] and bradycardia. Most studies, however, have found that the hypotension is readily amenable to treatment. An additional side effect is maternal sedation.[131,132,138] High epidural doses (>150 µg) may be associated with FHR changes,[130] although no adverse fetal effects have been observed with lower doses.

Clonidine is not often used for labor analgesia in North America, but it is more widely used in some European countries. It may be particularly useful in women in whom other epidural analgesics are contraindicated; in those who have breakthrough pain with standard local anesthetic/opioid solutions, despite a functioning epidural catheter; or in those with opioid tolerance. In this circumstance, additional local anesthetic will result in motor blockade but clonidine will not.

Dexmedetomidine. Dexmedetomidine is a selective alpha$_2$-adrenergic receptor agonist. Administered systemically, it has sedative, anxiolytic, and mild analgesia effects. Investigators have explored its use as an adjuvant to epidural local anesthetics. Studies performed largely in China in which dexmedetomidine (doses 0.5 to 1.0 µg/kg) has primarily been combined with epidural ropivacaine have demonstrated lower pain scores, but a higher incidence of bradycardia in women randomized to receive epidural dexmedetomidine compared to plain ropivacaine.[139] Heterogeneity among studies was high. Dexmedetomidine is not approved for neuraxial administration by the US FDA and rigorous neurotoxicity studies have not been performed. Further investigation is required before dexmedetomidine can be recommended for routine labor analgesia.

Neostigmine. Neostigmine inhibits the breakdown of acetylcholine within the spinal cord. Acetylcholine binds to both nicotinic (amplifying neurotransmitter release) and muscarinic receptors (inhibiting neurotransmitter release). On balance, the net effect of acetylcholine appears to be inhibitory, resulting in analgesia (see Chapter 21). Roelants et al.[140] randomly assigned parturients to receive either epidural ropivacaine (20 mg) alone or epidural neostigmine (4 µg/kg) combined with ropivacaine 10 mg, with or without sufentanil 10 µg for initiation of labor analgesia. The magnitude and duration of analgesia in the ropivacaine/neostigmine group were similar to that of the plain ropivacaine group but less than in the ropivacaine/sufentanil group. Neostigmine is hydrophilic, and the researchers hypothesized that only a small portion of the epidural dose penetrates the spinal cord.[140] In a subsequent study, the same researchers compared epidural sufentanil 20 µg with sufentanil 10 µg combined with neostigmine 250, 500, or 750 µg for initiation of analgesia in women in early labor.[141] Neostigmine 250 µg with sufentanil was ineffective, but both 500 and 750 µg of neostigmine produced effective analgesia similar in duration to that obtained with sufentanil alone.

Because animal studies suggest a synergistic antinociceptive effect of spinal alpha$_2$-adrenergic receptor agonists and cholinesterase inhibitors,[142] researchers have also investigated epidural neostigmine combined with clonidine.[136,137,143] The combination of clonidine 75 µg with neostigmine 500 or 750 µg for initiation of epidural labor analgesia provided acceptable analgesia in approximately 80% of parturients.[136] Epidural neostigmine 500 µg combined with clonidine 75 µg prolonged labor analgesia initiated with spinal ropivacaine and sufentanil.[137,143] In another study, maintenance of epidural analgesia with a solution of neostigmine 4 µg/mL combined with bupivacaine 0.125% resulted in a 19% reduction in bupivacaine consumption compared with administration of bupivacaine alone.[144] Booth et al.[145] randomized laboring women to receive initiation and maintenance of epidural analgesia with 0.125% bupivacaine, combined with fentanyl 2 µg/mL or neostigmine 2, 4, or 8 µg/mL. Hourly bupivacaine consumption and patient satisfaction did not differ among groups.

Taken together, the studies have not identified any significant adverse maternal or neonatal effects of epidural neostigmine, but neither is there compelling evidence to suggest a benefit for its use compared with the usual local anesthetic and lipid-soluble opioid combination typically used for labor analgesia. It may be useful for the treatment of breakthrough pain during maintenance epidural analgesia with local anesthetic and opioid. Neostigmine is not approved for neuraxial administration in the United States.

Summary

Epidural labor analgesia is usually initiated with the bolus injection of a local anesthetic combined with a lipid-soluble opioid. The advantages of the addition of an opioid to an epidural solution of local anesthetic include (1) lower total dose of anesthetic, (2) decreased motor blockade, and (3) greater patient satisfaction. Some anesthesia providers contend that local anesthetic–opioid techniques result in a lower risk for hypotension, but this belief is unproven. There are no clinically significant differences among the three commonly used, long-acting amide local anesthetics (bupivacaine, ropivacaine, levobupivacaine), or between fentanyl and sufentanil. Other adjuvants (e.g., epinephrine, clonidine) may prove useful in selected patients. High-volume/low-concentration local anesthetic solutions compared with low-volume/high-concentration solutions are associated with a lower dose requirement and better analgesia.

INITIATION OF SPINAL ANALGESIA

Initiation of neuraxial analgesia with the intrathecal injection of an opioid, or an opioid combined with a local anesthetic, usually performed as part of a CSE technique, results in a rapid onset of analgesia with a low dose of drug(s) (see Table 24.2). The onset of effective spinal analgesia occurs faster than epidural analgesia, and more women have effective analgesia at 10 minutes.[20] Intrathecal opioids can provide complete analgesia during early labor when the pain stimuli are primarily visceral. An intrathecal local anesthetic without an opioid is not commonly used for labor analgesia. Doses high enough to provide analgesia are associated with significant motor blockade, and lower doses either do not provide satisfactory analgesia or are associated with an unacceptably short duration of analgesia.[146,147] A lipid-soluble opioid is combined with a local anesthetic (bupivacaine, ropivacaine, or levobupivacaine) when sacral analgesia is necessary for complete analgesia (e.g., initiation of analgesia during the active first stage or the second stage of labor). The interaction between intrathecal local anesthetics and opioids is synergistic.[148] Like the combination of an epidural local anesthetic with an opioid, the combination of an intrathecal opioid with a local anesthetic results in better quality and longer duration of analgesia,[149,150] as well as a lower dose requirement for both drugs, compared with either drug used alone.[146,147,151]

Choice of Drugs

Opioids

Fentanyl and sufentanil. The two opioids most commonly used for initiation of spinal labor analgesia are fentanyl and sufentanil. When administered alone in early labor, intrathecal fentanyl and sufentanil provide complete analgesia without a sympathectomy or motor blockade. This is a particularly useful technique for patients in whom a sudden decrease in preload (secondary to neuraxial local anesthetic–induced sympathectomy) might not be well tolerated (e.g., patient with a stenotic heart lesion).

Studies have reported the ED_{50} of intrathecal fentanyl for labor analgesia varying from 5.5 to 18 µg.[152–154] The wide range of published values may be explained by differences in patient population (e.g., parity), cervical dilation at initiation of analgesia, and the definition of successful analgesia. Herman et al.[154] determined that the ED_{95} of intrathecal fentanyl for parturients of mixed parity in early labor (cervical dilation ≤ 5 cm) was 17.4 µg (95% CI, 13.8 to 27.1 µg). The duration of analgesia is dose dependent but plateaus at 80 to 90 minutes after administration of 15 to 25 µg of fentanyl (Fig. 24.3).[152] There does not appear to be any reason to administer doses higher than 25 µg because side effects (e.g., pruritus, respiratory depression) are also dose dependent.[146,152,154]

The reported ED_{50} of intrathecal sufentanil for labor analgesia varies from 1.8 to 4.1 µg,[155–158] and the ED_{95} varies from 8 to 10 µg.[155,158] A comparison of the potencies of fentanyl and sufentanil using ED_{50} estimates from different studies is difficult because of the differences in patient populations and the definition of efficacy. In a single-center study, the relative potency ratio of intrathecal sufentanil to fentanyl for labor analgesia was estimated to be 4.4:1.[153] When the drugs were administered at twice the ED_{50} (fentanyl 36 µg, sufentanil 8 µg), the duration of sufentanil analgesia was 25 minutes

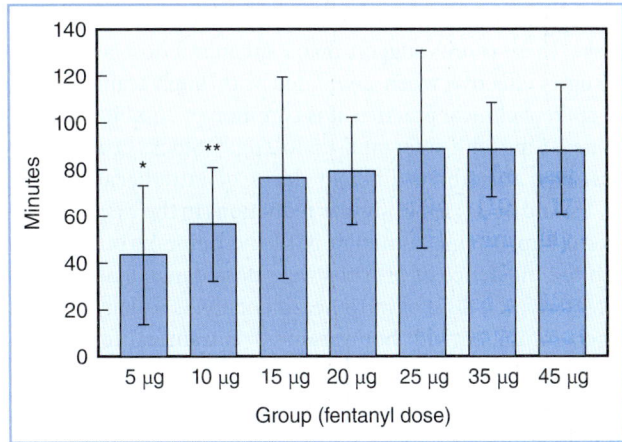

Fig. 24.3 Duration of intrathecal fentanyl analgesia (mean ± SD) among nulliparous women in active labor who received 5, 10, 15, 20, 25, 35, or 45 µg. Duration of analgesia (time from intrathecal dose to first request for additional analgesia) differed significantly among the groups (analysis of variance, $P < .005$). *$P < .05$ versus groups 15 to 45 µg; **$P < .05$ versus groups 25 to 45 µg. From Palmer CM, Cork RC, Hays R, et al. The dose-response relationship of intrathecal fentanyl for labor analgesia. *Anesthesiology*. 1998;88:355–361.

longer than that of fentanyl analgesia (104 versus 79 minutes), although the incidence of side effects was not different.[153]

Investigators have studied whether genetic variability in the µ-opioid receptor *OPRM1* influences intrathecal opioid analgesia. Data are conflicting. Landau et al.[159] found that nulliparous women who were heterozygous or homozygous for A118G had a lower ED_{50} for intrathecal fentanyl (18 µg, 95% CI, 13 to 22 µg) than women homozygous for the wild-type allele (A118) (27 µg, 95% CI, 23 to 31 µg). However, in two other studies assessing the duration of intrathecal fentanyl labor analgesia,[160,161] no difference in the duration of analgesia in women with the A118G allele compared with women who were homozygous for the wild-type allele was identified. Thus, the clinical implications of genetic polymorphisms of *OPRM1* on labor analgesia remain unclear.[162]

Typically, an intrathecal opioid injection for labor analgesia is administered as part of a CSE technique. Maintenance epidural analgesia is usually initiated soon after initiation of spinal analgesia. Therefore, the duration of intrathecal analgesia is relatively less important. Nelson et al.[153] concluded, and we concur, that the longer duration of sufentanil analgesia in comparison with fentanyl analgesia does not necessarily justify the former's use. Other factors, such as cost and the greater risk for a drug dose error with sufentanil (because of its greater potency), should be considered. In some European countries, sufentanil is available in a dilute concentration (5 µg/mL), possibly making it easier and safer to use.

Intrathecal fentanyl (or sufentanil) is often coadministered with an amide local anesthetic (see later discussion) (see Table 24.2). The addition of a local anesthetic to intrathecal fentanyl or sufentanil markedly decreases the dose of opioid necessary to produce analgesia. Wong et al.[146] randomly assigned parous women to receive intrathecal bupivacaine 2.5 mg and intrathecal sufentanil 0, 2.5, 5, 7.5, or 10 µg, followed by a standard epidural test dose. There were no differences among the sufentanil groups in quality and duration of analgesia. These results suggest that a sufentanil dose as small as 2.5 µg is effective when combined with bupivacaine 2.5 mg. In current clinical practice, it is common to combine bupivacaine 2.5 mg with sufentanil 1.5 to 2 µg.[163] Stocks et al.[150] demonstrated that three different doses of intrathecal fentanyl (5, 15, and 25 µg) led to similar reductions in the ED_{50} of intrathecal bupivacaine, although both the duration of analgesia and the incidence of pruritus were dose dependent. As with sufentanil, the dose of intrathecal fentanyl is usually reduced when combined with bupivacaine.[147] Intrathecal fentanyl 10 to 15 µg, combined with bupivacaine 1.25 to 2.5 mg, provides effective analgesia for most parturients.

Other opioids. Early studies demonstrated that the intrathecal administration of 0.5 to 2 mg of **morphine** reliably produced analgesia during the first stage of labor, but the analgesia was less reliable during the second stage of labor and during operative vaginal delivery.[164,165] However, intrathecal administration of these relatively large doses of morphine resulted in a high incidence of side effects, including somnolence, nausea and vomiting, pruritus, and respiratory depression. In addition, the onset of analgesia is slower with intrathecal morphine than with lipid-soluble opioids, and the long duration of action may be a disadvantage (e.g., side effects may persist for many hours after delivery). Abouleish[166] reported a case of life-threatening respiratory depression 1 hour after delivery and 7 hours after the administration of 1 mg of hyperbaric intrathecal morphine.

In several studies,[167–169] *low-dose* morphine (0.1 to 0.25 mg) was successfully combined with intrathecal bupivacaine (2 to 2.5 mg) and fentanyl (12.5 to 25 µg); the combination resulted in short latency of onset and a prolonged duration of analgesia. In contrast, a single study from Sweden[170] found no advantage to adding morphine 0.05 or 0.1 mg to bupivacaine 1.25 mg and sufentanil 5 µg. The addition of low-dose morphine to intrathecal bupivacaine and a lipid-soluble opioid may be useful in low-resource settings in which CEI techniques are impractical (see Chapter 15).[29,171]

When used as part of a CSE technique, the addition of intrathecal morphine to bupivacaine and fentanyl has been shown to result in less breakthrough pain during labor[167–169] as well as decreased analgesic use in the first 24 hours postpartum, compared with intrathecal bupivacaine and fentanyl without morphine.[167,168] The incidence of intrapartum side effects was similar[167,169]; however, the morphine group had a higher incidence of postpartum nausea (17% versus 0% for no morphine).[167]

An alternative drug is **meperidine**. Meperidine is unique among the opioids in that it possesses weak local anesthetic properties at analgesic doses,[102] and it has been used in large doses (e.g., 1 mg/kg) as the sole agent to provide spinal anesthesia for surgical procedures. Intrathecal administration of meperidine (10 to 20 mg) results in effective labor analgesia within 2 to 12 minutes, with a duration of 1 to 3 hours. Honet et al.[172] compared the efficacy of intrathecal meperidine 10 mg, fentanyl 10 µg, and sufentanil 5 µg in 65 laboring women. The three drugs were similar in onset of analgesia (<5 minutes)

and duration of effective analgesia (80 to 100 minutes). However, the meperidine group had significantly lower pain scores after cervical dilation had progressed beyond 6 cm. As labor advances, somatic pain plays an increasing role. Only meperidine also functions as a local anesthetic, perhaps explaining why meperidine provided more effective analgesia during advanced labor, including the second stage. However, intrathecal meperidine is associated with a significantly higher incidence of nausea and vomiting than a combination of fentanyl and bupivacaine for labor analgesia.[173] Therefore, intrathecal meperidine does not seem to offer any advantages over bupivacaine-fentanyl for routine intrathecal analgesia, although it may be useful for the rare patient with a contraindication to bupivacaine-fentanyl administration.

In the United Kingdom, some anesthesia providers have advocated the intrathecal administration of **diamorphine** for labor analgesia, although it is not commonly used for this purpose. This drug is not available for clinical use in the United States. Kestin et al.[174] observed that the intrathecal administration of diamorphine (0.2 to 0.5 mg) provided good to excellent analgesia in 90% of laboring women. The mean duration of analgesia was approximately 100 minutes. However, 75% of patients had pruritus, nausea, and vomiting. In contrast, Vaughan et al.[175] randomly assigned parturients to receive intrathecal bupivacaine 2.5 mg with either fentanyl 25 µg or diamorphine 0.25 mg. The duration of analgesia was longer in the diamorphine group, but the incidence of side effects was low in both groups.

Local Anesthetics

In the late first stage and the second stage of labor, a local anesthetic must be added to the spinal opioid to block somatic stimuli from the vagina and perineum caused by descent of the fetus. The local anesthetic works synergistically with the opioid, so lower doses of both drugs can be used.[146–148,150,176] **Bupivacaine** is most commonly combined with fentanyl or sufentanil. The ED_{95} of bupivacaine was 3.3 mg when combined with sufentanil 1.5 µg[163] and 1.7 mg when combined with fentanyl 15 µg.[177] Intrathecal bupivacaine doses between 1.25 and 2.5 mg are commonly used. Levobupivacaine and ropivacaine are not usually used for intrathecal injection in the United States. They are less potent than bupivacaine for intrathecal labor analgesia (Fig. 24.4).[163,178] Spinal lidocaine has not been studied for use in labor analgesia, but it is unlikely to have any advantages compared with other, longer-acting amide local anesthetics. Common doses of spinal local anesthetics are shown in Table 24.2.

Controversy exists as to whether the lower incidence and degree of motor blockade associated with ropivacaine and levobupivacaine[59,178] are a result of their inherent difference in potency or of greater sensory-motor separation with the S(−)-enantiomer drugs.[163] Camorcia et al.[178] have suggested that, especially during intrathecal use, ropivacaine may be associated with less motor blockade than bupivacaine, even when equipotent doses (e.g., 3.6-mg ropivacaine and 2.4-mg bupivacaine) are administered. However, this difference, even if it exists, is unlikely to have any clinical significance during

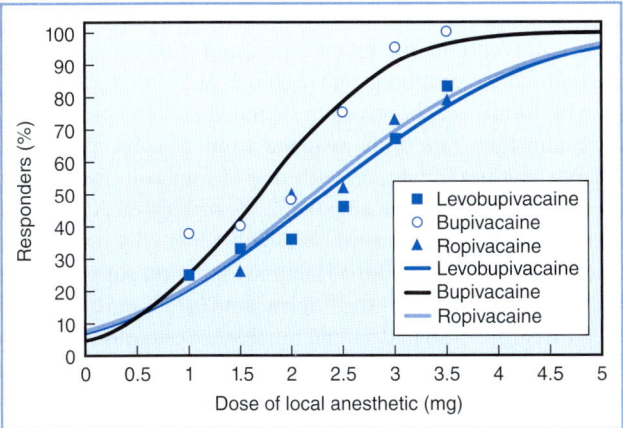

Fig. 24.4 Predicted *(lines)* and observed *(symbols)* dose-response of intrathecal bupivacaine, levobupivacaine, and ropivacaine combined with sufentanil 1.5 μg in 450 laboring women. The dose-response curves were constructed using probit regression and compared using likelihood ratio tests. No difference was observed between ropivacaine and levobupivacaine. Significant differences were observed between bupivacaine and ropivacaine ($P = .003$) and bupivacaine and levobupivacaine ($P < .001$). From Van de Velde M, Dreelinck R, Dubois J, et al. Determination of the full dose-response relation of intrathecal bupivacaine, levobupivacaine, and ropivacaine, combined with sufentanil, for labor analgesia. *Anesthesiology.* 2007;106:149–156.

spinal labor analgesia because all local anesthetics administered for this purpose are administered in low doses that lead to minimal motor blockade.

Data are conflicting as to whether there is a dose-response relationship between hypotension and intrathecal local anesthetics when these drugs are administered in low doses for labor analgesia. Palmer et al.[179] found no difference in blood pressure in women randomly assigned to receive intrathecal fentanyl combined with either 1.25 or 2.5 mg of bupivacaine. In contrast, Lee et al.[180] noted a greater decrease in blood pressure at 10 minutes in women who received bupivacaine 2.5 mg than in women who received 1.25 mg.

Baricity of the intrathecal solution. The plain local anesthetic/opioid solutions commonly injected for intrathecal labor analgesia have lower specific gravity relative to that of CSF and hence are hypobaric.[181] The extent of cephalad sensory blockade is higher for spinal analgesia initiated with the parturient in the sitting position than in the lateral position.[182] Adding dextrose to the solution (opioid alone or opioid with local anesthetic) to make the solution hyperbaric results in less extensive sensory blockade but also in inadequate analgesia.[183-185] It is probably necessary for the opioid to penetrate the spinal cord rather than just the nerve roots; therefore, injection of a hyperbaric solution of opioid and local anesthetic below the level of the spinal cord may lead to inadequate analgesia, even though the local anesthetic provides sensory blockade to the T10 dermatome.

Intrathecal Adjuvants

Several drugs have been investigated as adjuvants to local anesthetics, opioids, or combinations of local anesthetics and opioids for intrathecal labor analgesia (see Table 24.4). In one study, the addition of **clonidine** 30 μg to sufentanil (2.5 to 5 μg)

prolonged the duration of analgesia from 104 to 145 minutes without a motor block.[186] Other investigators have had similar results when clonidine was combined with sufentanil,[187] bupivacaine/ropivacaine, and sufentanil.[188,189] Intrathecal clonidine alone also provides analgesia.[190] A disadvantage of clonidine is the high incidence of maternal hypotension and sedation as well as FHR abnormalities. The slightly longer duration of analgesia provided by the addition of clonidine to bupivacaine and sufentanil is not an advantage when maintenance analgesia is provided via a catheter sited in the epidural space. Therefore, at present, intrathecal clonidine cannot be recommended for routine spinal labor analgesia, although it might be considered in parturients with tolerance to opioids or contraindications to the use of other drugs.

Adding intrathecal **neostigmine** to sufentanil, bupivacaine/sufentanil, or clonidine has been found to potentiate the analgesia and prolong its duration.[191,192] However, intrathecal neostigmine was associated with a markedly higher incidence of severe nausea that was unresponsive to standard antiemetics.[191,192] Therefore, neostigmine cannot be recommended as an adjuvant for intrathecal labor analgesia.

Analgesia is prolonged by 15 to 40 minutes when **epinephrine** is added to intrathecal bupivacaine-opioid.[193-195] Even an epinephrine dose as low as 2.25 μg prolonged analgesia by 15 minutes.[194] However, epinephrine 200 μg combined with bupivacaine 2.5 mg and sufentanil 10 μg resulted in a significant incidence of motor blockade[193]; epinephrine doses between 12.5 and 100 μg prolonged analgesia without any difference in the quality of analgesia.[195]

In summary, no adjuvant studied to date prolongs the duration of intrathecal fentanyl or sufentanil/bupivacaine analgesia long enough to avoid the use of maintenance epidural analgesia for most parturients, and no adjuvant reduces or eliminates the side effects associated with the analgesic drugs used clinically. Therefore, it makes little sense to routinely add adjuvant drugs because they are associated with higher cost, higher rate or severity of side effects, and probably an increased risk for drug error.

MAINTENANCE OF ANALGESIA

Epidural Analgesia

Painful labor lasts several hours in most parturients; therefore, a single intrathecal or epidural injection of local anesthetic and/or opioid usually does not provide adequate analgesia for the duration of labor and supplemental doses are needed. Neuraxial analgesia is maintained with the intermittent or continuous administration of analgesics, usually a combination of a long-acting amide local anesthetic and a lipid-soluble opioid. By far the most common technique is administration of drugs via a catheter into the epidural space. It is occasionally advantageous to administer drugs via a catheter placed in the subarachnoid space.

Drugs for the Maintenance of Epidural Analgesia

In the past, epidural labor analgesia was maintained with the intermittent injection or continuous infusion of a neuraxial

TABLE 24.5 Anesthetic Solutions for Maintenance of Epidural Analgesia: Continuous Infusion, Programmed-bolus, or Patient-Controlled Epidural Analgesia[a]

Drug[b]	Concentration
Local Anesthetics	
Bupivacaine	0.05%–0.125%
Ropivacaine	0.08%–0.2%
Levobupivacaine	0.05%–0.125%
Opioids	
Fentanyl	1.5–3 µg/mL
Sufentanil	0.2–0.4 µg/mL

[a]Local anesthetic is most often combined with an opioid.
[b]Continuous infusions are usually administered at a rate of 8–15 mL/h into the lumbar epidural space.

local anesthetic alone. In contemporary practice, most anesthesia providers maintain analgesia with a combination of a low-dose, long-acting amide local anesthetic and a lipid-soluble opioid (Table 24.5). In practice, neither lidocaine nor 2-chloroprocaine is used for maintenance of analgesia. Both have a short duration of action, and tachyphylaxis possibly may develop more quickly with these local anesthetics than with the longer-acting local anesthetics.[196,197] Lidocaine crosses the placenta to a greater extent than bupivacaine and there is less differentiation between the dose required for sensory and motor blockade.[198] There is no evidence that any one of the long-acting local anesthetics (bupivacaine, ropivacaine, levobupivacaine) or lipid-soluble opioids (fentanyl, sufentanil) has any advantages in terms of maternal or neonatal outcomes over the others.[59,61,62]

As with the induction dose, the combination of a local anesthetic with a lipid-soluble opioid allows administration of a lower concentration and a smaller total dose of local anesthetic for maintenance of analgesia. This approach improves safety and leads to less motor blockade and greater patient satisfaction. Chestnut et al.[89] demonstrated that maintenance of epidural analgesia by a continuous infusion of 0.0625% bupivacaine with fentanyl 2 µg/mL resulted in similar maternal and neonatal outcomes, with a lower incidence of motor blockade, compared with maintenance of analgesia by a CEI of 0.125% bupivacaine alone. When administered as manual intermittent epidural boluses for the maintenance of analgesia, the addition of sufentanil to bupivacaine resulted in better-quality analgesia and decreased motor blockade at delivery.[86]

In contemporary clinical practice, the bupivacaine concentration of maintenance bupivacaine/opioid solutions ranges from 0.05% to 0.125%. Hess et al.[199] retrospectively analyzed the use of three solutions at their institution: bupivacaine 0.125% and bupivacaine 0.0625%, both with fentanyl 2 µg/mL, administered at 8 to 12 mL/h, and bupivacaine 0.04% with fentanyl 1.7 µg/mL and epinephrine 1.7 µg/mL, administered at 15 mL/h. There were more interventions for

breakthrough pain in the two low-concentration groups and more interventions for hypotension and motor blockade in the high-concentration group. Beilin et al.[200] initiated analgesia with intrathecal bupivacaine/fentanyl and an epidural test dose, and then randomly assigned women to receive maintenance epidural analgesia with one of four solutions: bupivacaine 0.125%, bupivacaine 0.0625%, or bupivacaine 0.04% with epinephrine 1.7 µg/mL (all with fentanyl 2 µg/mL) or placebo (saline) at 10 mL/h. The time to request supplemental analgesia was longest in the bupivacaine 0.125% group; however, this group also had a higher incidence of motor blockade than the other groups. Therefore, to avoid motor blockade, it would seem reasonable to use a bupivacaine concentration less than 0.125%, especially if it is administered via CEI (see later discussion).

Several studies that compared equal concentrations of ropivacaine and bupivacaine given by patient-controlled epidural analgesia (PCEA) have not found any significant difference in clinical efficacy between the two local anesthetics.[58,59,201–203] Other studies that adjusted for the potency difference and compared equipotent concentrations (e.g., 0.0625% bupivacaine versus 0.1% ropivacaine) also found no difference in clinical efficacy.[204,205] It is important to recognize that potency is an unchanging property of a drug, whereas clinical efficacy is influenced by multiple variables. For example, ropivacaine has a longer duration of analgesia than bupivacaine,[52] which may offset its lesser potency when it is administered by CEI.

The dose-response relationships for fentanyl and sufentanil combined with a local anesthetic for the maintenance of epidural analgesia have not been well studied. The concentration range of fentanyl typically used in clinical practice is 1.5 to 3 µg/mL, and that of sufentanil, 0.2 to 0.33 µg/mL. Bernard et al.[206] combined sufentanil 0, 0.078, 0.156, 0.312, or 0.468 µg/mL with bupivacaine 0.125% and epinephrine 1.25 µg/mL. Each solution was administered as a 12-mL bolus via PCEA. Sufentanil concentrations less than 0.156 µg/mL did not provide adequate analgesia for the second stage of labor, and higher doses were associated with an increased incidence of pruritus. The optimal opioid concentration probably varies according to the local anesthetic concentration, the mode of drug delivery (i.e., bolus versus infusion), the presence of epinephrine, and the stage of labor, among other factors.

Both fentanyl and sufentanil undergo systemic absorption when administered into the epidural space, although the quantity of drug absorption with modern epidural solutions does not appear to have clinically significant maternal or perinatal effects. Bader et al.[207] infused epidural bupivacaine 0.125% with fentanyl 2 µg/mL at 10 mL/h for 1 to 15 hours. Maternal and neonatal fentanyl concentrations, and their ratio, remained constant over the infusion period, and no adverse maternal or neonatal outcomes were noted. Porter et al.[208] compared neonatal outcomes in women randomly assigned to receive epidural bupivacaine with fentanyl 2.5 µg/mL or bupivacaine alone to maintain analgesia. There were no differences between groups in measures of neonatal well-being at birth or 24 hours after delivery. Loftus et al.[209] compared bupivacaine with sufentanil 0.25 µg/mL or fentanyl

1.5 µg/mL as a CEI at 10 mL/h. Neonates in the fentanyl group had slightly lower 24-hour neuroadaptive capacity scores (NACS) than those in the sufentanil group.

Similar to the initiation of epidural analgesia, higher infusion rates of dilute local anesthetic solutions are superior to lower infusion rates of high-concentration solutions for maintenance of analgesia. Ginosar et al.[210] randomized parturients to receive maintenance of analgesia with an epidural infusion of either bupivacaine 0.25% at 5 mL/h or bupivacaine 0.0625% at 20 mL/h (10 mg/h in both groups). The median bupivacaine dose was lower and patient satisfaction was greater with bupivacaine 0.0625% than with bupivacaine 0.25%.

Administration Techniques

Several techniques or combinations of techniques are used to maintain epidural labor analgesia. As epidural infusion pump technology has evolved, the role of clinician-administered boluses is increasingly restricted to the treatment of breakthrough pain. Modern epidural infusion pumps have multiple settings, including CEI, PCEA, and programmed intermittent epidural bolus (PIEB). The PCEA setting allows the patient to press a button to direct the infusion pump to administer a bolus dose. With PIEB, the pump is programmed to automatically deliver a bolus dose at a set interval. In modern practice, the two technologies are frequently combined (see later discussion).

Intermittent bolus. Before the introduction of infusion pumps, epidural analgesia was routinely maintained by the intermittent administration of an additional therapeutic bolus dose of local anesthetic when analgesia began to wane. When the patient began to experience recurrent pain, the anesthesia provider assessed the pain relative to the stage of labor and the extent of sensory blockade and then administered another epidural bolus of local anesthetic. Analgesia was usually reestablished with the bolus injection of 8 to 12 mL of a local anesthetic/opioid solution.

The spread and quality of analgesia may change with repeated lumbar epidural injections of local anesthetic. After several injections, blockade of the sacral segments, intense motor blockade, or both may develop.[121] The sensory level and the intensity of motor blockade should be assessed and recorded before and after each bolus injection of local anesthetic.

This intermittent bolus technique has several disadvantages, the most salient of which is that pain relief is constantly interrupted by the regression of analgesia. The patient must notify the labor nurse or midwife that she is again uncomfortable and request additional analgesia. In the United States, labor nurses are not allowed to administer additional epidural analgesic drugs[211]; therefore, the nurse must call the anesthesia provider, resulting in unavoidable delays in administration of additional analgesic drugs and additional pain for the patient.

Continuous infusion. Administration of a CEI of a dilute solution of local anesthetic combined with an opioid for the maintenance of epidural labor analgesia reduces, but does not eliminate, the need for bolus doses of local anesthetic,

compared with manual intermittent bolus administration.[212–214] The continuous infusion technique lengthens the time between bolus injections and leads to greater patient satisfaction.[214,215]

Most studies suggest that the CEI technique leads to the administration of a larger total dose of bupivacaine.[213–216] The increased total bupivacaine dose does not seem to result in higher maternal venous or umbilical venous bupivacaine concentrations at delivery.[214,216] Unfortunately, a prolonged epidural infusion of 0.125% bupivacaine at 10 to 14 mL/h may cause significant motor blockade.[72,212,213,215,216] More dilute solutions of local anesthetic reduce the risk of significant motor blockade, but increase the likelihood of breakthrough pain. *In vitro*, animal, and human cadaveric data, along with clinical experience with modern drug delivery systems (see later discussion), suggest that distribution of the epidural solution in the epidural space may be limited when administered by infusion under low pressure.[217,218]

Patient-controlled epidural analgesia. The method of delivering the anesthetic solution into the epidural space influences the density of neuroblockade. Given the same concentration of local anesthetic, analgesia maintained by infusion results in greater drug use, a higher degree of motor blockade,[213,219] and a higher incidence of operative vaginal delivery than intermittent boluses.[216] However, intermittent manual bolus administration by the anesthesia provider results in more breakthrough pain, less patient satisfaction, and more work for the anesthesia provider. PCEA is a method of delivering anesthetic solution to the epidural space that overcomes these disadvantages. Since its first description in 1988 by Gambling et al.,[220] many studies have consistently found that the analgesia with PCEA is comparable to that with continuous infusion techniques.[221,222]

Van der Vyver et al.[222] reported a metaanalysis of nine randomized controlled trials ($n = 640$) comparing PCEA (without a background infusion) with CEI analgesia. There were fewer anesthetic interventions in the PCEA group and the total bupivacaine dose was lower, as was the incidence of motor blockade. There were no differences in pain scores, patient satisfaction, and maternal and neonatal outcomes between groups.

Although patients can self-administer effective epidural labor analgesia using PCEA alone, the addition of a CEI allows for ongoing drug administration, which may be important for women who wish to sleep. Bupivacaine consumption is higher in PCEA with a background infusion than in a pure PCEA technique without a background infusion,[222] but the addition of a background infusion provides better analgesia than pure PCEA.[15] A 2015 metaanalysis that included seven studies identified a lower requirement for physician-administered rescue bolus doses in patients who receive a background infusion.[223] There is no evidence that the higher local anesthetic dose associated with a background infusion has adverse effects on obstetric outcome when low-concentration infusion solutions are used.

A typical background infusion provides one-third to one-half of the total hourly dose.[221] Sng et al.[224] described a

TABLE 24.6   Examples of Patient-Controlled Epidural Analgesia (PCEA) Settings[a]

PCEA Technique	Basal Infusion Rate (mL/h)	Bolus Dose (mL)	Lockout Interval (min)
Without background infusion	0	8–12	10–20
With background infusion	4–8	5–8	10–15

[a]Anesthetic solutions are shown in Table 24.5.

PCEA system in which they used a computer-integrated infusion pump to modify the background infusion rate based on the previous hour's requirement for patient-administered bolus doses. Future pump technology will likely incorporate machine learning to tailor the administered anesthetic dose more closely to patient need.

A wide variety of PCEA regimens have been described (Table 24.6). The anesthesia provider can manipulate the infusion solution (local anesthetic/opioid concentration), patient-controlled bolus volume, lockout interval, background infusion rate, and maximum allowable dose per hour. Patient-controlled bolus doses from 2 to 20 mL and lockout intervals from 5 to 30 minutes have been reported[225–232]; most studies have evaluated patient-controlled bolus volumes of 5 to 12 mL.

Evidence suggests that a larger patient-controlled bolus volume is superior to a smaller volume. In a randomized controlled trial using bupivacaine 0.125% with sufentanil, a low-volume patient-controlled bolus (4 mL, 8-minute lockout) was compared with a high-volume bolus (12 mL, 25-minute lockout).[233] The high-volume group had lower pain scores at 6- and 9-cm cervical dilation, greater patient satisfaction with analgesia, and no differences in obstetric outcomes. In the first of a pair of experiments, Roofthooft et al.[234] compared maintenance analgesia with PCEA alone (5-mL bolus, 12-minute lockout interval, no background infusion) with PIEB plus PCEA (PIEB, 10-mL bolus every hour; PCEA, 5-mL bolus, 20-minute lockout interval). Analgesia was superior with the PIEB technique (less breakthrough pain, less motor block). In the second study by the same research team,[235] PCEA with a larger bolus volume and longer lockout interval (10-mL bolus, 30-minute lockout interval, no background infusion) was compared with the same PIEB technique. In contrast to the findings of the first study, breakthrough pain and motor block were not different between the groups. These studies suggest that larger patient-controlled bolus volumes (approximately 10 mL) are more efficacious than smaller bolus volumes (approximately 5 mL), even when total medication administration is similar. An experiment in a swine model confirmed that the epidural solution spread in the epidural space improves with a bolus administration compared with continuous infusion, and with larger bolus volumes.[217] The investigators administered radiopaque dye,

either as a 10-mL/h CEI, a 2-mL bolus every 12 minutes (total 10 mL), or a single 10-mL bolus. The spread of the solution averaged 5.6, 7.9, and 10.4 spinal levels, respectively.

Various local anesthetic concentrations also have been studied. No studies have reported any differences in analgesia efficacy. The use of more-concentrated local anesthetic solutions results in higher local anesthetic consumption[236–238] and greater motor blockade than the use of less-concentrated solutions.[151,225,237] Thus, as with continuous infusion epidural analgesia, administration of a dilute local anesthetic solution combined with an opioid results in less local anesthetic consumption and motor blockade without a reduction in analgesia efficacy.

In summary, solutions used for PCEA are identical to those used for CEI analgesia (see Table 24.5). It is suggested that larger bolus volumes be used if PCEA is administered without a background infusion. Early PCEA studies investigated higher-concentration local anesthetic solutions (i.e., 0.125% to 0.25% bupivacaine), smaller bolus volumes (≤5 mL), and low background infusion rates (3 to 5 mL/h). Given the more recent data supporting the efficacy of epidural administration of higher volumes of more dilute solutions of local anesthetic, it appears reasonable to apply this principle to PCEA. The safety of large-volume boluses (>10 mL) has not been determined.

Programmed intermittent epidural bolus injection. Bolus administration of a large volume of epidural solution into the epidural space results in better analgesia than CEI or administration of small bolus volumes.[217,218] However, both provider-administered bolus dosing and PCEA are associated with inconsistent analgesia as pain relief wanes and is then reestablished with a bolus dose. PIEB may overcome this disadvantage.

Wong et al.[239] randomly assigned patients to receive either a CEI of a dilute bupivacaine/fentanyl solution at 12 mL/h or 6 mL of the same solution delivered as a programmed bolus every 30 minutes. All patients in both studies were allowed PCEA for the treatment of breakthrough pain. The total dose of local anesthetic was smaller, breakthrough pain was less, and patient satisfaction was greater in the PIEB group than in the continuous infusion groups.

A 2023 systematic review of 18 randomized studies and 4590 women comparing PIEB with continuous infusion suggested that PIEB (5 to 10 mL every 30 to 60 minutes) administered via a programmable pump results in improved patient satisfaction, less drug use, longer duration of analgesia, and less breakthrough pain.[240] Data were insufficient to determine if the incidences of operative vaginal (RR, 0.85; 95% CI, 0.71 to 1.01) and cesarean delivery (RR, 0.85; 95% CI, 0.69 to 1.06) were different between the groups.

Studies of the PIEB technique have attempted to ascertain the optimal bolus volume and administration interval. Wong et al.[241] randomized nulliparous women to receive 1 of 3 PIEB regimens: 10-mL bolus every 60 minutes, 5-mL bolus every 30 minutes, 2.5-mL bolus every 15 minutes. The epidural solution was 0.0625% bupivacaine with fentanyl 2 μg/mL and all patients had access to PCEA. Although analgesia was not different between groups, local anesthetic consumption was lowest in the group that received a 10-mL bolus every

60 minutes. Using the same bupivacaine/fentanyl solution administered at 40-minute intervals, Zakus et al.[242] reported an effective analgesia volume in 90% of women (defined as no breakthrough pain requiring a patient-controlled or clinician-administered bolus) of 10.7 mL (95% CI, 10.3 to 11.0 mL). In a network metaanalysis that included 30 trials,[243] a PIEB volume of 10 mL every 60 minutes was ranked higher than 5 mL every 30 minutes for the outcome of total local anesthetic dose and incidence of motor block. The authors concluded that future research should focus on PIEB volume of 5 mL or greater and an administration interval of 30 minutes or greater.

Investigators have studied the optimal bolus delivery interval using a fixed volume of local anesthetic/opioid solution. Using a biased-coin up-and-down sequential allocation trial design with bupivacaine 0.0625% and fentanyl 2 µg/mL, Epsztein Kanczuk et al.[244] found an interval of 42.6 minutes (95% CI, 38.9 to 46.4 minutes) provided effective analgesia in 90% of women (defined as no breakthrough pain requiring a patient-controlled or clinician-administered bolus). Yao et al.,[245] using ropivacaine 0.1% and sufentanil 0.5 µg/mL, found an effective interval in 90% of patients of 37.0 minutes (95% CI, 28.4 to 40.9 minutes).

Finally, using an innovative mathematical modeling tool, response surface methodology, Munro et al.[246] aimed to estimate the optimal PIEB next bolus interval (interval between initiation bolus and first pump-administered bolus), the PIEB interval, and the PIEB volume that maximizes patient-centered outcomes (patient satisfaction, the number of clinician-administered boluses, and patient-administered boluses). The study solution was ropivacaine 0.1% with fentanyl 2 µg/mL. The suggested PIEB parameters to maximize these outcomes were next bolus 29.4 minutes, PIEB interval 59.8 minutes, and PIEB volume 6.2 mL. Overall, these trials suggest that the optimal interval ranges from 30 to 60 minutes and the optimal volume from 6 to 10 mL. The optimal values likely vary depending on the local anesthetic and opioid concentrations of the maintenance solution, and on individual patient preference, whether to minimize the need for PCEA demand doses (e.g., to facilitate sleep), or to allow for more control and analgesic titration using PCEA.

The design of the distal end of the epidural catheter and the infusion/bolus rate may influence the distribution of anesthetic solution in the epidural space (see Chapter 12). At low infusion rates, the epidural solution exits only the most proximal hole of a multiorifice catheter; thus, the multiorifice catheters behave like single-orifice catheters.[247] In an *in vitro* study,[247] an infusion rate > 300 mL/h was necessary to engage all three orifices of a multiorifice catheter. Higher infusion rates, such as those used with PIEB, will more consistently use all three orifices, depending on flow rate. The catheter design and infusion rate may also influence the "distance traveled" of the epidural solution[248] as well as the pressure generated during a bolus injection.[249] Most commercial epidural pumps administer bolus doses (PCEA or PIEB) at a default infusion rate 200 to 250 mL/h, although some pump manufacturers allow this rate to be manipulated by the user.

Using single-orifice epidural catheters, Lange et al.[250] randomized nulliparous women to PIEB maintenance analgesia with a bolus delivery rate of 100 mL/h or 300 mL/h and found no differences in analgesic outcomes between group. In contrast, in a study of PIEB using a high bolus delivery rate (480 mL/h), women randomized to single-orifice epidural catheters had better analgesia and sacral coverage with fewer PCEA boluses and less local anesthetic consumption compared with women randomized to multiorifice catheters.[251] Additional studies are needed with the PIEB technique to fully delineate the influence of catheter type and bolus delivery rate on analgesia characteristics.

A schematic diagram demonstrating the use of PIEB is shown in Fig. 24.5, and examples of PIEB pump parameters are shown in Table 24.7.

Patient Monitoring During Maintenance Epidural Analgesia

The use of a CEI, PCEA, or PIEB technique does not abolish the need for frequent assessment of the patient by the anesthesia provider at regular intervals. Regular assessment may be particularly important for the PIEB technique in which unwitnessed bolus doses are administered independent of breakthrough pain. Indeed, a 2017 case report describes the migration of a properly sited epidural catheter into the subarachnoid space after several hours of uneventful PIEB analgesia.[252] The patient became acutely hypotensive with new-onset nausea and dyspnea; CSF was easily aspirated from the neuraxial catheter.

Regular assessments should involve determining the quality of analgesia and progress of labor, recording the sensory level and intensity of motor block, and reviewing maternal vital signs and FHR tracings for the previous hour. An inappropriately high level of anesthesia signals the administration of an excessive dose of local anesthetic, or subdural or subarachnoid migration of the catheter. A low level of anesthesia may signal intravenous migration of the catheter, movement of the catheter outside the epidural space, or administration of an inadequate dose of local anesthetic.

Equipment

Anesthesia providers should consider the safety of their equipment when choosing a maintenance technique. The use of an infusion pump identical to that used for the intravenous administration of other drugs increases the chance of a nurse or physician administering the wrong drug (e.g., oxytocin, magnesium sulfate) into the epidural space. Thus, the use of an infusion pump that is used exclusively for epidural analgesia and that differs in appearance from the pumps used for intravenous drug and fluid administration is recommended. The pump should be easy to use, reliable, adjustable, and sturdy. PCEA pumps should differ from patient-controlled intravenous analgesia (PCIA) pumps. The PCEA "buttons" should be labeled with instructions that only the patient (not medical providers or family members) should push the button. If possible, pumps should be preprogrammed with maximum safe limits to prevent errors in clinician pump programming.

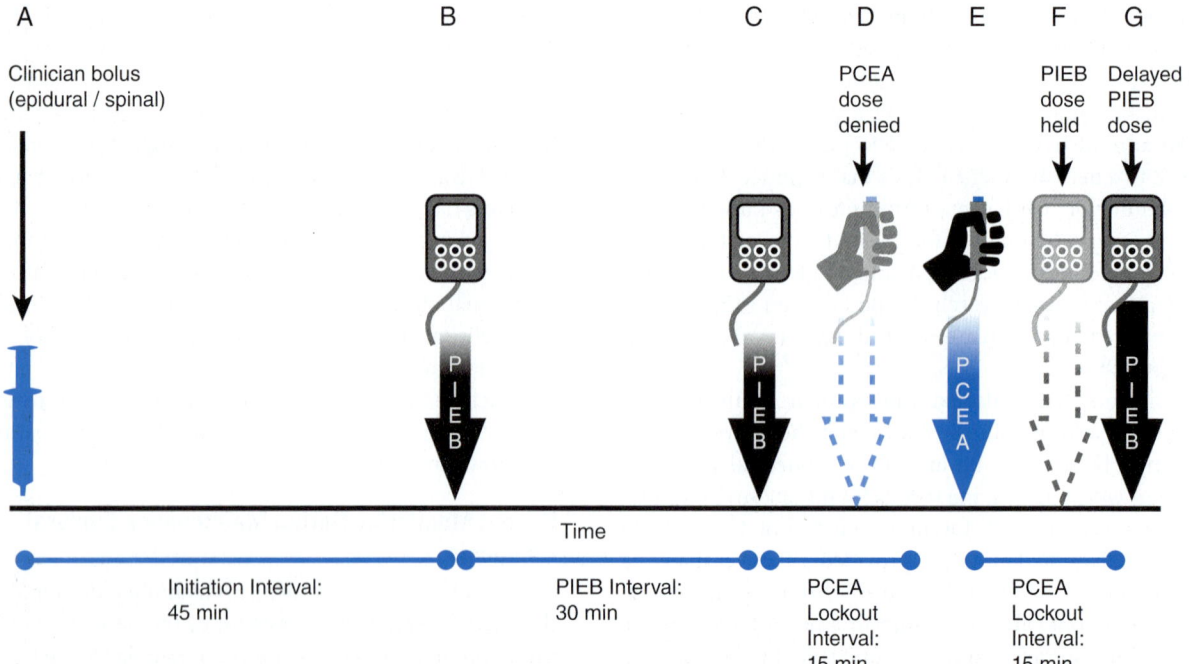

Fig. 24.5 Programmed Intermittent Epidural Bolus (PIEB) Schematic Diagrams. The PIEB pump is programmed with the following parameters: initiation interval = 45 min (time from initial clinician-administered neuraxial analgesia loading dose to first PIEB dose), PIEB interval = 30 min (interval between each PIEB dose), patient-controlled epidural analgesia (PCEA) lockout interval = 15 min (interval after PIEB dose or PCEA dose during which a bolus request by the patient or a PIEB dose will not be administered by the pump). On figure time line, A: Clinician-administered initial neuraxial (epidural/spinal) analgesia loading dose, B: First PIEB dose administered, C: Second PIEB dose administered 30 min later, D: PCEA dose is requested, but the dose is not administered because it is within the 15-min lockout interval of the PIEB dose at Time C, E: PCEA requested and administered, F: PIEB dose delayed because it was programmed to occur within the 15-min lockout interval of the PCEA dose administered at Time E, G: Delayed PIEB dose is administered 15 min after the PCEA dose (Time E) at end of 15-min lockout interval. Illustration by Naveen Nathan, M.D., NorthShore University HealthSystem, University of Chicago Pritzker School of Medicine, Evanston, IL.

TABLE 24.7 **Examples of Programmed Intermittent Epidural Bolus (PIEB) Settings**[a]	
PIEB initial bolus time[b]	15–45 min
PIEB bolus volume	5–10 mL
PIEB bolus interval	30–60 min
PCEA bolus volume	5–10 mL
PCEA lockout interval	10–15 min

[a]Anesthetic solutions are shown in Table 24.5.
[b]Interval from initial neuraxial analgesia loading dose (spinal or epidural) to first programmed bolus dose.
PCEA, Patient-controlled epidural analgesia.

The anesthesia provider should use infusion tubing (which connects the pump to the epidural catheter) that is unique to the epidural administration of drugs. Some tubing is color-coded (yellow). The use of tubing that does not have an injection side port is recommended. The epidural catheter and tubing should be clearly labeled with the word "epidural." Patient safety experts[253] have recommended that syringes, needles, and catheters used for neuraxial injections be modified so that it is not possible to use this equipment for intravenous injections, thus making

the possibility of drug administration error less likely. The use of this equipment has been mandated in the United Kingdom beginning in 2025.[254] The equipment is available in Europe, but is not yet widely used, and is not available in the United States.

Each labor unit must have a clear policy as to who may administer and adjust epidural infusion parameters. Anesthesia personnel should be responsible for changes in the content or rate of the infusion and the volume of bolus doses or develop protocols that allow nurses and midwives to make changes within the guidelines of the protocol or by order of the anesthesia provider. In the presence of maternal distress or fetal bradycardia, the nurse or obstetric provider may discontinue the epidural infusion, but the anesthesia provider should be notified immediately.

Solutions for maintenance of neuraxial analgesia require careful preparation. A hospital pharmacist or compounding pharmacy should prepare the solution in a clean or sterile environment. Preservative-free drugs and saline should be used to prepare the solutions. The solutions should be clearly labeled for epidural use, and solution contents should always be double-checked for content and expiration date by the anesthesia provider before analgesia is initiated.

Spinal Analgesia

The placement of a catheter in the subarachnoid space allows the anesthesia provider to administer continuous spinal analgesia by intermittent bolus injection or continuous infusion of a local anesthetic combined with an opioid. Continuous spinal analgesia is an option when unintentional dural puncture has occurred (see later discussion). The technique has also been described for use in patients in whom placement of an epidural catheter is difficult (e.g., in patients with morbid obesity or abnormal vertebral anatomy, such as kyphoscoliosis, or in patients with severe cardiac disease who require careful titration of analgesia).[255]

Reports of this technique usually describe the use of a standard epidural catheter placed through an 18- or 19-gauge epidural needle. Over 30 years ago, to reduce the incidence of post–dural puncture headache, very small (e.g., 28- to 32-gauge) catheters were developed for insertion through small (e.g., 22- to 26-gauge) spinal needles. Unfortunately, several cases of cauda equina syndrome (associated with the use of spinal microcatheters during surgery in nonpregnant patients) prompted the US FDA to remove these microcatheters from the market in 1992.[256] The etiology of these neurologic deficits is unclear. Some authors have suggested that neurologic injury may result from the maldistribution of local anesthetic within the subarachnoid space.[257] The very slow rate of injection through a caudally directed microcatheter may lead to the pooling of local anesthetic solution in the terminal part of the dural sac. If the local anesthetic solution is hyperbaric, the neighboring elements of the cauda equina experience prolonged exposure to a high concentration of local anesthetic and a hyperglycemic, hyperosmotic (e.g., 550 to 800 mOsm/L) marinade. Permanent neural damage may occur from the combination of tissue dehydration and a toxic concentration of local anesthetic. It is unclear whether this complication is unique to the use of microcatheters.

Arkoosh et al.[258] reported a randomized multicenter study that compared continuous spinal labor analgesia (via a 28-gauge catheter) with continuous epidural analgesia. The incidence of neurologic complications was not different between the two groups, and patients in the spinal group had better early analgesia, less motor blockade, and better patient satisfaction. The study was underpowered to determine if the incidence of post–dural puncture headache differed between the two groups. The spinal catheter was associated with a higher incidence of technical difficulties and catheter failures.

A 23-gauge, FDA-approved, spinal catheter is now available in the United States. The catheter is inserted using a "catheter-over-needle" technique. Initial observational study found that this catheter may have clinical utility[259]; however, similar to the Arkoosh et al. study,[258] the study was not large enough to assess the risk for complications. Several commercial spinal catheters are available in Europe.

Continuous spinal analgesia can be initiated with the same drug combination and dose used to initiate CSE analgesia (see Table 24.2).[255] For maintenance of analgesia, my colleagues and I administer our standard epidural solution (0.08% bupivacaine with fentanyl 2 μg/mL) at an initial rate of 2 mL/h.

The infusion is then titrated to patient needs. We prefer to use our standard PCEA pumps for the continuous infusion, with the PCEA function disabled. A separate "recipe" for continuous spinal analgesia is preprogrammed in the pump. This approach allows the anesthesia provider to administer a small (1 to 3 mL) bolus from the infusion bag without disconnecting the spinal catheter from the infusion tubing. Alternatively, the infusion pump can be programmed to administer 1-mL patient-controlled bolus doses. The catheter and pump should be clearly labeled so that all care providers know that the catheter is a spinal, not an epidural, catheter.

Continuous spinal analgesia with opioids has also been described for patients with obstructive cardiac lesions.[260,261] If intrathecal local anesthetics are used for intrapartum analgesia, the sensory level and the intensity of motor blockade should be monitored. Moreover, the anesthesia provider must be prepared to treat hypotension and other complications associated with high spinal anesthesia.

Ambulatory "Walking" Neuraxial Analgesia

The term "walking" or "mobile" epidural analgesia was first coined to describe low-dose CSE opioid analgesia because motor function was maintained and the ability to walk was not impaired.[262] However, the term is more accurately applied to any neuraxial analgesic technique that allows safe ambulation. Initial studies using clinical testing to assess sensory and motor impairment and dorsal column function produced conflicting results. After initiation of epidural analgesia with 15 mL of 0.1% bupivacaine/fentanyl 2 μg/mL, Buggy et al.[263] demonstrated that 66% of women had altered proprioception and 38% had impaired vibration sense. In contrast, Parry et al.[264] found that dorsal column function was impaired in only 7% of laboring women who received low-dose epidural or CSE analgesia. The same group of investigators then used computerized dynamic posturography to assess balance in nonpregnant women, term pregnant women not in labor, and laboring women after initiation of CSE analgesia with bupivacaine 2.5 mg and fentanyl 5 μg.[265] Pregnancy significantly affected balance function, but initiation of CSE analgesia did not further impair function. However, further supplementation of analgesia with the epidural injection of 10 mL of 0.1% bupivacaine/fentanyl 2 μg/mL in a subgroup of patients resulted in impaired balance function. The investigators concluded that the results supported the safety of allowing ambulation after low-dose CSE analgesia, but further studies are required to understand the relative contributions of dorsal column function, proprioception, and lower limb motor strength to overall balance and ability to ambulate.[265]

Several studies have shown that an epidural test dose containing lidocaine 45 mg and epinephrine 15 μg adversely affects the ability to ambulate after initiation of CSE or low-dose epidural analgesia.[266,267]

The concept of the "walking epidural" is popular in the lay press; however, many women, once comfortable, prefer to rest rather than ambulate. The ability to walk to the toilet or sit in a chair at the bedside, however, remains desirable to many laboring women.[268] In a small study, the ability to walk to the toilet to void resulted in lower postvoid residual volume than voiding on a bedpan.[269] Although ambulation *per se* has not been shown to affect the progress or outcome of labor positively or negatively, dense motor blockade may adversely affect the spontaneous vaginal delivery rate (see later discussion). Thus, the intent of the "walking epidural"—minimization of motor blockade—should be the goal of the anesthesia provider, whether or not the patient wishes to ambulate.[268]

Safe ambulation during labor requires several safeguards (Box 24.5). Before ambulation, orthostatic blood pressure and heart rate should be measured, and motor function and balance must be assessed. The patient should not ambulate alone.

ANALGESIA/ANESTHESIA FOR VAGINAL DELIVERY

During the second stage of labor, pain results from distention of the pelvic floor, vagina, and perineum. Pain impulses are transmitted to the spinal cord by means of somatic nerve fibers that enter the cord at S2 to S4. These somatic nerve fibers are larger than the visceral afferent nerve fibers that transmit the pain of the first stage of labor. A blockade of these larger nerve fibers may require administration of a more concentrated solution and/or a greater volume of local anesthetic than is required during the first stage of labor[46]; this need often creates a dilemma for the anesthesia provider. Administration of a more concentrated solution of local anesthetic results in more intense motor blockade at a time when maternal expulsive efforts are helpful.

The continous epidural infusion of bupivacaine often leads to the gradual development of sacral analgesia. Likewise, several lumbar epidural injections of local anesthetic (given every 60 to 90 minutes) may result in sacral analgesia.[121] If analgesia is not adequate for the second stage of labor and delivery, the anesthesia provider can give additional doses of local anesthetic to augment perineal analgesia (Box 24.6). Some anesthesia providers contend that the use of the sitting position helps facilitate the onset of perineal analgesia.

Published studies suggest that maternal position does not consistently affect the spread of local anesthetic in the epidural space[270,271]; rather, the administration of a larger volume of local anesthetic solution facilitates the onset of sacral analgesia.[272] Unfortunately, the larger volume also results in a higher (i.e., more cephalad) sensory level of analgesia, so the patient should be observed for evidence of hemodynamic or respiratory compromise.

Dense anesthesia is often required for operative vaginal delivery, especially if the obstetric provider performs an episiotomy or uses forceps. In most circumstances, the anesthesia provider administers 5 to 10 mL of the epidural local anesthetic solution typically used for epidural cesarean delivery anesthesia. In the event of failed operative vaginal delivery, dense sensory blockade anesthesia can be extended with the additional administration of the high-concentration local anesthetic solution. We inject this "delivery dose" (3-mL test dose followed by the remaining dose) when the fetal head is visible on the perineum during pushing or when the obstetric provider has decided to proceed with operative vaginal delivery. The anesthesia provider should monitor the maternal blood pressure carefully, especially if excessive blood loss occurs.

Occasionally a parturient tolerates the pain of labor until late in the first stage (i.e., more than 8 cm cervical dilation) and then requests analgesia. Advanced labor does not preclude initiation of neuraxial analgesia, especially in a nulliparous woman, in whom the second stage of labor may last 2 to 3 hours. However, initiation of lumbar epidural analgesia in the late first stage of labor often results in inadequate sacral analgesia unless large volumes of a concentrated local anesthetic solution are administered. This leads to higher cephalad sensory blockade than necessary and dense motor blockade. Single-shot spinal or CSE analgesia may be a better alternative that provides a rapid onset of analgesia with sacral coverage for advanced labor. When delivery is imminent, the single-shot spinal technique is frequently adequate. If anticipating prolonged labor or cesarean delivery, the CSE technique is preferred, but it is also reasonable to follow single-shot spinal analgesia with epidural catheter insertion in a second procedure, once the patient is comfortable.

Additional local anesthetic can be administered through the epidural catheter if the extent or duration of spinal analgesia is inadequate.

Single-shot spinal anesthesia for vaginal delivery may be indicated in a parturient who does not have epidural anesthesia and who requires rapid perineal anesthesia. A so-called saddle block can be administered to achieve blockade of the sacral spinal segments; a small dose of a hyperbaric local anesthetic solution is adequate for this purpose. A saddle block may be advantageous in the patient with a preterm fetus or a vaginal breech presentation. In these cases, dense perineal relaxation may facilitate an atraumatic vaginal delivery. A saddle block performed with the patient in the sitting position with hyperbaric local anesthetic solution provides excellent anesthesia for an outlet/low forceps delivery. A higher level (T10) of anesthesia often is required for a mid-forceps delivery.

Clear communication between the obstetric and anesthesia providers is essential. If the obstetric provider is certain that the application of forceps (or vacuum extraction) will result in a successful delivery, a saddle block will likely provide satisfactory anesthesia. However, in some cases, the obstetric provider will perform a *trial* of forceps. If the trial fails, cesarean delivery must follow. We alter our technique when giving spinal anesthesia for a trial of forceps. In some cases, we give a dose of local anesthetic appropriate for cesarean delivery. Alternatively, a saddle block can be administered via the CSE technique. If spinal anesthesia is inadequate for the planned procedure, additional local anesthetic can be given through the epidural catheter.

SIDE EFFECTS OF NEURAXIAL ANALGESIA

Hypotension

Neuraxial anesthesia–induced sympathetic blockade leads to peripheral vasodilation and increased venous capacitance. Hypotension that occurs after extensive neuroblockade primarily reflects decreased systemic vascular resistance.[273] Hypotension is often defined as a 20% to 30% decrease in systolic blood pressure (compared with baseline) or a systolic blood pressure < 90 to 100 mm Hg. Modest hypotension rarely has adverse consequences in young, nonpregnant patients. However, placental circulation has limited autoregulation; thus, maintenance of uteroplacental perfusion largely depends on maintenance of maternal blood pressure (see Chapter 3). Uncorrected hypotension results in decreased uteroplacental perfusion. If hypotension is severe and prolonged, hypoxia and acidosis will develop in the fetus. Blood pressure should be monitored frequently (every 2 to 3 minutes) after initiation of analgesia, until stable blood pressure is ascertained.

The incidence of hypotension after initiation of neuraxial analgesia *during labor* is approximately 14%.[20] Kinsella and Black[274] reported that maternal position and the position of the blood pressure cuff markedly influence the measured blood pressure. With laboring patients in the full lateral position,

the mean difference in systolic blood pressure between the dependent and upper arm was 10 mm Hg; the mean difference in diastolic pressure was 14 mm Hg.

A metaanalysis of studies comparing low-dose epidural analgesia with CSE analgesia found no difference in the incidence of hypotension between the two techniques.[20]

The prevention of hypotension includes avoidance of aortocaval compression. Preston et al.[38] noted a higher incidence of severe FHR decelerations in women placed in the supine-lateral tilt position than in those in the full lateral position after initiation of epidural analgesia. In contrast, Beilin et al.[275] found no difference in maternal blood pressure and FHR decelerations between the two positions.

Traditionally, intravenous "preload" (also known as "prehydration") with 0.5 to 1.5 L of crystalloid solution was used to reduce the incidence and severity of hypotension after the initiation of neuraxial labor analgesia. However, several randomized controlled trials have shown that the incidence of hypotension after preload with 0.5 to 1.0 L of fluid is no lower than that after no preload.[31,35] In women undergoing spinal anesthesia for cesarean delivery, there is no difference in the incidence of hypotension when crystalloid is administered as a rapid bolus before the initiation of neuroblockade (preload) compared with administration concurrently with the initiation of anesthesia (coload).[36] Data are inconsistent as to whether a fluid bolus decreases the risk for nonreassuring FHR changes associated with the initiation of neuraxial analgesia (see earlier discussion). Many anesthesia providers omit a fluid bolus, especially in patients at risk for pulmonary edema (e.g., women with preeclampsia), or in women who have maintained hydration with clear liquid oral intake during labor. In our practice, my colleagues and I usually administer approximately 500 mL of intravenous crystalloid (coload) at the time of initiation of neuraxial labor analgesia.

The hypotension associated with neuraxial analgesia is usually easily treated. Treatment includes the administration of additional intravenous crystalloid, placement of the mother in the full lateral position, and administration of an intravenous vasopressor. Traditionally, ephedrine 5 to 10 mg has been administered; however, studies in women undergoing spinal anesthesia for elective cesarean delivery have shown that phenylephrine is equally or more efficacious in restoring blood pressure and is associated with higher umbilical arterial blood pH measurements at birth.[276] No differences in neonatal outcome have been noted. Because there is no evidence that the choice of vasopressor influences maternal or neonatal outcome, the use of either drug is acceptable. The FHR should be monitored continuously, and treatment should be more aggressive if nonreassuring FHR patterns are noted or if the mother is symptomatic (e.g., presence of presyncope or nausea). Ephedrine crosses the placenta and may increase both FHR and FHR variability (e.g., saltatory FHR pattern).[277,278]

Pruritus

Pruritus is the most common side effect of epidural or intrathecal opioid administration (see Chapter 27).[279] Intrathecal opioid administration is associated with a higher incidence and severity of pruritus than epidural opioid administration.[20] The incidence of pruritus after intrathecal opioid administration is close to 100% in some studies, although the need for treatment is much lower.[146] The incidence and severity of pruritus are dose dependent for both epidural[90] and spinal[146,154] opioid administration. The coadministration of local anesthetic decreases the incidence of pruritus,[176] whereas the coadministration of epinephrine may worsen pruritus.[280]

The cause of the neuraxial opioid–induced pruritus is incompletely understood. In contrast to peripheral morphine administration, mast cell degranulation and release of histamine likely do not play a role. Current evidence suggests that neuraxial morphine causes sensitization of central itch-signaling pathways, leading to an enhanced response to peripheral stimulation.[281] Neuraxial opioids may cause itching through the inhibition of inhibitory neurons in the dorsal horn of the spinal cord as a result of dysregulation of opioid-sensitive pathways involving μ- and κ-opioid receptor signaling.[281]

Few studies have addressed the *treatment* of established pruritus (see Chapter 27). Most studies have addressed pruritus after intrathecal morphine, not lipid-soluble opioids such as fentanyl and sufentanil. The most effective treatment is a centrally acting μ-opioid antagonist (e.g., **naloxone** or **naltrexone**) or a partial agonist-antagonist, such as **nalbuphine** (Table 24.8). However, the use of these agents in a bolus or continuous infusion may reverse the analgesia. Antihistamines (e.g., diphenhydramine), low-dose propofol, 5-HT$_3$ receptor antagonists (e.g., ondansetron), pentazocine (a κ-opioid and partial μ-opioid receptor agonist), and dopamine-2 receptor antagonists have been studied for the treatment of pruritus after spinal morphine, but not the lipid-soluble opioids fentanyl and sufentanil.[281] Results of published studies are inconsistent and these drugs are not considered first-line treatment of neuraxial opioid–induced pruritus.

Several drugs have been investigated for *prophylaxis* against neuraxial opioid–induced pruritus, primarily coincident with neuraxial morphine administration. A 2016 metaanalysis included six randomized controlled trials of prophylactic ondansetron for prevention of intrathecal fentanyl- or sufentanil-induced pruritus in both obstetric and nonobstetric patients.[282] Ondansetron 8 mg did not decrease the incidence of pruritus. A single trial in obstetric patients who received ondansetron 4 or 8 mg before intrathecal fentanyl 25 μg found no benefit compared with a placebo.[283]

We do not routinely administer prophylaxis for the pruritus associated with neuraxial administration of opioids for labor analgesia. The pruritus is typically self-limiting; the severity of pruritus usually diminishes markedly in the first hour after opioid administration, and most women do not require treatment. For moderate to severe pruritus that requires treatment, we usually administer **nalbuphine** 2.5 mg and repeat the dose in 10 to 15 minutes if no improvement is noted. The advantage of nalbuphine is that it is less likely to reverse the intrathecal or epidural opioid analgesia than a pure μ-opioid receptor agonist.[284]

Nausea and Vomiting

Nausea and vomiting occur frequently during labor. It is difficult to determine the incidence of nausea and vomiting directly related to epidural and intrathecal opioid administration. Nausea and vomiting may also be secondary to neuraxial analgesia–induced hypotension. Maternal blood pressure should be measured when the patient complains of nausea in the presence of neuroblockade. Other causes of nausea and vomiting during labor are pregnancy itself, pain, opioid-induced delay of gastric emptying (see later discussion), and systemic opioids, which are sometimes administered before intrathecal or epidural opioids. In one study, the incidences of nausea (7% versus 44%) and vomiting (2% versus 17%) were significantly lower in women randomly assigned to receive intrathecal fentanyl than in those assigned to receive systemic hydromorphone analgesia in early labor.[285]

The etiology of neuraxial opioid–associated nausea is unclear, but it may be caused by the modulation of afferent input at the area postrema (i.e., the chemoreceptor trigger zone) or at the nucleus of the tractus solitarius, which is a key relay station in the visceral sensory network.[286] Of interest, nausea is less common after epidural or intrathecal opioid administration during labor than after the administration of the same drugs for post–cesarean delivery analgesia. Norris et al.[287] noted that women who received epidural or intrathecal opioid analgesia during labor had an incidence of nausea of only 1.0% and 2.4%, respectively.

Although the incidence of nausea is low, treatment should be available. No studies, however, have specifically addressed the *treatment* of neuraxial analgesia–associated nausea and vomiting during labor. We do not routinely administer prophylactic antiemetics before the administration of neuraxial lipid-soluble opioids for labor analgesia.

Fever

Both observational and randomized controlled trials have consistently noted a gradual rise in core temperature over several hours in a subset of laboring women receiving epidural analgesia that is not observed in women receiving no analgesia, inhaled nitrous oxide, or parenteral opioids.[288] The mean increase in core temperature is typically small (<1.0°C); however, women with epidural analgesia are more likely to have clinical fever (usually defined as core temperature ≥ 38°C) than those without epidural analgesia (odds ratio [OR], 4.17; 95% CI, 2.93 to 5.94). The incidence epidural-related

TABLE 24.8 Treatment of Neuraxial Opioid–Induced Pruritus

Drug	Dose
Naloxone	40–80 μg intravenous bolus
	1–2 μg/kg/h continuous intravenous infusion
Nalbuphine	2.5–5 mg intravenous bolus
Naltrexone	6 mg orally

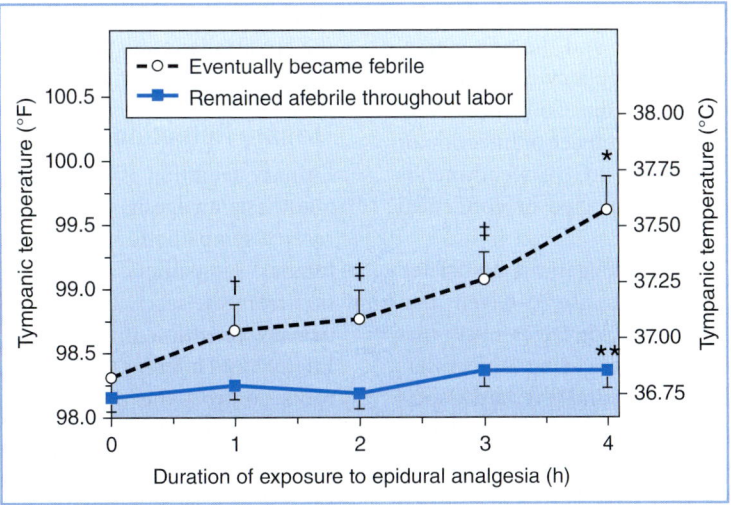

Fig. 24.6 Maternal tympanic temperature in the 4 h immediately after initiation of epidural analgesia, stratified by ultimate intrapartum fever status (temperature ≥ 38.0°C or <38°C). *P < .001; †P < .05; ‡P < .01 (repeated measures analysis, febrile versus afebrile); **P = .26 (repeated measures analysis, afebrile group temperature change over time). Modified from Goetzl L, Rivers J, Zighelboim I, et al. Intrapartum epidural analgesia and maternal temperature regulation. *Obstet Gynecol.* 2007;109:687–690.

maternal fever (ERMF) ranges from 15% to 25%.[288] The variability may be attributed to differences in study design, study populations, and the definition of fever.

In the subset of women who eventually develop clinical fever, core temperature begins to rise within 1 hour of initiation of epidural analgesia at a rate of approximately 0.18°C/h.[289] For these women, the development of fever is likely directly related to the duration of epidural analgesia. Others do not demonstrate this hourly increase in temperature (Fig. 24.6). It is unclear why some women receiving epidural analgesia develop a fever, whereas most do not. Genetic factors (polymorphisms in genes that produce proteins controlling the immune response) may play a role, but further research is needed to explore this hypothesis.[288] ERMF is not observed in nonlaboring women undergoing cesarean delivery with epidural anesthesia, nor is it observed in nonpregnant patients receiving epidural anesthesia for nonobstetric surgery. This suggests that there is something unique about the physiologic state of labor and its interaction with epidural analgesia and maternal genetics or other unidentified risk factors that leads to fever.

The neuraxial technique, specific local anesthetic agents, and inclusion of opioids used to initiate and maintain analgesia have not been shown to influence the risk for ERMF. The incidence of fever does not differ in women who receive epidural compared with CSE analgesia,[290] in early compared with late labor initiation of neuraxial analgesia,[285] or with bupivacaine epidural analgesia with and without fentanyl.[291] Likewise, delayed initiation of the epidural infusion does not affect the incidence of fever.[292]

Two mechanisms are proposed to explain ERMF: (1) epidural analgesia influences maternal immunomodulation, the so-called **sterile inflammation hypothesis**; and (2) epidural analgesia, via sympathetic nervous system blockade, inhibits

heat dissipation in laboring parturients, the so-called **thermoregulation hypothesis**.[288] Sterile inflammation is a state of noninfectious inflammation—labor itself is a state of sterile inflammation. Concentrations of both pro- and antiinflammatory cytokines increase during labor.[293] The prophylactic administration of glucocorticoids inhibits this rise in proinflammatory cytokines and lowers the incidence of ERMF.[294] There is evidence of an inhibitory effect of bupivacaine on the release of the antipyrogenic factor IL-1 receptor antagonist (IL-1ra) from circulating leukocytes by reducing the activation of caspase-1.[295] This finding supports the theory that epidural analgesia may cause fever by disrupting leukocyte immune function, and proinflammatory cytokines may cause fever if the release of the antipyrogenic IL-1ra is inhibited.[288]

During labor, heat production is increased. The thermoregulatory hypothesis suggests that epidural labor analgesia may reduce heat loss by several mechanisms, including decreased sweating (cholinergic blockade), increased thermoregulatory vasoconstriction, baroreceptor-mediated reflex vasoconstriction (physiologic response to a decrease in blood pressure), an elevated vasoconstriction set point, blockade of active cutaneous vasodilation, decreased heat-dissipating activities such as hyperventilation, and a reduced shivering threshold.[288] The current preponderance of evidence suggests that sterile inflammation is the most likely explanation of ERMF.[288]

The significance of ERMF during labor is unclear. At issue is the diagnosis of ERMF and its differentiation from chorioamnionitis. Currently, there is no reliable intrapartum method for differentiating the two entities. The ACOG defines three categories of maternal fever: (1) isolated maternal fever (single oral maternal temperature of 39°C or greater, or sustained oral temperature between 38°C and 38.9°C when rechecked after 30 minutes); (2) suspected intraamniotic infection; and

(3) confirmed intraamniotic infection.[296] Suspected chorioamnionitis is defined as maternal fever and the presence of one or more of the following criteria: leukocytosis, purulent cervical discharge, and/or fetal tachycardia. Confirmed diagnosis requires positive amniotic fluid evidence of infection or placental histopathologic diagnosis. The ACOG recommends intrapartum antibiotic therapy for suspected or confirmed chorioamnionitis.[296]

Studies have found that epidural analgesia is associated with increased intrapartum antibiotic use.[288] Given that ERMF does not have an infectious etiology, it is likely that women with ERMF (and their fetuses) are being unnecessarily exposed to antibiotics. Inflammation and fever are associated with abnormal labor curves, fetal intolerance to labor, and an increased rate of operative vaginal delivery. It is not clear whether these adverse outcomes are associated with all types of inflammation and fever (i.e., including ERMF) or are limited to infectious fever.

Fetal and neonatal outcomes are also of concern. The US Centers for Disease Control and the American Academy of Pediatrics recommend laboratory studies and empiric antibiotic therapy for neonates whose mothers have suspected or confirmed chorioamnionitis.[297] Similar to maternal antibiotic therapy, these measures are unnecessary if ERMF is misdiagnosed as chorioamnionitis. At a minimum, this care is stressful for parents and neonates, separates neonates from their parents shortly after birth, and adds unnecessary healthcare costs. More worrisome is the finding that maternal fever in the presence of fetal acidosis is associated with a markedly increased risk for neonatal encephalopathy, suggesting that fever may lower the threshold for fetal hypoxic brain injury.[298] Greenwell et al.[299] demonstrated that women with epidural analgesia who developed intrapartum fever had increased risk for adverse neonatal outcomes (including assisted ventilation, lower Apgar scores, and early onset seizures) compared with women who did not develop a fever. Again, because of the difficulty in diagnosing ERMF, it is not clear whether fever, *per se*, is the culprit, or infectious or noninfectious inflammation interact to play a role in adverse neonatal outcome.

Shivering

Several factors, including hormonal factors, likely influence thermoregulatory response during labor and delivery. Shivering is frequently observed during labor and may occur more commonly after administration of epidural analgesia, although its incidence and intensity are less than during cesarean delivery with epidural anesthesia.[300] Panzer et al.[301] performed an observational study of shivering during labor. Before delivery, 18% of women shivered, and 15% of these episodes were associated with normothermia and vasodilation, suggesting a nonthermoregulatory cause of the shivering. After delivery, shivering was observed in 16% of women, and in 28% of them it was nonthermoregulatory. There was no difference in the incidence of shivering between women who chose epidural (bupivacaine/fentanyl) analgesia and those who chose systemic meperidine analgesia. The addition of an opioid to the local anesthetic solution may affect the

shivering response.[104,302] At least one study has suggested that the epidural administration of epinephrine increases shivering[302]; the etiology of this response is unknown.

Urinary Retention

Urinary retention is a troublesome side effect of neuraxial anesthesia/analgesia. The bladder and urethral sphincters receive sympathetic innervation from the low thoracic/high lumbar sympathetic fibers and parasympathetic innervation from the sacral fibers. Neuraxial local anesthetics cause urinary retention through blockade of sacral nerve roots. Efferent and afferent nerve traffic via the S2, S3, and S4 nerve roots controls the detrusor muscle (responsible for urine storage and micturition) and internal and external sphincter function. Intrathecal opioids cause dose-dependent suppression of detrusor muscle contractility and decreased urge sensation via inhibition of sacral parasympathetic nervous system outflow.[286,303] The onset of urinary retention appears to parallel the onset of analgesia.

It is difficult to determine the magnitude of this problem during labor because parturients often require catheterization for other reasons. Postpartum bladder dysfunction was observed in 14% of women who had a normal spontaneous vaginal delivery and in 38% of women who underwent operative vaginal delivery, all without epidural analgesia.[304]

Several observational studies suggest that there is a higher risk for intrapartum and postpartum urinary retention in women who receive epidural labor analgesia than in those who receive nonepidural or no analgesia.[305,306] Similarly, a metaanalysis of four small randomized controlled trials that compared neuraxial with systemic opioid analgesia, in which urinary retention was reported as a secondary outcome, also identified this association.[3] Whether this higher risk reflects a cause-and-effect relationship or patient selection bias is not clear. Wilson et al.[307] found that women randomized to receive neuraxial labor analgesia with low-concentration bupivacaine with opioid more often retained the ability to void spontaneously than women who received epidural analgesia with 0.25% bupivacaine (approximately 31% versus 11%), which suggests a dose-response relationship.

Any difference in bladder function appears to be short-lived; differences between groups in one study had resolved by postpartum day 1.[305] In two studies, patients were randomly assigned to receive epidural analgesia with or without an opioid; there was no difference between groups in the incidence of intrapartum[308] or postpartum[306] urinary retention.

Parturients should be regularly observed during labor for evidence of bladder distention, especially if they complain of suprapubic pain during contractions. The differential diagnosis of breakthrough pain during neuraxial labor analgesia should include bladder distention. Personal observation suggests that many women can void in the presence of low-dose neuroblockade if placed on a bedpan or escorted to the toilet, even if they do not perceive a full bladder. The inability to void and bladder distention should prompt catheterization to empty the bladder.

Recrudescence of Herpes Simplex Virus

The common cold sore or fever blister is a manifestation of the reactivation of latent herpes simplex virus (HSV) infection. Reactivation can occur after exposure to ultraviolet light, fever, immunosuppression, or trauma. Prospective randomized studies have demonstrated a higher incidence of postpartum *oral* HSV reactivation in women randomly assigned to receive neuraxial morphine than among women assigned to receive systemic morphine for post–cesarean delivery analgesia.[309,310] We are unaware of any study that has investigated whether epidural or intrathecal opioid administration during labor increases the incidence of recurrent oral HSV infection after vaginal delivery. Therefore, we do not withhold neuraxial opioids during labor in women with a history of oral herpes.

Delayed Gastric Emptying

Labor may result in delayed gastric emptying, which may be exacerbated by opioid administration (see Chapter 28).[311,312] Intravenous or intramuscular opioid administration results in delayed gastric emptying in laboring women. Data are inconsistent on whether neuraxial opioids delay gastric emptying. Early studies assessed gastric emptying using acetaminophen absorption. Several studies suggest that epidural fentanyl combined with bupivacaine and administered as part of a CEI does not result in delayed gastric emptying compared with infusion of bupivacaine alone[313,314]; however, a third study found a small delay in gastric emptying following the infusion of epidural fentanyl after a cumulative fentanyl dose > 100 µg (after approximately 4 hours of infusion).[313] Two studies found delayed gastric emptying with epidural fentanyl administered as a bolus (50 to 100 µg) with bupivacaine.[315,316] In another study, intrathecal fentanyl 25 µg resulted in delayed gastric emptying compared with epidural fentanyl 50 µg plus bupivacaine or bupivacaine alone.[317]

In a study using gastric ultrasonography and measurement of antral cross-sectional area (CSA) in women who received epidural labor analgesia with ropivacaine and sufentanil, median CSA decreased between the preepidural initiation assessment and assessment at full cervical dilation (the median interval between the measurements was 188 minutes).[318] Another study using gastric ultrasonography identified solid food in the stomach of 9 of 10 laboring parturients without epidural analgesia fed a light meal; in contrast, only 3 of 10 parturients with epidural analgesia (ropivacaine with sufentanil) had solid food in the stomach.[319] Finally, a study comparing low (<100 µg) to high (>100 µg) cumulative fentanyl dose 2 hours after initiation of epidural analgesia with ropivacaine found no difference in antral CSA between the two groups.[320] Overall, these data do not suggest a clinically significant delay in gastric emptying when neuraxial local anesthetics are combined with opioids for labor analgesia.

Sensory Changes

In one of the early studies of intrathecal opioid administration during labor, Cohen et al.[279] observed decreased sensation to cold and pinprick in women who received intrathecal sufentanil. Subsequent studies have demonstrated that these sensory changes do not result from a local anesthetic effect of sufentanil. Sensory changes do not predict the quality or duration of analgesia or the extent of hemodynamic change.[321] Further, intrathecal sufentanil does not cause a sympathectomy.[322] Intrathecal opioids do not affect the efferent limb of the nervous system and so do not impair motor function. Thus, affected patients should be reassured that respiratory efforts are not compromised and that the symptoms will subside in 30 to 60 minutes.[323]

In addition to sensory changes, case reports have described mental status changes, aphasia, and automatisms after the intrathecal injection of fentanyl[324] and sufentanil.[325] These symptoms seem to be related to an opioid effect. In one case, the symptoms were partially reversed by naloxone.[324]

COMPLICATIONS OF NEURAXIAL ANALGESIA

Inadequate Analgesia

The reported failure rate for neuraxial analgesia varies according to the definition of "failure."[326–328] In survey studies, the rate of epidural catheter replacement has ranged from 5% to 13%.[22,326–328] Successful siting of the epidural space is not always possible, and satisfactory analgesia does not always occur, even when the epidural space has been identified correctly. Factors such as patient age and weight, the specific technique, the type of epidural catheter, and the skill of the anesthesia provider are associated with the rate of failure of neuraxial analgesia.[326,328] Failure to provide adequate analgesia not only results in a dissatisfying experience for the patient but also may lead to litigation.[329] The risk for failed anesthesia and the potential need to place a second epidural catheter should be discussed with the patient during the preanesthetic evaluation, before placement of the first epidural catheter.

Pan et al.[326] used quality assurance data to retrospectively assess the failure rate among more than 12,000 neuraxial procedures performed for labor analgesia over a 3-year period (Table 24.9). The overall failure rate of 12% included procedures that resulted in no or inadequate analgesia, unintentional dural puncture with an epidural needle or catheter, intravenous cannulation with the epidural catheter, or replacement of the catheter for any reason. The rate of failed analgesia was significantly lower after CSE than after epidural analgesia (10% versus 14%, respectively; $P < .001$). In a follow-up study from the same group of investigators,[22] the rate of epidural catheter failure was 6.6% after CSE analgesia and 11.6% after epidural analgesia ($P = .001$). Other studies have also found a higher epidural catheter failure rate when analgesia is initiated with a traditional epidural approach compared with a CSE technique.[328,330] Of note, these studies were performed in academic institutions where the neuraxial procedures were performed primarily by trainees. In a randomized trial comparing CSE with epidural analgesia in a large maternity hospital staffed by private practice anesthesiologists,[331] the epidural catheter replacement rate was lower and there was no difference between CSE and epidural analgesia (2% and 1.2% incidence, respectively; 95% CI of difference, −3.3% to 1.8%).

TABLE 24.9   Characteristics of Neuraxial Analgesia Failures[a]

Characteristic	RATE ACCORDING TO TYPE OF ANALGESIA (%)			
	Epidural (n = 7849)	Combined Spinal-Epidural (n = 4741)	Total (n = 12,590)	P Value
Overall Failure Rate	14	10	12	<.001
Initial Catheter Failure				
Intravenous catheter	7	5	6	<.001
Recognized dural puncture[b]	1.4	0.8	1.2	<.002
Other Failure				
No cerebrospinal fluid or spinal analgesia	NA	2.4	NA	
Inadequate analgesia with epidural catheter	8.4	4.2	6.8	<.001
Catheter replacement for inadequate analgesia[c]	7.1	3.2	5.6	<.001
Multiple replacements of epidural catheter	1.9	0.7	1.5	<.001

[a]Retrospective audit of all neuraxial analgesic procedures for labor analgesia at a single teaching institution over a 3-y period. Most of the procedures were performed by residents.
[b]Dural puncture with epidural needle or catheter.
[c]Epidural catheter initially functional but was replaced during the course of labor.
NA, Not applicable.
Modified from Pan PH, Bogard TD, Owen MD. Incidence and characteristics of failures in obstetric neuraxial analgesia and anesthesia: a retrospective analysis of 19,259 deliveries. *Int J Obstet Anesth.* 2004;13:227–233.

Typically, failed analgesia after injection of intrathecal or epidural anesthetics results in no neuroblockade, unilateral or asymmetric blockade, missed segments, or inadequate density of neuroblockade. Patient complaints of pain should prompt timely evaluation and treatment (Box 24.7). The progress of labor should be assessed, and the patient should be queried as to the nature of the pain. Typically, pain becomes more intense as labor progresses; for example, an epidural block that was adequate at 4-cm cervical dilation may not be adequate at 8-cm cervical dilation. Expectations and treatment may be different for women in latent versus active or second-stage labor. The bladder should be checked and emptied if distended. The position of the epidural catheter at the skin should be assessed to exclude the possibility of catheter migration out of the epidural space. Inadequate analgesia may also result from migration of the epidural catheter into a vein or movement of the catheter outside the epidural space. Before giving a large bolus dose of local anesthetic, the anesthesia provider should give a test dose to exclude intravenous migration of the catheter.

The extent of neuroblockade should be assessed with a cold or sharp stimulus that starts over the lateral thighs (the dermatomal level at which the tip of the epidural catheter is sited) and moves both *cephalad* and *caudad* on both sides. Inexperienced anesthesia providers often fail to check for the presence of a sacral blockade. In the case of no sensory blockade, the epidural catheter should be replaced. If the extent of neuroblockade is inadequate (in either the cephalad or caudad direction), or if there is unilateral blockade or missed segments, the injection of a large volume (10 to 15 mL) of a dilute local anesthetic solution (e.g., 0.0625% to 0.125% bupivacaine) may result in satisfactory analgesia. An advantage of using a more dilute solution of local anesthetic is the ability to increase the administered volume to ensure adequate spread of analgesia.

Some anesthesia providers advocate withdrawing the epidural catheter 1 to 2 cm out of the epidural space before administering the bolus injection. However, flexible epidural catheters begin to coil after being inserted into the epidural space. A study in young male patients used fluoroscopy to track the advancement of lumbar epidural catheters[332]; only 13% of catheters were threaded 4 cm beyond the tip of the epidural needle without coiling. Therefore, unless the epidural catheter is threaded deeply into the epidural space (e.g., beyond 6 to 8 cm), pulling the epidural catheter back 1 to 2 cm likely pulls out the coil, but does not change the location of the tip of the epidural catheter.

Some women appear to have pain despite adequate *distribution* of sensory blockade. These women may require more dense analgesia; a larger dose of local anesthetic (10- to 15-mL bolus of 0.125% bupivacaine or a 5- to 10-mL bolus of 0.25% bupivacaine) often successfully reestablishes analgesia. Alternatively, a lipid-soluble opioid (e.g., fentanyl 50 μg) may be added to the solution. Reynolds and O'Sullivan[85] showed that epidural bupivacaine 10 mg combined with fentanyl 100 μg was more effective for the treatment of breakthrough pain and had a faster onset and longer duration of action than either bupivacaine 25 mg or fentanyl 100 μg administered alone. The opioid is especially helpful if the parturient is experiencing back pain because the fetus is in the occiput posterior position. Epidural clonidine (75 μg) may be used to treat breakthrough pain that occurs during/after epidural administration of the standard local anesthetic-opioid solution.

Although available data are inconsistent, it appears that maternal position has little effect on the development of an asymmetric block after a *bolus* dose of anesthetic solution into

> **BOX 24.7 Assessment and Management of Inadequate Neuraxial Analgesia**
>
> - Complete a comprehensive assessment:
>   - Assess the distribution and density of any neuroblockade, and the distribution and timing of residual pain.
>   - Assess progress of labor and rule out other causes of pain (distended bladder, ruptured uterus).
>   - Trace the tubing from the epidural infusion pump to the skin insertion site to ensure no disconnections.
>   - Compare the skin insertion depth to the depth documented on the neuraxial block procedure note.
>   - Consider the distribution and density of the neuroblockade in the context of previously administered neuraxial medications (by epidural infusion pump or manual bolus).
>   - If in doubt, replace the catheter.
> - If the extent of neuroblockade is inadequate (does not extend from T10 to S4, as is required for late labor):
>   - Inject a dilute solution of local anesthetic (5 to 15 mL), with or without an opioid.
>   - Alter maintenance technique (e.g., increase volume, decrease concentration).
>   - If this maneuver is unsuccessful, replace the catheter.
> - If the block is asymmetric:
>   - Place the less-blocked side in the dependent position.
>   - Inject a dilute solution of local anesthetic (5 to 15 mL), with or without an opioid.
>   - Alter maintenance technique (e.g., increase volume, decrease concentration).
>   - If this maneuver is unsuccessful, replace the catheter.
> - If the patient has breakthrough pain despite adequate distribution of neuroblockade:
>   - Inject a more concentrated solution of local anesthetic, with or without an opioid.
>   - Consider administration of epidural clonidine (75 to 100 µg).
>   - Alter maintenance technique (e.g., increase concentration of local anesthetic).

the epidural space.[271,333–335] It is likely that the position of the epidural catheter in relation to other epidural space structures (e.g., connective tissue, fatty tissue, blood vessels) affects the spread and quality of analgesia to a greater extent than maternal position. Anatomic barriers (e.g., a longitudinal connective tissue band between the dura and ligamentum flavum) or placement of the catheter tip in the anterior epidural space or paravertebral space may explain some cases of single nerve root, unilateral, or asymmetric blockade.[336–339]

The response to the bolus dose should be assessed in a timely fashion, and the epidural catheter should be replaced (with the patient's consent) if satisfactory analgesia is not obtained.

Unintentional Dural Puncture

In a metaanalysis of 13 studies that involved more than 300,000 obstetric patients, Choi et al.[340] determined that the rate of unintentional dural puncture with an epidural needle or catheter was 1.5% (95% CI, 1.5% to 1.5%) (see Chapter 30).

Dural puncture may be detected at the time of insertion of the epidural needle or after placement of the catheter. If dural puncture is detected with the epidural needle, it is best to replace the stylet to stop the loss of CSF while considering next steps. The anesthesia provider has two primary options. The epidural needle may be withdrawn, and an epidural catheter may be sited at another interspace (intrathecal analgesia may be initiated by injecting a spinal analgesic dose through the epidural needle before it is removed and resited at a different interspace). Alternatively, the anesthesia provider may place a catheter in the subarachnoid space through the "epidural" needle and administer continuous spinal analgesia for labor and delivery. This latter technique is particularly advantageous for patients at high risk for repeat dural puncture on a second attempt or in cases in which it may be difficult to enter either the epidural or subarachnoid space successfully at an alternative interspace (e.g., in obese women or in patients with abnormal anatomy of the lumbar spine). It is very important to append a label that clearly identifies the catheter as a spinal catheter to decrease the risk for injecting an epidural dose of local anesthetic into the subarachnoid space. The parturient and all providers on the obstetric unit, including nurses, midwives, and other anesthesia providers, must be made aware of the intrathecal catheter, and this information must be communicated during any hand-off of care to another provider. Particular care must be taken if the catheter is used to extend the block for cesarean delivery.

Resiting the epidural catheter in a different interspace eliminates the problem of mistaking an intrathecal catheter for an epidural catheter. However, local anesthetic or opioid injected through the epidural catheter may pass through the dural puncture site and into the subarachnoid space, resulting in an unexpectedly high neuroblockade.[341] This complication is more likely to occur with the bolus injection of local anesthetic than with an epidural infusion of local anesthetic.

If dural puncture is not recognized until CSF is aspirated from the catheter, or if administration of the test dose results in spinal anesthesia, the anesthesia provider has the following two options: (1) replace the epidural catheter at an alternative interspace or (2) provide continuous spinal analgesia through the existing catheter.

Respiratory Depression

The administration of opioids by any route entails a risk for respiratory depression. Factors that affect the risk for respiratory depression after neuraxial opioid administration include the choice and dose of drug and its interaction with systemically administered opioids and other central nervous system depressants. The most important factor affecting the onset of respiratory depression is the lipid solubility of the drug.[286] In general, if respiratory depression is going to occur, it will do so within 2 hours of the injection of a lipid-soluble opioid such as fentanyl or sufentanil. When a lipid-soluble opioid gains access to the CSF, it is quickly absorbed by lipophilic body tissues. Subsequent clearance and elimination are similar to those associated with intravenous injection of the same drug. Thus, with a spinal or epidural injection of a lipid-soluble opioid, the "time window" for respiratory depression is short. Conversely, with a hydrophilic drug such as morphine, the onset of respiratory depression is delayed. Once a hydrophilic drug such as morphine enters the CSF, it tends to stay in the CSF. Rostral migration and absorption into the respiratory centers occur over several hours, so respiratory depression may not occur until 6 to 12 hours after injection of the drug (see Fig. 13.12).

A risk factor for respiratory depression is previous parenteral opioid administration. Several reports have implicated prior intravenous opioid administration as a contributing factor to the respiratory arrest that occurred after intrathecal sufentanil 10 μg administration in laboring women.[342,343] (This dose is higher than the currently recommended intrathecal dose range.) For this reason, we refrain from administering a bolus dose of epidural or spinal opioid to women who have recently received systemic opioid analgesia.

Intravascular Injection of Local Anesthetic

The incidence of fatal LAST appears to have declined since initial reports in the early 1980s.[344] In a prospective audit from the United Kingdom of more than 145,000 obstetric epidural procedures (1987 to 2003), the incidence of intravascular injection was 1 in 5000[345] (Table 24.10). Bupivacaine 0.75% is no longer used for epidural anesthesia in obstetric patients. In the United States, lidocaine or 2-chloroprocaine is most often used when a high-concentration local anesthetic is required for operative epidural anesthesia, but in other countries bupivacaine 0.5%, levobupivacaine 0.5%, and ropivacaine 0.75% are often used; low concentrations of local anesthetic are now routinely used for labor analgesia. Nonetheless, LAST remains a serious potential complication during the administration of epidural anesthesia in obstetric patients. Steps to decrease the risk of LAST are outlined in Box 12.3.

Intravenous injection of a large dose of local anesthetic causes central nervous system symptoms (e.g., restlessness, dizziness, tinnitus, perioral paresthesia, difficulty speaking, seizures, loss of consciousness) (see Chapter 13). Cardiovascular effects may progress from increased blood pressure (as a result of sympathetic stimulation) to bradycardia, depressed ventricular function, and ventricular tachycardia and fibrillation. The extension of epidural labor analgesia to epidural anesthesia, whether for intrapartum cesarean delivery or another procedure such as postpartum tubal sterilization, may be a particularly vulnerable risk period for LAST.[346] Bupivacaine cardiotoxicity may be fatal in pregnant women,[347] and robust institutional policies and procedures for safe medication handling are essential to prevent a medication error in which local anesthetic solution intended for the epidural space is inadvertently administered intravenously.[348]

Steps for the management of LAST are listed in Box 24.8.[349] They include treatment of convulsions, supporting oxygenation and ventilation, and initiating advanced cardiac life support, if indicated. Lidocaine should not be administered for the treatment of life-threatening ventricular arrhythmias.

The early administration of lipid emulsion for the management of LAST has been incorporated into guidelines from

---

TABLE 24.10 Incidence of Unintentional Intravascular, Intrathecal, and Subdural Injections During Attempted Epidural Labor Analgesia[a]

Event	Incidence	Rate (%)[b]
Intravascular injection	1:5000	0.020 (0.014 to 0.029)
Intrathecal injection	1:2900	0.035 (0.027 to 0.046)
Subdural injection	1:4200	0.025 (0.017 to 0.033)
High/total spinal anesthesia	1:16,200	0.006 (0.003 to 0.012)

[a]Prospective data collection of 145,550 epidural procedures for obstetric patients in 14 maternity units in the South West Thames Region (United Kingdom) over a 17-y period (1987–2003).
[b]95% confidence intervals shown in parentheses.
Modified from Jenkins JG. Some immediate serious complications of obstetric analgesia and anaesthesia: a prospective study of 145,550 epidurals. *Int J Obstet Anesth.* 2005;14:37–42.

BOX 24.8 Management of Local Anesthetic Systemic Toxicity

- Stop injecting local anesthetic.
- Call for help.
- Position patient with left uterine displacement.
- Prepare for emergency delivery. In women at 20 or more weeks' gestation, initiate delivery of the infant if the mother is not resuscitated within several minutes because this may facilitate successful resuscitation of the mother.
- Consider calling extracorporeal life support team.
- Administer 20% intravenous lipid emulsion administration at the first sign of LAST.
  - Bolus dose: Approximately 100 mL (1.5 mL/kg)
  - Infusion: Approximately 250 mL over 15–20 min (0.25 mL/kg/min)
  - Repeat bolus dose for persistent cardiovascular collapse.
  - Double the infusion rate if patient remains unstable.
  - Continue lipid emulsion infusion for at least 15 min once stable.
  - Maximum dose: 12 mL/kg
- Administer 100% oxygen to maintain maternal oxygenation.
- Stop the seizure with a benzodiazepine. Be aware that hypoxemia and acidosis develop rapidly during a seizure.
- Monitor maternal vital signs and fetal heart rate. Support maternal blood pressure with fluids and vasopressors.
- Initiate advanced cardiac life support if necessary, including modifications for pregnancy (see Chapters 41 and 53).
  - Avoid vasopressin, calcium entry-blocking agents, beta-adrenergic receptor antagonists, and local anesthetics.
  - Reduce individual epinephrine doses to 1 μg/kg or less.

LAST, Local anesthetic systemic toxicity.
Modified from Neal JM, Neal EJ, Weinberg GL. American Society of Regional Anesthesia and Pain Medicine local anesthetic systemic toxicity checklist: 2020 version. *Reg Anesth Pain Med.* 2021;46:81–82.

both the American Society of Regional Anesthesia and Pain Medicine[349] and the Association of Anaesthetists of Great Britain and Ireland.[350] A 2024 scoping review identified 15 pregnant women with presumed LAST who received resuscitation with lipid emulsion[351]; all survived.

High Neuroblockade and Total Spinal Anesthesia

An unexpectedly high level of anesthesia may result in one of several situations. High (or total) spinal blockade may occur after the unintentional and unrecognized injection of local anesthetic (via a needle or catheter) into either the subarachnoid or subdural space during the planned initiation of epidural analgesia/anesthesia. Alternatively, the epidural catheter may migrate into the subarachnoid or subdural space during the course of labor and delivery. Finally, high spinal blockade may result from an overdose of local anesthetic in the epidural space. Crawford[341] reported 6 cases of high or total spinal anesthesia in a series of nearly 27,000 cases of lumbar epidural anesthesia administered during labor (an incidence of approximately 1 in 4500). Paech et al.[327] reported eight cases of unexpectedly high neuroblockade in a series of 10,995 epidural blocks in obstetric patients (an incidence of approximately 1 in 1400). Two patients required tracheal intubation and mechanical ventilation. Jenkins[345] reported an incidence of 1 in 16,200 procedures (see Table 24.10). High spinal or epidural anesthesia contributed to 16% of anesthesia-related maternal deaths in the United States between 1997 and 2002.[344]

The lack of ability to withdraw CSF with aspiration, particularly through a single-orifice catheter, is not a completely reliable method of excluding subarachnoid placement of the catheter. Administration of an appropriate test dose and careful assessment of the patient's response to the test dose should minimize the chance of unintentional injection of a large dose of local anesthetic into the subarachnoid space (see Box 12.3).

High or total spinal anesthesia results in agitation, profound hypotension, dyspnea, the inability to speak, and loss of consciousness. Loss of consciousness usually results from hypoperfusion of the brain and brain stem, not from brain anesthesia. Evidence of spinal anesthesia may be apparent shortly after intrathecal injection of a local anesthetic, but the maximal spread may not be evident for several minutes. This delay underscores the need for the anesthesia provider to carefully assess the effects of both the test and therapeutic doses of local anesthetic. If total spinal anesthesia should occur, the anesthesia provider must be prepared to maintain oxygenation, ventilation, and circulation (Box 24.9). Immediate management consists of avoidance of aortocaval compression, ventilation with 100% oxygen, tracheal intubation, and administration of intravenous fluids and vasopressors to support the blood pressure as needed. The FHR should be monitored continuously.

Extensive neuroblockade may also result from subdural injection of a local anesthetic.[352–354] A subdural injection may be difficult to diagnose because onset is later than that with an intrathecal injection and more closely resembles that associated with epidural neuroblockade.

BOX 24.9 Management of High and Total Spinal Anesthesia

- High spinal anesthesia may occur several minutes after the injection of excessive intrathecal or epidural local anesthetic. Communication with the patient is important. Agitation, dyspnea, difficulty speaking, and profound hypotension may herald the onset of total spinal anesthesia.
- Avoid aortocaval compression; use manual left uterine displacement.
- Administer 100% oxygen.
- Provide positive-pressure ventilation, preferably through an endotracheal tube.
- Monitor maternal vital signs, electrocardiogram, and fetal heart rate.
- Support maternal circulation with intravenous fluids and vasopressors as needed. Do not hesitate to give epinephrine if needed.
- Maintain verbal communication with the mother or administer a sedative-hypnotic (after treating any hypotension and hypoxemia) because total spinal anesthesia does not signal brain anesthesia. Patients may lose consciousness and stop breathing because of central nervous system hypoperfusion, not brain anesthesia.

The subdural space is a potential space between the dura mater and the arachnoid mater. The incidence of subdural catheter placement and injection is not known. Subdural injection of local anesthetic typically results in unexpectedly high (but patchy) blockade with an onset time that is intermediate between that of spinal anesthesia and epidural anesthesia (i.e., 10 to 20 minutes) (Table 24.11).[355] Cranial spread is more extensive than caudal spread of the local anesthetic, so sacral analgesia typically is absent. The block may involve the cranial nerves. (The subdural space, unlike the epidural space, extends intracranially.) Thus, apnea and unconsciousness can occur during a subdural block. Horner's syndrome has been reported.[353]

A subdural block usually results in a less intense motor blockade than the blockade that occurs with high or total spinal anesthesia. This difference may reflect the limited spread of the local anesthetic within the subdural space, which helps spare the anterior motor fibers.[354] Subdural block results in less severe hypotension than that with high or total spinal anesthesia, most likely because subdural injection leads to less sympathetic blockade than spinal anesthesia. The unpredictable spread of local anesthetic, the slower onset of maximal spread (compared with spinal anesthesia), the patchy nature of the block, the potential for laceration of the arachnoid membrane with uncontrolled induction of spinal anesthesia, and the sacral sparing make it difficult to use a subdural catheter safely during labor and delivery. If it is suspected that a catheter is positioned within the subdural space, it should be replaced with an epidural catheter.

An unexpectedly high neuroblockade may result from the migration of an epidural catheter into the subdural or subarachnoid space.[354] The mechanism by which a soft epidural

TABLE 24.11	Clinical Features of Epidural, Subdural, and Spinal Blocks		
	Epidural Block	**Subdural Block**	**Spinal Block**
Onset time	Slow	Intermediate	Rapid
Spread	As expected	Higher than expected; may extend intracranially, but sacral sparing is common	Higher than expected; may extend intracranially, and a sacral block is typically present
Nature of block	Segmental	Patchy	Dense
Motor block	Minimal	Minimal	Dense
Hypotension	Less than spinal, and dependent on the extent of the block	Intermediate between spinal and epidural, and dependent on the extent of the block	Likely

catheter penetrates the dura or dura-arachnoid is unclear. Disposable epidural needles are sharp, and insertion of the needle into the epidural space may result in an unrecognized nick in the dura, which may create a site for delayed migration of the catheter into the subdural or subarachnoid space. Subdural or subarachnoid injection of local anesthetic also may occur if a multiorifice catheter is used, and one orifice is located within the epidural space while another is located within the subdural or subarachnoid space. In this situation, the force of injection determines the ultimate destination of the local anesthetic. Thus, each bolus injection of local anesthetic should serve as a test dose. During the continuous infusion of a local anesthetic, a gradual increase in the level of anesthesia and intensity of motor blockade may indicate the intrathecal infusion of the local anesthetic solution.

Extensive Motor Blockade

Clinically significant motor block may occur after repeated bolus doses, particularly if using high-concentration local anesthetic solutions (>0.125% bupivacaine)[121] or after many hours of a continuous infusion of local anesthetic into the epidural space. The administration of bupivacaine with epinephrine may result in a greater likelihood of motor blockade than the administration of bupivacaine alone.[121]

Extensive motor blockade is often bothersome for the patient, and it may impair maternal expulsive efforts during the second stage of labor and increase the likelihood of operative vaginal delivery (see later discussion). Some obstetricians argue that pelvic floor relaxation prevents rotation of the fetal head and increases the likelihood of an abnormal position of the vertex at delivery.

In contemporary practice, extensive motor blockade is frequently a consequence of breakthrough pain when local anesthetic solutions fail to distribute evenly, and subsequent PCEA and manual bolus doses increase anesthetic density without improving the distribution of the neuroblockade. Replacement of the neuraxial catheter with a CSE technique can frequently remediate breakthrough pain in such cases.

If an intense motor blockade develops during the continuous epidural infusion of local anesthetic, migration of the catheter to the subdural or subarachnoid space should be ruled out. The infusion can be discontinued for a short period (e.g., 30 minutes) and then restarted at a reduced rate or with a more dilute solution of local anesthetic. Extensive motor blockade does not occur with administration of a very dilute solution of local anesthetic combined with an opioid and is less likely with intermittent boluses compared with continuous infusion of local anesthetic into the epidural space (see earlier discussion).

Prolonged Neuroblockade

Rarely, the duration of neuraxial analgesia/anesthesia exceeds the time expected. Most cases of unexpectedly prolonged neuroblockade follow the epidural administration of a high concentration of local anesthetic with epinephrine.[356] Abnormal neurologic findings after the administration of neuraxial anesthesia should prompt the anesthesia provider to look for evidence to distinguish between peripheral nerve injury, radiculopathy, or epidural hematoma (see Chapter 31). Factors that argue against the presence of an epidural hematoma include (1) the absence of back pain, (2) a unilateral block, and (3) regression (rather than progression) of the symptoms. An injury to a nerve root typically presents as a sensory and motor deficit that follows a dermatomal distribution (see Figs. 31.1 and 31.2). Peripheral nerve injuries typically result in a neurologic deficit in the distribution of a specific peripheral nerve (see Fig. 31.1). Neurologic or neurosurgical consultation and immediate imaging studies should be obtained if there is any suspicion of a space-occupying lesion of the neuraxial canal. Avoiding the use of a high concentration of local anesthetic should help minimize the incidence of prolonged neuroblockade during and after labor and vaginal delivery.

Back Pain

Approximately 50% of women complain of back pain during pregnancy and the puerperium.[357,358] The most significant risk factors for postpartum back pain are antepartum back pain and the inability to reduce weight to prepregnancy levels.[357,359,360] Early retrospective studies identified an association between epidural anesthesia and an increased risk for postpartum back pain.[361,362] However, retrospective studies suffer not only from patient recall bias (i.e., patients with a problem are much more likely to complete and return the questionnaire) but also from selection bias in the epidural and nonepidural groups. Patients who select epidural analgesia for labor may have obstetric, orthopedic, social, or other unidentified factors that predispose them to postpartum back pain.

In an attempt to assess anesthetic factors that might contribute to postpartum backache (e.g., motor blockade), Russell et al.[360] randomly assigned laboring women requesting epidural analgesia to receive either bupivacaine alone or bupivacaine plus an opioid. Despite the expected differences in motor blockade, the incidence of backache did not differ between the two anesthetic groups (bupivacaine alone, 39%; bupivacaine plus an opioid, 30%). In addition, the incidence of backache in both epidural groups was similar to that found in a nonrandomized control group of women who labored without epidural analgesia (31%).

Prospective reports have not shown a significant relationship between the use of epidural analgesia and long-term backache.[359,363] Several randomized controlled trials have identified no difference in the incidence of postpartum back pain (at 6 months,[364] 3 and 12 months,[365] and several years[366]) in women randomized to epidural compared with nonepidural analgesia. Thus, prospective studies have consistently shown that no causal relationship exists between epidural analgesia and the development of long-term postpartum backache. Short-term backache (several days) may be related to local tissue trauma at the site of skin puncture. In patients with chronic low back pain, spine manipulation can trigger muscle spasms; this may be alleviated postpartum with a muscle relaxant such cyclobenzaprine or methocarbamol.

EFFECTS OF NEURAXIAL ANALGESIA ON THE PROGRESS OF LABOR AND OBSTETRIC OUTCOMES

Neuraxial analgesia during labor is associated with a prolonged labor and operative delivery. (The term *operative delivery* refers to both cesarean delivery and operative vaginal delivery [i.e., forceps delivery or vacuum extraction]). Controversy exists as to whether there is a cause-and-effect relationship between the use of these analgesic techniques and prolonged labor or operative delivery. The understanding of this subject has been limited by the difficulty of performing controlled trials in which parturients are randomly assigned to neuraxial analgesia or a control group. Ideally, if one wants to study the effect of neuraxial analgesia on the progress and outcome of labor, the control group would receive no analgesia. However, such a study is not ethical, and even if it were and women volunteered to participate in it, the crossover rate would probably be high, and the data consequently would not be interpretable. Therefore, controlled trials have randomly assigned parturients to receive neuraxial analgesia or an alternative form of pain relief, usually systemic opioid analgesia. However, even when the control group receives some type of analgesia, the crossover rate may be high because the quality

of neuraxial analgesia is markedly superior to that of all other modes of labor analgesia.[367]

The difficulty in performing and interpreting the results of labor analgesia trials was aptly described by Noble et al.,[368] who assessed obstetric outcome in 245 patients randomly assigned to receive either epidural analgesia or "conventional" analgesia (i.e., meperidine, nitrous oxide, or no analgesia). The investigators made the following comments[368]:

> *Of 245 selected patients, 43 had to be removed from the trial after labour ensued....Most of the patients removed from the non-epidural group were apparently experiencing severe pain; they were usually primigravidae whose baby presented in the occipito-posterior position....The majority of patients removed from the epidural group were apparently normal and usually multigravidas; their labours were so rapid it was not possible to arrange for an epidural block.*

In other words, patients at low risk for operative delivery were excluded from the epidural group and patients at high risk were excluded from the nonepidural group. The investigators' candid comments illustrate that, even when a prospective, randomized study is performed, it is difficult to maintain conditions that allow for the comparison of women at equal risk for abnormal labor and operative delivery.

Ironically, the effect of systemic opioids on the progress and outcome of labor has not been well studied. Furthermore, there may be differences among the opioids.[369] Finally, neuraxial analgesia is not a generic procedure. Conclusions about the effect of one technique on the progress of labor may not be applicable to other techniques (see later discussion).

Additional factors prevent rigorous scientific study of this issue. Ideally, a randomized controlled trial should be double blinded. This is not possible for studies that compare neuraxial analgesia with another mode of analgesia because of the marked difference in the quality of analgesia. Therefore, the potential for bias on the part of the parturient, nurses, and anesthesia and obstetric providers is substantial. Additionally, other factors are known to affect or to be associated with the progress and outcome of labor, including parity, artificial rupture of membranes, use of oxytocin, and payer status; these factors should be controlled in well-conducted studies.

One factor known to markedly influence the outcome of labor is the obstetric provider. Neuhoff et al.[370] retrospectively reviewed the records of 607 nulliparous women at term gestation and compared the mode of delivery in "clinic" patients (whose care was given primarily by trainees) and private patients (whose care was provided primarily by private obstetricians). Approximately 42% of patients received epidural analgesia during labor. Five percent of patients in the clinic group and 17% of patients in the private group underwent cesarean delivery (P < .001). More striking was the difference between groups in the incidence of cesarean delivery for dystocia (0.5% versus 13.7%, respectively; P < .001). Similarly, Guillemette and Fraser[371] observed marked obstetrician variation in cesarean delivery rates, despite similarities in the use of oxytocin and epidural analgesia. In Japan, the primary cesarean delivery rate was higher in regions with a lower density of obstetricians.[372]

Several groups of investigators have noted that the timing of cesarean delivery conforms to a "circadian" rhythm.[373,374] For example, investigators in Japan noted a delivery time rhythm in hospitals, but not birthing centers, suggesting that obstetric intervention, not biologic rhythm, partly determines the timing of delivery.[375]

Retrospective studies are difficult to interpret because they suffer from selection bias. In some cases, distinguishing between anesthesia administered for pain relief during labor and anesthesia administered in preparation for operative delivery is difficult. Moreover, women at higher risk for prolonged labor and operative delivery are more likely to request and receive epidural analgesia during labor than women who have a rapid, uncomplicated labor.[376] Wuitchik et al.[376] observed a relationship between pain and cognitive activity during early labor and the subsequent progress of labor in 115 healthy nulliparous women. During the latent phase, higher levels of pain were predictive of longer latent and active phases of labor. Those women who reported "horrible" or "excruciating" pain during the latent phase were more than twice as likely to require operative vaginal delivery as women who only had "discomfort." In addition, women who reported "distress" rather than "coping" had a fivefold higher incidence of abnormal FHR patterns and a fourfold higher requirement for assistance from pediatricians during neonatal resuscitation.

Greater pain intensity during labor appears to be a risk factor for operative delivery. This fact will significantly bias observational studies of labor analgesia because women with greater pain intensity request analgesia, specifically neuraxial analgesia, at a higher rate than women with less intense pain. Alexander et al.[377] performed a secondary analysis of data from a randomized controlled trial in which one group of laboring women received patient-controlled intravenous meperidine analgesia. The rate of cesarean delivery for dystocia was 14% in women who self-administered 50 mg/h or more of meperidine, compared with 1.4% in women who self-administered less than 50 mg/h. In a retrospective study of factors that predict operative delivery in laboring women, Hess et al.[378] found that the cesarean delivery rate in women who had significant breakthrough pain during low-dose bupivacaine/fentanyl epidural analgesia was more than twice as high as the rate in women with less breakthrough pain (OR, 2.62; 95% CI, 2.01 to 3.43). Panni and Segal[379] showed that women who subsequently deliver by cesarean for dystocia have a 30% increase in the median local anesthetic concentration of epidural bupivacaine required to induce analgesia at the beginning of labor compared with women who ultimately deliver vaginally.

Taken together, these studies suggest that the early onset of severe pain and the requirement of high doses of analgesic agents predict higher risks for abnormal labor, FHR abnormalities, and operative delivery. These findings may explain the observed association between neuraxial analgesia and operative delivery.

Cesarean Delivery Rate
Randomized Controlled Trials

Randomized controlled trials have studied the effect of neuraxial (primarily epidural) and systemic opioid (primarily meperidine) analgesia on the cesarean delivery rate.[3] These trials differ in a number of ways, including (1) the population studied (e.g., nulliparous women or women of mixed parity); (2) onset of labor (spontaneous labor alone or a mix of spontaneous and induced labors); (3) type of neuraxial analgesia; (4) density of neuraxial analgesia; (5) route of administration of systemic analgesia; (6) the crossover rate; and (7) management of labor (e.g., active management of labor, including electronic FHR monitoring, artificial rupture of membranes, and oxytocin infusion). A 2018 systematic review and meta-analysis included 10,350 women (33 studies) randomized to neuraxial labor analgesia (mostly epidural) or nonneuraxial or systemic opioid analgesia (mostly meperidine), and found no difference in the cesarean delivery rate between groups (Table 24.12).[3]

Among trials with a high crossover rate, the outcomes for all randomized participants, regardless of treatment received, should be included in an **intention-to-treat analysis**. Biased conclusions can be drawn from a **protocol compliant analysis**, in which data are analyzed only for those participants who received their assigned treatments. The influence of trial crossover and the method of analysis is illustrated by a series of four prospective, randomized trials performed at the University of Texas Southwestern Medical Center, Parkland Hospital, in Dallas.[367,380-382] This institution is unique among many others who have performed randomized trials, in that the population is composed largely of indigent women whose labor is managed by the same group of trainee physicians and midwives, supervised by the same core group of attending obstetricians. In the first study, 1330 women of mixed parity were randomly assigned to receive either epidural bupivacaine/fentanyl or intravenous meperidine for labor analgesia.[367] Approximately one-third of the women did not receive the assigned treatment. The cesarean delivery rates were 9.0% in women who were randomized to receive epidural analgesia and received it and 3.9% in women who were randomized to receive intravenous meperidine and received it (i.e., protocol compliant). However, the investigators did not report an intention-to-treat analysis of these data; they excluded from analysis those study participants who crossed over to the other treatment as well as those who received neither treatment. Subsequently, the investigators published a reanalysis of the data that included an intention-to-treat analysis of all participant data (Table 24.13).[383] The cesarean delivery rate in both groups was approximately 6% and did not differ between groups.

In an attempt to lower the rate of crossover by providing better analgesia to the control (meperidine) group, the Parkland Hospital investigators performed another study in which meperidine was administered by PCIA.[381] A significant number of women in both groups did not receive their assigned treatment, although the reason in all cases was rapid

TABLE 24.12 Labor Outcomes in Women Randomized to Receive Neuraxial Versus Systemic Opioid Labor Analgesia

Outcome	Neuraxial Analgesia	Systemic Opioid Analgesia		
Mode of Delivery	***n/N***	***n/N***	**Risk Ratio**	**95% Confidence Interval**
Cesarean delivery	699/5401	566/4949	1.07	0.96 to 1.18
Operative vaginal delivery	705/5186	470/4762	1.44	1.29 to 1.60
Duration of Labor	***N***	***N***	**Mean Difference (min)**	**95% Confidence Interval**
First stage	1139	1120	32.3	18.3 to 46.2
Second stage[a]	2694	2285	15.4	9.0 to 21.8
Other Outcomes	***n/N***	***n/N***	**Risk Ratio**	**95% Confidence Interval**
Oxytocin augmentation[b]	1851/4350	1608/4001	1.12	1.00 to 1.26
Perineal trauma requiring suturing	141/184	135/185	1.05	0.93 to 1.18

[a]High heterogeneity (I^2, 88.5%).
[b]High heterogeneity (I^2, 80.0%).
Data from Amin-Somuah M, Smyth RM, Cyna AM, Cuthbert A. Epidural versus non-epidural or no analgesia for pain management in labour. *Cochrane Database Syst Rev.* 2018;(5):CD000331.

TABLE 24.13 Parkland Hospital Randomized Controlled Trial of Epidural Versus Systemic Opioid Analgesia and Rate of Cesarean Delivery: Actual Treatment Versus Intention-to-Treat Analysis

	CESAREAN DELIVERY RATE (%)	
Type of Analysis	Epidural Analgesia	Systemic Opioid Analgesia
Received assigned treatment[a]	9.0 (39/432)	3.9 (17/437)
Intention-to-treat[b]	6.5 (43/664)	5.4 (36/666)

[a]The initial analysis was published in 1995, and excluded a total of 461 patients with protocol violations from the analysis, including 103 women in the systemic opioid group who requested and received epidural analgesia because opioid analgesia was inadequate. The difference was significant ($P < .05$).
[b]The intention-to-treat analysis of the same data was published in 2000 (no significant difference between groups).
Data from Ramin SM, Gambling DR, Lucas MJ, et al. Randomized trial of epidural versus intravenous analgesia during labor. *Obstet Gynecol.* 1995;86:783–789; Sharma SK, Leveno KJ. Update: epidural analgesia does not increase cesarean births. *Curr Anesthesiol Rep.* 2000;2:18–24.

labor. Only 5 of 357 women randomly assigned to the meperidine group crossed over to receive epidural analgesia. Using an intention-to-treat analysis, the investigators observed no difference between the groups in the incidence of cesarean delivery (4% in the epidural group and 5% in the PCIA group). There was no difference between the two groups in neonatal outcome, except that more neonates of women in the PCIA group received naloxone to reverse respiratory depression at birth.

Only one randomized trial from Parkland Hospital compared CSE and systemic opioid analgesia.[380] In this large study ($n = 1223$), patients of mixed parity were randomly assigned to receive CSE analgesia (intrathecal sufentanil 10 μg, followed by epidural bupivacaine with fentanyl at the second request for analgesia) or intravenous meperidine (50 mg every hour on request). An intention-to-treat analysis showed that there was no difference between groups in the rate of cesarean delivery (CSE 6%, systemic opioid 5.5%).

In an individual patient metaanalysis of all four studies performed at Parkland Hospital ($n = 4465$),[384] the OR for cesarean delivery between the neuraxial and systemic opioid analgesia groups was 1.04 (95% CI, 0.81 to 1.34).

Together, these analyses support the conclusion that women who choose epidural analgesia have an inherent risk factor(s) for cesarean delivery and that the administration of neuraxial analgesia *per se* does not alter this risk. The apparent association between epidural analgesia and cesarean delivery is an example of **confounding by indication**, in which a difficult childbirth increases the likelihood of both the selection of epidural analgesia and eventual delivery by cesarean.

Mode and density of neuraxial analgesia and effect on cesarean delivery rate. If neuraxial analgesia adversely affects the outcome of labor, one would expect to observe a dose-response effect. The COMET (Comparative Obstetric Mobile Epidural Trial) study randomly assigned more than 1000 parturients to one of three groups: (1) "high-dose" epidural analgesia (traditional epidural analgesia with bupivacaine 0.25%); (2) "low-dose" epidural analgesia (bupivacaine 0.1%/fentanyl 2 μg/mL bolus, followed by a CEI); and (3) "low-dose" CSE analgesia (intrathecal bupivacaine/fentanyl followed by intermittent boluses of epidural bupivacaine 0.1%/fentanyl 2 μg/mL).[385] There was no difference in cesarean delivery rates among groups (Fig. 24.7).

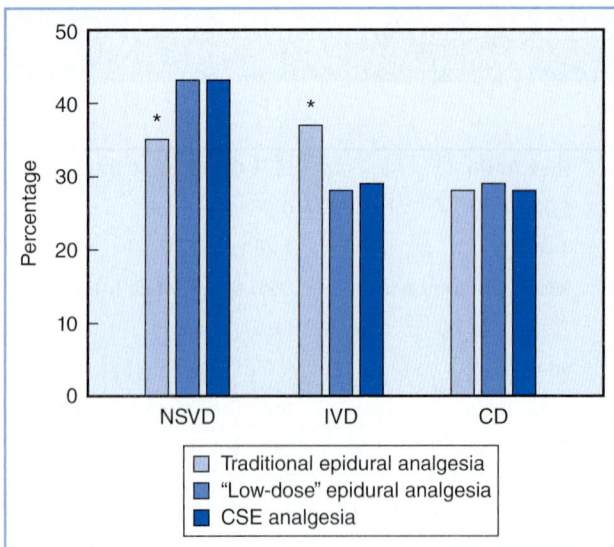

Fig. 24.7 Outcome of Labor in the COMET (Comparative Obstetric Mobile Epidural Trial) Study. Parturients were randomly assigned to traditional epidural analgesia or to one of two "low-dose" neuraxial techniques (see text). There was no difference among groups in the cesarean delivery (CD) rate. *Women who received traditional epidural analgesia had a higher rate of instrumental (operative) vaginal delivery (IVD) than those who received a "low-dose" technique (*P* = .04). *CSE*, Combined spinal-epidural; *NSVD*, normal spontaneous vaginal delivery. Data from Comparative Obstetric Mobile Epidural Trial Study Group UK. Effect of low-dose mobile versus traditional epidural techniques on mode of delivery: a randomised controlled trial. *Lancet*. 2001;358:19–23.

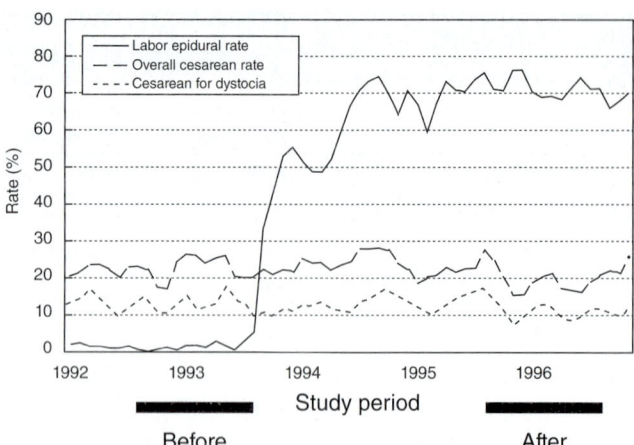

Fig. 24.8 Labor epidural rate, overall rate of cesarean delivery, and rate of cesarean delivery for dystocia in nulliparous women before and after the introduction of epidural labor analgesia to the Tripler Army Hospital, 1992–96. The epidural rate increased markedly, but the cesarean delivery rate remained unchanged. From Zhang J, Yancey MK, Klebanoff MA, et al. Does epidural analgesia prolong labor and increase risk of cesarean delivery? A natural experiment. *Am J Obstet Gynecol*. 2001;185:128–134.

There is no evidence that CSE analgesia influences the mode of delivery compared with epidural analgesia alone. A metaanalysis that compared CSE with low-dose epidural analgesia included 15 trials with 1960 women[20]; the risk ratio for cesarean delivery was 0.98 (95% CI, 0.82 to 1.16).

Finally, a metaanalysis included trials in which women were randomized to receive a high-concentration local anesthetic solution for maintenance of epidural analgesia (bupivacaine > 0.1%, ropivacaine > 0.17%). There was no difference between groups in the cesarean delivery rate (OR, 1.05; 95% CI, 0.82 to 1.33).[386] The results of these studies suggest that a "high-dose" neuraxial analgesia technique does not entail a higher risk for cesarean delivery than a "low-dose" technique; in other words, no dose-response effect has been observed.

Impact Studies

Some physicians have questioned whether prospective, randomized studies provide an accurate representation of the effect of neuraxial analgesia on the mode of delivery in actual clinical practice. They have suggested the possibility that prospective studies may introduce a Hawthorne effect (which may be defined as the appearance or disappearance of a phenomenon on initiation of a study to confirm or exclude its existence). An alternative study design is to assess the obstetric outcome immediately before and after a key event, such as the introduction of an epidural analgesia service. The results of these impact studies may be generalizable to the general population because patients have not chosen to participate in a study. It also eliminates the problem of treatment group crossover because

epidural analgesia was not available in the control period. One limitation of this study design is that it assumes that there were no other changes in obstetric management in the "after" period.

In 1999, Yancey et al.[387] published an impact study using data from the Tripler Army Medical Center in Hawaii. Because of relative homogeneity in socioeconomic status, universal access to healthcare, and the availability of dedicated healthcare providers in the population served by this hospital, its rate of cesarean delivery may not be subject to influences common to other hospitals. Before 1993, the rate of epidural analgesia was less than 1% at the center. In 1993, a policy change within the US Department of Defense mandated on-demand availability of neuraxial labor analgesia in military hospitals. In nulliparous women in spontaneous labor with a singleton infant with a vertex presentation, the rate of epidural labor analgesia rose from less than 1% to approximately 80% in a 1-year period.[388] Despite this, the rate of cesarean delivery was unchanged during the same period (14.4% versus 12.1%, respectively; adjusted RR, 0.8; 95% CI, 0.6 to 1.2) (Fig. 24.8).

Socol et al.[389] evaluated the impact of three initiatives to reduce the cesarean delivery rate in their hospital. First, they strongly encouraged a trial of labor and vaginal birth after cesarean delivery. Second, after the 1988 calendar year, they circulated data showing the cesarean delivery rate of every obstetrician to all obstetricians. Third, they recommended the active management of labor as the preferred method of labor management for term nulliparous women. The rates of total, primary, and repeat cesarean deliveries decreased from 27%, 18%, and 9% in 1986 to 17%, 11%, and 6%, respectively, in 1991 (*P* < .001 for all three comparisons). Meanwhile, the use of epidural analgesia rose from 28% in 1986 to 48% in 1991 (*P* < .001). There was no change in the incidence of operative vaginal delivery (13% in 1986 versus 13% in 1991).

In a metaanalysis, Segal et al.[390] identified impact studies involving a total of 37,753 patients that compared the rate of

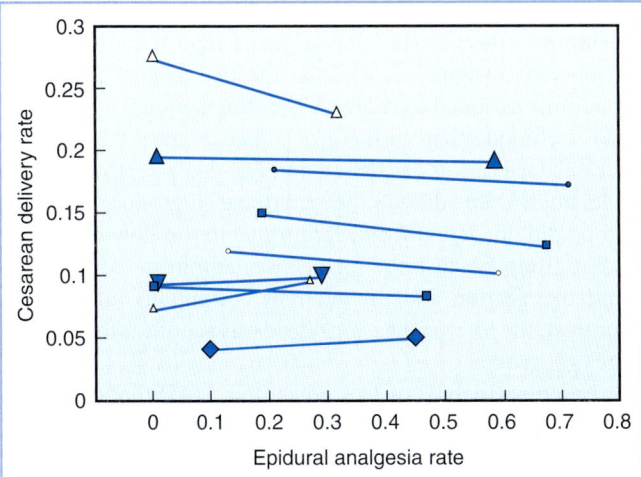

Fig. 24.9 Rates of cesarean delivery during periods of higher and lower availability of epidural analgesia in nine studies (*n* = 37,753) subjected to metaanalysis. Each pair of symbols shows data from one investigation (the *left symbol* is the epidural analgesia rate and cesarean delivery rate during the period of low epidural analgesia availability, and the *right symbol* is the epidural analgesia rate and cesarean delivery rate during the period of high epidural availability). The size of the plot symbol is proportional to the number of patients in the analysis. Modified from Segal S, Su M, Gilbert P. The effect of a rapid change in availability of epidural analgesia on the cesarean delivery rate: a meta-analysis. *Am J Obstet Gynecol.* 2000;183:974–978.

cesarean delivery before and after the introduction of neuraxial labor analgesia to nine obstetric units. The researchers found no increase in the rate of cesarean delivery with the increase in availability of epidural analgesia (Fig. 24.9). Thus, the before-after impact studies support the results of randomized controlled trials—namely, that neuraxial analgesia does not cause an increase in the cesarean delivery rate.

Several studies have assessed whether there is a relationship between an individual obstetrician's cesarean delivery rate and the rate of epidural analgesia for their patients.[391,392] For example, Lagrew and Adashek[391] divided obstetricians into two groups according to whether their individual cesarean delivery rates were more than 15% (the control group) or less than 15% (the target group). Obstetricians in the target group used epidural analgesia more often than obstetricians in the control group. In other words, the target group of obstetricians was able to achieve a lower cesarean delivery rate despite their greater use of epidural analgesia.

Timing of Initiation of Neuraxial Analgesia

A review of observational data suggests an association between cesarean delivery and the initiation of neuraxial analgesia during early labor (often defined as a cervical dilation < 4 to 5 cm).[393] For example, in a retrospective study of 1917 nulliparous women, the rate of cesarean delivery was twice as high in women who received neuraxial analgesia at a cervical dilation < 4 cm than in those in whom neuraxial analgesia was initiated at a cervical dilation ≥ 4 cm (18.9% versus 8.9%, respectively).[393] As a result of these data, for many years the ACOG suggested that women delay requesting epidural analgesia

"when feasible, until the cervix is dilated to 4 to 5 cm."[394] However, as with the cause-and-effect question raised by the association of neuraxial labor analgesia and cesarean delivery, the question arises as to whether the early initiation of neuraxial labor analgesia *causes* a higher risk for cesarean delivery or whether the request for early labor analgesia is a marker for some other risk factor(s) for cesarean delivery.

A number of randomized controlled trials have addressed the question of whether initiation of neuraxial analgesia during early labor adversely affects the mode of delivery. For example, Wong et al.[285] and Ohel et al.[395] reported randomized trials that compared early labor neuraxial analgesia with systemic opioid analgesia; the median cervical dilation at initiation of analgesia was 2 cm. There was no difference between the two groups in the rate of cesarean delivery or in the rate of operative vaginal delivery. The study protocols differed in that the treatment group in one study received *CSE* analgesia in early labor,[285] whereas the treatment group in the second study received *epidural* analgesia alone.[395] The use of oxytocin augmentation was markedly different in the two studies (94%[285] and 29%[395]). A 2014 metaanalysis of nine randomized controlled trials including over 15,000 women[19] found that early initiation of neuraxial analgesia does not increase the rate of cesarean delivery compared with delayed initiation (RR, 1.02; 95% CI, 0.96 to 1.08).

Subsequent to the publication of these studies, the ACOG[396] updated their guidelines. The 2024 ACOG clinical practice guideline states[397]:

> *Regional anesthesia is a highly effective mode of pain relief for individuals in labor. For pregnant women electing regional pain management in labor, a systematic review demonstrated that neither type of neuraxial analgesia (epidural vs combined spinal epidural) nor timing affected the risk of cesarean delivery.*

Operative Vaginal Delivery Rate

Observational data associate neuraxial labor analgesia with a higher rate of operative (forceps or vacuum extraction) vaginal delivery. The effect of neuraxial analgesia on mode of vaginal delivery has not been assessed as a primary outcome in randomized controlled trials, although it has been assessed as a secondary outcome in multiple trials. Interpretation of these results is clouded by the fact that most studies have not assessed the quality of analgesia during the second stage of labor. Further, most investigators did not define the criteria for the performance of operative vaginal delivery. In clinical practice, and in study interpretation, it is often difficult to distinguish "indicated" operative deliveries from elective operative deliveries. Indeed, we have observed that indications for operative vaginal delivery vary markedly among obstetric providers. An obstetric provider is more likely to perform an elective operative delivery in a patient with satisfactory anesthesia than in a patient without analgesia. In addition, most randomized controlled trials are conducted in teaching institutions that have an obligation to teach obstetric trainees how to perform operative vaginal deliveries. Operative vaginal deliveries performed for the purpose of teaching are more likely to be done in women with adequate analgesia.

Multiple randomized, controlled studies comparing epidural analgesia with systemic opioid analgesia have assessed the rate of operative vaginal delivery as a secondary outcome variable. Systematic reviews have concluded that epidural analgesia is associated with a higher risk for operative vaginal delivery than systemic analgesia (see Table 24.12).[3,384]

In contrast to these studies, many of the impact studies observed no difference in the operative vaginal delivery rate between the control and study periods. For example, despite a rise in the epidural analgesia rate from 1% to 84% at Tripler Army Medical Center, the rate of operative vaginal delivery did not change (22.1% versus 23.5%) among nulliparous women.[388] A systematic review of seven impact studies[390] involving more than 28,000 patients did not identify a difference in operative vaginal delivery rates between periods of low and periods of high epidural analgesia rates (mean change, 0.76%; 95% CI, −1.2% to 2.8%).

Studies of early versus late initiation of neuraxial labor analgesia have not identified an increased risk for operative vaginal delivery in the early analgesia group.[19]

Obstetricians and anesthesiologists have suggested that multiple factors (e.g., station and position of the fetal vertex, maternal pain and the urge to bear down, and neuraxial analgesia–induced motor blockade) may contribute to the outcome of the second stage of labor. The contribution of these factors to the mode of vaginal delivery, and their interactions, are not well understood, and these factors have not been well controlled in many studies.

Several studies have specifically assessed the role of second-stage neuraxial labor analgesia on the mode of delivery. For example, in a 2017 study from China,[398] 400 women receiving an epidural infusion of 0.08% ropivacaine with sufentanil 0.4 μg/mL for labor analgesia were randomized to continue the same infusion or to receive a saline-placebo at the onset of the second stage of labor. The rate of operative vaginal delivery did not differ between groups; more women in the placebo-control group had low satisfaction scores.

The effect of neuraxial analgesia on the outcome of the second stage of labor may be influenced by the density of neuraxial analgesia. High concentrations of epidural local anesthetic may cause maternal motor blockade, leading to relaxation of the pelvic floor musculature, which in turn may interfere with fetal head rotation into the occiput anterior position during descent. Pelvic floor analgesia also decreases involuntary pushing; abdominal muscle relaxation may decrease the effectiveness of maternal expulsive efforts. The effects of specific analgesic techniques, concentration of local anesthetic, total dose of local anesthetic, and degree of motor blockade on the risk for operative vaginal delivery are overlapping and difficult to study. For example, some studies suggest that the administration of epidural analgesia using higher concentrations of bupivacaine is associated with a higher risk for operative vaginal delivery compared with use of lower concentrations.[385,399–401] In contrast, Collis et al.[402] observed no difference in mode of delivery between women randomly

assigned to receive either a high-dose or a low-dose neuraxial technique. The COMET investigators reported a lower rate of operative vaginal delivery in the two groups of women randomly assigned to receive either the low-dose epidural or CSE technique than in the group that received 0.25% bupivacaine (see earlier discussion and Fig. 24.7).[385] However, the total bupivacaine dose in the traditional "high-dose" epidural group did not actually differ from that in the "low-dose" epidural group because the former was administered by intermittent injection and the latter by continuous infusion. In contrast, the total bupivacaine dose was significantly lower in the CSE group.

In a metaanalysis of 11 studies ($n = 1145$) that compared maintenance of epidural analgesia with high-concentration (bupivacaine > 0.1%, ropivacaine > 0.17%) with low-concentration local anesthesia solutions,[386] the odds of operative vaginal delivery were lower in the low-concentration group (OR, 0.70; 95% CI, 0.56 to 0.86), as was the duration of the second stage of labor. A 2017 metaanalysis[403] compared parturients randomized to low-concentration epidural analgesia (defined as bupivacaine ≤ 0.1% or equipotent alternative) with non-epidural or no analgesia. In contrast to the findings from a prior metaanalysis that included all epidural local anesthetic concentrations (Table 24.12), there was no difference in the rate of operative vaginal delivery (RR, 1.52; 95% CI, 0.97 to 2.4), although the confidence intervals are wide. Finally, in a metaanalysis of studies that compared CSE and epidural analgesia,[20] the operative vaginal delivery rate was lower in the CSE group than the traditional "high-dose" epidural analgesia group, but there was no difference between "low-dose" epidural and CSE analgesia. Taken together, these data suggest that the specific analgesia technique may influence the risk for operative vaginal delivery.

In general, the dose of bupivacaine is significantly lower if epidural analgesia is maintained with an intermittent bolus technique rather than a continuous infusion technique (see earlier discussion). Most investigators have noted a difference in motor blockade between the two techniques; higher total bupivacaine doses (i.e., continuous infusion techniques) are associated with a greater degree of motor blockade. However, the relationship between motor blockade and operative vaginal delivery is inconsistent. Smedstad and Morison[216] reported a higher incidence of operative vaginal delivery when bupivacaine 0.25% was administered as a CEI than as intermittent bolus injections. In contrast, the COMET investigators observed no difference in the operative vaginal delivery rate in the two groups that received "low-dose" bupivacaine/fentanyl, one by infusion and the other by intermittent bolus.[385] Similarly, in a metaanalysis of PCEA (without background infusion) compared with CEI analgesia,[222] the dose of bupivacaine and degree of motor blockade were significantly lower in the PCEA group, but the rates of operative vaginal delivery did not differ.

It is possible that the inconsistent results can be explained by the actual absolute differences in bupivacaine dose and motor blockade. For example, the differences in dose and motor blockade may have clinically significant adverse effects on the outcome of the second stage of labor if bupivacaine 0.25% is compared with bupivacaine 0.125% but not if bupivacaine 0.125% is compared with bupivacaine 0.0625%. Many of the randomized controlled trials included in the metaanalysis that compared an epidural with systemic opioid analgesia used concentrated solutions of bupivacaine for both the loading and infusion doses (e.g., bupivacaine 0.25% for the loading dose, bupivacaine 0.125% by continuous infusion for maintenance of analgesia).[3]

Motor blockade may increase the risk for malrotation of the fetal vertex. Robinson et al.[404] and Le Ray et al.[405] observed a higher incidence of occiput malposition at delivery in patients who received epidural analgesia before engagement of the fetal head. In contrast, Yancey et al.[406] and Sheiner et al.[407] noted that the administration of on-demand epidural analgesia did not increase the frequency of malposition of the fetal head at delivery; the incidence of operative vaginal delivery was not related to fetal station at initiation of analgesia. In a prospective cohort study using ultrasonography, Lieberman et al.[408] reported that fetal position changed frequently during labor but that epidural analgesia was associated with a higher incidence of occiput posterior position at delivery (13% versus 3%, $P < .002$). However, these results should be interpreted with caution as women were not randomly assigned to the treatment group. Factors that cause women to request analgesia when the fetal head is high may also be independent risk factors for operative vaginal delivery. A study from Italy,[409] in which ultrasonography was used to assess fetal head position, found no association between use of early labor neuraxial analgesia and fetal head position at delivery.

In an editorial, Chestnut[410] concluded that *effective* second-stage analgesia increases the risk for operative vaginal delivery. However, effective analgesia is a spectrum that ranges from complete absence of sensory input (dense analgesia) to perception of uterine contraction "pressure" without pain (less dense analgesia). Minimizing the risk for operative vaginal delivery while maximizing analgesia is both an art and a science and requires the attention of the anesthesia provider to the individual needs of the patient. A single analgesic technique or single dose/concentration of drug(s) is not likely to have optimal results for everyone.

Why should anesthesia providers give attention to the effects of analgesia on the method of vaginal delivery? Lack of effective maternal effort associated with inadequate progress of labor (descent of the fetus) is an indication for operative vaginal delivery.[411] Studies suggest that vacuum extraction may be associated with a higher neonatal risk for cephalohematoma, subgaleal hemorrhage, and intraventricular hemorrhage than spontaneous vaginal, forceps, or cesarean delivery, whereas forceps delivery is associated with an increased risk for facial trauma.[411,412] However, there is some evidence that these injuries may be attributed to the indication for delivery, rather than the specific delivery technique.[411] There is no evidence of adverse long-term neonatal outcome with operative vaginal compared with spontaneous vaginal or cesarean delivery.

The risk for maternal trauma is also greater with operative vaginal delivery (e.g., third- and fourth-degree vaginal lacerations). Robinson et al.[413] observed that epidural analgesia was associated with an increased rate of severe perineal trauma because of the more frequent use of operative vaginal delivery and episiotomy in nulliparous women who received epidural analgesia. In contrast, several large observational studies suggest that epidural analgesia is associated with a decreased risk for anal sphincter laceration in nulliparous women.[414,415] Regardless of the presence or magnitude of the risks for maternal or neonatal injury, many women want to minimize the likelihood of operative delivery, and they perceive that a higher risk for operative vaginal delivery is undesirable. Of concern is a decline in the number of obstetric providers skilled at operative vaginal delivery.[412] The concern is that loss of these skills will lead to an increase in second-stage cesarean delivery rates.

Duration of Labor

First Stage of Labor

The effect of neuraxial labor analgesia on the duration of the first stage of labor has been addressed as a secondary outcome variable in many of the randomized controlled trials. A 2018 metaanalysis[3] of nine studies found that the first stage of labor was longer in women who were randomly assigned to receive epidural analgesia than those assigned to receive systemic opioid analgesia (see Table 24.12). In the individual metaanalysis of the Parkland Hospital, data also showed a significant prolongation of the first stage of labor (approximately 30 minutes) in nulliparous women who were randomly assigned to receive epidural analgesia.[384]

Wong et al.[285] and Ohel et al.[395] assessed duration of labor as a secondary outcome in their randomized controlled trials of the initiation of neuraxial analgesia during early labor. Both groups of investigators determined that the duration of the first stage of labor, and thus consequently the overall duration of labor, were significantly *shorter* in women randomly assigned to receive early labor neuraxial analgesia than in those assigned to receive early systemic opioid analgesia and delayed neuraxial analgesia. In the Wong et al. study,[285] the median difference in the overall duration of the first stage of labor between the early and late neuraxial analgesia groups was −90 minutes (95% CI, −123 to −35 minutes) (Fig. 24.10).

Determining the duration of labor requires that investigators document start and end times. The definition of the start time varies among studies but is usually consistent between groups within a study. The end of the first stage of labor is defined as the time of full (10 cm) cervical dilation. This time point can be determined only with manual cervical examination. Most studies do not mandate regular cervical examinations by study protocol, or if they do, the intervals are fairly long (e.g., 1 to 2 hours). In clinical practice, full cervical dilation is usually diagnosed when a cervical examination is performed because the patient complains of rectal pressure, begins involuntarily grunting, or develops an urge to push. It is likely that women with effective epidural analgesia

First Stage of Labor Before Vaginal Delivery

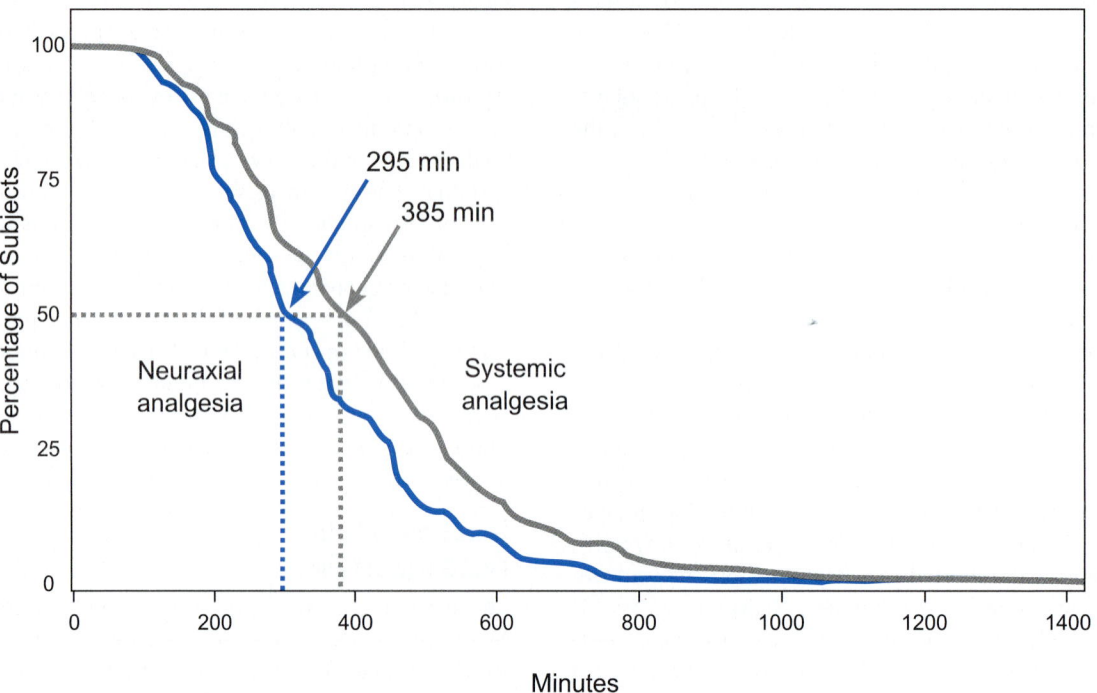

Fig. 24.10 Kaplan-Meier survival curves (percentage of subjects undelivered) for duration of the first stage of labor before vaginal delivery. The duration of the first stage of labor was a median of 90 min shorter (95% confidence interval −123 to −35 min) in women randomized to receive early neuraxial labor analgesia compared with women who received early systemic opioid analgesia and delayed epidural analgesia. From Wong CA, Scavone BM, Peaceman AM, et al. The risk of cesarean delivery with neuraxial analgesia given early versus late in labor. *N Eng J Med.* 2005;352:655–665.

will develop these signs and symptoms at a later time (and lower fetal station) than women with systemic opioid analgesia. In other words, the patient may be fully dilated for a significant period of time before cervical examination verifies full cervical dilation. This difference serves to artificially prolong the duration of the first stage of labor in the epidural group, although it shortens the apparent duration of the second stage of labor. Obstetric providers occasionally request epidural analgesia for women in advanced first-stage labor to limit involuntary Valsalva maneuvers when the cervix is not yet fully dilated, as this can lead to cervical edema that necessitates cesarean delivery.

Other factors may also influence the duration of the first stage of labor. Some clinicians have noted enhanced uterine activity in some patients for approximately 30 minutes after the initiation of neuraxial analgesia, whereas uterine activity appears to be reduced in other patients. Cheek et al.[416] noted that uterine activity decreased after the intravenous infusion of 1 L of crystalloid solution, but not after the infusion of 0.5 L or maintenance fluid alone. Miller[417] hypothesized that a fluid bolus might inhibit antidiuretic hormone (vasopressin) release from the posterior pituitary gland. Because this organ also releases oxytocin, the production of that hormone might also be transiently suppressed; this possible decrease in oxytocin release may partially explain the transient changes in uterine contractility observed in association with epidural analgesia.

In a prospective but nonrandomized study, Rahm et al.[418] observed that epidural analgesia (bupivacaine with sufentanil) was associated with lower plasma oxytocin levels at 60 minutes after the initiation of analgesia than in healthy controls who did not receive epidural analgesia. Behrens et al.[419] noted that epidural analgesia during the first stage of labor significantly reduced the release of prostaglandin $F_{2\alpha}$ and "impede[d] the normal progressive increase in uterine activity." In contrast, Nielsen et al.[420] measured upper and lower uterine segment intrauterine pressures for 50 minutes before and after the administration of epidural bupivacaine analgesia in 11 nulliparous women during spontaneous labor. No significant difference in the number of contractions before and after epidural analgesia was observed.

Increased uterine activity after the initiation of neuraxial analgesia has been hypothesized to be an indirect effect of neuraxial analgesia (see later discussion).[421] Initiation of neuraxial analgesia is associated with an acute decrease in the maternal plasma concentration of circulating epinephrine (see Fig. 24.1).[4] Epinephrine is a tocolytic, and the acute decrease in maternal concentration may result in greater uterine activity. This may be an explanation for the salutary effect on the progress of labor that is observed in some women with dysfunctional labor after the initiation of neuraxial analgesia[422] or in women who are extremely anxious.[423]

The epidural administration of a local anesthetic with epinephrine is followed by systemic absorption of both drugs.

Some physicians have expressed concern that the epinephrine may exert a systemic beta-adrenergic tocolytic effect and slow labor. Early studies, which used large doses of epinephrine, suggested that the caudal epidural administration of local anesthetic with epinephrine prolonged the first stage of labor and increased the number of patients who required oxytocin augmentation of labor.[424] Subsequently, most studies have suggested that the addition of epinephrine 1.25 to 5 µg/mL (1:800,000 to 1:200,000) to the local anesthetic solution does not affect the progress of labor or method of delivery.[113,114,116,425,426]

There is no evidence that the specific local anesthetic or opioid used for neuraxial analgesia directly or indirectly affects the duration of labor.[72,427] Randomized controlled trials that compared CSE and epidural analgesia have not found a difference in the duration of labor between the two techniques.[331,385,399,402]

In summary, neuraxial analgesia appears to have a variable effect on the duration of the first stage of labor. It may shorten labor in some women and lengthen it in others. However, analgesia-related prolongation of the first stage of labor, if it occurs, is short, has not been shown to have adverse maternal or neonatal effects, and is probably of minimal clinical significance.

Second Stage of Labor

There is little doubt that effective neuraxial analgesia prolongs the second stage of labor. Metaanalyses of randomized controlled trials that compared neuraxial with systemic opioid analgesia support this clinical observation (see Table 24.12).[3,384] The mean duration of the second stage was 15 to 20 minutes longer in women randomly assigned to receive neuraxial analgesia than in women assigned to receive systemic opioid analgesia.[3,384]

Historically, the ACOG has defined a prolonged second stage in nulliparous women as lasting more than 3 hours with neuraxial analgesia and more than 2 hours without neuraxial analgesia; for parous women, it is more than 2 hours in those with neuraxial analgesia and more than 1 hour in those without neuraxial analgesia.[428] Zhang et al.[429] performed a secondary analysis of data from the Consortium on Safe Labor, a large, multicenter study from 19 hospitals across the United States, to characterize the duration of labor in a contemporary cohort of American women. The 95th percentiles for duration of the second stage of labor were 3.6 and 2.8 hours for nulliparous women with and without epidural analgesia, respectively. These and other data[430] suggest that a significant proportion of women will have a "prolonged" second stage, as defined by the historical ACOG criteria. An observation study demonstrated that, even with more than 4 hours of pushing during the second stage of labor, the chance of vaginal delivery for a nulliparous parturient was 78%.[431] However, prolonged second stage of labor is associated with an increased risk for maternal morbidity, including chorioamnionitis, postpartum hemorrhage, cesarean and operative vaginal delivery, and third- and fourth-degree perineal lacerations, although it is not clear whether these relationships are causal.[431-433]

Data on the association between prolonged second stage and neonatal outcomes are conflicting. Data from several trials (secondary analyses of prospective trials[433,434] and retrospective cohort data[435]) have not identified an increased risk for adverse neonatal outcomes associated with the duration of the second stage of labor. In contrast, several retrospective trials have found an increased risk for 5-minute Apgar score < 7 and intensive care unit admission in neonates delivered after 3[436] and 2 hours[437] second-stage duration, respectively.

The 2024 ACOG clinical practice guideline[397] defines prolonged second stage as more than 3 hours of second-stage pushing in nulliparous women and more than 2 hours of pushing in multiparous women. However, the guideline states that an individual approach should be used to diagnose second-stage arrest of labor. Considerations should include the presence of factors that may influence the likelihood of vaginal delivery, a risk-benefit discussion of the alternatives to further expectant management of the second stage, and individual preferences. Given the risks to the alternatives to spontaneous vaginal delivery (i.e., operative delivery), it may be reasonable to continue expectant management if electronic FHR monitoring confirms the absence of nonreassuring fetal status, the mother is well hydrated and has adequate analgesia, and there is ongoing progress in the descent of the fetal head.

Second-stage management: immediate versus "delayed" pushing. There has been considerable discussion of the roles of immediate (as soon as full cervical dilation is confirmed) versus delayed pushing (allowing the fetus to descend in the birth canal without active maternal pushing) in the management of the second stage of labor. Some practitioners have suggested that "delayed" pushing might result in less maternal exhaustion and better maternal and fetal outcomes. A 2017 metaanalysis that included 13 studies that compared early and delayed pushing in women with epidural analgesia[438] concluded that delayed pushing resulted in an increase in the rate of spontaneous vaginal delivery (RR, 1.07; 95% CI, 1.03 to 1.12) and shorter duration of pushing at the expense of an increase in the total duration of the second stage of labor (mean difference 56 minutes). The authors judged that the evidence ranged from moderate to very low quality.[438] In 2018, Cahill et al.[439] reported the results of a multicenter randomized controlled trial of immediate versus delayed pushing in nulliparous women with neuraxial analgesia. The rate of spontaneous vaginal delivery was not different between groups (immediate group 85.9%, delayed group 86.5%), nor were there differences in the composite neonatal outcome measure. However, the immediate pushing group had a significantly shorter mean second-stage duration (102 versus 134 minutes), a lower rate of chorioamnionitis (6.7% versus 9.1%), and less postpartum hemorrhage. The 2024 ACOG clinical practice guideline[397] recommends that pushing commence immediately (strong recommendation, high-quality evidence) after full cervical dilation is confirmed. Although some practitioners have advocated for discontinuing neuraxial analgesia in an effort to improve pushing efforts (see earlier discussion), this is rarely indicated; it does not improve the rate of spontaneous vaginal delivery,[398] and analgesia/anesthesia may be difficult to reestablish if the need for operative delivery arises. If dense neuraxial analgesia is present (i.e., the mother has no sensation of contraction), the maintenance dose can be adjusted downward, but not discontinued.

Third Stage of Labor

Rosaeg et al.[440] retrospectively reviewed the outcomes of 7468 women who underwent vaginal delivery at their hospital between 1996 and 1999. Epidural analgesia was not associated with a prolonged third stage of labor. The duration of the third stage of labor was shorter in women who received epidural analgesia and subsequently required manual removal of the placenta. The researchers suggested that epidural analgesia "provided a 'permissive' role"—in other words, epidural analgesia likely facilitated and/or encouraged earlier intervention by the obstetrician.

Other Factors and Progress of Labor

Oxytocin

The ACOG recommends oxytocin augmentation when labor dystocia is diagnosed.[397] This practice is associated with a small increase in the rate of spontaneous vaginal delivery (RR, 1.09; 95% CI, 1.03 to 1.17).[441] Oxytocin augmentation is associated with increased pain and an increased risk for uterine tachysystole but without adverse neonatal outcomes.[441]

In randomized controlled trials that compared the effects of neuraxial and systemic opioid analgesia on the outcome of labor, women who received neuraxial opioids had a higher rate of oxytocin augmentation (see Table 24.12).[3,384] The reason(s) for this observation are not clear.

Randomized controlled trials that compared early and late initiation of neuraxial analgesia have used markedly different oxytocin protocols, yet all have concluded that early initiation of neuraxial analgesia does not have an adverse effect on the outcome of labor. In the study of early CSE analgesia by Wong et al.,[285] the rate of oxytocin use was high in both groups (approximately 93%). However, the maximum oxytocin infusion rate in the control (early systemic opioid) group was significantly higher than that in the early CSE group even though the median duration of labor was 81 minutes shorter in the CSE group. In a study of early epidural analgesia by Ohel et al.,[395] the rate of oxytocin use in both groups was much lower (approximately 29%); however, as in the study by Wong et al.,[285] the duration of labor was significantly shorter in the early neuraxial analgesia group. Taken together, these data do not support a hypothesis that oxytocin augmentation significantly interacts with neuraxial labor analgesia in the progress of labor.

Maternal Ambulation and Positioning

Observational studies suggest that ambulation may be associated with less pain and a shorter duration of labor.[442] However, randomized controlled trials that compared ambulation and bed rest during the first stage of labor in women with neuraxial analgesia have not demonstrated any advantages of ambulation with regard to the progress or outcome of labor. In a metaanalysis that reviewed five randomized controlled trials involving 1161 women with epidural analgesia, there were no differences in the mode of delivery (cesarean delivery RR, 0.91; 95% CI, 0.70 to 1.19), operative vaginal delivery (RR, 1.16; 95% CI, 0.93 to 1.44), use of oxytocin augmentation, satisfaction with analgesia, or Apgar scores.[443] No adverse effects were reported. These results are similar to those of trials that compared ambulation and bed rest in women without neuraxial analgesia.[444]

No studies have evaluated maternal position and the outcome of labor exclusively in women with neuraxial labor analgesia. In a 2013 metaanalysis,[445] upright and ambulating positions compared with recumbent and bed care positions were associated with shorter first-stage labor. There were no differences in second-stage duration, use of epidural analgesia, and neonatal outcomes; however, the authors cautioned that the quality of included studies was variable. Frequent position changes during labor may enhance maternal comfort and should be supported unless contraindicated by maternal or fetal conditions.[446]

Pelvic Floor Injury

Several studies have evaluated the possible effects of epidural analgesia on postpartum pelvic floor function. Retrospective studies have not identified an association between epidural analgesia and risk for perineal lacerations[447] or pelvic floor dysfunction.[448] A metaanalysis of studies that compared epidural analgesia versus nonepidural or no analgesia did not identify a difference in the risk for perineal trauma requiring suturing (see Table 24.12).[3] Epidural labor analgesia was not a risk factor for anal sphincter injury in a 2023 metaanalysis.[449]

Any factor that increases the likelihood of operative vaginal delivery might be expected to increase the risk for pelvic floor injury and subsequent pelvic floor dysfunction (see earlier discussion). However, there is no evidence that epidural analgesia *per se* predisposes to pelvic floor injury.

EFFECTS OF NEURAXIAL ANALGESIA ON THE FETUS AND NEONATE

Neuraxial analgesia may affect the fetus directly and/or indirectly. First, systemic absorption of the anesthetic agents may be followed by transplacental transfer of the drug, which has a direct effect on the fetus. Second, the effects of neuraxial blockade on the mother may affect the fetus indirectly. Effects of local anesthetics and opioids on the fetus and neonate are discussed in detail in Chapter 13.

Direct Effects

Direct fetal effects include intrapartum drug effects on the FHR as well as possible respiratory depression after delivery. The determinants of maternal plasma drug concentration, transfer across the placenta, and effects on the neonate are discussed in Chapters 4 and 13. Determinants of maternal plasma drug concentration include dose, site of administration, metabolism and excretion of the drug, and the presence of adjuvants (e.g., epinephrine); the degree of protein binding determines the free (unbound) drug concentration, the drug fraction which crosses the placenta. Factors that influence placental transfer include maternal and fetal placental perfusion, the physicochemical characteristics of the drug, concentration of the free drug in maternal plasma, and permeability of the placenta. Most anesthetic and analgesic drugs, including local anesthetics and opioids, readily cross the placenta.

Fetal Heart Rate

Effects of local anesthetics and opioids on FHR may be direct and indirect (see earlier discussion)[421,427]; however, there is little evidence for a direct effect when these drugs are administered as components of neuraxial analgesia. Transient changes in FHR variability and periodic decelerations have been observed during epidural labor analgesia with bupivacaine and other local anesthetics.[427,450,451] These FHR decelerations were not associated with maternal hypotension. However, Loftus et al.[452] did not observe FHR decelerations in women who received epidural bupivacaine for elective cesarean delivery, despite the use of larger doses of bupivacaine and the occurrence of more extensive sympathetic blockade in comparison with epidural labor analgesia. Of interest, one study noted that the administration of either epidural bupivacaine or intrathecal sufentanil was followed by a similar incidence of FHR decelerations (23% and 22%, respectively) in laboring women.[453] Other studies have not observed a higher incidence of FHR decelerations associated with epidural administration of bupivacaine during labor.[454] Further, the reports of FHR decelerations after bupivacaine did not demonstrate adverse neonatal outcome; thus, the significance of these decelerations is unclear. There are no published data on the relationship between the concentration of bupivacaine used for intrapartum epidural analgesia and the incidence of FHR decelerations. Altogether, these data suggest that epidural local anesthetics have minimal, if any, direct effect on FHR.

Similarly, neuraxial opioid administration has little direct effect on the FHR.[209,455,456] In contrast, systemic opioid analgesia is associated with a greater reduction of FHR variability and fewer FHR accelerations than epidural bupivacaine analgesia.[457] Spinal administration of local anesthetics and opioids results in lower maternal plasma concentrations of drug(s) than epidural administration and is therefore even less likely to cause a direct fetal effect.

Neonatal Depression

Systemic absorption of local anesthetic or opioid may have neonatal effects. This occurs more often after the systemic administration of opioid for labor analgesia.[285,458] The neonatal depressant effects of drugs administered to the mother in the intrapartum period are usually assessed with neurobehavioral testing. Unfortunately, these tests are quite subjective and lack specificity. Additionally, scientifically rigorous studies are lacking, and most of the local anesthetic studies were performed in the era when high-dose epidural analgesia was common.

When given by continous epidural infusion, epidural opioid administration rarely results in accumulation of the drug and subsequent neonatal respiratory depression.[88,97,207,208] Bader et al.[207] noted that an epidural infusion of 0.125% bupivacaine with fentanyl 2 µg/mL over a period of 1 to 15 hours did not result in significant fetal drug accumulation or adverse neonatal effects (in this study, the maximal cumulative dose of fentanyl was 300 µg). Porter et al.[208] reported no adverse effect of fentanyl on neurobehavioral scores or other indices of fetal welfare when patients received an epidural infusion of 0.0625% bupivacaine with or without fentanyl 2.5 µg/mL. Vertommen et al.[88] observed no difference in Apgar scores or NACS in neonates whose mothers were randomly assigned to receive epidural sufentanil (up to 30 µg) during the course of labor and a control group that did not receive sufentanil.[88] Maternal sufentanil levels were below the sensitivity of the assay (0.1 ng/mL) after an epidural bolus of 10 µg.[97]

When administered as a bolus dose to initiate epidural labor analgesia (fentanyl 50 to 100 µg,[87] sufentanil 5 to 50 µg[97]), no adverse neonatal effects were noted. Intrathecal administration of an opioid during labor would be expected to have even fewer direct effects on the fetus than epidural administration. Smaller doses of opioid are administered, and less drug is absorbed systemically.

Breastfeeding

The effect of epidural fentanyl administered for labor analgesia on breastfeeding in the postpartum period has been investigated. In a randomized controlled trial that compared epidural analgesia with no fentanyl, intermediate-dose fentanyl (<150 µg), and high-dose fentanyl (>150 µg), women who were randomized to receive high-dose fentanyl had a lower rate of breastfeeding at 6 weeks.[459] In contrast, a second randomized controlled trial compared three bupivacaine solutions with fentanyl 0, 1, or 2 µg/mL used to maintain CSE analgesia. No differences in the rate of breastfeeding at 6 weeks of age were identified.[460] Similarly, a secondary analysis of a randomized trial comparing neuraxial techniques with and without fentanyl found no differences in breastfeeding after delivery and at 12 months.[461] A 2021 systematic review that included 15 studies (14 observational studies and 1 secondary analysis of a randomized controlled trial) that compared women with neuraxial labor analgesia with women with nonneuraxial or no analgesia[462] found highly disparate results.

Indirect Effects

The indirect fetal effects of epidural and intrathecal opioids may be more significant than the direct effects. In a meta-analysis of randomized controlled trials that compared neuraxial with systemic opioid analgesia, the neonates of women randomized to neuraxial analgesia had a lower incidence of low umbilical artery pH (i.e., neuraxial analgesia was protective against fetal acidemia) and naloxone administration (presumably because systemic opioid analgesia is associated

TABLE 24.14 Neonatal Outcomes in Offspring of Women Randomized to Receive Neuraxial Versus Systemic Opioid Labor Analgesia

Outcome	Neuraxial Analgesia (n/N)	Systemic Opioid Analgesia (n/N)	Risk Ratio	95% Confidence Interval
Umbilical artery pH < 7.2	268/2590	305/2193	0.81	0.69 to 0.94
Naloxone administration	21/1302	151/1343	0.15	0.10 to 0.23
5-min Apgar score < 7	61/4538	72/4214	0.73	0.52 to 1.02
Neonatal intensive care unit admission	465/2228	461/2260	1.03	0.95 to 1.12

Data from Amin-Somuah M, Smyth RM, Cyna AM, Cuthbert A. Epidural versus non-epidural or no analgesia for pain management in labour. *Cochrane Database Syst Rev.* 2018;(5):CD000331.

with fetal depression from transfer of opioids across the placenta) (Table 24.14). There were no differences in the incidence of low Apgar scores (<7) or neonatal intensive care unit admission.

Fetal bradycardia is sometimes observed within the first 30 minutes of initiation of neuraxial analgesia. The presumed cause is that the rapid onset of analgesia results in decreased plasma concentrations of circulating catecholamines.[421] Epinephrine causes uterine relaxation by stimulating uterine beta$_2$-adrenergic receptors. A reduced circulating concentration of epinephrine may result in increased uterine tone. Because uteroplacental perfusion occurs during periods of uterine diastole (i.e., uterine relaxation), uterine tachysystole may result in decreased uteroplacental perfusion and fetal hypoxia.

Published observations suggest that uterine tachysystole and fetal bradycardia may follow the administration of either intrathecal or epidural analgesia during labor. Abrão et al.[463] randomized 72 laboring women to receive either CSE or epidural analgesia, and observed the incidences of FHR abnormalities (prolonged deceleration or bradycardia) and elevation in uterine tone (defined as an increase of 10 mm Hg or more in basal uterine pressure). The incidences of FHR abnormalities (32% versus 6%), and FHR abnormalities combined with an increase in uterine pressure (27% versus 3%), were significantly higher in the CSE group than in the epidural group. However, an important limitation of this study is that the outcomes were assessed for only 15 minutes after the initiation of analgesia and the analgesic techniques were not equipotent.[464] The overall high incidence of FHR abnormalities noted in the study may have been caused by the initiation of analgesia in women in advanced labor.

Fortunately, fetal bradycardia after labor analgesia does not appear to increase the overall risk for adverse outcome. Albright and Forster[465] retrospectively reviewed outcomes for 2560 women who delivered at their hospital between March 1995 and April 1996. Approximately half of the patients received CSE analgesia (10 to 15 µg of intrathecal sufentanil), and the other half received either systemic opioids or no medication. There was no difference between the two groups in the incidence of emergency cesarean delivery (1.3% versus 1.4%, respectively).

Mardirosoff et al.[466] performed a systematic review of reports of randomized comparisons of intrathecal opioid analgesia with any nonintrathecal opioid regimen in laboring women. The investigators noted that intrathecal opioid analgesia was associated with a significant increase in the risk for fetal bradycardia (OR, 1.8; 95% CI, 1.0 to 3.1). However, the risk for cesarean delivery for FHR abnormalities was similar in the two groups (6.0% versus 7.8%, respectively). Data are conflicting regarding an opioid dose-response for fetal bradycardia. Van de Velde et al.[467] randomly assigned laboring women to one of three treatment regimens: intrathecal sufentanil 7.5 µg, intrathecal sufentanil 1.5 µg/bupivacaine 2.5 mg/epinephrine 2.5 µg, or epidural bupivacaine 12.5 mg/sufentanil 7.5 µg/epinephrine 12.5 µg. Although the incidence of FHR abnormalities was higher in the high-dose intrathecal sufentanil group, there was no difference among groups in the need for emergency cesarean delivery. Wong et al.,[146,147] in two separate studies, randomized multiparous women to receive intrathecal fentanyl 0, 5, 10, 15, 20, or 25 µg, or sufentanil 0, 2.5, 5, 7.5, or 10 µg, combined with bupivacaine 2.5 mg. There was no difference in the incidence of fetal bradycardia among groups. Abrão et al.[463] and Cheng et al.[468] noted an association with the extent of decrease in pain scores after the initiation of analgesia and the incidence of fetal bradycardia. These data suggest that the incidence of bradycardia is associated with the rate of onset of analgesia; faster onset of analgesia is associated with the CSE technique and may be related to the dose/potency of the neuraxial drugs.

In a randomized controlled study, Gambling et al.[469] tested the hypothesis that prophylactic administration of ephedrine would decrease the incidence of fetal bradycardia (via its beta$_2$-adrenergic effects). They found no difference between groups in the incidence of fetal bradycardia, uterine tachysystole, or need for urgent delivery.

Given the risk for fetal bradycardia with neuraxial analgesia in laboring women, the FHR should be monitored during and after the administration of either epidural or intrathecal analgesia. Treatment of fetal bradycardia includes (1) relief of aortocaval compression; (2) discontinuation of intravenous oxytocin; (3) treatment of maternal hypotension, if present; and (4) fetal scalp stimulation. Persistent uterine tachysystole should also prompt the administration of a tocolytic drug (e.g., terbutaline or nitroglycerin).

CONCLUSIONS AND RECOMMENDATIONS

Philosophy of Labor Analgesia

An unacceptably high number of women involuntarily experience severe pain during labor. As noted by the ACOG, "There is no other circumstance where it is considered acceptable for a person to experience severe pain, amenable to safe intervention, while under a physician's care."[18] Unfortunately, labor represents one of the few circumstances in which the provision of effective analgesia is alleged to interfere with the parturient's and obstetric provider's goal of spontaneous vaginal delivery. Dense neuraxial anesthesia may adversely affect the progress of labor in some patients. Indeed, given the complicated neurohumoral and mechanical processes involved in childbirth, it would be unreasonable to expect that neuroblockade of the lower half of the body would *not* have an effect on this process, whether positive or negative. However, maternal-fetal factors and obstetric management—not the use of neuraxial analgesia—are the most important determinants of the outcome of labor. Anesthesia providers should identify those methods of analgesia that provide the most effective pain relief without unduly increasing the risk for obstetric intervention. Operative delivery increases the risk for maternal morbidity and mortality and is more expensive than spontaneous vaginal delivery. Randomized trials suggest that the use of neuraxial analgesia does not increase the cesarean delivery rate but may adversely influence the operative vaginal delivery rate.[3] Further, neuraxial analgesia may occasionally, either directly or indirectly, have adverse—usually temporary—effects on the fetus.

Despite these risks, many women opt for neuraxial analgesia because no other method of labor analgesia provides its benefits (almost complete analgesia), and the risks are acceptably low. Even no analgesia may be more hazardous to some women than neuraxial analgesia (e.g., patients with an anticipated difficult airway or those at high risk for emergency cesarean delivery). Therefore, it is the duty of the anesthesia provider to provide appropriate (albeit not always total) pain relief during the first and second stages of labor. Analgesia should be tailored to the individual patient's labor, medical condition, preferences, and goals. Most women strongly dislike dense motor blockade, and many prefer to maintain some sensation of uterine contractions and perineal pressure, especially during the second stage of labor. However, a few women may accept the probable increase in risk for operative vaginal delivery in exchange for dense analgesia.

A Practical Guide to Neuraxial Labor Analgesia

Initiation of Analgesia

Neuraxial labor analgesia may be initiated with either the intrathecal (CSE) or the epidural injection of analgesic/anesthetic agents. The decision regarding the specific technique and choice of drugs and doses is individualized for each parturient. Parity, stage and phase of labor, use of intravenous oxytocin, and the presence of any coexisting disease(s), as well as the status of the fetus, are all considered in the decision.

In healthy *nulliparous* women in *early* labor (<4- to 5-cm cervical dilation), my colleagues and I often initiate CSE analgesia with an intrathecal opioid alone (e.g., fentanyl 25 µg or sufentanil 5 µg), followed by placement of an epidural catheter and administration of a standard lidocaine 45 mg/epinephrine 15 µg epidural test dose. Some anesthesia providers initiate intrathecal analgesia with both an opioid and a local anesthetic. At another editor's institution, CSE analgesia is initiated with the bupivacaine/fentanyl solution that is used for maintenance of analgesia (0.0625% bupivacaine with fentanyl 2 µg/mL). The dose (volume) is escalated, depending on the stage of labor. For a nulliparous woman in early labor, intrathecal analgesia is initiated with 2 mL of the solution. If delivery is imminent, 4 mL is administered.

Alternatively, epidural analgesia can be initiated with injection of a low-concentration local anesthetic solution (bupivacaine 0.0625% to 0.125%) combined with an opioid (fentanyl 50 to 100 µg). The epidural catheter is sited and a standard epidural test dose is injected, followed by administration of 5 to 15 mL of the local anesthetic/opioid solution, injected in 5-mL increments. Ten to 15 mL provides satisfactory analgesia for most nulliparous women in early labor; injection of 20 mL may be necessary if a dilute solution (e.g., 0.0625% bupivacaine) is used. A smaller dose is necessary if administered after a standard test dose.

We typically give an epinephrine-containing test dose before initiation of epidural analgesia in laboring women. Some anesthesia providers elect to omit the epidural test dose when initiating epidural labor analgesia, particularly if a woman wishes to ambulate in early labor. The omission of the epidural test dose requires that the therapeutic dose of local anesthetic be injected slowly, incrementally, and cautiously, because the therapeutic dose functions as the test dose. These precautions should be followed with every bolus injection of local anesthetic through an epidural catheter.

For *nulliparous* women in the active phase of the first stage of labor, CSE analgesia is usually initiated with the intrathecal injection of an opioid combined with a local anesthetic (fentanyl 15 µg and bupivacaine 1.25 to 2.5 mg). Alternatively, epidural analgesia can be initiated with a local anesthetic (bupivacaine 0.125%) combined with an opioid (fentanyl 100 µg) with or without a dural puncture (DPE analgesia). Women in active labor may require a higher total volume of epidural local anesthetic solution (15 to 20 mL) than women in early labor (10 to 15 mL) as well as a higher local anesthetic concentration (e.g., 0.125% rather than 0.0625% bupivacaine).

Labor typically progresses at a faster rate in *parous* women, who often require a more rapid onset of analgesia and more extensive neuroblockade than nulliparous women when neuraxial analgesia is initiated at the same cervical dilation. Therefore, in healthy parous women, CSE analgesia is usually initiated with an intrathecal opioid combined with a local anesthetic, regardless of the stage and phase of labor. Alternatively, epidural analgesia is initiated with bupivacaine 0.125% combined with fentanyl 100 µg with a dural puncture (DPE analgesia).

CSE analgesia with both a local anesthetic and an opioid is particularly advantageous for parous women in the late active phase of the first stage of labor and in all women in whom neuraxial analgesia is initiated in the second stage of labor. Sacral neuroblockade is required for complete analgesia during the second stage of labor; this neuroblockade is difficult to accomplish in a timely fashion with an initial (*de novo*) lumbar epidural injection of analgesic/anesthetic agents. (For initiation of lumbar epidural anesthesia in late labor, the injection of a large volume [≥20 mL] of local anesthetic solution may be required to achieve sacral analgesia, and this injection often results in a mid- or high-thoracic neuroblockade that is more extensive than desired. Therefore, when initiating neuraxial analgesia in late labor, a CSE technique is preferred.)

Maintenance of Analgesia

Maintenance epidural analgesia is typically initiated soon after the initiation of analgesia (within 15 to 30 minutes) rather than waiting for the neuroblockade to regress. There are several advantages to this technique. Most women experience seamless analgesia (i.e., there is no window of pain as the initial block regresses). The workload for the anesthesia provider is lessened because they can set up and initiate the epidural infusion while monitoring the patient for hypotension after initiation of neuroblockade. Finally, an epidural bolus of local anesthetic is not required to reestablish or extend neuroblockade, possibly enhancing safety.

Analgesia is typically maintained with a dilute solution of an amide local anesthetic and an opioid, administered by continuous infusion or PIEB, combined with PCEA. My colleagues and I use PCEA because it allows patient titration of neuroblockade and entails less risk for breakthrough pain. Patient satisfaction is better and the workload for the anesthesia provider is decreased. At our institution, the PIEB and PCEA infusion pump parameters are the same for all laboring women, so there are fewer errors in pump setup. However, when a continuous infusion is used without PCEA to maintain analgesia, it may be necessary to titrate the continuous infusion rate to individual patient needs. For example, women in early labor require less drug to maintain analgesia (6 to 10 mL/h), whereas women in more advanced labor may require a higher infusion rate (8 to 15 mL/h). Similarly, a parous patient may require a higher infusion rate than a nulliparous patient, even though analgesia is initiated at the same stage of labor.

Some parturients experience breakthrough pain. After evaluating the nature of the pain, the extent of neuroblockade, and the progress of labor, we usually treat breakthrough pain with a bolus epidural injection of bupivacaine 0.125%, 10 to 15 mL, administered in 5-mL increments. The patient may benefit from additional instruction about the optimal use of PCEA. Rarely, we may elect to use a more concentrated local anesthetic solution (e.g., bupivacaine 0.25%), particularly in the presence of an abnormal fetal position or dysfunctional labor. Another alternative to treat this breakthrough pain is the administration of epidural clonidine 75 to 100 μg.

This maintenance technique usually results in satisfactory perineal analgesia for delivery. Occasionally, women with epidural analgesia require additional (more dense) analgesia for delivery, particularly if an operative vaginal delivery is planned. In this case, we often administer 5 to 12 mL of 1% to 2% lidocaine or 2% to 3% 2-chloroprocaine. This usually results in satisfactory sacral anesthesia in a patient with preexisting epidural labor analgesia.

There is no single correct way to provide neuraxial labor analgesia, although for particular patients and specific clinical conditions some methods may have advantages over others. Frequent communication among members of the anesthesia, obstetric, and nursing teams is essential to the safe and satisfactory provision of neuraxial labor analgesia. In addition, within each labor and delivery unit, consistency among anesthesia providers in their choice of techniques, specific drugs, and drug doses/concentrations is likely to result in fewer errors and higher satisfaction among other caregivers and patients.

KEY POINTS

- Neuraxial analgesia is the most effective form of intrapartum analgesia currently available.
- In most cases, maternal request for pain relief represents a sufficient indication for the administration of neuraxial analgesia.
- The safe administration of neuraxial analgesia requires a thorough (albeit directed) preanesthetic evaluation and the immediate availability of appropriate resuscitation equipment.
- Neuraxial labor analgesia is not a generic procedure. The procedure should be tailored to individual patient needs.
- The administration of the epidural test dose should allow the anesthesia provider to recognize most cases of unintentional intravascular or intrathecal placement of the epidural catheter. All therapeutic doses of local anesthetic should be administered incrementally.

- Bupivacaine is the local anesthetic most often used for epidural analgesia during labor in the United States. Ropivacaine and levobupivacaine are satisfactory alternatives. Most anesthesia providers reserve 2-chloroprocaine and lidocaine for cases that require the rapid extension of epidural anesthesia for vaginal or cesarean delivery.
- The addition of a lipid-soluble opioid to a neuraxial local anesthetic allows the anesthesia provider to provide excellent analgesia while reducing the total dose of local anesthetic and minimizing the side effects of each agent. Perhaps the major advantage of this technique is that the severity of motor block can be minimized during labor.
- Intrathecal opioids alone may provide complete analgesia during the early first stage of labor. Epidural opioids without local anesthetic do not provide complete analgesia during labor.

- Administration of a local anesthetic (with or without an opioid) is necessary to provide complete neuraxial analgesia for the late first stage and the second stage of labor. Although a neuraxial local anesthetic alone can provide complete analgesia, the required dose is often associated with an undesirably dense degree of motor blockade.
- Hypotension is a common side effect of neuraxial analgesia. Prophylaxis and treatment involve the avoidance of aortocaval compression and the administration of a vasopressor as needed. The administration of an intravenous fluid "preload" does not significantly decrease the incidence of hypotension in euvolemic patients.
- Other potential side effects of neuraxial analgesia include pruritus, shivering, urinary retention, delayed gastric emptying, maternal fever, and fetal heart rate changes.
- Complications of neuraxial analgesia include inadequate analgesia, unintentional dural puncture, respiratory depression, unintentional intravenous injection, and extensive or total spinal anesthesia.
- The presence of severe pain during early labor—and/or an increase in local anesthetic/opioid dose requirement—may signal a higher risk for prolonged labor and operative delivery.
- Neuraxial labor analgesia does not result in a higher rate of cesarean delivery than systemic opioid analgesia.
- Initiation of neuraxial analgesia in early labor (cervical dilation < 4 to 5 cm) does not increase the rate of cesarean delivery or prolong the duration of labor.
- Effective neuraxial analgesia likely results in a modest prolongation of the second stage of labor.
- Controversy exists as to whether there is a cause-and-effect relationship between neuraxial labor analgesia and risk for operative vaginal delivery. Dense neuroblockade (e.g., presence of significant motor blockade) and complete analgesia during the second stage of labor probably increase the rate of operative vaginal delivery. The use of a dilute solution of local anesthetic and opioid is less likely to adversely affect the progress of labor.
- Maternal-fetal factors and obstetric management—not the use of neuraxial analgesia—are the most important determinants of mode of delivery.

REFERENCES

1. Jones L, Othman M, Dowswell T, et al. Pain management for women in labour: an overview of systematic reviews. *Cochrane Database Syst Rev*. 2012;(3):CD009234.
2. Paech MJ. The King Edward Memorial Hospital 1,000 mother survey of methods of pain relief in labour. *Anaesth Intensive Care*. 1991;19:393–399.
3. Anim-Somuah M, Smyth RM, Cyna AM, Cuthbert A. Epidural versus non-epidural or no analgesia for pain management in labour. *Cochrane Database Syst Rev*. 2018;(5):CD000331.
4. Shnider SM, Abboud TK, Artal R, et al. Maternal catecholamines decrease during labor after lumbar epidural anesthesia. *Am J Obstet Gynecol*. 1983;147:13–15.
5. Lederman RP, Lederman E, Work B Jr, McCann DS. Anxiety and epinephrine in multiparous women in labor: relationship to duration of labor and fetal heart rate pattern. *Am J Obstet Gynecol*. 1985;153:870–877.
6. Jouppila R, Hollmén A. The effect of segmental epidural analgesia on maternal and foetal acid-base balance, lactate, serum potassium and creatine phosphokinase during labour. *Acta Anaesthesiol Scand*. 1976;20:259–268.
7. Levinson G, Shnider SM, DeLorimier AA, Steffenson JL. Effects of maternal hyperventilation on uterine blood flow and fetal oxygenation and acid-base status. *Anesthesiology*. 1974;40:340–347.
8. Peabody JL. Transcutaneous oxygen measurement to evaluate drug effects. *Clin Perinatol*. 1979;6:109–121.
9. Capogna G, Camorcia M, Stirparo S. Expectant fathers' experience during labor with or without epidural analgesia. *Int J Obstet Anesth*. 2007;16:110–115.
10. Traynor AJ, Aragon M, Ghosh D, et al. Obstetric Anesthesia Workforce Survey: a 30-year update. *Anesth Analg*. 2016;122:1939–1946.
11. Butwick AJ, Bentley J, Wong CA, et al. United States state-level variation in the use of neuraxial analgesia during labor for pregnant women. *JAMA Netw Open*. 2018;1:e186567.
12. Le Ray C, Lelong N, Cinelli H, Blondel B. Results of the 2021 French National Perinatal Survey and trends in perinatal health in metropolitan France since 1995. *J Gynecol Obstet Hum Reprod*. 2022;51102509.
13. Mu Y, Wang X, Wang Y, et al. The trends and associated adverse maternal and perinatal outcomes of labour neuraxial analgesia among vaginal deliveries in China between 2012 and 2019: a real-world observational evidence. *BMC Med*. 2021;19:74.
14. Toledo P, Sun J, Grobman WA, et al. Racial and ethnic disparities in neuraxial labor analgesia. *Anesth Analg*. 2012;114:172–178.
15. American Society of Anesthesiologists Practice guidelines for obstetric anesthesia: an updated report by the American Society of Anesthesiologists Task Force on Obstetric Anesthesia and the Society for Obstetric Anesthesia and Perinatology. *Anesthesiology*. 2016;124:270–300.
16. National Institute for Health and Care Excellence. Intrapartum care for healthy women and babies: Clinical guidance CG190 (updated 4 December 2022); 2014. https://www.nice.org.uk/guidance/cg190/chapter/recommendations. Accessed December 8, 2024.
17. Guasch E, Brogly N, Mercier FJ, et al. European minimum standards for obstetric analgesia and anaesthesia departments: an experts' consensus. *Eur J Anaesthesiol*. 2020;37:1115–1125.
18. American College of Obstetricians and Gynecologists Practice Bulletin No. 209: Obstetric analgesia and anesthesia (reaffirmed 2024). *Obstet Gynecol*. 2019;133:e208–e225.
19. Sng BL, Leong WL, Zeng Y, et al. Early versus late initiation of epidural analgesia for labour. *Cochrane Database Syst Rev*. 2014;(10):CD007238.

20. Simmons SW, Taghizadeh N, Dennis AT, et al. Combined spinal-epidural versus epidural analgesia in labour. *Cochrane Database Syst Rev*. 2012;(10):CD003401.

21. Sia AT, Chong JL, Tay DH, et al. Intrathecal sufentanil as the sole agent in combined spinal-epidural analgesia for the ambulatory parturient. *Can J Anaesth*. 1998;45:620–625.

22. Booth JM, Pan JC, Ross VH, et al. Combined spinal epidural technique for labor analgesia does not delay recognition of epidural catheter failures: a single-center retrospective cohort survival analysis. *Anesthesiology*. 2016;125:516–524.

23. Lee S, Lew E, Lim Y, Sia AT. Failure of augmentation of labor epidural analgesia for intrapartum cesarean delivery: aretrospective review. *Anesth Analg*. 2009;108:252–254.

24. Segal S, Pan PH. Dural puncture epidural for labor analgesia: is it really an improvement over conventional labor epidural analgesia? *Anesthesiology*. 2022;136:667–669.

25. Yin H, Tong X, Huang H. Dural puncture epidural versus conventional epidural analgesia for labor: a systematic review and meta-analysis of randomized controlled studies. *J Anesth*. 2022;36:413–427.

26. Chau A, Bibbo C, Huang CC, et al. Dural puncture epidural technique improves labor analgesia quality with fewer side effects compared with epidural and combined spinal epidural techniques: a randomized clinical trial. *Anesth Analg*. 2017;124:560–569.

27. Sharawi N, Williams M, Athar W, et al. Effect of dural-puncture epidural vs standard epidural for epidural extension on onset time of surgical anesthesia in elective cesarean delivery: a randomized clinical trial. *JAMA Netw Open*. 2023;6:e2326710.

28. NYSORA. Ultrasound-guided caudal epidural injections. https://www.nysora.com/pain-management/ultrasound-guided-caudal-epidural-injections/. Accessed December 8, 2024.

29. Kähkönen K, Väänänen A. Labour analgesia by single shot spinal for any parturient?—a retrospective one-year single centre audit. *Acta Anaesthesiol Scand*. 2023;67:1079–1084.

30. Al-Kazwini H, Sandven I, Dahl V, Rosseland LA. Prolonging the duration of single-shot intrathecal labour analgesia with morphine: a systematic review. *Scand J Pain*. 2016;13:36–42.

31. Kinsella SM, Pirlet M, Mills MS, et al. Randomized study of intravenous fluid preload before epidural analgesia during labour. *Br J Anaesth*. 2000;85:311–313.

32. Collins KM, Bevan DR, Beard RW. Fluid loading to reduce abnormalities of fetal heart rate and maternal hypotension during epidural analgesia in labour. *Br Med J*. 1978;2:1460–1461.

33. Zamora JE, Rosaeg OP, Lindsay MP, Crossan ML. Haemodynamic consequences and uterine contractions following 0.5 or 1.0 litre crystalloid infusion before obstetric epidural analgesia. *Can J Anaesth*. 1996;43:347–352.

34. Hawthorne L, Slaymaker A, Bamber J, Dresner M. Effect of fluid preload on maternal haemodynamics for low-dose epidural analgesia in labour. *Int J Obstet Anesth*. 2001;10:312–315.

35. Kubli M, Shennan AH, Seed PT, O'Sullivan G. A randomised controlled trial of fluid pre-loading before low dose epidural analgesia for labour. *Int J Obstet Anesth*. 2003;12:256–260.

36. Banerjee A, Stocche RM, Angle P, Halpern SH. Preload or coload for spinal anesthesia for elective cesarean delivery: ameta-analysis. *Can J Anaesth*. 2010;57:24–31.

37. Shapiro A, Fredman B, Zohar E, et al. Alternating patient position following the induction of obstetric epidural analgesia does not affect local anaesthetic spread. *Int J Obstet Anesth*. 1998;7:153–156.

38. Preston R, Crosby ET, Kotarba D, et al. Maternal positioning affects fetal heart rate changes after epidural analgesia for labour. *Can J Anaesth*. 1993;40:1136–1141.

39. Norris MC, Ferrenbach D, Dalman H, et al. Does epinephrine improve the diagnostic accuracy of aspiration during labor epidural analgesia? *Anesth Analg*. 1999;88:1073–1076.

40. Chestnut DH, Owen CL, Brown CK, et al. Does labor affect the variability of maternal heart rate during induction of epidural anesthesia? *Anesthesiology*. 1988;68:622–625.

41. Guay J. The epidural test dose: a review. *Anesth Analg*. 2006;102:921–929.

42. Gaiser RR. The epidural test dose in obstetric anesthesia: it is not obsolete. *J Clin Anesth*. 2003;15:474–477.

43. Pert CB, Kuhar MJ, Snyder SH. Opiate receptor: autoradiographic localization in rat brain. *Proc Natl Acad Sci U S A*. 1976;73:3729–3733.

44. Justins DM, Francis D, Houlton PG, Reynolds F. A controlled trial of extradural fentanyl in labour. *Br J Anaesth*. 1982;54:409–414.

45. Belfrage P, Berlin A, Raabe N, Thalme B. Lumbar epidural analgesia with bupivacaine in labor. Drug concentration in maternal and neonatal blood at birth and during the first day of life. *Am J Obstet Gynecol*. 1975;123:839–844.

46. Capogna G, Celleno D, Lyons G, et al. Minimum local analgesic concentration of extradural bupivacaine increases with progression of labour. *Br J Anaesth*. 1998;80:11–13.

47. Polley LS, Columb MO, Wagner DS, Naughton NN. Dose-dependent reduction of the minimum local analgesic concentration of bupivacaine by sufentanil for epidural analgesia in labor. *Anesthesiology*. 1998;89:626–632.

48. Pace NL, Stylianou MP. Advances in and limitations of up-and-down methodology: a précis of clinical use, study design, and dose estimation in anesthesia research. *Anesthesiology*. 2007;107:144–152.

49. Christiaens F, Verborgh C, Dierick A, Camu F. Effects of diluent volume of a single dose of epidural bupivacaine in parturients during the first stage of labor. *Reg Anesth Pain Med*. 1998;23:134–141.

50. Lyons GR, Kocarev MG, Wilson RC, Columb MO. A comparison of minimum local anesthetic volumes and doses of epidural bupivacaine (0.125% w/v and 0.25% w/v) for analgesia in labor. *Anesth Analg*. 2007;104:412–415.

51. Santos AC, Arthur GR, Wlody D, et al. Comparative systemic toxicity of ropivacaine and bupivacaine in nonpregnant and pregnant ewes. *Anesthesiology*. 1995;82:734–740.

52. Polley LS, Columb MO, Naughton NN, et al. Relative analgesic potencies of ropivacaine and bupivacaine for epidural analgesia in labor: implications for therapeutic indexes. *Anesthesiology*. 1999;90:944–950.

53. Capogna G, Celleno D, Fusco P, et al. Relative potencies of bupivacaine and ropivacaine for analgesia in labour. *Br J Anaesth*. 1999;82:371–373.

54. Ngan Kee WD, Ng FF, Khaw KS, et al. Determination and comparison of graded dose-response curves for epiduralbupivacaine and ropivacaine for analgesia in laboring nulliparous women. *Anesthesiology*. 2010;113:445–453.

55. Brockway MS, Bannister J, McClure JH, et al. Comparison of extradural ropivacaine and bupivacaine. *Br J Anaesth.* 1991;66:31–37.

56. Griffin RP, Reynolds F. Extradural anaesthesia for caesarean section: a double-blind comparison of 0.5% ropivacaine with 0.5% bupivacaine. *Br J Anaesth.* 1995;74:512–516.

57. Lacassie HJ, Habib AS, Lacassie HP, Columb MO. Motor blocking minimum local anesthetic concentrations of bupivacaine, levobupivacaine, and ropivacaine in labor. *Reg Anesth Pain Med.* 2007;32:323–329.

58. Owen MD, D'Angelo R, Gerancher JC, et al. 0.125% ropivacaine is similar to 0.125% bupivacaine for labor analgesia using patient-controlled epidural infusion. *Anesth Analg.* 1998;86:527–531.

59. Beilin Y, Guinn NR, Bernstein HH, et al. Local anesthetics and mode of delivery: bupivacaine versus ropivacaine versus levobupivacaine. *Anesth Analg.* 2007;105:756–763.

60. Halpern SH, Breen TW, Campbell DC, et al. A multicenter, randomized, controlled trial comparing bupivacaine with ropivacaine for labor analgesia. *Anesthesiology.* 2003;98:1431–1435.

61. Halpern SH, Walsh V. Epidural ropivacaine versus bupivacaine for labor: a meta-analysis. *Anesth Analg.* 2003;96:1473–1479.

62. Beilin Y, Halpern S. Focused review: ropivacaine versus bupivacaine for epidural labor analgesia. *Anesth Analg.* 2010;111:482–487.

63. Yoshida M, Matsuda H, Fukuda I, Furuya K. Sudden cardiac arrest during cesarean section due to epidural anaesthesia using ropivacaine: a case report. *Arch Gynecol Obstet.* 2008;277:91–94.

64. Bardsley H, Gristwood R, Baker H, et al. A comparison of the cardiovascular effects of levobupivacaine and rac-bupivacaine following intravenous administration to healthy volunteers. *Br J Clin Pharmacol.* 1998;46:245–249.

65. Vanhoutte F, Vereecke J, Verbeke N, Carmeliet E. Stereoselective effects of the enantiomers of bupivacaine on the electrophysiological properties of the Guinea-pig papillary muscle. *Br J Pharmacol.* 1991;103:1275–1281.

66. Lyons G, Columb M, Wilson RC, Johnson RV. Epidural pain relief in labour: potencies of levobupivacaine and racemic bupivacaine. *Br J Anaesth.* 1998;81:899–901.

67. Polley LS, Columb MO, Naughton NN, et al. Relative analgesic potencies of levobupivacaine and ropivacaine for epidural analgesia in labor. *Anesthesiology.* 2003;99:1354–1358.

68. Benhamou D, Ghosh C, Mercier FJ. A randomized sequential allocation study to determine the minimum effective analgesic concentration of levobupivacaine and ropivacaine in patients receiving epidural analgesia for labor. *Anesthesiology.* 2003;99:1383–1386.

69. Lacassie HJ, Columb MO. The relative motor blocking potencies of bupivacaine and levobupivacaine in labor. *Anesth Analg.* 2003;97:1509–1513.

70. Kennedy RL, Bell JU, Miller RP, et al. Uptake and distribution of lidocaine in fetal lambs. *Anesthesiology.* 1990;72:483–489.

71. Scanlon JW, Brown WU Jr, Weiss JB, Alper MH. Neurobehavioral responses of newborn infants after maternal epidural anesthesia. *Anesthesiology.* 1974;40:121–128.

72. Abboud TK, Afrasiabi A, Sarkis F, et al. Continuous infusion epidural analgesia in parturients receiving bupivacaine, chloroprocaine, or lidocaine–maternal, fetal, and neonatal effects. *Anesth Analg.* 1984;63:421–428.

73. Kuhnert BR, Harrison MJ, Linn PL, Kuhnert PM. Effects of maternal epidural anesthesia on neonatal behavior. *Anesth Analg.* 1984;63:301–308.

74. Vella LM, Willatts DG, Knott C, et al. Epidural fentanyl in labour. An evaluation of the systemic contribution to analgesia. *Anaesthesia.* 1985;40:741–747.

75. D'Angelo R, Gerancher JC, Eisenach JC, Raphael BL. Epidural fentanyl produces labor analgesia by a spinal mechanism. *Anesthesiology.* 1998;88:1519–1523.

76. Polley LS, Columb MO, Naughton NN, et al. Effect of intravenous versus epidural fentanyl on the minimum local analgesic concentration of epidural bupivacaine in labor. *Anesthesiology.* 2000;93:122–128.

77. Ginosar Y, Columb MO, Cohen SE, et al. The site of action of epidural fentanyl infusions in the presence of local anesthetics: a minimum local analgesic concentration infusion study in nulliparous labor. *Anesth Analg.* 2003;97:1439–1445.

78. Ginosar Y, Riley ET, Angst MS. The site of action of epidural fentanyl in humans: the difference between infusion and bolus administration. *Anesth Analg.* 2003;97:1428–1438.

79. Capogna G, Parpaglioni R, Lyons G, et al. Minimum analgesic dose of epidural sufentanil for first-stage labor analgesia: a comparison between spontaneous and prostaglandin-inducedlabors in nulliparous women. *Anesthesiology.* 2001;94:740–744.

80. Conell-Price J, Evans JB, Hong D, et al. The development and validation of a dynamic model to account for the progress of labor in the assessment of pain. *Anesth Analg.* 2008;106:1509–1515.

81. Capogna G, Camorcia M, Columb MO. Minimum analgesic doses of fentanyl and sufentanil for epidural analgesia in the first stage of labor. *Anesth Analg.* 2003;96:1178–1182.

82. Steinberg RB, Dunn SM, Dixon DE, et al. Comparison of sufentanil, bupivacaine, and their combination for epidural analgesia in obstetrics. *Reg Anesth.* 1992;17:131–138.

83. Connelly NR, Parker RK, Vallurupalli V, et al. Comparison of epidural fentanyl versus epidural sufentanil for analgesia in ambulatory patients in early labor. *Anesth Analg.* 2000;91:374–378.

84. Connelly NR, Parker RK, Pedersen T, et al. Diluent volume for epidural fentanyl and its effect on analgesia in early labor. *Anesth Analg.* 2003;96:1799–1804.

85. Reynolds F, O'Sullivan G. Epidural fentanyl and perineal pain in labour. *Anaesthesia.* 1989;44:341–344.

86. Van Steenberge A, Debroux HC, Noorduin H. Extradural bupivacaine with sufentanil for vaginal delivery. A double-blind trial. *Br J Anaesth.* 1987;59:1518–1522.

87. Celleno D, Capogna G. Epidural fentanyl plus bupivacaine 0.125 per cent for labour: analgesic effects. *Can J Anaesth.* 1988;35:375–378.

88. Vertommen JD, Vandermeulen E, Van Aken H, et al. The effects of the addition of sufentanil to 0.125% bupivacaine on the quality of analgesia during labor and on the incidence of instrumental deliveries. *Anesthesiology.* 1991;74:809–814.

89. Chestnut DH, Owen CL, Bates JN, et al. Continuous infusion epidural analgesia during labor: a randomized, double-blind comparison of 0.0625% bupivacaine/0.0002% fentanyl versus 0.125% bupivacaine. *Anesthesiology.* 1988;68:754–759.

90. Lyons G, Columb M, Hawthorne L, Dresner M. Extradural pain relief in labour: bupivacaine sparing by extradural fentanyl is dose dependent. *Br J Anaesth.* 1997;78:493–497.

91. Robinson AP, Lyons GR, Wilson RC, et al. Levobupivacaine for epidural analgesia in labor: the sparing effect of epidural fentanyl. *Anesth Analg.* 2001;92:410–414.

92. Buyse I, Stockman W, Columb M, et al. Effect of sufentanil on minimum local analgesic concentrations of epidural bupivacaine, ropivacaine and levobupivacaine in nullipara in early labour. *Int J Obstet Anesth.* 2007;16:22–28.

93. Palm S, Gertzen W, Ledowski T, et al. Minimum local analgesic dose of plain ropivacaine vs. ropivacaine combined with sufentanil during epidural analgesia for labour. *Anaesthesia.* 2001;56:526–529.

94. Polley LS, Columb MO, Lyons G, Nair SA. The effect of epidural fentanyl on the minimum local analgesic concentration of epidural chloroprocaine in labor. *Anesth Analg.* 1996;83:987–990.

95. Herman NL, Sheu KL, Van Decar TK, et al. Determination of the analgesic dose-response relationship for epidural fentanyl and sufentanil with bupivacaine 0.125% in laboring patients. *JClin Anesth.* 1998;10:670–677.

96. Yau G, Gregory MA, Gin T, et al. The addition of fentanyl to epidural bupivacaine in first stage labour. *Anaesth Intensive Care.* 1990;18:532–535.

97. Steinberg RB, Powell G, Hu XH, Dunn SM. Epidural sufentanil for analgesia for labor and delivery. *Reg Anesth.* 1989;14:225–228.

98. Sinatra RS, Eige S, Chung JH, et al. Continuous epidural infusion of 0.05% bupivacaine plus hydromorphone for labor analgesia: an observational assessment in 1830 parturients. *Anesth Analg.* 2002;94:1310–1311.

99. Parker RK, Connelly NR, Lucas T, et al. The addition of hydromorphone to epidural fentanyl does not affect analgesia in early labour. *Can J Anaesth.* 2002;49:600–604.

100. Mhyre JM. Strategies to induce labor analgesia with epidural hydromorphone. *Int J Obstet Anesth.* 2008;17:81–82.

101. Liu S, Carpenter R. Lipid solubility and epidural opioid efficacy. *Anesthesiology.* 1995;83:427–428.

102. Jaffe RA, Rowe MA. A comparison of the local anesthetic effects of meperidine, fentanyl, and sufentanil on dorsal root axons. *Anesth Analg.* 1996;83:776–781.

103. Handley G, Perkins G. The addition of pethidine to epidural bupivacaine in labour–effect of changing bupivacaine strength. *Anaesth Intensive Care.* 1992;20:151–155.

104. Brownridge P. Shivering related to epidural blockade with bupivacaine in labour, and the influence of epidural pethidine. *Anaesth Intensive Care.* 1986;14:412–417.

105. Massad IM, Khadra MM, Alkazaleh FA, et al. Bupivacaine with meperidine versus bupivacaine with fentanyl for continuous epidural labor analgesia. *Saudi Med J.* 2007;28:904–908.

106. Hill DA, McCarthy G, Bali IM. Epidural infusion of alfentanil or diamorphine with bupivacaine in labour—a dose finding study. *Anaesthesia.* 1995;50:415–419.

107. Cooper RA, Devlin E, Boyd TH, Bali IM. Epidural analgesia for labour using a continuous infusion of bupivacaine and alfentanil. *Eur J Anaesthesiol.* 1993;10:183–187.

108. Abboud TK, Afrasiabi A, Zhu J, et al. Epidural morphine or butorphanol augments bupivacaine analgesia during labor. *Reg Anesth.* 1989;14:115–120.

109. Hunt CO, Naulty JS, Malinow AM, et al. Epidural butorphanol-bupivacaine for analgesia during labor and delivery. *Anesth Analg.* 1989;68:323–327.

110. Hatjis CG, Meis PJ. Sinusoidal fetal heart rate pattern associated with butorphanol administration. *Obstet Gynecol.* 1986;67:377–380.

111. McLeod GA, Munishankar B, Columb MO. An isobolographic analysis of diamorphine and levobupivacaine for epidural analgesia in early labour. *Br J Anaesth.* 2007;98:497–502.

112. Lowson SM, Eggers KA, Warwick JP, et al. Epidural infusions of bupivacaine and diamorphine in labour. *Anaesthesia.* 1995;50:420–422.

113. Eisenach JC, Grice SC, Dewan DM. Epinephrine enhances analgesia produced by epidural bupivacaine during labor. *Anesth Analg.* 1987;66:447–451.

114. Abboud TK, Sheik-ol-Eslam A, Yanagi T, et al. Safety and efficacy of epinephrine added to bupivacaine for lumbar epidural analgesia in obstetrics. *Anesth Analg.* 1985;64:585–591.

115. Polley LS, Columb MO, Naughton NN, et al. Effect of epidural epinephrine on the minimum local analgesic concentration of epidural bupivacaine in labor. *Anesthesiology.* 2002;96:1123–1128.

116. Abboud TK, David S, Nagappala S, et al. Maternal, fetal, andneonatal effects of lidocaine with and without epinephrine for epidural anesthesia in obstetrics. *Anesth Analg.* 1984;63:973–979.

117. Reynolds F, Taylor G. Plasma concentrations of bupivacaine during continuous epidural analgesia in labour: the effect of adrenaline. *Br J Anaesth.* 1971;43:436–440.

118. Reynolds F, Laishley R, Morgan B, Lee A. Effect of time and adrenaline on the feto-maternal distribution of bupivacaine. *Br J Anaesth.* 1989;62:509–514.

119. Craft JB Jr, Epstein BS, Coakley CS. Effect of lidocaine with epinephrine versus lidocaine (plain) on induced labor. *Anesth Analg.* 1972;51:243–246.

120. Matadial L, Cibils LA. The effect of epidural anesthesia on uterine activity and blood pressure. *Am J Obstet Gynecol.* 1976;125:846–854.

121. Yarnell RW, Ewing DA, Tierney E, Smith MH. Sacralization of epidural block with repeated doses of 0.25% bupivacaine during labor. *Reg Anesth.* 1990;15:275–279.

122. Soetens FM, Soetens MA, Vercauteren MP. Levobupivacaine-sufentanil with or without epinephrine during epidural labor analgesia. *Anesth Analg.* 2006;103:182–186.

123. Albright GA, Jouppila R, Hollmén AI, et al. Epinephrine does not alter human intervillous blood flow during epidural anesthesia. *Anesthesiology.* 1981;54:131–135.

124. Skjöldebrand A, Garle M, Gustafsson LL, et al. Extradural pethidine with and without adrenaline during labour: wide variation in effect. *Br J Anaesth.* 1982;54:415–420.

125. Chabot-Doré AJ, Schuster DJ, Stone LS, Wilcox GL. Analgesic synergy between opioid and α2-adrenoceptors. *Br J Pharmacol.* 2015;172:388–402.

126. Landau R, Schiffer E, Morales M, et al. The dose-sparing effect of clonidine added to ropivacaine for labor epidural analgesia. *Anesth Analg.* 2002;95:728–734.

127. Tremlett MR, Kelly PJ, Parkins J, et al. Low-dose clonidine infusion during labour. *Br J Anaesth.* 1999;83:257–261.

128. Dewandre PY, Kirsch M, Bonhomme V, et al. Impact of the addition of sufentanil 5 µg or clonidine 75 µg on the minimum local analgesic concentration of ropivacaine for epidural analgesia in labour: a randomized comparison. *Int J Obstet Anesth.* 2008;17:315–321.

129. Dewandre PY, Decurninge V, Bonhomme V, et al. Side effects of the addition of clonidine 75 μg or sufentanil 5 μg to 0.2% ropivacaine for labour epidural analgesia. *Int J Obstet Anesth.* 2010;19:149–154.

130. Chassard D, Mathon L, Dailler F, et al. Extradural clonidine combined with sufentanil and 0.0625% bupivacaine for analgesia in labour. *Br J Anaesth.* 1996;77:458–462.

131. Paech MJ, Pavy TJ, Orlikowski CE, Evans SF. Patient-controlled epidural analgesia in labor: the addition of clonidine to bupivacaine-fentanyl. *Reg Anesth Pain Med.* 2000;25:34–40.

132. Claes B, Soetens M, Van Zundert A, Datta S. Clonidine added to bupivacaine-epinephrine-sufentanil improves epidural analgesia during childbirth. *Reg Anesth Pain Med.* 1998;23:540–547.

133. Wallet F, Clement HJ, Bouret C, et al. Effects of a continuous low-dose clonidine epidural regimen on pain, satisfaction and adverse events during labour: a randomized, double-blind, placebo-controlled trial. *Eur J Anaesthesiol.* 2010;27:441–447.

134. Bazin M, Bonnin M, Storme B, et al. Addition of clonidine to a continuous patient-controlled epidural infusion of low-concentration levobupivacaine plus sufentanil in primiparous women during labour. *Anaesthesia.* 2011;66:769–779.

135. Buggy DJ, MacDowell C. Extradural analgesia with clonidine and fentanyl compared with 0.25% bupivacaine in the first stage of labour. *Br J Anaesth.* 1996;76:319–321.

136. Roelants F, Lavand'homme PM, Mercier-Fuzier V. Epidural administration of neostigmine and clonidine to induce labor analgesia: evaluation of efficacy and local anesthetic-sparing effect. *Anesthesiology.* 2005;102:1205–1210.

137. Van de Velde M, Berends N, Kumar A, et al. Effects of epidural clonidine and neostigmine following intrathecal labour analgesia: a randomised, double-blind, placebo-controlled trial. *Int J Obstet Anesth.* 2009;18:207–214.

138. Aveline C, El Metaoua S, Masmoudi A, et al. The effect of clonidine on the minimum local analgesic concentration of epidural ropivacaine during labor. *Anesth Analg.* 2002;95:735–740.

139. Zhang D, Sun Y, Li J. Application of dexmedetomidine in epidural labor analgesia: a systematic review and meta-analysis on randomized controlled trials. *Clin J Pain.* 2024;40:57–65.

140. Roelants F, Rizzo M, Lavand'homme P. The effect of epidural neostigmine combined with ropivacaine and sufentanil on neuraxial analgesia during labor. *Anesth Analg.* 2003;96:1161–1166.

141. Roelants F, Lavand'homme PM. Epidural neostigmine combined with sufentanil provides balanced and selectiveanalgesia in early labor. *Anesthesiology.* 2004;101:439–444.

142. Naguib M, Yaksh TL. Antinociceptive effects of spinal cholinesterase inhibition and isobolographic analysis of the interaction with μ and $α_2$ receptor systems. *Anesthesiology.* 1994;80:1338–1348.

143. Boogmans T, Vertommen J, Valkenborgh T, et al. Epidural neostigmine and clonidine improves the quality of combined spinal epidural analgesia in labour: a randomised, double-blind controlled trial. *Eur J Anaesthesiol.* 2014;31:190–196.

144. Ross VH, Pan PH, Owen MD, et al. Neostigmine decreases bupivacaine use by patient-controlled epidural analgesia during labor: a randomized controlled study. *Anesth Analg.* 2009;109:524–531.

145. Booth JL, Ross VH, Nelson KE, et al. Epidural neostigmine versus fentanyl to decrease bupivacaine use in patient-controlled epidural analgesia during labor: a randomized, double-blind, controlled study. *Anesthesiology.* 2017;127:50–57.

146. Wong CA, Scavone BM, Loffredi M, et al. The dose-response of intrathecal sufentanil added to bupivacaine for labor analgesia. *Anesthesiology.* 2000;92:1553–1558.

147. Wong CA, Scavone BM, Slavenas JP, et al. Efficacy and side effect profile of varying doses of intrathecal fentanyl added to bupivacaine for labor analgesia. *Int J Obstet Anesth.* 2004;13:19–24.

148. Ngan Kee WD, Khaw KS, Ng FF, et al. Synergistic interaction between fentanyl and bupivacaine given intrathecally for labor analgesia. *Anesthesiology.* 2014;120:1126–1136.

149. Campbell DC, Camann WR, Datta S. The addition of bupivacaine to intrathecal sufentanil for labor analgesia. *Anesth Analg.* 1995;81:305–309.

150. Stocks GM, Hallworth SP, Fernando R, et al. Minimum local analgesic dose of intrathecal bupivacaine in labor and the effect of intrathecal fentanyl. *Anesthesiology.* 2001;94:593–598.

151. Sia AT, Chong JL, Chiu JW. Combination of intrathecal sufentanil 10 μg plus bupivacaine 2.5 mg for labor analgesia: is half the dose enough? *Anesth Analg.* 1999;88:362–366.

152. Palmer CM, Cork RC, Hays R, et al. The dose-response relation of intrathecal fentanyl for labor analgesia. *Anesthesiology.* 1998;88:355–361.

153. Nelson KE, Rauch T, Terebuh V, D'Angelo R. A comparison of intrathecal fentanyl and sufentanil for labor analgesia. *Anesthesiology.* 2002;96:1070–1073.

154. Herman NL, Choi KC, Affleck PJ, et al. Analgesia, pruritus, and ventilation exhibit a dose-response relationship in parturients receiving intrathecal fentanyl during labor. *Anesth Analg.* 1999;89:378–383.

155. Herman NL, Calicott R, Van Decar TK, et al. Determination of the dose-response relationship for intrathecal sufentanil in laboring patients. *Anesth Analg.* 1997;84:1256–1261.

156. Nelson KE, D'Angelo R, Foss ML, et al. Intrathecal neostigmine and sufentanil for early labor analgesia. *Anesthesiology.* 1999;91:1293–1298.

157. Arkoosh VA, Cooper M, Norris MC, et al. Intrathecal sufentanil dose response in nulliparous patients. *Anesthesiology.* 1998;89:364–370.

158. Camann W, Abouleish A, Eisenach J, et al. Intrathecal sufentanil and epidural bupivacaine for labor analgesia: dose-response of individual agents and in combination. *Reg Anesth Pain Med.* 1998;23:457–462.

159. Landau R, Kern C, Columb MO, et al. Genetic variability of the μ-opioid receptor influences intrathecal fentanyl analgesia requirements in laboring women. *Pain.* 2008;139:5–14.

160. Wong CA, McCarthy RJ, Blouin J, Landau R. Observational study of the effect of μ-opioid receptor genetic polymorphism on intrathecal opioid labor analgesia and post-cesarean delivery analgesia. *Int J Obstet Anesth.* 2010;19:246–253.

161. Ginosar Y, Birnbach DJ, Shirov TT, et al. Duration of analgesia and pruritus following intrathecal fentanyl for labour analgesia: no significant effect of A118G μ-opioid receptor polymorphism, but a marked effect of ethnically distinct hospital populations. *Br J Anaesth.* 2013;111:433–444.

162. Wong CA. The promise of pharmacogenetics in labor analgesia…tantalizing, but not there yet. *Int J Obstet Anesth.* 2012;21:105–108.

163. Van de Velde M, Dreelinck R, Dubois J, et al. Determination of the full dose-response relation of intrathecal bupivacaine, levobupivacaine, and ropivacaine, combined with sufentanil, for labor analgesia. *Anesthesiology*. 2007;106:149–156.

164. Baraka A, Noueihid R, Hajj S. Intrathecal injection of morphine for obstetric analgesia. *Anesthesiology*. 1981;54:136–140.

165. Abboud TK, Shnider SM, Dailey PA, et al. Intrathecal administration of hyperbaric morphine for the relief of pain in labour. *Br J Anaesth*. 1984;56:1351–1360.

166. Abouleish E. Apnoea associated with the intrathecal administration of morphine in obstetrics. A case report. *Br J Anaesth*. 1988;60:592–594.

167. Vasudevan A, Snowman CE, Sundar S, et al. Intrathecal morphine reduces breakthrough pain during labour epidural analgesia. *Br J Anaesth*. 2007;98:241–245.

168. Hess PE, Vasudevan A, Snowman C, Pratt SD. Small dose bupivacaine-fentanyl spinal analgesia combined with morphine for labor. *Anesth Analg*. 2003;97:247–252.

169. Yeh HM, Chen LK, Shyu MK, et al. The addition of morphine prolongs fentanyl-bupivacaine spinal analgesia for the relief of labor pain. *Anesth Analg*. 2001;92:665–668.

170. Hein A, Rösblad P, Norman M, et al. Addition of low-dose morphine to intrathecal bupivacaine/sufentanil labour analgesia: a randomised controlled study. *Int J Obstet Anesth*. 2010;19:384–389.

171. Minty RG, Kelly L, Minty A, Hammett DC. Single-dose intrathecal analgesia to control labour pain: is it a useful alternative to epidural analgesia? *Can Fam Physician*. 2007;53:437–442.

172. Honet JE, Arkoosh VA, Norris MC, et al. Comparison among intrathecal fentanyl, meperidine, and sufentanil for labor analgesia. *Anesth Analg*. 1992;75:734–739.

173. Booth JV, Lindsay DR, Olufolabi AJ, et al. Subarachnoid meperidine (Pethidine) causes significant nausea and vomiting during labor. *Anesthesiology*. 2000;93:418–421.

174. Kestin IG, Madden AP, Mulvein JT, Goodman NW. Analgesia for labour and delivery using incremental diamorphine and bupivacaine via a 32-gauge intrathecal catheter. *Br J Anaesth*. 1992;68:244–247.

175. Vaughan DJ, Ahmad N, Lillywhite NK, et al. Choice of opioid for initiation of combined spinal epidural analgesia in labour–fentanyl or diamorphine. *Br J Anaesth*. 2001;86:567–569.

176. Asokumar B, Newman LM, McCarthy RJ, et al. Intrathecal bupivacaine reduces pruritus and prolongs duration of fentanyl analgesia during labor: a prospective, randomized controlled trial. *Anesth Analg*. 1998;87:1309–1315.

177. Whitty R, Goldszmidt E, Parkes RK, Carvalho JC. Determination of the ED95 for intrathecal plain bupivacaine combined with fentanyl in active labor. *Int J Obstet Anesth*. 2007;16:341–345.

178. Camorcia M, Capogna G, Columb MO. Minimum local analgesic doses of ropivacaine, levobupivacaine, and bupivacaine for intrathecal labor analgesia. *Anesthesiology*. 2005;102:646–650.

179. Palmer CM, Van Maren G, Nogami WM, Alves D. Bupivacaine augments intrathecal fentanyl for labor analgesia. *Anesthesiology*. 1999;91:84–89.

180. Lee BB, Ngan Kee WD, Hung VY, Wong EL. Combined spinal-epidural analgesia in labour: comparison of two doses of intrathecal bupivacaine with fentanyl. *Br J Anaesth*. 1999;83:868–871.

181. Richardson MG, Wissler RN. Densities of dextrose-free intrathecal local anesthetics, opioids, and combinations measured at 37°C. *Anesth Analg*. 1997;84:95–99.

182. Richardson MG, Thakur R, Abramowicz JS, Wissler RN. Maternal posture influences the extent of sensory block produced by intrathecal dextrose-free bupivacaine with fentanyl for labor analgesia. *Anesth Analg*. 1996;83:1229–1233.

183. Ferouz F, Norris MC, Arkoosh VA, et al. Baricity, needle direction, and intrathecal sufentanil labor analgesia. *Anesthesiology*. 1997;86:592–598.

184. Gage JC, D'Angelo R, Miller R, Eisenach JC. Does dextrose affect analgesia or the side effects of intrathecal sufentanil? *Anesth Analg*. 1997;85:826–830.

185. Rofaeel A, Lilker S, Fallah S, et al. Intrathecal plain vs hyperbaric bupivacaine for labour analgesia: efficacy and side effects. *Can J Anaesth*. 2007;54:15–20.

186. Gautier PE, De Kock M, Fanard L, et al. Intrathecal clonidine combined with sufentanil for labor analgesia. *Anesthesiology*. 1998;88:651–656.

187. Mercier FJ, Dounas M, Bouaziz H, et al. The effect of adding a minidose of clonidine to intrathecal sufentanil for labor analgesia. *Anesthesiology*. 1998;89:594–601.

188. Missant C, Teunkens A, Vandermeersch E, Van de Velde M. Intrathecal clonidine prolongs labour analgesia but worsensfetal outcome: a pilot study. *Can J Anaesth*. 2004;51:696–701.

189. Sia AT. Optimal dose of intrathecal clonidine added to sufentanil plus bupivacaine for labour analgesia. *Can J Anaesth*. 2000;47:875–880.

190. Chiari A, Lorber C, Eisenach JC, et al. Analgesic and hemodynamic effects of intrathecal clonidine as the sole analgesic agent during first stage of labor: a dose-response study. *Anesthesiology*. 1999;91:388–396.

191. D'Angelo R, Dean LS, Meister GC, Nelson KE. Neostigmine combined with bupivacaine, clonidine, and sufentanil for spinal labor analgesia. *Anesth Analg*. 2001;93:1560–1564.

192. Owen MD, Ozsaraç O, Sahin S, et al. Low-dose clonidine and neostigmine prolong the duration of intrathecal bupivacaine-fentanyl for labor analgesia. *Anesthesiology*. 2000;92:361–366.

193. Campbell DC, Banner R, Crone LA, et al. Addition of epinephrine to intrathecal bupivacaine and sufentanil for ambulatory labor analgesia. *Anesthesiology*. 1997;86:525–531.

194. Vercauteren MP, Jacobs S, Jacquemyn Y, Adriaensen HA. Intrathecal labor analgesia with bupivacaine and sufentanil: the effect of adding 2.25 µg epinephrine. *Reg Anesth Pain Med*. 2001;26:473–477.

195. Gurbet A, Turker G, Kose DO, Uckunkaya N. Intrathecal epinephrine in combined spinal-epidural analgesia for labor: dose-response relationship for epinephrine added to a local anesthetic-opioid combination. *Int J Obstet Anesth*. 2005;14:121–125.

196. Moir DD, Slater PJ, Thorburn J, et al. Extradural analgesia in obstetrics: a controlled trial of carbonated lignocaine and bupivacaine hydrochloride with or without adrenaline. *Br J Anaesth*. 1976;48:129–135.

197. Mogensen T, Simonsen L, Scott NB, et al. Tachyphylaxis associated with repeated epidural injections of lidocaine is not related to changes in distribution or the rate of elimination from the epidural space. *Anesth Analg*. 1989;69:180–184.

198. Palmer SK, Bosnjak ZJ, Hopp FA, et al. Lidocaine and bupivacaine differential blockade of isolated canine nerves. *Anesth Analg*. 1983;62:754–757.

199. Hess PE, Pratt SD, Oriol NE. An analysis of the need for anesthetic interventions with differing concentrations of labor epidural bupivacaine: an observational study. *Int J Obstet Anesth*. 2006;15:195–200.

200. Beilin Y, Nair A, Arnold I, et al. A comparison of epidural infusions in the combined spinal/epidural technique for labor analgesia. *Anesth Analg*. 2002;94:927–932.

201. Owen MD, Thomas JA, Smith T, et al. Ropivacaine 0.075% and bupivacaine 0.075% with fentanyl 2 µg/mL are equivalent for labor epidural analgesia. *Anesth Analg*. 2002;94:179–183.

202. Meister GC, D'Angelo R, Owen M, et al. A comparison of epidural analgesia with 0.125% ropivacaine with fentanyl versus 0.125% bupivacaine with fentanyl during labor. *Anesth Analg*. 2000;90:632–637.

203. Chua NP, Sia AT, Ocampo CE. Parturient-controlled epidural analgesia during labour: bupivacaine vs. ropivacaine. *Anaesthesia*. 2001;56:1169–1173.

204. Fernández-Guisasola J, Serrano ML, Cobo B, et al. A comparison of 0.0625% bupivacaine with fentanyl and 0.1% ropivacaine with fentanyl for continuous epidural labor analgesia. *Anesth Analg*. 2001;92:1261–1265.

205. Parpaglioni R, Capogna G, Celleno D. A comparison between low-dose ropivacaine and bupivacaine at equianalgesic concentrations for epidural analgesia during the first stage of labor. *Int J Obstet Anesth*. 2000;9:83–86.

206. Bernard JM, Le Roux D, Barthe A, et al. The dose-range effects of sufentanil added to 0.125% bupivacaine on the quality of patient-controlled epidural analgesia during labor. *Anesth Analg*. 2001;92:184–188.

207. Bader AM, Fragneto R, Terui K, et al. Maternal and neonatal fentanyl and bupivacaine concentrations after epidural infusion during labor. *Anesth Analg*. 1995;81:829–832.

208. Porter J, Bonello E, Reynolds F. Effect of epidural fentanyl on neonatal respiration. *Anesthesiology*. 1998;89:79–85.

209. Loftus JR, Hill H, Cohen SE. Placental transfer and neonatal effects of epidural sufentanil and fentanyl administered with bupivacaine during labor. *Anesthesiology*. 1995;83:300–308.

210. Ginosar Y, Davidson EM, Firman N, et al. A randomized controlled trial using patient-controlled epidural analgesia with 0.25% versus 0.0625% bupivacaine in nulliparous labor: effect on analgesia requirement and maternal satisfaction. *Int J Obstet Anesth*. 2010;19:171–178.

211. Association of Women's Health Obstetric and Neonatal Nurses. Role of the registered nurse in the care of the pregnant woman receiving analgesia and anesthesia by catheter techniques. *Nurs Womens Health*. 2020;24:149–151.

212. Lamont RF, Pinney D, Rodgers P, Bryant TN. Continuous versus intermittent epidural analgesia. A randomised trial to observe obstetric outcome. *Anaesthesia*. 1989;44:893–896.

213. Bogod DG, Rosen M, Rees GA. Extradural infusion of 0.125% bupivacaine at 10 ml h⁻¹ to women during labour. *Br J Anaesth*. 1987;59:325–330.

214. Li DF, Rees GA, Rosen M. Continuous extradural infusion of 0.0625% or 0.125% bupivacaine for pain relief in primigravid labour. *Br J Anaesth*. 1985;57:264–270.

215. Hicks JA, Jenkins JG, Newton MC, Findley IL. Continuous epidural infusion of 0.075% bupivacaine for pain relief in labour. A comparison with intermittent top-ups of 0.5% bupivacaine. *Anaesthesia*. 1988;43:289–292.

216. Smedstad KG, Morison DH. A comparative study of continuous and intermittent epidural analgesia for labour and delivery. *Can J Anaesth*. 1988;35:234–241.

217. Cole J, Hughey S. Bolus epidural infusion improves spread compared with continuous infusion in a cadaveric porcine spine model. *Reg Anesth Pain Med*. 2019.

218. Hogan Q. Distribution of solution in the epidural space: examination by cryomicrotome section. *Reg Anesth Pain Med*. 2002;27:150–156.

219. Boutros A, Blary S, Bronchard R, Bonnet F. Comparison of intermittent epidural bolus, continuous epidural infusion and patient controlled-epidural analgesia during labor. *Int J Obstet Anesth*. 1999;8:236–241.

220. Gambling DR, Yu P, Cole C, et al. A comparative study of patient controlled epidural analgesia (PCEA) and continuous infusion epidural analgesia (CIEA) during labour. *Can J Anaesth*. 1988;35:249–254.

221. Halpern SH, Carvalho B. Patient-controlled epidural analgesia for labor. *Anesth Analg*. 2009;108:921–928.

222. van der Vyver M, Halpern S, Joseph G. Patient-controlled epidural analgesia versus continuous infusion for labour analgesia: a meta-analysis. *Br J Anaesth*. 2002;89:459–465.

223. Heesen M, Böhmer J, Klöhr S, et al. The effect of adding a background infusion to patient-controlled epidural labor analgesia on labor, maternal, and neonatal outcomes: a systematic review and meta-analysis. *Anesth Analg*. 2015;121:149–158.

224. Sng BL, Sia AT, Lim Y, et al. Comparison of computer-integrated patient-controlled epidural analgesia and patient-controlled epidural analgesia with a basal infusion for labour and delivery. *Anaesth Intensive Care*. 2009;37:46–53.

225. Lim Y, Ocampo CE, Supandji M, et al. A randomized controlled trial of three patient-controlled epidural analgesia regimens for labor. *Anesth Analg*. 2008;107:1968–1972.

226. Brogly N, Schiraldi R, Vazquez B, et al. A randomized control trial of patient-controlled epidural analgesia (PCEA) with and without a background infusion using levobupivacaine and fentanyl. *Minerva Anestesiol*. 2011;77:1149–1154.

227. Gambling DR, Huber CJ, Berkowitz J, et al. Patient-controlled epidural analgesia in labour: varying bolus dose and lockout interval. *Can J Anaesth*. 1993;40:211–217.

228. Okutomi T, Saito M, Mochizuki J, et al. A double-blind randomized controlled trial of patient-controlled epidural analgesia with or without a background infusion following initial spinal analgesia for labor pain. *Int J Obstet Anesth*. 2009;18:28–32.

229. Siddik-Sayyid SM, Aouad MT, Jalbout MI, et al. Comparison of three modes of patient-controlled epidural analgesia during labour. *Eur J Anaesthesiol*. 2005;22:30–34.

230. Stratmann G, Gambling DR, Moeller-Bertram T, et al. A randomized comparison of a five-minute versus fifteen-minute lockout interval for PCEA during labor. *Int J Obstet Anesth*. 2005;14:200–207.

231. Carvalho B, Cohen SE, Giarrusso K, et al. "Ultra-light" patient-controlled epidural analgesia during labor: effects of varying regimens on analgesia and physician workload. *Int J Obstet Anesth*. 2005;14:223–229.

232. Bernard JM, Le Roux D, Frouin J. Ropivacaine and fentanyl concentrations in patient-controlled epidural analgesia during labor: a volume-range study. *Anesth Analg*. 2003;97:1800–1807.

233. Bernard JM, Le Roux D, Vizquel L, et al. Patient-controlled epidural analgesia during labor: the effects of the increase in bolus and lockout interval. *Anesth Analg*. 2000;90:328–332.

234. Roofthooft E, Barbé A, Schildermans J, et al. Programmed intermittent epidural bolus vs. patient-controlled epidural analgesia for maintenance of labour analgesia: a two-centre, double-blind, randomised study. *Anaesthesia*. 2020;75:1635–1642.

235. Roofthooft E, Filetici N, Van Houwe M, et al. High-volume patient-controlled epidural vs. programmed intermittent epidural bolus for labour analgesia: a randomised controlled study. *Anaesthesia*. 2023;78:1129–1138.

236. Boselli E, Debon R, Duflo F, et al. Ropivacaine 0.15% plus sufentanil 0.5 µg/mL and ropivacaine 0.10% plus sufentanil 0.5 µg/mL are equivalent for patient-controlled epidural analgesia during labor. *Anesth Analg*. 2003;96:1173–1177.

237. Gogarten W, Van de Velde M, Soetens F, et al. A multicentre trial comparing different concentrations of ropivacaine plus sufentanil with bupivacaine plus sufentanil for patient-controlled epidural analgesia in labour. *Eur J Anaesthesiol*. 2004;21:38–45.

238. Nikkola E, Läärä A, Hinkka S, et al. Patient-controlled epidural analgesia in labor does not always improve maternal satisfaction. *Acta Obstet Gynecol Scand*. 2006;85:188–194.

239. Wong CA, Ratliff JT, Sullivan JT, et al. A randomized comparison of programmed intermittent epidural bolus with continuous epidural infusion for labor analgesia. *Anesth Analg*. 2006;102:904–909.

240. Tan HS, Zeng Y, Qi Y, et al. Automated mandatory bolus versus basal infusion for maintenance of epidural analgesia in labour. *Cochrane Database Syst Rev*. 2023;(6):CD011344.

241. Wong CA, McCarthy RJ, Hewlett B. The effect of manipulation of the programmed intermittent bolus time interval and injection volume on total drug use for labor epidural analgesia: a randomized controlled trial. *Anesth Analg*. 2011;112:904–911.

242. Zakus P, Arzola C, Bittencourt R, et al. Determination of the optimal programmed intermittent epidural bolus volume of bupivacaine 0.0625% with fentanyl 2 µg.ml⁻¹ at a fixed interval of forty minutes: a biased coin up-and-down sequential allocation trial. *Anaesthesia*. 2018;73:459–465.

243. Howle R, Ragbourne S, Zolger D, et al. Influence of different volumes and frequency of programmed intermittent epidural bolus in labor on maternal and neonatal outcomes: a systematic review and network meta-analysis. *J Clin Anesth*. 2024;93:111364.

244. Epsztein Kanczuk M, Barrett NM, Arzola C, et al. Programmed intermittent epidural bolus for labor analgesia during first stage of labor: a biased-coin up-and-down sequential allocation trial to determine the optimum interval time between boluses of a fixed volume of 10 mL of bupivacaine 0.0625% with fentanyl 2 µg/mL. *Anesth Analg*. 2017;124:537–541.

245. Yao HQ, Huang JY, Deng JL, et al. Randomized assessment of the optimal time interval between programmed intermittent epidural boluses when combined with the dural puncture epidural technique for labor analgesia. *Anesth Analg*. 2023;136:532–539.

246. Munro A, George RB, Andreou P. An innovative approach to determine programmed intermittent epidural bolus pump settings for labor analgesia: a randomized controlled trial. *Anesth Analg*. 2024;139:545–554.

247. Fegley AJ, Lerman J, Wissler R. Epidural multiorifice catheters function as single-orifice catheters: an in vitro study. *Anesth Analg*. 2008;107:1079–1081.

248. Du W, Song Y, Zhao Q, et al. The effect of open-end versus closed-end epidural catheter design on injection pressure and dye diffusion under various programmed intermittent epidural delivery rates: an in vitro study. *Int J Obstet Anesth*. 2022;51103252.

249. Krawczyk P, Piwowar P, Sałapa K, et al. Do epidural catheter size and flow rate affect bolus injection pressure in different programmed intermittent epidural bolus regimens? An in vitro study. *Anesth Analg*. 2019;129:1587–1594.

250. Lange EMS, Wong CA, Fitzgerald PC, et al. Effect of epidural infusion bolus delivery rate on the duration of labor analgesia: a randomized clinical trial. *Anesthesiology*. 2018;128:745–753.

251. Yi J, Li Y, Yuan Y, et al. Comparison of labor analgesia efficacy between single-orifice and multiorifice wire-reinforced catheters during programmed intermittent epidural boluses: a randomized controlled clinical trial. *Reg Anesth Pain Med*. 2023;48:61–66.

252. Betti F, Carvalho B, Riley ET. Intrathecal migration of an epidural catheter while using a programmed intermittent epidural bolus technique for labor analgesia maintenance: a case report. *A A Case Rep*. 2017;9:357–359.

253. Birnbach DJ, Vincent CA. A matter of conscience: a call to action for system improvements involving epidural and spinal catheters. *Anesth Analg*. 2012;114:494–496.

254. NHS England. National Patient Safety Alert: Transition to NRFit™ connectors for intrathecal and epidural procedure, and delivery of regional blocks; 2024. https://www.england.nhs.uk/publication/national-patient-safety-alert-transition-to-nrfit-connectors-for-intrathecal-and-epidural-procedures-and-delivery-of-regional-blocks/. Accessed November 16, 2024.

255. Palmer CM. Continuous spinal anesthesia and analgesia in obstetrics. *Anesth Analg*. 2010;111:1476–1479.

256. Rigler ML, Drasner K, Krejcie TC, et al. Cauda equina syndrome after continuous spinal anesthesia. *Anesth Analg*. 1991;72:275–281.

257. Rigler ML, Drasner K. Distribution of catheter-injected local anesthetic in a model of the subarachnoid space. *Anesthesiology*. 1991;75:684–692.

258. Arkoosh VA, Palmer CM, Yun EM, et al. A randomized, double-masked, multicenter comparison of the safety of continuous intrathecal labor analgesia using a 28-gauge catheter versus continuous epidural labor analgesia. *Anesthesiology*. 2008;108:286–298.

259. Tao W, Grant EN, Craig MG, et al. Continuous spinal analgesia for labor and delivery: an observational study with a 23-gauge spinal catheter. *Anesth Analg*. 2015;121:1290–1294.

260. Van de Velde M, Budts W, Vandermeersch E, Spitz B. Continuous spinal analgesia for labor pain in a parturient with aortic stenosis. *Int J Obstet Anesth*. 2003;12:51–54.

261. Okutomi T, Kikuchi S, Amano K, et al. Continuous spinal analgesia for labor and delivery in a parturient with hypertrophic obstructive cardiomyopathy. *Acta Anaesthesiol Scand*. 2002;46:329–331.

262. Collis RE, Baxandall ML, Srikantharajah ID, et al. Combined spinal epidural analgesia with ability to walk throughout labour. *Lancet*. 1993;341:767–768.

263. Buggy D, Hughes N, Gardiner J. Posterior column sensory impairment during ambulatory extradural analgesia in labour. *Br J Anaesth*. 1994;73:540–542.

264. Parry MG, Fernando R, Bawa GP, Poulton BB. Dorsal column function after epidural and spinal blockade: implications for

the safety of walking following low-dose regional analgesia for labour. *Anaesthesia*. 1998;53:382–387.

265. Davies J, Fernando R, McLeod A, et al. Postural stability following ambulatory regional analgesia for labor. *Anesthesiology*. 2002;97:1576–1581.

266. Calimaran AL, Strauss-Hoder TP, Wang WY, et al. The effect of epidural test dose on motor function after a combined spinal-epidural technique for labor analgesia. *Anesth Analg*. 2003;96:1167–1172.

267. Cohen SE, Yeh JY, Riley ET, Vogel TM. Walking with labor epidural analgesia: the impact of bupivacaine concentration and a lidocaine-epinephrine test dose. *Anesthesiology*. 2000;92:387–392.

268. Preston R. Walking epidurals for labour analgesia: do they benefit anyone? *Can J Anaesth*. 2010;57:103–106.

269. Weiniger CF, Yaghmour H, Nadjari M, et al. Walking reduces the post-void residual volume in parturients with epidural analgesia for labor: a randomized-controlled study. *Acta Anaesthesiol Scand*. 2009;53:665–672.

270. Merry AF, Cross JA, Mayadeo SV, Wild CJ. Posture and the spread of extradural analgesia in labour. *Br J Anaesth*. 1983;55:303–307.

271. Park WY, Hagins FM, Massengale MD, Macnamara TE. The sitting position and anesthetic spread in the epidural space. *Anesth Analg*. 1984;63:863–864.

272. Erdemir HA, Soper LE, Sweet RB. Studies of factors affecting peridural anesthesia. *Anesth Analg*. 1965;44:400–404.

273. Dyer RA, Reed AR, van Dyk D, et al. Hemodynamic effects of ephedrine, phenylephrine, and the coadministration of phenylephrine with oxytocin during spinal anesthesia for elective cesarean delivery. *Anesthesiology*. 2009;111: 753–765.

274. Kinsella SM, Black AM. Reporting of 'hypotension' after epidural analgesia during labour. Effect of choice of arm and timing of baseline readings. *Anaesthesia*. 1998;53:131–135.

275. Beilin Y, Abramovitz SE, Zahn J, et al. Improved epidural analgesia in the parturient in the 30 degree tilt position. *Can J Anaesth*. 2000;47:1176–1181.

276. Lee A, Ngan Kee WD, Gin T. A quantitative, systematic review of randomized controlled trials of ephedrine versus phenylephrine for the management of hypotension during spinal anesthesia for cesarean delivery. *Anesth Analg*. 2002;94:920–926.

277. Hughes SC, Ward MG, Levinson G, et al. Placental transfer of ephedrine does not affect neonatal outcome. *Anesthesiology*. 1985;63:217–219.

278. Wright RG, Shnider SM, Levinson G, et al. The effect of maternal administration of ephedrine on fetal heart rate and variability. *Obstet Gynecol*. 1981;57:734–738.

279. Cohen SE, Cherry CM, Holbrook RH Jr, et al. Intrathecal sufentanil for labor analgesia–sensory changes, side effects, and fetal heart rate changes. *Anesth Analg*. 1993;77: 1155–1160.

280. Douglas MJ, Kim JH, Ross PL, McMorland GH. The effect of epinephrine in local anaesthetic on epidural morphine-induced pruritus. *Can Anaesth Soc J*. 1986;33:737–740.

281. Nguyen E, Lim G, Ross SE. Evaluation of therapies for peripheral and neuraxial opioid-induced pruritus based on molecular and cellular discoveries. *Anesthesiology*. 2021;135:350–365.

282. Prin M, Guglielminotti J, Moitra V, Li G. Prophylactic ondansetron for the prevention of intrathecal fentanyl- or sufentanil-mediated pruritus: a meta-analysis of randomized trials. *Anesth Analg*. 2016;122:402–409.

283. Wells J, Paech MJ, Evans SF. Intrathecal fentanyl-induced pruritus during labour: the effect of prophylactic ondansetron. *Int J Obstet Anesth*. 2004;13:35–39.

284. Cohen SE, Ratner EF, Kreitzman TR, et al. Nalbuphine is better than naloxone for treatment of side effects after epidural morphine. *Anesth Analg*. 1992;75:747–752.

285. Wong CA, Scavone BM, Peaceman AM, et al. The risk of cesarean delivery with neuraxial analgesia given early versus late in labor. *N Engl J Med*. 2005;352:655–665.

286. Chaney MA. Side effects of intrathecal and epidural opioids. *Can J Anaesth*. 1995;42:891–903.

287. Norris MC, Grieco WM, Borkowski M, et al. Complications of labor analgesia: epidural versus combined spinal epidural techniques. *Anesth Analg*. 1994;79:529–537.

288. Patel S, Ciechanowicz S, Blumenfeld YJ, Sultan P. Epidural-related maternal fever: incidence, pathophysiology, outcomes, and management. *Am J Obstet Gynecol*. 2023;228:S1283–S1304.e1.

289. Goetzl L, Rivers J, Zighelboim I, et al. Intrapartum epidural analgesia and maternal temperature regulation. *Obstet Gynecol*. 2007;109:687–690.

290. Pascual-Ramirez J, Haya J, Pérez-López FR, et al. Effect of combined spinal-epidural analgesia versus epidural analgesia on labor and delivery duration. *Int J Gynaecol Obstet*. 2011;114:246–250.

291. Camann WR, Hortvet LA, Hughes N, et al. Maternal temperature regulation during extradural analgesia for labour. *Br J Anaesth*. 1991;67:565–568.

292. Wang LZ, Chang XY, Hu XX, et al. The effect on maternal temperature of delaying initiation of the epidural component of combined spinal-epidural analgesia for labor: a pilot study. *Int J Obstet Anesth*. 2011;20:312–317.

293. Goetzl L, Evans T, Rivers J, et al. Elevated maternal and fetal serum interleukin-6 levels are associated with epidural fever. *Am J Obstet Gynecol*. 2002;187:834–838.

294. Goetzl L, Zighelboim I, Badell M, et al. Maternal corticosteroids to prevent intrauterine exposure to hyperthermia and inflammation: a randomized, double-blind, placebo-controlled trial. *Am J Obstet Gynecol*. 2006;195: 1031–1037.

295. Del Arroyo AG, Sanchez J, Patel S, et al. Role of leucocyte caspase-1 activity in epidural-related maternal fever: a single-centre, observational, mechanistic cohort study. *Br J Anaesth*. 2019;122:92–102.

296. American College of Obstetricians and Gynecologists Committee Opinion No. 712: Intrapartum management of intraamniotic infection (reaffirmed 2022). *Obstet Gynecol*. 2017;130:e95–e101.

297. Brady MT, Polin RA. Prevention and management of infants with suspected or proven neonatal sepsis. *Pediatrics*. 2013;132:166–168.

298. Goetzl L. Maternal fever in labor: etiologies, consequences, and clinical management. *Am J Obstet Gynecol*. 2023;228:S1274–S1282.

299. Greenwell EA, Wyshak G, Ringer SA, et al. Intrapartum temperature elevation, epidural use, and adverse outcome in term infants. *Pediatrics*. 2012;129:e447–e454.

300. Kapusta L, Confino E, Ismajovich B, et al. The effect of epidural analgesia on maternal thermoregulation in labor. *Int J Gynaecol Obstet*. 1985;23:185–189.

301. Panzer O, Ghazanfari N, Sessler DI, et al. Shivering and shivering-like tremor during labor with and without epidural analgesia. *Anesthesiology*. 1999;90:1609–1616.

302. Shehabi Y, Gatt S, Buckman T, Isert P. Effect of adrenaline, fentanyl and warming of injectate on shivering following extradural analgesia in labour. *Anaesth Intensive Care*. 1990;18:31–37.

303. Kuipers PW, Kamphuis ET, van Venrooij GE, et al. Intrathecal opioids and lower urinary tract function: a urodynamic evaluation. *Anesthesiology*. 2004;100:1497–1503.

304. Grove LH. Backache, headache and bladder dysfunction after delivery. *Br J Anaesth*. 1973;45:1147–1149.

305. Weiniger CF, Wand S, Nadjari M, et al. Post-void residual volume in labor: a prospective study comparing parturients with and without epidural analgesia. *Acta Anaesthesiol Scand*. 2006;50:1297–1303.

306. Olofsson CI, Ekblom AO, Ekman-Ordeberg GE, Irestedt LE. Post-partum urinary retention: a comparison between two methods of epidural analgesia. *Eur J Obstet Gynecol Reprod Biol*. 1997;71:31–34.

307. Wilson MJ, Macarthur C, Shennan A. Urinary catheterization in labour with high-dose vs mobile epidural analgesia: a randomized controlled trial. *Br J Anaesth*. 2009;102:97–103.

308. Evron S, Muzikant G, Rigini N, et al. Patient-controlled epidural analgesia: the role of epidural fentanyl in peripartum urinary retention. *Int J Obstet Anesth*. 2006;15:206–211.

309. Van de Putte P, Jahr JS, Gieraerts R, et al. Pruritus, neuraxial morphine and recrudescence of oral herpes simplex and treatment: an educational review in obstetric patients. *Reg Anesth Pain Med*. 2022;47:484–486.

310. Bauchat JR. Focused review: neuraxial morphine and oral herpes reactivation in the obstetric population. *Anesth Analg*. 2010;111:1238–1241.

311. Murphy DF, Nally B, Gardiner J, Unwin A. Effect of metoclopramide on gastric emptying before elective and emergency caesarean section. *Br J Anaesth*. 1984;56:1113–1116.

312. Carp H, Jayaram A, Stoll M. Ultrasound examination of thestomach contents of parturients. *Anesth Analg*. 1992;74:683–687.

313. Porter JS, Bonello E, Reynolds F. The influence of epidural administration of fentanyl infusion on gastric emptying in labour. *Anaesthesia*. 1997;52:1151–1156.

314. Zimmermann DL, Breen TW, Fick G. Adding fentanyl 0.0002% to epidural bupivacaine 0.125% does not delay gastric emptying in laboring parturients. *Anesth Analg*. 1996;82:612–616.

315. Ewah B, Yau K, King M, et al. Effect of epidural opioids on gastric emptying in labour. *Int J Obstet Anesth*. 1993;2:125–128.

316. Wright PM, Allen RW, Moore J, Donnelly JP. Gastric emptying during lumbar extradural analgesia in labour: effect of fentanyl supplementation. *Br J Anaesth*. 1992;68:248–251.

317. Kelly MC, Carabine UA, Hill DA, Mirakhur RK. A comparison of the effect of intrathecal and extradural fentanyl on gastric emptying in laboring women. *Anesth Analg*. 1997;85:834–838.

318. Bataille A, Rousset J, Marret E, Bonnet F. Ultrasonographic evaluation of gastric content during labour under epidural analgesia: a prospective cohort study. *Br J Anaesth*. 2014;112:703–707.

319. Bouvet L, Schulz T, Piana F, et al. Pregnancy and labor epidural effects on gastric emptying: a prospective comparative study. *Anesthesiology*. 2022;136:542–550.

320. Fiszer E, Aptekman B, Baar Y, Weiniger CF. The effect of high-dose versus low-dose epidural fentanyl on gastric emptying in nonfasted parturients: a double-blinded randomised controlled trial. *Eur J Anaesthesiol*. 2022;39:50–57.

321. Riley ET, Ratner EF, Cohen SE. Intrathecal sufentanil for labor analgesia: do sensory changes predict better analgesia and greater hypotension? *Anesth Analg*. 1997;84:346–351.

322. Riley ET, Walker D, Hamilton CL, Cohen SE. Intrathecal sufentanil for labor analgesia does not cause a sympathectomy. *Anesthesiology*. 1997;87:874–878.

323. Abu Abdou W, Aveline C, Bonnet F. Two additional cases of excessive extension of sensory blockade after intrathecal sufentanil for labor analgesia. *Int J Obstet Anesth*. 2000;9:48–50.

324. Scavone BM. Altered level of consciousness after combined spinal-epidural labor analgesia with intrathecal fentanyl and bupivacaine. *Anesthesiology*. 2002;96:1021–1022.

325. Fragneto RY, Fisher A. Mental status change and aphasia after labor analgesia with intrathecal sufentanil/bupivacaine. *Anesth Analg*. 2000;90:1175–1176.

326. Pan PH, Bogard TD, Owen MD. Incidence and characteristics of failures in obstetric neuraxial analgesia and anesthesia: a retrospective analysis of 19,259 deliveries. *Int J Obstet Anesth*. 2004;13:227–233.

327. Paech MJ, Godkin R, Webster S. Complications of obstetric epidural analgesia and anaesthesia: a prospective analysis of 10,995 cases. *Int J Obstet Anesth*. 1998;7:5–11.

328. Eappen S, Blinn A, Segal S. Incidence of epidural catheter replacement in parturients: a retrospective chart review. *Int J Obstet Anesth*. 1998;7:220–225.

329. Davies JM, Posner KL, Lee LA, et al. Liability associated with obstetric anesthesia: a closed claims analysis. *Anesthesiology*. 2009;110:131–139.

330. Groden J, Gonzalez-Fiol A, Aaronson J, et al. Catheter failure rates and time course with epidural versus combined spinal-epidural analgesia in labor. *Int J Obstet Anesth*. 2016;26:4–7.

331. Gambling D, Berkowitz J, Farrell TR, et al. A randomized controlled comparison of epidural analgesia and combined spinal-epidural analgesia in a private practice setting: pain scores during first and second stages of labor and at delivery. *Anesth Analg*. 2013;116:636–643.

332. Lim YJ, Bahk JH, Ahn WS, Lee SC. Coiling of lumbar epidural catheters. *Acta Anaesthesiol Scand*. 2002;46:603–606.

333. Husemeyer RP, White DC. Lumbar extradural injection pressures in pregnant women. An investigation of relationships between rate of infection, injection pressures and extent of analgesia. *Br J Anaesth*. 1980;52:55–60.

334. Apostolou GA, Zarmakoupis PK, Mastrokostopoulos GT. Spread of epidural anesthesia and the lateral position. *Anesth Analg*. 1981;60:584–586.

335. Norris MC, Leighton BL, DeSimone CA, Larijani GE. Lateral position and epidural anesthesia for cesarean section. *Anesth Analg*. 1988;67:788–790.

336. Savolaine ER, Pandya JB, Greenblatt SH, Conover SR. Anatomy of the human lumbar epidural space: new insights using CT-epidurography. *Anesthesiology*. 1988;68:217–220.

337. Asato F, Goto F. Radiographic findings of unilateral epidural block. *Anesth Analg*. 1996;83:519–522.

338. Blomberg RG, Olsson SS. The lumbar epidural space in patients examined with epiduroscopy. *Anesth Analg.* 1989;68:157–160.

339. McCrae AF, Whitfield A, McClure JH. Repeated unilateral epidural blockade. *Anaesthesia.* 1992;47:859–861.

340. Choi PT, Galinski SE, Takeuchi L, et al. PDPH is a common complication of neuraxial blockade in parturients: a meta-analysis of obstetrical studies. *Can J Anaesth.* 2003;50:460–469.

341. Crawford JS. Some maternal complications of epidural analgesia for labour. *Anaesthesia.* 1985;40:1219–1225.

342. Ferouz F, Norris MC, Leighton BL. Risk of respiratory arrest after intrathecal sufentanil. *Anesth Analg.* 1997;85:1088–1090.

343. Lu JK, Manullang TR, Staples MH, et al. Maternal respiratory arrests, severe hypotension, and fetal distress after administration of intrathecal, sufentanil, and bupivacaine after intravenous fentanyl. *Anesthesiology.* 1997;87:170–172.

344. Hawkins JL, Chang J, Palmer SK, et al. Anesthesia-related maternal mortality in the United States: 1979-2002. *Obstet Gynecol.* 2011;117:69–74.

345. Jenkins JG. Some immediate serious complications of obstetric epidural analgesia and anaesthesia: a prospective study of 145,550 epidurals. *Int J Obstet Anesth.* 2005;14:37–42.

346. Regan KJ, O'Sullivan G. The extension of epidural blockade for emergency caesarean section: a survey of current UK practice. *Anaesthesia.* 2008;63:136–142.

347. Albright GA. Cardiac arrest following regional anesthesia with etidocaine or bupivacaine. *Anesthesiology.* 1979;51:285–287.

348. Smetzer J, Baker C, Byrne FD, Cohen MR. Shaping systems for better behavioral choices: lessons learned from a fatal medication error. *Jt Comm J Qual Patient Saf.* 2010;36:152–163.

349. Neal JM, Neal EJ, Weinberg GL. American Society of Regional Anesthesia and Pain Medicine local anesthetic systemic toxicity checklist: 2020 version. *Reg Anesth Pain Med.* 2021;46:81–82.

350. Association of Anaesthetists of Great Britian and Ireland. 3-10 Local anaesthetic toxicity; 2023. https://anaesthetists.org/Portals/0/PDFs/QRH/QRH_3-10_Local_anaesthetic_toxicity_v2_June%202023.pdf?ver=2023-06-23-141010-760. Accessed December 9, 2024.

351. Tsuji M, Nii M, Furuta M, et al. Intravenous lipid emulsion for local anaesthetic systemic toxicity in pregnant women: a scoping review. *BMC Pregnancy Childbirth.* 2024;24:138.

352. Lubenow T, Keh-Wong E, Kristof K, et al. Inadvertent subdural injection: a complication of an epidural block. *Anesth Analg.* 1988;67:175–179.

353. Rodríguez J, Bárcena M, Taboada-Muñiz M, Alvarez J. Horner syndrome after unintended subdural block. A report of 2 cases. *J Clin Anesth.* 2005;17:473–477.

354. Abouleish E, Goldstein M. Migration of an extradural catheter into the subdural space. A case report. *Br J Anaesth.* 1986;58:1194–1197.

355. Hoftman N. Unintentional subdural injection: a complication of neuraxial anesthesia/analgesia. *Anesthesiol Clin.* 2011;29:279–290.

356. Cuerden C, Buley R, Downing JW. Delayed recovery after epidural block in labour. A report of four cases. *Anaesthesia.* 1977;32:773–776.

357. To WW, Wong MW. Factors associated with back pain symptoms in pregnancy and the persistence of pain 2 yearsafter pregnancy. *Acta Obstet Gynecol Scand.* 2003;82:1086–1091.

358. Malmqvist S, Kjaermann I, Andersen K, et al. Prevalence oflow back and pelvic pain during pregnancy in a Norwegianpopulation. *J Manipulative Physiol Ther.* 2012;35:272–278.

359. Breen TW, Ransil BJ, Groves PA, Oriol NE. Factors associatedwith back pain after childbirth. *Anesthesiology.* 1994;81:29–34.

360. Russell R, Dundas R, Reynolds F. Long term backache after childbirth: prospective search for causative factors. *BMJ.* 1996;312:1384–1388.

361. MacArthur C, Lewis M, Knox EG, Crawford JS. Epidural anaesthesia and long term backache after childbirth. *BMJ.* 1990;301:9–12.

362. MacArthur C, Lewis M, Knox EG. Investigation of long term problems after obstetric epidural anaesthesia. *BMJ.* 1992;304:1279–1282.

363. Macarthur A, Macarthur C, Weeks S. Epidural anaesthesia and low back pain after delivery: a prospective cohort study. *BMJ.* 1995;311:1336–1339.

364. Loughnan BA, Carli F, Romney M, et al. Epidural analgesia and backache: a randomized controlled comparison with intramuscular meperidine for analgesia during labour. *Br J Anaesth.* 2002;89:466–472.

365. Howell CJ, Kidd C, Roberts W, et al. A randomised controlled trial of epidural compared with non-epidural analgesia in labour. *BJOG.* 2001;108:27–33.

366. Howell CJ, Dean T, Lucking L, et al. Randomised study of long term outcome after epidural versus non-epidural analgesia during labour. *BMJ.* 2002;325:357.

367. Ramin SM, Gambling DR, Lucas MJ, et al. Randomized trial of epidural versus intravenous analgesia during labor. *Obstet Gynecol.* 1995;86:783–789.

368. Noble AD, Craft IL, Bootes JA, et al. Continuous lumbar epidural analgesia using bupivacaine: a study of the fetus andnewborn child. *J Obstet Gynaecol Br Commonw.* 1971;78:559–563.

369. Yoo KY, Lee J, Kim HS, Jeong SW. The effects of opioids on isolated human pregnant uterine muscles. *Anesth Analg.* 2001;92:1006–1009.

370. Neuhoff D, Burke MS, Porreco RP. Cesarean birth for failed progress in labor. *Obstet Gynecol.* 1989;73:915–920.

371. Guillemette J, Fraser WD. Differences between obstetricians in caesarean section rates and the management of labour. *Br J Obstet Gynaecol.* 1992;99:105–108.

372. Ueda A, Nakakita B, Chigusa Y, et al. Regional disparities in primary cesarean delivery rates in Japan: the role of obstetrician availability. *AJOG Glob Rep.* 2024;4 100366.

373. Goldstick O, Weissman A, Drugan A. The circadian rhythm of "urgent" operative deliveries. *Isr Med Assoc J.* 2003;5:564–566.

374. Fraser W, Usher RH, McLean FH, et al. Temporal variation in rates of cesarean section for dystocia: does "convenience" play a role? *Am J Obstet Gynecol.* 1987;156:300–304.

375. Morita N, Matsushima N, Ogata N, et al. Nationwide description of live Japanese births by day of the week, hour, and location. *J Epidemiol.* 2002;12:330–335.

376. Wuitchik M, Bakal D, Lipshitz J. The clinical significance of pain and cognitive activity in latent labor. *Obstet Gynecol.* 1989;73:35–42.

377. Alexander JM, Sharma SK, McIntire DD, et al. Intensity of labor pain and cesarean delivery. *Anesth Analg.* 2001;92:1524–1528.

378. Hess PE, Pratt SD, Soni AK, et al. An association between severe labor pain and cesarean delivery. *Anesth Analg.* 2000;90:881–886.

379. Panni MK, Segal S. Local anesthetic requirements are greater in dystocia than in normal labor. *Anesthesiology.* 2003;98:957–963.

380. Gambling DR, Sharma SK, Ramin SM, et al. A randomized study of combined spinal-epidural analgesia versus intravenous meperidine during labor: impact on cesarean delivery rate. *Anesthesiology.* 1998;89:1336–1344.

381. Sharma SK, Sidawi JE, Ramin SM, et al. Cesarean delivery: a randomized trial of epidural versus patient-controlled meperidine analgesia during labor. *Anesthesiology.* 1997;87:487–494.

382. Sharma SK, Alexander JM, Messick G, et al. Cesarean delivery: a randomized trial of epidural analgesia versus intravenous meperidine analgesia during labor in nulliparous women. *Anesthesiology.* 2002;96:546–551.

383. Sharma SK, Leveno KJ. Update: epidural analgesia does not increase cesarean births. *Curr Anesthesiol Rep.* 2000;2:18–24.

384. Sharma SK, McIntire DD, Wiley J, Leveno KJ. Labor analgesia and cesarean delivery: an individual patient meta-analysis of nulliparous women. *Anesthesiology.* 2004;100:142–148.

385. Comparative Obstetric Mobile Epidural Trial (COMET) Study Group UK Effect of low-dose mobile versus traditional epidural techniques on mode of delivery: a randomised controlled trial. *Lancet.* 2001;358:19–23.

386. Sultan P, Murphy C, Halpern S, Carvalho B. The effect of low concentrations versus high concentrations of local anesthetics for labour analgesia on obstetric and anesthetic outcomes: a meta-analysis. *Can J Anaesth.* 2013;60:840–854.

387. Yancey MK, Pierce B, Schweitzer D, Daniels D. Observations on labor epidural analgesia and operative delivery rates. *Am J Obstet Gynecol.* 1999;180:353–359.

388. Zhang J, Yancey MK, Klebanoff MA, et al. Does epidural analgesia prolong labor and increase risk of cesarean delivery? A natural experiment. *Am J Obstet Gynecol.* 2001;185:128–134.

389. Socol ML, Garcia PM, Peaceman AM, Dooley SL. Reducing cesarean births at a primarily private university hospital. *Am J Obstet Gynecol.* 1993;168:1748–1754.

390. Segal S, Su M, Gilbert P. The effect of a rapid change in availability of epidural analgesia on the cesarean delivery rate: a meta-analysis. *Am J Obstet Gynecol.* 2000;183:974–978.

391. Lagrew DC Jr, Adashek JA. Lowering the cesarean section rate in a private hospital: comparison of individual physicians' rates, risk factors, and outcomes. *Am J Obstet Gynecol.* 1998;178:1207–1214.

392. Segal S, Blatman R, Doble M, Datta S. The influence of the obstetrician in the relationship between epidural analgesia and cesarean section for dystocia. *Anesthesiology.* 1999;91:90–96.

393. Seyb ST, Berka RJ, Socol ML, Dooley SL. Risk of cesarean delivery with elective induction of labor at term in nulliparous women. *Obstet Gynecol.* 1999;94:600–607.

394. American College of Obstetricians and Gynecologists Practice Bulletin No. 36: Obstetric analgesia and anesthesia. *Obstet Gynecol.* 2002;100:177–191.

395. Ohel G, Gonen R, Vaida S, et al. Early versus late initiation of epidural analgesia in labor: does it increase the risk of cesarean section? A randomized trial. *Am J Obstet Gynecol.* 2006;194:600–605.

396. American College of Obstetricians and Gynecologists. Committee Opinion No. 339: Analgesia and cesarean delivery rates. *Obstet Gynecol.* 2006;107:1487–1488.

397. American College of Obstetricians and Gynecologists Clinical Practice Guideline No. 8: First and second stage labor management. *Obstet Gynecol.* 2024;143:144–162.

398. Shen X, Li Y, Xu S, et al. Epidural analgesia during the second stage of labor: a randomized controlled trial. *Obstet Gynecol.* 2017;130:1097–1103.

399. Nageotte MP, Larson D, Rumney PJ, et al. Epidural analgesia compared with combined spinal-epidural analgesia during labor in nulliparous women. *N Engl J Med.* 1997;337:1715–1719.

400. Olofsson C, Ekblom A, Ekman-Ordeberg G, Irestedt L. Obstetric outcome following epidural analgesia with bupivacaine-adrenaline 0.25% or bupivacaine 0.125% with sufentanil—a prospective randomized controlled study in 1000 parturients. *Acta Anaesthesiol Scand.* 1998;42:284–292.

401. James KS, McGrady E, Quasim I, Patrick A. Comparison of epidural bolus administration of 0.25% bupivacaine and 0.1% bupivacaine with 0.0002% fentanyl for analgesia during labour. *Br J Anaesth.* 1998;81:507–510.

402. Collis RE, Davies DW, Aveling W. Randomised comparison of combined spinal-epidural and standard epidural analgesia in labour. *Lancet.* 1995;345:1413–1416.

403. Wang TT, Sun S, Huang SQ. Effects of epidural labor analgesia with low concentrations of local anesthetics on obstetric outcomes: a systematic review and meta-analysis ofrandomized controlled trials. *Anesth Analg.* 2017;124:1571–1580.

404. Robinson CA, Macones GA, Roth NW, Morgan MA. Does station of the fetal head at epidural placement affect the position of the fetal vertex at delivery? *Am J Obstet Gynecol.* 1996;175:991–994.

405. Le Ray C, Carayol M, Jaquemin S, et al. Is epidural analgesia a risk factor for occiput posterior or transverse positions during labour? *Eur J Obstet Gynecol Reprod Biol.* 2005;123:22–26.

406. Yancey MK, Zhang J, Schweitzer DL, et al. Epidural analgesia and fetal head malposition at vaginal delivery. *Obstet Gynecol.* 2001;97:608–612.

407. Sheiner E, Sheiner EK, Segal D, et al. Does the station of the fetal head during epidural analgesia affect labor and delivery? *Int J Gynaecol Obstet.* 1999;64:43–47.

408. Lieberman E, Davidson K, Lee-Parritz A, Shearer E. Changes in fetal position during labor and their association with epidural analgesia. *Obstet Gynecol.* 2005;105:974–982.

409. Malvasi A, Tinelli A, Brizzi A, et al. Intrapartum sonography head transverse and asynclitic diagnosis with and without epidural analgesia initiated early during the first stage of labor. *Eur Rev Med Pharmacol Sci.* 2011;15:518–523.

410. Chestnut DH. Epidural anesthesia and instrumental vaginal delivery. *Anesthesiology.* 1991;74:805–808.

411. American College of Obstetricians and Gynecologists Practice Bulletin Number 219: Operative vaginal birth (reaffirmed 2021). *Obstet Gynecol.* 2020;135:e149–e159.

412. Goetzinger KR, Macones GA. Operative vaginal delivery: current trends in obstetrics. *Womens Health (Lond).* 2008;4:281–290.

413. Robinson JN, Norwitz ER, Cohen AP, et al. Episiotomy, operative vaginal delivery, and significant perinatal trauma in

nulliparous women. *Am J Obstet Gynecol.* 1999;181: 1180–1184.

414. Baumann P, Hammoud AO, McNeeley SG, et al. Factors associated with anal sphincter laceration in 40,923 primiparous women. *Int Urogynecol J Pelvic Floor Dysfunct.* 2007;18:985–990.

415. Dahl C, Kjølhede P. Obstetric anal sphincter rupture in older primiparous women: a case-control study. *Acta Obstet Gynecol Scand.* 2006;85:1252–1258.

416. Cheek TG, Samuels P, Miller F, et al. Normal saline i.v. fluid load decreases uterine activity in active labour. *Br J Anaesth.* 1996;77:632–635.

417. Miller AC. The effects of epidural analgesia on uterine activity and labor. *Int J Obstet Anesth.* 1997;6:2–18.

418. Rahm VA, Hallgren A, Högberg H, et al. Plasma oxytocin levels in women during labor with or without epidural analgesia: a prospective study. *Acta Obstet Gynecol Scand.* 2002;81:1033–1039.

419. Behrens O, Goeschen K, Luck HJ, Fuchs AR. Effects of lumbarepidural analgesia on prostaglandin $F_{2\alpha}$ release and oxytocin secretion during labor. *Prostaglandins.* 1993;45: 285–296.

420. Nielsen PE, Abouleish E, Meyer BA, Parisi VM. Effect of epidural analgesia on fundal dominance during spontaneous active-phase nulliparous labor. *Anesthesiology.* 1996;84: 540–544.

421. Clarke VT, Smiley RM, Finster M. Uterine hyperactivity after intrathecal injection of fentanyl for analgesia during labor: a cause of fetal bradycardia? *Anesthesiology.* 1994;81:1083.

422. Moir DD, Willocks J. Management of incoordinate uterine action under continuous epidural analgesia. *Br Med J.* 1967;3:396–400.

423. Lederman RP, Lederman E, Work BA Jr, McCann DS. The relationship of maternal anxiety, plasma catecholamines, and plasma cortisol to progress in labor. *Am J Obstet Gynecol.* 1978;132:495–500.

424. Gunther RE, Bauman J. Obstetrical caudal anesthesia: I. A randomized study comparing 1% mepivacaine with 1% lidocaine plus epinephrine. *Anesthesiology.* 1969;31:5–19.

425. Grice SC, Eisenach JC, Dewan DM. Labor analgesia with epidural bupivacaine plus fentanyl: enhancement with epinephrine and inhibition with 2-chloroprocaine. *Anesthesiology.* 1990;72:623–628.

426. Yau G, Gregory MA, Gin T, Oh TE. Obstetric epidural analgesia with mixtures of bupivacaine, adrenaline and fentanyl. *Anaesthesia.* 1990;45:1020–1023.

427. Abboud TK, Khoo SS, Miller F, et al. Maternal, fetal, andneonatal responses after epidural anesthesia with bupivacaine, 2-chloroprocaine, or lidocaine. *Anesth Analg.* 1982;61:638–644.

428. Spong CY, Berghella V, Wenstrom KD, et al. Preventing the first cesarean delivery: summary of a joint Eunice Kennedy Shriver National Institute of Child Health and Human Development, Society for Maternal-Fetal Medicine, and American College of Obstetricians and Gynecologists Workshop. *Obstet Gynecol.* 2012;120:1181–1193.

429. Zhang J, Landy HJ, Branch DW, et al. Contemporary patterns of spontaneous labor with normal neonatal outcomes. *Obstet Gynecol.* 2010;116:1281–1287.

430. Cheng YW, Shaffer BL, Nicholson JM, Caughey AB. Second stage of labor and epidural use: a larger effect than previously suggested. *Obstet Gynecol.* 2014;123:527–535.

431. Grobman WA, Bailit J, Lai Y, et al. Association of the duration of active pushing with obstetric outcomes. *Obstet Gynecol.* 2016;127:667–673.

432. Laughon SK, Berghella V, Reddy UM, et al. Neonatal and maternal outcomes with prolonged second stage of labor. *Obstet Gynecol.* 2014;124:57–67.

433. Rouse DJ, Weiner SJ, Bloom SL, et al. Second-stage labor duration in nulliparous women: relationship to maternal and perinatal outcomes. *Am J Obstet Gynecol.* 2009;201: 357.e1–e7.

434. Le Ray C, Audibert F, Goffinet F, Fraser W. When to stop pushing: effects of duration of second-stage expulsion effortson maternal and neonatal outcomes in nulliparous women with epidural analgesia. *Am J Obstet Gynecol.* 2009;201:361.e1–e7.

435. Cheng YW, Hopkins LM, Caughey AB. How long is too long: does a prolonged second stage of labor in nulliparous women affect maternal and neonatal outcomes? *Am J Obstet Gynecol.* 2004;191:933–938.

436. Cheng YW, Hopkins LM, Laros RK Jr, Caughey AB. Duration of the second stage of labor in multiparous women: maternal and neonatal outcomes. *Am J Obstet Gynecol.* 2007;196: 585.e1–e6.

437. Allen VM, Baskett TF, O'Connell CM, et al. Maternal and perinatal outcomes with increasing duration of the second stage of labor. *Obstet Gynecol.* 2009;113:1248–1258.

438. Lemos A, Amorim MM, Dornelas de Andrade A, et al. Pushing/bearing down methods for the second stage of labour. *Cochrane Database Syst Rev.* 2017;(3):CD009124.

439. Cahill AG, Srinivas SK, Tita ATN, et al. Effect of immediate vs delayed pushing on rates of spontaneous vaginal delivery among nulliparous women receiving neuraxial analgesia: arandomized clinical trial. *JAMA.* 2018;320:1444–1454.

440. Rosaeg OP, Campbell N, Crossan ML. Epidural analgesia does not prolong the third stage of labour. *Can J Anaesth.* 2002;49:490–492.

441. Wei SQ, Luo ZC, Xu H, Fraser WD. The effect of early oxytocin augmentation in labor: a meta-analysis. *Obstet Gynecol.* 2009;114:641–649.

442. Lupe PJ, Gross TL. Maternal upright posture and mobility in labor—a review. *Obstet Gynecol.* 1986;67:727–734.

443. Roberts CL, Algert CS, Olive E. Impact of first-stage ambulation on mode of delivery among women with epidural analgesia. *Aust N Z J Obstet Gynaecol.* 2004;44:489–494.

444. Bloom SL, McIntire DD, Kelly MA, et al. Lack of effect of walking on labor and delivery. *N Engl J Med.* 1998;339:76–79.

445. Lawrence A, Lewis L, Hofmeyr GJ, Styles C. Maternal positions and mobility during first stage labour. *Cochrane Database Syst Rev.* 2013;(10):CD003934.

446. American College of Obstetricians and Gynecologists. Committee Opinion No. 766: Approaches to limit intervention during labor and birth (reaffirmed 2021). *Obstet Gynecol.* 2019;133:e164–e173.

447. Loewenberg-Weisband Y, Grisaru-Granovsky S, Ioscovich A, et al. Epidural analgesia and severe perineal tears: a literature review and large cohort study. *J Matern Fetal Neonatal Med.* 2014;27:1864–1869.

448. Sartore A, Pregazzi R, Bortoli P, et al. Effects of epidural analgesia during labor on pelvic floor function after vaginal delivery. *Acta Obstet Gynecol Scand.* 2003;82:143–146.

449. Packet B, Page AS, Cattani L, et al. Predictive factors for obstetric anal sphincter injury in primiparous women:

systematic review and meta-analysis. *Ultrasound Obstet Gynecol.* 2023;62:486–496.

450. Lavin JP, Samuels SV, Miodovnik M, et al. The effects of bupivacaine and chloroprocaine as local anesthetics for epidural anesthesia of fetal heart rate monitoring parameters. *Am J Obstet Gynecol.* 1981;141:717–722.

451. Boehm FH, Woodruff LF Jr, Growdon JH Jr. The effect of lumbar epidural anesthesia on fetal heart rate baseline variability. *Anesth Analg.* 1975;54:779–782.

452. Loftus JR, Holbrook RH, Cohen SE. Fetal heart rate after epidural lidocaine and bupivacaine for elective cesarean section. *Anesthesiology.* 1991;75:406–412.

453. Nielsen PE, Erickson JR, Abouleish EI, et al. Fetal heart rate changes after intrathecal sufentanil or epidural bupivacaine for labor analgesia: incidence and clinical significance. *Anesth Analg.* 1996;83:742–746.

454. Pello LC, Rosevear SK, Dawes GS, et al. Computerized fetalheart rate analysis in labor. *Obstet Gynecol.* 1991;78: 602–610.

455. Viscomi CM, Hood DD, Melone PJ, Eisenach JC. Fetal heart rate variability after epidural fentanyl during labor. *Anesth Analg.* 1990;71:679–683.

456. Wilhite AO, Moore CH, Blass NH, Christmas JT. Plasma concentration profile of epidural alfentanil. Bolus followed by continuous infusion technique in the parturient: effect of epidural alfentanil and fentanyl on fetal heart rate. *Reg Anesth.* 1994;19:164–168.

457. Hill JB, Alexander JM, Sharma SK, et al. A comparison of the effects of epidural and meperidine analgesia during labor on fetal heart rate. *Obstet Gynecol.* 2003;102:333–337.

458. Smith CV, Rayburn WF, Allen KV, et al. Influence of intravenous fentanyl on fetal biophysical parameters during labor. *J Matern Fetal Med.* 1996;5:89–92.

459. Beilin Y, Bodian CA, Weiser J, et al. Effect of labor epidural analgesia with and without fentanyl on infant breast-feeding: a prospective, randomized, double-blind study. *Anesthesiology.* 2005;103:1211–1217.

460. Lee AI, McCarthy RJ, Toledo P, et al. Epidural labor analgesia-fentanyl dose and breastfeeding success: a randomized clinical trial. *Anesthesiology.* 2017;127:614–624.

461. Wilson MJ, MacArthur C, Cooper GM, et al. Epidural analgesia and breastfeeding: a randomised controlled trial of epidural techniques with and without fentanyl and a non-epidural comparison group. *Anaesthesia.* 2010;65:145–153.

462. Heesen P, Halpern SH, Beilin Y, et al. Labor neuraxial analgesia and breastfeeding: an updated systematic review. *JClin Anesth.* 2021;68 110105.

463. Abrão KC, Francisco RP, Miyadahira S, et al. Elevation of uterine basal tone and fetal heart rate abnormalities after labor analgesia: a randomized controlled trial. *Obstet Gynecol.* 2009;113:41–47.

464. Landau R, Carvalho B, Wong C, et al. Elevation of uterine basal tone and fetal heart rate abnormalities after labor analgesia: a randomized controlled trial. *Obstet Gynecol.* 2009;113:1374–1375.

465. Albright GA, Forster RM. Does combined spinal-epidural analgesia with subarachnoid sufentanil increase the incidence of emergency cesarean delivery? *Reg Anesth.* 1997;22:400–405.

466. Mardirosoff C, Dumont L, Boulvain M, Tramèr MR. Fetal bradycardia due to intrathecal opioids for labour analgesia: a systematic review. *BJOG.* 2002;109:274–281.

467. Van de Velde M, Teunkens A, Hanssens M, et al. Intrathecal sufentanil and fetal heart rate abnormalities: a double-blind, double placebo-controlled trial comparing two forms of combined spinal epidural analgesia with epidural analgesia in labor. *Anesth Analg.* 2004;98:1153–1159.

468. Cheng SL, Bautista D, Leo S, Sia TH. Factors affecting fetal bradycardia following combined spinal epidural for labor analgesia: a matched case-control study. *J Anesth.* 2013;27:169–174.

469. Gambling DR, Bender M, Faron S, et al. Prophylactic intravenous ephedrine to minimize fetal bradycardia after combined spinal-epidural labour analgesia: a randomized controlled study. *Can J Anaesth.* 2015;62:1201–1208.

25

Postpartum Tubal Sterilization

Joy L. Hawkins, MD

Many women choose tubal sterilization for permanent contraception. It is the most common contraceptive method, currently used by 18% of women. Of the approximately 3.7 million births occurring annually in the United States, data from 2009 to 2021 found that the incidence of postpartum permanent contraception was approximately 6% to 7% of all live births.[1] The incidence varies by age, with 21% of women ages 30 to 39 years and 39% of women ages 40 to 49 years choosing permanent contraception compared with only 3% of women aged 20 to 29 years. The considerations and controversies regarding the administration of anesthesia for postpartum tubal sterilization and other postpartum procedures are discussed in this chapter.

AMERICAN SOCIETY OF ANESTHESIOLOGISTS GUIDELINES

The American Society of Anesthesiologists (ASA) has published "Practice Guidelines for Obstetric Anesthesia,"[2] which includes a discussion of postpartum tubal ligation. The Task Force recommendations can be summarized as follows:

1. Before a postpartum tubal ligation, the patient should have no oral intake of solid foods within 6 to 8 hours of the surgery, depending on the type of food ingested (e.g., fat content).
2. Consider aspiration prophylaxis.
3. Both the timing of the procedure and the decision to use a specific anesthetic technique (i.e., neuraxial versus general) should be individualized, based on anesthetic and obstetric risk factors (e.g., blood loss at delivery) and patient preferences.

4. Consider selecting neuraxial techniques in preference to general anesthesia for most postpartum tubal ligations.
5. Be aware that gastric emptying will be delayed in patients who have received opioids during labor.
6. Be aware that an epidural catheter placed for labor may be more likely to fail with longer postdelivery time intervals.
7. If a postpartum tubal ligation is to be performed before the patient is discharged from the hospital, do not attempt the procedure at a time when it might compromise other aspects of patient care on the labor and delivery unit.

SURGICAL CONSIDERATIONS

Tubal sterilization can be performed satisfactorily at any time, but the early postpartum period has several advantages for women who have had an uncomplicated vaginal delivery.[3] The patient avoids the cost and inconvenience of a second hospital visit. The uterine fundus remains near the umbilicus for several days postpartum, which allows easy access to the fallopian tubes via a mini-laparotomy. Mini-laparotomy and laparoscopy have similar rates of serious complications (e.g., bowel laceration, vascular injury), although postpartum tubal ligation is associated with lower failure rates than interval laparoscopic tubal ligation.[4,5] Finally, costs may be lower with postpartum mini-laparotomy.

There are at least two potential disadvantages to immediate postpartum sterilization. First, parous women are at increased risk for uterine atony and postpartum hemorrhage. This risk decreases substantially 12 hours after delivery. Second, immediate surgery results in sterilization before the assessment of the newborn is complete. Postpartum tubal ligation is not wise if the patient is ambivalent regarding permanent sterilization. The probability of regret diminishes steadily with increased interval between delivery and sterilization.[5] The key indicators for future regret are younger age, less than 30 years; having less access to information about alternative contraceptive methods; and having made the decision under pressure from a partner or because of medical indications.[5] Women should be counseled about failure, regret, and alternatives such as long-acting, reversible contraceptives (e.g., intrauterine device [IUD], subdermal implants), but younger age and lower parity should not be a barrier to sterilization.[5]

Several techniques are used for postpartum tubal sterilization (Fig. 25.1).[6] Postpartum sterilization has a failure rate that is lower than most interval procedures, and the failure rate is lowest (approximately 0.75%) if some form of tubal resection occurs.[5,7] With the Irving procedure, the obstetrician buries the cut ends of the tubes in the myometrium and mesosalpinx. This technique is least likely to fail, but it requires more extensive exposure and increases the risk for hemorrhage. The Pomeroy procedure is simplest. The surgeon ligates a loop of oviduct and excises the loop above the suture. With the Parkland procedure, the obstetrician ligates the tube proximally and distally and then excises the mid-segment. The last two methods are most commonly performed during postpartum tubal ligations. Regardless of the technique, the obstetrician should document that fimbriae are present to preclude ligation of another structure, such as the round ligament. The excised portions are typically sent to a pathologist for verification.

Recently, surgical technique has changed, and instead of performing a tubal ligation alone for sterilization, some surgeons are recommending bilateral salpingectomy. Ovarian cancer often arises from the fallopian tubes, and bilateral salpingectomy reduces the incidence of ovarian cancer by 64%, an estimated 422 fewer ovarian cancer diagnoses and 252 fewer deaths over 10 years.[8] Postpartum salpingectomy is a cost-effective procedure without additional complications compared with tubal ligation.

NONMEDICAL ISSUES

Nonmedical issues affect decisions regarding the timing of tubal sterilization. The obstetrician must obtain and document informed consent for surgery.[5] Tubal ligation should be considered an irreversible procedure. Therefore, most obstetricians require a discussion with the patient before labor and delivery. Physicians should be aware of state laws or insurance regulations that may require a specific interval between obtaining consent and performance of sterilization procedures. Regulations may not allow the woman to give consent while in labor or immediately after delivery. For example, the Colorado Medicaid reimbursement program includes the following requirements for sterilization[9]:

- The patient must be at least 21 years of age and mentally competent when consent is obtained.
- Informed consent may not be obtained while the patient is in labor or during childbirth.
- Consent may not be obtained while the patient is undergoing an abortion or under the influence of alcohol or other substances.
- A total of 30 days must pass between the date the consent is signed and the date the procedure is performed. (Exceptions to the 30-day waiting period can be made for preterm delivery or emergency abdominal surgery.)
- Consent is valid for only 180 days.

An ethical analysis of the Medicaid sterilization consent requirements suggests they merit revision because they present a barrier to desired sterilization for some women.[10] Women with private insurance are not required to follow these requirements, creating a two-tiered system based on the ability to pay. Factors that may decrease the likelihood of a patient obtaining desired postpartum sterilization include patient-related factors, obstetrician-related factors, lack of

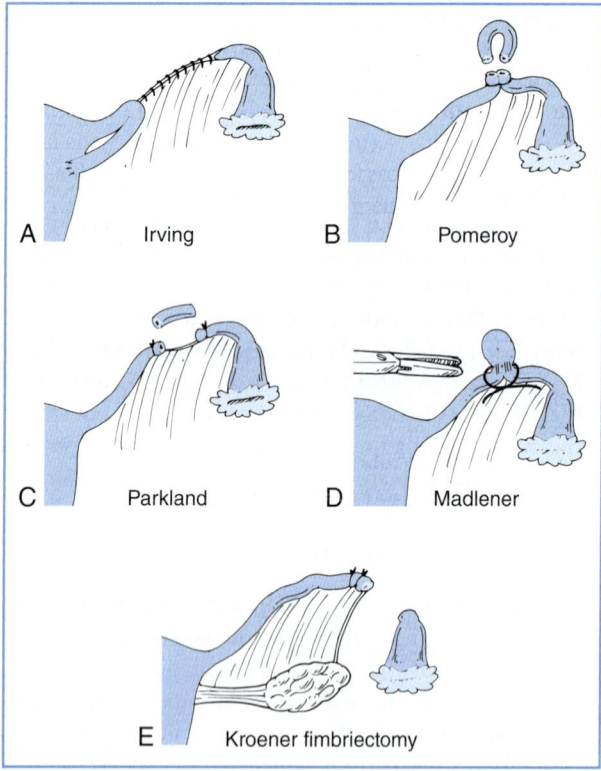

Fig. 25.1 Techniques for Tubal Sterilization. (A) Irving procedure. The medial cut end of the oviduct is buried in the myometrium posteriorly, and the distal cut end is buried in the mesosalpinx. (B) Pomeroy procedure. A loop of oviduct is ligated, and the knuckle of tube above the ligature is excised. (C) Parkland procedure. A mid-segment of tube is separated from the mesosalpinx at an avascular site, and the separated tubal segment is ligated proximally and distally and then excised. (D) Madlener procedure. A knuckle of oviduct is crushed and then ligated without resection; this technique has an unacceptably high failure rate of approximately 7%. (E) Kroener procedure. The tube is ligated across the ampulla, and the distal portion of the ampulla, including all of the fimbria, is resected; some studies have reported an unacceptably high failure rate with this technique. From Cunningham FG, Leveno KJ, Bloom SL, et al. *Williams Obstetrics.* 24th ed. McGraw-Hill Education; 2014:720–727.

Figure labels: A Irving, B Pomeroy, C Parkland, D Madlener, E Kroener fimbriectomy available operating rooms and anesthesia coverage, federal consent requirements as discussed above, and receiving care in some religiously affiliated hospitals.[11] The requirements create disparities and inequity for minority women, women with less education, and those who are economically disadvantaged by resulting in a disproportionate incidence of unplanned pregnancy.

In some cases, the obstetrician may schedule a patient for a postpartum tubal sterilization because of a fear that the patient will not return for interval tubal sterilization 6 weeks after delivery. Concerns regarding patient compliance should not prompt the performance of postpartum tubal sterilization in patients with significant medical or obstetric complications. However, women who request postpartum tubal sterilization but do not receive it are more likely to become pregnant within 1 year of delivery (46.7%) than are women who did not request the procedure (22.3%).[12]

The American College of Obstetricians and Gynecologists (ACOG) has stated that given the consequences of a missed procedure and the limited time frame in which it may be performed, institutions should consider designating postpartum sterilizations as nonelective procedures, which indicates its high priority to staff and schedulers.[11] They also stated that obstetrician-gynecologists should identify and eliminate barriers that restrict access to postpartum sterilization. The ACOG concluded that obstetrician-gynecologists should be champions or patient advocates for postpartum sterilization in their respective hospitals and help to coordinate administration and healthcare staff in streamlining access to the procedure. If individual physicians or institutions will not provide sterilization because of personal religious beliefs or institutional policy, patients must be informed as early as possible and transfer of care for the remainder of pregnancy should be offered.[10,11] Increasing access and availability of postpartum sterilization may not only directly improve outcomes for women desiring the procedure, but may decrease overall costs to the healthcare system.[11]

PREOPERATIVE EVALUATION

The patient scheduled for postpartum tubal sterilization requires a thorough preoperative evaluation, and a reevaluation should be performed even if the patient is known to the anesthesia provider because of the provision of labor analgesia. A cursory evaluation should not be performed simply because the patient is young and healthy. Patients with preeclampsia may safely receive neuraxial or general anesthesia for postpartum tubal sterilization, provided that there is no evidence of pulmonary edema, oliguria, or thrombocytopenia.[13]

Physicians and nurses often underestimate blood loss during delivery and some form of quantitative measurement of blood loss should be used.[14] Excessive blood loss from uterine atony is not uncommon in parous women. Orthostatic changes in blood pressure and heart rate should be excluded, especially if an immediate postpartum

procedure is to be performed. At the University of Colorado, for surgery performed the day after delivery, the patient's hematocrit is determined several hours after delivery (to allow for equilibration) and compared with the antepartum measurement. A hematocrit is not obtained before an immediate postpartum tubal sterilization (performed less than 8 hours after delivery), provided that the antepartum hematocrit was acceptable, there are no orthostatic vital sign changes, and there was no evidence of excessive blood loss during delivery.

No absolute value of hematocrit requires a delay of surgery, but physical signs of hypovolemia—such as hemodynamic instability or laboratory evidence of excessive blood loss—should prompt postponement of the procedure until 6 to 8 weeks postpartum. Fever may signal the presence of endometritis or urinary tract infection and may also require postponement of surgery until a later date. Finally, the condition of the neonate should be confirmed before surgery to exclude any unexpected problems.

Mothers may be concerned that medications administered during surgery might affect their ability to breastfeed or that these medications might harm the newborn. Any drug present in the mother's blood will be present in breast milk, with the concentration dependent on factors such as protein binding, lipid solubility, and degree of ionization.[15] Typically, the amount of drug present in breast milk is small and clinically insignificant. Opioids, benzodiazepines, and propofol administered during anesthesia are excreted in insignificant amounts. (See Chapter 16 for a detailed discussion of interactions between drugs and breastfeeding.)

RISK FOR ASPIRATION

Historically, anesthesiologists have considered maternal aspiration the major risk associated with anesthesia for postpartum tubal sterilization, although the evidence for this is scant and conflicting. A review of anesthesia-related maternal mortality found no maternal deaths associated with aspiration during postpartum tubal ligation, despite tracking deaths for an entire year after delivery.[16] A review of serious complications related to obstetric anesthesia sponsored by the Society for Obstetric Anesthesia and Perinatology also did not identify any cases of aspiration during postpartum tubal ligation.[17] However, several factors may place the pregnant woman at increased risk for aspiration. Some but not all risk factors for aspiration are resolved at delivery. For example, the placenta is the primary site of progesterone production, and progesterone concentrations fall rapidly after delivery of the placenta (Fig. 25.2).[18] Typically, progesterone concentrations decline within 2 hours of delivery; and by 24 hours postpartum, progesterone concentrations are similar to those found during the luteal phase of the menstrual cycle.

Important questions to address during the preanesthetic evaluation are: (1) What is the duration of the fast for solid foods? (2) Were parenteral opioids administered during labor? (3) If epidural labor analgesia was used, was the patient satisfied with their pain control?

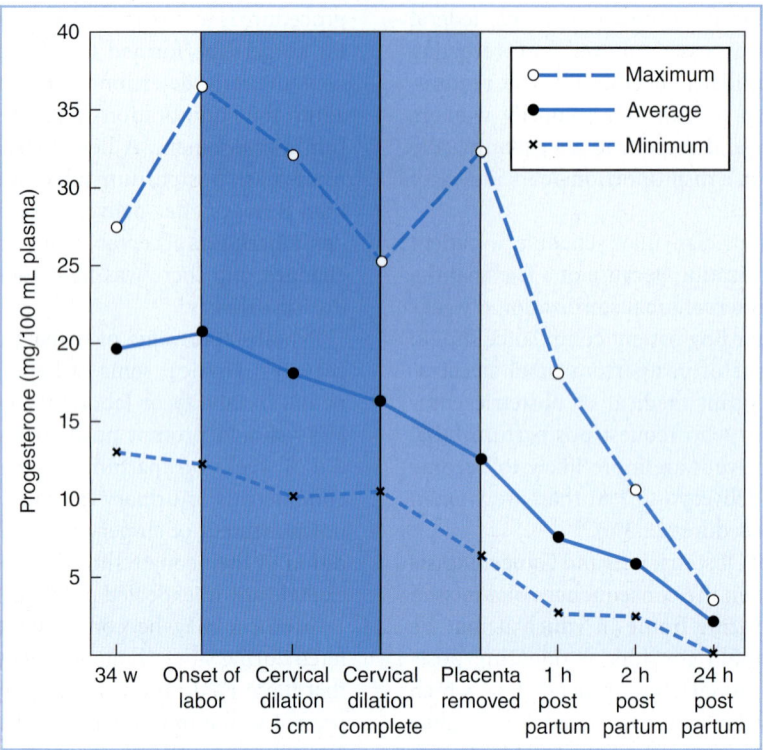

Fig. 25.2 Average progesterone concentrations with the highest and lowest measurements of 13 pregnant women at given time intervals. From Llauro JL, Runnebaum B, Zander J. Progesterone in human peripheral blood before, during, and after labor. *Am J Obstet Gynecol.* 1968;101:867–873.

Gastric Emptying, Reflux, and Aspiration Risk

Several studies have assessed gastric emptying in pregnant and postpartum women. Vial et al. used ultrasonographic assessment of gastric contents in laboring women after epidural analgesia was initiated and again after delivery in the immediate postpartum period.[19] Using an antral cross-sectional area of less than or equal to 381 mm^2 to define an empty stomach, 65% of women had stomach contents after epidural catheter placement and 48% after delivery. No risk factors, such as pain, anxiety, diabetes, or smoking, were associated with the occurrence of a full stomach postdelivery. Bouvet et al. compared four groups of women: nonpregnant, term pregnant, parturients with no labor analgesia, and parturients with epidural labor analgesia to determine the fraction of gastric emptying at 90 minutes following a light meal using serial gastric ultrasound.[20] They found the median fraction of gastric emptying was 52% in nonpregnant women, 45% in term pregnant women, 7% in women laboring with no analgesia, and 31% in laboring women with epidural analgesia ($P < .0001$) (Fig. 25.3). They concluded that gastric emptying is delayed in laboring compared with nonpregnant women and compared with pregnant women at term not in labor, but epidural labor analgesia facilitates emptying during labor compared with no epidural analgesia.

During the preoperative assessment of any woman scheduled for postpartum tubal sterilization, the anesthesia provider should determine when the patient last consumed solid food and whether opioids were administered by any route. Systemic absorption of an opioid occurs after epidural administration. However, published studies have provided conflicting results regarding the effect of epidural opioid administration on gastric emptying. Taking these findings into account, the ASA Committee on Obstetric Anesthesia made the following statements and recommendations[21]: (1) gastric emptying in labor is delayed; it is further delayed by systemic opioids and high-dose neuraxial opioids; (2) lower esophageal sphincter tone is reduced and 50% of women have reflux symptoms by the third trimester; (3) no benefits have been shown for solid food compared with clear liquid intake during labor, although maternal satisfaction may be adversely affected; (4) both the ASA and ACOG guidelines state that consumption of solid food in active labor should be avoided; (5) because strict NPO (*nil per os*; nothing by mouth) policies can cause patient distress, clear liquids should be encouraged during uncomplicated labor; and (6) neuraxial analgesia should not be denied, regardless of fasting status or stomach contents.[21] In contrast to these recommendations, other experts feel restrictions on oral intake during labor should be relaxed given the minimal risk of aspiration in the setting of modern obstetric practice.[22]

In summary, the preponderance of evidence suggests that (1) administration of an opioid during labor increases the likelihood of delayed gastric emptying during the early postpartum period, (2) gastric emptying of solid food is delayed during labor and in the immediate postpartum period in all parturients, and (3) gastric emptying of clear liquids is

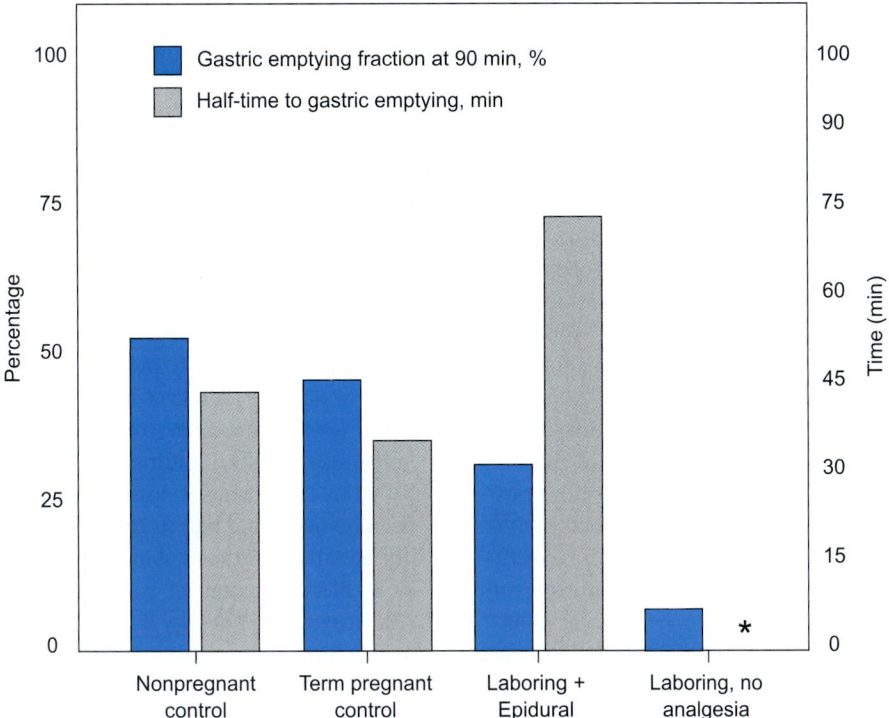

Fig. 25.3 Gastric Emptying Fractions and Halftime of Gastric Emptying in Four Groups. Gastric emptying is delayed in laboring compared with nonpregnant women and compared with pregnant women at term not in labor, but epidural labor analgesia facilitates emptying during labor compared with no epidural analgesia. *Unable to estimate Data from Bouvet L, Schulz T, Piana F, et al. Pregnancy and labor epidural effects on gastric emptying: a prospective comparative study. *Anesthesiology.* 2022;136:542–550. Illustration by Naveen Nathan, MD, NorthShore University HealthSystem, University of Chicago Pritzker School of Medicine, Evanston, IL.

probably not delayed unless intrapartum parenteral opioids were administered.

Summary of Aspiration Risk and Prevention

No data indicate that the postpartum patient's safety is enhanced by delaying surgery or is compromised by proceeding with surgery immediately after delivery. The lack of data has led to confusion and inconsistency in the development of policies for the performance of postpartum tubal sterilization. No particular waiting interval guarantees that the postpartum patient is free of risk for aspiration. It is probably prudent to use some form of aspiration prophylaxis in all patients undergoing postpartum tubal sterilization. However, significant aspiration pneumonitis is so rare that it will be difficult to document cost-effectiveness and decreased rates of morbidity and mortality from the use of these measures. H_2-receptor antagonists and antacids do not reduce the possibility of regurgitation and aspiration, but they may make the consequences less severe. Metoclopramide (a prokinetic agent) may decrease the incidence of reflux by increasing lower esophageal sphincter tone and hastening gastric emptying. None of these medications can guarantee that gastric contents will not enter the lungs. Aspiration is best prevented by an experienced anesthesia provider using careful airway management or by use of a neuraxial anesthetic technique.

TIMING OF POSTPARTUM TUBAL LIGATION SURGERY

Performance of an immediate postpartum tubal sterilization (within 8 hours of delivery) may decrease both length of hospital stay and hospital costs. In this era of healthcare cost-containment, any decision to postpone surgery that requires an extra day of hospitalization must be evaluated carefully. Possible reasons to consider a delay after delivery are as follows: (1) women may remain at increased risk for gastroesophageal reflux immediately after delivery; (2) delays in gastric emptying due to the antepartum administration of opioids will resolve during this period; (3) an 8-hour delay allows the administration of aspiration prophylaxis drugs, although they might also be given during labor; (4) maximal hemodynamic stress and potential instability occur immediately postpartum when central blood volume suddenly increases because of contraction of the evacuated uterus, relief of aortocaval compression, and loss of the low-resistance placental circuit (although unlikely to affect healthy parturients, the patient with cardiovascular disease is at greatest risk for hemodynamic decompensation immediately postpartum); (5) if there are concerns about excessive blood loss at delivery, an 8-hour delay allows the physician to assess serial hemodynamic measurements (including the presence or absence of orthostatic changes), obtain an equilibrated postpartum hematocrit, and, if necessary, restore intravascular volume; (6) delay allows a more thorough evaluation of the infant; and (7) delay allows the woman more time to assess her decision and minimize the possibility of regret. However, it is important to remember that women who request postpartum tubal sterilization but do not receive it before discharge from the hospital are twice as likely to become pregnant within 1 year of delivery than women who did not request the procedure.[12] The ACOG has stated that given the consequences of a missed procedure, postpartum sterilization should be considered an urgent surgical procedure.[11] Anesthesia providers should be aware of their role in advocating with obstetricians for completion of the procedure in a timely fashion.[23]

At the University of Colorado, we follow standard NPO guidelines (i.e., no solid foods for 6 to 8 hours [depending on fat content] and no clear liquids for 2 hours) before postpartum tubal sterilization. NPO policies for postpartum tubal sterilization should not differ from those used for elective surgery in the main operating rooms. Immediate postpartum tubal sterilization may be performed in patients who have a functioning epidural catheter in place. These patients are given an H_2-receptor antagonist and metoclopramide intravenously prior to surgery, and a clear (nonparticulate) antacid is administered just before taking the patient to the operating room. In other patients who did not want (or were unable to receive) epidural analgesia for labor, similar precautions are used. Before surgery, quantitative blood loss from delivery is reviewed and orthostatic vital signs may be assessed. Most patients without preexisting epidural analgesia receive spinal anesthesia for postpartum tubal sterilization, with sedation if requested. However, if the patient strongly prefers, general anesthesia can be provided using rapid-sequence induction of anesthesia with cricoid pressure.

ANESTHETIC MANAGEMENT

Local, general, or neuraxial anesthesia may be used successfully for postpartum tubal sterilization. Physiology remains altered in the postpartum patient and requires some modification in anesthetic technique. It seems reasonable to give all postpartum patients some form of aspiration prophylaxis.[2] This may include a clear (nonparticulate) antacid, an H_2-receptor antagonist, and/or metoclopramide to increase lower esophageal sphincter tone and hasten gastric emptying. Metoclopramide also may reduce emesis during and after surgery. Patients with additional risk factors for aspiration (e.g., morbid obesity, diabetes mellitus) warrant prophylaxis with all three classes of drugs. Tubal sterilization does not require administration of preoperative antibiotics.[24]

Local Anesthesia

Local anesthesia is used widely for tubal sterilizations worldwide, although neuraxial anesthesia is most often administered for postpartum tubal sterilization in the United States. Several reports have documented the efficacy and safety of local anesthesia for postpartum or laparoscopic tubal ligation in the hospital operating room or a freestanding outpatient facility. Cruikshank et al.[25] described the use of intraperitoneal lidocaine for postpartum tubal ligation. After intravenous (IV) administration of diazepam, lidocaine 100 mg was used to infiltrate the skin and subcutaneous tissue. The peritoneum was entered, and 400 mg of lidocaine (80 mL of 0.5% solution) was instilled into the peritoneal cavity. A Pomeroy tubal ligation was performed 5 minutes later. All patients had complete peritoneal anesthesia, and all patients stated they would have the same procedure again. None recalled any pain or discomfort 24 hours later. There were no signs of lidocaine toxicity in any patient, and the maximum lidocaine blood level obtained was 5.3 µg/mL (the toxic blood level is generally considered greater than 5 µg/mL). Surgeons rated the conditions excellent. This study was published in 1973, when anesthesiologists may or may not have been involved and before ASA monitoring standards such as pulse oximetry existed. An alternative local anesthetic might be 2-chloroprocaine, an ester local anesthetic which has less risk of systemic toxicity, thus allowing a greater intraperitoneal volume to be used.

Poindexter et al.[26] described almost 3000 *laparoscopic* tubal sterilization procedures performed with local anesthesia in an ambulatory surgical facility. After IV sedation with large doses of midazolam (5 to 10 mg) and additional fentanyl (50 to 100 µg), the skin was infiltrated with 10 mL of 0.5% bupivacaine. After insertion of the trocar, the abdomen was insufflated with nitrous oxide. Each tube was sprayed with 5 mL of 0.5% bupivacaine, and a Silastic ring was applied. Patients were discharged home after approximately 1 hour in the postanesthesia care unit. The authors reported a technical failure rate of 0.14% and no unintended laparotomies or intraoperative complications. They reported that this technique reduced surgical time by 33% and cost by 68% to 85% compared with general anesthesia. The investigators presented no data regarding patient satisfaction, and they made no comment on the use of pulse oximetry or blood pressure monitors. Four percent of patients, however, required oxygen therapy for "adequate tissue perfusion." This study was done in the 1980s before many ambulatory surgery facilities had institutional guidelines for sedation.

General Anesthesia

Much of the impetus for performing sterilization procedures under local anesthesia came from two reports in 1983 indicating that morbidity and mortality were much higher when general anesthesia was used. It is important to realize that these reports preceded the mandatory use of pulse oximetry and capnography and do not reflect modern anesthesia care. The first report involved 3500 interval (not postpartum) laparoscopic tubal sterilizations at nine university medical centers.[27] Among all patients, the risk for intraoperative or postoperative complications was 1.75%, but the risk was five times higher with general anesthesia than with local anesthesia. (In this report, local anesthesia included local, epidural, and spinal anesthesia.) The reason(s) for the difference was unclear. In the second report, the US Centers for Disease Control and Prevention examined deaths attributed to tubal sterilization procedures from 1977 to 1981.[28] Both immediate postpartum laparotomies and interval laparoscopic procedures were included. Of the 29 deaths, 11 followed complications of general anesthesia and were caused by hypoventilation or cardiorespiratory arrest. Aspiration was not reported as a cause of death. Of the six patients whose deaths were definitely attributed to hypoventilation, none had undergone tracheal intubation. Five of the 11 deaths attributed to general anesthesia occurred during postpartum laparotomy. Of these, only one woman had undergone tracheal intubation; all others underwent mask ventilation. The investigators concluded, "It appears that for tubal sterilization, like abortion, the greatest risk for death is that associated with the anesthesia used during the procedure."[28]

In the 40 years since those reports, appropriate airway management with tracheal intubation has become standard practice during general anesthesia. Adherence to ASA standards for basic anesthesia monitoring (including use of pulse oximetry and capnography to monitor oxygenation and ventilation) reduces morbidity and mortality associated with general anesthesia. At the University of Colorado, rapid-sequence induction (with cricoid pressure) is performed, and all patients undergo tracheal intubation during the administration of general anesthesia for postpartum tubal sterilization.

Volatile anesthetic agents cause uterine relaxation and could potentially increase the risk for postpartum hemorrhage if administered to women in the immediate postpartum period. Therefore, the question arises whether the anesthesia provider should use an inhalation or an IV technique to maintain general anesthesia for postpartum tubal sterilization. Marx et al.[29] measured postpartum uterine activity and the response to

oxytocin with different concentrations of halothane or enflurane (Fig. 25.4). Impairment of spontaneous uterine activity occurred at 0.5 minimum alveolar concentration (MAC) of both agents, and loss of the response to oxytocin occurred near 1 MAC. Spontaneous contractions reappeared when anesthetic concentrations were reduced below these levels. Parous women are at risk for postpartum uterine atony and administration of a high concentration of a volatile halogenated agent may precipitate postpartum hemorrhage.

Two studies have determined the MAC of isoflurane during the postpartum period. Chan and Gin[30] found a positive correlation between MAC and the length of time after delivery, with return to higher nonpregnant values achieved by 72 hours postpartum. Zhou et al.[31] determined that the MAC of isoflurane was approximately 0.75% in the first 12 hours postpartum and 1.04% in patients who were 12 to 24 hours postpartum. No significant difference in MAC existed between the latter group and a control group of nonpregnant gynecologic patients. Together these results demonstrate that the reduced MAC observed during pregnancy persists for a variable period between 12 and 36 hours postpartum.

Propofol has advantages (e.g., rapid awakening, decreased incidence of emesis) that make it attractive as an induction agent for short sterilization procedures. When propofol was used for induction and maintenance of anesthesia for cesarean delivery, breast milk samples obtained at 4 and 8 hours postpartum had a low concentration of the drug, which suggested a negligible newborn exposure to propofol.[15,32]

Alterations occur in the activity of both depolarizing and nondepolarizing muscle relaxants during the postpartum period. Evans and Wroe[33] described the changes in plasma cholinesterase activity during pregnancy. A rapid decline in activity occurred during the first trimester. This low level of

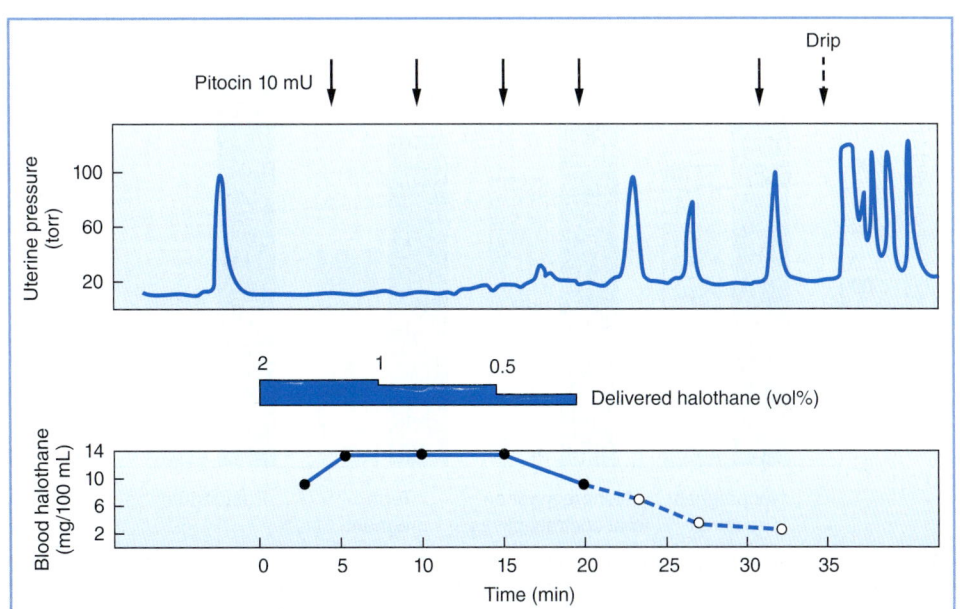

Fig. 25.4 Halothane anesthesia blocked the normal response to oxytocin when arterial blood levels exceeded 10.5 mg/100 mL or approximately 0.8 minimum alveolar concentration. From Marx GF, Kim YI, Lin CC, et al. Postpartum uterine pressures under halothane or enflurane anesthesia. *Obstet Gynecol*. 1978;51:695–698.

activity was maintained until delivery and was followed by an even lower level of activity during the first week postpartum. Leighton et al.[34] studied four groups of patients: nonpregnant, nonpregnant using oral contraceptives, term pregnant, and postpartum women. Cholinesterase activity was significantly lower in both term pregnant and postpartum women, and recovery time was 25% longer in the postpartum patients than in other groups (685 seconds versus approximately 500 seconds) (Fig. 25.5). Although a 3-minute prolongation of paralysis may not seem clinically significant, it could be important if airway difficulties occur. Metoclopramide prolongs neuromuscular block with succinylcholine by 135% to 228% because of its inhibition of plasma cholinesterase.[35]

Several studies have evaluated the use of the nondepolarizing muscle relaxants rocuronium, vecuronium, and cisatracurium in postpartum patients. Rocuronium's duration of action is prolonged by approximately 25% in postpartum patients,[36] and the duration of action of vecuronium is prolonged by more than 50%.[37] In contrast, the duration of action for cisatracurium is significantly shorter in the postpartum period.[38] Prolongation of neuromuscular block could be clinically significant during a short procedure. Khuenl-Brady et al.[37] suggested that a relative decrease in hepatic blood flow and/or competition between vecuronium and steroid hormones for hepatic uptake may interfere with the hepatic clearance of vecuronium in postpartum women. Alternatively, Gin et al.[39] concluded that the duration of

action for rocuronium is not prolonged in postpartum women if lean body mass—rather than total body weight—is used to calculate dose. These researchers speculated that the prolonged duration noted earlier[36] might be explained by relative drug overdose if the dose of rocuronium is based on the patient's gravid body weight.[39] Although it is unlikely a nondepolarizing muscle relaxant would be necessary for a short procedure such as postpartum tubal ligation, its duration may be less predictable in this setting and neuromuscular blockade monitoring should be used. Sugammadex has been used to reverse neuromuscular blockade with rocuronium after cesarean delivery, and it can be used to reverse neuromuscular blockade after postpartum tubal sterilization as well.[40] It is compatible with breastfeeding, as transfer into human breast milk is predicted to be minimal and infant enteral absorption unlikely.[41]

Neuraxial Anesthesia

Spinal and epidural anesthesia both provide excellent operating conditions for postpartum tubal sterilization. Airway obstruction, hypoventilation, and aspiration are much less likely during and after neuraxial anesthesia. A sensory level of T4 is needed to block visceral pain during exposure and manipulation of the fallopian tubes. Sedation can be provided if requested. The choice between spinal and epidural anesthesia is a matter of personal preference for the patient and the anesthesia provider.

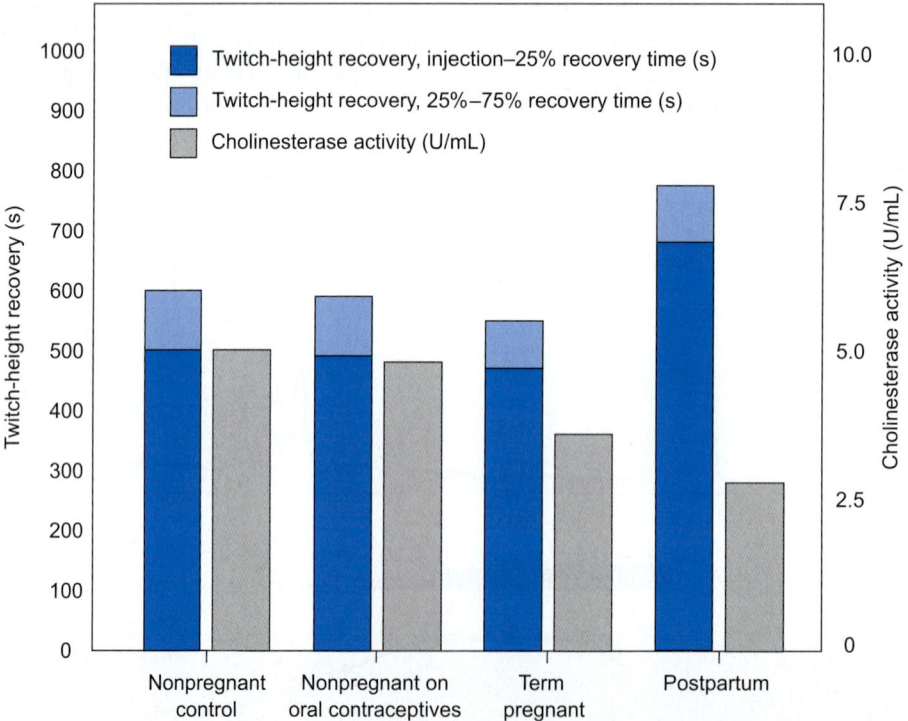

Fig. 25.5 Twitch-Height Recovery and Cholinesterase Activity After Succinylcholine 1 mg/kg. Cholinesterase activity was significantly lower in both term pregnant and postpartum women, and recovery time was 25% longer in the postpartum patients than in other groups. Data from Leighton BL, Cheek TG, Gross JB, et al. Succinylcholine pharmacodynamics in peripartum patients. *Anesthesiology.* 1986;64:202–205. Illustration by Naveen Nathan, MD, NorthShore University HealthSystem, University of Chicago Pritzker School of Medicine, Evanston, IL.

Epidural Anesthesia

When the performance of postpartum tubal sterilization is anticipated in a parous patient, we encourage the administration of epidural analgesia for labor and delivery. The epidural anesthetic can be extended for immediate postpartum tubal sterilization if appropriate. We avoid administration of parenteral opioids during labor if immediate postpartum tubal sterilization is planned. Immediate postpartum tubal sterilization may save the patient the cost and inconvenience of an extra day in the hospital, allow her to eat shortly after delivery (and surgery), and avoid the apprehension of undergoing a surgical procedure the following day. The avoidance of opioids helps maintain normal gastric emptying, which should decrease risk for aspiration during postpartum surgery. If the patient is stable and personnel are available, the procedure may be performed soon after delivery. The obstetrician and anesthesiologist must exclude excessive intrapartum blood loss and document that the patient has given informed consent.[5] Before going to the operating room, the patient should also be asked whether the epidural catheter provided adequate analgesia for the delivery. A catheter that was inadequate for labor analgesia is unlikely to provide adequate surgical anesthesia and an alternative anesthetic should be discussed.

At the time the patient is moved to the operating room, an epidural test dose is given to rule out intrathecal or intravascular migration of the epidural catheter, and the sensory level is extended with a surgical concentration of local anesthetic. A short-acting local anesthetic (e.g., 3% 2-chloroprocaine) is usually appropriate because the procedure is short in duration. An alternative choice is 2% lidocaine with epinephrine 1:200,000, although this may prolong the postanesthesia care unit stay while the block resolves. The addition of 100 μg epidural fentanyl may also improve the quality of the block and provide brief postoperative analgesia. Appropriate sedative drugs also may be given, if the patient requests.[42]

If surgery is not performed immediately after delivery, the catheter may be left in place for later postpartum tubal sterilization. Several studies have evaluated success rates when using a previously placed epidural catheter for a tubal ligation performed several hours after delivery and found their reliability decreased with increasing time since delivery. Vincent and Reid[43] found that the mean delivery-to-surgery interval was shorter in those patients who had adequate epidural anesthesia than in those without adequate anesthesia (10.6 versus 14.8 hours), but adequate anesthesia was achieved in only 78% of women overall after reinjection of the epidural catheter. The chance of successful epidural anesthesia was greatest if the catheter was used within 4 hours of delivery. A prospective, observational study addressed several risk factors that might decrease the success rate of epidural reactivation.[44] Overall success rate was again only 78%. The authors found that poor patient satisfaction with the epidural during labor, increasing time from delivery to epidural anesthesia reactivation, and the need for supplemental anesthesia during labor were associated with an increased risk of failure. No correlation was found with body mass index (BMI) or depth to loss of resistance (distance from skin to epidural space). A retrospective review of a single institution's anesthetic technique found that its success rate for epidural catheter reactivation was 74% (i.e., a 26% failure rate) and that time from catheter insertion until surgery was a significant factor associated with failure.[45] Failure of epidural anesthesia also corresponded to significantly longer times to provide surgical anesthesia than successful reactivation or spinal anesthesia. A survey of obstetric anesthesiology fellowship directors found 58% of respondents routinely leave the epidural catheter *in situ* if postpartum tubal ligation is planned, but 65% would not attempt reactivation after 8 hours postdelivery and only 7% would attempt to use the catheter after 24 hours.[45]

Clinical experience suggests that if the anesthesia provider plans to use an epidural catheter placed for labor, the risk for anesthesia failure is greater the longer surgery is delayed. To ensure maximal success in retaining efficacy when using a multiorifice epidural catheter, the anesthesia provider should thread the catheter 4 to 6 cm into the epidural space[46] and have the patient assume a deflexed position before taping the catheter to the skin.[47] After a prolonged interval from delivery, or if the patient was not satisfied with analgesia during labor, the anesthesia provider should consider spinal anesthesia rather than attempt reactivation of the epidural catheter.

Spinal Anesthesia

Spinal anesthesia for postpartum tubal sterilization has several advantages over epidural anesthesia. Epidural anesthesia requires the use of a large volume of concentrated local anesthetic and thereby introduces the risk for intravascular injection and cardiotoxicity.[48] The time to achieve adequate surgical anesthesia with epidural anesthesia may delay surgery; the induction of epidural anesthesia may require more time than the tubal sterilization itself. Spinal anesthesia is simple to perform, is rapid in onset, and provides dense sensory and motor block. In one study, spinal anesthesia for postpartum tubal ligation was associated with lower professional fees and operating room charges than attempted reactivation of an epidural catheter placed during labor.[49] There is no need to reinject a catheter intraoperatively for a short procedure such as postpartum tubal sterilization, and there is no need for prolonged postoperative analgesia. The risk for post–dural puncture headache (PDPH) is extremely low if a small-gauge (25- or 27-gauge) pencil-point or noncutting spinal needle is used. Although needle-gauge is significantly correlated with PDPH when cutting-bevel needles are used, selection of a larger-gauge pencil-point needle does not significantly increase rates of PDPH.[50] Nonetheless, most would choose a 25- or 27-gauge spinal needle for the procedure.

Local anesthetic requirements for spinal and epidural anesthesia are decreased during pregnancy, but studies have demonstrated a return to nonpregnant requirements by 36 hours postpartum.[51] Abouleish[52] prospectively compared the dose of spinal bupivacaine required for cesarean delivery with that required for postpartum tubal ligation. He noted that 30% more bupivacaine was required to achieve a T4 dermatomal level in women who were 8 to 24 hours postpartum.

The reason for the rapid decrease in sensitivity to local anesthetics is unclear but may be related to the rapid fall in progesterone levels after delivery of the placenta[18] (see Fig. 25.2). Datta et al.[53] examined plasma and cerebrospinal fluid (CSF) progesterone concentrations and spinal lidocaine requirements in nonpregnant, term pregnant, and postpartum women 12 to 18 hours after delivery. Plasma progesterone levels in pregnant women were 60 times higher than in nonpregnant women but only 7 times higher than those in postpartum women. CSF progesterone concentrations were eight times higher in term pregnant women and three times higher in postpartum women than in nonpregnant women. Significantly less lidocaine was needed for comparable segmental levels of spinal anesthesia in term and postpartum patients than in nonpregnant individuals. There was a significant correlation between lidocaine dose requirement for spinal anesthesia (mg/segment) and CSF progesterone concentration. The authors suggested "that a minimum level of progesterone in the CSF and/or plasma is necessary for this heightened local anesthetic activity" associated with progesterone. Together these studies suggest that local anesthetic requirements return to nonpregnant requirements 12 to 36 hours after delivery.[51–53]

Huffnagle et al.[54] gave hyperbaric intrathecal lidocaine 75 mg to postpartum women to determine whether age, weight, height, BMI, vertebral column length, or time from delivery to placement of the block correlated with the spread of sensory block. Only patient height had a weak positive correlation and it accounted for less than 15% of the variance in height of the block. Because of the large variation in the spread of sensory block among patients of the same height, the investigators concluded that there was little use in adjusting the dose of local anesthetic on the basis of height.

Many anesthesia providers discontinued the use of hyperbaric lidocaine for spinal anesthesia because of concern about transient neurologic symptoms (TNS) or transient radicular irritation (TRI), but obstetric patients may be at lower risk for this complication (see Chapter 31). A prospective, nonrandomized study of 303 obstetric patients who received spinal anesthesia during a 9-month period observed a 0% incidence of TRI (95% confidence interval, 0% to 4.5%) in those receiving 5% lidocaine.[55] Patients underwent a variety of procedures, including cesarean delivery, postpartum tubal ligation, cerclage, and other cases. The number of patients was too small to determine the true incidence of TRI in obstetric patients, but the investigators concluded that the true incidence is likely less than 5%. In a randomized, controlled trial, Philip et al.[56] compared spinal administration of hyperbaric 5% lidocaine with that of hyperbaric 0.75% bupivacaine for postpartum tubal ligation. They observed a 3% incidence of TNS with the use of lidocaine, compared with a 7% incidence with bupivacaine, a nonsignificant difference. In an editorial accompanying their report, Schneider and Birnbach[57] acknowledged that "there are no very short-acting hyperbaric spinal local anesthetics that have taken the place of lidocaine for these short procedures [and many believe that spinal bupivacaine lasts too long to be a reasonable choice of anesthetic

for a procedure that will last less than 20 minutes." However, they concluded, "Because pregnant patients represent a population that lies to the extreme in terms of the criteria for safety and lack of morbidity, we believe that for the present, there is still insufficient safety evidence to suggest that spinal hyperbaric 5% lidocaine be routinely used in obstetrics." Some anesthesia providers use 5% lidocaine because of its short duration of action, whereas others prefer to avoid spinal lidocaine despite the low risk for TNS in obstetric patients. Some continue to use hyperbaric bupivacaine despite its longer duration. Alternative shorter-acting spinal local anesthetics might be 2-chloroprocaine[58] or mepivacaine. Although there is less literature about the dosing or efficacy of these alternative local anesthetics in obstetric procedures, they could provide faster block resolution and improve throughput in the postoperative period on the labor and delivery unit.

Preservative-free intrathecal meperidine can be used as an alternative to local anesthetic for postpartum tubal sterilization if allergies to ester and amide local anesthetics are suspected or proven. The suggested dose is 1 mg/kg prepregnant weight (50 to 80 mg) for cesarean delivery or tubal sterilization. With an onset time of 3 to 5 minutes and a duration of 30 to 60 minutes, intrathecal meperidine compares favorably with 5% lidocaine. In a study that compared intrathecal lidocaine 70 mg with intrathecal meperidine 60 mg for postpartum tubal ligation, patients who received meperidine had more pruritus but longer postoperative analgesia (448 versus 83 minutes, respectively).[59] There was no difference between groups in rates of nausea, oxygen desaturation, or patient satisfaction. Intrathecal meperidine may be an alternative to local anesthetics for postpartum tubal sterilization.

Postpartum women seem to be at lower risk for hypotension during spinal anesthesia than pregnant women, and maintenance of uteroplacental perfusion is not a concern after delivery. Abouleish[52] gave ephedrine to correct maternal hypotension in 83% of pregnant women who received spinal bupivacaine anesthesia for cesarean delivery. In contrast, only 7% of postpartum women who received spinal anesthesia for tubal ligation required ephedrine. An autotransfusion of blood occurs immediately after delivery. Greater intravascular volume and the lack of aortocaval compression may help protect postpartum patients from hypotension during spinal anesthesia. Suelto et al.[60] compared normotensive and hypertensive patients receiving hyperbaric lidocaine for postpartum tubal ligation and found no difference in the use or dose of ephedrine for treatment of hypotension.

Box 25.1 summarizes anesthetic management for postpartum tubal sterilization.

POSTOPERATIVE ANALGESIA

Postpartum tubal sterilization produces modest postoperative pain of short duration. Patients may receive one dose of parenteral opioid postoperatively, or only oral analgesics. Providing optimal analgesia encourages early ambulation, interaction with the newborn including breastfeeding, and early discharge from the hospital. Nonsteroidal antiinflammatory

BOX 25.1 Anesthetic Management for Postpartum Tubal Sterilization

Management during labor
- Encourage use of epidural analgesia.
- Avoid administration of parenteral opioids.
- Keep patient on *nil per os* status except for clear liquids.
- Give aspiration prophylaxis if the procedure is to be performed immediately after delivery.

Timing of surgery
- Consider performing surgery immediately postpartum if the patient is hemodynamically stable and has received aspiration prophylaxis.
- An epidural catheter placed for labor may provide more reliable anesthesia if used within 8 h of delivery.

General anesthesia
- Perform a rapid-sequence induction with cricoid pressure.
- Intubate the trachea and control ventilation.
- Avoid high concentrations (>0.5 minimum alveolar concentration) of a volatile anesthetic agent.
- Monitor neuromuscular blockade if a nondepolarizing muscle relaxant is used.

Epidural anesthesia
- Requires a T4 sensory level of anesthesia.
- After a negative test dose result, consider using 3% 2-chloroprocaine unless a longer procedure is planned.
- If an epidural catheter placed during labor is used, beware of a higher risk for failure if the epidural placement-to-surgery interval is prolonged.
- Assure that the catheter functioned well for labor analgesia.
- Give fentanyl 50–100 µg via the epidural catheter for intraoperative and postoperative analgesia.

Spinal anesthesia
- Requires a T4 sensory level of anesthesia.
- It is the preferred technique for delayed postpartum tubal sterilization, or for immediate surgery in patients who did not have epidural labor analgesia, or in whom epidural analgesia during labor and delivery was ineffective.
- Use a small-gauge noncutting, pencil-point spinal needle to prevent post–dural puncture headache.
- Give bupivacaine 10–12 mg with fentanyl 10–25 µg. Consider lidocaine 75 mg with fentanyl 10–25 µg for a shorter-duration anesthetic.

Postoperative pain management
- Encourage the surgeon to infiltrate the skin and the mesosalpinx with bupivacaine.
- Administer acetaminophen and a nonsteroidal antiinflammatory drug such as ketorolac or ibuprofen perioperatively.
- Begin oral analgesics before complete block regression after spinal or epidural anesthesia.

drugs (NSAIDs) improve postoperative pain control. The manufacturer of ketorolac has stated that ketorolac is contraindicated in nursing mothers because of the possible adverse effects of prostaglandin synthetase inhibitors, including ductal closure and gastrointestinal bleeding on neonates.

In contrast, the American Academy of Pediatrics considers NSAIDs to be compatible with breastfeeding.[15,61] Either IV ketorolac or an oral NSAID such as ibuprofen should be given with acetaminophen for multimodal analgesia to minimize the need for opioid analgesics.

Adjuncts to neuraxial anesthesia can also be used to optimize postoperative pain control. When epinephrine 0.2 mg was added to lidocaine with fentanyl 10 µg for spinal anesthesia, the duration of complete and effective analgesia was prolonged and the incidence of pruritus was decreased, but the time to complete motor recovery was also prolonged.[62] Habib et al.[63] reported that adding intrathecal morphine 50 µg to intrathecal bupivacaine and fentanyl for postpartum tubal ligation resulted in less intense pain at rest and with movement at 4 hours after surgery than with saline control. However, patients who received morphine had more vomiting and pruritus. Despite side effects, the patients who received morphine were significantly more satisfied. Marcus et al.[64] also found that epidural morphine 2 mg provided better analgesia than control, but without increasing the need to treat side effects, when compared to a regimen of oral opioids and NSAIDs without epidural morphine. Although effective, spinal and epidural morphine analgesia should be used with caution because these patients could be discharged within hours after postpartum tubal sterilization, before the risk for delayed respiratory depression has lapsed. The method of postoperative analgesia chosen should not delay patient discharge because of side effects or the need for postoperative respiratory monitoring.

Local anesthetic infiltration of the skin incision and the mesosalpinx with bupivacaine, and topical application of a local anesthetic to the fallopian tubes, significantly decreases opioid requirements postoperatively.[65] These are simple, rapid techniques that can be used routinely by the obstetrician. A systematic review and metaanalysis of the application of topical or injectable local anesthetic during laparoscopic tubal ligation found that use of local anesthetic decreased pain substantially for up to 8 hours after surgery.[66]

OTHER POSTPARTUM PROCEDURES

Anesthesia for Removal of Retained Products, Postpartum Dilation, and Curettage

Therapeutic dilation and curettage (D&C) may be required for removal of retained products of conception in the postpartum period.[67] This is a short but painful procedure done in lithotomy position. It may be required for a patient with postpartum bleeding who had an unmedicated birth without epidural analgesia. It may be performed in a labor room or in the operating room. If the procedure is to be done in the labor room, emergency medications and airway equipment as well as a functioning suction device should be available in the room. There should be a low threshold for moving to the operating room, especially if hemodynamic instability is present or if general anesthesia is likely. Equipment, monitoring, lighting, and optimizing lithotomy position are likely better in the operating room, making both obstetric intervention and anesthetic induction safer.

Preoperative evaluation should include assessment of hemodynamic stability and blood loss since delivery. The patient should be considered to have a full stomach, and aspiration prophylaxis with at least a nonparticulate antacid should be administered prior to initiation of anesthesia. Anesthetic management may be sedation, neuraxial block, or general anesthesia depending on the situation and the patient's wishes. Standard ASA monitors should be applied and adequate IV access obtained. The patient's admission hematocrit should be reviewed and a blood sample for type and screen should be obtained in case of hemorrhage and need for transfusion. The need for prophylactic antibiotics should be discussed with the obstetrician.

If the patient has a well-functioning epidural catheter used for labor analgesia, a supplemental dose of a short-acting local anesthetic (e.g., 3% 2-chloroprocaine 10 to 15 mL or 2% lidocaine with epinephrine 10 to 15 mL) can provide dense surgical anesthesia to T10 with sacral coverage. This can generally be accomplished in the labor and delivery room.

If the patient did not have neuraxial labor analgesia, the patient should usually be moved to the operating room. If the obstetrician feels the placenta can be rapidly and easily removed with a manual sweep, inhaled nitrous oxide or IV sedation with midazolam and ketamine 0.25 to 0.5 mg/kg may be adequate. Oxygen by nasal cannula or mask should be administered prior to administering sedative medications. If the obstetrician feels the placenta will not be easy to remove, spinal or general anesthesia is indicated. Spinal anesthesia will provide a dense block with good sacral coverage. We typically administer hyperbaric bupivacaine 7.5 mg for this procedure. Prior to initiation of spinal anesthesia, it is important to assure blood loss has not been excessive and there is no concern for significant evolving coagulopathy. If these are present, general anesthesia may be the best option. This is usually accomplished with a rapid-sequence induction, securing the airway with an endotracheal tube, and limiting volatile agents to less than 0.5 MAC to prevent uterine atony.

Regardless of anesthetic technique, a tocolytic agent such as IV nitroglycerin should be available in case transient uterine relaxation is needed. After the uterus is evacuated, oxytocin is typically administered. After the procedure, the patient should recover in an appropriate monitored area.

Anesthesia for Examination Under Anesthesia and Repair of Lacerations

Lacerations are common after vaginal birth and can occur on the cervix, vagina, and vulva.[68] Of interest, neuraxial labor analgesia may decrease the incidence of lacerations by allowing for a more controlled delivery.[69] First- and second-degree lacerations may be repaired with local anesthesia or pudendal nerve block administered by the obstetrician, usually without sedation. Cervical and severe perineal lacerations extending into or through the anal sphincter (third-degree and fourth-degree lacerations) will likely require anesthesia rather than analgesia for repair. The obstetrician may also require anesthesia for a thorough examination to assess the extent of the injury prior to repair. Adequate exposure in lithotomy position and adjustable lighting are essential to a thorough examination. Although most lacerations can be repaired in the delivery room with the patient's legs in stirrups, severe lacerations may require an operating room to optimize lighting, positioning, and aseptic conditions. Antibiotic administration may be indicated and should be discussed with the obstetrician. The anesthetic considerations are similar to those for D&C.

Postprocedure, multimodal analgesia that includes neuraxial morphine, acetaminophen, and NSAIDs, with the goal of minimizing systemic opioid administration, can minimize constipation, thus preventing the Valsalva maneuver against the fresh surgical repair.

KEY POINTS

- Postpartum tubal sterilization should be considered a nonelective procedure to be accomplished during the delivery hospitalization. No data indicate that the postpartum patient's safety is enhanced by a delay of surgery or compromised by the performance of tubal sterilization immediately after delivery.
- Postpartum tubal sterilization (versus interval laparoscopic tubal sterilization) offers several advantages, including convenience for the patient and technical simplicity for the surgeon.
- Postpartum patients have similar gastric pH and gastric volumes as nonpregnant patients undergoing elective surgery. Studies suggest that gastric emptying is delayed postpartum only if the patient has received opioid analgesics during labor.
- Modern anesthetic drugs do not appear in breast milk in amounts that affect the newborn.

- The duration of succinylcholine-, rocuronium-, and vecuronium-induced neuromuscular blockade may be prolonged during the postpartum period. In contrast, the duration of action for cisatracurium is shorter.
- An epidural catheter placed for labor may be used for postpartum tubal sterilization if it functioned well for labor analgesia, but the risk of inadequate surgical anesthesia may be greater if surgery is delayed, especially more than 8 hours after delivery.
- Spinal anesthesia is preferred if postpartum tubal sterilization is not performed soon after delivery, regardless of whether an epidural catheter was placed for labor analgesia.
- The local anesthetic dose for spinal anesthesia returns to nonpregnant requirements by 12 to 36 hours postpartum.
- Use of postoperative multimodal analgesia, including local anesthetic infiltration of the skin and fallopian tubes,

improves maternal mobilization and may facilitate earlier hospital discharge.

- Retained products of conception may require dilation and curettage in the postpartum period. There should be ongoing assessment for hemorrhage. Depending on the circumstances, and with attention to monitoring and aspiration prophylaxis, anesthesia can be provided using preexisting epidural anesthesia, sedation, spinal anesthesia, or general anesthesia.

- Anesthesia for perineal examination and repair of significant obstetric lacerations after vaginal delivery is ideally managed with supplementation of a preexisting epidural anesthetic or spinal anesthesia. Multimodal analgesia that includes neuraxial morphine will provide optimal postoperative analgesia and minimize constipation from systemic opioid use.

REFERENCES

1. Fang NZ, Advaney SP, Castaño PM, et al. Female permanent contraception trends and updates. *Am J Obstet Gynecol*. 2022;226:773–780.

2. American Society of Anesthesiologists. Practice guidelines for obstetric anesthesia: an updated report by the American Society of Anesthesiologists Task Force on Obstetric Anesthesia and the Society for Obstetric Anesthesia and Perinatology. *Anesthesiology*. 2016;124:270–300.

3. Clark NV, Endicott SP, Jorgensen EM, et al. Review of sterilization techniques and clinical updates. *J Minim Invasive Gynecol*. 2018;25:1157–1164.

4. Kulier R, Boulvain M, Walker D, et al. Minilaparotomy and endoscopic techniques for tubal sterilisation. *Cochrane Database Syst Rev*. 2004;(3):CD001328.

5. American College of Obstetricians and Gynecologists. ACOG Practice Bulletin No. 208: Benefits and risks of sterilization (reaffirmed 2023). *Obstet Gynecol*. 2019;133:e194–e207.

6. Corton M, Leveno K, Bloom S, et al. *Williams Obstetrics*. 24th ed. McGraw-Hill Education; 2014.

7. Lawrie TA, Kulier R, Nardin JM. Techniques for the interruption of tubal patency for female sterilisation. *Cochrane Database Syst Rev*. 2016;(8):CD003034.

8. Zamorano AS, Mutch DG. Postpartum salpingectomy: a procedure whose time has come. *Am J Obstet Gynecol*. 2019;220:8–9.

9. Code of Colorado Regulations, Secretary of State, Colorado So. Department of Health Care Policy and Financing, Medical Services Board: Medical Assistance—Section 8.700. https://www.sos.state.co.us/CCR/GenerateRulePdf.do?ruleVersionId=7405&fileName=10%20CCR%202505-10%208.700. Accessed 1 August.

10. American College of Obstetricians and Gynecologists. Committee Statement No. 8: Permanent contraception: Ethical issues and considerations. *Obstet Gynecol*. 2024;143:e31–e39.

11. American College of Obstetricians and Gynecologists. ACOG Committee Opinion Number 827: Access to postpartum sterilization (reaffirmed 2024). *Obstet Gynecol*. 2021;137:e169–e176.

12. Thurman AR, Janecek T. One-year follow-up of women with unfulfilled postpartum sterilization requests. *Obstet Gynecol*. 2010;116:1071–1077.

13. Vincent RD Jr, Martin RW. Postpartum tubal ligation after pregnancy complicated by preeclampsia or gestational hypertension. *Obstet Gynecol*. 1996;88:119–122.

14. American College of Obstetricians and Gynecologists. Committee Opinion 794: Quantitative blood loss in obstetric hemorrhage (reaffirmed 2022). *Obstet Gynecol*. 2019;134:e150–e156.

15. Mitchell J, Jones W, Winkley E, Kinsella SM. Guideline on anaesthesia and sedation in breastfeeding women 2020: guideline from the Association of Anaesthetists. *Anaesthesia*. 2020;75:1482–1493.

16. Hawkins JL, Chang J, Palmer SK, et al. Anesthesia-related maternal mortality in the United States: 1979-2002. *Obstet Gynecol*. 2011;117:69–74.

17. D'Angelo R, Smiley RM, Riley ET, Segal S. Serious complications related to obstetric anesthesia: the serious complication repository project of the Society for Obstetric Anesthesia and Perinatology. *Anesthesiology*. 2014;120:1505–1512.

18. Löfgren M, Bäckström T. Serum concentrations of progesterone and 5 alpha-pregnane-3,20-dione during labor and early post partum. *Acta Obstet Gynecol Scand*. 1990;69:123–126.

19. Vial F, Hime N, Feugeas J, et al. Ultrasound assessment of gastric content in the immediate postpartum period: a prospective observational descriptive study. *Acta Anaesthesiol Scand*. 2017;61:730–739.

20. Bouvet L, Schulz T, Piana F, et al. Pregnancy and labor epidural effects on gastric emptying: a prospective comparative study. *Anesthesiology*. 2022;136:542–550.

21. American Society of Anesthesiologists' Committee on Obstetric Anesthesia. Statement on oral intake in labor; 2022. www.asahq.org/Guidelines. Accessed 1 August.

22. Sperling JD, Dahlke JD, Sibai BM. Restriction of oral intake during labor: whither are we bound? *Am J Obstet Gynecol*. 2016;214:592–596.

23. Richardson MG, Hall SJ, Zuckerwise LC. Postpartum tubal sterilization: making the case for urgency. *Anesth Analg*. 2018;126:1225–1231.

24. American College of Obstetricians and Gynecologists. Practice Bulletin No. 195: Prevention of infection after gynecologic procedures (reaffirmed 2022). *Obstet Gynecol*. 2018;131:e172–e189.

25. Cruikshank DP, Laube DW, De Backer LJ. Intraperitoneal lidocaine anesthesia for postpartum tubal ligation. *Obstet Gynecol*. 1973;42:127–130.

26. Poindexter AN 3rd, Abdul-Malak M, Fast JE. Laparoscopic tubal sterilization under local anesthesia. *Obstet Gynecol*. 1990;75:5–8.

27. Destefano F, Greenspan JR, Dicker RC, et al. Complications of interval laparoscopic tubal sterilization. *Obstet Gynecol*. 1983;61:153–158.

28. Peterson HB, DeStefano F, Rubin GL, et al. Deaths attributable to tubal sterilization in the United States, 1977 to 1981. *Am J Obstet Gynecol*. 1983;146:131–136.

29. Marx GF, Kim YI, Lin CC, et al. Postpartum uterine pressures under halothane or enflurane anesthesia. *Obstet Gynecol*. 1978;51:695–698.

30. Chan MT, Gin T. Postpartum changes in the minimum alveolar concentration of isoflurane. *Anesthesiology*. 1995;82:1360–1363.

31. Zhou HH, Norman P, DeLima LG, et al. The minimum alveolar concentration of isoflurane in patients undergoing bilateral tubal ligation in the postpartum period. *Anesthesiology*. 1995;82:1364–1368.

32. Dailland P, Cockshott ID, Lirzin JD, et al. Intravenous propofol during cesarean section: placental transfer, concentrations in breast milk, and neonatal effects. A preliminary study. *Anesthesiology*. 1989;71:827–834.

33. Evans RT, Wroe JM. Plasma cholinesterase changes during pregnancy. Their interpretation as a cause of suxamethonium-induced apnoea. *Anaesthesia*. 1980;35:651–654.

34. Leighton BL, Cheek TG, Gross JB, et al. Succinylcholine pharmacodynamics in peripartum patients. *Anesthesiology*. 1986;64:202–205.

35. Kao YJ, Turner DR. Prolongation of succinylcholine block by metoclopramide. *Anesthesiology*. 1989;70:905–908.

36. Pühringer FK, Sparr HJ, Mitterschiffthaler G, et al. Extended duration of action of rocuronium in postpartum patients. *Anesth Analg*. 1997;84:352–354.

37. Khuenl-Brady KS, Koller J, Mair P, et al. Comparison of vecuronium- and atracurium-induced neuromuscular blockade in postpartum and nonpregnant patients. *Anesth Analg*. 1991;72:110–113.

38. Pan PH, Moore C. Comparison of cisatracurium-induced neuromuscular blockade between immediate postpartum and nonpregnant patients. *J Clin Anesth*. 2001;13:112–117.

39. Gin T, Chan MT, Chan KL, Yuen PM. Prolonged neuromuscular block after rocuronium in postpartum patients. *Anesth Analg*. 2002;94:686–689.

40. Pühringer FK, Kristen P, Rex C. Sugammadex reversal of rocuronium-induced neuromuscular block in Caesarean section patients: a series of seven cases. *Br J Anaesth*. 2010;105:657–660.

41. Richardson MG, Raymond BL. Sugammadex administration in pregnant women and in women of reproductive potential: a narrative review. *Anesth Analg*. 2020;130:1628–1637.

42. Aaronson J, Goodman S. Obstetric anesthesia: not just for cesareans and labor. *Semin Perinatol*. 2014;38:378–385.

43. Vincent RD Jr, Reid RW. Epidural anesthesia for postpartum tubal ligation using epidural catheters placed during labor. *J Clin Anesth*. 1993;5:289–291.

44. Powell MF, Wellons DD, Tran SF, et al. Risk factors for failed reactivation of a labor epidural for postpartum tubal ligation: a prospective, observational study. *J Clin Anesth*. 2016;35: 221–224.

45. McKenzie C, Akdagli S, Abir G, Carvalho B. Postpartum tubal ligation: a retrospective review of anesthetic management at a single institution and a practice survey of academic institutions. *J Clin Anesth*. 2017;43:39–46.

46. Beilin Y, Bernstein HH, Zucker-Pinchoff B. The optimal distance that a multiorifice epidural catheter should be threaded into the epidural space. *Anesth Analg*. 1995;81: 301–304.

47. Hamilton CL, Riley ET, Cohen SE. Changes in the position of epidural catheters associated with patient movement. *Anesthesiology*. 1997;86:778–784.

48. Macfarlane AJR, Gitman M, Bornstein KJ, et al. Updates in our understanding of local anaesthetic systemic toxicity: a narrative review. *Anaesthesia*. 2021;76(suppl 1):27–39.

49. Viscomi CM, Rathmell JP. Labor epidural catheter reactivation or spinal anesthesia for delayed postpartum tubal ligation: a cost comparison. *J Clin Anesth*. 1995;7:380–383.

50. Zorrilla-Vaca A, Mathur V, Wu CL, Grant MC. The impact of spinal needle selection on postdural puncture headache: a meta-analysis and metaregression of randomized studies. *Reg Anesth Pain Med*. 2018;43:502–508.

51. Assali NS, Prystowsky H. Studies on autonomic blockade. I. Comparison between the effects of tetraethylammonium chloride (TEAC) and high selective spinal anesthesia on blood pressure of normal and toxemic pregnancy. *J Clin Invest*. 1950;29:1354–1366.

52. Abouleish EI. Postpartum tubal ligation requires more bupivacaine for spinal anesthesia than does cesarean section. *Anesth Analg*. 1986;65:897–900.

53. Datta S, Hurley RJ, Naulty JS, et al. Plasma and cerebrospinal fluid progesterone concentrations in pregnant and nonpregnant women. *Anesth Analg*. 1986;65:950–954.

54. Huffnagle SL, Norris MC, Leighton BL, et al. Do patient variables influence the subarachnoid spread of hyperbaric lidocaine in the postpartum patient? *Reg Anesth*. 1994;19: 330–334.

55. Wong CA, Slavenas P. The incidence of transient radicular irritation after spinal anesthesia in obstetric patients. *Reg Anesth Pain Med*. 1999;24:55–58.

56. Philip J, Sharma SK, Gottumukkala VN, et al. Transient neurologic symptoms after spinal anesthesia with lidocaine in obstetric patients. *Anesth Analg*. 2001;92:405–409.

57. Schneider MC, Birnbach DJ. Lidocaine neurotoxicity in the obstetric patient: is the water safe? *Anesth Analg*. 2001;92: 287–290.

58. Mandalia S, Dinges E, Bollag L, Delgado C. Spinal chloroprocaine for obstetrical non-delivery procedures: a retrospective analysis at a single academic center. *Int J Obstet Anesth*. 2021;45:158–159.

59. Norris MC, Honet JE, Leighton BL, Arkoosh VA. A comparison of meperidine and lidocaine for spinal anesthesia for postpartum tubal ligation. *Reg Anesth*. 1996;21:84–88.

60. Suelto MD, Vincent RD Jr, Larmon JE, et al. Spinal anesthesia for postpartum tubal ligation after pregnancy complicated by preeclampsia or gestational hypertension. *Reg Anesth Pain Med*. 2000;25:170–173.

61. Sachs HC. The transfer of drugs and therapeutics into human breast milk: an update on selected topics. *Pediatrics*. 2013;132:e796–e809.

62. Malinow AM, Mokriski BL, Nomura MK, et al. Effect of epinephrine on intrathecal fentanyl analgesia in patients undergoing postpartum tubal ligation. *Anesthesiology*. 1990;73:381–385.

63. Habib AS, Muir HA, White WD, et al. Intrathecal morphine for analgesia after postpartum bilateral tubal ligation. *Anesth Analg*. 2005;100:239–243.

64. Marcus RL, Wong CA, Lehor A, et al. Postoperative epidural morphine for postpartum tubal ligation analgesia. *Anesth Analg*. 2005;101:876–881.

65. Wittels B, Faure EA, Chavez R, et al. Effective analgesia after bilateral tubal ligation. *Anesth Analg*. 1998;87:619–623.

66. Harrison MS, DiNapoli MN, Westhoff CL. Reducing postoperative pain after tubal ligation with rings or clips: a systematic review and meta-analysis. *Obstet Gynecol*. 2014;124:68–75.

67. Fujita K, Ushida T, Imai K, et al. Manual removal of the placenta and postpartum hemorrhage: a multicenter retrospective study. *J Obstet Gynaecol Res.* 2021;47:3867–3874.

68. American College of Obstetricians and Gynecologists. ACOG Practice Bulletin No. 198: Prevention and management of obstetric lacerations at vaginal delivery (reaffirmed 2022). *Obstet Gynecol.* 2018;132:e87–e102.

69. Baumann P, Hammoud AO, McNeeley SG, et al. Factors associated with anal sphincter laceration in 40,923 primiparous women. *Int Urogynecol J Pelvic Floor Dysfunct.* 2007;18:985–990.

PART VII

Cesarean Delivery

26

Anesthesia for Cesarean Delivery

Lawrence C. Tsen, MD and Brian T. Bateman, MD, MSc

CHAPTER OUTLINE

HISTORY

Cesarean delivery (also known as **cesarean section** and **cesarean birth**) is defined as the birth of an infant through incisions in the abdomen (laparotomy) and uterus (hysterotomy). Although the technique is commonly associated with the birth of the Roman Emperor Julius Caesar, this is questioned by medical historians given that his birth was in an era (100 BCE) when such operations were invariably fatal and yet Caesar's mother was present in his later life.[1]

Morbidity and mortality, most often associated with hemorrhage and infection, limited the use of cesarean delivery until the 20th century, when advances in aseptic, surgical, and anesthetic techniques improved the safety for both mother and baby. Today, cesarean delivery is the most common major surgical procedure performed worldwide, with projections indicating that by 2030, 38 million women will use this method of birth each year. However, cesarean delivery rates are affected by a myriad of maternal, fetal, obstetric, social, medicolegal, and health system factors,[2] resulting in a range from 7.1% in sub-Saharan Africa to 63.4% in eastern Asia.[3] In high-resource countries, an optimal cesarean delivery rate of 19% has been suggested to minimize maternal and neonatal morbidity.[4] In low-resource countries, the World Health Organization (WHO) is focused on decreasing unmet need, unsafe provision, and even the relative overuse of the procedure when it depletes limited available resources.[3]

INDICATIONS

Indications for cesarean delivery can be maternal or fetal (Box 26.1).[5] An *elective* (scheduled) cesarean delivery can

> ### BOX 26.1 Indications for Cesarean Delivery
>
> **Maternal**
> - Antepartum or intrapartum hemorrhage
> - Arrest of labor
> - Breech presentation
> - Chorioamnionitis
> - Deteriorating maternal condition (e.g., severe preeclampsia)
> - Dystocia
> - Failure of induction of labor
> - Genital herpes (active lesions)
> - High-order multiple gestation (or twin gestation in which twin A has a breech presentation)
> - Maternal request
> - Placenta previa
> - Placental abruption
> - Previous myomectomy
> - Prior classical uterine incision
> - Uterine rupture
>
> **Fetal**
> - Breech presentation or other malpresentation
> - Fetal intolerance of labor
> - Suspected macrosomia
> - Nonreassuring fetal status
> - Prolapsed umbilical cord
>
> **Obstetric Provider**
> - Desire to avoid difficult forceps or vacuum delivery

> ### BOX 26.2 Complications of Cesarean Delivery
>
> **Intraoperative Complications**
> *Hemorrhage*
> - Uterine atony
> - Uterine lacerations
> - Broad ligament hematoma
>
> *Infection*
> - Endometritis
> - Wound infection
>
> **Postoperative Complications**
> - Cardiovascular: venous thromboembolism
> - Gastrointestinal: ileus, adhesions, injury
> - Genitourinary: bladder or ureteral injury
> - Respiratory: atelectasis, aspiration pneumonia
> - Chronic pain
>
> **Future Pregnancy Risks**
> - Placenta previa
> - Placenta accreta
> - Uterine rupture
> - Obstetric hysterectomy

be performed for obstetric or medical indications or at the request of a patient, and it is typically planned and performed *before* the onset of labor.[6] A cesarean delivery performed during labor for a planned vaginal delivery can also occur for a wide range of maternal and fetal indications but may need to be conducted in an urgent manner as an emergency. A prior cesarean delivery does not necessitate cesarean delivery in a subsequent pregnancy. A trial of labor after cesarean (TOLAC), which if successful is called a vaginal birth after cesarean (VBAC), is an alternative option; validated algorithms for predicting the probability of successful VBAC have been developed.[7] An elective repeat cesarean delivery is typically recommended in women with more than one previous cesarean delivery, a previous upper uterine vertical incision or full thickness scar, a previous history of uterine rupture, or a strong indicator for cesarean delivery (e.g., abnormal placentation; see Chapter 20).[8]

OPERATIVE TECHNIQUE

The technical aspects of performing a cesarean delivery are comparable worldwide, with minor variation. A midline vertical *abdominal* incision allows rapid access and greater surgical exposure; however, the horizontal *suprapubic* (Pfannenstiel) incision offers better cosmesis and wound strength. Similarly, a low transverse *uterine* incision, compared with a vertical incision, lowers the incidence of uterine dehiscence and rupture in subsequent pregnancies, and reduces the risks for

infection, blood loss, and bowel and omental adhesions. A vertical uterine incision is most often used in the following situations: (1) if the lower uterine segment is underdeveloped (typically before 34 weeks' gestation), (2) for delivery of a preterm infant in a woman who has not labored, and (3) in selected patients with multiple gestation and/or malpresentation. In some cases, a vertical uterine incision is performed high on the anterior uterine wall (i.e., classical incision), especially in the patient with a low-lying anterior placenta previa or when a cesarean hysterectomy is planned.

Uterine exteriorization may be performed following delivery to facilitate visualization and repair of the uterine incision, particularly when the incision has been extended laterally. In a systematic review and metaanalysis, uterine exteriorization had no significant effect on blood loss, transfusion requirement, duration of surgery or hospital stay, time to return of bowel function, fever, endometritis, or wound infection; however, higher rates of intraoperative nausea, venous air embolism, and postoperative pain have been reported.[9]

MORBIDITY AND MORTALITY

Complications of cesarean delivery include hemorrhage, infection, thromboembolism, ureteral and bladder injury, abdominal pain, and increased risk for abnormal placentation and uterine rupture in subsequent pregnancies (Box 26.2).[10] Maternal morbidity and mortality vary widely from country to country (see Chapter 39). Most developed nations have a similar experience to the United States, where the rate of maternal death associated with cesarean delivery (odds ratio [OR], 3.21; 95% confidence interval [CI], 2.80 to 3.61), particularly primary cesarean delivery (OR, 5.72; 95% CI, 4.92 to 6.51) remains higher than that associated with vaginal delivery.[11] Planned cesarean delivery is also associated with a higher risk for maternal morbidity compared with planned vaginal delivery, although the absolute differences in risk are small.[12] These differences in mortality and morbidity rates are largely attributable to the underlying conditions that necessitate cesarean delivery, although performance of cesarean delivery also increases maternal and neonatal morbidity (and perhaps mortality) in subsequent pregnancies and cesarean deliveries.[13] Neonatal and pediatric morbidity, particularly involving the respiratory system, is also greater with elective cesarean delivery than with vaginal delivery.[14]

PREVENTION OF CESAREAN DELIVERY

Some cesarean deliveries may be avoided through the provision of (1) adequate labor analgesia, especially for TOLAC and instrumental vaginal delivery; (2) analgesia for external cephalic version (ECV) (see Chapter 34); and (3) intrauterine resuscitation, including pharmacologic uterine relaxation in cases of uterine tachysystole. Neuraxial labor analgesia is not associated with a higher cesarean delivery rate compared with the use of systemic opioids (see Chapter 24)[15]; this finding includes the combined spinal-epidural (CSE) technique, despite its association with fetal bradycardia.[16]

Maternal Labor Analgesia

The National Institutes of Health State-of-the-Science statement on cesarean delivery on maternal request emphatically concluded that "maternal request for cesarean delivery should not be motivated by unavailability of effective [labor] pain management."[6] While most hospitals in the United States now offer labor epidural analgesia,[17] this is not the case in many parts of the world, and studies suggest that the introduction of labor epidural analgesia may be an effective approach to decrease the cesarean delivery rate in these settings.[18]

Adequate maternal analgesia and perineal relaxation are also important for instrumental (forceps, vacuum) vaginal delivery. Neuraxial techniques can optimize anesthetic conditions for these obstetric procedures (see Chapter 24).

External Cephalic Version

Singleton breech presentation occurs in 3% to 4% of term pregnancies. The Royal College of Obstetricians and Gynaecologists[19] and the American College of Obstetricians and Gynecologists (ACOG)[20] caution against vaginal breech delivery, given poorer neonatal outcomes compared with planned cesarean delivery. ECV is a procedure by which manual external pressure is applied to the maternal abdomen to change the fetal presentation from breech to cephalic. ECV is usually performed between 36 and 39 weeks' gestation (see Chapter 34).

Metaanalyses of available trial data support the finding that neuraxial, intravenous, or inhalation analgesia/anesthesia increases the success rate of attempted ECV.[21] Moreover, these studies show that the use of neuraxial blockade does not appear to compromise maternal and fetal safety, nor increase the risk for placental abruption, fetal bradycardia or death, or cesarean delivery. ACOG supports the use of neuraxial analgesia, in combination with tocolytic therapy, to increase ECV success.[22]

> **BOX 26.3   Obstetric Management of Nonreassuring Fetal Status**
>
> - Optimize maternal position:
>   - To avoid or relieve aortocaval compression.
>   - To relieve umbilical cord compression.
> - Administer supplemental oxygen.
> - Maintain maternal circulation:
>   - Perform rapid intravenous administration of a nondextrose-containing balanced salt solution.
>   - Treat hypotension with either ephedrine or phenylephrine.
> - Discontinue oxytocin.
> - Consider administration of a tocolytic agent for treatment of uterine tachysystole.

Intrauterine Resuscitation

Evidence of intrapartum fetal compromise (nonreassuring fetal status) should prompt the obstetric team (including obstetric, anesthesia, and nursing providers) to attempt intrauterine fetal resuscitation (Box 26.3). These actions include changing maternal position to relieve aortocaval compression, administering vasopressors and intravenous fluid to treat maternal hypotension, discontinuing exogenous oxytocin administration, and, in cases of uterine tachysystole, administration of a tocolytic agent such as terbutaline or nitroglycerin (see Chapter 8).

PREPARATION FOR ANESTHESIA

The anesthetic management of cesarean delivery may depend in part on the obstetric indication for operative delivery. The anesthesia provider should consider the patient's medical, surgical, and obstetric history, the presence or absence of labor, the urgency of the delivery, and the resources available in preparing for a cesarean delivery.

Preanesthetic Evaluation

All women admitted for labor and delivery are potential candidates for the emergency administration of anesthesia, and an anesthesia provider ideally should evaluate every woman shortly after admission. Optimally, for high-risk patients, preanesthesia consultation should occur in the late second or early third trimester, even if a vaginal delivery is planned. This practice, which can be accomplished remotely via video communication (i.e., "telemedicine"), offers the opportunity to provide patients with information, solicit further consultations, optimize medical conditions, and discuss plans and preparations for the upcoming delivery.[23] Early communication among the members of the multidisciplinary team is encouraged. In some cases, the urgent nature of the situation limits the time for evaluation before induction of anesthesia and commencement of surgery; nonetheless, essential information must be obtained and risks and benefits of alternative anesthetic management decisions should be considered.

A focused preanesthetic history and physical examination includes (1) a review of maternal health and anesthetic history, relevant obstetric history, allergies, and baseline blood pressure and heart rate measurements; and (2) performance of an airway, heart, and lung examination consistent with the American Society of Anesthesiologists (ASA) guidelines.[24]

BOX 26.4 Selected Risk Factors for Peripartum Hemorrhage

- Abnormal placentation
- Advanced maternal age
- Anticoagulation
- Bleeding disorder
- Chorioamnionitis
- Fetal demise
- Fetal malpresentation
- General anesthesia
- Increased parity/grand multiparity
- Instrumental vaginal delivery
- Internal trauma (e.g., curettage, internal version)
- Oxytocin augmentation of labor
- Placental abruption
- Precipitous delivery
- Preeclampsia
- Premature rupture of membranes
- Previous uterine surgery (e.g., cesarean delivery, myomectomy)
- Prolonged labor
- Retained placenta
- Tocolytic therapy
- Trauma
- Uterine distention (e.g., macrosomia, multiple gestation, polyhydramnios)
- Uterine leiomyoma

BOX 26.5 Suggested Resources for Obstetric Anesthesia

Monitors
- Electrocardiogram
- Noninvasive blood pressure
- Pulse oximetry
- Capnography
- Oxygen and volatile anesthetic analyzers
- Ventilator (with appropriate pressure and disconnection sensors/alarms)
- Peripheral nerve stimulator

For Hemorrhage
- Large-bore intravenous catheters
- Fluid warmer
- Forced-air body warmer
- Availability of blood bank resources
- Equipment for infusing intravenous fluids and blood products rapidly (e.g., hand-squeezed fluid chambers, hand-inflated pressure bags, automatic infusion devices)
- Availability of interventional radiology service
- Cell salvage equipment

For Routine Airway Management
- Laryngoscope and assorted blades
- Videolaryngoscope
- Oral airways of assorted sizes
- Endotracheal tubes of assorted sizes (6.5 and 7.0 mm) with stylets
- Oxygen source
- Suction source with tubing and catheters
- Self-inflating bag and mask for positive-pressure ventilation
- Medications for blood pressure support, hypnosis, and muscle relaxation

For Difficult Airway Management
- Rigid laryngoscope blades of alternative design and size from those routinely used
- Supraglottic airway devices (e.g., laryngeal mask airway)
- Endotracheal tube guides (e.g., semirigid stylets with or without hollow cores for jet ventilation, light wands, and forceps designed to manipulate the distal portion of the endotracheal tube)
- Retrograde intubation equipment
- At least one device suitable for emergency nonsurgical airway ventilation (e.g., hollow jet ventilation stylet with a transtracheal jet ventilator; supraglottic airway device, such as a Combitube [Sheridan Catheter Corporation, Argyle, NY] or intubating LMA [Fastrach LMA, LMA North America, San Diego, CA])
- Fiberoptic intubation equipment
- Equipment suitable for emergency surgical airway access (e.g., cricothyrotomy)
- Topical anesthetics and vasoconstrictors

LMA, Laryngeal mask airway.
Modified from the American Society of Anesthesiologists, Society for Obstetric Anesthesia and Perinatology. Practice guidelines for obstetric anesthesia: an updated report by the American Society of Anesthesiologists Task Force on Obstetric Anesthesia and the Society for Obstetric Anesthesia and Perinatology. *Anesthesiology.* 2016;124:270–300.

Blood Products

Peripartum hemorrhage remains a leading cause of maternal mortality worldwide (see Chapters 37 and 39).[25] There is little difference in blood loss between an uncomplicated elective cesarean delivery and an uncomplicated planned vaginal birth; however, a cesarean delivery performed during labor or in the setting of abnormal placentation is associated with greater blood loss.[26] Risk factors for peripartum hemorrhage are listed in Box 26.4.

Preparation for obstetric hemorrhage includes: (1) reviewing the patient's history for anemia or risk factors for hemorrhage; (2) consulting with the obstetric team regarding the presence of risk factors; (3) reviewing reports of ultrasonographic or magnetic resonance imaging (MRI) of placentation; (4) obtaining a blood sample for a type and screen or cross-match; (5) contacting the blood bank to ensure the availability of blood products; (6) obtaining and checking the necessary equipment (blood filters and warmers, infusion pumps and tubing), compatible fluids and medications, and standard clinical laboratory collection tubes; and (7) consulting with a blood bank pathologist, hematologist, and/or interventional radiologist in selected cases (Box 26.5).

Currently, there is a lack of consensus as to which patients require a blood type and screen and which patients require a cross-match. The maternal history (previous transfusion, existence of known red blood cell antibodies) and anticipated hemorrhagic complications, as well as local institutional policies, should guide decision-making. In certain high-risk cases (e.g., suspected placenta accreta), blood products (e.g., 2 to 4 units of packed red blood cells) should be physically present near or in the operating room before making the surgical incision, if possible.

Monitoring

Attention should be given to the availability and proper functioning of equipment and monitors for the provision of anesthesia and the management of potential complications (e.g., failed tracheal intubation, cardiopulmonary arrest).[24] Equipment should be checked on a daily basis and serviced at recommended intervals. The equipment and facilities available in the labor and delivery operating room suite should be comparable to those available in the main operating room.[24]

The ASA standards for basic monitoring apply to the provision of anesthesia for all patients.[27] Within obstetrics, basic monitoring consists of maternal pulse oximetry, electrocardiography (ECG), and noninvasive blood pressure monitoring,[a] as well as fetal heart rate (FHR) monitoring.

ECG abnormalities are often observed in late pregnancy and are believed to be caused by hyperdynamic circulation, circulating catecholamines, and/or altered estrogen and progesterone concentration ratios (see Chapter 2). During cesarean delivery with neuraxial anesthesia, ECG changes, including ST segment depression, have been reported at a high frequency (64%), but are almost always associated with normal (nonischemic) echocardiographic wall motion. The administration of **droperidol**, **ondansetron**, **oxytocin**, and **carbetocin** may be associated with prolongation of the QTc interval, and ST-segment depression.[28] The significance of these ECG findings as an indicator of cardiac pathology remains unclear, because only a small minority of parturients experience myocardial ischemia as measured by elevated serum cardiac troponin levels or echocardiographic wall motion abnormalities.[29,30] The placement of five ECG leads improves the sensitivity of detecting ischemic events; combining leads II, V_4, and V_5 resulted in a sensitivity of 96% for detecting ST-segment changes in a nonobstetric population.[31] In a prospective study of 254 healthy women undergoing cesarean delivery with spinal anesthesia, Shen et al.[32] determined the incidence of first- and second-degree atrioventricular block (3.5% for each), severe bradycardia defined as a heart rate < 50 beats/min (6.7%), and multiple premature ventricular contractions (1.2%). The investigators speculated that a relative increase in parasympathetic activity occurred as a result of spinal blockade of cardiac sympathetic activity. Most of the dysrhythmias were transient and resolved spontaneously.

Processed electroencephalogram monitors used to indicate the depth of anesthesia have received only limited evaluation in women undergoing cesarean delivery.[33] Whether routine use of these monitors can reduce the incidence of intraoperative awareness during general anesthesia for cesarean delivery is unclear (see discussion below).

An indwelling urinary catheter is used in almost all women undergoing cesarean delivery.[34] A urinary catheter helps avoid overdistention of the bladder during and after surgery. In cases associated with hypovolemia and/or oliguria, or anticipated significant blood loss, a collection system that allows precise measurement of urine volume is helpful.

The FHR is often assessed by a qualified individual before and after administration of anesthesia. However, data are insufficient to determine the value of FHR monitoring before elective cesarean delivery in patients without risk factors. Our practice is to monitor FHR until the abdominal skin preparation for cesarean delivery has begun.

In some cases of *emergency* cesarean delivery, a previously placed fetal scalp (or buttock) ECG electrode can be used to monitor the FHR before, during, and after the initiation of anesthesia. Typically, the fetal scalp electrode is removed when the surgical drapes are applied to the abdomen, but in some cases the scalp electrode may be left in place until just before delivery, when the circulating nurse reaches under the drapes to disconnect the electrode. Continuous FHR monitoring is useful in this setting for at least three reasons. First, the FHR abnormality often resolves; in some cases the obstetric provider may then elect to forgo the performance of a cesarean delivery, and in other cases continuous FHR monitoring may facilitate the administration of neuraxial anesthesia (e.g., extension of epidural anesthesia or administration of spinal anesthesia) for cesarean delivery. Second, continuous FHR monitoring may guide management in cases of failed tracheal intubation; if there is no evidence of fetal compromise, both the anesthesia provider and the obstetric provider may have greater confidence to awaken the patient and proceed with an alternative anesthetic technique, or alternatively, if there is evidence of ongoing fetal compromise, the anesthesia provider may decide to provide general anesthesia for cesarean delivery with a facemask or supraglottic airway (see Chapter 29). Third, intraoperative FHR monitoring allows the obstetric provider to modify the surgical technique according to the urgency of delivery.

Invasive monitoring (e.g., an intraarterial catheter), noninvasive cardiac output monitoring, or echocardiography may be indicated for individual patients at high risk for cardiopulmonary compromise.

Equipment

Labor and delivery units may be adjacent to or remote from the main operating rooms. In some facilities, the unit is located on a separate floor but shares a common operating room facility (used for other surgical procedures), whereas in others it is a geographically separate, self-contained unit with its own operating room facilities. Regardless of location, the equipment, facilities, and support personnel available in the labor and delivery operating room should be comparable to those available in the main operating room.[24] In addition, personnel and equipment should be available to care for obstetric patients recovering from major neuraxial or general anesthesia.

Resources for the conduct and support of neuraxial anesthesia and general anesthesia should include those necessary for the basic delivery of anesthesia and airway management as well as those required to manage complications (e.g., failed tracheal intubation). The *immediate* availability of these resources is particularly important, given the frequency and urgency of anesthesia care. Consideration should be given to having some of the equipment and supplies immediately available in one location

---

[a]Outside the operating room, and before the onset of labor, maternal blood pressure is ideally measured (using an appropriately sized cuff with a bladder length that is 80% and a width that is at least 46% of the arm circumference) after a rest period of 10 minutes or more, with the pregnant woman sitting or lying on her left side with her arm at the level of the right atrium. The onset (phase 1) and disappearance (phase 5) of Korotkoff sounds correspond to systolic and diastolic pressures, respectively.

or in a cart (e.g., difficult airway cart, massive hemorrhage cart, malignant hyperthermia box) specifically located on the labor and delivery unit. Equipment and supplies should be checked on a frequent and regular basis. Securing special-situation equipment and supplies in a cart with a single-use breakthrough tie helps ensure that the cart is kept in a fully stocked state.

Aspiration Prophylaxis

The patient should be asked about oral intake, although insufficient evidence exists regarding the relationship between recent ingestion and subsequent aspiration pneumonitis (see Chapter 28). Gastric emptying of clear liquids during pregnancy occurs relatively quickly; the residual content of the stomach (as measured by ultrasonographic assessment of the cross-sectional area of the gastric antrum 60 minutes after the ingestion of 300 mL of water) does not appear to be different from baseline fasting levels in either lean or obese nonlaboring pregnant women.[35,36] Wong et al.,[35] using serial gastric ultrasonographic examinations and acetaminophen (paracetamol) absorption, reported that gastric emptying half-time was shorter after ingestion of 300 mL of water (24 [SD 6] minutes) compared with 50 mL of water (33 [8] minutes) in healthy, nonlaboring, nonobese pregnant women. Bouvet et al.[37] reported that the gastric emptying fraction at 90 minutes after a light meal was lower in laboring women receiving epidural analgesia compared with nonpregnant and nonlaboring pregnant women; furthermore, the gastric emptying fraction was lower in laboring women not receiving epidural analgesia compared with laboring women receiving epidural analgesia.

The healthy patient undergoing *elective* cesarean delivery may drink modest amounts of clear liquids up to 2 hours before induction of anesthesia.[24] Examples of clear liquids are water, fruit juice without pulp, carbonated beverages, clear tea, black coffee, and sport drinks. The volume of liquid ingested is less important than the absence of particulate matter. Patients with additional risk factors for aspiration (e.g., morbid obesity, diabetes, difficult airway) or laboring patients at increased risk for cesarean delivery (e.g., nonreassuring FHR pattern) may have further restrictions of oral intake, determined on a case-by-case basis.[24]

Ingestion of solid foods should be avoided in laboring patients and patients undergoing elective surgery (e.g., scheduled cesarean delivery or postpartum tubal sterilization). A fasting period for solids of 6 to 8 hours, depending on the fat content of the food, has been recommended.[24]

A reduction in gastric content acidity and volume is believed to decrease the risk for damage to the respiratory epithelium should aspiration occur. Oral administration of a nonparticulate antacid (e.g., 0.3 M **sodium citrate**, pH 8.4) causes the mean gastric pH to increase to greater than 6 for 1 hour; it does not affect gastric volume.[38] **Histamine-2 (H$_2$)-receptor antagonists** (e.g., **ranitidine, famotidine**), **proton pump inhibitors** (e.g., **omeprazole**), and **metoclopramide** reduce gastric acid secretion and volume but require at least 30 to 40 minutes to exert their effects.[39] A systematic review of interventions used to reduce the risk for aspiration pneumonitis in women undergoing cesarean delivery found that there were significant reductions in the risk for gastric pH < 2.5 with antacids (relative risk [RR], 0.17; 95% CI, 0.09 to 0.32), H$_2$-receptor antagonists (RR, 0.09; 95% CI, 0.05 to 0.18), and proton-pump inhibitors (RR, 0.26; 95% CI, 0.14 to

0.46), compared with no treatment or placebo.[40] The combined use of an antacid and an H$_2$-receptor antagonist was found to be more effective in reducing gastric acidity than administration of placebo or an antacid alone.[40] However, in a randomized evaluation, sodium citrate was associated with a higher incidence and severity of nausea than an H$_2$-receptor antagonist (famotidine), suggesting that a H$_2$-receptor antagonist may be the preferred agent in selected patients.[41] **Metoclopramide** is a promotility agent that hastens gastric emptying, increases lower esophageal sphincter tone, and decreases nausea and vomiting.[42] Before surgical procedures, the timely administration of a nonparticulate antacid, an H$_2$-receptor antagonist, and metoclopramide should be considered, especially for nonelective procedures.[24]

Prophylactic Antibiotics

Prophylactic antibiotic administration results in a 60% decrease in the incidence of endometritis, a 25% to 65% decrease in the incidence of wound infection, and fewer episodes of fever and urinary tract infections for both elective (nonlaboring) and nonelective (laboring) cesarean deliveries.[43] The ACOG[44] has recommended the prophylactic administration of a narrow-spectrum antibiotic, such as a first-generation cephalosporin, within 1 hour of the start of cesarean delivery.

Antibiotics with efficacy against gram-positive, gram-negative, and some anaerobic bacteria are commonly used for prophylaxis for cesarean delivery. Appropriate antibiotics include IV ampicillin 2 g, cefazolin 2 g, or ceftriaxone 1 g. Appropriate antibiotic coverage should last for 3 to 4 hours; therefore, ampicillin may be less appropriate owing to a shorter half-life than the cephalosporins.[44,45] In parturients with a significant allergy to beta-lactam antibiotics (e.g., history of anaphylaxis, angioedema, respiratory distress, or urticaria), intravenous clindamycin with gentamicin is a reasonable alternative.

Higher doses of antibiotics may be considered in women with a body mass index (BMI) > 30 kg/m^2 or an absolute weight > 120 kg because of a greater volume of distribution.[44,46] After administration of cephazolin 2 g, Pevzner et al.[46] observed that the minimum inhibitory tissue concentration for gram-negative rods was not achieved at the time of skin incision or closure in 20% of obese women and 33% of morbidly obese women.

A randomized controlled trial addressed whether surgical site infection prophylaxis should be broadened to cover species commonly associated with postcesarean infection (e.g., ureaplasma).[47] Women undergoing cesarean delivery after labor or rupture of membranes were randomized to receive standard antibiotics with or without the addition of azithromycin (500 mg). Although the addition of azithromycin decreased the rate of the composite infection endpoint by half (6.1% versus 12.0%), almost three-fourths of the trial participants were obese, raising concern that the standard antibiotics may have been underdosed.[47] The 2018 ACOG guidelines suggest that prophylactic azithromycin administration may be considered for nonelective cesarean delivery.[44]

In the past, prophylactic antibiotics were typically administered after umbilical cord clamping because of concern that fetal antibiotic exposure might mask a nascent infection and/or increase the likelihood of a neonatal sepsis evaluation. However, a metaanalysis demonstrated that preincision antibiotic prophylaxis reduces the incidence of postcesarean endometritis and total maternal infectious morbidity, without evidence of adverse neonatal effects.[48]

Thus, current guidelines recommend administration of prophylactic antibiotics, including azithromycin (when indicated), within 60 minutes before the start of the cesarean delivery.[44]

Aseptic Technique

In the early 19th century, Ignác Semmelweis observed that puerperal fever, known as "childbed fever," was most likely transmitted when the first stage of labor was prolonged and multiple individuals performed vaginal examinations with contaminated hands. Since that time, the practice of hand hygiene has caused a significant reduction in maternal and neonatal infectious morbidity.

The immunologic changes of pregnancy may impair clearance of infections.[49] Epidural abscess and meningitis have been reported as complications of neuraxial procedures in obstetric patients (see Chapter 31). As a consequence, obstetric anesthesia providers should always give careful attention to aseptic technique, especially during the performance of a neuraxial procedure. Proper sterile technique for neuraxial procedures includes wearing a facemask, performing hand hygiene, and donning sterile gloves (see Chapter 12).[50] Although wearing sterile gowns is common in many countries, there is little available evidence addressing this practice and wearing gowns is controversial and less common in the United States.[51] Attention should also be given to the careful preparation of anesthetic drugs during administration of either general or neuraxial anesthesia. An increasing number of institutions are using premixed solutions of local anesthetic and opioid (prepared under aseptic conditions in a hospital or compounding pharmacy) to limit breaches in aseptic technique during the administration of neuraxial anesthesia.

Intravenous Access and Fluid Management

The establishment of functional intravenous access is of critical importance to the successful outcome of many clinical situations in obstetric anesthesia practice. According to the Hagen-Poiseuille equation, laminar flow of fluid through a cylindrical tube is directly proportional to the pressure gradient of the fluid and the fourth power of the tube's radius, and inversely proportional to the viscosity of the fluid and the tube's length. Extrapolation to intravenous catheters indicates that the size of the catheter, more than the size of the vein, dictates the flow rate; the use of a short, large-diameter catheter (e.g., 18-, 16-, or 14-gauge) is associated with the best flow.[52]

In general, a smaller but functional catheter is likely to be more effective than a larger catheter that is unreliable or requires frequent manipulation. In an emergency situation, if only a 20- or 22-gauge intravenous catheter is present, high flow rates for volume resuscitation can be achieved (without evidence of greater red blood cell destruction) by application of a pressure bag and diluting red blood cells with normal saline.[53] Devices are available to change a small-gauge intravenous catheter to a large-gauge intravenous catheter using a Seldinger technique. In situations when large blood loss is anticipated, or administration of multiple blood products is required, the anesthesia provider may choose to insert a central venous catheter.

Although the administration of intravenous fluids may decrease the incidence of neuraxial anesthesia-associated hypotension, initiation of anesthesia should not be delayed to administer a fixed volume of fluid,[24] particularly in the case of an emergency cesarean delivery, in which the life and health of the mother and the infant are best preserved with timely delivery. The type of fluid (crystalloid, colloid) and the volume, rate, and timing of administration are relevant factors in the prevention and treatment of hypotension.[54,55] In most situations, a balanced salt solution such as lactated Ringer's solution is acceptable. Blood products are most often administered with normal saline. Crystalloid or colloid solutions that contain calcium or glucose should not be administered with blood products, owing to the risks for clotting (caused by reversal of the citrate anticoagulant) and clumping of red blood cells, respectively.

Traditionally, approximately 1 L of crystalloid solution has been administered intravenously before induction of neuraxial anesthesia (as "preload" or "prehydration") to prevent or reduce the incidence and severity of hypotension. However, preload, even with large volumes (30 mL/kg), is minimally effective in preventing neuraxial anesthesia-induced hypotension. Although an initial study found that administering crystalloid solution at the time of the intrathecal injection ("coload" or "cohydration") was more efficacious than preload in preventing hypotension,[56] later studies did not support this finding,[57] likely because the infusion rate was too slow.[55] Colloid preload or coload is more effective than crystalloid for preventing hypotension.[58] Colloid coload is equally efficacious as preload.[57] In healthy patients, we rapidly administer approximately 1 L of crystalloid starting at the time of initiation of neuraxial anesthesia. For patients at high risk for hypotension or its consequences, colloid preload or coload may be considered.[55] Regardless of fluid administration, hypotension is best prevented and treated using vasopressors (see discussion below).

Supplemental Medications for Anxiety

The administration of benzodiazepines, even low doses (e.g., **midazolam** 0.02 mg/kg), may result in amnesia[59]; therefore, benzodiazepines are typically avoided during awake cesarean delivery. However, on occasion, particularly in women with severe anxiety or undergoing an emergency cesarean delivery, the use of low doses of intravenous midazolam or an opioid may facilitate performance of a neuraxial technique, awake tracheal intubation, or the induction of general anesthesia. Anxiolytics may also assist in mitigating the feelings of distress during the birthing experience, which may lessen the risk for developing posttraumatic stress disorder.[60] The use of low doses of sedative or anxiolytic agents has minimal to no neonatal effects. In a trial of healthy women randomized to receive intravenous midazolam (0.02 mg/kg) and fentanyl (1 μg/kg[b]) or saline before administration of spinal

---

[b]The Institute for Safe Medicine Practices has recommended that healthcare providers never use μg as an abbreviation for micrograms, but rather they should use mcg (http://www.ismp.org/tools/errorproneabbreviations.pdf, Accessed 4 August 2024). The use of the symbol μg is frequently misinterpreted and involved in harmful medication errors. The abbreviation may be mistaken for mg (milligrams), which would result in a 1000-fold overdose. The symbol μg should never be used when communicating medical information, including pharmacy and prescriber computer order entry screens, computer-generated labels, labels for drug storage bins, and medication administration records. However, most scholarly publications have continued to use the abbreviation μg. The editors have chosen to retain the use of the abbreviation μg throughout this text. However, the editors recommend the use of the abbreviation mcg in clinical practice.

anesthesia for cesarean delivery, no differences in neonatal Apgar scores, neurobehavioral scores, or oxygen saturation were observed between the two treatment groups.[61]

Positioning

After 20 weeks' gestation, most practitioners position patients with left uterine displacement to minimize aortocaval compression. The **supine hypotension syndrome**, which is caused by compression of the inferior vena cava and the aorta by the gravid uterus, can manifest as pallor, tachycardia, sweating, nausea, hypotension, and dizziness.[62] Uteroplacental blood flow is compromised by decreased venous return and cardiac output, increased uterine venous pressure, and compression of the aorta or common iliac arteries.[63]

The full lateral position minimizes aortocaval compression but does not allow performance of cesarean delivery. Fifteen degrees of **left lateral tilt (left uterine displacement)** has been proposed to significantly reduce the adverse hemodynamic consequences of the supine position, although both the aorta and inferior vena cava may remain partially compressed.[64] However, most anesthesia providers overestimate the degree of lateral tilt applied. These elements may explain the results of a 2013 systematic review that concluded that left compared with right lateral tilt was associated with some maternal and fetal benefit, but outcomes were not dramatically different among different positions.[65] Overall, data were insufficient to prove or disprove the benefits of tilting or flexing the operating room table or using wedges or mechanical displacers during positioning for cesarean delivery.[65]

Whether left uterine displacement is necessary in the context of patients receiving a coload of fluid and a prophylactic phenylephrine infusion at the time of induction of spinal anesthesia has been questioned.[66] In healthy, term women undergoing elective cesarean delivery, there was no difference in neonatal acid-base status in women randomized to the supine position versus left uterine displacement, despite mean maternal cardiac output being lower in the supine group.[66] The trial excluded women at increased risk for aortocaval compression (e.g., polyhydramnios, multiple gestation, obesity) or women with impaired placental perfusion (e.g., fetal growth restriction, preeclampsia). Given these limitations, and the apparent absence of adverse maternal or fetal effects with lateral uterine displacement, the routine use of this technique should not be abandoned.[67] Anesthesia providers should recognize that (1) susceptibility to aortocaval compression varies among individuals[68]; (2) visual estimates of lateral tilt may be in error[69]; and (3) in symptomatic women, increasing the extent of left uterine displacement may be beneficial. Lateral tilt should be used in all women in mid- to late pregnancy after the administration of neuraxial or general anesthesia, with greater tilt used when feasible if aortocaval compression is suspected as the cause for maternal or fetal compromise.[70]

The use of a slight (10 degrees) **head-up position** may help reduce the incidence of hypotension after initiation of hyperbaric spinal anesthesia.[71] A 30-degree head-up position significantly increases functional residual capacity compared with the supine position in term parturients, although this effect diminishes with increasing BMI.[72] In morbidly obese patients receiving general anesthesia, a 25-degree head-up position may be particularly useful to improve denitrogenation and glottic view during direct laryngoscopy[73]; this position can be accomplished with blankets or commercially available devices (see Chapters 29 and 48). If blankets are used to create the ramp position, they should be stacked rather than interlaced, to allow for rapid removal and readjustment of the head and neck position, if necessary. The ideal position aligns the external auditory meatus and the sternal notch in a horizontal plane; this position (1) aligns the oral, pharyngeal, and tracheal axes ("sniffing position") and (2) facilitates insertion of the laryngoscope blade.[74]

Theoretically, the **Trendelenburg (head-down) position** may augment venous return and increase cardiac output. The value of this approach in *preventing* hypotension during neuraxial anesthesia has been questioned.[65] After the initiation of hyperbaric spinal anesthesia, the Trendelenburg position was reported to result in more cephalad spread of anesthesia in one study[75] but not in others.[76,77] However, this position had no effect on the incidence of hypotension after the administration of hyperbaric spinal anesthesia.[75,77]

The optimal patient position for initiation of neuraxial anesthesia may depend on clinical circumstances and the preferences and skills of the anesthesia provider (see Chapter 12). Whether the use of the **lateral** or the **sitting position** is best for routine initiation of neuraxial anesthesia is controversial.[78,79] Advocates of the lateral position cite reduced vagal reflexes, which can result in dizziness, diaphoresis, pallor, bradycardia, and hypotension,[80] and improved uteroplacental blood flow, compared with the sitting position.[81] The lateral position may also be associated with a small increase in maternal cardiac index, stroke volume index, heart rate, and systolic blood pressure compared with the sitting or supine positions.[82] Further, in a randomized controlled trial, the severity and duration of hypotension were greater in women randomly assigned to receive CSE anesthesia (hyperbaric spinal bupivacaine with fentanyl) in the sitting position than the lateral position, despite no differences in the level of sensory blockade.[83]

Some parturients find the lateral position more comfortable during administration of neuraxial anesthesia, whereas others find the sitting position more comfortable.[84] Moreover, because uterine compression of the vena cava diverts blood into the epidural venous plexus,[85] the use of the lateral position can reduce hydrostatic pressure and engorgement of the epidural venous plexus.[86] Studies suggest that epidural catheter placement in the lateral recumbent head-down position results in lower risk for lumbar epidural venous plexus cannulation than the sitting or the lateral recumbent horizontal position in both obese and nonobese parturients.[87,88]

MRI and computed tomography studies have shown that the cross-sectional area and the anteroposterior diameter of the dural sac at the level of the L3 to L4, L4 to L5, and L5 to S1 interspaces are significantly influenced by posture.[89] Lumbar cerebrospinal fluid (CSF) pressure is lower and the dural sac cross-sectional area smaller in the recumbent compared with the upright position. Theoretically, the lateral position may be of value during advancement of an epidural needle because it minimizes the prominence of the dural sac. By contrast, a bulging dural sac might be preferable during administration of spinal, dural puncture epidural (DPE), or CSE anesthesia. Bulging of the lumbar dural sac—particularly in the sitting position—may decrease the force required to create a dural puncture with a Tuohy epidural needle, but this possibility is unproven.

The sitting position also has some advantages, including easier landmark recognition in obese parturients and ease of positioning patients in a symmetrical position (the spine is often rotated in the lateral position because the bottom shoulder is fixed).[79] Given that there is no evidence that one position is universally better than the other, patient position for initiating neuraxial anesthesia is largely a matter of practitioner preference. However, anesthesia providers should be facile with the placement of needles for neuraxial techniques in both the sitting and lateral positions because the sitting position should not be used in some situations (e.g., umbilical cord prolapse, footling breech presentation).[78]

Supplemental Oxygen

The routine administration of supplemental oxygen during elective cesarean delivery with neuraxial anesthesia is controversial. It became a common practice following the 1971 report by Fox and Houle[90] that demonstrated improved oxygenation, better umbilical cord blood acid-base measurements, and less time to sustained respiration in the neonate when mothers undergoing cesarean delivery with neuraxial anesthesia breathed 100% oxygen instead of air for at least 10 minutes. However, this practice has not been supported by subsequent work. A 2021 metaanalysis of randomized trials performed in low-risk women undergoing elective cesarean delivery with singleton, nonanomalous pregnancies, found that the administration of supplemental oxygen compared with room air was associated with higher umbilical arterial (UA) Pao_2, and no significant differences in UA base excess, UA pH < 7.2, Apgar scores, or neonatal intensive care unit (ICU) admissions.[91]

The use of a fractional inspired concentration of oxygen (Fio_2) of 0.35 to 0.4, which cannot be obtained by using a nasal cannula or a simple face mask with a flow rate < 6 L/ min,[92] does not improve fetal oxygenation during labor or elective cesarean delivery. Although respiratory function can deteriorate in parturients receiving neuraxial anesthesia, maternal or fetal hypoxemia does not normally occur when parturients breathe room air.[93] An Fio_2 of 0.6 in nonlaboring women undergoing elective cesarean delivery with spinal anesthesia was shown to increase umbilical venous (UV) oxygen content by only 12%; an increase in oxygen content was not observed when the uterine incision-to-delivery (U-D) interval exceeded 180 seconds.[94]

Supplemental oxygen may have detrimental effects.[95] High levels of maternal Fio_2 are necessary for significant maternal-fetal oxygen transfer, but also result in the formation of reactive oxygen species and subsequent peroxidation of lipids, alteration of cellular enzymatic functions, and destruction of genetic material.[96] Known to extend ischemia-reperfusion injury, deplete antioxidants, and suppress immune function,[95] free radicals have also been implicated in the pathogenesis of disorders related to prematurity, including neonatal retinopathy, bronchopulmonary dysplasia, necrotizing enterocolitis, and intraventricular hemorrhage.

Nonetheless, the emergency cesarean delivery of the compromised fetus should include maternal oxygen administration of high Fio_2, particularly in the setting of uterine contractions, which can exacerbate fetal compromise; in these situations, supplemental oxygen may reduce the severity of fetal hypoxia with limited oxygen free-radical effects.[97] Term (but not preterm) fetuses may be able to withstand the adverse effects of these reactive oxygen species through a compensatory increase in antioxidants during labor.[98,99] Antioxidants, the defense against reactive oxygen species, consist of enzymatic inactivators (superoxide dismutase, catalase, peroxidase) and scavengers (ascorbate, glutathione, transferrin, lactoferrin, ceruloplasmin). The activity of these compensatory mechanisms and their relationship to gestational age and labor suggest that the highest risk for ischemia-reperfusion injury occurs in preterm fetuses before the onset of labor.[95,99]

The use of high Fio_2 (>0.6) improves oxygen transfer to hypoxic fetuses for a limited period (approximately 10 minutes); beyond this time, continued hyperoxia, especially in the setting of restored perfusion, increases reactive oxygen species, placental vasoconstriction, and fetal acidosis.[100,101] A lower Fio_2 may be of benefit in some situations. Of interest, when asphyxiated infants are immediately resuscitated at birth with air instead of 100% oxygen, better short-term outcomes have been observed[102,103]; this finding may be a result of the shift in the balance between beneficial oxygenation and detrimental free radicals.

All women who are at risk for requiring general anesthesia for emergency cesarean delivery should receive an Fio_2 of 1.0 after transfer to the operating table to simultaneously promote maternal oxygenation and denitrogenation; denitrogenation significantly reduces the risk for maternal hypoxemia during apnea before tracheal intubation.

Although the value of supplemental oxygen use during *elective* cesarean delivery with neuraxial anesthesia of a noncompromised fetus is questionable, some obstetric anesthesia providers place nasal cannulae or a mask to monitor ventilation using expired carbon dioxide analysis.

ANESTHETIC TECHNIQUE

Providing anesthesia to the parturient is a dynamic, multistep process (Table 26.1). The most appropriate anesthetic technique for cesarean delivery depends on maternal, fetal, and obstetric factors (Table 26.2). The urgency and anticipated duration of the operation play an important role in the selection of an anesthetic technique. A standardized four-grade classification system, originally proposed in the United

TABLE 26.1 Provision of Anesthesia for Cesarean Delivery[a]

Phase	Issues	Specific Concerns
Preparation	Preanesthetic evaluation	History and physical examination
		Indicated laboratory measurements
		Imaging studies
	Oral intake	No clear liquids and solid foods for 2 h and 6–8 h respectively, before elective surgery (the presence of comorbid conditions may warrant a longer fasting interval)
	Communication with obstetric team	Indication(s) for cesarean delivery, including degree of urgency
		Anticipated surgical complications
	Informed consent	Threshold, information, and consent elements
		Informed refusal
	Blood products	Risk factors for hemorrhage
		Baseline hematocrit or hemoglobin measurement
		Blood type and screen or cross-match
		Equipment for rapid transfusion
	Monitoring	Pulse oximetry, electrocardiogram, blood pressure, fetal heart rate, urinary catheter
		Consider electroencephalographic (bispectral index) monitoring during general anesthesia (controversial)
		Invasive monitoring in selected patients
	Medication availability	Anesthetic (general and neuraxial anesthetic drugs, vasopressors)
		Obstetric (uterotonic agents)
		Emergency (advanced cardiac life support, malignant hyperthermia)
	Equipment availability	Anesthesia, airway management
	Aspiration prophylaxis	Fasting guidelines, nonparticulate antacid, H_2-receptor antagonist, metoclopramide
	Prophylactic antibiotics[b]	Within 60 min *before* incision
	Intravenous access and fluid management	Intravenous catheter: 18-gauge or larger
		Fluid type, volume, and rate
	Supplemental medications	Consider anxiolysis for severe anxiety
	Positioning	Lateral or sitting position for neuraxial needle/catheter placement
		Left uterine displacement, slight head up for surgery
		"Sniffing" position if general anesthesia is planned
	Supplemental oxygen	Preoxygenation/denitrogenation required before general anesthesia
		Of unclear benefit during neuraxial anesthesia for elective delivery of a noncompromised fetus
Selection of anesthetic technique	Neuraxial	Adequate sacral and cephalad spread (T4) and density of neuroblockade
		Prevention or treatment of hypotension
	General	Airway management
		Prevention of awareness and recall
		Prevention of anesthesia-associated uterine atony
	Local	Usually a supplement for inadequate neuraxial anesthesia
		Can facilitate emergency delivery in absence of an anesthesia provider
		Rarely provides satisfactory anesthesia as a primary technique

(Continued)

TABLE 26.1 Provision of Anesthesia for Cesarean Delivery[a]—cont'd

Phase	Issues	Specific Concerns
Recovery	Oral intake	Fluids and foods allowed within 4-8 h of surgery, in absence of complications
	Removal of urinary catheter	Typically within 24 h
	Postoperative assessment and discharge	Hemodynamic stability
		Resolution of neuroblockade
		Effective analgesia
		Recognition and treatment of surgical and anesthetic complications

[a]Procedures, techniques, and drugs may need to be modified for individual patients and circumstances.
[b]Evidence suggests that administration of prophylactic antibiotics *before* incision (rather than after cord clamping) reduces the incidence of postcesarean endometritis and total maternal infectious morbidity.[44]

TABLE 26.2 Selection of Anesthetic Technique for Cesarean Delivery

Indication(s)	Comments/Examples
For Neuraxial Anesthesia[a]	
Maternal desire to witness birth and/or avoid general anesthesia	Most common maternal preference
Risk factors for difficult airway or aspiration	Physical examination predicts possible difficult airway
	History of difficult tracheal intubation
	High body mass index (obesity)
	History of gastroesophageal reflux (common in pregnancy)
Presence of comorbid conditions	Malignant hyperthermia history
	Pulmonary disease
General anesthesia intolerance or failure	History of significant side effects with general anesthesia
	Attempted general anesthesia with failed intubation; patient awakened
Other benefits	Plan for neuraxial analgesia after surgery
	Less fetal drug exposure
	Less blood loss
	Allows presence of husband or support person
For General Anesthesia[a]	
Maternal refusal or failure to cooperate with neuraxial technique	Strong maternal preference, in the absence of factors that predict a difficult airway
	Severe psychiatric disorder
	Severe developmental delay
	Severe emotional immaturity or lability
Presence of comorbid conditions that contraindicate a neuraxial technique	Coagulopathy
	Local infection at neuraxial insertion site
	Sepsis
	Severe uncorrected hypovolemia (e.g., hemorrhage from placenta previa or uterine rupture)
	Intracranial mass with increased intracranial pressure
	Known allergy to local anesthetic (rare)
Insufficient time to induce neuraxial anesthesia for urgent delivery	Umbilical cord prolapse with persistent fetal bradycardia
Failure of neuraxial technique	Multiple needle placement failures
	Missed spinal segments
	Persistent intraoperative pain that is not treated successfully
Fetal issues	Planned *ex utero* intrapartum treatment (EXIT) procedure

[a]Many indications for or contraindications to specific anesthesia techniques are relative, and the choice of anesthetic must be tailored to individual circumstances.

Kingdom in 2000, may be used to communicate the degree of urgency among providers (Table 26.3).[104] Using such a classification system also facilitates comparing data and outcomes among providers and institutions.[104]

In cases of dire fetal compromise, the anesthesia provider may need to perform a preanesthetic evaluation simultaneously with other tasks (i.e., establishing intravenous access and placing a blood pressure cuff, pulse oximeter probe, and ECG electrodes). Regardless of the urgency, the anesthesia provider should not compromise maternal safety by failing to obtain critical information about previous medical and anesthetic history, allergies, and the airway. Effective communication with the obstetric team is critical to establish the degree of urgency, which helps guide decisions regarding anesthetic management. Further, contemporary standards for patient safety require that all members of the surgical team participate in a preoperative "time-out" to verify (1) the correct patient identity, position, and operative site; (2) agreement on the procedure to be performed; and (3) the availability of special equipment, if needed.

In cases of emergency cesarean delivery, the emotional needs of the mother and father are also important. Parental distress commonly occurs in this setting, and the anesthesia provider is often the best person to give reassurance. All members of the obstetric care team should remember that chaos does not need to accompany urgency.

TABLE 26.3 Classification for Urgency of Cesarean Delivery

Grade	Label	Definition	Example
1	Emergency	Immediate threat to life of mother or fetus	Prolonged fetal bradycardia
2	Urgent	Maternal or fetal compromise that is not immediately life threatening	Deep variable decelerations with cervical dilation of 3 cm
3	Scheduled	Needing early delivery but no maternal or fetal compromise	Ruptured membranes with previously undiagnosed breech presentation
4	Elective	At a time to suit the mother and delivery team	Elective repeat cesarean delivery

Modified from Lucas DN, Yentis SM, Kinsella SM, et al. Urgency of caesarean section: a new classification. *J R Soc Med.* 2000;93: 346–350.

Neuraxial Versus General Anesthesia

Overall, neuraxial (epidural, spinal, CSE) techniques are the preferred method for providing anesthesia for cesarean delivery; specific benefits and risks of each technique dictate the eventual choice. In contemporary practice, neuraxial anesthesia is administered to some patients who would have received general anesthesia in the past. Umbilical cord prolapse, placenta previa, and preeclampsia with severe features are no longer considered absolute indications for general anesthesia. For example, in some cases, a prolapsed umbilical cord can be decompressed, and if fetal status is reassuring, a neuraxial technique can be used. In an analysis of obstetric anesthesia trends in the United States between 1981 and 2012, a progressive increase was noted in the use of neuraxial anesthesia, especially spinal anesthesia, for both elective and emergency cesarean deliveries.[17] Neuraxial anesthesia is now used for more than 95% of elective cesarean deliveries and 80% of emergency cesarean deliveries in the United States,[17,105] with progress in a similar direction among high- and low-resource countries.

The greater use of neuraxial anesthesia for cesarean delivery has been attributed to several factors, including (1) the growing use of epidural techniques for labor analgesia, (2) an awareness of the possibility that an *in situ* epidural catheter may decrease the necessity for general anesthesia in an urgent situation, (3) improvement in the quality of neuraxial anesthesia with the addition of an opioid to the local anesthetic, (4) appreciation of the risks of airway complications during general anesthesia in parturients, (5) the desire for limited neonatal drug transfer, and (6) the ability of the mother to remain awake to experience childbirth and to have a support person present in the operating room. Spinal anesthesia is considered an appropriate technique even in the most urgent settings; in a tertiary care institution with an average of 9500 cesarean deliveries annually, neuraxial anesthesia was used in more than 99% of cesarean deliveries over a 6-year period.[106] In the setting of a category 1 (immediate threat to life of woman or fetus) cesarean delivery, Kinsella et al.[107] described a "rapid-sequence spinal" technique, by which skin preparation, spinal drug combinations, and the spinal technique were simplified; the median time from positioning until satisfactory neuroblockade was 8 minutes (interquartile range [IQR], 7 to 8 minutes; range, 6 to 8 minutes).

Maternal *mortality* following general anesthesia has been a primary motivator for the transition toward greater use of neuraxial anesthesia for cesarean delivery. Hawkins et al.[108] compared the anesthesia-related maternal mortality rate from 1979 to 1984 with that for the period from 1985 to 1990 in the United States. The estimated case-fatality risk ratio for general versus neuraxial anesthesia was as high as 16.7 in the years 1985 to 1990. However, a subsequent analysis by the same group found a nonsignificant risk ratio of 1.7 in the years 1991 to 2002.[109] Possible explanations for this change include better anesthetic monitoring, published standards for anesthetic care, and technological advances in the devices available for airway management and their widespread dissemination (e.g., supraglottic airways, fiberoptic bronchoscopes). It is possible that the relative risk associated with general anesthesia may be overstated because general anesthesia is mainly used when medical reasons or time constraints preclude the use of neuraxial anesthesia.

The type of maternal *morbidity* differs between neuraxial anesthetic techniques and general anesthesia. A systematic review of randomized and quasirandomized controlled trials comparing major maternal and neonatal outcomes with the use of neuraxial anesthesia and general anesthesia for cesarean delivery found less maternal blood loss and shivering but more nausea in the neuraxial anesthesia group.[110] The intraoperative "perception" of pain was greater in the neuraxial group, but the time elapsed before the first postoperative request for analgesia was longer. Prospective audits of postcesarean delivery outcomes have indicated that in the first postoperative week, patients who received neuraxial anesthesia had less pain, gastrointestinal stasis, coughing, fever, and depression and were able to breastfeed and ambulate more quickly than patients who received general anesthesia.[111]

Neonatal outcomes associated with maternal anesthetic selection require further study. Apgar and neonatal neurobehavioral scores are relatively insensitive measures of neonatal well-being, and umbilical cord blood gas and pH measurements may reflect the reason for the cesarean delivery rather than differences related to the anesthetic technique. In a metaanalysis, lower umbilical cord blood pH measurements were associated with spinal, but not epidural, anesthesia compared with general anesthesia.[112] However, the study included both randomized and nonrandomized trials and both elective and nonelective procedures, and most trials were conducted in an era when ephedrine was used to support maternal blood pressure (see discussion below). In a systematic review of randomized trials in which the indication for cesarean delivery was not urgent, no differences in umbilical cord arterial blood pH measurements were found among general and neuraxial anesthetic techniques[110]; similar findings were observed when the anesthesia induction-to-delivery interval was prolonged, such as in more complex obstetric surgeries (e.g., placenta accreta spectrum, higher-order cesarean deliveries, and morbid obesity).[113]

Overview of Neuraxial Anesthetic Techniques

Table 26.4 outlines the relative advantages and disadvantages of the various neuraxial anesthetic techniques for cesarean delivery. With all neuraxial techniques, an adequate sensory level of anesthesia is necessary to minimize maternal pain and avoid the urgent need for administration of general anesthesia. Because motor nerve fibers are typically larger and more difficult to block, the complete absence of hip flexion and ankle dorsiflexion most likely indicates that a functional sensory and sympathetic block is also present in a similar (primarily lumbosacral) distribution. However, because afferent nerves innervating abdominal and pelvic organs accompany sympathetic fibers that ascend and descend in the sympathetic trunk (T5 to L1), a sensory block that extends rostrally from the sacral dermatomes to T4 should be the goal for cesarean delivery anesthesia.

TABLE 26.4 Advantages and Disadvantages of Neuraxial Anesthetic Techniques for Cesarean Delivery

Neuraxial Technique	Advantages	Disadvantages
Epidural	No dural puncture required Can use *in situ* catheter placed for earlier administration of labor analgesia Ability to titrate extent of sensory blockade Continuous intraoperative anesthesia Continuous postoperative analgesia	Slow onset of anesthesia. Larger drug doses required than for spinal techniques: • Greater risk for maternal local anesthetic systemic toxicity • Greater fetal drug exposure
Combined spinal-epidural	May be technically easier than spinal anesthesia in obese patients Low doses of local anesthetic and opioid Rapid onset of dense lumbosacral and thoracic anesthesia Ability to titrate extent of sensory blockade Continuous intraoperative anesthesia Continuous postoperative analgesia	Delayed verification of functioning epidural catheter
Continuous spinal	Low doses of local anesthetic and opioid Rapid onset of dense anesthesia Ability to titrate extent of sensory blockade Continuous intraoperative anesthesia	Large dural puncture increases risk for postdural puncture headache Possibility of overdose and total spinal anesthesia if the spinal catheter is mistaken for an epidural catheter
Single-shot spinal	Technically simple Low doses of local anesthetic and opioid Rapid onset of dense lumbosacral and thoracic anesthesia	Limited duration of anesthesia Limited ability to titrate extent of sensory blockade

The manner in which the level of sensory blockade is assessed has implications for the success of a neuraxial technique. The different methods of assessing the extent of sensory blockade (i.e., sensation to light touch, pinprick, cold) may indicate levels of blockade that differ by several spinal segments. A prospective study of 102 women undergoing cesarean delivery with spinal anesthesia indicated that although sensory blockade to light touch differed from sensory blockade to pinprick or cold sensation by 0 to 11 spinal segments, no constant relationship among these levels could be determined.[114] The investigators concluded that a T6 blockade to touch would likely provide a pain-free cesarean delivery for most women.

Sensory examination should move caudad to cephalad in the midaxillary line on the lower extremities but can be performed in the midclavicular line on the torso. The time at which an adequate block is achieved, as well as the cephalad level of the block and the presence of surgical anesthesia of the lower abdomen, should be documented on the anesthetic record.

Because the undersurface of the diaphragm (C3 to C5) and the vagus nerve may be stimulated by surgical manipulation during cesarean delivery,[115] maternal discomfort (including shoulder pain) and other symptoms (e.g., nausea and vomiting) may occur despite a T4 level of blockade. Neuraxial or systemic opioids help prevent or alleviate these symptoms (see discussion below).

Spinal Anesthesia

Spinal anesthesia is a simple and reliable technique that allows visual confirmation of correct needle placement (by visualization of CSF) and is technically easier to perform than epidural anesthesia. Spinal anesthesia provides rapid onset of dense neuroblockade that is typically more profound than that provided with epidural anesthesia, resulting in a reduced need for supplemental intravenous analgesics or conversion to general anesthesia.[116,117] Only a small amount of local anesthetic is needed to establish functional spinal blockade; therefore, spinal anesthesia is associated with negligible maternal risk for local anesthetic systemic toxicity (LAST) and with minimal drug transfer to the fetus. Given these advantages, spinal anesthesia is the most commonly used anesthetic technique for cesarean delivery in the developed world.[17] Spinal anesthesia is also associated with predictable and relatively prompt recovery that enables patients to quickly transition through the postanesthesia care unit (PACU); in some settings, such a recovery may result in a cost savings to the institution.[116]

Spinal anesthesia is usually administered as a single-injection procedure ("single-shot" technique) through a non-cutting, pencil-point needle that is 25-gauge or smaller. A number of different needle designs are available (see Chapter 12); the size and design of the needle tip affect the incidence and severity of postdural puncture headache (see Chapter 30).

The spinal technique should be performed at the L3 to L4 interspace or below (see Chapter 12). This space is used to avoid the potential for spinal cord trauma; although the spinal cord ends at L1 in most adults, it extends to the L2 to L3 interspace in a small minority (see Chapter 31). Additionally, anesthesia providers often misidentify the location of the needle insertion site on the spinal column, and the needle is frequently introduced at a higher level than intended.[118]

On occasion, a continuous spinal anesthetic technique is used, particularly in the setting of an unintentional dural puncture with an epidural needle followed by the intentional threading of the epidural catheter into the intrathecal space.[119] Planned continuous spinal anesthesia may be desirable in certain settings, when the reliability of a spinal technique and the ability to precisely titrate the initiation and duration of anesthesia are strongly desired (e.g., a morbidly obese patient with a difficult airway). Continuous spinal anesthesia may be administered through purpose-intended spinal catheters or using equipment designed for epidural anesthesia (see Chapter 12).

Local Anesthetic Agents

The choice of local anesthetic agent (and adjuvants) used to provide spinal anesthesia depends on the expected duration of the surgery, the postoperative analgesia plan, the preferences of the anesthesia provider, and availability. For cesarean delivery, the local anesthetic agent of choice is typically **bupivacaine** (Table 26.5). In the United States, spinal bupivacaine is formulated as a 0.75% solution in dextrose 8.25%; in other countries, use of a 0.5% concentration is common.

The dose of intrathecal bupivacaine that has been successfully used for cesarean delivery ranges from 4.5 to 15 mg. In general, pregnant patients require smaller doses of spinal local anesthetic than nonpregnant patients. Reasons include (1) a smaller CSF volume in pregnancy, (2) cephalad movement of hyperbaric local anesthetic in the supine pregnant patient, and (3) greater sensitivity of nerve fibers to the local anesthetic during pregnancy.[120] Overall, the mass of local anesthetic, rather than the concentration or volume, is thought to be the most important factor influencing the spread of the resulting blockade[121]; however, the specific influence of the dose/concentration and baricity on the efficacy of the block is controversial. The required dose may be influenced by other factors, such as coadministration of neuraxial opioids and surgical technique (e.g., exteriorization of the uterus during closure of the uterus is more stimulating than closure *in situ*).

A dose-finding study in 48 women undergoing cesarean delivery demonstrated that the ED_{50} and ED_{95} values (effective dose in 50% and 95% of patients, respectively) for plain bupivacaine with fentanyl 10 µg and morphine 0.2 mg were 7.25 and 13 mg, respectively.[122] However, other studies have shown that lower doses of hyperbaric or plain bupivacaine can be used successfully, particularly when coadministered with an opioid (e.g., 9 mg with fentanyl 20 µg,[123] and 6.6 mg with sufentanil 3.3 µg[124]). Use of lower doses of local anesthetic has been shown to decrease the incidence of hypotension and nausea.[125] Whether hyperbaric or plain bupivacaine provides better anesthesia remains unclear. Finally, in a comparison of plain bupivacaine 4.5 mg with hyperbaric bupivacaine 12 mg (both with fentanyl 50 µg and morphine 0.2 mg), similar cephalad sensory levels (C8), incidence of hypotension (approximately

TABLE 26.5   Drugs Used for Spinal Anesthesia for Cesarean Delivery

Drug	Dose Range	Duration (min)[a]
Local Anesthetic Agents		
Lidocaine	60–80 mg	45–75
Bupivacaine	7.5–15 mg	60–120
Levobupivacaine	7.5–15 mg	60–120
Ropivacaine	15–25 mg	60–120
Opioids		
Fentanyl	10–25 μg	180–240
Sufentanil	2.5–5 μg	180–240
Morphine	100–200 μg (0.1–0.2 mg)	720–1440
Hydromorphone	60–75 μg (0.060–0.075 mg)	720–875
Meperidine[b]	60–70 mg	60
Adjuvant Drugs		
Epinephrine[c]	100–200 μg (0.1–0.2 mg)	

[a]For the local anesthetic agents, the duration is defined as the time to two-segment regression. For opioids, the duration is defined as the period of analgesia (or time to first request for a supplemental analgesic drug).

[b]Meperidine (pethidine) has both local anesthetic and opioid properties and can provide surgical anesthesia without the addition of a local anesthetic. The dose indicated represents meperidine used without a local anesthetic.

[c]The addition of epinephrine may augment the duration of local anesthetics by 15–20 min.

75%), side effects, and patient satisfaction scores were found with the two approaches.[126] Five of 27 (19%) patients in the bupivacaine 4.5-mg group and 1 of 25 (4%) patients in the bupivacaine 12-mg group required supplemental analgesia; no conversion to general anesthesia occurred. Altogether, while these data indicate that lower anesthetic doses *can* be used, whether they *should* be used is controversial. The anesthesia provider should consider whether adjuvant drugs will be used and whether the risks of giving supplemental analgesia or conversion to general anesthesia that are associated with low doses of bupivacaine outweigh the potential benefits (i.e., less hypotension, faster recovery). However, using lower doses of bupivacaine facilitated by higher doses of opioids is generally not an advisable strategy given the side effects (e.g., pruritis, nausea) associated with higher doses of opioids.

For a single-shot spinal technique, most clinicians use a dose of bupivacaine between 10 and 15 mg, in combination with an opioid. Most studies of hyperbaric bupivacaine (12 to 15 mg) have shown that the patient's age, height, weight, and BMI do not have an important influence on the resulting neuraxial blockade, although a weak correlation has been shown between vertebral column length and cephalad spread.[127,128] The use of the larger dose (15 mg) results in a longer duration

of surgical anesthesia; however, cervical sensory blockade is achieved more frequently (Fig. 26.1). In patients with extremes of height (<5 feet/152 cm or >6 feet/183 cm), some anesthesia providers alter the dose of local anesthetic. The baricity of the local anesthetic *does* appear to be associated with an increase in the speed of onset with hyperbaric solutions, and can affect the extent of blockade spread. When the cephalad spread of hyperbaric local anesthetic is desired, the patient can be placed in a slight head-down position; the blockade spread is malleable, particularly with longer duration local anesthetic agents such as bupivacaine.

Ropivacaine is approximately 40% less potent than bupivacaine after spinal injection in nonpregnant individuals.[129] In a dose-finding study of 72 patients undergoing elective cesarean delivery with CSE anesthesia randomly assigned to receive plain ropivacaine 10, 15, 20, or 25 mg,[130] the ED_{50} and ED_{95} were determined to be 16.7 and 26.8 mg, respectively. Subsequently, the same investigators demonstrated that hyperbaric spinal ropivacaine 25 mg produced a more rapid block with faster recovery and less requirement for supplemental epidural anesthesia compared with the same dose of plain ropivacaine in women undergoing cesarean delivery with spinal anesthesia.[131]

Whether ropivacaine has advantages over bupivacaine for spinal anesthesia is questionable. Given the low doses used for spinal anesthesia the risk for LAST is not an important consideration. Studies that have compared ropivacaine and bupivacaine for spinal anesthesia have not always used doses that accounted for differences in potency.[132]

Similarly, it is unclear whether spinal **levobupivacaine** is as effective as bupivacaine. A randomized trial assigned 90 parturients to receive bupivacaine 8 mg, levobupivacaine 8 mg, or ropivacaine 12 mg (all with sufentanil 2.5 μg); effective anesthesia was achieved in 97%, 80%, and 87% of patients, respectively.[133] The duration of levobupivacaine and ropivacaine sensory and motor blockade was shorter than that with bupivacaine.[133] The US Food and Drug Administration (FDA) has not approved ropivacaine or levobupivacaine for

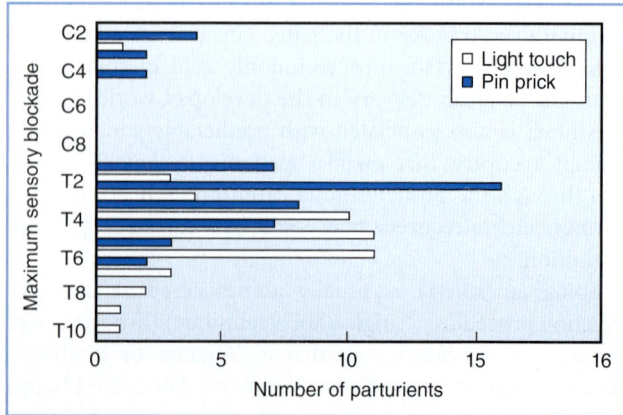

Fig. 26.1 Maximum cephalad sensory level for analgesia or anesthesia in 52 term parturients after spinal injection of hyperbaric bupivacaine 15 mg with morphine 0.15 mg. Modified from Norris MC. Patient variables and the subarachnoid spread of hyperbaric bupivacaine in the term patient. *Anesthesiology.* 1990;72:478–482.

intrathecal administration. Thus, in the United States, bupivacaine remains the most commonly used agent for spinal anesthesia for cesarean delivery.

Hyperbaric spinal **lidocaine** or **mepivacaine** (60 to 80 mg) may be used when the obstetric provider can reliably perform cesarean delivery in less than 45 minutes. The use of hyperbaric lidocaine for spinal anesthesia remains controversial because of concerns about transient neurologic symptoms (see Chapter 31).

Adjuvant Agents

Adjuvant medications contribute to spinal anesthesia by different mechanisms from those of local anesthetics. For cesarean delivery, adjuvant agents can improve the quality of intraoperative anesthesia, prolong postoperative analgesia, and reduce the dose, and therefore the side effects, of local anesthetics. It is important that the use of novel or untested agents in the neuraxial space should be studied initially in animal models with rigorous assessment of safety and efficacy, and avoided in routine clinical care until fully validated.

Opioids have been shown to improve intraoperative and postoperative comfort for patients undergoing spinal anesthesia for cesarean delivery. Intraoperatively, this effect can be observed through a reduction in local anesthetic drug doses and the need for analgesic supplementation. In a systematic review of intraoperative and postoperative analgesic efficacy and adverse effects of intrathecal opioids, 24% of patients undergoing cesarean delivery with spinal hyperbaric bupivacaine alone required supplemental intraoperative analgesia compared with 4% who also received intrathecal opioids.[134] Opioids augment the quality and prolong the duration of local anesthetic–induced blockade, an effect most likely modulated by A-delta (pinprick) and C (cold) nerve fibers; muscle function (A-alpha nerve fibers) does not appear to be affected.[135] The mechanism for the opioid-induced prolongation of sensory block remains unclear but may include modulation of sensory input at the spinal and supraspinal level as well as an alteration of consciousness of peripheral sensations.[136]

An additional advantage of intrathecal opioid administration is its salutary effect on the incidence of *intraoperative* nausea and vomiting. During periods of visceral stimulation (i.e., exteriorization of the uterus and fascial stimulation during closure), patients often complain of nausea; the incidence of nausea is decreased by the addition of spinal fentanyl (10–25 μg) to lidocaine or bupivacaine.[137,138]

Clinicians commonly add both a lipid- and water-soluble opioid to the local anesthetic for spinal anesthesia for cesarean delivery. This practice takes advantage of the fast onset of the lipid-soluble agent and the prolonged duration of the water-soluble agent (Fig. 26.2) (see Chapter 13). However, there is some evidence that the administration of a lipid-soluble agent (e.g., fentanyl, sufentanil) with a water-soluble agent (e.g., morphine) may lead to acute spinal opioid tolerance. In a study of 60 patients undergoing cesarean delivery, there was no difference in intravenous patient-controlled analgesia (PCA) morphine consumption within the first 6 hours in patients randomized to receive spinal fentanyl 25 μg or saline

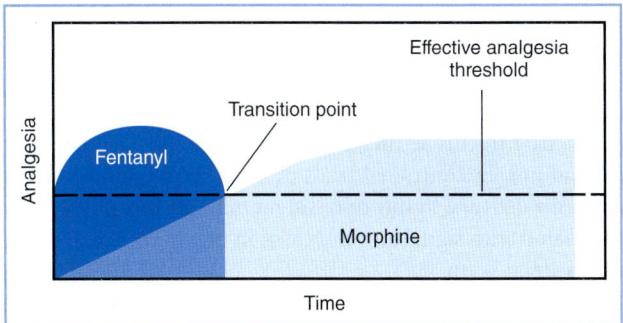

Fig. 26.2 Schematic illustration of the pharmacokinetic and pharmacodynamic activities resulting from the neuraxial administration of a lipid-soluble opioid (e.g., fentanyl) and a water-soluble opioid (e.g., morphine) for analgesia. The transition point varies according to the opioid drugs and doses administered. For most commonly used opioids, this transition point occurs in the postoperative period.

added to plain bupivacaine 10 mg.[139] However, between 6 and 23 hours, there was a 63% increase in morphine use in the group that received fentanyl.[139] In another a study of 40 women undergoing cesarean delivery using intrathecal fentanyl (0, 5, 10, or 25 μg) combined with hyperbaric bupivacaine 12 mg and morphine 0.2 mg, higher postoperative pain scores were observed in the patients who received fentanyl, but no differences were observed among groups in postoperative intravenous PCA morphine consumption.[140] Women who did not receive fentanyl had a higher incidence of intraoperative nausea and vomiting, suggesting that fentanyl is an important adjunct for *intraoperative* anesthesia.[140] In general, we believe the improvement of intraoperative analgesia outweighs the potential for acute opioid tolerance. We therefore recommend the administration of both a lipid- and a water-soluble opioid when spinal anesthesia is administered for cesarean delivery.

The optimal dose of spinal opioids is influenced by the type, dose, and baricity of the accompanying local anesthetic and the presence of other adjuvants. A systematic review and metaanalysis showed that addition of **fentanyl** (10 to 25 μg) to intrathecal bupivacaine for cesarean delivery reduced the need for supplemental analgesia by 82%, and reduced the incidence of intraoperative nausea/vomiting by 59%.[141] Intrathecal fentanyl increased intraoperative pruritus; the incidence was 8%, although there was insufficient evidence to establish whether this was dose related.[141] In contemporary practice, spinal doses of fentanyl 10 to 25 μg are commonly used for cesarean delivery anesthesia (see Table 26.5).

Spinal **sufentanil** 2.5 to 20 μg has been used with bupivacaine for cesarean delivery. A study of 37 parturients undergoing elective cesarean delivery with sufentanil (0, 10, 15, or 20 μg) added to hyperbaric bupivacaine 10.5 mg found better quality and longer duration of analgesia in all sufentanil groups than in the control group; Apgar scores, umbilical cord blood gas measurements, and Early Neonatal Neurobehavioral Scale scores were similar among groups.[142] No cases of respiratory depression occurred. A randomized study assigned parturients to receive hyperbaric bupivacaine

12.5 mg with sufentanil (0, 2.5, 5, or 7.5 μg).[143] Analgesia lasted longer with sufentanil 5 and 7.5 μg, and pruritus and somnolence were more pronounced with 7.5 μg. Thus, there appears to be little justification for giving a dose of sufentanil > 5 μg in this setting. A Bayesian network metaanalysis of randomized controlled trials of intrathecal opioids during cesarean delivery found only sufentanil and morphine were associated with significant increases in the incidence of respiratory depression.[144]

Spinal **morphine**, **hydromorphone**, and **diamorphine** are primarily used for providing prolonged (12 to 24 hours) postcesarean analgesia (see Chapter 27). Spinal morphine has a latency of 30 to 60 minutes for onset of analgesia,[145] and it produces significant analgesia with acceptable side-effect profiles when given in doses ranging from 0.05 to 0.25 mg. In a dose-response study of morphine added to hyperbaric bupivacaine 12.75 mg, morphine 0.1 mg provided analgesia comparable to that provided by doses as high as 0.5 mg.[146] The incidence of pruritus, but not nausea and vomiting, appeared to be dose related. In patients randomized to receive morphine 0.05, 0.10, or 0.15 mg combined with hyperbaric bupivacaine 12 mg and fentanyl 15 μg, and intravenous ketorolac, no difference in measures of analgesia were found among the three groups; pruritus was more common at doses of 0.10 and 0.15 than 0.05 mg.[147] **Hydromorphone**, while used less commonly than morphine, also appears to provide effective postcesarean analgesia, with an intrathecal potency ratio of 2:1 compared with morphine.[148]

Intrathecal **diamorphine** is used in the United Kingdom for postoperative analgesia. It is metabolized to the two active compounds 6-acetyl morphine and morphine. Diamorphine is more lipophilic than morphine, enabling a rapid onset (6 to 9 minutes, similar to fentanyl) but a potentially shorter duration of action.[149] In a study of intrathecal diamorphine 0.4 mg combined with bupivacaine 12.5 mg, the intraoperative supplementation rate was less than 5%; however, the incidence of nausea and vomiting was 56% and the incidence of pruritus was 80%.[150]

Neuraxial administration of water-soluble opioids such as morphine may be associated with delayed respiratory depression (6 to 18 hours after administration; see Chapter 27).[144] Postoperative monitoring protocols should include observation for respiratory depression, which although infrequent, can lead to mortality, particularly in high-risk patients (e.g., those with sleep apnea or obesity).[134,151,152] The respiratory depressant effects of many opioids, including morphine and diamorphine, outlast the antagonism provided by naloxone (approximately 90 minutes).[153] The Society for Obstetric Anesthesia and Perinatology consensus statement for monitoring for respiratory depression associated with neuraxial morphine for cesarean delivery promotes perioperative risk assessment and stratification to determine and adjust the intensity, frequency, and duration of respiratory monitoring.[151]

Spinal local anesthetics are often prepared in **dextrose** to make the injectate hyperbaric. For example, commercially available hyperbaric bupivacaine contains 8.25% dextrose (82.5 mg/mL). The amount of dextrose required to make a meaningful clinical difference in a spinal technique with local anesthetic agents has not been well characterized. *Baricity* is defined as the ratio of the density of the local anesthetic solution to the density of CSF measured at the same temperature. The density of CSF is lower in women than in men, particularly during pregnancy and the immediate postpartum period[154]; even so, CSF density is significantly greater than that of local anesthetics and opioids in the absence of dextrose.[154]

The intrathecal administration of an alpha-adrenergic receptor agonist (e.g., epinephrine [adrenaline], clonidine) increases the density of sensory and motor blockade and may prolong the duration of blockade as well as contribute to postcesarean analgesia. A randomized trial involving 63 women undergoing elective cesarean delivery showed that intrathecal **epinephrine** 0.1 to 0.2 mg, when combined with hyperbaric bupivacaine, improved the quality of intraoperative analgesia and prolonged both sensory and motor blockade by approximately 15% compared with bupivacaine alone.[155] However, another study found that the addition of epinephrine 0.3 mg to hyperbaric bupivacaine 12.5 mg for elective cesarean delivery increased the incidence of nausea.[156]

Spinal **clonidine**, in doses of 30 to 150 μg, improves intraoperative analgesia, decreases shivering, and reduces peri-incisional hyperalgesia in women undergoing cesarean delivery; however, it has been associated with hypotension and sedation.[157] This agent is not used commonly in the United States, although it may be considered in specific circumstances (e.g., when patients are expected to be tolerant to the effects of neuraxial opioid analgesia). The FDA has issued a "black box" warning against its use in obstetric patients because of concern for hypotension. A metaanalysis showed that intrathecal dexmedetomidine, an alpha-2 adrenergic receptor agonist similar to clonidine, prolonged the postcesarean pain-free period and reduced the occurrence of postoperative shivering, but not nausea and vomiting, bradycardia, or hypotension; importantly, there were no significant differences in UA oxygen or carbon dioxide, cord blood pH, or Apgar scores.[158] Safety data are lacking and dexmedetomidine has not been approved by the FDA for neuraxial administration.

In women undergoing cesarean delivery, spinal **neostigmine** in doses up to 100 μg reduced postoperative pain with no effect on FHR or Apgar scores. However, its clinical use is limited by a high incidence of nausea and vomiting refractory to treatment with antiemetic agents.[159]

At many institutions, the spinal agents and doses are standardized so that consistent results are obtained during the provision of spinal anesthesia for cesarean delivery. Such standardization enables the anesthesia, obstetric, and nursing staff to anticipate predictable onset and recovery characteristics and respond to physiologic responses that are outside the norm. Standardization of drugs and doses may also result in fewer errors. At the authors' institutions, spinal anesthesia for cesarean delivery is provided with 0.75% hyperbaric bupivacaine 12 mg, fentanyl 10 μg, and morphine 0.1 mg. Intrathecal opioids are drawn in a tuberculin or insulin syringe to ensure measurement accuracy. A common practice elsewhere is the administration of 0.75% hyperbaric bupivacaine 12 mg, fentanyl 15 µg, and morphine 0.15 mg.

Epidural Anesthesia

The use of epidural anesthesia for nonelective cesarean delivery has increased, primarily because of the greater use of epidural analgesia during labor. However, the use of epidural anesthesia is less common for *elective* cesarean delivery when an epidural catheter is not already *in situ*, in part because the resulting block is less reliable than that with spinal anesthesia.

Epidural local anesthetic and opioid doses are generally 5 to 10 times greater than doses given intrathecally; this difference results from the requirement for penetration of nerve roots as they traverse the epidural space, the greater capacity of the epidural space, and the presence of the epidural venous plexus, which becomes progressively more engorged during pregnancy. Greater systemic absorption of anesthetic agents occurs with epidural anesthesia than with spinal anesthesia, and the risk for LAST is a real possibility during epidural anesthesia, but not spinal anesthesia.

A possible advantage of epidural anesthesia is a slower onset of sympathetic blockade; this may allow compensatory mechanisms to attenuate the severity of hypotension. This approach has utility in the care of patients with severe cardiac disease for whom even transient hypotension may be poorly tolerated. A catheter-based technique also allows titration of the level, density, and duration of anesthesia, and continuous postcesarean analgesia.

Local Anesthetic Agents

The most common local anesthetic used in the United States for the initiation and maintenance of epidural anesthesia for cesarean delivery is 2% **lidocaine with epinephrine** (Table 26.6). The epidural administration of lidocaine in concentrations less than 2%, or without the addition of epinephrine, which augments the analgesia through alpha-adrenergic receptor blockade,[160] may result in anesthesia that is inadequate for surgery.[161]

The epidural administration of a 3% solution of **2-chloroprocaine** has the most rapid onset and the shortest duration of action of available local anesthetics. These characteristics make it an excellent choice for emergency cesarean delivery (see discussion below) because the dose is administered rapidly, and even if unintentional intravenous administration of drug were to occur, the maternal and fetal sequelae are likely to be less severe than the similar administration of an amide local anesthetic agent.[162] Administration of 2-chloroprocaine has historically been associated with neurologic sequelae, possibly associated with the antioxidant sodium bisulfite, and paralumbar muscle spasms and pain, believed to be a result of calcium chelation by the preservative ethylenediaminetetraacetic acid. Current preparations of 2-chloroprocaine do not contain an antioxidant or a preservative (see Chapter 13). Epidural administration of 2-chloroprocaine may be associated with a rapid onset of hypotension and an apparent reduction in the clinical efficacy of subsequently administered epidural opioids (see Chapter 13).[163] The pharmacokinetic

TABLE 26.6 Drugs Used for Epidural Anesthesia for Cesarean Delivery		
Drug	**Dose Range**[a]	**Duration (min)**[b]
Local Anesthetics		
Lidocaine 2% with epinephrine 5 µg/mL	300–500 mg	75–100
2-Chloroprocaine 3%	450–750 mg	40–50
Bupivacaine 0.5%	75–125 mg	120–180
Ropivacaine 0.5%	75–125 mg	120–180
Opioids		
Fentanyl	50–100 µg	120–240
Sufentanil	10–20 µg	120–240
Morphine	3–4 mg	720–1440
Hydromorphone	0.6–1.5 mg	780–1090
Meperidine	50–75 mg	240–720

[a]Both the mass and volume of local anesthetic affect the extent and quality of anesthesia. The usual volume of local anesthetic solution administered into the epidural space at the indicated concentrations is 15–25 mL. More mass/volume is required for initiating epidural anesthesia *de novo*; conversely, less is required if epidural labor analgesia is being extended to surgical anesthesia.
[b]For the local anesthetics, the duration is defined as the time to two-segment regression. For the opioids, the duration is defined as the period of analgesia (or time to first request for a supplemental analgesic drug).

characteristics of the drug likely play a role. The analgesic effect of epidural morphine administered 30 minutes *before* 2-chloroprocaine does not appear to be mitigated; however, such timing in the setting of emergency cesarean delivery is not possible.[163] These considerations limit the use of 2-chloroprocaine to those situations in which the rapid onset of anesthesia is paramount. Epidural administration of 3% 2-chloroprocaine 20 mL was demonstrated to be noninferior for rapidly converting labor analgesia to anesthesia to the T7 level for cesarean delivery compared with the combination of 2% lidocaine 20 mL, epinephrine 150 µg, 8.4% bicarbonate 2 mL, and fentanyl 100 µg.[164] This avoids the disadvantage of needing to mix multiple drugs, which is likely helpful in an emergency situation; moreover, an even faster blockade onset is achieved when 3% 2-chloroprocaine 20 mL is administered in the epidural space mixed with 8.4% bicarbonate 2 mL.

Surgical anesthesia can be produced with epidural administration of 0.5% **bupivacaine**; however, the slow onset of neuroblockade and the risk for cardiovascular sequelae (i.e., LAST) from unintentional intravascular injection (or systemic absorption) have limited the contemporary use of this agent in the United States. The risk for cardiovascular sequelae resulted in a earlier proscription against the epidural administration of 0.75% bupivacaine in obstetric patients by the FDA.[165] The single-isomer, levorotatory local anesthetics 0.5% and 0.75% **ropivacaine** and 0.5% **levobupivacaine** may be preferable to racemic bupivacaine because of their better safety profiles and earlier recovery, although a significant portion of the improved safety profile is caused by the lower potency of these agents (0.5% bupivacaine is more potent than 0.5% levobupivacaine and 0.5% ropivacaine).[166] A randomized controlled trial of 60 patients compared 30 mL of epidural 0.5% levobupivacaine with racemic 0.5% bupivacaine in women undergoing elective cesarean delivery; no differences in the block onset or resolution, signal-averaged ECG results, complications, or maternal and fetal plasma pharmacokinetic profiles between the treatment groups were found.[167] Another study involving 62 patients undergoing cesarean delivery with epidural anesthesia reported no difference in onset, spread, or duration of sensory block in women who received 25 mL of 0.5% levobupivacaine or 0.5% racemic bupivacaine,[168] although levobupivacaine produced lower limb motor blockade of longer duration and less intensity. Finally, a study of 60 patients demonstrated that the onset, duration, and regression of sensory blockade with 0.5% ropivacaine was similar to that provided by 0.5% bupivacaine, although a faster onset and longer duration of motor blockade was observed with bupivacaine.[169] The free concentrations of ropivacaine were approximately twice those of bupivacaine in both maternal and neonatal blood at delivery; however, these measurements were less than the concentrations shown to be toxic in animals.

Adjuvant Agents

As with spinal anesthesia, adjuvant medications are used for their intrinsic analgesic properties and to reduce the dose and side effects of local anesthetic agents. The use of epidural adjuvants can improve the quality of intraoperative anesthesia and result in less motor blockade as well as enhance postoperative analgesia (see Chapter 27).

Although some anesthesia providers administer an epidural opioid with the initial therapeutic dose of local anesthetic, others delay opioid administration until confirmation of an appropriate local anesthetic agent-induced blockade (so a less-than-optimal blockade is not obscured), or until clamping of the umbilical cord (to prevent transfer of opioid to the fetus). The onset of analgesia is dictated by complex pharmacokinetics; however, the lipid-soluble opioids (e.g., **fentanyl**, **sufentanil**) have more rapid onset and more rapid clearance than the water-soluble opioids (e.g., **morphine**).[170]

The administration of epidural **fentanyl** (50 to 100 μg) results in activity at both spinal and supraspinal sites of action,[171] improves the intraoperative quality of anesthesia during cesarean delivery,[172,173] and does not appear to adversely affect the neonate.[174] The optimal dose of epidural fentanyl has not been determined for patients undergoing cesarean delivery; however, in an experimental pain study in nonpregnant patients, there was an analgesic effect at the segmental level of injection for epidural fentanyl 100 μg, but not 50 μg.[175]

Epidural **sufentanil** (10 to 20 μg) added to 0.5% bupivacaine with epinephrine 5 μg/mL provides significantly better intraoperative anesthesia and longer postoperative analgesia than bupivacaine and epinephrine alone, with minimal maternal side effects and no adverse neonatal effects.[176] Epidural sufentanil is approximately five times more potent than epidural fentanyl, but when equipotent doses are administered, no differences between the agents in onset, quality, or duration of analgesia have been observed.[177,178]

Epidural administration of the hydrophilic opioid **morphine** provides prolonged postcesarean analgesia. A dose-response study of epidural morphine (1.25, 2.5, 3.75, and 5 mg) found 3.75 mg to be an optimal dose, above which postcesarean analgesia (as measured by PCA morphine demands) was no better.[179] Extended-release epidural morphine 10 mg provides better postoperative analgesia than epidural morphine 4 mg, with no differences in nausea, pruritus, or sedation scores.[180]

Epidural **hydromorphone** is sometimes used as an alternative to morphine. Doses of 0.6 to 1.5 mg are commonly used. Studies suggest a similar analgesia effect and side-effect profile compared with epidural morphine analgesia, although the duration of analgesia may be slightly shorter.[181–183]

Epidural **diamorphine** (2.5 to 3 mg) is commonly used in the United Kingdom for providing prolonged postcesarean analgesia.[184] Optimal dose-finding studies of epidural diamorphine have not been performed; however, the duration and quality of analgesia from epidural diamorphine 3 mg appears to be similar to that provided by spinal diamorphine 0.3 mg, with significantly less pruritus.[185]

Epidural **clonidine** (75 to 200 μg) combined with morphine or fentanyl reduces the requirement for postcesarean morphine analgesia.[186] The effect of coadministering clonidine and fentanyl appears to be additive rather than synergistic in producing postcesarean analgesia. Common side effects include hypotension and sedation. Currently, epidural clonidine has only one specific neuraxial indication in the United States (intractable cancer pain), and the package insert has a "black box" warning from the FDA stating that "epidural clonidine is not recommended for obstetrical, postpartum and perioperative pain management."

Epidural **neostigmine** produces a modest amount of postcesarean analgesia when given after umbilical cord clamping. A dose-finding study investigated the administration of 75, 150, or 300 μg of epidural neostigmine in women undergoing elective cesarean delivery.[187] An increase in intraoperative shivering and sedation was observed in the 300-μg group only; a dose-independent reduction in postoperative pain and sedation was observed in all groups.

Epinephrine may be added to the local anesthetic agent to minimize systemic absorption and peak blood level of the local anesthetic, increase the density of sensory and motor blockade, and prolong the duration of anesthesia.[160,188,189] The pharmacokinetic effects of epinephrine coadministered with an opioid vary with the opioid and the sampling site. In the lumbar epidural space, epinephrine lengthened the mean residence time of morphine but shortened that of fentanyl and sufentanil.[190]

The epidural administration of epidural epinephrine in preeclamptic women has been considered controversial because of the potential risks of exacerbating hypertension[191] and decreasing uteroplacental blood flow[192] when large doses of local anesthetic are given for cesarean delivery. However, many practitioners consider the risk/benefit ratio for the addition of epinephrine to lidocaine to be favorable in pre-eclamptic women (see Chapter 35).

When combined with local anesthetic for epidural anesthesia, the usual epinephrine concentration is 2.5 or 5 µg/mL (i.e., 1 : 400,000 or 1 : 200,000). The addition of epinephrine to a solution of plain local anesthetic just before administration results in a solution that has a higher pH than commercially prepared epinephrine-containing products, which use (low-pH) antioxidants to preserve the efficacy of the epinephrine (see Chapter 13). Thus, use of freshly prepared solutions hastens the onset of anesthesia.

The addition of **sodium bicarbonate** results in a solution with more local anesthetic molecules in a nonionized state, which hastens the onset and augments the quality of the local anesthetic blockade, particularly if sodium bicarbonate is added to a low-pH solution (see discussion below).

Combined Spinal-Epidural Anesthesia

The CSE technique incorporates the rapid and predictable onset of spinal blockade with the ability to augment or prolong anesthesia by injection of additional drug through the epidural catheter (see Chapter 12). Compared with a conventional epidural anesthesia for cesarean delivery, further advantages of the CSE technique include: (1) faster onset and lower pain scores at delivery,[193] (2) use of the epidural needle as an introducer for a longer spinal needle when attempts with a traditional introducer and spinal needle have failed, and (3) use of a spinal needle (and return of CSF through the needle) to "confirm" the correct positioning of the epidural needle in the epidural space.

Conventional spinal doses (e.g., 12 mg) of hyperbaric bupivacaine are most often used to provide CSE anesthesia for cesarean delivery; however, a satisfactory block has been reported with plain bupivacaine drug doses as low as 4.5 mg.[126] Although the use of lower doses of local anesthetic is enabled by the presence of the epidural catheter (because additional agents can be administered if discomfort occurs), the block achieved with the CSE technique may be inherently different from the block achieved with a single-shot spinal technique with the same dose(s) of medication. One study, in which men undergoing surgery were positioned in the right lateral position for initiation of neuraxial anesthesia, demonstrated that the ED_{50} values for intrathecal hyperbaric bupivacaine (to achieve a T6 sensory level of anesthesia for 60 minutes) for the CSE and spinal techniques were 9.2 and 11.4 mg, respectively.[194] The investigators speculated that the use of the loss-of-resistance to air (during introduction of the epidural needle) resulted in a reduction in lumbar CSF volume and a subsequently higher sensory blockade. Similarly, in another study that initiated neuraxial analgesia with intrathecal bupivacaine 10 mg in parturients undergoing *elective* cesarean delivery, median sensory levels were C6 and T3 with the CSE and spinal techniques, respectively.[195] The CSE technique was performed with loss-of-resistance

to air (2 mL); however, after administration of the spinal medications, the epidural catheter was not inserted. The investigators speculated that the loss of negative pressure in the epidural space created by the introduction of the epidural needle was responsible for the observed differences. However, when investigators from the same institution performed the same anesthetic techniques for cesarean delivery in *laboring* women, no differences in the block characteristics were observed.[196] The reasons for these differences are unclear.

The *sequential* CSE technique uses a lower dose of spinal bupivacaine (7.5 to 10 mg) followed by incremental injection of local anesthetic through the epidural catheter to achieve a T4 level of anesthesia.[197,198] The advantage of this approach is a lower incidence of hypotension. In a study comparing sequential CSE anesthesia using 1.5 mL of 0.5% of hyperbaric bupivacaine (followed by extension with fractionated doses of 0.5% bupivacaine administered through the epidural catheter as needed) versus single-shot spinal anesthesia using 2.5 mL of 0.5% of hyperbaric bupivacaine, there was more gradual onset of hypotension and a lower initial sensory level with the CSE technique (T7) compared with the single-shot spinal technique (T4).[198] The sequential CSE technique may be of particular advantage in high-risk parturients (e.g., significant cardiac disease) in whom avoidance of severe hypotension is vitally important.

Another CSE technique is the *extradural volume extension* (EVE) technique.[197,199] Intrathecal administration of a small dose of local anesthetic is followed by the administration of saline through the epidural catheter. Studies have observed a higher cephalad spread of one to four dermatomal segments associated with the use of this technique, presumably because of thecal compression.[197] However, the effect of EVE may depend on the initial dose and baricity of local anesthetic, the time interval between spinal and epidural injection, the volume of epidural saline, and the outcomes measured, as several studies have failed to find a difference in sensory blockade using this technique.[199,200]

Potential drawbacks of CSE techniques include an untested epidural catheter (although the rates of successful function of epidural catheters placed as part of a CSE technique is very high) and hypotension, which can be generally treated easily with vasopressors. Administering the CSE technique in the sitting position may result in greater severity and duration of hypotension than the left lateral decubitus position.[83] The hypotension may be related to the delay in moving the patient from the sitting to the supine (with leftward tilt) position.

Dural Puncture Epidural Anesthesia

The DPE and CSE techniques use similar methods for insertion, by which a spinal needle is placed through the shaft of a positioned epidural needle to obtain CSF (see Chapter 12). Although the DPE technique then introduces all medications via the epidural catheter, a portion of the epidural medications is subsequently translocated via the conduit from the epidural to the subarachnoid space.[201] Rao et al. reported that for elective cesarean delivery, the DPE technique was associated with a faster onset of anesthesia and less intraoperative pain compared with epidural anesthesia, and a slower onset of anesthesia with less hypotension and less phenylephrine requirement compared with CSE anesthesia.[202] Sharawi et al.[203] randomized women having scheduled cesarean delivery to first have a T10 sensory block established using DPE or standard epidural anesthesia, and then epidural extension to T6 using 3% chloroprocaine. They found that the time to achieve surgical anesthesia was faster in the DPE group (422 versus 655 seconds; $P < .001$), with a more favorable quality of anesthesia blockade.

Extension of Epidural Labor Analgesia

The extension of epidural labor *analgesia* to surgical *anesthesia* sufficient for cesarean delivery can be accomplished with several local anesthetic agents. The selection of agent often depends on the urgency of the case. Extension of epidural analgesia can be initiated as preparations are being made to move the patient from the labor room to the operating room. Whether an *in situ* epidural catheter should be used for an extension attempt depends on several factors, including the quality of the existing labor analgesia. If obtaining satisfactory epidural labor analgesia has been problematic (e.g., one-sided or "patchy" analgesia), removing the catheter and administering spinal or CSE anesthesia may be a better method to attain rapid and effective anesthesia. A systematic review and metaanalysis found that the risk for failed conversion of labor epidural analgesia to anesthesia is increased by the following factors: (1) a higher number of boluses administered during labor, (2) greater urgency for cesarean delivery, and (3) care being provided by a nonobstetric anesthesiologist.[204]

Specific local anesthetic and adjuvant solutions may influence whether the quality and level of epidural anesthesia is adequate for cesarean delivery. A metaanalysis of 11 randomized controlled trials examining the type of local anesthetic used to "top-up" epidural labor analgesia for emergency cesarean delivery[205] compared 0.5% bupivacaine or 0.5% levobupivacaine, lidocaine with epinephrine (with and without fentanyl), and 0.75% ropivacaine. The pooled analysis suggested that lidocaine with epinephrine resulted in the fastest onset of sensory block; the addition of fentanyl further hastened block onset, but not quality as measured by the need for intraoperative supplementation. Compared with 0.5% bupivacaine or 0.5% levobupivacaine, 0.75% ropivacaine was associated with a lower need for intraoperative supplementation. The epidural administration of 2% lidocaine with freshly added epinephrine 5 µg/mL was compared with 3% 2-chloroprocaine in a randomized trial involving 40 women undergoing elective cesarean delivery.[206] There was no significant difference in the onset of anesthesia between the two groups, although the study was likely underpowered; the median onset was 8 minutes (range, 4 to 13 minutes) in the 2-chloroprocaine group and 5 minutes (range, 2 to 22 minutes) in the lidocaine group. However, given the time taken to prepare the lidocaine with epinephrine solution, the investigators concluded that use

of a preprepared solution, such as 2-chloroprocaine, may be preferred.

Alkalinization of the local anesthetic solution not only increases the speed of onset but also improves the quality and prolongs the duration of neuroblockade.[207] Alkalinization shifts more of the local anesthetic molecules to the nonionized, lipid-soluble form, which allows the local anesthetic to pass more easily through the lipophilic neuronal membrane. Although this phenomenon can be demonstrated for all local anesthetics, alkalinization is most often performed with local anesthetic agents of short and medium duration (e.g., 2-chloroprocaine, lidocaine). Typically, 1 mL of 8.4% sodium bicarbonate (1 mEq/mL) is added to each 10 mL of lidocaine or 2-chloroprocaine. Longer-acting agents (e.g., bupivacaine, ropivacaine, levobupivacaine) easily precipitate with the addition of sodium bicarbonate; this occurs even with the addition of 0.2 mEq of bicarbonate to 20 mL of 0.5% bupivacaine.[208] Alkalinization exerts the greatest effect when it is freshly mixed with the local anesthetic solution; however, the mixture is relatively stable.[209] The addition of sodium bicarbonate to local anesthetics has been demonstrated to result in a clinically significant reduction in the time until an adequate anesthetic level is obtained (Fig. 26.3). In a randomized trial, 40 women with functioning epidural labor analgesia received a 3-mL epidural test dose of 2% lidocaine with epinephrine, followed by 12 mL of premixed 2% lidocaine with epinephrine 5 µg/mL (1 : 200,000) and fentanyl 75 µg with 1.2 mL of 8.4% sodium bicarbonate or saline.[207] The mean times to attain a T6 anesthesia level with and without bicarbonate were 5.2 and 9.7 minutes, respectively.

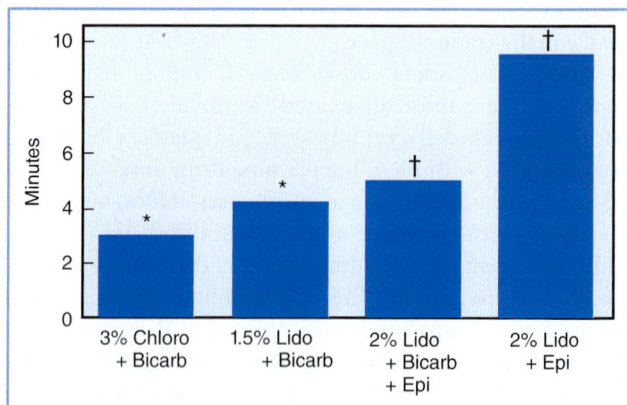

Fig. 26.3 Onset Time for Extension of Existing Labor Analgesia Blockade (T10 Sensory Level) With Different Local Anesthetic Preparations. Results between the two studies cannot be directly compared owing to differences in labor analgesia regimens, different sensory testing methods and target levels, and presence of epidural opioids. The 2% lidocaine with epinephrine solution was premixed. The epinephrine concentration was 5 µg/mL. *Bicarb,* Bicarbonate; *Chloro,* 2-chloroprocaine; *Epi,* epinephrine 5 µg/mL; *Lido,* lidocaine. **To T4 sensory level.* Data modified from Gaiser RR, Cheek TG, Gutsche BB. Epidural lidocaine versus 2-chloroprocaine for fetal distress requiring urgent cesarean section. *Int J Obstet Anesth.* 1994;3:20–210. †*To T6 sensory level.* Data modified from Lam DT, Ngan Kee WD, Khaw KS. Extension of epidural blockade in labour for emergency Caesarean section using 2% lidocaine with epinephrine and fentanyl, with or without alkalinisation. *Anaesthesia.* 2001;56:790–794.

Extension of a T10 level of *analgesia* to a T4 level of *anesthesia* typically requires a volume of 15 to 20 mL of local anesthetic with one or more adjuvants. At our institutions, the extension of epidural labor analgesia begins with assessment of the quality of analgesia. For emergency cesarean delivery, we initiate the extension of epidural anesthesia in the labor room by giving 10 mL of alkalinized 2% lidocaine (with epinephrine) or 3% 2-chloroprocaine. The sensory blockade is assessed after transfer of the patient to the operating room; if the blockade is bilateral and moving in a cephalad direction, an additional 5 to 10 mL is administered to bring the sensory level to T4. The use of this fractionated dosing schedule offers several advantages, including (1) greater hemodynamic stability during patient transfer; (2) assessment of the evolving sensory level before administration of the full dose of local anesthetic; (3) minimization of dural sac compression (by a large-volume epidural injection),[210] which enables a less difficult and safer conversion to spinal anesthesia if extension of epidural anesthesia is not successful (see discussion below); and (4) early sensory blockade at the incision site, so that surgery can be initiated in emergency cases before establishment of a full T4 sensory level.

The extension of epidural analgesia to anesthesia in the labor room is controversial.[211] Some anesthesia providers delay epidural administration of additional local anesthetic until the patient has arrived in the operating room. However, this practice may increase the risk for failed epidural anesthesia, necessitating the induction of general anesthesia with its attendant risks (see discussion below).

General Anesthesia

Although neuraxial anesthesia is usually preferred for cesarean delivery, in some situations general anesthesia is considered more appropriate (see Table 26.2). In addition, general anesthesia offers an advantage in cases in which uterine relaxation would be beneficial (e.g., cesarean delivery as part of an *ex utero* intrapartum treatment [EXIT] procedure; see Chapter 7).

The basic elements for preparation and care of the obstetric patient undergoing cesarean delivery apply to the patient undergoing general anesthesia (Box 26.6; see Table 26.1). The preanesthetic evaluation should focus on assessment of physical characteristics (e.g., airway) and comorbidities. The consent process should feature the risks associated with airway management, aspiration, and awareness. The importance of a careful airway evaluation cannot be overemphasized (see Chapter 29); pregnancy-induced changes in the upper airway may be exacerbated during labor. Acoustic reflectometry showed that soft tissue mucosal edema in both the oral (incisor teeth to oropharyngeal junction) and pharyngeal (oropharyngeal junction to the glottis) tissue increases during labor and results in worsening of the airway classification compared with the prelabor evaluation.[212] Failed tracheal intubation, failed ventilation and oxygenation, and pulmonary aspiration of gastric contents are important potential causes of anesthesia-related maternal death (see Chapters 29 and 39).[109] If the airway evaluation suggests the possibility of a difficult intubation, consideration should be given to the placement of a neuraxial catheter during early labor, even if it is not used to provide labor analgesia.[24]

Preparation

All pregnant patients requiring surgical anesthesia should be considered at risk for pulmonary aspiration of gastric contents (see Chapter 28). Attempts should be made to minimize both the risk for maternal aspiration and the risk for pulmonary injury if aspiration occurs. Fasting policies should be shared with all members of the obstetric care team. The authors administer **metoclopramide** 10 mg and **ranitidine** 50 mg IV 30 to 60 minutes before induction of general anesthesia, when possible, to diminish gastric volume and gastric acid secretion, respectively.[40] A clear, nonparticulate antacid (sodium citrate 30 mL) should also be administered within 30 minutes of surgery to neutralize gastric acid[38]; the antacid may be particularly important in emergency situations when metoclopramide and ranitidine have not had the necessary time to exert their pharmacologic effects.

Although less common in the era of videolaryngoscopy, in situations where highly difficult or impossible mask ventilation or intubation is anticipated (e.g., neck mass), **awake tracheal intubation** may be considered (see Chapter 29). Preparations include administering an antisialagogue (e.g., **glycopyrrolate**), judicious sedation (e.g., **midazolam**), and topical airway anesthesia (e.g., aerosolized **lidocaine** or **benzocaine**). **Glossopharyngeal** and **laryngeal nerve blocks** may also be considered, although these should be avoided in patients at excess risk for bleeding (e.g., hemolysis, elevated liver enzymes, and low platelet count [HELLP] syndrome).

The patient should be placed supine with left uterine displacement. The head, neck, and shoulders should be optimally positioned for airway management (i.e., the sniffing position). Routine monitoring should be established, including ECG, pulse oximetry, blood pressure, and capnography. Preoxygenation (denitrogenation) with 100% oxygen should be performed to delay the onset of hypoxemia during apnea; this hypoxemia occurs more rapidly because of the pregnancy-induced decrease in functional residual capacity and increase in oxygen consumption. In a computer simulation of the respiratory and cardiovascular systems during pregnancy, the presence of labor, high BMI, and sepsis further accelerated oxyhemoglobin desaturation during apnea; by contrast, multiple gestation and hemorrhage appeared to have minimal effect.[213] Ideally, preoxygenation is accomplished by 3 minutes of tidal-volume breathing with a tight-fitting face mask. Although four maximal deep breaths of 100% oxygen over 30 seconds can achieve a similar Pao_2, the same protection against rapid oxyhemoglobin desaturation is not afforded, owing to differences in tissue and venous compartment oxygen reserves.[213] The method of eight deep breaths over 1 minute appears to provide better protection from oxyhemoglobin desaturation during apnea than the method of four deep breaths over 30 seconds.[214] Recently, the use of high-flow nasal oxygen (HFNO) has been used as a method to provide efficient, prolonged oxygenation (longer apneic time with oxygen saturation > 90%) prior to intubation in women

BOX 26.6 Steps for Initiating General Anesthesia for Cesarean Delivery[a]

1. Discuss the operative plan with the multidisciplinary team.
2. Perform preanesthetic assessment, and obtain informed consent.
3. Prepare necessary medications and equipment.
4. Place patient supine with left uterine displacement.
5. Secure 18-gauge or larger intravenous access. Send blood specimen for baseline laboratory measurements; consider type and screen (or cross-match) if risk factors for peripartum hemorrhage are present.
6. Give metoclopramide 10 mg and/or ranitidine 50 mg intravenously more than 30 min before induction, if possible.
7. Give a nonparticulate antacid orally less than 30 min before induction.[b]
8. Administer antibiotic prophylaxis (with 60 min before incision).[c] [4444]
9. Initiate monitoring.
10. Perform a team "time-out" to verify patient identity, position, and operative site; procedure to be performed; and availability of special equipment, if needed.
11. Provide 100% oxygen with a tight-fitting face mask for 3 min or longer, when possible, for denitrogenation/preoxygenation. Otherwise, instruct the patient to take four to eight vital-capacity breaths immediately before induction of anesthesia.
12. After the abdomen has been prepared and operative drapes are in place, verify that the surgeon and assistant are ready to begin surgery.
13. Initiate rapid-sequence induction:
    a. Apply cricoid pressure 10 N while awake; increase to 30 N after loss of consciousness.
    b. Give thiopental 4–6 mg/kg or propofol 2–2.8 mg/kg and succinylcholine 1–1.5 mg/kg intravenously; wait 30–40 s.[d]
14. Perform tracheal intubation. Confirm correct placement of endotracheal tube.
15. Provide maintenance of anesthesia:
    a. Use isoflurane, sevoflurane, or desflurane (approximately 1 MAC) in 100% oxygen or oxygen/nitrous oxide (up to 50%).
    b. Treat hypotension (e.g., phenylephrine, ephedrine).
    c. If additional muscle relaxant (e.g., rocuronium, vecuronium) is necessary, titrate dose according to response to peripheral nerve stimulator.
16. Observe delivery of infant.
17. Administer a bolus and/or a continuous infusion of oxytocin; consider other uterotonic agents (e.g., methylergonovine, 15-methyl prostaglandin $F_{2\alpha}$) if uterine tone is inadequate. Monitor blood loss and respond as necessary.
18. Adjust maintenance technique after delivery of the infant:
    a. Administer a reduced concentration of a volatile halogenated agent (0.5–0.75 MAC).
    b. Supplement anesthesia with nitrous oxide and an intravenous opioid.
    c. Give attention to risk for awareness and recall. Consider administration of a benzodiazepine (e.g., midazolam).
19. Perform tracheal extubation when neuromuscular blockade is fully reversed and the patient is awake and responds to commands.
20. Evaluate postoperative issues (e.g., pain, nausea).

[a]The events and sequence of events may need to be modified and tailored to individual circumstances. In an emergency, some tasks may have to be performed simultaneously.

[b]Some anesthesiologists suggest that sodium citrate should be administered within 20 min of induction of general anesthesia (see Chapter 28).

[c]Evidence suggests that administration of prophylactic antibiotics before incision (rather than after umbilical cord clamping) reduces the incidence of postcesarean endometritis and total maternal infectious morbidity.

[d]Drugs and doses may have to be modified for individual patients and circumstances.

MAC, Minimum alveolar concentration.

undergoing general anesthesia for cesarean delivery.[215] The effect of HFNO on gastric distention and regurgitation needs further exploration, particularly in pregnant women.

In contrast to most surgical procedures, the patient's abdomen is prepared and draped *before* induction of general anesthesia to minimize fetal exposure to general anesthesia. After the surgical drapes have been applied and the operating personnel are ready at the tableside, the surgeon should be instructed to delay the incision until the anesthesia provider confirms correct placement of the endotracheal tube and gives verbal instructions to proceed with surgery.

Induction

A rapid-sequence induction is initiated with denitrogenation/preoxygenation followed by administration of an induction agent, paralysis, and cricoid pressure. Traditionally, mask ventilation is not performed, because when it is applied with inspiratory pressure > 20 cm H_2O without the application of cricoid pressure with pressures, insufflation of the stomach can occur (see Chapter 29). However, some guidelines[216] have recommended modification of the rapid-sequence induction to include gentle, low-pressure (<20 cm H_2O) mask ventilation to confirm that ventilation is possible and to maximize oxygen reserve while awaiting induction and paralysis. Whether rapid-sequence induction with or without modification should be employed, particularly in an appropriately fasted, nonlaboring patient having elective cesarean delivery, has been questioned.[217] Further, the value of cricoid pressure has been challenged owing to (1) physiologic evidence demonstrating that cricoid pressure reduces lower esophageal sphincter pressure, (2) anatomic investigations showing an inability to completely occlude the esophagus, (3) a lack of clinical outcome data that confirm that cricoid pressure reduces the incidence of aspiration, and (4) the frequent misapplication of the technique itself.[218] The technique for cricoid pressure begins with an assistant applying 10 newtons (N) of force, 1 N being the force required to accelerate a mass of 1 kg by 1 m/s² (as a practical guide to the amount of force to apply, 10 N is approximately equivalent to the downward gravitational force exerted by a weight of 1 kg). Following loss of consciousness, the amount of force is increased to 30 N. Application of the full amount of force while the patient is still awake can provoke active retching and regurgitation. In some cases, cricoid pressure may be briefly released to enable a successful intubation; not infrequently the benefit of release outweighs the risk for regurgitation. Cricoid pressure should then be reapplied until the correct endotracheal tube position is confirmed.

Historically, **thiopental (thiopentone)** (4 to 6 mg/kg) was the most frequently used induction agent for cesarean delivery. Because of recent lack of availability, it is now rarely used in the United States, although it is still used in other countries. **Propofol** (2 to 2.8 mg/kg) is now commonly used. In the presence of hemodynamic instability, **ketamine** (1 to 1.5 mg/kg) or **etomidate** (0.3 mg/kg) should be substituted for propofol. Paralysis is achieved by **succinylcholine (suxamethonium)** (1 to 1.5 mg/kg) in 30 to 40 seconds. Administration of a defasciculating dose of a nondepolarizing muscle relaxant is *not* recommended because it may delay the onset of neuromuscular blockade with succinylcholine. Pregnancy appears to be associated with less severe succinylcholine-induced fasciculations and muscle pain.[219]

Rocuronium (1 mg/kg) may provide intubating conditions similar to those provided with succinylcholine (1 mg/kg)[220,221] and is a suitable alternative when succinylcholine should be avoided (e.g., malignant hyperthermia susceptibility, myotonic dystrophy, spastic paraparesis). Some data suggest its use in cesarean delivery may be associated with a lower frequency of myalgia compared with succinylcholine.[221] The use of a priming preinduction dose of a nondepolarizing muscle relaxant is not recommended during pregnancy because it may result in complete paralysis and increase the risk for aspiration.[222] Enhanced activity of nondepolarizing agents may also be observed in patients receiving magnesium sulfate (e.g., for seizure prophylaxis in women with preeclampsia or for fetal neuroprotection).[223]

Sugammadex, a modified gamma-cyclodextrin, has been demonstrated to be effective in providing rapid recovery (a train-of-four ratio > 0.9) without recurarization from moderate and profound rocuronium-induced neuromuscular blockade in parturients undergoing cesarean delivery.[224]

A small-diameter cuffed endotracheal tube (i.e., 6.5 or 7.0 mm) should be used during pregnancy; the use of a videolaryngoscopy device (e.g., C-MAC, Glidescope), a flexible stylet within the endotracheal tube, and a bougie on standby allows a "first and best" attempt at tracheal intubation. Tissue trauma and airway edema may occur with repeated attempts at intubation. Correct endotracheal tube placement should be confirmed by checking for a normal capnographic tracing.

Auscultation should be performed to rule out inadvertent endobronchial intubation. The anesthesia provider should also observe ongoing evidence of adequate maternal oxyhemoglobin saturation as well as bilateral thoracic movement and breath sounds. If there is doubt, fiberoptic bronchoscopy can confirm the correct placement of the endotracheal tube in the trachea. If incorrect endotracheal tube placement is promptly recognized, extubation (with continued cricoid pressure) will often allow another attempt without the need for additional muscle relaxant. Anticipation of a difficult tracheal intubation, or a failed intubation attempt, should invoke the difficult airway algorithm and a call for assistance (see Chapter 29). Options include (1) allowing the patient to awaken, (2) using alternative techniques to place an endotracheal tube, and (3) using alternative airway devices. Emergency airway equipment (including equipment for surgical airway access) should be immediately available in all obstetric operating rooms.[24]

Some authors have suggested that a supraglottic airway device (e.g., **laryngeal mask airway** [**LMA**]) can be used routinely for general anesthesia for cesarean delivery. One series reported clinically effective airway management with a classic LMA that was placed successfully on the first attempt in 98% of 1067 healthy parturients undergoing elective cesarean delivery with general anesthesia.[225] Cricoid pressure was maintained throughout the cesarean delivery and no adverse sequelae occurred. Another study utilized an LMA with a higher seal pressure than a classic LMA and a built-in gastric draining tube, and reported successful placement in 98% of 3000 healthy parturients undergoing elective cesarean delivery.[226] Cricoid pressure was not maintained after confirmation of successful airway placement; there was one case of regurgitation without aspiration. In both of these studies, patients were excluded if they had symptoms of gastropharyngeal reflux, known/predicted difficult airway, and a prepregnancy BMI > 30 kg/m². As supraglottic airway devices do not prevent pulmonary soiling with gastric contents as efficiently as an endotracheal tube, and high morbidity rate is associated with aspiration, the authors do not routinely use these devices for cesarean delivery. However, any device that can facilitate ventilation should be used as a lifesaving device in situations of failed intubation. A number of variations to the classic LMA have been developed that may facilitate airway management in specific situations (see Chapter 29).

Maintenance

The goals for anesthetic maintenance include (1) adequate maternal and fetal oxygenation, with maintenance of normocapnia for pregnancy; (2) appropriate depth of anesthesia to promote maternal comfort and a quiescent surgical field and to prevent awareness and recall; (3) minimal effects on uterine tone after delivery; and (4) minimal adverse effects on the neonate. These goals can be accomplished using low concentration inhalational anesthesia or, less commonly, total intravenous anesthesia.

In the absence of fetal compromise, an F_{IO_2} of 0.3 appears to provide sufficient oxygenation while minimizing the production of oxygen free radicals (see discussion above). Although the use of a higher F_{IO_2} can increase maternal arterial (MA) and UV blood oxygen content, this action has not been observed to result in differences in 1- or 5-minute Apgar or neurobehavioral scores.[227,228] As a consequence, in the absence of fetal compromise, inspired oxygen concentrations should be guided by pulse oximetry rather than provision of an arbitrarily set level of F_{IO_2}.

Maternal ventilation should maintain normocapnia, which at term gestation is a $Paco_2$ of 30 to 32 mm Hg (4.0 to 4.3 kPa). Excessive ventilation can cause uteroplacental vasoconstriction and a leftward shift of the oxyhemoglobin dissociation curve, which may result in compromised fetal oxygenation.[229] On the other hand, hypercapnia can lead to maternal tachycardia and is also undesirable.

Initially, high fresh-gas flows should be used to ensure an adequate end-tidal concentration of the volatile halogenated agent. No specific volatile halogenated agent has been demonstrated to be superior. The anesthetic requirement for volatile halogenated agents is diminished 25% to 40% during pregnancy.[230] A **bispectral index (BIS)** < 60 typically requires greater than 0.75 minimum alveolar concentration (MAC) of a volatile halogenated agent combined with 50% nitrous oxide and has been suggested to prevent intraoperative awareness and recall in parturients undergoing general anesthesia[231]; however, this target BIS value requires further study in pregnant women. Several studies suggest the need for a lower volatile agent requirement to maintain a target BIS value in women with prior labor compared with women without prior labor[232,233]; these results could not be explained by differences in plasma concentrations of progesterone, prolactin, or cortisol.[233]

In clinical practice, approximately 1.0 MAC of a volatile halogenated agent is typically administered between tracheal intubation and delivery. Volatile halogenated agents cause dose-dependent depression of uterine contractility,[232,234,235] which may lead to greater blood loss after delivery.[236] Therefore, the concentration of the volatile agent is reduced to 0.5 to 0.75 MAC after delivery. Nitrous oxide 50% in oxygen is often added to reduce the required concentration of the volatile agent, thereby mitigating adverse effects on uterine tone; intravenous **propofol** or **ketamine** can also be administered to maintain an appropriate depth of anesthesia. The administration of a benzodiazepine (e.g., **midazolam**) after delivery may reduce the risk for maternal awareness.

Intravenous opioids are often withheld until after delivery to minimize the potential for neonatal respiratory depression; however, there may be circumstances in which maternal hemodynamic stability or blunting of responses to airway manipulation and surgical stimulation favor the administration of opioids during the induction of general anesthesia. Rapidly acting lipid soluble opioids (e.g., **remifentanil** and **alfentanil**) are ideal for mitigating the responses to laryngoscopy and intubation.[237] Intraoperatively, the prolonged activity of hydrophilic agents (e.g., morphine, hydromorphone) can be useful to minimize volatile agent use and for the provision of intraoperative and postoperative analgesia (see Chapter 27).

Because of pregnancy-induced stretching of the abdominal wall, additional neuromuscular blockade may not be necessary in the parturient who has an adequate depth of anesthesia (with administration of both a volatile agent and an opioid). A small dose of a short-acting nondepolarizing agent (or an infusion of succinylcholine) may be administered, with maternal response monitored with a peripheral nerve stimulator, if additional muscle relaxation is indicated.

General anesthetic agents can redistribute from the neonatal fat to the central circulation and lead to secondary depression of neonatal ventilatory effort; thus, the presence of a pediatrician (or another neonatal provider) is advisable until a normal ventilatory pattern is observed. Although differences in maternal and umbilical artery acid-base status have been observed in women who underwent elective general anesthesia compared with epidural anesthesia for cesarean delivery, similar neonatal outcomes were demonstrated.[238] Similarly, epidemiologic data suggest that brief exposure to general anesthetic agents at the time of cesarean delivery is not associated with an increased risk for abnormal neonatal neurodevelopment and later learning difficulties.[239]

Emergence and Tracheal Extubation

When the patient awakens, tracheal extubation should be performed with the patient in a semirecumbent position. The patient should demonstrate purposeful response to verbal commands and return of protective airway reflexes before tracheal extubation. In a review of anesthesia-related maternal deaths between 1985 and 2003 in the state of Michigan,[240] deaths associated with hypoventilation or airway obstruction did not occur at induction and tracheal intubation but rather during emergence, extubation, or recovery from anesthesia. Risk factors associated with mortality were obesity and African-American race, which may have delayed the visual recognition of cyanosis; medical management and medication issues were also identified. The ASA Practice Guidelines for Postanesthetic Care[241] suggest that pulse oximetry is associated with early detection of hypoxemia; the guidelines recommend periodic assessment of airway patency, respiratory rate, and oxygen saturation during emergence and recovery. If repeated airway manipulation, massive hemorrhage, or emergency hysterectomy has occurred, delayed extubation and/or transfer to an ICU should be considered.

Pharmacology

Thiopental Historically, the barbiturates (e.g., **thiopental**, **methohexital**, **thiamylal**) have been the induction agents most commonly used for cesarean delivery. Extensive published data have confirmed the safety and efficacy of thiopental for induction of anesthesia in patients undergoing cesarean delivery at various gestational ages. Thiopental 4 to 6 mg/kg provides a rapid and reliable induction of anesthesia. As a negative inotrope and vasodilator, thiopental can cause decreased cardiac output and blood pressure,[242] which may result in significant hypotension in hypovolemic patients. Some investigators have attempted to minimize this effect by using a lower dose of thiopental in combination with ketamine or propofol, with varying success.

Thiopental rapidly crosses the placenta. In 11 healthy subjects who underwent induction of general anesthesia with thiopental, the mean umbilical venous-to-maternal venous (UV/MV) ratio was 1.08 with an induction-to-delivery (I-D) interval that ranged from 8 to 22 minutes.[243] Fetal-to-maternal concentration ratios after a single thiopental dose exposure in other studies in term infants exhibited a range of 0.43 to 0.96.[244] The equilibration of thiopental occurs relatively rapidly in the fetus; however, fetal brain concentrations rarely exceed the threshold required for neonatal depression. With a maternal induction dose of 4 mg/kg, umbilical vein concentrations of thiopental are well below the arterial plasma concentrations necessary to produce anesthesia in adults.[245] However, with large induction doses (8 mg/kg), thiopental can produce significant neonatal depression.[246]

Several theories have been proposed to explain the clinical occurrence of an unconscious mother but an awake neonate: (1) preferential uptake of thiopental by the fetal liver, which is the first organ perfused by blood coming from the umbilical vein[246]; (2) the higher relative water content of the fetal brain[247]; (3) rapid redistribution of the drug into the maternal tissues, which causes a rapid reduction in the maternal-to-fetal concentration gradient; (4) nonhomogeneity of blood flow in the intervillous space; and (5) progressive dilution by admixture with the various components of the fetal circulation. Because of this rapid equilibration of thiopental and the low fetal brain concentration of thiopental, there is no advantage in delaying delivery until thiopental concentrations decline. There is no evidence that thiopental causes adverse fetal effects when the incision-to-delivery interval is prolonged.

Propofol Propofol is an induction agent with a rapid onset, rapid recovery, and favorable side-effect profile, which includes a low incidence of nausea and vomiting. Induction with propofol can result in pain on injection and a reduction in maternal blood pressure and cardiac output. The pharmacokinetics of propofol are similar in pregnant and nonpregnant women, except for a more rapid clearance observed during pregnancy, which may partially reflect drug removal through blood loss and the delivery of the infant and placenta.

When given as an intravenous bolus, by continuous infusion, or both, propofol rapidly crosses the placenta and results in an UV/MV ratio of approximately 0.7.[248] In an *in vitro* human placenta study,[249] propofol produced vasodilation of fetal placental blood vessels and decreased the effect of various vasoconstrictors, most likely through the inhibition of calcium influx through the smooth muscle sarcolemma; lipid emulsion, the propofol carrier solution, was not responsible for these effects. One randomized trial of women undergoing cesarean delivery with general anesthesia reported lower Apgar and neurobehavioral scores in neonates delivered of mothers who received propofol compared with thiopental[250]; however, this finding was not replicated in a more recent randomized trial.[251] Other studies have found no effect of propofol on neurobehavioral scores or the time to sustained spontaneous respiration with an induction bolus dose of propofol 2.5 mg/kg or with infusion doses < 6 mg/kg/h.[252,253] However, higher doses of propofol (9 mg/kg/h) have been correlated with a low Neurologic and Adaptive Capacity Score (NACS).[254]

Compared with thiopental, propofol results in a greater incidence of maternal hypotension,[255] which may more effectively attenuate the response to laryngoscopy and tracheal intubation at the risk for reduced uteroplacental blood flow. Care must be given to closely monitor maternal blood pressure following induction with propofol and, if needed, supporting the blood pressure with vasopressors. Maternal heart rate needs to also be carefully monitored; one report noted a transient but severe episode of maternal bradycardia after administration of propofol followed by succinylcholine for rapid-sequence induction.[256] This effect has also been demonstrated in pregnant ewes; one animal experienced severe bradycardia that led to a sinus arrest.[257]

In a study of nonpregnant women, the interaction of propofol and ketamine was found to be additive at hypnotic and anesthetic endpoints; the cardiostimulant effects of ketamine appear to offset the cardiodepressant effects of propofol.[258]

Ketamine The sympathomimetic properties of ketamine make it an ideal induction agent in the setting of an urgent cesarean delivery in a patient with hypotension or an acute exacerbation of asthma.[259] Ketamine is an analgesic, hypnotic, and amnestic agent associated with minimal respiratory depression; it is often used to supplement a neuraxial technique that may not be providing optimal anesthesia. Ketamine's effect is likely related to antagonism of the N-methyl-D-aspartate (NMDA) receptor.

An induction dose of ketamine 1 mg/kg is associated with an increase in blood pressure and heart rate immediately after induction, and a further increase is observed after laryngoscopy and tracheal intubation.[260] Such an increase can be desirable in the bleeding hypotensive patient but should be avoided in the parturient with hypertension (e.g., preeclampsia) or heart disease in which tachycardia or hypertension may not be well tolerated. In experimental animal models, ketamine was sometimes associated with direct myocardial depression and decreased cardiac output[242]; care must therefore be exercised when using this medication to induce patients with severe shock or impaired cardiac function.

Studies in pregnant ewes suggest that the use of ketamine is not associated with a reduction in uterine blood flow.[261] Ketamine is associated with dose-dependent increases in uterine tone, but a single induction dose does not increase uterine tone at term gestation.[262] Using an induction dose of ketamine 0.7 mg/kg in gravid ewes, a 39% increase in resting uterine tone with no effect on uterine blood flow was observed.[261]

Ketamine rapidly crosses the placenta. No neonatal depression is observed with doses < 1 mg/kg.[263] At higher doses, low Apgar scores, neonatal respiratory depression, and need for resuscitation have been reported.[263] Apgar scores and umbilical cord blood gas and pH measurements at delivery with ketamine are similar to those with thiopental.[264,265] A formulation of the S(+) stereoisomer of ketamine is available for clinical use in some countries outside the United States. In chronically instrumented pregnant sheep, Strumper et al.[266] found that the effects of S(+) ketamine were similar to those of the racemic mixture in terms of maternal and fetal hemodynamics and uterine perfusion; however, S(+) ketamine was associated with a smaller increase in maternal and fetal Pco_2 than that seen with racemic ketamine in spontaneously breathing animals.

The emergence delirium and hallucinations experienced with ketamine, particularly in the unpremedicated patient, have limited the adoption of this drug as a routine induction agent for cesarean delivery. If ketamine is used, a benzodiazepine may be administered to decrease the incidence of these psychomimetic effects.[267] Maternal awareness may still occur after an induction dose of ketamine 1 to 1.5 mg/kg,[268] but the incidence is lower than with thiopental 4 mg/kg or a mixture of ketamine 0.5 mg/kg and thiopental 2 mg/kg.[269] The incidence of maternal awareness can also be diminished with the coadministration of a benzodiazepine.

When used to maintain general anesthesia with 50% nitrous oxide in oxygen for cesarean delivery, a continuous infusion of ketamine (70 μg/kg/min) was followed by a higher incidence of factual recall and postoperative pain than seen with a volatile anesthetic technique, suggesting this approach is not preferred for the maintenance of anesthesia.[270] Whether ketamine, given as a bolus or infusion initiated after infant delivery, can provide postcesarean analgesia and pain modulation remains controversial (see discussion below). One study found that patients who received ketamine 1 mg/kg for induction had lower postoperative morphine consumption than patients who received thiopental 4 mg/kg (anesthesia was maintained with nitrous oxide and isoflurane).[264]

Etomidate Etomidate is an induction agent that produces rapid onset of anesthesia with minimal effects on cardiorespiratory function. This property makes it ideal for parturients who are hemodynamically unstable or who would not tolerate hemodynamic aberrations (e.g., patients with severe cardiac disease).[271] With an induction dose of 0.2 to 0.3 mg/kg, etomidate undergoes rapid hydrolysis, thereby allowing rapid recovery.[272] Intravenous administration of etomidate may cause pain and involuntary muscle movements in unpremedicated patients; etomidate is also associated with nausea and vomiting, potential activation of seizures in patients with an epileptogenic foci, and an impaired glucocorticoid response to stress.[273]

Etomidate crosses the placenta rapidly; however, large variations in the UV/MV ratio (0.04 to 0.5) have been reported.[272] An induction dose of etomidate 0.3 mg/kg was associated with better neonatal acid-base measurements and overall clinical condition than with thiopental 3.5 mg/kg.[274] A transient (<6 hours) reduction in neonatal cortisol production was observed when an induction dose of etomidate was used for cesarean delivery[275]; however, the clinical relevance of this finding is unclear.

Midazolam Midazolam is a short-acting, water-soluble benzodiazepine that has few adverse hemodynamic effects and provides hypnosis and amnesia. It is commonly used as a premedicant before anesthesia but also can be used as an induction agent for cesarean delivery, although there are few indications for this purpose (e.g., when there are relative or absolute contraindications to the use of other agents). Data suggest that compared with thiopental, midazolam (at a dose of 0.2 mg/kg) for induction of anesthesia results in a higher incidence of low Apgar scores and longer time to neonatal spontaneous respiration, as well as lower neurobehavioral scores, body temperature, general body tone, and arm recoil.[276] However, these differences are short lived and do not persist beyond 4 hours after delivery.

Muscle relaxants Muscle relaxants are commonly used before delivery to provide optimal tracheal intubation and operating conditions. These drugs are highly ionized with low lipid solubility and do not undergo significant placental transfer.

The depolarizing agent **succinylcholine** at a dose of 1 to 1.5 mg/kg is the muscle relaxant of choice for most parturients undergoing rapid-sequence induction of general anesthesia. Maternal administration provides adequate intubating conditions within approximately 45 seconds of intravenous administration. Succinylcholine is highly ionized and water-soluble and only small amounts cross the placenta. Although high doses of succinylcholine (2 to 3 mg/kg) can result in detectable levels in umbilical cord blood, animal experiments indicate that neonatal muscle weakness only occurs when very large doses many times higher than usual clinical doses are given.[277]

Succinylcholine is rapidly metabolized by plasma pseudocholinesterase, the concentration of which is decreased during pregnancy; however, in most patients this effect is offset by the pregnancy-induced increase in volume of distribution. Thus, recovery from succinylcholine is not prolonged unless the patient has extremely low levels of pseudocholinesterase or atypical pseudocholinesterase.[278] The administration of metoclopramide may also prolong succinylcholine-induced neuromuscular blockade, perhaps by inhibiting plasma pseudocholinesterase[279]; this effect is rarely (if ever) clinically significant. The return of neuromuscular function should be confirmed before additional doses of muscle relaxant are given.

Rocuronium is a suitable alternative to succinylcholine when a nondepolarizing agent is preferred for rapid-sequence induction (e.g., history of malignant hyperthermia), particularly with the option of rapid reversal using **sugammadex** (16 mg/kg). Abouleish et al.[280] reported that in women having cesarean delivery, rocuronium (0.6 mg/kg) provided good to excellent intubating conditions after a mean interval of 79 seconds, and maximal effect intubating conditions in 98 seconds. Magorian et al.[281] reported that rocuronium 0.9 and 1.2 mg/kg resulted in onset of paralysis similar to that of succinylcholine (55 seconds), but with a significantly longer clinical duration of action. Rocuronium does not appear to adversely affect Apgar scores, acid-base measurements, time to sustained respiration, or neurobehavioral scores.[280]

Although its onset of action is slower than that of rocuronium,[281] **vecuronium** 0.1 mg/kg is another alternative to succinylcholine. However, its onset of action is significantly slower than succinylcholine, even after a priming dose is administered.[282] The mean duration of action of vecuronium is significantly longer in peripartum patients compared with nonpregnant controls.[283] Vecuronium crosses the placenta in small amounts; however, neonatal outcome, as assessed by Apgar scores and NACS, does not appear to be adversely affected.[284]

Atracurium is a less desirable agent for rapid-sequence induction because the high dose required for a rapid onset of action may result in significant histamine release, which may cause hypotension. **Cisatracurium** does not have these undesirable side effects, but its relatively slow onset makes it less optimal than other alternatives.[285]

Regardless of the choice of agent, laryngoscopy and tracheal intubation should not be attempted until adequate muscle relaxation has occurred. The use of a quantitative nerve stimulator allows an objective assessment of the onset and duration of the neuromuscular blockade. Residual neuromuscular blockade can be reversed with **neostigmine** (with **atropine** or **glycopyrrolate**) or **sugammadex**. To diminish the risk for aspiration, the anesthesia provider should confirm that the patient responds appropriately to verbal commands before tracheal extubation.

Nitrous oxide Nitrous oxide is commonly used for cesarean delivery because of its minimal effects on maternal blood pressure and uterine tone. The use of nitrous oxide allows for a reduction in the concentration of the volatile halogenated agent (high concentrations of which decrease uterine tone). Administration of 50% to 67% nitrous oxide in oxygen *without* another anesthetic agent does not provide complete anesthesia and was reported to result in maternal awareness in 12% to 26% of cases.[286,287]

Nitrous oxide rapidly crosses the placenta, where fetal tissue uptake reduces the fetal arterial concentration for the first 20 minutes. In an evaluation of the relationship between duration of exposure to 67% nitrous oxide and the resulting UV/MA concentration ratios, the observed ratios differed according to duration of exposure, as follows: 2 to 9 minutes (0.37), 9 to 14 minutes (0.61), and 14 to 50 minutes (0.70).[288] Apgar scores at 1 minute inversely correlated with duration of anesthesia, an effect observed in other animal studies.[289] The use of a lower concentration (e.g., 50%) of nitrous oxide may reduce but not eliminate these neonatal effects. A randomized trial of parturients undergoing general anesthesia compared 100% oxygen with 50% nitrous oxide in oxygen, both supplemented by isoflurane (1.5 MAC for the first 5 minutes and 1.0 MAC thereafter).[290] Neonates exposed to nitrous oxide required more resuscitation, although no significant differences were observed in Apgar scores.

Volatile halogenated agents Volatile halogenated agents are the most commonly used agents for maintaining general anesthesia for cesarean delivery. Volatile halogenated agents produce central nervous system and cardiovascular effects in a dose-dependent manner; of particular concern for the obstetric patient are the resulting decreases in blood pressure (which may result in reduced uterine blood flow) and uterine tone. The uptake and delivery of volatile agents is determined by inspired partial pressure, blood flow, and the blood/gas/

tissue partition coefficient. The alveolar partial pressure of volatile agents during pregnancy follows known patterns of equilibration; the following commonly used agents are listed in order of more rapid to slower equilibration: **desflurane**, **sevoflurane**, and **isoflurane**. Volatile halogenated agents cross the placenta rapidly and equilibrate quickly with fetal tissues.[291] Neonatal depression may occur. This is typically not a clinical issue when volatile agents are used for emergency cesarean delivery, because the delivery usually occurs before much of the volatile agent crosses the placenta (particularly if uteroplacental insufficiency is the reason for emergency delivery). Volatile halogenated agents cause dose-dependent depression of uterine contractility. These effects may influence maternal blood loss after delivery.

Lower concentrations of volatile halogenated agents are required during pregnancy, with an approximately 30% reduction in MAC compared with nonpregnant women.[292,293] These findings were correlated with an increase in progesterone level. Animal models demonstrate that long-term administration of progesterone is associated with a reduction in MAC.[294] This reduction in MAC persists for 24 to 36 hours postpartum, with a gradual return to normal values by 72 hours.[295]

Opioids All opioids, particularly those with high lipid solubility (e.g., remifentanil, fentanyl, sufentanil), readily pass through the placenta to the fetus. Consequently, the administration of opioids is usually avoided until after delivery to reduce the risk for neonatal depression. However, the hemodynamic stability provided by opioids during airway manipulation and surgery may be valuable in select settings, particularly in the presence of maternal cardiac disease, neurologic conditions, and preeclampsia or hypertension.

Remifentanil administration has been observed to mitigate the hemodynamic responses to tracheal intubation and surgery. Ngan Kee et al.[237] reported that a single dose of remifentanil 1 µg/kg at induction attenuated the increase in blood pressure and heart rate after laryngoscopy and tracheal intubation in patients having elective cesarean delivery. These authors found that remifentanil crossed the placenta with UV/MA and UA/UV concentration ratios of 0.73 and 0.60, respectively.[237] In patients having elective cesarean delivery under general anesthesia, Draisci et al.[296] reported that when remifentanil was administered as a 0.5 µg/kg bolus followed by a 0.15 µg/kg/min continuous infusion until peritoneal incision there was transitory but significant neonatal depression; compared with infants of mothers who received fentanyl 5 µg/kg after delivery, infants exposed to remifentanil had lower Apgar scores and UVpH, and some required tracheal intubation.

Fentanyl rapidly crosses the placenta. It is 60% to 80% protein bound; thus, approximately one-third is available for transfer across the placenta.[297]

Morphine, despite its low lipid solubility, has a UV/MV concentration ratio of 0.96 at 5 minutes[298]; this rate of equilibration and the production of active metabolites are relevant considerations in the use and timing of intravenous morphine administration.

Meperidine (pethidine) is highly lipid soluble and is 50% to 70% protein bound; maternal administration results in a mean UV/MV blood concentration ratio of 0.75.[299] The production of the active metabolite normeperidine, which can accumulate in both the mother and neonate and result in respiratory and neurobehavioral alterations, limits the use of meperidine as a principal analgesic agent during cesarean delivery; however, after delivery of the neonate, an intravenous dose of 12.5 to 25 mg is useful for treatment of shivering in the mother.

Maternal respiratory depression, as well as nausea and emesis during the intraoperative and postoperative periods, represent significant concerns in parturients given IV opioids.

Local Anesthesia

As a method used primarily for supplementation of neuraxial anesthesia, local anesthetic infiltration can be used to facilitate an emergency cesarean delivery. This technique has been well described and is used predominantly in low-resource settings, where contemporary anesthesia techniques may not be readily available. Few contemporary obstetric providers are familiar or proficient with this technique in developed countries.

The success of local infiltration depends on the surgeon making a midline abdominal incision, avoiding the use of retractors, and not exteriorizing the uterus. In settings in which an anesthesia provider might not be readily available, the surgeon might begin surgery with the aid of local infiltration; after delivery of the infant, the achievement of temporary hemostasis, and the arrival of the anesthesia provider, surgery may be completed once general anesthesia has been induced.

Local infiltration is performed in sequential steps as the operation progresses (Box 26.7).[300] The use of 0.5% lidocaine with epinephrine is recommended; the use of a more concentrated solution may result in LAST. A 25-gauge spinal needle is used to make the intracutaneous injection; the needle is inserted just below the umbilicus and is directed in the midline toward the symphysis pubis. Approximately 10 mL of local anesthetic is required to create a skin wheal that extends from the symphysis pubis to the umbilicus. The subcutaneous injection is also performed for the full length of the planned incision with 10 to 20 mL of local anesthetic. Ideally, the surgeon should then wait 3 to 4 minutes to allow the local anesthetic agent to exert its effect before making the skin incision.

A vertical skin incision is made between the umbilicus and the symphysis pubis and is extended down to the rectus fascia. The surgeon then infiltrates local anesthetic into the rectus fascia and rectus muscles by making three to five laterally directed injections on each side. The needle should be passed between the rectus sheath and the transversus muscle at an angle of 10 to 15 degrees and a depth of 3 to 5 cm; aspiration is performed and 2 to 3 mL of local anesthetic is injected at each site, with an additional 1 mL injected with needle withdrawal. The surgeon should also make oblique injections at the upper and lower poles of the incision. The local anesthetic will spread freely in the rectus sheath, but it takes 4 to 5 minutes for anesthesia to be complete. The suprapubic area must also be generously infiltrated to ensure blockade of the branches of the iliohypogastric nerve. The disadvantage of the rectus sheath block is the large volume (40 to 50 mL) of local anesthetic required; a less effective alternative that requires less volume and time is to raise a longitudinal paramedian wheal in the rectus fascia on each side of the midline and to infiltrate the suprapubic region.

The surgeon then extends the incision through the rectus sheath, and the peritoneum is grasped with forceps clamps. If the patient has pain, the parietal peritoneum may be infiltrated with 5 to 10 mL of local anesthetic and then incised. The visceral peritoneum overlying the area of the uterine incision is injected with 10 mL of local anesthetic and is then incised and reflected appropriately. Paracervical infiltration with 5 to 10 mL of local anesthetic may block pain impulses from the uterus and cervix.

A uterine incision is made, and the infant is delivered. The surgeon must avoid forceful retraction and blunt dissection of tissue planes and uterine manipulation should be kept to a minimum. A support person at the head of the table who can provide coaching and reassurance to the mother is invaluable.

The major disadvantages of local infiltration anesthesia are patient discomfort and the potential for LAST, given that as much as 100 mL of local anesthetic solution is required. The risk for LAST may be especially problematic in the absence of a skilled anesthesia provider to assist with maternal resuscitation. Another disadvantage is the amount of time required for maximal anesthesia to develop; maternal discomfort often accompanies an urgent delivery performed with this form of anesthesia. Finally, local infiltration does not provide satisfactory operating conditions in the event of a surgical complication (e.g., uterine laceration, broad ligament hematoma).

Cesarean delivery with use of local infiltration, if successful, has the advantages of preserving maternal cardiovascular stability and a patent airway while allowing the initiation of surgery in emergency cases. However, the technique is frequently associated with incomplete maternal anesthesia, which subsequently presents significant management issues

---

BOX 26.7   Steps for Initiating Local Infiltration Anesthesia for Cesarean Delivery

1. Professional support person with patient
2. Infiltration with 0.5% lidocaine with epinephrine (total dose should not exceed 500 mg)
3. Intracutaneous injection in the midline from the umbilicus to the symphysis pubis
4. Subcutaneous injection
5. Incision down to the rectus fascia
6. Rectus fascia blockade
7. Parietal peritoneum infiltration and incision
8. Visceral peritoneum infiltration and incision
9. Paracervical injection
10. Uterine incision and delivery
11. Administration of general anesthesia for uterine repair and abdominal closure, if needed

because the surgical procedure has commenced, positioning options are limited, and the consequences of the operative procedure (e.g., hemorrhage) may require immediate attention.

Additional peripheral nerve blockade techniques (e.g., transversus abdominis plane blockade[301]) may successfully augment local anesthesia infiltration; however, the degree to which the maternal experience is enhanced and the timing required to place these blocks deserve further investigation.

RECOVERY FROM ANESTHESIA

Cesarean delivery is a major abdominal surgical procedure with significant anatomic, physiologic, and hormonal sequelae, even when it is performed electively without complications in a healthy parturient. The risk for adverse outcomes is greater in the presence of maternal comorbidity or in the setting of surgical complications (e.g., massive blood loss, cesarean hysterectomy).[302]

A study at a single tertiary care center found that the majority of patients who received neuraxial anesthesia for cesarean delivery could meet revised discharge criteria (i.e., presence of a normal level of consciousness, stable vital signs, adequate analgesia, and ability to flex the knees) within 60 minutes, which could shorten the average duration of PACU stay and result in cost savings.[303] However, 26% to 36% of patients remained in the PACU for up to 180 minutes because of pain, sedation, nausea and vomiting, pruritus, prolonged neuroblockade, and/or drug treatment. In addition, 16% to 22% remained in the PACU for up to 210 minutes for cardiovascular (e.g., bleeding, hypertension, hypotension, tachycardia) or respiratory events. Moreover, the study did not include the most seriously ill or highest-risk patients, who were transferred directly to an ICU.

The 2001 National Sentinel Caesarean Section Audit in the United Kingdom reported that 10% of women undergoing cesarean delivery required admission to a high-dependency unit.[304] Moreover, 3.5% of these women required subsequent transfer to an ICU. Preexisting comorbid conditions accounted for the majority (80%) of these ICU admissions; a smaller fraction were caused by the medical emergency (e.g., uterine rupture, placental abruption) that prompted the cesarean delivery.[304] Although ICU admission is uncommon in obstetric patients, it occurs more frequently (approximately 9 per 1000 patients) after cesarean delivery; the risk for ICU admission following cesarean delivery is greater in patients with a high BMI.[304]

Of concern, inadequate postoperative care has been cited as a recurring factor in maternal deaths (see Chapter 39). The ASA Practice Guidelines for Obstetric Anesthesia state that "appropriate equipment and personnel should be available to care for obstetric patients recovering from neuraxial or general anesthesia."[24] Similarly, the Guidelines for the Provision of Anaesthesia Services for an Obstetric Population from the Royal College of Anaesthetists state that postoperative recovery care of the patient undergoing cesarean delivery should meet the same standard of care as required for the nonobstetric postoperative population.[305]

The use of **enhanced recovery after surgery (ERAS)** protocols for women undergoing cesarean delivery appears to reduce the length of hospital stay, postpartum opioid consumption, pain scores, time to mobilization and urinary catheter removal, and hospitalization costs, with minimal maternal readmission rates.[306] Although there are inconsistencies among ERAS protocols, common components include the use of multimodal analgesia such as scheduled acetaminophen started preoperatively or intraoperatively and nonsteroidal antiinflammatory drugs after peritoneal closure, with early ambulation, oral intake, and removal of urinary catheters.

Oral Intake

A systematic review of six randomized clinical trials that compared early with delayed oral intake of fluid and food after cesarean delivery found that the early oral consumption (within 4 to 8 hours) was associated with a shorter time to return of bowel sounds and a shorter hospital stay.[307] No differences were reported in nausea and vomiting, abdominal distention, time to bowel activity, paralytic ileus, or need for analgesia. Guidelines from the National Institute for Health and Clinical Excellence state: "If women are recovering well after caesarean birth and do not have complications, they can eat and drink as normal."[308]

Removal of Urinary Catheter

There are no differences in the incidence of urinary retention after general anesthesia and epidural anesthesia following cesarean delivery.[309] Risk factors for postpartum urinary retention after cesarean delivery include the use of postoperative opioid analgesia (particularly when given via an epidural catheter), multiple gestation, and a low BMI.[310] Most urinary catheters are removed either immediately after cesarean delivery or within 24 hours; there are no differences between these two options in regard to postoperative urinary retention, dysuria, urgency, fever, positive microscopy, or length of hospital stay[311]; immediate removal does appear to decrease the risk for urinary infection and lead to earlier ambulation.[312] In obstetric patients, the return of bladder sensation of fullness after neuraxial techniques appears to be a function of time, rather than urinary volume.[313] The return of bladder sensation after spinal anesthesia for cesarean delivery (with hyperbaric bupivacaine and fentanyl) was shown to take longer (mean, 374 [IQR, 172 to 692 minutes]) than return of sensation after patient-controlled epidural analgesia for vaginal delivery (mean, 234 [IQR, 95 to 382] minutes).[313]

Postoperative Assessment and Discharge

The anesthesia provider should assess for recovery of motor and sensory function if a neuraxial technique was administered. Women should be reassured that breastfeeding is safe, even after general anesthesia, and that postoperative analgesics have a favorable safety profile. Early mobility and ambulation should be encouraged.

ANESTHETIC COMPLICATIONS

Awareness and Recall

Cesarean delivery is a high-risk procedure for the occurrence of intraoperative awareness, defined as the spontaneous postoperative recall of an event that occurred during general anesthesia.[33] The following factors contribute to the risk for maternal awareness during cesarean delivery: (1) avoidance of sedative premedication, (2) deliberate use of a low concentration of a volatile halogenated agent, (3) use of muscle relaxants, (4) reduction in dose of anesthetic agents during hypotension or hemorrhage, (5) presence of partial neuraxial blockade in parturients requiring conversion to general anesthesia after failed neuraxial anesthesia, and (6) the (mistaken) assumption that high baseline sympathetic tone is responsible for intraoperative tachycardia in parturients.

Concern for neonatal depression and uterine atony has led to the practice of administering relatively low doses of volatile halogenated agents. Historical studies showed that when general anesthesia for cesarean delivery was induced with thiopental followed by nitrous oxide/oxygen without a volatile agent, there was a high incidence of maternal awareness.[286,287] Using an isolated forearm technique, King et al.[314] assessed 30 women undergoing cesarean delivery with thiopental 250 mg, succinylcholine infusion, and 0.5% halothane in 50% nitrous oxide; the majority of patients signaled pain in the first minute. Other studies using the same anesthetic regimen have reported an incidence of recall of approximately 0% to 2%.[315] The use of higher concentrations of volatile has subsequently become a more common practice, leading to an incidence of maternal awareness of approximately 0.26%.[33] However, the result of increasing the depth of maternal anesthesia is that neonates born to women who receive general anesthesia tend to have lower Apgar and neurobehavioral scores, particularly when the incision-to-delivery interval exceeds 8 minutes.[316]

The optimal doses and concentrations of anesthetic agents to prevent awareness remain unclear, in part because of the difficulty in assessing awareness. Studies have evaluated several tools for assessment of depth of maternal anesthesia, including the electroencephalogram, brainstem auditory evoked potentials, and BIS monitoring.[33,232,269] BIS is an empirically derived electroencephalographic parameter in which values less than 60 are suggested to predict a low probability of intraoperative recall and awareness (although its utility remains controversial).[317] With each of these monitoring devices, the threshold for awareness will need further validation, particularly during pregnancy[318]; some data suggest that these types of monitors are not reliable for monitoring anesthesia depth in the setting of cesarean delivery.[319] Moreover, many of these devices may not be suitable for use during the emergency conditions under which most general anesthetics for cesarean delivery are administered.

Although pregnancy decreases anesthetic requirement by 25% to 40%,[230] administration of 0.5 MAC of a volatile halogenated agent may not reliably provide adequate depth of anesthesia to prevent maternal awareness. Therefore, some recommendations have included the following: (1) the use of larger doses of induction agents than are administered to nonpregnant patients (e.g., thiopental 5 to 7 mg/kg instead of 3 to 4 mg/kg); (2) an end-tidal volatile agent concentration > 0.8 MAC; (3) the highest concentration of nitrous oxide compatible with adequate oxygenation; and (4) the administration of an opioid and a benzodiazepine after delivery.[33] Intravenous induction or infusion techniques that may reduce the risk for maternal awareness include the administration of repeat doses of induction agents,[320] the use of ketamine,[268] or a combination of these.[321] Midazolam 0.075 mg/kg provides 30 to 60 minutes of anterograde amnesia when given to women undergoing elective cesarean delivery under epidural anesthesia.[322] Propofol exhibits an amnestic effect that is not dependent on the degree of sedation; however, the effect is significantly less than that with midazolam.[323]

The psychological morbidity associated with awareness should not be underestimated.[33] Further investigations into the anesthetic regimens and monitoring necessary to prevent awareness and recall in pregnant women undergoing operative procedures are needed. These studies should incorporate the growing data on sex- and pregnancy-related differences in pharmacokinetics and pharmacodynamics of drugs used for anesthesia.[324,325]

Paradoxically, the issue of recall is not limited to the administration of general anesthesia. In women undergoing cesarean delivery with a neuraxial technique who desire treatment for anxiety, the administration of anxiolytic or hypnotic agents may result in a lack of recall of delivery, which is typically undesirable.

Dyspnea

After the initiation of neuraxial anesthesia, the patient may complain of dyspnea. A common cause of this complaint is hypotension (causing hypoperfusion of the brainstem); therefore, the complaint of difficulty in breathing should prompt immediate assessment of blood pressure and treatment, if appropriate. Other causes of dyspnea are blunting of thoracic proprioception, partial blockade of abdominal and intercostal muscles, and the recumbent position, which increases the pressure of the abdominal contents against the diaphragm. The sensation of dyspnea appears related to the cephalad extent of the sensory blockade and may be mitigated by using a low-dose hyperbaric spinal bupivacaine technique in women undergoing cesarean delivery.[326]

Despite these changes, significant respiratory compromise is unlikely, primarily because the neuraxial blockade rarely affects the cervical nerves that control the diaphragm. A study examining the pulmonary effects of various spinal regimens including bupivacaine 10 mg, ropivacaine 20 mg, and levobupivacaine 10 mg, all with fentanyl 15 μg, in women undergoing cesarean delivery reported small reductions in the functional vital capacity (3% to 6%) and peak expiratory flow rate (6% to 13%).[327] However, the findings had no apparent clinical significance, were similar for all local anesthetics, and did not differ for sensory blockade that extended higher, versus no higher, than the T4 dermatome.

If the patient loses the ability to vocalize, demonstrate a strong hand grip, and/or maintain normal oxyhemoglobin saturation (e.g., symptoms suggestive of high spinal anesthesia), general anesthesia with tracheal intubation should be administered to maintain ventilation and prevent aspiration of gastric contents.

Hypotension

Hypotension is a common sequela of neuraxial anesthesia and, if severe and sustained, may lead to impairment of uteroplacental perfusion and result in fetal hypoxia, acidosis, and neonatal depression or injury.[328] Severe maternal hypotension can also have adverse maternal outcomes, including altered consciousness, pulmonary aspiration, apnea, and cardiac arrest.

Commonly accepted definitions for maternal hypotension are (1) a decrease in systolic blood pressure by more than 20% to 30% below baseline measurements or (2) a systolic blood pressure < 90 to 100 mm Hg.[329] Neuraxial anesthesia causes hypotension through blockade of sympathetic nerve fibers, which control vascular smooth muscle tone. Several studies using noninvasive measures of cardiac output have demonstrated that cardiac output commonly *increases* after spinal anesthesia, even in the presence of a phenylephrine infusion and fluid administration.[330-332] These studies emphasize that spinal anesthesia–induced hypotension is principally related to a marked decrease in systemic vascular resistance, rather than decreased cardiac output. The rate and extent of the sympathetic involvement, and subsequently the severity of hypotension, are determined by the onset and extent of the neuraxial blockade[333]; hypotension may be less common with epidural anesthesia than with spinal anesthesia because of the slower onset of neuroblockade and the earlier recognition and treatment.[334]

Risk Factors for Hypotension

A number of studies have attempted to identify pregnant women at increased risk for development of hypotension. Of interest, women with severe preeclampsia[335] or in established labor appear less likely to experience hypotension during administration of spinal anesthesia for cesarean delivery (see Chapter 35).

Studies using a modified orthostatic challenge (i.e., "tilt test") have been unable to establish a correlation in the observed change in orthostatic blood pressure or heart rate with hypotension after spinal anesthesia.[336,337] However, investigators found that patients with a baseline heart rate > 90 beats/min had an 83% chance (positive predictive value) of experiencing marked hypotension (decrease in blood pressure > 30%), whereas patients with a baseline heart rate < 90 beats/min had a 75% chance (negative predictive value) of *not* experiencing marked hypotension.[337]

One study found that the response of pregnant women to a preoperative *supine stress test* (i.e., placing the patient in the supine position to potentially cause aortocaval compression) predicted the occurrence of symptomatic hypotension, the need for ephedrine, and a decrease in systolic blood pressure

< 80 mm Hg during administration of spinal anesthesia for cesarean delivery.[338] The supine stress test was considered positive if it was associated with (1) an increase in maternal heart rate > 10 beats/min, (2) a decrease in systolic blood pressure > 15 mm Hg, or (3) signs and symptoms related to the supine position (e.g., nausea, dizziness). These investigators found that the preoperative stress test had a sensitivity of 69% and a specificity of 92% in identifying women who would have symptomatic hypotension.

Investigators have used other methods, including assessment of heart rate variability[339,340] and noninvasive measurements of systemic vascular resistance (e.g., thoracic impedance[341]) in an attempt to identify parturients at risk for neuraxial anesthesia–induced hypotension for cesarean delivery. To date, predicting which parturients will have hypotension after neuraxial anesthesia for cesarean delivery has not proven clinically feasible and will likely require more sophisticated studies that employ a number of different methodologies. Such a prediction is likely to be challenging given the myriad of factors that control the autonomic, physiologic, and hormonal changes and hemodynamic responses that occur during pregnancy.

Prevention and Treatment of Hypotension

A number of methods have been described for the prevention and treatment of hypotension during spinal anesthesia for cesarean delivery, including spinal dose modification, intravenous fluid loading, vasopressor administration, and various nonpharmacologic physical techniques (Table 26.7).[329] To achieve optimal outcomes for both mother (e.g., minimizing nausea and vomiting) and fetus (e.g., minimizing fetal acidosis), frequent measurement of blood pressure and aggressive management to prevent and treat hypotension are recommended.[342]

Spinal dose modification Spinal dose requirement is affected by many factors that vary according to individual circumstances.[342] The incidence of hypotension can be reduced by the use of lower doses of spinal local anesthetic, particularly if coadministered with a lipophilic opioid.[343] However, this needs to be balanced against the potential disadvantage of a decrease in quality and duration of block and the consequent risk for intraoperative pain that may require supplemental analgesia and sedation or the need to convert to general anesthesia.[342,344] It has been recommended that when low doses of spinal anesthetic are administered, a catheter-based technique such as CSE be used.[343]

Intravenous fluid loading The use of **intravenous fluid** to prevent hypotension can be manipulated by (1) the timing of administration, either before (preload or prehydration) or coincident with (coload or cohydration) the intrathecal injection; and (2) the type of fluid, either crystalloid or colloid. Rate of fluid administration may also play a role. Crystalloid preload is minimally effective, even when volumes as great as 30 mL/kg are infused.[55] By contrast, colloid preload has consistently been shown to reduce the incidence and severity of hypotension. A randomized trial of 36 healthy women undergoing elective cesarean delivery compared the administration of 1500 mL of lactated Ringer's solution and

TABLE 26.7   Methods for the Prevention and Treatment of Hypotension in Women Undergoing Cesarean Delivery with Neuraxial Anesthesia

	Intervention	Agent	Comments
Prevention			
	Left uterine displacement	15–30-degree tilt	May diminish IVC compression Limited by surgical exposure needs
	Fluids	Crystalloid	Preload: limited efficacy and intravascular duration Coload: greater efficacy
		Colloid	Greater efficacy and duration than crystalloids Anaphylaxis and AKI can occur
	Vasopressors	Phenylephrine	Infusion (25–50 µg/min) initially, started immediately after intrathecal injection Titrated to maintain systolic blood pressure ≥ 90% of baseline
		Ephedrine	Bolus (5–10 mg)
		Norepinephrine	Infusion (2–4 µg/min) initially Less bradycardia than with phenylephrine Limited data available
	Compression leg stockings		Not commonly used
Treatment			
	Vasopressors	Phenylephrine	Agent of choice, titrated in bolus doses (50 µg) to desired effect Infusion can be started
		Ephedrine	Bolus (5–10 mg) Useful to treat hypotension with bradycardia
	Fluids	Crystalloid	Guided by volume deficit or blood loss, of limited intravascular duration
		Colloids	Less commonly used Anaphylaxis and AKI can occur

AKI, Acute kidney injury; *IM*, intramuscularly; *IVC*, inferior vena cava.

500 mL and 1000 mL of hydroxyethyl starch solution (HES) 6% before spinal anesthesia for cesarean delivery.[345] The frequency of hypotension (systolic blood pressure < 100 mm Hg and < 80% of baseline) was 75%, 58%, and 17%, respectively. Significant increases in intravascular volume and cardiac output, as measured by indocyanine green spectrophotometry, were observed in the HES groups (Fig. 26.4). At 30 minutes, 100% of the HES volume, versus 28% of the lactated Ringer's volume, remained within the intravascular space.

Whether crystalloid fluid is given as a preload or coload does not appear to affect the frequency of hypotension. A metaanalysis of randomized trials comparing crystalloid preload with coload did not find a difference in the incidence of hypotension.[57] Similarly, no difference in the incidence of hypotension is observed with a colloid preload versus coload, likely reflecting the intravascular dwell time of colloid.[57]

Both preload and coload of colloid are more effective than coload of crystalloid in mitigating hypotension.[330] However, the cost and associated pruritus, mild coagulation abnormalities, and potential for allergic reaction to colloid starch solutions, particularly with first-generation agents, have tempered their widespread use. Possible fetal and neonatal effects related to the type and timing of maternal fluid administration deserve further investigation; for example, the rapid administration of 1500 to 2000 mL of fluid can release atrial

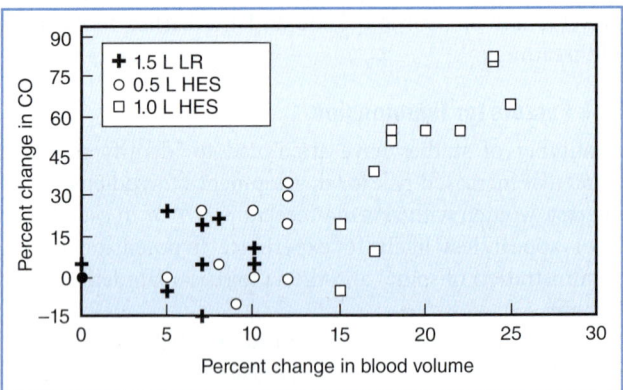

Fig. 26.4 The relationship between the changes (%) in blood volume and cardiac output after volume preload in parturients undergoing spinal anesthesia. Cardiac output (CO) was estimated with indocyanine green pulse spectrophotometry methodology. *HES*, Hydroxyethyl starch solution; *LR*, lactated Ringer's solution. Modified from Ueyama H, He Y, Tanigami H, et al. Effects of crystalloid and colloid preload on blood volume in the parturient undergoing spinal anesthesia for elective cesarean section. *Anesthesiology*. 1999;91:1571–1576.

natriuretic peptide, which may result in vasodilation and reduced sensitivity to vasoconstrictors.[346]

Our current practice is to administer rapid crystalloid coload (approximately 15 mL/kg) to healthy parturients undergoing elective cesarean delivery with spinal anesthesia. Parturients at high risk for hypotension (e.g., history of supine hypotension syndrome) or at high risk for the adverse consequences of hypotension (e.g., hypertrophic cardiomyopathy) receive colloid preload (500 mL).

Vasopressors Regardless of the method of intravenous fluid loading, vasopressor drugs are usually required for preventing and/or treating hypotension. Half a century ago, **ephedrine**, an indirect acting mixed alpha- and beta-adrenergic receptor agonist, was recommended as the vasopressor of choice in obstetric patients based on experiments that showed apparent superiority over direct-acting alpha adrenergic receptor agonists for protecting and restoring uterine blood flow in gravid animal models.[347] This was supported by *in vitro* studies that compared the effects of ephedrine versus vasopressors such as **metaraminol** on blood vessels from pregnant and nonpregnant sheep; these studies showed that the vasoconstrictor activity of ephedrine was more selective for systemic blood vessels than uterine blood vessels,[348] an effect postulated to be related to stimulation of nitric oxide synthase activity in the uterine arteries by ephedrine.[349]

However, subsequent clinical studies showed that alpha adrenergic receptor agonists such as **phenylephrine** and **metaraminol** have equal or greater efficacy to ephedrine for the prevention and treatment of hypotension, and are less likely to depress UA pH and base excess.[350,351] Differences between the results of clinical and animal studies may reflect interspecies differences in vascular smooth muscle physiology and control of blood flow but the fetal effects of placental transfer of drugs are also likely important. Cooper et al.[352] found that an index of fetal carbon dioxide generation, calculated by subtracting UV P_{CO_2} from UA P_{CO_2}, was greater when mothers received ephedrine versus phenylephrine; they postulated that this reflected higher fetal metabolic production of carbon dioxide when mothers received ephedrine. Ngan Kee et al.[353] found that ephedrine crosses the placenta to a greater extent than phenylephrine (median UV/MA concentration ratio 1.13 versus 0.17) and undergoes less early metabolism and/or redistribution. Fetal concentrations of lactate, glucose, and catecholamines were greater when parturients received ephedrine, which supported the hypothesis that the depression of fetal pH and base excess observed with ephedrine is related to metabolic effects secondary to stimulation of fetal beta-adrenergic receptors.[353]

Administration of ephedrine may lead to tachycardia, as well as tachyphylaxis. By contrast, reflex decreases in heart rate and cardiac output may occur with phenylephrine, although this does not appear to affect umbilical cord blood gas values or Apgar scores in uncompromised infants delivered electively.[354] Bradycardia occurring with phenylephrine is usually transient and resolves with stopping phenylephrine administration. Caution should be exercised with the use of **anticholinergic agents** because their administration in the absence of hypotension may result in marked hypertension.

Regardless of the agent used, vasopressors should be administered prophylactically or as soon as the blood pressure begins to decrease, rather than after the occurrence of clinically significant hypotension.[355] In addition, vasopressor administration strategies can optimize maternal, and potentially fetal, hemodynamics and well-being by maintaining blood pressure near baseline.[356]

Vasopressors can be administered by intermittent boluses or by titrated continuous intravenous infusion. Use of closed-loop feedback computer-controlled vasopressor infusions has also been described.[357] The use of intermittent boluses has the advantage of simplicity and may be associated with a smaller total dose of vasopressor.[358] When given by intermittent intravenous boluses, ephedrine is usually administered in doses of 5 to 10 mg and phenylephrine in doses of 50 to 100 μg. The effective phenylephrine *bolus* dose for *preventing* hypotension in 95% of patients (ED_{95}) was estimated at 159 (95% CI, 122 to 371) μg.[359]

An international consensus guideline recommended the use of a variable-rate prophylactic phenylephrine infusion using a syringe pump started at 25 to 50 μg/min immediately after intrathecal injection and titrated to maintain systolic blood pressure $\geq$ 90% of baseline. Small doses of ephedrine are recommended to treat hypotension when the heart rate is low.[360]

The combination of a vasopressors and intravenous fluid loading may be the most effective regimen to prevent hypotension. In a randomized study of women having spinal anesthesia for cesarean delivery, Ngan Kee et al.[361] found that in women who received a prophylactic phenylephrine infusion (beginning at 100 μg/min) combined with rapid crystalloid coload, only 1/53 (1.9%, 95% CI, 0.3% to 9.9%) experienced hypotension compared with 15/53 (28.3%, 95% CI, 18.0% to 41.6%) of women who received phenylephrine infusion without coload. No difference in neonatal outcome was observed between groups.

Although most studies of vasopressors have been performed in healthy, normotensive parturients, studies comparing phenylephrine and ephedrine in patients with preeclampsia have shown no difference in fetal acid-base status or Apgar scores.[362,363]

As an alternative to phenylephrine, a number of studies have investigated the use of dilute norepinephrine (noradrenaline), given by intermittent boluses,[364] titrated infusion,[365] and computer-controlled infusion.[366] Similar to phenylephrine, norepinephrine is a potent alpha-adrenergic receptor agonist. However, in contrast to phenylephrine, norepinephrine is also a relatively weak agonist at beta-adrenergic receptors, which makes it potentially an effective vasopressor for maintaining blood pressure with less tendency to decrease heart rate during spinal anesthesia. Norepinephrine is typically administered via a central venous line in the ICU setting, but similar to phenylephrine, short-term administration of dilute solutions via peripheral venous catheters appears safe.[367]

In a randomized controlled trial of computer-controlled infusions of norepinephrine (5 μg/mL) compared with phenylephrine (100 μg/mL), Ngan Kee al.[366] found that women who received norepinephrine had higher cardiac output (primary outcome) and a lower incidence of bradycardia, with similar neonatal outcomes. The median norepinephrine infusion rate required to maintain maternal blood pressure was 2.35 μg/min (IQR, 1.95 to 2.90 μg/min).[366] A metaanalysis of 15 studies comparing norepinephrine and phenylephrine showed that the drugs had comparable efficacy for management of hypotension but there was a lower risk of bradycardia with norepinephrine (OR, 0.39; 95% CI, 0.31 to 0.49; $P < .00001$).[368] A pragmatic study of norepinephrine versus phenylephrine in 668 patients having spinal anesthesia for elective and nonelective cesarean delivery found that norepinephrine was noninferior to phenylephrine for neonatal outcome assessed by UA pH.[369]

Nonpharmacologic and physical methods Physical methods to prevent hypotension include the use of left lateral tilt (see above) and lower limb compression using bandages or pneumatic compression devices, which have demonstrated some success and may assist in preventing thromboembolic complications.[370]

Failure of Neuraxial Blockade

"Failed" neuraxial anesthesia can be defined as neuroblockade insufficient in extent, density, or duration to provide anesthesia for cesarean delivery. Failure to provide sufficient anesthesia for the initiation or completion of cesarean delivery occurs in 4% to 13% of epidural anesthetics and 0.5% to 4% of spinal anesthetics.[204,371] Epidural techniques are more often associated with failure, possibly because epidural catheters placed during labor may migrate out of the epidural space over time. Factors that correlate with failed extension of labor epidural anesthesia for cesarean delivery include a higher number of bolus doses for the provision of labor analgesia (i.e., treatment of breakthrough pain), patient characteristics (e.g., obesity, distance from the skin to the epidural space), and the time elapsed between placement of the epidural catheter and cesarean delivery.[204]

The causes of failure of neuraxial techniques include anatomic, technical, and obstetric factors. Steps to reduce the likelihood of epidural block failure include meticulous attention to technical detail, the administration of a solution that contains both a local anesthetic and an opioid, and a better understanding of the characteristics of epidural versus spinal blockade. The patient should be informed that she should expect the sensation of deep pressure and movement, and she should be reassured that discomfort or pain will be addressed promptly. Initiation of surgery should be delayed until adequate thoracic and sacral sensory blockade have been achieved; on rare occasions, in the setting of an urgent procedure for which a developing epidural block is present at T10 but has yet to achieve a T4 level, surgery can commence with the understanding that adjuvant treatments or alternative forms of anesthesia may be required.

Evaluation of intraoperative pain requires (1) determination of the location and extent of discomfort, (2) evaluation of the sensory level of anesthesia, (3) assessment of the current status of the surgery (e.g., incision, delivery, uterine repair, skin closure), and (4) assessment of the presence of confounding factors (e.g., hemorrhage, anxiety). Shoulder pain can originate from irritation of the diaphragm (usually by amniotic fluid or blood) and is mediated by the phrenic nerve (C3 to C5); prolonged abduction and extension of the arms can also cause discomfort. Additional discomfort can occur from visceral stimulation, such as uterine manipulation, which often involves the greater splanchnic nerve (T5 to T10). Alternatively, the extent of the block may be adequate but the density of neuroblockade of the large nerve fibers in the lumbosacral plexus may be inadequate. Inadequate anesthesia can result from regression of the block from a cephalad or caudad direction.

Management of a failed neuraxial block should include consideration of the fetal (e.g., presence of nonreassuring fetal status), surgical (e.g., ongoing or anticipation of prolonged surgery), and anesthetic (e.g., maternal airway examination, BMI) implications, as well as the anesthesia provider's experience. Emergency or ongoing surgery may require administration of general anesthesia. If no block exists, the surgery has not begun, and time allows, neuraxial anesthesia can be repeated; whether an epidural or spinal technique is attempted depends on the previously mentioned factors. If an inadequate, partial block exists in an elective situation, either the surgery can be postponed (to allow resolution of the partial block) or a second neuraxial technique may be performed *with caution.*

The disadvantages of replacing a failed neuraxial block with epidural anesthesia include (1) the potential for LAST (particularly after epidural administration of a large dose of local anesthetic for the initial attempt), (2) the time required to establish an adequate block, and (3) the unpredictable reliability and quality of the resulting block. Therefore, after a failed neuraxial block, some practitioners suggest the *cautious* use of a technique with an intrathecal component (i.e., spinal, CSE, or continuous spinal technique).[372] The performance of a spinal technique in the setting of a partial but failed epidural or spinal anesthetic technique is controversial. In this setting, intrathecal administration of a standard intrathecal dose of bupivacaine may result in a high spinal block.[373–375] Radiographic evidence suggests that the dural sac is compressed by prior epidural drug administration.[210] Thus, when performing a spinal anesthetic technique after failed epidural or spinal anesthesia, strategies that the anesthesia provider can consider include: (1) using a different interspace to avoid possible anatomic distortions (e.g., from the loss of resistance to saline or previous needle passes) or abnormalities; (2) reducing the dose of bupivacaine (with the chosen dose depending on the extent of existing neuroblockade); (3) placing the patient in a semisitting (Fowler) position to limit cephalad spread of the local anesthetic; (4) using a CSE technique with a small intrathecal dose of local anesthetic, and, if necessary, titrating the sensory level with additional drugs administered through the epidural catheter; and/or (5) intentionally placing a catheter into the intrathecal space for administration of continuous spinal anesthesia. This last strategy may be especially useful in obese patients in whom the technical difficulty of the neuraxial approach may otherwise limit success.

If discomfort is reported after the start of surgery, it is often helpful to ask the surgeons to halt the operation while an assessment is made. If an epidural catheter is in place, an alkalinized local anesthetic with an opioid (e.g., 3% 2-chloroprocaine with fentanyl) should be administered. The density of epidural anesthesia may be improved by "repainting the fence." An additional dose of local anesthetic (20% to 30% of the initial dose [e.g., 4 to 7 mL]) can be administered approximately 20 minutes after the initial dose. This second dose serves to improve the density of neuroblockade without extending the sensory level. Some anesthesia providers routinely administer this supplemental dose, without waiting for a patient's complaint of breakthrough pain. If the anesthesia provider anticipates that the duration of the surgical procedure will be longer than the predicted duration of epidural or CSE anesthesia, additional local anesthetic (with or without an opioid) should be administered *before* anticipated regression of neuroblockade. The usual dose to maintain neuroblockade is one-third to half of the initial dose.

Intraoperative pain can occur despite careful sensory testing.[376] A prospective observational study reported that during elective cesarean delivery under spinal anesthesia (using 12 mg hyperbaric bupivacaine with 20 µg fentanyl and 0.1 mg morphine) intraoperative pain occurred in 11.9% and severe intraoperative pain occurred in 1.11% of parturients.[376] The authors highlighted that both the anesthesia and obstetric providers underestimated the pain experienced by patients.

Management of intraoperative pain should begin with acknowledgment of the patient's discomfort. Treatment can include intravenous administration of a rapidly acting opioid (e.g., **fentanyl**) and/or inhalation of **nitrous oxide** (40% to 50% in oxygen). **Ketamine** (intravenous increments of 5 to 10 mg) may be useful to manage severe pain. **Midazolam** given in small intravenous boluses may be useful for anxiolysis but does not have analgesic properties. Care should be exercised when administering multiple agents because of the risks of heavy sedation, loss of consciousness, and psychomimetic and amnestic effects. If necessary, the obstetric provider can infiltrate the wound or instill the peritoneal cavity with local anesthetic. In some instances, the induction of general anesthesia with tracheal intubation is appropriate. Recent published guidelines on the prevention and management of intraoperative pain during cesarean delivery under neuraxial anesthesia have recommended that a request for general anesthesia should be honored if possible and that it is good practice for the anesthesia provider to recommend general anesthesia if effective analgesia is unlikely to be achieved using other methods.[377] The importance of follow-up before the patient leaves the hospital was also emphasized.

High Neuraxial Blockade

It is not uncommon for the parturient to report mild dyspnea or reduced ability to cough, especially if the neuraxial blockade has achieved a T2 sensory level or higher. If impaired phonation, unconsciousness, respiratory depression, or significant impairment of ventilation occurs, general anesthesia should be induced. High neuraxial blockade may also result in cardiovascular sequelae, including bradycardia and hypotension. An easy method to diagnose clinically significant high neuraxial blockade is to ask the patient to make a fist ("squeeze your fingers"). A weak hand grasp indicates high thoracic and cervical motor blockade.

High neuraxial block can be caused by several mechanisms, including an exaggerated spread of spinal or epidural drugs and unintentional intrathecal or subdural administration of an "epidural dose" of local anesthetic. The rapid epidural administration of a large volume of local anesthetic solution in the presence of a large-bore dural puncture (e.g., after a "wet tap") may also result in high neuroblockade.

A 2024 review of total spinal anesthesia following obstetric neuraxial blockade reported that fatalities and neurologic injury continue to occur from high neuraxial blockade. The review highlighted that the performance of spinal anesthesia after a failed epidural block is a risk of particular concern.[375]

Nausea and Vomiting

Nausea and vomiting are regulated by the chemoreceptor trigger zone and the vomiting center, which are located in the area postrema and the medullary lateral reticular formation, respectively. The vomiting center receives impulses from the vagal sensory fibers in the gastrointestinal tract, the semicircular canals and ampullae (labyrinth) of the inner ear, higher cortical centers, the chemoreceptor trigger zone, and intracranial pressure receptors. Impulses from these structures are influenced by dopaminergic, muscarinic, tryptaminergic, histaminic, and opioid receptors, which are subsequently the targets for antiemetic agents. Efferent impulses from the vomiting center are transmitted through the vagus, phrenic, and spinal nerves to the abdominal muscles, which causes the physical act of vomiting.

Preoperative Nausea and Vomiting

Nausea and vomiting may occur separately or in combination and are not uncommon during pregnancy. A number of metabolic, endocrine, and anatomic changes have been implicated in the genesis of gestational nausea and vomiting, including human chorionic gonadotropin, estrogen, progesterone, prostaglandins, and immune system dysregulation.[378] When vomiting is sufficiently severe to produce weight loss, dehydration, acidosis from starvation, alkalosis from loss of hydrochloric acid in vomitus, and hypokalemia, it is referred to as *hyperemesis gravidarum* (see Chapter 17). This disorder most commonly occurs in early pregnancy, but as many as 10% of pregnant women have nausea and vomiting that persist beyond 22 weeks' gestation.[378] Severe and persistent hyperemesis may result in maternal and fetal morbidity. The presence of delayed gastric emptying during labor and administration of opioids are risk factors for nausea and vomiting before cesarean delivery.

Intraoperative Nausea and Vomiting

Intraoperative nausea and vomiting associated with cesarean delivery can be variable in incidence and presentation, depending on preexisting symptoms, anesthetic and obstetric techniques, and preventive and therapeutic measures. The incidence of nausea may be as high as 80%, particularly when the anesthesia provider specifically assesses for the presence of intraoperative symptoms. Symptoms occur frequently with exteriorization of the uterus.[379] Anesthetic causes of intraoperative nausea and vomiting include hypotension and increased vagal activity; nonanesthetic causes include surgical stimuli, bleeding, medications (e.g., uterotonic agents, antibiotics), and motion at the end of surgery.[380] Many of these elements occur simultaneously.

Hypotension is a particularly common cause of intraoperative nausea and vomiting. Centrally, hypotension may lead to cerebral and brainstem hypoperfusion, which results in stimulation of the medullary vomiting center. Peripherally, hypotension may cause gut ischemia with release of emetogenic substances (e.g., serotonin) from the intestine.[381] Strict maintenance of intraoperative blood pressure can reduce the occurrence of emesis; Datta et al.[355] observed that the incidence of intraoperative nausea and vomiting was 66% when the blood pressure decreased greater than 30% from baseline, but the incidence was less than 10% when blood pressure was maintained at baseline with ephedrine. Ngan Kee et al.[356] demonstrated progressive increases in intraoperative nausea and vomiting during spinal anesthesia for cesarean delivery when blood pressure control with an infusion of phenylephrine was less aggressive; the incidence of nausea and vomiting was 4% when blood pressure control targeted 100% of baseline, 16% for 90% of baseline, and 40% for 80% of baseline.

Uterotonic agents may also contribute to intraoperative nausea and vomiting. Ergot alkaloids (e.g., methylergonovine maleate) may cause nausea and vomiting by interacting with dopaminergic and serotoninergic receptors. Oxytocin causes nausea and vomiting primarily as a result of the hypotension produced through release of nitric oxide and atrial natriuretic peptide.[382] A 29% incidence of nausea and a 9% incidence of vomiting have been reported with an intravenous bolus of oxytocin 5 units during elective cesarean delivery with neuraxial anesthesia.[383] Administration of 15-methyl prostaglandin $F_{2\alpha}$ causes nausea through the stimulation of smooth muscles of the gastrointestinal tract; a 10% incidence of nausea and vomiting has been observed after administration of 250 µg intramuscularly.[380] Likewise, misoprostol is associated with a high risk for nausea and vomiting.[384]

Surgical stimuli, including exteriorization of the uterus, intraabdominal manipulation, and peritoneal traction, can cause visceral pain and subsequent nausea through the stimulation of vagal fibers and activation of the vomiting center. Despite high levels of thoracic sensory block obtained for cesarean delivery anesthesia, visceral pain may still occur, particularly after the neuraxial administration of a local anesthetic without opioid.[385] The administration of neuraxial opioids reduces visceral pain–induced nausea and vomiting. Neuraxial fentanyl

both improves the quality of neuraxial anesthesia and decreases intraoperative nausea; the minimal effective intrathecal and epidural doses were found to be 6.25 and 50 µg, respectively.[134]

Postoperative Nausea and Vomiting

Risk factors for postoperative nausea and vomiting have not been specifically studied in obstetric patients; however, studies have identified risk factors in nonobstetric patients receiving general or neuraxial anesthesia (Box 26.8).[386,387] A multicenter observational study identified the following four highly predictive factors for postoperative nausea and vomiting in nonobstetric patients after general anesthesia, which may also have relevance in the obstetric population: (1) female sex, (2) history of motion sickness or postoperative nausea and vomiting, (3) nonsmoking status, and (4) the use of perioperative opioids.[387] The incidence of postoperative nausea and vomiting was 10% if the patient had no risk factors, 21% for one, 39% for two, 61% for three, and 79% for four. A subset of pregnant women may have a lower threshold for nausea and vomiting associated with motion.[378] Changes in position and transfer to and on the stretcher may stimulate afferent neural pathways that trigger emesis. Because the histamine-1 (H_1) and muscarinic cholinergic pathways play primary roles in this response, antihistamine and anticholinergic agents should be considered first-line treatments.[388] Postoperative nausea and vomiting may be related to postoperative ileus, which in turn is influenced by the effect of opioids on the gastrointestinal tract, the activation of the sympathetic nervous system, the occurrence of intestinal wall inflammation, and the presence of volume overload or edema.[378]

Prophylaxis and Treatment of Nausea and Vomiting

Preventing maternal hypotension may be the best means of preventing nausea and vomiting (see discussion above). Several options exist for the pharmacologic prophylaxis of nausea and vomiting, and several different classes of drugs are available (Table 26.8). Although various algorithms have been

---

BOX 26.8   Risk Factors for Nausea and Vomiting

General Anesthesia–Related Factors
- Female sex
- History of motion sickness or postoperative nausea and vomiting
- Nonsmoking status
- Use of perioperative opioids

Spinal Anesthesia–Related Factors
- Block height of T5 or higher
- History of motion sickness
- Hypotension
- Omission of neuraxial opioids

Data from Gan TJ. Risk factors for postoperative nausea and vomiting. *Anesth Analg.* 2006;102:1884–1898; Apfel CC, Laara E, Koivuranta M, et al. A simplified risk score for predicting postoperative nausea and vomiting: conclusions from cross-validations between two centers. *Anesthesiology.* 1999;91:693–700.

developed to prevent postoperative nausea and vomiting, primarily targeting nonpregnant patients, none has been universally successful.[389] However, the prophylactic use of these agents either before or after umbilical cord clamping during cesarean delivery with neuraxial anesthesia has been demonstrated to be highly effective. Balki and Carvalho[380] suggested an algorithm consisting of metoclopramide as a first-line agent, dimenhydrinate (a combination of diphenhydramine and 8-chlorotheophylline) as a second-line agent, and ondansetron or granisetron as a third-line agent. Multimodal therapies may eventually prove the most effective, as has been demonstrated in nonpregnant patients.[390]

Metoclopramide is the agent most frequently given, owing to its favorable prokinetic effects. Common side effects include dizziness, drowsiness, and fatigue; rarer side effects include extrapyramidal reactions and acute dystonias. A metaanalysis of 11 studies of 702 patients undergoing cesarean delivery found that compared with placebo, intravenous metoclopramide 10 mg administered before neuraxial blockade is associated with a significant reduction in intraoperative nausea (RR, 0.27; 95% CI, 0.16 to 0.45) and vomiting (RR, 0.14; 95% CI, 0.03 to 0.56).[42] This approach was more effective than administering the metoclopramide after delivery, although administration after delivery also resulted

in a significant reduction in perioperative nausea and vomiting. Early postoperative nausea (RR, 0.47; 95% CI, 0.26 to 0.87) and vomiting (RR, 0.45; 95% CI, 0.21 to 0.93) were also reduced with metoclopramide.

Ondansetron has been found to be more effective than placebo for the prevention of intraoperative nausea and vomiting during cesarean delivery with spinal anesthesia.[391] A study that compared ondansetron 4 mg with metoclopramide 10 mg administered after umbilical cord clamping found ondansetron to be more effective in preventing nausea (26% versus 51%) but not vomiting (15% versus 18%).[392] A systematic review concluded that the use of a serotonin receptor antagonist (e.g., ondansetron, granisetron) in women undergoing neuraxial anesthesia for cesarean delivery was associated with a reduction in intraoperative nausea, but not vomiting, and postoperative nausea and vomiting, compared with placebo.[393] Furthermore, serotonin (5-HT) receptor antagonists were found to be more effective in reducing postoperative nausea than dopamine receptor antagonists (e.g., metoclopramide, droperidol).[393] Some studies have suggested that the administration of ondansetron decreases the incidence of hypotension following spinal anesthesia, potentially by blocking the Bezold-Jarisch reflex, which is mediated by serotonin receptors.[394]

TABLE 26.8 **Agents for Prevention of Nausea and Vomiting in Women Undergoing Cesarean Delivery with Neuraxial Anesthesia[a]**

Drug	Dose	Optimal or Recommended Timing	Comments
Dexamethasone	4–8 mg IV	Unknown for patients undergoing cesarean delivery[b]	Delayed onset of action; used infrequently in patients undergoing cesarean delivery
Dimenhydrinate[c]	25–50 mg IV	Unknown for patients undergoing cesarean delivery	Antihistamine
Dolasetron	12.5 mg IV	After umbilical cord clamping	Serotonin antagonist; not effective in the single published randomized controlled trial
Droperidol	0.625–1.25 mg IV	End of surgery	Butyrophenone with a package insert that contains an FDA "black box" warning regarding prolongation of corrected QT interval on electrocardiogram
Ephedrine[c]	0.5 mg/kg IM	End of surgery	Vasopressor
Granisetron	40 µg/kg IV	After umbilical cord clamping	Serotonin antagonist
Metoclopramide	10 mg IV	Before surgery or after umbilical cord clamping	Benzamide
Ondansetron	4 mg IV	After umbilical cord clamping	Serotonin antagonist
Scopolamine	1.5 mg transdermal patch	Unknown	Muscarinic antagonist

FDA, US Food and Drug Administration; *IM*, intramuscularly; *IV*, intravenously.
[a]If nausea and vomiting occur despite prophylaxis, the anesthesia provider should consider administration of a drug from a different pharmacologic class. There is no evidence that a second administration of the same drug within 6 hours provides additional benefit.
[b]Studies in nonobstetric patients suggest that administration of dexamethasone at induction of anesthesia results in better efficacy, but the optimal timing in obstetric patients is unclear.
[c]Has not been studied in patients undergoing cesarean delivery with neuraxial anesthesia; however, this drug has proved effective for prophylaxis of postoperative nausea and vomiting in studies of nonobstetric patients after administration of general anesthesia.

Animal toxicology studies suggest that the epidural administration of ondansetron may be safe.[395] In a study of 80 women undergoing elective cesarean delivery with CSE anesthesia, the incidence of postoperative nausea was lower in women randomized to receive an epidural infusion of ondansetron than in women who received an intravenous infusion (8 mg over 48 hours) at both 24 and 48 hours.[395] However, future investigations are needed to validate the safety of the neuraxial administration of ondansetron before this route of administration can be recommended.

A metaanalysis of aggregated data suggested that a single intravenous dose of **dexamethasone** 5 to 10 mg (but not 2.5 mg) compared with placebo reduces the incidence of postoperative nausea (23% versus 41%, respectively) and vomiting (20% versus 36%, respectively) in women who received neuraxial morphine for cesarean delivery.[396] In a subgroup analysis, the authors identified a lower incidence of postoperative nausea and vomiting in women who received epidural morphine; however, they were unable to draw definitive conclusions regarding the effect of dexamethasone on postoperative nausea and vomiting in women who received spinal morphine because of the small sample size. In a later study, women randomized to receive preincision dexamethasone 10 mg after spinal anesthesia with bupivacaine and morphine 0.06 mg had a lower 24-hour cumulative incidence of both nausea and vomiting compared with a control group.[397]

Administration of a **transdermal scopolamine** 1.5 mg patch after umbilical cord clamping was shown to be as effective as ondansetron 4 mg in the prevention of nausea and vomiting after cesarean delivery with spinal anesthesia (bupivacaine 12 mg with fentanyl 10 μg and morphine 0.2 mg); compared with placebo, both drugs resulted in a reduction in the incidence of postoperative emesis from approximately 60% to approximately 40%.[398] The use of scopolamine may be limited by side effects, particularly dry mouth and blurred vision. The results of a systematic review suggested that the use of an anticholinergic agent (e.g., scopolamine, glycopyrrolate) in women undergoing neuraxial anesthesia for cesarean delivery results in a significant reduction in intraoperative nausea but not vomiting.[393]

Alternative therapies may play a role in preventing or treating perioperative nausea and vomiting. Several studies have found a favorable effect of **acupressure** on the P6 acupoint (on the anterior aspect of the wrist). Harmon et al.[399] reported that after spinal anesthesia for cesarean delivery, acupressure decreased the incidence of intraoperative nausea or vomiting from 53% to 23% compared with placebo. Two systematic reviews of randomized controlled trials involving a total of 649 women undergoing neuraxial anesthesia for cesarean delivery concluded that despite heterogeneity in the data, P6 stimulation (compared with placebo) appears to reduce intraoperative nausea but not intraoperative vomiting or postoperative nausea or vomiting.[393,400]

One study found that the administration of **supplemental oxygen** (FIO$_2$ 0.7) between umbilical cord clamping and the end of cesarean delivery with neuraxial anesthesia was not associated with a lower incidence of nausea and vomiting compared with room air.[401] This finding is consistent with the results of a metaanalysis of randomized controlled trials in the nonobstetric population[402]; there was no difference in the incidence of nausea and vomiting with the use of supplemental oxygen (FIO$_2$ 0.8) compared with the use of lower oxygen concentrations (FIO$_2$ 0.3 to 0.4).

A systematic review[393] suggested that the administration of subhypnotic doses of **propofol** (0.5 to 1.5 mg/kg/h) for the reduction of intraoperative and postoperative nausea and vomiting in women undergoing neuraxial anesthesia for cesarean delivery is more effective than placebo; however, there are insufficient data to compare this method with other therapies.[393]

Perioperative Pain

In contrast to surveys performed in the general surgical patient population, in which nausea and vomiting ranked as patients' primary concern, a survey performed in obstetric patients during their expectant parent class found that pain during and after cesarean delivery was their greatest concern.[403] Inadequate neuraxial anesthesia leading to pain during labor or cesarean delivery was the most frequent "damaging event" in obstetric claims (31%) against the National Health Service in the United Kingdom from 1995 to 2007.[404]

A preoperative discussion about pain and discomfort can help allay patient concerns. The anesthesia provider should (1) explain that there may be some deep pressure or discomfort during cesarean delivery performed with a neuraxial technique; (2) reassure the patient that the anesthesia provider will be present throughout the operation to administer additional analgesics or general anesthesia if necessary; (3) ensure and document adequacy of neuraxial blockade before the start of surgery; (4) communicate with the patient frequently during the procedure, specifically about pain or discomfort; and (5) treat pain when it arises, in agreement with the patient's wishes. During the postoperative visit, the anesthesia provider should address any concerns that may have arisen during or after surgery.

The anesthetic technique for the cesarean delivery may be altered because of postoperative pain management considerations. For example, an epidural catheter–based technique may be optimal for the patient with a significant pain history (e.g., sickle cell vasoocclusive crises, chronic pain syndromes, opioid use disorder) so that the epidural catheter may be used for postoperative pain management. Intrathecal and epidural morphine are commonly administered for postoperative analgesia (see Chapter 27). The epidural administration of 2-chloroprocaine has been observed to adversely affect the subsequent efficacy of epidural morphine analgesia, although this remains a matter of some dispute.[163,405] The mechanism for this potential interaction remains unknown (see Chapter 13); however, the use of 2-chloroprocaine should be limited to emergency situations in which rapid augmentation of epidural anesthesia is desired (see discussion above).

Pruritus

The incidence of pruritus with the administration of neuraxial opioids can be as high as 30% to 100%. Pruritus is more commonly observed when opioids are administered intrathecally than epidurally. It may be generalized or localized to regions of the nose, face, and chest and is typically self-limited in duration. The particular combination and dose of opioid and local anesthetic may influence the incidence and severity of pruritus, and the addition of epinephrine to an opioid-local anesthetic solution has been observed to worsen pruritus.[406] Pruritus does not represent an allergic reaction to the neuraxial opioid. If flushing, urticaria, rhinitis, bronchoconstriction, or cardiac symptoms also occur, an allergic reaction to another substance should be considered.

The cause of neuraxial opioid-induced pruritus is not known, although multiple theories have been proposed. They include μ-opioid receptor stimulation at the medullary dorsal horn, antagonism of inhibitory transmitters, and activation of an "itch center" in the central nervous system.[407] Pharmacologic prophylaxis or treatment of pruritus may include an opioid receptor antagonist or agonist/antagonist, droperidol, a serotonin receptor antagonist (e.g., **ondansetron**), and/or a subhypnotic dose of propofol (Table 26.9).[407] In a comparison of prophylactic **granisetron** 3 mg versus **ondansetron** 8 mg in women having spinal anesthesia for cesarean delivery that included 150 μg of intrathecal morphine, Tan et al.[408] reported that the severity of pruritus and the use of antipruritic medication were less with granisetron but the overall incidence of pruritus was similar between groups. **Dexamethasone** in doses of 2.5 to 10 mg has not been found to reduce the incidence of pruritus associated with neuraxial morphine in women undergoing cesarean delivery.[396] Although opioid receptor antagonists, such as **naltrexone** and **naloxone**, and partial agonist/antagonists, such as **nalbuphine**, are currently the most effective treatments for pruritus, a single dose or continuous intravenous infusion of any of these agents may reverse analgesia. Because the primary mechanism of opioid-induced pruritus appears unrelated to histamine release, **antihistamines** are seldom effective, although some benefit may be derived from accompanying sedation.

Hypothermia and Shivering

Perioperative hypothermia and shivering are commonly observed in women undergoing cesarean delivery, with reported incidences of 66% and 85%, respectively.[409,410] Hypothermia has been associated with a number of adverse outcomes in nonpregnant surgical patients, including wound infection, coagulopathy, increased blood and transfusion requirements, increased oxygen consumption, decreased metabolism, and prolonged recovery.[411] In a systematic evaluation of randomized trials of normothermic and mildly hypothermic (34°C to 36°C) nonpregnant surgical patients, Rajagopalan et al.[412] observed that even hypothermia less than 1°C below normal body temperature was associated with a 16% increase in blood loss (95% CI, 4% to 26%) and a 22% increase in risk for transfusion (95% CI, 3% to 37%).

Normally, core body temperature is tightly regulated within a narrow range of 36°C to 37°C. During pregnancy, despite an increase in maternal basal metabolic rate and energy released by the developing fetal and uteroplacental unit, maternal core temperature decreases, reaching a nadir at 12 weeks postpartum (36.4°C).[413] Major causes of hypothermia during cesarean delivery are most likely related to core-to-periphery heat redistribution caused by diminished vasoconstriction and shivering, particularly after neuraxial blockade, and impairment of centrally mediated thermoregulatory control.[411]

The onset and severity of hypothermia and shivering are associated with the patient's baseline thermal status, the perioperative environment, and the anesthetic technique and agents selected. In patients randomized to receive spinal or epidural anesthesia for cesarean delivery, Saito et al.[414] reported that core temperature initially decreased more rapidly during spinal anesthesia. Although the onset and incidence of shivering were similar between groups, with spinal anesthesia the shivering severity was less and the shivering threshold was lower, suggesting that spinal anesthesia impaired autonomic thermoregulation more than epidural anesthesia.

The effect of neuraxial opioids on thermoregulation and shivering in patients undergoing cesarean delivery is not fully understood. Intravenous **meperidine** 12.5 to 25 mg is one of the most effective antishivering drugs and is unique among opioids in producing this effect at doses not typically associated with respiratory depression. The mechanism of this effect does not appear to be related to κ-opioid receptor activity or inhibition of cholinergic receptors; rather, central α_{2B}-adrenergic

TABLE 26.9 Agents for Prevention or Treatment of Pruritus in Women Undergoing Cesarean Delivery

Drug Class	Drug and Dose	Comments
Opioid antagonists	Naloxone infusion 1–2 μg/kg/h IV Naltrexone 6–9 mg PO	May reverse analgesia Contraindicated in patients who are opioid dependent
Opioid agonist/ antagonist	Nalbuphine 2.5–5 mg IV	Contraindicated in patients who are opioid dependent or on buprenorphine, methadone, or naltrexone
Sedative/ hypnotic agent	Propofol 10–20 mg IV	Subhypnotic dose with conflicting evidence regarding efficacy in treating pruritus
Serotonin antagonist	Ondansetron 0.1 mg/kg IV	Conflicting evidence regarding efficacy in treating pruritus

IV, Intravenously; *PO,* orally.

receptor stimulation may be involved.[415] The α_2-adrenergic receptor agonists **clonidine** (150 μg) and **dexmedetomidine** (0.5 μg/kg) are effective antishivering agents that can lower the shivering threshold,[415] although both agents may have limited use during pregnancy because of the potential to cause sedation, bradycardia, and hypotension. Dexmedetomidine has been used effectively in small intravenous doses (e.g., 10 μg) to diminish shivering, typically after the delivery of the infant.[416]

Other modalities have been used to prevent and treat hypothermia and shivering. Preoperative patient warming using forced air has been shown to reduce the incidence of perioperative and postoperative core hypothermia and shivering in patients undergoing cesarean delivery with *epidural* anesthesia.[417] In contrast, a subsequent study found that perioperative forced-air warming did not prevent maternal hypothermia after cesarean delivery with *spinal* anesthesia.[409] The ambient operating room temperature has also been shown to impact the risk for hypothermia. One study showed that increasing the set temperature from 20°C (67°F) to 23°C (73°F) resulted in significant reduction in maternal hypothermia on arrival in the postoperative care area.[418] Lower limb wrapping has been observed to have no effect on the incidence of hypothermia or shivering.[419]

OBSTETRIC COMPLICATIONS

Postpartum Hemorrhage

The ACOG defines postpartum hemorrhage (PPH) at cesarean delivery as blood loss $\geq$ 1000 mL.[420] PPH is a leading cause of maternal and fetal morbidity and mortality worldwide. Mild to moderate obstetric hemorrhage can be masked by pregnancy-related physiologic changes. Underestimation of blood loss and inadequacy of resuscitation are common problems. PPH is covered in detail in Chapter 37.

Uterine atony (failure of the uterus to contract) after delivery accounts for most cases of PPH and remains a leading cause of postpartum hysterectomy and blood transfusion. Uterine atony occurs more commonly after cesarean delivery than after vaginal delivery, perhaps as a reflection of the condition(s) that prompted the cesarean delivery or possibly because surgery disrupts the normal postpartum response to uterotonic hormones and pharmacologic agents. Risk factors for uterine atony are shown in Box 37.3. Initial efforts to control uterine atony include **uterine massage** and administration of **oxytocic (uterotonic) drugs**, which include **oxytocin, carbetocin, ergot alkaloids**, and **prostaglandins**. The pharmacology of oxytocic drugs and dosing recommendations are described in Chapter 37.

Preparation for blood loss when risk factors for hemorrhage are identified may include consideration of several preparatory steps. These include the use of **iron supplementation, recombinant human erythropoietin, autologous blood donation, acute normovolemic hemodilution**, and **intraoperative red blood cell salvage** (see Chapter 37).

The **response to blood loss** includes **intravenous volume replacement**, and **transfusion of blood and blood products**. Other interventions that may be considered include the use of **intravascular balloon occlusion catheters, uterine tamponade balloon catheters**, and **cesarean hysterectomy** (see Chapter 37).

Thromboembolic Events

Thromboembolic events constitute a major reason for peripartum maternal mortality, and risks for the development of pregnancy-associated thrombosis include an operative delivery, physiologic changes of pregnancy, and medical history and comorbidities (e.g., obesity, hemoglobinopathies, hypertension, smoking).[421] The risk for venous thromboembolism appears highest in the first postpartum week.[421] A number of prophylactic interventions have been evaluated; however, the trials have been small and have not provided robust results.[422] Recommended thromboprophylaxis measures include hydration, early mobilization, pneumatic compression devices, and, in high-risk patients, pharmacologic prophylaxis (see Chapter 38).

KEY POINTS

- Cesarean delivery is the most common major surgical procedure performed worldwide. The rate of cesarean delivery is increasing.
- Some cesarean deliveries might be avoided through the provision of satisfactory neuraxial analgesia for labor (including a trial of labor after cesarean delivery), instrumental vaginal delivery, and external cephalic version.
- Gastric emptying is unchanged during pregnancy. The parturient without complications may drink modest amounts of clear liquids up to 2 hours before induction of anesthesia for *elective* cesarean delivery. The fasting period for solids should be 6 to 8 hours. Slower digestion is observed for foods with high fat content, during labor, and with the administration of opioid analgesic agents.

- An H_2-receptor antagonist or a proton-pump inhibitor may be given intravenously to increase gastric fluid pH, and IV metoclopramide may be given to both accelerate gastric emptying and increase lower esophageal sphincter tone. If possible, these agents should be administered *more than* 30 minutes before induction of anesthesia. Oral sodium citrate, which also increases gastric fluid pH, should be administered *less than* 30 minutes before induction.
- Antibiotic prophylaxis, administered within 60 minutes before abdominal incision, decreases the risk for maternal infectious complications after cesarean delivery.
- Although the use of intravenous fluids may reduce the frequency of maternal hypotension, initiation of neuraxial anesthesia should not be delayed to administer a fixed volume of fluid.

- The value of supplemental maternal oxygen during neuraxial anesthesia for the elective cesarean delivery of a noncompromised fetus is questionable.
- Left uterine displacement should be applied during cesarean delivery, regardless of the anesthetic technique.
- Umbilical cord prolapse (without fetal bradycardia), placenta previa, and severe preeclampsia (in a patient with an acceptable platelet count) are not absolute indications for general anesthesia.
- Among women receiving general anesthesia for cesarean delivery, maternal deaths associated with hypoventilation or airway obstruction are occurring with greater frequency during emergence, tracheal extubation, or recovery, rather than during induction and tracheal intubation; attention to airway and ventilation management should focus on both of these critical time periods.
- The combined spinal-epidural technique offers the benefits of both spinal and epidural anesthesia while minimizing the disadvantages of either technique alone. Advantages include the fast onset of dense anesthesia with a small dose of local anesthetic and the ability to provide prolonged anesthesia and continuous postoperative analgesia.
- Alkalinization of the local anesthetic solution not only increases the speed of onset but also improves the quality and prolongs the duration of neuroblockade. Administration of 3% 2-chloroprocaine with 8.4% sodium bicarbonate (1 mL [1 mEq] of bicarbonate added to each 10 mL of 2-chloroprocaine) produces the fastest onset of epidural anesthesia.
- The application of cricoid pressure to prevent passive regurgitation during induction of general anesthesia is controversial. If used, pressure should be initiated with a force of 10 N on the cricoid cartilage and increased to 30 N once the patient loses consciousness.
- When choosing the concentration of a volatile halogenated agent to maintain general anesthesia, the anesthesia provider must consider the uterine relaxation caused by these agents as well as the reduced MAC of pregnancy and the potential for maternal awareness.
- Vasopressors should be administered early or prophylactically to prevent and treat hypotension during neuraxial anesthesia for cesarean delivery. Current international consensus recommends a phenylephrine infusion started at 25 to 50 µg/min and titrated to maintain systolic blood pressure ≥ 90% of baseline. Small doses of ephedrine are suitable to treat hypotension with low maternal heart rate. The use of norepinephrine has recently been described.
- Underestimation of blood loss and inadequate intravascular volume resuscitation during peripartum hemorrhage are common occurrences that contribute to maternal morbidity and mortality.

REFERENCES

1. Todman D. A history of caesarean section: from ancient world to the modern era. *Aust N Z J Obstet Gynaecol.* 2007;47:357–361.
2. Crespo FA, Verma U. High primary cesarean section rates: strategies for improvement. *Jt Comm J Qual Patient Saf.* 2022;48:617–624.
3. Betran AP, Ye J, Moller AB, et al. Trends and projections of caesarean section rates: global and regional estimates. *BMJ Glob Health.* 2021;6:e005671.
4. Bruno AM, Metz TD, Grobman WA, Silver RM. Defining a cesarean delivery rate for optimizing maternal and neonatal outcomes. *Obstet Gynecol.* 2022;140:399–407.
5. de Vries BS, Morton R, Burton AE, et al. Attributable factors for the rising cesarean delivery rate over 3 decades: an observational cohort study. *Am J Obstet Gynecol MFM.* 2022;4:100555.
6. National Institutes of Health state-of-the-science conference statement. Cesarean delivery on maternal request March 27-29, 2006. *Obstet Gynecol.* 2006;107:1386–1397.
7. Grobman WA, Lai Y, Landon MB, et al. Development of a nomogram for prediction of vaginal birth after cesarean delivery. *Obstet Gynecol.* 2007;109:806–812.
8. Turner MJ. Delivery after a previous cesarean section reviewed. *Int J Gynaecol Obstet.* 2023;163:757–762.
9. Tan HS, Taylor CR, Sharawi N, et al. Uterine exteriorization versus in situ repair in Cesarean delivery: a systematic review and meta-analysis. *Can J Anaesth.* 2022;69:216–233.
10. Belizán JM, Althabe F, Cafferata ML. Health consequences of the increasing caesarean section rates. *Epidemiology.* 2007;18:485–486.
11. Balayla J, Lasry A, Badeghiesh A, et al. Mode of delivery is an independent risk factor for maternal mortality: a case-control study. *J Matern Fetal Neonatal Med.* 2022;35:1962–1968.
12. Liu S, Liston RM, Joseph KS, et al. Maternal mortality and severe morbidity associated with low-risk planned cesarean delivery versus planned vaginal delivery at term. *CMAJ.* 2007;176:455–460.
13. Van Winsen KD, Savvidou MD, Steer PJ. The effect of mode of delivery and duration of labour on subsequent pregnancy outcomes: a retrospective cohort study. *BJOG.* 2021;128:2132–2139.
14. Słabuszewska-Jóźwiak A, Szymański JK, Ciebiera M, et al. Pediatrics consequences of caesarean section—a systematic review and meta-analysis. *Int J Environ Res Public Health.* 2020;17:8031.
15. Anim-Somuah M, Smyth RM, Cyna AM, Cuthbert A. Epidural versus non-epidural or no analgesia for pain management in labour. *Cochrane Database Syst Rev.* 2018;(5):CD000331.

16. Mardirosoff C, Dumont L, Boulvain M, Tramèr MR. Fetal bradycardia due to intrathecal opioids for labour analgesia: a systematic review. *BJOG*. 2002;109:274–281.

17. Traynor AJ, Aragon M, Ghosh D, et al. Obstetric Anesthesia Workforce Survey: a 30-year update. *Anesth Analg*. 2016;122:1939–1946.

18. Hu LQ, Zhang J, Wong CA, et al. Impact of the introduction of neuraxial labor analgesia on mode of delivery at an urban maternity hospital in China. *Int J Gynaecol Obstet*. 2015;129:17–21.

19. Royal College of Obstetricians and Gynaecologists. Management of breech presentation. Green-top Guideline No. 20b. Available at https://www.rcog.org.uk/en/guidelines-research-services/guidelines/gtg20b/. Accessed 24 August 2024.

20. American College of Obstetricians and Gynecologists. Committee Opinion No. 745: Mode of term singleton breech delivery (reaffirmed 2023). *Obstet Gynecol*. 2018;132:e60–e63.

21. Hao Q, Hu Y, Zhang L, et al. A systematic review and meta-analysis of clinical trials of neuraxial, intravenous, and inhalational anesthesia for external cephalic version. *Anesth Analg*. 2020;131:1800–1811.

22. External cephalic version: ACOG Practice Bulletin, Number 221. *Obstet Gynecol*. 2020;135:e203–e212.

23. Duarte SS, Nguyen TT, Koch C, et al. Remote obstetric anesthesia: leveraging telemedicine to improve fetal and maternal outcomes. *Telemed J E Health*. 2020;26:967–972.

24. American Society of Anesthesiologists, Society for Obstetric Anesthesia and Perinatology. Practice guidelines for obstetric anesthesia: an updated report by the American Society of Anesthesiologists Task Force on Obstetric Anesthesia and the Society for Obstetric Anesthesia and Perinatology. *Anesthesiology*. 2016;124:270–300.

25. WHO. *Trends in maternal mortality 2000 to 2020: estimates by WHO, UNICEF, UNFPA, World Bank Group and UNDESA/Population Division*. World Health Organization; 2023 Licence: CC BY-NC-SA 3.0 IGO.

26. Giouleka S, Tsakiridis I, Kalogiannidis I, et al. Postpartum hemorrhage: a comprehensive review of guidelines. *Obstet Gynecol Surv*. 2022;77:665–682.

27. American Society of Anesthesiologists. Standards for basic anesthetic monitoring. https://www.asahq.org/standards-and-practice-parameters/standards-for-basic-anesthetic-monitoring. Accessed 24 August 2024.

28. Bruyere M, Ait Hamou N, Benhamou D, et al. QT interval prolongation following carbetocin in prevention of post-cesarean delivery hemorrhage. *Int J Obstet Anesth*. 2014;23:88–89.

29. Zakowski MI, Ramanathan S, Baratta JB, et al. Electrocardiographic changes during cesarean section: a cause for concern? *Anesth Analg*. 1993;76:162–167.

30. Moran C, Ni Bhuinneain M, Geary M, et al. Myocardial ischaemia in normal patients undergoing elective caesarean section: a peripartum assessment. *Anaesthesia*. 2001;56:1051–1058.

31. London MJ, Hollenberg M, Wong MG, et al. Intraoperative myocardial ischemia: localization by continuous 12-lead electrocardiography. *Anesthesiology*. 1988;69:232–241.

32. Shen CL, Ho YY, Hung YC, Chen PL. Arrhythmias during spinal anesthesia for cesarean section. *Can J Anaesth*. 2000;47:393–397.

33. Robins K, Lyons G. Intraoperative awareness during general anesthesia for cesarean delivery. *Anesth Analg*. 2009;109:886–890.

34. Tully L, Gates S, Brocklehurst P, et al. Surgical techniques used during caesarean section operations: results of a national survey of practice in the UK. *Eur J Obstet Gynecol Reprod Biol*. 2002;102:120–126.

35. Wong CA, Loffredi M, Ganchiff JN, et al. Gastric emptying of water in term pregnancy. *Anesthesiology*. 2002;96:1395–1400.

36. Wong CA, McCarthy RJ, Fitzgerald PC, et al. Gastric emptying of water in obese pregnant women at term. *Anesth Analg*. 2007;105:751–755.

37. Bouvet L, Schulz T, Piana F, et al. Pregnancy and labor epidural effects on gastric emptying: a prospective comparative study. *Anesthesiology*. 2022;136:542–550.

38. Hauptfleisch JJ, Payne KA. An oral sodium citrate-citric acid non-particulate buffer in humans. *Br J Anaesth*. 1996;77:642–644.

39. Babaei A, Bhargava V, Aalam S, et al. Effect of proton pump inhibition on the gastric volume: assessed by magnetic resonance imaging. *Aliment Pharmacol Ther*. 2009;29:863–870.

40. Paranjothy S, Griffiths JD, Broughton HK, et al. Interventions at caesarean section for reducing the risk of aspiration pneumonitis. *Cochrane Database Syst Rev*. 2010;(1):CD004943.

41. Kjaer K, Comerford M, Kondilis L, et al. Oral sodium citrate increases nausea amongst elective cesarean delivery patients. *Can J Anaesth*. 2006;53:776–780.

42. Mishriky BM, Habib AS. Metoclopramide for nausea and vomiting prophylaxis during and after Caesarean delivery: a systematic review and meta-analysis. *Br J Anaesth*. 2012;108:374–383.

43. Smaill F, Hofmeyr GJ. Antibiotic prophylaxis for cesarean section. *Cochrane Database Syst Rev*. 2002;(3):CD000933.

44. American College of Obstetricians and Gynecologists. Practice Bulletin No. 199: Use of prophylactic antibiotics in labor and delivery (reaffirmed 2025). *Obstet Gynecol*. 2018;132:e103–e119.

45. Alfirevic Z, Gyte GM, Dou L. Different classes of antibiotics given to women routinely for preventing infection at caesarean section. *Cochrane Database Syst Rev*. 2010;(10):CD008726.

46. Pevzner L, Swank M, Krepel C, et al. Effects of maternal obesity on tissue concentrations of prophylactic cefazolin during cesarean delivery. *Obstet Gynecol*. 2011;117:877–882.

47. Tita AT, Szychowski JM, Boggess K, et al. Adjunctive azithromycin prophylaxis for cesarean delivery. *N Engl J Med*. 2016;375:1231–1241.

48. Costantine MM, Rahman M, Ghulmiyah L, et al. Timing of perioperative antibiotics for cesarean delivery: a metaanalysis. *Am J Obstet Gynecol*. 2008;199:301.e1–e6.

49. Kourtis AP, Read JS, Jamieson DJ. Pregnancy and infection. *N Engl J Med*. 2014;370:2211–2218.

50. American Society of Anesthesiologists, American Society of Regional Anesthesia and Pain Medicine. Practice advisory for the prevention, diagnosis, and management of infectious complications associated with neuraxial techniques: an updated report by the American Society of Anesthesiologists Task Force on Infectious Complications Associated with Neuraxial Techniques and the American Society of Regional Anesthesia and Pain Medicine. *Anesthesiology*. 2017;126:585–601.

51. Aleman-Ortega H, Lee R, Shambo L, Czinn E. Neuraxial anesthesia and the use of sterile gowning. *AORN J.* 2017;105:184–192.

52. Scott DA, Fox JA, Cnaan A, et al. Resistance to fluid flow in veins. *J Clin Monit.* 1996;12:331–337.

53. de la Roche MR, Gauthier L. Rapid transfusion of packed red blood cells: effects of dilution, pressure, and catheter size. *Ann Emerg Med.* 1993;22:1551–1555.

54. Hepner DL, Tsen LC. eds. *Fluid Management in Obstetrics.* Informa Healthcare; 2007.

55. Mercier FJ. Fluid loading for cesarean delivery under spinal anesthesia: have we studied all the options? *Anesth Analg.* 2011;113:677–680.

56. Dyer RA, Farina Z, Joubert IA, et al. Crystalloid preload versus rapid crystalloid administration after induction of spinal anaesthesia (coload) for elective caesarean section. *Anaesth Intensive Care.* 2004;32:351–357.

57. Banerjee A, Stocche RM, Angle P, Halpern SH. Preload or coload for spinal anesthesia for elective cesarean delivery: a meta-analysis. *Can J Anaesth.* 2010;57:24–31.

58. Morgan PJ, Halpern SH, Tarshis J. The effects of an increase of central blood volume before spinal anesthesia for cesarean delivery: a qualitative systematic review. *Anesth Analg.* 2001;92:997–1005.

59. Sohn HM, Na HS, Lim D, et al. Immediate retrograde amnesia induced by midazolam: a prospective, nonrandomized cohort study. *Int J Clin Pract.* 2021;75(11):e14745.

60. Olde E, van der Hart O, Kleber R, van Son M. Posttraumatic stress following childbirth: a review. *Clin Psychol Rev.* 2006;26:1–16.

61. Frölich MA, Burchfield DJ, Euliano TY, Caton D. A single dose of fentanyl and midazolam prior to cesarean section have no adverse neonatal effects. *Can J Anaesth.* 2006;53:79–85.

62. Massoth C, Chappell D, Kranke P, Wenk M. Supine hypotensive syndrome of pregnancy: a review of current knowledge. *Eur J Anaesthesiol.* 2022;39:236–243.

63. Pirhonen JP, Erkkola RU. Uterine and umbilical flow velocity waveforms in the supine hypotensive syndrome. *Obstet Gynecol.* 1990;76:176–179.

64. Kinsella SM. Lateral tilt for pregnant women: why 15 degrees? *Anaesthesia.* 2003;58:835–836.

65. Cluver C, Novikova N, Hofmeyr GJ, Hall DR. Maternal position during caesarean section for preventing maternal and neonatal complications. *Cochrane Database Syst Rev.* 2013;(3):CD007623.

66. Lee AJ, Landau R, Mattingly JL, et al. Left lateral table tilt for elective cesarean delivery under spinal anesthesia has no effect on neonatal acid-base status: a randomized controlled trial. *Anesthesiology.* 2017;127:241–249.

67. Farber MK, Bateman BT. Phenylephrine infusion: driving a wedge in our practice of left uterine displacement? *Anesthesiology.* 2017;127:212–214.

68. Morgan DJ, Paull JD, Toh CT, Blackman GL. Aortocaval compression and plasma concentrations of thiopentone at caesarean section. *Br J Anaesth.* 1984;56:349–354.

69. Jones SJ, Kinsella SM, Donald FA. Comparison of measured and estimated angles of table tilt at caesarean section. *Br J Anaesth.* 2003;90:86–87.

70. Paech MJ. Should we take a different angle in managing pregnant women at delivery? Attempting to avoid the 'supine hypotensive syndrome'. *Anaesth Intensive Care.* 2008;36:775–777.

71. Loke GP, Chan EH, Sia AT. The effect of 10 degrees head-up tilt in the right lateral position on the systemic blood pressure after subarachnoid block for caesarean section. *Anaesthesia.* 2002;57:169–172.

72. Hignett R, Fernando R, McGlennan A, et al. A randomized crossover study to determine the effect of a 30 degrees head-up versus a supine position on the functional residual capacity of term parturients. *Anesth Analg.* 2011;113:1098–1102.

73. Dixon BJ, Dixon JB, Carden JR, et al. Preoxygenation is more effective in the 25 degrees head-up position than in the supine position in severely obese patients: a randomized controlled study. *Anesthesiology.* 2005;102:1110–1115.

74. Mhyre JM. Anesthetic management for the morbidly obese pregnant woman. *Int Anesthesiol Clin.* 2007;45:51–70.

75. Miyabe M, Namiki A. The effect of head-down tilt on arterial blood pressure after spinal anesthesia. *Anesth Analg.* 1993;76:549–552.

76. Miyabe M, Sato S. The effect of head-down tilt position on arterial blood pressure after spinal anesthesia for cesarean delivery. *Reg Anesth.* 1997;22:239–242.

77. Sinclair CJ, Scott DB, Edstrom HH. Effect of the Trendelenberg position on spinal anaesthesia with hyperbaric bupivacaine. *Br J Anaesth.* 1982;54:497–500.

78. Tsen LC. Neuraxial techniques for labor analgesia should be placed in the lateral position. *Int J Obstet Anesth.* 2008;17:146–149.

79. Polley LS. Neuraxial techniques for labor analgesia should be placed in the lateral position. *Int J Obstet Anesth.* 2008;17:149–152.

80. Jones AY, Dean E. Body position change and its effect on hemodynamic and metabolic status. *Heart Lung.* 2004;33:281–290.

81. Suonio S, Simpanen AL, Olkkonen H, Haring P. Effect of the left lateral recumbent position compared with the supine and upright positions on placental blood flow in normal late pregnancy. *Ann Clin Res.* 1976;8:22–26.

82. Armstrong S, Fernando R, Columb M, Jones T. Cardiac index in term pregnant women in the sitting, lateral, and supine positions: an observational, crossover study. *Anesth Analg.* 2011;113:318–322.

83. Yun EM, Marx GF, Santos AC. The effects of maternal position during induction of combined spinal-epidural anesthesia for cesarean delivery. *Anesth Analg.* 1998;87:614–618.

84. Vincent RD, Chestnut DH. Which position is more comfortable for the parturient during identification of the epidural space? *Int J Obstet Anesth.* 1991;1:9–11.

85. Igarashi T, Hirabayashi Y, Shimizu R, et al. The fiberscopic findings of the epidural space in pregnant women. *Anesthesiology.* 2000;92:1631–1636.

86. Hirabayashi Y, Shimizu R, Fukuda H, et al. Effects of the pregnant uterus on the extradural venous plexus in the supine and lateral positions, as determined by magnetic resonance imaging. *Br J Anaesth.* 1997;78:317–319.

87. Bahar M, Chanimov M, Cohen ML, et al. Lateral recumbent head-down posture for epidural catheter insertion reduces intravascular injection. *Can J Anaesth.* 2001;48:48–53.

88. Bahar M, Chanimov M, Cohen ML, et al. The lateral recumbent head-down position decreases the incidence of epidural venous puncture during catheter insertion in obese parturients. *Can J Anaesth.* 2004;51:577–580.

89. Hirasawa Y, Bashir WA, Smith FW, et al. Postural changes of the dural sac in the lumbar spines of asymptomatic individuals using positional stand-up magnetic resonance imaging. *Spine.* 2007;32:E136–E140.

90. Fox GS, Houle GL. Acid-base studies in elective caesarean sections during epidural and general anaesthesia. *Can Anaesth Soc J.* 1971;18:60–71.

91. Raghuraman N, Temming LA, Doering MM, et al. Maternal oxygen supplementation compared with room air for intrauterine resuscitation: a systematic review and meta-analysis. *JAMA Pediatr.* 2021;175:368–376.

92. Ryerson EG, Block AJ, eds. *Oxygen as a Drug.* JB Lippincott; 1991.

93. Kelly MC, Fitzpatrick KT, Hill DA. Respiratory effects of spinal anaesthesia for caesarean section. *Anaesthesia.* 1996;51:1120–1122.

94. Khaw KS, Ngan Kee WD, Lee A, et al. Supplementary oxygen for elective caesarean section under spinal anaesthesia: useful in prolonged uterine incision-to-delivery interval? *Br J Anaesth.* 2004;92:518–522.

95. Khaw KS, Wang CC, Ngan Kee WD, et al. Effects of high inspired oxygen fraction during elective caesarean section under spinal anaesthesia on maternal and fetal oxygenation and lipid peroxidation. *Br J Anaesth.* 2002;88:18–23.

96. McCord JM. The evolution of free radicals and oxidative stress. *Am J Med.* 2000;108:652–659.

97. Khaw KS, Wang CC, Ngan Kee WD, et al. Supplementary oxygen for emergency caesarean section under regional anaesthesia. *Br J Anaesth.* 2009;102:90–96.

98. Yamada T, Yoneyama Y, Sawa R, Araki T. Effects of maternal oxygen supplementation on fetal oxygenation and lipid peroxidation following a single umbilical cord occlusion in fetal goats. *J Nippon Med Sch.* 2003;70:165–171.

99. Buhimschi IA, Buhimschi CS, Pupkin M, Weiner CP. Beneficial impact of term labor: nonenzymatic antioxidant reserve in the human fetus. *Am J Obstet Gynecol.* 2003;189:181–188.

100. Thorp JA, Trobough T, Evans R, et al. The effect of maternal oxygen administration during the second stage of labor on umbilical cord blood gas values: a randomized controlled prospective trial. *Am J Obstet Gynecol.* 1995;172:465–474.

101. Khazin AF, Hon EH, Hehre FW. Effects of maternal hyperoxia on the fetus. I. Oxygen tension. *Am J Obstet Gynecol.* 1971;109:628–637.

102. Vento M, Asensi M, Sastre J, et al. Resuscitation with room air instead of 100% oxygen prevents oxidative stress in moderately asphyxiated term neonates. *Pediatrics.* 2001;107:642–647.

103. Saugstad OD, Ramji S, Soll RF, Vento M. Resuscitation of newborn infants with 21% or 100% oxygen: an updated systematic review and meta-analysis. *Neonatology.* 2008;94:176–182.

104. Lucas DN, Yentis SM, Kinsella SM, et al. Urgency of caesarean section: a new classification. *J R Soc Med.* 2000;93:346–350.

105. Juang J, Gabriel RA, Dutton RP, et al. Choice of anesthesia for cesarean delivery: an analysis of the National Anesthesia Clinical Outcomes Registry. *Anesth Analg.* 2017;124:1914–1917.

106. Palanisamy A, Mitani AA, Tsen LC. General anesthesia for cesarean delivery at a tertiary care hospital from 2000 to 2005: a retrospective analysis and 10-year update. *Int J Obstet Anesth.* 2011;20:10–16.

107. Kinsella SM, Girgirah K, Scrutton MJ. Rapid sequence spinal anaesthesia for category-1 urgency caesarean section: a case series. *Anaesthesia.* 2010;65:664–669.

108. Hawkins JL, Koonin LM, Palmer SK, Gibbs CP. Anesthesia-related deaths during obstetric delivery in the United States, 1979-1990. *Anesthesiology.* 1997;86:277–284.

109. Hawkins JL, Chang J, Palmer SK, et al. Anesthesia-related maternal mortality in the United States: 1979-2002. *Obstet Gynecol.* 2011;117:69–74.

110. Afolabi BB, Lesi FE. Regional versus general anaesthesia for caesarean section. *Cochrane Database Syst Rev.* 2012;(10):CD004350.

111. Morgan BM, Aulakh JM, Barker JP, et al. Anaesthetic morbidity following caesarean section under epidural or general anaesthesia. *Lancet.* 1984;1:328–330.

112. Reynolds F, Seed PT. Anaesthesia for caesarean section and neonatal acid-base status: a meta-analysis. *Anaesthesia.* 2005;60:636–653.

113. Cojocaru L, Salvatori C, Sharon A, et al. General versus regional anesthesia and neonatal data: a propensity-score-matched study. *Am J Perinatol.* 2023;40:227–234.

114. Russell IF. A comparison of cold, pinprick and touch for assessing the level of spinal block at caesarean section. *Int J Obstet Anesth.* 2004;13:146–152.

115. Burns SM, Barclay PM. Regional anaesthesia for caesarean section. *Curr Anaesth Crit Care.* 2000;11:73–79.

116. Riley ET, Cohen SE, Macario A, et al. Spinal versus epidural anesthesia for cesarean section: a comparison of time efficiency, costs, charges, and complications. *Anesth Analg.* 1995;80:709–712.

117. Garry M, Davies S. Failure of regional blockade for caesarean section. *Int J Obstet Anesth.* 2002;11:9–12.

118. Schlotterbeck H, Schaeffer R, Dow WA, et al. Ultrasonographic control of the puncture level for lumbar neuraxial block in obstetric anaesthesia. *Br J Anaesth.* 2008;100:230–234.

119. Orbach-Zinger S, Jadon A, Lucas DN, et al. Intrathecal catheter use after accidental dural puncture in obstetric patients: literature review and clinical management recommendations. *Anaesthesia.* 2021;76:1111–1121.

120. Kestin IG. Spinal anaesthesia in obstetrics. *Br J Anaesth.* 1991;66:596–607.

121. Greene NM. Distribution of local anesthetic solutions within the subarachnoid space. *Anesth Analg.* 1985;64:715–730.

122. Carvalho B, Durbin M, Drover DR, et al. The ED_{50} and ED_{95} of intrathecal isobaric bupivacaine with opioids for cesarean delivery. *Anesthesiology.* 2005;103:606–612.

123. Sarvela PJ, Halonen PM, Korttila KT. Comparison of 9 mg of intrathecal plain and hyperbaric bupivacaine both with fentanyl for cesarean delivery. *Anesth Analg.* 1999;89:1257–1262.

124. Vercauteren MP, Coppejans HC, Hoffmann VL, et al. Small-dose hyperbaric versus plain bupivacaine during spinal anesthesia for cesarean section. *Anesth Analg.* 1998;86:989–993.

125. Ben-David B, Miller G, Gavriel R, Gurevitch A. Low-dose bupivacaine-fentanyl spinal anesthesia for cesarean delivery. *Reg Anesth Pain Med.* 2000;25:235–239.

126. Bryson GL, Macneil R, Jeyaraj LM, Rosaeg OP. Small dose spinal bupivacaine for cesarean delivery does not reduce hypotension but accelerates motor recovery. *Can J Anaesth.* 2007;54:531–537.

127. Norris MC. Height, weight, and the spread of subarachnoid hyperbaric bupivacaine in the term parturient. *Anesth Analg.* 1988;67:555–558.

128. Hartwell BL, Aglio LS, Hauch MA, Datta S. Vertebral column length and spread of hyperbaric subarachnoid bupivacaine in the term parturient. *Reg Anesth.* 1991;16:17–19.

129. McDonald SB, Liu SS, Kopacz DJ, Stephenson CA. Hyperbaric spinal ropivacaine: a comparison to bupivacaine in volunteers. *Anesthesiology.* 1999;90:971–977.

130. Khaw KS, Ngan Kee WD, Wong EL, et al. Spinal ropivacaine for cesarean section: a dose-finding study. *Anesthesiology.* 2001;95:1346–1350.

131. Khaw KS, Ngan Kee WD, Wong M, et al. Spinal ropivacaine for cesarean delivery: a comparison of hyperbaric and plain solutions. *Anesth Analg.* 2002;94:680–685.

132. Oğün CO, Kirgiz EN, Duman A, et al. Comparison of intrathecal isobaric bupivacaine-morphine and ropivacaine-morphine for caesarean delivery. *Br J Anaesth.* 2003;90:659–664.

133. Gautier P, De Kock M, Huberty L, et al. Comparison of the effects of intrathecal ropivacaine, levobupivacaine, and bupivacaine for caesarean section. *Br J Anaesth.* 2003;91:684–689.

134. Dahl JB, Jeppesen IS, Jørgensen H, et al. Intraoperative and postoperative analgesic efficacy and adverse effects of intrathecal opioids in patients undergoing cesarean section with spinal anesthesia: a qualitative and quantitative systematic review of randomized controlled trials. *Anesthesiology.* 1999;91:1919–1927.

135. Dickenson AH. Spinal cord pharmacology of pain. *Br J Anaesth.* 1995;75:193–200.

136. Ginosar Y, Columb MO, Cohen SE, et al. The site of action of epidural fentanyl infusions in the presence of local anesthetics: a minimum local analgesic concentration infusion study in nulliparous labor. *Anesth Analg.* 2003;97:1439–1445.

137. Palmer CM, Voulgaropoulos D, Alves D. Subarachnoid fentanyl augments lidocaine spinal anesthesia for cesarean delivery. *Reg Anesth.* 1995;20:389–394.

138. Dahlgren G, Hultstrand C, Jakobsson J, et al. Intrathecal sufentanil, fentanyl, or placebo added to bupivacaine for cesarean section. *Anesth Analg.* 1997;85:1288–1293.

139. Cooper DW, Lindsay SL, Ryall DM, et al. Does intrathecal fentanyl produce acute cross-tolerance to i.v. morphine? *Br J Anaesth.* 1997;78:311–313.

140. Carvalho B, Drover DR, Ginosar Y, et al. Intrathecal fentanyl added to bupivacaine and morphine for cesarean delivery may induce a subtle acute opioid tolerance. *Int J Obstet Anesth.* 2012;21:29–34.

141. Uppal V, Retter S, Casey M, et al. Efficacy of intrathecal fentanyl for cesarean delivery: a systematic review and meta-analysis of randomized controlled trials with trial sequential analysis. *Anesth Analg.* 2020;130:111–125.

142. Courtney MA, Bader AM, Hartwell B, et al. Perioperative analgesia with subarachnoid sufentanil administration. *Reg Anesth.* 1992;17:274–278.

143. Braga Ade F, Braga FS, Poterio GM, et al. Sufentanil added to hyperbaric bupivacaine for subarachnoid block in caesarean section. *Eur J Anaesthesiol.* 2003;20:631–635.

144. Seki H, Shiga T, Mihara T, et al. Effects of intrathecal opioids on cesarean section: a systematic review and Bayesian network meta-analysis of randomized controlled trials. *J Anesth.* 2021;35:911–927.

145. Fournier R, Van Gessel E, Macksay M, Gamulin Z. Onset and offset of intrathecal morphine versus nalbuphine for postoperative pain relief after total hip replacement. *Acta Anaesthesiol Scand.* 2000;44:940–945.

146. Palmer CM, Emerson S, Volgoropolous D, Alves D. Dose-response relationship of intrathecal morphine for postcesarean analgesia. *Anesthesiology.* 1999;90:437–444.

147. Berger JS, Gonzalez A, Hopkins A, et al. Dose-response of intrathecal morphine when administered with intravenous ketorolac for post-cesarean analgesia: a two-center, prospective, randomized, blinded trial. *Int J Obstet Anesth.* 2016;28:3–11.

148. Sviggum HP, Arendt KW, Jacob AK, et al. Intrathecal hydromorphone and morphine for postcesarean delivery analgesia: determination of the ED$_{90}$ using a sequential allocation biased-coin method. *Anesth Analg.* 2016;123:690–697.

149. Husaini SW, Russell IF. Intrathecal diamorphine compared with morphine for postoperative analgesia after caesarean section under spinal anaesthesia. *Br J Anaesth.* 1998;81:135–139.

150. Saravanan S, Robinson AP, Qayoum Dar A, et al. Minimum dose of intrathecal diamorphine required to prevent intraoperative supplementation of spinal anaesthesia for caesarean section. *Br J Anaesth.* 2003;91:368–372.

151. Bauchat JR, Weiniger CF, Sultan P, et al. Society for Obstetric Anesthesia and Perinatology consensus statement: monitoring recommendations for prevention and detection of respiratory depression associated with administration of neuraxial morphine for cesarean delivery analgesia. *Anesth Analg.* 2019;129:458–474.

152. Carvalho B. Respiratory depression after neuraxial opioids in the obstetric setting. *Anesth Analg.* 2008;107:956–961.

153. Kaufman RD, Gabathuler ML, Bellville JW. Potency, duration of action and pA2 in man of intravenous naloxone measured by reversal of morphine-depressed respiration. *J Pharmacol Exp Ther.* 1981;219:156–162.

154. Lui AC, Polis TZ, Cicutti NJ. Densities of cerebrospinal fluid and spinal anaesthetic solutions in surgical patients at body temperature. *Can J Anaesth.* 1998;45:297–303.

155. Abouleish EI. Epinephrine improves the quality of spinal hyperbaric bupivacaine for cesarean section. *Anesth Analg.* 1987;66:395–400.

156. Randalls B, Broadway JW, Browne DA, Morgan BM. Comparison of four subarachnoid solutions in a needle-through-needle technique for elective caesarean section. *Br J Anaesth.* 1991;66:314–318.

157. Lavand'homme PM, Roelants F, Waterloos H, et al. An evaluation of the postoperative antihyperalgesic and analgesic effects of intrathecal clonidine administered during elective cesarean delivery. *Anesth Analg.* 2008;107:948–955.

158. Sun S, Wang J, Wang J, et al. Fetal and maternal responses to dexmedetomidine intrathecal application during cesarean section: a meta-analysis. *Med Sci Monit.* 2020;26:e918523.

159. Cossu AP, De Giudici LM, Piras D, et al. A systematic review of the effects of adding neostigmine to local anesthetics for neuraxial administration in obstetric anesthesia and analgesia. *Int J Obstet Anesth.* 2015;24:237–246.

160. Sakura S, Sumi M, Morimoto N, Saito Y. The addition of epinephrine increases intensity of sensory block during epidural anesthesia with lidocaine. *Reg Anesth Pain Med.* 1999;24:541–546.

161. Sakura S, Sumi M, Kushizaki H, et al. Concentration of lidocaine affects intensity of sensory block during lumbar epidural anesthesia. *Anesth Analg.* 1999;88:123–127.

162. Kuhnert BR, Kuhnert PM, Philipson EH, et al. The half-life of 2-chloroprocaine. *Anesth Analg.* 1986;65:273–278.

163. Toledo P, McCarthy RJ, Ebarvia MJ, et al. The interaction between epidural 2-chloroprocaine and morphine: a randomized controlled trial of the effect of drug administration timing on the efficacy of morphine analgesia. *Anesth Analg.* 2009;109:168–173.

164. Sharawi N, Bansal P, Williams M, et al. Comparison of chloroprocaine versus lidocaine with epinephrine, sodium bicarbonate, and fentanyl for epidural extension anesthesia in elective cesarean delivery: a randomized, triple-blind, noninferiority study. *Anesth Analg.* 2021;132:666–675.

165. Albright GA. Cardiac arrest following regional anesthesia with etidocaine or bupivacaine. *Anesthesiology.* 1979;51:285–287.

166. Santos AC, DeArmas PI. Systemic toxicity of levobupivacaine, bupivacaine, and ropivacaine during continuous intravenous infusion to nonpregnant and pregnant ewes. *Anesthesiology.* 2001;95:1256–1264.

167. Bader AM, Tsen LC, Camann WR, et al. Clinical effects and maternal and fetal plasma concentrations of 0.5% epidural levobupivacaine versus bupivacaine for cesarean delivery. *Anesthesiology.* 1999;90:1596–1601.

168. Faccenda KA, Simpson AM, Henderson DJ, et al. A comparison of levobupivacaine 0.5% and racemic bupivacaine 0.5% for extradural anesthesia for caesarean section. *Reg Anesth Pain Med.* 2003;28:394–400.

169. Datta S, Camann W, Bader A, VanderBurgh L. Clinical effects and maternal and fetal plasma concentrations of epidural ropivacaine versus bupivacaine for cesarean section. *Anesthesiology.* 1995;82:1346–1352.

170. Bernards CM, Shen DD, Sterling ES, et al. Epidural, cerebrospinal fluid, and plasma pharmacokinetics of epidural opioids (part 1): differences among opioids. *Anesthesiology.* 2003;99:455–465.

171. Ginosar Y, Riley ET, Angst MS. The site of action of epidural fentanyl in humans: the difference between infusion and bolus administration. *Anesth Analg.* 2003;97:1428–1438.

172. Helbo-Hansen HS, Bang U, Lindholm P, Klitgaard NA. Maternal effects of adding epidural fentanyl to 0.5% bupivacaine for caesarean section. *Int J Obstet Anesth.* 1993;2:21–26.

173. Gaffud MP, Bansal P, Lawton C, et al. Surgical analgesia for cesarean delivery with epidural bupivacaine and fentanyl. *Anesthesiology.* 1986;65:331–334.

174. Helbo-Hansen HS, Bang U, Lindholm P, Klitgaard NA. Neonatal effects of adding epidural fentanyl to 0.5% bupivacaine for caesarean section. *Int J Obstet Anesth.* 1993;2:27–33.

175. Eichenberger U, Giani C, Petersen-Felix S, et al. Lumbar epidural fentanyl: segmental spread and effect on temporal summation and muscle pain. *Br J Anaesth.* 2003;90:467–473.

176. Vertommen JD, Van Aken H, Vandermeulen E, et al. Maternal and neonatal effects of adding epidural sufentanil

to 0.5% bupivacaine for cesarean delivery. *J Clin Anesth.* 1991;3:371–376.

177. Madej TH, Strunin L. Comparison of epidural fentanyl with sufentanil. Analgesia and side effects after a single bolus dose during elective caesarean section. *Anaesthesia.* 1987;42:1156–1161.

178. Grass JA, Sakima NT, Schmidt R, et al. A randomized, double-blind, dose-response comparison of epidural fentanyl versus sufentanil analgesia after cesarean section. *Anesth Analg.* 1997;85:365–371.

179. Palmer CM, Nogami WM, Van Maren G, Alves DM. Postcesarean epidural morphine: a dose-response study. *Anesth Analg.* 2000;90:887–891.

180. Carvalho B, Roland LM, Chu LF, et al. Single-dose, extended-release epidural morphine (DepoDur) compared to conventional epidural morphine for post-cesarean pain. *Anesth Analg.* 2007;105:176–183.

181. Chestnut DH, Choi WW, Isbell TJ. Epidural hydromorphone for postcesarean analgesia. *Obstet Gynecol.* 1986;68:65–69.

182. Halpern SH, Arellano R, Preston R, et al. Epidural morphine vs hydromorphone in post-caesarean section patients. *Can J Anaesth.* 1996;43:595–598.

183. Marroquin B, Feng C, Balofsky A, et al. Neuraxial opioids for post-cesarean delivery analgesia: can hydromorphone replace morphine? A retrospective study. *Int J Obstet Anesth.* 2017;30:16–22.

184. Hallworth SP, Fernando R, Bell R, et al. Comparison of intrathecal and epidural diamorphine for elective caesarean section using a combined spinal-epidural technique. *Br J Anaesth.* 1999;82:228–232.

185. Bloor GK, Thompson M, Chung N. A randomised, double-blind comparison of subarachnoid and epidural diamorphine for elective caesarean section using a combined spinal-epidural technique. *Int J Obstet Anesth.* 2000;9:233–237.

186. Eisenach JC, D'Angelo R, Taylor C, Hood DD. An isobolographic study of epidural clonidine and fentanyl after cesarean section. *Anesth Analg.* 1994;79:285–290.

187. Kaya FN, Sahin S, Owen MD, Eisenach JC. Epidural neostigmine produces analgesia but also sedation in women after cesarean delivery. *Anesthesiology.* 2004;100:381–385.

188. Mather LE, Tucker GT, Murphy TM, et al. The effects of adding adrenaline to etidocaine and lignocaine in extradural anaesthesia II: pharmacokinetics. *Br J Anaesth.* 1976;48:989–994.

189. Murphy TM, Mather LE, Stanton-Hicks M, et al. The effects of adding adrenaline to etidocaine and lignocaine in extradural anaesthesia I: block characteristics and cardiovascular effects. *Br J Anaesth.* 1976;48:893–898.

190. Bernards CM, Shen DD, Sterling ES, et al. Epidural, cerebrospinal fluid, and plasma pharmacokinetics of epidural opioids (part 2): effect of epinephrine. *Anesthesiology.* 2003;99:466–475.

191. Hadzic A, Vloka J, Patel N, Birnbach D. Hypertensive crisis after a successful placement of an epidural anesthetic in a hypertensive parturient. Case report. *Reg Anesth.* 1995;20:156–158.

192. Alahuhta S, Räsänen J, Jouppila P, et al. Uteroplacental and fetal circulation during extradural bupivacaine-adrenaline and bupivacaine for caesarean section in hypertensive pregnancies with chronic fetal asphyxia. *Br J Anaesth.* 1993;71:348–353.

193. Davies SJ, Paech MJ, Welch H, et al. Maternal experience during epidural or combined spinal-epidural anesthesia for cesarean section: a prospective, randomized trial. *Anesth Analg.* 1997;85:607–613.

194. Goy RW, Chee-Seng Y, Sia AT, et al. The median effective dose of intrathecal hyperbaric bupivacaine is larger in the single-shot spinal as compared with the combined spinal-epidural technique. *Anesth Analg.* 2005;100:1499–1502.

195. Ithnin F, Lim Y, Sia AT, Ocampo CE. Combined spinal epidural causes higher level of block than equivalent single-shot spinal anesthesia in elective cesarean patients. *Anesth Analg.* 2006;102:577–580.

196. Lim Y, Teoh W, Sia AT. Combined spinal epidural does not cause a higher sensory block than single shot spinal technique for cesarean delivery in laboring women. *Anesth Analg.* 2006;103:1540–1542.

197. McNaught AF, Stocks GM. Epidural volume extension and low-dose sequential combined spinal-epidural blockade: two ways to reduce spinal dose requirement for caesarean section. *Int J Obstet Anesth.* 2007;16:346–353.

198. Thorén T, Holmström B, Rawal N, et al. Sequential combined spinal epidural block versus spinal block for cesarean section: effects on maternal hypotension and neurobehavioral function of the newborn. *Anesth Analg.* 1994;78:1087–1092.

199. Kucukguclu S, Unlugenc H, Gunenc F, et al. The influence of epidural volume extension on spinal block with hyperbaric or plain bupivacaine for caesarean delivery. *Eur J Anaesthesiol.* 2008;25:307–313.

200. Loubert C, O'Brien PJ, Fernando R, et al. Epidural volume extension in combined spinal epidural anaesthesia for elective caesarean section: a randomised controlled trial. *Anaesthesia.* 2011;66:341–347.

201. Cappiello E, O'Rourke N, Segal S, Tsen LC. A randomized trial of dural puncture epidural technique compared with the standard epidural technique for labor analgesia. *Anesth Analg.* 2008;107:1646–1651.

202. Rao WY, Xu F, Dai SB, et al. Comparison of dural puncture epidural, epidural and combined spinal-epidural anesthesia for cesarean delivery: a randomized controlled trial. *Drug Des Devel Ther.* 2023;17:2077–2085.

203. Sharawi N, Williams M, Athar W, et al. Effect of dural-puncture epidural vs standard epidural for epidural extension on onset time of surgical anesthesia in elective cesarean delivery: a randomized clinical trial. *JAMA Netw Open.* 2023;6:e2326710.

204. Bauer ME, Kountanis JA, Tsen LC, et al. Risk factors for failed conversion of labor epidural analgesia to cesarean delivery anesthesia: a systematic review and meta-analysis of observational trials. *Int J Obstet Anesth.* 2012;21:294–309.

205. Hillyard SG, Bate TE, Corcoran TB, et al. Extending epidural analgesia for emergency caesarean section: a meta-analysis. *Br J Anaesth.* 2011;107:668–678.

206. Bjørnestad E, Iversen OL, Raeder J. Similar onset time of 2-chloroprocaine and lidocaine + epinephrine for epidural anesthesia for elective cesarean section. *Acta Anaesthesiol Scand.* 2006;50:358–363.

207. Lam DT, Ngan Kee WD, Khaw KS. Extension of epidural blockade in labour for emergency caesarean section using 2% lidocaine with epinephrine and fentanyl, with or without alkalinisation. *Anaesthesia.* 2001;56:790–794.

208. Peterfreund RA, Datta S, Ostheimer GW. pH adjustment of local anesthetic solutions with sodium bicarbonate: laboratory evaluation of alkalinization and precipitation. *Reg Anesth.* 1989;14:265–270.

209. Tuleu C, Allam J, Gill H, Yentis SM. Short term stability of pH-adjusted lidocaine-adrenaline epidural solution used for emergency caesarean section. *Int J Obstet Anesth.* 2008;17:118–122.

210. Higuchi H, Adachi Y, Kazama T. Effects of epidural saline injection on cerebrospinal fluid volume and velocity waveform: a magnetic resonance imaging study. *Anesthesiology.* 2005;102:285–292.

211. Regan KJ, O'Sullivan G. The extension of epidural blockade for emergency caesarean section: a survey of current UK practice. *Anaesthesia.* 2008;63:136–142.

212. Kodali BS, Chandrasekhar S, Bulich LN, et al. Airway changes during labor and delivery. *Anesthesiology.* 2008;108:357–362.

213. McClelland SH, Bogod DG, Hardman JG. Pre-oxygenation and apnoea in pregnancy: changes during labour and with obstetric morbidity in a computational simulation. *Anaesthesia.* 2009;64:371–377.

214. Soro Domingo M, Belda Nácher FJ, Aguilar G, et al. [Preoxygenation for anesthesia]. *Rev Esp Anestesiol Reanim.* 2004;51:322–327.

215. Sjöblom A, Hedberg M, Johansson S, et al. Pre-oxygenation using high-flow nasal oxygen in parturients undergoing caesarean section in general anaesthesia: a prospective, multi-centre, pilot study. *Acta Anaesthesiol Scand.* 2023;67:1028–1036.

216. Mushambi MC, Kinsella SM, Popat M, et al. Obstetric Anaesthetists' Association and Difficult Airway Society guidelines for the management of difficult and failed tracheal intubation in obstetrics. *Anaesthesia.* 2015;70:1286–1306.

217. de Souza DG, Doar LH, Mehta SH, Tiouririne M. Aspiration prophylaxis and rapid sequence induction for elective cesarean delivery: time to reassess old dogma? *Anesth Analg.* 2010;110:1503–1505.

218. Paech MJ. "Pregnant women having caesarean delivery under general anaesthesia should have a rapid sequence induction with cricoid pressure and be intubated." Can this 'holy cow' be sent packing? *Anaesth Intensive Care.* 2010;38:989–991.

219. Thind GS, Bryson TH. Single dose suxamethonium and muscle pain in pregnancy. *Br J Anaesth.* 1983;55:743–745.

220. Perry JJ, Lee JS, Sillberg VA, Wells GA. Rocuronium versus succinylcholine for rapid sequence induction intubation. *Cochrane Database Syst Rev.* 2008;(2):CD002788.

221. Stourac P, Adamus M, Seidlova D, et al. Low-dose or high-dose rocuronium reversed with neostigmine or sugammadex for cesarean delivery anesthesia: a randomized controlled noninferiority trial of time to tracheal intubation and extubation. *Anesth Analg.* 2016;122:1536–1545.

222. Cherala S, Eddie D, Halpern M, Shevde K. Priming with vecuronium in obstetrics. *Anaesthesia.* 1987;42:1021.

223. Guay J, Grenier Y, Varin F. Clinical pharmacokinetics of neuromuscular relaxants in pregnancy. *Clin Pharmacokinet.* 1998;34:483.

224. Pühringer FK, Kristen P, Rex C. Sugammadex reversal of rocuronium-induced neuromuscular block in caesarean section patients: a series of seven cases. *Br J Anaesth.* 2010;105:657–660.

225. Han TH, Brimacombe J, Lee EJ, Yang HS. The laryngeal mask airway is effective (and probably safe) in selected healthy parturients for elective cesarean section: a prospective study of 1067 cases. *Can J Anaesth.* 2001;48:1117–1121.

226. Halaseh BK, Sukkar ZF, Hassan LH, et al. The use of Proseal laryngeal mask airway in caesarean section–experience in 3000 cases. *Anaesth Intensive Care*. 2010;38:1023–1028.

227. Matthews P, Dann WL, Cartwright DP, Taylor E. Inspired oxygen concentration during general anaesthesia for caesarean section. *Eur J Anaesthesiol*. 1989;6:295–301.

228. Parpaglioni R, Capogna G, Celleno D, Fusco P. Intraoperative fetal oxygen saturation during caesarean section: general anaesthesia using sevoflurane with either 100% oxygen or 50% nitrous oxide in oxygen. *Eur J Anaesthesiol*. 2002;19:115–118.

229. Levinson G, Shnider SM, DeLorimier AA, Steffenson JL. Effects of maternal hyperventilation on uterine blood flow and fetal oxygenation and acid-base status. *Anesthesiology*. 1974;40:340–347.

230. Palahniuk RJ, Shnider SM, Eger EI 2nd. Pregnancy decreases the requirement for inhaled anesthetic agents. *Anesthesiology*. 1974;41:82–83.

231. Chin KJ, Yeo SW. A BIS-guided study of sevoflurane requirements for adequate depth of anaesthesia in caesarean section. *Anaesthesia*. 2004;59:1064–1068.

232. Yoo KY, Jeong CW, Kang MW, et al. Bispectral index values during sevoflurane-nitrous oxide general anesthesia in women undergoing cesarean delivery: a comparison between women with and without prior labor. *Anesth Analg*. 2008;106:1827–1832.

233. Erden V, Erkalp K, Yangin Z, et al. The effect of labor on sevoflurane requirements during cesarean delivery. *Int J Obstet Anesth*. 2011;20:17–21.

234. Munson ES, Embro WJ. Enflurane, isoflurane, and halothane and isolated human uterine muscle. *Anesthesiology*. 1977;46:11–14.

235. Dogru K, Yildiz K, Dalgiç H, et al. Inhibitory effects of desflurane and sevoflurane on contractions of isolated gravid rat myometrium under oxytocin stimulation. *Acta Anaesthesiol Scand*. 2003;47:472–474.

236. Butwick AJ, Ramachandran B, Hegde P, et al. Risk factors for severe postpartum hemorrhage after cesarean delivery: case-control studies. *Anesth Analg*. 2017;125:523–532.

237. Ngan Kee WD, Khaw KS, Ma KC, et al. Maternal and neonatal effects of remifentanil at induction of general anesthesia for cesarean delivery: a randomized, double-blind, controlled trial. *Anesthesiology*. 2006;104:14–20.

238. Petropoulos G, Siristatidis C, Salamalekis E, Creatsas G. Spinal and epidural versus general anesthesia for elective cesarean section at term: effect on the acid-base status of the mother and newborn. *J Matern Fetal Neonatal Med*. 2003;13:260–266.

239. Sprung J, Flick RP, Wilder RT, et al. Anesthesia for cesarean delivery and learning disabilities in a population-based birth cohort. *Anesthesiology*. 2009;111:302–310.

240. Mhyre JM, Riesner MN, Polley LS, Naughton NN. A series of anesthesia-related maternal deaths in Michigan, 1985-2003. *Anesthesiology*. 2007;106:1096–1104.

241. American Society of Anesthesiologists. Practice guidelines for postanesthetic care: an updated report by the American Society of Anesthesiologists Task Force on Postanesthetic Care. *Anesthesiology*. 2013;118:291–307.

242. Horwitz LD. Effects of intravenous anesthetic agents on left ventricular function in dogs. *Am J Physiol*. 1977;232:H44–H48.

243. Morgan DJ, Blackman GL, Paull JD, Wolf LJ. Pharmacokinetics and plasma binding of thiopental. II: studies at cesarean section. *Anesthesiology*. 1981;54:474–480.

244. Norman E, Westrin P, Fellman V. Placental transfer and pharmacokinetics of thiopentone in newborn infants. *Arch Dis Child Fetal Neonatal Ed*. 2010;95:F277–F282.

245. Kosaka Y, Takahashi T, Mark LC. Intravenous thiobarbiturate anesthesia for cesarean section. *Anesthesiology*. 1969;31:489–506.

246. Finster M, Morishima HO, Mark LC, et al. Tissue thiopental concentrations in the fetus and newborn. *Anesthesiology*. 1972;36:155–158.

247. Flowers CE Jr. The placental transmission of barbiturates and thiobarbiturates and their pharmacological action on the mother and the infant. *Am J Obstet Gynecol*. 1959;78:730–742.

248. Gin T, Gregory MA, Chan K, Oh TE. Maternal and fetal levels of propofol at caesarean section. *Anaesth Intensive Care*. 1990;18:180–184.

249. Soares de Moura R, Silva GA, Tano T, Resende AC. Effect of propofol on human fetal placental circulation. *Int J Obstet Anesth*. 2010;19:71–76.

250. Celleno D, Capogna G, Tomassetti M, et al. Neurobehavioural effects of propofol on the neonate following elective caesarean section. *Br J Anaesth*. 1989;62:649–654.

251. Tumukunde J, Lomangisi DD, Davidson O, et al. Effects of propofol versus thiopental on apgar scores in newborns and peri-operative outcomes of women undergoing emergency cesarean section: a randomized clinical trial. *BMC Anesthesiol*. 2015;15:63.

252. Yau G, Gin T, Ewart MC, et al. Propofol for induction and maintenance of anaesthesia at caesarean section. A comparison with thiopentone/enflurane. *Anaesthesia*. 1991;46:20–23.

253. Gin T, Gregory MA, Chan K, et al. Pharmacokinetics of propofol in women undergoing elective caesarean section. *Br J Anaesth*. 1990;64:148–153.

254. Gregory MA, Gin T, Yau G, et al. Propofol infusion anaesthesia for caesarean section. *Can J Anaesth*. 1990;37:514–520.

255. Grounds RM, Twigley AJ, Carli F, et al. The haemodynamic effects of intravenous induction. Comparison of the effects of thiopentone and propofol. *Anaesthesia*. 1985;40:735–740.

256. Baraka A. Severe bradycardia following propofol-suxamethonium sequence. *Br J Anaesth*. 1988;61:482–483.

257. Alon E, Ball RH, Gillie MH, et al. Effects of propofol and thiopental on maternal and fetal cardiovascular and acid-base variables in the pregnant ewe. *Anesthesiology*. 1993;78:562–576.

258. Hui TW, Short TG, Hong W, et al. Additive interactions between propofol and ketamine when used for anesthesia induction in female patients. *Anesthesiology*. 1995;82:641–648.

259. Corssen G, Gutierrez J, Reves JG, Huber FC Jr. Ketamine in the anesthetic management of asthmatic patients. *Anesth Analg*. 1972;51:588–596.

260. McDonald JS, Mateo CV, Reed EC. Modified nitrous oxide or ketamine hydrochloride for cesarean section. *Anesth Analg*. 1972;51:975–985.

261. Craft JB Jr, Coaldrake LA, Yonekura ML, et al. Ketamine, catecholamines, and uterine tone in pregnant ewes. *Am J Obstet Gynecol*. 1983;146:429–434.

262. Oats JN, Vasey DP, Waldron BA. Effects of ketamine on the pregnant uterus. *Br J Anaesth*. 1979;51:1163–1166.

263. Little B, Chang T, Chucot L, et al. Study of ketamine as an obstetric anesthetic agent. *Am J Obstet Gynecol.* 1972;113:247–260.

264. Ngan Kee WD, Khaw KS, Ma ML, et al. Postoperative analgesic requirement after cesarean section: a comparison of anesthetic induction with ketamine or thiopental. *Anesth Analg.* 1997;85:1294–1298.

265. Peltz B, Sinclair DM. Induction agents for caesarean section. A comparison of thiopentone and ketamine. *Anaesthesia.* 1973;28:37–42.

266. Strümper D, Gogarten W, Durieux ME, et al. The effects of S+-ketamine and racemic ketamine on uterine blood flow in chronically instrumented pregnant sheep. *Anesth Analg.* 2004;98:497–502.

267. Dich-Nielsen J, Holasek J. Ketamine as induction agent for caesarean section. *Acta Anaesthesiol Scand.* 1982;26:139–142.

268. Baraka A, Louis F, Dalleh R. Maternal awareness and neonatal outcome after ketamine induction of anaesthesia for caesarean section. *Can J Anaesth.* 1990;37:641–644.

269. Gaitini L, Vaida S, Collins G, et al. Awareness detection during caesarean section under general anaesthesia using EEG spectrum analysis. *Can J Anaesth.* 1995;42:377–381.

270. Mankowitz E, Downing JW, Brock-Utne JG, et al. Total intravenous anaesthesia using low-dose ketamine infusion for caesarean section. A comparison with a standard inhalation anaesthetic technique. *S Afr Med J.* 1984;65:246–250.

271. Orme RM, Grange CS, Ainsworth QP, Grebenik CR. General anaesthesia using remifentanil for caesarean section in parturients with critical aortic stenosis: a series of four cases. *Int J Obstet Anesth.* 2004;13:183–187.

272. Esener Z, Sarihasan B, Güven H, Ustün E. Thiopentone and etomidate concentrations in maternal and umbilical plasma, and in colostrum. *Br J Anaesth.* 1992;69:586–588.

273. Bergen JM, Smith DC. A review of etomidate for rapid sequence intubation in the emergency department. *J Emerg Med.* 1997;15:221–230.

274. Downing JW, Buley RJ, Brock-Utne JG, Houlton PC. Etomidate for induction of anaesthesia at caesarean section: comparison with thiopentone. *Br J Anaesth.* 1979;51:135–140.

275. Reddy BK, Pizer B, Bull PT. Neonatal serum cortisol suppression by etomidate compared with thiopentone, for elective caesarean section. *Eur J Anaesthesiol.* 1988;5:171–176.

276. Bland BA, Lawes EG, Duncan PW, et al. Comparison of midazolam and thiopental for rapid sequence anesthetic induction for elective cesarean section. *Anesth Analg.* 1987;66:1165–1168.

277. Kvisselgaard N, Moya F. Investigation of placental thresholds to succinylcholine. *Anesthesiology.* 1961;22:7–10.

278. Shnider SM. Serum chlonesterase activity during pregnancy, labor and the puerperium. *Anesthesiology.* 1965;26:335–339.

279. Kao YJ, Turner DR. Prolongation of succinylcholine block by metoclopramide. *Anesthesiology.* 1989;70:905–908.

280. Abouleish E, Abboud T, Lechevalier T, et al. Rocuronium (Org 9426) for caesarean section. *Br J Anaesth.* 1994;73: 336–341.

281. Magorian T, Flannery KB, Miller RD. Comparison of rocuronium, succinylcholine, and vecuronium for rapid-sequence induction of anesthesia in adult patients. *Anesthesiology.* 1993;79:913–918.

282. Hawkins JL, Johnson TD, Kubicek MA, et al. Vecuronium for rapid-sequence intubation for cesarean section. *Anesth Analg.* 1990;71:185–190.

283. Hawkins JL, Adenwala J, Camp C, Joyce TH 3rd. The effect of H_2-receptor antagonist premedication on the duration of vecuronium-induced neuromuscular blockade in postpartum patients. *Anesthesiology.* 1989;71:175–177.

284. Dailey PA, Fisher DM, Shnider SM, et al. Pharmacokinetics, placental transfer, and neonatal effects of vecuronium and pancuronium administered during cesarean section. *Anesthesiology.* 1984;60:569–574.

285. Eikermann M, Peters J. Nerve stimulation at 0.15 Hz when compared to 0.1 Hz speeds the onset of action of cisatracurium and rocuronium. *Acta Anaesthesiol Scand.* 2000;44:170–174.

286. Warren TM, Datta S, Ostheimer GW, et al. Comparison of the maternal and neonatal effects of halothane, enflurane, and isoflurane for cesarean delivery. *Anesth Analg.* 1983;62: 516–520.

287. Crawford JS. Awareness during operative obstetrics under general anaesthesia. *Br J Anaesth.* 1971;43:179–182.

288. Karasawa F, Takita A, Fukuda I, Kawatani Y. Nitrous oxide concentrations in maternal and fetal blood during caesarean section. *Eur J Anaesthesiol.* 2003;20:555–559.

289. Palahniuk RJ, Cumming M. Foetal deterioration following thiopentone-nitrous oxide anaesthesia in the pregnant ewe. *Can Anaesth Soc J.* 1977;24:361–370.

290. Piggott SE, Bogod DG, Rosen M, et al. Isoflurane with either 100% oxygen or 50% nitrous oxide in oxygen for caesarean section. *Br J Anaesth.* 1990;65:325–329.

291. Dwyer R, Fee JP, Moore J. Uptake of halothane and isoflurane by mother and baby during caesarean section. *Br J Anaesth.* 1995;74:379–383.

292. Gin T, Chan MT. Decreased minimum alveolar concentration of isoflurane in pregnant humans. *Anesthesiology.* 1994;81:829–832.

293. Chan MT, Mainland P, Gin T. Minimum alveolar concentration of halothane and enflurane are decreased in early pregnancy. *Anesthesiology.* 1996;85:782–786.

294. Datta S, Migliozzi RP, Flanagan HL, Krieger NR. Chronically administered progesterone decreases halothane requirements in rabbits. *Anesth Analg.* 1989;68:46–50.

295. Chan MT, Gin T. Postpartum changes in the minimum alveolar concentration of isoflurane. *Anesthesiology.* 1995;82:1360–1363.

296. Draisci G, Valente A, Suppa E, et al. Remifentanil for cesarean section under general anesthesia: effects on maternal stress hormone secretion and neonatal well-being: a randomized trial. *Int J Obstet Anesth.* 2008;17:130–136.

297. Craft JB Jr, Coaldrake LA, Bolan JC, et al. Placental passage and uterine effects of fentanyl. *Anesth Analg.* 1983;62: 894–898.

298. Gerdin E, Rane A, Lindberg B. Transplacental transfer of morphine in man. *J Perinat Med.* 1990;18:305–312.

299. Nation RL. Meperidine binding in maternal and fetal plasma. *Clin Pharmacol Ther.* 1981;29:472–479.

300. Bonica JJ, ed. *Local-Regional Analgesia for Abdominal Delivery.* FA Davis; 1967.

301. Mei W, Jin C, Feng L, et al. Bilateral ultrasound-guided transversus abdominis plane block combined with ilioinguinal-iliohypogastric nerve block for cesarean delivery anesthesia. *Anesth Analg.* 2011;113:134–137.

302. Bewley Waterstone M, Wolfe S. C. Incidence and predictors of severe obstetric morbidity: case-control study. *BMJ.* 2001;322:1089–1093.

303. Cohen SE, Hamilton CL, Riley ET, et al. Obstetric postanesthesia care unit stays: reevaluation of discharge criteria after regional anesthesia. *Anesthesiology.* 1998;89:1559–1565.

304. Thomas J, Paranjothy S, Royal College of Obstetricians and Gynaecologies Clinical Effectiveness Support Unit. *The National Sentinel Caesarean Section Audit Report.* RCOG Press; 2001.

305. Bamber JL, Kimber-Craig S, Lucas N, Platt F. Guidelines for the Provision of Anaesthesia Services (GPAS). Chapter 9: Guidelines for the Provision of Anaesthesia Services for an Obstetric Population 2025. Royal College of Anaesthetists.

306. Patel K, Zakowski M. Enhanced recovery after cesarean: current and emerging trends. *Curr Anesthesiol Rep.* 2021;11:136–144.

307. Mangesi L, Hofmeyr GJ. Early compared with delayed oral fluids and food after caesarean section. *Cochrane Database Syst Rev.* 2002:CD003516.

308. National Institute for Health and Clinical Excellence. Caesarean birth. NICE guideline [NG192]; 2021. Available at https://www.nice.org.uk/guidance/ng192/chapter/Recommendations#recovery-after-caesarean-birth. Accessed 11 August 2024.

309. Sharma KK, Mahmood TA, Smith NC. The short term effect of obstetric anaesthesia on bladder function. *J Obstet Gynaecol.* 1994;14:254–264.

310. Liang CC, Chang SD, Chang YL, et al. Postpartum urinary retention after cesarean delivery. *Int J Gynaecol Obstet.* 2007;99:229–232.

311. Onile TG, Kuti O, Orji EO, Ogunniyi SO. A prospective randomized clinical trial of urethral catheter removal following elective cesarean delivery. *Int J Gynaecol Obstet.* 2008;102:267–270.

312. El-Mazny A, El-Sharkawy M, Hassan A. A prospective randomized clinical trial comparing immediate versus delayed removal of urinary catheter following elective cesarean section. *Eur J Obstet Gynecol Reprod Biol.* 2014;181:111–114.

313. Foon R, Toozs-Hobson P, Millns P, Kilby M. The impact of anesthesia and mode of delivery on the urinary bladder in the postdelivery period. *Int J Gynaecol Obstet.* 2010;110:114–117.

314. King H, Ashley S, Brathwaite D, et al. Adequacy of general anesthesia for cesarean section. *Anesth Analg.* 1993;77:84–88.

315. Moir DD. Anaesthesia for caesarean section. An evaluation of a method using low concentrations of halothane and 50 per cent of oxygen. *Br J Anaesth.* 1970;42:136–142.

316. Datta S, Ostheimer GW, Weiss JB, et al. Neonatal effect of prolonged anesthetic induction for cesarean section. *Obstet Gynecol.* 1981;58:331–335.

317. Glass PS, Bloom M, Kearse L, et al. Bispectral analysis measures sedation and memory effects of propofol, midazolam, isoflurane, and alfentanil in healthy volunteers. *Anesthesiology.* 1997;86:836–847.

318. Sanders RD, Avidan MS. Evidence is lacking for interventions proposed to prevent unintended awareness during general anesthesia for cesarean delivery. *Anesth Analg.* 2010;110:972–973.

319. Zand F, Hadavi SM, Chohedri A, Sabetian P. Survey on the adequacy of depth of anaesthesia with bispectral index and isolated forearm technique in elective caesarean section under general anaesthesia with sevoflurane. *Br J Anaesth.* 2014;112:871–878.

320. Yeo SN, Lo WK. Bispectral index in assessment of adequacy of general anaesthesia for lower segment caesarean section. *Anaesth Intensive Care.* 2002;30:36–40.

321. Krissel J, Dick WF, Leyser KH, et al. Thiopentone, thiopentone/ketamine, and ketamine for induction of anaesthesia in caesarean section. *Eur J Anaesthesiol.* 1994;11:115–122.

322. Kanto J, Aaltonen L, Erkkola R, Äärimaa L. Pharmacokinetics and sedative effect of midazolam in connection with caesarean section performed under epidural analgesia. *Acta Anaesthesiol Scand.* 1984;28:116–118.

323. Polster MR, Gray PA, O'Sullivan G, et al. Comparison of the sedative and amnesic effects of midazolam and propofol. *Br J Anaesth.* 1993;70:612–616.

324. Dahan A, Kest B, Waxman AR, Sarton E. Sex-specific responses to opiates: animal and human studies. *Anesth Analg.* 2008;107:83–95.

325. Hoymork SC, Raeder J. Why do women wake up faster than men from propofol anaesthesia? *Br J Anaesth.* 2005;95:627–633.

326. Fan SZ, Susetio L, Wang YP, et al. Low dose of intrathecal hyperbaric bupivacaine combined with epidural lidocaine for cesarean section—a balance block technique. *Anesth Analg.* 1994;78:474–477.

327. Lirk P, Kleber N, Mitterschiffthaler G, et al. Pulmonary effects of bupivacaine, ropivacaine, and levobupivacaine in parturients undergoing spinal anaesthesia for elective caesarean delivery: a randomised controlled study. *Int J Obstet Anesth.* 2010;19:287–292.

328. Corke BC, Datta S, Ostheimer GW, et al. Spinal anaesthesia for caesarean section. The influence of hypotension on neonatal outcome. *Anaesthesia.* 1982;37:658–662.

329. Chooi C, Cox JJ, Lumb RS, et al. Techniques for preventing hypotension during spinal anaesthesia for caesarean section. *Cochrane Database Syst Rev.* 2020;(7):CD002251.

330. McDonald S, Fernando R, Ashpole K, Columb M. Maternal cardiac output changes after crystalloid or colloid coload following spinal anesthesia for elective cesarean delivery: a randomized controlled trial. *Anesth Analg.* 2011;113:803–810.

331. Dyer RA, Piercy JL, Reed AR, et al. Hemodynamic changes associated with spinal anesthesia for cesarean delivery in severe preeclampsia. *Anesthesiology.* 2008;108:802–811.

332. Langesaeter E, Dyer RA. Maternal haemodynamic changes during spinal anaesthesia for caesarean section. *Curr Opin Anaesthesiol.* 2011;24:242–248.

333. Mark JB, Steele SM. Cardiovascular effects of spinal anesthesia. *Int Anesthesiol Clin.* 1989;27:31–39.

334. Ng K, Parsons J, Cyna AM, Middleton P. Spinal versus epidural anaesthesia for caesarean section. *Cochrane Database Syst Rev.* 2004;(2):CD003765.

335. Aya AG, Vialles N, Tanoubi I, et al. Spinal anesthesia-induced hypotension: a risk comparison between patients with severe preeclampsia and healthy women undergoing preterm cesarean delivery. *Anesth Analg.* 2005;101:869–875.

336. Kinsella SM, Norris MC. Advance prediction of hypotension at cesarean delivery under spinal anesthesia. *Int J Obstet Anesth.* 1996;5:3–7.

337. Frölich MA, Caton D. Baseline heart rate may predict hypotension after spinal anesthesia in prehydrated obstetrical patients. *Can J Anaesth.* 2002;49:185–189.

338. Dahlgren G, Granath F, Wessel H, Irestedt L. Prediction of hypotension during spinal anesthesia for cesarean section and

its relation to the effect of crystalloid or colloid preload. *Int J Obstet Anesth.* 2007;16:128–134.

339. Hanss R, Bein B, Francksen H, et al. Heart rate variability-guided prophylactic treatment of severe hypotension after subarachnoid block for elective cesarean delivery. *Anesthesiology.* 2006;104:635–643.

340. Chamchad D, Arkoosh VA, Horrow JC, et al. Using heart rate variability to stratify risk of obstetric patients undergoing spinal anesthesia. *Anesth Analg.* 2004;99:1818–1821.

341. Ouzounian JG, Masaki DI, Abboud TK, Greenspoon JS. Systemic vascular resistance index determined by thoracic electrical bioimpedance predicts the risk for maternal hypotension during regional anesthesia for cesarean delivery. *Am J Obstet Gynecol.* 1996;174:1019–1025.

342. Benhamou D, Wong C. Neuraxial anesthesia for cesarean delivery: what criteria define the "optimal" technique? *Anesth Analg.* 2009;109:1370–1373.

343. Van de Velde M, Van Schoubroeck D, Jani J, et al. Combined spinal-epidural anesthesia for cesarean delivery: dose-dependent effects of hyperbaric bupivacaine on maternal hemodynamics. *Anesth Analg.* 2006;103:187–190.

344. Rucklidge MW, Paech MJ. Limiting the dose of local anaesthetic for caesarean section under spinal anaesthesia—has the limbo bar been set too low? *Anaesthesia.* 2012;67:347–351.

345. Ueyama H, He YL, Tanigami H, et al. Effects of crystalloid and colloid preload on blood volume in the parturient undergoing spinal anesthesia for elective cesarean section. *Anesthesiology.* 1999;91:1571–1576.

346. Pouta AM, Karinen J, Vuolteenaho OJ, Laatikainen TJ. Effect of intravenous fluid preload on vasoactive peptide secretion during caesarean section under spinal anaesthesia. *Anaesthesia.* 1996;51:128–132.

347. Ralston DH, Shnider SM, DeLorimier AA. Effects of equipotent ephedrine, metaraminol, mephentermine, and methoxamine on uterine blood flow in the pregnant ewe. *Anesthesiology.* 1974;40:354–370.

348. Tong C, Eisenach JC. The vascular mechanism of ephedrine's beneficial effect on uterine perfusion during pregnancy. *Anesthesiology.* 1992;76:792–798.

349. Li P, Tong C, Eisenach JC. Pregnancy and ephedrine increase the release of nitric oxide in ovine uterine arteries. *Anesth Analg.* 1996;82:288–293.

350. Lee A, Ngan Kee WD, Gin T. A quantitative, systematic review of randomized controlled trials of ephedrine versus phenylephrine for the management of hypotension during spinal anesthesia for cesarean delivery. *Anesth Analg.* 2002;94:920–926.

351. Ngan Kee WD, Lau TK, Khaw KS, Lee BB. Comparison of metaraminol and ephedrine infusions for maintaining arterial pressure during spinal anesthesia for elective cesarean section. *Anesthesiology.* 2001;95:307–313.

352. Cooper DW, Carpenter M, Mowbray P, et al. Fetal and maternal effects of phenylephrine and ephedrine during spinal anesthesia for cesarean delivery. *Anesthesiology.* 2002;97:1582–1590.

353. Ngan Kee WD, Khaw KS, Tan PE, et al. Placental transfer and fetal metabolic effects of phenylephrine and ephedrine during spinal anesthesia for cesarean delivery. *Anesthesiology.* 2009;111:506–512.

354. Stewart A, Fernando R, McDonald S, et al. The dose-dependent effects of phenylephrine for elective cesarean delivery under spinal anesthesia. *Anesth Analg.* 2010;111:1230–1237.

355. Datta S, Alper MH, Ostheimer GW, Weiss JB. Method of ephedrine administration and nausea and hypotension during spinal anesthesia for cesarean section. *Anesthesiology.* 1982;56:68–70.

356. Ngan Kee WD, Khaw KS, Ng FF. Comparison of phenylephrine infusion regimens for maintaining maternal blood pressure during spinal anaesthesia for caesarean section. *Br J Anaesth.* 2004;92:469–474.

357. Ngan Kee WD, Tam YH, Khaw KS, et al. Closed-loop feedback computer-controlled infusion of phenylephrine for maintaining blood pressure during spinal anaesthesia for caesarean section: a preliminary descriptive study. *Anaesthesia.* 2007;62:1251–1256.

358. Doherty A, Ohashi Y, Downey K, Carvalho JC. Phenylephrine infusion versus bolus regimens during cesarean delivery under spinal anesthesia: a double-blind randomized clinical trial to assess hemodynamic changes. *Anesth Analg.* 2012;115:1343–1350.

359. Tanaka M, Balki M, Parkes RK, Carvalho JC. ED$_{95}$ of phenylephrine to prevent spinal-induced hypotension and/or nausea at elective cesarean delivery. *Int J Obstet Anesth.* 2009;18:125–130.

360. Kinsella SM, Carvalho B, Dyer RA, et al. International consensus statement on the management of hypotension with vasopressors during caesarean section under spinal anaesthesia. *Anaesthesia.* 2018;73:71–92.

361. Ngan Kee WD, Khaw KS, Ng FF. FF. Prevention of hypotension during spinal anesthesia for cesarean delivery: an effective technique using combination phenylephrine infusion and crystalloid cohydration. *Anesthesiology.* 2005;103:744–750.

362. Higgins N, Fitzgerald PC, van Dyk D, et al. The effect of prophylactic phenylephrine and ephedrine infusions on umbilical artery blood pH in women with preeclampsia undergoing cesarean delivery with spinal anesthesia: a randomized, double-blind trial. *Anesth Analg.* 2018;126:1999–2006.

363. Dyer RA, Emmanuel A, Adams SC, et al. A randomised comparison of bolus phenylephrine and ephedrine for the management of spinal hypotension in patients with severe preeclampsia and fetal compromise. *Int J Obstet Anesth.* 2018;33:23–31.

364. Onwochei DN, Ngan Kee WD, Fung L, et al. Norepinephrine intermittent intravenous boluses to prevent hypotension during spinal anesthesia for cesarean delivery: a sequential allocation dose-finding study. *Anesth Analg.* 2017;125:212–218.

365. Ngan Kee WD, Lee SWY, Ng FF, Khaw KS. Prophylactic norepinephrine infusion for preventing hypotension during spinal anesthesia for cesarean delivery. *Anesth Analg.* 2018;126:1989–1994.

366. Ngan Kee WD, Lee SW, Ng FF, et al. Randomized double-blinded comparison of norepinephrine and phenylephrine for maintenance of blood pressure during spinal anesthesia for cesarean delivery. *Anesthesiology.* 2015;122:736–745.

367. Pancaro C, Shah N, Pasma W, et al. Risk of major complications after perioperative norepinephrine infusion through peripheral intravenous lines in a multicenter study. *Anesth Analg.* 2020;131:1060–1065.

368. Kumari K, Chaudhary K, Sethi P, et al. Norepinephrine versus phenylephrine for postspinal hypotension in parturients undergoing cesarean section: a systematic review and meta-analysis. *Minerva Anestesiol.* 2022;88:1043–1056.

369. Ngan Kee WD, Lee SWY, Ng FF, Lee A. Norepinephrine or phenylephrine during spinal anaesthesia for Caesarean delivery: a randomised double-blind pragmatic non-inferiority study of neonatal outcome. *Br J Anaesth.* 2020;125:588–595.

370. Cyna AM, Andrew M, Emmett RS, et al. Techniques for preventing hypotension during spinal anaesthesia for caesarean section. *Cochrane Database Syst Rev.* 2006;(4):CD002251.

371. Pan PH, Bogard TD, Owen MD. Incidence and characteristics of failures in obstetric neuraxial analgesia and anesthesia: a retrospective analysis of 19,259 deliveries. *Int J Obstet Anesth.* 2004;13:227–233.

372. Carvalho B. Failed epidural top-up for cesarean delivery for failure to progress in labor: the case against single-shot spinal anesthesia. *Int J Obstet Anesth.* 2012;21:357–359.

373. Furst SR, Reisner LS. Risk of high spinal anesthesia following failed epidural block for cesarean delivery. *J Clin Anesth.* 1995;7:71–74.

374. D'Angelo R, Smiley RM, Riley ET, Segal S. Serious complications related to obstetric anesthesia: the Serious Complication Repository Project of the Society for Obstetric Anesthesia and Perinatology. *Anesthesiology.* 2014;120:1505–1512.

375. Radwan MA, O'Carroll L, McCaul CL. Total spinal anaesthesia following obstetric neuraxial blockade: a narrative review. *Int J Obstet Anesth.* 2024;59:104208.

376. Keltz A, Heesen P, Katz D, et al. Intraoperative pain during caesarean delivery: incidence, risk factors and physician perception. *Eur J Pain.* 2022;26:219–226.

377. Plaat F, Stanford SER, Lucas DN, et al. Prevention and management of intra-operative pain during caesarean section under neuraxial anaesthesia: a technical and interpersonal approach. *Anaesthesia.* 2022;77:588–597.

378. Lee NM, Saha S. Nausea and vomiting of pregnancy. *Gastroenterol Clin North Am.* 2011;40:309–334.

379. Siddiqui M, Goldszmidt E, Fallah S, et al. Complications of exteriorized compared with in situ uterine repair at cesarean delivery under spinal anesthesia: a randomized controlled trial. *Obstet Gynecol.* 2007;110:570–575.

380. Balki M, Carvalho JC. Intraoperative nausea and vomiting during cesarean section under regional anesthesia. *Int J Obstet Anesth.* 2005;14:230–241.

381. Borgeat A, Ekatodramis G, Schenker CA. Postoperative nausea and vomiting in regional anesthesia: a review. *Anesthesiology.* 2003;98:530–547.

382. Pinder AJ, Dresner M, Calow C, et al. Haemodynamic changes caused by oxytocin during caesarean section under spinal anaesthesia. *Int J Obstet Anesth.* 2002;11:156–159.

383. Dansereau J, Joshi AK, Helewa ME, et al. Double-blind comparison of carbetocin versus oxytocin in prevention of uterine atony after cesarean section. *Am J Obstet Gynecol.* 1999;180:670–676.

384. Gibbins KJ, Albright CM, Rouse DJ. Postpartum hemorrhage in the developed world: whither misoprostol? *Am J Obstet Gynecol.* 2013;208:181–183.

385. Alahuhta S, Kangas-Saarela T, Hollmén AI, Edström HH. Visceral pain during caesarean section under spinal and epidural anaesthesia with bupivacaine. *Acta Anaesthesiol Scand.* 1990;34:95–98.

386. Gan TJ. Risk factors for postoperative nausea and vomiting. *Anesth Analg.* 2006;102:1884–1898.

387. Apfel CC, Laara E, Koivuranta M, et al. A simplified risk score for predicting postoperative nausea and vomiting: conclusions from cross-validations between two centers. *Anesthesiology.* 1999;91:693–700.

388. Kreis ME. Postoperative nausea and vomiting. *Auton Neurosci.* 2006;129:86–91.

389. Kranke P, Eberhart LH, Gan TJ, et al. Algorithms for the prevention of postoperative nausea and vomiting: an efficacy and efficiency simulation. *Eur J Anaesthesiol.* 2007;24:856–867.

390. Apfel CC, Korttila K, Abdalla M, et al. A factorial trial of six interventions for the prevention of postoperative nausea and vomiting. *N Engl J Med.* 2004;350:2441–2451.

391. Abouleish EI, Rashid S, Haque S, et al. Ondansetron versus placebo for the control of nausea and vomiting during caesarean section under spinal anaesthesia. *Anaesthesia.* 1999;54:479–482.

392. Pan PH, Moore CH. Comparing the efficacy of prophylactic metoclopramide, ondansetron, and placebo in cesarean section patients given epidural anesthesia. *J Clin Anesth.* 2001;13:430–435.

393. Griffiths JD, Gyte GM, Paranjothy S, et al. Interventions for preventing nausea and vomiting in women undergoing regional anaesthesia for caesarean section. *Cochrane Database Syst Rev.* 2012;(9):CD007579.

394. Zheng G, Zhang J, Liu J, et al. A meta-analysis of randomized controlled trials: efficiency and safety of ondansetron in preventing post-anesthesia shivering during cesarean section. *Arch Gynecol Obstet.* 2023;307:223–231.

395. Han DW, Hong SW, Kwon JY, et al. Epidural ondansetron is more effective to prevent postoperative pruritus and nausea than intravenous ondansetron in elective cesarean delivery. *Acta Obstet Gynecol Scand.* 2007;86:683–687.

396. Allen TK, Jones CA, Habib AS. Dexamethasone for the prophylaxis of postoperative nausea and vomiting associated with neuraxial morphine administration: a systematic review and meta-analysis. *Anesth Analg.* 2012;114:813–822.

397. Cardoso MM, Leite AO, Santos EA, et al. Effect of dexamethasone on prevention of postoperative nausea, vomiting and pain after caesarean section: a randomised, placebo-controlled, double-blind trial. *Eur J Anaesthesiol.* 2013;30:102–105.

398. Harnett MJ, O'Rourke N, Walsh M, et al. Transdermal scopolamine for prevention of intrathecal morphine-induced nausea and vomiting after cesarean delivery. *Anesth Analg.* 2007;105:764–769.

399. Harmon D, Ryan M, Kelly A, Bowen M. Acupressure and prevention of nausea and vomiting during and after spinal anaesthesia for caesarean section. *Br J Anaesth.* 2000;84:463–467.

400. Allen TK, Habib AS. P6 stimulation for the prevention of nausea and vomiting associated with cesarean delivery under neuraxial anesthesia: a systematic review of randomized controlled trials. *Anesth Analg.* 2008;107:1308–1312.

401. Phillips TW Jr, Broussard DM, Sumrall WD 3rd, Hart SR. Intraoperative oxygen administration does not reduce the incidence or severity of nausea or vomiting associated with neuraxial anesthesia for cesarean delivery. *Anesth Analg.* 2007;105:1113–1117.

402. Orhan-Sungur M, Kranke P, Sessler D, Apfel CC. Does supplemental oxygen reduce postoperative nausea and vomiting? A meta-analysis of randomized controlled trials. *Anesth Analg.* 2008;106:1733–1738.

403. Carvalho B, Cohen SE, Lipman SS, et al. Patient preferences for anesthesia outcomes associated with cesarean delivery. *Anesth Analg.* 2005;101:1182–1187.

404. Szypula K, Ashpole KJ, Bogod D, et al. Litigation related to regional anaesthesia: an analysis of claims against the NHS in England 1995-2007. *Anaesthesia.* 2010;65:443–452.

405. Hess PE, Snowman CE, Hahn CJ, et al. Chloroprocaine may not affect epidural morphine for postcesarean delivery analgesia. *J Clin Anesth.* 2006;18:29–33.

406. Douglas MJ, Kim JH, Ross PL, McMorland GH. The effect of epinephrine in local anaesthetic on epidural morphine-induced pruritus. *Can Anaesth Soc J.* 1986;33:737–740.

407. Szarvas S, Harmon D, Murphy DF. Neuraxial opioid-induced pruritus: a review. *J Clin Anesth.* 2003;15:234–239.

408. Tan T, Ojo R, Immani S, et al. Reduction of severity of pruritus after elective caesarean section under spinal anaesthesia with subarachnoid morphine: a randomised comparison of prophylactic granisetron and ondansetron. *Int J Obstet Anesth.* 2010;19:56–60.

409. Butwick AJ, Lipman SS, Carvalho B. Intraoperative forced air-warming during cesarean delivery under spinal anesthesia does not prevent maternal hypothermia. *Anesth Analg.* 2007;105:1413–1419.

410. Roy JD, Girard M, Drolet P. Intrathecal meperidine decreases shivering during cesarean delivery under spinal anesthesia. *Anesth Analg.* 2004;98:230–234.

411. Sessler DI. Temperature monitoring and perioperative thermoregulation. *Anesthesiology.* 2008;109:318–338.

412. Rajagopalan S, Mascha E, Na J, Sessler DI. The effects of mild perioperative hypothermia on blood loss and transfusion requirement. *Anesthesiology.* 2008;108:71–77.

413. Hartgill TW, Bergersen TK, Pirhonen JP. Core body temperature and the thermoneutral zone: a longitudinal study of normal human pregnancy. *Acta Physiol (Oxf).* 2011;201:467–474.

414. Saito T, Sessler DI, Fujita K, et al. Thermoregulatory effects of spinal and epidural anesthesia during cesarean delivery. *Reg Anesth Pain Med.* 1998;23:418–423.

415. Sessler DI. Thermoregulatory defense mechanisms. *Crit Care Med.* 2009;37:S203–S210.

416. Sween LK, Xu S, Li C, et al. Low-dose intravenous dexmedetomidine reduces shivering following cesarean delivery: a randomized controlled trial. *Int J Obstet Anesth.* 2021;45:49–55.

417. Horn EP, Schroeder F, Gottschalk A, et al. Active warming during cesarean delivery. *Anesth Analg.* 2002;94:409–414.

418. Duryea EL, Nelson DB, Wyckoff MH, et al. The impact of ambient operating room temperature on neonatal and maternal hypothermia and associated morbidities: a randomized controlled trial. *Am J Obstet Gynecol.* 2016;214:505.e1–e7.

419. Sun HL, Ling QD, Sun WZ, et al. Lower limb wrapping prevents hypotension, but not hypothermia or shivering, after the introduction of epidural anesthesia for cesarean delivery. *Anesth Analg.* 2004;99:241–244.

420. American College of Obstetricians and Gynecologists. ACOG Practice Bulletin No. 183: Postpartum hemorrhage (reaffirmed 2024). *Obstet Gynecol.* 2017;130:e168–e186.

421. American College of Obstetricians and Gynecologists' committee on Practice Bulletins—Obstetrics. ACOG Practice Bulletin No. 196: Thromboembolism in pregnancy (reaffirmed 2022). *Obstet Gynecol.* 2018;132:e1–e17.

422. Middleton P, Shepherd E, Gomersall JC. Venous thromboembolism prophylaxis for women at risk during pregnancy and the early postnatal period. *Cochrane Database Syst Rev.* 2021;(3):CD001689.

27

Postoperative Analgesia

Ronald B. George, MD, FRCPC, Hon Sen Tan, MD, MMed, MHSc, and Ashraf S. Habib, MBBCh, MSc, MHSc, FRCA

The cesarean delivery rate in the United States and around the world has been on an upward trajectory for over 50 years.[1] With cesarean delivery accounting for 32% of all deliveries in the United States, strategies for reducing adverse postcesarean maternal outcomes, including postoperative pain, have important clinical and public health implications.[2]

Pain is a potential harm that can occur during and after any surgical procedure. Inadequately treated pain can cause numerous undesirable physiologic and psychologic consequences in women undergoing cesarean delivery, including impaired recovery, persistent and chronic pain, and increased cost.[3]

PAIN AFTER CESAREAN DELIVERY

Management of postoperative pain is frequently substandard, with 30% to 80% of patients experiencing moderate to severe postoperative pain.[4,5] This pain is not the same for all patients as there are racial and ethnic disparities. Hispanic and Black women are more likely to experience severe pain and receive less treatment in the postpartum period.[6] Pain following cesarean delivery may be equivalent to that reported after a hysterectomy.[7] Postoperative pain results from direct tissue trauma and subsequent inflammation. Local and systemic inflammatory cytokines act to sensitize the peripheral nerves and enhance pain perception.[8] Inflammation likely plays a particularly important role in pain after delivery because inflammatory cytokines are increased as a part of the normal labor and delivery process.[9,10] After cesarean delivery, wound cytokine concentration is positively correlated with analgesic drug consumption.[11] The range of pain reported after cesarean delivery is greater than after vaginal delivery, but the pain burden and duration are remarkably similar (Fig. 27.1).[12,13] A sample of expectant mothers attending birthing classes identified pain during and after cesarean delivery as their most important concern.[14] Measuring pain intensity and satisfaction with simple tools has not met the goals of preventing and treating moderate and severe pain.[5,12–15]

Severe acute postoperative pain is one of the most prominent factors associated with chronic postoperative pain.[16–19] Some studies suggest that the use of perioperative neuraxial blockade may prevent central sensitization and chronic pain.[20] Additional mechanistic and clinical research is needed to improve our understanding of persistent pain after cesarean delivery (see Chapter 42). Multimodal pharmacologic and nonpharmacologic treatment for pain is the optimal approach and should be offered whenever feasible and medically indicated.

SYSTEMIC ANALGESIA

Opioid Analgesia

In the United States, most women who undergo cesarean delivery with neuraxial anesthesia receive neuraxial opioids for postoperative analgesia. However, many women require systemic analgesia to augment neuraxial therapy, and some women are unable to receive neuraxial anesthesia. In the United States it is common practice to prescribe oral opioids on discharge from the hospital, although this is not usual in other parts of the world.[21]

Choice of Opioid

Factors that affect the choice of opioid include speed of onset, duration of action, efficacy, type and frequency of side effects, and availability. If side effects prevent adequate analgesia,

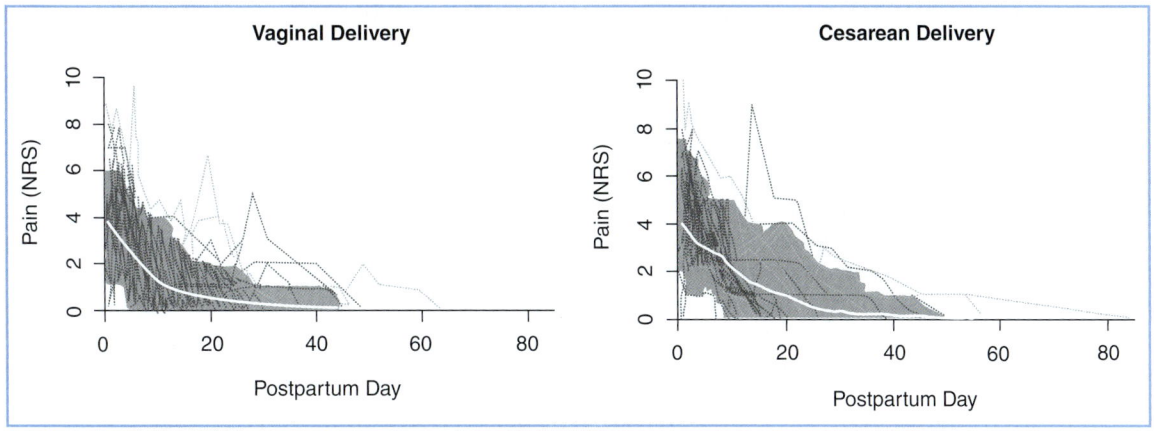

Fig. 27.1 Pain Trajectory After Vaginal and Cesarean Delivery. Dotted lines represent pain reports from individual subjects, and the solid white line is a moving average. Shaded area covers the range from the 5th to 95th percentile of the data. *NRS*, Verbal numerical rating scale from 0 to 10, with 0 = no pain and 10 = worst pain imaginable. From Komatsu R, Carvalho B, Flood PD. Recovery after nulliparous birth: a detailed analysis of pain analgesia and recovery of function. *Anesthesiology.* 2017;127:684–694.

TABLE 27.1　Opioid Equianalgesic Doses

Drug	Oral (mg)	Subcutaneous/Intravenous (mg)
Morphine	30	10
Oxycodone	20	N/A
Hydrocodone	20	N/A
Hydromorphone	7.5	1.5
Fentanyl	N/A A 25-µg/h transdermal patch is equianalgesic to approximately 50 mg of oral morphine per day	0.1 (100 µg)
Oxymorphone	10	1

N/A, Not applicable.
Courtesy The Dana Farber Cancer Institute Pain and Palliative Care Program and the Brigham and Women's Hospital Pain Committee. Modified with permission from Bridget C. Fowler, Pharm. D., Clinical Pharmacy Manager, Dana Farber Cancer Institute.

other opioids or nonopioid adjuvants should be used. Patient preferences based on past experiences and desired analgesia should also be considered.[22]

Historically, **meperidine (pethidine)** has been a popular opioid for postoperative analgesia. However, the American College of Obstetricians and Gynecologists[23] has discouraged the use of meperidine in obstetric patients because of the accumulation of the metabolite normeperidine in the neonate and its subsequent effect on neurobehavioral scores. Table 27.1 shows commonly used alternatives to meperidine with equianalgesic doses.

Oral Opioid Analgesia

The use of **oral analgesics** has been advocated as there is seldom a requirement for a prolonged fasting period after cesarean delivery.[24,25] Most evidence suggests that intravenous (IV) administration of opioids is not superior to oral opioids for postoperative analgesia.[26] Davis et al.[25] reported that patients randomized to receive oral **oxycodone** experienced less pain at 6 and 24 hours, and less nausea and drowsiness at 6 hours after cesarean delivery, compared with patients who received **morphine** by IV patient-controlled analgesia (PCA). Dieterich et al.[27] found IV PCA and oral opioids provided similar satisfaction and pain scores after cesarean delivery. Therefore, when tolerated, oral administration of opioids may be the preferred route. Advantages of this approach are cost savings and facilitation of early mobility. Long-acting oral opioids are not recommended in the immediate postoperative period.[26]

Intravenous Patient-Controlled Analgesia

Intramuscular (IM) and subcutaneous opioids are inexpensive, easy to administer, and associated with a long history of safety but are not commonly used in the United States because of the need for repeated painful injections, delayed (and sometimes erratic) absorption of drug, and an inconsistent analgesic response caused by variation in plasma opioid concentration. IV PCA allows patients to control their own pain management by self-administering small doses of IV opioids. A 2015 metaanalysis concluded that PCA is often preferred by patients compared with nurse-administered analgesia on request, and PCA was shown to provide better pain control and increased patient satisfaction compared with non-patient-controlled methods.[28] The American Society of Anesthesiologists (ASA) Task Force for Acute Pain Management in the Perioperative Setting recommended that "these modalities [epidural or intrathecal opioids, systemic opioid PCA, and peripheral regional techniques] should be used in preference to IM opioids ordered "as needed."[29] The American Pain Society has recommended the use of IV opioid PCA when parenteral administration of analgesics is necessary and the oral route is not available.[26]

PCA has been used via the IV and epidural routes after cesarean delivery. A study that compared IV and epidural

PCA using **fentanyl** reported higher pain scores and greater fentanyl consumption with the IV route, although patient satisfaction was similar in the two groups.[30] In another study that compared IV versus epidural PCA using **hydromorphone**, drug requirement was threefold to fourfold higher in the IV group; the two groups had similar pain and sedation scores, but patients in the IV group reported more frequent drowsiness and less pruritus.[31] Studies that compared IV **morphine** PCA to *single-shot* epidural morphine administration for postcesarean analgesia showed that analgesia and patient satisfaction were better and sedation was less with epidural morphine, although the incidence of pruritus was higher.[32,33]

Side Effects and Safety Considerations

The goal of opioid administration is to achieve maximal analgesia with minimal side effects. It is important to monitor the respiratory rate and sedation level before giving an additional dose or adjusting the PCA bolus dose. Patients with comorbidities such as hepatic or renal dysfunction (e.g., occurring with severe preeclampsia), morbid obesity, and/or obstructive sleep apnea are particularly susceptible to the respiratory depressant effects of opioids; these patients may need special alterations to pain management, including the use of multimodal analgesia (see later discussion).

Healthcare professionals who prescribe PCA should (1) evaluate candidates for PCA (e.g., mental state, level of consciousness, patient understanding); (2) know drug selection criteria, dosing schedules, lockout intervals, and infusion devices; (3) provide patient education on pain management and the use of PCA; (4) understand when to alter PCA settings and when to give or withhold additional (rescue) doses of medications; and (5) be able to respond to side effects and adverse events. Observational studies of nonobstetric patients have reported an incidence of respiratory depression with IV PCA of 0% to 11.5%, which is equivalent to or higher than that reported for neuraxial opioids.[34–38]

In 2004 The Joint Commission on the Accreditation of Healthcare Organizations (JCAHO) issued a Sentinel Event Alert on PCA "by proxy" (i.e., when other individuals, including family members, become involved in drug administration by PCA).[39] The JCAHO acknowledged that PCA is a safe and effective method of controlling pain when used as prescribed; however, serious adverse events, including oversedation, respiratory depression, and death, can result when analgesia is delivered "by proxy." The following recommendations were made: (1) develop criteria for selecting appropriate candidates for PCA, (2) carefully monitor patients, (3) teach patients and family members about the proper use of PCA and the dangers of others pressing the button for the patient, (4) alert staff to the dangers of administering a dose outside a prescribed protocol, and (5) consider placing warning tags on all PCA delivery pendants stating "only the patient should press this button." The PCA settings (drug, demand dose, lockout interval, 4-hour [or other time] limit, and the rate of continuous infusion [if used]) are documented on a flow sheet, and any changes in PCA settings clearly documented.

Infusion Pump Settings

Programmable PCA parameters include drug choice, bolus dose, maximum dose, and lockout interval (Table 27.2). Owen et al.[40–42] performed several PCA investigations in patients undergoing abdominal surgery. In an assessment of PCA morphine demand bolus doses (0.5, 1, or 2 mg with a 5-minute lockout interval), more patients in the 0.5-mg group had inadequate pain relief, whereas those in the 2-mg group had more side effects, including respiratory depression (respiratory rate < 10 breaths/min).[42] These outcomes correlated with the total dose of self-administered morphine.

The American Pain Society does not recommend routine use of basal infusions of opioid in opioid-naïve patients; most evidence does not demonstrate improved analgesia compared with patients who receive no basal infusion.[26] Basal infusions of opioids are associated with an increased incidence of nausea and vomiting, and some studies have shown an increased risk for respiratory depression.[26]

During PCA, the ratio of patient demands to delivered bolus doses appears to be a good measure of analgesia and is strongly correlated with pain scores.[43] A high ratio likely reflects patient misunderstanding or inadequate analgesia; a ratio close to 1 signifies adequate pain relief. Analgesia may be improved by an increase in the bolus dose, a shorter lockout interval, or a change of opioid.

Because of the significant morbidity associated with high doses of opioids, use of these drugs should invoke the application of algorithms for pain assessment, management, and monitoring. Acute postoperative pain is limited in duration; therefore, a plan should be devised for the transition from IV opioids to oral analgesic agents when pain is controlled and the patient is able to take medication by mouth.

Multimodal Analgesia

Multimodal analgesia combines the effectiveness of individual analgesics, thereby maximizing their efficacy while attempting to minimize side effects. The rationale for multimodal analgesia is the optimization of additive or synergistic effects of different modes of analgesia or drug classes, while reducing the dose and minimizing the side effects of individual drugs. Although analgesic efficacy is the primary goal, important secondary goals include minimizing transfer of drugs to breast milk and reducing maternal side effects that may interfere with breastfeeding or infant care. Various combinations of **opioids, nonsteroidal antiinflammatory drugs (NSAIDs), acetaminophen (paracetamol),** and **local anesthetics** are among drugs that have been used with varying degrees of success.[44–46] Several studies have demonstrated superior analgesia when oral analgesics are administered at a predetermined fixed interval rather than on demand.[24,47]

Acetaminophen

Acetaminophen is estimated to provide an opioid-sparing effect of approximately 10% to 20%.[48–50] However, the efficacy of IV perioperative acetaminophen in reducing postoperative opioid utilization has not yet been clearly established. A metaanalysis showed that perioperative IV acetaminophen

TABLE 27.2   General Patient-Controlled Analgesia Settings in Opioid-Naïve Patients

Drug	Morphine	Hydromorphone	Fentanyl
Concentration	1 mg/mL	1 mg/mL	10 µg/mL
PCA bolus dose	1–1.5 mg	0.2 mg	20 µg
Lockout interval (min)	5–10	5–10	5
4-h (or other time) dose limit	Calculated by settings	Calculated by settings	Calculated by settings
Typical PCA dose change	0.5 mg	0.1 mg	5 µg
Rescue doses	2 mg IV q 5 min (up to three doses)	0.3 mg IV q 5 min (up to three doses)	25 µg IV q 5 min (up to three doses)
Remarks	Relatively contraindicated in patients with impaired renal function	More potent than morphine	Shorter clinical effect than morphine

Recorded as: PCA bolus dose/lockout interval/4-h limit/continuous infusion rate. A continuous background infusion is typically avoided except in selected cases (e.g., opioid tolerance).

IV, Intravenous; *PCA*, patient-controlled analgesia.

Courtesy The Dana Farber Cancer Institute Pain and Palliative Care Program and the Brigham and Women's Hospital Pain Committee. Modified with permission from Bridget C. Fowler, PharmD, Clinical Pharmacy Manager, Dana Farber Cancer Institute.

was associated with similar opioid utilization compared with placebo. The authors concluded that the review was limited by small numbers and heterogeneity, as well as the absence of long-acting neuraxial opioids, which differed from contemporary anesthetic practice.[51] Nonetheless, based on its relative safety, minimal breast milk transfer, and potential opioid-sparing effects, administration of acetaminophen at scheduled intervals is recommended for postcesarean delivery analgesia.[45]

The use of IV acetaminophen is gaining popularity, supported by studies demonstrating faster and higher plasma and cerebrospinal fluid drug levels compared with oral acetaminophen.[52] However, there is little evidence that IV acetaminophen is superior to oral acetaminophen, especially given the additional costs of the IV formulation. A randomized controlled trial reported no significant difference in 24- and 48-hour opioid consumption, time to first opioid rescue, pain scores, satisfaction, side effects, and times to ambulation and discharge after cesarean delivery in patients who received IV acetaminophen at 8-hour intervals compared with those who received the oral formulation, following neuraxial anesthesia with intrathecal fentanyl (15 µg) and morphine (0.2 mg), plus IV ketorolac.[53]

Avoiding opioid/acetaminophen combination medication is recommended to decrease unnecessary opioid use and avoid exceeding recommended maximum doses of acetaminophen. Valentine et al.[54] performed a retrospective medical record review of women who underwent cesarean delivery before and after a change in clinical practice at their institution. All patients received spinal anesthesia with intrathecal morphine 0.2 mg and scheduled NSAIDs for 48 hours postoperatively. After the change, the women received oral acetaminophen 650 mg every 6 hours for 48 hours postoperatively with oral oxycodone administered as needed for breakthrough pain.[54] The scheduled acetaminophen group used less opioid in the first 48 hours than the historical as-needed group (Fig. 27.2).[54]

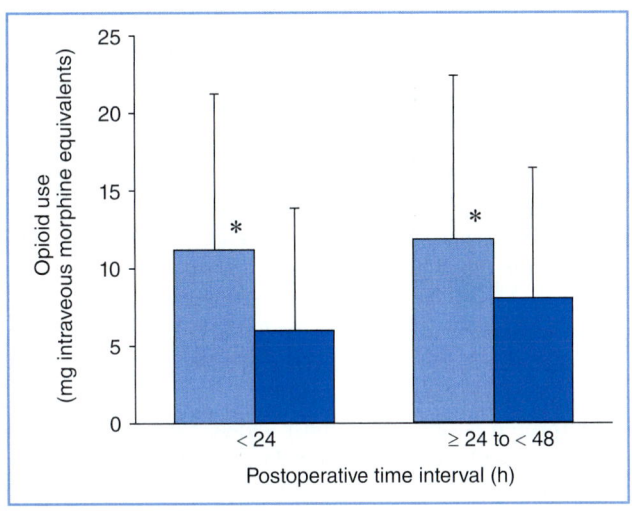

Fig. 27.2 Opioid use in milligram intravenous morphine equivalents after cesarean delivery in 24-h increments in patients who received scheduled oral acetaminophen with as-needed opioid *(dark shading)* versus patients who received as-needed combination opioid-acetaminophen *(light shading)*. Data are mean *(bar)* and standard deviation *(whisker)*. *Significant difference between groups (*P* < .001). Redrawn from Valentine AR, Carvalho B, Lazo TA, Riley ET. Scheduled acetaminophen with as-needed opioids compared to as-needed acetaminophen plus opioids for postcesarean pain management. *Int J Obstet Anesth.* 2015;24:210–216.

Nonsteroidal Antiinflammatory Drugs

NSAIDs suppress inflammation by inhibition of the cyclooxygenase (COX) enzymes and are a key component of multimodal analgesia. They are effective for perineal pain after vaginal delivery and postcesarean abdominal pain; when coadministered with opioids, they produce a 30% to 50% opioid-sparing effect[50] that can reduce opioid-related side effects.[55] A 2016 systematic review and metaanalysis showed that the use of NSAIDs resulted in lower pain scores up to 24 hours postoperatively, less opioid consumption, and less

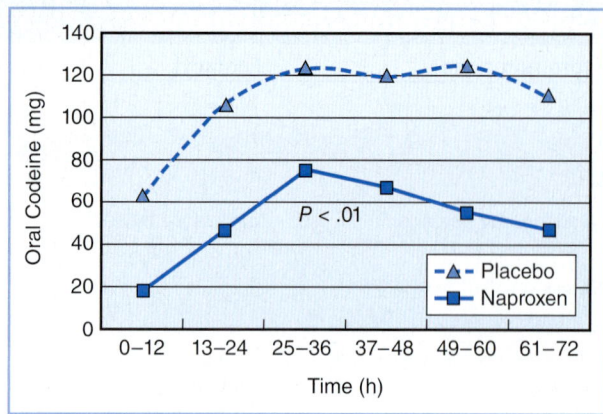

Fig. 27.3 Effect of naproxen on requirement for oral codeine after cesarean delivery: oral codeine use in milligram equivalents (expressed as mean) over time by group. From Angle PJ, Halpern SH, Leighton BL, et al. A randomized controlled trial examining the effect of naproxen on analgesia during the second day after cesarean delivery. *Anesth Analg.* 2002;95:741–745.

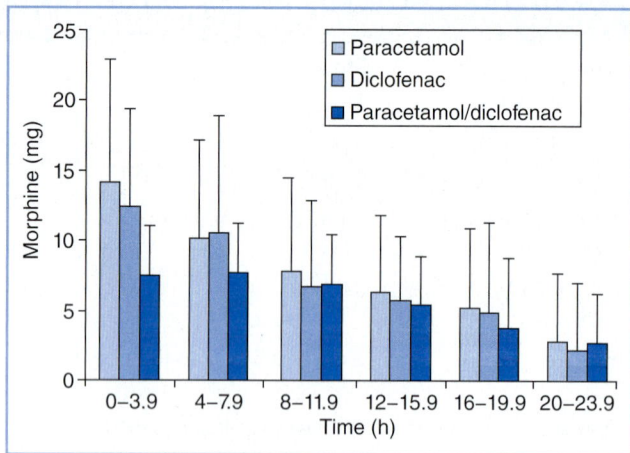

Fig. 27.4 Morphine consumption in milligrams in consecutive 4-h periods after cesarean delivery in women randomized to receive acetaminophen (paracetamol), diclofenac, or both. Data were analyzed using repeated measures analysis of variance; patients in the acetaminophen/diclofenac group used less morphine per 4-h period than patients in the acetaminophen but not the diclofenac group. Redrawn from Munishankar B, Fettes P, Moore C, McLeod GA. A double-blind randomised controlled trial of paracetamol, diclofenac, or the combination for pain relief after caesarean section. *Int J Obstet Anesth.* 2008;17:9–14.

sedation after cesarean delivery.[56] The combination of NSAIDs and acetaminophen has been shown to be more effective than either drug alone, with some evidence for a synergistic interaction.[57,58] In addition to antiinflammatory, analgesic, and antipyretic properties, nonselective NSAIDs that inhibit both COX-1 and COX-2 isoenzymes also inhibit platelet adhesion and cause renal artery vasoconstriction and gastrointestinal irritation. Therefore, NSAID use in patients at risk for hemorrhage and renal failure warrants caution. Nonetheless, in most parturients without these risk factors, use of NSAIDs is considered safe. Because of limited transfer to breast milk, NSAIDs are particularly beneficial for lactating mothers. The American Academic of Pediatrics considers NSAIDs safe for nursing mothers (see Chapter 16).[59]

Ibuprofen is one of the most widely used NSAIDs that is available without prescription. In a small study (oral ibuprofen 400 mg every 6 hours for 24 hours), less than 1 mg of ibuprofen was excreted in breast milk in a 36-hour period.[60] Many centers administer 600 to 800 mg every 6 to 8 hours as a standard dose. Oral **naproxen** 500 mg every 12 hours has been shown to reduce incisional pain compared with placebo and decrease opioid consumption (Fig. 27.3).[61] **Diclofenac** has also been extensively studied; rectal suppositories (100 mg twice a day) decreased morphine consumption compared with placebo (14 mg versus 22 mg in 32 hours) after cesarean delivery.[62] A single rectal dose of diclofenac 100 mg prolonged the mean time to first analgesic administration by more than 5 hours in patients who received intrathecal morphine.[63] Patients who received intrathecal morphine doses as small as 25 µg required no rescue analgesic when IM diclofenac 75 mg was administered every 8 hours.[64] Munishankar et al.[65] randomized patients who received spinal anesthesia with bupivacaine and fentanyl to receive one of three analgesic modalities: acetaminophen, diclofenac, or diclofenac plus acetaminophen. Women who received both diclofenac and acetaminophen required less morphine than those who received acetaminophen alone (Fig. 27.4).[65] Lowder et al.[66]

showed that **ketorolac** decreased pain scores at 2, 3, 4, 6, 12, and 24 hours after cesarean delivery and also decreased opioid consumption. Ketorolac previously had a "black box" warning that it was "contraindicated in nursing mothers," but current recommendations are to use it with caution.

Cyclooxygenase-2-Selective Inhibitors

COX-2–selective inhibitors have a potential benefit compared with traditional nonselective NSAIDs in that they have minimal effects on platelet adhesion and thus are less likely to interfere with blood clot formation and contribute to hemorrhage. This category of NSAIDs has similar analgesic effectiveness and opioid dose-sparing compared to traditional NSAIDs in nonobstetric settings.[67] However, in the setting of cesarean delivery, they do not appear to be as effective as nonselective NSAIDs.[68] Additionally, concerns about the potential to increase the risk for cardiovascular and thrombotic events, combined with the baseline elevated risk for these events during pregnancy and postpartum, have prevented COX-2 inhibitors from playing a major role in postpartum analgesia. **Celecoxib** is the only widely available COX-2–selective inhibitor in the United States. The breast milk content of **parecoxib** and its primary active metabolite **valdecoxib** was very low, and neonatal neurologic and adaptive capacity scores were normal, after a single 40-mg IV dose following cesarean delivery.[69]

Alpha₂-Adrenergic Receptor Agonists

Alpha₂-adrenergic receptor agonists have been used for the treatment of acute and chronic pain in nonobstetric patients. IV **dexmedetomidine** has been used as an adjunct to opioids as a component of general anesthesia for cesarean delivery.[70] Dexmedetomidine is excreted in breast milk in extremely small concentrations; one study observed a relative infant dose of 0.034%.[71] In a three-arm randomized controlled trial of patients who underwent cesarean delivery under spinal anesthesia without intrathecal morphine, one group received a single IV dexmedetomidine dose perioperatively and sufentanil PCA, a second received the same perioperative dexmedetomidine dose plus postoperative dexmedetomidine added to sufentanil PCA, and a third group received placebo and sufentanil PCA.[72] The group of patients who received both perioperative and postoperative dexmedetomidine had reduced sufentanil PCA requirement compared with the other groups. There was no significant difference in side effects among groups.[72] Neuraxial **clonidine** has been used for labor analgesia but is not commonly used for postcesarean analgesia. The epidural formulation of clonidine carries a "black box" warning from the US Food and Drug Administration (FDA) because of the risk for hypotension at higher neuraxial doses.[73] Nonetheless, Fernandes et al.[74] compared intrathecal clonidine, IV clonidine, and a placebo in patients undergoing cesarean delivery with intrathecal morphine and found no significant difference in 24-hour dynamic pain scores between the groups, although both clonidine groups had greater maternal sedation.

Magnesium Sulfate

Peripartum magnesium sulfate therapy is used for tocolysis for preterm labor, seizure prophylaxis in women with preeclampsia, and fetal neuroprotection in women at risk for preterm delivery.[75] Some studies have shown a small (likely not clinically significant) reduction in opioid consumption at 24 hours following magnesium sulfate administration prior to induction of general anesthesia for cesarean delivery, compared with placebo.[76,77] In patients undergoing cesarean delivery under neuraxial anesthesia without intrathecal morphine, Paech et al.[78] found no difference in pain scores, time to breakthrough analgesic dose, and total opioid consumption following a magnesium sulfate bolus and 24-hour postoperative infusion compared with placebo, although patients who received magnesium sulfate had a 15% to 20% greater median estimated blood loss.

Gabapentin

Gabapentin is an anticonvulsant that has analgesic properties, particularly in the setting of neuropathic pain. It has been extensively studied in the management of chronic pain and for postoperative analgesia, where it is associated with more rapid opioid cessation. Gabapentin's role in opioid-naïve patients undergoing cesarean delivery is less clear. As part of a multimodal analgesic regimen in patients undergoing cesarean delivery, a preoperative dose of oral gabapentin 600 mg was associated with lower pain scores with movement and at rest; however, the incidence of sedation was greater in the gabapentin group than in the placebo group (19% versus 0%).[79] A metaanalysis of six placebo-controlled trials showed significant reduction in 24-hour pain scores with movement (mean difference, –11.58 mm [95% CI, –23.04 to –0.12 mm] [scale: 0 to 100 mm]) in patients who received gabapentin

compared with placebo.[80] No significant difference in pain scores at other time points, analgesia consumption, or maternal and neonatal adverse effects were detected. Gabapentin has a high umbilical vein-to-maternal vein ratio and breast milk transfer.[81] Given the lack of clear analgesic benefit and concerns of maternal and neonatal adverse effects, routine use of gabapentin is not recommended for postcesarean analgesia, although it may play a role in patients with chronic pain and those with opioid tolerance.

Ketamine

Ketamine, an N-methyl-D-aspartate (NMDA) antagonist, is a potent analgesic and may play a role in the treatment of acute postoperative pain and prevention or reversal of central sensitization.[82] An evaluation of low-dose ketamine for postcesarean analgesia compared IV ketamine 0.15 mg/kg, intrathecal fentanyl, and a placebo.[83] The study demonstrated prolonged duration of analgesia in both the fentanyl and ketamine groups compared with the placebo group (time to first analgesic request was 145 minutes in the placebo group, 165 minutes in the fentanyl group, and 199 minutes in the ketamine group). Ketamine was superior to fentanyl and placebo for reducing pain scores at 90 and 180 minutes, and for reducing analgesic requirements in the first 24 hours, but not in the second 24 hours, after cesarean delivery.[83] A systematic review and metaanalysis of 20 randomized controlled studies (6 with general anesthesia and 14 with spinal anesthesia) of ketamine use for postcesarean delivery analgesia showed minimally reduced pain scores (mean difference, –1.10 [95% CI, –1.61 to –0.59] [scale: 0 to 10]), decreased morphine consumption (mean difference, –6.11 mg [95% CI, –9.93 to –2.29 mg]), and a longer interval before first analgesia request (mean difference 72.5 minutes [95% CI, 50.9 to 94.1 minutes]) with ketamine compared with controls.[84]

NEURAXIAL ANALGESIA

Efficacy and Benefits of Neuraxial Analgesia

Most cesarean deliveries in the developed world are performed with neuraxial anesthesia (spinal, epidural, or combined spinal-epidural [CSE] techniques).[85–87] This allows the administration of neuraxial drugs for postoperative analgesia.

Neuraxial opioid administration currently represents the "gold standard" for providing effective postcesarean delivery analgesia. A 2010 systematic review found that a single dose of epidural morphine provided better analgesia than parenteral opioids after cesarean delivery.[88] A metaanalysis of studies involving a broad population of patients undergoing a variety of surgical procedures confirmed that opioids delivered by either patient-controlled epidural analgesia (PCEA) or continuous epidural infusion (CEI) provided postoperative pain relief that is superior to that provided by IV PCA.[89] Similar results have been reported in studies comparing intrathecal and epidural opioid administration with IV opioid PCA or IM opioid administration after cesarean delivery (Fig. 27.5).[32,90]

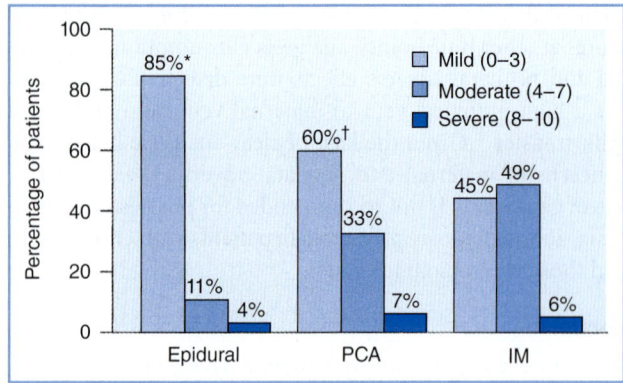

Fig. 27.5 Randomized trial of postcesarean analgesia with epidural analgesia, intravenous patient-controlled analgesia (*PCA*), or intramuscular (*IM*) administration of morphine. Percentage of patients reporting mild, moderate, or severe discomfort during a 24-h study period. *P < .05, epidural versus PCA and IM; †P = NS, PCA versus IM. From Harrison DM, Sinatra RS, Morgese L, Chung JH. Epidural narcotic and patient-controlled analgesia for postcesarean section pain relief. *Anesthesiology.* 1988;68:454–457.

Neuraxial opioids also provide superior postcesarean analgesia compared with nonneuraxial regional techniques (e.g., transversus abdominis plane [TAP] block, quadratus lumborum block [QLB], local wound infiltration, and oral analgesics [NSAIDs, opioids]).[91–93] Although neuraxial analgesia offers important benefits in optimizing postoperative analgesia, the analgesic effects can be augmented by multimodal analgesic strategies.[94] Most commonly, neuraxial opioid analgesia serves as the central component of multimodal analgesia.

Although analgesia is superior, some opioid–related side effects (e.g., pruritus) are more common after neuraxial opioid administration. Both higher[95] and lower[90,96] maternal satisfaction scores have been reported with neuraxial compared with systemic opioid analgesia. This variability in reported maternal satisfaction scores may be influenced by patients' relative value of analgesic quality versus side effects (e.g., pruritus, nausea, and vomiting). Depending on individual priorities, women may choose to receive a lower intrathecal morphine dose if they wish to avoid side effects, or they may choose a higher dose if they wish to optimize postcesarean delivery.[22]

Neuraxial techniques may confer other benefits in addition to better postoperative analgesia, including increased functional ability, earlier ambulation, and earlier return of bowel function.[97–100] Other potential benefits include a lower incidence of pulmonary infection and pulmonary embolism, fewer cardiovascular and coagulation disturbances, and a reduction in inflammatory and stress-induced responses to surgery.[97–99] Although a wealth of data from clinical studies and metaanalyses has shown a reduction in postoperative pain, there is less consistent evidence linking neuraxial anesthesia with a reduction in postoperative morbidity and mortality.[97,101]

The incidence of obstetric thromboembolism increased 72% during hospitalizations for childbirth between 1998 and 2009.[102] Risk factors for thromboembolism, including obesity,

advanced maternal age, and major medical comorbidities, are increasingly common in the obstetric population.[103–105] In theory, early ambulation and avoidance of prolonged immobility may reduce the risk for postpartum deep vein thrombosis and pulmonary embolism. Effective postoperative analgesia can reduce pain on movement, thereby facilitating deep breathing, coughing, and early ambulation.

Neuraxial analgesic techniques may be particularly useful for reducing perioperative morbidity in high-risk obstetric patients. Women with severe preeclampsia, cardiovascular disease, and morbid obesity may benefit from the reduction in cardiovascular stress and improved pulmonary function associated with effective postcesarean analgesia.[106,107] Investigators have found that CEI of a solution of opioid and dilute local anesthetic attenuates coagulation abnormalities, hemodynamic fluctuation, and stress hormone responses in nonpregnant patients.[108] Some studies suggest that opioid-based PCEA may improve postoperative outcome.[109,110] However, continuous postoperative neuraxial analgesia techniques also have disadvantages, including reduced mobility because of the infusion pump, more complicated management of postoperative thromboprophylaxis, and increased nursing workload.[44]

Mechanism of Action of Neuraxial Opioids

The discovery that opioid receptors are localized within discrete areas of the spinal cord (laminae I, II, and V of the dorsal horn) suggested that exogenous opioids could be administered into the neuraxis to produce antinociception. Opioids administered to superficial layers of the dorsal horn produce selective analgesia of prolonged duration without affecting motor function, sympathetic tone, or proprioception.[111] In 1979 Wang et al.[112] published the first report of intrathecal morphine administration in humans, which was followed shortly thereafter by a report of intrathecal meperidine. Intrathecal morphine (0.5 to 1 mg) produced complete pain relief for 12 to 24 hours in six of eight patients suffering from intractable cancer pain, with no evidence of sedation, respiratory depression, or impairment of motor function.[112] Opioids administered epidurally must penetrate the dura, pia, and arachnoid membranes to reach the dorsal horn and activate the spinal opioid receptors. The arachnoid layer is the primary barrier to drug transfer into the spinal cord.[113] Drug movement through this layer is passive and depends on the physicochemical properties of the opioid (see Chapter 13). Drugs penetrating this arachnoid layer must first move into a lipid bilayer membrane, then traverse the hydrophilic cell, and finally partition into other cell membranes before entering the cerebrospinal fluid (CSF). Opioids that are highly lipid soluble (e.g., sufentanil, fentanyl) can easily pass through the hydrophobic cell membrane. However, these drugs have difficulty crossing through the hydrophilic cellular fluid. In contrast, drugs that are less lipid soluble (e.g., morphine) have a greater challenge crossing the cell membrane but can easily traverse the cell interior. Thus, opioid penetration of the arachnoid mater is dependent on the drug's lipid solubility.[114] Highly lipid-soluble drugs have poor CSF bioavailability because of (1) poor penetration through the arachnoid layer, (2) rapid absorption and sequestration by epidural fat, and (3) rapid uptake by epidural veins.

Some investigators have suggested that parenteral fentanyl provides analgesia equivalent to that provided by epidural fentanyl,[115,116] but more recent evidence suggests that epidural fentanyl provides analgesia via a spinal mechanism.[117–119] Cohen et al.[120] compared a continuous infusion of IV fentanyl with epidural fentanyl after cesarean delivery and reported improved analgesia and less supplemental analgesic consumption despite lower plasma fentanyl levels with epidural administration. The difference may relate to speed of administration. There is evidence that bolus administration of lipophilic opioids has both spinal and supraspinal effects.[117–119,121] After the administration of an epidural bolus of sufentanil 50 μg in a dog model, CSF concentration of sufentanil was 140 times greater than that found in plasma, and the amount detected in cisternal CSF was only 5% of that measured in lumbar CSF.[122]

Hydrophilic morphine has greater CSF bioavailability, with better penetration into the CSF and less systemic absorption than the lipid-soluble opioids.[123] A bolus dose of epidural morphine 6 mg resulted in a peak plasma concentration of 34 ng/mL at 15 minutes after administration and a peak CSF concentration of approximately 1000 ng/mL at 1 hour.[124] A poor correlation between the analgesic effect and plasma levels of morphine has been observed after epidural administration, indicating a predominantly spinal location of action.[125,126] Intrathecal administration is a more efficient method of delivering opioid to spinal cord receptors than epidural or parenteral administration. A bolus dose of intrathecal morphine 0.5 mg resulted in a CSF concentration greater than 10,000 ng/mL, with barely detectable plasma concentration.[127]

Within the epidural space (and subsequently epidural fat or veins), lipophilic agents are more likely to be absorbed and transported from the epidural space to the systemic circulation. Rostral spread in the CSF is determined by CSF drug bioavailability and the drug concentration gradient; hydrophilic opioids (e.g., morphine) are associated with more rostral spread.[122,128] Although opioid dose, volume of injectate, and degree of ionization are important variables, lipid solubility plays the key role in determining the onset of analgesia, the dermatomal spread, and the duration of activity (Table 27.3).[129,130] Highly lipid-soluble opioids penetrate the spinal cord more rapidly and have a quicker onset of action than more water-soluble agents. The gain in potency is inversely proportional to the lipid solubility of the agent used. Hydrophilic opioids exhibit the greatest gain in potency; the potency ratio for intrathecal to systemic morphine is approximately 1:100.[130,131]

The duration of activity is affected by the rate of clearance of the drug from the sites of activity. Lipid-soluble opioids are rapidly absorbed from the epidural space, whereas hydrophilic agents remain in the CSF and spinal tissues for a longer time.[129,130]

Epidural Opioids

The provision of cesarean delivery anesthesia using an epidural catheter (placed during labor or as part of a CSE technique) has prompted an extensive evaluation of epidural opioids to facilitate postoperative analgesia (Table 27.4).

Morphine

Preservative-free morphine received FDA approval for neuraxial administration in 1984, and subsequently epidural morphine administration has been widely investigated and extensively used.[132] Compared with systemic opioids, epidural morphine provides superior postcesarean analgesia, prolonging the time to first analgesic request, decreasing pain scores, and reducing postoperative analgesic requests during the first 24 hours.[88]

Onset and duration. After epidural administration, plasma morphine concentration is similar to that observed after IM injection. Epidural morphine has a relatively slow onset of action as a result of its low lipid solubility and slower

TABLE 27.3 Spinal Opioid Physiochemistry and Pharmacodynamics

Opioid	Molecular Weight	Lipid Solubility[a]	Parenteral Potency	pKa	μ-Opioid Receptor Affinity	Dissociation Kinetics	Potency Gain (Epidural vs. IV or SC)	Onset of Analgesia	Duration of Analgesia
Morphine	285	0.7	1	7.9	Moderate	Slow	10	Delayed	Prolonged
Meperidine	247	39	0.1	8.5	Moderate	Moderate	2–3	Rapid	Intermediate
Methadone	309	116	2	9.3	High	Slow	2–3	Rapid	Intermediate
Hydromorphone	285	1.28	10		High	Slow	5	Rapid	Prolonged
Alfentanil	417	129	25	6.5	High	Very rapid	1–2	Very rapid	Short
Fentanyl	336	717	80	8.4	High	Rapid	1–2	Very rapid	Short
Sufentanil	386	2842	800	8.0	Very high	Moderate	1–1.5	Very rapid	Short

IV, Intravenous; *SC,* subcutaneous.
[a]Octanol-water partition coefficient at pH 7.4.

TABLE 27.4   Epidural Opioids for Cesarean Delivery

Drug(s)	Dose	Onset (min)	Peak Effect (min)	Duration (h)	Advantages	Disadvantages
Morphine	2–4 mg	30–60	60–90	12–24	Long duration	Delayed onset Side-effect profile Potential for delayed respiratory depression
Fentanyl	50–100 μg	5	20	2–3	Rapid onset	Short duration
Sufentanil	10–25 μg	5	15–20	2–4	Rapid onset	Short duration
Meperidine	25–50 mg	15	30	4–6	Rapid onset	Nausea and vomiting
Hydromorphone	0.4–1 mg	15	45–60	10–20	Intermediate onset and duration	Side-effect profile similar to that of morphine
Morphine/fentanyl	3 mg/50 μg	10	15	12–24	Rapid onset Long duration Fewer side effects than morphine 5-mg dose	
Morphine/sufentanil	3 mg/10 μg	5	15	12–24	Rapid onset Long duration Fewer side effects than morphine 5-mg dose	

penetration into spinal tissue.[129,130,133,134] The peak analgesic effect is observed 60 to 90 minutes after administration.[124] Many clinicians prefer to delay epidural morphine administration until immediately after delivery of the infant.

Morphine has a prolonged duration, analgesia typically persisting long after plasma concentration has declined to subtherapeutic levels.[129,130] Epidural morphine provides pain relief for approximately 24 hours after cesarean delivery[135–137]; however, there is wide variation in analgesic duration and efficacy among patients. Within the narrow range of doses studied, investigators have not demonstrated a correlation between the dose of morphine and the duration of analgesia.[138,139]

The volume of the diluent does not appear to affect the pharmacokinetics or clinical activity of epidural morphine. The quality and duration of analgesia, the need for supplemental analgesics, and the incidence of side effects were similar when epidural morphine 4 mg was diluted with saline to a volume of 2, 10, or 20 mL.[140]

In a prospective dose-response study, Palmer et al.[139] observed that postcesarean analgesia (assessed by need for supplemental IV morphine by PCA) improved as the dose of epidural morphine increased from 0 to 3.75 mg. A further increase in dose (to 5 mg) did not significantly improve analgesia or reduce the amount of supplemental IV morphine used in the first 24 postoperative hours (Fig. 27.6).[139] Chumpathong et al.[136] did not observe any difference in pain relief, patient satisfaction, or side effects in women receiving epidural morphine 2.5, 3, or 4 mg for postcesarean analgesia. Rosen et al.[137] found that epidural morphine 5 and 7.5 mg provided similar analgesic efficacy, but a 2-mg dose provided ineffective analgesia. Fuller et al.[138] recommended epidural morphine 3 mg after a large retrospective study of epidural

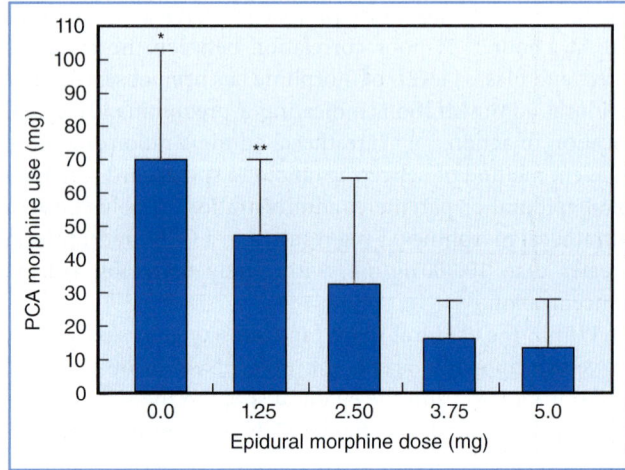

Fig. 27.6 Random allocation dose-response trial of epidural morphine 0, 1.25, 2.5, 3.75, and 5.0 mg for postcesarean delivery analgesia. Breakthrough pain as assessed by total 24-h patient-controlled analgesia (PCA) morphine use. Data are mean ± 95% confidence interval. Groups were significantly different (P < .001). *Group 0.0 mg was significantly different from groups 2.5, 3.75, and 5.0 mg. **Group 1.25 mg was significantly different from groups 3.75 and 5.0 mg. From Palmer CM, Nogami WM, Van Maren G, Alves DM. Postcesarean epidural morphine: a dose-response study. *Anesth Analg.* 2000;90:887–891.

morphine in doses ranging from 2 to 5 mg for postcesarean analgesia.

In contemporary clinical practice, doses of epidural morphine 2 to 4 mg are most commonly used. Lower doses may not provide effective analgesia, and women may require additional supplemental analgesia,[137,139] whereas higher doses may increase opioid-related side effects without improving analgesia. Singh et al.[141] conducted a randomized, noninferiority trial in which all women received scheduled ketorolac and acetaminophen as well as epidural morphine. Morphine 1.5 mg was noninferior to 3 mg for postcesarean delivery analgesia. They found no difference in 24-hour opioid consumption between the 1.5- and 3-mg epidural morphine groups.[141] Thus, lower epidural morphine doses may be appropriate when multimodal analgesia is used and minimizing side effects is a priority. The Society for Obstetric Anesthesia and Perinatology (SOAP) recommends the use of epidural morphine 1 to 3 mg.[142]

Fentanyl

Fentanyl is not approved by the FDA for neuraxial administration, but it is very commonly administered for short-term analgesia. Commercial preparations of fentanyl contain no preservative, are suitable for epidural or intrathecal administration, and have an excellent safety record. Grass et al.[143] reported that the 50% and 95% effective doses (ED_{50} and ED_{95}, respectively) of epidural fentanyl to reduce postcesarean visual analog scale pain scores to less than 10 mm (scale: 0 to 100 mm) were 33 and 92 µg, respectively. An epidural fentanyl dose of 1 µg/kg has also been suggested to optimize *intra*operative analgesia.[144] In clinical practice, doses of 50 to 100 µg are given alone or in combination with epidural morphine.

The slow onset of action of morphine limits its ability to provide optimal intraoperative analgesia, and more lipophilic opioids (e.g., fentanyl) with a faster onset of analgesia are more appropriate for supplementation of intraoperative anesthesia (see Table 27.3). Although single-dose epidural fentanyl improves intraoperative anesthesia, no meaningful postoperative pain relief occurs beyond 4 hours; duration is variable and dose dependent.[145] A dose-response study of epidural fentanyl 25, 50, 100, and 200 µg, administered at the time of first complaint of postoperative pain following epidural anesthesia using lidocaine (lignocaine) with epinephrine (adrenaline), found that the duration of analgesia ranged from 1 to 2 hours.[143]

Local anesthetics may have a synergistic interaction with neuraxial opioids.[146] The concurrent administration of local anesthetic reduces epidural fentanyl dose requirements after cesarean delivery.[147] Epidural fentanyl, administered either as a single dose or as a continuous or patient-controlled infusion, generally has fewer side effects than epidural morphine.[148] Some investigators have suggested that the administration of epidural fentanyl before incision may provide preemptive analgesia and improve postoperative analgesia.[144]

Sufentanil

Epidural administration of the lipid-soluble opioid sufentanil provides a rapid onset of effective postcesarean analgesia. The potency ratio of epidural sufentanil to epidural fentanyl is approximately 5:1.[143] No differences in onset, quality, or duration of analgesia were found after epidural administration of equianalgesic doses of sufentanil and fentanyl.[143] Like fentanyl, epidural sufentanil does not provide postoperative analgesia of long duration. Rosen et al.[149] compared epidural morphine

5 mg with epidural sufentanil 30, 45, or 60 µg. Although most patients who received sufentanil reported pain relief within 15 minutes, the duration of analgesia was 4 to 5 hours, in contrast to 26 hours of analgesia with epidural morphine.[149] The duration of analgesia is dose-dependent; an epidural bolus of sufentanil 25 µg produced less than 2 hours of analgesia, whereas 60 µg provided 5 hours of pain relief.[143,149]

Meperidine

Meperidine is an opioid agonist that also has local anesthetic properties at usual clinical doses. Epidural meperidine has been used for postcesarean analgesia. Two clinical trials compared the safety and efficacy of epidural meperidine 50 mg and IM meperidine 100 mg administered to patients after cesarean delivery.[150,151] Epidural meperidine provided a faster onset of analgesia with a duration (2 to 4 hours) similar to that provided by IM meperidine. Paech[152] evaluated the quality of analgesia and side effects produced by a single epidural bolus of meperidine 50 mg or fentanyl 100 µg. The onset of pain relief was slightly faster with fentanyl; however, the duration of analgesia was longer with meperidine. Ngan Kee et al.[153] compared different doses of epidural meperidine (12.5, 25, 50, 75, and 100 mg) and concluded that meperidine 25 mg was superior to 12.5 mg and that doses > 50 mg offered no improvement in the quality or duration of analgesia. Studies that have compared a single bolus dose of epidural or intrathecal morphine with PCEA meperidine have reported superior analgesia with morphine, but with a higher incidence of opioid-related side effects such as nausea, pruritus, and sedation.[154,155]

Other Epidural Opioids

Hydromorphone is a hydroxylated derivative of morphine with a lipid solubility intermediate between that of morphine and meperidine.[156] The quality of epidural hydromorphone analgesia after cesarean delivery appears to be similar to that observed with epidural morphine; however, its onset is faster and its duration shorter.[157-159] Evidence suggests a potency ratio of 3:1 to 5:1 between epidural morphine and epidural hydromorphone.[156] Halpern et al.[160] found no overall difference in quality of postcesarean analgesia or severity of side effects between patients who received epidural hydromorphone 0.6 mg or epidural morphine 3 mg. A metaanalysis suggested that epidural morphine and hydromorphone provide analgesia with similar efficacy and side effects when given for the treatment of acute or chronic pain.[161]

Diamorphine (heroin) is a lipid-soluble diacetylated derivative of morphine that is commonly administered neuraxially in the United Kingdom.[162] The lipid solubility of diamorphine provides rapid-onset analgesia, and its principal metabolite (morphine) facilitates prolonged duration of analgesia, although less than that of morphine. Roulson et al.[163] found that epidural diamorphine 2.5 mg provided postcesarean analgesia for 16 hours. Other investigators have found a duration of postcesarean analgesia of 6 to 12 hours after epidural diamorphine 5 mg.[164,165] In the United Kingdom, the National Institute for Health and Care Excellence (NICE) recommends doses of epidural diamorphine up to 3 mg for postcesarean analgesia.[166]

Epidural Opioid Combinations

Theoretically, the epidural administration of a lipophilic opioid combined with morphine should provide analgesia of rapid onset and prolonged duration. The use of a lipophilic opioid administered intrathecally (e.g., fentanyl 15 µg) or epidurally (e.g., fentanyl 100 µg) in combination with epidural morphine 3.5 mg improves intraoperative anesthesia and reduces nausea and vomiting during cesarean delivery.[167,168] Some investigators have expressed concern that opioid interactions might reduce analgesic efficacy after epidural administration and that neuraxial fentanyl might initiate acute tolerance or affect the pharmacokinetic and receptor-binding characteristics of morphine. However, these concerns have not been confirmed in subsequent studies.[168,169] Epidural fentanyl, administered immediately after delivery of the infant, improved the quality of intraoperative analgesia without worsening epidural morphine analgesia after cesarean delivery.[168]

Studies of combined epidural morphine and sufentanil have produced mixed results. Dottrens et al.[170] compared a single epidural dose of either morphine 4 mg, sufentanil 50 µg, or morphine 2 mg with sufentanil 25 µg. The addition of sufentanil to epidural morphine provided a more rapid onset and similar duration of postcesarean analgesia than morphine alone.[170] In another study, morphine alone or in combination with sufentanil provided analgesia of longer duration than sufentanil alone. Sinatra et al.[171] were unable to show any potentiation when epidural sufentanil 30 µg was added to morphine 3 mg, and the duration of this combination was shorter than that of epidural morphine 5 mg alone.

Patient-Controlled Epidural Analgesia

Better analgesia at rest and with movement has been reported in reviews of studies that compared continuous epidural analgesia with IV PCA after nonobstetric surgery.[4] However, PCEA is less frequently used for analgesia after cesarean delivery compared with single-dose epidural morphine.

Fanshawe[172] compared PCEA meperidine with single-dose epidural morphine and found that postoperative pain scores were better with epidural morphine at 6, 8, and 24 hours. However, lipophilic opioids have been widely evaluated for PCEA after cesarean delivery and can be used when requirement for long-lasting analgesia is anticipated.[173] Epidural morphine's prolonged latency and risk for delayed respiratory depression make it a less safe option for CEI. Previous investigations have compared meperidine PCEA with other routes of parenteral administration (PCA, IM). Paech et al.[174] performed a crossover study comparing PCEA with IV PCA meperidine after cesarean delivery; patients were randomly assigned to either PCEA or IV PCA for 12 hours before crossing over to the other route of drug administration for the next 12 hours. The PCEA and PCA meperidine protocols in this study were identical (20-mg bolus, 5-minute lockout interval).

Patients receiving meperidine PCEA had lower pain scores at rest and with coughing than patients receiving IV PCA. Ngan Kee et al.[30] observed that PCEA (fentanyl or meperidine) regimens were associated with lower pain scores compared with the respective IV PCA regimens. Goh et al.[175] observed similar analgesic profiles among patients receiving fentanyl and meperidine PCEA but noted more favorable side-effect profiles and better patient satisfaction among patients receiving meperidine PCEA.

Cooper et al.[109] postulated that the combination of epidural fentanyl with local anesthetic (fentanyl 2 µg/mL with 0.05% bupivacaine) would provide better analgesia than that provided by a single-drug PCEA regimen (fentanyl 4 µg/mL or 0.1% bupivacaine). The combination drug regimen was associated with lower pain scores at rest and significantly lower total drug requirements. However, no significant differences in pain scores during coughing were reported among the three groups. Cohen et al.[173] compared four different concentrations of ropivacaine (0.025%, 0.05%, 0.1%, 0.2%) with fentanyl 3 µg/mL and epinephrine 0.5 µg/mL. The lowest-dose group (0.025%) received the largest volume in the epidural space and had the lowest 24-hour pain scores and highest satisfaction scores with no immobility or urinary retention.

Parker and White[31] compared hydromorphone PCEA with IV PCA; no differences in pain scores were found between the two treatment groups. In a follow-up study, these investigators assessed hydromorphone PCEA, with and without a background infusion, and hydromorphone combined with 0.08% bupivacaine, with and without a background infusion.[110] No differences in pain scores, PCEA usage, or 24-hour PCEA requirements were noted, and the combination of hydromorphone-bupivacaine PCEA with a background infusion was associated with a greater degree of lower extremity numbness and weakness.

Cohen et al.[176] compared PCEA using 0.01% bupivacaine and epinephrine 0.5 µg/mL with either fentanyl 2 µg/mL or sufentanil 0.8 µg/mL after cesarean delivery. Pain scores and side effects (nausea, pruritus, and sedation) were similar in the two groups; however, vomiting occurred more commonly in the sufentanil group. Vercauteren et al.[177] compared sufentanil PCEA (bolus 5 µg, lockout 10 minutes) with or without a background infusion of sufentanil 4 µg/h.[177] Pain was lower at 6 hours in the group receiving a background infusion, but no other differences in analgesia were reported between 6 and 24 hours. The background infusion group received considerably more sufentanil and had a higher incidence and severity of sedation.

Chang et al.[178] reported a network metaanalysis of 23 studies that compared opioids administered via IV PCA or PCEA for postcesarean delivery analgesia. They found that, in general, delivery of opioids via PCEA was associated with better analgesic outcomes than delivery via IV PCA. In particular, PCEA fentanyl was associated with significantly lower pain scores at 4 and 8 hours, and it reduced the odds of developing nausea/vomiting and sedation/drowsiness compared with IV PCA morphine, but at the cost of increased odds of developing pruritus.

Although CEI or PCEA can provide satisfactory postoperative analgesia, these techniques may diminish maternal satisfaction because of local anesthetic–induced motor block in lower limbs and the lack of physical independence from infusion devices in the postpartum period. They increase cost and potentially increase the risk for catheter-related complications (e.g., hematoma, infection) in comparison with single-dose administration of neuraxial morphine.[86,179] In contrast, a single dose of neuraxial morphine may facilitate early discharge after elective cesarean delivery, a strategy suggested by the NICE guidelines, which state that "women who are recovering well, are apyrexial and do not have complications following cesarean should be offered early discharge."[166]

Extended-Release Epidural Morphine

Extended-release epidural morphine (EREM) is an FDA-approved preparation that delivers standard morphine sulfate via DepoFoam (Pacira Pharmaceuticals, Inc., San Diego, CA). DepoFoam is a drug-delivery system composed of multivesicular lipid particles containing nonconcentric aqueous chambers that encapsulate the active drug.[180] These naturally occurring lipids are broken down by erosion and reorganization, resulting in a sustained release of morphine for up to 48 hours after epidural administration of a single dose.[180,181] After treatment with EREM, lower pain scores and lower requirement for supplemental analgesia over 48 hours were reported compared with standard epidural morphine.[135] Supplemental analgesia consumption was reduced by 60% in women who received a single dose of EREM 10 mg compared with standard epidural morphine 4 mg after cesarean delivery.[135] However, caution is required, as pooled data from EREM studies for nonobstetric surgery suggest that EREM is associated with more opioid-related side effects, especially with higher doses, including a significantly higher risk for respiratory depression compared with IV opioid PCA (odds ratio [OR], 5.8; 95% CI, 1.1 to 31.9; $P = .04$).[180,182,183] Use of EREM requires extended monitoring for respiratory depression (48 hours compared with 24 hours with standard epidural morphine).[184] Any analgesic advantage must be weighed against the potential risk for serious side effects associated with EREM administration.

Epidural Versus Intrathecal Opioids

Several studies have compared the analgesic efficacy of epidural and intrathecal administration of opioids. Sarvela et al.[185] compared epidural morphine 3 mg with intrathecal morphine 0.1 and 0.2 mg; the two routes of administration provided postcesarean analgesia with similar efficacy and equal duration. Duale et al.[186] observed modest improvements in pain scores and lower morphine consumption with epidural morphine 2 mg compared with intrathecal morphine 0.075 mg. In both studies, the incidence of side effects (e.g., sedation, pruritus, nausea, and vomiting) was not different between the epidural and intrathecal routes.[185,186] A metaanalysis concluded that both epidural and intrathecal techniques provide effective postcesarean analgesia and neither technique is superior in terms of analgesic efficacy.[187] However, intrathecal

administration results in less systemic drug exposure and less potential fetal drug exposure and has a faster onset of action than epidural administration of morphine. Profound sedation and respiratory depression requiring opioid reversal and intensive care monitoring have been reported after unintentional subdural or intrathecal administration of a dose intended for epidural administration.[188] If a CSE anesthetic is planned, intrathecal administration of the opioid may be preferable.

Intrathecal Opioids

Spinal anesthesia has become the preferred anesthetic technique for patients undergoing elective cesarean delivery.[85,87] Intrathecal opioids are commonly administered with a local anesthetic to improve intraoperative anesthesia and postoperative analgesia (see Chapter 26). The potency difference between intrathecal and epidural opioids accounts for the smaller doses of intrathecal opioid used for cesarean delivery. A network metaanalysis of 66 randomized controlled trials investigating the effects of intrathecal opioids for cesarean delivery estimated that duration of complete analgesia (defined as time to pain score > 0) was prolonged the most with intrathecal morphine (190 minutes), followed by a combination of morphine and fentanyl (140 minutes), fentanyl (96 minutes), and sufentanil (96 minutes), compared with placebo. However, there was no statistically significant difference in the duration of complete analgesia between the various intrathecal opioids studied.[189] Similar results were obtained when time to first analgesic use was assessed: intrathecal morphine (660 minutes), morphine and fentanyl combination (520 minutes), and sufentanil (230 minutes), compared with placebo. In addition, intrathecal morphine and diamorphine were associated with significantly lower 24-hour postoperative opioid consumption compared with fentanyl or placebo.[189]

Morphine

Intrathecal morphine 0.075 to 0.2 mg is equivalent to epidural morphine 2 to 3 mg.[185,186] The analgesic efficacy, duration of action, and side-effect profile of intrathecal morphine are similar to that of epidural morphine (see earlier discussion).[185,186] A systematic review and metaanalysis found that the median time to first analgesic request after cesarean delivery was 27 hours (range, 11 to 29 hours) after intrathecal morphine administration.[96] The duration of analgesia is dose-dependent.[96,190,191] A 2016 metaanalysis comparing low-dose (0.05 to 0.1 mg) and high-dose (>0.1 to 0.25 mg) intrathecal morphine found mean time to first analgesic request was longer (mean difference, 4.5 hours; 95% CI, 1.8 to 7.1 hours; $P = .0008$) for the high-dose group compared with the low-dose group.[191]

Dose. Several studies have attempted to determine the optimal dose of intrathecal morphine for postcesarean analgesia. Palmer et al.[192] assessed IV PCA morphine use after doses of intrathecal morphine ranging from 0.025 to 0.5 mg and found no decrease in PCA morphine use with morphine doses >0.075 mg.[192] Uchiyama et al.[193] performed a dose-response study with intrathecal morphine 0, 0.05, 0.1, and 0.2 mg. They observed that 0.1 mg and 0.2 mg provided comparable and effective postcesarean analgesia for 28 hours. The 0.05-mg dose was less effective, and the incidence of side effects was greater with the 0.2-mg dose; therefore, the investigators concluded that intrathecal morphine 0.1 mg is the optimal dose for postcesarean analgesia.[193] Berger et al.[194] compared 0.05, 0.1, and 0.15 mg of intrathecal morphine in women who received multimodal analgesia with IV ketorolac; all doses provided similar analgesia after cesarean delivery. There were no differences in 24-hour morphine consumption or reported pain or nausea scores, but pruritus scores were lower at 6 and 12 hours in the 0.05-mg group. Sultan et al.[191] performed a metaanalysis to determine whether low-dose (0.05 to 0.1 mg) intrathecal morphine provides comparable duration and quality of analgesia with fewer side effects than a high-dose (>0.1 to 0.25 mg). Pain scores at 12 hours and morphine consumption at 24 hours were not significantly different, but duration of analgesia was longer with the higher doses. The incidence of opioid-related side effects, including nausea or vomiting (OR 0.4; 95% CI, 0.3 to 0.7) and pruritus (OR 0.3; 95% CI, 0.2 to 0.6) were lower in the low-dose group.[191] Thus, there is a trade-off between incidence of side effects and duration of analgesia.

The analgesic efficacy and side-effect profile of intrathecal morphine with those of PCEA after cesarean delivery have been compared. Vercauteren et al.[179] reported that intrathecal morphine 0.15 mg provided superior analgesia and fewer side effects compared with PCEA using 0.06% bupivacaine and sufentanil 1 µg/mL. Paech et al.[155] reported that patients who received intrathecal morphine 0.2 mg had lower pain scores, offset by a higher incidence of pruritus, nausea, and drowsiness, compared with patient who received PCEA meperidine. In another study in which intrathecal morphine (0, 0.05, and 0.1 mg) was combined with CEI (0.2% ropivacaine at 6 mL/h), inclusion of intrathecal morphine improved postcesarean analgesia compared with placebo.[195]

In summary, the intrathecal administration of a small dose of morphine (0.05 to 0.2 mg) provides effective analgesia for 14 to 36 hours after cesarean delivery. Higher doses (>0.1 mg) may slightly increase the *duration* of analgesia but are associated with increasing side effects and limited improvement in analgesic *quality* in the typical patient. Because of the variability in patient response to intrathecal morphine, some patients treated with low doses may experience inadequate postoperative analgesia and/or opioid-related side effects. Thus, the use of low-dose intrathecal morphine as a component of multimodal analgesia may provide optimal analgesia with a low risk for side effects. SOAP recommends the use of a long-acting opioid such as intrathecal morphine 0.05 to 0.15 mg (50 to 150 µg) whenever feasible.[142]

There is a need for more study of the relationship between patients' expectations for pain after cesarean delivery and their analgesic needs and use. Carvalho et al.[22] investigated the relationship between patients' choice of dose of intrathecal morphine, postcesarean pain scores, and opioid use. Patients were randomly assigned to a choice of 0.1 or 0.2 mg

of intrathecal morphine or no choice. Women assigned a choice were read a standardized script that discussed the trade-off of pain relief with increased risk for the most common intrathecal morphine side effects (nausea, vomiting, and pruritus). Participants who requested the larger dose of intrathecal morphine required more supplemental opioids and reported more pain with movement regardless of the intrathecal morphine dose they actually received. Thus, patients may correctly anticipate a greater postoperative opioid need. Using a higher dose of intrathecal morphine in patients predicted to be at risk for high acute postpartum pain after cesarean delivery may result in less acute postoperative pain.[22,196] Shared decision-making, involvement of both the patient and anesthesia provider in a sharing of information to build a consensus about preferred dose, and reaching an agreement about which dose to use may result in improved analgesia.[197]

Fentanyl

Intrathecal fentanyl improves intraoperative anesthesia (especially during uterine exteriorization), reduces intraoperative nausea and vomiting (IONV), decreases local anesthetic dose requirement, and provides a better postoperative transition to other pain medications during recovery from spinal anesthesia for cesarean delivery.[198–201] However, intrathecal fentanyl provides a limited duration of postoperative analgesia, with a median time to first request for additional analgesia of 4 hours (range, 2 to 13 hours).[96] A study that compared intrathecal morphine 0.1 mg with fentanyl 25 µg found that morphine provided better and longer postoperative analgesia after cesarean delivery.[202]

The analgesic effects, duration of analgesia, and side effects after intrathecal fentanyl are dose-related.[96,198,199] Belzarena[198] found that the mean duration of postcesarean analgesia ranged from 305 to 787 minutes with intrathecal fentanyl doses of 0.25 to 0.75 µg/kg; however, patients who received the higher doses experienced decreased respiratory rate and a high incidence of side effects (e.g., pruritus, nausea). Dahlgren et al.[199] reported that intrathecal fentanyl 10 µg added to bupivacaine increased the mean time of effective analgesia from 121 to 181 minutes. Similarly, Wilwerth et al.[203] found that intrathecal fentanyl 25 µg added to bupivacaine resulted in a median duration of analgesia of 187 minutes (interquartile range [IQR], 151 to 230 minutes). Hunt et al.[204] compared intrathecal fentanyl doses of 2.5 to 50 µg combined with intrathecal bupivacaine for cesarean delivery and found that doses greater than 6.25 µg were associated with better intraoperative anesthesia and a longer time to first request for additional analgesia than administration of bupivacaine alone (72 minutes versus 192 minutes, respectively).[204] Chu et al.[205] found that fentanyl doses of 12.5 to 15 µg were required to increase the duration of effective analgesia.

In summary, intrathecal fentanyl optimizes intraoperative anesthesia and provides immediate postoperative analgesia. However, intrathecal fentanyl (10 to 25 µg) provides a limited duration of postcesarean analgesia (2 to 4 hours) and does not decrease subsequent postoperative analgesic requirements.

Sufentanil

Sufentanil has a fast onset of action, which may improve intraoperative anesthesia and reduce the dose of local anesthetic required for cesarean anesthesia.[206] However, its pharmacokinetic properties limit the duration of effective postoperative analgesia after intrathecal administration.[96] Courtney et al.[207] found that intrathecal sufentanil 10, 15, or 20 μg resulted in a mean duration of postcesarean analgesia of approximately 3 hours. More than 90% of patients reported pruritus, but only one patient required treatment. Dahlgren et al.[199] compared the safety and efficacy of sufentanil 2.5 or 5 μg, fentanyl 10 μg, or placebo added to hyperbaric bupivacaine 12.5 mg for cesarean delivery and found that the duration of effective analgesia was longer with inclusion of opioids and was longest with sufentanil 5 μg, although this dose also had the highest incidence of pruritus. Patients receiving intrathecal sufentanil had *lower* requirements for intraoperative antiemetics and postoperative IV morphine rescue. In another study, increasing the dose of intrathecal sufentanil to 7.5 μg did not increase the duration of postoperative analgesia compared with 5 μg but increased the incidence of pruritus.[208] Karaman et al.[209] found that intrathecal sufentanil 5 μg delayed the time to first analgesic request to 6 hours, compared with 20 hours for intrathecal morphine 0.2 mg. A study that compared intrathecal fentanyl 20 μg and sufentanil 2.5 μg added to bupivacaine found no difference in the quality of intraoperative and postoperative analgesia, as well as no difference in the frequency of nausea and pruritus.[210] Wilwerth et al.[203] added intrathecal fentanyl 25 μg, sufentanil 2.5 μg, or sufentanil 5 μg to hyperbaric bupivacaine 10 mg. Effective analgesia was defined as time from spinal injection to first IV morphine administered. Median duration of analgesia was longer with sufentanil 2.5 μg (214 minutes) and 5 μg (236 minutes) compared with fentanyl 25 μg (187 minutes).[203] The incidence of pruritus and postoperative nausea and vomiting (PONV) was similar among groups.

In summary, intrathecal sufentanil, similar to fentanyl, enhances intraoperative anesthesia and provides postoperative analgesia of limited duration. The duration of analgesia is not prolonged with doses > 5 μg and higher doses are associated with greater pruritus.

Other Intrathecal Opioids

Intrathecal **meperidine** reduces the intensity of pain associated with the regression of spinal anesthesia and provides postoperative analgesia of intermediate duration (4 to 5 hours).[211,212] Yu et al.[213] found that the addition of meperidine 10 mg to hyperbaric bupivacaine 10 mg prolonged the mean duration of postcesarean analgesia (234 minutes for meperidine versus 125 minutes for placebo); however, the incidence of IONV was greater in the meperidine group. Imarengiaye et al.[214] reported that meperidine 7.5 mg added to bupivacaine 10 mg resulted in mean duration of postoperative analgesia of 257 minutes compared with 161 minutes with saline-placebo. Unlike other opioids, meperidine possesses local anesthetic properties at usual clinical doses. Although the use of larger intrathecal meperidine doses (e.g., 1 mg/kg) as the sole agent

for spinal anesthesia for cesarean delivery has been described, experience with this technique is limited.[211,212]

Diamorphine has physicochemical properties that are of value in providing intrathecal analgesia as well as epidural analgesia. A high lipophilicity (octanol-water partition coefficient, 280) results in a rapid onset of analgesia, and diamorphine's active metabolite (morphine) provides prolonged duration of analgesia. The rapid onset of diamorphine is an advantage in the provision of intraoperative as well as postoperative analgesia. Saravanan et al.[215] concluded that the ED$_{95}$ for intrathecal diamorphine to prevent intraoperative discomfort was 0.4 mg when combined with hyperbaric bupivacaine 12.5 mg.

Kelly et al.[216] compared intrathecal diamorphine 0.125, 0.25, and 0.375 mg for postcesarean analgesia. The 0.25- and 0.375-mg doses provided effective analgesia; the incidence of both vomiting and pruritus was dose-related. Stacey et al.[217] reported that the duration of analgesia was dose-dependent and found that intrathecal diamorphine 1 mg provided 10 hours of postcesarean analgesia, compared with 7 hours for 0.5 mg. A dose-response study of intrathecal diamorphine 0.1, 0.2, or 0.3 mg reported a dose-dependent enhancement of analgesia and an increase in pruritus.[15] Husaini and Russell[218] observed that intrathecal diamorphine 0.2 mg and intrathecal morphine 0.2 mg provided similar postcesarean analgesia as assessed by rescue postoperative IV PCA morphine requirement. However, the patients who received intrathecal morphine had a higher incidence of pruritus and drowsiness. Hallworth et al.[219] reported that *intrathecal* diamorphine 0.25 mg produced the same duration and quality of postcesarean analgesia as *epidural* diamorphine 5 mg, with less nausea and vomiting.

Diamorphine is commonly used in the United Kingdom, but it is not available for clinical use in the United States and Canada. In the United Kingdom, NICE recommends the use of an intrathecal diamorphine dose up to 0.3 mg (300 μg) for postcesarean analgesia.[166]

Intrathecal **hydromorphone** has been used to provide analgesia following cesarean delivery as an alternative to morphine; its use increased with shortages of intrathecal morphine in the United States. Two retrospective studies found an analgesic advantage in favor of intrathecal morphine. Marroquin et al.[220] retrospectively compared intrathecal morphine 0.2 mg or epidural morphine 3 mg with intrathecal hydromorphone 60 μg or epidural hydromorphone 0.6 mg. Time to first opioid request was 17 to 21 hours with neuraxial morphine compared with 13 to 15 hours for neuraxial hydromorphone.[220] Beatty et al.[221] compared intrathecal morphine 0.1 mg with intrathecal hydromorphone 40 μg and found 24-hour supplemental opioid use favored intrathecal morphine (8 versus 33 mg). The side effects of intrathecal morphine and hydromorphone are similar.[220,221]

The optimal intrathecal hydromorphone dose has not been fully elucidated. Using an up-down sequential allocation method, Lynde[222] estimated that the ED$_{50}$ of intrathecal hydromorphone was 4.6 μg. In a dose-response study, Sviggum et al.[223] randomized 80 participants to intrathecal morphine or intrathecal hydromorphone in a biased-coin, up-down sequential allocation study. The ED_{90} for achieving a numeric pain score (scale, 0 to 10) ≤ 3 for a duration of 12 hours was 75 μg for intrathecal hydromorphone compared with 150 μg for intrathecal morphine.[223] Further research is needed to help refine the optimal dose of intrathecal hydromorphone for postcesarean analgesia.

Intrathecal Opioid Combinations

Intrathecal administration of morphine in combination with a lipophilic opioid (e.g., fentanyl, sufentanil) may offer some advantages, similar to their combination in the epidural space. Intrathecal morphine has a delayed onset; therefore, the coadministration of a lipophilic opioid may serve to improve intraoperative anesthesia and reduce the intensity of pain associated with the regression of spinal anesthesia in the postanesthesia care unit. Chung et al.[224] found that the combination of intrathecal meperidine 10 mg and morphine 0.15 mg provided better intraoperative analgesia, less need for supplemental analgesia, and greater satisfaction than intrathecal morphine alone following cesarean delivery. Intrathecal sufentanil 5 μg coadministrated with morphine 0.15 mg provided better and longer pain relief than intrathecal sufentanil plus a single injection of subcutaneous morphine; however, a higher incidence of side effects, such as nausea and vomiting, was observed with intrathecal morphine.[225]

Some investigators have suggested that intrathecal morphine may be less effective when concurrently administered with intrathecal fentanyl, suggesting acute spinal opioid tolerance.[226] This claim is controversial, and study results are inconsistent. Cooper et al.[226] reported that patients who received intrathecal fentanyl 25 μg with bupivacaine had higher postoperative IV morphine PCA requirements than patients who received bupivacaine alone. By contrast, Sibilla et al.[227] found that the intrathecal combination of fentanyl 25 μg and morphine 0.1 mg provided similar postoperative analgesia to that provided by intrathecal morphine alone. Carvalho et al.[228] found no difference in postoperative analgesia requirements but small increases in postoperative pain scores with the addition of increasing doses of intrathecal fentanyl (5, 10, or 25 μg) to intrathecal morphine 0.2 mg for cesarean delivery. The authors suggested that intrathecal fentanyl may induce subtle acute tolerance to intrathecal morphine. The clinical significance of this finding is unclear, however, especially because of widespread evidence that intrathecal lipid-soluble opioids decrease the incidence of *intraoperative* visceral pain and nausea. Many anesthesia providers currently administer both intrathecal morphine and fentanyl with a local anesthetic for spinal anesthesia for cesarean delivery (see Chapter 26).[86] The coadministration of intrathecal fentanyl does *not* appear to significantly compromise the postoperative analgesia provided by intrathecal morphine.

Despite the administration of neuraxial opioid analgesia, the quality and duration of analgesia after cesarean delivery are often incomplete. Thus, neuraxial opioid analgesia is rarely the sole analgesic technique used for postcesarean analgesia. Rather, neuraxial opioids should be considered as part of a multimodal analgesic approach for the treatment of postcesarean pain.[91,94,100]

Side Effects of Neuraxial Opioids

Careful evaluation of the potential adverse effects of neuraxial pharmacologic agents is important before making the decision to administer these drugs. In obstetric patients, adverse maternal effects as well as potential neonatal effects should be considered.

Maternal Safety

Neurotoxicity (safety) studies suggest that **morphine, fentanyl, sufentanil, hydromorphone, meperidine, clonidine,** and **neostigmine** are safe for neuraxial administration.[229,230] Morphine and clonidine are approved by the FDA for neuraxial administration. Although unlicensed for neuraxial administration, fentanyl and sufentanil have been used for many years without evidence of neurotoxicity. Studies in sheep have reported potential neurotoxicity with intrathecal **butorphanol.**[231] Culebras et al.[232] reported potential toxic interactions with the coadministration of **nalbuphine** and local anesthetic. However, Rawal et al.[231] evaluated the behavioral and histopathologic effects of butorphanol, sufentanil, and nalbuphine after intrathecal administration in sheep and found that nalbuphine caused the least evidence of neural tissue damage.

Clinicians should avoid neuraxial administration of any agent before adequate evaluation for potential neurotoxicity has been completed.[233-235] Drugs and diluents that are proven safe for parenteral use may have adverse effects when administered intrathecally. Despite these valid concerns, a number of opioid analgesics, including fentanyl and sufentanil, have been administered intrathecally to healthy obstetric patients without prior adequate investigation of their safety profile in animal and clinical volunteer studies.[235]

Preservatives added to many commercial preparations may be hazardous if administered to the neuraxis. Examples are **sodium (meta)bisulfite** and **disodium ethylenediaminetetraacetic acid (EDTA)**, which are known to incite inflammatory and fibrotic changes in pia-arachnoid and spinal tissue after intrathecal administration. **Dezocine** has been shown to cause neuropathologic changes in the dog spinal cord.[236] Similarly, **glycine**, a neurotransmitter, is added as a preservative to **remifentanil** preparations and is specifically contraindicated for neuraxial injection.

Neonatal Effects

All opioids have the potential for placental transfer and neonatal effects. Minimal neonatal effects have been found after the administration of epidural morphine 2 to 7.5 mg for cesarean delivery.[237] This is not surprising given the slow increase in plasma concentration after epidural administration and active transport of morphine out of the blood-brain barrier[238] and placenta[239] by P-glycoproteins. Some clinicians prefer to administer neuraxial opioids after umbilical cord clamping to avoid placental transfer, although it is minimal. Lipophilic opioids are associated with faster systemic uptake;

if indicated (e.g., for treatment of intraoperative pain before delivery), the smallest necessary dose should be administered. Courtney et al.[207] found that intrathecal sufentanil (10, 15, or 20 µg) did not affect neonatal outcome as assessed by umbilical cord blood gas measurements and Apgar and neurobehavioral scores. Smaller doses of intrathecal opioids are associated with less neonatal drug transfer than epidural or IV opioid administration.[240]

Respiratory Depression

Neuraxial opioids can depress the respiratory center in the brainstem via direct and/or indirect mechanisms.[128–130,134] Respiratory depression after neuraxial morphine administration is biphasic.[241] Early respiratory depression can occur 30 to 90 minutes after epidural morphine administration following systemic vascular absorption from the epidural space,[130] whereas delayed respiratory depression can occur 6 to 18 hours after epidural or intrathecal morphine administration following rostral spread in CSF and slow penetration into the brainstem.[242,243] In contrast, lipophilic opioids do not cause delayed respiratory depression but may cause early respiratory depression, typically within 30 minutes, because of vascular uptake and rostral spread in CSF and, potentially, direct transit in epidural veins.[244]

The incidence of respiratory depression, which can lead to death or permanent brain damage, after neuraxial morphine administration in obstetric patients is very low, with a reported range from 8.67 per 10,000 to 5.96 per 10,000.[245] The Serious Complication Repository project of SOAP systematically tracked complications related to obstetric anesthesia between 2004 and 2009.[246] Among 90,795 reported cases of neuraxial anesthesia for cesarean delivery, no cases of respiratory arrest secondary to neuraxial opioid administration were reported. No studies in the obstetric setting have reported serious morbidity, although some patients have required naloxone administration for treatment of respiratory depression.[138] Early reports suggested that intrathecal morphine was more likely to cause delayed respiratory depression than epidural morphine.[130] However, this likely reflected the relatively high intrathecal morphine doses (1 to 10 mg) used in early clinical studies.[247] Subsequently, lower doses of intrathecal morphine have been found to provide effective analgesia with a low risk for clinically significant respiratory depression. No maternal deaths attributable to maternal neuraxial opioid administration were reported in the United Kingdom and Ireland Confidential Enquiries into Maternal Deaths and Morbidity 2018–2020.[248] In a retrospective study of 5036 postpartum women who received low-dose neuraxial morphine for cesarean delivery, no instances of respiratory depression were identified (defined as clinically relevant episodes of respiratory depression requiring naloxone administration or a rapid-response team call).[249] Thus, clinicians have concluded that the analgesic benefits derived from neuraxial opioids outweigh the risks associated with respiratory depression in most patients. The incidence of respiratory depression associated with systemic (IV or IM) opioids is likely to be equivalent or higher than that observed with neuraxial opioids.[36,250]

There are very few case reports of respiratory depression after neuraxial administration of lipophilic opioids in the obstetric setting. In one report, respiratory depression occurred 25 minutes after intrathecal fentanyl 15 µg and morphine 0.2 mg and required reversal with naloxone.[251] Respiratory depression has been described after administration of epidural fentanyl 90 to 100 µg for cesarean delivery.[252,253] Cohen et al.[244] reported that epidural sufentanil 30 to 50 µg depressed the ventilatory response to CO_2 after cesarean delivery. Although overt respiratory depression did not occur, the highest sedation scores and depression of CO_2 response occurred 45 minutes after administration. Another group reported that epidural fentanyl 100 µg or sufentanil 10 to 50 µg added to lidocaine for cesarean delivery caused significant changes in respiratory rate and end-tidal CO_2 but no adverse clinical events.[254]

Historically, respiratory depression was more common because patients received greater doses of neuraxial opioid than those currently used in modern practice. For cesarean delivery, neuraxial morphine appears to have a limit or "ceiling" in analgesic efficacy. More specifically, effective doses of intrathecal and epidural morphine are 0.075 to 0.2 mg and 2 to 4 mg, respectively, in opioid-naïve patients.[96,139,192,255] Sultan et al.[191] performed a systematic review of studies of low-dose compared with high-dose intrathecal morphine administered for postoperative analgesia following elective cesarean delivery; there were no reported episodes of respiratory depression. Thus, avoiding high doses of neuraxial morphine may improve safety without compromising analgesia.[255]

Monitoring and Detection of Respiratory Depression

All patients who receive neuraxial opioids should be monitored for adequacy of ventilation, oxygenation, and level of consciousness. Opioid effects on respiration include reduced minute ventilation (decrease in respiratory rate, tidal volume, or both) and decreased response to hypoxemia and changes in $PaCO_2$.[247,256] In nearly two-thirds of cases of respiratory depression following general anesthesia in the Anesthesia Closed Claims Project database, somnolence was present, but not addressed, before the respiratory depression event.[257]

Guidelines for the prevention, detection, and management of respiratory depression associated with neuraxial opioid administration have been published by the ASA and the American Society of Regional Anesthesia and Pain Medicine (ASRA).[184] The duration of respiratory monitoring corresponds to the expected duration of action of the administered opioid. The onset of respiratory depression after neuraxial opioids is variable and has been reported to range from 2 to 12 hours.[250] CO_2 responsiveness is depressed for up to 24 hours after the administration of epidural morphine 5 mg.[258] The ASA recommends that respiratory monitoring after neuraxial administration of morphine should occur at least every hour for the first 12 hours and then every 2 hours for the next 12 hours.[184] However, these guidelines do not specifically address obstetric patients and are likely overly prescriptive given the low risk for clinically significant neuraxial opioid–induced respiratory depression with conventional dosing in this patient population.[259] The SOAP has commissioned a consensus statement specific to the obstetric population following cesarean delivery, whereby the frequency and modality of respiratory monitoring should be based on patient risk stratification and neuraxial morphine dose.[260] In summary, patients who receive **high-dose** neuraxial morphine (intrathecal > 0.15 mg or epidural > 3 mg) or those with risk factors, including cardiopulmonary or neurological comorbidity, body mass index (BMI) ≥ 40 kg/m², obstructive sleep apnea, chronic opioid use, hypertension, general anesthesia, supplemental IV opioid, concomitant use of sedating medications or magnesium, and postanesthesia desaturation, should be monitored according to the ASA guidelines.[184] In contrast, patients without these risk factors who receive **ultra-low-dose** neuraxial morphine (intrathecal ≤ 0.05 mg or epidural ≤ 1 mg) do not require additional respiratory monitoring apart from routine postoperative vital sign assessments. Respiratory rate and sedation assessments should be performed every 2 hours for 12 hours in patients who received **low-dose** neuraxial morphine (intrathecal 0.05 to 0.15 mg or epidural 1 to 3 mg).[260]

Early-onset respiratory depression associated with lipophilic opioids usually occurs within 30 minutes of administration and is likely to occur in a high-visibility, controlled setting (e.g., operating or labor room). The ASA and ASRA recommend that respiratory monitoring after administration of neuraxial fentanyl should continue for a minimum of 2 hours.[184]

Nausea and Vomiting

Nausea and vomiting are common complaints after cesarean delivery, and the causes are likely multifactorial. It was hypothesized that neuraxial opioids increase the risk for PONV after cesarean delivery in a non–dose-dependent manner via rostral spread of opioid in the CSF to the brainstem or from vascular uptake and delivery to the vomiting center and chemoreceptor trigger zone.[261] However, the link between intrathecal opioids and PONV after cesarean delivery is unclear. Palmer et al.[192] found no difference in PONV between intrathecal morphine (0.025 to 0.5 mg) and placebo, nor a relationship between PONV and morphine dose. A similar study by the same group found no difference in the severity of PONV in patients receiving increasing doses of epidural morphine (1.25 to 5 mg).[139] However, neither study was adequately powered to investigate the absence of PONV as a primary outcome measure. A 2021 network metaanalysis investigating the effects of intrathecal morphine, morphine and fentanyl combination, fentanyl, diamorphine, sufentanil, and meperidine for cesarean delivery found that, compared with a placebo, intrathecal opioids did not significantly increase the incidence of nausea or vomiting when assessed as separate outcomes.[189] When assessed as a combined outcome of PONV, only meperidine was associated with increased risk for nausea and vomiting.

Many studies have investigated different regimens to reduce PONV in patients receiving neuraxial opioids for cesarean delivery, but these studies did not standardize PONV outcome measures and did not stratify patients according to risk for PONV. It is notable that PONV is mainly triggered by the emetogenic effects of opioids and severe pain,[262] hence underscoring the importance of optimal neuraxial opioid dosing and the use of a multimodal opioid-sparing strategy to provide adequate analgesia while minimizing opioid use.

Single antiemetic agents. Older antiemetics, such as **metoclopramide** and **droperidol**, have been used to prevent or treat neuraxial opioid–induced emesis in the obstetric setting. Metoclopramide antagonizes dopamine receptors in the chemoreceptor trigger zone. It is often administered preoperatively owing to its favorable gut prokinetic properties. In a metaanalysis of studies that assessed efficacy of antiemetic prophylaxis, metoclopramide was associated with a reduced incidence of IONV and early PONV compared with placebo.[263]

The use of a transdermal **scopolamine** patch may also lower the incidence of PONV after cesarean delivery. A transdermal scopolamine patch (1.5 mg) provided efficacy similar to that provided by **ondansetron** 4 mg in reducing emesis among parturients receiving spinal anesthesia (incidence of 40% and 42%, respectively, versus 59% in the control group).[264] However, transdermal scopolamine has a latency period of 3 to 4 hours, and side effects, including dry mouth, visual disturbances, dizziness, and agitation, are common.

Serotonin (5-HT$_3$) receptor antagonists have been used for both prophylaxis and treatment of PONV. These drugs bind to 5-HT$_3$ receptors in the chemoreceptor trigger zone and at vagal afferents in the gastrointestinal tract. Prophylactic administration of **ondansetron** 4 to 8 mg has been shown to have a better antiemetic profile in the first 24 hours after intrathecal and epidural opioid administration compared with placebo (Fig. 27.7).[265] A metaanalysis of six trials found that the use of serotonin receptor antagonists reduced the incidence of PONV and the need for rescue antiemetic treatment in women who received intrathecal opioids for cesarean delivery.[266]

Corticosteroid receptors have been identified in areas important to the signal processing of nausea and vomiting, including the nucleus of the solitary tract, the nucleus of raphe, and the area postrema. Tzeng et al.[267] reported that IV **dexamethasone** 8 mg and **droperidol** 1.25 mg provided similar efficacy in the prevention of PONV. Wang et al.[268] suggested that dexamethasone 5 mg is the minimum effective dose for preventing PONV. In both studies, patients received epidural morphine 3 mg.[267,268] In a 2012 metaanalysis of studies of obstetric and gynecologic patients who received neuraxial morphine, prophylactic dexamethasone (2.5 to 10 mg) was associated with a reduced risk for PONV and need for antiemetic rescue therapy compared with placebo.[269] Administration of **cyclizine** 50 mg has been reported to be associated with fewer episodes of PONV (0 to 12 hours after cesarean delivery) than administration of dexamethasone 8 mg after intrathecal opioid (fentanyl and morphine) administration.[270]

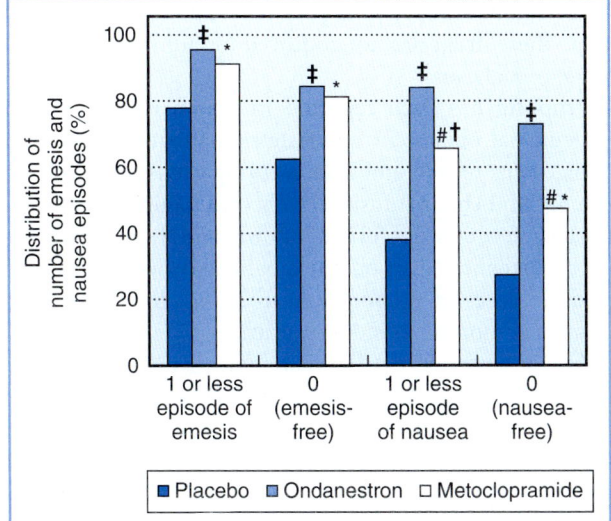

Fig. 27.7 Randomized trial of postoperative nausea and emesis in patients undergoing cesarean delivery with epidural anesthesia (2% lidocaine with epinephrine and fentanyl) who received prophylactic ondansetron, metoclopramide, or placebo. Distribution of nausea and emesis episodes (0 [nausea or emesis free] or 1 or less) in the first 24 h. Values are given as percentages of each patient group. #Group metoclopramide versus ondansetron; $P < .05$. *Group metoclopramide versus placebo; $P < .05$. †Group metoclopramide versus placebo; $P < .005$. ‡Group ondansetron versus placebo; $P < .005$. Data from Pan PH, Moore CM. Comparing the efficacy of prophylactic metoclopramide, ondansetron, and placebo in cesarean section patients given epidural anesthesia. *J Clin Anesth.* 2001;13:430–435.

Combination antiemetic regimens. Administration of drugs acting at more than one different receptor sites may improve antiemetic efficacy through additivity or synergism.[271] Drug combinations may also facilitate a concomitant reduction in drug doses limiting individual side effects. Wu et al.[272] reported lower rates of PONV after intrathecal morphine administration with use of a combination of dexamethasone 8 mg and droperidol 0.625 mg than with the use of dexamethasone 8 mg or droperidol 1.25 mg alone. In a multicenter study, Habib et al.[273] randomized women to one of three groups: placebo, metoclopramide 10 mg plus placebo, or a combination of metoclopramide 10 mg plus ondansetron 4 mg. Spinal anesthesia–induced hypotension was managed prophylactically with a phenylephrine infusion to maintain the systolic blood pressure within 20% of baseline or more than 90 mm Hg. The combination of metoclopramide and ondansetron reduced IONV and PONV compared with placebo.[273]

Nonpharmacologic techniques. Several studies have investigated the prophylactic use of **acupressure** (using wrist bands with a plastic bead placed bilaterally on the P6 [HG-6] acupoint) for reducing PONV after neuraxial anesthesia for cesarean delivery. A metaanalysis of six studies (649 patients) that assessed the effect of P6 stimulation versus placebo to reduce IONV and PONV revealed inconsistent results, thereby limiting any definitive conclusions regarding the efficacy of this intervention.[274] Based on very limited evidence in patients undergoing cesarean delivery, supplemental oxygen

and generous IV fluid administration do not appear to reduce IONV or PONV.[275]

Pruritus

Pruritus is a common side effect of neuraxial opioids. In a retrospective review of 4880 patients undergoing cesarean delivery who received epidural morphine 2 to 5 mg, pruritus was reported by 58% of patients.[138] However, a sample of patients who received spinal anesthesia for cesarean delivery ranked pain, nausea, and vomiting as more undesirable than pruritus.[14] The incidence and severity of pruritus are likely influenced by the opioid dose, route of administration (more common after intrathecal administration), and method of assessment.[191,276] The incidence of pruritus after intrathecal morphine is as high as 70% to 90%, with approximately 25% to 40% of patients requesting treatment.[138,185,277–280]

Pruritus may manifest in the dermatomal distribution of neuraxial opioid spread as well as nonspecific areas of the head and neck; specific symptoms and severity vary among patients.[281] Opioid-induced histamine release from mast cells does not appear to be the causative mechanism for pruritus after *neuraxial* opioid administration. Plasma opioid and histamine levels are clinically insignificant at the time of symptom presentation (3 to 6 hours after intraspinal morphine administration).[130,242,282] At present, the mechanisms of spinal and epidural opioid–induced pruritus remain unclear. Postulated theories include: (1) direct or indirect excitatory effects on central μ-opioid receptors; (2) cephalad migration of the opioid within the CSF to the trigeminal nucleus (which contains the subnucleus caudalis, integrates facial sensory input, and exhibits high opioid receptor density); (3) excitatory effects on dorsal or ventral horn neurons; and (4) other mechanisms (e.g., effects on dopamine-2 [D_2] receptors, prostaglandin system, serotonin receptors, and CNS gamma-aminobutyric acid and glycine receptors).[282] Pregnant patients may be more susceptible as a result of estrogen interaction with opioid receptors.[283] The incidence of moderate-to-severe pruritus with epidural morphine administered for postcesarean analgesia has been reported to be lower in patients homozygous for the G118G polymorphism in the μ-opioid receptor gene *(OPRM1)* than in patients with the A118G or A118A genotype (incidence 5%, 42%, and 53%, respectively).[284] In a study of 63 women who received morphine 0.1 mg during spinal anesthesia for elective cesarean delivery, Pettini et al.[285] reported an incidence of pruritus of 50% in patients homozygous for the G118G polymorphism and 82% in patients with the A118G or A118A genotype.

There is little consensus regarding the prevention and treatment of neuraxial opioid–induced pruritus after cesarean delivery.[286] Further, there are currently no validated or consistent methods for assessing pruritus, which limits the analysis of data from studies investigating the efficacy of antipruritic regimens.

Studies comparing **opioid antagonists** for the treatment of pruritus have demonstrated mixed results. **Nalbuphine** (5 mg) significantly reduced the severity of pruritus after epidural morphine, and fewer patients required additional treatment of persistent pruritus.[279] Smaller doses of nalbuphine (2 to 3 mg) were effective for treating moderate-to-severe pruritus after intrathecal morphine administration.[287] Wu et al.[288] found that **butorphanol** 1 mg followed by an infusion of 0.2 mg/h was associated with reduced pruritus compared with a saline-control group in patients who received intrathecal morphine.

Prophylactic treatment with **opioid antagonists** has also been investigated as a method of reducing the incidence of opioid-induced pruritus. Morgan et al.[289] reported that pretreatment with IV nalbuphine (20 mg at skin closure) with subsequent postoperative administration (20 mg in divided doses) was ineffective in reducing pruritus in patients receiving epidural morphine. Similarly, pretreatment with subcutaneous **naloxone** (0.4 mg) did not reduce the incidence of pruritus in patients receiving intrathecal fentanyl and morphine for elective cesarean delivery.[290] This is not surprising given the short half-life of naloxone. However, naloxone and nalbuphine administered via patient-controlled bolus doses with a continuous background infusion have been found to reduce the incidence of pruritus after cesarean delivery in patients who received epidural morphine 5 mg.[278] The long-acting oral opioid antagonist **naltrexone** reduced pruritus compared with placebo after cesarean delivery in patients who received epidural or intrathecal morphine.[291,292] Paech et al.[277] compared **methylnaltrexone**, a peripherally acting µ-opioid receptor antagonist developed to antagonize the peripheral side effects of opioids while preserving centrally mediated analgesia, with placebo. Women undergoing elective cesarean delivery under spinal anesthesia with intrathecal morphine 0.1 mg were randomized to receive subcutaneous methylnaltrexone 12 mg or placebo after delivery. The incidence and severity of pruritus were not statistically different between groups, although the study may have been underpowered to identify a small effect. **Pentazocine**, a κ-opioid receptor agonist and partial µ-opioid receptor agonist, may be a useful drug for treating opioid-induced pruritus.[293–295] Hirabayashi et al.[296] randomized women scheduled for cesarean delivery with spinal anesthesia containing fentanyl 10 µg and morphine 0.1 mg to receive pentazocine 15 mg or saline-placebo. Pentazocine reduced the overall incidence of pruritus within the first 24 hours compared with saline.[296]

The effects of neuraxially administered opioid antagonists have also been investigated. Jeon et al.[297] reported less pruritus in patients who received epidural naloxone (1.2 mg over 48 hours) with epidural 0.1% bupivacaine and morphine (6 mg over 48 hours) than in patients in a control group. Similarly, Culebras et al.[232] investigated the effects of three different doses of intrathecal nalbuphine (0.2, 0.8, and 1.6 mg) and found a significantly lower incidence of pruritus in all of the nalbuphine groups compared with a control group that received intrathecal morphine without nalbuphine. However, the duration of analgesia was shorter among patients in the nalbuphine groups.[232] It is not clear whether an optimal dose of µ-opioid receptor antagonists

can be found that prevents pruritus without reducing analgesia. These drugs are not approved for administration into the neuraxial canal.

Propofol has been reported to relieve pruritus caused by neuraxial opioids in nonobstetric patients after a single 10-mg bolus dose[298] and after a 10-mg bolus dose followed by a 30 mg/24 hour infusion.[299] The mechanism of the antipruritic effect of propofol is unknown, and these results have not been replicated in obstetric patients who received subhypnotic doses of propofol (10 to 20 mg) for treatment of intrathecal morphine–induced pruritus.[300,301] A comparative study demonstrated that IV nalbuphine 3 mg is superior to propofol 20 mg for treating pruritus after administration of intrathecal morphine.[302]

Stimulation of 5-HT$_3$ receptors found in the dorsal horn of the spinal cord and in the nucleus of the spinal tract of the trigeminal nerve in the medulla may occur after subarachnoid opioid administration. A metaanalysis of studies of surgical patients receiving neuraxial opioids concluded that prophylaxis with a **5-HT$_3$ antagonist** results in a reduced risk for postoperative pruritus compared with placebo (OR, 0.44; 95% CI, 0.29 to 0.68).[303] IV **ondansetron** 4 to 8 mg has been shown to be more effective than placebo for reducing the incidence of postcesarean pruritus after intrathecal administration of morphine 0.15 to 0.2 mg.[304,305] However, other studies that compared ondansetron 8 mg with placebo found no significant reduction in pruritus after intrathecal administration of morphine (0.1 to 0.2 mg) alone[306] or in combination with a lipophilic opioid (sufentanil or fentanyl).[307,308] The lack of antipruritic effect in these studies may be caused by the peak effect of ondansetron occurring sooner (15 minutes after IV administration) than that of intrathecal morphine. The antipruritic effects associated with ondansetron may depend on the dose, lipophilicity, and duration of action of the intrathecal opioid.[309] Siddik-Sayyid et al.[306] found no significant difference in the incidence or severity of pruritus among patients who received **granisetron** 3 mg or ondansetron 8 mg or saline. In contrast, Tan et al.[310] observed that the severity of pruritus was reduced at 8 and 24 hours after cesarean delivery in patients who received granisetron 3 mg compared with those who received ondansetron 8 mg.

George et al.[266] reported a metaanalysis of studies of women who received spinal anesthesia with morphine for cesarean delivery; *prophylactic* administration of a 5-HT$_3$ antagonist did not reduce the risk for pruritus compared with the placebo-control group. However, administration of a 5-HT$_3$ antagonist reduced the severity of pruritus and the need for rescue treatment compared with a placebo. Heterogeneity and small sample sizes in the studies included in this systematic review limited detailed analysis of the efficacy of prophylactic administration of a 5-HT$_3$ antagonist. Few studies have assessed the *therapeutic* effect of 5-HT$_3$ antagonists for managing postcesarean pruritus induced by neuraxial opioids. In one study, ondansetron 4 mg had a high rate of success for the treatment of moderate-to-severe pruritus compared with placebo (80% and 36%, respectively).[311]

Historically, **antihistamines** have been a popular first choice for treatment of pruritus. However, the efficacy of these agents has been questioned in patients receiving neuraxial opioids, as histamine release is not the mechanism of pruritus. Alhashemi et al.[312] demonstrated that **diphenhydramine** was less effective than nalbuphine (higher itching scores and more treatment failures) after administration of intrathecal morphine 0.2 mg. Yeh et al.[305] found that the incidence of pruritus was comparable among patients receiving diphenhydramine 30 mg and placebo (80% and 85%, respectively); however, both groups had a higher incidence of pruritus compared with a group that received ondansetron 0.1 mg/kg (25%). In contrast, Siddik-Sayyid et al.[313] found that the therapeutic success rates for ondansetron 4 mg and diphenhydramine 25 mg were identical (70% for each drug), with similar recurrence rates in successfully treated patients (28% versus 35%, respectively). Differences in study methodology and antihistamine-induced sedation may explain the inconsistent antipruritic effect of diphenhydramine observed in these studies.

Urinary Retention

The mechanisms by which neuraxial opioids affect specific components of micturition (urge sensation, detrusor and sphincter function) are not fully understood, although spinal and supraspinal sites of action are likely to be involved. Kuipers et al.[314] performed urodynamic studies in healthy male volunteers who received intrathecal sufentanil or morphine. Both opioids caused dose-dependent decreases in detrusor contractility and the urgency to void. Volunteers who received intrathecal sufentanil had earlier recovery of lower urinary tract function than those who received intrathecal morphine. Intrathecal local anesthetics (bupivacaine and lidocaine) have also been shown to ablate detrusor contractility and urge sensation until the dermatomal block regresses to the S2 to S3 level, with no partial recovery until this regression has occurred.[315]

Evron et al.[316] performed an observational study investigating the urinary effects of epidural morphine and methadone in 120 women undergoing cesarean delivery. Not surprisingly given the longer duration of action, difficulty in micturition and need for bladder catheterization were greater in the morphine group (58%) compared with the methadone group (3%).[316] A similar study by Liang et al.[317] reported a higher incidence of postcesarean urinary retention and urinary catheterization (22%) among patients receiving epidural morphine compared with other analgesia modalities (PCEA with ropivacaine-fentanyl [7%] and IV meperidine [3%]). In a study of male volunteers, naloxone reversed the impact of neuraxial morphine on urodynamic function.[318]

To avoid impairment of bladder/detrusor function, urinary catheterization should be considered if voiding has not occurred within 6 hours.[319] Risk factors for postcesarean urinary retention include low BMI, multiparity, emergency cesarean delivery, prolonged operation time, perineal injury, and postoperative analgesia.[320,321] Transient postpartum voiding difficulty is not detrimental to urinary function and does not subsequently lead to voiding difficulties.[320] Reversal with systemic naloxone may be considered in problematic cases.

Neuraxial Nonopioid Analgesic Adjuvants

The search for improved analgesia from nonopioid medications has led to a search for neuraxial nonopioid adjuvants that may be additive or synergistic with standard cesarean anesthesia drugs. Potential advantages of neuraxial drug combinations include a reduction in dose of individual drugs (with subsequent reductions in dose-dependent side effects), in particular a reduction in postoperative opioid requirement and opioid-related side effects.[322]

Alpha$_2$-Adrenergic Receptor Agonists

Epidural and intrathecal alpha$_2$-adrenergic receptor agonists provide analgesia by activating the descending noradrenergic system, binding to presynaptic and postsynaptic alpha$_2$-adrenergic receptors at the spinal dorsal horn.[323,324] This process subsequently leads to norepinephrine release, which in turn modulates pain processing in the dorsal horn by inhibiting the release of substance P and increasing acetylcholine levels to produce analgesia.[325,326] **Clonidine**, an alpha$_2$-adrenergic receptor agonist, provides a more potent analgesic response with fewer side effects when administered neuraxially than systemically. Clonidine also potentiates sensory and motor block when administered with epidural local anesthetics and acts additively or synergistically with intraspinal opioids.[322,326] Pregnancy may enhance the analgesic effects of alpha$_2$-adrenergic receptor agonists, thus making them particularly valuable in this setting.[327] In combination with an intrathecal local anesthetic, intrathecal clonidine may prolong the regression of sensory block, improve postoperative analgesia, and decrease intraoperative pain.[328] However, a combination of intrathecal clonidine and local anesthetic may also increase the risk for hypotension in a non–dose-dependent manner.[328] Mendez et al.[329] compared the analgesic efficacy of low-dose epidural clonidine (400-μg bolus) versus high-dose clonidine (800-μg bolus), followed by epidural infusion at 10 or 20 μg/h after cesarean delivery. They observed short-lived, dose-dependent analgesia and sedation, and prolonged motor block, which might lead to delays in the discharge of patients from the postanesthesia care unit.

Several studies have investigated epidural clonidine in combination with epidural opioids for optimizing postcesarean analgesia. An isobolographic evaluation of epidural clonidine (in doses ranging from 50 to 400 μg) with fentanyl (15 to 135 μg) demonstrated nonsynergistic, additive effects between clonidine and fentanyl in patients recovering from cesarean delivery.[330] However, marked variability in drug response and failure of high doses to produce complete analgesia limited the validity of dose-response and ED$_{50}$ analyses. Capogna et al.[331] observed that the addition of clonidine 75 to 50 μg to epidural morphine 2 mg lengthened the duration of postcesarean analgesia without increasing the incidence of side effects.

A number of studies have evaluated the potential role of intrathecal clonidine for postcesarean analgesia. Ginosar et al.[332] administered intrathecal clonidine (0 to 100 µg) to healthy volunteers to assess the analgesic effect of doses less than 100 µg; analgesia to experimental heat pain was detected for doses greater than 25 µg.[332] Van Tuijl et al.[333] assessed postcesarean analgesia in patients who received intrathecal clonidine 75 µg combined with bupivacaine compared with intrathecal bupivacaine alone. Early postoperative analgesia (for 1 to 2 hours) was improved in patients who received clonidine; however, no difference was found in 24-hour morphine consumption between the groups, likely reflecting the short duration of action of a bolus dose of clonidine.

Interaction studies of intrathecal opioids combined with clonidine have investigated the contribution of each drug to analgesia and side effects. Benhamou et al.[334] evaluated postcesarean analgesic outcomes in patients who received hyperbaric bupivacaine alone, or bupivacaine and clonidine 75 µg, or bupivacaine with clonidine and fentanyl 12.5 µg. Patients who received the bupivacaine-clonidine-fentanyl combination reported less intraoperative pain and more prolonged postcesarean analgesia (time to first analgesia request 215 minutes) than those who received bupivacaine-clonidine and bupivacaine alone (183 and 137 minutes, respectively). However, higher rates of pruritus and sedation were reported for the bupivacaine-clonidine-fentanyl group. Paech et al.[335] performed a six-arm study assessing postcesarean analgesia after intrathecal bupivacaine 12.5 mg with fentanyl 15 µg and one of the following regimens: clonidine 150 µg; morphine 0.1 mg; morphine 0.1 mg with clonidine 30, 60, 90, or 150 µg. They concluded that the morphine-clonidine regimens provided optimal analgesia with lower pain scores at rest and with coughing in the first 4 hours. The minimum effective intrathecal dose of clonidine was 30 to 60 µg combined with bupivacaine, fentanyl 15 µg, and morphine 0.1 mg. However, an increase in intraoperative sedation was observed in all groups receiving clonidine.

Lavand'homme et al.[336] compared antihyperalgesic effects in patients receiving intrathecal clonidine 150 µg with bupivacaine, clonidine 75 µg with bupivacaine-sufentanil, or bupivacaine-sufentanil. The bupivacaine-clonidine 150-µg group had a smaller area of periincisional hyperalgesia and a lower incidence of hyperalgesia compared with the other study groups. However, no between-group differences were observed in postoperative morphine consumption or in pain scores before and after discharge. Carvalho et al.[337] randomized 195 women to receive intrathecal hyperbaric bupivacaine with morphine 0.05 mg, morphine 0.1 mg, or morphine 0.05 mg combined with clonidine 75 µg for surgical anesthesia. Pain intensity at rest or while coughing did not differ among groups.[337] During recovery, the incidences of hypotension, bradycardia, and sedation were similar among groups.

Allen et al.[338] performed a systematic review and metaanalysis evaluating the effect of neuraxial clonidine on 24-hour morphine consumption and time to first analgesic request in women undergoing elective cesarean delivery.

Eighteen studies were included in the analysis (12 intrathecal administration, 6 epidural administration). Neuraxial clonidine reduced 24-hour morphine consumption by 7.2 mg and prolonged time to first analgesic request by 135 minutes compared with the control group.[338] Intraoperative hypotension and intraoperative sedation were more frequent with neuraxial clonidine.

In summary, neuraxial clonidine may offer a small improvement in postcesarean analgesia in addition to that provided by neuraxial morphine. Epidural clonidine (150 to 800 µg) may prolong postcesarean analgesia when given in combination with epidural opioids. Intrathecal clonidine (75 to 450 µg) has modest efficacy and a relatively short duration of action. Ongoing concern about the adverse side-effect profile of epidural and intrathecal clonidine—notably sedation and hypotension—limit the neuraxial administration of this agent in most patients undergoing cesarean delivery. Additionally, in the United States, epidural clonidine has a "black box" warning stating that it is not recommended for obstetric, postpartum, or perioperative pain management because of the risk for hypotension and bradycardia that were identified after high doses. In selected cases, the anesthesia provider may conclude that the potential benefits outweigh the risks.

Dexmedetomidine is a highly selective alpha$_2$-adrenergic receptor agonist that provides some analgesic effects mediated at the spinal level. Its systemic administration is widespread in anesthesia and critical care; however, its use in peripheral nerve blocks and neuraxial anesthesia is off-label.[339] In one of the few studies evaluating neuraxial dexmedetomidine, 80 healthy women were randomly assigned to a control group (intrathecal hyperbaric bupivacaine 5 mg and an epidural mixture of 10 mL plain bupivacaine 0.25% and fentanyl 50 µg) or a study group who received the same drugs with the addition of *epidural* dexmedetomidine (0.5 µg/kg).[340] The dexmedetomidine group required less intraoperative and postoperative fentanyl than the control group (4/40 and 18/40, respectively). There was no difference between the groups in block characteristics or sedation.[340] In a study of *intrathecal* dexmedetomidine for cesarean anesthesia, Qi et al.[341] compared bupivacaine 10 mg, bupivacaine 10 mg combined with dexmedetomidine 5 µg, and bupivacaine 10 mg combined with morphine 0.1 mg. Sensory blockade was longer in the dexmedetomidine group than in other groups. Intrathecal dexmedetomidine provided similar analgesia and less pruritus and shivering compared with morphine.[341] Dexmedetomidine via the neuraxial route is currently not approved by any regulatory body.

Epinephrine has a direct analgesic effect by activating alpha$_2$-adrenergic receptors and may potentiate local anesthetics by inducing local vasoconstriction through alpha$_1$-adrenergic activation, resulting in slower drug clearance. Several clinical studies have investigated epinephrine as a spinal or epidural adjunct. Robertson et al.[97] reported that *epidural* epinephrine 25 µg prolonged the duration of analgesia with epidural fentanyl 100 µg but increased the incidence of pruritus. Similar prolongation of analgesia has been observed when epinephrine (5 to 30 µg/mL) was combined with epidural diamorphine or sufentanil; however, the incidence of side effects (including vomiting that required treatment) was also increased.[164,342] In contrast, McMorland et al.[343] did not replicate this finding, although their study was not powered to demonstrate noninferiority. Importantly, studies of the addition of epidural epinephrine (5 μg/mL) to 2% lidocaine or 0.5% bupivacaine have not demonstrated any detrimental effects of epinephrine on umbilical artery blood-flow velocity waveforms, uteroplacental or fetal vascular resistance, fetal myocardial function, or fetal heart rate or neonatal outcomes.[344,345]

The use of *intrathecal* epinephrine as an adjunct to local anesthetics, with or without opioids, has been evaluated in several studies. The addition of epinephrine 200 μg to hyperbaric spinal bupivacaine improved perioperative analgesia but was associated with a longer duration of residual sensory and motor block.[346] In a separate study, a combined intrathecal regimen of epinephrine 200 μg with morphine 0.2 mg improved intra- and postoperative analgesia compared with intrathecal morphine 0.2 mg alone.[347] Zakowski et al.[348] found earlier and higher peak plasma bupivacaine concentrations with the addition of spinal epinephrine 200 μg to spinal bupivacaine in patients undergoing cesarean delivery. In contrast, plasma levels of morphine were approximately 66% *lower* in the epinephrine group than in the control group.[348] The investigators concluded that the enhanced efficacy of intrathecal bupivacaine combined with morphine and epinephrine was not caused by vasoconstriction alone.

In summary, the use of epidural epinephrine (2.5 to 30 μg/mL) seems to prolong the duration of analgesia with epidural opioids but may increase side effects. The use of intrathecal epinephrine 200 μg does seem to enhance neuraxial opioid analgesia but is associated with prolonged sensory and motor block.

Neostigmine

By interfering with the breakdown of acetylcholine, neostigmine indirectly stimulates spinal nicotinic and muscarinic receptors and the release of nitric oxide. As both nicotinic and muscarinic receptors are important to central and peripheral pain transmission, the resulting analgesia may be caused by central and/or peripheral alterations in pain modulation and transmission. Initial studies of *intrathecal* neostigmine in animals and human volunteers have demonstrated analgesic effects without neurotoxic effects.[349–351] However, despite producing dose-dependent analgesia, intrathecal neostigmine results in nausea that is particularly resistant to traditional antiemetic treatment, and therefore the use of intrathecal neostigmine is generally not recommended.

Kaya et al.[352] assessed the analgesic efficacy of *epidural* neostigmine administration after cesarean delivery. A CSE technique was employed with intrathecal bupivacaine 8 mg and fentanyl 10 μg, and patients subsequently received epidural neostigmine doses of 75, 150, or 300 μg after delivery. The investigators reported modest, short-lived, and dose-independent reductions in postoperative pain in the neostigmine groups.[352] No differences among groups in 24-hour morphine consumption after surgery were observed.

Epidural neostigmine is not currently recommended for routine use until additional studies substantiate clinically significant postcesarean analgesic benefits with fewer side effects compared with alternatives. Data regarding the maternal and fetal safety profile of epidural neostigmine are reassuring.[353]

N-Methyl-ᴅ-Aspartate Receptor Antagonists

Ketamine. Limited data exist regarding the role of neuraxial ketamine in the provision of postcesarean analgesia. Anesthetic and subanesthetic doses of ketamine have analgesic properties via noncompetitive antagonism of NMDA receptors. In patients undergoing cesarean delivery randomly assigned to receive intrathecal bupivacaine alone or in combination with S(+) ketamine 0.05 mg/kg or fentanyl 25 μg, significantly prolonged and better quality analgesia was observed in the fentanyl group.[354] It is unclear whether the S(+) or R(-) isomers of ketamine have analgesic advantages over the racemate. No published studies have evaluated perioperative epidural ketamine administration in patients undergoing cesarean delivery. At this time, neuraxial use cannot be recommended for patients undergoing cesarean delivery because there is a lack of data regarding the safety of neuraxial administration.

Magnesium. **Magnesium** is a noncompetitive antagonist of the NMDA receptor and may alter pain signaling by preventing central sensitization after nociceptive stimulation.[355] Magnesium blocks NMDA ion channels in a voltage-dependent manner. Studies investigating intrathecal and epidural magnesium have shown variable analgesic effects after cesarean delivery. Sun et al.[356] compared the postcesarean analgesic profile of four different *epidural* solutions administered in the perioperative period. All patients received 0.1% bupivacaine 10 mL with one of the following: morphine 1.5 mg, magnesium 500 mg, morphine 1.5 mg and magnesium 500 mg, or placebo. Patients who received magnesium and morphine had lower postoperative pain scores at rest and with movement, an increased time to first analgesic request, and increased satisfaction at 24 hours after surgery compared with women who received only one drug or placebo. Albrecht et al.[357] reviewed 18 trials (including some trials in women undergoing cesarean delivery) of the efficacy and safety of neuraxial magnesium sulfate for postoperative analgesia. They observed an overall increase in the interval to first analgesic request (mean difference of 40 minutes after intrathecal administration and 110 minutes after epidural administration). However, only four trials assessed neurologic complications, and the authors concluded that there were not enough patients ($n = 140$) to evaluate the risk for neurologic complications.

Intrathecal magnesium sulfate 50 mg prolonged the duration of spinal anesthesia and improved postoperative analgesia in patients undergoing nonobstetric surgery with bupivacaine and fentanyl spinal anesthesia.[358,359] In women undergoing cesarean delivery, no difference in the first request for postcesarean analgesia was found among patients who were randomized to receive intrathecal magnesium sulfate 50 mg compared with placebo (median time, 100 versus

105 minutes, respectively); patients who received intrathecal fentanyl 25 µg had a longer time to first request for analgesia (132 minutes) compared with those who received magnesium.[360]

In summary, neuraxial administration of magnesium may have a favorable analgesic effect in patients after cesarean delivery. However, more research, including dose-response studies and comparison with systemic administration, are needed to formally assess the analgesic efficacy of epidural and intrathecal magnesium.

Experimental Agents

In the future, newer agents and adjuvants may enhance postoperative pain management strategies in patients receiving neuraxial anesthesia for cesarean delivery. **Adenosine** (and adenosine analogues) have been proposed to have antinociceptive activity related to activation of spinal adenosine A_1 receptors.[361] However, studies have not demonstrated improved analgesia with intrathecal adenosine administration in patients undergoing hysterectomy[362,363] or for labor analgesia.[364]

Intrathecal **midazolam** may have a favorable pharmacologic profile for cesarean anesthesia. After cesarean delivery, patients who received intrathecal midazolam 2 mg (without neuraxial opioids) had prolonged postoperative analgesia, reduced requirement for rescue analgesic, and lower pain scores for 6 hours after surgery compared with patients who received either intrathecal midazolam 1 mg or no midazolam.[365] Dodawad et al.[366] randomly assigned 60 women with pregnancy-induced hypertension undergoing cesarean delivery to receive intrathecal bupivacaine 10 mg (control group) or bupivacaine combined with midazolam 2 mg (study group). Postoperative analgesia was longer in the midazolam group than in the control group (202 and 358 minutes, respectively). A systematic review and metaanalysis by Hung et al.[367] demonstrated that adjuvant intrathecal midazolam prolonged the time to the first analgesic and decreased perioperative maternal nausea and vomiting but with more sedation. It is unknown whether intrathecal midazolam has any benefit compared with intrathecal morphine or in addition to morphine.

Several neuraxially administered drugs have been shown to produce antinociceptive effects by altering calcium channel conductance in the spinal cord. Intrathecal **gabapentin** reduced incision-induced allodynia in rats,[368,369] and epidural **verapamil** lowered postoperative opioid consumption after lower abdominal surgery.[370] **Ziconotide**, a neuronal N-type-selective voltage-sensitive calcium entry–blocking agent, has been shown to have analgesic effects after intrathecal administration in chronic pain patients.[371]

Before recommendations can be made about the potential use of new adjunct agents, neurotoxicity studies are necessary to ensure these agents' safety for neuraxial administration. In addition, studies assessing analgesic efficacy, side effects, and toxicity must demonstrate that these agents result in significant improvement over the neuraxial local anesthetic and opioid regimens currently used in clinical practice.

NONNEURAXIAL REGIONAL ANALGESIC TECHNIQUES

Although neuraxial opioids are commonly recommended for postcesarean analgesia, there may be a role for regional analgesic techniques in patients whose neuraxial blocks are contraindicated or who are at elevated risk of opioid-related adverse effects.

Fascial Sheath Blocks

The TAP block, the QLB, and the erector spinae plane (ESP) block are fascial sheath blocks that have been investigated for postcesarean analgesia. In clinical practice, the blocks are usually performed using ultrasonography to verify correct needle position and site of injection. In the TAP block, infiltration is between the internal oblique and the transversus abdominis muscle layers (Fig. 27.8), in the QLB (Fig. 27.9), infiltration is adjacent to the anterolateral aspect of the quadratus lumborum muscle, and in the ESP block, infiltration is within the plane deep to the erector spinae muscle. Those techniques block the plexus of nerves supplying the anterior abdominal wall. Some have suggested the possibility that the QLB and ESP block may have greater efficacy than the TAP block because of spread of the local anesthetic solution beyond the muscle fascia into an interfascial plane close to the paravertebral space,[372] thereby providing some visceral analgesia, whereas TAP block provide mainly analgesia for incisional pain.[373] Chin et al.[374] provided a detailed review of the anatomy of abdominal wall blocks.

Several systematic reviews and metaanalyses of TAP blocks for postcesarean analgesia have been completed and reported similar findings. Mishriky et al.[92] reviewed the efficacy of TAP blocks after cesarean delivery with primary outcomes of pain intensity scores and opioid consumption at 24 hours. Nine studies compared TAP blocks with inactive controls, seven of them done in combination with spinal anesthesia for cesarean delivery. In women who did not receive intrathecal morphine, TAP blocks reduced opioid consumption (mean difference, –20.2 mg morphine equivalents; 95% CI, –33.7 to –6.8 mg) and opioid-related side effects.[92] In patients who received intrathecal morphine, there was no difference between TAP blocks and inactive controls in pain scores at 24 hours, and the impact on opioid consumption was inconclusive. Three studies directly compared TAP blocks with intrathecal morphine (two with 0.1 mg and one with 0.2 mg). Intrathecal morphine provided lower pain scores on movement (mean difference, –0.98; 95% CI, –1.91 to –0.06) and reduced 24-hour opioid consumption (mean difference, –8.4 mg morphine equivalents; 95% CI, –15.1 to –1.7 mg).[92] In a subsequent metaanalysis, Champaneria et al.[375] confirmed that TAP blocks are effective but do not confer additional analgesia when intrathecal morphine is included as part of a multimodal analgesia regimen.

The QLB is an abdominal fascial block similar to the TAP block, but with potential for the local anesthetic to spread into the paravertebral space, therefore providing more visceral analgesia because the point of injection is more posterior.

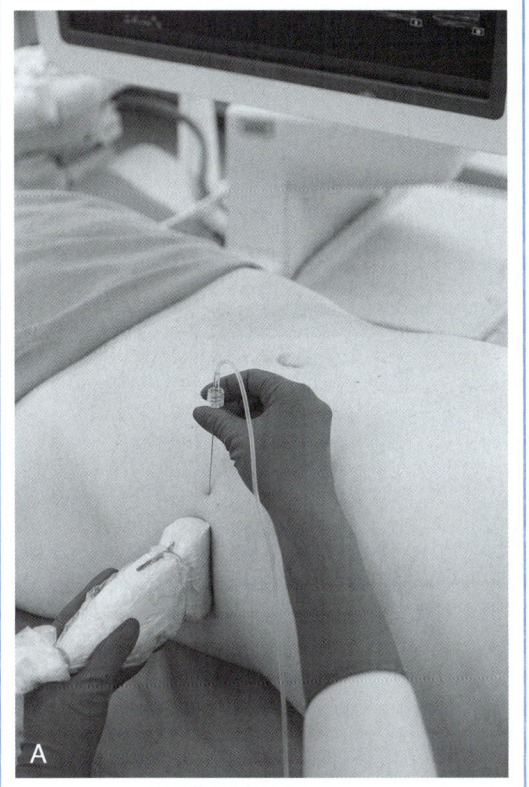
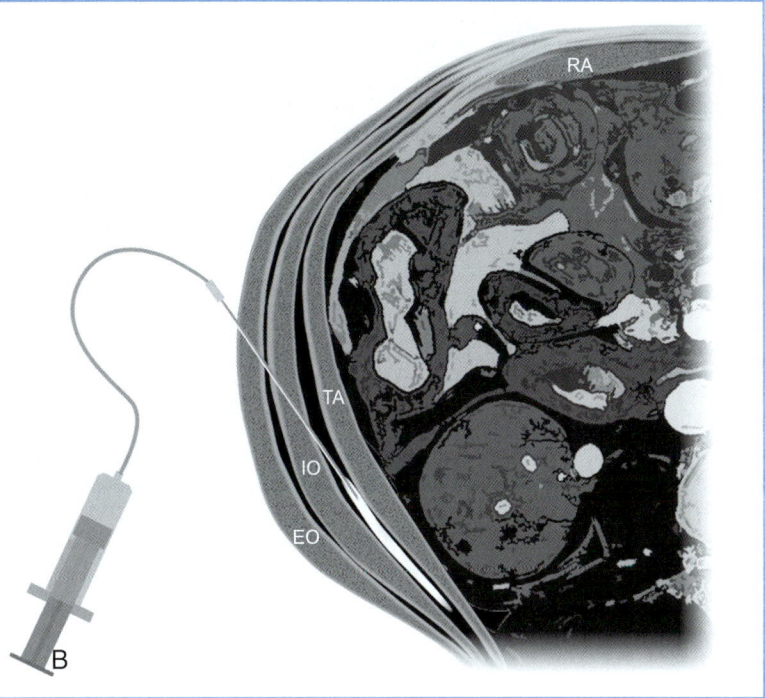

Fig. 27.8 Midaxillary Transversus Abdominis Plane (TAP) Block. (A) With the patient in the supine position, the transducer is placed near the midaxillary line between the costal margin and pelvic brim for a transverse imaging plane. (B) Line drawing of a transverse section through the abdominal wall with local anesthetic injected in the transversus abdominis plane. *EO*, External oblique; *IO*, internal oblique; *RA*, rectus abdominis; *TA*, transversus abdominis. The transversus abdominis plane lies between the internal oblique and transversus abdominis muscles. Visualization of an elliptical distribution of the local anesthetic with well-defined margins provides evidence for the proper injection of the solution into the plane between the internal oblique and transversus abdominis muscles. From Gray AT. *Atlas of Ultrasound-Guided Regional Anesthesia*. 2nd ed. Elsevier; 2013.

QLB types 1, 2, and 3 are described based on the location of local anesthetic administration relative to the quadratum lumborum muscle; consensus on the best approach is lacking.[374] Tan et al.[93] performed a systematic review with metaanalysis and trial sequential analysis of 10 studies to assess the efficacy of QLBs for postcesarean analgesia. In the absence of neuraxial morphine, QLBs were associated with a significant reduction in 24-hour opioid consumption (mean difference −10.6 mg morphine equivalents; 95% CI, −16.0 to −5.3 mg), as well as lower opioid consumption at 6 and 12 hours; lower pain scores at rest and on movement at 12 hours; and lower pain scores on movement at 6 hours. There was no benefit of QLBs in the presence of neuraxial morphine or when used in conjunction with neuraxial morphine.

It is unclear if QLBs provide improved analgesia compared with TAP blocks. A systematic review and network metaanalysis suggested that QLBs and TAP blocks provided comparable postoperative analgesia and opioid-sparing effects, with both techniques being superior to inactive control in the absence of intrathecal morphine, but they provided no additional benefit when intrathecal morphine was used.[376] This review was, however, limited by a modest quality of evidence, the fact that all QLB approaches (lateral, posterior, and

anterior/transmuscular) and TAP block approaches (posterior and lateral) were combined, and several indirect comparisons were included; therefore, the conclusions should be interpreted with caution. On the other hand, a few studies directly compared QLBs with TAP blocks and suggested some benefit associated with QLBs. Blanco et al.[377] reported a randomized placebo-controlled trial of QLBs after cesarean delivery; 25 women who did not receive neuraxial morphine received QLBs with 0.125% bupivacaine 0.2 mL/kg, and outcomes were compared with 25 women who received a placebo block with saline. Patients in the QLB group used less morphine at 6 and 12 hours postoperatively; the difference was not significant at 24 hours (median dose, 11 mg [IQR 5 to 18 mg] and 19 mg [IQR 11 to 36 mg], respectively; $P = .11$).[377] Similarly, Blanco et al.[372] compared QLBs and TAP blocks in women scheduled for elective cesarean delivery under spinal anesthesia with bupivacaine and fentanyl. Women in the QLB group used less morphine than those in the TAP block group, with no difference in pain scores between groups. Jadon et al.[378] also compared QLBs with TAP blocks in women undergoing scheduled cesarean delivery under spinal anesthesia with bupivacaine. Performance of QLBs was associated with longer time to first analgesia, lower analgesic

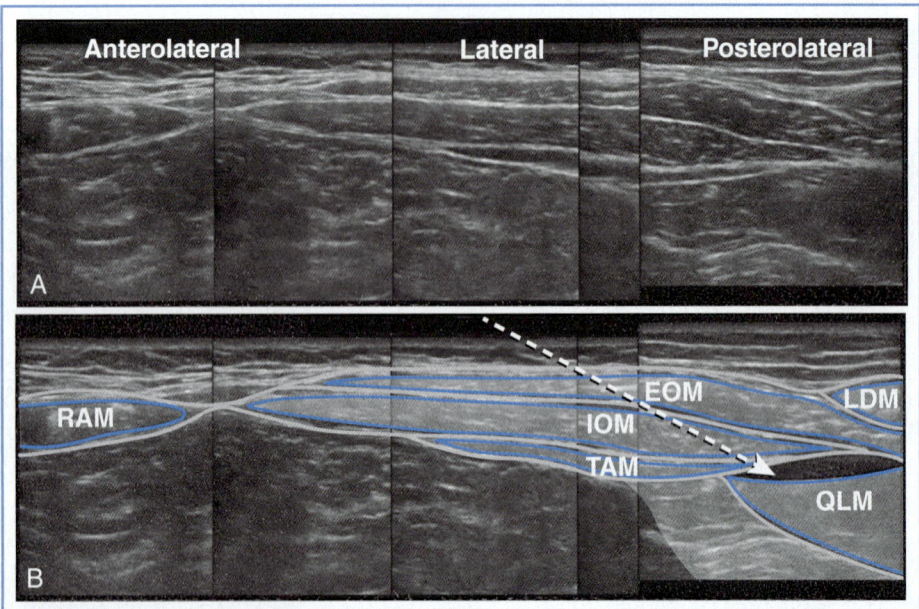

Fig. 27.9 Ultrasonographic Image of the Quadratus Lumborum Block-1 (QLB-1). (A) With the patient in the supine position, the three muscle layers of the abdomen and the quadratus lumborum muscle are visualized with a high-frequency linear probe. (B) The abdominal fascial planes and the infiltration site for the QLB-1 between the quadratus lumborum muscle and the medial layer of the thoracolumbar fascia are clearly outlined. The *broken arrow* shows the needle path and point of injection. *EOM*, External oblique muscle; *IOM*, internal oblique muscle; *LDM*, latissimus dorsi muscle; *QLM*, quadratus lumborum muscle; *RAM*, rectus abdominus muscle; *TAM*, transversus abdominus muscle. Modified from Murouchi T, Iwasaki S, Yamakage M. Quadratus lumborum block: analgesic effects and chronological ropivacaine concentrations after laparoscopic surgery. *Reg Anesth Pain Med.* 2016;41:146–150.

consumption, lower pain scores, and higher satisfaction compared with TAP blocks. Future research should assess if QLBs add benefit to current multimodal analgesia practices.

Data regarding the ESP block are very limited. A metaanalysis including only three studies concluded that ESP blocks may be associated with reduced postoperative opioid consumption with no difference in pain scores compared with control, but the quality of evidence was very low.[379] Similar to QLBs, the analgesia provided with ESP blocks might be superior to that provided by TAP blocks in the absence of neuraxial morphine,[373,380] but data are limited. Boules et al.[373] randomized women undergoing scheduled cesarean delivery to receive TAP blocks or ESP blocks following spinal anesthesia with bupivacaine. The ESP block group had longer duration to first request for analgesia, lower pain scores, and lower opioid consumption compared with the TAP block group ($n = 30$ per group). Similarly, Malawat et al.[380] found longer time to first rescue analgesia and lower opioid consumption with ESP blocks compared with TAP blocks following spinal anesthesia with bupivacaine ($n = 30$ per group). In contrast, two studies compared QLBs and ESP blocks for analgesia following cesarean delivery. Priya et al.[381] found no differences in postoperative opioid consumption, pain scores, or quality of recovery scores between patients who received QLB type 2 or ESP blocks following spinal anesthesia with intrathecal bupivacaine ($n = 26$ per group). Similarly, Bakshi et al.[382] reported no differences in time to first request for analgesia, pain scores, and analgesic consumption in women who received spinal anesthesia with bupivacaine and fentanyl and

were randomized to receive QLBs or ESP blocks ($n = 30$ per group).

Current data support the conclusion that abdominal fascial sheath blocks may represent a reasonable alternative for patients who are unable to receive neuraxial morphine, and they may serve as a rescue technique in special cases.[92,93,383] However, they are not superior to neuraxial opioid analgesia–based multimodal techniques, which remain the gold standard for postcesarean analgesia. Additionally, because analgesia from TAP blocks may be comparable to that provided by simple wound infiltration or a continuous wound infiltration catheter (see later discussion), the value of TAP blocks in postcesarean analgesia remains unclear.

The use of liposomal bupivacaine however might confer some benefits, even in the presence of neuraxial morphine. Habib et al.[384] randomized women undergoing cesarean delivery to three groups: TAP blocks with liposomal bupivacaine (no intrathecal morphine), TAP blocks with liposomal bupivacaine and low dose intrathecal morphine (50 μg), and intrathecal bupivacaine 150 μg (no TAP block). Opioid consumption in morphine milligram equivalents through 72 hours was noninferior in both the TAP block-alone group (least squares mean, 19.2 [SE 1.2]) and the TAP block-with-low-dose intrathecal morphine group (14.6 [1.2]) versus the intrathecal morphine-alone group (16.4 [1.2]). The severity of pruritus was higher in the intrathecal morphine-alone group compared with the other two groups. When examining opioid consumption in the first 24 hours, the TAP block-alone group was inferior to the other two groups.

Complications of the fascial plane blocks are infrequent and include local anesthetic systemic toxicity (LAST) from systemic absorption of local anesthetic or intravascular injection, and bowel perforation. The described potential benefit of QLB, spread to the paravertebral space, may also result in unintended motor blockade. Wikner[385] described a patient with hip flexion and knee extension weakness that led to unplanned overnight admission following QLB with 20 mL of 0.25% levobupivacaine for a laparoscopic gynecologic procedure. Presumably, paravertebral spread to the lumbar spinal nerves led to weakness of the psoas and quadriceps muscles.

The relationships between local anesthetic dose, volume, concentration, and response have not been well studied, and consensus on the optimal volume and concentration of local anesthetic for single-shot abdominal fascial plane blocks is lacking. Griffiths et al.[386] performed a bilateral TAP block with a total ropivacaine dose of 2.5 mg/kg (diluted with 0.9% saline to a total volume of 40 mL) in women who had spinal anesthesia for elective cesarean delivery (dose corresponding to 20 mL of 0.5% ropivacaine on each side for an 80-kg patient). The mean ($\pm$ SD) peak plasma ropivacaine concentration 30 minutes after injection was $1.82 \pm 0.69\,\mu g/mL$. Although this concentration is below the reported threshold for LAST ($2.2\,\mu g/mL$), 12 of 30 patients had peak concentration measurements above this threshold (maximum, $3.76\,\mu g/mL$), and 3 patients had symptoms of mild LAST (perioral tingling, metallic taste).[386] Similarly, Trabelsi et al.[387] demonstrated that bilateral TAP block with bupivacaine 100 mg (total dose) led to plasma concentrations above the reported toxic threshold in 3 of 17 women; plasma bupivacaine concentration above the threshold value persisted for as long as 90 minutes. The addition of epinephrine to the local anesthetic solution decreases local anesthetic peak plasma concentration.[388] Clinically significant LAST (seizures) has been reported following TAP block in obstetric patients.[389–391]

The concentration of local anesthetic (ropivacaine, bupivacaine, levobupivacaine) has ranged from 0.125% to 0.5% for QLBs and TAP blocks. A 2018 metaanalysis comparing high (>50 mg) versus low doses ($\leq$50-mg bupivacaine equivalents per side) for TAP blocks in women undergoing cesarean delivery found no difference in opioid consumption, time to first analgesia, pain scores, or satisfaction between doses.[392] Given current reports, we suggest that a local anesthetic dose less than 2.5 mg/kg should be used and that patients should be observed for LAST for at least 30 minutes after these blocks are performed.[393]

Ilioinguinal and iliohypogastric blocks also reduced cumulative morphine consumption at 6 and 24 hours, in addition to pain scores at 6, 12, and 24 hours during movement compared with controls.[394] A network metaanalysis investigated the analgesic effectiveness of regional analgesia with or without intrathecal morphine and found that combined ilioinguinal nerve and anterior TAP block in conjunction with intrathecal morphine was the most effective in reducing postcesarean pain and 24-hour morphine consumption, compared with the other techniques. Of the regional analgesic techniques studied, only the combined ilioinguinal nerve and anterior TAP block was associated with reduced rest pain at 6 hours, compared with intrathecal morphine alone.[395]

Wound Infusion Catheters

Continuous wound infusion of local anesthetic can provide effective adjunctive analgesia after cesarean delivery, reducing postoperative opioid consumption and increasing the time to rescue analgesia. This is principally true in patients who do not receive neuraxial morphine. Adesope et al.[396] conducted a systematic review of randomized trials to assess the efficacy of local anesthetic wound infusion in women undergoing cesarean delivery. Wound infusion reduced opioid consumption at 24 hours (morphine equivalent –9.7 mg), as well as pain scores at rest and on movement at 24 hours, although the reduction in pain scores was small and might not be clinically relevant and did not reduce opioid-related side effects.[396] The opioid-sparing effect was seen in patients who did not receive neuraxial morphine, but not in those who received neuraxial morphine, although the data in patients who received neuraxial morphine were limited to only two studies.

In a study comparing pain control and prevention of persistent postcesarean pain, Gómez-Ríos et al.[397] assessed secondary hyperalgesia following cesarean delivery. In elective cesarean delivery with spinal anesthesia (0.5% hyperbaric bupivacaine with fentanyl) patients had a multihole wound catheter placed beneath the fascia and were randomized to receive continuous 0.35% levobupivacaine 7 mL/h for 48 hours or an equal volume of saline. There was no difference in secondary hyperalgesia using a dynamic hyperalgesia test for punctate mechanical stimuli at 24, 48, or 72 hours, nor was there any difference in somatic or visceral postoperative pain on movement or at rest.[397]

Lalmand et al.[398] randomly allocated patients undergoing elective cesarean delivery into three groups: control, intrathecal morphine, and wound catheter infusion. All patients received spinal anesthesia with bupivacaine and sufentanil, and a multiorifice catheter was inserted into the wound. The control group received saline intrathecally, the intrathecal morphine group received intrathecal morphine 0.1 mg and saline infusion through the wound catheter, and the wound catheter infusion group received intrathecal saline and 0.2% ropivacaine infused through the catheter (15-mL bolus followed by a 10-mL/h infusion). The results showed that intrathecal morphine and wound catheter infusion increased the time to the first oral morphine request and reduced morphine consumption compared with the control group. Wound infusion was not superior to intrathecal morphine for analgesia and had a similar side-effect profile.[398] Barney et al.[399] randomized 71 women who had elective cesarean delivery with a multimodal postoperative analgesic regimen incorporating intrathecal morphine 150 µg to receive wound infiltration with ropivacaine with ketorolac or placebo. There were no differences between the groups in the primary endpoint of pain scores on movement at 24 hours or in any of the secondary outcomes of opioid consumption or pain scores over 48 hours.

A network metaanalysis of randomized controlled trials by Singh et al.[400] compared avenues of injection of local anesthetics for pain-related outcomes after cesarean delivery. Compared with ilioinguinal, TAP, and erector spinae blocks, continuous wound infiltration was less successful at reducing postoperative morphine equivalents (mean reduction 8 mg).[400] Confidence in the results was very low based upon small sample sizes and extensive heterogeneity in methodologies.

Continuous wound infusion below the fascia has been shown to be more effective in reducing postcesarean morphine consumption compared with infusion above the fascia.[396,401] Klasen et al.[402] evaluated a multimodal analgesic regimen for cesarean delivery and found no difference between TAP blocks and continuous subfascial wound infiltration. Several studies compared wound infusion with TAP blocks. A systematic review and network metaanalysis found no differences in analgesic efficacy between the two techniques, with both being more effective than inactive controls in patients who did not receive neuraxial morphine.[403] Although some centers use wound-infusion catheters, the additional cost of the pump and some minor inconveniences, such as wound leakage, may have discouraged widespread use.

Ilioinguinal-Iliohypogastric Block

Ilioinguinal-iliohypogastric nerve block is useful for postoperative analgesia after lower abdominal surgery. Similar to TAP blocks, the block can be performed with ultrasonographic guidance. Evidence is inconsistent as to whether ilioinguinal-iliohypogastric blocks improve analgesia provided by neuraxial morphine.[404,405] A metaanalysis reported that the ilioinguinal-iliohypogastric nerve blocks were associated with a significant reduction in 24-hour opioid consumption (−15.57 mg [95% CI, −19.87 to −11.28 mg] morphine equivalents) and pain scores, a decrease in the risk of PONV (OR 0.45 [95% CI, 0.27 to 0.75]), and a longer time to first request for analgesia (mean difference 6.29 hours [95% CI, 3.56 to 9.01 hours]) compared with a placebo or no block.[406] The quality of evidence was, however, low owing to the significant heterogeneity of included studies.

The **ilioinguinal-TAP (I-TAP) block** is a combination of ilioinguinal block with TAP block to address sparing of the L1 dermatome that may occur in up to 50% of TAP blocks.[407] In a randomized controlled trial, the addition of the I-TAP block to a multimodal analgesia regimen that incorporated 150 µg intrathecal morphine resulted in a 59% reduction in opioid consumption (fentanyl PCA) over the first 24 hours, together with a reduction in pain scores at rest and on movement.[408] Further studies are needed to confirm these findings.

Subcutaneous Infiltration of Local Anesthetic

Subcutaneous local wound infiltration is a relatively simple component of multimodal postoperative analgesia. In a study of patients who did not receive neuraxial morphine for postcesarean analgesia, infiltration of 0.25% bupivacaine

with epinephrine (40 mL) before wound closure was associated with decreased opioid requirement in the first 12 hours compared with a saline-placebo.[409] Similarly, in another study of 288 women undergoing scheduled cesarean delivery under spinal anesthesia without intrathecal morphine, Garmi et al.[410] reported that single infiltration of 30 mL of 0.25% bupivacaine with epinephrine 1:200,000 at the end of surgery significantly reduced pain scores and need for rescue opioids and increased patient satisfaction compared with a control group that received no wound infiltration. In the absence of intrathecal morphine, a systematic review and network metaanalysis suggested that wound infiltration may confer similar analgesia to bilateral TAP blocks following cesarean delivery with spinal anesthesia.[403] Simavli et al.[411] randomized patients who had general anesthesia for cesarean delivery to receive bupivacaine-soaked absorbable gelatin sponges or placebo, placed in the wound. Pain scores were lower in the sponge group compared with the control group, and fewer patients required rescue opioid. Adesope et al.[396] conducted a systematic review to assess the efficacy of local anesthetic wound infiltration in women undergoing cesarean delivery. Wound infiltration reduced opioid consumption at 24 hours (−8.9 mg morphine equivalents) and was associated with a small non–clinically relevant reduction in pain scores at rest at 24 hours, but did not reduce opioid-related side effects.[396] Of interest, this metaanalysis suggested that there were no differences in opioid consumption and pain scores in the first 24 hours between single infiltration and wound infusion techniques. In contrast, wound infiltration with 40 mL liposomal bupivacaine at the end of cesarean delivery was not effective in reducing pain scores or opioid consumption in the first 48 hours in women who received neuraxial morphine and scheduled NSAIDs and acetaminophen.[412]

Intraperitoneal Local Anesthetic

Intraperitoneal administration of local anesthetic has been investigated as a component of multimodal analgesia, as well as a method for the management of severe pain occurring intraoperatively. Patel et al.[413] investigated intraperitoneal administration of 20 mL lidocaine 2% in epinephrine 1:200,000 or saline-placebo before peritoneal or fascial closure in 204 women who received a multimodal analgesic regimen incorporating 100 µg intrathecal morphine with scheduled NSAIDs and acetaminophen. There were no differences between the groups in pain scores on movement (primary outcome) or at rest at 24 hours. Pain scores on movement and at rest were, however, lower at 2 hours in the intraperitoneal local anesthetic group, and fewer patients required opioids in this group compared with the saline group (40% versus 65%, P = .001). Peritoneal closure was not standardized, but a subgroup analysis suggested a reduction in the primary outcome of pain score on movement in women who underwent peritoneal closure (n = 64), but not in those without peritoneal closure. Werntz et al.[414] described a case series of 32 patients who received intraperitoneal chloroprocaine for the management of severe pain during cesarean delivery after delivery of the baby. The doses of 3% chloroprocaine ranged from 20 to 60 mL 3% chloroprocaine, with the most common dose given being 40 mL (mean dose 11.8 mg/kg). The authors reported improvement of pain scores in 17 of those patients, with no signs of LAST or need for conversion to general anesthesia. The same group performed a prospective study of 15 women who had spinal anesthesia and received 40 mL of intraperitoneal chloroprocaine (1%, 2%, or 3%) after delivery of the baby.[415] There were no clinical symptoms of LAST. The time to maximum plasma chloroprocaine concentration was 5 minutes and the half-life was 5.3 minutes, with a peak plasma concentration of 799.2 ng/mL (79.9 µg/kg), which was well below the authors' predefined safe level of exposure (970 µg/kg) and levels associated with clinical symptoms (2.6 to 2.9 mg/kg).

KEY POINTS

- Cesarean deliveries account for nearly one-third of all deliveries in the United States; therefore, strategies for reducing adverse postcesarean maternal outcomes, including postoperative pain, have important clinical and public health implications.
- Effective postoperative analgesia confers many physiologic and psychological benefits and may improve maternal and neonatal outcomes after cesarean delivery.
- Multimodal techniques provide efficient postcesarean analgesia by acting on different pain pathways to maximize analgesia while limiting side effects.
- Neuraxial morphine administration currently represents the "gold standard" for providing effective postcesarean analgesia and is the most important component of multimodal analgesia.
- Morphine has the longest duration of action among available neuraxial opioids. Neuraxial administration of opioids provides better postoperative pain relief than systemic administration.
- Single-dose epidural (2 to 4 mg) or intrathecal (0.075 to 0.2 mg) morphine administration is most commonly administered for postcesarean analgesia. Higher doses may increase opioid-related side effects without improving analgesia.

- Nonopioid neuraxial adjuncts (e.g., alpha$_2$-adrenergic receptor agonists, anticholinesterases) may be considered as alternatives to, or combined with, neuraxial opioids. However, these adjuncts are associated with modest analgesic benefits, and the related risk for spinal neurotoxicity remains to be determined.
- Opioids are the most common systemic medications administered for postcesarean analgesia. Adverse effects, which often limit their use, include respiratory depression, sedation, constipation, nausea and vomiting, urinary retention, and pruritus.
- Oral analgesic adjuvants (acetaminophen, NSAIDs) should be prescribed at scheduled intervals, rather than on patient request.
- Abdominal fascial sheath blocks may represent a reasonable alternative for patients who are unable to receive longer acting neuraxial opioids, or they may be used as a rescue technique in selected cases.
- Local wound instillation may be considered in addition to neuraxial opioids, acetaminophen, and NSAIDs to provide further multimodal analgesia.

REFERENCES

1. Stephenson J. Rate of first-time cesarean deliveries on the rise in the US. *JAMA Health Forum*. 2022;3:e222824.
2. Osterman MJK, Hamilton BE, Martin JA, et al. Births: final data for 2021. *Natl Vital Stat Rep*. 2023;72:1–53.
3. Sun KW, Pan PH. Persistent pain after cesarean delivery. *Int J Obstet Anesth*. 2019;40:78–90.
4. Dolin SJ, Cashman JN, Bland JM. Effectiveness of acute postoperative pain management: I. Evidence from published data. *Br J Anaesth*. 2002;89:409–423.
5. Houle TT, Miller S, Lang JE, et al. Day-to-day experience in resolution of pain after surgery. *Pain*. 2017;158:2147–2154.
6. Badreldin N, Grobman WA, Yee LM. Racial disparities in postpartum pain management. *Obstet Gynecol*. 2019;134:1147–1153.
7. Fassoulaki A, Gatzou V, Petropoulos G, Siafaka I. Spread of subarachnoid block, intraoperative local anaesthetic requirements and postoperative analgesic requirements in caesarean section and total abdominal hysterectomy. *Br J Anaesth*. 2004;93:678–682.
8. Woolf CJ. Pain: moving from symptom control toward mechanism-specific pharmacologic management. *Ann Intern Med*. 2004;140:441–451.
9. Smith R. Parturition. *N Engl J Med*. 2007;356:271–283.
10. Unal ER, Cierny JT, Roedner C, et al. Maternal inflammation in spontaneous term labor. *Am J Obstet Gynecol*. 2011;204:223.e1–e5.
11. Carvalho B, Clark DJ, Angst MS. Local and systemic release of cytokines, nerve growth factor, prostaglandin E2, and substance P in incisional wounds and serum following cesarean delivery. *J Pain*. 2008;9:650–657.
12. Eisenach JC, Pan PH, Smiley R, et al. Severity of acute pain after childbirth, but not type of delivery, predicts persistent pain and postpartum depression. *Pain*. 2008;140:87–94.
13. Komatsu R, Carvalho B, Flood PD. Recovery after nulliparous birth: a detailed analysis of pain analgesia and recovery of function. *Anesthesiology*. 2017;127:684–694.
14. Carvalho B, Cohen SE, Lipman SS, et al. Patient preferences for anesthesia outcomes associated with cesarean delivery. *Anesth Analg*. 2005;101:1182–1187.

15. Wrench IJ, Sanghera S, Pinder A, et al. Dose response to intrathecal diamorphine for elective caesarean section and compliance with a national audit standard. *Int J Obstet Anesth.* 2007;16:17–21.

16. Nikolajsen L, Sørensen HC, Jensen TS, Kehlet H. Chronic pain following caesarean section. *Acta Anaesthesiol Scand.* 2004;48:111–116.

17. Kainu JP, Sarvela J, Tiippana E, et al. Persistent pain after caesarean section and vaginal birth: a cohort study. *Int J Obstet Anesth.* 2010;19:4–9.

18. Lavand'homme P. Chronic pain after vaginal and cesarean delivery: a reality questioning our daily practice of obstetric anesthesia. *Int J Obstet Anesth.* 2010;19:1–2.

19. Kehlet H, Jensen TS, Woolf CJ. Persistent postsurgical pain: risk factors and prevention. *Lancet.* 2006;367:1618–1625.

20. Lavand'homme P, De Kock M, Waterloos H. Intraoperative epidural analgesia combined with ketamine provides effective preventive analgesia in patients undergoing major digestive surgery. *Anesthesiology.* 2005;103:813–820.

21. Wong CA, Girard T. Under- or overtreated? Opioids for postdelivery analgesia. *Br J Anaesth.* 2018;121:339–342.

22. Carvalho B, Mirza F, Flood PD. Patient choice compared with no choice of intrathecal morphine dose for caesarean analgesia: a randomized clinical trial. *Br J Anaesth.* 2017;118:762–771.

23. American College of Obstetricians and Gynecologists' Committee on Practice Bulletins—Obstetrics. ACOG Practice Bulletin No. 209: Obstetric analgesia and anesthesia (reaffirmed 2024). *Obstet Gynecol.* 2019;133:e208–e225.

24. Jakobi P, Solt I, Tamir A, Zimmer EZ. Over-the-counter oral analgesia for postcesarean pain. *Am J Obstet Gynecol.* 2002;187:1066–1069.

25. Davis KM, Esposito MA, Meyer BA. Oral analgesia compared with intravenous patient-controlled analgesia for pain after cesarean delivery: a randomized controlled trial. *Am J Obstet Gynecol.* 2006;194:967–971.

26. Chou R, Gordon DB, de Leon-Casasola OA, et al. Management of postoperative pain: a clinical practice guideline from the American Pain Society, the American Society of Regional Anesthesia and Pain Medicine, and the American Society of Anesthesiologists' Committee on Regional Anesthesia, Executive Committee, and Administrative Council. *J Pain.* 2016;17:131–157.

27. Dieterich M, Muller-Jordan K, Stubert J, et al. Pain management after cesarean: a randomized controlled trial of oxycodone versus intravenous piritramide. *Arch Gynecol Obstet.* 2012;286:859–865.

28. McNicol ED, Ferguson MC, Hudcova J. Patient controlled opioid analgesia versus non-patient controlled opioid analgesia for postoperative pain. *Cochrane Database Syst Rev.* 2015;(6):CD003348.

29. American Society of Anesthesiologists. Practice guidelines for acute pain management in the perioperative setting. An updated report by the American Society of Anesthesiologists Task Force on Acute Pain Management. *Anesthesiology.* 2012;116:248–273.

30. Ngan Kee WD, Lam KK, Chen PP, Gin T. Comparison of patient-controlled epidural analgesia with patient-controlled intravenous analgesia using pethidine or fentanyl. *Anaesth Intensive Care.* 1997;25:126–132.

31. Parker RK, White PF. Epidural patient-controlled analgesia: an alternative to intravenous patient-controlled analgesia for pain relief after cesarean delivery. *Anesth Analg.* 1992;75:245–251.

32. Harrison DM, Sinatra R, Morgese L, Chung JH. Epidural narcotic and patient-controlled analgesia for post-cesarean section pain relief. *Anesthesiology.* 1988;68:454–457.

33. Rapp-Zingraff N, Bayoumeu F, Baka N, et al. Analgesia after caesarean section: patient-controlled intravenous morphine vs epidural morphine. *Int J Obstet Anesth.* 1997;6:87–92.

34. Kopka A, Wallace E, Reilly G, Binning A. Observational study of perioperative $PtcCO_2$ and SpO_2 in non-ventilated patients receiving epidural infusion or patient-controlled analgesia using a single earlobe monitor (TOSCA). *Br J Anaesth.* 2007;99:567–571.

35. McCormack JG, Kelly KP, Wedgwood J, Lyon R. The effects of different analgesic regimens on transcutaneous CO_2 after major surgery. *Anaesthesia.* 2008;63:814–821.

36. Cashman JN, Dolin SJ. Respiratory and haemodynamic effects of acute postoperative pain management: Evidence from published data. *Br J Anaesth.* 2004;93:212–223.

37. Gwirtz KH, Young JV, Byers RS, et al. The safety and efficacy of intrathecal opioid analgesia for acute postoperative pain: Seven years' experience with 5969 surgical patients at Indiana University Hospital. *Anesth Analg.* 1999;88:599–604.

38. Pattinson KT. Opioids and the control of respiration. *Br J Anaesth.* 2008;100:747–758.

39. Joint Commission on the Accreditation of Healthcare Organizations, JCAHO alert gives new recommendations for PCA. *Hosp Peer Rev.* 2005;30:24–25.

40. Owen H, Brose WG, Plummer JL, Mather LE. Variables of patient-controlled analgesia. 3: test of an infusion-demand system using alfentanil. *Anaesthesia.* 1990;45:452–455.

41. Owen H, Kluger MT, Plummer JL. Variables of patient-controlled analgesia 4: the relevance of bolus dose size to supplement a background infusion. *Anaesthesia.* 1990;45:619–622.

42. Owen H, Plummer JL, Armstrong I, et al. Variables of patient-controlled analgesia. 1. Bolus size. *Anaesthesia.* 1989;44:7–10.

43. McCoy EP, Furness G, Wright PM. Patient-controlled analgesia with and without background infusion. Analgesia assessed using the demand: delivery ratio. *Anaesthesia.* 1993;48:256–260.

44. Carvalho B, Butwick AJ. Postcesarean delivery analgesia. *Best Pract Res Clin Anaesthesiol.* 2017;31:69–79.

45. Roofthooft E, Joshi G, Rawal N, et al. PROSPECT guideline for elective caesarean section: updated systematic review and procedure-specific postoperative pain management recommendations. *Anaesthesia.* 2021;76:665–680.

46. Sen Tan H, Diomede O, Habib AS. Postoperative analgesia after cesarean delivery. *Int Anesthesiol Clin.* 2021;59:90–97.

47. Yefet E, Taha H, Salim R, et al. Fixed time interval compared with on-demand oral analgesia protocols for post-caesarean pain: a randomised controlled trial. *BJOG.* 2017;124:1063–1070.

48. Remy C, Marret E, Bonnet F. Effects of acetaminophen on morphine side-effects and consumption after major surgery: meta-analysis of randomized controlled trials. *Br J Anaesth.* 2005;94:505–513.

49. Maund E, McDaid C, Rice S, et al. Paracetamol and selective and non-selective non-steroidal anti-inflammatory drugs for the reduction in morphine-related side-effects after major surgery: a systematic review. *Br J Anaesth.* 2011;106:292–297.

50. Elia N, Lysakowski C, Tramer MR, Phil D. Does multimodal analgesia with acetaminophen, nonsteroidal antiinflammatory drugs, or selective cyclooxygenase-2 inhibitors and patient-controlled analgesia morphine offer advantages over morphine alone? *Anesthesiology.* 2005;103:1296–1304.

51. Felder L, Riegel M, Quist-Nelson J, Berghella V. Perioperative intravenous acetaminophen and postcesarean pain control: a systematic review and meta-analysis of randomized controlled trials. *Am J Obstet Gynecol MFM.* 2021;3:100338.

52. Singla NK, Parulan C, Samson R, et al. Plasma and cerebrospinal fluid pharmacokinetic parameters after single-dose administration of intravenous, oral, or rectal acetaminophen. *Pain Pract.* 2012;12:523–532.

53. Wilson SH, Wolf BJ, Robinson SM, et al. Intravenous vs oral acetaminophen for analgesia after cesarean delivery: a randomized trial. *Pain Med.* 2019;20:1584–1591.

54. Valentine AR, Carvalho B, Lazo TA, Riley ET. Scheduled acetaminophen with as-needed opioids compared to as-needed acetaminophen plus opioids for post-cesarean pain management. *Int J Obstet Anesth.* 2015;24:210–216.

55. Bloor M, Paech M. Nonsteroidal anti-inflammatory drugs during pregnancy and the initiation of lactation. *Anesth Analg.* 2013;116:1063–1075.

56. Zeng AM, Nami NF, Wu CL, Murphy JD. The analgesic efficacy of nonsteroidal anti-inflammatory agents (NSAIDs) in patients undergoing cesarean deliveries: a meta-analysis. *Reg Anesth Pain Med.* 2016;41:763–772.

57. Ing Lorenzini K, Besson M, Daali Y, et al. A randomized, controlled trial validates a peripheral supra-additive antihyperalgesic effect of a paracetamol-ketorolac combination. *Basic Clin Pharmacol Toxicol.* 2011;109:357–364.

58. Ong CK, Seymour RA, Lirk P, Merry AF. Combining paracetamol (acetaminophen) with nonsteroidal antiinflammatory drugs: a qualitative systematic review of analgesic efficacy for acute postoperative pain. *Anesth Analg.* 2010;110:1170–1179.

59. American Academy of Pediatrics Committee on Drugs. Transfer of drugs and other chemicals into human milk. *Pediatrics.* 2001;108:776–789.

60. Townsend RJ, Benedetti TJ, Erickson SH, et al. Excretion of ibuprofen into breast milk. *Am J Obstet Gynecol.* 1984;149:184–186.

61. Angle PJ, Halpern SH, Leighton BL, et al. A randomized controlled trial examining the effect of naproxen on analgesia during the second day after cesarean delivery. *Anesth Analg.* 2002;95:741–745.

62. Dahl V, Hagen IE, Sveen AM, et al. High-dose diclofenac for postoperative analgesia after elective caesarean section in regional anaesthesia. *Int J Obstet Anesth.* 2002;11:91–94.

63. Dennis AR, Leeson-Payne CG, Hobbs GJ. Analgesia after caesarean section. The use of rectal diclofenac as an adjunct to spinal morphine. *Anaesthesia.* 1995;50:297–299.

64. Cardoso MM, Carvalho JC, Amaro AR, et al. Small doses of intrathecal morphine combined with systemic diclofenac for postoperative pain control after cesarean delivery. *Anesth Analg.* 1998;86:538–541.

65. Munishankar B, Fettes P, Moore C, McLeod GA. A double-blind randomised controlled trial of paracetamol, diclofenac or the combination for pain relief after caesarean section. *Int J Obstet Anesth.* 2008;17:9–14.

66. Lowder JL, Shackelford DP, Holbert D, Beste TM. A randomized, controlled trial to compare ketorolac tromethamine versus placebo after cesarean section to reduce pain and narcotic usage. *Am J Obstet Gynecol.* 2003;189:1559–1562.

67. Rømsing J, Møiniche S. A systematic review of COX-2 inhibitors compared with traditional NSAIDs, or different COX-2 inhibitors for post-operative pain. *Acta Anaesthesiol Scand.* 2004;48:525–546.

68. Murdoch I, Carver A, Sultan P, et al. Comparison of different nonsteroidal anti-inflammatory drugs for cesarean section: a systematic review and network meta-analysis. *Korean J Anesthesiol.* 2023;76:597–616.

69. Paech MJ, Salman S, Ilett KF, et al. Transfer of parecoxib and its primary active metabolite valdecoxib via transitional breastmilk following intravenous parecoxib use after cesarean delivery: a comparison of naive pooled data analysis and nonlinear mixed-effects modeling. *Anesth Analg.* 2012;114:837–844.

70. Palanisamy A, Klickovich RJ, Ramsay M, et al. Intravenous dexmedetomidine as an adjunct for labor analgesia and cesarean delivery anesthesia in a parturient with a tethered spinal cord. *Int J Obstet Anesth.* 2009;18:258–261.

71. Yoshimura M, Kunisawa T, Suno M, et al. Intravenous dexmedetomidine for cesarean delivery and its concentration in colostrum. *Int J Obstet Anesth.* 2017;32:28–32.

72. Nie Y, Liu Y, Luo Q, Huang S. Effect of dexmedetomidine combined with sufentanil for post-caesarean section intravenous analgesia: a randomised, placebo-controlled study. *Eur J Anaesthesiol.* 2014;31:197–203.

73. Package insert: Duraclon (clonidine hydrochloride) injection, solution. Available at: https://www.accessdata.fda.gov/drugsatfda_docs/label/2010/020615s003lbl.pdf. Accessed 18 July 2024.

74. Fernandes HS, Bliacheriene F, Vago TM, et al. Clonidine effect on pain after cesarean delivery: a randomized controlled trial of different routes of administration. *Anesth Analg.* 2018;127:165–170.

75. Pryde PG, Mittendorf R. Contemporary usage of obstetric magnesium sulfate: Indication, contraindication, and relevance of dose. *Obstet Gynecol.* 2009;114:669–673.

76. Rezae M, Naghibi K, Taefnia AM. Effect of pre-emptive magnesium sulfate infusion on the post-operative pain relief after elective cesarean section. *Adv Biomed Res.* 2014;3:164.

77. Mireskandari SM, Pestei K, Hajipour A, et al. Effects of preoperative magnesium sulphate on post-cesarean pain, a placebo controlled double blind study. *J Family Reprod Health.* 2015;9:29.

78. Paech MJ, Magann EF, Doherty DA, et al. Does magnesium sulfate reduce the short-and long-term requirements for pain relief after caesarean delivery? A double-blind placebo-controlled trial. *Am J Obstet Gynecol.* 2006;194:1596–1602.

79. Moore A, Costello J, Wieczorek P, et al. Gabapentin improves postcesarean delivery pain management: a randomized, placebo-controlled trial. *Anesth Analg.* 2011;112:167–173.

80. Felder L, Saccone G, Scuotto S, et al. Perioperative gabapentin and post cesarean pain control: a systematic review and meta-analysis of randomized controlled trials. *Eur J Obstet Gynecol Reprod Biol.* 2019;233:98–106.

81. Hovinga CA, Pennell PB. Antiepileptic drug therapy in pregnancy II: Fetal and neonatal exposure. *Int Rev Neurobiol.* 2008;83:241–258.

82. Schmid RL, Sandler AN, Katz J. Use and efficacy of low-dose ketamine in the management of acute postoperative pain: a review of current techniques and outcomes. *Pain.* 1999;82:111–125.

83. Sen S, Ozmert G, Aydin ON, et al. The persisting analgesic effect of low-dose intravenous ketamine after spinal anaesthesia for caesarean section. *Eur J Anaesthesiol.* 2005;22:518–523.

84. Wang J, Xu Z, Zhou F, et al. Impact of ketamine on pain management in cesarean section: a systematic review and meta-analysis. *Pain Physician.* 2020;23:135.

85. Jenkins JG, Khan MM. Anaesthesia for caesarean section: a survey in a UK region from 1992 to 2002. *Anaesthesia.* 2003;58:1114–1118.

86. Aiono-Le Tagaloa L, Butwick AJ, Carvalho B. A survey of perioperative and postoperative anesthetic practices for cesarean delivery. *Anesthesiol Res Pract.* 2009;2009:510642.

87. Traynor AJ, Aragon M, Ghosh D, et al. Obstetric Anesthesia Workforce Survey: a 30-year update. *Anesth Analg.* 2016;122:1939–1946.

88. Bonnet MP, Mignon A, Mazoit JX, et al. Analgesic efficacy and adverse effects of epidural morphine compared to parenteral opioids after elective caesarean section: a systematic review. *Eur J Pain.* 2010;14:894.e1–e9.

89. Wu CL, Cohen SR, Richman JM, et al. Efficacy of postoperative patient-controlled and continuous infusion epidural analgesia versus intravenous patient-controlled analgesia with opioids: a meta-analysis. *Anesthesiology.* 2005;103:1079–1088.

90. Eisenach JC, Grice SC, Dewan DM. Patient-controlled analgesia following cesarean section: a comparison with epidural and intramuscular narcotics. *Anesthesiology.* 1988;68:444–448.

91. Pan PH. Post cesarean delivery pain management: multimodal approach. *Int J Obstet Anesth.* 2006;15:185–188.

92. Mishriky BM, George RB, Habib AS. Transversus abdominis plane block for analgesia after cesarean delivery: a systematic review and meta-analysis. *Can J Anaesth.* 2012;59:766–778.

93. Tan HS, Taylor C, Weikel D, et al. Quadratus lumborum block for postoperative analgesia after cesarean delivery: a systematic review with meta-analysis and trial-sequential analysis. *J Clin Anesth.* 2020;67:110003.

94. Lavand'homme P. Postcesarean analgesia: effective strategies and association with chronic pain. *Curr Opin Anaesthesiol.* 2006;19:244–248.

95. Terajima K, Onodera H, Kobayashi M, et al. Efficacy of intrathecal morphine for analgesia following elective cesarean section: comparison with previous delivery. *J Nippon Med Sch.* 2003;70:327–333.

96. Dahl JB, Jeppesen IS, Jorgensen H, et al. Intraoperative and postoperative analgesic efficacy and adverse effects of intrathecal opioids in patients undergoing cesarean section with spinal anesthesia: a qualitative and quantitative systematic review of randomized controlled trials. *Anesthesiology.* 1999;91:1919–1927.

97. Tziavrangos E, Schug SA. Regional anaesthesia and perioperative outcome. *Curr Opin Anaesthesiol.* 2006;19:521–525.

98. Guay J. The benefits of adding epidural analgesia to general anesthesia: a metaanalysis. *J Anesth.* 2006;20:335–340.

99. Richman JM, Wu CL. Epidural analgesia for postoperative pain. *Anesthesiol Clin North America.* 2005;23:125–140.

100. Rosaeg OP, Lui AC, Cicutti NJ, et al. Peri-operative multimodal pain therapy for caesarean section: analgesia and fitness for discharge. *Can J Anaesth.* 1997;44:803–809.

101. Kettner SC, Willschke H, Marhofer P. Does regional anaesthesia really improve outcome? *Br J Anaesth.* 2011;107:i90–i95.

102. Ghaji N, Boulet SL, Tepper N, Hooper WC. Trends in venous thromboembolism among pregnancy-related hospitalizations, United States, 1994-2009. *Am J Obstet Gynecol.* 2013;209: e1–e8.

103. Callaghan WM, Creanga AA, Kuklina EV. Severe maternal morbidity among delivery and postpartum hospitalization in the United States. *Obstet Gynecol.* 2012;120: 1029–1036.

104. Jacobsen AF, Skjeldestad FE, Sandset PM. Incidence and risk patterns of venous thromboembolism in pregnancy and puerperium—a register-based case-control study. *Am J Obstet Gynecol.* 2008;198:233.e1–e7.

105. Sultan AA, Tata LJ, West J, et al. Risk factors for first venous thromboembolism around pregnancy: a population-based cohort study from the United Kingdom. *Blood.* 2013;121:3953–3962.

106. Ramanathan J, Coleman P, Sibai B. Anesthetic modification of hemodynamic and neuroendocrine stress responses to cesarean delivery in women with severe preeclampsia. *Anesth Analg.* 1991;73:772–779.

107. Rawal N, Sjöstrand U, Christoffersson E, et al. Comparison of intramuscular and epidural morphine for postoperative analgesia in the grossly obese: influence on postoperative ambulation and pulmonary function. *Anesth Analg.* 1984;63:583–592.

108. Yeager MP, Glass DD, Neff RK, Brinck-Johnsen T. Epidural anesthesia and analgesia in high-risk surgical patients. *Anesthesiology.* 1987;66:729–736.

109. Cooper DW, Ryall DM, McHardy FE, et al. Patient-controlled extradural analgesia with bupivacaine, fentanyl, or a mixture of both, after caesarean section. *Br J Anaesth.* 1996;76: 611–615.

110. Parker RK, Sawaki Y, White PF. Epidural patient-controlled analgesia: influence of bupivacaine and hydromorphone basal infusion on pain control after cesarean delivery. *Anesth Analg.* 1992;75:740–746.

111. Yaksh TL, Rudy TA. Analgesia mediated by a direct spinal action of narcotics. *Science.* 1976;192:1357–1358.

112. Wang JK, Nauss LA, Thomas JE. Pain relief by intrathecally applied morphine in man. *Anesthesiology.* 1979;50:149–151.

113. Bernards CM, Hill HF. Morphine and alfentanil permeability through the spinal dura, arachnoid, and pia mater of dogs and monkeys. *Anesthesiology.* 1990;73:1214–1219.

114. Bernards CM, Hill HF. Physical and chemical properties of drug molecules governing their diffusion through the spinal meninges. *Anesthesiology.* 1992;77:750–756.

115. Glass PS, Estok P, Ginsberg B, et al. Use of patient-controlled analgesia to compare the efficacy of epidural to intravenous fentanyl administration. *Anesth Analg.* 1992;74:345–351.

116. Ellis DJ, Millar WL, Reisner LS. A randomized double-blind comparison of epidural versus intravenous fentanyl infusion for analgesia after cesarean section. *Anesthesiology.* 1990;72:981–986.

117. D'Angelo R, Gerancher JC, Eisenach JC, Raphael BL. Epidural fentanyl produces labor analgesia by a spinal mechanism. *Anesthesiology.* 1998;88:1519–1523.

118. Liu SS, Gerancher JC, Bainton BG, et al. The effects of electrical stimulation at different frequencies on perception and pain in human volunteers: epidural versus intravenous administration of fentanyl. *Anesth Analg.* 1996;82:98–102.

119. Ginosar Y, Riley ET, Angst MS. The site of action of epidural fentanyl in humans: the difference between infusion and bolus administration. *Anesth Analg.* 2003;97:1428–1438.

120. Cohen S, Pantuck CB, Amar D, et al. The primary action of epidural fentanyl after cesarean delivery is via a spinal mechanism. *Anesth Analg.* 2002;94:674–679.

121. Sadurní M, Beltrán de Heredia S, Dürsteler C, et al. Epidural vs. intravenous fentanyl during colorectal surgery using a double-blind, double-dummy design. *Acta Anesthesiol Scand.* 2013;57:1103–1110.

122. Stevens RA, Petty RH, Hill HF, et al. Redistribution of sufentanil to cerebrospinal fluid and systemic circulation after epidural administration in dogs. *Anesth Analg.* 1993;76:323–327.

123. Bujedo BM. Spinal opioid bioavailability in postoperative pain. *Pain Pract.* 2014;14:350–364.

124. Nordberg G, Hedner T, Mellstrand T, Dahlström B. Pharmacokinetic aspects of epidural morphine analgesia. *Anesthesiology.* 1983;58:545–551.

125. Youngstrom PC, Cowan RI, Sutheimer C, et al. Pain relief and plasma concentrations from epidural and intramuscular morphine in post-cesarean patients. *Anesthesiology.* 1982;57:404–409.

126. Weddel SJ, Ritter RR. Serum levels following epidural administration of morphine and correlation with relief of postsurgical pain. *Anesthesiology.* 1981;54:210–214.

127. Nordberg G, Hedner T, Mellstrand T, Dahlström B. Pharmacokinetic aspects of intrathecal morphine analgesia. *Anesthesiology.* 1984;60:448–454.

128. Gourlay GK, Murphy TM, Plummer JL, et al. Pharmacokinetics of fentanyl in lumbar and cervical CSF following lumbar epidural and intravenous administration. *Pain.* 1989;38:253–259.

129. Gourlay GK, Cherry DA, Plummer JL, et al. The influence of drug polarity on the absorption of opioid drugs into CSF and subsequent cephalad migration following lumbar epidural administration: application to morphine and pethidine. *Pain.* 1987;31:297–305.

130. Cousins MJ, Mather LE. Intrathecal and epidural administration of opioids. *Anesthesiology.* 1984;61:276–310.

131. van den Hoogen RH, Colpaert FC. Epidural and subcutaneous morphine, meperidine (pethidine), fentanyl and sufentanil in the rat: analgesia and other in vivo pharmacologic effects. *Anesthesiology.* 1987;66:186–194.

132. Brill S, Gurman GM, Fisher A. A history of neuraxial administration of local analgesics and opioids. *Eur J Anaesthesiol.* 2003;20:682–689.

133. Bernards CM, Shen DD, Sterling ES, et al. Epidural, cerebrospinal fluid, and plasma pharmacokinetics of epidural opioids (part 2): effect of epinephrine. *Anesthesiology.* 2003;99:466–475.

134. Bernards CM, Shen DD, Sterling ES, et al. Epidural, cerebrospinal fluid, and plasma pharmacokinetics of epidural opioids (part 1): differences among opioids. *Anesthesiology.* 2003;99:455–465.

135. Carvalho B, Roland LM, Chu LF, et al. Single-dose, extended-release epidural morphine (DepoDur) compared to conventional epidural morphine for post-cesarean pain. *Anesth Analg.* 2007;105:176–183.

136. Chumpathong S, Santawat U, Saunya P, et al. Comparison of different doses of epidural morphine for pain relief following cesarean section. *J Med Assoc Thai.* 2002;85:S956–S962.

137. Rosen MA, Hughes SC, Shnider SM, et al. Epidural morphine for the relief of postoperative pain after cesarean delivery. *Anesth Analg.* 1983;62:666–672.

138. Fuller JG, McMorland GH, Douglas MJ, Palmer L. Epidural morphine for analgesia after caesarean section: a report of 4880 patients. *Can J Anaesth.* 1990;37:636–640.

139. Palmer CM, Nogami WM, Van Maren G, Alves DM. Postcesarean epidural morphine: a dose-response study. *Anesth Analg.* 2000;90:887–891.

140. Asantila R, Eklund P, Rosenberg PH. Epidural analgesia with 4 mg of morphine following caesarean section: effect of injected volume. *Acta Anaesthesiol Scand.* 1993;37:764–767.

141. Singh SI, Rehou S, Marmai KL, Jones PM. The efficacy of 2 doses of epidural morphine for postcesarean delivery analgesia: a randomized noninferiority trial. *Anesth Analg.* 2013;117:677–685.

142. Bollag L, Lim G, Sultan P, et al. Society for Obstetric Anesthesia and Perinatology: consensus statement and recommendations for enhanced recovery after cesarean. *Anesth Analg.* 2021;132:1362–1377.

143. Grass JA, Sakima NT, Schmidt R, et al. A randomized, double-blind, dose-response comparison of epidural fentanyl versus sufentanil analgesia after cesarean section. *Anesth Analg.* 1997;85:365–371.

144. Preston PG, Rosen MA, Hughes SC, et al. Epidural anesthesia with fentanyl and lidocaine for cesarean section: maternal effects and neonatal outcome. *Anesthesiology.* 1988;68:938–943.

145. King MJ, Bowden MI, Cooper GM. Epidural fentanyl and 0.5% bupivacaine for elective caesarean section. *Anaesthesia.* 1990;45:285–288.

146. Ngan Kee WD, Khaw KS, Ng FF, et al. Synergistic interaction between fentanyl and bupivacaine given intrathecally for labor analgesia. *Anesthesiology.* 2014;120:1126–1136.

147. Cohen S, Lowenwirt I, Pantuck CB, et al. Bupivacaine 0.01% and/or epinephrine 0.5 μg/mL improve epidural fentanyl analgesia after cesarean section. *Anesthesiology.* 1998;89:1354–1361.

148. Robertson K, Douglas MJ, McMorland GH. Epidural fentanyl, with and without epinephrine for post-caesarean section analgesia. *Can Anaesth Soc J.* 1985;32:502–505.

149. Rosen MA, Dailey PA, Hughes SC, et al. Epidural sufentanil for postoperative analgesia after cesarean section. *Anesthesiology.* 1988;68:448–454.

150. Perriss BW, Latham BV, Wilson IH. Analgesia following extradural and i.m. pethidine in post-caesarean section patients. *Br J Anaesth.* 1990;64:355–357.

151. Brownridge P, Frewin DB. A comparative study of techniques of postoperative analgesia following caesarean section and lower abdominal surgery. *Anaesth Intensive Care.* 1985;13:123–130.

152. Paech MJ. Epidural pethidine or fentanyl during caesarean section: a double-blind comparison. *Anaesth Intensive Care.* 1989;17:157–165.

153. Ngan Kee WD, Lam KK, Chen PP, Gin T. Epidural meperidine after cesarean section. A dose-response study. *Anesthesiology.* 1996;85:289–294.

154. Rosaeg OP, Lindsay MP. Epidural opioid analgesia after caesarean section: a comparison of patient-controlled analgesia with meperidine and single bolus injection of morphine. *Can J Anaesth.* 1994;41:1063–1068.

155. Paech MJ, Pavy TJ, Orlikowski CE, et al. Postoperative intraspinal opioid analgesia after caesarean section; a randomised comparison of subarachnoid morphine and epidural pethidine. *Int J Obstet Anesth.* 2000;9:238–245.

156. de Leon-Casasola OA, Lema MJ. Postoperative epidural opioid analgesia: what are the choices? *Anesth Analg.* 1996;83:867–875.

157. Dougherty TB, Baysinger CL, Henenberger JC, Gooding DJ. Epidural hydromorphone with and without epinephrine for post-operative analgesia after cesarean delivery. *Anesth Analg.* 1989;68:318–322.

158. Henderson SK, Matthew EB, Cohen H, Avram MJ. Epidural hydromorphone: a double-blind comparison with intramuscular hydromorphone for postcesarean section analgesia. *Anesthesiology.* 1987;66:825–830.

159. Chestnut DH, Choi WW, Isbell TJ. Epidural hydromorphone for postcesarean analgesia. *Obstet Gynecol.* 1986;68:65–69.

160. Halpern SH, Arellano R, Preston R, et al. Epidural morphine vs hydromorphone in post-caesarean section patients. *Can J Anaesth.* 1996;43:595–598.

161. Quigley C. Hydromorphone for acute and chronic pain. *Cochrane Database Syst Rev.* 2002;(1):CD003447.

162. Rawal N, Allvin R. Acute pain services in Europe: a 17-nation survey of 105 hospitals. The EuroPain Acute Pain Working Party. *Eur J Anaesthesiol.* 1998;15:354–363.

163. Roulson CJ, Bennett J, Shaw M, Carli F. Effect of extradural diamorphine on analgesia after caesarean section under subarachnoid block. *Br J Anaesth.* 1993;71:810–813.

164. Semple AJ, Macrae DJ, Munishankarappa S, et al. Effect of the addition of adrenaline to extradural diamorphine analgesia after caesarean section. *Br J Anaesth.* 1988;60:632–638.

165. Macrae DJ, Munishankrappa S, Burrow LM, et al. Double-blind comparison of the efficacy of extradural diamorphine, extradural phenoperidine and i.m. diamorphine following caesarean section. *Br J Anaesth.* 1987;59:354–359.

166. National Institute for Health and Care Excellence. Caesarean birth. 2021. https://www.nice.org.uk/guidance/ng192. Accessed 18 July 2024.

167. Palmer CM, Voulgaropoulos D, Alves D. Subarachnoid fentanyl augments lidocaine spinal anesthesia for cesarean delivery. *Reg Anesth.* 1995;20:389–394.

168. Vincent RD Jr, Chestnut DH, Choi WW, et al. Does epidural fentanyl decrease the efficacy of epidural morphine after cesarean delivery? *Anesth Analg.* 1992;74:658–663.

169. Cooper DW, Garcia E, Mowbray P, Millar MA. Patient-controlled epidural fentanyl following spinal fentanyl at caesarean section. *Anaesthesia.* 2002;57:266–270.

170. Dottrens M, Rifat K, Morel DR. Comparison of extradural administration of sufentanil, morphine and sufentanil-morphine combination after caesarean section. *Br J Anaesth.* 1992;69:9–12.

171. Sinatra RS, Sevarino FB, Chung JH, et al. Comparison of epidurally administered sufentanil, morphine, and sufentanil-morphine combination for postoperative analgesia. *Anesth Analg.* 1991;72:522–527.

172. Fanshawe MP. A comparison of patient controlled epidural pethidine versus single dose epidural morphine for analgesia after caesarean section. *Anaesth Intensive Care.* 1999;27:610–614.

173. Cohen S, Chhokra R, Stein MH, et al. Ropivacaine 0.025% mixed with fentanyl 3.0 μg/ml and epinephrine 0.5 μg/ml is effective for epidural patient-controlled analgesia after cesarean section. *J Anaesthesiol Clin Pharmacol.* 2015;31:471–477.

174. Paech MJ, Moore JS, Evans SF. Meperidine for patient-controlled analgesia after cesarean section. Intravenous versus epidural administration. *Anesthesiology.* 1994;80:1268–1276.

175. Goh JL, Evans SF, Pavy TJ. Patient-controlled epidural analgesia following caesarean delivery: a comparison of pethidine and fentanyl. *Anaesth Intensive Care.* 1996;24:45–50.

176. Cohen S, Amar D, Pantuck CB, et al. Postcesarean delivery epidural patient-controlled analgesia. Fentanyl or sufentanil? *Anesthesiology.* 1993;78:486–491.

177. Vercauteren MP, Coppejans HC, ten Broecke PW, et al. Epidural sufentanil for postoperative patient-controlled analgesia (PCA) with or without background infusion: a double-blind comparison. *Anesth Analg.* 1995;80:76–80.

178. Chang C-Y, Tu Y-K, Kao M-C, et al. Effects of opioids administered via intravenous or epidural patient-controlled analgesia after caesarean section: a network meta-analysis of randomised controlled trials. *EClinicalMedicine.* 2023;56:101787.

179. Vercauteren M, Vereecken K, La Malfa M, et al. Cost-effectiveness of analgesia after caesarean section. A comparison of intrathecal morphine and epidural PCA. *Acta Anaesthesiol Scand.* 2002;46:85–89.

180. Angst MS, Drover DR. Pharmacology of drugs formulated with DepoFoam: a sustained release drug delivery system for parenteral administration using multivesicular liposome technology. *Clin Pharmacokinet.* 2006;45:1153–1176.

181. Viscusi ER, Gambling DR, Hughes TL, Manvelian GZ. Pharmacokinetics of extended-release epidural morphine sulfate: pooled analysis of six clinical studies. *Am J Health Syst Pharm.* 2009;66:1020–1030.

182. Nagle PC, Gerancher JC. DepoDur®: extended-release epidural morphine: a review of an old drug in a new vehicle. *Tech Reg Anesth Pain Manag.* 2007;11:9–18.

183. Sumida S, Lesley MR, Hanna MN, et al. Meta-analysis of the effect of extended-release epidural morphine versus intravenous patient-controlled analgesia on respiratory depression. *J Opioid Manag.* 2009;5:301–305.

184. American Society of Anesthesiologists Task Force on Neuraxial Opioids, American Society of Regional Anesthesia and Pain Medicine, Practice guidelines for the prevention, detection, and management of respiratory depression associated with neuraxial opioid administration. An updated report by the American Society of Anesthesiologists Task Force on Neuraxial Opioids and the American Society of Regional Anesthesia and Pain Medicine. *Anesthesiology.* 2016;124:535–552.

185. Sarvela J, Halonen P, Soikkeli A, Korttila K. A double-blinded, randomized comparison of intrathecal and epidural morphine for elective cesarean delivery. *Anesth Analg.* 2002;95:436–440.

186. Duale C, Frey C, Bolandard F, et al. Epidural versus intrathecal morphine for postoperative analgesia after caesarean section. *Br J Anaesth.* 2003;91:690–694.

187. Ng K, Parsons J, Cyna AM, Middleton P. Spinal versus epidural anaesthesia for caesarean section. *Cochrane Database Syst Rev.* 2004;(2):CD003765.

188. Chadwick HS, Bernards CM, Kovarik DW, Tomlin JJ. Subdural injection of morphine for analgesia following cesarean section: a report of three cases. *Anesthesiology.* 1992;77:590–594.

189. Seki H, Shiga T, Mihara T, et al. Effects of intrathecal opioids on cesarean section: a systematic review and Bayesian network meta-analysis of randomized controlled trials. *J Anesth.* 2021;35:911–927.

190. Abboud TK, Dror A, Mosaad P, et al. Mini-dose intrathecal morphine for the relief of post-cesarean section pain: safety, efficacy, and ventilatory responses to carbon dioxide. *Anesth Analg.* 1988;67:137–143.

191. Sultan P, Halpern SH, Pushpanathan E, et al. The effect of intrathecal morphine dose on outcomes after elective cesarean delivery: a meta-analysis. *Anesth Analg.* 2016;123:154–164.

192. Palmer CM, Emerson S, Volgoropolous D, Alves D. Dose-response relationship of intrathecal morphine for postcesarean analgesia. *Anesthesiology.* 1999;90:437–444.

193. Uchiyama A, Nakano S, Ueyama H, et al. Low dose intrathecal morphine and pain relief following caesarean section. *Int J Obstet Anesth.* 1994;3:87–91.

194. Berger JS, Gonzalez A, Hopkins A, et al. Dose-response of intrathecal morphine when administered with intravenous ketorolac for post-cesarean analgesia: a two-center, prospective, randomized, blinded trial. *Int J Obstet Anesth.* 2016;28:3–11.

195. Mikuni I, Hirai H, Toyama Y, et al. Efficacy of intrathecal morphine with epidural ropivacaine infusion for postcesarean analgesia. *J Clin Anesth.* 2010;22:268–273.

196. Booth JL, Harris LC, Eisenach JC, Pan PH. A randomized controlled trial comparing two multimodal analgesic techniques in patients predicted to have severe pain after cesarean delivery. *Anesth Analg.* 2016;122:1114–1119.

197. Charles C, Gafni A, Whelan T. Shared decision-making in the medical encounter: what does it mean? (or it takes at least two to tango). *Soc Sci Med.* 1997;44:681–692.

198. Belzarena SD. Clinical effects of intrathecally administered fentanyl in patients undergoing cesarean section. *Anesth Analg.* 1992;74:653–657.

199. Dahlgren G, Hultstrand C, Jakobsson J, et al. Intrathecal sufentanil, fentanyl, or placebo added to bupivacaine for cesarean section. *Anesth Analg.* 1997;85:1288–1293.

200. Siddik-Sayyid SM, Aouad MT, Jalbout MI, et al. Intrathecal versus intravenous fentanyl for supplementation of subarachnoid block during cesarean delivery. *Anesth Analg.* 2002;95:209–213.

201. Meyer RA, Macarthur AJ, Downey K. Study of equivalence: spinal bupivacaine 15 mg versus bupivacaine 12 mg with fentanyl 15 μg for cesarean delivery. *Int J Obstet Anesth.* 2012;21:17–23.

202. Siti Salmah G, Choy YC. Comparison of morphine with fentanyl added to intrathecal 0.5% hyperbaric bupivacaine for analgesia after caesarean section. *Med J Malaysia.* 2009;64:71–74.

203. Wilwerth M, Majcher JL, Van der Linden P. Spinal fentanyl vs. sufentanil for post-operative analgesia after c-section: a double-blinded randomised trial. *Acta Anaesthesiol Scand.* 2016;60:1306–1313.

204. Hunt CO, Naulty JS, Bader AM, et al. Perioperative analgesia with subarachnoid fentanyl-bupivacaine for cesarean delivery. *Anesthesiology.* 1989;71:535–540.

205. Chu CC, Shu SS, Lin SM, et al. The effect of intrathecal bupivacaine with combined fentanyl in cesarean section. *Acta Anaesthesiol Sin.* 1995;33:149–154.

206. Chen X, Qian X, Fu F, et al. Intrathecal sufentanil decreases the median effective dose (ED$_{50}$) of intrathecal hyperbaric ropivacaine for caesarean delivery. *Acta Anaesthesiol Scand.* 2010;54:284–290.

207. Courtney MA, Bader AM, Hartwell B, et al. Perioperative analgesia with subarachnoid sufentanil administration. *Reg Anesth.* 1992;17:274–278.

208. Braga Ade F, Braga FS, Potério GM, et al. Sufentanil added to hyperbaric bupivacaine for subarachnoid block in caesarean section. *Eur J Anaesthesiol.* 2003;20:631–635.

209. Karaman S, Kocabas S, Uyar M, et al. The effects of sufentanil or morphine added to hyperbaric bupivacaine in spinal anaesthesia for caesarean section. *Eur J Anaesthesiol.* 2006;23:285–291.

210. Lee JH, Chung KH, Lee JY, et al. Comparison of fentanyl and sufentanil added to 0.5% hyperbaric bupivacaine for spinal anesthesia in patients undergoing cesarean section. *Korean J Anesthesiol.* 2011;60:103–108.

211. Kafle SK. Intrathecal meperidine for elective caesarean section: a comparison with lidocaine. *Can J Anaesth.* 1993;40:718–721.

212. Nguyen Thi TV, Orliaguet G, Ngû TH, Bonnet F. Spinal anesthesia with meperidine as the sole agent for cesarean delivery. *Reg Anesth.* 1994;19:386–389.

213. Yu SC, Ngan Kee WD, Kwan AS. Addition of meperidine to bupivacaine for spinal anaesthesia for caesarean section. *Br J Anaesth.* 2002;88:379–383.

214. Imarengiaye CO, Asudo FD, Akpoguado DD, et al. Subarachnoid bupivacaine and pethidine for caesarean section: assessment of quality of perioperative analgesia and side effects. *Niger Postgrad Med J.* 2011;18:200–204.

215. Saravanan S, Robinson AP, Qayoum Dar A, et al. Minimum dose of intrathecal diamorphine required to prevent intraoperative supplementation of spinal anaesthesia for caesarean section. *Br J Anaesth.* 2003;91:368–372.

216. Kelly MC, Carabine UA, Mirakhur RK. Intrathecal diamorphine for analgesia after caesarean section. A dose finding study and assessment of side-effects. *Anaesthesia.* 1998;53:231–237.

217. Stacey R, Jones R, Kar G, Poon A. High-dose intrathecal diamorphine for analgesia after caesarean section. *Anaesthesia.* 2001;56:54–60.

218. Husaini SW, Russell IF. Intrathecal diamorphine compared with morphine for postoperative analgesia after caesarean section under spinal anaesthesia. *Br J Anaesth.* 1998;81:135–139.

219. Hallworth SP, Fernando R, Bell R, et al. Comparison of intrathecal and epidural diamorphine for elective caesarean section using a combined spinal-epidural technique. *Br J Anaesth.* 1999;82:228–232.

220. Marroquin B, Feng C, Balofsky A, et al. Neuraxial opioids for post-cesarean delivery analgesia: can hydromorphone replace morphine? A retrospective study. *Int J Obstet Anesth.* 2017;30:16–22.

221. Beatty NC, Arendt KW, Niesen AD, et al. Analgesia after cesarean delivery: a retrospective comparison of intrathecal

hydromorphone and morphine. *J Clin Anesth.* 2013;25: 379–383.

222. Lynde GC. Determination of ED50 of hydromorphone for postoperative analgesia following cesarean delivery. *Int J Obstet Anesth.* 2016;28:17–21.

223. Sviggum HP, Arendt KW, Jacob AK, et al. Intrathecal hydromorphone and morphine for postcesarean delivery analgesia: determination of the ED$_{90}$ using a sequential allocation biased-coin method. *Anesth Analg.* 2016;123: 690–697.

224. Chung JH, Sinatra RS, Sevarino FB, Fermo L. Subarachnoid meperidine-morphine combination. An effective perioperative analgesic adjunct for cesarean delivery. *Reg Anesth.* 1997;22:119–124.

225. Draisci G, Frassanito L, Pinto R, et al. Safety and effectiveness of coadministration of intrathecal sufentanil and morphine in hyperbaric bupivacaine-based spinal anesthesia for cesarean section. *J Opioid Manag.* 2009;5:197–202.

226. Cooper DW, Lindsay SL, Ryall DM, et al. Does intrathecal fentanyl produce acute cross-tolerance to i.v. morphine? *Br J Anaesth.* 1997;78:311–313.

227. Sibilla C, Albertazz P, Zatelli R, Martinello R. Perioperative analgesia for caesarean section: comparison of intrathecal morphine and fentanyl alone or in combination. *Int J Obstet Anesth.* 1997;6:43–48.

228. Carvalho B, Drover DR, Ginosar Y, et al. Intrathecal fentanyl added to bupivacaine and morphine for cesarean delivery may induce a subtle acute opioid tolerance. *Int J Obstet Anesth.* 2012;21:29–34.

229. Yaksh TL, Grafe MR, Malkmus S, et al. Studies on the safety of chronically administered intrathecal neostigmine methylsulfate in rats and dogs. *Anesthesiology.* 1995;82: 412–427.

230. Sabbe MB, Grafe MR, Mjanger E, et al. Spinal delivery of sufentanil, alfentanil, and morphine in dogs. Physiologic and toxicologic investigations. *Anesthesiology.* 1994;81:899–920.

231. Rawal N, Nuutinen L, Raj PP, et al. Behavioral and histopathologic effects following intrathecal administration of butorphanol, sufentanil, and nalbuphine in sheep. *Anesthesiology.* 1991;75:1025–1034.

232. Culebras X, Gaggero G, Zatloukal J, et al. Advantages of intrathecal nalbuphine, compared with intrathecal morphine, after cesarean delivery: an evaluation of postoperative analgesia and adverse effects. *Anesth Analg.* 2000;91:601–605.

233. Hodgson PS, Neal JM, Pollock JE, Liu SS. The neurotoxicity of drugs given intrathecally (spinal). *Anesth Analg.* 1999;88: 797–809.

234. Eisenach JC, Yaksh TL. Safety in numbers: how do we study toxicity of spinal analgesics? *Anesthesiology.* 2002;97: 1047–1049.

235. Yaksh TL, Collins JG. Studies in animals should precede human use of spinally administered drugs. *Anesthesiology.* 1989;70:4–6.

236. Coombs DW, Colburn RW, Allen CD, et al. Toxicity of chronic spinal analgesia in a canine model: neuropathologic observations with dezocine lactate. *Reg Anesth.* 1990;15:94–102.

237. Hughes SC, Rosen MA, Shnider SM, et al. Maternal and neonatal effects of epidural morphine for labor and delivery. *Anesth Analg.* 1984;63:319–324.

238. Xie R, Hammarlund-Udenaes M, de Boer AG, de Lange EC. The role of P-glycoprotein in blood-brain barrier transport of morphine: transcortical microdialysis studies in *mdr1a* (−/−) and *mdr1a* (+/+) mice. *Br J Pharmacol.* 1999;128:563–568.

239. Hemauer SJ, Patrikeeva SL, Nanovskaya TN, et al. Opiates inhibit paclitaxel uptake by P-glycoprotein in preparations of human placental inside-out vesicles. *Biochem Pharmacol.* 2009;78:1272–1278.

240. Baraka A, Noueihid R, Hajj S. Intrathecal injection of morphine for obstetric analgesia. *Anesthesiology.* 1981;54:136–140.

241. Kafer ER, Brown JT, Scott D, et al. Biphasic depression of ventilatory responses to CO_2 following epidural morphine. *Anesthesiology.* 1983;58:418–427.

242. Bromage PR, Camporesi EM, Durant PA, Nielsen CH. Rostral spread of epidural morphine. *Anesthesiology.* 1982;56:431–436.

243. Bailey PL, Lu JK, Pace NL, et al. Effects of intrathecal morphine on the ventilatory response to hypoxia. *New Engl J Med.* 2000:1228–1234.

244. Cohen SE, Labaille T, Benhamou D, Levron JC. Respiratory effects of epidural sufentanil after cesarean section. *Anesth Analg.* 1992;74:677–682.

245. Sharawi N, Carvalho B, Habib AS, et al. A systematic review evaluating neuraxial morphine and diamorphine-associated respiratory depression after cesarean delivery. *Anesth Analg.* 2018;127:1385–1395.

246. D'Angelo R, Smiley RM, Riley ET, Segal S. Serious complications related to obstetric anesthesia: the serious complication repository project of the Society for Obstetric Anesthesia and Perinatology. *Anesthesiology.* 2014;120:1505–1512.

247. Etches RC, Sandler AN, Daley MD. Respiratory depression and spinal opioids. *Can J Anaesth.* 1989;36:165–185.

248. Knight M, Bunch K, Patel R, et al. *MBRRACE-UK. Saving Lives, Improving Mothers' Care Core Report – Lessons Learned to Inform Maternity Care From the UK and Ireland Confidential Enquiries Into Maternal Deaths and Morbidity 2018-20.* National Perinatal Epidemiology Unit; 2022. https://www.npeu.ox.ac.uk/assets/downloads/mbrrace-uk/reports/maternal-report-2022/MBRRACE-UK_Maternal_MAIN_Report_2022_UPDATE.pdf. Accessed 8 August 2023.

249. Crowgey TR, Dominguez JE, Peterson-Layne C, et al. A retrospective assessment of the incidence of respiratory depression after neuraxial morphine administration for postcesarean delivery analgesia. *Anesth Analg.* 2013;117: 1368–1370.

250. Shapiro A, Zohar E, Zaslansky R, et al. The frequency and timing of respiratory depression in 1524 postoperative patients treated with systemic or neuraxial morphine. *J Clin Anesth.* 2005;17:537–542.

251. Palmer CM. Early respiratory depression following intrathecal fentanyl-morphine combination. *Anesthesiology.* 1991;74:1153–1155.

252. Brockway MS, Noble DW, Sharwood-Smith GH, McClure JH. Profound respiratory depression after extradural fentanyl. *Br J Anaesth.* 1990;64:243–245.

253. Noble DW, Morrison LM, Brockway MS, McClure JH. Adrenaline, fentanyl or adrenaline and fentanyl as adjuncts to bupivacaine for extradural anaesthesia in elective caesarean section. *Br J Anaesth.* 1991;66:645–650.

254. Madej TH, Strunin L. Comparison of epidural fentanyl with sufentanil. Analgesia and side effects after a single bolus dose during elective caesarean section. *Anaesthesia.* 1987;42: 1156–1161.

255. Sultan P, Gutierrez MC, Carvalho B. Neuraxial morphine and respiratory depression: finding the right balance. *Drugs*. 2011;71:1807–1819.

256. Bauchat JR, McCarthy R, Fitzgerald P, et al. Transcutaneous carbon dioxide measurements in women receiving intrathecal morphine for cesarean delivery: a prospective observational study. *Anesth Analg*. 2017;124:872–878.

257. Lee LA, Caplan RA, Stephens LS, et al. Postoperative opioid-induced respiratory depression: a closed claims analysis. *Anesthesiology*. 2015;122:659–665.

258. Abboud TK, Moore M, Zhu J, et al. Epidural butorphanol or morphine for the relief of post-cesarean section pain: Ventilatory responses to carbon dioxide. *Anesth Analg*. 1987;66:887–893.

259. Carvalho B. Respiratory depression after neuraxial opioids in the obstetric setting. *Anesth Analg*. 2008;107:956–961.

260. Bauchat JR, Weiniger CF, Sultan P, et al. Society for Obstetric Anesthesia and Perinatology consensus statement: monitoring recommendations for prevention and detection of respiratory depression associated with administration of neuraxial morphine for cesarean delivery analgesia. *Anesth Analg*. 2019;129:458–474.

261. Chaney MA. Side effects of intrathecal and epidural opioids. *Can J Anaesth*. 1995;42:891–903.

262. Goodwin TM. Nausea and vomiting of pregnancy: an obstetric syndrome. *Am J Obstet Gynecol*. 2002;186:S184–S189.

263. Mishriky BM, Habib AS. Impact of data by Fujii and colleagues on the meta-analysis of metoclopramide for antiemetic prophylaxis in women undergoing caesarean delivery under neuraxial anaesthesia. *Br J Anaesth*. 2012;109:826.

264. Harnett MJ, O'Rourke N, Walsh M, et al. Transdermal scopolamine for prevention of intrathecal morphine-induced nausea and vomiting after cesarean delivery. *Anesth Analg*. 2007;105:764–769.

265. Pan PH, Moore CH. Comparing the efficacy of prophylactic metoclopramide, ondansetron, and placebo in cesarean section patients given epidural anesthesia. *J Clin Anesth*. 2001;13:430–435.

266. George RB, Allen TK, Habib AS. Serotonin receptor antagonists for the prevention and treatment of pruritus, nausea, and vomiting in women undergoing cesarean delivery with intrathecal morphine: a systematic review and meta-analysis. *Anesth Analg*. 2009;109:174–182.

267. Tzeng JI, Wang JJ, Ho ST, et al. Dexamethasone for prophylaxis of nausea and vomiting after epidural morphine for post-caesarean section analgesia: comparison of droperidol and saline. *Br J Anaesth*. 2000;85:865–868.

268. Wang JJ, Ho ST, Wong CS, et al. Dexamethasone prophylaxis of nausea and vomiting after epidural morphine for post-cesarean analgesia. *Can J Anaesth*. 2001;48:185–190.

269. Allen TK, Jones CA, Habib AS. Dexamethasone for the prophylaxis of postoperative nausea and vomiting associated with neuraxial morphine administration: a systematic review and meta-analysis. *Anesth Analg*. 2012;114:813–822.

270. Nortcliffe SA, Shah J, Buggy DJ. Prevention of postoperative nausea and vomiting after spinal morphine for caesarean section: comparison of cyclizine, dexamethasone and placebo. *Br J Anaesth*. 2003;90:665–670.

271. Heffernan AM, Rowbotham DJ. Postoperative nausea and vomiting—time for balanced antiemesis? *Br J Anaesth*. 2000;85:675–677.

272. Wu JI, Lo Y, Chia YY, et al. Prevention of postoperative nausea and vomiting after intrathecal morphine for cesarean section: a randomized comparison of dexamethasone, droperidol, and a combination. *Int J Obstet Anesth*. 2007;16:122–127.

273. Habib AS, George RB, McKeen DM, et al. Antiemetics added to phenylephrine infusion during cesarean delivery: a randomized controlled trial. *Obstet Gynecol*. 2013;121:615–623.

274. Allen TK, Habib AS. P6 stimulation for the prevention of nausea and vomiting associated with cesarean delivery under neuraxial anesthesia: a systematic review of randomized controlled trials. *Anesth Analg*. 2008;107:1308–1312.

275. Griffiths JD, Gyte GM, Paranjothy S, et al. Interventions for preventing nausea and vomiting in women undergoing regional anaesthesia for caesarean section. *Cochrane Database Syst Rev*. 2012;(5):CD007579.

276. Slappendel R, Weber EW, Benraad B, et al. Itching after intrathecal morphine. Incidence and treatment. *Eur J Anaesthesiol*. 2000;17:616–621.

277. Paech M, Sng B, Ng L, et al. Methylnaltrexone to prevent intrathecal morphine-induced pruritus after caesarean delivery: a multicentre, randomized clinical trial. *Br J Anaesth*. 2015;114:469–476.

278. Kendrick WD, Woods AM, Daly MY, et al. Naloxone versus nalbuphine infusion for prophylaxis of epidural morphine-induced pruritus. *Anesth Analg*. 1996;82:641–647.

279. Cohen SE, Ratner EF, Kreitzman TR, et al. Nalbuphine is better than naloxone for treatment of side effects after epidural morphine. *Anesth Analg*. 1992;75:747–752.

280. Kung AT, Yang X, Li Y, et al. Prevention versus treatment of intrathecal morphine-induced pruritus with ondansetron. *Int J Obstet Anesth*. 2014;23:222–226.

281. Morgan M. The rational use of intrathecal and extradural opioids. *Br J Anaesth*. 1989;63:165–188.

282. Ganesh A, Maxwell LG. Pathophysiology and management of opioid-induced pruritus. *Drugs*. 2007;67:2323–2333.

283. LaBella FS, Kim RS, Templeton J. Opiate receptor binding activity of 17-alpha estrogenic steroids. *Life Sci*. 1978;23:1797–1804.

284. Tsai FF, Fan SZ, Yang YM, et al. Human opioid μ-receptor A118G polymorphism may protect against central pruritus by epidural morphine for post-cesarean analgesia. *Acta Anaesthesiol Scand*. 2010;54:1265–1269.

285. Pettini E, Micaglio M, Bitossi U, et al. Influence of OPRM1 polymorphism on postoperative pain after intrathecal morphine administration in Italian patients undergoing elective cesarean section. *Clin J Pain*. 2018;34:178–181.

286. Kjellberg F, Tramèr MR. Pharmacological control of opioid-induced pruritus: a quantitative systematic review of randomized trials. *Eur J Anaesthesiol*. 2001;18:346–357.

287. Somrat C, Oranuch K, Ketchada U, et al. Optimal dose of nalbuphine for treatment of intrathecal-morphine induced pruritus after caesarean section. *J Obstet Gynaecol Res*. 1999;25:209–213.

288. Wu Z, Kong M, Wang N, et al. Intravenous butorphanol administration reduces intrathecal morphine-induced pruritus after cesarean delivery: a randomized, double-blind, placebo-controlled study. *J Anesth*. 2012;26:752–757.

289. Morgan PJ, Mehta S, Kapala DM. Nalbuphine pretreatment in cesarean section patients receiving epidural morphine. *Reg Anesth*. 1991;16:84–88.

290. Lockington PF, Fa'aea P. Subcutaneous naloxone for the prevention of intrathecal morphine induced pruritus in elective caesarean delivery. *Anaesthesia.* 2007;62:672–676.

291. Abboud TK, Afrasiabi A, Davidson J, et al. Prophylactic oral naltrexone with epidural morphine: effect on adverse reactions and ventilatory responses to carbon dioxide. *Anesthesiology.* 1990;72:233–237.

292. Abboud TK, Lee K, Zhu J, et al. Prophylactic oral naltrexone with intrathecal morphine for cesarean section: effects on adverse reactions and analgesia. *Anesth Analg.* 1990;71:367–370.

293. Ko MC, Lee H, Song MS, et al. Activation of kappa-opioid receptors inhibits pruritus evoked by subcutaneous or intrathecal administration of morphine in monkeys. *J Pharmacol Exp Ther.* 2003;305:173–179.

294. Shu H, Hayashida M, Arita H, et al. Pentazocine-induced antinociception is mediated mainly by mu-opioid receptors and compromised by kappa-opioid receptors in mice. *J Pharmacol Exp Ther.* 2011;338:579–587.

295. Tamdee D, Charuluxananan S, Punjasawadwong Y, et al. A randomized controlled trial of pentazocine versus ondansetron for the treatment of intrathecal morphine-induced pruritus in patients undergoing cesarean delivery. *Anesth Analg.* 2009;109:1606–1611.

296. Hirabayashi M, Doi K, Imamachi N, et al. Prophylactic pentazocine reduces the incidence of pruritus after cesarean delivery under spinal anesthesia with opioids: a prospective randomized clinical trial. *Anesth Analg.* 2017;124:1930–1934.

297. Jeon Y, Hwang J, Kang J, et al. Effects of epidural naloxone on pruritus induced by epidural morphine: a randomized controlled trial. *Int J Obstet Anesth.* 2005;14:22–25.

298. Borgeat A, Wilder-Smith OH, Saiah M, Rifat K. Subhypnotic doses of propofol relieve pruritus induced by epidural and intrathecal morphine. *Anesthesiology.* 1992;76:510–512.

299. Torn K, Tuominen M, Tarkkila P, Lindgren L. Effects of sub-hypnotic doses of propofol on the side effects of intrathecal morphine. *Br J Anaesth.* 1994;73:411–412.

300. Beilin Y, Bernstein HH, Zucker-Pinchoff B, et al. Subhypnotic doses of propofol do not relieve pruritus induced by intrathecal morphine after cesarean section. *Anesth Analg.* 1998;86:310–313.

301. Warwick JP, Kearns CF, Scott WE. The effect of subhypnotic doses of propofol on the incidence of pruritus after intrathecal morphine for caesarean section. *Anaesthesia.* 1997;52:270–275.

302. Charuluxananan S, Kyokong O, Somboonviboon W, et al. Nalbuphine versus propofol for treatment of intrathecal morphine-induced pruritus after cesarean delivery. *Anesth Analg.* 2001;93:162–165.

303. Bonnet MP, Marret E, Josserand J, Mercier FJ. Effect of prophylactic 5-HT3 receptor antagonists on pruritus induced by neuraxial opioids: a quantitative systematic review. *Br J Anaesth.* 2008;101:311–319.

304. Charuluxananan S, Kyokong O, Somboonviboon W, et al. Nalbuphine versus ondansetron for prevention of intrathecal morphine-induced pruritus after cesarean delivery. *Anesth Analg.* 2003;96:1789–1793.

305. Yeh HM, Chen LK, Lin CJ, et al. Prophylactic intravenous ondansetron reduces the incidence of intrathecal morphine-induced pruritus in patients undergoing cesarean delivery. *Anesth Analg.* 2000;91:172–175.

306. Siddik-Sayyid SM, Aouad MT, Taha SK, et al. Does ondansetron or granisetron prevent subarachnoid morphine-induced pruritus after cesarean delivery? *Anesth Analg.* 2007;104:421–424.

307. Yazigi A, Chalhoub V, Madi-Jebara S, et al. Prophylactic ondansetron is effective in the treatment of nausea and vomiting but not on pruritus after cesarean delivery with intrathecal sufentanil-morphine. *J Clin Anesth.* 2002;14:183–186.

308. Sarvela PJ, Halonen PM, Soikkeli AI, et al. Ondansetron and tropisetron do not prevent intraspinal morphine- and fentanyl-induced pruritus in elective cesarean delivery. *Acta Anaesthesiol Scand.* 2006;50:239–244.

309. Yazigi A, Chalhoub V, Madi-Jebara S, Haddad F. Ondansetron for prevention of intrathecal opioids-induced pruritus, nausea and vomiting after cesarean delivery. *Anesth Analg.* 2004;98:264.

310. Tan T, Ojo R, Immani S, et al. Reduction of severity of pruritus after elective caesarean section under spinal anaesthesia with subarachnoid morphine: a randomised comparison of prophylactic granisetron and ondansetron. *Int J Obstet Anesth.* 2010;19:56–60.

311. Charuluxananan S, Somboonviboon W, Kyokong O, Nimcharoendee K. Ondansetron for treatment of intrathecal morphine-induced pruritus after cesarean delivery. *Reg Anesth Pain Med.* 2000;25:535–539.

312. Alhashemi JA, Crosby ET, Grodecki W, et al. Treatment of intrathecal morphine-induced pruritus following caesarean section. *Can J Anaesth.* 1997;44:1060–1065.

313. Siddik-Sayyid SM, Yazbeck-Karam VG, Zahreddine BW, et al. Ondansetron is as effective as diphenhydramine for treatment of morphine-induced pruritus after cesarean delivery. *Acta Anaesthesiol Scand.* 2010;54:764–769.

314. Kuipers PW, Kamphuis ET, van Venrooij GE, et al. Intrathecal opioids and lower urinary tract function: a urodynamic evaluation. *Anesthesiology.* 2004;100:1497–1503.

315. Kamphuis ET, Ionescu TI, Kuipers PW, et al. Recovery of storage and emptying functions of the urinary bladder after spinal anesthesia with lidocaine and with bupivacaine in men. *Anesthesiology.* 1998;88:310–316.

316. Evron S, Samueloff A, Simon A, et al. Urinary function during epidural analgesia with methadone and morphine in post-cesarean section patients. *Pain.* 1985;23:135–144.

317. Liang CC, Chang SD, Wong SY, et al. Effects of postoperative analgesia on postpartum urinary retention in women undergoing cesarean delivery. *J Obstet Gynaecol Res.* 2010;36:991–995.

318. Rawal N, Mollefors K, Axelsson K, et al. An experimental study of urodynamic effects of epidural morphine and of naloxone reversal. *Anesth Analg.* 1983;62:641–647.

319. Rathmell JP, Lair TR, Nauman B. The role of intrathecal drugs in the treatment of acute pain. *Anesth Analg.* 2005;101:S30–S43.

320. Liang CC, Wu MP, Chang YL, et al. Voiding dysfunction in women following cesarean delivery. *Taiwan J Obstet Gynecol.* 2015;54:678–681.

321. Buchanan J, Beckmann M. Postpartum voiding dysfunction: Identifying the risk factors. *Aust N Z J Obstet Gynaecol.* 2014;54:41–45.

322. Walker SM, Goudas LC, Cousins MJ, Carr DB. Combination spinal analgesic chemotherapy: a systematic review. *Anesth Analg.* 2002;95:674–715.

323. Kitahata LM. Spinal analgesia with morphine and clonidine. *Anesth Analg.* 1989;68:191–193.

324. Taiwo YO, Fabian A, Pazoles CJ, Fields HL. Potentiation of morphine antinociception by monoamine reuptake inhibitors in the rat spinal cord. *Pain.* 1985;21:329–337.

325. Kuraishi Y, Hirota N, Sato Y, et al. Noradrenergic inhibition of the release of substance P from the primary afferents in the rabbit spinal dorsal horn. *Brain Res.* 1985;359:177–182.

326. Eisenach JC, De Kock M, Klimscha W. Alpha(2)-adrenergic agonists for regional anesthesia. A clinical review of clonidine (1984-1995). *Anesthesiology.* 1996;85:655–674.

327. Iwasaki H, Collins JG, Saito Y, et al. Low-dose clonidine enhances pregnancy-induced analgesia to visceral but not somatic stimuli in rats. *Anesth Analg.* 1991;72:325–329.

328. Elia N, Culebras X, Mazza C, et al. Clonidine as an adjuvant to intrathecal local anesthetics for surgery: systematic review of randomized trials. *Reg Anesth Pain Med.* 2008;33:159–167.

329. Mendez R, Eisenach JC, Kashtan K. Epidural clonidine analgesia after cesarean section. *Anesthesiology.* 1990;73:848–852.

330. Eisenach JC, D'Angelo R, Taylor C, Hood DD. An isobolographic study of epidural clonidine and fentanyl after cesarean section. *Anesth Analg.* 1994;79:285–290.

331. Capogna G, Celleno D, Zangrillo A, et al. Addition of clonidine to epidural morphine enhances postoperative analgesia after cesarean delivery. *Reg Anesth.* 1995;20:57–61.

332. Ginosar Y, Riley ET, Angst MS. Analgesic and sympatholytic effects of low-dose intrathecal clonidine compared with bupivacaine: a dose-response study in female volunteers. *Br J Anaesth.* 2013;111:256–263.

333. van Tuijl I, van Klei WA, van der Werff DB, Kalkman CJ. The effect of addition of intrathecal clonidine to hyperbaric bupivacaine on postoperative pain and morphine requirements after caesarean section: a randomized controlled trial. *Br J Anaesth.* 2006;97:365–370.

334. Benhamou D, Thorin D, Brichant JF, et al. Intrathecal clonidine and fentanyl with hyperbaric bupivacaine improves analgesia during cesarean section. *Anesth Analg.* 1998;87:609–613.

335. Paech MJ, Pavy TJ, Orlikowski CE, et al. Postcesarean analgesia with spinal morphine, clonidine, or their combination. *Anesth Analg.* 2004;98:1460–1466.

336. Lavand'homme PM, Roelants F, Waterloos H, et al. An evaluation of the postoperative antihyperalgesic and analgesic effects of intrathecal clonidine administered during elective cesarean delivery. *Anesth Analg.* 2008;107:948–955.

337. Carvalho FA, Tenorio SB, Shiohara FT, et al. Randomized study of postcesarean analgesia with intrathecal morphine alone or combined with clonidine. *J Clin Anesth.* 2016;33:395–402.

338. Allen TK, Mishriky BM, Klinger RY, Habib AS. The impact of neuraxial clonidine on postoperative analgesia and perioperative adverse effects in women having elective caesarean section-a systematic review and meta-analysis. *Br J Anaesth.* 2018;120:228–240.

339. Marhofer P, Brummett CM. Safety and efficiency of dexmedetomidine as adjuvant to local anesthetics. *Curr Opin Anaesthesiol.* 2016;29:632–637.

340. Yousef AA, Salem HA, Moustafa MZ. Effect of mini-dose epidural dexmedetomidine in elective cesarean section using combined spinal-epidural anesthesia: a randomized double-blinded controlled study. *J Anesth.* 2015;29:708–714.

341. Qi X, Chen D, Li G, et al. Comparison of intrathecal dexmedetomidine with morphine as adjuvants in cesarean sections. *Bio Pharm Bull.* 2016;39:1455–1460.

342. Leicht CH, Kelleher AJ, Robinson DE, Dickerson SE. Prolongation of postoperative epidural sufentanil analgesia with epinephrine. *Anesth Analg.* 1990;70:323–325.

343. McMorland GH, Douglas MJ, Kim JH, et al. Epidural sufentanil for post-caesarean section analgesia: lack of benefit of epinephrine. *Can J Anaesth.* 1990;37:432–437.

344. McLintic AJ, Danskin FH, Reid JA, Thorburn J. Effect of adrenaline on extradural anaesthesia, plasma lignocaine concentrations and the feto-placental unit during elective caesarean section. *Br J Anaesth.* 1991;67:683–689.

345. Alahuhta S, Räsänen J, Jouppila R, et al. Effects of extradural bupivacaine with adrenaline for caesarean section on uteroplacental and fetal circulation. *Br J Anaesth.* 1991;67:678–682.

346. Abouleish EI. Epinephrine improves the quality of spinal hyperbaric bupivacaine for cesarean section. *Anesth Analg.* 1987;66:395–400.

347. Abouleish E, Rawal N, Tobon-Randall B, et al. A clinical and laboratory study to compare the addition of 0.2 mg of morphine, 0.2 mg of epinephrine, or their combination to hyperbaric bupivacaine for spinal anesthesia in cesarean section. *Anesth Analg.* 1993;77:457–462.

348. Zakowski MI, Ramanathan S, Sharnick S, Turndorf H. Uptake and distribution of bupivacaine and morphine after intrathecal administration in parturients: effects of epinephrine. *Anesth Analg.* 1992;74:664–669.

349. Bouaziz H, Tong C, Eisenach JC. Postoperative analgesia from intrathecal neostigmine in sheep. *Anesth Analg.* 1995;80:1140–1144.

350. Hood DD, Eisenach JC, Tuttle R. Phase I safety assessment of intrathecal neostigmine methylsulfate in humans. *Anesthesiology.* 1995;82:331–343.

351. Hood DD, Eisenach JC, Tong C, et al. Cardiorespiratory and spinal cord blood flow effects of intrathecal neostigmine methylsulfate, clonidine, and their combination in sheep. *Anesthesiology.* 1995;82:428–435.

352. Kaya FN, Sahin S, Owen MD, Eisenach JC. Epidural neostigmine produces analgesia but also sedation in women after cesarean delivery. *Anesthesiology.* 2004;100:381–385.

353. Ross VH, Pan PH, Owen MD, et al. Neostigmine decreases bupivacaine use by patient-controlled epidural analgesia during labor: a randomized controlled study. *Anesth Analg.* 2009;109:524–531.

354. Unlugenc H, Ozalevli M, Gunes Y, et al. A double-blind comparison of intrathecal S(+) ketamine and fentanyl combined with bupivacaine 0.5% for caesarean delivery. *Eur J Anaesthesiol.* 2006;23:1018–1024.

355. Tramèr MR, Schneider J, Marti RA, Rifat K. Role of magnesium sulfate in postoperative analgesia. *Anesthesiology.* 1996;84:340–347.

356. Sun J, Wu X, Xu X, et al. A comparison of epidural magnesium and/or morphine with bupivacaine for postoperative analgesia after cesarean section. *Int J Obstet Anesth.* 2012;21:310–316.

357. Albrecht E, Kirkham KR, Liu SS, Brull R. The analgesic efficacy and safety of neuraxial magnesium sulphate: a quantitative review. *Anaesthesia.* 2013;68:190–202.

358. Ozalevli M, Cetin TO, Unlugenc H, et al. The effect of adding intrathecal magnesium sulphate to bupivacaine-fentanyl

spinal anaesthesia. *Acta Anaesthesiol Scand.* 2005;49: 1514–1519.

359. Arcioni R, Palmisani S, Tigano S, et al. Combined intrathecal and epidural magnesium sulfate supplementation of spinal anesthesia to reduce post-operative analgesic requirements: a prospective, randomized, double-blind, controlled trial in patients undergoing major orthopedic surgery. *Acta Anaesthesiol Scand.* 2007;51:482–489.

360. Unlugenc H, Ozalevli M, Gunduz M, et al. Comparison of intrathecal magnesium, fentanyl, or placebo combined with bupivacaine 0.5% for parturients undergoing elective cesarean delivery. *Acta Anaesthesiol Scand.* 2009;53:346–353.

361. Gan TJ, Habib AS. Adenosine as a non-opioid analgesic in the perioperative setting. *Anesth Analg.* 2007;105:487–494.

362. Rane K, Sollevi A, Segerdahl M. Intrathecal adenosine administration in abdominal hysterectomy lacks analgesic effect. *Acta Anaesthesiol Scand.* 2000;44:868–872.

363. Sharma M, Mohta M, Chawla R. Efficacy of intrathecal adenosine for postoperative pain relief. *Eur J Anaesthesiol.* 2006;23:449–453.

364. Rane K, Sollevi A, Segerdahl M. A randomised double-blind evaluation of adenosine as adjunct to sufentanil in spinal labour analgesia. *Acta Anaesthesiol Scand.* 2003;47:601–603.

365. Prakash S, Joshi N, Gogia AR, et al. Analgesic efficacy of two doses of intrathecal midazolam with bupivacaine in patients undergoing cesarean delivery. *Reg Anesth Pain Med.* 2006;31:221–226.

366. Dodawad R, Sumalatha GB, Pandarpurkar S, Jajee P. Intrathecal midazolam as an adjuvant in pregnancy-induced hypertensive patients undergoing an elective caesarean section: a clinical comparative study. *Anesth Pain Med.* 2016;6:e38550.

367. Hung TY, Huang YS, Lin YC. Maternal and neonatal outcomes with the addition of intrathecal midazolam as an adjuvant to spinal anesthesia in cesarean delivery: a systematic review and meta-analysis of randomized controlled trials. *J Clin Anesth.* 2022;80:110786.

368. Cheng JK, Chen CC, Yang JR, Chiou LC. The antiallodynic action target of intrathecal gabapentin: Ca2+ channels, KATP channels or N-methyl-D-aspartic acid receptors? *Anesth Analg.* 2006;102:182–187.

369. Cheng JK, Lai YJ, Chen CC, et al. Magnesium chloride and ruthenium red attenuate the antiallodynic effect of intrathecal gabapentin in a rat model of postoperative pain. *Anesthesiology.* 2003;98:1472–1479.

370. Choe H, Kim JS, Ko SH, et al. Epidural verapamil reduces analgesic consumption after lower abdominal surgery. *Anesth Analg.* 1998;86:786–790.

371. Schug SA, Saunders D, Kurowski I, Paech MJ. Neuraxial drug administration: a review of treatment options for anaesthesia and analgesia. *CNS Drugs.* 2006;20:917–933.

372. Blanco R, Ansari T, Riad W, Shetty N. Quadratus lumborum block versus transversus abdominis plane block for postoperative pain after cesarean delivery: a randomized controlled trial. *Reg Anesth Pain Med.* 2016;41:757–762.

373. Boules ML, Goda AS, Abdelhady MA, et al. Comparison of analgesic effect between erector spinae plane block and transversus abdominis plane block after elective cesarean section: a prospective randomized single-blind controlled study. *J Pain Res.* 2020;13:1073–1080.

374. Chin KJ, McDonnell JG, Carvalho B, et al. Essentials of our current understanding: abdominal wall blocks. *Reg Anesth Pain Med.* 2017;42:133–183.

375. Champaneria R, Shah L, Wilson MJ, Daniels JP. Clinical effectiveness of transversus abdominis plane (TAP) blocks for pain relief after caesarean section: a meta-analysis. *Int J Obstet Anesth.* 2016;28:45–60.

376. El-Boghdadly K, Desai N, Halpern S, et al. Quadratus lumborum block vs. transversus abdominis plane block for caesarean delivery: a systematic review and network meta-analysis. *Anaesthesia.* 2021;76:393–403.

377. Blanco R, Ansari T, Girgis E. Quadratus lumborum block for postoperative pain after caesarean section: a randomised controlled trial. *Eur J Anaesthesiol.* 2015;32:812–818.

378. Jadon A, Amir M, Sinha N, et al. Quadratus lumborum or transversus abdominis plane block for postoperative analgesia after cesarean: a double-blinded randomized trial. *Braz J Anesthesiol.* 2022;72:472–478.

379. Ribeiro Junior IDV, Carvalho VH, Brito LGO. Erector spinae plane block for analgesia after cesarean delivery: a systematic review with meta-analysis. *Braz J Anesthesiol.* 2022;72: 506–515.

380. Malawat A, Verma K, Jethava D, Jethava DD. Erector spinae plane block and transversus abdominis plane block for postoperative analgesia in cesarean section: a prospective randomized comparative study. *J Anaesthesiol Clin Pharmacol.* 2020;36:201–206.

381. Priya TK, Singla D, Talawar P, et al. Comparative efficacy of quadratus lumborum type-II and erector spinae plane block in patients undergoing caesarean section under spinal anaesthesia: a randomised controlled trial. *Int J Obstet Anesth.* 2023;53:103614.

382. Bakshi A, Srivastawa S, Jadon A, et al. Comparison of the analgesic efficacy of ultrasound-guided transmuscular quadratus lumborum block versus thoracic erector spinae block for postoperative analgesia in caesarean section parturients under spinal anaesthesia – a randomised study. *Indian J Anaesth.* 2022;66:S213–S219.

383. Mirza F, Carvalho B. Transversus abdominis plane blocks for rescue analgesia following cesarean delivery: a case series. *Can J Anaesth.* 2013;60:299–303.

384. Habib AS, Nedeljkovic SS, Horn JL, et al. Randomized trial of transversus abdominis plane block with liposomal bupivacaine after cesarean delivery with or without intrathecal morphine. *J Clin Anesth.* 2021;75:110527.

385. Wikner M. Unexpected motor weakness following quadratus lumborum block for gynaecological laparoscopy. *Anaesthesia.* 2017;72:230–232.

386. Griffiths JD, Le NV, Grant S, et al. Symptomatic local anaesthetic toxicity and plasma ropivacaine concentrations after transversus abdominis plane block for caesarean section. *Br J Anaesth.* 2013;110:996–1000.

387. Trabelsi B, Charfi R, Bennasr L, et al. Pharmacokinetics of bupivacaine after bilateral ultrasound-guided transversus abdominis plane block following cesarean delivery under spinal anesthesia. *Int J Obstet Anesth.* 2017;32:17–20.

388. Kitayama M, Wada M, Hashimoto H, et al. Effects of adding epinephrine on the early systemic absorption kinetics of local anesthetics in abdominal truncal blocks. *J Anesth.* 2014;28:631–634.

389. Chandon M, Bonnet A, Burg Y, et al. Ultrasound-guided transversus abdominis plane block versus continuous wound infusion for post-caesarean analgesia: a randomized trial. *PLoS ONE.* 2014;9:e103971.

390. Weiss E, Jolly C, Dumoulin JL, et al. Convulsions in 2 patients after bilateral ultrasound-guided transversus abdominis plane blocks for cesarean analgesia. *Reg Anesth Pain Med*. 2014;39:248–251.

391. Scherrer V, Compere V, Loisel C, Dureuil B. Cardiac arrest from local anesthetic toxicity after a field block and transversus abdominis plane block: a consequence of miscommunication between the anesthesiologist and surgeon. *A A Case Rep*. 2013;1:75–76.

392. Ng SC, Habib AS, Sodha S, et al. High-dose versus low-dose local anaesthetic for transversus abdominis plane block post-caesarean delivery analgesia: a meta-analysis. *Br J Anaesth*. 2018;120:252–263.

393. Wong CA. Editorial comment: Cardiac arrest from local anesthetic toxicity after a field block and transversus abdominis plane block: a consequence of miscommunication between the anesthesiologist and surgeon and probable local anesthetic systemic toxicity in a postpartum patient with acute fatty liver of pregnancy after a transversus abdominis plane block. *A A Case Rep*. 2013;1:77–78.

394. Wang J, Zhao G, Song G, Liu J. The efficacy and safety of local anesthetic techniques for postoperative analgesia after cesarean section: a Bayesian network meta-analysis of randomized controlled trials. *J Pain Res*. 2021:1559–1572.

395. Ryu C, Choi GJ, Jung YH, et al. Postoperative analgesic effectiveness of peripheral nerve blocks in cesarean delivery: a systematic review and network meta-analysis. *J Pers Med*. 2022;12:634.

396. Adesope O, Ituk U, Habib AS. Local anaesthetic wound infiltration for postcaesarean section analgesia: a systematic review and meta-analysis. *Eur J Anaesthesiol*. 2016;33:731–742.

397. Gómez-Ríos MÁ, Codesido-Barreiro P, Seco-Vilariño C, et al. Wound infusion of 0.35% levobupivacaine reduces mechanical secondary hyperalgesia and opioid consumption after cesarean delivery: a prospective, randomized, triple-blind, placebo-controlled trial. *Anesth Analg*. 2022;134:791–801.

398. Lalmand M, Wilwerth M, Fils JF, Van der Linden P. Continuous ropivacaine subfascial wound infusion compared with intrathecal morphine for postcesarean analgesia: a prospective, randomized controlled, double-blind study. *Anesth Analg*. 2017;125:907–912.

399. Barney EZ, Pedro CD, Gamez BH, et al. Ropivacaine and ketorolac wound infusion for post-cesarean delivery analgesia: a randomized controlled trial. *Obstet Gynecol*. 2020;135:427–435.

400. Singh NP, Monks D, Makkar JK, et al. Efficacy of regional blocks or local anaesthetic infiltration for analgesia after caesarean delivery: a network meta-analysis of randomised controlled trials. *Anaesthesia*. 2022;77:463–474.

401. Rackelboom T, Le Strat S, Silvera S, et al. Improving continuous wound infusion effectiveness for postoperative analgesia after cesarean delivery: a randomized controlled trial. *Obstet Gynecol*. 2010;116:893–900.

402. Klasen F, Bourgoin A, Antonini F, et al. Postoperative analgesia after caesarean section with transversus abdominis plane block or continuous infiltration wound catheter: a randomized clinical trial. TAP vs. infiltration after caesarean section. *Anaesth Crit Care Pain Med*. 2016;35:401–406.

403. Sultan P, Patel SD, Jadin S, et al. Transversus abdominis plane block compared with wound infiltration for postoperative analgesia following Cesarean delivery: a systematic review and network meta-analysis. *Can J Anaesth*. 2020;67:1710–1727.

404. Vallejo MC, Steen TL, Cobb BT, et al. Efficacy of the bilateral ilioinguinal-iliohypogastric block with intrathecal morphine for postoperative cesarean delivery analgesia. *ScientificWorldJournal*. 2012;2012:107316.

405. Wolfson A, Lee AJ, Wong RP, et al. Bilateral multi-injection iliohypogastric-ilioinguinal nerve block in conjunction with neuraxial morphine is superior to neuraxial morphine alone for postcesarean analgesia. *J Clin Anesth*. 2012;24:298–303.

406. Singh NP, Makkar JK, Bhatia N, Singh PM. The analgesic effectiveness of ilioinguinal-iliohypogastric block for caesarean delivery: a meta-analysis and trial sequential analysis. *Eur J Anaesthesiol*. 2021;38:S87–S96.

407. Lee TH, Barrington MJ, Tran TM, et al. Comparison of extent of sensory block following posterior and subcostal approaches to ultrasound-guided transversus abdominis plane block. *Anaesth Intensive Care*. 2010;38:452–460.

408. Staker JJ, Liu D, Church R, et al. A triple-blind, placebo-controlled randomised trial of the ilioinguinal-transversus abdominis plane (I-TAP) nerve block for elective caesarean section. *Anaesthesia*. 2018;73:594–602.

409. Niklasson B, Börjesson A, Carmnes UB, et al. Intraoperative injection of bupivacaine-adrenaline close to the fascia reduces morphine requirements after cesarean section: a randomized controlled trial. *Acta Obstet Gynecol Scand*. 2012;91:1433–1439.

410. Garmi G, Parasol M, Zafran N, et al. Efficacy of single wound infiltration with bupivacaine and adrenaline during cesarean delivery for reduction of postoperative pain: a randomized clinical trial. *JAMA Netw Open*. 2022;5:e2242203.

411. Simavli S, Kaygusuz I, Kinay T, et al. Bupivacaine-soaked absorbable gelatin sponges in caesarean section wounds: Effect on postoperative pain, analgesic requirement and haemodynamic profile. *Int J Obstet Anesth*. 2014;23:302–308.

412. Prabhu M, Clapp MA, McQuaid-Hanson E, et al. Liposomal bupivacaine block at the time of cesarean delivery to decrease postoperative pain: a randomized controlled trial. *Obstet Gynecol*. 2018;132:70–78.

413. Patel R, Carvalho JC, Downey K, et al. Intraperitoneal instillation of lidocaine improves postoperative analgesia at cesarean delivery: a randomized, double-blind, placebo-controlled trial. *Anesth Analg*. 2017;124:554–559.

414. Werntz M, Burwick R, Togioka B. Intraperitoneal chloroprocaine is a useful adjunct to neuraxial block during cesarean delivery: a case series. *Int J Obstet Anesth*. 2018;35:33–41.

415. Togioka BM, Zarnegarnia Y, Bleyle LA, et al. Pharmacokinetics and tolerability of intraperitoneal chloroprocaine after fetal extraction in women undergoing cesarean delivery. *Anesth Analg*. 2022;135:777–786.

PART VIII

Anesthesia Complications

28

Aspiration: Risk, Prophylaxis, and Treatment

Michaela K. Farber, MD, MS

CHAPTER OUTLINE

HISTORY

In 1848, Sir James Simpson first suggested aspiration as a cause of death during anesthesia. Hannah Greener, a 15-year-old given chloroform for a toenail extraction, became cyanotic and "sputtered" during the anesthetic. A "rattling in her throat" then developed, and she soon died. Her physician had administered water and brandy by mouth. Simpson[1] contended that it was the aspiration of water and brandy and not the adverse effects from the chloroform that caused her death. In 1940, Hall published a report of 15 cases of aspiration, 14 of which occurred in mothers receiving inhalation anesthesia for a vaginal or cesarean delivery.[2] Among the 14 obstetric cases, 5 mothers died.

In a subsequent landmark paper, Mendelson reported a series of animal experiments that clearly described the clinical course and pathology of pulmonary acid aspiration.[3] In the same paper, Mendelson audited 44,016 deliveries at the New York Lying-In Hospital between 1932 and 1945. He identified 66 (0.15%) cases of aspiration, of which the aspirated material was recorded in 45 cases; 40 mothers aspirated liquid and 5 aspirated solid food. Importantly, no mothers died from aspirated liquid, but two mothers died from asphyxiation caused by the aspiration of solid food. At this time general

anesthesia usually involved the inhalation of ether, often as Mendelson observed, by "a new and inexperienced intern." Mendelson therefore advocated (1) the withholding of food during labor, (2) the greater use of regional anesthesia, (3) the administration of antacids, (4) the emptying of the stomach before administration of general anesthesia, and (5) the competent administration of general anesthesia. This advice, meant to minimize the risk of pulmonary aspiration of gastric contents in parturients, has endured as a foundation of obstetric anesthesia practice.

INCIDENCE, MORBIDITY, AND MORTALITY

Maternal mortality from pulmonary aspiration of gastric contents has declined to almost negligible levels over the last several decades (Fig. 28.1).[4–9] This decline can likely be attributed to the following factors: (1) the greater use of neuraxial anesthesia; (2) the use of antacids, histamine-2 (H_2) receptor antagonists, and/or proton-pump inhibitors (PPIs); (3) the use of rapid-sequence induction of general anesthesia; (4) improved training of anesthesia providers; and (5) the establishment and enforcement of nil per os (NPO) policies during labor and delivery. Arguably, the common use of neuraxial analgesic/anesthetic techniques, both during

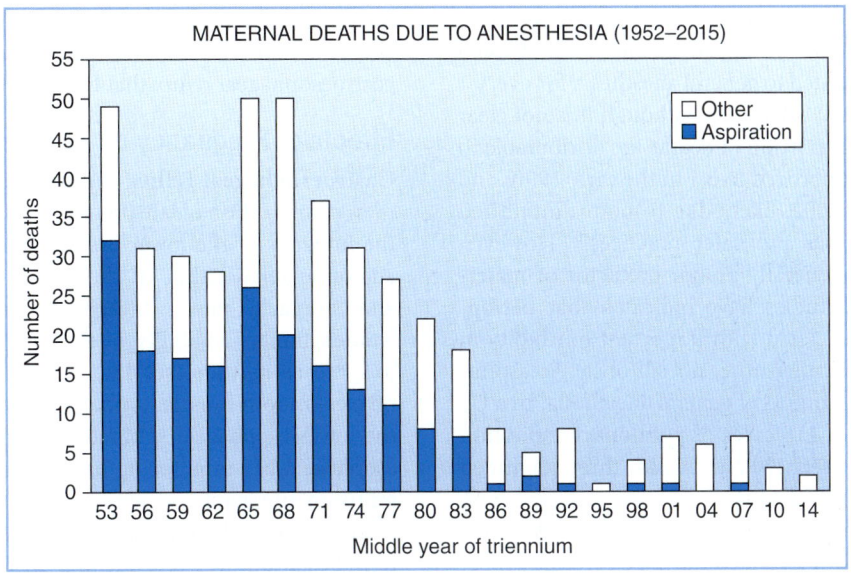

Fig. 28.1 Maternal mortality from anesthesia and pulmonary aspiration in the United Kingdom, 1952–2015 (each year on the *y*-axis represents the middle year of triennial data). Data from Turnbull A, Tindall VR, Beard RW, et al. Report on confidential enquiries into maternal deaths in England and Wales 1982–1984. *Rep Health Soc Subj (Lond)*. 1989;34:1–166; Bamber J, Lucas N, on behalf of the MBRRACE-UK Anaesthesia Chapter Writing Group. Messages for anaesthetic care In: Knight M, Nair M, Tuffnell D, Shakespeare J, Kenyon S, Kurinczuk JJ, eds., on behalf of MBRRACE-UK. Saving Lives, Improving Mothers' Care—Lessons Learned to Inform Maternity Care From the UK and Ireland Confidential Enquiries Into Maternal Deaths and Morbidity 2013-15. National Perinatal Epidemiology Unit, University of Oxford; 2017:67–73. Available at https://www.npeu.ox.ac.uk/mbrrace-uk/reports. Accessed 2 September 2024.

labor and for cesarean delivery, is the single most important factor in this remarkable decline in maternal mortality from pulmonary aspiration.

The reported incidence of aspiration pneumonitis depends on the criteria used for making the diagnosis. The relative risk for aspiration in pregnant versus nonpregnant women can best be estimated from comparisons within single-study populations. Olsson et al.[7] reported an overall incidence of aspiration of 1 in 2131 in the general population undergoing anesthesia and 1 in 661 in women undergoing cesarean delivery (i.e., a threefold higher aspiration risk). In two other surveys (a retrospective review of 172,334 consecutive patients undergoing general anesthesia[8] and a review of 133 cases of aspiration from the Australian Anaesthetic Incident Monitoring Study [AIMS][9]), there were no cases of pulmonary aspiration in women undergoing either elective or emergency cesarean delivery. However, in the latter two studies,[8,9] emergency surgery was a significant predisposing factor for aspiration; this finding may be relevant for the practice of obstetric anesthesia, given that many obstetric surgical procedures are performed on an urgent or emergency basis. The AIMS study also implicated obesity as a significant risk factor for aspiration.[9]

Morbidity and mortality associated with aspiration vary according to (1) the physical status of the patient, (2) the contents and volume of aspirate, (3) the therapy administered, and (4) the criteria used for making the diagnosis. Since 1952, organizations in the United Kingdom have published detailed triennial reports on all maternal deaths. Data

from these reports, now administered by the body *Mothers and Babies—Reducing Risk through Audits and Confidential Enquiries across the UK* (MBRRACE-UK), indicate that death from pulmonary aspiration in obstetrics is rare (see Fig. 28.1).[4–6,10,11] In the MBRRACE-UK reports from 2009 to 2015, there were no reported maternal deaths from aspiration. Prior reports from 2006 to 2008 identified three maternal deaths from aspiration[10]; one was an obese parturient, the second was a mother anesthetized 3 days after delivery, and the third was a woman with a placenta previa who required an emergency cesarean delivery after eating a full meal and aspirated on emergence from general anesthesia. The UK Obstetric Surveillance System identified nine cases of aspiration in 1,496,720 maternities between September 2013 and August 2015, for an incidence of 6.0 per 1,000,000 maternities (95% confidence interval [CI] 2.18 to 11.4) and one mortality (case fatality 11%).[11] Seven cases occurred in association with general anesthesia and two in women semiconscious for other reasons. Of the cases associated with anesthesia, one occurred during difficult tracheal intubation, one while intubated, one following tracheal extubation, two had a supraglottic (laryngeal mask) airway in place, and two had an oropharyngeal airway at the time of the event.

Data on pulmonary aspiration in obstetrics in the United States are less comprehensive. The Serious Complication Registry from the Society for Obstetric Anesthesia and Perinatology (SOAP) review of 307,000 deliveries from 30 US centers between 2004 and 2009 reported a failed tracheal intubation rate of 1 in 533, but no related cases of pulmonary aspiration.[12] Prior to 1990, aspiration was the most common cause of anesthesia-related maternal death in the United States, with 17 deaths related to general anesthesia for every 1 death related to neuraxial anesthesia, although it is not clear from these data what proportion of deaths are attributable to aspiration.[13] This ratio improved to 6:1 in the early 1990s and nearly equilibrated by 2002, likely due to both diminished use of general anesthesia and safer practices.[14] However, mortality statistics are generally a poor predictor of maternal morbidity; several studies have indicated that perioperative aspiration is associated with important morbidity in obstetric patients.[15–17] Furthermore, not all obstetric aspiration events occur in the context of general anesthesia. In a US closed claims analysis of 115 cases of pulmonary aspiration of gastric contents between 2000 and 2014, three identified obstetric patients were undergoing cesarean delivery with only one of the three receiving general anesthesia.[18] A fourth identified obstetric patient aspirated during a cerclage procedure, prompting emergency cesarean delivery under general anesthesia.

A retrospective study of 48,619 patients undergoing cesarean delivery from 2007 to 2018 at two high-volume centers in Israel (general anesthesia rate 46.7%) reported three cases of suspected pulmonary aspiration.[19] Two cases occurred during induction of general anesthesia for emergency cesarean delivery associated with a difficult airway, and one under deep sedation as an adjunct to spinal anesthesia. This represents an incidence of aspiration of 1 in 11,345 with general anesthesia and 1 in 25,929 with neuraxial anesthesia. There were no associated deaths. Taken together, these data reinforce that, while pulmonary aspiration in obstetric patients is rare, all possible measures must be taken to prevent it and vigilance must be maintained during both neuraxial and general anesthesia.

GASTROESOPHAGEAL ANATOMY AND FUNCTION DURING PREGNANCY

Esophagus

In adults, the esophagus is approximately 25 cm long and the esophagogastric junction is approximately 40 cm from the incisor teeth. In humans, the proximal one-third of the esophagus is composed of striated muscle, but the distal end contains only smooth muscle. Muscular sphincters at both ends are normally closed. The cricopharyngeal or upper esophageal sphincter prevents the entry of air into the esophagus during respiration, and the gastroesophageal or lower esophageal sphincter prevents the reflux of gastric contents. The lower esophageal sphincter is characterized anatomically and manometrically as a 3-cm zone of specialized muscle that maintains tonic activity. The end-expiratory pressure in the sphincter is 8 to 20 mm Hg above the end-expiratory gastric pressure. The lower esophageal sphincter is kept in place by the phrenoesophageal ligament, which inserts into the esophagus approximately 3 cm above the diaphragmatic

opening (Fig. 28.2). The lower esophageal sphincter is not always closed; transient relaxations occur that account for the gastroesophageal reflux that healthy people experience.

Effects of Pregnancy on Gastric Function

Gastroesophageal reflux, resulting in heartburn, is a common complication of late pregnancy. Pregnancy compromises the integrity of the lower esophageal sphincter; it alters the anatomic relationship of the esophagus to the diaphragm and stomach, raises intragastric pressure, and in some women limits the ability of the lower esophageal sphincter to increase its tone (see Fig. 28.2).[20–23] Progesterone, which relaxes smooth muscle, probably accounts for the inability of the lower esophageal sphincter to increase its tone.[24] Lower esophageal pH monitoring has shown a higher incidence of reflux in pregnant women at term, even in those who are asymptomatic, than in nonpregnant controls.[23] Therefore, at term gestation the pregnant woman who requires anesthesia should be regarded as having an **incompetent lower esophageal sphincter**. These physiologic changes return to their prepregnancy levels by 48 hours after delivery.[23]

Serial studies assessing **gastric acidity** during pregnancy have proved difficult to perform because they require repeated placement of a nasogastric tube. However, in the most comprehensive study of gastric acid secretion during pregnancy, basal and histamine-augmented gastric acid secretion was measured in 10 controls and 30 pregnant women equally distributed throughout the three trimesters of pregnancy.[25] No significant differences in basal gastric acid secretion were seen between the pregnant and nonpregnant women. The plasma concentration of the gastrointestinal hormone motilin is decreased during pregnancy.[26] Studies have shown either no change[20,22,27] or an increase[28] in the plasma concentration of gastrin. A variety of techniques have been used to study **gastric emptying** during pregnancy and labor (Table 28.1).[29–44,46–49] Overall, the data suggest that pregnancy does not significantly alter the rate of gastric emptying.[32,50] Moreover, gastric emptying has not been found to be delayed in either obese or nonobese term pregnant women who ingested 300 mL of water after an overnight fast.[46,47] However, management of obese parturients should take into account the possible presence of other associated problems in this group of patients (e.g., hiatal hernia, difficult airway).

Gastric emptying appears to be normal in early labor but becomes delayed as labor advances; the cause is uncertain. Parenteral opioids cause a significant delay in gastric emptying, as do bolus doses of epidural and intrathecal opioids.[35,37,41,42,48] Gastric emptying measured by acetaminophen absorption in laboring parturients receiving an epidural infusion of bupivacaine/fentanyl demonstrated delay when the cumulative fentanyl dose exceeded 100 μg.[41] However, in a randomized controlled trial of 80, nonfasted, laboring women comparing low-dose (cumulative fentanyl < 100 μg) and high-dose (cumulative fentanyl > 100 μg) epidural fentanyl, the ultrasonographically determined rate of gastric emptying (assessment of change in antral cross-sectional area

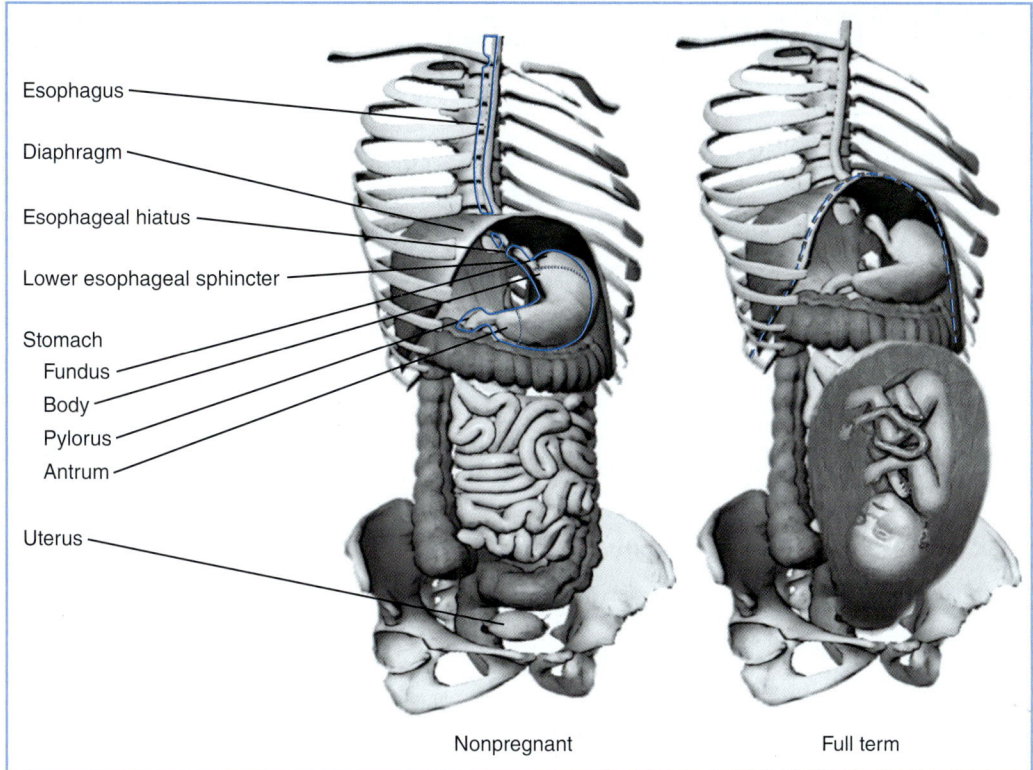

Fig. 28.2 The Stomach and Its Relationship to the Diaphragm in Nonpregnancy *(Left)* and Pregnancy *(Right)*. The stomach consists of a fundus, body, antrum, and pylorus. The function of the lower esophageal sphincter depends on the chronic contraction of circular muscle fibers, the wrapping of the esophagus by the crus of the diaphragm at the esophageal hiatus, and the length of the esophagus exposed to intraabdominal pressure. The gravid uterus may encroach on the stomach and alter the effectiveness of the lower esophageal sphincter. Illustration by Naveen Nathan, MD, NorthShore University HealthSystem, University of Chicago Pritzker School of Medicine, Evanston, IL.

[CSA]) was not different between groups.[45] While previous studies evaluated gastric emptying by pharmacokinetic timing of paracetamol absorption in the duodenum, this study used direct ultrasonographic assessment of gastric contents and is likely more relevant for the real-time assessment of aspiration risk.

RISK FACTORS FOR ASPIRATION PNEUMONITIS

Mendelson[3] categorized aspiration pneumonitis into two types: liquid and solid. Whereas the aspiration of solids could result in asphyxiation, Mendelson demonstrated that the sequelae from the aspiration of liquids resulted in more severe pathology and clinical severity when the liquid was highly acidic. His observations and other investigations[51-56] suggest that the morbidity and mortality of aspiration depend on the following three variables: (1) the chemical nature of the aspirate, (2) the physical nature of the aspirate, and (3) the volume of the aspirate. Aspirates with a pH < 2.5 cause a granulocytic reaction that continues beyond the acute phase.[56] Aspiration of particulate material can yield a clinical picture

with severity on par or worse than that caused by the aspiration of acidic liquid.[55] Aspiration of small volumes of neutral liquid results in a low rate of mortality. However, aspiration of large volumes of neutral liquid results in a high mortality rate, presumably as a result of the disruption of surfactant by the large volume of liquid or from a mechanism similar to that seen in "near drowning."[52]

Historically, anesthesia providers have considered a nonparticulate gastric fluid with a pH < 2.5 and a gastric volume > 25 mL (i.e., 0.4 mL/kg) as risk factors for aspiration pneumonitis.[51,53,54] No human study has directly addressed the relationship between preoperative fasting, gastric acidity and volume, and the risk for pulmonary aspiration during anesthesia.[57,58] There appears to be a reasonable scientific basis to use a gastric pH threshold value of less than 2.5 as a risk factor. In animal experiments, the risk for aspiration pneumonitis clearly increased with decreasing pH of the tracheal aspirate (Fig. 28.3).[51,52]

Animal studies have also demonstrated that an increase in the volume of tracheal aspirate is associated with a higher risk for aspiration pneumonitis.[52] However, the volume of aspirated material associated with risk has been disputed. The commonly accepted volume of 0.4 mL/kg (approximately

TABLE 28.1   Studies of Gastric Emptying During Pregnancy and Labor (1982–Present)

Method of Assessment	Study	Study Period and Subjects	Gastric Emptying
Epigastric impedance	O'Sullivan et al. (1987)[29]	Nonpregnant controls, third trimester, 60 min postpartum	No delay
Applied potential tomography	Sandhar et al. (1992)[30]	Sequential study 10 mothers: 37–40 weeks' gestation, 2–3 d postpartum, 6 w postpartum	No delay
Acetaminophen absorption	Simpson et al. (1988)[31]	Nonpregnant controls, 8–11 weeks' gestation, 12–14 weeks' gestation	8–11 w: no delay 12–14 w: delay
	Macfie et al. (1991)[32]	Nonpregnant controls, first, second, and third trimesters	No delay in any trimester
	Geddes et al. (1991)[33]	Postcesarean delivery Epidural fentanyl 100 µg	Delay
	Gin et al. (1991)[34]	Postpartum: day 1 and day 3, 6 w	No delay
	Wright et al. (1992)[35]	Labor, epidural bolus: (1) bupivacaine 0.375%; (2) bupivacaine 0.375% + fentanyl 100 µg	Epidural opioids: delay
	Whitehead et al. (1993)[36]	Nonpregnant controls, first, second, and third trimesters Postpartum: 2, 18–24, and 24–48 h	Pregnancy: No change Postpartum: • 2 h: delay • 18–24 h: no delay • 24–48 h: no delay
	Ewah et al. (1993)[37]	Labor with epidural infusion: (1) bupivacaine 0.25%; (2) bupivacaine 0.25% + fentanyl 50 or 100 µg, or diamorphine 2.5 or 5 mg	Epidural opioids: delay
	Levy et al. (1994)[38]	Nonpregnant controls, 8–12 weeks' gestation	Delay
	Stanley et al. (1995)[39]	Second and third trimesters and 8 w postpartum	No delay
	Zimmermann et al. (1996)[40]	Labor with epidural infusion: (1) bupivacaine 0.125%; (2) bupivacaine 0.125% + fentanyl 2 µg/mL	No delay
	Porter et al. (1997)[41]	Labor with epidural infusion: (1) bupivacaine 0.125%; (2) bupivacaine 0.125% + fentanyl 2.5 µg/mL	Epidural fentanyl total: • <100 µg: no delay • >100 µg: delay
	Kelly et al. (1997)[42]	Labor with neuraxial bolus: (1) epidural bupivacaine 0.375%; (2) epidural bupivacaine 0.25% + fentanyl 50 µg; (3) intrathecal bupivacaine 2.5 mg + fentanyl 25 µg	Epidural fentanyl: no delay Intrathecal fentanyl: delay
Real-time ultrasonography	Carp et al. (1992)[43]	Nonpregnant controls, third trimester	No delay
	Chiloiro et al. (2001)[44]	Serial study in 11 women: first and third trimesters, 4–6 mo postpartum	No delay
	Fiszer et al. (2022)[45]	80 low-risk nonfasted parturients in labor randomized to receive high dose versus low-dose epidural fentanyl	Epidural fentanyl > 100 µg versus < 100 µg: no difference
Real-time ultrasonography and acetaminophen absorption	Wong et al. (2002)[46]	Third trimester crossover study	50- or 300-mL water: no delay Faster gastric emptying with 300 mL
	Wong et al. (2007)[47]	10 obese parturients Third-trimester crossover study	50- or 300-mL water: no delay

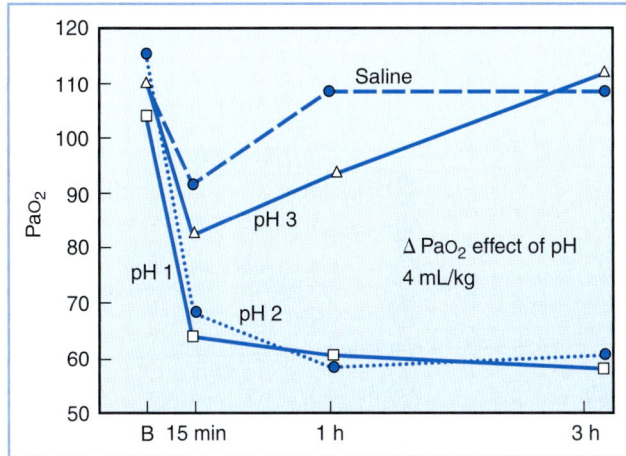

Fig. 28.3 Relationship Between Acidity and Pao$_2$. In this study, 4 mL/kg of fluid of varying pH was instilled into the tracheas of dogs. The severity of the hypoxemia correlated with the pH of the aspirate. A maximal decrease in Pao$_2$ occurred with aspirates with a pH < 2.5. *B*, Baseline. From Awe WC, Fletcher WS, Jacob SW. The pathophysiology of aspiration pneumonitis. *Surgery*. 1966;60: 232–239.

25 mL in a 70-kg adult) originated from an experiment in a single rhesus monkey in which 0.4 mL/kg of an acidic liquid was administered into the right mainstem bronchus and resulted in the animal's death.[54,56] The investigators made the assumption that this entire volume, if contained in the stomach, could be aspirated. However, Raidoo et al.[59] demonstrated variability in the response of juvenile monkeys to different volumes of an acidic tracheal aspirate. Death was seen with aspirate volumes of 0.8 and 1.0 mL/kg but not with volumes of 0.4 and 0.6 mL/kg. Similarly, Plourde and Hardy[60] refuted the assumption that all the gastric contents will be aspirated and demonstrated that gastric volumes of 0.4 mL/ kg did not increase the risk for aspiration. Hence, the gastric volume that puts a patient at risk for aspiration pneumonitis has not been determined. However, a reasonable goal of prophylactic therapy would be a gastric pH > 2.5 and a gastric volume as low as possible.

PATHOPHYSIOLOGY

Aspiration pneumonitis (Mendelson syndrome) describes a chemical injury to the tracheobronchial tree and alveoli caused by the inhalation of sterile acidic gastric contents, whereas **aspiration pneumonia** may be regarded as an infectious process of the respiratory tract caused by the inhalation of oropharyngeal secretions that are colonized by pathogenic bacteria. Aspiration of gastric contents could therefore result in acid injury to the lung with or without bacterial and particulate matter–related effects.

Aspiration of acidic liquid injures the alveolar epithelium and results in an alveolar exudate composed of edema, albumin, fibrin, cellular debris, and red blood cells, whereas the aspiration of neutral, nonparticulate liquid leads to an alveolar exudate with minimal damage to the alveoli. The phospholipid and apoprotein composition of surfactant

changes, exerting a negative effect on its surface-active properties.[61] This effect leads to an increase in intra-alveolar water and protein content and a loss of lung volume, resulting in a decrease in pulmonary compliance and intrapulmonary shunting of blood. The cellular debris and bronchial denuding cause bronchial obstruction. The exudative pulmonary edema, bronchial obstruction, reduced lung compliance, and shunting result in hypoxemia, increased pulmonary vascular resistance, and increased work of breathing. After the direct acid-mediated injury of the respiratory tract, an intense inflammatory response ensues from macrophage activation and secretion of cytokines.[62] These inflammatory mediators lead to the chemotaxis, accumulation, and activation of neutrophils in the alveolar exudate, upregulation of adhesion molecules within the pulmonary vasculature, and activation of the complement pathways. The neutrophils subsequently release oxidants, proteases, leukotrienes, and other proinflammatory molecules.[62] Amplification of these inflammatory processes may result in the development of acute lung injury or acute respiratory distress syndrome (ARDS) (Fig. 28.4).[61–63]

The acidic contents of the stomach prevent the growth of bacteria under normal conditions. However, gastric contents may become colonized with pathogenic gram-negative bacteria in patients receiving antacid therapy (e.g., PPI or H$_2$-receptor antagonist) or patients with gastroparesis or intestinal obstruction. The bacterial content adds to the inflammatory response of acid aspiration.[64]

Aspiration of particulate matter in the supine position most commonly involves injury to the posterior segments of the upper lobes and the apical segments of the lower lobes, whereas aspiration in the semirecumbent or upright position typically leads to injury to the lower lobes. The right lower lobe is the most common site of aspiration injury because the right mainstem bronchus has larger and more vertical architecture compared with the left mainstem bronchus. Obstruction of the bronchus or bronchioles results in bronchial denudation and collapse of the bronchopulmonary segments. Persistent or unresolved collapse can lead to lung abscesses and cavitation.[64]

After the acute period, the process resolves through the proliferation and differentiation of surviving type II pneumocytes in the alveolar epithelial cells.[62,63] The type II pneumocytes actively transport sodium out of the alveolus, and water follows passively. Soluble proteins are removed by paracellular diffusion and endocytosis, and insoluble proteins are removed by macrophages. Neutrophils are removed by programmed cell death and subsequent phagocytosis by macrophages. Type II pneumocytes gradually restore the normal composition of the surfactant. In a subset of patients with ARDS, the injury progresses to fibrosing alveolitis—an accumulation of mesenchymal cells, their products, and new blood vessels.

Bronchospasm and disruption of surfactant likely account for the decrease in Pao$_2$ and increase in shunting that are observed.[56] Aspiration of large solid particles may cause atelectasis by obstructing large airways.[3] Aspiration of

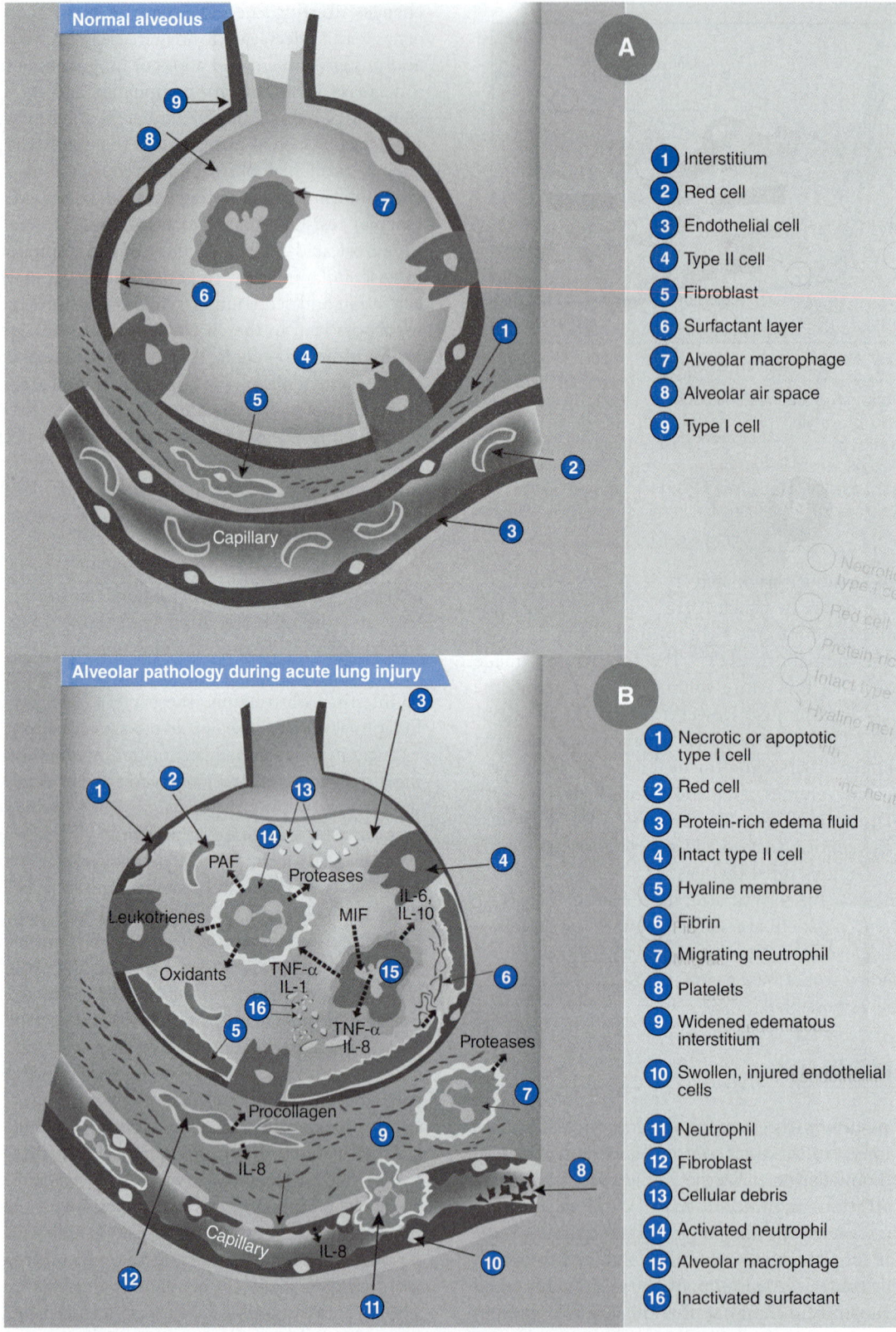

Normal alveolus

A

1. Interstitium
2. Red cell
3. Endothelial cell
4. Type II cell
5. Fibroblast
6. Surfactant layer
7. Alveolar macrophage
8. Alveolar air space
9. Type I cell

Capillary

Alveolar pathology during acute lung injury

B

PAF
Proteases
IL-6, IL-10
Leukotrienes
MIF
Oxidants
TNF-α IL-1
TNF-α IL-8
Proteases
Procollagen
IL-8
Capillary
IL-8

1. Necrotic or apoptotic type I cell
2. Red cell
3. Protein-rich edema fluid
4. Intact type II cell
5. Hyaline membrane
6. Fibrin
7. Migrating neutrophil
8. Platelets
9. Widened edematous interstitium
10. Swollen, injured endothelial cells
11. Neutrophil
12. Fibroblast
13. Cellular debris
14. Activated neutrophil
15. Alveolar macrophage
16. Inactivated surfactant

Fig. 28.4 Illustration Showing the Normal Alveolus (A) and the Injured Alveolus (B) During Acute Lung Injury. In the acute phase of acute lung injury, there is formation of protein-rich hyaline membranes on the denuded basement membrane. Neutrophils are marginating through the interstitium into the air space. Alveolar macrophages secrete interleukin (IL)-1, 6, 8, and 10, as well as tumor necrosis factor-alpha (TNF-α), which stimulate and activate neutrophils. Neutrophils release proinflammatory molecules (oxidants, proteases, leukotrienes, platelet-activating factor [PAF]). The influx of protein-rich edema fluid into the alveolus has led to the inactivation of surfactant and, together with unresolved fibrin depositions, fibrin-rich hyaline membranes are formed. *MIF*, Mullerian inhibiting factor. From Dahlem P, van Aalderen WMC, Bos AP. Pediatric acute lung injury. *Paediatr Respir Rev.* 2007;8:348–362.

smaller particulate matter causes an exudative neutrophilic response at the level of the bronchioles and alveolar ducts; the clinical picture is similar after the aspiration of acidic liquid.[55,56]

CLINICAL COURSE

In most cases of aspiration during anesthesia, the anesthesia provider witnesses regurgitation of gastric contents into the hypopharynx.[3] Patients who aspirate while breathing spontaneously have a brief period of breath-holding followed by tachypnea, tachycardia, and a slight respiratory acidosis. Significant aspiration always results in hypoxemia caused by an increase in shunting and, frequently, bronchospasm.

An abnormality on a chest radiograph can be seen in 85% to 90% of patients who aspirate gastric contents.[65] Because these chest radiographic findings may lag behind clinical signs by as much as 12 to 24 hours, the initial radiograph may appear normal.[65] In mild cases, alveolar infiltrates are seen in the dependent portions of the lungs. Severe aspiration results in diffuse bilateral infiltrates without signs of heart failure (i.e., without engorged pulmonary vasculature and/or enlarged cardiac silhouette) (Fig. 28.5).

These symptoms and signs may progress to satisfy the Berlin Definition for ARDS. The criteria are as follows[66]:

- *Clinical:* within 1 week of known clinical insult
- *Chest imaging:* bilateral opacities not explained by effusions
- *Biochemical:* Pao_2/Fio_2 ratio ≤ 300 mm Hg with continuous positive airway pressure (CPAP) or positive end-expiratory pressure (PEEP) > 5 cm H_2O
- *Origin of pulmonary edema:* not explained by cardiac failure or fluid overload

A new global definition of ARDS builds upon the Berlin Definition to include high-flow nasal oxygen with a minimum flow rate ≥ 30 L/min, Pao_2/Fio_2 ratio ≤ 300 mm Hg, or $Spo_2/Fio_2 \geq 315$ to identify hypoxemia, the addition of lung ultrasonography as an imaging modality along with chest radiography, and not mandating specific respiratory support devices in low-resource settings.[67]

TREATMENT

Management principles for the treatment of pulmonary aspiration include (1) tracheal suction; (2) rigid bronchoscopy in cases of aspiration of large, solid particles; and (3) management of hypoxemia with CPAP in nonintubated patients. Treatments that lack evidence to support their use are the administration of corticosteroids, routine use of prophylactic antibiotics, and lung lavage with saline and bicarbonate.[64]

Initial Management

Pulmonary aspiration of gastric contents must be instantly recognized and trigger a rapid, systematic response.[68] Critical management steps include positioning the patient in a head-down position and prompt suction of the upper airway followed by tracheal intubation and suction of the primary bronchi with a soft suction catheter. Fiberoptic bronchoscopy can be useful for evaluating the extent of aspiration and whether solid particles are present, and for the removal of liquid contents. Rigid bronchoscopy is useful for removing large food particles that cause airway obstruction. Lung lavage with saline or bicarbonate does *not* reduce the parenchymal damage caused by acid aspiration and can worsen hypoxemia.[64]

Antibiotics

Prophylactic antibiotics are *not* efficacious for treatment of aspiration and may lead to the development of infection with resistant organisms. Infection is not a component of acute pulmonary aspiration of sterile gastric contents.[64] Antibiotics should be administered only in the presence of clinical findings that suggest infection (e.g., fever, worsening infiltrates on chest radiographs, leukocytosis, positive result of Gram stain of sputum, clinical deterioration).

In patients who are intubated, a nonbronchoscopic bronchoalveolar lavage sample can be sent for laboratory analysis. Tracheal sputum samples may be insufficient to identify a bacterial pathogen, and some authorities recommend sampling of the lower respiratory tract with a protected specimen brush.[64]

Empirical antibiotic therapy is appropriate in patients with suspected bacterial colonization of gastric contents. The "at-risk" group (see earlier discussion) includes patients who have gastroparesis or bowel obstruction and those who are receiving antacid therapy. The use of PPIs and H_2-receptor antagonists is common in late pregnancy, given the prevalence of gastroesophageal reflux disease. Reduced gastric acidity from long-term antacid therapy increases the incidence of community-acquired and ventilation-associated pneumonia,[69,70] but it is uncertain whether parturients on long-term acid-suppression therapy are at higher risk for developing bacterial pneumonia after aspiration. Nonetheless, empirical antibiotic therapy is also appropriate for parturients on long-term antacid therapy and for those with aspiration pneumonitis

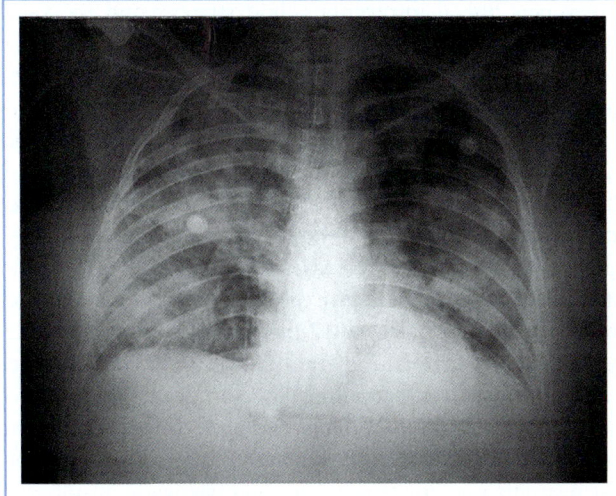

Fig. 28.5 Radiographic changes after pulmonary aspiration of gastric contents in pregnancy.

that fails to resolve within 48 hours. The choice of antibiotic depends on the observed local patterns of antibiotic resistance. The target pathogens are gram-positive organisms (e.g., *Streptococcus pneumoniae, Staphylococcus aureus*) and some gram-negative organisms (e.g., *Haemophilus influenzae, Escherichia coli,* Enterobacteriaceae) when the diagnosis is made less than 48 hours after hospital admission (i.e., community-acquired pneumonia). *Pseudomonas aeruginosa* is a common pathogen in cases of nosocomial (hospital-acquired) aspiration pneumonia. Anaerobes are no longer believed to be present in the majority of cases.[64] Pharmacologic therapy should be altered when specific pathogens and their antibiotic sensitivities are determined.

Treatment of Hypoxemia

Exudation of fluid into the alveoli, decreased surface activity of surfactant, and atelectasis all result in intrapulmonary shunting and hypoxemia. The administration of CPAP in patients breathing spontaneously or the administration of PEEP in patients undergoing mechanical ventilation restores functional residual capacity, reduces pulmonary shunting, and reverses hypoxemia. Supplemental oxygen should be given as required.

Corticosteroids

Despite decades-long use of corticosteroids in the management of aspiration pneumonitis, animal and human studies have failed to demonstrate a beneficial effect on pulmonary function, lung injury, alveolar-capillary permeability, or clinical outcomes after acid aspiration.[64] Thus, the administration of corticosteroids for aspiration pneumonitis is not recommended. Further consideration of corticosteroids for aspiration complicated by ARDS is discussed below.

Management of Respiratory Failure

Aspiration of gastric contents can result in activation of inflammatory intrapulmonary pathways[64] consistent with the pathophysiology observed in ARDS.[63,66] The basic tenets of management of ARDS include the use of lung-protective ventilation strategies, the judicious management of fluids, and the application of basic critical care algorithms. The management of severe ARDS and hypoxemia resistant to conventional management involves the use of rescue therapies (e.g., prone positioning, high-frequency oscillatory ventilation, extracorporeal membrane oxygenation) usually used in the critical care setting (see Chapter 53).[71,72]

Mechanical Ventilation

The key principles governing mechanical ventilation in ARDS involve limiting the inspiratory plateau pressure to 30 cm H_2O and providing the lowest effective tidal volume to prevent alveolar overdistention and tidal (cyclic) recruitment-derecruitment. Such lung-protective strategies correlated with improved outcomes in a prospective multicenter trial of the management of ARDS in which the use of low tidal volumes and plateau pressure (6 mL/kg and 30 cm H_2O or less) was compared with traditional ventilation strategy (12 mL/kg and

50 cm H_2O or less).[73] Patients in the lower tidal volume group had a 22% reduction in mortality and an increase in ventilator-free days. Current recommendations for the treatment of ARDS include mechanical ventilation that minimizes ventilator-induced lung injury (low target tidal volume [6 mL/kg], plateau pressure < 30 cm H_2O, prone positioning for severe ARDS, and higher PEEP in moderate and severe ARDS).[72] In addition, guidelines support the use of high-frequency oscillatory ventilation for those with severe hypoxemia and limiting extracorporeal membrane oxygenation to a subset of patients who have defined dead space and static lung compliance values.[71,72]

Positive End-Expiratory Pressure

PEEP is a recommended component of the initial ventilatory support in the setting of ARDS. A randomized clinical trial of ARDS (n = 549) compared the effects of low and intermediate PEEP levels set according to predetermined combinations of PEEP and Fio_2 in the setting of a lung-protective mechanical ventilation strategy.[74] There were no significant differences in hospital mortality (24.9% versus 27.5%, respectively) or days to unassisted breathing (14.5 versus 13.8 days, respectively) between the two groups. However, the role of comparatively higher levels of PEEP in protective ventilation strategies for ARDS is far from clear.[75-77] An experimental model for acute lung injury from acid aspiration demonstrated that the titration of PEEP improved arterial oxygenation but was associated with lung inflammation, as evidenced by histopathologic evaluation.[78] This study supports the concept of best PEEP as a compromise between alveolar recruitment, lung inflammation, and hyperinflation. Current PEEP strategies focus on degree of recruitability of the lungs, given the finding that higher PEEP benefits patients with high recruitability (severe lung injury), while the injurious effects of high PEEP outweigh the benefit in those with low recruitability (mild lung injury).[79]

Fluid Management

In a 2 × 2 factorial trial design, the ARDS Clinical Trials Network Research Group evaluated the use of a conservative versus liberal intravenous fluid strategy and the value of guiding this intervention with central venous pressure or pulmonary artery occlusion pressure measurements.[80] The group that received conservative fluid management, whether guided by central venous pressure and/or pulmonary capillary occlusion pressure measurements, had much lower net fluid balance, better lung function, and a shorter duration of mechanical ventilation and intensive care unit stay. Further, there appeared to be no increase in the incidence or duration of shock or need for dialysis in the conservative fluid management arm of the trial. A 2017 metaanalysis of studies comparing conservative and liberal fluid resuscitation strategies found increased ventilator-free days and decreased intensive care unit stay among patients managed with conservative fluid strategies.[81] Thus, early management of ARDS (after initial resuscitation) focuses on limiting iatrogenic insult with conservative fluid management.

Basic Critical Care Algorithms

To minimize the risk for sepsis, central venous catheters and other invasive hemodynamic monitors should be discontinued as early as is clinically feasible. Aseptic precautions should be used during care, and infections should be treated with antibiotics specific to the bacterial pathogen. Whether tight and rigorous glycemic control should be employed is controversial. Occasional withdrawal of sedation and the use of prophylaxis for gastrointestinal bleeding and thromboembolic events are currently considered the standard of care in any critically ill patient (see Chapter 53).[82]

Corticosteroids

Recovery from ARDS depends on the functional resolution of the underlying pulmonary disorder, which may follow one of two courses: (1) rapid improvement in lung function with an uncomplicated recovery or (2) slow improvements in lung function, oxygenation, and ventilation with prolonged weaning and recovery. The corticosteroid controversy in ARDS in the context of aspiration is still unresolved.[64] Although a 2009 systematic review suggested potential benefit from corticosteroids,[83] their use did *not* appear to improve lung function or recovery in patients with ARDS in two well-conducted randomized clinical trials[84,85] and may be associated with long-term side effects. A 2007 randomized controlled trial reported shortened duration of mechanical ventilation but no impact on mortality in patients with ARDS randomized to receive a methylprednisolone infusion versus placebo.[86] A 2014 metaanalysis of corticosteroid therapy among 1474 patients in 18 studies showed no impact on mortality. While there was no specific analysis of cases of ARDS from aspiration-related lung injury, corticosteroid therapy increased mortality in a subgroup of patients with influenza-related ARDS. At the current time, while data do not support the routine use of high-dose corticosteroids in ARDS for the attenuation of lung injury after pulmonary aspiration,[87] management algorithms support consideration of their use for nonresolving ARDS early in the nonresolving phase (between days 4 and 14).[88]

PROPHYLAXIS

The risk for aspiration is extremely low when gastric emptying is normal and patients, including parturients, are appropriately fasted. Factors predisposing to regurgitation, particularly in obstetrics, include emergency surgery, difficult/failed tracheal intubation, light anesthesia, and gastroesophageal reflux. The risk for failed intubation is 3 to 11 times greater in pregnant patients than in nonpregnant patients, reported as 1 in 250 at the end of a 17-year audit in the United Kingdom (1978 to 1994)[89] and as 1 in 232 in an 8-year audit in the United States (2006 to 2013)[90] (see Chapter 29). An analysis of the Multicenter Perioperative Outcomes Group Database of patients undergoing general anesthesia for cesarean delivery from 2004 to 2019 revealed a lower failed intubation rate of 1 in 808, which may reflect the integration of video laryngoscopy into obstetric anesthesia practice.[91] Nonetheless,

airway edema, breast enlargement, obesity, and the high rate of emergency surgery can all contribute to the risk for failed tracheal intubation in pregnant women. Aspiration pneumonitis is often associated with difficult or failed intubation during the induction of general anesthesia. In a survey conducted by SOAP, intubation was recorded as difficult in 14 of 19 cases of aspiration in which tracheal intubation was required.[92] Moreover, Warner et al.[8] reported that the risk for aspiration during emergence from anesthesia was almost as high as that during induction of anesthesia. Furthermore, the most recent US closed claims analysis and UK reports highlighted aspiration during cesarean delivery with both general and neuraxial anesthesia.[6,18] Thus, prophylactic regimens must provide protection during both induction of, and emergence from, general anesthesia. A high degree of vigilance for universal pharmacologic aspiration prophylaxis and careful surveillance must be maintained for all patients undergoing cesarean delivery or other obstetric procedures with general or neuraxial anesthesia.

Because the incidence of aspiration pneumonitis is low, the efficacy of prophylactic regimens is measured by their ability to alter gastric pH and volume. In 30% to 43% of pregnant women, the fasting gastric volume is greater than 25 mL and the gastric fluid pH is less than 2.5.[93,94] However, the percentage of term parturients at risk may not differ from that of patients undergoing elective abortion, postpartum sterilization, or gynecologic surgery (Table 28.2).[95–97] Gastric volume and acidity at term gestation are similar to gastric volume and acidity during early pregnancy and the postpartum period, and in nonpregnant patients.[93–100] Decreased lower esophageal sphincter tone and a higher risk for difficult tracheal intubation are the primary factors that increase the risk for aspiration during pregnancy and the immediate postpartum period, and these are the factors that mandate the need for pharmacologic prophylaxis.

Preoperative Oral Fluid Administration

Multiple studies have described no increase in gastric volume or acidity after the oral administration of 150 mL of fluid (e.g., coffee, tea, water, other clear liquids, orange juice without pulp) in nonpregnant adults 2 hours before elective surgery.[58] The patients in these studies all fasted overnight

TABLE 28.2 Prevalence of Fasting Gastric Findings in Various Populations (%)

Population	pH < 2.5	Volume > 25 mL	pH < 2.5 and Volume > 25 mL
Pregnant[92–94]	57–80	51–54	31–43
Nonpregnant[95,96]	75–95	45–67	45–60
Postpartum[95,97,98]	54–93	61	60
Children[99]	93–100	64–78	64–77
Obese, nonpregnant[100]	88	86	75

and were expected to have a low gastric volume when the test meal was given. Lewis and Crawford[101] noted that allowing women undergoing elective cesarean delivery to consume a meal of both tea and toast 2 to 4 hours preoperatively increased gastric volume and decreased gastric pH compared with a fasted control group. Consumption of tea without toast resulted in an increase in gastric volume, but it did not alter gastric pH. Particulate material was aspirated from the stomachs of 2 of the 11 patients who consumed both tea and toast. The investigators did not state the volume of tea consumed by these patients.

When gastric emptying of both 50 and 300 mL of water was assessed in nonlaboring term parturients, the gastric emptying half-time for 300 mL was significantly shorter than that for 50 mL.[46] When a similar study was conducted in obese nonlaboring term parturients (mean [± standard deviation] prepregnancy body mass index $41 \pm 9 \, kg/m^2$), the gastric emptying time for 300 mL was not longer than that for 50 mL.[47] The latter finding suggests that the American Society of Anesthesiologists (ASA) Guidelines for Obstetric Anesthesia,[57] which state that "the uncomplicated patient undergoing elective cesarean delivery may have modest amounts of clear liquids up to 2 h before induction of anesthesia," could also be applied to healthy, *obese* pregnant women presenting for elective surgery. However, factors other than the rate of gastric emptying can influence the rate of pulmonary aspiration, particularly in obese subjects. Obesity is associated with a higher incidence of gastroesophageal reflux and difficult airway management (both intraoperatively and postoperatively; see Chapter 48). Moreover, the cesarean delivery rate is higher and the success rate of trial of labor after cesarean delivery is lower in obese parturients.[102,103]

Choice of Anesthesia

The US Obstetric Anesthesia Work Force Survey demonstrated that general anesthesia was used for less than 5% of elective cesarean procedures by 2011.[104] Two sequential analyses performed at a large tertiary care obstetric facility showed that the use of general anesthesia for cesarean delivery decreased from 7.2% to 3.6% from 1990 to 1995[105] with a further decline from 1% to 0.8% from 2000 to 2005.[106] One maternal death resulted from a failed tracheal intubation in the first cohort, with no reported anesthesia-related mortality during the second study period. Hawkins et al.[13] reported 67 maternal deaths resulting from complications of general anesthesia and 33 maternal deaths resulting from complications of neuraxial anesthesia in the United States during the years 1979 to 1990. Approximately 73% of general anesthesia–related maternal deaths were caused by airway difficulty, primarily failed intubation and/or aspiration. In contrast, data from the more recent period spanning the years 1997 to 2002 indicate that the mortality rates for cesarean delivery are similar for general and neuraxial anesthesia.[14] Studies reviewing failed tracheal intubation during the periods 1993 to 1998, 1999 to 2003, and 2013 to 2015 in the United Kingdom showed that, while the rate of failed intubation during this period had not declined, there were no deaths from

this potentially fatal complication.[107–109] Although this relative change in maternal mortality from the complications of general anesthesia is very encouraging, other global factors such as obesity have increased the challenges presented to anesthesia providers, particularly with respect to emergency operative deliveries. Therefore, techniques for preventing pulmonary aspiration of gastric contents will remain or even become increasingly relevant to clinical practice.

Antacids

The ASA Practice Guidelines for Obstetric Anesthesia state: "Before surgical procedures (e.g., cesarean delivery and postpartum tubal ligation), consider timely administration of nonparticulate antacids, H_2-receptor antagonist, and/or metoclopramide for aspiration prophylaxis."[57] Particulate antacids should not be used as prophylaxis because, when aspirated, they cause pulmonary shunting and hypoxemia of magnitude similar to that caused by acid aspiration and greater than that caused by saline, alkalinized saline, or sodium citrate.[110] Therefore, nonparticulate antacids (e.g., 0.3 M sodium citrate, Bicitra, Alka-Seltzer effervescent) should be used. Efficacy of sodium citrate depends on the baseline gastric volume and acidity. A volume of 30 mL of sodium citrate neutralizes 255 mL of hydrochloric acid with a pH of 1.0.[111,112] The duration of action of sodium citrate is variable and depends on the rate of gastric emptying. O'Sullivan and Bullingham assessed the efficacy of sodium citrate in pregnant women using noninvasive radiotelemetry pH pills.[113,114] After the administration of 15 mL of sodium citrate to women in the third trimester of pregnancy, pH remained greater than 3.0 for less than 30 minutes.[113] When the same study was repeated in laboring women,[114] the mean time that gastric pH remained greater than 3.0 was 57 minutes in subjects who had received no analgesia and 166 minutes in those who had received meperidine. Nonparticulate antacids should be administered within 20 minutes of the induction of general anesthesia, particularly if the procedure is an emergency and there is insufficient time for a coadministered H_2-receptor antagonist to be effective.

Histamine-2 Receptor Antagonists

The ASA Task Force on Obstetric Anesthesia concluded that H_2-receptor antagonists are efficacious in reducing gastric acidity and volume.[57] H_2-receptor antagonists block histamine receptors on the oxyntic cell, diminishing gastric acid production and slightly reducing gastric volume in the fasting patient. When given intravenously, an H_2-receptor antagonist begins to take effect in as little as 30 minutes, but 60 to 90 minutes are required for maximal effect.[94] After oral administration, gastric pH is higher than 2.5 in approximately 60% of patients at 60 minutes and in 90% at 90 minutes.[115] The duration of action is sufficiently long to cover emergence from general anesthesia for a cesarean delivery.

While **cimetidine** (200 to 400 mg intravenously or orally) reduces gastric acidity within 60 to 90 minutes with plasma concentrations sustained for approximately 4 hours,[94,115] its side effect profile has limited its use in obstetric patients. Specifically, cimetidine may decrease the rate of plasma clearance of lidocaine by binding to the cytochrome P450 system in the hepatocyte and by reducing hepatic blood flow.[116] Cimetidine crosses the placenta, but this does not appear to have harmful effects.[117] Because arrhythmias and cardiac arrest have been reported with the rapid intravenous administration of cimetidine,[118] a slow rate of intravenous administration or the oral route of administration is recommended. The use of cimetidine in obstetric anesthesia has largely been replaced by other H_2-receptor antagonists.

Ranitidine, a chemically substituted amino-alkyl furan, has been evaluated after the administration of an intravenous or intramuscular dose of 50 to 100 mg or an oral dose of 150 mg.[119-121] These studies demonstrated a gastric pH > 2.5 within 1 hour and sustained therapeutic concentrations for approximately 8 hours.[119-121] Ranitidine does not have any major interaction with the cytochrome P450 system[122] and does not alter plasma concentrations of lidocaine or bupivacaine after their epidural administration.[123] **Nizatidine** (given in doses of 150 to 300 mg orally) and **famotidine** (given in doses of 20 to 40 mg orally or intravenously) are alternative H_2-receptor antagonists.[124] Both have a duration of action > 10 hours and do not interfere with the metabolism of other drugs by the cytochrome P450 system.[124]

Proton-Pump Inhibitors

Omeprazole (20 to 40 mg orally) and **lansoprazole** (15 to 30 mg orally) are substituted benzimidazoles that inhibit the hydrogen ion pump on the gastric surface of the oxyntic cell. Purported advantages of PPIs are a long duration of action, low toxicity, and the potential for low maternal and fetal blood concentrations at the time of delivery.[125,126] However, a metaanalysis has indicated that premedication with ranitidine is more effective than PPIs in reducing the volume of gastric secretion and increasing gastric pH.[127]

Metoclopramide

Metoclopramide is a procainamide derivative that is a peripheral cholinergic agonist and a central dopamine-2 receptor antagonist. An intravenous dose of metoclopramide 10 mg increases lower esophageal sphincter tone and reduces gastric volume by increasing gastric peristalsis. Metoclopramide can have a significant effect on gastric volume in as little as 15 minutes.[93] Unfortunately, prior administration of an opioid or atropine antagonizes the effect of metoclopramide.[128] Extrapyramidal effects are a major potential side effect of metoclopramide. Metoclopramide crosses the placenta, but no significant effects on the fetus or neonate have been reported.[129]

A systematic review of antacid prophylaxis concluded that there was no evidence to support the routine administration of drugs to women in labor to reduce the incidence of pulmonary aspiration or Mendelson syndrome.[130] This conclusion reflects the low incidence of pulmonary aspiration of gastric contents and the absence of high-quality studies of antacid prophylaxis, rather than the presence of studies demonstrating negative results; the review cited only three studies, published in 1971, 1980, and 1984.[130] One study assessed the use of metoclopramide and perphenazine in women receiving

meperidine in labor, and the other two studies focused on the use of particulate antacids. A 2004 audit of acid aspiration prophylaxis during labor in the United Kingdom showed a decreasing number of institutions with policies to administer routine antacid prophylaxis to all laboring women.[131] However, many institutions attempted to identify women at high risk for an emergency cesarean delivery, to whom they gave oral ranitidine 150 mg at 6-hour intervals throughout labor. A 2005 audit of French obstetric units revealed that at least one medication to prevent gastric content aspiration was used in every patient in 93% of institutions before cesarean delivery, but the frequency of prophylaxis administration for laboring parturients was not assessed.[132]

Combination Prophylaxis Therapy

A systematic review of interventions for reducing the risk for aspiration pneumonitis in women who received general anesthesia for cesarean delivery (22 studies) showed that each assessed therapy, including antacids, H_2-receptor antagonists, and PPIs, achieved significant reduction of intragastric pH below 2.5.[133] H_2-receptor antagonists showed superior gastric acid pH reduction compared with PPIs at the time of tracheal intubation. Compared with placebo or with antacids alone, the combined use of antacids and H_2-receptor antagonists yielded a significantly greater reduction in intragastric pH.

Prevention of Intraoperative and Postoperative Nausea and Vomiting

Prevention of intraoperative and postoperative nausea and vomiting (IONV, PONV) is recommended to minimize the associated peridelivery risk of regurgitation of gastric contents. The SOAP Consensus Statement and Recommendations for Enhanced Recovery after Cesarean include the following steps to prevent IONV and PONV[134]:

- Prophylactic vasopressor infusion at the time of initiation of spinal anesthesia
- Limit or avoid uterine exteriorization and abdominal saline irrigation during surgery
- Combine at least two prophylactic antiemetics with different mechanisms of action, such as a serotonin 5-HT_3-receptor antagonist (e.g., ondansetron 4 mg), a glucocorticoid (e.g., dexamethasone 4 mg), or a dopamine$_2$-receptor antagonist (e.g., metoclopramide 10 mg).

Sellick Maneuver and Induction of Anesthesia

Sellick demonstrated that the occlusion of the esophagus by downward cricoid pressure in supine cadavers prevented the flow of barium from the stomach to the pharynx.[135] He also reported the successful use of this maneuver in 26 cases to prevent the passive regurgitation of gastric contents into the airway. For proper application of cricoid pressure, the head should be fully extended; it may help to have a trained assistant place a hand behind the patient's neck, so that the cervical vertebrae and esophagus are brought forward, making it easier to occlude the latter. The trained assistant should place the thumb and middle finger on either side of the cricoid cartilage; no more than light pressure should be applied while the patient is awake, to prevent coughing, straining, retching, and esophageal rupture. After denitrogenation (preoxygenation) and administration of an induction agent, an increasingly firm downward pressure is applied to the cricoid cartilage as loss of consciousness occurs. Full application of cricoid pressure requires a force of 30 N, 1 N being the force required to accelerate a mass of 1 kg by 1 m/s². As a practical clinical guide to the amount of force to apply, 10 N is approximately equivalent to the downward force exerted by a mass of 1 kg (see Chapters 26 and 29). Vanner and Pryle[136] demonstrated that 30 N of cricoid force prevented regurgitation of saline in cadavers with esophageal pressures as high as 40 mm Hg. The research team recommended a modest cricoid force (10 N) before loss of consciousness, increasing to 30 N after loss of consciousness; their data suggested that such pressure should be sufficient to prevent passive regurgitation of esophageal contents during induction of general anesthesia in most patients.[137] Cricoid pressure is maintained until the endotracheal tube cuff is inflated and correct endotracheal tube position is confirmed.

The value of cricoid pressure has been questioned. A study employing magnetic resonance imaging of 22 healthy volunteers of both genders noted that the resting position of the esophagus was lateral relative to the cricoid cartilage in 53% of the subjects without cricoid pressure and in 91% with cricoid pressure.[138] In addition, cricoid pressure displaced the esophagus relative to its initial resting position to the left and right in 68% and 21% of the subjects, respectively. The authors suggested that cricoid pressure may lead to airway displacement and an inability to reliably produce midline esophageal compression; these factors could limit the protective effect of the maneuver against passive reflux and make the intubation process more difficult. However, Rice et al.[139] challenged these conclusions in a subsequent magnetic resonance imaging study investigating the efficacy of cricoid pressure. They demonstrated that the hypopharynx, rather than the esophagus, lies behind the cricoid cartilage (Fig. 28.6). The relationship of the cricoid and laryngeal cartilages is constant and is maintained by their connecting ligaments and muscles. Because the cricoid cartilage and postcricoid hypopharynx are constantly related, they will behave as a unit when compressed against

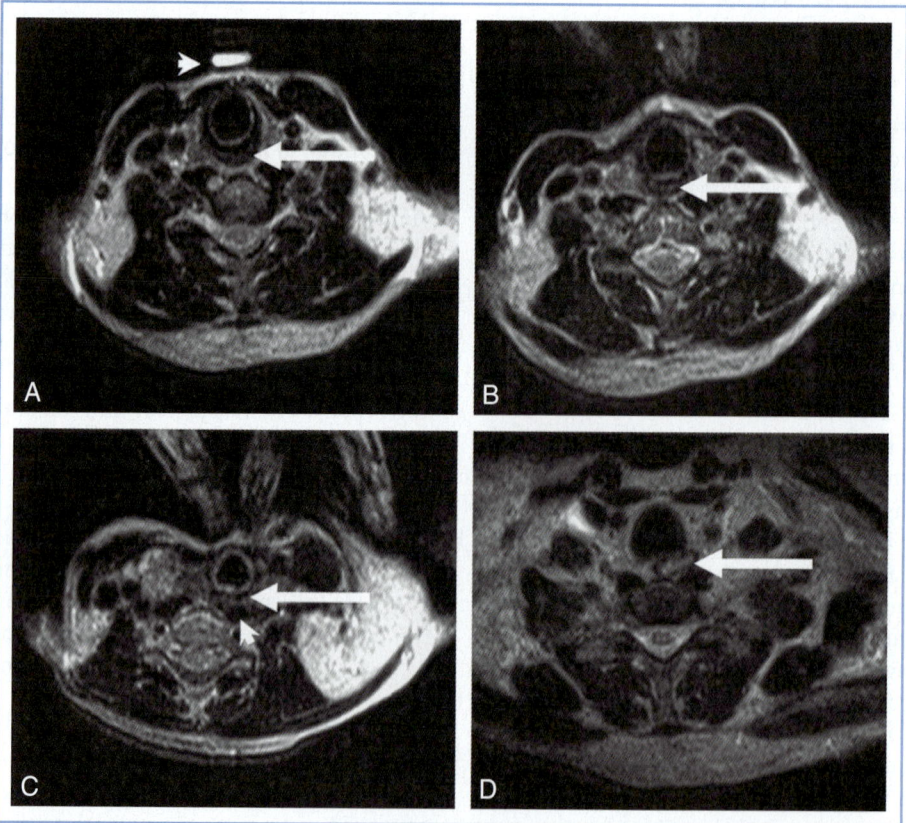

Fig. 28.6 Axial Magnetic Resonance Images in the Sniffing Position, Without (A) and With (B) Cricoid Pressure. (A) Postcricoid hypopharynx *(arrow)* and the cricoid cartilage skin marker *(arrowhead)* placed by the anesthesiologist before imaging. (C) Example of postcricoid hypopharynx compression *(arrow)* lateral to the vertebral body with cricoid pressure. In this image, the postcricoid hypopharynx is compressed against the longus colli muscle group *(arrowhead)*. (D) Image 2 cm inferior to the cricoid ring distinctly shows the cervical esophagus *(arrow)* lateral to the vertebral body. In (B) and (C) the anesthesiologist's thumb and index finger can be seen pushing on the cricoid cartilage. The axial image chosen for each study (A to C) was the image at the most inferior level of the cricoid cartilage. From Rice MJ, Mancuso AA, Gibbs C, et al. Cricoid pressure results in compression of the postcricoid hypopharynx: the esophageal position is irrelevant. *Anesth Analg.* 2009;109:1546–1552.

the cervical spine. The investigators contended that the sealing of the hypopharynx is therefore independent of the position of the esophagus, and the actual position of the esophagus is irrelevant to the successful application of cricoid pressure.

When the technique of rapid-sequence induction of anesthesia with tracheal intubation was first described in detail, it was recommended that the trunk be elevated 30 degrees to prevent reflux and aspiration.[140] Hignett et al.[141] demonstrated that the functional residual capacity of healthy term parturients was increased in the 30-degree head-up position compared with the supine position. Moreover, in the 30-degree head-up position, the esophageal pressure is lower and thus the force applied to the cricoid could be reduced to 20 N[142]; this reduction in force may reduce the incidence of airway complications because these complications are often proportional to the force applied.[143] Further work is required to determine whether the increase in functional residual capacity in the 30-degree head-up position prolongs the time to oxygen desaturation during the apnea phase of rapid-sequence induction and whether this position should be routinely adopted for induction of general anesthesia in obstetric patients. Should the incorrect application of cricoid pressure distort the laryngeal inlet and cause difficulty with laryngoscopy and/or intubation, the cricoid pressure should be promptly released.

RECOMMENDATIONS FOR CESAREAN DELIVERY

When possible, all mothers should be encouraged to have neuraxial anesthesia for cesarean delivery (see Chapter 26). Awake fiberoptic intubation should be considered for parturients with a potentially difficult airway who require general anesthesia. For **elective cesarean delivery**, a suitable antacid regimen may include the oral or intravenous administration of an H_2-receptor antagonist (e.g., famotidine 20 mg) 60 to 120 minutes before the induction of anesthesia and oral sodium citrate 30 mL within 30 minutes before surgery. Some

practitioners also give metoclopramide 10 mg orally at the same time as the H_2-receptor antagonist or intravenously at least 15 minutes before the induction of anesthesia.

For **emergency cesarean delivery under general anesthesia**, 30 mL of sodium citrate should be administered just after transfer of the patient to the operating room. This timing is important because sodium citrate has a relatively short duration of action, except in those mothers in whom gastric emptying has been delayed by the administration of an opioid. In addition, ranitidine 50 mg (or famotidine 20 mg or omeprazole 40 mg) and metoclopramide 10 mg should be given intravenously when time allows. Administration of these drugs may not reduce gastric volume or acidity at the time of tracheal intubation but will decrease the risk for aspiration at the time of extubation. For further protection against aspiration upon emergence from general anesthesia, an orogastric tube can be utilized to empty the stomach contents before extubation.

Some units administer an H_2-receptor antagonist orally every 6 hours during labor to all mothers considered to be at risk for an operative delivery. The evidence that the prophylactic use of H_2-receptor antagonists or PPIs reduces maternal morbidity and mortality has not been conclusively demonstrated; however, increasing the pH and reducing the volume of gastric contents should assist in limiting damage if pulmonary aspiration occurs. The use of cricoid pressure as part of a rapid-sequence induction technique remains standard practice.

Gastric Ultrasonography

Real-time assessment of gastric contents using gastric ultrasonography may have clinical utility for cases in which non-fasted parturients require urgent cesarean delivery. The use of gastric ultrasonography to assess peripartum aspiration risk and guide anesthetic management has evolved since its first reported use in studies of gastric emptying during pregnancy.[43,44,46,47] The gastric antrum can be visualized in a sagittal plane between the liver anteriorly and the pancreas

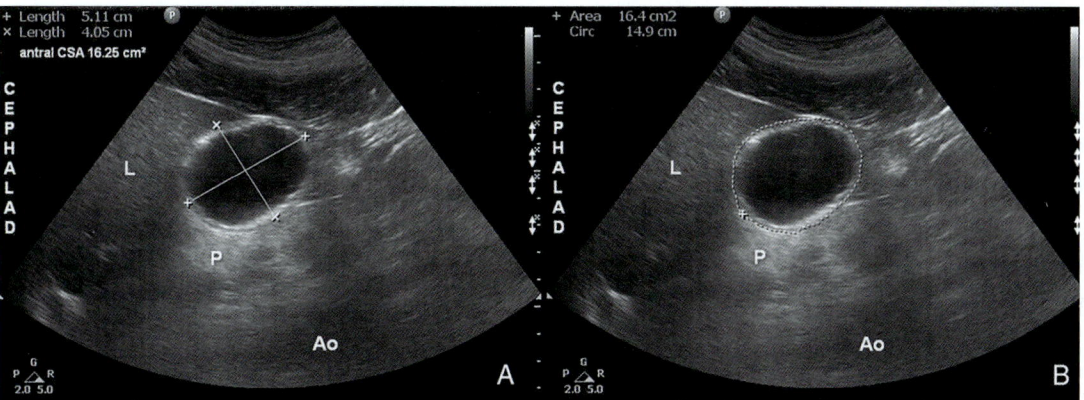

Fig. 28.7 Two Alternate Methods to Measure Antral Cross-Sectional Area (CSA). (A) Illustrates a method based on two perpendicular diameters (anteroposterior [AP] and craniocaudal [CC]). The diameters are used to calculate the CSA (CSA = [AP × CC × π]/4). (B) Illustrates a free-tracing method following the outer border of the antrum at the level of the gastric serosa. *Ao,* aorta; *L,* Liver; *P,* pancreas. From Van de Putte P, Perlas A. Ultrasound assessment of gastric content and volume. *Br J Anaesth.* 2014;13:12–22.

posteriorly and the antral CSA can be measured (Fig. 28.7).[144] Two mathematical models have been reported to predict gastric volume based on antral CSA.[145,146] Additionally, a qualitative three-point grading system, which assesses gastric antrum contents in both the supine and right lateral decubitus (RLD) positions, has been described[144]: grade 0 antrum is defined as the absence of fluid content in both the supine and RLD positions, grade 1 antrum is defined as the observation of fluid in only the RLD position, and grade 2 antrum is defined if fluid is observed in both positions. The upper 95th percentile limit of antral CSA for fasting term, nonlaboring pregnant women was $10.3\,cm^2$ in the RLD position.[144] In a randomized controlled trial with blinded assessors, fasted third-trimester pregnant women ingested apple juice, 0, 50, 100, 200, 300, or 400 mL; antral CSA measures correlated well with the ingested volume.[147] Further studies are warranted to validate the use of gastric ultrasonography for assessment of aspiration risk and anesthetic management for obstetric patients. Ultrasonographic detection of delayed gastric emptying or a full stomach may serve as a trigger to avoid the use of general anesthesia or prompt administration of prophylactic neutralizing and promotility agents.

ORAL INTAKE DURING LABOR

The recognition of Mendelson syndrome and the principle of "nil per os" was applied to surgical patients and laboring women starting in the 1950s. Since that time, fasting protocols for obstetric patients have remained, although some liberalization of these policies has occurred in the past two decades consistent with changes in preoperative fasting protocols for nonobstetric patients. Both US and French guidelines allow clear liquid consumption and light meals 2 and 6 hours prior to elective cesarean delivery, respectively.[57,148] In the United States, clear fluids are permissible during labor for women, barring the presence of risk factors for aspiration such as diabetes mellitus or morbid obesity.[57] The French guidelines specify no restriction except in parturients at increased risk of general anesthesia.[148] Conversely, since 2007, the UK National Institute for Health and Care Excellence guidelines allow a woman to eat a light diet during labor "unless she has received opioids or she develops risk factors that make a cesarean birth more likely."[149] Despite more liberal guidelines in the United Kingdom in the past two decades, the overall incidence of pulmonary aspiration has remained low (6 cases per 1,000,000 pregnancies).[11]

Impact of Fasting During Labor on Maternal Physiology and Outcomes

Women in the third trimester of pregnancy exhibit a state of "accelerated starvation" if denied food and drink.[150] Fasting results in the production of ketones, primarily beta-hydroxybutyrate and acetoacetic acid, and the nonesterified fatty acids from which they are derived. These changes are exacerbated by the metabolic demands of childbirth.

A randomized study examined the effect of a light diet on the maternal metabolic profile, the residual gastric volume, and

the outcome of labor.[151] Women presenting in early, uncomplicated labor at term were stratified by parity and randomized to receive a light diet or water only. Women who consumed a light diet did not have the increase in beta-hydroxybutyrate and nonesterified acid levels seen in the mothers who consumed water only. However, the gastric volumes as measured by ultrasonography were significantly larger in those who had eaten. Thus, mothers who consume a light diet during labor may be at greater risk for aspiration if general anesthesia is required. The same study design was used in another group of women, but isotonic "sports drinks" were administered instead of solid food[152]; these drinks reduced ketosis without increasing intragastric volume. Neither of these studies demonstrated a difference in maternal or newborn outcomes between ketotic or nonketotic laboring subjects.

O'Sullivan et al.[153] evaluated the effect of food intake during labor on obstetric outcomes in a randomized controlled study. A total of 2443 low-risk nulliparous women in labor were randomly assigned to either an "eating" or a "water-only" group. Intention-to-treat analysis was performed. No significant differences were found in (1) the spontaneous vaginal delivery rate, (2) the operative vaginal delivery rate, (3) the cesarean delivery rate, or (4) the incidence of vomiting (Fig. 28.8). Similarly, there was no difference between groups in the duration of labor; the geometric mean (GM) labor duration was 597 minutes in the "eating" group and 612 minutes in the "water-only" group (ratio of GM, 0.975; 95% CI, 0.927 to 1.025).

Impact of Neuraxial Analgesia on Gastric Emptying and Aspiration Risk

Maternal death from Mendelson syndrome is now extremely rare, and its decline probably owes more to the widespread use of neuraxial anesthesia than to NPO policies. The use of neuraxial analgesia has decreased the use of systemic opioids for labor analgesia, resulting in fewer women at risk for opioid-induced delayed gastric emptying and its inherent

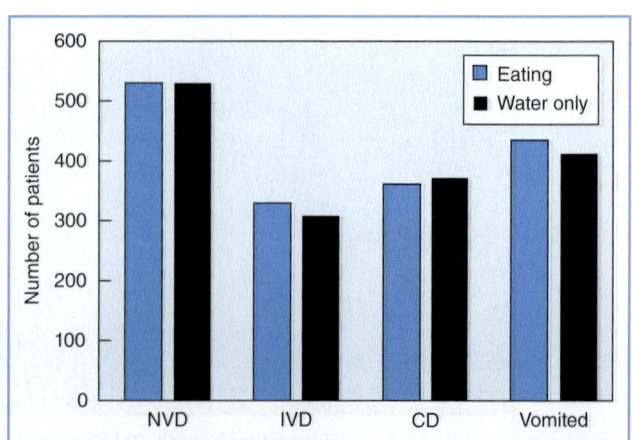

Fig. 28.8 The Effect of Eating During Labor on Maternal Obstetric Outcome. *CD*, Cesarean delivery; *IVD*, instrumental vaginal delivery; *NVD*, normal vaginal delivery. Based on data from O'Sullivan G, Liu B, Hart D, et al. Effect of food intake during labour on obstetric outcome: randomised controlled trial. *BMJ.* 2009;338:b784.

potential for aspiration.[104] Gastric ultrasonography studies over the past decade have increased our understanding of gastric emptying kinetics during labor with various oral intake and analgesic exposures. A randomized trial of high- versus low-dose epidural fentanyl in labor demonstrated no delay in gastric emptying or greater gastric content with high-dose fentanyl in women who were allowed to eat during labor.[45] In an observational study of parturients with epidural labor analgesia (ropivacaine and sufentanil) who fasted during labor,[154] the proportion of parturients with CSA > 320 mm^2 was greater at the time of initiation of epidural analgesia than at full cervical dilation. Conversely, in a randomized trial, women who were or were not allowed to drink clear fluids in labor had similar gastric volumes at the time of full cervical dilation.[155] In an observational study, four groups of 10 patients each—nonpregnant, pregnant not in labor, laboring with epidural analgesia (ropivacaine and sufentanil), and laboring without analgesia—were fed a light meal.[156] Gastric emptying was delayed in pregnant compared with nonpregnant subjects, and in subjects in labor compared to those not in labor. Gastric emptying was facilitated in subjects in labor with epidural analgesia compared to those without epidural analgesia.[156] Given the results of these studies, and that some laboring women and women requiring intrapartum cesarean delivery are likely to have full stomachs (and thus be at increased risk for pulmonary aspiration), the integration of point-of-care gastric ultrasonography may enable clinical assessment of aspiration risk in real time for a tailored anesthetic approach to anesthetic care, regardless of NPO status.

Adherence to Guidelines for Oral Intake During Labor and Delivery

Global guidelines for oral intake during labor and delivery remain variable in their degree of restriction of oral intake during childbirth; thus, it is important for clinicians to understand and adhere to local guidelines as they evolve. The American College of Obstetricians and Gynecologists,[157] as well as the ASA, SOAP[57] and French guidelines,[148] agree that moderate amounts of *clear liquid* may be allowed during labor, but that *solid food should be avoided in laboring patients*. In contrast, European and Australian guidelines are more liberal, allowing women with low risk to consume low-residue foods such as biscuits, toast, and cereals during labor.[158,159] To date, countries with a more liberal attitude toward eating during labor have not witnessed a higher incidence of maternal deaths from pulmonary aspiration. Further audit, research, and observation will continue to inform guidelines for oral intake during labor.

KEY POINTS

- Airway management complications associated with general anesthesia are a common cause of anesthesia-related maternal deaths.
- Reduced lower esophageal sphincter tone and a higher risk for difficult tracheal intubation are the primary factors that increase the risk for aspiration during pregnancy and the immediate postpartum period.
- Although pulmonary aspiration of gastric contents is rare in contemporary obstetric anesthesia practice, fatal aspiration may occur during cesarean delivery, during difficult or failed tracheal intubation, or after extubation.
- The most effective way to decrease the risk for aspiration is to avoid the administration of general anesthesia. The risk for aspiration also exists with the use of sedation as an adjunct to neuraxial anesthesia.
- Women undergoing elective cesarean delivery should fast from solid food. Clear liquids may be consumed up until 2 hours before the scheduled cesarean delivery.
- Preoperative prophylaxis before emergency cesarean delivery under general anesthesia should include a nonparticulate antacid administration immediately prior to the induction of anesthesia. Strong consideration should also be given to the administration of an H$_2$-receptor antagonist (or a proton pump inhibitor) and metoclopramide. These drugs may be administered after the induction of anesthesia if time does not permit their administration before induction.
- Hypoxemia is the hallmark of aspiration pneumonitis. Mechanical ventilation with positive end-expiratory pressure is the most effective treatment for severe hypoxemia. Lung-protective ventilation strategies (i.e., lower tidal volumes and inspiratory pressures) should be employed.
- The oral intake of clear fluids may be allowed during labor. Although some units allow solid food during labor, this practice should be limited in parturients at high risk for intrapartum cesarean delivery.
- Eating during labor results in larger residual gastric volume. Eating during labor does not improve obstetric outcomes.
- Point-of-care gastric ultrasonography may allow assessment of risk for aspiration prior to administration of general or neuraxial anesthesia in obstetric patients.

REFERENCES

1. Simpson JY. Remarks on the alleged case of death from the action of chloroform. *Lancet.* 1848;51:175–176.
2. Hall C. Aspiration pneumonitis: an obstetric hazard. *JAMA.* 1940;114:728–733.
3. Mendelson CL. The aspiration of stomach contents into the lungs during obstetric anesthesia. *Am J Obstet Gynecol.* 1946;52:191–205.
4. Turnbull A, Tindall VR, Beard RW, et al. Report on confidential enquiries into maternal deaths in England and Wales 1982-1984. *Rep Health Soc Subj (Lond).* 1989;34:1–166.
5. Bamber J, Lucas N, on behalf of the MBRRACE-UK Anaesthesia Chapter Writing Group *Messages for anaesthetic care. Saving Lives, Improving Mothers' Care—Lessons Learned to Inform Maternity Care From the UK and Ireland Confidential Enquiries Into Maternal Deaths and Morbidity 2013-15.* National Perinatal Epidemiology Unit, University

of Oxford; 2017:67–73. https://www.npeu.ox.ac.uk/assets/downloads/mbrrace-uk/reports/MBRRACE-UK%20Maternal%20Report%202017%20-%20Web.pdf. Accessed December 28, 2024.

6. Lucas DN, Bamber J, Felker A, et al. *4. Improving anaesthetic care. Saving Lives, Improving Mothers' Care Core Report—Lessons Learned to Inform Maternity Care From the UK and Ireland Confidential Enquiries Into Maternal Deaths and Morbidity 2019-21.* National Perinatal Epidemiology Unit, University of Oxford; 2023. https://www.npeu.ox.ac.uk/assets/downloads/mbrrace-uk/reports/maternal-report-2023/MBRRACE-UK_Maternal_Compiled_Report_2023.pdf. Accessed December 28, 2024.

7. Olsson GL, Hallen B, Hambraeus-Jonzon K. Aspiration during anaesthesia: a computer-aided study of 185,358 anaesthetics. *Acta Anaesthesiol Scand.* 1986;30:84–92.

8. Warner MA, Warner ME, Weber JG. Clinical significance of pulmonary aspiration during the perioperative period. *Anesthesiology.* 1993;78:56–62.

9. Kluger MT, Short TG. Aspiration during anaesthesia: a review of 133 cases from the Australian Anaesthetic Incident Monitoring Study (AIMS). *Anaesthesia.* 1999;54:19–26.

10. Cantwell R, Clutton-Brock T, Cooper G, et al. Saving Mothers' Lives: Reviewing maternal deaths to make motherhood safer: 2006-2008. The eighth report on Confidential Enquiries into Maternal Deaths in the United Kingdom. *BJOG.* 2011;118:1–203.

11. Knight M, Bogod D, Lucas DN, et al. Pulmonary aspiration during pregnancy or immediately postpartum in the UK: a two-year national descriptive study. *Int J Obstet Anesth.* 2016;15:S6–S54.

12. D'Angelo R, Smiley RM, Riley ET, Segal S. Serious complications related to obstetric anesthesia: the serious complication repository project of the Society for Obstetric Anesthesia and Perinatology. *Anesthesiology.* 2014;120:1505–1512.

13. Hawkins JL, Koonin LM, Palmer SK, Gibbs CP. Anesthesia-related deaths during obstetric delivery in the United States, 1979-1990. *Anesthesiology.* 1997;86:277–284.

14. Hawkins JL, Chang J, Palmer SK, et al. Anesthesia-related maternal mortality in the United States: 1979-2002. *Obstet Gynecol.* 2011;117:69–74.

15. Catanzarite V, Willms D, Wong D, et al. Acute respiratory distress syndrome in pregnancy and the puerperium: causes, courses, and outcomes. *Obstet Gynecol.* 2001;97:760–764.

16. Soreide E, Bjornestad E, Steen PA. An audit of perioperative aspiration pneumonitis in gynaecological and obstetric patients. *Acta Anaesthesiol Scand.* 1996;40:14–19.

17. Mhyre JM, Tsen LC, Einav S, et al. Cardiac arrest during hospitalization for delivery in the United States, 1998-2011. *Anesthesiology.* 2014;120:810–818.

18. Warner MA, Meyerhoff KL, Warner ME, et al. Pulmonary aspiration of gastric contents: a closed claims analysis. *Anesthesiology.* 2021;135:284–291.

19. Binyamin Y, Orbach-Zinger S, Ioscovich A, et al. Incidence and clinical impact of aspiration during cesarean delivery: a multi-center retrospective study. *Anaesth Crit Care Pain Med.* 2024;43 101347.

20. Hey VM, Cowley DJ, Ganguli PC, et al. Gastro–oesophageal reflux in late pregnancy. *Anaesthesia.* 1977;32:372–377.

21. Lind JF, Smith AM, McIver DK, et al. Heartburn in pregnancy—a manometric study. *Can Med Assoc J.* 1968;98:571–574.

22. Van Thiel DH, Gavaler JS, Joshi SN, et al. Heartburn of pregnancy. *Gastroenterology.* 1977;72:666–668.

23. Vanner RG, Goodman NW. Gastro-oesophageal reflux in pregnancy at term and after delivery. *Anaesthesia.* 1989;44:808–811.

24. Van Thiel DH, Gavaler JS, Stremple J. Lower esophageal sphincter pressure in women using sequential oral contraceptives. *Gastroenterology.* 1976;71:232–234.

25. Murray FA, Erskine JP, Fielding J. Gastric secretion in pregnancy. *J Obstet Gynaecol Br Emp.* 1957;64:373–381.

26. Christofides ND, Ghatei MA, Bloom SR, et al. Decreased plasma motilin concentrations in pregnancy. *Br Med J (Clin Res Ed).* 1982;285:1453–1454.

27. O'Sullivan G, Sear JW, Bullingham RE, Carrie LE. The effect of magnesium trisilicate mixture, metoclopramide and ranitidine on gastric pH, volume and serum gastrin. *Anaesthesia.* 1985;40:246–253.

28. Attia RR, Ebeid AM, Fischer JE, Goudsouzian NG. Maternal fetal and placental gastrin concentrations. *Anaesthesia.* 1982;37:18–21.

29. O'Sullivan GM, Sutton AJ, Thompson SA, et al. Noninvasive measurement of gastric emptying in obstetric patients. *Anesth Analg.* 1987;66:505–511.

30. Sandhar BK, Elliott RH, Windram I, Rowbotham DJ. Peri-partum changes in gastric emptying. *Anaesthesia.* 1992;47:196–198.

31. Simpson KH, Stakes AF, Miller M. Pregnancy delays paracetamol absorption and gastric emptying in patients undergoing surgery. *Br J Anaesth.* 1988;60:24–27.

32. Macfie AG, Magides AD, Richmond MN, Reilly CS. Gastric emptying in pregnancy. *Br J Anaesth.* 1991;67:54–57.

33. Geddes SM, Thorburn J, Logan RW. Gastric emptying following caesarean section and the effect of epidural fentanyl. *Anaesthesia.* 1991;46:1016–1018.

34. Gin T, Cho AM, Lew JK, et al. Gastric emptying in the post-partum period. *Anaesth Intensive Care.* 1991;19:521–524.

35. Wright PM, Allen RW, Moore J, Donnelly JP. Gastric emptying during lumbar extradural analgesia in labour: effect of fentanyl supplementation. *Br J Anaesth.* 1992;68:248–251.

36. Whitehead EM, Smith M, Dean Y, O'Sullivan G. An evaluation of gastric emptying times in pregnancy and the puerperium. *Anaesthesia.* 1993;48:53–57.

37. Ewah B, Yau K, King M, et al. Effect of epidural opioids on gastric emptying in labour. *Int J Obstet Anesth.* 1993;2:125–128.

38. Levy DM, Williams OA, Magides AD, Reilly CS. Gastric emptying is delayed at 8-12 weeks' gestation. *Br J Anaesth.* 1994;73:237–238.

39. Stanley K, Magides A, Arnot M, et al. Delayed gastric emptying as a factor in delayed postprandial glycaemic response in pregnancy. *Br J Obstet Gynaecol.* 1995;102:288–291.

40. Zimmermann DL, Breen TW, Fick G. Adding fentanyl 0.0002% to epidural bupivacaine 0.125% does not delay gastric emptying in laboring parturients. *Anesth Analg.* 1996;82:612–616.

41. Porter JS, Bonello E, Reynolds F. The influence of epidural administration of fentanyl infusion on gastric emptying in labour. *Anaesthesia.* 1997;52:1151–1156.

42. Kelly MC, Carabine UA, Hill DA, Mirakhur RK. A comparison of the effect of intrathecal and extradural fentanyl on gastric emptying in laboring women. *Anesth Analg.* 1997;85:834–838.

43. Carp H, Jayaram A, Stoll M. Ultrasound examination of the stomach contents of parturients. *Anesth Analg.* 1992;74:683–687.

44. Chiloiro M, Darconza G, Piccioli E, et al. Gastric emptying and orocecal transit time in pregnancy. *J Gastroenterol.* 2001;36:538–543.

45. Fiszer E, Aptekman B, Baar Y, Weiniger CF. The effect of high-dose versus low-dose epidural fentanyl on gastric emptying in nonfasted parturients: a double-blinded randomised controlled trial. *Eur J Anaesthesiol.* 2022;39:50–57.

46. Wong CA, Loffredi M, Ganchiff JN, et al. Gastric emptying of water in term pregnancy. *Anesthesiology.* 2002;96:1395–1400.

47. Wong CA, McCarthy RJ, Fitzgerald PC, et al. Gastric emptying of water in obese pregnant women at term. *Anesth Analg.* 2007;105:751–755.

48. Nimmo WS, Wilson J, Prescott LF. Narcotic analgesics and delayed gastric emptying during labour. *Lancet.* 1975;1:890–893.

49. Nimmo W, Wilson J, Prescott LF. Further studies of gastric emptying during labour. *Anaesthesia.* 1977;32:100–101.

50. Davison JS, Davison MC, Hay DM. Gastric emptying time in late pregnancy and labour. *J Obstet Gynaecol Br Commonw.* 1970;77:37–41.

51. Awe W, Fletcher W, Jacob S. The pathophysiology of aspiration pneumonitis. *Surgery.* 1966;60:323–329.

52. James CF, Modell JH, Gibbs CP, et al. Pulmonary aspiration—effects of volume and pH in the rat. *Anesth Analg.* 1984;63:665–668.

53. Roberts RB, Shirley MA. Reducing the risk of acid aspiration during cesarean section. *Anesth Analg.* 1974;53:859–868.

54. Roberts RB, Shirley MA. Antacid therapy in obstetrics. *Anesthesiology.* 1980;53:83.

55. Schwartz DJ, Wynne JW, Gibbs CP, et al. The pulmonary consequences of aspiration of gastric contents at pH values greater than 2.5. *Am Rev Respir Dis.* 1980;121:119–126.

56. Teabeaut JR 2nd. Aspiration of gastric contents; an experimental study. *Am J Pathol.* 1952;28:51–67.

57. American Society of Anesthesiologists Practice guidelines for obstetric anesthesia: an updated report by the American Society of Anesthesiologists Task Force on Obstetric Anesthesia and the Society for Obstetric Anesthesia and Perinatology. *Anesthesiology.* 2016;124:270–300.

58. American Society of Anesthesiologists Practice guidelines for preoperative fasting and the use of pharmacologic agents to reduce the risk of pulmonary aspiration: application to healthy patients undergoing elective procedures: an updated report by the American Society of Anesthesiologists Task Force on Preoperative Fasting and the Use of Pharmacologic Agents to Reduce the Risk of Pulmonary Aspiration. *Anesthesiology.* 2017;126:376–393.

59. Raidoo DM, Rocke DA, Brock-Utne JG, et al. Critical volume for pulmonary acid aspiration: reappraisal in a primate model. *Br J Anaesth.* 1990;65:248–250.

60. Plourde G, Hardy JF. Aspiration pneumonia: assessing the risk of regurgitation in the cat. *Can Anaesth Soc J.* 1986;33:345–348.

61. Gunther A, Ruppert C, Schmidt R, et al. Surfactant alteration and replacement in acute respiratory distress syndrome. *Respir Res.* 2001;2:353–364.

62. Matthay MA. Conference summary: acute lung injury. *Chest.* 1999;116:119S–126S.

63. Ware LB, Matthay MA. The acute respiratory distress syndrome. *N Engl J Med.* 2000;342:1334–1349.

64. Marik PE. Pulmonary aspiration syndromes. *Curr Opin Pulm Med.* 2011;17:148–154.

65. Landay MJ, Christensen EE, Bynum LJ. Pulmonary manifestations of acute aspiration of gastric contents. *AJR Am J Roentgenol.* 1978;131:587–592.

66. Ranieri VM, Rubenfeld GD, Thompson BT, et al. Acute respiratory distress syndrome: the Berlin definition. *JAMA.* 2012;307:2526–2533.

67. Matthay MA, Arabi Y, Arroliga AC, et al. A new global definition of acute respiratory distress syndrome. *Am J Respir Crit Care Med.* 2024;209:37–47.

68. Kluger MT, Visvanathan T, Myburgh JA, Westhorpe RN. Crisis management during anaesthesia: regurgitation, vomiting, and aspiration. *Qual Saf Health Care.* 2005;14:e4.

69. Miano TA, Reichert MG, Houle TT, et al. Nosocomial pneumonia risk and stress ulcer prophylaxis: a comparison of pantoprazole vs ranitidine in cardiothoracic surgery patients. *Chest.* 2009;136:440–447.

70. Laheij RJ, Sturkenboom MC, Hassing RJ, et al. Risk of community-acquired pneumonia and use of gastric acid-suppressive drugs. *JAMA.* 2004;292:1955–1960.

71. Alessandri F, Pugliese F, Ranieri VM. The role of rescue therapies in the treatment of severe ARDS. *Respir Care.* 2018;63:92–101.

72. Fan E, Brodie D, Slutsky AS. Acute respiratory distress syndrome: advances in diagnosis and treatment. *JAMA.* 2018;319:698–710.

73. Brower RG, Matthay MA, Morris A, et al. Ventilation with lower tidal volumes as compared with traditional tidal volumes for acute lung injury and the acute respiratory distress syndrome. *N Engl J Med.* 2000;342:1301–1308.

74. Brower RG, Lanken PN, MacIntyre N, et al. Higher versus lower positive end-expiratory pressures in patients with the acute respiratory distress syndrome. *N Engl J Med.* 2004;351:327–336.

75. Briel M, Meade M, Mercat A, et al. Higher vs lower positive end-expiratory pressure in patients with acute lung injury and acute respiratory distress syndrome: systematic review and meta-analysis. *JAMA.* 2010;303:865–873.

76. Meade MO, Cook DJ, Guyatt GH, et al. Ventilation strategy using low tidal volumes, recruitment maneuvers, and high positive end-expiratory pressure for acute lung injury and acute respiratory distress syndrome: a randomized controlled trial. *JAMA.* 2008;299:637–645.

77. Mercat A, Richard JC, Vielle B, et al. Positive end-expiratory pressure setting in adults with acute lung injury and acute respiratory distress syndrome: a randomized controlled trial. *JAMA.* 2008;299:646–655.

78. Ambrosio AM, Luo R, Fantoni DT, et al. Effects of positive end-expiratory pressure titration and recruitment maneuver on lung inflammation and hyperinflation in experimental acid aspiration-induced lung injury. *Anesthesiology.* 2012;117:1322–1334.

79. Del Sorbo L, Goligher EC, McAuley DF, et al. Mechanical ventilation in adults with acute respiratory distress syndrome. Summary of the experimental evidence for the clinical practice guideline. *Ann Am Thorac Soc.* 2017;14:S261–S270.

80. Wiedemann HP, Wheeler AP, Bernard GR, et al. Comparison of two fluid-management strategies in acute lung injury. *N Engl J Med*. 2006;354:2564–2575.

81. Silversides JA, Major E, Ferguson AJ, et al. Conservative fluid management or deresuscitation for patients with sepsis or acute respiratory distress syndrome following the resuscitation phase of critical illness: a systematic review and meta-analysis. *Intensive Care Med*. 2017;43:155–170.

82. Chang SY, Sevransky J, Martin GS. Protocols in the management of critical illness. *Crit Care*. 2012;16:306.

83. Tang BM, Craig JC, Eslick GD, et al. Use of corticosteroids in acute lung injury and acute respiratory distress syndrome: a systematic review and meta-analysis. *Crit Care Med*. 2009;37:1594–1603.

84. Bernard GR, Luce JM, Sprung CL, et al. High-dose corticosteroids in patients with the adult respiratory distress syndrome. *N Engl J Med*. 1987;317:1565–1570.

85. Steinberg KP, Hudson LD, Goodman RB, et al. Efficacy and safety of corticosteroids for persistent acute respiratory distress syndrome. *N Engl J Med*. 2006;354:1671–1684.

86. Meduri GU, Golden E, Freire AX, et al. Methylprednisolone infusion in early severe ARDS: results of a randomized controlled trial. *Chest*. 2007;131:954–963.

87. Ruan SY, Lin HH, Huang CT, et al. Exploring the heterogeneity of effects of corticosteroids on acute respiratory distress syndrome: a systematic review and meta-analysis. *Crit Care*. 2014;18:R63.

88. Bos LDJ, de Grooth HJ, Tuinman PR. A structured diagnostic algorithm for patients with ARDS. *Crit Care*. 2023;27:94.

89. Hawthorne L, Wilson R, Lyons G, Dresner M. Failed intubation revisited: 17-yr experience in a teaching maternity unit. *Br J Anaesth*. 1996;76:680–684.

90. Rajagopalan S, Suresh M, Clark SL, et al. Airway management for cesarean delivery performed under general anesthesia. *Int J Obstet Anesth*. 2017;29:64–69.

91. Reale SC, Bauer ME, Klumpner TT, et al. Frequency and risk factors for difficult intubation in women undergoing general anesthesia for cesarean delivery: a multicenter retrospective cohort analysis. *Anesthesiology*. 2022;136:697–708.

92. Gibbs CP, Rolbin SH, Norman P. Cause and prevention of maternal aspiration. *Anesthesiology*. 1984;61:111–112.

93. Cohen SE, Jasson J, Talafre ML, et al. Does metoclopramide decrease the volume of gastric contents in patients undergoing cesarean section? *Anesthesiology*. 1984;61:604–607.

94. McCaughey W, Howe JP, Moore J, Dundee JW. Cimetidine in elective caesarean section. Effect on gastric acidity. *Anaesthesia*. 1981;36:167–172.

95. Blouw R, Scatliff J, Craig DB, Palahniuk RJ. Gastric volume and pH in postpartum patients. *Anesthesiology*. 1976;45:456–457.

96. Wyner J, Cohen SE. Gastric volume in early pregnancy: effect of metoclopramide. *Anesthesiology*. 1982;57:209–212.

97. James CF, Gibbs CP, Banner T. Postpartum perioperative risk of aspiration pneumonia. *Anesthesiology*. 1984;61:756–759.

98. Rennie AL, Richard JA, Milne MK, Dalrymple DG. Post-partum sterilisation—an anaesthetic hazard? *Anaesthesia*. 1979;34:267–269.

99. Cote CJ, Goudsouzian NG, Liu LM, et al. Assessment of risk factors related to the acid aspiration syndrome in pediatric patients-gastric pH and residual volume. *Anesthesiology*. 1982;56:70–72.

100. Vaughan RW, Bauer S, Wise L. Volume and pH of gastric juice in obese patients. *Anesthesiology*. 1975;43:686–689.

101. Lewis M, Crawford JS. Can one risk fasting the obstetric patient for less than 4 hours? *Br J Anaesth*. 1987;59:312–314.

102. Barau G, Robillard PY, Hulsey TC, et al. Linear association between maternal pre-pregnancy body mass index and risk of caesarean section in term deliveries. *BJOG*. 2006;113:1173–1177.

103. Durnwald CP, Ehrenberg HM, Mercer BM. The impact of maternal obesity and weight gain on vaginal birth after cesarean section success. *Am J Obstet Gynecol*. 2004;191:954–957.

104. Traynor AJ, Aragon M, Ghosh D, et al. Obstetric anesthesia workforce survey: a 30-year update. *Anesth Analg*. 2016;122:1939–1946.

105. Tsen LC, Pitner R, Camann WR. General anesthesia for cesarean section at a tertiary care hospital 1990–1995: indications and implications. *Int J Obstet Anesth*. 1998;7:147–152.

106. Palanisamy A, Mitani AA, Tsen LC. General anesthesia for cesarean delivery at a tertiary care hospital from 2000 to 2005: a retrospective analysis and 10-year update. *Int J Obstet Anesth*. 2011;20:10–16.

107. Barnardo PD, Jenkins JG. Failed tracheal intubation in obstetrics: a 6-year review in a UK region. *Anaesthesia*. 2000;55:690–694.

108. Rahman K, Jenkins JG. Failed tracheal intubation in obstetrics: no more frequent but still managed badly. *Anaesthesia*. 2005;60:168–171.

109. Knight M BD, Lucas DN, Quinn A, Kurinczuk JJ. Pulmonary aspiration during pregnancy or immediately postpartum in the UK: a two-year national descriptive study. *Int J Obstet Anesth*. 2016;26:54.

110. Gibbs CP, Schwartz DJ, Wynne JW, et al. Antacid pulmonary aspiration in the dog. *Anesthesiology*. 1979;51:380–385.

111. Chen CT, Toung TJ, Haupt HM, et al. Evaluation of the efficacy of alka-seltzer effervescent in gastric acid neutralization. *Anesth Analg*. 1984;63:325–329.

112. Gibbs CP, Spohr L, Schmidt D. The effectiveness of sodium citrate as an antacid. *Anesthesiology*. 1982;57:44–46.

113. O'Sullivan GM, Bullingham RE. The assessment of gastric acidity and antacid effect in pregnant women by a non-invasive radiotelemetry technique. *Br J Obstet Gynaecol*. 1984;91:973–978.

114. O'Sullivan GM, Bullingham RE. Noninvasive assessment by radiotelemetry of antacid effect during labor. *Anesth Analg*. 1985;64:95–100.

115. Johnston JR, McCaughey W, Moore J, Dundee JW. Cimetidine as an oral antacid before elective caesarean section. *Anaesthesia*. 1982;37:26–32.

116. Somogyi A, Gugler R. Drug interactions with cimetidine. *Clin Pharmacokinet*. 1982;7:23–41.

117. Howe JP, McGowan WA, Moore J, et al. The placental transfer of cimetidine. *Anaesthesia*. 1981;36:371–375.

118. Lineberger AS 3rd, Sprague DH, Battaglini JW. Sinus arrest associated with cimetidine. *Anesth Analg*. 1985;64:554–556.

119. Dammann HG, Muller P, Simon B. Parenteral ranitidine: onset and duration of action. *Br J Anaesth*. 1982;54:1235–1236.

120. Francis RN, Kwik RS. Oral ranitidine for prophylaxis against Mendelson's syndrome. *Anesth Analg*. 1982;61:130–132.

121. Maile CJ, Francis RN. Pre-operative ranitidine. Effect of a single intravenous dose on pH and volume of gastric aspirate. *Anaesthesia*. 1983;38:324–326.

122. Kirch W, Hoensch H, Janisch HD. Interactions and non-interactions with ranitidine. *Clin Pharmacokinet*. 1984;9:493–510.

123. Dailey PA, Hughes SC, Rosen MA, et al. Effect of cimetidine and ranitidine on lidocaine concentrations during epidural anesthesia for cesarean section. *Anesthesiology*. 1988;69:1013–1017.

124. Howden CW, Tytgat GN. The tolerability and safety profile of famotidine. *Clin Ther*. 1996;18:36–54.

125. Ewart MC, Yau G, Gin T, et al. A comparison of the effects of omeprazole and ranitidine on gastric secretion in women undergoing elective caesarean section. *Anaesthesia*. 1990;45:527–530.

126. Levack ID, Bowie RA, Braid DP, et al. Comparison of the effect of two dose schedules of oral omeprazole with oral ranitidine on gastric aspirate pH and volume in patients undergoing elective surgery. *Br J Anaesth*. 1996;76:567–569.

127. Clark K, Lam LT, Gibson S, Currow D. The effect of ranitidine versus proton pump inhibitors on gastric secretions: a meta-analysis of randomised control trials. *Anaesthesia*. 2009;64:652–657.

128. Hey VM, Ostick DG, Mazumder JK, Lord WD. Pethidine, metoclopramide and the gastro-oesophageal sphincter. A study in healthy volunteers. *Anaesthesia*. 1981;36:173–176.

129. Bylsma-Howell M, Riggs KW, McMorland GH, et al. Placental transport of metoclopramide: assessment of maternal and neonatal effects. *Can Anaesth Soc J*. 1983;30:487–492.

130. Gyte GM, Richens Y. Routine prophylactic drugs in normal labour for reducing gastric aspiration and its effects. *Cochrane Database Syst Rev*. 2006;(3):CD005298.

131. Calthorpe N, Lewis M. Acid aspiration prophylaxis in labour: a survey of UK obstetric units. *Int J Obstet Anesth*. 2005;14:300–304.

132. Benhamou D, Bouaziz H, Chassard D, et al. Anaesthetic practices for scheduled caesarean delivery: a 2005 French national survey. *Eur J Anaesthesiol*. 2009;26:694–700.

133. Paranjothy S, Griffiths JD, Broughton HK, et al. Interventions at caesarean section for reducing the risk of aspiration pneumonitis. *Cochrane Database Syst Rev*. 2014;(2):CD004943.

134. Bollag L, Lim G, Sultan P, et al. Society for Obstetric Anesthesia and Perinatology: consensus statement and recommendations for enhanced recovery after cesarean. *Anesth Analg*. 2021;132:1362–1377.

135. Sellick BA. Cricoid pressure to control regurgitation of stomach contents during induction of anaesthesia. *Lancet*. 1961;2:404–406.

136. Vanner RG, Pryle BJ. Regurgitation and oesophageal rupture with cricoid pressure: a cadaver study. *Anaesthesia*. 1992;47:732–735.

137. Vanner RG, O'Dwyer JP, Pryle BJ, Reynolds F. Upper oesophageal sphincter pressure and the effect of cricoid pressure. *Anaesthesia*. 1992;47:95–100.

138. Smith KJ, Dobranowski J, Yip G, et al. Cricoid pressure displaces the esophagus: an observational study using magnetic resonance imaging. *Anesthesiology*. 2003;99:60–64.

139. Rice MJ, Mancuso AA, Gibbs C, et al. Cricoid pressure results in compression of the postcricoid hypopharynx: the esophageal position is irrelevant. *Anesth Analg*. 2009;109:1546–1552.

140. Stept WJ, Safar P. Rapid induction-intubation for prevention of gastric-content aspiration. *Anesth Analg*. 1970;49:633–636.

141. Hignett R, Fernando R, McGlennan A, et al. A randomized crossover study to determine the effect of a 30 degrees head-up versus a supine position on the functional residual capacity of term parturients. *Anesth Analg*. 2011;113:1098–1102.

142. Vanner RG, Pryle BJ, O'Dwyer JP, Reynolds F. Upper oesophageal sphincter pressure and the intravenous induction of anaesthesia. *Anaesthesia*. 1992;47:371–375.

143. Hartsilver EL, Vanner RG. Airway obstruction with cricoid pressure. *Anaesthesia*. 2000;55:208–211.

144. Van de Putte P, Perlas A. Ultrasound assessment of gastric content and volume. *Br J Anaesth*. 2014;113:12–22.

145. Bouvet L, Mazoit JX, Chassard D, et al. Clinical assessment of the ultrasonographic measurement of antral area for estimating preoperative gastric content and volume. *Anesthesiology*. 2011;114:1086–1092.

146. Perlas A, Mitsakakis N, Liu L, et al. Validation of a mathematical model for ultrasound assessment of gastric volume by gastroscopic examination. *Anesth Analg*. 2013;116:357–363.

147. Arzola C, Perlas A, Siddiqui NT, et al. Gastric ultrasound in the third trimester of pregnancy: a randomised controlled trial to develop a predictive model of volume assessment. *Anaesthesia*. 2018;73:295–303.

148. Ducloy-Bouthors AS, Keita-Meyer H, Bouvet L, et al. Normal childbirth: physiologic labor support and medical procedures. Guidelines of the French National Authority for Health (HAS) with the collaboration of the French College of Gynaecologists and Obstetricians (CNGOF) and the French College of Midwives (CNSF)—Mother's wellbeing and regional or systemic analgesia for labor. *Gynecol Obstet Fertil Senol*. 2020;48:891–906.

149. National Institute for Health and Care Excellence. Intrapartum care; 2023. https://www.nice.org.uk/guidance/ng235. Accessed December 28, 2024.

150. Metzger BE, Ravnikar V, Vileisis RA, Freinkel N. "Accelerated starvation" and the skipped breakfast in late normal pregnancy. *Lancet*. 1982;1:588–592.

151. Scrutton MJ, Metcalfe GA, Lowy C, et al. Eating in labour. A randomised controlled trial assessing the risks and benefits. *Anaesthesia*. 1999;54:329–334.

152. Kubli M, Scrutton MJ, Seed PT, O'Sullivan G. An evaluation of isotonic "sport drinks" during labor. *Anesth Analg*. 2002;94:404–408.

153. O'Sullivan G, Liu B, Hart D, et al. Effect of food intake during labour on obstetric outcome: randomised controlled trial. *BMJ*. 2009;338:b784.

154. Bataille A, Rousset J, Marret E, Bonnet F. Ultrasonographic evaluation of gastric content during labour under epidural analgesia: a prospective cohort study. *Br J Anaesth*. 2014;112:703–707.

155. Rousset J, Clariot S, Tounou F, et al. Oral fluid intake during the first stage of labour: a randomised trial. *Eur J Anaesthesiol*. 2020;37:810–817.

156. Bouvet L, Schulz T, Piana F, et al. Pregnancy and labor epidural effects on gastric emptying: a prospective comparative study. *Anesthesiology*. 2022;136:542–550.

157. American College of Obstetricians and Gynecologists. Committee Opinion No. 766: Approaches to limit intervention during labor and birth (reaffirmed 2021). *Obstet Gynecol*. 2019;133:e164–e173.

158. Smith I, Kranke P, Murat I, et al. Perioperative fasting in adults and children: guidelines from the European Society of Anaesthesiology. *Eur J Anaesthesiol.* 2011;28:556–569.

159. Department for Health and Wellbeing, Government of South Australia. South Australian Perinatal Practice Guideline: Labour and birth care. Routine care in normal labour and birth; 2021. https://www.sahealth.sa.gov.au/wps/wcm/connect/b754c4d4-273b-47d9-86ed-e6d28eb6656f/Labour+and+Birth.+Routine+care+in+normal+labour+_birth_PPG_V1_1.pdf?MOD=AJPERES&CACHEID=ROOTWORKSPACE-b754c4d4-273b-47d9-86ed-e6d28eb6656f-ocQNBqF. Accessed January 5, 2025.

29

The Difficult Airway: Risk, Assessment, Prophylaxis, and Management

Sharon C. Reale, MD

CHAPTER OUTLINE

RISK

Definitions

The American Society of Anesthesiologists (ASA) Task Force on Management of a Difficult Airway defines a **difficult airway** as the clinical situation in which anticipated or unanticipated difficulty or failure is experienced by a physician trained in anesthesia care, including difficulty with one or more of the following: face mask ventilation, laryngoscopy, ventilation using a supraglottic airway (SGA) device, tracheal intubation, extubation, or invasive airway.[1] Difficulty with airway management can lead to hypoventilation, hypoxemia, or soiling of the tracheobronchial tree.

The prevalence of **difficult face mask ventilation** is dependent on the definition. In one study,[2] 5% of 1502 nonpregnant patients experienced difficulty in face mask ventilation, which was defined as an oxyhemoglobin saturation < 92% when using FIO_2 1.0. **Impossible face mask ventilation**, defined as an inability to exchange air during bag-and-mask ventilation despite multiple providers, airway adjuncts, and neuromuscular blockade, was reported in 77 of 50,000 (0.15%) nonobstetric anesthetic procedures.[3] **Difficult laryngeal**

mask ventilation may be defined as the inability after three attempts of device insertion to produce expired tidal volumes > 7 mL/kg (leak pressure > 15 to 20 cm H_2O).[4] In a study of 11,910 nonobstetric patients,[5] the incidence of difficult laryngeal mask ventilation was 0.19%.

The definition of **failed tracheal intubation** varies widely, ranging from tracheal intubation not accomplished with a single dose of succinylcholine to inability to intubate during general anesthesia. Such variation inevitably leads to heterogeneity in the reported rate of failed intubation.[6,7] Defining **difficult tracheal intubation** is even more complex. Difficulty may be encountered because of failure to visualize the glottis (difficult laryngoscopy) or due to an anatomic laryngeal or tracheal abnormality. Difficulty has been variously defined by (1) the time required to intubate, (2) the number of attempts, (3) the view at laryngoscopy, and (4) the requirement for special equipment or procedures.

Although a dramatic decrease in the number of anesthesia-related maternal deaths has been reported in the UK Confidential Enquiries into Maternal Deaths over the past 40 years,[8] complications from general anesthesia, primarily in the form of complications of airway management,

TABLE 29.1 Incidence of Failed Intubation in Obstetrics

Study	Year	Country	Number	Incidence
Lyons[12]	1985	United Kingdom	2331	1:291
Samsoon[17]	1987	United Kingdom	1980	1:280
Rocke[13]	1992	South Africa	1500	1:750
Hawthorne[18]	1996	United Kingdom	5802	1:250
Barnardo[19]	2000	United Kingdom	8970	1:249
Rahman[20]	2005	United Kingdom	4768	1:238
Saravanakumar[14]	2006	United Kingdom	5968	1:543
McDonnell[21]	2008	Australia	1095	1:274
Djabatey[15]	2009	United Kingdom	3430	0
Bullough[23]	2009	United Kingdom	19,762	1:309
McKeen[16]	2011	Canada	2633	1:1300
Quinn[22]	2013	United Kingdom	12,800	1:224
D'Angelo[24]	2014	United States	5332	1:533
Reale[7]	2022	United States	14,748	1:808

continue to be a leading cause of anesthesia-related maternal mortality. Similarly, data from the United States have demonstrated ongoing risks of failed airway management in obstetric anesthesia.[9] Although the development of national guidelines[1,10,11] has resulted in a more systematic approach to the management of the difficult airway, deaths directly resulting from anesthesia still occur due to failures in ventilation, tracheal intubation, or airway management following extubation. Despite the widespread use of neuraxial anesthesia for operative delivery, general anesthesia may still be required in emergency situations or in the setting of contraindications to neuraxial anesthesia, patient refusal, or, most commonly, inadequate neuraxial anesthesia.

Incidence and Epidemiology

The incidence of failed intubation in obstetrics has long been considered to be approximately 1 in 250 to 300 (Table 29.1).[12–24] A 2015 systematic review including data from published studies, abstracts, and databases reported a failed intubation rate at cesarean delivery of 1 in 433.[6] The incidence of failed intubation for all obstetric procedures was slightly higher at 1 in 390, which likely reflects intubation difficulties resulting from airway swelling following crystalloid resuscitation in postpartum hemorrhage. The authors noted no increase in incidence from 1985 to 2014. However, there was significant heterogeneity among reports. In 2022, a large, multicenter, retrospective investigation reported a difficult intubation rate of 1 in 49 based on an analysis of nearly 15,000 cases of cesarean delivery performed under general anesthesia in 45 medical centers enrolled in the Multicenter Perioperative Outcomes Group.[7] Difficult intubation was defined as Cormack-Lehane view grade 3 ≥, three or more intubation attempts, or the requirement of rescue fiberoptic intubation, rescue SGA, or surgical airway. Failed intubation was defined as any attempt at intubation without successful endotracheal tube (ETT) placement; the rate of failed intubation was 1 in 808.

The failed intubation rate in obstetric patients is approximately eight times higher than estimates of the rate in nonobstetric surgical populations.[17] A number of reasons have been proposed to explain the increased difficulty with obstetric airway management. Significant physiologic and anatomic changes of pregnancy (see later discussion) affect the airway, oxygenation, and metabolism. The majority of obstetric general anesthetics are administered for emergency deliveries, often during off-hours,[25] when there are likely to be fewer personnel available for assistance. Excessive cricoid pressure applied by a poorly trained assistant can worsen the glottic view at laryngoscopy,[26] as can positioning the parturient with left lateral tilt. With an increasing focus on neuraxial anesthesia and a concomitant decrease in the number of cesarean deliveries performed under general anesthesia, trainees also have fewer opportunities to become familiar with challenges of the obstetric difficult airway.[27–29]

Changes in maternal characteristics, most notably an increase in the prevalence of maternal obesity, may increase the risk for complications from general anesthesia, especially when performed for emergency procedures. Women with obesity are at increased risk for obstetric interventions requiring anesthesia[30] and are also at increased risk for failed neuraxial anesthesia,[31] necessitating the use of general anesthesia for emergency delivery (see Chapter 48). In the large Multicenter Perioperative Outcomes Group cohort, a body mass index (BMI) ≥ 40 kg/m² was found to be associated with a 1 in 28 risk of difficult intubation, and had an odds ratio of 2.02 for difficult intubation compared with women with a BMI < 25 kg/m².[7] Poor head and neck positioning at induction of anesthesia, inappropriately applied cricoid pressure, macromastia, and shorter interval from start of apnea until significant oxygen desaturation[32,33] may be responsible for a higher incidence of difficult airway management in obese patients.[7,14]

The presence of experienced anesthesia staff during induction of general anesthesia is recommended to reduce the morbidity and mortality, and perhaps the frequency, of difficulty with airway management.[25] The introduction and widespread acceptance of simulation training in obstetrics[34] may also lead to improvement in staff performance during critical events such as difficult airway management (see Chapter 11). It is critical to maintain situational awareness and recognition of the risk for fixation error, especially when dealing with emergency airway issues and the perceived need for tracheal intubation.

Avoidable General Anesthesia

Given the multitude of risks inherent in general anesthesia, along with the maternal morbidity associated with the difficult and failed airway management, avoiding general anesthesia when possible is critically important (see Chapter 26). The rate of general anesthesia for cesarean delivery is a notable quality and safety metric; the Society for Obstetric Anesthesia and Perinatology Centers of Excellence criteria call for an overall rate of general anesthesia less than 5% of all cesarean deliveries.[35] The Royal College of Anaesthetists has recommended a threshold greater than 99% for conversion of neuraxial labor analgesia to neuraxial anesthesia for elective cesarean delivery, greater than 95% for urgent deliveries, and greater than 85% for emergency deliveries.[36] When general anesthesia rates are high, it is likely that at least some of the general anesthetics are avoidable with high-quality obstetric anesthesia care.

In an analysis of 60,000 general anesthetics for cesarean delivery, Guglielminotti et al.[37] deemed 44% of general anesthetics to be avoidable; these cases had no known indication for general anesthesia or contraindication to neuraxial anesthesia. Avoidable general anesthetics were associated with an increased risk of anesthesia-related complications, surgical site infection, and venous thromboembolism, suggesting that an overreliance on general anesthesia is associated with multiple poor processes that compromise maternal safety. The authors found that low hospital-level rates of neuraxial analgesia were among the strongest predictors of avoidable general anesthesia.

To decrease the frequency of avoidable general anesthesia, several strategies are necessary. High rates of neuraxial labor analgesia use are required, along with successful conversion of neuraxial analgesia to surgical anesthesia for cesarean delivery (see below discussion). Close communication among anesthesia providers, obstetricians, midwives, and labor and delivery nurses maximizes the likelihood of successful conversion of epidural analgesia to intrapartum cesarean delivery anesthesia.[38] Frequent multidisciplinary communication is necessary to allow the anesthesia provider to understand the likelihood of emergency cesarean delivery and to plan for appropriate anesthesia techniques in these eventualities. Furthermore, regular collaboration between obstetric teams and obstetric anesthesia providers throughout the peripartum period to discuss high-risk parturients may also help reduce rates of general anesthesia.[39]

Neuraxial Labor Analgesia as Prophylaxis

The widespread acceptance and use of neuraxial analgesic and anesthetic techniques for obstetric patients can significantly reduce the need for general anesthesia and airway manipulation for cesarean delivery. In obstetric patients in whom difficult airway management or neuraxial anesthesia administration is anticipated, or when risk factors for an urgent or emergency cesarean delivery are present, early or prophylactic placement of an epidural catheter should be encouraged. A *prophylactic* epidural catheter is one that is placed either before the onset of labor, or early in labor, is dosed with a low-dose infusion of

local anesthetic and is monitored regularly to verify a bilateral block. The epidural catheter provides a readily available conduit for rapidly inducing neuraxial surgical anesthesia, especially in the setting of emergency cesarean delivery. Early epidural catheter placement also allows the neuraxial procedure to take place in a controlled setting and allows time for catheter manipulation and replacement, if necessary, before further pathophysiologic changes (e.g., decreasing platelet count, worsening airway edema) occur. The correct placement of the epidural catheter in the epidural space should be tested with the injection of a local anesthetic test dose and careful bilateral sensory testing to confirm the presence of bilateral neural blockade. It should, however, be remembered that catheters may become dislodged, leading to delays in analgesia or anesthesia when conversion to epidural anesthesia is required. Starting a low-dose local anesthetic infusion after insertion of a prophylactic epidural catheter serves to verify that the catheter remains in position in the epidural space, facilitating timely extension to surgical anesthesia, if necessary.

Unfortunately, labor *analgesia* cannot always be successfully converted to surgical *anesthesia* for an operative delivery; reported failure rates are as high as 8%.[40] A 2012 metaanalysis demonstrated the need for conversion to general anesthesia in 5% of women who receive epidural analgesia in labor[41]; higher failure rates are observed among women requiring more clinician-administered bolus doses for inadequate epidural labor analgesia, in settings of need for urgent delivery, and when an anesthesiologist without subspecialty training or experience in obstetric anesthesia is providing care. Another 2019 single-center, retrospective analysis also demonstrated higher rates of general anesthesia among patients receiving care from an anesthesiologist without subspecialty training.[42] Women receiving labor epidural analgesia must be evaluated at regular intervals; standardized evaluations can both enhance labor analgesic quality and expedite the detection of nonfunctioning catheters that must be replaced in order to provide successful surgical anesthesia in the event of an intrapartum cesarean delivery.[43]

When the obstetric anesthesia providers work alongside the obstetric providers, and there is early and ongoing communication about the possible need for intrapartum cesarean delivery, it is possible to begin rapid administration of the epidural solution for cesarean anesthesia as the decision for intrapartum cesarean is made. For emergency cesarean delivery, a common strategy is to administer half the planned dose in the labor room as soon as the obstetrician calls for cesarean delivery, and the remaining dose upon entering the operating room as the block sensory level and density are reassessed.

A metaanalysis of studies comparing different local anesthetic solutions for conversion of epidural analgesia to anesthesia found that lidocaine with epinephrine has a faster onset than bupivacaine, levobupivacaine, or ropivacaine.[44] The addition of bicarbonate to chloroprocaine or lidocaine with epinephrine further hastens the onset of local anesthetic action (see Chapter 26). A 2021 randomized, triple-blinded, noninferiority study compared the onset time of a lidocaine mixture (20 mL of 2% lidocaine, epinephrine 150 µg, 2 mL of 8.4% sodium bicarbonate, fentanyl 100 µg) versus 3% chloroprocaine for extension of labor analgesia to surgical anesthesia for cesarean delivery.[45] The authors found insufficient evidence to confirm the noninferiority of 3% chloroprocaine (655 seconds to achieve a T7 level) compared to the lidocaine mixture (558 seconds) (the recorded times did not include the time it takes to prepare each solution). Thus, both solutions provided a rapid conversion to surgical anesthesia from labor analgesia.

In situations in which conversion of epidural analgesia to surgical anesthesia is not possible, general anesthesia may still be avoided if time permits the replacement of the epidural catheter or administration of single-shot spinal anesthesia, or combined spinal-epidural anesthesia. When the epidural space contains a large volume of solution, spinal dose reduction is necessary to limit the risk of total spinal anesthesia, which necessitates induction of general anesthesia with tracheal intubation (see Chapter 26). A combined spinal-epidural anesthetic technique with a reduced dose of intrathecal local anesthesia allows for epidural extension in the event that the reduced spinal dose is insufficient to provide acceptable anesthesia for cesarean delivery. Nevertheless, both high-spinal and inadequate neuraxial anesthesia require conversion to general anesthesia. An airway management plan must always be in place, even if the primary plan is for the administration of neuraxial anesthesia.

Maternal Morbidity and Mortality

Although rare, maternal morbidity from airway-related issues remains an important problem. In the report covering the 2012 to 2014 triennium, the UK Confidential Enquiries into Maternal Deaths reported that pregnancy-related mortality from anesthetic causes was the 11th most common cause of maternal mortality, accounting for 1% of maternal deaths.[8] In the United States, 1.6% of maternal deaths between 1991 and 2002 were related to complications of anesthesia care, representing a 59% reduction in anesthesia-related mortality compared with data from 1979 to 1990.[9] These data demonstrate dramatic improvements in anesthesia-related maternal mortality in the past three decades, likely reflecting efforts by national anesthesia organizations in defining standards of care that lead to improved maternal safety.

Compared with neuraxial anesthesia, general anesthesia has historically been associated with a greater risk for maternal mortality (Table 29.2; see Chapter 39).[9] Using data from the Centers for Disease Control and Prevention from 1985 to 1990, the estimated case-fatality risk ratio for general anesthesia versus neuraxial anesthesia was 16.7.[46] However, the estimated risk ratio for the period between 1997 and 2002 was only 1.7 (95% confidence interval [CI], 0.6 to 4.6; $P = .2$).[9] Improvements in monitoring and rescue airway equipment, and the publication of algorithms for difficult airway management, may account for the reduction in mortality from general anesthesia over time.[47] Unfortunately, maternal deaths directly attributable to general anesthesia are still reported,[48,49] and although protocols for the management of a difficult airway are now widespread, they may not be uniformly followed.[19,50,51]

Hypoventilation and airway obstruction after extubation are now increasingly recognized as causes of maternal mortality.[8,52] In Michigan between 1985 and 2003, eight maternal deaths were believed to be related to anesthesia care; all deaths occurred during emergence from general anesthesia or the recovery period, and six of the eight patients were obese. System errors in which the care of the patient did not meet recognized standards were identified in five of the eight cases.[52] These errors included inadequate supervision by an anesthesiologist and lapses in postoperative monitoring.

Physiologic and Anatomic Changes in Pregnancy

Many anatomic and physiologic changes occur in pregnancy (see Chapter 2) and several have significant effects on the difficult airway (Box 29.1).

Airway Edema

Fluid retention makes the tissues of the head and neck less compliant and may lead to narrowing of the upper airway, especially in the supine position. Nasal congestion, snoring, and voice changes all occur more frequently in advanced pregnancy.[53] A 34% increase in Mallampati class IV scores[54] from the first to the third trimester of pregnancy has been observed[55] (see later). Difficulty with intubation has been shown to be almost four times more common in obstetric patients with Mallampati class IV compared with class I or II scores, and the risk of difficult intubation in women with a Mallampati class IV score was 1 in 12.[7]

Although changes in the airway develop gradually during pregnancy, more acute changes may be observed during labor. Mallampati class scores are known to deteriorate during

TABLE 29.2 Case-Fatality Rates and Risk Ratios of Anesthesia-Related Mortality During Cesarean Delivery in the United States: 1979–2002

| Year Range | CASE-FATALITY RATES[a] | | Risk Ratio |
	General Anesthesia	Neuraxial Anesthesia	
1979–84	20.0	8.6	2.3 (95% CI, 1.9 to 2.9)
1985–90	32.3	1.9	16.7 (95% CI, 12.9 to 21.8)
1991–96	16.8	2.5	6.7 (95% CI, 3.0 to 14.9)
1997–2002	6.5	3.8	1.7 (95% CI, 0.6 to 4.6)

CI, Confidence interval.
[a]Deaths per million anesthetics.
From Hawkins JL, Chang J, Palmer SK, et al. Anesthesia-related maternal mortality in the United States: 1979–2002. *Obstet Gynecol.* 2011;117:69–74.

BOX 29.1 Anatomic and Physiologic Risk Factors for Airway Complications During Pregnancy

- Airway edema
- Decreased functional residual capacity
- Increased oxygen consumption
- Weight gain
- Breast enlargement
- Full dentition
- Decreased lower esophageal sphincter tone
- Delayed gastric emptying in labor

labor.[56,57] Decreases in upper airway volume during labor have been demonstrated by acoustic reflectometry.[56] Soft tissue edema contributes to airway narrowing, which may be more significant in women with preeclampsia. The airway edema that has been observed during labor may be exacerbated by expulsive efforts during the second stage of labor,[58] after extubation following cesarean delivery,[13] or by fluid resuscitation for obstetric hemorrhage. Therefore, it is prudent to reevaluate the airway before induction of general anesthesia rather than relying solely on a prelabor assessment.[56]

Nasal capillary engorgement during pregnancy increases the risk for epistaxis after nasal instrumentation and has led many practitioners to believe that nasal instrumentation and intubation are relatively contraindicated in pregnancy. In a 2011 review, Arendt et al.[59] challenged this opinion, suggesting that nasal fiberoptic intubation is acceptable after careful and appropriate preparation of the nasal mucosa with topical vasoconstrictors. However, the effects of topical agents for the prevention of epistaxis on maternal hemodynamic parameters and uteroplacental perfusion must be considered, and the relative risk (RR) versus benefit associated with this procedure should be assessed on an individual basis.

Respiratory and Metabolic Changes

As pregnancy progresses, the gravid uterus increasingly encroaches on the diaphragm and lung volumes are reduced (see Chapter 2). By term, expiratory reserve volume decreases by 25% and residual volume decreases by 15%, resulting in a 20% reduction in functional residual capacity (FRC). This decrease is most notable with the patient in the supine position, as well as in the obese patient. Closing volume is unchanged in pregnancy, but the decrease in FRC results in airway closure in 50% of women in the supine position.[60] Metabolic requirements for oxygen increase by nearly 60% during pregnancy, predominantly because of fetal demands. This oxygen requirement is further increased during labor. Taken together, these changes contribute to a greater likelihood that pregnant women will become hypoxemic during periods of apnea, such as during the induction of general anesthesia.[61] Therefore, adequate denitrogenation/preoxygenation is vital to delay the onset of hypoxemia during periods of apnea (see later discussion).

Preoxygenation and the rate of hemoglobin desaturation have been investigated by computer modeling.[33,62,63] In these models, labor, morbid obesity, and sepsis all hasten preoxygenation; however, desaturation also occurs more rapidly in moderately ill and obese women (Fig. 29.1). Importantly, the time to life-threatening hypoxemia is significantly shorter than that for recovery from paralysis from succinylcholine.[62] Therefore, should ventilation be impossible, it cannot be assumed that the patient will recommence breathing before dangerously low levels of oxygen saturation have been reached. If rocuronium is used instead of succinylcholine, and ventilation and oxygenation are impossible, emergency reversal of neuromuscular blockade with sugammadex 16 mg/kg is recommended and may allow for reversal of neuromuscular blockade faster than spontaneous recovery of ventilation after succinylcholine 1 mg/kg administration.[64] Studies of emergency sugammadex reversal in obstetric patients are currently lacking.

Weight Gain

During pregnancy, most women gain at least 10 to 15 kg (22 to 33 lb) due to increases in fat deposition, blood and interstitial fluid volume, and uterine and fetal mass. An elevated BMI is associated with difficulty in mask ventilation and tracheal intubation,[3,7,14] in part due to the more rapid oxygen desaturation that occurs during induction of general anesthesia in obese women. Elevated BMI is also associated with a greater risk for requiring emergency cesarean delivery, another contributing factor for difficulty with airway management.[30]

Breast Enlargement

Breast enlargement during pregnancy may impede intubation by interfering with oral insertion of the laryngoscope blade and laryngoscopic manipulation to improve visualization of the larynx. Various strategies can minimize this problem, the most important of which is optimizing the patient's position. With both arms abducted, breast tissue falls away from the chest. Ensuring that the patient is in the ideal intubating position (see later discussion and Chapter 48) further facilitates laryngoscope blade insertion; a short-handled laryngoscope is recommended. The handle can be directed toward the shoulder on insertion of the blade and then redirected once the blade is in the oropharynx.

Gastroesophageal Changes

Given the increased risk for aspiration from the second trimester onward (see Chapters 2 and 28), rapid-sequence induction of general anesthesia is advocated for almost all parturients, thus potentially increasing the risk for difficult airway management. Antacid prophylaxis is recommended if induction of general anesthesia is required. Gastric ultrasonography, performed shortly before the induction of anesthesia, is increasingly used to assess the volume and nature (liquid or solid) of gastric contents, and therefore risk of aspiration (see Chapter 28).

AIRWAY ASSESSMENT

Preanesthetic assessment of the airway is necessary before both general and neuraxial anesthesia, in order to establish plans for airway management. A variety of bedside tests have been used to attempt to predict airway difficulty. Despite having both reasonably high sensitivity and specificity, many predictive tests have limited accuracy in the clinical environment because failed intubation is rare; the number of false-positive tests (those predicted to be difficult that are not) will always be significantly higher than the number of true-positive tests (those predicted to be difficult that actually are).[65] The positive predictive value for individual difficult airway tests is typically less than 50%; that is, fewer than one-half of the procedures predicted to be difficult will actually be difficult.[65] Despite these shortcomings in difficult airway prediction, airway assessment remains a vital part of anesthetic management. Combining bedside tests can elevate the index of suspicion for difficulty with airway management. Preanesthetic assessment allows for the consideration of potential airway

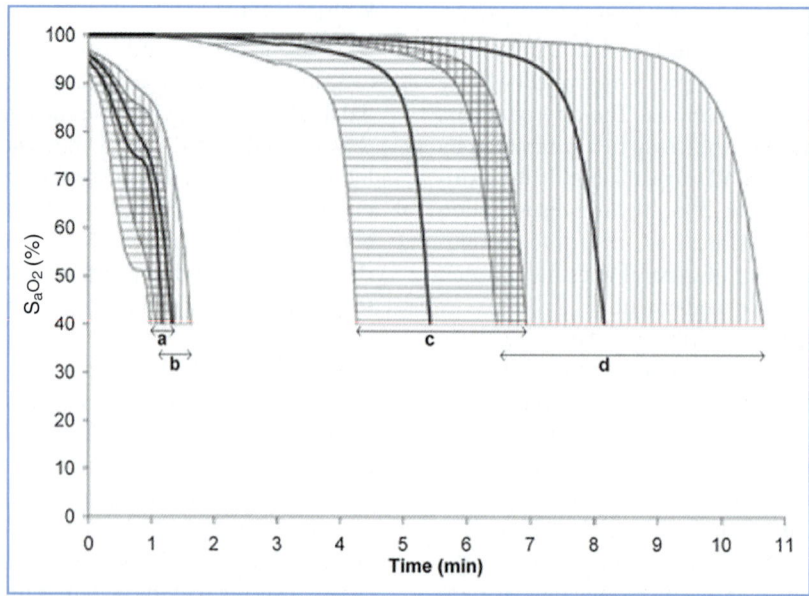

Fig. 29.1 Time course of Sao_2 during apnea in pregnant (horizontal hatching) and nonpregnant (vertical hatching) virtual subjects predicted to tolerate short, average, and long periods of apnea. Heavy lines represent average subjects. (a) Pregnant subjects, no preoxygenation; (b) nonpregnant subjects, no preoxygenation; (c) pregnant subjects, 99% complete denitrogenation; (d) nonpregnant subjects, 99% complete denitrogenation. From McClelland SH, Bogod DG, Hardman JG. Apnoea in pregnancy: an investigation using physiological modelling. *Anaesthesia.* 2008;63:264–269.

problems and the creation of a stepwise plan for dealing with difficulties should they arise.

Cormack and Lehane Grade

Cormack and Lehane[66] devised a glottic view grading system in 1984; the original purpose of the system was to grade the glottic view obtained with direct laryngoscopy to help train for difficult airways during obstetric general anesthesia. Thus, the Cormack and Lehane grade is a classification method to describe the relative difficulty with subsequent tracheal intubation. The original description includes four grades of laryngoscopy (Fig. 29.2):

- Grade 1: Full view of glottis
- Grade 2: Partial view of glottis or arytenoids
- Grade 3: Only epiglottis visible
- Grade 4: Neither glottis nor epiglottis visible

Subsequent modifications have been proposed: grade 2 may be divided into 2A (part of vocal cords visible) and 2B (only arytenoids or very posterior origin of vocal cords visible).[67,68] Grade 3 may be divided into those in whom the epiglottis is visible and is able to be lifted, such as with a gum elastic bougie (Grade 3A), and those in which the epiglottis is visible but not able to be lifted (Grade 3B).[68,69]

Because of the widespread acceptance of the Cormack and Lehane grading system, useful information about the potential for difficulty with intubation can be gained by reviewing previous anesthetic records. However, prior reports should be treated with caution because grades given in the nonpregnant state will likely differ from those determined during pregnancy, and the potential for interobserver and intraobserver variability exists.

Mallampati Class

In 1985, Mallampati et al.[54] described a 3-point scale of the oropharyngeal view of the open mouth; the more the view was obscured, the greater the difficulty with laryngoscopy and intubation. Samsoon and Young[17] later modified the scoring system into a 4-point scale (Fig. 29.3):

- Class I: Visualization of soft palate, uvula, and tonsillar pillars
- Class II: Visualization of soft palate and base of uvula
- Class III: Visualization of soft palate only
- Class IV: Visualization of hard palate only

The test should be performed with the patient sitting upright with her head in the neutral position; the patient should open her mouth as wide as possible and protrude her tongue as far as possible *without* phonation. Increasing difficulty with laryngoscopy and tracheal intubation has been demonstrated with greater Mallampati scores in both obstetric[7,13] and nonobstetric populations.[54]

Mallampati scores are frequently used as part of an assessment to predict difficult intubation. However, scores change both during pregnancy[55] and during labor.[56,57] When used as the sole predictor of a difficult airway, the incidence of both false-positive and false-negative results is high[70] due to the use of phonation, poor patient positioning, involuntary arching of the tongue, and interobserver variability in interpretation. A metaanalysis of the Mallampati score concluded that the test had limited accuracy for predicting a difficult airway and was not a useful screening test,[71] and as such it is best used in combination with other tests.

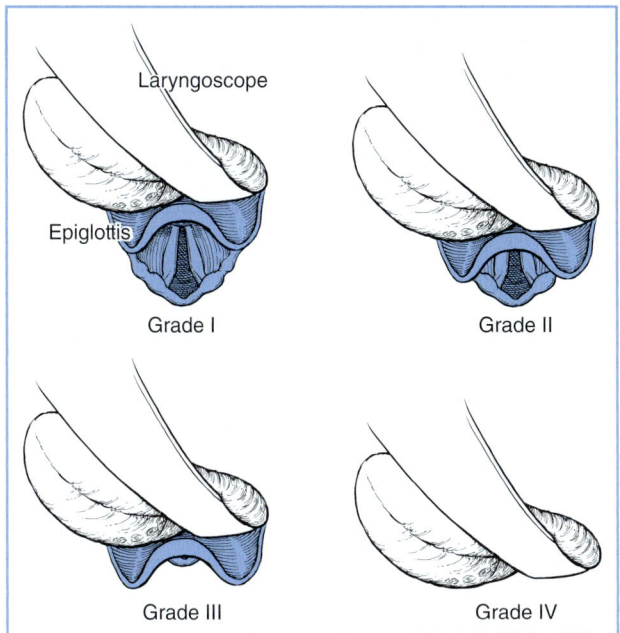

Fig. 29.2 Cormack and Lehane Laryngoscopic View Grades. Grade I is visualization of the entire laryngeal aperture. Grade II is visualization of only the posterior portion of the laryngeal aperture. Grade III is visualization of only the epiglottis. Grade IV is visualization of only the soft palate. From Cormack RS, Lehane J. Difficult tracheal intubation in obstetrics. *Anaesthesia*. 1984;39:1105–1111.

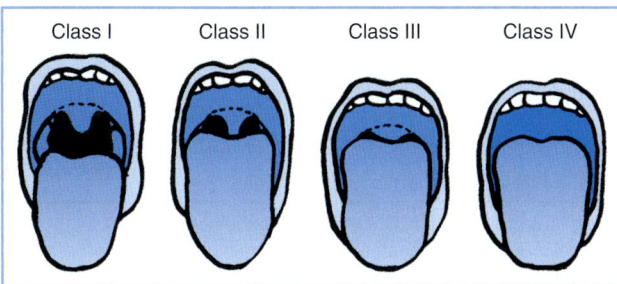

Fig. 29.3 Modified Mallampati Classification of the Oropharynx. Classification of the upper airway in terms of the size of the tongue and the pharyngeal structures that are visible with the mouth open. In class I, the soft palate, uvula, and anterior and posterior tonsillar pillars can be seen. In class II, the soft palate and uvula can be seen; the tonsillar pillars are hidden by the tongue. In class III, the soft palate and the base of the uvula can be seen. In class IV, only the hard palate can be seen. From Mallampati SR, Gatt SP, Gugino LD, et al. A clinical sign to predict difficult tracheal intubation: a prospective study. *Can Anaesth Soc J*. 1985;32:429–434.

Thyromental Distance

During laryngoscopy, the tongue is normally pushed into the mandibular space. The thyromental distance, the distance from the tip of the chin to the notch of the thyroid cartilage, can be used to estimate the volume of this space and whether the tongue can easily be displaced to facilitate laryngoscopy.[72] A thyromental distance < 6 cm suggests an increased risk for airway difficulty.[70]

Atlanto-occipital Joint Extension

Extension of the atlanto-occipital joint is necessary for the patient to be in the ideal intubating position in which the oral,

pharyngeal, and laryngeal axes are aligned (see later discussion). Movement can be assessed with the patient seated with the head and neck in the neutral position facing forward and then with the joint maximally extended (Fig. 29.4). Normal extension should be 35 degrees or more; difficulty with intubation can be expected when joint movement is decreased.[72]

Mandibular Protrusion

The patient's ability to extend the mandibular teeth anteriorly beyond the line of the maxillary teeth may predict adequate visualization of the larynx during direct laryngoscopy. In the mandibular protrusion test, patients are asked to protrude their mandible as far as possible (Fig. 29.5); one of three classes is assigned[73,74]:

- Class A: The lower incisors can protrude anterior to the upper incisors
- Class B: The lower incisors can be brought edge to edge with the upper incisors
- Class C: The lower incisors cannot be brought edge to edge with the upper incisors

Class A predicts a good glottic view with direct laryngoscopy, whereas class C is associated with poor glottic view.[73]

The **upper lip bite test** (ULBT) is similar to mandibular protrusion. In class I, the lower incisors can bite the upper lip above the vermillion border; in class II, the lower incisors can bite the upper lip below the vermillion border; and in class III, the lower incisors cannot bite the upper lip.[75] The ULBT has been shown to be a better predictor than a Mallampati score for predicting ease with laryngoscopy and intubation.[75]

Other Assessments

Limited mouth opening impedes the introduction of a laryngoscope blade or other airway devices; an interincisor distance < 5 cm may predict difficult intubation. Mouth opening

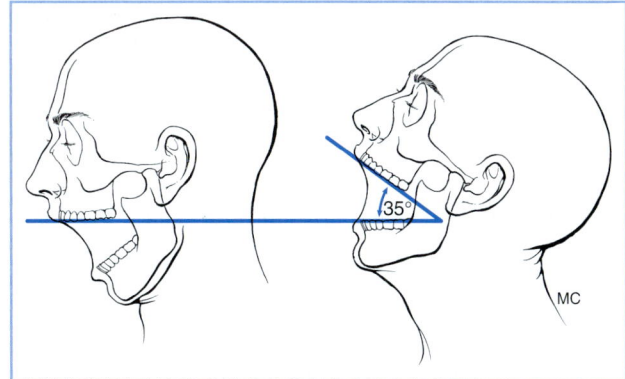

Fig. 29.4 Clinical Method for Quantifying Atlanto-occipital Joint Extension. When the head is held erect and faces forward, the plane of the occlusal surface of the upper teeth is horizontal and parallel to the floor. When the atlanto-occipital joint is extended, the occlusal surface of the upper teeth forms an angle with the plane parallel to the floor. The angle between the erect and the extended planes of the occlusal surface of the upper teeth quantifies the atlanto-occipital joint extension. A normal person can produce 35 degrees of atlanto-occipital joint extension. From Bellhouse CP, Dore C. Criteria for estimating likelihood of difficulty of endotracheal intubation with Macintosh laryngoscope. *Anaesth Intensive Care*. 1988;16:329–337.

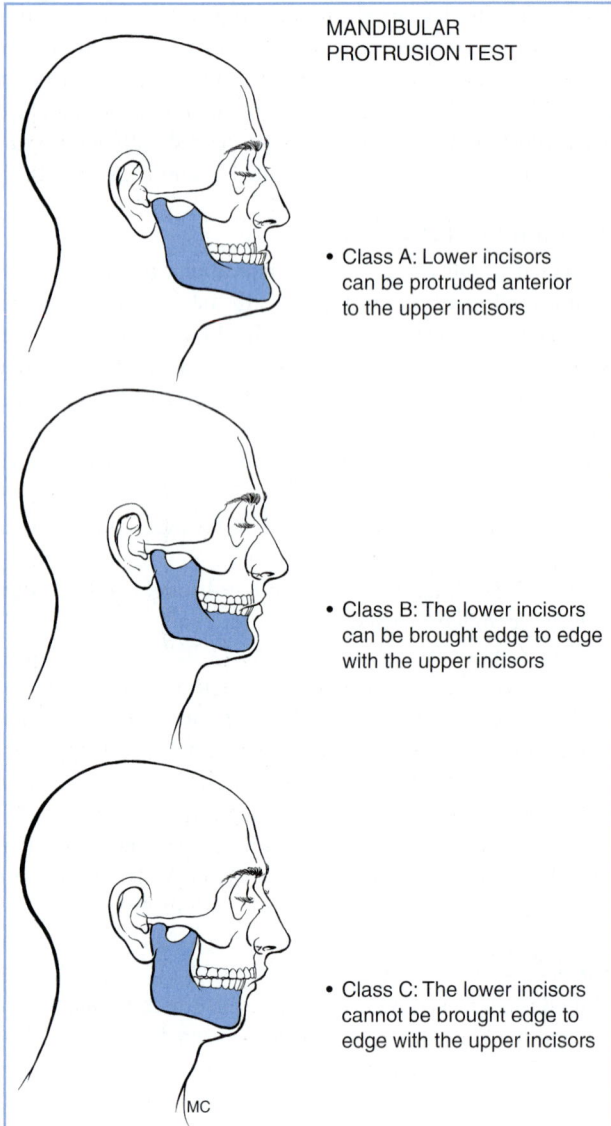

MANDIBULAR PROTRUSION TEST

- Class A: Lower incisors can be protruded anterior to the upper incisors

- Class B: The lower incisors can be brought edge to edge with the upper incisors

- Class C: The lower incisors cannot be brought edge to edge with the upper incisors

MC

Fig. 29.5 Mandibular Protrusion Test. Three classifications are based on the test. Class A predicts a good glottic view with direct laryngoscopy, whereas class C is associated with a poor view. Redrawn from Munnur U, de Boisblanc B, Suresh MS. Airway problems in pregnancy. *Crit Care Med.* 2005;33:S259–S268.

TABLE 29.3   Components of Preoperative Airway Examination

Airway Examination Component	Nonreassuring Findings
1. Length of upper incisors	Relatively long
2. Relation of maxillary and mandibular incisors during normal jaw closure	Prominent overbite (maxillary incisors anterior to mandibular incisors)
3. Relation of maxillary and mandibular incisors during voluntary protrusion or upper lip bite test	Patient cannot bring mandibular incisors anterior to maxillary incisors
4. Interincisor distance	<3 cm
5. Visibility of uvula	Not visible when tongue protruded with patient sitting (e.g., Mallampati class > II)
6. Shape of palate	Highly arched or very narrow
7. Compliance of mandibular space	Stiff, indurated, occupied by mass, or nonresilient
8. Thyromental distance	< three ordinary fingerbreadths
9. Length of neck	Short
10. Thickness of neck	Thick
11. Range of motion of head and neck	Patient cannot touch tip of chin to chest or cannot extend neck
12. Presence of beard	Beard present

Modified from American Society of Anesthesiologists. 2022 American Society of Anesthesiologists practice guidelines for the management of the difficult airway. *Anesthesiology.* 2022;136:31–81.

< two fingerbreadths has been shown to reduce the prevalence of easy intubation from 95% to 62%.[76] Mouth opening also is influenced by cervical spine movement; if movement is limited, mouth opening may also be restricted.[77] Protruding maxillary incisors, a single maxillary incisor, and missing maxillary incisors have been shown to be predictive of difficult intubation in obstetric patients.[13] Components of a comprehensive preoperative airway evaluation are listed in Table 29.3.

Multivariable Assessments

Individual tests are poorly predictive of airway difficulty; therefore, investigators have combined assessments in an effort to improve specificity. In a study of 400 pregnant women scheduled for elective cesarean delivery, Honarmand and Safavi[78] evaluated Mallampati class score, ratio of height to thyromental distance, and the ULBT, both in isolation and combination. A total of 8.75% of patients had a Cormack and Lehane grade 3 or 4 laryngoscopic view; the ratio of height to thyromental distance was the best predictor of this outcome.[78] Reale et al. assessed the following factors for a composite risk of difficult intubation: age ≥ 35 years, BMI ≥ 25 kg/m², ASA physical status score III or IV, Mallampati score III or IV, small hyoid-to-mentum distance, limited jaw protrusion, limited mouth opening, altered neck anatomy, cervical spine limitations, and presence of preeclampsia or eclampsia.[7] The frequency of difficult intubation increased from 0.8% for women with one risk factor for difficult intubation, to 3.7% for women with three risk factors, to 8.8% for women with five or more risk factors.

Recommendations

The thoroughness of the airway assessment may be limited by the urgency of surgery. For emergency procedures, relatively little time is available; thus, all women in the obstetric unit should be assessed soon after their arrival, focusing on those with the greatest number of risk factors for difficult intubation and those with the greatest risk for surgical intervention.[79] However, changes in assessment during the course of labor must be anticipated, and reevaluation before inducing anesthesia is vital to the safe care of these patients.

The assessment should start with a history and physical examination to detect factors that may indicate the presence of a difficult airway, as well as the potential risk for pulmonary aspiration. Examination of previous anesthetic records, if available, may indicate problems with ventilation or intubation. Comorbidities may influence airway management and should be considered before anticipated airway management. Most notably, maternal obesity is associated with an increased incidence of airway problems (see earlier discussion).[7,14,30,31,80] Similarly, difficulties in airway management should be anticipated in patients with preeclampsia with severe features,[7] or those who receive large volume fluid resuscitation for obstetric hemorrhage.

Asssessing and documenting mouth opening, the Mallampati class, atlanto-occipital mobility, thyromental distance, and mandibular protrusion may be performed relatively quickly and should identify most patients who will present difficulties with airway management. When risk factors are identified, appropriate plans for airway management, such as the availability of additional equipment and personnel (e.g., individuals experienced with airway management and the creation of a surgical airway) should be made. The proposed plan should consider that the administration of a neuraxial anesthetic technique may be the safest option for both mother and infant, even in the presence of nonreassuring fetal status. The use of ultrasonography to identify the cricothyroid membrane before the induction of general anesthesia may improve landmark identification should emergency surgical (front-of-neck) access be required to rescue failed tracheal intubation.[81] The risks and benefits of various alternatives should be discussed with the patient and the obstetric, neonatal, and nursing teams and documented in the patient's medical record.

STANDARD AIRWAY MANAGEMENT

Fasting and Antacid Prophylaxis

All obstetric patients requiring surgical anesthesia are at risk for pulmonary aspiration of gastric contents, particularly if airway difficulties are encountered (see Chapter 28). Because conversion from neuraxial to general anesthesia may be required for any patient, either before or during surgery, strategies must be adopted to minimize this risk. The ASA and the American College of Obstetricians and Gynecologists recommendations allow modest amounts of clear liquids throughout an uncomplicated labor, with the avoidance of solid foods in laboring women.[82] Clear liquids and solids are allowed up to 2 hours and 6 to 8 hours, respectively, before an elective operative procedure.[83,84] The UK National Institute for Health and Clinical Excellence allows more liberal policies on oral intake in labor and suggests that women be allowed to drink

isotonic fluids in labor and eat a light diet unless they develop risk factors that make general anesthesia more likely.[85] All laboring women should be assessed and oral intake restricted if surgical intervention appears likely.

Once surgical intervention is required, antacids such as intravenous histamine-2 (H_2)-receptor antagonists or proton-pump inhibitors should be administered (if not recently administered), in case general anesthesia is necessary. However, these drugs take up to 30 minutes to become effective. If emergency general anesthesia is required, oral administration of a nonparticulate antacid such as sodium citrate is used to increase the pH of gastric contents. A dose of sodium citrate (0.3 molar) 30 mL is effective for approximately 30 minutes and should be administered shortly before the induction of general anesthesia.[86]

Metoclopramide promotes gastric emptying and increases lower esophageal sphincter tone, although its efficacy is decreased by concurrent use of opioids. It may be given orally in labor or intravenously before general anesthesia.

A number of deaths and complications from presumed aspiration after tracheal extubation have been reported in the UK Confidential Enquiries into Maternal Deaths as well as the National Audit Project of the Royal College of Anaesthetists and the Difficult Airway Society.[48,87] When general anesthesia is administered to a woman with a potentially full stomach, reports have recommended that consideration be given to passing an "in and out" orogastric tube before extubation, and delaying extubation until the patient is awake and protective airway reflexes have returned.

Patient Positioning

The optimal laryngoscopic view yielding the best chance for successful intubation requires appropriate patient positioning. The sniffing position, with 35 degrees of neck flexion and 15 degrees of head extension, has been considered the ideal position for facilitating a view of the glottis by aligning the oral, pharyngeal, and laryngeal axes (Fig. 29.6).[88] In pregnancy, a ramped sniffing position, where the external auditory meatus and sternum are in horizontal alignment, optimizes first pass airway management success (Fig. 29.7). The anteroposterior chest diameter is increased in obese patients, making 35 degrees of neck flexion unachievable in the supine position. Consequently, the shoulders and upper torso need to be raised; this can be achieved with the use of multiple blankets or pillows, or one of the many commercially available, wedge-shaped positioning cushions. Optimal elevation is verified by checking that the external auditory meatus and sternoclavicular joint are in horizontal alignment. Elevating the back of the operating table by 25 degrees may make laryngoscopy easier and also aids preoxygenation by increasing FRC and delaying time to oxygen desaturation.[89,90] Some video laryngoscopes (see later discussion) do not require the patient's head and neck to be in the sniffing position to obtain a view of the glottic opening. Nevertheless, even with video laryngoscopy, the ramped sniffing position facilitates oral insertion and manipulation of airway equipment to ensure timely intubation, particularly for the patient with obesity and macromastia.

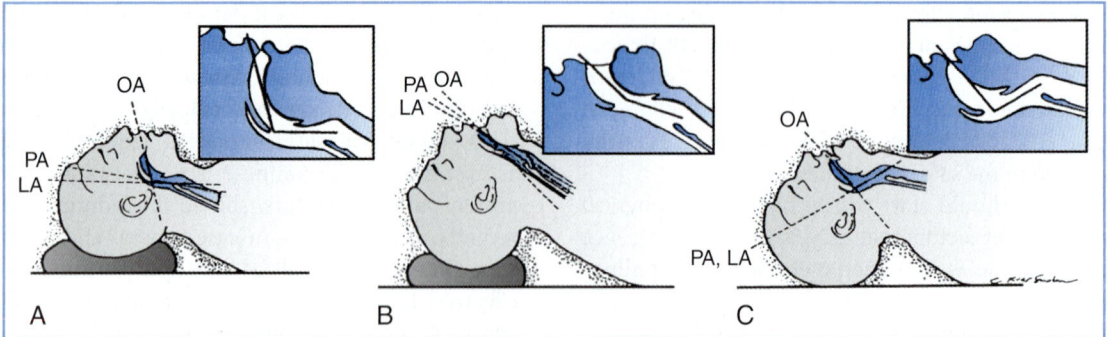

Fig. 29.6 Head and Neck Position During Laryngoscopy. As the head position changes from neutral, the alignment of the oral axis (OA), pharyngeal axis (PA), and laryngeal axis (LA) changes within the upper airway. (A) The head is resting on a large pad that flexes the neck on the chest and aligns the LA with the PA (the neutral position). (B) The head is resting on a pad (which flexes the neck on the chest) and concomitant extension of the head on the neck can be seen, which brings all three axes into alignment (the sniffing position). (C) Extension of the head on the neck without concomitant elevation of the head on a pad, which results in nonalignment of the PA and LA with the OA. From Benumof JL. Conventional [laryngoscopic] orotracheal and nasotracheal intubation [single-lumen type]. In: Benumof JL, ed. *Clinical Procedures in Anesthesia and Intensive Care.* JB Lippincott; 1991:115–148.

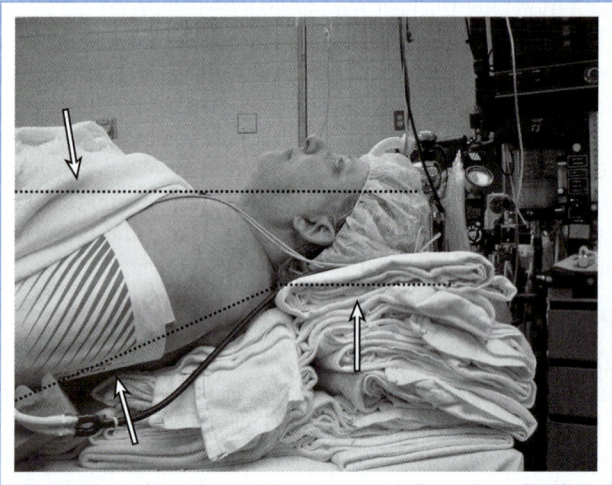

Fig. 29.7 A morbidly obese patient is in an optimal position for direct laryngoscopy when an imaginary horizontal line can be drawn from the sternal notch through (or slightly anterior to) the external auditory meatus. To achieve this, the upper back and shoulders should be significantly elevated with pads or blankets (or a commercial elevation wedge/pillow) to allow the head to be extended at the atlantooccipital joint. Additional blankets should be used to support the head in this position.

Left uterine displacement to minimize aortocaval compression should be maintained during preparation for, and induction of, general anesthesia. This may be achieved by tilting the operating table or by placing a wedge under the right hip.

Denitrogenation (Preoxygenation)

In pregnancy, the decrease in FRC and increase in oxygen requirement result in rapid oxygen desaturation during periods of apnea (e.g., during induction of general anesthesia). The FRC is the primary reservoir for oxygen during apnea. Therefore, effective denitrogenation, or preoxygenation, of the FRC is vital to delay the onset of hypoxemia. Some authors suggest that the end-tidal oxygen fraction ($F_{ET}O_2$) should be greater than 0.8 before anesthesia is induced.[91]

The standard technique for preoxygenation has been to breathe 100% oxygen through a tight-fitting face mask at normal tidal volumes for 3 to 5 minutes. Given the urgent nature of obstetric general anesthesia, attention has focused on whether several maximal deep breaths over a shorter period can be as effective. Chiron et al.[92] compared a traditional 3-minute technique with either eight deep breaths over 1 minute (8 DB/1 min) or four deep breaths over 30 seconds (4 DB/30 s). By monitoring the $F_{ET}O_2$, a marker of lung denitrogenation, the authors found that both the 3 minutes of tidal volume breathing and the 8 DB/1 min technique were more effective than the 4 DB/30 s technique. They suggested using the 8 DB/1 min technique in the setting of emergency obstetric anesthesia.

The use of maximal deep breaths to achieve denitrogenation may cause maternal hypocarbia and, therefore, should be limited to situations in which time does not allow normal tidal volume breathing of 100% oxygen to maximize oxygen storage in tissue and vascular body compartments. Indeed, during apnea, the time to desaturation depends on (1) the amount of oxygen stored in the lungs, tissue, and blood; (2) the mixed venous oxyhemoglobin saturation; and (3) the presence of intrapulmonary shunting.

A tight-fitting face mask is necessary to prevent room air entrainment, which reduces the efficiency of preoxygenation. With normal tidal volume breathing, preoxygenation is best achieved with oxygen flow rates in excess of 10 L/min for 3 minutes,[93] although this may still be inadequate due to air entrainment. A 20-degree to 30-degree head-up tilt increases the FRC[90] and delays the time to desaturation, especially in obese patients.[89]

There has been recent interest in the use of high-flow nasal oxygen (HFNO) to prolong time to desaturation.[94] Using flow rates of up to 70 L/min of oxygen, desaturation was not observed despite a mean apnea time of 248 seconds in nonobstetric patients undergoing rapid-sequence induction of anesthesia.[95] Computer modeling of the effects of HFNO in the pregnant patient has shown that with an F_{IO_2} of 1.0 and a patent airway, apnea times in excess of 30 minutes are predicted without maternal desaturation to less than 90%.[96] However, long apnea times should be avoided as much as possible due to a concomitant increase in $Paco_2$ and a fall in pH. It has also been suggested that HFNO may be used for preoxygenation of pregnant women. However, a prospective, observational study of 73 pregnant women found that a HFNO protocol of 30 L/min for 30 seconds, then 50 L/min for the next 150 seconds, was inadequate for preoxygenation (i.e., $Feto_2 \geq 0.9$) compared to face mask preoxygenation.[97] With this protocol, only 60% of women achieved $Feto_2 \geq 0.9$ after 3 minutes. Further work is required to determine the role of HFNO in obstetric airway management.

Rapid-Sequence Induction and Cricoid Pressure

In an attempt to minimize the risk for aspiration, rapid-sequence induction has become the standard technique for induction of obstetric general anesthesia. It usually consists of preoxygenation, rapid intravenous injection of a predetermined dose of induction agent followed immediately by succinylcholine administration, application of cricoid pressure, and avoidance of positive-pressure ventilation before tracheal intubation with a cuffed ETT. The urgency of intubation, coupled with avoidance of ventilation, may increase the likelihood of intubation failure.

Although in widespread use, the implementation of rapid-sequence induction is not uniform. Ideally, induction agents should provide rapid loss of consciousness, minimal hemodynamic instability, and optimal quality of intubating conditions.[98] Propofol is a frequently used induction agent (see Chapter 26) and provides excellent suppression of pharyngeal and laryngeal reflexes. Opioids have traditionally not been part of rapid-sequence induction because of concerns about respiratory depression should intubation fail. Moreover, in the obstetric population, the potential for neonatal depression is greater if opioids are used, given rapid placental transfer of these drugs.[99]

Because of its rapid onset, **succinylcholine** has traditionally been the muscle relaxant of choice for rapid-sequence induction of anesthesia in obstetric patients. Succinylcholine is associated with several undesirable side effects, most notably the potential for triggering malignant hyperthermia and anaphylaxis, and a prolonged duration of action in patients with cholinesterase deficiency. Despite reduced levels of plasma pseudocholinesterase in pregnancy, the duration of action of succinylcholine remains clinically unchanged in the obstetric patient.[100] The ideal dose of succinylcholine, traditionally 1 mg/kg, remains controversial[101]; when combined with opioids in nonobstetric patients, succinylcholine 1 mg/kg fails to produce good intubating conditions at 1 minute in up to 8% of cases.[102] Naguib et al.[102] found that succinylcholine doses as high as 2 mg/kg still do not guarantee excellent intubating conditions in all patients; however, the authors

found little extra benefit from using doses above 1.5 mg/kg. In a study of succinylcholine in nonobstetric obese patients,[103] a dose of 1 mg/kg total body weight was found to provide more predictable laryngoscopic conditions than 1 mg/kg ideal or lean body weight.

The potential disadvantage of an increased succinylcholine dose is delayed return of spontaneous respiration, which is vital should intubation fail. Reducing the succinylcholine dose to 0.5 mg/kg slightly shortens recovery time and does not appear to compromise intubating conditions when administered with propofol and fentanyl in the nonobstetric population.[104] In pregnancy, however, the reduced FRC and increased oxygen consumption make significant desaturation likely before the return of spontaneous respiration, no matter the succinylcholine dose. Because opioids are not commonly administered at induction, continued use of succinylcholine 1 to 1.5 mg/kg is recommended.

The use of alternative muscle relaxants for rapid-sequence intubation may be considered given the side-effect profile of succinylcholine. **Rocuronium** is often used when succinylcholine is contraindicated. In a study of 240 women undergoing rapid-sequence induction of general anesthesia for cesarean delivery,[105] rocuronium did not prolong time to tracheal intubation, and it provided less resistance to laryngoscopy and a lower incidence of postoperative myalgia than succinylcholine. However, its prolonged duration of action is a significant concern when failure to ventilate or intubate occurs. **Sugammadex**, with its ability to rapidly reverse the effects of rocuronium, may address this concern (see earlier discussion). Authors of a 2015 metaanalysis[106] concluded that succinylcholine (≥ 1 mg/kg), when used with propofol for rapid-sequence induction, produced superior intubating conditions than rocuronium (0.6 to 0.7 mg/kg) (relative risk, 0.86; 95% CI, 0.81 to 0.92). However, no significant difference was observed between the two agents when a larger dose of rocuronium (1.2 mg/kg) was used.[106]

Although the effectiveness of cricoid pressure in preventing pulmonary aspiration of gastric contents has been challenged,[107,108] it is frequently used during the induction of obstetric general anesthesia (see Chapters 26 and 28). However, the use of cricoid pressure can adversely affect the ease of ventilation, laryngoscopy, and intubation. In a comparison of cricoid pressure with 20, 30, and 44 N of force, increasing pressure was more likely to lead to cricoid deformity and esophageal occlusion, particularly in women.[109] Difficulty with ventilation is less likely when 30 N is applied (currently accepted practice) than with 44 N (the previously suggested optimum value).[110] When correctly applied, with an increase in force from 10 to 30 N with the induction of general anesthesia, there is little evidence of harm. However, when difficulty with intubation or ventilation is encountered, cricoid pressure may need to be adjusted, reduced, or released (see later discussion).

Although the cricoid pressure technique originally described by Sellick[111] was a one-handed technique, the placement of a second hand behind the patient's neck to prevent excessive neck flexion has been observed to provide a superior laryngoscopic view.[112] However, the two-handed cricoid pressure technique does not allow the assistant to aid in other procedures, such as holding additional equipment necessary for difficult airway management.

Finally, although the traditional rapid-sequence induction technique avoids mask ventilation (to avoid introducing air into the stomach), this contributes to oxygen desaturation during the period of apnea. The current Obstetric Anaesthetists' Association (OAA)/Difficult Airway Society (DAS) algorithm suggests that face mask ventilation (limiting P_{max} to 20 cm H_2O) can be considered.

COMPLEX AIRWAY MANAGEMENT

Planning

The approach to the difficult airway in the obstetric patient depends on the clinical situation as well as the skill set of the anesthesia provider. A suggested approach for management of obstetric patients with an anticipated difficult airway is outlined in Fig. 29.8. After an initial assessment of the patient, an airway management plan should be created and shared with the patient and other members of the multidisciplinary team. In extreme cases, anesthetic considerations may influence the mode and timing of delivery. Despite a thorough airway assessment and management plan, unanticipated or unrecognized airway issues and complications may arise; alternative algorithms and equipment should be readily available to ensure oxygenation and ventilation. Emergence and extubation should also be planned in advance. Lack of forethought and planning can lead to poor decision-making in crisis situations.

Neuraxial Anesthesia

The value of establishing and confirming a functional epidural catheter during labor in patients with an anticipated difficult airway has been described (see earlier discussion). Neuraxial anesthesia may also be preferable in patients with an anticipated difficult airway undergoing urgent or elective cesarean delivery. The choice of anesthetic technique (e.g., single-shot spinal, epidural, combined spinal-epidural [CSE], sequential CSE, continuous spinal techniques) depends on the circumstances and preferences of the anesthesia provider. Neuraxial techniques do not obviate the necessity of planning for airway management, as both inadequate neuraxial anesthesia and high spinal anesthesia may complicate any neuraxial technique and necessitate urgent airway intervention. Therefore, plans for securing the airway must always be preformulated, and standard and alternative airway equipment should be readily available.

Awake Intubation Before General Anesthesia

Performing an awake intubation may be the safest option for the patient with an anticipated difficult airway, particularly if difficult face mask ventilation is anticipated or if neuraxial anesthesia is contraindicated or fails. Induction of general anesthesia with paralysis can distort airway anatomy by allowing soft tissue relaxation and movement of the larynx in an anterior direction, making attempts at direct laryngoscopy more difficult. Therefore, it may be optimal to secure the airway of these patients while they are awake and spontaneously breathing, before induction of general anesthesia.[113] In skilled hands, the awake intubation can be accomplished quickly and comfortably with a high success rate.[114]

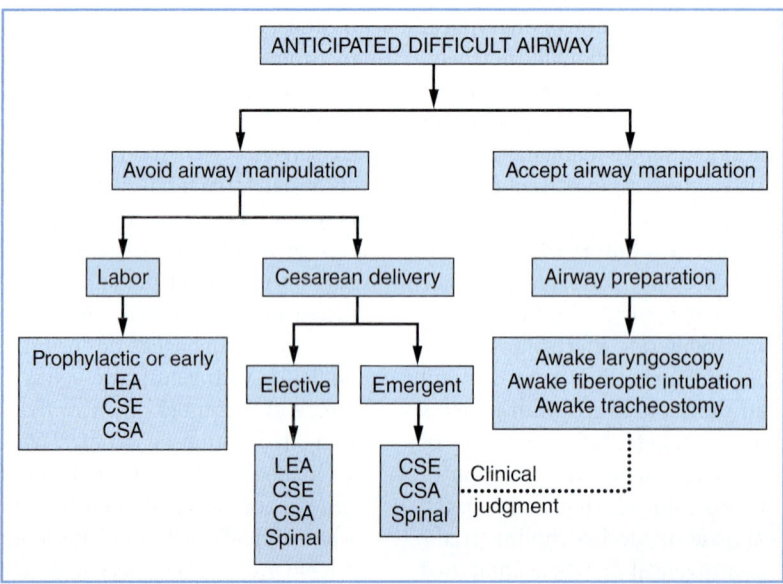

Fig. 29.8 Algorithm for Anticipated Difficult Airway. This algorithm is not intended to provide comprehensive guidance that addresses every contingency. Rather, it should help anesthesia providers consider the various options that are available. Management should be individualized, and the anesthesia provider's clinical skills and judgment should guide decision-making. For additional information, the reader is referred to the American Society of Anesthesiologists practice guidelines.[1] *CSA*, Continuous spinal anesthesia technique; *CSE*, combined spinal-epidural technique; *LEA*, lumbar epidural analgesia or anesthesia technique; *spinal*, spinal anesthesia technique.

Awake intubation can be performed with a variety of airway management devices, but the flexible fiberoptic bronchoscope offers unique advantages (Box 29.2). Proper planning and execution, with attention to detail, are key to a high success rate. It is useful to have two anesthesia providers: one to perform the endoscopy and another to monitor the patient.[87] Pulse oximetry, capnography, continuous electrocardiography, and blood pressure monitoring are mandatory. The level of conscious sedation must be constantly monitored to obtain the desired level for the procedure (see later discussion). Supplemental oxygen should be administered, with HFNO (see discussion above) as an optional adjunctive oxygenation technique.

When possible, an unhurried, thorough explanation of the technique to the patient helps allay anxiety. Pharmacologic premedication should include prophylaxis for pulmonary aspiration and an **antisialagogue** such as intravenous glycopyrrolate 0.2 mg. A dry mouth improves topical oral anesthesia by ensuring better contact between the local anesthetic and the mucosa.[115] Secretions may also cause internal reflection from the light source and distort the fiberoptic view. Performing the procedure with the patient in the upright, rather than supine, position minimizes airway obstruction and aortocaval occlusion, enhances drainage of secretions, and allows better acceptance of topical anesthesia by the patient.

Conscious Sedation

Although termed *awake intubation*, most patients receive some form of sedation to relieve anxiety, produce amnesia, and reduce pain and discomfort during the procedure. With moderate sedation/analgesia, also termed *conscious sedation*, the patient can respond purposefully to verbal or tactile stimulation, no interventions are required to maintain a patent airway, and spontaneous ventilation is adequate.[116] An overdose of the sedative/hypnotic or analgesic drugs can result in airway obstruction, hypoxemia, and cardiorespiratory depression; maintenance of continuous verbal contact is the optimal method for avoiding oversedation.[117]

The choice of drugs to produce conscious sedation depends on the preference and experience of the anesthesia provider.

Small boluses of intravenous midazolam (0.5 to 1 mg) and fentanyl (25 to 50 µg) are usually adequate[118]; the use of a propofol infusion has also been described.[113] Remifentanil may confer some advantages over fentanyl in providing rapid onset, more precise titration with the ability to use an infusion, and rapid metabolism and dissipation of effects; decreased respiratory rate or apnea may be quickly reversed by stopping the infusion. Remifentanil infusion rates between 0.05 and 0.175 µg/kg/min have been used for awake fiberoptic intubation in nonobstetric patients[119]; target-controlled infusions of remifentanil, with or without propofol, can also provide ideal conditions.[120] The use of intravenous dexmedetomidine infusion to facilitate awake fiberoptic intubation at cesarean delivery has also been described; benefits include minimal depression of respiratory function or hemodynamic status.[121,122] Neonatal effects of the drugs used for sedation are usually minimal; however, the neonatologist should be informed of the drugs administered to the mother before delivery.

Topical Anesthesia

Providing adequate topical anesthesia of the upper respiratory tract is critical to a successful awake fiberoptic intubation. Local anesthetic agents can be used in two basic ways to provide topical upper airway anesthesia: direct application to the mucosa or the injection for laryngeal nerve blocks. Topical application of local anesthetic is the most commonly used technique owing to its ease and effectiveness. A variety of techniques can be successfully employed. For example, the patient can be asked to gargle and slowly swallow viscous lidocaine (2% or 4%), or lidocaine (2%, 4%, or 10%) can be aerosolized and sprayed onto the tongue and oropharynx.

Commercially available devices, which are produced in a variety of shapes and sizes, can aerosolize and spray local anesthetic solutions in a jetlike stream. The Mackenzie technique uses an intravenous cannula with an injection port (e.g., 20- or 18-gauge) connected to oxygen tubing via a three-way connector (Fig. 29.9). Administration of local anesthetic from a syringe through the connector, with the oxygen flowing at 2 L/min, creates a jetlike spray.[123] An additional method uses a nebulizer mask or mouthpiece, with 4% lidocaine (4 to 6 mL) placed in the nebulizer bowl and connected to an oxygen source at a flow rate of 8 L/min. This method is easy to administer, noninvasive, and comfortable for the patient, with minimal or absent coughing. Each of these techniques may be insufficient as a single entity and may be combined with other methods, including instillation of local anesthetic through the working channel of the fiberoptic bronchoscope channel.

The "spray as you go" (SAYGO) technique uses the working channel of the fiberoptic bronchoscope to instill local anesthetic onto the mucous membranes of the airway. The working channel of an intubating fiberoptic bronchoscope, such as the Olympus LF-2 (Olympus America Inc., Centre Valley, PA), is 600 mm long and 1.5 mm in diameter. If a small syringe is directly attached to the working channel port and the solution is merely injected, the local anesthetic is likely to stay in the channel rather than be sprayed onto the mucosa. This problem can be overcome by placing an epidural catheter

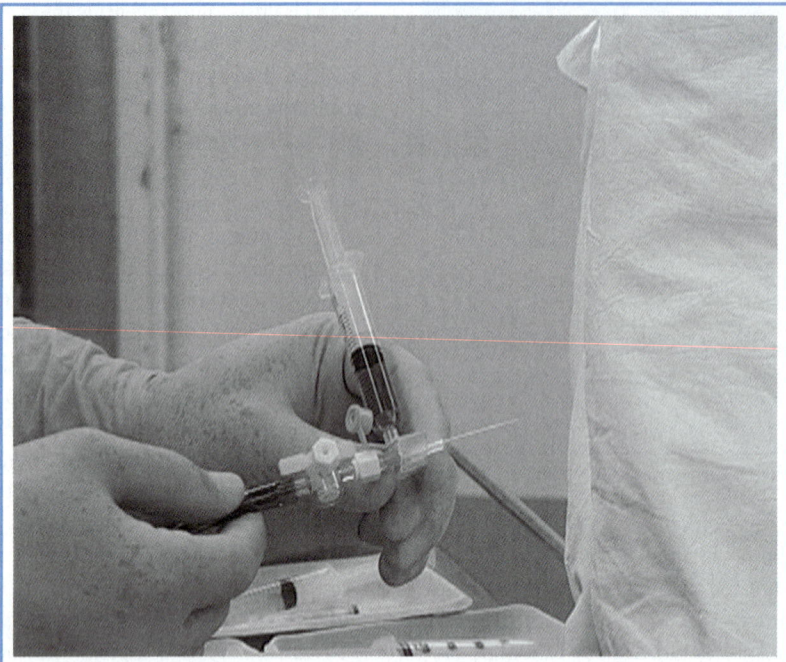

Fig. 29.9 Topical Airway Anesthesia. The MacKenzie technique[123] uses a 20-gauge intravenous cannula with an injection port connected to oxygen tubing via a three-way connector to produce a jetlike spray of local anesthetic administered from a syringe connected to the cannula with the oxygen flowing at 2 L/min.

through the working channel; using a Luer-Lok connector for the epidural catheter allows a direct and tight connection with the local anesthetic syringe and avoids leakage. The local anesthetic agent is drawn up in a 2-mL syringe and "dripped" on the mucus membranes; this instillation can be better targeted if the distal tip of the epidural catheter is allowed to protrude approximately 1 cm from the tip of the fiberoptic bronchoscope.

Nerve Blocks

The nerve supply to the upper airway is derived from branches of cranial nerves V, VII, IX, and X. The lingual branch of the glossopharyngeal nerve (IX), which innervates the submucosal pressure receptors at the base of the tongue, can be blocked with the bilateral administration of 1% lidocaine (2 mL) just under the mucosa at the base of the anterior tonsillar pillars. The necessity of this block during performance of awake intubation in obstetric patients is controversial.[124] Laryngeal and tracheal sensation can be minimized with blockade of the internal branch of the superior laryngeal nerve and transtracheal administration of lidocaine, respectively. Blockade of the superior laryngeal nerve may be performed by locating the greater cornu of the hyoid bone, advancing a small-bore needle until the bone is contacted, walking the needle off the edge of the bone into the thyrohyoid membrane, and injecting 1% lidocaine, approximately 3 mL. The injection is then repeated on the other side of the neck.

Historically, nerve blocks were an essential part of preparing the upper airway; today, meticulous topical application is easier to perform, less invasive, and provides effective intubating conditions. A technique for topical anesthesia for oral awake fiberoptic intubation is described in Box 29.3.

BOX 29.3   Suggested Airway Anesthesia for Awake Fiberoptic Intubation

Topical Anesthesia
- Tongue and oropharynx: 2% lidocaine gargle (5–10 mL) plus 4% lidocaine (3–4 mL) sprayed using the Mackenzie technique[a]
- Supraglottic region: SAYGO through an epidural catheter,[b] 4% lidocaine (1–2 mL)
- Glottic/infraglottic region: SAYGO through an epidural catheter,[b] 4% lidocaine (1–2 mL)

Supplemental Anesthesia
- The gag reflex is tested before endoscopy with gentle suction; if it is not obtunded, transtracheal anesthesia is performed (cricothyroid puncture and injection of 4% lidocaine [3–4 mL])

SAYGO, Spray as you go (see text).
[a]See Fig. 29.9.
[b]An epidural catheter is inserted through the working channel of the fiberoptic scope. A syringe with local anesthetic is attached to the proximal end (see text).

Airway Anesthesia and Risk for Aspiration

Some anesthesia providers are concerned that local anesthesia of the larynx might obtund airway protective reflexes, particularly after a transtracheal block.[125,126] However, in a series of 129 patients, both the transtracheal injection and SAYGO techniques were effective and safe, with no evidence of regurgitation or aspiration in any patient.[127] It has been suggested that topical anesthesia of the larynx does not impair voluntary motor function of the vocal cords, such as coughing on request,[128] thus allowing the patient to protect their airway.

The SAYGO technique may be preferred because the interval between topical anesthesia and endoscopy is minimal and if gastric reflux occurs during endoscopy it can be visualized and the gastric juice aspirated through the fiberoptic bronchoscope. The key to minimizing the risk for aspiration, however, is avoidance of oversedation. Nonetheless, administration of aspiration prophylaxis is advised, and the patient should be monitored for possible reflux or emesis.

Fiberoptic Intubation

Fiberoptic laryngoscopy can be performed orally or nasally, but the oral route is more common because of the potential for epistaxis due to engorgement of the nasal mucosa. However, in very specific situations (i.e., when the oral aperture is insufficient to allow fiberoptic bronchoscope passage), the nasal route can be successfully used in the obstetric patient with careful topical preparation of the nasal mucosa with agents that provide anesthesia and vasoconstriction.[59]

A common impediment to successful fiberoptic laryngoscopy is the inability to blindly advance the ETT into the correct position. The ETT most commonly arrests at the right arytenoid cartilage.[129] In a review of the causes, incidence, and solutions to this issue, Asai and Shingu[130] noted that impingement can be minimized by selecting the appropriate size and type of ETT and by using proper advancement technique. Smaller-diameter tracheal tubes (6- to 7-mm internal diameter [ID]) that fit more snugly onto the bronchoscope generally advance more easily. The design and flexibility of the tube and tip may also determine success; for example, the intubating laryngeal mask airway (LMA) ETT with its Huber tip is easier to advance than a flexometallic ETT during nasal fiberoptic intubation, probably owing to the acute angle of the Huber tip (Fig. 29.10).[131]

The lubricated ETT is loaded over the fiberoptic bronchoscope in its normal position (curve facing anterior, leading edge [tip] on the right, bevel facing left) and the fiberoptic bronchoscope is advanced into the airway. After the tip of the fiberoptic bronchoscope is positioned above the carina, the ETT is advanced over the fiberoptic bronchoscope into the airway. If impingement occurs, the ETT is withdrawn approximately 1 cm and rotated 90 degrees counterclockwise to bring the tip of the ETT anteriorly, and the ETT is reinserted. If this does not work, the ETT is rotated a further 90 degrees counterclockwise, and advancement is reattempted. Alternatively, the tube can be loaded on the fiberoptic bronchoscope with the tip facing anteriorly or other maneuvers may be employed, such as keeping the airway patent with jaw thrust and application of pressure on the neck to shift the vocal cords posteriorly.

Awake direct laryngoscopy results in more noxious stimulation than fiberoptic laryngoscopy, but a well-prepared and highly motivated patient may tolerate the procedure surprisingly well. Awake intubation also has been described using indirect or video laryngoscopes (see later discussion), but their role in awake intubation in the obstetric setting has yet to be determined. Other techniques for awake intubation, such as blind-nasal intubation and retrograde intubation, are performed infrequently in obstetric patients.

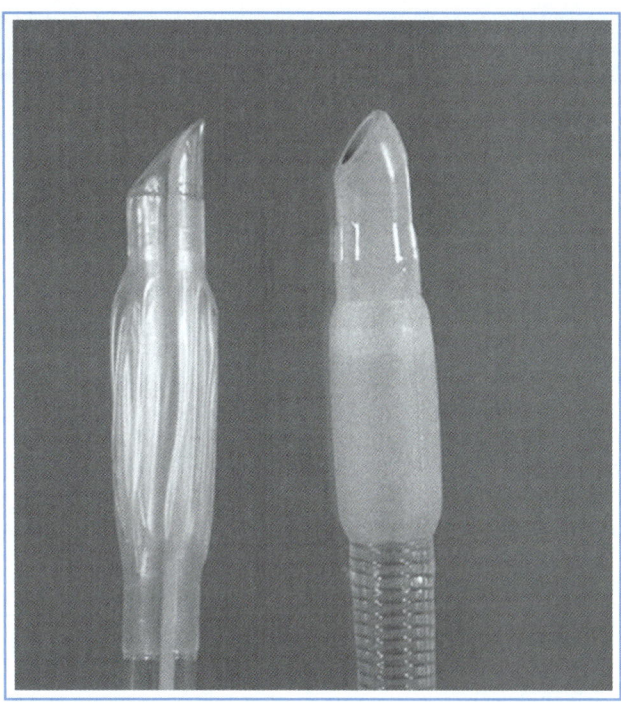

Fig. 29.10 Endotracheal Tube Tips. *Left,* The tip of a conventional endotracheal tube. *Right,* The tip of an endotracheal tube used with an intubating laryngeal mask airway (LMA). The Huber tip of the intubating LMA endotracheal tube is less likely to impinge on other structures, thus increasing the success of advancement and correct placement in the trachea.

Video Laryngoscopy

A number of rigid, indirect-optical laryngoscopes have been developed; these capture an image of the glottis in real time and transmit it to a video screen via a video camera eye near the tip of the laryngoscope blade.[132] Video laryngoscopes offer several advantages over conventional direct laryngoscopy (Box 29.4). To obtain a good view of the glottis with a direct laryngoscope, a line of sight from the oral opening to the glottis must be obtained by neck flexion and head extension (see earlier discussion). With video laryngoscopes, a direct line of sight to the glottis is unnecessary. Furthermore, if laryngeal pressure is required to improve the view, the assistant may watch the screen image to directly assess the effect of the pressure.

A 2016 systematic review,[133] which included more than 7000 adult patients, found significantly fewer failed intubations when a video laryngoscope was used (odds ratio [OR] 0.35) compared with direct laryngoscopy, and fewer failed intubations in both anticipated (OR 0.28) and simulated (OR 0.18) difficult airways. However, in patients not predicted to have a difficult airway, no significant reduction in failed intubation rate was observed. Of note, laryngeal or airway trauma was reduced when a video laryngoscope was used.

Video laryngoscopes may be classified into three categories (Fig. 29.11)[134]:
1. *Macintosh type* (e.g., C-MAC, Karl Storz Endoscopy, Tuttlingen, Germany). These devices have a Macintosh-type blade, and the glottis may be visualized either directly or on the video screen. In the setting of anticipated

BOX 29.4 Advantages and Disadvantages of Video Laryngoscopes

Advantages

- Improvement in Cormack and Lehane grade view
- Fewer failed intubations in anticipated and simulated difficult airways
- Reduced requirement for bougie and external laryngeal manipulation
- Utility as a rescue technique in patients with a difficult airway
- Assistant can view glottis and facilitate view with external glottic manipulation
- Useful teaching tool
- Possible advantage in patients with cervical spine pathology because of less need to manipulate neck
- Reduced risk for dental trauma because less force is required to align oropharyngeal axes
- Increased rates of successful tracheal intubation for inexperienced providers

Disadvantages

- Various models with different characteristics requiring different positioning
- Limited data comparing efficacy of different models
- Learning required to become familiar with technique
- Difficulty passing endotracheal tube despite good glottic view
- Increased rate of successful intubation only in those familiar with technique
- Adequate mouth opening required
- Possibly increased time to achieve intubation

Modified from Scott-Brown S, Russell R. Video laryngoscopes and the obstetric airway. *Int J Obstet Anesth.* 2015;24:137–146.

difficult airway, the success rate is generally higher with these devices than with direct laryngoscopy, but external pressure and an ETT introducer are more frequently required.[135]

2. *Anatomically shaped without a tube guide* (e.g., GlideScope video laryngoscope, Verathon Inc., Bothell, WA; McGrath video laryngoscope, LMA North America, San Diego, CA, United States). The curved shape of the blade allows a view of the glottis without flexing or extending the head and neck; however, directing the ETT toward the glottis may be difficult, resulting in trauma. Several reports have described pharyngeal and palatal injury with use of the GlideScope.[136,137] Injury is more likely when the GlideScope or ETT is inserted blindly through the mouth, when a rigid stylet is used, and when undue force is employed during ETT insertion.

3. *Anatomically shaped blade with tube guide* (e.g., Airtraq, King Systems Corporation, Noblesville, IN; The Airway Scope AWS-S100, Hoya-Pentax, Tokyo, Japan). The tip of the tube is captured on the video screen even before the device is inserted, and its location can be continuously confirmed during the entire course of intubation. Palatal injury has also been reported with the Pentax Airway Scope.[138]

New, low-profile versions of these video laryngoscopes may be of benefit in the obstetric setting, as they can aid in maneuverability in the mouth when mucosal edema might otherwise hinder placement of the laryngoscope. Although there are a number of studies comparing different video laryngoscopes in patients with normal airways,[139-141] there are few studies that compare the use of different video laryngoscopes in patients with an anticipated difficult airway.[142,143] Furthermore, it is not known whether the preoperative assessments used to predict difficult direct laryngoscopy are valid predictors of difficult video laryngoscopy.

Evidence of benefit of video laryngoscopy in the obstetric population remains limited.[134] Arici et al.[144] performed a randomized study comparing the McGrath Series 5 with a Macintosh blade in 80 women undergoing cesarean delivery with general anesthesia. Video laryngoscopy resulted in a significantly better view of the glottic opening but a longer apnea interval. All intubation attempts were successful on the first attempt. Dhonneur et al.[145] reported the successful use of a difficult airway algorithm in which the Airtraq device was used in parturients as a rescue device if tracheal intubation failed after 2 minutes of direct laryngoscopy. During a 6-month period, 69 parturients underwent emergency cesarean delivery with general anesthesia; 2 morbidly obese parturients required the Airtraq device for successful tracheal intubation. The investigators suggested that the device might be an acceptable primary airway management tool in cases of emergency cesarean delivery in parturients with an anticipated difficult airway. Aziz et al.[146] retrospectively analyzed 180 tracheal intubations over a 3-year period in their obstetric unit. Traditional direct laryngoscopy resulted in 157 of 163 successful intubations on first attempt, with one failed intubation (95% CI, 92% to 99%). Video laryngoscopy with a GlideScope resulted in 18 of 18 successful intubations on the first attempt (95% CI, 81% to 100%) and a successful intubation in the patient with the failed direct laryngoscopy. In their study of almost 15,000 cases of general anesthesia for cesarean delivery, Reale et al.[7] identified 295 difficult intubations; 49 involved failed direct laryngoscopy and 26 involved failed video laryngoscopy. Of 18 failed intubations, 14 involved failed direct laryngoscopy and 10 involved failed video laryngoscopy; all cases were rescued with an SGA.

The use of video laryngoscopy has become increasing more common,[147] as evidence demonstrating its potential advantages continues to be published. Literature in the obstetric population is, however, sparse, although extrapolation of studies in nonpregnant patients, especially the obese, suggests use of video laryngoscopy is of benefit. Moreover, the 2015 OAA/DAS guidelines for the management of failed intubation state that a video laryngoscope should be immediately available for all obstetric general anesthetics.[10]

Awake Tracheostomy or Surgery Standby

It is possible to perform an awake tracheostomy with local anesthesia, a technique that may be required in some situations in which airway management is anticipated to be extremely difficult and dangerous.[148] In some cases,

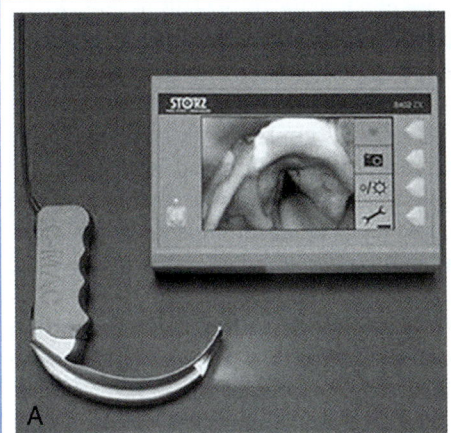 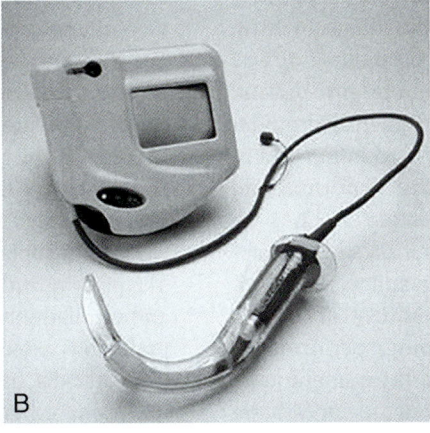 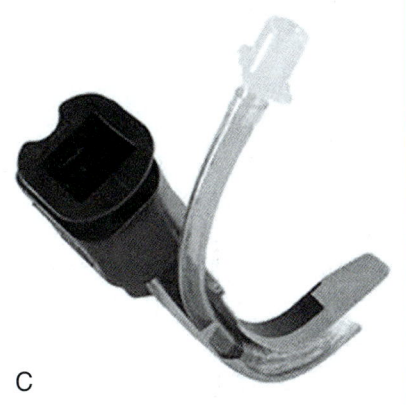

Fig. 29.11 The Three Categories of Video Laryngoscope. (A) The C-MAC video laryngoscope with a Macintosh-type blade. (B) The Glidescope video laryngoscope with an anatomically shaped blade without a tube guide. (C) The Airtraq video laryngoscope with an anatomically shaped blade and a tube guide. A, Illustration Karl Storz Endoscopy, Tuttlingen, Germany; B and C, Illustration Verathon Inc., Bothell, WA.

particularly if there is a known pathologic airway condition, it is prudent to request that a surgical team proficient in emergency surgical airway management be immediately available before the induction of anesthesia for cesarean delivery.

Local Anesthesia for Cesarean Delivery

Rarely, the infiltration of local anesthesia may be used as a *primary* anesthetic technique for emergency cesarean delivery in the patient with an anticipated difficult airway. This technique, which has been well described, is most often used in developing countries, where contemporary anesthetic techniques may not be readily available (see Chapter 26).[149] Few obstetricians today are familiar or proficient with this technique, but some resident training programs still provide instruction on its use.[74] A large volume (i.e., 75 to 100 mL) of a dilute local anesthetic solution, such as 0.5% lidocaine, is often required.[150] Administration of such a large volume entails a risk for systemic local anesthetic toxicity (LAST). Mei et al.[151] described four cases in which cesarean delivery was performed with bilateral transversus abdominis plane block and ilioinguinal-iliohypogastric nerve blocks using 0.5% ropivacaine 40 mL.

In some cases, it is possible to perform the entire surgical procedure with local infiltration, provided the obstetrician makes a midline abdominal incision, makes minimal use of retractors, and does not exteriorize the uterus. Alternatively, the obstetrician might begin surgery and deliver the infant with the aid of local infiltration. Temporary hemostasis may be achieved until the airway is secured and then surgery completed after the induction of general anesthesia.[149]

Intraperiotoneal chloroprocaine is another analgesic option that has shown to be a safe and useful adjunct to an inadequate neuraxial block. In a 2022 study, Togioka et al.[152] reported 15 women who received 40 mL of 1%, 2%, or 3% intraperitoneal chloroprocaine. No patients had any symptoms consistent with LAST, and peak plasma levels for all groups remained well below thresholds for risk of LAST. Similarly, a 2018 single-center, retrospective review found that among 32 women receiving intraperitoneal chloroprocaine, none experienced

signs of LAST or required conversion to general anesthesia, and 17 of 32 patients experienced improved pain scores after chloroprocaine instillation.[153] These data suggest that intraperitoneal chloroprocaine is well tolerated when used to manage breakthrough pain during cesarean delivery.

Cesarean delivery performed with local infiltration or intraperitoneal chloroprocaine, if successful, has the advantages of preserving maternal hemodynamic stability and a patent airway while allowing emergency delivery of the infant, particularly in the setting of an emergency delivery when venous access is unobtainable. However, the local infiltration technique requires a skilled and patient obstetrician; thus, it may often not be suitable in rushed, emergency settings. Maternal anesthesia is typically incomplete and often inadequate, and thus local infiltration does not obviate the need to obtain venous access, particularly given that complications such as hemorrhage may arise. Intraosseous access may be appropriate in these types of extreme circumstances if venous access cannot be obtained.

Finally, the possibility of development of psychological trauma should be considered, particularly if anesthesia is inadequate or the neonatal outcome is poor; in such cases, appropriate counselling and services should be offered to the parturient after delivery.

THE UNANTICIPATED DIFFICULT AIRWAY

Obstetric Anesthesia Failed Intubation Guidelines

Despite best attempts to adequately risk-stratify parturients preoperatively, cases of unanticipated difficulty with airway management will occur. Therefore, both the anesthesia providers and the entire operating team should have a plan to manage unanticipated difficult airways *before* administering general anesthesia to obstetric patients. Historically, guidelines on difficult airway management specific to the obstetric patient did not exist. New guidelines have been developed that reflect the unique difficulties inherent to obstetric general anesthesia, in which difficulties in airway management may threaten the life of the mother as well as the infant. In 2013, Law et al.[154] published recommendations on difficult airway management that contained a section on the obstetric patient. Subsequently, in 2015, the OAA and DAS published guidelines on the management of difficult and failed intubation in obstetrics.[10] These guidelines consist of three algorithms and two tables; the master algorithm is shown in Fig. 29.12.

Algorithm 1 covers safe obstetric general anesthesia practice, emphasizing the need for planning and preparation. The algorithm includes preoperative assessment of mother and fetus, multidisciplinary team planning, performance of a rapid-sequence induction, and up to three attempts at laryngoscopy. Before induction of anesthesia, the anesthesia provider and obstetrician should discuss whether to awaken the woman or continue with surgery if tracheal intubation is not possible. Patient position should be optimized, effective preoxygenation performed (see earlier discussion), and appropriate doses of drugs administered. If the first attempt at laryngoscopy produces a poor view of the larynx, consideration should be given to reducing or removing cricoid pressure, applying external laryngeal manipulation, repositioning

the head, and the use of a bougie. If this fails to improve the view, the guidelines recommend gentle face mask ventilation. For a second attempt at laryngoscopy, consideration should be given to using an alternative laryngoscope and removing cricoid pressure. If this is also unsuccessful, a third attempt should only be attempted by an experienced colleague.

Algorithm 2 summarizes the initial management of obstetric failed intubation. Failure to intubate is communicated to the operating room team, who should summon help. The priority at this stage is to maintain maternal oxygenation and ventilation. This may be achieved by insertion of an SGA, preferably a second-generation device with a gastric drain (see later discussion) with cricoid pressure removed during insertion; or by face mask, with or without an oropharyngeal airway. If oxygenation is possible, a decision must then be made regarding whether to proceed with surgery.

If oxygenation is not possible, **Algorithm 3** should be followed. This final algorithm provides details of management of a *"cannot intubate, cannot oxygenate"* scenario. The situation should be declared to all members of the operating room team, and specialist help (e.g., otolaryngologist, trauma surgeon, intensivist) should be summoned. Laryngospasm

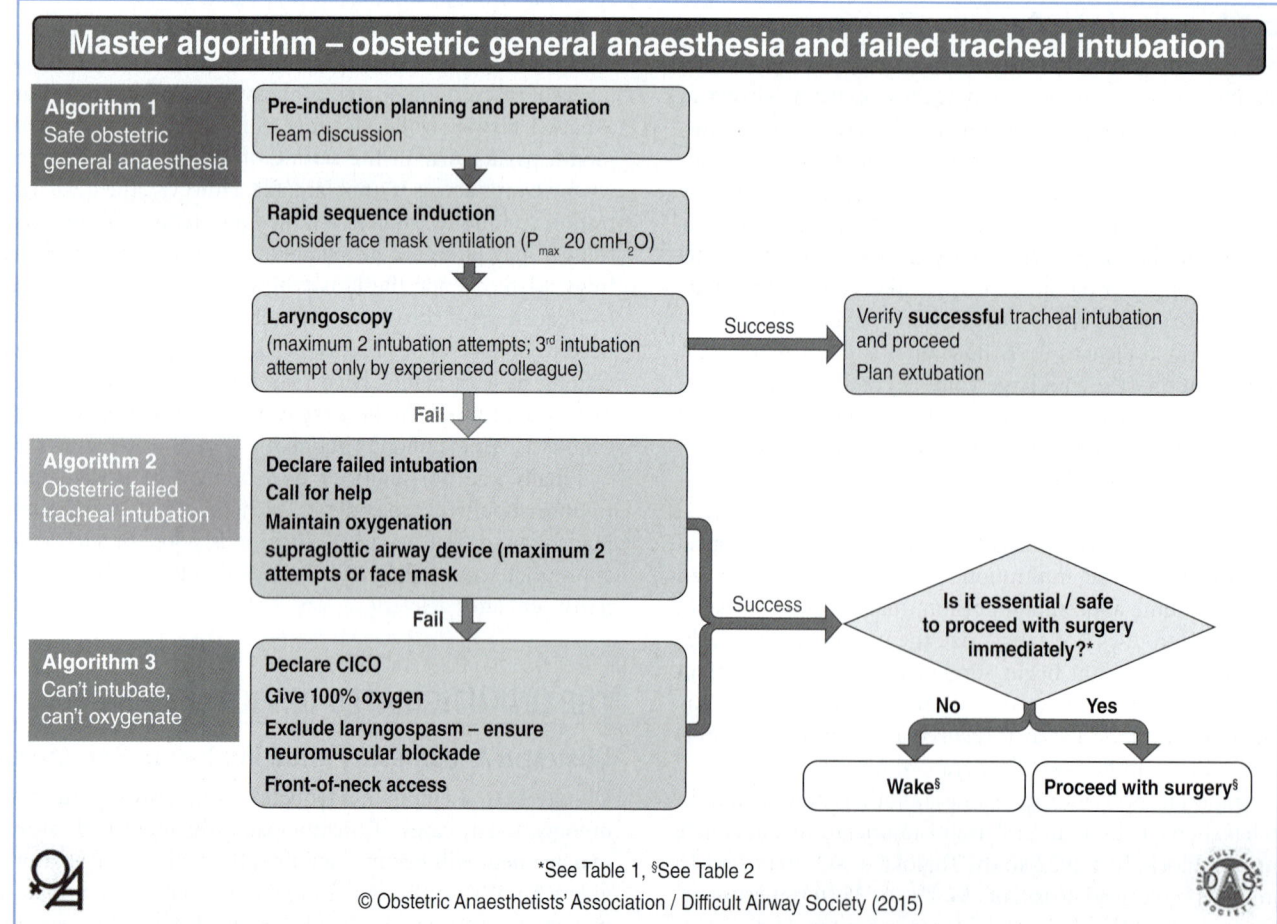

Fig. 29.12 Obstetric Anaesthetists' Association and Difficult Airway Society master algorithm for the management of difficult and failed tracheal intubation in obstetrics. *CICO*, Can't intubate, can't oxygenate; P_{max}, maximal inflation pressure. From Mushambi MC, Kinsella SM, Popat M, et al. Obstetric Anaesthetists' Association and Difficult Airway Society guidelines for the management of difficult and failed tracheal intubation in obstetrics. *Anaesthesia.* 2015;70:1286–1306, with permission from Obstetric Anaesthetists' Association/Difficult Airway Society.

should be excluded and adequate neuromuscular blockade ensured. Front-of-neck access (see later discussion), with either a needle or surgical cricothyroidotomy, may be necessary. If successful, a decision is made on whether to proceed with cesarean delivery. If front-of-neck access fails to restore oxygenation, maternal advanced life support and perimortem cesarean delivery (see Chapter 53) may be required.

Table 1 of the OAA/DAS algorithm (Fig. 29.13) provides a structure of individual factors that should aid in the decision of whether to proceed with surgery. Factors such as the maternal and fetal conditions, experience of the anesthesia provider, maternal obesity, anticipated surgical difficulty, aspiration risk, and possible alternative anesthetic techniques should be addressed before induction of anesthesia. The availability of airway devices facilitating ventilation and the presence of airway hazards such as edema, stridor, or bleeding should be assessed after failed intubation. Although some criteria may suggest proceeding with delivery and others with waking the mother, the final decision depends on the anesthesia provider's judgment. If the mother and fetus are not in immediate jeopardy, the safest course is to awaken the mother. Once this is accomplished, other anesthetic options, such as an awake intubation or a neuraxial

anesthetic technique, should be considered. The risk associated with proceeding with surgery in this scenario represents an understanding of the possibility of mask airway failure, the requirement of additional airway manipulation, the risk for aspiration, and possible progression to a *"cannot oxygenate"* scenario.

If the situation is immediately life threatening to the mother for reasons such as hemorrhage due to uterine rupture or placental abruption, it may be necessary to proceed with cesarean delivery to optimize outcomes for both the mother and infant. Significant angst and controversy often accompany decision-making in the situation of a stable mother with evidence of life-threatening fetal compromise, such as a prolapsed umbilical cord causing fetal bradycardia. In such cases, if mask ventilation is easy and adequate, the risk-benefit ratio of proceeding with an unsecured airway and an increased risk for aspiration should be weighed against the benefits of prompt delivery of the infant. In cases in which the maternal risk for aspiration is considered low and mask ventilation is easy, it may be reasonable to continue mask ventilation and avoid further intubation attempts. It is unclear whether continued mask ventilation or repeated intubation attempts represent the greater risk to the mother; even

	Table 1 – proceed with surgery?			
Factors to consider	**WAKE** ⟵		⟶	**PROCEED**
Before induction — Maternal condition	• No compromise	• Mild acute compromise	• Haemorrhage responsive to resuscitation	• Hypovolaemia requiring corrective surgery • Critical cardiac or respiratory compromise, cardiac arrest
Fetal condition	• No compromise	• Compromise corrected with intrauterine resuscitation, pH < 7.2 but > 7.15	• Continuing fetal heart rate abnormality despite intrauterine resuscitation, pH < 7.15	• Sustained bradycardia • Fetal haemorrhage • Suspected uterine rupture
Anaesthetist	• Novice	• Junior trainee	• Senior trainee	• Consultant / specialist
Obesity	• Supermorbid	• Morbid	• Obese	• Normal
Surgical factors	• Conplex surgery or major haemorrhage anticipated	• Multiple uterine scars • Some surgical difficulties expected	• Single uterine scar	• No risk factors
Aspiration risk	• Recent food	• No recent food • In labour • Opioids given • Antacids not given	• No recent food • In labour • Opioids not given • Antacids given	• Fasted • Not in labour • Antacids given
Alternative anaesthesia • regional • securing airway awake	• No anticipated difficulty	• Predicted difficulty	• Relatively contraindicated	• Absolutely contraindicated or has failed • Surgery started
After failed intubation — Airway device / ventilation	• Difficult face mask ventilation • Front-of-neck	• Adequate face mask ventilation	• First generation supraglottic airway device	• Second generation supraglottic airway device
Airway hazards	• Laryngeal oedema • Stridor	• Bleeding • Trauma	• Secretions	• None evident

Criteria to be used in the decision to wake or proceed following failed tracheal intubation. In any individual patient, some factors may suggest waking and others proceeding. The final decision will depend on the anaesthetist's clinical judgement.
© Obstetric Anaesthetists' Association /Difficult Airway Soeciety (2015)

Fig. 29.13 OAA/DAS guidance for the management of difficult and failed tracheal intubation in obstetrics: Table 1—proceed with surgery? From Mushambi MC, Kinsella SM, Popat M, et al. Obstetric Anaesthetists' Association and Difficult Airway Society guidelines for the management of difficult and failed tracheal intubation in obstetrics. *Anaesthesia.* 2015;70:1286–1306, with permission from OAA/DAS.

insertion of an SGA may further traumatize the airway or precipitate regurgitation.

The anesthesia provider should carefully consider the maternal risks of proceeding with cesarean delivery in a mother with an unsecured and unprotected airway, especially if no urgency exists and/or mask ventilation is difficult. Some obstetric anesthesiologists argue that even a nonreassuring (but not life-threatening) fetal heart rate tracing does not always justify proceeding with cesarean delivery under general anesthesia in a patient with an unsecured airway. Alternatively, in some of these cases, proceeding with cesarean delivery via mask ventilation or with an SGA may be a better option than awakening the patient, especially in those in whom neuraxial techniques are contraindicated. In these cases, the importance of communication between the obstetric and anesthesia teams cannot be overemphasized.

Table 2 from the OAA/DAS guidelines (Fig. 29.14) provides information on management after a failed intubation with information on awakening the patient and proceeding with surgery. If the patient is to be awakened, oxygenation should be maintained, and cricoid pressure continued unless it impedes ventilation. The patient is positioned head-up or in the left-lateral position, and, if necessary, neuromuscular blockade is reversed. Further airway difficulty should be anticipated. Once awake, the urgency for delivery should be reviewed and alternative anesthetic options considered. In situations in which surgery is to proceed via face mask or SGA ventilation, aspiration risk should be minimized by maintaining cricoid pressure, emptying the stomach, minimizing fundal pressure, and administering antacids. Surgery should be performed by the senior obstetrician, and the neonatal team should be informed of the failed tracheal intubation attempt. If uterine tone is poor, propofol may be substituted for volatile agents to maintain anesthesia. Throughout surgery, the anesthetist must anticipate further airway problems.

The publication of the OAA/DAS guidelines[10] and the associated narrative review[6] are welcome additions to the armamentarium of the obstetric anesthesia provider. These important documents address problems specific to the obstetric patient; an accompanying editorial by Preston[155] highlights some important management features. The emphasis is now on *oxygenation* rather than *ventilation*, with bag-and-mask ventilation no longer forbidden. The decision to awaken the patient and perform another technique is often a difficult

---

Table 2 – management after failed tracheal intubation

Wake	**Proceed with surgery**

• Maintain oxygenation
• Maintain cricoid pressure if not impeding ventilation
• Either maintain head-up position or turn left lateral recumbent
• If rocuronium used, reverse with sugammadex
• Assess neuromuscular blockade and manage awareness if paralysis is prolonged
• Anticipate laryngospasm / can't intubate, can't oxygenate
	• Maintain anaesthesia
	• Maintain ventilation - consider merits of:
	  □ controlled or spontaneous ventilation
	  □ paralysis with rocuronium if sugammadex available
	• Anticipate laryngospasm / can't intubate, can't oxygenate
	• Minimise aspiration risk:
	  □ maintain cricoid pressure until delivery (if not impeding ventilation)
	  □ after delivery maintain vigilance and reapply cricoid pressure if signs of regurgitation
	  □ empty stomach with gastric drain tube if using second-generation supraglottic airway device
	  □ minimise fundal pressure
	  □ administer H$_2$ receptor blocker i.v. if not already given
	• Senior obstetrician to operate
	• Inform neonatal team about failed intubation
	• Consider total intravenous anaesthesia

After waking	

• Review urgency of surgery with obstetric team
• Intrauterine fetal resuscitation as appropriate
• For repeat anaesthesia, manage with two anaesthetists
• Anaesthetic options:
  □ Regional anaesthesia preferably inserted in lateral position
  □ Secure airway awake before repeat general anaesthesia	

© Obstetric Anaesthetists' Association / Difficult Airway Society (2015)

Fig. 29.14 OAA/DAS guidance for the management of difficult and failed tracheal intubation in obstetrics: Table 2—management after failed tracheal intubation. *i.v.*, Intravenous; *H$_2$*, histamine-2. From Mushambi MC, Kinsella SM, Popat M, et al. Obstetric Anaesthetists' Association and Difficult Airway Society guidelines for the management of difficult and failed tracheal intubation in obstetrics. *Anaesthesia.* 2015;70:1286–1306, with permission from OAA/DAS.

one. Kinsella et al.[6] concluded that there has been increasing willingness to continue with general anesthesia rather than awakening the patient over the last 40 years. Hopefully, with routine preinduction discussion and with the guidance offered in Table 1 of the OAA/DAS guidelines, this decision will be more informed. Finally, front-of-neck access (attaining a surgical airway) is not an easy rescue technique and one that is unfamiliar to many obstetric anesthesia providers and obstetricians. If it is to be recommended, obstetric anesthesia providers will need to master this skill.

Laryngeal Mask Airway

The LMA is arguably the SGA with which anesthesia providers are most familiar. The introduction of the LMA into anesthetic practice was a significant advance in airway management that resulted in major updates to the difficult airway algorithms of the ASA and other societies.[1] Insertion of an SGA in an obstetric patient who can easily be ventilated by face mask is controversial because little additional ventilation benefit is obtained and placement can induce vomiting and aspiration in this setting. However, if the anethesia provider is a solo provider, then SGA insertion may be necessary to allow the provider to perform other necessary tasks. In any situation in which conventional face mask ventilation is difficult or impossible, an SGA is the rescue device of choice.

The LMA has many advantages, most notably its ease of use and a very high initial success rate.[156] Moreover, the LMA need not be perfectly positioned over the larynx to allow adequate ventilation. When assessed by flexible fiberoptic endoscopy, radiography, and magnetic resonance imaging, placement of the LMA around the larynx is variable[156]; however, 94% to 99% of patients with an LMA have little or no difficulty with ventilation.

In a prospective study, an LMA was inserted by experienced users in 1067 healthy parturients undergoing *elective* cesarean delivery under general anesthesia.[157] The investigators demonstrated that a clinically effective and acceptable airway was obtained on the first attempt in 98% of patients and on the second or third attempt in an additional 1%. Fewer than 1% of patients required tracheal intubation for failure to obtain satisfactory LMA placement within 90 seconds, or for an $SpO_2 < 94\%$, or an end-tidal $CO_2 > 45$ mm Hg. Moreover, the airway management (which was accomplished with the LMA, maintenance of cricoid pressure until delivery, and mechanical tidal-volume ventilation of 8 to 12 mL/kg) was associated with no episodes of hypoxemia ($SpO_2 < 90\%$), regurgitation, aspiration, laryngospasm, bronchospasm, or gastric insufflation. The investigators concluded that, in experienced hands, an LMA is effective and "probably safe" for ventilation and the administration of a volatile anesthetic agent for general anesthesia in selected healthy patients undergoing elective cesarean delivery.

Many case reports have described the use of an LMA as a rescue device for obstetric patients in whom conventional methods of securing the airway have failed. In a national case control study performed in the United Kingdom from 2007 to 2009, 39 of 57 patients with a failed intubation were managed with a classic LMA.[22] In the multicenter study by Reale et al.,[7] 18 of 18 failed intubations were managed with an LMA. An LMA may also act as a conduit for intubation (see later discussion).

Despite these benefits, the LMA has been associated with the following disadvantages: (1) placement can induce vomiting; (2) aspiration of gastric contents is not prevented; (3) improper positioning can lead to gastric insufflation; (4) multiple insertion attempts may be required for correct placement, which may result in airway trauma; and (5) use of positive-pressure ventilation may be limited. In 0.4% to 0.6% of patients with normal airway findings, the placement of an LMA leads to inadequate ventilation[156]; reasons for this outcome have been reported to include (1) backfolding of the distal cuff, (2) occlusion of the glottis by the distal cuff, (3) complete downfolding of the epiglottis, and (4) 90- to 180-degree rotation of the mask around its long axis.

Most of these data pertain to the use of the original classic LMA; several variations in LMA design have since become available. Updated designs that have been found to be useful in difficult airway management of parturients are the ProSeal LMA (LMA North America), the Fastrach LMA (LMA North America), and the Air-Q LMA (Cookgas LLC, Mercury Medical, Clearwater, FL, United States). The ProSeal LMA has a specialized high-volume/low-pressure cuff that allows the device to achieve a better fit over the glottis than a classic LMA (Fig. 29.15).[158] This design allows the use of higher ventilation pressures (up to 30 to 40 cm H_2O) with less air leakage around the cuff and a lower risk for air entry into the stomach. The ProSeal LMA also contains a specialized drainage conduit that bypasses the bowl of the LMA to minimize the entry of gastric fluid into the glottis, which has been shown to be effective in venting both passive and active regurgitation[159,160] and can accommodate the passage of a gastric tube.

Halaseh et al.[161] described the use of the ProSeal LMA in 3000 patients undergoing cesarean delivery who had fasted for more than 4 hours and were not thought to have

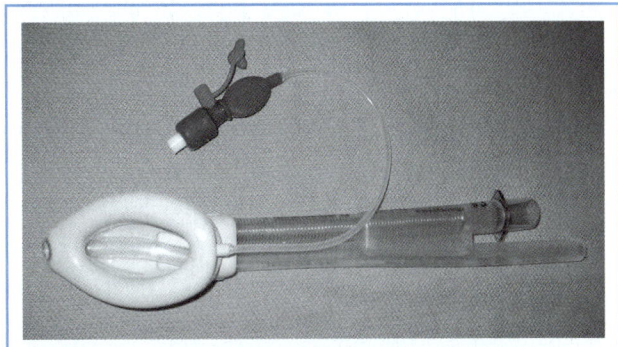

Fig. 29.15 The ProSeal LMA (Laryngeal Mask Airway). This LMA device has a specialized high-volume/low-pressure cuff, which allows glottis coverage that enables the use of higher ventilation pressures (up to 30–40 cm H_2O) with less air leakage around the cuff and a lower risk for entry of air into the stomach than a conventional LMA. The ProSeal LMA also contains a specialized drainage tube that bypasses the bowl of the LMA and prevents gastric fluid from entering the glottic area. A gastric tube can be passed down this drainage lumen to assist in emptying the stomach contents.

a difficult airway. They established an "effective" airway on the first attempt in 2992 (99.7%) women, with only 8 patients (0.3%) requiring a change to a different LMA size. None of the patients required tracheal intubation, and only one patient experienced regurgitation of gastric contents into the mouth. Minor side effects such as a sore throat occurred in 21 patients (0.7%).[161] Case reports have described the successful use of the ProSeal LMA after failed intubation in obstetric patients.[162–164]

A disadvantage of use of the ProSeal LMA in an emergency is that it requires practice and experience to use correctly. High rates of successful first-pass insertion can be achieved by loading the drainage conduit with a lubricated gum elastic bougie[165] or orogastric tube[166] and using direct laryngoscopy to position the conduit in the esophagus, and then railroading the ProSeal LMA into position. Given its complexity, this technique may not be appropriate when inserting an LMA to rescue failed intubation. A disposable, single-use version of the ProSeal LMA—the LMA Supreme—has a rigid design that facilitates high rates of successful first-pass insertion. Yao et al.[167] described the successful use of the LMA Supreme in 700 nonobese women undergoing cesarean delivery under general anesthesia. However, both the ProSeal LMA and LMA Supreme have a large esophageal drain that decreases the size of the airway conduit, and thereby impedes direct passage of an ETT. Intubating conduits (e.g., fiberoptic scopes) are also difficult to insert through the LMA Supreme due to their rigid design.

Although designed specifically to facilitate blind tracheal intubation, the Fastrach or Air-Q intubating LMA can also be combined with fiberoptic bronchoscopy (Fig. 29.16).[168] However, neither has a gastric drainage conduit. When properly placed, the Fastrach intubating LMA allows ventilation similar to that of the original LMA; however, a more rigid J-shaped design improves the alignment of the mask over the glottic opening and better accommodates a special soft-tipped tracheal tube for blind intubation (see Fig. 29.10). The Air-Q LMA includes an ETT ramp that helps facilitate passage of the ETT anteriorly into the trachea. The successful use of the intubating LMA during a failed intubation at emergency cesarean delivery has been reported.[169]

Laryngeal Mask Airway and Cricoid Pressure

With the possible exception of the ProSeal, an LMA does not protect against pulmonary aspiration of gastric contents, and its placement may precipitate regurgitation in a lightly anesthetized patient.[170] Therefore, it is generally recommended that continuous cricoid pressure be maintained after the placement of an LMA in obstetric patients. Although a correctly placed LMA does not appear to compromise the effectiveness of cricoid pressure,[171] the use of cricoid pressure can inhibit proper insertion of the LMA and, in some cases, may make correct insertion impossible (Fig. 29.17).[172–175] The application of cricoid pressure can prevent the tip of the LMA from fully occupying the hypopharynx behind the arytenoid and cricoid cartilages. Therefore, if difficulty with insertion of an LMA is encountered during an obstetric airway emergency, consideration should be given to releasing cricoid pressure temporarily while a second insertion attempt is made.[174] The risk for hypoxemia after failed LMA placement is most likely greater than the small risk for aspiration due to the temporary release of cricoid pressure. Once the LMA is in place, cricoid pressure can be reapplied.[171] However, in

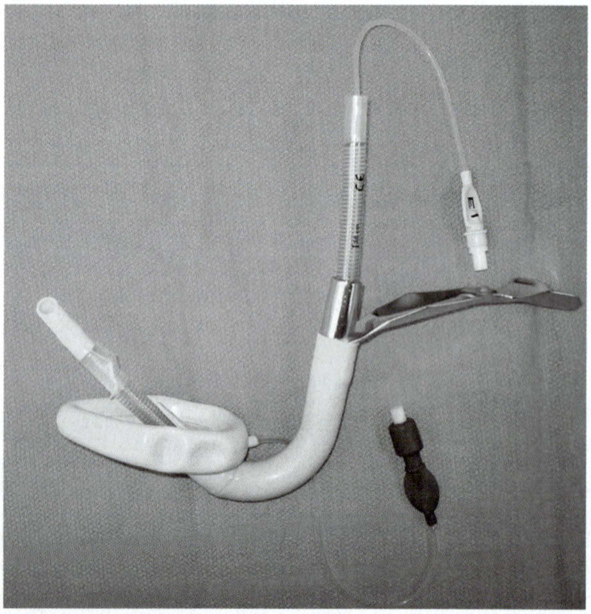

Fig. 29.16 Intubating Laryngeal Mask Airway (LMA). This device features a more rigid J-shaped design than the conventional LMA to facilitate the alignment of the mask over the glottic opening and better accommodate a special soft-tipped tracheal tube for blind intubation (see Fig. 29.10).

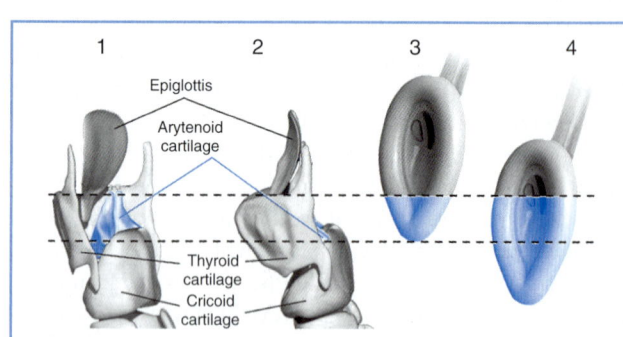

Fig. 29.17 The Position of the Laryngeal Mask Airway (LMA) With and Without Cricoid Pressure. The blue-shaded area indicates the distal part of the LMA that occupies the hypopharynx. The dashed lines indicate anatomic correlation. *1*, Posterior view of the larynx. *2*, Lateral view of the larynx. *3*, Position of the tip of the LMA when cricoid pressure is applied. When cricoid pressure is applied before placement, the LMA, in theory, might be wedged in the hypopharynx but is more likely to occupy the space behind the arytenoid cartilages. The LMA is positioned at least 2 cm more proximal than usual. *4*, Position of the LMA when no cricoid pressure is applied. When the LMA is placed correctly, the distal tip is at the distal end of C5 (fifth cervical vertebra), and the distal part of the LMA should fully occupy the hypopharynx and the pharyngeal space behind both the arytenoid and cricoid cartilages. Illustration by Naveen Nathan, MD, NorthShore University HealthSystem, University of Chicago Pritzker School of Medicine.

some patients, reapplication of cricoid pressure may decrease tidal volumes during positive-pressure ventilation through an LMA.[176] In such cases, a reduction in cricoid pressure typically allows adequate ventilation.

Laryngeal Mask Airway as a Conduit for Intubation

Intubation through an LMA can be achieved blindly, especially with an intubating LMA, or with the assistance of a fiberoptic bronchoscope. While passage of an ETT without visualization has a low success rate,[177] fiberoptic-guided intubation through the LMA has a success rate that has approached 100% in some studies.[156] Before starting this maneuver, the risks and benefits of an intubation attempt must be weighed.[178] Intubation attempts should never supersede or compromise active ventilation; furthermore, many emergency cesarean deliveries have relatively quick operating times and intubation may not be a priority if ventilation is satisfactorily achieved via an LMA. However, in certain situations, such as a patient at significant risk for aspiration, if ventilation is marginal, or in the setting of postpartum hemorrhage or critical illness, securing the airway with an ETT may take precedence. The use of a fiberoptic bronchoscope through an LMA has been reported to be nearly 100% successful in achieving intubation.[178] A 6-mm ID, cuffed ETT may be passed over the fiberoptic bronchoscope and through the shaft of a size 3 or 4 classic or intubating LMA; of note, a nasal right-angle endotracheal tube (Nellcor, Boulder, CO) is a suitable match for this purpose, owing to its adequate length and widespread availability.[179] A 7-mm ID, cuffed ETT may be passed in a similar manner through the shaft of a size 5 classic or intubating LMA.

When a fiberoptic bronchoscope is passed through an LMA, the bronchoscope should be introduced through the self-sealing diaphragm of an elbow adapter attached to the ETT and the airway circuit to allow continuous ventilation. Alternatively, a two-stage method can be employed, in which a fiberoptic bronchoscope is placed through the lumen of an Aintree Intubation Catheter (Cook Critical Care, Bloomington, IN) and the stem of a size 3 or 4 LMA. With the LMA in the oropharynx, the fiberoptic bronchoscope and Aintree Catheter are advanced through the vocal cords, the fiberoptic bronchoscope withdrawn, and then an ETT is guided over the Aintree Catheter.[180] There are no studies assessing the success rate of these advanced techniques that use the LMA as a conduit for tracheal intubation; however, these techniques take time and skill and should be performed by anesthesia providers experienced in their use.

Laryngeal Tube and Esophageal-Tracheal Combitube

The laryngeal tube (VBM Medizintechnik GmbH, Sulz, Germany) is another SGA device that has ventilation apertures between a proximal oropharyngeal cuff and a distal esophageal cuff.[181,182] The laryngeal tube is inserted into the oropharynx until resistance is met, which should result in positioning of the ventilation apertures directly above the glottic opening.

These devices are reported to provide seal pressures similar to those with the ProSeal LMA (40 cm H_2O) and insertion times and success rates comparable to those of the LMA.[183] The Laryngeal Tube-S (LTS) contains a second lumen that can be used for drainage of the stomach.[184] The LTS has been used successfully after a failed intubation and ventilation in a patient undergoing emergency cesarean delivery.[185]

The esophageal-tracheal combitube (ETC; Sheridan Catheter Corporation, Argyle, NY) has two lumens, one with an open distal end resembling a tracheal tube (i.e., the tracheal lumen), and the other with a closed distal end (i.e., the esophageal lumen). When the ETC is correctly positioned, a 100-mL pharyngeal balloon fills the space between the tongue base and soft palate, sealing the oral and nasal cavities. The ETC can be inserted with or without the aid of a laryngoscope, and its insertion does not require visualization of the larynx. The ETC enters the esophagus 96% of the time, allowing ventilation through perforations in the esophageal lumen.[186] If the ETC enters the trachea, the patient's lungs can be ventilated directly through the tracheal lumen. Therefore, regardless of whether the distal end of the ETC enters the trachea or esophagus, the anesthesia provider can ventilate the lungs, assuming correct identification of which lumen should be used for ventilation.

The ETC can allow adequate ventilation while preventing aspiration of gastric contents. If the distal end of the ETC enters the esophagus, the ETC can assist in removing gastric fluids through suction applied to the "tracheal" lumen. However, when long-term ventilation is anticipated or required, the ETC should be exchanged for an ETT. Of note, the stiffness and anterior curvature of the ETC, along with the potential for balloon overinflation, represent potential sources of airway and esophageal injury.[187]

Cannula and Surgical Cricothyrotomy

The anesthesia provider must promptly diagnose the failure of oxygenation and ventilation with conventional airway devices and decide that direct tracheal access is necessary. A delay in performing cricothyrotomy results in greater morbidity and mortality than complications resulting from the attempt.[50,188] Several techniques for cricothyrotomy are available, including narrow-bore cricothyrotomy (using a purpose-designed cannula less than 2-mm ID), wide-bore cricothyrotomy (using a purposed-designed cannula greater than 4-mm ID), and surgical cricothyrotomy (using a small, less than 6-mm ID, standard tracheal or tracheostomy tube).[189]

Narrow-bore cannula cricothyrotomy requires the use of a high-pressure ventilation source (e.g., Manujet) for transtracheal jet ventilation (TTJV). A patent upper airway and minimum pressure of 20 to 30 psi is required in most patients to inflate the chest and provide appropriate tidal volumes and minute ventilation.[190] During TTJV, it is critical that the operator allow time for exhalation of inspired gas to avoid hyperinflation of the lungs, potential air trapping, and barotrauma.[191-193] Exhalation can be facilitated by keeping the airway patent by some means (e.g., nasal/oral airway, jaw thrust, LMA). There are numerous reports of the use of TTJV as a means to prevent hypoxemia during life-threatening airway emergencies[193-195] and as a temporizing measure before a more definitive surgical airway can be established.

Although cannula cricothyrotomy is faster, its success rate is lower than that of surgical cricothyrotomy.[87,189] As highlighted by Preston,[155] the anesthesia provider should evaluate and practice various airway techniques to maximize success during an emergency. The role of ultrasound in locating the cricothyroid membrane has recently received attention[196]; further research is required to assess its benefit in emergency front-of-neck access.

EXTUBATION OF THE PATIENT WITH A DIFFICULT AIRWAY

General Principles

Tracheal extubation is a critical step during emergence from general anesthesia, and the airway condition at the time of tracheal extubation may be less favorable than at induction of anesthesia. The patient's disease process (e.g., preeclampsia) may contribute to worsening airway edema, as do fluid and blood products that have been administered during the procedure. Comorbidities, such as obesity and obstructive sleep apnea, may contribute to an increased risk for airway compromise after extubation of the trachea. Although the majority of extubations occur without incident, a number of serious adverse events, including hypoxic brain injury, can occur during emergence from general anesthesia and tracheal extubation or in the postoperative period.[52,197]

After publication of the first ASA guidelines for management of the difficult airway in 1993, a statistically significant reduction in airway claims arising from injury at *induction* of anesthesia was observed.[198] However, the number of claims arising from intraoperative events and those at extubation and during recovery did not change. Death and brain injury occurred more commonly after extubation and during recovery than during induction of anesthesia.[198] Not surprisingly, extubation complications are more common in obese patients and in those with obstructive sleep apnea.[198] In the fourth National Audit Project of the Royal College of Anaesthetists and DAS, major airway complications in patients receiving anesthesia occurred during emergence or recovery in approximately one-third of the reported cases.[87]

Extubation is an elective procedure that should always have a management strategy.[199-201] The goals of extubation management are to ensure uninterrupted oxygen delivery, to avoid airway stimulation, and to allow ventilation and possibly reintubation with minimum difficulty and delay should extubation fail. Importantly, obstetric patients are at risk for extubation complications, given their risk for pulmonary aspiration.[11] A crucial decision is to determine whether it is safe to extubate the trachea or to postpone the extubation. If the surgical procedure was long, or massive bleeding and significant fluid replacement has occurred, consideration should be given to transferring the patient to the intensive care unit and delaying tracheal extubation. The decision to remove the ETT should follow a full assessment of the patient (i.e., ability to follow commands, appropriate level of consciousness, recovery from neuromuscular blockade). The head of the bed can be elevated during emergence.

KEY POINTS

- Morbidity and mortality associated with airway management are key concerns for obstetric anesthesia providers.
- Difficulties with airway management occur with both intubation and extubation of the trachea.
- Physiologic and anatomic changes of pregnancy—such as airway edema, respiratory and metabolic changes, weight gain, breast enlargement, and the risk for gastroesophageal reflux—contribute to difficult airway management.
- All parturients receiving either general or neuraxial anesthesia must undergo airway assessment; plans should be devised for airway management.
- Airway difficulty is best predicted using a combination of assessments, including Mallampati class, thyromental distance, atlanto-occipital extension, and protrusion of the mandible.
- Early administration of neuraxial labor analgesia is recommended for laboring parturients with an anticipated difficult airway.
- Antacid prophylaxis should be given to all parturients who require general or neuraxial anesthesia.

- Correct positioning of the parturient on the operating table is necessary to maximize the chance of successful tracheal intubation, especially in the obese parturient.
- Securing the airway before inducing general anesthesia may be the safest option in patients in whom airway management is expected to be difficult.
- Maintenance of maternal and fetal oxygenation is the primary objective in the management of an unanticipated difficult airway.
- If conventional mask ventilation is difficult or impossible, a supraglottic airway (e.g., laryngeal mask airway) is the rescue device of choice.
- Needle cricothyrotomy with transtracheal jet ventilation can be life sustaining when other means to achieve adequate oxygenation have failed.
- In parturients known to be difficult to intubate or with risk factors for a difficult airway, caution must be employed with both intubation and extubation of the trachea.
- Potential or actual airway difficulties should be discussed with obstetricians, and management decisions should incorporate multidisciplinary communication and cooperation.

REFERENCES

1. Apfelbaum JL, Hagberg CA, Connis RT, et al. 2022 American Society of Anesthesiologists practice guidelines for management of the difficult airway. *Anesthesiology*. 2022;136:31–81.

2. Langeron O, Masso E, Huraux C, et al. Prediction of difficult mask ventilation. *Anesthesiology*. 2000;92:1229–1236.

3. Kheterpal S, Martin L, Shanks AM, Tremper KK. Prediction and outcomes of impossible mask ventilation: a review of 50,000 anesthetics. *Anesthesiology*. 2009;110:891–897.

4. Pearce A. Evaluation of the airway and preparation for difficulty. *Best Pract Res Clin Anaesthesiol*. 2005;19:559–579.

5. Verghese C, Brimacombe JR. Survey of laryngeal mask airway usage in 11,910 patients: safety and efficacy for conventional and nonconventional usage. *Anesth Analg*. 1996;82:129–133.

6. Kinsella SM, Winton AL, Mushambi MC, et al. Failed tracheal intubation during obstetric general anaesthesia: a literature review. *Int J Obstet Anesth*. 2015;24:356–374.

7. Reale SC, Bauer ME, Klumpner TT, et al. Frequency and risk factors for difficult intubation in women undergoing general anesthesia for cesarean delivery: a multicenter retrospective cohort analysis. *Anesthesiology*. 2022;136:697–708.

8. Knight M, Nair M, Tuffnell D, et al. Saving Lives, Improving Mother's Care: Surveillance of Maternal Deaths in the UK 2012-14 and Lessons Learned to Inform Maternity Care From the UK and Ireland Confidential Enquiries into Maternal Deaths and Morbidity 2009-14. 2016. Available at https://www.npeu.ox.ac.uk/assets/downloads/mbrrace-uk/reports/MBRRACE-UK%20Maternal%20Report%202016%20-%20website.pdf. Accessed 15 July 2024.

9. Hawkins JL, Chang J, Palmer SK, et al. Anesthesia-related maternal mortality in the United States: 1979-2002. *Obstet Gynecol*. 2011;117:69–74.

10. Mushambi MC, Kinsella SM, Popat M, et al. Obstetric Anaesthetists' Association and Difficult Airway Society guidelines for the management of difficult and failed tracheal intubation in obstetrics. *Anaesthesia*. 2015;70:1286–1306.

11. Popat M, Mitchell V, Dravid R, et al. Difficult airway society guidelines for the management of tracheal extubation. *Anaesthesia*. 2012;67:318–340.

12. Lyons G. Failed intubation. Six years' experience in a teaching maternity unit. *Anaesthesia*. 1985;40:759–762.

13. Rocke DA, Murray WB, Rout CC, Gouws E. Relative risk analysis of factors associated with difficult intubation in obstetric anesthesia. *Anesthesiology*. 1992;77:67–73.

14. Saravanakumar K, Rao SG, Cooper GM. Obesity and obstetric anaesthesia. *Anaesthesia*. 2006;61:36–48.

15. Djabatey EA, Barclay PM. Difficult and failed intubation in 3430 obstetric general anaesthetics. *Anaesthesia*. 2009;64:1168–1171.

16. McKeen DM, George RB, O'Connell CM, et al. Difficult and failed intubation: incident rates and maternal, obstetrical, and anesthetic predictors. *Can J Anaesth*. 2011;58:514–524.

17. Samsoon GL, Young JR. Difficult tracheal intubation: a retrospective study. *Anaesthesia*. 1987;42:487–490.

18. Hawthorne L, Wilson R, Lyons G, Dresner M. Failed intubation revisited: 17-yr experience in a teaching maternity unit. *Br J Anaesth*. 1996;76:680–684.

19. Barnardo PD, Jenkins JG. Failed tracheal intubation in obstetrics: a 6-year review in a UK region. *Anaesthesia*. 2000;55:690–694.

20. Rahman K, Jenkins JG. Failed tracheal intubation in obstetrics: no more frequent but still managed badly. *Anaesthesia*. 2005;60:168–171.

21. McDonnell NJ, Paech MJ, Clavisi OM, Scott KL. Difficult and failed intubation in obstetric anaesthesia: an observational study of airway management and complications associated with general anaesthesia for caesarean section. *Int J Obstet Anesth*. 2008;17:292–297.

22. Quinn AC, Milne D, Columb M, et al. Failed tracheal intubation in obstetric anaesthesia: 2 yr national case-control study in the UK. *Br J Anaesth*. 2013;110:74–80.

23. Bullough AS, Carraretto M. A United Kingdom national obstetric intubation equipment survey. *Int J Obstet Anesth*. 2009;18:342–345.

24. D'Angelo R, Smiley RM, Riley ET, Segal S. Serious complications related to obstetric anesthesia: the serious complication repository project of the society for obstetric anesthesia and perinatology. *Anesthesiology*. 2014;120:1505–1512.

25. Palanisamy A, Mitani AA, Tsen LC. General anesthesia for cesarean delivery at a tertiary care hospital from 2000 to 2005: a retrospective analysis and 10-year update. *Int J Obstet Anesth*. 2011;20:10–16.

26. Haslam N, Parker L, Duggan JE. Effect of cricoid pressure on the view at laryngoscopy. *Anaesthesia*. 2005;60:41–47.

27. Tsen LC, Pitner R, Camann WR. General anesthesia for cesarean section at a tertiary care hospital 1990-1995: indications and implications. *Int J Obstet Anesth*. 1998;7:147–152.

28. Searle RD, Lyons G. Vanishing experience in training for obstetric general anaesthesia: an observational study. *Int J Obstet Anesth*. 2008;17:233–237.

29. Panni MK, Camann WR, Tsen LC. Resident training in obstetric anesthesia in the United States. *Int J Obstet Anesth*. 2006;15:284–289.

30. Dresner M, Brocklesby J, Bamber J. Audit of the influence of body mass index on the performance of epidural analgesia in labour and the subsequent mode of delivery. *BJOG*. 2006;113:1178–1181.

31. Tonidandel A, Booth J, D'Angelo R, et al. Anesthetic and obstetric outcomes in morbidly obese parturients: a 20-year follow-up retrospective cohort study. *Int J Obstet Anesth*. 2014;23:357–364.

32. Jense HG, Dubin SA, Silverstein PI, O'Leary-Escolas U. Effect of obesity on safe duration of apnea in anesthetized humans. *Anesth Analg*. 1991;72:89–93.

33. McClelland SH, Bogod DG, Hardman JG. Pre-oxygenation and apnoea in pregnancy: changes during labour and with obstetric morbidity in a computational simulation. *Anaesthesia*. 2009;64:371–377.

34. Pratt SD. Focused review: Simulation in obstetric anesthesia. *Anesth Analg*. 2012;114:186–190.

35. Carvalho B, Mhyre JM. Centers of Excellence for anesthesia care of obstetric patients. *Anesth Analg*. 2019;128:844–846.

36. Purva M, Kinsella M. Caesarean section anaesthesia: technique and failure rate. In: Lucas N, ed. *Raising the Standards: RCoA Quality Improvement Compendium*. 4th ed. Royal College of Anaesthetists; 2020.

37. Guglielminotti J, Landau R, Li G. Adverse events and factors associated with potentially avoidable use of general anesthesia in cesarean deliveries. *Anesthesiology*. 2019;130:912–922.

38. Bauer ME, Mhyre JM. Active management of labor epidural analgesia Is the key to successful conversion of epidural analgesia to cesarean delivery anesthesia. *Anesth Analg.* 2016;123:1074–1076.

39. Ikeda T, Kato A, Bougaki M, et al. A retrospective review of 10-year trends in general anesthesia for cesarean delivery at a university hospital: the impact of a newly launched team on obstetric anesthesia practice. *BMC Health Serv Res.* 2020;20:421.

40. Riley ET, Papasin J. Epidural catheter function during labor predicts anesthetic efficacy for subsequent cesarean delivery. *Int J Obstet Anesth.* 2002;11:81–84.

41. Bauer ME, Kountanis JA, Tsen LC, et al. Risk factors for failed conversion of labor epidural analgesia to cesarean delivery anesthesia: a systematic review and meta-analysis of observational trials. *Int J Obstet Anesth.* 2012;21:294–309.

42. Cobb BT, Lane-Fall MB, Month RC, et al. Anesthesiologist specialization and use of general anesthesia for cesarean delivery. *Anesthesiology.* 2019;130:237–246.

43. Ende HB, Tran B, Thampy M, et al. Standardization of epidural top-ups for breakthrough labor pain results in a higher proportion of catheter replacements within 30 min of the first bolus dose. *Int J Obstet Anesth.* 2021;47:103161.

44. Hillyard SG, Bate TE, Corcoran TB, et al. Extending epidural analgesia for emergency caesarean section: a meta-analysis. *Br J Anaesth.* 2011;107:668–678.

45. Sharawi N, Bansal P, Williams M, et al. Comparison of chloroprocaine versus lidocaine with epinephrine, sodium bicarbonate, and fentanyl for epidural extension anesthesia in elective cesarean delivery: a randomized, triple-blind, noninferiority study. *Anesth Analg.* 2021;132:666–675.

46. Hawkins JL, Koonin LM, Palmer SK, Gibbs CP. Anesthesia-related deaths during obstetric delivery in the United States, 1979-1990. *Anesthesiology.* 1997;86:277–284.

47. Schroeder RA, Pollard R, Dhakal I, et al. Temporal trends in difficult and failed tracheal intubation in a regional community anesthetic practice. *Anesthesiology.* 2018;128: 502–510.

48. Knight M, Kenyon S, Brocklehurst P, et al. *Saving Lives, Improving Mother's Care – Lessons Learned to Inform Future Maternity Care From the UK and Ireland Confidential Enquiries Into Maternal Deaths and Morbidity 2009-12.* https://www.npeu.ox.ac.uk/assets/downloads/mbrrace-uk/reports/Saving%20Lives%20Improving%20Mothers%20Care%20report%202014%20Full.pdf. Accessed 14 July 2024.

49. Creanga AA, Syverson C, Seed K, Callaghan WM. Pregnancy-related mortality in the United States, 2011-2013. *Obstet Gynecol.* 2017;130:366–373.

50. Cook TM, McCrirrick A. A survey of airway management during induction of general anaesthesia in obstetrics: are the recommendations in the confidential enquiries into maternal deaths being implemented? *Int J Obstet Anesth.* 1994;3:143–145.

51. Kovacheva VP, Brovman EY, Greenberg P, et al. A contemporary analysis of medicolegal issues in obstetric anesthesia between 2005 and 2015. *Anesth Analg.* 2019;128:1199–1207.

52. Mhyre JM, Riesner MN, Polley LS, Naughton NN. A series of anesthesia-related maternal deaths in Michigan, 1985-2003. *Anesthesiology.* 2007;106:1096–1104.

53. Izci B, Riha RL, Martin SE, et al. The upper airway in pregnancy and pre-eclampsia. *Am J Respir Crit Care Med.* 2003;167:137–140.

54. Mallampati SR, Gatt SP, Gugino LD, et al. A clinical sign to predict difficult tracheal intubation: a prospective study. *Can Anaesth Soc J.* 1985;32:429–434.

55. Pilkington S, Carli F, Dakin MJ, et al. Increase in mallampati score during pregnancy. *Br J Anaesth.* 1995;74:638–642.

56. Kodali BS, Chandrasekhar S, Bulich LN, et al. Airway changes during labor and delivery. *Anesthesiology.* 2008;108:357–362.

57. Boutonnet M, Faitot V, Katz A, et al. Mallampati class changes during pregnancy, labour, and after delivery: can these be predicted? *Br J Anaesth.* 2010;104:67–70.

58. Jouppila R, Jouppila P, Hollmen A. Laryngeal oedema as an obstetric anaesthesia complication: case reports. *Acta Anaesthesiol Scand.* 1980;24:97–98.

59. Arendt KW, Khan K, Curry TB, Tsen LC. Topical vasoconstrictor use for nasal intubation during pregnancy complicated by cardiomyopathy and preeclampsia. *Int J Obstet Anesth.* 2011;20:246–249.

60. Russell IF, Chambers WA. Closing volume in normal pregnancy. *Br J Anaesth.* 1981;53:1043–1047.

61. Archer GW Jr, Marx GF. Arterial oxygen tension during apnoea in parturient women. *Br J Anaesth.* 1974;46:358–360.

62. Benumof JL, Dagg R, Benumof R. Critical hemoglobin desaturation will occur before return to an unparalyzed state following 1 mg/kg intravenous succinylcholine. *Anesthesiology.* 1997;87:979–982.

63. McClelland SH, Bogod DG, Hardman JG. Apnoea in pregnancy: an investigation using physiological modelling. *Anaesthesia.* 2008;63:264–269.

64. Naguib M, Brewer L, LaPierre C, et al. The myth of rescue reversal in "can't intubate, can't ventilate" scenarios. *Anesth Analg.* 2016;123:82–92.

65. Yentis SM. Predicting difficult intubation – worthwhile exercise or pointless ritual? *Anaesthesia.* 2002;57:105–109.

66. Cormack RS, Lehane J. Difficult tracheal intubation in obstetrics. *Anaesthesia.* 1984;39:1105–1111.

67. Yentis SM, Lee DJ. Evaluation of an improved scoring system for the grading of direct laryngoscopy. *Anaesthesia.* 1998;53:1041–1044.

68. Rutter JM, Murphy PG. Cormack and Lehane revisited. *Anaesthesia.* 1997;52:927.

69. Cook TM, Nolan JP, Gabbott DA. Cricoid pressure–are two hands better than one? *Anaesthesia.* 1997;52:179–180.

70. Shiga T, Wajima Z, Inoue T, Sakamoto A. Predicting difficult intubation in apparently normal patients: a meta-analysis of bedside screening test performance. *Anesthesiology.* 2005;103:429–437.

71. Lee A, Fan LT, Gin T, et al. A systematic review (meta-analysis) of the accuracy of the Mallampati tests to predict the difficult airway. *Anesth Analg.* 2006;102:1867–1878.

72. Bellhouse CP, Dore C. Criteria for estimating likelihood of difficulty of endotracheal intubation with the Macintosh laryngoscope. *Anaesth Intensive Care.* 1988;16:329–337.

73. Calder I, Calder J, Crockard HA. Difficult direct laryngoscopy in patients with cervical spine disease. *Anaesthesia.* 1995;50:756–763.

74. Munnur U, de Boisblanc B, Suresh MS. Airway problems in pregnancy. *Crit Care Med.* 2005;33:S259–S268.

75. Khan ZH, Mohammadi M, Rasouli MR, et al. The diagnostic value of the upper lip bite test combined with sternomental distance, thyromental distance, and interincisor distance for prediction of easy laryngoscopy and intubation: a prospective study. *Anesth Analg.* 2009;109:822–824.

76. Rose DK, Cohen MM. The airway: problems and predictions in 18,500 patients. *Can J Anaesth*. 1994;41:372–383.

77. Calder I, Picard J, Chapman M, et al. Mouth opening: a new angle. *Anesthesiology*. 2003;99:799–801.

78. Honarmand A, Safavi MR. Prediction of difficult laryngoscopy in obstetric patients scheduled for caesarean delivery. *Eur J Anaesthesiol*. 2008;25:714–720.

79. Morgan BM, Magni V, Goroszenuik T. Anaesthesia for emergency caesarean section. *Br J Obstet Gynaecol*. 1990;97:420–424.

80. Juvin P, Lavaut E, Dupont H, et al. Difficult tracheal intubation is more common in obese than in lean patients. *Anesth Analg*. 2003;97:595–600.

81. You-Ten KE, Desai D, Postonogova T, Siddiqui N. Accuracy of conventional digital palpation and ultrasound of the cricothyroid membrane in obese women in labour. *Anaesthesia*. 2015;70:1230–1234.

82. American College of Obstetricians and Gynecologists. ACOG Committee Opinion No. 766: Approaches to limit intervention during labor and birth (reaffirmed 2021). *Obstet Gynecol*. 2019;133:e164–e173.

83. American College of Obstetricians and Gynecologists. Committee Opinion No. 441: Oral intake during labor (reaffirmed 2017). *Obstet Gynecol*. 2009;114:714.

84. American Society of Anesthesiologists. Practice guidelines for obstetric anesthesia: an updated report by the American Society of Anesthesiologists Task Force on Obstetric Anesthesia and the Society for Obstetric Anesthesia and Perinatology. *Anesthesiology*. 2016;124:270–300.

85. National Institute for Health and Clinical Excellence. Clinical guideline [CG190]. Intrapartum care: Care of healthy women and their babies during childbirth. 2014. Updated February 2017. https://www.nice.org.uk/guidance/cg190. Accessed 15 July 2024.

86. O'Sullivan GM, Bullingham RE. The assessment of gastric acidity and antacid effect in pregnant women by a non-invasive radiotelemetry technique. *Br J Obstet Gynaecol*. 1984;91:973–978.

87. Cook TM, Woodall N, Frerk C, 4th National Audit Project *Major Complications of Airway Management in the UK*. 2011. Available at https://www.rcoa.ac.uk/research/research-projects/national-audit-projects-naps/nap4-major-complications-airway-management. Accessed 15 July 2024.

88. El-Orbany M, Woehlck H, Salem MR. Head and neck position for direct laryngoscopy. *Anesth Analg*. 2011;113:103–109.

89. Dixon BJ, Dixon JB, Carden JR, et al. Preoxygenation is more effective in the 25 degrees head-up position than in the supine position in severely obese patients: a randomized controlled study. *Anesthesiology*. 2005;102:1110–1115.

90. Hignett R, Fernando R, McGlennan A, et al. A randomized crossover study to determine the effect of a 30 degrees head-up versus a supine position on the functional residual capacity of term parturients. *Anesth Analg*. 2011;113:1098–1102.

91. Porter R, Wrench IJ, Freeman R. Preoxygenation for general anaesthesia in pregnancy: is it adequate? *Int J Obstet Anesth*. 2011;20:363–365.

92. Chiron B, Laffon M, Ferrandiere M, et al. Standard preoxygenation technique versus two rapid techniques in pregnant patients. *Int J Obstet Anesth*. 2004;13:11–14.

93. Russell EC, Wrench I, Feast M, Mohammed F. Pre-oxygenation in pregnancy: the effect of fresh gas flow rates within a circle breathing system. *Anaesthesia*. 2008;63:833–836.

94. Patel A, Nouraei SA. Transnasal humidified rapid-insufflation ventilatory exchange (THRIVE): a physiological method of increasing apnoea time in patients with difficult airways. *Anaesthesia*. 2015;70:323–329.

95. Mir F, Patel A, Iqbal R, et al. A randomised controlled trial comparing transnasal humidified rapid insufflation ventilatory exchange (THRIVE) pre-oxygenation with face mask pre-oxygenation in patients undergoing rapid sequence induction of anaesthesia. *Anaesthesia*. 2017;72: 439–443.

96. Pillai A, Chikhani M, Hardman JG. Apnoeic oxygenation in pregnancy: a modelling investigation. *Anaesthesia*. 2016;71:1077–1080.

97. Tan PCF, Millay OJ, Leeton L, Dennis AT. High-flow humidified nasal preoxygenation in pregnant women: a prospective observational study. *Br J Anaesth*. 2019;122:86–91.

98. El-Orbany M, Connolly LA. Rapid sequence induction and intubation: current controversy. *Anesth Analg*. 2010;110: 1318–1325.

99. Ngan Kee WD, Khaw KS, Ma KC, et al. Maternal and neonatal effects of remifentanil at induction of general anesthesia for cesarean delivery: a randomized, double-blind, controlled trial. *Anesthesiology*. 2006;104:14–20.

100. Blitt CD, Petty WC, Alberternst EE, Wright BJ. Correlation of plasma cholinesterase activity and duration of action of succinylcholine during pregnancy. *Anesth Analg*. 1977;56:78–83.

101. Donati F. The right dose of succinylcholine. *Anesthesiology*. 2003;99:1037–1038.

102. Naguib M, Samarkandi AH, El-Din ME, et al. The dose of succinylcholine required for excellent endotracheal intubating conditions. *Anesth Analg*. 2006;102:151–155.

103. Lemmens HJ, Brodsky JB. The dose of succinylcholine in morbid obesity. *Anesth Analg*. 2006;102:438–442.

104. Naguib M, Samarkandi A, Riad W, Alharby SW. Optimal dose of succinylcholine revisited. *Anesthesiology*. 2003;99:1045–1049.

105. Stourac P, Adamus M, Seidlova D, et al. Low-dose or high-dose rocuronium reversed with neostigmine or sugammadex for cesarean delivery anesthesia: a randomized controlled noninferiority trial of time to tracheal intubation and extubation. *Anesth Analg*. 2016;122:1536–1545.

106. Tran DT, Newton EK, Mount VA, et al. Rocuronium versus succinylcholine for rapid sequence induction intubation. *Cochrane Database Syst Rev*. 2015;(10):CD002788.

107. Fenton PM, Reynolds F. Life-saving or ineffective? An observational study of the use of cricoid pressure and maternal outcome in an African setting. *Int J Obstet Anesth*. 2009;18:106–110.

108. Paech MJ. Pregnant women having caesarean delivery under general anaesthesia should have a rapid sequence induction with cricoid pressure and be intubated." Can this 'holy cow' be sent packing? *Anaesth Intensive Care*. 2010;38:989–991.

109. Ball Mac GPJH. DR. The effect of cricoid pressure on the cricoid cartilage and vocal cords: an endoscopic study in anaesthetised patients. *Anaesthesia*. 2000;55:263–268.

110. Hartsilver EL, Vanner RG. Airway obstruction with cricoid pressure. *Anaesthesia*. 2000;55:208–211.

111. Sellick BA. Cricoid pressure to control regurgitation of stomach contents during induction of anaesthesia. *Lancet*. 1961;2:404–406.

112. Yentis SM. The effects of single-handed and bimanual cricoid pressure on the view at laryngoscopy. *Anaesthesia*. 1997;52:332–335.

113. Popat M, Russell R. Awake fibreoptic intubation following previous failed intubation. *Int J Obstet Anesth.* 2001;10:332–333.

114. Ovassapian A. Fiberoptic tracheal intubation in adults. In: Ovassapian A, ed. *Fiberoptic Endoscopy and the Difficult Airway.* 2nd ed. Lippincott-Raven; 1996:72–103.

115. Watanabe H, Lindgren L, Rosenberg P, Randell T. Glycopyrronium prolongs topical anaesthesia of oral mucosa and enhances absorption of lignocaine. *Br J Anaesth.* 1993;70:94–95.

116. American Society of Anesthesiologists. Continuum of depth of sedation: definition of general anesthesia and levels of sedation/analgesia. 2019. Available at https://www.asahq.org/standards-and-practice-parameters/statement-on-continuum-of-depth-of-sedation-definition-of-general-anesthesia-and-levels-of-sedation-analgesia. Accessed 15 July 2024.

117. Benumof JL. Management of the difficult airway. *Ann Acad Med Singapore.* 1994;23:589–591.

118. Popat MT, Chippa JH, Russell R. Awake fibreoptic intubation following failed regional anaesthesia for caesarean section in a parturient with Still's disease. *Eur J Anaesthesiol.* 2000;17:211–214.

119. Puchner W, Egger P, Puhringer F, et al. Evaluation of remifentanil as single drug for awake fiberoptic intubation. *Acta Anaesthesiol Scand.* 2002;46:350–354.

120. Rai MR, Parry TM, Dombrovskis A, Warner OJ. Remifentanil target-controlled infusion vs propofol target-controlled infusion for conscious sedation for awake fibreoptic intubation: a double-blinded randomized controlled trial. *Br J Anaesth.* 2008;100:125–130.

121. Shah TH, Badve MS, Olajide KO, et al. Dexmedetomidine for an awake fiber-optic intubation of a parturient with Klippel-Feil syndrome, Type I Arnold Chiari malformation and status post released tethered spinal cord presenting for repeat cesarean section. *Clin Pract.* 2011;1:e57.

122. Neumann MM, Davio MB, Macknet MR, Applegate RL 2nd. Dexmedetomidine for awake fiberoptic intubation in a parturient with spinal muscular atrophy type III for cesarean delivery. *Int J Obstet Anesth.* 2009;18:403–407.

123. Mackenzie I. A new method of drug application to the nasal passage. *Anaesthesia.* 1998;53:309–310.

124. Sitzman BT, Rich GF, Rockwell JJ, et al. Local anesthetic administration for awake direct laryngoscopy. Are glossopharyngeal nerve blocks superior? *Anesthesiology.* 1997;86:34–40.

125. Claeys DW, Lockhart CH, Hinkle JE. The effects of translaryngeal block and innovar on glottic competence. *Anesthesiology.* 1973;38:485–486.

126. Walts LF, Kassity KJ. Spread of local anesthesia after upper airway block. *Arch Otolaryngol.* 1965;81:77–79.

127. Ovassapian A, Krejcie TC, Yelich SJ, Dykes MH. Awake fibreoptic intubation in the patient at high risk of aspiration. *Br J Anaesth.* 1989;62:13–16.

128. Mahajan RP, Murty GE, Singh P, Aitkenhead AR. Effect of topical anaesthesia on the motor performance of vocal cords as assessed by tussometry. *Anaesthesia.* 1994;49:1028–1030.

129. Marfin AG, Iqbal R, Mihm F, et al. Determination of the site of tracheal tube impingement during nasotracheal fibreoptic intubation. *Anaesthesia.* 2006;61:646–650.

130. Asai T, Shingu K. Difficulty in advancing a tracheal tube over a fibreoptic bronchoscope: incidence, causes and solutions. *Br J Anaesth.* 2004;92:870–881.

131. Rai MR, Scott SH, Marfin AG, et al. A comparison of a flexometallic tracheal tube with the intubating laryngeal mask tracheal tube for nasotracheal fibreoptic intubation using the two-scope technique. *Anaesthesia.* 2009;64:1303–1306.

132. Asai T. Videolaryngoscopes: do they truly have roles in difficult airways? *Anesthesiology.* 2012;116:515–517.

133. Lewis SR, Butler AR, Parker J, et al. Videolaryngoscopy versus direct laryngoscopy for adult patients requiring tracheal intubation. *Cochrane Database Syst Rev.* 2016;(3):CD011136.

134. Scott-Brown S, Russell R. Video laryngoscopes and the obstetric airway. *Int J Obstet Anesth.* 2015;24:137–146.

135. Aziz MF, Dillman D, Fu R, Brambrink AM. Comparative effectiveness of the C-MAC video laryngoscope versus direct laryngoscopy in the setting of the predicted difficult airway. *Anesthesiology.* 2012;116:629–636.

136. Pham Q, Lentner M, Hu A. Soft palate injuries during orotracheal intubation with the videolaryngoscope. *Ann Otol Rhinol Laryngol.* 2017;126:132–137.

137. Greer D, Marshall KE, Bevans S, et al. Review of videolaryngoscopy pharyngeal wall injuries. *Laryngoscope.* 2017;127:349–353.

138. Ogino Y, Uchiyama K, Hasumi M, et al. [A pitfall of airway scope – an experience of distinctive airway edema after palatal laceration caused by airway scope]. *Masui.* 2008;57:1245–1248.

139. Teoh WH, Saxena S, Shah MK, Sia AT. Comparison of three videolaryngoscopes: pentax airway scope, C-MAC, Glidescope vs the macintosh laryngoscope for tracheal intubation. *Anaesthesia.* 2010;65:1126–1132.

140. Teoh WH, Shah MK, Sia AT. Randomised comparison of pentax airwayscope and glidescope for tracheal intubation in patients with normal airway anatomy. *Anaesthesia.* 2009;64:1125–1129.

141. Maassen R, Lee R, Hermans B, et al. A comparison of three videolaryngoscopes: the macintosh laryngoscope blade reduces, but does not replace, routine stylet use for intubation in morbidly obese patients. *Anesth Analg.* 2009;109:1560–1565.

142. Liu EH, Goy RW, Tan BH, Asai T. Tracheal intubation with videolaryngoscopes in patients with cervical spine immobilization: a randomized trial of the airway scope and the GlideScope. *Br J Anaesth.* 2009;103:446–451.

143. Malik MA, Maharaj CH, Harte BH, Laffey JG. Comparison of macintosh, Truview EVO2, Glidescope, and airwayscope laryngoscope use in patients with cervical spine immobilization. *Br J Anaesth.* 2008;101:723–730.

144. Arici S, Karaman S, Dogru S, et al. The McGrath series 5 video laryngoscope versus the macintosh laryngoscope: a randomized trial in obstetric patients. *Turk J Med Sci.* 2014;44:387–392.

145. Dhonneur G, Ndoko S, Amathieu R, et al. Tracheal intubation using the airtraq in morbid obese patients undergoing emergency cesarean delivery. *Anesthesiology.* 2007;106:629–630.

146. Aziz MF, Kim D, Mako J, et al. A retrospective study of the performance of video laryngoscopy in an obstetric unit. *Anesth Analg.* 2012;115:904–906.

147. Cook TM, Kelly FE. A national survey of videolaryngoscopy in the United Kingdom. *Br J Anaesth.* 2017;118:593–600.

148. Benumof JL. Management of the difficult adult airway. With special emphasis on awake tracheal intubation. *Anesthesiology.* 1991;75:1087–1110.

149. Cooper MG, Feeney EM, Joseph M, McGuinness JJ. Local anaesthetic infiltration for caesarean section. *Anaesth Intensive Care*. 1989;17:198–201.

150. Ranney B, Stanage WF. Advantages of local anesthesia for cesarean section. *Obstet Gynecol*. 1975;45:163–167.

151. Mei W, Jin C, Feng L, et al. Bilateral ultrasound-guided trans- versus abdominis plane block combined with ilioinguinal-iliohypogastric nerve block for cesarean delivery anesthesia. *Anesth Analg*. 2011;113:134–137.

152. Togioka BM, Zarnegarnia Y, Bleyle LA, et al. Pharmacokinetics and tolerability of intraperitoneal chloroprocaine after fetal extraction in women undergoing cesarean delivery. *Anesth Analg*. 2022;135:777–786.

153. Werntz M, Burwick R, Togioka B. Intraperitoneal chloroprocaine is a useful adjunct to neuraxial block during cesarean delivery: a case series. *Int J Obstet Anesth*. 2018;35:33–41.

154. Law JA, Broemling N, Cooper RM, et al. The difficult airway with recommendations for management – part 1 – difficult tracheal intubation encountered in an unconscious/induced patient. *Can J Anaesth*. 2013;60:1089–1118.

155. Preston R. Management of the obstetric airway – time for a paradigm shift (or two). *Int J Obstet Anesth*. 2015;24:293–296.

156. Benumof JL. Laryngeal mask airway and the ASA difficult airway algorithm. *Anesthesiology*. 1996;84:686–699.

157. Han TH, Brimacombe J, Lee EJ, Yang HS. The laryngeal mask airway is effective (and probably safe) in selected healthy parturients for elective cesarean section: a prospective study of 1067 cases. *Can J Anaesth*. 2001;48:1117–1121.

158. Brimacombe J, Keller C. The ProSeal laryngeal mask airway: a randomized, crossover study with the standard laryngeal mask airway in paralyzed, anesthetized patients. *Anesthesiology*. 2000;93:104–109.

159. Evans NR, Gardner SV, James MF. ProSeal laryngeal mask protects against aspiration of fluid in the pharynx. *Br J Anaesth*. 2002;88:584–587.

160. Keller C, Brimacombe J, Kleinsasser A, Loeckinger A. Does the ProSeal laryngeal mask airway prevent aspiration of regurgitated fluid? *Anesth Analg*. 2000;91:1017–1020.

161. Halaseh BK, Sukkar ZF, Hassan LH, et al. The use of ProSeal laryngeal mask airway in caesarean section – experience in 3000 cases. *Anaesth Intensive Care*. 2010;38:1023–1028.

162. Awan R, Nolan JP, Cook TM. Use of a ProSeal laryngeal mask airway for airway maintenance during emergency caesarean section after failed tracheal intubation. *Br J Anaesth*. 2004;92:144–146.

163. Keller C, Brimacombe J, Lirk P, Puhringer F. Failed obstetric tracheal intubation and postoperative respiratory support with the ProSeal laryngeal mask airway. *Anesth Analg*. 2004;98:1467–1470.

164. Sharma B, Sahai C, Sood J, Kumra VP. The ProSeal laryngeal mask airway in two failed obstetric tracheal intubation scenarios. *Int J Obstet Anesth*. 2006;15:338–339.

165. Brimacombe J, Keller C. Gum elastic bougie-guided insertion of the ProSeal laryngeal mask airway. *Anaesth Intensive Care*. 2004;32:681–684.

166. Nagata T, Kishi Y, Tanigami H, et al. Oral gastric tube-guided insertion of the ProSeal laryngeal mask is an easy and noninvasive method for less experienced users. *J Anesth*. 2012;26:531–535.

167. Yao WY, Li SY, Sng BL, et al. The LMA supreme in 700 parturients undergoing cesarean delivery: an observational study. *Can J Anaesth*. 2012;59:648–654.

168. Joo HS, Rose DK. The intubating laryngeal mask airway with and without fiberoptic guidance. *Anesth Analg*. 1999;88:662–666.

169. Minville V, N'Guyen L, Coustet B, et al. Difficult airway in obstetric using ILMA-Fastrach. *Anesth Analg*. 2004;99:1873.

170. Asai T, Appadurai I. LMA for failed intubation. *Can J Anaesth*. 1993;40:802.

171. Strang TI. Does the laryngeal mask airway compromise cricoid pressure? *Anaesthesia*. 1992;47:829–831.

172. Asai T, Barclay K, Power I, Vaughan RS. Cricoid pressure impedes placement of the laryngeal mask airway. *Br J Anaesth*. 1995;74:521–525.

173. Aoyama K, Takenaka I, Sata T, Shigematsu A. Cricoid pressure impedes positioning and ventilation through the laryngeal mask airway. *Can J Anaesth*. 1996;43:1035–1040.

174. Brimacombe J, White A, Berry A. Effect of cricoid pressure on ease of insertion of the laryngeal mask airway. *Br J Anaesth*. 1993;71:800–802.

175. Harry RM, Nolan JP. The use of cricoid pressure with the intubating laryngeal mask. *Anaesthesia*. 1999;54:656–659.

176. Asai T, Barclay K, McBeth C, Vaughan RS. Cricoid pressure applied after placement of the laryngeal mask prevents gastric insufflation but inhibits ventilation. *Br J Anaesth*. 1996;76:772–776.

177. Heath ML, Allagain J. Intubation through the laryngeal mask. A technique for unexpected difficult intubation. *Anaesthesia*. 1991;46:545–548.

178. Benumof JL. Laryngeal mask airway. Indications and contraindications. *Anesthesiology*. 1992;77:843–846.

179. Henderson JJ, Popat MT, Latto IP, Pearce AC. Difficult airway society guidelines for management of the unanticipated difficult intubation. *Anaesthesia*. 2004;59:675–694.

180. Atherton DP, O'Sullivan E, Lowe D, Charters P. A ventilation-exchange bougie for fibreoptic intubations with the laryngeal mask airway. *Anaesthesia*. 1996;51:1123–1126.

181. Asai T, Shingu K. The laryngeal tube. *Br J Anaesth*. 2005;95:729–736.

182. Agro F, Cataldo R, Alfano A, Galli B. A new prototype for airway management in an emergency: the laryngeal tube. *Resuscitation*. 1999;41:284–286.

183. Figueredo E, Martinez M, Pintanel T. A comparison of the ProSeal laryngeal mask and the laryngeal tube in spontaneously breathing anesthetized patients. *Anesth Analg*. 2003;96:600–605.

184. Genzwurker H, Finteis T, Hinkelbein J, Ellinger K. First clinical experiences with the new LTS. A laryngeal tube with an oesophageal drain. *Anaesthesist*. 2003;52:697–702.

185. Zand F, Amini A. Use of the laryngeal tube-S for airway management and prevention of aspiration after a failed tracheal intubation in a parturient. *Anesthesiology*. 2005;102:481–483.

186. Lefrancois DP, Dufour DG. Use of the esophageal tracheal combitube by basic emergency medical technicians. *Resuscitation*. 2002;52:77–83.

187. Vezina MC, Trepanier CA, Nicole PC, Lessard MR. Complications associated with the esophageal-tracheal combitube in the pre-hospital setting. *Can J Anaesth*. 2007;54:124–128.

188. Frerk C, Frampton C. Cricothyroidotomy; time for change. *Anaesthesia*. 2006;61:921–923.

189. Frerk C, Cook TM. Management of the "can't intubate can't ventilate" situation and the emergency surgical airway. Report on the findings of the 4th National Audit Project of the Royal College of Anaesthetists. In: Cook T, Woodall N, Frerk C, eds.

4th National Audit Project of the Royal College of Anaesthetists and the Difficult Airway Society. Major complications of airway management in the United Kingdom; 2011:105–113. http://www.rcoa.ac.uk/nap4/. Accessed 15 July 2024.

190. Benumof JL, Scheller MS. The importance of transtracheal jet ventilation in the management of the difficult airway. *Anesthesiology.* 1989;71:769–778.

191. Cook TM, Bigwood B, Cranshaw J. A complication of transtracheal jet ventilation and use of the aintree intubation catheter during airway resuscitation. *Anaesthesia.* 2006;61:692–697.

192. Craft TM, Chambers PH, Ward ME, Goat VA. Two cases of barotrauma associated with transtracheal jet ventilation. *Br J Anaesth.* 1990;64:524–527.

193. McLellan I, Gordon P, Khawaja S, Thomas A. Percutaneous transtracheal high frequency jet ventilation as an aid to difficult intubation. *Can J Anaesth.* 1988;35:404–405.

194. Chandradeva K, Palin C, Ghosh SM, Pinches SC. Percutaneous transtracheal jet ventilation as a guide to tracheal intubation in severe upper airway obstruction from supraglottic oedema. *Br J Anaesth.* 2005;94:683–686.

195. McHugh R, Kumar M, Sprung J, Bourke D. Transtracheal jet ventilation in management of the difficult airway. *Anaesth Intensive Care.* 2007;35:406–408.

196. Talati C, Arzola C, Carvalho JC. The use of ultrasonography in obstetric anesthesia. *Anesthesiol Clin.* 2017;35:35–58.

197. Auroy Y, Benhamou D, Pequignot F, et al. Mortality related to anaesthesia in France: analysis of deaths related to airway complications. *Anaesthesia.* 2009;64:366–370.

198. Peterson GN, Domino KB, Caplan RA, et al. Management of the difficult airway: a closed claims analysis. *Anesthesiology.* 2005;103:33–39.

199. Cooper R. Extubation and reintubation of the difficult airway. In: Hagberg C, Artime C, Aziz MF, eds. *Hagberg and Benumof's Airway Management.* 4th ed. Elsevier; 2018: 844–867.

200. Calder I, Pearce A. Basic principles of airway management. In: Calder I, Pearce A, eds. *Core Topics in Airway Management.* 2nd ed. Cambridge University Press; 2011:43–52.

201. Dravid R, Lee G. Extubation and re-intubation strategy. In: Popat M, ed. *Difficult Airway Management.* Oxford University Press; 2009:131–144.

Postpartum Headache

Feyce M. Peralta, MD, MS

Postpartum headache is the complaint of cephalic, neck, or shoulder pain occurring during the first 6 weeks after delivery. The incidence of postpartum headache throughout the 6-week postpartum period has not been followed in a prospective manner. However, information is available from several sources, including an evaluation of women during the first week postpartum,[1] from a secondary analysis of parturients followed for postpartum pain,[2] and from a survey of women at 5 months and 1 year postpartum.[3] Goldszmidt et al.[1] evaluated 985 women during the first week postpartum and found a 38.7% incidence of headache. The median time to onset of symptoms was 2 days, and the median duration of headache was 4 hours. Turner et al.[2] evaluated patients at four university hospitals in the United States and Europe and found that a history of headache before pregnancy was predictive of headache during pregnancy and at 8 weeks postpartum but not at 72 hours. Saurel-Cubizolles et al.[3] surveyed 1286 women on their general health following their first or second delivery and found the incidence of headache was 22% and 42% at 5 and 12 months, respectively.

Post–dural puncture headache (PDPH) is one of the most common postpartum complications of neuraxial anesthesia. However, healthcare providers should be aware that a dural puncture is only one of many causes of postpartum headache (Table 30.1). Most headaches are benign and do not require immediate attention; however, the timely diagnosis of some headaches (e.g., cortical vein thrombosis, subdural hematoma) is critical to good outcomes. Knowledge of both benign and nonbenign headaches is important for the anesthesia provider, who is frequently the first provider to evaluate patients with postpartum headache. Difficult diagnostic problems may require a consultation with a neurologist or imaging studies. The purpose of this chapter is to discuss the differential diagnosis of postpartum headache with a focus on PDPH.

DIFFERENTIAL DIAGNOSIS OF POSTPARTUM HEADACHE

The classification of headaches follows the International Classification of Headache Disorders (ICHD), created in 1988 by the Headache Classification Committee of the International Headache Society. This classification system, which was updated in 2018 (3rd edition), identifies two broad categories of headaches: primary and secondary (Box 30.1).[4] Primary headaches are classified as migraine, tension-type headaches, trigeminal autonomic cephalalgia, or other primary headache disorders associated with recurring activities (e.g., coughing, strenuous exertion, sexual activity). Secondary headaches are attributable to a specific underlying pathologic process. Primary headaches are 20 times more common than secondary headaches among women in the first week postpartum.[1]

Primary Headaches

The postpartum patient can present with a recurrence of a known primary disorder or with the first manifestation of a primary condition. The most common postpartum headaches are tension-type and migraine headaches, which account for almost two-thirds of headaches during this period.[1,6,7] **Tension-type headaches** are often circumferential and constricting, can be associated with scalp tenderness, and are usually of mild to moderate severity.

TABLE 30.1   Differential Diagnosis of Postpartum Headache

Headache Etiology	Primary Symptoms/Signs	Diagnostic Modality
Tension headache	Mild to moderate headache, lasting 30 min to 7 d Often bilateral, nonpulsating, and not aggravated by physical activity	History and physical examination
Migraine	Recurrent moderate to severe headache, lasting 4–72 h Often unilateral, pulsating, and aggravated by physical activity Associated with nausea, photophobia, and phonophobia	History and physical examination
Musculoskeletal	Mild to moderate headache accompanied by neck and/or shoulder pain	History and physical examination
Preeclampsia/eclampsia	Hypertension and/or hemolysis, elevated liver enzymes, low platelet count syndrome Headache often bilateral, pulsating, and aggravated by physical activity	History and physical examination Laboratory evaluation (alanine aminotransferase, aspartate transaminase, uric acid, platelet count, urine protein)
Posterior reversible (leuko) encephalopathy syndrome	Severe and diffuse headache with an acute or gradual onset Possible focal neurologic deficits and seizures	History and physical examination MRI
Stroke	Ischemic or hemorrhagic *Cerebral infarction/ischemia:* new headache that is overshadowed by focal signs and/or disorders of consciousness *Subarachnoid hemorrhage:* abrupt onset of an intense and incapacitating headache Often unilateral accompanied by nausea, nuchal rigidity, and altered consciousness	History and physical examination CT without contrast or MRI (FLAIR sequence)
Subarachnoid hemorrhage	Sudden onset of severe headache ("worst headache of my life"). Accompanied by neck stiffness, nausea, vomiting, decreased level of consciousness, and focal neurologic deficits	History and physical examination CT imaging
Subdural hematoma	Headache usually without typical features Often overshadowed by focal neurologic signs and/or altered consciousness	History and physical examination CT or MRI
Carotid artery dissection	Late-developing headache that is constant in nature Bilateral or unilateral location	History and physical examination Carotid ultrasonography or MRA
Cerebral venous and sinus thrombosis	Nonspecific headache that may have a postural component Often accompanied by focal neurologic signs and seizures	History and physical examination MRV Possible angiography
Brain tumor	Progressive and often localized headache Often worse in the morning Aggravated by coughing/straining	History and physical examination CT or MRI
Idiopathic intracranial hypertension (pseudotumor cerebri/benign intracranial hypertension)	Progressive nonpulsating headache Aggravated by coughing/straining Associated with increased CSF pressure and normal CSF chemistry	History and physical examination Lumbar puncture
Spontaneous intracranial hypotension	No history of dural trauma Diffuse, dull headache worsening within 15 min of sitting or standing Associated with neck stiffness, nausea, tinnitus, and photophobia CSF opening pressure < 60 mm H_2O in the sitting position	History and physical examination Lumbar puncture Radioisotope cisternography CT myelography

TABLE 30.1 Differential Diagnosis of Postpartum Headache—cont'd

Headache Etiology	Primary Symptoms/Signs	Diagnostic Modality
Pneumocephalus	Frontal headache Often an abrupt onset immediately after dural puncture Symptoms can worsen with upright posture	History and physical examination CT or MRI
Meningitis	Headache is most frequent symptom Often diffuse Intensity increases with time Associated with nausea, photophobia, phonophobia, general malaise, and fever	History and physical examination Lumbar puncture
Sinusitis	Frontal headache with accompanying facial pain Development of headache coincides with nasal obstruction Purulent nasal discharge, anosmia, and fever	History and physical examination Nasal endoscopy CT or MRI
Caffeine withdrawal	Onset of headache within 24 h of cessation of regular caffeine consumption[a] Often bilateral and pulsating Relieved within 1 h of ingestion of caffeine 100 mg	History and physical examination
Lactation headache	Mild to moderate headache associated temporally with onset of breastfeeding or with breast engorgement	History and physical examination
Ondansetron headache	Mild to moderate headache associated with ondansetron intake	History and physical examination
Post–dural puncture headache	Headache within 5 d of dural puncture Worsens within 15 min of sitting or standing Associated with neck stiffness, tinnitus, photophobia, and nausea	History and physical examination Possible MRI

CSF, Cerebrospinal fluid; *CT*, computed tomography; *FLAIR*, fluid-attenuated inversion recovery; *MRA*, magnetic resonance angiogram; *MRI*, magnetic resonance imaging; *MRV*, magnetic resonance venography.

[a]The International Classification of Headache Disorders criterion states that caffeine-withdrawal headache occurs on cessation of daily caffeine ≥ 200 mg for more than 2 w.[4] However, others have suggested that caffeine-withdrawal headache may occur after as little as 3 days' exposure to 300 mg/d or 7 days' exposure to 100 mg/d.[5]

BOX 30.1 International Classification of Headache Disorders, 3rd Edition (ICHD-3)

Primary
- Migraine
- Tension-type headache
- Trigeminal autonomic cephalalgias
  - Cluster headache
- Other primary headaches

Secondary
- Headache attributed to:
  - Head and/or neck trauma
  - Cranial or cervical vascular disorder
  - Nonvascular intracranial disorder
  - A substance or its withdrawal
  - Infection
  - Disorder of homeostasis
  - Disorder of the cranial structures (e.g., eyes, ears, nose, sinuses, teeth, mouth)
  - Psychiatric disorder
- Lesions of cranial neuralgias and other facial pain
- Other headache disorders

Modified from Headache Classification Committee of the International Headache Society (IHS). The international classification of headache disorders, 3rd edition. *Cephalalgia*. 2018;38:1–211.

Migraine headaches are defined as recurring cranial pain lasting 4 to 72 hours, often with typical features such as pulsating pain in a unilateral location, nausea, and photophobia.[4] In the United States, the estimated overall age-adjusted prevalence of migraine is 15.9%. Migraine headache is more common in females (21%) than males (10.7%) and is most common between 18 and 44 years of age.[8] Pregnancy has an ameliorating effect on migraine frequency in the majority of sufferers. However, symptoms may recur soon after delivery, with reports of 34% within the first week postpartum and 55% within the first month.[9] Generally, the symptoms are similar to their typical pattern, although often milder and less often unilateral. It is rare for a migraine to manifest for the first time during the postpartum period. Pregnant women with severe migraines experience higher rates of adverse labor and delivery outcomes (e.g., preterm delivery, preeclampsia, low birth weight), but a lower rate of cesarean delivery than the general population.[10] The higher rates of preeclampsia may reflect an underlying predisposition to cerebral ischemic injury.

Secondary Headaches

A common secondary headache in the postpartum period is the **musculoskeletal headache**, exacerbated by the maternal physical exertion of labor and associated sleep deprivation.

This headache has accompanying neck and shoulder pain without a history of dural puncture. Approximately 11% to 14% of postpartum headaches are diagnosed as musculoskeletal.[1] Other causes of secondary headaches are discussed in the following paragraphs.

Hypertension

Hypertensive disorders of pregnancy, including preeclampsia, are commonly associated with headaches. Eclampsia is a form of hypertensive encephalopathy that includes headache, visual disturbances, nausea, vomiting, seizures, stupor, and coma. Seizures may occur in the absence of severe hypertension. A headache is a serious premonitory sign, present in more than 50% of women in whom eclampsia develops.[11] About one-half of the cases of postpartum eclampsia occur within 48 hours after delivery, and the remainder occur between 2 days and 4 weeks after delivery. Occipital or frontal thunderclap headache, blurred vision, scotomas, photophobia, and altered mental status are some of the potential presenting symptoms. Other hypertensive disorders, with or without superimposed preeclampsia, are also associated with headaches both antepartum and postpartum and may lead to encephalopathy.

Posterior Reversible Leukoencephalopathy Syndrome

Posterior reversible (leuko)encephalopathy syndrome (PRES) is a neuroclinical syndrome with specific imaging findings characterized by headaches, seizures, encephalopathy, visual disturbances, and focal neurologic deficits.[12] Conditions associated with PRES include preeclampsia, uremia, hemolytic-uremic syndrome, infection, malignancy, exposure to immunosuppressant drugs, and SARS-CoV-2 infection.[13,14] Approximately 25% of cases of PRES occur during pregnancy or in the immediate postpartum period. Mayama et al.[15] conducted a retrospective cohort study to assess the incidence of PRES in women with eclampsia and preeclampsia with neurologic symptoms. PRES occurred in 92.3% of women with eclampsia and in 19.2% of women with preeclampsia with neurologic symptoms.

The pathophysiology of PRES is believed to be similar to that of hypertensive encephalopathy in that altered cerebrovascular regulation causes loss of blood-brain barrier integrity. The accompanying vasogenic edema can be reversed by prompt recognition and supportive therapy (e.g., cessation of provocative medications, aggressive treatment of hypertension, seizure prophylaxis) in 70% to 90% of cases.[16] However, irreversible cytotoxic edema with permanent neurologic damage can occur if the initial disorder is not diagnosed early.[17]

The neuroradiologic features of PRES typically include symmetric areas of cerebral edema, predominantly involving the white matter regions of the posterior circulation (occipital lobes, posterior parietal and temporal lobes) (Fig. 30.1). Magnetic resonance imaging (MRI) is the "gold standard" for diagnosing PRES because it can provide information about cerebral involvement earlier than computed tomography (CT).[18]

Stroke

The physiologic changes that occur during pregnancy and the postpartum period (e.g., venous stasis, edema, and hypercoagulability) render these patients susceptible to stroke, and a headache is a common presenting symptom. Strokes can be ischemic or hemorrhagic.

The evaluation and treatment of stroke during pregnancy should mimic that performed for nonpregnant patients. Treatment will depend on the etiology. In addition to supportive care, acute reperfusion therapy with fibrinolytic agents (recombinant tissue plasminogen activator) and intra-arterial mechanical thrombectomy should be considered in pregnant women with qualifying strokes.[19–21]

Ischemic strokes account for approximately 87% of all strokes.[22] Causes of ischemic stroke include cerebral venous sinus thrombosis, preeclampsia/eclampsia, thromboembolism related to valvular heart disease, and profound and persistent hypotension (e.g., cervical arterial dissection and amniotic fluid embolism).[19] The clinical presentation often comprises a new-onset headache that is overshadowed by focal neurologic signs and/or disorders of consciousness.

Hemorrhagic strokes can be subclassified into intracerebral hemorrhage (ICH) or subarachnoid hemorrhage (SAH), with a 10% and 3% incidence, respectively.[22] Hemorrhagic stroke in pregnancy and the postpartum period is relatively more common than in the nonpregnant state. Conditions associated with hemorrhagic stroke include preeclampsia/eclampsia, aneurysms, and arteriovenous malformations.[19]

Subarachnoid Hemorrhage

SAH usually occurs secondary to a ruptured aneurysm or arteriovenous malformation. The classic presentation is a sudden onset of a severe headache that is unlike any previous headache ("worst headache of my life"). Associated symptoms may include neck stiffness, nausea, vomiting, decreased level of consciousness, and focal neurologic deficits. Suspicion of SAH necessitates urgent investigation by CT imaging; nonsurgical therapies (e.g., endovascular ablation) are available, and long-term sequelae can be minimized with early therapy.

Subdural Hematoma

Although usually associated with head trauma, subdural hematomas can occur spontaneously during pregnancy or can be associated with dural puncture (see later discussion). In several case reports, identification of the subdural hematoma was preceded by symptoms of PDPH.[23] Dural puncture results in cerebrospinal fluid (CSF) leakage and decreased intracranial pressure (ICP). Presumably, the reduction in ICP causes stress on bridging cerebral vessels, which precipitates tearing and bleeding. Spontaneous subdural hematomas have been reported in parturients with diseases associated with angiopathy, such as preeclampsia and fatty liver disease of pregnancy.[24] Neurologic signs of subdural hematoma are variable but include evidence of increased ICP (e.g., headache, somnolence, vomiting, confusion) and focal abnormalities.

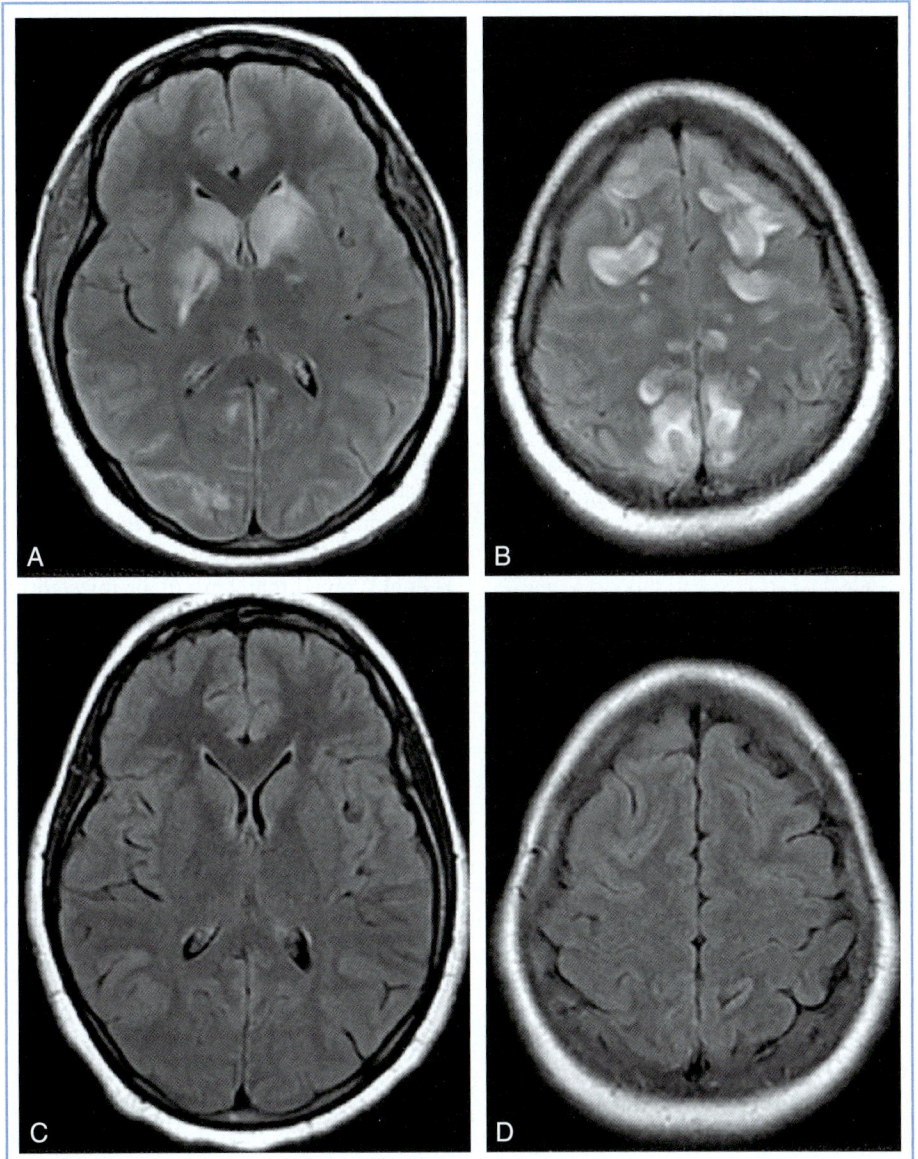

Fig. 30.1 **Posterior Reversible (Leuko)Encephalopathy Syndrome.** MR images of a 19-year-old pregnant woman at 31 weeks' gestation who presented with a urinary tract infection. She developed eclampsia, hemolysis, elevated liver enzymes, low platelet count syndrome, confusion, seizures, and a blood pressure of 190/140 mm Hg. Axial T2 fluid-attenuated inversion recovery images demonstrate cortical/subcortical vasogenic edema in the frontal lobes (the superior frontal sulci), parietal lobes, and occipital lobes as well as deep gray structures such as caudate nuclei and lentiform nuclei (A, B). With magnesium sulfate, blood pressure control, and cesarean delivery, the patient had complete resolution of imaging findings (C, D) and symptoms. From Brady E, Parikh NS, Navi BB, et al. The imaging spectrum of posterior reversible encephalopathy syndrome: a pictorial review. Clin Imaging. 2018;47:80–89.

Carotid Artery Dissection

Trager et al.[25] queried a US research network and compared, using propensity matching, the incidence of spontaneous cervical artery dissection (sCeAD) in pregnant and nonpregnant women. They included more than 460,000 women per group; pregnant women had a twofold increased risk of sCeAD (relative risk [RR], 2.06; 95% confidence interval [CI], 1.17 to 3.61; $P = .0104$) compared to nonpregnant women (8% versus 3.9% in pregnant and nonpregnant women, respectively). Most cases occurred during the pregnancy, not postpartum.

Abdelnour et al.[26] performed a systematic review of all published cases of sCeAD in the peripartum period. The identified 77 patients had a mean age of 33.7 years. Risk factors included migraine, hyperlipidemia, connective tissue disorders, preeclampsia and eclampsia, HELLP syndrome (hemolysis, elevated liver enzymes, and low platelet count), and prolonged second stage of labor. The most common symptom was a headache followed by neck pain. The diagnosis was commonly made after carotid vessel ultrasonography or magnetic resonance angiography.

Cerebral Venous and Sinus Thrombosis

Cerebral venous and sinus thrombosis (CVST) is an uncommon cause of stroke (<1% of all strokes) that results from thrombosis of the cerebral venous system, including dural venous sinuses, and deep and superficial cerebral veins.[27] The most common clinical presentations are signs of intracranial hypertension and parenchymal drainage: headache (70% to 90%), seizure (30% to 40%), papilledema (30% to 60%), focal neurological deficits (30% to 50%), aphasia (15% to 20%), altered level of consciousness (15% to 25%), coma (5% to 15%), and rarely, movement disorder. Diagnosis is best confirmed by MRI in combination with venography. Treatment of cortical vein thrombosis includes anticoagulation and treatment of seizures and increased ICP.[28]

Anticoagulation therapy is recommended for patients with acute CVST, even in selected patients with intracranial hemorrhage. Thrombolysis may be a therapeutic option in a select group of patients with small hemorrhagic infarct and continued neurologic deterioration. Steroid therapy is not recommended.[28]

Brain Tumor

Intracranial tumors may manifest as a postpartum headache. A headache that is dull rather than throbbing may be an early feature of a brain tumor. Nausea, vomiting, seizures, and/or focal neurologic signs may be present. Neurologic examination may reveal evidence of increased ICP.

Idiopathic Intracranial Hypertension

Parturients with idiopathic intracranial hypertension (i.e., increased ICP in the absence of a mass lesion, also known as pseudotumor cerebri or benign intracranial hypertension) have headaches and visual disturbances, usually in the antepartum period (see Chapter 47). The features of postpartum pseudotumor cerebri mimic the usual chronic headache symptoms experienced by the patient (i.e., nonspecific and varying in type, location, and frequency) and associated symptoms (e.g., visual loss, diplopia, nausea, vomiting, pulsatile tinnitus). The diagnosis is largely one of exclusion. Treatment involves reduction of CSF pressure, either with glucocorticoids, carbonic anhydrase inhibitors, diuretics, or surgical interventions (e.g., optic nerve sheath fenestration, CSF diversion via lumboperitoneal or ventriculoperitoneal shunt, or intracranial venous sinus stenting). Since CSF volume is rapidly replaced, serial lumbar punctures are of limited value and should be reserved for patients who refuse or cannot undergo conventional medical or surgical therapy. Case reports describe the use of an intrathecal catheter for labor analgesia[29] and the administration of an epidural blood patch (EBP) for PDPH in patients with idiopathic intracranial hypertension.[30]

Spontaneous Intracranial Hypotension

Spontaneous intracranial hypotension is an uncommon cause of a headache that develops following CSF leakage secondary to dural tears. The tears usually occur at the thoracic spinal level and are not associated with prior spinal intervention.[31]

An MRI of the brain with contrast will confirm the diagnosis of intracranial hypotension. An MRI of the spine, CT cisternography, or CT myelography with contrast or radioisotope can help identify the exact location of the CSF leak. Presentation of this disorder is identical to that of PDPH because the pathophysiology is the same. The only difference is the lack of a prior neuraxial procedure. Spontaneous intracranial hypotension has been reported during pregnancy and in the postpartum period.[32]

Pneumocephalus

The subdural or subarachnoid injection of air used to identify the epidural space may be associated with the sudden onset of a severe frontotemporal headache, sometimes accompanied by neck pain, back pain, or changes in mental status.[33] A headache is caused by meningeal irritation by air, and symptoms can mimic those of PDPH in that they are worse in the sitting position and may be relieved by lying down. Roderick et al.[34] noted that 2 mL of air injected into the subarachnoid space was sufficient to provoke a symptomatic pneumocephalus. A CT is more sensitive than an MRI to confirm the presence of air within the cranial cavity.[35] The headache typically occurs soon after air enters into the intrathecal space and resolves within 3 to 5 days with reabsorption of the air.[36] Treatment is symptomatic. Administration of oxygen by nasal cannula or face mask may hasten resorption of the air and speed recovery, although this therapy has yet to be proven for pneumocephalus after neuraxial anesthesia.[37]

Meningitis

Meningitis is a complication of neuraxial procedures, and the associated severe headache typically manifests within 12 hours to several days following the procedure (see Chapter 31). A headache is accompanied by fever, nuchal rigidity, and the presence of Kernig and Brudzinski signs. Lethargy, confusion, vomiting, seizures, and a rash also may occur. Various strains of *Streptococcus*, organisms typically found in the upper airway and vagina, have been linked to bacterial meningitis after neuraxial procedures.[38,39] In several cluster cases, the organisms in the patients' CSF were matched with the proceduralists' nasopharyngeal swabs, confirming that these cases of post–dural puncture bacterial meningitis were the result of droplet contamination.[40] Aseptic technique during the neuraxial procedure, including donning of a face mask by the proceduralist, is of paramount importance. The diagnosis of meningitis is confirmed by examination and CSF culture and warrants immediate treatment with antibiotics.

Sinusitis

A headache caused by inflamed paranasal sinuses is associated with purulent nasal discharge and, occasionally, fever. Pain may be unilateral or bilateral, depending on the extent of the disease, and the skin over the affected sinus may be tender. The sinuses fill overnight, and the pain typically is worse on awakening. Pain improves in the upright position, which assists drainage.[41]

Caffeine Withdrawal

Caffeine withdrawal may lead to headache, increased fatigue, and anxiety. Caffeine-withdrawal headaches may occur after just 3 days' exposure to 300 mg/day or 7 days' exposure to 100 mg/day of caffeine.[5] The average daily dose of caffeine is estimated at 135 mg, which corresponds to 1.5 standard cups of brewed coffee.[42] Although a caffeine-withdrawal headache has not been documented as a cause of postpartum headache, the diagnosis should be considered if the parturient has been drinking caffeinated beverages during the pregnancy.

Lactation Headache

Askmark and Lundberg[43] reported episodes of intense headache during periods of breastfeeding in a woman known to suffer from migraines. The onset of headaches occurred within the first few minutes of breastfeeding, and the headaches resolved after cessation of nursing. The headaches were associated with an increase in plasma vasopressin concentration. Headaches have also been described in women with breast engorgement who have elected not to breastfeed or have reduced the frequency of breastfeeding.[44]

Ondansetron

Sharma and Panda[45] reported a case in which a woman received ondansetron for nausea and vomiting after uneventful spinal anesthesia for cesarean delivery. Several hours later, the patient developed a severe frontal headache that was worse in the upright position and in the morning and evening hours. The symptoms abruptly stopped after the discontinuation of ondansetron. A headache is a common side effect of ondansetron (incidence, 3% to 17%), owing to its antagonism of serotonin 5-HT$_3$ receptors, and should be considered in the differential diagnosis of postpartum headache.

POST–DURAL PUNCTURE HEADACHE

Incidence

PDPH may occur after an intentional dural puncture with a spinal needle or an unintentional dural puncture (UDP) with an epidural or other needle. In a 10-year, single-center, retrospective study of 7718 women who received neuraxial anesthesia published in 2023, the rate of UDP was 1.25% and the rate of PDPH in women with UDP was 53.6%.[46] A metaanalysis of studies of PDPH in obstetric patients ($n = 328,769$) calculated a pooled risk for UDP with any epidural needle of 1.5% (95% CI, 1.5% to 1.5%).[47] After a dural puncture with an epidural needle, the risk for PDPH was 52.1% (95% CI, 51.4% to 52.8%) (Fig. 30.2). The rate of PDPH after dural puncture with spinal needles ranged between 1.5% and 11.2%, depending on the needle size and type of

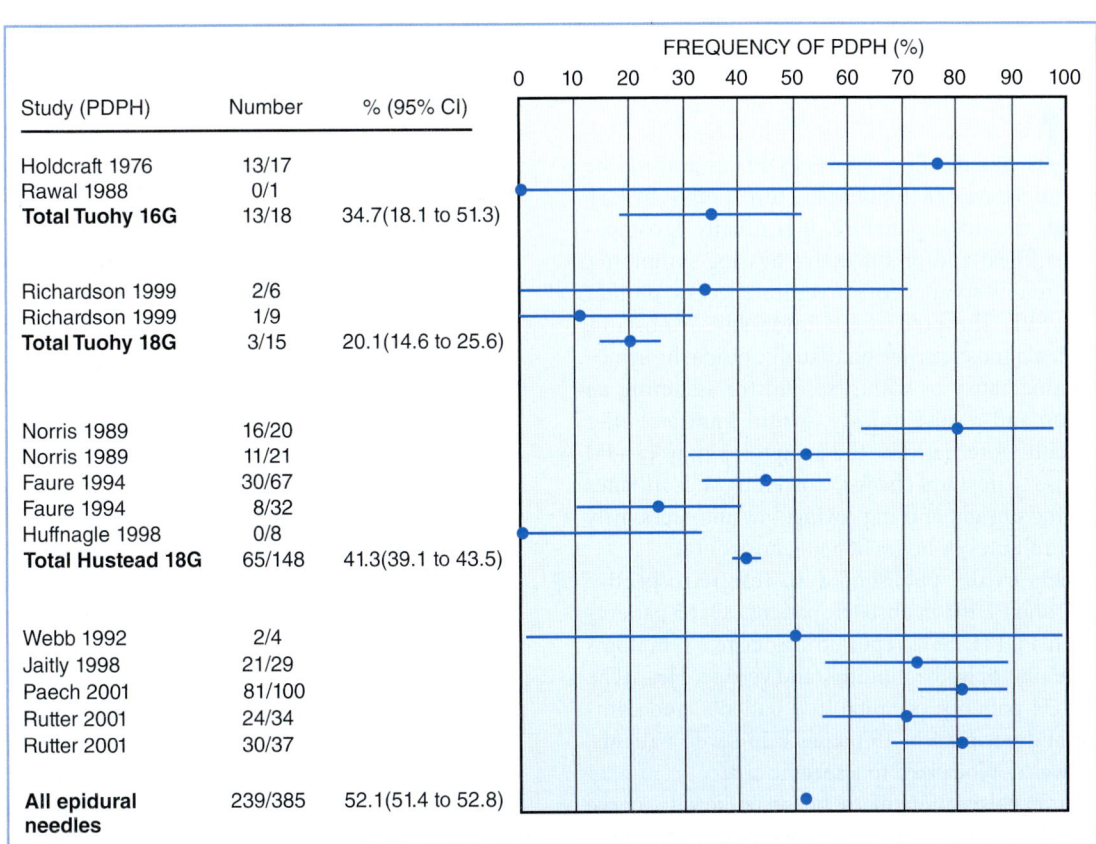

Fig. 30.2 Metaanalysis of Post–Dural Puncture Headache (PDPH) Frequency for Epidural Needles in the Obstetric Population. The *dots* represent the percentages of patients experiencing the event. The *horizontal lines* represent the 95% confidence interval (CI). From Choi PT, Galinski SE, Takeuchi L, et al. PDPH is a common complication of neuraxial blockade in parturients: a meta-analysis of obstetric studies. *Can J Anaesth.* 2003;50:460–469.

TABLE 30.2   Frequency of Post–Dural Puncture Headache in Obstetric Patients According to Spinal Needle Design

Needle Design	Gauge	n/N	Frequency of PDPH (%)[a]	95% Confidence Interval[b]
Quincke	24	15/238	11.2	10.2 to 12.2[47,48]
	25	114/1792	6.4	5.3 to 7.6[47,48]
	26	139/2467	5.6	5.6 to 5.7[47]
	27	34/1167	2.9	2.0 to 4.0[47,48]
Atraucan	26	16/350	4.6	2.6 to 7.3[49–51]
Whitacre	22	1/68	1.5	1.2 to 2.8[47]
	25	137/6992	2.0	1.6 to 2.3[47–50]
	27	13/820	1.6	0.08 to 2.7[47,48]
Sprotte	24	57/1767	3.5	3.5 to 3.5[47]
Polymedic	25	22/292	6.6	5.9 to 7.4[47]
BD	26	205/2560	5.8	5.6 to 5.9[47]
Gertie Marx	24	8/201	4.0	1.7 to 7.7[51]

n, Number of headaches; N, total number of procedures; PDPH, post–dural puncture headache.
[a]Estimates based on binomial probability estimation.
[b]Superscript numbers indicate reference citations at the end of the chapter.

needle (see later discussion) (Table 30.2).[47–51] PDPH was the cause of 12% of obstetric claims in the American Society of Anesthesiologists (ASA) Closed-Claims Project database,[52] and growing evidence suggests an increased association with long-term sequelae and major neurologic complications (see later discussion).[53,54]

Symptoms

The ICHD-3 beta classification defines PDPH as a headache occurring within 5 days of a lumbar puncture, caused by CSF leakage through the dural puncture. It is usually accompanied by neck stiffness and/or subjective hearing symptoms. PDPH usually remits spontaneously within 2 weeks, or after an autologous EBP. The headache is invariably orthostatic, but this is not a diagnostic criterion. Usually, headache symptoms occur immediately or within seconds of assuming an upright position and resolve quickly (within 1 minute) after lying horizontally. Alternatively, the symptoms may exhibit delayed response to postural change, worsening after minutes or hours of being upright and improving, but not necessarily resolving, after minutes or hours of being horizontal.[4]

Van de Velde et al.[55] published a 10-year retrospective review of UDP and PDPH in obstetric patients. Of 65 patients diagnosed with PDPH, 55% reported associated symptoms such as nausea, photophobia, tinnitus, and vertigo. Headache was frontal in 34 patients, occipital in 9 patients, and combined frontal and occipital in 15 patients. In seven patients, the headache was not localized to a specific area.

Cranial nerve palsy, thought to be secondary to nerve traction caused by low CSF volume, is associated with PDPH. The sixth cranial nerve (abducens) is most susceptible to traction during its long and tortuous intracranial course. Injuries to this nerve constitute 92% to 95% of cranial nerve injuries associated with intracranial hypotension.[56] The traction results in failure of the involved eye to abduct, and patients may have diplopia or extraocular muscle paralysis. In a literature review, Hofer and Scavone[56] concluded that early administration of an EBP may decrease morbidity or prevent the progression of ocular symptoms if PDPH is present with symptoms of nerve palsy. Corrective surgery may be necessary in persistent or permanent cases.

Hearing loss is also associated with PDPH. The deficit is usually in the low-frequency range and may be secondary to endolymph and perilymph imbalance and alteration of hair cell position in the inner ear.[57] Therapeutic EBP improves hearing within 1 hour in most patients with severe PDPH.[58]

Other rare symptoms associated with PDPH include seizures,[59] vertigo,[60] bilateral forearm pain,[61] abdominal pain, and diarrhea.[62] In these rare case reports, the headache and associated symptoms resolved after therapy with an EBP.

Onset and Duration

In a prospective study of 75 nonobstetric patients with PDPH, 65% developed symptoms within 24 hours of the lumbar puncture, and 92% developed symptoms within 48 hours.[63] By ICHD-3 beta criteria, headache must appear within 5 days of dural puncture.[4] However, a systematic review of PDPH in obstetric patients reported that the onset of a headache can occur up to 7 days after dural puncture,[47] and one case report described a woman who developed a PDPH 12 days after labor neuraxial analgesia.[64] Headaches caused by dural puncture with a spinal needle ranged in duration from 1 to 7 days.[47] The duration of headache after dural puncture with an epidural needle has not been well studied, but is likely longer than that for a spinal needle.[47,65] In a systematic review and metaanalysis, women who had a PDPH following an UDP had an increased risk for persistent headache that lasted more than 12 months compared to women who had uneventful neuraxial procedures.

Imaging

Imaging investigations are not routinely recommended for the postpartum patient with a PDPH unless the symptoms suggest other diagnoses or the diagnosis of PDPH is in doubt. Contrast-enhanced MRI is the method of choice to study the meninges and has revealed characteristic findings of intracranial hypotension.[66,67] These findings include (1) marked, diffuse pachymeningeal thickening and enhancement; (2) compression of the ventricles; (3) caudal displacement of the brain, brainstem, and optic chiasm; (4) cerebellar ectopia; (5) pituitary enlargement and enhancement; and (6) expansion of the superior sagittal sinus. The enlarged venous sinus may represent compensatory venous expansion in response to low CSF pressure. At times, imaging is needed to differentiate PDPH from other causes of headache.

Pathophysiology

Debate continues regarding the precise etiology of PDPH symptoms. The original theory was that pain-sensitive nerve fibers were stimulated by a downward shift of the brain secondary to a loss of CSF volume. German surgeon August Bier[68] is credited with the first description of successful spinal anesthesia and PDPH after his pioneering work on spinal anesthesia with cocaine. Bier and his assistant, Hildebrandt, performed spinal anesthesia on each other with cocaine; using blows to the shin with an iron hammer and application of a burning cigar to the skin, they demonstrated dense sensory blockade.[68] Both experienced severe PDPH. The assistant forced himself to work the next day, but Bier stayed home for 9 days. Bier suggested the PDPH might be caused by CSF loss. Today there is no doubt that leakage of CSF initiates the syndrome. Kunkle et al.[69] consistently produced PDPH by draining 20 mL of CSF from volunteers. Symptoms were immediately relieved by subarachnoid injection of saline to restore initial CSF pressure.

Total CSF volume is approximately 150 mL, and the production rate is approximately 0.35 mL/min or a daily volume of 500 mL. The rate of CSF leakage through a dural hole may exceed the rate of CSF production. If this occurs, low CSF pressure results in a loss of the cushioning effect provided by intracranial fluid.

CSF pressure during labor is normal between contractions but increases significantly during painful contractions and expulsive efforts. Effective epidural analgesia attenuates this increase in CSF pressure.[70] In a study of five women with UDP, epidural pressures were normal preceding the development of a headache.[71] However, with the development of headache symptoms, the mean epidural pressure measurements were found to decrease significantly.

Not all patients with PDPH symptoms have decreased CSF pressure, and not all patients with a significant CSF leak experience symptoms. The pain of PDPH may be caused, in part, by an increase in cerebral blood flow (and cerebral vasodilation) as a consequence of low CSF pressure or volume. This phenomenon has been observed in animals.[72,73] The inverse relationship between intracranial blood volume and CSF volume reflects the body's effort to maintain a constant intracranial volume.[74] The lumbar CSF compartment is a dynamic structure and acts as a reservoir for intracranial CSF volume adjustment.[75] In a descriptive study of cerebral blood flow measured by middle cerebral artery transcranial Doppler in 15 postpartum women with UDP following labor epidural analgesia, the authors demonstrated that women with PDPH symptoms had lower pulsatility indices compared with women without headaches.[76] The pulsatility index is inversely related to cerebral blood flow. The occurrence of cerebral vasodilation may explain the relief of headache symptoms with treatment with vasoconstrictors such as caffeine, theophylline, and sumatriptan.

Risk Factors

In a classic study of 10,098 spinal anesthetics published in 1956, Vandam and Dripps[77] noted that three patient factors influenced the incidence of PDPH: age, gender, and pregnancy. The analysis did not allow determination of whether these factors were independent risk factors. Subsequently, other risk factors for development of PDPH have been identified.

Age

Extensive evidence supports the observation that PDPH is uncommon in patients older than 60 years of age and is most common in patients younger than 40 years of age.[78] In older people, the dura may be inelastic and less likely to gape after puncture. CSF leakage may be impeded by adhesions and calcification. The cerebrovascular system also may be less reactive in older patients. Further, this group is less active physically, and older patients may be less likely to complain.

Gender

Amorim et al.[78] observed a gender difference with respect to the incidence of PDPH after spinal anesthesia (11.1% female versus 3.6% male). This difference may be related to differences in cerebrovascular reactivity; it is well known that migraine headaches occur predominantly in females and are influenced by hormonal changes. Women may have enhanced vascular reactivity, or perhaps changes in cerebral blood flow are more likely to produce pain in women than in men. A metaanalysis of randomized clinical trials identified a twofold higher risk for PDPH in nonpregnant females than in males.[79]

Vaginal Delivery

In a database study of 1,752,243 privately insured patients in the United States, women who had a vaginal delivery following neuraxial labor analgesia had a higher rate of PDPH (0.58%) compared to those who underwent a cesarean delivery following a neuraxial procedure (0.47%).[80] This may be due to pushing during the second stage of labor in women undergoing vaginal delivery. In a retrospective study of 235 parturients who suffered an UDP during epidural catheter placement, the rate of PDPH was lower in women who delivered via cesarean compared with those that delivered vaginally (53% versus 74%).[81] This difference may also be a result of the mechanical consequences of expulsive efforts during the second stage of labor and/or postpartum hormonal changes in cerebrovascular reactivity. Expulsive efforts in the second stage may increase CSF leakage. This possibility has prompted some physicians to restrict maternal pushing after UDP and to use forceps to shorten the second stage of labor. The evidence supporting this practice, however, is conflicting.[82,83]

Morbid Obesity

Data are conflicting regarding the relationship between obesity and PDPH. In a retrospective study of 518 women, Peralta et al.[83] demonstrated that higher body mass index (BMI) was associated with a lower rate of PDPH. Using a threshold BMI of $31.5 \, kg/m^2$, the incidence of PDPH was 39% and 56% in those with BMI greater than and less than the threshold, respectively. However, pain intensity at headache presentation and the highest reported pain score were similar between high and low BMI groups. In contrast, Song et al.,[84] in a retrospective study of 164 women with UDP, did not identify a protective effect of obesity. Possible but unproven explanations of a lower incidence of PDPH in obese patients include increased abdominal pressure, which may reduce the extent of CSF leakage, and/or reduced physical activity in these patients. Other confounding factors, such as differences in the mode of delivery (higher rate of cesarean delivery) and neuraxial opioid administration, may also play a role.

History of Previous Post–Dural Puncture Headache

A history of PDPH after previous spinal anesthesia is associated with the development of PDPH with subsequent spinal anesthesia. In a cross-sectional study of nonobstetric patients who underwent spinal anesthesia for elective surgery, those with a previous history of PDPH were 4.3 times more likely (95% CI, 1.99 to 9.31) to have a second PDPH than patients without a history of PDPH (26.4% versus 6.2%, respectively).[78] This finding suggests that certain individuals are predisposed to the development of PDPH.

Multiple Dural Punctures

Seeberger et al.[85] found that multiple dural punctures significantly increased the risk for PDPH. Surgical patients who received a second spinal injection owing to failure of the initial spinal puncture had a 4.2% incidence of PDPH compared with a 1.6% incidence among patients who had a single dural puncture.

Neuraxial Anesthetic Technique

Technical factors related to the neuraxial technique influence the incidence of PDPH.

Spinal needle design. Historically, the beveled Quincke needle, a needle with a cutting bevel (Fig. 30.3), was widely used for dural puncture for both diagnostic and anesthetic purposes. In 1951 Hart and Whitacre[86] introduced a solid-tipped, pencil-point spinal needle with a lateral injection port, which is now known as the Whitacre design. They believed

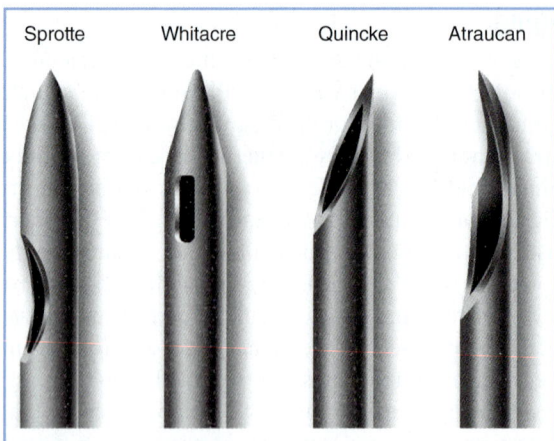

Fig. 30.3 Designs of Spinal Needle Tips (Not to Scale). Illustration by Naveen Nathan, MD, NorthShore University HealthSystem, University of Chicago Pritzker School of Medicine, Evanston, IL.

that the new needle tip would stretch and separate rather than cut the dural fibers and result in a lower incidence of PDPH. Studies have confirmed the anticipated lower incidence of PDPH with the pencil-point tip (see Table 30.2).[47,87] *In vitro* data suggest that fluid leak through the dural puncture site is slower with a pencil-point needle compared with a beveled needle.[88] With the recognition that pencil-point spinal needle tips reduce the incidence of PDPH, other tip designs have appeared. In 1987 Sprotte et al.[89] reported experience with the use of a new needle that has a solid oval tip and a longer orifice than the Whitacre needle. The incidence of PDPH was 0.02% with its use in a heterogeneous patient population of almost 35,000 patients.[89] Subsequent studies have shown the incidence of PDPH with the Sprotte needle is lower than that with Quincke needles of smaller gauge.[47] A 2017 metaanalysis of eight randomized clinical trials including 1324 women undergoing cesarean delivery confirmed that spinal needles with cutting bevels were more likely to cause PDPH than pencil-point needles (RR 3.12; 95% CI, 1.60 to 6.10).[90]

A modification of the Quincke needle, the Atraucan needle, has a cutting tip and a double bevel, which is intended to cut a small dural hole and then dilate it.[49] Studies suggest that the use of this needle is associated with a higher risk for PDPH than the use of a noncutting, pencil-point needle.[51]

Spinal needle size. With the Quincke needle, the incidence and severity of PDPH are directly related to the size of the needle. The incidence of PDPH is lower with a 27-gauge needle than with 25- and 26-gauge needles (see Table 30.2).[47] A similar relationship may exist with pencil-point needles but findings are inconsistent.[90] Because of the morbidity associated with PDPH, every effort should be made to use a needle associated with a low incidence of PDPH (e.g., a small-gauge, noncutting needle).

Direction of bevel of the cutting spinal needle. It was originally thought that the dural fibers ran in a longitudinal direction and therefore inserting the needle parallel to the long axis of the spine caused less trauma to the dura. However, electron microscopy has revealed that the dura consists of multidirectional interlacing collagen fibers with both transverse and longitudinal elastic fibers.[91] Some authors have suggested that the insertion of the needle with the bevel parallel to the long axis of the spine most likely results in less tension on the dural hole and, therefore, a smaller aperture with less CSF leak. *In vitro* studies of bevel orientation and fluid leak have provided conflicting results.[92,93] However, despite confusing anatomic evidence, clinical experience strongly supports insertion of the Quincke needle with the bevel parallel to the long axis of the spine[94] or perhaps facing the caudad but not the cephalad direction.[95]

Epidural needle size and design. The high rate of PDPH after UDP with an epidural needle has led investigators to alter the epidural needle design and size in an attempt to reduce headache incidence and severity. Data on the success of this endeavor are conflicting. In an *in vitro* study using cadaver dura, no differences were found in fluid leak rate among punctures made with Hustead, Tuohy, Crawford, and Sprotte epidural needles.[96] In contrast, in an *in vivo* study, Morley-Forster et al.[97] observed a risk difference of −0.44 (95% CI, −0.67 to −0.21) in the incidence of PDPH with the use of an 18-gauge Sprotte needle compared with the standard 17-gauge Tuohy needle despite no difference in the UDP rate. However, the Sprotte epidural needle, with its lateral orifice, is not commonly used as an introducer of epidural catheters.

The incidence of PDPH is greater when the UDP occurs with a 16-gauge compared with an 18-gauge epidural needle (RR 2.21; 95% CI, 1.4 to 2.6).[98]

Direction of the bevel of the Tuohy needle. Norris et al.[99] examined two groups of women who received epidural anesthesia with a Tuohy needle. In one group, the bevel was advanced with the orifice perpendicular to the long axis of the spine. In the other group, the needle entered the epidural space with the bevel parallel to the long axis and the needle was then rotated 90 degrees before insertion of the catheter. The authors observed a decreased incidence of PDPH in the latter group. However, some anesthesiologists argue that rotation of the needle within the epidural space may increase the risk for UDP. Richardson and Wissler[100] randomized laboring women to a cephalad or lateral orientation of the Tuohy bevel during epidural needle insertion. The needle was not rotated before insertion of the epidural catheter. There was no difference in dural puncture or PDPH rates, but catheter insertion was easier with a cephalad orientation of the bevel.

Midline or paramedian approach. There is conflicting evidence as to whether the spinal needle approach affects the incidence of PDPH. Hatfalvi[101] reported no cases of PDPH in a retrospective survey of 4465 spinal anesthesia procedures. This investigator used a paramedian approach with a 20-gauge Quincke needle, and the skin was punctured 3 cm from the midline. He suggested that tangential dural puncture creates a dural flap and prevents PDPH. In contrast, Viitanen et al.,[102] prospectively monitoring obstetric patients after administration of single-shot spinal analgesia for labor (27-gauge Quincke needle), observed PDPH in 3 of 85 (3.5%) patients in whom the midline approach was used, compared with 15 of 127 (11.8%) patients in whom the paramedian approach was used. Using a rigid paper cylinder model of the

dura, Kempen and Mocek[103] studied median and paramedian punctures with a 22-gauge Quincke needle in different orientations. With midline punctures, all entry and exit holes were of uniform size regardless of bevel orientation, and no "dural" flaps were seen. After paramedian punctures, flaps formed when the needle bevel faced the cylinder surface with a near-tangential angle of perforation, suggesting it may be beneficial to insert the needle via the paramedian approach to reduce the incidence of PDPH. Currently, data are insufficient to recommend either the median or paramedian approach.

Air versus saline method of locating the epidural space. The medium (air or saline) used for the loss-of-resistance technique to identify the epidural space has not clearly been shown to influence the incidence of PDPH. Many anesthesia providers have adopted the loss-of-resistance-to-saline technique in the belief that it is associated with a lower incidence of UDP and PDPH than the use of air.[104] However, the data are inconsistent, and not all studies have found a difference.[105]

Segal and Arendt[106] suggested that a randomized study of air versus saline to identify the epidural space may lead to overestimation of the difference between air and saline, should one exist, because it is impossible to blind the anesthesia provider to the technique, and the study design forces the provider to use a less preferred technique. In a retrospective study, they found that the rate of UDP was not different between the saline versus air technique.[106] However, among anesthesia providers who had a preference for one technique, the use of their preferred technique was associated with fewer UDPs than the use of the nonpreferred technique. A 2014 Cochrane review also did not find a difference in UDP or headache with air versus saline.[107] Thus, current data do not support a difference in the incidence of PDPH between the loss-of-resistance-to-air versus the loss-of-resistance-to-saline technique to identify the epidural space, and providers who currently use air to identify the epidural space should not change techniques hoping it may decrease the rate of PDPH.

Choice of local anesthetic drug for spinal anesthesia. Naulty et al.[108] reported that the use of bupivacaine-glucose or lidocaine-glucose for spinal anesthesia was associated with a higher incidence of PDPH than the use of tetracaine-procaine. They postulated that osmotic, cerebral irritant, and/or cerebrovascular effects of the glucose could be responsible for these findings. Whether this finding is applicable to other nonglucose-containing local anesthetic preparations, such as plain bupivacaine, is unknown.

Continuous spinal anesthesia. A multicenter randomized clinical trial compared analgesia and safety of 28-gauge spinal microcatheters to epidural catheters for labor analgesia.[109] There was no difference in the incidence of PDPH (9% versus 4%, respectively) or EBP (5% versus 2%, respectively) between women randomly assigned to receive an intrathecal catheter and those who received an epidural catheter; however, the study was insufficiently powered to assess these outcomes. Spinal microcatheters are not currently available in North America.

Some investigators have evaluated a 23-gauge spinal catheter for labor analgesia or cesarean delivery.[110,111] The PDPH rate ranged from 3% to 29%. This range is greater than that reported in other studies using traditional epidural or combined spinal-epidural (CSE) techniques.

Combined spinal-epidural anesthesia. The CSE technique is widely used for both labor analgesia and cesarean delivery. Intuitively, it seems that the incidence of PDPH should be identical to, or greater than, that observed after single-shot spinal anesthesia with the same size and type of needle. However, this does not appear to be the case. A systematic review and metaanalysis of 18 prospective randomized studies did not find a difference in headache rate between those who received a single-shot spinal anesthetic versus CSE anesthesia (RR 0.83; 95% CI, 0.32 to 2.15).[112] Initial placement of the epidural needle facilitates precise dural puncture and the subsequent increase in epidural space pressure after the epidural injection of local anesthetic may reduce CSF leakage. If the anesthesia provider is in doubt about correct epidural needle placement, a needle-through-needle dural puncture might resolve the issue and prevent UDP with a large-gauge epidural needle.

Complications

The immediate problems associated with PDPH include (1) the inability to perform activities of daily living, such as providing care for the newborn; (2) an extended duration of hospitalization; and (3) a higher number of emergency department visits. The National Obstetric Anaesthesia Database project of the Obstetric Anaesthetists' Association reported that 75% of 975 women with PDPH had difficulty performing activities of daily living.[113] In a retrospective study, Angle et al.[114] reported that hospital length of stay increased by a mean of 17 hours. Rare but serious complications may occur following dural puncture and PDPH, including subdural hematoma, cerebral venous sinus thrombosis, chronic headache, diplopia, and hearing loss.

In a large retrospective cohort study using State Inpatient Databases, Guglielminotti et al.[54] found that the incidence of cerebral venous thrombosis and subdural hematoma was significantly higher in women with PDPH than in women without PDPH (3.12 per 1000 neuraxial [1:320] versus 0.16 per 1000 [1:6250], respectively; $P < .001$). The incidences of bacterial meningitis, depression, headache and migraine, and low back pain were also significantly higher in women with PDPH than in women without PDPH. The adjusted odds ratio (aOR) associated with PDPH was 19.0 (95% CI, 11.2 to 32.1) for the composite of cerebral venous thrombosis and subdural hematoma. Seventy percent of cerebral venous thrombosis and subdural hematoma were identified during a readmission with a median time to readmission of 5 days.

Diplopia or **hearing loss** after dural puncture, secondary to cranial nerve dysfunction, may be permanent, even after successful treatment of the PDPH with an EBP.[58] A review of 95 cases of neurapraxia or axonotmesis of the ocular cranial nerves (oculomotor, trochlear, and abducens nerves)

concluded that symptoms may last from 2 weeks to 8 months but that almost 90% of patients recover.[115]

Several studies have described the **persistence of headache, backache, or cranial nerve symptoms** after PDPH.[116-119] Ranganathan et al.[116] conducted a retrospective case-control study over a 5-year period in which parturients with an UDP were contacted by telephone to assess acute and long-term residual symptoms. Compared with a control group, patients with an UDP were more prone to acute headache (87% versus 8.7%) and chronic headache (34.9% versus 2.2%) as well as backache and neck ache.

In a 1:1 case-control study of women who sustained an UDP during epidural catheter placement for labor analgesia, Lacombe et al.[118] observed that these parturients had a higher risk of developing chronic headaches (14.3% versus 4.8%; aOR 3.67; 95% CI, 1.05 to 12.82; $P = .057$) and chronic back pain (39.7% versus 19.1%; aOR 2.67; 95% CI, 1.25 to 5.72; $P = .009$) than women who did not sustain a dural puncture. The incidence of chronic auditory impairment was also higher in the UDP group (14.3% versus 1.6%, $P = .01$). Chronicity in this study was defined as a symptom that lasted or recurred for greater than 3 months.

In a prospective observational study, Ansari et al.[119] also observed that the prevalence of a disabling headache was greater among patients with UDP than matched controls (2 months, 74% versus 38%, RR 1.9; 95% CI, 1.2 to 2.9; $P = .009$; 6 months, 56% versus 25%, RR 2.1; 95% CI, 1.1 to 4.0; $P = .033$). These findings reinforce the concept that long-term sequelae from dural puncture occur.

Orbach-Zinger et al.,[120] in a matched cohort study design, found that those with a PDPH had a greater incidence of postpartum depression (52.3% versus 11.2%) and posttraumatic stress disorder (12.8% versus 0.4%) and a lower incidence of breastfeeding (54.5% versus 76.8%) than those who did not experience a PDPH. These results, combined with the previously mentioned metaanalysis[53] and database study,[54] emphasize the need for close follow-up in patients who experience PDPH.

Prevention

Many practices and maneuvers have been used in an attempt to reduce the incidence of PDPH after UDP, most with limited success. A 2005 survey of British obstetric anesthesiologists quantified the frequency of such practices.[121] These included encouraging postpartum fluid intake (91%), regular analgesia (83%), caffeine administration (30%), and using an intrathecal catheter (15%) at the time of UDP. Older practices, such as avoiding pushing during the second stage, restricting postpartum mobility, abdominal binders, and prophylactic epidural saline or autologous blood administration, appear to be declining in use. A 2010 systematic review of prevention strategies summarized the evidence from comparative studies and concluded that studies were heterogeneous and that "no clinical recommendation can be made until the superiority of one preventative intervention over another has been unequivocally proven in a definitive multicenter RCT (randomized controlled trial)."[122]

Bed Rest

In a 2016 systematic review, Arevalo-Rodriguez et al.[123] reviewed the evidence for prolonged bed rest combined with different body and head positions, as well as supplementary fluid administration, for the prevention of PDPH after dural puncture. The review included 24 trials with 2996 patients; 26% of study participants randomized to bed rest experienced PDPH compared with 21% in women who were allowed to mobilize immediately after dural puncture. Given these data, and the knowledge that pregnant women are hypercoagulable and at increased risk for deep vein thrombosis and pulmonary embolism, immobility should not be used as a maneuver to prevent PDPH (see Chapter 38).

Hydration

Despite the widespread practice of encouraging women to increase oral fluid intake after UDP, there is little evidence that greater hydration prevents PDPH. A 2016 systematic review identified only one randomized trial in 100 nonobstetric patients. There was no difference in the incidence of PDPH in patients randomized to receive 3 L or 1.5 L of fluid per day.[123]

Caffeine

Two clinical trials in nonobstetric patients have evaluated the efficacy of oral or intravenous caffeine to prevent PDPH, but neither study showed a reduction in the incidence of headaches.[124,125] Based on these results, prophylactic caffeine is not advocated for prevention of PDPH.

Cosyntropin

Cosyntropin has been studied for the prevention of PDPH after UDP, yielding mixed results. Liu et al.[126] conducted a propensity-matched retrospective analysis of parturients with UDP ($n = 115$). Intravenous cosyntropin was administered to 65 patients (55.6%). Among those who received cosyntropin, 37 (57%) developed PDPH compared with 29 patients (58%) in the no-cosyntropin group. EBP was performed in 21 patients (56.8%) who received cosyntropin and 13 patients (61.7%) who did not. These findings were corroborated by Pancaro et al.[127] in another retrospective study in which the benefits of cosyntropin for the prevention and treatment of PDPH after UDP were assessed. The authors did not find a significant difference in the incidence of PDPH between those exposed to cosyntropin (19/32, 59%) and unexposed patients (17/32, 53%; OR 1.37; 95% CI, 0.48 to 3.98; $P = .56$), or in the incidence of EBP between exposed (12/32, 38%) and unexposed patients (6/32, 19%; OR 2.6; 95% CI, 0.83 to 8.13; $P = .095$). Both groups of investigators concluded that prophylactic administration of cosyntropin is not associated with a reduced incidence of PDPH.

In contrast to these findings, in an RCT, Hakim[128] found that prophylactic cosyntropin was effective in reducing the incidence of PDPH after UDP in parturients, 33% versus 69%, in the cosyntropin and placebo groups, respectively. The mechanism of cosyntropin is unknown but may be related to an aldosterone-stimulating effect on volume expansion, modulation of pain perception via central endorphin-like action, or increased CSF production by enhanced sodium ion transport.

Adequate dose-response and safety studies have yet to be performed. With the existing evidence, we do not recommend routine use of cosyntropin for the prevention of PDPH after UDP in parturients.

Neuraxial Opioids

The prophylactic administration of neuraxial hydrophilic or lipophilic opioid for the prevention of PDPH after UDP has yielded conflicting results. In a randomized, blinded trial published in 2008, 50 parturients with UDP and subsequent epidural analgesia were randomized to receive epidural morphine 3 mg or saline-placebo after delivery and again 24 hours later, before removal of the epidural catheter.[129] The incidence of PDPH was 48% in the saline-placebo group and 12% in the morphine group.

In 2020 Peralta et al.[130] published a randomized, double-blind trial that assessed whether prophylactic administration of intrathecal morphine decreases the incidence of PDPH and/or need for EBP after UDP. Parturients who had an intrathecal catheter placed after UDP with a 17-gauge Tuohy needle during intended epidural catheter placement for labor analgesia were enrolled. After delivery, subjects were randomized to receive intrathecal morphine 150 µg or normal saline before the catheter was removed. The incidence of PDPH was 21 of 27 (78%) in the intrathecal morphine group and 27 of 34 (79%) in the intrathecal saline group (difference, −1%; 95% CI, −25% to 24%). There were no differences between groups in the onset, duration, or severity of headache, or presence of cranial nerve symptoms. EBP was administered to 10 of 27 (37%) of subjects in the intrathecal morphine and 11 of 21 (52%) of the intrathecal saline group (difference 15%; 95% CI, −18% to 48%). This study does not support the clinical use of prophylactic intrathecal morphine after an UDP.

Intrathecal Catheters

Placing a 19- or 20-gauge epidural catheter into the intrathecal space after UDP with an epidural needle has become an increasingly popular technique.[131–133] The immediate benefits of an intrathecal catheter are continuous labor analgesia using low doses of local anesthetic and opioid, and rapid-onset surgical anesthesia should it be required. Some experts have speculated that the intrathecal catheter might reduce the immediate CSF leak into the epidural space by mechanical obstruction as well as inducing an inflammatory fibrous reaction in the dura rent, thus facilitating closure of the puncture after removal of the catheter. Most studies are retrospective and observational and lack rigorous outcome definitions and follow-up. Data from these studies are conflicting but suggest that intrathecal catheters do not significantly reduce the incidence of PDPH, even if left in place for at least 24 hours after delivery (Table 30.3).[81,98,131–136] Russell[98] conducted a prospective, nonblinded, quasirandomized multicenter study in

TABLE 30.3 **Rate of Post–Dural Puncture Headache After Unintentional Dural Puncture and Prophylactic Intrathecal Catheter Placement**

Study[a]	Year	Study Design	Intrathecal Catheter, *n/N* (%)	No Intrathecal Catheter, *n/N* (%)
Jagannathan et al.[81]	2016	Retrospective cohort	117/173 (68)	49/63 (78)
Paech et al.[133]	2001	Prospective cohort; catheter discontinued immediately after delivery	21/24 (87)	60/76 (79)
Rutter et al.[132]	2001	Retrospective cohort; catheter left in place for unknown duration	24/34 (71)	30/37 (81)
Ayad et al.[131]	2003	Retrospective cohort:		34/37 (92)
		Catheter discontinued immediately after delivery	18/35 (51)[b]	
		Catheter left in place for 24 h	2/31 (6)[b]	
Russell[98]	2012	Prospective, randomized in 6-mo blocks, nonblinded intrathecal catheter for 24–36 h	36/50 (72)	29/47 (62)
Verstraete et al.[134]	2014	Retrospective cohort; catheter left in place for at least 24 h	37/89 (42)	24/39 (62)
Bolden and Gebre[135]	2016	Retrospective cohort; catheters were either removed immediately after delivery or removed at variable periods up to 30 h after delivery.[c]	66/118 (56)	68/100 (68)
Binyamin et al.[136]	2023	Retrospective cohort; Catheters were either removed immediately after delivery or removed at variable periods up to 30 h after delivery.[c]	219/550 (40)	331/550 (60)

[a]Superscript numbers indicate reference citations at the end of the chapter.
[b]Different from no catheter, $P < .05$.
[c]A subset of those with an intrathecal catheter also received an injection of preservative-free normal saline through the intrathecal catheter.

parturients who had an UDP during epidural needle placement. Participating institutions were randomized in 6-month blocks to either repeating the epidural procedure with placement of an epidural catheter, or placement of a spinal catheter through the dural puncture if UDP occurred during initiation of epidural labor analgesia. Spinal catheters were left *in situ* for 24 to 36 hours. The incidence of PDPH was not significantly different between women in the epidural (62%) and spinal (72%) catheter groups.

Some studies have evaluated the effect of intrathecal catheter placement on the severity of PDPH. Heesen et al.[137] conducted a metaanalysis that included nine studies of various quality. The authors concluded that placement of an intrathecal catheter did not significantly reduce the incidence of PDPH

compared with placement of an epidural catheter.[137] However, they did observe a significant reduction in the need for EBP (RR 0.64; 95% CI, 0.49 to 0.84) after intrathecal catheter placement. These results were reconfirmed in a follow-up metaanalysis 2020.[138] Similar results were reported in another retrospective study that compared laboring patients with UDP who had the epidural resited or had an intrathecal catheter placed.[136] Use of an intrathecal catheter versus resiting the epidural catheter did not decrease the odds of PDPH (aOR 0.91; 95% CI, 0.81 to 1.01), but was associated with a lower need for EBP (aOR 0.82; 95% CI, 0.73 to 0.91; $P < .001$). The authors found no benefit in leaving the intrathecal catheter for 24 hours for postpartum PDPH (aOR 1.01; 95% CI, 1.00 to 1.02; $P = .015$) or need for EBP (aOR 1.00; 95% CI, 0.99 to 1.01; $P = .40$).[136]

The current evidence suggests that advancing a traditional epidural catheter into the intrathecal space after UDP does *not* appear to reduce the incidence of PDPH but may reduce its severity or the need for an EBP. Leaving the spinal catheter *in situ* after the patient leaves the birthing unit may increase the risk for drug error or infection. Further studies are required before a definitive conclusion can be reached about the benefits and safety of this technique.

Prophylactic Epidural or Intrathecal Saline

Trivedi et al.[139] randomly assigned patients with UDP to receive either a prophylactic epidural saline bolus (40 to 60 mL) or blood patch (15 mL) just before epidural catheter removal, or conservative therapy without a saline bolus or blood patch. The incidence of PDPH was not different between the saline and control groups (88% versus 67%, respectively). Shah[71] studied 17 patients who received an epidural saline infusion (at a rate of approximately 40 mL/h) for 24 to 36 hours after UDP. Four patients complained of severe intrascapular pain, which resolved when the infusion rate was reduced. Severe PDPH developed in 47% of patients after the infusion was stopped. In contrast, in a nonrandomized, nonblinded study of patients with UDP, Charsley and Abram[140] reported that *intrathecal* injection of 10 mL of saline immediately before needle or catheter withdrawal resulted in a lower incidence of PDPH (32%) than in a control group who did not receive the saline (62%), as well as a less frequent need for an EBP. In a large retrospective study, Binyamin et al.[136] also found an added benefit of injecting intrathecal saline (10 mL) as it decreased the incidence of PDPH (aOR 0.85; 95% CI, 0.73 to 0.99; $P = .04$) and the need for EBP (aOR 0.75; 95% CI, 0.64 to 0.87; $P < .001$). The intrathecal injection of saline after UDP deserves further study. Intrathecal or epidural saline should not be administered until residual local anesthetic effects have resolved.

Prophylactic Blood Patch

Interest in the use of prophylactic EBP before the removal of a labor epidural catheter arose after early observational studies suggested that the incidence of PDPH was lower with such treatment.[141] A 2010 systematic review[142] identified five studies in 221 obstetric patients; four studies found a reduction in the headache rate, and one did not.[143] Scavone et al.,[143] in the largest study included in the review, reported a double-blind trial in which 64 parturients with UDP were randomly assigned to receive 20 mL of autologous blood (prophylactic EBP) or a sham procedure. Both groups had a 56% incidence of PDPH; however, the duration of headache was shorter in the prophylactic EBP group. The systematic review highlighted the difficulty in estimating the risks and benefits of prophylactic EBP. Because of the low incidence of UDP, studies are small; therefore, reliable conclusions about the technique cannot be made based on current evidence.[142]

Because UDP with a 16- or 18-gauge epidural needle results in a high incidence of PDPH, some anesthesiologists believe that prophylactic EBP is always justified. Others argue that with such an approach, a significant number of patients will receive unnecessary treatment and that an EBP is not devoid of complications. These latter anesthesiologists call attention to the potential for epidural catheters to become contaminated after prolonged use. The injection of blood through a contaminated epidural catheter may be associated with a higher risk for infection than injection through an epidural needle placed *de novo* for a therapeutic blood patch. A case report of a parturient who received a prophylactic EBP and was subsequently diagnosed with streptococcal septicemia highlights the potential risk for maternal infection using this technique.[144]

If performed, a prophylactic EBP should be delayed until resolution of residual neuroblockade. Additionally, evidence suggests that lidocaine may inhibit coagulation.[145] The occurrence of pain during injection is a signal for the anesthesia provider to stop the injection of blood. Finally, Leivers[146] reported a case of total spinal anesthesia after the epidural injection of 15 mL of blood before epidural anesthesia had regressed. The investigator speculated that residual lidocaine in the lumbar CSF was transferred to the brain as a consequence of an increase in lumbar CSF pressure and reduced CSF volume produced by the patch. (*Editors' note:* One of us [DHC] has observed one case of transient, total blindness after the rapid, bolus injection of 30 mL of epidural saline after vaginal delivery in a patient who had experienced UDP during labor. The blindness resolved after 15 to 20 minutes, and subsequent ophthalmologic and neurologic examinations were normal. The etiology of the transient blindness was unclear. Nonetheless, it seems prudent to delay administration of prophylactic epidural saline or blood until the block has regressed and to avoid rapid epidural administration of blood or saline at any time.)

It is important to avoid the direct intrathecal injection of blood. Aldrete and Brown[147] reported a case of intrathecal hematoma and arachnoiditis with prolonged neurologic sequelae after prophylactic EBP. Nineteen milliliters of blood were injected through an epidural catheter that, in retrospect, was positioned in the subarachnoid space. There was considerable resistance to injection of the blood, and severe lower back pain with tinnitus accompanied the procedure.

Prophylactic Dextran Patch

Salvador et al.[148] reported the prophylactic epidural injection of 20 mL of dextran-40 in 17 patients who had experienced UDP with a 17- or 18-gauge needle. Three of the patients were parturients, and none of the 17 patients experienced PDPH. This injection was performed before regression of the local anesthetic effect. No additional studies of this technique have been reported; its safety and efficacy remain unclear.

Treatment

Early treatment of PDPH is indicated. Not only does this avert the vicious cycle of immobility, weakness, and depression, but it also may help prevent the rare case of subdural hematoma, chronic headache, or cranial nerve palsy in patients with persistent PDPH.

Psychological Support

The patient is aware that PDPH is an iatrogenic problem, and may be angry and resentful as well as depressed and tearful. It is imperative to include disclosure of the risk during the preoperative interview. A headache makes it more difficult to care for the newborn and to interact with other family members. Severe PDPH may delay discharge from the hospital and have economic consequences.[114] Unlike patients who have PDPH after nonobstetric surgery, these patients typically are healthy and do not expect to feel ill. Two patients have eloquently described their own miserable experiences with postpartum PDPH.[149,150] Not surprisingly, a retrospective study of 43 obstetric patients with PDPH showed that this complication leads to a negative attitude toward epidural anesthesia.[151]

It is essential that anesthesia providers visit the patient at least once daily to explain symptoms and prognosis, give support, and offer therapeutic options. If feasible, the patient's partner should attend these discussions. Nurses can help the patient by ensuring adequate analgesics are given on a regular schedule and by teaching alternative breastfeeding techniques, such as the lateral horizontal position.

The anesthesia provider and nurses should write detailed notes in the patient's record. After discharge, follow-up telephone conversations should be documented. A headache associated with neuraxial anesthesia was the third most common reason for litigation among obstetric cases in the ASA Closed-Claims Project database after maternal death and neonatal brain damage.[52] This fact should dispel any notion that postpartum PDPH is a trivial complaint.

Posture

In most cases, PDPH presents with a postural component. Significant relief should occur when the patient assumes the horizontal position. However, there is no evidence that remaining supine for a prolonged period treats or shortens the duration of the headache. The prone position relieves PDPH in some patients, presumably because increased intraabdominal pressure results in an increase in CSF pressure. Unfortunately, this position is not comfortable for many patients, especially those who had a cesarean delivery.

Hydration

Enhanced oral hydration remains a popular therapy initiated by most anesthesiologists for parturients with PDPH, but there is no evidence that vigorous hydration has any therapeutic benefit in a patient with normal fluid intake. However, no patient with PDPH should be allowed to become dehydrated because of the increased fluid demands of breast milk formation and CSF production.

Pharmacologic Treatment

A safe and effective drug therapy for PDPH would be very useful, even if relief is transient. The current gold standard therapy, an EBP, is not appropriate or effective in all patients. Katz and Beilin[152] published a detailed review regarding alternatives to EBP for treatment of PDPH; a consensus report from a multisociety international working group, summarizing the diagnosis and management of PDPH was published in 2024.[153]

A 2015 systematic review of pharmacologic therapies for treatment of PDPH evaluated studies using caffeine, gabapentin, hydrocortisone, theophylline, sumatriptan, adrenocorticotropic hormone, pregabalin, and cosyntropin.[154] Participants in the studies were not limited to obstetric patients. Of the drugs included in this study, caffeine and theophylline seemed most beneficial for the treatment of PDPH. The evidence was inconclusive for sumatriptan, adrenocorticotropic hormone, pregabalin, and cosyntropin. The authors noted that the results of the analysis should be interpreted with caution because of the inability to assess risk for bias and the small sample sizes of the studies included in their study.[154]

Caffeine

Caffeine has been used to treat PDPH for many years. In the systematic review,[154] two randomized trials comparing caffeine with placebo with different routes of administration but at equipotent doses were identified. Caffeine transiently reduced the number of participants with PDPH at 4 hours compared with placebo but not beyond, and also decreased the need for a conservative supplementary therapeutic medication.

Caffeine is a cerebral vasoconstrictor, and one study demonstrated a reduction of cerebral blood flow after intravenous administration of caffeine sodium benzoate for the treatment of PDPH.[155] Caffeine also increases CSF production by stimulating sodium-potassium pumps.[156] However, caffeine is also a potent central nervous system stimulant. Published case reports have described seizures after intravenous[157] and oral administration[158] of caffeine for the treatment of PDPH in postpartum patients.

To our knowledge, there are no reports of adverse effects on the infant after maternal administration of one or two doses of caffeine for the treatment of PDPH. Out of caution, one author recommended limiting the total dose of caffeine to 900 mg in a 24-hour period.[159] The US Centers for Disease Control and Prevention recommend limiting the dose to 300 mg in breastfeeding women.[160] Long-term caffeine therapy cannot be recommended.

Theophylline

Theophylline, a methylxanthine, has also been used for the management of PDPH. Although several studies have demonstrated that theophylline results in lower pain scores than either placebo or acetaminophen, none have included obstetric patients.[154] Additionally, theophylline is not commonly used for the management of PDPH because of its narrow safety profile.

Sumatriptan

Sumatriptan is a serotonin receptor agonist with cerebral vasoconstrictor properties that is administered subcutaneously for the treatment of migraine headaches. Side effects include pain at the injection site and, uncommonly, chest tightness and coronary artery vasospasm. Carp et al.[161] reported that the administration of sumatriptan 6 mg resulted in complete resolution of PDPH in four of six patients. Connelly et al.[162] randomized 10 patients with severe PDPH scheduled for EBP to receive sumatriptan 6 mg or placebo. After 1 hour, only one patient in each group had significant relief; the authors concluded that sumatriptan was not effective in treating PDPH.

Adrenocorticotropic Hormone and Analogs

The use of adrenocorticotropic hormone (ACTH) for the treatment of PDPH was first reported in a 1994 letter.[163] Subsequently, anecdotal reports have described different regimens of either intramuscular or intravenously administered ACTH or the synthetic drugs cosyntropin or tetracosactrin acetate. Mood elevation, antiinflammatory effects, increased endorphin levels, and augmented intravascular volume are postulated as possible mechanisms of action in the relief of headache following ACTH administration. To date, the only randomized clinical trial of ACTH treatment in parturients involved 18 postpartum women who had PDPH after spinal anesthesia or UDP.[164] There was no difference in the severity of headache or the requirement for EBP between women receiving tetracosactrin acetate 1 mg intramuscularly and those who received saline-placebo.

In a small, prospective, nonblinded, randomized trial of 28 nonpregnant patients with severe PDPH, Hanling et al.[165] evaluated the efficacy of intravenous cosyntropin as an alternative to EBP for the treatment of refractory or severe PDPH. An EBP showed a significant reduction of pain and improved function compared with cosyntropin on day 1; however, cosyntropin demonstrated similar efficacy to EBP immediately after treatment and at days 3 and 7 after treatment. The number of patients who returned to the emergency department for further treatment was greater in the cosyntropin group than the EBP group (60% versus 8%, respectively).[165] Pancaro et al.[127] also assessed the need for EBP after treatment of PDPH with cosyntropin following UDP. In patients exposed to cosyntropin, the incidence of EBP was significantly higher than in those not exposed to cosyntropin (56% versus 28%; OR 3.20; 95% CI, 1.52 to 6.74; $P = .002$). Given current evidence, we do not recommend ACTH therapy as the first-line treatment of PDPH.

Miscellaneous Medications

Other agents evaluated for their effectiveness in reducing PDPH symptoms include pregabalin, methylergonovine, hydrocortisone, and gabapentin. Randomized clinical trials have been conducted with intravenous hydrocortisone[166] and oral pregabalin.[167] In a nonblinded study, Noyan et al.[166] evaluated 60 parturients who developed PDPH after spinal anesthesia and were randomly assigned to receive intravenous hydrocortisone (200-mg loading dose followed by 100 mg three times daily for 2 days) or conventional therapy (bed rest, hydration, and scheduled acetaminophen with meperidine). Patients who received hydrocortisone had a 50% reduction in headache severity as assessed by visual analog scale (VAS)

pain scores at 6 to 48 hours. Huseyinoglu et al.[167] randomized 40 patients with PDPH after lumbar puncture to receive pregabalin (150 mg daily for 2 days followed by 300 mg for 3 days) or a placebo; pain scores and oral analgesic requirements were lower in the treatment group.

Use of gabapentin or methylergonovine has been reported only in case series.[168] Efficacy and side effects (maternal and neonatal) are unclear. All four drugs require further study before they can be recommended for therapy for PDPH.

Epidural Morphine

Eldor et al.[169] reported six nonobstetric patients whose PDPH headaches were successfully treated with epidural morphine 3.5 to 4.5 mg. The study has not been repeated and there are not enough data to support its use.

Epidural or Intrathecal Saline

The use of epidural or intrathecal fluids to treat PDPH preceded the use of EBP. Intrathecal injection of fluid was first described by Jacobaeus and Frumerie[170] in 1923, and epidural injection of saline was reported by Rice and Dabbs in 1950.[171] These first reports were in conjunction with research attempting to understand the pathophysiology of PDPH, and they demonstrated transient elevations of CSF pressure after fluid injection. Subsequently, there has been sporadic interest in using injections of fluids (other than blood) into the neuraxial space to treat PDPH.

Usubiaga et al.[172] injected 10 to 30 mL of saline through a lumbar epidural catheter in 11 nonobstetric patients with a PDPH after spinal anesthesia in whom 48 hours of conservative therapy had failed. Immediate relief of headache was observed in 10 patients, and the relief was permanent in 8 patients. However, the investigators did not comment whether other therapies (e.g., supine posture, abdominal binder, analgesics) were continued. In a quasirandomized trial, 43 parturients with PDPH after UDP during an epidural procedure or after spinal anesthesia with a 25-gauge needle were assigned to receive a 30-mL lumbar epidural saline bolus or a 10-mL lumbar EBP.[173] Forty-two patients had dramatic relief of their symptoms in the first hour after the intervention; however, 12 of the 21 (57%) patients who had received saline had return of the PDPH in the next 24 hours.

Prolonged epidural saline infusion may provide better therapy for PDPH symptoms than therapy with a single bolus. In a retrospective study that included both obstetric and nonobstetric patients, patients who received a continuous epidural saline infusion for 4 days had a lower incidence of PDPH, and the headache was less severe, than patients who received conservative therapy.[174] This therapy, however, may not be practical in hospital settings in which women are discharged 1 or 2 days after delivery. Two case reports described the use of epidural saline infusion for parturients with an UDP whose PDPH symptoms returned after EBP therapy.[175,176] The rate of infusion (15 to 25 mL/h) was limited by the onset of pain in the back, legs, and eyes. Although both saline techniques offer only temporary relief, these options might be considered for patients who have a contraindication to EBP therapy.

Epidural Blood Patch

Efficacy. The EBP is regarded by many as the gold standard therapy for PDPH. Although reported in third person, Gormley, in 1960, is credited with performing the first successful EBP.[177] He described relief of PDPH symptoms in seven patients after epidural administration of only 2 to 3 mL of blood. However, this report was largely ignored until 1970, when DiGiovanni and Dunbar[178] described the immediate and permanent cure of PDPH in 41 of 45 patients in whom 10 mL of autologous blood was injected into the epidural space. Their success led to the widespread adoption of this technique for the relief of PDPH.

In early case series, the reported success rate of EBP therapy for PDPH was between 89% and 91%.[178,179] Safa-Tisseront et al.[180] reviewed their experience with EBP therapy over a 12-year period ($n = 504$ patients, including 78 obstetric patients). Complete relief of PDPH was obtained in 75%, partial relief occurred in 18%, and treatment failed in 7% of patients. The investigators noted a significantly higher failure rate of EBP after large-gauge needle puncture of the dura. The difference in early reports and more modern audits of PDPH and EBP success may be related to differences in the studied population, timing of EBP, blood volume injected, or the duration of follow-up after EBP therapy.

In studies limited to obstetric patients, the published success rates of EBP have been even less encouraging. Stride and Cooper[82] noted complete and permanent relief of PDPH in 64% of patients after one EBP procedure. In a retrospective study, Tomala et al.[181] identified 212 patients requiring an EBP. Of these, 55 (25.9%) had a failed EBP. Factors associated with a failed EBP were EBP performed less than 48 hours following injury and distance from the skin to the epidural space > 5.5 cm. In a prospective, multicenter, international cohort study, Gupta et al.[182] evaluated factors associated with failed EBP for the treatment of PDPH in parturients who had UDP. Failed EBP was defined as headache intensity numeric rating scale (NRS) score ≥ 7 in the upright position at 4, 24, or 48 hours, or the need for a second EBP; and complete success was defined by NRS score = 0 at 0 to 48 hours after EBP. Data analysis was done on 591 (91.9%) women. Failed EBP occurred in 167 (28.3%) patients; EBP was completely successful in 195 (33.0%) patients and was partially successful in 229 (38.7%) patients; 126 women (19.8%) received a second EBP. The authors found a statistically significant association with failure in patients with a history of migraines, when the UDP occurred between lumbar levels L1 to L3 as compared with L3 to L5, and when the EBP was performed less than 48 hours compared with 48 hours or more after UDP (Box 30.2).

A 2010 systematic review[142] identified three randomized trials comparing EBP to either a sham procedure or conservative treatment. All three studies found a reduction in headache rate in the treatment group. Seebacher et al.[183] randomized 12 heterogeneous patients with PDPH to receive an EBP with 10 to 20 mL of blood or a sham patch procedure. Five of six patients receiving an EBP had complete relief of

> **BOX 30.2   Risk Factors for Failed Epidural Blood Patch After Unintentional Dural Puncture in Parturients**
>
> History of migraine headaches
> Short interval between accidental dural puncture and epidural blood patch (<24–48 h)
> Skin to epidural space distance > 5.5 cm
> Unintentional dural puncture at cephalad lumbar levels (L1–L3)

From Gupta A, Van de Velde M, Magnuson A, et al. Factors associated with failed epidural blood patch after accidental dural puncture in obstetrics: a prospective, multicentre, international cohort study. *Br J Anaesth*. 2022;129:758–766.

headache symptoms at 24 hours, while none of the sham procedure patients had relief. Sandesc et al.[184] described a randomized trial of 32 obstetric and nonobstetric patients with PDPH symptoms for a minimum of 24 hours; subjects were randomly assigned to receive conservative therapy or an EBP. The primary outcome was headache VAS pain scores at 2 and 24 hours. At 2 hours, the mean ± standard deviation (SD) VAS score for the conservative therapy group was 8.2 ± 1.4 cm compared with 1.0 ± 0.2 cm for the group receiving an EBP. This difference remained at 24 hours. In the largest trial to date, van Kooten et al.[185] randomized 40 subjects with PDPH for 1 to 7 days to receive either conservative therapy or an EBP using 15 to 20 mL of autologous blood. The primary outcome was headache 24 hours after intervention, but patients were observed for 1 week after therapy. The incidence of headache at 24 hours was 58% in the EBP group compared with 90% in the conservative therapy group. At 1 week, the difference widened, with a 16% incidence of headache in the EBP group compared with 86% in the conservative group. In summary, administration of an autologous EBP, although not perfect, often dramatically relieves this debilitating condition and, at present, it is the therapy with the greatest likelihood of success.

Epidural blood patch volume. The optimal volume of injected blood remains controversial. Szeinfeld et al.[186] used a gamma camera to observe the epidural spread of technetium-labeled red blood cells during and after EBP. They injected blood until pain occurred in the back, buttocks, or legs. The mean ± SD blood volume injected was 14.8 ± 1.7 mL and the mean ± SD spread was 9.0 ± 2.0 spinal segments. Blood spread more readily in the cephalad than in the caudad direction. The EBP relieved the headache in all 10 patients. The investigators concluded that 12 to 15 mL of blood should be a sufficient patch volume for most patients.

The best evidence to date is an international, multicenter study by Paech et al.,[187] who randomized 121 women after UDP with a Tuohy needle (16- to 18-gauge) to receive an EBP with 15, 20, or 30 mL of blood. Partial or complete relief of headache (the primary outcome) occurred in 61%, 73%, and 67% of those who received 15, 20, or 30 mL of blood, respectively. However, complete relief of headache was achieved by only 10%, 32%, and 26% of women in these same groups. The rate of complete headache relief was greater in the 20-mL than in the 15-mL group; there was no difference between the 20- and 30-mL groups. Thus, the investigators concluded that 20 mL of autologous blood is the optimal volume for an EBP. This suggestion is supported by a single-institution review of 466 epidural patches performed over 15 years in obstetric patients in which the mean ± SD blood patch volume was 20.5 ± 5.4 mL.[188] A 2011 survey demonstrated that most North American anesthesiologists inject 20 mL of blood.[189]

Beards et al.[190] performed MRI studies after the performance of an EBP (18 to 20 mL) in five patients. Similar to Szeinfeld et al.,[186] they noted that the injected blood spread over three to five segments in a predominantly cephalad direction. All patients had an extensive hematoma in subcutaneous fat, and some also had displacement of nerve roots and/or evidence of intrathecal blood. A thick layer of mature clot had formed by 7 hours, but the clot had broken up into smaller clots by 18 hours. These findings may help explain the back pain and occasional nerve root pain that occur after EBP therapy.

In another MRI study, Vakharia et al.[191] noted compression of the thecal sac and a mean spread over 4.6 spinal segments after a lumbar epidural injection of 20 mL of blood. Djurhuus et al.[192] employed CT epidurography in four patients immediately and 24 hours after an 18-mL EBP. Initial images showed adherence of clot to the dura in three patients as well as dural compression in two patients, but there was no evidence of compression at 24 hours.

Using a goat model, DiGiovanni et al.[193] examined the microscopic appearance of the dura as late as 6 months after dural puncture. Some study animals received a 2-mL EBP in addition to dural puncture. The investigators concluded that the EBP acted as a gelatinous tampon that produced no harmful tissue reaction.

Mechanism of action.
The mechanism of EBP for relief of PDPH is unclear. Pain relief is often rapid, but CSF volume is not restored immediately. Thus, there must be another explanation for the immediate relief of headache besides "patching" of the dural puncture. Carrie[194] hypothesized that epidural injection of blood increases lumbar CSF pressure, an action that restores intracranial CSF pressure and decreases symptoms. Increased CSF pressure also may result in reflex cerebral vasoconstriction. Coombs and Hooper[195] demonstrated that EBP resulted in a threefold increase in lumbar CSF pressure. Further, they noted that 15 minutes later, lumbar CSF pressure was sustained at greater than 70% of the peak pressure observed after the injection of blood. Ultrasonographic examination of the optic nerve sheath diameter (a noninvasive measurement that correlates with ICP) in 10 patients with PDPH demonstrated increased measurements after EBP.[196] The sheath diameter increased 10 minutes after an EBP with 17 to 26 mL of blood and was sustained over the 20-hour study period. The only patient whose EBP failed to successfully relieve the PDPH did not have the same increase in optic nerve sheath diameter.

MRI and CT studies have shown that the epidural blood is largely resorbed or broken up 18 to 24 hours after the procedure.[190] It is unlikely that the increase in CSF pressure is sustained or that the blood acts as a mechanical plug to block CSF leak for a prolonged duration. The blood applied to the hole in the dura may initiate an inflammatory reaction that facilitates puncture site repair and closure. It is possible, and even likely, that an EBP ameliorates PDPH by several mechanisms.

Timing.
The optimal timing for administration of an EBP has not been adequately studied. Observational studies suggest that failure is more likely if the EBP is performed within 24[180] or 48 hours[182,187] of the dural puncture. Booth et al.[188] demonstrated a strong positive correlation between success of the EBP and the interval from the dural puncture or onset of PDPH to performance of the EBP. It is unclear, however, whether this finding is a result of selection bias. Early-onset PDPH (often resulting from dural puncture with a large-gauge needle) is likely to be more severe and more difficult to treat. Alternatively, a large CSF leak may displace the clot. Partial healing of the dura may have already occurred if an EBP is delayed, a possibility that may explain the better outcome of a delayed patch procedure.

Technique.
The anesthesia provider should thoroughly explain the risks and benefits of the blood patch procedure to the patient, and the patient should give consent for the procedure. An EBP can be accomplished on an outpatient basis. Ideally, the environment for the procedure is one conducive to postpartum patients who may have accompanying family and a newborn. Contraindications to the administration of an EBP are related to complications of placing a needle in the central neuraxis or the injection of blood into the epidural space; they include (1) known coagulopathy (e.g., concurrent pharmacologic anticoagulation), (2) local cutaneous infection or untreated systemic infection, (3) increased ICP caused by a space-occupying lesion, and (4) patient refusal. Transient bradycardia has been observed after administration of an EBP, and some anesthesia providers may choose to establish intravenous access and monitor the electrocardiogram in selected patients.[197]

The EBP procedure should employ sterile measures equivalent to those used for the administration of any neuraxial procedure. The lateral position is usually more comfortable than the sitting position for patients with severe PDPH. If the anesthesia provider is uncertain about the location of the dural puncture, the more caudad interspace should be chosen. The epidural space is identified in the usual manner. Using meticulous sterile technique (including skin preparation and draping, and donning of a face mask and sterile gloves), an assistant withdraws the desired volume of blood (usually 10 to 25 mL) into a syringe. This autologous blood is injected slowly into the epidural space through the epidural needle; the injection is terminated if severe back, leg, or neck pain or pressure occurs. Sometimes slowing the injection rate leads to resolution of the back pain. Jehovah's Witness patients may accept an EBP procedure if a technique is used that keeps blood in continuity with the circulation.[198]

Occasionally a few drops of CSF are encountered on entering the epidural space, leading to doubt about correct needle placement.[199] One can either repeat the epidural needle placement, or a small test dose of a local anesthetic agent can be administered, sufficient to cause a rapid onset of spinal anesthesia. If no block results, the EBP can be performed. Real-time ultrasound-guided and fluoroscopically guided EBP has been described and should be considered when difficulty with epidural needle placement is anticipated.[200]

After the procedure, the patient should rest quietly in the supine position for 1 to 2 hours.[201] Subsequently, the patient may resume ambulation, but should avoid vigorous physical activity for several days. It would be wise for the patient to avoid the Valsalva maneuver and heavy lifting. A stool softener should be considered. Most patients report almost instantaneous relief of headache symptoms, although relief is delayed for 6 to 8 hours in some patients. The patient may continue to have neck and back fullness over the next 24 hours.[187] The back pain can continue up to 5 days after the procedure. Patients should be counseled to immediately report fever, severe back pain, or radiating lower extremity pain. The anesthesia provider should contact the patient after the EBP procedure.

The EBP may be repeated if the initial patch fails to relieve pain. Often the second patch is successful. Although not adequately studied, it seems reasonable to wait 24 hours before repeating an EBP procedure to allow the first procedure adequate time to work. The diagnosis should be reconsidered if headache persists after two failed EBP procedures. Consultation by a neurologist may be appropriate when a PDPH fails to respond to two EBP procedures and should definitely be requested if there is any doubt about the diagnosis. Imaging of the head should be considered to exclude other causes of a headache.

Complications. Ong et al.[202] reported that the success of neuraxial anesthesia/analgesia was impaired in women with a prior history of UDP with or without EBP therapy. However, this conclusion has been refuted by follow-up studies in both obstetric patients[203] and nonobstetric patients.[204]

Although EBP therapy is the most reliable method of relieving PDPH symptoms, adverse outcomes are associated with the procedure. These adverse events can be categorized into two broad groups: infectious/hematologic and neurologic.

Infectious/hematologic complications. Conventional wisdom holds that the patient should be afebrile at the time of the EBP procedure. Many anesthesia providers believe that it is wise to avoid the epidural injection of blood in the presence of systemic infection. Meningitis has been reported after an EBP procedure.[39] After conservative measures have failed, the optimal treatment of a febrile patient with severe, persistent PDPH is controversial. Epidural infusion of saline involves the use of an indwelling epidural catheter for many hours, which also may be undesirable in a febrile patient. A patch using dextran-40 may be an alternative in febrile patients, but further experience is needed in healthy patients before this technique can be recommended.

The presence of high fever and/or other evidence of sepsis contraindicate the performance of an EBP procedure. However, we do not believe that a low-grade fever of known etiology is an absolute contraindication to EBP, provided the patient is receiving appropriate antibiotic therapy. Management should be individualized, and the known benefits of EBP should be weighed against the unknown risk for infection.

The risks associated with EBP therapy in the presence of human immunodeficiency virus (HIV) infection have been debated (see Chapter 36). However, the central nervous system is infected with HIV at the time of primary infection; therefore, it seems unlikely that the injection of autologous blood into the epidural space would alter progression of the disease. Successful use of EBP therapy, without sequelae, has been reported in patients with acquired immunodeficiency syndrome (AIDS) or who are HIV positive.[205]

The incidence of cancer during pregnancy is increasing, likely secondary to advancing maternal age. The development of PDPH in this population has raised a theoretical concern about seeding the neuraxial space with neoplastic cells if a blood patch procedure is performed. This concern should be discussed with the patient and her oncologist before the procedure. Bucklin et al.[206] reported the conservative management of a woman with acute leukemia and PDPH; the investigators discussed the therapeutic options for this immunocompromised patient. The use of epidural fibrin glue was reported in a nonobstetric patient with metastatic breast cancer and PDPH,[207] whereas an EBP was performed for PDPH in a young woman with rhabdomyosarcoma.[208]

Neurologic complications. Serious or permanent problems after EBP therapy are rare. Diaz and Weed[209] summarized case reports of adverse neurologic complications after EBP procedures. These authors identified 26 reports published between 1966 and 2004 and stratified the complications into neurologic, neurovascular, or inflammatory events. The events occurring in obstetric patients included lumbovertebral syndrome (defined as low back pain with neurologic impairment of the lower extremities), subdural hematoma, arachnoiditis, radicular back pain, pneumocephalus, seizures, and acute meningeal irritation. Compressive complications (e.g., lumbovertebral syndrome, subdural hematoma, cauda equina syndrome) were associated with larger EBP volume (mean of 35 mL) than noncompressive complications (mean 17 mL). Cranial nerve palsy symptoms that were present before EBP administration did not uniformly resolve. The delay in performing the EBP may have been a significant factor. Two patients who were treated within 4 days of the onset of PDPH symptoms recovered within 6 weeks, whereas three patients treated on days 9 to 11 had palsy that persisted for 3 to 4 months. Two obstetric patients experienced new facial nerve palsies, which manifested as facial weakness after the administration of an EBP.[209]

Abouleish et al.[179] reported the results of the long-term evaluation of 118 patients who had received an EBP. Back pain was the most common complication; it occurred during the first 48 hours in 35% of patients and persisted in 16% of patients, with a mean duration of 27 days. These investigators also noted cases of neck pain, lower extremity radicular pain, and transient temperature elevation.

Epidural space scarring is also a possibility after placement of an EBP. Although subsequent epidural analgesia is generally successful (see earlier discussion),[204] Collier[210] reported two cases of unsuccessful epidural analgesia related to suspected scarring of the epidural space. In both women, the initial epidural catheter placement was complicated by UDP and PDPH treated with EBP. During a subsequent pregnancy, epidural catheter placement was complicated by inadequate analgesia, and an epidurogram revealed limited spread of the contrast media, suggesting epidural space scarring.

The development of an inflammatory reaction to epidural blood can cause acute arachnoiditis, an entity that can present several days after EBP.[211] This phenomenon is believed to be caused by free radical damage to spinal root nerves in the intrathecal space after hemoglobin degradation. Obstetric patients with this entity who required analgesic therapy for prolonged periods have been reported.[212] The diagnosis is made with a presenting history of severe back pain, often with radicular pain, and characteristic MRI findings such as nerve root clumping in the intrathecal space and adhesions between nerve roots.

The occurrence of new neurologic symptoms appearing after an EBP should prompt consideration of the presence of other intracranial pathology such as cortical vein thrombosis or subdural hematoma.[54] Other symptoms may include (1) mental deterioration caused by increased ICP from an intracranial tumor[213] and (2) seizures caused by late-onset eclampsia or PRES.[214]

Diaz[215] described a woman in whom permanent paraparesis and cauda equina syndrome developed after an EBP with 30 mL of blood injected slowly and without symptoms. Low back pain and leg pain developed after the EBP procedure, and later the patient also experienced incontinence. Twelve days after the procedure, a subdural hematoma at L2 to L4 was diagnosed and surgically treated. Six months later, the patient still had marked symptoms. Although a larger volume of blood than usual was injected, the technique appears to have been within normal practice standards. Other long-term sequelae reported in obstetric patients include a cerebral ischemic event after two blood patches that resulted in permanent hemianopsia[216] and a calcified EBP leading to chronic back pain.[217]

Alternatives to Epidural Blood Patch

Alternatives to an EBP may be considered if a blood patch is contraindicated or fails. In extreme cases, surgery may be needed to close the dural tear.[152]

Sphenopalatine ganglion block. The sphenopalatine ganglion (SPG) block has become a useful adjunct in the treatment of cluster and migraine headaches. This parasympathetic ganglion is located in the pterygopalatine fossa, immediately adjacent to the posterior component of the middle turbinate of the nose (Fig. 30.4).[218] Blocking the ganglion inhibits

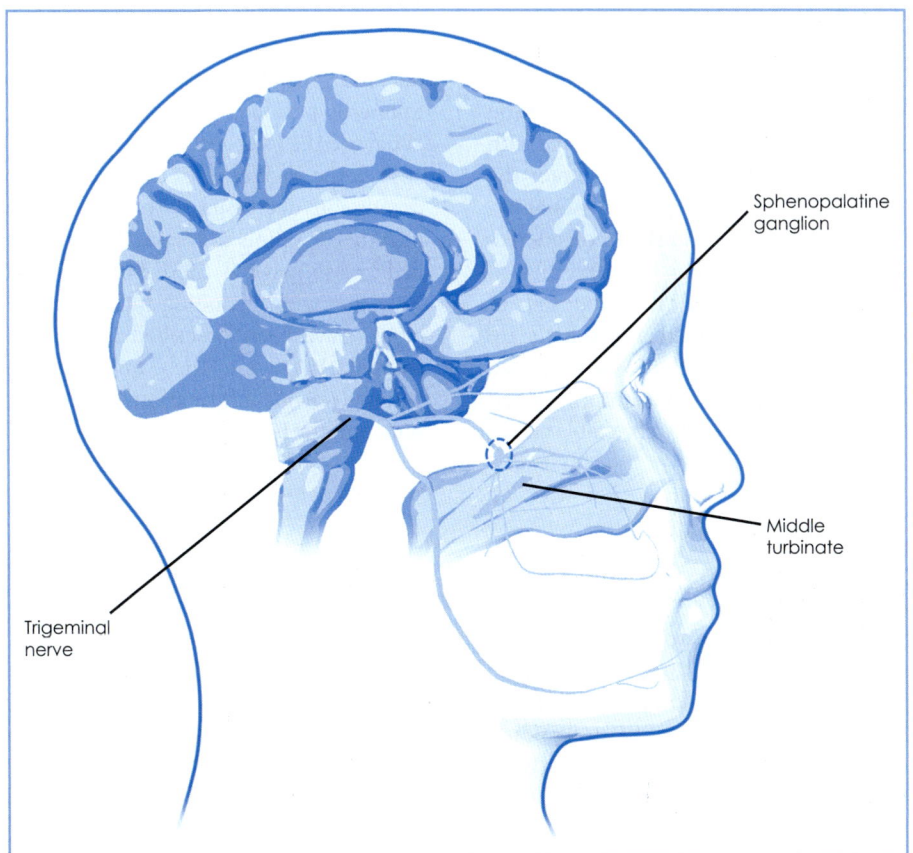

Fig. 30.4 Anatomy of the Sphenopalatine Ganglion Block. Illustration by Naveen Nathan, MD, NorthShore University HealthSystem, University of Chicago Pritzker School of Medicine, Evanston, IL.

parasympathetic outflow to cerebral vasculature and prevents vasodilation. A simple technique, the operator places a cotton pledget soaked with local anesthetic in the nose and allows diffusion across the nasal mucosa. Data on the efficacy of SPG block to treat PDPH are inconsistent. Cohen et al.[219] retrospectively compared women who received EBP ($n = 39$) with those who received SPG block ($n = 42$). They found better relief in the SPG block group at 30 and 60 minutes and similar difference in relief at 1, 2, and 7 days later. Prospective study is required to evaluate the role of SPG block in the treatment of PDPH,[153] although it is a low-risk procedure that may be useful in providing symptom relief for those with severe, early symptoms following dural puncture.

Dextran or gelatin patch.   Dextran-40 and gelatin-based solutions, including Gelfoam and Plasmion, have been substituted for blood in epidural patches.[148,220] These solutions were chosen as alternatives to blood owing to relative contraindications to injection of blood. The use of these agents appears to be more common in countries outside North America. In an observational study of 56 patients, Barrios-Alarcon et al.[221] reported that epidural administration of 20 to 30 mL of dextran-40 was safe and effective for the relief of PDPH; all headaches were relieved permanently. The only side effect was a transient discomfort or burning sensation at the time of injection in six patients. Some physicians have treated intractable PDPH successfully by performing a dextran-40 patch followed by epidural infusion of dextran at 3 mL/h for 5 to 12 hours.[222]

Information on neurotoxicity of these materials is scant; Chanimov et al.[223] did not observe neurotoxicity after infusion of dextran-40 or polygeline, a gelatin powder, into the rat intrathecal space. However, further information is needed before these materials can be widely adopted for epidural administration in humans. From MRI studies in patients with an EBP, we can anticipate that some dextran will enter the subarachnoid space. The small but definite risk for anaphylaxis after the injection of dextran also must be considered, although the risk appears minimal with dextran-40.

Fibrin sealant patch.   Fibrin sealant is composed of fibrinogen and thrombin. Several commercial products are prepared from human pooled plasma. Products may also contain antifibrinolytics, such as animal aprotinin.[224] When injected, these products form a firm, nonretractable fibrin clot. Epidural injection of fibrin glue in rats produces a sustained rise in CSF pressure comparable to the increase that occurs after injection of blood.[225] Fibrin sealant has been evaluated for its effectiveness in preventing dural leaks after spinal surgery.[226] An epidural fibrin glue patch has been used successfully to treat recurrent PDPH, spontaneous intracranial hypotension,[227] and CSF leak after long-term intrathecal catheterization.[228] In the future, fibrin glue may have a role in patients with intractable PDPH, but further study is required before it can be recommended for routine use.

Surgery.   There are rare reports of curative surgical closure of a dural rent for intractable PDPH. In one case, the interval between dural puncture and surgery was 5 years.[229]

Summary of Treatment

The parturient with PDPH should be actively managed with scheduled analgesics and should receive psychological support as the mother cares for the newborn and manages her symptoms. If the headache is severe, the physician can consider additional agents, such as caffeine, or proceed directly to an EBP. Epidural administration of fluids other than blood, such as saline or dextran, typically is not first-line therapy but may be considered if there are contraindications to the epidural injection of autologous blood or if an EBP procedure fails. The accuracy of PDPH diagnosis must always be considered when atypical symptoms present or when therapy fails.

UNANSWERED QUESTIONS

Important knowledge about PDPH is still lacking. A large, detailed prospective study of PDPH and EBP, with a long follow-up period (e.g., 1 year), is needed in obstetric patients. What are the long-term effects of both PDPH and EBP therapy? Is the incidence of chronic symptoms and postpartum depression decreased with the performance of EBP? Can intrathecal saline decrease the incidence of PDPH and/or EBP? If so, what is the optimal volume of administration? New therapies, including intravenous cosyntropin and SPG block, have been described, but have not been rigorously studied. Answers to these questions are needed to give our patients reliable information, a sound basis for informed consent, and the best possible care.

KEY POINTS

- Dural puncture is only one of many causes of postpartum headache, although many are quick to blame postpartum headaches on dural puncture. A detailed history and physical examination, as well as indicated neuroimaging, should ensure diagnostic accuracy.
- A patient with PDPH experiences an exacerbation of symptoms when moved from the horizontal to the upright position, possibly owing to decreased intracranial pressure and secondary cerebral vasodilation, which affect pain-sensitive intracranial structures.

- Anesthesia providers should use a small-gauge (24-gauge or smaller), noncutting (pencil-point) spinal needle whenever possible to decrease the risk for PDPH.
- PDPH has been associated with long-term sequelae and major complications.
- No therapies reliably prevent the development of PDPH after unintentional dural puncture with an epidural needle.
- The initial therapy for PDPH consists of psychological support and scheduled oral analgesics. Although dehydration

should be avoided, no evidence supports a role for vigorous hydration for prophylaxis or therapy for PDPH.

- The gold standard therapy for PDPH headache is an autologous epidural blood patch (EBP). A second EBP may be performed—and typically is successful—if the first one fails. If the second procedure fails, alternative diagnoses should be excluded. Other therapies have not proved as safe or as effective as the EBP for treatment of PDPH.

REFERENCES

1. Goldszmidt E, Kern R, Chaput A, Macarthur A. The incidence and etiology of postpartum headaches: a prospective cohort study. *Can J Anaesth*. 2005;52:971–977.
2. Turner DP, Smitherman TA, Eisenach JC, et al. Predictors of headache before, during, and after pregnancy: a cohort study. *Headache*. 2012;52:348–362.
3. Saurel-Cubizolles MJ, Romito P, Lelong N, Ancel PY. Women's health after childbirth: a longitudinal study in France and Italy. *BJOG*. 2000;107:1202–1209.
4. Headache Classification Committee of the International Headache Society (IHS). The international classification of headache disorders, 3rd edition. *Cephalalgia*. 2018;38:1–211.
5. Shapiro RE. Caffeine and headaches. *Neurol Sci*. 2007;28:S179–S183.
6. Benhamou D, Hamza J, Ducot B. Postpartum headache after epidural analgesia without dural puncture. *Int J Obstet Anesth*. 1995;4:17–20.
7. Stella CL, Jodicke CD, How HY, et al. Postpartum headache: is your work-up complete? *Am J Obstet Gynecol*. 2007;196:e1–e7.
8. Burch R, Rizzoli P, Loder E. The prevalence and impact of migraine and severe headache in the United States: updated age, sex, and socioeconomic-specific estimates from government health surveys. *Headache*. 2021;61:60–68.
9. Sances G, Granella F, Nappi RE, et al. Course of migraine during pregnancy and postpartum: a prospective study. *Cephalalgia*. 2003;23:197–205.
10. Grossman TB, Robbins MS, Govindappagari S, Dayal AK. Delivery outcomes of patients with acute migraine in pregnancy: a retrospective study. *Headache*. 2017;57:605–611.
11. Sibai BM. Diagnosis, prevention, and management of eclampsia. *Obstet Gynecol*. 2005;105:402–410.
12. Pande AR, Ando K, Ishikura R, et al. Clinicoradiological factors influencing the reversibility of posterior reversible encephalopathy syndrome: a multicenter study. *Radiat Med*. 2006;24:659–668.
13. Hinchey J, Chaves C, Appignani B, et al. A reversible posterior leukoencephalopathy syndrome. *N Engl J Med*. 1996;334:494–500.
14. Lin E, Lantos JE, Strauss SB, et al. Brain imaging of patients with COVID-19: findings at an academic institution during the height of the outbreak in New York City. *AJNR Am J Neuroradiol*. 2020;41:2001–2008.
15. Mayama M, Uno K, Tano S, et al. Incidence of posterior reversible encephalopathy syndrome in eclamptic and patients with preeclampsia with neurologic symptoms. *Am J Obstet Gynecol*. 2016;215:e1–e5.
16. Brady E, Parikh NS, Navi BB, et al. The imaging spectrum of posterior reversible encephalopathy syndrome: a pictorial review. *Clin Imaging*. 2017;47:80–89.
17. Torrillo TM, Bronster DJ, Beilin Y. Delayed diagnosis of posterior reversible encephalopathy syndrome (PRES) in a parturient with preeclampsia after inadvertent dural puncture. *Int J Obstet Anesth*. 2007;16:171–174.
18. Tetsuka S, Nonaka H. Importance of correctly interpreting magnetic resonance imaging to diagnose posterior reversible encephalopathy syndrome associated with HELLP syndrome: a case report. *BMC Med Imaging*. 2017;17:35.
19. Grear KE, Bushnell CD. Stroke and pregnancy: clinical presentation, evaluation, treatment, and epidemiology. *Clin Obstet Gynecol*. 2013;56:350–359.
20. Berkhemer OA, Fransen PS, Beumer D, et al. A randomized trial of intraarterial treatment for acute ischemic stroke. *N Engl J Med*. 2015;372:11–20.
21. Goyal M, Demchuk AM, Menon BK, et al. Randomized assessment of rapid endovascular treatment of ischemic stroke. *N Engl J Med*. 2015;372:1019–1030.
22. Benjamin EJ, Blaha MJ, Chiuve SE, et al. Heart disease and stroke statistics–2017 update: a report from the American Heart Association. *Circulation*. 2017;135:e146–e603.
23. Gomez-Rios MA, Kuczkowski KM. Bilateral subdural intracranial hematoma after accidental dural puncture. *Anesthesiology*. 2012;117:646.
24. Wayhs SY, Wottrich J, Uggeri DP, Dias FS. Spontaneous acute subdural hematoma and intracerebral hemorrhage in a patient with thrombotic microangiopathy during pregnancy. *Rev Bras Ter Intensiva*. 2013;25:175–180.
25. Trager RJ, Daniels CJ, Scott ZE, Perez JA. Pregnancy and spontaneous cervical artery dissection: a propensity-matched retrospective cohort study. *J Stroke Cerebrovasc Dis*. 2023;32:107384.
26. Abdelnour LH, Kurdy M, Idris A. Systematic review of postpartum and pregnancy-related cervical artery dissection. *J Matern Fetal Neonatal Med*. 2022;35:10287–10295.
27. Ranjan R, Ken-Dror G, Sharma P. Pathophysiology, diagnosis and management of cerebral venous thrombosis: a comprehensive review. *Medicine (Baltimore)*. 2023;102:e36366.
28. Saposnik G, Barinagarrementeria F, Brown RD Jr, et al. Diagnosis and management of cerebral venous thrombosis: a statement for healthcare professionals from the American Heart Association/American Stroke Association. *Stroke*. 2011;42:1158–1192.
29. Gragasin FS, Chiarella AB. Use of an intrathecal catheter for analgesia, anesthesia, and therapy in an obstetric patient with pseudotumor cerebri syndrome. *A A Case Rep*. 2016;6:160–162.
30. Shiwlochan D, Ohanyan S, Rajput K. It is just a blood patch: considerations for patients with preexisting intracranial hypertension. *Case Rep Anesthesiol*. 2020;2020:8365296.
31. Mokri B. Spontaneous low cerebrospinal pressure/volume headaches. *Curr Neurol Neurosci Rep*. 2004;4:117–124.
32. Rohatgi VK, Robbins MS, Roytman M, Chazen JL. Spontaneous intracranial hypotension in pregnancy. *Curr Pain Headache Rep*. 2023;27:685–693.
33. Smarkusky L, DeCarvalho H, Bermudez A, Gonzalez-Quintero VH. Acute onset headache complicating labor epidural caused by intrapartum pneumocephalus. *Obstet Gynecol*. 2006;108:795–798.

34. Roderick L, Moore DC, Artru AA. Pneumocephalus with headache during spinal anesthesia. *Anesthesiology*. 1985;62:690–692.

35. Ahmad M, Bellamy S, Ott W, Mekhail R. Pneumocephalus secondary to epidural analgesia: a case report. *J Med Case Rep*. 2023;17:217.

36. Aida S, Taga K, Yamakura T, et al. Headache after attempted epidural block: the role of intrathecal air. *Anesthesiology*. 1998;88:76–81.

37. Siegel JL, Hampton K, Rabinstein AA, et al. Oxygen therapy with high-flow nasal cannula as an effective treatment for perioperative pneumocephalus: case illustrations and pathophysiological review. *Neurocrit Care*. 2018;29:366–373.

38. Hebl JR. The importance and implications of aseptic techniques during regional anesthesia. *Reg Anesth Pain Med*. 2006;31:311–323.

39. Beilin Y, Spitzer Y. Presumed group b streptococcal meningitis after epidural blood patch. *A A Case Rep*. 2015;4:163–165.

40. Baer ET. Post-dural puncture bacterial meningitis. *Anesthesiology*. 2006;105:381–393.

41. Sobol SE, Frenkiel S, Nachtigal D, et al. Clinical manifestations of sinonasal pathology during pregnancy. *J Otolaryngol*. 2001;30:24–28.

42. van Dam RM, Hu FB, Willett WC. Coffee, caffeine, and health. *N Engl J Med*. 2020;383:369–378.

43. Askmark H, Lundberg PO. Lactation headache—a new form of headache? *Cephalalgia*. 1989;9:119–122.

44. Thorley V. Lactational headache: a lactation consultant's diary. *J Hum Lact*. 1997;13:51–53.

45. Sharma R, Panda A. Ondansetron-induced headache in a parturient mimicking postdural puncture headache. *Can J Anaesth*. 2010;57:187–188.

46. Poma S, Bonomo MC, Gazzaniga G, et al. Complications of unintentional dural puncture during labour epidural analgesia: a 10-year retrospective observational study. *J Anesth Analg Crit Care*. 2023;3:42.

47. Choi PT, Galinski SE, Takeuchi L, et al. PDPH is a common complication of neuraxial blockade in parturients: a meta-analysis of obstetrical studies. *Can J Anaesth*. 2003;50: 460–469.

48. Shaikh JM, Memon A, Memon MA, Khan M. Postdural puncture headache after spinal anaesthesia for caesarean section: a comparison of 25 g Quincke, 27 g Quincke and 27 g Whitacre spinal needles. *J Ayub Med Coll Abbottabad*. 2008;20:10–13.

49. Sharma SK, Gambling DR, Joshi GP, et al. Comparison of 26-gauge Atraucan and 25-gauge Whitacre needles: insertion characteristics and complications. *Can J Anaesth*. 1995;42:706–710.

50. Pan PH, Fragneto R, Moore C, Vernon R. Incidence of postdural puncture headache and backache, and success rate of dural puncture: comparison of two spinal needle designs. *South Med J*. 2004;97:359–363.

51. Vallejo MC, Mandell GL, Sabo DP, Ramanathan S. Postdural puncture headache: a randomized comparison of five spinal needles in obstetric patients. *Anesth Analg*. 2000;91:916–920.

52. Davies JM, Posner KL, Lee LA, et al. Liability associated with obstetric anesthesia: a closed claims analysis. *Anesthesiology*. 2009;110:131–139.

53. Mims SC, Tan HS, Sun K, et al. Long-term morbidities following unintentional dural puncture in obstetric patients: a systematic review and meta-analysis. *J Clin Anesth*. 2022;79:110787.

54. Guglielminotti J, Landau R, Li G. Major neurologic complications associated with postdural puncture headache in obstetrics: a retrospective cohort study. *Anesth Analg*. 2019;129:1328–1336.

55. Van de Velde M, Schepers R, Berends N, et al. Ten years of experience with accidental dural puncture and post-dural puncture headache in a tertiary obstetric anaesthesia department. *Int J Obstet Anesth*. 2008;17:329–335.

56. Hofer JE, Scavone BM. Cranial nerve VI palsy after dural-arachnoid puncture. *Anesth Analg*. 2015;120:644–646.

57. Erol A, Topal A, Arbag H, et al. Auditory function after spinal anaesthesia: the effect of differently designed spinal needles. *Eur J Anaesthesiol*. 2009;26:416–420.

58. Lybecker H, Andersen T, Helbo-Hansen HS. The effect of epidural blood patch on hearing loss in patients with severe postdural puncture headache. *J Clin Anesth*. 1995;7:457–464.

59. Shearer VE, Jhaveri HS, Cunningham FG. Puerperal seizures after post-dural puncture headache. *Obstet Gynecol*. 1995;85:255–260.

60. Vazquez R, Johnson DW, Ahmed SU. Epidural blood patch for postdural puncture positional vertigo. *Pain Med*. 2011;12:148–151.

61. Schabel JE, Wang ED, Glass PS. Arm pain as an unusual presentation of postdural puncture intracranial hypotension. *Anesth Analg*. 2000;91:910–912.

62. Yang CP, Lee CH, Borel CO, et al. Postdural puncture headache with abdominal pain and diarrhea. *Anesth Analg*. 2005;100:879–881.

63. Lybecker H, Djernes M, Schmidt JF. Postdural puncture headache (PDPH): onset, duration, severity, and associated symptoms. An analysis of 75 consecutive patients with PDPH. *Acta Anaesthesiol Scand*. 1995;39:605–612.

64. Reamy BV. Post-epidural headache: how late can it occur? *J Am Board Fam Med*. 2009;22:202–205.

65. MacArthur C, Lewis M, Knox EG. Accidental dural puncture in obstetric patients and long term symptoms. *BMJ*. 1993;306:883–885.

66. Bakshi R, Mechtler LL, Kamran S, et al. MRI findings in lumbar puncture headache syndrome: abnormal dural-meningeal and dural venous sinus enhancement. *Clin Imaging*. 1999;23:73–76.

67. Corbonnois G, O'Neill T, Brabis-Henner A, et al. Unrecognized dural puncture during epidural analgesia in obstetrics later confirmed by brain imaging. *Ann Fr Anesth Reanim*. 2010;29:584–588.

68. Bier A. Versuche ueber cocainisirung des rueckenmarkes. *Dtsch Zeitschr Chir*. 1899;51:361–369.

69. Kunkle EC, Ray BS, Wolff HG. Experimental studies on headache: analysis of the headache associated with changes in intracranial pressure. *Arch Neurol Psychiatry*. 1943;49: 323–358.

70. Marx GF, Zemaitis MT, Orkin LR. Cerebrospinal fluid pressures during labor and obstetrical anesthesia. *Anesthesiology*. 1961;22:348–354.

71. Shah JL. Epidural pressure and postdural puncture headache in the parturient. *Int J Obstet Anesth*. 1993;2:187–189.

72. Boezaart AP. Effects of cerebrospinal fluid loss and epidural blood patch on cerebral blood flow in swine. *Reg Anesth Pain Med*. 2001;26:401–406.

73. Hattingh J, McCalden TA. Cerebrovascular effects of cerebrospinal fluid removal. *S Afr Med J*. 1978;54:780–781.

74. Grant R, Condon B, Patterson J, et al. Changes in cranial CSF volume during hypercapnia and hypocapnia. *J Neurol Neurosurg Psychiatry*. 1989;52:218–222.

75. Martins AN, Wiley JK, Myers PW. Dynamics of the cerebrospinal fluid and the spinal dura mater. *J Neurol Neurosurg Psychiatry*. 1972;35:468–473.

76. Vadhera RB, Babazade R, Suresh MS, et al. Role of transcranial Doppler measurements in postpartum patients with post-dural puncture headache: a pilot study. *Int J Obstet Anesth*. 2017;29:90–91.

77. Vandam LD, Dripps RD. Long-term follow-up of patients who received 10,098 spinal anesthetics; syndrome of decreased intracranial pressure (headache and ocular and auditory difficulties). *J Am Med Assoc*. 1956;161:586–591.

78. Amorim JA, Gomes de Barros MV, Valenca MM. Post-dural (post-lumbar) puncture headache: risk factors and clinical features. *Cephalalgia*. 2012;32:916–923.

79. Wu CL, Rowlingson AJ, Cohen SR, et al. Gender and post-dural puncture headache. *Anesthesiology*. 2006;105:613–618.

80. Delgado C, Bollag L, Van Cleve W. Neuraxial labor analgesia utilization, incidence of postdural puncture headache, and epidural blood patch placement for privately insured parturients in the United States (2008–2015). *Anesth Analg*. 2020;131:850–856.

81. Jagannathan DK, Arriaga AF, Elterman KG, et al. Effect of neuraxial technique after inadvertent dural puncture on obstetric outcomes and anesthetic complications. *Int J Obstet Anesth*. 2016;25:23–29.

82. Stride PC, Cooper GM. Dural taps revisited. A 20-year survey from Birmingham Maternity Hospital. *Anaesthesia*. 1993;48:247–255.

83. Peralta F, Higgins N, Lange E, et al. The relationship of body mass index with the incidence of postdural puncture headache in parturients. *Anesth Analg*. 2015;121:451–456.

84. Song J, Zhang T, Choy A, et al. Impact of obesity on post-dural puncture headache. *Int J Obstet Anesth*. 2017;30:5–9.

85. Seeberger MD, Kaufmann M, Staender S, et al. Repeated dural punctures increase the incidence of postdural puncture headache. *Anesth Analg*. 1996;82:302–305.

86. Hart JR, Whitacre RJ. Pencil-point needle in prevention of postspinal headache. *J Am Med Assoc*. 1951;147:657–658.

87. Santanen U, Rautoma P, Luurila H, et al. Comparison of 27-gauge (0.41-mm) Whitacre and Quincke spinal needles with respect to post-dural puncture headache and non-dural puncture headache. *Acta Anaesthesiol Scand*. 2004;48:474–479.

88. Westbrook JL, Uncles DR, Sitzman BT, Carrie LE. Comparison of the force required for dural puncture with different spinal needles and subsequent leakage of cerebrospinal fluid. *Anesth Analg*. 1994;79:769–772.

89. Sprotte G, Schedel R, Pajunk H, Pajunk H. An "atraumatic" universal needle for single-shot regional anesthesia: clinical results and a 6 year trial in over 30,000 regional anesthesias. *Reg Anaesth*. 1987;10:104–108.

90. Arevalo-Rodriguez I, Munoz L, Godoy-Casasbuenas N, et al. Needle gauge and tip designs for preventing post-dural puncture headache (PDPH). *Cochrane Database Syst Rev*. 2017;(4):CD010807.

91. Fink BR, Walker S. Orientation of fibers in human dorsal lumbar dura mater in relation to lumbar puncture. *Anesth Analg*. 1989;69:768–772.

92. Ready LB, Cuplin S, Haschke RH, Nessly M. Spinal needle determinants of rate of transdural fluid leak. *Anesth Analg*. 1989;69:457–460.

93. Cruickshank RH, Hopkinson JM. Fluid flow through dural puncture sites. An in vitro comparison of needle point types. *Anaesthesia*. 1989;44:415–418.

94. Richman JM, Joe EM, Cohen SR, et al. Bevel direction and postdural puncture headache: a meta-analysis. *Neurologist*. 2006;12:224–228.

95. Bicak M, Salik F, Akelma H. Is there an effect on the development of postdural puncture headache of dural punction made with the spinal needle in three different orientations during spinal anaesthesia applied to pregnant patients? *J Pain Res*. 2019;12:3167–3174.

96. Angle PJ, Kronberg JE, Thompson DE, et al. Dural tissue trauma and cerebrospinal fluid leak after epidural needle puncture: effect of needle design, angle, and bevel orientation. *Anesthesiology*. 2003;99:1376–1382.

97. Morley-Forster PK, Singh S, Angle P, et al. The effect of epidural needle type on postdural puncture headache: a randomized trial. *Can J Anaesth*. 2006;53:572–578.

98. Russell IF. A prospective controlled study of continuous spinal analgesia versus repeat epidural analgesia after accidental dural puncture in labour. *Int J Obstet Anesth*. 2012;21:7–16.

99. Norris MC, Leighton BL, DeSimone CA. Needle bevel direction and headache after inadvertent dural puncture. *Anesthesiology*. 1989;70:729–731.

100. Richardson MG, Wissler RN. The effects of needle bevel orientation during epidural catheter insertion in laboring parturients. *Anesth Analg*. 1999;88:352–356.

101. Hatfalvi BI. Postulated mechanisms for postdural puncture headache and review of laboratory models. Clinical experience. *Reg Anesth*. 1995;20:329–336.

102. Viitanen H, Porthan L, Viitanen M, et al. Postpartum neurologic symptoms following single-shot spinal block for labour analgesia. *Acta Anaesthesiol Scand*. 2005;49:1015–1022.

103. Kempen PM, Mocek CK. Bevel direction, dura geometry, and hole size in membrane puncture: laboratory report. *Reg Anesth*. 1997;22:267–272.

104. Gleeson CM, Reynolds F. Accidental dural puncture rates in UK obstetric practice. *Int J Obstet Anesth*. 1998;7:242–246.

105. Evron S, Sessler D, Sadan O, et al. Identification of the epidural space: loss of resistance with air, lidocaine, or the combination of air and lidocaine. *Anesth Analg*. 2004;99:245–250.

106. Segal S, Arendt KW. A retrospective effectiveness study of loss of resistance to air or saline for identification of the epidural space. *Anesth Analg*. 2010;110:558–563.

107. Antibas PL, do Nascimento Junior P, Braz LG, et al. Air versus saline in the loss of resistance technique for identification of the epidural space. *Cochrane Database Syst Rev*. 2014;(7):CD008938.

108. Naulty JS, Hertwig L, Hunt CO, et al. Influence of local anesthetic solution on postdural puncture headache. *Anesthesiology*. 1990;72:450–454.

109. Arkoosh VA, Palmer CM, Yun EM, et al. A randomized, double-masked, multicenter comparison of the safety of continuous intrathecal labor analgesia using a 28-gauge

catheter versus continuous epidural labor analgesia. *Anesthesiology*. 2008;108:286–298.

110. Alonso E, Gilsanz F, Gredilla E, et al. Observational study of continuous spinal anesthesia with the catheter-over-needle technique for cesarean delivery. *Int J Obstet Anesth*. 2009;18:137–141.

111. Tao W, Grant EN, Craig MG, et al. Continuous spinal analgesia for labor and delivery: an observational study with a 23-gauge spinal catheter. *Anesth Analg*. 2015;121:1290–1294.

112. Simmons SW, Dennis AT, Cyna AM, et al. Combined spinal-epidural versus spinal anaesthesia for caesarean section. *Cochrane Database Syst Rev*. 2019;(10):CD008100.

113. Chan TM, Ahmed E, Yentis SM, Holdcroft A. Postpartum headaches: summary report of the National Obstetric Anaesthetic Database (NOAD) 1999. *Int J Obstet Anesth*. 2003;12:107–112.

114. Angle P, Tang SL, Thompson D, Szalai JP. Expectant management of postdural puncture headache increases hospital length of stay and emergency room visits. *Can J Anaesth*. 2005;52:397–402.

115. Nishio I, Williams BA, Williams JP. Diplopia: a complication of dural puncture. *Anesthesiology*. 2004;100:158–164.

116. Ranganathan P, Golfeiz C, Phelps AL, et al. Chronic headache and backache are long-term sequelae of unintentional dural puncture in the obstetric population. *J Clin Anesth*. 2015;27:201–206.

117. Webb CA, Weyker PD, Zhang L, et al. Unintentional dural puncture with a Tuohy needle increases risk of chronic headache. *Anesth Analg*. 2012;115:124–132.

118. Lacombe A, Downey K, Ye XY, Carvalho JCA. Long-term complications of unintentional dural puncture during labor epidural analgesia: a case-control study. *Reg Anesth Pain Med*. 2022;47:364–369.

119. Ansari JR, Barad M, Shafer S, Flood P. Chronic disabling postpartum headache after unintentional dural puncture during epidural anaesthesia: a prospective cohort study. *Br J Anaesth*. 2021;127:600–607.

120. Orbach-Zinger S, Eidelman LA, Livne MY, et al. Long-term psychological and physical outcomes of women after postdural puncture headache: a retrospective, cohort study. *Eur J Anaesthesiol*. 2021;38:130–137.

121. Baraz R, Collis RE. The management of accidental dural puncture during labour epidural analgesia: a survey of UK practice. *Anaesthesia*. 2005;60:673–679.

122. Apfel CC, Saxena A, Cakmakkaya OS, et al. Prevention of postdural puncture headache after accidental dural puncture: a quantitative systematic review. *Br J Anaesth*. 2010;105:255–263.

123. Arevalo-Rodriguez I, Ciapponi A, Roque i Figuls M, et al. Posture and fluids for preventing post-dural puncture headache. *Cochrane Database Syst Rev*. 2016;(3):CD009199.

124. Yucel A, Ozyalcin S, Talu GK, et al. Intravenous administration of caffeine sodium benzoate for postdural puncture headache. *Reg Anesth Pain Med*. 1999;24:51–54.

125. Esmaoglu A, Akpinar H, Ugur F. Oral multidose caffeine-paracetamol combination is not effective for the prophylaxis of postdural puncture headache. *J Clin Anesth*. 2005;17:58–61.

126. Liu M, Mitchell A, Palanisamy A, Singh PM. Role of cosyntropin in the prevention of post-dural puncture headache: a propensity-matched retrospective analysis. *Int J Obstet Anesth*. 2023;56:103922.

127. Pancaro C, Balonov K, Herbert K, et al. Role of cosyntropin in the management of postpartum post-dural puncture headache: a two-center retrospective cohort study. *Int J Obstet Anesth*. 2023;56:103917.

128. Hakim SM. Cosyntropin for prophylaxis against postdural puncture headache after accidental dural puncture. *Anesthesiology*. 2010;113:413–420.

129. Al-Metwalli RR. Epidural morphine injections for prevention of post dural puncture headache. *Anaesthesia*. 2008;63:847–850.

130. Peralta FM, Wong CA, Higgins N, et al. Prophylactic intrathecal morphine and prevention of post-dural puncture headache: a randomized double-blind trial. *Anesthesiology*. 2020;132:1045–1052.

131. Ayad S, Demian Y, Narouze SN, Tetzlaff JE. Subarachnoid catheter placement after wet tap for analgesia in labor: Influence on the risk of headache in obstetric patients. *Reg Anesth Pain Med*. 2003;28:512–515.

132. Rutter SV, Shields F, Broadbent CR, et al. Management of accidental dural puncture in labour with intrathecal catheters: an analysis of 10 years' experience. *Int J Obstet Anesth*. 2001;10:177–181.

133. Paech M, Banks S, Gurrin L. An audit of accidental dural puncture during epidural insertion of a Tuohy needle in obstetric patients. *Int J Obstet Anesth*. 2001;10:162–167.

134. Verstraete S, Walters MA, Devroe S, et al. Lower incidence of post-dural puncture headache with spinal catheterization after accidental dural puncture in obstetric patients. *Acta Anaesthesiol Scand*. 2014;58:1233–1239.

135. Bolden N, Gebre E. Accidental dural puncture management: 10-year experience at an academic tertiary care center. *Reg Anesth Pain Med*. 2016;41:169–174.

136. Binyamin Y, Azem K, Heesen M, et al. The effect of placement and management of intrathecal catheters following accidental dural puncture on the incidence of postdural puncture headache and severity: a retrospective real-world study. *Anaesthesia*. 2023;78:1256–1261.

137. Heesen M, Klohr S, Rossaint R, et al. Insertion of an intrathecal catheter following accidental dural puncture: a meta-analysis. *Int J Obstet Anesth*. 2013;22:26–30.

138. Heesen M, Hilber N, Rijs K, et al. Intrathecal catheterisation after observed accidental dural puncture in labouring women: update of a meta-analysis and a trial-sequential analysis. *Int J Obstet Anesth*. 2020;41:71–82.

139. Trivedi NS, Eddi D, Shevde K. Headache prevention following accidental dural puncture in obstetric patients. *J Clin Anesth*. 1993;5:42–45.

140. Charsley MM, Abram SE. The injection of intrathecal normal saline reduces the severity of postdural puncture headache. *Reg Anesth Pain Med*. 2001;26:301–305.

141. Colonna-Romano P, Shapiro BE. Unintentional dural puncture and prophylactic epidural blood patch in obstetrics. *Anesth Analg*. 1989;69:522–523.

142. Boonmak P, Boonmak S. Epidural blood patching for preventing and treating post-dural puncture headache. *Cochrane Database Syst Rev*. 2010;(1):CD001791.

143. Scavone BM, Wong CA, Sullivan JT, et al. Efficacy of a prophylactic epidural blood patch in preventing post dural puncture headache in parturients after inadvertent dural puncture. *Anesthesiology*. 2004;101:1422–1427.

144. Allen DL, Berenguer JV, White JB. A potential complication of early blood patching following inadvertent dural puncture. *Int J Obstet Anesth*. 1993;2:202–203.

145. Tobias MD, Pilla MA, Rogers C, Jobes DR. Lidocaine inhibits blood coagulation: implications for epidural blood patch. *Anesth Analg.* 1996;82:766–769.

146. Leivers D. Total spinal anesthesia following early prophylactic epidural blood patch. *Anesthesiology.* 1990;73:1287–1289.

147. Aldrete JA, Brown TL. Intrathecal hematoma and arachnoiditis after prophylactic blood patch through a catheter. *Anesth Analg.* 1997;84:233–234.

148. Salvador L, Carrero E, Castillo J, et al. Prevention of post dural puncture headache with epidural-administered dextran 40. *Reg Anesth.* 1992;17:357–358.

149. Magides AD. A personal view of postdural puncture headache. *Anaesthesia.* 1991;46:694.

150. Weir EC. The sharp end of the dural puncture. *BMJ.* 2000;320:127.

151. Costigan SN, Sprigge JS. Dural puncture: the patients' perspective. A patient survey of cases at a DGH maternity unit 1983-1993. *Acta Anaesthesiol Scand.* 1996;40:710–714.

152. Katz D, Beilin Y. Review of the alternatives to epidural blood patch for treatment of postdural puncture headache in the parturient. *Anesth Analg.* 2017;124:1219–1228.

153. Uppal V, Russell R, Sondekoppam RV, et al. Evidence-based clinical practice guidelines on postdural puncture headache: a consensus report from a multisociety international working group. *Reg Anesth Pain Med.* 2024;49:471–501.

154. Basurto Ona X, Osorio D, Bonfill Cosp X. Drug therapy for treating post-dural puncture headache. *Cochrane Database Syst Rev.* 2015;(7):CD007887.

155. Mathew RJ, Wilson WH. Caffeine induced changes in cerebral circulation. *Stroke.* 1985;16:814–817.

156. Choi A, Laurito CE, Cunningham FE. Pharmacologic management of postdural puncture headache. *Ann Pharmacother.* 1996;30:831–839.

157. Cohen SM, Laurito CE, Curran MJ. Grand mal seizure in a postpartum patient following intravenous infusion of caffeine sodium benzoate to treat persistent headache. *J Clin Anesth.* 1992;4:48–51.

158. Paech M. Unexpected postpartum seizures associated with post-dural puncture headache treated with caffeine. *Int J Obstet Anesth.* 1996;5:43–46.

159. Russell R, Laxton C, Lucas DN, et al. Treatment of obstetric post-dural puncture headache. Part 1: conservative and pharmacological management. *Int J Obstet Anesth.* 2019;38:93–103.

160. US Centers for Disease Control. Maternal diet and breastfeeding; 2024. https://www.cdc.gov/breastfeeding-special-circumstances/hcp/diet-micronutrients/maternal-diet.html?CDC_AAref_Val=https://www.cdc.gov/breastfeeding/breastfeeding-special-circumstances/diet-and-micronutrients/maternal-diet.html. Accessed July 23, 2024.

161. Carp H, Singh PJ, Vadhera R, Jayaram A. Effects of the serotonin-receptor agonist sumatriptan on postdural puncture headache: report of six cases. *Anesth Analg.* 1994;79:180–182.

162. Connelly NR, Parker RK, Rahimi A, Gibson CS. Sumatriptan in patients with postdural puncture headache. *Headache.* 2000;40:316–319.

163. Foster P. ACTH treatment for post-lumbar puncture headache. *Br J Anaesth.* 1994;73:429.

164. Rucklidge MW, Yentis SM, Paech MJ. Synacthen depot for the treatment of postdural puncture headache. *Anaesthesia.* 2004;59:138–141.

165. Hanling SR, Lagrew JE 2nd, Colmenar DH, et al. Intravenous cosyntropin versus epidural blood patch for treatment of postdural puncture headache. *Pain Med.* 2016;17:1337–1342.

166. Noyan Ashraf MA, Sadeghi A, Azarbakht Z, et al. Evaluation of intravenous hydrocortisone in reducing headache after spinal anesthesia: a double blind controlled clinical study [corrected]. *Middle East J Anaesthesiol.* 2007;19:415–422.

167. Huseyinoglu U, Huseyinoglu N, Hamurtekin E, et al. Effect of pregabalin on post-dural-puncture headache following spinal anesthesia and lumbar puncture. *J Clin Neurosci.* 2011;18:1365–1368.

168. Erol DD. The analgesic and antiemetic efficacy of gabapentin or ergotamine/caffeine for the treatment of postdural puncture headache. *Adv Med Sci.* 2011;56:25–29.

169. Eldor J, Guedj P, Cotev S. Epidural morphine injections for the treatment of postspinal headache. *Can J Anaesth.* 1990;37:710–711.

170. Jacobaeus HC, Frumerie K. About the leakage of spinal fluid after lumbar puncture and its treatment. *Acta Med Scand.* 1923;58:102–108.

171. Rice GG, Dabbs CH. The use of peridural and subarachnoid injections of saline solution in the treatment of severe postspinal headache. *Anesthesiology.* 1950;11:17–23.

172. Usubiaga JE, Usubiaga LE, Brea LM, Goyena R. Effect of saline injections on epidural and subarachnoid space pressures and relation to postspinal anesthesia headache. *Anesth Analg.* 1967;46:293–296.

173. Bart AJ, Wheeler AS. Comparison of epidural saline placement and epidural blood placement in the treatment of post-lumbar-puncture headache. *Anesthesiology.* 1978;48:221–223.

174. Che X, Zhang W, Xu M. Continuous epidural pumping of saline contributes to prevent and treat postdural puncture headache. *J Clin Anesth.* 2016;34:154–158.

175. Baysinger CL, Menk EJ, Harte E, Middaugh R. The successful treatment of dural puncture headache after failed epidural blood patch. *Anesth Analg.* 1986;65:1242–1244.

176. Stevens RA, Jorgensen N. Successful treatment of dural puncture headache with epidural saline infusion after failure of epidural blood patch. Case report. *Acta Anaesthesiol Scand.* 1988;32:429–431.

177. Cullen S. Current comment. *Anesthesiology.* 1960;21:564–568.

178. DiGiovanni AJ, Dunbar BS. Epidural injections of autologous blood for postlumbar-puncture headache. *Anesth Analg.* 1970;49:268–271.

179. Abouleish E, Vega S, Blendinger I, Tio TO. Long-term follow-up of epidural blood patch. *Anesth Analg.* 1975;54:459–463.

180. Safa-Tisseront V, Thormann F, Malassine P, et al. Effectiveness of epidural blood patch in the management of post-dural puncture headache. *Anesthesiology.* 2001;95:334–339.

181. Tomala S, Savoldelli GL, Pichon I, Haller G. Risk factors for recurrence of post-dural puncture headache following an epidural blood patch: a retrospective cohort study. *Int J Obstet Anesth.* 2023;56:103925.

182. Gupta A, Van de Velde M, Magnuson A, et al. Factors associated with failed epidural blood patch after accidental dural puncture in obstetrics: a prospective, multicentre, international cohort study. *Br J Anaesth.* 2022;129:758–766.

183. Seebacher J, Ribeiro V, LeGuillou JL, et al. Epidural blood patch in the treatment of post dural puncture headache: a double blind study. *Headache.* 1989;29:630–632.

184. Sandesc D, Lupei MI, Sirbu C, et al. Conventional treatment or epidural blood patch for the treatment of different etiologies of post dural puncture headache. *Acta Anaesthesiol Belg.* 2005;56:265–269.

185. van Kooten F, Oedit R, Bakker SL, Dippel DW. Epidural blood patch in post dural puncture headache: a randomised, observer-blind, controlled clinical trial. *J Neurol Neurosurg Psychiatry.* 2008;79:553–558.

186. Szeinfeld M, Ihmeidan IH, Moser MM, et al. Epidural blood patch: evaluation of the volume and spread of blood injected into the epidural space. *Anesthesiology.* 1986;64:820–822.

187. Paech MJ, Doherty DA, Christmas T, et al. The volume of blood for epidural blood patch in obstetrics: a randomized, blinded clinical trial. *Anesth Analg.* 2011:126–133.

188. Booth JL, Pan PH, Thomas JA, et al. A retrospective review of an epidural blood patch database: the incidence of epidural blood patch associated with obstetric neuraxial anesthetic techniques and the effect of blood volume on efficacy. *Int J Obstet Anesth.* 2017;29:10–17.

189. Baysinger CL, Pope JE, Lockhart EM, Mercaldo ND. The management of accidental dural puncture and postdural puncture headache: a North American survey. *J Clin Anesth.* 2011;23:349–360.

190. Beards SC, Jackson A, Griffiths AG, Horsman EL. Magnetic resonance imaging of extradural blood patches: appearances from 30 min to 18 h. *Br J Anaesth.* 1993;71:182–188.

191. Vakharia SB, Thomas PS, Rosenbaum AE, et al. Magnetic resonance imaging of cerebrospinal fluid leak and tamponade effect of blood patch in postdural puncture headache. *Anesth Analg.* 1997;84:585–590.

192. Djurhuus H, Rasmussen M, Jensen EH. Epidural blood patch illustrated by CT-epidurography. *Acta Anaesthesiol Scand.* 1995;39:613–617.

193. DiGiovanni AJ, Galbert MW, Wahle WM. Epidural injection of autologous blood for postlumbar-puncture headache. II. Additional clinical experiences and laboratory investigation. *Anesth Analg.* 1972;51:226–232.

194. Carrie LE. Epidural blood patch: why the rapid response? *Anesth Analg.* 1991;72:129–130.

195. Coombs DW, Hooper D. Subarachnoid pressure with epidural blood patch. *Reg Anesth Pain Med.* 1979;4

196. Dubost C, Le Gouez A, Zetlaoui PJ, et al. Increase in optic nerve sheath diameter induced by epidural blood patch: a preliminary report. *Br J Anaesth.* 2011;107:627–630.

197. Andrews PJ, Ackerman WE, Juneja M, et al. Transient bradycardia associated with extradural blood patch after inadvertent dural puncture in parturients. *Br J Anaesth.* 1992;69:401–403.

198. Brimacombe J, Clarke G, Craig L. Epidural blood patch in the Jehovah's Witness. *Anaesth Intensive Care.* 1994;22:319.

199. Cucchiara RF, Wedel DJ. Finding cerebrospinal fluid during epidural blood patch: how to proceed. *Anesth Analg.* 1984;63:1121–1123.

200. Khayata I, Lance Lichtor J, Amelin P. Ultrasound-guided epidural blood patch. *Anesthesiology.* 2011;114:1453.

201. Martin R, Jourdain S, Clairoux M, Tetrault JP. Duration of decubitus position after epidural blood patch. *Can J Anaesth.* 1994;41:23–25.

202. Ong BY, Graham CR, Ringaert KR, et al. Impaired epidural analgesia after dural puncture with and without subsequent blood patch. *Anesth Analg.* 1990;70:76–79.

203. Blanche R, Eisenach JC, Tuttle R, Dewan DM. Previous wet tap does not reduce success rate of labor epidural analgesia. *Anesth Analg.* 1994;79:291–294.

204. Hebl JR, Horlocker TT, Chantigian RC, Schroeder DR. Epidural anesthesia and analgesia are not impaired after dural puncture with or without epidural blood patch. *Anesth Analg.* 1999;89:390–394.

205. Parris WC. Post-dural puncture headache and epidural blood patch in an AIDS patient. *J Clin Anesth.* 1997;9:87–88.

206. Bucklin BA, Tinker JH, Smith CV. Clinical dilemma: a patient with postdural puncture headache and acute leukemia. *Anesth Analg.* 1999;88:166–167.

207. Decramer I, Fuzier V, Franchitto N, Samii K. Is use of epidural fibrin glue patch in patients with metastatic cancer appropriate? *Eur J Anaesthesiol.* 2005;22:724–725.

208. Scher CS, Amar D, Wollner N. Extradural blood patch for post-lumbar puncture headaches in cancer patients. *Can J Anaesth.* 1992;39:203–204.

209. Diaz JH, Weed JT. Correlation of adverse neurological outcomes with increasing volumes and delayed administration of autologous epidural blood patches for postdural puncture headaches. *Pain Pract.* 2005;5:216–222.

210. Collier CB. Blood patches may cause scarring in the epidural space: two case reports. *Int J Obstet Anesth.* 2011;20:347–351.

211. Rice I, Wee MY, Thomson K. Obstetric epidurals and chronic adhesive arachnoiditis. *Br J Anaesth.* 2004;92:109–120.

212. Riley CA, Spiegel JE. Complications following large-volume epidural blood patches for postdural puncture headache. Lumbar subdural hematoma and arachnoiditis: initial cause or final effect? *J Clin Anesth.* 2009;21:355–359.

213. Eede HV, Hoffmann VL, Vercauteren MP. Post-delivery postural headache: not always a classical post-dural puncture headache. *Acta Anaesthesiol Scand.* 2007;51:763–765.

214. Marfurt D, Lyrer P, Ruttimann U, et al. Recurrent postpartum seizures after epidural blood patch. *Br J Anaesth.* 2003;90:247–250.

215. Diaz JH. Permanent paraparesis and cauda equina syndrome after epidural blood patch for postdural puncture headache. *Anesthesiology.* 2002;96:1515–1517.

216. Mercieri M, Mercieri A, Paolini S, et al. Postpartum cerebral ischaemia after accidental dural puncture and epidural blood patch. *Br J Anaesth.* 2003;90:98–100.

217. Willner D, Weissman C, Shamir MY. Chronic back pain secondary to a calcified epidural blood patch. *Anesthesiology.* 2008;108:535–537.

218. Robbins MS, Robertson CE, Kaplan E, et al. The sphenopalatine ganglion: anatomy, pathophysiology, and therapeutic targeting in headache. *Headache.* 2016;56:240–258.

219. Cohen S, Levin D, Mellender S, et al. Topical sphenopalatine ganglion block compared with epidural blood patch for postdural puncture headache management in postpartum patients: a retrospective review. *Reg Anesth Pain Med.* 2018;43:880–884.

220. Ambesh SP, Kumar A, Bajaj A. Epidural gelatin (Gelfoam) patch treatment for post dural puncture headache. *Anaesth Intensive Care.* 1991;19:444–447.

221. Barrios-Alarcon J, Aldrete JA, Paragas-Tapia D. Relief of post-lumbar puncture headache with epidural dextran 40: a preliminary report. *Reg Anesth*. 1989;14:78–80.

222. Reynvoet ME, Cosaert PA, Desmet MF, Plasschaert SM. Epidural dextran 40 patch for postdural puncture headache. *Anaesthesia*. 1997;52:886–888.

223. Chanimov M, Berman S, Cohen ML, et al. Dextran 40 (Rheomacrodex) or polygeline (Haemaccel) as an epidural patch for post dural puncture headache: a neurotoxicity study in a rat model of dextran 40 and polygeline injected intrathecally. *Eur J Anaesthesiol*. 2006;23:776–780.

224. Spotnitz WD, Burks S. Hemostats, sealants, and adhesives: components of the surgical toolbox. *Transfusion*. 2008;48:1502–1516.

225. Kroin JS, Nagalla SK, Buvanendran A, et al. The mechanisms of intracranial pressure modulation by epidural blood and other injectates in a postdural puncture rat model. *Anesth Analg*. 2002;95:423–429.

226. Nakamura H, Matsuyama Y, Yoshihara H, et al. The effect of autologous fibrin tissue adhesive on postoperative cerebrospinal fluid leak in spinal cord surgery: a randomized controlled trial. *Spine*. 2005;30:E347–E351.

227. Kamada M, Fujita Y, Ishii R, Endoh S. Spontaneous intracranial hypotension successfully treated by epidural patching with fibrin glue. *Headache*. 2000;40:844–847.

228. Gerritse BM, van Dongen RT, Crul BJ. Epidural fibrin glue injection stops persistent cerebrospinal fluid leak during long-term intrathecal catheterization. *Anesth Analg*. 1997;84:1140–1141.

229. Harrington H, Tyler HR, Welch K. Surgical treatment of post-lumbar puncture dural CSF leak causing chronic headache. Case report. *J Neurosurg*. 1982;57:703–707.

31

Neurologic Complications of Pregnancy and Neuraxial Anesthesia

Hans P. Sviggum, MD

CHAPTER OUTLINE

Neurologic complications of childbirth may be associated with neuraxial analgesia and anesthesia or may result from childbirth itself. Complications of neuraxial anesthesia may be immediate, such as an unexpectedly high spinal block or seizures after unintentional intravenous injection of local anesthetic, or they may be delayed. Immediate complications of neuraxial anesthesia are described in Chapter 24; here, the discussion is focused on neurologic sequelae.

Although neurologic disorders after childbirth are more likely to have obstetric than anesthetic causes, neuraxial anesthesia may be suspected. For example, Tubridy and Redmond[1] described seven women referred with neurologic symptoms after childbirth, all of which had been attributed to epidural analgesia. The women suffered from brachial neuritis, peroneal neuropathy, femoral neuropathy, neck strain, and leg symptoms for which there was no obvious physical cause. In such circumstances, a careful history and neurologic examination, together with diagnostic aids such as electromyography, nerve conduction studies, and imaging techniques, can localize the lesion and differentiate obstetric from anesthetic causes. For example, it should be possible to distinguish by simple clinical means between a mononeuropathy, which is likely to have an obstetric cause, and a radiculopathy, which might result from neuraxial blockade. An accurate and prompt diagnosis is essential to increase the likelihood of the best possible outcome.

THE INCIDENCE OF NEUROLOGIC SEQUELAE

Patients frequently ask obstetricians and anesthesia providers about the incidence of complications of neuraxial anesthesia. However, even if accurate data were available, the question is difficult to answer. The incidence of neurologic complications varies widely according to local practice, the skill and training of the practitioners, and individual patient characteristics—many of which may be unknown or unrecognized at the point of care. Some older surveys are based on accurate local records, but the data relate to a time when obstetric and anesthetic practices, equipment, and drugs were radically different. The incidence of serious complications is now too low to be estimated accurately on a local basis. Nonetheless, anesthesia providers have a duty to inform patients of the possible complications associated with a proposed procedure and are expected to give some estimate of the level of risk.

Obstetric Surveys

The reported incidence of neurologic deficits in obstetric patients varies widely depending on the source and the complications that are being measured. Many surveys have attempted to assess the incidence of neurologic complications of neuraxial anesthesia, but these surveys share common limitations, including low response rates, lack of control groups that did not receive neuraxial anesthesia, and inaccurate diagnosis (Box 31.1). Moreover, bias is created when more attention is paid to patients who received neuraxial blockade than to those who did not. Some of the more relevant surveys are listed in Table 31.1.[2-17] Although each survey is distinct in its population, measurements, and reporting, some generalizations can be made. Most of the neurologic complications in these reports were transient, most occurred in patients who labored, and only a very small minority were attributable to neuraxial anesthesia. Peripheral nerve damage was more common than central cord or plexus damage.

One of these reports from Leeds in the United Kingdom involved 3991 women who delivered in one center in a 1-year period.[10] Twenty-one women who self-reported neurologic symptoms, defined as areas of numbness or motor weakness in the lower extremities, after neuraxial blockade were matched with 21 patients who reported no symptoms after neuraxial blockade and a third group of 21 patients who did not receive neuraxial blockade for delivery and also did not report any neurologic symptoms. Among the women in the first group reporting symptoms, typical peripheral neuropathies occurred among those who delivered vaginally; sacral numbness was most commonly detected after cesarean delivery. All changes were transient, and none could be attributed to neuraxial anesthesia. Interestingly, similar neurologic deficits were detected on physical examination among the groups of patients who did not report symptoms, regardless of whether they had received a neuraxial block or not. These results demonstrate that minor neurologic deficits are frequently found postpartum, if sought, regardless of anesthetic intervention. Permanent or significant neurologic deficits after childbirth are rare with or without the use of neuraxial anesthesia.

A prospective survey among 6057 women who delivered in 1 year in Chicago corroborates the findings of the Leeds study.[10,13] The incidence of lower limb nerve injuries was approximately 1% (24 lateral femoral cutaneous nerve, 22 femoral nerve, 3 peroneal nerve, 3 lumbosacral plexus, 2 sciatic nerve, 3 obturator nerve, and 5 radicular injuries).[13] Significant risk factors identified by logistic regression

analysis included nulliparity and a prolonged second stage of labor but *not* neuraxial anesthesia.

A national audit of neuraxial blocks from the United Kingdom, without controls, published in 2009, found that the risk for major complications was 6- to 14-fold higher for perioperative than for obstetric procedures. Among the obstetric patients, the risk was highest for combined spinal-epidural (CSE), intermediate for spinal, and lowest for epidural procedures.[14] Finally, the Serious Complication Repository (SCORE) project sponsored by the Society for Obstetric Anesthesia and Perinatology collected data from 30 institutions and more than 250,000 neuraxial blocks in the United States over a 5-year period (2004 to 2009); the incidence of anesthesia-related nerve injury for obstetric patients was approximately 1 in 35,000 deliveries.[15] Four cases of epidural abscess/meningitis and a single case of epidural hematoma were reported.

Several conclusions can be drawn from these surveys. Despite an increased cesarean delivery rate in the past several decades, obstetric palsies still occur. Additionally, the reported frequency of neurologic sequelae depends on how hard one seeks them. The risk for transient mild deficits after childbirth may be quite high.[10,13] Permanent or persistent injury is extremely rare. A 2006 review, which included some of the previously mentioned surveys, reported an incidence of persistent neurologic injury of four per million.[18] However, a completely accurate figure for anesthetic complications cannot be calculated, even from thorough surveys because (1) the diagnosis is rarely accurate and (2) definitions, severity, and duration are often ill defined. Although we have some reliable data of neurologic complications after neuraxial anesthesia in nonobstetric populations, this cannot accurately extrapolated to the obstetric population due to confounding variables.[11,12,14,17] Table 31.1 demonstrates a variation in the incidence of neurologic sequelae from 1 in 3 for mild symptoms with no neuraxial block[10] to 1 in 250,000 for epidural hematoma.[15]

PERIPHERAL NERVE PALSIES

Postpartum nerve injury is often assumed to be caused by neuraxial anesthesia, but peripheral nerve palsies, which generally have obstetric causes,[19] are much more common than anesthesia-related injury, with a reported incidence between 0.6 and 92 per 10,000.[20] They may arise from compression in the pelvis by the fetal head or from more distal compression, the symptoms and signs of which may be overlooked in the presence of neuraxial anesthesia. Risk factors for postpartum neuropathies include a prolonged second stage of labor, difficult operative vaginal delivery, nulliparity, and prolonged use of the lithotomy position.[20]

Reference to the distribution of spinal dermatomes and peripheral nerve sensory innervation demonstrates the distinction between peripheral and central lesions (Fig. 31.1). Central lesions are most often bilateral, create weakness or paralysis from the site of the lesion distally, are often associated with autonomic dysfunction, and may be associated with upper motor neuron signs such as spasticity, brisk reflexes, and bowel and bladder dysfunction. In contrast, peripheral nerve

---

> ### BOX 31.1 Limitations of Surveys of Neurologic Sequelae of Neuraxial Anesthesia in Obstetrics
>
> - Poor response rate
> - Positive reporting bias
> - Absence of controls without neuraxial anesthesia
> - Greater attention/evaluation given to those who received neuraxial anesthesia
> - Inadequate investigation and lack of accurate diagnosis
> - Variable skill and care of obstetric and anesthetic providers
> - Older surveys relate to outdated obstetric and anesthetic practices
> - Lack of statistical power to assess incidence of rare disorders
> - Inaccurate counting of numerator and denominator
> - Likelihood of missing cases that arise after hospital discharge

TABLE 31.1   Surveys of Neurologic Complications of Childbirth and of Neuraxial Blocks in Obstetrics

Study	Type of Study	Population	Number of Neurologic Deficits (Risk Ratio)
Ong et al., 1987[2]	Medical record review of all patients, interview of those receiving anesthesia in one center (1975–83)	23,827 deliveries	45, all transient (1/530)
		12,964 inhalational or no analgesia	5 (1/2593)
		9403 epidural procedures	34 (1/277)
		1460 general anesthetics and other	6 (1/243)
Scott and Hibbard, 1990[3]	Retrospective multicenter review (1982–86), no control group	505,000 epidural procedures	47 (1/10,745) 1 anterior spinal artery syndrome 1 epidural abscess, 1 epidural hematoma (unconfirmed) 38 mononeuropathies, 5 cranial nerve palsies 1 subdural hematoma
MacArthur et al., 1992[4]	Questionnaire sent in 1987 to mothers delivering in one center (1978–85)	11,701 women (39%) who responded	Tingling/paresthesias
		4766 epidural procedures	143 upper limb, 23 lower limb
		6935 no epidural procedures	150 upper limb, 3 lower limb
Palot et al., 1994[5]	Questionnaire listing possible complications sent to hospitals with obstetric beds (1988–93), no control group	288,351 epidural procedures	92 (1/3134) 1 cranial subdural hematoma 88 temporary radiculopathy (1/3277) 3 meningitis (1/96,117) (also reported negligence cases: 1 sciatic nerve palsy, 1 intracranial hematoma)
Scott and Tunstall, 1995[6]	Prospective multicenter review (1990–91), no control group	467,491 deliveries 108,133 epidural procedures 14,856 spinal procedures	46 neuropathies (details for procedures not given) 38 (1/2846) 8 (1/1857)
Holdcroft et al., 1995[7]	Regional community and hospital-based audit (1991–92)	48,066 deliveries	10 new neurologic complications (1/4807)
		34,430 no neuraxial block	1 foot drop, 1 cervical nerve lesion (1/17,215)
		13,007 epidural procedures	1 paresthesia of nerve root distribution (1/13,007) (disorders unrelated to anesthesia: 2 cranial nerve palsies, 1 hypotensive cord damage; 5 peripheral nerve lesions)
		629 spinal procedures	0
Paech et al., 1998[8]	Prospective local audit (1989–94), no control group	10,995 epidural procedures	1 traumatic "mononeuropathy" (1/10,995)
Holloway et al., 2000[9]	Retrospective multicenter audit, elastic time frame, no control group	29,698 spinal procedures	4 unrelated to anesthesia (3 meralgia paresthetica, 1 peroneal neuropathy), 10?root damage, 1 conus damage, 22 uncertain (overall incidence? 1/986)
		12,254 CSE procedures	5 unrelated to anesthesia (1 femoral neuropathy, 2 foot drop, 2 paresthesia), 6 root damage, 1 meningitis, 1 conus damage, 6 uncertain (overall incidence? 1/901)
Dar et al., 2002[10]	Prospective local audit of immediate symptoms (1998–99)	1376 vaginal deliveries without anesthesia (random sample of 21 examined + 1 complaint)	4 peripheral neuropathy, 1 foot drop, 2 vague (1/3)
		2615 regional blocks (all followed up)	21 had neurologic symptoms
		1782 vaginal deliveries	7 peripheral neuropathies, 1 foot drop, 3 vague (1/162)
		833 cesarean deliveries	8 numb areas, 2 vague (1/83)

Continued

TABLE 31.1   Surveys of Neurologic Complications of Childbirth and of Neuraxial Blocks in Obstetrics—cont'd

Study	Type of Study	Population	Number of Neurologic Deficits (Risk Ratio)
Auroy et al., 2002[11]	Prospective multicenter survey, no control group	29,732 epidural procedures	0
		5640 spinal procedures	2 "peripheral neuropathy"
Moen et al., 2004[12]	National postal survey and search of administrative files (1990–99), no control group	205,000 epidural procedures	1 epidural hematoma (HELLP), 1 epidural abscess, 2 cord damage, 2 intracranial subdural hematoma, 1 abducent nerve palsy (1/29,286)
		50,000 spinal procedures	1 spinal hematoma (HELLP), 1 cord damage (1/25,000)
Wong et al., 2003[13]	Prospective 1-y survey (1997–98) at a single institution	5603 laboring patients (72% with neuraxial blocks) and 454 nonlaboring patients	66 nerve injuries (63 in laboring, 3 in nonlaboring). Lateral femoral cutaneous nerve (24) and femoral nerve (22) injuries most common
Cook et al., 2009[14]	National audit of major complications of neuraxial blockade over 1 y (unstated), obstetric and nonobstetric, no control group	329,425 obstetric procedures	1 epidural abscess, 2 nerve injury, 1 unknown
		161,550 epidural procedures	Possible harm per 100,000 (95% CI), 0.6 (0–3.4)
		133,525 spinal procedures	Possible harm per 100,000 (95% CI), 1.5 (1–5.4)
		25,350 CSE procedures	Possible harm per 100,000 (95% CI), 3.9 (1–22)
D'Angelo et al., 2014[15]	Prospective multicenter survey (2004–09)	307,495 deliveries 131,460 epidural procedures 35,369 spinal procedures 84,634 CSE procedures	27 cases of serious neurologic injury (1/11,389); 7 related to anesthesia (1/35,923), 1 epidural hematoma, 4 epidural abscess/meningitis
Richards et al., 2017[16]	Prospective observational single-center study (2016)	1019 deliveries 752 neuraxial procedures	23 cases of neurologic injury (19 in laboring, 4 in nonlaboring); majority were lumbar or lumbosacral plexopathies
Tournier et al., 2020[17]	Single-center observational study (2013–15)	10,569 vaginal deliveries 76% received neuraxial block (type not defined)	31 cases of neurologic injury; 66% were sensory; 84% were in femoral nerve distribution; all with follow-up recovered completely

CI, Confidence interval; *CSE,* combined spinal-epidural; *HELLP,* hemolysis, elevated liver enzymes, and low platelet count.

lesions are typically unilateral, with weakness or paralysis limited to a single muscle or muscle group that the peripheral nerve innervates. Peripheral injuries create sensory deficits in the distribution of the specific nerve, while central lesions typically involve multiple dermatomes with a defined sensory level. Spinal nerve root lesions are also manifested by weakness that involves several lower extremity joints and movements (Fig. 31.2). Obstetric peripheral nerve injuries include compression of the lumbosacral trunk and palsies of the obturator, femoral, lateral femoral cutaneous, sciatic, and peroneal nerves.

Compression of the Lumbosacral Trunk

Compression of the lumbosacral trunk by the fetal head at the pelvic brim (Fig. 31.3) preferentially affects the more medial fibers that make up the peroneal rather than the tibial nerve.[20] In addition to weakness that predominantly affects ankle dorsiflexion (foot drop), compression of the lumbosacral trunk produces sensory disturbance mainly involving the L5 dermatome (see Fig. 31.1). This palsy most often results from cephalopelvic disproportion and is therefore typically seen after prolonged labor and difficult vaginal delivery.[8–10,13]

Obturator Nerve Palsy

The obturator nerve is susceptible to compressive injury as it crosses the brim of the pelvis and within the obturator canal (see Fig. 31.3). The patient may complain of pain when the damage occurs, followed by weakness of hip adduction and internal rotation, with sensory disturbance over the medial thigh (see Fig. 31.1) and may have an abnormal gait secondary to weakness of thigh adduction. Cases are reported after both labor and cesarean delivery[21,22]; three of 66 new nerve injuries detected in a prospective study by Wong et al.[13] were obturator nerve injuries. The most likely cause of obturator nerve palsy is compression of the nerve between the pelvis and fetal head or forceps applied to the fetal head.

Femoral Nerve Palsy

The femoral nerve does not enter the true pelvis and is therefore not vulnerable to compression by the fetal head but rather is vulnerable to stretch injury as it passes beneath the inguinal ligament. The femoral nerve may be injured proximal to or at the inguinal ligament. Proximal injuries are associated

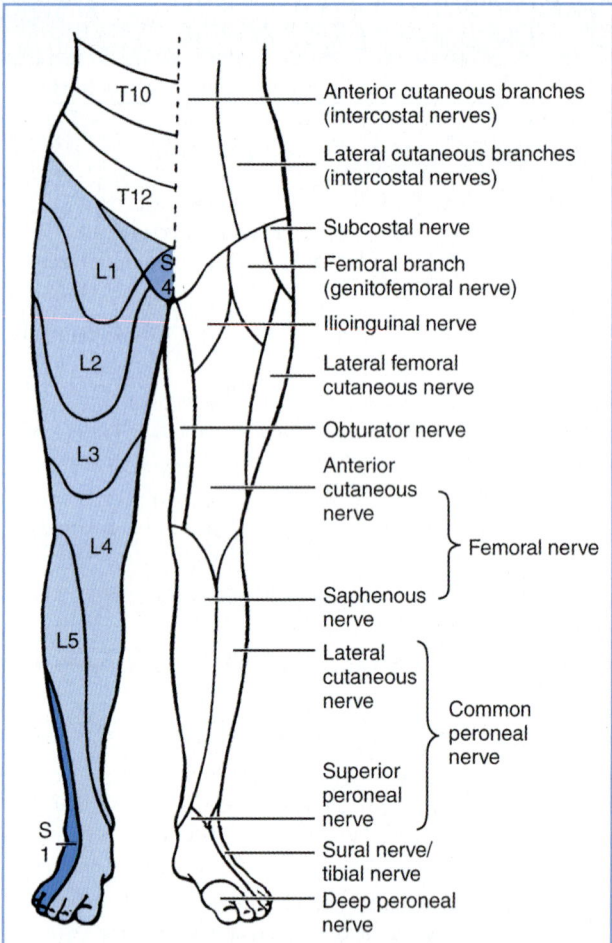

Fig. 31.1 Segmental *(right leg)* and peripheral *(left leg)* sensory nerve distributions useful in distinguishing central from peripheral nerve lesions. From Redick LF. Maternal perinatal nerve palsies. *Postgrad Obstet Gynecol.* 1992;12:1–6.

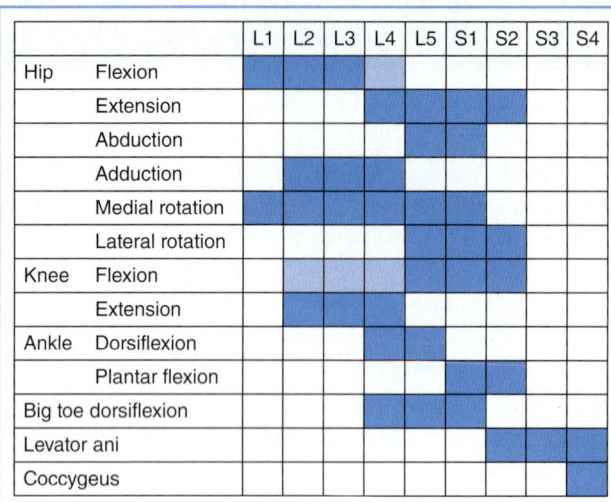

		L1	L2	L3	L4	L5	S1	S2	S3	S4
Hip	Flexion	■	■	■	▨					
	Extension				■	■	■			
	Abduction				■	■	■			
	Adduction		■	■	■					
	Medial rotation	■	■	■			■	■		
	Lateral rotation				■	■	■	■		
Knee	Flexion			▨	▨	■	■			
	Extension		■	■	■					
Ankle	Dorsiflexion				■	■				
	Plantar flexion						■	■		
Big toe dorsiflexion						■	■			
Levator ani									■	■
Coccygeus										■

Fig. 31.2 The Spinal Segments Involved in Movements of Joints in the Leg. Lighter shading denotes a minor contribution. Data from Russell R. Assessment of motor blockade during epidural analgesia in labour. *Int J Obstet Anesth.* 1992;4:230–234.

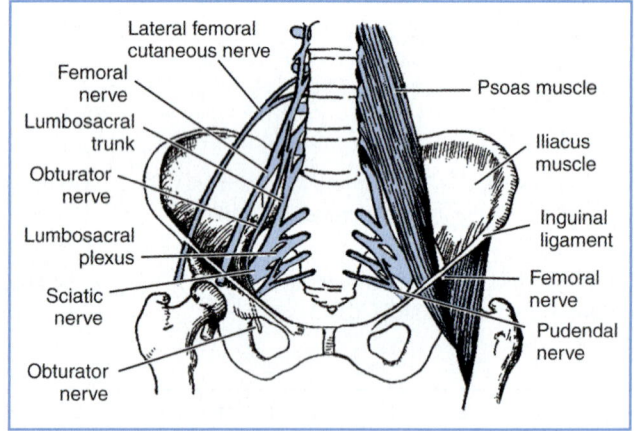

Fig. 31.3 The Principal Nerves in the Pelvis. The lumbosacral trunk (L4 to L5) and obturator nerve (L2 to L4) are vulnerable to pressure as they cross the pelvic brim, particularly in cases of cephalopelvic disproportion. The femoral (L2 to L4) and lateral femoral cutaneous (L2 to L3) nerves are particularly vulnerable in the lithotomy position, where they pass beneath the inguinal ligament. Modified from Cole JT. Maternal obstetric paralysis. *Am J Obstet Gynecol.* 1946;52:374.

with weakness of hip flexion, whereas more distal injuries spare the motor supply to the iliopsoas muscle. The patient with a femoral neuropathy may walk satisfactorily on a level surface but may be unable to climb stairs; the patellar reflex is diminished or absent. Although the incidence of femoral nerve palsy has decreased because of changes in obstetric management (e.g., fewer deliveries with prolonged second stage), it is still one of the most common obstetric nerve injuries. Approximately one-third of the postpartum palsies detected by Wong et al.[13] were femoral nerve palsies. Dar et al.[10] detected five cases in their small population, although the symptoms were transient. Damage may result from prolonged flexion, abduction, and external rotation of the hips during the second stage of labor and also during procedures conducted in an excessive lithotomy position.[23] To avoid this injury, the hips should never remain continuously flexed during the second stage of labor and position changes or breaks should be encouraged.

Meralgia Paresthetica

Meralgia paresthetica is a neuropathy of the lateral femoral cutaneous nerve, a purely sensory nerve also known as the lateral cutaneous nerve of the thigh. First described more

than 100 years ago, meralgia paresthetica is commonly encountered in pregnancy and childbirth.[10,13] It is the most common nerve injury of pregnancy.[13] The palsy may arise both during pregnancy, typically at about 30 weeks' gestation, and intrapartum.[13,24] The distribution is unlike that of a nerve root lesion (see Fig. 31.1), yet the disturbance is commonly misattributed to neuraxial blockade. Meralgia paresthetica manifests as numbness, tingling, burning, or other paresthesias affecting the anterolateral aspect of the thigh. The most likely cause is entrapment of the nerve as it passes around the anterior superior iliac spine beneath or through the inguinal ligament, where its vulnerability is increased by a gravid uterus or by retractors used during pelvic surgery.

The compressive effect of edema may also contribute. The condition can be expected to resolve after childbirth.

Sciatic Nerve Palsy

Sciatic nerve palsy arises from compression of the nerve, usually in the buttock. It is not commonly mentioned in surveys or generally recognized as a complication of childbirth, possibly because it is mistaken for a lesion of the lumbosacral trunk. It gives rise to loss of sensation below the knee with sparing of the medial leg, and loss of movement below the knee. Posterior cutaneous nerve and gluteal function are preserved, implying damage distal to the lumbosacral plexus, where the gluteal nerves branch off the sciatic nerve (Fig. 31.4). Three cases out of 66 new nerve injuries were detected by Wong et al.[13] It has occurred during childbirth with neuraxial blockade, either from sitting in one position too long[25] or from a hip wedge misplaced during cesarean delivery.[25–27] It has also been reported after iliac artery balloon placement for cesarean delivery in a woman with placenta accreta spectrum.[28]

Peroneal Nerve Palsy

The common peroneal nerve is vulnerable to compression as it passes around the head of the fibula below the knee. It is also susceptible to damage while it still forms part of the sciatic nerve as it leaves the pelvis. When the peroneal nerve is damaged at the knee, there is sensory impairment on the anterolateral calf and the dorsum of the foot. Foot drop may be profound, with steppage gait and weak ankle eversion, but plantar flexion and inversion at the ankle are preserved. Peroneal nerve palsy may be caused by prolonged squatting,[29]

sometimes popular in "natural childbirth," by excessive knee flexion for any reason, by compression of the lateral side of the knee against any hard object, even the patient's hand,[30] by prolonged use of the lithotomy position, and even by tight compression stockings in patients under spinal anesthesia.[31] The incidence of peroneal nerve palsy is lower than that of lateral femoral cutaneous and femoral nerve palsy.[13]

Compression as a Risk Factor for Peripheral Neuropathy

During pregnancy, nerve compression caused by edema may be a factor in the genesis of several peripheral neuropathies, such as carpal tunnel syndrome, Bell's palsy, and meralgia paresthetica.[24,32,33] Neuraxial blockade may indirectly contribute to compression injuries because it may decrease the ability of a woman to perceive that their legs are in a position that contributes to compression-induced neuropathy. Practices that providers should observe to lessen the risk for compression-induced neuropathy are listed in Box 31.2.

POSTPARTUM BLADDER DYSFUNCTION

There are several mechanisms by which bladder function may be disturbed postpartum (Fig. 31.5). In theory, neuraxial blockade (1) may necessitate bladder catheterization with subsequent increased risk for infection, (2) may allow bladder distention to go undetected, and (3) on very rare occasions, may be associated with cauda equina syndrome (see later discussion). However, several postpartum studies of bladder function have found no association with neuraxial analgesia[34,35] or only a weak correlation between epidural analgesia and an increased residual volume immediately postpartum.[36] In contrast, a prolonged second stage of labor, operative vaginal delivery, and perineal damage have been identified as significant factors for postpartum bladder dysfunction.[34,36] No association has been found between epidural analgesia and stress incontinence or urinary frequency.[6,37]

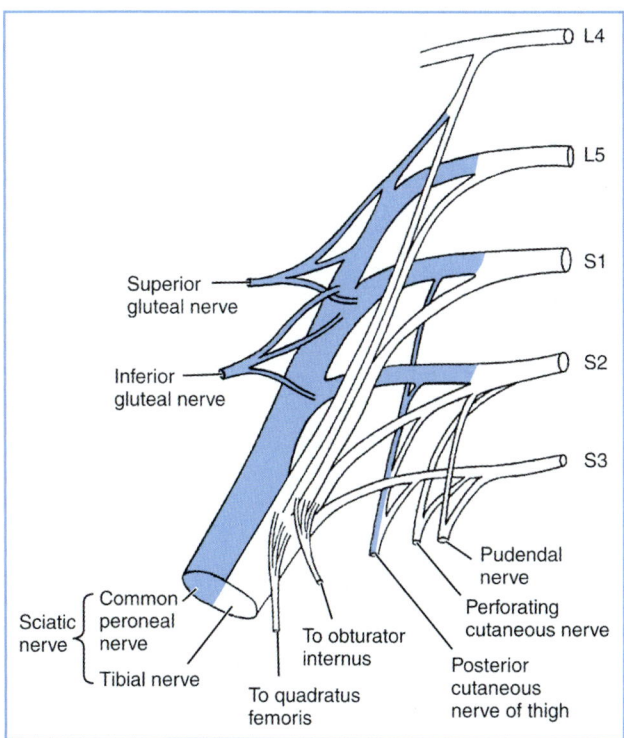

Fig. 31.4 The Sacral Plexus. The dorsal divisions of the anterior primary rami are shaded. From Silva M, Mallinson C, Reynolds F. Sciatic nerve palsy following childbirth. *Anaesthesia.* 1996;51:1144–1148.

BOX 31.2 Safeguards to Minimize Peripheral Nerve Compression

- Be mindful of patient positioning that could contribute to nerve compression, particularly with neuraxial blockade.
- Avoid prolonged use of the lithotomy position; regularly reduce hip flexion and abduction.
- Avoid prolonged positioning that may cause compression of the sciatic or peroneal nerve.
- Place the hip wedge under the bony pelvis rather than the buttock.
- Use low-dose local anesthetic/opioid combinations during labor to allow maximum mobility.
- Encourage the parturient to change position regularly.
- Ensure that those caring for women receiving low-dose local anesthetic/opioid combinations understand that numbness or weakness may be signs of nerve compression; such symptoms should prompt an immediate change of position.

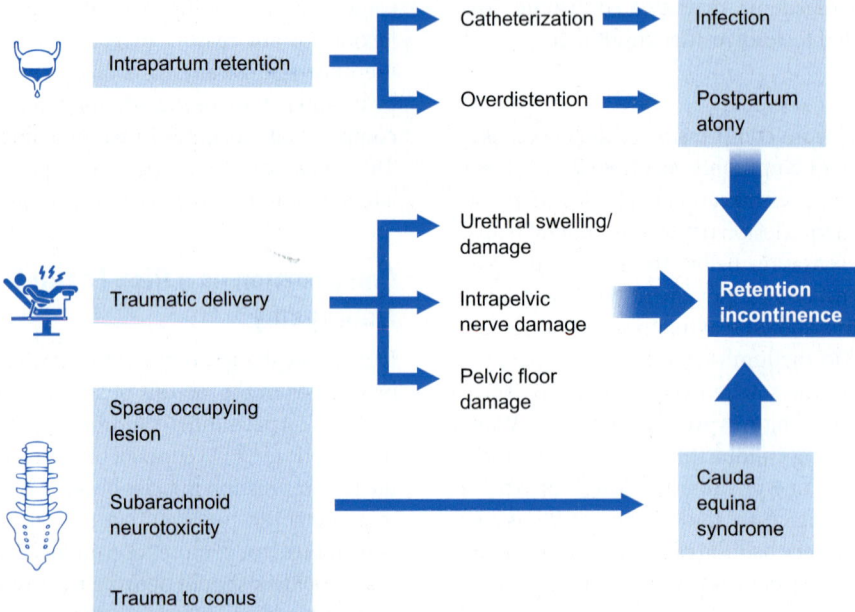

Fig. 31.5 Mechanisms by which bladder function may be disturbed after parturition.

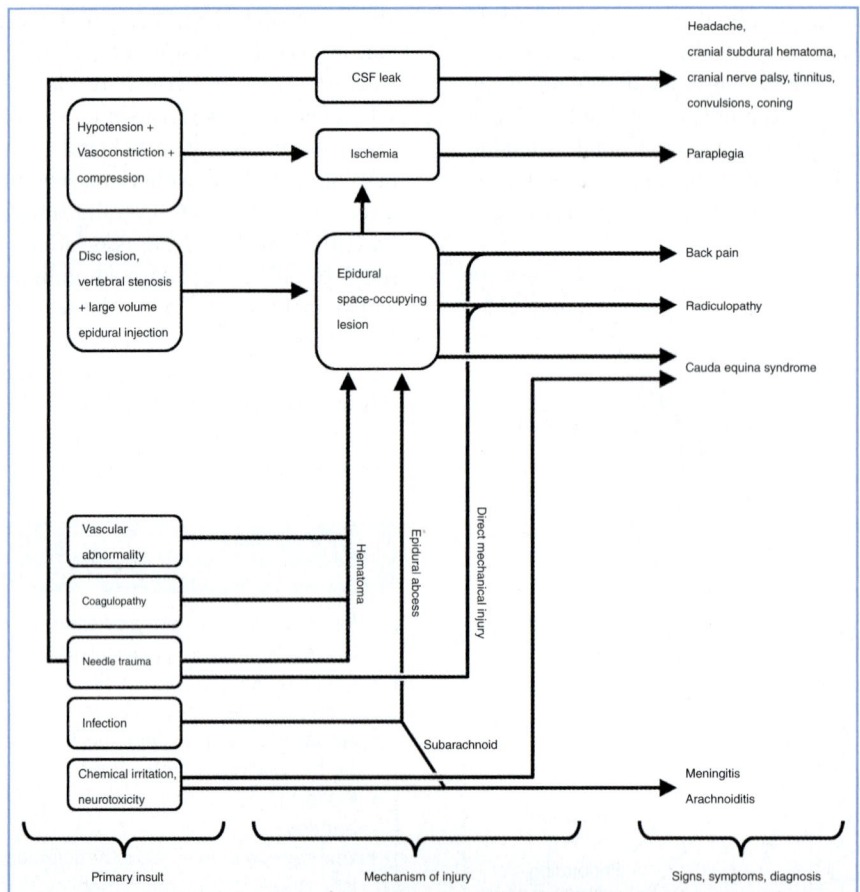

Fig. 31.6 Mechanisms by which lesions of the central nervous system may arise in parturients. *CSF,* Cerebrospinal fluid.

CENTRAL NERVOUS SYSTEM LESIONS

Lesions of the central nervous system (CNS) after childbirth have complex causes (Fig. 31.6) and may be classified as traumatic (to nervous tissue, meninges, or blood vessels), infectious, ischemic, or chemical (to nervous tissue or meninges). Anesthesia providers should bear in mind that even central lesions may have causes other than neuraxial block (e.g., a prolapsed intervertebral disc). Apart from sequelae of dural puncture, serious iatrogenic complications related to neuraxial analgesia and anesthesia are remarkably rare.

Neurologic Sequelae of Dural Puncture

The subject of postdural puncture headache (PDPH) is discussed in detail in Chapter 30. Other neurologic sequelae of dural puncture include meningitis (see later discussion), cranial nerve palsies, and subdural hematoma. These often present as a headache but are distinct from disorders that should be included in the differential diagnosis for postpartum headache, including tension/stress and migraine headaches, cortical vein and venous sinus thrombosis, preeclampsia, hypertensive encephalopathy, intracerebral or subarachnoid hemorrhage, internal carotid artery dissection, and posterior reversible encephalopathy syndrome.[38] It can be difficult to distinguish PDPH from other serious causes of a headache because signs and symptoms overlap.

Cranial Nerve Palsy

Substantial loss of cerebrospinal fluid (CSF), usually following unintentional dural puncture with a large-bore needle, may cause a number of cranial nerve palsies; palsies of cranial nerves VI, VII, and VIII are the most frequently reported.[39–45] Because of its long course within the cranium, the abducens nerve (VI) is the most vulnerable. PDPH associated with cranial nerve palsies should be promptly treated (e.g., epidural blood patch) to reverse neurologic symptoms, but even after the blood patch recovery may be delayed. In the case of cranial nerve VIII dysfunction, tinnitus may not resolve.[44,45] Trigeminal nerve dysfunction is usually a transient effect of high neuraxial blockade, but trigeminal and facial nerve palsies have also been reported in relation to PDPH and subdural hematoma.[46] A review of 43 cases of cranial nerve palsy following central neuraxial blockage concluded that intracranial hypotension is the most common etiology (27).[47] The abducens (17) and trigeminal (12) nerves were most affected, and the majority (35) resolved over a period of 2 months.

Cranial Subdural Hematoma

More seriously, reduced CSF pressure may cause rupture of bridge meningeal veins and result in cranial subdural hematoma, a rare but potentially fatal condition.[48] Palot et al.[5] identified one case in 288,351 obstetric epidural procedures. In 2000, Loo et al.[19] identified eight cases in their systematic review of published cases of neurologic complications in obstetric regional anesthesia. While more commonly associated with dural puncture with a large-bore needle or a cutting spinal needle, subdural hematoma requiring craniotomy has been reported after puncture with a small-gauge, pencil-point spinal needle[49] and after an unintentional dural puncture that had been appropriately treated with an epidural blood patch.[50] A thorough review of 56 cases of subdural hematoma in obstetric patients who received neuraxial blocks (34 epidural, 20 spinal, 2 CSE) published in 2016 concluded that predisposing risk factors such as coagulation disorders, aneurysms or arteriovenous malformations, or head trauma were present in only a minority of patients.[51] Persistent headache was present in more than 80% of cases, and focal neurologic signs were present in nearly 70%. Whenever headache persists after treatment with an epidural blood patch (particularly if the headache is accompanied by altered consciousness, seizures, or other focal neurologic findings), magnetic resonance imaging (MRI) is warranted to exclude subdural hematoma, which may be fatal without urgent surgery.

Cerebral venous thrombosis is a rare complication that can mimic a PDPH. It nearly always presents with a severe headache. A review of 58 cases concluded that the key clinical features to help distinguish cerebral venous thrombosis from a PDPH were a change in character of headache with loss of postural component, failure of an epidural blood patch to relieve a headache, and focal neurologic signs such as cranial nerve palsy or motor deficit.[52]

Trauma to Nerve Roots and the Spinal Cord

Insertion of a spinal needle or epidural catheter may be accompanied by paresthesia that is sometimes painful. However, such a paresthesia is neither sensitive nor specific for nerve injury.[53] If a paresthesia is encountered, advancement of the needle or catheter should be halted. It is generally deemed appropriate to continue spinal or epidural catheter placement after the paresthesia subsides. Continued paresthesias should prompt removal and redirection of the needle. Although a flexible catheter is unlikely to do lasting damage to a nerve root in the epidural space, nerve roots in the subarachnoid space may be more vulnerable.

Trauma Associated With Attempted Epidural Catheter Insertion

An epidural catheter may injure nerve roots either because it is rigid[54] or because an undue length is advanced and ensnares a root.[55] A catheter seemingly advanced into the epidural space may lodge in an intervertebral foramen or even pass into the paravertebral space. In rare instances, the epidural catheter and the artery of Adamkiewicz share the same foramen. If the epidural catheter is stiff enough to compress the artery within the unyielding foramen, the blood supply to the spinal cord may be impaired. This is a possible cause of anterior spinal artery syndrome resulting in bilateral lower extremity paresis with loss of pain and temperature sensation. Clinical reports indicate that the condition resolves rapidly and completely if the catheter is withdrawn before permanent damage has occurred.[56,57]

Injury to the spinal cord may result from attempted identification of the epidural space in the presence of a tethered spinal cord[58] or as a result of unintentional dural puncture

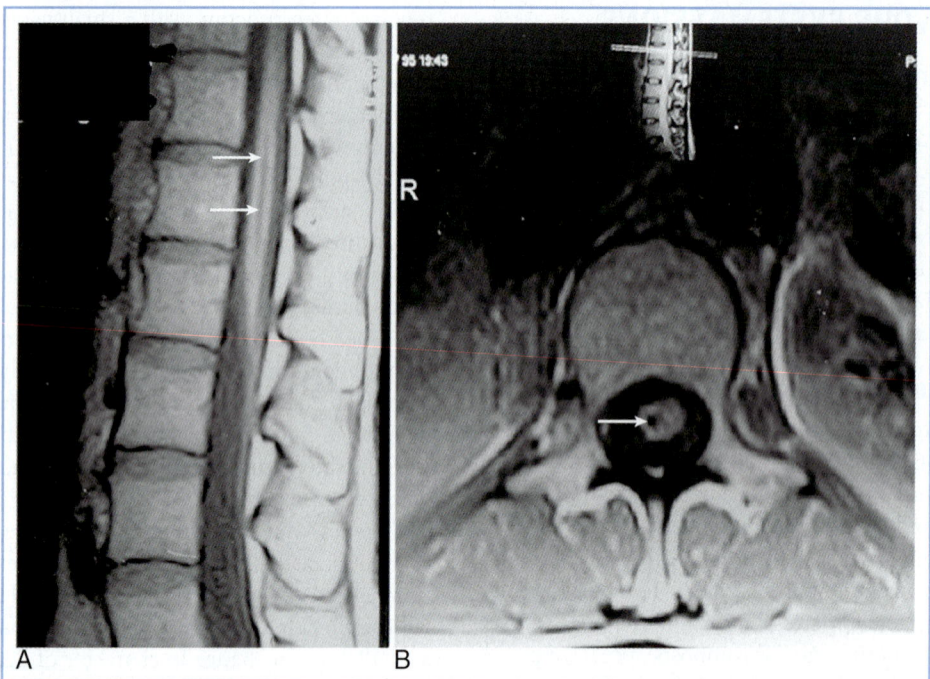

Fig. 31.7 (A and B) Magnetic resonance images of a conus medullaris lesion *(arrows)*. From Reynolds F. Damage to the conus medullaris following spinal anaesthesia. *Anaesthesia*. 2001;56:238–247.

at a higher-than-anticipated interspace (see later discussion). Patients with spina bifida occulta may safely undergo both epidural and spinal anesthesia as the spinal cord is rarely tethered in true spina bifida occulta (see Chapter 46). However, if there is concern for occult spinal dysmorphism, which is more frequently associated with a tethered cord, it is prudent to obtain a lumbar MRI before initiating a neuraxial procedure.[59] Insertion of an epidural catheter in an anesthetized patient increases the risk for spinal cord damage, and catastrophic injury may occur with injection of fluid into the substance of the spinal cord.[60]

Trauma Associated With Spinal Anesthesia

Insertion of a spinal needle below the level of the spinal cord sometimes causes brief radiating pain or paresthesia, which may be associated with persistent paresthesia in the same dermatomal distribution. Prolonged symptoms involving more than one spinal segment suggest damage to the spinal cord itself. Damage to the terminal portion of the cord (the conus medullaris) without intracord injection has also been reported in healthy conscious parturients receiving spinal or CSE anesthesia using a pencil-point needle.[9,12,61,62] Typically, the patient complains of pain on needle insertion before any fluid is injected, often followed by the normal appearance of CSF from the needle hub, easy injection of the local anesthetic agent, and a normal onset of neural blockade. On recovery, there is unilateral numbness, which is followed by pain and paresthesia in the L5 to S1 distribution and foot drop, and in some cases urinary symptoms; sensory symptoms may last for months or years. The MRI appearance is one of a small syrinx or hematoma within the conus on the same side as the pain at insertion and subsequent leg symptoms (Fig. 31.7).[62]

In most reported cases, the anesthesia provider believed the interspace selected was L2 to L3. In one patient who subsequently died of other causes, hematomyelia was confirmed at autopsy.[63] After a rash of cases of conus damage in the 1990s, increasing awareness of this phenomenon may have led providers to conscientiously choose a lower interspace than they otherwise might have, but an abnormally long cord may still be damaged with the best of techniques.[64]

These injuries may have occurred for the following reasons:

- Identification of lumbar interspaces is far from accurate. Studies showed that it is common to select a space that is higher than assumed by one, two, or even more segments (Fig. 31.8).[65,66] In a study of 125 obese women, 21% of epidural and intrathecal catheters were unintentionally placed at the L1 to L2 interspace level or above. Even the use of ultrasound did not improve accuracy of level placement.[67]
- Although the spinal cord typically ends level with the lower body of L1 or the L1 to L2 interspace, the length varies (Fig. 31.9).[68] From the L1 to L2 interspace, the needle tip can easily reach the conus in 27% of men and 43% of women.[68,69]
- The standard method of identifying lumbar interspaces involves the use of Tuffier's line, the imaginary line joining the two iliac crests. This method can be inaccurate, however, particularly in obese or pregnant women (Fig. 31.10). Moreover, even when accurately assessed, Tuffier's line is an inconstant landmark.[70] Although typically at the level of the L4 spinous process, it may lie anywhere between the L3 to L4 and L5 to S1 interspaces.
- Pencil-point spinal needles must be advanced further than cutting needles before the orifice is within the subarachnoid space, at which point the tip may impinge on the spinal cord.

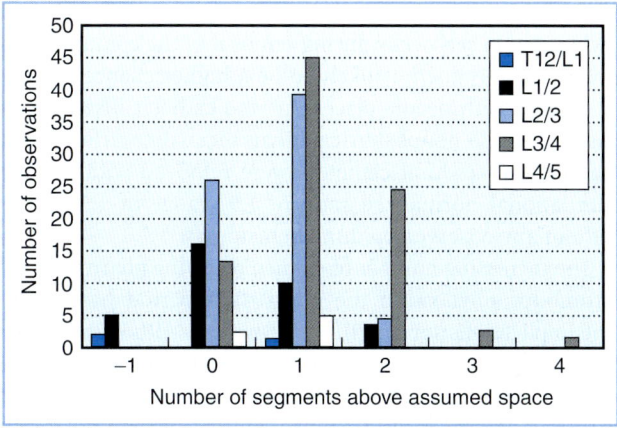

Fig. 31.8 Identification of Lumbar Interspaces by Oxford Anesthetists. The horizontal axis shows the position of the actual interspace identified on magnetic resonance imaging, relative to the assumed space, in 200 observations. Data from Broadbent CR, Maxwell WB, Ferrie R, et al. Ability of anaesthetists to identify a marked lumbar interspace. *Anaesthesia.* 2000;55:1122–1126.

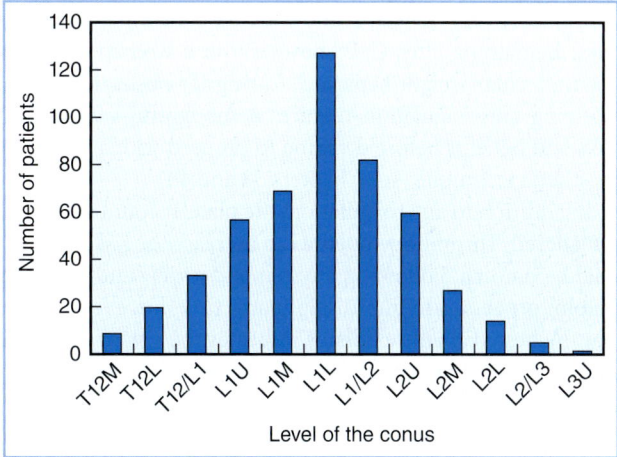

Fig. 31.9 Variation in the level of the tip of the conus medullaris assessed by magnetic resonance imaging of the lumbar spine among 504 consecutive adults. *L,* Lower third of vertebral body listed; *M,* middle third of vertebral body listed; *T12/L1,* interspace between T12 and L1; *U,* upper third of vertebral body listed. Data derived from Saifuddin A, Burnett SJ, White J. The variation of position of the conus medullaris in an adult population: a magnetic resonance imaging study. *Spine.* 1998;23:1452–1456.

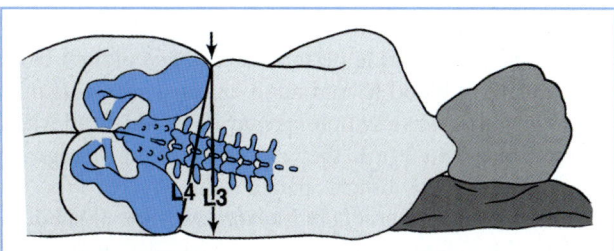

Fig. 31.10 Error that may arise if Tuffier's line is judged in a pregnant patient in the lateral position, when a line is drawn perpendicularly from the upper iliac crest rather than through both iliac crests. In pregnant patients at term, the hips may have a greater width than the shoulders. The resulting cephalad pelvic tilt may lead to an error in the cephalad direction.

Given the inaccuracy of identification of lumbar interspaces and the variability of the position of the conus, it is both logical and prudent to insert a spinal needle into a lower lumbar interspace. Although entry into the intrathecal space is frequently accompanied by a transient paresthesia, injection of spinal medication should not occur if there is a persistent paresthesia or pain with initial injection. Box 31.3 summarizes the problems and precautions in identifying lumbar interspaces and avoiding damage to the conus medullaris. In cases in which there is doubt about the level of lumbar interspace for injection, ultrasound guidance may be useful in accurately identifying the correct interspace.[71]

Catheters advanced into the intrathecal space theoretically would seem to place patients at risk for traumatic nerve injury. However, a retrospective study of 761 short-term intrathecal catheters placed over a 12-year period found no neurologic or serious complications.[72] Transient paresthesias with catheter placement into the intrathecal space have been reported, but do not appear to be associated with long-term consequences.[73]

Space-Occupying Lesions of the Vertebral Canal

Space-occupying lesions of the vertebral canal include intraspinal hematoma (epidural or subdural), epidural abscess, and intraspinal tumors, any of which, within the rigid confines of the bony spinal canal, can cause dangerous compression of nervous tissue and its blood supply. Urgent laminectomy is required to avoid permanent neurologic damage. Delayed recognition and treatment (>8 to 12 hours after onset of symptoms) may have a catastrophic outcome.

Epidural analgesia in labor does not normally behave like a space-occupying lesion and produces no lasting deformation of the thecal sac on MRI.[74] Nevertheless, in the presence of vertebral stenosis or lumbar disc protrusion, a large volume injected into the epidural space may tip the balance and produce signs of nervous tissue compression that normally resolve in a few hours.[75,76]

The neurologic deficit that may arise from a compressive lesion depends on the vertebral level; lower thoracic lesions are associated with leg weakness or paraplegia, and lumbar lesions with cauda equina syndrome, including urinary

---

BOX 31.3 Points to Remember to Reduce Risk for Damage to the Conus Medullaris During Spinal Anesthesia

- Tuffier's line is not in a constant position relative to the spine.
- The interspace chosen is usually higher than supposed.
- The spinal needle should be inserted into a lower lumbar level.
- Advancement of the spinal needle should be halted immediately, and the stylet removed to check for CSF, if entry of the needle tip into the subarachnoid space is suspected.
- The procedure should be abandoned if the patient is unable to cooperate.

CSF, Cerebrospinal fluid.

retention and incontinence. Back pain (often radiating to the legs) is a common feature.

Neuraxial Hematoma

Epidural Hematoma After Neuraxial Blockade

Incidence. Neuraxial hematoma is fortunately very rare, and even rarer in pregnant patients than in the general population. During pregnancy and the peripartum period, spontaneous neuraxial hematoma is reported more frequently than hematoma associated with neuraxial blockade. Only a handful of cases have been reported in the past two decades.[77–81] Epidural hematoma in pregnancy associated with coagulopathy but not neuraxial anesthesia has also been reported.[82,83] Ten surveys, including 1,462,631 obstetric epidural procedures, identified three cases (see Table 31.1), two without confirmatory details[3,15] and the other in a patient with HELLP (hemolysis, elevated liver enzymes, low platelets) syndrome.[12] This gives an estimated incidence of 0.205 per 100,000 epidural procedures.

Risk factors. Risk factors for epidural hematoma identified from comprehensive reviews of case reports include (1) difficult or traumatic epidural needle/catheter placement, (2) coagulopathy or therapeutic anticoagulation, (3) spinal deformity, and (4) spinal tumor.[19,84,85] Antiplatelet therapy with nonsteroidal antiinflammatory drugs does not appear to be associated with an increased risk for hematoma after neuraxial anesthesia.[86]

Of the five cases of epidural hematoma in obstetric patients identified by Loo et al.,[19] four were without details and the other was associated with coagulopathy. In the most recent analysis from the American Society of Anesthesiologists' (ASA) Closed-Claims Project database,[87] there were four cases of epidural hematoma, of which only one had coagulopathy; again, other details were not provided. The SCORE project reported a single case of epidural hematoma in more than 215,000 epidural and CSE procedures.[15] Two further case reports are of interest. A patient with eclampsia and thrombocytopenia suffered a persistent lower limb deficit after a traumatic epidural catheter insertion using the loss-of-resistance-to-air technique.[88] Laminectomy revealed multiple bubbles and a 4-mL blood clot, the exact site of which was not stated. Such a small volume could have caused neurologic deficit only if it was subdural rather than epidural. In another case, an epidural hematoma was reported presenting 9 days after removal of an epidural catheter that had been sited and used uneventfully for labor analgesia.[89] Apparently the only risk factor was a traumatic insertion. The coagulation assessment was normal, but the hematoma was extensive and required decompressive surgery. It is possible that this was a spontaneous hematoma and neuraxial analgesia was coincidental.

Both vessel damage and coagulopathy (whether inherited, acquired, or caused by anticoagulation) are usually necessary to produce a hematoma large enough to cause a neurologic deficit in the parturient. Safe epidural catheter insertion in coagulopathic parturients has often been recorded, but the frequency of vessel trauma is rarely mentioned.[90–92] Although vessel trauma can occur during removal of the epidural catheter, intuitively there is likely to be a higher chance for vessel trauma with needle placement and catheter insertion. In a series of 4365 nonobstetric patients receiving warfarin anticoagulation, epidural catheters were removed with a mean international normalized ratio of 1.9 (range of 1.5 to 7.1) without any observed epidural hematomas.[93]

The increasing number of women receiving pharmacologic thromboprophylaxis in the peripartum period has important implications for anesthesia providers. Although there is obvious concern that these patients may be at increased risk for bleeding complications, a systematic review published in 2017 revealed no cases of spinal-epidural hematoma associated with neuraxial anesthesia and thromboprophylaxis with unfractionated or low-molecular-weight heparin in obstetric patients.[94] Since then, Pujic et al.[95] reported a case of spinal-epidural hematoma on the third postoperative day in a patient who received a prophylactic dose of low-molecular-weight heparin 14 hours before spinal anesthesia for cesarean delivery and then twice daily postpartum (starting 9 hours after the cesarean delivery) as well as another case of delayed spinal epidural hematoma after CSE anesthesia in a woman receiving low-molecular-weight heparin.[96] Caring for obstetric patients receiving anticoagulation requires a thoughtful weighing of risks and benefits before deciding to proceed with a neuraxial anesthetic technique (see Chapters 38 and 44).

In addition to anticoagulation, the platelet count should be considered. Thrombocytopenia can increase the risk for neuraxial hematoma. Following a systematic review and modified Delphi process, an interdisciplinary task force concluded that the best available evidence indicates the risk of neuraxial hematoma associated with a platelet count > 70,000/μL is very low in the absence of other risk factors.[97] If the platelet count is less than 50,000/μL, it may be reasonable to avoid neuraxial procedures. It is important to consider the risks and benefits of proceeding or withholding neuraxial anesthesia in each individual situation.

Protective factors. Some epidural hematomas may be too small to cause neurologic deficit. One factor limiting the incidence of epidural hematomas may be the hypercoagulable state of parturients. Another is the ease with which a large volume of anticoagulated blood may flow out of the unrestricting intervertebral foramina in young patients. Injected blood is known to disappear from the epidural space rapidly in the parturient.[74,98] During performance of an epidural blood patch, 20 mL of blood is commonly injected with impunity. Although compressive symptoms may be experienced with a volume larger than 20 mL, they do not normally presage any neurologic deficit in obstetric patients.

Subdural and subarachnoid hematoma. Spinal subdural hematoma has been reported in obstetric patients: one in association with an ependymoma[19]; one after spinal anesthesia and an epidural blood patch[99]; and another in a woman with preeclampsia, known vessel puncture during epidural catheter insertion, and mild coagulopathy.[100] A subarachnoid hematoma after spinal anesthesia was reported in a patient with HELLP syndrome.[101] A fourth report described a healthy woman who suffered major subarachnoid hematoma after apparently straightforward CSE anesthesia.[102] All four patients developed cauda equina syndrome; laminectomy was required in three.

Inadvertent continuous administration of subdural local anesthetic has been reported to produce nerve compression resulting in permanent nerve damage.[103] Although MRI in this case did not show a hematoma, laminectomy was needed to relieve the fluid accumulation. Subdural injection may be as frequent as 1 in 4200[104]; the typical course is complete resolution of sensory and motor symptoms within hours.

Dural puncture is a prerequisite for subdural and subarachnoid hematoma. However, coagulopathy may *not* be a prerequisite because the extravasated blood is confined in a small space in which even a small volume may compress adjacent nerve roots.

Prevention, diagnosis, and management. It is clearly important to assess the coagulation status in an at-risk parturient before initiating a neuraxial procedure, and possibly when removing the epidural catheter as well. If a neuraxial blockade is found to have been conducted in the presence of risk factors for spinal hematoma, it is a responsibility of the anesthesia provider to examine the lower extremities after delivery, to confirm and document the return of normal motor and sensory function, and to request subsequent regular checks of lower extremity neurologic function by the nursing staff, typically for 24 hours. Severe back pain and a significant delay in normal recovery or deterioration of lower extremity or bladder function signal the need for emergency imaging of the spine. If intraspinal compression is confirmed by MRI, a neurosurgical consultation must be emergently sought. Even though neuraxial hematomas are rare, they may require emergency neurosurgical intervention as recovery is dependent on how quickly decompression can be achieved (e.g., treatment within 8 to 12 hours for epidural hematoma).[105]

Infection

Neuraxial infection (epidural abscess and meningitis) was identified as the most common cause of neuraxial injury in obstetric cases in the ASA Closed-Claims Project database between 1980 and 1999.[106] Infections that have been reported include epidural abscess, paraspinal and other epidural-related infection, and meningitis.

Epidural Abscess

Frequency. Epidural abscess may occur spontaneously in pregnancy and the puerperium as at other times.[19,107] An analysis of 915 reports of spinal-epidural abscess published between 1954 and 1997 found that epidural blockade had been performed in only 5.5% of cases.[108] Epidural abscess, like neuraxial hematoma, appears to be rare after neuraxial blockade in obstetric patients. Seven cases were found among 1,462,631 epidural procedures listed in ten surveys summarized in Table 31.1, a frequency of 0.479 per 100,000. The incidence among general surgical patients has been reported as 10-fold[12] to 100-fold[109] higher, with most cases arising in elderly and immunocompromised patients. A 4-year Australian study of 9482 obstetric patients who underwent childbirth in a center where correct sterile procedures were used found 49 epidural catheter–related infections (0.52%): 45 superficial, 2 epidural, and 2 paraspinal, giving an epidural infection rate of 21 per 100,000,[110] which was 100-fold higher than the calculated frequency from larger, but potentially less sensitive, surveys.

Multiple case reports of epidural abscess after epidural analgesia in obstetric patients illustrate that even when the principal risk factors of prolonged catheterization, suboptimal aseptic technique, and traumatic insertion are avoided, epidural abscess still may occur.[111-118] A comprehensive review of epidural abscess cases after neuraxial anesthesia found that all cases occurred after epidural catheterization, with three following CSE anesthesia; none followed spinal anesthesia alone.[119]

Risk factors identified from these cases are summarized in Table 31.2. An epidural abscess typically follows prolonged epidural catheterization, usually between 1 and 4 days in obstetric cases. Other possible etiologic factors are traumatic or difficult insertion of the catheter,[112,114] and diabetes or immunosuppression from any cause.[109,116] Inflammation at the epidural catheter entry point may presage epidural space infection.[110,112,115] In light of these reports, it may be prudent to avoid epidural catheterization of more than 2 days in the patient with other risk factors for infection.

Clinical presentation. In contrast to epidural hematoma, symptoms of epidural abscess are more insidious.[120] Backache (with local tenderness) and fever, with or without radiating or root pain, are the presenting features. The catheter entry point may be inflamed with some fluid leak, and a hematology screen typically reveals leukocytosis and increased C-reactive protein. Fever, neck stiffness, headache, and signs of inflammation serve to differentiate epidural abscess from hematoma. These signs and symptoms should prompt MRI, which may allow early diagnosis before the onset of neurologic symptoms (Fig. 31.11).[121] If untreated, symptoms may progress to leg weakness, paresthesias, bladder dysfunction, and other evidence of cauda equina syndrome. A blood culture may identify the organism before or without surgical drainage.

Etiology. *Staphylococcus aureus* is the most common causative organism in cases of epidural abscess, with the occasional infection with *Streptococcus* and *Pseudomonas* species. The skin appears to be the most likely source of infection.[19]

The skin is commonly colonized by *Staphylococcus epidermidis* and other weakly pathogenic bacteria and occasionally by *S. aureus*. The highest concentration of colonies is found in hair follicles,[122] where organisms may be protected from poorly applied disinfectants. Infectious organisms from the skin can reach deeper tissue planes via the needle track or an implanted epidural catheter to create a localized abscess in the paraspinal or epidural space. Despite all aseptic precautions, some level of detectable bacterial colonization of the epidural catheter is very common, but robust host defenses normally prevent infection. When defenses are weak and infection containment breaks down, epidural abscess formation begins.

TABLE 31.2   Possible Etiologic Factors for Epidural Abscess and Meningitis

	Epidural Abscess	Meningitis
Entry point	Through the epidural catheter or along its track	Via dural puncture
Usual causative organism	*Staphylococcus aureus*	*Streptococcus salivarius*
Possible source of infection	Patient's skin, tracking along the catheter entry point Epidural equipment contaminated by operator's skin Body fluids in the bed Injectate without racemic local anesthetic	Operator's mouth Talking without a mask Blood-borne Vagina
Risk factors	Prolonged catheterization Poor aseptic technique Multiple attempts at insertion, traumatic insertion No bacterial filter Lying in a wet, contaminated bed Polyurethane occlusive dressing Immunocompromise: corticosteroids, diabetes, acquired immunodeficiency syndrome	Dural puncture Labor No proceduralist face mask Manual removal of the placenta Vaginal infection Bacteremia Immunocompromise

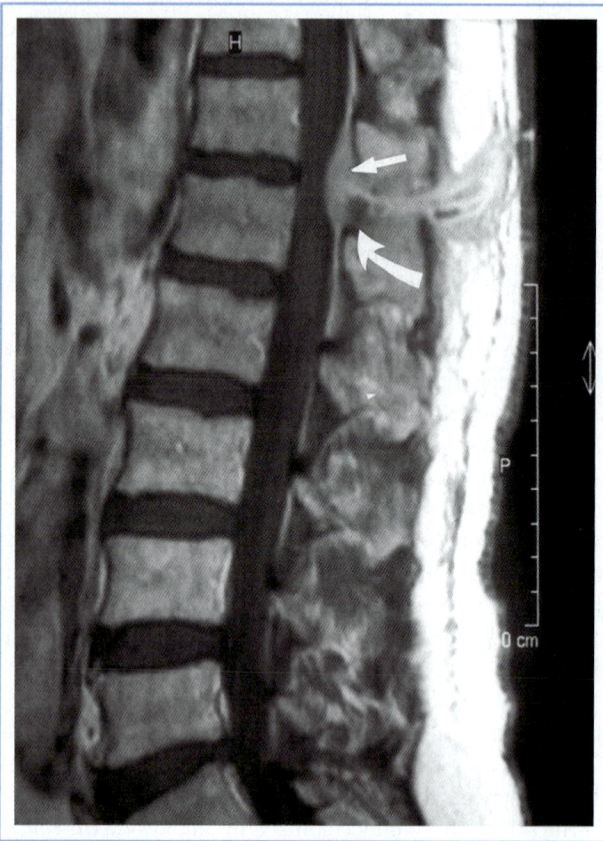

Fig. 31.11 Epidural Abscess. Midsagittal T1-weighted magnetic resonance image of the lumbar and lower thoracic region after intravenous gadolinium-DTPA. Note the dorsal epidural mass located at T12–L1 *(arrows)*, convex anteriorly but not compressing the conus. Normal epidural fat is flat anteriorly. From Royakers AA, Willigers H, van der Ven AJ, et al. Catheter-related epidural abscesses—don't wait for neurological deficits. *Acta Anaesthesiol Scand.* 2002;46:611–615.

Management. As with spinal hematoma, once neurologic signs are present, early diagnosis with prompt laminectomy is essential to recovery. In the presence of mild symptoms without neurologic changes, successful conservative treatment

with antibiotics[113] and successful percutaneous needle drainage[123] of epidural abscesses have also been reported, although only a laminectomy can ensure that all loculations are drained under direct vision. Prompt identification of the infectious organism(s) and directed antibiotic therapy are mandatory. The duration of antibiotic therapy should be determined on a case-by-case basis but is usually 4 to 6 weeks.

Other Epidural-Related Infections

Paraspinal abscess and osteomyelitis after epidural analgesia[124,125] and discitis after spinal blockade[126] have been reported in obstetric patients. Catheter-site inflammation is relatively common with prolonged postoperative epidural analgesia.[110,127] One report described both a subdural abscess after CSE anesthesia and infection in the subcutaneous tissues after an apparently misplaced epidural blood patch.[128]

A variety of organisms have been associated with epidural-related infections.[119] All such conditions are associated with back pain and signs of inflammation and pose a threat of spread to the epidural space. Moreover, paraspinal abscess may itself cause neurologic deficit.[129]

Meningitis

Although not consistently included in surveys, post–spinal meningitis has become a cause for concern[130] and is a serious neurologic complication of neuraxial labor analgesia. It was suspected in two cases in the prospective survey of 108,133 epidural procedures and 14,865 spinal anesthetic procedures reported by Scott and Tunstall,[6] although the specific type of anesthesia was not stated. Palot et al.[5] reported three cases of meningitis among 288,351 obstetric epidural procedures but did not state whether they followed dural puncture. One case was identified in a survey of spinal and CSE anesthesia (1/42,000 procedures).[9] A 2008 review found an incidence derived from surveys of spinal and CSE anesthesia in obstetrics of 1 in 39,000.[119] Table 31.3 summarizes 55 published reports of post–spinal meningitis in obstetric patients.[130–158]

Causative organisms. Community-acquired meningitis may occur in pregnancy as at other times. It is commonly caused by *Neisseria meningitidis, Streptococcus pneumoniae,* or *Haemophilus influenzae,* while occasional cases caused by tuberculosis, several β-hemolytic streptococci, and viruses are also reported in pregnancy. Post–spinal meningitis, by contrast, is most commonly caused by streptococci of the viridans type (α-hemolytic streptococci such as *Streptococcus salivarius, Streptococcus sanguis,* and *Streptococcus uberis*) (see Table 31.3). These organisms are found in the upper airway and the vagina. *Pseudomonas* meningitis has also been reported.[133] Neither *Pseudomonas* nor α-hemolytic streptococci are normally virulent; they do not, for example, cause a wound infection, but they thrive in a watery medium and flourish if introduced into CSF. In several early cases (before the use of the polymerase chain reaction), no organisms were grown on culture and chemical meningitis was diagnosed. In most cases, however, there were features of bacterial meningitis, including low CSF glucose concentration. Streptococci of the viridans type do not grow readily in conventional culture media and may well have been present but not detected.

Risk factors. Dural puncture is probably a prerequisite for iatrogenic meningitis. A retrospective review of surgical patients in one hospital in Brazil found three cases among 38,128 patients receiving spinal anesthesia and none among 12,822 patients receiving other types of anesthesia.[159] Among 73 women with β-hemolytic streptococcal infections in the puerperium identified in a survey from Iowa,[160] the only woman who suffered meningitis had received spinal anesthesia. In normal circumstances, the blood-brain barrier (the endothelial lining of the capillaries, which are continuous with tight junctions and no pinocytotic vesicles) protects the CNS against weakly pathogenic bacteria. The dura mater should not be confused with the blood-brain barrier, but dural puncture is commonly associated with vascular trauma,[161] which allows blood to enter the CSF.

Of the 55 published cases of meningitis after neuraxial anesthesia for which details are available (see Table 31.3), 49 occurred after known dural puncture. Among the six cases that followed apparently uncomplicated epidural analgesia, one was viral and may have been a chance event,[153] one was probably an epidural abscess,[154] and two were blood-borne from vaginal infection caused by group B streptococcus.[155,156] Uncomplicated epidural catheterization itself is unlikely to increase the risk for puerperal meningitis. Although spinal analgesia is used less commonly than epidural analgesia during labor, case reports of meningitis after spinal analgesia far outnumber those after epidural analgesia. A causative relationship between epidural catheterization and meningitis after vaginal delivery may be attributed to unrecognized dural puncture, which may occur during multiple attempts at epidural catheter insertion or even with apparently uncomplicated catheter insertion.

Labor may also be a risk factor for meningitis, as the great majority of parturients developing meningitis had labored (see Table 31.3). Meningitis appears surprisingly rare after elective cesarean delivery, despite the extensive use of spinal anesthesia in this context.

The possible reasons why meningitis is reported more commonly in laboring women than among those undergoing elective cesarean delivery are as follows:

- The vagina may be colonized by streptococci, and vaginal delivery is commonly followed by mild bacteremia. Thus, labor, with its potential for vaginal trauma, is clearly an important risk factor. Unlike vaginal delivery, elective cesarean delivery is not normally associated with streptococcal bacteremia.
- For elective cesarean delivery, spinal anesthesia is administered in the operating room, which is a cleaner environment than the labor and delivery room.
- The anesthesia provider is more likely to wear a face mask in the operating room.
- The nonlaboring patient is not thrashing about in a (possibly) contaminated bed.
- An antibiotic is usually administered immediately before cesarean delivery.

Systemic infection may also be a risk factor for meningitis (see Chapter 36). Bacteremia has been detected in approximately 8% of women with chorioamnionitis,[162] although two small studies found no evidence of spinal infection among 12 women with bacteremia who received epidural blockade without antibiotic treatment.[163,164] There are no studies detailing the risk of meningitis when performing spinal anesthesia in a parturient with systemic infection. Human immunodeficiency virus (HIV) infection and acquired immunodeficiency syndrome (AIDS) should not be regarded as contraindications to neuraxial analgesia, given the presence of the virus within the CNS early in the course of disease.[165] Performing an epidural blood patch in the presence of bacteremia is also a theoretical risk for both meningitis and abscess, but neither has been reported.

Other risk factors for meningitis include faulty technique, in particular failure to wear a mask (see later discussion). Manual removal of the placenta is a postulated risk factor for meningitis, and one such case has been reported,[144] although given the popularity of spinal anesthesia for this indication, one would expect a higher frequency. It may be postulated that use of the CSE technique, with the presence of a foreign body next to a dural hole, may increase the risk for meningitis.

Clinical presentation and management. Fever, headache, photophobia, nausea, vomiting, and neck stiffness are typical symptoms of meningitis; when they are accompanied by confusion, drowsiness, and Kernig sign (inability to straighten the knee when the hip is flexed), meningitis should be strongly suspected. The onset of symptoms may be a few hours to a few days after delivery. Diagnostic lumbar puncture (best avoided in the presence of raised intracranial pressure or suspicion of epidural abscess) shows increased CSF pressure, increases in CSF protein level and white blood cell count (mainly polymorphonuclear leukocytes in patients with bacterial meningitis), and a CSF glucose concentration that is lower than that in the blood. Because of the nature of the *Streptococcus viridans* group, culture on plates rather than in broth may have negative results, particularly if antibiotics have been given.[130] Treatment with an appropriate antibiotic should not await the microbiology results and should result

TABLE 31.3   Case Reports of Post–Dural Puncture Meningitis Among Obstetric Patients

	References	Number of Cases	Organism; Comments
Spinal Analgesia for Labor (11 cases)	Gibbons, 1969[131]	3	Case cluster, no growth, "chemical meningitis," CSF findings suggested bacterial etiology
	Phillips, 1970[132]	1	No growth, CSF findings suggested bacterial etiology
	Corbett and Rosenstein, 1971[133]	3	Case cluster, single anesthesiologist, unsterile technique, *Pseudomonas aeruginosa*
	Newton et al., 1994[134]	1	*S. salivarius*
	Lurie et al., 1999[135]	1	*Streptococcus viridans*
	Centers for Disease Control and Prevention, 2010[137]	2	Case cluster, single anesthesiologist, *S. salivarius*, one death
Spinal Anesthesia for Cesarean Delivery (24 cases)	Bugedo et al., 1991[136]	1	Signs of bacterial meningitis following cesarean delivery, labor unknown
	Lee and Parry, 1991[137]	1	No growth, CSF findings suggested bacterial etiology, in labor, three attempts at epidural analgesia
	Stallard and Barry, 1995[138]	1	No growth, CSF findings suggested bacterial etiology, in labor, three attempts at epidural analgesia, spinal anesthesia at same interspace
	Donnelly et al., 1998[139]	1	No growth, CSF findings suggested bacterial etiology, membranes ruptured
	Thomas and Cooper, 2001[140]	1	Preeclampsia, labor unknown, patient died
	Rodrigo et al., 2007[141]	6	*Aspergillus*, five elective cesarean deliveries, one in labor, three patients died
	Celik et al., 2014[142]	1	No growth, CSF findings suggested aseptic meningitis
	Ersoz et al., 2014[143]	12	*Serratia marcescens*, elective cesarean deliveries, extrinsic vial contamination
Spinal Anesthesia for Retained Placenta (1 case)	Roberts and Petts, 1990[144]	1	Two attempts at spinal anesthesia, no growth, CSF findings suggested bacterial etiology
CSE Analgesia for Labor (9 cases)	Harding et al., 1994[145]	2	No growth, CSF findings suggested bacterial etiology
	Cascio and Heath, 1996[146]	1	*S. salivarius* (dismissed as contaminant)
	Bouhemad et al., 1998[147]	1	*S. salivarius*
	Duflo et al., 1998[148]	1	*S. viridans*
	Vernis et al., 2004[149]	1	One case in the course of a randomized trial
	Centers for Disease Control and Prevention, 2010[137]	3	Cluster, single anesthesiologist, *S. salivarius*
CSE Anesthesia for Cesarean Delivery (1 case)	Gordon et al., 2022[150]	1	CSF-cutaneous fistula, recognized on postoperative day 2
Unintentional Dural Puncture in Labor (3 cases)	Berga and Trierweiler, 1989[151]	1	*Streptococcus sanguis*
	Sansome et al., 1991[152]	1	No growth, CSF findings ambivalent
	Baer, 2006[130]	1	*S. simulans* and *S. salivarius*; patient died
"Uncomplicated" Epidural Analgesia for Labor (6 cases)	Neumark et al., 1980[153]	1	Coxsackievirus B
	Ready and Helfer, 1989[154]	2	1 *Streptococcus uberis* 1 *Streptococcus faecalis* (epidural inflammation)
	Davis et al., 1993[155]	1	Group B streptococcus
	Goldstein et al., 1996[156]	1	Group B streptococcus
	Choy, 2000[157]	1	Two attempts at epidural analgesia, no growth, CSF findings suggested bacterial etiology, patient died
Total (55 cases)	49 known dural punctures 18 elective cesarean deliveries, all with extrinsic contamination of medication or equipment 7 deaths		

CSE, Combined spinal-epidural anesthesia; *CSF*, cerebrospinal fluid.

in full recovery.[19] Vancomycin and third-generation cephalosporins have been recommended as first-line treatment.[159] The treatment regimen should be adjusted according to the results of culture and sensitivity testing.

Prevention of Neuraxial Infection

Measures to prevent intraspinal infection are summarized in Box 31.4. Means of preventing meningitis and epidural abscess are not identical, because abscess usually follows epidural catheterization and is commonly caused by *S. aureus*, which enters via the skin, whereas meningitis classically follows dural puncture, is caused by vaginal or nasal organisms, may be blood-borne, and is usually caused by streptococcus and never by *S. aureus*.

Because adverse outcomes are rare, the use of sterile precautions can rarely be supported by evidence from randomized trials. The components of good sterile technique should be guided by common sense and the best available indirect evidence. It is notable that in many case reports of neuraxial infection, sterile precautions used in initiating neuraxial blockade receive no mention.

A practice advisory published in 2017 by the ASA Task Force on Infectious Complications Associated with Neuraxial Techniques[166] concerns prevention, diagnosis, and management of infectious complications. Key aspects are discussed here.

Mask. Several surveys indicate widespread disregard of surgical masks for infection control during neuraxial block administration.[159,167,168] Among case reports of nosocomial meningitis, a mask was not mentioned[132,144,151,153,154] or was not worn ("as it is of doubtful value"[137] or because it "contributes little to prevent infection during spinal or epidural anesthesia,"[135] or is not considered part of "full aseptic technique"[155]).

Confusion has arisen because randomized trials have demonstrated that omission of masks in the operating room does not increase the occurrence of wound infection.[169] This is not surprising, however, because organisms from the upper airway do not cause wound infection, but they certainly do cause nosocomial meningitis. The effect of wearing a mask in the prevention of such rare complications cannot readily be ascertained by a randomized controlled trial. Nevertheless, the obvious value of masks in reducing the dispersion of bacteria from the mouth and nose has been well demonstrated.[170,171] A mask is an essential part of aseptic precautions that should be taken for neuraxial needle and catheter insertion.[130,166]

Sterile gown. Although undeniably part of "full aseptic precautions" employed by surgeons, a sterile gown is rarely worn for spinal needle placement. For insertion of an epidural catheter, a gown is commonly worn in the United Kingdom, although rarely in the United States. The value of wearing a gown is not supported by evidence, but some postulate that wearing one may be safer than not doing so.

Sterilizing the skin. Evidence from laboratory and clinical studies shows that chlorhexidine in 70% alcohol consistently outperforms povidone-iodine for skin disinfection.[122,127,172] The concentration of chlorhexidine used varies from 0.5% to 2%. It is superior in speed of onset and duration of action and is less likely to provoke a skin reaction. Unlike povidone-iodine, it is effective in the presence of blood or pus, it stays sterile in the container, and bacterial resistance is unlikely.[119] Alcohol provides the rapid onset, and chlorhexidine provides the longer duration of action.

Concerns have been raised about chlorhexidine neurotoxicity. Both chlorhexidine and iodine have been shown to damage neuronal cells during *in vitro* experiments.[173] Neither chlorhexidine nor iodine is licensed for skin sterilization before neuraxial block administration. Although there are a few case reports of adhesive arachnoiditis in which chlorhexidine was suspected as a possible cause, the only clinical study performed supports its safety for use before spinal anesthesia.[174] Additionally, the risk for infection usually outweighs that for neurotoxicity, and the superiority of chlorhexidine as an antiseptic is clear. It is appropriate, nevertheless, to take precautions, such as using the lowest effective concentration available and not allowing the solution to come into contact with other solutions or equipment that will enter the patient's neuraxis. Use of a single application "swab stick" overcomes this concern; if such an applicator is not used, the aqueous chlorhexidine container must be removed from the immediate area before equipment for neuraxial insertion is deployed. Adequate drying time should be allowed after application of the antiseptic solution to the skin.[166]

Maintaining sterility of the epidural catheter, its contents, and the entry point. The entry point of the epidural catheter clearly needs to be protected from contamination by a suitable dressing.[175] Although it would seem logical, there is no evidence to support or discourage the use of a bacterial filter during a short-term (1 to 2 days) epidural infusion.[175] Prolonged catheterization of more than 2 days is best avoided after dural puncture, whether unintentional or deliberate, and when sepsis or immunocompromise is present or suspected.

BOX 31.4   Procedures to Decrease the Risk for Infection After Neuraxial Anesthesia

- Wear an effective mask.
- Remove hand jewelry and watches, and wash hands with an alcohol-based scrub solution.
- Use sterile gloves in correct manner.
- Apply chlorhexidine-in-alcohol solution to the patient's skin, following the package instructions, and allow the skin to dry after application.
- Make sure the back is securely draped.
- Avoid contaminating any equipment and drugs that are used in the procedure.
- Minimize touching parts of the equipment that will enter the patient.
- After the procedure, apply a suitable dressing to the catheter entry point.
- Bacterial filters may be considered during extended continuous epidural infusion.
- Remove the epidural catheter shortly after delivery unless there are specific indications for not doing so.

Vascular Disorders

Ischemic Injury to the Spinal Cord

Ischemic injury to the spinal cord is rare. It is more likely to be seen in older patients than in the obstetric population, in whom arterial disease is unusual and hypotension is treated aggressively. It can occur after neuraxial anesthesia or after general anesthesia with accompanying hypotension.

The blood supply to the spinal cord depends on a single anterior spinal artery and bilateral posterior spinal arteries. The arteries arise from the circle of Willis and receive reinforcements during their descent in the spinal canal. The posterior spinal arteries receive regular contributions from radicular arteries, but the single anterior spinal artery, which supplies the anterior two-thirds of the spinal cord, receives only sporadic reinforcement. Anterior spinal artery syndrome, which may result from arterial compression or hypotension, is characterized by a predominantly motor deficit, with or without loss of pain and temperature sensation, but with sparing of vibration and joint sensations, which are transmitted in the posterior columns. The condition has been reported among obstetric patients with particular risk factors (see later discussion).[3,19,176] In one report[177] a parous woman received epidural analgesia with lidocaine, then bupivacaine with epinephrine, followed by 2-chloroprocaine when she required urgent cesarean delivery. Hypotension caused by blood loss from a placenta previa and a ruptured uterus was followed by irreversible anterior spinal artery syndrome.

Chemical Injury

Many substances, primarily drugs, have been injected in error in the neuraxial canal. In a review covering the years 1950 to 2014, 29 case reports of drug errors during obstetric neuraxial procedures were identified.[178] Drugs injected in error included ephedrine, magnesium sulfate, antibiotics, labetalol, ondansetron, tranexamic acid, and chlorhexidine, among others.

The Epidural Space

The epidural space is remarkably tolerant of foreign and potentially neurotoxic substances because of two protective factors. First, vascular uptake and outward flow via the intervertebral foramina remove a large proportion of solutions deposited in the epidural space. Second, nerve roots within the epidural space are protected by a cuff of dura and arachnoid as well as pia mater. Severe neuraxial damage occurs only when these defenses are overwhelmed either by gross overdose or if there is unintentional contamination of the subarachnoid space. There are many case reports of unintentional epidural injection of the wrong substance, including the following:

1. **Vasopressors (ephedrine and metaraminol)**. Epidural administration resulted in severe hypertension.[179]
2. **Potassium chloride**. At least four well-documented cases have been reported.[180,181] All patients had profound motor and sensory block with pain or depolarizing spasms. Only one, who received the largest epidural dose (15 mL of 11.25% KCl), remained permanently paraplegic.[181]

3. **Other potentially noxious substances**. Administration of an unknown substance, possibly paraldehyde, given in error as an epidural bolus injection during labor, resulted in permanent painful quadriplegia and the largest monetary award for damages in the United Kingdom at that time.[182] Additionally, the inadvertent administration of a large volume of chlorhexidine resulted in severe adhesive arachnoiditis.[183] Unintentional misconnections of intravenous and epidural infusion systems have led to large-volume epidural infusions of potentially harmful substances, including total parenteral nutrition solutions with a high osmolality[184] and ranitidine in a phenol-containing solution.[185] Fortunately, in most cases of this type of drug error, neurologic sequelae have not been reported.

With these few exceptions, the epidural space appears to be tolerant of most inadvertent administrations. Nevertheless, the possibility of occult dural puncture means that unintentional administration of a potentially neurotoxic substance (e.g., traces of alcohol, antioxidant, or preservative) may migrate into the subarachnoid space. Vigilance and systems to avoid these errors are mandatory.

The Subarachnoid Space

The subarachnoid space, with its exposed nerve roots and direct communication with intracranial structures, presents a greater risk than the epidural space for adverse outcome after unintentional injection of toxic substances. Intrathecal potassium can be lethal.[186] A 2015 review of neuraxial drug administration errors[178] identified four reports of intrathecal injection of tranexamic acid (all caused by misidentification of the drug ampule). All four cases were fatal; the patients ultimately died from refractory ventricular tachycardia and fibrillation. Further cases of severe neurologic injury and death when tranexamic acid was administered intrathecally continue to be reported.[187] Inadvertent intrathecal administration of magnesium at many times higher than the typical clinical dose has led to hemodynamic and respiratory instability and prolonged motor blockade, but no permanent neurologic sequelae.

Nerve roots within the subarachnoid space are highly vulnerable to chemical damage, particularly the sacral roots, which are poorly myelinated. Irritant solutions may cause neurotoxicity and arachnoiditis. Neurotoxicity may manifest as **cauda equina syndrome** or, if more extensive, as paraplegia or quadriplegia. For example, in 1937, 14 cases of severe cauda equina syndrome were reported after spinal anesthesia using a solution called "heavy duracaine," a mixture (in 15% ethanol) of procaine, glycerin, and gliadin or gum acacia, which presumably was added in an attempt to prolong the action of procaine.[188] In the 1940s and 1950s in the United Kingdom, spinal injection of 10 mL of hypoosmolar dibucaine was associated with paraplegia, but whether the paraplegia resulted from disturbance of the intrathecal milieu or contamination with phenol is argued.

More recently, there were numerous reports of cauda equina syndrome after intrathecal injection of lidocaine (all types of administration, both intended and unintended, most commonly hyperbaric 5%)[189-191] and occasionally after intrathecal administration of other local anesthetics.[192,193] None of these cases involved obstetric patients. In all cases, other causes of neurologic deficit (trauma, ischemia, infection, compression, contamination, and adverse positioning) were excluded. An upper safe dose limit for intrathecal lidocaine of 60 mg[190,194] has been recommended. More concerning, cauda equina syndrome has also been reported after CSE anesthesia with spinal levobupivacaine for cesarean delivery.[195] Postpartum MRI showed contrast enhancement in the cauda equina fibers concordant with arachnoiditis; the patient made a complete recovery after 8 weeks of rehabilitation therapy. A similar presentation has also been reported after CSE anesthesia with hyperbaric bupivacaine for cesarean delivery.[196] These case reports should not deter the use of spinal bupivacaine, but rather highlight that cauda equina syndrome is rare and is most likely to occur without an apparent anesthetic error. Potential risk factors for neurotoxic damage are summarized in Box 31.5.

Conus damage and cauda equina syndrome may appear similar—back pain, leg weakness and numbness, and/or bowel and bladder dysfunction. Although conus damage may involve upper motor neuron signs, these are not always present, and both conditions may have unilateral or bilateral features.[62] However, the causation is different. Whereas conus damage may result from ischemia or trauma, cauda equina syndrome typically results from either compression or chemical damage within the lumbar spinal canal.

Transient Neurologic Syndrome

Transient neurologic syndrome (also called transient radicular irritation) is not associated with any detectable neurologic deficit, but the distribution of pain in the back, buttocks, and thighs mirrors the distribution of nerve damage in cauda equina syndrome sufficiently to support the theory that the nerves are indeed irritated by a noxious intrathecal injection. Like cauda equina syndrome, it follows spinal anesthesia, most commonly with lidocaine. Moreover, other risk factors for cauda equina syndrome and transient neurologic syndrome are similar (see Box 31.5), although transient

neurologic syndrome may be less dependent on lidocaine dose or the presence of a vasoconstrictor.[197] Transient neurologic syndrome occurs more than four times more frequently with spinal lidocaine than with other local anesthetics.[198] It is, however, much more common in nonobstetric patients, with a median frequency, according to one review, of 22%.[197] Reported frequencies after spinal anesthesia in obstetric patients are 0%,[199] 4.2%,[200] 5.3%,[201] and 8.9%.[202]

Arachnoiditis

Arachnoiditis is a disastrous condition, usually with a delayed onset of permanent quadriplegia. It is extremely rare and has not been detected in any surveys of neurologic sequelae of obstetric neuraxial blockade. Among parturients, chronic adhesive arachnoiditis of chemical origin has arisen after unintentional intrathecal injection of a large dose of 2-chloroprocaine with antioxidant and preservative intended for the epidural space,[203] while seven cases have been reported after epidural analgesia for childbirth with 2% lidocaine, probably with preservative.[204] Six cases were reported among Italian surgical patients after apparently standard epidural anesthesia with bupivacaine and/or mepivacaine, usually with epinephrine.[205] The local anesthetic agents, however, were obtained from multidose vials containing parabens as preservative, and the glass syringes used for loss-of-resistance identification of the epidural space had been washed in detergent. With earlier publications, it is not always possible to distinguish the cause of arachnoiditis, but it seemed to appear in clusters, suggesting that there may have been shortcomings in anesthetic technique. In a more recent case, a woman suffered severe arachnoiditis after spinal anesthesia for elective cesarean delivery.[206] Her skin had been cleaned with iodine and then chlorhexidine in alcohol and allowed to dry. It was unclear whether the tray containing antiseptic solutions was removed before the rest of the procedure. Because of pain during attempted insertion of the spinal needle, the skin was infiltrated at least three times with lidocaine before intrathecal bupivacaine was given. Shortly thereafter, she became disturbed and experienced a severe headache, and general anesthesia was administered. Postpartum, she developed obstructive hydrocephalus and extensive adhesive arachnoiditis. The judge in the subsequent lawsuit determined that, on balance of probabilities, there must have been contact in some way between the chlorhexidine and the local anesthetic solution.

Vulnerable Patients

Various conditions may render some women more vulnerable than normal to neurologic injury precipitated by neuraxial anesthesia. The following discussion of conditions is not exhaustive.

Vertebral Abnormality

Skeletal abnormalities involving the spine, including congenital anomaly, trauma, and back surgery, can make epidural or spinal needle insertion difficult. Patients with spinal dysraphism are at risk for accidental dural puncture and nerve root damage unless the needle is inserted above the defect (see

---

BOX 31.5 Risk Factors for Chemical Damage to the Cauda Equina

- Poor spread of local anesthetic in the subarachnoid space
  - Block failure, followed by repeat injection
  - Fine-gauge or pencil-point needle
  - Microbore spinal catheter
  - Continuous infusion
  - Hyperbaric solution
  - Lithotomy position
- Unintentional intrathecal injection of a large volume intended for the epidural space
- Incorrect formulation, with unsuitable preservative or antioxidant
- Intrathecal injection of lidocaine, particularly 5% (possibly also tetracaine or dibucaine)

Chapter 46). Those with tethered cord syndrome are at risk for cord damage if the spinal or epidural needle is inserted at a vertebral level that would normally be expected to be below the conus.[58] Occasionally, a low-lying conus may be present without any premonitory signs.[64] Pressure from spinal stenosis or prolapsed intervertebral disc, coupled with a large-volume epidural injection, may result in spinal cord compression and neurologic deficit.[76]

Vascular Abnormalities

Vascular disease and malformation are risk factors for spinal cord ischemia, hematoma, and compression. The major supply to the lumbar enlargement of the spinal cord is the artery of Adamkiewicz, a unilateral structure that typically arises from the lower thoracic or upper lumbar portion of the aorta between T9 and L2. Compression of this single vessel may therefore jeopardize the blood supply to the lower cord in susceptible individuals. In 15% of individuals, a secondary blood supply to the spinal cord that ascends from the internal iliac arteries[207] assumes a major role. These ascending arteries lie close to the lumbosacral trunk and are, in theory, vulnerable to pressure from the fetal head or damage by obstetric instrumentation, thus causing conus ischemia.

A neuraxial arteriovenous malformation is an obvious cause for concern for the obstetric anesthesia provider.[208] Small arterial feeders from a segmental intercostal artery supply dilated serpiginous epidural veins that may extend over many segments of the spinal canal.[209] The resulting hemangioma raises the pressure on epidural veins and reduces spinal cord blood flow. Oxygen delivery to local tissues is reduced, and the risk for spinal hematoma or ischemic damage and compression is increased. Pregnancy and epidural analgesia have been known to precipitate paraplegia in previously asymptomatic patients[210,211]; aortocaval compression, a large blood volume, and a large epidural injection (which may cause severe pain) all increase epidural pressure.

The preanesthesia examination should include inspection of the back for cutaneous angiomas or macular areas of skin discoloration, which may suggest the presence of an underlying spinal angioma at the same segmental level. Because spinal cord capillary flow is compromised in the drainage area of an arteriovenous malformation, systemic arterial pressure should be kept close to normal throughout the peripartum period, regardless of anesthetic technique.

Spinal Tumor

Epidural blockade has been reported to precipitate neurologic symptoms in the presence of previously undiagnosed spinal tumors. Spinal tumors also predispose to spinal hematoma after neuraxial blockade,[19] and epidural analgesia may precipitate extreme pain.[212]

Coagulopathy or Anticoagulation

The risk associated with neuraxial procedures in patients with a preexisting coagulopathy or anticoagulation therapy is discussed earlier in this chapter and in Chapters 38 and 44.

Immunocompromise. Most cases of epidural infection that have been reported in surveys involve older patients with immunocompromise.[12,109] It is advisable to avoid prolonged epidural catheterization in immunocompromised patients, although prophylactic antibiotic therapy is not warranted.

Preexisting neurologic disorder. Patients with hereditary neuropathy with liability to pressure palsy are particularly sensitive to compression neuropathy during the course of labor and delivery.[213]

It is postulated that patients with preexisting peripheral neuropathies may be more susceptible to nerve injury when exposed to a second insult, the so-called *double crush phenomenon*.[214] To explore whether neuraxial anesthesia represented such an insult, Hebl et al.[214] reviewed the medical records of 567 patients with peripheral neuropathies who had spinal or epidural blockade, including 12 obstetric patients. There were two instances of worsening neurologic status, both in older patients with diabetes. There were no control patients, but clearly, if there is a risk that neuraxial anesthesia will exacerbate a neuropathy, it is very small. The exception may be patients with **spinal stenosis**. Reports of worsening neurologic status after spinal anesthesia should cause providers to consider the risks and benefits before initiating a neuraxial blockade in patients with known spinal stenosis.[215] Fortunately, spinal stenosis is rare in the obstetric population.

Patients with multiple sclerosis often suffer relapses in the postpartum period and neuraxial blockade may be blamed erroneously (see Chapter 47).[216] Epidural rather than spinal anesthesia has traditionally been recommended in patients with multiple sclerosis because the concentration of local anesthetic in the white matter of the spinal cord is less after epidural than after spinal injection, and exposing demyelinated spinal cord to local anesthetics could theoretically worsen the disease.[217] However, although many providers are reluctant to perform spinal anesthesia in patients with multiple sclerosis, there is no good evidence that it will worsen the neurologic conditions in these patients.[218] In fact, the most recent study showed no new or worsening symptoms in 35 patients with multiple sclerosis undergoing a variety of surgical procedures.[219] Similarly, no association between worsening multiple sclerosis symptoms and any form of neuraxial anesthesia was found in a study cohort limited to obstetric patients.[217] It is clearly important to document neurologic status and to discuss relapse rates with the mother before and after any anesthetic intervention, but patients can be reassured that no type of anesthesia has been shown to increase postpartum relapse risk or negatively influence long-term disease progression.

Diabetes. Patients with diabetes are vulnerable to neurologic injury for three reasons. They are susceptible to infection, they may have vascular disease, and they may have a peripheral neuropathy. Diabetic spinal artery syndrome has also been described in parturients,[176] and worsening neuropathy has been observed in surgical patients with diabetes.[214] Patients with gestational diabetes alone are unlikely to have developed chronic vascular or neurologic sequelae that place them at high risk for neurologic injury.

RISK MANAGEMENT AND FOLLOW-UP

Women at high risk for neurologic injury should be referred to the obstetric anesthesia clinic during pregnancy so that an anesthesia provider can obtain a thorough history, examine the patient, organize consultations or imaging studies as needed, and discuss the anesthetic plan with the patient and their obstetric providers. The recommended aspects of the history and physical examination that should be explored are summarized in Boxes 31.6 and 31.7.

In addition to minimizing risk by adhering to standard practices and precautions, vigilance must be extended to the postpartum period to detect, diagnose, and treat any disorders that may arise. It is important that those caring for women in the puerperium are taught to look for signs of neurologic pathology and that the women themselves, once home, are taught to recognize symptoms that might be attributable to anesthetic complications, and to contact an anesthesia provider if they experience them.

Diagnosis of Possible Neurologic Injury

Clinical examination coupled with knowledge of basic neuroanatomy outlined in this chapter should make it possible to distinguish peripheral from central lesions. Preanesthesia history (see Box 31.6) and physical examination (see Box 31.7) may reveal some helpful clues, and any preexisting signs or deficits documented in the record will narrow the search or even provide an immediate answer. Patient history and physical examination are integral to establishing associations between the complaint and the manifested physical signs and symptoms as well as helping to determine the site and cause of injury.

The basic physical examination should be repeated postpartum (see Box 31.7), and the results should be compared with the preanesthesia findings. Additionally, nerve conduction studies can be helpful in localizing and differentiating injuries. Significant back pain with unexplained fever, worsening neurologic symptoms, coagulopathy, and immunosuppression are red flags that suggest spine imaging is indicated.[220] Pain radiating to the legs or buttocks is a late and urgent sign of spinal cord or cauda equina compression. Headache, fever, and neck stiffness suggest meningitis.

MRI has revolutionized the speed and precision with which intraspinal lesions can be identified, and gadolinium enhancement further improves its sensitivity. An MRI cannot distinguish clearly between blood and other fluid, although the distinction can usually be made on other grounds. In the presence of meningitis, an MRI with gadolinium enhancement shows swelling of the cord and punctate areas of increased density, reflecting inflammatory cell infiltrates. Arteriovenous malformations of the cord or dura may be visible, and the enlarged veins draining them may be seen as serpiginous signal voids.

BOX 31.6 Topics to Explore in the Preanesthesia History

- Allergies, medications, and use of recreational drugs
- Diabetes or cardiovascular disorder
- Previous spinal or epidural anesthetics (what was the outcome?)
- Preexisting neurologic signs or symptoms (e.g., sciatica, leg weakness)
- Skeletal abnormality or back surgery
- Anticoagulant medication or easy bleeding/bruising
- Possibility of immunocompromise

BOX 31.7 Preanesthesia Neurologic Examination

- If there is a question of neurologic disorder, examine the lower limbs:
  - Sensation to pinprick or ice, and vibration sense
  - Knee and ankle tendon reflexes and Babinski reflex
  - Motor power of hips, knees, and ankles
- Examine the back for:
  - Signs of infection (pustules to be avoided)
  - Nevi suggestive of arteriovenous malformation
  - Midline hair tuft or fat pad, suggesting dysraphism (e.g., spina bifida occulta)
  - Scoliosis
  - If the spine anatomy is abnormal, as in severe scoliosis, is there an easily palpable sacral hiatus as an alternative to the lumbar epidural space?
  - Range of motion and maneuvers that might aggravate radicular pain
- Look for signs of bleeding tendency
- Document:
  - The history and physical examination
  - Abnormalities and treatment decisions
  - Differences of opinion
  - The reasons the anesthetic is administered despite a relative contraindication

---

KEY POINTS

- The vast majority of maternal nerve injuries can be attributed to the process of labor and delivery. Some patients may have a preexisting disease that predisposes them to nerve injury.
- Intrapartum symptoms of nerve compression may go unnoticed, particularly when neuraxial analgesia/anesthesia is used. Therefore, neurologic status should be regularly assessed, and the patient should be encouraged to change positions frequently.
- Postpartum neurologic deficit is most often transient in nature and likely to be a result of causes other than anesthesia. Nevertheless, there is a tendency to attribute neurologic deficits to neuraxial anesthesia.

- The exact incidence of neurologic complications caused by neuraxial anesthesia is difficult to determine because of wide variations in practice, criteria for diagnosis, accuracy of records, and overall low frequency of serious injury.
- Neuraxial anesthesia is more likely to cause central injuries, while peripheral nerve injuries are more likely to have obstetric causes.
- Proper sterile technique involves wearing a face mask, hand washing, donning sterile gloves, and cleansing the skin with chlorhexidine in alcohol and allowing it to dry before initiating neuraxial blockade.
- Choosing a lower lumbar interspace (L2–L3 or below) for insertion of the spinal needle minimizes the risk for trauma to the spinal cord. Using surface landmarks, anesthesia providers often identify an interspinous space that is one or even two lumbar levels higher than they believe.
- The risk for meningitis may be decreased by avoiding dural puncture during labor in a patient with systemic infection who has not received appropriate antibiotic treatment.
- The anesthesia provider should clearly document the preoperative history and physical examination, the rationale for the anesthetic procedure, and the details of each procedure.
- Rapid diagnosis and treatment are essential to minimizing neurologic sequelae and reducing the chance for permanent injury. Compressive intraspinal lesions with neurologic changes require urgent laminectomy within 8 to 12 hours of the onset of symptoms.

REFERENCES

1. Tubridy N, Redmond JM. Neurological symptoms attributed to epidural analgesia in labour: an observational study of seven cases. *Br J Obstet Gynaecol*. 1996;103:832–833.
2. Ong BY, Cohen MM, Esmail A, et al. Paresthesias and motor dysfunction after labor and delivery. *Anesth Analg*. 1987;66:18–22.
3. Scott DB, Hibbard BM. Serious non-fatal complications associated with extradural block in obstetric practice. *Br J Anaesth*. 1990;64:537–541.
4. MacArthur C, Lewis M, Knox EG. Investigation of long term problems after obstetric epidural anaesthesia. *BMJ*. 1992;304:1279–1282.
5. Palot M, Visseaux H, Botmans C, Pire JC. Epidemiology of complications of obstetrical epidural analgesia. *Cah Anesthesiol*. 1994;42:229–233.
6. Scott DB, Tunstall ME. Serious complications associated with epidural/spinal blockade in obstetrics: a two-year prospective study. *Int J Obstet Anesth*. 1995;4:133–139.
7. Holdcroft A, Gibberd FB, Hargrove RL, et al. Neurological complications associated with pregnancy. *Br J Anaesth*. 1995;75:522–526.
8. Paech MJ, Godkin R, Webster S. Complications of obstetric epidural analgesia and anaesthesia: a prospective analysis of 10,995 cases. *Int J Obstet Anesth*. 1998;7:5–11.
9. Holloway J, Seed PT, O'Sullivan G, Reynolds F. Paraesthesiae and nerve damage following combined spinal epidural and spinal anaesthesia: a pilot survey. *Int J Obstet Anesth*. 2000;9:151–155.
10. Dar AQ, Robinson AP, Lyons G. Postpartum neurological symptoms following regional blockade: a prospective study with case controls. *Int J Obstet Anesth*. 2002;11:85–90.
11. Auroy Y, Benhamou D, Bargues L, et al. Major complications of regional anesthesia in France: the SOS Regional Anesthesia Hotline Service. *Anesthesiology*. 2002;97:1274–1280.
12. Moen V, Dahlgren N, Irestedt L. Severe neurological complications after central neuraxial blockades in Sweden 1990-1999. *Anesthesiology*. 2004;101:950–959.
13. Wong CA, Scavone BM, Dugan S, et al. Incidence of postpartum lumbosacral spine and lower extremity nerve injuries. *Obstet Gynecol*. 2003;101:279–288.
14. Cook TM, Counsell D, Wildsmith JA. Major complications of central neuraxial block: report on the Third Audit Project of the Royal College of Anaesthetists. *Br J Anaesth*. 2009;102:179–190.
15. D'Angelo R, Smiley RM, Riley ET, Segal S. Serious complications related to obstetric anesthesia: the serious complication repository project of the Society for Obstetric Anesthesia and Perinatology. *Anesthesiology*. 2014;120:1505–1512.
16. Richards A, McLaren T, Paech MJ, et al. Immediate postpartum neurological deficits in the lower extremity: a prospective observational study. *Int J Obstet Anesth*. 2017;31:5–12.
17. Tournier A, Doremieux AC, Drumez E, et al. Lower-limb neurologic deficit after vaginal delivery: a prospective observational study. *Int J Obstet Anesth*. 2020;41:35–38.
18. Ruppen W, Derry S, McQuay H, Moore RA. Incidence of epidural hematoma, infection, and neurologic injury in obstetric patients with epidural analgesia/anesthesia. *Anesthesiology*. 2006;105:394–399.
19. Loo CC, Dahlgren G, Irestedt L. Neurological complications in obstetric regional anaesthesia. *Int J Obstet Anesth*. 2000;9:99–124.
20. Wong CA. Nerve injuries after neuraxial anaesthesia and their medicolegal implications. *Best Pract Res Clin Obstet Gynaecol*. 2010;24:367–381.
21. Haas DM, Meadows RS, Cottrell R, Stone WJ. Postpartum obturator neurapraxia. A case report. *J Reprod Med*. 2003;48:469–470.
22. Hong BY, Ko YJ, Kim HW, et al. Intrapartum obturator neuropathy diagnosed after cesarean delivery. *Arch Gynecol Obstet*. 2010;282:349–350.
23. Peirce C, O'Brien C, O'Herlihy C. Postpartum femoral neuropathy following spontaneous vaginal delivery. *J Obstet Gynaecol*. 2010;30:203–204.
24. Van Diver T, Camann W. Meralgia paresthetica in the parturient. *Int J Obstet Anesth*. 1995;4:109–112.
25. Silva M, Mallinson C, Reynolds F. Sciatic nerve palsy following childbirth. *Anaesthesia*. 1996;51:1144–1148.
26. Roy S, Levine AB, Herbison GJ, Jacobs SR. Intraoperative positioning during cesarean as a cause of sciatic neuropathy. *Obstet Gynecol*. 2002;99:652–653.

27. Postaci A, Karabeyoglu I, Erdogan G, et al. A case of sciatic neuropathy after caesarean section under spinal anaesthesia. *Int J Obstet Anesth.* 2006;15:317–319.

28. Teare J, Evans E, Belli A, Wendler R. Sciatic nerve ischaemia after iliac artery occlusion balloon catheter placement for placenta percreta. *Int J Obstet Anesth.* 2014;23:178–181.

29. Babayev M, Bodack MP, Creatura C. Common peroneal neuropathy secondary to squatting during childbirth. *Obstet Gynecol.* 1998;91:830–832.

30. Radawski MM, Strakowski JA, Johnson EW. Acute common peroneal neuropathy due to hand positioning in normal labor and delivery. *Obstet Gynecol.* 2011;118:421–423.

31. Kulkarni S, Koshy L, Babu AR, Eldesoky A. Iatrogenic bilateral foot drop after uneventful cesarean section. *Int J Obstet Anesth.* 2021;46102971

32. LeBlanc KE, Cestia W. Carpal tunnel syndrome. *Am Fam Physician.* 2011;83:952–958.

33. Farrar D, Raoof N. Bell's palsy, childbirth and epidural analgesia. *Int J Obstet Anesth.* 2001;10:68–70.

34. Weissman A, Grisaru D, Shenhav M, et al. Postpartum surveillance of urinary retention by ultrasonography: the effect of epidural analgesia. *Ultrasound Obstet Gynecol.* 1995;6:130–134.

35. Chien PFW, Khan KS, Agustsson P, et al. The determinants of residual bladder volume following spontaneous vaginal delivery. *J Obstet Gynaecol.* 1996;16:146–150.

36. Liang CC, Wong SY, Tsay PT, et al. The effect of epidural analgesia on postpartum urinary retention in women who deliver vaginally. *Int J Obstet Anesth.* 2002;11:164–169.

37. MacArthur C, Lewis M, Knox EG. Health after childbirth. *Br J Obstet Gynaecol.* 1991;98:1193–1195.

38. Negro A, Delaruelle Z, Ivanova TA, et al. Headache and pregnancy: a systematic review. *J Headache Pain.* 2017;18:106.

39. Heyman HJ, Salem MR, Klimov I. Persistent sixth cranial nerve paresis following blood patch for postdural puncture headache. *Anesth Analg.* 1982;61:948–949.

40. Dunbar SA, Katz NP. Failure of delayed epidural blood patching to correct persistent cranial nerve palsies. *Anesth Analg.* 1994;79:806–807.

41. Chohan U, Khan M, Saeed Uz Z. Abducent nerve palsy in a parturient with a 25-gauge sprotte needle. *Int J Obstet Anesth.* 2003;12:235–236.

42. Perez M, Olmos M, Garrido FJ. Facial nerve paralysis after epidural blood patch. *Reg Anesth.* 1993;18:196–198.

43. Carrero EJ, Agusti M, Fabregas N, et al. Unilateral trigeminal and facial nerve palsies associated with epidural analgesia in labour. *Can J Anaesth.* 1998;45:893–897.

44. Martin-Hirsch DP, Martin-Hirsch PL. Vestibulocochlear dysfunction following epidural anaesthesia in labour. *Br J Clin Pract.* 1994;48:340–341.

45. Viale M, Narchi P, Veyrac P, Benhamou D. Chronic tinnitus and hearing loss caused by cerebrospinal fluid leak treated with success with peridural blood patch. Apropos of 2 cases. *Ann Otolaryngol Chir Cervicofac.* 1996;113:175–177.

46. Richa F, Chalhoub V, El-Hage C, et al. Subdural hematoma with cranial nerve palsies after obstetric epidural analgesia. *Int J Obstet Anesth.* 2015;24:390–391.

47. Chambers DJ, Bhatia K. Cranial nerve palsy following central neuraxial block in obstetrics – a review of the literature and analysis of 43 case reports. *Int J Obstet Anesth.* 2017;31:13–26.

48. Reynolds F. Dural puncture and headache. *BMJ.* 1993;306:874–876.

49. Cantais E, Behnamou D, Petit D, Palmier B. Acute subdural hematoma following spinal anesthesia with a very small spinal needle. *Anesthesiology.* 2000;93:1354–1356.

50. Davies JM, Murphy A, Smith M, O'Sullivan G. Subdural haematoma after dural puncture headache treated by epidural blood patch. *Br J Anaesth.* 2001;86:720–723.

51. Cuypers V, Van de Velde M, Devroe S. Intracranial subdural haematoma following neuraxial anaesthesia in the obstetric population: a literature review with analysis of 56 reported cases. *Int J Obstet Anesth.* 2016;25:58–65.

52. Poteau S, Genis A, Kumaraswami S. Postdural puncture headache and cerebral venous thrombosis in obstetric anaesthesia. *Br J Anaesth.* 2023;130:e196–e198.

53. Neal JM, Barrington MJ, Brull R, et al. The second ASRA practice advisory on neurologic complications associated with regional anesthesia and pain medicine: executive summary 2015. *Reg Anesth Pain Med.* 2015;40:401–430.

54. Yoshii W, Rottman R, Rosenblatt R, et al. Epidural catheter induced traumatic radiculopathy in obstetrics: one center's experience. *Reg Anesth Pain Med.* 1994;19:132–135.

55. Loo CC, Cheong KF. Monoplegia following obstetric epidural anaesthesia. *Ann Acad Med Singapore.* 1997;26:232–234.

56. Richardson J, Bedder M. Transient anterior spinal cord syndrome with continuous postoperative epidural analgesia. *Anesthesiology.* 1990;72:764–766.

57. Ben-David B, Vaida S, Collins G, et al. Transient paraplegia secondary to an epidural catheter. *Anesth Analg.* 1994;79:598–600.

58. Reynolds F. Litigation in obstetric regional anaesthesia. In: Van Zurdert A, ed. *Highlights in Pain Therapy and Regional Anaesthesia V.* Publicidad Permanyer; 1996:39–43.

59. Ali L, Stocks GM. Spina bifida, tethered cord and regional anaesthesia. *Anaesthesia.* 2005;60:1149–1150.

60. Bromage PR, Benumof JL. Paraplegia following intracord injection during attempted epidural anesthesia under general anesthesia. *Reg Anesth Pain Med.* 1998;23:104–107.

61. Rajakulendran Y, Rahman S, Venkat N. Long-term neurological complication following traumatic damage to the spinal cord with a 25-gauge Whitacre spinal needle. *Int J Obstet Anesth.* 1999;8:62–66.

62. Reynolds F. Damage to the conus medullaris following spinal anaesthesia. *Anaesthesia.* 2001;56:238–247.

63. Greaves JD. Serious spinal cord injury due to haematomyelia caused by spinal anaesthesia in a patient treated with low-dose heparin. *Anaesthesia.* 1997;52:150–154.

64. Ahmad FU, Pandey P, Sharma BS, Garg A. Foot drop after spinal anesthesia in a patient with a low-lying cord. *Int J Obstet Anesth.* 2006;15:233–236.

65. Van Gessel EF, Forster A, Gamulin Z. Continuous spinal anesthesia: Where do spinal catheters go? *Anesth Analg.* 1993;76:1004–1007.

66. Broadbent CR, Maxwell WB, Ferrie R, et al. Ability of anaesthetists to identify a marked lumbar interspace. *Anaesthesia.* 2000;55:1122–1126.

67. Arnolds D, Hofer J, Scavone B. Inadvertent neuraxial block placement at or above the L1-L2 interspace in the super-obese parturient: a retrospective study. *Int J Obstet Anesth.* 2020;42:20–25.

68. Saifuddin A, Burnett SJ, White J. The variation of position of the conus medullaris in an adult population. A magnetic resonance imaging study. *Spine*. 1998;23:1452–1456.

69. Thomson A. Fifth annual report of the Committee of Collective Investigation of the Anatomical Society of Great Britain and Ireland for the year 1893-94. *J Anat Physiol*. 1894;29:35–60.

70. Render CA. The reproducibility of the iliac crest as a marker of lumbar spine level. *Anaesthesia*. 1996;51:1070–1071.

71. Lee AJ, Ranasinghe JS, Chehade JM, et al. Ultrasound assessment of the vertebral level of the intercristal line in pregnancy. *Anesth Analg*. 2011;113:559–564.

72. Cohn J, Moaveni D, Sznol J, Ranasinghe J. Complications of 761 short-term intrathecal macrocatheters in obstetric patients: A retrospective review of cases over a 12-year period. *Int J Obstet Anesth*. 2016;25:30–36.

73. McKenzie CP, Carvalho B, Riley ET. The Wiley spinal catheter-over-needle system for continuous spinal anesthesia: a case series of 5 cesarean deliveries complicated by paresthesias and headaches. *Reg Anesth Pain Med*. 2016;41:405–410.

74. Davidson EM, Sklar E, Bhatia R, et al. Magnetic resonance imaging findings after uneventful continuous infusion neuraxial analgesia: a prospective study to determine whether epidural infusion produces pathologic magnetic resonance imaging findings. *Anesth Analg*. 2010;110:233–237.

75. Horlocker TT. Neuraxial blockade in patients with spinal stenosis: Between a rock and a hard place. *Anesth Analg*. 2010;110:13–15.

76. Forster MR, Nimmo GR, Brown AG. Case report: Prolapsed intervertebral disc after epidural analgesia in labour. *Anaesthesia*. 1996;51:773–775.

77. Case AS, Ramsey PS. Spontaneous epidural hematoma of the spine in pregnancy. *Am J Obstet Gynecol*. 2005;193:875–877.

78. Bose S, Ali Z, Rath GP, Prabhakar H. Spontaneous spinal epidural haematoma: a rare cause of quadriplegia in the post-partum period. *Br J Anaesth*. 2007;99:855–857.

79. Tada S, Yasue A, Nishizawa H, et al. Spontaneous spinal epidural hematoma during pregnancy: three case reports. *J Obstet Gynaecol Res*. 2011;37:1734–1738.

80. Matsubara S, Inoue H, Takamura K, et al. Spontaneous spinal epidural hematoma at the 16th week of a twin pregnancy. *J Obstet Gynaecol Res*. 2011;37:1466–1469.

81. Jo YY, Lee D, Chang YJ, Kwak HJ. Anesthetic management of a spontaneous spinal-epidural hematoma during pregnancy. *Int J Obstet Anesth*. 2012;21:185–188.

82. Forsnes E, Occhino A, Acosta R. Spontaneous spinal epidural hematoma in pregnancy associated with using low molecular weight heparin. *Obstet Gynecol*. 2009;113:532–533.

83. Doblar DD, Schumacher SD. Spontaneous acute thoracic epidural hematoma causing paraplegia in a patient with severe preeclampsia in early labor. *Int J Obstet Anesth*. 2005;14:256–260.

84. Wulf H. Epidural anaesthesia and spinal haematoma. *Can J Anaesth*. 1996;43:1260–1271.

85. Esler MD, Durbridge J, Kirby S. Epidural haematoma after dural puncture in a parturient with neurofibromatosis. *Br J Anaesth*. 2001;87:932–934.

86. Horlocker TT, Wedel DJ, Schroeder DR, et al. Preoperative antiplatelet therapy does not increase the risk of spinal hematoma associated with regional anesthesia. *Anesth Analg*. 1995;80:303–309.

87. Davies JM, Posner KL, Lee LA, et al. Liability associated with obstetric anesthesia: a closed claims analysis. *Anesthesiology*. 2009;110:131–139.

88. Yuen TS, Kua JS, Tan IK. Spinal haematoma following epidural anaesthesia in a patient with eclampsia. *Anaesthesia*. 1999;54:350–354.

89. Guffey PJ, McKay WR, McKay RE. Epidural hematoma nine days after removal of a labor epidural catheter. *Anesth Analg*. 2010;111:992–995.

90. Beilin Y, Zahn J, Comerford M. Safe epidural analgesia in thirty parturients with platelet counts between 69,000 and 98,000 mm-3. *Anesth Analg*. 1997;85:385–388.

91. Chi C, Lee CA, England A, et al. Obstetric analgesia and anaesthesia in women with inherited bleeding disorders. *Thromb Haemost*. 2009;101:1104–1111.

92. Goodier CG, Lu JT, Hebbar L, et al. Neuraxial anesthesia in parturients with thrombocytopenia: a multisite retrospective cohort study. *Anesth Analg*. 2015;121:988–991.

93. Liu SS, Buvanendran A, Viscusi ER, et al. Uncomplicated removal of epidural catheters in 4365 patients with international normalized ratio greater than 1.4 during initiation of warfarin therapy. *Reg Anesth Pain Med*. 2011;36:231–235.

94. Leffert LR, Dubois HM, Butwick AJ, et al. Neuraxial anesthesia in obstetric patients receiving thromboprophylaxis with unfractionated or low-molecular-weight heparin: a systematic review of spinal epidural hematoma. *Anesth Analg*. 2017;125:223–231.

95. Pujic B, Holo-Djilvesi N, Djilvesi D, Palmer CM. Epidural hematoma following low molecular weight heparin prophylaxis and spinal anesthesia for cesarean delivery. *Int J Obstet Anesth*. 2019;37:118–121.

96. Svelato A, Rutili A, Bertelloni C, et al. Case report: Difficulty in diagnosis of delayed spinal epidural hematoma in puerperal women after combined spinal epidural anaesthesia. *BMC Anesthesiol*. 2019;19:54.

97. Bauer ME, Arendt K, Beilin Y, et al. The Society for Obstetric Anesthesia and Perinatology interdisciplinary consensus statement on neuraxial procedures in obstetric patients with thrombocytopenia. *Anesth Analg*. 2021;132:1531–1544.

98. Beards SC, Jackson A, Griffiths AG, Horsman EL. Magnetic resonance imaging of extradural blood patches: appearances from 30 min to 18 h. *Br J Anaesth*. 1993;71:182–188.

99. Verduzco LA, Atlas SW, Riley ET. Subdural hematoma after an epidural blood patch. *Int J Obstet Anesth*. 2012;21:189–192.

100. Lao TT, Halpern SH, MacDonald D, Huh C. Spinal subdural haematoma in a parturient after attempted epidural anaesthesia. *Can J Anaesth*. 1993;40:340–345.

101. Koyama S, Tomimatsu T, Kanagawa T, et al. Spinal subarachnoid hematoma following spinal anesthesia in a patient with HELLP syndrome. *Int J Obstet Anesth*. 2010;19:87–91.

102. Walters MA, Van de Velde M, Wilms G. Acute intrathecal haematoma following neuraxial anaesthesia: diagnostic delay after apparently normal radiological imaging. *Int J Obstet Anesth*. 2012;21:181–185.

103. Chen J, Hu Y, Lv L. Paraplegia after accidental continuous subdural analgesia. *Int J Obstet Anesth*. 2017;30:61–64.

104. Jenkins JG. Some immediate serious complications of obstetric epidural analgesia and anaesthesia: a prospective study of 145,550 epidurals. *Int J Obstet Anesth*. 2005;14:37–42.

105. Yentis SM, Lucas DN, Brigante L, et al. Safety guideline: Neurological monitoring associated with obstetric neuraxial block 2020: a joint guideline by the Association of Anaesthetists and the Obstetric Anaesthetists' Association. *Anaesthesia.* 2020;75:913–919.

106. Lee LA, Posner KL, Domino KB, et al. Injuries associated with regional anesthesia in the 1980s and 1990s: a closed claims analysis. *Anesthesiology.* 2004;101:143–152.

107. Anderson BL, Nau GJ, Simhan HN. Idiopathic vertebral abscess in pregnancy: case report and literature review. *Am J Perinatol.* 2007;24:377–379.

108. Reihsaus E, Waldbaur H, Seeling W. Spinal epidural abscess: a meta-analysis of 915 patients. *Neurosurg Rev.* 2000;23:175–204.

109. Wang LP, Hauerberg J, Schmidt JF. Incidence of spinal epidural abscess after epidural analgesia: a national 1-year survey. *Anesthesiology.* 1999;91:1928–1936.

110. Green LK, Paech MJ. Obstetric epidural catheter-related infections at a major teaching hospital: a retrospective case series. *Int J Obstet Anesth.* 2010;19:38–43.

111. Borum SE, McLeskey CH, Williamson JB, et al. Epidural abscess after obstetric epidural analgesia. *Anesthesiology.* 1995;82:1523–1526.

112. Kindler C, Seeberger M, Siegemund M, Schneider M. Extradural abscess complicating lumbar extradural anaesthesia and analgesia in an obstetric patient. *Acta Anaesthesiol Scand.* 1996;40:858–861.

113. Dysart RH, Balakrishnan V. Conservative management of extradural abscess complicating spinal-extradural anaesthesia for caesarean section. *Br J Anaesth.* 1997;78:591–593.

114. Dhillon AR, Russell IF. Epidural abscess in association with obstetric epidural analgesia. *Int J Obstet Anesth.* 1998;6:118–121.

115. Rathmell JP, Garahan MB, Also from GF. Epidural abscess following epidural analgesia. *Reg Anesth Pain Med.* 2000;25:79–82.

116. Rohrbach M, Plotz J. Epidural abscess following delivery with peridural analgesia. The question of prevention. *Anaesthesist.* 2001;50:411–415.

117. Schroeder TH, Krueger WA, Neeser E, et al. Spinal epidural abscess—a rare complication after epidural analgesia for labour and delivery. *Br J Anaesth.* 2004;92:896–898.

118. Chiang HL, Chia YY, Chen YS, et al. Epidural abscess in an obstetric patient with patient-controlled epidural analgesia—a case report. *Int J Obstet Anesth.* 2005;14:242–245.

119. Reynolds F. Neurological infections after neuraxial anesthesia. *Anesthesiol Clin.* 2008;26:23–52. v.

120. Grewal S, Hocking G, Wildsmith JA. Epidural abscesses. *Br J Anaesth.* 2006;96:292–302.

121. Royakkers AA, Willigers H, van der Ven AJ, et al. Catheter-related epidural abscesses – don't wait for neurological deficits. *Acta Anaesthesiol Scand.* 2002;46:611–615.

122. Sato S, Sakuragi T, Dan K. Human skin flora as a potential source of epidural abscess. *Anesthesiology.* 1996;85:1276–1282.

123. Tabo E, Ohkuma Y, Kimura S, et al. Successful percutaneous drainage of epidural abscess with epidural needle and catheter. *Anesthesiology.* 1994;80:1393–1395.

124. Huang YY, Zuo Z, Yuan HB, et al. A paraspinal abscess following spinal anaesthesia for caesarean section and patient-controlled epidural analgesia for postoperative pain. *Int J Obstet Anesth.* 2005;14:252–255.

125. Yang YW, Chen WT, Chen JY, et al. Bacterial infection in deep paraspinal muscles in a parturient following epidural analgesia. *Acta Anaesthesiol Taiwan.* 2011;49:75–78.

126. Bajwa ZH, Ho C, Grush A, et al. Discitis associated with pregnancy and spinal anesthesia. *Anesth Analg.* 2002;94:415–416.

127. Cameron CM, Scott DA, McDonald WM, Davies MJ. A review of neuraxial epidural morbidity: experience of more than 8,000 cases at a single teaching hospital. *Anesthesiology.* 2007;106:997–1002.

128. Collis RE, Harries SE. A subdural abscess and infected blood patch complicating regional analgesia for labour. *Int J Obstet Anesth.* 2005;14:246–251.

129. Raj V, Foy J. Paraspinal abscess associated with epidural in labour. *Anaesth Intensive Care.* 1998;26:424–426.

130. Baer ET. Post-dural puncture bacterial meningitis. *Anesthesiology.* 2006;105:381–393.

131. Gibbons RB. Chemical meningitis following spinal anesthesia. *JAMA.* 1969;210:900–902.

132. Phillips OC. Aseptic meningitis following spinal anesthesia. *Anesth Analg.* 1970;49:866–871.

133. Corbett JJ, Rosenstein BJ. Pseudomonas meningitis related to spinal anesthesia. Report of three cases with a common source of infection. *Neurology.* 1971;21:946–950.

134. Newton JA Jr, Lesnik IK, Kennedy CA. *Streptococcus salivarius* meningitis following spinal anesthesia. *Clin Infect Dis.* 1994;18:840–841.

135. Lurie S, Feinstein M, Heifetz C, Mamet Y. Iatrogenic bacterial meningitis after spinal anesthesia for pain relief during labor. *J Clin Anesth.* 1999;11:438–439.

136. Bugedo G, Valenzuela J, Munoz H. Aseptic meningitis following spinal anesthesia. Report of a case. *Rev Med Chil.* 1991;119:440–442.

137. Lee JJ, Parry H. Bacterial meningitis following spinal anaesthesia for caesarean section. *Br J Anaesth.* 1991;66:383–386.

138. Stallard N, Barry P. Another complication of the combined extradural-subarachnoid technique. *Br J Anaesth.* 1995;75:370–371.

139. Donnelly T, Koper M, Mallaiah S. Meningitis following spinal anaesthesia - a coincidental infection? *Int J Obstet Anesth.* 1998;7:170–172.

140. Thomas T, Cooper G. *Why Mothers Die 1997-1999. Confidential Enquiries Into Maternal Deaths in the United Kingdom.* RCOG Press; 2001:147.

141. Rodrigo N, Perera KN, Ranwala R, et al. Aspergillus meningitis following spinal anaesthesia for caesarean section in Colombo, Sri Lanka. *Int J Obstet Anesth.* 2007;16:256–260.

142. Celik M, Kizilkaya M, Dostbil A, et al. Meningitis following spinal anaesthesia in an obstetric patient. *Trop Doct.* 2014;44:179–181.

143. Ersoz G, Uguz M, Aslan G, et al. Outbreak of meningitis due to serratia marcescens after spinal anaesthesia. *J Hosp Infect.* 2014;87:122–125.

144. Roberts SP, Petts HV. Meningitis after obstetric spinal anaesthesia. *Anaesthesia.* 1990;45:376–377.

145. Harding SA, Collis RE, Morgan BM. Meningitis after combined spinal-extradural anaesthesia in obstetrics. *Br J Anaesth.* 1994;73:545–547.

146. Cascio M, Heath G. Meningitis following a combined spinal-epidural technique in a labouring term parturient. *Can J Anaesth.* 1996;43:399–402.

147. Bouhemad B, Dounas M, Mercier FJ, Benhamou D. Bacterial meningitis following combined spinal-epidural analgesia for labour. *Anaesthesia*. 1998;53:292–295.

148. Duflo F, Allaouchiche B, Mathon L, Chassard D. Bacterial meningitis following combined obstetric spinal and peridural anesthesia. *Ann Fr Anesth Reanim*. 1998;17:1286.

149. Vernis L, Duale C, Storme B, et al. Perispinal analgesia for labour followed by patient-controlled infusion with bupivacaine and sufentanil: combined spinal-epidural vs. epidural analgesia alone. *Eur J Anaesthesiol*. 2004;21:186–192.

150. Gordon C, Fry C, Salman M, Desai N. Meningitis following cerebrospinal fluid-cutaneous fistula secondary to combined spinal-epidural anaesthesia for elective caesarean delivery. *Int J Obstet Anesth*. 2022;49 103241.

151. Berga S, Trierweiler MW. Bacterial meningitis following epidural anesthesia for vaginal delivery: a case report. *Obstet Gynecol*. 1989;74:437–439.

152. Sansome AJ, Barnes GR, Barrett RF. An unusual presentation of meningitis as a consequence of inadvertent dural puncture. *Int J Obstet Anesth*. 1991;1:35–37.

153. Neumark J, Feichtinger W, Gassner A. Epidural block in obstetrics followed by aseptic meningoencephalitis. *Anesthesiology*. 1980;52:518–519.

154. Ready LB, Helfer D. Bacterial meningitis in parturients after epidural anesthesia. *Anesthesiology*. 1989;71:988–990.

155. Davis L, Hargreaves C, Robinson PN. Postpartum meningitis. *Anaesthesia*. 1993;48:788–789.

156. Goldstein MJ, Parker RL, Dewan DM. Status epilepticus amauroticus secondary to meningitis as a cause of postpartum cortical blindness. *Reg Anesth*. 1996;21:595–598.

157. Choy JC. Mortality from peripartum meningitis. *Anaesth Intensive Care*. 2000;28:328–330.

158. Centers for Disease Control and Prevention. Bacterial meningitis after intrapartum spinal anesthesia – New York and Ohio, 2008-2009. *MMWR Morb Mortal Wkly Rep*. 2010;59:65–69.

159. Videira RL, Ruiz-Neto PP, Brandao Neto M. Post spinal meningitis and asepsis. *Acta Anaesthesiol Scand*. 2002;46: 639–646.

160. White CA, Koontz FP. β-hemolytic streptococcus infections in postpartum patients. *Obstet Gynecol*. 1973;41:27–32.

161. Knowles PR, Randall NP, Lockhart AS. Vascular trauma associated with routine spinal anaesthesia. *Anaesthesia*. 1999;54:647–650.

162. Gibbs RS, Castillo MS, Rodgers PJ. Management of acute chorioamnionitis. *Am J Obstet Gynecol*. 1980;136:709–713.

163. Bader AM, Gilbertson L, Kirz L, Datta S. Regional anesthesia in women with chorioamnionitis. *Reg Anesth*. 1992;17:84–86.

164. Goodman EJ, DeHorta E, Taguiam JM. Safety of spinal and epidural anesthesia in parturients with chorioamnionitis. *Reg Anesth*. 1996;21:436–441.

165. Gershon RY, Manning-Williams D. Anesthesia and the HIV infected parturient: a retrospective study. *Int J Obstet Anesth*. 1997;6:76–81.

166. American Society of Anesthesiologists. Practice advisory for the prevention, diagnosis, and management of infectious complications associated with neuraxial techniques: an updated report by the American Society Task Force on Infectious Complications Associated with Neuraxial Techniques and the American Society of Regional Anesthesia and Pain Medicine. *Anesthesiology*. 2017;126:585–601.

167. Panikkar KK, Yentis SM. Wearing of masks for obstetric regional anaesthesia. A postal survey. *Anaesthesia*. 1996;51:398–400.

168. Sellors JE, Cyna AM, Simmons SW. Aseptic precautions for inserting an epidural catheter: a survey of obstetric anaesthetists. *Anaesthesia*. 2002;57:593–596.

169. Tunevall TG. Postoperative wound infections and surgical face masks: a controlled study. *World J Surg*. 1992;16: 147–148.

170. Philips BJ, Fergusson S, Armstrong P, et al. Surgical face masks are effective in reducing bacterial contamination caused by dispersal from the upper airway. *Br J Anaesth*. 1992;69:407–408.

171. McLure HA, Talboys CA, Yentis SM, Azadian BS. Surgical face masks and downward dispersal of bacteria. *Anaesthesia*. 1998;53:624–626.

172. Sakuragi T, Yanagisawa K, Dan K. Bactericidal activity of skin disinfectants on methicillin-resistant *Staphylococcus aureus*. *Anesth Analg*. 1995;81:555–558.

173. Doan L, Piskoun B, Rosenberg AD, et al. In vitro antiseptic effects on viability of neuronal and Schwann cells. *Reg Anesth Pain Med*. 2012;37:131–138.

174. Sviggum HP, Jacob AK, Arendt KW, et al. Neurologic complications after chlorhexidine antisepsis for spinal anesthesia. *Reg Anesth Pain Med*. 2012;37:139–144.

175. Hebl JR. The importance and implications of aseptic techniques during regional anesthesia. *Reg Anesth Pain Med*. 2006;31:311–323.

176. Eastwood DW. Anterior spinal artery syndrome after epidural anesthesia in a pregnant diabetic patient with scleredema. *Anesth Analg*. 1991;73:90–91.

177. Ackerman WE, Juneja MM, Knapp RK. Maternal paraparesis after epidural anesthesia and cesarean section. *South Med J*. 1990;83:695–697.

178. Patel S, Loveridge R. Obstetric neuraxial drug administration errors: a quantitative and qualitative analytical review. *Anesth Analg*. 2015;121:1570–1577.

179. Savage R, Beattie C. Inadvertent epidural administration of metaraminol. *Anaesthesia*. 2004;59:624–625.

180. Shanker KB, Palkar NV, Nishkala R. Paraplegia following epidural potassium chloride. *Anaesthesia*. 1985;40:45–47.

181. Lin D, Becker K, Shapiro HM. Neurologic changes following epidural injection of potassium chloride and diazepam: a case report with laboratory correlations. *Anesthesiology*. 1986;65:210–212.

182. Brahams D. Record award for personal injuries sustained as a result of negligent administration of epidural anaesthetic. *Lancet*. 1982;1:159.

183. Bogod D. The sting in the tail: Antiseptics and the neuraxis revisited. *Anaesthesia*. 2012;67:1305–1309.

184. Patel PC, Sharif AM, Farnando PU. Accidental infusion of total parenteral nutrition solution through an epidural catheter. *Anaesthesia*. 1984;39:383–384.

185. McGuinness JP, Cantees KK. Epidural injection of a phenol-containing ranitidine preparation. *Anesthesiology*. 1990;73:553–555.

186. Meel B. Inadvertent intrathecal administration of potassium chloride during routine spinal anesthesia: case report. *Am J Forensic Med Pathol*. 1998;19:255–257.

187. Moran NF, Bishop DG, Fawcus S, et al. Tranexamic acid at cesarean delivery: drug-error deaths. *Am J Obstet Gynecol*. 2023;228:1–4.

188. Ferguson FR, Watkins KH. Paralysis of the bladder and associated neurological sequelae of spinal anaesthesia (cauda equina syndrome). *Br J Surg.* 1937;25:735–752.

189. Rigler ML, Drasner K, Krejcie TC, et al. Cauda equina syndrome after continuous spinal anesthesia. *Anesth Analg.* 1991;72:275–281.

190. Loo CC, Irestedt L. Cauda equina syndrome after spinal anaesthesia with hyperbaric 5% lignocaine: a review of six cases of cauda equina syndrome reported to the Swedish pharmaceutical insurance 1993-1997. *Acta Anaesthesiol Scand.* 1999;43:371–379.

191. Cheng AC. Intended epidural anesthesia as possible cause of cauda equina syndrome. *Anesth Analg.* 1994;78:157–159.

192. Yamauchi Y, Nomoto Y. Irreversible damage to the cauda equina following repeated intrathecal injection of hyperbaric dibucaine. *J Anesth.* 2002;16:176–178.

193. Chabbouh T, Lentschener C, Zuber M, et al. Persistent cauda equina syndrome with no identifiable facilitating condition after an uneventful single spinal administration of 0.5% hyperbaric bupivacaine. *Anesth Analg.* 2006;101:1847–1848.

194. Drasner K. Local anesthetic neurotoxicity: clinical injury and strategies that may minimize risk. *Reg Anesth Pain Med.* 2002;27:576–580.

195. Sarifakioglu AB, Yemisci OU, Yalbuzdag SA, et al. Cauda equina syndrome after cesarean section. *Am J Phys Med Rehabil.* 2013;92:179–182.

196. Chen X, Xu Z, Lin R, Liu Z. Persistent cauda equina syndrome after cesarean section under combined spinal-epidural anesthesia: a case report. *J Clin Anesth.* 2015;27:520–523.

197. Pollock JE. Transient neurologic symptoms: etiology, risk factors, and management. *Reg Anesth Pain Med.* 2002;27:581–586.

198. Zaric D, Christiansen C, Pace NL, Punjasawadwong Y. Transient neurologic symptoms after spinal anesthesia with lidocaine versus other local anesthetics: a systematic review of randomized, controlled trials. *Anesth Analg.* 2005;100:1811–1816.

199. Wong CA, Slavenas P. The incidence of transient radicular irritation after spinal anesthesia in obstetric patients. *Reg Anesth Pain Med.* 1999;24:55–58.

200. Viitanen H, Porthan L, Viitanen M, et al. Postpartum neurologic symptoms following single-shot spinal block for labour analgesia. *Acta Anaesthesiol Scand.* 2005;49:1015–1022.

201. Philip J, Sharma SK, Gottumukkala VN, et al. Transient neurologic symptoms after spinal anesthesia with lidocaine in obstetric patients. *Anesth Analg.* 2001;92:405–409.

202. Rorarius M, Suominen P, Haanpaa M, et al. Neurologic sequelae after caesarean section. *Acta Anaesthesiol Scand.* 2001;45:34–41.

203. Reisner LS, Hochman BN, Plumer MH. Persistent neurologic deficit and adhesive arachnoiditis following intrathecal 2-chloroprocaine injection. *Anesth Analg.* 1980;59:452–454.

204. Sklar EM, Quencer RM, Green BA, et al. Complications of epidural anesthesia: MR appearance of abnormalities. *Radiology.* 1991;181:549–554.

205. Sghirlanzoni A, Marazzi R, Pareyson D, et al. Epidural anaesthesia and spinal arachnoiditis. *Anaesthesia.* 1989;44:317–321.

206. Bogod D. The truth, the whole truth? *Anaesthesia News.* 2010;271:7–8.

207. Lazorthes G, Poulhes J, Bastide G, et al. La vascularization de la moelle épinière (étude anatomique et physiologique). *Rev Neurol.* 1962;106:535–537.

208. Ong BY, Littleford J, Segstro R, et al. Spinal anaesthesia for caesarean section in a patient with a cervical arteriovenous malformation. *Can J Anaesth.* 1996;43:1052–1058.

209. Doppman JL, Wirth FP Jr, Di Chiro G, Ommaya AK. Value of cutaneous angiomas in the arteriographic localization of spinal-cord arteriovenous malformations. *N Engl J Med.* 1969;281:1440–1444.

210. Hirsch NP, Child CS, Wijetilleka SA. Paraplegia caused by spinal angioma—possible association with epidural analgesia. *Anesth Analg.* 1985;64:937–940.

211. Liu CL, Yang DJ. Paraplegia due to vertebral hemangioma during pregnancy. A case report. *Spine.* 1988;13:107–108.

212. Martin HB, Gibbons JJ, Bucholz RD. An unusual presentation of spinal cord tumor after epidural anesthesia. *Anesth Analg.* 1992;75:844–846.

213. Chilvers RJ, Salman MM. Hereditary neuropathy with a liability to pressure palsies presenting as a case of sensory neuropathy following spinal anaesthesia for caesarean delivery. *Int J Obstet Anesth.* 2011;20:95–96.

214. Hebl JR, Kopp SL, Schroeder DR, Horlocker TT. Neurologic complications after neuraxial anesthesia or analgesia in patients with preexisting peripheral sensorimotor neuropathy or diabetic polyneuropathy. *Anesth Analg.* 2006;103:1294–1299.

215. Kopp SL, Peters SM, Rose PS, et al. Worsening of neurologic symptoms after spinal anesthesia in two patients with spinal stenosis. *Reg Anesth Pain Med.* 2015;40:502–505.

216. Drake E, Drake M, Bird J, Russell R. Obstetric regional blocks for women with multiple sclerosis: a survey of UK experience. *Int J Obstet Anesth.* 2006;15:115–123.

217. Kopp SL, Jacob AK, Hebl JR. Regional anesthesia in patients with preexisting neurologic disease. *Reg Anesth Pain Med.* 2015;40:467–478.

218. Hopkins AN, Alshaeri T, Akst SA, Berger JS. Neurologic disease with pregnancy and considerations for the obstetric anesthesiologist. *Semin Perinatol.* 2014;38:359–369.

219. Hebl JR, Horlocker TT, Schroeder DR. Neuraxial anesthesia and analgesia in patients with preexisting central nervous system disorders. *Anesth Analg.* 2006;103:223–228.

220. O'Neal MA, Chang LY, Salajegheh MK. Postpartum spinal cord, root, plexus and peripheral nerve injuries involving the lower extremities: a practical approach. *Anesth Analg.* 2015;120:141–148.

32

Shared Decision-Making and Informed Consent in Obstetric Anesthesia

Joanna A. Kountanis, MD, Tracey M. Vogel, MD, FASA, and Jessica M. Meister Berger, MD, JD

CHAPTER OUTLINE

INFORMED CONSENT

Informed consent is a foundational element of the ethical practice of modern medicine.[1] Its purpose is to facilitate care in a manner that honors the autonomy of the patient while incorporating the medical expertise of the clinician. Informed consent is a process in which a patient and healthcare provider engage in information exchange and discussion about the patient's condition and the nature of the proposed treatment. The clinician should identify the risks, benefits, and alternatives, including lack of treatment, thereby empowering the patient to be an active participant in her medical care.[2] When engendered by a strong informed consent process, patient–physician communication has been associated with more realistic patient expectations, improved satisfaction, and a lower rate of medical malpractice claims.[3-5]

Evidence of the physician's engagement with the informed consent process may be found among consultation notes (paper or electronic), informational aids shared with patients, and signed consent forms acknowledging that the discussion has occurred.[6] The act of reviewing and signing a written consent form ensures an opportunity for the patient to ask questions. It also provides additional documentation that consent was obtained. A signed consent form is not necessary for valid informed consent to exist; verbal consent from the patient is valid and sufficient.[7] However, in instances in which the patient has not signed an informed consent form, anesthesia providers should nevertheless carefully document that a discussion of risks and benefits of anesthesia occurred, and that verbal informed consent was obtained before administration of anesthesia.

A robust and meaningful informed consent process[8] includes the following hallmarks:

1. **Disclosure of information:** The physician must disclose the proposed treatment, its alternatives, including no treatment, as well as the risks and benefits.
2. The disclosure should be tailored to the patient and clinical situation.
3. The discussion should be provided in the patient's preferred language and using accessible terminology rather than medical jargon.
4. A patient must have the capacity to understand the nature and consequences of the proposed treatments and their alternatives, and the ability to weigh the information to make a decision.
5. The patient's decision must be given voluntarily, free from coercion.
6. Consent can be withdrawn at any time before the therapy/procedure has occurred.

WHAT RISKS MUST BE DISCLOSED?

Legal precedent established through case law provides guidance as to which risks ought to be disclosed, applying a standard that has come to be known as the "reasonable person" test. This standard, applicable in most states in the United States, requires disclosure of those risks that a "reasonable patient would consider material to the decision of whether to consent to a procedure offered."[9] In practical terms, this has been held to require disclosure of commonly occurring risks, as well as those risks that are rare but severe.[10] Dornette[11] suggested that significant risk is one that poses a high (10% or greater) incidence of a transient complication or a low (0.5% to 1% or less) incidence of permanent consequences. Broaddus and Chandrasekhar[12] have recommended discussion of risks with high incidence, high morbidity, or adverse fetal effects.[12] Investigation into the nature and prevalence of risks associated with obstetric anesthesia have been explored in a 5-year, multicenter study that examined 257,000 anesthetics.[13] Of 187 serious complications that were identified, 85 were related to anesthesia. The most frequent serious events included high neuraxial blockade, unrecognized spinal catheter, and respiratory arrest.

Adequate informed consent does not require disclosure of every possible risk no matter how slight; overdisclosure can produce patient anxiety and confusion, and may overwhelm and have effects of negative suggestion, termed the "nocebo" effect.[14] Some clinicians have questioned whether such detailed risk disclosure is even consistent with the dictum *primum non nocere*, and have suggested the impetus for thorough risk disclosure stems predominantly from medicolegal threat and fear of liability rather than truly exchanging relevant information in the interest of patient autonomy.[15,16] These are complex questions, and clinical nuance precludes a universally applicable directive of how to provide optimal information disclosure in the clinical setting.

Therapeutic options and their associated risks and benefits should be disclosed to the patient; however, when a patient's clinical condition strongly favors a particular course of treatment, that information should be clearly communicated.[10] Increasingly, as the patient–physician model evolves away from a paternalistic structure to one of shared decision-making, uncertainty may arise regarding what limits, if any, ought to exist regarding patient decision-making. It can be difficult to balance competing interests, and there may be clinical scenarios in which a patient's expressed wishes conflict with medically recommended care. It is important to recognize that patient autonomy in medical decision-making does not compel clinicians to offer or perform therapies/procedures that are unreasonable or not within the standard of care.[17]

SHARED DECISION-MAKING

Shared decision-making is a process by which the physician expands upon the requirements of informed consent to establish a collaborative decision-making partnership with the patient.[18] The shared decision-making approach involves medical providers and patients making healthcare decisions together.[19] This communication technique is central to patient- and family-centered care; it is a major component of healthcare quality and safety and is embraced as a quality indicator.[20–22] The medical providers explain the risks and benefits of each intervention and ensure that patients are fully informed about their options. They also help the patient elucidate her values and preferences. Explicitly asking "what matters to you?" can help the team align its interventions. Patients will reach a decision with their

medical provider that aligns with what they feel is most congruent with their preferences. Meaningful dialogue is at the core of this relationship.[23] The Agency for Healthcare Research and Quality outlines a five-step SHARE approach (Table 32.1).[19]

Conversations may also involve family members, friends, and other members of the care team, according to the preferences of the patient. Clear communication is critical and requires careful attention to both verbal and nonverbal cues. Explanations must avoid language that is overly technical and clinical but also remain specific enough to meaningfully provide an understanding of the complex clinical decisions faced by the patient. Through this approach, providers can develop a trusting connection with the patient and more effectively communicate the evidence for healthcare decisions.

Frequently, **decision aids** are utilized during the conversation to facilitate the patient's understanding of the medical information presented. Decision aids used to facilitate shared decision-making are available online, on paper, or on video. A metaanalysis of 105 trials published through 2015 demonstrated that the use of decision aids resulted in increased patient knowledge, more accurate perceptions of treatment risks, better alignment of treatments with patient values, a decreased sense of conflict for patients, and greater patient participation.[20,24] Most notably, decision aids improve outcomes for those with socioeconomic disadvantage, low literacy, and low education. These aids serve to increase knowledge, participation in decision-making, decision self-efficacy, and preference for collaborative decision-making; inform choice; and reduce decisional conflict.[25] Just as cognitive aids can help guide operating room teams through the critical steps of a crisis, decision aids help patients absorb clinical evidence and communicate their preferences. The use of decision aids also helps clinicians set aside their traditional paternalistic role to be partners and coaches in the patient-centered process, and to present information that is easier for patients to understand. Decision aids can facilitate properly informing patients so that they can choose between various options (e.g., between different methods of pain management, between neuraxial and general anesthesia) based on their own values and preferences, even when the decision differs from their clinician's preferred decision.[20]

The process of shared decision-making appears to increase patients' subsequent participation, compliance, and self-monitoring.[9] According to observations, focus groups,

TABLE 32.1 **The SHARE Approach**	
Step 1	**S**eek your patient's participation
Step 2	**H**elp your patient explore and compare treatment options
Step 3	**A**ssess your patient's values and preferences
Step 4	**R**each a decision with your patient
Step 5	**E**valuate your patient's decision

From Agency of Healthcare Research and Quality. The SHARE approach: A model for shared decision making—fact sheet. 2020. Available from https://www.ahrq.gov/health-literacy/professional-training/shared-decision/tools/factsheet.html. Accessed 24 July 2024.

and questionnaires conducted as part of the Making Good Decisions in Collaboration (MAGIC) program in the United Kingdom, even when shared decision-making conversations are imperfect or when there is a lack of complete agreement on best choices, the process of bringing perspectives together improves the likelihood that decisions are more informed and better accepted by patients, families, and staff.[26] Using a "plan-do-study-act" rapid-cycle approach, MAGIC researchers determined that incorporating effective shared decision-making requires a holistic bundle of interventions to drive culture change and to establish a supportive healthcare delivery system.[26] Younger patients, women, and those with more education are most likely to prefer shared decision-making, according to a study of anesthesia decision-making in Germany that measured preferences using the autonomy preference index and the preference for involvement in care scale.[27] Based on a Swiss study of 197 clinician-patient dyads, anesthesia clinicians frequently overestimate how much shared decision-making occurs. In this study, Flierler et al.[28] showed that 94% of surgical patients wanted to be involved in preoperative anesthetic management decisions. Patients had a stronger desire for a "balanced" decision-making process, wherein each party would have an equal contribution to decision-making (desired by 65% of patients versus 32% of clinicians). Satisfaction decreased when patients perceived insufficient opportunity for involvement, and when anesthesia providers underestimated patient preference for shared decision-making.

Shared decision-making not only improves provider–patient communication but has also been shown to promote desirable clinical outcomes. In a study by Prabhu et al.,[29] 90% of participants reported being satisfied with their pain management through a shared decision-making approach, even though providers ultimately reduced opioid prescribing by 50%. Patients cited the education regarding expectations and the risks and benefits of oxycodone as the most helpful part of the process. A 2015 systematic review of shared decision-making identified a positive relationship between shared decision-making and patient outcomes for 42 of 97 unique outcomes among 39 studies that met inclusion criteria.[30] The authors noted differences in the way shared decision-making was measured (patient-reported, observer-reported, and clinician-reported). Regardless of measurement methods, 54% of affective-cognitive outcomes were positively associated with the patient's perception that shared decision-making had occurred; such outcomes included improved patient satisfaction, resolved concerns and anxieties about illness, resolved decisional conflict, improved knowledge, and enhanced confidence in the decision. Thirty-seven percent of the behavioral outcomes studied were improved with the presence of shared decision-making, including greater medication adherence. Twenty-five percent of the clinical outcomes studied were improved when there was shared decision-making, with specific improvements in patient ratings of overall health, quality of life, depressive symptoms, and physiologic measures such as blood pressure. Evidence for improved clinical outcomes appears most robust for patients with chronic conditions that require self-management,[31] such as hypertension.[32] Certainly, unsatisfactory communication with patients has been associated with treatment noncompliance in diabetes mellitus,[33] asthma,[34] and chronic disease.[35]

A potential disadvantage to a shared decision-making approach is that it takes time to engage patients in a lengthy discussion. An anesthesia provider may not be able to accomplish such a consultation while on a busy obstetric unit, or when consulted to facilitate emergency obstetric interventions. Patients who are in severe pain or active labor may not want to engage in the shared decision-making process and feel burdened by making multiple medical decisions at that time. Long-standing practices of medical paternalism and unethical practices by the medical establishment, particularly in people of color, may hamper true shared decision-making.

Ideally, patients with complex needs are referred to an anesthesia clinic during the antepartum period. However, even when meeting the patient for the first time on the obstetric unit, it is frequently possible to employ a shared decision-making approach at the time of hospital admission for a high-risk antepartum condition, for an induction of labor or early in labor, or prior to any need for labor analgesia. Shared decision-making is a particularly useful way to empower women who experience an unplanned birth outcome; examples include decisions about the primary anesthetic type for dilation and curettage, therapeutic management of post–dural puncture headache, or management of inadequate labor epidural analgesia.

TRAUMA-INFORMED CARE

Trauma-informed care is shared decision-making with an awareness and understanding of how previous individual or collective trauma impacts an individual's mental, physical, social, or emotional health. The US Substance Abuse and Mental Health Services Administration (SAMHSA) defines trauma-informed care using four general principles of care: (1) *realize* the pervasive and widespread nature of trauma in our society; (2) *recognize* what unresolved trauma looks like in survivors (patients, family members, staff); (3) *respond* by incorporating knowledge into new practices, policies, and protocols; and (4) *resist retraumatization* of survivors.[36] More recently, the US Centers for Disease Control and Prevention expanded on these concepts to establish six guiding principles for a trauma-informed approach to care, including a focus on (1) safety; (2) trustworthiness and transparency; (3) peer support; (4) collaboration and mutuality; (5) empowerment, voice, and choice; and (6) respect and understanding for an individual's cultural, historical, and gender identity.[37] Trauma-informed care involves an approach to care, including physical and behavioral healthcare, which commits to these principles, while also supporting an individual's resilience and recovery when possible.

One of the first crucial steps in becoming a trauma-informed provider is to become trauma-aware.[38] Providers must realize that trauma not only exists, but is pervasive in society, and that certain types of interpersonal trauma disproportionately affect women, especially Indigenous women and women of color, members of the LGBTQIA+ community, and individuals with intellectual or physical disabilities. These include childhood sexual trauma, adult sexual assault and rape, military sexual trauma, physical violence from intimate partner violence, loss of bodily autonomy due to state-mandated pregnancy where abortion is illegal, and birth trauma. The statistics regarding these types of trauma are sobering: approximately 20% to 33% of women will be the victims of childhood sexual trauma,[39–41] approximately 33% of female veterans will self-report a history of military sexual trauma,[42] and approximately 25% of women will experience severe physical violence from an intimate partner in their lifetimes.[43] Pregnant adolescent patients have a mean Adverse Childhood Experience score of 5.1/10 when screened for 10 common types of childhood maltreatment identified in previous research.[44] Birthing women who have a history of interpersonal trauma are at an increased risk of having a negative birth experience and developing postpartum mental health conditions, such as childbirth-related posttraumatic stress disorder (PTSD).[45]

Trauma, however, is not limited to an individual's life experience before pregnancy. It can occur de novo during childbirth. It is imperative that providers recognize the various types of birth trauma an individual may experience—up to 44% of birthing women report their birth experiences as traumatic.[46] Numerous studies have identified intrapartum events associated with a traumatic birth experience and an increased risk for postpartum PTSD, including operative birth, obstetric emergencies, and infant complications.[47–49] Postpartum hemorrhage, emergency responses, and early pregnancy loss have also been identified as predictors of postpartum mental health disorders,[47–49] in addition to anesthesia-related events such as intraoperative pain, traumatic neuraxial block placement, severe post–dural puncture headache, and neurologic injuries.[50] Importantly, an identifiable complication need not occur for an individual to perceive childbirth as traumatic. Recent studies suggest that a patient's negative subjective experience of childbirth is a significant contributor to a traumatic experience and the subsequent development of postpartum PTSD. Other intrapartum factors such as minimal support during labor and delivery, loss of control, and fear of childbirth have also been identified as significant predictors of postpartum PTSD.[47,48,51] Shared decision-making in subsequent pregnancies with individuals who have experienced birth trauma requires a thorough understanding of the traumatic nature of these events and the negative impact they may have on the patient's current psychological state.

Awareness of the impact of trauma is essential for shared decision-making, but it is also crucial that providers apply this knowledge to clinical practice. SAMHSA's fourth pillar of trauma-informed care states that all providers should resist retraumatizing survivors of trauma; however, the role of the anesthesia provider in preventing retraumatization has not been clearly elucidated. Adding to the challenge of avoiding retraumatization to this patient population is the fact that identification of survivors is not straightforward. Although universal screening for trauma is either required or recommended for obstetric providers by multiple agencies and organizations, including the American College of Obstetricians and Gynecologists (ACOG),[52] it is not routinely performed, and many survivors of trauma have never

voluntarily disclosed their history. Furthermore, there is no universally accepted screening tool to facilitate this process. However, various physical, psychological, and behavioral conditions have been associated with unresolved traumatic stress, and these can serve as an indicator of patients who may have suffered trauma (Box 32.1).[38,41,45,53–59] Although these conditions can raise suspicion for the presence of trauma in an individual's life, they are not always accompanied by trauma and therefore should only be used to guide further conversations.

Inquiring about a history of trauma is not exclusively the responsibility of obstetricians, and anesthesia providers may find themselves in a position to either elicit this history or receive a patient disclosure. The National Health Service England and the UK Center for Early Child Development, in an effort to implement trauma-informed care practices, put forth general guidelines to help any provider when eliciting a trauma history or responding to a disclosure.[60] These include:

- Ask birthing women how their traumatic past continues to affect them generally and what they might need from you;
- Avoid triggering PTSD reactions by learning potential triggers;
- Assume, in the absence of disclosure, but in the presence of PTSD reactions (e.g., exaggerated startle, agitation, panic with the use of restraints, avoidance of male providers) that the birthing woman could be a survivor; and
- Acknowledge the long-term effects of trauma, and that they are not alone and that you and/or others can help.

An alternative approach is for providers to assume that all birthing women have a history of trauma, thereby eliminating the need for screening. Shifting a patriarchal approach to care from "this is what we are doing today" to "what can we do together to achieve a mutually agreeable goal," while

---

BOX 32.1 Physical, Psychological, and Behavioral Manifestations of Chronic Unresolved Traumatic Stress

Physical
- Hypertension, cardiovascular disease
- Gastrointestinal problems
- Chronic pain states, including chronic migraines, fibromyalgia syndrome, interstitial cystitis/bladder pain syndrome
- Poor immune function
- Fatigue

Psychological
- Depression/suicidal ideation
- Posttraumatic stress disorder
- Anxiety
- Extreme fear of childbirth

Behavioral
- Substance use disorders
- Eating disorders
- Sleeping difficulties
- Request for no male providers

Content copied with permission Vogel TM, Coffin E. Trauma-informed care on labor and delivery. *Anesthesiol Clin.* 2021;39:779–791.

focusing on what makes individuals feel safe, building trust, allowing them some choice and control, and respecting their autonomy, is applicable and valuable for all birthing women. Although available research is limited, the application of trauma-informed care principles in obstetric settings is not known to be associated with any negative consequences. Further, recent studies have shown that offering trauma-focused interventions such as psychotherapy and eye movement desensitization and reprocessing during pregnancy do not increase risk for maternal or fetal harm.[61]

Trauma is unique to each individual; thus, it is crucial to direct shared decision-making and trauma-informed care approaches appropriately to the patient's needs. Practice recommendations surrounding the peripartum period are based on general trauma-informed care principles and the authors' extensive work with trauma survivors (Box 32.2).

BOX 32.2   Trauma-informed Care Principles to Prevent Retraumatization in Obstetric Patients

Antepartum period
- Plan for early consultation during pregnancy.
  - Elucidate fears or concerns regarding the upcoming delivery.
  - Identify known triggers, history of panic, and any successful nonpharmacologic and pharmacologic coping mechanisms for stressful situations.
- Explain the risks and benefits of low-dose anxiolytics.
- Discuss pain expectations and pain management options, opioid maintenance and withdrawal prevention strategies, and nicotine management (especially for women with substance use disorder).
- Discuss the role of the partner, the level of social support, and any need for private preoperative and/or recovery space.
- Offer an opportunity for patients to familiarize themselves with the hospital environment, including the operating room (live or virtual tours), so they can process information and ask questions in advance of delivery.
- Plan for early selection and introduction of team members to foster trusting, positive, therapeutic relationships.
- Establish best practice for communicating the patient's history and plan to her care team when she presents to the obstetric unit.

Intrapartum and intraoperative periods
- Minimize the number of providers assigned to the patient.
- Eliminate positions that promote the authoritative hierarchy between patient and provider (i.e., sit at eye level with the patient) to foster a more collaborative relationship; sitting also implies that the clinician is taking time to listen to a patient.
- Focus on culturally sensitive, compassionate, and respectful language at all times.
- Perform frequent "check-ins" to inquire about the patient's emotional state and planned use of nonpharmacologic (e.g., breathing techniques, music) or pharmacologic anxiolysis.
- Minimize harsh and loud stimuli, and allow for compassionate measures (e.g., warm blankets, mouth swabs, and clear surgical drapes) if desired.

- Communicate with a calm voice with a focus on the patient; avoid nonrelevant sidebar discussions with other staff members.
- Avoid separation of the patient and her partner, the use of arm straps (unless she meets criteria for restraints), unnecessary oxygen masks, severe nausea and vomiting, and severe shaking; these events can all trigger acute stress responses.
- Respect a patient's modesty and privacy by keeping her body covered as much as possible and asking before entering the room.
- Designate the most advanced anesthesia provider to perform any neuraxial procedures.
- Insist on vigilance and consistency with neuraxial block evaluation for surgery, and rapidly convert to other forms of anesthesia when neuraxial block is deemed inadequate.
- Support an environment that allows for early skin-to-skin contact with the neonate.

Postpartum period
- Observe for any changes in affect or mood, and refer early to perinatal mental health specialists.
- Recognize that any complications, including difficult neuraxial block placement or conversion to general anesthesia, could be perceived as a traumatic experience. Acknowledge any such reports with understanding, validation, and support, and offer referrals for mental health experts.

Content copied with permission. Vogel TM, Coffin E. Trauma-informed care on labor and delivery. *Anesthesiol Clin.* 2021;39:779–791.

CLINICAL CAPACITY, LEGAL COMPETENCE, AND SURROGATE DECISION-MAKING

For the informed consent process to be both meaningful and legally adequate, the clinician needs to confirm that the patient has the **capacity** to make autonomous decisions about her care. Capacity requires the ability to (1) understand the relevant information, (2) appreciate the situation and its consequences, and (3) appreciate the reason for treatment options, and (4) communicate a choice.[62] **Competence** to participate in legal proceedings is distinct from capacity to make medical decisions, though the two terms are often erroneously conflated.

Characteristics such as an individual's level of education, preferred conversational language, and cultural background may influence how the individual processes information, but do not impair capacity to consent. It is the clinician's responsibility to make the information accessible and understandable. Plain language should be utilized and technical medical jargon minimized (Table 32.2). The consent process should occur in the patient's preferred language with the use of a certified medical translator. Translation services are a federal legal requirement for healthcare in the United States (Title VI of the Civil Rights Act of 1964).[63]

A patient's decision-making capacity may be compromised temporarily or permanently by her condition, medications, or a combination of the two.[64] Capacity to make a medical

TABLE 32.2. Plain Language Alternatives to Medical Terms Patients May Not Understand

Medical Term	Translation Into Plain Language
Analgesic	Pain killer
Antepartum	Before birth
Antiinflammatory	Lessens swelling and irritation
Bolus	A large amount given all at once
Cardiac disease	Heart problem
Contraception	Birth control
Enlarge	Get bigger
Epidural space	Space surrounding the spinal cord
Heart failure	Heart is not pumping well
Hypertension	High blood pressure
Infertility	Cannot get pregnant
Intrathecal	Into the spinal fluid
Intravenous	Into a vein
Lateral	Outside
Menses	Period
Monitor	Keep track of, keep an eye on
Occluded	Blocked
Oral	By mouth
Postpartum	After birth
Referral	Send you to another doctor

Adapted, in part, from Agency for Healthcare Research and Quality. Health Literacy Toolkit, 3rd edition. Plan language words. Available at https://www.ahrq.gov/health-literacy/improve/precautions/tool4e.html. Accessed 26 July 2024.

decision is decision-specific and context-specific; a patient may have capacity to make some medical decisions but might lack the capacity to make more complex medical decisions.[64] Frequent capacity reassessment will maximize patient autonomy, particularly in cases of temporary impairment.

Any determination of clinical incapacity should be clearly documented in the medical record, including the clinical factors supporting the determination.[65,66] State requirements vary; however, they commonly require the consensus of at least two treating clinicians.[67] By definition, incapacitated patients cannot give informed consent. In emergency situations, physicians can provide necessary care under the doctrine of **implied consent**, which presumes that a reasonable person would have consented to the anticipated treatment (see later discussion).[68]

Absent an emergency situation, incapacitated patients require a **surrogate decision-maker** who can engage with the informed consent process as if they were the patient.[68] Legally, it is necessary both to establish the need for a surrogate decision-maker and to identify the most appropriate

person to serve in this role. In some circumstances, the patient may have an advanced directive document that identifies a surrogate decision-maker. Frequently, people of child-bearing age do not have an advanced directive, and the surrogate decision-maker must be identified according to state statutory guidance. Some states provide clear statutory algorithms, typically reflecting relational hierarchy, while others provide only vague guidance as to appropriate surrogate decision-makers.

In cases of prolonged or permanent impairment, a court may make a determination of legal incompetence,[69] and vest a surrogate with authority to make many kinds of decisions on behalf of the patient. The scope of decision-making authority varies, but often includes medical decision-making. Such legal determinations are usually made in the course of a petition for guardianship filed on behalf of the allegedly incapacitated individual, supported by evidence of clinical incapacity.[69,70] If a court has determined that a person is legally incompetent and has named a surrogate decision-maker, decision-making authority can be revoked only if the patient or some other third party goes back to court and challenges the determination, either because circumstances have changed and the patient has regained capacity, or because the patient or third party appeals the initial determination of the court.[71]

Surrogate decision-makers use a **"substituted judgment" standard** when making decisions on behalf of the patient. This standard obligates the surrogate to make the decision they believe the patient would have made, rather than the decision the surrogate prefers, and rather than the decision that might be otherwise deemed in the patient's best interest.[69] "The surrogate decision-maker (judge or guardian) should attempt to determine what the incapacitated person would decide regarding the proposed treatment or procedure were he or she competent."[71] When it is impossible to determine what decision the patient would have made, and there is little or no collateral information to help guide the surrogate, it may be necessary to switch to a **"best interest" standard**.[66] If the surrogate appears to be unable to carry out this obligation, the surrogate's authority for decision-making may be challenged, either through institutional processes or through the courts.[72] Institutional ethics committees may be a useful resource in navigating questions of surrogate decision-making.

Highly complex decisions, such as those pertaining to withdrawal of life-sustaining treatment, change in resuscitation/code status, or major surgery, may be considered as "extraordinary" measures, and in some instances may warrant a multidisciplinary evaluation, occasionally even necessitating court involvement.[73,74] The necessity to return to court to request specific authority for these "extraordinary" decisions is driven by state law, and so it is important to determine the breadth of a surrogate decision-maker's authority to consent to various treatments and care plans within the laws of the state in which the treatment is being provided.[75] Some patients may have identified a surrogate decision-maker through prior establishment of an advanced directive document, such as a durable healthcare power of attorney. Some advanced directives provide very specific guidance and limitations on the authority of the surrogate decision-maker, while others do not. It is important to determine whether an advanced directive exists and to consult the document for guidance.[75]

DECISION-MAKING IN OBSTETRIC ANESTHESIA

There are unique challenges to obtaining consent and engaging in shared decision-making in the labor and delivery setting. These include balancing competing interests of the mother and fetus, the interaction with distressed patients who can be part of a complex family system, and interdisciplinary collaboration during rapidly evolving clinical situations. The anesthesia provider must work quickly to establish trust, elicit preferences for information and decision-making, and tailor shared decision-making to the patient, while coordinating decisions with other members of the interdisciplinary care team. This is no easy task. Misunderstandings, unmet expectations, patient dissatisfaction, and liability are potential outcomes.

Most women prefer to learn about labor analgesia options from their healthcare providers in the second or third trimester.[76] However, not all obstetric providers are able to provide robust discussions regarding analgesia and anesthesia for labor and delivery in the prenatal period. Historically, consent for anesthesia was incorporated into consent for surgery, and direct participation of the anesthesia provider in the consent conversation was not mandated. Now, most states require separate consent conversations (and forms) for surgery and anesthesia procedures.[9] Regardless of state mandate, a personalized consent conversation with the patient is important for optimal care and helps to establish the therapeutic patient–physician relationship. A good therapeutic relationship has been shown to protect against future medicolegal liability.[77] This separate, focused discussion on the benefits and risks of anesthesia provides a unique opportunity to address misconceptions. In a survey study of 509 English-speaking parturients (63% White, 23% Hispanic, 14% African-American) admitted to a single institution, Toledo et al.[78] showed that 39% of participants expressed concerns regarding neuraxial anesthesia. These ranged from general misunderstandings about the anesthetic (e.g., epidural analgesia slows down labor or causes cerebral palsy), fears about long-term complications of the procedure, and lack of trust in providers, to concerns regarding fetal effects of medications administered in the epidural space.[78] Ideally, informed consent discussions about anesthesia services begin with an antepartum consultation or with the admission history and physical examination, and address possible delivery scenarios and corresponding anesthetic options in general terms. This conversation opens an ongoing dialogue to support shared decision-making, which continues throughout the hospitalization for delivery.

Some have questioned whether receiving information during labor influences a patient's ability to understand and recall the discussion, and what mode of communication is most effective. To evaluate the ability of laboring women to recall the details of a preanesthetic discussion, and to determine whether verbal consent alone or a combination of verbal and written consent provided better recall, Gerancher et al.[79] randomly assigned 113 laboring patients to one of two groups, those from whom verbal consent alone was obtained and those from whom verbal consent plus written consent was obtained. The verbal-plus-written consent group had significantly higher median (range) recall scores (90 [80 to 100]) than the verbal-only group (80 [70 to 90]). Only two patients (both in the verbal group) believed that they were unable (because of either inadequate information or situational stress) to give valid consent.

Clark et al.[80] randomly assigned hospital inpatients to receive either a verbal anesthesia discussion alone or both a verbal anesthesia discussion and a preprinted anesthesia consent form. In contrast with the results of Gerancher et al.,[79] these investigators found that "patients remembered less of the information concerning anesthetic risks discussed during the preoperative interview if they received a preprinted, risk-specific anesthesia consent form at the beginning of the interview." They speculated that "patients who see an anesthesia consent form for the first time during the preoperative interview may try to read and listen simultaneously, and with their attention divided, may remember less of the preoperative discussion."

Many patients have strong opinions about their analgesic options, based on information gathered from their obstetric provider, websites, books, magazines, classes, and friends and family.[78] In addition, factors such as patient-provider racial and ethnic discordance, implicit bias, structural racism, and maternal distrust of the healthcare system influence any discussion (see Chapter 14). The nature of the consent process will differ depending on the level of prior knowledge, health literacy, decision-making preferences, and clinical circumstances, but a paternalistic approach, grounded on the premise that patients cannot have the same clinical knowledge of the clinicians, can no longer be justified.[81]

SPECIAL CONSIDERATIONS IN OBSTETRIC ANESTHESIA

Patient Who Is in Pain

Anesthesia providers often first encounter pregnant patients during labor when they are in pain. Some have questioned whether patients who are in pain can be truly informed in any meaningful way during the consenting process.[82]

While acute pain has been shown in nonobstetric contexts to impact cognition,[83] the suggestion that the pain of labor constitutes duress, and thus invalidates any consent provided under such circumstance, is not supported in the medical literature or in case law. A survey of 60 Canadian women revealed their strong preference to be informed of all possible complications of epidural anesthesia, even those with low likelihood of occurrence, despite experiencing labor pain.[84] This study queried individuals up to 2 months after delivery and found the level of patient satisfaction with the neuraxial consent process was high (8.1/10) and not affected by pain

($r = 0.013$) or anxiety ($r = 0.048$).[84] Further, a study conducted by Gerancher et al.[79] demonstrated no difference in patient satisfaction with the consent process, whether or not the patient had received opioid premedication before obtaining consent. A 2005 study evaluated whether labor pain and neuraxial fentanyl administration affect the intellectual function of birthing women.[85] The Mini-Mental Status Examination (MMSE) was used to evaluate orientation, registration, attention, calculation, recall, and language both before and after initiation of analgesia in 41 laboring women. There was no difference in MMSE scores before and after administration of neuraxial analgesia. Thus, these studies support the notion that women who are laboring should not receive an abbreviated consenting process nor is it essential to provide analgesia prior to obtaining consent. Courts have also held that labor and its associated pain does not nullify a pregnant woman's capacity to make medical decisions,[86] finding the onset of labor did not by itself render a woman incompetent to engage in decision-making.

Labor pain does not diminish a birthing woman's capacity to provide informed consent. A clinician is still required to obtain informed consent prior to therapies or procedures despite the presence of maternal pain, and maternal pain is not a defense for inadequate informed consent. In navigating how to conduct an informed consent discussion with the patient in pain, the provider should recognize that patients experience and respond to pain differently. Some laboring patients may desire to engage in discussion consistently, while other patients may prefer to pause conversation during painful contractions. Inquiring "May we continue to talk, or would you prefer to pause until the end of the contraction?" applies the shared decision-making construct by simultaneously acknowledging the patient's pain and respecting their preference for when and how to continue the dialogue. Verbal consent in lieu of a written signature is acceptable in circumstances where an urgent neuraxial procedure is required due to the patient's level of need. Written documentation can be obtained once the patient is more comfortable; however, this does not obviate the requirement for an antecedent informed discussion regarding the procedure. Clear documentation of the conversation and context for the circumstances should be recorded in the medical record.

Patient Who Has Received Sedatives or Opioids

Many anesthetic medications as well as medications administered during labor and childbirth have the potential to impact maternal cognition, memory, and consciousness.[87] These effects have implications for the patient's ability to engage in shared decision-making and to provide informed consent. However, the mere administration of medications, including anxiolytics or opioids, does not necessarily preclude a patient from providing informed consent. Judicious use of medications to alleviate significant anxiety, or opioids to treat severe pain, can enhance the patient's ability to interact and participate in shared decision-making without compromising their ability to comprehend and process critical information. In a randomized, prospective, placebo-controlled trial, there

was no difference in maternal recall during cesarean delivery between the control group and those premedicated with fentanyl 1 µg/kg and midazolam 0.02 mg/kg.[88]

Nevertheless, it is inappropriate to use sedatives to manipulate the patient's decision or to eliminate their decision-making capacity. The use of drugs with amnestic potential merits thoughtful consideration as the patient may not recall the informed consent process afterward, especially with high or cumulative doses of benzodiazepines. However, even when a patient cannot recall the details of the informed consent discussion, that does not necessarily mean that they did not, at the time consent was obtained, understand the risks, benefits, and alternatives presented.[89]

Patient With a Birth Plan

The birth plan is a document wherein patients state their wishes and preferences for the management of certain aspects of their labor and delivery course. The practice of using a formal, written birth plan dates back to the 1970s. Its intended purpose was to enhance communication between the expectant mother and healthcare provider.[90–92] The premise was that patient participation in childbirth decision-making would result in a positive labor and delivery experience for the mother. To investigate the association between presence of a birth plan, mode of delivery, obstetric intervention, and patient satisfaction, Afshar et al.[93] prospectively studied a cohort of 300 patients in a tertiary care center. Compared with the group that did not have a birth plan ($n = 157$), the 143 patients with a birth plan experienced fewer intrapartum obstetric interventions, such as oxytocin augmentation (61% versus 78%, $P < .01$) and artificial rupture of membranes (15% versus 29%, $P < .01$). There was no difference in the cesarean delivery rate between the groups. Interestingly, parturients with a birth plan reported less satisfaction with their birth experience compared with parturients without one. A possible explanation for this finding may be that a departure from the expected plan may be met with disappointment, irrespective of the outcome.[94]

The birth plan is a written expression of the patient's wishes. It is not a legally binding document and does not constitute legal consent; instead, it should be understood as an expression of a patient's wishes at the time it was created, and that a patient may choose something different in the course of labor.[95] As such, it provides a good starting point for a thoughtful discussion that dispels myths, addresses anxieties, and educates the patient on the evidence-based risks and benefits of analgesia and anesthesia for labor and delivery. For some, the creation of a birth plan is an individual's attempt to maintain a sense of control over an otherwise unpredictable and vulnerable situation. Maintaining control, for many, is a surrogate for safety. As a birth plan is typically drafted before admission to the labor and delivery unit, it is possible that a patient may change her mind regarding her wishes. The birth plan reflects the patient's best assessment of the balance between risks and benefits before the onset of labor. This highlights an important aspect of informed consent: it must be contemporaneous with the actual clinical situation. It is incumbent on healthcare providers to read this document and use it as a tool to facilitate communication using shared decision-making techniques.

EMERGENCY PROCEDURES

Generally, in emergency situations, healthcare professionals provide treatment under a **"presumed consent"** model. Absent any collateral information to the contrary from the patient or a surrogate decision-maker, a patient should receive care in their "best interest" in emergency situations, even if such a patient cannot provide informed consent.[96] In many jurisdictions, family or the decision-making surrogate can refuse emergency care on behalf of the incapacitated patient if they can genuinely state that they know the patient would refuse such care were the patient able to consent themself.[96] When in doubt as to the accuracy of the family's refusal, it may be necessary to preserve the best interest of the patient in the face of uncertainty as to the patient's wishes. If the healthcare providers treatment was authorized under a medical emergency, the emergency determination should be carefully documented.[96] The documentation in the patient's medical record should contain a description of the patient's presenting condition, its immediacy, its magnitude, and the nature of the immediate threat or harm to the patient.[97]

MINORS AS VULNERABLE POPULATIONS

Traditionally, minors have not been allowed to provide informed consent, based on concerns that they may lack the experience or capacity to inform judgments related to healthcare decisions.[98] Consequently, in most states, a minor child needs a parent or guardian to make legal decisions, including informed consent for treatment.[98] In many states, pregnancy is an exception to this rule, and pregnant women less than 18 years of age may consent for procedures related to prenatal, intrapartum, and postpartum care, as well as interventions that benefit the fetus.[99–103] Pregnant minors still need medical assessment for capacity to make medical decisions (see earlier discussion). Because state laws vary substantially and can evolve rapidly, specific laws will not be covered here, and clinicians should consult the current statutory and case law of their state for specific guidance. Institutional legal departments can provide practical interpretation if needed. Despite nuanced differences, many states have some form of statutory exemption for pregnant minors, often utilizing an **"emancipated minor"** or **"mature minor"** standard, which are terms defined by individual state statute.[101]

Some states additionally recognize circumstances such as being married/divorced, being in the military, and living independently, to confer decision-making authority to minors. These legal theories permit minors, in applicable situations, to make their own medical decisions wholly or partially. Furthermore, medical care provided to minors under these doctrines may be considered confidential and prohibited from disclosure to parents and guardians.[104–107] Institutional legal counsel should be consulted for case-specific concerns.

Many states allow minors to consent to their own contraception-oriented healthcare services.[108] Title X under US federal law explicitly stipulates that family planning services must be provided to minors on a confidential basis, and the ACOG stresses the importance of confidentiality in counseling adolescents about contraception.[109] Rules governing consent for permanent sterilization tend to be more restrictive,[110] and may require involvement of parents or guardians on behalf of minor patients.[111] In most states, the adolescent parturient may petition a court for the ability to consent to permanent sterilization, without the involvement of their parent or guardian.[110]

Procedures to end pregnancy receive special legal treatment in the United States. In 2022, the US Supreme Court overturned a long-standing precedent that recognized federal protection of previability pregnancy termination. Following the *Dobbs v. Jackson Women's Health Organization* decision,[112] many state legislatures moved to make abortion illegal or to impose gestational age limits in the first or second trimester of pregnancy. In states where abortion remains legal, access to abortion care for minors may require parental or guardian consent, although some states allow for judicial bypass in situations of incest or sexual abuse by a parent.[111] Most states allow for termination of pregnancy threatening the life of the mother; however, there is sparse guidance on how grave of a threat must exist for this exception to apply. Some states permit termination of pregnancy in instances of severe fetal anomalies, with varying limits as to gestational age. Current individual state laws should be consulted for definitive guidance.

LANGUAGE AND HEALTH LITERACY CONSIDERATIONS

In 2014, more than 900,000 births in the United States were to immigrant mothers, a threefold increase since 1970.[113] In 2018, immigrants accounted for 13.7% of the US population, and the birth rate among immigrant women (7.5%) was higher than those born in the United States (5.7%).[114] If current immigration trends continue, immigrants and their descendants will account for 88% of US population growth through 2065.[114] This rise in diversity challenges the ability of healthcare providers and institutions to appropriately care for immigrant obstetric patients. Some studies have shown poorer obstetric and perinatal outcomes in immigrant versus native individuals.[115] Limited language proficiency is associated with significant risk for poor maternal outcomes,[116] which highlights the importance of native language communication in healthcare.

The language gap between a patient and healthcare provider is commonly bridged using an interpreter. The use of bilingual family members, especially children, is discouraged as their unfamiliarity with medical terminology and emotional ties to the patient may hinder the accurate transfer of information from patient to doctor and vice versa.[117,118] Suboptimal interpretation not only impairs information exchange but can undermine the shared decision-making and informed consent processes.[119] The use of professional medical interpreters is a resource-intensive tool not always available for all languages or after regular work hours. However, there is a growing industry of HIPAA-compliant (Health Insurance Portability and Accountability Act) video or phone interpreter services offered 24 hours a day, 7 days a week that may be an alternative option for some health systems.

In addition to language discordance, low levels of health literacy can impair patients' ability to understand the information provided by their healthcare provider. Unlike functional literacy, which refers to an individual's operational capacity to function in daily life through use of basic reading, writing, and computational skills,[120] health literacy demands the use of more complex language skills as well as the ability to process numerical information.[121] Health literacy is defined as the "degree to which individuals have capacity to obtain, process, and understand basic health information and services needed to make appropriate health decisions."[122] In 2004 the Institute of Medicine reported that "nearly half of all American adults—90 million people—have difficulty understanding and using health information, and there is a higher rate of hospitalization and use of emergency services among patients with limited health literacy."[122]

The 2003 National Assessment of Adult Literacy, conducted by the US Department of Education, assessed literacy in a representative sample of 19,000 US adults (ages 16 years and older) who spoke either English or Spanish with at least some English. The report found individuals at higher risk of having low health literacy are those who (1) identify with a minority ethnicity (Hispanic ethnicity and those speaking only Spanish at home prior to schooling had the lowest rates identified), (2) have government insurance (Medicaid/Medicare) without a high school degree, and (3) obtain medical information from nonprint media.[123–125] Low health literacy also affects immigrants with limited English proficiency.[126] In a prospective, matched cohort design investigation, Brice et al.[121] compared the health literacy level of adult English-speaking patients to Spanish-speaking patients presenting to an emergency department in suburban North Carolina. The Test of Functional Health Literacy in Adults was administered to both groups. The results revealed that 74% of Spanish-speaking participants possess less-than-adequate functional health literacy, compared with 7% of the English-speaking cohort.[121] In a 2017 survey of medically trained interpreters and anesthesia providers at a major teaching hospital in Boston, 43% of interpreters felt that "less than half of their patient population was sufficiently literate to read and consent in their native language."[127]

Unfortunately, many published materials available for public education in anesthesia are written at a level higher than what the public can understand. In a review of educational material downloaded from 24 national anesthesiology society websites, Govender et al.[128] discovered all material was above an eighth-grade level, which is too complex for lay comprehension. The US Agency for Healthcare Research and Quality published a health literacy universal precautions toolkit for clinicians.[129] Strategies for patient communication include (1) using plain, nonmedical language (see Table 32.2); (2) adopting the patient's words to describe their condition; (3) limiting information to 3 to 5 points and repeating them; (4) being concrete and avoiding terms that could be interpreted in different ways; and (5) using graphics designed to demonstrate the most important concepts.[129]

Educational aids such as written material (brochures, illustrations, models) and video-assisted patient education can be invaluable in the transfer of information to patients, particularly if the material is presented in the patient's own language with minimal use of medical jargon.[130–133] Additionally, the use of educational videos has been shown to decrease patient anxiety and increase patient satisfaction with medical care.[134] Obstetric patients frequently need to make complex healthcare decisions in unfamiliar surroundings when their healthcare providers are burdened by time constraints. By standardizing the information presented on specific topics, supplemental educational aids can help minimize misleading information, censoring of information, or devaluing of information.

CULTURE CONSIDERATIONS

The Institute of Medicine in the United States describes patient-centered care as care that honors the individual patient and respects their choices, culture, ethnicity, social context, values, and informational needs.[21] Effective communication between patients and care providers is a building block of patient-centered care and a cornerstone of patient safety and optimal healthcare delivery. Using interviews of pregnant individuals of Mexican origin to explore their expectations of healthcare providers, Baxley and Ibitayo[135] noted that patients "wanted to hear everything, hear it directly, and have it presented to them as if from a friend." For these study participants, faith was a major component of their culture and a strong influence on their perceptions of health outcomes.[135] Similarly, newly arrived Somali couples expressed the importance of their beliefs and cultural values during perinatal interviews.[136] In their culture, having many children is considered desirable. Thus, a high value is placed on a vaginal delivery; a cesarean delivery can limit the number of children and, in their culture, cesarean delivery is also believed to be associated with death.[136]

Patient autonomy is an important principle to uphold in decision-making. In many cultures and social contexts, this autonomy is preserved even when power to make medical decisions is passed on to another individual. For example, a competent patient may choose to allow a partner or other family member to make "first-order" decisions regarding medical care. If their decision to defer to the judgment of another person is truly free and voluntary, then this "second-order" decision is authentic and autonomous.[137] Although justified in principle, this can be difficult to carry out in practice. One can imagine a situation in which a nulliparous individual has decided that she does not want epidural analgesia for labor pain management and that medical management decisions have been willingly relinquished to her partner. If the patient changes her mind once labor pains have started, but the surrogate, with all good intentions, insists on the predetermined plan, the patient's wishes are no longer being properly represented. In this setting, the will of the patient needs to be confirmed and takes priority over predetermined proxy arrangements.[138] Strong-willed family members, intending to advocate for their loved ones, may seem angry and even threatening. Often, they respond to patience and empathy, nonconfrontational communication, and input from the laboring patient and other parties.

RELIGIOUS-BASED OR CULTURALLY BASED OBJECTIONS TO CARE

When a provider is aware that a patient has expressed a religious or culturally based objection to certain aspects of medical care (e.g., blood transfusion for a Jehovah's Witness), that aspect of the care should not be provided even in an emergency context.[139] If a blood transfusion would be required to save the life of an individual who has expressed objection to blood transfusion, absent any collateral information to the contrary, it is appropriate to withhold the blood transfusion.[139] Detailed lists of blood products and blood conservation therapies are available[140,141] to facilitate shared decision-making and to clarify the specific interventions individual patients will and will not accept. Certain therapies (e.g., cell salvage with a continuous circuit) may be acceptable to some individuals.[142] It is also helpful to explicitly consider likely clinical scenarios in advance. Patients can change their minds about receiving life-saving interventions at any time point, but severe hemorrhage can impact decision-making capacity, so it is important to confirm the four elements of capacity to make medical decisions, including the ability to express a choice. An incapacitated patient with a previously documented clear objection to the provision of some or all care should not receive undesired interventions just because they do not have the capacity in an emergency situation.[139]

Although an adult patient can decline life-saving medical treatment on their own behalf, parental refusal of care for their child is more complex. The courts generally recognize that the state's interest in protecting the life and well-being of a child outweighs the parents' right to make decisions for the child when that decision could result in a significantly poor outcome.[143] In some jurisdictions, the default is that the parents retain such rights and providers must go to court to overcome that presumption.[144] In other jurisdictions, providers faced with a similar situation have the right to provide care to the child over the objection of the parents, and the parents or guardians must go to court to attempt to obtain an injunction to bar the provision of such care.

GESTATIONAL CARRIER OR SURROGATES

A gestational carrier is a person contracted to carry a pregnancy with a fetus created from a donated ovum (rather than her own) on behalf of another family.[145] The gestational carrier is considered the patient at all times throughout the pregnancy, regardless of the level of involvement of the intended parents during such time. Although gestational carriers may, and likely do, have a formal contract with the intended parents that specifies the gestational carrier's obligations, any agreement is only applicable between the gestational carrier and the intended parents.[145] Healthcare providers are not parties to such agreements and are not bound to any provisions contained therein.[145] If a gestational carrier violates a provision, the intended parents may have a contractual recourse against the gestational carrier. This has no effect on the healthcare providers' obligation to treat the gestational carrier as the patient and allow the gestational carrier to remain the sole decision-maker. Healthcare providers should always remember that the gestational carrier is their patient, and it is their obligation to only provide care to which the gestational carrier consents, irrespective of the intended parents' position.

This arrangement is distinguished from a traditional surrogate, who carries a fetus originating from her own ovum on behalf of another family. In these situations, the surrogate is a legal parent to the child even after birth, until a traditional adoption has taken place.

CONFLICTS ARISING OUT OF THE MATERNAL–FETAL RELATIONSHIP

During pregnancy, situations may arise in which the interests of the pregnant woman and those of the fetus appear to diverge, or even to conflict. Common scenarios in which maternal autonomy may impact fetal well-being include parental substance use, declining recommended antenatal diagnostic testing or treatment, and delaying indicated delivery.[146] Pregnancy may compromise maternal health and well-being in a variety of situations, including abstinence from otherwise routine medications or activities, exacerbation of medical comorbidities such as severe cardiac disease or pulmonary hypertension, and deferring standard medical treatment such as chemotherapy and/or radiation for cancer.

Numerous examples of maternal–fetal conflict have risen to the level of judicial review. Typically, appellate courts' decisions have prioritized the pregnant woman's decisions over the presumed fetal consequences.[147] An index case is illustrative. In 1987 at 25 weeks' gestation, Angela Carder, a survivor of Ewing's sarcoma, developed back pain and shortness of breath. A chest x-ray revealed a large, inoperable lung tumor, and subsequent evaluation confirmed terminal cancer recurrence. Initially, she consented to treatments that could prolong her life to 28 weeks' gestation, at which point she would consent to cesarean delivery. Unfortunately, her condition deteriorated rapidly, and within a week, she elected palliative care. She declined delivery, deciding the risks to her own health and comfort were not worth the small chance of producing a viable infant in the context of ongoing intrauterine hypoxia and extreme preterm birth. Her husband, mother, and obstetrician agreed. With Angela Carder intubated and sedated on mechanical ventilation and deteriorating rapidly, the hospital sought judicial review of this course of action, asking whether a surgical delivery should be authorized to save the potentially viable fetus. The judge in the case decided in favor of the fetus. A cesarean delivery was performed at 26 weeks' gestation by a hospital-appointed obstetrician, and the infant died approximately 2 hours after delivery while the mother died 2 days later. This case spawned extensive debate as to whether coercive intervention to protect the fetus is ever morally or legally justifiable.[148] With the assistance of the American Civil Liberties Union, Angela's parents sued the hospital, administrators, and physicians for claims, including battery, false imprisonment, discrimination, and medical malpractice. These civil lawsuits were settled and the hospital adopted a written policy concerning decision-making for pregnant patients.[149] The court later reversed its initial decision authorizing the surgical delivery and ultimately issued an opinion setting forth the legal principles that should govern the doctor–parturient relationship. The court stated: "In virtually all cases the question of what is to be done is to be decided by the patient—the pregnant woman—on behalf of herself and the fetus. If the patient is incompetent … her decision must be ascertained through substituted judgment." The court affirmed that the patient's wishes, once ascertained, must be followed in "virtually all cases" unless there are "truly extraordinary or compelling reasons to override them."[150]

Many contemporary medical ethicists agree that a pregnant individual's informed refusal of medical intervention should prevail as long as they have the capacity to make medical decisions.[151] In the case of an incapacitated patient, a legal surrogate decision maker has the right to speak for the patient in refusing such medical intervention. Newer legislation and some high-profile legal cases (some involving criminal prosecution) have challenged this notion, indicating there are circumstances in which a pregnant individual's rights to informed consent and bodily integrity may be subordinated to protect the unborn child. For example, in 2004, Melissa Rowland was charged by the state of Utah with murder for the stillbirth of one twin because she initially refused cesarean delivery, even though she later accepted delivery by cesarean and her second twin survived. She pleaded guilty to child endangerment in order to avoid more serious charges.[152]

Many cases have focused on prosecuting pregnant women with substance use disorders. In 1991 Regina McKnight was convicted of homicide by child abuse, and served 8 years in jail, after she delivered a stillborn infant. The state of South Carolina blamed the stillbirth on her use of cocaine. In 2008 the South Carolina Supreme Court unanimously reversed her conviction on the grounds that she did not receive a fair trial, primarily on the basis that her attorney failed to challenge the science that was used to convict her.[153]

In a similar case, Shekelia Ward delivered a live infant in 2008, and both she and her newborn tested positive for cocaine.[154] The facility reported it to authorities for possible child abuse, and she was arrested, imprisoned, and charged with a felony—chemical endangerment of a child. Prosecutors cited an Alabama state statute enacted in 2006 for the purpose of prosecuting parents who exposed children to the toxins associated with methamphetamine production; the statute did not mention pregnant women or their fetuses.[155]

These cases reflect the concept that a fetus can and should be treated as separate and legally, philosophically, and essentially independent from the mother.[147] The refinement of techniques of intrauterine fetal imaging, testing, and treatment prompted the view that fetuses are independent patients who can be treated directly while in utero.[156] The prominence of some ethical models with assertions that physicians have moral obligations to fetal patients separate from their obligations to pregnant women also contributed to these developments.[157] Finally, a number of laws (primarily passed at the state level) were enacted with the aim of defining fetal rights separate from a pregnant woman's rights. In 2011 (reaffirmed in 2022) the ACOG Committee on Healthcare for Underserved Women issued a statement addressing the role of the obstetrician in reporting substance use.[158] This document described a "disturbing trend" in legal actions and policies that criminalize drug use during pregnancy when thought to be associated with fetal harm or adverse outcomes. Noting that women seeking obstetric care should not be exposed to criminal or civil penalties and that few treatment facilities are available to effectively treat substance use disorders in pregnancy, the ACOG concluded that the use of the legal system to address alcohol and substance use issues is inappropriate and urged that policy makers and legislators instead focus on strategies to address the needs of pregnant women with substance use disorders.

The American Medical Association (AMA) has taken a similar position, stating that (1) substance use disorder is a disease amenable to treatment, rather than criminal activity; and (2) there is a pressing need for maternal drug treatment and supportive child protective services.[159] Any legislation that criminalizes maternal substance use disorders or requires physicians to function as agents of law enforcement will be opposed by the AMA.[159]

There has been an evolution in the approach of the ACOG and medical ethicists on the best means to address maternal–fetal conflict. A 1999 ACOG opinion offered the following three options: (1) respect the patient's autonomy and not proceed with the recommended intervention regardless of the consequences, (2) offer the patient the option of obtaining medical care from another individual before conditions become emergent, and (3) request that the court issue an order to permit the recommended treatment.[160] In 2004 the ACOG addressed the situation in which healthcare providers may consider this last option (i.e., legal intervention against a pregnant woman).[149] Specifically, the ACOG stated that the following criteria should be satisfied: (1) "there is a high probability of serious harm to the fetus in respecting the patient's decision"; (2) "there is a high probability that the recommended treatment will prevent or substantially reduce harm to the fetus"; (3) "there are no comparably effective, less intrusive options to prevent harm to the fetus"; and (4) "there is a high probability that the recommended treatment [will] also benefit the pregnant woman or that the risks to the pregnant woman are relatively small." The most recent 2016 ACOG recommendations emphasize the key principles of shared decision-making and discourage external coercion from the court system.[161]

In summary, two approaches are available to the practitioner dealing with maternal–fetal conflict. One approach is to honor a competent pregnant patient's refusal of care. The other approach, less favored by many medical ethicists and the ACOG, is to seek judicial authorization of treatment, which overrides a competent pregnant woman's refusal of care.[162] Institutional ethics committees may be a useful resource for navigating the perceived conflict while also supporting shared decision-making.

In honoring a competent patient's desire to refuse medically recommended treatment, the healthcare providers should carefully document the woman's competency and ability to provide informed consent. Every attempt should be made to counsel the patient to follow the treatment recommendations. Documentation should include how, when, and what information was provided to the patient and family regarding the significant risks to both the patient and fetus if the recommended care was not provided. If time permits, the treatment options should be reevaluated with the patient at frequent intervals, with detailed documentation in the patient's medical record. Additionally, legal counsel for the healthcare providers and medical facility may wish to prepare an "assumption of risk" form for the patient to sign. This form represents another level of documentation (beyond the detailed notes in the patient's medical record) demonstrating that the patient was fully informed about the risks associated with her refusal of treatment and that the patient voluntarily elected to accept those risks. However, such a release signed by the parents may not protect the physician and medical facility from a claim brought on behalf of the child who suffers an injury as a result of nonintervention. In some cases, the court has found that physicians have a duty to provide care to the unborn child.[163]

Before deciding whether to seek court review, healthcare providers should identify what issue they want the court to resolve. Is it whether the pregnant woman is competent? Is it whether there is a superior state interest in preserving the life of the viable fetus and/or the pregnant woman despite the (competent) patient's desire to refuse recommended care? Healthcare providers also should consider whether a court is the proper forum for resolving these issues or whether another forum (e.g., an institutional ethics committee) may be a better choice. If a patient care dilemma is put before a judge, the healthcare providers give up a large amount of control over the disposition of the case. Nonetheless, in the absence of a legally authorized decision-maker, if a patient's competency is at issue and there is adequate time, court review to settle the patient's competency may be beneficial and is supported by both the ACOG guidelines[146] and the *Angela Carder* decision (see earlier discussion).[150] It is beneficial to obtain authorization for the provision of medically recommended care without waiting until the situation becomes an emergency. If the patient is deemed incompetent, the court may either appoint a surrogate decision-maker or directly authorize (by court order) the provision of medically indicated care.

It is not unusual for physicians to disagree with their patients' healthcare decisions, and such differences are expected. In some cases, physicians conclude that providing the requested care would present a personal moral problem—a conflict of conscience, which prompts them to refuse to provide the requested care. Conscientious refusals have become especially prevalent in the practice of reproductive medicine, an area characterized by deep societal divisions regarding the morality of contraception and pregnancy termination. The ACOG Committee on Ethics has acknowledged that "respect for conscience is one of many values important to the ethical practice of reproductive medicine."[164] The ACOG stated that when conscience implores physicians to refuse to perform abortion, sterilization, and/or provision of contraceptives, "they must provide potential patients with accurate and prior notice of their personal moral commitments." The ACOG committee opinion also emphasized that providers have an obligation to provide medically indicated care in an emergency that threatens the patient's health, in which referral is not possible.[164]

UNANTICIPATED OUTCOMES AND MEDICAL ERRORS

Medical Liability

Medical malpractice is a form of tort law that is based on negligence. As with all negligence claims, the plaintiff (either the patient or the patient's legal surrogate) must prove four elements: (1) duty, (2) breach of such duty, (3) injury, and (4) proximate causation (meaning that the "breach" was the "cause" of the "injury"). If the plaintiff is unable to prove even one of these elements, then the claim will fail as a matter of law.

In a malpractice case, the "duty" that must be proven to have been "breached" is the duty to provide care that meets a minimum level of competence as determined by expert opinion on both sides of the case. It does not need to be the highest level of care, nor does it even need to be the level of care provided by most clinicians. However, it must not be beneath the minimum standard of care expected of a licensed provider. The standard of care is generally defined as "that care which a reasonable, similarly situated professional would have provided to the patient."[165,166] Proving that such a standard of care has been breached is the role of experts.[167] Because medicine is a complex, continuously evolving discipline, it is the province of experts in the field to weigh in on whether the standard of care was met.[166] In making these judgments, experts can rely on their own knowledge, developed through education and practice, and on authoritative sources such as pharmaceutical publications and US Food and Drug Administration–approved inserts; scientific journals; and professional organizational standards, guidelines, and practice advisories.[168] Ultimately, expert testimony and other evidence presented by both parties will be evaluated by judges or juries for their persuasiveness. If either the judge or jury determines that the standard of care was not met, then the plaintiff will still need to prove that there was an "injury" that was "caused" by the "breach."[166]

It is important to remember that the burden of proof lies with the plaintiff (i.e., the injured patient) to show that the standard of care was not met, and that such breach caused the injury from which the patient suffers.[166] The plaintiff must prove by a "preponderance of the evidence" (meaning it is more than 50% likely) that each element of the claim has been proven.[166] Although this "preponderance of the evidence" standard is significantly lower than the criminal law standard of "proof beyond a reasonable doubt," it is still a relatively high burden to meet. The evidence presented, including the expert testimony, must be significant and objectively strong.

Some of the most common standards of care that are evaluated in a medical malpractice claim include whether an appropriate diagnosis was made, whether there was a surgical error, or whether pharmaceuticals have been prescribed and/or administered appropriately.[169]

It is also important to remember that an unanticipated outcome does not mean that malpractice has occurred. In fact, most unanticipated outcomes in medical care are a result of known risks, and despite the plaintiff's wish to establish fault through a medical malpractice claim, it is often established that the standard of care was met even though the outcome was not the desired one.

Sometimes, a physician makes a promise of a specific outcome to the patient, which could create a cause of action against the physician if such an outcome is not met.[170] But such cases are a rarity and require the plaintiff to make the case that a reasonable patient would have understood the words of the physician to indicate a promise of that specific outcome. It is more often the case that the process of care is being evaluated, rather than the outcome. A physician is liable for a misjudgment or mistake only when it is proved to have occurred through a failure to act in accordance with the "care and skill of a reasonably prudent practitioner."[170]

Many potential plaintiffs struggle to file a medical malpractice claim in a timely manner.[171] Numerous factors may interfere with bringing timely claims, not the least of which is the awareness that an unanticipated outcome has occurred.[171] Even when a medical error leads to iatrogenic injury, this may never be disclosed to the patient and family, and knowing the cause of any particular outcome can be difficult for the average patient (or their legal surrogates) to discern. Injured patients may serve notice of the intent to sue for malpractice as a strategy to find out what happened and use legal procedures to require disclosure of the details of care that may otherwise be inaccessible. Statutes of limitations, legal time frames in which legal claims must be brought for such claims to be valid, vary from state to state but are generally 2 to 3 years.[172] Most laws establish that this time frame begins when a reasonable person becomes aware of an injury that might be the result of a breach of the standard of care.[169] If this acknowledgment occurs right after care has been provided, then the time frame has begun; if it is years later (such as when the patient tries to conceive and discovers that she suffers from sterility), then the time frame will begin at the point of discovery of the injury. If a plaintiff can show that she would have been aware of an injury if not for fraudulent concealment by the provider, then the time frame may be extended to take such fraudulent behavior into account.[173] Additionally, if the plaintiff was a minor when the alleged breach occurred, then the statute of limitations does not usually begin until she reaches the age of majority.

Disclosure of Unanticipated Outcomes and Medical Errors

Most practitioners strive to provide the highest quality of care, but even with the growing focus on patient safety, unintended consequences—including patient injury and death—do occur. Unfortunately, most physicians remain largely unprepared to engage patients and their families in a timely, truthful, and candid manner in the aftermath of such events. Although some providers and medical malpractice insurers might want potential breaches of the standard of care to go unnoticed or unrecognized, emerging evidence suggests that timely disclosure may reduce legal risk.[174] In cases of unanticipated adverse outcomes, patients and families most commonly seek truthfulness, empathy, and a plan to ensure similar patients will not face similar risks in the future. Transparency, as well as a culture of accountability that includes providing apologies after such events, can mitigate distrust between the patient and provider, and ameliorate the desire to find someone to blame.[175] Many states have laws that protect providers from having disclosure and apology held against them should a malpractice claim be subsequently brought. Statutes of limitation for medical malpractice claims vary by state, but generally span from 2 to 3 years.[173] Some states even require reporting of medical errors.[176]

The ethical imperative to disclose is captured in the following passage from the *Charter on Medical Professionalism*, published by the American Board of Internal Medicine (ABIM) Foundation[177]:

> *Physicians should also acknowledge that in healthcare, medical errors that injure patients do sometimes occur. Whenever patients are injured as a consequence of medical care, patients should be informed promptly because failure to do so seriously compromises patient and societal trust. Reporting and analyzing medical mistakes provide the basis for appropriate prevention and improvement strategies and for appropriate compensation for injured parties.*

The AMA's *Code of Medical Ethics* contains the following statement: "It is a fundamental ethical requirement that a physician should at all times deal honestly and openly with patients.... Concern regarding legal liability, which might result following truthful disclosure, should not affect the physician's honesty with a patient."[178] The Joint Commission standard requires that "the hospital provides the patient or surrogate decision-maker with information about ... unanticipated outcomes of the patient's care treatment, and services that are sentinel events..."[179]

In 2006, the Harvard teaching hospitals and their associated Risk Management Foundation developed a document entitled "When Things Go Wrong: Responding to Adverse Events."[180] This white paper acknowledged the presence of many barriers to disclosure, including the fear of being sued, but the authors insisted that communication with patients and their families must be timely, open, and ongoing. In addition to stressing the imperative of providing support for the patient and family involved in the unexpected outcome, the paper emphasized the need to provide support to the healthcare providers involved. This concern is reflected in a 2008 survey that indicated that as many as 75% of obstetricians felt that caring for a patient with an unanticipated stillbirth exacted a large toll on them, with almost 10% of those affected considering giving up their obstetric practice.[181]

Even in the absence of laws requiring prompt disclosure of patient harm, some healthcare entities and their insurers have adopted disclosure policies that also contain early settlement or "offer" programs.[182] These types of programs encourage patients or their families to accept an early, modest payment for an unanticipated outcome that will eliminate the need for complex, expensive, and uncertain litigation that could take years to resolve.[182] Such offers are often protected from legal discovery, meaning the fact of such an offer cannot be used against the providers in any future litigation.[182]

Regardless, team debriefing can be used to establish the need for disclosure, to clarify what is known about the event, and to decide who will lead the disclosure process. Experts advise limiting disclosure to factual information that is known at the time of the discussion, and stating that discovery is ongoing and that information may evolve as the discovery process unfolds. A simple apology (e.g., "I am sorry this happened") conveys empathy without laying blame or fault. It is important to maintain open dialogue with the patient and family as information is clarified, but this requires careful coordination among different members of the healthcare team. Conflicting information and speculation, especially speculation that places blame on other members of the healthcare team, can raise concerns that the entire team may be hiding the truth. The process is analogous to shared decision-making; effective communication established before a patient safety incident or adverse outcome will carry over into the communication that must continue after the event.

KEY POINTS

- Effective communication with the parturient and their family is an important component of obstetric anesthesia practice.
- Informed consent may be either verbal or both verbal and written. Written consent provides documentation that the consent process has occurred. If possible, it is best to obtain consent early in labor, before the onset of severe pain.
- Shared decision-making is a best practice for communication in which the clinician partners with the patient to address a series of decisions throughout the healthcare encounter. In addition to standard disclosure of risks, benefits, and alternatives, the clinician elicits questions, values, and preferences from the patient, and guides the discussion toward a decision that is consistent with both the patient's preferences and current evidence.
- Trauma-informed care is shared decision-making with an understanding of the role of trauma on an individual's life and development. It emphasizes the "4 R" principles: (1) realizing the pervasive nature of trauma in our society, (2) recognizing what trauma looks like in survivors, (3) responding by changing our protocols and procedures to address the needs of survivors, and (4) resisting retraumatization with our clinical practice.

- Techniques to ensure understanding and avoid coercion are particularly important for vulnerable populations, including pregnant adolescents, non-English speakers, and individuals from diverse cultural backgrounds.
- Honest, caring, and comprehensive discussion with the patient before the administration of anesthesia meets legal and ethical standards, improves the image of the anesthesia provider, and reduces the likelihood of dissatisfaction and possible litigation after unanticipated complications.
- Refusal of care by pregnant patients may raise unique legal and ethical concerns. In such situations, the woman's competency or ability to make an informed medical decision may be an issue. When the patient is competent, the healthcare providers should attempt to resolve treatment conflicts through additional patient education and discussion. Rarely, it may be advisable to seek a court order to resolve competency or medical treatment issues.
- Effective interprofessional team communication is essential to ensure optimal team performance and to maintain consistent communication with the patient and family, all of which serve to mitigate the risk for medical liability in the event of an unanticipated adverse outcome.

REFERENCES

1. Gillon R. Ethics needs principles – four can encompass the rest – and respect for autonomy should be "first among equals". *J Med Ethics*. 2003;29:307–312.
2. *See* Salgo v. Leland Stanford Jr University Board of Trustees. California Appellate Court 1957.
3. Chen JY, Tao ML, Tisnado D, et al. Impact of physician-patient discussions on patient satisfaction. *Med Care*. 2008;46: 1157–1162.
4. Iversen MD, Daltroy LH, Fossel AH, Katz JN. The prognostic importance of patient pre-operative expectations of surgery for lumbar spinal stenosis. *Patient Educ Couns*. 1998;34: 169–178.

5. Levinson W, Roter DL, Mullooly JP, et al. Physician-patient communication. The relationship with malpractice claims among primary care physicians and surgeons. *JAMA*. 1997;277:553–559.

6. Burkle CM, Olsen DA, Sviggum HP, Jacob AK. Parturient recall of neuraxial analgesia risks: impact of labor pain vs no labor pain. *J Clin Anesth*. 2017;36:158–163.

7. *See* 38 CFR § 17.32.

8. CRICO. General informed consent guidelines 2016. https://www.rmf.harvard.edu/Risk-Prevention-and-Education/Guidelines-and-Algorithms-Catalog-Page/Guidelines-Algorithms/2011/General-Informed-Consent-Guidelines. Accessed 24 July 2024.

9. Hoehner PJ. Ethical aspects of informed consent in obstetric anesthesia—new challenges and solutions. *J Clin Anesth*. 2003;15:587–600.

10. *See* Canterbury v. Spence, 464 F.2d 772, 788-89 (D.C. Cir.1972); Restatement (Second) of Torts: Privileges § 890 (Am. Law Inst. 1979); Restatement (Second) of Torts: Emergency Action Without Consent § 892D (Am. Law Inst. 1979).

11. Dornette WH. Informed consent and anesthesia. *Anesth Analg*. 1974;53:832–837.

12. Broaddus BM, Chandrasekhar S. Informed consent in obstetric anesthesia. *Anesth Analg*. 2011;112:912–915.

13. D'Angelo R, Smiley RM, Riley ET, Segal S. Serious complications related to obstetric anesthesia: the serious complication repository project of the Society for Obstetric Anesthesia and Perinatology. *Anesthesiology*. 2014;120:1505–1512.

14. Fortunato JT, Wasserman JA, Menkes DL. When respecting autonomy is harmful: a clinically useful approach to the nocebo effect. *Am J Bioeth*. 2017;17:36–42.

15. Krauss BS. "This may hurt": Predictions in procedural disclosure may do harm. *BMJ*. 2015;350:h649.

16. Cyna AM, Simmons SW. Guidelines on informed consent in anaesthesia: unrealistic, unethical, untenable. *Br J Anaesth*. 2017;119:1086–1089.

17. Benjamin R. Informed refusal: Toward a justice-based bioethics. *Sci Technol Human Values*. 2016;41:967–990.

18. Chhabra KR, Sacks GD, Dimick JB. Surgical decision making: Challenging dogma and incorporating patient preferences. *JAMA*. 2017;317:357–358.

19. Agency for Healthcare Research and Quality. The SHARE approach: A model for shared decision making – fact sheet. 2020. cited 2023. https://www.ahrq.gov/health-literacy/professional-training/shared-decision/tools/factsheet.html. Accessed 24 July 2024.

20. Barry MJ, Edgman-Levitan S. Shared decision making – pinnacle of patient-centered care. *N Engl J Med*. 2012;366:780–781.

21. Institute of Medicine Committee on Quality of Healthcare in America. *Crossing the Quality Chasm: A New Health System for the 21st Century*. National Academies Press; 2001.

22. Gerteis M, Edgman-Levitan S, Daley J, Delbanco T. *Through the Patient Eyes: Understanding and Promoting Patient-Centered Care*. 1st ed. Jossey-Bass Publishers; 1993.

23. American College of Obstetricians and Gynecologists. Committee Opinion No. 490: Partnering with patients to improve safety (reaffirmed 2019). *Obstet Gynecol*. 2011;117:1247–1249.

24. Stacey D, Legare F, Lewis K, et al. Decision aids for people facing health treatment or screening decisions. *Cochrane Database Syst Rev*. 2017;(4):CD001431.

25. Durand MA, Carpenter L, Dolan H, et al. Do interventions designed to support shared decision-making reduce health inequalities? A systematic review and meta-analysis. *PLoS One*. 2014;9:e94670.

26. Joseph-Williams N, Lloyd A, Edwards A, et al. Implementing shared decision making in the NHS: lessons from the MAGIC programme. *BMJ*. 2017;357:j1744.

27. Spies CD, Schulz CM, Weiss-Gerlach E, et al. Preferences for shared decision making in chronic pain patients compared with patients during a premedication visit. *Acta Anaesthesiol Scand*. 2006;50:1019–1026.

28. Flierler WJ, Nubling M, Kasper J, Heidegger T. Implementation of shared decision making in anaesthesia and its influence on patient satisfaction. *Anaesthesia*. 2013;68:713–722.

29. Prabhu M, McQuaid-Hanson E, Hopp S, et al. A shared decision-making intervention to guide opioid prescribing after cesarean delivery. *Obstet Gynecol*. 2017;130:42–46.

30. Shay LA, Lafata JE. Where is the evidence? A systematic review of shared decision making and patient outcomes. *Med Decis Making*. 2015;35:114–131.

31. Michie S, Miles J, Weinman J. Patient-centredness in chronic illness: what is it and does it matter? *Patient Educ Couns*. 2003;51:197–206.

32. Stewart MA. Effective physician-patient communication and health outcomes: a review. *CMAJ*. 1995;152:1423–1433.

33. Hulka BS, Kupper LL, Cassel JC, Mayo F. Doctor-patient communication and outcomes among diabetic patients. *J Community Health*. 1975;1:15–27.

34. Wissow LS, Roter D, Bauman LJ, et al. Patient-provider communication during the emergency department care of children with asthma. The National Cooperative Inner-City Asthma Study, National Institute of Allergy and Infectious Diseases, NIH, Bethesda, MD. *Med Care*. 1998;36:1439–1450.

35. Bartlett EE, Grayson M, Barker R, et al. The effects of physician communications skills on patient satisfaction; recall, and adherence. *J Chronic Dis*. 1984;37:755–764.

36. Substance Abuse and Mental Health Services Administration (SAMHSA). Concept of trauma and guidance for a trauma-informed approach. 2014. https://store.samhsa.gov/product/samhsas-concept-trauma-and-guidance-trauma-informed-approach/sma14-4884?referer=from_search_result. Accessed 24 July 2024.

37. US Centers for Disease Control and Prevention. 6 guiding principles to a trauma-informed approach. 2018. https://stacks.cdc.gov/view/cdc/56843. Accessed 1 June 2025.

38. Vogel TM, Coffin E. Trauma-informed care on labor and delivery. *Anesthesiol Clin*. 2021;39:779–791.

39. Singh MM, Parsekar SS, Nair SN. An epidemiological overview of child sexual abuse. *J Family Med Prim Care*. 2014;3:430–435.

40. Seng JS, Sperlich M, Low LK, et al. Childhood abuse history, posttraumatic stress disorder, postpartum mental health, and bonding: a prospective cohort study. *J Midwifery Womens Health*. 2013;58:57–68.

41. Felitti VJ, Anda RF, Nordenberg D, et al. Relationship of childhood abuse and household dysfunction to many of the leading causes of death in adults. The Adverse Childhood Experiences (ACE) study. *Am J Prev Med*. 1998;14:245–258.

42. Sadler AG, Mengeling MA, Syrop CH, et al. Lifetime sexual assault and cervical cytologic abnormalities among military women. *J Womens Health (Larchmt)*. 2011;20:1693–1701.

43. Centers for Disease Control and Prevention (CDC). Fast Facts: Preventing Intimate Partner Violence. Centers for Disease Control and Prevention (CDC); 2024. https://www.cdc.gov/intimate-partner-violence/about/?CDC_AAref_Val=https://www.cdc.gov/violenceprevention/intimatepartnerviolence/fastfact.html. Accessed 24 July 2024.

44. Millar HC, Lorber S, Vandermorris A, et al. "No, you need to explain what you are doing": obstetric care experiences and preferences of adolescent mothers with a history of childhood trauma. *J Pediatr Adolesc Gynecol*. 2021;34:538–545.

45. Vogel TM, Homitsky S. Antepartum and intrapartum risk factors and the impact of PTSD on mother and child. *BJA Educ*. 2020;20:89–95.

46. de Graaff LF, Honig A, van Pampus MG, Stramrood CAI. Preventing post-traumatic stress disorder following childbirth and traumatic birth experiences: a systematic review. *Acta Obstet Gynecol Scand*. 2018;97:648–656.

47. Ayers S, Bond R, Bertullies S, Wijma K. The aetiology of post-traumatic stress following childbirth: a meta-analysis and theoretical framework. *Psychol Med*. 2016;46:1121–1134.

48. Andersen LB, Melvaer LB, Videbech P, et al. Risk factors for developing post-traumatic stress disorder following childbirth: a systematic review. *Acta Obstet Gynecol Scand*. 2012;91:1261–1272.

49. Soet JE, Brack GA, DiIorio C. Prevalence and predictors of women's experience of psychological trauma during childbirth. *Birth*. 2003;30:36–46.

50. Lopez U, Meyer M, Loures V, et al. Post-traumatic stress disorder in parturients delivering by caesarean section and the implication of anaesthesia: a prospective cohort study. *Health Qual Life Outcomes*. 2017;15:118.

51. Dekel S, Stuebe C, Dishy G. Childbirth induced posttraumatic stress syndrome: a systematic review of prevalence and risk factors. *Front Psychol*. 2017;8:560.

52. American College of Obstetricians and Gynecologists. Committee Opinion Summary, No. 825. Caring for patients who have experienced trauma (reaffirmed 2024). *Obstet Gynecol*. 2021;137:757–758.

53. Simpkin P, Klaus P. *When Survivors Give Birth*. Classic Day Publishing; 2004.

54. Herman JL. *Trauma and Recovery*. 2015 ed. BasicBooks; 2015.

55. Van der Kolk BA, McFarlane AC, Weisæth L. *Traumatic Stress: The Effects of Overwhelming Experience on Mind, Body, and Society*. 1st ed. Guilford Press; 2007.

56. Hellou R, Hauser W, Brenner I, et al. Self-reported childhood maltreatment and traumatic events among Israeli patients suffering from fibromyalgia and rheumatoid arthritis. *Pain Res Manag*. 2017;2017:3865249.

57. Gerber MR, Bogdan KM, Haskell SG, Scioli ER. Experience of childhood abuse and military sexual trauma among women veterans with fibromyalgia. *J Gen Intern Med*. 2018;33:2030–2031.

58. Tietjen GE, Peterlin BL. Childhood abuse and migraine: epidemiology, sex differences, and potential mechanisms. *Headache*. 2011;51:869–879.

59. McKernan LC, Johnson BN, Reynolds WS, et al. Posttraumatic stress disorder in interstitial cystitis/bladder pain syndrome: relationship to patient phenotype and clinical practice implications. *Neurourol Urodyn*. 2019;38:353–362.

60. Centre for Early Childhood Development. Trauma informed care in the perinatal period. https://www.england.nhs.uk/publication/a-good-practice-guide-to-support-implementation-of-trauma-informed-care-in-the-perinatal-period/. Accessed 18 February 2025.

61. Baas MAM, van Pampus MG, Braam L, et al. The effects of PTSD treatment during pregnancy: systematic review and case study. *Eur J Psychotraumatol*. 2020;11:1762310.

62. *See* generally 21 C.F.R. §§ 50.20-50.27 (1999); Norwood Hosp. v. Munoz, 409 Mass. 116 1991.

63. *See* Mass. Ann. Laws ch. 111, § 70E. See generally Civil Rights Act of 1964, Title VI, 42 U.S.C. § 2000D et seq. (prohibiting discrimination on the basis of race, color or national origin in any program or activity that receives Federal funds or other Federal financial assistance); Exec. Order No. 13166, 65 Fed. Reg. 50121 (Aug. 16, 2000) (improving access to services for persons with limited English proficiency).

64. *See* 42 C.F.R. §§ 483.10(b)(4), (b)(7) (2016); Superintendent of Belchertown State Sch. v. Saikewicz, 370 N.E.2d 417, 430 (Mass. 1977). 2016.

65. See Minn. Stat. Ann. § 144.651 (requiring that all conditions and circumstances must be documented within the medical record).

66. Howe E. Ethical aspects of evaluating a patient's mental capacity. *Psychiatry (Edgmont)*. 2009;6:15–23.

67. *See* Mass. Ann. Laws ch. 201D, §§ 6, 17 (LexisNexis 1990).

68. Berg JW, Appelbaum PS, Lidz CW, Parker L. *Informed Consent: Legal Theory and Clinical Practice*. 2nd ed. Oxford University Press; 2001.

69. *See, e.g.,* Mass. Ann. Laws ch. 201D, § 5-306A (LexisNexis 2012); Fla. Stat. Ann. § 765.205(1)(b) (LexisNexis 2015); Guardianship of L.H., 3 N.E.3d 92, 102 (Mass. App. Ct. 2014). See generally Lisa M. Cukier et al., Substituted Judgment and Extraordinary Treatment, Massachusetts guardianship and conservatorship under the MCLE § 7.2 (2017).

70. *See* Mass. Ann. Laws ch. 190B, § 5-106 (LexisNexis 2008).

71. *See* Mass. Ann. Laws ch. 201D, §§ 6, 17 (LexisNexis 1990).

72. *See, e.g.,* N.Y. Pub. Health Law § 2994-d (Consol. 2010); 20 Pa. Stat. and Cons. Stat. Ann. § 5461 (LexisNexis 2006); W. Va.Code Ann. § 16-30-9 (LexisNexis 2000).

73. *See, e.g.,* Mass. Ann. Laws ch. 190B, § 5-311; Cruzan v. Dir., Mo. Dep't of Health, 497 U.S. 261, 325 (1990).

74. *See, e.g.,* Mass. Ann. Laws ch. 190B, § 5-311 (LexisNexis 2008); Cruzan v. Dir., Mo. Dept of Health, 497 U.S. 261, 325 (1990).

75. *See* Superintendent of Belchertown State Sch. v. Saikewicz, 370 N.E.2d 417, 432-33 (Mass. 1977). See also Guardianship of L.H., 3 N.E.3d at 101. 1977.

76. Toledo P, Pumarino J, Grobman WA, et al. Patients' preferences for labor analgesic counseling: a qualitative analysis. *Birth*. 2017;44:345–351.

77. Schleiter KE. Difficult patient-physician relationships and the risk of medical malpractice litigation. *Virtual Mentor*. 2009;11:242–246.

78. Toledo P, Sun J, Peralta F, et al. A qualitative analysis of parturients' perspectives on neuraxial labor analgesia. *Int J Obstet Anesth*. 2013;22:119–123.

79. Gerancher JC, Grice SC, Dewan DM, Eisenach J. An evaluation of informed consent prior to epidural analgesia for labor and delivery. *Int J Obstet Anesth*. 2000;9:168–173.

80. Clark SK, Leighton BL, Seltzer JL. A risk-specific anesthesia consent form may hinder the informed consent process. *J Clin Anesth*. 1991;3:11–13.

81. Ingelfinger FJ. Informed (but uneducated) consent. *N Engl J Med*. 1972;287:465–466.

82. Almand AI. A mother's worst nightmare, what's left unsaid: the lack of informed consent in obstetrical practices. *Wm & Mary J Women & L.* 2012;18:565.

83. Morogiello J, Murray NG, Hunt TN, et al. The effect of acute pain on executive function. *J Clin Transl Res.* 2019;4:113–121.

84. Pattee C, Ballantyne M, Milne B. Epidural analgesia for labour and delivery: informed consent issues. *Can J Anaesth.* 1997;44:918–923.

85. Siddiqui M, Siddiqui S, Ranasinghe S, et al. Does labor pain and labor epidural analgesia impair decision capabilities of parturients. *Int J Anesthesiol.* 2005;10:1–7.

86. *See* Bankert v. United States, 937 F. Supp. 1169, 1174 (D. Md. 1996) 1996.

87. Ghia N, Spong CY, Starbuck VN, et al. Magnesium sulfate therapy affects attention and working memory in patients undergoing preterm labor. *Am J Obstet Gynecol.* 2000;183:940–944.

88. Frölich MA, Burchfield DJ, Euliano TY, Caton D. A single dose of fentanyl and midazolam prior to Cesarean section have no adverse neonatal effects. *Can J Anaesth.* 2006;53:79–85.

89. *See* Rizzo v. Schiller, 445 S.E.2d 153, 155 (Va. 1994) (finding the plaintiff was capable of making medical decisions even after being medicated with delivery drugs) 1994.

90. Simkin P. Birth plans: after 25 years, women still want to be heard. *Birth.* 2007;34:49–51.

91. Simkin P, Reinke C. *Planning Your Baby's Birth.* International Childbirth Education Association; 1980.

92. Kaufman T. Evolution of the birth plan. *J Perinat Educ.* 2007;16:47–52.

93. Afshar Y, Mei JY, Gregory KD, et al. Birth plans-Impact on mode of delivery, obstetrical interventions, and birth experience satisfaction: a prospective cohort study. *Birth.* 2018;45:43–49.

94. Adler NE, Snibbe AC. The role of psychosocial processes in explaining the gradient between socioeconomic status and health. *Curr Dir Psychol Sci.* 2003;12:119–123.

95. Christensen-Szalanski JJ. Discount functions and the measurement of patients' values. Women's decisions during childbirth. *Med Decis Making.* 1984;4:47–58.

96. *See* Canterbury v. Spence, 464 F.2d 772, 788-89 (D.C. Cir. 1972); Restatement (Second) of Torts: Privileges § 890 (Am. Law Inst. 1979); Restatement (Second) of Torts: Emergency Action Without Consent § 892D (Am. Law Inst. 1979) 1979.

97. *See* S.D. Codified Laws § 34-12D-3 (2007); Ky. Rev. Stat. Ann. § 311.625 (LexisNexis 2013).

98. *See* Bellotti v. Baird, 443 U.S. 622, 635 (1979) ("[D]uring the formative years of childhood and adolescence, minors often lack the experience, perspective, and judgment to recognize and avoid choices that could be detrimental to them") 1979.

99. *See* Mass. Ann. Laws ch. 112 § 12F (LexisNexis 1975); Bellotti, 443 U.S. at 635.

100. *See*, e.g., Mass. Ann. Laws ch. 112, § 12F (LexisNexis 1975); Cal. Fam. Code § 6925 (Deering 1996); Md. Code Ann., Health-General § 20-102 (LexisNexis 2017).

101. Guttmacher Institute. Minors' access to prenatal care. 2023. https://www.guttmacher.org/state-policy/explore/minors-access-prenatal-care. Accessed 29 July 2024.

102. *See*, e.g., In re E.G., 549 N.E.2d 322 (Ill. 1989); Bellotti v. Baird, 443 U.S. 622 (1979) 1979.

103. *See*, e.g., Ala. Code § 22-8-4 (LexisNexis 2017); Nev. Rev. Stat. Ann. § 129.030 (LexisNexis 2013); S.C. Code Ann. § 63-5-350 (2008).

104. Will JF. My God my choice: the mature minor doctrine and adolescent refusal of life-saving or sustaining medical treatment based upon religious beliefs. *J Contemp Health Law Policy.* 2006;22:233–300.

105. *See* N.Y. Pub. Health Law § 18(3)(c) (Consol. 2017) 2017.

106. *See* 45 C.F.R. § 164.502(g) (2013) 2013.

107. *See*, e.g., Fla. Stat. Ann. § 743.065 (LexisNexis 1999); Ala. Code § 22-8-6 (LexisNexis 2017).

108. Guttmacher Institute. Minors' Access to Contraceptive Services. Guttmacher Institute; 2023. https://www.guttmacher.org/state-policy/explore/minors-access-contraceptive-services#:~:text=24%20states%20explicitly%20permit%20minors,not%20provided%20with%20contraceptive%20services. Accessed 24 July 2024.

109. American College of Obstetricians and Gynecologists. Committee Opinion No. 710: Counseling adolescents about contraception (reaffirmed 2021). *Obstet Gynecol.* 2017;130:e74–e80.

110. *See*, e.g., Mass. Ann. Laws ch. 112, § 12F (LexisNexis 1975); N.C. Gen. Stat. § 90-21.5 (2009).

111. Guttmacher Institute. Parental involvement in minors' abortions. 2023. https://www.guttmacher.org/state-policy/explore/parental-involvement-minors-abortions. Accessed 24 July 2024.

112. Dobbs v. Jackson Women's Health Organization, 597 U.S. 215 (2022).

113. Pew Research Center. Births outside of marriage decline for immigrant women. 2016. https://www.pewresearch.org/social-trends/2016/10/26/births-outside-of-marriage-decline-for-immigrant-women/. Accessed 24 July 2024.

114. Pew Research Center. Key findings about U.S. immigrants. 2020. https://www.pewresearch.org/short-reads/2020/08/20/key-findings-about-u-s-immigrants/. Accessed 24 July 2024.

115. Bollini P, Pampallona S, Wanner P, Kupelnick B. Pregnancy outcome of migrant women and integration policy: a systematic review of the international literature. *Soc Sci Med.* 2009;68:452–461.

116. Hayes I, Enohumah K, McCaul C. Care of the migrant obstetric population. *Int J Obstet Anesth.* 2011;20:321–329.

117. Cantwell R, Clutton-Brock T, Cooper G, et al. Saving Mothers' Lives: reviewing maternal deaths to make motherhood safer: 2006-2008. The Eighth Report of the Confidential Enquiries into Maternal Deaths in the United Kingdom. *BJOG.* 2011;118(suppl 1):1–203.

118. Gerrish K, Chau R, Sobowale A, Birks E. Bridging the language barrier: the use of interpreters in primary care nursing. *Health Soc Care Community.* 2004;12:407–413.

119. Woloshin S, Bickell NA, Schwartz LM, et al. Language barriers in medicine in the United States. *JAMA.* 1995;273:724–728.

120. Parker RM, Baker DW, Williams MV, Nurss JR. The test of functional health literacy in adults: a new instrument for measuring patients' literacy skills. *J Gen Intern Med.* 1995;10:537–541.

121. Brice JH, Travers D, Cowden CS, et al. Health literacy among Spanish-speaking patients in the emergency department. *J Natl Med Assoc.* 2008;100:1326–1332.

122. Nielsen-Bohlman L, Panzer AM, Kindig DA. *Health Literacy: A Prescription to End Confusion. Institute of Medicine Committee on Health Literacy.* National Academies Press; 2004.

123. Kutner M, Greenberg E, Jin Y, Paulsen C. *The Health Literacy of America's Adults: Results From the 2003 National Assessment of Adult Literacy.* U. S. Department of Education, National Center for Education Statistics; 2006. https://nces.ed.gov/pubsearch/pubsinfo.asp?pubid=2006483. Accessed 24 July 2024.

124. U.S. Department of Education National Center for Education Statistics. National Assessment of Adult Literacy: Key Findings. U.S. Department of Education, National Center for Education Statistics; 2003. https://nces.ed.gov/naal/kf_demographics.asp. Accessed 29 July 2024.

125. Lopez C, Bumyang K, Sacks K. *Health Literacy in the United States: Enhancing Assessments and Reducing Disparities.* Milken Institute; 2022. https://milkeninstitute.org/report/health-literacy-us-assessments-disparities. Accessed 24 July 2024.

126. Guerra CE, Krumholz M, Shea JA. Literacy and knowledge, attitudes and behavior about mammography in Latinas. *J Healthcare Poor Underserved.* 2005;16:152–166.

127. Shapeton A, O'Donoghue M, VanderWielen B, Barnett SR. Anesthesia lost in translation: perspective and comprehension. *J Educ Perioper Med.* 2017;19:E505.

128. Govender D, Villafranca A, Hamlin C, et al. Appropriateness of language used in patient educational materials from 24 national anesthesiology associations. *Anesthesiology.* 2016;125:1221–1228.

129. Agency for Healthcare Research and Quality. Health Literacy University Precautions Toolkit, 3rd edition: Communicate clearly: Tool #4. https://www.ahrq.gov/health-literacy/improve/precautions/tool4.html. Accessed 24 July 2024.

130. Courtney MJ. The effect of a preanaesthetic information booklet on patient understanding and satisfaction. *N Z Med J.* 1997;110:212–214.

131. Salzwedel C, Petersen C, Blanc I, et al. The effect of detailed, video-assisted anesthesia risk education on patient anxiety and the duration of the preanesthetic interview: a randomized controlled trial. *Anesth Analg.* 2008;106:202–209.

132. Cowan EA, Calderon Y, Gennis P, et al. Spanish and English video-assisted informed consent for intravenous contrast administration in the emergency department: a randomized controlled trial. *Ann Emerg Med.* 2007;49:221–230, 230.e1–e3.

133. Snyder-Ramos SA, Seintsch H, Bottiger BW, et al. Patient satisfaction and information gain after the preanesthetic visit: a comparison of face-to-face interview, brochure, and video. *Anesth Analg.* 2005;100:1753–1758.

134. West AM, Bittner EA, Ortiz VE. The effects of preoperative, video-assisted anesthesia education in Spanish on Spanish-speaking patients' anxiety, knowledge, and satisfaction: a pilot study. *J Clin Anesth.* 2014;26:325–329.

135. Baxley SM, Ibitayo K. Expectations of pregnant women of Mexican origin regarding their healthcare providers. *J Obstet Gynecol Neonatal Nurs.* 2015;44:389–396.

136. Wojnar DM. Perinatal experiences of Somali couples in the United States. *J Obstet Gynecol Neonatal Nurs.* 2015;44:358–369.

137. Dworkin G. Autonomy and behavior control. *Hastings Cent Rep.* 1976;6:23–28.

138. Scott WE. Anaesthesia and pregnancy. *Ethical Issues in Anaesthesia.* Butterworth-Heinemann Ltd; 1994:73–85.

139. Pope TM. Clinicians may not administer life-sustaining treatment without consent: civil, criminal, and disciplinary sanctions. *J Health Biomed Law.* 2013;9:213.

140. Main E, The California Maternal Quality Care Collaborative (CMQCC). Planning for Women (Jehovah's Witnesses and Others) Who May Decline Blood and Blood Products. The California Maternal Quality Care Collaborative (CMQCC); 2015. https://www.cmqcc.org/resource/3316/download. Accessed 24 July 2024.

141. Jorgenson TD, Golbaba B, Guinn NR, et al. When blood is not an option: the case for a standardized blood transfusion consent form. *ASA Monitor.* 2017;81:48–50.

142. Waters JH, Potter PS. Cell salvage in the Jehovah's Witness patient. *Anesth Analg.* 2000;90:229–230.

143. *See* Commonwealth v. Nixon, 761 A.2d 1151 (Pa. 2000); Jehovah's Witnesses v. King County Hospital, 278 F. Supp. 488 (W.D. Wash. 1967), aff'd. per curiam, 390 U.S. 598 (1968); Prince v. Massachusetts, 321 U.S. 158, 170 (1944) ("Parents may be free to become martyrs themselves. But it does not follow that they are free, in identical circumstances, to make martyrs of their children before they have reached the age of full and legal discretion when they can make that choice for themselves.") Courts generally do not recognize a fetus as a child, even if the fetus is viable. See In re A.C., 573 A.2d 1235 (D.C. 1990); in re Doe 632 N.E.2d 326 (Ill. App. Ct. 1st Dist. 1994), cert. denied, 114 S. Ct. 1198 (1994). See also Planned Parenthood v. Casey, 505 U.S. 833, 860 (1992), for a discussion regarding the viability of a fetus in the context of abortion. 2000.

144. *See* Niebla v. County of San Diego, 1992 U.S. App. LEXIS 15049 (9th Cir. 1992); In re McCauley, 565 N.E.2d 411 (Mass. 1991) 1991.

145. American College of Obstetricians and Gynecologists. Committee Opinion No. 660: Family building through gestational surrogacy (reaffirmed 2019). *Obstet Gynecol.* 2016;127:e97–e013.

146. American College of Obstetricians and Gynecologists. Committee Opinion No. 390: Ethical decision making in obstetrics and gynecology (reaffirmed 2019). *Obstet Gynecol.* 2007;110:1479–1487.

147. *See* Superintendent of Belchertown State Sch. v. Saikewicz, 370 N.E.2d 417, 429 (Mass. 1977). See also Mass. Ann. Laws ch. 201D, § 5 (LexisNexis 1990); Vt. Stat. Ann tit. 18, § 9702 (2005); Tenn. Code Ann. § 68-11-1803 (2014) 1977.

148. Neale H. Mother's rights prevail: In re A.C. and the status of forced obstetrical intervention in the District of Columbia. *J Health Hosp Law.* 1990;23:208–213.

149. Mishkin DB, Povar GJ. Decision making with pregnant patients: a policy born of experience. *Jt Comm J Qual Improv.* 1993;19:291–302.

150. *See* In re: A.C., 573 A.2d 1235, 1237 (D.C. App. 1990) 1990.

151. Annas GJ. Protecting the liberty of pregnant patients. *N Engl J Med.* 1987;316:1213–1214.

152. Minkoff H, Paltrow LM. Melissa Rowland and the rights of pregnant women. *Obstet Gynecol.* 2004;104:1234–1236.

153. Drug Policy Alliance Network. South Carolina Supreme Court Reverses 20-year Homicide Conviction of Regina McKnight. Drug Policy Alliance Network; 2008. https://drugpolicy.org/news/south-carolina-supreme-court-reverses-20-year-homicide-conviction-regina-mcknight/. Accessed 24 July 2024.

154. Private Officer Breaking News. New Alabama law that puts some new mothers in jail causing controversy. Private Officer Breaking News; 2008. http://privateofficerbreakingnews.blogspot.com/2008/02/new-alabama-law-that-puts-some-new.html. Accessed 24 July 2024.

155. *See* Ala. Stat. Ann § 26-15-3.2.

156. Bianchi DW, Crombleholme TM, D'Alton ME. *Fetology: Diagnosis and Management of the Fetal Patient.* McGraw-Hill; 2000.

157. McCullough L, Chervenak F. *Ethics in Obstetrics and Gynecology.* Oxford University Press; 1994.

158. American College of Obstetricians and Gynecologists. Committee Opinion No. 473: Substance abuse reporting

and pregnancy: the role of the obstetrician-gynecologist (reaffirmed 2022). *Obstet Gynecol.* 2011;117:200–201.

159. American Medical Association. *Treatment versus criminalization—physician role in drug addiction during pregnancy. H-420.970. Reaffirmed: CSAPH Rep. 01, A-20.* American Medical Association; 2020. https://policysearch.ama-assn.org/policyfinder/detail/addiction%20pregnancy?uri=%2FAMADoc%2FHOD.xml-0-3713.xml. Accessed 24 July 2024.

160. American College of Obstetricians and Gynecologists. Committee Opinion No. 214: Patient choice and the maternal-fetal relationship. *Int J Gynaecol Obstet.* 1999;65:213–215.

161. American College of Obstetricians and Gynecologists. Committee Opinion No. 664: Refusal of medically recommended treatment during pregnancy (reaffirmed 2019). *Obstet Gynecol.* 2016;127:e175–e182.

162. Jonsen AR, Siegler M, Winslade WJ. *Clinical Ethics: A Practical Approach to Ethical Decisions in Clinical Medicine.* 3rd ed. McGraw-Hill; 1992.

163. McCullough LB, Chervenak FA, Coverdale JH. Managing care of an intrapartum patient with agitation and psychosis: ethical and legal implications. *AMA J Ethics.* 2016;18:209–214.

164. American College of Obstetricians and Gynecologists. Committee Opinion No. 385: The limits of conscientious refusal in reproductive medicine (reaffirmed 2019). *Obstet Gynecol.* 2007;110:1203–1208.

165. Peters PG. Resuscitating hospital enterprise liability. *Missouri Law Rev.* 2008;73:369.

166. Bal BS. An introduction to medical malpractice in the United States. *Clin Orthop Relat Res.* 2009;467:339–347.

167. *See* Cox v. M.A. Primary & Urgent Care Clinic, 313 S.W.3d 240, 259 (Tenn. 2010); Weymers v. Khera, 563 N.W.2d 647, 655 (Mich. 1997). 1997.

168. Bal BS. The expert witness in medical malpractice litigation. *Clin Orthop Relat Res.* 2009;467:383–391.

169. Munoz VE. University of Texas Medical Branch at Galveston v. York: Information is not tangible personal property for the purpose of waiving sovereign immunity *Baylor L Rev.* 1995;47:265.

170. *See Grossman v. Barke*, 868 A.2d 561, 566-67 (Pa. Super. Ct. 2005). 2005.

171. Wait CF. The statute of limitations governing medical malpractice claims: rules, problems, and solutions. *S Tex L Rev.* 1999;41:371.

172. *See*, e.g., Mass. Ann. Laws ch. 201D, § 5-306A (LexisNexis 2012); Fla. Stat. Ann. § 765.205(1)(b) (LexisNexis 2015); Guardianship of L.H., 3 N.E.3d 92, 102 (Mass. App. Ct. 2014).

See generally Lisa M. Cukier et al., Substituted Judgment and Extraordinary Treatment, Massachusetts guardianship and conservatorship under the MCLE § 7.2 (2017) [hereinafter, Cukier, Substituted Judgment]. 2015.

173. Statutes of limitation for medical malpractice claims vary by state, but generally span from two to three years. See, e.g., Iowa Code § 614.1(9)(a) (2013) ("[Actions shall be brought] within two years after the date on which the claimant knew, or through the use of reasonable diligence should have known, or received notice in writing of the existence of, the injury or death…."); Cal. Civ. Proc. Code § 340.5 (Deering 1975) ("[T]he time for the commencement of action shall be three years after the date of injury or one year after the plaintiff discovers, or through the use of reasonable diligence should have discovered, the injury, whichever occurs first."); Fla. Stat. Ann. § 95.11(4)(b) ("An action for medical malpractice shall be commenced within 2 years from the time the incident giving rise to the action occurred or within 2 years from the time the incident is discovered, or should have been discovered with the exercise of due diligence.").

174. Cohen JR. The path between Sebastian's hospitals: fostering reconciliation after a tragedy. *Barry L Rev.* 2011;17:89.

175. Robbennolt JK. Apologies and medical error. *Clin Orthop Relat Res.* 2009;467:376–382.

176. *See* CA legislative mandates: Senate Bill ("SB") 739 (2006), SB 1058 (2008), and SB 158 (2008). 2008.

177. ABIM Foundation, ACP-ASIM Foundation, European Federation of Internal Medicine. Medical professionalism in the new millennium: a physician charter. *Ann Intern Med.* 2002;136:243–246.

178. American Medical Association. AMA code of medical ethics. 2024. https://code-medical-ethics.ama-assn.org/. Accessed 24 July 2024.

179. The Joint Commission. *2024 Comprehensive Accreditation Manual.* Joint Commission Resources; 2023:Standard RI.01.02.01.

180. Massachusetts Coalition for the Prevention of Medical Errors. When things go wrong: Responding to adverse events. A consensus statement of the Harvard hospitals. 2006. http://psnet.ahrq.gov/resource.aspx?resourceID=3474. Accessed 24 July 2024.

181. Gold KJ, Kuznia AL, Hayward RA. How physicians cope with stillbirth or neonatal death: a national survey of obstetricians. *Obstet Gynecol.* 2008;112:29–34.

182. Bell SK, Smulowitz PB, Woodward AC, et al. Disclosure, apology, and offer programs: stakeholders' views of barriers to and strategies for broad implementation. *Milbank Q.* 2012;90:682–705.

PART IX

Obstetric Complications

33

Preterm Labor and Delivery

Alyssa L. Trochtenberg, MD and Erika F. Werner, MD

CHAPTER OUTLINE

DEFINITIONS

A preterm infant is defined as one who is born between 20 0/7 and 36 6/7 weeks' gestation. *Early preterm birth* is defined as birth prior to 34 0/7 weeks' gestation, and *late preterm birth* is defined as birth from 34 0/7 to 36 6/7 weeks' gestation. Early preterm births may be further classified as *extremely preterm* in the event of delivery prior to 28 0/7 weeks' gestation. The American College of Obstetricians and Gynecologists (ACOG) has defined *periviable birth* as birth between 20 0/7 and 25 6/7 weeks' gestation.[1] The guidelines for this gestational window are constantly evolving. Currently neonatal resuscitation is not recommended prior to 22 weeks' gestation, and shared decision-making is often used to determine

resuscitation plans from 22 to 24 weeks. During the periviable period, there is a high risk of neonatal mortality with significant risk of both early and long-term morbidity among survivors. Survival and neurocognitive outcomes improve with advancing periviable gestational age, although outcomes remain guarded. Neonatal death occurs in the overwhelming majority (94% to 95%) of neonates born before 23 weeks, and an estimated 1% of these neonates survive without long-term neurodevelopmental impairment. In contrast, 55% of neonates born between 24 0/7 and 24 6/7 weeks' gestation survive, approximately one-third of whom will have no neurodevelopmental disability.[1] Further classification of deliveries based on gestational age is outlined in Table 33.1.

TABLE 33.1 Classification of Deliveries Based on Gestational Age

Classification	Gestational Age
Extremely preterm	<28 w
Late preterm	34 0/7–36 6/7 w
Early term	37 0/7–38 6/7 w
Full term	39 0/7–40 6/7 w
Late term	41 0/7–41 6/7 w
Postterm	≥42 0/7 w and beyond

Definitions from Spong CY. Defining "term" pregnancy: Recommendations from the defining "term" pregnancy workgroup. *JAMA.* 2013;309:2445–2446; American College of Obstetricians and Gynecologists. Committee Opinion No. 579: Definition of term pregnancy (reaffirmed 2025). *Obstet Gynecol.* 2013;122:1139–1140; World Health Organization. *Born Too Soon: Decade of Action on Preterm Birth.* World Health Organization; 2023. https://www.who.int/publications/i/item/9789240073890. Accessed 26 July 2024.

Preterm birth may be classified as either spontaneous or medically indicated. Spontaneous preterm birth occurs following preterm labor, preterm premature rupture of membranes (PPROM), or painless cervical dilation (cervical insufficiency). Medically indicated, provider-initiated preterm birth occurs following induction of labor or cesarean delivery necessitated by maternal or fetal pregnancy complications (Table 33.2).

EPIDEMIOLOGY

The incidence of preterm birth has increased significantly over the past two generations, notably increasing by 25% from 1981 to 2005.[2] Following a transient 1% decline in the US preterm birth rate between 2019 and 2020, the preterm birth rate further rose 4% in 2021 to 10.5% (Fig. 33.1).[3] These increases are driven largely by growing rates of late preterm deliveries, which comprise roughly 70% of preterm births. There are striking racial, ethnic, and economic disparities in the frequency of preterm birth in the United States. In 2021,

TABLE 33.2 Common Medical Indications for Preterm Delivery

Medical Condition	Recommended Gestational Age at Delivery (Weeks' Gestation)
Obstetric Conditions	
Preterm premature rupture of membranes	34 0/7–36 6/7
Maternal Conditions	
Intrahepatic cholestasis of pregnancy (with bile acids > 100 µmol/L)	36 0/7, or at time of diagnosis if later
Chronic hypertension, poorly controlled	36 0/7–37 6/7
Pregestational diabetes, poorly controlled or with vascular complications	36 0/7–38 6/7
Preeclampsia with severe features	34 0/7, or at time of diagnosis if later
HELLP syndrome/preeclampsia with severe features with contraindications to expectant management[a]	At time of diagnosis following maternal stabilization
Fetal Growth Restriction (Singleton) With Abnormal Umbilical Artery Doppler Measurements	
Absent end-diastolic flow	33 0/7–34 0/7, or at time of diagnosis if later
Reversed end-diastolic flow	30 0/7–32 0/7, or at time of diagnosis if later
Multifetal Gestation	
Monochorionic-diamniotic twins, uncomplicated	34 0/7–37 6/7
Monochorionic-monoamniotic twins, uncomplicated	32 0/7–34 0/7
Dichorionic-diamniotic twins, complicated by fetal growth restriction	36 0/7–37 6/7
Monochorionic-diamniotic twins, complicated by fetal growth restriction	32 0/7–34 6/7
Placental Conditions	
Placenta accreta spectrum	34 0/7–35 6/7
Vasa previa	34 0/7–37 0/7
Placenta previa	36 0/7–37 0/7
History of classical cesarean	36 0/7–37 0/7

[a]Contraindications to expectant management of preeclampsia with severe features include eclamptic seizure, persistent severe headache, visual disturbances, severe right upper quadrant pain, pulmonary edema, elevated liver function tests to greater than or equal to twice the upper limit of normal, creatinine > 1.1 mg/dL or greater than or equal to twice the patient's known baseline creatinine, platelet count < 150,000/µL. Modified from American College of Obstetricians and Gynecologists. Committee Opinion No. 831: Medically indicated late-preterm and early-term deliveries. *Obstet Gynecol.* 2021;138:e35–e39.

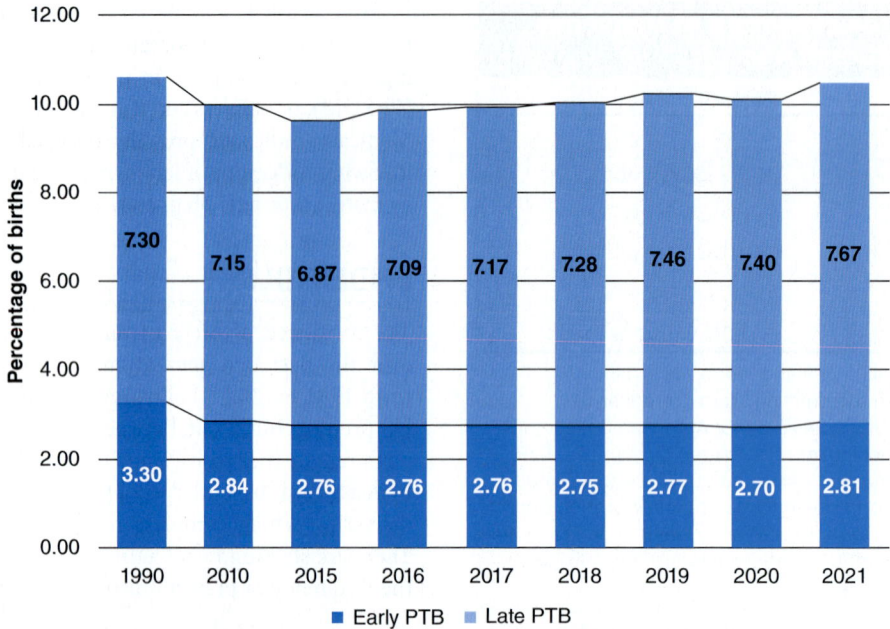

Fig. 33.1 Total, Early, and Late Preterm Birth Rates: United States, 1990 and 2010–21. Preterm birth is defined as less than 37 weeks' completed gestation. Early preterm birth is defined as less than 34 weeks' completed gestation. Late preterm birth is defined as 34–36 weeks' completed gestation. *Early PTB*, Early preterm birth; *Late PTB*, late preterm birth. Data from Martin JA, Hamilton BE, Ventura SJ, et al. Births: final data for 2000. *Natl Vital Stat Rep.* 2002;50:1–101; Martin JA, Hamilton BE, Ventura SJ, et al. Births: final data for 2010. *Natl Vital Stat Rep.* 2012;61: 1–72; Osterman MJK, Hamilton BE, Martin JA, et al. Births: final data for 2021. *Natl Vital Stat Rep.* 2023;72:1–53.

9.5% of non-Hispanic White, 10.2% of Hispanic, and 14.8% of non-Hispanic Black patients delivered preterm.[4]

The World Health Organization (WHO) and other non-governmental organizations have identified the frequency of preterm birth as a critical global health issue (see Chapter 15). The global preterm birth rate in 2020 was 9.9%, amounting to 13.4 million preterm births worldwide, with 900,000 newborn deaths due to complications of prematurity. The majority of preterm births occur in low- and middle-income nations with the highest rates in sub-Saharan Africa and South Asia.[5] The global neonatal mortality rate is 19 per 1000 live births, and significant economic disparity exists in the neonatal mortality rate of infants born preterm. In higher-income countries in Northern America, Europe, Australia, and New Zealand, only 3% of preterm births in 2020 resulted in neonatal death, in contrast to a preterm neonatal death rate of 11% in sub-Saharan Africa.[5]

COMPLICATIONS OF PREMATURITY

Neonatal Morbidity

Prematurity affects multiple organ systems, resulting in both immediate neonatal and sometimes lifelong adverse health sequelae. Though some infants born late preterm do not require intensive care, the majority of preterm infants require admission to the neonatal intensive care unit (NICU) for management of prematurity. The earlier the gestational age at delivery, the longer the anticipated duration of NICU admission. The economic costs for the care of surviving preterm infants (especially very low-birthweight infants) can be enormous, and the annual US healthcare costs of medical care for preterm infants are estimated at approximately $25 billion.[6]

Respiratory immaturity is a common complication of prematurity, with risk of respiratory distress syndrome,

bronchopulmonary dysplasia, apneic episodes, and need for mechanical ventilation. Smaller brain volume, immaturity of neurologic structures, and altered sensory experiences related to NICU admission may have profound neurodevelopmental consequences in preterm infants, including cerebral palsy, intraventricular hemorrhage, retinopathy of prematurity, hearing impairment, and delayed motor and speech development. Additional neonatal sequelae of prematurity include feeding immaturity, hypoglycemia, hyperbilirubinemia, anemia, thrombocytopenia, persistent patent ductus arteriosus, pulmonary hypertension of the newborn, necrotizing enterocolitis, and heightened risk of sepsis.

The risks for severe morbidity and mortality decrease with advancing gestational age at delivery. For example, the incidence of high-grade (III or IV) intraventricular hemorrhage diminishes rapidly after 27 weeks' gestation, rarely occuring after 32 weeks' gestation. Likewise, neonatal morbidity from patent ductus arteriosus and necrotizing enterocolitis diminishes significantly after 32 weeks' gestation.[7] Lower birthweight, which is often a function of earlier gestational age at delivery, has additionally been associated with more severe neonatal morbidity. Data from the National Institute of Child Health and Development (NICHD) Neonatal Research Network sites from 1997 to 2002 indicate that survival without complications (e.g., bronchopulmonary dysplasia, severe intraventricular hemorrhage, necrotizing enterocolitis, or a combination of these disorders) ranged from 20% for infants with a birth weight of 501 to 750 g to 89% for those with a birth weight of 1251 to 1500 g.[8]

Neonatal Mortality

The survival rate among neonates increases as the birth weight and gestational age at delivery increase (Fig. 33.2; Table 33.3).[9] Excess mortality risk for infants born preterm is concentrated

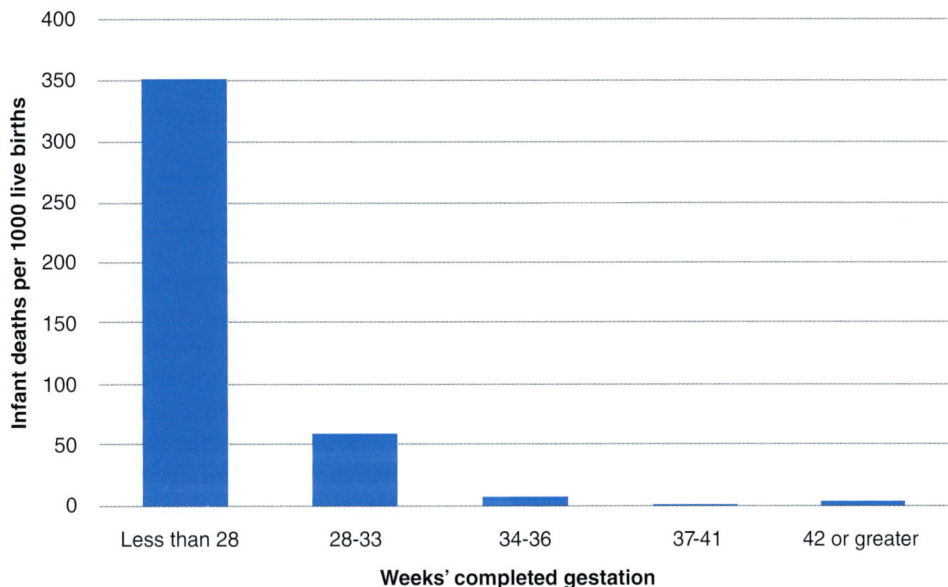

Fig. 33.2 Infant Mortality Rates by Gestational Age—United States, 2021. Data from Osterman MJK, Hamilton BE, Martin JA, et al. Births: final data for 2021. *Natl Vital Stat Rep.* 2023;72:1–53.

TABLE 33.3 Neonatal Deaths by Gestational Age

Completed Weeks' Gestation	Percentage of Deaths Prior to Hospital Discharge	
	2008–12[a]	2013–18[b]
22	93	89
23	68	51
24	38	30
25	23	21
26	15	12
27	10	11
28	6	6

[a]Data from Stoll BJ, Hansen N, Bell EF, et al. Trends in care practices, morbidity, and mortality of extremely preterm neonates, 1993–2012. *JAMA.* 2015;314:1039–1051.
[b]Data from Bell EF, Hintz SR, Hansen NI, et al.; Eunice Kennedy Shriver National Institute of Child Health and Human Development Neonatal Research Network. Mortality, in-hospital morbidity, care practices, and 2-year outcomes for extremely preterm infants in the US, 2013–2018. *JAMA.* 2022;327:248–263.
Impact of gestational age at birth on neonatal mortality rate over time among extremely preterm infants born at Neonatal Research Network centers.

TABLE 33.4 Selected Outcomes for Extremely Preterm Infants[a]

Outcome	Percent
Maternal corticosteroid administration	64
Maternal antibiotic administration	66
Cesarean delivery	38
Male gender	52
Multiple birth	27
Surfactant therapy after birth	66
Death before discharge	64
Survival without neurodevelopmental impairment[b]	20
Survival without neurosensory impairment[c]	29

[a]Gestational age between 22 and 24 weeks' gestation, born from 2008 to 2011.
[b]Neurodevelopmental impairment defined as at least one of the following conditions: moderate or severe cerebral palsy, Gross Motor Function Classification System ≥ level 2, profound hearing loss requiring amplification in both ears, profound visual impairment with visual acuity of less than 20/200 in both eyes, or cognitive impairment.
[c]Neurosensory impairment defined as moderate or severe cerebral palsy, Gross Motor Function Classification System ≥ level 2, profound hearing loss, or profound visual impairment.
Total *N* = 1348.
Data from Younge N, Goldstein RF, Bann CM, et al. Survival and neurodevelopmental outcomes among periviable infants. *N Engl J Med.* 2017;376:617–628.

in the first year of life.[10] After data are controlled for gestational age and weight, male infants have a higher mortality risk than female infants.[11] During the past three decades, there has been a significant improvement in the survival rate for preterm infants, with the greatest improvement occurring in the subgroup with a birth weight between 501 and 1250 g.[12] The rate of neonatal survival is now approximately 94% for extremely preterm infants born at 28 weeks' gestation.[9]

Infants born at the threshold of viability (22 to 24 weeks' gestation) continue to have the greatest risk for poor outcomes.[1] A retrospective cohort study assessed survival rates for infants delivered between 22 and 28 weeks' gestation from 1993 to

2012.[9] Neonatal survival was 9% at 22 weeks; 33% at 23 weeks; and then 65%, 81%, and 87% at 24, 25, and 26 weeks' gestation, respectively.[9] Another retrospective study examined trends in neonatal mortality outcomes for infants born between 22 and 24 weeks' gestation from 2000 to 2011 (Table 33.4).[13] While the overall mortality rate decreased over the study period, the mortality rate did not improve for 22-week infants. As expected, the greatest decrease in mortality was seen in the 24-week group (55% from 2000 to 2003 to 18% from 2008 to 2011).[13]

Long-Term Health Outcomes

Preterm birth is associated with multiple long-term adverse neurodevelopmental outcomes, including cerebral palsy, motor delay, cognitive impairment, speech delay, and learning disabilities. Neuropsychiatric disorders are also more prevalent among children born preterm, particularly attention-deficit hyperactivity disorder and autism spectrum disorder. As with neonatal morbidity, the risk of persistent disability increases with earlier gestational age at delivery.

The EPIPAGE cohort, a large population-based cohort study of infants born between 22 and 32 weeks' gestation in France in 1997, showed that at 2 years of age, 20% of children born between 24 and 26 weeks' gestation had cerebral palsy compared with only 4% of children born at 32 weeks' gestation.[14] While persistent disability is certainly more common among children born extremely preterm, developmental outcomes have improved over time with advancements in newborn medicine. The EPICure study group assessed the association between extreme preterm delivery and long-term physical and mental disability in a cohort of infants delivered between 22 and 25 weeks' gestation during a 10-month period in 1995.[15] These investigators noted rates of severe disability of 54%, 52%, and 45% among surviving infants delivered at 23, 24, and 25 weeks' gestation, respectively. A 6-year follow-up to the EPICure study cohort reported persistent severe disability in 25%, 29%, and 18% of infants born at 23, 24, and 25 weeks' gestation, respectively.[16] In a later cohort of preterm infants born between 1997 and 2002, improvement was noted in the rates of severe disability, which were 33%, 21%, and 12% for infants delivered at 23, 24, and 25 weeks' gestation, respectively.[17]

Researchers have additionally examined the association between late preterm birth and neurocognitive performance in late adulthood; 919 Finnish men and women born preterm were evaluated at a mean age of 68.2 years.[18] When controlling for confounders, those who were born between 34 and 37 weeks' gestation had lower scores on tests evaluating neurocognitive performance than those born after 37 weeks' gestation.[18]

PHYSIOLOGY OF PRETERM BIRTH

The process of normal parturition involves anatomic, physiologic, and biochemical changes that lead to (1) greater uterine contractility, (2) cervical ripening, and (3) membrane/decidual activation.[19] The fetus also appears to play a role in parturition. It is hypothesized that the mature fetal hypothalamus secretes more corticotropin-releasing hormone (CRH), which in turn stimulates fetal adrenal production of adrenocorticotropic hormone and cortisol.[19] Preterm labor results from the pathologic activation of one or more of these components (Fig. 33.3). Preterm delivery results from (1) PPROM in approximately 25% of cases, (2) spontaneous preterm labor in approximately 45% of cases, and (3) maternal or fetal indications for early delivery in approximately 30% of cases (Fig. 33.4).[2,20] However, the "spontaneous" causes do not have a uniform underlying pathophysiology, and it appears that preterm labor is a syndrome with multiple causes influenced by a number of genetic, biologic, biophysical, psychosocial, and environmental factors (Fig. 33.5).

Two factors of interest are the influences of infection and uterine distention on initiation of myometrial contractility. Infection is thought to be present in up to 40% of preterm deliveries.[2] Commonly identified organisms include *Ureaplasma urealyticum*, *Bacteroides* species, *Neisseria gonorrhoeae*, *Chlamydia trachomatis*, group B streptococci, *Staphylococcus aureus*, *Treponema pallidum*, and enteropharyngeal bacteria.[21-23]

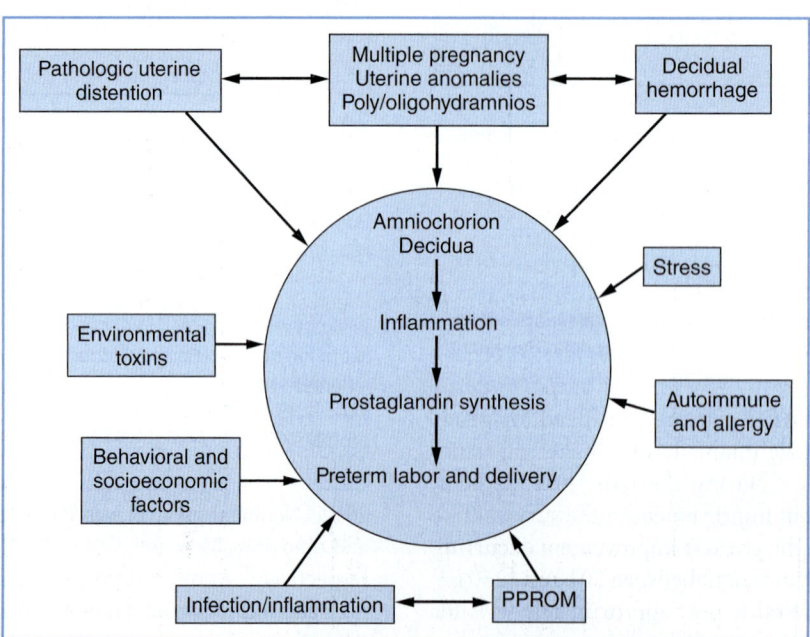

Fig. 33.3 **Major Etiologic Factors in Preterm Birth.** Pathways include activation of the maternal or fetal hypothalamic-pituitary axis (stress), inflammation, decidual hemorrhage, and pathologic distension of the myometrium. The pathways are not mutually exclusive and may overlap, and they share a common biochemical pathway. *PPROM*, Preterm premature rupture of membranes. From Menon R. Spontaneous preterm birth, a clinical dilemma: etiologic, pathophysiologic and genetic heterogeneities and racial disparity. *Acta Obstet Gynecol Scand.* 2008;87:590–600.

Although approximately 50% of preterm deliveries occur in women with no apparent risk factors, subclinical infection may precipitate preterm labor in some of these cases.[22]

Myometrial smooth muscle consists of thick (myosin) and thin (actin) filaments that slide past one another and thereby lead to the contractile force of uterine contractions. The myometrium also has pacemaker cells; electrical activity is spread by gap junctions between myometrial cells. A rise in intracellular calcium concentration from influx across the sarcolemma and/or release from internal calcium stores leads to contractions. Hormones and neurotransmitters also may regulate uterine activity through agonist-induced entry of calcium or other ions by means of receptor-controlled channels and the release of internally stored calcium.[24] Calcium binds to calmodulin, which then activates myosin light-chain kinase (MLCK), leading to phosphorylation of the light-chain subunit of myosin. This phosphorylation allows actin to bind to myosin, with the subsequent activation of myosin adenosine triphosphatase. Adenosine triphosphate (ATP) is then hydrolyzed, and muscle shortening or contraction results. Increases in intracellular cyclic adenosine monophosphate (cAMP) cause muscle relaxation by (1) activation of a cAMP-dependent protein kinase, which decreases the activity of MLCK and (2) a reduction of the intracellular calcium concentration.[24]

The actual signals for the onset of contractions and labor, however, are complex and incompletely understood. Before labor, the uterus is in a state of functional quiescence due to various inhibitors, including progesterone, prostacyclin, relaxin, nitric oxide, parathyroid hormone–related peptide, CRH, human placental lactogen, calcitonin gene–related peptide, adrenomedullin, and vasoactive intestinal peptide (Fig. 33.5). Before term, the uterus goes through an activation phase characterized by (1) greater expression of a series of contraction-associated proteins (including myometrial receptors for prostaglandins and oxytocin), (2) activation of certain ion channels, and (3) an increase in connexin-43 concentration. Expression of the oxytocin receptor in the human myometrium is tightly regulated during pregnancy. Its levels increase during gestation, with a relative paucity of receptors in mid-gestation, accumulation in the third trimester, and peak at labor onset. The receptor levels fall sharply in advanced labor and the postpartum period.[25]

There is evidence, albeit from animal models, that the fetus may contribute to changes in uterine activity through (1) its influence on the production of placental steroid hormones, (2) mechanical distention of the uterus, and (3) secretion of neurohypophyseal hormones and other stimulators of prostaglandin synthesis. The final common pathway for labor is thought to be activation of the fetal hypothalamic-pituitary-adrenal axis. Of interest, however, is the observation that spontaneous labor occurs in women even if a fetus is anencephalic (without a functioning pituitary gland), suggesting that intact fetal neurohypophyseal function is not a prerequisite for the onset of human labor.[26]

In recent years, the hormonal control of human parturition has been linked to progesterone signaling. It appears that human parturition may be triggered by a functional progesterone withdrawal, mediated at least in part by changes in progesterone receptor transcriptional activity. It is also thought

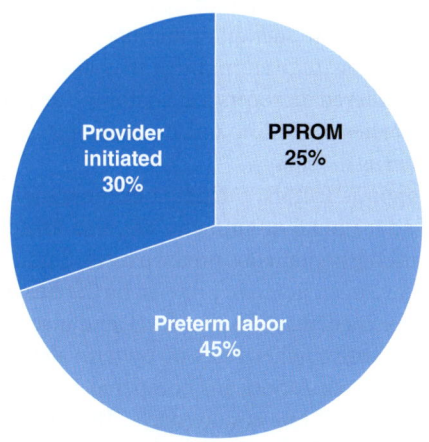

Fig 33.4 Antecedent Causes of Preterm Birth. *PPROM*, Preterm premature rupture of membranes. From Goldenberg RL, Culhane JF, Iams JD, Robero R. Epidural and causes of preterm birth. *Lancet.* 2008:371:75–84.

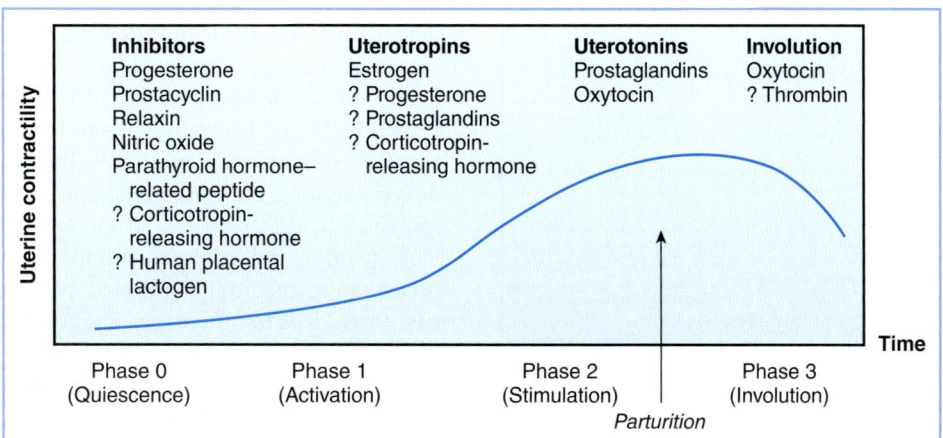

Fig. 33.5 The Regulation of Uterine Activity. The regulation of uterine activity during pregnancy and labor can be divided into four distinct physiologic phases—quiescence, activation, stimulation, and involution—that are, or may be, influenced by a number of stimulatory and inhibitory factors. From Liao JB, Buhimschi CS, Norwitz ER. Normal labor: mechanism and duration. *Obstet Gynecol Clin North Am.* 2005;32:145–164; modified from Challis JRG, Gibb W. Control of parturition. *Prenat Neonat Med.* 1996;1:283.

that parturition may be related to changes in inflammation, which itself is linked to functional progesterone withdrawal.[27]

Risk Factors for Preterm Delivery

Multiple maternal health, socioeconomic, and obstetric factors have been identified as potential risk factors for preterm birth. Box 33.1 lists factors associated with preterm labor.[2,28] The most important predictor of risk for preterm birth is a history of spontaneous preterm birth in a prior pregnancy. After one preterm birth, the risk of recurrent preterm birth in the subsequent pregnancy is approximately 35%.[6] An individual's risk of recurrent preterm birth increases with the number of prior preterm deliveries and earlier gestational age at delivery.

Several additional maternal health history factors are associated with an increased risk for preterm birth. Low prepregnancy body mass index ($<18.5\,kg/m^2$), tobacco use, and substance use are additional risk factors for spontaneous preterm delivery. Studies have repeatedly demonstrated an association between periodontal disease and preterm birth; however, randomized trials have not shown reduced preterm birth risk following treatment of periodontal disease in pregnancy.[6] Infectious exposures during pregnancy, including urinary tract infections (UTIs) and bacterial vaginitis, may also increase preterm birth risk.

Short cervical length, as assessed by transvaginal ultrasonography and defined as cervical length < 25 mm, is associated with a greater risk for preterm delivery. In a 2006 systematic analysis, Kagan et al.[29] concluded that shorter cervical length is associated with preterm birth in *symptomatic* women. Furthermore, multiple studies have shown an increased risk for preterm delivery in *asymptomatic* women

with a shortened cervix. A Maternal-Fetal Medicine Units Network study of nearly 3000 women found that the risk for spontaneous preterm delivery is increased in women with evidence of a short cervix detected by transvaginal ultrasonography between 24 and 28 weeks' gestation.[30] A cervical length below the 10th percentile had a sensitivity of 37% and a specificity of 92% in predicting preterm birth before 35 weeks' gestation, with a corresponding positive predictive value of 18% and a negative predictive value of 97%.[31]

A history of cervical surgery, including conization and loop electrosurgical excision procedure (LEEP), has traditionally been identified as a risk factor for preterm birth because of associated cervical injury and/or shortening. However, this relationship may be related to environmental or behavioral factors that underlie the progression of cervical dysplasia rather than cervical structural changes. A systematic review and metaanalysis of patients both with and without a history of LEEP showed that while LEEP was associated with greater risk of preterm birth before 37 weeks' gestation, the risk was equivalent to those patients with a history of cervical dysplasia without LEEP.[32] Uterine instrumentation, such as dilation and curettage, has also been associated with an increased risk for preterm birth in some studies, possibly secondary to endometrial injury or introduction of microbes into the intrauterine space.[6] The risk of preterm birth may also be heightened in those with altered uterocervical anatomy due to congenital uterine anomalies, including unicornuate uterus, bicornuate uterus, or uterus didelphys.

Socioeconomic factors, including economic disadvantage and lower educational attainment, are also associated with increased risk of spontaneous preterm birth. Significant racial disparities have been noted in preterm birth rates. Even when controlling for income, education level, and insurance status, there are markedly higher rates of preterm delivery among non-Hispanic Black Americans compared to their Hispanic and non-Hispanic White counterparts. The ACOG proposes that this disparity is likely a reflection of exposure of this population to systemic structural racism,[6] and efforts to address racial inequities are an active area of focus in the obstetric community (see Chapter 14).

Obstetric factors associated with increased risk of spontaneous preterm birth include multifetal gestation, vaginal bleeding in pregnancy, and short interpregnancy interval (<18 months between consecutive pregnancies). In the United States, 62.1% of twins were born preterm compared to 8.76% of singletons in 2021.[33] The high rate of preterm delivery among multiple gestations is attributable to both spontaneous preterm labor in the setting of increased uterine distention and increased risk for obstetric complications necessitating medically indicated preterm delivery. In the past three decades, there was a significant rise in the incidence of multiple gestation (see Chapter 34) due to a shift toward older maternal age at conception and increased utilization of assisted reproductive technology (ART).[34] The twin birth rate rose 76% from 1980 to 2009 (from 18.9 twins per 1000 total births to 33.2 per 1000). In 2015 ART contributed to 1.7% of all infants born in the United States and 17.0% of

---

BOX 33.1 Factors Associated With Spontaneous Preterm Labor

Demographic and Medical Characteristics
Non-White race
Extremes of age (<17 y or >35 y)
Low socioeconomic status
Low prepregnancy body mass index
Periodontal disease
Abnormal uterine anatomy (e.g., myomas, Mullerian anomalies)
Trauma
Abdominal surgery during pregnancy

Behavioral Factors
Tobacco use
Substance use disorder

Obstetric Factors
Previous preterm birth
Vaginal bleeding
Infection (systemic, genital tract, periodontal)
Short cervical length
Multiple gestation
Interpregnancy interval < 6 m
Assisted reproductive technology
Preterm premature rupture of membranes
Polyhydramnios

all multiple-birth infants.[35] Recently, rates of multifetal pregnancies have started to decline. The twin birth rate peaked at 33.9 twins per 1000 births in 2014 and has since decreased to 31.2 per 1000 births in 2021.[33] Likewise, the triplet and higher-order multiple birth rate has fallen 59% since the 1998 peak (193.5 per 100,000 births) to a rate of 80.0 per 100,000 births in 2021.[33] Modifications in ART may be contributing to changes in the preterm birth rate and recent declines in multiple gestation.[35]

SCREENING STRATEGIES FOR PRETERM BIRTH RISK STRATIFICATION

Various screening approaches have been investigated to accurately predict which asymptomatic patients are at highest risk for spontaneous preterm delivery, with the goal of offering effective interventions to prevent preterm birth.

Cervical Length Screening

No History of Preterm Birth

Dedicated screening ultrasonography for cervical length measurement is not recommended in asymptomatic patients without a prior preterm birth. A prospective cohort study by Orzechowski et al.[36] investigated a universal cervical length screening program for mid-trimester patients without a history of preterm delivery. Among 1569 patients who underwent transvaginal cervical length measurement between 18 0/7 and 23 6/7 weeks' gestation, only 1.1% of patients had a short cervix measuring less than or equal to 20 mm; there was no difference in the incidence of spontaneous preterm birth between screened and unscreened patients. Nevertheless, transabdominal sonographic visualization of the cervix is recommended at the time of the fetal anatomic survey, typically performed between 18 and 22 weeks' gestation. If the cervix cannot be adequately visualized transabdominally or appears short on transabdominal view, transvaginal ultrasonography for further cervical length assessment is indicated.

Prior Preterm Birth

Cervical length screening ultrasonography is recommended for all patients with a history of one or more spontaneous preterm births. Transvaginal ultrasonography is performed for cervical length measurement starting at 16 weeks' gestation. Serial cervical length surveillance ultrasonography should be continued every 2 weeks until 24 weeks' gestation.

Although studies have demonstrated higher risk of spontaneous preterm birth in subsequent pregnancy in those patients with a history of medically indicated preterm delivery, serial cervical length surveillance is not presently recommended in this population. Cervix visualization at the time of fetal anatomy ultrasonography is recommended in alignment with the recommendation for women without a history of preterm birth.

Special Populations

In the absence of prior preterm birth, serial cervical length surveillance is not recommended solely for the indications of multifetal gestation, uterine anomaly, or history of cervical excisional procedure. A prospective cohort study showed that while the mean cervical length was decreased in patients with a history of cervical excisional procedure compared to those without (33 mm versus 39 mm, respectively), there were no significant differences in frequency of short cervix measuring less than 25 mm or preterm birth before 34 weeks' gestation between groups.[37] Cervix visualization at the time of fetal anatomy ultrasonography is recommended in these patient populations.

Infection Screening

UTIs and infectious vaginitis have been associated with increased risk of preterm birth. While treatment of symptomatic UTIs has not been shown to reduce the risk of preterm birth,[38] universal screening and treatment for asymptomatic bacteriuria is recommended in early pregnancy to prevent morbidity related to progression to pyelonephritis. Bacterial vaginosis (BV) is a common bacterial vaginitis caused by *Gardnerella vaginalis* which has been associated with increased risk of preterm birth. A systematic review and metaanalysis showed that while antibiotics effectively clear BV in pregnancy, treatment was not associated with reduced risk of preterm labor or PPROM.[39] Universal screening and treatment for BV in pregnancy is therefore not recommended for asymptomatic patients.

Biomarkers

Fetal fibronectin (FFN) is an extracellular matrix protein found at the uteroplacental interface that has been suggested as a biomarker for preterm labor when detected in cervicovaginal fluid. While the presence of elevated FFN levels in cervicovaginal fluid of symptomatic patients is both highly sensitive (93%) and specific (82%), this test has overall poor positive predictive value (29%) for preterm delivery within 7 days. However, negative FFN testing has a remarkably high negative predictive value (99.5%), rendering the likelihood of preterm delivery within 7 days of a negative test extremely low.[40] Given the limited positive predictive value of FFN testing for preterm delivery, performing FFN screening is not recommended for *asymptomatic* patients. For *symptomatic* patients at high risk of preterm delivery, FFN testing with concurrent cervical length measurement may have utility in the appropriate clinical context.[41]

Other novel proteomic biomarkers are being investigated for their ability to predict preterm birth. A 2016 study found that two serum proteins (insulin-like growth factor-binding protein 4 [IBP4] and sex hormone–binding globulin) identified asymptomatic pregnant women at risk for spontaneous preterm delivery[42]; these findings were replicated in a subsequent independent multicenter observational study.[43] Proteomic analysis of cervicovaginal fluid samples obtained from high-risk asymptomatic patients has identified multiple additional biomarker candidates, including human interleukin−1 receptor antagonist protein, γ-glutamyl hydrolase, extracellular matrix protein 1, vitamin D−binding protein, metalloproteinase inhibitor 1, human laminin subunit gamma-2, and pigment epithelium-derived factor.[44,45] Although promising, these markers have yet to be used in clinical practice.

PREVENTION OF SPONTANEOUS PRETERM BIRTH

Screening for any disease is of greatest benefit when there are interventions available to decrease the incidence of said disease. Unfortunately, few, if any, interventions have been shown to definitively reduce the incidence of preterm labor and delivery. Interventions that have been studied include progesterone supplementation, cervical cerclage, cervical pessary, low-dose aspirin, prophylactic antibiotics, and bedrest.

Progesterone Supplementation

Evidence suggests that progesterone therapy may be effective in reducing the rate of preterm birth in select patient populations. Multiple formulations and routes of administration of supplemental progesterone have been studied. Though vaginal progesterone has consistently been shown to reduce the incidence of preterm birth in patients diagnosed with a short cervix without a history of preterm birth, the benefit of supplemental progesterone for prevention of recurrent spontaneous preterm birth remains controversial.

Intramuscular Progesterone

Until recently, prophylactic administration of intramuscular 17α-hydroxyprogesterone caproate (17-OHPC), sold under the brand-name Makena, was a mainstay in the obstetric management of subsequent pregnancy in patients with a history of spontaneous preterm delivery. The treatment regimen entailed weekly injections of 17-OHPC beginning at 16 to 20 weeks' gestation and continued until 36 weeks' gestation.

In collaboration with the Maternal-Fetal Medicine Units Network, Meis et al.[46] performed a multicenter, double-blind randomized controlled trial comparing 17-OHPC to placebo in patients with a history of spontaneous preterm delivery; 310 patients were randomized to receive 17-OHPC and 153 patients were randomized to receive placebo. Assuming a baseline recurrent preterm birth rate of 37%, the study was powered to detect a 33% reduction in the incidence of preterm birth before 37 weeks' gestation in the 17-OHPC group compared to placebo. The 17-OHPC group had a significantly lower incidence of the primary outcome of recurrent delivery before 37 weeks' gestation compared with placebo (36.3% versus 54.9%).[46] In 2011 the US Food and Drug Administration (FDA) granted accelerated approval for 17-OHPC for the prevention of recurrent preterm birth based on the promising results of the trial, with the stipulation that a postapproval confirmatory trial must be performed.

The Meis et al. trial[46] results were questioned given the disproportionately high rate of recurrent preterm delivery in the placebo group. Critics of the study noted that "the rate of recurrent preterm birth in the 17-OHPC treated cohort matched the baseline *a priori* expected rate and was only significant compared with the 54.9% unexpected rate in the

placebo arm."[47] The high rate of preterm birth in the placebo arm was postulated to be related to the high proportion of patients with more than one prior preterm delivery (41.2% in the placebo group compared to 27.7% in the 17-OHPC group).[46] Concerns were also raised about the generalizability of these results, as more than half of the study participants identified as non-Hispanic Black race, a population known to have elevated risk of preterm birth.

In 2019 the results of the long-awaited confirmatory PROLONG trial[48] were published, an international multicenter double-blind, randomized controlled trial evaluating the efficacy of 17-OHPC compared to placebo in over 1700 participants. In contrast to the Meis et al. trial,[46] the PROLONG study demonstrated that 17-OHPC use did not reduce the incidence of recurrent preterm birth before 35 weeks' gestation (17-OHPC 11.0% versus placebo 11.5%). Furthermore, 17-OHPC use was not associated with lower composite neonatal morbidity compared with placebo.[48] Following publication, the FDA performed secondary analyses of the PROLONG trial data to evaluate if there were differences in the efficacy of 17-OHPC by nationality, race, and number of preterm deliveries. No differences in the coprimary outcomes of recurrent preterm birth or composite neonatal morbidity were noted in the US versus non-US, Black versus non-Black, and one versus greater than one prior preterm birth subgroups.[47]

Following the results of the PROLONG trial, the FDA recommended withdrawal of 17-OHPC from the market in October 2020. After an appeal by the manufacturer of Makena, an FDA advisory panel voted 14-1 to remove Makena from the market, and the drug's FDA approval was officially withdrawn in April 2023.

Vaginal Progesterone

Vaginal progesterone therapy has been shown to be beneficial in reducing the incidence of preterm delivery in the subset of patients with short cervix and no history of spontaneous preterm birth. In two double-blind, placebo-controlled trials, women with a mid-trimester diagnosis of a short cervix (<15 mm in one trial[49] and 10 to 20 mm in the other[50]) were randomized to receive either vaginal progesterone or placebo. Women who received vaginal progesterone experienced a significant reduction in the frequency of preterm delivery before 33 weeks' gestation.[49,50] Metaanalyses have further demonstrated that vaginal progesterone treatment in patients with a sonographic short cervix is associated with significantly reduced risk of neonatal morbidity and mortality.[51]

The OPPTIMUM study was a multicenter, double-blind, randomized controlled trial evaluating the efficacy of prophylactic vaginal progesterone for reducing the incidence of preterm birth before 34 weeks' gestation and composite neonatal morbidity in a heterogeneous cohort of women at risk for preterm birth. While vaginal progesterone exposure caused no identifiable adverse neurodevelopmental outcomes in exposed offspring, vaginal progesterone treatment did not reduce the risk of preterm birth or composite neonatal morbidity in this cohort.[52] However, interpretation of these results is limited due to the inclusion of patients with nonequivalent risk factors for preterm birth into a single cohort, which included those with history of spontaneous preterm birth at or before 34 weeks' gestation, short cervical length ≤ 25 mm, and positive FFN in the setting of other clinical risk factors, without planned subgroup analysis.

The Evaluating Progestogens for Preventing Preterm birth International Collaborative (EPPPIC) metaanalysis pooled individual patient data from randomized controlled trials for 11,644 women to compare the effectiveness of vaginal progesterone, intramuscular 17-OHPC, and oral progesterone for preventing preterm birth in a heterogeneous population of women at high risk for preterm delivery (primarily due to history of preterm birth or short cervix).[53] Notably, this analysis included both the Meis et al.[46] and PROLONG[48] trials. This study found that both vaginal progesterone and 17-OHPC prophylactic treatment were associated with a lower rate of preterm birth before 34 weeks' gestation, although the effect was more robust for vaginal progesterone. Subgroup analysis showed no benefit of vaginal progesterone or 17-OHPC for patients with history of preterm birth with cervical length > 30 mm.[53] Furthermore, in the absence of other clinical risk factors, neither vaginal progesterone nor 17-OHPC have been shown to reduce the risk of preterm delivery in unselected multifetal gestations.[53] Supplemental progesterone has also not been found to increase pregnancy latency following PPROM.[54]

A recent metaanalysis conducted by Conde-Agudelo and Romero[55] investigated prophylactic vaginal progesterone treatment specifically in patients with a history of spontaneous preterm birth, including 10 studies with a total of 2958 participants. Vaginal progesterone use was associated with a significantly lower incidence of preterm birth before 37 weeks' gestation, preterm birth before 34 weeks' gestation, and NICU admission. However, the authors concluded that these results were biased by small-study effect, and efficacy of vaginal progesterone for prevention of recurrent preterm birth was no longer demonstrated when their analysis was adjusted for small-study effect.[55]

Cervical Cerclage

Cervical cerclage placement is a surgical procedure, typically performed via a vaginal approach, in which the cervix is sutured circumferentially to provide structural support to the cervix, thereby preventing cervical shortening and dilation (see Chapter 17). Candidacy for cerclage placement is dependent on the patient's obstetric history and cervical length.

History-indicated cerclage is typically performed at 12 to 14 weeks' gestation for patients with an established history of cervical insufficiency. History of adverse obstetric outcomes consistent with cervical insufficiency include one or more mid-trimester pregnancy losses resulting from painless cervical dilation and/or need for cerclage placement in prior pregnancy. A multicenter, randomized controlled trial conducted by the Royal College of Obstetricians and Gynaecologists Working Party on Cervical Cerclage[56] found that history-indicated cerclage placement was associated with a significantly lower risk of preterm birth before 33 weeks' gestation

with a number needed to treat of 25 patients. However, the efficacy and cost-effectiveness of history-indicated cerclage compared to serial cervical length surveillance has been less convincing in other studies,[57] leading many providers to instead recommend a surveillance strategy for prevention of recurrent preterm birth.

Patients with a history of spontaneous preterm birth undergoing serial cervical length surveillance with sonographic cervical length < 25 mm are candidates for **ultrasound-indicated cerclage**. In a metaanalysis including patients with a prior preterm birth and cervical length < 25 mm before 24 weeks' gestation, cerclage placement was associated with a 39% reduction in the risk of preterm delivery before 35 weeks.[58] No studies have directly compared the efficacy of cerclage versus vaginal progesterone for patients with short cervical length and a history of spontaneous preterm birth. However, a metaanalysis including randomized controlled trials that compared (1) cerclage versus expectant management or (2) vaginal progesterone versus placebo suggests that vaginal progesterone therapy may be equally effective to cerclage in this population.[59]

The benefit of ultrasound-indicated cerclage in patients with a short cervix has been consistently demonstrated only for those with prior preterm delivery. Among patients with a cervical length < 25 mm but *no* history of preterm birth, cerclage placement has not been shown in randomized trials to reduce the risk of preterm delivery.[58] Some studies have, however, suggested that cerclage placement reduces the risk of preterm delivery for the subset of patients without prior preterm birth with a very short cervical length < 10 mm.[6]

In contrast to history-indicated and ultrasound-indicated cerclages, a **physical examination-indicated cerclage** is placed to prolong gestation in asymptomatic patients incidentally found to have mid-trimester cervical dilation prior to 24 weeks' gestation, regardless of past obstetric history. A metaanalysis demonstrated that, compared with expectant management, examination-indicated cerclage placement resulted in mean pregnancy prolongation of approximately 34 days and a 65% increase in neonatal survival.[60] Contraindications include established preterm labor with impending preterm birth, chorioamnionitis, heavy vaginal bleeding, PPROM, fetal compromise, life-limiting fetal anomalies, and fetal demise. Prior to cerclage placement, amniocentesis can be performed as clinically indicated to evaluate the amniotic fluid for evidence of subclinical infection. Data are mixed regarding mandating a waiting period before placement. Some experts advocate for immediate placement, while others recommend delaying placement for up to 24 hours with monitoring for evidence of preterm labor; there is no single evidence-based standard to define best practice regarding the timing of examination-indicated cerclage placement.

When placing the cerclage, prolapsing membranes, if present, need to be replaced in the uterine cavity to reduce the risk for iatrogenic PPROM. The surgical technique typically involves the lithotomy position with steep Trendelenburg tilt and applying tension circumferentially around the external os by placing ring forceps or stay sutures to ease the membranes back into the uterus. Invasive methods may also be used, including using a Foley catheter balloon to directly push the membranes back into the uterus. However, this practice may be associated with increased risk for iatrogenic PPROM. Some evidence suggests a course of perioperative antibiotic and tocolytic administration is beneficial in patients undergoing examination-indicated cerclage placement.[61]

Other Experimental Methods

Low-dose aspirin prophylaxis has been studied as a possible low-cost, readily accessible intervention for the prevention of preterm birth. The spirin in the prevention of recurrent spontaneous preterm labor (APRIL) study,[62] a double-bind randomized controlled trial including patients with a history of spontaneous singleton preterm birth, did not observe a decreased incidence of recurrent preterm birth in patients taking aspirin compared to placebo. However, the aspirin supplementation for pregnancy indicated risk reduction in nulliparas (ASPIRIN) study,[63] an international, double-blind, randomized controlled trial that enrolled nulliparous patients in six low- and middle-income countries, found a 25% decrease in the incidence of spontaneous preterm delivery in patients taking aspirin compared to controls. Data are currently insufficient to recommend aspirin use for the indication of spontaneous preterm birth risk reduction.

Vaginal pessaries have not been shown to decrease the risk of preterm delivery in singleton or multifetal gestations in multiple studies.[6] Evidence does *not* support the administration of **prophylactic antibiotics** in asymptomatic women at risk for preterm labor.[64] Likewise, evidence does not support the prophylactic use of **beta-adrenergic receptor agonists** to prevent preterm labor in high-risk women.[65,66] Strict bed rest has not been shown to reduce the risk of preterm delivery, and may increase the risk of adverse maternal health consequences, including deconditioning, mood disturbances, and venous thromboembolism (VTE).

MANAGEMENT OF PRETERM LABOR

Diagnosis

Determining whether a woman is in early preterm labor or in false labor is often difficult. Criteria for the diagnosis of preterm labor include gestational age between 20 0/7 and 36 6/7 weeks and regular uterine contractions accompanied by a change in cervical dilation, effacement, or both (or initial presentation with regular contractions and cervical dilation ≥ 2 cm). Compared to approximately 50% of patients with PPROM,[67] less than 10% of women diagnosed with preterm labor progress to delivery within 7 days of presentation.[68]

Assessment and Therapy

Initial assessment of the patient with possible preterm labor includes physical examination and external monitoring of contractions with a tocodynamometer (and fetal heart rate [FHR] monitoring if indicated by gestational age). Acute conditions associated with preterm labor should be considered, including intrauterine infection and placental abruption. Maternal physical examination may include a sterile speculum examination to evaluate the cervix and exclude PPROM, as well as a sterile digital cervical examination. Transabdominal ultrasonography should be performed to evaluate fetal presentation, amniotic fluid level, and estimated fetal weight. Laboratory evaluation may include complete blood count with differential, urine culture, vaginitis swabs, and vaginal/rectal culture for Group B streptococcus (GBS). In many women who have preterm uterine contractions, these contractions will cease spontaneously. In the past, clinicians assumed that intravenous hydration was a useful component of therapy. However, there is no evidence that intravenous hydration reduces the chance of preterm delivery.[69]

Once the diagnosis of preterm labor is established, the obstetric care provider must decide whether intervention is warranted, including administration of antenatal corticosteroids for fetal lung maturation,[68] magnesium sulfate for fetal neuroprotection,[70] or tocolysis.

Antenatal Corticosteroids

Antenatal corticosteroids are recommended for all singleton and multifetal gestations from 24 0/7 to 33 6/7 weeks' gestation in which there is a high likelihood of preterm delivery within 7 days. Typical steroid regimens for **betamethasone** and **dexamethasone** are listed in Table 33.5. Maximal steroid effect is reached 48 hours after the first dose, though beneficial effects for the fetus begin within a few hours of exposure.

The neonatal benefits of corticosteroid administration before preterm delivery have been clearly demonstrated in large clinical trials. The NICHD Neonatal Research Network evaluated outcomes for 11,718 preterm infants delivered after antenatal maternal corticosteroid administration between 1988 and 1992.[71] Antenatal corticosteroid treatment significantly reduced the incidence of neonatal respiratory distress syndrome, intraventricular hemorrhage, and neonatal death in all subgroups of the population studied (including male and female infants, Black and White infants, and infants delivered before 30 weeks' gestation). The reduction in neonatal morbidity and mortality from antenatal corticosteroid administration is additive to the reduction observed with the use of neonatal surfactant alone.[72] Although antenatal corticosteroids had historically been reserved for pregnancies at risk for preterm delivery prior to 34 weeks' gestation, the Antenatal Late Preterm Steroids (ALPS) trial demonstrated

TABLE 33.5 Antenatal Corticosteroid Therapy		
Drug	Dose and Route	Frequency/Duration
Betamethasone	12 mg IM	Every 24 h × 2 doses
Dexamethasone	6 mg IM	Every 12 h × 4 doses

IM, Intramuscular.
From National Institutes of Health Consensus Development Panel. Antenatal corticosteroids revisited: Repeat courses—National Institutes of Health Consensus Development Conference Statement, August 17–18, 2000. *Obstet Gynecol.* 2001;98:144–150.

that these benefits extend to neonates born after 34 weeks' gestation.[73] A single course of corticosteroids administered to women with singleton pregnancies at risk for preterm birth between 34 and 37 weeks' gestation resulted in a significantly lower incidence of severe neonatal respiratory morbidity for appropriately selected patients.[73] Women with prior antenatal steroid exposure, pregestational diabetes mellitus, multifetal gestation, and anticipated delivery within 12 hours were notably excluded from the ALPS trial. Given the potential risks of steroid-induced maternal hyperglycemia in the absence of data demonstrating neonatal benefit, administration of late-preterm corticosteroids to patients with pregestational diabetes is not presently recommended.

Although there is little controversy about the efficacy of a single course of antenatal corticosteroids, there remains debate over the use of multiple courses of corticosteroids for women who remain undelivered 7 days after the initial dose of corticosteroids. A large study performed by the Maternal-Fetal-Medicine Units Network randomly assigned women at risk for preterm delivery between 23 and 32 weeks' gestation to receive either a single course or repeated (weekly) courses of antenatal corticosteroids.[74] Weekly corticosteroid administration did not significantly reduce the composite primary morbidity outcome, but it significantly reduced the need for neonatal surfactant, mechanical ventilation, and continuous positive airway pressure, as well as the incidence of pneumothorax. However, weekly corticosteroid administration was associated with an increase in the delivery of small for gestational age infants, and there was a significant reduction in the birth weight of the infants whose mothers received four or more courses of corticosteroids. Studies have also identified an association between repeated antenatal steroid exposure and small head circumference.

To balance the potential beneficial effects and risks of additional courses of corticosteroids, some have advocated a single **"rescue" course** (i.e., a second course of corticosteroids), which is administered at the time of a clinical status change with an associated high probability of preterm delivery. A large randomized placebo-controlled trial found neonatal benefit in administering an additional course of corticosteroids.[75] Criteria for administration included absence of rupture of membranes, prior corticosteroid administration at least 2 weeks earlier, gestational age < 33 weeks, and a change in clinical scenario such that it was believed that preterm birth was likely to occur within 1 week. A metaanalysis concluded that a single rescue course of antenatal corticosteroids should be considered in women whose prior course of antenatal corticosteroids was administered at least 7 days previously and who are at acute risk for preterm delivery before 34 weeks' gestation.[76] The ACOG[77] has stated that one rescue course of corticosteroids may be considered in these specific populations. However, regularly scheduled repeat courses or multiple courses of corticosteroids (>2) are not currently recommended.

Antibiotic Therapy

The results of a large, multicenter, randomized controlled trial[78] and a metaanalysis[79] do *not* support the use of prophylactic antibiotic therapy in the management of preterm labor in patients with intact membranes as a method to reduce the likelihood of preterm birth. In fact, there was an increase in cerebral palsy in children born to mothers in preterm labor with intact membranes who received any prophylactic antibiotics versus no antibiotics (relative risk [RR] 1.82; 95% confidence interval [CI], 0.99 to 3.34; 3173 children).[80] Accordingly, the ACOG does not recommend empirical antibiotic therapy in this population.[81] Prophylactic antibiotic administration remains appropriate, however, in women who are GBS positive or with unknown GBS status who are thought to be in preterm labor.[81]

Fetal Neuroprotection

Several clinical trials have provided evidence that maternal administration of magnesium sulfate provides fetal neuroprotection when administered to women at risk for imminent preterm delivery prior to 32 weeks' gestation. It is hypothesized that magnesium decreases inflammation at the fetal blood-brain barrier and suppresses the excitotoxic activity of glutamate, although the precise neuroprotective mechanism of magnesium remains unknown.[82]

Magnesium administered with neuroprotective intent has been studied in patients at risk for imminent preterm birth due to PPROM, preterm labor with cervical dilation between 4 and 8 cm (with or without ruptured membranes), or planned medically indicated delivery within 2 to 24 hours. In 2003 the Australasian collaborative trial of magnesium sulphate (ACTOMgSO4) study group[83] reported the results of a multicenter, randomized, placebo-controlled study of 1062 women (1255 infants) at less than 30 weeks' gestation in whom delivery was planned or expected within 24 hours. The investigators observed no significant difference between groups in the primary outcomes, which included total pediatric mortality, cerebral palsy, or both, at a corrected age of 2 years. However, they observed a significantly reduced rate of substantial gross-motor dysfunction, as well as a reduced combined rate of death or substantial gross-motor dysfunction, in the children exposed to magnesium sulfate *in utero*.[83] Similarly, the PREterm brain protection by MAGnesium sulfate (PREMAG) study, a randomized controlled trial of magnesium sulfate administration to 573 pregnant women at less than 33 weeks' gestation in whom delivery was planned or expected within 24 hours found that infants exposed to magnesium sulfate had a reduced rate of total neonatal mortality, severe cerebral white matter injury (which is associated with cerebral palsy), and the combination of severe white matter injury and/or death; however, the differences were not statistically significant.[84] In the beneficial effects of antenatal magnesium sulfate (BEAM) study, the largest randomized controlled trial to date,[85] 2241 women at imminent risk for delivery before 32 weeks' gestation were randomized to receive magnesium sulfate or placebo. The offspring who had been exposed to magnesium sulfate *in utero* were significantly less likely to develop moderate/severe cerebral palsy (1.9% versus 3.5%; RR, 0.55; 95% CI, 0.32 to 0.95).[85]

A metaanalysis of these clinical trials suggests that prenatal administration of magnesium sulfate for the indication of fetal neuroprotection reduces the occurrence of cerebral palsy (RR, 0.68; 95% CI, 0.54 to 0.87).[82,86] The ACOG has stated that, based on available evidence, magnesium sulfate—given before anticipated *early* preterm birth—reduces the risk for cerebral palsy in surviving infants.[70] The recently published magnesium sulphate at 30 to 34 weeks' gestational age: neuroprotection (MAGENTA) trial suggests magnesium may not have a neuroprotective benefit in preterm infants after 30 weeks' gestation. This randomized controlled trial of magnesium sulfate administration to 1433 patients between 30 and 34 weeks' gestation at risk for imminent delivery demonstrated no differences in death or cerebral palsy at age 2 years between study groups.[87]

Of note, the gestational age ranges and magnesium dosage protocols utilized in the available literature differ widely; some study protocols called for administering a single magnesium sulfate bolus (4 to 6 g given intravenously over 20 to 30 minutes), and other studies called for administering an intravenous bolus followed by intravenous infusion of varying duration (4 to 6 g given intravenously over 20 to 30 minutes followed by a 1 to 2 g per hour infusion continued for 12 to 24 hours). Because the best regimen of magnesium sulfate administration remains unclear, physicians electing to use magnesium sulfate for fetal neuroprotection should develop specific guidelines regarding inclusion criteria, treatment regimens, concurrent tocolysis, and monitoring based on the protocols of the larger published trials.[70]

Tocolysis

Although widely used before 34 weeks' gestation, acute tocolytic therapy remains a source of controversy due to lack of consistent evidence that tocolysis reduces the likelihood of preterm birth or improves neonatal outcome. However, because acute tocolysis has been associated with a short (approximately 48 hours) prolongation of pregnancy, it may be beneficial to facilitate transfer of the patient from a community hospital to a tertiary care facility that can provide optimal care for the preterm neonate. Moreover, a short course of tocolytic therapy may delay delivery for 24 to 48 hours, allowing maternal administration of antenatal steroids to accelerate fetal lung maturity. Thus the ACOG[68] supports the use of acute tocolysis to allow administration of a complete first course of antenatal corticosteroids prior to 34 weeks' gestation but discourages the continued use of tocolysis after corticosteroid administration is complete. Furthermore, tocolysis is not recommended to facilitate administration of a rescue course of corticosteroids or late-preterm corticosteroids after 34 weeks' gestation. Tocolytics should not be administered if there is clinical evidence of intrauterine infection or active placental abruption, as the risk of both maternal and neonatal morbidity with delayed delivery in these settings outweigh the potential fetal benefit of pregnancy prolongation (Box 33.2).

BOX 33.2   Contraindications to Tocolytic Therapy for Preterm Labor

- Fetal death
- Fetal anomalies incompatible with life
- Nonreassuring fetal status
- Chorioamnionitis
- Severe hemorrhage

Once the obstetrician has decided to begin tocolytic therapy, an appropriate agent must be selected (Table 33.6). A 2003 analysis of studies that compared the four classes of tocolytic agents (i.e., beta-adrenergic receptor agonists, calcium entry–blocking agents, magnesium sulfate, and cyclooxygenase inhibitors) concluded that all are more effective than placebo in prolonging pregnancy, but the investigators found no evidence of a beneficial effect on neonatal morbidity or mortality.[88]

Although **beta-adrenergic receptor agonists** (e.g., ritodrine, terbutaline), which relax smooth muscle via beta$_2$-adrenergic receptor stimulation, were used as tocolytic agents for many years, they are utilized less in current practice than other tocolytic agents that are equally efficacious with fewer side effects.[89,90] A 2014 metaanalysis that compared beta-adrenergic receptor agonists with a placebo concluded that the use of beta-adrenergic receptor agonists reduced the number of women who delivered within 48 hours and decreased the number of births within 7 days.[91] However, there was no reduction in overall preterm birth rate or in perinatal/neonatal death or neonatal morbidity. Tocolysis was significantly associated with adverse maternal side effects (see Table 33.6).

Given safety concerns, ritodrine is no longer available in the United States, although it remains in use as a first-line tocolytic agent in several Asian countries. In 2011 the FDA issued a warning regarding terbutaline use.[92] Specifically, it stated that *injectable* terbutaline should not be used in pregnant women for prolonged treatment (beyond 48 to 72 hours) of preterm labor in either the hospital or outpatient setting because of the potential for maternal cardiac complications and death. It also noted that oral terbutaline should not be used for prevention or treatment of preterm labor because it had not been shown to be effective and was associated with similar safety concerns.[92]

A metaanalysis has suggested that **calcium entry–blocking agents** (e.g., nifedipine), which block calcium inflow into cells through voltage-dependent calcium channels, have benefits over beta-adrenergic receptor agonists with respect to prolongation of pregnancy, serious neonatal morbidity, and maternal adverse effects.[90]

Prostaglandins, which are produced by cyclooxygenase (COX) enzymes, are mediators in the final pathways of uterine contraction. They increase intracellular calcium concentrations, increase activation of MLCK, and promote gap junction formation. The nonselective **COX inhibitor** indomethacin is the agent in this class most often studied as a tocolytic agent. Serious maternal side effects are uncommon. Fetal concerns, particularly in the setting of prolonged use (>48 hours), include a risk for premature closure of the ductus arteriosus and oligohydramnios (caused by fetal renal dysfunction). A 2015 metaanalysis concluded that COX inhibitors have no clear benefit compared with a placebo or any other tocolytic agents.[93]

The **oxytocin receptor antagonist** atosiban has also been used as a tocolytic agent. Although available in Europe, the drug was not approved by the FDA due to safety concerns following a randomized trial showing a higher rate of fetal

TABLE 33.6 Tocolytic Drugs for Preterm Labor

Drug	Contraindications	Maternal Side Effects	Fetal/Neonatal Side Effects
Calcium entry–blocking agents	Cardiac disease Renal disease (use with caution) Maternal hypotension	Transient hypotension, flushing, headache, dizziness, nausea	None identified
Cyclooxygenase inhibitors (NSAIDs)	Significant renal or hepatic impairment Active peptic ulcer disease Coagulation disorders or thrombocytopenia NSAID-sensitive asthma Other NSAID sensitivities	Nausea, heartburn	Constriction of the ductus arteriosus, pulmonary hypertension, reversible renal dysfunction (leading to oligohydramnios), IVH, hyperbilirubinemia, necrotizing enterocolitis
Beta-adrenergic receptor agonists	Cardiac dysrhythmias Poorly controlled thyroid disease Poorly controlled diabetes mellitus	*Cardiopulmonary:* dysrhythmias, pulmonary edema, myocardial ischemia, hypotension, tachycardia *Metabolic:* hyperglycemia, hyperinsulinemia, hypokalemia, antidiuresis, altered thyroid function *Other:* tremor, palpitations, nervousness, nausea/vomiting, fever, hallucinations	*Fetal:* tachycardia, hyperinsulinemia, hyperglycemia, myocardial and septal hypertrophy, myocardial ischemia *Neonatal:* tachycardia, hypoglycemia, hypocalcemia, hyperbilirubinemia, hypotension, IVH
Magnesium sulfate	Myasthenia gravis Myotonic dystrophy	Flushing, lethargy, headache, muscle weakness, diplopia, dry mouth, pulmonary edema, cardiac arrest	Lethargy, hypotonia, respiratory depression, demineralization (prolonged use)

IVH, Intraventricular hemorrhage; *NSAIDs*, nonsteroidal antiinflammatory drugs.
Modified from Hearne AE, Nagey DA. Therapeutic agents in preterm labor: tocolytic agents. *Clin Obstet Gynecol.* 2000;43:787–801.

death in patients treated with atosiban.[94] A 2014 metaanalysis did not demonstrate superiority of oxytocin receptor antagonists (largely atosiban) compared with placebo, beta-adrenergic receptor agonists, or calcium entry–blocking agents (largely nifedipine) for pregnancy prolongation or neonatal outcomes, although treatment with oxytocin receptor antagonists was associated with fewer adverse maternal effects than treatment with the other two drug classes.[90] A subsequent large randomized controlled trial comparing atosiban with nifedipine found that 48 hours of tocolysis with nifedipine or atosiban resulted in similar perinatal outcomes.[95]

Historically, **magnesium sulfate** has also been used as a tocolytic agent in patients presenting with threatened preterm labor with cervical dilation < 4 cm. A 2014 metaanalysis of 37 heterogeneous trials that compared magnesium with placebo, no treatment, or other tocolytic drugs[96] concluded that magnesium is ineffective in delaying or preventing preterm birth. While the benefit of magnesium for fetal neuroprotection and maternal seizure prophylaxis in preeclampsia has been established, magnesium treatment had no benefit for a range of neonatal and maternal outcomes when used solely for the purpose of tocolysis. Furthermore, its use for this indication may be associated with an increased risk for total fetal, neonatal, or infant mortality. A secondary tocolytic agent should therefore be utilized concurrently for patients who require tocolysis who are receiving magnesium for the indication of fetal neuroprotection.

The **nitric oxide donor** nitroglycerin has also been evaluated for its efficacy as a tocolytic. However, findings from metaanalyses indicate that nitroglycerin results in neither significantly later gestational age at delivery nor better neonatal outcome compared with a placebo or other tocolytic drugs.[97]

The ACOG[68] has stated that evidence supports the use of tocolytic treatment with beta-adrenergic receptor agonist therapy, calcium entry–blocking agents, or COX inhibitors for short-term prolongation of pregnancy (up to 48 hours) to allow for antenatal maternal corticosteroid administration. Multiple clinical trials have demonstrated that prolonged use of tocolytic agents (as prophylactic therapy or after completion of acute treatment) does not alter pregnancy outcome. Regardless of which tocolytic agent is chosen, the risk for side effects appears to increase when more than one tocolytic agent is administered simultaneously.[98] It is unclear whether a combination of tocolytic drugs for preterm labor is more effective for women and/or newborns because there is a lack of large, well-designed trials that include the outcomes of interest.[98]

MANAGEMENT OF PRETERM PREMATURE RUPTURE OF MEMBRANES

Diagnosis

PPROM is diagnosed based on the following three findings on sterile speculum examination: (1) pooling of fluid in the posterior fornix of the vagina; (2) alkaline pH of the vaginal fluid, typically assessed by blue color change of nitrazine paper; and (3) the presence of "ferning" on microscopic evaluation of the dried vaginal fluid. Digital cervical examination is generally avoided in PPROM to limit introduction of genital tract pathogens into the amniotic space. Assessment of cervical dilation is therefore typically performed visually with sterile speculum examination. As for patients presenting with preterm labor symptoms, external FHR and contraction monitoring, obstetric ultrasonography, and laboratory evaluation are recommended.

Intrauterine infection accompanies an estimated 15% to 35% of cases of PPROM.[67] Close monitoring should therefore be performed to detect any fever, maternal and/or fetal tachycardia, tenderness of the uterine fundus, mucopurulent and/or malodorous amniotic fluid, and leukocytosis, any of which may indicate intrauterine infection.

Latency Antibiotics

In contrast to patients presenting with preterm labor, antibiotic therapy in patients with PPROM has been shown to increase pregnancy latency and reduce both maternal and neonatal morbidity.[99,100] Thus the ACOG[67] recommends a 7-day course of antimicrobial therapy when PPROM is diagnosed. The best antibiotic regimen is not known with certainty, although intravenous ampicillin and erythromycin (48 hours), followed by oral amoxicillin and erythromycin (5 days), is a commonly used regimen for women with PPROM who are receiving expectant management; a single dose of oral azithromycin can be used as an alternative to erythromycin.[67] Regardless of exposure to latency antibiotics, prolonged expectant management for PPROM is a known risk for chorioamnionitis and maternal sepsis (see Chapter 36).

Fetal Well-Being

If not previously administered, a single course of antenatal steroids is recommended for patients diagnosed with PPROM between 24 0/7 and 33 6/7 weeks' gestation; a single course of late-preterm antenatal corticosteroids can also be offered to appropriately selected patients with PPROM diagnosed between 34 0/7 and 36 6/7 weeks' gestation in whom delivery is planned in greater than 24 hours but no more than 7 days from the time of diagnosis.[67] The benefit of a rescue course of antenatal steroids in the setting of PPROM remains uncertain. In a 2023 double-blind, randomized controlled trial that included 386 patients with PPROM, administration of rescue steroids did not improve neonatal morbidity or mortality, but was well tolerated without increased rates of maternal chorioamnionitis or neonatal sepsis.[101]

Magnesium is recommended for fetal neuroprotection for patients with PPROM at less than 32 weeks' gestation in which delivery is imminent. Intrapartum antibiotics for GBS prophylaxis are additionally indicated for patients in preterm labor following PPROM.[67]

Tocolysis

Historically, obstetricians have worried that tocolytic therapy in patients with PPROM may suppress labor in the setting of subclinical infection, thereby increasing the risk for maternal and neonatal infectious morbidity. A systematic review and metaanalysis demonstrated that while tocolysis prolongs pregnancy latency following PPROM, it was associated with increased rates of maternal chorioamnionitis without measurable improvement in neonatal outcomes.[102] However, interpretation of these data is limited by inconsistent administration of latency antibiotics and antenatal steroids in the included studies. Data remain insufficient to guide recommendations regarding the use of tocolytic agents in patients with PPROM.

Delivery Timing

Over half of patients diagnosed with PPROM will deliver within 7 days of membrane rupture. For patients remaining pregnant, the length of pregnancy latency following PPROM is inversely correlated with the gestational age at diagnosis.[67] PPROM is associated with increased risk of intrauterine infection and placental abruption. Contraindications to expectant management of PPROM include chorioamnionitis, significant placental abruption, and nonreassuring fetal testing. PPROM is also associated with increased risk for umbilical cord prolapse, particularly in the setting of fetal malpresentation, which necessitates emergency cesarean delivery.

In the absence of contraindications, patients diagnosed with PPROM between 24 0/7 and 33 6/7 weeks' gestation should be offered expectant management in a monitored inpatient setting. Historically, delivery has been recommended at 34 0/7 weeks' gestation (or at the time of diagnosis if after 34 weeks) for patients with PPROM. However, the landmark immediate delivery versus expectant care of women with preterm prelabour rupture of membranes close to term (PPROMT) trial[103] provides compelling evidence that there may be neonatal benefit to prolonging expectant management of PPROM past 34 weeks. The PPROMT study was an international, multicenter, randomized controlled trial including 1839 patients, in which participants with PPROM between 34 0/7 and 36 6/7 weeks' gestation without evidence of chorioamnionitis were randomized to immediate delivery or expectant management.[103] Approximately 20% of participants in both study arms were diagnosed with PPROM prior to 34 weeks' gestation and were expectantly managed per typical obstetric guidelines prior to eligibility for randomization at 34 0/7 weeks' gestation. While there were no differences in incidence of neonatal sepsis (2% immediate delivery versus 3% expectant management), the incidence of neonatal respiratory distress syndrome and need for mechanical ventilation was significantly lower in the expectant management group. Although the incidence of adverse maternal events was overall low, the rates of maternal hemorrhage and intrapartum fever were significantly higher in the expectant management group.[103] Based on these data, the ACOG states both immediate delivery and expectant management are reasonable strategies for patients with PPROM between 34 0/7 and 36 6/7 weeks' gestation.[67] For patients electing expectant management of PPROM past 34 weeks' gestation, latency antibiotics are not recommended, and delivery no later than 37 0/7 weeks' gestation is advised.

Previable and Periviable Preterm Premature Rupture of Membranes

PPROM prior to fetal viability is rare, occurring in fewer than 1% of pregnancies.[67] Rupture of membranes prior to 22 weeks' gestation carries a particularly guarded pregnancy prognosis, with high rates of intrauterine fetal demise and neonatal demise. The presence of adequate amniotic fluid volume in the second trimester plays a critical role in normal fetal development. Pregnancies complicated by PPROM occurring prior to 22 weeks' gestation are therefore at increased vulnerability for serious fetal complications, including pulmonary hypoplasia and Potter sequence.

The risks of early PPROM are not limited to fetal morbidity. In a study of 174 patients diagnosed with previable PPROM between 14 0/7 and 22 6/7 weeks' gestation, 14% experienced at least one component of composite maternal morbidity, including sepsis, intensive care unit (ICU) admission, acute kidney injury (AKI), need for surgical intervention (uterine curettage or hysterectomy), VTE, blood transfusion, readmission, or maternal death.[104] A retrospective cohort study of patients with PPROM between 14 0/7 and 23 6/7 weeks' gestation evaluated outcomes among 100 patients who elected for immediate termination of pregnancy compared to 108 patients who elected for expectant management.[105] Expectantly managed patients had 3.57-fold greater odds of composite maternal morbidity compared to patients who terminated their pregnancy, including systemic infection (chorioamnionitis, endometritis, or sepsis), unplanned operative procedure (dilation and curettage, laparoscopy, laparotomy, hysterotomy unrelated to cesarean delivery, or hysterectomy), uterine rupture, hemorrhage, blood transfusion, ICU admission, AKI, VTE, and readmission.

When balancing the high likelihood of adverse fetal/neonatal outcomes against the potentially severe maternal risks of expectant management, many patients diagnosed with previable and periviable PPROM elect for pregnancy termination. However, following the enactment of several statewide abortion bans in the United States, affected states have reported dramatic changes in expectant management of periviable PPROM. The impact of new abortion legislation that mandates expectant management of patients at less than 22 weeks' gestation presenting with severe pregnancy complications, including periviable PPROM, was analyzed at two major Texas hospitals in 2021.[106] Notably, expectant management of these pregnancies resulted in a 57% incidence of composite maternal morbidity compared to a 33% incidence of morbidity among medically comparable patients undergoing immediate pregnancy interruption in states without restrictive abortion legislation. In 2022 the United States Supreme Court *Dobbs v. Jackson Women's Health Organization (Dobbs)* ruling reversed the long-standing *Roe v. Wade* decision, rescinding the constitutional right to abortion.[107] A decision analytical modeling study based on publicly available data projected that compulsory expectant management of periviable PPROM would result in at least 454 additional cases of maternal morbidity and 202 additional cases of hemorrhage annually in the United States.[108]

Available studies regarding neonatal outcomes following previable and periviable PPROM are subject to selection bias, as they include only patients who elected to continue their pregnancy. In the setting of PPROM prior to 22 weeks' gestation, the rate of neonatal survival is estimated at only 14% to 22% compared to 58% in the setting of membrane rupture between 22 0/7 and 23 6/7 weeks' gestation (see earlier discussion). While the ACOG states that latency antibiotics can be considered as early as 20 0/7 weeks' gestation for patients with previable PPROM electing for expectant management, the administration of antenatal corticosteroids, magnesium for fetal neuroprotection, GBS prophylaxis, and tocolytics are not recommended before viability.[67]

CERCLAGE REMOVAL

Cerclage removal does not routinely precipitate the labor process in asymptomatic patients. When term vaginal delivery is planned, cerclage removal at 36 to 37 weeks' gestation is recommended. By contrast, in cases of planned cesarean delivery, it is permissible to defer cerclage removal until the time of delivery. However, labor may occur before the planned delivery date, and removal may need to be performed urgently to prevent injury to the cervix.

Cerclage removal is usually a straightforward procedure. With the patient in the dorsal lithotomy position, a speculum is inserted. The suture is grasped with ringed forceps, and the suture beneath the knot is transected with scissors. In most cases, bedside removal of a cerclage in either the ambulatory or inpatient setting is appropriate.[109] Occasionally, the entire stitch becomes embedded within the cervical mucosa (i.e., "buried"), and neuraxial anesthesia (see later discussion) may be required to facilitate cervical dissection and cerclage removal.

There is a paucity of data to guide management of women with a cerclage who subsequently experience PPROM or preterm labor. Patients presenting with preterm contractions should have a sterile speculum examination to evaluate if the cerclage is on tension. For patients with isolated preterm contractions in whom the cerclage remains off tension, the decision to remove the cerclage can be a difficult one, as cerclage retention may prolong pregnancy if the patient's symptoms arrest without delivery. However, management of preterm labor should not be influenced by the presence of a cerclage; if the patient demonstrates cervical change, persistent painful contractions, or vaginal bleeding, the cerclage should be promptly removed.[109]

Cerclage retention in the setting of stable PPROM without subsequent onset of preterm labor remains controversial. In some studies, cerclage retention following PPROM has been associated with increased incidence of both maternal and neonatal infectious morbidity, as well as neonatal respiratory distress syndrome. However, other studies have not identified these associations. Given current evidence, it is reasonable to either remove or retain the cerclage after diagnosis of PPROM through shared decision-making. However, evidence of intrauterine infection is a strict contraindication to continued cerclage retention.

DELIVERY OF THE PRETERM INFANT

Mode of Delivery

In the absence of contraindications to vaginal delivery, preterm birth at any gestational age is not considered a contraindication for a trial of labor. A retrospective analysis of 2466 very low birth weight (VLBW) preterm infants (<1500 g) delivered in the state of Washington between 1994 and 2003 did not demonstrate any benefit of cesarean delivery for improving survival.[110] In a study published in 2012, Reddy et al.[111] examined neonatal outcomes by mode of delivery for singleton pregnancies with a fetus in cephalic presentation delivering between 24 0/7 and 31 6/7 weeks' gestation. Even among extremely preterm infants, no differences were observed in neonatal mortality or other adverse neonatal outcomes between neonates born vaginally and those born by elective cesarean. Vacuum-assisted operative vaginal delivery should not be routinely performed prior to 34 weeks' gestation; forceps-assisted delivery is preferred in this population if operative vaginal delivery is indicated.

In the setting of progressing preterm labor or medically indicated preterm delivery, cesarean delivery is recommended for fetal malpresentation or nonreassuring fetal status after 25 weeks' gestation, although it can be considered as early as 23 weeks' gestation after appropriate counseling.[1] A systematic review of seven studies involving more than 3500 women concluded that cesarean delivery reduces neonatal morbidity compared with vaginal delivery for breech presentation.[112] Compared to breech infants delivered vaginally at term, head entrapment behind an incompletely dilated cervix is more common in breech preterm infants because the head measures disproportionately larger than the wedge formed by the buttocks and thighs. Similarly, cesarean delivery has been recommended for preterm twins in whom the presenting fetus has a nonvertex presentation.[113] Vaginal delivery can be offered for appropriately selected twin pregnancies in which the presenting twin is cephalic.

Notably, cesarean delivery likely offers minimal long-term neonatal benefit compared to vaginal delivery for breech presentation in the periviable period. A systematic review and metaanalysis compared neonatal outcomes for breech infants delivered vaginally compared with cesarean delivery between 23 0/7 and 24 6/7 weeks' gestation. While short-term survival was improved for breech neonates delivered by cesarean, major neonatal morbidity events were more common following cesarean delivery; there was no survival benefit to cesarean delivery for neonates with birthweight < 500 g, and 6-month survival outcomes were equivalent between the vaginal and cesarean delivery groups.[114]

Patients delivering by cesarean at early gestational ages and/or with VLBW infants are more likely to require a classical uterine incision (vertical hysterotomy involving the contractile portion of the uterus) due to underdevelopment of the lower uterine segment. Compared to cesarean delivery via a low-transverse uterine incision, cesarean delivery by classical uterine incision may result in increased intraoperative blood loss and longer operative time due to the need for a multilayer uterine closure. Aside from operative risks in the index pregnancy, a history of classical cesarean delivery increases the risk for complications in subsequent pregnancies. Due to elevated risk of uterine rupture following a classical cesarean delivery, future trial of labor is contraindicated, and earlier repeat cesarean delivery at 36 to 37 weeks' gestation is indicated in subsequent pregnancies (see Chapter 20). A history of preterm low transverse cesarean delivery is not associated with increased risk of uterine rupture in subsequent pregnancy compared to patients with a history of low transverse cesarean delivery at term.[115]

In balancing maternal risks against the guarded outcomes for neonates born at periviability, decision-making regarding whether to perform cesarean delivery for fetal indications in the periviable period involves complex shared decision-making between patients and their obstetric providers (see Chapter 32). The neonatologist is frequently asked to speak with the patient about the risk for neonatal morbidity and mortality so that the patient can make an informed decision about the method of delivery. For patients electing for full fetal intervention, fetal indications for periviable cesarean encompass emergency obstetric conditions associated with high risk of intrauterine fetal demise, such as prolonged fetal bradycardia, category III FHR tracing, advanced preterm labor with fetal malpresentation, or umbilical cord prolapse. For patients declining periviable cesarean delivery, fetal assessment should be limited to intermittent FHR checks. When a gestational age is reached at which the patient desires cesarean delivery for fetal indications, external FHR monitoring may be initiated to evaluate fetal well-being. It is important for anesthesia providers to be aware of plans regarding both fetal monitoring and mode of delivery in these clinical scenarios so emergency cesarean delivery can be safely facilitated, if indicated.

Ethical Considerations

The antenatal maternal administration of corticosteroids, the application of advanced neonatal ventilation techniques, the use of neonatal surfactant therapy and extracorporeal membrane oxygenation have reduced mortality and morbidity for preterm neonates.[9] Unfortunately, these interventions are often futile for preventing neonatal mortality at extremely early gestational ages (i.e., less than 22 0/7 to 23 0/7 weeks). For infants born at the cusp of viability, the chance of survival, and particularly survival without long-term major adverse outcomes, remains low and difficult to predict for any individual neonate. These uncertainties often lead to controversy about the decision to provide resuscitation versus comfort care for the periviable infant. Parents, obstetricians, and neonatologists should all be involved in the decision-making process.[1]

Anesthesia providers may find themselves in the middle of these ethical dilemmas if they are practicing at a location in which the anesthesia provider is responsible for neonatal resuscitation. Although no firm rules exist, some basic principles can be applied. First, the parents should have a critical role in the decision-making process. Second, as much data as possible should be obtained to provide a prognostic assessment. The NICHD Extremely Preterm Birth Outcomes Tool allows providers to input readily available patient data to estimate preterm birth outcomes based on US hospital birth data collected from 2006 to 2012.[116] Third, discussion of these issues ideally should be held before delivery, not in the moment of crisis. The ACOG[1] has published general recommendations about the care of infants on the threshold of viability but has not made specific recommendations for neonatal resuscitation on the basis of gestational age.

Withholding and/or discontinuation of life-sustaining treatment during or following resuscitation are considered by many to be ethically equivalent; it is considered reasonable to withdraw support when the possibility of functional survival is highly unlikely. In cases of very early gestation (gestational age < 22 to 23 weeks), extremely low birth weight (<400 g), and life-limiting anomalies, resuscitation is generally not advised. Resuscitation is nearly always indicated in conditions associated with a high survival rate and acceptable morbidity, which generally includes infants with a gestational age ≥ 25 weeks. In conditions associated with uncertain prognosis, parental desires regarding resuscitation should be supported.[117]

Fetal Monitoring

Most obstetricians use continuous electronic FHR monitoring once preterm labor becomes established if the gestational age and circumstances are consistent with the possibility of neonatal survival. Preterm gestation may complicate the interpretation of FHR patterns, given that the FHR pattern of preterm fetuses may have relatively decreased variability and magnitude of accelerations compared with the FHR pattern of term fetuses.[118]

The value of continuous electronic FHR monitoring over intermittent auscultation of the FHR remains controversial. Luthy et al.[119] performed a randomized trial comparing continuous electronic FHR monitoring (with selective fetal blood gas assessment) with periodic auscultation of the FHR during preterm labor in women with fetuses weighing between 700 and 1750 g. There was no significant difference between groups in the incidence of cesarean delivery, low 5-minute Apgar scores, intrapartum acidosis, intracranial hemorrhage, or perinatal death. A metaanalysis, which added a second trial, also showed no benefit to continuous FHR monitoring in preventing cerebral palsy (RR, 1.75; 95% CI, 0.84 to 3.63).[80] In a follow-up study of the infants included in the Luthy et al. study[119] at 18 months of age, the incidence of cerebral palsy was significantly higher in the electronic FHR group than in the intermittent auscultation group (20% versus 8%, respectively).[120]

ANESTHETIC MANAGEMENT

Anesthesia providers often participate in the care of women with preterm delivery. Many women who deliver preterm request neuraxial analgesia for labor and vaginal delivery. These patients may also require cesarean delivery (e.g., nonreassuring fetal status, cord prolapse) and may require urgent administration of anesthesia. For patients admitted to the inpatient antepartum unit at risk for unscheduled preterm delivery, additional anesthetic considerations may include exposure to VTE chemoprophylaxis and maintenance of adequate long-term peripheral venous access.

Conventional wisdom holds that the preterm fetus is more vulnerable than the term fetus to the depressant effects of analgesic and anesthetic drugs, for the following reasons: (1) less fetal serum protein available for drug binding and reduced protein-drug affinity, leading to increased circulating free drug levels; (2) higher levels of bilirubin, which may compete with the drug for protein binding, also leading to increased circulating drug levels; (3) greater drug access to the central nervous system because of the presence of an incomplete blood-brain barrier; (4) decreased ability to metabolize and excrete drugs; and (5) a higher incidence of acidosis during labor and delivery.[121-123] However, few controlled studies have documented the maternal and fetal pharmacokinetics and pharmacodynamics of anesthetic agents throughout gestation. The preterm fetus may be less vulnerable to the depressant effects of local anesthetics than originally thought. The human fetal liver cytochrome P450 system is present as early as 14 weeks' gestation and has the capability to oxidize several drugs.[124,125]

Perinatal Effects of Maternal Local Anesthetic Administration

Information about the fetal effects of maternal exposure to local anesthetics is largely extrapolated from studies in animal models. Teramo et al.[126] noted that higher doses of lidocaine were necessary to produce seizure activity in preterm fetal lambs than in later gestation fetal lambs. These investigators also observed that the cardiovascular response to lidocaine (i.e., increases in blood pressure and heart rate) was less severe in preterm fetuses.

Pedersen et al.[127] evaluated the effects of gestational age on the pharmacokinetics and pharmacodynamics of lidocaine in gravid ewes and fetal lambs. They studied two groups of animals, preterm (mean 119 days' gestation or 0.8 of term pregnancy) and near-term (mean 138 days' gestation or 0.95 of term pregnancy). They administered an intravenous infusion of lidocaine to obtain a maternal steady-state plasma concentration of 2 μg/mL. Transplacental transfer of lidocaine did not adversely affect fetal cardiac output, organ blood flow, or blood gas and acid-base measurements in either group. Tissue uptake of lidocaine was overall similar in the two groups of fetal lambs, although uptake was greater in the lungs and liver of the term fetuses. The investigators concluded that there was no significant difference in the pharmacokinetics and pharmacodynamics of lidocaine between preterm and near-term fetal lambs.[127] Smedstad et al.[128] also concluded that there was no difference in fetal blood pressure, heart rate, or blood gas measurements in response to maternal intravenous infusion of lidocaine or bupivacaine between early-preterm (119 days' gestation) and late-preterm (132 days' gestation) fetal lambs. In addition, the plasma concentrations of bupivacaine and lidocaine and the fetal-to-maternal ratios of both drugs were similar in the two groups of fetuses.

Notably, these studies did not evaluate the effects of anesthetic agents on the acidotic preterm fetus. Asphyxia may increase the risk for adverse effects by causing the following changes in the fetal environment: (1) increased drug ionization in the fetal circulation due to interaction with excess ionized hydrogen in the setting of fetal acidemia; (2) "ion trapping" of the ionized drug in fetal tissue causing impaired drug diffusion with resultant diminished drug clearance[129]; (3) increased maternal-to-fetal transplacental drug transfer, likely due to widened maternal-to-fetal unionized drug concentration gradient secondary to fetal ion trapping[129]; and (4) enhanced susceptibility to the myocardial depressant effects of local anesthetics.[130,131] Morishima et al.[130] subjected a group of preterm fetal lambs (0.8 of term gestation) to asphyxia by causing partial occlusion of the umbilical cord. They subsequently administered either lidocaine or saline-control intravenously to the gravid ewes for 180 minutes. The mean ($\pm$ standard deviation) maternal and fetal steady-state plasma lidocaine concentrations were 2.32 ± 0.12 and $1.23 \pm 0.17\,\mu g/mL$, respectively, which are concentrations comparable to those achieved during administration of epidural anesthesia in humans. Umbilical cord occlusion resulted in the typical fetal compensatory response to hypoxia (i.e., decreased FHR and increased blood flow to the fetal brain, heart, and adrenal glands). Maternal administration of saline-control did not result in additional deterioration of the fetus. However, maternal administration of lidocaine resulted in a significant increase in $Paco_2$, and decreases in pH; mean arterial pressure (MAP); and blood flow to the brain, myocardium, and adrenal glands. Thus lidocaine attenuated the normal fetal compensatory response to asphyxia.

In an earlier study, the same investigators observed that lidocaine did not affect the fetal compensatory response to asphyxia in term fetuses.[131] They concluded that "the immature fetus loses its cardiovascular adaptation to asphyxia when exposed to clinically acceptable plasma concentrations of lidocaine obtained transplacentally from the mother."[130] Limitations of this study include (1) a failure to compare the fetal response to lidocaine with the response to other anesthetic, analgesic, or sedative drugs and (2) consideration of only the effects of a steady-state concentration of lidocaine in the presence of asphyxia. Furthermore, the investigators did not evaluate the potential benefits derived from epidural anesthesia, such as reduced maternal concentrations of catecholamines and the ability of epidural anesthesia to facilitate a controlled, atraumatic delivery of the preterm infant.

Bupivacaine has a low fetal-to-maternal plasma concentration ratio because of its high (96%) maternal protein binding and therefore was hypothesized to have lower potential for fetal toxicity.[122] However, studies of the impact of bupivacaine on the compensatory response to asphyxia in preterm fetal lambs have demonstrated detrimental effects similar to those seen with lidocaine. Santos et al.[132] observed that bupivacaine abolished the compensatory increase in blood flow to vital organs in asphyxiated preterm fetal lambs but did not affect FHR, blood pressure, or acid-base measurements. The investigators suggested that these changes were less severe than those seen with lidocaine in earlier studies.[130,132]

Ropivacaine may have a more favorable safety profile than bupivacaine with respect to the preterm fetus. Ropivacaine and bupivacaine have almost identical dissociation constants (pK_a of 8.0 and 8.2, respectively). However, in contrast to bupivacaine, ropivacaine has slightly lower protein binding (92% ropivacaine versus 96% bupivacaine) and is substantially less lipid soluble (see Chapter 13).[133] These differences may affect maternal and fetal free plasma concentrations of drug. Investigators have documented higher maternal and fetal plasma concentrations with ropivacaine than with bupivacaine.[134,135] Studies suggest that ropivacaine is less cardiotoxic than bupivacaine. However, no study has evaluated the effect of ropivacaine on the fetal compensatory response to hypoxia.

2-Chloroprocaine is also a suitable local anesthetic to use for the mother of a preterm fetus because it is rapidly metabolized in both the maternal plasma and fetal plasma.[136] Further, placental transfer of 2-chloroprocaine is not increased by fetal acidosis.[137]

Vaginal Delivery

Neuraxial labor analgesia decreases maternal concentrations of catecholamines, ameliorating cycles of maternal hypoventilation and hyperventilation, and may thereby improve uteroplacental perfusion as long as hypotension is avoided.[138] No prospective, controlled studies have evaluated the effect of neuraxial labor analgesia on preterm infant outcomes. The timing of the intrapartum administration of neuraxial analgesia in preterm parturients may be problematic for several reasons. First, there may be uncertainty as to whether patients presenting with preterm contractions are in labor. Second, even women with a clear diagnosis of preterm labor often have a prolonged latent phase of labor, independent of the use of tocolytic agents. Third, once active labor is established, patients' labor often progresses rapidly. Thus in some cases, it may be appropriate to establish neuraxial analgesia even before knowing that a preterm delivery will soon occur. An advantage of early initiation of neuraxial analgesia is the ability to rapidly convert labor analgesia to surgical anesthesia if emergency cesarean delivery should be necessary.

Cesarean Delivery

If cesarean delivery is necessary, conventional wisdom holds that it is preferable to administer either epidural or spinal anesthesia to avoid the depressant effects of agents given for general anesthesia. Rolbin et al.[139] observed that preterm infants exposed to epidural anesthesia for cesarean delivery had higher 1- and 5-minute Apgar scores than similar infants exposed to general anesthesia. Laudenbach et al.[140] performed a secondary analysis of prospectively gathered data from a population-based cohort study of all deliveries before 33 weeks' gestation in nine regions in France in 1997 ($n = 1338$). Of concern, after controlling for known confounders, infants born by cesarean delivery to mothers who received spinal anesthesia had a higher mortality rate than those born to mothers who received general or epidural anesthesia (adjusted odd ratio [OR] 1.7; 95% CI, 1.1 to 2.6).[140] However, the authors noted that the secondary analysis of a preexisting database did not allow them to adjust for confounders known to affect anesthetic and fetal outcomes (e.g., intraoperative hypotension, choice of vasopressor, fluid management). Nonetheless, it seems reasonable that anesthesia providers should pay meticulous attention to maternal hemodynamic variables for these high-risk births, regardless of the type of anesthesia that is administered.

The administration of general anesthesia for preterm cesarean delivery is similar to that for parturients at term (see Chapter 26). Most anesthetic agents that are used for induction and maintenance of general anesthesia cross the placenta. Data from animal studies suggest that exposure of the immature brain to anesthetic agents such as propofol, thiopental, ketamine, and inhalation agents can trigger significant brain cell apoptosis in the developing fetal/neonatal brain and cause functional learning deficits in later life.[141,142] However, in these animal studies, the duration of exposure to anesthetic agents was much longer than is typical for cesarean delivery in humans. Whether clinical exposure to anesthetic agents during general anesthesia for cesarean delivery results in clinically significant brain cell apoptosis in humans remains to be determined (see Chapter 10).

The term pregnant patient requires significantly less local anesthetic to achieve adequate surgical anesthesia than nonpregnant women (see Chapter 2). There are limited data about spinal dose requirements for cesarean delivery in preterm parturients. A retrospective study of over 5000 patients investigated the association between gestational age and the risk for inadequate spinal anesthesia for cesarean delivery.[143] The incidence of neuraxial block failure correlated inversely with gestational age, decreasing from 10.8% for women who were less than 28 weeks' gestation, to 7.7% for those between 28 and 32 weeks, and 5.3% or less for those beyond 32 weeks. In multivariable analysis, the association of gestational age with block failure was not significant; however, birth weight < 2500 g was associated with a 2.5-fold increased odds of failed neuraxial anesthesia.[143]

In summary, there is insufficient evidence to support altering the anesthetic technique for cesarean delivery of the preterm infant. Further study is necessary to determine whether one technique or medication has specific risks or benefits relative to the preterm infant.

Anesthesia for Cerclage Placement and Cerclage Removal

Cerclage placement requires a T10 level of surgical anesthesia (see Chapter 17). Frequently, cerclage placement is a brief surgical procedure lasting less than 30 minutes, although increased surgical complexity related to atypical cervical anatomy or need for cervical dissection can extend the procedure. For patients undergoing placement of an examination-indicated cerclage, the presence of advanced cervical dilation or prolapsing membranes can pose surgical challenges that may increase operative time. In addition, patient characteristics (e.g., class III obesity) may extend the duration required for positioning and increase the risks associated with unplanned

induction of general anesthesia. The optimal anesthetic technique also depends on the obstetric plan, specifically whether the patient will be admitted for prolonged observation or will be discharged home. Shorter-acting spinal anesthetics may accelerate recovery and discharge for those going home. For those who will be admitted for postprocedural monitoring, a longer-duration spinal anesthetic or a catheter-based neuraxial technique may be appropriate.

Cerclage removal does not typically require anesthesia, but surgical anesthesia may be necessary if the stitch is embedded (i.e., "buried") under the cervical mucosa. In this circumstance, spinal anesthesia for cerclage removal requires a T10 sensory level and, depending on gestational age and fetal weight, may result in excessive blockade if doses typically used for early second-trimester cerclage placement are used. The decision to utilize a catheter-based technique or single-shot spinal anesthesia depends on the obstetric plan, specifically, whether the patient will remain in hospital for delivery or will be discharged home to await spontaneous labor.

Venous Thromboembolism Prophylaxis

Obstetric VTE is a leading cause of maternal morbidity and mortality (see Chapter 38). Antepartum hospitalization and prolonged immobility increase the risk for VTE, particularly among obese women. Several professional societies recommend pharmacologic VTE prophylaxis for prolonged antepartum admissions, although the suggested dosing regimens are not uniform.[144] For example, the National Partnership for Maternal Safety recommends daily thromboprophylaxis with low-molecular-weight heparin, or twice-daily thromboprophylaxis with unfractionated heparin, for all antepartum patients hospitalized for more than 72 hours deemed low risk for acute bleeding or imminent delivery. With wider adoption of these VTE guidelines, an increasing number of pregnant women will present for neuraxial analgesia or anesthesia having received pharmacologic anticoagulation. Strategies to ensure safe neuraxial blockade for women receiving anticoagulant drugs are discussed in Chapter 38 and are addressed by consensus documents from the Society for Obstetric Anesthesia and Perinatology[145] and the American Society of Regional Anesthesia.[146] Regular, ongoing communication between obstetricians and anesthesia providers to discuss women admitted to the hospital for antepartum care is required to ensure that evolving plans for delivery or surgical intervention appropriately inform optimal anticoagulation and anesthetic management.[145]

Intravenous Access

Antenatal patients admitted for management of threatened preterm labor, PPROM, and other pregnancy complications that may result in preterm delivery (e.g., preeclampsia, fetal growth restriction, placental abruption) may remain in the hospital for several weeks. Maintaining appropriate intravenous access for these patients throughout hospitalization can sometimes be challenging. Although subject to infiltration, occlusion, and need for frequent replacement, peripheral venous access should be maintained in hospitalized antepartum patients. Although central venous catheters are commonly used to maintain long-term intravenous access in nonpregnant inpatients, their routine use should be avoided in pregnancy due to a high risk of catheter-associated infectious morbidity.[147]

INTERACTIONS BETWEEN TOCOLYTIC THERAPY AND ANESTHESIA

Indications for Anesthesia During and After Tocolytic Therapy

There are several situations in which obstetric patients require analgesia or anesthesia during or after tocolytic therapy. First, preterm labor may progress, and delivery may occur despite tocolysis. In this case, the patient may desire pain relief during labor and vaginal delivery or may require anesthesia for cesarean delivery. Second, some obstetricians advocate the bolus injection of a tocolytic agent when there is a tetanic uterine contraction or tachysystole in the setting of FHR abnormality. Third, a tocolytic may be administered for uterine relaxation when attempting external cephalic version (a procedure that may also involve neuraxial analgesia) or during fetal surgery. Finally, magnesium, although no longer routinely used for tocolysis, is commonly administered to obstetric patients for fetal neuroprotection and maternal seizure prophylaxis. Typical dose regimens for drugs used for tocolysis are listed in Table 33.7.

TABLE 33.7   Tocolytic Dose Regimens for Preterm Labor

Drug	Initiation Dose	Maintenance Dose
Nifedipine (immediate release)	20–30 mg PO	10–20 mg every 4–6 h
Cyclooxygenase inhibitors (NSAIDs)[a]:		
Indomethacin	50–100 mg PO or PR	25–50 mg every 6 h
Ketorolac	60 mg IM	30 mg every 6 h
Sulindac	200 mg PO	200 mg every 12 h
Terbutaline[b]	0.25 mg SQ	0.25 mg every 20 min to 3 h
Magnesium sulfate	4–6 g IV bolus over 20 min	2 g/h continuous IV infusion

IM, Intramuscularly; *IV*, intravenously; *NSAIDs*, nonsteroidal antiinflammatory drugs; *PO*, per os (orally); *PR*, per rectum; *SQ*, subcutaneously.
[a]NSAID administration should be limited to 48–72 h and restricted to gestations < 32 w.
[b]Treatment with terbutaline should not be used beyond 48–72 h. In particular, injectable terbutaline should not be used in the outpatient or home setting.

Calcium Entry–Blocking Agents

The calcium entry–blocking agent **nifedipine** has undergone the most extensive evaluation in this class; it has been proposed by some as a first-line therapy for treatment of preterm labor.

Mechanism of Action

Calcium entry–blocking agents block the aqueous voltage-dependent cell membrane channels that are selective for calcium and prevent calcium release from the sarcoplasmic reticulum. The net result is a decrease in available intracellular calcium, which inhibits MLCK activity. This inhibition leads to decreased actin-myosin interaction, which results in the relaxation of smooth muscle (including myometrial smooth muscle).[148]

Side Effects

Nifedipine has fewer side effects than beta-adrenergic receptor agonists (see Table 33.6). Common side effects include headache, flushing, dizziness, palpitations, and nausea.[149] Most effects are mild, but pulmonary edema[150] has been reported. Nifedipine induces significant afterload reduction. This triggers a compensatory increase in cardiac output, which is usually well tolerated,[151] but may increase the risk for demand myocardial ischemia or heart failure in women with underlying cardiac disease.

Although some initial animal studies raised concern that nifedipine and nicardipine could decrease uterine blood flow and increase fetal hypoxemia and acidosis, clinical studies have not demonstrated these outcomes.[151–153]

Anesthetic Management

Nifedipine has fewer effects on cardiac conduction than some of the other calcium entry–blocking agents; however, it may cause vasodilation, hypotension, myocardial depression, and conduction defects when used in combination with volatile halogenated anesthetic agents.[154] One report noted that administration of both nifedipine and magnesium sulfate was associated with neuromuscular blockade in a patient with preeclampsia at 28 weeks' gestation.[155]

Cyclooxygenase Inhibitors

Indomethacin is the cyclooxygenase inhibitor most typically used for tocolysis, although other agents, such as **sulindac** and **ketorolac**, have been evaluated.

Mechanism of Action

Cyclooxygenase inhibitors inhibit the enzyme cyclooxygenase, and thereby prevent the conversion of arachidonic acid to prostaglandins, which stimulate uterine contractions.

Side Effects

Maternal side effects from indomethacin are minimal when it is used for tocolytic therapy; nausea and heartburn are the most common complaints.[156] Indomethacin is often used to promote closure of the ductus arteriosus in the preterm neonate, causing concern that maternal administration may result in premature ductus closure in the fetus.[156] Moise et al.[157] used fetal echocardiography to evaluate the fetal response to short-term (<72 hours) indomethacin therapy between 26 and 31 weeks' gestation. They observed evidence of transient ductal constriction in 7 of 14 fetuses. Tricuspid regurgitation was also noted in three fetuses. These changes, however, were reversed within 24 hours of discontinuation of indomethacin, and are less likely at earlier gestational ages.[156,158–160] Additionally, studies suggest that clinically significant adverse neonatal effects are unlikely if indomethacin is used in short courses (e.g., 24 to 48 hours).[156,159,160]

Indomethacin administration also may result in fetal oligohydramnios secondary to decreased fetal urine output.[161–163] One proposed mechanism for the decrease in fetal urine output is an enhanced antidiuretic hormone effect.[164] Oligohydramnios secondary to indomethacin administration typically resolves within 1 week after its discontinuation. Wurtzel[165] showed that maternal administration of indomethacin did not significantly alter neonatal renal function. There is no consistent evidence that transient prenatal administration of indomethacin results in poorer neonatal outcomes.[166]

Anesthetic Management

The effects of indomethacin on platelet function are transient. Several large studies have demonstrated the safety of epidural and spinal anesthesia in patients receiving low-dose aspirin or one of a variety of cyclooxygenase inhibitors.[145] Consensus statements from professional anesthesiology societies have concluded that such therapy is not a contraindication to administration of neuraxial anesthesia, but that additional caution is recommended for patients receiving NSAIDs in combination with other pharmacologic anticoagulation (see Chapter 38).[145]

NSAIDs and acetaminophen are key components of effective postcesarean delivery pain management. Administration of ketorolac or other NSAIDs for postoperative analgesia should consider the timing and dose of any previously administered indomethacin.

Beta-Adrenergic Receptor Agonists

The use of the beta-adrenergic receptor agonists, **ritodrine** and **terbutaline**, for tocolysis has declined substantially because of maternal side effects.[91]

Mechanism of Action

Beta$_2$-adrenergic receptors are found in smooth muscle (uterus, blood vessels, bronchi, intestine, detrusor, and spleen capsule) as well as a variety of other tissues. Ritodrine and terbutaline are relatively selective for beta$_2$-adrenergic receptors. Stimulation of these receptors in the myometrium results in relaxation of uterine smooth muscle. Unfortunately, other undesired beta$_2$-adrenergic agonist effects (e.g., vasodilation) and beta$_1$-adrenergic agonist effects (e.g., maternal tachycardia and increased cardiac output) still occur.[167]

Beta-adrenergic agonists interact with beta$_2$-adrenergic receptors on the outer membrane of uterine myometrial cells, activating the enzyme adenyl cyclase, which catalyzes the conversion of ATP to cAMP and causes a decrease in intracellular calcium.[161]

Treatment Regimen

Before initiation of treatment, the provider should obtain baseline maternal vital signs and weight and exclude significant cardiovascular or pulmonary disease. Although terbutaline infusion is now rarely used in US obstetric practice, an individual dose of subcutaneous terbutaline 0.25 mg may be administered as a uterine relaxant to treat tetanic contractions with fetal compromise or to facilitate obstetric procedures such as external cephalic version.

Side Effects

The administration of beta-adrenergic receptor agonist tocolytic therapy has resulted in the following maternal side effects: (1) hypotension; (2) tachycardia, with or without cardiac arrhythmias and myocardial ischemia; (3) pulmonary edema; (4) hyperglycemia; and (5) hypokalemia.[161] The reported frequency of these side effects varies from 0.5% to 9%.[168–170] While the risk of adverse effects is increased by prolonged intravenous infusion, these effects may also be observed following administration of a single dose. Other uncommon maternal side effects reported with the use of beta-adrenergic receptor agonists are elevations in serum transaminase levels,[171] paralytic ileus,[172] cerebral vasospasm in patients with a previous history of migraine,[173] and respiratory arrest caused by increased muscle weakness in a patient with myasthenia gravis.[174]

Anesthetic Management

Ideally, the initiation of anesthesia should be delayed until beta-adrenergic receptor agonist–induced maternal tachycardia subsides. A delay of 15 minutes often results in slowing of the maternal heart rate, although this may not be possible in emergency scenarios. For example, subcutaneous terbutaline is commonly administered to abate tachysystole or tetanic contractions resulting in significant fetal decelerations or bradycardia. If fetal bradycardia persists despite treatment, emergency cesarean delivery may be required. Published reports of anesthetic management after administration of a beta-adrenergic receptor agonist are scarce.[175–179] Ravindran et al.[177] reported one case each of intraoperative pulmonary edema, sinus tachycardia, and ventricular arrhythmia during general anesthesia in patients who had received terbutaline therapy immediately before or 15 minutes after the induction of anesthesia.

Theoretically, induction of epidural analgesia or anesthesia after beta-adrenergic receptor agonist therapy may cause less hemodynamic compromise than spinal anesthesia because of the slower onset of sympathetic blockade. However, this theory remains unproven. Patients receiving beta-adrenergic receptor agonist therapy are at risk for development of pulmonary edema. Therefore, aggressive hydration should be avoided before and during the induction of anesthesia in these patients.

If general anesthesia is required in a patient who has recently received tocolysis with a beta-adrenergic receptor agonist, agents that might exacerbate maternal tachycardia (e.g., atropine, glycopyrrolate, ephedrine, norepinephrine) should be avoided. Residual maternal tachycardia may make it more difficult to assess volume status and depth of anesthesia. Hyperventilation should be avoided because it may exacerbate hypokalemia and potentiate the hyperpolarization of the cell membrane. In nonpregnant patients, Slater et al.[180] found that terbutaline pretreatment shortened the onset time and recovery of succinylcholine-induced neuromuscular blockade. It seems prudent to monitor neuromuscular function with a peripheral nerve stimulator during general anesthesia.

Oxytocin Receptor Antagonists

Atosiban (1-deamino-2-D-Tyr-[OEt]-4-Thr-8-Orn-vasotocin/oxytocin) is an oxytocin receptor antagonist. It is a competitive inhibitor of oxytocin that binds to both myometrial and decidual receptors. It does not alter the subsequent sensitivity of the myometrium to oxytocin.[181] Clinically, this feature represents a major advantage; it should reduce the risk for postpartum uterine atony and hemorrhage.

Studies have suggested that atosiban has efficacy similar to that of beta-adrenergic receptor agonists and nifedipine in obtaining and maintaining uterine quiescence. Phase II and III studies have shown that atosiban has few maternal side effects, undergoes minimal placental transfer, and does not increase maternal blood loss at delivery.[94,95,182] The FDA has not approved atosiban for use in the United States because of a higher rate of perinatal deaths in the atosiban arm of the study that it reviewed.[94]

There are no data on the interaction between atosiban and anesthetic agents. However, given the hemodynamic profile of this agent, one would not expect significant interactions. Atosiban is widely used in Europe.

Magnesium Sulfate

Mechanism of Action

Extracellular magnesium functions as a competitive antagonist of calcium, thus reducing calcium influx into the uterine myocyte.[161]

Side Effects

Magnesium sulfate results in less frequent and less severe cardiovascular side effects than beta-adrenergic receptor agonist tocolytic agents.[183–185] Nonetheless, magnesium sulfate may lead to chest pain and tightness, palpitations, nausea, transient hypotension, blurred vision, sedation, dampened deep tendon reflexes, and pulmonary edema.[184,185] Magnesium

overdose can have serious consequences for both the mother and fetus, including hypotonia, respiratory depression, hypotension, cardiac arrhythmias, and cardiac arrest. It has been hypothesized that intrapartum magnesium exposure may increase the risk of uterine atony resulting in postpartum hemorrhage; however, this has not been demonstrated in metaanalyses.[82,186,187]

Magnesium is eliminated almost entirely by renal excretion. Therefore, patients with abnormal renal function should be monitored carefully. Consideration should be given to administering a lower maintenance dose (i.e., infusion rate) in women with renal dysfunction.

Magnesium infusion is contraindicated for patients with myasthenia gravis due to an inhibitory effect on acetylcholine release.

Anesthetic Management

It has been suggested that magnesium sulfate should be discontinued before the administration of neuraxial analgesia or anesthesia because magnesium may increase the likelihood of hypotension through its generalized vasodilating properties. Vincent et al.[188] observed that magnesium sulfate reduced maternal MAP but not uterine blood flow or fetal oxygenation during epidural lidocaine anesthesia in gravid ewes. This study suggests that hypermagnesemia may increase the likelihood of modest hypotension during neuraxial anesthesia in normotensive parturients. Clinical relevance in humans is debatable; any effect on hemodynamic parameters may be managed with appropriate fluid and vasopressor therapy. Thus routine discontinuation of magnesium therapy is not recommended at the time of induction of analgesia or anesthesia. Magnesium sulfate administered for the purpose of fetal neuroprotection may be discontinued immediately following delivery of the neonate.

Magnesium potentiates the action of both depolarizing and nondepolarizing muscle relaxants.[189] A defasciculating dose of a nondepolarizing muscle relaxant should not be given before administration of succinylcholine in women with hypermagnesemia. A standard intubating dose of muscle relaxant (e.g., succinylcholine 1 mg/kg) should be used because the extent of potentiation by magnesium sulfate is variable.[190] Subsequent nondepolarizing neuromuscular muscle relaxants should be administered only if necessary, at the lowest required dose to facilitate surgery, and with quantitative neuromuscular blockade monitoring.

Parturients receiving magnesium sulfate often appear sedated. Thompson et al.[191] evaluated the anesthetic effects of magnesium sulfate and ritodrine on the minimum alveolar concentration of halothane in pregnant and nonpregnant rats and reported a 20% decrease with serum magnesium levels of 7 to 11 mg/dL. A more detailed discussion of magnesium sulfate, its interactions with anesthetic agents, and management of overdose is found in Chapter 35.

KEY POINTS

- Despite improved antenatal care, the incidence of preterm delivery in the United States remains approximately 10%.
- Preterm birth is a leading cause of neonatal mortality. Survivors have an increased chance of disability.
- Spontaneous preterm labor or preterm premature rupture of membranes account for the majority of preterm births.
- Treatment with tocolytic therapy may prolong pregnancy by up to 48 hours, and thereby facilitate transfer of the patient from a small community hospital to a tertiary care facility, maternal administration of a corticosteroid to accelerate fetal lung maturity, and maternal administration of magnesium for fetal neuroprotection. Long-term tocolytic therapy does not improve neonatal outcome.
- Nifedipine and indomethacin are used commonly to treat preterm labor in the United States; oxytocin receptor antagonists are used in Europe. Magnesium sulfate is not an effective tocolytic but is considered beneficial when used specifically for neuroprotection in reducing rates of cerebral palsy in preterm infants.
- Terbutaline is associated with a high incidence of maternal and fetal side effects, including hypotension, tachycardia (with or without cardiac arrhythmias and myocardial ischemia), pulmonary edema, hyperglycemia, and hypokalemia. Pulmonary edema is the most serious complication, and it may be life threatening.
- Cyclooxygenase inhibitors reversibly inhibit cyclooxygenase, resulting in a transient effect on platelet function. However, their use does not necessitate the assessment of platelet or coagulation function before administration of neuraxial analgesia/anesthesia in a patient whose only risk factor for bleeding is recent ingestion of a cyclooxygenase inhibitor.
- Prior administration of a tocolytic agent, regardless of drug class, does not contraindicate the administration of neuraxial anesthesia.

REFERENCES

1. American College of Obstetricians and Gynecologists. Obstetric Care Consensus No. 6: Periviable birth (reaffirmed 2021). *Obstet Gynecol*. 2017;130:e187–e199.
2. Goldenberg RL, Culhane JF, Iams JD, Romero R. Epidemiology and causes of preterm birth. *Lancet*. 2008;371:75–84.
3. Martin JAHB, Osterman MJK. Births in the United States, 2021. *NCHS Data Brief*. 2022:442.
4. Martin JA, Hamilton BE, Osterman MJK. Births in the United States, 2021. *NCHS Data Brief, No. 442*. National Center for Health Statistics; 2022. https://dx.doi.org/10.15620/cdc:119632.
5. World Health Organization. *Born too soon: decade of action on preterm birth*. World Health Organization; 2023. https://www.who.int/publications/i/item/9789240073890. Accessed 26 July 2024.
6. American College of Obstetricians and Gynecologists. Practice Bulletin No. 234: Prediction and prevention of spontaneous preterm birth (reaffirmed 2025). *Obstet Gynecol*. 2021;138:e65–e90.
7. Wilson-Costello D, Friedman H, Minich N, et al. Improved neurodevelopmental outcomes for extremely low birth weight infants in 2000-2002. *Pediatrics*. 2007;119:37–45.
8. Eichenwald EC, Stark AR. Management and outcomes of very low birth weight. *N Engl J Med*. 2008;358:1700–1711.
9. Stoll BJ, Hansen NI, Bell EF, et al. Trends in care practices, morbidity, and mortality of extremely preterm neonates, 1993-2012. *JAMA*. 2015;314:1039–1051.
10. Srinivasjois R, Nembhard W, Wong K, et al. Risk of mortality into adulthood according to gestational age at birth. *J Pediatr*. 2017;190:185–191.e1.
11. Lemons JA, Bauer CR, Oh W, et al. Very low birth weight outcomes of the National Institute of Child Health and Human Development Neonatal Research Network, January 1995 through December 1996. NICHD Neonatal Research Network. *Pediatrics*. 2001;107:E1.
12. Horbar JD, Carpenter JH, Badger GJ, et al. Mortality and neonatal morbidity among infants 501 to 1500 grams from 2000 to 2009. *Pediatrics*. 2012;129:1019–1026.
13. Younge N, Goldstein RF, Bann CM, et al. Survival and neurodevelopmental outcomes among periviable infants. *N Engl J Med*. 2017;376:617–628.
14. Ancel PY, Livinec F, Larroque B, et al. Cerebral palsy among very preterm children in relation to gestational age and neonatal ultrasound abnormalities: the EPIPAGE cohort study. *Pediatrics*. 2006;117:828–835.
15. Wood NS, Marlow N, Costeloe K, et al. Neurologic and developmental disability after extremely preterm birth. EPICure Study Group. *N Engl J Med*. 2000;343:378–384.
16. Marlow N, Wolke D, Bracewell MA, Samara M. Neurologic and developmental disability at six years of age after extremely preterm birth. *N Engl J Med*. 2005;352:9–19.
17. Keogh J, Sinn J, Hollebone K, et al. Delivery in the 'grey zone': collaborative approach to extremely preterm birth. *Aust N Z J Obstet Gynaecol*. 2007;47:273–278.
18. Heinonen K, Eriksson JG, Lahti J, et al. Late preterm birth and neurocognitive performance in late adulthood: a birth cohort study. *Pediatrics*. 2015;135:e818–e825.
19. Menon R, Bonney EA, Condon J, et al. Novel concepts on pregnancy clocks and alarms: redundancy and synergy in human parturition. *Hum Reprod Update*. 2016;22:535–560.
20. American College of Obstetricians and Gynecologists. Committee Opinion No. 831: Medically indicated late-preterm and early-term deliveries. *Obstet Gynecol*. 2021;138:e35–e39.
21. Goldenberg RL, Hauth JC, Andrews WW. Intrauterine infection and preterm delivery. *N Engl J Med*. 2000;342:1500–1507.
22. Gibbs RS, Romero R, Hillier SL, et al. A review of premature birth and subclinical infection. *Am J Obstet Gynecol*. 1992;166:1515–1528.

23. Boyle AK, Rinaldi SF, Norman JE, Stock SJ. Preterm birth: inflammation, fetal injury and treatment strategies. *J Reprod Immunol.* 2017;119:62–66.

24. Wray S. Uterine contraction and physiological mechanisms of modulation. *Am J Physiol.* 1993;264:C1–C18.

25. Yulia A, Johnson MR. Myometrial oxytocin receptor expression and intracellular pathways. *Minerva Ginecol.* 2014;66:267–280.

26. Lopez Bernal A. Overview. Preterm labour: Mechanisms and management. *BMC Pregnancy Childbirth.* 2007;7:S2.

27. Talati AN, Hackney DN, Mesiano S. Pathophysiology of preterm labor with intact membranes. *Semin Perinatol.* 2017;41:420–426.

28. Behrman RE, Butler AS, Institute of Medicine (U.S.) Committee on Understanding Premature Birth and Assuring Healthy Outcomes. *Preterm Birth: Causes, Consequences, and Prevention.* National Academies Press (US); 2007. http://www.ncbi.nlm.nih.gov/books/NBK11362/. Accessed 24 July 2024.

29. Kagan KO, To M, Tsoi E, Nicolaides KH. Preterm birth: The value of sonographic measurement of cervical length. *BJOG.* 2006;113:52–56.

30. Iams JD, Cebrik D, Lynch C, et al. The rate of cervical change and the phenotype of spontaneous preterm birth. *Am J Obstet Gynecol.* 2011;205:130.e1–e6.

31. Iams JD, Goldenberg RL, Meis PJ, et al. The length of the cervix and the risk of spontaneous premature delivery. *N Engl J Med.* 1996;334:567–572.

32. Conner SN, Frey HA, Cahill AG, et al. Loop electrosurgical excision procedure and risk of preterm birth: a systematic review and meta-analysis. *Obstet Gynecol.* 2014;123:752–761.

33. Osterman MJK, Hamilton BE, Martin JA, et al. Births: final data for 2021. *Natl Vital Stat Rep.* 2021;72:1–53.

34. American College of Obstetricians and Gynecologists. Practice Bulletin No. 231: Multifetal gestations: twin, triplet, and higher-order multifetal pregnancies (reaffirmed 2024). *Obstet Gynecol.* 2021;137:e145–e162.

35. Sunderam S, Kissin DM, Crawford SB, et al. Assisted reproductive technology surveillance—United States, 2015. *MMWR Surveill Summ.* 2018;67:1–22.

36. Orzechowski KM, Boelig RC, Baxter JK, Berghella V. A universal transvaginal cervical length screening program for preterm birth prevention. *Obstet Gynecol.* 2014;124:520–525.

37. Fischer RL, Sveinbjornsson G, Hansen C. Cervical sonography in pregnant women with a prior cone biopsy or loop electrosurgical excision procedure. *Ultrasound Obstet Gynecol.* 2010;36:613–617.

38. Vazquez JC, Abalos E. Treatments for symptomatic urinary tract infections during pregnancy. *Cochrane Database Syst Rev.* 2011;(1):CD002256.

39. Brocklehurst P, Gordon A, Heatley E, Milan SJ. Antibiotics for treating bacterial vaginosis in pregnancy. *Cochrane Database Syst Rev.* 2013;(1):CD000262.

40. Iams JD, Casal D, McGregor JA, et al. Fetal fibronectin improves the accuracy of diagnosis of preterm labor. *Am J Obstet Gynecol.* 1995;173:141–145.

41. Kiefer DG, Vintzileos AM. The utility of fetal fibronectin in the prediction and prevention of spontaneous preterm birth. *Rev Obstet Gynecol.* 2008;1:106–112.

42. Saade GR, Boggess KA, Sullivan SA, et al. Development and validation of a spontaneous preterm delivery predictor in asymptomatic women. *Am J Obstet Gynecol.* 2016;214:633.e1–e24.

43. Burchard J, Polpitiya AD, Fox AC, et al. Clinical validation of a proteomic biomarker threshold for increased risk of spontaneous preterm birth and associated clinical outcomes: a replication study. *J Clin Med.* 2021;10:5088.

44. Parry S, Leite R, Esplin MS, et al. Cervicovaginal fluid proteomic analysis to identify potential biomarkers for preterm birth. *Am J Obstet Gynecol.* 2020;222:493.e1–e13.

45. Leow SM, Di Quinzio MKW, Ng ZL, et al. Preterm birth prediction in asymptomatic women at mid-gestation using a panel of novel protein biomarkers: the Prediction of PreTerm Labor (PPeTaL) study. *Am J Obstet Gynecol MFM.* 2020;2:100084.

46. Meis PJ, Klebanoff M, Thom E, et al. Prevention of recurrent preterm delivery by 17 alpha-hydroxyprogesterone caproate. *N Engl J Med.* 2003;348:2379–2385.

47. Nelson DB, McIntire DD, Leveno KJ. A chronicle of the 17-alpha hydroxyprogesterone caproate story to prevent recurrent preterm birth. *Am J Obstet Gynecol.* 2021;224:175–186.

48. Blackwell SC, Gyamfi-Bannerman C, Biggio JR Jr, et al. 17-OHPC to Prevent Recurrent Preterm Birth in Singleton Gestations (PROLONG Study): a multicenter, international, randomized double-blind trial. *Am J Perinatol.* 2020;37:127–136.

49. Fonseca EB, Celik E, Parra M, et al. Progesterone and the risk of preterm birth among women with a short cervix. *N Engl J Med.* 2007;357:462–469.

50. Hassan SS, Romero R, Vidyadhari D, et al. Vaginal progesterone reduces the rate of preterm birth in women with a sonographic short cervix: a multicenter, randomized, double-blind, placebo-controlled trial. *Ultrasound Obstet Gynecol.* 2011;38:18–31.

51. Romero R, Conde-Agudelo A, Da Fonseca E, et al. Vaginal progesterone for preventing preterm birth and adverse perinatal outcomes in singleton gestations with a short cervix: a meta-analysis of individual patient data. *Am J Obstet Gynecol.* 2018;218:161–180.

52. Norman JE, Marlow N, Messow CM, et al. Vaginal progesterone prophylaxis for preterm birth (the OPPTIMUM study): a multicentre, randomised, double-blind trial. *Lancet.* 2016;387:2106–2116.

53. Epppic Group. Evaluating Progestogens for Preventing Preterm birth International Collaborative (EPPPIC): meta-analysis of individual participant data from randomised controlled trials. *Lancet.* 2021;397:1183–1194.

54. Quist-Nelson J, Parker P, Mokhtari N, et al. Progestogens in singleton gestations with preterm prelabor rupture of membranes: a systematic review and metaanalysis of randomized controlled trials. *Am J Obstet Gynecol.* 2018;219:346–355.e2.

55. Conde-Agudelo A, Romero R. Does vaginal progesterone prevent recurrent preterm birth in women with a singleton gestation and a history of spontaneous preterm birth? Evidence from a systematic review and meta-analysis. *Am J Obstet Gynecol.* 2022;227:440–461.e2.

56. Medical Research Council, Royal College of Obstetricians and Gynaecologists. Final report of the Medical Research Council/Royal College of Obstetricians and Gynaecologists multicentre randomised trial of cervical cerclage. *Br J Obstet Gynaecol.* 1993;100:516–523.

57. Nehme L, Huang JC, Abuhamad A, et al. Cost-effectiveness of history-indicated cerclage vs cervical length assessment for prevention of preterm birth. *Am J Obstet Gynecol.* 2023;229:674.e1–e9.

58. Berghella V, Keeler SM, To MS, et al. Effectiveness of cerclage according to severity of cervical length shortening: a meta-analysis. *Ultrasound Obstet Gynecol.* 2010;35:468–473.

59. Conde-Agudelo A, Romero R, Da Fonseca E, et al. Vaginal progesterone is as effective as cervical cerclage to prevent preterm birth in women with a singleton gestation, previous spontaneous preterm birth, and a short cervix: updated indirect comparison meta-analysis. *Am J Obstet Gynecol.* 2018;219:10–25.

60. Ehsanipoor RM, Seligman NS, Saccone G, et al. Physical examination-indicated cerclage: a systematic review and meta-analysis. *Obstet Gynecol.* 2015;126:125–135.

61. Miller ES, Grobman WA, Fonseca L, Robinson BK. Indomethacin and antibiotics in examination-indicated cerclage: a randomized controlled trial. *Obstet Gynecol.* 2014;123:1311–1316.

62. Landman A, de Boer MA, Visser L, et al. Evaluation of low-dose aspirin in the prevention of recurrent spontaneous preterm labour (the APRIL study): a multicentre, randomised, double-blinded, placebo-controlled trial. *PLoS Med.* 2022;19:e1003892.

63. Hoffman MK, Goudar SS, Kodkany BS, et al. Low-dose aspirin for the prevention of preterm delivery in nulliparous women with a singleton pregnancy (ASPIRIN): a randomised, double-blind, placebo-controlled trial. *Lancet.* 2020;395:285–293.

64. Thinkhamrop J, Hofmeyr GJ, Adetoro O, et al. Antibiotic prophylaxis during the second and third trimester to reduce adverse pregnancy outcomes and morbidity. *Cochrane Database Syst Rev.* 2015;(6):CD002250.

65. Whitworth M, Quenby S. Prophylactic oral betamimetics for preventing preterm labour in singleton pregnancies. *Cochrane Database Syst Rev.* 2008;(1):CD006395.

66. Yamasmit W, Chaithongwongwatthana S, Tolosa JE, et al. Prophylactic oral betamimetics for reducing preterm birth in women with a twin pregnancy. *Cochrane Database Syst Rev.* 2015:CD004733.

67. American College of Obstetricians and Gynecologists. Practice Bulletin No. 217: Prelabor rupture of membranes (reaffirmed 2023). *Obstet Gynecol.* 2020;135:e80–e97.

68. American College of Obstetricians and Gynecologists. Practice Bulletin No. 171: Management of preterm labor (reaffirmed 2022). *Obstet Gynecol.* 2016;128:e155–e164.

69. Stan CM, Boulvain M, Pfister R, Hirsbrunner-Almagbaly P. Hydration for treatment of preterm labour. *Cochrane Database Syst Rev.* 2013;(11):CD003096.

70. American College of Obstetricians and Gynecologists. Committee Opinion No. 455: Magnesium sulfate before anticipated preterm birth for neuroprotection (reaffirmed 2023). *Obstet Gynecol.* 2010;115:669–671.

71. Wright LL, Verter J, Younes N, et al. Antenatal corticosteroid administration and neonatal outcome in very low birth weight infants: the NICHD Neonatal Research Network. *Am J Obstet Gynecol.* 1995;173:269–274.

72. Andrews EB, Marcucci G, White A, Long W. Associations between use of antenatal corticosteroids and neonatal outcomes within the Exosurf Neonatal Treatment Investigational New Drug Program. *Am J Obstet Gynecol.* 1995;173:290–295.

73. Gyamfi-Bannerman C, Thom EA, Blackwell SC, et al. Antenatal betamethasone for women at risk for late preterm delivery. *N Engl J Med.* 2016;374:1311–1320.

74. Wapner RJ, Sorokin Y, Thom EA, et al. Single versus weekly courses of antenatal corticosteroids: evaluation of safety and efficacy. *Am J Obstet Gynecol.* 2006;195:633–642.

75. Garite TJ, Kurtzman J, Maurel K, Clark R. Impact of a 'rescue course' of antenatal corticosteroids: a multicenter randomized placebo-controlled trial. *Am J Obstet Gynecol.* 2009;200:248.e1–e9.

76. Crowther CA, McKinlay CJ, Middleton P, Harding JE. Repeat doses of prenatal corticosteroids for women at risk of preterm birth for improving neonatal health outcomes. *Cochrane Database Syst Rev.* 2015;(7):CD003935.

77. American College of Obstetricians and Gynecologists. Committee Opinion No. 713: Antenatal corticosteroid therapy for fetal maturation (reaffirmed 2024). *Obstet Gynecol.* 2017;130:e102–e109.

78. Kenyon SL, Taylor DJ, Tarnow-Mordi W. ORACLE Collaborative Group. Broad-spectrum antibiotics for spontaneous preterm labour: the ORACLE II randomised trial. *Lancet.* 2001;357:989–994.

79. Flenady V, Hawley G, Stock OM, et al. Prophylactic antibiotics for inhibiting preterm labour with intact membranes. *Cochrane Database Syst Rev.* 2013;(12):CD000246.

80. Shepherd E, Salam RA, Middleton P, et al. Antenatal and intrapartum interventions for preventing cerebral palsy: an overview of Cochrane systematic reviews. *Cochrane Database Syst Rev.* 2017;(8):CD012077.

81. American College of Obstetricians and Gynecologists. Practice Bulletin No. 199: Use of prophylactic antibiotics in labor and delivery (reaffirmed 2021). *Obstet Gynecol.* 2018;132:e103–e119.

82. Doyle LW, Crowther CA, Middleton P, et al. Magnesium sulphate for women at risk of preterm birth for neuroprotection of the fetus. *Cochrane Database Syst Rev.* 2009;(1):CD004661.

83. Crowther CA, Hiller JE, Doyle LW, Haslam RR. Effect of magnesium sulfate given for neuroprotection before preterm birth: a randomized controlled trial. *JAMA.* 2003;290:2669–2676.

84. Marret S, Marpeau L, Zupan-Simunek V, et al. Magnesium sulphate given before very-preterm birth to protect infant brain: the randomised controlled PREMAG trial. *BJOG.* 2007;114:310–318.

85. Rouse DJ, Hirtz DG, Thom E, et al. A randomized, controlled trial of magnesium sulfate for the prevention of cerebral palsy. *N Engl J Med.* 2008;359:895–905.

86. Crowther CA, Middleton PF, Voysey M, et al. Assessing the neuroprotective benefits for babies of antenatal magnesium sulphate: an individual participant data meta-analysis. *PLoS Med.* 2017;14:e1002398.

87. Crowther CA, Ashwood P, Middleton PF, et al. Prenatal intravenous magnesium at 30-34 weeks' gestation and neurodevelopmental outcomes in offspring: the MAGENTA randomized clinical trial. *JAMA.* 2023;330:603–614.

88. Berkman ND, Thorp JM Jr, Lohr KN, et al. Tocolytic treatment for the management of preterm labor: a review of the evidence. *Am J Obstet Gynecol.* 2003;188:1648–1659.

89. Haas DM, Caldwell DM, Kirkpatrick P, et al. Tocolytic therapy for preterm delivery: systematic review and network meta-analysis. *BMJ*. 2012;345:e6226.

90. Flenady V, Wojcieszek AM, Papatsonis DN, et al. Calcium channel blockers for inhibiting preterm labour and birth. *Cochrane Database Syst Rev*. 2014;(6):CD002255.

91. Anotayanonth S, Subhedar NV, Garner P, et al. Betamimetics for inhibiting preterm labour. *Cochrane Database Syst Rev*. 2004;(2):CD004352.

92. U.S. Food and Drug Administration. FDA drug safety communication: new warnings against use of terbutaline to treat preterm labor; 2011. http://www.fda.gov/drugs/drugsafety/ucm243539.htm. Accessed 25 July 2025.

93. Reinebrant HE, Pileggi-Castro C, Romero CL, et al. Cyclo-oxygenase (COX) inhibitors for treating preterm labour. *Cochrane Database Syst Rev*. 2015:CD001992.

94. Romero R, Sibai BM, Sanchez-Ramos L, et al. An oxytocin receptor antagonist (atosiban) in the treatment of preterm labor: a randomized, double-blind, placebo-controlled trial with tocolytic rescue. *Am J Obstet Gynecol*. 2000;182:1173–1183.

95. van Vliet EOG, Nijman TAJ, Schuit E, et al. Nifedipine versus atosiban for threatened preterm birth (APOSTEL III): a multicentre, randomised controlled trial. *Lancet*. 2016;387:2117–2124.

96. Crowther CA, Brown J, McKinlay CJ, Middleton P. Magnesium sulphate for preventing preterm birth in threatened preterm labour. *Cochrane Database Syst Rev*. 2014;(8):CD001060.

97. Duckitt K, Thornton S, O'Donovan OP, Dowswell T. Nitric oxide donors for treating preterm labour. *Cochrane Database Syst Rev*. 2014:CD002860.

98. Vogel JP, Nardin JM, Dowswell T, et al. Combination of tocolytic agents for inhibiting preterm labour. *Cochrane Database Syst Rev*. 2014;(5):CD006169.

99. Mercer BM, Miodovnik M, Thurnau GR, et al. Antibiotic therapy for reduction of infant morbidity after preterm premature rupture of the membranes. A randomized controlled trial. National Institute of Child Health and Human Development Maternal-Fetal Medicine Units Network. *JAMA*. 1997;278:989–995.

100. Kenyon SL, Taylor DJ, Tarnow-Mordi W. Broad-spectrum antibiotics for preterm, prelabour rupture of fetal membranes: the ORACLE I randomised trial. ORACLE Collaborative Group. *Lancet*. 2001;357:979–988.

101. Porreco R, Garite TJ, Combs CA, et al. Booster course of antenatal corticosteroids after preterm prelabor rupture of membranes: a double-blind randomized trial. *Am J Obstet Gynecol MFM*. 2023;5:100896.

102. Mackeen AD, Seibel-Seamon J, Muhammad J, et al. Tocolytics for preterm premature rupture of membranes. *Cochrane Database Syst Rev*. 2014;(2):CD007062.

103. Morris JM, Roberts CL, Bowen JR, et al. Immediate delivery compared with expectant management after preterm pre-labour rupture of the membranes close to term (PPROMT trial): a randomised controlled trial. *Lancet*. 2016;387:444–452.

104. Dotters-Katz SK, Panzer A, Grace MR, et al. Maternal morbidity after previable prelabor rupture of membranes. *Obstet Gynecol*. 2017;129:101–106.

105. Sklar A, Sheeder J, Davis AR, et al. Maternal morbidity after preterm premature rupture of membranes at <24 weeks' gestation. *Am J Obstet Gynecol*. 2022;226:558.e1–e11.

106. Nambiar A, Patel S, Santiago-Munoz P, et al. Maternal morbidity and fetal outcomes among pregnant women at 22 weeks' gestation or less with complications in 2 Texas hospitals after legislation on abortion. *Am J Obstet Gynecol*. 2022;227:648–650.e1.

107. Dobbs v. Jackson Women's Health Org., 142 S. Ct. 2228, 213 L. Ed. 2d 545, 2022 U.S. LEXIS 3057, 29 Fla. L. Weekly Fed. S 486, 2022 WL 2276808.

108. Gaffney A, Himmelstein DU, Dickman S, et al. Projected health outcomes associated with 3 US Supreme Court decisions in 2022 on COVID-19 workplace protections, handgun-carry restrictions, and abortion rights. *JAMA Netw Open*. 2023;6:e2315578.

109. American College of Obstetricians and Gynecologists. Practice Bulletin No. 142: Cerclage for the management of cervical insufficiency (reaffirmed 2024). *Obstet Gynecol*. 2014;123:372–379.

110. Wylie BJ, Davidson LL, Batra M, Reed SD. Method of delivery and neonatal outcome in very low-birthweight vertex-presenting fetuses. *Am J Obstet Gynecol*. 2008;198:640.e1–e7.

111. Reddy UM, Zhang J, Sun L, et al. Neonatal mortality by attempted route of delivery in early preterm birth. *Am J Obstet Gynecol*. 2012;207:117.e1–e8.

112. Bergenhenegouwen LA, Meertens LJ, Schaaf J, et al. Vaginal delivery versus caesarean section in preterm breech delivery: a systematic review. *Eur J Obstet Gynecol Reprod Biol*. 2014;172:1–6.

113. Chervenak FA, Johnson RE, Youcha S, et al. Intrapartum management of twin gestation. *Obstet Gynecol*. 1985;65:119–124.

114. Tucker Edmonds B, McKenzie F, Macheras M, et al. Morbidity and mortality associated with mode of delivery for breech periviable deliveries. *Am J Obstet Gynecol*. 2015;213:70.e1–e12.

115. Mantel A, Ajne G, Lindblad Wollmann C, Stephansson O. Previous preterm cesarean delivery and risk of uterine rupture in subsequent trial of labor-a national cohort study. *Am J Obstet Gynecol*. 2021;224:380.e1–e13.

116. National Institute of Child Health and Human Development Pregnancy and Perinatology Branch. Extremely preterm birth outcomes tool; 2020. https://www.nichd.nih.gov/research/supported/EPBO. Accessed 26 July 2024.

117. Wyllie J, Bruinenberg J, Roehr CC, et al. European Resuscitation Council guidelines for resuscitation 2015: Section 7. Resuscitation and support of transition of babies at birth. *Resuscitation*. 2015;95:249–263.

118. Westgren M, Holmquist P, Svenningsen NW, Ingemarsson I. Intrapartum fetal monitoring in preterm deliveries: prospective study. *Obstet Gynecol*. 1982;60:99–106.

119. Luthy DA, Shy KK, van Belle G, et al. A randomized trial of electronic fetal monitoring in preterm labor. *Obstet Gynecol*. 1987;69:687–695.

120. Shy KK, Luthy DA, Bennett FC, et al. Effects of electronic fetal-heart-rate monitoring, as compared with periodic auscultation, on the neurologic development of premature infants. *N Engl J Med*. 1990;322:588–593.

121. Low JA, Wood SL, Killen HL, et al. Intrapartum asphyxia in the preterm fetus less than 2000 gm. *Am J Obstet Gynecol*. 1990;162:378–382.

122. Thomas J, Long G, Moore G, Morgan D. Plasma protein binding and placental transfer of bupivacaine. *Clin Pharmacol Ther*. 1976;19:426–434.

123. Mattingly JE, D'Alessio J, Ramanathan J. Effects of obstetric analgesics and anesthetics on the neonate: a review. *Paediatr Drugs*. 2003;5:615–627.

124. Rane A, Sjoqvist F, Orrenius S. Cytochrome P-450 in human fetal liver microsomes. *Chem Biol Interact*. 1971;3:305.

125. Rane A, Sjoqvist F, Orrenius S. Drugs and fetal metabolism. *Clin Pharmacol Ther*. 1973;14:666–672.

126. Teramo K, Benowitz N, Heymann MA, Rudolph AM. Gestational differences in lidocaine toxicity in the fetal lamb. *Anesthesiology*. 1976;44:133–138.

127. Pedersen H, Santos AC, Morishima HO, et al. Does gestational age affect the pharmacokinetics and pharmacodynamics of lidocaine in mother and fetus? *Anesthesiology*. 1988;68:367–372.

128. Smedstad KG, Morison DH, Harris WH, Pascoe P. Placental transfer of local anaesthetics in the premature sheep fetus. *Int J Obstet Anesth*. 1993;2:34–38.

129. Johnson RF, Herman NL, Johnson HV, et al. Effects of fetal pH on local anesthetic transfer across the human placenta. *Anesthesiology*. 1996;85:608–615.

130. Morishima HO, Pedersen H, Santos AC, et al. Adverse effects of maternally administered lidocaine on the asphyxiated preterm fetal lamb. *Anesthesiology*. 1989;71:110–115.

131. Morishima HO, Santos AC, Pedersen H, et al. Effect of lidocaine on the asphyxial responses in the mature fetal lamb. *Anesthesiology*. 1987;66:502–507.

132. Santos AC, Yun EM, Bobby PD, et al. The effects of bupivacaine, L-nitro-L-arginine-methyl ester, and phenylephrine on cardiovascular adaptations to asphyxia in the preterm fetal lamb. *Anesth Analg*. 1997;85:1299–1306.

133. Arthur GR, Feldman HS, Covino BG. Comparative pharmacokinetics of bupivacaine and ropivacaine, a new amide local anesthetic. *Anesth Analg*. 1988;67:1053–1058.

134. Datta S, Camann W, Bader A, VanderBurgh L. Clinical effects and maternal and fetal plasma concentrations of epidural ropivacaine versus bupivacaine for cesarean section. *Anesthesiology*. 1995;82:1346–1352.

135. Ala-Kokko TI, Alahuhta S, Jouppila P, et al. Feto-maternal distribution of ropivacaine and bupivacaine after epidural administration for cesarean section. *Int J Obstet Anesth*. 1997;6:147–152.

136. Kuhnert BR, Kuhnert PM, Reese AL, et al. Maternal and neonatal elimination of CABA after epidural anesthesia with 2-chloroprocaine during parturition. *Anesth Analg*. 1983;62:1089–1094.

137. Philipson EH, Kuhnert BR, Syracuse CD. Fetal acidosis, 2-chloroprocaine, and epidural anesthesia for cesarean section. *Am J Obstet Gynecol*. 1985;151:322–324.

138. Hollmen AI, Jouppila R, Jouppila P, et al. Effect of extradural analgesia using bupivacaine and 2-chloroprocaine on intervillous blood flow during normal labour. *Br J Anaesth*. 1982;54:837–842.

139. Rolbin SH, Cohen MM, Levinton CM, et al. The premature infant: anesthesia for cesarean delivery. *Anesth Analg*. 1994;78:912–917.

140. Laudenbach V, Mercier FJ, Roze JC, et al. Anaesthesia mode for caesarean section and mortality in very preterm infants: an epidemiologic study in the EPIPAGE cohort. *Int J Obstet Anesth*. 2009;18:142–149.

141. Jevtovic-Todorovic V, Olney JW. PRO: anesthesia-induced developmental neuroapoptosis: status of the evidence. *Anesth Analg*. 2008;106:1659–1663.

142. De Tina A, Palanisamy A. General anesthesia during the third trimester: any link to neurocognitive outcomes? *Anesthesiol Clin*. 2017;35:69–80.

143. Adesope OA, Einhorn LM, Olufolabi AJ, et al. The impact of gestational age and fetal weight on the risk of failure of spinal anesthesia for cesarean delivery. *Int J Obstet Anesth*. 2016;26:8–14.

144. D'Alton ME, Friedman AM, Smiley RM, et al. National Partnership for Maternal Safety: consensus bundle on venous thromboembolism. *Anesth Analg*. 2016;123:942–949.

145. Leffert L, Butwick A, Carvalho B, et al. The Society for Obstetric Anesthesia and Perinatology consensus statement on the anesthetic management of pregnant and postpartum women receiving thromboprophylaxis or higher dose anticoagulants. *Anesth Analg*. 2018;126:928–944.

146. Kopp SL, Vandermeulen E, McBane RD, et al. Regional anesthesia in the patient receiving antithrombotic or thrombolytic therapy: American Society of Regional Anesthesia and Pain Medicine Evidence-Based Guidelines. 5th ed. *Reg Anesth Pain Med*. 2025:rapm-2024-105766. Online ahead of print.

147. Nuthalapaty FS, Beck MM, Mabie WC. Complications of central venous catheters during pregnancy and postpartum: a case series. *Am J Obstet Gynecol*. 2009;201:311.e1–e5.

148. Struyker-Boudier HA, Smits JF, De Mey JG. The pharmacology of calcium antagonists: a review. *J Cardiovasc Pharmacol*. 1990;15:S1–S10.

149. Glock JL, Morales WJ. Efficacy and safety of nifedipine versus magnesium sulfate in the management of preterm labor: a randomized study. *Am J Obstet Gynecol*. 1993;169:960–964.

150. Bal L, Thierry S, Brocas E, et al. Pulmonary edema induced by calcium-channel blockade for tocolysis. *Anesth Analg*. 2004;99:910–911.

151. Cornette J, Duvekot JJ, Roos-Hesselink JW, et al. Maternal and fetal haemodynamic effects of nifedipine in normotensive pregnant women. *BJOG*. 2011;118:510–540.

152. Mari G, Kirshon B, Moise KJ Jr, et al. Doppler assessment of the fetal and uteroplacental circulation during nifedipine therapy for preterm labor. *Am J Obstet Gynecol*. 1989;161:1514–1518.

153. Pirhonen JP, Erkkola RU, Ekblad UU, Nyman L. Single dose of nifedipine in normotensive pregnancy: nifedipine concentrations, hemodynamic responses, and uterine and fetal flow velocity waveforms. *Obstet Gynecol*. 1990;76:807–811.

154. Tosone SR, Reves JG, Kissin I, et al. Hemodynamic responses to nifedipine in dogs anesthetized with halothane. *Anesth Analg*. 1983;62:903–908.

155. Ben-Ami M, Giladi Y, Shalev E. The combination of magnesium sulphate and nifedipine: a cause of neuromuscular blockade. *Br J Obstet Gynaecol*. 1994;101:262–263.

156. Niebyl JR, Witter FR. Neonatal outcome after indomethacin treatment for preterm labor. *Am J Obstet Gynecol*. 1986;155:747–749.

157. Moise KJ Jr, Huhta JC, Sharif DS, et al. Indomethacin in the treatment of premature labor. Effects on the fetal ductus arteriosus. *N Engl J Med*. 1988;319:327–331.

158. Dudley DK, Hardie MJ. Fetal and neonatal effects of indomethacin used as a tocolytic agent. *Am J Obstet Gynecol*. 1985;151:181–184.

159. Vermillion ST, Scardo JA, Lashus AG, Wiles HB. The effect of indomethacin tocolysis on fetal ductus arteriosus constriction with advancing gestational age. *Am J Obstet Gynecol.* 1997;177:256–259.

160. Moise KJ Jr. Effect of advancing gestational age on the frequency of fetal ductal constriction in association with maternal indomethacin use. *Am J Obstet Gynecol.* 1993;168:1350–1353.

161. Hearne AE, Nagey DA. Therapeutic agents in preterm labor: tocolytic agents. *Clin Obstet Gynecol.* 2000;43:787–801.

162. Kirshon B, Moise KJ Jr, Mari G, Willis R. Long-term indomethacin therapy decreases fetal urine output and results in oligohydramnios. *Am J Perinatol.* 1991;8:86–88.

163. Kirshon B, Moise KJ Jr, Wasserstrum N, et al. Influence of short-term indomethacin therapy on fetal urine output. *Obstet Gynecol.* 1988;72:51–53.

164. Anderson RJ, Berl T, McDonald KM, Schrier RW. Prostaglandins: effects on blood pressure, renal blood flow, sodium and water excretion. *Kidney Int.* 1976;10:205–215.

165. Wurtzel D. Prenatal administration of indomethacin as a tocolytic agent: effect on neonatal renal function. *Obstet Gynecol.* 1990;76:689–692.

166. Hammers AL, Sanchez-Ramos L, Kaunitz AM. Antenatal exposure to indomethacin increases the risk of severe intraventricular hemorrhage, necrotizing enterocolitis, and periventricular leukomalacia: a systematic review with metaanalysis. *Am J Obstet Gynecol.* 2015;212:505.e1–e13.

167. Kleinman G, Nuwayhid B, Rudelstorfer R, et al. Circulatory and renal effects of beta-adrenergic-receptor stimulation in pregnant sheep. *Am J Obstet Gynecol.* 1984;149:865–874.

168. Benedetti TJ, Hargrove JC, Rosene KA. Maternal pulmonary edema during premature labor inhibition. *Obstet Gynecol.* 1982;59:33s–37s.

169. Hatjis CG, Swain M. Systemic tocolysis for premature labor is associated with an increased incidence of pulmonary edema in the presence of maternal infection. *Am J Obstet Gynecol.* 1988;159:723–728.

170. Perry KG Jr, Morrison JC, Rust OA, et al. Incidence of adverse cardiopulmonary effects with low-dose continuous terbutaline infusion. *Am J Obstet Gynecol.* 1995;173:1273–1277.

171. Lotgering FK, Lind J, Huikeshoven FJ, Wallenburg HC. Elevated serum transaminase levels during ritodrine administration. *Am J Obstet Gynecol.* 1986;155:390–392.

172. Nair GV, Ghosh AK, Lewis BV. Bowel distension during treatment of premature labour with beta-receptor agonists. *Lancet.* 1976;1:907.

173. Rosene KA, Featherstone HJ, Benedetti TJ. Cerebral ischemia associated with parenteral terbutaline use in pregnant migraine patients. *Am J Obstet Gynecol.* 1982;143:405–407.

174. Catanzarite VA, McHargue AM, Sandberg EC, Dyson DC. Respiratory arrest during therapy for premature labor in a patient with myasthenia gravis. *Obstet Gynecol.* 1984;64:819–822.

175. Schoenfeld A, Joel-Cohen SJ, Duparc H, Levy E. Emergency obstetric anaesthesia and the use of beta2-sympathomimetic drugs. *Br J Anaesth.* 1978;50:969–971.

176. Crowhurst JA. Salbutamol, obstetrics and anaesthesia: a review and case discussion. *Anaesth Intensive Care.* 1980;8:39–43.

177. Ravindran R, Viegas OJ, Padilla LM, LaBlonde P. Anesthetic considerations in pregnant patients receiving terbutaline therapy. *Anesth Analg.* 1980;59:391–392.

178. Shin YK, Kim YD. Ventricular tachyarrhythmias during cesarean section after ritodrine therapy: Interaction with anesthetics. *South Med J.* 1988;81:528–530.

179. Suppan P. Tocolysis and anaesthesia for caesarean section. *Br J Anaesth.* 1982;54:1007.

180. Slater RM, From RP, Sum Ping JS, Pank JR. Changes in plasma potassium and neuromuscular blockade following suxamethonium in patients pre-treated with terbutaline. *Eur J Anaesthesiol.* 1991;8:281–286.

181. Phaneuf S, Asboth G, MacKenzie IZ, et al. Effect of oxytocin antagonists on the activation of human myometrium in vitro: atosiban prevents oxytocin-induced desensitization. *Am J Obstet Gynecol.* 1994;171:1627–1634.

182. Goodwin T, Millar L, North L, et al. The pharmacokinetics of the oxytocin antagonist atosiban in pregnant women with preterm uterine contractions. *Am J Obstet Gynecol.* 1995;173:913–917.

183. Beall MH, Edgar BW, Paul RH, Smith-Wallace T. A comparison of ritodrine, terbutaline, and magnesium sulfate for the suppression of preterm labor. *Am J Obstet Gynecol.* 1985;153:854–859.

184. Hollander DI, Nagey DA, Pupkin MJ. Magnesium sulfate and ritodrine hydrochloride: a randomized comparison. *Am J Obstet Gynecol.* 1987;156:631–637.

185. Chau AC, Gabert HA, Miller JM Jr. A prospective comparison of terbutaline and magnesium for tocolysis. *Obstet Gynecol.* 1992;80:847–851.

186. Ende HB, Lozada MJ, Chestnut DH, et al. Risk factors for atonic postpartum hemorrhage: a systematic review and meta-analysis. *Obstet Gynecol.* 2021;137:305–323.

187. Pergialiotis V, Bellos I, Constantinou T, et al. Magnesium sulfate and risk of postpartum uterine atony and hemorrhage: a meta-analysis. *Eur J Obstet Gynecol Reprod Biol.* 2021;256:158–164.

188. Vincent RD Jr, Chestnut DH, Sipes SL, et al. Magnesium sulfate decreases maternal blood pressure but not uterine blood flow during epidural anesthesia in gravid ewes. *Anesthesiology.* 1991;74:77–82.

189. De Vore JS, Asrani R. Magnesium sulfate prevents succinylcholine-induced fasciculations in toxemic parturients. *Anesthesiology.* 1980;52:76–77.

190. James MF, Cork RC, Dennett JE. Succinylcholine pretreatment with magnesium sulfate. *Anesth Analg.* 1986;65:373–376.

191. Thompson SW, Moscicki JC, DiFazio CA. The anesthetic contribution of magnesium sulfate and ritodrine hydrochloride in rats. *Anesth Analg.* 1988;67:31–34.

34

Abnormal Presentation and Multiple Gestation

Holly B. Ende, MD

CHAPTER OUTLINE

Multiple gestation and abnormal fetal presentation represent major challenges in obstetric and obstetric anesthesia care. Operative vaginal and cesarean deliveries are more commonly required, and an obstetric emergency may necessitate immediate intervention. All members of the perinatal care team must communicate directly and clearly to ensure the best possible outcome for both the mother and neonate(s).

How one or multiple fetuses are arranged within the uterus is communicated using a series of descriptors denoting presentation, lie, and position. **Presentation** describes the portion of the fetus that overlies the pelvic inlet and may be **cephalic**, **breech**, or **shoulder**. Cephalic presentations are further subdivided into **vertex**, **brow**, and **face** according to the degree of flexion of the neck. With an **asynclitic** presentation, the fetal head is tilted toward one shoulder and the opposite parietal eminence enters the pelvic inlet first. Breech and shoulder presentations occur with increased frequency in patients with multiple gestation. In most cases, the fetal presenting part is determined via ultrasonography or palpation through the cervix during a vaginal examination.

The **position** of the fetus denotes the relationship of a specific fetal bony point to the maternal pelvis. The orientation of the **occiput** defines the position for vertex presentation (Fig. 34.1). Other markers for position are the **sacrum** for breech presentation, the **mentum** for face presentation, and the **acromion** for shoulder presentation. The **attitude** of the fetus describes the relationship of the fetal parts with one another; the term is typically used to refer to the position of the head with regard to the trunk, as in flexed, military, or hyperextended.

The **lie** refers to the alignment of the fetal spine with the maternal spine. The fetal lie can be **longitudinal**, **transverse**, or **oblique**. A fetus with a vertex or breech presentation has a longitudinal lie. A persistent oblique or transverse lie typically requires cesarean delivery.

ABNORMAL POSITION

Obstetric providers diagnose fetal head position with ultrasonography or palpation of the sagittal suture during vaginal examination. During normal labor, the fetal occiput rotates to a direct **occiput anterior** position (Fig. 34.1). In a minority of patients with a right or left occiput posterior position, the occiput rotates directly posteriorly and results in a **persistent occiput posterior** position. The occiput posterior position may lead to a prolonged labor that is associated with increased maternal discomfort. Less often, the vertex remains in the **occiput transverse** position. This condition is known as **deep transverse arrest**.

Obstetric providers may perform manual or forceps rotation to hasten delivery and lessen perineal trauma in women with an abnormal position of the vertex. Rotational forceps are uncommonly performed owing to concern for excessive maternal and/or fetal trauma; however, manual rotation of the vertex is often attempted to facilitate vaginal birth.[1] Prophylactic manual rotation of occiput transverse and posterior positions during the early second stage of labor reduces the likelihood of operative delivery and shortens the second stage of labor.[2] Some cases of persistent occiput posterior position and many cases of deep transverse arrest require cesarean delivery because of dystocia.[3]

During administration of epidural analgesia to a patient with an abnormal fetal position, the addition of a lipid-soluble opioid to a dilute solution of local anesthetic provides

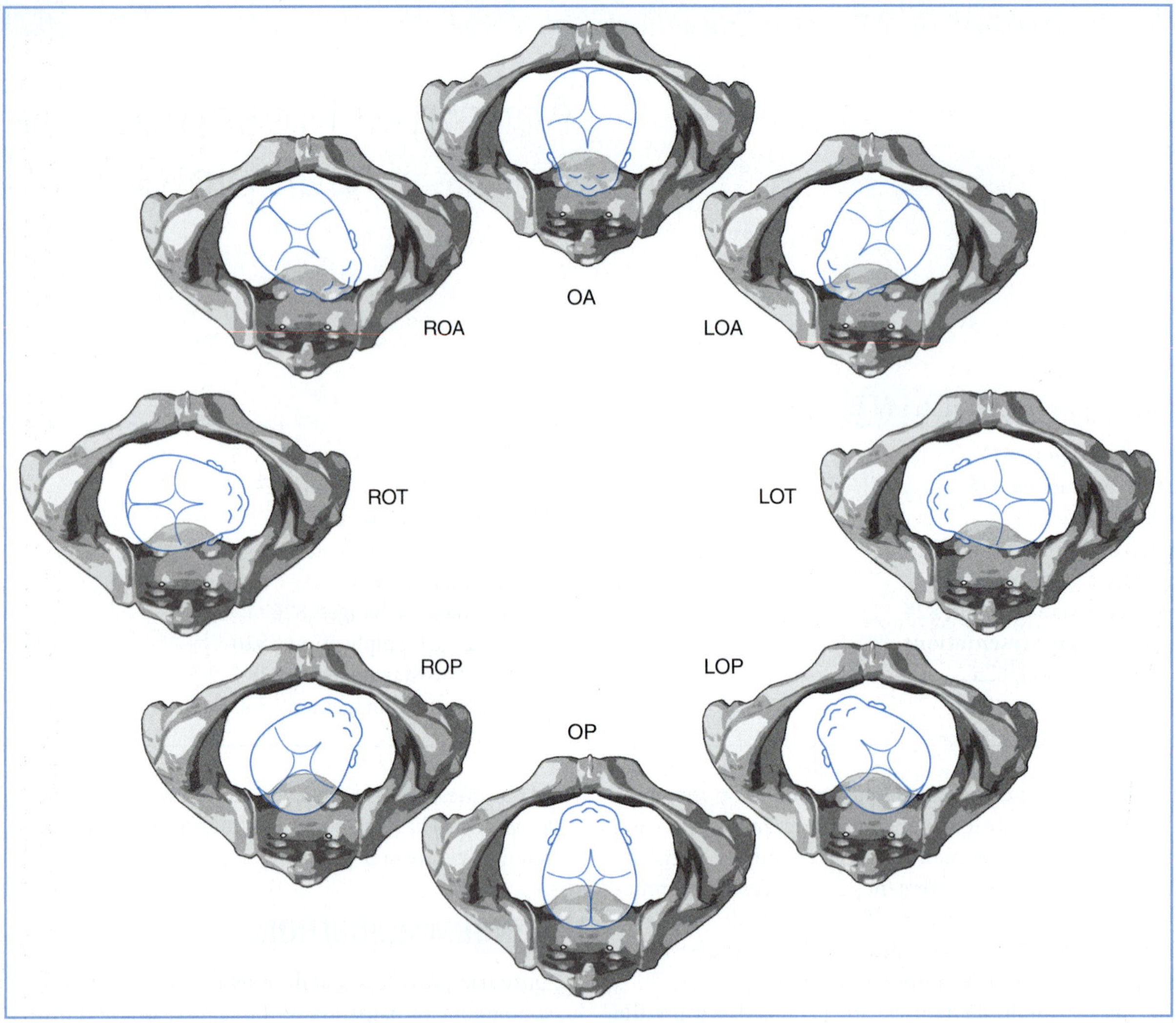

Fig. 34.1 Fetal Head Position in the Maternal Pelvis. *OA*, Occiput anterior; *LOA*, left occiput anterior; *LOP*, left occiput posterior; *LOT*, left occiput transverse; *OP*, occiput posterior; *ROA*, right occiput anterior; *ROP*, right occiput posterior; *ROT*, right occiput transverse.

analgesia while preserving pelvic muscle tone. This is particularly useful given that relaxation of the pelvic floor and perineum may prevent the spontaneous rotation of the vertex during labor.[4] In contrast, if operative vaginal delivery is later attempted, profound pelvic floor relaxation is required to facilitate forceps placement.

BREECH PRESENTATION

Breech presentation describes a longitudinal lie in which the fetal buttocks and/or lower extremities overlie the pelvic inlet. There are three types of breech presentation (Fig. 34.2):
- **Complete breech**—lower extremities flexed at both the hips and the knees
- **Incomplete breech**—one or both of the lower extremities extended at the hips
- **Frank breech**—lower extremities flexed at the hips and extended at the knees

Ultrasonographic or radiographic examination typically allows the obstetric provider to confirm the type of breech

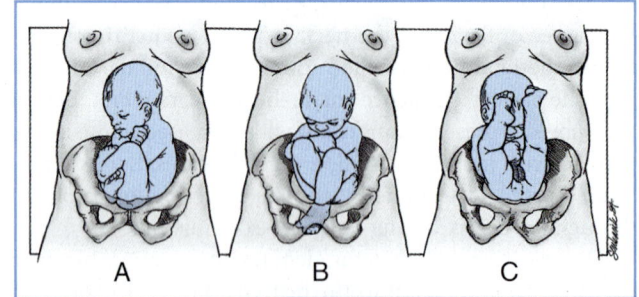

Fig. 34.2 Three Possible Breech Presentations. (A) The *complete breech* demonstrates flexion of the hips and flexion of the knees. (B) The *incomplete breech* demonstrates intermediate deflexion of one or both hips and knees. (C) The *frank breech* shows flexion of the hips and extension of both knees. From Barth WH. Malpresentations. In: Landon MB, Galan HL, Jauniaux ERM, et al., eds. *Gabbe's Obstetrics: Normal and Problem Pregnancies.* 8th ed. Elsevier; 2021:319–342.

presentation and to exclude the presence of associated severe congenital anomalies (e.g., anencephaly). The fetus with a frank breech presentation tends to remain in that presentation throughout labor. In contrast, a complete breech presentation may change to an incomplete breech presentation at any time before or during labor.

Epidemiology

Breech presentation is the most common type of abnormal presentation. Both the incidence and the type of breech presentation vary with gestational age (Table 34.1). Before 28 weeks' gestation, approximately 25% of fetuses are in a breech presentation.[5] Most change to a vertex presentation by 34 weeks' gestation, but 3% to 4% of fetuses remain in a breech presentation at term.[5]

Many factors predispose to breech presentation, including fetal, pelvic, and uterine abnormalities (Box 34.1).[5] Breech presentation may allow more room for fetal growth and movement in the setting of pelvic or uterine anomalies.

TABLE 34.1 Types and Incidences of Breech Presentation

Type of Breech	Percentage of All Breech Presentations	Percentage of Preterm Breech Presentations
Complete	5%–12%	12%
Incomplete	12%–38%	50%
Frank	48%–73%	38%

Modified from Barth WH. Malpresentations. In: Landon MB, Galan HL, Jauniaux ERM, et al., eds. *Gabbe's Obstetrics: Normal and Problem Pregnancies*. 8th ed. Elsevier; 2021:319–342.

BOX 34.1 Factors Associated With Breech Presentation

Uterine Distention or Relaxation
- Multiparity
- Multiple gestation
- Polyhydramnios
- Macrosomia

Abnormalities of the Uterus or Pelvis
- Pelvic tumors
- Uterine anomalies
- Pelvic contracture

Abnormalities of the Fetus
- Hydrocephalus
- Anencephaly

Obstetric Conditions
- Previous breech delivery
- Preterm gestation
- Oligohydramnios
- Cornual-fundal placenta
- Placenta previa

Modified from Singleton breech delivery. In: Cunningham FG, Leveno KJ, Dashe JS, et al., eds. *Williams Obstetrics*. 26th ed. McGraw-Hill Education; 2022; Barth WH. Malpresentations. In: Landon MB, Galan HL, Jauniaux ERM, et al., eds. *Gabbe's Obstetrics: Normal and Problem Pregnancies*. 8th ed. Elsevier; 2021:319–342.

Hydrocephalic fetuses are also more likely to assume a breech presentation. Multiparity, multiple gestation, polyhydramnios, and anencephaly additionally predispose to breech presentation. These conditions may interfere with the normal process of accommodation among the fetal head, the uterine cavity, and maternal pelvis.

Obstetric Complications

Obstetric complications are more likely in the setting of breech presentation (Table 34.2). Cesarean delivery decreases the risk for some of these complications. Vaginal breech delivery entails a higher risk for neonatal trauma than delivery of an infant with a vertex presentation, but cesarean delivery does not eliminate the risk for trauma to the infant.[6] Rather, cesarean delivery of a breech presentation can be difficult and traumatic, especially if the skin and uterine incisions are insufficient or maternal muscle relaxation is inadequate.

The risk for umbilical cord prolapse varies with the type of breech presentation (Table 34.3). With incomplete breech presentation, the presenting part does not occlude the cervix to the same extent as the vertex or buttocks, thus allowing the possibility of umbilical cord prolapse before delivery. Umbilical cord prolapse typically necessitates emergency cesarean delivery.

TABLE 34.2 Incidences of Complications Associated With Breech Presentation

Complication	Incidence
Intrapartum fetal death	Increased 16-fold[a]
Intrapartum asphyxia	Increased 3.8-fold[a]
Umbilical cord prolapse	Increased 5–20-fold[a]
Birth trauma	Increased 13-fold[a]
Arrest of aftercoming head	5%–9%
Spinal cord injuries with deflexion	21%
Major congenital anomalies	6%–18%
Preterm delivery	16%–33%
Hyperextension of head	5%
Fetal heart rate abnormalities	15%

[a]Compared with cephalic presentation.
Modified from Barth WH. Malpresentations. In: Landon MB, Galan HL, Jauniaux ERM, et al., eds. *Gabbe's Obstetrics: Normal and Problem Pregnancies*. 8th ed. Elsevier; 2021:319–342.

TABLE 34.3 Risk for Umbilical Cord Prolapse in Breech Presentation

Type of Breech	Risk for Cord Prolapse
Frank	0.5%
Complete	4%–6%
Incomplete	15%–18%

Modified from Barth WH. Malpresentations. In: Landon MB, Galan HL, Jauniaux ERM, et al., eds. *Gabbe's Obstetrics: Normal and Problem Pregnancies*. 8th ed. Elsevier; 2021:319–342.

Morbidity and Mortality

There is a higher risk for perinatal morbidity and mortality with breech presentation, even when the risk is adjusted for preterm gestation. The factors that cause breech presentation are often more important than the presentation itself. For example, hydrocephalus and anencephaly predispose to breech presentation and significantly contribute to neonatal morbidity and mortality. Relative perinatal mortality rates (calculated from data for linked siblings from the Medical Birth Registry of Norway) confirm that breech presentation is a marker of perinatal risk, regardless of the mode of delivery.[7] Even after successful external cephalic version (ECV), women are at increased risk for cesarean delivery because of dystocia or an abnormal fetal heart rate (FHR) tracing, compared with women with natural cephalic presentation.[8]

Vaginal breech delivery entails a higher risk for **maternal morbidity** (e.g., infection, perineal trauma, hemorrhage) than vertex delivery.[5] However, among women with breech presentation, maternal outcomes are similar between women who have a planned cesarean delivery and those who have a trial of labor.[6,9] At 2 years postpartum, maternal morbidity assessed by questionnaire (917 responses for a 79% response rate) did not differ for urinary incontinence, breastfeeding, pain, depression, menstrual problems, fatigue, and distressing memories of the birth experience.[9] In a single-center study of 846 singleton breech deliveries, Schiff et al.[10] did not find a higher risk for maternal morbidity in women who had intrapartum cesarean delivery compared with women who had elective cesarean delivery.

Obstetric Management

External Cephalic Version

The process of ECV converts a breech or shoulder presentation to a vertex presentation by the application of pressure to the maternal abdomen to reposition the fetus. The average success rate for this procedure is 58%, with a wide range reported in published studies.[11,12] ECV is most likely to be successful if (1) the presenting part has not entered the pelvis, (2) amniotic fluid volume is normal, (3) the fetal back is not positioned posteriorly, (4) the patient is not obese, (5) the patient is parous, and (6) the presentation is either frank breech or transverse.[13] Early labor does not preclude successful ECV, but ECV is rarely successful when the cervix is fully dilated or when the membranes have ruptured. Multivariable predictive models may allow clinicians to improve prediction of successful ECV, with published models showing moderate discrimination and good calibration.[14,15]

ECV should ideally occur between 37 and 39 weeks' gestation for multiple reasons.[12,16] First, spontaneous version to vertex presentation most often occurs by 37 weeks' gestation. Second, successful performance of ECV after 37 weeks' gestation decreases the likelihood of spontaneous reversion from vertex to breech presentation. Third, if complications occur during ECV performed after 37 weeks' gestation, emergency delivery will not result in delivery of a preterm infant.

Successful ECV helps reduce the risk for perinatal morbidity and mortality associated with breech delivery. The American College of Obstetricians and Gynecologists (ACOG) has suggested that "because the risk of an adverse event occurring as a result of ECV is small and the cesarean birth rate is significantly lower among women who have undergone successful ECV, all women who are near term with breech presentations should be offered an ECV attempt if there are no contraindications."[11] There is no general consensus on eligibility for ECV, and contraindications vary among published guidelines.[17] Labor and vaginal delivery occur in the majority of patients who undergo successful ECV, but anesthesia providers should remain vigilant because of the increased risk for intrapartum cesarean delivery necessitated by dystocia or a nonreassuring FHR tracing.[8]

ECV is associated with a low rate of morbidity in contemporary obstetric practice, although placental abruption and preterm labor are potential complications.[11] Safe ECV requires FHR monitoring and access to cesarean delivery services. In a systematic review of 84 studies that included 12,955 women, complications included transient (6.14%) and persistent (0.22%) FHR abnormalities, vaginal bleeding (0.30%), placental abruption (0.08%), emergency cesarean delivery (0.35%), and stillbirth (0.09%).[12] Fetal-maternal hemorrhage is another potential complication of ECV.[12] In one study, 16 of 89 (18%) patients undergoing ECV had Kleihauer-Betke stains indicating fetal-maternal hemorrhage.[18]

The success of ECV is improved with the administration of a tocolytic agent (e.g., terbutaline or nitroglycerin) prior to the procedure. A randomized placebo-controlled trial found that the success rate of ECV doubled with use of terbutaline compared with placebo.[18] A randomized controlled trial of intravenous nitroglycerin for tocolysis (100 to 300 µg bolus doses, up to a maximum total dose of 1000 µg) demonstrated a success rate of 24% in nulliparous women receiving nitroglycerin versus 8% in those receiving placebo.[19] In parous women, the success rate was higher (43%) compared with nulliparous women and there was no difference between the nitroglycerin and placebo groups.[19] Of interest, the rates of hypotension were similar between groups. A Cochrane review found that tocolysis with a beta-adrenergic receptor agonist prior to ECV increased the number of women with a cephalic presentation at the onset of labor (relative risk [RR], 1.68; 95% confidence interval [CI], 1.14 to 2.48) and reduced the number of cesarean deliveries (RR, 0.77; 95% CI, 0.67 to 0.88).[20] Women with a prior cesarean delivery are also candidates for ECV, with studies showing similar rates of successful version compared with women without a prior cesarean delivery.[21]

Another potential method to improve the success of ECV is neuraxial analgesia or anesthesia, likely via reducing maternal discomfort and relaxing abdominal wall musculature. Maternal discomfort can be significant during ECV, and greater pain during the procedure is associated with a lower chance of success.[22] While historically some worried that anesthesia would facilitate the use of excessive force during the procedure and increase adverse perinatal events, these concerns are not supported by published evidence. In fact, spinal anesthesia reduces the force required for successful version.[23]

Numerous studies now support the use of neuraxial analgesia for ECV.[24] For example, Weiniger et al.[25] randomly assigned 70 nulliparous women undergoing ECV to receive either spinal anesthesia with bupivacaine 7.5 mg or no anesthesia. The success rate was 67% in those who received spinal anesthesia, 32% in those without analgesia, and 42% in those who did not consent to enroll in the study; multivariable logistic regression modeling showed that the odds of successful ECV were 4.0-fold higher with spinal analgesia. A similar study in parous women by the same investigators also found an increased success rate with spinal anesthesia (87% versus 58%).[26] A metaanalysis of nine trials that included 934 women found that, compared with control, neuraxial anesthesia increased the ECV success rate, increased the occurrence of cephalic presentation in labor, increased the vaginal delivery rate, decreased the cesarean delivery rate, and decreased maternal discomfort.[27] There were no differences in the incidences of emergency cesarean delivery, transient fetal bradycardia, nonreassuring fetal testing, or placental abruption.

Additionally, several investigators have reported successful outcomes with neuraxial analgesia for ECV in women in whom a first attempt at ECV without neuraxial analgesia had been unsuccessful.[25,28] Weiniger et al.[25] found that failure of ECV was attributable to pain in 15 women in their control group, 11 of whom (73%) subsequently underwent successful ECV with spinal analgesia.

The optimal dose of intrathecal local anesthetic for ECV remains controversial. A metaanalysis of seven studies using neuraxial blockade to facilitate ECV concluded that administration of an *anesthetic* dose of local anesthetic doubles the success rate of ECV (RR, 1.95; 95% CI, 1.46 to 2.60), whereas an *analgesic* dose does not have any effect (RR, 1.18; 95% CI, 0.94 to 1.49).[29] A subsequent prospective, randomized, blinded trial addressed the question of optimal intrathecal bupivacaine dose to facilitate ECV success.[30] Patients were randomized to receive intrathecal bupivacaine doses of 2.5, 5, 7.5, or 10 mg with fentanyl 15 μg as part of a combined spinal-epidural (CSE) technique. Overall ECV success rate was 51.5% with no difference in success rates or cesarean delivery rates between the groups, demonstrating that intrathecal bupivacaine doses > 2.5 mg are not necessary and may only increase the incidence of hypotension. The obstetricians in that study did not perceive a difference in abdominal wall relaxation between the groups, even though pain scores were higher in the 2.5 mg bupivacaine group (median visual analog scale pain score 12 mm versus 4 to 5 mm in the other groups [scale 0 to 100 mm]). Patient satisfaction was high and not different between groups. Overall, optimal spinal local anesthetic dose likely varies according to the clinical situation.[31] If the goal is timely discharge whether or not the ECV is successful, a lower spinal dose allows faster resolution of the block. If the patient will be admitted for delivery regardless of whether the version is successful, a higher dose will not affect the length of stay and could facilitate emergency cesarean delivery should that become necessary.[31]

In contrast to neuraxial analgesia or anesthesia, the benefit of intravenous analgesia for ECV remains unclear. Khaw et al.[28] randomized women with breech presentations to receive either spinal anesthesia with hyperbaric bupivacaine 9 mg plus fentanyl 15 μg, intravenous remifentanil infusion 0.1 μg/kg/min, or control (no anesthetic or analgesic intervention) before attempted ECV. On the first attempt, success rates were 83% in the spinal anesthesia group, 64% in the remifentanil group, and 64% in the control group. Cases in the control group who failed were rerandomized to spinal anesthesia or remifentanil for a second attempt, which resulted in success rates of 78% with spinal anesthesia versus 0% with remifentanil. There was no significant difference in the occurrence of fetal bradycardia requiring cesarean delivery. A recent systematic review of remifentanil's effectiveness for ECV demonstrated a 43% increased chance of success compared with placebo (RR, 1.43; 95% CI, 1.14 to 1.78).[32]

Overall, evidence suggests that neuraxial anesthesia helps to facilitate successful ECV and vaginal delivery and should therefore be used routinely. Intrathecal administration of 2.5 mg bupivacaine combined with fentanyl provides sufficient analgesia and abdominal wall relaxation while avoiding side effects such as hypotension associated with higher doses. Higher local anesthetic doses may be appropriate on a case-by-case basis.

Mode of Delivery

Most parturients with a breech presentation now undergo cesarean delivery since the publication of the Term Breech Trial in 2000.[6] In this trial, 2088 women with a singleton fetus in frank or complete breech presentation were enrolled from 26 countries and were randomly to undergo planned cesarean or planned vaginal delivery. While the study did not demonstrate any significant differences in maternal morbidity or mortality between groups during the delivery admission or the first 6 postpartum weeks, the finding of considerable differences in neonatal outcomes prompted important changes to contemporary obstetric practice, with nearly all planned breech deliveries now occurring via cesarean delivery. Using intention-to-treat analysis, the investigators demonstrated a lower rate of perinatal mortality, neonatal mortality, and serious neonatal morbidity in the planned cesarean delivery group (1.6% versus 5.0%, RR, 0.33 [95% CI, 0.19 to 0.56]). This difference was greatest in the 16 countries with a low perinatal mortality rate.[6] The lowest risk for adverse perinatal outcomes occurred with prelabor cesarean delivery performed at term.[33] The risk for adverse perinatal outcomes progressively increased with cesarean delivery performed during early labor, cesarean delivery performed during active labor, and vaginal birth. Labor augmentation and longer second stage of labor were associated with an increased risk for adverse perinatal outcomes, whereas the presence of an experienced clinician at delivery was associated with a reduced risk.[33] A subsequent metaanalysis of 27 studies including 258,953 deliveries confirmed higher perinatal morbidity and mortality with planned vaginal breech delivery compared with planned cesarean delivery, although absolute risks were relatively low in both groups.[34]

Despite the results of the Term Breech Trial, multicenter data from 2003 to 2011 showed an increase in vaginal delivery in Canadian women with breech presentation of non-anomalous singleton infants at term.[35] The vaginal breech delivery rate increased from 2.7% to 3.9% over the studied time period, and the rate of cesarean breech delivery in labor increased from 8.7% to 9.8%. Composite neonatal morbidity and mortality rates, however, were significantly higher after vaginal delivery compared with cesarean delivery without labor, with an adjusted rate ratio of 3.6 (95% CI, 2.50 to 5.15). This difference was even more pronounced among women with a gestational age greater than 40 weeks (adjusted rate ratio 5.39; 95% CI, 2.68 to 10.80). Thus, the Canadian data support the results of the Term Breech Trial.

In many regions of the world, the number of planned vaginal breech deliveries has decreased because of the Term Breech Trial. For example, in Denmark, the proportion of singleton term breech infants delivered vaginally decreased abruptly from 20% before 1999 to 6% after 2001.[36] At the same time, intrapartum or early neonatal mortality among all term breech infants decreased from 0.13% to 0.05% (RR, 0.38; 95% CI, 0.15 to 0.98).[36] The downward trend in rates of vaginal breech delivery is likely to continue. As the number of practitioners with experience in performing vaginal breech delivery has decreased, the number of vaginal breech deliveries available to teach obstetric residents may no longer be adequate. Unintended results of this practice change include a generation of obstetricians who have lost the skills to practice vaginal breech deliveries and medicolegal concerns that now discourage the practice of vaginal breech delivery.[37]

Nevertheless, obstetric providers in some regions of the world retain a strong tradition of offering vaginal breech delivery for selected patients. Published in 2006, the PREMODA (PREsentation et MODe d'Accouchement: presentation and mode of delivery) study[38] described birth outcomes for all term breech deliveries in 12-month periods during 2001 to 2002 in 174 centers in France and Belgium. The study included 2526 women who planned vaginal breech delivery, of whom 1794 delivered vaginally, and 5579 women who planned cesarean breech delivery.[38] The primary outcome captured a composite of fetal and neonatal mortality and serious morbidity and was not statistically different between women who planned to undergo vaginal delivery (1.60%; 95% CI, 1.14 to 2.17) and women who planned to undergo cesarean delivery (1.45%; 95% CI, 1.16 to 1.81), with odds ratio (OR) 1.10 (95% CI, 0.75 to 1.61).[38] The authors suggested that rigorous adherence to protocols for patient selection, intrapartum fetal surveillance, and management of the second stage of labor contributed to improved outcomes for women attempting vaginal breech delivery.

Acknowledging the potential for acceptable patient outcomes with vaginal breech delivery in the setting of appropriate provider training and hospital resources, the ACOG makes the following recommendations about mode of singleton breech delivery at term[39]:

- "The decision regarding the mode of delivery should consider patient wishes and the experience of the healthcare provider."
- "Obstetrician-gynecologists and other obstetric care providers should offer ECV as an alternative to planned cesarean for a woman who has a term singleton breech fetus, desires a planned vaginal delivery of a vertex-presenting fetus, and has no contraindications. ECV should be attempted only in settings in which cesarean delivery services are readily available."
- "Planned vaginal delivery of a term singleton breech fetus may be reasonable under hospital-specific protocol guidelines for eligibility and labor management."
- "If a vaginal breech delivery is planned, a detailed informed consent should be documented—including risks that perinatal or neonatal mortality or short-term serious neonatal morbidity may be higher than if a cesarean delivery is planned."

Vaginal Breech Delivery

Owing to the concerns regarding adverse perinatal outcomes, planned vaginal breech delivery occurs uncommonly in most hospitals in North America and the United Kingdom[40]; however, vaginal breech delivery does occur, rarely, when patients present in advanced labor. In cases where vaginal breech delivery is considered, criteria listed in Box 34.2 may be used to determine appropriate patient eligibility.[5] Personnel experienced in obstetric anesthesia and neonatal resuscitation are prerequisites for a trial of breech labor. Hyperextension of the fetal head remains an absolute contraindication to a trial of labor in the patient with a breech presentation.[5] Many obstetric providers delay maternal expulsive efforts for 30 minutes

---

BOX 34.2 Criteria for Trial of Labor and Vaginal Delivery for Patients With Breech Presentation

- Frank breech presentation
- Adequate pelvis by imaging pelvimetry
- Absence of a fetal anomaly that could cause dystocia
- Estimated fetal weight between 2000 g and 3500 g by ultrasonography or by two experienced examiners
- Flexion of the fetal head (the neutral position is also acceptable)
- Continuous electronic fetal heart rate monitoring
- Spontaneous progression of labor, with timely effacement and dilation of the cervix and timely descent of the breech
- Availability of an individual skilled in vaginal breech delivery and an assistant
- Availability of an individual skilled in the administration of obstetric anesthesia
- Spontaneous delivery to the level of the umbilicus
- Ability to perform an abdominal delivery promptly
- Availability of an individual with skills in neonatal resuscitation

after full cervical dilation. Others delay expulsive efforts until the breech is at the perineum.

There are three techniques for vaginal breech delivery. **Spontaneous breech delivery** avoids any traction or manipulation other than support of the infant's body. With **assisted breech delivery** (also known as partial breech extraction), the infant is delivered spontaneously as far as the umbilicus; at that time, the obstetric provider assists delivery of the chest and the aftercoming head. With **total breech extraction**, the obstetric provider applies traction on the feet and ankles to deliver the entire body of the infant. Except for vaginal delivery of a second twin, obstetric providers almost never perform total breech extraction. Total breech extraction increases the likelihood of difficult, traumatic delivery, including entrapment of the fetal head. During assisted breech delivery or total breech extraction, the obstetric provider attempts to maintain flexion of the cervical spine during delivery of the head. This may be accomplished manually or by the application of Piper forceps (Figs. 34.3 to 34.5). The obstetric provider commonly performs a generous episiotomy to prevent perineal obstruction of the aftercoming head.

Cesarean Delivery

For patients with persistent breech presentation at term, elective cesarean delivery should be offered between 39 and 41 weeks' gestation. Cesarean delivery at or near 39 weeks' gestation reduces perinatal mortality not only through avoiding the risks of vaginal breech birth, but also by avoiding stillbirth after 39 weeks' gestation and intrapartum risks should labor begin spontaneously before scheduled cesarean delivery.[41] Obstetric providers should confirm breech presentation via ultrasonographic examination immediately prior to surgery to ensure spontaneous version has not occurred. Generous

skin and uterine incisions should be made based on estimated fetal size, to minimize the likelihood of traumatic delivery. In preterm deliveries, a vertical uterine incision may need to be performed if the lower uterine segment is poorly developed. When such incisions extend to the body of the uterus (classical uterine incision), this confers a 1% to 12% risk for uterine rupture in subsequent pregnancies (see Chapter 20).

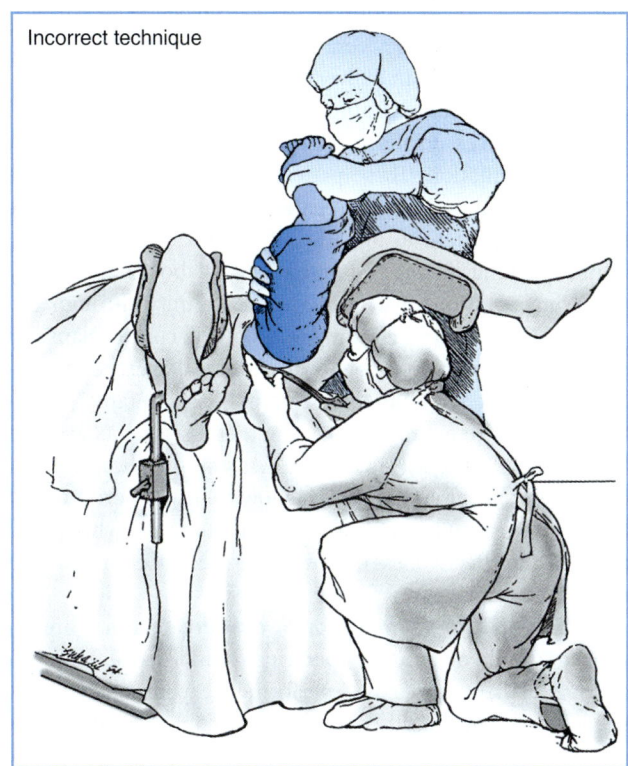

Fig. 34.4 Vaginal Breech Delivery. Demonstration of ***incorrect assistance*** during the application of Piper forceps; the assistant hyperextends the fetal neck. Such positioning increases the risk for neurologic injury. From Barth WH. Malpresentations. In: Landon MB, Galan HL, Jauniaux ERM, et al., eds. *Gabbe's Obstetrics: Normal and Problem Pregnancies.* 8th ed. Elsevier; 2021:319–342.

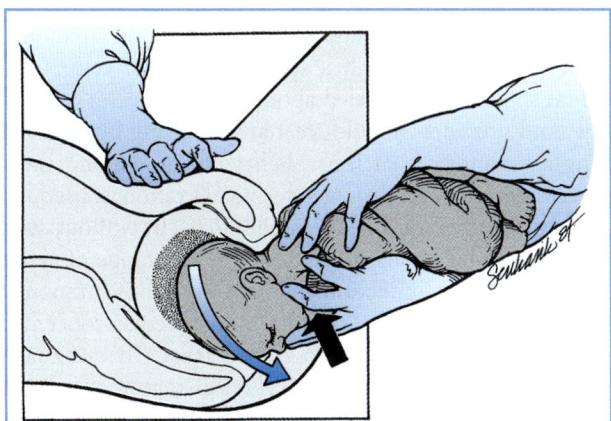

Fig. 34.3 Vaginal Breech Delivery. The *black arrow* indicates the direction of pressure from two fingers of the operator's right hand on the fetal maxilla (not the mandible). This maneuver assists in maintaining appropriate flexion of the fetal vertex *(direction of blue arrow)*, as does moderate suprapubic pressure from an assistant. Delivery of the head may be accomplished with continued maternal expulsive forces and gentle downward traction. From Barth WH. Malpresentations. In: Landon MB, Galan HL, Jauniaux ERM, et al., eds. *Gabbe's Obstetrics: Normal and Problem Pregnancies.* 8th ed. Elsevier; 2021:319–342.

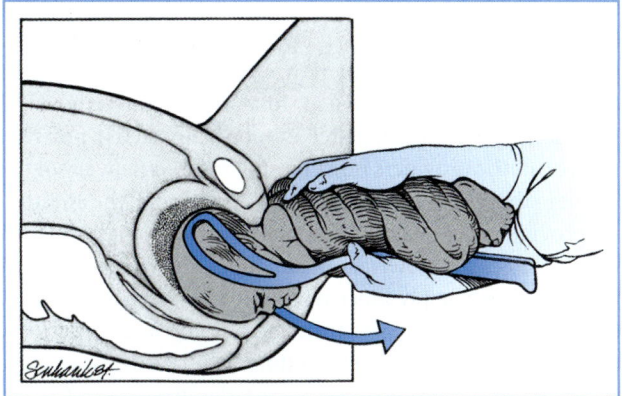

Fig. 34.5 Vaginal Breech Delivery. Once the Piper forceps are applied, the fetal trunk is supported by one hand, and gentle traction on the forceps *(arrow)* in the direction of the pelvic axis results in a controlled delivery. From Barth WH. Malpresentations. In: Landon MB, Galan HL, Jauniaux ERM, et al., eds. *Gabbe's Obstetrics: Normal and Problem Pregnancies.* 8th ed. Elsevier; 2021:319–342.

Anesthetic Management

Analgesia for Labor

Benefits of neuraxial analgesia during breech labor include (1) pain relief, (2) inhibition of early pushing by blocking the perineal reflex, (3) ability of the parturient to push during the second stage and spontaneously deliver the infant to the level of the umbilicus, (4) a relaxed pelvic floor and perineum at delivery, and (5) the option to extend analgesia to surgical anesthesia for emergency cesarean delivery if needed.

Emergency cesarean delivery may be required at any time during a trial of labor. Both epidural and CSE analgesia are excellent choices during a trial of labor in patients with a breech presentation. These patients often have earlier complaints of rectal pressure than patients with a vertex presentation. It is important to provide sufficient sacral analgesia to inhibit pushing during the first stage of labor, which could result in expulsion of a fetal lower extremity through the partially dilated cervix, leading to umbilical cord prolapse or fetal head entrapment. A bolus dose of local anesthetic solution that includes a lipid-soluble opioid (e.g., fentanyl, sufentanil) may be required to block the sacral segments and the reflex urge to push during the late first stage of labor. Use of a local anesthetic alone to eliminate low back and perineal discomfort may result in extensive motor blockade, which may decrease the effectiveness of maternal expulsive efforts during the second stage.

Anesthesia for vaginal breech delivery. Vaginal breech delivery should occur in an operating room where emergency abdominal delivery can be performed expeditiously when needed. Umbilical cord compression is common during the second stage of labor in a patient with a breech presentation, and the anesthesia provider should be prepared for emergency administration of general anesthesia at any time. For this reason, consideration should be given to the administration of a nonparticulate antacid at the time of transfer to the operating room.

Provision of effective analgesia and anesthesia for vaginal breech delivery represents a true challenge in obstetric anesthesia. In contrast to the *vertex* presentation, where obstetric providers may perform operative vaginal delivery to assist expulsive efforts when needed, total breech extraction of a singleton fetus is unacceptable in modern obstetric practice. Most obstetric providers insist on spontaneous delivery of the infant to the level of the umbilicus. Furthermore, the anesthesia provider may be asked to quickly provide anesthesia for vaginal or cesarean delivery at any time. Many obstetric providers routinely apply Piper forceps to the aftercoming head, a maneuver that requires adequate anesthesia and perineal muscle relaxation. Because a dilute solution of local anesthetic has been administered during the first stage of labor, it is often necessary to administer a more concentrated local anesthetic at the time of delivery. Either 3% 2-chloroprocaine or 2% lidocaine with epinephrine and bicarbonate may be used to rapidly extend epidural analgesia to anesthesia for operative delivery (see Chapter 26).

Probably the obstetric provider's greatest fear is the risk for **fetal head entrapment**. Most cases of this complication involve entrapment of the fetal head behind a partially dilated cervix, but the head may also be entrapped by the perineum. Fetal head entrapment is more likely to occur in patients at less than 32 weeks' gestation, when the fetal head is larger than the wedge formed by the fetal buttocks and thighs. If this complication occurs, the obstetric provider may choose one of the following three options: (1) performance of Dührssen incisions in the cervix, (2) relaxation of skeletal and cervical smooth muscle, or (3) cesarean delivery.

The performance of **Dührssen incisions** involves two or three radial incisions in the cervix at the 2-, 6-, and 10-o'clock positions.[5] This procedure is associated with a high risk for maternal morbidity (e.g., genitourinary trauma, hemorrhage), and substantial blood loss, which may be concealed within the peritoneal cavity.

More often, the obstetric provider requests that the anesthesia provider establish **relaxation of the cervix** via pharmacologic means or induction of general anesthesia. Intravenous or sublingual nitroglycerin (coupled with neuraxial local anesthetic if an epidural catheter is *in situ*) is often successful in achieving uterine and cervical relaxation.[42] Administration of nitroglycerin results in the release of nitric oxide, which mediates the relaxation of smooth muscle. While transient hypotension is common, the administration of nitroglycerin for the purpose of uterine relaxation appears safe for both the mother and the infant.[43] Published case reports have described clinically apparent uterine relaxation achieved with cumulative intravenous nitroglycerin doses ranging from 50 to 1500 μg. The actual dose required for specific clinical situations is unknown. Sublingual tablets or sprays of metered-dose nitroglycerin (400 μg) may provide a more convenient means of administration, whereas intravenous administration may allow for more rigorous titration. Both routes of administration appear to provide rapid onset of uterine relaxation with a short duration of action. The patient should be counseled about the acute onset of headache, and providers should treat any resulting hypotension using a vasopressor such as phenylephrine. Should nitroglycerin not provide adequate uterine relaxation, subsequent conversion to general anesthesia should occur without delay.

If general anesthesia is required, the technique of choice is rapid-sequence induction followed by administration of a high concentration (2 to 3 minimum alveolar concentration [MAC]) of a volatile halogenated agent. This technique typically results in uterine and cervical relaxation in 2 to 3 minutes. Immediately after delivery, the anesthesia provider should discontinue administration of the volatile halogenated agent and substitute alternative anesthetic agents with lower risk for uterine atony. Anesthesia should be maintained until the placenta is delivered, the episiotomy and lacerations are repaired, and hemostasis is achieved.

The use of epidural analgesia likely lowers the incidence of fetal head entrapment during vaginal breech delivery for at least two reasons. First, epidural analgesia inhibits early pushing during the first stage of labor. Second, although epidural analgesia does not relax the cervix at delivery, it provides effective pain relief and skeletal muscle relaxation. A relaxed pelvic floor and perineum facilitates placement of Piper forceps and delivery of the aftercoming head. Moreover, effective analgesia and skeletal muscle relaxation allow an assistant to provide maternal suprapubic pressure, which helps maintain flexion of the fetal cervical spine during delivery.

Anesthesia for Cesarean Delivery

Spinal, epidural, or general anesthesia can be administered for breech cesarean delivery. Because breech delivery can be more challenging than delivery of a vertex fetus, even during cesarean birth, uterine relaxation may be required. Certain fetal malformations, such as sacral teratoma or hydrocephalus, can present additional challenges to fetal extraction. When general anesthesia is used, the anesthesia provider can increase the concentration of volatile halogenated agent to facilitate uterine relaxation. When neuraxial anesthesia is used, intravenous or sublingual administration of nitroglycerin or intravenous administration of a beta-2-adrenergic receptor agonist such as terbutaline typically provides adequate uterine relaxation. It is rarely necessary to perform intraoperative induction of general anesthesia followed by administration of a high concentration of a volatile halogenated agent to facilitate delivery.

Regardless of the route of delivery, newborn infants with a breech presentation are typically born more depressed than infants with a vertex presentation. An individual skilled in neonatal resuscitation should be immediately available.

OTHER ABNORMAL PRESENTATIONS

Face Presentation

Face presentation, in which the neck is deflexed (extended backward) occurs in 1 in 600 to 800 live births. Vaginal delivery can be achieved in 70% to 80% of infants with a face presentation if the mentum rotates to an anterior position, but FHR abnormalities are common.[5] Manual efforts to flex the fetal cervical spine or convert an unfavorable mentum posterior position to a more favorable mentum anterior position are rarely successful and may result in significant maternal complications including uterine rupture, as well as adverse neonatal complications including spinal cord injury and difficult ventilation due to tracheal and laryngeal edema.[44]

Brow Presentation

In patients with a brow presentation, the cervical spine position is intermediate between the full flexion of a normal vertex presentation and the full extension of a face presentation. On vaginal examination, the obstetric provider can palpate the brow, orbits, and saddle of the nose, but not the mouth or chin. Brow presentation occurs in approximately 1 in 500 to 4000 deliveries. Persistent brow presentation typically requires cesarean delivery because of dystocia. Spontaneous flexion or extension of the neck may occur during labor, which may allow vaginal delivery.[5]

Compound Presentation

Compound presentation (where an extremity is prolapsed alongside the main presenting fetal part) occurs in 1 in 300 to 1000 deliveries. Most often, an upper extremity presents with the vertex. Umbilical cord prolapse is more common (10% to 20%) in deliveries with a compound presentation, as is neurologic or musculoskeletal damage to the involved extremity.[5] Labor and delivery may occur safely, but abdominal delivery is needed in patients with cord prolapse or arrest of labor. Expectant management rather than manipulation of the prolapsed extremity is the most common practice.[5]

Shoulder Presentation

A shoulder presentation (also known as a transverse lie) mandates performance of cesarean delivery except in two circumstances. First, successful ECV will allow vaginal delivery. Second, the obstetric provider may perform internal podalic version and total breech extraction of a second twin with a shoulder presentation.

Transverse lie can present as back down or back up. Cesarean delivery of a fetus with a back-down transverse lie can be especially difficult with no presenting part to grasp. If intraabdominal version cannot be accomplished before hysterotomy, this presentation represents an indication for a classical or low vertical uterine incision.

MULTIPLE GESTATION

Epidemiology

Monozygotic twins (which occur when a single fertilized ovum divides into two distinct individuals after a variable number of cell divisions) exhibit a constant incidence of approximately 4 per 1000 births. The incidence of **dizygotic twins** (which occur when two separate ova are fertilized) varies among races and by maternal age. In the United States, twin births occur most frequently among non-Hispanic Black and non-Hispanic White Americans (40.7 and 32.6 per 1000 live births, respectively) and less frequently among Asian Americans, Native Americans, Hispanics, or Native Hawaiians (23.1 to 26.3 per 1000 live births).[45] The incidence increases with parity, independent of maternal age.[46] In the United States, the twin birth rate rose 76% between 1980 and 2009 (from 19 to 33 per 1000 live births), peaked in 2014 at 34 per 1000 live births, and has been steadily declining in recent years to a low of 31 per 1000 live births in 2020.[45] Twin birth rates have risen most dramatically (>200%) among women 40 years of age and older. Delayed childbearing and spontaneous twinning among older women appear to explain one-third of the increase in the rate of multiple gestation between 1980 and 2010, with the remainder attributed to greater use of assisted reproductive technologies.[47]

Placentation

Placentas in multiple gestation may be (1) **monochorionic monoamniotic**, (2) **monochorionic diamniotic**, or (3) **dichorionic diamniotic** (Fig. 34.6). In all occurrences of dizygotic twins, the placenta is dichorionic diamniotic. A dichorionic diamniotic placenta is also present if monozygotic twinning occurs during the first 2 to 3 days after fertilization. Twinning between 3 and 8 days commonly results in a monochorionic diamniotic placenta. Monochorionic monoamniotic placentas are found when twinning occurs at 8 to 13 days. Embryonic cleavage between 13 and 15 days results in conjoined twins with a monochorionic monoamniotic placenta. Chorionicity is best determined by ultrasonography in the first or early second trimester.[48]

It is important to know the type of placentation because it determines the likelihood of vascular communications. Vascular communications occur in nearly all monochorionic placentas and are rare in dichorionic placentas.[49] Vascular communications may result in twin-to-twin transfusion syndrome and intrauterine fetal death. Monochorionic placentation also increases the risk for intrauterine fetal death from other causes (e.g., cord accident).[49]

Physiologic Changes

Multiple gestation accelerates and may exaggerate the physiologic and anatomic changes of pregnancy. Of interest to the anesthesia provider, multiple gestation intensifies the cardiovascular and pulmonary changes of pregnancy. However, the renal, hepatic, and central nervous system changes resemble those that occur in women with a singleton fetus.

Increased uterine size, especially near term, may result in a reduction in both total lung capacity and functional residual capacity. During periods of hypoventilation or apnea, hypoxemia develops more rapidly because of decreased functional residual capacity and increased maternal metabolic rate. However, one cross-sectional study demonstrated no significant difference in pulmonary function tests between 68 women with a twin pregnancy and 140 women with a singleton pregnancy.[50] Maternal weight increases at a greater rate after 30 weeks' gestation in women with multiple gestation.[51] Greater uterine size displaces the stomach cephalad, decreasing the competence of the lower esophageal sphincter and increasing the risk for passive regurgitation and potential pulmonary aspiration of gastric contents. All these physiologic and anatomic factors, plus increased breast size, combine to potentially increase the risk for difficult tracheal intubation and ventilation.

The increase in plasma volume at term in twin gestation pregnancy is approximately 750 mL more than in singleton pregnancy.[52] Relative or actual anemia often occurs. Multiple gestation also results in a 20% greater increase in cardiac output compared with singleton pregnancy, owing to a greater stroke volume (15%) and higher heart rate (3.5%). In a longitudinal study that compared uncomplicated twin pregnancies to singleton pregnancies, cardiac output was higher at all time points with twins while total vascular resistance was lower.[53] The greater fetal weight and larger volume of amniotic fluid predispose the mother with multiple gestation to aortocaval compression and supine hypotension syndrome.

Obstetric Complications
Fetal Complications

Fetal complications include those related solely to multiple gestation (e.g., twin-to-twin transfusion syndrome) and those related to abnormal presentation (e.g., prolapsed umbilical cord) (Box 34.3).

Twin-to-twin transfusion. Nearly all monochorionic twin placentas have vascular anastomoses, but most of these have little fetal consequence. Deep arteriovenous vascular

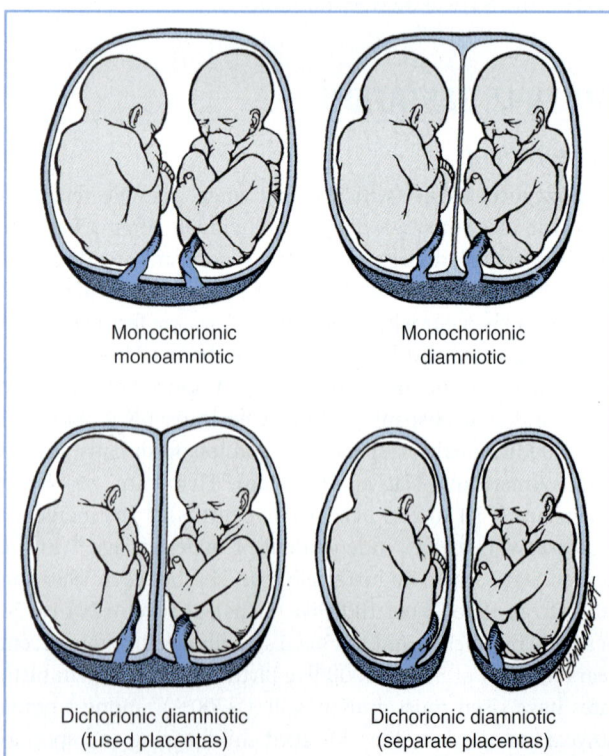

Fig. 34.6 **Placentation in Twin Pregnancies.** From Unal ER, Newman RB. Multiple gestations. In: Landon MB, Galan HL, Jauniaux ERM, et al., eds. *Gabbe's Obstetrics: Normal and Problem Pregnancies.* 8th ed. Elsevier; 2021:751–783.

Monochorionic
monoamniotic

Monochorionic
diamniotic

Dichorionic diamniotic
(fused placentas)

Dichorionic diamniotic
(separate placentas)

BOX 34.3   Fetal Complications Associated With Multiple Gestation

- Twin-to-twin transfusion
- Fetal growth restriction
- Preterm delivery
- Malpresentation
- Congenital anomalies
- Polyhydramnios
- Cord entanglement
- Umbilical cord prolapse

communications create a common villous compartment in about one-half of monochorionic twin placentas and can result in twin-to-twin transfusion,[54] in which one twin becomes the donor and the other twin becomes the recipient. The donor twin is smaller and is at risk for fetal growth restriction and anemia. The recipient twin is plethoric and is at risk for volume overload and cardiac failure. Alternative explanations for the syndrome include unequal blood volumes secondary to compression of a velamentous umbilical cord insertion and higher arterial blood pressure in the donor twin than in the recipient. Twin-to-twin transfusion increases both the perinatal mortality rate and the risk for adverse neurodevelopmental outcome in survivors.[55]

Potential therapeutic options include decompression amniocentesis, amniotic septostomy, interruption of the placental vessel communications, and selective feticide.[56] Decompression amniocentesis or serial amnioreduction to treat polyhydramnios in the recipient twin may improve circulation to a "stuck" donor twin (the term refers to such severe oligohydramnios in the donor twin that the fetus is wedged in the corner of the uterus and appears "stuck"). Amnioreduction restores normal amniotic fluid volume and improves fetal growth in the donor twin. Compared with serial amnioreduction, septostomy has the advantage of requiring only a single procedure.[57] Selective fetoscopic laser photocoagulation reduces vascular anastomoses and may improve perinatal outcomes.[58–61] Anesthetic management of these procedures focuses on maintaining uteroplacental circulation, achieving profound uterine relaxation, optimizing surgical conditions, monitoring fetal hemodynamics, and minimizing maternal and fetal risk.[62]

Fetal growth restriction. Twin-to-twin transfusion represents only one of the potential causes of fetal growth restriction in multiple gestation. The polyhydramnios within one fetal sac may limit the growth of the other fetus. In patients with three or more fetuses, limited intrauterine size may restrict fetal growth. In addition, factors that cause fetal growth restriction in singleton pregnancies also cause fetal growth restriction in multiple gestation (e.g., uteroplacental insufficiency, chromosomal abnormalities).

Preterm labor. Patients with multiple gestation are at high risk for preterm labor and delivery. Preterm labor occurs in 52% of women with twins resulting from *in vitro* fertilization compared with 22% of women with spontaneous twins.[48,63] Sixty percent of women with twins deliver before 37 weeks' gestation, and only 6.4% of triplet pregnancies reach term.[64] Routine use of bed rest, prophylactic cerclage, vaginal progesterone, and tocolytic therapy have not been shown to improve perinatal outcome in multiple gestation pregnancies.[65] When preterm labor occurs, the patient may receive parenteral tocolytic therapy to facilitate administration of betamethasone for fetal lung maturation, magnesium sulfate for fetal neuroprotection, or both. The side effects of magnesium and other tocolytic agents may affect the response to anesthesia (see Chapter 33) and may increase the risk for postpartum hemorrhage. Multiple gestation also increases the risk for pulmonary edema associated with tocolytic therapy.[66]

Abnormal presentation. Multiple gestation is associated with a higher incidence of abnormal presentation, which results in part from the need to accommodate two or more fetuses within the uterine cavity. Malpresentation increases the risk for umbilical cord prolapse, which may occur either before or after delivery of the first infant.

Morbidity and mortality. In 2020, 6.6% of fetal deaths occurred in multiple gestation pregnancies.[67] The perinatal mortality rate in twin pregnancies is two times greater than that associated with singleton pregnancies (12.1 deaths per 1000 births versus 5.5 per 1000 births, respectively) and is five-fold higher in triplet or higher-order gestations (28.7 per 1000 births).[68] Preterm delivery accounts for most of this increase, although twins and triplets also have a higher weight-specific mortality, which may be related to twin-to-twin transfusion, congenital malformations, preeclampsia, malpresentation, or prolapsed umbilical cord. Some maternal-fetal medicine specialists advocate selective multifetal reduction to reduce the risk for maternal morbidity and perinatal morbidity and mortality associated with three or more fetuses. This issue is a moral and ethical dilemma for some patients and physicians; however, studies have shown that women who undergo pregnancy reduction from triplets to twins have rates of pregnancy complications, including preterm birth, low-birth-weight infants, stillbirth, and neonatal deaths, that are lower than in those who continue with triplets and are similar to those observed in women with spontaneously conceived twin gestations.[48]

Intensive inpatient monitoring improves perinatal survival of monoamniotic twins. A literature review of studies comparing inpatient and outpatient monitoring of monoamniotic twins suggested a 10-fold reduction in fetal death with inpatient monitoring after 28 weeks' gestation.[69] In addition to the risks faced by all twins, monoamniotic twins face the unique risk for cord entanglement. Three-times daily fetal monitoring and nonstress tests are used to check for multiple deep variable decelerations that could be related to cord entanglement. Intensive surveillance may also benefit monochorionic diamniotic twins.[70]

In multiple gestation pregnancies, death of one fetus can occur well before term. Johnson and Zhang[71] evaluated outcomes for 150,386 sets of twins and 5240 sets of triplets born between 1995 and 1997. Fetal death at 20 weeks' gestation or later occurred in 2.6% of twin gestations and 4.3% of triplet gestations. The investigators noted that survival of remaining fetuses declined with greater elapsed time from the fetal demise. Opposite-sex twins were more likely to survive, possibly reflecting the absence of monochorionic placentation. Obstetric management decisions are based on the cause of death and the status of both the surviving fetus and the mother. In monochorionic twin gestations complicated by twin-to-twin transfusion and fetal death, approximately 40% of the surviving twins experience mortality or serious neurodevelopmental morbidity.[72] If the cause of death was an abnormality of the fetus rather than maternal or uteroplacental pathology, expectant management of the pregnancy may be warranted.[48,49] Development of maternal pulmonary edema from **mirror syndrome** or disseminated intravascular coagulation from dead fetal tissue are theoretical complications that occur rarely.[48]

Multiple gestation is also associated with increased morbidity and mortality during the neonatal period. Triplet and quadruplet pregnancies have significantly higher risks than twin pregnancies for neonatal complications.[73]

Order of Delivery

Compared with first-born twins, the second-born has a higher incidence of adverse outcomes owing to lower birth weight and a higher frequency of malpresentation, umbilical cord prolapse, and placental abruption.[48,74,75] Placental abruption can occur when rapid decompression of the uterus following delivery of the first twin leads to shearing forces through the basal plate of the placenta. Internal podalic version of a second twin due to nonvertex presentation can also lead to abruption.

Administration of neuraxial anesthesia may improve the outcome of the second twin. In 1987 Crawford[76] observed that among women who received epidural analgesia, the two twins had similar umbilical cord blood pH measurements. In contrast, among women who received general anesthesia, the second twin tended to be more acidotic than the first. Likewise, Jarvis and Whitfield[77] reported no difference in outcome for first and second twins when the mother received epidural analgesia. Administration of general anesthesia is increasingly rare for cesarean delivery in women with multiple gestation.[78]

Maternal Complications

Multiple gestation increases the incidence of maternal morbidity and mortality (Box 34.4), even when adjusting for confounding factors.[79] A population-based cohort study in the Netherlands found the incidence of severe acute maternal morbidity was 7.0 per 1000 deliveries overall, but was 6.5 and 28.0 per 1000 for singleton and multiple pregnancies, respectively. The RR for severe acute maternal morbidity in twins compared with singleton pregnancies was 4.3 (95% CI, 3.7 to 5.0) and increased to 6.2 (95% CI, 2.5 to 15.3) in triplet pregnancies. Risk factors for morbidity included age > 40 years, nulliparity, use of assisted reproductive technology, and nonspontaneous onset of labor.[79] The increased incidence of

cesarean delivery as well as higher rates of preeclampsia also contribute to the higher risk for maternal morbidity and mortality associated with multiple gestation.[80]

The incidence of maternal complications increases in proportion to the number of fetuses.[81] Compared with mothers of twins, mothers of triplets and quadruplets are more likely to: (1) have preterm premature rupture of membranes, hypertension, and/or excessive bleeding; (2) require tocolysis; (3) require cesarean delivery at less than 29 weeks' gestation; and (4) have one or more infants die.[73] Abdominal distention and diaphragmatic elevation can cause respiratory distress and may necessitate early delivery in some patients with three or more fetuses.

Blood loss at delivery is approximately 500 mL greater in multiple gestation pregnancies than in singleton pregnancies.[49] Uterine distention increases the risk for uterine atony and postpartum hemorrhage. Most cases of atony respond to standard pharmacologic therapy (e.g., oxytocin, methylergonovine, 15-methyl prostaglandin $F_{2\alpha}$ [carboprost]). Persistent uterine atony may require the performance of interventions such as a uterine brace, B-Lynch suture, or emergency hysterectomy (see Chapter 37).

Obstetric Management

Based on the balance between risks of prematurity and increasing perinatal mortality at later gestational ages, the ACOG makes the following recommendations for timing of delivery[48]:

- Uncomplicated dichorionic-diamniotic twin gestation: 38 0/7 to 38 6/7 weeks' gestation
- Uncomplicated monochorionic-diamniotic twin gestation: 34 0/7 to 37 6/7 weeks' gestation
- Uncomplicated monochorionic-monoamniotic twin gestation: 32 0/7 to 34 0/7 weeks' gestation

Twin gestation itself does not contraindicate labor and vaginal delivery. However, multiple gestation is associated with a higher incidence of cesarean delivery. Most obstetric providers favor cesarean delivery for all patients with three or more fetuses.[49]

Several studies have investigated outcomes for twin delivery by planned cesarean or trial of labor.[82] Barrett et al.[83] randomized 2804 women with twin pregnancy and the first twin in cephalic presentation to planned cesarean delivery (1398 women) or planned vaginal delivery (1406 women). The rate of cesarean delivery was 90.7% in the planned-cesarean-delivery group and 43.8% in the planned-vaginal-delivery group. The authors found that planned cesarean delivery did not significantly affect the risk for fetal or neonatal death or serious neonatal morbidity, compared with planned vaginal delivery.[83] A 2-year neurodevelopmental follow-up of these children found no significant difference in the outcome of death or neurodevelopmental delay: 5.99% in the planned cesarean delivery group versus 5.83% in the planned vaginal delivery group (OR, 1.04; 95% CI, 0.77 to 1.41; P = .79).[84]

Observational data suggest that perinatal outcomes may be improved with planned vaginal delivery when the presenting

---

BOX 34.4   Maternal Complications Associated With Multiple Gestation

- Preterm premature rupture of membranes
- Preterm labor
- Prolonged labor
- Preeclampsia
- Placental abruption
- Operative delivery (operative vaginal and cesarean)
- Uterine atony
- Obstetric trauma
- Antepartum and/or postpartum hemorrhage

twin is in a vertex position. A large cohort study of 5915 twin deliveries in France compared planned cesarean delivery with planned vaginal delivery.[85] Of the women with a cephalic presentation of the first twin at or beyond 32 weeks' gestation, 75.4% had planned vaginal delivery, of whom 80.3% delivered both twins vaginally. Planned cesarean delivery compared with planned vaginal delivery before 37 weeks' gestation was associated with increased composite neonatal mortality and morbidity, and the authors recommended planned vaginal delivery rather than cesarean delivery between 32 and 37 weeks' gestation.[85] Another cohort study of 2597 twin deliveries at or after 34 weeks' gestation, with the first twin in a cephalic presentation, assessed a composite outcome of neonatal complications, defined as intrapartum or postpartum death, neonatal transfer to intensive or special care, or trauma of one or both twins.[86] The authors found that the rate of neonatal complications was lower for planned vaginal delivery compared with planned cesarean delivery (26.5% versus 31.7%, $P = .005$) and concluded that their findings do not support a policy of planned cesarean delivery for twin pregnancies at or after 34 weeks' gestation. A metaanalysis of 39,571 twin pregnancies found that neonatal morbidity was lower after vaginal delivery than after cesarean delivery for twin A (fetus closest to the birth canal), but there was no significant difference in neonatal morbidity between the two modes of delivery for twin B.[87] When outcomes were stratified for both presentation and mode of delivery, the mortality rate was lower after vaginal delivery than after cesarean delivery for both vertex and nonvertex twin B. If twin A is in a vertex presentation, the evidence supports a planned vaginal delivery after 32 weeks' gestation. Retrospective data support a similar policy for twin delivery before 32 weeks' gestation. In an analysis of data from centers with differing management policies for preterm twins, a policy of planned vaginal delivery of very preterm twins from 26 to 32 weeks' gestation with the first twin in cephalic presentation did not increase either severe neonatal morbidity or mortality compared with planned cesarean delivery.[88]

Maternal morbidity depends on the likelihood of achieving vaginal birth for both twins. A 7-year retrospective cohort study compared maternal morbidity in women with twins at or beyond 32 weeks' gestation who underwent trial of labor or elective cesarean delivery.[89] Vaginal delivery of both twins was successful in 74% of those having a trial of labor, but postpartum hemorrhage was more common among women who attempted vaginal delivery compared with those electing cesarean delivery (9.1% versus 4.9%; $P < .01$; adjusted OR, 2.2 [95% CI, 1.4 to 3.6]). Hemorrhage was responsible for the difference in the composite morbidity rate between groups. The authors noted that the trade-off for a 74% chance of vaginal delivery is a 4% absolute increase in the rate of serious postpartum hemorrhage, a discussion that should occur between the patient and her obstetric provider during delivery planning. The ACOG recommends a trial of labor for women with twin gestation when the first twin is in cephalic presentation as one method of safe reduction of the rate of primary cesarean deliveries.[90]

Both fetuses have a vertex presentation in 30% to 50% of twin gestations, and in 25% to 40% of cases the presentation is a vertex/breech combination. The remaining patients have various combinations of vertex, breech, and transverse lie.

Twin A

Decisions regarding the mode of delivery typically begin with the gestational age and presentation of twin A. Most obstetric providers allow a trial of labor if both twins have a vertex presentation. Similarly, most obstetric providers opt for cesarean delivery if the twin A has a breech or shoulder presentation. If twin A has a breech presentation and twin B has a vertex presentation, the chins may become interlocked during labor and delivery. This complication occurs infrequently, but the consequences can be devastating.[49] The unanticipated case of head entrapment, deflexed head, or locked twins may necessitate emergency abdominal delivery of both twins. The obstetric provider proceeds with cesarean delivery while an assistant supports the exteriorized body of twin A. The obstetric provider applies gentle traction on the head while the infant's body is guided back into the uterus.[49]

When twin A has a cephalic presentation, decisions about mode of delivery must account for the relative size, presentation, and position of twin B. Antepartum ultrasonographic examination allows the obstetric provider to assess the presentation, position, head size, and weight of both fetuses. Indications for planned cesarean delivery of twins include (1) evidence of discordant growth (especially if twin B is larger than twin A), (2) twin-to-twin transfusion syndrome, (3) selected congenital anomalies, and (4) evidence of uteroplacental insufficiency.[49]

A trial of labor mandates continuous FHR monitoring of both fetuses. After amniotomy, an electrocardiography lead may be placed on the scalp of twin A and Doppler ultrasonography may be used to monitor twin B.

Twin B

After vaginal delivery of twin A, the obstetric provider must decide about the method of delivery of twin B. Presentation and position should be verified, because these can change after delivery of twin A. If twin B has a vertex presentation and the head is well applied to the cervix, or if the amniotic membranes are still intact in a diamniotic pregnancy, the obstetric provider may allow the patient to resume labor and await spontaneous vaginal delivery.

For twin B with nonvertex presentation, options include (1) ECV followed by a resumption of labor, (2) internal podalic version and total breech extraction, and (3) cesarean delivery. Real-time ultrasonography facilitates the performance of ECV. Parturients receiving epidural anesthesia will be more relaxed and should tolerate the procedure better than those without neuraxial anesthesia.[48] Internal podalic version and total breech extraction may increase the likelihood of vaginal birth compared with attempted ECV. Total breech extraction is considered appropriate if twin A is the same size or larger than twin B, which ensures that the pelvis and cervical dilation are adequate for vaginal delivery of twin B, and if delivery is attempted early after delivery of twin A which ensures that the cervix has not begun to contract.[49] In a retrospective cohort study of women who labored with twin pregnancies with twin A in vertex presentation, patients with nonvertex twin B had comparable, if not higher, rates of vaginal delivery than their vertex-presenting counterparts.[91] Vaginal birth of both twins was associated with labor induction and the physician's years in practice, leading the authors to suggest a role for provider selection and delivery planning. Indications for emergency cesarean delivery of twin B include malpresentation not amenable to obstetric maneuvers, nonreassuring FHR tracing, and umbilical cord prolapse.

In the past, obstetric providers favored the delivery of twin B within 15 to 30 minutes of delivery of twin A. However, most data supporting this practice were obtained before the use of intrapartum FHR monitoring. In a 2002 review of 118 twin deliveries, Leung et al.[92] showed that umbilical cord blood gas and pH measurements of twin B deteriorated with increasing twin-to-twin delivery interval. In this study, 73% of second twins not delivered by 30 minutes required operative delivery because of a nonreassuring FHR tracing. A German retrospective analysis of 4110 twin pregnancies suggested that an increasing interval between delivery of twins is an independent risk factor for adverse short-term outcomes for twin B.[93] Continuous FHR monitoring of twin B is essential.

Anesthetic Management

Labor and Vaginal Delivery

Epidural analgesia provides optimal pain control and flexibility for subsequent anesthetic needs. The anesthesia provider must be vigilant, because obstetric conditions are dynamic and anesthetic requirements may change rapidly. Given the greater risk for cesarean delivery in patients with multiple gestation, the anesthesia provider should ensure that the epidural catheter is functioning throughout labor. If there is any question regarding the location of the catheter or the quality of the block, the catheter should be removed and replaced.

Patients with multiple gestation may be at higher risk than singleton pregnancies for aortocaval compression and hypotension during the administration of neuraxial analgesia and anesthesia. Use of the full left or right lateral position after induction of epidural analgesia reduces this risk. Because these patients are at increased risk for uterine atony and postpartum hemorrhage, establishment of large-bore intravenous access is recommended before delivery.

Patients with multiple gestation should deliver in an area where an emergency abdominal delivery can be performed immediately. As the time for delivery of twin A nears, the epidural analgesia should be evaluated once more and augmented, if necessary, although motor block should be avoided so that the patient can continue to push effectively. Effective anesthesia facilitates the performance of internal podalic version and total breech extraction of twin B, if necessary, and enables the extension to anesthesia for cesarean delivery when needed. Concentrated local anesthetic (e.g., 3% 2-chloroprocaine or 2% lidocaine with epinephrine) should

be immediately available for use if emergency cesarean delivery is required. Nitroglycerin may also be urgently required if uterine relaxation is needed acutely for delivery of twin B. At least one member of the anesthesia team should remain with the patient until twin A is delivered, and twin B is either delivered or the vertex is well applied in the pelvis.

CSE anesthesia is a reasonable alternative for vaginal delivery in patients with multiple gestation who do not already have a functioning epidural catheter *in situ*. An analgesic spinal dose can be administered for the second stage of labor and vaginal delivery, while the epidural catheter can be used to extend the block if cesarean delivery is required. Single-shot spinal anesthesia for vaginal delivery in these patients is not recommended because of its lack of flexibility in rapidly changing conditions. If an analgesic spinal dose is administered, it will not be adequate if cesarean delivery is required, and if an anesthetic spinal dose is administered, it will cause too much motor block for effective pushing and vaginal delivery.

Vaginal Delivery of Twin A/Operative Delivery of Twin B

The flexibility of epidural analgesia is especially advantageous if the obstetric provider delivers twin A vaginally, but twin B requires operative delivery. Once the obstetric provider determines that cesarean delivery will be necessary, additional local anesthetic should be administered to extend the surgical sensory level to approximately the T4 dermatome using a rapid-acting local anesthetic such as 3% 2-chloroprocaine or 2% lidocaine with epinephrine. In cases of prolonged fetal bradycardia or umbilical cord prolapse, it may be necessary to administer general anesthesia if adequate neuraxial anesthesia cannot be achieved rapidly. This problem can usually be avoided if (1) both the level and density of analgesia are optimized at the time of delivery of twin A, and (2) the anesthesia provider is present in the room and gives attention to both the FHR tracing and the obstetric provider.

If the obstetric provider opts for internal podalic version and total breech extraction of twin B, it is better to perform the procedure shortly after delivery of twin A, before the uterus and the cervix begin to contract. Pain relief and skeletal muscle relaxation (both provided by epidural anesthesia) facilitate internal version and total breech extraction of twin B. In some cases, pharmacologic uterine relaxation may be required. Sublingual (400 μg) or intravenous (150 to 250 μg) nitroglycerin or intravenous or subcutaneous terbutaline (250 μg) should provide adequate uterine relaxation for internal podalic version.[94,95] If this maneuver is unsuccessful, rapid-sequence induction of general anesthesia, followed by administration of a high concentration of a volatile halogenated agent, may be needed.

Cesarean Delivery

Epidural, spinal, or general anesthesia can be used for elective cesarean delivery for multiple gestation. Historically, epidural anesthesia was preferred to spinal anesthesia because of concern for higher risk for hemodynamic instability during administration of neuraxial anesthesia in women with multiple gestation. However, Ngan Kee et al.[96] compared the incidence of hypotension and vasopressor requirement in multiple versus singleton gestations undergoing cesarean delivery with spinal anesthesia and found no differences between groups in maternal and neonatal outcomes. Thus, spinal anesthesia is increasingly preferred by many anesthesia providers owing to the reliability of dense sensory blockade and rapidity of onset.

Whether spinal anesthetic doses should be decreased in patients with multiple gestation remains unclear. Jawan et al.[97] found that women with multiple gestation had a greater cephalad spread of local anesthetic with spinal anesthesia (10 mg hyperbaric bupivacaine) than women with a singleton gestation, whereas Ngan Kee et al.[96] found no difference. Similarly, Behforouz et al.[98] found no difference in the extent of sensory blockade after administration of epidural anesthesia between women with higher-order multiple gestation pregnancies and women with a singleton gestation. Any difference that may exist is likely to be of little clinical significance. If dose reduction is desired, a CSE technique allows use of a lower dose of local anesthetic for the spinal anesthesia component, while retaining the capability to raise the anesthetic level via the epidural catheter if needed.

Vallejo and Ramanathan[99] reported that umbilical venous and arterial lidocaine concentrations were 35% to 53% higher in twin newborns than in singleton newborns during epidural lidocaine anesthesia for cesarean delivery. Mean fetal-to-maternal lidocaine ratios were also up to 18% higher in the twin newborns. The investigators speculated that this difference may be a result of greater maternal cardiac output and plasma volume associated with twin gestation as well as the decreased total plasma protein concentration, which leads to an increase in the free lidocaine concentration. The clinical relevance of these findings is unclear.

Patients with multiple gestation are additionally at greater risk of supine hypotension syndrome. Comparison of brachial artery (arm) and popliteal artery (leg) blood pressures could allow the detection of occult supine hypotension and reduced uteroplacental perfusion in the presence of a normal brachial artery pressure. A nonreassuring FHR tracing for either infant should also prompt additional efforts to optimize uteroplacental perfusion, which may include additional left uterine displacement or transition to right uterine displacement.

When general anesthesia is used, greater oxygen consumption and decreased functional residual capacity associated with multiple gestation increases the risk for maternal hypoxemia during periods of apnea. Adequate preoxygenation prior to induction is essential.

The presence of two or more fetuses can result in a prolonged uterine incision-to-delivery interval because of the longer time required to deliver multiple infants. A prolonged interval increases the risk for fetal acidosis and neonatal depression. Neonatal depression, especially of twin B, is less likely with neuraxial anesthesia than with general anesthesia.[76,77] Regardless of the method of anesthesia, an individual skilled in neonatal resuscitation should be immediately available during the delivery.

KEY POINTS

- Breech presentation occurs more frequently at earlier gestational ages. There is a higher risk for perinatal morbidity and mortality with breech presentation, even when adjusted for preterm gestation.

- External cephalic version converts a breech or shoulder presentation to a vertex presentation and is recommended by the American College of Obstetricians and Gynecologists for most women with a singleton breech presentation near term.

- Successful external cephalic version reduces perinatal morbidity and mortality associated with breech delivery and lowers the cesarean delivery rate. Neuraxial anesthesia improves the success rate of external cephalic version, even after an initial attempt failed without neuraxial anesthesia.

- Advantages of epidural analgesia during a trial of labor in the patient with breech presentation include: (1) effective pain relief; (2) inhibition of early pushing; (3) relaxation of the pelvic floor and perineum, facilitating atraumatic delivery of the aftercoming head; (4) provision of anesthesia for emergency cesarean delivery by injecting additional local anesthetic through the epidural catheter.

- Multiple gestation exaggerates the physiologic and anatomic changes of pregnancy, with cardiovascular and pulmonary changes being most pronounced.

- Many fetal and maternal complications occur more commonly in multiple gestation pregnancies. Fetal complications include twin-to-twin transfusion, fetal growth restriction, preterm labor, abnormal presentation, congenital anomalies, and umbilical cord prolapse. Maternal complications include uterine atony, postpartum hemorrhage, placental abruption, preeclampsia, and operative delivery.

- Neuraxial analgesia is the analgesic technique of choice during labor in the patient with multiple gestation. Pain relief and skeletal muscle relaxation facilitate the vaginal delivery of twin B, and an *in situ* epidural catheter facilitates the administration of anesthesia for emergency cesarean delivery, if needed.

- The obstetric provider may request drugs for uterine or cervical relaxation to facilitate vaginal delivery of twin B or, in cases of breech presentation, to facilitate the delivery of the aftercoming fetal head. Intravenous or sublingual nitroglycerin provides rapid uterine relaxation of short duration. Alternatively, rapid-sequence induction of general anesthesia followed by administration of a high concentration of a volatile halogenated agent also reliably provides uterine and cervical relaxation.

REFERENCES

1. Masturzo B, Farina A, Attamante L, et al. Sonographic evaluation of the fetal spine position and success rate of manual rotation of the fetus in occiput posterior position: a randomized controlled trial. *J Clin Ultrasound.* 2017;5:472–476.

2. Blanc J, Castel P, Mauviel F, et al. Prophylactic manual rotation of occiput posterior and transverse positions to decrease operative delivery: the PROPOP randomized clinical trial. *Am J Obstet Gynecol.* 2021;225:444.e1–e8.

3. Shaffer BL, Cheng YW, Vargas JE, Caughey AB. Manual rotation to reduce caesarean delivery in persistent occiput posterior or transverse position. *J Matern Fetal Neonatal Med.* 2011;24:65–72.

4. Lieberman E, Davidson K, Lee-Parritz A, Shearer E. Changes in fetal position during labor and their association with epidural analgesia. *Obstet Gynecol.* 2005;105:974–982.

5. Barth WH. Malpresentations. In: Landon MB, Galan HL, Jauniaux ERM, et al., eds. *Gabbe's Obstetrics: Normal and Problem Pregnancies.* 8th ed. Elsevier; 2021:319–342.

6. Hannah ME, Hannah WJ, Hewson SA, et al. Planned caesarean section versus planned vaginal birth for breech presentation at term: a randomised multicentre trial. *Lancet.* 2000;356:1375–1383.

7. Albrechtsen S, Rasmussen S, Dalaker K, Irgens LM. Perinatal mortality in breech presentation sibships. *Obstet Gynecol.* 1998;92:775–780.

8. De Hundt M, Velzel J, DeGroot CJ, et al. Mode of delivery after successful external cephalic version: a systematic review and meta-analysis. *Obstet Gynecol.* 2014;123:1327–1334.

9. Hannah ME, Whyte H, Hannah WJ, et al. Maternal outcomes at 2 years after planned cesarean section versus planned vaginal birth for breech presentation at term: the international randomized Term Breech Trial. *Am J Obstet Gynecol.* 2004;191:917–927.

10. Schiff E, Friedman SA, Mashiach S, et al. Maternal and neonatal outcome of 846 term singleton breech deliveries: seven-year experience at a single center. *Am J Obstet Gynecol.* 1996;175:18–23.

11. American College of Obstetricians and Gynecologists. Practice Bulletin No. 221: External cephalic version (reaffirmed 2023). *Obstet Gynecol.* 2020;135:1239–1241.

12. Grootscholten K, Kok M, Oei SG, et al. External cephalic version-related risks: a meta-analysis. *Obstet Gynecol.* 2008;112:1143–1151.

13. Kok M, Cnossen J, Gravendeel L, et al. Clinical factors to predict the outcome of external cephalic version: a meta-analysis. *Am J Obstet Gynecol.* 2008;199:630.e1–e7.

14. Dahl CM, Zhang Y, Ong JX, et al. A multivariable predictive model for success of external cephalic version. *Obstet Gynecol.* 2021;138:426–433.

15. Dong T, Chen X, Zhao B, et al. Development of prediction models for successful external cephalic version and delivery outcome. *Arch Gynecol Obstet.* 2022;305:63–75.

16. Hutton EK, Hannah ME, Ross SJ, et al. The early external cephalic version (ECV) 2 trial: an international multicentre randomised controlled trial of timing of ECV for breech pregnancies. *BJOG.* 2011;118:564–577.

17. Rosman AN, Guijt A, Vlemmix F, et al. Contraindications for external cephalic version in breech position at term: a systematic review. *Acta Obstet Gynecol Scand.* 2012;91:137–142.

18. Fernandez CO, Bloom SL, Smulian JC, et al. A randomized placebo-controlled evaluation of terbutaline for external cephalic version. *Obstet Gynecol.* 1997;90:775–779.

19. Hilton J, Allan B, Swaby C, et al. Intravenous nitroglycerin for external cephalic version: a randomized controlled trial. *Obstet Gynecol.* 2009;114:560–567.

20. Cluver C, Gyte GML, Sinclair M, et al. Interventions for helping to turn term breech babies to head first presentation when using external cephalic version. *Cochrane Database Syst Rev.* 2015;(2):CD000184.

21. Homafar M, Gerard J, Turrentine M. Vaginal delivery after external cephalic version in patients with a previous cesarean delivery: a systematic review and meta-analysis. *Obstet Gynecol.* 2020;136:965–971.

22. Fok WY, Chan LW, Leung TY, Lau TK. Maternal experience of pain during external cephalic version at term. *Acta Obstet Gynecol Scand.* 2005;84:748–751.

23. Suen SS, Khaw KS, Law LW, et al. The force applied to successfully turn a foetus during reattempts of external cephalic version is substantially reduced when performed under spinal analgesia. *J Matern Fetal Neonatal Med.* 2012;25:719–722.

24. Goetzinger KR, Harper LM, Tuuli MG, et al. Effect of regional anesthesia on the success rate of external cephalic version: a systematic review and meta-analysis. *Obstet Gynecol.* 2011;118:1137–1144.

25. Weiniger CF, Ginosar Y, Elchalal U, et al. External cephalic version for breech presentation with or without spinal analgesia in nulliparous women at term: a randomized controlled trial. *Obstet Gynecol.* 2007;110:1343–1350.

26. Weiniger CF, Ginosar Y, Elchalal U, et al. Randomized controlled trial of external cephalic version in term multiparawith or without spinal analgesia. *Br J Anaesth.* 2010;104:613–618.

27. Magro-Malosso ER, Saccone G, Di Tommaso M, et al. Neuraxial analgesia to increase the success rate of external cephalic version: a systematic review and meta-analysis of randomized controlled trials. *Am J Obstet Gynecol.* 2016;215:276–286.

28. Khaw KS, Lee SWY, Ngan Kee WD, et al. Randomized trial of anaesthetic interventions in external cephalic version for breech presentation. *Br J Anaesth.* 2015;114:944–950.

29. Lavoie A, Guay J. Anesthetic dose neuraxial blockade increases the success rate of external fetal version: a meta-analysis. *Can J Anaesth.* 2010;57:408–414.

30. Chalifoux LA, Bauchat JR, Higgins N, et al. Effect of intrathecal bupivacaine dose on the success of external cephalic version for breech presentation. *Anesthesiology.* 2017;127:625–632.

31. Carvalho B, Bateman BT. Not too little, not too much. *Anesthesiology.* 2017;127:596–598.

32. Lomas S, Minton Z, Daniels JP. Systematic review of the effectiveness of remifentanil in term breech pregnancies undergoing external cephalic version. *Int J Obstet Anesth.* 2023;54:103649.

33. Su M, McLeod L, Ross S, et al. Factors associated with adverse perinatal outcome in the term breech trial. *Am J Obstet Gynecol.* 2003;189:740–745.

34. Berhan Y, Haileamlak A. The risks of planned vaginal breech delivery versus planned caesarean section for term breech birth: a meta-analysis including observational studies. *BJOG.* 2016;123:49–57.

35. Lyons J, Pressey T, Bartholomew S, et al. Delivery of breech presentation at term gestation in Canada, 2003-2011. *Obstet Gynecol.* 2015;125:1153–1161.

36. Hartnack Tharin JE, Rasmussen S, Krebs L. Consequences of the term breech trial in Denmark. *Acta Obstet Gynecol Scand.* 2011;90:767–771.

37. Weiniger CF, Carvalho B. The dilemma of vaginal breech delivery worldwide. *Lancet.* 2014;384:1183.

38. Goffinet F, Carayol M, Foidart JM, et al. Is planned vaginal delivery for breech presentation at term still an option? Results of an observational prospective survey in France and Belgium. *Am J Obstet Gynecol.* 2006;194:1002–1011.

39. American College of Obstetricians and Gynecologists. Committee Opinion No. 745: Mode of term singleton breech delivery (reaffirmed 2023). *Obstet Gynecol.* 2018;132:531–532.

40. Joseph KS, Pressey T, Lyons J, et al. Once more into the breech: planned vaginal delivery compared with planned cesarean delivery. *Obstet Gynecol.* 2015;125:1162–1167.

41. Management of breech presentation: Green-top Guideline No. 20b. *BJOG.* 2017;124:e151–e177.

42. Practice guidelines for obstetric anesthesia: an updated report by the American Society of Anesthesiologists Task Force on Obstetric Anesthesia and the Society for Obstetric Anesthesia and Perinatology. *Anesthesiology.* 2016;124:270–300.

43. Caponas G. Glyceryl trinitrate and acute uterine relaxation: aliterature review. *Anaesth Intensive Care.* 2001;29:163–177.

44. Bashiri A, Burstein E, Bar-David J, et al. Face and brow presentation: independent risk factors. *J Matern Fetal Neonatal Med.* 2008;21:357–360.

45. Osterman M, Hamilton B, Martin JA, et al. Births: final data for 2020. *Natl Vital Stat Rep.* 2021;70:1–50.

46. Hrubec Z, Robinette CD. The study of human twins in medical research. *N Engl J Med.* 1984;310:435–441.

47. Martin JA, Hamilton BE, Osterman MJK. Three decades of twin births in the United States, 1980-2009. *NCHS Data Brief.* 2012(80):1–8.

48. American College of Obstetricians and Gynecologists. Practice Bulletin No. 231: Multifetal gestations: twin, triplet, and higher-order multifetal pregnancies (reaffirmed 2024). *Obstet Gynecol.* 2021;137:1140–1143.

49. Unal ER, Newman RB. Multiple gestations. In: Landon MB, Galan HL, Jauniaux ERM, et al., eds. *Gabbe's Obstetrics: Normal and Problem Pregnancies.* 8th ed. Elsevier; 2021:751–783.

50. McAuliffe F, Kametas N, Costello J, et al. Respiratory functionin singleton and twin pregnancy. *BJOG.* 2002;109:765–769.

51. Hickok DE, Pederson AL, Worthington-Roberts B. Weight gain patterns during twin gestation. *J Am Diet Assoc.* 1989;89:642–646.

52. Thomsen JK, Fogh-Andersen N, Jaszczak P. Atrial natriuretic peptide, blood volume, aldosterone, and sodium excretion during twin pregnancy. *Acta Obstet Gynecol Scand.* 1994;73: 14–20.

53. Kuleva M, Youssef A, Maroni E, et al. Maternal cardiac function in normal twin pregnancy: a longitudinal study. *Ultrasound Obstet Gynecol.* 2011;38:575–580.

54. Bermúdez C, Becerra CH, Bornick PW, et al. Placental types and twin-twin transfusion syndrome. *Am J Obstet Gynecol.* 2002;187:489–494.

55. Lopriore E, Nagel HT, Vandenbussche FP, Walther FJ. Long-term neurodevelopmental outcome in twin-to-twin transfusion syndrome. *Am J Obstet Gynecol.* 2003;189:1314–1319.

56. Society for Maternal-Fetal Medicine Simpson LL. Twin-twin transfusion syndrome. *Am J Obstet Gynecol.* 2013;208:3–18.

57. Moise KJ Jr, Dorman K, Lamvu G, et al. A randomized trial of amnioreduction versus septostomy in the treatment of twin-twin transfusion syndrome. *Am J Obstet Gynecol.* 2005;193:701–707.

58. Roberts D, Neilson JP, Kilby MD, Gates S. Interventions for the treatment of twin-twin transfusion syndrome (review). *Cochrane Database Syst Rev.* 2014;(1):CD002073.

59. Crombleholme TM, Shera D, Lee H, et al. A prospective, randomized, multicenter trial of amnioreduction vs selective fetoscopic laser photocoagulation for the treatment of severe twin-twin transfusion syndrome. *Am J Obstet Gynecol.* 2007;197:396.e1–e9.

60. Chmait RH, Quintero RA. Operative fetoscopy in complicated monochorionic twins: current status and future direction. *Curr Opin Obstet Gynecol.* 2008;20:169–174.

61. Emery SP, Hasley SK, Catov JM, et al. North American Fetal Therapy Network: intervention vs expectant management for stage I twin-twin transfusion syndrome. *Am J Obstet Gynecol.* 2016;215:346.e1–e7.

62. Hoagland MA, Chatterjee D. Anesthesia for fetal surgery. *Pediatric Anesth.* 2017;27:346–357.

63. Nassar AH, Usta IM, Rechdan JB, et al. Pregnancy outcome in spontaneous twins versus twins who were conceived through in vitro fertilization. *Am J Obstet Gynecol.* 2003;189:513–518.

64. Martin JA, Hamilton BE, Osterman MJK, et al. Births: final data for 2015. *Natl Vital Stat Rep.* 2017;66:1–71.

65. Norman JE, Mackenzie F, Owen P, et al. Progesterone for the prevention of preterm birth in twin pregnancy (STOPPIT): a randomised, double-blind, placebo-controlled study and meta-analysis. *Lancet.* 2009;373:2034–2040.

66. American College of Obstetricians and Gynecologists. Practice Bulletin No. 171: Management of preterm labor (reaffirmed 2022). *Obstet Gynecol.* 2016;128:e155–e164.

67. Gregory EC, Valenzuela CP, Hoyert DL. Fetal mortality: United States, 2020. *Natl Vital Stat Rep.* 2022;71:1–20.

68. MacDorman MF, Gregory ECW. Fetal and perinatal mortality: United States, 2013. *Natl Vital Stat Rep.* 2015;64:1–23.

69. Post A, Heyborne K. Managing monoamniotic twin pregnancies. *Clin Obstet Gynecol.* 2015;58:643–653.

70. Simões T, Amaral N, Lerman R, et al. Prospective risk of intrauterine death of monochorionic-diamniotic twins. *Am J Obstet Gynecol.* 2006;195:134–139.

71. Johnson CD, Zhang J. Survival of other fetuses after a fetal death in twin or triplet pregnancies. *Obstet Gynecol.* 2002;99:698–703.

72. Hillman SC, Morris RK, Kilby MD. Co-twin prognosis after single fetal death: a systematic review and meta-analysis. *Obstet Gynecol.* 2011;118:928–940.

73. Luke B, Brown MB. Maternal morbidity and infant death in twin vs triplet and quadruplet pregnancies. *Am J Obstet Gynecol.* 2008;198:401.e1–e10.

74. Armson BA, O'Connell C, Persad V, et al. Determinants of perinatal mortality and serious neonatal morbidity in the second twin. *Obstet Gynecol.* 2006;108:556–564.

75. Luo ZC, Ouyang F, Zhang J, Klebanoff M. Perinatal mortality in second- vs firstborn twins: a matter of birth size or birth order? *Am J Obstet Gynecol.* 2014;211:153.e1–e8.

76. Crawford JS. A prospective study of 200 consecutive twin deliveries. *Anaesthesia.* 1987;42:33–43.

77. Jarvis GJ, Whitfield MF. Epidural analgesia and the delivery of twins. *J Obstet Gynaecol.* 1981;2:90–92.

78. Marino T, Goudas LC, Steinbok V, et al. The anesthetic management of triplet cesarean delivery: a retrospective case series of maternal outcomes. *Anesth Analg.* 2001;93:991–995.

79. Witteveen T, Van den Akker T, Zwart JJ, et al. Severe acute maternal morbidity in multiple pregnancies: a nationwide cohort study. *Am J Obstet Gynecol.* 2016;214:641.e1–e10.

80. Lynch A, McDuffie R Jr, Murphy J, et al. Preeclampsia in multiple gestation: the role of assisted reproductive technologies. *Obstet Gynecol.* 2002;99:445–451.

81. Malone FD, Kaufman GE, Chelmow D, et al. Maternal morbidity associated with triplet pregnancy. *Am J Perinatol.* 1998;15:73–77.

82. Hogle KL, Hutton EK, McBrien KA, et al. Cesarean delivery for twins: a systematic review and meta-analysis. *Am J Obstet Gynecol.* 2003;188:220–227.

83. Barrett JFR, Hannah ME, Hutton EK, et al. A randomized trial of planned cesarean or vaginal delivery for twin pregnancy. *N Engl J Med.* 2013;369:1295–1305.

84. Asztalos EV, Hannah ME, Hutton EK, et al. Twin birth study: 2-year neurodevelopmental follow-up of the randomized trial of planned cesarean or planned vaginal delivery for twin pregnancy. *Am J Obstet Gynecol.* 2016;214:371.e1–e19.

85. Schmitz T, Prunet C, Azria E, et al. Association between planned cesarean delivery and neonatal mortality and morbidity in twin pregnancies. *Obstet Gynecol.* 2017;129:986–995.

86. Vendittelli F, Rivière O, Crenn-Hébert C, et al. Is a planned cesarean necessary in twin pregnancies? *Acta Obstet Gynecol Scand.* 2011;90:1147–1156.

87. Rossi AC, Mullin PM, Chmait RH. Neonatal outcomes of twins according to birth order, presentation and mode of delivery: a systematic review and meta-analysis. *BJOG.* 2011;118:523–531.

88. Sentilhes L, Oppenheimer A, Bouhours AC, et al. Neonatal outcome of very preterm twins: policy of planned vaginal or cesarean delivery. *Am J Obstet Gynecol.* 2015;213:73.e1–e7.

89. Easter SR, Robinson JN, Lieberman E, Carusi D. Association of intended route of delivery and maternal morbidity in twin pregnancy. *Obstet Gynecol.* 2017;129:305–310.

90. American College of Obstetricians and Gynecologists, Society for Maternal-Fetal Medicine. Obstetric Care Consensus No. 1: Safe prevention of the primary cesarean delivery. *Obstet Gynecol.* 2014;123:693–711.

91. Easter SR, Lieberman E, Carusi D. Fetal presentation and successful twin vaginal delivery. *Am J Obstet Gynecol.* 2016;214:116.e1–e10.

92. Leung TY, Tam WH, Leung TN, et al. Effect of twin-to-twin delivery interval on umbilical cord blood gas in the second twins. *BJOG.* 2002;109:63–67.

93. Stein W, Misselwitz B, Schmidt S. Twin-to-twin delivery time interval: influencing factors and effect on short-term outcomeof the second twin. *Acta Obstet Gynecol Scand.* 2008;87:346–353.

94. Dufour P, Vinatier D, Vanderstichele S, et al. Intravenous nitroglycerin for internal podalic version of the second twin in transverse lie. *Obstet Gynecol.* 1998;92:416–419.

95. Vinatier D, Dufour P, Berard J. Utilization of intravenous nitroglycerin for obstetrical emergencies. *Int J Gynaecol Obstet.* 1996;55:129–134.

96. Ngan Kee WD, Khaw KS, Ng FF, et al. A prospective comparison of vasopressor requirement and hemodynamic changes during spinal anesthesia for cesarean delivery in patients with multiple gestation versus singleton pregnancy. *Anesth Analg.* 2007;104:407–411.

97. Jawan B, Lee JH, Chong ZK, Chang CS. Spread of spinal anaesthesia for caesarean section in singleton and twin pregnancies. *Br J Anaesth.* 1993;70:639–641.

98. Behforouz N, Dounas M, Benhamou D. Epidural anaesthesia for caesarean delivery in triple and quadruple pregnancies. *Acta Anaesthesiol Scand.* 1998;42:1088–1091.

99. Vallejo MC, Ramanathan S. Plasma lidocaine concentrations are higher in twin compared to singleton newborns following epidural anesthesia for cesarean delivery. *Can J Anaesth.* 2002;49:701–705.

Hypertensive Disorders

Philip E. Hess, MD

INTRODUCTION

Hypertension is the most common medical disorder of pregnancy, affecting approximately 18 million women and 6% to 10% of pregnancies worldwide.[1] Hypertensive disorders of pregnancy can significantly impact both mother and fetus. Almost 50,000 women worldwide die from hypertensive disorders of pregnancy each year, and while the vast majority occur in low-resource settings, these disorders account for up to one-in-six maternal deaths in high-resource countries.[2] Being diagnosed with a hypertensive disorder also carries an increased future risk of cardiovascular diseases, renal failure, and diabetes. Hypertensive disorders also heavily impact the fetus, leading to fetal growth restriction, preterm birth, and over 500,000 perinatal deaths worldwide each year. The immediate financial impact of neonatal care for these pregnancies is estimated to be greater than $1 billion annually in the United States alone.[3,4]

Preeclampsia represents a clinically significant form of the hypertension spectrum. Although important advances have been made in understanding the pathophysiology, the proximal cause of preeclampsia remains unknown. Risk factor assessment aids in identifying patients for closer monitoring or prophylactic treatment; however, most cases of preeclampsia occur in nulliparous mothers without known risk factors.[2] Once preeclampsia has been diagnosed, medications can be

used to temporize the disease with blood pressure control or prevention of seizures; however, delivery of the fetus is the only definitive treatment.

Anesthesia providers play an important role in the management of women with preeclampsia; they are well positioned, with a thorough understanding of pathophysiology, to assist with assessment and management of complications, cardiovascular monitoring, and critical care. Working as part of a multidisciplinary team that includes obstetricians, nurses, cardiologists, neonatologists, midwives, and critical care specialists, anesthesia providers can play a critical role in ensuring optimal outcomes for women with preeclampsia.[5,6]

CLASSIFICATION

Hypertensive disorders of pregnancy encompass a range of conditions that may differ in their prognoses but can be difficult to differentiate because the clinical presentations are often similar. The classification of hypertensive disorders of pregnancy was updated by the American College of Obstetricians and Gynecologists (ACOG) Taskforce on Hypertension in Pregnancy in 2013 and has been substantially adopted by other major societies.[4,7] Hypertension in pregnancy is defined as either (1) systolic blood pressure $\geq$ 140 mm Hg and/or (2) diastolic blood pressure $\geq$ 90 mm Hg; this must be confirmed

---

BOX 35.1   Classification of Hypertensive Disorders in Pregnancy

- Gestational hypertension
- Preeclampsia without severe features
- Preeclampsia with severe features
- Chronic hypertension
- Chronic hypertension with superimposed preeclampsia
- White coat hypertension
- Masked hypertension
- Eclampsia

Adapted from the American College of Obstetricians and Gynecologists. Hypertension in pregnancy: report of the American College of Obstetricians and Gynecologists' Task Force on Hypertension in Pregnancy. *Obstet Gynecol.* 2013;122:1122–1131; and Magee LA, Brown MA, Hall DR, et al. The 2021 International Society for the Study of Hypertension in Pregnancy classification, diagnosis & management recommendations for international practice. *Pregnancy Hypertens.* 2022;27:148–169.

BOX 35.2   Diagnostic Criteria for Preeclampsia

Preeclampsia Without Severe Features
- Blood pressure ≥ 140/90 mm Hg after 20 weeks' gestation
- Proteinuria (≥300 mg/24 h, protein-creatinine ratio ≥ 0.3, or urine dipstick specimen ≥ 1+)

Preeclampsia With Severe Features
- Blood pressure ≥ 160 mm Hg systolic, or ≥ 110 mm Hg diastolic, or both
- Thrombocytopenia (platelet count < 100,000/mm^3)
- Serum creatinine concentration > 1.1 mg/dL or greater than two times the baseline serum creatinine concentration
- Pulmonary edema
- New-onset, persistent cerebral or visual disturbances
- Twofold increase in AST or ALT, or persistent right upper quadrant or epigastric pain

ALT, Alanine transaminase; *AST,* aspartate transferase.
Modified from American College of Obstetricians and Gynecologists. ACOG Practice Bulletin Number 222: Gestational hypertension and preeclampsia (reaffirmed 2023). *Obstet Gynecol.* 2020;135:e237–e260.

---

on at least two measurements. The classification of hypertensive disorders consists of gestational hypertension, chronic hypertension, chronic hypertension with superimposed preeclampsia, and preeclampsia with or without severe features (Box 35.1). The International Society for the Study of Hypertension in Pregnancy (ISSHP) includes the categories of **white coat hypertension** and **masked hypertension**.[4] White coat hypertension can be associated with normal blood pressures when not in the physician's office and may not need to be treated; however, it can progress to preeclampsia and should be closely monitored.[8] Masked hypertension is associated with normal blood pressures in the clinic, but high blood pressures in the ambulatory setting—it is suspected when there is evidence of end-organ disease, but no elevated blood pressure when assessed in the clinic.[4]

Gestational hypertension is the most common hypertensive disorder of pregnancy, affecting approximately 5% of parturients.[2] This disorder presents as hypertension after 20 weeks' gestation that resolves by 12 weeks postpartum. Approximately one-fourth of patients diagnosed with gestational hypertension will develop preeclampsia.

Chronic hypertension involves hypertension presenting before pregnancy or before 20 weeks' gestation, or hypertension that fails to resolve after delivery. Chronic hypertension develops into preeclampsia in approximately 20% to 25% of affected patients. However, even in the absence of preeclampsia, chronic hypertension is an important risk factor for unfavorable maternal and fetal pregnancy outcomes.[9]

Chronic hypertension with superimposed preeclampsia occurs when a woman with chronic hypertension develops new onset or a sudden increase in proteinuria and/or hypertension, or when other manifestations of preeclampsia with severe features appear. Morbidity is increased for both the mother and fetus compared with preeclampsia alone.[10]

Preeclampsia is defined as the new onset of hypertension and proteinuria after 20 weeks' gestation. The diagnosis of preeclampsia should also be considered in the absence of proteinuria when signs or symptoms of end-organ involvement are present.[2] Preeclampsia is classified as **preeclampsia with or without severe features**. Both the ACOG and ISSHP discourage use of the term *mild preeclampsia* for women without severe features because preeclampsia may be rapidly progressive, and appropriate management involves frequent reevaluation for severe features. The diagnostic set of features that identify severe disease are manifestations of end-organ injury (Box 35.2). Evidence of uteroplacental insufficiency (e.g., intrauterine growth restriction, abnormal uterine artery doppler flow velocities) is no longer considered a severe feature in the ACOG classification,[2] but remains present in the ISSHP diagnostic set of features due to the association with angiogenic imbalance.[4] The ISSHP diagnostic set of severe features also includes other evidence of hematologic or neurologic dysfunction.

Early-onset preeclampsia, with symptom onset before 34 weeks' gestation, is more often associated with abnormal placentation, has a high rate of recurrence, and may have a stronger genetic component. Early-onset preeclampsia also results in greater fetal and maternal morbidity.

Late-onset preeclampsia more often occurs in women metabolically predisposed to the disease, and abnormal placentation may feature less prominently in the pathogenesis. These women may have long-standing hypertension, obesity, diabetes, or other forms of microvascular disease. They are challenged to meet the demands of the growing fetoplacental unit and decompensate near term.

HELLP syndrome refers to the development of hemolysis, elevated liver enzymes, and low platelet count in a woman with preeclampsia. Women with HELLP syndrome may not have the classical findings of preeclampsia and often do not have hypertension at the time of diagnosis.

Eclampsia is defined as a new onset of seizures in a pregnant woman without an identifiable cause. Eclampsia most often occurs in woman who have been diagnosed with preeclampsia, but rarely may also appear as the first sign of a hypertensive disorder.

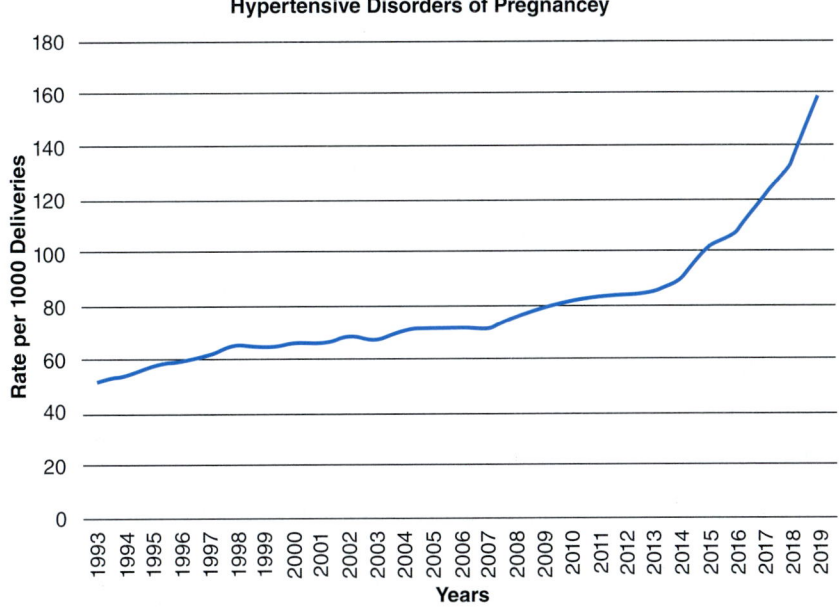

Fig. 35.1 Rate of hypertensive disorders per 1000 delivery hospitalizations, 1993–2019. Data from US Centers for Disease Control and Prevention: https://www.cdc.gov/index.html.

EPIDEMIOLOGY

The incidence of all hypertensive disorders of pregnancy has tripled in the United States in the past quarter century, reaching almost 16% of all births (Fig. 35.1).[11] The highest prevalence occurs among women over the age of 35 years, and among racial and ethnic minorities. The recent increase is primarily driven by higher rates of pregnancy-related hypertension, while the frequency of chronic hypertension increased modestly. The rapid rise in incidence after the publication of the 2013 ACOG guidelines suggests that more aggressive screening and diagnosis contributed to the reported rise. The increased incidence is primarily due to major shifts in the demographic characteristics and medical comorbidities among pregnant women. Preeclampsia occurs in 3% to 4% of pregnancies in the United States. Eclampsia is significantly more common in underresourced settings, while the incidence in high-resource countries is likely less than 0.1% of pregnancies.[12]

Risk Factors

Numerous preconception and pregnancy-related risk factors associated with the development of preeclampsia have been identified (Box 35.3). Risk factors for preeclampsia can be divided into maternal demographic factors, genetic factors, medical and obstetric conditions, behavioral factors, and partner-related factors.

Demographic Factors

Advanced maternal age has consistently been shown to be a risk factor for preeclampsia, with women who are 40 years of age or older having an approximately twofold increase in risk compared with women between 20 and 29 years of age.[13] This risk may be independent of the increased prevalence of medical conditions and obesity that accompany advancing age.

Race and ethnicity are associated with hypertensive disorders of pregnancy. Black women have increased rates of

---

BOX 35.3 Risk Factors for Preeclampsia

Demographic Factors
- Advanced maternal age > 35 y
- Black race
- Hispanic ethnicity

Maternal Factors
- Nulliparity
- History of preeclampsia in previous pregnancy
- Family history of preeclampsia
- History of placental abruption, fetal growth restriction, or fetal death

Medical Conditions
- Obesity
- Chronic hypertension
- Diabetes mellitus
- Chronic renal disease
- Antiphospholipid antibody syndrome
- Systemic lupus erythematosus

Obstetric Conditions
- Multiple gestation
- Hydatidiform mole

Behavioral Factor
- Cigarette smoking (risk reduction)
- Regular exercise (risk reduction)

---

chronic hypertension, preexisting diabetes, and obesity; however, after adjusting for these preexisting conditions, there remains a higher incidence of preeclampsia, with more extreme hypertension requiring greater amounts of antihypertensive medication.[4,14,15] Black women are also more likely to develop eclampsia[16] and have higher rates of both morbidity and mortality due to their hypertensive disorder of pregnancy.[14] Women of Native American descent and Hispanic ethnicity may also have a small increased risk for developing preeclampsia and eclampsia compared to White women.[14]

Genetic Factors

Maternal genetic factors are known to be important risk factors for the development of preeclampsia. Pregnant women with a family history of preeclampsia are approximately twice as likely to develop the disorder.[17,18] It is estimated that approximately one-third of the variance in liability to preeclampsia is caused by maternal genetic factors.[19]

In a study of 1.7 million births in the Medical Birth Registry of Norway, men who fathered one preeclamptic pregnancy were found to be nearly twice as likely to father a preeclamptic pregnancy with a different woman, irrespective of her previous obstetric history.[20] Therefore, **paternal genes** (in the fetus) contribute significantly to a pregnant woman's risk for preeclampsia. It is estimated that approximately one-fifth of the variance in liability for preeclampsia is conferred through the fetal genes.[19]

Women with a history of preeclampsia in a previous pregnancy are at increased risk for preeclampsia in a subsequent pregnancy, particularly if the preeclampsia was of early onset.[21,22] Risk for recurrence increases with multiple affected pregnancies. In addition, women with a history of previous placental abruption and fetal growth restriction are at increased risk for preeclampsia in a subsequent pregnancy,[23] and women with a history of preeclampsia are at risk for these outcomes even in the absence of recurrent preeclampsia.[24] These associations suggest that some women harbor a susceptibility (potentially genetically mediated) to obstetric conditions caused by placental dysfunction, which manifests differently in different pregnancies.

It is estimated that approximately one-fifth of the variance in disease risk is attributable to fetal genetic effects, and one-third is attributable to maternal genetic factors.[19] A genome-wide association study in offspring from preeclamptic pregnancies reported that variants in the fetal genome near fms-like tyrosine kinase-1 gene (*FLT1*) are associated with risk for preeclampsia.[25] With the possible exception of thrombophilia genes, no genetic variants in the maternal genome have been robustly associated with preeclampsia.[26]

Medical and Obstetric Conditions

Metabolic syndrome occurs in about one-fifth of women of childbearing age in the United States and is characterized by the presence of obesity, hyperglycemia, insulin resistance, and hypertension.[27] Women with chronic hypertension are at a 10- to 12-fold increased risk for developing preeclampsia.[4] When associated with other risk factors, including diabetes, renal disease, and collagen vascular disease, chronic hypertension confers even greater risk.[4] Obesity is also a major independent risk factor; an increase in body mass index (BMI) of 5 to 7 kg/m^2 is associated with a twofold increased risk for preeclampsia.[28] Diabetes mellitus is associated with an approximately twofold increase in the risk for development of preeclampsia.[4,7] Other maternal medical conditions that are well-recognized risk factors for preeclampsia include chronic renal disease, antiphospholipid antibody syndrome, and systemic lupus erythematosus.[4,7]

Behavioral Factors

Paradoxically, cigarette smoking during pregnancy confers a 30% to 40% lower risk for developing preeclampsia, an effect consistently observed across studies in various countries.[29,30] A possible mechanism is that nicotine restores endothelial function by stimulating placental growth factor (PlGF) and inhibiting the antiangiogenic impact of soluble fms-like tyrosine kinase-1 and soluble endoglin.[31]

Recreational Physical Activity

Recreational physical activity during pregnancy has been associated with a decrease in the risk for gestational hypertensive disorder, particularly in nonobese women.[32,33] Exercise in pregnancy is strongly recommended due to the health benefits that may result.[4]

Pregnancy-Related Risk Factors

Nulliparity is a leading risk factor for hypertensive disorders of pregnancy; first-time mothers are three times more likely to be diagnosed compared to parous women.[7] Preeclampsia is also more common in parous women who have conceived with a new partner. It is not clear whether this is the impact of exposure to a new partner or the length of time between pregnancies, which often accompanies births with different partners.[34] Multifetal gestation[35] and hydatidiform mole[36] are associated with higher rates of preeclampsia, likely due to an increased placental oxygen demand that exceeds supply. Additionally, assisted reproductive techniques and the use of donated gametes increase the risk for hypertensive disorders, potentially by altering the maternal-fetal immune reaction and by its association with an increased incidence of multiple gestation.[37]

PATHOGENESIS

The exact pathogenic mechanisms responsible for the initiation of preeclampsia are not known, but significant advances in knowledge of the disease have been made in recent years. The current description of the pathophysiology of preeclampsia focuses on chronic placental hypoxia inducing the release of antiangiogenic proteins, leading to widespread maternal endothelial injury. The placenta is central to the development of the disease, as evidenced by delivery resulting in its resolution. Further, the disease can occur in the absence of a fetus (e.g., a molar pregnancy).[38] Angiogenic imbalance is a fundamental characteristic of women with preeclampsia, notably demonstrated by a decrease in the proangiogenic and increase in antiangiogenic factors.

Placental-Derived Angiogenic Imbalance

In a healthy pregnancy, embryo-derived cytotrophoblasts invade the decidual and myometrial segments of the spiral arteries, replacing endothelium and causing remodeling of vascular smooth muscle and the inner elastic lamina (Fig. 35.2).[39,40] The luminal diameter of the spiral arteries increases fourfold, resulting in the creation of flaccid tubes that provide a low-resistance vascular pathway to the intervillous space. Furthermore, the remodeled arteries are unresponsive to vasoactive stimuli. These alterations in maternal vasculature ensure adequate blood flow to nourish the growing fetus and placenta.

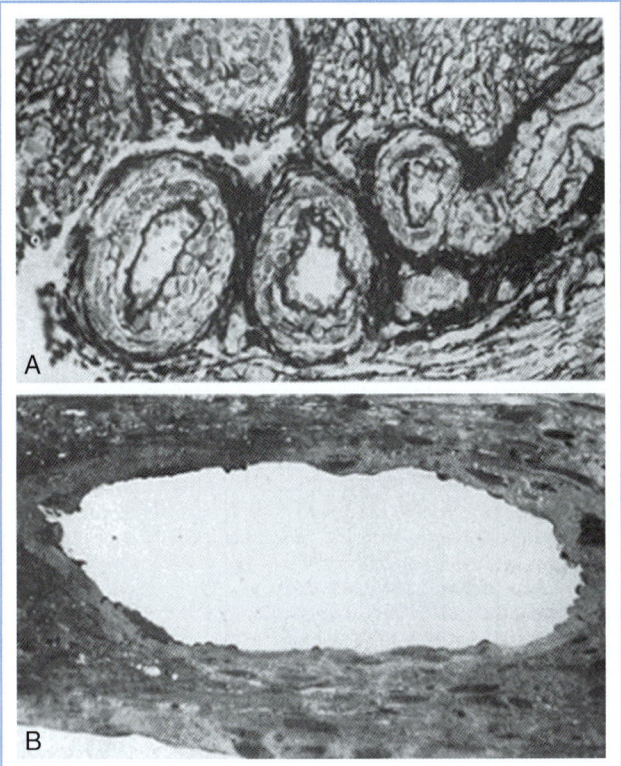

Fig. 35.2 Sections through spiral arteries (A) at the myometrial-endometrial junction of the nonpregnant uterus and (B) at the myometrial-decidual junction in late normal pregnancy (×150). From Sheppard BL, Bonnar J. Uteroplacental arteries and hypertensive pregnancy. In: Bonnar J, MacGillivray I, Symonds G, eds. *Pregnancy Hypertension.* University Park Press; 1980:205.

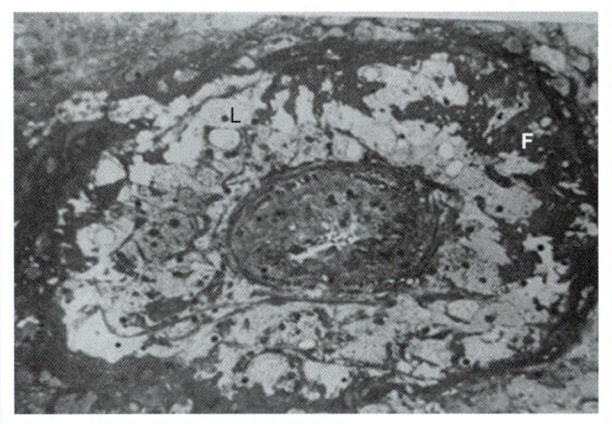

Fig. 35.3 This figure shows lipid-laden cells *(L)* and fibrin deposition *(F)* in this occluded decidual vessel characteristic of both severe preeclampsia and severe fetal growth restriction (×150). From Sheppard BL, Bonnar J. Uteroplacental arteries and hypertensive pregnancy. In: Bonnar J, MacGillivray I, Symonds G, eds. *Pregnancy Hypertension.* University Park Press; 1980:205.

Healthy endothelium prevents platelet activation, activates circulating anticoagulants, buffers the response to vasopressors, and maintains fluid in the intravascular compartment.

In women with early-onset preeclampsia, cytotrophoblast invasion is incomplete and only the decidual segments undergo change; the myometrial spiral arteries are not invaded and remodeled and thus remain small, constricted, and hyperresponsive to vasomotor stimuli.[41,42] Abnormal placentation results in decreased placental perfusion and placental infarcts, predisposing the fetus to growth restriction (Fig. 35.3). The cellular stress and damage in the nascent placental cytotrophoblasts can be detected by the increased release of extracellular vesicles as early as 11 to 14 weeks' gestation.[43] Moreover, the contents of extracellular vesicles derived from the placenta of near-term women with preeclampsia are able to induce vascular dysfunction in both animal and human cell cultures.[44] Placental ischemia worsens throughout pregnancy as restricted vessels are increasingly unable to meet the needs of the growing fetoplacental unit. In later-onset preeclampsia, placental ischemia may result from other factors, such as a preexisting maternal disease, infarction, or twin pregnancy.

The fetal cytotrophoblasts release key antiangiogenic factors when exposed to chronic hypoxia.[45] Thus, as the placenta becomes relatively hypoxic with progression of the pregnancy, placentally derived, antiangiogenic factors are overexpressed and released into the maternal circulation. **Soluble fms-like tyrosine kinase-1 (sFlt-1)** and **soluble endoglin (sEng)** are

among the most studied antiangiogenic factors.[38,46] Each of these factors is a partial receptor for the angiogenic hormone, which normally binds angiogenic hormone leading to angiogenesis. sFlt-1 antagonizes the angiogenic growth factors, **vascular endothelial growth factor (VEGF)** and **placental growth factor (PlGF)** (a member of the VEGF family due to the sharing of structure and receptors).[47,48] The release of these antiangiogenic factors from the intervillous space into the maternal circulation causes widespread maternal endothelial dysfunction and an accentuated systemic inflammatory response. Studies have demonstrated that sFlt-1 increases several weeks prior to the diagnosis of preeclampsia, and that both VEGF and PlGF are reduced.[49]

Evidence for a central role of sFlt-1 in the pathogenesis of preeclampsia comes from both animal and human studies. Maynard et al.[47] demonstrated that sFlt-1 levels increase during gestation and fall after delivery and that increased circulating sFlt-1 levels reduce circulating levels of free VEGF and PlGF, causing endothelial dysfunction that can be rescued by exogenous VEGF and PlGF. Furthermore, these investigators found that the administration of sFlt-1 to pregnant rats induced hypertension, proteinuria, and glomerular endotheliosis, the classic renal lesion of preeclampsia.[47] When administered *in vitro*, VEGF and PlGF cause rat renal arteriolar relaxation, which is blocked by sFlt-1.[47] In response to increased circulating levels of sFlt-1, VEGF and PlGF levels are reduced, resulting in endothelial dysfunction in maternal vessels (Fig. 35.4).[50] Importantly, elevated sFlt-1 levels and reduced levels of PlGF not only predict the subsequent development of preeclampsia, but do so with a "dose-response effect"—a greater ratio is found with more severe disease.[49] The use of this information for early screening and diagnosis has been examined extensively and endorsed by the UK National Institute for Health and Care Excellence, but is currently hampered by lack of standardization of measurement. Knowledge of the state of angiogenic biomarkers can lead to earlier diagnosis of preeclampsia,[51] and may help identify women who will develop adverse outcomes due to their disease.[52,53]

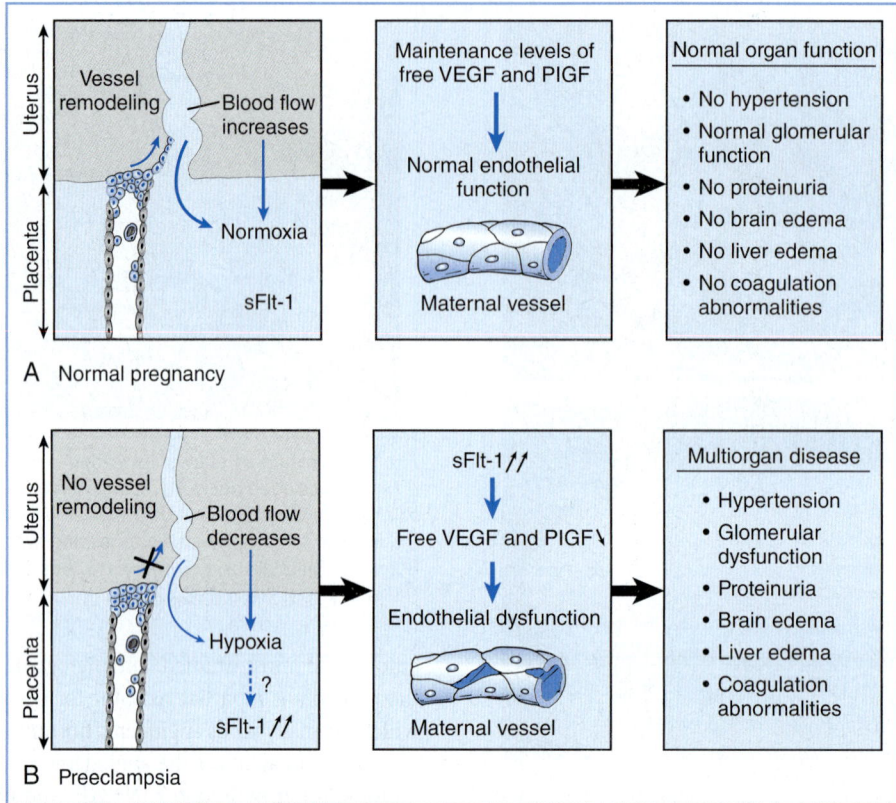

Fig. 35.4 Hypothesis on the Role of Soluble fms-Like Tyrosine Kinase (sFlt-1) in Preeclampsia. (A) During normal pregnancy, the uterine spiral arteries are infiltrated and remodeled by endovascular invasive trophoblasts, thereby increasing blood flow significantly to meet the oxygen and nutrient demands of the fetus. (B) In the placenta of preeclamptic women, trophoblast invasion does not occur and blood flow is reduced, resulting in placental hypoxia. In addition, increased amounts of soluble sFlt-1 are produced by the placenta and scavenge vascular endothelial growth factor (VEGF) and placental growth factor (PIGF), thereby lowering circulating levels of unbound VEGF and PIGF. This altered balance causes generalized endothelial dysfunction, resulting in multiorgan disease. From Luttun A, Carmeliet P. Soluble VEGF receptor Flt1: the elusive preeclampsia factor discovered? *J Clin Invest.* 2003;111:600–602.

Abnormal Placentation

The basis for abnormal uteroplacental development has not been fully elucidated and is likely due to a complex interaction of immunologic, vascular, environmental, and genetic factors. Hypothetically, immune maladaptation may play a central role in predisposing to abnormal placentation. Immune cells present in the decidua, derived from the endometrium in the nonpregnant state, include macrophages, dendritic cells, and natural killer (NK) cells. Macrophages and dendritic cells are found in greater density in preeclamptic placentas than in control placentas.[54,55] Similarly, levels of chemokines that attract these immune cells are also elevated.[54,55] Excess macrophages in the decidua are associated with impaired trophoblast invasion, suggesting that excess inflammation may be one of the causal components of impaired placentation.[55] NK cells may also be important in regulating vascular development during placentation. NK cells interact with fetal trophoblast cell markers via killer immunoglobulin receptors (KIR) to influence trophoblastic invasion. Specific genotypic combinations of maternal KIR and trophoblastic human leukocyte antigen C (HLA-C) may mediate the risk for preeclampsia.[56,57]

Aberrant hemostatic activation during placental development has also been proposed to contribute to the abnormal placentation that is a hallmark of pregnancies destined to develop preeclampsia.[58] Increased tissue factor expression may cause inappropriate activation of clotting pathways, which in turn may impair trophoblast invasion of the decidua. Abnormal protease-activated receptor 1 (PAR 1) may also play a role in the failure of trophoblasts to convert to an endothelial phenotype.

Agonistic autoantibodies to the angiotensin type 1 receptor (AT$_1$) are present in many women with preeclampsia in association with defective remodeling of the uteroplacental vasculature.[59,60] These autoantibodies activate AT$_1$ receptors on trophoblast cells, endothelial cells, and vascular smooth muscle cells.[61–63] They appear to block trophoblastic invasion[62] and may induce the production of reactive oxygen species[63] and thus play a significant role in the pathophysiology of preeclampsia (Fig. 35.5). Furthermore, introduction of these autoantibodies into pregnant mice increases production of sFlt-1 and results in hypertension and proteinuria.[64] Thus, these autoantibodies may play an important role in the pathogenesis of preeclampsia at several different stages.

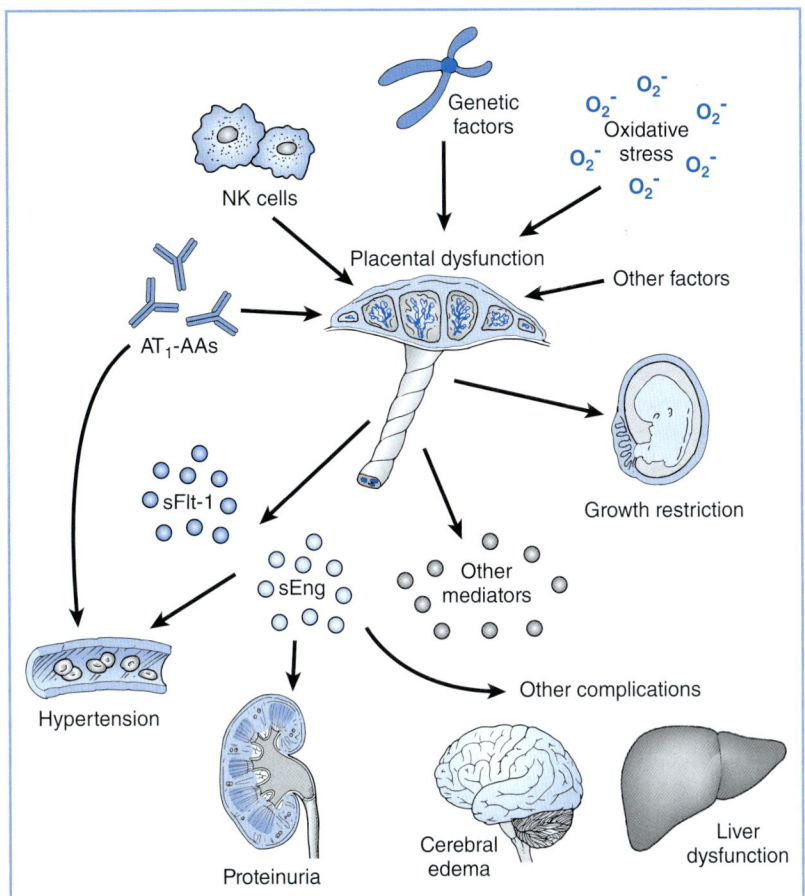

Fig. 35.5 Angiotensin Receptor Autoantibodies (AT$_1$-AAs) in Preeclampsia. AT$_1$-AAs and other factors (e.g., oxidative stress and genetic factors) may cause placental dysfunction, which, in turn, leads to the release of anti-angiogenic factors (e.g., soluble fms-like tyrosine kinase-1 [sFlt-1] and soluble endoglin [sEng]) and other inflammatory mediators to induce preeclampsia. AT$_1$-AAs may also act directly on the maternal vasculature to enhance angiotensin II sensitivity and hypertension. *NK*, Natural killer. From Parikh SM, Karumanchi SA. Putting pressure on preeclampsia. *Nat Med.* 2008;14:810–812.

CLINICAL PRESENTATION AND COMPLICATIONS

Hypertensive disorders of pregnancy can present simply as increased blood pressure (chronic and gestational hypertension) or preeclampsia, which is a multisystem disease unique to human pregnancy characterized by diffuse endothelial dysfunction.[12] Preeclampsia can manifest as a **maternal syndrome** consisting of hypertension and proteinuria with or without other systemic abnormalities. Women with the disease may develop multisystem injury, and preeclampsia is leading indication for maternal peripartum admission to an intensive care unit.[65,66] The disease may also be associated with a **fetal syndrome** (fetal growth restriction, oligohydramnios),[4] which carries a high rate of medically indicated, preterm delivery in developed countries,[67] and is the most common indication for admission to the neonatal intensive care unit.[68] Preeclampsia can occur any time after 20 weeks' gestation until 1 to 2 weeks after delivery[69]; onset before 34 weeks' gestation is associated with increased disease severity and poorer outcomes for both the mother and fetus. The disease typically regresses within 48 hours after delivery.

Cardiovascular

Women with preeclampsia have pathophysiologic changes to the cardiovascular system directly caused by dysfunction of the endothelium. These changes include hypertension characterized by increased vascular resistance and sensitivity to vasoconstrictors and circulating catecholamines.[70] In addition, alterations of endothelial permeability impact fluid balance and tissue edema. The added load on the heart also alters myocardial structure and function.

Arterial Vascular Function

Compared to a woman with a normotensive pregnancy, a woman with preeclampsia has higher blood pressure on average as early as the 9th week of gestation, as well as subtle measures of arterial stiffness.[71,72] Two physiologic hypothesis explaining the hypertension are proposed: (1) constricted physiology (elevated vascular resistance, reduced central volume and cardiac index), or (2) a hyperdynamic state (elevated myocardial mass, systolic function, and cardiac output, with marginally increased resistance). Data from the landmark study by Visser and Wallenburg[73] showed that women with severe preeclampsia had dramatically elevated systemic vascular resistance with a reduced cardiac index compared to normotensive women. Importantly, the authors also recorded hemodynamic values from a cohort of women with severe preeclampsia who had started receiving treatment (fluids, antihypertensive, and antiseizure medications), who had only a slightly elevated resistance compared to normotensive women. Some data suggest that the increase in arterial resistance is primarily due to the decrease in capillary bed volume, with later increases due to decreased arterial compliance.[74,75]

An alternative hypothesis holds that the underlying arterial vascular resistance may not be elevated, even in the untreated patient, but that the hypertension is a result of a hyperdynamic state.[76] For example, echocardiographic studies of both treated and untreated women with preeclampsia show only mildly elevated vascular resistance in a setting of increased left ventricular mass, normal-to-increased cardiac output, and left ventricular contractility.[77–79] One possible reason for these different findings may be the duration of symptomatic preeclampsia, as pregnant women are more carefully observed and diagnosed earlier in the current era. Further, studies using pulmonary artery catheterization or echocardiography have reported variations in patient population, definition of preeclampsia, disease severity, prior treatment, and the presence or absence of concomitant comorbid disease.[73,78,80,81] Finally, the gestational age at onset of preeclampsia may be associated with different hemodynamic patterns. For example, a prospective series of transthoracic echocardiography (TTE) in 1345 normotensive nulliparous women at 24 weeks' gestation subsequently identified 107 women who developed preeclampsia, 75 of whom were early onset and 32 late onset. Systemic vascular resistance was considerably higher, and cardiac output lower among women with early- compared to late-onset preeclampsia, suggesting varying cardiovascular responses.[82]

Myocardial Structure and Function

The left ventricle of women with preeclampsia is characterized by echocardiographic evidence of increased left ventricular mass, increased global systolic function, and evidence of a hyperdynamic state.[79] Microscopically, there is evidence of decreased capillary bed volume, suggesting the antiangiogenic stress results in compensatory hypertrophy. The edematous and hypertrophied myocardium can be visualized on cardiac magnetic resonance imaging (MRI)[83]; the hypertrophy leads to diastolic dysfunction and subclinical systolic dysfunction.[77,84] Overt systolic dysfunction, however, is less common but occurs more frequently in early- than late-onset disease,[85] and in some cases may present as severe cardiac failure with a low ejection fraction.[79,86] A well-documented relationship between severe preeclampsia and peripartum cardiomyopathy may be mediated by the antiangiogenic milieu in women with pre-existing genetic risk.[87–89] Of interest, TTE in women with peripartum cardiomyopathy, higher sFlt-1 levels are associated with worse outcomes, while elevated relaxin-2, which

promotes VEGF activity, is associated with improved postpartum outcome.[90]

Circulating Blood Volume

The central blood volume status of women with preeclampsia varies considerably and is impacted by both the severity of the disease and the degree of fetal involvement. Among women with a reduced plasma volume, body water is redistributed to the extracellular space, leading to nondependent edema.[91] Pathologic endothelial cell permeability further contributes to nondependent edema. Several studies have demonstrated that the maternal plasma volume is reduced proportionately with fetal birth weight.[91,92]

Determining a patient's central blood volume status can be challenging. Previous guidelines recommended the placement of a pulmonary artery catheter to inform management decisions in women with pulmonary edema or renal failure. No randomized trials have evaluated the use of the pulmonary artery catheter for fluid management in women with preeclampsia.[93] Further, interpretation of the data is challenging as left ventricular compliance and cardiovascular conditions vary widely, and a poor correlation exists between pulmonary capillary wedge pressure and left ventricular end-diastolic volume, especially in women with diastolic dysfunction. The placement of a pulmonary artery catheter is not a benign procedure; risks are well recognized.[94] Both immediate and delayed maternal deaths have been attributed to the use of central venous catheters.[95] The insertion of pulmonary artery catheters for management of preeclampsia should be done only after careful consideration of risks and benefits.

Point-of-care TTE may be useful for assessing cardiopulmonary status in the peripartum period.[77,96] Valuable information about volume status, chamber size, wall thickness, and ventricular function may be gleaned. In the setting of low urine output, TTE assessment of stroke volume changes occurring with passive leg raise may predict fluid responsiveness but further work is needed to understand the clinical impact of this finding.[97]

Pulmonary edema **Pulmonary edema** is a severe complication that occurs in approximately 3% of women with preeclampsia.[98] The risk increases in older multigravid women, among women with preeclampsia superimposed on chronic hypertension, and among those with acute or chronic renal disease. The clinical presentation is characterized by worsening dyspnea and orthopnea with concomitant signs of respiratory compromise, including tachypnea, rales, and hypoxemia. A large proportion of cases of pulmonary edema occur postpartum, usually within 2 to 3 days after delivery, and management is directed toward the underlying cause.[99] Initial treatment includes standard treatments such as supplemental oxygen, fluid restriction, and diuretic therapy (e.g., furosemide).

Preeclampsia is associated with multiple factors that promote pulmonary edema: decreased colloid osmotic pressure, increased vascular permeability due to pulmonary endothelial dysfunction, increased intravascular hydrostatic pressure due to arterial hypertension, and increased venous pressure from diastolic dysfunction.[100,101] Plasma colloid osmotic pressure, which is reduced in normal pregnancy because of decreased plasma albumin concentration, decreases even further in women with preeclampsia, likely due to proteinuria.[102] Women with normal pregnancies have a mean osmotic pressure of approximately 22 mm Hg in the third trimester and approximately 17 mm Hg during the early postpartum period. In contrast, a study of women with preeclampsia demonstrated a mean colloid osmotic pressure of approximately 18 mm Hg before delivery and 14 mm Hg after delivery.[103]

TTE may be helpful in distinguishing the etiology of heart failure with low ejection fraction, and in the identification of other cardiac comorbidities contributing to pulmonary edema.[77] Lung ultrasonography may be a useful adjunct to identify lung pathology. In the absence of respiratory symptoms, women with preeclampsia and healthy women have similar appearing lung ultrasonography images.[104] In a study of 20 asymptomatic women with severe preeclampsia and healthy controls,[105] interstitial edema, which precedes alveolar edema, was identified by sonographic B-line artifacts in 25% of the cases. High lung "echo comet scores" were associated with increased left ventricular end-diastolic pressure. Another investigation in women with preeclampsia found echo comet scores were higher before delivery than 4 days after delivery, although tissue Doppler indices did not change after delivery.[106] The authors concluded that increased extravascular lung water before delivery may be associated with increased pulmonary capillary permeability and cardiac dysfunction.

Pulmonary

Obstructive sleep apnea (OSA) is a sleep-related breathing disorder characterized by recurrent episodes of upper airway collapse leading to hypoxia and sleep disturbance. Even in nonpregnant persons, OSA is strongly associated with hypertension. A metaanalysis of cohort studies suggests that pregnant women with OSA have a twofold increased risk for developing preeclampsia.[107] The precise nature of this relationship is not known, and several mechanisms have been proposed.[108] Further studies examining the impact of OSA treatment on maternal and neonatal outcomes are needed.

A review of anesthesia-related maternal deaths in Michigan described a series of postoperative and postpartum deaths attributed to **airway obstruction** or **hypoventilation**.[109] One death was complicated by severe preeclampsia and sleep-disordered breathing likely associated with opioid analgesia-related respiratory depression after cesarean delivery. Such findings highlight the need for close monitoring and consistent vigilance in the postoperative care of women with severe preeclampsia—particularly those with generalized edema, known OSA, airway swelling, snoring, and obesity.

Central Nervous System

Central nervous system manifestations of preeclampsia include persistent or severe headache, hyperexcitability, hyperreflexia, eclampsia, and coma. Approximately 25% of women with preeclampsia have visual disturbances, such as scotoma, amaurosis, and blurred vision; these symptoms may be the initial presenting finding.[110]

Noninvasive measurements of cerebral blood flow and resistance, along with other neuroimaging approaches, suggest that the loss of cerebral vascular autoregulation and vascular barotrauma occur.[111,112] Hyperperfusion of the brain, particularly in the setting of the endothelial dysfunction, causes vasogenic edema. Consequently, these changes may result in the **posterior reversible leukoencephalopathy syndrome (PRES)**.[111,113-115] Measures of cerebrospinal fluid content have demonstrated stark changes in protein content among women with preeclampsia, especially those with neurologic symptoms.[116] Eclampsia is believed to be the manifestation of vasogenic brain edema; MRI findings mimic those of nonpregnant patients with PRES. One review of MRI findings in women with eclampsia found signs consistent with PRES in 46 of 47 women.[115]

Obtaining improved assessment of central nervous system injury would be helpful. **Optic nerve sheath diameter (ONSD)** is a marker for increased intracranial pressure in the nonobstetric population. In a study that compared women with preeclampsia and healthy controls, the median ONSD was greater in women with disease.[117] Nineteen percent of women with preeclampsia had ONSD > 5.8 mm, a value that had previously been associated with a 95% risk for raised intracranial pressure in nonobstetric settings. However, this study found no association between ONSD and the severity of preeclampsia. Understanding the clinical impact of this finding, given the lack of an accurate, alternate measure of intracranial pressure, requires further investigation. Regional cerebral hemoglobin oxygen saturation ($rcSO_2$) has been measured using near-infrared spectroscopy in women with severe preeclampsia and was found to be lower in women with preeclampsia compared with healthy women.[118] The $rcSO_2$ increased after the administration of magnesium sulfate; the percent increase indirectly correlated with blood pressure.

Stroke and Other Intracranial Pathology

Although the absolute risk for pregnancy-associated stroke is low, the risk for intracerebral and subarachnoid hemorrhage and ischemic stroke are markedly increased in women with preeclampsia.[119] Pregnant women with stroke are more likely to have had preeclampsia with severe features, eclampsia, or chronic hypertension.[120] Stroke remains a leading cause of death in women with preeclampsia.[121] Most strokes occur postpartum, and have a high mortality rate because the stroke is likely to be hemorrhagic.

Reversible cerebral edema is a common CNS feature of preeclampsia or eclampsia. The loss of cerebral autoregulation causes hyperperfusion that, compounded by endothelial disruption, leads to interstitial or vasogenic edema.[38,122,123] The vascular hyperreactivity can lead to vasospasm, which can be seen on angiographic exams as segmental narrowing in some women with severe preeclampsia and eclampsia.[124] Calle-Fleming syndrome is a **reversible cerebral vasoconstriction**

syndrome (RCVS), also known **postpartum angiopathy** when it occurs within 1 week of delivery.[125] RCVS may cause recurrent, severe headaches in these women, and when severe, can result in cerebral ischemia. Microvascular hemorrhage is a common feature of preeclampsia and can lead to intracranial hemorrhage.

Mean arterial blood pressure and diastolic blood pressure may not reflect the true risk for stroke. A review of 28 case histories of women with severe preeclampsia who suffered a stroke revealed that (1) systolic blood pressure in excess of 160 mm Hg was a far superior predictor of stroke than diastolic hypertension or elevated mean arterial pressure, (2) the majority of strokes were hemorrhagic (93%) as opposed to thrombotic (7%), and (3) the majority of strokes (57%) occurred in the postpartum period.[126] Close attention to blood pressure control throughout the peripartum period is the mainstay of stroke prevention.[2] In keeping with this goal, ergot alkaloids should generally be avoided in hypertensive patients because their administration can result in severe hypertension.[127]

Hematologic

Several hematologic changes occur in women with preeclampsia. Most common is a relative increase in plasma hemoglobin concentration due to hemoconcentration. In addition, the oxyhemoglobin dissociation curve is shifted to the left compared to healthy pregnancies, with a mean (± standard deviation) P_{50} of 25.1 ± 0.38 mm Hg versus 30.4 ± 0.20 mm Hg, at near-term gestation.[128] Despite a higher hemoglobin concentration, the red blood cells of women with severe preeclampsia have less deformability and are prone to destruction under sheer forces,[129] which makes these patients prone to hemolysis.

Thrombocytopenia, defined as a platelet count < 150,000/mm³, occurs in approximately 10% of uncomplicated pregnancies,[130] but impacts roughly 50% of patients with preeclampsia with severe features.[2] Platelet counts < 100,000/mm³ occur rarely in women with uncomplicated pregnancies, but are a hallmark of HELLP syndrome. More than a quarter of patients with HELLP syndrome have a platelet count < 80,000/mm³.[129] Platelets contribute to coagulation by exposing a phospholipid surface as a catalytic site, and through adhesive and cohesive functions, facilitate the formation of the hemostatic plug. Studies using thromboelastography have found that women with preeclampsia without severe features have measurements similar to women with normal blood pressures, and that those with severe disease and thrombocytopenia (platelet count < 100,000/mm³) have relatively decreased maximum amplitude.[131] In contrast to healthy pregnancies and other hypertensive disorders, platelets are activated in preeclampsia[132]; activated platelets release adenosine diphosphate, serotonin, thromboxane A₂, adhesive proteins and coagulation factors, and growth factors (see Chapter 44). Platelet degranulation is believed to account for some of the decrease in platelet function, while the decrease in platelet count is explained by splenic sequestration[133] and possibly placental sequestration.[134]

Hepatic

Hepatic manifestations of preeclampsia include periportal hemorrhage and fibrin deposition in hepatic sinusoids. Hepatic involvement frequently presents as right upper quadrant or epigastric pain, which may represent pathologies ranging from mild hepatocellular necrosis to subcapsular bleeding.

Subcapsular Hematoma

Rupture of a subcapsular hematoma of the liver is a life-threatening complication of severe preeclampsia and HELLP syndrome that manifests as abdominal pain, nausea and vomiting, and headache.[135] The pain worsens over time and becomes localized to the epigastric area or right upper quadrant. Hypotension and shock typically develop with rupture.[136] Diagnosis is confirmed with ultrasonography, computed tomography, or MRI of the liver (Fig. 35.6). Subcapsular hematoma rupture *with shock* is a surgical emergency that requires immediate multidisciplinary treatment that includes intravascular volume resuscitation and blood and plasma transfusions.[136] In some circumstances, selective arterial embolization by an interventional radiologist may be useful.[135,137,138] Patients with fulminant hepatic failure may require liver transplantation.[135] Prompt surgical intervention and refinements in surgical technique have substantially reduced the maternal mortality rate associated with spontaneous hepatic rupture to less than 20%.[135] The most common causes of death are coagulopathy and exsanguination.[139,140]

HELLP Syndrome

In 1982 Weinstein[141] described a series of 29 cases and coined the acronym HELLP syndrome, characterized by hemolysis, elevated levels of liver enzymes, and a low platelet count. Sibai[142] proposed standardized laboratory diagnostic

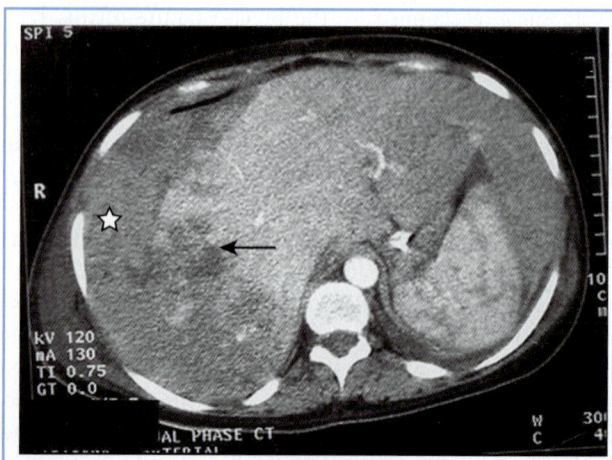

Fig. 35.6 Contrast-enhanced computed tomography scan showing a large area of parenchymal hemorrhage with hepatic rupture (*arrow*) and subcapsular hematoma (*star*) in the right lobe of the liver. From Das CJ, Srivastava DN, Debnath J, et al. Endovascular management of hepatic hemorrhage and subcapsular hematoma in HELLP syndrome. *Indian J Gastroenterol.* 2007;26:244–245.

criteria (Table 35.1). Diagnosis can be especially challenging because other medical and surgical disorders can mimic HELLP syndrome, including acute fatty liver of pregnancy, hemolytic-uremic syndrome, thrombotic thrombocytopenic purpura, idiopathic thrombocytopenic purpura, and lupus (Box 35.4).

HELLP syndrome is associated with increased maternal morbidity and preterm delivery; the degree of thrombocytopenia is associated with outcome (Table 35.2).[139] Most cases of HELLP syndrome are diagnosed after 34 weeks' gestation.[139] Hemolysis, defined as the presence of microangiopathic hemolytic anemia, is the classic hallmark of HELLP syndrome; the peripheral blood smear demonstrates schistocytes, burr cells, and echinocytes.[142] Common histopathologic findings are periportal hepatic necrosis and hemorrhage.[143] Maternal signs and symptoms include right upper quadrant

TABLE 35.1 Diagnostic Criteria for Hemolysis, Elevated Liver Enzymes, and Low Platelets Syndrome

Criteria	Laboratory Tests
Hemolysis	Abnormal peripheral blood smear
	Increased bilirubin > 1.2 mg/dL
	Increased LDH > 600 IU/L
Elevated liver enzyme levels	Increased AST ≥ 70 IU/L
	Increased LDH > 600 IU/L
Thrombocytopenia	Platelet count < 100,000/mm³

AST, Aspartate transferase; *LDH*, lactic dehydrogenase.
Modified from Sibai BM. The HELLP syndrome (hemolysis, elevated liver enzymes, and low platelets): Much ado about nothing? *Am J Obstet Gynecol*. 1990;162:311–316.

BOX 35.4 Differential Diagnosis of Hemolysis, Elevated Liver Enzymes, and Low Platelets Syndrome

- Acute fatty liver of pregnancy
- Appendicitis
- Cholestasis of pregnancy
- Diabetes insipidus
- Cholecystitis
- Gastroenteritis
- Glomerulonephritis
- Hemolytic-uremic syndrome
- Hepatic encephalopathy
- Hyperemesis gravidarum
- Idiopathic thrombocytopenia
- Nephrolithiasis
- Peptic ulcer disease
- Systemic lupus erythematosus
- Thrombotic thrombocytopenic purpura
- Viral hepatitis

From O'Brien JM, Barton JR. Controversies with the diagnosis and management of HELLP syndrome. *Clin Obstet Gynecol*. 2005;48:460–477.

TABLE 35.2 Serious Maternal Complications in a Series of 442 Patients With Hemolysis, Elevated Liver Enzymes, and Low Platelets Syndrome

Complication[a]	Number of Patients	Percent
Disseminated intravascular coagulation	92	21
Placental abruption	69	16
Acute renal failure	33	8
Severe ascites	32	8
Pulmonary edema	26	6
Pleural effusion	26	6
Cerebral edema	4	1
Retinal detachment	4	1
Laryngeal edema	4	1
Subcapsular liver hematoma	4	1
Acute respiratory distress syndrome	3	1
Maternal death	4	1

[a]Some women had multiple complications.
Modified from Sibai BM, Ramadan MK, Usta I, et al. Maternal morbidity and mortality in 442 pregnancies with hemolysis, elevated liver enzymes, and low platelets (HELLP syndrome). *Am J Obstet Gynecol*. 1993;169:1000–1006.

or epigastric pain, nausea and vomiting, headache, hypertension, and proteinuria. Notably, clinical presentation varies; 12% to 18% of women may be normotensive, and proteinuria is absent in approximately 13% of affected women.[2]

Patients with HELLP syndrome are poor candidates for expectant management[2,144]; however, deferred delivery for 24 to 48 hours to allow for corticosteroid administration to accelerate fetal lung maturity may be appropriate for women less than 34 weeks' gestation if the maternal and fetal condition remain stable.[7] Women with HELLP syndrome who have not yet reached 34 weeks' gestation should be managed in a tertiary care facility with a neonatal intensive care unit capable of caring for a compromised preterm neonate.[7] Clinical management aligns with that for preeclampsia with severe features and includes intravenous magnesium sulfate for seizure prophylaxis and antihypertensive medications to maintain systolic blood pressure < 160 mm Hg and a diastolic blood pressure < 110 mm Hg.[2,142]

The platelet count can fall precipitously and may remain depressed up to 48 hours after delivery. The decision to initiate neuraxial analgesia or anesthesia is complex and must take into account the rate of change in platelet count and other factors such as signs and symptoms of bleeding or bruising.[145] Women with a platelet count < 50,000/mm³ may be at risk for bleeding,[146] and for spinal epidural hematoma with neuraxial anesthesia.

Platelet transfusions are indicated in the presence of significant bleeding and in all parturients with a platelet count < 20,000/mm³. For women with a platelet count < 40,000/mm³ who are scheduled for cesarean delivery, the preincision administration of platelets has been recommended.[147] As the risk for postpartum hemorrhage is significantly increased in patients with HELLP syndrome, large-bore intravenous access should be obtained, and compatible red blood cell units should be available.

Renal

Renal manifestations of preeclampsia include **proteinuria, changes in the glomerular filtration rate (GFR), and hyperuricemia**. Proteinuria is found in 75% of women with preeclampsia and is a defining element, but its presence is no longer considered essential for diagnosis when other evidence of end-organ injury is evident. Additionally, the presence of proteinuria may be challenging to interpret among women with preexisting renal dysfunction. The characteristic renal histologic lesion of preeclampsia is glomerular capillary endotheliosis, which manifests as glomerular enlargement and endothelial and mesangial cell swelling. Increasing urinary excretion of protein likely results from changes in the pore size or charge selectivity of the glomerular filter and impaired proximal tubular reabsorption.[148]

During normal pregnancy, the GFR *increases* by 40% to 60% during the first trimester,[149,150] with a resulting decrease in the serum markers of renal clearance, including blood urea nitrogen (BUN), creatinine, and uric acid (see Chapter 2). In preeclampsia, this increase in GFR is blunted compared with normal pregnancy.[148] Notably, women with preeclampsia may have BUN and creatinine measurements in the normal range for nonpregnant women.

The association between preeclampsia and hyperuricemia was recognized as early as 1917.[151] Most evidence suggests that decreased renal clearance is the primary mechanism for elevated uric acid levels.[152] Because levels of serum uric acid begin to increase as early as 25 weeks' gestation,[153] it has been investigated as a possible early marker of preeclampsia.

Renal Failure

Acute renal failure is a rare but serious complication of severe preeclampsia.[154] The true incidence remains unknown. Acute renal failure is divided into three categories: (1) **prerenal**, which refers to renal hypoperfusion; (2) **intrarenal**, which suggests intrinsic renal parenchymal damage; and (3) **postrenal**, which implies obstructive uropathy. The majority of cases (83% to 90%) of acute renal failure in preeclampsia result from prerenal and intrarenal pathologic processes (most commonly acute tubular necrosis) and resolve completely after delivery.[155,156] In contrast, bilateral renal cortical necrosis is a rare and serious condition associated with considerable maternal and perinatal morbidity and mortality. It occurs most commonly in association with known renal parenchymal disease, chronic hypertension with superimposed preeclampsia, placental abruption, disseminated intravascular coagulation (DIC), HELLP syndrome, sepsis, or fetal death.[157,158]

Oliguria is a possible late manifestation of severe preeclampsia and parallels the severity of disease. Persistent oliguria requires immediate assessment of intravascular volume status; however, hypovolemia should not be assumed. Progression to renal failure is rare and is typically preceded by hypovolemia, placental abruption, or DIC.

CLINICAL AND OBSTETRIC MANAGEMENT

Obstetric management of preeclampsia centers on (1) fetal and maternal surveillance, (2) treatment of hypertension, (3) seizure prophylaxis, and (4) timing and route of delivery.

Maternal and Fetal Surveillance

Maternal surveillance is indicated for all women with preeclampsia.[159] In women with preeclampsia without severe features, the goal is early detection of progression to severe disease. In women with severe disease, the goal is detection of worsening organ dysfunction. Initial laboratory investigations for the pregnant woman who develops hypertension after 20 weeks' gestation are listed in Table 35.3. The admission platelet count is an excellent predictor of subsequent thrombocytopenia.[160] For women with a platelet count exceeding 100,000/mm³, further coagulation testing is not required because coagulopathy is rarely present in severely

TABLE 35.3 **Initial Laboratory Investigations for Women in Whom Hypertension Develops After 20 Weeks' Gestation**	
Test	**Rationale**
Hemoglobin and hematocrit	Hemoconcentration supports diagnosis of preeclampsia and is an indicator of severity. Values are decreased if hemolysis is present.
Platelet count	Thrombocytopenia suggests preeclampsia with severe features.
Urine protein-creatinine ratio or 24-h urine protein excretion	Presence of proteinuria distinguishes preeclampsia from gestational hypertension.
Serum creatinine level	Abnormal or rising creatinine level suggests preeclampsia with severe features, especially in presence of oliguria.
Serum aminotransferase levels	Elevated serum aminotransferase levels suggest preeclampsia with severe features with hepatic involvement.

Modified from Report of the National High Blood Pressure Education Program Working Group on High Blood Pressure in Pregnancy. *Am J Obstet Gynecol.* 2000;183:S1–S22; and American College of Obstetricians and Gynecologists Taskforce on Hypertension in Pregnancy. *Hypertension in Pregnancy.* American College of Obstetricians and Gynecologists; 2013.

preeclamptic women who have a normal platelet count.[160] If the platelet count is less than 100,000/mm^3, other hemostatic abnormalities (e.g., prolonged prothrombin time [PT] and activated partial thromboplastin time [aPTT], reduced fibrinogen concentration) may be present.[160] Further coagulation studies may be useful, particularly if risk factors for DIC are present (e.g., placental abruption, liver dysfunction, HELLP syndrome). Liver function tests are obtained in all women with preeclampsia because abnormal levels indicate severe disease and may prompt delivery. Approximately 20% of women with preeclampsia have elevated serum aminotransferase levels.[161] The value of uric acid testing is controversial, with conflicting evidence regarding its association with increased fetal or maternal risk for complications.[162–164]

The frequency of subsequent laboratory evaluation is guided by the initial findings and the severity of illness and disease progression.[144] A diagnosis of preeclampsia without severe features should prompt at least weekly laboratory investigations, with the frequency modified based on subsequent clinical findings.[7] In the expectant management of preeclampsia with severe features, hemoglobin, platelet count, liver function tests, creatinine, and coagulation function should be assessed daily or every other day.[7,165] For women undergoing induction of labor for whom initial laboratory measurement or platelet counts are suspicious for HELLP syndrome, serial platelet counts at least every 6 hours may guide decision-making about the timing of delivery and analgesic or anesthetic technique. Finally, for women with indicated delivery, an active blood type and screen is indicated with consideration of type and cross-match of red blood cells for patients with thrombocytopenia or other abnormalities in coagulation tests.[166]

Preeclampsia is a known risk factor for perinatal death. The ACOG Taskforce on Hypertension in Pregnancy recommended daily fetal movement counts with either nonstress testing or biophysical profile testing at the time of diagnosis (see Chapter 6) and at regular intervals thereafter.[7] Ultrasonography is used to estimate fetal weight and amniotic fluid volume. Doppler ultrasonography is used to measure fetal blood flow velocimetry if fetal growth restriction is suspected.[7,167]

Corticosteroid Administration

To accelerate fetal lung maturity, all women who develop preeclampsia with severe features or HELLP syndrome between 24 and 34 weeks' gestation should receive a course of corticosteroid therapy. A randomized double-blind trial of 218 women with severe preeclampsia at 26 to 34 weeks' gestation found that the infants of those receiving betamethasone, compared with the infants of those receiving placebo, exhibited a significant reduction in the rate of the neonatal respiratory distress syndrome and reduced rates of neonatal intraventricular hemorrhage, infection, and death.[168] The available data also suggest that treatment with corticosteroids results in improvement in the maternal platelet count in women with HELLP syndrome, with dexamethasone being more efficacious than betamethasone.[169] However, these studies do not show a clear benefit of corticosteroid treatment on the endpoints of severe maternal morbidity or mortality.[169]

Uteroplacental Perfusion

Uteroplacental perfusion may be impaired in pregnancies complicated by preeclampsia. In contrast with normal pregnancy, fetal umbilical artery flow waveforms demonstrate an increase in downstream resistance, a decrease in diastolic flow velocity, and an increase in the systolic-to-diastolic flow velocity ratio.[170] The systolic-to-diastolic ratio, calculated from Doppler ultrasonographic determination of blood flow velocities, reflects intrinsic arterial resistance in the chorionic plate of the placenta.[167] Pathophysiologic changes can result in fetal growth restriction (the fetal syndrome) in some pregnancies complicated by severe preeclampsia.

Placental Abruption

Placental abruption occurs in approximately 2% of women with preeclampsia and results in increased perinatal morbidity and mortality. A 2006 retrospective case-control study of 161 women with placental abruption and 2000 women without abruption found a threefold increased risk for placental abruption in women with preeclampsia.[171] The incidence is also increased in women with underlying chronic hypertension. Management depends on the extent of abruption and associated hypotension, coagulopathy, or fetal compromise (see Chapter 37). Placental abruption is also associated with the development of DIC (see Chapter 44).

Treatment of Acute Hypertension

Antihypertensive medications are used to treat severe hypertension (systolic blood pressure ≥ 160 mm Hg or diastolic blood pressure ≥ 110 mm Hg) with the goal of preventing adverse maternal sequelae such as hypertensive encephalopathy, cerebrovascular hemorrhage, myocardial ischemia, and congestive heart failure.[2]

Although acute control of maternal blood pressure is critical, rapid changes in maternal perfusion pressure may adversely affect uteroplacental perfusion and oxygen delivery to the fetus. Antihypertensive medications should be carefully titrated to avoid abrupt changes in maternal blood pressure. The ISSHP targets treatment to a diastolic blood pressure of 85 mm Hg or less, regardless of systolic pressure, while the ACOG does not provide specific targets due to lack of evidence of benefit.[2,4,7] In either case, blood pressure in the severe range (≥160/110 mg Hg) is considered an emergency and treatment should be administered within 30 to 60 minutes.[2] Commonly used drugs include labetalol, hydralazine, and nifedipine (Table 35.4). Nicardipine and esmolol may be considered second-line agents. Historically, sodium nitroprusside was also a second-line agent. However, because it is a highly potent smooth muscle vasodilator, and careful titration is required to avoid acute hypotension, it is seldom used in the current management of preeclampsia.

Systematic review and metaanalysis of available studies show insufficient data regarding the relative efficacy of these commonly used agents and recommend selection based on

TABLE 35.4   Treatment of Acute Severe Hypertension in Preeclampsia/Eclampsia[a]

Medication	Onset of Action (min)	Dose
Labetalol[b]	1–2	10–20 mg IV, then 20–80 mg every 10–30 min if needed, up to a maximum cumulative dose of 300 mg
Hydralazine[b]	10–20	5 mg IV or IM, then 5–10 mg IV every 20–40 min if needed, up to a maximum cumulative dose of 20 mg
Nifedipine[b]	5–10	10–20 mg orally, repeat in 20 min if needed; then 10–20 mg every 2–6 h; maximum daily dose of 180 mg
Nicardipine[c]	10–15	Initial infusion 5 mg/h, increase by 2.5 mg/h every 5 min if needed; maximum dose of 15 mg/h
Esmolol[c]	1–2	500 μg/kg loading dose, infusion 50 μg/kg/min, titrate upward by 50 μg/kg/min increments if needed; maximum dose 200 μg/kg/min

IM, Intramuscularly; *IV,* intravenously.
[a]Treatment of systolic blood pressure ≥ 160 mm Hg, diastolic blood pressure ≥ 110 mm Hg, or both, if sustained.
[b]First-line therapy.
[c]Second-line therapy.
Modified from American College of Obstetricians and Gynecologists. ACOG Practice Bulletin, Number 222: Gestational hypertension and preeclampsia (reaffirmed 2023). *Obstet Gynecol.* 2020;135:e237–e260.

clinician familiarity and adverse effects.[172] The authors of the systematic review do, however, suggest that some agents are inferior and recommend avoiding diazoxide, ketanserin, nimodipine, and magnesium sulfate for the treatment of severe hypertension in pregnancy (although magnesium is recommended for maternal seizure prophylaxis).[172] The ACOG practice bulletin on the treatment of acute hypertension recommends intravenous labetalol, intravenous or intramuscular hydralazine, or oral nifedipine as a first-line treatment for acute-onset, severe hypertension in pregnant or postpartum patients.[2]

Specific Medications

Labetalol is a combined alpha- and beta-adrenergic receptor antagonist with a 1:7 ratio of alpha- to beta-adrenergic receptor antagonism when administered intravenously. Labetalol should be avoided in women with severe asthma or congestive heart failure.[173]

A metaanalysis concluded that intravenous labetalol has efficacy similar to intravenous hydralazine but with fewer maternal side effects, although evidence was limited to four small, randomized controlled trials.[172] Neonates born to mothers exposed to beta-adrenergic receptor antagonists during delivery, including labetalol, demonstrate increased rates of neonatal hypoglycemia and bradycardia.[174]

Hydralazine has been used safely in pregnant women for decades and is also considered a first-line drug for treating severe hypertension in pregnancy.[2] Hydralazine exerts a potent direct vasodilating effect. Plasma volume expansion before administration decreases the risk for maternal hypotension. Other side effects include tachycardia, palpitations, headache, and neonatal thrombocytopenia. In a randomized clinical trial, hydralazine was associated with more maternal tachycardia and palpitations and less neonatal bradycardia and hypotension than labetalol.[175]

Nifedipine is a calcium entry–blocking agent that lowers blood pressure by relaxing arterial and arteriolar smooth muscle. It can be administered as a long-acting oral medication once the severe hypertension has stabilized. Nifedipine immediate-release capsules should not be administered to women with known coronary artery disease, long-standing diabetes mellitus or aortic stenosis, or to women older than 45 years of age because of an increased risk for sudden cardiac death.[46] In the absence of contraindications, nifedipine is now recommended as a first-line agent in women for whom intravenous access is difficult to secure.[2]

Although earlier reports suggested that the coadministration of nifedipine with magnesium sulfate causes adverse effects in both the mother and fetus, including severe maternal hypotension,[176] neuromuscular blockade,[177] and nonreassuring fetal heart rate (FHR) patterns,[176] subsequent data suggest that these drugs can be used together safely.[178] Oral nifedipine has been found to be as efficacious and safe as intravenous labetalol.[179]

Nicardipine is a calcium entry–blocking agent that can be administered by intravenous infusion and has been shown to achieve rapid decreases in systolic and diastolic blood pressures in pregnant women.[180] It is an excellent option for treating severe hypertension that is not responsive to labetalol or hydralazine.[181]

Esmolol is a short-acting beta-adrenergic receptor antagonist that can be used to treat acute hypertension accompanied by maternal tachycardia. Concerns regarding the use of esmolol during pregnancy arose in 1989 after a report of dose-dependent prolonged fetal bradycardia in a study of gravid ewes receiving esmolol by stepped infusion.[182] Subsequent human case reports have reported variable responses,[183,184] but in most cases fetal bradycardia was transient and FHR returned to baseline after discontinuation of the drug. Placental transfer is rapid, and clinicians should expect to observe the effects of beta-adrenergic receptor blockade in the fetus. Maternal administration of esmolol produces a greater degree of beta-adrenergic receptor blockade in the fetal lamb than that observed after maternal administration of an equipotent dose of labetalol.[182,185]

Seizure Prophylaxis and Treatment

In the setting of preeclampsia and eclampsia, magnesium sulfate is indicated for both seizure prophylaxis and treatment.

Seizure Prophylaxis

The routine use of magnesium sulfate for seizure prophylaxis in women with preeclampsia with *severe features* is an established obstetric practice. There is clear evidence that magnesium sulfate is the best available agent for prevention of recurrent seizures in women with eclampsia.[186,187]

A metaanalysis of the available data identified six trials involving 11,444 women that compared magnesium sulfate for prevention of eclampsia with either placebo or no anticonvulsant.[188] Magnesium decreased the risk for developing eclampsia (relative risk [RR], 0.41; 95% confidence interval [CI], 0.29 to 0.58); there was also a trend toward lower risk for maternal death (RR, 0.54; 95% CI, 0.26 to 1.10), but no effect on serious maternal morbidity.[188] Additionally, magnesium therapy reduced the risk for placental abruption. It did not adversely affect fetal and/or neonatal outcomes, including stillbirth, perinatal death, or neurosensory disability.[188] Treatment with magnesium increased the risk for maternal respiratory depression (RR, 1.98; 95% CI, 1.24 to 3.15) and cesarean delivery (RR, 1.05; 95% CI, 1.01 to 1.10).[188] Other side effects that were significantly more common in those treated with magnesium included feeling warm or flushed, nausea/vomiting, muscle weakness, hypotension, dizziness, drowsiness/confusion, and headache.[188] Magnesium sulfate is not indicated for seizure prevention in preeclampsia without severe features.[7] Studies have failed to show a difference in the number of women who progressed to severe preeclampsia.[189,190]

The mechanism of the anticonvulsant effect of magnesium is not well understood. It was previously believed that eclamptic seizures were the result of cerebral vasospasm and that the cerebral vasodilating properties of magnesium reduced the rate of eclamptic seizures by relieving vasospasm.[191] However, there is evidence that abrupt, sustained blood pressure elevation overwhelms myogenic vasoconstriction and causes forced dilation of the cerebral vessels, hyperperfusion, and cerebral edema.[112,191–193] This raises the question of how magnesium sulfate—a vasodilator—could be effective in seizure prophylaxis, as magnesium would be expected to worsen cerebral hyperperfusion and edema. Using a rat model, Euser and Cipolla[191] demonstrated that the mesenteric vessels are more sensitive to magnesium-induced vasodilation than are cerebral vessels, suggesting that part of the effect may be mediated through decreasing peripheral vascular resistance. Further animal studies suggest that magnesium may ameliorate neuroinflammation and brain edema in an eclampsia-like seizure model.[194] Magnesium may also protect the blood-brain barrier, or act centrally at *N*-methyl-D-aspartate receptors to raise the seizure threshold.[195]

No consensus exists regarding (1) the ideal time to initiate treatment with magnesium sulfate, (2) the best loading and maintenance doses, or (3) the optimal duration of therapy. Many obstetricians administer a loading dose of 4 to 6 g over 20 to 30 minutes, followed by a maintenance infusion of 1 to 2 g/h. The infusion is commonly initiated once the decision is made to deliver the fetus and is continued for 24 hours postpartum.[196] Expert opinion recommends that women with preeclampsia with severe features undergoing cesarean delivery should receive magnesium sulfate at least 2 hours before the procedure, during surgery, and for 24 hours postpartum.[7,189]

Magnesium sulfate is eliminated almost entirely by renal excretion,[197] and serum levels may become dangerously high in the presence of renal insufficiency. Side effects of hypermagnesemia include chest pain and tightness, palpitations, nausea, blurred vision, sedation, transient hypotension, and, rarely, pulmonary edema.[198,199] In untreated patients, the normal range for serum magnesium concentrations is 1.7 to 2.4 mg/dL. The therapeutic range lies between 5 and 9 mg/dL.[200] Reflex testing is used as a clinical screen for hypermagnesemia; when deep tendon reflexes are preserved, the more serious side effects are usually avoided. Patellar reflexes are lost at serum magnesium levels of approximately 12 mg/dL. Respiratory arrest occurs at levels between 15 and 20 mg/dL, and asystole occurs when the level exceeds 25 mg/dL.[2] Serial measurement of serum magnesium levels may be helpful in the management of women with renal dysfunction because magnesium toxicity can occur with usual dosing regimens.

Treatment of suspected magnesium toxicity includes immediate discontinuation of the infusion and the intravenous administration of **calcium gluconate** (1 g) over 10 minutes. In the rare event of respiratory compromise, the patient may require tracheal intubation and mechanical ventilation until spontaneous ventilation returns.[2]

Seizure Treatment

Immediate goals are to stop convulsions, establish a patent airway, and prevent major complications (e.g., hypoxemia, aspiration). Further obstetric management includes antihypertensive therapy, induction or augmentation of labor, and expeditious (preferably vaginal) delivery. Fetal bradycardia typically begins during or immediately after a seizure but does not mandate immediate delivery unless it is persistent.

During the seizure, oxygenation may prove impossible, but supplemental oxygen should be delivered by means of a face mask (Box 35.5). Attempts to insert an oral airway should be withheld until the seizure abates. As soon as breathing resumes, ventilation may be gently augmented with a bag-and-mask device. Pulse oximetry should be used to assess maternal oxygenation. Blood pressure and the electrocardiogram should be monitored to identify hypertension, arrhythmia, or cardiac arrest. While initial resuscitation is underway, an assistant should establish intravenous access, which may be difficult in a combative postictal woman. Judicious sedation may be required to allow further treatment in some patients.

Magnesium sulfate is preferred to diazepam for the prevention of further seizures in eclampsia.[186,187] The administration of magnesium sulfate in women with eclampsia is associated with significantly lower maternal death rates. An

BOX 35.5   Eclampsia: The ABCs of Eclamptic Seizure Control

Airway
- Turn patient to the left side; apply jaw thrust.
- Attempt bag-and-mask ventilation ($FIO_2 = 1.0$) or administer oxygen by face mask.
- Insert oral airway if necessary.

Breathing
- Continue bag-and-mask ventilation ($FIO_2 = 1.0$) or administer oxygen by face mask.
- Apply pulse oximeter and monitor SpO_2.

Circulation
- Secure intravenous access.
- Check blood pressure at frequent intervals.
- Monitor electrocardiogram.

Drugs
- Magnesium sulfate
  - 4–6 g IV over 20 min
  - 1–2 g/h IV for maintenance therapy
  - 2–4 g IV over 10 min for recurrent seizures
- Antihypertensive agents
  - Labetalol or hydralazine as needed to treat hypertension (see Table 35.4)

IV, Intravenously.

initial intravenous bolus of 4 to 6 g is administered, followed by an infusion at 1 to 2 g/h, assuming the patient has adequate renal function.[2,201] Recurrent convulsions should prompt administration of an additional bolus of 2 to 4 g, infused over 5 to 10 minutes. The patient should be carefully monitored for signs of magnesium toxicity. Should there be recurrent uncontrolled seizures, small doses of midazolam or diazepam may be used to raise the seizure threshold.

Decision and Route of Delivery

Delivery remains the only cure for preeclampsia; however, the delivery of women with preeclampsia without severe features is not urgent. Data suggest that induction of labor for pregnancies beyond 37 weeks' gestation in women with gestational hypertension or preeclampsia without severe features is associated with improved maternal outcomes compared with expectant management.[7,202] Outcomes in these pregnancies are similar to those in uncomplicated pregnancies.[7,46,203] In general, delivery is recommended for women presenting with preeclampsia with severe features at 34 weeks' gestation or later.[2,7]

For women with preeclampsia with severe features at less than 34 weeks' gestation (Fig. 35.7), expectant management may improve fetal outcomes without substantially endangering the mother,[2,7,46,204] but data are few.[205] Delay of delivery for 24 to 48 hours allows for the administration of corticosteroids to facilitate fetal lung maturity and transfer to a facility with maternal and neonatal intensive care resources. Expedited delivery, regardless of corticosteroid administration, is indicated for patients with eclampsia, pulmonary edema, DIC,

placental abruption, abnormal fetal surveillance, a previable or nonviable fetus, or intrauterine fetal demise.[4,7] If a woman develops refractory severe hypertension despite maximum doses of antihypertensive agents *or* persistent cerebral symptoms (e.g., headache, visual disturbance) while receiving magnesium sulfate, delivery should occur within 24 to 48 hours, regardless of gestational age or corticosteroid administration.[2,7,144] Expectant management before 34 weeks' gestation should be undertaken at facilities with neonatal and maternal intensive care resources.[2,7]

Vaginal delivery should be attempted in all women with preeclampsia without severe features, assuming no other indications for cesarean delivery exist. Vaginal delivery should also be attempted in most women with severe disease, especially those beyond 34 weeks' gestation. Cesarean delivery is appropriate when the maternal or fetal condition mandates immediate delivery or when other indications for cesarean delivery exist.

Postpartum venous thromboembolism (VTE) is a leading cause of maternal mortality in pregnancy. Both cesarean delivery[206,207] and preeclampsia[206,208] are independent risk factors for postpartum VTE. Prophylaxis and treatment of VTE are discussed in Chapter 38.

ANESTHETIC MANAGEMENT

The anesthetic management of the woman with hypertensive disorder of pregnancy must consider pathophysiologic changes in the maternal airway and cardiovascular system, and increased potential for complications such as pulmonary edema. Additionally, the potential for rapid progression to the severe form of preeclampsia or eclampsia mandates continual reassessment of the patient.

Preanesthetic Evaluation

The preanesthetic assessment of women with confirmed or suspected preeclampsia should assess, at a minimum, the airway, maternal hemodynamic parameters and fluid balance, and coagulation status. Laboratory analysis should include a complete blood count, including hemoglobin concentration and platelet count. Other assessments of coagulation (e.g., PT, PTT, fibrinogen concentration) should be considered if the patient demonstrates thrombocytopenia or severe features. In addition, the clinician should assess renal function (creatinine concentration, recent urine output, and fluid administration over the last 24 to 48 hours). The clinician should reassess the airway prior to the initiation of anesthesia for a surgical procedure, as the appearance can change rapidly during labor. Finally, the patient should be assessed for the presence of pulmonary edema. Placement of an arterial catheter for invasive blood pressure monitoring may be considered.

Blood Pressure Assessment

The assessment and management of blood pressure is vital to the care of patients with hypertensive disorders of pregnancy. Noninvasive blood pressure monitoring is appropriate in patients with hypertensive disorder without severe disease,

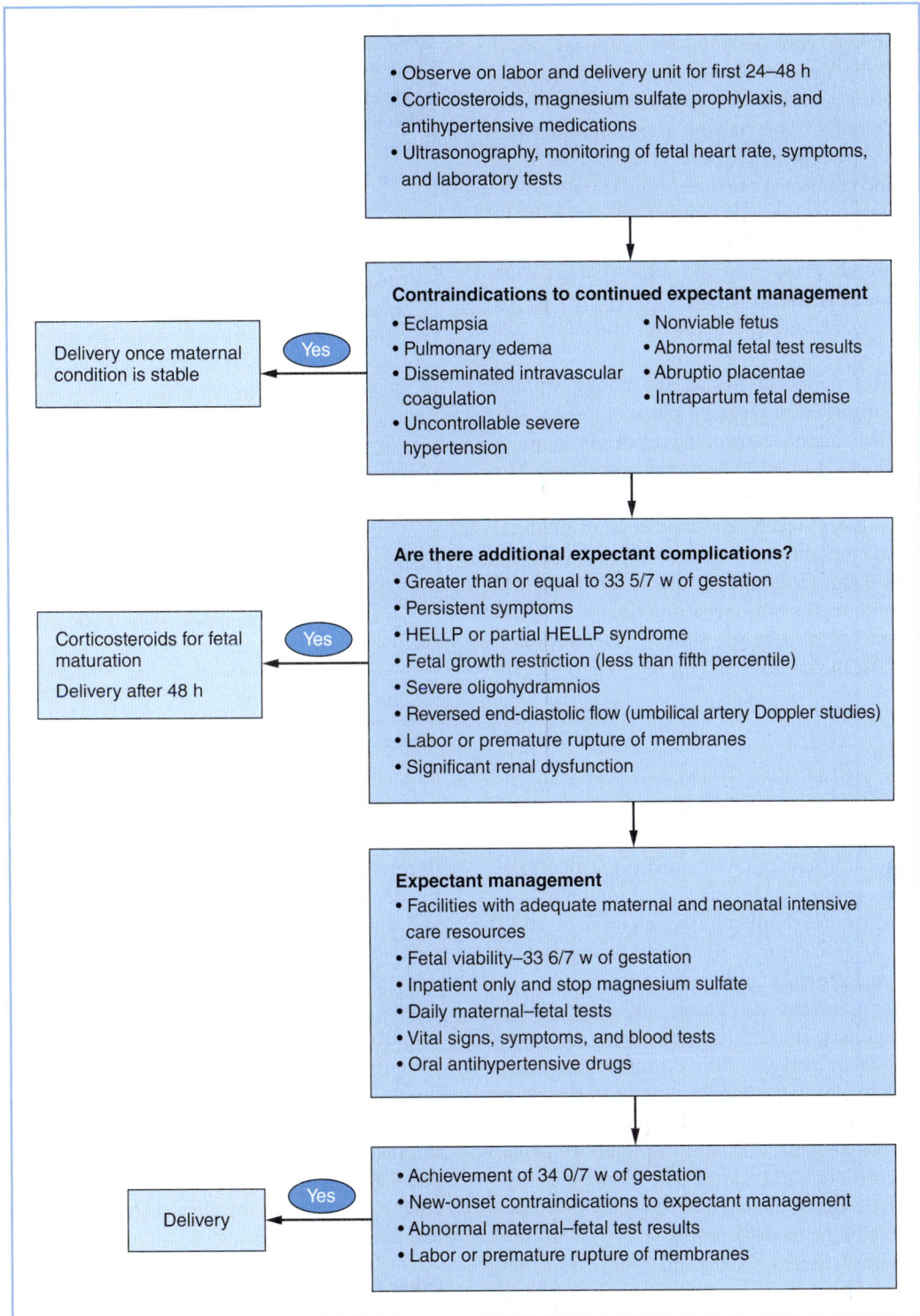

Fig. 35.7 Suggested algorithm for the management of severe preeclampsia at less than 34 weeks' gestation. *HELLP*, Hemolysis, elevated liver enzymes, and low platelet count. From American College of Obstetricians and Gynecologists Taskforce on Hypertension in Pregnancy. *Hypertension in Pregnancy*. American College of Obstetricians and Gynecologists; 2013.

although automated devices may underestimate blood pressure in preeclampsia.[209,210] The clinician may consider insertion of an intraarterial catheter for (1) accurate, continuous blood pressure monitoring, especially with poorly controlled hypertension; (2) frequent venous or arterial sampling, especially in patients with difficult venous access or in the context of pulmonary edema; and (3) to estimate intravascular volume status using calculated systolic pressure variation.[211] Pulse waveform analysis has been suggested as a minimally invasive method to measure cardiac output and has been shown to closely match those obtained from thermodilution in women with preeclampsia.[212]

Coagulation Status

Among the hematologic considerations for neuraxial procedures in women with hypertensive disorders of pregnancy are the platelet count and trend over time, along with any coexisting coagulopathy. Women with preeclampsia without severe features are typically hypercoagulable relative to women with an uncomplicated pregnancy and should not be denied neuraxial labor analgesia.[131] Women with preeclampsia with severe features and those with HELLP syndrome may develop thrombocytopenia and other coagulation abnormalities, which increases the risk for bleeding into the epidural or spinal space during a neuraxial procedure (see Chapter 31).

The incidence of neuraxial hematoma among women with hypertensive disorders of pregnancy cannot be precisely stated due to the challenge of determining the denominator of all such women who have received neuraxial procedures. The low incidence of coagulopathy combined with careful screening has led to an exceptionally low incidence of epidural hematoma in contemporary obstetric anesthesia practice, estimated at 0.4 to 0.6 per 100,000.[213,214] The risk for **epidural hematoma** formation exists not only at the time of epidural catheter placement but also at the time of its removal.[215] Clinicians should use the same criteria for removal as they do for placement.

Platelet Count

While the precise platelet count at which risk of a spinal-epidural hematoma increases is unknown, in the absence of preeclampsia with severe features, a recent platelet count > 100,000/mm³ is sufficient prior to initiating a neuraxial procedure. Women with preeclampsia with thrombocytopenia or other severe features should be assessed more carefully prior to a neuraxial procedure. A recent reassuring platelet count may help avoid general anesthesia.[216]

The Society for Obstetric Anesthesia and Perinatology (SOAP) interdisciplinary consensus statement on neuraxial procedures in obstetric patients with thrombocytopenia[145] suggests a low risk of bleeding complications when the platelet count is greater than 70,000/mm³ among patients with gestational thrombocytopenia, idiopathic thrombocytopenia, and preeclampsia without HELLP syndrome. Consensus suggests that a platelet count < 50,000/mm³ typically precludes the administration of neuraxial anesthesia.[145] For women with a platelet count between 50,000 and 70,000/mm³, the risks and benefits of neuraxial anesthesia must be weighed against the risks associated with general anesthesia for the individual patient if emergency cesarean delivery is required, including whether anatomic features of the patient's airway are favorable. A neuraxial procedure may be considered with careful documentation of the decision-making process and best practices for the procedure; an example of such a pathway is presented in Box 35.6. Among patients with HELLP syndrome, the SOAP statement recommends determination of the platelet count within 6 hours of the neuraxial procedure due to the rapid decrease that is often observed with this disease.

> ### BOX 35.6   Suggested Actions for Neuraxial Procedures in Women With Preeclampsia If Thrombocytopenia Is Present[a]
>
> - The most skilled anesthesia provider available should perform the neuraxial procedure to minimize the number of needle passes.
> - Neuraxial ultrasonography may be considered to reduce the number of needle passes.
> - A single-shot spinal technique may be preferable to an epidural technique (when appropriate) because of the smaller needle size (supporting data are lacking).
> - Use of a flexible wire–embedded epidural catheter may reduce epidural vein trauma.
> - Careful monitoring after delivery for neurologic signs that may signal spinal-epidural hematoma, which may present up to 48 h after the procedure.
> - Check platelet count within 6 h of initiating neuraxial procedure in women with HELLP syndrome or high risk of coagulopathy.
> - Check platelet count postpartum in women with HELLP syndrome before removing epidural catheter for evidence of return toward normal (at least 75,000–80,000/mm³).
> - Immediate neurologic or neurosurgical consultation and neuraxial imaging are necessary if there is any suspicion of epidural hematoma.

[a]Platelet count < 70,000/mm³.

Trend over time In certain cases, the platelet count decreases rapidly and the nadir in the platelet count cannot be identified prospectively. If serial platelet counts are stable and remain in the normal range, a platelet count measurement every 24 to 48 hours is adequate to monitor women undergoing expectant management of severe preeclampsia remote from term; the platelet count is unlikely to decrease if thrombocytopenia is absent on the admission assessment.[7,217] Among women with confirmed or suspected HELLP syndrome, early epidural catheter placement may be recommended in anticipation of worsening thrombocytopenia if the platelet count is greater than 70,000/mm³. The platelet count should be assessed after delivery, before removal of the epidural catheter, as the platelet count nadir often occurs several days after delivery.[218]

Other Coagulation Disorders

Women with severe preeclampsia, with or without thrombocytopenia, may have other hemostatic abnormalities.[160] Additional risk factors include placental abruption, intrauterine fetal demise, and HELLP syndrome. In these scenarios, the PT, aPTT, and serum fibrinogen concentration should be assessed before the initiation of neuraxial anesthesia.[160,219] Viscoelastic assessment of coagulation has demonstrated some benefit in the management of hemorrhage and trauma, but its use for assessment of women with preeclampsia-related hemostatic dysfunction remains unproven. Although thromboelastography has shown some promise in the assessment of coagulation status in pregnant patients with thrombocytopenia,[131] it is not yet recommended as an adjunct for decision-making.[145] Platelet function analysis (PFA-100) appears to be sensitive to platelet dysfunction in women with severe preeclampsia,[134] but is not a widely available technology. Both viscoelastic testing and PFA require further study to determine their utility in assessing the risk of epidural hematoma after the administration of neuraxial anesthesia.[220]

Neuraxial Analgesia and Anesthesia

Continuous antepartum epidural infusion of local anesthetic has been suggested to optimize uteroplacental blood flow and prolong pregnancy in women with preeclampsia remote from term. In one study, women with severe preeclampsia between 28 and 32 weeks' gestation who received an epidural local anesthetic infusion had delayed delivery and improved blood pressure and platelet counts compared with women who received standard treatment.[221] A second study found a unilateral decrease in uterine artery vascular resistance (in the artery with highest baseline resistance) during the period of epidural ropivacaine infusion compared with saline infusion in women with early-onset preeclampsia.[222] Although promising, this technique for prolonging pregnancy requires further study, as the risk of infection due to prolonged neuraxial catheterization increases with longer insertion time.

Continuous lumbar epidural or combined spinal-epidural (CSE) analgesia is the preferred method of pain management during labor in women with preeclampsia. Advantages include (1) provision of high-quality analgesia, which attenuates the hypertensive response to pain; (2) a reduction in levels of circulating catecholamines and stress-related hormones[223]; (3) provision of a means for rapid initiation of epidural anesthesia for emergency cesarean delivery, obviating the need for general anesthesia and its associated risk for airway catastrophe and critical hypertension during laryngoscopy; and (4) improvement in intervillous blood flow.[224]

Early initiation of neuraxial labor analgesia is recommended in the absence of contraindications in all patients with preeclampsia with severe features, particularly in women with HELLP syndrome, obesity, a concerning airway assessment, or a concern for fetal status. Placement of an epidural catheter prior to labor onset may be indicated to avoid general anesthesia if urgent cesarean delivery is indicated. The choice of technique and administration of neuraxial labor analgesia to women with preeclampsia does not differ from that in healthy women (see Chapter 24). However, clinicians must assess coagulation status, ensure appropriate hydration to avoid sudden hypotension, and administer vasopressors for the treatment of hypotension judiciously.

Neuraxial Anesthesia-Induced Hypotension

The principles and management of hypotension are similar for both labor analgesia or cesarean anesthesia; however, the more rapid and complete sympathetic blockade associated with spinal and epidural anesthesia for cesarean delivery is more likely to result in hypotension than neuraxial analgesia initiated for labor. Because placental perfusion is impaired in preeclampsia, correcting blood pressure is important for maintaining fetal well-being. Clinicians should expect to maintain a higher target pressure in women with hypertensive disorders to ensure fetal well-being than in women with healthy pregnancies. The contemporary practice of labor analgesia using low concentrations of local anesthetic solutions, in combination with an opioid, results in low incidence of hypotension in patients with a hypertensive disorder. Fluid administration during the initiation of neuraxial labor analgesia may not be necessary unless the patient is judged to be hypovolemic, as this practice has little impact on the risk for hypotension.[225]

Historically, it was believed that spinal anesthesia is relatively contraindicated in women with severe preeclampsia because of the possibility of marked hypotension as a result of the rapid onset of spinal anesthesia–induced sympathetic blockade. However, this concern is not supported by evidence; multiple studies have demonstrated that the incidence of hypotension during spinal anesthesia is similar to that observed with epidural and general anesthesia; maternal outcomes may be improved with spinal anesthesia.[226-229] Berends et al.[230] randomized women with severe preeclampsia to receive either conventional epidural anesthesia or CSE anesthesia for cesarean delivery. There was no difference between groups in the incidence of hypotension.

In contrast, a randomized multicenter study comparing the hemodynamic effects of spinal anesthesia with epidural anesthesia for cesarean delivery in women with severe preeclampsia found that significantly more women in the spinal anesthesia group experienced hypotension.[231] However, the duration of hypotension was less than 1 minute in both groups and, although more ephedrine was used in the spinal group than in the epidural group, hypotension was easily treated in both groups. In addition, there was no significant difference in neonatal outcome between infants whose mothers received spinal anesthesia compared with those whose mothers received epidural anesthesia.

Treatment of hypotension Consistent with contemporary practice, vasopressors can be used as either continuous infusion or intermittent bolus administration. Available data suggest that women with severe preeclampsia require less vasopressor for treatment of blood pressure, and typical doses administered to normotensive women might result in a sharp increase in blood pressure if administered to women with preeclampsia.[232-234] As women with preeclampsia are typically tachycardic, phenylephrine (intermittent bolus of 25 to 50 μg or infusion 0.2 to 0.5 μg/kg/min) is recommended for treatment of hypotension and has a demonstrated record of safety in this population. A metaanalysis examined vasopressor use for women with preeclampsia undergoing spinal anesthesia for cesarean delivery.[235] Eight randomized studies involving 712 women were included in the analysis. The authors did not identify a difference in fetal acidosis between phenylephrine and ephedrine for prophylaxis and treatment of hypotension. Further, no difference in maternal outcomes such as nausea and vomiting, bradycardia, hypertension, or hypotension were noted. Thus, while phenylephrine is appropriate for treatment, ephedrine may be used when the maternal heart rate is below 80 to 90 beats per minute. Limited data on the use of nor-epinephrine for the prophylaxis and treatment of spinal anes-thesia-induced hypotension exists in hypertensive obstetric patients. One study found a marginally higher maternal heart rate with norepinephrine compared to phenylephrine, with no other significant differences in the mother or neonate.[236]

Medications Containing Epinephrine

Women with preeclampsia demonstrate an increased demon-strable sensitivity to vasopressors, including angiotensin II,[237,238] norepinephrine and epinephrine,[239,240] and a thrombox-ane A_2-mimetic agent.[241] Some clinicians have raised a concern of administering epinephrine as part of a local anesthetic solu-tion. Inadvertent intravenous administration of epinephrine as part of an epidural test dose poses theoretical risk of severe blood pressure response, but this scenario does not appear to have been realized clinically. In contrast, patients who have received beta-adrenergic receptor antagonists (e.g., labet-alol) may not demonstrate the tachycardic response typically observed after intravascular administration of epinephrine.[242] This lack of response decreases the sensitivity of the epineph-rine test dose. Alternative testing strategies to detect intravas-cular catheter location may be considered (see Chapter 12).[243]

The standard practice of adding epinephrine as an adjunct for epidural lidocaine anesthesia for cesarean anesthesia may have a favorable risk/benefit ratio. Epinephrine enhances the quality of epidural lidocaine anesthesia for surgery, and when administering a large dose of lidocaine, the addition of epi-nephrine likely reduces the risk of local anesthetic systemic toxicity. Only one case report described a hypertensive crisis in a woman with preeclampsia after the incremental adminis-tration of 30 mL of freshly mixed 2% lidocaine with epineph-rine 5 μg/mL for planned cesarean delivery.[244] However, the onset and duration of hypertension were atypical, and a drug error could not be excluded. In contrast, several other case series and prospective studies have used the same solution without adverse effects in women with preeclampsia.[245]

General Anesthesia for Cesarean Delivery

Neuraxial anesthesia is the preferred technique, when possi-ble, due to its benefits on hemodynamic control, pain control, and avoidance of maternal airway manipulation. The presence of preeclampsia minimally impacts the choice of local anes-thetic agent, technical aspects of neuraxial anesthesia, and the maintenance of anesthesia (see Chapter 26). Nonetheless, in some situations, general anesthesia may be the best option. The most common conditions associated with preeclampsia that may prohibit neuraxial anesthesia are severe thrombo-cytopenia and coagulopathy, severe fetal compromise due to placental abruption or reduced uteroplacental blood flow, and maternal conditions such as acute stroke with thrombolysis therapy or pulmonary edema. The safe administration of general anesthesia in women with preeclampsia requires an advanced state of readiness and careful preparation.

General anesthesia in patients with a hypertensive disor-der presents several challenges, including the hypertensive response to direct laryngoscopy and tracheal intubation and potential difficulty in securing the airway due to airway edema. The risk for intracranial hemorrhage from the hypertensive response to both tracheal intubation and extubation is high-lighted in a study involving more than 300,000 women in Taiwan.[246] Women with preeclampsia who received general anesthesia experienced a greater than twofold increase in the incidence of stroke after adjusting for confounders compared with women who received neuraxial anesthesia. In addition, the clinician must be aware of the effects of magnesium sulfate on neuromuscular transmission. A suggested technique for the administration of general anesthesia is outlined in Box 35.7.

Airway Management

In pregnant women, the internal diameter of the trachea is reduced because of mucosal capillary engorgement. These changes may be exaggerated in women with preeclampsia because of **pharyngolaryngeal edema**, which may compro-mise visualization of airway landmarks during direct laryn-goscopy.[247] The edematous tissue is easily friable and can bleed with manipulation. Signs of severe airway obstruc-tion, including dysphonia, hoarseness, snoring, stridor, and hypoxemia, are exceedingly rare.[248,249]

One observational study found that women with hyperten-sion were twice as likely to have arterial oxygen desaturation, defined as $SpO_2 < 90\%$, than women without hypertension during the induction of general anesthesia.[250] Related factors included increasing BMI, low baseline room-air oxygen satura-tion, the presence of airway edema, increasing Mallampati class, and the number of attempts required for tracheal intubation. Low room-air oxygen saturation may reflect the finding that approximately one-quarter of women with severe preeclampsia have ultrasonographic evidence of pulmonary congestion.[105]

When tracheal intubation is necessary, the procedure should be optimized to achieve success on the first attempt, given the likelihood for increasing difficulty on subsequent attempts (see Chapter 29). Thus, use of video laryngoscopy should be considered a first-line technique for tracheal intuba-tion. A small-diameter endotracheal tube should be inserted due to the expectation of tracheal edema. If tracheal intuba-tion cannot be rapidly achieved, a supraglottic airway device should be placed to facilitate oxygenation and ventilation while additional steps are taken to gain definitive control of the airway.[251] Some modern supraglottic airway devices allow the passage of a small-diameter endotracheal tube to obtain definitive airway access. In rare circumstances, an awake fiber-optic tracheal intubation or a surgical airway may be necessary.

Response to laryngoscopy The hemodynamic instabil-ity associated with rapid-sequence induction and tracheal intubation presents a serious problem in women with severe preeclampsia. The transient, but severe, hypertension that may accompany tracheal intubation can result in cerebral hemorrhage or pulmonary edema, both potentially fatal complications.[252] Invasive arterial blood pressure monitor-ing should be considered for patients with poorly controlled and severe hypertension. This allows continuous monitoring of the effects of antihypertensive drugs administered before

BOX 35.7 A Suggested Technique for Administration of General Anesthesia in Women With Preeclampsia With Severe Features

1. Place a radial arterial cannula for continuous blood pressure monitoring in women with severe hypertension.
2. Verify that smaller-sized endotracheal tubes and supraglottic airway devices are immediately available. Equipment needed for difficult airway management should also be immediately available.
3. Consider the administration of an intravenous H_2-receptor antagonist and IV metoclopramide between 30 and 60 min before induction of anesthesia.
4. Administer 0.3 M sodium citrate 30 mL PO immediately before induction of anesthesia.
5. Denitrogenate (3 min of tidal-volume breathing or eight vital capacity breaths with an F_{IO_2} of 1.0 and a tight-fitting face mask).
6. Give labetalol (10-mg bolus doses) IV to titrate systolic blood pressure between 140/90 and 160/110 mm Hg before the induction of anesthesia.
7. Continue to monitor FHR during labetalol administration.
8. Consider alternative antihypertensive agents for patients who do not respond to labetalol (or those with a contraindication to labetalol) (see Table 35.4). A remifentanil bolus (0.5 μg/kg) is an effective adjunct.
9. Perform rapid-sequence induction with propofol 2.0–2.8 mg/kg and succinylcholine 1.0–1.5 mg/kg (avoid ketamine as an induction agent given its sympathomimetic properties). For patients with severe heart failure, titrate propofol carefully or use etomidate and avoid beta-adrenergic antagonists. Consider the administration of a bolus dose of labetalol, esmolol, remifentanil, or magnesium sulfate to blunt the hemodynamic response to laryngoscopy.
10. Maintain anesthesia with a volatile halogenated agent and 40%–50% oxygen as required, together with 50%–60% nitrous oxide, before delivery. After delivery, decrease the concentration of the volatile halogenated agent to prevent uterine atony, and administer an opioid. Consider administering a propofol infusion and/or a benzodiazepine if there is concern for awareness and recall.
11. Avoid giving additional muscle relaxants; if absolutely required, administer a small repeat dose of succinylcholine with a small dose of anticholinergic agent, or a *low dose* of a short-acting nondepolarizing muscle relaxant because of the exaggerated effect of this class of drug when coadministered with magnesium sulfate.
12. At the end of surgery, reverse neuromuscular blockade if appropriate and consider the administration of labetalol 5–10 mg IV bolus, titrated to effect, to prevent hypertension during emergence and tracheal extubation.

FHR, Fetal heart rate; *IV,* intravenously; *PO,* per os.
Modified from Ramanathan J, Bennett K. Pre-eclampsia: fluids, drugs, and anesthetic management. *Anesthesiol Clin North Am.* 2003;21:145–163.

and after tracheal intubation and facilitates rapid detection of adverse hemodynamic responses to laryngoscopy. The goal of treatment is to reduce the arterial blood pressure to less than 160/110 mm Hg before the induction of general anesthesia and to maintain the systolic blood pressure between 140 and 160 mm Hg and the diastolic blood pressure between 90 and 100 mm Hg throughout laryngoscopy and tracheal intubation.[7]

Several medications have been recommended to blunt the hemodynamic response during general anesthesia, including remifentanil, sodium nitroprusside, nitroglycerin, hydralazine, and magnesium sulfate; each has limitations.[253,254] A network metaanalysis of 12 studies found that high-dose remifentanil (1.0 to 1.25 μg/kg and continuous infusion at a rate of 0.5 μg/kg/min, administered 3 minutes prior to tracheal intubation) ranked highest in blunting the hypertensive response to intubation in hypertensive parturients.[253] Nitroglycerin and labetalol were similarly effective in blunting mean arterial pressure, but labetalol was the most effective medication for control of heart rate.

The short-acting opioid, **remifentanil**, is rapidly metabolized by both the mother and neonate by nonspecific blood and tissue esterases and has been administered to women with preeclampsia to prevent the hypertensive response to tracheal intubation.[255] An advantage of remifentanil compared with other opioids is the short duration of action of the drug; the limited duration of action should not interfere with the resumption of spontaneous ventilation if tracheal intubation is unsuccessful. Remifentanil may be associated with low initial Apgar scores and respiratory depression in the neonate.[255,256]

Ramanathan et al. **esmolol**[257] compared **labetalol** (initial 20-mg dose followed by 10-mg increments to a total of 1 mg/kg) with no treatment in a randomized study of women with preeclampsia who received general anesthesia for cesarean delivery. Labetalol blunted, but did not prevent, the hypertensive response after tracheal intubation, and it prevented the tachycardia that occurred in the control group. Labetalol can be administered using either a bolus technique or a continuous intravenous infusion, or both.[174]

There is also evidence for the safe, short-term administration of **esmolol** in this setting. A randomized, double-blind study of 80 women with hypertension presenting for cesarean delivery demonstrated that intravenous esmolol—carefully titrated to doses as high as 2 mg/kg—can be safely used to dampen the hemodynamic response to laryngoscopy and tracheal intubation, particularly if hypertension and tachycardia are present.[252] Maternal beta-adrenergic receptor blockade may be associated with fetal bradycardia or hypoglycemia.[174] Esmolol has been associated with fetal bradycardia, at least when administered by infusion.**nebulized lidocaine**[256]

Intravenous lidocaine has been shown to reduce the response to intubation,[252] as has **nebulized lidocaine** prior to intubation.[256]

A bolus dose of **magnesium sulfate** 30 to 40 mg/kg administered immediately after the induction agent, with or without alfentanil, has been found to suppress maternal catecholamine release and effectively obtund the hypertensive response to tracheal intubation in women with preeclampsia.[259–262] Adverse maternal or neonatal effects attributable to bolus magnesium were not observed, although caution is advised in women with renal insufficiency and those already receiving this medication. Magnesium sulfate may interact with neuromuscular blocking drugs (see later discussion).

Sodium nitroprusside and nitroglycerin have been used but are more difficult to titrate and are associated with tachycardia. The former can cause precipitous hypotension in the volume-depleted patient, and the hemodynamic effects of the latter are also dependent on intravascular volume.

Effects of Magnesium Sulfate

Most women with severe preeclampsia will present to the labor or operating room while receiving magnesium sulfate for seizure prophylaxis. Magnesium sulfate, when appropriately administered, is a safe drug, but systems should be in place to avoid inadvertent infusion of large boluses of the drug. The magnesium infusion should continue throughout surgery to minimize the risk for eclampsia.[2]

Even though succinylcholine mimics acetylcholine at the nerve terminal, the onset and duration of a single intubating dose are not clinically prolonged when administered concurrently with a magnesium sulfate infusion[263]; a routine intubating dose of 1 to 1.5 mg/kg should be used during rapid-sequence induction of general anesthesia.

Magnesium sulfate can also interact with nondepolarizing muscle relaxants by inhibiting the presynaptic release of acetylcholine at the neuromuscular junction, decreasing the sensitivity of the postsynaptic receptor to acetylcholine, and depressing the excitability of the muscle fiber membrane. Magnesium sulfate increases the potency and duration of vecuronium, rocuronium, and mivacurium.[264–266] Several case reports have described a requirement for overnight mechanical ventilation after administration of routine doses of vecuronium in women receiving magnesium sulfate.[267] For this reason, many practitioners avoid the use of nondepolarizing neuromuscular blocking agents in women with preeclampsia.

Airway management guidelines discuss the use of sugammadex for the reversal of neuromuscular blockade when rocuronium has been used for rapid-sequence induction. Studies in nonpregnant populations showed that peri-induction administration of magnesium sulfate 40 to 60 mg/kg did not delay reversal of neuromuscular blockade with sugammadex.[268,269] No cases of recurarization were observed. Although these studies did not address the patient with preeclampsia who is receiving magnesium, several case reports of magnesium use in women with severe preeclampsia support the assertion that magnesium does not influence reversal with sugammadex.[270]

Although some reports have suggested that coadministration of a calcium entry–blocking agent and magnesium may cause hypotension and/or neuromuscular blockade,[176–178,271] more recent information suggests that these medications can be used safely together.[178] Although magnesium sulfate has been used for tocolysis, it is relatively ineffective, and postpartum uterine tone is unlikely to be altered.[272]

Anesthetic Considerations in Eclampsia

The anesthetic management of a woman with eclampsia is similar to that of a patient with preeclampsia with severe features. Eclampsia, *per se*, is not an indication for urgent or emergency delivery. The FHR during and shortly after a seizure will be depressed, but usually recovers with time and adequate maternal oxygenation. Considerations[273,274] specific to the woman with eclampsia are as follows:

1. **Assessment of seizure control and neurologic function**. The possibility of increased intracranial pressure is not a cause for concern if the patient remains conscious, alert, and free of seizures. Persistent coma and localizing signs may indicate a major intracranial pathologic process or PRES that may affect anesthetic management.
2. **Maintenance of fluid balance**. Intake should be restricted to 1 mL/kg/h to minimize the risk of exacerbating cerebral and pulmonary edema.
3. **Continuous pulse oximetry monitoring of maternal oxygen saturation**.

The anesthetic plan is tailored to each individual case. In stable eclamptic women (fully conscious, no recent seizures, treated with magnesium sulfate, and no organ failure), neuraxial analgesia/anesthesia can be considered. In a retrospective review of 66 South African women with stable eclampsia, Moodley et al.[275] found no difference in maternal and neonatal outcomes in women who received epidural anesthesia compared with general anesthesia for cesarean delivery. Another series describing spinal anesthesia in 12 stable eclamptic women reported only one episode of hypotension and no major complications.[276]

Most women with eclampsia are suspected of having elevated intracranial pressure.[115] Intravenous induction agents such as propofol and thiopental will reduce the cerebral metabolic rate and cerebral blood flow, with a consequent decrease in cerebral blood volume and intracranial pressure.[277] These agents are also effective in terminating seizures.[278] Because hyperventilation reduces cerebral blood flow without a reduction in cerebral metabolic rate, it should be employed with caution. Conversely, hypoventilation should be avoided because hypercarbia can lower the seizure threshold. Blood pressure should be managed to maintain cerebral perfusion pressure (the difference between mean arterial pressure and intracranial pressure). Avoidance of hypoxemia, hyperthermia, and hyperglycemia is also important in avoiding an exacerbation of neurologic injury.[279] Mechanical ventilation should be continued after cesarean delivery in patients who have not recovered neurologically, and these patients should be monitored in an intensive care unit. Sedation during ventilation should include a sedative with anticonvulsant activity. Although benzodiazepine infusions have often been used in this setting, recent evidence in the nonobstetric population suggests that nonbenzodiazepine options are associated with less drug accumulation, a shorter period of mechanical ventilation, and shorter hospital stay.[280] An infusion of propofol supplemented with judicious doses of an opioid is an acceptable alternative, carefully titrated to maintain adequate cerebral perfusion pressure in view of cerebral edema. If unconsciousness persists after discontinuation of sedation, further neurologic evaluation with electroencephalography and brain imaging to rule out persistent seizures and/or other underlying neurologic disorders should be performed.

POSTPARTUM MANAGEMENT

Care of the obstetric patient with a hypertensive disorder does not end with the delivery of the neonate. The patient must be observed carefully to ensure that her condition is resolving. The anesthetic considerations include providing postoperative analgesia, avoiding complications, and assessment and treatment of complications.

Provision of postoperative analgesia is similar to that in the patient with an uncomplicated pregnancy and includes acetaminophen (paracetamol), nonsteroidal antiinflammatory drugs (NSAIDs), oral or intravenous opioids, neuraxial opioids (single injection), and continuous epidural infusion of analgesic agents. Many anesthesia providers prefer neuraxial opioid administration for postcesarean analgesia (see Chapter 27). NSAIDs should be avoided in women who have evidence of acute renal insufficiency, as these medications constrict the afferent glomerular arterioles in a setting where the efferent arterioles are already constricted. In the past, the ACOG has suggested that NSAIDs be replaced by alternative analgesics if hypertension persists beyond the first postpartum day, as these drugs might contribute to hypertension.[7] However, this recommendation was based on data from elderly hypertensive patients on chronic NSAID therapy; more recent data have called this recommendation into question in the hypertensive parturient, and current ACOG guidelines do not suggest withholding NSAID therapy in this population.[2] Regardless of the postoperative analgesic technique, all women should be carefully monitored for signs of respiratory depression, pulmonary edema, and further progression of the disease.

LONG-TERM OUTCOMES

Women who experience a hypertensive disorder of pregnancy are at increased risk for diabetes, obesity, and several cardiovascular diseases, including ischemic heart disease, renal failure, stroke, and diabetes, later in life.[281,282] These women are prone to earlier onset of cardiovascular disease than women with healthy pregnancies.[283,284] As expected, women with more severe hypertensive disease during pregnancy are at greater future risk. One systematic review, including almost 29 million patients in 84 studies, found that the odds ratio of cardiovascular disease was 1.7 (95% intrinsic CI, 1.3 to 2.2) in women with a history of gestational hypertension, and 2.7 (95% intrinsic CI, 2.5 to 3.0) in women with a history of preeclampsia.[285] Women with preeclampsia in both their first and second pregnancies are at even greater risk for future ischemic heart disease.[284]

The mechanism of increased risk for cardiovascular disease in women with a history of preeclampsia is unclear. It is possible that preeclampsia causes permanent damage to the endothelium and hastens the onset of cardiovascular disease. Women with a history of preeclampsia have persistent impairment of brachial artery endothelium-dependent vascular relaxation at 1 to 3 years after delivery compared with healthy control women, and they also have persistent moderate to severe abnormalities of left ventricular function as demonstrated using echocardiography 1 year postpartum.[85,286,287] Alternately, preeclampsia may be a cardiovascular risk marker in women with an underlying predisposition to vascular disease; the hemodynamic and metabolic stress of pregnancy causes the predisposition to manifest as preeclampsia. After pregnancy, women return to a normal state until the threshold for disease development is exceeded in later life.

The experience of severe preeclampsia (particularly with early-onset disease and preterm delivery) reflects a serious complication that threatens the mother's life and the life of her child. In one study, approximately one-fourth of women developed posttraumatic stress disorder (PTSD) after early-onset preeclampsia.[288] This association may be mediated by the condition of the offspring after preterm delivery.[289-291] Further research is required to characterize women at risk for PTSD and to investigate strategies for PTSD prevention and intervention.

KEY POINTS

- The hypertensive disorders of pregnancy are a spectrum of conditions that increase maternal and fetal risk.
- The hypertensive disorders of pregnancy include chronic hypertension, gestational hypertension, preeclampsia, and chronic hypertension with superimposed preeclampsia and eclampsia. White coat hypertension and masked hypertension are additional categories of hypertension during pregnancy.
- Preeclampsia is associated with severe maternal and fetal manifestations.
- Eclampsia, or hypertension-associated seizures, is one of the more dangerous forms of preeclampsia.
- The three most common organs affected by preeclampsia are the brain, kidney, and liver.

- HELLP syndrome (hemolysis, elevated liver enzymes, low platelets) is a severe form of preeclampsia.
- Severely elevated blood pressure ($\geq 160/110$ mm Hg) should be treated urgently with labetalol, hydralazine, or nifedipine as first-line antihypertensive agents.
- Neuraxial analgesia/anesthesia is preferred for labor and vaginal or cesarean delivery and can be safely used in patients with hypertensive disorders in the absence of contraindications.
- When performing general anesthesia, anesthesia providers must be aware of the potential for airway edema and an exaggerated hypertensive response to tracheal intubation and extubation.
- Preeclampsia is associated with a future risk of cardiovascular disease.

REFERENCES

1. Wang W, Xie X, Yuan T, et al. Epidemiological trends of maternal hypertensive disorders of pregnancy at the global, regional, and national levels: a population-based study. *BMC Pregn Childb*. 2021;21:364.

2. American College of Obstetricians and Gynecologists. Practice Bulletin, Number 222: Gestational hypertension and preeclampsia (reaffirmed 2023). *Obstet Gynecol*. 2020;135:e237–e260.

3. Stevens W, Shih T, Incerti D, et al. Short-term costs of preeclampsia to the United States health care system. *Am J Obstet Gynecol*. 2017;217:237–248.e16.

4. Magee LA, Brown MA, Hall DR, et al. The 2021 International Society for the Study of Hypertension in Pregnancy classification, diagnosis & management recommendations for international practice. *Pregnancy Hypertens*. 2022;27:148–169.

5. Hofmeyr R, Matjila M, Dyer R. Preeclampsia in 2017: obstetric and anaesthesia management. *Best Pract Res Clin Anaesthesiol*. 2017;31:125–138.

6. Bernstein PS, Martin JN Jr, Barton JR, et al. National Partnership for Maternal Safety: consensus bundle on severe hypertension during pregnancy and the postpartum period. *Obstet Gynecol*. 2017;130:347–357.

7. American College of Obstetricians and Gynecologists. Hypertension in pregnancy. Report of the American College of Obstetricians and Gynecologists' Task Force on Hypertension in Pregnancy. *Obstet Gynecol*. 2013;122:1122–1131.

8. Rodrigues A, Barata C, Marques I, Almeida MC. Diagnosis of white coat hypertension and pregnancy outcomes. *Pregnancy Hypertens*. 2018;14:121–124.

9. Bramham K, Parnell B, Nelson-Piercy C, et al. Chronic hypertension and pregnancy outcomes: systematic review and meta-analysis. *BMJ*. 2014;348:g2301.

10. Giannubilo SR, Dell'Uomo B, Tranquilli AL. Perinatal outcomes, blood pressure patterns and risk assessment of superimposed preeclampsia in mild chronic hypertensive pregnancy. *Eur J Obstet Gynecol Reprod Biol*. 2006;126:63–67.

11. Ford ND, Cox S, Ko JY, et al. Hypertensive disorders in pregnancy and mortality at delivery hospitalization—United States, 2017-2019. *Morb Mortal Wkly Rep*. 2022;71:585–591.

12. Abalos E, Cuesta C, Grosso AL, et al. Global and regional estimates of preeclampsia and eclampsia: a systematic review. *Eur J Obstet Gynecol Reprod Biol*. 2013;170:1–7.

13. Redman CW. Hypertension in pregnancy: the NICE guidelines. *Heart*. 2011;97:1967–1969.

14. Minhas AS, Ogunwole SM, Vaught AJ, et al. Racial disparities in cardiovascular complications with pregnancy-induced hypertension in the United States. *Hypertension*. 2021;78:480–488.

15. Breathett K, Muhlestein D, Foraker R, Gulati M. Differences in preeclampsia rates between African American and Caucasian women: trends from the National Hospital Discharge Survey. *J Womens Health (Larchmt)*. 2014;23:886–893.

16. Esakoff TF, Rad S, Burwick RM, Caughey AB. Predictors of eclampsia in California. *J Matern Fetal Neonatal Med*. 2016;29:1531–1535.

17. Mogren I, Hogberg U, Winkvist A, Stenlund H. Familial occurrence of preeclampsia. *Epidemiology*. 1999;10:518–522.

18. Esplin MS, Fausett MB, Fraser A, et al. Paternal and maternal components of the predisposition to preeclampsia. *N Engl J Med*. 2001;344:867–872.

19. Cnattingius S, Reilly M, Pawitan Y, Lichtenstein P. Maternal and fetal genetic factors account for most of familial aggregation of preeclampsia: a population-based Swedish cohort study. *Am J Med Genet A*. 2004;130A:365–371.

20. Lie RT, Rasmussen S, Brunborg H, et al. Fetal and maternal contributions to risk of pre-eclampsia: population based study. *BMJ*. 1998;316:1343–1347.

21. van Oostwaard MF, Langenveld J, Schuit E, et al. Recurrence of hypertensive disorders of pregnancy: an individual patient data metaanalysis. *Am J Obstet Gynecol*. 2015;212:624.e1–e17.

22. Klungsoyr K, Morken NH, Irgens L, et al. Secular trends in the epidemiology of pre-eclampsia throughout 40 years in Norway: prevalence, risk factors and perinatal survival. *Paediatr Perinat Epidemiol*. 2012;26:190–198.

23. Ananth CV, Peltier MR, Chavez MR, et al. Recurrence of ischemic placental disease. *Obstet Gynecol*. 2007;110:128–133.

24. Wikstrom AK, Stephansson O, Cnattingius S. Previous preeclampsia and risks of adverse outcomes in subsequent nonpreeclamptic pregnancies. *Am J Obstet Gynecol*. 2011;204:148.e1–e6.

25. McGinnis R, Steinthorsdottir V, Williams NO, et al. Variants in the fetal genome near FLT1 are associated with risk of preeclampsia. *Nat Genet*. 2017;49:1255–1260.

26. Fong FM, Sahemey MK, Hamedi G, et al. Maternal genotype and severe preeclampsia: a HuGE review. *Am J Epidemiol*. 2014;180:335–345.

27. Aguilar M, Bhuket T, Torres S, et al. Prevalence of the metabolic syndrome in the United States, 2003-2012. *JAMA*. 2015;313:1973–1974.

28. O'Brien TE, Ray JG, Chan WS. Maternal body mass index and the risk of preeclampsia: a systematic overview. *Epidemiology*. 2003;14:368–374.

29. England LJ, Levine RJ, Qian C, et al. Smoking before pregnancy and risk of gestational hypertension and preeclampsia. *Am J Epidemiol*. 2002;186:1035–1040.

30. Conde-Agudelo A, Althabe F, Belizan JM, Kafury-Goeta AC. Cigarette smoking during pregnancy and risk of preeclampsia: a systematic review. *Am J Epidemiol*. 1999;181:1026–1035.

31. Mimura K, Tomimatsu T, Sharentuya N, et al. Nicotine restores endothelial dysfunction caused by excess sFlt1 and sEng in an in vitro model of preeclamptic vascular endothelium: a possible therapeutic role of nicotinic acetylcholine receptor (nAChR) agonists for preeclampsia. *Am J Epidemiol*. 2010;202:464.e1–e6.

32. Davenport MH, Ruchat SM, Poitras VJ, et al. Prenatal exercise for the prevention of gestational diabetes mellitus and hypertensive disorders of pregnancy: a systematic review and meta-analysis. *Br J Sports Med*. 2018;52:1367–1375.

33. Magro-Malosso ER, Saccone G, Di Tommaso M, et al. Exercise during pregnancy and risk of gestational hypertensive disorders: a systematic review and meta-analysis. *Acta Obstet Gynecol Scand*. 2017;96:921–931.

34. Skjaerven R, Wilcox AJ, Lie RT. The interval between pregnancies and the risk of preeclampsia. *N Engl J Med*. 2002;346:33–38.

35. Bdolah Y, Lam C, Rajakumar A, et al. Twin pregnancy and the risk of preeclampsia: bigger placenta or relative ischemia? *Am J Obstet Gynecol*. 2008;198:428.e1–e6.

36. Koga K, Osuga Y, Tajima T, et al. Elevated serum soluble fms-like tyrosine kinase 1 (sFlt1) level in women with hydatidiform mole. *Fertil Steril.* 2010;94:305–308.

37. Masoudian P, Nasr A, de Nanassy J, et al. Oocyte donation pregnancies and the risk of preeclampsia or gestational hypertension: a systematic review and metaanalysis. *Am J Obstet Gynecol.* 2016;214:328–339.

38. Powe CE, Levine RJ, Karumanchi SA. Preeclampsia, a disease of the maternal endothelium: the role of antiangiogenic factors and implications for later cardiovascular disease. *Circulation.* 2011;123:2856–2869.

39. Brosens I, Robertson WB, Dixon HG. The physiological response of the vessels of the placental bed to normal pregnancy. *J Pathol Bacteriol.* 1967;93:569–579.

40. Keogh RJ, Harris LK, Freeman A, et al. Fetal-derived trophoblast use the apoptotic cytokine tumor necrosis factor-alpha-related apoptosis-inducing ligand to induce smooth muscle cell death. *Circ Res.* 2007;100:834–841.

41. Brosens IA, Robertson WB, Dixon HG. The role of the spiral arteries in the pathogenesis of preeclampsia. *Obstet Gynecol Annu.* 1972;1:177–191.

42. Meekins JW, Pijnenborg R, Hanssens M, et al. A study of placental bed spiral arteries and trophoblast invasion in normal and severe pre-eclamptic pregnancies. *Br J Obstet Gynaecol.* 1994;101:669–674.

43. Salomon C, Guanzon D, Scholz-Romero K, et al. Placental exosomes as early biomarker of preeclampsia: potential role of exosomal microRNAs across gestation. *J Clin Endocrinol Metab.* 2017;102:3182–3194.

44. Murugesan S, Hussey H, Saravanakumar L, et al. Extracellular vesicles from women with severe preeclampsia impair vascular endothelial function. *Anesth Analg.* 2022;134:713–723.

45. Nagamatsu T, Fujii T, Kusumi M, et al. Cytotrophoblasts up-regulate soluble fms-like tyrosine kinase-1 expression under reduced oxygen: an implication for the placental vascular development and the pathophysiology of preeclampsia. *Endocrinology.* 2004;145:4838–4845.

46. Steegers EA, von Dadelszen P, Duvekot JJ, Pijnenborg R. Pre-eclampsia. *Lancet.* 2010;376:631–644.

47. Maynard SE, Min JY, Merchan J, et al. Excess placental soluble fms-like tyrosine kinase 1 (sFlt1) may contribute to endothelial dysfunction, hypertension, and proteinuria in preeclampsia. *J Clin Invest.* 2003;111:649–658.

48. Venkatesha S, Toporsian M, Lam C, et al. Soluble endoglin contributes to the pathogenesis of preeclampsia. *Nat Med.* 2006;12:642–649.

49. Levine RJ, Maynard SE, Qian C, et al. Circulating angiogenic factors and the risk of preeclampsia. *N Engl J Med.* 2004;350:672–683.

50. Luttun A, Carmeliet P. Soluble VEGF receptor Flt1: the elusive preeclampsia factor discovered? *J Clin Invest.* 2003;111:600–602.

51. Cerdeira AS, O'Sullivan J, Ohuma EO, et al. Randomized interventional study on prediction of preeclampsia/eclampsia in women with suspected preeclampsia: INSPIRE. *Hypertension.* 2019;74:983–990.

52. Lim S, Li W, Kemper J, et al. Biomarkers and the prediction of adverse outcomes in preeclampsia: a systematic review and meta-analysis. *Obstet Gynecol.* 2021;137:72–81.

53. Lopes Perdigao J, Chinthala S, Mueller A, et al. Angiogenic factor estimation as a warning sign of preeclampsia-related peripartum morbidity among hospitalized patients. *Hypertension.* 2019;73:868–877.

54. Young BC, Levine RJ, Karumanchi SA. Pathogenesis of preeclampsia. *Annu Rev Pathol.* 2010;5:173–192.

55. Lockwood CJ, Matta P, Krikun G, et al. Regulation of monocyte chemoattractant protein-1 expression by tumor necrosis factor-alpha and interleukin-1beta in first trimester human decidual cells: implications for preeclampsia. *Am J Pathol.* 2006;168:445–452.

56. Hiby SE, Walker JJ, O'Shaughnessy KM, et al. Combinations of maternal KIR and fetal HLA-C genes influence the risk of preeclampsia and reproductive success. *J Exp Med.* 2004;200:957–965.

57. Nakimuli A, Chazara O, Hiby SE, et al. A KIR B centromeric region present in Africans but not Europeans protects pregnant women from pre-eclampsia. *Proc Natl Acad Sci USA.* 2015;112:845–850.

58. Gardiner C, Vatish M. Impact of haemostatic mechanisms on pathophysiology of preeclampsia. *Thromb Res.* 2017;151:S48–S52.

59. Wallukat G, Homuth V, Fischer T, et al. Patients with preeclampsia develop agonistic autoantibodies against the angiotensin AT1 receptor. *J Clin Invest.* 1999;103:945–952.

60. Walther T, Wallukat G, Jank A, et al. Angiotensin II type 1 receptor agonistic antibodies reflect fundamental alterations in the uteroplacental vasculature. *Hypertension.* 2005;46:1275–1279.

61. Dechend R, Homuth V, Wallukat G, et al. AT(1) receptor agonistic antibodies from preeclamptic patients cause vascular cells to express tissue factor. *Circulation.* 2000;101:2382–2387.

62. Xia Y, Wen H, Bobst S, et al. Maternal autoantibodies from preeclamptic patients activate angiotensin receptors on human trophoblast cells. *J Soc Gynecol Investig.* 2003;10:82–93.

63. Dechend R, Viedt C, Muller DN, et al. AT1 receptor agonistic antibodies from preeclamptic patients stimulate NADPH oxidase. *Circulation.* 2003;107:1632–1639.

64. Zhou CC, Zhang Y, Irani RA, et al. Angiotensin receptor agonistic autoantibodies induce pre-eclampsia in pregnant mice. *Nat Med.* 2008;14:855–862.

65. Umo-Etuk J, Lumley J, Holdcroft A. Critically ill parturient women and admission to intensive care: a 5-year review. *Int J Obstet Anesth.* 1996;5:79–84.

66. Small MJ, James AH, Kershaw T, et al. Near-miss maternal mortality: cardiac dysfunction as the principal cause of obstetric intensive care unit admissions. *Obstet Gynecol.* 2012;119:250–255.

67. Basso O, Rasmussen S, Weinberg CR, et al. Trends in fetal and infant survival following preeclampsia. *JAMA.* 2006;296:1357–1362.

68. Lee SK, McMillan DD, Ohlsson A, et al. Variations in practice and outcomes in the Canadian NICU Network: 1996-1997. *Pediatrics.* 2000;106:1070–1079.

69. Matthys LA, Coppage KH, Lambers DS, et al. Delayed postpartum preeclampsia: an experience of 151 cases. *Am J Obstet Gynecol.* 2004;190:1464–1466.

70. Mol BWJ, Roberts CT, Thangaratinam S, et al. Pre-eclampsia. *Lancet.* 2016;387:999–1011.

71. Reiss RE, O'Shaughnessy RW, Quilligan TJ, Zuspan FP. Retrospective comparison of blood pressure course during preeclamptic and matched control pregnancies. *Am J Obstet Gynecol.* 1987;156:894–898.

72. Malberg H, Bauernschmitt R, Voss A, et al. Analysis of cardiovascular oscillations: a new approach to the early prediction of pre-eclampsia. *Chaos*. 2007;17:015113.

73. Visser W, Wallenburg HC. Central hemodynamic observations in untreated preeclamptic patients. *Hypertension*. 1991;17:1072–1077.

74. Hibbard JU, Korcarz CE, Nendaz GG, et al. The arterial system in pre-eclampsia and chronic hypertension with superimposed pre-eclampsia. *BJOG*. 2005;112:897–903.

75. Hibbard JU, Shroff SG, Lang RM. Cardiovascular changes in preeclampsia. *Semin Nephrol*. 2004;24:580–587.

76. Easterling TR, Benedetti TJ. Preeclampsia: a hyperdynamic disease model. *Am J Obstet Gynecol*. 1989;160:1447–1453.

77. Dennis AT. Transthoracic echocardiography in women with preeclampsia. *Curr Opin Anaesthesiol*. 2015;28:254–260.

78. Dennis AT, Castro J, Carr C, et al. Haemodynamics in women with untreated pre-eclampsia. *Anaesthesia*. 2012;67:1105–1118.

79. Dennis AT, Dyer RA, Gibbs M, et al. Transthoracic echocardiographic assessment of haemodynamics in severe pre-eclampsia and HIV in South Africa. *Anaesthesia*. 2015;70:1028–1038.

80. Cotton DB, Lee W, Huhta JC, Dorman KF. Hemodynamic profile of severe pregnancy-induced hypertension. *Am J Obstet Gynecol*. 1988;158:523–529.

81. Mabie WC, Ratts TE, Sibai BM. The central hemodynamics of severe preeclampsia. *Am J Obstet Gynecol*. 1989;161:1443–1448.

82. Valensise H, Vasapollo B, Gagliardi G, Novelli GP. Early and late preeclampsia: two different maternal hemodynamic states in the latent phase of the disease. *Hypertension*. 2008;52:873–880.

83. Chen SSM, Leeton L, Castro JM, Dennis AT. Myocardial tissue characterisation and detection of myocardial oedema by cardiovascular magnetic resonance in women with pre-eclampsia: a pilot study. *Int J Obstet Anesth*. 2018;36:56–65.

84. Shahul S, Rhee J, Hacker MR, et al. Subclinical left ventricular dysfunction in preeclamptic women with preserved left ventricular ejection fraction: a 2D speckle-tracking imaging study. *Circ Cardiovasc Imaging*. 2012;5:734–739.

85. Melchiorre K, Sharma R, Thilaganathan B. Cardiovascular implications in preeclampsia: an overview. *Circulation*. 2014;130:703–714.

86. Desai DK, Moodley J, Naidoo DP, Bhorat I. Cardiac abnormalities in pulmonary oedema associated with hypertensive crises in pregnancy. *Br J Obstet Gynaecol*. 1996;103:523–528.

87. Patten IS, Rana S, Shahul S, et al. Cardiac angiogenic imbalance leads to peripartum cardiomyopathy. *Nature*. 2012;485:333–338.

88. Gammill HS, Chettier R, Brewer A, et al. Cardiomyopathy and preeclampsia. *Circulation*. 2018;138:2359–2366.

89. Sheppard R, Hsich E, Damp J, et al. GNB3 C825T polymorphism and myocardial recovery in peripartum cardiomyopathy: results of the Multicenter Investigations of Pregnancy-Associated Cardiomyopathy Study. *Circ Heart Fail*. 2016;9:e002683.

90. Damp J, Givertz MM, Semigran M, et al. Relaxin-2 and soluble Flt1 levels in peripartum cardiomyopathy: results of the multicenter IPAC study. *JACC Heart Fail*. 2016;4:380–388.

91. Brown MA, Zammit VC, Mitar DM. Extracellular fluid volumes in pregnancy-induced hypertension. *J Hypertens*. 1992;10:61–68.

92. Sibai BM, Anderson GD, Spinnato JA, Shaver DC. Plasma volume findings in patients with mild pregnancy-induced hypertension. *Am J Obstet Gynecol*. 1983;147:16–19.

93. Li YH, Novikova N. Pulmonary artery flow catheters for directing management in pre-eclampsia. *Cochrane Database Syst Rev*. 2012;(6):CD008882.

94. American Society of Anesthesiologists Task Force on Pulmonary Artery Catheterization. Practice guidelines for pulmonary artery catheterization. *Anesthesiology*. 2003;99:988–1014.

95. Chestnut DH, Lumb PD, Jelovsek F, Killam AP. Nonbacterial thrombotic endocarditis associated with severe preeclampsia and pulmonary artery catheterization. A case report. *J Reprod Med*. 1985;30:497–500.

96. Botker MT, Vang ML, Grofte T, et al. Implementing point-of-care ultrasonography of the heart and lungs in an anesthesia department. *Acta Anaesthesiol Scand*. 2017;61:156–165.

97. Brun C, Zieleskiewicz L, Textoris J, et al. Prediction of fluid responsiveness in severe preeclamptic patients with oliguria. *Intensive Care Med*. 2013;39:593–600.

98. Sibai BM, Mabie BC, Harvey CJ, Gonzalez AR. Pulmonary edema in severe preeclampsia-eclampsia: analysis of thirty-seven consecutive cases. *Am J Obstet Gynecol*. 1987;156:1174–1179.

99. Dildy GA 3rd, Cotton DB. Management of severe preeclampsia and eclampsia. *Crit Care Clin*. 1991;7:829–850.

100. Benedetti TJ, Kates R, Williams V. Hemodynamic observations in severe preeclampsia complicated by pulmonary edema. *Am J Obstet Gynecol*. 1985;152:330–334.

101. Dennis AT, Solnordal CB. Acute pulmonary oedema in pregnant women. *Anaesthesia*. 2012;67:646–659.

102. Zinaman M, Rubin J, Lindheimer MD. Serial plasma oncotic pressure levels and echoencephalography during and after delivery in severe pre-eclampsia. *Lancet*. 1985;1:1245–1247.

103. Benedetti TJ, Carlson RW. Studies of colloid osmotic pressure in pregnancy-induced hypertension. *Am J Obstet Gynecol*. 1979;135:308–311.

104. Pachtman Shetty SL, Koenig S, Tenenbaum S, Meirowitz N. Point-of-care lung ultrasound patterns in late third-trimester gravidas with and without preeclampsia. *Am J Obstet Gynecol MFM*. 2021;3:100310.

105. Zieleskiewicz L, Contargyris C, Brun C, et al. Lung ultrasound predicts interstitial syndrome and hemodynamic profile in parturients with severe preeclampsia. *Anesthesiology*. 2014;120:906–914.

106. Ambrozic J, Brzan Simenc G, Prokselj K, et al. Lung and cardiac ultrasound for hemodynamic monitoring of patients with severe pre-eclampsia. *Ultrasound Obstet Gynecol*. 2017;49:104–109.

107. Xu T, Feng Y, Peng H, et al. Obstructive sleep apnea and the risk of perinatal outcomes: a meta-analysis of cohort studies. *Sci Rep*. 2014;4:6982.

108. Dominguez JE, Habib AS, Krystal AD. A review of the associations between obstructive sleep apnea and hypertensive disorders of pregnancy and possible mechanisms of disease. *Sleep Med Rev*. 2018;42:37–46.

109. Mhyre JM, Riesner MN, Polley LS, Naughton NN. A series of anesthesia-related maternal deaths in Michigan, 1985-2003. *Anesthesiology*. 2007;106:1096–1104.

110. Roos NM, Wiegman MJ, Jansonius NM, Zeeman GG. Visual disturbances in (pre)eclampsia. *Obstet Gynecol Surv*. 2012;67:242–250.

111. Zeeman GG. Neurologic complications of pre-eclampsia. *Semin Perinatol.* 2009;33:166–172.

112. Belfort MA, Varner MW, Dizon-Townson DS, et al. Cerebral perfusion pressure, and not cerebral blood flow, may be the critical determinant of intracranial injury in preeclampsia: a new hypothesis. *Am J Obstet Gynecol.* 2002;187:626–634.

113. Liman TG, Bohner G, Heuschmann PU, et al. Clinical and radiological differences in posterior reversible encephalopathy syndrome between patients with preeclampsia-eclampsia and other predisposing diseases. *Eur J Neurol.* 2012;19:935–943.

114. Wagner SJ, Acquah LA, Lindell EP, et al. Posterior reversible encephalopathy syndrome and eclampsia: pressing the case for more aggressive blood pressure control. *Mayo Clin Proc.* 2011;86:851–856.

115. Brewer J, Owens MY, Wallace K, et al. Posterior reversible encephalopathy syndrome in 46 of 47 patients with eclampsia. *Am J Obstet Gynecol.* 2013;208:468.e1–e6.

116. Ciampa E, Li Y, Dillon S, et al. Cerebrospinal fluid protein changes in preeclampsia. *Hypertension.* 2018;72:219–226.

117. Dubost C, Le Gouez A, Jouffroy V, et al. Optic nerve sheath diameter used as ultrasonographic assessment of the incidence of raised intracranial pressure in preeclampsia: a pilot study. *Anesthesiology.* 2012;116:1066–1071.

118. Guerci P, Vial F, Feugeas J, et al. Cerebral oximetry assessed by near-infrared spectrometry during preeclampsia: an observational study: impact of magnesium sulfate administration. *Crit Care Med.* 2014;42:2379–2386.

119. Liu S, Chan W, Ray JG, et al. Stroke and cerebrovascular disease in pregnancy: incidence, temporal trends, and risk factors. *Stroke.* 2019;50:8.

120. Miller EC, Gatollari HJ, Too G, et al. Risk factors for pregnancy-associated stroke in women with preeclampsia. *Stroke.* 2017;48:1752–1759.

121. Ijas P. Trends in the incidence and risk factors of pregnancy-associated stroke. *Front Neurol.* 2022;13:833215.

122. Zeeman GG, Fleckenstein JL, Twickler DM, Cunningham FG. Cerebral infarction in eclampsia. *Am J Obstet Gynecol.* 2004;190:714–720.

123. Schaefer PW, Buonanno FS, Gonzalez RG, Schwamm LH. Diffusion-weighted imaging discriminates between cytotoxic and vasogenic edema in a patient with eclampsia. *Stroke.* 1997;28:1082–1085.

124. Garcia-Reitboeck P, Al-Memar A. Images in clinical medicine: reversible cerebral vasoconstriction after preeclampsia. *N Engl J Med.* 2013;369:e4.

125. Konstantinopoulos PA, Mousa S, Khairallah R, Mtanos G. Postpartum cerebral angiopathy: an important diagnostic consideration in the postpartum period. *Am J Obstet Gynecol.* 2004;191:375–377.

126. Martin JN Jr, Thigpen BD, Moore RC, et al. Stroke and severe preeclampsia and eclampsia: a paradigm shift focusing on systolic blood pressure. *Obstet Gynecol.* 2005;105:246–254.

127. Cantwell R, Clutton-Brock T, Cooper G, et al. Saving mothers' lives: reviewing maternal deaths to make motherhood safer: 2006-2008. The eighth report of the Confidential Enquiries into Maternal Deaths in the United Kingdom. *BJOG.* 2011;118:1–203.

128. Kambam JR, Handte RE, Brown WU, Smith BE. Effect of normal and preeclamptic pregnancies on the oxyhemoglobin dissociation curve. *Anesthesiology.* 1986;65:426–427.

129. Heilmann L, Rath W, Pollow K. Hemorheological changes in women with severe preeclampsia. *Clin Hemorheol Microcirc.* 2004;31:49–58.

130. Reese JA, Peck JD, Deschamps DR, et al. Platelet counts during pregnancy. *N Engl J Med.* 2018;379:32–43.

131. Sharma SK, Philip J, Whitten CW, et al. Assessment of changes in coagulation in parturients with preeclampsia using thromboelastography. *Anesthesiology.* 1999;90:385–390.

132. Harlow FH, Brown MA, Brighton TA, et al. Platelet activation in the hypertensive disorders of pregnancy. *Am J Obstet Gynecol.* 2002;187:688–695.

133. Aster RH. Pooling of platelets in the spleen: role in the pathogenesis of "hypersplenic" thrombocytopenia. *J Clin Invest.* 1966;45:645–657.

134. Davies JR, Fernando R, Hallworth SP. Hemostatic function in healthy pregnant and preeclamptic women: an assessment using the platelet function analyzer (PFA-100) and thromboelastograph. *Anesth Analg.* 2007;104:416–420.

135. Vigil-De Gracia P, Ortega-Paz L. Pre-eclampsia/eclampsia and hepatic rupture. *Int J Gynaecol Obstet.* 2012;118:186–189.

136. Sheikh RA, Yasmeen S, Pauly MP, Riegler JL. Spontaneous intrahepatic hemorrhage and hepatic rupture in the HELLP syndrome: four cases and a review. *J Clin Gastroenterol.* 1999;28:323–328.

137. Boulleret C, Chahid T, Gallot D, et al. Hypogastric arterial selective and superselective embolization for severe postpartum hemorrhage: a retrospective review of 36 cases. *Cardiovasc Intervent Radiol.* 2004;27:344–348.

138. Chauleur C, Fanget C, Tourne G, et al. Serious primary post-partum hemorrhage, arterial embolization and future fertility: a retrospective study of 46 cases. *Hum Reprod.* 2008;23:1553–1559.

139. Sibai BM, Ramadan MK, Usta I, et al. Maternal morbidity and mortality in 442 pregnancies with hemolysis, elevated liver enzymes, and low platelets (HELLP syndrome). *Am J Obstet Gynecol.* 1993;169:1000–1006.

140. Onrust S, Santema JG, Aarnoudse JG. Pre-eclampsia and the HELLP syndrome still cause maternal mortality in the Netherlands and other developed countries; can we reduce it? *Eur J Obstet Gynecol Reprod Biol.* 1999;82:41–46.

141. Weinstein L. Syndrome of hemolysis, elevated liver enzymes, and low platelet count: a severe consequence of hypertension in pregnancy. *Am J Obstet Gynecol.* 1982;42:159–167.

142. Sibai BM. Diagnosis, controversies, and management of the syndrome of hemolysis, elevated liver enzymes, and low platelet count. *Obstet Gynecol.* 2004;103:981–991.

143. Barton JR, Riely CA, Adamec TA, et al. Hepatic histopathologic condition does not correlate with laboratory abnormalities in HELLP syndrome (hemolysis, elevated liver enzymes, and low platelet count). *Am J Obstet Gynecol.* 1992;167:1538–1543.

144. Society for Maternal-Fetal Medicine Publications Committee, Sibai BM. Evaluation and management of severe preeclampsia before 34 weeks' gestation. *Am J Obstet Gynecol.* 2011;205:191–198.

145. Bauer ME, Arendt K, Beilin Y, et al. The Society for Obstetric Anesthesia and Perinatology interdisciplinary consensus statement on neuraxial procedures in obstetric patients with thrombocytopenia. *Anesth Analg.* 2021;132:1531–1544.

146. Douglas M. The use of neuraxial anesthesia in parturients with thrombocytopenia: what is an adequate platelet count?. In: Halpern S, Douglas M, eds. *Evidence-Based Obstetric Anaesthesia.* Blackwell Publishing; 2005:165–177.

147. Barton JR, Sibai BM. Diagnosis and management of hemolysis, elevated liver enzymes, and low platelets syndrome. *Clin Perinatol.* 2004;31:807–833.

148. Moran P, Baylis PH, Lindheimer MD, Davison JM. Glomerular ultrafiltration in normal and preeclamptic pregnancy. *J Am Soc Nephrol.* 2003;14:648–652.

149. Sims EA, Krantz KE. Serial studies of renal function during pregnancy and the puerperium in normal women. *J Clin Invest.* 1958;37:1764–1774.

150. Davison JM, Dunlop W. Renal hemodynamics and tubular function normal human pregnancy. *Kidney Int.* 1980;18:152–161.

151. Siemens J, Bogert L. The uric acid content of maternal and fetal blood. *J Biol Chem.* 1917;32:63–67.

152. Schaffer NK, Dill LV, Cadden JF. Uric acid clearance in normal pregnancy and pre-eclampsia. *J Clin Invest.* 1943;22:201–206.

153. Powers RW, Bodnar LM, Ness RB, et al. Uric acid concentrations in early pregnancy among preeclamptic women with gestational hyperuricemia at delivery. *Am J Obstet Gynecol.* 2006;194:160.

154. Abraham KA, Kennelly M, Dorman AM, Walshe JJ. Pathogenesis of acute renal failure associated with the HELLP syndrome: a case report and review of the literature. *Eur J Obstet Gynecol Reprod Biol.* 2003;108:99–102.

155. Sibai BM, Villar MA, Mabie BC. Acute renal failure in hypertensive disorders of pregnancy. Pregnancy outcome and remote prognosis in thirty-one consecutive cases. *Am J Obstet Gynecol.* 1990;162:777–783.

156. Drakeley AJ, Le Roux PA, Anthony J, Penny J. Acute renal failure complicating severe preeclampsia requiring admission to an obstetric intensive care unit. *Am J Obstet Gynecol.* 2002;186:253–256.

157. Stratta P, Canavese C, Colla L, et al. Acute renal failure in preeclampsia-eclampsia. *Gynecol Obstet Invest.* 1987;24:225–231.

158. Ganesan C, Maynard SE. Acute kidney injury in pregnancy: the thrombotic microangiopathies. *J Nephrol.* 2011;24:554–563.

159. Preventive Services Task Force US, Bibbins-Domingo K, Grossman DC, et al. Screening for preeclampsia: U.S. Preventive Services Task Force recommendation statement. *JAMA.* 2017;317:1661–1667.

160. Leduc L, Wheeler JM, Kirshon B, et al. Coagulation profile in severe preeclampsia. *Obstet Gynecol.* 1992;79:14–18.

161. Romero R, Vizoso J, Emamian M, et al. Clinical significance of liver dysfunction in pregnancy-induced hypertension. *Am J Perinatol.* 1988;5:146–151.

162. Hawkins TL, Roberts JM, Mangos GJ, et al. Plasma uric acid remains a marker of poor outcome in hypertensive pregnancy: a retrospective cohort study. *BJOG.* 2012;119:484–492.

163. Thangaratinam S, Ismail KM, Sharp S, et al. Accuracy of serum uric acid in predicting complications of pre-eclampsia: a systematic review. *BJOG.* 2006;113:369–378.

164. Koopmans CM, van Pampus MG, Groen H, et al. Accuracy of serum uric acid as a predictive test for maternal complications in pre-eclampsia: bivariate meta-analysis and decision analysis. *Eur J Obstet Gynecol Reprod Biol.* 2009;146:8–14.

165. Haddad B, Sibai BM. Expectant management of severe preeclampsia: proper candidates and pregnancy outcome. *Clin Obstet Gynecol.* 2005;48:430–440.

166. Bateman BT, Berman MF, Riley LE, Leffert LR. The epidemiology of postpartum hemorrhage in a large, nationwide sample of deliveries. *Anesth Analg.* 2010;110:1368–1373.

167. Kane SC, Dennis AT. Doppler assessment of uterine blood flow in pre-eclampsia: a review. *Hypertens Pregnancy.* 2015;34:400–421.

168. Amorim MM, Santos LC, Faundes A. Corticosteroid therapy for prevention of respiratory distress syndrome in severe preeclampsia. *Am J Obstet Gynecol.* 1999;180:1283–1288.

169. Woudstra DM, Chandra S, Hofmeyr GJ, Dowswell T. Corticosteroids for HELLP (hemolysis, elevated liver enzymes, low platelets) syndrome in pregnancy. *Cochrane Database Syst Rev.* 2010;(9):CD008148.

170. Trudinger BJ, Giles WB, Cook CM, et al. Fetal umbilical artery flow velocity waveforms and placental resistance: clinical significance. *Br J Obstet Gynaecol.* 1985;92:23–30.

171. Lindqvist PG, Happach C. Risk and risk estimation of placental abruption. *Eur J Obstet Gynecol Reprod Biol.* 2006;126:160–164.

172. Duley L, Meher S, Jones L. Drugs for treatment of very high blood pressure during pregnancy. *Cochrane Database Syst Rev.* 2013;(7):CD001449.

173. MacCarthy EP, Bloomfield SS. Labetalol: a review of its pharmacology, pharmacokinetics, clinical uses and adverse effects. *Pharmacotherapy.* 1983;3:193–219.

174. Bateman BT, Patorno E, Desai RJ, et al. Late pregnancy beta blocker exposure and risks of neonatal hypoglycemia and bradycardia. *Pediatrics.* 2016;138

175. Vigil-De Gracia P, Lasso M, Ruiz E, et al. Severe hypertension in pregnancy: hydralazine or labetalol. A randomized clinical trial. *Eur J Obstet Gynecol Reprod Biol.* 2006;128:157–162.

176. Impey L. Severe hypotension and fetal distress following sublingual administration of nifedipine to a patient with severe pregnancy induced hypertension at 33 weeks. *Br J Obstet Gynaecol.* 1993;100:959–961.

177. Ben-Ami M, Giladi Y, Shalev E. The combination of magnesium sulphate and nifedipine: a cause of neuromuscular blockade. *Br J Obstet Gynaecol.* 1994;101:262–263.

178. Magee LA, Miremadi S, Li J, et al. Therapy with both magnesium sulfate and nifedipine does not increase the risk of serious magnesium-related maternal side effects in women with preeclampsia. *Am J Obstet Gynecol.* 2005;193:153–163.

179. Shekhar S, Gupta N, Kirubakaran R, Pareek P. Oral nifedipine versus intravenous labetalol for severe hypertension during pregnancy: a systematic review and meta-analysis. *BJOG.* 2016;123:40–47.

180. Nij Bijvank SW, Duvekot JJ. Nicardipine for the treatment of severe hypertension in pregnancy: a review of the literature. *Obstet Gynecol Surv.* 2010;65:341–347.

181. American College of Obstetricians and Gynecologists. Committee Opinion No. 692: Emergent therapy for acute-onset, severe hypertension during pregnancy and the postpartum period. *Obstet Gynecol.* 2017;129:e90–e95.

182. Eisenach JC, Castro MI. Maternally administered esmolol produces fetal beta-adrenergic blockade and hypoxemia in sheep. *Anesthesiology.* 1989;71:718–722.

183. Losasso TJ, Muzzi DA, Cucchiara RF. Response of fetal heart rate to maternal administration of esmolol. *Anesthesiology.* 1991;74:782–784.

184. Ducey JP, Knape KG. Maternal esmolol administration resulting in fetal distress and cesarean section in a term pregnancy. *Anesthesiology.* 1992;77:829–832.

185. Eisenach JC, Mandell G, Dewan DM. Maternal and fetal effects of labetalol in pregnant ewes. *Anesthesiology.* 1991;74:292–297.

186. Duley L, Henderson-Smart DJ, Chou D. Magnesium sulphate versus phenytoin for eclampsia. *Cochrane Database Syst Rev.* 2010;(10):CD000128.

187. Duley L, Henderson-Smart DJ, Walker GJ, Chou D. Magnesium sulphate versus diazepam for eclampsia. *Cochrane Database Syst Rev.* 2010;(12):CD000127.

188. Duley L, Gulmezoglu AM, Henderson-Smart DJ, Chou D. Magnesium sulphate and other anticonvulsants for women with pre-eclampsia. *Cochrane Database Syst Rev.* 2010;(11):CD000025.

189. Sibai BM. Magnesium sulfate prophylaxis in preeclampsia: lessons learned from recent trials. *Am J Obstet Gynecol.* 2004;190:1520–1526.

190. Cahill AG, Macones GA, Odibo AO, Stamilio DM. Magnesium for seizure prophylaxis in patients with mild preeclampsia. *Obstet Gynecol.* 2007;110:601–607.

191. Euser AG, Cipolla MJ. Resistance artery vasodilation to magnesium sulfate during pregnancy and the postpartum state. *Am J Physiol Heart Circ Physiol.* 2005;288:H1521–H1525.

192. Manfredi M, Beltramello A, Bongiovanni LG, et al. Eclamptic encephalopathy: imaging and pathogenetic considerations. *Acta Neurol Scand.* 1997;96:277–282.

193. Engelter ST, Provenzale JM, Petrella JR. Assessment of vasogenic edema in eclampsia using diffusion imaging. *Neuroradiology.* 2000;42:818–820.

194. Li X, Han X, Yang J, et al. Magnesium sulfate provides neuroprotection in eclampsia-like seizure model by ameliorating neuroinflammation and brain edema. *Mol Neurobiol.* 2017;54:7938–7948.

195. Cotton DB, Hallak M, Janusz C, et al. Central anticonvulsant effects of magnesium sulfate on N-methyl-D-aspartate-induced seizures. *Am J Obstet Gynecol.* 1993;168:974–978.

196. Okusanya BO, Oladapo OT, Long Q, et al. Clinical pharmacokinetic properties of magnesium sulphate in women with pre-eclampsia and eclampsia. *BJOG.* 2016;123:356–366.

197. Cruikshank DP, Pitkin RM, Donnelly E, Reynolds WA. Urinary magnesium, calcium, and phosphate excretion during magnesium sulfate infusion. *Obstet Gynecol.* 1981;58:430–434.

198. Elliott JP, O'Keeffe DF, Greenberg P, Freeman RK. Pulmonary edema associated with magnesium sulfate and betamethasone administration. *Am J Obstet Gynecol.* 1979;134:717–719.

199. Altman D, Carroli G, Duley L, et al. Do women with pre-eclampsia, and their babies, benefit from magnesium sulphate? The Magpie Trial: a randomised placebo-controlled trial. *Lancet.* 2002;359:1877–1890.

200. Livingston JC, Livingston LW, Ramsey R, et al. Magnesium sulfate in women with mild preeclampsia: a randomized controlled trial. *Obstet Gynecol.* 2003;101:217–220.

201. Aagaard-Tillery KM, Belfort MA. Eclampsia: morbidity, mortality, and management. *Clin Obstet Gynecol.* 2005;48:12–23.

202. Koopmans CM, Bijlenga D, Groen H, et al. Induction of labour versus expectant monitoring for gestational hypertension or mild pre-eclampsia after 36 weeks' gestation (HYPITAT): a multicentre, open-label randomised controlled trial. *Lancet.* 2009;374:979–988.

203. Hauth JC, Ewell MG, Levine RJ, et al. Pregnancy outcomes in healthy nulliparas who developed hypertension. Calcium for Preeclampsia Prevention Study Group. *Obstet Gynecol.* 2000;95:24–28.

204. Magee LA, Yong PJ, Espinosa V, et al. Expectant management of severe preeclampsia remote from term: a structured systematic review. *Hypertens Pregnancy.* 2009;28:312–347.

205. Churchill D, Duley L, Thornton JG, Jones L. Interventionist versus expectant care for severe pre-eclampsia between 24 and 34 weeks' gestation. *Cochrane Database Syst Rev.* 2013;(7):CD003106.

206. Jacobsen AF, Skjeldestad FE, Sandset PM. Incidence and risk patterns of venous thromboembolism in pregnancy and puerperium—a register-based case-control study. *Am J Obstet Gynecol.* 2008;198:233.e1–e7.

207. Simpson EL, Lawrenson RA, Nightingale AL, Farmer RD. Venous thromboembolism in pregnancy and the puerperium: incidence and additional risk factors from a London perinatal database. *BJOG.* 2001;108:56–60.

208. Lindqvist P, Dahlback B, Marsal K. Thrombotic risk during pregnancy: a population study. *Obstet Gynecol.* 1999;94:595–599.

209. Natarajan P, Shennan AH, Penny J, et al. Comparison of auscultatory and oscillometric automated blood pressure monitors in the setting of preeclampsia. *Am J Obstet Gynecol.* 1999;181:1203–1210.

210. Bello NA, Woolley JJ, Cleary KL, et al. Accuracy of blood pressure measurement devices in pregnancy: a systematic review of validation studies. *Hypertension.* 2018;71:326–335.

211. Preisman S, Pfeiffer U, Lieberman N, Perel A. New monitors of intravascular volume: a comparison of arterial pressure waveform analysis and the intrathoracic blood volume. *Intensive Care Med.* 1997;23:651–657.

212. Dyer RA, Piercy JL, Reed AR, et al. Comparison between pulse waveform analysis and thermodilution cardiac output determination in patients with severe pre-eclampsia. *Br J Anaesth.* 2011;106:77–81.

213. D'Angelo R, Smiley RM, Riley ET, Segal S. Serious complications related to obstetric anesthesia: the serious complication repository project of the Society for Obstetric Anesthesia and Perinatology. *Anesthesiology.* 2014;120:1505–1512.

214. Rosero EB, Joshi GP. Nationwide incidence of serious complications of epidural analgesia in the United States. *Acta Anaesthesiol Scand.* 2016;60:810–820.

215. Bos EME, Haumann J, de Quelerij M, et al. Haematoma and abscess after neuraxial anaesthesia: a review of 647 cases. *Br J Anaesth.* 2018;120:693–704.

216. Seymour LM, Fernandes NL, Dyer RA, et al. General anesthesia for cesarean delivery for thrombocytopenia in hypertensive disorders of pregnancy: findings from the Obstetric Airway Management Registry. *Anesth Analg.* 2023;136:992–998.

217. Beilin Y, Katz DJ. Analgesia use among 984 women with preeclampsia: a retrospective observational single-center study. *J Clin Anesth.* 2020;62:109741.

218. Martin JN Jr, Blake PG, Lowry SL, et al. Pregnancy complicated by preeclampsia-eclampsia with the syndrome of hemolysis, elevated liver enzymes, and low platelet count: how rapid is postpartum recovery? *Obstet Gynecol.* 1990;76:737–741.

219. Leffert L, Butwick A, Carvalho B, et al. The Society for Obstetric Anesthesia and Perinatology consensus statement on the anesthetic management of pregnant and postpartum women receiving thromboprophylaxis or higher dose anticoagulants. *Anesth Analg.* 2018;126:928–944.

220. Watson HG. Thromboelastography should be available in every labour ward. *Int J Obstet Anesth.* 2005;14:325–327.

221. Kanayama N, Belayet HM, Khatun S, et al. A new treatment of severe pre-eclampsia by long-term epidural anaesthesia. *J Hum Hypertens.* 1999;13:167–171.

222. Ginosar Y, Nadjari M, Hoffman A, et al. Antepartum continuous epidural ropivacaine therapy reduces uterine artery vascular resistance in pre-eclampsia: a randomized, dose-ranging, placebo-controlled study. *Br J Anaesth.* 2009;102:369–378.

223. Ramanathan J, Coleman P, Sibai B. Anesthetic modification of hemodynamic and neuroendocrine stress responses to cesarean delivery in women with severe preeclampsia. *Anesth Analg.* 1991;73:772–779.

224. Jouppila P, Jouppila R, Hollmen A, Koivula A. Lumbar epidural analgesia to improve intervillous blood flow during labor in severe preeclampsia. *Obstet Gynecol.* 1982;59:158–161.

225. Karinen J, Rasanen J, Alahuhta S, et al. Maternal and uteroplacental haemodynamic state in pre-eclamptic patients during spinal anaesthesia for caesarean section. *Br J Anaesth.* 1996;76:616–620.

226. Wallace DH, Leveno KJ, Cunningham FG, et al. Randomized comparison of general and regional anesthesia for cesarean delivery in pregnancies complicated by severe preeclampsia. *Obstet Gynecol.* 1995;86:193–199.

227. Neme D, Aweke Z, Jemal B, et al. Effect of anesthesia choice on hemodynamic stability and fetomaternal outcome of the preeclamptic patient undergoing cesarean section. *Ann Med Surg (Lond).* 2022;77:103654.

228. Sharwood-Smith G, Clark V, Watson E. Regional anaesthesia for caesarean section in severe preeclampsia: spinal anaesthesia is the preferred choice. *Int J Obstet Anesth.* 1999;8:85–89.

229. Hood DD, Curry R. Spinal versus epidural anesthesia for cesarean section in severely preeclamptic patients: a retrospective survey. *Anesthesiology.* 1999;90:1276–1282.

230. Berends N, Teunkens A, Vandermeersch E, Van de Velde M. A randomized trial comparing low-dose combined spinal-epidural anesthesia and conventional epidural anesthesia for cesarean section in severe preeclampsia. *Acta Anaesthesiol Belg.* 2005;56:155–162.

231. Visalyaputra S, Rodanant O, Somboonviboon W, et al. Spinal versus epidural anesthesia for cesarean delivery in severe preeclampsia: a prospective randomized, multicenter study. *Anesth Analg.* 2005;101:862–868.

232. Aya AG, Vialles N, Tanoubi I, et al. Spinal anesthesia-induced hypotension: a risk comparison between patients with severe preeclampsia and healthy women undergoing preterm cesarean delivery. *Anesth Analg.* 2005;101:869–875.

233. Dyer RA, Piercy JL, Reed AR, et al. Hemodynamic changes associated with spinal anesthesia for cesarean delivery in severe preeclampsia. *Anesthesiology.* 2008;108:802–811.

234. Hu LJ, Mei Z, Shen YP, et al. Comparative dose-response study of phenylephrine bolus for the treatment of the first episode of spinal anesthesia-induced hypotension for cesarean delivery in severe preeclamptic versus normotensive parturients. *Drug Des Devel Ther.* 2022;16:2189–2198.

235. Heesen M, Rijs K, Hilber N, et al. Ephedrine versus phenylephrine as a vasopressor for spinal anaesthesia-induced hypotension in parturients undergoing high-risk caesarean section: meta-analysis, meta-regression and trial sequential analysis. *Int J Obstet Anesth.* 2019;37:16–28.

236. Guo L, Qin R, Ren X, et al. Prophylactic norepinephrine or phenylephrine infusion for bradycardia and post-spinal anaesthesia hypotension in patients with preeclampsia during Caesarean delivery: a randomised controlled trial. *Br J Anaesth.* 2022;128:e305–e307.

237. Gant NF, Daley GL, Chand S, et al. A study of angiotensin II pressor response throughout primigravid pregnancy. *J Clin Invest.* 1973;52:2682–2689.

238. Baker PN, Kilby MD, Broughton Pipkin F. The effect of angiotensin II on platelet intracellular free calcium concentration in human pregnancy. *J Hypertens.* 1992;10:55–60.

239. VanWijk MJ, Boer K, van der Meulen ET, et al. Resistance artery smooth muscle function in pregnancy and preeclampsia. *Am J Obstet Gynecol.* 2002;186:148–154.

240. Nisell H, Hjemdahl P, Linde B. Cardiovascular responses to circulating catecholamines in normal pregnancy and in pregnancy-induced hypertension. *Clin Physiol.* 1985;5:479–493.

241. Vedernikov YP, Belfort MA, Saade GR, Garfield RE. Inhibition of cyclooxygenase but not nitric oxide synthase influences effects on the human omental artery of the thromboxane A2 mimetic U46619 and 17beta-estradiol. *Am J Obstet Gynecol.* 2001;185:182–189.

242. Guinard JP, Mulroy MF, Carpenter RL, Knopes KD. Test doses: optimal epinephrine content with and without acute beta-adrenergic blockade. *Anesthesiology.* 1990;73:386–392.

243. Guay J. The epidural test dose: a review. *Anesth Analg.* 2006;102:921–929.

244. Hadzic A, Vloka J, Patel N, Birnbach D. Hypertensive crisis after a successful placement of an epidural anesthetic in a hypertensive parturient. Case report. *Reg Anesth.* 1995;20:156–158.

245. Heller PJ, Goodman C. Use of local anesthetics with epinephrine for epidural anesthesia in preeclampsia. *Anesthesiology.* 1986;65:224–226.

246. Huang CJ, Fan YC, Tsai PS. Differential impacts of modes of anaesthesia on the risk of stroke among preeclamptic women who undergo caesarean delivery: a population-based study. *Br J Anaesth.* 2010;105:818–826.

247. Munnur U, de Boisblanc B, Suresh MS. Airway problems in pregnancy. *Crit Care Med.* 2005;33:S259–S268.

248. Rout CC. Anaesthesia and analgesia for the critically ill parturient. *Best Pract Res Clin Obstet Gynaecol.* 2001;15:507–522.

249. Perlow JH, Kirz DS. Severe preeclampsia presenting as dysphonia secondary to uvular edema. A case report. *J Reprod Med.* 1990;35:1059–1062.

250. Smit MI, du Toit L, Dyer RA, et al. Hypoxaemia during tracheal intubation in patients with hypertensive disorders of pregnancy: analysis of data from an obstetric airway management registry. *Int J Obstet Anesth.* 2021;45:41–48.

251. Mushambi MC, Kinsella SM, Popat M, et al. Obstetric Anaesthetists' Association and Difficult Airway Society guidelines for the management of difficult and failed tracheal intubation in obstetrics. *Anaesthesia.* 2015;70:1286–1306.

252. Bansal S, Pawar M. Haemodynamic responses to laryngoscopy and intubation in patients with pregnancy-induced hypertension: effect of intravenous esmolol with or without lidocaine. *Int J Obstet Anesth.* 2002;11:4–8.

253. Yoon SW, Choi GJ, Seong HK, et al. Pharmacological strategies to prevent haemodynamic changes after intubation in parturient women with hypertensive disorders of pregnancy: a network meta-analysis. *Int J Med Sci.* 2021;18:1039–1050.

254. Pant M, Fong R, Scavone B. Prevention of peri-induction hypertension in preeclamptic patients: a focused review. *Anesth Analg.* 2014;119:1350–1356.

255. Yoo KY, Kang DH, Jeong H, et al. A dose-response study of remifentanil for attenuation of the hypertensive response to laryngoscopy and tracheal intubation in severely preeclamptic women undergoing caesarean delivery under general anaesthesia. *Int J Obstet Anesth*. 2013;22:10–18.

256. Noskova P, Blaha J, Bakhouche H, et al. Neonatal effect of remifentanil in general anaesthesia for caesarean section: a randomized trial. *BMC Anesthesiol*. 2015;15:38.

257. Ramanathan J, Sibai BM, Mabie WC, et al. The use of labetalol for attenuation of the hypertensive response to endotracheal intubation in preeclampsia. *Am J Obstet Gynecol*. 1988;159:650–654.

258. Nabil F, Gharib AA, Gadelrab NA, Osman HM. Preoperative lignocaine nebulisation for attenuation of the pressor response of laryngoscopy and tracheal intubation in patients with severe preeclampsia undergoing caesarean section delivery: a randomised double-blind controlled trial. *Indian J Anaesth*. 2023;67:515–522.

259. James MF, Dyer RA. Prevention of peri-induction hypertension in pre-eclamptic patients. *Anesth Analg*. 2015;121:1678–1679.

260. James MF, Beer RE, Esser JD. Intravenous magnesium sulfate inhibits catecholamine release associated with tracheal intubation. *Anesth Analg*. 1989;68:772–776.

261. Allen RW, James MF, Uys PC. Attenuation of the pressor response to tracheal intubation in hypertensive proteinuric pregnant patients by lignocaine, alfentanil and magnesium sulphate. *Br J Anaesth*. 1991;66:216–223.

262. Ashton WB, James MF, Janicki P, Uys PC. Attenuation of the pressor response to tracheal intubation by magnesium sulphate with and without alfentanil in hypertensive proteinuric patients undergoing caesarean section. *Br J Anaesth*. 1991;67:741–747.

263. Baraka A, Yazigi A. Neuromuscular interaction of magnesium with succinylcholine-vecuronium sequence in the eclamptic parturient. *Anesthesiology*. 1987;67:806–808.

264. Sinatra RS, Philip BK, Naulty JS, Ostheimer GW. Prolonged neuromuscular blockade with vecuronium in a patient treated with magnesium sulfate. *Anesth Analg*. 1985;64:1220–1222.

265. Kussman B, Shorten G, Uppington J, Comunale ME. Administration of magnesium sulphate before rocuronium: effects on speed of onset and duration of neuromuscular block. *Br J Anaesth*. 1997;79:122–124.

266. Hodgson RE, Rout CC, Rocke DA, Louw NJ. Mivacurium for caesarean section in hypertensive parturients receiving magnesium sulphate therapy. *Int J Obstet Anesth*. 1998;7:12–17.

267. Yoshida A, Itoh Y, Nagaya K, et al. Prolonged relaxant effects of vecuronium in patients with deliberate hypermagnesemia: time for caution in cesarean section. *J Anesth*. 2006;20:33–35.

268. Germano Filho PA, Cavalcanti IL, Barrucand L, Vercosa N. Effect of magnesium sulphate on sugammadex reversal time for neuromuscular blockade: a randomised controlled study. *Anaesthesia*. 2015;70:956–961.

269. Czarnetzki C, Tassonyi E, Lysakowski C, et al. Efficacy of sugammadex for the reversal of moderate and deep rocuronium-induced neuromuscular block in patients pretreated with intravenous magnesium: a randomized controlled trial. *Anesthesiology*. 2014;121:59–67.

270. Song S, Yoo BH, Kim KM, Lee S. Reversal of rocuronium induced neuromuscular blockade using sugammadex in a patient with eclampsia treated by magnesium intraoperatively. *Korean J Anesthesiol*. 2014;67:S102–S103.

271. Snyder SW, Cardwell MS. Neuromuscular blockade with magnesium sulfate and nifedipine. *Am J Obstet Gynecol*. 1989;161:35–36.

272. Navathe R, Berghella V. Tocolysis for acute preterm labor: where have we been, where are we now, and where are we going? *Am J Perinatol*. 2016;33:229–235.

273. Sibai BM. Diagnosis, prevention, and management of eclampsia. *Obstet Gynecol*. 2005;105:402–410.

274. Brodie H, Malinow AM. Anesthetic management of preeclampsia/eclampsia. *Int J Obstet Anesth*. 1999;8:110–124.

275. Moodley J, Jjuuko G, Rout C. Epidural compared with general anaesthesia for caesarean delivery in conscious women with eclampsia. *BJOG*. 2001;108:378–382.

276. Singh R, Kumar N, Jain A, Chakraborty M. Spinal anesthesia for lower segment cesarean section in patients with stable eclampsia. *J Clin Anesth*. 2011;23:202–206.

277. Oshima T, Karasawa F, Satoh T. Effects of propofol on cerebral blood flow and the metabolic rate of oxygen in humans. *Acta Anaesthesiol Scand*. 2002;46:831–835.

278. Wood PR, Browne GP, Pugh S. Propofol infusion for the treatment of status epilepticus. *Lancet*. 1988;1:480–481.

279. Bissonnette B. Cerebral protection. *Paediatr Anaesth*. 2004;14:403–406.

280. Fraser GL, Devlin JW, Worby CP, et al. Benzodiazepine versus nonbenzodiazepine-based sedation for mechanically ventilated, critically ill adults: a systematic review and meta-analysis of randomized trials. *Crit Care Med*. 2013;41:S30–S38.

281. Ray JG, Vermeulen MJ, Schull MJ, Redelmeier DA. Cardiovascular health after maternal placental syndromes (CHAMPS): population-based retrospective cohort study. *Lancet*. 2005;366:1797–1803.

282. Bellamy L, Casas JP, Hingorani AD, Williams DJ. Pre-eclampsia and risk of cardiovascular disease and cancer in later life: systematic review and meta-analysis. *BMJ*. 2007;335:974.

283. Funai EF, Friedlander Y, Paltiel O, et al. Long-term mortality after preeclampsia. *Epidemiology*. 2005;16:206–215.

284. Wilson BJ, Watson MS, Prescott GJ, et al. Hypertensive diseases of pregnancy and risk of hypertension and stroke in later life: results from cohort study. *BMJ*. 2003;326:845.

285. Grandi SM, Filion KB, Yoon S, et al. Cardiovascular disease-related morbidity and mortality in women with a history of pregnancy complications. *Circulation*. 2019;139:1069–1079.

286. Chambers JC, Fusi L, Malik IS, et al. Association of maternal endothelial dysfunction with preeclampsia. *JAMA*. 2001;285:1607–1612.

287. Hamad RR, Eriksson MJ, Silveira A, et al. Decreased flow-mediated dilation is present 1 year after a pre-eclamptic pregnancy. *J Hypertens*. 2007;25:2301–2307.

288. Engelhard IM, van Rij M, Boullart I, et al. Posttraumatic stress disorder after pre-eclampsia: an exploratory study. *Gen Hosp Psychiatry*. 2002;24:260–264.

289. Furuta M, Sandall J, Bick D. A systematic review of the relationship between severe maternal morbidity and post-traumatic stress disorder. *BMC Pregnancy Childbirth*. 2012;12:125.

290. Hoedjes M, Berks D, Vogel I, et al. Symptoms of post-traumatic stress after preeclampsia. *J Psychosom Obstet Gynaecol*. 2011;32:126–134.

291. Stramrood CA, Wessel I, Doornbos B, et al. Posttraumatic stress disorder following preeclampsia and PPROM: a prospective study with 15 months follow-up. *Reprod Sci*. 2011;18:645–653.

36

Infection

Melissa E. Bauer, DO and Catherine M. Albright, MD, MS

CHAPTER OUTLINE

NORMAL TEMPERATURE RANGE AND FEVER

Definition and Pathophysiology

The normal range of temperature for adults is 36.2°C to 37.0°C (mean ± 2 standard deviations), with an average temperature of 36.6°C, according to a metaanalysis of prospectively measured temperatures.[1] Temperature measurements greater than 38°C represent fever. The fetus, by virtue of its intraabdominal location, has a unique problem with heat elimination. Evidence suggests that the fetus relies on heat exchange across the uteroplacental circulation to dissipate most of its metabolic heat. The normal fetus maintains a temperature that is approximately 0.5°C to 0.75°C higher than the maternal temperature.[2,3]

Maternal Effects of Fever

Fever produces significant maternal effects. Elevated temperature is associated with increased maternal heart rate, cardiac output, oxygen consumption, and catecholamine production. Women who develop a fever are more likely to shiver and experience uncomfortable rigors.[4,5] Not surprisingly, obstetric providers, fearing infection, are more likely to treat febrile women with antibiotics.[6,7]

Neonatal Effects of Maternal Fever

Infection is the most common cause of fever and involves liberation of inflammatory cytokines, which are implicated in the pathogenesis of many fetal and neonatal injuries (see Chapter 10).[8,9] The mechanism linking neonatal neurologic injuries to maternal fever likely involves the inflammatory cytokines.[8-10] Animal models of chorioamnionitis suggest that fetal brain lesions can be induced by infection and blocked by antiinflammatory cytokines.[11] Infants developing neonatal encephalopathy in the setting of maternal fever do not generally exhibit positive blood cultures, implying that it is neuroinflammation, rather than infection, that causes damage.[12,13] Fever alone has a limited effect, but when combined with acidosis, inflammation, and/or infection, it appears to exacerbate neurologic injury.[14]

Studies have suggested that maternal intrapartum fever may not be benign. Intrapartum fever is associated with neonatal morbidity. Many studies focused only on the presence or absence of fever and did not specifically comment on a clinical or pathologic diagnosis of chorioamnionitis. In studies that reported clinical or pathologic chorioamnionitis, there are high rates in all groups with fever, so it is difficult to determine whether morbidity is a result of the fever, infection, or both.[15,16] Hensel et al.[17] found a correlation with maternal fever and composite neonatal morbidity (umbilical artery pH < 7.1, mechanical ventilation, respiratory distress, meconium aspiration with pulmonary hypertension, hypoglycemia, neonatal intensive care unit (ICU) admission, and Apgar score < 7 at 5 minutes), with higher fever associated with greater odds of neonatal morbidity in a dose-dependent fashion. In this study, almost all patients with fever were diagnosed with clinical chorioamnionitis and treated accordingly.

Hyperthermia

Hot tub and sauna use in pregnancy have been linked epidemiologically to neural tube defects in the fetus.[18] Spontaneous abortion[19] and major structural birth defects[20] have similarly been associated with the frequency of use of hot tubs and saunas. Neonatal hypoxic encephalopathy has been observed after prolonged immersion in 39.7°C water during otherwise uncomplicated labor.[21]

Noninfectious Inflammatory Fever

Neuraxial labor analgesia is associated with intrapartum fever (so-called "epidural-related maternal fever"). The predominant theory is that noninfectious inflammation is responsible for epidural analgesia–associated fever (see Chapter 24). The incidence of fever in parturients with neuraxial analgesia ranges from 15% to 25% compared with 5% to 7% in parturients without neuraxial analgesia.[22] Why some women with neuraxial analgesia develop fever, but others do not, is not understood. There is insufficient evidence to evaluate whether epidural analgesia–associated fever contributes to neonatal brain injury.

BACTERIAL INFECTIONS IN PREGNANCY

Clinical Chorioamnionitis

Clinical chorioamnionitis is primarily caused by intraamniotic infection, which is an infection of the amniotic fluid, fetal membranes, placenta, or fetus. It is a common condition encountered in the labor and delivery room, affecting 1% to 6% of term gestations, almost 40% of deliveries between 25 and 28 weeks' gestation, and over 90% of deliveries before 24 weeks' gestation.[23,24] In 2015, an expert panel was convened by the Eunice Kennedy Shriver National Institute of Child Health and Human Development (NICHD) to review the criteria for diagnosis and management of chorioamnionitis.[25] It proposed that the phrase "intrauterine inflammation, infection, or both" (abbreviated "Triple I") be used instead of the term "chorioamnionitis" because of the diverse range of conditions, both infectious and inflammatory, that it was used to describe. Throughout this chapter, the phrase "clinical chorioamnionitis" is used in place of "Triple I" because most clinicians continue to use the term "chorioamnionitis" in clinical practice. The word "clinical" differentiates this diagnosis from histologic chorioamnionitis, which is diagnosed via placental pathology.

The American College of Obstetricians and Gynecologists (ACOG) defines clinical chorioamnionitis (suspected intraamniotic infection) as a maternal temperature ≥ 39.0°C, or 38.0°C to 38.9°C with one additional clinical risk factor present (maternal leukocytosis, purulent cervical drainage, or fetal tachycardia).[26] The NICHD expert panel defined maternal leukocytosis as a white blood cell count > 15,000/μL $(15 \times 10^9/L)$ in the absence of corticosteroids, and fetal tachycardia > 160 beats/min for at least 10 minutes.[25] The expert workshop executive summary defined isolated maternal fever as a temperature ≥ 39°C with no other clinical risk factors. The ACOG recommends that these patients be given

the diagnosis of clinical chorioamnionitis because infection is the most likely cause of markedly elevated maternal temperature.[26]

Independent risk factors for clinical chorioamnionitis include low parity, a history of chorioamnionitis in a prior delivery, the number of vaginal examinations, duration of total labor, duration of ruptured membranes, and the use of internal monitors.[26]

In most cases, bacteria gain access to the amniotic cavity and the fetus by ascending through the cervix after rupture of the membranes. Alternatively, infectious agents present in the maternal circulation may undergo transplacental transport and gain access to the amniotic cavity.[26] Similar to other pelvic infections, histologic chorioamnionitis often is polymicrobial in origin, and bacteria normally present in the genital tract are most likely responsible for infections.[26] Maternal bacteremia occurs in approximately 10% of women with clinical chorioamnionitis.[27,28]

Maternal complications of clinical chorioamnionitis include preterm labor, placental abruption, postpartum infection, uterine atony, postpartum hemorrhage, peripartum hysterectomy, adult respiratory distress syndrome, sepsis, ICU admission, and death.[25,26,29–31] In addition, several studies have noted an increased incidence of cesarean delivery for labor dystocia in parturients with clinical chorioamnionitis.[32–35] Some investigators have suggested that infection adversely affects uterine contractility and contributes to an increased risk for cesarean delivery.[36] However, in some cases, clinical chorioamnionitis may represent an ascending infection developing late in labor that is already prolonged and dysfunctional.[33]

Neonatal complications of clinical chorioamnionitis include pneumonia, meningitis, sepsis, and death.[26,34] Importantly, the use of intrapartum antibiotic therapy given in response to maternal Group B streptococcal colonization or in response to signs of chorioamnionitis has significantly decreased the incidence of neonatal infection and sepsis.[37–40] An association between clinical chorioamnionitis and cerebral palsy has been identified. However, in a recent metaanalysis, once studies were separated by gestational age, excluded if they did not have an evaluation of postnatal causes of cerebral palsy, and potential sources of bias and confounding were accounted for, the relative risk (RR) was much lower than in previous analyses.[41] The link between maternal infection and neurologic injury in the neonate appears to be related to intraamniotic infection or inflammation, particularly when there is evidence of fetal systemic inflammation or inflammation of the umbilical cord (funisitis).[42]

Historically, prompt delivery was the cornerstone of obstetric management of patients with clinical chorioamnionitis. However, Gibbs et al.[43] did not identify a correlation between poor maternal or neonatal outcome and the time interval from diagnosis of clinical chorioamnionitis to delivery. They performed cesarean delivery only for standard obstetric indications and not for the diagnosis of clinical chorioamnionitis alone.[43] Similarly, a large prospective observational study found no relationship between the duration of suspected infection and most measures of adverse neonatal outcome among 1965 gestations complicated by clinical chorioamnionitis, although low 5-minute Apgar scores and neonatal mechanical ventilation were correlated with the duration of chorioamnionitis.[34] Many fetuses will exhibit tachycardia during maternal fever and infection, but this pattern is not highly predictive of neonatal acidemia and, therefore by itself, is not an indication for immediate delivery.[44] Neonatal adverse outcomes are associated with any exposure to clinical chorioamnionitis and not the length of time until delivery.[45]

Treatment for clinical chorioamnionitis prior to delivery results in decreased maternal and neonatal morbidity compared with postpartum treatment.[26] With clinical chorioamnionitis, a combination of **ampicillin** and **gentamicin** should cover most relevant pathogens and is the recommended primary antibiotic regimen.[26] The early use of antibiotics also may affect the anesthesia provider's decision regarding the administration of neuraxial labor analgesia or anesthesia (see discussion below). If a cesarean delivery is performed, additional anaerobic coverage with **clindamycin** or **metronidazole** may decrease the risk for endometritis.[26] Additionally, **azithromycin** is indicated during intrapartum cesarean delivery to reduce the risk of endometritis.[46] Many providers also administer azithromycin at the time of cesarean delivery in this scenario in order to ensure *Ureaplasma* coverage; however, it has not been studied in patients with clinical chorioamnionitis. Continuation of antimicrobial agents postpartum should not be automatic, but rather based on risk factors for postpartum endometritis. In general, women who have a vaginal delivery are less likely to develop postpartum endometritis, and therefore may be candidates for discontinuing antimicrobial therapy after delivery. Even in women undergoing cesarean delivery, studies have shown only preoperative or one single postoperative dose appears to have the same efficacy as continuing antibiotics for a longer duration.[26,47-49]

Urologic Infection

Urinary tract infections are common during pregnancy, although the incidence of asymptomatic bacteriuria may not be higher than in nonpregnant women. Increased concentration of progesterone causes the relaxation of ureteral smooth muscle. In addition, the gravid uterus causes partial ureteral obstruction. Both factors cause urinary stasis, which increases the risk for urinary tract infection.[50] Furthermore, these physiologic changes increase the likelihood that asymptomatic bladder infection will ascend into the kidneys and produce pyelonephritis. Approximately 2% to 7% of pregnant women will develop symptomatic cystitis, and up to 25% of women with untreated bacteriuria in pregnancy may develop pyelonephritis.[51]

Acute pyelonephritis is a serious threat to maternal and fetal well-being and complicates approximately 1% to 2.5% of pregnancies.[50] Symptoms of acute pyelonephritis include fever, chills, flank pain, and other symptoms of lower urinary tract infection. Approximately 14% to 17% of pregnant women with pyelonephritis will develop bacteremia during the course of this infection.[52,53] The most common causative organisms are *Escherichia coli*, gram-positive organisms,

Klebsiella, *Enterobacter*, and *Proteus* species.[53] Complications may also include anemia, renal insufficiency, respiratory insufficiency, sepsis, and septic shock.[53,54]

Patients with pyelonephritis may also experience pulmonary injury. Cunningham et al.[55] suggested that "this syndrome was probably caused by permeability pulmonary edema, likely mediated by endotoxin-induced alveolar-capillary membrane injury."[55] Towers et al.[56] compared 11 pregnant women who had pyelonephritis and pulmonary injury with 119 women who had pyelonephritis only. They observed that fluid overload and the use of tocolytic therapy were the most significant predictive factors associated with pulmonary injury. The authors suggested that "strict management of fluids should occur so that patients do not have fluid overload."[56] Contemporary authors, however, have questioned fluid restriction in pyelonephritis and instead suggest fluid administration sufficient to generate urine output of 30 to 50 mL/h, while observing respiratory rate, oxygen saturation, and symptoms of dyspnea to identify impending respiratory compromise. Respiratory failure should be investigated with chest radiography and arterial blood gas analysis and managed with appropriate respiratory support.[50]

Hospitalization is indicated to initiate aggressive parenteral antibiotic treatment of this serious maternal infection, although limited data support outpatient treatment for carefully selected patients in the first and second trimester.[57] However, treatment failures and septic complications have been reported in patients randomized to outpatient therapy in clinical trials.[58]

Bacterial Respiratory Tract Infection

Pregnancy results in many changes that may predispose the pregnant woman to the development of serious respiratory tract infection. Hyperemia and hypersecretion are characteristic of the respiratory tract mucosa during pregnancy, and these changes may intensify the effect of the initial infection.[59] In the case of a viral infection, the excess secretions may predispose the patient to bacterial superinfection. Immunologic modulation during pregnancy may also predispose to pulmonary infection.[60] Furthermore, the increased oxygen consumption, elevation of the diaphragm, and decreased functional residual capacity characteristic of pregnancy may increase the likelihood that infection will result in maternal hypoxemia.

Fortunately, most respiratory tract infections during pregnancy are upper respiratory tract viral infections that do not pose a serious threat to the mother or fetus. Most lower respiratory tract infections are also viral and self-limiting; pneumonia occurs during pregnancy with an incidence approximating that of the nonpregnant population.[61]

Benedetti et al.[62] emphasized the importance of early diagnosis and treatment as well as the direct measurement of maternal oxygenation in cases of pneumonia during pregnancy. Most community-acquired pneumonias in healthy young women are bacterial in origin. *Streptococcus pneumoniae* is the most common pathogen.[62] *Mycoplasma pneumoniae* and influenza are other common pathogens. *Legionella pneumophila*, *Chlamydia*, and varicella are less common pathogens in this population.

Postpartum Endometritis and Surgical Site Infection

The most common source of postpartum infection is the **genital tract**. Postpartum endometritis occurs in 2% to 16% of patients who have cesarean delivery[63] and typically presents with a combination of fever, malaise, abdominal pain, and/or purulent discharge or lochia. Although obstetric providers typically refer to postpartum uterine infection as *endometritis*, this infection involves the decidua, myometrium, and parametrial tissues. Bacteria that colonize the cervix and vagina gain access to the amniotic fluid during labor, and they may invade devitalized uterine tissue postpartum. Surgical site infection (SSI) is another increasingly common postpartum infection and appears to occur in 2% to 7% of patients after cesarean delivery.[63] SSI is defined by the US Centers for Disease Control and Prevention (CDC) as infection related to an operative procedure that occurs at or near the surgical incision within 30 days of the procedure.[64]

Cesarean delivery, prolonged rupture of membranes, and prolonged duration of labor are risk factors for postpartum endometritis.[50] Similarly, risk factors for SSI following cesarean delivery include patient-level factors such as obesity, prior cesarean delivery, hypertension, diabetes, and tobacco use; pregnancy-related factors such as emergency delivery, labor or rupture of membranes, and chorioamnionitis; and surgical factors such as operative time and surgeon experience.[65]

Prophylactic administration of antibiotics decreases the incidence of postpartum uterine infection and wound infection after cesarean delivery, whether performed electively or as an emergency.[66] Antibiotic prophylaxis should be administered up to 60 minutes before skin incision for cesarean delivery.[67] A first-generation cephalosporin is effective against gram-positive bacteria, gram-negative bacteria, and some anaerobic bacteria, and is the first-line antibiotic for cesarean delivery prophylaxis. In women with a history of cephalosporin allergy, clindamycin with an aminoglycoside is an appropriate alternative.[68] However, it has shown that patients receiving alternative antibiotics have higher rates of SSIs.[69] Allergy skin testing is considered safe in pregnancy and is recommended to allow for appropriate antibiotic administration.[70] Extended-spectrum antibiotics, such as azithromycin, used in addition to first-generation cephalosporins for cesarean delivery prophylaxis, have been shown to reduce the rates of endometritis and wound infection in women undergoing nonelective cesarean delivery during labor or after a membrane rupture.[46]

A single intravenous dose of **cefazolin** is appropriate for most women undergoing cesarean delivery, as a therapeutic level is maintained for 3 to 4 hours. However, obese women may require a higher dose, although the specific appropriate dose has yet to be identified.[68,71–73] Consistent with surgical prophylaxis principles, patients with prolonged surgical procedures or those with significant blood loss (>1500 mL) should receive an additional intraoperative dose of the antibiotic used for preincision prophylaxis.[74]

Additional preventative measures for endometritis and SSI include the avoidance of perioperative hyperglycemia and hypothermia.[74]

A systematic review reported that skin preparation using chlorhexidine gluconate was slightly more effective than povidone iodine for reducing the incidence of SSI after cesarean delivery (RR, 0.72; 95% CI, 0.58 to 0.91).[75] Vaginal preparation before cesarean delivery has been evaluated in a metaanalysis of 16 trials.[76] These trials demonstrate an overall reduction in postcesarean endometritis, especially for women in labor or with ruptured membranes. More data are needed to evaluate the effect of this intervention on women not in labor or with intact membranes. A metaanalysis evaluating the effect of bundles of at least three evidence-based interventions (such as antibiotic prophylaxis selection or dose, hair removal with clippers, and chlorhexidine skin preparation) showed a significant reduction in SSI rates with a reduction in risk of 67%.[77] There is insufficient evidence to recommend prophylactic antibiotics for operative vaginal delivery, dilation and curettage, placement of an indwelling intrauterine balloon, or manual removal of the placenta after vaginal delivery; however, consideration may be given to prophylactic antibiotics in the setting of complex perineal repairs.[68,78-80]

Parenteral, broad-spectrum antibiotic therapy with a combination of **gentamicin** and **clindamycin** is recommended to treat postpartum endometritis. Ampicillin is added in refractory cases and often in cases in which the patient was colonized with group B streptococcus before delivery.[81] Endometritis typically responds to this antibiotic therapy regimen, and outcomes are generally excellent. However, serious complications (e.g., peritonitis, abscess, septic thrombophlebitis) may rarely occur.[82,83] Puerperal group A streptococcal infection has high rates of morbidity and mortality. Early wound debridement and/or hysterectomy may be lifesaving in the setting of clinical deterioration.[84,85] For SSI treatment, debridement, wound exploration, wet to dry packing, or negative pressure therapy may be required for treatment. Antimicrobial treatment is also recommended. If the obstetric provider is unable to determine the depth of infection at bedside and the wound requires exploration, it is best practice to provide anesthesia in the operating room allowing use of American Society of Anesthesiologists (ASA) standard monitors and administration of regional anesthesia, if possible.

VIRAL INFECTIONS IN PREGNANCY

Respiratory Infections

Influenza

Pregnant women are disproportionately represented when evaluating mortality from influenza, and a significant number of women have been treated with extracorporeal membrane oxygenation (ECMO) (see Chapter 53).[86,87] Because morbidity and mortality from influenza are increased in pregnancy, influenza vaccination is strongly recommended for pregnant women or those who will be pregnant during influenza season.[88] In the Confidential Enquiries into Maternal Deaths and Morbidity in the United Kingdom and Ireland 2009 to 2012 report, of the women who died, 1 in 11 died from influenza and more than half of the deaths from influenza could have been prevented by vaccination.[89] The risk for fetal death is increased by maternal influenza infection and is reduced by vaccination.[90] The infant is also passively protected for up to 20 weeks after birth.[91] Aggressive treatment with antiviral drugs (**oseltamivir, zanamivir**) reduces the severity of the ensuing illness; in the 2009 to 2010 H1N1 influenza pandemic, initiation of therapy in the first 2 days of the infection reduced hospitalization and ICU admission; however, benefits have also been seen if antiviral drugs are started up to 4 days after onset of symptoms.[86,92] Antiviral drugs appear to be safe in pregnancy, with no reported increase in adverse pregnancy or neonatal outcomes.[93,94]

COVID-19

Coronavirus disease 2019 (COVID-19) is caused by the SARS-CoV-2 virus. While it remains unclear whether pregnancy increases susceptibility to SARS-CoV-2, it has been well documented that pregnancy increases the risk for morbidity and mortality. Data from the COVID-19 surveillance system from the CDC have demonstrated that, compared with nonpregnant women with COVID-19, pregnant women with COVID-19 were more likely to be admitted to an ICU (10.5 versus 3.9 per 1000), to require invasive ventilation (2.9 versus 1.1 per 1000), to require ECMO (0.7 versus 0.3 per 1000), and to die (1.5 versus 1.2 per 1000).[95]

In addition to an increase in morbidity and mortality related to SARS-CoV-2 during pregnancy, it is also likely that SARS-CoV-2 infection increases the risk of adverse pregnancy outcomes. Multiple studies as well as a systematic review and metaanalysis have demonstrated an increased risk of preterm birth, preeclampsia, and stillbirth among pregnant persons with SARS-CoV-2.[96-98] A few cases of intrauterine transmission have been reported; however, this appears to be rare.[99]

Clinical management of SARS-CoV-2 infection during pregnancy should mirror management outside of pregnancy, and appropriate medical therapy should not be withheld (including treatment with **remdesivir** and **monoclonal antibodies**). Additionally, **nirmatrelvir** and **ritonavir** may be considered for use in patients at high risk for severe disease.[100] Like other infections, COVID-19 in and of itself is not an indication for delivery; with a clinically stable patient, it may be helpful to delay delivery to reduce the possibility of transmission to the neonate after delivery. The Society for Maternal and Fetal Medicine (SMFM) and the National Institutes of Health have developed and regularly update clinical guidelines for the management of pregnant patients with COVID-19.[101,102]

Vaccination for patients during pregnancy or those who plan to become pregnant is strongly recommended by the ACOG, SMFM, and the Royal College of Obstetricians and Gynaecologists, given the known risks of COVID-19 during pregnancy.[102-104] There are no concerns regarding the safety of the three COVID-19 vaccines currently available in the United States during pregnancy or lactation. Maternal IgG crosses the placenta and results in detectable antibody titers in the neonate; however, whether and for how long this correlates with neonatal protection from SARS-CoV-2 infection is unclear.[105-109]

Anesthetic Management. For patients with active COVID-19 infection, numerous anesthetic neuraxial procedures have been reported without neurologic complications.[110-112] If a patient meets criteria for tracheal intubation, this should be completed without delay. Performing cesarean delivery is not an effective strategy to avoid intubation for the patient with respiratory failure; delivery has been shown to delay the deterioration of the Pao_2/Fio_2 ratio but not substantially improve it.[113] If cesarean delivery is indicated, the optimal anesthetic technique depends on the patient's clinical condition (i.e., the level of hemodynamic stability, the ability to lay flat, Pao_2/Fio_2 ratio, and recent anticoagulation) and airway examination. Difficult intubation has been reported to occur in 1 in 49 patients and failed intubation in 1 in 808 patients who undergo general anesthesia for cesarean delivery.[114] For the patient with significant respiratory compromise, planned tracheal intubation may be more appropriate than an urgent intraoperative conversion to general anesthesia.

In patients with COVID-19 who experience a post–dural puncture headache (PDPH), there is little evidence to guide management. There are case reports of uneventful epidural blood patch placement with no neurologic sequelae.[115,116] There are also case reports of encephalitis, encephalomyelitis, and meningoencephalitis associated with COVID-19 infection, although the mechanism for these neurologic complications is unclear. Cerebrospinal fluid (CSF) testing for SARS-CoV-2 has been variably reported as either positive or negative in patients with and without neurologic symptoms. Given few data, and the unknown mechanism for neurologic sequelae, it seems prudent to assess the patient for urgency of the epidural blood patch procedure (such as neurologic symptoms, inability to perform activities of daily living or care for the infant) and engage with the patient in shared decision-making to decide on whether to perform an epidural blood patch procedure or delay the procedure until the acute COVID-19 infection resolves. (See Chapter 31 for more details about the epidural blood patch procedure.)

Genital Herpes

Herpes simplex virus type 2 (HSV-2) causes locally recurring disease that is characterized by asymptomatic periods interrupted by episodes of viral reactivation from sites in the sensory ganglia, resulting in painful vesicular lesions on the skin or mucous membranes of the genital tract or mouth.[117] **Primary maternal HSV-2 infection** is associated with transient viremia, and up to 2% of pregnant women will be primarily infected during gestation.[117] Patients with primary infection may have systemic symptoms, including fever, headache, and lymphadenopathy, although asymptomatic primary infection is common. Epidemiologic evidence suggests that HSV-1, formerly associated only with perioral lesions (herpes labialis), is the predominant cause of new genital herpes infections in some populations.[118] During recurrent (i.e., secondary) infection, maternal antibodies prevent the recurrence of viremia. Thus, systemic symptoms are less severe—or do not occur at all—during episodes of recurrent infection. However, recurrent infection may result in severe symptoms localized to the site of the lesions on the external genitalia. Prodromal symptoms, including vulvar pain or burning, often precede development of recurrent lesions. Unfortunately, asymptomatic shedding of the virus also may occur in the genital tract.[117]

Interaction With Pregnancy

The major obstetric concern is the potential for transmission of the virus to the infant at the time of birth. The infant may become infected in one of two ways: intrauterine infection can occur by ascent of the organism after rupture of membranes, or neonatal infection can occur as the fetus comes in direct contact with the virus during vaginal delivery.[117] Neonatal HSV infection is a life-threatening infection with the potential for permanent central nervous system (CNS) sequelae.[117]

Obstetric Management

Metaanalysis of seven randomized trials of antepartum antiviral therapy with **acyclovir** or **valacyclovir** demonstrated a reduction in the presence of active genital lesions at delivery (RR, 0.28) and requirement for cesarean delivery (RR, 0.30).[119] However, these trials could not demonstrate a reduction in neonatal HSV infection (there were no cases in any trial), and failure of suppressive therapy to prevent such transmission has been reported.[120]

Retrospective studies have suggested that the risk for neonatal HSV infection associated with a primary maternal infection is much greater than that associated with recurrent maternal infection or asymptomatic viral shedding.[117] The risk for transmission is 30% to 60% in the setting of a primary HSV outbreak, 3% in the setting of active recurrent HSV, and 0.02% without genital lesions at the time of delivery.[117] Most likely, there is a greater risk that the infant will be exposed to the virus during episodes of primary maternal infection; the lower incidence in cases of recurrent herpes is likely caused by passive transfer of antibodies to HSV from the mother to the fetus.[121]

A large epidemiologic study of 58,362 women provided direct evidence that cesarean delivery dramatically reduces the overall risk for HSV transmission to the neonate when HSV cultures of the cervix and external genitalia taken at the time of labor were positive (odds ratio [OR], 0.14).[121] Other risk factors for neonatal transmission included primary maternal HSV infection, use of invasive obstetric monitoring, and HSV-1 (compared with HSV-2) infection.[121]

The ACOG recommends cesarean delivery in parturients with active lesions or prodromal symptoms, regardless of whether it is a primary or recurrent infection.[117] In the setting of an active HSV lesion and rupture of membranes near term, cesarean delivery should be performed as soon as logistically feasible. There is no consensus regarding when the risk for HSV outweighs the risk for preterm delivery in the setting of preterm premature rupture of membranes[117];

however, in general, expectant management has become standard.

Anesthetic Management

There are at least five published retrospective studies of the use of neuraxial anesthesia in patients with genital HSV infection. These studies reported no serious neurologic sequelae related to the use of neuraxial anesthesia.[122-126] However, most of the patients in these studies had recurrent (secondary) infection. Two studies[123,124] were limited to patients with recurrent infection, a third report had a recurrent infection,[126] and a fourth report[122] did not indicate whether the patients had primary or recurrent infection. Bader et al.[125] reported outcomes for 169 women with genital herpes infection who underwent cesarean delivery. Five of the 169 women in this study had primary infections, and three of these women received spinal anesthesia. Of the three women, one had transient, postoperative weakness of the left leg. The authors stated, "None of the cases of primary infection had associated systemic symptom; it is therefore possible that some of these cases were actually misdiagnosed recurrent infections. The safety of regional anesthesia in patients with primary HSV infection remains unclear."[125]

Viremia rarely complicates recurrent episodes of genital herpes infection. Therefore, it is unlikely that a spinal or epidural needle could introduce virus into the CNS in patients with recurrent genital herpes infection. A consensus exists that it is safe to administer spinal or epidural anesthesia to women with recurrent genital herpes infection and no systemic symptoms. There are insufficient data to allow a definitive recommendation regarding the safety of neuraxial anesthesia in patients with primary infection who may be viremic. If the anesthesia provider is confronted with a patient with primary infection, the theoretical risk for CNS infection should be weighed against the risks associated with alternative methods of analgesia and anesthesia.

Finally, several studies have suggested that spinal or epidural administration of morphine for postcesarean delivery analgesia increases the incidence of **recurrence of oral HSV infection**. This phenomenon was confirmed in prospective randomized trials for both epidural[127] and intrathecal[128] morphine. The cause is unknown, but some investigators have speculated that pruritus and scratching play a role in reactivation of oral lesions. Boyle[129] concluded that facial pruritus is a marker of the migration of morphine to the trigeminal nucleus but not the cause of HSV recrudescence. She suggested that immunologic modulation by the opioid within this ganglion is the primary cause of the viral reactivation. Substantial evidence now supports this mechanism.[130] A case of HSV-1 meningitis after unintentional dural puncture and passage of an intrathecal catheter has been reported.[131] The patient underwent cesarean delivery with spinal bupivacaine, fentanyl, and morphine; the authors suggested that reactivation of HSV-1 caused by morphine, and the presence of the intrathecal catheter, may have contributed to the infection.[131] To our knowledge, there are no reports suggesting that epidural or intrathecal administration of opioids increases the risk for recurrent *genital* herpes infection. However, a possible case of postnatal transmission secondary to maternal reactivation of oral HSV from intrathecal morphine has been reported.[132]

Human Immunodeficiency Virus

Human immunodeficiency virus (HIV) is a member of the lentivirus subfamily of human retroviruses (i.e., it carries the enzyme reverse transcriptase). This enzyme converts the single-stranded viral RNA into double-stranded DNA, which subsequently can be integrated into the DNA of the infected cell. This process is error prone, leading to rapid mutation of the virus, which significantly complicates drug therapy. Immune suppression is mainly caused by infection of helper T cells, $CD4^+$ monocytes, and macrophages. Abnormalities of these elements of the immune system render the HIV patient vulnerable to bacterial, viral, fungal, parasitic, and mycobacterial infection. In addition, for reasons that are not entirely clear, patients infected with HIV are susceptible to several malignancies (e.g., Kaposi's sarcoma, B-cell lymphoma, invasive cervical carcinoma). Clinical manifestations can affect every organ system and result from the HIV infection itself, opportunistic infection, secondary malignancy, or long-term exposure to antiretroviral therapy (ART).

In the United States, the estimated number of live births to women with diagnosed HIV decreased from approximately 4500 in 2010 to approximately 3500 in 2019.[133] In the setting of opt-out HIV screening in pregnancy as well

as risk-reducing strategies such as ART, scheduled cesarean delivery, and avoidance of breastfeeding, the number of perinatal transmissions of HIV in the United States has decreased dramatically.[133] The number of infants who acquired HIV perinatally in the United States decreased from 216 in 2002 to 74 in 2010 to 32 in 2019.[133,134]

Interaction With Pregnancy

Available data are mixed on whether HIV infection increases the risk for adverse pregnancy outcomes (e.g., low birth weight, small for gestational age, and preterm delivery).[135,136] ART, especially protease inhibitor–based ART, may increase the risk for preterm delivery,[137-139] but does not appear to lead to low birth weight, small for gestational age, or stillbirth.[139,140] Likewise, no evidence suggests that pregnancy accelerates clinical deterioration in the HIV-infected patient or that the viral RNA load changes significantly during pregnancy.[135,141,142]

Obstetric Management

Antenatal testing for HIV is part of routine prenatal screening, ideally completed in the first trimester of pregnancy, or as early as possible during the pregnancy, using an opt-out approach.[143] Repeat HIV testing is recommended in the third trimester for patients at high risk for acquiring HIV infection or who live in areas with elevated HIV incidence.[144] Women with undocumented HIV status should have rapid HIV testing upon presentation for delivery to guide appropriate treatment to prevent vertical transmission (Fig. 36.1).[143] For those diagnosed with HIV, serial plasma HIV RNA levels, $CD4^+$

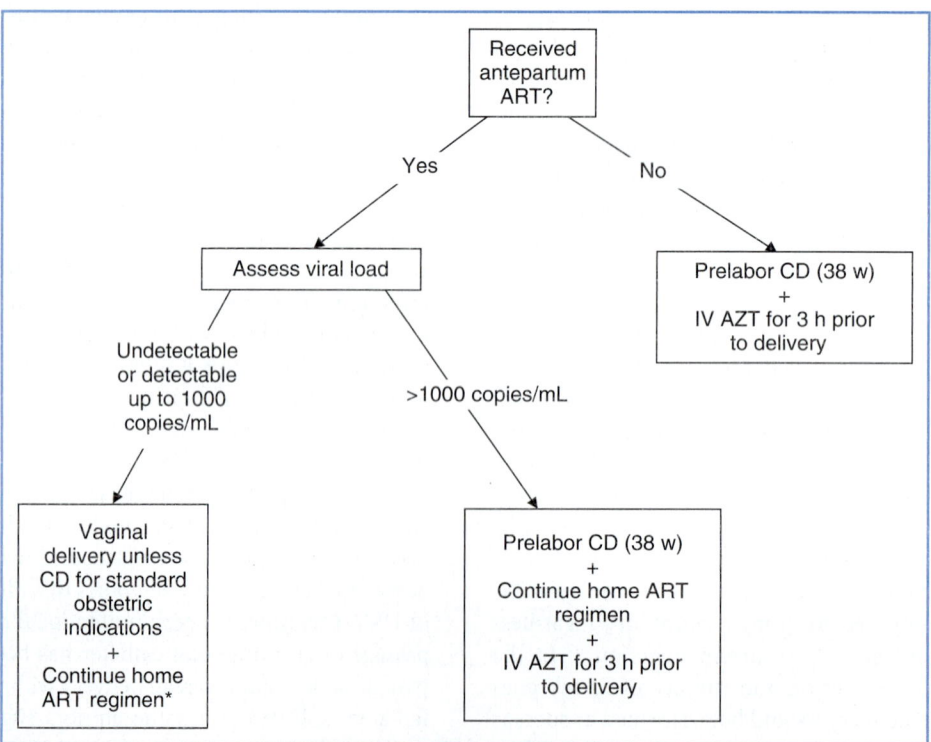

Fig. 36.1 Intrapartum Management for HIV-Infected Pregnant Women. *ART,* Antiretroviral therapy; *AZT,* azidothymidine, also known as zidovudine; *CD,* cesarean delivery; *IV,* intravenous. *IV AZT may be considered at the discretion of the provider.

T lymphocyte cell counts, and HIV drug-resistance assays are used to optimize ART throughout pregnancy, and plasma HIV RNA levels repeated at 34 to 36 weeks' gestation are used to guide decisions about mode of delivery and treatment of the newborn.

Intrapartum Antiretroviral Therapy/Prophylaxis

Pregnant women should continue their antepartum ART drug regimen without interruption during labor and delivery to provide maximal virologic suppression and to minimize the chance of development of drug resistance.[139] Additionally, to minimize vertical transmission, IV **zidovudine (AZT)** should be administered as soon as possible upon arrival for delivery to HIV-infected women with a viral load that is high (HIV RNA > 1000 copies/mL) or unknown, with a goal of at least 3 hours of administration before delivery.[139] For women with an HIV RNA ≤ 1000 copies/mL but still with a detectable viral load (50 to 1000 copies/mL), IV AZT is not necessary but may be considered, especially in cases of unclear compliance with medications or a recent increase in viral load.[139] Multiple studies have demonstrated that in the setting of virologic suppression (i.e., HIV RNA < 50 copies/mL), the addition of IV AZT did not provide additional protection against vertical transmission and therefore is not recommended.[145-148] Irrespective of viral load, the clinician may use intrapartum IV AZT based on clinical judgment.[139]

Mode of Delivery

For women with plasma HIV RNA > 1000 copies/mL near term, the ACOG recommends scheduled cesarean delivery at 38 weeks' gestation to reduce the risk for labor or rupture of membranes before delivery. IV AZT administration (loading dose followed by infusion) should be started 3 hours before the scheduled cesarean delivery, allowing adequate time to reach equilibrium across the placenta, although cord blood zidovudine levels required to prevent perinatal transmission of HIV are currently unknown.[149] Similar to women delivering vaginally, if the viral load is 1000 copies/mL or less at the time of cesarean delivery (i.e., the cesarean delivery is not performed for the indication of maternal HIV), IV AZT is not necessary, but may be considered[139] (see Fig. 36.1).

After membrane rupture or onset of labor in women with a detectable viral load, the optimal strategies for zidovudine administration and mode of delivery are not established. There have been similar rates of vertical transmission reported for cesarean delivery performed for obstetric indications after labor and membrane rupture as for vaginal delivery; however, there appear to be increasing rates of transmission for every additional hour after membrane rupture.[150,151] The duration after the onset of labor or the rupture of membranes at which there is no longer a benefit to performing cesarean delivery is unclear.[146,152-154]

Additional Intrapartum and Postpartum Management Considerations

In the setting of ART and an undetectable viral load, artificial rupture of membranes (AROM) is not associated with increased risk for perinatal transmission.[146,153] AROM should be avoided in women with detectable viral loads unless there is a strong clinical indication. Invasive obstetric procedures (e.g., fetal scalp electrode, intrauterine pressure catheter, operative vaginal delivery, episiotomy) that increase the chance of fetal exposure to maternal blood may increase the risk for vertical transmission. While this risk has not been well studied in women receiving suppressive ART, obstetric providers should avoid the routine use of these procedures in women with HIV.[155-158]

Medical management of postpartum hemorrhage in the setting of uterine atony may need to be modified based on the ART regimen. Based on manufacturer recommendations, the use of **methylergonovine maleate**, which is a major substrate of cytochrome P450 CYP3A4, should be avoided, if possible, in women receiving CYP3A4 enzyme inhibitors. CYP3A4 enzyme inhibitors include protease inhibitors (e.g., **ritonavir**, **indinavir**, **nelfinavir**), certain nonnucleoside reverse transcriptase inhibitors (e.g., **delavirdine**), and **cobicistat**. There have been reports of severe vasospasm leading to cerebral and extremity ischemia with concurrent use of ergot alkaloid drugs and CYP3A4 inhibitors.[159] Conversely, in women taking a CYP3A4 enzyme inducer (e.g., **nevirapine**, **efavirenz**, or **etravirine**), the efficacy of methylergonovine may be decreased.[159]

Finally, there has been considerable focus on infant feeding for patients living with HIV in the United States, and a call for a patient-centered approach to counseling to allow for and support shared decision-making. Using formula or pasteurized donor milk are the only feeding options that eliminate the risk of HIV transmission, and because of the risk of perinatal HIV transmission and the general availability and safety of formula or pasteurized donor milk in the United States, feeding a child using milk from an HIV-infected mother was previously discouraged. However, the risk of HIV transmission through breastfeeding for patients with **a sustained, undetectable viral load on ART** is very low (<1%),[160-162] and breastfeeding has known benefits. Importantly, individuals with a sustained, undetectable viral load on ART should be supported, regardless of whether they chose to breastfeed or to feed their infant with formula or pasteurized donor milk.[139] Patients with HIV who are not on ART and/or those with a detectable viral load should be counseled to feed their infant with formula or pasteurized donor milk.[139]

Anesthetic Management

Whether HIV-infected pregnant women are prone to the occurrence of infection after administration of neuraxial anesthesia is an important concern. In a study of 30 HIV-positive parturients, of whom 18 received neuraxial anesthesia and 12 did not, Hughes et al.[163] found no evidence of accelerated disease progression in either group, and no neurologic or infectious complications in either group immediately after delivery and at 4 to 6 months postpartum.[163] A later study demonstrated no postoperative changes in viral load or CD4+/CD8+ lymphocyte ratio and no increased hemodynamic instability or blood loss in HIV-infected patients undergoing elective cesarean delivery with spinal anesthesia.[164] The prevention of infectious complications of neuraxial anesthesia depends on strict aseptic technique, which should include handwashing with an alcohol-based antiseptic solution; removal of jewelry (e.g., rings, watches); and wearing sterile gloves, a face mask, and a hat (see Chapters 12 and 31). The CDC recommends that "universal blood and body-fluid precautions" should be used in the care of all patients, including goggles when anticipating contact with blood or bodily fluids.[165,166] For cases of occupational exposure, CDC or other guidelines for the management of healthcare worker exposures to HIV and recommendations for postexposure prophylaxis should be consulted.[166,167]

Neurologic involvement can occur at any time during HIV infection. Viral particles can be isolated from CSF at the time of primary infection.[168] Patients with HIV infection typically have CSF abnormalities, including the local synthesis of HIV antibody and the presence of HIV particles or viral nucleic acid.[168] This is an important consideration when determining the risk for introducing virus into the CNS during the performance of neuraxial anesthesia in an asymptomatic patient. It is almost certain that CNS infection has already occurred. There may be neurologic deficits associated with HIV infection. Prior to the performance of the neuraxial procedure, it is prudent to complete a thorough history and physical examination to document preexisting deficits and to conduct a postanesthesia evaluation to assess for any changes from baseline.

Despite the use of small-gauge, pencil-point spinal needles, and despite careful technique during administration of epidural anesthesia, PDPH remains a problem in pregnant patients (see Chapter 30). Clearly, the onset of headache and photophobia in an immunosuppressed patient who has recently received neuraxial anesthesia can be worrisome, but the typical postural nature of a PDPH should allay fears of bacterial meningitis. Once the diagnosis of PDPH is made, conservative therapy and pharmacologic interventions may be used. However, the "gold standard" for treatment of PDPH is an autologous epidural blood patch. Some physicians have expressed concern that the introduction of HIV-infected blood into the neuraxis might lead to the introduction of HIV into a previously uninfected CNS.[169] Even though CNS infection occurs quite early in the course of HIV disease, even in asymptomatic patients, it seems prudent to acknowledge the possibility that an epidural blood patch could accelerate the CNS manifestations of the disease. This question was addressed in a study of six seropositive patients who experienced PDPH after diagnostic lumbar puncture and who subsequently received an epidural blood patch.[170] These patients subsequently underwent serial neuropsychological testing for as long as 2 years. The investigators stated that "none of these six subjects had a decline in neurocognitive performance or other adverse neurologic or infectious sequelae" during the period of the study. Although these numbers are small and this study has never been repeated, it provides the best evidence to date of the safety of epidural blood patch in an HIV-infected patient.

As with neuraxial anesthesia, it is appropriate to ask whether patients with HIV might be more susceptible to the infectious (e.g., pulmonary) complications of general anesthesia. No published study has addressed this question.

However, it seems appropriate to handle the endotracheal tube in as sterile a manner as possible and to minimize the duration of postoperative ventilation. Care should also be taken to maintain sterility of intravenous lines by scrubbing injection ports with alcohol, placing caps on stopcocks when not in use, and not allowing the IV line to touch the floor.

Another question involves the effect of general anesthesia on immune function. Several studies have suggested that general anesthesia can transiently depress immune function; this depression appears to be clinically insignificant in healthy patients but has not been studied in patients with HIV disease.[171] At present, it would be inappropriate to recommend one anesthetic technique over another on the basis of unknown effects on immune function.[172]

SEPSIS AND SEPTIC SHOCK

Definition

Sepsis is defined by the Society of Critical Care Medicine and the European Society of Intensive Care Medicine as "life-threatening organ dysfunction caused by a dysregulated host response to infection."[173] The term "severe sepsis" is no longer used because of redundancy. **Septic shock** is defined as "a subset of sepsis in which profound circulatory, cellular, and metabolic abnormalities are associated with a greater risk for mortality than with sepsis alone." It can be identified clinically in patients with a vasopressor requirement and a lactic acid level greater than 2 mmol/L despite adequate fluid resuscitation.[173]

Sepsis remains an important cause of maternal mortality and morbidity, with an incidence that has not meaningfully changed over the past few decades. Between 2017 and 2019 in the United States, infection accounted for 14.3% of all maternal deaths, with a cause-specific mortality ratio of 2.5 deaths per 100,000 live births.[174] In a population-based study of sepsis in delivery hospitalizations, Bauer et al.[82] reported that the most common infections were pneumonia, genitourinary infection, and chorioamnionitis. Although only 40.4% reported a specific organism, the most common organisms were *E. coli*, staphylococcus, streptococcus, and gram-negative organisms. While multiple independent risk factors have been reported in the literature, authors have noted that sepsis often occurs in the absence of risk factors.[82] Sepsis occurs more commonly with postpartum readmissions (compared with delivery hospitalization) and is a leading cause of postpartum maternal deaths.[175,176]

Screening and Diagnosis

Given the importance of early identification and treatment, prompt recognition is key. Clinically, sepsis is now defined as the combination of infection with end-organ injury. If end-organ injury is suspected, it is essential to assess for infection. If a patient has a suspected infection, it is essential to monitor closely for end-organ injury. Serial bedside evaluation is desirable to detect trends in vital signs and clinical status and to more rapidly assess and reassess for signs of sepsis.[173]

Several **screening tools** exist to help in the identification of sepsis (Table 36.1). Maternal Early Warning criteria were proposed by the National Partnership for Maternal Safety as a set of criteria to identify impending maternal morbidity from a variety of causes.[177] These were then modified slightly by the Safe Motherhood Initiative.[178] The California Maternal Quality Care Collaborative (CMQCC) and the UK Obstetric Surveillance System (UKOSS) both use modified systemic inflammatory response syndrome (SIRS) criteria.[179,180] Previous diagnostic criteria using two or more abnormal values of the SIRS criteria were nonspecific; patients with noninfectious inflammatory processes exhibit these signs, including healthy pregnant patients.[181] The Maternal Early Warning Trigger tool has been shown to reduce severe maternal morbidity when combined with protocols for treatment.[182] A study by Bauer et al.[183] demonstrated that using a nonpregnancy adjusted tool prior to 20 weeks' gestation and after 3 days postpartum will have improved sensitivity to identify patients at risk for sepsis. During delivery hospitalizations, UKOSS and CMQCC criteria have sensitivity > 90% with the lowest false-positive rates for screening.[184] Given the rarity of maternal sepsis, utilizing a screening tool to assess multiple types of morbidity at once rather than using a separate tool for each may be the best approach. It is recommended that if

TABLE 36.1	Pregnancy-Adjusted Screening Tools for Sepsis and Severe Maternal Morbidity
Organization/ Named Criteria	**Criteria**
California Maternal Quality Care Collaborative[a]	• Oral temperature < 36°C or > 38°C • Heart rate > 110 beats/min • Respiratory rate > 24/min • WBC > 15,000/µL (15 × 10⁹/L) or < 4000/µL (4 × 10⁹/L) or > 10% bands Positive if any two of four criteria are met (sustained for 15 min)
Maternal Early Warning Trigger Tool[b]	**Red criteria (any one sustained > 20 min)** • Heart rate < 50 beats/min or > 130 beats/min • Respiratory rate < 10/min or > 30/min • Oxygen saturation < 90% • Blood pressure > 160/110 mm Hg • Mean arterial pressure < 55 mm Hg **Yellow Criteria (any two sustained > 20 min)** • Heart rate > 110 beats/min • Respiratory rate > 24/min • Oxygen saturation < 93% • Blood pressure < 85/45 mm Hg • Temperature < 36°C or > 38°C
Safe Motherhood Initiative[c]	• Systolic BP < 90 mm Hg or > 160 mm Hg • Diastolic BP > 100 mm Hg • Heart rate < 50 beats/min or > 120 beats/min • Respiratory rate < 10/min or > 24/min • Oxygen saturation on room air < 95% • Oliguria < 35 mL/h × 2 h • Temperature < 36°C or > 38°C • WBC < 4000/µL (4 × 10⁹/L) or > 15,000/µL (15 × 10⁹/L) • Maternal agitation, confusion, or unresponsiveness Positive if any one criterion is met (sustained for 20 min)
UK Obstetric Surveillance System[d]	• Temperature < 36°C or > 38°C • Heart rate > 100 beats/min • Respiratory rate > 20/min • WBC > 17 × 10⁹/L (17,000/µL) or < 4 × 10⁹/L (4000/µL) or with 10% immature band forms Positive if any two of four criteria are met if measured on two occasions (at least 4 h apart for temperature, heart rate, and respiratory rate)

BP, Blood pressure; *WBC*, white blood cell count.

[a]Criteria from Gibbs R, Bauer M, Olvera L, et al. Improving diagnosis and treatment of maternal sepsis: a quality improvement toolkit. California Maternal Quality Care Collaborative; 2019. Available at: https://www.cmqcc.org/sites/default/files/Sepsis%20Toolkit_FINAL.2_Errata_7.1.22.pdf. Accessed 27 December 2024.

[b]Criteria from Shields LE, Wiesner S, Klein C, et al. Use of maternal early warning trigger tool reduces maternal morbidity. *Am J Obstet Gynecol.* 2016;214:527.e1–e6.

[c]Criteria from American College of Obstetricians and Gynecologists District II. Safe Motherhood Initiative: maternal safety bundle for sepsis in pregnancy. Available at: https://www.acog.org/community/districts-and-sections/district-ii/programs-and-resources/safe-motherhood-initiative. Accessed 13 December 2024.

[d]Criteria from National Perinatal Epidemiology Unit. UK Obstetric Surveillance System (UKOSS). Available at: https://www.npeu.ox.ac.uk/ukoss/completed-surveillance/ss. Accessed 13 December 2024.

a patient meets any screening tool criteria, the patient should receive prompt evaluation by a physician or other practitioner to assess for end-organ injury (to make the diagnosis of sepsis) with ability to escalate care.

In two case series of maternal deaths due to sepsis in Michigan and California, the authors found that deaths were preceded by delays in seeking care, provider recognition, treatment, and escalation of care.[185,186] Additionally, patient education of warning signs and provider education of the signs of sepsis should be improved. Presentation of sepsis during pregnancy and postpartum is different than in the general population; only 25% of patients who ultimately die of sepsis present with fever or hypothermia.[185] A diagnosis of pulmonary, genital tract, or other systemic infection should prompt close monitoring for end-organ injury, and therefore sepsis.

Organ dysfunction is required for **diagnosis** of sepsis, characterized by a score of 2 points or more on the Sequential Organ Failure Assessment (SOFA) score (Table 36.2).[173]

It is not known how SOFA performs in the identification of sepsis in pregnant patients. Parameters have not been adjusted for pregnancy. Pregnancy-adjusted changes such as lower creatinine levels, lower blood pressure (which nadirs at 20 weeks' gestation), and lower platelet count are not accounted for in the SOFA criteria; no standardized pregnancy-adjusted criteria to indicate end-organ injury are available. Any change in markers for end-organ injury should prompt concern for sepsis and the need for escalation of care.

The Sepsis in Obstetrics Score (SOS) may be useful for assessing the severity of illness, and to identify patients requiring ICU admission (Table 36.3). In a retrospective cohort of 850 women with clinical suspicion of sepsis, an SOS $\geq$ 6 was independently associated with ICU admission.[187] A

prospective validation study confirmed the threshold score of 6, making it the first score derived and validated in an obstetric population. The specificity of the score was 88%, but the sensitivity was only 64%. Additionally, given the low incidence of ICU admission, the negative predictive value of the score was excellent (98.6%), but the positive predictive value was poor (15%). It did not perform statistically better than other validated sepsis scoring systems.[188] A screening tool that consistently facilitates rapid diagnosis of sepsis as well as the need for escalation of care in pregnancy remains an unmet need.

Initial Treatment

Once diagnosis has been established, prompt treatment is of paramount importance. In nonobstetric patients, there is an increase in mortality of 7.6% for each hour delay in appropriate antibiotic administration.[189] Similarly, a multicenter case control study demonstrated a mortality rate of 8% in pregnant patients who received antibiotics within 1 hour and a mortality rate of 20% in patients who received antibiotics after 1 hour.[190] Care should be escalated to accommodate the resources and requirements to treat critically ill patients. Surviving Sepsis Campaign (SSC) Guidelines[191] were created to define best practice in the management of sepsis based on available evidence, with strong recommendations worded as "recommended" and weak recommendations as "suggested." The SSC guidelines *recommend* IV antimicrobial administration as soon as possible, ideally within 1 hour for patients with septic shock or a high likelihood for sepsis. The antibiotic regimen chosen should provide empiric coverage for common obstetric infections; a combination of **vancomycin** and **pipercillin/ tazobactam** should be considered if the cause is unknown or

TABLE 36.2	Sequential Organ Failure Assessment Score (SOFA)			
SOFA Score	**1**	**2**	**3**	**4**
Respiration				
Pao_2/Fio_2 (mm Hg)	<400	<300	<200 with respiratory support	<100 with respiratory support
Coagulation				
Platelets ($\times 10^3/\mu L$ [$\times 10^9/L$])	<150	<100	<50	<20
Liver				
Bilirubin (mg/dL [μmol/L])	1.2–1.9 [20–32]	2.0–5.9 [33–101]	6.0–11.9 [102–204]	>12.0 [>204]
Cardiovascular				
Hypotension	MAP < 70 mm Hg	Dopamine $\leq$ 5 or dobutamine (any dose)[a]	Dopamine 6–15, epinephrine $\leq$ 0.1, or norepinephrine $\leq$ 0.1[a]	Dopamine > 15 or epinephrine > 0.1 or norepinephrine > 0.1[a]
Central Nervous System				
Glasgow Coma Score	13–14	10–12	6–9	<6
Renal				
Creatinine (mg/dL [μmol/L]) or urine output	1.2–1.9 [110–170]	2.0–3.4 [171–299]	3.5–4.9 [300–440] or <500 mL/day	>5.0 [>440] or <200 mL/day

Fio₂, Fraction of inspired oxygen; *MAP*, mean arterial pressure; *Pao₂*, partial pressure of oxygen in arterial blood.
[a]Adrenergic agonist agents administered for at least 1 h (doses are in μg/kg/min).
From Vincent JL, Moreno R, Takala J, et al. The SOFA (Sepsis-related Organ Failure Assessment) score to describe organ dysfunction/failure. On behalf of the Working Group on Sepsis-Related Problems of the European Society of Intensive Care Medicine. *Intensive Care Med.* 1996;22:707–710.

TABLE 36.3 Sepsis in Obstetrics Score

Variable	High Abnormal Range				Normal Range	Low Abnormal Range			
Score	+4	+3	+2	+1	0	+1	+2	+3	+4
Temperature (°C)	>40.9	39–40.9		38.5–38.9	36–38.4	34–35.9	32–33.9	30–31.9	<30
Systolic blood pressure (mm Hg)					>90		70–90		<70
Heart rate (beats/min)	>179	150–179	130–149	120–129	≤119				
Respiratory rate (breaths/min)	>49	35–49		25–34	12–24	10–11	6–9		≤5
SpO$_2$ (%)					≥92%	90%–91%		85%–89%	<85%
White blood cell count (/µL) [× 10^9/L]	>39,900 [>39.9]		25,000–39,900 [25–39.9]	17,000–24,900 [17–24.9]	5700–16,900 [5.7–16.9]	3000–5600 [3–5.6]	1000–2900 [1–2.9]		<1000 [<1]
% Immature neutrophils			≥10%		<10%				
Lactic acid (mmol/L)			≥4		<4				

Spo$_2$, Blood oxygen saturation.
From Albright CM, Ali TN, Lopes V, et al. The Sepsis in Obstetrics Score: a model to identify risk of morbidity from sepsis in pregnancy. *Am J Obstet Gynecol*. 2014;211:39.e1–e8.

in cases of septic shock. Both the CMQCC sepsis toolkit and the Society for Maternal-Fetal Medicine Consult Series for Maternal Sepsis provide first-line antimicrobial selection for pregnant and postpartum common conditions.[180,192] Within the first 3 hours it is *suggested* to give 30 mL/kg (ideal body weight) of IV crystalloid fluid to treat sepsis-induced hypotension or septic shock. It is *recommended* to set an initial target mean arterial blood pressure of 65 mm Hg, with norepinephrine used as the first-line vasopressor, and the *suggested* addition of vasopressin to achieve hemodynamic goals. It is *suggested* that trends in serum lactate may be used to guide resuscitation.[191] In the Confidential Enquiries into Maternal Deaths and Morbidity in the United Kingdom and Ireland 2009 to 2012 report, it was also recommended to consult with an infectious disease specialist.[89] Further discussion of sepsis management is found in Chapter 53.

Although the effects of maternal therapy on the fetus should be considered, treatment of the mother has first priority. Fetal status is best optimized by meeting maternal treatment goals. For nonreassuring fetal heart rate patterns in the setting of maternal sepsis, fetal resuscitation *in utero* and maternal medical therapy are frequently successful in delaying delivery.[193] Nevertheless, in some cases, maternal sepsis may require delivery, even before viability, particularly if chorioamnionitis is present. In a 2013 series of maternal admissions for sepsis, 40% of women diagnosed with severe sepsis and all with septic shock required delivery during the same hospitalization and most required emergency delivery for worsening maternal respiratory status.[194] Maternal sepsis also increases the risk for perinatal mortality, with the rate of stillbirth approaching 33% when maternal sepsis requires ICU admission.[194-197] A multidisciplinary team should consider the mother's response to initial therapeutic interventions; vasopressor, oxygen, and ventilatory requirements; and the gestational age and fetal well-being when considering the optimal timing and route of delivery.

NEURAXIAL ANESTHESIA IN THE FEBRILE OR INFECTED PATIENT

Clinicians have long suspected an association between the performance of dural puncture during a period of bacteremia and the subsequent development of meningitis. Some clinicians have feared that diagnostic lumbar puncture may cause meningitis rather than aid in its diagnosis. They reasoned that lumbar puncture may disrupt the rich venous plexus surrounding the spinal cord and allow the direct introduction of infected blood into the CNS by the needle. Alternatively, others have speculated that disruption of the dural barrier may permit hematogenous spread of infection into the CNS without direct vessel trauma. Administration of continuous epidural analgesia often results in blood vessel trauma, and it includes the introduction of a foreign body. Theoretically, this technique could produce a nidus for subsequent infection.

This section focuses on the additional risk for CNS infection in the setting of bacteremia. The epidemiology of iatrogenic meningitis or epidural abscess as well as the discussion of lapses in sterile technique contributing to CNS infection are discussed in Chapter 31.

Laboratory Studies

Carp and Bailey[198] performed a study to assess the risk for meningitis after the performance of dural puncture in bacteremic rodents. In this study, rats were made bacteremic by producing a flank abscess using *E. coli*. The bacteremia was similar in magnitude to that which occurs during the early phase of sepsis in humans. Cisternal dural puncture was performed after the onset of bacteremia. After 24 hours, the cisterna magna was drained surgically, and the CSF was cultured for evidence of meningitis. Of the 40 animals that underwent dural puncture during *E. coli* bacteremia, 12 developed meningitis. None of the 40 bacteremic animals *not* subjected to dural puncture developed meningitis. Furthermore, dural puncture did not result in infection in the 30 animals without bacteremia. Importantly, *none* of the 30 bacteremic animals given a dose of gentamicin 15 minutes before dural puncture developed meningitis[198] (Table 36.4).

This study is consistent with earlier laboratory studies that observed the development of meningitis after the performance of dural puncture in bacteremic laboratory animals.[199,200] Although animal models of disease permit careful control of experimental conditions, these studies do not duplicate clinical conditions. Thus, there are limitations in the application of the rat study[198] to clinical practice. First, the level of bacteremia produced in the rats exceeded the transient, low-grade bacteremia that often occurs clinically. Second, although *E. coli* is a common cause of bacteremia in surgical and obstetric patients, it is an uncommon cause of meningitis. Third, the relative size of the dural tear produced by the 26-gauge needle used in this study is greater in rats than in humans. Fourth, the cisternal site of dural puncture

is not used clinically. Fifth, spinal and epidural anesthesia involves the injection of local anesthetic agents, and these drugs appear to be bacteriostatic.[201] Finally, the investigators knew the identity of the organism (*E. coli*) and also knew that it was susceptible to gentamicin.

In summary, this study suggests that high-grade bacteremia may increase the risk for meningitis after dural puncture. However, antibiotic therapy before dural puncture appears to reduce, if not eliminate, this risk.

Clinical Studies

At least six retrospective clinical studies have evaluated *diagnostic lumbar puncture* and the risk for meningitis.[202-207] (These studies did not evaluate the risk associated with neuraxial anesthesia or analgesia.) These reports provided conflicting conclusions regarding the risk for meningitis after the performance of dural puncture in bacteremic patients. Two studies suggested an association between dural puncture and meningitis.[202,205] However, both studies had serious methodologic flaws. A study performed during an epidemic of meningitis reported five cases of meningitis with initial negative CSF cultures (with positive blood cultures) and subsequent bacterial meningitis after lumbar puncture. However, they did not evaluate a comparable control group who did not undergo lumbar puncture.[202] Teele et al.[205] reported an association between lumbar puncture and meningitis only in bacteremic children younger than 1 year of age. Although there is a theoretical risk that a lumbar puncture seeded the meninges at the time of the procedure, it is also possible in both studies that diagnostic lumbar puncture was performed early in the progression of the disease before the CSF provided diagnostic evidence of infection. The remaining four studies clearly did not support an association between dural puncture and meningitis.[203,204,206,207]

Undoubtedly some parturients are bacteremic during the administration of epidural or spinal anesthesia, given the frequency with which parturients develop fever and infection during labor. For example, Blanco et al.[208] found a 1% incidence of bacteremia in a random sample of patients on the labor ward. Other studies have noted an incidence of bacteremia ranging from 5% to 12% in parturients with chorioamnionitis.[27,28,43,209] Although bacteremia is common, epidural abscess and meningitis rarely present after neuraxial blockade, and no epidemiologic study has clearly established a causal relationship between the performance of dural puncture during bacteremia and the subsequent development of meningitis or an epidural abscess.[210]

Bader et al.[211] retrospectively observed no cases of CNS infection after the administration of epidural or spinal anesthesia for labor or cesarean delivery in 279 patients with chorioamnionitis. Only 43 of these 279 women received antibiotic therapy before the administration of neuraxial anesthesia. At least three women had positive blood cultures consistent with bacteremia, and none of these three women received antibiotics before the administration of anesthesia. Similarly, Goodman et al.[27] found no cases of meningitis or epidural abscess among 531 patients with chorioamnionitis (proven by culture or pathologic examination) who received

TABLE 36.4   The Association Between Bacteremia and the Recovery of *Escherichia coli* From the Cerebrospinal Fluid After Dural Puncture in Rats

n	Bacteremia (CFU/mL)[a]	Gentamicin[b]	Dural Puncture	CSF *E. coli*[c]
40	40 ± 22 (5–100)	No	Yes	12/40[d]
40	48 ± 25[e] (2–100)	No	No	0/40
30	0 (0)	No	Yes	0/30
30	49 ± 35 (5–110)	Yes	Yes	0/30

CFU, Colony-forming units; *CSF*, cerebrospinal fluid.
[a]Mean ± standard deviation (range in parentheses).
[b]Gentamicin administered before dural puncture.
[c]Number of animals in which *E. coli* was cultured from spinal fluid per total number of animals in that group.
[d]*P* < .05 compared with other groups.
[e]Not significantly different from that in the bacteremia groups undergoing cisternal puncture.
Modified from Carp H, Bailey S. The association between meningitis and dural puncture in bacteremic rats. *Anesthesiology* 1992; 76:739–742.

epidural ($n = 517$) or spinal ($n = 14$) anesthesia. Eleven of 45 patients with fever before initiation of the neuraxial procedure, and 174 of 229 patients with preexisting leukocytosis, received no antibiotics before instrumentation of the epidural or subarachnoid space.

Together, these clinical studies (combined with evidence in nonfebrile women, presented in Chapter 31) suggest that meningitis and epidural abscess are rare complications of epidural or spinal anesthesia. Furthermore, bacteremia itself does not appear to increase the risk for CNS infection after the administration of neuraxial anesthesia. However, published studies of neuraxial anesthesia in patients with chorioamnionitis were small and retrospective. Given the infrequent occurrence of CNS infection among noninfected patients undergoing neuraxial anesthesia, none of these studies was sufficiently large to exclude the possibility that chorioamnionitis increases the risk for meningitis or epidural

abscess. Moreover, the retrospective study design introduces the possibility of selection bias; anesthesia providers may have avoided neuraxial anesthesia in the sickest patients with chorioamnionitis.

Recommendations

The 2017 ASA Practice Advisory for the Prevention, Diagnosis, and Management of Infectious Complications Associated with Neuraxial Techniques recommended performing a complete history, physical examination (including vital signs), and review of laboratory studies to identify patients at risk for infectious complications.[212] There is no specific laboratory parameter that precludes the use of neuraxial techniques. In pregnancy, C-reactive protein and erythrocyte sedimentation rate are elevated.[213,214] In a metaanalysis of more than 4500 healthy pregnant women, many women had a white blood cell count $> 12,000/\mu L$ ($12 \times 10^9/L$) in the

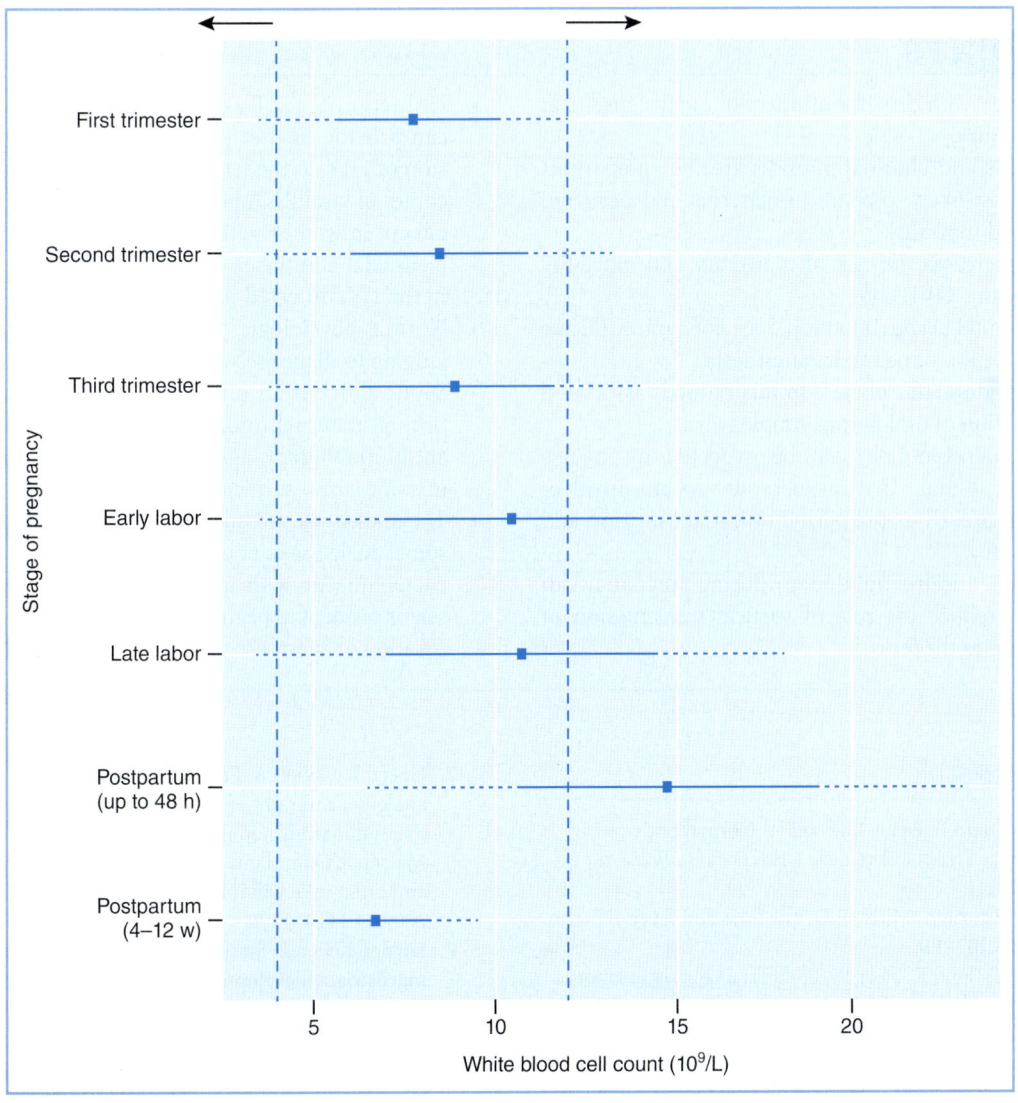

Fig. 36.2 Normal White Blood Cell Count Variation During Pregnancy and Postpartum. The mean is indicated by the center of each forest plot, 1 standard deviation (SD) is indicated by a *solid line*, and a *dotted line* indicates 2 SDs from the mean. *Vertical dotted lines* indicate systemic inflammatory response syndrome criteria. From Bauer ME, Bauer ST, Rajala B, et al. Maternal physiologic parameters in relationship to systemic inflammatory response syndrome criteria. *Obstet Gynecol.* 2014;124:535–541.

absence of infection (Fig. 36.2).[181] These tests are unreliable to determine infection or severity of infection in pregnant women. We recommend an evaluation of the patient's entire clinical picture to weigh the risks and benefits for performing a neuraxial technique. In our judgment, the anesthesia provider may safely administer spinal or epidural anesthesia to healthy patients at risk for low-grade bacteremia. Appropriate antibiotic therapy may lessen the risk for meningitis or epidural abscess in patients with established infection. Thus, it often is appropriate for the anesthesia provider to request the initiation of antibiotic therapy before administration of neuraxial blockade in accordance with the ASA practice advisory.[212] Finally, the choice of anesthesia must be individualized; it seems prudent to avoid spinal or epidural anesthesia in untreated patients who are hemodynamically unstable. During the COVID-19 pandemic, many patients met the criteria for sepsis (e.g., respiratory dysfunction, renal dysfunction, requirement for low-dose vasopressors) and safely received neuraxial anesthetic procedures. The risk-benefit ratio should be assessed with each patient to determine the optimal anesthetic technique for the clinical situation.

POSTINFECTIOUS ILLNESS

There are a number of postviral or postbacterial illnesses that cause long-term effects after acute illness (e.g., long COVID). There are reports of patients who are receiving intravenous long-term antibiotic therapy for conditions such as posttreatment Lyme disease syndrome. There is no known benefit to long-term antibiotic therapy and it may be harmful.[215] The long-term effects, such as fatigue, pain, and joint and muscle aches, are not thought to be related to a current infection. Neuraxial anesthetic procedures are appropriate in these patients after assessment and treatment of the acute illness.

KEY POINTS

- Maternal fever, with or without infection, may cause fetal neurologic injury.
- Pyelonephritis and chorioamnionitis are the antepartum infections most likely to result in maternal and perinatal morbidity and mortality.
- Pregnancy increases the risk of morbidity and mortality associated with COVID-19.
- Recurrent genital herpes infection does not contraindicate the administration of neuraxial anesthesia.
- Spinal and epidural morphine administration is associated with reactivation of oral herpes simplex virus.
- HIV infection eventually can be expected to involve every organ system. Central nervous system involvement occurs as early as the period of initial infection and seroconversion.
- Highly active antiretroviral therapy during pregnancy can significantly reduce the rate of vertical transmission of HIV infection to the fetus.

- Utilization of AZT as well as scheduled cesarean delivery can provide further protection against vertical transmission of HIV to the fetus in women with greater than 1000 copies of viral RNA per mL of plasma, and AZT may be of benefit in women with lower viral loads as well.
- Neuraxial anesthesia and autologous blood patch are safe in the HIV-infected parturient.
- Normal physiologic changes in pregnancy make it challenging to diagnose sepsis.
- Septic shock is an uncommon but devastating complication of maternal infection that demands broad-spectrum antibiotic therapy, aggressive hemodynamic support, and in some cases, surgical intervention.
- The anesthesia provider may safely administer epidural or spinal analgesia or anesthesia to patients at risk for transient bacteremia or with an established infection. However, it seems prudent to begin antibiotic therapy before the administration of anesthesia in patients with established infection.

REFERENCES

1. Geneva II, Cuzzo B, Fazili T, Javaid W. Normal body temperature: a systematic review. *Open Forum Infect Dis.* 2019;6:ofz032.
2. Laburn HP, Faurie A, Mitchell D. The fetus and fever. *J Therm Biol.* 2003;28:107–116.
3. Macaulay JH, Bond K, Steer PJ. Epidural analgesia in labor and fetal hyperthermia. *Obstet Gynecol.* 1992;80:665–669.
4. Benson MD, Haney E, Dinsmoor M, Beaumont JL. Shaking rigors in parturients. *J Reprod Med.* 2008;53:685–690.
5. Gleeson NC, Nolan KM, Ford MR. Temperature, labour, and epidural analgesia. *Lancet.* 1989;2:861–862.
6. Mayer DC, Chescheir NC, Spielman FJ. Increased intrapartum antibiotic administration associated with epidural analgesia in labor. *Am J Perinatol.* 1997;14:83–86.
7. Goetzl L, Cohen A, Frigoletto F Jr, et al. Maternal epidural analgesia and rates of maternal antibiotic treatment in a low-risk nulliparous population. *J Perinatol.* 2003;23:457–461.
8. Malaeb S, Dammann O. Fetal inflammatory response and brain injury in the preterm newborn. *J Child Neurol.* 2009;24:1119–1126.
9. Snyder-Keller A, Stark PF. Prenatal inflammatory effects on nigrostriatal development in organotypic cultures. *Brain Res.* 2008;1233:160–167.
10. Yoon BH, Romero R, Park JS, et al. Fetal exposure to an intra-amniotic inflammation and the development of cerebral palsy at the age of three years. *Am J Obstet Gynecol.* 2000;182:675–681.
11. Rodts-Palenik S, Wyatt-Ashmead J, Pang Y, et al. Maternal infection-induced white matter injury is reduced by treatment with interleukin-10. *Am J Obstet Gynecol.* 2004;191:1387–1392.

12. Impey L, Greenwood C, MacQuillan K, et al. Fever in labour and neonatal encephalopathy: a prospective cohort study. *BJOG.* 2001;108:594–597.

13. Impey LW, Greenwood CE, Black RS, et al. The relationship between intrapartum maternal fever and neonatal acidosis as risk factors for neonatal encephalopathy. *Am J Obstet Gynecol.* 2008;198:49.e1–e6.

14. Goetzl L, Korte JE. Interaction between intrapartum maternal fever and fetal acidosis increases risk for neonatal encephalopathy. *Am J Obstet Gynecol.* 2008;199:e9.

15. Dior UP, Kogan L, Eventov-Friedman S, et al. Very high intrapartum fever in term pregnancies and adverse obstetric and neonatal outcomes. *Neonatology.* 2016;109:62–68.

16. Petrova A, Demissie K, Rhoads GG, et al. Association of maternal fever during labor with neonatal and infant morbidity and mortality. *Obstet Gynecol.* 2001;98:20–27.

17. Hensel D, Zhang F, Carter EB, et al. Severity of intrapartum fever and neonatal outcomes. *Am J Obstet Gynecol.* 2022;227:513.e1–e8.

18. Milunsky A, Ulcickas M, Rothman KJ, et al. Maternal heat exposure and neural tube defects. *JAMA.* 1992;268:882–885.

19. Li DK, Janevic T, Odouli R, Liu L. Hot tub use during pregnancy and the risk of miscarriage. *Am J Epidemiol.* 2003;158:931–937.

20. Duong HT, Shahrukh Hashmi S, Ramadhani T, et al. Maternal use of hot tub and major structural birth defects. *Birth Defects Res A Clin Mol Teratol.* 2011;91:836–841.

21. Rosevear SK, Fox R, Marlow N, Stirrat GM. Birthing pools and the fetus. *Lancet.* 1993;342:1048–1049.

22. Patel S, Ciechanowicz S, Blumenfeld YJ, Sultan P. Epidural-related maternal fever: Incidence, pathophysiology, outcomes, and management. *Am J Obstet Gynecol.* 2023;228:S1283–S1304.

23. Jung E, Romero R, Suksai M, et al. Clinical chorioamnionitis at term: definition, pathogenesis, microbiology, diagnosis, and treatment. *Am J Obstet Gynecol.* 2024;230:S807–S840.

24. Kim CJ, Romero R, Chaemsaithong P, et al. Acute chorioamnionitis and funisitis: definition, pathologic features, and clinical significance. *Am J Obstet Gynecol.* 2015;213:S29–S52.

25. Higgins RD, Saade G, Polin RA, et al. Evaluation and management of women and newborns with a maternal diagnosis of chorioamnionitis: summary of a workshop. *Obstet Gynecol.* 2016;127:426–436.

26. American College of Obstetricians and Gynecologists. Committee Opinion No. 712: Intrapartum management of intraamniotic infection (reaffirmed 2022). *Obstet Gynecol.* 2017;130:e95–e101.

27. Goodman EJ, DeHorta E, Taguiam JM. Safety of spinal and epidural anesthesia in parturients with chorioamnionitis. *Reg Anesth.* 1996;21:436–441.

28. Yoder PR, Gibbs RS, Blanco JD, et al. A prospective, controlled study of maternal and perinatal outcome after intra-amniotic infection at term. *Am J Obstet Gynecol.* 1983;145:695–701.

29. Romero R, Espinoza J, Gonçalves LF, et al. The role of inflammation and infection in preterm birth. *Semin Reprod Med.* 2007;25:21–39.

30. Nath CA, Ananth CV, Smulian JC, et al. Histologic evidence of inflammation and risk of placental abruption. *Am J Obstet Gynecol.* 2007;197:319.e1–e6.

31. Rouse DJ, Leindecker S, Landon M, et al. The MFMU Cesarean Registry: uterine atony after primary cesarean delivery. *Am J Obstet Gynecol.* 2005;193:1056–1060.

32. Mark SP, Croughan-Minihane MS, Kilpatrick SJ. Chorioamnionitis and uterine function. *Obstet Gynecol.* 2000;95:909–912.

33. Satin AJ, Maberry MC, Leveno KJ, et al. Chorioamnionitis: a harbinger of dystocia. *Obstet Gynecol.* 1992;79:913–915.

34. Rouse DJ, Landon M, Leveno KJ, et al. The Maternal-Fetal Medicine Units cesarean registry: chorioamnionitis at term and its duration-relationship to outcomes. *Am J Obstet Gynecol.* 2004;191:211–216.

35. Bommarito KM, Gross GA, Willers DM, et al. The effect of clinical chorioamnionitis on cesarean delivery in the United States. *Health Serv Res.* 2016;51:1879–1895.

36. Duff P, Sanders R, Gibbs RS. The course of labor in term patients with chorioamnionitis. *Am J Obstet Gynecol.* 1983;147:391–395.

37. Escobar GJ, Puopolo KM, Wi S, et al. Stratification of risk of early-onset sepsis in newborns ≥34 weeks' gestation. *Pediatrics.* 2014;133:30–36.

38. Bizzarro MJ, Raskind C, Baltimore RS, Gallagher PG. Seventy-five years of neonatal sepsis at Yale: 1928-2003. *Pediatrics.* 2005;116:595–602.

39. Puopolo KM, Draper D, Wi S, et al. Estimating the probability of neonatal early-onset infection on the basis of maternal risk factors. *Pediatrics.* 2011;128:e1155–e1163.

40. Schrag SJ, Farley MM, Petit S, et al. Epidemiology of invasive early-onset neonatal sepsis, 2005 to 2014. *Pediatrics.* 2016;138:e20162013.

41. Shi Z, Ma L, Luo K, et al. Chorioamnionitis in the development of cerebral palsy: a meta-analysis and systematic review. *Pediatrics.* 2017;139:e20163781.

42. Gaudet LM, Smith GN. Cerebral palsy and chorioamnionitis: the inflammatory cytokine link. *Obstet Gynecol Surv.* 2001;56:433–436.

43. Gibbs RS, Castillo MS, Rodgers PJ. Management of acute chorioamnionitis. *Am J Obstet Gynecol.* 1980;136:709–713.

44. American College of Obstetricians and Gynecologists Practice Bulletin No. 116: Management of intrapartum fetal heart rate tracings (reaffirmed 2025). *Obstet Gynecol.* 2010;116:1232–1240.

45. Venkatesh KK, Jackson W, Hughes BL, et al. Association of chorioamnionitis and its duration with neonatal morbidity and mortality. *J Perinatol.* 2019;39:673–682.

46. Tita AT, Szychowski JM, Boggess K, et al. Adjunctive azithromycin prophylaxis for cesarean delivery. *N Engl J Med.* 2016;375:1231–1241.

47. Edwards RK, Duff P. Single additional dose postpartum therapy for women with chorioamnionitis. *Obstet Gynecol.* 2003;102:957–961.

48. Turnquest MA, How HY, Cook CR, et al. Chorioamnionitis: is continuation of antibiotic therapy necessary after cesarean section? *Am J Obstet Gynecol.* 1998;179:1261–1266.

49. Black LP, Hinson L, Duff P. Limited course of antibiotic treatment for chorioamnionitis. *Obstet Gynecol.* 2012;119:1102–1105.

50. Wylie B. Bacterial and parasitic infections in pregnancy. In: Lockwood C, Moore T, Copel J, et al., eds. *Creasy and Resnik's Maternal-Fetal Medicine: Principles and Practice.* 9th ed. Elsevier; 2022:879–907.

51. Gilstrap LC 3rd, Ramin SM. Urinary tract infections during pregnancy. *Obstet Gynecol Clin North Am.* 2001;28:581–591.

52. Angel JL, O'Brien WF, Finan MA, et al. Acute pyelonephritis in pregnancy: a prospective study of oral versus intravenous antibiotic therapy. *Obstet Gynecol.* 1990;76:28–32.

53. Hill JB, Sheffield JS, McIntire DD, Wendel GD Jr. Acute pyelonephritis in pregnancy. *Obstet Gynecol.* 2005;105:18–23.

54. Barry R, Houlihan E, Knowles SJ, et al. Antenatal pyelonephritis: a three-year retrospective cohort study of two Irish maternity centres. *Eur J Clin Microbiol Infect Dis.* 2023;42:827–833.

55. Cunningham FG, Lucas MJ, Hankins GD. Pulmonary injury complicating antepartum pyelonephritis. *Am J Obstet Gynecol.* 1987;156:797–807.

56. Towers CV, Kaminskas CM, Garite TJ, et al. Pulmonary injury associated with antepartum pyelonephritis: can patients at risk be identified? *Am J Obstet Gynecol.* 1991;164:974–978.

57. Wing DA. Pyelonephritis in pregnancy: treatment options for optimal outcomes. *Drugs.* 2001;61:2087–2096.

58. Wing DA, Hendershott CM, Debuque L, Millar LK. Outpatient treatment of acute pyelonephritis in pregnancy after 24 weeks. *Obstet Gynecol.* 1999;94:683–688.

59. Toppozada H, Michaels L, Toppozada M, et al. The human respiratory nasal mucosa in pregnancy. An electron microscopic and histochemical study. *J Laryngol Otol.* 1982;96:613–626.

60. Brito V, Niederman MS. Pneumonia complicating pregnancy. *Clin Chest Med.* 2011;32:121–132.

61. Lim WS, Macfarlane JT, Colthorpe CL. Treatment of community-acquired lower respiratory tract infections during pregnancy. *Am J Respir Med.* 2003;2:221–233.

62. Benedetti TJ, Valle R, Ledger WJ. Antepartum pneumonia in pregnancy. *Am J Obstet Gynecol.* 1982;144:413–417.

63. Kawakita T, Landy HJ. Surgical site infections after cesarean delivery: epidemiology, prevention and treatment. *Matern Health Neonatol Perinatol.* 2017;3:12.

64. Horan TC, Gaynes RP, Martone WJ, et al. CDC definitions of nosocomial surgical site infections, 1992: a modification of CDC definitions of surgical wound infections. *Am J Infect Control.* 1992;20:271–274.

65. Temming LA, Raghuraman N, Carter EB, et al. Impact of evidence-based interventions on wound complications after cesarean delivery. *Am J Obstet Gynecol.* 2017;217:449.e1–e9.

66. Smaill FM, Grivell RM. Antibiotic prophylaxis versus no prophylaxis for preventing infection after cesarean section. *Cochrane Database Syst Rev.* 2014;(10):CD007482.

67. van Schalkwyk J, Van Eyk N. Antibiotic prophylaxis in obstetric procedures. *J Obstet Gynaecol Can.* 2010;32:878–892.

68. American College of Obstetricians and Gynecologists. Practice Bulletin No. 199: Use of prophylactic antibiotics in labor and delivery (reaffirmed 2025). *Obstet Gynecol.* 2018;132;(3):e103–e119. Erratum in: *Obstet Gynecol.* 2019 Oct;134:883–884.

69. Kawakita T, Huang CC, Landy HJ. Choice of prophylactic antibiotics and surgical site infections after cesarean delivery. *Obstet Gynecol.* 2018;132:948–955.

70. Gill MM, Gasner S, Banken A, et al. Improving routine prenatal penicillin allergy testing for reported penicillin allergy. *BMJ Open Qual.* 2022;11:e001859.

71. Maggio L, Nicolau DP, DaCosta M, et al. Cefazolin prophylaxis in obese women undergoing cesarean delivery: a randomized controlled trial. *Obstet Gynecol.* 2015;125:1205–1210.

72. Young OM, Shaik IH, Twedt R, et al. Pharmacokinetics of cefazolin prophylaxis in obese gravidae at time of cesarean delivery. *Am J Obstet Gynecol.* 2015;213:e1–e7.

73. Swank ML, Wing DA, Nicolau DP, McNulty JA. Increased 3-gram cefazolin dosing for cesarean delivery prophylaxis in obese women. *Am J Obstet Gynecol.* 2015;213:e1–e8.

74. American College of Obstetricians and Gynecologists. Practice Bulletin No. 195: Prevention of infection after gynecologic procedures (reaffirmed 2022). *Obstet Gynecol.* 2018;131:e172–e189.

75. Hadiati DR, Hakimi M, Nurdiati DS, et al. Skin preparation for preventing infection following caesarean section. *Cochrane Database Syst Rev.* 2020;(6):CD007462.

76. Caissutti C, Saccone G, Zullo F, et al. Vaginal cleansing before cesarean delivery: a systematic review and meta-analysis. *Obstet Gynecol.* 2017;130:527–538.

77. Carter EB, Temming LA, Fowler S, et al. Evidence-based bundles and cesarean delivery surgical site infections: a systematic review and meta-analysis. *Obstet Gynecol.* 2017;130:735–746.

78. Chongsomchai C, Lumbiganon P, Laopaiboon M. Prophylactic antibiotics for manual removal of retained placenta in vaginal birth. *Cochrane Database Syst Rev.* 2014;(10):CD004904.

79. Chibueze EC, Parsons AJ, Ota E, et al. Prophylactic antibiotics for manual removal of retained placenta during vaginal birth: a systematic review of observational studies and meta-analysis. *BMC Pregnancy Childbirth.* 2015;15:313.

80. Liabsuetrakul T, Choobun T, Peeyananjarassri K, Islam QM. Antibiotic prophylaxis for operative vaginal delivery. *Cochrane Database Syst Rev.* 2017;(8):CD004455.

81. AAP Committee of Fetus and Newborn and ACOG Committee on Obstetric Practice. *Guidelines for Perinatal Care.* 8th ed. American Academy of Pediatrics and American College of Obstetricians and Gynecologists; 2017.

82. Bauer ME, Bateman BT, Bauer ST, et al. Maternal sepsis mortality and morbidity during hospitalization for delivery: temporal trends and independent associations for severe sepsis. *Anesth Analg.* 2013;117:944–950.

83. Barton JR, Sibai BM. Severe sepsis and septic shock in pregnancy. *Obstet Gynecol.* 2012;120:689–706.

84. Anderson BL. Puerperal group A streptococcal infection: beyond Semmelweis. *Obstet Gynecol.* 2014;123:874–882.

85. Harris K, Proctor LK, Shinar S, et al. Outcomes and management of pregnancy and puerperal group A streptococcal infections: a systematic review. *Acta Obstet Gynecol Scand.* 2023;102:138–157.

86. Siston AM, Rasmussen SA, Honein MA, et al. Pandemic 2009 influenza A(H1N1) virus illness among pregnant women in the United States. *JAMA.* 2010;303:1517–1525.

87. Saad AF, Rahman M, Maybauer DM, et al. Extracorporeal membrane oxygenation in pregnant and postpartum women with H1N1-related acute respiratory distress syndrome: a systematic review and meta-analysis. *Obstet Gynecol.* 2016;127:241–247.

88. Grohskopf LA, Sokolow LZ, Broder KR, et al. Prevention and control of seasonal influenza with vaccines: recommendations of the advisory committee on immunization practices—United States, 2017–18 influenza season. *MMWR Recomm Rep.* 2017;66:1–20.

89. Knight M, Kenyon S, Brocklehurst P, et al. *Saving Lives, Improving Mothers' Care—Lessons Learned to Inform Future Maternity Care From the UK and Ireland Confidential Enquiries Into Maternal Deaths and Morbidity 2009–2012.*

National Perinatal Epidemiology Unit, University of Oxford; 2014.

90. Håberg SE, Trogstad L, Gunnes N, et al. Risk of fetal death after pandemic influenza virus infection or vaccination. *N Engl J Med*. 2013;368:333–340.

91. Steinhoff MC, Omer SB, Roy E, et al. Influenza immunization in pregnancy-antibody responses in mothers and infants. *N Engl J Med*. 2010;362:1644–1646.

92. Hansen C, Desai S, Bredfeldt C, et al. A large, population-based study of 2009 pandemic influenza A virus subtype H1N1 infection diagnosis during pregnancy and outcomes for mothers and neonates. *J Infect Dis*. 2012;206:1260–1268.

93. Wollenhaupt M, Chandrasekaran A, Tomianovic D. The safety of oseltamivir in pregnancy: an updated review of post-marketing data. *Pharmacoepidemiol Drug Saf*. 2014;23: 1035–1042.

94. Ghulmiyyah LM, Alame MM, Mirza FG, et al. Influenza and its treatment during pregnancy: a review. *J Neonatal Perinatal Med*. 2015;8:297–306.

95. Zambrano LD, Ellington S, Strid P, et al. Update: characteristics of symptomatic women of reproductive age with laboratory-confirmed SARS-CoV-2 infection by pregnancy status—United States, January 22-October 3, 2020. *MMWR Morb Mortal Wkly Rep*. 2020;69:1641–1647.

96. Metz TD, Clifton RG, Hughes BL, et al. Disease severity and perinatal outcomes of pregnant patients with coronavirus disease 2019 (COVID-19). *Obstet Gynecol*. 2021;137:571–580.

97. Wei SQ, Bilodeau-Bertrand M, Liu S, Auger N. The impact of COVID-19 on pregnancy outcomes: a systematic review and meta-analysis. *CMAJ*. 2021;193:e540–e548.

98. Villar J, Ariff S, Gunier RB, et al. Maternal and neonatal morbidity and mortality among pregnant women with and without COVID-19 infection: the INTERCOVID multinational cohort study. *JAMA Pediatr*. 2021;175:817–826.

99. Vivanti AJ, Vauloup-Fellous C, Prevot S, et al. Transplacental transmission of SARS-CoV-2 infection. *Nat Commun*. 2020; 11:3572.

100. Garneau WM, Jones-Beatty K, Ufua MO, et al. Analysis of clinical outcomes of pregnant patients treated with nirmatrelvir and ritonavir for acute SARS-CoV-2 infection. *JAMA Netw Open*. 2022;5:e2244141.

101. Gulick RM, Pau AK, Daar E, et al. National Institutes of Health COVID-19 Treatment Guidelines Panel: perspectives and lessons learned. *Ann Intern Med*. 2024;177:1547–1557.

102. Society for Maternal-Fetal Medicine. Coronavirus (COVID-19) publications & clinical guidance. Available at: https://www. smfm.org/clincial-guidance. Accessed December 22, 2024.

103. Royal College of Obstetricians and Gynaecologists. *Coronavirus (COVID-19) Infection in Pregnancy. Information for healthcare professionals. Version 16*. December 2022. https://www.rcog.org.uk/media/0qune0d3/covid-19-infection-in-pregnancy-v161-final.pdf. Accesssed August 3, 2025.

104. American College of Obstetricians and Gynecologists. Practice advisory: COVID-19 vaccination considerations for obstetric-gynecologic care (updated June 4, 2025). Available at: https:// www.acog.org/clinical/clinical-guidance/practice-advisory/ articles/2020/12/covid-19-vaccination-considerations-for-obstetric-gynecologic-care. Accessed June 15, 2025.

105. Gray KJ, Bordt EA, Atyeo C, et al. Coronavirus disease 2019 vaccine response in pregnant and lactating women: a cohort study. *Am J Obstet Gynecol*. 2021;225:303.e1–e17.

106. Beharier O, Plitman Mayo R, Raz T, et al. Efficient maternal to neonatal transfer of antibodies against SARS-CoV-2 and BNT162b2 mRNA COVID-19 vaccine. *J Clin Invest*. 2021;131:e154834.

107. Collier AY, McMahan K, Yu J, et al. Immunogenicity of COVID-19 mRNA vaccines in pregnant and lactating women. *JAMA*. 2021;325:2370–2380.

108. Prabhu M, Murphy EA, Sukhu AC, et al. Antibody response to coronavirus disease 2019 (COVID-19) messenger RNA vaccination in pregnant women and transplacental passage into cord blood. *Obstet Gynecol*. 2021;138:278–280.

109. Rottenstreich A, Zarbiv G, Oiknine-Djian E, et al. Efficient maternofetal transplacental transfer of anti-severe acute respiratory syndrome coronavirus 2 (SARS-CoV-2) spike antibodies after antenatal SARS-CoV-2 BNT162b2 messenger RNA vaccination. *Clin Infect Dis*. 2021;73:1909–1912.

110. Katz D, Bateman BT, Kjaer K, et al. The Society for Obstetric Anesthesia and Perinatology Coronavirus Disease 2019 Registry: an analysis of outcomes among pregnant women delivering during the initial severe acute respiratory syndrome coronavirus-2 outbreak in the United States. *Anesth Analg*. 2021;133:462–473.

111. Bauer ME, Chiware R, Pancaro C. Neuraxial procedures in COVID-19-positive parturients: a review of current reports. *Anesth Analg*. 2020;131:c22–e24.

112. Bauer ME, Bernstein K, Dinges E, et al. Obstetric anesthesia during the COVID-19 pandemic. *Anesth Analg*. 2020;131:7–15.

113. Pineles BL, Stephens A, Narendran LM, et al. The relationship between delivery and the PaO_2/FiO_2 ratio in COVID-19: a cohort study. *BJOG*. 2022;129:493–499.

114. Reale SC, Bauer ME, Klumpner TT, et al. Frequency and risk factors for difficult intubation in women undergoing general anesthesia for cesarean delivery: a multicenter retrospective cohort analysis. *Anesthesiology*. 2022;136:697–708.

115. Ibrahim M, Darling R, Oaks N, et al. Epidural blood patch for a post-dural puncture headache in a COVID-19 positive patient following labor epidural analgesia. *Int J Obstet Anesth*. 2021;46:102970.

116. Norris MC, Kalustian A, Salavati S. Epidural blood patch for postdural puncture headache in a patient with coronavirus disease 2019: a case report. *A A Pract*. 2020;14:e01303.

117. American College of Obstetricians and Gynecologists. Practice Bulletin Number 220: Management of genital herpes in pregnancy (reaffirmed 2023). *Obstet Gynecol*. 2020;135:e193–e202.

118. Roberts CM, Pfister JR, Spear SJ. Increasing proportion of herpes simplex virus type 1 as a cause of genital herpes infection in college students. *Sex Transm Dis*. 2003;30:797–800.

119. Hollier LM, Wendel GD. Third trimester antiviral prophylaxis for preventing maternal genital herpes simplex virus (HSV) recurrences and neonatal infection. *Cochrane Database Syst Rev*. 2008;(1):CD004946.

120. Pinninti SG, Angara R, Feja KN, et al. Neonatal herpes disease following maternal antenatal antiviral suppressive therapy: a multicenter case series. *J Pediatr*. 2012;161(1):134–138.e1–e3.

121. Brown ZA, Wald A, Morrow RA, et al. Effect of serologic status and cesarean delivery on transmission rates of herpes simplex virus from mother to infant. *JAMA*. 2003;289:203–209.

122. Ravindran RS, Gupta CD, Stoops CA. Epidural analgesia in the presence of herpes simplex virus (type 2) infection. *Anesth Analg*. 1982;61:714–715.

123. Ramanathan S, Sheth R, Turndorf H. Anesthesia for cesarean section in patients with genital herpes infections: a retrospective study. *Anesthesiology*. 1986;64:807–809.

124. Crosby ET, Halpern SH, Rolbin SH. Epidural anaesthesia for caesarean section in patients with active recurrent genital herpes simplex infections: a retrospective review. *Can J Anaesth*. 1989;36:701–704.

125. Bader AM, Camann WR, Datta S. Anesthesia for cesarean delivery in patients with herpes simplex virus type-2 infections. *Reg Anesth*. 1990;15:261–263.

126. Birnbach DJ, Bourlier RA, Choi R, Thys DM. Anaesthetic management of caesarean section in a patient with active recurrent genital herpes and AIDS-related dementia. *Br J Anaesth*. 1995;75:639–641.

127. Boyle RK. Herpes simplex labialis after epidural or parenteral morphine: a randomized prospective trial in an Australian obstetric population. *Anaesth Intensive Care*. 1995;23:433–437.

128. Davies PW, Vallejo MC, Shannon KT, et al. Oral herpes simplex reactivation after intrathecal morphine: a prospective randomized trial in an obstetric population. *Anesth Analg*. 2005;100:1472–1476.

129. Boyle RK. A review of anatomical and immunological links between epidural morphine and herpes simplex labialis in obstetric patients. *Anaesth Intensive Care*. 1995;23:425–432.

130. Bauchat JR. Focused review: neuraxial morphine and oral herpes reactivation in the obstetric population. *Anesth Analg*. 2010;111:1238–1241.

131. Hoesni S, Bhinder R, Tan T, et al. Herpes simplex meningitis after accidental dural puncture during epidural analgesia for labour. *Int J Obstet Anesth*. 2010;19:466–467.

132. De Guzman MC, Chawla R, Duttchen K. Possible neonatal herpes simplex virus (HSV) acquired postpartum from maternal oral HSV reactivation after neuraxial morphine. *A A Case Rep*. 2014;2:103–105.

133. Lampe MA, Nesheim SR, Oladapo KL, et al. Achieving elimination of perinatal HIV in the United States. *Pediatrics*. 2023;151:e2022059604.

134. Taylor AW, Nesheim SR, Zhang X, et al. Estimated perinatal HIV infection among infants born in the United States, 2002–2013. *JAMA Pediatr*. 2017;171:435–442.

135. Alger LS, Farley JJ, Robinson BA, et al. Interactions of human immunodeficiency virus infection and pregnancy. *Obstet Gynecol*. 1993;82:787–796.

136. Temmerman M, Chomba EN, Ndinya-Achola J, et al. Maternal human immunodeficiency virus-1 infection and pregnancy outcome. *Obstet Gynecol*. 1994;83:495–501.

137. Kourtis AP, Schmid CH, Jamieson DJ, Lau J. Use of antiretroviral therapy in pregnant HIV-infected women and the risk of premature delivery: a meta-analysis. *AIDS*. 2007;21:607–615.

138. Powis KM, Kitch D, Ogwu A, et al. Increased risk of preterm delivery among HIV-infected women randomized to protease versus nucleoside reverse transcriptase inhibitor-based HAART during pregnancy. *J Infect Dis*. 2011;204:506–514.

139. U.S. Department of Health and Human Services. Recommendations for the use of antiretroviral drugs during pregnancy and interventions to reduce perinatal HIV transmission in the United States; 2024. Available at: https://clinicalinfo.hiv.gov/en/guidelines/perinatal/whats-new. Accessed December 22, 2024.

140. Tuomala RE, Shapiro DE, Mofenson LM, et al. Antiretroviral therapy during pregnancy and the risk of an adverse outcome. *N Engl J Med*. 2002;346:1863–1870.

141. Burns DN, Landesman S, Minkoff H, et al. The influence of pregnancy on human immunodeficiency virus type 1 infection: antepartum and postpartum changes in human immunodeficiency virus type 1 viral load. *Am J Obstet Gynecol*. 1998;178:355–359.

142. Bessinger R, Clark R, Kissinger P, et al. Pregnancy is not associated with the progression of HIV disease in women attending an HIV outpatient program. *Am J Epidemiol*. 1998;147:434–440.

143. American College of Obstetricians and Gynecologists. Committee Opinion No. 752: Prenatal and perinatal human immunodeficiency virus testing (reaffirmed 2024). *Obstet Gynecol*. 2018;132:e138–e142.

144. Branson BM, Handsfield HH, Lampe MA, et al. Revised recommendations for HIV testing of adults, adolescents, and pregnant women in healthcare settings. *MMWR Recomm Rep*. 2006;55:1–17.

145. Briand N, Warszawski J, Mandelbrot L, et al. Is intrapartum intravenous zidovudine for prevention of mother-to-child HIV-1 transmission still useful in the combination antiretroviral therapy era? *Clin Infect Dis*. 2013;57:903–914.

146. Cotter AM, Brookfield KF, Duthely LM, et al. Duration of membrane rupture and risk of perinatal transmission of HIV-1 in the era of combination antiretroviral therapy. *Am J Obstet Gynecol*. 2012;207:482.e1–e5.

147. Chiappini E, Galli L, Giaquinto C, et al. Use of combination neonatal prophylaxis for the prevention of mother-to-child transmission of HIV infection in European high-risk infants. *AIDS*. 2013;27:991–1000.

148. Wong VV. Is peripartum zidovudine absolutely necessary for patients with a viral load less than 1,000 copies/ml? *J Obstet Gynaecol*. 2011;31:740–742.

149. Rodman JH, Flynn PM, Robbins B, et al. Systemic pharmacokinetics and cellular pharmacology of zidovudine in human immunodeficiency virus type 1-infected women and newborn infants. *J Infect Dis*. 1999;180:1844–1850.

150. Townsend CL, Cortina-Borja M, Peckham CS, et al. Low rates of mother-to-child transmission of HIV following effective pregnancy interventions in the United Kingdom and Ireland, 2000-2006. *AIDS*. 2008;22:973–981.

151. International Perinatal HIV Group. Duration of ruptured membranes and vertical transmission of HIV-1: a meta-analysis from 15 prospective cohort studies. *AIDS*. 2001;15:357–368.

152. Jamieson DJ, Read JS, Kourtis AP, et al. Cesarean delivery for HIV-infected women: recommendations and controversies. *Am J Obstet Gynecol*. 2007;197:S96–S100.

153. Peters H, Byrne L, De Ruiter A, et al. Duration of ruptured membranes and mother-to-child HIV transmission: a prospective population-based surveillance study. *BJOG*. 2016;123:975–981.

154. Eppes C. Is it time to leave the avoidance of rupture of membranes for women infected with HIV and receiving cart in the past? *BJOG*. 2016;123:982.

155. Boyer PJ, Dillon M, Navaie M, et al. Factors predictive of maternal-fetal transmission of HIV-1. Preliminary analysis of

zidovudine given during pregnancy and/or delivery. *JAMA*. 1994;271:1925–1930.

156. Mandelbrot L, Mayaux MJ, Bongain A, et al. Obstetric factors and mother-to-child transmission of human immunodeficiency virus type 1: the French perinatal cohorts. SEROGEST French Pediatric HIV Infection Study Group. *Am J Obstet Gynecol*. 1996;175:661–667.

157. Mofenson LM, Lambert JS, Stiehm ER, et al. Risk factors for perinatal transmission of human immunodeficiency virus type 1 in women treated with zidovudine. Pediatric AIDS Clinical Trials Group Study 185 Team. *N Engl J Med*. 1999;341:385–393.

158. Shapiro DE, Sperling RS, Mandelbrot L, et al. Risk factors for perinatal human immunodeficiency virus transmission in patients receiving zidovudine prophylaxis. Pediatric AIDS Clinical Trials Group Protocol 076 Study Group. *Obstet Gynecol*. 1999;94:897–908.

159. Novartis. Methergine package insert. Available at: https://www.accessdata.fda.gov/drugsatfda_docs/label/2012/006035s078lbl.pdf. Accessed December 22, 2024.

160. Behrens GMN, Aebi-Popp K, Babiker A. Close to zero, but not zero: what is an acceptable HIV transmission risk through breastfeeding? *J Acquir Immune Defic Syndr*. 2022;89:e42.

161. Malaba TR, Nakatudde I, Kintu K, et al. 72 weeks post-partum follow-up of dolutegravir versus efavirenz initiated in late pregnancy (DolPHIN-2): an open-label, randomised controlled study. *Lancet HIV*. 2022;9:e534–e543.

162. Flynn PM, Taha TE, Cababasay M, et al. Prevention of HIV-1 transmission through breastfeeding: efficacy and safety of maternal antiretroviral therapy versus infant nevirapine prophylaxis for duration of breastfeeding in HIV-1-infected women with high CD4 cell count (IMPAACT PROMISE): a randomized, open-label, clinical trial. *J Acquir Immune Defic Syndr*. 2018;77:383–392.

163. Hughes SC, Dailey PA, Landers D, et al. Parturients infected with human immunodeficiency virus and regional anesthesia. Clinical and immunologic response. *Anesthesiology*. 1995;82:32–37.

164. Avidan MS, Groves P, Blott M, et al. Low complication rate associated with cesarean section under spinal anesthesia for HIV-1-infected women on antiretroviral therapy. *Anesthesiology*. 2002;97:320–324.

165. US Centers for Disease Control and Prevention. Recommendations for prevention of HIV transmission in healthcare settings. *MMWR Suppl*. 1987;36:1S–18S.

166. US Centers for Disease Control and Prevention. HIV occupational transmission. Available at: https://www.cdc.gov/hiv/causes/occupational-transmission.html?CDC_AAref_Val=https://www.cdc.gov/hiv/workplace/healthcareworkers.html. Accessed December 22, 2024.

167. Kuhar DT, Henderson DK, Struble KA, et al. Updated US public health service guidelines for the management of occupational exposures to human immunodeficiency virus and recommendations for postexposure prophylaxis. *Infect Control Hosp Epidemiol*. 2013;34:875–892.

168. García F, Niebla G, Romeu J, et al. Cerebrospinal fluid HIV-1 RNA levels in asymptomatic patients with early stage chronic HIV-1 infection: support for the hypothesis of local virus replication. *AIDS*. 1999;13:1491–1496.

169. Gibbons JJ. Post-dural puncture headache in the HIV-positive patient. *Anesthesiology*. 1991;74:953.

170. Tom DJ, Gulevich SJ, Shapiro HM, et al. Epidural blood patch in the HIV-positive patient. Review of clinical experience. San Diego HIV Neurobehavioral Research Center. *Anesthesiology*. 1992;76:943–947.

171. Schneemilch CE, Schilling T, Bank U. Effects of general anaesthesia on inflammation. *Best Pract Res Clin Anaesthesiol*. 2004;18:493–507.

172. Gershon RY, Manning-Williams D. Anesthesia and the HIV infected parturient: a retrospective study. *Int J Obstet Anesth*. 1997;6:76–81.

173. Singer M, Deutschman CS, Seymour CW, et al. The third international consensus definitions for sepsis and septic shock (Sepsis-3). *JAMA*. 2016;315:801–810.

174. United States Centers for Disease Control and Prevention. Pregnancy mortality surveillance system; 2024. Available at: https://www.cdc.gov/maternal-mortality/php/pregnancy-mortality-surveillance/?CDC_AAref_Val=https://www.cdc.gov/reproductivehealth/maternal-mortality/pregnancy-mortality-surveillance-system.htm. Accessed December 22, 2024.

175. Liu LY, Wen T, Reddy UM, et al. Risk factors, trends, and outcomes associated with postpartum sepsis readmissions. *Obstet Gynecol*. 2024;143:346–354.

176. Petersen EE, Davis NL, Goodman D, et al. Vital signs: pregnancy-related deaths, United States, 2011-2015, and strategies for prevention, 13 states, 2013-2017. *MMWR Morb Mortal Wkly Rep*. 2019;68:423–429.

177. Mhyre JM, D'Oria R, Hameed AB, et al. The maternal early warning criteria: a proposal from the national partnership for maternal safety. *Obstet Gynecol*. 2014;124:782–786.

178. American College of Obstetricians and Gynecologists District II. Safe Motherhood Initiative: maternal safety bundle for sepsis in pregnancy. Available at: https://www.acog.org/community/districts-and-sections/district-ii/programs-and-resources/safe-motherhood-initiative. Accessed December 22, 2024.

179. Acosta CD, Kurinczuk JJ, Lucas DN, et al. Severe maternal sepsis in the UK, 2011-2012: a national case-control study. *PLoS Med*. 2014;11:e1001672.

180. Gibbs R, Bauer M, Olvera L, et al. Improving diagnosis and treatment of maternal sepsis: a CMQCC quality improvement toolkit. California Maternal Quality Care Collaborative; 2020. https://www.cmqcc.org/sites/default/files/Sepsis%20Toolkit_FINAL.2_Errata_7.1.22.pdf. Accessed December 27, 2024.

181. Bauer ME, Bauer ST, Rajala B, et al. Maternal physiologic parameters in relationship to systemic inflammatory response syndrome criteria: a systematic review and meta-analysis. *Obstet Gynecol*. 2014;124:535–541.

182. Shields LE, Wiesner S, Klein C, et al. Use of maternal early warning trigger tool reduces maternal morbidity. *Am J Obstet Gynecol*. 2016;214:527.e1–e6.

183. Bauer ME, Fuller M, Kovacheva V, et al. Performance characteristics of sepsis screening tools during antepartum and postpartum admissions. *Obstet Gynecol*. 2024;143:336–345.

184. Main EK, Fuller M, Kovacheva VP, et al. Performance characteristics of sepsis screening tools during delivery admissions. *Obstet Gynecol*. 2024;143:326–335.

185. Bauer ME, Lorenz RP, Bauer ST, et al. Maternal deaths due to sepsis in the state of Michigan, 1999–2006. *Obstet Gynecol*. 2015;126:747–752.

186. Seacrist MJ, Morton CH, VanOtterloo LR, Main EK. Quality improvement opportunities identified through case review of pregnancy-related deaths from sepsis. *J Obstet Gynecol Neonatal Nurs.* 2019;48:311–320.

187. Albright CM, Ali TN, Lopes V, et al. The sepsis in obstetrics score: a model to identify risk of morbidity from sepsis in pregnancy. *Am J Obstet Gynecol.* 2014;211:39.e1–e8.

188. Albright CM, Has P, Rouse DJ, Hughes BL. Internal validation of the sepsis in obstetrics score to identify risk of morbidity from sepsis in pregnancy. *Obstet Gynecol.* 2017;130:747–755.

189. Kumar A, Roberts D, Wood KE, et al. Duration of hypotension before initiation of effective antimicrobial therapy is the critical determinant of survival in human septic shock. *Crit Care Med.* 2006;34:1589–1596.

190. Bauer ME, Housey M, Bauer ST, et al. Risk factors, etiologies, and screening tools for sepsis in pregnant women: a multi-center case-control study. *Anesth Analg.* 2019;129:1613–1620.

191. Evans L, Rhodes A, Alhazzani W, et al. Executive summary: Surviving Sepsis Campaign: international guidelines for the management of sepsis and septic shock 2021. *Crit Care Med.* 2021;49:1974–1982.

192. Society for Maternal-Fetal Medicine, Shields A, Plante LA, et al. Society for Maternal-Fetal Medicine Consult Series #67: Maternal sepsis. *Am J Obstet Gynecol.* 2023;229:B2–B19.

193. American College of Obstetricians and Gynecologists. Practice Bulletin No. 211: Critical care in pregnancy (reaffirmed 2025). *Obstet Gynecol.* 2019;133:e303–e319.

194. Snyder CC, Barton JR, Habli M, Sibai BM. Severe sepsis and septic shock in pregnancy: indications for delivery and maternal and perinatal outcomes. *J Matern Fetal Neonatal Med.* 2013;26:503–506.

195. Knowles SJ, O'Sullivan NP, Meenan AM, et al. Maternal sepsis incidence, aetiology and outcome for mother and fetus: a prospective study. *BJOG.* 2015;122:663–671.

196. Chau A, Tsen LC. Fetal optimization during maternal sepsis: relevance and response of the obstetric anesthesiologist. *Curr Opin Anaesthesiol.* 2014;27:259–266.

197. Timezguid N, Das V, Hamdi A, et al. Maternal sepsis during pregnancy or the postpartum period requiring intensive care admission. *Int J Obstet Anesth.* 2012;21:51–55.

198. Carp H, Bailey S. The association between meningitis and dural puncture in bacteremic rats. *Anesthesiology.* 1992;76:739–742.

199. Weed LH, Wegeforth P, Ayer JB, Felton LD. The production of meningitis by release of cerebrospinal fluid during an experimental septicemia: preliminary note. *JAMA.* 1919;72:190–193.

200. Petersdorf RG, Swarner DR, Garcia M. Studies on the pathogenesis of meningitis. II. Development of meningitis during pneumococcal bacteremia. *J Clin Invest.* 1962;41:320–327.

201. James FM, George RH, Naiem H, White GJ. Bacteriologic aspects of epidural analgesia. *Anesth Analg.* 1976;55:187–190.

202. Wegefroth P, Lastham JR. Lumbar puncture as a factor in the causation of meningitis. *Am J Med Sci.* 1919;158:183–185.

203. Pray L. Lumbar puncture as a factor in the pathogenesis of meningitis. *Am J Dis Child.* 1941;295:62–68.

204. Eng RH, Seligman SJ. Lumbar puncture-induced meningitis. *JAMA.* 1981;245:1456–1459.

205. Teele DW, Dashefsky B, Rakusan T, Klein JO. Meningitis after lumbar puncture in children with bacteremia. *N Engl J Med.* 1981;305:1079–1081.

206. Smith KM, Deddish RB, Ogata ES. Meningitis associated with serial lumbar punctures and post-hemorrhagic hydrocephalus. *J Pediatr.* 1986;109:1057–1060.

207. Shapiro ED, Aaron NH, Wald ER, Chiponis D. Risk factors for development of bacterial meningitis among children with occult bacteremia. *J Pediatr.* 1986;109:15–19.

208. Blanco JD, Gibbs RS, Castaneda YS. Bacteremia in obstetrics: clinical course. *Obstet Gynecol.* 1981;58:621–625.

209. Sperling RS, Ramamurthy RS, Gibbs RS. A comparison of intrapartum versus immediate postpartum treatment of intra-amniotic infection. *Obstet Gynecol.* 1987;70:861–865.

210. Chestnut DH. Spinal anesthesia in the febrile patient. *Anesthesiology.* 1992;76:667–669.

211. Bader AM, Gilbertson L, Kirz L, Datta S. Regional anesthesia in women with chorioamnionitis. *Reg Anesth.* 1992;17:84–86.

212. American Society of Anesthesiologists. Practice advisory for the prevention, diagnosis, and management of infectious complications associated with neuraxial techniques: an updated report by the American Society of Anesthesiologists Task Force on Infectious Complications Associated with Neuraxial Techniques and the American Society of Regional Anesthesia and Pain Medicine. *Anesthesiology.* 2017;126:585–601.

213. Keski-Nisula L, Suonio S, Makkonen M, et al. Infection markers during labor at term. *Acta Obstet Gynecol Scand.* 1995;74:33–39.

214. Dapper DV, Ibe CJ, Nwauche CA. Haematological values in pregnant women in Port Harcourt, Nigeria. *Niger J Med.* 2006;15:237–240.

215. National Institute of Allergy and Infectious Diseases. Chronic Lyme disease. Available at: https://www.niaid.nih.gov/diseases-conditions/chronic-lyme-disease. Accessed December 22, 2024.

37

Antepartum and Postpartum Hemorrhage

Jennifer M. Banayan, MD and Alexander J. Butwick, MBBS, FRCA, MS

CHAPTER OUTLINE

Obstetric hemorrhage is the most common cause of maternal mortality worldwide, accounting for 27% of maternal deaths.[1] Data from a World Health Organization (WHO) global systematic analysis estimates that 44,190 (95% uncertainty interval: 39,275 to 50,819) maternal deaths from hemorrhage occurred in 2013.[2] In the United States, hemorrhage is the leading cause of preventable maternal mortality and accounted for 13.7% of maternal deaths from 2017 to 2019,[3] with a case-fatality rate of 0.8 deaths per 100,000 live births in 2018.[4] In contrast, France has witnessed a decrease in the maternal mortality rate from hemorrhage over time (from 2.3 per 100,000 live births between 2001 and 2003 to 0.8 per 100,000 live births between 2013 and 2015).[5]

Hemorrhage is also a well-recognized cause of severe maternal morbidity. Transfusion is the most common indicator for severe maternal morbidity, which includes a composite of birth-related injuries defined by the US Centers for Disease Control and Prevention (CDC).[6] Survivors of severe postpartum hemorrhage (PPH) can incur severe morbidity,

including organ failure from hypoperfusion, disseminated intravascular coagulation (DIC), hysterectomy, and intensive care unit (ICU) admission.[7-9] Of concern, the rates of PPH and hemorrhage-related morbidity have increased over time in the United States and other high-resource countries.[7,10-14] For example, in the United States, the rate of PPH increased from 2.7% in 2000 to 4.3% in 2019.[15]

ANTEPARTUM HEMORRHAGE

Antepartum hemorrhage affects 2% to 5% of pregnancies, and is defined as genital tract bleeding occurring after 24 weeks' gestation.[16] It is an important cause of perinatal and maternal mortality. Bleeding can occur from cervical or vaginal lesions, including cervical ectropion, cervicitis, cervical polyps, and cervical carcinoma; from the placental site, including placental abruption and placenta previa; and occasionally, from the fetus. There are no consistent definitions for the magnitude of blood loss for classifying antepartum hemorrhage.

Placenta Previa

Placenta previa occurs when the placenta covers the cervix. In the past, the classification was based on the relationship between the placenta and the cervical os, using terms such as *total*, *partial*, and *marginal*. Use of this terminology is decreasing due to advances in transvaginal ultrasonography that enable evaluation of the placental edge relative to the cervical os. Current approaches for classification are typically based on whether the placenta overlies the os (referred to as a *previa*), and if any placenta extends to the lower uterine segment but does not reach the os (referred to as *low lying*).[17,18] Based on data from a systematic review, the pooled prevalence of antepartum hemorrhage (52%) is high among patients with placenta previa.[19]

Epidemiology

The incidence of placenta previa varies worldwide, with rates ranging from 2 to 12 per 1000 pregnancies.[20] The exact cause is unclear, but prior uterine trauma (e.g., scar from prior cesarean delivery) is a common finding. The placenta may implant in the scarred area, which typically includes the lower uterine segment. Conditions associated with placenta previa include multiparity, advanced maternal age, smoking history, male fetus, previous cesarean delivery or other uterine surgery, and previous placenta previa.[21,22] There is a "dose-response" relation between the risk of placenta previa and the number of prior cesarean deliveries; the relative risk (RR) increases from 4.5 (95% confidence interval [CI], 3.6 to 5.5) with one prior cesarean to 44.9 (95% CI, 13.5 to 149.5) with four prior cesarean deliveries.[23] In the United States, Asian patients are at increased risk for placenta previa compared with White patients.[24] Placenta previa can lead to antepartum hemorrhage and PPH, and it is associated with perinatal and neonatal morbidities, including preterm birth, fetal anomalies, neurodevelopmental delay, and sudden infant death syndrome.[25–27]

Diagnosis

Most patients are initially diagnosed during routine transabdominal ultrasonography. Due to its superior diagnostic accuracy, transvaginal ultrasonography is typically performed for diagnostic confirmation. Measuring the distance from the placental edge to the internal os predicts the likelihood of antepartum hemorrhage and the need for cesarean delivery.[28,29] Magnetic resonance imaging (MRI) may be useful for the diagnosis of placenta previa, but its use is not practical in most cases of antepartum hemorrhage.

The classic clinical sign of placenta previa is **painless vaginal bleeding** during the second or third trimester. All parturients with painless vaginal bleeding after 20 weeks' gestation should be assumed to have placenta previa until proven otherwise. Digital examination may cause catastrophic hemorrhage and should be avoided. Placenta previa diagnosed in asymptomatic patients before the third trimester frequently resolves as pregnancy progresses; 90% of low-lying placentas diagnosed in early pregnancy normalize by the third trimester.[30] The lack of abdominal pain does not exclude placental abruption, and patients with placenta previa are at risk for coexisting placental abruption.

Obstetric Management

Obstetric management is based on the severity of vaginal bleeding, the gestational age, and fetal status. Active labor, persistent bleeding, a mature fetus (gestational age ≥ 36 weeks), or nonreassuring fetal status should prompt delivery.[31] The fetus is at risk for two distinct pathophysiologic processes: (1) progressive or sudden placental separation that causes uteroplacental insufficiency and (2) preterm delivery and its sequelae. The first episode of bleeding characteristically stops spontaneously and rarely causes maternal shock or fetal compromise. Expectant management in the hospital has been reported to prolong pregnancy by an average of 4 weeks after the initial bleeding episode.[31] Maternal vital signs and hemoglobin concentration should be assessed frequently. Fetal evaluation involves nonstress tests, biophysical profiles, and ultrasonographic assessments of fetal growth (see Chapter 6). Traditionally, limited physical activity and avoidance of vaginal examinations and coitus has been recommended, although the evidence supporting these measures is limited.

Outpatient management is associated with favorable outcomes in select patients, such as stable patients without bleeding in the previous 48 hours who have both telephone access and the ability to be transported quickly to the hospital.[32] Expectant management requires immediate access to a medical center with 24-hour obstetric and anesthesia coverage and a neonatal ICU.[31]

For patients with placenta previa diagnosed between 24 and 34 weeks' gestation, a corticosteroid (e.g., betamethasone) is typically administered. This is done to accelerate fetal lung maturity due to concern for preterm delivery.[31] To mitigate this concern, short-term tocolytic therapy may be used to treat patients with preterm uterine contractions. Tocolytic therapy is not recommended for patients with uncontrolled hemorrhage or those with evidence of maternal or fetal compromise.

If the placental edge–to–internal os distance is greater than 1 cm, patients may be offered a trial of labor—the risk of antepartum hemorrhage and the need for cesarean delivery during labor are low.[28] Conversely, patients require cesarean delivery if the placental edge–to–internal os distance is less than 1 cm, total placenta previa is present, fetal status is nonreassuring, or if significant bleeding is present.

Anesthetic Management

Typically, stable patients with a placenta previa without significant antepartum vaginal bleeding or uterine contractions will undergo a scheduled cesarean delivery between 36 and 37 weeks' gestation.

All patients presenting with antepartum vaginal bleeding or uterine contractions should undergo urgent anesthesia evaluation in anticipation of expedited delivery. Special consideration should be given to the airway examination, intravascular volume assessment, and history of previous cesarean delivery or other procedures that create a uterine scar. Large-bore intravenous access should be obtained. For patients with significant or active bleeding, hematologic and coagulation indices should be urgently evaluated, red blood cells

(RBCs) ordered, and intravenous fluid resuscitation initiated. Activation of a massive transfusion protocol (MTP) is advised for patients with severe or massive antepartum hemorrhage (see later discussion).

Patients without significant vaginal bleeding may require antepartum hospitalization. Vascular access with at least one intravenous catheter should be maintained if bleeding is recurrent or imminent delivery is anticipated. The use of lower-extremity sequential compression devices may decrease the risk for venous thromboembolism in patients on bed rest.

The choice of anesthetic technique depends on the indication and urgency for delivery, the severity of maternal hypovolemia, laboratory indices, and the obstetric history (e.g., prior cesarean delivery, risk for placenta accreta). Few reliable data exist to guide anesthetic choice in the context of abnormal placentation. Survey data reveal that most anesthesia providers prefer neuraxial anesthesia in patients with placenta previa without active bleeding or intravascular volume deficit.[33] A large cohort study examined the mode of anesthesia in patients with placenta previa and reported outcomes for 1234 patients.[34] Neuraxial anesthesia and general anesthesia were performed in 59.7% and 40.3% of cases, respectively. Blood transfusion was less common in the neuraxial anesthesia group (19.8% versus 76.7%). After adjustment for confounders, findings from regression analyses suggested that neuraxial anesthesia was associated with less blood loss, a lower transfusion requirement, and less neonatal morbidity (neonatal asphyxia and neonatal ICU admission). However, these findings may be explained by residual confounding.

Patients who have placenta previa—even without active preoperative bleeding—remain at risk for increased intraoperative blood loss for three reasons. First, an anteriorly located placenta may be surgically transected during a uterine incision. Second, after delivery, the lower uterine segment implantation site, lacking uterine muscle compared with the fundus, does not contract as well as the fundal implantation site. Third, a patient with placenta previa is at increased risk for placenta accreta, especially if there is a history of previous cesarean delivery (Table 37.1).[22] Therefore, anesthesia providers should be prepared for severe or massive intraoperative hemorrhage in all patients with placenta previa (see later discussion). Before delivery, intravenous access should be established with at least two large-bore intravenous catheters and two cross-matched RBC units should be immediately available.

If the placenta does not separate easily from the uterine wall, placenta accreta should be suspected, and massive blood loss and cesarean hysterectomy should be anticipated.

Placental Abruption

Placental abruption is defined as complete or partial separation of the placenta from the decidua basalis before delivery of the fetus. There are two main types of placental abruption: *revealed* (65% to 80% of cases), in which bleeding tracks from the site of placental separation resulting in vaginal bleeding, and *concealed*, in which a retroplacental clot is formed with no vaginal bleeding.

Epidemiology

Placental abruption complicates 0.6% to 1.2% of pregnancies,[35] with an incidence of 3 to 10 per 1000 births worldwide.[36] The causes of abruption are not well understood, but several conditions are known risk factors for abruption (Box 37.1).[37,38] Patients with abruption are also at risk for PPH from uterine atony and coagulopathy.[7]

Diagnosis

For an acute revealed abruption, the classic clinical features are vaginal bleeding in 70% to 80% of cases, abdominal pain or uterine tenderness in two-thirds of cases, and increased uterine contractions in one-third of cases. In cases of concealed abruption (20% of cases), vaginal bleeding and pain may be absent, but fetal death and coagulopathy can still occur.[39] In nearly a third of concealed cases, abruption may manifest as idiopathic preterm labor. Uterine contractions may be difficult to distinguish from the pain associated with placental abruption. Patients may have a variety of nonreassuring fetal heart rate (FHR) patterns, including late or

TABLE 37.1 Risk for Placenta Accreta in Patients With Placenta Previa: Relationship to Number of Prior Cesarean Deliveries

Number of Prior Cesarean Deliveries	% of Patients With Placenta Accreta
0	3
1	11
2	40
3	61
≥4	67

Modified from Silver RM, Landon MB, Rouse DJ, et al. Maternal morbidity associated with multiple repeat cesarean deliveries. *Obstet Gynecol.* 2006;107:1226–1232.

BOX 37.1 Conditions Associated With Placental Abruption

Obstetric conditions
- Advanced maternal age
- Multiparity
- Preeclampsia
- Premature rupture of membranes
- Chorioamnionitis

Maternal comorbidities
- Hypertension
- Acute or chronic respiratory illness
- Substance use disorder
- Maternal cocaine use
- Maternal or paternal tobacco use

Trauma
- Direct (e.g., blunt abdominal)
- Indirect (e.g., acceleration/deceleration injury)

variable decelerations, fetal tachycardia, and loss of variability. The severity of FHR changes may correspond with the severity of abruption. For example, with profound fetal hypoxia, sinusoidal patterns can occur before terminal bradycardia. For a chronic abruption, the clinical features include light to moderate vaginal bleeding only.

In a subset of cases, ultrasonography may help confirm the diagnosis, which appears as large abnormal blood collections close to or within the placenta. Ultrasonography is highly specific for placental abruption (96% to 100%) but assessment of sensitivity varies between studies, ranging from 24% to 57%.[40,41] Ultrasonography is also useful for determining placental location to exclude placenta previa, a retroplacental hematoma, and subchorionic hematoma. However, normal ultrasonographic findings do not exclude placental abruption.

Obstetric Management

The initial management of placental abruption should focus on maternal stabilization and appropriate resuscitation.

Delivery may be necessary, especially in patients presenting with severe bleeding, to minimize the risks of severe hemorrhage, coagulopathy, fetal compromise, and maternal hypoperfusion.

Current evidence is insufficient to guide the timing of delivery for patients with acute or chronic abruption. A suggested obstetric management algorithm has been published (Fig. 37.1).[35] After an initial period of observation for noncompromised patients, decision-making regarding the need and timing of delivery versus inpatient or outpatient management is necessary. These decisions should consider the patients' gestational age and other complicating factors (e.g., oligohydramnios, ongoing vaginal bleeding, FHR abnormalities). A course of corticosteroids may be administered to promote fetal lung maturity for patients presenting preterm, but delivery should not be deferred to administer corticosteroids in the late preterm period. Vaginal delivery is preferred for patients with intrauterine fetal demise unless they are at increased risk for uterine rupture.[42]

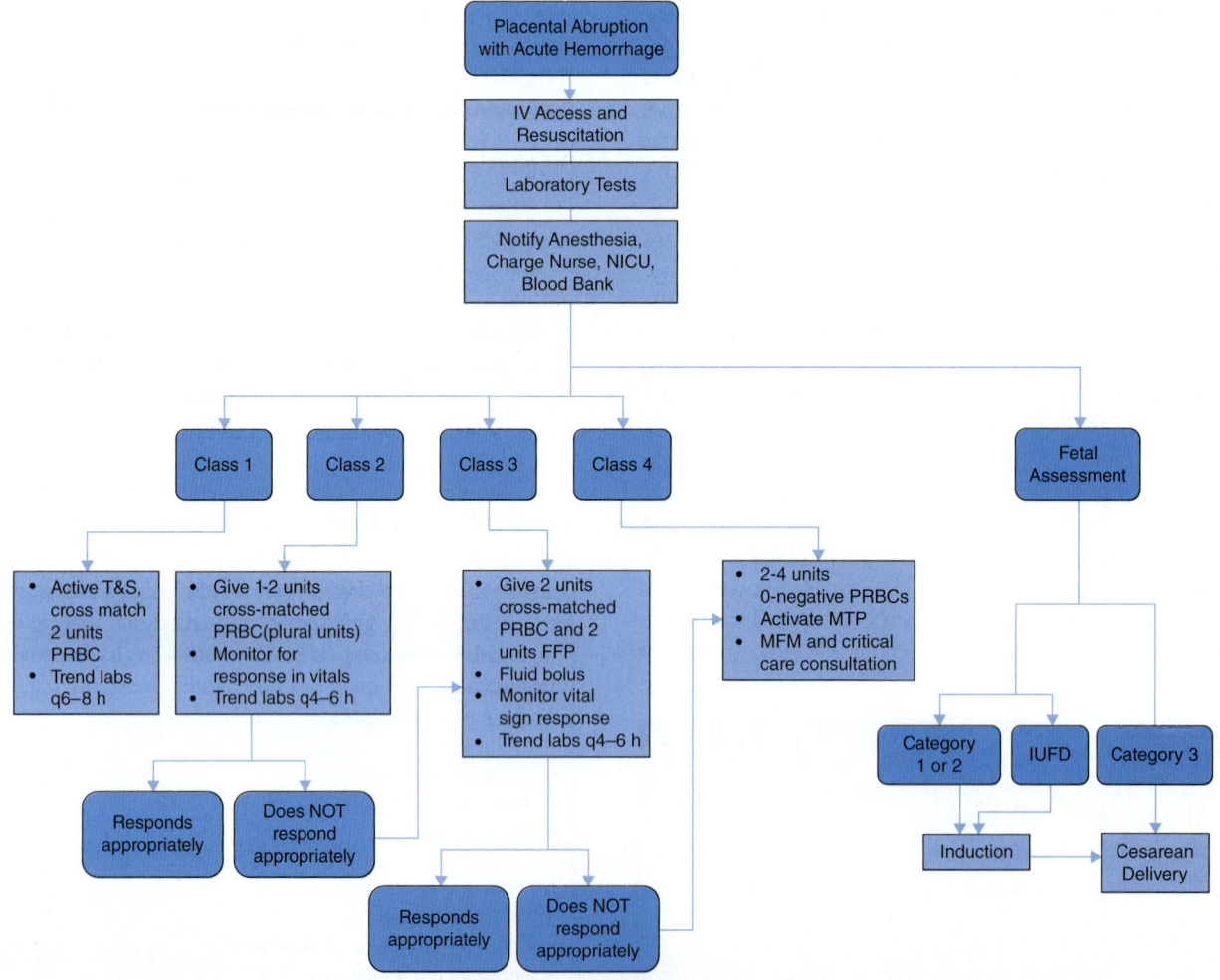

Fig. 37.1 Management Algorithm for Placental Abruption. The algorithm for the management of placental abruption with acute hemorrhage employs the Advanced Trauma Life Support classification of hypovolemic shock, which has not been validated in pregnancy. *FFP*, Fresh frozen plasma; *IUFD*, intrauterine fetal death; *IV*, intravenous; *MFM*, maternal-fetal medicine; *MTP*, massive transfusion protocol; *NICU*, neonatal intensive care unit; *PRBCs*, packed red blood cells; *T&S*, type and screen. Placental abruption at near-term and term gestations. From Brandt JS, Ananth CV. Placental abruption at near-term and term gestations: pathophysiology, epidemiology, diagnosis, and management. *Am J Obstet Gynecol.* 2023;228(5S):S1313–S1329.

Coagulopathy and abruption. Accumulating observational data indicate that abruption is the most frequent cause of **acute obstetric coagulopathy**, a highly morbid condition characterized by accelerated thrombin generation and fibrinolysis. In a study examining hemostatic changes in 518 patients with obstetric hemorrhage, a subgroup of 12 patients developed acute obstetric coagulopathy, of whom 5 (41.6%) had placental abruption.[43] Findings from several observational cohorts report a high prevalence of hypofibrinogenemia (fibrinogen level < 200 mg/dL [2 g/L]) in patients with abruption (22% to 40%),[43–45] with a higher prevalence among those with severe or massive PPH. The risk of massive hemorrhage and coagulopathy may be particularly high in patients with abruption and fetal demise. In a small cohort study of 16 patients with both abruption and fetal death, a massive transfusion was required in most patients—71% received at least 20 units of plasma and 64% patients received at least 10 units of RBCs.[42] Due to concern for coagulopathy, hematologic and coagulation indices, including fibrinogen concentration levels, should be assessed at admission and at regular time intervals (e.g., 4 to 6 hourly) during the peripartum period using laboratory testing and, if available, point-of-care testing. Either cryoprecipitate or fibrinogen concentrate is appropriate to treat hypofibrinogenemia (plasma fibrinogen concentration < 200 mg/dL).

Anesthetic Management

If abruption is suspected, initial interventions should focus on maternal stabilization, including large-bore intravenous access, intravenous fluid resuscitation, and assessment of hemoglobin, coagulation status, and the need for blood products. Clinicians must be vigilant for hypovolemic shock, even in the absence of external blood loss (presence of concealed abruption).

Neuraxial techniques for labor analgesia or cesarean anesthesia may be offered for patients who are hemodynamically stable without coagulopathy. Intravenous patient-controlled opioid analgesia should be considered for patients in labor, and general anesthesia should be administered for cesarean delivery in patients with severe thrombocytopenia or coagulopathy. General anesthesia (see Chapter 26) may also be necessary for emergency cesarean delivery in the setting of severe fetal compromise or severe antepartum hemorrhage.

Uterine Rupture

Rupture of the gravid uterus can be disastrous for both the mother and the fetus. Because of variation in nomenclature and severity, accurate determination of maternal and fetal morbidity secondary to uterine rupture is difficult. The most common variety of uterine scar disruption is separation or dehiscence; some cases are asymptomatic. **Uterine scar dehiscence** is defined as a uterine wall defect that does not lead to excessive hemorrhage, FHR abnormalities, emergency cesarean delivery, or postpartum laparotomy. Its frequency is between 2.2% and 6.3%.[46] In contrast, **uterine rupture** refers to a uterine wall defect with maternal hemorrhage and/or fetal compromise sufficient to require emergency cesarean delivery or postpartum laparotomy. The rupture of a classical uterine incision scar (a vertical incision involving the muscular uterine fundus) is associated with greater morbidity and mortality than rupture of a low transverse uterine incision scar because the anterior uterine wall is highly vascular and may include the area of placental implantation. Nevertheless, even a transverse uterine incision may underlie the placenta, and lateral extension of the rupture can involve the major uterine vessels with the potential for massive bleeding.

Epidemiology

Uterine rupture is rare (1:16,849)[47] among patients with an unscarred uterus.[48] Previous uterine surgery (e.g., cesarean delivery, myomectomy) increases the risk (<1% for patients with one previous cesarean delivery, 3.9% for those with more than one cesarean delivery).[49] Box 37.2 lists other conditions associated with uterine rupture.[48,49]

Among patients who have undergone a prior cesarean delivery, the presence or absence of labor influences their risk of uterine rupture (see Chapter 20). A population-based retrospective analysis of more than 20,000 patients demonstrated that the risk among nonlaboring versus laboring patients was 1.6 per 1000 versus 5.2 per 1000.[50] Among patients undergoing induction of labor, the risk increased nearly fivefold to 7.7 per 1000 and was highest among those undergoing prostaglandin induction (24.5 per 1000).[50,51] Additional risk factors for uterine rupture during a trial of labor after cesarean (TOLAC) include an interdelivery interval of less than 12 to 16 months, multiple previous cesarean deliveries, postterm gestation, birth weight > 4000 g, maternal age > 35 years, and previous delivery with severe PPH.[52,53] Decreased thickness of the lower uterine segment on ultrasonographic examination increases rupture risk, but a precise threshold value below

---

BOX 37.2   Conditions Associated With Uterine Rupture

Obstetric conditions
- Prior uterine surgery
- Induction of labor
- High-dose oxytocin induction
- Prostaglandin induction
- Grand multiparity (>5)
- Morbidly adherent placenta
- Congenital uterine anomaly (e.g., bicornuate uterus)

Maternal comorbidities
- Connective tissue disorder (e.g., Ehlers-Danlos syndrome)

Trauma
Obstetric
- Forceps application/rotation
- Internal podalic version
- Excessive fundal pressure

Nonobstetric
- Blunt
- Penetrating

which TOLAC should not be offered because the risk of rupture is too high is unclear.[54]

Maternal death secondary to uterine rupture is rare, although there were three deaths attributed to uterine rupture in the 2006 to 2008 triennial report from the United Kingdom.[55] Rupture-associated neonatal hypoxic-ischemic encephalopathy or mortality occurs at a rate of less than one per 1000 TOLACs in the United States.[49]

Diagnosis

An FHR abnormality is the first sign of uterine rupture in more than 80% of patients (see Chapter 20).[56] Breakthrough pain and need for frequent neuraxial labor analgesia redosing may also indicate impending or evolving uterine rupture.[57] Other presenting signs include vaginal bleeding, uterine hypertonia, cessation of labor, maternal hypotension, loss of the fetal station, decrease in cervical dilation, or a change in fetal presentation.

Obstetric Management

Treatment options for uterine rupture include repair of the uterus, arterial ligation, and hysterectomy. Uterine repair is appropriate for most cases of separation of a prior low transverse uterine scar and for some cases of rupture of a classical incision. However, the risk for rupture in a future pregnancy remains.[49]

Anesthetic Management

Patient evaluation and resuscitation should be initiated while the patient is being prepared for emergency laparotomy. If antepartum rupture has occurred, fetal compromise is likely. Rapid induction of general anesthesia is likely to be necessary, but neuraxial anesthesia may be possible in stable maternal patients with a functioning epidural catheter that allows timely conversion from labor analgesia to surgical anesthesia. In many cases, major hemorrhage requiring massive transfusion and hemostatic support may be required (see later discussion).

Vasa Previa

Vasa previa occurs when the fetal blood vessels traverse the fetal membranes covering the internal cervical os. Consequently, the fetal vessels are not protected by the placenta or the umbilical cord, and rupture of membranes can be accompanied by tearing of a fetal vessel and exsanguination of the fetus.

Three types of vasa previa exist. Type 1, the most common, occurs when the vessels are associated with a velamentous umbilical cord. Type 2 occurs when the vessels connect the lobes of a multilobed placenta or the placenta and a succenturiate lobe.[58] Type 3 occurs when unprotected fetal vessels run from one placental edge through the membranes to another edge. Although no universal definition exists regarding the exact distance between fetal vessels and internal os that constitutes vasa previa, many clinicians use a threshold of 2 cm.[59] This distance is based on a case series that demonstrated that all emergency deliveries caused by vasa previa had a fetal vessel within 2 cm of the cervical os.[60] However, there are no data confirming the safety of a 2-cm distance if unprotected vessels are in close proximity to the cervix for patients undergoing a trial of labor.

Epidemiology

Vasa previa occurs rarely (1 in 2500 to 1 in 5000 deliveries).[31] Because it involves the loss of fetal blood, vasa previa is associated with a high fetal mortality rate (nearly 60% if vasa previa is unrecognized and the unprotected vessels tear).[61] The blood volume of the fetus at term is approximately 80 to 100 mL/kg; thus, the loss of small amounts of blood can have devastating fetal consequences. In addition, the presence of vasa previa exposes the vulnerable fetal vessels to compression by the fetal presenting part, resulting in fetal hypoxia and death. Risk factors for vasa previa include the presence of velamentous cord insertion, placenta previa or low-lying placenta in the second trimester, placental accessory lobes, *in vitro* fertilization, and multiple gestation.[31]

Diagnosis

Prenatal ultrasonography can be used to visualize the velamentous insertion of the vessels and leads to improved perinatal outcomes.[31,61] Vasa previa should be suspected whenever bleeding occurs with intrapartum rupture of membranes, particularly if the rupture is accompanied by FHR decelerations (e.g., a sinusoidal pattern, fetal bradycardia). Hemorrhage can also occur without the rupture of membranes, making the diagnosis challenging.

Obstetric Management

Prenatal diagnosis is critical for neonatal survival. Antenatal diagnosis reduces neonatal mortality to 3%, while undiagnosed cases have a mortality rate of 56%.[61] Any patient at risk for vasa previa should have an ultrasonographic examination with transvaginal color Doppler.[61] The management of vasa previa is directed toward ensuring fetal survival.

The timing of delivery reflects a balance between the risks associated with preterm delivery and the risk for vessel rupture if the pregnancy is allowed to continue. Cesarean delivery should occur before labor or membrane rupture to prevent vessel rupture. Experts advocate antenatal corticosteroid administration between 30 and 32 weeks' gestation to promote fetal lung maturity, and antepartum maternal hospitalization between 30 and 34 weeks' gestation to ensure prompt delivery in the event of rupture of membranes.[62] Findings from a decision analysis suggest scheduling a cesarean delivery between 34 and 35 weeks' gestation.[63] This overlaps with the Society for Maternal-Fetal Medicine guidelines for delivery between 34 and 37 weeks' gestation.[58] However, recommendations for delivery at 34 weeks were made prior to published data, highlighting the perinatal morbidity risks of preterm delivery. Recent expert opinion suggests that delivery be considered at 36 to 37 weeks in asymptomatic patients.[64] Amniocentesis to evaluate fetal lung maturity is not recommended because delaying delivery is typically not an option.[58]

Ruptured vasa previa in the presence of FHR abnormalities (bradycardia, late decelerations, sinusoidal pattern) is an obstetric emergency that requires immediate cesarean delivery. Neonatal resuscitation requires attention to neonatal blood volume status.

Anesthetic Management

The choice of anesthetic technique depends on the urgency of the cesarean delivery. Patients with prenatally diagnosed vasa previa will typically undergo scheduled cesarean delivery before labor or rupture of membranes, with a lower-segment transverse uterine incision. Assuming no contraindications, neuraxial anesthesia is recommended for these patients. Neuraxial anesthesia may also be considered for patients in labor or with membrane rupture but without vessel rupture or fetal compromise. In these scenarios, continuous fetal monitoring in the case of vessel rupture and fetal compromise is required before, during, and after the initiation of neuraxial anesthesia. General anesthesia may be necessary for emergency cesarean delivery if there is acute, potentially life-threatening fetal compromise from a vessel rupture.

POSTPARTUM HEMORRHAGE

PPH refers to excessive bleeding after delivery. PPH definitions vary across international medical and obstetric societies.[65] The American College of Obstetricians and Gynecologists (ACOG) defines PPH as blood loss ≥ 1000 mL or blood loss accompanied by signs or symptoms of hypovolemia within 24 hours of birth.[66] Primary PPH occurs during the first 24 hours, and secondary PPH occurs between 24 hours and 6 weeks after delivery.[66]

Epidemiology

The global prevalence of PPH and severe PPH is estimated to be 10.8% and 2.8%, respectively.[67] Wide variation exists worldwide, with the PPH prevalence ranging from 7.2% in Oceania to 25.7% in Africa. Among many developed countries, there has been an increase in national PPH rates over time.[7,10–14] An increase in the number of cesarean deliveries as well as the proportion of patients with PPH risk factors, in part, explains this increase. Among deliveries with PPH, the rate of blood transfusion was 16.7% in 2011, but decreased from 2.1% to 0.9% from 2016 to 2019.[15] Advances in clinical care may have mitigated progressive increases in rates of severe PPH and the accompanying morbidity over time.

Quantitative Blood Loss Measurement and Postpartum Hemorrhage Diagnosis

Blood loss assessment is an established practice after delivery, with blood loss volume considered the most common variable for defining PPH. Blood loss can be assessed using several methods: visual estimation, gravimetric assessment (weighing blood-soaked laps or sponges), or volumetric assessment (measuring the volume of blood in volumetric drapes after vaginal delivery or suction canisters during cesarean delivery).[68] Clinical and simulation studies have shown that quantitative blood loss (QBL) measurement, calculated with gravimetric and/or volumetric assessment, is more accurate than visual estimation, which can miss up to 30% of actual blood loss.[69–71]

A commonly held belief is that measuring QBL can lead to timely PPH diagnosis and subsequent treatment, but published evidence suggests that in clinical practice, QBL rarely accomplishes this task. A large randomized trial compared the use of blood collection bags to visual estimation in 25,381 vaginal deliveries and reported similar rates of severe PPH (1.7% versus 2.1%, respectively).[72] One possible reason for this finding is that accurate blood loss measurement may not change or improve PPH management. In a two-phase, sequential, mixed-methods study incorporating focus groups, interviews, and a cross-over study, investigators explored how clinicians evaluate blood loss and the detection of excessive bleeding using simulations of "rapid" and "slow" blood loss.[73] Key study findings were that clinicians initiate treatment when bleeding is recognized as abnormal. Based on these findings, QBL measurement may not improve reaction speed in rapid blood loss scenarios. However, it may be valuable for diagnosing PPH during slow blood loss, for helping clinicians account for blood loss that cumulates over multiple phases of care (i.e., intrapartum and postpartum), and for documentation. Because blood loss quantification typically occurs after the arrest of postpartum bleeding and not during active bleeding, research is needed to evaluate how the timing of QBL measurement relates to the timing of PPH diagnosis and management.[74] New approaches to blood loss measurement have been investigated, such as colorimetric approaches.[75–78] Large prospective trials are needed to determine whether these or other approaches result in timelier detection of PPH and clinically meaningful improvements in short- and long-term maternal outcomes.[79]

In summary, QBL measurement remains an established approach for evaluating the magnitude of blood loss after delivery. However, in scenarios of acute and evolving hemorrhage, clinicians should not rely solely on QBL values or arbitrary blood loss threshold values before making a diagnosis of PPH and escalating care. QBL assessment should be integrated into a multidimensional approach for diagnosing PPH that accounts for dynamic changes in physiologic parameters, laboratory values, and the clinical status of a patient experiencing acute postpartum blood loss.

Uterine Atony

Epidemiology

Uterine atony is the most common cause of PPH, accounting for 80% of all PPH events.[7,10] Atony is associated with other causes of PPH, such as genital tract trauma, placenta previa, and placental abruption. The mechanism of this association is unclear but suggests that atony may not always be the primary cause of PPH, but rather an exacerbating complication (Box 37.3).[80]

Uterine smooth muscle physiology. Several reviews provide comprehensive information about the physiology of myometrial smooth muscle.[81–84] Briefly, the uterus is a myogenic

BOX 37.3   Conditions Associated With Uterine Atony

Asian race
Prior postpartum hemorrhage
Preexisting or gestational diabetes
Placental disorders (placenta previa and placental abruption)
Prolonged labor
Genital tract trauma during delivery

Conditions likely associated with uterine atony
Hispanic ethnicity
Nulliparity
Hypertensive disease of pregnancy
Multiple gestation
Chorioamnionitis
Uterine rupture
Predelivery oxytocin exposure
Induction of labor
Operative vaginal delivery

Modified from Ende HB, Lozada MJ, Chestnut DH, et al. Risk factors for atonic postpartum hemorrhage: a systematic review and meta-analysis. *Obstet Gynecol.* 2021;137(2):305–323.

organ that provides a critical protective environment for the fetus before delivery. Smooth muscle, or **myometrium**, within the uterine wall is responsible for generating the electrical activity and uterine contractions during labor and the elevated uterine tone after delivery. Myometrial smooth muscle cells have a phasic pattern of contractile activity, comprising maintenance of a resting tone with discrete, intermittent contractions of varying amplitude, duration, and frequency. The contractile activity of these cells is regulated predominantly by intracellular calcium (Ca^{2+}). Ca^{2+} regulation has three phases: maintenance of basal contractions, which influence the resting smooth muscle tone; a marked increase in cytosolic Ca^{2+}, which induces a contractile response; and the restoration of cytosolic Ca^{2+} concentrations to a resting state after smooth muscle contraction.

The **excitation-contraction coupling process** is modulated through membrane potential changes, ion channel regulation, and protein phosphorylation via specific signaling pathways.[82] Myometrial contractions occur in direct response to action potentials generated in smooth muscle cells. When the membrane potential of the smooth muscle cell reaches a threshold of depolarization, voltage-dependent channels are activated, which ultimately leads to opening of voltage-dependent L-type Ca^{2+} channels and Ca^{2+} influx. Receptor agonists, such as oxytocin, bind to G-protein coupled receptors on the cell membrane. Through a second messenger system, inositol triphosphate releases Ca^{2+} from sarcoplasmic reticulum. Intracellular Ca^{2+}, liberated from intracellular stores as well as from the extracellular space, binds to calmodulin and activates myosin light chain kinase (MLCK). MLCK phosphorylates a regulatory protein (serine 19) on myosin light chain, which triggers interaction of phosphorylated myosin with actin. This results in a cross-bridging cycle and smooth

muscle contraction. Smooth muscle cell relaxation occurs when the intracellular Ca^{2+} decreases, leading to the deactivation of MLCK and eventual dissociation of the actin-myosin cross-bridges. The decrease in Ca^{2+} occurs through the activity of calcium ATPases and sodium-calcium exchangers that extrude Ca^{2+} from the cell. The activity of myosin light chain phosphatase also contributes to smooth muscle relaxation by dephosphorylating the myosin light chain, which inhibits an actin-myosin interaction.

Pathophysiology of Uterine Atony

Although molecular phenotypes or signatures for uterine atony are not fully known, studies have improved our understanding of the pathophysiology of uterine atony. In cultured human uterine smooth muscle cells, decreased oxytocin receptor mRNA and a 50% to 60% reduction in oxytocin-induced calcium occur after 48 hours of oxytocin pretreatment.[85,86] In addition, oxytocin-induced desensitization of smooth muscle cells occurred after 4 hours of oxytocin exposure, although the cells continued to respond to prostaglandin $F_{2\alpha}$ stimulation.[87] In an *in vitro* study of contractility patterns in isolated human myometrium from nonlaboring patients undergoing elective caesarean delivery, decreased contractility was observed in response to oxytocin when preexposed to a higher versus lower oxytocin concentration (10^{-5} to 10^{-8} M versus 10^{-10} M).[88]

Based on the totality of these research findings, oxytocin pretreatment attenuates increases in intracellular Ca^{2+} and myometrial contractility in response to exogenous oxytocin in a dose- and duration-dependent manner. Oxytocin receptor desensitization may not impair the pre- or postreceptor signaling of other drugs that potentiate myometrial contractility, such as prostaglandins or ergot alkaloids. These findings provide a scientific rationale for the association between prolonged or augmented labor and poor uterine responsiveness to oxytocin after delivery.

Clinical Diagnosis

A poorly contractile uterus and excessive blood loss are the most common clinical features of uterine atony. The diagnosis is typically based on bimanual uterine assessment after vaginal delivery or direct evaluation of uterine tone during cesarean delivery. The absence of vaginal bleeding does not exclude this disorder because an atonic, engorged uterus may contain more than 1000 mL of blood. Unrecognized bleeding may manifest initially as tachycardia, with worsening hypovolemia eventually leading to hypotension.[89]

Uterine Atony Prophylaxis

The prophylactic administration of oxytocic agents, most commonly oxytocin or carbetocin, is a critical component of the active management of the third stage of labor.[66,90,91] When uterine atony occurs, additional oxytocic supplementation can be considered. In the setting of refractory uterine atony, prostaglandins and ergot alkaloids are recommended for second-line treatment (Table 37.2).[66] Based on data from a nationwide sample of US delivery hospitalizations between

TABLE 37.2 Second-Line Uterotonic Drugs for the Treatment of Uterine Atony

Agent	Dose and Route	Relative Contraindications	Side Effects	Notes
Ergonovine or methylergonovine	0.2 mg IM	Hypertension Preeclampsia Coronary artery disease	Nausea and vomiting Arteriolar constriction Hypertension	Long duration of action May be repeated once after 30 min
15-Methylprostaglandin $F_{2\alpha}$	0.25 mg IM	Reactive airway disease Pulmonary hypertension Hypoxemia	Fever Chills Nausea and vomiting Diarrhea Bronchoconstriction	May be repeated every 15 min up to 2 mg
Misoprostol	600–1000 µg PR, sublingual, or buccal	None	Fever Chills Nausea and vomiting Diarrhea	Off-label use. May not provide benefit in treating PPH in patients who have been treated with high-dose oxytocin.

IM, Intramuscular; *PPH*, postpartum hemorrhage; *PR*, per rectum.

2007 and 2011, the median hospital-level frequency of second-line uterotonic use was 7.1%; the most frequently used second-line uterotonics were methylergonovine maleate, misoprostol, and carboprost.[92]

Oxytocics

Oxytocin. The WHO and the ACOG recommend oxytocin as a first-line agent after all births for PPH prevention.[66,93] A 2018 Cochrane network metaanalysis reported that oxytocin was more effective than a placebo or no treatment for preventing a blood loss ≥ 1000 mL (RR, 0.61; 95% CI, 0.5 to 0.7).[94] Similar findings were observed in a 2019 Cochrane systematic review; prophylactic oxytocin resulted in a 49% reduced risk of PPH compared with a placebo or no treatment (RR, 0.5; 95% CI, 0.4 to 0.7).[91]

The exogenous preparation of the hormone (Pitocin, Syntocinon) is a synthetic formulation with a rapid onset of action (immediate after intravenous injection, and 3 to 5 minutes after intramuscular injection) and short half-life (3 to 12 minutes) due to rapid metabolism by hepatic oxytocinases and clearance in the urine and bile.

To initiate adequate uterine tone after delivery, oxytocin is routinely administered as a *prophylactic* bolus (intramuscular or intravenous) or as an intravenous rapid infusion. In the setting of elective cesarean delivery, several studies have reported that a low-dose oxytocin bolus is sufficient for initiating adequate uterine tone. In a prospective study of patients undergoing elective cesarean delivery, the minimum effective dose in 90% of patients (ED90) was 0.35 IU (95% CI, 0.18 to 0.52).[95] In a randomized dose-response study, high rates of adequate uterine tone were observed across a range of low to moderate bolus doses of 0, 0.5, 1, 3, and 5 IU (73%, 100%, 93%, 100%, and 93%, respectively).[96] Similar findings were observed in a study comparing 5, 10, 15, and 20 IU.[97] Several studies have investigated the ED90 of an oxytocin infusion

and observed similar results ([0.29 IU/min for 3 minutes; 95% CI, 0.15 to 0.43][98] and [0.27/min IU for 4 minutes; 95% CI, 0.21 to 0.32][99]). Higher ED90 doses have been reported for morbidly obese patients (ED90, 0.75 IU; 95% CI, 0.5 to 0.93),[100] and for those with twin gestation (ED90, 4.38 IU; 95% CI, 3.68 to 4.86).[101]

For patients undergoing intrapartum cesarean delivery, data from prospective studies indicate that higher oxytocin doses are required to initiate adequate uterine tone. Among a cohort who underwent intrapartum cesarean delivery for labor arrest, the oxytocin bolus-dose ED90 was 2.99 IU (95% CI, 2.32 to 3.67); this dose is nine times higher than the ED90 for a prelabor singleton cesarean delivery.[102] Similarly, the ED90 for an oxytocin infusion is also higher (0.74 IU/min for 4 minutes; 95% CI, 0.56 to 0.93).[99] These findings provide clinical evidence in support of oxytocin receptor desensitization from exogenous oxytocin augmentation during labor.

Maintenance oxytocin infusions are typically used to sustain adequate uterine tone and reduce the likelihood of patients experiencing delayed PPH or requiring additional uterotonics. In a randomized controlled trial, patients who received a maintenance oxytocin infusion for 4 hours after a 5 IU bolus dose required less additional uterotonics compared to patients who received the bolus dose followed by a placebo infusion (12.2% versus 18.4%).[103] Less information is available on the optimal rate of infusion for maintaining adequate uterine tone. In a randomized trial comparing a low-rate to a high-rate oxytocin infusion (2.5 IU/h versus 15 IU/h), no significant between-group differences were observed in uterine tone or blood loss, suggesting that a low maintenance infusion rate may be sufficient.[104]

Dose-dependent *side effects* of oxytocin include vasodilation, tachycardia, and hypotension.[105–111] Exposure to high-dose oxytocin regimens in hemodynamically compromised patients or patients with cardiac dysfunction increases the risk of cardiovascular collapse and cardiac arrest.[109,112]

TABLE 37.3   Oxytocin and Carbetocin Dosing Recommendations for Uterine Atony Prophylaxis During Elective and Intrapartum Cesarean Delivery

	Elective Cesarean Delivery	Intrapartum Cesarean Delivery
Oxytocin bolus for *initiating* adequate uterine tone	1 IU	3 IU
Oxytocin infusion for *maintenance* of adequate uterine tone	2.5–7.5 IU/h (0.04–0.125 IU/min)	7.5–15 IU/h (0.125–0.25 IU/min)
Carbetocin	20–100 µg over at least 30 s (lower doses possible; maximum dose, 100 µg)	100 µg over at least 30 s (careful monitoring for hypotension and tachycardia is recommended with doses >100 µg; maximum dose, 120 µg)

From Heesen M, Carvalho B, Carvalho JCA, et al. International consensus statement on the use of uterotonic agents during caesarean section. *Anaesthesia.* 2019;74:1305–1319; Lagrew D, McNulty J, Sakowski C, et al. Improving healthcare response to obstetric hemorrhage, a California Maternal Quality Care Collaborative toolkit; 2022. https://www.cmqcc.org/sites/default/files/HEMToolkit_03252022%20Errata%207.2022%20%282%29.pdf. Accessed 31 December 2024.

Concomitant administration of a vasopressor, such as phenylephrine, can mitigate hypotension associated with a bolus dose of oxytocin.[113]

Recommendations for oxytocin dosing based on published data, a 2019 expert consensus statement for oxytocin dosing for cesarean delivery, and the California Maternal Quality Care Collaborative (CMQCC) hemorrhage toolkit are found in Table 37.3.[114,115]

Carbetocin. Carbetocin (1-deamino-1-carba-2-tyrosine (*O*-methyl)-oxytocin) is an alternative synthetic oxytocin-receptor agonist. It is not available in the United States. Latency is short after IV or IM administration (2 minutes). Because its half-life is 4 to 10 times longer than oxytocin, a continuous maintenance infusion is not required after bolus administration.

Dose-finding studies report that a low dose of *prophylactic* carbetocin is sufficient for initiating adequate uterine tone at elective cesarean delivery. Based on data from two randomized trials and one noninferiority study reporting the effects of carbetocin doses ranging from 20 to 100 µg, a dose < 100 µg is likely sufficient for initiating adequate tone during elective cesarean delivery.[116–118] For patients who undergo intrapartum cesarean delivery for labor arrest after oxytocin augmentation, the ED90 of carbetocin is 121 µg (95% CI, 111 to 130 µg).[119] The ED90 in women with morbid obesity undergoing elective cesarean delivery (body mass index [BMI] > 40 kg/m²) was 68 µg (95% CI, 52 to 77 µg),[120] approximately four times higher than in women with a BMI < 40 kg/m², also undergoing elective cesarean (14.8 µg; 95% CI, 13.7 to 15.8).[121]

Side effects associated with carbetocin are similar to those with oxytocin. Carbetocin 100 µg has a similar side-effect profile to oxytocin 5 IU, with respect to hypotension, tachycardia, vomiting, flushing, shortness of breath, chest pain, and abdominal pain.[122,123] A 37% incidence of hypotension was reported in a dose-response study for elective cesarean delivery.[121] No differences in hypotension incidence among doses were reported in dose-ranging studies.[116,117] In the dose-finding study of carbetocin administration in patients requiring intrapartum cesarean delivery for labor arrest, the overall incidence of hypotension and tachycardia was high (45% and 57.5%, respectively).[119] At a dose of 140 µg, the incidence of tachycardia and intraoperative arrhythmias was 76% and 14%, respectively. Therefore, the routine use of high doses of carbetocin (≥140 µg) is not recommended. Patients receiving doses between 100 and 140 µg should be carefully monitored.

Studies comparing oxytocin and carbetocin for postpartum hemorrhage prevention. A large multinational randomized noninferiority trial of 29,645 patients who underwent vaginal delivery found that carbetocin 100 µg was noninferior to oxytocin 10 IU for prevention of blood loss ≥ 500 mL (14.5% versus 14.5%, carbetocin versus oxytocin) and the need for additional uterotonic agents (10.4% versus 10.4%).[124] Data from a randomized trial suggest that there are no differences in the need for additional uterotonics, estimated blood loss, change in hemoglobin level, or need for transfusion in patients receiving carbetocin 100 µg compared to oxytocin 5 IU.[125] Following a medication shortage in Canada, a before-and-after study compared carbetocin and oxytocin after both vaginal and cesarean deliveries; no between-group differences in the need for additional uterotonics, estimated blood loss, and calculated blood loss at cesarean delivery were identified.[126] Based on data from four metaanalyses,[94,127–129] carbetocin compared to oxytocin reduced the need for additional uterotonics by 55% among all delivery modes and between 53% and 78% for those undergoing cesarean delivery. However, no clinically meaningful or significant differences were reported between patients receiving oxytocin and carbetocin in the risk of PPH or in the volume of blood loss after delivery. These findings suggest that carbetocin is noninferior to oxytocin in preventing PPH and is likely more effective in reducing the need for additional uterotonics.

Ergot Alkaloids

The natural ergot alkaloids are produced by a fungus that commonly infests rye and other grains. Ergonovine and methylergonovine (a semisynthetic preparation with an identical pharmacologic profile) are the two ergot alkaloids currently available for use. Their uterotonic effect is most likely mediated by serotonergic agonism; the ergot alkaloids are also weak dopamine and alpha-adrenergic receptor agonists.[130] Both drugs have similar pharmacologic properties and are dispensed in ampules containing 0.2 mg. When administered via the intramuscular route, both drugs have a rapid onset (1 to 3 minutes), long half-lives (30 to 120 minutes), and reach maximal plateau concentrations in 40 minutes.[131] Ergot alkaloids are stable at room temperature for prolonged periods.[132]

Postpartum hemorrhage prevention. Based on data from metaanalyses,[94,127] ergometrine does not reduce the risk of PPH or the need for additional uterotonics compared with oxytocin. In addition, there was no between-group difference in blood loss. Several randomized trials have examined whether prophylaxis with methylergonovine combined with oxytocin reduces the need for additional uterotonics compared with oxytocin alone in patients undergoing intrapartum cesarean delivery. In a study of 80 patients, patients who received intramuscular methylergonovine 0.2 mg and an oxytocin infusion (0.3 IU/min) had a lower need for additional uterotonics (20% versus 55%; RR, 0.4; 95% CI, 0.2 to 0.6), and a lower incidence of PPH (35% versus 59%; RR, 0.6; 95% CI, 0.4 to 0.9) than those who received oxytocin alone.[133] In another study of 105 patients comparing prophylaxis with intravenous oxytocin (5 IU) alone, or with intravenous ergonovine (0.25 mg) or intramuscular carboprost (0.25 mg), no differences were observed in the need for additional uterotonics (37% versus 33% versus 34%, respectively) or total calculated blood loss (1180 mL versus 1145 mL versus 1242 mL).[134] Between-study differences in the characteristics of study populations, prophylactic oxytocin regimens, and approaches for determining the need for additional uterotonics may explain these divergent findings. Notably, in both studies, the need for an additional uterotonic in patients who underwent intrapartum cesarean delivery who received combined oxytocin and ergonovine prophylaxis was at least 20% across all study groups, highlighting the concern for refractory uterine atony in this high-risk subpopulation.

Postpartum hemorrhage treatment. Population-based and randomized trial data provide insight into the effectiveness of methylergonovine compared with carboprost for the treatment of PPH. In a propensity-score matched secondary analysis of 1335 patients who underwent cesarean delivery, the risk of hemorrhage-related morbidity (transfusion, need for additional uterotonics, surgical interventions) was 1.7-fold higher in patients who received carboprost compared with methylergonovine, after adjustment for relevant confounders.[135] A randomized trial of 100 patients who experienced refractory uterine atony during nonemergency cesarean delivery compared the effect of methylergonovine to carboprost on uterine tone, which was evaluated using a 0 to 10 numerical scale 10 minutes after drug administration.[136] After administration of methylergonovine or carboprost, there were no between-group differences in uterine tone scores (mean [standard deviation (SD)], 7.3 [1.7] versus 7.6 [2.1]), need for additional second-line uterotonics, or PPH rate. Given that this study was not powered to examine differences in second-line uterotonic use

or hemorrhage-related morbidity, we routinely use methylergonovine as the preferred second-line uterotonic in the absence of contraindications.

Side effects. Ergot alkaloids are associated with nausea and vomiting, arteriolar vasoconstriction, and hypertension.[130] In the 2018 metaanalysis, ergometrine compared with oxytocin was associated with an increased risk of nausea (RR, 2.4; 95% CI, 1.65 to 3.49) and vomiting (RR, 2.4; 95% CI, 1.6 to 3.6).[94] Intravenous bolus administration is not recommended because of the propensity to cause serious cardiovascular system derangements. Intramuscular administration may cause vasoconstriction, hypertension, myocardial ischemia and infarction caused by coronary vasospasm,[137,138] cerebrovascular accident,[139] seizures,[139] and death.[137,140] Fortunately, these serious adverse effects occur rarely.[141] Relative contraindications to the use of ergot alkaloids include hypertension, preeclampsia, peripheral vascular disease, and ischemic heart disease. Treatment of ergot-induced vasoconstriction and hypertension may require administration of a potent vasodilator, such as nitroglycerin or sodium nitroprusside. Blood pressure and the electrocardiogram should be monitored closely after administration.

Prostaglandins

Prostaglandins of the E and F families have gained wide acceptance as second-line therapy when high-dose oxytocin is inadequate for the treatment of uterine atony. Concentrations of endogenous prostaglandins increase during labor, and levels peak at the time of placental separation. It is hypothesized that uterine atony may represent a failure of prostaglandin concentrations to increase during the third stage of labor in some women.[142,143] Prostaglandins increase myometrial intracellular free calcium concentration, ultimately leading to an increase in myosin light-chain kinase activity. Common side effects noted after prostaglandin administration include fever, chills, diarrhea, nausea, and vomiting.[130]

15-Methyl prostaglandin $F_{2\alpha}$. 15-Methyl prostaglandin $F_{2\alpha}$, or carboprost tromethamine (Hemabate), is manufactured as 0.25 mg (250 µg) per 1-mL vial and requires refrigeration for storage. After intramuscular administration, the time to peak effect is between 15 and 60 minutes and the half-life is 8 minutes. The drug may be repeated every 15 to 30 minutes; the total dose should not exceed 2 mg (eight doses).

In a 2018 metaanalysis evaluating uterotonic agents for *prevention* of PPH, injectable prostaglandins compared to oxytocin were not associated with a reduced risk of PPH (RR, 1.43; 95% CI, 0.20 to 10.31); the quality of evidence was deemed uncertain.[94] Based on low-certainty evidence, injectable prostaglandins were associated with a reduced likelihood of additional uterotonics compared with oxytocin (RR, 0.29; 95% CI, 0.09 to 0.94). The wide confidence interval indicated the uncertainty about the accuracy of the risk estimates.[94]

Rare *side effects* of carboprost may include bronchospasm, abnormal ventilation-perfusion ratio, increased intrapulmonary shunt fraction, and hypoxemia in susceptible patients.[144,145] Carboprost is relatively contraindicated in patients with a history of bronchospasm or asthma.

Misoprostol. Misoprostol is a prostaglandin E_1 analog that has been used successfully for cervical ripening and induction of labor. Furthermore, misoprostol is thermostable in tropical conditions and does not require intravenous access for administration. These characteristics make it an attractive alternative to oxytocin and other injectable uterotonics in low-resource areas with high rates of death from hemorrhage.[146] Although less effective than oxytocin, prophylactic misoprostol administration reduces the incidence of PPH compared with placebo.[147] Misoprostol can be administered via different routes, including sublingual, rectal, vaginal, and oral. Based on pharmacokinetic data, the onset time is relatively slow for all routes of administration (oral, 8 minutes; sublingual, 11 minutes; vaginal, 20 minutes; and rectal, 100 minutes) and the duration of action is relatively long (approximately 2, 3, 4, and 4 hours, respectively).[148]

Data from two metaanalyses indicate that, compared with oxytocin, misoprostol use has a slightly higher risk for PPH, but no difference in the need for additional uterotonics when used to *prevent PPH*.[94,127]

Based on outcome data from several high-quality randomized trials, the use of misoprostol for *treating PPH* has been questioned.[149] In a double-blind noninferiority trial, patients with PPH who received prophylactic oxytocin were randomized to receive sublingual misoprostol 800 μg or an additional 40 IU of oxytocin (in 1-L intravenous solution administered over 15 minutes).[150] A similar proportion of patients in each group had control of active bleeding within 20 minutes (misoprostol, 89%; oxytocin, 90%). However, women in the misoprostol group were more likely to experience serious ongoing hemorrhage (3% versus 1%). In addition, the women in the misoprostol group were more likely to undergo intrauterine clinical exploration under anesthesia.

In a second randomized controlled trial, the combination of misoprostol and oxytocin for PPH management was not more effective than oxytocin alone.[151] Patients with a PPH diagnosis who received prophylactic oxytocin were randomized to receive additional oxytocin 10 IU or oxytocin 10 IU combined with sublingual misoprostol 600 μg. Women who received combined misoprostol and oxytocin were no less likely to have additional hemorrhage compared with those receiving only oxytocin (14% versus 14%). Moreover, misoprostol use was associated with an increase in adverse events such as intense shivering, hyperthermia, and vomiting. In a third randomized trial, patients who experienced PPH in the absence of prophylactic oxytocin were randomized to receive sublingual misoprostol 800 μg versus oxytocin (40 IU in 1-L normal saline over 15 minutes).[152] The proportion of women in whom bleeding resolved within 20 minutes of the study drug administration was lower in the misoprostol group compared with the oxytocin group (90% versus 96%). More women in the misoprostol group experienced additional blood loss (30% versus 17%) and required additional uterotonics (13% versus 6%). Overall, these data suggest that misoprostol should only be considered for the first-line treatment of PPH if oxytocin is not available.

In the randomized trials, patients who received misoprostol experienced substantially higher rates of *side effects*. In a systematic review of randomized trials with misoprostol in at least one intervention arm for PPH prevention, the incidence and risk of misoprostol-induced fever were related to its dosage and route of administration.[153] The highest reported incidence of fever was for the sublingual route (15%), with lower rates with the oral (11.4%) and rectal routes (4%). In a separate systematic review of uterotonic agents, the risk of fever was 3.4-fold higher in patients receiving misoprostol compared with oxytocin (two trials) and 3.1-fold higher in patients receiving misoprostol and oxytocin compared with oxytocin only (four trials).[154] In the same review,[154] the risk of vomiting associated with misoprostol was increased 2.5-fold (two trials) for misoprostol alone and 1.9-fold (two trials) for misoprostol combined with oxytocin compared with oxytocin alone.

Given current evidence of the limited effectiveness of misoprostol as a second-line agent in patients who have already received oxytocin for PPH prophylaxis or treatment, and considering the adverse side-effect profile, misoprostol should *not* be considered as a second-line uterotonic unless absolute contraindications prevent the use of other second-line uterotonic drugs.

Calcium. Calcium may be a viable adjunct for the treatment of refractory uterine atony. *In vitro* studies have shown that spontaneous and oxytocin-induced myometrial contractility is reduced in the setting of low extracellular calcium.[155–157] A randomized trial compared the effects of calcium chloride 1 g to a placebo on blood loss in 120 patients undergoing intrapartum cesarean delivery who had received an oxytocin infusion during labor (for induction or augmentation).[158] The between-group difference in median blood loss was not significant (211 mL; 95% CI, −33 to 410). A planned subgroup analysis that excluded cases of nonatonic bleeding suggested that calcium exposure may result in less blood loss. Adequately powered studies are needed to determine whether calcium supplementation for refractory atonic PPH reduces the transfusion rate or the need for more invasive intervention.

Genital Trauma

The most common childbirth injuries are lacerations and hematomas of the perineum, vagina, and cervix. Most injuries have minimal consequence, but some puerperal lacerations and hematomas are associated with significant hemorrhage, either immediate or delayed.[159] Prompt recognition and treatment can minimize morbidity and mortality.[159] Genital tract lacerations should be suspected in all patients who have vaginal bleeding. The cervix and vagina must be carefully inspected; the index of suspicion for cervical laceration should be high after forceps-assisted delivery.[160] Computed tomography (CT) and/or MRI may be useful in detecting the presence, location, and extent of suspected hematoma in hemodynamically stable patients.[161]

Pelvic hematomas may be divided into three types: vaginal, vulvar, and retroperitoneal.[159] **Vaginal hematomas** result from bleeding from the descending branch of the uterine artery due to soft tissue injury from a complicated or operative vaginal delivery.[159,162] In a population-based study of deliveries in Sweden between 1987 and 2000, the prevalence of vaginal hematomas was 1 in 1240 deliveries.[163] Risk factors for vaginal hematomas include nulliparity, advanced maternal age, neonatal birth weight exceeding 4000 g, prolonged second stage of labor, multiple gestation, preeclampsia, and vulvovaginal varicosities.[159] Vaginal hematomas larger than 4 cm may need exploration and evacuation to ligate bleeding vessels.[164] Vaginal packing with povidone-iodine gauze may be helpful for achieving tamponade.

Vulvar hematomas are blood collections in the vulva; the incidence is 1:300 to 1:1000 deliveries.[164] Due to its rich blood supply and soft tissue friability, the vulva is vulnerable to hematoma formation secondary to childbirth-related trauma.[159] Most hematomas occur after an uncomplicated delivery[165]; however, direct injury can occur from an episiotomy, vaginal laceration repair, or operative vaginal delivery. Indirect injury can occur from extensive stretching of the birth canal during vaginal delivery. The source of blood can be venous or arterial in origin; arterial bleeding originates from a branch of the pudendal artery.

Perineal, abdominal, or buttock pain is the most common presenting feature of a vulvar or vaginal hematoma. Other clinical features include intermittent bleeding, urinary retention or dysfunction (from mechanical obstruction), and, in severe cases, hemodynamic instability. Depending on acuity and severity, symptoms can occur within a few hours to days after delivery. A hematoma is typically visualized on physical examination. Pelvic ultrasound, CT, or MRI may be necessary to evaluate the hematoma size and location.

Small, nonenlarging vaginal or vulvar hematomas can be treated conservatively with ice packs and oral analgesics. Large or expanding hematomas, especially in patients with hemodynamic instability, urologic dysfunction, or neurologic signs, require urgent surgical drainage; ligation of bleeding vessels; evaluation for bleeding that tracks posteriorly, vaginally, or into the retroperitoneum; and surveillance for pressure necrosis. In anticipation of severe blood loss, blood products should be available before surgery. In some cases, arterial embolization may be considered to decrease bleeding and aid the surgical management of genital tract hematomas.[162]

Cervical lacerations are tears or cuts to the cervix that most typically occur after a vaginal delivery. The cervix is a very vascular organ, supplied mainly by descending branches of the uterine arteries. Due to the rich vasculature, cervical tears can result in significant blood loss, although most cervical lacerations are small and do not require repair. Clinically significant cervical lacerations are rare, occurring in 0.2% to 0.5% of deliveries.[166–170] Risk factors for cervical laceration include cervical cerclage, precipitous labor, operative vaginal delivery, induction of labor, oxytocin use, and episiotomy.[166,167,169,170] A systematic review reported that the risk of cervical laceration was between two- and five-fold greater for a forceps-assisted than vacuum-assisted delivery.[171] However,

the certainty of the evidence was very low to moderate. Patients with posterior tears may be at risk for greater morbidity, including DIC, prolonged hospitalization, and transfer to the operating room, than those with lateral or anterior tears.[172]

Proper lighting, visualization, and analgesia are important when evaluating the location of the cervical laceration and for achieving adequate hemostasis. Anesthetic options include augmentation of epidural analgesia or low-dose spinal anesthesia to ensure that patients can undergo adequate evaluation and repair without experiencing undue pain or distress. The magnitude of blood loss associated with a cervical laceration may be underappreciated. Close monitoring of vital signs as well as hematologic and coagulation indices are recommended, especially if there is more than one etiology for blood loss, such as cervical laceration with uterine atony. Given these obstetric and anesthetic concerns, transfer to the operating room to expedite resuscitation and surgical treatment is recommended for patients with cervical lacerations with active bleeding.

Retroperitoneal hematomas are the least common and most dangerous hematomas associated with childbirth. A retroperitoneal hemorrhage occurs after laceration of one of the branches of the hypogastric artery. Vessel injury can occur during cesarean delivery, peripartum hysterectomy, or after the rupture of a low-transverse uterine scar during labor. A hematoma that originates in the broad ligament may dissect into the retroperitoneal space along the lateral pelvic sidewalls and may extend as far as the kidneys.

Symptoms of concealed bleeding depend on the size and growth rate of the hematoma. Because a retroperitoneal hematoma is not associated with external bleeding, it is important to consider the diagnosis in patients with unexplained and worsening tachycardia and hypotension, acute decreases in hematocrit, or acute coagulopathy. Other signs and symptoms are restlessness, lower abdominal pain, a tender mass above the inguinal ligament that displaces a firm uterus to the contralateral side, and vaginal bleeding with hypotension out of proportion to the external blood loss. Ileus, unilateral leg edema, urinary retention, and hematuria also may occur.[159] In obese women, it may be especially difficult to examine the abdomen for signs of retroperitoneal hematoma.

When a retroperitoneal hematoma is suspected, urgent and close evaluation is necessary. Clinicians must be prepared for immediate transfer to the operating room if there is ongoing hemodynamic instability in the postpartum period. Life-threatening hematomas require exploratory laparotomy with experienced obstetric, anesthesia, and surgical staff providing direct care. Blood products should be immediately available; one study reported that 38 of 39 patients with a broad ligament hematoma required a blood transfusion and 8 patients required a hysterectomy.[173] Abdominal imaging such as CT scan or interventional radiology treatment may be considered for hemodynamically stable patients.

Ultrasonographic imaging can be used to identify intraabdominal or intrauterine blood but may not be sufficient to rule out a retroperitoneal hematoma. Therefore, a negative scan result should not obviate the need for urgent surgical exploration in a patient with symptoms and signs of hypovolemic shock, acute anemia, and/or coagulopathy in the absence of external bleeding.

Anesthetic Management

Choice of anesthetic technique for the repair of genital lacerations and evacuation of pelvic hematomas depends on the affected area, surgical requirements, the patient's intravascular volume and hemodynamic status, and urgency of the procedure. Local infiltration and a small dose of intravenous opioid may suffice for the drainage of small vulvar hematomas; however, repair of extensive lacerations and drainage of large vaginal hematomas require a greater depth of surgical anesthesia. A pudendal nerve block may not be technically feasible because of anatomic distortion or severe pain from the hematoma. Spinal or epidural anesthesia may be indicated for patients requiring surgical anesthesia beyond a localized area. However, clinicians should exercise caution initiating (or extending) a neuraxial block in a patient with significant hypovolemia due to concern for precipitating cardiovascular collapse. For patients with severe hemodynamic instability or severe and evolving hemorrhage, general anesthesia with tracheal intubation may be necessary. Exploratory laparotomy for a retroperitoneal hematoma typically requires general anesthesia with anticipation for severe or massive intrabdominal hemorrhage requiring a massive transfusion and hemostatic support (see later discussion).

Retained Placenta

A retained placenta is defined as the failure to deliver the placenta completely within 30 minutes of delivery of the infant and occurs in approximately 3% of vaginal deliveries.[174–176] A retained placenta typically results from one of three causes: (1) the placenta may be blocked behind a contracted lower uterus/cervix (incarcerated placenta), (2) it may be adhered to the uterine wall (placenta adherens), or (3) it may be invading the myometrium (placenta accreta). The severity of bleeding ranges from minimal to severe, requiring transfusion.[175] The risk for PPH increases significantly if the interval between delivery of the infant and the placenta exceeds 30 minutes.[174,176] Prophylactic oxytocin facilitates placental separation from the uterine wall and is not associated with retained placenta after vaginal birth.[177,178] Risk factors for retained placenta include history of retained placenta, preterm delivery, oxytocin use during labor, preeclampsia, and nulliparity.[174,175]

Obstetric Management

Treatment of retained placenta during the early postpartum period often involves gentle cord traction, uterine massage, manual removal, and inspection of the placenta. If manual extraction is not successful, curettage may be required. The clinician may need to discontinue oxytocin during curettage and then, once the placenta has fully delivered, restart it to augment uterine tone. The eventual removal of the placenta typically promotes uterine contraction and reduces bleeding.

However, close observation for signs of recurrent hemorrhage is warranted. Because manual extraction of the placenta increases the risk for endometritis, the WHO recommends prophylactic antibiotic administration,[179] but published studies neither support nor refute this recommendation.[180]

Anesthetic Management

Manual extraction of the placenta is painful and requires analgesia. In some cases, intravenous analgesia may be adequate to allow examination and manual placental extraction by a skilled obstetrician. However, in many cases, administration of local anesthetic through an indwelling epidural catheter provides better quality analgesia.[181] In the absence of an indwelling epidural catheter, *de novo* spinal anesthesia should be considered in patients who are not bleeding severely and are hemodynamically stable in the operating room. General anesthesia with a rapid sequence induction may be necessary for patients experiencing severe breakthrough pain or who are hemodynamically unstable. Caution should be exercised in using sedation or "monitored anesthesia care" because many patients will not meet "nil by mouth" precautions and thus be at risk for pulmonary aspiration. Additionally, the depth of analgesia with sedatives and/or opioids is typically not sufficient to ensure that patients can safely experience manual placental removal without incurring significant periprocedural pain and psychological distress.

To facilitate manual placental removal, nitroglycerin may be administered for uterine relaxation. Nitroglycerin provides a rapid onset of smooth muscle relaxation and a short plasma half-life (2 to 3 minutes).[182] Successful removal of retained placenta was observed in 15 parturients after administration of intravenous nitroglycerin 500 μg.[183] Others have used substantially lower doses of nitroglycerin (50 to 100 μg) with similar results.[184] Nitroglycerin may also be administered sublingually via spray or tablet. A double-blind, randomized controlled study compared sublingual nitroglycerin with a placebo for management of retained placenta; the placenta was delivered successfully within 5 minutes in all 12 of the parturients who received nitroglycerin compared with only 1 of the 12 who received a placebo.[185] Nitroglycerin most likely produces uterine smooth muscle relaxation by releasing nitric oxide, which temporarily decreases systemic blood pressure. Because of its short plasma half-life, sustained hypotension after bolus administration is rare. Nevertheless, administration of nitroglycerin necessitates vigilant blood pressure monitoring and treatment when indicated.

Uterine Inversion

Uterine inversion is a rare but potentially disastrous event. It is associated with severe PPH and hemodynamic instability may be worsened by concurrent vagal reflex–mediated bradycardia. The reported incidence of this disorder varies widely; recent reports suggest an incidence of approximately 1 in 3400 deliveries.[186] Cervical dilation and uterine relaxation are key etiologic factors necessary for the uterus to prolapse through the cervical ring.

Risk factors for uterine inversion include uterine atony, a short umbilical cord, uterine anomalies, and overly aggressive management of the third stage of labor, including inappropriate fundal pressure or excessive umbilical cord traction.[186] However, 15% to 50% of inversions occur in patients with no associated risk factors, implying congenital abnormalities of the uterine musculature or innervation may be contributing factors. Uterotonic therapy can convert a partial inversion to a complete inversion. An abnormally implanted placenta (i.e., placenta accreta) may be first recognized when uterine inversion occurs.

Diagnosis

Uterine inversion should be suspected when severe hemorrhage occurs in the presence of a mass in the vagina and a nonpalpable fundus. Inversion should be suspected in all cases of PPH. Ultrasonographic examination may show characteristic findings, such as an echolucent zone within an echogenic mass filling the uterine cavity on transverse view.[187] Historically, obstetricians have observed that the shock is out of proportion to the blood loss, which may be mediated by parasympathetic stimulation caused by tissue stretching. An incomplete inversion not protruding through the introitus is more likely to result in missed or delayed diagnosis.[159]

Obstetric Management

Replacement of the uterus and resuscitation, even before removal of the placenta, are the immediate treatment goals.[188] All uterotonic drugs should be discontinued immediately. The obstetrician should attempt to reduce the inversion by applying pressure through the vagina to the uterine fundus; ring forceps may be used on the cervix to apply countertraction. Once the uterus is repositioned, uterine atony often follows, especially if tocolytics have been used. It is therefore important to treat uterine atony early and establish uterine contractility to avoid any likelihood of reinversion. Therapeutic measures to treat uterine atony include fundal massage and second-line uterotonic agents. Insertion of an intrauterine balloon may prove useful during treatment to prevent reinversion.[189]

Anesthetic Management

Hemorrhage in the setting of uterine inversion can be abrupt, severe, and life threatening. Immediate resuscitation is needed by the anesthesia team. Closure of the cervical os and uterine smooth muscle contraction precludes reducing the uterus. Thus, relaxation of both the cervical ring and uterus is a prerequisite for successful treatment. Nitroglycerin can facilitate uterine relaxation and replacement, with reports describing an intravenous bolus dose between 200 and 250 µg.[190,191] Given that the vasodilatory effect of nitroglycerin can compound maternal hemodynamic instability, the anesthesia provider should closely support the maternal circulation with intravenous fluids and vasopressors. If early attempts to reposition the uterus fail following tocolysis, general anesthesia with a volatile halogenated agent is indicated to facilitate uterine relaxation and/or a laparotomy.

Placenta Accreta Spectrum

Placenta accreta spectrum (PAS) disorders constitute highly morbid conditions characterized by direct attachment of villous tissue to superficial myometrium and fibrinoid deposition at the uteroplacental interface.[192] There are three subtypes of placenta accreta, together referred to as **PAS** (Fig. 37.2). **Placenta accreta vera** is defined as adherence of the basal plate of the placenta directly to uterine myometrium without an intervening decidual layer. **Placenta increta** refers to a placenta in which chorionic villi invade the myometrium. **Placenta percreta** represents invasion through the myometrium into serosa and sometimes into adjacent organs, most often the bladder.[193] Newer clinical and pathological grading schemes have been proposed to categorize the PAS severity based on the degree of surgical complexity during delivery and correlate these data to the histopathologic findings. The goal of these schemes is to ensure consistency in the reporting of PAS data in the international literature.[194]

Epidemiology

The incidence of PAS has increased over the last several decades in association with increasing rates of cesarean delivery. In the United States, the incidence has increased from 1 in 30,000 pregnancies in the 1960s to 1 in 300 pregnancies in the 2010s.[195,196] In a systematic review of PAS in general population studies, the pooled prevalence was 0.17% (95% CI, 0.14 to 0.19).[197]

Previous cesarean delivery or other uterine surgery increases the risk for both placenta previa and PAS. The combination of placenta previa with previous cesarean delivery increases the risk for PAS, particularly if the placenta is anterior and overlies the uterine scar. A prospective multicenter observational study found that for patients with a placenta previa and prior cesarean delivery, the risk of PAS was 3%, 11%, 40%, 61%, and 67% for the first, second, third, fourth,

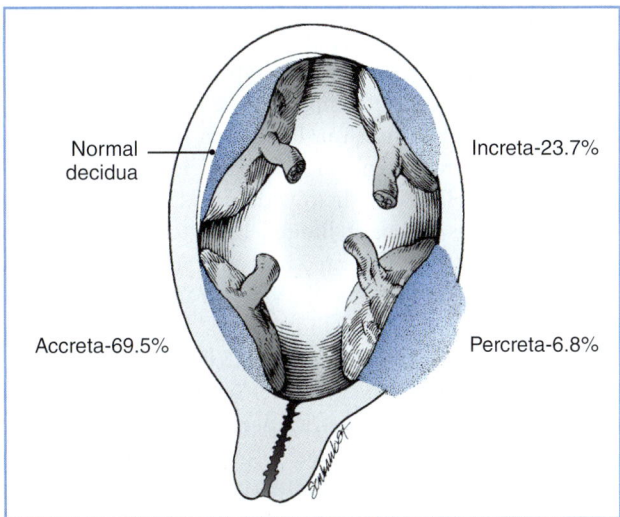

Fig. 37.2 Uteroplacental Relationships Found in Abnormal Placentation. From Francois KE, Foley MR. Antepartum and postpartum hemorrhage. In: Landon MB, Galan HL, Jauniaux ERM, et al., eds. *Gabbe's Obstetrics: Normal and Problem Pregnancies.* 9th ed. Elsevier; 2021:351.

and fifth or more prior cesareans, respectively (see Table 37.1).[22] A systematic review of 3889 patients with one or more prior cesarean deliveries with placenta previa or low-lying placenta in the index pregnancy (identified by ultrasonography) found that the incidence of placenta accreta was 4.1% in patients with one prior cesarean and 13.3% in patients with two or more prior cesareans.[198] Based on data from pathologic studies, the distribution of accreta subtype in descending order of frequency is accreta (69.5%), increta (23.7%), and percreta (6.8%).[199]

Diagnosis

Ultrasonography is the primary diagnostic modality for the antenatal diagnosis of placenta accreta.[193] Ideally, patients with risk factors for placenta accreta should be evaluated by obstetricians experienced in the ultrasonographic diagnosis of placenta accreta. Features of placenta accreta may be visible on ultrasonography as early as the first trimester. However, in most cases, the diagnosis is made in the second or third trimesters. Placenta previa is typically detected in more than 80% of PAS cases in the second and third trimesters. Other key ultrasonographic features include multiple placental vascular lacunae, loss of the normal hypoechoic zone between the placenta and myometrium, reduced retroplacental myometrial thickness (<1 mm), an abnormal uterine serosa-bladder interface, and extension of the placenta into myometrium, serosa, or bladder. No clear ultrasonographic features reliably predict the depth of placental invasion or PAS subtype.

Ultrasonography has very high sensitivity (91%) and specificity (97%) in the diagnosis of PAS.[200] MRI is another well-described modality for identifying PAS. Findings from a systematic review indicate MRI has comparable predictive accuracy to ultrasonography, with high sensitivity (94%) and moderate-to-high specificity (84%).[201] The accuracy of these modalities may be overestimated because studies typically involve patients with risk factors for PAS who undergo imaging in high-volume specialist centers. Although patients with indeterminate ultrasonographic findings or who are at high risk for more invasive accreta subtypes may undergo MRI, the extent to which MRI improves the diagnostic accuracy of ultrasonography is unclear. Prediction models that incorporate clinical, radiologic, and/or biologic data have been explored.[202,203] However, their widespread integration into clinical practice has been limited by heterogeneity across studies in terms of the selected potential predictors for PAS, the classification of PAS, and the variable accuracy of prediction models upon external validation.[204]

While antenatal identification of PAS is crucial for optimizing outcomes, a 2011 survey of ACOG members revealed that only one in four general obstetricians refered patients with suspected PAS to a specialist center.[205] Therefore, all facilities that provide obstetric care should have an action plan or checklist for the delivery care of patients with suspected or unexpected PAS.[206] In such cases, mobilization of essential resources and experienced staff is critical. Numerous studies have shown that antenatal compared to intrapartum diagnosis of PAS leads to less blood loss at delivery and optimized maternal outcomes.[207]

BOX 37.4   Criteria for a Placenta Accreta Spectrum Center of Excellence

- Multidisciplinary team
  - Experienced maternal-fetal medicine physician or obstetrician
  - Imaging experts (ultrasonography)
  - Pelvic surgeon (e.g., gynecologic oncologist, urogynecologist)
  - Anesthesiologist (e.g., obstetric, cardiac anesthesiologist)
  - Urologist
  - Trauma or general surgeon
  - Interventional radiologist
  - Neonatologist
- Intensive care unit and facilities
  - Interventional radiology capability
  - Surgical or medical intensive care unit
  - Neonatal intensive care unit
- Blood banking services
  - Massive transfusion capabilities
  - Cell salvage device and perfusionists
  - Experts in blood banking pathology or transfusion medicine specialists

Modified from Silver RM, Fox KA, Barton JR, et al. Center of excellence for placenta accreta. *Am J Obstet Gynecol* 2015;212: 561–568.

Obstetric Management

The ACOG and the Society for Maternal-Fetal Medicine (SMFM) recommend that patients with PAS be referred to and managed at a center with available resources of a Maternal Level of Care III (subspecialty) or IV facility (see Table 11.3).[193] Observational data suggest that patients who deliver in centers with a multidisciplinary team that includes a 24-hour in-house obstetrician and anesthesia provider, immediate availability of a gynecologic oncologist, a fully stocked blood bank, and interventional radiology services, experience less morbidity than those treated at hospitals without these services.[208] Criteria for a PAS center of excellence have been described (Box 37.4).[207]

Antenatal bleeding may necessitate emergency preterm delivery, although some cases of vaginal bleeding remote from term resolve spontaneously, and expectant management may prolong the duration of pregnancy into the third trimester. The risk for severe antenatal bleeding increases as gestational age increases.[208] The timing of delivery involves balancing the risk of emergency delivery for hemorrhage against the neonatal risks associated with preterm delivery. Decision analysis suggests that 34 weeks' gestation is the preferred time for planned delivery.[209] Professional organizations, including the ACOG and SMFM, recommend delivery between 34 0/7 and 35 6/7 weeks' gestation in a stable patient without additional medical, surgical, or fetal comorbidity and in the absence of labor or bleeding.[193]

Most patients with known PAS should undergo planned preterm cesarean delivery and hysterectomy with the placenta left *in situ*. Manual attempts to remove the placenta are strongly discouraged. For patients with an uncertain antenatal diagnosis, spontaneous placental separation may be appropriate if resources are available to manage severe hemorrhage. Preoperative placement of ureteral stents may minimize urinary tract injury.[193] Preoperative cystoscopy may also be considered to visualize placental involvement in the bladder wall. A midline vertical skin incision can improve surgical exposure. To avoid cutting through the placenta, surgeons may modify the uterine incision, such as selecting a fundal location to avoid a low-lying accreta.

Balloon occlusion. Balloon occlusion can be considered at different anatomic levels: uterine arteries, internal iliac arteries, common iliac arteries, and the distal abdominal aorta. Data are conflicting on the benefits of internal iliac artery balloon catheterization, the most well-described approach.[210–213] A small, single-center randomized trial of 27 patients comparing preoperative internal iliac balloon catheters to a control group reported no between-group difference in transfusion use (RBC units, 5.2 versus 4.1 U).[214] Multiple complications have been reported, including serious disruptions of the vasculature, infection, and lower extremity ischemia.[211,213,215,216] Introduction of the arterial catheters, even without balloon inflation, may cause fetal bradycardia necessitating emergency delivery.[217] If employed, internal iliac artery balloon catheters should be placed in the operating room after neuraxial block administration to avoid dislodgement and to allow for rapid delivery should fetal compromise occur. The SMFM recommends prophylactic intraarterial balloon catheters for well-counseled women with a strong desire for fertility preservation, those who decline blood products, and those with unresectable placenta percreta.[218]

Originally conceived to manage noncompressible torso hemorrhage, resuscitative endovascular balloon occlusion of the aorta (REBOA) has been deployed for the intraoperative management of hemorrhage in patients with PAS. The intended effect of REBOA is to reduce distal arterial pulse pressure and reduce perfusion to the uterus to minimize blood loss. Findings from a 2022 metaanalysis suggest that prophylactic aortic balloon occlusion may be the most effective balloon technique for lowering blood loss, transfusion volume, and the likelihood of hysterectomy.[219] However, these data were predominantly based on retrospective studies with varied inclusion criteria and indications for use. As with iliac balloon catheters, insertion through the femoral artery may lead to arterial dissection with lower extremity ischemia. Overall, any decision to use endovascular balloon approaches should be a local decision based on the expertise of the care team, the suspected degree of placental invasion, and anticipated surgical complexity for each case.

Conservative surgical approaches. Conservative management has been described as an approach for potentially preserving the uterus for future pregnancy and to reduce surgical morbidity. During cesarean delivery, the intact placenta is left *in situ* and the uterus and abdomen are closed to allow time for complete placental resorption.[220] Observational studies report reductions of up to 70% in the odds of transfusion, blood loss, and operative injury compared with immediate

hysterectomy.[221] However, conservatively managed patients often require additional therapies such as internal iliac artery balloon inflation or embolization, or administration of methotrexate. Some patients treated in this way have had successful subsequent pregnancies.[222] However, complications have been reported, including secondary hemorrhage, coagulopathy, endometritis, hysterectomy, and sepsis.[221–224] Therefore, these patients require prolonged and intensive postpartum follow-up. Although there is a lack of clear recommendations for the duration of follow-up, residual villous tissue in the uterine wall may require up to 6 months to be completely resorbed.[225] Based on expert opinion, weekly follow-up visits during the first 2 months, followed by monthly visits, in the absence of complications, is suggested.[225] Logistical issues and barriers to care may limit the availability of this approach to patients who live close to a specialist center that can rapidly manage any complications.[204] The ACOG considers planned peripartum hysterectomy to be the preferred management choice for patients with PAS and suggests limiting the use of uterine conservation strategies to hemodynamically stable patients who strongly desire future fertility.[193]

Interval hysterectomy. One proposed strategy to minimize risks associated with both immediate hysterectomy and conservative management of PAS is to perform an interval hysterectomy weeks after delivery. This approach allows for definitive treatment of PAS while potentially mitigating the risks associated with immediate hysterectomy, especially in severe cases. Prior to cesarean delivery, the surgical team systematically evaluates the abdomen and pelvis to document the extent of the disease, including remodeled uterus, bladder, parametria, adhesive disease, and other pelvic organ involvement. Based on this evaluation, a surgical decision is made to perform either an immediate or delayed hysterectomy. The latter involves systematic evaluations after delivery to ensure hysterotomy integrity and absence of significant vaginal bleeding. While delayed hysterectomy remains investigational, small retrospective, single-center studies suggest that delayed hysterectomy has potential benefits such as lower estimated blood loss and reduced transfusion volume compared to immediate hysterectomy.[226,227] Further investigation is warranted to determine the value of adjunctive procedures for delayed hysterectomy.

Partial myometrial resection and uterine reconstruction. An alternative treatment approach involves single-surgery partial myometrial resection and uterus reconstruction, primarily practiced in select regions of the world such as Brazil and various countries in Europe and Asia.[228–230] This strategy entails en bloc resection of the placenta and attached myometrium, followed by repair and reconstruction of the remaining uterus and cervix during cesarean delivery. Success relies on the surgical team's ability to assess, in real time, whether to attempt resection or proceed directly to hysterectomy based on the presence of characteristics such as viable myometrial tissue, hypervascularity, and pelvic adhesive disease. Some practitioners incorporate pelvic devascularization procedures, compression suturing, cervix integration, and/or tourniquet placement to reduce blood loss during reconstruction.

Patients should be informed that resection may not be possible or could result in significant bleeding necessitating hysterectomy. Outcome data are limited to uncontrolled case series with unclear selection criteria, and this approach remains experimental.[193]

Anesthetic Management

Patients diagnosed with PAS should receive anesthetic management in specialist centers (ACOG Maternal Level of Care III or IV), with 24-hour availability of anesthesia providers. However, consensus on best approaches to anesthetic management is lacking because most studies of anesthesia practices are based on small samples from single obstetric centers.[231] Further, sparse information is available on the level of subspecialist experience of anesthesia staff that manage PAS cases, as well as the location for delivery, whether an operating room on the labor and delivery unit, the main operating room complex, or a hybrid room in the interventional radiology suite.[232]

Options for the primary mode of anesthesia for cesarean delivery include neuraxial anesthesia, general anesthesia, or both (Table 37.4).[231] A review of anesthetic practices from published studies revealed a wide range in the reported frequency of general anesthesia (5% to 100%), neuraxial anesthesia (0% to 72%), and intraoperative conversion from neuraxial to general anesthesia (7% to 70%).[231]

Nearly half of patients with suspected PAS experience hemorrhage requiring blood transfusion.[197] Therefore, anticipatory planning for massive intraoperative hemorrhage is critical. Key considerations for hemorrhage management include location and size of intravenous access (peripheral and/or central), blood product ordering (number and types of blood components), resources for facilitating massive transfusion (e.g., institution-specific MTP, rapid infusion devices, intraoperative use of cell salvage), and point-of-care devices (e.g., transthoracic echocardiography for assessing intracardiac volume and contractility, viscoelastic testing devices). Based on a metaanalysis of studies that reported transfusion volumes in the surgical management of patients with PAS, a minimum of six units of RBCs should be available.[233]

In all cases, anesthesia providers should prepare for the potential for massive hemorrhage. The SMFM has developed an emergency checklist, planning worksheet, and system preparedness bundle to assist anesthesia and obstetric providers in system and team preparedness for peripartum management.[206] For all PAS cases, the anesthesia care should be directed by an experienced obstetric anesthesiologist, and preparations made for large volume blood loss (Box 37.5). In our current practice, we prefer neuraxial anesthesia (combined spinal-epidural anesthesia or single-shot spinal and thoracic epidural catheter placement) for the cesarean

---

TABLE 37.4   **Advantages and Disadvantages of Neuraxial, General, and Combined Neuraxial-General Anesthesia for Cesarean Hysterectomy**

Anesthetic Mode	Advantages	Disadvantages
Neuraxial anesthesia	• Awake patient • Maternal-infant bonding possible • Lower incidence of Apgar scores < 7 • Minimal effect on uterine tone • Possibly lower blood loss • Possibly superior postoperative analgesia[a] • Reduced ICU admission	• Possible need for emergency conversion to GA • Inferior operating conditions • Intraoperative nausea and vomiting • Risk of neuraxial block failure • Need for maternal anxiolysis or sedation • Concern for epidural hematoma in a high-blood-loss surgery associated with coagulopathy • Risk of post–dural puncture headache
General anesthesia	• Airway secured • Controlled ventilation • Superior operating conditions	• Failed tracheal intubation/airway disasters • Unwarranted use of GA if PAS not identified at surgery • Fetal exposure to general anesthetic medications • Volatile anesthetic agent decreases uterine tone • Higher magnitude of blood loss • Higher incidence of Apgar scores < 7 • Negative effect on neonatal bonding and breastfeeding • Postoperative nausea and vomiting • May require high-dose systemic opioid for postoperative analgesia
Elective conversion from neuraxial to GA after delivery	• No fetal exposure to general anesthetic agents • Patient awake for delivery, opportunity to bond with neonate • Airway secured for the resuscitation phase of procedure	• Timing of laryngoscopy and intubation may not be ideal • Hemodynamic instability after induction of GA in the presence of a neuraxial sympathectomy and/or possible hemorrhage

GA, General anesthesia; *ICU,* intensive care unit; *PAS,* placenta accreta spectrum.
[a]Depends on the site of surgical incision relative to the site of epidural catheter.
Modified from Warrick CM, Markley JC, Farber MK, et al. Placenta accreta spectrum disorders: knowledge gaps in anesthesia care. *Anesth Analg.* 2022;135(1):191–197.

BOX 37.5 Anesthetic Management of Placenta Accreta Spectrum

- Anesthesia provider: Experienced in the management of PAS
- Intravenous access: At least two large-bore venous cannulas (central or peripheral, 16-gauge or larger)
- Arterial cannula for invasive blood pressure monitoring and obtaining blood samples for laboratory testing
- Laboratory testing: Availability of rapid testing of hemoglobin/hematocrit, platelet count, coagulation indices
- Rapid infusion device(s)
- Warming device(s)
- Epidural catheter: For intraoperative anesthesia and/or postoperative analgesia[a]
- Blood products: Minimum six units RBC units, availability of other blood products
- Focused echocardiography[b]

PAS, Placenta accreta spectrum; *RBC*, red blood cells.
[a] A low-mid-thoracic catheter can be sited for postoperative analgesia.
[b] Focused transesophageal echocardiography is useful for monitoring rapid ventricle filling volume changes during a major hemorrhage.

delivery, with planned conversion to general anesthesia for patients requiring hysterectomy.

Limited information exists regarding postpartum outcomes and analgesia use after cesarean hysterectomy. In a single-center study of 39 patients with suspected PAS who underwent cesarean delivery, postoperative opioid consumption varied according to anesthesia mode.[234] Compared to patients who received general anesthesia only, mean-adjusted postoperative opioid consumption was lower (at least 150 oral morphine mg equivalents) for patients who had neuraxial anesthesia only, or neuraxial anesthesia with conversion to general anesthesia following delivery.

Postoperative analgesia options include long-acting neuraxial opioids, an epidural infusion of local anesthetic with or without opioids, intravenous patient-controlled analgesia, abdominal wall field blocks, and intravenous or oral analgesia (see Chapter 27). Because patients who undergo cesarean hysterectomy typically have a midline vertical skin incision, multimodal postoperative analgesia is suggested.

PREVENTION AND MITIGATION OF HEMORRHAGE-RELATED MORBIDITY

National maternal mortality reviews from the United States, France, and the United Kingdom indicate that hemorrhage is one of the most preventable causes of maternal death, with estimated rates of preventability of hemorrhage-related deaths between 60% and 70%.[55,235–237] Suboptimal care has been recognized as a major contributory factor.[181,235] Facility-related factors linked to severe morbidity or death from hemorrhage include (1) hospitals with no policies, protocols, or staff training; (2) absence of an onsite rapid response team or interventional care teams (e.g., interventional radiology, gynecologic oncology surgeons); and (3) a lack of key resources or equipment failure.[238] Provider-related factors include (1) a lack of knowledge about

PPH management; (2) limited familiarity with key equipment; (3) lack of response to clinical warning signs; (4) suboptimal or delayed medical, surgical, or radiologic intervention after ineffective pharmacologic treatment; (5) inadequate blood product use; (6) fixation errors; (7) delays in summoning physicians to the bedside of bleeding patients; (8) poor clinician communication; (9) poor care coordination among clinicians; and (10) delays in transferring patients to a higher level of care within or outside of the primary institution.[236]

Team-Based Approaches to Postpartum Hemorrhage Management

To address the rising rate of PPH in the United States, maternal safety agencies have focused their attention on approaches that standardize high-quality care to improve patient safety and maternal outcomes. Specifically, bundles, including checklists, algorithms, and simulations, have been developed to standardize and systematize multidisciplinary team-based protocols for anticipatory planning and the acute management of PPH. Multistakeholder multidisciplinary quality collaboratives, such as the National Partnership for Maternal Safety, The CMQCC, and the ACOG Safe Motherhood Initiative, have published patient safety bundles comprising toolkits of evidence-based practices, educational tools, and implementation aides.[239–241] In the United States, The Joint Commission, a private nonprofit organization that awards hospitals accreditation, developed new requirements for PPH prevention and treatment for hospitals providing obstetric services that were based on previously published PPH bundles.[242] In 2023, the WHO updated its PPH guidelines to include recommendations to perform objective blood loss measurement for improving PPH diagnosis and to standardize PPH management approaches through implementation of a PPH treatment bundle.[243]

Obstetric hemorrhage bundles are typically divided into five domains: (1) readiness, (2) recognition and prevention, (3) response, (4) reporting and systems learning, and (5) respectful care. Key aspects of the domains are illustrated in the bundle published by the Alliance for Innovation in Maternal Health (Box 37.6).[244] Common themes described in these bundles include (1) ongoing hemorrhage risk assessment in all patients; (2) access to a hemorrhage cart containing important supplies, surgical instruments, and medications; (3) a system for ensuring rapid availability of blood products, such as a MTP; (4) QBL measurement; (5) implementation of a PPH treatment protocol; (6) team-based approaches to PPH management; and (7) audit and feedback processes such as huddles, debriefing sessions, multidisciplinary reviews, and quality improvement committees.

Randomized trials and observational studies have examined whether the implementation of standardized bundles for PPH prevention or treatment is associated with reductions in hemorrhage-related morbidity. Within a large California healthcare system, investigators observed that, over a 10-month period, a standardized hemorrhage bundle was associated with a moderate decrease in total blood product use (35.9 versus 26.6 blood products per 1000 births) and a nonsignificant decrease in the hysterectomy rate (1.2 versus

BOX 37.6   Obstetric Hemorrhage Patient Safety Bundle

Readiness—Every Unit/Team

Develop processes for the management of patients with obstetric hemorrhage, including:

- A designated rapid response team co-led by nursing, obstetrics, and anesthesia with membership appropriate to the facility's level of maternal care.
- A standardized, facility-wide, stage-based obstetric hemorrhage emergency management plan with checklists and escalation policy.
- Emergency release and massive transfusion protocols to ensure immediate access to blood products.
- A protocol, including education and consent practices, to collaborate with patients who decline blood products, but may accept alternative approaches.
- Review of policies to identify and address organizational root causes of racial and ethnic disparities in outcomes related to the diagnosis, management, and surveillance of obstetric hemorrhage.
- Maintain a hemorrhage cart or equivalent with supplies, checklists, and instruction cards for devices or procedures where antepartum, laboring, and postpartum patients are located.
- Ensure immediate access to first- and second-line hemorrhage medications in a kit or equivalent.
- Conduct interprofessional and interdepartmental team-based drills with timely debriefs that include the use of simulated patients.

Recognition and Prevention—Every Patient

- Assess and communicate hemorrhage risk to all team members as clinical conditions change or high-risk conditions are identified (at a minimum, on admission, during the peripartum period, and on transition to postpartum care).
- Measure and communicate cumulative blood loss to all team members using quantitative approaches.
- Actively manage the third stage of labor per department protocols.
- Provide ongoing education to all patients on obstetric hemorrhage risk and causes, early warning signs, and risk for postpartum complications.

Response—Every Event

- Utilize a standardized, facility-wide, stage-based, obstetric hemorrhage emergency management plan, with checklists and escalation policies for stage-based management of patients with obstetric hemorrhage, including:
  - Advance preparations made based on hemorrhage risk (e.g., cell salvage, blood bank notification).
  - Evaluating patients for etiology of hemorrhage.
  - Use of obstetric rapid response team.
  - Evidence-based medication administration or use of nonpharmacological interventions.
  - Appropriate activation of expanded care team and clinical resources as necessary.
- Provide trauma-informed support for patients, identified support network, and staff for all obstetric hemorrhages, including discussions regarding birth events, follow-up care, resources, and appointments.

Reporting and Systems Learning—Every Unit

- Establish a culture of multidisciplinary planning, huddles, and postevent debriefs for every obstetric hemorrhage.
  - Identify successes, opportunities for improvement, and action planning for future events.
  - Perform multidisciplinary reviews of serious complications per established facility criteria to identify system issues.
- Monitor outcomes and process measures related to obstetric hemorrhage, with disaggregation by race and ethnicity due to known racial and ethnic disparities in obstetric hemorrhage outcomes.
- Establish processes for data reporting and the sharing of data with the obstetric rapid response team, care providers, and facility stakeholders to inform care and change care systems, as necessary.

Respectful, Equitable, and Supportive Care—Every Unit/Provider/Team Member

- Include each patient who experienced an obstetric hemorrhage and their identified support network as respected members of and contributors to the multidisciplinary care team and as participants in patient-centered huddles and debriefs.
- Engage in open, transparent, and empathetic communication with pregnant and postpartum women and their identified support network to understand diagnoses, options, and treatment plans, including consent regarding blood products and blood product alternatives.

From Alliance for Innovation on Maternal Health. Obstetric hemorrhage patient safety bundle. ACOG; 2022. https://saferbirth.org/psbs/obstetric-hemorrhage/. Accessed 31 December 2024.

1.0 per 1000 births) compared with a 2-month preimplementation period.[245] At a state level, implementation of a quality improvement hemorrhage toolkit across 99 California hospitals was associated with a 20% reduction in the rate of hemorrhage-related severe maternal morbidity.[246]

These types of programs also have positive effects on sentinel events and malpractice payments.[247] In low- and middle-income countries, these bundles are beneficial. A large, multicenter, cluster, randomized trial conducted in four African countries (the E-MOTIVE trial) showed that the use of a calibrated drape for PPH detection and a PPH treatment bundle, supported with an implementation strategy, resulted in a 60% decrease in the risk of severe hemorrhage, laparotomy for bleeding, or death from PPH after vaginal birth.[248] A systematic review evaluated the effectiveness of bundles for PPH prevention and treatment.[249] The authors concluded that the E-MOTIVE trial provided the highest-certainty evidence for a treatment-only bundle in reducing the morbidity risk in secondary facilities in lower- and middle-income countries. In contrast, for other treatment or combination prevention and treatment bundles, the evidence was found to be less certain because of a lack of high-quality randomized trials.

Maintaining protocol adherence may be a concern after implementation of a standardized protocol or set of guidelines. For example, in a study that used prospective video analysis to evaluate PPH guideline adherence in 16 Dutch hospitals, key aspects of care were frequently not performed, with care gaps in heart rate and blood pressure monitoring and active management during active bleeding.[250] Therefore, lead clinicians should continually assess bundle effectiveness and identify deficiencies in the implementation, acceptability, and sustainability of each bundle element, and how to best tailor bundles according to individual hospitals' resources, staff availability and experience, as well as systemwide approaches to education and quality improvement.[251,252] Further research is needed to determine whether simulation training leads to sustained improvements in care and maternal outcomes.[253]

Risk Assessment

PPH risk assessment is an essential starting point for informing decisions about risk management. It allows clinicians to identify patients at risk for severe PPH, optimize predelivery blood product ordering, and allocate limited resources to those at greatest risk. PPH risk assessment tools, developed by maternal health organizations, including the CMQCC, Association for Women's Health, Obstetric and Neonatal Nurses (AWHONN), and the ACOG Safe Motherhood Initiatives, have been integrated in clinical obstetric practice.[240,241,254] Each of these tools assigns PPH risk factors into medium- or high-risk categories. Use of these risk assessment tools has been endorsed by The Joint Commission in their perinatal standards of care for US maternity units.[242] Although these tools may have face validity and are easy to use, validation studies have shown poor predictive validity, with more than 40% of all PPH events occurring in patients classified as low risk (i.e., with no risk factors).[255–260] These studies have reported very low rates of RBC transfusions in medium-risk patients (2.0% to 4.5%) and relatively low rates in high-risk patients (7.3% to 22.6%), meaning that the majority of patients classified as medium or high risk do not experience severe PPH (low specificity).[260] An alternative approach to risk categorization is calculating individual probabilities of PPH risk using risk prediction models. However, based on systematic reviews, studies examining PPH prediction models have important limitations, including high risk of bias, overfitting, and suboptimal or no external validation, and thus cannot be used in clinical practice.[261,262]

An important reason for the challenges in predicting PPH is that knowledge of PPH risk factors remains incomplete. A metaanalysis of risk factors for PPH secondary to uterine atony identified only 15 clinical variables deemed definite or likely risk factors (see Box 37.3), and many of the risk factors with the strongest association with uterine atony are other causes of PPH, such as abruption and cervical laceration.[80] The risk of PPH remains unknown in many patients up to the time of delivery. In addition, evidence suggests that risk profiles likely vary by delivery mode.[263,264] Emerging research suggests that predictive models that rely on automated, real-time data from electronic health records have greater accuracy than risk categorization.[265] Future research is needed to externally validate these models in different obstetric populations and to evaluate the value of quantifying individual probabilities of risk compared to risk categorization into low-, medium-, and high-risk groups. Despite their limitations, current risk assessment tools may be useful as cognitive aids to inform, but not drive, multidisciplinary discussions about risk management decision-making.[260]

LABORATORY AND COAGULATION MONITORING DURING AN OBSTETRIC HEMORRHAGE

In patients with severe PPH, identification of coagulation abnormalities and coagulopathy is critical for mitigating the risk of morbidity. Making a diagnosis of coagulopathy during PPH can be challenging. Laboratory tests, such as the activated partial thromboplastin time (aPTT), prothrombin time (PT), and Clauss fibrinogen level, have slow turnaround times, and prolongations in aPTT and PT often occur late during severe PPH. Although the International Society on Thrombosis and Hemostasis has developed a modified obstetric DIC score, there is no clear clinical or laboratory phenotype for DIC in obstetric hemorrhage.[266] Experts have suggested that three broad categories may exist for PPH-related coagulopathy: (1) *late dilutional coagulopathy* (hypofibrinogenemia develops before other coagulation abnormalities in patients with severe atonic PPH); (2) *early coagulopathy* (hypofibrinogenemia develops rapidly with or without abnormal aPTT/PT values during placental abruption); and (3) rare cases of *generalized coagulation failure and thrombocytopenia* caused by an amniotic fluid embolism, hemolysis, elevated liver enzymes, and low platelets (HELLP) syndrome, severe placental abruption, or PPH complicated by sepsis.[267] The incidences of hypofibrinogenemia, thrombocytopenia, and abnormal laboratory coagulation indices grouped by severity of hemorrhage or hemorrhage-related morbidity are presented in Table 37.5.

Coagulation Testing
Hypofibrinogenemia

Fibrinogen levels increase during pregnancy up to 4 to 6 g/L by term.[272] Observational studies have reported an inverse nonlinear relationship between the magnitude of blood loss and nadir plasma fibrinogen level.[269,273] Among patients with 1000- to 1500-mL blood loss, the incidence of hypofibrinogenemia is between 4% and 5%.[44,268,274] In a cohort of patients with major PPH ($\geq$5-unit RBC over 4 hours or $\geq$8-unit total RBC transfusion), 40% to 50% have a fibrinogen level < 200 mg/dL.[270]

In cohorts of patients who experience moderate-to-severe PPH, retrospective and prospective studies have shown that the fibrinogen level is a predictive biomarker for morbidity or progression to more severe PPH. A landmark study from France first reported that a fibrinogen level < 200 mg/dL during the early phase of PPH had a 100% positive predictive value for subsequent RBC transfusion greater than four units or a reduction in hemoglobin levels by 4 g/dL or more.[275] Subsequent observational studies have confirmed that a fibrinogen level < 200 mg/dL is an important predictor of severe PPH.[276,277]

Thrombocytopenia

Thrombocytopenia is a less common abnormality, occurring in 1% to 5% of patients with mild to moderate PPH.[44] The incidence increases up to 50% during severe or life-threatening PPH. In a cohort study of patients with PPH, investigators observed that a platelet transfusion was only required with large-volume blood loss (>5 L) or if hemorrhage was associated with placental abruption or a preexisting thrombocytopenia.[278]

Other Clotting Factor Abnormalities

The presence, type, and severity of coagulopathy vary according to the primary hemorrhage etiology and the volume of blood lost. Coagulopathy is very uncommon when PPH is due to uterine atony or genital tract trauma, unless there is massive hemorrhage. Observational data indicate that hypofibrinogenemia occurs in only 2% to 3% of cases of hemorrhage of approximately of 1000 mL caused by uterine atony or genital tract trauma.[44,274] For a hemorrhage greater than 2500 mL, the incidence was approximately 14%. In patients with PAS, large-volume hemorrhage is more common, but the presence of coagulopathy correlates with the severity of blood loss. For example, in one observational study, 60% of PAS cases with massive hemorrhage (median blood loss, 6 L) had fibrinogen levels < 200 mg/dL at the time of initial blood sampling.[271]

For hemorrhage due to uterine atony and birth trauma, the incidence of a prolonged PT or aPTT is rare with blood loss < 3000 mL, and correlates with the volume of bleeding (see Table 37.5). In a prospective cohort study of 518 patients with PPH, a linear fall in nearly all clotting factors levels, except platelets and factor VIII, was reported with increasing volume of blood loss.[43]

In contrast, for PPH associated with placental abruption and amniotic fluid embolism, coagulopathy can occur early, is severe, and is unrelated to blood loss severity; severe hypofibrinogenemia and hyperfibrinolysis are common features.[279-282] Several observational studies have found that cases with placental abruption or amniotic fluid embolism had the greatest proportion of patients with hypofibrinogenemia.[44,271] **Acute obstetric coagulopathy**, a distinct coagulopathic phenotype, is characterized by markedly elevated markers of fibrinolysis, hypofibrinogenemia, dysfibrinogenemia, and reduced factor V and VIII levels.[43] This particular phenotype is rare, is not correlated with blood loss volume, is most commonly seen with placental abruption and amniotic fluid embolism, but can occur with any PPH etiology, and often requires massive hemostatic support.

In summary, the likelihood of coagulopathy is most common with placental abruption and amniotic fluid embolism, but can still occur regardless of hemorrhage etiology, and is usually related to the severity of blood loss. Therefore, patients with a known coagulopathy, suspected abruption, amniotic fluid embolism, or a PPH greater than 2000 mL should undergo an evaluation for coagulopathy, especially during the setting of ongoing severe blood loss.

TABLE 37.5 **Incidence of Hypofibrinogenemia, Thrombocytopenia, and Abnormal Laboratory Coagulation Indices by the Severity of Hemorrhage or Hemorrhage-Related Morbidity**

| | Netherlands (N = 391)[268] | UK | | Netherlands (N = 1312)[269] | Australia/NZ (N = 249)[270] | UK (N = 181)[271] |
		(N = 2111)[44]	(N = 349)[45]			
Study entry criteria	800–1500 mL	>1500 mL or any blood product transfused	>2500 mL or ≥5 units RBCs transfused	Median 3000 mL	>5 units RBCs transfused within 4 h of PPH or ≥8 units RBCs transfused total	Median 6000 mL
Incidence of hypofibrinogenemia (<200 mg/dL)	4%	5.4%	17.1%	26%	52%	>60%
Incidence of thrombocytopenia (<75,000/μL)	ND	1.3%	5.1%	ND	16%[a]	50%
Incidence of abnormal (PT/INR or aPTT > 1.5 times nonpregnant reference range)	ND	PT 0.5% aPTT 0.2%	PT 3.4% aPTT 3.0%	ND	PT/INR 18% aPTT 13%	ND

aPTT, Activated partial thromboplastin time; *INR,* international normalized ratio; *ND,* no data; *NZ,* New Zealand; *PPH,* postpartum hemorrhage; *PT,* prothrombin time; *RBC,* red blood cells; *UK,* United Kingdom.
[a]<50,000/μL.

Viscoelastic Testing

Viscoelastic testing, including thromboelastography (TEG) and rotational thromboelastometry (ROTEM), can be used to detect coagulopathy, observe trends in abnormal coagulation, and differentiate between surgical and coagulopathic bleeding during ongoing hemorrhage.[283,284] These assays reflect cell-based models of hemostasis; provide data on specific aspects of hemostasis, such as clot initiation, fibrin polymerization, and clot lysis; and have several benefits over standard laboratory tests of coagulation, including faster turnaround times and more nuanced information on clot formation and lysis. Sequential testing of viscoelastic parameters allows cliniciansto evaluate for coagulation abnormalities, consider goal-directed or targeted approaches to treatment, and evaluate the effectiveness of therapeutic interventions. Suggested TEG- and ROTEM-based algorithms for PPH management have been described.[284,285]

Studies have examined TEG and ROTEM profiles in patients with PPH. In a case control study assessing TEG changes in 49 patients with major obstetric hemorrhage, clot stability was decreased (decreased alpha angle and maximum amplitude), fibrinolysis was decreased (decreased LY30 values), and clot initiation was increased (shorter reaction [R] times) compared to 49 women without hemorrhage.[286]

Studies of patients with PPH using ROTEM also reveal important changes in the maternal coagulation profile. In a study of 37 patients with severe PPH, ROTEM parameters of the FIBTEM test were altered, namely prolonged clotting times, reduced clot amplitude at 5 and 15 minutes (A5 and A15), and reduced maximum clot firmness. These parameters correlated well with plasma fibrinogen levels.[287] In another study of 356 patients with PPH, a FIBTEM A5 < 10 mm was associated with more prolonged bleeding, blood transfusion, and prolonged duration of stay in the high-dependency unit.[274]

The ROTEM FIBTEM and TEG functional fibrinogen (FF) parameters can be used to detect fibrinogen levels < 200 mg/dL.[288] Values derived from the newer generation of cartridge-based devices—the TEG 6S and ROTEM sigma—have similar utility.[44,289] Stronger correlations have been reported between Clauss fibrinogen levels with FIBTEM A5 values obtained using the ROTEM sigma device compared to the ROTEM delta device.[290] Of note, a prolonged EXTEM clotting time or citrated kaolin R time is often observed with a low FIBTEM or FF value before fibrinogen supplementation. Therefore, repeat testing is advised before deciding whether to administer other clotting factors in a patient with hypofibrinogenemia detected using these monitors. Further, EXTEM and R time thresholds for guiding clotting factor replacement have yet to be determined.

Emerging observational data suggests that goal-directed therapy using TEG and ROTEM is associated with a lower use of plasma and reduced transfusion-related morbidity. In a study assessing the impact of replacing a fixed-ratio massive transfusion approach (4 units plasma:4 units RBC:1 unit platelets) with a ROTEM-based algorithm to guide fibrinogen and blood product administration, reduced plasma, platelet, and cryoprecipitate use and a reduction in transfusion-associated circulatory overload (TACO) was found in the goal-directed therapy group.[291] Another study comparing outcomes before and after implementation of a viscoelastic testing-based algorithm found a reduction in blood product use, overall blood loss, and rates of hysterectomy, length of hospital stay, and ICU admission after protocol implementation.[292] A third study examining the impact of a ROTEM-based PPH bundle in the United Kingdom observed a progressive reduction in rates of severe PPH, RBC, and plasma use, with no increase in postpartum coagulopathy.[293] An unblinded, randomized trial of 60 patients with PPH suggested that a ROTEM-guided protocol may have a plasma-sparing effect compared with conventional treatment.[294]

MEDICAL AND SURGICAL APPROACHES TO HEMORRHAGE MANAGEMENT

Invasive Treatment Options

Regardless of the cause of obstetric hemorrhage, first-line conservative measures may fail to control bleeding. In these cases, invasive procedures must be performed promptly to avoid severe morbidity and mortality. Second-line interventions, including intrauterine balloon tamponade, vacuum-induced hemorrhage control devices, uterine compression sutures, angiographic arterial embolization, and uterine artery and/or internal iliac artery ligation, may help to avoid hysterectomy.[295,296] Unfortunately, no randomized controlled trials comparing the relative efficacy and safety of these options exist. In cases of intractable hemorrhage, a hysterectomy may become necessary.

Intrauterine balloon tamponade is a conservative method for controlling PPH, especially when refractory uterine atony or lower uterine segment bleeding is suspected.[66] A systematic review that included data from randomized and observational trials reported a high rate of treatment success (87.9%).[297] Additionally, two before-and-after studies in single obstetric centers reported a decrease in invasive interventions after the introduction of intrauterine balloon tamponade into the institutional PPH protocol.[298,299] An intrauterine balloon can be deployed quickly, requires minimal analgesia for both insertion and removal, and preserves fertility. However, caution must be taken as continued bleeding may be concealed behind the balloon. Failure may also be attributed to prolapse through a partially open cervix. Few complications have been reported with intrauterine balloons, although concerns for infection exist.[300]

Vacuum-induced hemorrhage control devices have been introduced into clinical practice. The Jada System is an intrauterine device that has an elliptical silicone loop placed in the uterus and uses low-level vacuum (approximately 80 mm Hg) to promote uterine contraction in patients with PPH attributed to uterine atony.[301] In a postmarket registry study of 800 patients who used the Jada device, the treatment success rate was 92.5% for vaginal births and 83.7% for cesarean deliveries.[302] Three serious adverse events were deemed possibly related to the device, including two cases of endometritis and one case of failure to control bleeding.

Uterine compression sutures (e.g., B-Lynch suture[303]) are most useful in cases of refractory uterine atony[304] when placed at the time of cesarean delivery or during exploratory laparotomy to treat PPH. A systematic review, based mostly on case reports and case series, and therefore subject to reporting bias, estimated a 92% success rate for this procedure.[304] A subsequent prospective population-based trial reported a 75% success rate in avoiding the need for hysterectomy.[305] The suture may slip off of the uterine fundus and fail to provide compression. Placement of compression sutures may preserve fertility, but data on the long-term effects on fertility and pregnancy outcomes are lacking. Complications include infection, uterine necrosis, and suture erosion,[304] and a case report described PAS and uterine rupture presumably caused by a uterine compression suture that had been placed after a previous delivery.[306]

Angiographic arterial embolization may be appropriate in the setting of continuing moderate blood loss if the patient is stable for transport to the interventional radiology suite. The uterine arteries, which are branches of the anterior trunk of the internal iliac arteries, provide the primary blood supply to the uterus. The ovarian and vaginal arteries also make a sizable contribution to uterine blood flow during pregnancy. During angiography, the radiologist can identify the vessels responsible for bleeding and embolize these vessels with gelatin sponge pledgets (Gelfoam). Some cases may require placement of a metallic coil in addition to gelatin sponges. The gelatin sponge is a temporary occlusive agent, and flow through these vessels returns over time, preserving both the uterus and fertility.[307] Published success rates in controlling PPH with this approach vary between 70% and 100%.[304] Successful treatment of acute PPH with this modality requires rapid access to an angiography facility and a skilled interventional radiologist. The patient must be observed and monitored carefully while undergoing the procedure. Ischemic complications of embolization therapy have been reported, but the risk is reduced with the use of selective techniques.[304,308,309]

Bilateral surgical ligation of the uterine arteries (O'Leary sutures) may be used to control bleeding during a laparotomy.[310] In the case of failure to control bleeding, the surgeon may proceed with a more complex procedure that involves ligation of the tuboovarian arteries and ascending and descending uterine arteries. Internal iliac artery ligation may also be considered, although it is more difficult to perform. Reported success rates are highly variable, and it appears that arterial ligation is being used less often than in the past.[66] The rich collateral circulation of the uterus at term most likely contributes to a failure to control bleeding, as does the challenging nature of the procedure itself. Engorgement of pelvic viscera, variability in vascular anatomy, and the increased blood flow during pregnancy may contribute to the challenges in performing this procedure. Successful surgical ligation permits the preservation of fertility. Ischemic complications and neuropathy have been reported.[304]

Peripartum hysterectomy is the definitive treatment for PPH unresponsive to medical and other invasive therapies. The three most common indications for this procedure are uterine atony, PAS, and uterine rupture.[311] Between 2009 and 2020, the overall rate of unplanned peripartum hysterectomy increased in the United States from 3.4 per 10,000 deliveries to 4.5 per 10,000 deliveries.[312] Parturients with a history of previous cesarean delivery are more than five times as likely to require a peripartum hysterectomy as those without this history, and the risk for hysterectomy rises progressively with an increasing number of previous cesarean deliveries.[8,22] The incidence of peripartum hysterectomy caused by a uterine rupture has declined in the United States because the rate of TOLAC has declined.[8] Elective peripartum hysterectomy may also be undertaken for concurrent gynecologic abnormalities, especially malignancies.

Peripartum hysterectomy is a technically challenging operation; the uterus is enlarged, exposure may be difficult, the vessels are engorged, and the pregnant uterus receives a rich collateral blood supply. The presence of dense adhesions from previous surgeries can further complicate the procedure. Compared with nonobstetric hysterectomy, patients undergoing obstetric hysterectomy are more likely to suffer PPH and require a blood transfusion; have an intraoperative urinary tract injury; and experience perioperative complications such as wound infection, venous thromboembolism, and cardiovascular and other medical complications.[313] Mortality is more than 25 times higher in a peripartum than nonperipartum hysterectomy.[313]

Emergency peripartum hysterectomy is associated with increased blood loss, worse coagulopathy, and increased transfusion rates compared with a planned peripartum hysterectomy.[314] A 2010 systematic review of emergency postpartum hysterectomies for hemorrhage revealed a perioperative morbidity rate of 56% and a mortality rate of 2.6%.[315] Transfusion is required in 44% or more of patients.[315] A multicenter review showed that the mean blood loss for an emergency obstetric hysterectomy was 2526 mL, with a mean transfusion requirement of 6.6 units of RBCs; in elective procedures, the mean blood loss was 1319 mL and the average transfusion requirement was 1.6 units of RBCs.[314]

Because of the challenging technical aspects of the procedure, the obstetrician may elect to perform a subtotal hysterectomy, wherein the cervix is left *in situ*. Subtotal approaches are associated with fewer urinary tract and other operative injuries and a shorter length of hospital stay,[313,315] but greater mean transfusion requirements and more frequent rates of reoperation than a total hysterectomy.[313] A subtotal hysterectomy is not appropriate for patients with bleeding from the cervix, lower uterine segment, or both (e.g., implantation of the placenta on the lower uterine segment).

Temporizing **manual compression of the aorta** can be a lifesaving procedure in the event of a catastrophic obstetric hemorrhage.[316] Effective aortic compression against a vertebral body in the upper abdomen should decrease blood flow to the pelvis, thereby allowing hemodynamic and hemostatic resuscitation and surgical control. An aortic cross-clamp requires vascular surgery expertise and retroperitoneal dissection but may be necessary to achieve hemostasis. Cardiac and renal dysfunction have been noted in nonobstetric patients if the aortic cross-clamp time exceeds 50 minutes.[317] If a prolonged clamp time is required, the anesthesia provider should prepare for lactic acidosis and significant hypotension at the time the clamp is released.

REBOA (see earlier discussion) may be considered in patients with severe and life-threatening PPH. The clinical team should consider the availability of this resource and the time needed to mobilize a surgical or radiology team. When used, partial inflation of the aortic balloon just below the renal arteries may be sufficient to facilitate surgical visualization by reducing uterine blood flow while preserving limited distal blood flow.[318] Complications associated with REBOA can be subdivided into complications from arterial access and balloon malposition and overinflation, and reperfusion complications after balloon deflation.[319] Access site complications can include vessel dissection, pseudoaneurysm, perforation, and peripheral ischemia from an occlusive thrombus or sheath. Vessel complications can be minimized by reducing the introducer sheath size (e.g., use of 4- to 7-French introducer sheaths) and by using ultrasonography to guide insertion. Close communication is required prior to balloon deflation to anticipate vasodilation and hypotension resulting from the acute reduction of afterload and the release of ischemic metabolites. The use of partial as opposed to complete REBOA inflation may mitigate the risk of ischemic complications and reperfusion injury.

Advanced surgical techniques to control friable, engorged blood vessels include felt or Teflon pledgets to buttress sutures, the rapid application of straight clamps, and the application of high-pressure surgical sealants.[320–322]

Anesthesia for Peripartum Hysterectomy

Anesthesia for a peripartum hysterectomy is frequently challenging because massive blood loss may occur unpredictably.[323] An experienced, skilled team is invaluable and critical to a successful outcome. As the magnitude of blood loss increases, general anesthesia becomes the preferred anesthetic technique. First, severely hypotensive patients may require tracheal intubation for airway protection. Second, large fluid shifts and TACO from massive transfusion may adversely affect oxygenation. Third, these same fluid shifts increase airway edema, potentially increasing the risk for failed ventilation/failed tracheal intubation as the surgical procedure progresses. Fourth, the massive transfusion of blood products often results in the need for coadministration of potent vasopressors and calcium chloride. The placement of a central venous catheter may be more easily accomplished after the induction of general anesthesia.

The induction of general anesthesia in the setting of severe hemorrhage requires careful dosing of noncardiodepressant induction agents such as ketamine or etomidate. The circulation should be supported with replacement of intravascular volume and vasopressors. A review of maternal deaths from PPH in France revealed that 5 of 38 deaths followed cardiac arrest on induction of general anesthesia.[324] Single-shot spinal anesthesia is unlikely to be of sufficient duration for an unanticipated hysterectomy. Patients who have delivered vaginally with an epidural catheter *in situ* can potentially be managed with augmentation/extension ofepidural anesthesia to initiate and maintain surgical anesthesia. However, the threshold for conversion to general anesthesia in the setting of severe hemorrhage or hemodynamic instability should be low. Animal models suggest that sympatholysis established before the onset of hemorrhage reduces excessive catecholamine response to blood loss and may improve survival.[325] However, induction of sympatholysis during hemorrhage may compromise end-organ perfusion and even precipitate cardiopulmonary arrest.[325]

Regardless of the anesthetic technique, at least two large-bore intravenous catheters should be inserted. Invasive blood pressure monitoring is valuable for the prompt recognition of hypotension and to provide access for frequent blood draws and laboratory testing. The blood bank should be alerted to the possible need for a massive transfusion by activating a MTP or the emergency blood release protocol. The ACOG recommends the consideration of intraoperative blood salvage in cases with massive transfusion potential.[66,193] Vasoactive drugs (e.g., phenylephrine, epinephrine), fluid warmers, a forced-air body warmer, and equipment for the rapid infusion of fluids and blood products should be accessible if the care team is anticipating and managing significant blood loss (see later discussion).

Pharmacologic Treatment

Tranexamic Acid

Tranexamic acid (TXA) binds to plasminogen, preventing the conversion of plasminogen to plasmin, thus inhibiting the fibrinolytic action of plasmin on fibrin clots. TXA is widely used in many perioperative settings to reduce blood loss.[326] In a large multicenter trial in adult trauma patients (CRASH-2 trial), TXA lowered the risk of death from bleeding by 9% compared to a placebo, without increasing the risk for thromboembolic events or deaths.[327] There has been increasing interest in the potential utility of TXA for PPH prevention and treatment. Although the WHO and the International Federation of Gynecology and Obstetrics both recommend TXA as part of the first response to PPH,[328,329] there is no consensus for its use in national obstetric society PPH guidelines. Pharmacokinetic data from obstetric patients indicate that a TXA infusion results in a peak plasma concentration within 3 minutes.[330] Pharmacodynamic data using ROTEM suggest that low-dose TXA (5 mg/kg) inhibits maximal lysis for at least 60 minutes.[330,331]

Tranexamic acid for treatment of postpartum hemorrhage. Several studies have evaluated the effectiveness of TXA for treatment of PPH. In a French open-label, randomized trial, patients with greater than 800-mL blood loss after a vaginal delivery who received TXA (4 g loading dose, 1 g/h infusion for 6 hours) had modestly lower blood loss than those who received a placebo (median blood loss TXA versus placebo, 170 versus 221 mL, respectively).[332] The WOMAN trial, a large multinational, placebo-controlled trial, investigated the effect of TXA compared to placebo in a cohort of

20,060 patients with PPH in predominantly low- and middle-income countries.[333] The mortality rate from PPH was lower among patients who received TXA than among those in the placebo group (1.5% versus 1.9%; RR, 0.81; 95% CI, 0.65 to 1.00; P = .045). No differences in adverse events (including venous and arterial thromboembolic events) between the two groups were reported. Secondary data suggested no benefit in reducing morbidity, including transfusion, hysterectomy, or a composite of all-cause mortality or hysterectomy. In a metaanalysis combining the CRASH-2 and WOMAN trial data from 40,138 patients, TXA was associated with improved survival by more than 70% if administered within 3 hours of the onset of hemorrhage, with the survival benefit decreasing by 10% for every 15 minutes of delayed treatment.[334]

Less clear is whether TXA is associated with survival or morbidity benefit in patients who deliver in well-resourced countries. In a cohort study of 1260 patients with PPH in the Netherlands, no reduction in the risk of morbidity (hysterectomy, vessel ligation, B-lynch suture, arterial embolization, or ICU admission) or death was reported in patients exposed to early TXA compared with those who had no TXA or late TXA exposure (adjusted odds ratio [aOR], 0.92; 95% CI, 0.66 to 1.27).[335]

Tranexamic acid for prophylaxis of postpartum hemorrhage. Three high-quality randomized trials have assessed whether prophylactic TXA, administered before vaginal or cesarean delivery, is effective in decreasing the risk of PPH. In a trial of 4057 patients who underwent vaginal delivery, the rate of PPH (blood loss > 500 mL) was similar between those receiving prophylactic TXA versus placebo (8.1% versus 9.8%; RR, 0.83; 95% CI, 0.68 to 1.01).[336] Although metaanalyses have been performed to compare the effect of prophylactic TXA versus placebo on PPH rates,[337,338] between-study differences in blood loss reporting, TXA dosing, and study quality limit the validity of findings from these analyses. Overall, available study data suggest that, for vaginal delivery, prophylactic TXA does not result in a clinically meaningful decrease in blood loss or PPH risk after delivery.

In the setting of elective cesarean delivery, two high-quality studies have investigated the effect of prophylactic TXA. In a multicenter study from France, 4551 patients were randomized to TXA (1 g) versus a placebo after umbilical cord clamping.[339] The primary outcome was PPH, defined as estimated blood loss > 1000 mL (calculated using the difference between pre- and postdelivery hematocrit values and estimated blood volume) or RBC transfusion within 2 days of delivery. The risk of PPH was 16% lower for the TXA group compared to the placebo group (26.7% versus 31.6%; adjusted RR [aRR], 0.84; 95% CI, 0.75 to 0.94). However, no between-group differences were reported for gravimetrically measured blood loss, the percentage of patients with a gravimetric blood loss > 1000 mL, and requirement for postpartum transfusion. In a secondary analysis of study data in patients with multiple gestation only, no differences in PPH or transfusion were reported.[340]

In the largest study to date, 11,000 patients delivering in the United States were randomized to TXA (1 g) versus a placebo; the primary outcome was death or transfusion by hospital discharge or postpartum day 7.[341] No between-group differences were reported in the rate of the primary outcome (TXA, 3.6% versus placebo, 4.3%; aRR, 0.89; 95% CI, 0.74 to 1.07) or other secondary hemorrhage-related morbidity outcomes, including the rate of PPH or surgical or radiologic intervention. A metaanalysis published in 2023 that incorporated data from 50 trials of prophylactic TXA during a cesarean delivery reported no reduced risk of blood loss > 1000 mL, total blood loss, or transfusion in low- or high-risk patients.[342] However, the quality of evidence was low and moderate in studies of low-risk and high-risk patients, respectively. The lack of strong evidence from recent metaanalyses and large randomized trials indicates that TXA should not be used for PPH prophylaxis for cesarean delivery.

Adverse effects of tranexamic acid. Data from randomized trials investigating TXA for PPH prophylaxis and treatment do not indicate that there is an increased risk of thrombosis associated with TXA. However, adequately powered studies are not available to fully evaluate potential differences in thrombotic risk between TXA and a placebo.

An additional patient safety concern is **inadvertent intrathecal injection** of TXA. Because TXA is a potent neurotoxin, and it may be packaged in vials or ampules that look similar to those of spinal anesthetic agents, there have been multiple reports of maternal deaths from accidental intrathecal injection of TXA.[343,344] In 2020 the US Food and Drug Administration (FDA) issued an alert that recommended revision of all TXA vial container and carton labeling to state "For Intravenous Use Only" and strengthened warnings in prescribing information about the risks of drug error from incorrect route of administration.[345] The FDA and expert reviews have published recommendations for drug storage, preparation, and use, such as verifying vial contents by a second provider and the barcode scanning of TXA vials prior to drug preparation and administration. Anesthesia providers are advised to check all drug vials before performing neuraxial anesthesia and ensure that TXA vials are stored in a separate location from vials of drugs used for neuraxial anesthesia.

A case cluster of renal cortical thrombosis and irreversible kidney damage developed among 18 women treated with TXA for PPH in France.[346] The doses used in these cases were higher (>2 g) than those employed in the WOMAN trial. Clinicians are cautioned not to exceed doses of 1 g administered slowly over 10 minutes; this dose may be repeated once if the bleeding continues after 30 minutes.[333]

Fibrinogen Concentrate

Fibrinogen concentrate is an alternative source of fibrinogen and has been used to restore fibrinogen levels in patients with PPH and hypofibrinogenemia.[347] Detailed information about the formulation, pharmacokinetics, and studies of effectiveness in nonobstetric settings has been published.[348,349] Fibrinogen concentrate is derived from human plasma, is virally inactivated, and is formulated as a pasteurized and lyophilized product that does not require cross-matching. It is reconstituted in sterile water. Each vial contains approximately

1 g fibrinogen (range, 900 to 1300 mg). It is typically administered as a slow injection (5 mL/min); however, it is possible to infuse it more quickly when severe bleeding occurs.[348]

Several studies have examined the potential impact of preemptive fibrinogen supplementation in patients with severe PPH. In a randomized trial of 249 women with early PPH, fibrinogen concentrate (2 g) was compared to saline as a preemptive treatment.[350] The frequency of RBC transfusion did not differ between women receiving fibrinogen concentrate and those receiving saline (20% versus 22%). The lack of effect may be because few patients (2.2%) had hypofibrinogenemia (fibrinogen concentration < 200 mg/dL) at baseline. Similar findings were observed in another randomized trial comparing preemptive fibrinogen concentrate with a placebo in 437 patients with severe PPH after vaginal delivery.[351] No significant between-group difference was observed in failure to respond to treatment, the primary outcome, in the treatment and placebo groups (40% versus 42%; OR, 0.99; 95% CI, 0.66 to 1.47).

Using ROTEM technology, a multicenter study compared the number of RBC units transfused among 55 women with PPH and a FIBTEM A5 ≤ 15 mm who were randomized to receive fibrinogen concentrate versus a placebo.[352] The rates of transfusion did not significantly differ between groups. A prespecified subgroup analysis suggested a potential benefit for patients with FIBTEM A5 < 12 mm or a fibrinogen level < 200 mg/dL, but the sample size was insufficient to confirm or exclude benefit for this group.

Several single-center observational studies of patients with severe PPH and a plasma fibrinogen level < 150 mg/dL suggest that fibrinogen concentrate use is associated with improved plasma fibrinogen levels and less blood loss and plasma transfusion.[353,354] Further research is needed to determine whether goal-directed fibrinogen replacement to target a fibrinogen concentration > 200 mg/dL, or a FIBTEM A5 value > 10 or 12 mm, will improve outcomes in patients with severe PPH. A dose of 2 to 4 g fibrinogen concentrate is a reasonable starting dose in patients with active and evolving severe PPH and hypofibrinogenemia (fibrinogen level < 200 mg/dL) or in patients with a major life-threatening hemorrhage requiring early and significant blood product support from an MTP. Additional and ongoing replacement should be guided by the results of laboratory or viscoelastic testing.

Recombinant Activated Factor VII

Factor VIIa binds not only to tissue factor but also with low affinity to the thrombin-activated platelet. This low-affinity binding to the activated platelet allows direct activation of factor X to Xa on the surface of the activated platelet, bypassing the normal need for factors VIIIa and IXa. The activation of factor X leads to a small thrombin burst. This thrombin, in turn, activates more platelets. Additionally, factor VIIa enhances platelet aggregation and adhesion.

Recombinant activated factor VII (rFVIIa) is currently approved in the United States for the treatment and prophylaxis of bleeding in patients with hemophilia A and B with inhibitors to factors VIII and IX, acquired hemophilia, and congenital factor VII deficiency. Its off-label use has been reported in multiple clinical scenarios, including PPH.[355] Very limited evidence exists examining the efficacy and safety of rFVIIa for severe PPH management. A 2024 review synthesized available data from one open-label randomized controlled trial and four observational studies.[356] Although the rate of invasive procedures was lower in rFVIIa-exposed versus nonexposed women in randomized trial data, the effect was not observed in observational studies. As part of this review, a metaanalysis of safety data from these studies suggests no increased risk of thrombotic complications, with similar frequencies of thromboembolic events in rFVIIa-exposed and nonexposed women (1.5% versus 1.6%).

The ASA guidelines recommend consideration of rFVIIa therapy "when traditional options for treating excessive bleeding due to coagulopathy have been exhausted."[357] A 2024 European expert consensus group advises earlier consideration of rFVIIa therapy as a second-line treatment for PPH after a vaginal or cesarean delivery or as part of the first-line treatment during or after a hysterectomy.[358] The initial dose range is between 60 and 90 µg/kg, with the possibility for a second dose in the event of an inadequate clinical or hemostatic response at least 30 minutes after the initial dose. Importantly, maintenance of normothermia and correction of acidosis are necessary for optimal rFVIIa activity. The optimization of platelet count, fibrinogen, and serum calcium are also advisable. Given the limited clinical effectiveness data and lack of pharmacoeconomic data, the indications, timing, and dosing of rFVIIa remain unclear.

TRANSFUSION

Knowing when and which blood components to transfuse is a highly complex and multifactorial decision. Although hemorrhage toolkits and bundles provide valuable information to aid transfusion decision making, clinical judgment remains essential. Key characteristics of commonly used blood components are summarized in Table 37.6.

Epidemiology of Transfusion

In obstetrics, national rates of RBC transfusions vary between 0.5% and 1.4% of deliveries.[359–361] Among US deliveries with PPH, blood transfusions increased from 5.4% to 16.7% between 2000 and 2011.[15] Similar trends of increasing transfusions have been reported in other well-resourced countries.[361–363] However, between 2011 and 2019, there has been a modest decrease in the US rate of transfusions associated with hemorrhage, decreasing from 16.7% to 12.6%.[15] The majority of transfusions (91%) occur during the birth admission, with 81% of these transfusions associated with a hemorrhage diagnosis.[361]

Indications for Red Blood Cell Transfusion

The indications for RBC transfusions include active hemorrhage or symptoms related to anemia (e.g., fatigue, dyspnea on exertion) with low hemoglobin concentration. While

TABLE 37.6   Characteristics of Blood Components

Component	Dose	Volume per Dose	Shelf Life	Storage Conditions	Expected Response
Packed red blood cells	1 unit	250–325 mL	21–42 d	1°C–6°C	1 g/dL increase in hemoglobin concentration
Plasma	10–15 mL/kg	200 mL	Frozen: 1 y Thawed: 24 h	Frozen: ≤ –18°C Thawed 1°C–10°C	Correction of PT, aPTT, INR by replacement of coagulation factors
Platelets	4–6 units of pooled whole blood–derived platelets or 1 unit of apheresis platelets	200–250 mL	5 d	20°C–24°C with continuous and gentle agitation	Increase in platelet count of 30,000–60,000/µL
Cryoprecipitate	10 pooled units	100 mL	Frozen: 1 y Thawed/pooled: 4 h	Frozen: ≤ –18°C Thawed: 1°C–10°C	Increase in levels of fibrinogen, von Willebrand factor, factor VIII, factor XIII

aPTT, Activated partial thromboplastin time; *INR*, international normalized ratio; *PT*, prothrombin time.
Modified from Sanford K, Roseff S. A surgeon's guide to blood banking and transfusion medicine. In: Spiess BD, Spence RK, Shander A, eds. *Perioperative Transfusion Medicine.* 2nd ed. Lippincott Williams and Wilkins; 2006:179–198.

patients who experience a hemorrhage may develop anemia, isolated anemia in the absence of hemorrhage is not an absolute indication for RBC transfusions. In contrast, RBC transfusions are a critical aspect of resuscitation during the acute management of severe ongoing hemorrhage, especially in patients with hemorrhagic shock.

Blood Product Ordering

Approaches for blood ordering typically rely on the clinical evaluation of PPH risk as well as the maternal hemoglobin level. The benefit of predelivery blood ordering is that it allows adequate time to ensure that sufficient types and quantities of blood products are available before delivery. The CMQCC, AWHONN, and Alliance for Innovation in Maternal Health risk assessment tools (see earlier discussion) have tied predelivery blood ordering to assigned PPH risk categories (low, medium, and high risk).[240,241,254] Recommendations include a hold specimen for low risk (so-called *draw and hold*), a *type and screen* for medium risk, and *type and cross-match* for high-risk patients. However, decisions about pretransfusion testing are complicated because of the challenges in predicting the timing of delivery, PPH risk, and the need for a transfusion. Predelivery blood ordering is beneficial for specific subpopulations, including very high-risk patients (e.g., placenta previa, PAS, known antibodies). Current recommendations from the ASA and the Society for Obstetric Anesthesia and Perinatology (SOAP) suggest that clinicians order intrapartum type and screen based on maternal history, anticipated hemorrhagic complications, and local institutional policies.[364] These guidelines also state that a routine blood cross-match is not necessary for healthy, uncomplicated parturients.

Reducing unnecessary pretransfusion testing can reduce hospital charges and costs. In a 2017 simulation study of 10,000 deliveries that assumed an overall transfusion rate of 1.6%, the total estimated cost of a type and cross-match for high-risk patients and a universal type and screen for other patients was $958,984; the cost for a universal type and screen policy was $913,161; and the cost for a selective type and screen in high-risk patients was $347,208.[365] Based on the ACOG guidelines, all pregnant patients should undergo testing at the first prenatal visit for ABO blood group and Rh-D type, and they should be screened for the presence of erythrocyte antibodies.[366] Additionally, the ACOG recommends that all patients be screened for anemia with a complete blood count in the first trimester and at 24 weeks' gestation.[367] Consideration of this information as well as the presence of risk factors for hemorrhage may allow selective type and screen policies, which are beneficial in reducing costs without significantly increasing the use of unmatched blood for transfusion.[368,369]

Massive Transfusion Protocols

In clinical scenarios in which the rate and magnitude of blood loss outpaces the time required to order and receive cross-matched blood products, activation of an institution-specific MTP ensures rapid mobilization and timely delivery of sufficient types and quantities of blood products to the medical care team.[370] Although data from single obstetric centers indicate that the transfusion rate of blood products from an MTP is low (0.09% to 0.21%),[371,372] the access to blood products from an MTP is particularly important when managing unanticipated and severe PPH. For example, in a single-center study of patients with PAS, 40% of patients who received RBC transfusion from an MTP did not have an antenatal PAS diagnosis.[373] In addition, the availability of type-specific or cross-matched blood components may not obviate the need for an MTP for patients with life threatening hemorrhage. The decision to activate an MTP is based on the severity and acuity of obstetric hemorrhage, the presence of hypoperfusion, the degree of cardiovascular support, and the likelihood of continued blood loss.[370]

The potential for alloimmunization in the recipient after exposure to uncross-matched Rh-negative RBCs is a theoretical concern. In the general population, new antierythrocyte antibodies have been identified in 1.8% to 3% of patients who receive uncross-matched RBC transfusions, comparable to the incidence of seroconversion after administration of cross-matched RBCs.[374] Notably, most cases of severe hemolytic disease of the fetus or newborn result from alloimmunization in prior pregnancies, with only 3% caused by prior exposure to a transfusion.[375]

Regardless of the availability of cross-matched blood components, clinicians should have access to an MTP or an equivalent emergency access protocol to ensure that sufficient quantity and types of blood components are rapidly available. This availability is vital during transfusion-based hemorrhagic shock resuscitation in scenarios of rapid and uncontrolled hemorrhage, especially when cross-matched products have already been transfused and bleeding remains active.

Transfusion Strategies for Managing Severe Postpartum Hemorrhage

Based on evidence from the trauma literature, the ACOG guidelines recommend *fixed ratios* of RBCs, plasma, and platelets.[66] However, no evidence is available from randomized clinical trials to determine whether fixed-ratio or *goal-directed* transfusion is superior for women with severe PPH. Extrapolating from the trauma literature is problematic because marked differences exist between the obstetric and trauma populations in baseline physiology and pathophysiology of coagulopathy related to hemorrhage.[376] Additionally, protocols that comprise high ratios of plasma:RBC transfusion may paradoxically lower plasma fibrinogen levels in women who have moderate PPH and normal coagulation indices.[377] Therefore, cryoprecipitate or fibrinogen concentrate is preferred to plasma transfusion for the treatment of hypofibrinogenemia; a large plasma volume is required to increase the fibrinogen level. Excessive plasma transfusion also increases the risk of hypervolemia, TACO, and transfusion-associated acute lung injury.[370] Further, in an observational study of 1216 women with persistent PPH, the transfusion of plasma within 60 minutes of PPH onset was not associated with reduced severe hemorrhage-related morbidity (defined as a composite of death, hysterectomy, or arterial embolization) compared with later or no plasma transfusion.[378] In patients with acute onset and major or life-threatening PPH, empiric plasma transfusion may be considered. In these scenarios, early and repeated laboratory evaluation of clotting factor function is strongly recommended to guide decision-making regarding plasma use after the initial phase of resuscitation has occurred (see later discussion).

The use of a fixed-ratio approach may also expose patients with a platelet count above a threshold level of 75,000/μL to unnecessary platelet transfusions. Most patients with severe PPH due to uterine atony in the setting of a 3- to 4-L blood loss have normal coagulation values and platelet counts when blood products are administered.[269,273–275] Thus, a plasma or platelet transfusion should be considered based on laboratory or relevant point-of-care data indicating significant clotting factor deficiency or severe thrombocytopenia. If the institutional protocols recommend a formulaic transfusion during the initial phase of active resuscitation during a severe hemorrhage, consideration should be given to transitioning to a goal-directed transfusion with laboratory or point-of-care-based approaches once the anesthesia team has ensured adequate intravenous access, invasive monitoring, blood component availability, and availability of sufficient staff to assist with hemostatic monitoring and resuscitation.

RECOMMENDED MANAGEMENT APPROACH TO MASSIVE HEMORRHAGE

Early Communication

Early communication among the obstetric, anesthesia, and nursing teams is vital to ensure that providers are updated on the evolving severity of PPH. During cesarean delivery, close and ongoing communication between the surgical and anesthesia teams is essential, and when concern escalates, the most senior or experienced anesthesiologist should be consulted. For cases of worsening hemorrhage after vaginal delivery, an automated notification system can be used to call the anesthesia team to the labor room expeditiously.[379] Local protocols should establish clinical thresholds for alerting anesthesia staff and should consider the prevalence of PPH and severe PPH, integrating both laboratory and clinical parameters and clinical judgment.

Initial Evaluation and Resuscitation

Considerations for the diagnosis and management of massive PPH are summarized in Fig. 37.3 and Box 37.7. Establishing large-bore intravenous access (ideally 16-gauge or greater) should be prioritized. Maternal vital signs should be monitored closely. Serial QBL measurements provide the anesthesia and surgical teams with information about the rate and cumulative magnitude of blood loss. Supplemental oxygen should be administered to the patient. After vaginal delivery, prompt transfer to the operating room allows the obstetric team adequate space and light to evaluate for genital tract lacerations, to place intrauterine devices for treating refractory atony, and to prepare for possible exploratory laparotomy if initial interventions fail. Additionally, the operating room enables access to critical anesthetic and resuscitation equipment, including drugs, a rapid infusion device, warming devices, temperature monitors, ultrasound machine, and urometer (for assessing urine output), and facilitates the rapid induction of general anesthesia, if indicated. An ultrasound machine should be available to expedite obtaining peripheral or central venous access. The use of transthoracic or transesophageal echocardiography can aid in assessing intravascular volume status and response to resuscitation efforts. Performing echocardiographic studies should not delay fluid and hemostatic resuscitation in an exsanguinating patient. Caution should be used in transferring patients to the interventional radiology suite when there is concern for major

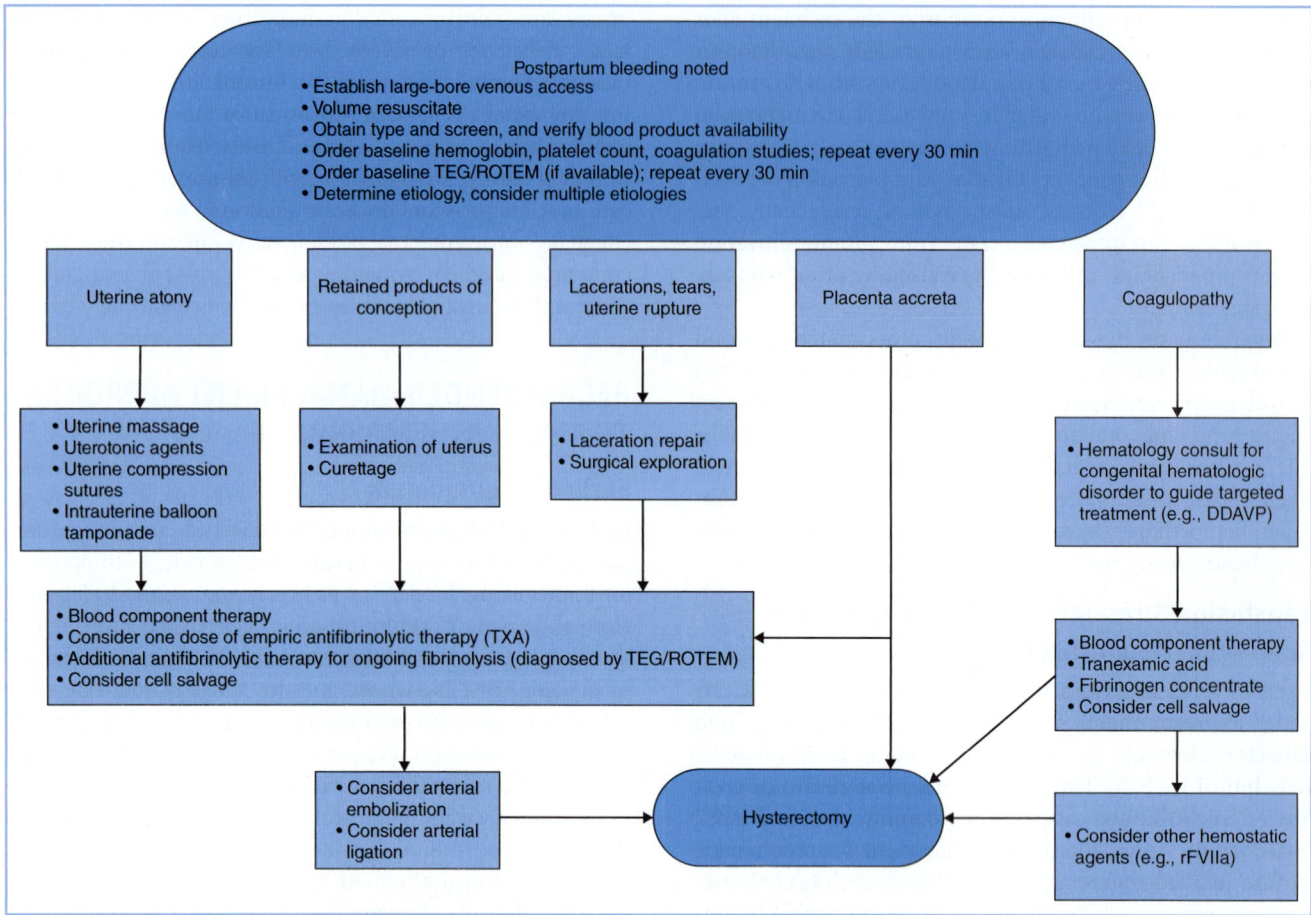

Fig. 37.3 Management Options for Postpartum Hemorrhage. *DDAVP*, 1-Desamino-8-D-arginine-vasopressin; *rFVIIa*, recombinant factor VIIa; *ROTEM*, rotational thromboelastometry; *TEG*, thromboelastography; *TXA*, tranexamic acid.

hemorrhage as these patients typically require urgent and immediate resuscitation and surgical intervention to control the source of bleeding.

Clinicians should initially identify the cause of PPH, which may involve a single or multiple etiologies (e.g., uterine atony, lacerations[380]). As PPH evolves from mild to moderate to severe, the workload necessary to deliver effective resuscitation will exceed the capacity of a sole anesthesia provider; therefore, early involvement of additional anesthesia staff is strongly recommended.

Resuscitation should commence with warmed non-dextrose-containing crystalloid (e.g., Plasma-lyte, lactated Ringer's, normal saline) and/or colloid (e.g., 5% albumin) solutions for intravascular volume replacement. TXA (1 g) should be administered (by 10-minute intravenous infusion) within the first 30 to 60 minutes of onset of PPH. Early activation of an MTP ensures timely access to sufficient blood products, essential even when cross-matched or type-specific RBCs are available, as these can quickly deplete during a major hemorrhage. Early placement of an arterial catheter allows continuous blood pressure monitoring and regular blood sampling (every 20 to 30 minutes) to assess hematologic, coagulation, biochemical, and arterial blood gas indices. Viscoelastic monitoring, if available, should be performed regularly to screen for hypofibrinogenemia, clotting factor deficiencies, and thrombocytopenia. Availability of point-of-care and laboratory indices are also critical for optimizing goal-directed approaches to hemostatic resuscitation with blood components and prohemostatic agents, notably fibrinogen concentrate.

For a patient experiencing a massive hemorrhage with active blood loss, an RBC transfusion should be considered for a hemoglobin level < 9 g/dL, fibrinogen replacement with a fibrinogen concentrate or cryoprecipitate for a fibrinogen concentration < 200 mg/dL, administration of plasma for a prothrombin or aPTT greater than 1.5 times the normal range, and platelet transfusion for a platelet count < 50,000/μL. Monitoring for hypocalcemia and hyperkalemia is vital in patients experiencing a major hemorrhage and a massive transfusion. Depending on availability, we advise obtaining multiple vials of calcium gluconate or calcium chloride to correct hypocalcemia as well as vials of insulin and 50% dextrose solution to correct hyperkalemia.

General Anesthesia

Depending on the extent of blood loss, etiology, bleeding control, and the hemodynamic status, the anesthesia team

BOX 37.7 Recommended Management Approach to Massive Hemorrhage

- Early communication: obstetric, anesthesia, nursing teams
- Low threshold for transferring patient to the operating room[a]
- Initial evaluation and resuscitation
  - Call for help.
  - Establish large-bore IV access (≥16-gauge).
  - Closely monitor vital signs.
  - Assess serial QBL.
  - Consider TTE or focused cardiac ultrasonography.
  - Initiate fluid resuscitation with crystalloid and colloid solutions.
  - Administer tranexamic acid 1 g.
  - Order emergency-release blood products (e.g., MTP).
  - Consider placement of arterial catheter.
  - Send blood for Hgb/Hct, platelet count, and coagulation studies at regular intervals during active hemorrhage.
  - Consider initiating blood product transfusion:
    - Hgb < 9 g/mL
    - Fibrinogen < 200 mg/dL (consider fibrinogen concentrate)
    - PT, aPTT > 1.5 times normal values
    - Platelet count < 50,000/µL
  - Closely monitor Ca^{+2} and K^+ at regular intervals and treat if indicated.
  - Warm patient actively.
- Induction of general anesthesia
  - Perform rapid sequence induction.[b]
  - Administer vasopressor(s) if indicated.
- Transfusion management
  - Consider fixed-ratio, goal-directed, or hybrid approach.
  - Administer warmed blood products through rapid infusion device.
  - Consider cell salvage.
- Treatment of cardiovascular collapse
  - Surgeons should manually compress or clamp the aorta.
  - Continue massive fluid/blood product resuscitation.
  - Close postpartum monitoring in a step-down unit or ICU after hemorrhage has been treated, and vital signs and coagulation status are stable.[c]

aPTT, Activated partial thromboplastin time; *Hct*, hematocrit; *Hgb*, hemoglobin; *ICU*, intensive care unit; *IV*, intravenous; *MTP*, massive transfusion protocol; *PT*, prothrombin time; *QBL*, quantitative blood loss; *TTE*, transthoracic echocardiography.

[a]For patient with hemorrhage outside of the operating room (e.g., labor and delivery room, postanesthesia care unit, postpartum unit).

[b]Consider induction ketamine or etomidate if the patient is hemodynamically unstable.

[c]Mechanical ventilation with prolonged sedation may be required during treatment for transfusion-associated circulatory overload or transfusion-associated lung injury.

should have a low threshold for inducing general anesthesia, especially if the surgical team is planning an exploratory laparotomy after a vaginal delivery or if prolonged surgical exploration or a hysterectomy is being considered after a cesarean delivery. A rapid-sequence induction agent such as etomidate or ketamine may be appropriate; vasoactive drugs

such as phenylephrine or norepinephrine may be necessary to support the central circulation. However, vasopressors do not substitute for aggressive treatment of hypovolemic shock with fluids and blood products. General anesthesia can be maintained in a variety of ways, including use of a volatile agent or a propofol infusion, with anesthetic depth, volume resuscitation, and vasopressor therapy adjusted to maintain systolic blood pressure and end-organ perfusion. Volatile halogenated agents should be administered with caution, if at all, in cases of PPH secondary to uterine atony.

Transfusion Management

Dynamic assessments of the intravascular fluid requirements and transfusion decision-making pose significant challenges during an ongoing massive hemorrhage. A liberal approach to a transfusion is recommended as underestimation of intravascular volume is common. Delayed recognition of severe hypovolemia (waiting until the patient is hypotensive) can lead to late decompensation in obstetric patients that can be challenging to treat, especially if severe hypoperfusion has occurred.

Aggressive transfusion strategies include fixed-ratio, goal-directed, and hybrid approaches (i.e., starting with a fixed-ratio approach and transitioning to a goal-directed approach; see earlier discussion), or clinical judgment-based approaches. A rapid infusion device is vital for ensuring the replacement of warmed blood components during a severe and rapid hemorrhage. Cell salvage and transfusion of autologous blood can be considered. Given the current lack of high-quality evidence, a tailored approach that accounts for an individual patient's physiologic, clinical, hematologic, and hemostatic indices is recommended. Dynamic evaluation of clinical and physiologic responses to transfusion is essential to gauge treatment effectiveness.

Real-Time Multidisciplinary Communication

Effective multidisciplinary communication among the obstetric, surgical, anesthesia, and nursing teams ensures that everyone providing care is aware of past, present, and anticipated concerns for surgical bleeding. This is particularly important during the management of an intraabdominal and pelvic hemorrhage during an exploratory laparotomy or peripartum hysterectomy. In cases of intraoperative cardiovascular collapse or cardiac arrest, the anesthesia team should assume that hypovolemia is the most likely cause and instruct the surgical team to compress or clamp the aorta temporarily until adequate cardiac output is restored.

Posthemorrhage Evaluation and Postpartum Care

Resuscitation endpoints should include cessation of surgical bleeding, hemodynamic stability, improved end-organ perfusion, and stabilization of hemoglobin and coagulation indices. Patients should be transferred to the ICU for close monitoring after a major hemorrhage event. Patients should remain in the operating room for ongoing evaluation if there is any clinical concern for ongoing bleeding or hemodynamic instability.

KEY POINTS

- Obstetric hemorrhage is the most common cause of maternal mortality worldwide and a leading contributor to maternal mortality in developed nations.
- Most severe morbidity and mortality that occurs secondary to obstetric hemorrhage is considered preventable.
- There has been an overall increase in PPH rates over time, which in part is attributed to the increase in the number of cesarean deliveries as well as the proportion of patients with PPH risk factors.
- PPH is increasing in both rate and severity in the developed world, primarily due to an increase in the incidence of uterine atony.
- Uterine atony is the most common cause of PPH, accounting for 80% of all PPH events.
- The increased incidence of PAS has paralleled increasing rates of cesarean delivery.
- Peripartum hysterectomy is increasing in frequency because of an increase in the incidence of both uterine atony and PAS.
- Patients with PAS are at high risk for massive hemorrhage and should be managed in facilities with multidisciplinary specialists, including interventional radiologists and a well-staffed blood bank.
- Multidisciplinary team responses that emphasize the accurate estimation of blood loss, early warning signs of shock, and rapid response to blood loss and coagulopathy are associated with less maternal morbidity.

- Prophylactic oxytocin is administered after delivery to decrease the rate of uterine atony.
- Methylergonovine and carboprost are second-line agents for the treatment of uterine atony after the use of oxytocin.
- Misoprostol has limited effectiveness as a second-line uterotonic agent in patients who have already received oxytocin for PPH prophylaxis or treatment and has an unfavorable side-effect profile.
- In both vaginal and cesarean deliveries, prophylactic tranexamic acid does not result in a clinically meaningful decrease in blood loss or PPH risk after delivery.
- Fibrinogen level < 200 mg/dL is an important predictor of severe PPH, but evidence is insufficient to confirm that this threshold represents a reasonable target for replacement.
- Transfusion protocols that comprise high ratios of plasma:RBC transfusion may paradoxically lower plasma fibrinogen levels in women who have moderate PPH and normal coagulation indices.
- Cryoprecipitate or fibrinogen concentrate, rather than plasma transfusion, is recommended for the treatment of hypofibrinogenemia.
- Viscoelastic monitors are useful for diagnosing or ruling out coagulopathy and assessing the potential effectiveness of hemostatic support in cases of severe or massive hemorrhage.

REFERENCES

1. Say L, Chou D, Gemmill A, et al. Global causes of maternal death: a WHO systematic analysis. *Lancet Glob Health.* 2014;2:e323–e333.
2. Kassebaum NJ, Bertozzi-Villa A, Coggeshall MS, et al. Global, regional, and national levels and causes of maternal mortality during 1990-2013: a systematic analysis for the Global Burden of Disease Study 2013. *Lancet.* 2014;384:980–1004.
3. Trost S, Beauregard J, Chandra G, et al. Pregnancy-related deaths: Data from Maternal Mortality Review Committees in 36 US States, 2017-2019; 2022. https://www.cdc.gov/maternal-mortality/php/data-research/mmrc-2017-2019.html. Accessed December 31, 2024.
4. Hoyert DL, Miniño AM. Maternal mortality in the United States: changes in coding, publication, and data release, 2018. *Natl Vital Stat Rep.* 2020;69:1–18.
5. Bonnet MP, de Vries PLM, Levet S, et al. Trends in maternal mortality from obstetric hemorrhage in France: 15 years of confidential enquiry into maternal deaths. *Anesth Analg.* 2024;139:1170–1180.
6. Fingar KR, Hambrick MM, Heslin KC, Moore JE. *Trends and Disparities in Delivery Hospitalizations Involving Severe Maternal Morbidity, 2006–2015.* Agency for Healthcare Research and Quality (US); 2018. www.hcup-us.ahrq.gov/reports/statbriefs/sb243-Severe-Maternal-Morbidity-Delivery-Trends-Disparities.pdf. Accessed December 31, 2024.
7. Bateman BT, Berman MF, Riley LE, Leffert LR. The epidemiology of postpartum hemorrhage in a large, nationwide sample of deliveries. *Anesth Analg.* 2010;110:1368–1373.
8. Bateman BT, Mhyre JM, Callaghan WM, Kuklina EV. Peripartum hysterectomy in the United States: nationwide 14 year experience. *Am J Obstet Gynecol.* 2012;206:63.e1–e8.
9. Wanderer JP, Leffert LR, Mhyre JM, et al. Epidemiology of obstetric-related ICU admissions in Maryland: 1999–2008. *Crit Care Med.* 2013;41:1844–1852.
10. Callaghan WM, Kuklina EV, Berg CJ. Trends in postpartum hemorrhage: United States, 1994–2006. *Am J Obstet Gynecol.* 2010;202:353.e1–e6.
11. Knight M, Callaghan WM, Berg C, et al. Trends in postpartum hemorrhage in high resource countries: a review and recommendations from the International Postpartum Hemorrhage Collaborative Group. *BMC Pregnancy Childbirth.* 2009;9:55.
12. Roberts CL, Ford JB, Algert CS, et al. Trends in adverse maternal outcomes during childbirth: a population-based study of severe maternal morbidity. *BMC Pregnancy Childbirth.* 2009;9:7.
13. Mehrabadi A, Liu S, Bartholomew S, et al. Temporal trends in postpartum hemorrhage and severe postpartum hemorrhage in Canada from 2003 to 2010. *J Obstet Gynaecol Can.* 2014;36:21–33.
14. Rossen J, Okland I, Nilsen OB, Eggebo TM. Is there an increase of postpartum hemorrhage, and is severe hemorrhage associated with more frequent use of obstetric interventions? *Acta Obstet Gynecol Scand.* 2010;89:1248–1255.

15. Corbetta-Rastelli CM, Friedman AM, Sobhani NC, et al. Postpartum hemorrhage trends and outcomes in the United States, 2000–2019. *Obstet Gynecol.* 2023;141:152–161.

16. Calleja-Agius J, Custo R, Brincat MP, Calleja N. Placental abruption and placenta praevia. *Eur Clin Obstet Gynaecol.* 2006;2:121–127.

17. Silver RM. Abnormal placentation: placenta previa, vasa previa, and placenta accreta. *Obstet Gynecol.* 2015;126: 654–668.

18. Dashe JS. Toward consistent terminology of placental location. *Semin Perinatol.* 2013;37:375–379.

19. Fan D, Wu S, Liu L, et al. Prevalence of antepartum hemorrhage in women with placenta previa: a systematic review and meta-analysis. *Sci Rep.* 2017;7:40320.

20. Cresswell JA, Ronsmans C, Calvert C, Filippi V. Prevalence of placenta praevia by world region: a systematic review and meta-analysis. *Trop Med Int Health.* 2013;18:712–724.

21. Faiz AS, Ananth CV. Etiology and risk factors for placenta previa: an overview and meta-analysis of observational studies. *J Matern Fetal Neonatal Med.* 2003;13:175–190.

22. Silver RM, Landon MB, Rouse DJ, et al. Maternal morbidity associated with multiple repeat cesarean deliveries. *Obstet Gynecol.* 2006;107:1226–1232.

23. Ananth CV, Wilcox AJ, Savitz DA, et al. Effect of maternal age and parity on the risk of uteroplacental bleeding disorders in pregnancy. *Obstet Gynecol.* 1996;88:511–516.

24. Taylor VM, Peacock S, Kramer MD, Vaughan TL. Increased risk of placenta previa among women of Asian origin. *Obstet Gynecol.* 1995;86:805–808.

25. Crane JM, Van den Hof MC, Dodds L, et al. Maternal complications with placenta previa. *Am J Perinatol.* 2000;17:101–105.

26. Li DK, Wi S. Maternal placental abnormality and the risk of sudden infant death syndrome. *Am J Epidemiol.* 1999;149:608–611.

27. Spinillo A, Fazzi E, Stronati M, et al. Early morbidity and neurodevelopmental outcome in low-birthweight infants born after third trimester bleeding. *Am J Perinatol.* 1994;11:85–90.

28. Vergani P, Ornaghi S, Pozzi I, et al. Placenta previa: distance to internal os and mode of delivery. *Am J Obstet Gynecol.* 2009;201:266.e1–e5.

29. Oppenheimer LW, Farine D. A new classification of placenta previa: measuring progress in obstetrics. *Am J Obstet Gynecol.* 2009;201:227–229.

30. Wexler P, Gottesfeld KR. Early diagnosis of placenta previa. *Obstet Gynecol.* 1979;54:231–234.

31. Rao KP, Belogolovkin V, Yankowitz J, Spinnato JA 2nd. Abnormal placentation: evidence-based diagnosis and management of placenta previa, placenta accreta, and vasa previa. *Obstet Gynecol Surv.* 2012;67:503–519.

32. Wing DA, Paul RH, Millar LK. Management of the symptomatic placenta previa: a randomized, controlled trial of inpatient versus outpatient expectant management. *Am J Obstet Gynecol.* 1996;175:806–811.

33. Bonner SM, Haynes SR, Ryall D. The anaesthetic management of caesarean section for placenta praevia: a questionnaire survey. *Anaesthesia.* 1995;50:992–994.

34. Fan D, Rao J, Lin D, et al. Anesthetic management in cesarean delivery of women with placenta previa: a retrospective cohort study. *BMC Anesthesiol.* 2021;21:247.

35. Brandt JS, Ananth CV. Placental abruption at near-term and term gestations: pathophysiology, epidemiology, diagnosis, and management. *Am J Obstet Gynecol.* 2023;228: S1313–S1329.

36. Lueth A, Blue N, Silver RM, et al. Prospective evaluation of placental abruption in nulliparous women. *J Matern Fetal Neonatal Med.* 2022;35:8603–8610.

37. Tikkanen M, Nuutila M, Hiilesmaa V, et al. Clinical presentation and risk factors of placental abruption. *Acta Obstet Gynecol Scand.* 2006;85:700–705.

38. Ananth CV, Oyelese Y, Srinivas N, et al. Preterm premature rupture of membranes, intrauterine infection, and oligohydramnios: risk factors for placental abruption. *Obstet Gynecol.* 2004;104:71–77.

39. Sylvester HC, Stringer M. Placental abruption leading to hysterectomy. *BMJ Case Rep.* 2017;2017

40. Glantz C, Purnell L. Clinical utility of sonography in the diagnosis and treatment of placental abruption. *J Ultrasound Med.* 2002;21:837–840.

41. Shinde GR, Vaswani BP, Patange RP, et al. Diagnostic performance of ultrasonography for detection of abruption and its clinical correlation and maternal and foetal outcome. *J Clin Diagn Res.* 2016;10:QC04–QC07.

42. Inoue A, Kondoh E, Suginami K, et al. Vaginal delivery after placental abruption with intrauterine fetal death: a 20-year single-center experience. *J Obstet Gynaecol Res.* 2017;43: 676–681.

43. de Lloyd L, Jenkins PV, Bell SF, et al. Acute obstetric coagulopathy during postpartum hemorrhage is caused by hyperfibrinolysis and dysfibrinogenemia: an observational cohort study. *J Thromb Haemost.* 2023;21:862–879.

44. Bell SF, Collis RE, Collins PW. Comparison of haematological indices and transfusion management in severe and massive postpartum haemorrhage: analysis of a two-year national prospective observational study. *Int J Obstet Anesth.* 2022;50:103547.

45. Bell SF, Collis RE, Bailey C, et al. The incidence, aetiology, and coagulation management of massive postpartum haemorrhage: a two-year national prospective cohort study. *Int J Obstet Anesth.* 2021;47:102983.

46. Vachon-Marceau C, Demers S, Bujold E, et al. Single versus double-layer uterine closure at cesarean: impact on lower uterine segment thickness at next pregnancy. *Am J Obstet Gynecol.* 2017;217:65.e1–e5.

47. Miller DA, Goodwin TM, Gherman RB, Paul RH. Intrapartum rupture of the unscarred uterus. *Obstet Gynecol.* 1997;89:671–673.

48. Gibbins KJ, Weber T, Holmgren CM, et al. Maternal and fetal morbidity associated with uterine rupture of the unscarred uterus. *Am J Obstet Gynecol.* 2015;213:382.e1–e6.

49. Holmgren CM. Uterine rupture associated with VBAC. *Clin Obstet Gynecol.* 2012;55:978–987.

50. Lydon-Rochelle M, Holt VL, Easterling TR, Martin DP. Risk of uterine rupture during labor among women with a prior cesarean delivery. *N Engl J Med.* 2001;345:3–8.

51. Harper LM, Cahill AG, Boslaugh S, et al. Association of induction of labor and uterine rupture in women attempting vaginal birth after cesarean: a survival analysis. *Am J Obstet Gynecol.* 2012;206:51.e1–e5.

52. Landon MB. Predicting uterine rupture in women undergoing trial of labor after prior cesarean delivery. *Semin Perinatol.* 2010;34:267–271.

53. Al-Zirqi I, Daltveit AK, Forsén L, et al. Risk facors for complete uterine rupture. *Am J Obstet Gynecol.* 2017;216: 165.e1–e8.

54. Kok N, Wiersma IC, Opmeer BC, et al. Sonographic measurement of lower uterine segment thickness to predict uterine rupture during a trial of labor in women with previous cesarean section: a meta-analysis. *Ultrasound Obstet Gynecol.* 2013;42:132–139.

55. Cantwell R, Clutton-Brock T, Cooper G, et al. Saving Mothers' Lives: reviewing maternal deaths to make motherhood safer: 2006-2008. The eighth report of the confidential enquiries into maternal deaths in the United Kingdom. *BJOG.* 2011;118:1–203.

56. Guiliano M, Closset E, Therby D, et al. Signs, symptoms and complications of complete and partial uterine ruptures during pregnancy and delivery. *Eur J Obstet Gynecol Reprod Biol.* 2014;2014:130–134.

57. Cahill AG, Odibo AO, Allsworth JE, Macones GA. Frequent epidural dosing as a marker for impending uterine rupture in patients who attempt vaginal birth after cesarean delivery. *Am J Obstet Gynecol.* 2010;202:355.e1–e5.

58. Society of Maternal-Fetal Medicine, Sinkey RG, Odibo AO, Dashe JS. #37: Diagnosis and management of vasa previa. *Am J Obstet Gynecol.* 2015;213:615–619.

59. Rebarber A, Dolin C, Fox NS, et al. Natural history of vasa previa across gestation using a screening protocol. *J Ultrasound Med.* 2014;33:141–147.

60. Bronsteen R, Whitten A, Balasubramanian M, et al. Vasa previa: clinical presentations, outcomes, and implications for management. *Obstet Gynecol.* 2013;122:352–357.

61. Oyelese Y, Catanzarite V, Prefumo F, et al. Vasa previa: the impact of prenatal diagnosis on outcomes. *Obstet Gynecol.* 2004;103:937–942.

62. Swank ML, Garite TJ, Maurel K, et al. Vasa previa: diagnosis and management. *Am J Obstet Gynecol.* 2016;215:223.e1–e6.

63. Robinson BK, Grobman WA. Effectiveness of timing strategies for delivery of individuals with vasa previa. *Obstet Gynecol.* 2011;117:542–549.

64. Oyelese Y, Javinani A, Shamshirsaz AA. Vasa previa. *Obstet Gynecol.* 2023;142:503–518.

65. Giouleka S, Tsakiridis I, Kalogiannidis I, et al. Postpartum hemorrhage: a comprehensive review of guidelines. *Obstet Gynecol Surv.* 2022;77:665–682.

66. American College of Obstetricians and Gynecologists. Practice Bulletin No. 183: Postpartum hemorrhage (reaffirmed 2024). *Obstet Gynecol.* 2017;130:923–925.

67. Calvert C, Thomas SL, Ronsmans C, et al. Identifying regional variation in the prevalence of postpartum haemorrhage: a systematic review and meta-analysis. *PLoS One.* 2012;7:e41114.

68. American College of Obstetricians and Gynecologists. Committee Opinion No. 794: Quantitative blood loss in obstetric hemorrhage (reaffirmed 2022). *Obstet Gynecol.* 2019;134:e150–e156.

69. Al Kadri HM, Al Anazi BK, Tamim HM. Visual estimation versus gravimetric measurement of postpartum blood loss: a prospective cohort study. *Arch Gynecol Obstet.* 2011;283:1207–1213.

70. Toledo P, McCarthy RJ, Hewlett BJ, et al. The accuracy of blood loss estimation after simulated vaginal delivery. *Anesth Analg.* 2007;105:1736–1740.

71. Patel A, Goudar SS, Geller SE, et al. Drape estimation vs. visual assessment for estimating postpartum hemorrhage. *Int J Gynaecol Obstet.* 2006;93:220–224.

72. Zhang WH, Deneux-Tharaux C, Brocklehurst P, et al. Effect of a collector bag for measurement of postpartum blood loss after vaginal delivery: cluster randomised trial in 13 European countries. *BMJ.* 2010;340:c293.

73. Hancock A, Weeks AD, Furber C, et al. The recognition of excessive blood loss at childbirth (REACT) study: a two-phase exploratory, sequential mixed methods inquiry using focus groups, interviews and a pilot, randomised crossover study. *BJOG.* 2021;128:1843–1854.

74. de Vries PLM, Deneux-Tharaux C, Baud D, et al. Postpartum haemorrhage in high-resource settings: variations in clinical management and future research directions based on a comparative study of national guidelines. *BJOG.* 2023;130:1639–1652.

75. Lumbreras-Marquez MI, Reale SC, Carusi DA, et al. Introduction of a novel system for quantitating blood loss after vaginal delivery: a retrospective interrupted time series analysis with concurrent control group. *Anesth Analg.* 2020;130:857–868.

76. Rubenstein AF, Zamudio S, Al-Khan A, et al. Clinical experience with the implementation of accurate measurement of blood loss during cesarean delivery: influences on hemorrhage recognition and allogeneic transfusion. *Am J Perinatol.* 2018;35:655–659.

77. Konig G, Waters JH, Javidroozi M, et al. Real-time evaluation of an image analysis system for monitoring surgical hemoglobin loss. *J Clin Monit Comput.* 2018;32:303–310.

78. Saoud F, Stone A, Nutter A, et al. Validation of a new method to assess estimated blood loss in the obstetric population undergoing cesarean delivery. *Am J Obstet Gynecol.* 2019;221:267.e1–e6.

79. Chau A, Farber MK. Do quantitative blood loss measurements and postpartum hemorrhage protocols actually make a difference? Yes, no, and maybe. *Int J Obstet Anesth.* 2020;42:1–3.

80. Ende HB, Lozada MJ, Chestnut DH, et al. Risk factors for atonic postpartum hemorrhage: a systematic review and meta-analysis. *Obstet Gynecol.* 2021;137:305–323.

81. Wray S, Prendergast C. The myometrium: from excitation to contractions and labour. In: Hashitani H, Lang R, eds. *Smooth Muscle Spontaneous Activity: Advances in Experimental Medicine and Biology.* Springer; 2019:233–263.

82. Aguilar HN, Mitchell BF. Physiological pathways and molecular mechanisms regulating uterine contractility. *Hum Reprod Update.* 2010;16:725–744.

83. Wray S. Insights into the uterus. *Exp Physiol.* 2007;92:621–631.

84. Koutras A, Fasoulakis Z, Syllaios A, et al. Physiology and pathology of contractility of the myometrium. *In Vivo.* 2021;35:1401–1408.

85. Phaneuf S, Asbóth G, MacKenzie IZ, et al. Effect of oxytocin antagonists on the activation of human myometrium in vitro: atosiban prevents oxytocin-induced desensitization. *Am J Obstet Gynecol.* 1994;171:1627–1634.

86. Phaneuf S, Asbóth G, Carrasco MP, et al. The desensitization of oxytocin receptors in human myometrial cells is accompanied by down-regulation of oxytocin receptor messenger RNA. *J Endocrinol.* 1997;154:7–18.

87. Robinson C, Schumann R, Zhang P, Young RC. Oxytocin-induced desensitization of the oxytocin receptor. *Am J Obstet Gynecol.* 2003;188:497–502.

88. Balki M, Erik-Soussi M, Kingdom J, Carvalho JC. Oxytocin pretreatment attenuates oxytocin-induced contractions in human myometrium in vitro. *Anesthesiology.* 2013;119:552–561.

89. Guly HR, Bouamra O, Little R, et al. Testing the validity of the ATLS classification of hypovolaemic shock. *Resuscitation.* 2010;81:1142–1147.

90. Begley CM, Gyte GM, Devane D, et al. Active versus expectant management for women in the third stage of labour. *Cochrane Database Syst Rev.* 2015;(3):CD007412.

91. Salati JA, Leathersich SJ, Williams MJ, et al. Prophylactic oxytocin for the third stage of labour to prevent postpartum haemorrhage. *Cochrane Database Syst Rev.* 2019;(4):CD001808.

92. Bateman BT, Tsen LC, Liu J, et al. Patterns of second-line uterotonic use in a large sample of hospitalizations for childbirth in the United States: 2007-2011. *Anesth Analg.* 2014;119:1344–1349.

93. Tunçalp O, Souza JP, Gülmezoglu M. New WHO recommendations on prevention and treatment of postpartum hemorrhage. *Int J Gynaecol Obstet.* 2013;123:254–256.

94. Gallos ID, Papadopoulou A, Man R, et al. Uterotonic agents for preventing postpartum haemorrhage: a network meta-analysis. *Cochrane Database Syst Rev.* 2018;(12):CD011689.

95. Carvalho JC, Balki M, Kingdom J, Windrim R. Oxytocin requirements at elective cesarean delivery: a dose-finding study. *Obstet Gynecol.* 2004;104:1005–1010.

96. Butwick AJ, Carvalho B. Minimum effective bolus dose of oxytocin during elective Caesarean delivery. *Br J Anaesth.* 2010;105:92–93.

97. Sarna MC, Soni AK, Gomez M, Oriol NE. Intravenous oxytocin in patients undergoing elective cesarean section. *Anesth Analg.* 1997;84:753–756.

98. George RB, McKeen D, Chaplin AC, McLeod L. Up-down determination of the ED(90) of oxytocin infusions for the prevention of postpartum uterine atony in parturients undergoing cesarean delivery. *Can J Anaesth.* 2010;57:578–582.

99. Lavoie A, McCarthy RJ, Wong CA. The ED90 of prophylactic oxytocin infusion after delivery of the placenta during cesarean delivery in laboring compared with nonlaboring women: an up-down sequential allocation dose-response study. *Anesth Analg.* 2015;121:159–164.

100. Peska E, Balki M, Maxwell C, et al. Oxytocin at elective caesarean delivery: a dose-finding study in women with obesity. *Anaesthesia.* 2021;76:918–923.

101. Peska E, Balki M, Pfeifer W, et al. Oxytocin at elective cesarean delivery: a dose-finding study in pregnant people with twin pregnancy. *Anesth Analg.* 2024;138:814–820.

102. Balki M, Ronayne M, Davies S, et al. Minimum oxytocin dose requirement after cesarean delivery for labor arrest. *Obstet Gynecol.* 2006;107:45–50.

103. Sheehan SR, Montgomery AA, Carey M, et al. Oxytocin bolus versus oxytocin bolus and infusion for control of blood loss at elective caesarean section: double blind, placebo controlled, randomised trial. *BMJ.* 2011;343:d4661.

104. Duffield A, McKenzie C, Carvalho B, et al. Effect of a high-rate versus a low-rate oxytocin infusion for maintaining uterine contractility during elective cesarean delivery: a prospective randomized clinical trial. *Anesth Analg.* 2017;124:857–862.

105. Pinder AJ, Dresner M, Calow C, et al. Haemodynamic changes caused by oxytocin during caesarean section under spinal anaesthesia. *Int J Obstet Anesth.* 2002;11:156–159.

106. Archer TL, Knape K, Liles D, et al. The hemodynamics of oxytocin and other vasoactive agents during neuraxial anesthesia for cesarean delivery: findings in six cases. *Int J Obstet Anesth.* 2008;17:247–254.

107. Svanstrom MC, Biber B, Hanes M, et al. Signs of myocardial ischaemia after injection of oxytocin: a randomized double-blind comparison of oxytocin and methylergometrine during caesarean section. *Br J Anaesth.* 2008;100:683–689.

108. Jonsson M, Hanson U, Lidell C, Norden-Lindeberg S. ST depression at caesarean section and the relation to oxytocin dose. A randomised controlled trial. *BJOG.* 2010;117:76–83.

109. Thomas TA, Cooper GM, Editorial board of the Confidential Enquiries into Maternal Deaths in the United Kingdom. Maternal deaths from anaesthesia. An extract from why mothers die 1997–1999, the Confidential Enquiries into Maternal Deaths in the United Kingdom. *Br J Anaesth.* 2002;89:499–508.

110. Thomas JS, Koh SH, Cooper GM. Haemodynamic effects of oxytocin given as i.v. bolus or infusion on women undergoing caesarean section. *Br J Anaesth.* 2007;98:116–119.

111. Sartain JB, Barry JJ, Howat PW, et al. Intravenous oxytocin bolus of 2 units is superior to 5 units during elective caesarean section. *Br J Anaesth.* 2008;101:822–826.

112. Langesæter E, Rosseland LA, Stubhaug A. Haemodynamic effects of oxytocin in women with severe preeclampsia. *Int J Obstet Anesth.* 2011;20:26–29.

113. Dyer RA, Reed AR, van Dyk D, et al. Hemodynamic effects of ephedrine, phenylephrine, and the coadministration of phenylephrine with oxytocin during spinal anesthesia for elective cesarean delivery. *Anesthesiology.* 2009;111:753–765.

114. Heesen M, Carvalho B, Carvalho JCA, et al. International consensus statement on the use of uterotonic agents during caesarean section. *Anaesthesia.* 2019;74:1305–1319.

115. Lagrew D, McNulty J, Sakowski C, et al. Improving healthcare response to obstetric hemorrhage, a California Maternal Quality Care Collaborative toolkit; 2022. https://www.cmqcc.org/sites/default/files/HEMToolkit_03252022%20Errata%207.2022%20%282%29.pdf. Accessed December 31, 2024.

116. Anandakrishnan S, Balki M, Farine D, et al. Carbetocin at elective Cesarean delivery: a randomized controlled trial to determine the effective dose, part 2. *Can J Anaesth.* 2013;60:1054–1060.

117. Cordovani D, Balki M, Farine D, et al. Carbetocin at elective Cesarean delivery: a randomized controlled trial to determine the effective dose. *Can J Anaesth.* 2012;59:751–757.

118. Tabl S, Balki M, Downey K, et al. Uterotonics in elective caesarean delivery: a randomised non-inferiority study comparing carbetocin 20 µg and 100 µg. *Anaesthesia.* 2019;74:190–196.

119. Nguyen-Lu N, Carvalho JC, Farine D, et al. Carbetocin at Cesarean delivery for labour arrest: a sequential allocation trial to determine the effective dose. *Can J Anaesth.* 2015;62:866–874.

120. Drew T, Balki M, Farine D, et al. Carbetocin at elective caesarean section: a sequential allocation trial to determine the minimum effective dose in obese women. *Anaesthesia.* 2020;75:331–337.

121. Khan M, Balki M, Ahmed I, et al. Carbetocin at elective Cesarean delivery: a sequential allocation trial to determine the minimum effective dose. *Can J Anaesth.* 2014;61:242–248.

122. Rosseland LA, Hauge TH, Grindheim G, et al. Changes in blood pressure and cardiac output during cesarean delivery: the effects of oxytocin and carbetocin compared with placebo. *Anesthesiology.* 2013;119:541–551.

123. Moertl MG, Friedrich S, Kraschl J, et al. Haemodynamic effects of carbetocin and oxytocin given as intravenous bolus on women undergoing caesarean delivery: a randomised trial. *BJOG.* 2011;118:1349–1356.

124. Widmer M, Piaggio G, Nguyen TMH, et al. Heat-stable carbetocin versus oxytocin to prevent hemorrhage after vaginal birth. *N Eng J Med.* 2018;379:743–752.

125. Whigham CA, Gorelik A, Loughnan TE, Trivedi A. Carbetocin versus oxytocin to reduce additional uterotonic use at non-elective caesarean section: a double-blind, randomised trial. *J Matern Fetal Neonatal Med.* 2016;29:3866–3869.

126. Ben Tareef A, Downey K, Ma B, et al. Carbetocin versus oxytocin following vaginal and Cesarean delivery: a before-after study. *Can J Anaesth.* 2022;69:97–105.

127. Jaffer D, Singh PM, Aslam A, et al. Preventing postpartum hemorrhage after cesarean delivery: a network meta-analysis of available pharmacologic agents. *Am J Obstet Gynecol.* 2022;226:347–365.

128. Onwochei DN, Owolabi A, Singh PM, Monks DT. Carbetocin compared with oxytocin in non-elective Cesarean delivery: a systematic review, meta-analysis, and trial sequential analysis of randomized-controlled trials. *Can J Anaesth.* 2020;67:1524–1534.

129. Onwochei DN, Van Ross J, Singh PM, et al. Carbetocin reduces the need for additional uterotonics in elective caesarean delivery: a systematic review, meta-analysis and trial sequential analysis of randomised controlled trials. *Int J Obstet Anesth.* 2019;40:14–23.

130. Vallera C, Choi LO, Cha CM, Hong RW. Uterotonic medications: oxytocin, methylergonovine, carboprost, misoprostol. *Anesthesiol Clin.* 2017;35:207–219.

131. Mäntylä R, Kanto J. Clinical pharmacokinetics of methylergometrine (methylergonovine). *Int J Clin Pharmacol Ther Toxicol.* 1981;19:386–391.

132. De Winter S, Vanbrabant P, Vi NT, et al. Impact of temperature exposure on stability of drugs in a real-world out-of-hospital setting. *Ann Emerg Med.* 2013;62:380–387.

133. Masse N, Dexter F, Wong CA. Prophylactic methylergonovine and oxytocin compared with oxytocin alone in patients undergoing intrapartum cesarean birth: a randomized controlled trial. *Obstet Gynecol.* 2022;140:181–186.

134. Balki M, Downey K, Walker A, et al. Prophylactic administration of uterotonics to prevent postpartum hemorrhage in women undergoing cesarean delivery for arrest of labor: a randomized controlled trial. *Obstet Gynecol.* 2021;137:505–513.

135. Butwick AJ, Carvalho B, Blumenfeld YJ, et al. Second-line uterotonics and the risk of hemorrhage-related morbidity. *Am J Obstet Gynecol.* 2015;212:642.e1–e7.

136. Cole NM, Kim JJ, Lumbreras-Marquez MI, et al. Second-line uterotonics for uterine atony: a randomized controlled trial. *Obstet Gynecol.* 2024;144:832–841.

137. Hayashi Y, Ibe T, Kawato H, et al. Postpartum acute myocardial infarction induced by ergonovine administration. *Intern Med.* 2003;42:983–986.

138. Satoh H, Sano M, Suwa K, et al. Pregnancy-related acute myocardial infarction in Japan: a review of epidemiology, etiology and treatment from case reports. *Circ J.* 2013;77:725–733.

139. Abouleish E. Postpartum hypertension and convulsion after oxytocic drugs. *Anesth Analg.* 1976;55:813–815.

140. Lin YH, Seow KM, Hwang JL, Chen HH. Myocardial infarction and mortality caused by methylergonovine. *Acta Obstet Gynecol Scand.* 2005;84:1022.

141. Bateman BT, Huybrechts KF, Hernandez-Diaz S, et al. Methylergonovine maleate and the risk of myocardial ischemia and infarction. *Am J Obstet Gynecol.* 2013;209:459.e1–e13.

142. Fuchs AR, Husslein P, Sumulong L, Fuchs F. The origin of circulating 13,14-dihydro-15-keto-prostaglandin F2 alpha during delivery. *Prostaglandins.* 1982;24:715–722.

143. Noort WA, van Bulck B, Vereecken A, et al. Changes in plasma levels of PGF2 alpha and PGI2 metabolites at and after delivery at term. *Prostaglandins.* 1989;37:3–12.

144. Harber CR, Levy DM, Chidambaram S, Macpherson MB. Life-threatening bronchospasm after intramuscular carboprost for postpartum haemorrhage. *BJOG.* 2007;114:366–368.

145. Andersen LH, Secher NJ. Pattern of total and regional lung function in subjects with bronchoconstriction induced by 15-me PGF2 alpha. *Thorax.* 1976;31:685–692.

146. Oladapo OT. Misoprostol for preventing and treating postpartum hemorrhage in the community: a closer look at the evidence. *Int J Gynaecol Obstet.* 2012;119:105–110.

147. Alfirevic Z, Blum J, Walraven G, et al. Prevention of postpartum hemorrhage with misoprostol. *Int J Gynaecol Obstet.* 2007;99:S198–S201.

148. Tang OS, Gemzell-Danielsson K, Ho PC. Misoprostol: pharmacokinetic profiles, effects on the uterus and side-effects. *Int J Gynaecol Obstet.* 2007;99:S160–S167.

149. Gibbins KJ, Albright CM, Rouse DJ. Postpartum hemorrhage in the developed world: whither misoprostol? *Am J Obstet Gynecol.* 2013;208:181–183.

150. Blum J, Winikoff B, Raghavan S, et al. Treatment of post-partum haemorrhage with sublingual misoprostol versus oxytocin in women receiving prophylactic oxytocin: a double-blind, randomised, non-inferiority trial. *Lancet.* 2010;375:217–223.

151. Widmer M, Blum J, Hofmeyr GJ, et al. Misoprostol as an adjunct to standard uterotonics for treatment of post-partum haemorrhage: a multicentre, double-blind randomised trial. *Lancet.* 2010;375:1808–1813.

152. Winikoff B, Dabash R, Durocher J, et al. Treatment of post-partum haemorrhage with sublingual misoprostol versus oxytocin in women not exposed to oxytocin during labour: a double-blind, randomised, non-inferiority trial. *Lancet.* 2010;375:210–216.

153. Elati A, Weeks A. Risk of fever after misoprostol for the prevention of postpartum hemorrhage: a meta-analysis. *Obstet Gynecol.* 2012;120:1140–1148.

154. Parry Smith WR, Papadopoulou A, Thomas E, et al. Uterotonic agents for first-line treatment of postpartum haemorrhage: a network meta-analysis. *Cochrane Database Syst Rev.* 2020;(11):CD012754.

155. Kawarabayashi T, Kishikawa T, Sugimori H. Effects of external calcium, magnesium, and temperature on spontaneous contractions of pregnant human myometrium. *Biol Reprod.* 1989;40:942–948.

156. Luckas MJ, Taggart MJ, Wray S. Intracellular calcium stores and agonist-induced contractions in isolated human myometrium. *Am J Obstet Gynecol.* 1999;181:468–476.

157. Talati C, Ramachandran N, Carvalho JC, et al. The effect of extracellular calcium on oxytocin-induced contractility in naive and oxytocin-pretreated human myometrium in vitro. *Anesth Analg.* 2016;122:1498–1507.

158. Ansari JR, Yarmosh A, Michel G, et al. Intravenous calcium to decrease blood loss during intrapartum cesarean delivery: a randomized controlled trial. *Obstet Gynecol.* 2024;143: 104–112.

159. You WB, Zahn CM. Postpartum hemorrhage: abnormally adherent placenta, uterine inversion, and puerperal hematomas. *Clin Obstet Gynecol.* 2006;49:184–197.

160. Fong A, Wu E, Pan D, et al. Temporal trends and morbidities of vacuum, forceps, and combined use of both. *J Matern Fetal Neonatal Med.* 2014;27:1886–1891.

161. Lee NK, Kim S, Lee JW, et al. Postpartum hemorrhage: clinical and radiologic aspects. *Eur J Radiol.* 2010;74:50–59.

162. Fargeaudou Y, Soyer P, Morel O, et al. Severe primary postpartum hemorrhage due to genital tract laceration after operative vaginal delivery: successful treatment with transcatheter arterial embolization. *Eur Radiol.* 2009;19: 2197–2203.

163. Saleem Z, Rydhstrom H. Vaginal hematoma during parturition: a population-based study. *Acta Obstet Gynecol Scand.* 2004;83:560–562.

164. Egan E, Dundee P, Lawrentschuk N. Vulvar hematoma secondary to spontaneous rupture of the internal iliac artery: clinical review. *Am J Obstet Gynecol.* 2009;200:e17–e18.

165. Rani S, Verma M, Pandher DK, et al. Risk factors and incidence of puerperal genital haematomas. *J Clin Diagn Res.* 2017;11:QC01–QC03.

166. Hamou B, Sheiner E, Coreanu T, et al. Intrapartum cervical lacerations and their impact on future pregnancy outcome. *J Matern Fetal Neonatal Med.* 2020;33:883–887.

167. Melamed N, Ben-Haroush A, Chen R, et al. Intrapartum cervical lacerations: characteristics, risk factors, and effects on subsequent pregnancies. *Am J Obstet Gynecol.* 2009;200:388.e1–e4.

168. Wong LF, Wilkes J, Korgenski K, et al. Intrapartum cervical laceration and subsequent pregnancy outcomes. *AJP Rep.* 2016;6:e318–e323.

169. Parikh R, Brotzman S, Anasti JN. Cervical lacerations: some surprising facts. *Am J Obstet Gynecol.* 2007;196:e17–e18.

170. Landy HJ, Laughon SK, Bailit JL, et al. Characteristics associated with severe perineal and cervical lacerations during vaginal delivery. *Obstet Gynecol.* 2011;117:627–635.

171. Hossein-Pour P, Rajasingham M, Muraca GM. Risk of cervical laceration in forceps vs vacuum delivery: a systematic review and meta-analysis. *Acta Obstet Gynecol Scand.* 2024;104:29–38.

172. Gluck O, David M, Kovo M, et al. The clinical significance of cervical tears' anatomical location—a retrospective study. *Eur J Obstet Gynecol Reprod Biol.* 2024;295:215–218.

173. Fliegner JR. Postpartum broad ligament haematomas. *J Obstet Gynaecol Br Commonw.* 1971;78:184–189.

174. Combs CA, Laros RKJ. Prolonged third stage of labor: morbidity and risk factors. *Obstet Gynecol.* 1991;77:863–867.

175. Endler M, Grunewald C, Saltvedt S. Epidemiology of retained placenta: oxytocin as an independent risk factor. *Obstet Gynecol.* 2012;119:801–809.

176. Magann EF, Evans S, Chauhan SP, et al. The length of the third stage of labor and the risk of postpartum hemorrhage. *Obstet Gynecol.* 2005;105:290–293.

177. Jackson KW Jr, Allbert JR, Schemmer GK, et al. A randomized controlled trial comparing oxytocin administration before and after placental delivery in the prevention of postpartum hemorrhage. *Am J Obstet Gynecol.* 2001;185:873–877.

178. Soltani H, Hutchon DR, Poulose TA. Timing of prophylactic uterotonics for the third stage of labour after vaginal birth. *Cochrane Database Syst Rev.* 2010;(8):CD006173.

179. World Health Organization. WHO recommendations for prevention and treatment of maternal peripartum infections; 2015. https://www.who.int/publications/i/item/9789241549363. Accessed November 25, 2024.

180. Chongsomchai C, Lumbiganon P, Laopaiboon M. Prophylactic antibiotics for manual removal of retained placenta in vaginal birth. *Cochrane Database Syst Rev.* 2014;(10):CD004904.

181. Driessen M, Bouvier-Colle MH, Dupont C, et al. Postpartum hemorrhage resulting from uterine atony after vaginal delivery: factors associated with severity. *Obstet Gynecol.* 2011;117:21–31.

182. Chandraharan E, Arulkumaran S. Acute tocolysis. *Curr Opin Obstet Gynecol.* 2005;17:151–156.

183. Peng AT, Gorman RS, Shulman SM, et al. Intravenous nitroglycerin for uterine relaxation in the postpartum patient with retained placenta. *Anesthesiology.* 1989;71:172–173.

184. DeSimone CA, Norris MC, Leighton BL. Intravenous nitroglycerin aids manual extraction of a retained placenta. *Anesthesiology.* 1990;73:787.

185. Bullarbo M, Tjugum J, Ekerhovd E. Sublingual nitroglycerin for management of retained placenta. *Int J Gynaecol Obstet.* 2005;91:228–232.

186. Coad SL, Dahlgren LS, Hutcheon JA. Risks and consequences of puerperal uterine inversion in the United States, 2004 through 2013. *Am J Obstet Gynecol.* 2017;217:377.e1–e6.

187. Smulian JC, DeFulvio JD, Diven L, Terrazas JL. Sonographic findings in acute uterine inversion. *J Clin Ultrasound.* 2013;41:453–456.

188. Wendel PJ, Cox SM. Emergent obstetric management of uterine inversion. *Obstet Gynecol Clin North Am.* 1995;22:261–274.

189. Haeri S, Rais S, Monks B. Intrauterine tamponade balloon use in the treatment of uterine inversion. *BMJ Case Rep.* 2015;2015:bcr2014206705.

190. Hong RW, Greenfield ML, Polley LS. Nitroglycerin for uterine inversion in the absence of placental fragments. *Anesth Analg.* 2006;103:511–512.

191. Dufour P, Vinatier D, Puech F. The use of intravenous nitroglycerin for cervico-uterine relaxation: a review of the literature. *Arch Gynecol Obstet.* 1997;261:1–7.

192. Jauniaux E, Hussein AM, Elbarmelgy RM, et al. Failure of placental detachment in accreta placentation is associated with excessive fibrinoid deposition at the utero-placental interface. *Am J Obstet Gynecol.* 2022;226:243.e1–e10.

193. American College of Obstetricians and Gynecologists, Society for Maternal-Fetal Medicine. Obstetric Care Consensus No. 7: Placenta accreta spectrum (reaffirmed 2021). *Obstet Gynecol.* 2018;132:e259–e275.

194. Jauniaux E, Ayres-de-Campos D, Langhoff-Roos J, et al. FIGO classification for the clinical diagnosis of placenta accreta spectrum disorders. *Int J Gynaecol Obstet.* 2019;146:20–24.

195. Matsuzaki S, Mandelbaum RS, Sangara RN, et al. Trends, characteristics, and outcomes of placenta accreta spectrum:

a national study in the United States. *Am J Obstet Gynecol.* 2021;225:534.e1–e38.

196. Miller DA, Chollet JA, Goodwin TM. Clinical risk factors for placenta previa-placenta accreta. *Am J Obstet Gynecol.* 1997;177:210–214.

197. Jauniaux E, Bunce C, Grønbeck L, Langhoff-Roos J. Prevalence and main outcomes of placenta accreta spectrum: a systematic review and meta-analysis. *Am J Obstet Gynecol.* 2019;221:208–218.

198. Jauniaux E, Bhide A. Prenatal ultrasound diagnosis and outcome of placenta previa accreta after cesarean delivery: a systematic review and meta-analysis. *Am J Obstet Gynecol.* 2017;217:27–36.

199. Jauniaux E, Chantraine F, Silver RM, et al. FIGO consensus guidelines on placenta accreta spectrum disorders: epidemiology. *Int J Gynaecol Obstet.* 2018;140:265–273.

200. D'Antonio F, Iacovella C, Bhide A. Prenatal identification of invasive placentation using ultrasound: systematic review and meta-analysis. *Ultrasound Obstet Gynecol.* 2013;42:509–517.

201. D'Antonio F, Iacovella C, Palacios-Jaraquemada J, et al. Prenatal identification of invasive placentation using magnetic resonance imaging: systematic review and meta-analysis. *Ultrasound Obstet Gynecol.* 2014;44:8–16.

202. Sargent W, Gerry S, Collins SL. A risk-prediction model for placenta accreta spectrum severity from standardized ultrasound markers. *Ultrasound Med Biol.* 2023;49:512–519.

203. Singh S, Carusi DA, Wang P, et al. External validation of a multivariable prediction model for placenta accreta spectrum. *Anesth Analg.* 2023;137:537–547.

204. Einerson BD, Gilner JB, Zuckerwise LC. Placenta accreta spectrum. *Obstet Gynecol.* 2023;142:31–50.

205. Wright JD, Silver RM, Bonanno C, et al. Practice patterns and knowledge of obstetricians and gynecologists regarding placenta accreta. *J Matern Fetal Neonatal Med.* 2013;26:1602–1609.

206. Society for Maternal-Fetal Medicine, Einerson BD, Healy AD, Lee A, et al. Society for Maternal-Fetal Medicine Special Statement: emergency checklist, planning worksheet, and system preparedness bundle for placenta accreta spectrum. *Am J Obstet Gynecol.* 2024;230:B2–B11.

207. Silver RM, Fox KA, Barton JR, et al. Center of excellence for placenta accreta. *Am J Obstet Gynecol.* 2015;212:561–568.

208. Eller AG, Bennett MA, Sharshiner M, et al. Maternal morbidity in cases of placenta accreta managed by a multidisciplinary care team compared with standard obstetric care. *Obstet Gynecol.* 2011;117:331–337.

209. Robinson BK, Grobman WA. Effectiveness of timing strategies for delivery of individuals with placenta previa and accreta. *Obstet Gynecol.* 2010;116:835–842.

210. Tan CH, Tay KH, Sheah K, et al. Perioperative endovascular internal iliac artery occlusion balloon placement in management of placenta accreta. *Am J Roentgenol.* 2007;189:1158–1163.

211. Shrivastava V, Nageotte M, Major C, et al. Case-control comparison of cesarean hysterectomy with and without prophylactic placement of intravascular balloon catheters for placenta accreta. *Am J Obstet Gynecol.* 2007;197:402.e1–e5.

212. Angstmann T, Gard G, Harrington T, et al. Surgical management of placenta accreta: a cohort series and suggested approach. *Am J Obstet Gynecol.* 2010;202:38.e1–e9.

213. Ballas J, Hull AD, Saenz C, et al. Preoperative intravascular balloon catheters and surgical outcomes in pregnancies complicated by placenta accreta: a management paradox. *Am J Obstet Gynecol.* 2012;207:216.e1–e5.

214. Salim R, Chulski A, Romano S, et al. Precesarean prophylactic balloon catheters for suspected placenta accreta: a randomized controlled trial. *Obstet Gynecol.* 2015;126:1022–1028.

215. Greenberg JI, Suliman A, Iranpour P, Angle N. Prophylactic balloon occlusion of the internal iliac arteries to treat abnormal placentation: a cautionary case. *Am J Obstet Gynecol.* 2007;197:470.e1–e4.

216. Bishop S, Butler K, Monaghan S, et al. Multiple complications following the use of prophylactic internal iliac artery balloon catheterisation in a patient with placenta percreta. *Int J Obstet Anesth.* 2011;20:70–73.

217. Sadashivaiah J, Wilson R, Thein A, et al. Role of prophylactic uterine artery balloon catheters in the management of women with suspected placenta accreta. *Int J Obstet Anesth.* 2011;20:282–287.

218. Society for Maternal-Fetal Medicine. Belfort MA. Placenta accreta. *Am J Obstet Gynecol.* 2010;203:430–439.

219. Dai M, Zhang F, Li K, et al. The effect of prophylactic balloon occlusion in patients with placenta accreta spectrum: a Bayesian network meta-analysis. *Eur Radiol.* 2022;32:3297–3308.

220. Fox KA, Shamshirsaz AA, Carusi D, et al. Conservative management of morbidly adherent placenta: expert review. *Am J Obstet Gynecol.* 2015;213:755–760.

221. Sentilhes L, Seco A, Azria E, et al. Conservative management or cesarean hysterectomy for placenta accreta spectrum: the PACCRETA prospective study. *Am J Obstet Gynecol.* 2022;226:839.e1–e24.

222. Kayem G, Davy C, Goffinet F, et al. Conservative versus extirpative management in cases of placenta accreta. *Obstet Gynecol.* 2004;104:531–536.

223. Sentilhes L, Ambroselli C, Kayem G, et al. Maternal outcome after conservative treatment of placenta accreta. *Obstet Gynecol.* 2010;115:526–534.

224. Judy AE, Lyell DJ, Druzin ML, Dorigo O. Disseminated intravascular coagulation complicating the conservative management of placenta percreta. *Obstet Gynecol.* 2015;126:1016–1018.

225. Sentilhes L, Kayem G, Chandraharan E, et al. FIGO consensus guidelines on placenta accreta spectrum disorders: conservative management. *Int J Gynaecol Obstet.* 2018;140:291–298.

226. Zuckerwise LC, Craig AM, Newton JM, et al. Outcomes following a clinical algorithm allowing for delayed hysterectomy in the management of severe placenta accreta spectrum. *Am J Obstet Gynecol.* 2020;222:179.e1–e9.

227. Gatta LA, Weber JM, Gilner JB, et al. Transfusion requirements with hybrid management of placenta accreta spectrum incorporating targeted embolization and a selectiveuse of delayed hysterectomy. *Am J Perinatol.* 2022;29:1503–1513.

228. Chandraharan E, Rao S, Belli AM, Arulkumaran S. The Triple-P procedure as a conservative surgical alternative to peripartum hysterectomy for placenta percreta. *Int J Gynaecol Obstet.* 2012;117:191–194.

229. Aryananda RA, Aditiawarman A, Gumilar KE, et al. Uterine conservative-resective surgery for selected placenta accreta spectrum cases: surgical-vascular control methods. *Acta Obstet Gynecol Scand.* 2022;101:639–648.

230. Palacios-Jaraquemada JM, Fiorillo A, Hamer J, et al. Placenta accreta spectrum: a hysterectomy can be prevented in almost 80% of cases using a resective-reconstructive technique. *J Matern Fetal Neonatal Med*. 2022;35:275–282.

231. Warrick CM, Markley JC, Farber MK, et al. Placenta accreta spectrum disorders: knowledge gaps in anesthesia care. *Anesth Analg*. 2022;135:191–197.

232. Einerson BD, Weiniger CF. Placenta accreta spectrum disorder: updates on anesthetic and surgical management strategies. *Int J Obstet Anesth*. 2021;46:102975.

233. Miller SE, Leonard SA, Meza PK, et al. Red blood cell transfusion in patients with placenta accreta spectrum: a systematic review and meta-analysis. *Obstet Gynecol*. 2023;141:49–58.

234. Panjeton GD, Reynolds PS, Saleem D, et al. Neuraxial anesthesia and postoperative opioid administration for cesarean delivery in patients with placenta accreta spectrum disorder: a retrospective cohort study. *Int J Obstet Anesth*. 2021:103220.

235. Bouvier-Colle MH, Ould El Joud D, Varnoux N, et al. Evaluation of the quality of care for severe obstetrical haemorrhage in three French regions. *BJOG*. 2001;108:898–903.

236. Main EK, McCain CL, Morton CH, et al. Pregnancy-related mortality in California: causes, characteristics, and improvement opportunities. *Obstet Gynecol*. 2015;125:938–947.

237. Zaharatos J, St Pierre A, Cornell A, et al. Building U.S. capacity to review and prevent maternal deaths. *J Womens Health (Larchmt)*. 2018;27:1–5.

238. Seacrist MJ, VanOtterloo LR, Morton CH, Main EK. Quality improvement opportunities identified through case review of pregnancy-related deaths from obstetric hemorrhage. *J Obstet Gynecol Neonatal Nurs*. 2019;48:288–299.

239. Main EK, Goffman D, Scavone BM, et al. National Partnership for Maternal Safety: consensus bundle on obstetric hemorrhage. *Obstet Gynecol*. 2015;126:155–162.

240. California Maternal Quality Care Collaborative. *Obstetric Hemorrhage Toolkit V 3.0*. CMQCC; 2022. https://www.cmqcc.org/ob_hemorrhage/ob_hemorrhage_compendium_of_best_practices. Accessed December 31, 2024.

241. American College of Obstetricians and Gynecologists. *Safe Motherhood Initiative: Obstetric Hemorrhage*. ACOG; 2024. https://www.acog.org/community/districts-and-sections/district-ii/programs-and-resources/safe-motherhood-initiative/obstetric-hemorrhage. Accessed December 31, 2024.

242. The Joint Commission. *R3 Report Issue 24: PC Standards For Maternal Safety*. The Joint Commission; 2019. https://www.jointcommission.org/-/media/tjc/documents/standards/r3-reports/r3-issue-24-maternal-12-7-2021.pdf. Accessed December 31, 2024.

243. World Health Organization. *WHO Recommendations on the Assessment of Postpartum Blood Loss and Treatment Bundles for Postpartum Haemorrhage*. World Health Organization; 2023. https://www.who.int/publications/i/item/9789240085398. Accessed December 31, 2024.

244. Alliance for Innovation on Maternal Health. Obstetric hemorrhage patient safety bundle. ACOG; 2022. https://saferbirth.org/psbs/obstetric-hemorrhage/. Accessed December 31, 2024.

245. Shields LE, Wiesner S, Fulton J, Pelletreau B. Comprehensive maternal hemorrhage protocols reduce the use of blood products and improve patient safety. *Am J Obstet Gynecol*. 2015;212:272–280.

246. Main EK, Cape V, Abreo A, et al. Reduction of severe maternal morbidity from hemorrhage using a state perinatal quality collaborative. *Am J Obstet Gynecol*. 2017;216:298.e1–e11.

247. Grunebaum A, Chervenak F, Skupski D. Effect of a comprehensive obstetric patient safety program on compensation payments and sentinel events. *Am J Obstet Gynecol*. 2011;204:97–105.

248. Gallos I, Devall A, Martin J, et al. Randomized trial of early detection and treatment of postpartum hemorrhage. *N Engl J Med*. 2023;389:11–21.

249. Vogel JP, Nguyen PY, Ramson J, et al. Effectiveness of care bundles for prevention and treatment of postpartum hemorrhage: a systematic review. *Am J Obstet Gynecol*. 2024;231:67–91.

250. Woiski M, de Visser S, van Vugt H, et al. Evaluating adherence to guideline-based quality indicators for postpartum hemorrhage care in the Netherlands using video analysis. *Obstet Gynecol*. 2018;132:656–667.

251. De Tina A, Chau A, Carusi DA, et al. Identifying barriers to implementation of the National Partnership for Maternal Safety obstetric hemorrhage bundle at a tertiary center: utilization of the Delphi method. *Anesth Analg*. 2019;124:1045–1050.

252. Duzyj CM, Boyle C, Mahoney K, et al. The postpartum hemorrhage patient safety bundle implementation at a single institution: successes, failures, and lessons learned. *Am J Perinatol*. 2021;38:1281–1288.

253. Baldvinsdóttir T, Blomberg M, Lilliecreutz C. Improved clinical management but not patient outcome in women with postpartum haemorrhage—an observational study of practical obstetric team training. *PLoS One*. 2018;13:e0203806.

254. Association of Women's Health Obstetric and Neonatal Nurses. *Postpartum Hemorrhage (PPH)*. AWHONN; 2024. https://www.awhonn.org/postpartum-hemorrhage-pph/. Accessed December 31, 2024.

255. Dilla AJ, Waters JH, Yazer MH. Clinical validation of risk stratification criteria for peripartum hemorrhage. *Obstet Gynecol*. 2013;122:120–126.

256. Ladfors LV, Butwick A, Stephansson O. A validation of The California Maternal Quality Care Collaborative obstetric hemorrhage risk assessment tool in a Swedish population. *Am J Obstet Gynecol*. 2024;6:101240.

257. Hussain SA, Guarini CB, Blosser C, Poole AT. Obstetric hemorrhage outcomes by intrapartum risk stratification at a single tertiary care center. *Cureus*. 2019;11:e6456.

258. Wu E, Jolley JA, Hargrove BA, et al. Implementation of an obstetric hemorrhage risk assessment: validation and evaluation of its impact on pretransfusion testing and hemorrhage outcomes. *J Matern Fetal Neonatal Med*. 2015;28:71–76.

259. Ruppel H, Liu VX, Gupta NR, et al. Validation of postpartum hemorrhage admission risk factor stratification in a large obstetrics population. *Am J Perinatol*. 2021;38:1192–1200.

260. Ende HB, Butwick AJ. Current state and future direction of postpartum hemorrhage risk assessment. *Obstet Gynecol*. 2021;138:924–930.

261. Carr BL, Jahangirifar M, Nicholson AE, et al. Predicting postpartum haemorrhage: a systematic review of prognostic models. *Aust N Z J Obstet Gynaecol*. 2022;62:813–825.

262. Neary C, Naheed S, McLernon DJ, Black M. Predicting risk of postpartum haemorrhage: a systematic review. *BJOG*. 2021;128:46–53.

263. Butwick AJ, Ramachandran B, Hegde P, et al. Risk factors for severe postpartum hemorrhage after cesarean delivery: case-control studies. *Anesth Analg*. 2017;125:523–532.

264. Miller CM, Cohn S, Akdagli S, et al. Postpartum hemorrhage following vaginal delivery: risk factors and maternal outcomes. *J Perinatol*. 2017;37:243–248.

265. Ende HB, Domenico HJ, Polic A, et al. Development and validation of an automated, real-time predictive model for postpartum hemorrhage. *Obstet Gynecol*. 2024;144:109–117.

266. Collins P, Abdul-Kadir R, Thachil J. Management of coagulopathy associated with postpartum hemorrhage: guidance from the SSC of the ISTH. *J Thromb Haemost*. 2016;14:205–210.

267. Collis RE, Kenyon C, Roberts TCD, McNamara H. When does obstetric coagulopathy occur and how do I manage it? *Int J Obstet Anesth*. 2021;46:102979.

268. Ramler PI, Gillissen A, Henriquez D, et al. Clinical value of early viscoelastometric point-of-care testing during postpartum hemorrhage for the prediction of severity of bleeding: a multicenter prospective cohort study in the Netherlands. *Acta Obstet Gynecol Scand*. 2021;100:1656–1664.

269. Gillissen A, van den Akker T, Caram-Deelder C, et al. Coagulation parameters during the course of severe postpartum hemorrhage: a nationwide retrospective cohort study. *Blood Adv*. 2018;2:2433–2442.

270. Lasica M, Sparrow RL, Tacey M, et al. Haematological features, transfusion management and outcomes of massive obstetric haemorrhage: findings from the Australian and New Zealand Massive Transfusion Registry. *Br J Haematol*. 2020;190:618–628.

271. Green L, Knight M, Seeney F, et al. The haematological features and transfusion management of women who required massive transfusion for major obstetric haemorrhage in the UK: a population based study. *Br J Haematol*. 2016;172:616–624.

272. Butwick AJ. Postpartum hemorrhage and low fibrinogen levels: the past, present and future. *Int J Obstet Anesth*. 2013;22:87–91.

273. de Lloyd L, Bovington R, Kaye A, et al. Standard haemostatic tests following major obstetric haemorrhage. *Int J Obstet Anesth*. 2011;20:135–141.

274. Collins PW, Lilley G, Bruynseels D, et al. Fibrin-based clot formation as an early and rapid biomarker for progression of postpartum hemorrhage: a prospective study. *Blood*. 2014;124:1727–1736.

275. Charbit B, Mandelbrot L, Samain E, et al. The decrease of fibrinogen is an early predictor of the severity of postpartum hemorrhage. *J Thromb Haemost*. 2007;5:266–273.

276. Cortet M, Deneux-Tharaux C, Dupont C, et al. Association between fibrinogen level and severity of postpartum haemorrhage: secondary analysis of a prospective trial. *Br J Anaesth*. 2012;108:984–989.

277. Gayat E, Resche-Rigon M, Morel O, et al. Predictive factors of advanced interventional procedures in a multicentre severe postpartum haemorrhage study. *Intensive Care Med*. 2011;37:1816–1825.

278. Jones RM, de Lloyd L, Kealaher EJ, et al. Platelet count and transfusion requirements during moderate or severe postpartum haemorrhage. *Anaesthesia*. 2016;71:648–656.

279. Kaur K, Bhardwaj M, Kumar P, et al. Amniotic fluid embolism. *J Anaesthesiol Clin Pharmacol*. 2016;32:153–159.

280. Levi M. Pathogenesis and management of peripartum coagulopathic calamities (disseminated intravascular coagulation and amniotic fluid embolism). *Thromb Res*. 2013;131:S32–S34.

281. Erez O, Othman M, Rabinovich A, et al. DIC in pregnancy—pathophysiology, clinical characteristics, diagnostic scores, and treatments. *J Blood Med*. 2022;13:21–44.

282. Schröder L, Hellmund A, Gembruch U, Merz WM. Amniotic fluid embolism-associated coagulopathy: a single-center observational study. *Arch Gynecol Obstet*. 2020;301:923–929.

283. Katz D, Farber M, Getrajdman C, et al. The role of viscoelastic hemostatic assays for postpartum hemorrhage management and bedside intrapartum care. *Am J Obstet Gynecol*. 2024;230:S1089–S1106.

284. Dias JD, Butwick AJ, Hartmann J, Waters JH. Viscoelastic haemostatic point-of-care assays in the management of postpartum haemorrhage: a narrative review. *Anaesthesia*. 2022;77:700–711.

285. Collis R, Bell S. The role of thromboelastography during the management of postpartum hemorrhage: background, evidence, and practical application. *Semin Thromb Hemost*. 2023;49:145–161.

286. Karlsson O, Jeppsson A, Hellgren M. Major obstetric haemorrhage: monitoring with thromboelastography, laboratory analyses or both? *Int J Obstet Anesth*. 2014;23:10–17.

287. Huissoud C, Carrabin N, Audibert F, et al. Bedside assessment of fibrinogen level in postpartum haemorrhage by thrombelastometry. *BJOG*. 2009;116:1097–1102.

288. Rigouzzo A, Louvet N, Favier R, et al. Assessment of coagulation by thromboelastography during ongoing postpartum hemorrhage: a retrospective cohort analysis. *Anesth Analg*. 2020;130:416–425.

289. Bell SF, Roberts TCD, Freyer Martins Pereira J, et al. The sensitivity and specificity of rotational thromboelastometry (ROTEM) to detect coagulopathy during moderate and severe postpartum haemorrhage: a prospective observational study. *Int J Obstet Anesth*. 2022;49:103238.

290. Gillissen A, van den Akker T, Caram-Deelder C, et al. Comparison of thromboelastometry by ROTEM(®) Delta and ROTEM(®) Sigma in women with postpartum haemorrhage. *Scand J Clin Lab Invest*. 2019;79:32–38.

291. McNamara H, Kenyon C, Smith R, et al. Four years' experience of a ROTEM((R))-guided algorithm for treatment of coagulopathy in obstetric haemorrhage. *Anaesthesia*. 2019;74:984–991.

292. Snegovskikh D, Souza D, Walton Z, et al. Point-of-care viscoelastic testing improves the outcome of pregnancies complicated by severe postpartum hemorrhage. *J Clin Anesth*. 2018;44:50–56.

293. Bell SF, Collis RE, Pallmann P, et al. Reduction in massive postpartum haemorrhage and red blood cell transfusion during a national quality improvement project, Obstetric Bleeding Strategy for Wales, OBS Cymru: an observational study. *BMC Pregnancy Childbirth*. 2021;21:377.

294. Jokinen S, Kuitunen A, Uotila J, Yli-Hankala A. Thromboelastometry-guided treatment algorithm in postpartum haemorrhage: a randomised, controlled pilot trial. *Br J Anaesth*. 2023;130:165–174.

295. Kong CW, To WWK. Trends in conservative procedures and peripartum hysterectomy rates in severe postpartum

haemorrhage. *J Matern Fetal Neonatal Med*. 2018;31: 2820–2826.

296. Revert M, Rozenberg P, Cottenet J, Quantin C. Intrauterine balloon tamponade for severe postpartum hemorrhage. *Obstet Gynecol*. 2018;131:143–149.

297. Suarez S, Conde-Agudelo A, Borovac-Pinheiro A, et al. Uterine balloon tamponade for the treatment of postpartum hemorrhage: a systematic review and meta-analysis. *Am J Obstet Gynecol*. 2020;222:293.e1–e52.

298. Laas E, Bui C, Popowski T, et al. Trends in the rate of invasive procedures after the addition of the intrauterine tamponade test to a protocol for management of severe postpartum hemorrhage. *Am J Obstet Gynecol*. 2012;207:281.e1–e7.

299. Gauchotte E, De La Torre M, Perdriolle-Galet E, et al. Impact of uterine balloon tamponade on the use of invasive procedures in severe postpartum hemorrhage. *Acta Obstet Gynecol Scand*. 2017;96:877–882.

300. Einerson BD, Son M, Schneider P, et al. The association between intrauterine balloon tamponade duration and postpartum hemorrhage outcomes. *Am J Obstet Gynecol*. 2017;216:300.e1–e5.

301. D'Alton M, Rood K, Simhan H, Goffman D. Profile of the Jada® System: the vacuum-induced hemorrhage control device for treating abnormal postpartum uterine bleeding and postpartum hemorrhage. *Expert Rev Med Devices*. 2021;18:849–853.

302. Goffman D, Rood KM, Bianco A, et al. Real-world utilization of an intrauterine, vacuum-induced, hemorrhage-control device. *Obstet Gynecol*. 2023;142:1006–1016.

303. B-Lynch C, Coker A, Lawal AH, et al. The B-Lynch surgical technique for the control of massive postpartum haemorrhage: an alternative to hysterectomy? Five cases reported. *Br J Obstet Gynaecol*. 1997;104:372–375.

304. Doumouchtsis SK, Papageorghiou AT, Arulkumaran S. Systematic review of conservative management of postpartum hemorrhage: what to do when medical treatment fails. *Obstet Gynecol Surv*. 2007;62:540–547.

305. Kayem G, Kurinczuk JJ, Alfirevic Z, et al. Uterine compression sutures for the management of severe postpartum hemorrhage. *Obstet Gynecol*. 2011;117:14–20.

306. Harlow FH, Smith RP, Nortje J, et al. Catastrophic uterine rupture associated with placenta accreta after previous B-Lynch sutures. *J Obstet Gynaecol*. 2018;38:282–284.

307. Eriksson LG, Mulic-Lutvica A, Jangland L, Nyman R. Massive postpartum hemorrhage treated with transcatheter arterial embolization: technical aspects and long-term effects on fertility and menstrual cycle. *Acta Radiol*. 2007;48: 635–642.

308. Porcu G, Roger V, Jacquier A, et al. Uterus and bladder necrosis after uterine artery embolisation for postpartum haemorrhage. *BJOG*. 2005;112:122–123.

309. Cottier JP, Fignon A, Tranquart F, Herbreteau D. Uterine necrosis after arterial embolization for postpartum hemorrhage. *Obstet Gynecol*. 2002;100:1074–1077.

310. O'Leary JL, O'Leary JA. Uterine artery ligation in the control of intractable postpartum hemorrhage. *Am J Obstet Gynecol*. 1966;94:920–924.

311. van den Akker T, Brobbel C, Dekkers OM, Bloemenkamp KWM. Prevalence, indications, risk indicators, and outcomes of emergency peripartum hysterectomy worldwide: a systematic review and meta-analysis. *Obstet Gynecol*. 2016;128:1281–1294.

312. Givens M, Einerson BD, Allshouse AA, et al. Trends in unplanned peripartum hysterectomy in the United States, 2009-2020. *Obstet Gynecol*. 2022;139:449–451.

313. Wright JD, Devine P, Shah M, et al. Morbidity and mortality of peripartum hysterectomy. *Obstet Gynecol*. 2010;115: 1187–1193.

314. Chestnut DH, Dewan DM, Redick LF, et al. Anesthetic management for obstetric hysterectomy: a multi-institutional study. *Anesthesiology*. 1989;70:607–610.

315. Rossi AC, Lee RH, Chmait RH. Emergency postpartum hysterectomy for uncontrolled postpartum bleeding: a systematic review. *Obstet Gynecol*. 2010;115:637–644.

316. Belfort MA, Zimmerman J, Schemmer G, et al. Aortic compression and cross clamping in a case of placenta percreta and amniotic fluid embolism: a case report. *AJP Rep*. 2011;1:33–36.

317. Georgakis P, Paraskevas KI, Bessias N, et al. Duration of aortic cross-clamping during elective open abdominal aortic aneurysm repair operations and postoperative cardiac/renal function. *Int Angiol*. 2010;29:244–248.

318. Stensaeth KH, Sovik E, Haig IN, et al. Fluoroscopy-free resuscitative endovascular balloon occlusion of the aorta (REBOA) for controlling life threatening postpartum hemorrhage. *PLoS ONE*. 2017;12:e0174520.

319. Webster LA, Little O, Villalobos A, et al. REBOA: expanding applications from traumatic hemorrhage to obstetrics and cardiopulmonary resuscitation. *Am J Roentgenol*. 2023;220:16–22.

320. Rasmussen TE, Tai NRM. *Rich's Vascular Trauma*. 4th ed. Elsevier Saunders; 2022.

321. Natour E, Suedkamp M, Dapunt OE. Assessment of the effect on blood loss and transfusion requirements when adding a polyethylene glycol sealant to the anastomotic closure of aortic procedures: a case-control analysis of 102 patients undergoing bentall procedures. *J Cardiothorac Surg*. 2012;7:105.

322. Manzano-Nunez R, Escobar-Vidarte MF, Naranjo MP, et al. Expanding the field of acute care surgery: a systematic review of the use of resuscitative endovascular balloon occlusion of the aorta (REBOA) in cases of morbidly adherent placenta. *Eur J Trauma Emerg Surg*. 2018;44:519–526.

323. Mhyre JM, Shilkrut A, Kuklina EV, et al. Massive blood transfusion during hospitalization for delivery in New York state, 1998-2007. *Obstet Gynecol*. 2013;122:1288–1294.

324. Bonnet MP, Deneux-Tharaux C, Bouvier-Colle MH. Critical care and transfusion management in maternal deaths from postpartum haemorrhage. *Eur J Obstet Gynecol Reprod Biol*. 2011;158:183–188.

325. Shibata K, Yamamoto Y, Murakami S. Effects of epidural anesthesia on cardiovascular response and survival in experimental hemorrhagic shock in dogs. *Anesthesiology*. 1989;71:953–959.

326. Patel PA, Wyrobek JA, Butwick AJ, et al. Update on applications and limitations of perioperative tranexamic acid. *Anesth Analg*. 2022;135:460–473.

327. CRASH Trial Collaborators, et al.Shakur H, Roberts I, et al. Effects of tranexamic acid on death, vascular occlusive events, and blood transfusion in trauma patients with significant haemorrhage (CRASH-2). A randomised, placebo-controlled trial. *Lancet*. 2010;376:23–32.

328. Escobar MF, Nassar AH, Theron G, et al. FIGO recommendations on the management of postpartum hemorrhage 2022. *Int J Gynaecol Obstet*. 2022;157:3–50.

329. World Health Organization. *WHO Recommendation on Tranexamic Acid for the Treatment of Postpartum Haemorrhage.* World Health Organization; 2017. https://www.who.int/publications/i/item/WHO-RHR-17.21. Accessed December 31, 2024.

330. Ahmadzia HK, Luban NLC, Li S, et al. Optimal use of intravenous tranexamic acid for hemorrhage prevention in pregnant women. *Am J Obstet Gynecol.* 2021;225:85.e1–e11.

331. Seifert SM, Lumbreras-Marquez MI, Goobie SM, et al. Tranexamic acid administered during cesarean delivery in high-risk patients: maternal pharmacokinetics, pharmacodynamics, and coagulation status. *Am J Obstet Gynecol.* 2022;227:763.e1–e10.

332. Ducloy-Bouthors AS, Jude B, Duhamel A, et al. High-dose tranexamic acid reduces blood loss in postpartum haemorrhage. *Crit Care.* 2011;15:R117.

333. WOMAN Trial Collaborators. Effect of early tranexamic acid administration on mortality, hysterectomy, and other morbidities in women with post-partum haemorrhage (WOMAN). An international, randomised, double-blind, placebo-controlled trial. *Lancet.* 2017;389:2105–2116.

334. Gayet-Ageron A, Prieto-Merino D, Ker K, et al. Effect of treatment delay on the effectiveness and safety of antifibrinolytics in acute severe haemorrhage: a meta-analysis of individual patient-level data from 40 138 bleeding patients. *Lancet.* 2018;391:125–132.

335. Gillissen A, Henriquez D, van den Akker T, et al. The effect of tranexamic acid on blood loss and maternal outcome in the treatment of persistent postpartum hemorrhage: a nationwide retrospective cohort study. *PLoS One.* 2017;12:e0187555.

336. Sentilhes L, Winer N, Azria E, et al. Tranexamic acid for the prevention of blood loss after vaginal delivery. *N Engl J Med.* 2018;379:731–742.

337. Saccone G, Della Corte L, D'Alessandro P, et al. Prophylactic use of tranexamic acid after vaginal delivery reduces the risk of primary postpartum hemorrhage. *J Matern Fetal Neonatal Med.* 2020;33:3368–3376.

338. Xia Y, Griffiths BB, Xue Q. Tranexamic acid for postpartum hemorrhage prevention in vaginal delivery: a meta-analysis. *Medicine.* 2020;99:e18792.

339. Sentilhes L, Sénat MV, Le Lous M, et al. Tranexamic acid for the prevention of blood loss after cesarean delivery. *N Engl J Med.* 2021;384:1623–1634.

340. Sentilhes L, Madar H, Le Lous M, et al. Tranexamic acid for the prevention of blood loss after cesarean among women with twins: a secondary analysis of the TRAnexamic acid for preventing postpartum hemorrhage following a cesarean delivery randomized clinical trial. *Am J Obstet Gynecol.* 2022;227:889.e1–e17.

341. Pacheco LD, Clifton RG, Saade GR, et al. Tranexamic acid to prevent obstetrical hemorrhage after cesarean delivery. *N Engl J Med.* 2023;388:1365–1375.

342. Cheema HA, Ahmad AB, Ehsan M, et al. Tranexamic acid for the prevention of blood loss after cesarean section: an updated systematic review and meta-analysis of randomized controlled trials. *Am J Obstet Gynecol MFM.* 2023;5:101049.

343. Moran NF, Bishop DG, Fawcus S, et al. Tranexamic acid at cesarean delivery: drug-error deaths. *Am J Obstet Gynecol.* 2023;228:1–4.

344. Patel S, Robertson B, McConachie I. Catastrophic drug errors involving tranexamic acid administered during spinal anaesthesia. *Anaesthesia.* 2019;74:904–914.

345. US Food and Drug Administration. FDA alerts healthcare professionals about the risk of medication errors with tranexamic acid injection resulting in inadvertent intrathecal (spinal) injection; 2020. https://www.fda.gov/drugs/drug-safety-and-availability/fda-alerts-healthcare-professionals-about-risk-medication-errors-tranexamic-acid-injection-resulting. Accessed December 31, 2024.

346. Frimat M, Decambron M, Lebas C, et al. Renal cortical necrosis in postpartum hemorrhage: a case series. *Am J Kidney Dis.* 2016;68:50–57.

347. Bell SF, Rayment R, Collins PW, Collis RE. The use of fibrinogen concentrate to correct hypofibrinogenaemia rapidly during obstetric haemorrhage. *Int J Obstet Anesth.* 2010;19:218–223.

348. Levy JH, Welsby I, Goodnough LT. Fibrinogen as a therapeutic target for bleeding: a review of critical levels and replacement therapy. *Transfusion.* 2014;54:1389–1405.

349. Fenger-Eriksen C, Ingerslev J, Sørensen B. Fibrinogen concentrate—a potential universal hemostatic agent. *Expert Opin Biol Ther.* 2009;9:1325–1333.

350. Wikkelsø AJ, Edwards HM, Afshari A, et al. Pre-emptive treatment with fibrinogen concentrate for postpartum haemorrhage: randomized controlled trial. *Br J Anaesth.* 2015;114:623–633.

351. Ducloy-Bouthors AS, Mercier FJ, Grouin JM, et al. Early and systematic administration of fibrinogen concentrate in postpartum haemorrhage following vaginal delivery: the FIDEL randomised controlled trial. *BJOG.* 2021;128:1814–1823.

352. Collins PW, Cannings-John R, Bruynseels D, et al. Viscoelastometric-guided early fibrinogen concentrate replacement during postpartum haemorrhage: OBS2, a double-blind randomized controlled trial. *Br J Anaesth.* 2017;119:411–421.

353. Matsunaga S, Takai Y, Nakamura E, et al. The clinical efficacy of fibrinogen concentrate in massive obstetric haemorrhage with hypofibrinogenaemia. *Sci Rep.* 2017;7:46749.

354. Seto S, Itakura A, Okagaki R, et al. An algorithm for the management of coagulopathy from postpartum hemorrhage, using fibrinogen concentrate as first-line therapy. *Int J Obstet Anesth.* 2017;32:11–16.

355. Yank V, Tuohy CV, Logan AC, et al. Systematic review: benefits and harms of in-hospital use of recombinant factor VIIa for off-label indications. *Ann Intern Med.* 2011;154:529–540.

356. Caram-Deelder C, McKinnon Edwards H, Zdanowicz JA, et al. Efficacy and safety analyses of recombinant factor VIIa in severe post-partum hemorrhage. *J Clin Med.* 2024;13.

357. American Society of Anesthesiologists. Practice guidelines for perioperative blood management: an updated report by the American Society of Anesthesiologists Task Force on Perioperative Blood Management. *Anesthesiology.* 2015;122:241–275.

358. Surbek D, Blatný J, Wielgos M, et al. Role of recombinant factor VIIa in the clinical management of severe postpartum hemorrhage: consensus among European experts. *J Matern Fetal Neonatal Med.* 2024;37:2332794.

359. Al-Zirqi I, Vangen S, Forsen L, Stray-Pedersen B. Prevalence and risk factors of severe obstetric haemorrhage. *BJOG.* 2008;115:1265–1272.

360. Kuklina EV, Meikle SF, Jamieson DJ, et al. Severe obstetric morbidity in the United States: 1998–2005. *Obstet Gynecol.* 2009;113:293–299.

361. Patterson JA, Roberts CL, Bowen JR, et al. Blood transfusion during pregnancy, birth, and the postnatal period. *Obstet Gynecol*. 2014;123:126–133.

362. Kramer MS, Dahhou M, Vallerand D, et al. Risk factors for postpartum hemorrhage: can we explain the recent temporal increase? *J Obstet Gynaecol Can*. 2011;33:810–819.

363. Lutomski JE, Byrne BM, Devane D, Greene RA. Increasing trends in atonic postpartum haemorrhage in Ireland: an 11-year population-based cohort study. *BJOG*. 2012;119:306–314.

364. American Society of Anesthesiologists Task Force on Obstetric Anesthesia. Practice guidelines for obstetric anesthesia. An updated report by the American Society of Anesthesiologists Task Force on Obstetric Anesthesia and the Society for Obstetric Anesthesia and Perinatology. *Anesthesiology*. 2016;124:270–300.

365. Einerson BD, Stehlikova Z, Nelson RE, et al. Transfusion preparedness strategies for obstetric hemorrhage: a cost-effectiveness analysis. *Obstet Gynecol*. 2017;130:1347–1355.

366. American College of Obstetricians and Gynecologists. Practice Bulletin No. 192: Management of alloimmunization during pregnancy (reaffirmed 2024). *Obstet Gynecol*. 2018;131:e82–e90.

367. American College of Obstetricians and Gynecologists. Practice Bulletin, No. 233: Anemia in pregnancy (reaffirmed 2024). *Obstet Gynecol*. 2021;138:e55–e64.

368. Benson AE, Metcalf RA, Cail K, et al. Transfusion preparedness in the labor and delivery unit: an initiative to improve safety and cost. *Obstet Gynecol*. 2021;138:788–794.

369. Goodnough LT, Daniels K, Wong AE, et al. How we treat: transfusion medicine support of obstetric services. *Transfusion*. 2011;51:2540–2548.

370. Butwick A, Lyell D, Goodnough L. How do I manage severe postpartum hemorrhage? *Transfusion*. 2020;60:897–907.

371. Gutierrez MC, Goodnough LT, Druzin M, Butwick AJ. Postpartum hemorrhage treated with a massive transfusion protocol at a tertiary obstetric center: a retrospective study. *Int J Obstet Anesth*. 2012;21:230–235.

372. Margarido C, Ferns J, Chin V, et al. Massive hemorrhage protocol activation in obstetrics: a 5-year quality performance review. *Int J Obstet Anesth*. 2019;38:37–45.

373. Panigrahi AK, Yeaton-Massey A, Bakhtary S, et al. A standardized approach for transfusion medicine support in patients with morbidly adherent placenta. *Anesth Analg*. 2017;125:603–608.

374. Boisen ML, Collins RA, Yazer MH, Waters JH. Pretransfusion testing and transfusion of uncrossmatched erythrocytes. *Anesthesiology*. 2015;122:191–195.

375. Delaney M, Wikman A, van de Watering L, et al. Blood group antigen matching influence on gestational outcomes (AMIGO) study. *Transfusion*. 2017;57:525–532.

376. Collis RE, Collins PW. Haemostatic management of obstetric haemorrhage. *Anaesthesia*. 2015;70(Suppl 1):78–86, e27–e28.

377. Collins PW, Solomon C, Sutor K, et al. Theoretical modelling of fibrinogen supplementation with therapeutic plasma, cryoprecipitate, or fibrinogen concentrate. *Br J Anaesth*. 2014;113:585–595.

378. Henriquez DDCA, Caram-Deelder C, le Cessie S, et al. Association of timing of plasma transfusion with adverse maternal outcomes in women with persistent postpartum hemorrhage. *JAMA Netw Open*. 2019;2:e1915628.

379. Abir G, Riley ET, Oakeson AM, et al. Automated alert system of second-line uterotonic drug administration. *A A Pract*. 2023;17:e01687.

380. Widmer M, Piaggio G, Hofmeyr GJ, et al. Maternal characteristics and causes associated with refractory postpartum haemorrhage after vaginal birth: a secondary analysis of the WHO CHAMPION trial data. *BJOG*. 2020;127:628–634.

38

Embolic Disorders

Paloma Toledo, MD, MPH, FASA and David Arnolds, MD, PhD

Embolic disease during pregnancy includes venous thromboembolism, amniotic fluid embolism (AFE), and venous air embolism (VAE). These vary in incidence, clinical course, and consequences and account for almost one-sixth of all maternal deaths in the United States.[1] Early recognition, diagnosis, and treatment are necessary to reduce associated morbidity and to avoid mortality.

THROMBOEMBOLIC DISORDERS

Incidence

Venous thromboembolic events (VTEs) in pregnancy refer to deep vein thrombosis (DVT) and pulmonary thromboembolism (PTE). Analysis of administrative data from US hospital admissions including 73,109,789 pregnancy-related hospitalizations (2000 to 2018) suggested a VTE event rate of 6.6 events per 10,000 deliveries.[2] Among these, the DVT event rate (5.1 per 10,000 deliveries) was higher than the PTE event rate (1.7 per 10,000 deliveries).[2] In the United States, 5.3% of maternal mortalities are related to VTE,[3] but the incidence is increasing,[4] as is the number of patients with related risk factors.[2]

The risk for thromboembolic events is elevated during pregnancy. Compared with nonpregnant patients, pregnant women have 5-fold greater odds of thromboembolic events during pregnancy (odds ratio [OR], 4.6; 95% confidence interval [CI], 2.7 to 7.8) and at 60-fold greater odds postpartum (OR, 60.1; 95% CI, 26.5 to 135.9).[5] DVTs are more likely to occur antepartum, with 21%, 23%, and 56% occurring in the first, second, and third trimester, respectively.[6] Most cases of PTE (60% to 80%) occur postpartum.[7,8] Analysis from a 30-year population-based cohort ($n = 50,080$ births) revealed the risk for both DVT and PTE was highest in the first week postpartum, with a progressive decline thereafter.[8] Risk is elevated until at least 12 weeks after delivery.[9]

Although VTE-related mortality, as reported by the Confidential Enquiries into Maternal Deaths and Morbidity in the United Kingdom and Ireland, appeared to have been decreasing a decade ago, more recently, the VTE-associated mortality rate has been stable.[10] VTE was the leading cause of direct maternal deaths with 1.6 deaths per 100,000 births in 2019 to 2021.[10] VTE-related maternal mortality appears to be stable in the United States, at 1.8 deaths per 100,000 births.[3]

Pathophysiology

Virchow's triad describes three factors that increase risk for thromboembolism: (1) **venous stasis**, (2) **hypercoagulability**, and (3) **vascular damage**. The incidence of each factor is increased during pregnancy, especially postpartum. Venous stasis occurs as a result of decreased venous flow velocity, venocaval compression, and possibly decreased mobility later in pregnancy.[11] Additionally, pregnancy is a relatively hypercoagulable state, associated with enhanced platelet turnover, coagulation, and fibrinolysis.[12,13] Thrombin generation and the concentration of clotting factors increase during pregnancy, including factors I (fibrinogen), V, VII, VIII, IX, X, and XII.[12] Fibrinolytic activity decreases during the 48 hours after delivery and enhances clot stability in the early postpartum period.[12] Vascular damage occurs at delivery. Placental separation from the uterine wall traumatizes the endometrium and accelerates the coagulation cascade. This vascular damage, in addition to delivery events that increase the risk of thromboembolism, explains the increased incidence of VTE events postpartum.

Risk Assessment

Awareness of VTE risk factors and frequent assessment of VTE risk are crucial for identification of patients who require thromboprophylaxis because the risk is not static throughout pregnancy. The assessment of risk should be performed antepartum, at hospital admission, and postpartum.[14,15] The VTE risk factors can be categorized into maternal characteristics, pregnancy and delivery characteristics, and obstetric complications.

The two most important risk factors for thromboembolic events during pregnancy and postpartum are a previous history of thromboembolism and a diagnosis of thrombophilia.[16] The increased risk is notable, with an increased odds of VTE of 24.8 (95% CI, 17.1 to 36) for women with a history of prior VTE and 51.8 (95% CI, 38.7 to 69.2) for women with thrombophilia.[16] Thrombophilias increase the risk for VTE in pregnancy, for example in women homozygous for the factor V Leiden mutation.[17] Other risk factors include advanced maternal age, race/ethnicity, obesity, anemia, hypertensive disorders, inflammatory bowel disease, and smoking status.[4,18,19] Multifetal gestation, hyperemesis, hypertensive disorders of pregnancy, antenatal hospitalization and prolonged bedrest, intrauterine fetal demise, and cesarean delivery also increase the risk for postpartum VTE.[4,20–22] In a metaanalysis of 28 studies (pooled $n > 53,000$ postpartum VTE events), the OR of postpartum VTE after cesarean delivery compared with vaginal delivery was 3.7 (95% CI, 3.0 to 4.6).[20] Greater increases occurred after emergency versus elective cesarean deliveries.[4,20] Obstetric complications, such as postpartum hemorrhage and postpartum infections, are also associated with increased risk, likely mediated via effects on maternal coagulation and inflammation.[4,19] The Nationwide Inpatient Sample showed that between 2000 and 2018, the average annual percent change in the proportion of deliveries with one, two, or three VTE risk factors increased by 2.7%, 5.0%, and 7.5%, respectively.[2] Patients with two or more risk factors accounted for over one-fourth of the VTE diagnoses.[2]

Deep Vein Thrombosis

Clinical Presentation

The signs and symptoms of DVT are nonspecific and often mimic normal pregnancy symptoms such as lower leg edema and pain,[22] necessitating a high degree of awareness for timely diagnosis. A systematic review of the anatomic distribution of DVT in symptomatic pregnant patients identified left leg thrombus in 88% of women in whom the side of the DVT was reported.[23] Most thrombi were proximally located in the iliac or femoral veins, or both. This differs from nonpregnant patients, who are more likely to have thrombi in the distal calf vessels.[23] A prospective observational study of serial ultrasonographic examinations in pregnant women found an increase in vessel diameter and a decrease in flow velocity in the proximal deep leg veins with increasing gestation, most notably in the common femoral vein.[11] The flow velocity was slower in the left leg than in the right leg, presumably caused by uterine compression of the left iliac vein where it crosses the right iliac artery.[11]

Diagnosis

For patients with new-onset signs or symptoms suggestive of DVT, the American College of Obstetricians and Gynecologists (ACOG) recommends compression ultrasonography of proximal veins as the initial diagnostic test.[15] If the test is negative, and involvement of the iliac vessels is not suspected, no further action other than routine surveillance is necessary. A positive result warrants treatment (see later discussion). If the results are negative or equivocal, or iliac vein thrombosis is suspected, Doppler ultrasonography of the iliac vein, venography, magnetic resonance imaging (MRI), or presumptive anticoagulation may be considered.[15] Alternatively, compression ultrasonography may be repeated after 3 to 7 days. The negative predictive value of serial compression duplex ultrasonography is 99.5% (95% CI, 96.9% to 100%).[24]

The D-dimer test has high sensitivity and high negative predictive value in nonpregnant patients. Unfortunately, D-dimer levels are increased in pregnancy, and levels may be further elevated in women with multiple gestation,[25] making interpretation of elevated levels difficult. In one prospective, longitudinal study, serial D-dimer levels were evaluated in healthy pregnant women ($n = 89$); values exceeded the normal nonpregnant reference range in all but one woman in the third trimester.[26] One study ($n = 16,127$ deliveries with 19 VTE events), suggested that a D-dimer threshold of greater than or equal to 3.7 mg/L could be used as an independent predictor of VTE (specificity 75.5%, sensitivity 73.7%)[27]; however, this has not been validated in prospective studies. Therefore, the D-dimer test is not recommended for diagnosis of DVT in pregnancy.[15,28]

Pulmonary Thromboembolism

Clinical Presentation

The clinical presentation and prognosis of PTE depend on: (1) the size and number of emboli, (2) concurrent cardiopulmonary function, (3) the rate of clot fragmentation and lysis, (4) the presence or absence of a source for recurrent emboli, and (5) the location of the embolism (proximal or main pulmonary artery embolism is more symptomatic than segmental embolization).[29] Massive PTE can occlude the pulmonary vasculature and precipitate cardiopulmonary arrest; smaller emboli may lead to cardiopulmonary failure by triggering pulmonary arterial vasospasm and secondary pulmonary edema.[30] Local platelets embedded in the clot release serotonin, adenosine diphosphate, and thrombin, which promote both vasoconstriction and bronchoconstriction.[31] Redistribution of pulmonary blood flow leads to "hyperperfusion" of otherwise low V/Q zones in unaffected areas of the lung; the resulting intrapulmonary shunts cause hypoxemia disproportionate to the cross-sectional area occluded by a clot.[32] Simultaneously, regional hypoxic pulmonary vasoconstriction exacerbates pulmonary hypertension initiated by mechanical and humoral factors. Intracardiac shunting may develop when elevated right ventricular pressure forces blood across a probe-patent foramen ovale. The increase in right ventricular pressure leads to right ventricular dilation, with increased wall tension and oxygen demand, and a leftward shift of the interventricular septum.[33] Compression of the left ventricle combined with a decrease in preload impairs left ventricular function, cardiac output, and coronary arterial perfusion, with eventual myocardial ischemia and cardiopulmonary failure.

Clinical suspicion for PTE is critical for timely diagnosis and treatment. Physical signs and symptoms may be subtle and limited to symptoms (e.g., shortness of breath) that mimic normal pregnancy (Table 38.1).[22] Palpitations, anxiety, pleuritic chest pain, cyanosis, diaphoresis, and cough with or without hemoptysis may all indicate PTE. Hypotension and syncope, though rare, may indicate massive PTE.[22] Examination commonly reveals tachypnea, crackles on chest auscultation, decreased breath sounds, and tachycardia. Signs of right ventricular failure, such as an accentuated or split second heart sound, jugular venous distention, a parasternal heave, or hepatic enlargement, may be apparent. Although the Pao_2 is commonly decreased to less than 80 mm Hg (10.7 kPa), in up to 30% of patients this is not apparent; thus, the diagnosis of PTE cannot be excluded on the basis of a normal Pao_2.[29,34] Left ventricular failure may occur secondary to poor left ventricular filling and arterial hypoxemia. One or more signs of DVT (calf or thigh edema, erythema, tenderness, palpable cord) generally accompany the pulmonary or cardiovascular findings.[29] The electrocardiogram may show signs of right ventricular strain, including a right-axis shift, P pulmonale, ST-segment abnormalities, and T-wave inversion, as well as supraventricular arrhythmias. Transthoracic echocardiography may reveal signs of right ventricular dysfunction or hypokinesis of the right ventricular free wall with normal contraction of the apical segment (McConnell's sign).[35]

Diagnosis

Diagnosing PTE in pregnancy is challenging given the lack of validated criteria specific for the peripartum period. The American Thoracic Society developed an evidence-based guideline for the evaluation of suspected PTE in pregnancy,[28] which has been endorsed by the ACOG.[15] A diagnostic algorithm for suspected PTE is shown in Fig. 38.1. If the pregnant patient has signs or symptoms suggestive of DVT, in addition to the signs or symptoms of PTE, compression ultrasonography should be performed. If the results are positive, treatment should ensue. However, if the results are negative, further imaging is necessary. If there are no signs or symptoms of DVT, a chest radiograph should be performed to exclude alternative diagnoses and to guide further decision making. If the chest radiograph is normal, V/Q scanning should be performed.[15] A retrospective study of 304 women who underwent computed tomographic angiography (CTA) or V/Q scanning at a single institution demonstrated that pregnant women with a normal chest radiograph have a fivefold higher rate of a nondiagnostic result from a CTA compared with a V/Q scan (relative risk [RR], 5.3; 95% CI, 2.1 to 13.8).[36] Screening with chest radiography may minimize radiation exposure if the patient is a candidate for V/Q scanning.[28] If the chest radiograph is abnormal, CTA is the next appropriate test because the proportion of nondiagnostic V/Q scans in the presence of an abnormal chest radiograph is reportedly as high as 48%.[37] If either the V/Q scan or CTA is positive, anticoagulation should ensue. In clinical practice, although a V/Q scan may be the most appropriate test for diagnosis of a PTE, CTA may be considered because it may inform an alternative diagnosis. Magnetic resonance pulmonary angiography has not been validated in pregnant patients and uses gadolinium, which crosses the placenta, and historically its use during pregnancy has been discouraged. However, in a study of 782 women who received gadolinium in pregnancy, there was no increased risk of fetal or infant death (adjusted RR, 0.73; 95% CI, 0.34 to 1.55).[38] As the impact of exposure on subacute and chronic outcomes is unknown, gadolinium-based imaging studies during pregnancy should be used when necessary for a diagnosis, in accordance with professional society guidelines.[39] Traditional pulmonary angiography is now rarely used because of high radiation doses and cost.

Single-photon emission computed tomography (SPECT) has been evaluated in pregnant women.[40,41] In a nonpregnant patient population, the V/Q SPECT demonstrated 100% sensitivity and 94% specificity compared with CTA as the "gold standard."[42] A retrospective analysis of 127 women who underwent evaluation for PTE with V/Q SPECT identified PTE in 11 women (9%).[43] The negative predictive value was 100%, and the calculated fetal and breast absorbed radiation doses were low (<0.014 and 0.25 mGy, respectively).[43]

A great concern with diagnostic imaging for PTE is maternal and fetal exposure to ionizing radiation,[44] (see Chapter 18). Both V/Q scanning and CTA are associated with low fetal radiation exposure (<1 mGy). V/Q scanning delivers a higher *fetal* dose of radiation than CTA; however, the *maternal* radiation exposure is higher with CTA, particularly radiation to breast tissue.[44] A patient's lifetime breast cancer risk may increase as much as 14% after CTA.[45] Maternal radiation exposure is lower with V/Q SPECT than

TABLE 38.1 Symptoms and Signs of Pulmonary Embolism During Pregnancy and Postpartum

Finding	Patients Affected (%)
Dyspnea	85
Chest pain	59
Oxygen saturation < 95%	32
Syncope	8
Hemoptysis	4

Data from Elgendy, IY, Fogerty A, Blanco-Molina Á, et al. Clinical characteristics and outcomes of women presenting with venous thromboembolism during pregnancy Obstet the postpartum period: findings from the RIETE registry. *Thromb Haemost.* 2020;120:1454–1462.

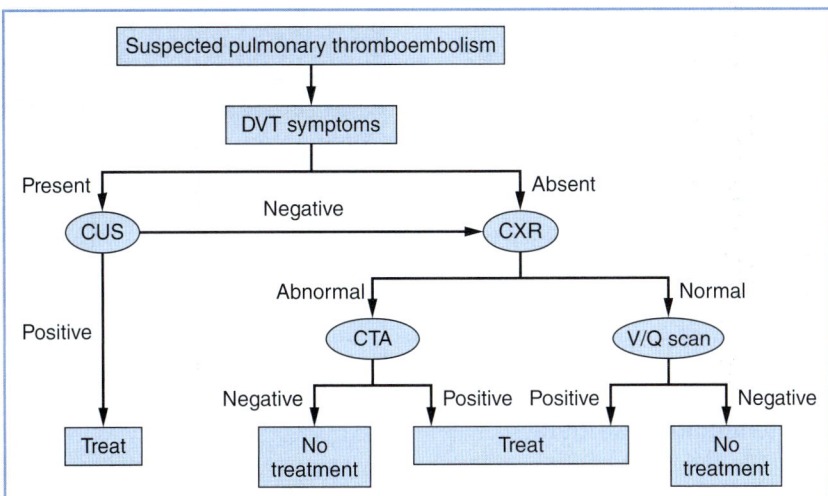

Fig. 38.1 Diagnostic algorithm for workup of suspected pulmonary thromboembolism during pregnancy. *CTA*, Computed tomography angiography; *CUS*, compression ultrasonography; *CXR*, chest radiograph; *DVT*, deep vein thrombosis; *V/Q scan*, ventilation-perfusion scan.

with CTA.[43,46] Two prospective studies used D-dimer testing in conjunction with prediction rules to determine whether diagnostic imaging is required.[47,48] Validation studies are necessary as the risk of a missed PTE has potentially catastrophic implications.

Prevention of Thromboembolic Events

Anesthesia and obstetric providers should work together to develop and implement strategies to reduce VTE. Systems should be developed to identify at-risk women for whom peripartum mechanical or pharmacologic thromboprophylaxis is indicated. Given the recent expansion of indications for pharmacologic thromboprophylaxis,[14] it is imperative that there is communication between anesthesia and obstetric providers regarding timing of delivery, plans for neuraxial analgesia and/or anesthesia, and plans for postpartum anticoagulation.

Several risk assessment tools provide guidance on antepartum and postpartum anticoagulation management.[14,15,49-51] Currently, there is not one validated and clinically accepted scoring tool, and controversy exists regarding the VTE risk level at which patients should be anticoagulated.[51] The ACOG Practice Bulletin on thromboembolism in pregnancy summarizes which patients should receive prophylactic versus therapeutic anticoagulation.[15] Patients with a previous history of thrombosis, certain high-risk populations (e.g., patients with acquired or inherited thrombophilia), or patients with a mechanical heart valve should be anticoagulated during pregnancy as well as postpartum. The American College of Chest Physicians has defined major and minor risk factors for postcesarean VTE (Box 38.1). The National Partnership for Maternal Safety published a consensus bundle on VTE in 2016.[14] This bundle broadens the indications for antepartum and postpartum pharmacologic anticoagulation beyond the ACOG practice guidelines,[15] including recommending daily thromboprophylaxis for antepartum patients hospitalized for longer than 72 hours.[14] This has anesthetic implications

BOX 38.1 Risk Factors for Venous Thromboembolism in the Postpartum Period

Major risk factors[a]
- Previous venous thromboembolism
- Thrombophilia
  - Antithrombin III deficiency
  - Factor V Leiden (homozygous or heterozygous)
  - Prothrombin G20210A (homozygous or heterozygous)
- Immobility (strict bed rest for 1 w or more in the antepartum period)
- Preeclampsia with fetal growth restriction
- Medical conditions (e.g., systematic lupus erythematous, heart disease, sickle cell disease)
- Postpartum hemorrhage ≥ 1000 mL *and* surgery
- Blood transfusion
- Postpartum infection

Minor risk factors[a]
- Body mass index > 30 kg/m²
- Emergency cesarean delivery
- Multiple pregnancy
- Postpartum hemorrhage > 1000 mL
- Smoking more than 10 cigarettes/d
- Fetal growth restriction
- Thrombophilia (Protein C or S deficiency)
- Preeclampsia

[a]The presence of at least one major risk factor or two minor risk factors is an indication for prophylactic therapy for venous thromboembolism (see text).

Modified from Bates SM, Greer IA, Middeldorp S, et al. VTE, thrombophilia, antithrombotic therapy, and pregnancy: antithrombotic therapy and prevention of thrombosis. 9th ed. American College of Chest Physicians evidence-based clinical practice guidelines. *Chest.* 2012;141(2 suppl):e691S–e736S.

(see later discussion). All women with a new-onset thromboembolic event in pregnancy should be therapeutically anticoagulated.[15]

Mechanical thromboprophylaxis should be initiated in women with contraindications to pharmacologic anticoagulation, and after all cesarean births.[15,49] Intermittent pneumatic compression stockings are cost-effective versus no thromboprophylaxis after cesarean delivery[52]; however, compliance has been shown to be suboptimal.[53] For women in whom significant risk factors persist after delivery, extended prophylaxis (6 to 8 weeks postpartum) is recommended.[14,15,49] Women are at the highest risk for thrombotic events in the first week postpartum[8]; therefore, careful postdischarge planning and evaluation of VTE risk are equally as important as inpatient management.

Management of Thromboembolic Disorders

Anticoagulation

Two classes of drugs are typically used to initiate anticoagulation in pregnancy and postpartum: **unfractionated heparin (UFH)** and **low-molecular-weight heparin (LMWH)**. Direct oral anticoagulants inhibit factor Xa (e.g., **dabigatran**, **rivaroxaban**, **apixaban**) and are preferred for nonpregnant patients; however, experience in pregnancy and postpartum is limited.[22,54] As they may cross the placenta and may be excreted in breastmilk,[54,55] their use in pregnancy is not recommended, but they may be used postpartum in patients who are not breastfeeding.[15] Table 38.2 lists anticoagulation regimens commonly used in pregnancy. The ACOG, the American College of Chest Physicians, and the American Society of Hematology recommend LMWH rather than UFH for prophylactic and therapeutic anticoagulation for pregnant women.[49,51] LMWH is preferred because of a more predictable anticoagulant response, better bioavailability, longer half-life, and fewer side effects.[51,56] The most appropriate dosing strategy remains controversial.[51] The Highlow study randomized 1110 women who had a history of VTE to either a fixed low dose of LMWH or a weight-adjusted intermediate dose of LMWH.[57] There was no difference in the incidence of VTE between the two groups (RR, 0.69; 95% CI, 0.32 to 1.47), and no difference in major bleeding, suggesting that a fixed low-dose LWMH strategy is preferred for antepartum anticoagulation.[57]

LMWH has an enhanced ratio of antithrombotic (anti–factor Xa) to anticoagulant (anti–factor IIa) activity compared with UFH and does not affect activated partial thromboplastin time (aPTT).[56] A systematic review (pooled $n = 2777$) evaluated the efficacy and safety of LMWH in pregnancy.[56] The rate of VTE in women receiving LMWH was 0.9% (95% CI, 0.6% to 1.3%), and the rate of significant bleeding was 2.0% (95% CI, 1.5% to 2.6%).

Pregnancy alters the pharmacokinetics of LMWH.[58] When LMWH is used for therapeutic anticoagulation, dosing can be adjusted based on anti–factor Xa activity. The desired peak level is 0.6 to 1.0 U/mL measured 4 hours after injection[15]; however, because of the cost, routine monitoring of anti–factor Xa activity is not recommended during therapy in pregnancy.[49] Viscoelastic monitoring provides an alternative method to assess LMWH activity. The delta reaction time (ΔR) measured by thromboelastography correlates with anti–factor Xa levels in pregnancy[59]; this allows LMWH doses to be

TABLE 38.2   Commonly Used Anticoagulation Regimens During Pregnancy

Drug	Dose
Prophylactic LMWH	Enoxaparin 40 mg SC once daily
	Dalteparin 5000 units SC once daily
	Tinzaparin 4500 units SC once daily
	Nadroparin 2850 units SC once daily
Intermediate-dose LMWH	Enoxaparin 40 mg SC every 12 h
	Dalteparin 5000 units SC every 12 h
Therapeutic LMWH (weight-adjusted treatment dose)[a]	Enoxaparin 1 mg/kg every 12 h
	Dalteparin 200 units/kg once daily
	Tinzaparin 175 units/kg once daily
	Dalteparin 100 units/kg every 12 h
Prophylactic UFH in the first trimester	UFH 5000–7500 units SC every 12 h
Prophylactic UFH in the second trimester	UFH 7500–10,000 units SC every 12 h
Prophylactic UFH in the third trimester	UFH 10,000 units SC every 12 h (unless aPTT is elevated)
Therapeutic (adjusted-dose) UFH[b]	UFH 10,000 units or more SC every 12 h
Postpartum anticoagulation[c]	Prophylactic LMWH for 6–8 w

aPTT, Activated partial thromboplastin time; LMWH, low-molecular-weight heparin; SC, subcutaneously; UFH, unfractionated heparin.
[a]Target anti-Xa level 4 h after last injection for twice-daily regimen: 0.6–1.0 unit/mL. Slightly higher doses may be necessary for once-daily dosing.
[b]Adjust dose to target aPTT (1.5–2.5 times the normal range 6 h after injection).
[c]Oral anticoagulants may be considered based on planned duration of therapy, lactation, and patient preference.
Modified from American College of Obstetricians and Gynecologists. Practice Bulletin No. 196: Thromboembolism in pregnancy (reaffirmed 2025). *Obstet Gynecol.* 2018;132:e1–e17.

adjusted to ensure anticoagulation or, conversely, confirm the absence of anticoagulation. LMWH is cleared by the kidney; therefore, dose reduction may be required in patients with renal failure.

UFH therapy may be used to initiate anticoagulation or to maintain therapy. UFH exerts its anticoagulant activity by binding to antithrombin III and potentiates inactivation of other coagulation factors, including thrombin (factor IIa); factors IXa, Xa, XIa, and XIIa; and kallikrein. Typically, UFH is administered as a subcutaneous injection for both prophylactic and therapeutic therapy. The aPTT measured 6 hours after an injection or dose adjustment should be maintained at 1.5 to 2.5 times the normal range.[15] In pregnancy, the bioavailability of UFH decreases because of an increase in heparin-binding proteins, increased plasma volume, increased renal clearance, and increased degradation by plasma heparinases.[60] Even a twice-daily dose of subcutaneous UFH is often inadequate to achieve *prophylactic* plasma heparin concentrations in the second half of pregnancy, possibly because of the presence of a heparin-neutralizing protein or the presence of increased factor VIII and fibrinogen levels in pregnancy.[61] For *therapeutic* anticoagulation, the ACOG currently recommends a subcutaneous, twice-daily UFH dose ≥ 10,000 units, with aPTT monitoring and dose adjustment.[15] In the event of antepartum massive PTE with hemodynamic instability, thrombolytic therapy is associated with high maternal and fetal survival.[51,62] However, in the postpartum period, other options, including thrombectomy, should be considered because thrombolysis is associated with a significant risk for hemorrhage.[62]

In patients who develop heparin-induced thrombocytopenia, or severe cutaneous reactions to heparin, **fondaparinux** is the preferred anticoagulant because it has minimal cross-reactivity with UFH.[15] Anticoagulation with other classes of drugs such as **vitamin K antagonists**, **thienopyridines**, **direct factor Xa inhibitors**, and **direct thrombin inhibitors** is possible in pregnancy, but the use of these medications is less common. **Inferior vena cava filters** may be considered for women with contraindications to anticoagulant therapy or DVT progression despite adequate anticoagulant therapy.[63]

Antithrombotic Therapy and Anesthetic Implications

In 2025, the American Society of Regional Anesthesia and Pain Medicine (ASRA) published its fifth edition guidelines for regional anesthesia in patients receiving antithrombotic or thrombolytic therapy.[64] The ASRA suggests following the guidelines for surgical patients when developing clinical policy for obstetric patients regarding initiation of neuraxial procedures and postpartum thromboprophylaxis.[64] The ASRA-recommended time intervals between anticoagulant administration and the initiation of neuraxial anesthesia are summarized in Table 38.3. Of note, it was once recommended that patients be transitioned from LWMH to UFH at 36 weeks' gestation to facilitate neuraxial procedures. In the third trimester, the ACOG-recommended prophylactic doses of UFH require a 12-hour delay prior to initiation of neuraxial anesthesia; therefore, there is no benefit to transitioning patients from LMWH to UFH.[15]

In 2018 the Society for Obstetric Anesthesia and Perinatology (SOAP) released a consensus statement with *pregnancy-specific* recommendations regarding neuraxial procedures in obstetric patients receiving thromboprophylaxis or therapeutic anticoagulation.[65] This integrated the ASRA guidelines, pharmacokinetic parameters of anticoagulants in pregnancy, and the risks associated with maternal airway management into decision-making algorithms intended to guide clinicians. The consensus statement emphasized the importance of weighing the risk associated with potential spinal or epidural hematoma versus the risk associated with general anesthesia in decision making.

Other anticoagulants sometimes administered to pregnant women include **aspirin**, **warfarin**, and newer anticoagulants. The ASRA recommends discontinuation of warfarin for 5 days and waiting for normalization of the international

TABLE 38.3 Recommended Time Intervals for Administration of Neuraxial Anesthesia After Anticoagulation and Initiation of Postpartum Anticoagulation

Therapy	TIME INTERVAL	
	Administration of Neuraxial Anesthesia After Anticoagulation	Initiation of Postpartum Anticoagulation
SC UFH, low-dose prophylactic[a]	>4–6 h or assessment of coagulation status[b]	≥1 h after neuraxial block or epidural catheter removal
SC UFH, intermediate dose[c]	≥12 h, and verify normal coagulation status[b,d]	≥1 h after neuraxial block or epidural catheter removal
SC UFH, therapeutic[e]	≥24 h, and verify normal coagulation status[b]	≥1 h after neuraxial block or epidural catheter removal
IV UFH	4–6 h, and verify normal coagulation status[b]	≥1 h after neuraxial block or epidural catheter removal
LMWH, prophylactic	≥12 h[b]	≥12 h after neuraxial block *and* ≥4 h after catheter removal
LMWH, therapeutic	≥24 h[b]	≥24 h after neuraxial block *and* ≥4 h after catheter removal

IV, Intravenous; *LMWH*, low-molecular-weight heparin; *SC*, subcutaneous; *UFH*, unfractionated heparin.
[a]UFH regimens of 5000 units SC two or three times a day.
[b]Check platelet count if either UFH or LMWH therapy for greater than 4 d.
[c]UFH regimens of 7500–10,000 units twice a day.
[d]If less than 12 h and aPTT is within normal range, may consider neuraxial procedure based on assessment of risks and benefits.
[e]UFH individual dose > 10,000 units SC or > 20,000 total units per day.
Modified from Kopp SL, Vandermeulen E, McBane RD, Perlas A, Leffert L, Horlocker T. Regional anesthesia in the patient receiving antithrombotic or thrombolytic therapy: American Society of Regional Anesthesia and Pain Medicine evidence-based guidelines (fifth edition). *Reg Anesth Pain Med.* 2025: Epub ahead of print Jan 29; https://doi.org/10.1136/rapm-2024-105766; Leffert L, Butwick A, Carvalho B, et al. The Society for Obstetric Anesthesia and Perinatology consensus statement on the anesthetic management of pregnant and postpartum women receiving thromboprophylaxis or higher dose anticoagulants. *Anesth Analg.* 2018;126:928–944.

normalized ratio.[64] Neuraxial catheters are *not* recommended in patients receiving fondaparinux, and neuraxial techniques are *not* recommended in patients anticoagulated with direct thrombin inhibitors. Treatment with thrombolytics is an absolute contraindication to neuraxial anesthesia.[64] By contrast, there is no contraindication to neuraxial anesthesia in patients receiving nonsteroidal antiinflammatory drugs or aspirin, if used alone.[64]

If neuraxial anesthesia is contraindicated, alternative analgesic methods (e.g., intravenous opioid) should be offered for labor, and general anesthesia should be performed for operative procedures. The anesthesia provider should note that placement of nasopharyngeal and oropharyngeal airways, gastric tubes, and other devices (e.g., temperature probes) carries a risk for traumatic hemorrhage. Emergency surgery may necessitate the administration of protamine or the transfusion of blood products (e.g., plasma) to reverse anticoagulation and reduce the risk for hemorrhage.

The timing of initiation of pharmacologic prophylaxis postpartum varies according to drug and dose. Both the ASRA and the SOAP consensus statements recommend at least a 1-hour delay after neuraxial blockade or epidural catheter removal before starting or restarting UFH, regardless of dose; at least a 12-hour delay after neuraxial blockade before the initiation of low-dose LWMH; and at least a 24-hour delay after neuraxial blockade before initiating therapeutic LMWH (see Table 38.3).[64,65]

The greatest concern with neuraxial procedures in anticoagulated patients is spinal or epidural hematoma. A meta-analysis estimated the incidence of epidural hematoma in obstetric patients to be 1:183,000.[66] An incidence of 1:251,643 (95% CI, 1:46,090 to 1:10,142,861) was identified in the SOAP Serious Complication Repository Project (SCORE).[67] The consequences of a spinal-epidural hematoma can be devastating. A systematic review and review of the American Society of Anesthesiologists Closed Claims Project Database (1990 to 2013) identified no cases of spinal or epidural hematoma in obstetric patients who received thromboprophylaxis consistent with the 2018 ASRA guidelines.[68] However, two case reports describe epidural hematoma following neuraxial anesthesia for cesarean delivery and administration of LMWH. In the first case, the initial dose of LMWH followed the onset of lower extremity weakness and sensory changes, and in the second case, symptoms began only after the initiation of therapeutic anticoagulation on postpartum day three.[64] Spontaneous epidural hematoma in pregnancy has been reported.[69]

Signs and symptoms of epidural hematoma include (1) severe, unremitting backache; (2) neurologic deficit, including bowel or bladder dysfunction or radiculopathy; (3) tenderness over the spinous or paraspinous area; and (4) unexplained fever (see Chapter 31).[70] Suspicion of epidural hematoma should lead to immediate spinal imaging and neurosurgical consultation. Neurologic recovery is a function of the severity of the deficits, the duration of maximum deficit, and the interval between symptom onset and surgery; better outcomes are associated with a shorter symptom onset-to-surgery interval.[71] A high index of suspicion is necessary because neurologic dysfunction may mimic local anesthetic–induced effects.[72]

AMNIOTIC FLUID EMBOLISM

Death attributable to AFE was first reported by Meyer in 1926.[73] Early reports described a syndrome of fatal peripartum shock attributed to emboli of amniotic fluid mechanically obstructing the maternal pulmonary circulation.[74] Although the pathophysiology of AFE is poorly understood, current evidence suggests that emboli alone are insufficient to precipitate it. Rather, fetal material in the maternal circulation has the potential to trigger a catastrophic cascade of inflammatory and hemostatic reactions that culminate in cardiopulmonary collapse and profound coagulopathy.

Epidemiology

The incidence of AFE is difficult to establish because (1) there are no universally accepted diagnostic criteria, (2) differing ascertainment methods yield divergent rates of AFE, and (3) there are no serum or histologic markers that are specific for AFE, making AFE a clinical diagnosis that is ultimately a diagnosis of exclusion. The dependence on clinical criteria has likely resulted in both over- and under-diagnosis; mild cases without permanent sequelae may not be reported, and many reports, particularly those based on administrative codes, likely include inappropriate diagnoses of AFE in women who become critically ill from other causes. As AFE is considered the least preventable cause of maternal mortality,[75] there may be medical-legal pressure to diagnose AFE in some cases of maternal mortality or severe morbidity. The lack of uniform diagnostic criteria is a significant barrier to furthering our understanding of AFE.

In an effort to standardize diagnosis and reporting of AFE for research purposes, in 2016 an expert panel convened by the Society for Maternal-Fetal Medicine (SMFM) and the AFE Foundation proposed diagnostic criteria for AFE.[76] Notably, this definition requires documentation of coagulopathy to confirm diagnosis and excludes patients who were febrile during labor. It is intentionally biased toward specificity in an effort to standardize reporting; thus, even some cases considered by experts to represent true cases of AFE do not meet all components of this definition.[77] Similar, but slightly more liberal definitions of AFE, have been established by the International Network of Obstetric Survey Systems (INOSS),[78] the UK Obstetric Surveillance System (UKOSS),[79] and by consensus in Japan[80] (see Table 38.4).

The challenges of applying definitions to AFE are evident from studies that have combined expert case review with application of various consensus criteria. In an analysis of cases submitted to the US AFE Registry, 12% of cases were considered atypical because they did not meet the full research criteria, but on expert review were considered to represent AFE.[77] A retrospective observational study confirmed that a larger number of cases are classified as AFE using Japanese criteria compared with US or UKOSS criteria.[81] In

TABLE 38.4 Commonly Used Amniotic Fluid Embolism Diagnostic Criteria

Society for Maternal-Fetal Medicine and the Amniotic Fluid Foundation Criteria[76]	International Network of Obstetric Survey Systems Criteria[78]	UK Obstetric Surveillance System Criteria[85]	Japanese Consensus Criteria[80]
1. Sudden onset of cardiorespiratory arrest, or both hypotension and respiratory compromise 2. Documentation of overt DIC, after the appearance of initial signs or symptoms, using the scoring system of Scientific and Standardization Committee on DIC of the International Society on Thrombosis and Hemostasis, modified for pregnancy. The coagulopathy must be detected before sufficient blood is lost to account for dilutional or shock-related consumptive coagulopathy. 3. Clinical onset during labor or within 30 min of delivery of the placenta 4. No fever (≥38.0°C) during labor	Acute cardiorespiratory collapse within 6 h after labor, delivery, or ruptured membranes, with no other identifiable cause, followed by acute coagulopathy in those women who survive the initial event	In the absence of any other clear cause, either: 1. Acute maternal collapse with one or more of the following features: acute fetal compromise, cardiac arrest, cardiac arrhythmias, coagulopathy, hypotension, maternal hemorrhage, premonitory symptoms, seizures, shortness of breath or: 2. Pathologic diagnosis of fetal squames or hair in the maternal lungs	1. Symptoms appeared during pregnancy or within 12 h of delivery. 2. Intensive medical intervention was conducted to treat one or more of the following symptoms/diseases: (a) cardiac arrest, (b) severe bleeding of unknown origin within 2 h of delivery (≥1500 mL) (c) DIC (d) respiratory failure 3. The findings or symptoms obtained cannot be explained by other diseases.

DIC, Disseminated intravascular coagulation.
Criteria from Clark SL, Romero R, Dildy GA, et al. Proposed diagnostic criteria for the case definition of amniotic fluid embolism in research studies. *Am J Obstet Gynecol.* 2016;215:408–412; Fitzpatrick KE, van den Akker T, Bloemenkamp KWM, et al. Risk factors, management, and outcomes of amniotic fluid embolism: a multicountry, population-based cohort and nested case-control study. *PLoS Med.* 2019;16:e1002962; Fitzpatrick KE, Tuffnell D, Kurinczuk JJ, Knight M. Incidence, risk factors, management and outcomes of amniotic-fluid embolism: a population-based cohort and nested case-control study. *BJOG.* 2016;123:100–109; Kanayama N, Tamura N. Amniotic fluid embolism: pathophysiology and new strategies for management. *J Obstet Gynaecol Res.* 2014;40:1507–1517.

an international cohort study that included a comparison of criteria,[78] the INOSS found that 31% of cases collected by member institutions met INOSS, but not SMFM criteria, with a lack of evidence for disseminated intravascular coagulation (DIC) being the most common reason for not meeting SMFM criteria. Similarly, in the French Confidential Enquiry into Maternal Deaths (2007 to 2011), documentation of coagulopathy was missing for 14 of 39 deaths.[82] Practically, while obtaining laboratory studies to assess coagulation status can be essential in the management of a critically ill patient, it may not occur in the appropriate time frame in the context of ongoing resuscitation.

While a rate of up to 6 per 100,000 pregnancies has been recently reported in the United States based on data from the National Inpatient Sample,[83] this discrepancy likely represents the result of ascertaining cases using administrative codes versus diagnostic criteria rather than geographical variation. Overdiagnosis of AFE in administrative data has been identified in studies from a regional surveillance system in Australia that has the capacity to systematically review records for all cases identified from administrative data. By only counting women using a validated case identification

system, the reported incidence of AFE decreased from 6.3 to 3.3 cases per 100,000 pregnancies.[84] The largest international study of the epidemiology of AFE suggested a much lower event rate of 0.8 to 1.8 per 100,000 pregnancies, with a lower rate when the SMFM criteria are applied and a higher rate using the more liberal UKOSS criteria.[78]

Risk Factors

Maternal demographic factors, including older age and maternal race or ethnicity, have been associated with AFE in population-based studies.[78,83,85,86] Other obstetric factors such as abnormal placentation, placenta previa, placental abruption, eclampsia, multiple gestation, induction of labor (particularly with prostaglandins), artificial or spontaneous rupture of membranes, fetal demise, and operative delivery have also been associated with AFE.[78,83–89] Notably, 66% of women in the US AFE registry had a history of atopy, latex, medication, or food allergy.[90] This potentially may reflect a predilection for immunologic hyperreactivity in patients with AFE.

Because nonreassuring fetal heart rate (FHR) tracings can complicate AFE in labor, cesarean delivery may be a consequence, rather than a cause, of intrapartum AFE.

Nonetheless, there was a strong association between cesarean birth and postpartum AFE in the INOSS data set, with an adjusted OR (aOR) of 14.02[78]; notably, 61% of women did not labor prior to their cesarean delivery, and 33% of cesarean deliveries complicated by postpartum AFE were elective. In the US registry, of the patients who had a cesarean delivery and AFE, only 27.5% underwent emergency cesarean delivery in response to AFE.[90] Overall these results suggest that the association between cesarean birth and AFE is not solely a consequence of emergency intrapartum cesarean delivery prompted by nonreassuring fetal well-being as a result of maternal hemodynamic collapse.

Despite possible association between AFE and maternal demographic characteristics, obstetric complications, and labor outcomes, the rarity of AFE and the tenuous nature of the described associations means that none of the potentially identified risk factors carry clinical utility for prediction or risk stratification of AFE.

Pathophysiology

In 1941, Steiner and Lushbaugh described eight autopsies after fatal intrapartum shock in which examination of lung tissue revealed embolic material of squamous cells, mucin, meconium, and amorphous eosinophilic material.[74] Because all of these patients were described as having tumultuous labors with stronger than usual uterine contractions, it was presumed that the forceful contractions loosened or tore the placenta and forced the emboli into the maternal circulation.[74] Yet, periods of uterine tachysystole are the least likely times for maternoplacental exchange of embolic material to occur as uterine blood flow ceases.[91] The tachysystole is probably a result of endogenous norepinephrine (noradrenaline) release and, therefore is likely temporally related to, but not causative for, embolic material transfer.[91]

Large intravenous boluses of human meconium suspended in human amniotic fluid can precipitate cardiovascular collapse in rabbits and dogs,[74] but injection of autologous amniotic fluid fails to reproduce the AFE syndrome in many animal models, including primates.[92] Passage of fetal squames, lanugo hair, and mucin into the maternal pelvic vasculature appears to be a common event at term,[93] and fetal material has been identified in pulmonary arterial samples aspirated from critically ill women who did not have AFE.[94,95] Furthermore, in a goat model of AFE, histopathologic analysis of the lungs after injection of autologous amniotic fluid failed to demonstrate evidence for amniotic debris in 19 of 29 animals.[96] Therefore, the presence of fetal tissue in the lungs is neither sensitive nor specific for the diagnosis of AFE.

The trigger for development of AFE, as well as the pathophysiology driving the associated cardiovascular collapse and coagulopathy, are all unknown. Given that AFE appears to be a systemic inflammatory response, its pathophysiology may include the inappropriate release of endogenous inflammatory mediators, such as arachidonic acid metabolites (i.e., thromboxane, prostaglandins, leukotrienes),[97] although a role for these inflammatory mediators in AFE has not yet been definitively established.

The large proportion of women in AFE registries with a history of allergy or atopy has led to suggestions of an anaphylactoid mechanism.[87] In support of this theory, the symptoms of AFE were blocked by the administration of a leukotriene inhibitor in a rabbit model.[98] However, a series of case reports suggested that levels of tryptase and histamine are not dramatically or universally elevated among women with AFE.[99,100] While mast cell degranulation may play a role in the pathophysiology of AFE, this may be a secondary product of the inflammatory cascade, rather than causal, and thus the term *anaphylactoid syndrome of pregnancy* may be a misnomer.[100]

Other immune-mediated mechanisms may be potential mediators of AFE. A case-control study demonstrated low levels of the complement components C3 and C4 among women diagnosed with AFE compared with controls, suggesting that complement activation may also contribute to the inflammatory cascade.[99] Levels of C1 esterase inhibitor (C1INH), a regulator of the complement pathway, have also been shown to be decreased in AFE compared with controls.[101] These studies should be considered preliminary; it is unknown whether complement plays a primary,[102] secondary,[103] or no role in AFE.

Coagulopathy develops in the majority of women who survive initial cardiovascular collapse.[85,87] *In vitro* studies using amniotic fluid and viscoelastic testing suggested that amniotic fluid may accelerate thrombin production and increase platelet activation,[104,105] leading to a consumptive coagulopathy, although the *in vivo* relevance of these findings has not been established. One proposed mechanism for the coagulopathy in AFE involves tissue factor. As pregnancy progresses, increasing amounts of tissue factor, a potent procoagulant, accumulates in the amniotic fluid.[106,107] Tissue factor binds factor VII, thus activating the extrinsic pathway and triggering clotting by activating factor X, with the subsequent development of a consumptive coagulopathy.[106] A second possible mechanism is that amniotic fluid has a thromboplastin-like effect, which induces platelet aggregation, releases platelet factor III, and activates the clotting cascade.[108] Other components of amniotic fluid, the amniochorion, and the placenta have also been implicated in contributing to the coagulopathy. Uterine atony, from a specific myometrial depressant or from uterine hypoperfusion, may exacerbate hemorrhage and the consumptive coagulopathy seen in AFE.[109] While these studies suggest that the bleeding seen in AFE is due primarily to a consumptive coagulopathy, conflicting evidence suggests that the coagulopathy may primarily be due to hypofibrinogenemia. Specifically, reports of viscoelastic testing conducted early in AFE suggest that, at least in some cases, the initial coagulopathy may result from isolated hyperfibrinolysis and hypofibrinogenemia.[110,111]

Clinical Presentation

AFE presents clinically as cardiorespiratory collapse and coagulopathy during labor, immediately postpartum, or very rarely after abdominal trauma or abortion.[112,113]

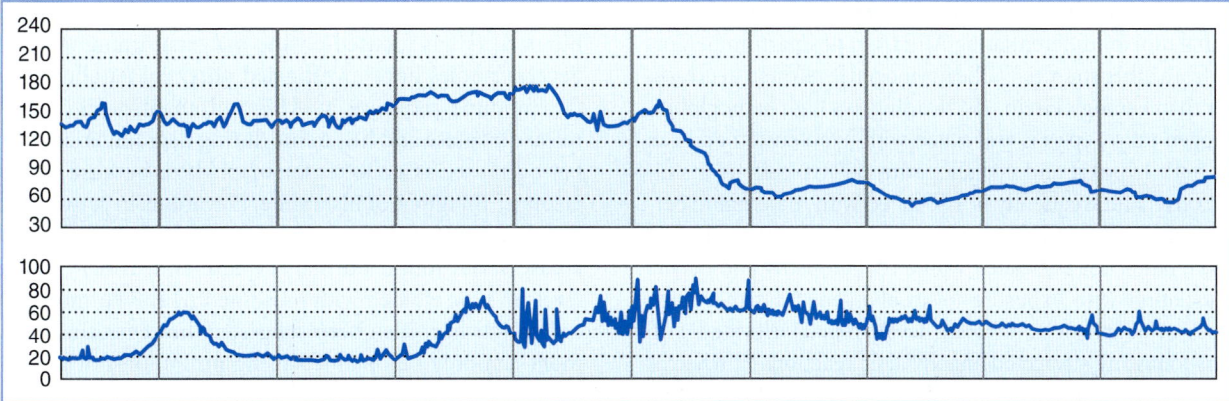

Fig. 38.2 Fetal Heart Rate Tracing in a Patient With Amniotic Fluid Embolism. Maternal symptoms began just before the onset of spontaneous uterine tachysystole and fetal bradycardia. Modified from Clark SL, Hankins GDV, Dudley DA, et al. Amniotic fluid embolism: analysis of the national registry. *Am J Obstet Gynecol.* 1995; 172:1158–1167.

AFE most often occurs during labor; intrapartum events comprised 46% of cases in the INOSS registry[78] and 70% of cases in the initial cohort of the US registry.[87] With the caveat that milder cases may not be as reliably reported, severe initial presentations are common: 50% of cases in the INOSS registry presented with cardiac arrest, 67% of cases in an Israeli retrospective study presented with sudden loss of consciousness,[114] and 97% of cases in the US registry presented with hypotension.[90] AFE may also be accompanied by cough, cyanosis, or seizures, and some cases are accompanied by nonspecific premonitory symptoms such as restlessness or agitation.[78,90] Maternal symptoms may precede FHR changes. Fetal bradycardia, or the abrupt onset of variable decelerations that progress to fetal bradycardia, may also herald AFE in labor (Fig. 38.2).[87]

Point-of-care echocardiography has established that the cardiovascular collapse that heralds the onset of AFE is typically accompanied, and likely caused, by acute right ventricular failure.[115] While right ventricular failure in AFE is thought to be mediated by acute pulmonary hypertension, the molecular mediators causing increased pulmonary vascular resistance are unknown. Echocardiographic findings include a dilated, akinetic right ventricle and a normally contracting left ventricle with a nearly obliterated cavity.[116–119] Right ventricular failure results in an underfilled left ventricle, decreased systemic cardiac output, and hypotension.

Patients who survive the initial cardiorespiratory collapse associated with AFE subsequently develop profound coagulopathy. This has classically been described as DIC,[76] and numerous reports document thrombocytopenia with prolonged prothrombin time and aPTT in addition to hypofibrinogenemia[87] or "flatline" viscoelastic testing suggesting global hemostatic failure.[120,121] More recent reports, however, suggest that hyperfibrinolysis and severe hypofibrinogenemia may be the hallmarks of coagulation failure in AFE, with less prominent decreases in factor V and preservation, at least initially, of other components of the coagulation cascade.[110,111,122–125] It is unclear whether the global hemostatic failure that has been described represents progression of the disease process or a more severe variant of AFE-induced coagulopathy.

BOX 38.2 Differential Diagnosis of Amniotic Fluid Embolism

Nonobstetric
- Myocardial infarction
- Pulmonary embolism
- Aspiration
- Sepsis
- Anaphylaxis
- Venous air embolism

Obstetric
- Placental abruption
- Eclampsia
- Uterine rupture or laceration
- Obstetric hemorrhage

Anesthetic
- High neuraxial blockade ("total spinal")
- Local anesthetic systemic toxicity
- Medication error

The coagulopathy described in some cases of AFE is indistinguishable from cases of severe placental abruption.[126] It is unclear whether they share a common inciting mechanism or whether this represents a common pathway in acute obstetric coagulopathy.

Because many of the signs and symptoms of AFE are nonspecific, AFE must be distinguished from other life-threatening causes of cardiovascular collapse in obstetric patients (Box 38.2). In an analysis of cases submitted to the US AFE Registry, obstetric hemorrhage was most commonly misdiag-nosed as AFE.[90] While severe obstetric hemorrhage may cause life-threatening hypotension and coagulopathy, it can be distinguished from AFE by the *sequence* of presentation; massive blood loss precedes cardiovascular collapse in hemorrhage, whereas cardiovascular collapse precedes blood loss in AFE. Furthermore, except in cases of placental abruption, massive blood loss typically precedes development of a coagulopathy in obstetric hemorrhage, whereas a coagulopathy precedes significant blood loss in AFE. Reflecting this, the hemoglobin/

fibrinogen ratio, when assessed early, has been suggested as a potential tool for differentiating AFE from postpartum hemorrhage from other sources.[127] The fibrinogen level often decreases earlier than hemoglobin in AFE, leading to a high hemoglobin/fibrinogen ratio Sepsis is associated with hypotension and can cause both hypoxia and coagulopathy, but typically is insidious in onset and frequently is associated with maternal hyper- or hypothermia. Anaphylaxis can cause hypotension and hypoxia, but is not associated with a coagulopathy and occurs in association with exposure to an allergen.[128] Furthermore, in cases of anaphylaxis, tryptase levels remain elevated 1 to 2 hours following suspected anaphylactic reactions,[129] whereas serum tryptase levels are not elevated in cases of AFE.[99] High neuraxial block can cause hypotension and respiratory compromise, but does not include coagulopathy. While pulmonary or air embolism can cause hypotension and hypoxia, they are not typically associated with coagulopathy. Similarly, hemodynamic collapse from a primary cardiac etiology, such as an acute myocardial infarction, does not present with coagulopathy and typically occurs in the clinical context of patients with known risk factors or recognized cardiac pathology.

Confirmatory Tests

There is no definitive diagnostic test for AFE. While the UKOSS considers fetal material in the maternal pulmonary vasculature at autopsy to be pathognomonic for AFE,[85] fetal squamous cells and trophoblasts are commonly found in the maternal circulation of healthy parturients.[95] Furthermore, differentiating between maternal and fetal cells histologically is challenging.[130] Therefore, the presence of fetal cells in the maternal pulmonary vasculature is neither sensitive nor specific for diagnosis of AFE.

The search for an AFE biochemical marker is a topic of intense interest. While several biochemical markers have been suggested based on suspected pathophysiology and results from small studies,[131] the rarity and unpredictability of AFE make validation of markers proposed from small studies extremely challenging. Most investigations have focused either on detection of markers typically enriched in amniotic fluid in maternal plasma or on identification of potential mediators of the maternal response. As an example, insulin-like growth factor binding protein-1 (IGFBP-1) is found at 100- to 500-fold higher concentrations in the amniotic fluid than in maternal plasma,[132] and was found in a small case-control study to potentially identify cases of AFE,[133] with a cutoff of 104.5 μg/L having sensitivity of 92% and specificity of 97.8% for AFE. Unfortunately, a validation study using a multicenter retrospective cohort suggested that IGFBP-1 is a not a useful diagnostic marker for AFE, as a value > 100 μg/L was associated with sensitivity of only 16% and specificity of 88%.[134] While these results are disappointing, the study is an excellent example of the rigorous study design that is necessary to evaluate possible biomarkers for AFE.[135] Additional potential biomarkers enriched in amniotic fluid or meconium that have been studied for diagnostic utility include zinc coproporphyrin,[136] sialyl Tn antigen,[99] and squamous cell carcinoma antigen.[137] While these markers have shown potential utility in small studies, validation studies are necessary.

A complementary line of investigation into potential biomarkers has focused on the maternal immune response. Several studies have investigated potential parallels between the immune response in AFE and anaphylaxis. Mast cells release tryptase and histamine during degranulation; tryptase has been used as a marker for anaphylaxis because its half-life is longer than that of histamine. Elevations in serum tryptase have been reported in some parturients with AFE.[100] However, a case series found normal tryptase and urinary histamine levels in nine women with presumed AFE.[99] Pulmonary mast cell counts have also been suggested; however, this measurement can only be obtained using immunohistochemistry at autopsy. In one observational study, the mean pulmonary mast cell count per fixed area for parturients who died of AFE was similar to that of parturients who died of anaphylactic shock but was higher than the mean counts in both pregnant and nonpregnant control patients.[138] These data, together with the finding of minimal to no elevation in serum tryptase, suggest that pulmonary mast cell degranulation may be a secondary process in AFE.[100]

Complement activation may cause mast cell degranulation, and there is some evidence supporting widespread complement activation, and subsequently depressed C3 and C4 levels in AFE.[99] However, because complement is activated during acute respiratory distress syndrome and other inflammatory states, these results are not specific for AFE. C1INH, which inhibits C1 as well as kallikrein and factors XIa and XIIa, has been suggested as a possible biomarker to support the clinical diagnosis of AFE.[101] C1INH levels were lower in women who were diagnosed with AFE compared with healthy pregnant controls (30% versus 62%, P < .001). C1INH levels were further decreased in fatal AFE cases compared with nonfatal cases (23% versus 32%, P < .05). Validation of C1INH as a possible biomarker supporting a diagnosis of AFE awaits validation in larger cohorts.

Management

Management of AFE is predicated on timely recognition and goal-directed treatment of the cardiovascular collapse and coagulopathy that are its hallmarks. There are no known treatments that reverse AFE, and therefore providing high-quality supportive care is critical to improving outcomes. Maternal resuscitation should focus on three priorities: (1) maintenance of oxygenation, (2) hemodynamic support, and (3) correction of coagulopathy (Box 38.3).

When AFE is suspected, 100% oxygen should be administered and large-bore intravenous access secured. An arterial line and central venous catheter may facilitate hemodynamic monitoring, blood sampling, fluid and blood administration, and vasopressor administration. Point-of-care transthoracic or transesophageal echocardiography is useful to guide resuscitation, particularly with right ventricular failure.

Some patients with AFE present with cardiac arrest; for these patients, initial management should focus on providing high-quality advanced cardiac life support.[139] Key considerations in patients at greater than 20 weeks' gestation include left uterine displacement, prioritization of oxygenation and

BOX 38.3 Management of Amniotic Fluid Embolism

Airway
- Administer 100% oxygen.
- Intubate trachea, support ventilation as needed.

Cardiovascular Support
- Start chest compressions if indicated.
- Ensure left uterine displacement to relieve aortocaval compression if appropriate.
- Administer fluids and vasopressors.
- Establish large-bore intravenous access.
- Consider invasive blood pressure monitoring.

Fetus
- Monitor fetal well-being.
- Expedite delivery for nonreassuring status in a viable fetus or in the event of maternal cardiopulmonary arrest in the second half of pregnancy (i.e., perimortem cesarean delivery).

Hemostatic Support
- Activate obstetric hemorrhage protocol and massive transfusion protocol.[a]
- Send blood for serial laboratory assessment to monitor for coagulopathy and electrolyte disturbances.
- Provide blood component therapy as indicated.
- Ensure normothermia.

Postresuscitation Care
- Notify intensive care unit of potential admission.
- Consider initiation of mild therapeutic hypothermia after cardiac arrest.

[a]See Chapter 37.

airway management, and perimortem cesarean delivery (resuscitative hysterotomy) (see Chapter 53). Although the operating room may provide a more favorable environment for surgery and resuscitation, simulation studies have suggested that resuscitation quality and the arrest-to-delivery interval both suffer with maternal transport[140,141]; therefore, if obstetric conditions do not support an immediate operative vaginal delivery (i.e., forceps or vacuum), a bedside perimortem cesarean delivery is indicated.

For patients with AFE who do not present with cardiac arrest or in whom return of spontaneous circulation is achieved, acute pulmonary hypertension and right ventricular failure are typically the primary cardiovascular pathophysiology.[115] The treatment of right ventricular failure is predicated on vasopressor support to maintain systemic perfusion, inotropic support for the failing right ventricle, and pulmonary vasodilators. All efforts should be made to avoid hypoxia, hypercarbia, and acidosis as these increase pulmonary vascular resistance. Pharmacologic therapy for hemodynamic collapse associated with acute right ventricular failure includes **norepinephrine** or **epinephrine** (**adrenaline**), depending on the extent of circulatory collapse, with consideration for the use of **dobutamine** or **milrinone** for inotropic support and inhaled **nitric oxide** or **epoprostenol**

as pulmonary vasodilators if clinically indicated.[142,143] If these agents are not immediately available, **phenylephrine** and **ephedrine** may be useful in initial resuscitation. Processes to rapidly obtain advanced inotropic support and pulmonary vasodilators should be identified in institutional-specific planning sessions and clearly featured on cognitive aids. **Extracorporeal membrane oxygenation (ECMO)** can be considered early if available, and cognitive aids should include ECMO contact information. Overzealous fluid administration may exacerbate right ventricular failure.

Patients who survive the initial cardiorespiratory collapse associated with AFE go on to develop profound coagulopathy. Close communication with the blood bank is essential. Viscoelastic testing may help guide rational management of blood products and clotting factor concentrates.[121] As discussed above, several case reports and case series suggest hyperfibrinolysis during AFE.[110,111,122–125] Therefore, based on extrapolation from the World Maternal Antifibrinolytic Trial (WOMAN),[144] intravenous **tranexamic acid** administration (1 g over 10 minutes, with the possibility of an additional 1 g dose after 30 minutes with ongoing bleeding) is recommended.[142] Administration of a concentrated source of **fibrinogen** (fibrinogen concentrate or cryoprecipitate) has been associated with improved outcomes.[78] Clotting factor concentrates (i.e., **prothrombin complex concentrate**) may be useful, particularly if a coagulopathy is present with a need to limit intravascular volume in the setting of right ventricular failure. There is no evidence that the use of **recombinant factor VII (rVIIa)** improves outcomes: A systematic review of case reports of women with AFE identified a twofold increase in risk for death or permanent disability among 16 women treated with rVIIa compared with 28 control patients who underwent surgery to control bleeding but did not receive rVIIa.[145] Furthermore, the use of rVIIa was not associated with improved survival in the INOSS cohort.[78]

Maternal and Perinatal Outcomes

AFE is responsible for 6.1% of maternal deaths in the United States and is the second most common cause of maternal mortality on the day of delivery.[146,147] Despite being the least preventable cause of maternal mortality,[75] maternal outcomes in AFE have improved substantially over the last several decades. Analysis of the US AFE registry revealed a decrease in maternal mortality from 61% in the cohort analyzed between 1988 and 1994 to 10% in the 2013 to 2017 cohort.[87,90] The mortality rate in the contemporaneous multinational INOSS cohort (2005 to 2018) was slightly higher, at 20%, when cases were classified using the SMFM criteria.[78] While maternal mortality from AFE has improved, severe morbidity remains common, highlighted by neurologically intact survival rates of only 46% in the US AFE registry,[77] and 61% of patients in the INOSS cohort.[78] Opportunities to improve care in AFE management were identified in 20 of the 36 AFE mortalities in the French Confidential Enquiry into Maternal Deaths (2007 to 2011), with contributing factors including delays in, or suboptimal, transfusion management, as well as delays or lack of performing indicated hysterectomies.[82]

There are ethnic disparities in mortality rates in AFE. Patients who died of AFE were more likely to be from ethnic minority groups than survivors, even after adjusting for confounders such as age, socioeconomic status, body mass index, parity, and induction of labor (aOR, 2.85; 95% CI, 1.02 to 8.00).[85] Similar findings have been observed in the United States.[148] Multidisciplinary reviews may reduce current racial/ethnic disparities[149] and are recommended following all cases of AFE to identify opportunities for systems improvement.[142]

Neonates have a high survival rate > 90%.[78,90] Intact neurologic survival is related to the arrest-to-delivery interval in women whose presentation includes cardiac arrest; delays > 15 minutes are associated with poor outcomes.[87]

While uncomplicated pregnancies have been reported amongst survivors of AFE, verified recurrent AFE has not been reported.[150,151] Given the rarity and severity of AFE, as well as the low number of pregnancies reported in survivors of AFE, it is not yet known whether survivors of AFE have an increased risk for AFE recurrence in subsequent pregnancies.

VENOUS AIR EMBOLISM

VAE may occur in many surgical procedures, including cesarean delivery.[152] Most air emboli are small, but volumes > 200 to 300 mL, or 3 to 5 mL/kg, may be lethal.[152] The true incidence of fatal VAE in obstetric patients is unknown. Early recognition and appropriate management are necessary for avoiding unfavorable outcomes.

Incidence

The reported incidence of VAE during cesarean delivery varies depending on the method used to ascertain the presence of air. The most sensitive monitors detect volumes of air as low as 0.02 mL/kg.[152] Studies using precordial Doppler monitoring during cesarean delivery with neuraxial anesthesia have found an incidence ranging from as low as 10%[153] to as high as 65%.[154] A study correlating precordial Doppler monitoring with transthoracic echocardiography in 42 patients having cesarean delivery with neuraxial anesthesia found that 11 (26%) had evidence of VAE, with perfect agreement between the Doppler and the echocardiographic monitoring (kappa = 1.0).[155] Another study of healthy parturients undergoing elective cesarean delivery with general anesthesia found that 29 of 30 parturients had evidence of intraoperative VAE.[156] The authors defined VAE as a 0.1% increase from the baseline of expired nitrogen concentration (equivalent to 0.25 to 1.0 mL/kg venous air).[156]

The incidence of VAE does not appear to vary with maternal position. Although the Trendelenburg position could produce a pressure gradient between the heart and open venous sinuses, a metaanalysis of two randomized controlled trials that compared 5 degrees with 10 degrees Trendelenburg positioning versus supine positioning for cesarean delivery (pooled $n = 130$) found no difference in the incidence of VAE (RR, 0.85; 95% CI, 0.28 to 2.57).[157]

Pathophysiology

A pressure gradient as small as -5 cm H_2O between the surgical field and the heart allows entrainment of air into the venous circulation. Immediately after placental separation, the raw endometrial surface appears to be a location of significant air entrainment; almost all episodes of VAE during cesarean delivery are noted after delivery of the placenta.[154] In the noncesarean delivery setting, pressurized air in the vagina is believed to traverse the cervical canal, dissect around fetal membranes (if present), and enter the maternal circulation via subplacental sinuses.[158]

Small volumes of air can precipitate pulmonary vasospasm via a pathophysiologic process that mimics that of other embolic phenomena. Vasoactive mediators or mechanical obstruction of small vessels appear to induce pulmonary vasoconstriction that leads to V/Q mismatch, hypoxemia, right-sided heart failure, arrhythmias, and hypotension. Fluid resuscitation and increased hydrostatic pressure may provoke interstitial pulmonary edema. Paradoxical air embolism into the arterial circulation (by means of a patent foramen ovale) can lead to cardiovascular and neurologic sequelae and morbidity. Large volumes of air (>3 mL/kg) can generate cardiovascular collapse by creating an "air lock" that causes right-ventricular outflow tract obstruction.

Clinical Presentation

Most air emboli are subclinical; however, massive VAE can manifest as a sudden, dramatic, and devastating event with hypotension, hypoxemia, and cardiac arrest.[159] In awake patients receiving neuraxial anesthesia, transient episodes of hypoxemia, dyspnea, or chest pain during uterine repair suggest VAE.[153,154,160] In the patient receiving general anesthesia, evidence of VAE may be limited to hypoxemia and a slight decrease in end-tidal CO_2.[152] VAE may be more frequent when the uterus is exteriorized, because of vertical elevation relative to the heart or traction on the uterus that opens venous sinuses.[153,160] Auscultation may reveal a pathognomonic "mill-wheel murmur." Transesophageal echocardiography may detect air in the right atrium or the pulmonary artery. Clinically significant air emboli may be associated with hypotension, heart rate or rhythm changes, evidence of right-sided heart strain on the electrocardiogram, an increase in central venous pressure, and/or an increase in pulmonary artery pressure. Although isolated ST-segment depression during cesarean delivery is common and once thought to be possibly related to VAE,[161] more recent evidence suggests that it may be associated with rapid oxytocin administration.[162] One small prospective observational study failed to identify VAE using echocardiography at the time of ST-segment depression during cesarean deliveries.[161]

Management

VAE should be considered in women who complain of intraoperative chest pain or dyspnea or experience sudden hypoxemia, hypotension, or arrhythmia during cesarean delivery. Although continuous precordial Doppler monitoring has been recommended,[152] the rarity of hemodynamically significant VAE suggests that targeted use in high-risk patients (e.g.,

BOX 38.4   Resuscitation of the Obstetric Patient With Massive Venous Air Embolism

Air
- Prevent further air entrainment (e.g., flood the surgical field with saline solution, lower the surgical field relative to the heart, if tolerated).

Airway
- Administer 100% oxygen, discontinue nitrous oxide, intubate the trachea, and support ventilation as needed.

Cardiovascular Support
- Support circulation with chest compressions, intravascular volume expansion, and vasopressors as needed.

Fetus
- Expedite delivery.

Postresuscitation Care
- Evaluate for intracerebral air and consider hyperbaric oxygen therapy if indicated.
- Avoid hyperthermia after cardiac arrest.

women with a known intracardiac shunt) may be more appropriate than routine application. Transthoracic or transesophageal echocardiography may help to confirm a diagnosis of VAE, to exclude alternative causes of hemodynamic instability, and to guide appropriate clinical management. Clinical suspicion of VAE should prompt appropriate management (Box 38.4).

Currently, no data support central line insertion for air aspiration from the right side of the heart, although it may be indicated to deliver potent vasopressors.[152] Maternal position changes to limit air entrainment are recommended; however, no human data support using the left lateral decubitus position to relieve the "air lock."[152] In a canine study of resuscitation positioning after a 2.5-mL/kg VAE, repositioning animals to direct air to the nondependent portion of the right side of the heart did not improve cardiac function or survival.[163] The use of the Valsalva maneuver and positive-end expiratory pressure should be avoided because an increase in right atrial pressure may result in a paradoxical embolism. In patients with delayed emergence from anesthesia, computed tomography or MRI may be considered to evaluate for intracerebral air. Hyperbaric oxygen may improve neurologic outcomes if instituted within 6 hours of intracerebral air embolism.[164]

KEY POINTS

- Embolic disorders are a major cause of maternal morbidity and mortality.
- Early recognition, diagnosis, and therapy may reduce the incidence of morbidity and mortality associated with embolic disorders.
- During pulmonary embolic phenomena, hemostatic and immunologic mediators may trigger a cascade of physiologic derangements disproportionate to the cross-sectional area of occluded lung tissue.
- Pregnant patients are at a fivefold higher risk than nonpregnant patients for thromboembolic events. The third trimester and first postpartum week are the periods of highest risk.
- Several prophylactic and therapeutic anticoagulation regimens exist for patients with venous thromboembolism or those at increased risk for thromboembolism; anesthesia providers should be aware of the safety implications of anticoagulation therapy on the timing of the initiation of neuraxial anesthesia and neuraxial catheter removal.
- Amniotic fluid embolism is a diagnosis of exclusion. It may occur at any time during labor or delivery, as well as antepartum or postpartum.
- Venous air embolism is a common occurrence during cesarean delivery. Most of the emboli are small, transient, and benign. Massive venous air embolism is rare during vaginal or cesarean delivery but can be fatal.

REFERENCES

1. Creanga AA, Syverson C, Seed K, Callaghan WM. Pregnancy-related mortality in the United States, 2011–2013. *Obstet Gynecol.* 2017;130:366–373.
2. Krenitsky N, Friedman AM, Yu K, et al. Trends in venous thromboembolism and associated risk factors during delivery hospitalizations from 2000 to 2018. *Obstet Gynecol.* 2022;139:223–234.
3. US Centers for Disease Control and Prevention. Pregnancy Mortality Surveillance System; 2022. https://www.cdc.gov/reproductivehealth/maternal-mortality/pregnancy-mortality-surveillance-system.htm. Accessed November 15, 2023.
4. Ghaji N, Boulet SL, Tepper N, Hooper WC. Trends in venous thromboembolism among pregnancy-related hospitalizations, United States, 1994-2009. *Am J Obstet Gynecol.* 2013;209:433.e1–e8.
5. Pomp ER, Lenselink AM, Rosendaal FR, Doggen CJ. Pregnancy, the postpartum period and prothrombotic defects: risk of venous thrombosis in the MEGA study. *J Thromb Haemost.* 2008;6:632–637.
6. Kourlaba G, Relakis J, Kontodimas S, et al. A systematic review and meta-analysis of the epidemiology and burden of venous thromboembolism among pregnant women. *Int J Gynaecol Obstet.* 2016;132:4–10.
7. Morris JM, Algert CS, Roberts CL. Incidence and risk factors for pulmonary embolism in the postpartum period. *J Thromb Haemost.* 2010;8:998–1003.
8. Heit JA, Kobbervig CE, James AH, et al. Trends in the incidence of venous thromboembolism during pregnancy or

postpartum: a 30-year population-based study. *Ann Intern Med.* 2005;143:697–706.

9. Kamel H, Navi BB, Sriram N, et al. Risk of a thrombotic event after the 6-week postpartum period. *N Engl J Med.* 2014;370:1307–1315.

10. Knight M, Bunch K, Felker A, et al. *Saving Lives, Improving Mothers' Care Core Report—Lessons Learned to Inform Maternity Care From the UK and Ireland Confidential Enquiries Into Maternal Deaths and Morbidity 2019–21.* National Perinatal Epidemiology Unit, University of Oxford; 2023.

11. Macklon NS, Greer IA, Bowman AW. An ultrasound study of gestational and postural changes in the deep venous system of the leg in pregnancy. *Br J Obstet Gynaecol.* 1997;104:191–197.

12. Gerbasi FR, Bottoms S, Farag A, Mammen E. Increased intravascular coagulation associated with pregnancy. *Obstet Gynecol.* 1990;75:385–389.

13. Gerbasi FR, Bottoms S, Farag A, Mammen EF. Changes in hemostasis activity during delivery and the immediate postpartum period. *Am J Obstet Gynecol.* 1990;162:1158–1163.

14. D'Alton ME, Friedman AM, Smiley RM, et al. National Partnership for Maternal Safety: consensus bundle on venous thromboembolism. *Anesth Analg.* 2016;123:942–949.

15. American College of Obstetricians and Gynecologists Practice Bulletin No. 196: Thromboembolism in pregnancy (reaffirmed 2025). *Obstet Gynecol.* 2018;132:e1–e17.

16. James AH, Jamison MG, Brancazio LR, Myers ER. Venous thromboembolism during pregnancy and the postpartum period: incidence, risk factors, and mortality. *Am J Obstet Gynecol.* 2006;194:1311–1315.

17. American College of Obstetricians and Gynecologists Practice Bulletin No. 197: Inherited thrombophilias in pregnancy (reaffirmed 2025). *Obstet Gynecol.* 2018;132:e18–e34.

18. Friedman AM, Ananth CV, Prendergast E, et al. Thromboembolism incidence and prophylaxis during vaginal delivery hospitalizations. *Am J Obstet Gynecol.* 2015;212:e1–e12.

19. Tepper NK, Boulet SL, Whiteman MK, et al. Postpartum venous thromboembolism: incidence and risk factors. *Obstet Gynecol.* 2014;123:987–996.

20. Blondon M, Casini A, Hoppe KK, et al. Risks of venous thromboembolism after cesarean sections: a meta-analysis. *Chest.* 2016;150:572–596.

21. Macklon NS, Greer IA. Venous thromboembolic disease in obstetrics and gynaecology: the Scottish experience. *Scott Med J.* 1996;41:83–86.

22. Elgendy IY, Fogerty A, Blanco-Molina Á, et al. Clinical characteristics and outcomes of women presenting with venous thromboembolism during pregnancy and postpartum period: findings from the RIETE registry. *Thromb Haemost.* 2020;120:1454–1462.

23. Chan WS, Spencer FA, Ginsberg JS. Anatomic distribution of deep vein thrombosis in pregnancy. *CMAJ.* 2010;182:657–660.

24. Chan WS, Spencer FA, Lee AY, et al. Safety of withholding anticoagulation in pregnant women with suspected deep vein thrombosis following negative serial compression ultrasound and iliac vein imaging. *CMAJ.* 2013;185:E194–E200.

25. Yamada T, Kawaguchi S, Araki N, et al. Difference in the D-dimer rise between women with singleton and multifetal pregnancies. *Thromb Res.* 2013;131:493–496.

26. Kovac M, Mikovic Z, Rakicevic L, et al. The use of D-dimer with new cutoff can be useful in diagnosis of venous thromboembolism in pregnancy. *Eur J Obstet Gynecol Reprod Biol.* 2010;148:27–30.

27. Hu W, Wang Y, Li J, et al. The predictive value of D-dimer test for venous thromboembolism during puerperium: a prospective cohort study. *Clin Appl Thromb Hemost.* 2020;26:1076029620901786.

28. Leung AN, Bull TM, Jaeschke R, et al. An official American Thoracic Society/Society of Thoracic Radiology clinical practice guideline: evaluation of suspected pulmonary embolism in pregnancy. *Am J Respir Crit Care Med.* 2011;184:1200–1208.

29. Stein PD, Beemath A, Matta F, et al. Clinical characteristics of patients with acute pulmonary embolism: data from PIOPED II. *Am J Med.* 2007;120:871–879.

30. Piazza G, Goldhaber SZ. Acute pulmonary embolism: part I: epidemiology and diagnosis. *Circulation.* 2006;114:e28–e32.

31. Stratmann G, Gregory GA. Neurogenic and humoral vasoconstriction in acute pulmonary thromboembolism. *Anesth Analg.* 2003;97:341–354.

32. Tsang JY, Hogg JC. Gas exchange and pulmonary hypertension following acute pulmonary thromboembolism: has the emperor got some new clothes yet? *Pulm Circ.* 2014;4:220–236.

33. Wood KE. Major pulmonary embolism. *Crit Care Clin.* 2011;27:885–906.

34. Stein PD, Goldhaber SZ, Henry JW, Miller AC. Arterial blood gas analysis in the assessment of suspected acute pulmonary embolism. *Chest.* 1996;109:78–81.

35. Kurnicka K, Lichodziejewska B, Goliszek S, et al. Echocardiographic pattern of acute pulmonary embolism: analysis of 511 consecutive patients. *J Am Soc Echocardiogr.* 2016;29:907–913.

36. Cahill AG, Stout MJ, Macones GA, Bhalla S. Diagnosing pulmonary embolism in pregnancy using computed-tomographic angiography or ventilation-perfusion. *Obstet Gynecol.* 2009;114:124–129.

37. Forbes KP, Reid JH, Murchison JT. Do preliminary chest X-ray findings define the optimum role of pulmonary scintigraphy in suspected pulmonary embolism? *Clin Radiol.* 2001;56:397–400.

38. Winterstein AG, Thai TN, Nduaguba S, et al. Risk of fetal or neonatal death or neonatal intensive care unit admission associated with gadolinium magnetic resonance imaging exposure during pregnancy. *Am J Obstet Gynecol.* 2023;228:465.e1–e11.

39. U.S. Food & Drug Administration. Gadolinium-based contrast agents for MRI: safety in pregnancy. https://www.fda.gov/drugs/regulatory-science-action/gadolinium-based-contrast-agents-mri-safety-pregnancy. Accessed November 20, 2024.

40. Gutte H, Mortensen J, Jensen CV, et al. Detection of pulmonary embolism with combined ventilation-perfusion SPECT and low-dose CT: head-to-head comparison with multidetector CT angiography. *J Nucl Med.* 2009;50:1987–1992.

41. Sostman HD, Miniati M, Gottschalk A, et al. Sensitivity and specificity of perfusion scintigraphy combined with chest radiography for acute pulmonary embolism in PIOPED II. *J Nucl Med.* 2008;49:1741–1748.

42. Bhatia KD, Ambati C, Dhaliwal R, et al. SPECT-CT/VQ versus CTPA for diagnosing pulmonary embolus and other lung pathology: pre-existing lung disease should not be a contraindication. *J Med Imaging Radiat Oncol*. 2016;60: 492–497.

43. Bajc M, Olsson B, Gottsäter A, et al. V/P SPECT as a diagnostic tool for pregnant women with suspected pulmonary embolism. *Eur J Nucl Med Mol Imaging*. 2015;42:1325–1330.

44. Baysinger CL. Imaging during pregnancy. *Anesth Analg*. 2010;110:863–867.

45. Bhalla S, Lopez-Costa I. MDCT of acute thrombotic and nonthrombotic pulmonary emboli. *Eur J Radiol*. 2007;64: 54–64.

46. Grüning T, Mingo RE, Gosling MG, et al. Diagnosing venous thromboembolism in pregnancy. *Br J Radiol*. 2016;89:20160021.

47. Righini M, Robert-Ebadi H, Elias A, et al. Diagnosis of pulmonary embolism during pregnancy: a multicenter prospective management outcome study. *Ann Intern Med*. 2018;169:766–773.

48. van der Pol LM, Tromeur C, Bistervels IM, et al. Pregnancy-adapted YEARS algorithm for diagnosis of suspected pulmonary embolism. *N Engl J Med*. 2019;380:1139–1149.

49. Bates SM, Greer IA, Middeldorp S, et al. VTE, thrombophilia, antithrombotic therapy, and pregnancy: antithrombotic therapy and prevention of thrombosis, 9th ed: American College of Chest Physicians Evidence-Based Clinical Practice Guidelines. *Chest*. 2012;141:e691S–e736S.

50. Royal College of Obstetricians and Gynaecologists. Thrombosis and embolism during pregnancy and the puerperium: acute management (Green-top guideline No. 37b). https://www.rcog.org.uk/en/guidelines-research-services/guidelines/gtg37b/. Accessed September 30, 2024.

51. Bates SM, Rajasekhar A, Middeldorp S, et al. American Society of Hematology 2018 guidelines for management of venous thromboembolism: venous thromboembolism in the context of pregnancy. *Blood Adv*. 2018;2:3317–3359.

52. Casele H, Grobman WA. Cost-effectiveness of thromboprophylaxis with intermittent pneumatic compression at cesarean delivery. *Obstet Gynecol*. 2006;108:535–540.

53. Brady MA, Carroll AW, Cheang KI, et al. Sequential compression device compliance in postoperative obstetrics and gynecology patients. *Obstet Gynecol*. 2015;125:19–25.

54. Lameijer H, Aalberts JJJ, van Veldhuisen DJ, et al. Efficacy and safety of direct oral anticoagulants during pregnancy; a systematic literature review. *Thromb Res*. 2018;169: 123–127.

55. Cutts BA, Dasgupta D, Hunt BJ. New directions in the diagnosis and treatment of pulmonary embolism in pregnancy. *Am J Obstet Gynecol*. 2013;208:102–108.

56. Greer IA, Nelson-Piercy C. Low-molecular-weight heparins for thromboprophylaxis and treatment of venous thromboembolism in pregnancy: a systematic review of safety and efficacy. *Blood*. 2005;106:401–407.

57. Bistervels IM, Buchmüller A, Wiegers HMG, et al. Intermediate-dose versus low-dose low-molecular-weight heparin in pregnant and post-partum women with a history of venous thromboembolism (Highlow study): an open-label, multicentre, randomised, controlled trial. *Lancet*. 2022;400:1777–1787.

58. Sephton V, Farquharson RG, Topping J, et al. A longitudinal study of maternal dose response to low molecular weight heparin in pregnancy. *Obstet Gynecol*. 2003;101:1307–1311.

59. Carroll RC, Craft RM, Whitaker GL, et al. Thrombelastography monitoring of resistance to enoxaparin anticoagulation in thrombophilic pregnancy patients. *Thromb Res*. 2007;120:367–370.

60. Barbour LA, Smith JM, Marlar RA. Heparin levels to guide thromboembolism prophylaxis during pregnancy. *Am J Obstet Gynecol*. 1995;173:1869–1873.

61. Brancazio LR, Roperti KA, Stierer R, Laifer SA. Pharmacokinetics and pharmacodynamics of subcutaneous heparin during the early third trimester of pregnancy. *Am J Obstet Gynecol*. 1995;173:1240–1245.

62. Kearon C, Akl EA, Ornelas J, et al. Antithrombotic therapy for VTE disease: CHEST guideline and expert panel report. *Chest*. 2016;149:315–352.

63. Bistervels IM, Buchmüller A, Tardy B. Inferior vena cava filters in pregnancy: safe or sorry? *Front Cardiovasc Med*. 2022;9:1026002.

64. Kopp SL, Vandermeulen RD, McBane RD, Perlas A, Leffert L, Horlocker T. Regional anesthesia in the patient receiving antithrombotic or thrombolytic therapy: American Society of Regional Anesthesia and Pain Medicine evidence-based guidelines (fifth edition). *Reg Anesth Pain Med*. 2025;Epub ahead of print Jan 29. https://doi.org/10.1136/rapm-2024-105766.

65. Leffert L, Butwick A, Carvalho B, et al. The Society for Obstetric Anesthesia and Perinatology consensus statement on the anesthetic management of pregnant and postpartum women receiving thromboprophylaxis or higher dose anticoagulants. *Anesth Analg*. 2018;126:928–944.

66. Ruppen W, Derry S, McQuay H, Moore RA. Incidence of epidural hematoma, infection, and neurologic injury in obstetric patients with epidural analgesia/anesthesia. *Anesthesiology*. 2006;105:394–399.

67. D'Angelo R, Smiley RM, Riley ET, Segal S. Serious complications related to obstetric anesthesia: the Serious Complication Repository Project of the Society for Obstetric Anesthesia and Perinatology. *Anesthesiology*. 2014;120:1505–1512.

68. Leffert LR, Dubois HM, Butwick AJ, et al. Neuraxial anesthesia in obstetric patients receiving thromboprophylaxis with unfractionated or low-molecular-weight heparin: a systematic review of spinal epidural hematoma. *Anesth Analg*. 2017;125:223–231.

69. Jea A, Moza K, Levi AD, Vanni S. Spontaneous spinal epidural hematoma during pregnancy: case report and literature review. *Neurosurgery*. 2005;56:E1156.

70. Bos EME, Haumann J, de Quelerij M, et al. Haematoma and abscess after neuraxial anaesthesia: a review of 647 cases. *Br J Anaesth*. 2018;120:693–704.

71. Lawton MT, Porter RW, Heiserman JE, et al. Surgical management of spinal epidural hematoma: relationship between surgical timing and neurological outcome. *J Neurosurg*. 1995;83:1–7.

72. Cheney FW, Domino KB, Caplan RA, Posner KL. Nerve injury associated with anesthesia: a closed claims analysis. *Anesthesiology*. 1999;90:1062–1069.

73. Meyer J. Embolia pulmonar amnio-caseosa. *Bras Med*. 1926;2:301–303.

74. Steiner PE, Lushbaugh CC. Maternal pulmonary embolism by amniotic fluid as a cause of obstetric shock and unexpected deaths in obstetrics. *JAMA*. 1941;117:1245–1254.

75. Main EK, McCain CL, Morton CH, et al. Pregnancy-related mortality in California: causes, characteristics, and improvement opportunities. *Obstet Gynecol.* 2015;125:938–947.

76. Clark SL, Romero R, Dildy GA, et al. Proposed diagnostic criteria for the case definition of amniotic fluid embolism in research studies. *Am J Obstet Gynecol.* 2016;215:408–412.

77. Stafford IA, Moaddab A, Dildy GA, et al. Evaluation of proposed criteria for research reporting of amniotic fluid embolism. *Am J Obstet Gynecol.* 2019;220:285–287.

78. Fitzpatrick KE, van den Akker T, Bloemenkamp KWM, et al. Risk factors, management, and outcomes of amniotic fluid embolism: a multicountry, population-based cohort and nested case-control study. *PLoS Med.* 2019;16:e1002962.

79. Knight M, Tuffnell D, Brocklehurst P, et al. Incidence and risk factors for amniotic-fluid embolism. *Obstet Gynecol.* 2010;115:910–917.

80. Kanayama N, Tamura N. Amniotic fluid embolism: pathophysiology and new strategies for management. *J Obstet Gynaecol Res.* 2014;40:1507–1517.

81. Kobayashi H, Akasaka J, Naruse K, et al. Comparison of the different definition criteria for the diagnosis of amniotic fluid embolism. *J Clin Diagn Res.* 2017;11:QC18–QC21.

82. Bonnet MP, Zlotnik D, Saucedo M, et al. Maternal death due to amniotic fluid embolism: a national study in France. *Anesth Analg.* 2018;126:175–182.

83. Mazza GR, Youssefzadeh AC, Klar M, et al. Association of pregnancy characteristics and maternal mortality with amniotic fluid embolism. *JAMA Netw Open.* 2022;5:e2242842.

84. Knight M, Berg C, Brocklehurst P, et al. Amniotic fluid embolism incidence, risk factors and outcomes: a review and recommendations. *BMC Pregnancy Childbirth.* 2012;12:7.

85. Fitzpatrick KE, Tuffnell D, Kurinczuk JJ, Knight M. Incidence, risk factors, management and outcomes of amniotic-fluid embolism: a population-based cohort and nested case-control study. *BJOG.* 2016;123:100–109.

86. Abenhaim HA, Azoulay L, Kramer MS, Leduc L. Incidence and risk factors of amniotic fluid embolisms: a population-based study on 3 million births in the United States. *Am J Obstet Gynecol.* 2008;199:49.e1–e8.

87. Clark SL, Hankins GD, Dudley DA, et al. Amniotic fluid embolism: analysis of the national registry. *Am J Obstet Gynecol.* 1995;172:1158–1167.

88. Kramer MS, Rouleau J, Liu S, et al. Amniotic fluid embolism: incidence, risk factors, and impact on perinatal outcome. *BJOG.* 2012;119:874–879.

89. Kramer MS, Rouleau J, Baskett TF, Joseph KS. Amniotic-fluid embolism and medical induction of labour: a retrospective, population-based cohort study. *Lancet.* 2006;368:1444–1448.

90. Stafford IA, Moaddab A, Dildy GA, et al. Amniotic fluid embolism syndrome: analysis of the Unites States International Registry. *Am J Obstet Gynecol MFM.* 2020;2:100083.

91. Paul RH, Koh KS, Bernstein SG. Changes in fetal heart rate-uterine contraction patterns associated with eclampsia. *Am J Obstet Gynecol.* 1978;130:165–169.

92. Clark SL. Amniotic fluid embolism. *Obstet Gynecol.* 2014;123:337–348.

93. Leong AS, Norman JE, Smith R. Vascular and myometrial changes in the human uterus at term. *Reprod Sci.* 2008;15:59–65.

94. Kuhlman K, Hidvegi D, Tamura RK, Depp R. Is amniotic fluid material in the central circulation of peripartum patients pathologic? *Am J Perinatol.* 1985;2:295–299.

95. Clark SL, Pavlova Z, Greenspoon J, et al. Squamous cells in the maternal pulmonary circulation. *Am J Obstet Gynecol.* 1986;154:104–106.

96. Hankins GD, Snyder R, Dinh T, et al. Documentation of amniotic fluid embolism via lung histopathology. Fact or fiction? *J Reprod Med.* 2002;47:1021–1024.

97. Clark SL. Amniotic fluid embolism. *Clin Obstet Gynecol.* 2010;53:322–328.

98. Azegami M, Mori N. Amniotic fluid embolism and leukotrienes. *Am J Obstet Gynecol.* 1986;155:1119–1124.

99. Benson MD, Kobayashi H, Silver RK, et al. Immunologic studies in presumed amniotic fluid embolism. *Obstet Gynecol.* 2001;97:510–514.

100. Benson MD. Current concepts of immunology and diagnosis in amniotic fluid embolism. *Clin Dev Immunol.* 2012;2012:946576.

101. Tamura N, Kimura S, Farhana M, et al. C1 esterase inhibitor activity in amniotic fluid embolism. *Crit Care Med.* 2014;42:1392–1396.

102. Benson MD. A hypothesis regarding complement activation and amniotic fluid embolism. *Med Hypotheses.* 2007;68:1019–1025.

103. Oikonomopoulou K, Ricklin D, Ward PA, Lambris JD. Interactions between coagulation and complement—their role in inflammation. *Semin Immunopathol.* 2012;34:151–165.

104. Harnett MJ, Hepner DL, Datta S, Kodali BS. Effect of amniotic fluid on coagulation and platelet function in pregnancy: an evaluation using thromboelastography. *Anaesthesia.* 2005;60:1068–1072.

105. Oda T, Tamura N, Shen Y, et al. Amniotic fluid as a potent activator of blood coagulation and platelet aggregation: study with rotational thromboelastometry. *Thromb Res.* 2018;172:142–149.

106. Lockwood CJ, Bach R, Guha A, et al. Amniotic fluid contains tissue factor, a potent initiator of coagulation. *Am J Obstet Gynecol.* 1991;165:1335–1341.

107. Zhou J, Liu S, Ma M, et al. Procoagulant activity and phosphatidylserine of amniotic fluid cells. *Thromb Haemost.* 2009;101:845–851.

108. Courtney LD, Allington M. Effect of amniotic fluid on blood coagulation. *Br J Haematol.* 1972;22:353–355.

109. Society for Maternal-Fetal Medicine, Pacheco LD, Saade G, et al. Amniotic fluid embolism: diagnosis and management. *Am J Obstet Gynecol.* 2016;215:B16–B24.

110. Schröder L, Hellmund A, Gembruch U, Merz WM. Amniotic fluid embolism-associated coagulopathy: a single-center observational study. *Arch Gynecol Obstet.* 2020;301:923–929.

111. Oliver C, Freyer J, Murdoch M, et al. A description of the coagulopathy characteristics in amniotic fluid embolism: a case report. *Int J Obstet Anesth.* 2022;51:103573.

112. Cromey MG, Taylor PJ, Cumming DC. Probable amniotic fluid embolism after first-trimester pregnancy termination. A case report. *J Reprod Med.* 1983;28:209–211.

113. Olcott C, Robinson AJ, Maxwell TM, Griffin HA. Amniotic fluid embolism and disseminated intravascular coagulation after blunt abdominal trauma. *J Trauma.* 1973;13:737–740.

114. Skolnik S, Ioscovich A, Eidelman LA, et al. Anesthetic management of amniotic fluid embolism—a multi-center,

retrospective, cohort study. *J Matern Fetal Neonatal Med.* 2017:1–5.

115. Wiseman D, Simard C, Yang SS, et al. Echocardiography findings in amniotic fluid embolism: a systematic review of the literature. *Can J Anaesth.* 2025;70:151–160.

116. Bernstein SN, Cudemus-Deseda GA, Ortiz VE, et al. Case 33-2019: a 35-year-old woman with cardiopulmonary arrest during cesarean section. *N Engl J Med.* 2019;381:1664–1673.

117. Acker LC, Jones RC, Rasouli MR, Bronshteyn YS. Focused cardiac ultrasound during amniotic fluid embolism. *Anesthesiology.* 2019;130:1032–1033.

118. Stanten RD, Iverson LI, Daugharty TM, et al. Amniotic fluid embolism causing catastrophic pulmonary vasoconstriction: diagnosis by transesophageal echocardiogram and treatment by cardiopulmonary bypass. *Obstet Gynecol.* 2003;102:496–498.

119. Shechtman M, Ziser A, Markovits R, Rozenberg B. Amniotic fluid embolism: early findings of transesophageal echocardiography. *Anesth Analg.* 1999;89:1456–1458.

120. Hurwich M, Zimmer D, Guerra E, et al. A case of successful thromboelastographic guided resuscitation after postpartum hemorrhage and cardiac arrest. *J Extra Corpor Technol.* 2016;48:194–197.

121. Loughran JA, Kitchen TL, Sindhakar S, et al. Rotational thromboelastometry (ROTEM®)-guided diagnosis and management of amniotic fluid embolism. *Int J Obstet Anesth.* 2019;38:127–130.

122. Annecke T, Geisenberger T, Kurzl R, et al. Algorithm-based coagulation management of catastrophic amniotic fluid embolism. *Blood Coagul Fibrinolysis.* 2010;21:95–100.

123. Collins NF, Bloor M, McDonnell NJ. Hyperfibrinolysis diagnosed by rotational thromboelastometry in a case of suspected amniotic fluid embolism. *Int J Obstet Anesth.* 2013;22:71–76.

124. Tanaka H, Katsuragi S, Osato K, et al. Value of fibrinogen in cases of maternal death related to amniotic fluid embolism. *J Matern Fetal Neonatal Med.* 2017;30:2940–2943.

125. Fudaba M, Tachibana D, Misugi T, et al. Excessive fibrinolysis detected with thromboelastography in a case of amniotic fluid embolism: fibrinolysis may precede coagulopathy. *J Thromb Thrombolysis.* 2021;51:818–820.

126. de Lloyd L, Jenkins PV, Bell SF, et al. Acute obstetric coagulopathy during postpartum hemorrhage is caused by hyperfibrinolysis and dysfibrinogenemia: an observational cohort study. *J Thromb Haemost.* 2023;21:862–879.

127. Oda T, Tamura N, Ide R, et al. Consumptive coagulopathy involving amniotic fluid embolism: the importance of earlier assessments for interventions in critical care. *Crit Care Med.* 2020;48:e1251–e1259.

128. McCall SJ, Bunch KJ, Brocklehurst P, et al. The incidence, characteristics, management and outcomes of anaphylaxis in pregnancy: a population-based descriptive study. *BJOG.* 2018;125:965–971.

129. Hopkins PM, Cooke PJ, Clarke RC, et al. Consensus clinical scoring for suspected perioperative immediate hypersensitivity reactions. *Br J Anaesth.* 2019;123:e29–e37.

130. Lee W, Ginsburg KA, Cotton DB, Kaufman RH. Squamous and trophoblastic cells in the maternal pulmonary circulation identified by invasive hemodynamic monitoring during the peripartum period. *Am J Obstet Gynecol.* 1986;155:999–1001.

131. Busardo FP, Frati P, Zaami S, Fineschi V. Amniotic fluid embolism pathophysiology suggests the new diagnostic armamentarium: beta-tryptase and complement fractions C3-C4 are the indispensable working tools. *Int J Mol Sci.* 2015;16:6557–6570.

132. Rutanen EM, Bohn H, Seppälä M. Radioimmunoassay of placental protein 12: levels in amniotic fluid, cord blood, and serum of healthy adults, pregnant women, and patients with trophoblastic disease. *Am J Obstet Gynecol.* 1982;144:460–463.

133. Legrand M, Rossignol M, Dreux S, et al. Diagnostic accuracy of insulin-like growth factor binding protein-1 for amniotic fluid embolism. *Crit Care Med.* 2012;40:2059–2063.

134. Bouvet L, Gariel C, Charvet A, et al. Contribution of blood detection of insulin-like growth factor binding protein-1 for the diagnosis of amniotic-fluid embolism: a retrospective multicentre cohort study. *BJOG.* 2021;128:1966–1973.

135. Clark SL. A biomarker for amniotic fluid embolism: the search continues. *BJOG.* 2021;128:1974.

136. Kanayama N, Yamazaki T, Naruse H, et al. Determining zinc coproporphyrin in maternal plasma—a new method for diagnosing amniotic fluid embolism. *Clin Chem.* 1992;38:526–529.

137. Koike N, Oi H, Naruse K, et al. Squamous cell carcinoma antigen as a novel candidate marker for amniotic fluid embolism. *J Obstet Gynaecol Res.* 2017;43:1815–1820.

138. Fineschi V, Gambassi R, Gherardi M, Turillazzi E. The diagnosis of amniotic fluid embolism: an immunohistochemical study for the quantification of pulmonary mast cell tryptase. *Int J Legal Med.* 1998;111:238–243.

139. Panchal AR, Bartos JA, Cabanas JG, et al. Part 3: adult basic and advanced life support: 2020 American Heart Association guidelines for cardiopulmonary resuscitation and emergency cardiovascular care. *Circulation.* 2020;142:S366–S468.

140. Lipman S, Daniels K, Cohen SE, Carvalho B. Labor room setting compared with the operating room for simulated perimortem cesarean delivery: a randomized controlled trial. *Obstet Gynecol.* 2011;118:1090–1094.

141. Lipman SS, Wong JY, Arafeh J, et al. Transport decreases the quality of cardiopulmonary resuscitation during simulated maternal cardiac arrest. *Anesth Analg.* 2013;116:162–167.

142. Combs CA, Montgomery DM, Toner LE, Dildy GA. Society for Maternal-Fetal Medicine Special Statement: checklist for initial management of amniotic fluid embolism. *Am J Obstet Gynecol.* 2021;224:B29–B32.

143. Pacheco LD, Clark SL, Klassen M, Hankins GDV. Amniotic fluid embolism: principles of early clinical management. *Am J Obstet Gynecol.* 2020;222:48–52.

144. Woman Trial Collaborators. Effect of early tranexamic acid administration on mortality, hysterectomy, and other morbidities in women with post-partum haemorrhage (WOMAN): an international, randomised, double-blind, placebo-controlled trial. *Lancet.* 2017;389:2105–2116.

145. Leighton BL, Wall MH, Lockhart EM, et al. Use of recombinant factor VIIa in patients with amniotic fluid embolism: a systematic review of case reports. *Anesthesiology.* 2011;115:1201–1208.

146. Centers for Disease Control and Prevention. Pregnancy Mortality Surveillance System; 2023. [updated March 23, 2023]. https://www.cdc.gov/reproductivehealth/maternal-mortality/pregnancy-mortality-surveillance-system.htm#causes. Accessed June 15, 2023.

147. Petersen EE, Davis NL, Goodman D, et al. Vital signs: pregnancy-related deaths, United States, 2011–2015, and strategies for prevention, 13 states, 2013–2017. *MMWR Morb Mortal Wkly Rep.* 2019;68:423–429.

148. Creanga AA, Syverson C, Seed K, Callaghan WM. Pregnancy-related mortality in the United States, 2011–2013. *Obstet Gynecol.* 2017;130:366–373.

149. Howell EA, Brown H, Brumley J, et al. Reduction of peripartum racial and ethnic disparities: a conceptual framework and maternal safety consensus bundle. *Obstet Gynecol.* 2018;131:770–782.

150. Moaddab A, Klassen M, Priester CD, et al. Reproductive decisions after the diagnosis of amniotic fluid embolism. *Eur J Obstet Gynecol Reprod Biol.* 2017;211:33–36.

151. Cahan T, Castro HD, Kalter A, Simchen MJ. Amniotic fluid embolism—implementation of international diagnosis criteria and subsequent pregnancy recurrence risk. *J Perinat Med.* 2021;49:546–552.

152. Mirski MA, Lele AV, Fitzsimmons L, Toung TJ. Diagnosis and treatment of vascular air embolism. *Anesthesiology.* 2007;106:164–177.

153. Handler JS, Bromage PR. Venous air embolism during cesarean delivery. *Reg Anesth Pain Med.* 1990;15:170–173.

154. Vartikar JV, Johnson MD, Datta S. Precordial Doppler monitoring and pulse oximetry during cesarean delivery: detection of venous air embolism. *Reg Anesth.* 1989;14:145–148.

155. Fong J, Gadalla F, Pierri MK, Druzin M. Are Doppler-detected venous emboli during cesarean section air emboli? *Anesth Analg.* 1990;71:254–257.

156. Lew TW, Tay DH, Thomas E. Venous air embolism during cesarean section: more common than previously thought. *Anesth Analg.* 1993;77:448–452.

157. Cluver C, Novikova N, Hofmeyr GJ, Hall DR. Maternal position during caesarean section for preventing maternal and neonatal complications. *Cochrane Database Syst Rev.* 2013;(3):CD007623.

158. Nelson PK. Pulmonary gas embolism in pregnancy and the puerperium. *Obstet Gynecol Surv.* 1960;15:449–481.

159. Epps SN, Robbins AJ, Marx GF. Complete recovery after near-fatal venous air embolism during cesarean section. *Int J Obstet Anesth.* 1998;7:131–133.

160. Karuparthy VR, Downing JW, Husain FJ, et al. Incidence of venous air embolism during cesarean section is unchanged by the use of a 5 to 10 degree head-up tilt. *Anesth Analg.* 1989;69:620–623.

161. Mathew JP, Fleisher LA, Rinehouse JA, et al. ST segment depression during labor and delivery. *Anesthesiology.* 1992;77:635–641.

162. Svanström MC, Biber B, Hanes M, et al. Signs of myocardial ischaemia after injection of oxytocin: a randomized double-blind comparison of oxytocin and methylergometrine during Caesarean section. *Br J Anaesth.* 2008;100:683–689.

163. Geissler HJ, Allen SJ, Mehlhorn U, et al. Effect of body repositioning after venous air embolism. An echocardiographic study. *Anesthesiology.* 1997;86:710–717.

164. Blanc P, Boussuges A, Henriette K, et al. Iatrogenic cerebral air embolism: importance of an early hyperbaric oxygenation. *Intensive Care Med.* 2002;28:559–563.

39

Maternal Mortality

Jill M. Mhyre, MD and David G. Bishop, MD, PhD, FCA

CHAPTER OUTLINE

GLOBAL MATERNAL MORTALITY

Globally, in 2023, an estimated 260,000 women died while pregnant or within 42 days of the end of pregnancy, equivalent to approximately one maternal death every 2 minutes (see Chapter 15).[1] This number corresponds to a ratio of 197 (80% uncertainty interval [UI], 174 to 234) maternal deaths per 100,000 live births and to a 1-in-272 lifetime risk for pregnancy-related death for a 15-year-old girl (Table 39.1).[1] According to the World Health Organization (WHO), "No issue is more central to global well-being than maternal and perinatal health. Every individual, every family and every community is at some point intimately involved in pregnancy and the success of childbirth."[2]

Definitions for terms used to measure maternal death are listed in Table 39.2, and measures of maternal mortality are listed in Table 39.3. More than 99% of maternal deaths occur in low- and middle-income countries (LMICs), with 87% in either sub-Saharan Africa or South Asia. Between 2000 and 2015,[3] the global **maternal mortality ratio (MMR)** fell by 33%, an impressive improvement, but less than the 75% reduction targeted by the United Nations Millennium Development Goals. In 2015 the United Nations issued 17 Sustainable Development Goals (SDGs), including a commitment to reduce the global MMR to less than 70 per 100,000 live births by 2030, with no single country having an MMR > 140. During the first 5 years of the SDG era, the MMR remained almost unchanged.[1] The average annual rate of reduction (ARR) in global MMR between 2000 and 2015 was 2.7% (80% UI, 2.0% to 3.2%), but between 2016 and 2020 this rate was −0.04% (80% UI, −1.6% to 1.1%), indicating a stagnation in the global MMR. To achieve the SDG target MMR of 70 per 100,000 births, an annual average ARR of 11.6% will be required over the next decade (2021 to 2030).[1]

Several regions still require substantial investment to meet this goal, most notably sub-Saharan Africa, where the lifetime risk for maternal death remains remarkably high, at 1 in 55 (MMR 454 per 100,000 births), compared with 1 in 21,248 in Australia and New Zealand (MMR 3 per 100,000 births).[1] There is considerable regional variation. Within sub-Saharan Africa, the highest MMRs in 2023 were in South Sudan (692 per 100,000 births), Central African Republic (692 per 100,000 births), Chad (748 per 100,000 births), and Nigeria (993 per 100,000 births),[1] and represent rates that are 10-fold higher than the lowest ratios in the region. Throughout the world, climate change, war, natural disaster, and political conflict can degrade health systems and trigger a rise in deaths caused by complications that would be treatable under stable conditions.[6]

Leading Causes

Hemorrhage, **hypertensive disorders of pregnancy**, and **sepsis** account for more than one-half of global maternal deaths and for slightly more than one-third of deaths in high-income countries (HICs) (Fig. 39.1).[7] Hemorrhage is the leading direct cause of maternal death worldwide, followed by hypertensive disorders, causing an estimated 27.1% and 14.0% of all deaths, respectively.[7] Infection and sepsis may be substantially underestimated in regions where laboratory diagnostic tests are unavailable.[8] In one Malawian hospital with full laboratory capabilities, infection played a primary role in almost three-fourths of all maternal deaths.[9]

Rarely, **anemia** can cause lethal congestive heart failure in pregnancy,[10] but more commonly, it increases the risk for maternal death from other complications, particularly hemorrhage and infection. Risk factors associated with anemia include (1) iron and other micronutrient deficiencies; (2) pregnancy interval < 1 year; (3) adolescent pregnancy; (4) hemoglobinopathy; (5) urinary tract infection; (6) human immunodeficiency virus (HIV) infection; (7) parasitic infections, including malaria; and (8) recurrent antepartum hemorrhage.[10–12]

TABLE 39.1   Estimates of Maternal Mortality Ratio, Number of Maternal Deaths, Lifetime Risk, and Proportion of Deaths Among Women of Reproductive Age That Are Due to Maternal Causes, by United Nations Sustainable Development Goal Region, Subregion and Other Grouping, 2020

SDG Region and Subregion[a]	MMR[b] POINT ESTIMATE AND RANGE OF 80% UI			Number of Maternal Deaths[c]	Lifetime Risk of Maternal Death (1 in)[d]	PM Point Estimate (%)
	Lower UI	Point Estimate	Upper UI			
World	174	197	234	260,000	272	8.9
Sub-Saharan Africa	387	454	572	182,000	55	16.9
Eastern Africa	223	263	317	42,000	93	14.1
Middle Africa	322	415	609	34,000	46	20.5
Southern Africa	113	137	159	1900	339	2.8
Western Africa	545	691	975	102,000	36	18.6
Northern Africa and Western Asia	61	78	105	9100	509	6.5
Northern Africa	72	101	146	5900	370	7.4
Western Asia	38	52	76	3000	807	5.0
Central and Southern Asia	97	112	134	44,000	410	6.0
Central Asia	17	21	28	410	1560	1.7
Southern Asia	101	117	140	43,000	399	6.2
Eastern and Southeastern Asia	53	65	88	13,000	1384	2.4
Eastern Asia	13	17	22	1800	7079	0.7
Southeastern Asia	89	114	158	12,000	501	3.9
Latin America and the Caribbean	68	77	88	7200	789	3.5
Caribbean	143	190	289	1200	296	7.8
Central America	42	49	55	1500	1063	2.5
South America	65	77	91	4400	842	3.3
Oceania (excluding Australia and New Zealand)	116	173	268	550	196	6.9
Melanesia	115	176	275	530	193	7.0
Micronesia	83	126	212	9	279	4.4
Polynesia	54	98	198	8	317	6.0
Australia and New Zealand	2	3	4	11	21,248	0.5
Europe and Northern America	9	11	12	1100	7410	0.5
Eastern Europe	7	9	12	210	10,302	0.3
Northern Europe	7		10	76	10,358	0.5
Southern Europe	5	6	7	66	16,139	0.5
Western Europe	5	5	6	96	14,337	0.5
Northern America	13	16	20	650	4322	0.8
Small island developing states	155	193	253	2300	260	8.2
Landlocked developing countries	244	284	343	50,000	95	14.8
Least developed countries	277	313	368	114,000	83	16.1

[a]The countries in each SDG regional grouping can be found at https://unstats.un.org/sdgs/indicators/regional-groups. Data are only included in this table for the 195 countries and territories that met the inclusion criteria for this analysis (193 WHO member states, Puerto Rico, and the occupied Palestinian territory).

[b]MMR (maternal deaths per 100,000 live births) estimates have been rounded to the nearest 1.

[c]Numbers of maternal deaths have been rounded according to the following scheme: <100 rounded to nearest 1; 100–999 rounded to nearest 10; 1000–9999 rounded to nearest 100; and ≥10,000 rounded to nearest 1000.

[d]Lifetime risk has been rounded according to the following scheme: <100 rounded to nearest 1; 100–999 rounded to nearest 10; 1000–9999 rounded to nearest 100; and ≥10,000 rounded to nearest 1000.

MMR, Maternal mortality ratio; *PM*, proportion of maternal deaths due to maternal causes; *SDG*, Sustainable Development Goal; *UI*, uncertainly interval.

Data summarized from World Health Organization. *Trends in Maternal Mortality 2020 to 2023: Estimates by WHO, UNICEF, UNFPA, World Bank Group and UNDESA/Population Division.* World Health Organization. https://www.who.int/publications/i/item/9789240108462. Accessed 16 June 2025.

TABLE 39.2   Glossary of Terms Used in Discussions of Maternal Mortality

Source	Term	Definition[a]
World Health Organization	Maternal death	Death of a woman while pregnant or within 42 d of termination of pregnancy, irrespective of the duration and site of the pregnancy, from any cause related to or aggravated by the pregnancy or its management, but not from accidental or incidental causes. ICD-10: A34, O00-O95, O98-O99[a] ICD-11: JB60, JB62-JB65, JB6Y, JB6Z[b]
	Direct maternal death	Death resulting from obstetric complications of the pregnant state (pregnancy, labor, and puerperium), and from interventions, omissions, incorrect treatment, or from a chain of events resulting from any of the above. ICD-10: A34, O00-O95[a] ICD-11: JB62[b]
	Indirect maternal death	Death resulting from previously existing disease or disease that developed during pregnancy, and that was not due to direct obstetric causes but was aggravated by the physiologic effects of pregnancy. ICD-10: O98-O99[a] ICD-11: JB63-JB64[b]
	Comprehensive maternal death	A grouping that combines maternal death and late maternal death. ICD-11: JB62-JB64[b]
	Late maternal death	Death of a woman from direct or indirect obstetric causes, more than 42 d but less than 1 y after termination of pregnancy. ICD-10: O96-O97[a] ICD-11: JB61[b]
US Centers for Disease Control and Prevention, Pregnancy Mortality Surveillance System[c]	Pregnancy-associated death	Death while pregnant or within 1 y of termination of pregnancy, irrespective of cause.
	Pregnancy-related death	Death while pregnant or within 1 y of termination of pregnancy, irrespective of the duration and site of the pregnancy, from any cause related to or aggravated by the pregnancy or its management, but not from accidental or incidental causes.
	Non–pregnancy-related death	Death while pregnant or within 1 y of termination of pregnancy, from a cause unrelated to pregnancy.

[a]ICD-10, International Statistical Classification of Diseases and Related Health Problems: 10th revision.
[b]ICD-11, International Statistical Classification of Diseases and Related Health Problems: 11th revision.
[c]From Berg CJ, Callaghan WM, Syverson C, Henderson Z. Pregnancy-related mortality in the United States, 1998 to 2005. *Obstet Gynecol.* 2010;116:1302–1309.

TABLE 39.3   Measures of Maternal Mortality

Maternal Mortality Measure	Definitions	Reports Using the Measure
Maternal mortality ratio	Direct and indirect maternal deaths, but not late maternal deaths, per 100,000 live births	WHO[1]
Maternal mortality rate (MMRate)	Direct and indirect maternal deaths, but not late maternal deaths, divided by person-years lived by women of reproductive age in a population. The MMRate captures both the risk of maternal death per pregnancy, and the level of fertility in the population.	UK CEMD[4]
Pregnancy-related mortality ratio	Pregnancy-related deaths per 100,000 live births	US CDC PMSS[5]
Lifetime risk for maternal death	The lifetime risk for maternal death takes into account both the probability of becoming pregnant and the probability of dying as a result of that pregnancy cumulated across a woman's reproductive years	

UK CEMD, The United Kingdom Confidential Enquiry into Maternal Death; *US CDC PMSS*, US Centers for Disease Control and Prevention Pregnancy Mortality Surveillance System; *WHO*, World Health Organization.

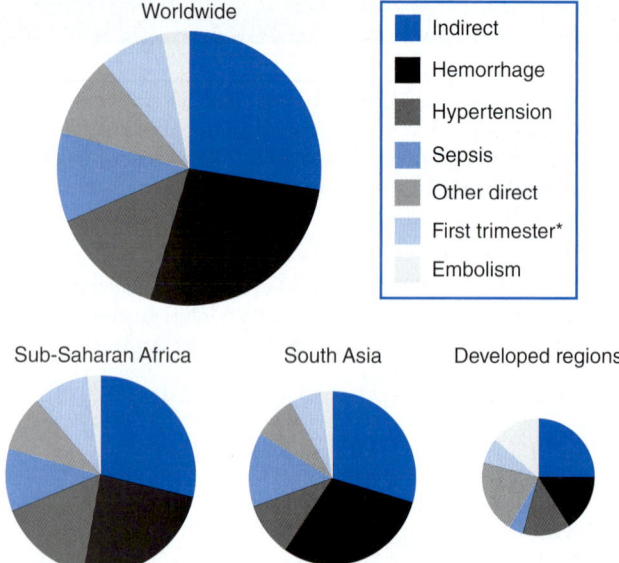

Fig. 39.1 Estimated Distribution for the Main Causes of Maternal Death Worldwide, and in Selected Regions. The relative size of each circle is illustrative but not directly proportional to the relative numbers of deaths in the three illustrated regions. *First-trimester deaths include those from induced abortion, miscarriage, and ectopic pregnancy. Data from Say L, Chou D, Gemmill, et al. Global causes of maternal death: a WHO systematic analysis. *Lancet Glob Health.* 2014;2:e323–e333.

Obstructed labor causes less than 10% of maternal deaths worldwide,[7] but it is an important cause of mortality in communities where early adolescent pregnancy is common, childhood malnutrition leads to small maternal pelvises, and operative delivery is unavailable.[13] Death from obstructed labor is largely the result of hemorrhage caused by uterine rupture or sepsis caused by ascending genital tract infection, and deaths may be coded under those categories.[13,14] Prolonged pressure on the pelvic outlet can lead to tissue necrosis and obstetric fistula, a complication that is thought to affect at least 2 million women worldwide.[15,16]

HIV/acquired immunodeficiency syndrome (AIDS) increases vulnerability to both nonobstetric infection (e.g., tuberculosis, malaria) and obstetric complications (e.g., pregnancy-related sepsis, septic abortion) (see Chapter 36).[17,18] Global mortality attributed to HIV/AIDS peaked in 2005 at 2.5%; by 2023 the WHO attributed approximately 0.5% of maternal deaths to HIV/AIDS.[1] In countries most severely affected (Botswana, Malawi, South Africa), the MMR increased between 1990 and 2000, but has subsequently declined with increasing availability of antiretroviral therapy.[3,6,18,19]

Deaths attributed to **unsafe abortion** account for 5% to 13% of maternal deaths worldwide.[7,20] Unsafe abortion is highest in countries with both restrictive laws and limited healthcare infrastructure.[21] Worldwide, 45% of abortions were unsafe between 2010 and 2014, compared with 44% in 1995.[22,23] Risk is highest in sub-Saharan Africa; between 2010 and 2014, 77% of the region's abortions were considered unsafe. Fortunately, increasing availability of medication abortion and postabortion care has improved abortion safety

over the past 20 years; the case-fatality rate has decreased from 315 to 185 maternal deaths per 100,000 abortions.[20,24] A WHO evidence-based protocol offers guidance for pregnant women less than 12 weeks' gestational age to manage their own medical abortions using mifepristone and misoprostol in combination or misoprostol alone.[25]

Early marriage (before 18 years of age) has been identified as a major health risk for girls, increasing their exposure to domestic violence, coercion, pregnancy, and sexually transmitted diseases such as HIV/AIDS.[26–28] Girls younger than 15 years of age are four times more likely to die in childbirth than women in their 20s,[29] and pregnancy is among the leading causes of death worldwide for girls 15 to 19 years of age.[30] Early childbearing also increases the likelihood of **high parity birth** (≥5) later in life. With a threefold increase in the MMR, high parity remains an important demographic risk for maternal death because it remains so common in countries with high maternal mortality rates.[31] **Advanced maternal age** is less common globally, but the MMR increases 3-fold by 35 years, 7-fold by 40 years, and 15-fold after 45 years of age.[32]

Cesarean delivery is the most common major surgical procedure in Africa,[33] but anesthesia providers working in LMICs often must contend with profound limitations in staffing, equipment, and other resources. Cesarean delivery rates should be approximately 15% to 20% to optimize maternal and neonatal outcomes,[34] but are less than 10% in more than half of African countries.[35] Low workforce density compounds resource deficiencies. An inflection point suggests that in settings with less than four specialist anesthesiologists per 100,000 population, maternal mortality increases dramatically.[36] Yet only five African countries have more than one physician anesthesia provider per 100,000 population.[37–42]

In addition, patients who labor at home may face a variety of social and environmental obstacles to reach a facility with the capacity to provide comprehensive emergency obstetric care,[43–45] and many arrive at these facilities in septic or hemorrhagic shock.[46–48] While complication rates following cesarean delivery are 2 to 3 times higher in LMICs, maternal mortality rates are 50 times higher than in HIC, indicating high rates of failure to rescue.[49]

Perioperative maternal mortality is estimated to be between 1.2% and 2%.[50–52] Based on a 2016 metaanalysis of studies that assessed anesthesia-related maternal death in LMICs, an estimated one in seven deaths associated with cesarean delivery is attributed to anesthesia.[53] Although general anesthesia is associated with a threefold increased risk for death compared with neuraxial anesthesia (5.9 per 1000 and 1.2 per 1000, respectively),[53] reports of high spinal anesthesia and hemodynamic collapse highlight potential hazards with neuraxial anesthesia.[53–55] Failed airway management (including bronchospasm and aspiration of gastric contents) accounts for three-quarters of anesthesia-related deaths reported from LMICs.[53] Peripartum deaths have also been attributed to limited availability or affordability of blood products,[47,50,56,57] cardiac arrest at induction of anesthesia, drug overdose, adverse medication reaction, and drug error.[53,58] The increased use of tranexamic acid for postpartum hemorrhage has led to an apparent increase in the number of cases of inadvertent intrathecal administration of tranexamic acid with planned spinal anesthesia, resulting in the release of a WHO drug safety alert.[59] Overall, the number of maternal perioperative deaths likely pales in comparison with maternal deaths that result from the unmet need for lifesaving obstetric procedures, including cesarean delivery.[60]

Strategies to reduce global maternal mortality include (1) improvement in family planning services and a reduction in the performance of an unsafe abortion[61,62]; (2) community-based education focused on safe birth practices and indications for transfer to a higher level of care[63,64]; and (3) development of the infrastructure needed to provide timely emergency obstetric care, including the performance of indicated cesarean delivery (and safe administration of anesthesia) by trained healthcare providers[65,66] who can also provide resuscitation of women in whom shock develops secondary to hemorrhage or infection.[67–71] Cluster randomized trials[72–74] and cost-effectiveness analyses[75,76] to evaluate these strategies are beginning to be published. When deployed as part of an integrated, context-specific, and culturally sensitive program,[68] interventions to reduce maternal and fetal mortality can be highly cost effective.[75,76]

MATERNAL MORTALITY IN HIGH-INCOME COUNTRIES

In HICs, the MMR decreased 57% from 23 per 100,000 births in 1990 to 10 (80% UI, 9 to 11) per 100,000 births in 2023.[1,6] The United States was the only HIC where the MMR increased over this time period.[6]

The most comprehensive maternal surveillance system in the world is the **Confidential Enquiry into Maternal Deaths (CEMD)** in the United Kingdom.[a] Triennial reports of CEMD in England and Wales extend back to 1952 and have included the entire United Kingdom since the 1985 to 1987 report. Since 2014, annual reports summarize overall mortality statistics and focus on specific clinical diagnoses on a rolling basis that covers all clinical conditions every 3 years. By government mandate, all maternal deaths are subject to this enquiry, and health professionals have a duty to provide all requested information.[77] Once a case is identified, practitioners are asked to provide (1) a full account of the circumstances leading up to the woman's death, (2) all supporting records, (3) any clinical or other lessons that have been learned, and (4) details of any actions that may have been taken as a result.[4,78] Regional assessors review the files

to ensure completeness before removing identifying information. Once data are complete, central assessors review the anonymized cases and produce the reports. The reports focus on both medical and nonmedical recommendations for action to improve safety for future pregnant women.

The CEMD reports include both the internationally defined MMR and the UK-defined maternal mortality rate (see Table 39.3).

National confidential enquiry reports are now published by many other countries, including France,[79] the Netherlands,[80] New Zealand,[81] and South Africa.[18]

In the United States, the **National Center for Health Statistics (NCHS)** has provided maternal death counts since 1900 and MMRs since 1915.[82] Accuracy is limited because (1) the system relies on death certificates rather than active surveillance, (2) the certification of death is the legal responsibility of individual states, and (3) the process of maternal death ascertainment varies by state.

The US MMR reported by the NCHS declined from more than 600 deaths per 100,000 live births in 1915 to fewer than 10 deaths per 100,000 live births by 1980 (Fig. 39.2).[82] Throughout the 1980s and 1990s, the MMR oscillated between 6.6 and 9.2 per 100,000 births. Then, in 1999, the MMR began to increase (Fig. 39.3).[83] Improvements in ascertainment explain some of the increase. In 1999 the *International Statistical Classification of Diseases and Related Health Problems, Tenth Revision* (ICD-10) replaced the ICD-9 as the coding system for US death certificates and liberalized the criteria by which pregnancy could be linked with death. Growing numbers of states perform electronic matches among women's death certificates, live birth certificates, and fetal death files. Perhaps most importantly, the 2003 revision of the US Standard Certificate of Death introduced questions about pregnancy status at the time of death (Box 39.1). Between 2003 and 2017, individual states implemented the new questions when revising their death certificates.[84] Staggered implementation allowed epidemiologists to estimate that the pregnancy checkbox identifies an additional 9.6 deaths per 100,000 live births, with greater increases noted for older women and non-Hispanic Black women.[84]

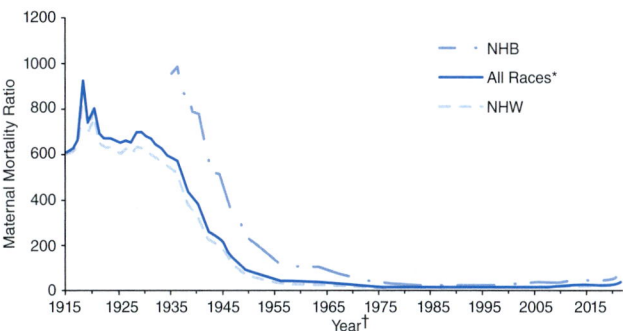

Fig. 39.2 US Maternal Mortality Ratios by Race, 1915–2021.[82,85] *Includes races other than White and Black. †For 1915–34, data on Black race were not available. *NHB*, Non-Hispanic Black; *NHW*, non-Hispanic White. Data are from the US Centers for Disease Control and Prevention. CDC Wonder. https://wonder.cdc.gov/. Accessed 5 October 2024.

---

[a]The Confidential Enquiry into Maternal Deaths has been overseen by a series of organizations in recent years, including the Confidential Enquiry into Maternal and Child Health (CEMACH), the Centre for Maternal and Child Enquiries (CMACE), and, currently, Mothers and Babies: Reducing Risk through Audits and Confidential Enquiries across the United Kingdom (MBRRACE-UK), led by the National Perinatal Epidemiology Unit (NPEU) at the University of Oxford (https://www.npeu.ox.ac.uk/mbrrace-uk).

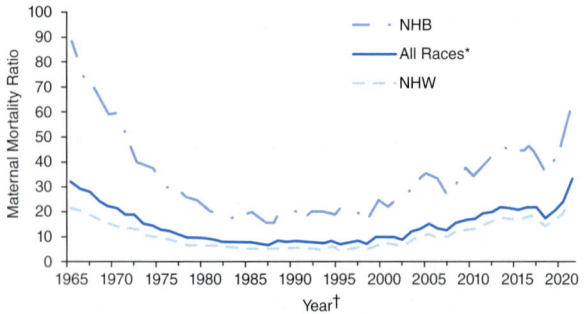

Fig. 39.3 US Maternal Mortality Ratios by Race, 1970–2021. *Includes races other than White and Black. †Beginning in 1989, race for live births tabulated according to race of mother, not child. *NHB*, Non-Hispanic Black; *NHW*, non-Hispanic White. Data are from the US Centers for Disease Control and Prevention. CDC Wonder. https://wonder.cdc.gov/. Accessed 5 October 2024.

BOX 39.1 Pregnancy Questions, US Standard Certificate of Death, 2003 Revision

If female:
- Not pregnant within the past year
- Pregnant at the time of death
- Not pregnant, but pregnant within 42 d of death
- Not pregnant, but pregnant 42 d to 1 y before death
- Unknown if pregnant within the past year

Reprinted from National Center for Health Statistics. United States Standard Certificate of Death—Rev. 11/2003. www.cdc.gov/nchs/data/dvs/DEATH11-03final-acc.pdf. Accessed 26 July 2025.

In 1987 the US Centers for Disease Control and Prevention (CDC) partnered with state health departments and the American College of Obstetricians and Gynecologists to form the **Pregnancy Mortality Surveillance System (PMSS)**.[5] To more completely capture maternal deaths, the PMSS recommended that states develop an active surveillance system and collect death certificates and matching live birth or fetal death certificates for all pregnancy-associated deaths (see Table 39.2). These certificates are forwarded to the CDC, where clinically experienced epidemiologists manually review the certificates to identify all pregnancy-related deaths (see Table 39.2). Similar surveillance enhancement procedures have been estimated to improve case ascertainment by between 22% and 93%.[86] The pregnancy-related mortality ratio includes deaths that occur up to 1 year after the end of pregnancy and, according to the PMSS, increased from 10.3 in 1991 to 18.7 in 2023.[87,88]

In response to an apparent doubling of the US MMR over two decades, a growing number of states have established maternal mortality review committees to analyze case records in detail and to publish recommendations to improve safety for future women. Ascertainment and review procedures vary by state,[89] so the CDC has created a national database to facilitate standardized review.[90,91] To move recommendations into practice, the US Alliance for Innovation on Maternal Health has partnered with state and regional healthcare collaboratives to identify and implement evidence-based practices and

systems solutions that will improve outcomes for the leading causes of maternal death.[92–94] Ongoing surveillance will determine whether these efforts are effective.

The MMR in the United States[83] soared in 2021 to 33.2 per 100,000 births,[88] likely due to the highly virulent coronavirus disease 2019 (COVID-2019) caused by the SARS-CoV-2 delta variant.[91] In particular, non-Hispanic Black American women were disproportionately affected. In 2021 the maternal mortality rate for non-Hispanic Black women was 69.9 deaths per 100,000 live births, 2.6 times the rate for non-Hispanic White women. With resolution of the COVID-19 pandemic, the MMR subsequently returned to levels consistent with a 2% annual increase between 1990 and 2023.[88]

The MMR in the United Kingdom was 10.9 deaths per 100,000 maternities between 2018 and 2020 (which included the first year of the COVID-19 pandemic), 24% higher than between 2017 and 2019. Excluding COVID-19 deaths, the MMR was 10.5 per 100,000 maternities, an increase of 19%. Ethnic minority groups remain disproportionately affected, although the disparity has decreased slightly; Black women were 3.7 times more likely to die than White women. Most women died in the postnatal period (86%), and maternal mental health factored into many of the deaths.

Leading Causes

According to a 2010 systematic review of data from HICs, **hypertensive disorders of pregnancy, embolic disorders**, and **hemorrhage** together account for 43% of maternal deaths in HICs (see Fig. 39.1).[7] **Indirect deaths** account for another 25%.[7]

Indirect deaths have exceeded direct deaths in the United Kingdom since 1997, with cardiac disease being the most common category of death. Similar patterns are seen in the United States, where the combination of cardiovascular conditions and cardiomyopathy comprised 20.6% of all pregnancy-related deaths in 2023, and cerebrovascular accidents and noncardiovascular medical conditions represented another 15.1%.[88] Cardiomyopathy, including both peripartum and other types of cardiomyopathy, is the leading diagnosis underlying maternal cardiac death in the United States. In the United Kingdom, sudden arrhythmia, ischemic cardiac disease, and cardiomyopathy are the leading causes of maternal cardiac death.[78]

Since 2015, psychiatric diseases have emerged in the United Kingdom, the United States, and France as a leading cause of death, equaling cardiac disease and cardiomyopathy in some reports.[77] In the United States, 36 state maternal mortality review committees following the standardized CDC review process identified the six most frequent underlying causes of pregnancy-related death for 2017 to 2019: mental health conditions (22.7%), hemorrhage (13.7%), cardiac and coronary conditions (12.8%), infection (9.2%), thrombotic embolism (8.7%), and cardiomyopathy (8.5%).[90] A preventability determination was made in 996 deaths; 839 (84%) were determined to be preventable. Data from France for the period between 2013 and 2015 revealed that the two leading causes of maternal deaths (suicides and cardiovascular disease) were also those with the highest proportion of preventable mortality, at 91.3% and 65.7% respectively.[95]

The COVID-19 pandemic had a significant impact on the global MMR (see Chapter 36). Increases in MMR were due to either an increase in indirect obstetric deaths (due to the SARS-CoV-2 infection) or a decrease in global healthcare as a result of disruption to services caused by the pandemic, leading to a failure to manage the complications of pregnancy.[1] In the United States, the COVID-19 pandemic seemed to heighten the existing racial disparities in MMR.[96] A rapid systematic review using data from Mexico, Peru, Uganda, South Africa, and Kenya also showed increases in MMR in these locations.[97] Early studies suggested pregnant patients were at increased risk of both severe morbidity and mortality following infection with SARS-CoV-2.[98] However, concerns about vaccine safety led to vaccine hesitancy, which persisted despite a lack of evidence for adverse outcomes linked to the vaccine.[99] A growing body of evidence subsequently confirmed that immunization protects both the mother and the neonate from adverse outcomes.[99-101]

Detailed descriptions of hypertensive disorders of pregnancy, infection, hemorrhage, embolic disorders, cardiovascular diseases, and psychiatric disorders in pregnancy are provided in Chapters 35, 36, 37, 38, 41, and 49, respectively. **Injury-related deaths** are considered pregnancy-associated but not pregnancy-related (see Chapter 53). Common clinical and sociodemographic factors that increase the risk for maternal death from all these complications are discussed in the following sections.

Risk Factors

Advanced maternal age increases maternal risk,[102] with a linear trend evident for each 5-year increase in maternal age beyond 34 years.[103] The MMR for women over 40 was 7.8 times higher than for women under 25 years of age in the United States between 2018 and 2020,[83] and three times higher in the United Kingdom than for women aged 20 to 24 years old.[77] Significant differences were seen between ethnic groups in both countries with respect to advanced maternal age. In the United States, the MMR among women 40 years of age and older was 223.5 per 100,000 births for Black women (compared with 20.8 per 100,000 births for Black women less than 25 years of age) and 81.4 per 100,000 births for White women (compared with 11.7 per 100,000 births for White women less than 25 years of age).[83] Based on data from the PMSS for 1991 to 1999, the association between age and mortality persisted after data were controlled for parity, prenatal care, race, and education.[103] Among older Black women (≥40 years), the excess risks were greatest for hypertensive disorders of pregnancy, infection, cerebrovascular accident, and other medical conditions. Among older White women, the greatest excess risks for death were caused by hemorrhage, cardiomyopathy, embolic disorders, and other medical conditions.[103]

In the United States, **Black or African-American race** significantly correlates with the risk for death. Non-Hispanic

Black women experience a MMR that is 2.9-fold higher than non-Hispanic White women.[83] In a case series of anesthesia-related maternal deaths in Michigan published in 2007, six of eight deaths occurred among non-Hispanic Black women in Detroit, suggesting a profound concentration of maternal risk.[104] The disparity in maternal mortality between Black women and White women persists after data are controlled for maternal age, income, and receipt of prenatal care[105] and appears to be related to a higher case-fatality rate.[106] In the United Kingdom, the relative risk (RR) for Black women was 3.68 (95% confidence interval [CI], 2.32 to 5.65) compared with White women.[77]

Other racial and ethnic groups also experience increased risk. In the United States between 2011 and 2016, the MMR was 240% higher for American Indian or Alaskan Native women compared with non-Hispanic White women.[107] In England, women from Asian backgrounds were at higher risk than White women (RR, 1.75; 95% CI, 1.13 to 2.62), as were women from mixed ethnic backgrounds (RR, 1.32; 95% CI, 0.35 to 3.47).[77]

Immigrants, asylum seekers, and nonnative language speakers appear to be particularly vulnerable to both maternal death and substandard care, based on data from the United Kingdom and the Netherlands.[4,77,80,108,109] In the United States, Hispanic and Asian/Pacific Islander immigrants face increased risk compared with women of these same racial/ethnic groups born in the United States.[110] Significant regional variation has been identified in France, with increased risk noted for women delivering in Paris (adjusted odds ratio [aOR], 1.6; 95% CI, 1.2 to 2.0) and the overseas districts (aOR, 3.5; 95% CI, 2.4 to 5.0) compared with continental France.[111] Differences in behavior, biology, environmental conditions, social circumstances, and the quality of clinical care may contribute to disparities in outcomes in sociodemographically vulnerable populations.[4,111,112]

Rural residence is an important risk factor for maternal mortality in the United States, with impacts across all age cohorts and racial and ethnic groups.[107] Workforce shortages and economic stress have accelerated obstetric unit closures in rural communities, increasing the distances rural women need to travel for obstetric care. Higher rates of substance use and mental health disorders further contribute to population risk.[113]

Maternal obesity increases the risk for maternal death from a variety of causes, including pulmonary embolism, infection, preeclampsia, and anesthesia-related complications. Remarkably, there are limited epidemiologic data to establish this connection. Obesity is a common feature in case series of maternal deaths. In the 2018 to 2020 CEMD report from the United Kingdom, 51% of women who died were overweight or obese, and admission to an ICU was more common in women with a body mass index (BMI) > 35 kg/m². [77]

Multifetal pregnancies increase maternal risk for a variety of complications, including preeclampsia, venous thromboembolism, heart failure, myocardial infarction, peripartum hemorrhage, and maternal death.[4,114-117] Compared with twin pregnancies, triplet and higher-order multiple pregnancies further increase maternal risk for preeclampsia, hemorrhage, and emergency peripartum hysterectomy.[115,116] In the United States between 1979 and 2000, the relative risk for death associated with a multifetal pregnancy compared with a singleton pregnancy was 3.6 (95% CI, 3.1 to 4.1) with threefold to fourfold increases in the cause-specific relative risk for death for embolism, hemorrhage, hypertensive disorders of pregnancy, infection, cardiomyopathy, and other medical conditions.[117]

Cesarean delivery has also been associated with an increased risk for maternal death; however, the association does not always reflect a causal relationship. Death can be a consequence of the indication for the operation rather than the mode of delivery itself. Confidential enquiry reports in the United Kingdom and United States do not routinely report maternal mortality data based on cesarean delivery versus vaginal delivery, possibly due to difficulties adjusting for the confounding influence of the indication for operative delivery. In an attempt to estimate the relative risk for death caused by cesarean delivery, a population-based case-control study from France focused on 65 maternal deaths after singleton births among low-risk women in whom complications developed only after delivery.[118] Cases were identified by the French National Confidential Enquiry on Maternal Deaths from 1996 through 2000.[118] These cases were compared with 10,244 singleton births to low-risk women identified through the French National Perinatal Survey conducted in 1998. After data were controlled for maternal age, nationality, parity, and preterm delivery, the aOR for increased risk for death with cesarean delivery was 3.64 (95% CI, 2.15 to 6.19). The increased risk was most dramatic for intrapartum cesarean deliveries (aOR, 4.58; 95% CI, 2.30 to 9.09) but was also present when cesarean delivery preceded labor (aOR, 2.42; 95% CI, 1.14 to 5.13).[118] Among women who underwent cesarean delivery, there was an increased risk for cause-specific maternal mortality from venous thromboembolism, puerperal infection, and complications of anesthesia, but not for risk for death from postpartum hemorrhage or amniotic fluid embolism. A more recent study in Brazil used similar methodology to examine the relationship between cesarean delivery and postpartum maternal mortality.[119] The authors showed that, after controlling for indication bias and confounders, cesarean delivery was associated with a higher risk of maternal death (OR, 2.87; 95% CI, 1.63 to 5.06). This risk was predominantly due to postpartum hemorrhage and complications of anesthesia.

A cohort study of deliveries in Canada between 1991 and 2005 compared 46,766 planned cesarean deliveries for breech presentation with 2,292,420 planned vaginal deliveries in which labor was either spontaneous or induced.[120] Planned cesarean delivery increased the risk for postpartum cardiac arrest (aOR, 5.1; 95% CI, 4.1 to 6.3), major puerperal infection (aOR, 3.0; 95% CI, 2.7 to 3.4), anesthesia complications (aOR, 2.3; 95% CI, 2.0 to 2.6), and puerperal venous thromboembolism (aOR, 2.2; 95% CI, 1.5 to 3.4).[120]

A medical record review of all in-hospital maternal deaths that occurred in a sample of US hospitals between 2000 and 2006 sought to identify evidence for a causal connection between mode of delivery and the mechanism of maternal death.[121] Among 1,461,270 live births, there were 95 maternal deaths (6.5 per 100,000). Although 61% of the deaths were associated with cesarean delivery, one-third of these were perimortem cesarean deliveries in which the surgical procedure followed maternal cardiac arrest. Four deaths were thought to have been directly caused by cesarean delivery (attributed to hemorrhage or infection), with an additional seven deaths attributed to pulmonary thromboembolism after cesarean delivery. Two deaths were thought to have been causally related to vaginal delivery (one case of uterine inversion and one case of rupture of an unrecognized cerebral berry aneurysm during labor), and two deaths were attributed to pulmonary thromboembolism after vaginal delivery. Another 16 deaths were thought to have been potentially preventable had a cesarean delivery or an earlier cesarean delivery been performed (12 caused by preeclampsia, 3 caused by hemorrhage, and 1 caused by sepsis).[121] The investigators concluded that a policy of universal thromboprophylaxis for all patients undergoing cesarean delivery would eliminate the increased risk for maternal death caused by cesarean delivery compared with vaginal delivery.[121]

Regardless of mode of delivery, risk appears to be particularly concentrated in women with preexisting medical conditions; pulmonary hypertension, malignancy, systemic lupus erythematosus, sickle cell disease, and major cardiovascular and renal disease all confer substantially increased risk for maternal death or end-organ injury.[102,122,123] Given the preponderance of indirect deaths documented in recent CEMD reports, assessors have repeatedly recommended both preconception counseling and intensive multidisciplinary antepartum and intrapartum care for women with serious medical or mental health conditions that may be aggravated by pregnancy.[4,78] These conditions include congenital or acquired cardiac disease, obesity with a BMI $\geq 30\,kg/m^2$, epilepsy, diabetes, asthma, autoimmune disorders, renal or liver disease, HIV infection, and a personal or family history of severe mental illness.[4,78] The "One Key Question Initiative"[124] encourages clinicians to ask women the question "Would you like to become pregnant in the next year?" as a way to open conversations about contraception and the need for preconception counseling.[125] It is further recommended that women at highest risk for adverse health events in future pregnancies be offered long-acting reversible contraception (LARC) as a strategy to improve maternal safety.[126] The placement of LARC in the immediate postpartum period may help avoid systemic barriers to contraceptive use.

Some **health system characteristics** have been associated with a higher risk for maternal death; they include (1) low maternal-fetal medicine specialist density[127] and (2) a single physician functioning as both the obstetrician and the anesthesia provider.[128]

Severe and Near-Miss Morbidity

Death is considered the extreme outcome of the following continuum of adverse pregnancy events: normal pregnancy

→ morbidity → severe morbidity → near-miss → death.[129] Approximately one-half of women experience some **morbidity** during pregnancy, most commonly anemia, urinary tract infection, mental health conditions, hypertensive disorders, and pelvic or perineal trauma.[130] Research has focused on severe morbidity, near-miss events, and maternal deaths to elucidate the patient, provider, and health system factors that lead to these adverse outcomes.

Severe maternal morbidity includes unexpected complications of childbirth that result in significant short- or long-term consequences to a woman's health[131]; its estimated incidence depends on the health system evaluated, the method of ascertainment, and the definition of severe morbidity used.[132–135]

Near-miss morbidity occurs when a woman survives a life-threatening complication that occurred during pregnancy, childbirth, or within 42 days of termination of pregnancy.[136] The concept of a near-miss event evolved from early studies of pregnant patients who required intensive care.[137–139] The WHO Working Group on Maternal Mortality and Morbidity Classification determined that end-organ injury represents the most epidemiologically sound way to identify near-miss morbidity.[140] In 2009 the WHO proposed a panel of clinical, laboratory-based, and management-based criteria to identify maternal end-organ injury.[136,141] Cecatti et al.[142] applied the WHO near-miss criteria to all ICU admissions in a tertiary care facility in Brazil between 2002 and 2007 and found a near-miss morbidity ratio of 14.7 events per 1000 live births, an MMR of 125 deaths per 100,000 live births, and a maternal near-miss–to–mortality ratio of 10.7:1. Subsequently, in 2011, the WHO released a maternal near-miss approach for "monitoring the implementation of critical interventions in maternal healthcare," which aims to provide a systematic process for assessing and improving the quality of healthcare.[143] The inclusion criteria for baseline assessment of quality of care are shown in Box 39.2.

A review assessing the applicability of the WHO near-miss criteria to sub-Saharan Africa showed that the tool is not uniformly applied, and suggested challenges with the laboratory and management-based criteria.[144] A broader systematic review focusing on LMICs confirmed multiple recommendations to adapt these laboratory and management-based criteria.[145]

Despite these concerns, a systematic review published in 2022 evaluated global maternal near-miss frequencies using the WHO tool from 2011 to 2018.[146] The global pooled near-miss estimate was 1.4% (95% CI, 0.4% to 2.5%). While there was not substantial between-study heterogeneity, the criteria were modified in some LMICs to exclude some laboratory tests and interventions due to resource restrictions.

Preventability has emerged as an important concept in maternal mortality and near-miss morbidity reviews because the opportunities for prevention identified from these reviews can be used to prioritize changes in clinical policy and health system improvements.[147–149] The Perinatal and Maternal Mortality Review Committee in New Zealand proposed a comprehensive list of contributory factors, including those

attributed to the healthcare organization, personnel, technology and equipment, the environment and geography, and patient-level barriers to accessing or engaging with care.[81] If

---

BOX 39.2 World Health Organization Inclusion Criteria for Baseline Assessment of Quality of Care

Severe Maternal Complications
- Severe postpartum hemorrhage
- Severe preeclampsia
- Eclampsia
- Sepsis or severe systemic infection
- Ruptured uterus
- Severe complications of abortion

Critical Interventions or Intensive Care Unit Use
- Admission to intensive care unit
- Interventional radiology
- Laparotomy (includes hysterectomy, excludes cesarean delivery)
- Use of blood products

Life-Threatening Conditions (Near-Miss Criteria)
- Cardiovascular dysfunction
  - Shock, cardiac arrest (absence of pulse/heart beat and loss of consciousness), use of continuous vasoactive drugs, cardiopulmonary resuscitation, severe hypoperfusion (lactate > 5 mmol/L or > 45 mg/dL), severe acidosis (pH < 7.1)
- Respiratory dysfunction
  - Acute cyanosis, gasping, severe tachypnea (respiratory rate > 40 breaths per minute), severe bradypnea (respiratory rate < 6 breaths per minute), tracheal intubation and ventilation not related to anesthesia, severe hypoxemia (O_2 saturation < 90% for greater than or equal to 60 min or $PaO_2/FiO_2 < 200$)
- Renal dysfunction
  - Oliguria nonresponsive to fluids or diuretics, dialysis for acute renal failure, severe acute azotemia (creatinine ≥ 300 μmol/mL or ≥ 3.5 mg/dL)
- Coagulation/hematologic dysfunction
  - Failure to form clots, massive transfusion of blood or red cells (≥5 units), severe acute thrombocytopenia (<50,000/μL)
- Hepatic dysfunction
  - Jaundice in the presence of preeclampsia, severe acute hyperbilirubinemia (bilirubin > 100 μmol/L or > 6.0 mg/dL)
- Neurologic dysfunction
  - Prolonged unconsciousness (lasting 12 h or more), coma (including metabolic coma), stroke, uncontrollable seizures/status epilepticus, total paralysis
- Uterine dysfunction
  - Uterine hemorrhage or infection leading to hysterectomy

Maternal Vital Status
- Maternal death

From World Health Organization. Evaluating the quality of care for severe pregnancy complications: The WHO near-miss approach for maternal health. https://iris.who.int/handle/10665/44692. Accessed 5 October 2024.

all these contributory factors are addressed, experts estimate that up to 80% of deaths could be prevented, but if changes are limited to modifications in clinical care, only 20% to 45% are likely preventable.[81,150–153]

Preventability is a key strategy aimed at achieving the SDG by 2030. The WHO has released a document entitled "Ending Preventable Maternal Mortality (EPMM): A Renewed Focus for Improving Maternal and Newborn Health and Well-being."[154] This report outlines a systems approach that is aimed to be context-specific, people-centric, and which prioritizes equity. Five targets were set as goals for 2025, including (1) antenatal care contacts, (2) skilled health personal attending births, (3) early routine postnatal care, (4) emergency care coverage, and (5) the proportion of women informed and empowered to make their own decisions regarding sexual relations, contraceptive use, and reproductive healthcare.[154]

Anesthesia-Related Maternal Mortality

Anesthesia-related maternal mortality has been defined as "death attributable to anesthesia, either as the result of medications used, method chosen, or the technical maneuvers performed, whether iatrogenic in origin or resulting from an abnormal patient response."[155] A death may be considered anesthesia-related if it can be uniquely attributed to an anesthetic complication.[104] Actual case reports often include layers of comorbidities, anesthetic complications, and problems with nonanesthetic care; these cases may be considered anesthesia-related if optimal anesthetic care would likely have averted the death.[104] If optimal anesthetic care in combination with improvements in obstetric or medical management would likely have saved the woman's life, then the death may be considered **anesthesia-contributing**.[104] In some cases, the anesthetic complication is tragic but incidental (e.g., failed tracheal intubation during advanced cardiac life support for massive pulmonary embolism).

Anesthesia-related maternal death is extremely rare in HICs. Table 39.4 shows recent MMRs attributed to anesthesia in the United States and the United Kingdom. Comparable ratios reported elsewhere include 1.4 per million live births in France for 2001 to 2006 and 1.0 per million in the Netherlands for 1993 to 2005.[80] Active surveillance in the United Kingdom may be particularly effective at comprehensive identification of anesthesia-related maternal deaths. In LMICs, the contribution of anesthesia to maternal mortality is likely higher. South Africa is one of few LMICs that conducts a CEMD. The 2017 to 2019 report on perioperative deaths included both anesthesia-related deaths (proportion of maternal deaths due directly to anesthesia [7%]) and cases with anesthesia-contribution (proportion of maternal deaths due to another cause but where action or inaction by the anesthetist likely contributed to the death [15%]). This means that in one in five cases (22%) of maternal death when a cesarean delivery was performed, there was a significant anesthetic contribution to the death. These numbers are supported by a systematic review which suggests that in LMICs, anesthesia accounted for 13.8% (95% CI, 9.0 to 20.7) of deaths after cesarean delivery, and 2.8% (95% CI, 2.4 to 3.4) of all maternal deaths.[53]

TABLE 39.4 Anesthesia-Related Maternal Mortality Ratios in the United States and the United Kingdom

Observation Period	MMR United States (95% CI)[a]	Triennium	MMR United Kingdom (95% CI)[a]
1979–81	4.3 (3.1 to 5.7)	1979–81	8.7 (5.5 to 13.2)[b]
1982–84	3.3 (2.3 to 4.5)	1982–84	7.2 (4.3 to 11.4)[b]
1985–87	2.3 (1.5 to 3.4)	1985–87	2.6 (1.2 to 5.8)
1988–90	1.7 (1.1 to 2.7)	1988–90	1.7 (0.7 to 4.4)
1991–93	1.4 (0.8 to 2.2)	1991–93	3.5 (1.8 to 6.8)
1994–96	1.1 (0.6 to 1.9)	1994–96	0.5 (0.1 to 2.6)
1997–99	1.2 (0.7 to 2.0)	1997–99	1.4 (0.5 to 4.2)
2000–02	1.0 (0.5 to 1.7)	2000–02	3.0 (1.4 to 6.6)
		2003–05	2.8 (1.3 to 6.2)
2007–16	0.8 (0.5 to 1.0)	2006–08	3.1 (1.5 to 6.4)
		2009–11	1.2 (0.3 to 3.7)
		2012–14	0.9 (0.1 to 3.1)
		2015–17	0.4 (0.01 to 2.4)
2017–19	0.4 (0.1 to 1.0)	2018–20	0.5 (0.01 to 2.7)

[a]Reported rates refer to the risk for anesthesia-related death during pregnancy per million live births in the United States[156] or per million maternities in the United Kingdom.[4,78]
[b]Rates for England and Wales only.
CI, Confidence interval.

Several clinical and sociodemographic factors commonly appear among cases of anesthesia-related maternal death and may play a causal role in the mechanism of death. These include (1) maternal obesity; (2) patient refusal of neuraxial anesthesia; (3) remote anesthetic location; (4) delay in anesthesia provider consultation; (5) insufficient multidisciplinary planning, communication, and coordination; and (6) inadequate supervision of care.[4,104,155,157–159] In the United States, the relative risk for anesthesia-related maternal death appears to be increased for African-American women.[104,155,156]

Anesthesia-related maternal deaths are distributed throughout the perioperative period and follow both neuraxial and general anesthesia, primarily administered for cesarean delivery, but occasionally for vaginal delivery or another obstetric or nonobstetric surgical procedure.[104,156,157,159] Case-fatality rates according to mode of anesthesia for cesarean delivery are presented in Table 39.5. To generate these estimates, cases were identified from death certificate data collected by the CDC PMSS, and the total number of anesthetics delivered was estimated based on the national incidence of cesarean delivery and the proportions of cesarean deliveries completed with neuraxial and general anesthesia according to national surveys of anesthesia providers.[156,160]

Anesthesia-related maternal deaths are almost always preventable,[4,104,148,157,159,161] as evidenced by both individual case analysis and review of historical trends. The relative risks of general and neuraxial anesthesia for cesarean delivery in the

United States have shifted over time (see Table 39.5), reflecting three major safety initiatives in anesthesia practice.[162] The first initiative addressed the hazard of **local anesthetic systemic toxicity (LAST)**, identified as a major problem in a series of editorials published in the early 1980s.[163,164] In response, in 1984 the US Food and Drug Administration recommended that bupivacaine 0.75% not be used for epidural anesthesia in obstetric patients. Also, anesthesiologists developed a series of safety procedures to avoid the unintentional intravascular administration of a toxic dose of local anesthetic through an epidural catheter (see Box 12.3). Case-fatality rates for neuraxial anesthesia subsequently declined 78% between 1979 to 1984 and 1985 to 1990 (see Table 39.5). Despite this improvement in prevention, LAST remains a rare and potentially lethal complication in obstetric anesthesia, with recent events attributed to drug error by nonanesthesia providers, cumulative dosing above the toxic threshold, epidural catheter migration, and single-shot transversus abdominis plane blocks.[157,165-167] Lipid emulsion is now recommended as part of a comprehensive resuscitation strategy (see Box 24.8).[168]

The second initiative involved a shift toward **greater use of neuraxial anesthesia for cesarean delivery**.[160] Between 1985 and 1990, the relative risk of anesthesia-related maternal mortality associated with general anesthesia compared with neuraxial anesthesia for cesarean delivery was 16.7 (see Table 39.5), and much of the increase in risk was attributed to failed tracheal intubation or aspiration of gastric contents during induction of general anesthesia, or both. In response, anesthesia providers now reserve general anesthesia for specific indications, including (1) emergency cesarean delivery with insufficient time to establish neuraxial anesthesia; (2) medical conditions that make neuraxial anesthesia unsafe, such as maternal coagulopathy, hemorrhagic shock, and septic shock; and (3) failed neuraxial anesthesia with intraoperative pain (see Chapter 26).[169]

The third initiative introduced a series of **protocols and devices to improve the safety of general anesthesia**.[162,170] Pulse oximetry and capnography have been widely credited with the decline in the incidence of unrecognized esophageal intubation.[171] Failed tracheal intubation algorithms, supraglottic airway devices (particularly the laryngeal mask airway), and a heightened focus on simulation and practice have driven a transformation in airway management toward a clear focus on effective oxygenation and ventilation as well as ongoing preparation for airway emergencies.[148,170,172] Consequently, the case-fatality rate for general anesthesia for cesarean delivery decreased by 80% between 1985 to 1990 and 1997 to 2002 (see Table 39.5).[156] Nevertheless, recent series continue to report deaths from difficult tracheal intubation, unrecognized esophageal intubation, pulmonary aspiration of gastric contents (both during anesthetic induction and emergence), postextubation airway obstruction, and postoperative respiratory arrest attributed to opioids or other respiratory depressants.[4,104,157,173,174] Strategies to limit the risk for airway complications are discussed in Chapters 28 and 29.

The relative risk associated with general anesthesia in comparison with neuraxial anesthesia has fallen since 1990

TABLE 39.5 Case-Fatality Rates per Million Anesthetics for Cesarean Delivery in the United States (95% CI)			
Year of Death	General	Neuraxial	Risk Ratios
1979–84	20.0 (17.7 to 22.7)	8.6 (7.8 to 9.4)	2.3 (1.9 to 2.9)
1985–90	32.3 (25.9 to 49.3)	1.9 (1.8 to 2.0)	16.7 (12.9 to 21.8)
1991–96	16.8 (8.9 to 28.7)	2.5 (1.2 to 4.5)	6.7 (3.0 to 14.9)
1997–2002	6.5 (2.1 to 15.3)	3.8 (2.3 to 6.1)	1.7 (0.6 to 4.6)

CI, Confidence interval.
Data from Hawkins JL, Chang J, Palmer SK, et al. Anesthesia-related maternal mortality in the United States: 1979-2002. *Obstet Gynecol.* 2011;117:69–74.

and was estimated to be 1.7 (95% CI, 0.6 to 4.6) between 1997 and 2002.[156] In contemporary anesthesia practice, both general anesthesia and neuraxial anesthesia carry remote, but tangible risks for maternal death.

High neuraxial block was the leading cause of anesthesia-related maternal death among women receiving neuraxial anesthesia for cesarean delivery in the United States between 1997 and 2002.[156] It was also the leading cause of legal claims for maternal death or permanent brain injury filed between 1990 and 2003 (n = 15/25; 60%), with the majority of these attributed to an unrecognized intrathecal catheters intended for the epidural space.[173] Single-shot spinal anesthesia administered after failed epidural anesthesia for cesarean delivery represents a second clinical scenario associated with high neuraxial block.[175] Details on high neuraxial block and its management may be found in Box 24.9 and Chapter 26.

Potentially lethal **infectious complications of neuraxial block** include meningitis, encephalitis, and neuraxial abscess (see Chapter 31).[176-178] The CEMD 2006 to 2008 report included a case of acute hemorrhagic disseminated leukoencephalitis attributed to thoracolumbar spinal canal empyema.[4] Current guidelines stress the importance of strict aseptic technique during neuraxial block administration, as well as appropriate monitoring and management for any infectious complications that may develop.[179,180]

Other series suggest that neuraxial cardiac arrest and hypotensive arrest may be important mechanisms by which neuraxial anesthesia can lead to maternal death.[55,181] Prevention likely depends on careful attention to intravascular volume status, as well as the prompt, aggressive treatment of maternal hypotension to prevent reflex-mediated bradycardia and cardiovascular collapse.[182] Finally, perioperative respiratory arrest can result from neuraxial opioids or intravenous opioids or other respiratory depressants administered during or after neuraxial anesthesia.[104,157]

Further efforts to improve maternal safety must include a comprehensive approach to **high-quality perioperative patient care**. Timely preanesthesia evaluation and ongoing communication with obstetric providers are essential to limit the number of patients who require emergency administration of anesthesia without sufficient evaluation and preparation. Problems with **postoperative care** have long been recognized[183] but appear to account for a growing proportion of perioperative maternal deaths,[157–159,184] particularly those attributed to respiratory events, hemorrhage, and maternal sepsis.[80,81,112,175,177] The physiology of pregnancy and the compensatory physiologic responses that occur in young pregnant women may obscure early signs of septic or hemorrhagic shock. **Early warning scoring systems** may facilitate the early identification of women who have, or are beginning to develop, a critical illness (see Chapter 11).[4,147,157,159,185] Postanesthesia and postpartum care are commonly provided by labor and delivery nurses (rather than perianesthesia care nurses[186]) with limited training and experience with major anesthetic complications, noninvasive ventilation, and advanced cardiopulmonary life support.

Fortunately, severe morbidity and mortality are rare in obstetrics; as an unfortunate consequence of this rarity, individual clinical experience with serious adverse events will always be limited. Simulation may be an effective strategy for all obstetric and anesthesia providers to prepare for a wide variety of obstetric emergencies, including postoperative airway obstruction, failed tracheal intubation, eclampsia, anaphylaxis, maternal cardiac arrest, and maternal hemorrhage. Chapter 11 details additional strategies to enhance patient safety.

KEY POINTS

- Ninety-nine percent of maternal deaths worldwide occur in LMICs. More than one-half of global maternal deaths are attributed to direct obstetric causes, including maternal hemorrhage, hypertensive disorders of pregnancy, and infection.
- In HICs, 10 women die per 100,000 live births. In the United States, the maternal mortality ratio is increasing by approximately 2% per year.
- Advanced maternal age, maternal obesity, multiple gestation, cesarean delivery, and non-White race increase the risk for maternal death.
- Hypertensive disorders of pregnancy, embolic disorders, and hemorrhage together account for just under one-half of maternal deaths in HICs but appear to be eclipsed by indirect deaths in some countries.
- Death is considered the extreme outcome of the following continuum of adverse pregnancy events: normal pregnancy → morbidity → severe morbidity → near-miss → death.
- In HICs, the anesthesia-related maternal mortality ratio is estimated to range between 0.5 and 3 per million live births.
- Anesthesia safety for obstetric patients depends on the provision of high-quality perioperative patient care.

REFERENCES

1. World Health Organization. *Trends in Maternal Mortality 2020 to 2023: Estimates by WHO, UNICEF, UNFPA, World Bank Group and UNDESA/Population Division*. World Health Organization; 2025. https://www.who.int/publications/i/item/9789240108462. Accessed June 16, 2025.
2. World Health Organization. *Making a Difference in Countries: Strategic Approach to Improving Maternal and Newborn Survival and Health: Ensuring Skilled Care for Every Birth*. World Health Organization; 2006. https://iris.who.int/handle/10665/69468. Accessed October 5, 2024.
3. World Health Organization. *Trends in Maternal Mortality 2000 to 2017: Estimates by WHO, UNICEF, UNFPA, World Bank Group and the United Nations Population Division*. World Health Organization; 2019. https://iris.who.int/handle/10665/327596. Accessed October 5, 2024.
4. Cantwell R, Clutton-Brock T, Cooper G, et al. Saving mothers' lives: reviewing maternal deaths to make motherhood safer: 2006-2008. The Eighth Report of the Confidential Enquiries into Maternal Deaths in the United Kingdom. *BJOG*. 2011;118:1–203.
5. Berg C, Danel I, Atrash H, et al. *Strategies to Reduce Pregnancy-Related Deaths: From Identification and Review to Action*. US Centers for Disease Control and Prevention; 2001. https://stacks.cdc.gov/view/cdc/6537/cdc_6537_DS1.pdf. Accessed October 5, 2024.
6. World Health Organization. *Trends in Maternal Mortality 1990-2015: Estimates Developed by WHO, UNICEF, UNFPA, World Bank Group and the United Nations Population Division, Executive Summary*. World Health Organization; 2015. https://data.unicef.org/wp-content/uploads/2015/12/Trends-in-MMR-1990-2015_Full-report_243.pdf. Accessed October 5, 2024.
7. Say L, Chou D, Gemmill A, et al. Global causes of maternal death: a WHO systematic analysis. *Lancet Glob Health*. 2014;2:e323–e333.
8. Costello A, Azad K, Barnett S. An alternative strategy to reduce maternal mortality. *Lancet*. 2006;368:1477–1479.
9. Lema VM, Changole J, Kanyighe C, Malunga EV. Maternal mortality at the Queen Elizabeth Central Teaching Hospital, Blantyre, Malawi. *East Afr Med J*. 2005;82:3–9.
10. Kavatkar AN, Sahasrabudhe NS, Jadhav MV, Deshmukh SD. Autopsy study of maternal deaths. *Int J Gynaecol Obstet*. 2003;81:1–8.
11. van den Broek N. Anaemia and micronutrient deficiencies. *Br Med Bull*. 2003;67:149–160.
12. Kagu MB, Kawuwa MB, Gadzama GB. Anaemia in pregnancy: a cross-sectional study of pregnant women in a Sahelian tertiary hospital in Northeastern Nigeria. *J Obstet Gynaecol*. 2007;27:676–679.
13. Neilson JP, Lavender T, Quenby S, Wray S. Obstructed labour. *Br Med Bull*. 2003;67:191–204.
14. Hofmeyr GJ, Say L, Gülmezoglu AM. WHO systematic review of maternal mortality and morbidity: the prevalence of uterine rupture. *BJOG*. 2005;112:1221–1228.
15. United National Population Fund and the University of Aberdeen. *Obstetric Fistula Needs Assessment Report: Findings from Nine African Countries*. UNFPA; 2003.

16. Wall LL. Obstetric vesicovaginal fistula as an international public-health problem. *Lancet.* 2006;368:1201–1209.

17. Moodley J, Pattinson RC, Baxter C, et al. Strengthening HIV services for pregnant women: an opportunity to reduce maternal mortality rates in Southern Africa/sub-Saharan Africa. *BJOG.* 2011;118:219–225.

18. Moodley J, Pattinson RC, Fawcus S, et al. The confidential enquiry into maternal deaths in South Africa: a case study. *BJOG.* 2014;121:53–60.

19. Kassebaum NJ, Bertozzi-Villa A, Coggeshall MS, et al. Global, regional, and national levels and causes of maternal mortality during 1990-2013: a systematic analysis for the Global Burden of Disease Study 2013. *Lancet.* 2014;384:980–1004.

20. World Health Organization. Unsafe abortion: Global and regional estimates of the incidence of unsafe abortion and associated mortality in 2008. World Health Organization; 2011. https://www.who.int/publications/i/item/9789241501118. Accessed October 5, 2024.

21. Bearak J, Popinchalk A, Ganatra B, et al. Unintended pregnancy and abortion by income, region, and the legal status of abortion: estimates from a comprehensive model for 1990-2019. *Lancet Glob Health.* 2020;8:e1152–e1161.

22. Ganatra B, Gerdts C, Rossier C, et al. Global, regional, and subregional classification of abortions by safety, 2010-14: estimates from a Bayesian hierarchical model. *Lancet.* 2017;390:2372–2381.

23. Sedgh G, Singh S, Shah IH, et al. Induced abortion: incidence and trends worldwide from 1995 to 2008. *Lancet.* 2012;379:625–632.

24. Bankole A, Remez L, Owolabi O, et al. *From Unsafe to Safe Abortion in Sub-Saharan Africa: Slow but Steady Progress.* Guttmacher Institute; 2020. https://www.guttmacher.org/report/from-unsafe-to-safe-abortion-in-subsaharan-africa. Accessed October 5, 2024.

25. World Health Organization. *WHO Guideline on Self-care Interventions for Health and Wellbeing, 2022 Revision.* World Health Organization; 2022. https://www.who.int/publications/i/item/9789240052192. Accessed October 10, 2024.

26. Clark S. Early marriage and HIV risks in sub-Saharan Africa. *Stud Fam Plann.* 2004;35:149–160.

27. Jain S, Kurz K. *New Insights on Preventing Child Marriage: A Global Analysis of Factors and Programs.* International Center for Research on Women; 2007.

28. Mathur S, Greene M, Malhotra A. *Too Young to Wed: The Lives, Rights, and Health of Young Married Girls.* International Center for Research on Women; 2003.

29. Conde-Agudelo A, Belizan JM, Lammers C. Maternal-perinatal morbidity and mortality associated with adolescent pregnancy in Latin America: cross-sectional study. *Am J Obstet Gynecol.* 2005;192:342–349.

30. Patton GC, Coffey C, Sawyer SM, et al. Global patterns of mortality in young people: a systematic analysis of population health data. *Lancet.* 2009;374:881–892.

31. Stover J, Ross J. How increased contraceptive use has reduced maternal mortality. *Matern Child Health J.* 2010;14:687–695.

32. Nove A, Matthews Z, Neal S, Camacho AV. Maternal mortality in adolescents compared with women of other ages: evidence from 144 countries. *Lancet Glob Health.* 2014;2:e155–e164.

33. Grimes CE, Law RS, Borgstein ES, et al. Systematic review of met and unmet need of surgical disease in rural sub-Saharan Africa. *World J Surg.* 2012;36:8–23.

34. Molina G, Weiser TG, Lipsitz SR, et al. Relationship between cesarean delivery rate and maternal and neonatal mortality. *JAMA.* 2015;314:2263–2270.

35. Sobhy S, Arroyo-Manzano D, Murugesu N, et al. Maternal and perinatal mortality and complications associated with caesarean section in low-income and middle-income countries: a systematic review and meta-analysis. *Lancet.* 2019;393:1973–1982.

36. Davies JI, Vreede E, Onajin-Obembe B, Morriss WW. What is the minimum number of specialist anaesthetists needed in low-income and middle-income countries? *BMJ Glob Health.* 2018;3:e001005.

37. Kempthorne P, Morriss WW, Mellin-Olsen J, Gore-Booth J. The WFSA global anesthesia workforce survey. *Anesth Analg.* 2017;125:981–990.

38. Dyer RA, Reed AR, James MF. Obstetric anaesthesia in low-resource settings. *Best Pract Res Clin Obstet Gynaecol.* 2010;24:401–412.

39. Enohumah KO, Imarengiaye CO. Factors associated with anaesthesia-related maternal mortality in a tertiary hospital in Nigeria. *Acta Anaesthesiol Scand.* 2006;50:206–210.

40. Linden AF, Sekidde FS, Galukande M, et al. Challenges of surgery in developing countries: a survey of surgical and anesthesia capacity in Uganda's public hospitals. *World J Surg.* 2012;36:1056–1065.

41. Hodges SC, Mijumbi C, Okello M, et al. Anaesthesia services in developing countries: defining the problems. *Anaesthesia.* 2007;62:4–11.

42. Epiu I, Tindimwebwa JV, Mijumbi C, et al. Challenges of anesthesia in low- and middle-income countries: a cross-sectional survey of access to safe obstetric anesthesia in East Africa. *Anesth Analg.* 2017;124:290–299.

43. Thaddeus S, Maine D. Too far to walk: maternal mortality in context. *Soc Sci Med.* 1994;38:1091–1110.

44. Essendi H, Mills S, Fotso JC. Barriers to formal emergency obstetric care services' utilization. *J Urban Health.* 2011;88:S356–S369.

45. Hirose A, Borchert M, Niksear H, et al. Difficulties leaving home: a cross-sectional study of delays in seeking emergency obstetric care in Herat, Afghanistan. *Soc Sci Med.* 2011;73:1003–1013.

46. Tumwebaze J. Lamula's story. *Anaesthesia.* 2007;62:4.

47. Okafor UV, Efetie ER, Amucheazi A. Risk factors for maternal deaths in unplanned obstetric admissions to the intensive care unit-lessons for sub-Saharan Africa. *Afr J Reprod Health.* 2011;15:51–54.

48. Lori JR, Starke AE. A critical analysis of maternal morbidity and mortality in Liberia, West Africa. *Midwifery.* 2012;28:67–72.

49. Bishop D, Dyer RA, Maswime S, et al. Maternal and neonatal outcomes after caesarean delivery in the African Surgical Outcomes Study: a 7-day prospective observational cohort study. *Lancet Glob Health.* 2019;7:e513–e522.

50. Ouro-Bang'na Maman AF, Tomta K, Ahouangbévi S, Chobli M. Deaths associated with anaesthesia in Togo, West Africa. *Trop Doct.* 2005;35:220–222.

51. Pereira C, Mbaruku G, Nzabuhakwa C, et al. Emergency obstetric surgery by non-physician clinicians in Tanzania. *Int J Gynaecol Obstet.* 2011;114:180–183.

52. Chilopora G, Pereira C, Kamwendo F, et al. Postoperative outcome of caesarean sections and other major emergency obstetric surgery by clinical officers and medical officers in Malawi. *Hum Resour Health.* 2007;5:17.

53. Sobhy S, Zamora J, Dharmarajah K, et al. Anaesthesia-related maternal mortality in low-income and middle-income countries: a systematic review and meta-analysis. *Lancet Glob Health*. 2016;4:e320–e327.

54. Farina Z, Rout C. But it's just a spinal: combating increasing rates of maternal death related to spinal anaesthesia. *S Afr Med J*. 2012;103:81–82.

55. Centre of Maternal, Fetal, Newborn and Child Healthcare Strategies. *Saving Mothers Reports. Saving Mothers 2005-2007: Fourth Report on Confidential Enquiries Into Maternal Deaths in South Africa*. Department of Health; 2008. https://www.up.ac.za/centre-for-maternal-fetal-newborn-and-child-healthcare/article/2929870/saving-mothers-reports-mammas. Accessed October 5, 2024.

56. Hansen D, Gausi SC, Merikebu M. Anaesthesia in Malawi: complications and deaths. *Trop Doct*. 2000;30:146–149.

57. Bates I, Chapotera GK, McKew S, van den Broek N. Maternal mortality in sub-Saharan Africa: the contribution of ineffective blood transfusion services. *BJOG*. 2008;115:1331–1339.

58. Al-Kadhimi S, Patel AD, Plaat F. Intrathecal tranexamic acid—an accident waiting to happen? *Int J Obstet Anesth*. 2018;34:116–117.

59. World Health Organization. Risk of medication errors with tranexamic acid injection resulting in inadvertent intrathecal injection; 2022. Available at: https://www.who.int/news/item/16-03-2022-risk-of-medication-errors-with-tranexamic-acid-injection-resulting-in-inadvertent-intrathecal-injection. Accessed October 5, 2024.

60. Ronsmans C. Severe acute maternal morbidity in low-income countries. *Best Pract Res Clin Obstet Gynaecol*. 2009;23:305–316.

61. Carvalho N, Salehi AS, Goldiem SJ. National and sub-national analysis of the health benefits and cost-effectiveness of strategies to reduce maternal mortality in Afghanistan. *Health Policy Plan*. 2013;28:62–74.

62. Goldie SJ, Sweet S, Carvalho N, et al. Alternative strategies to reduce maternal mortality in India: a cost-effectiveness analysis. *PLoS Med*. 2010;7:e1000264.

63. Kavi A, Kinshella MW, Ramadurg UY, et al. Community engagement for birth preparedness and complication readiness in the Community Level Interventions for Pre-eclampsia (CLIP) Trial in India: a mixed-method evaluation. *BMJ Open*. 2022;12:e060593.

64. Molina RL, Bobanski L, Dhingra-Kumar N, et al. The WHO safe childbirth checklist after 5 years: future directions for improving outcomes. *Lancet Glob Health*. 2022;10:e324–e325.

65. Olufolabi AJ, Atito-Narh E, Eshun M, et al. Teaching neuraxial anesthesia techniques for obstetric care in a Ghanaian referral hospital: achievements and obstacles. *Anesth Analg*. 2015;120:1317–1322.

66. Potisek MG, Hatch DM, Atito-Narh E, et al. Where are they now? Evolution of a nurse anesthesia training school in Ghana and a survey of graduates. *Front Public Health*. 2017;5:78.

67. Nyamtema AS, Pemba SK, Mbaruku G, et al. Tanzanian lessons in using non-physician clinicians to scale up comprehensive emergency obstetric care in remote and rural areas. *Hum Resour Health*. 2011;9:28.

68. Nyamtema AS, Urassa DP, van Roosmalen J. Maternal health interventions in resource limited countries: a systematic review of packages, impacts and factors for change. *BMC Pregnancy Childbirth*. 2011;11:30.

69. Bangoura IF, Hu J, Gong X, et al. Availability and quality of emergency obstetric care, an alternative strategy to reduce maternal mortality: experience of Tongji Hospital, Wuhan, China. *J Huazhong Univ Sci Technol Med Sci*. 2012;32:151–158.

70. Liang J, Li X, Dai L, et al. The changes in maternal mortality in 1000 counties in mid-Western China by a government-initiated intervention. *PLoS One*. 2012;7:e37458.

71. Holmer H, Oyerinde K, Meara JG, et al. The global met need for emergency obstetric care: a systematic review. *BJOG*. 2015;122:183–189.

72. Lassi ZS, Bhutta ZA. Community-based intervention packages for reducing maternal and neonatal morbidity and mortality and improving neonatal outcomes. *Cochrane Database Syst Rev*. 2015;(3):CD007754.

73. Kaplan LC, Ichsan I, Diba F, et al. Effects of the World Health Organization Safe Childbirth Checklist on quality of care and birth outcomes in Aceh, Indonesia: a cluster-randomized clinical trial. *JAMA Netw Open*. 2021;4:e2137168.

74. Seim AR, Alassoum Z, Souley I, et al. The effects of a peripartum strategy to prevent and treat primary postpartum haemorrhage at health facilities in Niger: a longitudinal, 72-month study. *Lancet Glob Health*. 2023;11:e287–e295.

75. Goodman DM, Ramaswamy R, Jeuland M, et al. The cost effectiveness of a quality improvement program to reduce maternal and fetal mortality in a regional referral hospital in Accra, Ghana. *PLoS One*. 2017;12:e0180929.

76. Willcox M, Harrison H, Asiedu A, et al. Incremental cost and cost-effectiveness of low-dose, high-frequency training in basic emergency obstetric and newborn care as compared to status quo: part of a cluster-randomized training intervention evaluation in Ghana. *Glob Health*. 2017;13:88.

77. Knight M, Bunch K, Patel R, et al. *Saving Lives, Improving Mothers' Care Core Report—Lessons Learned to Inform Maternity Care From the UK and Ireland Confidential Enquiries Into Maternal Deaths and Morbidity 2018-20*. National Perinatal Epidemiology Unit, University of Oxford; 2022. https://www.npeu.ox.ac.uk/mbrrace-uk/reports/maternal-reports/maternal-report-2018-2020. Accessed October 5, 2024.

78. Knight M, Nair M, Tuffnell D, on behalf of MBRRACE-UK. *Saving Lives, Improving Mothers' Care—Surveillance of Maternal Deaths in the UK 2012-14 and Lessons Learned to Inform Maternity Care From the UK and Ireland Confidential Enquiries Into Maternal Deaths and Morbidity 2009-14*. National Perinatal Epidemiology Unit, University of Oxford; 2016. https://www.npeu.ox.ac.uk/mbrrace-uk/reports/maternal-reports/maternal-report-2012-2014. Accessed October 5, 2024.

79. Saucedo M, Deneux-Tharaux C, Bouvier-Colle MH. Ten years of confidential inquiries into maternal deaths in France, 1998–2007. *Obstet Gynecol*. 2013;122:752–760.

80. Schutte JM, Steegers EA, Schuitemaker NW, et al. Rise in maternal mortality in the Netherlands. *BJOG*. 2010;117:399–406.

81. Farquhar C, Sadler L, Masson V, et al. Beyond the numbers: classifying contributory factors and potentially avoidable maternal deaths in New Zealand, 2006-2009. *Am J Obstet Gynecol*. 2011;205:331.e1–e8.

82. Hoyert DL. Maternal mortality and related concepts. *Vital Health Stat*. 2007;3:1–13.

83. Hoyert DL. Maternal mortality rates in the United States, 2020. *NCHS Health E-Stats*. 2022

84. Rossen L, Womack L, Hoyert D, et al. The impact of the pregnancy checkbox and misclassification on maternal mortality trends in the United States, 1999-2017; 2020. https://stacks.cdc.gov/view/cdc/84767. Accessed October 5, 2024.

85. US Centers for Disease Control and Prevention. CDC wonder. Available at: http://wonder.cdc.gov/. Accessed October 5, 2024.

86. Deneux-Tharaux C, Berg C, Bouvier-Colle MH, et al. Underreporting of pregnancy-related mortality in the United States and Europe. *Obstet Gynecol.* 2005;106:684–692.

87. Chang J, Elam-Evans LD, Berg CJ, et al. Pregnancy-related mortality surveillance—United States, 1991–1999. *MMWR Surveill Summ.* 2003;52:1–8.

88. US Centers for Disease Control and Prevention. *Data from the Pregnancy Mortality Surveillance System.* Centers for Disease Control and Prevention; 2025. https://www.cdc.gov/maternal-mortality/php/pregnancy-mortality-surveillance-data/. Accessed June 17, 2025.

89. St Pierre A, Zaharatos J, Goodman D, Callaghan WM. Challenges and opportunities in identifying, reviewing, and preventing maternal deaths. *Obstet Gynecol.* 2018;131: 138–142.

90. Trost SL, Beauregard J, Njie F, et al. *Pregnancy-Related Deaths: Data From Maternal Mortality Review Committees in 36 US States, 2017-2019.* Centers for Disease Control and Prevention; 2022. https://www.cdc.gov/maternal-mortality/php/data-research/mmrc-2017-2019.html. Accessed October 5, 2024.

91. Hoyert DL. Maternal mortality rates in the United States, 2021. *NCHS Health E-Stats.* 2023

92. Main EK, Goffman D, Scavone BM, et al. National Partnership for Maternal Safety: consensus bundle on obstetric hemorrhage. *Anesth Analg.* 2015;121:142–148.

93. D'Alton ME, Friedman AM, Smiley RM, et al. National partnership for maternal safety: consensus bundle on venous thromboembolism. *Anesth Analg.* 2016;123:942–949.

94. Bernstein PS, Martin JN Jr, Barton JR, et al. National Partnership for Maternal Safety: consensus bundle on severe hypertension during pregnancy and the postpartum period. *Anesth Analg.* 2017;125:540–547.

95. Saucedo M, Deneux-Tharaux C. Pour le Comite National d'Experts sur la Mortalite M. [Maternal mortality, frequency, causes, women's profile and preventability of deaths in France, 2013-2015]. *Gynecol Obstet Fertil Senol.* 2021;49:9–26.

96. Thoma ME, Declercq ER. All-cause maternal mortality in the US before vs during the COVID-19 pandemic. *JAMA Netw Open.* 2022;5:e2219133.

97. Calvert C, John J, Nzvere FP, et al. Maternal mortality in the COVID-19 pandemic: findings from a rapid systematic review. *Glob Health Action.* 2021;14:1974677.

98. Badr DA, Mattern J, Carlin A, et al. Are clinical outcomes worse for pregnant women at >/=20 weeks' gestation infected with coronavirus disease 2019? A multicenter case-control study with propensity score matching. *Am J Obstet Gynecol.* 2020;223:764–768.

99. Badell ML, Dude CM, Rasmussen SA, Jamieson DJ. COVID-19 vaccination in pregnancy. *BMJ.* 2022;378:e069741.

100. Halasa NB, Olson SM, Staat MA, et al. Maternal vaccination and risk of hospitalization for COVID-19 among infants. *N Engl J Med.* 2022;387:109–119.

101. Thoma ME, Declercq ER. Changes in pregnancy-related mortality associated with the coronavirus disease 2019 (COVID-19) pandemic in the United States. *Obstet Gynecol.* 2023.

102. Nair M, Knight M, Kurinczuk JJ. Risk factors and newborn outcomes associated with maternal deaths in the UK from 2009 to 2013: a national case-control study. *BJOG.* 2016;123:1654–1662.

103. Callaghan WM, Berg CJ. Pregnancy-related mortality among women aged 35 years and older, United States, 1991–1997. *Obstet Gynecol.* 2003;102:1015–1021.

104. Mhyre JM, Riesner MN, Polley LS, Naughton NN. A series of anesthesia-related maternal deaths in Michigan, 1985–2003. *Anesthesiology.* 2007;106:1096–1104.

105. Harper MA, Espeland MA, Dugan E, et al. Racial disparity in pregnancy-related mortality following a live birth outcome. *Ann Epidemiol.* 2004;14:274–279.

106. Tucker MJ, Berg CJ, Callaghan WM, Hsia J. The Black-White disparity in pregnancy-related mortality from 5 conditions: differences in prevalence and case-fatality rates. *Am J Public Health.* 2007;97:247–251.

107. Merkt PT, Kramer MR, Goodman DA, et al. Urban-rural differences in pregnancy-related deaths, United States, 2011–2016. *Am J Obstet Gynecol.* 2021;225:183.e1–e16.

108. Kayem G, Kurinczuk J, Lewis G, et al. Risk factors for progression from severe maternal morbidity to death: a national cohort study. *PLoS One.* 2011;6:e29077.

109. Schutte JM, de Jonge L, Schuitemaker NW, et al. Indirect maternal mortality increases in the Netherlands. *Acta Obstet Gynecol Scand.* 2010;89:762–768.

110. Hopkins FW, MacKay AP, Koonin LM, et al. Pregnancy-related mortality in Hispanic women in the United States. *Obstet Gynecol.* 1999;94:747–752.

111. Saucedo M, Deneux-Tharaux C, Bouvier-Colle MH. Understanding regional differences in maternal mortality: a national case-control study in France. *BJOG.* 2012;119:573–581.

112. Bryant AS, Worjoloh A, Caughey AB, Washington AE. Racial/ethnic disparities in obstetric outcomes and care: prevalence and determinants. *Am J Obstet Gynecol.* 2010;202:335–343.

113. Kozhimannil KB, Interrante JD, Tuttle MKS, Henning-Smith C. Changes in hospital-based obstetric services in rural US counties, 2014-2018. *JAMA.* 2020;324:197–199.

114. Walker M, Murphy KE, Pan S, et al. Adverse maternal outcomes in multifetal pregnancies. *BJOG.* 2004;111:1294–1296.

115. Day MC, Barton JR, O'Brien JM, et al. The effect of fetal number on the development of hypertensive conditions of pregnancy. *Obstet Gynecol.* 2005;106:927–931.

116. Francois K, Ortiz J, Harris C, et al. Is peripartum hysterectomy more common in multiple gestations? *Obstet Gynecol.* 2005;105:1369–1372.

117. MacKay AP, Berg CJ, King JC, et al. Pregnancy-related mortality among women with multifetal pregnancies. *Obstet Gynecol.* 2006;107:563–568.

118. Deneux-Tharaux C, Carmona E, Bouvier-Colle MH, Breart G. Postpartum maternal mortality and cesarean delivery. *Obstet Gynecol.* 2006;108:541–548.

119. Esteves-Pereira AP, Deneux-Tharaux C, Nakamura-Pereira M, et al. Caesarean delivery and postpartum maternal mortality: a population-based case control study in Brazil. *PLoS One.* 2016;11:e0153396.

120. Liu S, Liston RM, Joseph KS, et al. Maternal mortality and severe morbidity associated with low-risk planned cesarean delivery versus planned vaginal delivery at term. *CMAJ.* 2007;176:455–460.

121. Clark SL, Belfort MA, Dildy GA, et al. Maternal death in the 21st century: causes, prevention, and relationship to cesarean delivery. *Am J Obstet Gynecol.* 2008;199:36.e1–e5.

122. Mhyre JM, Bateman BT, Leffert LR. Influence of patient comorbidities on the risk of near-miss maternal morbidity or mortality. *Anesthesiology.* 2011;115:963–972.

123. Karamlou T, Diggs BS, McCrindle BW, Welke KF. A growing problem: maternal death and peripartum complications are higher in women with grown-up congenital heart disease. *Ann Thorac Surg.* 2011;92:2193–2198.

124. Bellanca HK, Hunter MS. ONE KEY QUESTION®: preventive reproductive health is part of high quality primary care. *Contraception.* 2013;88:3–6.

125. American College of Obstetricians and Gynecologists. Committee Opinion No. 762: Prepregnancy counseling (reaffirmed 2024). *Obstet Gynecol.* 2019;133:e78–e89.

126. Vricella LK, Gawron LM, Louis JM. Society for Maternal-Fetal Medicine (SMFM) Consult Series No. 48: Immediate postpartum long-acting reversible contraception for women at high risk for medical complications. *Am J Obstet Gynecol.* 2019;220:B2–B12.

127. Sullivan SA, Hill EG, Newman RB, Menard MK. Maternal-fetal medicine specialist density is inversely associated with maternal mortality ratios. *Am J Obstet Gynecol.* 2005;193:1083–1088.

128. Nagaya K, Fetters MD, Ishikawa M, et al. Causes of maternal mortality in Japan. *JAMA.* 2000;283:2661–2667.

129. Geller SE, Rosenberg D, Cox SM, Kilpatrick S. Defining a conceptual framework for near-miss maternal morbidity. *J Am Med Womens Assoc.* 2002;57:135–139.

130. Bruce FC, Berg CJ, Hornbrook MC, et al. Maternal morbidity rates in a managed care population. *Obstet Gynecol.* 2008;111:1089–1095.

131. Kilpatrick SK, Ecker JL. Severe maternal morbidity: screening and review. *Am J Obstet Gynecol.* 2016;215:B17–B22.

132. Waterstone M, Bewley S, Wolfe C. Incidence and predictors of severe obstetric morbidity: case-control study. *BMJ.* 2001;322:1089–1093.

133. Zhang WH, Alexander S, Bouvier-Colle MH, Macfarlane A. Incidence of severe pre-eclampsia, postpartum haemorrhage and sepsis as a surrogate marker for severe maternal morbidity in a European population-based study: the MOMS-B survey. *BJOG.* 2005;112:89–96.

134. Wen SW, Huang L, Liston R, et al. Severe maternal morbidity in Canada, 1991-2001. *CMAJ.* 2005;173:759–764.

135. Callaghan WM, Mackay AP, Berg CJ. Identification of severe maternal morbidity during delivery hospitalizations, United States, 1991–2003. *Am J Obstet Gynecol.* 2008;199:133.e1–e8.

136. Say L, Souza JP, Pattinson RC. Maternal near miss—towards a standard tool for monitoring quality of maternal healthcare. *Best Pract Res Clin Obstet Gynaecol.* 2009;23:287–296.

137. Bouvier-Colle MH, Salanave B, Ancel PY, et al. Obstetric patients treated in intensive care units and maternal mortality. Regional teams for the survey. *Eur J Obstet Gynecol Reprod Biol.* 1996;65:121–125.

138. Baskett TF, Sternadel J. Maternal intensive care and near-miss mortality in obstetrics. *Br J Obstet Gynaecol.* 1998;105:981–984.

139. Wheatley E, Farkas A, Watson D. Obstetric admissions to an intensive therapy unit. *Int J Obstet Anesth.* 1996;5:221–224.

140. Say L, Pattinson RC, Gulmezoglu AM. WHO systematic review of maternal morbidity and mortality: the prevalence of severe acute maternal morbidity (near miss). *Reprod Health.* 2004;1:3.

141. Pattinson R, Say L, Souza JP, et al. WHO maternal death and near-miss classifications. *Bull World Health Organ.* 2009;87:734.

142. Cecatti JG, Souza JP, Oliveira Neto AF, et al. Pre-validation of the WHO organ dysfunction based criteria for identification of maternal near miss. *Reprod Health.* 2011;8:22.

143. World Health Organization. *Evaluating the Quality of Care for Severe Pregnancy Complications: The WHO Near-Miss Approach for Maternal Health.* World Health Organization; 2011. https://iris.who.int/handle/10665/44692. Accessed October 5, 2024.

144. Tura AK, Trang TL, van den Akker T, et al. Applicability of the WHO maternal near miss tool in sub-Saharan Africa: a systematic review. *BMC Pregnancy Childbirth.* 2019;19:79.

145. Heitkamp A, Meulenbroek A, van Roosmalen J, et al. Maternal mortality: near-miss events in middle-income countries, a systematic review. *Bull World Health Organ.* 2021;99:693–707F.

146. Firoz T, Trigo Romero CL, Leung C, et al. Global and regional estimates of maternal near miss: a systematic review, meta-analysis and experiences with application. *BMJ Glob Health.* 2022;7.

147. The Joint Commission, Preventing Maternal Death. *Sentinel Event Alert.* 2010;44:1–4.

148. McClure JH, Cooper GM, Clutton-Brock TH. Saving mothers' lives: reviewing maternal deaths to make motherhood safer, 2006-8: a review. *Br J Anaesth.* 2011;107:127–132.

149. Main EK. Maternal mortality: new strategies for measurement and prevention. *Curr Opin Obstet Gynecol.* 2010;22:511–516.

150. Geller SE, Rosenberg D, Cox S, et al. A scoring system identified near-miss maternal morbidity during pregnancy. *J Clin Epidemiol.* 2004;57:716–720.

151. National Expert Committee on Maternal Mortality (CNEMM) F. *Report of the National Expert Committee on Maternal Mortality (CNEMM), France, 2001-2006.* Institut de Veille Sanitaire; 2011.

152. Berg CJ, Harper MA, Atkinson SM, et al. Preventability of pregnancy-related deaths: results of a state-wide review. *Obstet Gynecol.* 2005;106:1228–1234.

153. Geller SE, Rosenberg D, Cox SM, et al. The continuum of maternal morbidity and mortality: factors associated with severity. *Am J Obstet Gynecol.* 2004;191:939–944.

154. World Health Organization. *Ending Preventable Maternal Mortality (EPMM): A Renewed Focus for Improving Maternal and Newborn Health and Well-Being.* World Health Organization; 2021. https://www.who.int/publications/i/item/9789240040519. Accessed October 5, 2024.

155. Endler GC, Mariona FG, Sokol RJ, Stevenson LB. Anesthesia-related maternal mortality in Michigan, 1972 to 1984. *Am J Obstet Gynecol.* 1988;159:187–193.

156. Hawkins JL, Chang J, Palmer SK, et al. Anesthesia-related maternal mortality in the United States: 1979-2002. *Obstet Gynecol.* 2011;117:69–74.

157. Lewis G. The Confidential Enquiry into Maternal and Child Health (CEMACH). *Saving Mothers' Lives: Reviewing Maternal Deaths to Make Motherhood Safer—2003–2005*; 2007. The Seventh Report of the Confidential Enquiries into Maternal Deaths in the United Kingdom. CEMACH. https://www.publichealth.hscni.net/sites/default/files/Saving%20

Mothers%27%20Lives%202003-05%20.pdf. Accessed October 5, 2024.

158. Cooper GM, McClure JH. Anaesthesia. In: Lewis G, ed. *Why Mothers Die 2000-2002: The Sixth Report of Confidential Enquiries Into Maternal Deaths in the United Kingdom.* RCOG Press; 2004:122–133.

159. Dob D, Cooper G, Holdcroft A, eds. *Crises in Childbirth—Why Mothers Survive: Lessons From the Confidential Enquiries Into Maternal Deaths.* Radcliffe Publishing Ltd; 2007.

160. Bucklin BA, Hawkins JL, Anderson JR, Ullrich FA. Obstetric anesthesia workforce survey: twenty-year update. *Anesthesiology.* 2005;103:645–653.

161. Wong CA. Saving mothers' lives: the 2006-8 anaesthesia perspective. *Br J Anaesth.* 2011;107:119–122.

162. D'Angelo R. Anesthesia-related maternal mortality: a pat on the back or a call to arms? *Anesthesiology.* 2007;106:1082–1084.

163. Albright GA. Cardiac arrest following regional anesthesia with etidocaine or bupivacaine. *Anesthesiology.* 1979;51:285–287.

164. Marx GF. Cardiotoxicity of local anesthetics—the plot thickens. *Anesthesiology.* 1984;60:3–5.

165. Spence AG. Lipid reversal of central nervous system symptoms of bupivacaine toxicity. *Anesthesiology.* 2007;107:516–517.

166. Smetzer J, Baker C, Byrne FD, Cohen MR. Shaping systems for better behavioral choices: lessons learned from a fatal medication error. *Jt Comm J Qual Patient Saf.* 2010;36:152–163.

167. Naidu RK, Richebe P. Probable local anesthetic systemic toxicity in a postpartum patient with acute fatty liver of pregnancy after a transversus abdominis plane block. *A A Case Rep.* 2013;1:72–74.

168. Neal JM, Neal EJ, Weinberg GL. American Society of Regional Anesthesia and Pain Medicine local anesthetic systemic toxicity checklist: 2020 version. *Reg Anesth Pain Med.* 2021;46:81–82.

169. Palanisamy A, Mitani AA, Tsen LC. General anesthesia for cesarean delivery at a tertiary care hospital from 2000 to 2005: a retrospective analysis and 10-year update. *Int J Obstet Anesth.* 2011;20:10–16.

170. Mushambi MC, Kinsella SM, Popat M, et al. Obstetric Anaesthetists' Association and Difficult Airway Society guidelines for the management of difficult and failed tracheal intubation in obstetrics. *Anaesthesia.* 2015;70:1286–1306.

171. Cheney FW, Posner KL, Lee LA, et al. Trends in anesthesia-related death and brain damage: a closed claims analysis. *Anesthesiology.* 2006;105:1081–1086.

172. Apfelbaum JL, Hagberg CA, Connis RT, et al. 2022 American Society of Anesthesiologists practice guidelines for management of the difficult airway. *Anesthesiology.* 2020;136:31–81.

173. Davies JM, Posner KL, Lee LA, et al. Liability associated with obstetric anesthesia: a closed claims analysis. *Anesthesiology.* 2009;110:131–139.

174. Warner MA, Meyerhoff KL, Warner ME, et al. Pulmonary aspiration of gastric contents: a closed claims analysis. *Anesthesiology.* 2021;135:284–291.

175. Dadarkar P, Philip J, Weidner C, et al. Spinal anesthesia for cesarean section following inadequate labor epidural analgesia: a retrospective audit. *Int J Obstet Anesth.* 2004;13:239–243.

176. US Centers for Disease Control and Prevention (CDC). Bacterial meningitis after intrapartum spinal anesthesia—New York and Ohio, 2008-2009. *MMWR Morb Mortal Wkly Rep.* 2010;59:65–69.

177. Baer ET. Post-dural puncture bacterial meningitis. *Anesthesiology.* 2006;105:381–393.

178. Rodrigo N, Perera KN, Ranwala R, et al. Aspergillus meningitis following spinal anaesthesia for caesarean section in Colombo, Sri Lanka. *Int J Obstet Anesth.* 2007;16:256–260.

179. American Society of Anesthesiologists. Practice advisory for the prevention, diagnosis, and management of infectious complications associated with neuraxial techniques: an updated report by the American Society of Anesthesiologists Task Force on Infectious Complications Associated with Neuraxial Techniques and the American Society of Regional Anesthesia and Pain Medicine. *Anesthesiology.* 2017;126:585–601.

180. Association of Anaesthetists of Great Britain and Ireland. Infection control in anaesthesia. *Anaesthesia.* 2008;63:1027–1036.

181. Lee LA, Posner KL, Domino KB, et al. Injuries associated with regional anesthesia in the 1980s and 1990s: a closed claims analysis. *Anesthesiology.* 2004;101:143–152.

182. Campagna JA, Carter C. Clinical relevance of the Bezold-Jarisch reflex. *Anesthesiology.* 2003;98:1250–1260.

183. Li XF, Fortney JA, Kotelchuck M, Glover LH. The postpartum period: the key to maternal mortality. *Int J Gynaecol Obstet.* 1996;54:1–10.

184. World Health Organization. *Maternal Mortality in 2005: Estimates Developed by WHO, UNICEF, and UNFPA;* 2007. Department of Reproductive Health and Research. https://www.who.int/publications/i/item/9789241596213. Accessed October 5, 2024.

185. Singh S, McGlennan A, England A, Simons R. A validation study of the CEMACH recommended modified early obstetric warning system (MEOWS). *Anaesthesia.* 2012;67:12–18.

186. Wilkins KK, Greenfield ML, Polley LS, Mhyre JM. A survey of obstetric perianesthesia care unit standards. *Anesth Analg.* 2009;108:1869–1875.

PART X

The Patient With Systemic Disease

40

Autoimmune Disorders

Phil Popham, BSc, MBBS, FRCA, MD, PG Cert US

CHAPTER OUTLINE

At the turn of the 20th century, Ehrlich proposed the dictum of *horror autotoxicus*, the belief that immunity is directed against foreign material and never against one's own body. The demonstration of autoantibodies in the 1950s disproved the theory and demonstrated the failure of self-tolerance.[1]

Autoimmunity has been described in more than 40 disorders and may result in chronic illness and severe disability. The classification of autoimmune diseases has been controversial because it is recognized that both genetic and epigenetic (potentially heritable changes in gene expression that are not associated with changes in DNA sequencing) factors play a role. The traditional clinical classification recognizes immune responses that are directed against a specific antigen and are limited to a specific organ or cell type (**organ-specific disease**), and those that are directed against a range of antigens that produce multisystem involvement (**systemic disease**). Classification now incorporates a "spectrum of autoimmunity" from low-level (possibly beneficial to self) to high-level (clearly detrimental to self) autoimmunity.[2]

The pathogenesis of autoimmunity is complex. A genetic predisposition underlies abnormal reactivity of B cells and immunoglobulins, T-cell receptors, and genes within the major histocompatibility complex (MHC).[3] Specific allotypes within the MHC are associated with certain diseases; for example, HLA-DR2 is strongly positively associated with **systemic lupus erythematosus (SLE)** but negatively associated with **diabetes mellitus type 1**. Genome-wide association studies have identified genetic associations between single-nucleotide polymorphisms (SNPs) and some autoimmune conditions.[4] Metaanalyses of HLA subclasses showed similar associations with autoimmunity.[5] Additionally, epigenetic factors, including dysregulation of DNA expression (but not of its sequencing), noncoding RNA, histone (a nucleosomal protein) modification, and immunoendocrine status, have been shown to influence immune status.[6,7]

Other factors (e.g., environmental conditions) may predispose individuals to autoimmunity. Parasitic infection may reduce the incidence of autoimmunity, whereas bacterial infection with *Klebsiella* may predispose individuals to ankylosing spondylitis. Drug-induced SLE is well described.

Sex hormones, notably the androgen–estrogen balance and its effect on cytokine production, have been implicated in the development of autoimmunity.[8]

BOX 40.1 Classification of Some Autoimmune Diseases

Organ-Specific Disease

Neurologic: Myasthenia gravis, autoimmune peripheral neuropathy, Hashimoto's encephalopathy, temporal arteritis

Hematologic: Autoimmune hemolytic anemia, idiopathic thrombocytopenic purpura, cold agglutinin disease

Skin: Vitiligo, pemphigus vulgaris, alopecia areata, autoimmune urticaria, psoriasis

Gastrointestinal: Crohn's disease, celiac disease, autoimmune hepatitis, primary biliary cirrhosis, ulcerative colitis

Endocrine: Hashimoto's thyroiditis, Addison's disease, diabetes mellitus type 1, Graves' disease

Skeleton: Ankylosing spondylitis, psoriatic arthropathy

Cardiovascular: Autoimmune cardiomyopathy

Renal: Goodpasture's syndrome

Systemic Disease

Systemic lupus erythematosus

Rheumatoid arthritis

Multiple sclerosis

Sjögren's syndrome

Dermatomyositis

Scleroderma

Polymyositis

Mixed connective tissue disease

Wegener's granulomatosis

Autoimmune disorders are more common in women than in men, with the highest incidence of several conditions occurring during childbearing years,[9] and occasionally the initial diagnosis is made during pregnancy. Altered immune function during pregnancy allows maternal tolerance of the fetal allograft, although the mechanisms are complex and poorly understood. The Th1 subset of lymphocytic T helper cells mediates cell-mediated immunity through the production of pro-inflammatory cytokines that may result in cytotoxic damage; in contrast, the Th2 subset produces antiinflammatory cytokines that may promote humoral immunity.[10] As pregnancy progresses, a change from Th1- to Th2-mediated cytokine production is well documented and may be implicated in preeclampsia and preterm labor.[11] Therefore, conditions with a predominant Th1 causation, such as **multiple sclerosis** (see Chapter 47) or **Hashimoto's thyroiditis** (see Chapter 43) may improve in pregnancy, while those with a predominantly Th2 causation (such as SLE or scleroderma) may worsen.[12]

Examples of autoimmune disorders are shown in Box 40.1. **SLE, lupus anticoagulant (LAC), scleroderma**, and **polymyositis/dermatomyositis** are discussed in this chapter. Other autoimmune disorders that are discussed elsewhere in this text include **diabetes mellitus type 1** (see Chapter 43) **autoimmune thrombocytopenic purpura** and **autoimmune hemolytic anemia** (see Chapter 44), **rheumatoid arthritis** and **ankylosing spondylitis** (see Chapter 46), and **myasthenia gravis** (see Chapter 47).

SYSTEMIC LUPUS ERYTHEMATOSUS

Definition and Epidemiology

SLE is a multisystem inflammatory disease of unknown etiology that is characterized by the production of autoantibodies against nuclear, cytoplasmic, and cell membrane antigens. Although its overall prevalence is about 50 per 100,000 population,[13] it is recognized most commonly in women during their childbearing years, with a female-to-male ratio of 9:1. Certain groups have a higher prevalence, including individuals of African ancestry, Asians, and Native Americans.[9]

Pathophysiology

The etiology of SLE remains unclear. The principal mechanism is thought to be immune complex–mediated, involving immunoglobulin G (IgG) antibodies to double-stranded DNA and other nuclear proteins. Intracellular autoantigens are released by necrotic and apoptotic cells, leading to aberrant sensitization against these antigens. Impaired clearance of apoptotic cells and prolonged exposure to nuclear autoantigens may be involved.[14] Affected individuals have both hyperactivity of the antibody-producing B cells and defects of the helper and suppressor T cells.[15] Genetic defects of immune regulation and possibly environmental triggers including viruses and bacteria lead to a proliferation of B cells capable of producing autoantibodies that may target more than 30 classes of antigens. A variety of antigen-antibody immune complexes are formed, followed by secondary inflammatory responses. Deposits may occur within the skin, choroid plexus, and other endothelial surfaces, with or without an inflammatory response. In certain locations (e.g., the renal glomerulus), deposition of immune complexes and continued inflammation may lead to irreversible injury. However, SLE is not simply an immune complex disorder because some autoantibodies actively bind to erythrocytes, granulocytes, lymphocytes, and macrophages, leading to their removal from the circulation.[16]

Diagnosis

Clinical manifestations of SLE are diverse, owing to the widespread antigenic targets. Box 40.2 outlines objective criteria for the diagnosis of SLE, which place emphasis on selected clinical and immunological features.[17] Not all epidemiologic studies use these criteria, and the clinical diagnosis may be suspected if fewer features are present without another explanation.[18] Typically, the diagnosis of SLE is made before conception, but in 20% of cases the initial diagnosis is made during pregnancy.[19]

Effect of Pregnancy

SLE disease activity may increase during pregnancy,[20] and some pregnancy-related complications may have long-term effects on women with SLE.[19,21,22] The PROMISSE study, an observational prospective outcome study of 385 women with SLE, with or without **antiphospholipid antibodies (aPLs)**, used formal measurements of disease activity to delineate

---

BOX 40.2   Diagnostic Criteria for Systemic Lupus Erythematosus (SLE)

Entry Criterion: Antinuclear antibodies at a specified titer
Additive criteria, each of which is assigned a weighted importance

Clinical
Constitutional: fever
Hematologic: leucopenia, thrombocytopenia, autoimmune hemolysis
Neuropsychiatric: delirium, psychosis, seizure
Mucocutaneous: nonscarring alopecia, oral ulcers, subacute cutaneous or discoid lupus, acute cutaneous lupus
Serosal: pleural or pericardial effusion, acute pericarditis
Musculoskeletal: joint involvement
Renal: proteinuria (>0.5 g/24 h), lupus nephritis demonstrable on renal biopsy

Immunologic
Antiphospholipid antibodies (anticardiolipin or anti-β_2GPI antibodies or lupus anticoagulant)
Complement proteins low
SLE-specific antibodies (anti-dsDNA or anti-Smith)

GPI, Glycoprotein I.
From: Aringer M, Costenbader K, Daikh D, et al. 2019 European League Against Rheumatism/American College of Rheumatology classification criteria for systemic lupus erythematosus. *Ann Rheum Dis.* 2019;78:1151–1159.

---

risk.[23] Renal disease, SLE disease activity, and the presence of aPLs are considered significant risk factors for maternal deterioration during pregnancy. Assessments using the SLE Disease Activity Index found that 50% to 65% of women with active disease had deterioration during pregnancy in both retrospective[24] and prospective[23] studies. Such flares occur most commonly in the second and third trimesters and the puerperium, are not more severe than those in nonpregnant patients and mostly respond to conservative management. The risk for significant disease activity during pregnancy is increased sevenfold if active disease is present in the 6 months before conception,[25] and a preconception history of nephritis predicts adverse maternal outcome.[26]

Women with SLE have a two- to fourfold increase in the overall rate of pregnancy complications, with increased rates of hypertension, renal disease, preeclampsia, preterm delivery, cesarean delivery, and maternal and neonatal death.[19] Nevertheless, maternal and fetal outcomes have improved with advances in disease management.[9]

Effect on the Mother

Most women with SLE do not have renal impairment at conception, possibly because renal insufficiency impairs fertility. If lupus nephritis preexists, deterioration in renal function may occur during pregnancy and may in some cases be irreversible.[27] Long-term glomerular filtration rate, with or without preexisting lupus nephritis, is usually preserved.[28]

Renal involvement is also associated with maternal hypertension. The presence of hypertension, edema, and proteinuria in both lupus nephritis and preeclampsia makes distinguishing between the two difficult. Although it is controversial whether preeclampsia is more common in patients with SLE, two metaanalyses showed a positive association between a history of lupus nephritis and preeclampsia.[29,30] Distinction between SLE and preeclampsia is critical because treatments are different (immunosuppressive therapy versus delivery, respectively). Increased serum uric acid concentration, proteinuria without active urinary sediment, and liver enzyme abnormalities suggest preeclampsia. The two conditions may also coexist.

SLE may cause thrombocytopenia in pregnancy. When thrombocytopenia occurs in a pregnant woman, preeclampsia, HELLP (hemolysis, elevated liver enzymes, and low platelets) syndrome, and disseminated intravascular coagulation must also be considered. Anemia associated with SLE must be differentiated from nutritional anemia and the physiologic anemia of pregnancy.

Ligamentous relaxation often occurs during late pregnancy and may worsen the pain of lupus arthritis. Patients with SLE occasionally require joint replacement, most commonly of the femoral head. These prostheses may become painful, dislocated, or infected during pregnancy.[31]

Effect on the Fetus

Maternal SLE impairs fetal survival and increases the risk for preterm delivery. The primary predictor for adverse pregnancy outcomes is the presence of LAC.[23] A systematic review of papers published up to 2016 showed that the pooled relative risk (RR) of preterm delivery for patients with SLE versus controls was 2.05 (95% confidence interval [CI], 1.72 to 3.32).[29] In the Hopkins Lupus Pregnancy Cohort, preterm birth occurred in 38 of 57 (67%) pregnancies in women with moderate to severe active SLE, compared with 68 of 210 (32%) pregnancies in women with inactive or mild active SLE.[32] Improved perinatal management and control of disease activity have reduced the rate of fetal loss from 43% (between 1960 and 1965) to 17% (between 2000 and 2003).[33] Data from California showed a preterm delivery rate in SLE that was six times higher than that found in the general population.[34]

Neonatal lupus erythematosus (NLE) is a syndrome resulting from maternal autoantibodies against Ro (SS-A) or La (SS-B) autoantigens crossing the placenta and binding to fetal tissue. Although these autoantibodies are found in up to 87% of patients with SLE,[35] NLE occurs in only a small proportion of patients. The condition is generally benign and self-limiting, and reversible manifestations such as cutaneous lupus, elevation in aminotransferase levels, and thrombocytopenia resolve as maternal antibodies disappear from the neonatal circulation within 8 months of birth. Anti-Ro/anti-La antibodies may bind to fetal cardiac conduction cells *in utero*, leading to cell death and irreversible fetal heart block. Neonatal congenital heart block occurs in 2% of neonates when anti-Ro antibody is detected in the mother, and mortality occurs in about 18% of affected babies.[13,36] Fetal echocardiography reveals atrioventricular dissociation, cardiac dilation, and pericardial effusion. Treatment includes prompt delivery, newborn cardiac pacing, antepartum administration of dexamethasone, and consideration of apheresis to remove maternal antibodies.[37]

Medical Management

Optimally, women with SLE should delay pregnancy until their disease has been quiescent for at least 6 months, and they should be taking "acceptably safe" medications at the time of conception.[20,23,26] Medications with acceptable safety are used to minimize disease activity during gestation.[38] Medications to treat SLE and other rheumatic diseases such as rheumatoid arthritis fall into four broad categories: nonfluorinated glucocorticoids, synthetic disease-modifying antirheumatic drugs (DMARDs), targeted DMARDs, and biologics.[39]

Corticosteroids may be used to treat flares of SLE disease activity. Antenatal exposure to low-dose **prednisone** (<20 mg daily) appears to be safe, and most children born to mothers who have used antenatal corticosteroids develop normally. However, fluorinated glucocorticoids such as **dexamethasone** or **betamethasone** readily cross the placenta and may cause fetal growth restriction and abnormal neuronal development; their use should be restricted to a single course for fetal lung maturation.[39] Prolonged corticosteroid therapy carries the risk of gestational diabetes, striae, gastrointestinal ulceration, and bone demineralization. Regular use of antacids may be required.

DMARDs and immunosuppressive agents form the mainstay of treatment. Synthetic DMARDs such as **hydroxychloroquinine (HCQ), azathioprine**, and **tacrolimus** are frequently used to reduce SLE activity, and their use is considered safe in pregnancy.[38,40] Discontinuation of HCQ just before conception or in early pregnancy leads to a significant increase in disease activity.[41] A systematic review found that antimalarial drugs, particularly HCQ, prevent lupus flares; increase long-term survival; contribute to protection against irreversible organ damage, thrombosis, and bone loss; and have low toxicity.[42] HCQ should be continued in all women who have been taking it before conception, and it may be used to treat flares during gestation. In contrast, **mycophenolate mofetil** should be discontinued before conception owing to the risk for teratogenicity. There is little evidence to support the use of targeted DMARDs such as apremilast and tofacitinib.

Immunosuppressive agents such as **azathioprine** and **tacrolimus** are considered safe for use in pregnancy and may be considered if corticosteroid avoidance is desirable.[19,39] Azathioprine should be continued if used before conception.[20,25] The fetal liver does not express the enzyme necessary to convert azathioprine to its active form, but maternal use of azathioprine has been associated with reversible neonatal lymphopenia, depressed serum immunoglobulin levels, and decreased thymic size in the newborn.[43] Transplant registries do not report increased risk for congenital abnormalities after its use.[44]

Biologic agents such as **rituximab** and **belimumab** are recombinant proteins that typically incorporate IgG antibodies or receptor-blocking proteins. They are being used more frequently,[45] but concerns exist about their duration of action, placental transfer, and teratogenic potential.[38] If used antenatally, consideration is given to their continuation during pregnancy. Data do not yet support their use as first-line medications during pregnancy.

Aspirin, nonsteroidal antiinflammatory drugs (NSAIDs), and stronger analgesics may be used to manage lupus arthritis.[46] Although there is no evidence of teratogenicity with these agents,[43] concern exists that NSAIDs may cause premature closure of the fetal ductus arteriosus, and high-dose aspirin and NSAIDs ideally should be discontinued by 30 weeks' gestation[19] (see Chapter 16). Pregabalin and gabapentin have limited safety data during pregnancy and are best avoided.

Obstetric Management

Patients with SLE are at increased risk for intrauterine fetal death and preterm delivery. Estimation of the gestational age is obtained with ultrasonography at the first prenatal visit and again at 20 weeks' gestation. Continued surveillance consists of nonstress testing, biophysical profile measurement, and/or umbilical artery Doppler velocimetry beginning at 26 to 28 weeks' gestation and performed weekly until delivery.[47]

The coexistence of aPLs (either LAC or triple-positive aPLs; see later discussion) predicts higher maternal and fetal risk. Patients with SLE have an increased risk of preeclampsia (RR 2.99; 95% CI, 2.31 to 3.88).[30] Maternal serologic markers are checked regularly, together with platelet count, creatinine clearance, 24-hour urine protein level, uric acid, and complement levels.[19] In normal pregnancy, serial complement levels gradually increase. However, declining levels of C3 and C4 suggest active disease and lupus nephritis.[20] Thromboprophylaxis is important in patients with **antiphospholipid syndrome** (see later discussion). Aspirin resistance may predict adverse maternal and neonatal outcomes.[48] Regular assessment of blood pressure, weight gain, and proteinuria is performed to detect the development of preeclampsia. Prediction of cardiovascular risk in women with SLE may be possible using the pulse-mass index.[49]

The timing and route of delivery are individualized. Although vaginal delivery is preferred, a cesarean delivery rate of 48% has been reported in parturients with SLE, primarily due to preeclampsia and maternal SLE activity.[50]

Anesthetic Management

The obstetric and anesthesia providers and the rheumatologist should formulate a joint plan for delivery. Maternal organ system involvement, current disease severity, and particularly the presence of flares must be assessed.[51]

Pericarditis is common in patients with SLE and is typically asymptomatic. A history of dyspnea on exertion or unexplained tachycardia may suggest pericarditis or **myocarditis. Cardiac tamponade** has been reported.[52] Prolongation of the PR interval or nonspecific T-wave changes may be seen on the electrocardiogram. Coronary artery vasculitis, accelerated atherosclerosis leading to **myocardial ischemia**, and even **myocardial infarction** in young women have been reported.[53]

An echocardiographic study showed a high incidence of **valvular abnormalities** in patients with SLE, including valvular thickening (51%), vegetation (43%), regurgitation (25%), and stenosis (4%).[54] The American Heart Association does not recommend prophylactic antibiotics for women with common valvular lesions undergoing genitourinary procedures, including vaginal delivery.[55] The recommendations are discussed in Chapter 41.

The prevalence and progression of **pulmonary hypertension** in 28 patients with SLE have been studied.[56] The prevalence increased from 14% at initial evaluation to 43% 5 years later. Epidural anesthesia for cesarean delivery in parturients with pulmonary hypertension has been reported (see Chapter 41).[57,58]

Subclinical **pleuritis** is common, but significant **pleural effusion** is rare. Patients may suffer from **infectious pneumonia** or **lupus pneumonitis**. The latter condition is characterized by fleeting hemorrhagic infiltrates that may become consolidated. **Pulmonary embolism** and **diaphragmatic dysfunction** have been reported.[59]

Central and peripheral sensorimotor and autonomic neuropathies are observed in as many as 25% of patients with SLE,[60] and **vocal cord palsy** has been reported.[51,61] These deficits should be documented before the administration of either neuraxial or general anesthesia. **Migraine headache** and **cerebral vasculitis** resulting from SLE must be considered in the differential diagnosis of a postpartum headache. **Psychological disorders** and frank **psychosis** can occur during disease flares.[62] **Seizures** can occur, especially if chronic anticonvulsant medications are discontinued inadvertently.

Hematologic abnormalities, including **anemia, thrombocytopenia**, and **coagulopathy**, should be documented. An abnormality of the activated partial thromboplastin time (aPTT), which is not corrected with a 1:1 control plasma mix, suggests the presence of either LAC (a coexistent but separate disease entity) or, more rarely, true autoantibodies against specific coagulation factors (e.g., VIII, IX, XII). LAC is a laboratory artifact that does not cause clinical coagulopathy. True coagulation factor autoantibodies (or inhibitors) may result in a significant bleeding diathesis, which contraindicates the administration of neuraxial anesthesia.

Long-term use of NSAIDs leads to qualitative platelet abnormalities, but their role in causing spinal epidural hematoma remains conjectural. In prospective studies of patients undergoing orthopedic procedures (924 patients receiving spinal or epidural anesthesia, of whom 39% were taking preoperative antiplatelet medications)[63] and epidural steroid injection for chronic pain management (1035 patients, of whom 32% reported NSAID use),[64] no cases of spinal epidural hematoma were observed. In the Collaborative Low-dose Aspirin Study in Pregnancy (CLASP), a large, multicenter randomized trial, 9364 pregnant women received either low-dose aspirin (60 mg daily) or placebo for prevention and treatment of preeclampsia. Of 5000 enrollees, at least 1069 patients received epidural analgesia, and no cases of epidural hematoma were observed.[65,66] Current recommendations are that neuraxial anesthesia should not be withheld from patients taking aspirin.[67]

Prosthetic orthopedic joints should be positioned carefully during vaginal or cesarean delivery. Lupus arthritis rarely involves the cervical spine. Women who have undergone long-term corticosteroid therapy should receive a peripartum stress dose of a corticosteroid.

ANTIPHOSPHOLIPID SYNDROME

Definition and Epidemiology

Antiphospholipid syndrome (APS, also known as Hughes' syndrome) was first recognized in the early 1980s[68,69] and classified by international consensus in 2006.[70,71] It is an autoimmune prothrombotic disorder characterized by the presence of three aPLs: LAC, anticardiolipin antibodies (aCL), and anti-beta$_2$-glycoprotein I (aβ_2GPI).[72] Affected patients are at risk for arterial and venous thrombosis and pregnancy-related complications.[73]

Although initially described as a subset of patients with SLE, it is now accepted that APS is a distinct and separate disease entity.[74] About 40% of patients with SLE may have aPLs (LAC in 34% and aCL in 44%),[75] but few will progress to develop thrombotic events. Long-term follow-up suggests that more than half of patients with SLE and aPLs will progress to APS, but few with APS progress to SLE.[74]

The prevalence of APS is unclear. Most information has been derived from the "Euro Phospholipid" cohort of 1000 patients.[76] Prevalence of aPLs in the general population is 1% to 5%, but APS occurs in only a small proportion of people with aPLs; the estimated population prevalence is 40 to 50 per 100,000.[77] Initially APS was thought to be uncommon,[78] but improved clinical recognition suggests that the prevalence of APS may exceed that of SLE.[69]

Pathophysiology

APS is associated with two important misnomers. First, the aPLs do not bind directly to phospholipids but to phospholipid-binding plasma proteins such as β_2GPI, prothrombin, and annexin V. Second, the LAC has no true anticoagulant activity *in vivo* but is a laboratory artifact that affects phospholipid-dependent coagulation assays: the aPTT, the kaolin clotting time (KCT), the tissue thromboplastin inhibition (TTI) test, and the dilute Russell viper venom time (dRVVT). These times remain prolonged even when the tests are repeated with a 1:1 mixture of the patient's plasma and control plasma. Typically the prothrombin time (PT) is normal. LAC appears to block *in vitro* assembly of prothrombinase (a phospholipid complex), thus preventing the conversion of prothrombin to thrombin. True bleeding associated with LAC is extremely rare and, in most cases, is caused by an underlying factor deficiency or inhibitor.[79]

Contrary to expectation, LAC and aCL are associated with both arterial and venous **thrombotic events**. The binding of aPL and aβ_2GPI to cellular β_2GPI receptors causes activation of endothelial cells, platelets, and monocytes, with complement activation and production of prothrombotic mediators that lead to thrombosis.[72,80] Complement activation may lead to inflammation, placental insufficiency, and fetal loss, while aPL interference with fibrinolysis may predispose patients to thrombotic events.[81]

Diagnosis

The diagnosis of APS depends on a clinical history of unexplained recurrent venous or arterial thrombosis, pregnancy loss, and laboratory evidence of aCL or LAC.[80] The latter is demonstrated by abnormal phospholipid-dependent coagulation (elevated aPTT), evidence that this abnormality is caused by an inhibitor rather than a factor deficiency (elevated aPTT with 1:1 mix), and proof that the inhibitor is directed against phospholipid rather than specific coagulation factors. Antibodies should be demonstrable on two occasions separated by 12 weeks.[82] The presence of LAC, aCL, and aβ_2GPI antibodies (triple positivity) with a clinical diagnosis of APS predicts severe disease, particularly if aPLs are present in high titer.[80,83] Results from different laboratories show considerable variability, and guidelines on diagnostic criteria have been published.[84]

Tests for syphilis detect the aPLs present in syphilis, and consequently, the Venereal Disease Research Laboratory (VDRL) and Wasserman test results may be falsely positive. Some 20% of patients with APS may present with an initial diagnosis of idiopathic thrombocytopenic purpura.[81]

Effect on the Mother

Pregnant women with APS are at risk for **venous and arterial thrombosis, pulmonary embolism, myocardial infarction, cerebral infarction**, and **fetal loss**. Cohort studies suggest that contemporary management strategies may improve maternal outcome. The PROMISSE study showed that higher risk was indicated by African or Hispanic descent, presence of LAC, moderate clinical disease activity when pregnancy was diagnosed, thrombocytopenia, and flare activity.[39]

Silver et al.[85] reported that of 130 women with APS followed over a 3-year period, 48% experienced at least one of the following disorders: **transient ischemic attack, peripheral thrombosis** (of which one-fourth occurred in pregnancy and the puerperium), **stroke, amaurosis fugax, autoimmune thrombocytopenia**, and **SLE**. Clark et al.[86] reported that women diagnosed with APS on the basis of recurrent pregnancy loss and evidence of aPLs, but without prior thrombotic events, rarely suffered thrombosis during pregnancy. A history of thromboembolic events significantly worsens prognosis and increases the likelihood of future events, an effect ameliorated by the use of oral anticoagulants.[87] A systematic review estimated an odds ratio of 33 for thrombosis with triple positivity (95% CI, 7.0 to 157.6),[88] while a metaanalysis identified the most important predictors of adverse pregnancy outcomes as previous thrombosis, triple positivity and the presence of LAC.[89]

Low-dose aspirin (ceased 4 weeks prior to delivery) plus low-molecular-weight heparin (LMWH) (e.g., enoxaparin 40 mg daily, continued for 3 to 6 weeks after delivery) is a typical standard regimen for thromboprophylaxis.[80,90] Thrombocytopenia, present in one-fourth of patients with APS, is generally mild and responds to prednisone therapy.

Direct oral anticoagulants (DOACs) such as rituximab and rivaroxaban[91] have been used as alternatives to warfarin in nonpregnant women. Two clinical trials, however, failed to demonstrate clinical advantage, and their use in obstetric patients is not recommended.[72]

The use of HCQ for women with pregnancies at particular risk, in the absence of study findings, has been the subject of expert consensus, with the conclusion that its use may be justified in certain cases or when treatment with aspirin and heparin has been ineffective.[92] Clinical trials for primary and secondary thromboprophylaxis continue.[90]

Catastrophic antiphospholipid syndrome (CAPS or Asherson's syndrome) occurs rarely and is discussed below.[93]

Effect on the Fetus

Pregnant women with APS are at high risk for intrauterine fetal death. Early studies showed that only 7.5% of pregnancies resulted in the delivery of a live newborn.[94] Outcomes have improved, but with a greater incidence of preterm birth.[95] Pregnant women with high positive aPL titers (four times the upper limit of normal) were found to have a 5.7 times higher risk of adverse fetal/neonatal outcome (fetal/neonatal loss, preterm birth and/or low birthweight).[96] The retrospective cohort PREGNANTS study recorded that only 30% of women with triple positivity had a live-born neonate.[97] Placental infarction is the apparent mechanism of fetal demise, of which most occur during mid and late pregnancy. Recommendations for the management of nonpregnant and pregnant patients with APS have been formulated and center around anticoagulation therapy (see later discussion).[98]

Most infants born to women with APS do not have an increased rate of neonatal or childhood complications.[99] Cases of antiphospholipid-related **fetal and neonatal thrombosis** (mainly cerebral thrombosis) and neurodevelopmental abnormalities have been reported.[100]

Medical and Obstetric Management

The mainstay of obstetric management is thromboprophylaxis.[81] Fetal survival and maternal thrombotic risk may be improved when affected pregnant women are treated with combined anticoagulation (low-dose unfractionated heparin) and antiplatelet (low-dose aspirin) medication.[101] Live-birth rates of 70% to 80% have been reported.[102] Neither type of heparin crosses the placental barrier.[103] Recommendations on investigation and management of APS have been made.[104] Women with more than three unexplained pregnancy losses before 10 weeks' gestation should be tested for aPLs; women with APS and recurrent pregnancy loss should receive prophylactic doses of **heparin** and **low-dose aspirin** throughout pregnancy, and administration for 6 to 8 weeks postpartum should be considered. A history of APS with thrombosis may require full anticoagulation throughout pregnancy and the postpartum period.

Catastrophic antiphospholipid syndrome occurs in 1% of patients with APS.[93] It is characterized by rapidly progressive thromboses with organ damage, thrombotic microangiopathy, and a systemic inflammatory response syndrome. Diagnosis requires the presence of aPLs with involvement of at least three organs and rapid onset and progression of disease. Urgent management strategies include elimination of precipitating causes, antibiotic cover for a precipitating bacterial infection, full anticoagulation, intravenous corticosteroids and immunoglobulin, and plasma exchange. **HCQ** and **rituximab** are increasingly used.[105] Mortality is as high as 50%.

Anesthetic Management

There are no large-scale studies describing anesthetic management of patients with APS, and management is similar to that of the patient with SLE. Coexisting autoimmune disorders, secondary organ involvement, and thrombotic phenomena should be evaluated. The term *lupus anticoagulant* is a misnomer (see earlier discussion) and does not warrant withholding neuraxial anesthesia. Infrequently, aPLs can cause coagulation factor deficiencies, and in such patients neuraxial anesthesia is relatively contraindicated. In the absence of an underlying coagulation deficit or anticoagulant therapy, the prolonged aPTT does not suggest a bleeding tendency, and neuraxial anesthesia may be administered safely.

The anesthetic management of pregnancies complicated by APS has been reviewed.[106] All subjects received aspirin (75 to 150 mg daily) throughout pregnancy. In parturients who received thromboprophylaxis with standard unfractionated heparin, spinal or epidural anesthesia was administered 4 hours after the last dose of heparin. The use of LMWH for thromboprophylaxis precludes administration of neuraxial anesthesia for 12 or 24 hours depending on the dose.[67] (see Chapters 38 and 44). The use of **thromboelastography** to document clearance of heparin before administration of neuraxial anesthesia in parturients with LAC has been described.[107]

Neuraxial anesthesia with an epidural, intrathecal, or combined spinal-epidural technique is not contraindicated provided that blood pressure is closely controlled. Parturients with APS who undergo general anesthesia are at risk for venous thrombosis. Compression stockings, warm intravenous fluids, and early ambulation should be used, whereas hypothermia and dehydration should be avoided.[106]

SYSTEMIC SCLEROSIS (SCLERODERMA)

Definition and Epidemiology

Systemic sclerosis or scleroderma is a rare chronic progressive autoimmune disease of unknown etiology characterized by deposition of fibrous connective tissue in the skin and other tissues, microvascular changes, and chronic inflammation. It is a heterogeneous disorder and may be in the form of **limited** or **diffuse cutaneous scleroderma**. A subset of patients exhibit systemic sclerosis without cutaneous involvement.[108] The annual incidence of scleroderma in the United States is 19 per million. The prevalence is 240 per million, which is four to nine times greater than the reported global prevalence. Scleroderma is almost five times more common in women and occurs primarily between 30 and 50 years of age.[109]

Pathophysiology

Epigenetic regulation of gene expression through cellular transcription, without changes in gene sequence, plays a key role in phenotypic expression and is a possible mechanism by which the same genotype can be expressed as different phenotypes.[110] Possible mechanisms include chemical modification of DNA (particularly methylation), histone coding, modification of RNA, and environmental influences. Although the stimulus for fibroblasts to produce excessive collagen and other matrix constituents is unknown, their accumulation leads to microvascular obliteration and fibrosis in the skin and other target organs. Endothelial cells undergo vasomotor and permeability changes, producing cyclic vasoconstriction–vasodilation and edema. Patients with scleroderma produce autoantibodies against nuclear and centromere structures, although their significance is unclear. Scleroderma exhibits a strong female predilection, a steep rise in incidence after the childbearing years, and features that are similar to graft-versus-host disease after bone marrow transplantation, prompting some to postulate that microchimerism may be involved in its pathogenesis. Fetal cells gain access to the maternal circulation during gestation and may be detected in maternal blood for decades after delivery. After some unknown stimulus but possibly including environmental factors, they may differentiate and initiate a reaction similar to graft-versus-host disease.

Diagnosis

Raynaud's phenomenon, characterized by cyclic pallor and cyanosis of the digits in response to cold or emotion, may be a prodrome to scleroderma, with 1% of patients progressing to scleroderma. The triad of Raynaud's phenomenon, non-pitting edema, and hidebound skin establishes the diagnosis of scleroderma. Limited cutaneous scleroderma, formerly termed **CREST syndrome**, involves calcinosis, Raynaud's phenomenon, esophageal dysfunction, sclerodactyly, and telangiectasia. Skin involvement is limited to the hands, face, and feet in this form of the disease. The classification of systemic sclerosis has been updated by The American College of Rheumatology/European League Against Rheumatism and is summarized in Box 40.3.[111]

Effect of Pregnancy

Progression of scleroderma tends to be slow. More than 70% of patients with diffuse cutaneous scleroderma and more than 90% of those with limited cutaneous scleroderma are alive 15 years after diagnosis.[112] Renal failure and malignant hypertension are the most common causes of death. Improvements in

BOX 40.3 Classification of Systemic Sclerosis From the 2013 American College of Rheumatology and European League Against Rheumatism

Proximal skin involvement
  Skin thickening of the fingers of both hands
Skin thickening of the fingers
  Puffy fingers
  Sclerodactyly of the fingers
Fingertip lesions (only count the higher score)
  Digital tip ulcers
  Fingertip pitting scars
Telangiectasia
Abnormal nailfold capillaries
Pulmonary arterial hypertension or interstitial lung disease
Raynaud's phenomenon
Systemic sclerosis-related autoantibodies
  Anticentromere
  Antitopoisomerase I
  Anti-RNA polymerase III

From Denton C, Khanna D. Systemic sclerosis. *Lancet*. 2017;390: 1685–1699.

management allow patients with scleroderma to have successful maternal and fetal outcomes.[113–115] Maternal symptoms were unchanged in 62% of pregnancies and improved in 20%. In the other 18% of pregnancies, esophageal reflux, cardiac arrhythmias, arthritis, skin thickening, and/or renal crisis occurred or worsened. Deterioration of renal function is of greatest concern.[116]

Effect on Pregnancy and the Fetus

In a retrospective study from a single center, the risk of adverse pregnancy outcomes (a composite endpoint that included fetal death, small-for-dates and growth-restricted babies, preeclampsia, preterm birth, and neonatal death) was increased compared with healthy controls and patients with scleroderma.[117,118] Preterm birth occurs in 25% of pregnancies (compared with 5% in control pregnancies), and most preterm deliveries occur in women with unstable diffuse scleroderma of less than 4 years' duration. Miscarriage occurs more commonly in women with long-standing diffuse scleroderma.

Medical Management

Management is symptomatic rather than curative and is directed toward slowing end-organ damage. When lifestyle alterations (e.g., avoidance of cold, cessation of smoking) are no longer effective, management may include **calcium entry–blocking agents** for skin manifestations; **proton-pump inhibitors**, and occasionally **esophageal dilation**, for gastrointestinal tract symptoms; and **phosphodiesterase inhibitors** and **prostaglandins** for pulmonary arterial hypertension. Recent work suggests that tyrosine kinase inhibitors may have a beneficial effect in slowing the development of interstitial lung disease.[119] No disease modification benefits have been shown by administration of **penicillamine**, **methotrexate**, or other immunosuppressive agents (other than the use of glucocorticoids for inflammatory myositis).[120,121]

Drugs with unproven or potential teratogenicity are relatively contraindicated during pregnancy. However, **angiotensin-converting enzyme (ACE) inhibitors** are the agents of choice for treating scleroderma-associated renal crisis and malignant hypertension, despite the potential for fetal teratogenicity, renal atresia, pulmonary hypoplasia, anhydramnios, and fetopathy; captopril is most favored.[116] ACE inhibitors provide the only effective control of hypertension during scleroderma-associated renal crisis and should be started immediately if maternal hypertension occurs. Their use should be avoided if hypertension or overt renal crisis is not present. **Nitric oxide donors** and possibly **heparin** may provide some protection against placental dysfunction in pregnant women with scleroderma.[122]

Obstetric Management

Pregnant women with scleroderma should be specifically evaluated for evidence of renal, pulmonary, and cardiac dysfunction. Preterm delivery or termination of pregnancy may be required in the presence of advanced or rapidly progressive disease. Frequent assessment of renal function and intensive observation for the onset of systemic or pulmonary hypertension, cardiac dysfunction, and fetal compromise, combined with improvements in monitoring and treatment, allow most mothers to deliver healthy infants. Although the prevalence of left ventricular diastolic dysfunction is known to be higher in patients with scleroderma than in the general population,[123] an association with pregnancy has not been noted. However, additional monitoring based on clinical findings may be indicated. Obstructive uropathy may result from an enlarging uterus trapped within a noncompliant abdomen.[124] Uterine and cervical wall thickening may lead to ineffective uterine contractions or cervical dystocia at delivery.[125] Even the tightest abdominal skin usually heals if cesarean delivery is necessary.

Anesthetic Management

Anesthetic management can be challenging and early multidisciplinary involvement is required. History and physical examination should be directed toward detection of underlying systemic dysfunction. Laboratory tests include complete blood cell count, coagulation screen, electrolyte concentrations and creatinine clearance, arterial blood gas analysis, urinalysis, and urine protein determination. An electrocardiogram and pulmonary function testing should be performed in all patients. Echocardiography is commonly used to assess ventricular dysfunction, pericardial and pleural effusions, and pulmonary hypertension.[126] Patients with scleroderma may develop pulmonary hypertension as a consequence of vascular changes, fibrosis, or left ventricular dysfunction. Administration of a pulmonary vasodilator may increase the likelihood of a favorable outcome.[127] Particular attention should be paid to arterial pulses, noninvasive blood pressure measurement, peripheral venous access, extent of Raynaud's phenomenon involvement, and special positioning requirements.

Severe limitation of mouth opening caused by hidebound perioral skin may make direct laryngoscopy impossible, mandates careful airway assessment[128] and may necessitate awake tracheal intubation.[129] The changes in airway assessment scores that occur during labor should also be borne in mind[130] (see Chapter 29).

If cesarean delivery is required, the decision to use neuraxial or general anesthesia depends on the urgency of delivery, anticipated airway difficulty, and operator skills. A report of two pregnant women with scleroderma and pulmonary hypertension described administration of neuraxial anesthesia in one and general anesthesia in the other, highlighting the complexity of management choices.[127] Gastric hypomotility increases the risk for esophageal reflux and aspiration. Early administration of epidural analgesia in laboring women is encouraged if tracheal intubation is likely to be difficult. Even when severe diffuse cutaneous involvement is present, the skin of the lumbar back is usually spared.

Prolonged duration of neuraxial anesthesia has been observed in some patients with scleroderma and may be caused by reduced uptake of the local anesthetic agent as a consequence of microvasculature changes. This is not a contraindication to neuraxial techniques but should prompt the use of small incremental boluses of the local anesthetic agent, and the patient should be warned of the possibility of prolonged neural blockade.[131]

Venous access may be difficult. Diffuse cutaneous involvement may indicate the need for central venous catheterization, and for invasive arterial monitoring if noninvasive blood pressure measurement is inaccurate. Radial artery catheterization is contraindicated in patients with Raynaud's phenomenon because of the risk for hand ischemia. Brachial artery catheterization may be necessary. Warming of the patient, and especially of the extremities affected by Raynaud's phenomenon, is required. Scleroderma reduces tear production, and the eyes should be protected against corneal abrasions.

POLYMYOSITIS AND DERMATOMYOSITIS

Definition and Epidemiology

Polymyositis and **dermatomyositis** represent two members of a larger disease group, the idiopathic inflammatory myopathies. Polymyositis is characterized by nonsuppurative inflammation of muscle, primarily skeletal muscles of the proximal limbs, neck, and pharynx. This inflammation leads to symmetrical weakness, atrophy, and fibrosis of affected muscle groups, with the hip and thigh muscles most frequently affected.[132] Dermatomyositis represents the same disorder, with the addition of a characteristic heliotrope eruption (blue-purple discoloration of the upper eyelid) and Gottron's papules (raised, scaly, violet eruptions over the knuckles). These disorders are rare and more common in women and with increasing age. A systematic review reported the incidence of inflammatory myopathies as a whole as 1.16 to 19/million/year with prevalence 2.4 to 33.8/100,000.[133]

Pathophysiology

Both polymyositis and dermatomyositis are associated with other autoimmune disorders, notably scleroderma. The etiology of inflammatory muscle disease is unknown and probably multifactorial. An initial insult mediated by viral or other infectious agents, or exposure to environmental substances, may lead to muscle damage in genetically susceptible individuals, which may then trigger an autoimmune response involving chronic muscle inflammation. A viral etiology is suggested by seasonal and geographic clustering of new cases. However, viral genomic material has not been identified in affected muscle tissue. Recent findings show that infection with SARS-Cov-2 (COVID-19) may induce myositis and trigger inflammation in patients with autoimmune conditions.[134] Many drugs, including lipid-lowering drugs in the statin group and antiretroviral drugs, are associated with the development of myopathy. The presence of cellular infiltrates within affected muscle tissue and complement-mediated capillary damage are features of inflammatory muscle diseases. More than 12 autoantibodies have been identified in affected individuals. Underlying malignancy has been associated with both conditions, although causality is unclear; the association is stronger for dermatomyositis than for polymyositis.[135]

Diagnosis

The diagnostic criteria proposed by Bohan and Peter remain the standard for classification of polymyositis and dermatomyositis (Box 40.4).[136] After exclusion of other conditions that can mimic polymyositis or dermatomyositis, clinical features together with electromyographic and laboratory evidence of myositis (both through blood tests and muscle biopsy) establish the diagnosis. Serum creatine kinase concentration correlates with disease activity. More recently the identification of myositis-specific autoantibodies may permit further refinement in classification.[132]

Systemic involvement may be variable. Pharyngeal muscle involvement leads to **dysphagia** and **reflux**, and most patients exhibit **impairment of gastric and esophageal motility**.[137] Pulmonary involvement is present in 50% of

---

> **BOX 40.4   Diagnostic Criteria for Polymyositis and Dermatomyositis**
>
> **Polymyositis**
> - Symmetric weakness of proximal muscles
> - Histologic evidence of muscle inflammation and necrosis
> - Elevation of serum skeletal muscle enzymes
> - Electromyographic evidence of myopathy
>
> **Dermatomyositis**
> - Three or four of the above, plus heliotrope eruption or Gottron's papules
>
> From Bohan A, Peter JB. Polymyositis and dermatomyositis (second of two parts). *N Engl J Med*. 1975;292:403–407.

patients with polymyositis/dermatomyositis, with **chronic aspiration pneumonitis** and **pneumonia** as the most common manifestations. **Interstitial lung disease** occurs in about 30% of patients and may rarely lead to **pulmonary hypertension**.[138] Myositis of the respiratory muscles may cause respiratory insufficiency. **Cardiac involvement** includes nonspecific repolarization abnormalities, conduction disturbances, arrhythmias, coronary artery vasculitis, and, rarely, heart failure.[139] **Arthritis** generally involves the small joints of the hands and fingers. Renal or hematologic involvement is rare. The onset of a pregnancy-associated form of dermatomyositis has been described postpartum.[140]

Effect of Pregnancy

There are limited reports of polymyositis or dermatomyositis during pregnancy. Ishii et al.[141] reviewed 12 reports of 29 pregnancies during a 30-year period. In 11 (40%) of the patients, the initial diagnosis was made during gestation or the immediate postpartum period. Among the 18 patients with previously diagnosed disease, the disease remained inactive in 11 (61%) of the patients, and two (11%) had an exacerbation of disease activity. Pregnancy may be a trigger for induction of dermatomyositis in some women.[142] Pregnant patients with inflammatory myopathies have increased risk for developing hypertensive disorders and an increased length of hospital admission compared with women who do not have myopathy.[143]

Effect on the Fetus

Fetal outcome is influenced by disease activity; it has been reported that 60% of women with minimal activity delivered healthy newborns at term,[141] but fetal survival is affected by concurrent polymyositis/dermatomyositis. Consequences may include fetal growth restriction, preterm delivery, and fetal death.[144] A similar correlation was noted between outcome and disease activity in four pregnant women with polymyositis/dermatomyositis: two with active disease and fetal death and two with disease remission and uneventful outcome. A large cohort study from Brazil documented 98 female patients (60 with dermatomyositis and 38 with polymyositis), of whom 78 women had an obstetric history; 57 women had been pregnant before their myositis diagnosis; 15 women became pregnant after the diagnosis was made; and six women were diagnosed with myositis while pregnant or in the postpartum period.[145] Adverse pregnancy outcomes (either as worsening of maternal condition or of fetal compromise) were associated with intercurrent clinical conditions such as diabetes mellitus, hypertension, and hypothyroidism, rather than as a direct consequence of dermatomyositis or polymyositis.

Medical and Obstetric Management

Pregnancy should be planned during periods of disease inactivity. Serum creatine kinase, glutamic oxaloacetic transaminase, and aldolase determinations can guide this decision. Obstetric management involves frequent monitoring of disease activity and fetal well-being.

Glucocorticoid treatment remains the mainstay of medical management of active disease. Efficacy of steroids has not been demonstrated in controlled studies, but improvement in muscle strength and decreased creatine kinase concentrations are usually seen after 1 to 2 months of either continuous or pulsed steroid therapy. **Methotrexate, azathioprine**, and **intravenous immunoglobulin** may be beneficial; their use and safety in pregnant patients are supported by a limited amount of evidence.[146,147] A recent systematic review suggested, but could not confirm, benefit from methotrexate, azathioprine, **cyclosporine, rituximab**, and intravenous immunoglobulin,[148] but very few data relate to pregnant patients. The first-line drug for treatment of skin manifestations is **HCQ**.[149]

Rituximab and tocilizumab (biologic agents that deplete a subset of B cells implicated in myositic infiltration) demonstrated some efficacy in patients with severe and refractory myositis, but failed to achieve specified endpoints in large trials.[150,151]

Anesthetic Management

Anesthetic management of the pregnant woman with polymyositis/dermatomyositis begins with the evaluation of disease activity and underlying cardiopulmonary involvement. If muscle weakness is present, spirometry should be performed to determine whether respiratory muscles are affected. Maximum breathing capacity and peak expiratory flow rate are the most helpful measurements. Pharyngeal weakness may cause chronic aspiration and pulmonary diffusion defects. Arterial blood gas analysis and a chest radiograph should be obtained in patients with a history of aspiration. An electrocardiogram should be obtained to exclude conduction abnormalities and arrhythmias.

Although neuraxial anesthesia has been used safely,[152] its use in patients with muscle weakness requires caution because excessive cephalad spread may further impair intercostal muscle function and lead to ventilatory failure. Abdominal muscle paralysis may slow progress of the second stage of labor. Careful epidural administration of a dilute solution of local anesthetic with a lipophilic opioid may provide effective pain relief without adverse effect on the progress of labor; intrathecal opioid administration is an attractive alternative in these patients.

Patients with polymyositis/dermatomyositis may exhibit an **atypical response to muscle relaxants**. Isolated case reports with the use of **succinylcholine (suxamethonium)** have described both short-lived (3 minutes) thumb contractures in a child with dermatomyositis,[153] and prolonged paralysis (50 minutes) in a patient who was also found to be homozygous for atypical pseudocholinesterase.[154] Of four other patients with dermatomyositis in whom the dibucaine number was measured, one was heterozygous for atypical pseudocholinesterase. The occurrence of benign contractures and the possibility of atypical pseudocholinesterase do not preclude the use of succinylcholine if it is required for cesarean delivery. Alternatively, rocuronium may be considered for rapid-sequence induction.

An atypical response to **nondepolarizing muscle relaxants** may also occur. A case of prolonged paralysis (9.5 hours) after administration of vecuronium in a patient with polymyositis has been reported.[155] However, underlying malignancy, to which patients with dermatomyositis and polymyositis are prone, may have an associated **myasthenic syndrome** that can prolong neuromuscular blockade. Other reports of nondepolarizing neuromuscular blockade in patients with polymyositis/dermatomyositis have described a normal response and recovery.[156] Parturients who have undergone long-term corticosteroid therapy should receive a peripartum stress dose of a corticosteroid.

Neuromuscular recovery should be verified before tracheal extubation. Some investigators have advocated the avoidance of agents known to trigger malignant hyperthermia in patients with polymyositis/dermatomyositis and elevated creatine kinase levels,[156] but the association is speculative and is not supported by published clinical experience.

KEY POINTS

- Pregnancy does not worsen the long-term course of autoimmune disorders.
- Autoimmune disorders can lead to renal, cardiac, and pulmonary dysfunction.
- Systemic lupus erythematosus can result in maternal thrombocytopenia.
- Systemic lupus erythematosus is associated with a higher incidence of spontaneous abortion, intrauterine fetal demise, and preterm delivery.
- Antiphospholipid syndrome is characterized by the presence of the autoantibodies lupus anticoagulant, anticardiolipin antibody, and anti-beta$_2$-glycoprotein I.
- The term *lupus anticoagulant* is a misnomer because it has no true anticoagulant activity *in vivo*.
- Patients with lupus anticoagulant do not have a bleeding tendency in the absence of an underlying coagulation disorder and can safely receive neuraxial anesthesia.
- Patients with scleroderma are at increased risk for difficult airway management.
- Scleroderma can prolong the duration of neuraxial anesthesia.
- The severity of polymyositis/dermatomyositis affects fetal survival.
- Patients with polymyositis/dermatomyositis may have an atypical response to succinylcholine.
- Neuraxial anesthesia must be administered cautiously to parturients with polymyositis/dermatomyositis and intercostal muscle weakness.

REFERENCES

1. Burnet F. A modification of Jerne's theory of antibody production using the concept of clonal selection. *Aust J Sci.* 1957;20:67–69.
2. McGonagle D, McDermott MF. A proposed classification of the immunological diseases. *PLoS Med.* 2006;3:e297.
3. Davidson A, Diamond B. Autoimmune diseases. *N Engl J Med.* 2001;345:340–350.
4. Cotsapas C, Voight BF, Rossin E, et al. Pervasive sharing of genetic effects in autoimmune disease. *PLoS Genet.* 2011;7:e1002254.
5. Cruz-Tapias P, Pérez-Fernández OM, Rojas-Villarraga A, et al. Shared HLA class II in six autoimmune diseases in Latin America: a meta-analysis. *Autoimmune Dis.* 2012;10:569728.
6. Long H, Yin H, Wang L, et al. The critical role of epigenetics in systemic lupus erythematosus and autoimmunity. *J Autoimmun.* 2016;74:118–138.
7. Lahita R. The immunoendocrinology of systemic lupus erythematosus. *Clin Immunol.* 2016;172:98–100.
8. Weckerle CE, Niewold TB. The unexplained female predominance of systemic lupus erythematosus: clues from genetic and cytokine studies. *Clin Rev Allergy Immunol.* 2011;40:42–49.
9. Marder W, Littlejohn EA, Somers EC. Pregnancy and autoimmune connective tissue diseases. *Best Pract Res Clin Rheumatol.* 2016;30:63–80.
10. Chau A, Markley JC, Juang J, Tsen LC. Cytokines in the perinatal period; Part II. *Int J Obstet Anesth.* 2016;26:48–58.
11. Chau A, Markley JC, Juang J, Tsen LC. Cytokines in the perinatal period; Part I. *Int J Obstet Anesth.* 2016;26:39–47.
12. Somers E. Pregnancy and autoimmune diseases. *Best Pract Res Clin Obstet Gynaecol.* 2020;64:3–10.
13. Yamamoto Y, Aoki S. Systemic lupus erythematosus: strategies to improve pregnancy outcomes. *Int J Womens Health.* 2016;8:265–272.
14. Munoz L, van Bavel C, Franz S, et al. Apoptosis in the pathogenesis of systemic lupus erythematosus. *Lupus.* 2008;17:371–375.
15. Varghese S, Crocker I, Bruce IN, Tower C. Systemic lupus erythematosus, regulatory T cells and pregnancy. *Expert Rev Clin Immunol.* 2011;7:635–648.
16. D'Cruz D, Khamashta M, Hughes G. Systemic lupus erythematosus. *Lancet.* 2007;369:587–596.
17. Aringer M, Costenbader K, Daikh D, et al. 2019 European League Against Rheumatism/American College of Rheumatology classification criteria for systemic lupus erythematosus. *Ann Rheum Dis.* 2019;78:1151–1159.
18. He X, Jiang D, Wang Z, et al. Clinical features of new-onset systemic lupus erythematosus during pregnancy in Central China: a retrospective study of 68 pregnancies. *Clin Rheumatol.* 2021;40:2121–2131.
19. Sammaritano LR. Management of systemic lupus erythematosus during pregnancy. *Annu Rev Med.* 2017;68:271–285.

20. Petri M. The Hopkins lupus pregnancy center: ten key issues in management. *Rheum Dis Clin North Am.* 2007;33:227–235.

21. Soh MC, Nelson-Piercy C. High-risk pregnancy and the rheumatologist. *Rheumatology (Oxford).* 2015;54:572–587.

22. Soh MC, Nelson-Piercy C, Dib F, et al. Brief report: Association between pregnancy outcomes and death from cardiovascular causes in parous women with systemic lupus erythematosus: a study using Swedish population registries. *Arthritis Rheumatol.* 2015;67:2376–2382.

23. Buyon JP, Kim MY, Guerra MM, et al. Predictors of pregnancy outcomes in patients with lupus: a cohort study. *Ann Intern Med.* 2015;163:153–163.

24. Kim JW, Jung JY, Kim HA, et al. Lupus low disease activity state achievement is important for reducing adverse outcomes in pregnant patients with systemic lupus erythematosus. *J Rheumatol.* 2021;48:707–716.

25. Clowse ME. Lupus activity in pregnancy. *Rheum Dis Clin North Am.* 2007;33:237–252.

26. Kwok LW, Tam LS, Zhu T, et al. Predictors of maternal and fetal outcomes in pregnancies of patients with systemic lupus erythematosus. *Lupus.* 2011;20:829–836.

27. Lazzaroni MG, Dall'Ara F, Fredi M, et al. A comprehensive review of the clinical approach to pregnancy and systemic lupus erythematosus. *J Autoimmun.* 2016;74:106–117.

28. Bramham K, Hunt BJ, Bewley S, et al. Pregnancy outcomes in systemic lupus erythematosus with and without previous nephritis. *J Rheumatol.* 2011;38:1906–1913.

29. Wei S, Lai K, Yang Z, Zeng K. Systemic lupus erythematosus and risk of preterm birth: a systematic review and meta-analysis of observational studies. *Lupus.* 2017;26:563–571.

30. Dong Y, Yuan F, Dai Z, et al. Preeclampsia in systemic lupus erythematosus pregnancy: a systematic review and meta-analysis. *Clin Rheumatol.* 2020;39:319–325.

31. Lockshin MD. Pregnancy associated with systemic lupus erythematosus. *Semin Perinatol.* 1990;14:130–138.

32. Clowse ME, Magder LS, Witter F, Petri M. The impact of increased lupus activity on obstetric outcomes. *Arthritis Rheum.* 2005;52:514–521.

33. Clark CA, Spitzer KA, Laskin CA. Decrease in pregnancy loss rates in patients with systemic lupus erythematosus over a 40-year period. *J Rheumatol.* 2005;32:1709–1712.

34. Yasmeen S, Wilkins EE, Field NT, et al. Pregnancy outcomes in women with systemic lupus erythematosus. *J Matern Fetal Med.* 2001;10:91–96.

35. Petri M, Watson R, Hochberg MC. Anti-Ro antibodies and neonatal lupus. *Rheum Dis Clin North Am.* 1989;15:335–360.

36. Brucato A, Doria A, Frassi M, et al. Pregnancy outcome in 100 women with autoimmune diseases and anti-Ro/SSA antibodies: a prospective controlled study. *Lupus.* 2002;11:716–721.

37. Buyon JP, Clancy RM. Neonatal lupus: basic research and clinical perspectives. *Rheum Dis Clin North Am.* 2005;31:299–313.

38. Tosounidou S, Gordon C. Medications in pregnancy and breastfeeding. *Best Pract Res Clin Obstet Gynaecol.* 2020;64:68–76.

39. Petri M. Pregnancy and systemic lupus erythematosus. *Best Pract Res Clin Obstet Gynaecol.* 2020;64:24–30.

40. Dima A, Jurcut C, Arnaud L. Hydroxychloroquine in systemic and autoimmune diseases: where are we now? *Joint Bone Spine.* 2021;88:105143.

41. Clowse ME, Magder L, Witter F, Petri M. Hydroxychloroquine in lupus pregnancy. *Arthritis Rheum.* 2006;54:3640–3647.

42. Ruiz-Irastorza G, Martín-Iglesias D, Soto-Peleteiro A. Update on antimalarials and systemic lupus erythematosus. *Curr Opin Rheumatol.* 2020;32:572–582.

43. Ostensen M, Ostensen H. Safety of nonsteroidal antiinflammatory drugs in pregnant patients with rheumatic disease. *J Rheumatol.* 1996;23:1045–1049.

44. Saavedra MA, Sanchez A, Morales S, et al. Azathioprine during pregnancy in systemic lupus erythematosus patients is not associated with poor fetal outcome. *Clin Rheumatol.* 2015;34:1211–1216.

45. Doria A, Gershwin ME, Selmi C. From old concerns to new advances and personalized medicine in lupus: the end of the tunnel is approaching. *J Autoimmun.* 2016;74:1–5.

46. Sammaritano LR, Bermas BL, Chakravarty EE, et al. American College of Rheumatology guideline for the management of reproductive health in rheumatic and musculoskeletal disease. *Arthritis Rheum.* 2020;72:529–556.

47. Witter FR. Management of the high-risk lupus pregnant patient. *Rheum Dis Clin North Am.* 2007;33:253–265.

48. Wojtowicz A, Undas A, Huras H, et al. Aspirin resistance may be associated with adverse pregnancy outcomes. *Neuro Endocrinol Lett.* 2011;32:334–339.

49. García-Villegas EA, Márquez-González H, Flores-Suárez LF, Villa-Romero AR. The pulse-mass index as a predictor of cardiovascular events in women with systemic lupus erythematosus. *Med Clin (Barc).* 2017;148:57–62.

50. Eudy AM, Jayasundara M, Haroun T, et al. Reasons for cesarean and medically indicated deliveries in pregnancies in women with systemic lupus erythematosus. *Lupus.* 2018;27:351–356.

51. Ben-Menachem E. Systemic lupus erythematosus: a review for anesthesiologists. *Anesth Analg.* 2010;111:665–676.

52. Averbuch M, Bojko A, Levo Y. Cardiac tamponade in the early postpartum period as the presenting and predominant manifestation of systemic lupus erythematosus. *J Rheumatol.* 1986;13:444–445.

53. Zahid S, Mohamed MS, Wassif H, et al. Analysis of cardiovascular complications during delivery admissions among patients with systemic lupus erythematosus, 2004-2019. *JAMA Netw Open.* 2022;5:e2243388.

54. Roldan C, Shively B, Crawford M. An echocardiographic study of valvular heart disease associated with systemic lupus erythematosus. *N Engl J Med.* 1996;335:1424–1430.

55. Wilson WR, Gewitz M, Lockhart PB, et al. Prevention of viridans group streptococcal infective endocarditis: a scientific statement from the American Heart Association. *Circulation.* 2021;143:e963–e978.

56. Winslow T, Ossipov M, Fazio GP, et al. Five-year follow-up study of the prevalence and progression of pulmonary hypertension in systemic lupus erythematosus. *Am Heart J.* 1995;129:510–515.

57. Cuenco J, Tzeng G, Wittels B. Anesthetic management of the parturient with systemic lupus erythematosus, pulmonary hypertension, and pulmonary edema. *Anesthesiology.* 1999;91:568–570.

58. McMillan E, Martin WL, Waugh J, et al. Management of pregnancy in women with pulmonary hypertension secondary to SLE and anti-phospholipid syndrome. *Lupus.* 2002;11:392–398.

59. Carette S. Cardiopulmonary manifestations of systemic lupus erythematous. *Rheum Dis Clin North Am*. 1988;14:135–147.

60. Huynh C, Ho S, Fong K, et al. Peripheral neuropathy in systemic lupus erythematosus. *J Clin Neurophysiol*. 1999;16:164–168.

61. Leszczynski P, Pawlak-Bus K. Vocal cords palsy in systemic lupus erythematosus patient: diagnostic and therapeutic difficulties. *Rheumatol Int*. 2013;33:1577–1580.

62. Brey RL, Holliday SL, Saklad AR, et al. Neuropsychiatric syndromes in lupus: prevalence using standardized definitions. *Neurology*. 2002;58:1214–1220.

63. Horlocker TT, Wedel DJ, Schroeder DR, et al. Preoperative antiplatelet therapy does not increase the risk of spinal hematoma associated with regional anesthesia. *Anesth Analg*. 1995;80:303–309.

64. Horlocker TT. Regional anaesthesia in the patient receiving antithrombotic and antiplatelet therapy. *Br J Anaesth*. 2011;107(suppl 1):i96–106.

65. de Swiet M, Redman CW. Aspirin, extradural anaesthesia and the MRC Collaborative Low-dose Aspirin Study in Pregnancy (CLASP). *Br J Anaesth*. 1992;69:109–110.

66. CLASP (Collaborative Low-dose Aspirin Study in Pregnancy) Collaborative Group CLASP: a randomised trial of low-dose aspirin for the prevention and treatment of pre-eclampsia among 9364 pregnant women. *Lancet*. 1994;343:619–629.

67. Horlocker TT, Vandermeulen E, Kopp SL, et al. Regional anesthesia in the patient receiving antithrombotic or thrombolytic therapy: American Society of Regional Anesthesia and Pain Medicine evidence-based guidelines (fourth edition). *Reg Anesth Pain Med*. 2018;43:263–309.

68. Hughes GR. Thrombosis, abortion, cerebral disease, and the lupus anticoagulant. *Br Med J (Clin Res Ed)*. 1983;287:1088–1089.

69. Hughes G. Hughes syndrome: the antiphospholipid syndrome – a clinical overview. *Clin Rev Allergy Immunol*. 2007;32:3–12.

70. Miyakis S, Lockshin MD, Atsumi T, et al. International consensus statement on an update of the classification criteria for definite antiphospholipid syndrome (APS). *J Thromb Haemost*. 2006;4:295–306.

71. Tripodi A, de Groot PG, Pengo V. Antiphospholipid syndrome: laboratory detection, mechanisms of action and treatment. *J Intern Med*. 2011;270:110–122.

72. Petri M. Antiphospholipid syndrome. *Transl Res*. 2020;225:70–81.

73. Gómez-Puerta JA, Cervera R. Diagnosis and classification of the antiphospholipid syndrome. *J Autoimmun*. 2014;48–49:20–25.

74. Pons-Estel GJ, Andreoli L, Scanzi F, et al. The antiphospholipid syndrome in patients with systemic lupus erythematosus. *J Autoimmun*. 2017;76:10–20.

75. Love PE, Santoro SA. Antiphospholipid antibodies: anticardiolipin and the lupus anticoagulant in systemic lupus erythematosus (SLE) and in non-SLE disorders. Prevalence and clinical significance. *Ann Intern Med*. 1990;112:682–698.

76. Cervera R, Piette JC, Font J, et al. Antiphospholipid syndrome: clinical and immunologic manifestations and patterns of disease expression in a cohort of 1,000 patients. *Arthritis Rheum*. 2002;46:1019–1027.

77. Arslan E, Branch DW. Antiphospholipid syndrome: diagnosis and management in the obstetric patient. *Best Pract Res Clin Obstet Gynaecol*. 2020;64:31–40.

78. Harris EN. A reassessment of the antiphospholipid syndrome. *J Rheumatol*. 1990;17:733–735.

79. Vermylen J, Carreras LO, Arnout J. Attempts to make sense of the antiphospholipid syndrome. *J Thromb Haemost*. 2007;5:1–4.

80. Sammaritano LR. Antiphospholipid syndrome. *Best Pract Res Clin Rheumatol*. 2020;34:101463.

81. Negrini S, Pappalardo F, Murdaca G, et al. The antiphospholipid syndrome: from pathophysiology to treatment. *Clin Exp Med*. 2017;17:257–267.

82. Sangle NA, Smock KJ. Antiphospholipid antibody syndrome. *Arch Pathol Lab Med*. 2011;135:1092–1096.

83. Pengo V. APS-controversies in diagnosis and management, critical overview of current guidelines. *Thromb Res*. 2011;127(suppl 3):S51–S52.

84. Devreese KMJ, de Groot PG, de Laat B, et al. Guidance from the Scientific and Standardization Committee for lupus anticoagulant/antiphospholipid antibodies of the International Society on Thrombosis and Haemostasis: update of the guidelines for lupus anticoagulant detection and interpretation. *J Thromb Haemost*. 2020;18:2828–2839.

85. Silver RM, Draper ML, Scott JR, et al. Clinical consequences of antiphospholipid antibodies: an historic cohort study. *Obstet Gynecol*. 1994;83:372–377.

86. Clark CA, Spitzer KA, Crowther MA, et al. Incidence of postpartum thrombosis and preterm delivery in women with antiphospholipid antibodies and recurrent pregnancy loss. *J Rheumatol*. 2007;34:992–996.

87. Pengo V, Ruffatti A, Legnani C, et al. Clinical course of high-risk patients diagnosed with antiphospholipid syndrome. *J Thromb Haemost*. 2010;8:237–242.

88. Reynaud Q, Lega JC, Mismetti P, et al. Risk of venous and arterial thrombosis according to type of antiphospholipid antibodies in adults without systemic lupus erythematosus: a systematic review and meta-analysis. *Autoimmun Rev*. 2014;13:595–608.

89. Walter IJ, Klein Haneveld MJ, Lely AT, et al. Pregnancy outcome predictors in antiphospholipid syndrome: a systematic review and meta-analysis. *Autoimmun Rev*. 2021;20:102901.

90. Radin M, Cecchi I, Rubini E, et al. Treatment of antiphospholipid syndrome. *Clin Immunol*. 2020;221:108597.

91. Cohen H, Hunt BJ, Efthymiou M, et al. Rivaroxaban versus warfarin to treat patients with thrombotic antiphospholipid syndrome, with or without systemic lupus erythematosus (RAPS): a randomised, controlled, open-label, phase 2/3, non-inferiority trial. *Lancet Haematol*. 2016;3:e426–e436.

92. Sciascia S, Branch DW, Levy RA, et al. The efficacy of hydroxychloroquine in altering pregnancy outcome in women with antiphospholipid antibodies. Evidence and clinical judgment. *Thromb Haemost*. 2016;115:285–290.

93. Asherson R. The catastrophic antiphospholipid (Asherson's) syndrome. *Autoimmun Rev*. 2006;6:64–67.

94. Lubbe WF, Liggins GC. Lupus anticoagulant and pregnancy. *Am J Obstet Gynecol*. 1985;153:322–327.

95. Strouse J, Donovan BM, Fatima M, et al. Impact of autoimmune rheumatic diseases on birth outcomes: a population-based study. *RMD Open*. 2019;5:e000878.

96. Simchen MJ, Dulitzki M, Rofe G, et al. High positive antibody titers and adverse pregnancy outcome in women with antiphospholipid syndrome. *Acta Obstet Gynecol Scand*. 2011;90:1428–1433.

97. Saccone G, Berghella V, Maruotti GM, et al. Antiphospholipid antibody profile based obstetric outcomes of primary antiphospholipid syndrome: the PREGNANTS study. *Am J Obstet Gynecol.* 2017;216:525.e1–e12.

98. Tektonidou MG, Andreoli L, Limper M, et al. EULAR recommendations for the management of antiphospholipid syndrome in adults. *Ann Rheum Dis.* 2019;78:1296–1304.

99. Nalli C, Iodice A, Andreoli L, et al. The effects of lupus and antiphospholipid antibody syndrome on foetal outcomes. *Lupus.* 2014;23:507–517.

100. Mekinian A, Lachassinne E, Nicaise-Roland P, et al. European registry of babies born to mothers with antiphospholipid syndrome. *Ann Rheum Dis.* 2013;72:217–222.

101. Empson M, Lassere M, Craig J, Scott J. Prevention of recurrent miscarriage for women with antiphospholipid antibody or lupus anticoagulant. *Cochrane Database Syst Rev.* 2005;(2):CD002859.

102. Schreiber K, Hunt BJ. Managing antiphospholipid syndrome in pregnancy. *Thromb Res.* 2019;181:S41–S46.

103. Ziakas PD, Pavlou M, Voulgarelis M. Heparin treatment in antiphospholipid syndrome with recurrent pregnancy loss: a systematic review and meta-analysis. *Obstet Gynecol.* 2010;115:1256–1262.

104. Keeling D, Mackie I, Moore GW, et al. Guidelines on the investigation and management of antiphospholipid syndrome. *Br J Haemat.* 2012;157:47–58.

105. Ünlü O, Zuily S, Erkan D. The clinical significance of antiphospholipid antibodies in systemic lupus erythematosus. *Eur J Rheumatol.* 2016;3:75–84.

106. Kim JW, Kim TW, Ryu KH, et al. Anaesthetic considerations for patients with antiphospholipid syndrome undergoing non-cardiac surgery. *J Int Med Res.* 2020;48:300060519896889.

107. Harnett M, Kodali BS. Thromboelastography assessment of coagulation status in parturients with lupus anticoagulant receiving heparin therapy. *Int J Obstet Anesth.* 2006;15:177–178.

108. Walker JG, Pope J, Baron M, et al. The development of systemic sclerosis classification criteria. *Clin Rheumatol.* 2007;26:1401–1409.

109. Mayes MD, Lacey JV, Beebe-Dimmer J, et al. Prevalence, incidence, survival, and disease characteristics of systemic sclerosis in a large US population. *Arthritis Rheum.* 2003;48:2246–2255.

110. Altorok N, Kahaleh B. Epigenetics and systemic sclerosis. *Semin Immunopathol.* 2015;37:453–462.

111. Denton CP, Khanna D. Systemic sclerosis. *Lancet.* 2017;390:1685–1699.

112. Scussel-Lonzetti L, Joyal F, Raynauld J-P, et al. Predicting mortality in systemic sclerosis: analysis of a cohort of 309 French Canadian patients with emphasis on features at diagnosis as predictive factors for survival. *Medicine (Baltimore).* 2002;81:154–167.

113. Deshauer S, Junek M, Baron M, et al. Effect of pregnancy on scleroderma progression. *J Scleroderma Relat Disord.* 2023;8:27–30.

114. Steen VD. Pregnancy in women with systemic sclerosis. *Obstet Gynecol.* 1999;94:15–20.

115. Steen VD. Pregnancy in scleroderma. *Rheum Dis Clin North Am.* 2007;33:345–358.

116. Clark KE, Etomi O, Ong VH. Systemic sclerosis in pregnancy. *Obstet Med.* 2020;13:105–111.

117. Barilaro G, Castellanos A, Gomez-Ferreira I, et al. Systemic sclerosis and pregnancy outcomes: a retrospective study from a single center. *Arthritis Res Ther.* 2022;24:91.

118. Taraborelli M, Ramoni V, Brucato A, et al. Brief report: Successful pregnancies but a higher risk of preterm births in patients with systemic sclerosis: an Italian multicenter study. *Arthritis Rheum.* 2012;64:1970–1977.

119. Distler O, Highland KB, Gahlemann M, et al. Nintedanib for systemic sclerosis–associated interstitial lung disease. *N Engl J Med.* 2019;380:2518–2528.

120. Seibold J, ed. *Scleroderma.* WB Saunders; 1989:1215–1244.

121. Tuffanelli DL. Systemic scleroderma. *Med Clin North Am.* 1989;73:1167–1180.

122. Carbonne B, Mace G, Cynober E, et al. Successful pregnancy with the use of nitric oxide donors and heparin after recurrent severe preeclampsia in a woman with scleroderma. *Am J Obstet Gynecol.* 2007;197:e6–e7.

123. Vemulapalli S, Cohen L, Hsu V. Prevalence and risk factors for left ventricular diastolic dysfunction in a scleroderma cohort. *Scand J Rheumatol.* 2017;46:281–287.

124. Moore M, Saffran JE, Baraf HS, Jacobs RP. Systemic sclerosis and pregnancy complicated by obstructive uropathy. *Am J Obstet Gynecol.* 1985;153:893–894.

125. Steen VD, Conte C, Day N, et al. Pregnancy in women with systemic sclerosis. *Arthritis Rheum.* 1989;32:151–157.

126. Plastiras SC, Papazefkos V, Pamboucas C, et al. Scleroderma heart: pericardial effusion with echocardiographic signs of tamponade during pregnancy. *Clin Exp Rheumatol.* 2010;28:447–448.

127. Moaveni D, Cohn J, Brodt J, et al. Scleroderma and pulmonary hypertension complicating two pregnancies: use of neuraxial anesthesia, general anesthesia, epoprostenol and a multidisciplinary approach for cesarean delivery. *Int J Obstet Anesth.* 2015;24:375–382.

128. Albilia JB, Lam DK, Blanas N, et al. Small mouths...Big problems? A review of scleroderma and its oral health implications. *J Can Dent Assoc.* 2007;73:831–836.

129. Foote J, Singh P, Stowers A. Oropharynx in scleroderma. *Anesthesiology.* 2019;131:149.

130. Boutonnet M, Faitot V, Katz A, et al. Mallampati class changes during pregnancy, labour, and after delivery: can these be predicted? *Br J Anaesth.* 2010;104:67–70.

131. Dempsey ZS, Rowell S, McRobert R. The role of regional and neuroaxial anesthesia in patients with systemic sclerosis. *Local Reg Anesth.* 2011;4:47–56.

132. Lundberg IE, Fujimoto M, Vencovsky J, et al. Idiopathic inflammatory myopathies. *Nat Rev Dis Primers.* 2021;7:86.

133. Meyer A, Meyer N, Schaeffer M, et al. Incidence and prevalence of inflammatory myopathies: a systematic review. *Rheumatology (Oxford).* 2015;54:50–63.

134. Saud A, Naveen R, Aggarwal R, Gupta L. COVID-19 and myositis: what we know so far. *Curr Rheumatol Rep.* 2021;23:63.

135. Bronner IM, van der Meulen MFG, de Visser M, et al. Long-term outcome in polymyositis and dermatomyositis. *Ann Rheum Dis.* 2006;65:1456–1461.

136. Bohan A, Peter JB. Polymyositis and dermatomyositis (second of two parts). *N Engl J Med.* 1975;292:403–407.

137. Horowitz M, McNeil JD, Maddern GJ, et al. Abnormalities of gastric and esophageal emptying in polymyositis and dermatomyositis. *Gastroenterology.* 1986;90:434–439.

138. Dickey BF, Myers AR. Pulmonary disease in polymyositis/dermatomyositis. *Semin Arthritis Rheum.* 1984;14:60–76.

139. Senechal M, Crete M, Couture C, Poirier P. Myocardial dysfunction in polymyositis. *Can J Cardiol.* 2006;22:869–871.

140. Yassaee M, Carrie L, Kovaric M, Werth VP. Pregnancy-associated dermatomyositis. *Arch Dermatol.* 2009;145:952–953.

141. Ishii N, Ono H, Kawaguchi T, Nakajima H. Dermatomyositis and pregnancy. Case report and review of the literature. *Dermatologica.* 1991;183:146–149.

142. Mateus S, Malheiro M, Santos MP, Costa R. Dermatomyositis onset in the puerperium period. *BMJ Case Rep.* 2015;2015:bcr2015211025.

143. Kolstad KD, Fiorentino D, Li S, et al. Pregnancy outcomes in adult patients with dermatomyositis and polymyositis. *Semin Arthritis Rheum.* 2018;47:865–869.

144. Silva CA, Sultan SM, Isenberg DA. Pregnancy outcome in adult-onset idiopathic inflammatory myopathy. *Rheumatology (Oxford).* 2003;42:1168–1172.

145. Missumi LS, Souza FH, Andrade JQ, Shinjo SK. Pregnancy outcomes in dermatomyositis and polymyositis patients. *Rev Bras Reumatol.* 2015;55:95–102.

146. Nozaki Y, Ikoma S, Funauchi M, Kinoshita K. Respiratory muscle weakness with dermatomyositis during pregnancy: successful treatment with intravenous immunoglobulin therapy. *J Rheumatol.* 2008;35:2289.

147. Williams L, Chang PY, Park E, et al. Successful treatment of dermatomyositis during pregnancy with intravenous immunoglobulin monotherapy. *Obstet Gynecol.* 2007;109:561–563.

148. Vermaak E, Tansley SL, McHugh NJ. The evidence for immunotherapy in dermatomyositis and polymyositis: a systematic review. *Clin Rheumatol.* 2015;34:2089–2095.

149. Wan J, Imadojemu S, Werth VP. Management of rheumatic and autoimmune blistering disease in pregnancy and postpartum. *Clin Dermatol.* 2016;34:344–352.

150. Oddis CV, Reed AM, Aggarwal R, et al. Rituximab in the treatment of refractory adult and juvenile dermatomyositis and adult polymyositis: a randomized, placebo-phase trial. *Arthritis Rheum.* 2013;65:314–324.

151. Oddis CV, Rockette HE, Zhu L, et al. Randomized trial of tocilizumab in the treatment of refractory adult polymyositis and dermatomyositis. *ACR Open Rheumatol.* 2022;4:983–990.

152. Kamal K, Bansal T, Saini S, Walia S. Anesthetic management of a pregnant female posted for caesarean section with biopsy proven polymyositis. *Saudi J Anaesth.* 2015;9:338–339.

153. Johns RA, Finholt DA, Stirt JA. Anaesthetic management of a child with dermatomyositis. *Can Anaesth Soc J.* 1986;33:71–74.

154. Eielsen O, Stovner J. Dermatomyositis, suxamethonium action and atypical plasmacholinesterase. *Can Anaesth Soc J.* 1978;25:63–64.

155. Flusche G, Unger-Sargon J, Lambert DH. Prolonged neuromuscular paralysis with vecuronium in a patient with polymyositis. *Anesth Analg.* 1987;66:188–190.

156. Saarnivaara LH. Anesthesia for a patient with polymyositis undergoing myectomy of the cricopharyngeal muscle. *Anesth Analg.* 1988;67:701–702.

41

Cardiovascular Disease

Katherine W. Arendt, MD, Kathryn J. Lindley, MD, and Mladen I. Vidovich, MD, FACC, FSCAI

Maternal mortality is increasing in the United States, and maternal cardiovascular deaths are increasing faster than the overall rate. Currently, cardiovascular disease is the leading cause of maternal mortality in the United States, accounting for one-quarter of maternal deaths. An increasing average age of pregnancy, along with increasing prevalence of cardiovascular risk factors among pregnant women, such as diabetes mellitus, hypertension, and obesity, may be contributing.

Historically, rheumatic mitral stenosis represented the most common cardiac condition encountered in pregnant women. This disease continues to be a major problem in low-resource countries and in certain immigrant populations in the United States. Acquired heart diseases, such as peripartum cardiomyopathy, account for the majority of cardiovascular maternal deaths in the United States.[1] Congenital heart disease in pregnancy has become increasingly common as a result of significant advances in the treatment of complex congenital heart conditions and survival of these patients to childbearing age.

For most women with heart disease, pregnancy is associated with favorable outcomes.[2,3] However, even with modern advances in monitoring and treatment, there remains a high incidence of morbidity and mortality for some diseases. There is significant individual variability in the severity of specific cardiovascular diseases. Several cardiovascular conditions may be simultaneously present in one individual. Management may be further complicated by the presence of pregnancy-related diseases such as preeclampsia, or noncardiovascular or obstetric pathologic processes. Thus, the anesthetic management of the parturient with cardiovascular disease should be individualized, and it is important that all patients with significant cardiovascular disease are cared for by a multidisciplinary pregnancy heart team.[4,5] Members of the pregnancy heart team include cardiologists, obstetric providers, maternal-fetal medicine subspecialists, and anesthesia providers.

Optimal analgesia and anesthesia care is an essential element of safe childbirth in cardiovascular patients. Case reports and small series describe the anesthetic management of patients with cardiovascular disease, but, in general, few data justify choosing one analgesic or anesthetic technique over another. With a thorough understanding of the normal physiologic changes of pregnancy and an individual parturient's unique cardiovascular pathophysiology, the anesthesia provider can plan anesthetic management that best achieves the desired hemodynamic goals.

CARDIOVASCULAR PHYSIOLOGIC CHANGES OF PREGNANCY

The cardiovascular system adapts to support the growing fetus throughout pregnancy (see Chapter 2). **Cardiac output** increases by approximately 50% by the second trimester of pregnancy and increases further in the peripartum period. Cardiac output is highest in the immediate hour following delivery and does not return to prepregnancy levels for 12 to 24 weeks after delivery (Box 41.1; see also Fig. 2.2). **Left ventricular mass** increases during normal pregnancy.[6] The increase in left ventricular mass is greater in multiple gestation than in singleton gestation[7] and in women with preeclampsia.[8] Changes in the **electrocardiogram (ECG)** are outlined in Box 41.2.[9,10] Oxytocin administration during the third stage of labor has been associated with ST-segment depression, which has not been shown to be related to myocardial damage.[11,12]

Brain natriuretic peptide (BNP) is a natriuretic hormone synthesized primarily in the heart ventricles. BNP levels increase as a response to increased filling pressures in patients with heart failure. Physiologically, BNP has vasodilatory, diuretic, and natriuretic effects. BNP levels change during normal pregnancy and even more during pregnancy associated with heart failure or preeclampsia (Box 41.3)[8,13–18] The role of serial BNP measurements for individual patient management remains unclear, although limits to detect disease in pregnancy have been proposed.[14–16] A normal BNP during pregnancy excludes cardiac decompensation.

Cardiac enzyme levels may be altered by pregnancy or pregnancy-associated disease.[19,20] Myocardial cell death is associated with elevation of specific and sensitive cardiac biomarkers: **cardiac troponins** and **creatine kinase MB**

isoenzyme **(CK-MB)** (Box 41.4).[20,21] Both cardiac troponins and CK-MB are sensitive, but not specific, markers for the diagnosis of myocardial infarction during pregnancy.[22]

RECOGNITION OF CARDIAC DISEASE IN PREGNANCY

Failure to recognize cardiac disease and heart failure in pregnancy is a major contributor to maternal cardiac deaths.[23] The anesthesia provider, as a peridelivery clinician on obstetric units, should actively work with the obstetric care team to enhance recognition of cardiac disease. Cardiovascular disease may not be recognized prior to pregnancy; the normal physiologic changes or pathologic changes in pregnancy (e.g., hypertensive disorders of pregnancy) may exacerbate preexisting disease, leading to symptom development. Still other women may develop pregnancy-related cardiovascular disease such as peripartum cardiomyopathy. Recognition

---

BOX 41.1   Cardiac Output Changes During Pregnancy

- Elevation begins at 5 weeks' gestation.
- Elevation continues throughout the first and second trimester.
- Peaks at 30%–50% greater than nonpregnant values in the early third trimester and remains elevated until after delivery.
- Some studies report a decrease at the end of the third trimester if measurements are made in the supine position because of aortocaval compression.
- Elevation is from increases in both heart rate and stroke volume.
- Distribution of cardiac output to the uterine circulation increases from 1% in nonpregnancy to 12% during the second half of pregnancy.
- During labor, cardiac output increases further with each contraction because of:
  - Catecholamine surges from pain (increasing heart rate and myocardial contractility)
  - Autotransfusion of 300–500 mL of blood back into the venous system from the contracting uterus
  - Aortocaval decompression with contraction
- Cardiac output peaks at the time of delivery (approximately 75% above predelivery values, which may be as high as 125% above prepregnancy values).

Modified from Nishimura RA, Otto CM, Bonow RO, et al. 2014 AHA/ACC guideline for the management of patients with valvular heart disease: a report of the American College of Cardiology/American Heart Association Task Force on Practice Guidelines. *Circulation.* 2014;129:e521–e643.

BOX 41.2   Electrocardiogram Changes During Pregnancy

- Variable QRS axis
  - Left-axis deviation of 15–20 degrees may occur in third trimester from gravid uterus pushing the heart upward with lateral rotation.
- ST-segment and T-wave changes[9]
  - ST-segment *elevation* is never seen in normal pregnancy and should always be considered pathologic.
  - ST-segment *depression* is seen in 25%–81% of parturients undergoing cesarean delivery, regardless of the type of anesthesia.[10]
  - Oxytocin administration during the third stage of labor has been associated with ST-segment depression, which has not been shown to be associated with myocardial damage.[11,12]

BOX 41.3   Brain Natriuretic Peptide (BNP) Levels During Pregnancy

- BNP levels increase approximately twofold during normal pregnancy.[13]
  - An upper limit of normal BNP in pregnancy has been proposed as 50 pg/mL.[14]
- BNP is increased above typical pregnancy levels in heart disease.[15]
  - BNP is a sensitive marker for heart failure in pregnancy (normal BNP excludes heart failure during pregnancy).
  - BNP > 100 pg/mL and > 111 pg/mL have been proposed as thresholds to detect or predict heart failure in pregnant women or women who are immediately postpartum.[15,16]
- BNP is further increased above typical pregnancy levels in women with preeclampsia.[17]
  - A correlation exists between increases in BNP and increases in left ventricular mass and end-diastolic and end-systolic volumes in women with preeclampsia.[8,18]
  - BNP returns to baseline approximately 3 d after delivery.[13]

BOX 41.4 Cardiac Enzymes During Pregnancy

Cardiac Troponin
- Normal in uncomplicated pregnancy
- Elevated in pregnancy-induced hypertension or preeclampsia[19,20]
- In preeclampsia with concurrent myocardial infarction, troponin is higher than expected for the underlying preeclampsia.[22]
- Heterophil antibody interference with the troponin assay may cause a false-positive increase in troponin levels during pregnancy.
- Cardiac troponin is a sensitive marker for myocardial infarction during pregnancy (normal troponin excludes myocardial infarction).

Creatine Kinase MB Isoenzyme
- Elevated two to four times the upper limit of normal during pregnancy
  - CK-MB is present in the uterus and placenta.
- Elevated CK-MB levels are not specific for the diagnosis of myocardial infarction during pregnancy.[20,21]
- CK-MB is a sensitive marker for myocardial infarction during pregnancy (normal CK-MB excludes diagnosis of myocardial infarction).

CK-MB, Creatine kinase MB isoenzyme.

and appropriate diagnosis of cardiovascular disease is a critical step in reducing maternal cardiovascular morbidity and mortality.

It can be difficult to differentiate normal from pathologic symptoms in pregnant patients. For example, healthy women frequently complain of mild dyspnea at rest and exertion during pregnancy. However, the following symptoms warrant a cardiac evaluation[4]: (1) new onset asthma, (2) persistent cough, (3) severe obstructive sleep apnea symptoms, (4) paroxysmal nocturnal dyspnea, (5) orthopnea, (6) refractory pneumonia, (7) palpitations lasting longer than a few seconds or associated with lightheadedness or syncope, or (8) chest pain not consistent with gastroesophageal reflux. Vital signs and physical examination signs that should prompt evaluation are summarized in Table 41.1.

ANTEPARTUM ANESTHESIOLOGY CLINIC EVALUATION

Anesthesia teams should have the ability to evaluate high-risk pregnant patients with cardiac disease in advance of delivery in a clinic setting. This allows the team to obtain a thorough anesthetic, obstetric, and cardiac history; perform a physical

TABLE 41.1 Recognizing Heart Disease in Pregnancy: Vital Signs and Cardiovascular Examination

Feature	Normal Pregnancy	Abnormal	Implication of Abnormal Findings
Heart rate	<90 beats/min	≥120 beats/min: evaluate urgently 90–119 beats/min: evaluate nonurgently	Differential diagnosis of tachycardia in pregnancy is vast[a]
Systolic blood pressure	120–139 mm Hg	≥160 mm Hg: evaluate urgently 140–159 mm Hg: evaluate nonurgently	Assess for hypertensive disorders of pregnancy
		Symptomatic low blood pressure: evaluate urgently	Differential diagnosis of hypotension in pregnancy is vast[a]
Respiratory rate	12–15 breaths/min	≥25 breaths/min: evaluate urgently 16–25 breaths/min: evaluate nonurgently	Differential diagnosis of tachypnea in pregnancy is vast[a]
Oxygen saturation	>97%	<95%: evaluate urgently 95%–97%: evaluate nonurgently	Differential diagnosis of tachypnea in pregnancy is vast[a]
Jugular venous pressure	Normal (not visible)	Elevated (visible greater than 2 cm above clavicle)	Evaluate for heart failure with chest x-ray and/or echocardiography
Carotid pulse	Normal upstroke Normal volume	Decreased, delayed, shudder, or bruit	Evaluate for aortic stenosis with echocardiography
		Bifid pulse	Evaluate for hypertrophic cardiomyopathy with echocardiography
Peripheral pulses	Well filled	Diminished or delayed	Evaluate for aortic stenosis or left ventricular outflow obstruction
Point of maximum impulse	Crisp, slightly laterally displaced	Any enlargement or more than slight lateral displacement	Evaluate for valvular diseases or cardiomyopathies with chest x-ray and/or echocardiography

(Continued)

TABLE 41.1   Recognizing Heart Disease in Pregnancy: Vital Signs and Cardiovascular Examination—cont'd

Feature	Normal Pregnancy	Abnormal	Implication of Abnormal Findings
S1 heart sound	Louder and widely split		
S2 heart sound	Unchanged	Soft/absent/paradoxically split	Evaluate for aortic stenosis with echocardiography
		Loud P2 heart sound, fixed split	Evaluate for pulmonary hypertension with echocardiography
S3 heart sound	Normally present		
S4 heart sound	Rarely heard	Heard	
Aortic stenosis murmur	Increased		Helpful to confirm physical examination findings with echocardiography
Aortic regurgitation murmur	Decreased	Any diastolic murmur is abnormal	
Mitral stenosis murmur	Increased	Any diastolic murmur is abnormal	
Mitral regurgitation murmur	Decreased		
Hypertrophic cardiomyopathy murmur	Decreased		Not all hypertrophic cardiomyopathies have obstructive murmurs; helpful to confirm with echocardiography
Peripheral edema	Mild edema	Moderate, marked, or asymmetric	Asymmetric edema warrants further evaluation for deep venous thrombosis
Stigmata of Marfan syndrome	N/A	Tall stature, large arm span	Assess for genetic disease because of increased risk for aortic dissection
Stigmata of Turner syndrome	N/A	Short stature, webbed neck	Assess for genetic disease because of increased risk for aortic dissection

[a]Consider assessing for bleeding/hypovolemia, sepsis, arrhythmias, pulmonary embolism, or heart failure with physical examination, electrocardiogram, blood laboratory evaluation, imaging, and/or echocardiogram.
N/A, Not applicable.
Summarized from American College of Obstetricians and Gynecologists' Presidential Task Force on Pregnancy and Heart Disease and Committee on Practice Bulletins—Obstetrics. ACOG Practice Bulletin No. 212: Pregnancy and heart disease (reaffirmed 2025). *Obstet Gynecol.* 2019;133:e320–e356.

examination; review cardiac testing; and make recommendations. The most important aspects of this consultation are summarized in Box 41.5.

Cardiac Examination During Pregnancy

It is important to recognize normal changes in vital signs and physical examination associated with pregnancy and those that require further evaluation (see Table 41.1). Central venous pressure remains unchanged during pregnancy, and any elevation of jugular venous pressure is an abnormal finding. Basilar rales may be heard on lung auscultation; however, these are no longer heard after deep inspiration, a brief breath-hold, or a cough. These evanescent rales likely result from basilar atelectasis.

New normal pregnancy-associated murmurs are heard in greater than 90% of pregnant women. The loudest murmurs are heard between 15 and 25 weeks' gestation; murmur intensity decreases toward term and increases again during labor

and the early postpartum period. Most pregnancy-associated murmurs are no longer appreciated by 6 weeks postpartum.[24]

The differentiation of normal from pathologic murmurs is important. Diastolic murmurs during pregnancy are almost always associated with an underlying pathologic process. The murmurs of aortic and mitral regurgitation generally decrease and may become inaudible during pregnancy owing to the decrease in systemic vascular resistance (SVR). However, administration of phenylephrine or development of hypertension during pregnancy—both of which raise SVR—increases the intensity of these murmurs.[25] The murmur associated with aortic stenosis increases in intensity during pregnancy from increased flow through the stenotic valve. A diminished carotid upstroke, soft or inaudible second heart sound (S2), and a grade 4/6 murmur are almost always indicative of severe aortic stenosis. An audible, physiologic split S2 almost invariably rules out severe aortic stenosis. The murmur of

History
- Anesthetic history
- Obstetric history
- Cardiac history with special attention to:
  - All prior cardiac testing (e.g., echocardiogram, ECG, Holter monitor)
  - Prior surgical history
  - Current cardiac medication regimen
  - Prior or current episodes of heart failure
  - Intracardiac shunting and cyanosis
  - Prior arrhythmias
  - Left heart obstructive lesions
  - Left and right heart function
  - Pacemaker or defibrillator management
  - Anticoagulation therapy

Physical Examination
- Airway
- Cardiac
- Pulmonary
- Back (to assess for ease of performing neuraxial techniques)

Consider/Discuss/Recommend
- Participate in multidisciplinary planning with the pregnancy heart team
- Risk stratify according to the modified World Health Organization criteria (see Box 41.6)
- With the pregnancy heart team, plan appropriate delivery location based on maternal levels of care (see Box 41.7)
- Determine optimal monitoring plans
  - ECG monitoring during labor
  - Intra-arterial blood pressure monitoring
  - Additional intravenous access
  - Potential central venous access, or rarely, pulmonary artery catheter
- Clarify plan for pacemaker or defibrillator
  - Automatic implantable cardioverter-defibrillator should be enabled during labor or cesarean delivery
- Partner with pregnancy heart team to plan for peripartum anticoagulation regimen
  - Consider timing relative to neuraxial procedures
- Consider risks, benefits, and alternatives of neuraxial techniques
- Consider and document which obstetric drugs may cause hemodynamic instability—use after risk/benefit discussion (e.g., methylergonovine, carboprost, terbutaline, rapid infusion of oxytocin) (see Table 41.3)
- Partner with pregnancy heart team to clarify postpartum monitoring plan (including location)

ECG, Electrocardiogram.

hypertrophic cardiomyopathy decreases in intensity because the pregnancy-associated increase in intravascular volume may result in decreased outflow tract obstruction. The murmur of an atrial septal defect (ASD) may become more audible during pregnancy.

Most pregnant women display some degree of peripheral edema, partly because compression of the inferior vena cava by the uterus impedes venous return from the lower extremities. This physiologic edema is symmetric and decreases with leg elevation and the left lateral decubitus position. Asymmetric lower extremity edema is almost invariably pathologic. A tender and warm lower extremity may suggest deep vein thrombosis or cellulitis.

It is also important to look for stigmata of genetic conditions that could result in significant pregnancy complications such as aortic dissection. For example, tall stature, large arm span, or other stigmata may alert the practitioner to the presence of previously undiagnosed Marfan syndrome. Patients with Marfan syndrome frequently demonstrate scoliosis and may have dural ectasia. Turner syndrome is characterized by short stature and a webbed neck. Both conditions predispose pregnant women to aortic dissection (see discussion below).

Cardiac Risk Prediction

Antepartum risk stratification is critical for identifying pregnancies at high risk for childbirth complications so that these patients can be triaged to deliver at appropriate hospitals. Several classifications have been proposed to specifically predict cardiac risk during pregnancy: The **ZAHARA I** (Zwangerschap bij vrouwen met een Aangeboren HARtAfwijking) model was developed from a retrospective cohort of patients with congenital heart disease.[26] The **CARPREG II** (CARdiac disease in PREGnancy) model was developed from a prospective cohort of patients with congenital, acquired structural, and arrhythmic heart disease.[27] The **modified World Health Organization** (mWHO) model was developed based upon lesion-specific risk (Box 41.6).[28,29] These classifications may help predict the individual pregnant woman's cardiac risk and, combined with the clinical constellation and results of cardiac imaging, may help guide clinical management.[28–31] Many anesthesia providers use the mWHO model[26] along with the American College of Obstetricians and Gynecologists levels of maternal care[32] (see Chapter 11) to inform a recommendation for delivery location (Box 41.7).[5]

Cardiovascular Imaging During Pregnancy
Echocardiography

Both transthoracic and transesophageal echocardiography can be performed at any stage of pregnancy. Expected physiologic changes in echocardiographic parameters during pregnancy are outlined in Table 41.2.[33] These parameters return to baseline within 3 to 6 months postpartum.[34] In normal pregnancy, left ventricular diastolic function is increased in the first two trimesters and declines in the third trimester.[35] Forty percent of patients with preeclampsia have evidence of global diastolic dysfunction, compared with 14% of normotensive pregnant patients (see Chapter 35).[36]

Although there are limited data regarding echocardiographic contrast agents during pregnancy and lactation, no evidence of fetal harm has been identified in animal studies.[37] Given the very brief half-life of these agents, no fetal or infant harm is expected and the use of these agents during pregnancy and lactation is acceptable if required for optimal maternal care.[37]

BOX 41.6   Modified World Health Organization Cardiac Risk Assessment

Class I (No Increase or a Mild Increase in Morbidity)
Mild pulmonary stenosis
PDA
Mitral valve prolapse
Repaired ASD, VSD, PDA, anomalous pulmonary venous return

Class II (Small Increase in Maternal Mortality, Moderate Increase in Maternal Morbidity)
Unrepaired ASD or VSD
Repaired tetralogy of Fallot
Most arrhythmias
Mild left ventricular dysfunction
Hypertrophic cardiomyopathy
Marfan syndrome without aortic dilation
Bicuspid aortic valve with aortic diameter < 45 mm

Class III (Significant Increase in Maternal Mortality and Severe Increase in Maternal Morbidity)
Mechanical valve(s)

Systemic right ventricle
Fontan circulation
Unrepaired cyanotic heart disease
Complex congenital heart disease
Marfan syndrome with aortic dilation 40–45 mm
Bicuspid aortic valve with aortic dilation 45–50 mm

Class IV (Pregnancy Is Not Recommended or Is Contraindicated)
Pulmonary hypertension of any cause
Severe left ventricular dysfunction
Previous peripartum cardiomyopathy with residual left ventricular dysfunction
Severe mitral stenosis
Severe aortic stenosis
Marfan syndrome with aortic dilation > 45 mm
Bicuspid aortic valve with aortic dilation > 50 mm
Severe unrepaired aortic coarctation

ASD, Atrial septal defect; *PDA*, patent ductus arteriosus; *VSD*, ventricular septal defect.
Modified from Thorne S, MacGregor A, Nelson-Piercy C. Risks of contraception and pregnancy in heart disease. *Heart.* 2006;92:1520–1525; Regitz-Zagrosek V, Roos-Hesselink JW, Bauersachs J, et al. 2018 ESC guidelines on the management of cardiovascular diseases during pregnancy. *Eur Heart J.* 2018;39:3165–3241.

BOX 41.7   Suggested Levels of Maternal Care for Pregnant Patients with Cardiac Disease[a] and Modified World Health Organization Risk[b]

Level	Title	Maternal Health	Hospital Capabilities	Anesthesia Staffing	Appropriate Patients (mWHO Class)
Birth center	Birth center	Low risk	Not applicable	None	None
Level I	Basic care	Low to moderate risk	Limited obstetric ultrasonography Blood bank	Anesthesiologist readily available at all times	Class I
Level II	Specialty care	Moderate to high risk	CT/MRI Maternal echocardiography Nonobstetric ultrasonography	Anesthesiologist readily available at all times	Class I or II
Level III	Subspecialty care	More complex maternal, obstetric, and fetal conditions	Interventional radiology In-house availability of all blood components	Board-certified anesthesiologist physically present at all times	Class I, II, or some III
Level IV	Regional perinatal health center	Most complex maternal conditions	ICU care with maternal-fetal medicine subspecialist comanagement Cardiovascular surgery, ECMO, and cardiac transplant capabilities	Board-certified anesthesiologist with obstetric anesthesiology fellowship or experience in obstetric anesthesia physically present at all times	Class I, II, III, or IV

[a]American College of Obstetricians and Gynecologist. Obstetric Care Consensus No. 9: Levels of maternal care (reaffirmed 2021). *Obstet Gynecol.* 2019;143:e41–e55.
[b]See Box 41.6.
CT, Computed tomography; *ECMO*, extracorporeal membrane oxygenation; *ICU*, intensive care unit; *MRI*, magnetic resonance imaging; *mWHO*, modified World Health Organization.
Modified from Meng ML, Arendt KW. Obstetric anesthesia and heart disease: practical clinical considerations. *Anesthesiology.* 2021;135:164–183.

TABLE 41.2 Physiologic Changes in Echocardiographic Imaging During Pregnancy

Anatomic Location	Parameter	Expected Change
Left ventricle	Left ventricular size	Increased
	Left ventricular mass	Increased
	Left ventricular ejection fraction	Unchanged
Right ventricle	Right ventricular size	Increased
	Right ventricular ejection fraction	Unchanged
Pulmonary vasculature	Pulmonary arterial pressure	Unchanged
	Pulmonary vascular resistance	Decreased
Left atrium	Size	Increased
Aortic root	Size	Unchanged
Pericardium	Pericardial effusion	Trace to small

Pregnant patients usually require anesthesia care for transesophageal echocardiography. The risk for pulmonary aspiration of gastric contents associated with sedation (with an unprotected airway) should be weighed against the risks associated with general anesthesia and tracheal intubation. Tracheal intubation is frequently for used for transesophageal echocardiography beyond 18 weeks' gestation to reduce the risk of aspiration.[33] If the uterine fundus is above the umbilicus, the patient should be positioned in the left lateral decubitus position to avoid inferior vena cava compression.[33]

Cardiac Magnetic Resonance Imaging

The risks associated with magnetic resonance imaging (MRI) in pregnant women are similar to those in nonpregnant patients, and there is no evidence that MRI causes harm to the fetus.[37] Given the quality of images and diagnostic yield, cardiac magnetic resonance (CMR) is typically preferable to any imaging modality that uses ionizing radiation. Gadolinium crosses the placenta and has been found to be teratogenic in animal models. Currently available human data suggest that gadolinium should not be used in pregnant women unless it significantly improves diagnostic performance and is expected to improve maternal or neonatal outcome.[37] There is minimal excretion of gadolinium into breast milk, and lactation should not be interrupted following its administration.[33]

Cardiac Catheterization

Coronary angiography remains the "gold standard" for diagnosis of coronary artery disease and can be performed at any time during pregnancy. Radial arterial access is preferable to femoral access because it is associated with earlier ambulation, increased patient comfort, and fewer access-related bleeding complications. The left lateral decubitus position can be more easily maintained with radial access. Pulmonary arterial catheterization may be required for mWHO class IV patients, including those with pulmonary hypertension, decompensated heart failure, or severe left-sided valvular obstruction. For all catheterization procedures, cardiologists should strictly adhere to the ALARA principle (as low as reasonably achievable) to limit both maternal and fetal ionizing radiation exposure (see Chapter 18). Typical ionizing radiation dose of a diagnostic or therapeutic cardiac catheterization is between 3 and 20 mGy, below the accepted fetal radiation threshold of 50 mGy.[33]

Computed Tomographic Angiography

Multidetector computed tomography (CT) allows noninvasive imaging of the coronary arteries along with cardiac structure and function. The use of contemporary CT with aggressive dose-reduction techniques can significantly limit the radiation dose. The overall radiation dose of chest CT imaging is 0.03 to 0.66 mGy.[33]

The use of iodinated contrast media in pregnant and lactating women appears safe.[37] To date, there has been no report of fetal teratogenic or mutagenic effects after maternal administration of iodinated contrast media. Minimal amounts of iodinated contrast media are excreted in breast milk; even smaller amounts are absorbed by the neonate's gastrointestinal tract. Therefore, interruption of breastfeeding after maternal administration of iodinated contrast media is not recommended.

Ionizing Radiation Risks to the Fetus

The ionizing radiation dose to the fetus can be limited by performing cardiac imaging with echocardiography or MRI techniques. If cardiac catheterization is necessary, the radiation dose can be limited by using reduced fluoroscopy frame rates and contemporary image noise-reduction technology. Because the fetus is not directly within the radiation beam for cardiac procedures, the fetal exposure occurs primarily through indirect scatter radiation. No deterministic radiation effects are expected at any gestational age for fetal radiation exposure < 50 mGy. Risks increase with doses > 100 mGy and with first-trimester exposure.[33] Risks and benefits of the cardiac imaging modality in pregnancy should always be considered with the aim to maximize diagnostic accuracy and therapeutic efficacy while minimizing potential risks of radiation exposure.[33]

CARDIOVASCULAR PHARMACOLOGY AND PREGNANCY

Cardiac Drugs and Pregnancy

Angiotensin-Converting Enzyme Inhibitors

Angiotensin-converting enzyme (ACE) inhibitors are the mainstay treatment of coronary artery disease, left ventricular dysfunction, and hypertension in nonpregnant patients. These drugs are particularly useful in nonpregnant patients

BOX 41.8   Angiotensin Converting Enzyme (ACE) Inhibitor Risks in Pregnancy

- First-trimester use: increased risk for fetal cardiovascular and central nervous system malformations
- Second- and third-trimester use: fetal kidney malfunction and decreased fetal urine output, which results in oligohydramnios
- ACE inhibitor–associated oligohydramnios has been shown to result in:
  - Positional limb deformities
  - Skull ossification retardation
  - Lung hypoplasia

with diabetes mellitus. However, they are contraindicated during pregnancy (Box 41.8).[38]

Angiotensin Receptor Blockers

Few data are available on the use of angiotensin receptor blockers in pregnancy. However, similar to ACE inhibitors, the use of these drugs is not recommended during pregnancy.[38]

Beta-Adrenergic Receptor Antagonists

Beta-adrenergic receptor antagonists are often used for treatment of coronary artery disease, myocardial infarction, hypertension, many arrhythmias, and a wide spectrum of cardiomyopathies. There is no evidence that beta-adrenergic receptor antagonists are teratogenic. Prolonged and high-dose use of these drugs has been associated with fetal growth restriction; however, the overall risk is likely small.[38] Neonatal bradycardia, hypotension, and hypoglycemia are rarely encountered.

Calcium Channel Blockers

All calcium channel blockers in typical clinical doses appear safe during pregnancy.[38] This includes nondihydropyridine calcium channel blockers such as **verapamil** and **diltiazem**, which are effective treatments for cardiac arrhythmias in the second and third trimesters.[38] Dihydropyridine calcium channel blockers are also considered safe (**amlodipine**, **nifedipine**, **nicardipine**, and **clevidipine**). Oral nifedipine is frequently used in pregnancy. It has been reported to lower blood pressure more quickly with greater reduction of cerebral perfusion pressure than IV **labetalol** and, therefore, has become a first-line agent to treat preeclampsia with severe features.[39] The use of both oral and IV nicardipine has also been described in pregnancy; infusion of IV nicardipine has been shown to achieve blood pressure control after failure of other antihypertensive agents in women with preeclampsia.[40]

In nonpregnant patients, many anesthesia providers consider clevidipine the drug of choice for acute and rapid control of hypertension since the ECLIPSE trials demonstrated the drug's superiority in cardiac surgery.[41] Animal studies show that it crosses the placenta; when administered for prolonged periods at supratherapeutic doses, it is associated with an increased incidence of intrauterine fetal death, reduced fetal weight, and delayed skeletal development.[42] There are no

data indicating harm at typical clinical doses, and there are few descriptions of its use in human pregnancy. In the setting of a maternal hypertensive emergency with failure of other agents, clevidipine's ultrashort half-life may make it a reasonable option for rapid arterial blood pressure reduction.

Calcium channel blockers have tocolytic effects by limiting calcium ion entry into myometrial smooth muscle cells.[43] *In vitro* testing indicates that diltiazem and verapamil display greater concentration-dependent inhibition of spontaneous human pregnant myometrium than nifedipine (i.e., nifedipine exhibits the least degree of tocolysis).[44]

Other Drugs

Amiodarone is generally avoided in pregnancy because animal studies have shown evidence of fetal toxicity at doses less than the maximum recommended human maintenance dose. Further, in humans, congenital goiter/hypothyroidism, hyperthyroidism, and neonatal bradycardia have been reported. However, its safe and effective use has been reported for the treatment of drug-refractory fetal tachycardia in the setting of hydrops fetalis or ventricular dysfunction.[45] Similarly, in the setting of an acute unstable maternal arrhythmia, the benefits of maternal amiodarone therapy may outweigh the risks.

Hydralazine is used in the treatment of cardiomyopathy and is also an excellent antihypertensive agent. It has a long track record of safe use during pregnancy, especially in women with preeclampsia (see Chapter 35).[38]

The use of **nitrates** for treatment of angina during pregnancy appears safe. They can be safely used long term in pregnant women with cardiomyopathy.[38] Nitrates can have profound acute tocolytic effects because nitric oxide directly inhibits myometrial contractions.[46]

Digoxin may be useful for the treatment of various cardiomyopathies and some arrhythmias. Digoxin freely crosses the placenta, but its use has not been associated with congenital abnormalities or untoward fetal effects.[38] Digoxin's pharmacokinetics are altered during pregnancy; monitoring of blood levels is recommended.

Various antiplatelet drugs may be prescribed for patients with coronary artery disease, after stent placement, with acute coronary syndrome (ACS), or after heart valve replacement. For example, **eptifibatide**, **tirofiban**, and **abciximab** are potent platelet aggregation inhibitors (IIB/IIIA receptor inhibitors) administered intravenously (IV) to inhibit platelet aggregation during percutaneous coronary intervention. Adenosine diphosphate receptor blockers such as **clopidogrel**, **ticagrelor**, **ticlopidine**, and **prasugrel** and phosphodiesterase inhibitors such as **dipyridamole** and **cilostazol** may also be used. Both the American Society of Regional Anesthesia and Pain Medicine and the European Society of Anaesthesiology guidelines strongly advise avoidance of neuraxial anesthesia until platelet function has recovered after administration of antiplatelet agents.[47,48]

Statins interrupt cholesterol synthesis and result in a lowering of plasma cholesterol levels. The widespread use of statins (which are associated with exceptionally robust cardiovascular outcome data) has transformed the treatment of coronary artery disease. Nonetheless, given the critical importance of cholesterol synthesis in the normal development of the embryo and placenta, statins are contraindicated in pregnancy, given their potential for teratogenicity.[38]

Thiazide diuretics do not appear to be teratogenic. Long-term use may result in a reduction in uteroplacental perfusion, which may be associated with fetal growth restriction and oligohydramnios.[38] Neonatal hypoglycemia and thrombocytopenia have been reported.

Loop diuretics are likely not teratogenic.[38] Similar to thiazide diuretics, fetal growth restriction may be associated with long-term use during pregnancy. **Spironolactone** is an aldosterone antagonist frequently used in the treatment of patients with congestive heart failure and cardiomyopathy, but because of its antiandrogenic potential, its use during pregnancy is not recommended.[38] Data are inadequate to determine the safety of **sacubitril**, **empagliflozin**, and **dapagliflozin** use during pregnancy.

Obstetric Drugs with Hemodynamic Effects

Both uterotonic (oxytocic) and tocolytic drugs can have profound hemodynamic consequences (Table 41.3). Because patients with cardiovascular disease are at increased risk of postpartum hemorrhage, uterotonic agents may be necessary and appropriate in the setting of uterine atony. **Oxytocin** is considered a first-line treatment for uterine atony, but it causes a decrease in SVR.[49] Thus, it should be administered as an infusion via an IV pump; hypotension can be treated with **phenylephrine** or **norepinephrine** in the setting of hemorrhage. Bolus dosing of oxytocin is not recommended in patients with cardiac disease.[50]

Methylergonovine and **carboprost** are typically considered second-line therapy for uterine atony (see Chapter 37). Because of their significant cardiovascular effects, they are relatively contraindicated in patients with cardiac disease. For example, methylergonovine is thought to stimulate alpha-adrenergic receptors and has been reported to increase SVR resulting in hypertension and stroke as well as coronary vasospasm, resulting in myocardial ischemia and death.[51,52] Carboprost has been shown to increase pulmonary vascular resistance (PVR) by over 100% and pulmonary artery pressure (PAP) by 125%.[53] It has been described as precipitating bronchospasm, abnormal ventilation perfusion ratios, increased intrapulmonary shunt fraction, hypoxemia, and death.[54-56] **Misoprostol** is an alternative second-line therapy for uterine atony, although it is important to note that there have been rare reports of cardiac events and coronary vasospasm with its use.[57]

Tocolytic therapy may also be administered by the obstetric team in the event of uterine tachysystole and fetal compromise. Drugs such as **ritodrine** or **terbutaline** are beta-adrenergic receptor agonists that may be administered in the setting of fetal bradycardia associated with uterine tachysystole. They can also cause significant elevation in maternal heart rate (HR) and decrease in SVR. Administration of beta-adrenergic receptor agonists to patients with hypertrophic obstructive cardiomyopathy may cause infundibular spasm and/or worsen the outflow tract gradient. Similarly, patients with cardiac disease who do not tolerate tachycardia, or patients with a history of tachyarrhythmias, should not receive beta-adrenergic receptor agonists. If these drugs are administered in the setting of uterine tachysystole and fetal distress, the decrease in SVR and increase in HR can be treated with the administration of phenylephrine.

PRINCIPLES OF LABOR ANALGESIA IN PATIENTS WITH CARDIAC DISEASE

Vaginal delivery is associated with less blood loss and a decreased risk of infection and venous thromboembolism than cesarean delivery. Therefore, vaginal delivery is the preferred mode of delivery for most women with cardiovascular

TABLE 41.3 Anticipated Adverse Effects of Uterotonic and Tocolytic Drugs in Patients With Cardiac Disease

Drug	Cardiopulmonary Effects	Notes
Oxytocin	↓ SVR Slight ↑ PAP	Administer cautiously and slowly (via infusion pump) in patients intolerant of hypotension Consider treating hypotension with phenylephrine infusion Do not administer an IV bolus dose
Methylergonovine	↑ SVR ↑ PVR coronary vasospasm	Generally avoided
Carboprost (15-methyl-prostaglandin F₂ alpha)	↑PAP Bronchospasm can cause ventilation/perfusion mismatch	Do not use in patients who cannot tolerate increased PAP
Misoprostol	Uncommon cardiovascular events reported	Can be used prophylactically
Terbutaline	↑HR ↓SVR	Avoid, if possible, in patients with HOCM, history of arrhythmia, or severe stenotic valvular lesions

HOCM, Hypertrophic obstructive cardiomyopathy; *HR*, heart rate; *IV*, intravenous; *PAP*, pulmonary artery pressure; *PVR*, pulmonary vascular resistance; *SVR*, systemic vascular resistance.

disease. Effective neuraxial labor analgesia is an important component of labor management in patients with moderate to severe cardiovascular disease. Neuraxial analgesia can minimize the pain of labor and delivery and its associated catecholamine surges, thus mitigating the risk for tachycardia, arrhythmias, hypertension, increases in cardiac output, and ventricular stress. The principles of neuraxial labor analgesia in women with cardiac disease are summarized in Box 41.9.

If neuraxial analgesia is not an option for a high-risk patient with cardiac disease, then the pregnancy heart team may wish to reconsider vaginal delivery. Many patients with cardiac disease are treated with anticoagulants or antiplatelet drugs, which may increase the risk for spinal epidural hematoma. In planning for labor and delivery, the pregnancy heart team should consider the benefits and risk of continuing or discontinuing these medications and the effect of these drugs on the risk for neuraxial hematoma (see Chapter 44).[47,58]

Traditional epidural analgesia, combined spinal-epidural (CSE) analgesia, and dural puncture epidural (DPE) analgesia are all reasonable techniques for patients with cardiac disease. For individual patients, the cardiac disease physiology should be weighed against the speed of the onset of neuroblockade, considering the direct cardiovascular effects associated with blockade of the sympathetic nervous system and the indirect effects associated with pain relief (see Chapter 24). In patients with intracardiac shunts, locating the epidural space using loss-of-resistance to saline (rather than air) may theoretically minimize the risk for paradoxical air embolism in the event of intravascular needle placement. Initiation of CSE analgesia with an intrathecal opioid without a local anesthetic

minimizes the risk for an acute sympathectomy. DPE analgesia compared with traditional epidural analgesia may offer greater reassurance that the epidural needle tip (and, therefore, the epidural catheter) is located in the epidural space. It may be prudent to avoid test doses containing epinephrine (adrenaline) in patients with a history of arrhythmias.

Neuraxial analgesia and anesthesia cause a sympathectomy, which decreases SVR and increases HR; overall there is a decrease in both preload and afterload. These hemodynamic changes during the onset of neuraxial labor analgesia in patients with cardiovascular disease need to be managed appropriately. Epidural local anesthetic should be administered slowly to allow time for hemodynamic compensation. There is no evidence that the administration of an IV crystalloid bolus (i.e., preload) prevents hypotension after initiation of neuraxial labor analgesia. Therefore, for patients with cardiovascular disease at high risk for pulmonary edema, it is reasonable to avoid a fluid bolus prior to initiation of neuraxial analgesia. Vasopressor medications such as phenylephrine and ephedrine should be immediately available. The anesthesia provider should closely monitor the HR and blood pressure during the initiation of neuraxial labor analgesia with rapid treatment of hypotension with fluids or vasopressors, as indicated.

Labor pain, neuraxial analgesia, the Valsalva maneuver during the second stage, delivery, hemorrhage, and the hemodynamic effects of obstetric medications have hemodynamic consequences. Therefore, women with cardiovascular disease should be appropriately monitored during labor and the postpartum period. In general, standard labor monitoring for women with moderate to severe cardiac disease is inadequate. Principles of appropriate hemodynamic monitoring during labor are summarized in Table 41.4.

Pulse oximetry in laboring women is often incorporated into the fetal heart rate (FHR) and tocodynamometer monitor but may provide neither a visible waveform nor audible tones. It may be prudent to monitor laboring women with heart disease with pulse oximetry with a visible waveform and audible alarms dedicated to detecting maternal bradycardia, tachycardia, and hypoxemia. If a patient has a history of a tachyarrhythmia, ischemic heart disease, aortic stenosis, or hypertrophic cardiomyopathy, or is at risk for ischemia or arrhythmia, a 5-lead ECG telemetry during labor may be utilized to monitor for cardiovascular compromise.

For high-risk patients with cardiovascular disease, invasive blood pressure monitoring with an intra-arterial catheter should be initiated for hemodynamic monitoring during labor. This can be critically important in patients at risk for rapid hemodynamic decompensation with hypotension, such as patients with severe aortic stenosis, severe left ventricular dysfunction, or pulmonary hypertension with right ventricular dysfunction. This is also important for patients at risk for urgent cesarean delivery. The beat-to-beat blood pressure measurements are useful for diagnosing acute hypo- and hypertension and response to treatment should the need for rapid induction of epidural or general anesthesia for urgent cesarean delivery arise. Finally, intermittent transthoracic

---

BOX 41.9   Principles of Neuraxial Labor Analgesia in Patients With Cardiac Disease

- Initiate neuraxial analgesia early in labor.
- Do not use a routine preload fluid bolus for patients at risk for pulmonary edema.
- Epidural, dural puncture epidural, or CSE analgesia are all reasonable options.
- Use a neuraxial technique that achieves gradual onset of labor analgesia.
  - If CSE analgesia is chosen, consider opioid-only intrathecal dose.
  - Titrate local anesthetic administration slowly.
- Monitor closely during onset of analgesia for hypotension.
  - Treat with goal-directed fluid administration.
  - Administer vasopressors (e.g., phenylephrine, ephedrine) to maintain normotension.
- Replace epidural catheter early if it is not functioning optimally.
- Density of neuroblockade should:
  - Eliminate pain
  - Minimize urge to push (bear down) during second stage of labor
  - Allow labor analgesia to be quickly transitioned to surgical anesthesia if urgent intrapartum cesarean delivery is necessary

CSE, Combined spinal-epidural.

TABLE 41.4 Suggested Cardiovascular Monitoring During Labor

Parameter	Low Risk for Cardiac Complications	Moderate Risk for Cardiac Complications	High Risk for Cardiac Complications
Pulse oximetry	Pulse oximetry without visual waveform[a]	Pulse oximetry with visual waveform	
ECG	None	5-lead continuous ECG	
Blood pressure	Noninvasive	Noninvasive blood pressure cycling every 15 min throughout labor and delivery	Intra-arterial, beat-to-beat blood pressure monitoring
Central venous pressure	Rarely indicated		
Pulmonary artery pressure	Rarely indicated		

[a]Usually available with fetal monitor.
ECG, Electrocardiography.

echocardiography (TTE) may be useful to assess baseline (prelabor) cardiac function and volume status, and to assess causes of hemodynamic instability during labor, should they occur. Rarely, a central venous line or pulmonary artery catheter may be necessary during labor. Specialized nursing may be necessary to interpret and manage ECG and invasive blood pressure monitoring.

PRINCIPLES OF CESAREAN DELIVERY ANESTHESIA IN PATIENTS WITH CARDIAC DISEASE

In general, neuraxial anesthesia is the technique of choice for most patients with cardiac disease undergoing cesarean delivery. The onset of neuraxial anesthesia-induced sympathectomy requires intense vigilance from the time of block initiation. Invasive blood pressure monitoring initiated prior to neuraxial anesthesia allows for the careful titration of prophylactic **phenylephrine**, **norepinephrine**, or other vasoactive drugs to maintain blood pressure and HR in appropriate doses.[59]

The hemodynamic changes associated with onset of **spinal anesthesia** are more rapid and pronounced than with epidural anesthesia.[60] **Single-shot spinal anesthesia** may hold additional risk for patients with cardiac lesions for which a rapid decrease in preload or afterload may cause acute decompensation (e.g., moderate-severe mitral stenosis, moderate-severe aortic stenosis, aortic coarctation, patients at risk for right-to-left shunting). In such cases, **epidural anesthesia** or **sequential CSE anesthesia** may be preferred (see discussion below and Chapter 26). Single-shot spinal anesthesia may be appropriate for patients with mild or moderate cardiovascular disease for whom a decrease in preload or afterload is not anticipated to be detrimental.

Sequential, low-dose CSE anesthesia has been used successfully in high-risk patients with cardiac disease.[61] An intrathecal dose of **bupivacaine** or **ropivacaine** (one-third to one-half of the dose used for single-shot spinal anesthesia) with a short-acting opioid (e.g., **fentanyl**, **sufentanil**) and a long-acting opioid (e.g., **morphine**) is injected and the epidural catheter is sited in the epidural space. After the patient is positioned supine with left uterine displacement, the sensory level is assessed and additional local anesthesia (e.g., **2% lidocaine**, 3-mL increments) is injected through the epidural catheter, titrated to achieve a T4-6 surgical level of neuroblockade. The benefits of the sequential CSE technique include slow onset of the neuraxial block, which allows the anesthesia provider to maintain preload and afterload during the onset of the sympathetic block, while also achieving greater block density and reliability compared with epidural anesthesia without an intrathecal injection.

General anesthesia may be a safer option than neuraxial anesthesia in some circumstances, for example: (1) the patient has recently received an anticoagulant, (2) rapid provision of surgical conditions is required because of catastrophic maternal or fetal compromise, (3) the patient has extreme cardiopulmonary compromise and cannot lie flat without respiratory support, or (4) there is potential for cardiovascular catastrophe during delivery.

If general anesthesia is planned, and time allows, an intra-arterial catheter for invasive blood pressure monitoring should be placed prior to induction of anesthesia. The ability to continuously monitor blood pressure measurements facilitates titration of the induction agent(s) and vasoactive medications used to counteract the adverse hemodynamic effects of the induction agent. A disadvantage of general anesthesia is newborn depression from placental transfer of general anesthetic agents. However, maternal hemodynamic stability should be prioritized. Furthermore, maternal hemodynamic instability also adversely affects the fetus/neonate. Therefore, the periinduction administration of **opioids** or **lidocaine** and slow titration of induction agents may be preferred to rapid sequence induction. Pediatric personnel should be available to provide support to the neonate after delivery.

SPECIFIC CARDIAC CONDITIONS

Aortic Diseases and Aortic Dissection

The cardiovascular changes of pregnancy may predispose the aorta to dissection during pregnancy,[62] owing to increased arterial wall tension and intimal shear forces. Further, estrogen-induced changes in collagen deposition, and circulating elastases and relaxin, may weaken the aortic media. Certain risk factors predispose women to aortic dissection during

---

BOX 41.10 Risk Factors for Aortic Dissection During Pregnancy

- Marfan syndrome
- Vascular Ehlers-Danlos syndrome (Type IV)
- Loeys-Dietz syndrome
- Bicuspid aortic valve
- Turner syndrome
- Non–Marfan syndrome–associated familial thoracic aneurysms
- Hypertension (hypertensive disorders of pregnancy and chronic hypertension)

BOX 41.11 General Management Strategies in Patients at High-Risk for Aortopathy and Management of Aortic Dissection

General Management Strategies
- Strict blood pressure management to target less than 140/90 mm Hg
- Beta-adrenergic receptor antagonist therapy throughout pregnancy, intrapartum, and the postpartum period
- Serial monitoring of aortic caliber via noncontrast MRI or transthoracic echocardiography
- Second trimester preferred for semielective aortic repair

Aortic Dissection Management
- Ascending aorta (Stanford type A or DeBakey type I or II)—surgical emergency:
  - During the first two trimesters, emergency surgery should be performed with cardiopulmonary bypass.
  - Modify anesthetic and perfusion technique to optimize fetal outcome after discussion of risks and benefit.
- Gestational age
  - Between 24 and 28 weeks' gestation, use multidisciplinary decision making to determine whether cesarean delivery should be performed followed by aortic surgery, or if aortic surgery should be performed with or without fetal monitoring.
  - Beyond 28 weeks' gestation, cesarean delivery should be performed, immediately followed by aortic surgery.
- Descending aorta (Stanford type B or DeBakey type III) is predominantly treated medically in all three trimesters.

MRI, Magnetic resonance imaging.
Summarized from Lindley KJ, Bairey Merz CN, Asgar AW, et al. Management of women with congenital or inherited cardiovascular disease from pre-conception through pregnancy and postpartum. *J Am Coll Cardiol.* 2021:77:1778–1798; Isselbacher EM, Preventza O, Hamilton Black J 3rd, et al. 2022 ACC/AHA Guideline for the diagnosis and management of aortic disease: a report of the American Heart Association/American College of Cardiology Joint Committee on Clinical Practice Guidelines. *J Am Coll Cardiol.* 2022:80; e223–e393.

---

pregnancy (Box 41.10).[63–66] Pregnancy-associated aortic dissections are predominantly type A (ascending aorta).[67,68] The risk of dissection increases with dilation. An aortic diameter ≥ 4.5 cm was reported to have a risk of dissection 6000 times greater compared with a diameter < 3.5 cm.[69] Dissections typically occur during late pregnancy: 39% third trimester and 26% postpartum.[67,68]

Patients with high-risk aortopathy should be managed at a center that has a pregnancy heart team.[69,70] The team should include cardiologists and maternal-fetal medicine physicians as well as cardiac and obstetric anesthesiologists with experience managing high-risk aortopathies during pregnancy. Further, the patient should have immediate access to a cardiothoracic surgeon with expertise in aortic endovascular repair techniques. The pregnancy and dissection management strategies are reviewed in Box 41.11. Both neuraxial[71,72] and general anesthesia[73] have been described. Dural ectasia and scoliosis may complicate neuraxial anesthetic techniques in parturients with heritable aortopathies such as Marfan syndrome.[74] It is reasonable to consider obtaining a lumbar spine MRI prior to delivery (preconception when possible). Emphasis should be placed on meticulous blood pressure stability and control throughout labor (Table 41.5). This includes typical cardiac labor analgesia techniques (see discussion below), continuing beta-adrenergic receptor blockade through the delivery and postpartum, and invasive blood pressure monitoring.

Congenital Heart Disease

Atrial Septal Defect

Patients with an undiagnosed ASD may remain asymptomatic until late in life, or they may become symptomatic for the first time during pregnancy. The most common defect is the secundum-type ASD (80%), whereas the primum, sinus venosus, and coronary sinus types of ASD are less common. Repaired ASD without long-term sequelae is a mWHO class I condition with no significantly increased risk of cardiovascular complications during pregnancy.[70] Unrepaired ASD is a mWHO class II lesion, with increased risk of right ventricular volume overload, atrial arrhythmias, and paradoxical embolism.[70] Less than 5% of patients with an ASD develop pulmonary hypertension, in which case pregnancy risk is considered prohibitively high.[70] Intravenous line bubble filters should be used in these patients recognizing that, at times, such as in

the setting of a propofol infusion or a massive transfusion requiring rapid transfusion, they may need to be removed. Typical obstetric and anesthetic management is generally recommended for patients with repaired and unrepaired ASD (see Table 41.5).[70]

Ventricular Septal Defect

There are four types of ventricular septal defects (VSDs); the most common type is a perimembranous VSD. Pregnancy is well tolerated (mWHO class I) in patients with a repaired or restrictive (small) VSD in the absence of pulmonary hypertension.[70] An unrepaired nonrestrictive VSD with Eisenmenger syndrome is associated with a prohibitively high risk for maternal cardiac complications (see discussion below). The risk of paradoxical embolism is minimal given the significant left-to-right pressure gradient between the left and right ventricle. Typical obstetric and anesthetic management (vaginal delivery with neuraxial analgesia) is generally recommended (see Table 41.5).[70]

TABLE 41.5 Anesthetic Considerations for Specific Cardiovascular Pathologic Processes

Disease	Modifier	Anesthetic Considerations	Monitoring
Ascending aortic dilation/aneurysm	Bicuspid aortic valve Marfan syndrome Turner syndrome	Meticulous attention to blood pressure control Maintain beta-adrenergic receptor antagonist therapy Consider imaging for dural ectasia in Marfan syndrome	Consider intra-arterial blood pressure monitoring
Unrepaired ASD or VSD	PAP < 40 mm Hg	Pregnancy/labor usually well tolerated Meticulous attention to de-airing all venous access tubing Consider potential for air embolism with loss-of-resistance-to-air epidural technique	
	PAP ≥ 40 mm Hg	Higher-risk group depending on degree of PAP elevation Maintain afterload (carefully titrate neuraxial anesthesia, treat hypotension with phenylephrine, titrate oxytocin, early recognition and aggressive treatment of hemorrhage) Minimize PVR (avoid carboprost, oversedation, and elevated airway pressures) Maintain adequate blood volume and venous return Avoid myocardial depressants (avoid beta-adrenergic receptor antagonists) Avoid and monitor for ischemia and arrhythmias	Consider intra-arterial blood pressure monitoring Consider 5-lead ECG monitoring in labor Consider PA catheter Consider partnership with cardiovascular anesthesiologist
Repaired ASD or VSD	PAP < 40 mm Hg	Pregnancy well tolerated	
	PAP ≥ 40 mm Hg	Higher-risk group depending on degree of PAP elevation Maintain afterload (carefully titrate neuraxial anesthesia, treat hypotension with phenylephrine, titrate oxytocin, early recognition and aggressive treatment of hemorrhage) Minimize PVR (avoid carboprost and oversedation) Maintain adequate blood volume and venous return Avoid myocardial depressants (avoid beta-adrenergic receptor antagonists) Avoid and monitor for ischemia and arrhythmias	Consider intra-arterial blood pressure monitoring Consider 5-lead ECG monitoring in labor Consider PA catheter Consider partnership with cardiovascular anesthesiologist
Patent ductus arteriosus		Pregnancy well tolerated	Echocardiographic evaluation to rule out pulmonary hypertension (rare)
Fontan repair		Meticulous attention to preload; low and high preload poorly tolerated Minimize PVR (avoid carboprost, oversedation, and elevated airway pressures)	Consider intra-arterial blood pressure monitoring Consider 5-lead ECG monitoring in labor
Transposition of the great arteries	Complete/repaired	Meticulous attention to preload and afterload because of propensity for systemic ventricular dysfunction	Consider intra-arterial blood pressure monitoring Consider 5-lead ECG monitoring in labor In decompensation, consider assessment of ventricular function with echocardiography or central venous access/filling pressure monitoring
	Congenitally corrected	Pregnancy well tolerated	Echocardiographic assessment of ventricular function is helpful

(Continued)

TABLE 41.5   **Anesthetic Considerations for Specific Cardiovascular Pathologic Processes—cont'd**

Disease	Modifier	Anesthetic Considerations	Monitoring
Ebstein anomaly		May have associated ASD detected by echocardiography (see above for ASD considerations) Pregnancy well tolerated with normal RV function If RV function is compromised, then minimize PVR (avoid carboprost, oversedation, and elevated airway pressures); avoid myocardial depressants and maintain coronary perfusion with adequate afterload	Consider 5-lead ECG monitoring in labor because of high incidence of arrhythmias In the setting of significantly compromised RV function, consider PA catheter and partnership with cardiovascular anesthesiologist
Tetralogy of Fallot (repaired)		Pregnancy well tolerated	Echocardiographic assessment of RV structure and function; look for evidence of pulmonary hypertension
Pulmonary hypertension	Mild to moderate	Maintain adequate blood volume and venous return Minimize PVR (avoid carboprost, oversedation, and elevated airway pressures) Avoid myocardial depressants Avoid and monitor for ischemia and arrhythmias	Consider 5-lead ECG monitoring in labor Consider intra-arterial blood pressure monitoring
	Severe	Very high-risk group Maintain afterload (carefully titrate neuraxial anesthesia, treat hypotension with phenylephrine, titrate oxytocin, early recognition and aggressive treatment of hemorrhage) Minimize PVR (avoid carboprost and oversedation/hypercapnia) May require pulmonary vasodilators Maintain adequate blood volume and venous return Avoid myocardial depressants (avoid beta-adrenergic receptor antagonists) Avoid and monitor for ischemia and arrhythmias	Multidisciplinary approach 5-lead ECG Intra-arterial blood pressure monitoring Ability to perform rapid echocardiography to direct management Consider central venous catheter and/or PA catheter but caution performing PA catheterization without fluoroscopic guidance Partner with cardiovascular anesthesiologist Monitor postpartum in cardiac ICU
Aortic stenosis	Transvalvular gradient < 25 mm Hg, valve area > 1.5 cm², normal LV function	Attentive preservation of preload and afterload Monitor closely for volume overload during the first 24 h after delivery	Consider 5-lead ECG in labor Consider intra-arterial blood pressure monitoring
	Transvalvular gradient ≥ 25 mm Hg, valve area < 1.0 cm², LV dysfunction	High-risk group Maintain afterload (carefully titrate neuraxial anesthesia, treat hypotension with phenylephrine, titrate oxytocin, early recognition and aggressive treatment of hemorrhage) Maintain normal HR (avoid tachycardia and respond rapidly to new-onset atrial fibrillation with rate control and potential cardioversion) Maintain normovolemia	5-lead ECG in labor Intra-arterial blood pressure monitoring

TABLE 41.5 Anesthetic Considerations for Specific Cardiovascular Pathologic Processes—cont'd

Disease	Modifier	Anesthetic Considerations	Monitoring
Mitral stenosis	Valve area > 1.5 cm², no pulmonary hypertension	Maintain normal HR (avoid tachycardia, continue beta-adrenergic receptor antagonists) Maintain sinus rhythm (respond to atrial fibrillation rapidly with rate control and/or cardioversion) Prevent and monitor for pulmonary edema	5-lead ECG in labor Intra-arterial blood pressure monitoring
	Valve area ≤ 1.5 cm², pulmonary hypertension	High-risk group Consider percutaneous mitral valvuloplasty before labor/delivery Manage pulmonary edema (consider diuretics and supplemental oxygen, labor in upright position, if needed consider intubation and positive-pressure ventilation with positive end-expiratory pressure)	5-lead ECG in labor Intra-arterial blood pressure monitoring
Pulmonary stenosis	Mild to moderate	Pregnancy well tolerated	
	Severe	High-risk group Consider balloon valvuloplasty Prevent tachycardia Mitigate increase in pulmonary artery resistance (e.g., hypoxemia, hypercarbia, positive-pressure ventilation)	5-lead ECG in labor Intra-arterial blood pressure monitoring
Hypertrophic cardiomyopathy	Without LVOT obstruction	Pregnancy well tolerated	
	With LVOT obstruction	Maintain beta-adrenergic receptor antagonist therapy Low preload and low afterload worsen outflow tract gradient Treat hypotension with phenylephrine Maintain sinus rhythm and prevent tachycardia Address new-onset atrial fibrillation (rate control, consider cardioversion) Avoid terbutaline, if possible	Low threshold for invasive blood pressure monitoring and central venous access/filling pressure monitoring Echocardiography helpful to follow outflow tract gradient
Cardiac tamponade		Meticulous attention to preload Maintain spontaneous ventilation Maintain heart rate Maintain afterload	Invasive blood pressure monitoring Central venous access/filling pressure monitoring

All patients with cardiovascular disease should labor in the lateral position to decrease aortocaval compression. Central venous pressure monitoring should be performed above the diaphragm.

ASD, Atrial septal defect; *ECG*, electrocardiogram; *HR*, heart rate; *ICU*, intensive care unit; *LV*, left ventricle; *LVOT*, left ventricular outflow tract; *PA*, pulmonary artery; *PAP*, pulmonary artery pressure; *PVR*, pulmonary vascular resistance; *RV*, right ventricle; *VSD*, ventricular septal defect.

Patent Ductus Arteriosus

Pregnancy is well tolerated in patients with a repaired, silent, or small patent ductus arteriosus (PDA), and complications are rare (mWHO class I).[70] Typical obstetric and anesthetic management (vaginal delivery with neuraxial analgesia) is generally recommended (see Table 41.5).[70] An unrepaired large PDA may cause pulmonary hypertension, and pregnancy is not recommended because of prohibitively high risk.[75,76]

Coarctation of the Aorta

Repaired coarctation of the aorta is generally considered a mWHO class II to III risk, depending on whether there is any residual gradient or aneurysm.[70] Severe unrepaired coarctation is considered mWHO class IV and pregnancy is

not recommended until the coarctation has been repaired. Systemic arterial hypertension is a common long-term sequela of coarctation even after repair, and several studies report increased risk of hypertensive disorders of pregnancy.[77,78] Coarctation is associated with a bicuspid aortic valve in more than half the patients, and 10% of adults develop intracranial aneurysms.[79,80] Prepregnancy evaluation of the coarctation, including residual degree of obstruction, evidence of aortic aneurysm and associated anomalies, is recommended.[75] Typical obstetric and anesthetic management (vaginal delivery with neuraxial analgesia) is generally recommended.[78] Blood pressure measurements should be obtained in the right arm as typically left arm pressures are falsely reduced, even in repaired patients.

Single Ventricle Palliation (Fontan Repair)

Single ventricle palliation is a multistep procedure that establishes blood flow from the venous system to the pulmonary artery by bypassing the right ventricle (Fig. 41.1). It is performed for cyanotic heart defects that cannot undergo a two-ventricle repair, typically related to severe underdevelopment of either the left or right ventricle. Common conditions leading to this type of repair include tricuspid or pulmonary atresia and hypoplastic left heart syndrome. Because there is no functional subpulmonic ventricle, right-sided filling pressures are chronically elevated and patients have limited capacity to augment cardiac output.[81] Common long-term complications include atrial arrhythmias (which are poorly tolerated), hepatic fibrosis with liver dysfunction, development of pulmonary collateral vessels with shunting and cyanosis, single ventricular systolic and diastolic dysfunction, atrioventricular (AV) valve regurgitation, lower extremity venous stasis, and protein-losing enteropathy.[81]

Pregnancy is considered mWHO class III for functional patients with single ventricle palliation and mWHO class IV for patients with evidence of Fontan failure (clinical cirrhosis, protein-losing enteropathy, symptomatic heart failure, plastic bronchitis).[70,81] Patients with a Fontan repair are at increased risk for arrhythmias, symptomatic heart failure, and thromboembolism during pregnancy. There is a high rate of fetal complications for patients with single ventricle palliation, including miscarriage, stillbirth, preterm birth, and fetal growth restriction.

Patients with a Fontan repair are preload dependent and should be adequately hydrated during labor and delivery (see Table 41.5).[70,81] Laboring in the left lateral decubitus position may be considered. A vaginal delivery with early, slowly titrated neuraxial anesthesia is generally recommended. The use of neuraxial anesthesia for operative delivery avoids the adverse effects of myocardial depression and positive-pressure ventilation on the Fontan circulation.[82,83] Patients may require a low threshold for assisted second stage of labor, given their dependence on preload.[70,81]

Intravenous bubble filters should be used if the patient has a patent Fontan fenestration or venovenous collaterals to reduce the risk of paradoxical embolism.[70,81] Oxygen saturation commonly decreases in the third trimester in these patients, owing to increased shunting through venovenous collaterals. The desaturation often does not respond to supplemental oxygen.[81]

Transposition of the Great Arteries

Transposition of the great arteries (TGA) comprises two distinct groups: complete TGA (D-transposition) and congenitally corrected TGA (L-transposition). In both conditions, the aorta originates from the right ventricle and the pulmonary artery originates from the left ventricle. Patients with L-TGA are not born cyanotic and often have not undergone previous cardiac surgery unless they were born with additional cardiac defects such as a VSD.

D-TGA manifests as neonatal cyanosis and patients born with this condition will have undergone surgical correction.

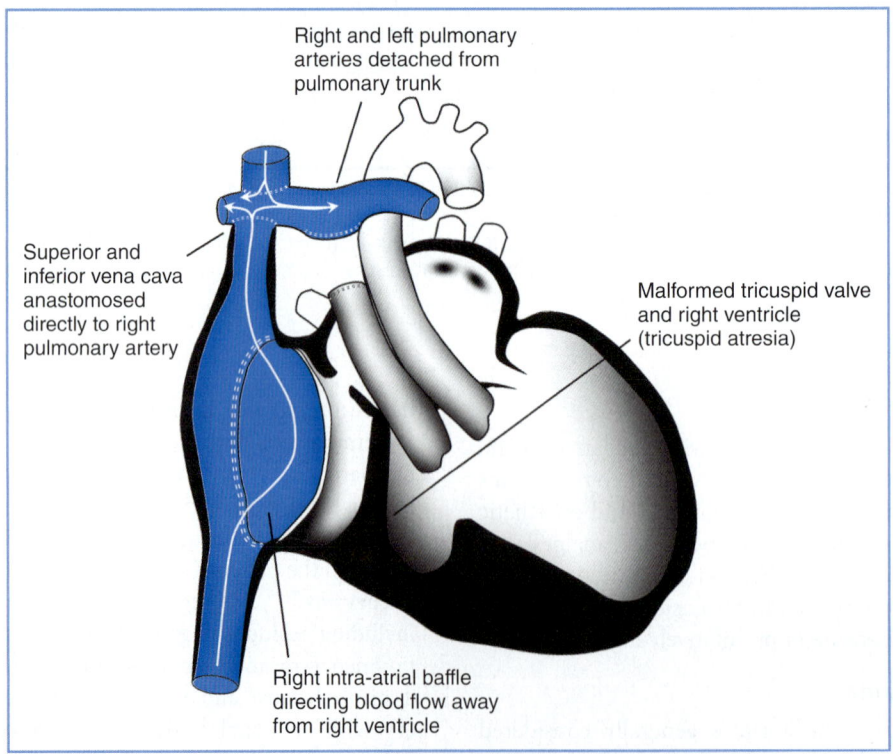

Right and left pulmonary arteries detached from pulmonary trunk

Superior and inferior vena cava anastomosed directly to right pulmonary artery

Malformed tricuspid valve and right ventricle (tricuspid atresia)

Right intra-atrial baffle directing blood flow away from right ventricle

Fig. 41.1 Schematic Depiction of a Fontan Repair. There is no functional right ventricle. The *white lines with arrows* represent the pathway of venous blood returning to the heart. Illustration by Naveen Nathan, MD, NorthShore University HealthSystem, University of Chicago Pritzker School of Medicine, Evanston, IL.

This was previously performed via an atrial switch procedure (Senning or Mustard), and the right ventricle functions as the systemic ventricle. Atrial arrhythmias, systemic right ventricular dysfunction, systemic tricuspid regurgitation, atrial baffle obstruction or leaks, and pulmonary hypertension are common long-term complications.[76]

In the contemporary era, an arterial switch procedure (Jatene) is performed and the left ventricle is the systemic ventricle. The most common complications include myocardial ischemia due to coronary button reimplantation and neoaortic regurgitation due to dilation of the neoaortic root.[84]

Pregnancy is considered mWHO class III for patients with a systemic right ventricle (L-TGA or D-TGA with atrial switch).[70] Patients with a systemic right ventricle carry increased risk for atrial arrhythmias (15%), symptomatic heart failure (10%), and worsening systemic tricuspid regurgitation during pregnancy.

All women with TGA require detailed echocardiography prior to planned pregnancy.[75,76] Typical obstetric and anesthetic management (vaginal delivery with neuraxial analgesia) is generally recommended for patients with a history of TGA (see Table 41.5).[70] Neuraxial anesthesia is recommended, with consideration of slowly titrated dosing for patients with systemic right ventricles because of their preload dependence. Patients with systemic right ventricular dysfunction or significant systemic tricuspid regurgitation are at increased risk for pulmonary edema, and volume status should be monitored closely. Telemetry monitoring is generally recommended because of the increased risk of atrial arrhythmias.[70]

Ebstein Anomaly

In Ebstein anomaly, the tricuspid valve is displaced toward the apex of the right ventricle, which can result in severe tricuspid regurgitation and right atrial enlargement (Figs. 41.2 and 41.3). It is commonly associated with an ASD and preexcitation syndromes. Accessory pathways result in arrhythmias in approximately 30% of patients; the most observed arrhythmias are atrial tachycardia, atrial flutter, and atrial fibrillation. Pregnancy appears to be well tolerated in patients with Ebstein anomaly (mWHO class II to III), especially in women with preserved ventricular function.[76,85] Typical obstetric and anesthetic management (vaginal delivery with neuraxial analgesia) is generally recommended (see Table 41.5).

Tetralogy of Fallot

Unrepaired tetralogy of Fallot consists of a VSD, an aorta that overrides the VSD, and right ventricular outflow tract obstruction (infundibular, valvular, or both), with resulting right ventricular hypertrophy.[75,86] Most adults born with tetralogy of Fallot in the United States have undergone surgical repair in childhood. During surgical repair, the VSD is closed and the right ventricular outflow obstruction is repaired. The common long-term sequelae are residual pulmonary valve insufficiency and resulting right ventricular dilation and dysfunction.[77] Patients with repaired tetralogy of Fallot are also at risk for atrial and ventricular arrhythmias.

The preanesthetic evaluation of these patients should include detailed echocardiographic evaluation of cardiac structure and function. Patients with repaired tetralogy of Fallot and no symptoms of right heart failure are considered mWHO class II.[87] Right ventricular dysfunction, severe right ventricular dilation, and/or severe pulmonary regurgitation increase the risk of arrhythmias and right-sided heart failure.[76,87,88] Typically, obstetric and anesthetic management (vaginal delivery with neuraxial analgesia) is generally recommended for patients with tetralogy of Fallot (see Table 41.5).[70]

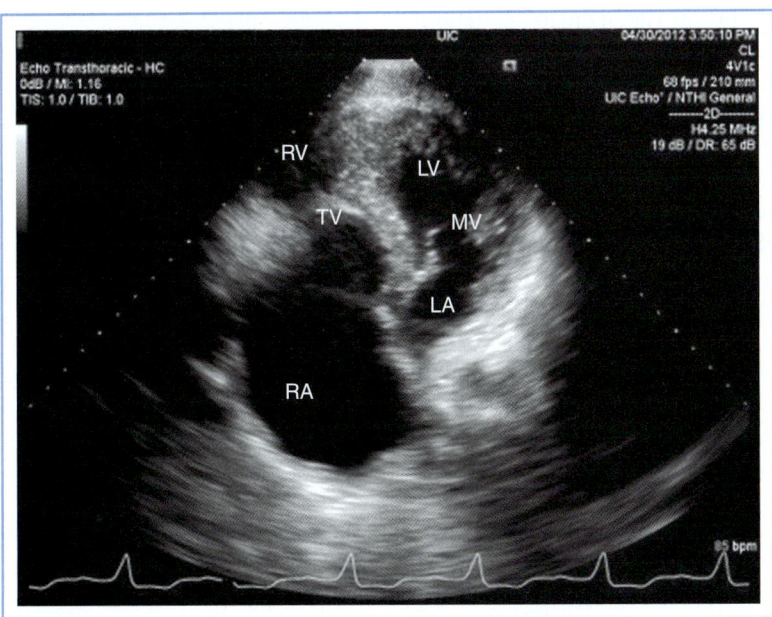

Fig. 41.2 Echocardiographic Image of Ebstein Anomaly. The right atrium is markedly enlarged. *LA*, Left atrium; *LV*, left ventricle; *MV*, mitral valve; *RA*, right atrium; *RV*, right ventricle; *TV*, tricuspid valve. Illustration Dr. Mayank Kansal, University of Illinois at Chicago, Chicago, IL.

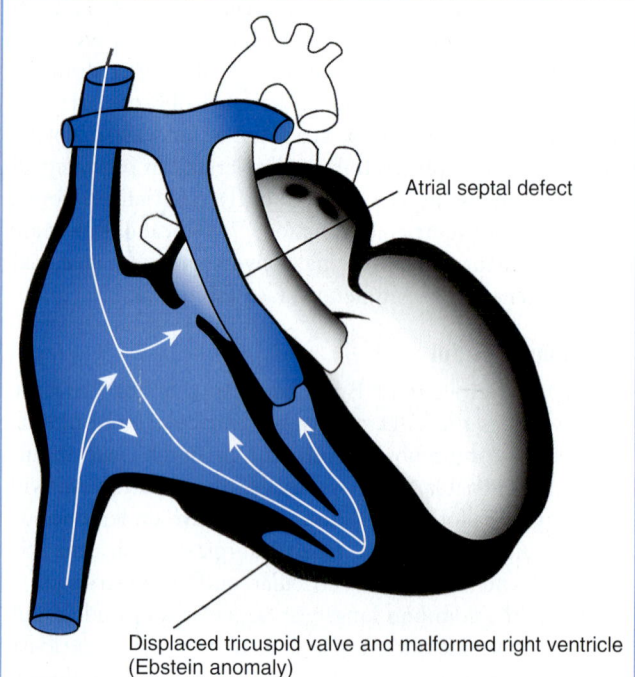

Fig. 41.3 Schematic Depiction of Ebstein Anomaly and Atrial Septal Defect. An atrial septal defect is present in more than one-third of patients with Ebstein anomaly. The *white lines with arrows* represent the pathway of venous blood returning to the heart. Illustration by Naveen Nathan, MD, NorthShore University HealthSystem, University of Chicago Pritzker School of Medicine, Evanston, IL.

Patients with significant right ventricular enlargement and dysfunction are preload dependent, so it is important to maintain adequate intravascular volume and venous return.

Pulmonary Hypertension

Normal mean PAP at rest is 14 mm Hg (standard deviation [SD], 3 mm Hg) in both pregnant and nonpregnant patients. Pulmonary hypertension was traditionally defined as a mean PAP > 25 mm Hg but is now defined as a mean PAP > 20 mm Hg, determined by right heart catheterization.[89,90] There are five broad categories of pulmonary hypertension based on the underlying cause of raised PAP: (1) pulmonary arterial hypertension (PAH), (2) left heart disease, (3) lung diseases and/or hypoxia, (4) pulmonary artery obstructions (e.g., thromboembolic disease), and (5) undifferentiated or multifactorial causes (e.g., sickle cell disease, sarcoidosis; Box 41.12).[89,90] Left heart and lung diseases are the most common causes. Classification of pulmonary hypertension, based on the pathophysiologic mechanisms, informs the clinical presentation, hemodynamic characteristics, and therapeutic management of the disease.

"Precapillary" pulmonary hypertension is caused by the pulmonary arterial system alone and is defined by pulmonary artery wedge pressure (PAWP) ≤ 15 mm Hg and PVR > 2 Wood units.[90]

"Postcapillary" pulmonary hypertension occurs secondary to elevations of the pulmonary venous system pressure

---

BOX 41.12   Classification of Pulmonary Hypertension

1. **Group 1 Pulmonary arterial hypertension**
   1.1. Idiopathic
      1.1.1. Nonresponders at vasoreactivity testing
      1.1.2. Acute responders at vasoreactivity testing
   1.2. Heritable
   1.3. Associated with drugs and toxins
   1.4. Associated with:
      1.4.1. Connective tissue disease
      1.4.2. HIV infection
      1.4.3. Portal hypertension
      1.4.4. Congenital heart disease
      1.4.5. Schistosomiasis
   1.5. Pulmonary arterial hypertension with features of PVOD/PCH involvement
   1.6. Persistent pulmonary hypertension of the newborn
2. **Group 2 Pulmonary hypertension associated with left heart disease**
   2.1. Heart failure:
      2.1.1. with preserved ejection fraction
      2.1.2. with reduced or mildly reduced ejection fraction
   2.2. Valvular heart disease
   2.3. Congenital/acquired cardiovascular conditions leading to postcapillary pulmonary hypertension
3. **Group 3 Pulmonary hypertension associated with lung diseases and/or hypoxia**
   3.1. Obstructive lung disease or emphysema
   3.2. Restrictive lung disease
   3.3. Lung disease with mixed restrictive/obstructive pattern
   3.4. Hypoventilation syndromes
   3.5. Hypoxia without lung disease (e.g., high altitude)
   3.6. Developmental lung disorders
4. **Group 4 Pulmonary hypertension associated with pulmonary artery obstruction**
   4.1. Chronic thromboembolic pulmonary hypertension
   4.2. Other pulmonary artery obstructions
5. **Group 5 Pulmonary hypertension with unclear and/or multifactorial mechanisms**
   5.1. Hematologic disorders
   5.2. Systemic disorders
   5.3. Metabolic disorders
   5.4. Chronic renal failure with or without hemodialysis
   5.5. Pulmonary tumor thrombotic microangiopathy
   5.6. Fibrosing mediastinitis

HIV, Human immunodeficiency virus; *PCH*, pulmonary capillary hemangiomatosis; *PVOD*, venous/capillary veno-occlusive disease. Modified from Humbert M, Kovacs G, Hoeper MM, et al. 2022 ESC/ERS guidelines for the diagnosis and treatment of pulmonary hypertension. *Eur Heart J.* 2022;43:3618–3731.

---

such as that caused by left-sided heart disease and is defined by PAWP > 15 mm Hg and PVR ≤ 2 Wood units.[90]

Severe pulmonary hypertension of all causes is associated with exceptionally high maternal mortality. Older studies reported maternal mortality rates as high as 56%[91]; however, more contemporary studies have demonstrated some improvement in maternal mortality, with rates ranging from 12% to 33%.[92,93] The cause of the pulmonary hypertension predicts the mortality rate; Group 1 pulmonary hypertension has the greatest risk of death from pregnancy.

The contemporary Registry of Pregnancy and Cardiac Disease reported the highest mortality associated with idiopathic pulmonary hypertension (43%), followed by left heart disease pulmonary hypertension (2.7%) and congenital heart disease pulmonary hypertension (2.7%).[94] Similarly, among 49 women with pulmonary hypertension who gave birth in one of four US institutions between 2001 and 2015, the overall mortality rate was 16%; seven of eight deaths occurred in women with idiopathic pulmonary hypertension (mortality rate 23%). A 2021 systematic review of births between 2008 and 2018 found a maternal mortality rate of 12% for all causes of pulmonary hypertension and a 20% mortality for idiopathic pulmonary hypertension.[93] Of note, all deaths in both studies occurred in the postpartum period.[93,94]

Physical examination findings consistent with pulmonary hypertension include (1) a loud pulmonary heart sound (P2), (2) a widely split S2 caused by delayed closure of the pulmonary valve secondary to high right-sided pressures (the pulmonary valve closes *after* the aortic valve), (3) a right-sided holosystolic murmur of tricuspid regurgitation, and (4) a classic right ventricular heave upon palpation of the precordium. ECG findings consistent with pulmonary hypertension include (1) right-axis deviation and (2) right ventricular hypertrophy.

Echocardiography helps establish the diagnosis and prognosis of pulmonary hypertension because it demonstrates the degree of right ventricular hypertrophy, the presence of right ventricular dysfunction, and an estimation of PAP by assessing the velocity of the tricuspid regurgitant jet (Fig. 41.4). The echocardiographic assessment of right-sided pressures may be inaccurate; therefore, invasive right-sided—and frequently

left-sided—heart catheterization is required for the definitive diagnosis of pulmonary hypertension. Right-sided heart catheterization allows for accurate pressure measurements to establish the diagnosis and severity, cardiac output measurement using thermodilution and the Fick equation, and vasoreactivity testing for prognosis and to define effective treatment regimens.

Vasoreactive testing is usually performed with inhaled **nitric oxide** or IV infusion of **sodium nitroprusside**, **epoprostenol**, or **adenosine** in the cardiac catheterization laboratory. Patients who achieve a decrease in mean PAP ≥ 10 mm Hg and achieve a mean PAP ≤ 40 mm Hg without a decrease in cardiac output are "positive acute responders."[95,96] Patients with a positive response have a better prognosis and may respond to oral therapy with a calcium channel blocker.[95]

Eisenmenger Syndrome

In patients with an anatomic shunt between the systemic and pulmonary circulations at the atrial, ventricular, or aortopulmonary artery level, a left-to-right shunt initially causes increased pulmonary blood flow. Over time, the pulmonary vasculature changes, PVR increases, and pulmonary hypertension develops. The development of pulmonary hypertension results, at least in part, from endothelial dysfunction and vascular remodeling of the pulmonary vascular bed. This increase in PVR causes reversal of the shunt (from left-to-right to right-to-left), which results in hypoxemia and cyanosis. This anatomic and physiologic scenario is referred to as Eisenmenger syndrome.

Pulmonary hypertension due to congenital heart disease can be caused by unrepaired congenital heart defects with a left-to-right shunt. Eisenmenger syndrome is associated with VSD, ASD, PDA, and AV septal defect (also referred to as endocardial cushion defect). More rarely encountered congenital heart defects (e.g., partial or total anomalous pulmonary venous return, TGA) may also lead to pulmonary hypertension and Eisenmenger syndrome.

Maternal mortality in women with Eisenmenger syndrome is exceptionally high (30% to 50%), although outcomes appear to have improved in the past two decades.[91,92] The cardiovascular physiologic changes of pregnancy present a significant hemodynamic challenge for women with pulmonary hypertension and may lead to development of right ventricular failure. The peripartum period, with its rapid fluid shifts and increased oxygen demand, is particularly challenging. Death usually occurs peripartum or postpartum. In a systematic review of case reports of pulmonary hypertension associated with congenital heart disease published between 1997 and 2007 (*n* = 29), all eight maternal deaths occurred postpartum (range, 0 to 24 days after delivery).[92]

Women with Eisenmenger syndrome often cannot respond to the increased oxygen demands of pregnancy. The normal pregnancy-related decrease in PVR does not occur because the PVR is fixed. In addition, the normal pregnancy-associated decrease in SVR tends to exacerbate the severity of the right-to-left shunt. These changes, together with the normal pregnancy-associated decrease in functional residual

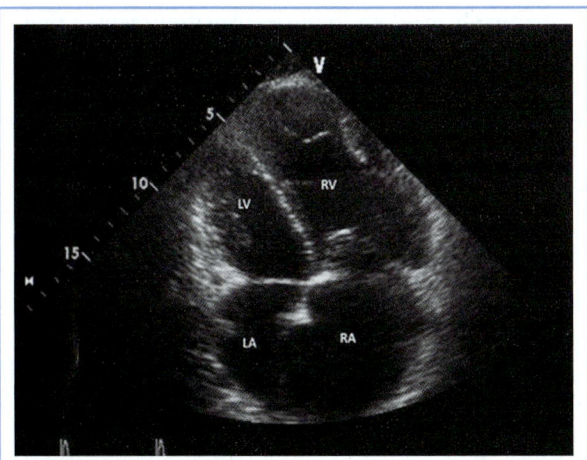

Fig. 41.4 Echocardiographic Image of Pulmonary Hypertension With Severe Right-Chamber Enlargement. The RV basal measurement is 55 mm (upper limit of normal 42 mm); the RA minor axis dimension is 70 mm (upper limit of normal 44 mm). *LA*, Left atrium; *LV*, left ventricle; *RA*, right atrium; *RV*, right ventricle. Illustration Dr. Mayank Kansal, University of Illinois at Chicago, Chicago, IL.

capacity, predispose women with Eisenmenger syndrome to hypoxemia. Maternal hypoxemia leads to a high incidence of fetal growth restriction and fetal demise. With contemporary drug therapy, cardiac imaging, and collaborative care, successful pregnancy has been described in patients with Eisenmenger syndrome.[92,97]

Medical and Obstetric Management

Pregnant women with pulmonary hypertension should receive multidisciplinary care in a referral center by a pregnancy heart team experienced in managing pulmonary hypertension in pregnancy.[90] The most recent European Society of Cardiology guidelines recommend discontinuing the endothelin receptor antagonists, **riociguat** and **selexipag**, because of potential or unknown teratogenicity.[90] Other endothelin receptor antagonists (e.g., **bosentan** and **ambrisentan**) are likely also teratogenic, and therefore their use is contraindicated during pregnancy. It is unclear whether pregnant patients with pulmonary hypertension should receive thromboprophylaxis during pregnancy and the peripartum period. Both hemorrhage and thromboembolism are causes of maternal mortality.[92] Box 41.13 summarizes therapies for pulmonary hypertension that are considered safe.[98–102,104–106]

The optimal mode of delivery in patients with pulmonary hypertension is unknown. A 2015 statement on pregnancy in patients with pulmonary hypertension from the Pulmonary Vascular Research Institute recommended cesarean delivery as the preferred mode of delivery unless it is not available or in cases of emergencies.[107] However, in a systematic review that included reports from 1978 to 1996,[91] operative delivery was an independent risk factor for maternal mortality. In contrast, the mode of delivery was not identified as a risk factor for maternal death in a more recent systematic review.[92] While vaginal delivery often involves the Valsalva maneuver, which increases intrathoracic pressure, as well as the potential for labor-induced vasovagal responses, cesarean delivery is associated with larger changes in intravascular volume, more bleeding complications and blood loss, and a greater risk for thromboembolism. Therefore, while it seems reasonable to reserve cesarean delivery for obstetric indications, unstable patients may require intubation and intensive care, thereby necessitating cesarean delivery.

Anesthetic Management

The goals of anesthetic management include (1) maintenance of adequate SVR; (2) maintenance of intravascular volume and venous return; (3) avoidance of aortocaval compression; (4) prevention of pain, hypoxemia, hypercarbia, and acidosis, which may increase PVR; and (5) avoidance of myocardial depression during general anesthesia (see Table 41.5).

Current evidence on choice of anesthetic technique for patients with pulmonary hypertension is based on case reports and series from high-volume referral centers. The use of general,[103,108] epidural,[109,110] and CSE anesthesia[111] has been reported. Neuraxial (epidural and CSE) anesthesia with use of pulmonary vasodilators in highly specialized centers appears to be associated with favorable overall outcomes.[112,113] In published case reports, cautious administration of epidural anesthesia did not affect the shunt flow in parturients with Eisenmenger syndrome. Slowly titrated epidural or CSE anesthesia eliminates the undesirable effects of positive-pressure ventilation associated with general anesthesia.

Because patients with pulmonary hypertension frequently require systemic anticoagulation, neuraxial anesthetic options may be limited. Invasive blood pressure monitoring is typically described in cases involving both neuraxial and general anesthesia.

Intravascular volume assessment in patients with severe pulmonary hypertension can be informed by central venous pressure monitoring. Pulmonary artery catheterization without the use of fluoroscopy is technically challenging owing to the frequent presence of tricuspid regurgitation and right-sided chamber enlargement and has not been shown to improve outcome. Either transthoracic (during neuraxial anesthesia) and transesophageal (during general anesthesia) echocardiography may be helpful.

Nitric oxide may be administered in the urgent setting and has been described during epidural anesthesia for emergency cesarean delivery using a noninvasive ventilation device.[114] Successful cesarean delivery with inhaled **iloprost** and slowly titrated epidural anesthesia has also been reported.[115,116] Given the high rate of postpartum mortality, patients with severe pulmonary hypertension should be monitored in an intensive care setting for a minimum of several days postpartum.

Infective Endocarditis

Endocarditis during pregnancy is most frequently associated with intravenous drug use or preexisting structural heart and valve abnormalities (e.g., rheumatic valvular disease, congenital heart disease). Maternal and fetal mortality rates are high (approximately 15% and 22%, respectively).[117] Currently, the American College of Cardiology (ACC) and the American Heart Association (AHA) do not recommend infective endocarditis antibiotic prophylaxis during vaginal or cesarean delivery for patients with any valvular heart condition (Class C recommendation [no benefit], level of

---

BOX 41.13 **Therapy for Pulmonary Hypertension During Pregnancy**

- Calcium channel blockers[90]
- Phosphodiesterase-5 inhibitors[90]
  - Sildenafil[98,99]
  - Milrinone infusion (for acute right ventricular afterload reduction)
- Inhaled/intravenous/subcutaneous prostacyclin analogs[90]
  - Epoprostenol[100–103]
  - Treprostinil
  - Iloprost
- Diuretics (to manage volume overload)
- Dobutamine, epinephrine, or norepinephrine infusion (to improve right ventricular function)
- Inhaled nitric oxide (to selectively dilate the pulmonary vasculature during vaginal or cesarean delivery)[104–106]

evidence B).[118] In the absence of active infection, endocarditis prophylaxis is currently only recommended for dental procedures in the highest-risk patients.[118] There is general agreement that patients with *untreated* **systemic infection** (i.e., bacteremia) should not receive neuraxial anesthesia. Animal studies suggest that spinal anesthesia may be safely administered in patients who have received antibiotic treatment and are responding to treatment at the time of dural puncture (see Chapter 36).[119] It is likely that epidural analgesia and anesthesia may be safely administered to patients with treated systemic infection.

Implantable Cardiac Devices

Permanent and temporary pacemakers, as well as automatic implantable cardioverter-defibrillators (ICDs) are generally well tolerated in pregnant patients.[120] Pregnancy does not increase the risk for ICD-related complications, and it does not increase the number of ICD discharges.[121] Rather, the severity of underlying structural heart disease determines the overall complication rate.[122] Case reports suggest that pregnant women tolerate ICD shocks as well as nonpregnant women.[122,123] Management principles for implantable cardiac devices that can help guide the pregnancy heart team during labor and delivery are shown in Box 41.14.

Maternal Arrhythmias

The incidence of arrhythmias is increased during pregnancy as a result of the elevated intravascular volume causing atrial[6] and ventricular stretch.[34] Additionally, autonomic and hormonal changes of pregnancy have been proposed as mechanisms. Palpitations are frequent during pregnancy. Of interest, there is no correlation between symptomatic palpitations in pregnancy and the frequency of underlying arrhythmias.[126] Holter monitoring often reveals premature atrial and ventricular contractions. No treatment is indicated in asymptomatic patients with premature atrial contractions (PACs) or premature ventricular contractions (PVCs). The frequency of ectopy decreases after delivery. Women who have been diagnosed with an arrhythmia before pregnancy frequently develop an exacerbation of arrhythmia during pregnancy. Recurrence of a preexisting arrhythmia during pregnancy is associated with adverse fetal events.[127]

Supraventricular Arrhythmias

Supraventricular tachycardia (SVT) is one of the more common arrhythmias to present in pregnancy, with an estimated 24 episodes/100,000 pregnancies.[128] Symptoms of SVT may be exacerbated during pregnancy.[129] Acute and chronic management of nonreentrant SVT in pregnancy is summarized in Box 41.15.[130] If the patient has a history of preexcitation, flecainide or procainamide should be used to avoid increasing conduction in the accessory pathway, which there may increase the risk of an AV reentrant tachycardia deteriorating.

Atrial fibrillation and **flutter** are not uncommon in pregnancy and frequently result from underlying structural heart disease (e.g., rheumatic mitral stenosis or congenital heart disease).[131] Therefore, a new diagnosis in pregnancy

BOX 41.14 Management Principles of Implantable Cardiac Devices in Pregnant Patients

- The indications for pacemaker placement (e.g., symptomatic bradycardia, periods of asystole > 3 s, escape rhythms below the atrioventricular node with rates < 40 beats/min) also apply in pregnancy.
- Pregnant patients who develop hemodynamic instability caused by bradycardia that is refractory to other therapies should receive a temporary venous pacemaker.
- For all procedures in patients with a pacemaker or ICD, a magnet should be immediately available.
- Pacemakers and ICDs should be interrogated before or during pregnancy and before delivery. The type of device, manufacturer, and model should be documented as well as the indication for the device, the patient's underlying rhythm, whether the patient is pacemaker dependent, and the device's response to magnet placement
- Pacemakers and ICDs should be left active in labor. A cesarean delivery occurs below the umbilicus; therefore, according to guidelines, disabling the defibrillation function of an ICD is not necessary.[124] If the anesthesia team chooses to disable an ICD for a surgical procedure in order to avoid the remote possibility of discharge from cautery interference, external defibrillation pads should be placed.
- If placement of a defibrillation device is indicated during pregnancy, the cardiology team may choose to utilize a wearable automatic defibrillator or a subcutaneous ICD. A subcutaneous system does not require heart leads or fluoroscopy-guided lead placement and has been described as an option during pregnancy.[125]
- In patients with a pacemaker or an ICD, central venous catheter placement in the upper body should be be performed with extreme caution so as not to damage or entangle device leads; this is particularly important in leads that were recently inserted (within the past 3 mo).
- For most pacemakers, the magnet will allow pacing in an asynchronous mode. The magnet will have no effect for leadless, single-chamber pacemakers.
- For most ICDs, the magnet will disable the tachycardia detection function (i.e., the device will not deliver a shock for ventricular tachycardia or ventricular fibrillation). The magnet will not alter the pacing mode or rate settings, or the bradycardia pacing settings.

ICD, Implantable cardioverter defibrillator.

should prompt an evaluation for structural heart disease. These arrhythmias occur most commonly at the end of the second trimester.[131] The acute and chronic management of atrial fibrillation and flutter in pregnancy are summarized in Box 41.15.[130] Anticoagulation with low-molecular-weight heparin (LMWH) may be indicated.[130]

Stroke risk stratification in pregnant patients is the same as that in nonpregnant patients.[29] The **CHADS₂** and **CHA₂DS₂-VASc scores** facilitate risk stratification for predicting stroke and thromboembolism associated with atrial fibrillation, thereby informing the choice of anticoagulation.[132] In the CHA₂DS₂-VASc score, points are assigned for **C**ongestive

BOX 41.15   Treatment of Cardiac Arrhythmias During Pregnancy

Nonreentrant supraventricular tachycardia
- Acute therapy
  - Vagal maneuvers
  - Adenosine
- Chronic therapy
  - First line: beta-adrenergic receptor antagonist (with or without digoxin)
  - Second line: calcium channel blocker

Supraventricular tachycardia with history of preexcitation
- Flecainide or procainamide

Atrial fibrillation and flutter
- Acute therapy
  - Synchronized DC cardioversion if unstable
  - First line: beta-adrenergic receptor antagonist (with or without digoxin)
  - Second line: calcium channel blocker
- Chronic therapy
  - First line: flecainide or procainamide
  - Second line: ablation[a]

Ventricular tachycardia
- Acute management
  - Synchronized DC cardioversion if unstable
  - Polymorphic ventricular tachycardia: IV magnesium sulfate
  - First line: lidocaine or beta-adrenergic receptor antagonist (e.g., sotalol)
  - Second line: procainamide or quinidine
  - Third line: amiodarone[b]
  - Fourth line: ablation (if refractory)

[a]Preferably deferred to the postpartum period.
[b]Fetal exposure to amiodarone has been associated with fetal hypothyroidism and growth restriction.[38]
DC, Direct current; IV, intravenous.
Summarized from Tamirisa KP, Elkayam U, Briller JE, et al. Arrhythmias in pregnancy. *JACC Clin Electrophysiol.* 2022;8:120–135.

heart failure, **H**ypertension, **A**ge 75 years or older (doubled), **D**iabetes mellitus, prior **S**troke or transient ischemic accident or thromboembolism (doubled), **V**ascular disease, **A**ge 65 to 74 years, and female **S**ex. The direct oral anticoagulants (e.g., **dabigatran**, **apixaban**, **rivaroxaban**) are not well studied in pregnancy and should not be used.

Ventricular preexcitation syndromes (e.g., **Wolff-Parkinson-White syndrome**) are rarely encountered in pregnancy; these patients are usually identified at a younger age and have undergone highly effective electrophysiologic treatment. A few case reports suggest that preexcitation syndromes may be associated with an increased rate of supraventricular arrhythmias during pregnancy.

Ventricular Arrhythmias

Ventricular arrhythmias occur at a rate of 2 per 100,000 delivery admissions and are often associated with congenital heart disease and underlying cardiomyopathies.[127] For example, sudden cardiac death caused by idiopathic ventricular tachycardia has been described in pregnant women with hypertrophic cardiomyopathy.[133–135] Idiopathic ventricular tachycardia is most commonly monomorphic, originating from the right ventricular outflow tract, and is catecholamine sensitive and responsive to treatment with a beta-adrenergic receptor antagonist,[136] **verapamil**,[137] or **isoproterenol (isoprenaline)**.[138] Polymorphic ventricular tachycardia[139] and electrical storm with **Brugada syndrome**[140] have also been reported during pregnancy. Management of ventricular tachycardia in pregnancy is summarized in Box 41.15.[130]

Congenital Long QT Syndrome

The congenital long QT syndrome is caused by mutations in cardiac ion channels resulting in prolongation of ventricular repolarization and a QTc > 470 ms. The clinical spectrum ranges from a lack of symptoms to arrhythmia-associated syncope and sudden cardiac death. Risk for cardiac events (syncope, arrhythmias, or death) is decreased during pregnancy, but increased in the 40 weeks following pregnancy.[141] Different long QT syndrome genotypes may have different risks associated with pregnancy. The LQT2 genotype is associated with a higher rate of cardiac events in the 9-month postpartum period than the LQT1 and LQT3 genotypes.[141,142] Prophylactic treatment with a beta-adrenergic receptor antagonist is recommended during pregnancy and postpartum in patients with long QT syndrome.[141,143] During delivery, it is important to minimize adrenergic stimuli (e.g., with effective labor analgesia) and avoid drugs that further prolong the QT interval, including antiemetic medications such as **droperidol**, **haloperidol**, or **phenothiazines**.

Electric Cardioversion

Life-threatening or hemodynamically unstable arrhythmias should be terminated by electric cardioversion.[132,143] **Defibrillation** refers to administration of electrical energy to terminate ventricular fibrillation. By contrast, **synchronized cardioversion** is delivery of an electric shock synchronized to the QRS complex. Synchronized cardioversion is administered for supraventricular rhythms (i.e., atrial fibrillation, atrial flutter, atrial tachycardia) as well as for monomorphic ventricular tachycardia with a pulse.[143] Pulseless ventricular tachycardia and polymorphic ventricular tachycardia should be treated with **unsynchronized cardioversion**.

Electric cardioversion can be performed safely throughout pregnancy without apparent adverse effects on fetal hemodynamic function.[144] Nonetheless, it is prudent to monitor the FHR before and after cardioversion.[145]

Patients usually require anesthesia care for cardioversion. The risk for pulmonary aspiration of gastric contents associated with sedation (with an unprotected airway) should be weighed against the risks associated with general anesthesia and tracheal intubation. For elective cardioversion in the setting of appropriate fasting, the judicious use of sedation rather than general anesthesia is usually preferred. A nonparticulate antacid followed by the administration of a benzodiazepine and/or propofol can provide satisfactory sedation and amnesia.

Myocardial Infarction

The term *myocardial infarction* signifies myocardial cell death caused by ischemia.[146] It is diagnosed by clinical signs and symptoms, ECG patterns, elevation of biomarkers (CK-MB, troponin), and various imaging modalities (echocardiography, radionuclide imaging, CMR imaging, CT). Pregnancy-associated myocardial infarction occurs in 2.8 to 8.1 per 100,000 deliveries and accounts for 20% of maternal cardiac deaths in the United States.[147] Risk factors include age > 35 years, cigarette smoking, hypertension, hyperlipidemia, and diabetes.[148] The current Universal Classification of Myocardial Infarction recognizes five types of myocardial infarction (Box 41.16),[146] and pregnancy-associated myocardial infarction occurs in the setting of both obstructive and nonobstructive coronary arteries. Approximately one-third of pregnancy-associated myocardial infarctions are a result of unstable obstructive atherosclerotic disease and one-third are a result of spontaneous coronary artery dissection. Other causes include *in situ* thrombus or thrombotic emboli because of the hypercoagulable state associated with pregnancy as well as coronary vasospasm, which has been described as a result of cocaine or ergot alkaloids.

ACS is an encompassing term used to describe unstable angina, non–ST-segment elevation myocardial infarction (NSTEMI), and ST-segment elevation myocardial infarction (STEMI). Unstable angina is differentiated from NSTEMI by lack of elevation of cardiac biomarkers. Compared with unstable angina or NSTEMI, STEMI is an emergency and requires early reperfusion; a "door-to-balloon" interval < 90 minutes for percutaneous coronary intervention is optimal. The standard of care for the nonpregnant patient with ACS should be the standard of care for the pregnant patient with ACS with certain modifications.[147] The diagnosis of ACS can be difficult in pregnancy. The following diagnostic principles should be considered:

- ST-segment depression is common in cesarean delivery and has been attributed, in part, to oxytocin administration.[11,12,149,150]
- ST-segment elevation is not a normal occurrence during labor and delivery or with any type of intrapartum anesthesia. Hence, ST-segment elevation should always be considered abnormal.
- CK-MB may be elevated during normal labor and the postpartum period (see discussion below and Box 41.4); thus, measurement of this enzyme is less useful for the diagnosis of myocardial infarction in women in the peripartum period.[21]
- An elevated troponin level is specific, although troponin may be elevated in patients with gestational hypertension and preeclampsia/eclampsia (which may be related to subclinical cardiac myofibrillary damage).[19,20]
- Symptoms and signs, such as chest pain, prominent jugular venous distension, pulmonary rales, and deep T-wave inversions, especially in leads V1 to V3, should also prompt further workup.

BOX 41.16 Universal Classification of Myocardial Infarction

Type 1 Spontaneous Myocardial Infarction
Caused by atherosclerosis and plaque rupture/erosion resulting in intracoronary thrombus formation

Type 2 Myocardial Infarction Caused by Ischemic Imbalance
Caused by conditions other than atherosclerosis (e.g., supply-demand mismatch, coronary vasospasm, coronary embolism, coronary dissection, stress of noncardiac surgery)

Type 3 Cardiac Death Caused by Myocardial Infarction
Cardiac death highly suggestive of myocardial infarction without the availability of biomarker confirmation

Type 4a Myocardial Infarction Related to Percutaneous Coronary Intervention
Caused by distal plaque embolization and side-branch occlusion; directly related to coronary intervention (e.g., stenting or balloon angioplasty)

Type 4b Myocardial Infarction Caused by Stent Thrombosis
Detected by autopsy or angiography

Type 4c Restenosis Associated With Percutaneous Coronary Intervention

Type 5 Myocardial Infarction Caused by Coronary Artery Bypass Grafting
Cardiac biomarker elevation associated with surgical revascularization procedure

Modified from Thygesen K, Alpert JS, Jaffe AS, et al. Fourth universal definition of myocardial infarction. *Circulation.* 2018;138:e618–e651.

Percutaneous Coronary Intervention

STEMI during pregnancy should be treated with primary percutaneous coronary intervention via radial arterial access and systemic anticoagulation with unfractionated heparin.[151] While conventional balloon angioplasty does not require ongoing dual antiplatelet therapy, placement of a stent is associated with a lower risk for abrupt vessel closure in the short term and a lower long-term risk for restenosis.

Dual antiplatelet therapy is mandatory after placement of a coronary artery stent to prevent stent thrombosis, the duration of which depends upon the type of stent (Table 41.6).[152] This therapy consists of both **aspirin** (81 to 325 mg daily) and **clopidogrel**. In pregnancy, clopidogrel should not be replaced by one of the newer agents (e.g., **prasugrel, ticagrelor**) because of limited safety data. There are few data on the optimal duration of dual antiplatelet therapy in this unique clinical setting. Clopidogrel should be discontinued 7 days before the performance of neuraxial anesthesia.[47] Aspirin, however, should be continued indefinitely in patients with any type of stent. Both spinal and epidural anesthesia can be performed safely in patients receiving aspirin.

Valvular Heart Disease

The risk of cardiovascular complications during pregnancy depends on the valvular lesion severity and location (Table 41.7). The highest-risk valvular lesions in pregnancy are

TABLE 41.6   Dual Antiplatelet Therapy Recommendations

		Bare-Metal Stent	Drug-Eluting Stent[a]
Stable coronary artery disease	Aspirin	Indefinitely	Indefinitely
	Clopidogrel	1 mo	3–6 mo
Acute coronary syndrome[b]	Aspirin	Indefinitely	Indefinitely
	Clopidogrel	12 mo	12 mo
High bleeding risk/ pregnancy	Aspirin	Indefinitely	—[a]
	Clopidogrel	1 mo	—[a]

[a]The placement of drug-eluting stents requires prolonged dual antiplatelet therapy; thus, drug-eluting stents are not recommended in pregnant women at high risk for bleeding. However, drug-eluting stent technology is advancing, and in the future, new-generation drug-eluting stents may allow for shorter durations of dual antiplatelet therapy.
[b]Acute coronary syndrome includes unstable angina, non–ST-segment elevation myocardial infarction, and ST-segment elevation myocardial infarction.
From Virani SS, Newby LK, Arnold SV, et al. 2023 AHA/ACC/ACCP/ASPC/NLA/PCNA guideline for the management of patients with chronic coronary disease: a report of the American Heart Association/American College of Cardiology Joint Committee on Clinical Practice Guidelines. *J Am Coll Cardiol.* 2023;82:833–955.

TABLE 41.7   Risk Stratification for Valvular Heart Disease in Pregnancy

Valvular Lesion	Severity of Disease	mWHO Classification[a]
Aortic stenosis	Bicuspid aortic value with mild to moderate stenosis	II–III
	Aortic value area < 1.0 cm² or peak gradient > 50 mm Hg	IV
Aortic regurgitation	Mild to moderate	II
	Moderate to severe	III
Mitral stenosis	Mild to moderate	III
	Mitral value area < 1.5 cm²	IV
Mitral regurgitation	Mild to moderate	II
	Moderate to severe	III
Pulmonary stenosis	Mild	I
	Moderate	II
	Severe	III
Pulmonary regurgitation	Mild to moderate	I
	Severe	II–III
Tricuspid regurgitation	Mild	I
	Moderate	II
	Severe	III

[a]Modified World Health Organization risk classification (see Box 41.6).

severe symptomatic aortic and mitral stenosis (mWHO IV). Pulmonary stenosis and regurgitant lesions are generally well tolerated.

Aortic Stenosis

The most common cause of aortic stenosis in pregnant women is a congenital bicuspid aortic valve.[70] Less common causes/types of aortic stenosis include rheumatic, supravalvular, and subvalvular aortic stenosis.[153] Patients with a bicuspid aortic valve often have associated aortopathy, predisposing to ascending aortic dissection.[67] Aortic valve pressure gradients increase during pregnancy secondary to physiologic changes in cardiac output, although the aortic valve area typically remains unchanged.[70] Thus, serial echocardiography is recommended to monitor valve gradients and left ventricular function. Symptomatic aortic stenosis can be managed with HR control and diuretics during pregnancy. Structural intervention should be considered for patients with symptoms refractory to medical management, with type and timing of intervention based on gestational age (Table 41.8).[153–155]

Even in patients with severe aortic stenosis, vaginal delivery is generally preferred and neuraxial labor analgesia is appropriate; however, cesarean delivery may be considered in patients with severe and symptomatic aortic stenosis .[70] Neuraxial anesthesia for cesarean delivery is reasonable if the maternal hemodynamic parameters are managed appropriately. The primary hemodynamic goal is the maintenance of afterload to maintain coronary perfusion pressure (see Table 41.5). Peripartum invasive arterial blood pressure monitoring is generally recommended for parturients with moderate and severe aortic stenosis. Telemetry monitoring is recommended as arrhythmias are poorly tolerated. Sinus rhythm should be promptly restored if new-onset atrial fibrillation results in hypotension or pulmonary edema. Diastolic dysfunction may be present in the setting of left ventricular hypertrophy and will render these patients more sensitive to the adverse effects of decreased preload, tachycardia, and the development of congestive heart failure.

Aortic Regurgitation

The most common etiology of chronic aortic regurgitation in pregnant patients is bicuspid aortic valve. Rheumatic aortic regurgitation occurs less frequently. Aortic root dilation may also result in aortic regurgitation. Common causes include Marfan syndrome and the related heritable aortopathies, or bicuspid aortic valve aortopathy.

Chronic aortic regurgitation is generally well tolerated during pregnancy (mWHO II to III, depending on severity of regurgitation), especially in patients with preserved left ventricular ejection fraction (LVEF) (see Table 41.7).[156] The

TABLE 41.8 Gestational Age and Interventions for Aortic and Mitral Valve Stenosis During Pregnancy

Gestational Age (w)	INTERVENTION	
	Aortic Stenosis	**Mitral Stenosis**
<22–24	Surgical AVR	Balloon valvuloplasty if favorable anatomy
	Transcatheter AVR	Surgical MVR
	Balloon valvuloplasty if favorable anatomy	Percutaneous MVR if favorable anatomy
24–28	Individual patient discussion of options	Individual patient discussion of options
	(1) Intervention during pregnancy	(1) Intervention during pregnancy
	(2) Cesarean delivery followed by intervention	(2) Cesarean delivery followed by intervention
>28	Cesarean delivery followed by surgical AVR	Cesarean delivery followed by surgical MVR

AVR, Aortic valve replacement; *MVR*, mitral value replacement.

physiologic changes of pregnancy (increased HR resulting in a shorter duration of diastole, as well as reduced SVR) contribute to an overall reduction in regurgitant aortic flow. Acute aortic regurgitation is typically poorly tolerated and may require urgent surgery. Endocarditis and ascending aortic dissection are the most common causes of acute aortic regurgitation during pregnancy.

Vaginal delivery with neuraxial anesthesia is generally preferred in the absence of decompensated heart failure.[70] The goals of anesthetic management include (1) maintenance of a normal to slightly elevated HR, (2) prevention of an increase in SVR, (3) avoidance of aortocaval compression, and (4) avoidance of myocardial depression during general anesthesia.

Severe aortic insufficiency with left ventricular dysfunction is not a contraindication for neuraxial anesthesia. Initiation of neuraxial analgesia during early labor may mitigate pain-associated increases in SVR that can be deleterious in patients with aortic regurgitation.

Mitral Stenosis

The most common cause of mitral stenosis in pregnant patients is rheumatic heart disease.[70] Patients with mitral stenosis are at increased risk for atrial arrhythmia and thromboembolism. Mitral valve pressure gradients increase during pregnancy secondary to physiologic changes in cardiac output, although the mitral valve area typically remains unchanged.[157] Thus, serial echocardiography is recommended to monitor valve gradient and PAP.[70]

Symptomatic mitral stenosis can be managed with HR control, diuretics, and activity reduction during pregnancy. Structural intervention should be considered for patients with symptoms refractory to medical management, with type and timing of intervention based on gestational age (see Table 41.8).[70,158–160] Percutaneous balloon mitral valvuloplasty is generally the procedure of choice for patients with favorable anatomy. The second trimester is the most optimal time for valve intervention.[161]

Vaginal delivery with neuraxial labor analgesia is generally preferred in the absence of decompensated heart failure.[70] The goals of anesthetic management include (1) maintenance of a low-normal HR and preservation of sinus rhythm; (2)

aggressive treatment of atrial fibrillation, if present; (3) avoidance of aortocaval compression; (4) maintenance of venous return; (5) maintenance of adequate SVR; and (6) prevention of pain, hypoxemia, hypercarbia, and acidosis, which may increase PVR (see Table 41.5).

Neuraxial anesthesia for cesarean delivery is generally appropriate for patients with stable respiratory status. When general anesthesia is chosen because of high maternal risk (decompensated heart failure, critical valvular disease, pulmonary hypertension), tachycardia should be prevented by administration of a beta-adrenergic receptor antagonist and/or an opioid; positive end-expiratory pressure is often needed to treat pulmonary edema. Peripartum invasive arterial blood pressure monitoring is generally recommended for parturients with moderate and severe mitral stenosis for both labor and cesarean delivery. Telemetry monitoring is also recommended as arrhythmias are poorly tolerated. If new-onset atrial fibrillation results in hypotension or pulmonary edema, sinus rhythm should be promptly restored.

Mitral Regurgitation

Mitral regurgitation is generally well tolerated during pregnancy (mWHO class II to III depending on severity of regurgitation) (see Table 41.5). Its severity may transiently worsen in late pregnancy and the early postpartum period, increasing the risk of pulmonary edema.[162] Chronic mitral regurgitation may be associated with left ventricular dysfunction; thus, echocardiographic assessment of left ventricular function may help guide anesthetic and fluid management.

Vaginal delivery with neuraxial anesthesia is generally preferred in the absence of decompensated heart failure.[70] Both neuraxial and general anesthesia are well tolerated. The goals of anesthetic management in patients with mitral regurgitation include (1) prevention of an increase in SVR, (2) maintenance of a normal to slightly increased HR, (3) maintenance of sinus rhythm, (4) aggressive treatment of acute atrial fibrillation, (5) avoidance of aortocaval compression, (6) maintenance of venous return, (7) prevention of an increase in central venous volume, (8) avoidance of myocardial depression during general anesthesia, and (9) prevention of pain, hypoxemia, hypercarbia, and acidosis, which may increase PVR.

Pulmonary Stenosis and Regurgitation

Pregnancy is generally well tolerated in patients with **pulmonary stenosis**, even when severe (mWHO class I to III, depending on severity of stenosis) (see Table 41.7).[163] Vaginal delivery with neuraxial analgesia is generally preferred (see Table 41.5).[70] In the setting of moderate to severe pulmonary stenosis, the overloaded right ventricle will be preload dependent.

Pulmonary regurgitation is most commonly associated with congenital heart disease, such as repaired tetralogy of Fallot[88] or repaired pulmonary stenosis. Pregnancy and labor are well tolerated in the presence of mild or moderate pulmonary regurgitation (mWHO class I) (see Table 41.7). Severe pulmonary regurgitation (mWHO II to III) is associated with increased risk of right-sided heart failure and arrhythmias during pregnancy, particularly in the setting of preexisting right ventricular systolic dysfunction.[164,165] Vaginal delivery with neuraxial anesthesia is generally preferred.[70]

Tricuspid Regurgitation

Mild functional tricuspid regurgitation is often observed in normal pregnancy with no clinical consequence. Severe tricuspid regurgitation is often associated with congenital heart disease (Ebstein anomaly, TGA) or prior endocarditis. Pregnancy is generally well tolerated in the presence of tricuspid regurgitation (mWHO I to III, depending on regurgitation severity) (see Table 41.7). Patients may be susceptible to hypotension with a decrease in preload or transient right-sided heart failure symptoms due to right-sided volume overload.[166] Vaginal delivery with neuraxial anesthesia is generally preferred.[70]

Prosthetic Heart Valves in Pregnancy

Bioprosthetic valves. It is unclear whether pregnancy accelerates bioprosthetic valve structural degeneration; studies report inconsistent results. Current guidelines from the AHA/ACC suggest that a bioprosthetic valve is preferred over mechanical heart valves for patients desiring pregnancy (Class 2a recommendation, level of evidence B).[118]

Mechanical valves. For patients with mechanical heart valves, the risk of valve thrombosis during pregnancy is approximately 5%.[118] Risk factors include mechanical or tricuspid mechanical valves, atrial arrhythmias, left ventricular dysfunction, and a history of thromboembolism.

Anticoagulation with **warfarin** is associated with lower rates of thromboembolic complications and maternal death compared with unfractionated heparin or LMWH.[167] However, warfarin is potentially teratogenic and crosses the placental barrier, resulting in fetal anticoagulation. Maternal daily doses ≤ 5 mg daily carry limited risk of embryopathy.[118] The fetal risk is substantially reduced after the first trimester.

The ACC/AHA guidelines recommend meticulous anticoagulation dosing with frequent monitoring throughout pregnancy.[118] The anticoagulation strategy is primarily dependent upon a routine daily therapeutic warfarin dose (Fig. 41.5). Patients requiring daily warfarin doses ≤ 5 mg should

continue warfarin throughout all three trimesters (Class 2a recommendation). Patients requiring daily warfarin doses > 5 mg should take dose-adjusted **LMWH** (with target peak anti-Xa levels 0.8 to 1.2 U/mL) during the first trimester and resume warfarin for the second and third trimesters (Class 2a recommendation).

Warfarin should be discontinued at least 1 week before delivery.[118] Because warfarin crosses the placenta, cesarean delivery is required if warfarin is ingested within 1 week of delivery, even in the setting of a normal international normalized ratio (INR), owing to the risk for fetal intracranial hemorrhage with vaginal delivery. Dose-adjusted LMWH or continuous IV **unfractionated heparin** should be substituted during this time. LMWH should be switched to continuous unfractionated IV heparin at least 24 to 36 hours prior to delivery.[58,118] IV heparin should be discontinued 4 to 6 hours before the initiation of a neuraxial procedure. The activated partial thromboplastin time (aPTT) should be measured to verify normalization of coagulation function and a platelet count should be checked to rule out heparin-induced thrombocytopenia.

Neuraxial catheters can be removed 4 to 6 hours after the last dose of unfractionated heparin.[58] Unfractionated heparin can be restarted 1 hour after removal of a neuraxial catheter. Anticoagulation is typically resumed 4 to 6 hours after a vaginal delivery or 6 to 12 hours after a cesarean delivery.[168] Dose-adjusted LMWH can be restarted 24 hours after neuraxial block and at least 4 hours after neuraxial catheter removal. Warfarin can be resumed 24 hours after delivery.

Cardiomyopathies
Heart Failure Nomenclature

Accurate description of patients with heart failure is important for diagnostic, therapeutic, and prognostic purposes. Heart failure is categorized as **new onset (acute)**, **chronic**, or **acute-on-chronic heart failure**; **left-sided** (predominantly pulmonary congestion and pulmonary edema), **right-sided** (predominantly peripheral edema), or **biventricular** heart failure; and **systolic** and/or **diastolic** heart dysfunction (preferably labeled **heart failure with reduced ejection fraction [hFrEF]** and **heart failure with preserved ejection fraction [hFpEF]**, respectively).[169] Arbitrarily, left ventricular dysfunction is defined by a LVEF < 45% to 50%.

The New York Heart Association (NYHA) classification describes patients' *functional status* (Box 41.17); this can change over time. In contrast, the *staging classification* of heart failure recognizes that heart failure is a progressive condition and may manifest as variable symptoms over time.[169,170] Both classifications remain useful in clinical practice and apply to pregnant patients.

Medical Management of Heart Failure

Principles of heart failure management for pregnant patients are similar to those for nonpregnant patients with two notable exceptions: **ACE inhibitors/angiotensin receptor–blocking agents** and **aldosterone antagonists (spironolactone,**

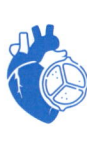 Pregnant patient with mechanical heart valve

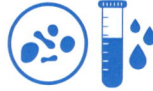 These patients should receive therapeutic anticoagulation with frequent monitoring during pregnancy.

Can therapeutic anticoagulation with frequent monitoring be maintained?

No — Counsel against pregnancy.

Yes

Patient counseled that there is no anticoagulation strategy that is perfectly safe for mother and fetus. Shared decision making is advised.

Warfarin dose > 5mg/day?

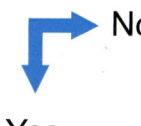

No ← → **Yes** → Dose adjusted LMWH with Factor Xa level monitoring available?

Yes ← → **No**

Dose-adjusted **LMWH** for the 1st trimester followed by **warfarin** for the 2nd and 3rd trimesters. OR **Warfarin** for all 3 trimesters.	Dose-adjusted **LMWH** for the 1st trimester followed by **warfarin** for the 2nd and 3rd trimesters. OR Dose-adjusted **LMWH** for all 3 trimesters.	Continuous dose-adjusted **UFH** for the 1st trimester. **Warfarin** for the 2nd and 3rd trimesters.

At least 1 week before delivery	Discontinue warfarin. Switch to continuous IV **UFH** or dose-adjusted **LMWH**.	If labor begins or urgent delivery is required in a woman therapeutically anticoagulated with a VKA, cesarean delivery should be performed after **reversal** of anticoagulation.
At least 36 hrs before delivery	Switch to continuous IV **UFH**.	
4-6 hrs before planned delivery	**Stop** IV UFH.	

Fig. 41.5 American College of Cardiology/American Heart Association Recommendations for Anticoagulation Management in Women With Mechanical Values During Pregnancy. *UFH*, unfractionated heparin; *LMWH*, low-molecular-weight heparin; *VKA*, vitamin K antagonist. From Otto CM, Nishimura RA, Bonow RO, et al. 2020 ACC/AHA guideline for the management of patients with valvular heart disease: a report of the American College of Cardiology/American Heart Association Joint Committee on Clinical Practice Guidelines. *J Am Coll Cardiol.* 2021;77:e25–e197.

eplerenone) should *not* be used in pregnant women. A beta-adrenergic receptor antagonist may be administered and **hydralazine** can be substituted for ACE inhibitors/angiotensin receptor–blocking agents. **Digoxin** use is safe in pregnancy. **Loop diuretics** and **sodium restriction** are indicated to prevent or treat volume overload. In patients with decompensated heart failure, treatment with IV **nitroglycerin** and **dopamine** or **dobutamine** is indicated.

Observational studies have reported two distinct peaks of exacerbation of heart failure during pregnancy. The first occurs between the second and third trimester and is more frequently seen in patients with pulmonary hypertension and mitral stenosis. The other peak occurs around the time of delivery with predominance of other cardiomyopathy etiologies.[171]

Peripartum Cardiomyopathy

Peripartum cardiomyopathy is a unique cardiomyopathy of unknown cause that occurs toward the end of pregnancy or in the postpartum period.[172,173] Its incidence is increasing in the United States.[174] The incidence of peripartum cardiomyopathy varies considerably by geography. For example, the incidence is as high as 1 in 300 live births in Haiti, 1 in 1000 to 4000 live births in the United States, and 1 in 20,000 births in Japan.[175-177] A possible genetic component has been identified, with overlap between genetic mutations linked to dilated cardiomyopathy and peripartum cardiomyopathy.[178]

Risk factors for peripartum cardiomyopathy include African race, multiparity, multiple gestation, preeclampsia, gestational hypertension, use of tocolytic agents, cocaine abuse, and age > 30 years.[178] The etiology remains unclear; proposed causes include underlying myocarditis, apoptosis, inflammation, pathologic maternal immune response to fetal antigens, effects of prolactin, viral triggers, and hereditary/familial factors.[179] In the United States, Black women have a greater incidence and more severe disease, and they are almost three times more likely to die of peripartum cardiomyopathy than White women.[176]

Peripartum cardiomyopathy is a diagnosis of exclusion and its symptoms may be difficult to differentiate from physiologic changes of pregnancy; thus, the use of echocardiography is needed to confirm the diagnosis (Fig. 41.6). The following three diagnostic criteria must be met: (1) development of heart failure toward the end of pregnancy (typically last month) or within 5 months following delivery, (2) absence of another identifiable cause of heart failure, and (3) left ventricular systolic dysfunction with a LVEF < 45%, with or without left ventricular dilation.

Cardiology management of peripartum cardiomyopathy rests on basic treatment paradigms for congestive heart failure and dilated cardiomyopathy (see discussion below). Obstetric management involves expedient delivery after stabilization of the mother; in most cases, cesarean delivery is reserved for obstetric indications. Neuraxial analgesia and anesthesia are appropriate for most patients, even with severe peripartum cardiomyopathy.[180-182] Neuraxial analgesia is recommended for labor and vaginal delivery. General anesthesia is reserved for patients who are unable to lie flat for a cesarean delivery as a result of pulmonary edema or who are markedly unstable. Preload increases in the immediate postpartum period because of autotransfusion (see Chapter 2). If a patient in heart failure has difficulty with lying flat at the initiation of anesthesia for cesarean delivery, she will likely need support with positive end-expiratory pressure immediately after delivery of the infant; therefore, administration of general anesthesia may be prudent. Invasive blood pressure monitoring is indicated for labor and vaginal delivery and cesarean delivery, as it provides beat-to-beat blood pressure assessments, allowing rapid and appropriate response to cardiac, obstetric, or anesthetic emergencies.

Other Nonischemic Cardiomyopathies

Hypertrophic cardiomyopathy. Hypertrophic cardiomyopathy is relatively common, with a prevalence estimated at 1 in 500. Complications of hypertrophic cardiomyopathy are mechanical or electrophysiologic. The mechanical consequences relate to left ventricular outflow tract obstruction,

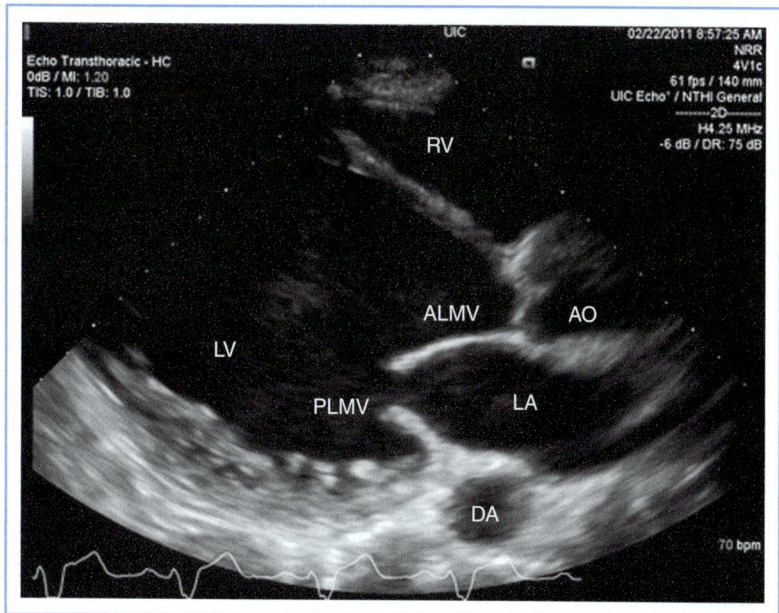

Fig. 41.6 Echocardiographic Image of Dilated Cardiomyopathy. *ALMV*, Anterior leaflet of the mitral valve; *AO*, aorta; *DA*, descending aorta; *LA*, left atrium; *LV*, left ventricle; *PLMV*, posterior leaflet of the mitral valve; *RV*, right ventricle. Illustration Dr. Mayank Kansal, University of Illinois at Chicago, Chicago, IL.

mitral regurgitation, diastolic dysfunction, and development of heart failure. The electrophysiologic complications include atrial and ventricular arrhythmias and, importantly, risk for sudden cardiac death.

Hypertrophic cardiomyopathy is associated with disorganized myocardial architecture, myocardial disarray, and fibrosis. Myocardial ischemia can occur because of supply-demand mismatch. Pregnant women with hypertrophic cardiomyopathy may have dyspnea, fatigue, angina, palpitations, and/or syncope.

Echocardiographic diagnostic criteria include septal thickness > 15 mm.[133] A wall thickness ≥ 30 mm is associated with a high risk for sudden cardiac death.[183] Patients with a gradient ≥ 50 mm Hg are at highest risk for complications.[133]

One of the hallmarks of hypertrophic cardiomyopathy is the dynamic left ventricular outflow tract obstruction. A gradient ≥ 30 mm Hg is clinically significant and is apparent during Doppler ultrasound interrogation; the continuous wave tracing has a classic "dagger-shaped" contour (Fig. 41.7).[184] The obstruction increases with drops in preload and afterload as well as increases in contractility. Fortuitously, the pregnancy-associated increase in blood volume allows most women with hypertrophic cardiomyopathy to tolerate pregnancy well.[135] However, acute hemodynamic collapse during the peripartum period may be caused by (1) atrial fibrillation, SVT, or sinus tachycardia, leading to the rapid onset of congestive heart failure; (2) decreased preload secondary to hemorrhage, sepsis, or neuraxial anesthetic initiation; or (3) decreased afterload secondary to the administration of a vasodilating drug (e.g., bolus dose of oxytocin or terbutaline) or induction of general anesthesia.

The anesthesia provider should be most concerned about patients with a gradient ≥ 50 mm Hg, those with symptoms of heart failure during pregnancy, and those with a history of arrhythmias (see Table 41.5). Beta-adrenergic receptor antagonists should be continued through labor and delivery because they decrease myocardial contractility and decrease the severity of left ventricular outflow tract obstruction. Slowly titrated neuraxial analgesia or anesthesia for labor or cesarean delivery is appropriate for most patients.[185–192]

Five-lead ECG monitoring during labor allows for early identification and treatment of arrhythmias during labor. In the setting of new-onset atrial fibrillation, the anesthesia provider should be prepared to respond with HR and rhythm control and direct current cardioversion if the patient is unstable (see discussion above). Invasive arterial blood pressure monitoring may facilitate rapid identification of hypotension, indicating a decrease in preload or afterload, which can increase the outflow tract obstruction. A second IV catheter allows for rapid fluid resuscitation in the setting of hemorrhage. TTE facilitates assessment of intravascular volume. **Phenylephrine** is the drug of choice for the treatment of hypotension. Inotropic agents such as **ephedrine, epinephrine**, or **terbutaline** should be avoided, if possible.[133] Rapid administration of IV **oxytocin** has been associated with a decrease in SVR, and slow administration via an infusion pump is recommended.

Stress-induced cardiomyopathy. Stress-induced cardiomyopathy, also known as *Takotsubo cardiomyopathy, broken heart syndrome*, and *apical ballooning syndrome*, is a transient cardiomyopathy with typical left ventricular systolic dysfunction of the apical and mid-cavity segments.[193] The basal ventricular segments are frequently hyperkinetic and may cause left ventricular outflow tract obstruction. Affected patients

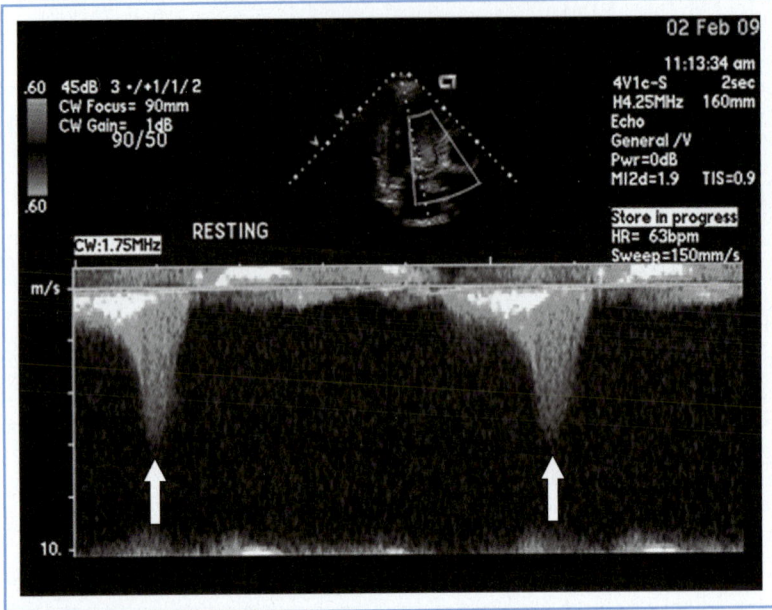

Fig. 41.7 Dynamic Left Ventricular Outflow Obstruction in Hypertrophic Cardiomyopathy. Continuous-wave Doppler tracing in left ventricular outflow tract displays typical late-peaking ("dagger-shaped") contour of dynamic outflow obstruction *(arrows).* Illustration Dr. Mayank Kansal, University of Illinois at Chicago, Chicago, IL.

typically do not have underlying coronary artery disease. Stress-induced cardiomyopathy occurs predominantly in postmenopausal women in the seventh and eight decades of life and is frequently associated with emotional and physical stressors. It has also been described during pregnancy in the setting of emotional and physical triggers, postpartum depression, and administration of pharmacologic triggers such as ergot alkaloids. It has also been reported in the absence of apparent triggers[194] and during otherwise uncomplicated spinal anesthesia for cesarean delivery.[195,196]

Clinically, patients have chest pain, dyspnea, and symptoms of left ventricular systolic dysfunction and heart failure. ECG abnormalities are frequently observed in the left precordial leads and may mimic STEMI. Coronary angiography is required to rule out STEMI; ventriculography and echocardiography allow recognition and characterization of wall motion abnormalities. The most critical differential diagnoses are STEMI and peripartum cardiomyopathy. When treating patients who develop shock, it is critically important to determine the degree of left ventricular outflow tract obstruction. Shock without left ventricular outflow tract obstruction can be treated in standard fashion with an inotropic agent. Patients with left ventricular outflow tract obstruction require optimization of intravascular volume and administration of a beta-adrenergic receptor antagonist; use of an intra-aortic balloon pump may be necessary to relieve the obstruction.

Dilated and other cardiomyopathies. In women with **idiopathic** or **anthracycline-induced cardiomyopathy**, pregnancy is associated with a high risk for adverse maternal, fetal, and neonatal outcomes. Pregnancy appears to unfavorably affect the short-term course of these cardiomyopathies. The NYHA functional status and ejection fraction may predict outcomes in this population.[197] Other causes of cardiomyopathy during pregnancy include **cocaine abuse** and **hemochromatosis**; the latter results in an infiltrative cardiomyopathy.

Rapid atrial or ventricular HR caused by arrhythmia can cause **tachycardia-induced cardiomyopathy**. This cardiomyopathy is a potentially reversible condition that has been described in pregnancy[198] and successfully treated with radiofrequency ablation.[199,200] Differentiation from other forms of cardiomyopathy may be difficult, but it is important from a prognostic standpoint.

Ventricular Assist Devices

Anecdotal reports have described ventricular assist device use during pregnancy. A successful completion of pregnancy with cesarean delivery in a patient with a ventricular assist device has been reported.[201] In another patient with myocardial infarction and subsequent severe left ventricular dysfunction, a ventricular assist device was placed, although pregnancy was not recognized at the time of placement; fetal death subsequently ensued.[202] The preconception presence of a ventricular assist device remains a contraindication to pregnancy.

Pericardial Disease

Asymptomatic trace to small pericardial effusions are frequently found in otherwise healthy pregnant patients.[203] Pericarditis remains a clinical diagnosis confirmed by ECG and echocardiography. Patients typically have pleuritic precordial pain that improves with sitting and leaning forward. A viral etiology is most common, with rates during pregnancy comparable to that of the general population. Treatment of pericarditis in pregnancy typically includes glucocorticoids, given potential fetal risks of nonsteroidal antiinflammatory drugs and colchicine. Immunosuppressant drugs may be indicated for pericarditis of autoimmune etiology.

Cardiac tamponade is a clinical diagnosis characterized by tachycardia, hypotension, and dyspnea. Physical examination reveals pulsus paradoxus > 10 mm Hg and elevated jugular venous pressure. Echocardiographic findings are consistent with a pericardial effusion with right ventricular diastolic collapse, distended inferior vena cava, and high variation in mitral and tricuspid valve inflow velocities. Echocardiographic-guided diagnostic and therapeutic pericardiocentesis or a surgical pericardial window can be safely performed during pregnancy.

Constrictive pericarditis is a condition in which a noncompliant pericardium prevents filling of the right- and left-sided heart chambers. Hemodynamic features include equalization and elevation of both left and right ventricular diastolic pressures, preserved systolic function, and a "dip and plateau" pattern of the ventricular pressure tracing. Patients present with symptoms of heart failure with preserved systolic function. Common causes include previous chest irradiation, recurrent pericarditis, and neoplasm.

Constrictive physiology and cardiac tamponade share some common pathophysiologic features that are important for the conduct of anesthesia (see Table 41.5). Impaired filling of the right side of the heart results from either a noncompliant pericardium (constrictive physiology) or pericardial fluid (tamponade physiology). Cardiac output is reduced by any intervention that reduces preload (e.g., aortocaval compression, sympathectomy with neuraxial anesthesia, positive-pressure ventilation with general anesthesia). Maintenance of preload is critically important; this goal can be achieved with central venous pressure monitoring, slowly titrated neuraxial anesthesia, and avoidance of positive-pressure ventilation. Invasive blood pressure monitoring is recommended in the setting of constrictive physiology from cardiac tamponade.

CARDIOPULMONARY RESUSCITATION DURING PREGNANCY

Cardiac arrest during pregnancy occurs in about 1 in every 12,000 admissions for delivery. Survival rates are greater than that of nonpregnant patients (Table 41.9).[204,205]

Standard Basic Life Support (BLS) and Advanced Cardiac Life Support (ACLS) principles apply to these patients with few modifications to the resuscitation protocol (Box 41.18; see also Box 53.5).[206,207] If the fundal height is at or above the umbilicus, early delivery should occur within 5 minutes after the time of the arrest.[207] This is referred to as a **perimortem cesarean delivery** or **resuscitative hysterotomy**. The primary purpose of cesarean delivery is to improve the chance of *maternal* survival, but timely delivery also improves the chances of infant survival. Perimortem cesarean delivery should be performed at the site of cardiac arrest.[208]

TABLE 41.9 Cause and Survival Rates of Maternal Cardiac Arrest

	Percentage of Maternal Cardiac Arrests (*n* = 4843) (%)	Percentage Survival (%)
Postpartum hemorrhage	27.9	55
Antepartum hemorrhage	16.8	53
Heart failure	15.6	71
Amniotic fluid embolism	13.3	53
Sepsis	11.2	47
Anesthesia complications	7.8	82
Aspiration pneumonitis	7.1	83
Venous thromboembolism	7.1	42
Eclampsia	6.1	77
Cerebrovascular disorder	4.4	40
Trauma	3.9	23
Acute myocardial infarction	3.1	56
Pulmonary edema	2.4	71
Magnesium toxicity	1.4	86
Asthma	1.1	54
Anaphylaxis	0.3	100
Aortic dissection/rupture	0.3	0

Data from the US Nationwide Inpatient Sample, 1998–2011. From Mhyre JM, Tsen LC, Einav S, et al. Cardiac arrest during hospitalization for delivery in the United States, 1998-2011. *Anesthesiology.* 2014;120:810–818.

Defibrillation should be performed based on current ACLS protocols.[206] Resuscitation should be continued until all resources or possibilities for survival have been exhausted. There are multiple reports of neurologically intact survival after cardiac arrest in pregnant women who have been resuscitated using extracorporeal life support (ECLS) or extracorporeal membrane oxygenation (ECMO) and survived. A systematic review of cases of ECLS rescue of pregnant patients after cardiac arrest reported a survival rate of 87.7%.[209] If available, the ECLS support team should be alerted as early as possible after the cardiac arrest. Intra-aortic balloon pumps, percutaneous left ventricular assist devices, and cardiopulmonary bypass have also been successfully used in pregnant women with cardiac arrest, and favorable outcomes have been reported. Therapeutic hypothermia has also been used after cardiac arrest during pregnancy, with successful delivery and favorable neonatal outcome.

BOX 41.18 Cardiopulmonary Resuscitation in Pregnancy

Basic Life Support

- Intravenous access established above the diaphragm
- Patient placed supine for chest compressions
  - If the uterus is palpated at or above the umbilicus, then continuous manual left uterine displacement
- Chest compressions: same standard as nonpregnant adults
  - Use of a firm backboard
  - Hand position: center of chest, lower half of sternum
  - Technique:
  - Rate: 100 compressions/min
  - Depth: at least 2 in (5 cm)
  - Compression-ventilation ratio: 30:2.
  - Minimize interruptions: limit to less than 10 s except for specific interventions such as insertion of an advanced airway or defibrillation
- Defibrillation and cardioversion: same standard as nonpregnant adults
  - Biphasic shock energy of 120–200 J with escalation of energy if the first shock is not effective
  - No need to remove FHR monitoring electrode
- Resuscitation and cesarean delivery performed at the location of the cardiac arrest
  - Do not transport to operating room for cesarean delivery

Advanced Cardiac Life Support

- Airway management mimics standards for nonpregnant adults
  - Experienced laryngoscopist
  - No more than two attempts, then use rescue supraglottic airway device
  - Continuous waveform capnography
  - Effective chest compressions should result in an end-tidal carbon dioxide > 10 mm Hg
- Medical therapy for cardiac arrest: same standard as nonpregnant adults
- Fetal assessment should not be performed during resuscitation
  - Fetal monitors should be removed or detached to facilitate cesarean delivery
- Perimortem cesarean delivery (resuscitative hysterotomy)
  - Perform if the fundal height is at or above the umbilicus
  - Perform at site of arrest (do not transfer to operating room)
  - Delivery should occur within 5 min of the cardiac arrest (requires only a scalpel)
- Continue resuscitation until all resources or possibilities for survival have been exhausted
  - Consider cardiopulmonary bypass or ECLS
  - Alert ECLS team as early as possible after the cardiac arrest

ECLS, Extracorporeal life support.

From Jeejeebhoy FM, Zelop CM, Lipman S, et al. Cardiac arrest in pregnancy: a scientific statement from the American Heart Association. *Circulation*. 2015;132:1747–1773; Merchant RM, Topjian AA, Panchal AR. Part 1: Executive summary: 2020 American Heart Association guidelines for cardiopulmonary resuscitation and emergency cardiovascular care. *Circulation*. 2020;142(16 suppl 2):S337–S357.

PREGNANCY AFTER HEART TRANSPLANTATION

The first successful pregnancy in a heart transplant recipient was described in 1988. Subsequently, several reports have documented the feasibility and relative safety of pregnancy and delivery in female heart transplant recipients.[210,211] Successful patient management requires an interdisciplinary team approach.[212] Baseline echocardiography allows assessment of ejection fraction and the presence of transplant valvulopathy. Peripartum immunosuppression therapy should be managed by a multidisciplinary team.

The transplanted heart is denervated; therefore, the increase in cardiac output observed with pregnancy results from an increase in stroke volume rather than HR. Changes in HR cannot be achieved with antimuscarinic agents (e.g., atropine or glycopyrrolate) or vagal maneuvers. Isoproterenol or epinephrine can be used to treat bradycardia.

Monitoring with a 5-lead ECG for ischemia should be maintained throughout the peripartum period. Cardiac transplant vasculopathy constitutes the second most common cause of death 1 year after heart transplantation. The patient may not present with classic anginal symptoms owing to denervation of the transplanted heart.

The risk for infection is greater in patients receiving immunosuppression therapy. The AHA considers valvulopathy in heart transplant recipients a high risk for the development of bacterial endocarditis. Thus, given the unfavorable outcomes in heart transplant recipients who develop endocarditis, it appears reasonable to recommend antibiotic endocarditis prophylaxis at the time of membrane rupture for these parturients undergoing labor and vaginal delivery.[213]

Generally, most parturients with a heart transplant with a normal ejection fraction and normal right-sided pressures tolerate labor and delivery well. Standard neuraxial analgesia and anesthesia are acceptable.

CARDIOPULMONARY BYPASS DURING PREGNANCY

In the modern era, maternal mortality associated with elective cardiopulmonary bypass during pregnancy is comparable to that in nonpregnant women.[214] Fetal mortality remains high (14% in a single-center retrospective study of cases from 1976 to 2009[214]), although some series report excellent fetal outcomes.[215] The optimal timing of cardiopulmonary bypass appears to be the second trimester of pregnancy. Procedures performed immediately after delivery and on an emergency basis appear to confer added risk for maternal mortality. The degree of hypothermia is associated with poor fetal outcome. There is no evidence that anesthesia *per se* contributes to adverse maternal or fetal outcomes in this setting.[214] The need for intraoperative FHR monitoring is universally accepted. Measures to lower fetal mortality include normothermic cardiopulmonary bypass with flow rates > 2.4 L/min/m² while maintaining mean arterial blood pressure > 70 to 75 mm Hg. Left uterine displacement and maintenance of a hematocrit > 28% are recommended.

KEY POINTS

- Cardiac disease is the leading cause of maternal mortality in the developed world.
- For most women with heart disease, pregnancy is associated with favorable outcomes.
- Cardiac output increases during pregnancy, increases even further during labor, and is highest immediately after delivery.
- The anesthetic management of the parturient with cardiovascular disease should be individualized. It is important that all patients with significant cardiovascular disease are cared for by a multidisciplinary pregnancy heart team.
- At a minimum, members of a pregnancy heart team should include a cardiologist, an obstetric provider, a maternal-fetal medicine specialist, and an anesthesia provider.
- Women with known cardiovascular disease should be risk stratified according to a cardiac risk prediction tool and subsequently triaged to a hospital with the appropriate level of maternal care.
- Recognition and correct diagnosis of cardiovascular disease on obstetric units is a critical step in reducing maternal cardiovascular morbidity and mortality.
- The anesthesia provider must be familiar with the pregnancy implications of cardiac medications and obstetric medications with cardiovascular effects.
- For most women with cardiovascular disease, a trial of labor with neuraxial labor analgesia is appropriate.
- Hemodynamic monitoring during labor for women with severe cardiovascular disease often includes continuous pulse oximetry monitoring with a visible waveform, 5-lead ECG monitoring, and intra-arterial blood pressure monitoring.
- For most women with cardiovascular disease undergoing cesarean delivery, neuraxial anesthesia is appropriate.
- The treatment of most arrhythmias during pregnancy mimics that for nonpregnant women.
- The indication and standards for percutaneous coronary intervention in pregnant patients with acute coronary syndrome are the same as those for nonpregnant patients.
- Standard advanced cardiac life support protocols should be used for cardiac arrest during pregnancy. The patient should be placed supine with manual left uterine displacement. Choice of drugs (and doses) as well as indications for defibrillation are the same as those for nonpregnant adult women. If the fundal height is above the umbilicus, hysterotomy and uterine evacuation should occur within 5 minutes of arrest.

REFERENCES

1. Briller J, Koch AR, Geller SE. Illinois Department of Public Health Maternal Mortality Review Committee Working Group. Maternal cardiovascular mortality in Illinois, 2002–2011. *Obstet Gynecol*. 2017;129:819–826.
2. Roos-Hesselink J, Baris L, Johnson M, et al. Pregnancy outcomes in women with cardiovascular disease: evolving trends over 10 years in the ESC Registry of Pregnancy and Cardiac disease (ROPAC). *Eur Heart J*. 2019;40:3848–3855.
3. Roos-Hesselink JW, Ruys TP, Stein JI, et al. Outcome of pregnancy in patients with structural or ischaemic heart disease: results of a registry of the European Society of Cardiology. *Eur Heart J*. 2013;34:657–665.
4. American College of Obstetricians and Gynecologists. Practice Bulletin No. 212: Pregnancy and heart disease (reaffirmed 2021). *Obstet Gynecol*. 2019;133:e320–e356.
5. Meng ML, Arendt KW, Banayan JM, et al. Anesthetic care of the pregnant patient with cardiovascular disease: a scientific statement from the American Heart Association. *Circulation*. 2023;147:e657–e673.
6. Desai DK, Moodley J, Naidoo DP. Echocardiographic assessment of cardiovascular hemodynamics in normal pregnancy. *Obstet Gynecol*. 2004;104:20–29.
7. Kametas NA, McAuliffe F, Krampl E, et al. Maternal cardiac function in twin pregnancy. *Obstet Gynecol*. 2003;102:806–815.
8. Borghi C, Esposti DD, Immordino V, et al. Relationship of systemic hemodynamics, left ventricular structure and function, and plasma natriuretic peptide concentrations during pregnancy complicated by preeclampsia. *Am J Obstet Gynecol*. 2000;183:140–147.
9. Oram S, Holt M. Innocent depression of the S-T segment and flattening of the T-wave during pregnancy. *J Obstet Gynaecol Br Emp*. 1961;68:765–770.
10. Burton A, Camann W. Electrocardiographic changes during cesarean section: a review. *Int J Obstet Anesth*. 1996;5:47–53.
11. Jonsson M, Hanson U, Lidell C, Nordén-Lindeberg S. ST depression at caesarean section and the relation to oxytocin dose. a randomised controlled trial. *BJOG*. 2010;117:76–83.
12. Svanström MC, Biber B, Hanes M, et al. Signs of myocardial ischaemia after injection of oxytocin: a randomized double-blind comparison of oxytocin and methylergometrine during caesarean section. *Br J Anaesth*. 2008;100:683–689.
13. Hameed AB, Chan K, Ghamsary M, Elkayam U. Longitudinal changes in the B-type natriuretic peptide levels in normal pregnancy and postpartum. *Clin Cardiol*. 2009;32:E60–E62.
14. Dockree S, Brook J, Shine B, et al. Pregnancy-specific reference intervals for BNP and NT-pro BNP-changes in natriuretic peptides related to pregnancy. *J Endocr Soc*. 2021;5:bvab091.
15. Tanous D, Siu SC, Mason J, et al. B-type natriuretic peptide in pregnant women with heart disease. *J Am Coll Cardiol*. 2010;56:1247–1253.
16. Malhamé I, Hurlburt H, Larson L, et al. Sensitivity and specificity of B-type natriuretic peptide in diagnosing heart failure in pregnancy. *Obstet Gynecol*. 2019;134:440–449.
17. Resnik JL, Hong C, Resnik R, et al. Evaluation of B-type natriuretic peptide (BNP) levels in normal and preeclamptic women. *Am J Obstet Gynecol*. 2005;193:450–454.
18. Eindhoven JA, van den Bosch AE, Jansen PR, et al. The usefulness of brain natriuretic peptide in complex congenital

heart disease: a systematic review. *J Am Coll Cardiol.* 2012;60:2140–2149.

19. Fleming SM, O'Gorman T, Finn J, et al. Cardiac troponin I in pre-eclampsia and gestational hypertension. *BJOG.* 2000;107:1417–1420.

20. Shivvers SA, Wians FH Jr, Keffer JH, Ramin SM. Maternal cardiac troponin I levels during normal labor and delivery. *Am J Obstet Gynecol.* 1999;180:122.

21. Abramov Y, Abramov D, Abrahamov A, et al. Elevation of serum creatine phosphokinase and its MB isoenzyme during normal labor and early puerperium. *Acta Obstet Gynecol Scand.* 1996;75:255–260.

22. Nabatian S, Quinn P, Brookfield L, Lakier J. Acute coronary syndrome and preeclampsia. *Obstet Gynecol.* 2005;106:1204–1206.

23. Main EK, McCain CL, Morton CH, et al. Pregnancy-related mortality in California: causes, characteristics, and improvement opportunities. *Obstet Gynecol.* 2015;125:938–947.

24. Goldberg LM, Uhland H. Heart murmurs in pregnancy: a phonocardiographic study of their development, progression and regression. *Dis Chest.* 1967;52:381–386.

25. Marcus FI, Ewy GA, O'Rourke RA, et al. The effect of pregnancy on the murmurs of mitral and aortic regurgitation. *Circulation.* 1970;41:795–805.

26. Drenthen W, Boersma E, Balci A, et al. Predictors of pregnancy complications in women with congenital heart disease. *Eur Heart J.* 2010;31:2124–2132.

27. Silversides CK, Grewal J, Mason J, et al. Pregnancy outcomes in women with heart disease: the CARPREG II study. *J Am Coll Cardiol.* 2018;71:2419–2430.

28. Thorne S, MacGregor A, Nelson-Piercy C. Risks of contraception and pregnancy in heart disease. *Heart.* 2006;92:1520–1525.

29. Regitz-Zagrosek V, Roos-Hesselink JW, Bauersachs J, et al. 2018 ESC guidelines on the management of cardiovascular diseases during pregnancy. *Eur Heart J.* 2018;39:3165–3241.

30. Siu SC, Sermer M, Colman JM, et al. Prospective multicenter study of pregnancy outcomes in women with heart disease. *Circulation.* 2001;104:515–521.

31. Drenthen W, Pieper PG, Roos-Hesselink JW, et al. Outcome of pregnancy in women with congenital heart disease: a literature review. *J Am Coll Cardiol.* 2007;49:2303–2311.

32. American College of Obstetricians and Gynecologists. Obstetric Care Consensus No. 9: Levels of maternal care (reaffirmed 2021). *Obstet Gynecol.* 2019;134:e41–e55.

33. Bello NA, Bairey Merz CN, Brown H, et al. Diagnostic cardiovascular imaging and therapeutic strategies in pregnancy: JACC Focus Seminar 4/5. *J Am Coll Cardiol.* 2021;77:1813–1822.

34. Savu O, Jurcuţ R, Giuşcă S, et al. Morphological and functional adaptation of the maternal heart during pregnancy. *Circ Cardiovasc Imaging.* 2012;5:289–297.

35. Kametas NA, McAuliffe F, Hancock J, et al. Maternal left ventricular mass and diastolic function during pregnancy. *Ultrasound Obstet Gynecol.* 2001;18:460–466.

36. Melchiorre K, Sutherland GR, Baltabaeva A, et al. Maternal cardiac dysfunction and remodeling in women with preeclampsia at term. *Hypertension.* 2011;57:85–93.

37. American College of Obstetricians and Gynecologists. Committee Opinion No. 723: Guidelines for diagnostic imaging during pregnancy and lactation (reaffirmed 2021). *Obstet Gynecol.* 2017;130:e210–e216.

38. Briggs GG, Freeman RK, Towers CV, Forinash AB. *Drugs in Pregnancy and Lactation. A Reference Guide to Fetal and Neonatal risk.* 12th ed. Wolters Kluwer; 2021:1648.

39. Tolcher MC, Fox KA, Sangi-Haghpeykar H, et al. Intravenous labetalol versus oral nifedipine for acute hypertension in pregnancy: effects on cerebral perfusion pressure. *Am J Obstet Gynecol.* 2020;223:441.e1–e8.

40. Nij Bijvank SW, Hengst M, Cornette JC, et al. Nicardipine for treating severe antepartum hypertension during pregnancy: nine years of experience in more than 800 women. *Acta Obstet Gynecol Scand.* 2022;101:1017–1025.

41. Aronson S, Dyke CM, Stierer KA, et al. The ECLIPSE trials: comparative studies of clevidipine to nitroglycerin, sodium nitroprusside, and nicardipine for acute hypertension treatment in cardiac surgery patients. *Anesth Analg.* 2008;107:1110–1121.

42. Clevidipine [FDA package insert, Reference ID: 4780628]. Chiesi USA, Inc.; 2021. https://www.accessdata.fda.gov/drugsatfda_docs/label/2021/022156s007lbl.pdf. Accessed August 25, 2024.

43. Godfraind T. Discovery and development of calcium channel blockers. *Front Pharmacol.* 2017;8:286.

44. Poli E, Merialdi A, Coruzzi G. Characterization of the spontaneous motor activity of the isolated human pregnant myometrium. *Pharmacol Res.* 1990;22:115–124.

45. Strasburger JF, Cuneo BF, Michon MM, et al. Amiodarone therapy for drug-refractory fetal tachycardia. *Circulation.* 2004;109:375–379.

46. Ekerhovd E, Weidegård B, Brännström M, Norström A. Nitric oxide-mediated effects on myometrial contractility at term during prelabor and labor. *Obstet Gynecol.* 1999;93:987–994.

47. Kopp SL, Vandermeulen E, McBane RD, Perlas A, Leffert L, Horlocker T. Regional anesthesia in the patient receiving antithrombotic or thrombolytic therapy: American Society of Regional Anesthesia and Pain Medicine evidence-based guidelines (fifth edition). *Reg Anesth Pain Med.* 2025; Epub ahead of print Jan 29. https://doi.org/10.1136/rapm-2024-105766.

48. Gogarten W, Vandermeulen E, Van Aken H, et al. Regional anaesthesia and antithrombotic agents: recommendations of the European Society of Anaesthesiology. *Eur J Anaesthesiol.* 2010;27:999–1015.

49. Rosseland LA, Hauge TH, Grindheim G, et al. Changes in blood pressure and cardiac output during cesarean delivery: the effects of oxytocin and carbetocin compared with placebo. *Anesthesiology.* 2013;119:541–551.

50. Meng ML, Arendt KW. Obstetric anesthesia and heart disease: practical clinical considerations. *Anesthesiology.* 2021;135:164–183.

51. Hayashi Y, Ibe T, Kawato H, et al. Postpartum acute myocardial infarction induced by ergonovine administration. *Intern Med.* 2003;42:983–986.

52. Lin YH, Seow KM, Hwang JL, Chen HH. Myocardial infarction and mortality caused by methylergonovine. *Acta Obstet Gynecol Scand.* 2005;84:1022.

53. Partridge BL, Key T, Reisner LS. Life-threatening effects of intravascular absorption of PGF2 alpha during therapeutic termination of pregnancy. *Anesth Analg.* 1988;67:1111–1113.

54. Hankins GD, Berryman GK, Scott RT Jr, Hood D. Maternal arterial desaturation with 15-methyl prostaglandin F_2 alpha for uterine atony. *Obstet Gynecol.* 1988;72:367–370.

55. Cates W Jr, Jordaan HV. Sudden collapse and death of women obtaining abortions induced with prostaglandin F2alpha. *Am J Obstet Gynecol*. 1979;133:398–400.

56. Cates W Jr, Grimes DA, Haber RJ, Tyler W Jr. Abortion deaths associated with the use of prostaglandin F$_{2\alpha}$. *Am J Obstet Gynecol*. 1977;127:219–222.

57. Matthesen T, Olsen RH, Bosselmann HS, Lidegaard Ø. [Cardiac arrest induced by vasospastic angina pectoris after vaginally administered misoprostol]. *Ugeskr Laeger*. 2017;179.

58. Leffert L, Butwick A, Carvalho B, et al. The Society for Obstetric Anesthesia and Perinatology consensus statement on the anesthetic management of pregnant and postpartum women receiving thromboprophylaxis or higher dose anticoagulants. *Anesth Analg*. 2018;126:928–944.

59. Liu P, He H, Zhang SS, et al. Comparative efficacy and safety of prophylactic norepinephrine and phenylephrine in spinal anesthesia for cesarean section: a systematic review and meta-analysis with trial sequential analysis. *Front Pharmacol*. 2022;13:1015325.

60. Arendt KW, Muehlschlegel JD, Tsen LC. Cardiovascular alterations in the parturient undergoing cesarean delivery with neuraxial anesthesia. *Expert Rev Obstet Gynecol*. 2012;7:59–75.

61. Hamlyn EL, Douglass CA, Plaat F, et al. Low-dose sequential combined spinal-epidural: an anaesthetic technique for caesarean section in patients with significant cardiac disease. *Int J Obstet Anesth*. 2005;14:355–361.

62. Sawlani N, Shroff A, Vidovich MI. Aortic dissection and mortality associated with pregnancy in the United States. *J Am Coll Cardiol*. 2015;65:1600–1601.

63. Anderson RA, Fineron PW. Aortic dissection in pregnancy: importance of pregnancy-induced changes in the vessel wall and bicuspid aortic valve in pathogenesis. *Br J Obstet Gynaecol*. 1994;101:1085–1088.

64. Hiratzka LF, Bakris GL, Beckman JA, et al. 2010 ACCF/AHA/AATS/ACR/ASA/SCA/SCAI/SIR/STS/SVM guidelines for the diagnosis and management of patients with thoracic aortic disease: a report of the American College of Cardiology Foundation/American Heart Association Task Force on Practice Guidelines, American Association for Thoracic Surgery, American College of Radiology, American Stroke Association, Society of Cardiovascular Anesthesiologists, Society for Cardiovascular Angiography and Interventions, Society of Interventional Radiology, Society of Thoracic Surgeons, and Society for Vascular Medicine. *Circulation*. 2010;121:e266–e369.

65. Wanga S, Silversides C, Dore A, et al. Pregnancy and thoracic aortic disease: managing the risks. *Can J Cardiol*. 2016;32:78–85.

66. Weissmann-Brenner A, Schoen R, Divon MY. Aortic dissection in pregnancy. *Obstet Gynecol*. 2004;103:1110–1113.

67. Immer FF, Bansi AG, Immer-Bansi AS, et al. Aortic dissection in pregnancy: analysis of risk factors and outcome. *Ann Thorac Surg*. 2003;76:309–314.

68. Kim SY, Wolfe DS, Taub CC. Cardiovascular outcomes of pregnancy in Marfan's syndrome patients: a literature review. *Congenit Heart Dis*. 2018;13:203–209.

69. Isselbacher EM, Preventza O, Hamilton Black J 3rd, et al. 2022 ACC/AHA Guideline for the diagnosis and management of aortic disease: a report of the American Heart Association/American College of Cardiology Joint Committee on Clinical Practice Guidelines. *J Am Coll Cardiol*. 2022;80:e223–e393.

70. Lindley KJ, Bairey Merz CN, Asgar AW, et al. Management of women with congenital or inherited cardiovascular disease from pre-conception through pregnancy and postpartum: JACC focus seminar 2/5. *J Am Coll Cardiol*. 2021;77:1778–1798.

71. Buser RT, Mordecai MM, Brull SJ. Combined spinal-epidural analgesia for labor in a patient with Marfan's syndrome. *Int J Obstet Anesth*. 2007;16:274–276.

72. Gordon CF 3rd, Johnson MD. Anesthetic management of the pregnant patient with Marfan syndrome. *J Clin Anesth*. 1993;5:248–251.

73. Singh SI, Brooks C, Dobkowski W. General anesthesia using remifentanil for Cesarean delivery in a parturient with Marfan's syndrome. *Can J Anaesth*. 2008;55:526–531.

74. Lacassie HJ, Millar S, Leithe LG, et al. Dural ectasia: a likely cause of inadequate spinal anaesthesia in two parturients with Marfan's syndrome. *Br J Anaesth*. 2005;94:500–504.

75. Warnes CA, Williams RG, Bashore TM, et al. ACC/AHA 2008 Guidelines for the management of adults with congenital heart disease: a report of the American College of Cardiology/American Heart Association Task Force on Practice Guidelines. *Circulation*. 2008;118:e714–e833.

76. Baumgartner H, Bonhoeffer P, De Groot NM, et al. ESC guidelines for the management of grown-up congenital heart disease. *Eur Heart J*. 2010;31:2915–2957.

77. Stout KK, Daniels CJ, Aboulhosn JA, et al. 2018 AHA/ACC guideline for the management of adults with congenital heart disease: a report of the American College of Cardiology/American Heart Association Task Force on Clinical Practice Guidelines. *J Am Coll Cardiol*. 2018;73:e81–e192.

78. Vriend JW, Drenthen W, Pieper PG, et al. Outcome of pregnancy in patients after repair of aortic coarctation. *Eur Heart J*. 2005;26:2173–2178.

79. Stout KK, Otto CM. Pregnancy in women with valvular heart disease. *Heart*. 2007;93:552–558.

80. Beauchesne LM, Connolly HM, Ammash NM, Warnes CA. Coarctation of the aorta: outcome of pregnancy. *J Am Coll Cardiol*. 2001;38:1728–1733.

81. Wolfe NK, Sabol BA, Kelly JC, et al. Management of Fontan circulation in pregnancy: a multidisciplinary approach to care. *Am J Obstet Gynecol MFM*. 2021;3:100257.

82. Carp H, Jayaram A, Vadhera R, et al. Epidural anesthesia for cesarean delivery and vaginal birth after maternal Fontan repair: report of two cases. *Anesth Analg*. 1994;78:1190–1192.

83. Ioscovich A, Briskin A, Fadeev A, et al. Emergency cesarean section in a patient with Fontan circulation using an indwelling epidural catheter. *J Clin Anesth*. 2006;18:631–634.

84. Warnes CA. Transposition of the great arteries. *Circulation*. 2006;114:2699–2709.

85. Donnelly JE, Brown JM, Radford DJ. Pregnancy outcome and Ebstein's anomaly. *Br Heart J*. 1991;66:368–371.

86. Actis Dato GM, Rinaudo P, Revelli A, et al. Atrial septal defect and pregnancy: a retrospective analysis of obstetrical outcome before and after surgical correction. *Minerva Cardioangiol*. 1998;46:63–68.

87. Meijer JM, Pieper PG, Drenthen W, et al. Pregnancy, fertility, and recurrence risk in corrected tetralogy of Fallot. *Heart*. 2005;91:801–805.

88. Veldtman GR, Connolly HM, Grogan M, et al. Outcomes of pregnancy in women with tetralogy of Fallot. *J Am Coll Cardiol*. 2004;44:174–180.

89. Maron BA. Revised definition of pulmonary hypertension and approach to management: a clinical primer. *J Am Heart Assoc.* 2023;12:e029024.

90. Humbert M, Kovacs G, Hoeper MM, et al. 2022 ESC/ERS guidelines for the diagnosis and treatment of pulmonary hypertension. *Eur Heart J.* 2022;43:3618–3731.

91. Weiss BM, Zemp L, Seifert B, Hess OM. Outcome of pulmonary vascular disease in pregnancy: a systematic overview from 1978 through 1996. *J Am Coll Cardiol.* 1998;31:1650–1657.

92. Bedard E, Dimopoulos K, Gatzoulis MA. Has there been any progress made on pregnancy outcomes among women with pulmonary arterial hypertension? *Eur Heart J.* 2009;30:256–265.

93. Low TT, Guron N, Ducas R, et al. Pulmonary arterial hypertension in pregnancy—a systematic review of outcomes in the modern era. *Pulm Circ.* 2021;11:20458940211013671.

94. Sliwa K, van Hagen IM, Budts W, et al. Pulmonary hypertension and pregnancy outcomes: data from the Registry of Pregnancy and Cardiac Disease (ROPAC) of the European Society of Cardiology. *Eur J Heart Fail.* 2016;18:1119–1128.

95. McLaughlin VV, Archer SL, Badesch DB, et al. ACCF/AHA 2009 expert consensus document on pulmonary hypertension. A report of the American College of Cardiology Foundation Task Force on Expert Consensus Documents and the American Heart Association. *J Am Coll Cardiol.* 2009;53:1573–1619.

96. Galiè N, Hoeper MM, Humbert M, et al. Guidelines for the diagnosis and treatment of pulmonary hypertension: the Task Force for the Diagnosis and Treatment of Pulmonary Hypertension of the European Society of Cardiology (ESC) and the European Respiratory Society (ERS). Endorsed by the International Society of Heart and Lung Transplantation (ISHLT). *Eur Heart J.* 2009;30:2493–2537.

97. Katsuragi S, Kamiya C, Yamanaka K, et al. Maternal and fetal outcomes in pregnancy complicated with Eisenmenger syndrome. *Taiwan J Obstet Gynecol.* 2019;58:183–187.

98. Goland S, Tsai F, Habib M, et al. Favorable outcome of pregnancy with an elective use of epoprostenol and sildenafil in women with severe pulmonary hypertension. *Cardiology.* 2010;115:205–208.

99. Ng WP, Yip WL. Successful maternal-foetal outcome using nitric oxide and sildenafil in pulmonary hypertension with atrial septal defect and HIV infection. *Singapore Med J.* 2012;53:e3–e5.

100. Bendayan D, Hod M, Oron G, et al. Pregnancy outcome in patients with pulmonary arterial hypertension receiving prostacyclin therapy. *Obstet Gynecol.* 2005;106:1206–1210.

101. Avila WS, Grinberg M, Snitcowsky R, et al. Maternal and fetal outcome in pregnant women with Eisenmenger's syndrome. *Eur Heart J.* 1995;16:460–464.

102. Geohas C, McLaughlin VV. Successful management of pregnancy in a patient with Eisenmenger syndrome with epoprostenol. *Chest.* 2003;124:1170–1173.

103. O'Hare R, McLoughlin C, Milligan K, et al. Anaesthesia for caesarean section in the presence of severe primary pulmonary hypertension. *Br J Anaesth.* 1998;81:790–792.

104. Robinson JN, Banerjee R, Landzberg MJ, Thiet MP. Inhaled nitric oxide therapy in pregnancy complicated by pulmonary hypertension. *Am J Obstet Gynecol.* 1999;180:1045–1046.

105. Lam GK, Stafford RE, Thorp J, et al. Inhaled nitric oxide for primary pulmonary hypertension in pregnancy. *Obstet Gynecol.* 2001;98:895–898.

106. Goodwin TM, Gherman RB, Hameed A, Elkayam U. Favorable response of Eisenmenger syndrome to inhaled nitric oxide during pregnancy. *Am J Obstet Gynecol.* 1999;180:64–67.

107. Hemnes AR, Kiely DG, Cockrill BA, et al. Statement on pregnancy in pulmonary hypertension from the Pulmonary Vascular Research Institute. *Pulm Circ.* 2015;5:435–465.

108. Monnery L, Nanson J, Charlton G. Primary pulmonary hypertension in pregnancy; a role for novel vasodilators. *Br J Anaesth.* 2001;87:295–298.

109. Olofsson C, Bremme K, Forssell G, Ohqvist G. Cesarean section under epidural ropivacaine 0.75% in a parturient with severe pulmonary hypertension. *Acta Anaesthesiol Scand.* 2001;45:258–260.

110. Martin JT, Tautz TJ, Antognini JF. Safety of regional anesthesia in Eisenmenger's syndrome. *Reg Anesth Pain Med.* 2002;27:509–513.

111. Blaise G, Langleben D, Hubert B. Pulmonary arterial hypertension: pathophysiology and anesthetic approach. *Anesthesiology.* 2003;99:1415–1432.

112. Kiely DG, Condliffe R, Webster V, et al. Improved survival in pregnancy and pulmonary hypertension using a multiprofessional approach. *BJOG.* 2010;117:565–574.

113. Bonnin M, Mercier FJ, Sitbon O, et al. Severe pulmonary hypertension during pregnancy: mode of delivery and anesthetic management of 15 consecutive cases. *Anesthesiology.* 2005;102:1133–1137.

114. Decoene C, Bourzoufi K, Moreau D, et al. Use of inhaled nitric oxide for emergency cesarean section in a woman with unexpected primary pulmonary hypertension. *Can J Anaesth.* 2001;48:584–587.

115. Weiss BM, Maggiorini M, Jenni R, et al. Pregnant patient with primary pulmonary hypertension: inhaled pulmonary vasodilators and epidural anesthesia for cesarean delivery. *Anesthesiology.* 2000;92:1191–1194.

116. Elliot CA, Stewart P, Webster VJ, et al. The use of iloprost in early pregnancy in patients with pulmonary arterial hypertension. *Eur Respir J.* 2005;26:168–173.

117. Campuzano K, Roque H, Bolnick A, et al. Bacterial endocarditis complicating pregnancy: case report and systematic review of the literature. *Arch Gynecol Obstet.* 2003;268:251–255.

118. Otto CM, Nishimura RA, Bonow RO, et al. 2020 ACC/AHA guideline for the management of patients with valvular heart disease: a report of the American College of Cardiology/American Heart Association Joint Committee onClinical Practice Guidelines. *J Am Coll Cardiol.* 2021;77:e25–e197.

119. Carp H, Bailey S. The association between meningitis and dural puncture in bacteremic rats. *Anesthesiology.* 1992;76:739–742.

120. Thaman R, Curtis S, Faganello G, et al. Cardiac outcome of pregnancy in women with a pacemaker and women with untreated atrioventricular conduction block. *Europace.* 2011;13:859–863.

121. Topf A, Bacher N, Kopp K, et al. Management of implantable cardioverter-defibrillators during pregnancy—a systematic review. *J Clin Med.* 2021:10.

122. Natale A, Davidson T, Geiger MJ, Newby K. Implantable cardioverter-defibrillators and pregnancy: a safe combination? *Circulation*. 1997;96:2808–2812.

123. Bonini W, Botto GL, Broffoni T, Dondina C. Pregnancy with an ICD and a documented ICD discharge. *Europace*. 2000;2:87–90.

124. American Society of Anesthesiologists. Practice advisory for the perioperative management of patients with cardiac implantable electronic devices: pacemakers and implantable cardioverter-defibrillators 2020: an updated report by the American Society of Anesthesiologists Task Force on Perioperative Management of Patients with Cardiac Implantable Electronic Devices. *Anesthesiology*. 2020;132:938.

125. Viani S, Zucchelli G, Paperini L, et al. Subcutaneous implantable defibrillator in an acromegalic pregnant woman for secondary prevention of sudden cardiac death: when (2) technologies save (2) lives. *Int J Cardiol*. 2016;223:313–315.

126. Shotan A, Ostrzega E, Mehra A, et al. Incidence of arrhythmias in normal pregnancy and relation to palpitations, dizziness, and syncope. *Am J Cardiol*. 1997;79:1061–1064.

127. Silversides CK, Harris L, Haberer K, et al. Recurrence rates of arrhythmias during pregnancy in women with previous tachyarrhythmia and impact on fetal and neonatal outcomes. *Am J Cardiol*. 2006;97:1206–1212.

128. Li JM, Nguyen C, Joglar JA, et al. Frequency and outcome of arrhythmias complicating admission during pregnancy: experience from a high-volume and ethnically-diverse obstetric service. *Clin Cardiol*. 2008;31:538–541.

129. Lee SH, Chen SA, Wu TJ, et al. Effects of pregnancy on first onset and symptoms of paroxysmal supraventricular tachycardia. *Am J Cardiol*. 1995;76:675–678.

130. Tamirisa KP, Elkayam U, Briller JE, et al. Arrhythmias in pregnancy. *JACC Clin Electrophysiol*. 2022;8:120–135.

131. Salam AM, Ertekin E, van Hagen IM, et al. Atrial fibrillation or flutter during pregnancy in patients with structural heart disease: data from the ROPAC (Registry on Pregnancy and Cardiac Disease). *JACC Clin Electrophysiol*. 2015;1:284–292.

132. January CT, Wann LS, Alpert JS, et al. 2014 AHA/ACC/ HRS guideline for the management of patients with atrial fibrillation. *Circulation*. 2014;130:2071–2104.

133. Gersh BJ, Maron BJ, Bonow RO, et al. 2011 ACCF/AHA guideline for the diagnosis and treatment of hypertrophic cardiomyopathy: a report of the American College of Cardiology Foundation/American Heart Association Task Force on Practice Guidelines. *J Am Coll Cardiol*. 2011;58:e212–e260.

134. Maron BJ. The electrocardiogram as a diagnostic tool for hypertrophic cardiomyopathy: revisited. *Ann Noninvasive Electrocardiol*. 2001;6:277–279.

135. Autore C, Conte MR, Piccininno M, et al. Risk associated with pregnancy in hypertrophic cardiomyopathy. *J Am Coll Cardiol*. 2002;40:1864–1869.

136. Brodsky M, Doria R, Allen B, et al. New-onset ventricular tachycardia during pregnancy. *Am Heart J*. 1992;123:933–941.

137. Cleary-Goldman J, Salva CR, Infeld JI, Robinson JN. Verapamil-sensitive idiopathic left ventricular tachycardia in pregnancy. *J Matern Fetal Neonatal Med*. 2003;14:132–135.

138. Mittadodla PS, Salen PN, Traub DM. Isoproterenol as an adjunct for treatment of idiopathic ventricular fibrillation storm in a pregnant woman. *Am J Emerg Med*. 2012;30: 251.e3–e5.

139. Burrows K, Fox J, Biblo LA, Roth JA. Pregnancy and short-coupled torsades de pointes. *Pacing Clin Electrophysiol*. 2013;36:e77–e79.

140. Sharif-Kazemi MB, Emkanjoo Z, Tavoosi A, et al. Electrical storm in Brugada syndrome during pregnancy. *Pacing Clin Electrophysiol*. 2011;34:e18–e21.

141. Seth R, Moss AJ, McNitt S, et al. Long QT syndrome and pregnancy. *J Am Coll Cardiol*. 2007;49:1092–1098.

142. Khositseth A, Tester DJ, Will ML, et al. Identification of a common genetic substrate underlying postpartum cardiac events in congenital long QT syndrome. *Heart Rhythm*. 2004;1:60–64.

143. Zipes DP, Camm AJ, et al. European Heart Rhythm Association. ACC/AHA/ESC 2006 Guidelines for management of patients with ventricular arrhythmias and the prevention of sudden cardiac death: a report of the American College of Cardiology/American Heart Association Task Force and the European Society of Cardiology Committee for Practice Guidelines. *Circulation*. 2006;114:e385–e484.

144. Wang YC, Chen CH, Su HY, Yu MH. The impact of maternal cardioversion on fetal haemodynamics. *Eur J Obstet Gynecol Reprod Biol*. 2006;126:268–269.

145. Barnes EJ, Eben F, Patterson D. Direct current cardioversion during pregnancy should be performed with facilities available for fetal monitoring and emergency caesarean section. *BJOG*. 2002;109:1406–1407.

146. Thygesen K, Alpert JS, Jaffe AS, et al. Fourth universal definition of myocardial infarction (2018). *Circulation*. 2018;138:e618–e651.

147. Tweet MS, Lewey J, Smilowitz NR, et al. Pregnancy-associated myocardial infarction: prevalence, causes, and interventional management. *Circ Cardiovasc Interv*. 2020;13:e008687.

148. Gibson P, Narous M, Firoz T, et al. Incidence of myocardial infarction in pregnancy: a systematic review and meta-analysis of population-based studies. *Eur Heart J Qual Care Clin Outcomes*. 2017;3:198–207.

149. Zakowski MI, Ramanathan S, Baratta JB, et al. Electrocardiographic changes during cesarean section: a cause for concern? *Anesth Analg*. 1993;76:162–167.

150. Palmer CM, Norris MC, Giudici MC, et al. Incidence of electrocardiographic changes during cesarean delivery under regional anesthesia. *Anesth Analg*. 1990;70:36–43.

151. Ismail S, Wong C, Rajan P, Vidovich MI. ST-elevation acute myocardial infarction in pregnancy: 2016 update. *Clin Cardiol*. 2017;40:399–406.

152. Virani SS, Newby LK, Arnold SV, et al. 2023 AHA/ACC/ ACCP/ASPC/NLA/PCNA guideline for the management of patients with chronic coronary disease: a report of the American Heart Association/American College of Cardiology Joint Committee on Clinical Practice Guidelines. *J Am Coll Cardiol*. 2023;82:833–955.

153. Silversides CK, Colman JM, Sermer M, et al. Early and intermediate-term outcomes of pregnancy with congenital aortic stenosis. *Am J Cardiol*. 2003;91:1386–1389.

154. Orwat S, Diller G-P, van Hagen IM, et al. Risk of pregnancy in moderate and severe aortic stenosis: from the multinational ROPAC Registry. *J Am Coll Cardiol*. 2016;68:1727–1737.

155. Hodson R, Kirker E, Swanson J, et al. Transcatheter aortic valve replacement during pregnancy. *Circ Cardiovasc Interv*. 2016;9:e004006.

156. Erturk E, Bostan H, Eroglu A. Epidural analgesia and vaginal delivery in a patient with aortic stenosis and insufficiency. *Med Princ Pract.* 2011;20:574–576.

157. Bryg RJ, Gordon PR, Kudesia VS, Bhatia RK. Effect of pregnancy on pressure gradient in mitral stenosis. *Am J Cardiol.* 1989;63:384–386.

158. Habib F, Mendel B, Fauzan R, Nasution AN. Revisiting percutaneous balloon mitral valvotomy technique and safety in various population: an evidence-based case report and literature review. *Front Cardiovasc Med.* 2024;11:1334444.

159. Cupido B, Zühlke L, Osman A, et al. Managing rheumatic heart disease in pregnancy: a practical evidence-based multidisciplinary approach. *Can J Cardiol.* 2021;37:2045–2055.

160. Lewey J, Andrade L, Levine LD. Valvular heart disease in pregnancy. *Cardiol Clin.* 2021;39:151–161.

161. de Souza JA, Martinez EE Jr, Ambrose JA, et al. Percutaneous balloon mitral valvuloplasty in comparison with open mitral valve commissurotomy for mitral stenosis during pregnancy. *J Am Coll Cardiol.* 2001;37:900–903.

162. Borges VT, Matsubara BB, Magalhaes CG, et al. Effect of physiological overload on pregnancy in women with mitral regurgitation. *Clinics (Sao Paulo).* 2011;66:47–50.

163. Hameed AB, Goodwin TM, Elkayam U. Effect of pulmonary stenosis on pregnancy outcomes—a case-control study. *Am Heart J.* 2007;154:852–854.

164. Khairy P, Ouyang DW, Fernandes SM, et al. Pregnancy outcomes in women with congenital heart disease. *Circulation.* 2006;113:517–524.

165. Greutmann M, Von Klemperer K, Brooks R, et al. Pregnancy outcome in women with congenital heart disease and residual haemodynamic lesions of the right ventricular outflow tract. *Eur Heart J.* 2010;31:1764–1770.

166. Nishimura RA, Otto CM, Bonow RO, et al. 2014 AHA/ACC guideline for the management of patients with valvular heart disease. *Circulation.* 2014;129:e521–e643.

167. Chan WS, Anand S, Ginsberg JS. Anticoagulation of pregnant women with mechanical heart valves: a systematic review of the literature. *Arch Intern Med.* 2000;160:191–196.

168. American College of Obstetricians and Gynecologists. Practice Bulletin No. 196: Thromboembolism in pregnancy (reaffirmed 2022). *Obstet Gynecol.* 2018;132:243–248.

169. Yancy CW, Jessup M, Bozkurt B, et al. 2013 ACCF/AHA guideline for the management of heart failure: a report of the American College of Cardiology Foundation/American Heart Association Task Force on Practice Guidelines. *Circulation.* 2013;128:e240–e327.

170. Dickstein K, Cohen-Solal A, Filippatos G, et al. ESC guidelines for the diagnosis and treatment of acute and chronic heart failure 2008: the Task Force for the Diagnosis and Treatment of Acute and Chronic Heart Failure 2008 of the European Society of Cardiology. *Eur J Heart Fail.* 2008;10:933–989.

171. Ruys TP, Roos-Hesselink JW, Hall R, et al. Heart failure in pregnant women with cardiac disease: data from the ROPAC. *Heart.* 2014;100:231–238.

172. Sliwa K, Hilfiker-Kleiner D, Petrie MC, et al. Current state of knowledge on aetiology, diagnosis, management, and therapy of peripartum cardiomyopathy: a position statement from the Heart Failure Association of the European Society of Cardiology Working Group on Peripartum Cardiomyopathy. *Eur J Heart Fail.* 2010;12:767–778.

173. Bauersachs J, Arrigo M, Hilfiker-Kleiner D, et al. Current management of patients with severe acute peripartum cardiomyopathy: practical guidance from the Heart Failure Association of the European Society of Cardiology Study Group on Peripartum Cardiomyopathy. *Eur J Heart Fail.* 2016;18:1096–1105.

174. Kolte D, Khera S, Aronow WS, et al. Temporal trends in incidence and outcomes of peripartum cardiomyopathy in the United States: a nationwide population-based study. *J Am Heart Assoc.* 2014;3:e001056.

175. Gunderson EP, Croen LA, Chiang V, et al. Epidemiology of peripartum cardiomyopathy: incidence, predictors, and outcomes. *Obstet Gynecol.* 2011;118:583–591.

176. Brar SS, Khan SS, Sandhu GK, et al. Incidence, mortality, and racial differences in peripartum cardiomyopathy. *Am J Cardiol.* 2007;100:302–304.

177. Isogai T, Kamiya CA. Worldwide incidence of peripartum cardiomyopathy and overall maternal mortality. *Int Heart J.* 2019;60:503–511.

178. Kamiya CA, Yoshimatsu J, Ikeda T. Peripartum cardiomyopathy from a genetic perspective. *Circ J.* 2016;80:1684–1688.

179. Ersbøll AS, Damm P, Gustafsson F, et al. Peripartum cardiomyopathy: a systematic literature review. *Acta Obstet Gynecol Scand.* 2016;95:1205–1219.

180. Velickovic IA, Leicht CH. Continuous spinal anesthesia for cesarean section in a parturient with severe recurrent peripartum cardiomyopathy. *Int J Obstet Anesth.* 2004;13:40–43.

181. Shnaider R, Ezri T, Szmuk P, et al. Combined spinal-epidural anesthesia for cesarean section in a patient with peripartum dilated cardiomyopathy. *Can J Anaesth.* 2001;48:681–683.

182. Pirlet M, Baird M, Pryn S, et al. Low dose combined spinal-epidural anaesthesia for caesarean section in a patient with peripartum cardiomyopathy. *Int J Obstet Anesth.* 2000;9:189–192.

183. Spirito P, Bellone P, Harris KM, et al. Magnitude of left ventricular hypertrophy and risk of sudden death in hypertrophic cardiomyopathy. *N Engl J Med.* 2000;342:1778–1785.

184. Maron MS, Olivotto I, Zenovich AG, et al. Hypertrophic cardiomyopathy is predominantly a disease of left ventricular outflow tract obstruction. *Circulation.* 2006;114:2232–2239.

185. Autore C, Brauneis S, Apponi F, et al. Epidural anesthesia for cesarean section in patients with hypertrophic cardiomyopathy: a report of three cases. *Anesthesiology.* 1999;90:1205–1207.

186. Dolbeau JB, Hebert T, Espitalier F, et al. Obstructive hypertrophic cardiomyopathy and caesarean section under combined spinal and epidural anaesthesia with prophylactic vascular ligation: regarding a case. *Ann Fr Anesth Reanim.* 2011;30:64–66.

187. Pryn A, Bryden F, Reeve W, et al. Cardiomyopathy in pregnancy and caesarean section: four case reports. *Int J Obstet Anesth.* 2007;16:68–73.

188. Deiml R, Hess W, Bahlmann E. Primary cesarean section. Use of phenylephrine during anesthesia in a patient with hypertrophic obstructive cardiomyopathy. *Anaesthesist.* 2000;49:527–531.

189. Thaman R, Varnava A, Hamid MS, et al. Pregnancy related complications in women with hypertrophic cardiomyopathy. *Heart.* 2003;89:752–756.

190. Ho KM, Ngan Kee WD, Poon MC. Combined spinal and epidural anesthesia in a parturient with idiopathic hypertrophic subaortic stenosis. *Anesthesiology*. 1997;87:168–169.

191. Okutomi T, Kikuchi S, Amano K, et al. Continuous spinal analgesia for labor and delivery in a parturient with hypertrophic obstructive cardiomyopathy. *Acta Anaesthesiol Scand*. 2002;46:329–331.

192. Ishiyama T, Oguchi T, Iijima T, et al. Combined spinal and epidural anesthesia for cesarean section in a patient with hypertrophic obstructive cardiomyopathy. *Anesth Analg*. 2003;96:629–630.

193. Akashi YJ, Goldstein DS, Barbaro G, Ueyama T. Takotsubo cardiomyopathy: a new form of acute, reversible heart failure. *Circulation*. 2008;118:2754–2762.

194. Brezina P, Isler CM. Takotsubo cardiomyopathy in pregnancy. *Obstet Gynecol*. 2008;112:450–452.

195. Zdanowicz JA, Utz AC, Bernasconi I, et al. "Broken heart" after cesarean delivery. Case report and review of literature. *Arch Gynecol Obstet*. 2011;283:687–694.

196. Crimi E, Baggish A, Leffert L, et al. Images in cardiovascular medicine. Acute reversible stress-induced cardiomyopathy associated with cesarean delivery under spinal anesthesia. *Circulation*. 2008;117:3052–3053.

197. Grewal J, Siu SC, Ross HJ, et al. Pregnancy outcomes in women with dilated cardiomyopathy. *J Am Coll Cardiol*. 2009;55:45–52.

198. Hasdemir C, Ulucan C, Yavuzgil O, et al. Tachycardia-induced cardiomyopathy in patients with idiopathic ventricular arrhythmias: the incidence, clinical and electrophysiologic characteristics, and the predictors. *J Cardiovasc Electrophysiol*. 2011;22:663–668.

199. Ferguson JD, Helms A, Mangrum JM, DiMarco JP. Ablation of incessant left atrial tachycardia without fluoroscopy in a pregnant woman. *J Cardiovasc Electrophysiol*. 2011;22:346–349.

200. Pagad SV, Barmade AB, Toal SC, et al. 'Rescue' radiofrequency ablation for atrial tachycardia presenting as cardiomyopathy in pregnancy. *Indian Heart J*. 2004;56:245–247.

201. LaRue S, Shanks A, Wang IW, et al. Left ventricular assist device in pregnancy. *Obstet Gynecol*. 2011;118:426–428.

202. Etz C, Welp H, Scheld HH, Schmid C. Near fatal infection of a patient with a left ventricular assist device due to unrecognized fetal death. *Eur J Cardiothorac Surg*. 2005;27:722–723.

203. Abduljabbar HS, Marzouki KM, Zawawi TH, Khan AS. Pericardial effusion in normal pregnant women. *Acta Obstet Gynecol Scand*. 1991;70:291–294.

204. Mhyre JM, Tsen LC, Einav S, et al. Cardiac arrest during hospitalization for delivery in the United States, 1998-2011. *Anesthesiology*. 2014;120:810–818.

205. Mogos MF, Salemi JL, Spooner KK, et al. Differences in mortality between pregnant and nonpregnant women after cardiopulmonary resuscitation. *Obstet Gynecol*. 2016;128:880–888.

206. Jeejeebhoy FM, Zelop CM, Lipman S, et al. Cardiac arrest in pregnancy: a scientific statement from the American Heart Association. *Circulation*. 2015;132:1747–1773.

207. Merchant RM, Topjian AA, Panchal AR, et al. Part 1: executive summary: 2020 American Heart Association guidelines for cardiopulmonary resuscitation and emergency cardiovascular care. *Circulation*. 2020;142:S337–S357.

208. Lipman SS, Wong JY, Arafeh J, et al. Transport decreases the quality of cardiopulmonary resuscitation during simulated maternal cardiac arrest. *Anesth Analg*. 2013;116:162–167.

209. Naoum EE, Chalupka A, Haft J, et al. Extracorporeal life support in pregnancy: a systematic review. *J Am Heart Assoc*. 2020;9:e016072.

210. Morini A, Spina V, Aleandri V, et al. Pregnancy after heart transplant: update and case report. *Hum Reprod*. 1998;13:749–757.

211. Armenti VT, Radomski JS, Moritz MJ, et al. Report from the National Transplantation Pregnancy Registry (NTPR): outcomes of pregnancy after transplantation. *Clin Transpl*. 2004:103–114.

212. Kittleson MM, DeFilippis EM, Bhagra CJ, et al. Reproductive health after thoracic transplantation: an ISHLT expert consensus statement. *J Heart Lung Transplant*. 2023;42:e1–e42.

213. Wilson W, Taubert KA, Gewitz M, et al. Prevention of infective endocarditis: a guideline from the American Heart Association Rheumatic Fever, Endocarditis, and Kawasaki Disease Committee, Council on Cardiovascular Disease in the Young, and the Council on Clinical Cardiology, Council on Cardiovascular Surgery and Anesthesia, and the Quality of Care and Outcomes Research Interdisciplinary Working Group. *Circulation*. 2007;116:1736–1754.

214. John AS, Gurley F, Schaff HV, et al. Cardiopulmonary bypass during pregnancy. *Ann Thorac Surg*. 2011;91:1191–1196.

215. Iscan ZH, Mavioglu L, Vural KM, et al. Cardiac surgery during pregnancy. *J Heart Valve Dis*. 2006;15:686–690.

42

Chronic Pain During and After Pregnancy

Ruth Landau, MD and Leena Mathew, MD

INTRODUCTION

According to 2021 data from the US Centers for Disease Control and Prevention (CDC), approximately 20.9% of US adults (51.6 million) have chronic pain, and 6.9% (17.1 million) have high-impact chronic pain.[1] There is a higher prevalence of chronic pain among women compared to men. New findings of high-impact chronic pain demonstrate it is more prevalent among non-Hispanic American Indian and Alaska Native adults, adults identifying as bisexual, and adults who are divorced or separated.[1]

The management of pain in pregnant patients is challenging because of the etiologic factors resulting in chronic pain and the unique limitations on certain therapeutic interventions during pregnancy and lactation. The coexistence of chronic pain with mood disorders such as anxiety and depression is common in the general population and pregnancy tends to exacerbate both. Recognizing the significant overlap of chronic pain and mood disorders among pregnant women is crucial to reducing mental health–related maternal morbidity and mortality.[2]

In the *2016 Health, United States Report*, 25% of women of childbearing age (18 to 44 years of age) reported migraine headaches, 26% reported low back pain (LBP), and 15% reported neck pain.[3] Common chronic pain conditions in women are migraine headaches, pelvic pain, back pain, and

fibromyalgia[4]; the most common chronic pain complaints in pregnant women include neck and back pain and headaches.[5] Although migraine and autoimmune disease–mediated symptoms often improve or even resolve during pregnancy, back pain and pelvic girdle pain (PGP) frequently worsen as a direct result of pregnancy.[6]

This chapter will review the interplay between chronic pain preceding pregnancy and patient-specific factors, obstetric considerations, and the relationship between acute and chronic pain after delivery (Fig. 42.1). Specifically, it will explore (1) the epidemiology and risk factors for chronic pain before and during pregnancy, (2) management strategies for pain conditions during pregnancy, (3) the peridelivery management of pregnant women with a spinal cord stimulator (SCS), (4) factors associated with persistent and chronic pain after delivery, and (5) strategies to prevent chronic pain after cesarean delivery.

EPIDEMIOLOGY AND RISK FACTORS FOR PAIN DURING PREGNANCY

When identifying the prevalence and risk factors for different pain conditions before, during, and after pregnancy, it is important to acknowledge that pain is a nuanced and complex phenotype. In 2020, the International Association for the Study of Pain (IASP) redefined pain as "an unpleasant sensory

Obstetric Considerations

- Pain prevalence and severity during pregnancy
- Maternal and fetal morbidity and mortality associated with chronic pain condition
- Management of chronic pain during pregnancy
- Specific considerations associated with chronic opioid use during pregnancy
- Specific consideration for pregnant women with spinal cord stimulator
- Labor analgesia, anesthesia for cesarean delivery

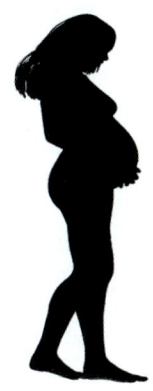

Chronic Pain Conditions

- Migraine headache
- Sickle cell disease
- Low back pain
- Pelvic girdle pain
- Fibromyalgia

Chronic Pain after Delivery

- Risk factors for chronic pain after delivery
- Management of intractable postpartum pain
- Factors associated with acute, persistent, and chronic pain

Fig. 42.1 Interplay between chronic pain preceding pregnancy and patient-specific factors, obstetric considerations, and the relationship between acute and chronic pain after delivery.

BOX 42.1 Pain Redefined According to the International Association for the Study of Pain

- Pain is always a personal experience that is influenced to varying degrees by biological, psychological, and social factors.
- Pain and nociception are different phenomena. Pain cannot be inferred solely from activity in sensory neurons.
- Through their life experiences, individuals learn the concept of pain.
- A person's report of an experience as pain should be respected.
- Although pain usually serves an adaptive role, it may have adverse effects on function and social and psychological well-being.
- Verbal description is only one of several behaviors to express pain; inability to communicate does not negate the possibility that a human or a nonhuman animal experiences pain.

From Raja SN, Carr DB, Cohen M, et al. The revised International Association for the Study of Pain definition of pain: concepts, challenges, and compromises. *Pain.* 2020;161:1976–1982.

---

and emotional experience associated with, or resembling that associated with, actual or potential tissue damage" and emphasized six additional key considerations in defining pain (Box 42.1).[7] Perhaps most applicable to pregnancy and childbirth pain is the conclusion that "pain is always a personal experience that is influenced to varying degrees by biological, psychological, and social factors" and "a person's report of an experience as pain should be respected." This understanding of pain as a personal experience helps explain why some women choose to experience "natural childbirth" without any form of analgesia, while chronic pain during pregnancy may

be poorly tolerated by other women. In this unique context, pain during or after cesarean delivery may result in traumatic childbirth experiences and is associated with an increased risk for postpartum depression and persistent pain.[8]

Quality of life (QoL) and maternal mental health issues during pregnancy and the postpartum period are key concerns in healthcare. The American College of Obstetrics and Gynecology (ACOG) emphasizes the importance of adequate screening and management of mental health conditions during pregnancy and the postpartum period.[9,10]

In a 2022 systematic review assessing the health-related QoL during pregnancy, obesity, LBP and PGP, and hyperemesis gravidarum were the three most frequent pathologies associated with poor QoL during pregnancy.[11] Health-related QoL during pregnancy is not often reported or assessed in clinical practice or research. However, symptoms that are associated with pain during pregnancy, such as fear of managing labor, poor sleep quality, headache or migraine, anxiety and depression, and LBP, should not be overlooked. Among factors associated with a better QoL in pregnancy are exercise, moderate physical activity in water, high exercise adherence, adopting low-to-moderate intensity resistance training, higher energy expenditures, Pilates exercises, better sleep quality, sexual satisfaction, and receiving lifestyle advice and social support.[11]

In a prospective study of 133 nulliparous women with uncomplicated singleton pregnancies recruited in the third trimester at a large perinatal center in Canada, 38% reported a chronic pain condition or pain before pregnancy, and 55% reported pain during the current pregnancy.[12] Forty-three percent of the cohort reported pain that persisted at 2 weeks postpartum and 25% at 3 months postpartum. Migraine was the most common source of chronic pain, and lower back pain was the most common source of pain overall.[12] Pain during pregnancy was primarily described as mild or discomforting; the lower back was the most common site of pain 3 months postpartum.[12]

Pain before and during pregnancy is predictive of pain after delivery, and severe acute pain during labor and delivery can presage pain that persists during the postpartum period and beyond.[8] The proposed mechanism linking acute pain with persistent pain is central sensitization; activity-dependent synaptic plasticity in the spinal cord generates postinjury pain hypersensitivity.[13] As a consequence, mild pain is augmented in the sensitized synapse and transmitted as severe pain (hyperalgesia); even touch can be transmitted as painful (allodynia). Drugs that specifically block pain sensitization in the context of postoperative pain are suggested as a strategy to prevent persistent postoperative pain (see later discussion).[14]

MANAGEMENT OF PAIN DURING PREGNANCY AND POSTPARTUM

During pregnancy, the primary goal of multimodal analgesia is to provide adequate pain relief while minimizing the risks to the fetus/neonate and side effects for pregnant women. The use of **nonpharmacologic interventions**, including pain psychology and physiotherapy techniques, may be useful for pregnant women with chronic pain.[15] **Interventional techniques**, including nerve blocks and radiofrequency techniques, are limited by the requirement to minimize radiation exposure from fluoroscopy. However, many of these procedures can now be accomplished with ultrasonographic guidance, and local anesthetic and corticosteroid injections are not contraindicated during pregnancy.[16]

In the postpartum period, minimizing the transfer of drugs to breast milk and reducing maternal side effects that may interfere with breastfeeding or caring for the neonate are key. In general, medications for which infant plasma concentration is less than 10% of maternal plasma concentration are considered safe for the breastfeeding infant (see Chapter 16). Acetaminophen and nonsteroidal antiinflammatory drugs (NSAIDs) are compatible with breastfeeding and should be the foundation for treating mild-to-moderate pain in postpartum patients.[17,18] An important resource for information about the interaction between specific drugs and breastfeeding can be found online at the Drugs and Lactation Database (LactMed).[19]

Nonopioid Analgesics

Acetaminophen

Long considered the safest drug in pregnancy, recent studies have raised concerns that the use of acetaminophen during pregnancy is linked to neurobehavioral disorders such as attention deficit hyperactivity disorder (ADHD) and autism spectrum disorder (ASD) in children.[20–23] The studies suggesting this association often have serious limitations, including relying on self-reported data and inadequate control for confounding factors. A rigorous analysis of all singleton liveborn children born in Sweden between 1995 and 2019

(n = 2,489,721), which controlled for a large number of confounders and included a sibling analysis, did not find a link between acetaminophen use during pregnancy and offspring risk for ADHD, ASD, or intellectual disability.[24]

Nonsteroidal Antiinflammatory Drugs

Despite a general recommendation to avoid the use of NSAIDs during pregnancy unless the maternal benefit is deemed to significantly outweigh the risk to the fetus, over-the-counter NSAID use is common during pregnancy. In one multicenter survey of more than 5000 pregnant women, 24% reported the use of ibuprofen, 5% reported the use of aspirin, and 4% reported the use of naproxen.[25]

Current data suggest no effect of NSAIDs use on early pregnancy loss. NSAIDs should be used sparingly and avoided if possible in the first trimester. Large observational studies have suggested a small increase in the risk for congenital defects, generally small cardiac septal defects, neural tube defects, and possibly gastroschisis.[26] Compared with neonates exposed to acetaminophen alone, neonates exposed to NSAIDs in the first trimester were found to have an increased risk for gastroschisis, hypospadias, cleft lip and palate, anencephaly, spina bifida, hypoplastic left heart syndrome, pulmonary valve stenosis, and tetralogy of Fallot.[27] An association does not demonstrate causation, and it is possible that the increased risk for congenital anomalies may be related to the indication for use rather than the pharmacologic effect of NSAIDs. The US Food and Drug Administration (FDA) warns against the use of NSAIDs at 20 weeks' gestation or later because they can cause fetal renal dysfunction and low amniotic fluid volume,[28] in addition to ductus arteriosus constriction.[29] Unless the maternal benefits significantly outweigh the risks, NSAIDs are generally contraindicated in the third trimester because of increased risk for premature closure of the ductus arteriosus as well as fetal renal dysfunction and oligohydramnios.

Historically, the ACOG warned against the postpartum use of NSAIDs in women recovering from preeclampsia with persistent postpartum hypertension; however, following a systematic review and metaanalysis showing that postpartum NSAID use among women with hypertensive disorders of pregnancy was not associated with maternal hypertension exacerbation,[30] this recommendation has been updated and the ACOG no longer discourages NSAID use in these women.[31]

NSAIDS are an important component in the multimodal management of postpartum pain in patients with chronic pain and opioid tolerance. They are widely utilized and extremely effective for postdelivery pain. Given the limited transfer of ibuprofen to breast milk, the Academy of Breastfeeding Medicine deems it a suitable analgesic drug in breastfeeding mothers.[18] Data on other NSAIDs (e.g., etodolac, fenoprofen, meloxicam, oxaprozin, piroxicam, sulindac, and tolmetin) are limited, and the FDA labeling discourages their use. Less than 1% of the maternal dose of ketorolac is excreted into human milk, and adverse events in nursing mothers have not been reported.[32]

Low-dose aspirin is increasingly used beginning at 12 weeks' gestation until delivery for preeclampsia prophylaxis in women at high risk for the disease (see Chapter 35). To date, no significant adverse fetal effects have been noted in the offspring of women allocated to aspirin compared with placebo therapy in large clinical trials.[33]

Selective Cyclooxygenase-2 Inhibitors

Cyclooxygenase-2 (COX-2) inhibitors are additive or synergistic with opioids and other analgesics. Compared with nonselective NSAIDs, COX-2 inhibitors have minimal effects on platelet adhesion and are less likely to be associated with bleeding and coagulopathy. However, concerns about potential increased risk for cardiovascular and thrombotic events, combined with the baseline elevated risk for these events during pregnancy and the postpartum period, have prevented COX-2 inhibitors from playing a major role in postpartum analgesia. In addition, the use of celecoxib in late pregnancy has been associated with an increased risk for preterm delivery (adjusted odds ratio [aOR], 2.46; 95% confidence interval [CI], 1.28 to 4.72).[34] In 2023, the Society for Maternal-Fetal Medicine consult series on systemic lupus erythematosus recommended that COX-2 inhibitors, as well as high-dose aspirin, be avoided during pregnancy.[35]

Gabapentinoids

Gabapentin is a mainstay in the management of chronic pain. It is thought to provide analgesia by binding to presynaptic voltage-gated calcium channels in the dorsal root ganglia of the spinal cord, thereby inhibiting the release of excitatory neurotransmitters. Perioperative gabapentin has been shown to decrease acute pain after a variety of surgical procedures, although recent data do not support its routine use to reduce acute or chronic postoperative pain in adult surgical patients.[36] Similarly, data from healthy women undergoing elective cesarean delivery are conflicting.[37,38]

Gabapentin crosses the placenta. Studies on its use during pregnancy show a wide range of fetal-to-maternal (F/M) drug ratios, likely reflecting the timing of sampling after delivery. The Gabapentin Pregnancy Registry examined the outcomes of 39 pregnancies in which mothers received gabapentin for epilepsy or chronic pain conditions.[39] Thirty-six of these mothers received gabapentin continuously throughout pregnancy; there was no evidence of increased risk for adverse maternal or fetal/neonatal effects compared with the general population.[39] The most recent population-based study evaluating the association between gabapentin exposure during pregnancy and risk of adverse neonatal and maternal outcomes used the US Medicaid Analytic eXtract (MAX) data set.[40] Gabapentin exposure during early pregnancy was not associated with major malformations, although a higher risk of cardiac malformations was identified. Late pregnancy gabapentin exposure was associated with preterm birth, small-for-gestational-age infants, and neonatal intensive care unit admission.

The milk/plasma (M/P) ratio of gabapentin was assessed in five lactating mothers whose chronic gabapentin dose ranged from 600 to 2100 mg/day; the mean ratio was 1.0 (sampling ranged from 2 weeks to 3 months of neonatal age).[41] The infant dose (mg/kg body weight) of gabapentin was estimated to be 1.3% to 3.8% of the maternal dose. The drug is rapidly metabolized by the newborn[41]; mean neonatal plasma concentrations were 27% of the umbilical artery plasma levels at 24 hours postpartum. No adverse effects were observed in the five mother-infant dyads.[41] Thus, current data suggest that gabapentin use by lactating mothers is safe.[32]

Pregabalin is not as well studied as gabapentin for the treatment of chronic pain in pregnancy. Although concerns were raised for a possible link between pregabalin use in the first trimester and increased risk for major fetal malformations, follow-up studies have proven more reassuring. A 2016 study included 116 pregnancies with first-trimester exposure; 6% (n = 7) of offspring had malformations compared with 2% (n = 2) in the nonexposed group.[42] Four of the six fetal malformations in the pregabalin group were cerebral ventriculomegaly.[42] By contrast, results from a subsequent larger cohort study from the MAX database (477 infants exposed to pregabalin in the first trimester) were reassuring.[43] After propensity score adjustment for indication, the relative risk (RR) for major fetal malformations in the pregabalin group was 1.16 (95% CI, 0.81 to 1.67). When limited to patients on pregabalin monotherapy, the relative risk for malformations was 1.0 (95% CI, 0.7 to 1.5). Additionally, none of the 477 pregabalin-exposed infants carried a diagnosis of cerebral ventriculomegaly or other brain anomalies reported in the initial smaller study.[42,43]

Pregabalin crosses into breast milk, as predicted by its low molecular weight and lack of plasma protein binding. In 10 lactating women receiving daily pregabalin 300 mg, the calculated amount of pregabalin present in 24-hour breast milk collections was 0.2% of the administered daily maternal dose, and no adverse effects were reported.[44]

Antidepressants

Antidepressants are commonly used to treat chronic pain conditions ranging from migraine disorders to fibromyalgia and neuropathic pain conditions. Two classes of antidepressants have demonstrated efficacy in the management of chronic pain: **tricyclic antidepressants** (TCAs) and **serotonin-norepinephrine reuptake inhibitors** (SNRIs). Both increase the synaptic concentrations of serotonin and norepinephrine.

Among TCAs, amitriptyline and nortriptyline have the largest body of reassuring safety data in pregnancy and lactation. TCAs cross the placenta; the approximate F/M ratio is 0.6.[45] The largest and most recent epidemiologic studies on the risk for major congenital malformation have yielded conflicting results.[46] Among the TCAs, clomipramine has been the most strongly implicated in increased risk for congenital anomalies[47] and postexposure withdrawal syndrome in neonates.

Duloxetine and venlafaxine are commonly used SNRIs for chronic pain conditions. In a recent Scandinavian study, the chronic use of SNRIs during pregnancy was not associated with adverse pregnancy outcomes, and duloxetine exposure was unlikely to increase the risk of small-for-gestational age.[48] Like the TCAs, neonates of mothers taking SNRIs at the end of pregnancy should be monitored for transient agitation and withdrawal symptoms; the risk is greater in drugs with shorter half-lives, such as venlafaxine.[49] The American Academy of Pediatrics (AAP) recommends using SNRIs with caution in lactating mothers because the long-term effects of chronic exposure on neurodevelopment are unknown.[32]

N-Methyl-D-aspartate Receptor Antagonists

Ketamine, an N-methyl-D-aspartate (NMDA) receptor antagonist, is used for the treatment of acute postoperative pain and prevention or reversal of central sensitization in the setting of chronic pain.[50]

Ketamine is contraindicated in pregnancy, given lack of safety data and its potential effects on the developing fetus. Animal studies suggest that prenatal and early postnatal exposure to ketamine can be neurotoxic to the developing brain, with long-term neurocognitive abnormalities in offspring of pregnant rats treated with ketamine.[51] Similar effects on the developing fetal brain after exposure to **esketamine** have recently been suggested.[52]

Ketamine is sometimes used for intraoperative analgesia as an adjuvant to neuraxial anesthesia or for induction of general anesthesia in cesarean deliveries (see Chapter 26); small intravenous doses provide significant analgesia with minimal respiratory depression. It is reasonable to consider using ketamine in a patient with chronic pain or to prevent conversion to chronic pain after cesarean delivery. In one study, patients undergoing cesarean delivery with spinal anesthesia and multimodal postoperative analgesia that included spinal morphine were randomized to receive ketamine 10 mg or placebo after delivery.[53] Women who received ketamine reported less pain at 2 weeks postpartum compared with women who received a placebo.

There are currently limited data regarding ketamine safety in lactation. Two studies on the pharmacokinetics of ketamine transfer in breast milk suggest that transfer of ketamine and its major metabolites (norketamine, dehydronorketamine, and hydroxynorketamine isomers) into human milk is minimal, with an estimated relative infant dose (RID) of less than 1% for ketamine and norketamine.[54,55]

Alpha₂-Adrenergic Receptor Agonists

The use of neuraxial **clonidine** and, more recently, **dexmedetomidine**, as adjuvants for intraoperative and postcesarean analgesia has been reported.[56–59] In a 2024 statement from the American Society of Anesthesiologists, consideration for the use of epidural clonidine and dexmedetomidine as adjuvants for the management of intraoperative pain during cesarean delivery with epidural anesthesia is suggested.[60] The epidural formulation of clonidine carries a black box warning from the US FDA stating the following: "Clonidine hydrochloride injection (epidural clonidine) is not recommended for obstetrical, postpartum or perioperative pain management. The risk of hemodynamic instability, especially hypotension and bradycardia, from epidural clonidine may be unacceptable in these patients. However, in a rare, obstetrical, postpartum

or perioperative patient, potential benefits may outweigh the possible risks."[61] The use of intrathecal clonidine is off-label.

Neuraxial clonidine may be beneficial in patients who are at risk for the development of neuropathic pain after cesarean delivery. One study reported that the combination of intrathecal clonidine (150 µg) and bupivacaine was associated with decreased wound hyperalgesia after cesarean delivery[62]; however, further study of the use of alpha₂-adrenergic agonists in women with chronic pain is warranted. The use of neuraxial (both epidural and intrathecal) dexmedetomidine is off-label for all patient populations and indications.

Opioids

Although opioids are commonly prescribed in the United States to pregnant women, long-term treatment with opioids for pain syndromes, including headache, fibromyalgia, and chronic back pain, or sickle cell disease (SCD), should be thoroughly discussed and weighed against the risks associated with *in utero* fetal exposure to opioids.

Significant regional variation in prescription practice exists within the United States. Depending on the state of residence, the prevalence of chronic opioid use in pregnancy among publicly insured women nearly doubled from 2008 to 2014 and was fivefold more common compared to women with commercial insurance.[63] The persistent use of opioids after cesarean delivery in opioid-naive women in the United States is also an area for concern; a systematic review of four studies reporting on data from 486,263 women who delivered between 2001 and 2016 reported persistent opioid use rates up to 12 months postpartum ranging from 0.12% to 2.2% (from 1:1000 to 1:50).[64]

Pregnant women who use illicit opioids or take medication for opioid use disorder (MOUD) often have concomitant chronic disease and life circumstances that may confound analyses of the effects of opioid use during pregnancy. These confounders include a higher incidence of tobacco use, frequent alcohol and/or polysubstance use disorder, and life stressors and experiences that may independently alter their pregnancy outcome (see Chapter 52).

A 2024 systematic review and metaanalysis of 12 studies used medication dispensing claim data (n = 6) or self-reporting (n = 6) to estimate first-trimester opioid use and teratogenic potential of opioid use during pregnancy.[65] Infants exposed to any opioid during the first trimester, relative to those unexposed, were not at an increased risk of major congenital malformations (RR, 1.04; 95% CI, 0.98 to 1.11). Although this systematic review and metaanalysis synthesized all the available evidence, the authors identified important methodologic issues, leading to the conclusion that the risk of major malformations following first-trimester exposure to opioids remains unclear, despite 50 years of observational research.

In utero opioid exposure after the first trimester may also adversely affect the fetus. Fetal growth restriction may occur later in gestation. The neonate is at risk for neonatal opioid withdrawal syndrome if opioids are used by the mother in the third trimester.[66,67] In a metaanalysis of studies of neurobehavioral outcomes in infants and preschool children who were chronically exposed to opioids *in utero*, no significant impairment was identified compared with nonexposed peers.[68] However, the subset of infants born to mothers with opioid use disorder (OUD) may have risks that are not directly attributable to *in utero* opioid exposure. Behavioral issues have been identified in children raised by mothers with untreated OUD.[68,69]

Interventional Treatments

Neuromodulation therapies have the potential to improve functional status in patients with chronic pain; these typically include SCS, dorsal root ganglion (DRG) stimulation, and other implantable treatments such as intrathecal pumps (ITPs). The higher rate of chronic pain among women of childbearing age makes it likely that obstetricians and obstetric anesthesiologists will need to treat increasing numbers of pregnant women with complex or chronic pain syndromes.[6]

Mechanism of Action of Neuromodulation

Neuromodulation, such as SCS, is a reversible analgesic therapy that is being more widely used because systemic adverse effects are minimal. The basis of neuromodulation was established by the gate theory of pain, highlighting the role of the dorsal spinal cord columns in pain perception.[70] In addition to altering pain perception, SCS also improves microcirculation and activates dorsal column afferent neurons while inhibiting sympathetic efferent neurons, resulting in modification of neurotransmitter activity at the segmental and supraspinal levels. In painful ischemic conditions, SCS is purported to improve oxygenation by vasodilation resulting from reduced sympathetic tone.[70]

SCS is based on stimulation of the dorsal column of the spinal cord through one or more electrodes (SCS leads) permanently implanted in the epidural space. A typical SCS lead has 8 to 16 contacts used to generate a customized electric field. Unilateral or bilateral leads are placed in the dorsal epidural space from C3 to T11 depending on the area and laterality of pain. The lead placement corresponds with the dermatomal distribution of pain: cervical for neck and upper extremity pain and mid- to low-thoracic for low back and lower extremity pain. These leads are anchored with sutures to the supraspinous ligament and tunneled to the implanted pulse generator in a subcutaneous pocket positioned in the patient's lower back. It is important to understand the number, type, and location of leads prior to considering any neuraxial procedure.

Safety and Concerns During Pregnancy

Despite the absence of Class 1 evidence for the effectiveness of neuromodulation in pain management, its use has increased.[71,72] The FDA has not approved neuromodulation systems during pregnancy, and there is no established consensus on managing patients with such devices during and after pregnancy, and during labor and delivery. Because evidence on the safety of SCS during pregnancy is scarce, out of an abundance of caution, current industry recommendations

are to deactivate SCSs throughout pregnancy and in the intraoperative period.[73,74]

There are two commonly cited concerns with SCS or DRG therapy in pregnancy. The first concern is the impact of the electromagnetic field (EMF) generation around the implanted leads on the developing fetus. Teratogenic effects and reduction in fertility from chronic exposure to EMF is a theoretical concern. Clinically, the magnitude and extent of the EMF are insignificant, and it is highly unlikely that it exerts any substantive ill effects on pregnancy.[75] Most studies suggest that neuromodulation systems produce minimal electrical currents, and the EMF is confined to the posterior spinal column and is insulated from vertebral bones and ligaments. More studies are needed to establish stimulation parameters of these devices and the miscarriage and teratogenic rates in pregnant patients.

A second concern is impairment of placental blood flow, although studies demonstrate that SCS improves microcirculation and produces peripheral vasodilation without compromising uteroplacental blood flow.[76] The uteroplacental circulation lacks autonomic innervation and lacks the regulatory mechanisms of the peripheral circulation. Thus, it seems unlikely that the autonomic effects of SCS will have any perceptible impact on placental or fetal blood flow. Ultrasonographic studies showed no notable differences in uteroplacental and fetal blood flows during the on and off phases of SCS therapy.[77] Human data on the lack of effect of SCS on the developing fetus are limited to a few case reports.

Ultimately, patients should be educated on the potential ramifications of neuromodulation and intrathecal drug therapy. Shared decision-making around care should be made with collaboration and communication among a multidisciplinary team consisting of the anesthesiologist, obstetrician, surgeon, nursing team, pharmacist, pain medicine physician, and the patient (see Chapter 32).

Technical Complications

A case series indicated that SCS lead breakage associated with pregnancy and childbirth was most likely due to increased mechanical stressors associated with increased abdominal pressure during pregnancy and delivery,[78] and that the abdominal wall should be avoided as a site for the pulse generator implantation in women planning pregnancy.[79] Switching off the SCS or DRG stimulator mitigates accidental reprogramming. Device manufacturers also recommend that patients with implanted SCS should avoid procedures that potentially interfere with device programming such as high-output ultrasound or lithotripsy. Manufacturers recommend (1) turning off the neuromodulation device, (2) avoiding the focus of high-output ultrasound or lithotripsy beam within 15 cm of the SCS, and (3) interrogating the device in the postoperative period before turning it back on.[73,74]

Turning off the SCS is not an inconsequential decision; poor analgesia may have deleterious consequences in pregnancy. Worsening pain can make pregnancy challenging; patients may have to judiciously resume or increase systemic analgesic intake or conversely, they may choose to endure pain to avoid potential analgesic side effects. Both these choices may have subtle or significant psychosocial and physiologic adverse effects on the mother and fetus.

Implanted Devices and Neuraxial Procedures

Lumbar neuromodulation devices in pregnant women create a unique problem for the anesthesia provider. SCS leads in the epidural space can make the administration of neuraxial analgesia and anesthesia challenging. There is a risk of accidental injury to epidural leads with neuraxial procedures, but the presence of neuromodulation devices should not dissuade the anesthesia provider from performing a neuraxial anesthetic. Antepartum referral to the anesthesia provider is optimal as it allows adequate time for review of records and appropriate planning. Review of the manufacturer's recommendations is essential.

A 2019 systematic review evaluated 18 publications reporting on 25 pregnant patients with 32 pregnancies with SCS; complex regional pain syndrome (CRPS) and failed back were the most common indications.[80] The first report of management of a SCS in a pregnant woman in 1999 was in the setting of CRPS after a traumatic brachial plexus injury. Prior to the pregnancy, she was treated with chronic systemic medications that she wanted to avoid during pregnancy.[81] The patient was offered a cervical SCS. The device was placed before pregnancy and resulted in excellent pain relief and discontinuation of all pain medications. The SCS was not turned off during the peripartum period. Since this initial report, there have been many additional reports of pregnant women with indwelling SCS, including cervical[82] and thoracic or lumbar SCS with descriptions of neuraxial analgesia and anesthesia management for vaginal or cesarean delivery.[83–86]

In one case series, one of four patients had failed neuraxial anesthesia.[85] The possibility of fibrosis created by the SCS leads forming an encapsulating sheath or scarring in the epidural space may increase technical challenges or suboptimal spread of epidural medication, even if the epidural catheter is correctly sited in the epidural space.[87] Spinal anesthesia is not impacted.

The anesthesia provider should review the device implantation procedure report to confirm the site of lead placement, power source location, and the path of the leads and extension wires. If the report or imaging is unavailable, a single X-ray of the lumbar spine may be considered to identify the details of the implanted device. A single plain X-ray exposes the patient and fetus to a minimal ionizing radiation (see Chapter 18).

Another concern during cesarean deliveries and other surgical procedures is complications stemming from the use of diathermy or electrocautery. This may damage the neuromodulator lead insulation, suppress stimulator output, and inadvertently reprogram the neurostimulator. Painful electric shocks have been reported; thus, most manufacturers recommend avoidance of monopolar diathermy when possible. Bipolar diathermy appears to be safe. Most practice guidelines suggest decreasing SCS amplitude to zero followed by powering off the device and using bipolar cautery in short, quick intermittent bursts at the lowest feasible energy levels.

The electrical dispersal pad should be placed close to the field and far from the SCS components.[87]

Implantable Devices and Intrathecal Pumps

Implantable intrathecal pumps (ITPs) are used for the treatment of severe chronic pain or intractable spasticity; medications such as opioids, clonidine, and baclofen are delivered directly into the cerebrospinal fluid. Rarely, the care team may encounter ITP drug delivery devices in pregnant patients. The advantage of these systems lies in the ability to administer high-potency medications while minimizing systemic side effects; the intrathecal dose is substantially smaller than the equipotent/equianalgesic systemic dose (100 to 1000 times more potent, depending on the medication). An ITP system usually consists of a programmable reservoir placed subcutaneously in the lower abdomen and a tunneled catheter of variable length communicating between the reservoir and intrathecal space. The catheter tip is sited in the low thoracic or high lumbar region. There is little evidence or clinical experience to inform the healthcare team of the safety of these systems in pregnant women. The few case reports describing pregnant patients with ITPs have not described any adverse effects on the fetus or significant plasma levels of the medication in the neonate or in breast milk.

The anesthesia team should be knowledgeable of the drugs delivered through the ITP to recognize and mitigate complications associated with ITP drug overdose or withdrawal. Abrupt discontinuation of intrathecal medication has serious consequences. For example, withdrawal from baclofen may cause hallucinations, seizure, hypertonicity, hypermetabolic emergency, multiorgan system failure, and death. It is essential to ensure the ITP has adequate battery life, the reservoir is filled with appropriate medication(s), and the logistics regarding ITP use through pregnancy and peripartum are well organized.

There are no absolute contraindications to the provision of neuraxial analgesia or anesthesia in the patient with an ITP. Awareness of the entry level of the intrathecal catheter will allow the anesthesia provider to identify a spinal interspace (usually the lowest feasible) for the neuraxial anesthetic procedure. The pump system and the level of the ITP catheter can be identified by reviewing the ITP procedure report, communicating with the implanting physician, and reviewing plain radiographs. Other potential concerns are localized discomfort at the reservoir site with increasing abdominal size in pregnancy. Care should be taken during cesarean delivery to prevent violation of the pump pocket. Meticulous sterile precautions during the performance of neuraxial blockade may help prevent infectious complications.

SPECIFIC PAIN CONDITIONS IN PREGNANT WOMEN

Migraine

Migraines are more common in women, with a 3:1 sex prevalence ratio, explained by the influence of female sex hormones.[88] Approximately 25% of women of reproductive age experience migraines, and up to 80% of these women continue to report migraines during pregnancy.[89] However, migraine attacks tend to be most common during the first trimester and improve as pregnancy progresses,[90] secondary to stabilization of estrogen levels.

Optimization of lifestyle factors, such as stress, sleep, diet, and physical activity, is key to reduce the migraine attack occurrence.[91] Prophylaxis is recommended in pregnancy if women continue to experience frequent or prolonged severe attacks, especially if there is limited response to symptomatic treatment or significant nausea, vomiting, or evidence of fetal compromise.[92] A history of prepregnancy migraine is associated with a higher risk for preterm delivery, gestational hypertension, and preeclampsia compared with no migraine history. These increased risks may be mitigated by prepregnancy aspirin intake.[93]

Pharmacologic Approaches for Management of Migraine Headaches

Pharmacologic treatment and prophylactic medications from a migraine headache are summarized in Table 42.1.

Acetaminophen. A recent survey among women's healthcare providers reported that a majority of respondents felt "somewhat or very comfortable" with recommending or continuing acute treatments for pregnant women with migraine, with the highest comfort levels for treatment with acetaminophen and caffeine and higher discomfort levels with triptans.[94] In a study evaluating medication use during pregnancy in a cohort of women with migraines, the most commonly filled prescription before pregnancy was for a triptan (43.2%), followed by opioids (26.7%), acetaminophen (26.2%), antidepressants (24.9%), antiepileptics (18.6%), and antihypertensives (12.3%).[95] Antiepileptics, antidepressants, and triptans were frequently discontinued early in pregnancy with few new users, and opioids and acetaminophen were used intermittently throughout pregnancy.

Acetaminophen is thought to be safe during pregnancy and in breastfeeding mothers and is the first-line therapy for migraine headaches. Magnesium, both oral and intravenous formulations, is also thought to be safe and often efficacious in both acute treatment and headache prophylaxis.[96] Opioids have limited efficacy in migraine headaches and create a risk for OUD and medication overuse.

Triptans. Triptans are effective for treating acute migraine headaches. Of the seven triptans available worldwide, sumatriptan has the longest clinical experience and the greatest body of literature demonstrating safety in pregnancy and breastfeeding.[92] In a large study using the Swedish birth registry, among 3286 women using ergot alkaloids or triptans (mostly sumatriptan) in the first trimester and 1394 women using these medications after the first trimester, there was no association with congenital malformations.[97] In five women who received subcutaneous sumatriptan 6 mg, breast milk was collected hourly for 8 hours; the mean M/P ratio was 4.9.[98] The calculated RID of sumatriptan was 3.5%. Oral bioavailability of sumatriptan is low (approximately 15%); thus, the amount of sumatriptan that reaches the infant circulation

TABLE 42.1 Migraine Management During Pregnancy and Lactation

Medications	Considerations During Pregnancy	Consideration During Lactation
Treatment		
Acetaminophen	First-line therapy	First-line therapy
Triptans	Sumatriptan preferred	Eletriptan or sumatriptan preferred
Ergot alkaloids	Contraindicated	Limited data
Prophylaxis		
Beta-adrenergic blocking agents	Metoprolol and propranolol at lowest effective doses are first-line prophylactic medications	Compatible with breastfeeding
Calcium channel blocking agents	Verapamil is second-line prophylactic medication	Compatible with breastfeeding
Tricyclic antidepressants	Amitriptyline is an alternative second-line prophylactic medication	Compatible with breastfeeding
Anticonvulsants	Valproic acid and topiramate are considered teratogens and should not be used	Valproic acid: compatible with breastfeeding Topiramate: compatible with breastfeeding, but other medications should be considered first

during breastfeeding is likely exceedingly low. Given the limited data on other triptan medications, sumatriptan is the first choice among triptans for use during pregnancy.[92]

Eletriptan may be even safer than sumatriptan for breastfeeding mothers because its high plasma protein binding results in even lower concentrations in breast milk (M/P ratio 0.25).[99] Oral bioavailability is approximately 50%, and the estimated RID is 0.02%. Because data regarding the safety of the use of other triptans during breastfeeding are lacking, sumatriptan and eletriptan should be selected for lactating mothers.

Ergot alkaloids. Ergotamine and other ergot alkaloids that are used for migraine treatment are contraindicated during pregnancy because of known vasoconstrictive and uterotonic effects; the closely related drug, methylergonovine, is commonly used as a second-line agent for the treatment of uterine atony.

No systematic evidence of increased risk for congenital malformations exists for ergot alkaloids, but there are case reports of sirenomelia (fusion of the lower limbs, lower spinal column defects, and malformations of the urogenital and gastrointestinal tracts), renal agenesis, and urethral atresia associated with methylergonovine use in the first weeks of pregnancy.[100,101] The association has causal biological plausibility, as it is hypothesized that sirenomelia results from vascular insufficiency. Pregnant women who use ergot alkaloids for migraine headache treatment in the first and second trimesters, usually because the pregnancy is not recognized, should be assessed carefully, and ergot alkaloid therapy should be avoided once pregnancy is diagnosed.

Breastfeeding data for ergot alkaloids are limited.

Migraine Prophylaxis

Beta-adrenergic blocking agents. **Metoprolol** and **propranolol** at the lowest possible effective doses have been suggested as first-line medications for migraine prophylaxis in pregnancy. Beta-adrenergic blocking agents are frequently used in pregnancy for a variety of indications. The largest and most recent population-based study in five Nordic countries and the US Medicaid database assessed the risks for major congenital malformations associated with first-trimester exposure to beta-adrenergic blocking agents and found no overall increase in the risk for major congenital malformations.[102]

The increased volume of distribution and clearance during pregnancy requires that metoprolol dose and dosing frequency be increased to maintain efficacy.[103] Transfer across the placenta to the fetus with subsequent risk for neonatal bradycardia and hypoglycemia has been observed when these agents are used in the peripartum period; however, these medications have a long safety record when used to treat hypertension in women with preeclampsia.[32]

The AAP considers beta-adrenergic blocking agents to be compatible with breastfeeding.[32] Although metoprolol concentrates in breast milk (approximate M/P ratio, 3), no adverse effects have been observed in nursing infants. The reported propranolol M/P ratio ranges widely from 0.2 to 1.5.[32]

Calcium channel blocking agents. **Verapamil** has been recommended as the second-line prophylactic medication for migraine headache in breastfeeding women if beta-adrenergic blocking agents are contraindicated or ineffective.[99] Retrospective and prospective studies have not identified increased risk for major malformations with first-trimester use.[32] Data suggest a possible increase in preterm birth in patients taking verapamil; however, poor placental perfusion caused by hypertension, rather than a direct effect of hypertensive therapy, explains this finding.[104]

The AAP considers verapamil to be compatible with breastfeeding. The estimated RID is less than 0.01%; no adverse effects have been reported.[32]

Data are lacking for safety in pregnancy and breastfeeding for the newer calcium channel blocking agents, flunarizine and cinnarizine.

Tricyclic antidepressants. **Amitriptyline** has been used effectively for migraine prevention and has been suggested as an alternative second-line agent for migraine prevention in pregnancy.[105] Although data are conflicting, the risk for teratogenicity from early gestational exposure is likely low.

Anticonvulsants. **Valproic acid** and **topiramate** are two anticonvulsant medications with demonstrated efficacy in migraine prophylaxis. However, they are considered teratogens and should *not* be used in pregnant women for migraine headache prophylaxis.[92] Studies have shown an 11% risk for major congenital malformations, primarily an increased risk for cleft palate and neural tube defects, in infants with *in utero* topiramate exposure.[106] In addition, valproic acid use in late pregnancy has been associated with ASD, lower cognitive function, and lower intelligence in offspring.[106]

Valproic acid can be resumed for migraine prophylaxis in the postpartum period; the AAP believes the drug is compatible with breastfeeding.[32] Valproic acid is almost completely bound to plasma proteins. In a study of six nursing mothers who were receiving valproate for epilepsy, breast milk concentrations were less than or equal to 15% of the maternal serum concentration.[107] Infant serum levels of valproate were 0.9% to 2.3% of maternal values. However, one report described neonatal thrombocytopenia, anemia, and purpura that resolved after maternal discontinuation of valproate.[108] Thus, nursing infants exposed to valproic acid who exhibit thrombocytopenia or jaundice should have serum valproate levels measured.[99]

Topiramate is excreted into the breast milk.[32] The estimated M/P ratio is 0.86, and the RID is 3% to 23%.[32] Breastfeeding mothers who are taking topiramate should be advised to watch for adverse effects in their infants, including decreased alertness, fatigue, anorexia, and weight loss. Although topiramate is considered safe in breastfeeding mothers, its use for migraine prophylaxis should be considered only if other medications are contraindicated or ineffective.

Sickle Cell Disease

Pregnancy in women with SCD is associated with increased maternal and fetal morbidity and mortality, contributing to racial disparities and the elevated risk for severe maternal morbidity among Black women with SCD in the United States.[109]

Pregnancy is associated with an increased incidence of acute, painful **vaso-occlusive crises**, occurring between 9% and 17% of pregnant women with SCD.[110] **Acute chest syndrome** is a serious vaso-occlusive crisis affecting between 10% and 23% of pregnant women with SCD.[111–113] Factors thought to be associated with the increased incidence of crises in pregnancy include physical and psychological stress; dehydration, particularly in early pregnancy when hyperemesis is common; gestational anemia; the procoagulant state of pregnancy; and the increased risk of infection (urinary tract or influenza), which can precipitate a sickle crisis.[110]

Hydroxyurea, which reduces pain crises, acute chest syndrome, and blood transfusions in SCD, may be safe up to the time of conception, but caution regarding its use during pregnancy is advised due to the risk of miscarriage.[114,115]

BOX 42.2 Care of the Pregnant Patient With Sickle Cell Disease

- Discontinue hydroxyurea during pregnancy
- Avoid dehydration
- Minimize physical and psychosocial stress
- Uncomplicated vaso-occlusive crisis
  - Oral or intravenous hydration
  - Oral or intravenous analgesia
- Complicated vaso-occlusive crisis
  - Intravenous hydration
  - Aggressive treatment of pain (often with opioids[a])
  - Broad spectrum antibiotics, if indicated
  - Supplemental oxygen
  - Red blood cell transfusion to decrease hemoglobin S below 30%

[a]A controlled substance agreement plan should be discussed with the patient.

Women with SCD require individualized care plans, including transfusion therapy and management of acute pain (Box 42.2).[114] Women presenting with uncomplicated vaso-occlusive crises should be managed with oral or intravenous hydration and analgesics. Pain caused by an uncomplicated vaso-occlusive crisis may last up to 2 weeks and red blood cell transfusion is usually not recommended.

Acute chest syndrome is diagnosed by imaging findings consistent with a new pulmonary infiltrate and one additional item (oxygen desaturation, cough, temperature $\geq$ 38.5°C, tachypnea, wheezing). Treatment of complicated vaso-occlusive crises, including acute chest syndrome, requires hydration and aggressive pain management (typically intravenous opioids), along with broad-spectrum antibiotics, supplemental oxygen, and blood transfusions to decrease hemoglobin S (HbS) to to less than 30%.

A tailored opioid-dosing plan and controlled substance agreement should be outlined to facilitate optimal pain management.[114] Findings from a retrospective analysis from the 2002 to 2014 National Inpatient Sample database suggest that pregnant women with SCD have a fourfold increased risk for OUD compared with pregnant women without SCD.[116] The risk of neonatal opioid withdrawal syndrome (NOWS) has been reported to be relatively high, likely due to the *in utero* exposure to opioids.[117]

Chronic Low Back Pain

Preexisting LBP is reported in 2% of women who become pregnant, but more than two-thirds of women complain of back pain during pregnancy.[118] Back pain persists postpartum in approximately 25% of women, and there is a significant relapse in subsequent pregnancies.[119] Three pregnancy-related changes have been suggested to contribute to lumbopelvic pain: (1) hormonal changes, resulting in ligament hyperlaxity and joint instability; (2) biomechanical changes causing postural changes; and (3) neuromuscular adaptation with a decrease in the endurance of the pelvic floor muscles.[120] Angles of lordosis and kyphosis of the spine may increase during pregnancy, and postural control is reduced.[121] Recent data suggest that pregnancy is a significant life event associated with a risk of functionally significant LBP, even decades after women gave birth.[122] Referral to transitional pain services, a new concept and framework to treat patients at risk of progressing from acute to chronic pain, has been proposed for pregnant women as well as other at-risk postsurgical patients, particularly in the setting of pregnancy-related PGP.[123]

Nonpharmacologic Interventions for Management of Low Back Pain

The use of nonpharmacologic interventions on LBP in pregnancy was evaluated in a 2021 systematic review and meta-analysis which included six randomized trials (693 pregnant participants); exercise, muscle relaxation exercises accompanied by music and transcutaneous electrical nerve stimulation (TENS) were more effective than the other types of interventions (kinesio tape, yoga, and ear acupuncture) in the treatment of pregnancy-related LBP.[124]

Exercise, stretching, and Pilates. In a 2015 Cochrane review combining the results from seven studies (645 women) comparing any land-based exercise with usual prenatal care, exercise interventions (lasting from 5 to 20 weeks) improved LBP and disability during pregnancy.[118] A 2023 systematic review and metaanalysis included 16 randomized controlled trials (1885 pregnant participants) with PGP or LBP; women randomized to the exercise group had lower pain scores, although the difference did not reach statistical significance.[125] In a single-center study, standardized postural stretching, a nondynamic technique using muscular contractions and stretches, appeared to be beneficial when practiced for a period of 8 weeks.[126] Reports on the effect of Pilates exercises on LBP in pregnancy seem promising, although the quality of these studies is low.[127–129]

Acupuncture. In a 2023 systematic review and metaanalysis of 12 randomized controlled trials involving 1302 pregnant women, the efficacy and safety of acupuncture, combined with other treatments for managing LBP, was evaluated; acupuncture significantly reduced pain scores.[130]

Chiropractic care. An expert panel convened in 2019 to develop the first best-practice consensus statement on chiropractic care for pregnant and postpartum patients with LBP or PGP.[131] Studies implementing the panel's recommendations are needed to determine whether chiropractic care is beneficial.

Pelvic Girdle Pain

Chronic PGP in women represents a diagnostic challenge as multiple pelvic pain syndromes often overlap in the same patient, along with other nonpelvic pain conditions, such as migraine, chronic fatigue, and fibromyalgia.[132]

The prevalence of pregnancy-related PGP is high; a systematic review and metaanalysis of 38 studies (n = 21,533 pregnant participants) estimated a pooled prevalence of 58%.[133] Ten percent of women with PGP continue to suffer up to 10 years later, with chronic LBP as a predictor for long-term

PGP.[134] Although common, the exact pathophysiology of PGP remains poorly understood, involving both hormonal and biomechanical changes that occur during pregnancy.[135] Pelvic pain can originate from various elements of the pelvic girdle, including the sacroiliac joints and pubic symphysis. These joints are stabilized by thick ligaments that usually do not allow much motion. Increasing estrogen and progesterone in pregnancy causes softening of the ligaments, allowing important skeletal reconfiguration to support the enlarging fetus and delivery. The FABER (flexion, abduction, and external rotation of the lower extremity) sign is commonly positive, and overextension during delivery, particularly in the setting of neuraxial analgesia (which can mask pain caused by maternal malposition) should be avoided. Similar to other persistent pain conditions in women, pregnancy may be the condition that initiates long-term lumbopelvic pain.

In a scoping review of risk factors for pregnancy-related PGP, a history of LBP or PGP, obesity, prior pregnancy, younger age, lower educational level, no prepregnancy exercise, physically demanding work, previous back trauma or disease, progestin-intrauterine device use, stress, depression, and anxiety were associated with experiencing PGP.[136] In a 2023 study evaluating risk factors for developing PGP, the most significant predictor of pregnancy-related pain in the second and third trimesters was the experience of similar pain in the first trimester.[137] Depressive symptoms identified early in pregnancy are associated with the onset and severity of PGP later in the pregnancy,[138] while generalized joint hypermobility does not increase the risk of PGP during or postpregnancy.[139] However, women with obesity in association with hypermobility reported greater pain intensity early in their pregnancy.[139]

Prevention and Management of Pelvic Girdle Pain

Exercise. Numerous studies have assessed the effect of stabilizing exercises in preventing pregnancy-related PGP, with limited evidence that it is effective.[119,140] The quality of six studies included in a 2023 systematic review and meta-analysis assessing prevention of PGP was judged very low to moderate, and no conclusions could be drawn regarding the efficacy of prevention measures.[141]

Acupuncture, transcutaneous electrical nerve stimulation, and complementary manual therapies. Management of PGP with acupuncture or TENS has been shown to help maintain function and physical activity, with decreased pain and concerns about pain, suggesting either intervention can be recommended as a nonpharmacologic approach.[142] However, there is limited evidence to support the use of complementary manual therapies for LBP or PGP.[143]

Fibromyalgia

Fibromyalgia is a common pain syndrome in young women associated with central nervous system sensitization to pain. In addition to pain, fibromyalgia presents with a broad range of symptoms, such as sleep disruption, chronic fatigue, brain fog, depression, muscle stiffness, and migraine.[144]

Fibromyalgia may be diagnosed if all of the following criteria are met: (1) generalized pain, defined as pain in at least four or five regions; (2) symptoms present at a similar level for at least 3 months, widespread pain index (WPI) $\geq$ 7, and symptom severity scale (SSS) score $\geq$ 5 or WPI of 4 to 6 and SSS score $\geq$ 9.[145] A diagnosis of fibromyalgia does not exclude the presence of other clinically important illnesses.[145]

Women with fibromyalgia usually experience an aggravation of symptoms in pregnancy, particularly during the third trimester and after childbirth.[144] LBP is the most common complaint and fatigue is the most common symptom in pregnant women with fibromyalgia, along with anxiety, fear of childbirth, and depression.[146] Symptoms of fibromyalgia, especially pain in various parts of the body and generalized fatigue, may be difficult to differentiate from normal symptoms of pregnancy; therefore, a definitive diagnosis of fibromyalgia should not be made during pregnancy.

Lifestyle modifications, including sleep hygiene and exercise, are mainstays for the treatment of fibromyalgia during and outside of pregnancy. Migraine headaches may occur in women with fibromyalgia, and migraine management is helpful. Duloxetine and pregabalin may be given to pregnant women diagnosed with severe forms of fibromyalgia after carefully weighing the benefits and risks for both mother and fetus.[147]

MANAGEMENT OF INTRACTABLE PAIN AFTER DELIVERY

Most healthy patients have low postdelivery pain scores and well-controlled postdelivery pain using the normal multimodal approaches to treat pain (see Chapter 27), making it difficult to identify benefits to adding adjuvant therapies.[148] However, patients with chronic pain syndromes may report more severe postdelivery pain than patients without chronic pain because of sensitization and tolerance to systemic opioids. Women with OUD receiving MOUD may also have pain not responsive to the usual multimodal approaches for postdelivery analgesia. Patient-specific tailored approaches with analgesic adjuvants should be considered in patients with a history of, or risk factors for, severe acute postpartum pain. Although not robustly evaluated, several strategies are proposed (Table 42.2).[149]

Opioid-sparing approaches should include: (1) stepwise, multimodal analgesia, with scheduled NSAIDs and acetaminophen, which is the mainstay for enhanced recovery in all women undergoing cesarean delivery; and (2) a shared decision-making, patient-driven model, with realistic analgesic goals, and appropriate patient-reported outcome measures.

Intravenous or Oral Opioids

Systemic opioids have been considered the usual "rescue" strategy for postoperative breakthrough pain, particularly in the United States; however, other modalities for an

TABLE 42.2 Enhanced Analgesic Strategies for Severe Acute Postcesarean Pain

Standard Multimodal Opioid-Sparing Analgesia	
Systemic Nonopioid Analgesia[a] • Acetaminophen 1 g every 6–8h • Ibuprofen 600mg every 6h	**Neuraxial Medication**[b] Morphine—enhanced or repeated dose • Intrathecal 150–300 µg • Epidural 3mg × one dose • Epidural 2–3mg every 12–18h Bupivacaine low concentration with fentanyl 2µg/mL ± clonidine 1–2µg/mL via PIEB + PCEA
Enhanced Analgesia With Systemic or Neuraxial Adjuvants, or Regional Blocks	
Systemic Analgesia—Rescue • Gabapentin oral 150–300mg every 8h • Ketamine IV 0.1–0.3mg/kg/h • Dexmedetomidine IV 0.2–0.7µg/kg/h • Hydromorphone IV PCA	**Neuraxial Adjuvant and Regional Nerve Blocks** Clonidine—Neuraxial • Intrathecal 30–60µg • Epidural 100µg TAP blocks (local anesthetic) • Consider catheters QL blocks (local anesthetic) Ilioinguinal and iliohypogastric nerve blocks (local anesthetic)

IV, Intravenous; *PCA,* patient-controlled analgesia; *PCEA,* patient-controlled epidural analgesia; *PIEB,* programmed intermittent epidural bolus; *QL,* quadratus lumborum; *TAP,* transversus abdominis plane.
[a]Systemic analgesia agents should be administered on a regular schedule.
[b]Epidural catheter may remain *in situ* for several days after cesarean delivery for continuous or intermittent medication delivery.

opioid-balanced (or even opioid-free) approach may be preferable to avoid persistent opioid use. In a 2023 systematic review of four studies from the United States, rates of persistent opioid use after cesarean delivery ranged from 0.12% to 2.2%, with the highest rate reported in patients with private insurance, emphasizing the significant number of women at risk (from 1:1000 to 1:50) for persistent opioid use up to 12 months postpartum.[64]

Neuraxial and Systemic Alpha$_2$-Adrenergic Agonist Adjuvants

Alpha$_2$-adrenergic agonists may be beneficial in women with OUD. **Epidural clonidine** in lieu of fentanyl has been used for postcesarean analgesia in women with OUD, in combination with a continuous infusion of low-concentration bupivacaine (bupivacaine 0.0625% or 0.1% with clonidine 1.2 to 2µg/mL) with good analgesic outcomes.[150] A retrospective observational study found intrathecal clonidine in patients with OUD was associated with a reduced 24-hour opioid use after cesarean delivery[151]; however, this has not been rigorously studied in women with chronic pain or OUD. A case report described the use of an intravenous dexmedetomidine infusion (titrated from 0.2 to 0.7µg/kg/h) to treat postcesarean pain in a woman receiving methadone (80mg/day) therapy, who, after receiving intrathecal morphine (200µg), experienced severe acute pain; the infusion was maintained for 20 hours.[152]

Intravenous Ketamine

Ketamine, a competitive NMDA-receptor antagonist, may be beneficial in patients with opioid tolerance, as it may prevent opioid-induced tolerance and opioid withdrawal.[153,154] The concurrent use of buprenorphine, methadone, or naltrexone does not appear to interact with the antidepressant effect of ketamine.[155]

Evidence of successful use of ketamine for postpartum analgesia is sparse, but has been reported in two pregnant women with SCD[156]; for burn surgery during pregnancy[157]; and after a cesarean delivery in a woman with buprenorphine maintenance therapy, for whom a ketamine infusion 2µg/kg/min was used for 12 hours.[158] In two systematic reviews, including women undergoing cesarean delivery, postoperative opioid use and pain severity were lower in patients receiving ketamine.[159,160]

Neuraxial Postcesarean Analgesia

Peripartum epidural analgesia is effective with low-concentration local anesthetics (e.g., bupivacaine 0.0625%) and adjuvants (e.g., fentanyl and/or clonidine). In two reports, two women with receiving chronic buprenorphine therapy were managed with lumbar and low-thoracic epidural analgesia after cesarean delivery[161]; in both cases, neuraxial opioids were omitted. A retrospective observational study reported the use of epidural clonidine in women on buprenorphine maintenance therapy.[150] Epidural hydromorphone was reported to be very effective in a patient using high doses of methadone for her second cesarean delivery.[162] Although not published, our institution uses intrathecal clonidine (0.5 to 1.0µg/kg) at the time of delivery and repeated doses of epidural morphine (2 mg every 12 hours or 3 mg every 18 hours) in opioid-tolerant patients; this technique provides prolonged and effective analgesia, without affecting the ability to ambulate.

Abdominal Wall Blocks

Regional anesthesia/analgesia techniques, including abdominal wall blocks, have been proposed as a component of multimodal postcesarean analgesia to improve postpartum recovery. These blocks may facilitate earlier hospital discharge and minimize opioid use as part of enhanced recovery protocols.[163] **Transversus abdominis plane (TAP), quadratus lumborum** and **erector spinae plane blocks** may be performed if neuraxial opioid analgesia is not possible or if rescue analgesia is needed (see Chapter 27).[164] The use of liposomal bupivacaine or the addition of dexmedetomidine to the local anesthetic used for the block has been suggested, but these techniques have not been evaluated in women with chronic pain or opioid tolerance.

The analgesic and antihyperalgesic effects of several classes of drugs, including NMDA antagonists and alpha$_2$-adrenergic agonists, warrant further studies to confirm their potential benefits to treat persistent pain after cesarean delivery and prevent the transition from acute to chronic pain.

TRANSITION FROM ACUTE TO CHRONIC PAIN AFTER CHILDBIRTH

In a new, 2019 classification by the International Association for the Study of Pain,[165] chronic postsurgical and posttraumatic pain was defined as: "pain that develops or increases in intensity after a surgical procedure or a tissue injury and persists beyond the healing process (i.e., at least 3 months after the surgery or tissue trauma)." This definition is included in the International Classification of Diseases (ICD-11). The classification distinguishes between tissue trauma arising from a controlled procedure in the delivery of healthcare (surgery) and forms of uncontrolled accidental damage (other traumas). A previous cesarean delivery is a risk factor for the development of chronic pain after a hysterectomy.[165]

It may be challenging to determine whether the postpartum pain experienced by some women is the result of tissue injury that occurred during delivery, and thus qualifies as persistent pain after childbirth, or whether the pain is better defined as chronic pelvic pain, pain that that existed prior to delivery, or pain at other locations.[123,166,167]

Epidemiology

The prevalence of persistent pain after abdominal hysterectomy with a Pfannenstiel incision is significantly higher after hysterectomy (up to 20% at 6 to 12 months after a hysterectomy) than after a cesarean delivery with the same incision (4% at 6 to 12 months).[168,169] This is a striking difference given that preoperative pain (abdominal or pelvic pain, as well as pain elsewhere in the body) and postoperative pain are significant risk factors in both populations. It has been proposed that the small number of patients with new and persistent pain after cesarean and vaginal delivery may be attributed to a protective effect of peripartum exposure to oxytocin on the transition of acute to chronic pain.[170–172]

Nonetheless, the reported number of women with persistent pain after childbirth varies widely, in part related to differences in study design (retrospective or prospective) and the population studied (all deliveries, scheduled cesarean deliveries). Some studies with very high estimates (up to 20%) used a retrospective cohort design that suffers from recall bias. Others with lower estimates (1% to 3%) discontinued prospective follow-up of enrolled patients at the first report of no pain and may have missed those with episodic symptoms.

Although most women have an uneventful recovery and use opioids only briefly in the peripartum period, a 2019 systematic review of 17 studies evaluating chronic pain up to 6 months after cesarean delivery reported rates that varied between 4% and 42%.[173] Severe acute pain was the strongest predictive factor for chronic pain. In a 2024 systematic review and metaanalysis evaluating studies published between January 2015 and September 2022 (50 studies involving 13,149 patients), the incidence of scar-specific chronic pain that interfered with daily life, work, social life, and personal care was 16.7% between 3 and 6 months after cesarean delivery, 11.4% between 6 and 12 months, and 8.8% after 12 months.[174] This updated metaanalysis shows that the incidence of chronic pain after cesarean delivery has remained unchanged for the past 20 years, despite efforts to improve management of acute postoperative pain with multimodal analgesia strategies. It also refutes early suggestions that chronic pain after cesarean delivery might not exist.[175,176]

Current research investigating patient-reported outcomes with validated tools should allow better evaluation of the incidence of persistent and chronic pain after childbirth.[177] The reported incidence of chronic pain will likely evolve with a better understanding of how to prevent acute and persistent postpartum pain and the ability to measure it more accurately.

Risk Factors and Predictors for Acute, Persistent, and Chronic Pain After Delivery

Risk factors associated with persistent pain after childbirth include maternal factors, obstetric factors, and anesthesia-related factors.[166] The presence of intrinsic (patient-specific) and extrinsic factors (surgical and anesthesia-specific) should help predict severe acute pain, persistent pain, and chronic pain since the transition from acute to chronic pain is associated with these factors (Box 42.3).[14]

Measurement of predictive factors with validated scales may be useful in identifying a subset of women for whom enhanced treatment of acute postsurgical pain with multimodal analgesia may prevent the transition from acute to chronic pain.[178] One such example of a predictive test is the evaluation of pain during local anesthesia infiltration before spinal anesthesia for cesarean delivery; the degree of pain during infiltration has been shown to be associated with acute postoperative pain and increased analgesic use,[179] and more recently, with persistent pain 1 month after cesarean delivery.[180]

BOX 42.3 Risk Factors for Pain During and After Pregnancy

Prepregnancy and During Pregnancy
- Chronic pain before pregnancy (migraine, back pain, pelvic girdle pain)
- Anxiety
- Depression
- Stress
- Sleep deprivation
- Genetics/epigenetic factors

Acute Pain Immediately After Delivery[a]
- Opioid use during pregnancy
- Sleep deprivation before delivery
- Residual scar hyperalgesia from previous cesarean delivery
- Pain during local anesthetic infiltration for neuraxial anesthesia
- Poor mental health
- Uterine exteriorization during repair
- General anesthesia
- Pfannenstiel incision

Persistent and Chronic Pain
- Prepregnancy pain (migraine, back pain)
- Pain during pregnancy
- Severe acute postpartum pain
- Recurrent Pfannenstiel incision
- Neuropathic pain present 1 w postpartum

[a]There is no evidence that acute postpartum pain and persistent pain are influenced by mode of delivery, but women who deliver by cesarean use more opioid analgesia for a longer period of time than women who delivery vaginally.

Depression, anxiety, sleep deprivation, and disability, in addition to being risk factors for the development of chronic pain, are predictable consequences of severe acute pain, thus creating a positive reinforcing cycle. Interruption of this cycle by predicting and treating severe pain after delivery may be critical to preventing the development of acute severe and chronic pain. Identification and treatment of coexisting psychological distress and sleep disorders are key to effective postoperative pain management and may prevent conversion of acute to chronic pain.

A large prospective study followed women after planned vaginal delivery until resolution of pain, opioid use, and functional recovery (composite outcome).[181] Factors predicting the longest resolution of the composite outcome were investigated. Even after a correction for mode of delivery, the induction of labor was strongly predictive of more severe pain, prolonged opioid use, and delayed functional recovery. Cesarean delivery was predictive of a longer use of opioid analgesics compared with a vaginal delivery.[181]

Previous Chronic Pain

The strongest predictor of postpartum pain is previous chronic pain, most often back pain and migraines.[167] Additionally, in women without a history of chronic pain, severe pain in the early postpartum period is associated with persistent pain after childbirth.[8] This association could result from inflammation and nerve injury causing long-term synaptic plasticity, amplifying and maintaining pain signaling (pain sensitization). Peripheral pain sensitization is associated with wound hyperalgesia and exaggerated acute postoperative pain.[13] Central sensitization causes secondary hyperalgesia, and chronic postsurgical pain occurs when there is an imbalance between pain inhibition and facilitation.[14]

Acute and Persistent Pain

There is growing evidence that acute pain, particularly with a neuropathic component, is associated with persistent and chronic pain. Central sensitization, identified as residual scar hyperalgesia from a previous cesarean delivery, was identified in up to 40% of women undergoing planned repeat cesarean delivery and was associated with severe acute postcesarean pain.[182] In a large prospective observational cohort study (n = 610), the incidence of persistent pain at 3 months and chronic pain at 12 months was 6.2% and 1%, respectively.[183] The presence of neuropathic pain 1 week after cesarean delivery was associated with an increased risk of chronic pain after cesarean delivery (aOR, 1.63; 95% CI, 1.26 to 2.11).[183]

Anxiety and Depression

The severity of postdelivery pain and the likelihood of developing chronic pain after childbirth are associated with maternal depression and anxiety.[166,178] Higher prenatal State Anxiety Scale scores are associated with higher mean pain scores and greater opioid consumption within the first several days after cesarean delivery.[184] Similarly, in a large French cohort, persistent pain 6 months after cesarean delivery was also associated with preoperative anxiety.[185]

Depression is also closely linked with chronic pain. Both prepregnancy anxiety and depression were predictive of pain symptoms (fatigue, back pain, muscle pain, dyspepsia, obstipation) during pregnancy and postpartum.[186] In a large, prospectively followed cohort, women with severe acute postpartum pain had a threefold increased risk for postpartum depression compared with women who had mild postpartum pain.[8]

Sleep Deprivation and Stress

Sleep deprivation accentuates pain, and pain, in turn, interrupts sleep, creating a vicious cycle that commonly exacerbates pain after delivery. Painful labor lasting many hours to days may precede delivery. In a study evaluating sleep quality in the week preceding a scheduled cesarean delivery, women with poor sleep (assessed using the Pittsburgh Sleep Quality Index score) reported significantly higher pain scores.[187]

Tissue Injury and Surgical Technique

Surgical technique, tissue injury, and nerve entrapment have been investigated in the setting of chronic pain after cesarean delivery.[188–192] The Misgav-Ladach incision is associated with a lower incidence of acute and chronic pain after a cesarean delivery than a Pfannenstiel incision.[188] A repeat Pfannenstiel incision is associated with an increased risk for chronic pain after cesarean delivery,[193] due to the greater risk for nerve entrapment and chronic inguinal pain. Nerve entrapment may be relieved with tender-point infiltration and surgical neurectomy.[188,190,194] Uterine exteriorization during repair of the uterus after cesarean delivery is also shown to increase the risk for chronic pain.[183] It is not known whether an emergency cesarean compared with a scheduled cesarean delivery increases the risk for chronic pain, although it may increase the risk of nerve damage in the incisional area.

Anesthesia Factors

Acute pain after delivery is significantly associated with persistent and chronic pain; general anesthesia compared with neuraxial anesthesia for cesarean delivery is also reported as a strong predictor.[8,167,173,178] This observation underscores the recommendations that multimodal, opioid-sparing analgesic strategies are important, not only for early recovery pathways, but likely also for long-term recovery after childbirth.

CHARACTERISTICS OF CHRONIC PAIN AFTER DELIVERY

In women with new-onset chronic pain after cesarean delivery, scar pain is the most commonly reported type of pain,[175] with a neuropathic component attributed to the suprapubic Pfannenstiel incision, which can entrap the ilioinguinal or iliohypogastric nerves.[195] In some instances, women report tingling and itching as their main symptoms, which may not be characterized as painful, but may nonetheless be very uncomfortable.[196]

In some women, new-onset pelvic pain is reported, as described in the Norwegian Mother and Child Cohort Study (1999 to 2008) cohort that included more than 20,000 women without preexisting pelvic pain in pregnancy. Acute pain associated with new-onset pelvic pain was reported by 4.5% of women 3 months after delivery.[197]

Another long-term complication of cesarean delivery is an unhealed defect in the uterine myometrium, which is referred to as a uterine niche or **cesarean scar defect**. This is defined as an "indentation in the uterine myometrium of at least 2 mm at the site of the cesarean scar assessed by transvaginal ultrasound," and is observed in 60% of women after a cesarean delivery.[198] In the newly established criteria to diagnose a cesarean scar disorder, chronic pelvic pain was defined as one important symptom.[198]

PREVENTION OF CHRONIC PAIN AFTER CESAREAN DELIVERY

In a 2023 systematic review and network metaanalysis of studies evaluating nonopioid analgesics for the prevention of chronic postsurgical pain in adults undergoing any surgical procedure, 132 randomized controlled trials that included 23,902 adult patients found intravenous lidocaine (OR, 0.32; 95% credible interval [CrI], 0.17 to 0.58), ketamine (OR, 0.64; 95% CrI, 0.44 to 0.92), gabapentinoids (OR, 0.67; 95% CrI, 0.47 to 0.92), and possibly dexmedetomidine (OR, 0.36; 95% CrI, 0.12 to 1.00) reduced the incidence of chronic postsurgical pain at 6 months.[50]

Regional anesthesia, including neuraxial adjuvants and abdominal wall blocks, has been proposed as a strategy to prevent central sensitization and, therefore, reduce the incidence of persistent postoperative pain by blocking the barrage of pain signals with a local anesthetic nerve blockade (Table 42.3).[62,195,199–203] In a 2019 update of a systematic review and metaanalysis on the effect of local anesthetics (by any route) or regional anesthesia versus any combination of systemic (opioid or nonopioid) analgesia in adults or children on any pain outcomes beyond 3 months, data from 39 studies were pooled; four studies were randomized controlled trials in women undergoing cesarean delivery (n = 551 cases).[204] Chronic pain after cesarean delivery was markedly lower when regional methods were used compared to control groups without the use or regional anesthesia (OR, 0.46; 95% CI, 0.28 to 0.78; P = .0004). Some trials have included analgesic adjuvants in the spinal anesthetic, including morphine[200] or clonidine[62] to reduce central sensitization and affect hyperalgesia. Another trial evaluated the effect of TAP blocks with or without clonidine to reduce wound hyperalgesia and potentially prevent chronic pain.[199] Spinal clonidine reduced wound hyperalgesia, but the addition of clonidine to a TAP block in healthy women undergoing cesarean delivery did not impact short- or long-term pain outcomes, although pain scores were low in all groups.

A 2024 systematic review and metaanalysis on the analgesic effects of quadratus lumborum block (QLB) on acute and chronic pain after cesarean delivery included 21 studies (n = 1976 patients); 4 studies reported the incidence of chronic pain after cesarean delivery at 3 months and 4 studies reported on the incidence of pain at 6 months. No beneficial effect of QLB in reducing acute pain was identified, but the analysis was inconclusive for the outcome of incidence of chronic pain.[202]

Ultrasound-guided bilateral ilioinguinal and iliohypogastric nerve blocks (bupivacaine) significantly reduced the incidence of pain at 3 and 6 months in one small randomized controlled trial,[195] and continuous wound infusion for 48 hours had a beneficial effect on wound hyperalgesia but did not impact the incidence of chronic pain.[205]

Due to the challenges in evaluating chronic pain, its relative rare occurrence, study methodologic issues (small sample sizes) and selection bias (scheduled cesarean deliveries in women at low risk for pain), no intervention has been reliably identified as having a protective effect on chronic pain after childbirth.

TABLE 42.3   Clinical Trials With Strategies to Reduce Postoperative Hyperalgesia and Prevent Chronic Pain After Cesarean Delivery[a]

Adjuvant or Technique	Study Type	Finding	Effect
Spinal morphine[200] • Placebo • Morphine 100 µg	Placebo-controlled RCT (n = 290)	*Pain at 3 mo:* 19% versus 18% (control) *Pain at 6 mo:* 16% versus 14% (control) (OR, 1.23; 95% CI, 0.63 to 2.38)	No measurable effect
Spinal clonidine[62] Bupivacaine with: • Sufentanil 2 µg • Sufentanil 2 µg + clonidine 75 µg • Clonidine 150 µg (no spinal morphine)	Placebo-controlled RCT (n = 96)	*Wound hyperalgesia at 48 h:* 41% without clonidine 34% with clonidine 75 µg 16% with clonidine 150 µg (P = .03) *Pain at 3 mo:* 17%, 22%, 3% (ns) *Pain at 6 mo:* 7%, 12%, 3% (ns)	Antihyperalgesic effect with clonidine 150 µg
TAP with clonidine[199] • Placebo • Bupivacaine • Bupivacaine ± clonidine 150 µg (spinal morphine 100 µg)	Placebo-controlled RCT (n = 90)	*Wound hyperalgesia at 48 h:* 20% with placebo 12% with bupivacaine 23% with bupivacaine/clonidine (ns) *Pain intensity (0–10 scale) at 3 mo:* 0.1, 0.24, 0 (ns) *Neuropathic pain descriptors at 3 mo:* 59%, 52%, 58% (ns) *Pain intensity (0–10 scale) at 6 mo:* 0.04, 0, 0 (ns) *Neuropathic pain descriptors at 6 mo:* 54%, 38%, 58% (ns) *Pain intensity (0–10 scale) at 12 mo:* 0, 0, 0 (ns) *Neuropathic pain descriptors at 12 mo:* 39%, 14%, 22% (ns)	No benefit of TAP block with or without clonidine 1 in 4 women reported some itching, tingling, or numbness at 12 mo
QLB versus TAP block (ropivacaine 0.375%) versus control[201] (no spinal opioid)	RCT (n = 105)	*Pain at 3 mo:* QLB 48% TAP 60% Control 61% (ns) *Pain at 6 mo:* QLB 32% TAP 45% Control 57% (ns)	Lower chronic pain intensity in QLB group at 6 mo (NPSI score)
QLB versus no/sham block[202]	Systematic review and metaanalysis 21 studies (n = 1976): five studies reported on chronic pain after cesarean delivery	*Pain at 3 mo:* No significant difference (OR, 0.41; 95% CI, 0.09 to 1.88) *Pain at 6 mo:* No significant difference (OR, 0.83; 95% CI, 0.33 to 2.07)	Underpowered to determine a difference between QLB and no/sham block
Ilioinguinal/iliohypogastric block (bupivacaine 0.25%) versus no block[195] (no spinal opioid)	Placebo-controlled RCT (n = 64)	*Pain at 3 mo:* 10% (block) versus 33% (P = .028) *Pain at 6 mo:* 3% (block) versus 20% (P = .044)	Lower incidence of chronic pain with block
Continuous wound infusion (levobupivacaine 0.35% for 48 h) versus saline placebo[203] (spinal fentanyl, no morphine)	Placebo-controlled RCT (n = 70)	*Pain at 3 mo:* 27% versus 19% (ns) *Pain at 6 mo:* 15% versus 3% (ns) *Pain at 12 mo:* 3% versus 5% (ns)	Antihyperalgesic effect at 24 and 48 h

CI, Confidence interval; *NPSI*, Neuropathic Pain Symptom Inventory; *ns*, nonsignificant; *OR*, odds ratio; *QLB*, quadratus lumborum block; *RCT*, randomized controlled trial; *TAP*, transversus abdominis plane.
[a]Trials were conducted in healthy women undergoing scheduled cesarean delivery with spinal anesthesia.

KEY POINTS

- The prevalence of chronic headache, back pain, pelvic girdle pain, and fibromyalgia is high in women of reproductive age; these conditions are common during pregnancy.
- Multimodal pain management, including medication, psychological support, and physical therapy, is key to support women with chronic pain throughout pregnancy.
- Transitional pain services may be helpful to establish referral criteria, pathways, and effective strategies to decrease the transition from acute to chronic pain during pregnancy, peripartum, and postpartum.
- Interventional pain injections may contribute to optimal pain control during pregnancy and can be guided by ultrasonography to minimize fetal exposure to ionizing radiation.
- Knowledge of the pharmacokinetics and pharmacodynamics of medications used for the management of chronic pain, as well as changes induced by pregnancy and possible interactions with pregnancy and breastfeeding, are important to tailoring medication management during pregnancy and the postpartum period.
- Management of patients with opioid use disorder throughout pregnancy and peripartum can be challenging and requires a multispecialty team that includes an addiction specialist.
- Women who take chronic opioids during pregnancy are at risk for tolerance, and the neonate is at risk for opioid withdrawal syndrome.
- Risk factors for chronic pain after delivery include chronic pain before pregnancy, pain during pregnancy, anxiety, depression, stress, sleep deprivation, and acute pain.
- Acute pain after delivery should be prevented, as this may decrease the risk for persistent and chronic pain (the transition from acute to chronic pain).

REFERENCES

1. Rikard SM, Strahan AE, Schmit KM, Guy GP Jr. Chronic pain among adults—United States, 2019–2021. *MMWR Morb Mortal Wkly Rep.* 2023;72:379–385.
2. Dalton VK, Pangori A, As-Sanie S, et al. Trends in chronic pain conditions among delivering women with and without mood and anxiety disorders. *Gen Hosp Psychiatry.* 2023;84:142–148.
3. U.S. Department of Health and Human Services, Centers for Disease Control and Prevention, National Center for Health Statistics. Health, United States, 2016: With chartbook on long-term trends in health; 2017. Available at: https://www.cdc.gov/nchs/data/hus/hus16.pdf. Accessed 2 February 2025.
4. Maurer AJ, Lissounov A, Knezevic I, et al. Pain and sex hormones: a review of current understanding. *Pain Manag.* 2016;6:285–296.
5. Ray-Griffith SL, Morrison B, Stowe ZN. Chronic pain prevalence and exposures during pregnancy. *Pain Res Manag.* 2019;2019:6985164.
6. Ray-Griffith SL, Wendel MP, Stowe ZN, Magann EF. Chronic pain during pregnancy: a review of the literature. *Int J Womens Health.* 2018;10:153–164.
7. Raja SN, Carr DB, Cohen M, et al. The revised International Association for the Study of Concepts, challenges, and compromises. *Pain.* 2020;161:1976–1982.
8. Eisenach JC, Pan PH, Smiley R, et al. Severity of acute pain after childbirth, but not type of delivery, predicts persistent pain and postpartum depression. *Pain.* 2008;140:87–94.
9. American College of Obstetricians and Gynecologists. Clinical Practice Guideline No. 5: Treatment and management of mental health conditions during pregnancy and postpartum. *Obstet Gynecol.* 2023;141:1262–1288.
10. American College of Obstetricians and Gynecologists. Clinical Practice Guideline No. 4: Screening and diagnosis of mental health conditions during pregnancy and postpartum. *Obstet Gynecol.* 2023;141:1232–1261.
11. Boutib A, Chergaoui S, Marfak A, et al. Quality of life during pregnancy from 2011 to 2021: systematic review. *Int J Womens Health.* 2022;14:975–1005.
12. Munro A, George RB, Chorney J, et al. Prevalence and predictors of chronic pain in pregnancy and postpartum. *J Obstet Gynaecol Can.* 2017;39:734–741.
13. Latremoliere A, Woolf CJ. Central sensitization: a generator of pain hypersensitivity by central neural plasticity. *J Pain.* 2009;10:895–926.
14. Richebe P, Capdevila X, Rivat C. Persistent postsurgical pain: pathophysiology and preventative pharmacologic considerations. *Anesthesiology.* 2018;129:590–607.
15. Shapiro M, Sujan AC, Guille C. A clinical trial of a program for pain management and opioid reduction during pregnancy. *Reprod Sci.* 2022;29:606–613.
16. Filippini C, Saran S, Chari B. Musculoskeletal steroid injections in pregnancy: a review. *Skeletal Radiol.* 2023;52:1465–1473.
17. Donaldson M, Goodchild JH. Analgesics in pregnancy and lactation: safe medication practices. *Compend Contin Educ Dent.* 2023;44:242–248.
18. Martin E, Vickers B, Landau R, Reece-Stremtan S. ABM Clinical Protocol #28, Peripartum analgesia and anesthesia for the breastfeeding mother. *Breastfeed Med.* 2018;13:164–171.
19. National Institute of Child Health and Human Development. Drugs and Lactation Database (LactMed®). https://www.ncbi.nlm.nih.gov/books/NBK501922/. Accessed 2 February 2025.
20. Alemany S, Avella-Garcia C, Liew Z, et al. Prenatal and postnatal exposure to acetaminophen in relation to autism spectrum and attention-deficit and hyperactivity symptoms in childhood: meta-analysis in six European population-based cohorts. *Eur J Epidemiol.* 2021;36:993–1004.
21. Gustavson K, Ystrom E, Ask H, et al. Acetaminophen use during pregnancy and offspring attention deficit hyperactivity disorder—a longitudinal sibling control study. *JCPP Adv.* 2021;1:e12020.
22. Khan FY, Kabiraj G, Ahmed MA, et al. A systematic review of the link between autism spectrum disorder and acetaminophen: a mystery to resolve. *Cureus.* 2022;14:e26995.
23. Sznajder KK, Teti DM, Kjerulff KH. Maternal use of acetaminophen during pregnancy and neurobehavioral problems in offspring at 3 years: a prospective cohort study. *PLoS One.* 2022;17:e0272593.

24. Ahlqvist VH, Sjoqvist H, Dalman C, et al. Acetaminophen use during pregnancy and children's risk of autism, ADHD, and intellectual disability. *JAMA*. 2024;331:1205–1214.

25. Price HR, Collier AC. Analgesics in pregnancy: an update on use, safety and pharmacokinetic changes in drug disposition. *Curr Pharm Des*. 2017;23:6098–6114.

26. Zafeiri A, Raja EA, Mitchell RT, et al. Maternal over-the-counter analgesics use during pregnancy and adverse perinatal outcomes: cohort study of 151 141 singleton pregnancies. *BMJ Open*. 2022;12:e048092.

27. Interrante JD, Ailes EC, Lind JN, et al. Risk comparison for prenatal use of analgesics and selected birth defects, National Birth Defects Prevention Study 1997–2011. *Ann Epidemiol*. 2017;27:645–653.e2.

28. U.S. Food and Drug Administration. FDA recommends avoiding use of NSAIDs in pregnancy at 20 weeks or later because they can result in low amniotic fluid (updated September 1, 2022); 2020. https://www.fda.gov/drugs/drug-safety-and-availability/fda-recommends-avoiding-use-nsaids-pregnancy-20-weeks-or-later-because-they-can-result-low-amniotic. Accessed 2 February 2025.

29. Safety update: NSAIDs in pregnancy. *Drug Ther Bull*. 2023;61:131.

30. Premkumar A, Ayala NK, Miller CH, et al. Postpartum NSAID use and adverse outcomes among women with hypertensive disorders of pregnancy: a systematic review and meta-analysis. *Am J Perinatol*. 2021;38:1–9.

31. American College of Obstetricians and Gynecologists. Clinical Consensus No. 1: Pharmacologic stepwise multimodal approach for postpartum pain management (reaffirmed 2025). *Obstet Gynecol*. 2021;138:507–517.

32. Briggs GG, Freeman RK, Towers CV, Forinash AB. *Drugs in Pregnancy and Lactation: a Reference Guide to Fetal and Neonatal Risk*. 12th ed. Wolters Kluwer; 2021.

33. Rolnik DL, Wright D, Poon LC, et al. Aspirin versus placebo in pregnancies at high-risk for preterm preeclampsia. *N Engl J Med*. 2017;377:613–622.

34. Berard A, Sheehy O, Girard S, et al. Risk of preterm birth following late pregnancy exposure to NSAIDs or COX-2 inhibitors. *Pain*. 2018;159:948–955.

35. Society for Maternal-Fetal Medicine, Silver R, Craigo S, et al. Society for Maternal-Fetal Medicine Consult Series #64: Systemic lupus erythematosus in pregnancy. *Am J Obstet Gynecol*. 2023;228:B41–B60.

36. Verret M, Lauzier F, Zarychanski R, et al. Perioperative use of gabapentinoids for the management of postoperative acute pain: a systematic review and meta-analysis. *Anesthesiology*. 2020;133:265–279.

37. Felder L, Saccone G, Scuotto S, et al. Perioperative gabapentin and post cesarean pain control: a systematic review and meta-analysis of randomized controlled trials. *Eur J Obstet Gynecol Reprod Biol*. 2019;233:98–106.

38. Fowler C, Chu AW, Guo N, et al. Outpatient treatment with gabapentin in women with severe acute pain after cesarean delivery is ineffective: a randomized, double-blind, placebo-controlled trial. *Anesth Analg*. 2023;136:1122–1132.

39. Montouris G. Gabapentin exposure in human pregnancy: results from the Gabapentin Pregnancy Registry. *Epilepsy Behav*. 2003;4:310–317.

40. Patorno E, Hernandez-Diaz S, Huybrechts KF, et al. Gabapentin in pregnancy and the risk of adverse neonatal and maternal outcomes: a population-based cohort study nested in the US Medicaid Analytic eXtract dataset. *PLoS Med*. 2020;17:e1003322.

41. Ohman I, Vitols S, Tomson T. Pharmacokinetics of gabapentin during delivery, in the neonatal period, and lactation: does a fetal accumulation occur during pregnancy? *Epilepsia*. 2005;46:1621–1624.

42. Winterfeld U, Merlob P, Baud D, et al. Pregnancy outcome following maternal exposure to pregabalin may call for concern. *Neurology*. 2016;86:2251–2257.

43. Patorno E, Bateman BT, Huybrechts KF, et al. Pregabalin use early in pregnancy and the risk of major congenital malformations. *Neurology*. 2017;88:2020–2025.

44. Lockwood PA, Pauer L, Scavone JM, et al. The pharmacokinetics of pregabalin in breast milk, plasma, and urine of healthy postpartum women. *J Hum Lact*. 2016;32:NP1–NP8.

45. Loughhead AM, Stowe ZN, Newport DJ, et al. Placental passage of tricyclic antidepressants. *Biol Psychiatry*. 2006;59:287–290.

46. Ornoy A, Koren G. Selective serotonin reuptake inhibitors during pregnancy: do we have now more definite answers related to prenatal exposure? *Birth Defects Res*. 2017;109:898–908.

47. Reis M, Källén B. Delivery outcome after maternal use of antidepressant drugs in pregnancy: an update using Swedish data. *Psychol Med*. 2010;40:1723–1733.

48. Ankarfeldt MZ, Petersen J, Andersen JT, et al. Duloxetine exposure during pregnancy and the risk of offspring being born small for gestational age or prematurely: a nationwide Danish and Swedish safety study. *Drugs Real World Outcomes*. 2023;10:69–81.

49. Carvalho AF, Sharma MS, Brunoni AR, et al. The safety, tolerability and risks associated with the use of newer generation antidepressant drugs: a critical review of the literature. *Psychother Psychosom*. 2016;85:270–288.

50. Doleman B, Mathiesen O, Sutton AJ, et al. Non-opioid analgesics for the prevention of chronic postsurgical pain: a systematic review and network meta-analysis. *Br J Anaesth*. 2023;130:719–728.

51. Guo R, Liu G, Du M, et al. Early ketamine exposure results in cardiac enlargement and heart dysfunction in Xenopus embryos. *BMC Anesthesiol*. 2016;16:23.

52. Huang R, Lin B, Tian H, et al. Prenatal exposure to general anesthesia drug esketamine impaired neurobehavior in offspring. *Cell Mol Neurobiol*. 2023;43:3005–3022.

53. Bauchat JR, Higgins N, Wojciechowski KG, et al. Low-dose ketamine with multimodal postcesarean delivery analgesia: a randomized controlled trial. *Int J Obstet Anesth*. 2011;20:3–9.

54. Majdinasab E, Datta P, Krutsch K, et al. Pharmacokinetics of ketamine transfer into human milk. *J Clin Psychopharmacol*. 2023;43:407–410.

55. Wolfson P, Cole R, Lynch K, et al. The pharmacokinetics of ketamine in the breast milk of lactating women: quantification of ketamine and metabolites. *J Psychoactive Drugs*. 2023;55:354–358.

56. Allen TK, Mishriky BM, Klinger RY, Habib AS. The impact of neuraxial clonidine on postoperative analgesia and perioperative adverse effects in women having elective Caesarean section-a systematic review and meta-analysis. *Br J Anaesth*. 2018;120:228–240.

57. Crespo S, Dangelser G, Haller G. Intrathecal clonidine as an adjuvant for neuraxial anaesthesia during caesarean delivery:

a systematic review and meta-analysis of randomised trials. *Int J Obstet Anesth*. 2017;32:64–76.

58. Giaccari LG, Coppolino F, Aurilio C, et al. Is intrathecal bupivacaine plus dexmedetomidine superior to bupivacaine in spinal anesthesia for a cesarean section? A systematic review and meta-analysis. *Eur Rev Med Pharmacol Sci*. 2024;28:4067–4079.

59. Mo X, Huang F, Wu X, et al. Intrathecal dexmedetomidine as an adjuvant to plain ropivacaine for spinal anesthesia during cesarean section: a prospective, double-blinded, randomized trial for ED(50) determination using an up-down sequential allocation method. *BMC Anesthesiol*. 2023;23:325.

60. American Society of Anesthesiologists Committee on Obstetric Anesthesia. Statement on the use of adjuvant medications and management of intraoperative pain during cesarean delivery; 2024. https://www.asahq.org/standards-and-practice-parameters/statement-on-the-use-of-adjuvant-medications-and-management-of-intraoperative-pain-during-cesarean-delivery. Accessed 2 February 2025.

61. Bioniche Pharma USA LLC. Package insert: Duraclon (clonidine hydrochloride) injection, solution; 2010. https://www.accessdata.fda.gov/drugsatfda_docs/label/2010/020615s003lbl.pdf. Accessed 2 February 2025.

62. Lavand'homme PM, Roelants F, Waterloos H, et al. An evaluation of the postoperative antihyperalgesic and analgesic effects of intrathecal clonidine administered during elective cesarean delivery. *Anesth Analg*. 2008;107:948–955.

63. Straub L, Huybrechts KF, Hernandez-Diaz S, et al. Chronic prescription opioid use in pregnancy in the United States. *Pharmacoepidemiol Drug Saf*. 2021;30:504–513.

64. Landau R, Cavanaugh PF, DiGiorgi M. Persistent opioid use after cesarean delivery in the United States of America: a systematic review. *Int J Obstet Anesth*. 2023;54:103644.

65. Varney B, Brett J, Zoega H, et al. Opioid analgesic exposure during the first trimester of pregnancy and the risk of major congenital malformations in infants: a systematic review and meta-analysis. *Anaesthesia*. 2024;79:967–977.

66. Desai RJ, Huybrechts KF, Hernandez-Diaz S, et al. Exposure to prescription opioid analgesics in utero and risk of neonatal abstinence syndrome: population based cohort study. *BMJ Open*. 2015;350:h2102.

67. Huybrechts KF, Bateman BT, Desai RJ, et al. Risk of neonatal drug withdrawal after intrauterine co-exposure to opioids and psychotropic medications: cohort study. *BMJ*. 2017;358:j3326.

68. Baldacchino A, Arbuckle K, Petrie DJ, McCowan C. Neurobehavioral consequences of chronic intrauterine opioid exposure in infants and preschool children: a systematic review and meta-analysis. *BMC Psychiatry*. 2014;14:104.

69. Baldacchino A, Balfour DJ, Matthews K. Impulsivity and opioid drugs: differential effects of heroin, methadone and prescribed analgesic medication. *Psychol Med*. 2015;45:1167–1179.

70. Linderoth B, Foreman RD. Conventional and novel spinal stimulation algorithms: hypothetical mechanisms of action and comments on outcomes. *Neuromodulation*. 2017;20:525–533.

71. Provenzano DA, Heller JA. Daring discourse: economics of neuromodulation for the treatment of persistent spinal pain syndrome and complex regional pain syndrome. *Reg Anesth Pain Med*. 2023;48:288–295.

72. Niyomsri S, Duarte RV, Eldabe S, et al. A systematic review of economic evaluations reporting the cost-effectiveness of spinal cord stimulation. *Value Health*. 2020;23:656–665.

73. Abbott. Neuromodulation products from Abbott for chronic pain, Parkinson's, essential tremor; 2025. https://www.neuromodulation.abbott/us/en/healthcare-professionals.html. Accessed 2 February 2025.

74. Metronic. Spinal cord stimulation: Indications, safety, and warnings; 2025. https://www.medtronic.com/us-en/healthcare-professionals/therapies-procedures/neurological/spinal-cord-stimulation/indications-safety-warnings.html. Accessed 2 February 2025.

75. Brent RL. Reproductive and teratologic effects of low-frequency electromagnetic fields: a review of in vivo and in vitro studies using animal models. *Teratology*. 1999;59:261–286.

76. Linderoth B, Herregodts P, Meyerson BA. Sympathetic mediation of peripheral vasodilation induced by spinal cord stimulation: animal studies of the role of cholinergic and adrenergic receptor subtypes. *Neurosurgery*. 1994;35:711–719.

77. Meier K, Glavind J, Milidou I, et al. Burst spinal cord stimulation in pregnancy: first clinical experiences. *Neuromodulation*. 2023;26:224–232.

78. Takeshima N, Okuda K, Takatanin J, et al. Trial spinal cord stimulator reimplantation following lead breakage after third birth. *Pain Physician*. 2010;13:523–526.

79. Saxena A, Eljamel MS. Spinal cord stimulation in the first two trimesters of pregnancy: case report and review of the literature. *Neuromodulation*. 2009;12:281–283.

80. Camporeze B, Simm R, Maldaun MVC, Pires de Aguiar PH. Spinal cord stimulation in pregnant patients: current perspectives of indications, complications, and results in pain control: a systematic review. *Asian J Neurosurg*. 2019;14:343–355.

81. Segal R. Spinal cord stimulation, conception, pregnancy, and labor: case study in a complex regional pain syndrome patient. *Neuromodulation*. 1999;2:41–45.

82. Hanson JL, Goodman EJ. Labor epidural placement in a woman with a cervical spinal cord stimulator. *Int J Obstet Anesth*. 2006;15:246–249.

83. Innamorato MA, Cascella M, Bignami EG, et al. Neurostimulation for chronic low back pain during pregnancy: implications for child and mother safety. *Int J Environ Res Public Health*. 2022;19:15488.

84. Jozwiak MJ, Wu H. Complex regional pain syndrome management: an evaluation of the risks and benefits of spinal cord stimulator use in pregnancy. *Pain Pract*. 2020;20:88–94.

85. Young AC, Lubenow TR, Buvanendran A. The parturient with implanted spinal cord stimulator: management and review of the literature. *Reg Anesth Pain Med*. 2015;40:276–283.

86. Zanfini BA, De Martino S, Frassanito L, et al. "Please mind the gap": successful use of ultrasound-assisted spinal anesthesia for urgent cesarean section in a patient with implanted spinal cord stimulation system for giant chest wall arteriovenous malformation—a case report. *BMC Anesthesiol*. 2020;20:122.

87. Harned ME, Gish B, Zuelzer A, Grider JS. Anesthetic considerations and perioperative management of spinal cord stimulators: literature review and initial recommendations. *Pain Physician*. 2017;20:319–329.

88. Burch R. Epidemiology and treatment of menstrual migraine and migraine during pregnancy and lactation: a narrative review. *Headache.* 2020;60:200–216.

89. Frederick IO, Qiu C, Enquobahrie DA, et al. Lifetime prevalence and correlates of migraine among women in a Pacific northwest pregnancy cohort study. *Headache.* 2014;54:675–685.

90. Kardes G, Hadimli A, Ergenoglu AM. Determination of the frequency of migraine attacks in pregnant women and the ways they cope with headaches: a cross-sectional study. *Healthcare (Basel).* 2023;11:2070.

91. Seng EK, Martin PR, Houle TT. Lifestyle factors and migraine. *Lancet Neurol.* 2022;21:911–921.

92. Amundsen S, Nordeng H, Nezvalová-Henriksen K, et al. Pharmacological treatment of migraine during pregnancy and breastfeeding. *Nat Rev Neurol.* 2015;11:209–219.

93. Purdue-Smithe AC, Stuart JJ, Farland LV, et al. Prepregnancy migraine, migraine phenotype, and risk of adverse pregnancy outcomes. *Neurology.* 2023;100:e1464–e1473.

94. Verhaak A, Bakaysa S, Johnson A, et al. Migraine treatment in pregnancy: a survey of comfort and treatment practices of women's healthcare providers. *Headache.* 2023;63:211–221.

95. Wood ME, Burch RC, Hernandez-Diaz S. Polypharmacy and comorbidities during pregnancy in a cohort of women with migraine. *Cephalalgia.* 2021;41:392–403.

96. Mazza GR, Solorio C, Stek AM, et al. Assessing the efficacy of magnesium oxide and riboflavin as preventative treatment of migraines in pregnancy. *Arch Gynecol Obstet.* 2023;308:1749–1754.

97. Källén B, Nilsson E, Otterblad Olausson P. Delivery outcome after maternal use of drugs for migraine: a register study in Sweden. *Drug Saf.* 2011;34:691–703.

98. Wojnar-Horton RE, Hackett LP, Yapp P, et al. Distribution and excretion of sumatriptan in human milk. *Br J Clin Pharmacol.* 1996;41:217–221.

99. Davanzo R, Bua J, Paloni G, Facchina G. Breastfeeding and migraine drugs. *Eur J Clin Pharmacol.* 2014;70:1313–1324.

100. Cozzolino M, Riviello C, Fichtel G, Tommaso MD. Exposure to methylergonovine maleate as a cause of sirenomelia. *Birth Defects Res A Clin Mol Teratol.* 2016;106:643–647.

101. Demirel G, Oguz SS, Erdeve O, Dilmen U. Unilateral renal agenesis and urethral atresia associated with ergotamine intake during pregnancy. *Ren Fail.* 2012;34:643–644.

102. Bateman BT, Heide-Jorgensen U, Einarsdottir K, et al. Beta-blocker use in pregnancy and the risk for congenital malformations: an international cohort study. *Ann Intern Med.* 2018;169:665–673.

103. Ansari J, Carvalho B, Shafer SL, Flood P. Pharmacokinetics and pharmacodynamics of drugs commonly used in pregnancy and parturition. *Anesth Analg.* 2016;122:786–804.

104. Jürgens TP, Schaefer C, May A. Treatment of cluster headache in pregnancy and lactation. *Cephalalgia.* 2009;29:391–400.

105. Pringsheim T, Davenport W, Mackie G, et al. Canadian Headache Society guideline for migraine prophylaxis. *Can J Neurol Sci.* 2012;39:S1–S59.

106. Banach R, Boskovic R, Einarson T, Koren G. Long-term developmental outcome of children of women with epilepsy, unexposed or exposed prenatally to antiepileptic drugs: a meta-analysis of cohort studies. *Drug Saf.* 2010;33:73–79.

107. Piontek CM, Baab S, Peindl KS, Wisner KL. Serum valproate levels in 6 breastfeeding mother-infant pairs. *J Clin Psychiatry.* 2000;61:170–172.

108. Stahl MM, Neiderud J, Vinge E. Thrombocytopenic purpura and anemia in a breast-fed infant whose mother was treated with valproic acid. *J Pediatr.* 1997;130:1001–1003.

109. Boghossian NS, Greenberg LT, Saade GR, et al. Association of sickle cell disease with racial disparities and severe maternal morbidities in black individuals. *JAMA Pediatr.* 2023;177:808–817.

110. Oteng-Ntim E, Pavord S, Howard R, et al. Management of sickle cell disease in pregnancy. a British Society for Haematology guideline. *Br J Haematol.* 2021;194:980–995.

111. Oteng-Ntim E, Ayensah B, Knight M, Howard J. Pregnancy outcome in patients with sickle cell disease in the UK—a national cohort study comparing sickle cell anaemia (HbSS) with HbSC disease. *Br J Haematol.* 2015;169:129–137.

112. Asare EV, DeBaun MR, Olayemi E, et al. Acute pain episodes, acute chest syndrome, and pulmonary thromboembolism in pregnancy. *Hematology Am Soc Hematol Educ Program.* 2022;2022:388–407.

113. Hachey SM, Joseph S, Dolin CD, et al. Contemporary obstetric and neonatal outcomes in sickle cell disease: a retrospective cohort study. *Am J Perinatol.* 2024;41(S 01):e2291–e2298.

114. Society for Maternal-Fetal Medicine, Sinkey RG, Ogunsile FJ, et al. Society for Maternal-Fetal Medicine Consult Series #68: Sickle cell disease in pregnancy. *Am J Obstet Gynecol.* 2024;230:B17–B40.

115. Kroner BL, Hankins JS, Pugh N, et al. Pregnancy outcomes with hydroxyurea use in women with sickle cell disease. *Am J Hematol.* 2022;97:603–612.

116. Darlington F, Acha BM, Roshan T, et al. Opioid-related disorders among pregnant women with sickle cell disease and outcomes. *Pain Med.* 2020;21:3087–3093.

117. Brown JA, Sinkey RG, Steffensen TS, et al. Neonatal abstinence syndrome among infants born to mothers with sickle cell hemoglobinopathies. *Am J Perinatol.* 2020;37:326–332.

118. Liddle SD, Pennick V. Interventions for preventing and treating low-back and pelvic pain during pregnancy. *Cochrane Database Syst Rev.* 2015;(9):CD001139.

119. Shiri R, Coggon D, Falah-Hassani K. Exercise for the prevention of low back and pelvic girdle pain in pregnancy: a meta-analysis of randomized controlled trials. *Eur J Pain.* 2018;22:19–27.

120. Daneau C, Abboud J, Marchand AA, et al. Mechanisms underlying lumbopelvic pain during pregnancy: a proposed model. *Front Pain Res (Lausanne).* 2021;2:773988.

121. Conder R, Zamani R, Akrami M. The biomechanics of pregnancy: a systematic review. *J Funct Morphol Kinesiol.* 2019;4:72.

122. Zhang M, Cooley C, Ziadni MS, et al. Association between history of childbirth and chronic, functionally significant back pain in later life. *BMC Womens Health.* 2023;23:4.

123. Blanco R, Ansari T. Transitional pain services updates and a novel service for the obstetric population. *Curr Opin Anaesthesiol.* 2024;37:513–519.

124. Koukoulithras Sr I, Stamouli A, Kolokotsios S, et al. The effectiveness of non-pharmaceutical interventions upon pregnancy-related low back pain: a systematic review and meta-analysis. *Cureus.* 2021;13:e13011.

125. Kandru M, Zallipalli SN, Dendukuri NK, et al. Effects of conventional exercises on lower back pain and/or pelvic girdle pain in pregnancy: a systematic review and meta-analysis. *Cureus.* 2023;15:e42010.

126. Barbier M, Blanc J, Faust C, et al. Standardized Stretching Postural postures to treat low-back pain in pregnancy: the GEMALODO randomized clinical trial. *Am J Obstet Gynecol MFM.* 2023;5:101087.

127. Ferraz VS, Peixoto C, Ferreira Resstel AP, et al. Effect of the pilates method on pain and quality of life in pregnancy: a systematic review and meta-analysis. *J Bodyw Mov Ther.* 2023;35:220–227.

128. Reis YA, Akay A, Aktan B, et al. The effect of clinical Pilates exercises and prenatal education on maternal and fetal health. *Z Geburtshilfe Neonatol.* 2023;227:354–363.

129. Yildirim P, Basol G, Karahan AY. Pilates-based therapeutic exercise for pregnancy-related low back and pelvic pain: a prospective, randomized, controlled trial. *Turk J Phys Med Rehabil.* 2023;69:207–215.

130. Li R, Chen L, Ren Y, et al. Efficacy and safety of acupuncture for pregnancy-related low back pain: a systematic review and meta-analysis. *Heliyon.* 2023;9:e18439.

131. Weis CA, Pohlman K, Barrett J, et al. Best-practice recommendations for chiropractic care for pregnant and postpartum patients: results of a consensus process. *J Manipulative Physiol Ther.* 2022;45:469–489.

132. Lamvu G, Carrillo J, Ouyang C, Rapkin A. Chronic pelvic pain in women: a review. *JAMA.* 2021;325:2381–2391.

133. Shanshan H, Liying C, Huihong Z, et al. Prevalence of lumbopelvic pain during pregnancy: a systematic review and meta-analysis of cross-sectional studies. *Acta Obstet Gynecol Scand.* 2024;103:225–240.

134. Elden H, Gutke A, Kjellby-Wendt G, et al. Predictors and consequences of long-term pregnancy-related pelvic girdle pain: a longitudinal follow-up study. *BMC Musculoskelet Disord.* 2016;17:276.

135. Sward L, Manning N, Murchison AB, et al. Pelvic girdle pain in pregnancy: a review. *Obstet Gynecol Surv.* 2023;78:349–357.

136. Wuytack F, Begley C, Daly D. Risk factors for pregnancy-related pelvic girdle pain: a scoping review. *BMC Pregnancy Childbirth.* 2020;20:739.

137. Ertmann RK, Nicolaisdottir DR, Kragstrup J, et al. The predictive value of common symptoms in early pregnancy for complications later in pregnancy and at birth. *Acta Obstet Gynecol Scand.* 2023;102:33–42.

138. Algard T, Kalliokoski P, Ahlqvist K, et al. Role of depressive symptoms on the development of pelvic girdle pain in pregnancy: a prospective inception cohort study. *Acta Obstet Gynecol Scand.* 2023;102:1281–1289.

139. Ahlqvist K, Bjelland EK, Pingel R, et al. Generalized joint hypermobility and the risk of pregnancy-related pelvic girdle pain: is body mass index of importance?—a prospective cohort study. *Acta Obstet Gynecol Scand.* 2023;102:1259–1268.

140. Almousa S, Lamprianidou E, Kitsoulis G. The effectiveness of stabilising exercises in pelvic girdle pain during pregnancy and after delivery: a systematic review. *Physiother Res Int.* 2018;23:e1699.

141. Santos FF, Lourenco BM, Souza MB, et al. Prevention of low back and pelvic girdle pain during pregnancy: a systematic review and meta-analysis of randomised controlled trials with GRADE recommendations. *Physiotherapy.* 2023;118:1–11.

142. Svahn Ekdahl A, Fagevik Olsen M, Jendman T, Gutke A. Maintenance of physical activity level, functioning and health after non-pharmacological treatment of pelvic girdle pain with either transcutaneous electrical nerve stimulation

or acupuncture: a randomised controlled trial. *BMJ Open.* 2021;11:e046314.

143. Hall H, Cramer H, Sundberg T, et al. The effectiveness of complementary manual therapies for pregnancy-related back and pelvic pain: a systematic review with meta-analysis. *Medicine (Baltimore).* 2016;95:e4723.

144. Mucci V, Demori I, Browne CJ, et al. Fibromyalgia in pregnancy: neuro-endocrine fluctuations provide insight into pathophysiology and neuromodulation treatment. *Biomedicines.* 2023;11:615.

145. Wolfe F, Clauw DJ, Fitzcharles MA, et al. 2016 Revisions to the 2010/2011 fibromyalgia diagnostic criteria. *Semin Arthritis Rheum.* 2016;46:319–329.

146. Genc H, Atasever M, Duyur Cakit B, et al. The effects of fibromyalgia syndrome on physical function and psychological status of pregnant females. *Arch Rheumatol.* 2017;32:129–140.

147. Gentile S, Fusco ML. Managing fibromyalgia syndrome in pregnancy no bridges between USA and EU. *Arch Womens Ment Health.* 2019;22:711–721.

148. Komatsu R, Carvalho B, Flood PD. Recovery after nulliparous birth: a detailed analysis of pain analgesia and recovery of function. *Anesthesiology.* 2017;127:684–694.

149. Landau R. Post-cesarean delivery pain. Management of the opioid-dependent patient before, during and after cesarean delivery. *Int J Obstet Anesth.* 2019;39:105–116.

150. Hoyt MR, Shah U, Cooley J, Temple M. Use of epidural clonidine for the management of analgesia in the opioid addicted parturient on buprenorphine maintenance therapy: an observational study. *Int J Obstet Anesth.* 2018;34:67–72.

151. Cook MI, Kushelev M, Coffman JH, Coffman JC. Analgesic outcomes in opioid use disorder patients receiving spinal anesthesia with or without intrathecal clonidine for cesarean delivery: a retrospective investigation. *J Pain Res.* 2022;15:1191–1201.

152. Wasiluk IM, Castillo D, Panni JK, et al. Postpartum analgesia with dexmedetomidine in opioid tolerance during pregnancy. *J Clin Anesth.* 2011;23:593–594.

153. Schwenk ES, Viscusi ER, Buvanendran A, et al. Consensus guidelines on the use of intravenous ketamine infusions for acute pain management from the American Society of Regional Anesthesia and Pain Medicine, the American Academy of Pain Medicine, and the American Society of Anesthesiologists. *Reg Anesth Pain Med.* 2018;43:456–466.

154. Colvin LA, Bull F, Hales TG. Perioperative opioid analgesia—when is enough too much? A review of opioid-induced tolerance and hyperalgesia. *Lancet.* 2019;393:1558–1568.

155. Marton T, Barnes DE, Wallace A, Woolley JD. Concurrent use of buprenorphine, methadone, or naltrexone does not inhibit ketamine's antidepressant activity. *Biol Psychiatry.* 2019;85:e75–e76.

156. Gimovsky AC, Fritton K, Viscusi E, Roman A. Evaluating the use of ketamine for pain control with sickle cell crisis in pregnancy: a report of 2 cases. *A A Pract.* 2018;10:20–22.

157. Roy AB, Hughes LP, West LA, et al. Meeting the challenge of analgesia in a pregnant woman with burn injury using subanesthetic ketamine: a case report and literature review. *J Burn Care Res.* 2020;41:913–917.

158. Tith S, Bining G, Bollag L. Management of eight labor and delivery patients dependent on buprenorphine (Subutex): a retrospective chart review. *F1000Research.* 2018;7:7.

159. Brinck EC, Tiippana E, Heesen M, et al. Perioperative intravenous ketamine for acute postoperative pain in adults. *Cochrane Database Syst Rev.* 2018;(12):CD012033.

160. Wang J, Xu Z, Feng Z, et al. Impact of ketamine on pain management in cesarean section: a systematic review and meta-analysis. *Pain Physician.* 2020;23:135–148.

161. Leighton BL, Crock LW. Case series of successful postoperative pain management in buprenorphine maintenance therapy patients. *Anesth Analg.* 2017;125:1779–1783.

162. Stanislaus MA, Reno JL, Small RH, et al. Continuous epidural hydromorphone infusion for post-cesarean delivery analgesia in a patient on methadone maintenance therapy: a case report. *J Pain Res.* 2020;13:837–842.

163. Sultan P, Sultan E, Carvalho B. Regional anaesthesia for labour, operative vaginal delivery and caesarean delivery: a narrative review. *Anaesthesia.* 2021;76(suppl 1):136–147.

164. El-Boghdadly K, Desai N, Halpern S, et al. Quadratus lumborum block vs. transversus abdominis plane block for caesarean delivery: a systematic review and network meta-analysis. *Anaesthesia.* 2021;76:393–403.

165. Schug SA, Lavand'homme P, Barke A, et al. The IASP classification of chronic pain for ICD-11: chronic postsurgical or posttraumatic pain. *Pain.* 2019;160:45–52.

166. Tan HS, Sng BL. Persistent pain after childbirth. *BJA Educ.* 2022;22:33–37.

167. Sng BL, Sia AT, Quek K, et al. Incidence and risk factors for chronic pain after caesarean section under spinal anaesthesia. *Anaesth Intensive Care.* 2009;37:748–752.

168. As-Sanie S, Till SR, Schrepf AD, et al. Incidence and predictors of persistent pelvic pain following hysterectomy in women with chronic pelvic pain. *Am J Obstet Gynecol.* 2021;225:568.e1–e11.

169. Sharma LR, Schaldemose EL, Alaverdyan H, et al. Perioperative factors associated with persistent postsurgical pain after hysterectomy, cesarean section, prostatectomy, and donor nephrectomy: a systematic review and meta-analysis. *Pain.* 2022;163:425–435.

170. Gutierrez S, Liu B, Hayashida K, et al. Reversal of peripheral nerve injury-induced hypersensitivity in the postpartum period: role of spinal oxytocin. *Anesthesiology.* 2013;118:152–159.

171. Monks DT, Palanisamy A. Oxytocin: at birth and beyond. A systematic review of the long-term effects of peripartum oxytocin. *Anaesthesia.* 2021;76:1526–1537.

172. Severino AL, Chen R, Hayashida K, et al. Plasticity and function of spinal oxytocin and vasopressin signaling during recovery from surgery with nerve injury. *Anesthesiology.* 2018;129:544–556.

173. Yimer H, Woldie H. Incidence and associated factors of chronic pain after caesarean section: a systematic review. *J Obstet Gynaecol Can.* 2019;41:840–854.

174. Ciechanowicz S, Reville Joy RC, Kasmirski J, et al. Incidence, severity and interference of chronic postsurgical pain after cesarean delivery: a systematic review and meta-analysis. *J Clin Anesth.* 2025;104:111832.

175. Eisenach JC, Pan P, Smiley RM, et al. Resolution of pain after childbirth. *Anesthesiology.* 2013;118:143–151.

176. Flood P, Wong CA. Chronic pain secondary to childbirth: does it exist? *Anesthesiology.* 2013;118:16–18.

177. Ciechanowicz S, Kim J, Mak K, et al. Outcomes and outcome measures utilised in randomised controlled trials of postoperative caesarean delivery pain: a scoping review. *Int J Obstet Anesth.* 2024;57:103927.

178. Komatsu R, Ando K, Flood PD. Factors associated with persistent pain after childbirth: a narrative review. *Br J Anaesth.* 2020;124:e117–e130.

179. Orbach-Zinger S, Aviram A, Fireman S, et al. Severe pain during local infiltration for spinal anaesthesia predicts post-caesarean pain. *Eur J Pain.* 2015;19:1382–1388.

180. Nimmaanrat S, Wongwiwattananon W, Siripreukpong S, et al. A prospective observational study to investigate the relationship between local anesthetic infiltration pain before spinal anesthesia and acute and chronic postsurgical pain in women undergoing elective cesarean delivery. *Int J Obstet Anesth.* 2021;45:56–60.

181. Komatsu R, Carvalho B, Flood P. Prediction of outliers in pain, analgesia requirement, and recovery of function after childbirth: a prospective observational cohort study. *Br J Anaesth.* 2018;121:417–426.

182. Ortner CM, Granot M, Richebe P, et al. Preoperative scar hyperalgesia is associated with post-operative pain in women undergoing a repeat Caesarean delivery. *Eur J Pain.* 2013;17:111–123.

183. Rodriguez Roca MC, Brogly N, Gredilla Diaz E, et al. Neuropathic component of postoperative pain for predicting post-cesarean chronic pain at three months: a prospective observational study. *Minerva Anestesiol.* 2021;87:1290–1299.

184. Gorkem U, Togrul C, Sahiner Y, et al. Preoperative anxiety may increase postcesarean delivery pain and analgesic consumption. *Minerva Anestesiol.* 2016;82:974–980.

185. Richez B, Ouchchane L, Guttmann A, et al. The role of psychological factors in persistent pain after cesarean delivery. *J Pain.* 2015;16:1136–1146.

186. Roomruangwong C, Kanchanatawan B, Sirivichayakul S, et al. Lower serum zinc and higher CRP strongly predict prenatal depression and physio-somatic symptoms, which all together predict postnatal depressive symptoms. *Mol Neurobiol.* 2017;54:1500–1512.

187. Orbach-Zinger S, Fireman S, Ben-Haroush A, et al. Preoperative sleep quality predicts postoperative pain after planned caesarean delivery. *Eur J Pain.* 2017;21:787–794.

188. Gizzo S, Andrisani A, Noventa M, et al. Caesarean section: could different transverse abdominal incision techniques influence postpartum pain and subsequent quality of life? A systematic review. *PLoS One.* 2015;10:e0114190.

189. Loos MJ, Scheltinga MR, Mulders LG, Roumen RM. The Pfannenstiel incision as a source of chronic pain. *Obstet Gynecol.* 2008;111:839–846.

190. Loos MJ, Scheltinga MR, Roumen RM. Surgical management of inguinal neuralgia after a low transverse Pfannenstiel incision. *Ann Surg.* 2008;248:880–885.

191. Verhagen T, Loos MJ, Mulders LG, et al. A step up therapeutic regimen for chronic post-Pfannenstiel pain syndrome. *Eur J Obstet Gynecol Reprod Biol.* 2018;231:248–254.

192. Belci D, Di Renzo GC, Stark M, et al. Morbidity and chronic pain following different techniques of caesarean section: a comparative study. *J Obstet Gynaecol.* 2015;35:442–446.

193. Wang LZ, Wei CN, Xiao F, et al. Incidence and risk factors for chronic pain after elective caesarean delivery under spinal anaesthesia in a Chinese cohort: a prospective study. *Int J Obstet Anesth.* 2018;34:21–27.

194. Farrell SA, Clermont ME. Surgical treatment of intractable pelvic, groin, and perineal neuropathic pain in a gynaecologic

patient: triple neurectomy. *J Obstet Gynaecol Can.* 2015;37:145–149.

195. Elahwal L, Elrahwan S, Elbadry AA. Ilioinguinal and iliohypogastric nerve block for acute and chronic pain relief after caesarean section: a randomized controlled trial. *Anesth Pain Med.* 2022;12:e121837.

196. Ortner CM, Turk DC, Theodore BR, et al. The Short-Form McGill Pain Questionnaire-Revised to evaluate persistent pain and surgery-related symptoms in healthy women undergoing a planned cesarean delivery. *Reg Anesth Pain Med.* 2014;39:478–486.

197. Bjelland EK, Owe KM, Pingel R, et al. Pelvic pain after childbirth: a longitudinal population study. *Pain.* 2016;157:710–716.

198. Klein Meuleman SJM, Murji A, van den Bosch T, et al. Definition and criteria for diagnosing cesarean scar disorder. *JAMA Netw Open.* 2023;6:e235321.

199. Bollag L, Richebe P, Siaulys M, et al. Effect of transversus abdominis plane block with and without clonidine on post-cesarean delivery wound hyperalgesia and pain. *Reg Anesth Pain Med.* 2012;37:508–514.

200. Subedi A, Schyns-van den Berg A, Thapa P, et al. Intrathecal morphine does not prevent chronic postsurgical pain after elective Caesarean delivery: a randomised controlled trial. *Br J Anaesth.* 2022;128:700–707.

201. Borys M, Zamaro A, Horeczy B, et al. Quadratus lumborum and transversus abdominis plane blocks and their impact on acute and chronic pain in patients after cesarean section: a randomized controlled study. *Int J Environ Res Public Health.* 2021;18:3500.

202. Du H, Luo X, Chen M, et al. Efficacy of quadratus lumborum block in the treatment of acute and chronic pain after cesarean section: a systematic review and meta-analysis based on randomized controlled trials. *Medicine (Baltimore).* 2024;103:e36652.

203. Gomez-Rios MA, Codesido-Barreiro P, Seco-Vilarino C, et al. Wound infusion of 0.35% levobupivacaine reduces mechanical secondary hyperalgesia and opioid consumption after cesarean delivery: a prospective, randomized, triple-blind, placebo-controlled trial. *Anesth Analg.* 2022;134:791–801.

204. Levene JL, Weinstein EJ, Cohen MS, et al. Local anesthetics and regional anesthesia versus conventional analgesia for preventing persistent postoperative pain in adults and children: a Cochrane systematic review and meta-analysis update. *J Clin Anesth.* 2019;55:116–127.

205. Chilkoti GT, Gaur D, Saxena AK, et al. Ultrasound-guided transversalis fascia plane block versus wound infiltration for both acute and chronic post-caesarean pain management—a randomised controlled trial. *Indian J Anaesth.* 2022;66:517–522.

43

Endocrine Disorders

Richard N. Wissler, MD, PhD, FASA

CHAPTER OUTLINE

The endocrine system has evolved to provide blood-borne communications between tissues and organs that improve the overall well-being of the individual. The interaction between the endocrine system and pregnancy is complex and can impact negatively on the pregnancy if not cared for properly. In this chapter we review the pathophysiology, clinical presentation, and management during pregnancy of three of the more common endocrine disorders: diabetes mellitus, thyroid disease, and pheochromocytoma.

DIABETES MELLITUS

Definition and Epidemiology

Diabetes mellitus (DM) is a common metabolic disorder with a prevalence of approximately 11% in the general adult population worldwide and is projected to increase in the future.[1] DM results from either an absolute deficiency in insulin secretion or a combination of resistance to insulin in target tissues and inadequate insulin secretion. There are four general categories of DM.[2] Type 1 is primarily an autoimmune disorder with an absolute insulin deficiency. Type 2 is primarily associated with obesity, accounts for 90% to 95% of adult DM, and is a combination of insulin resistance and decreased insulin secretion. The third category includes monogenic syndromes, diseases of the exocrine pancreas, and chemically induced DM. The fourth category is gestational DM (GDM): newly diagnosed DM during the second or third trimester of pregnancy.[3] GDM represents 86% of DM in pregnant women and has an estimated prevalence of 6% in pregnancy, although the true prevalence is controversial given variations in screening test strategies.[4]

Pathophysiology

Insulin is a peptide hormone secreted by the beta cells of the islets of Langerhans in the pancreas, which binds to specific cell-surface receptors in insulin-responsive target tissues (e.g., liver, skeletal muscle, fat). The intracellular effects of insulin are mediated by tyrosine kinase in the beta-subunit of the receptor through a cascade of distal protein kinase–mediated phosphorylations.[5] Normal hepatic glucose metabolism represents a balance between the effects of insulin and several "counterregulatory" hormones (e.g., glucagon, cortisol, epinephrine [adrenaline], growth hormone).[6] This control system for glucose homeostasis permits rapid adjustments in glucose metabolism in the fed and fasted states. Insulin is also an important anabolic regulator of lipid and amino acid metabolism (Fig. 43.1). Insulin deficiency (absolute or relative) associated with DM results in abnormal metabolism of carbohydrates, lipids, and amino acids.

Acute and chronic complications occur in patients with DM (Box 43.1). The three major acute complications are **diabetic ketoacidosis (DKA)**, **hyperosmolar hyperglycemic state (HHS)**, and **hypoglycemia. DKA** occurs predominantly in patients with type 1 DM but is increasingly identified in patients with type 2 DM.[7] It may develop with a new source of insulin resistance (e.g., infection, trauma, stress) and/or as a result of failure to administer usual insulin doses. DKA results from decreased uptake of glucose by insulin-responsive

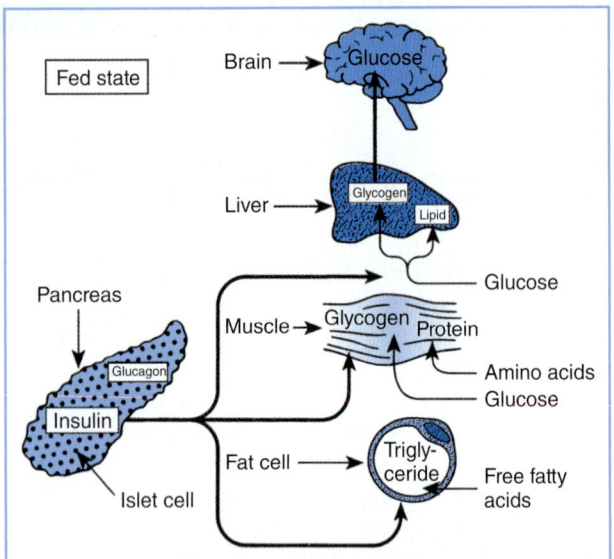

Fig. 43.1 Substrate use in the fed state, showing the role of insulin in the promotion of fuel storage. From Kitabchi AE, Murphy MB. *Diabetic ketoacidosis and hyperosmolar hyperglycemic nonketotic coma. Med Clin North Am.* 1988;72:1545–1563.

BOX 43.1   Major Complications of Diabetes Mellitus

Acute
- Diabetic ketoacidosis
- Hyperosmolar hyperglycemic state
- Hypoglycemia

Chronic
Macrovascular (Atherosclerosis)
- Coronary
- Cerebrovascular
- Peripheral vascular

Microvascular
- Retinopathy
- Nephropathy

Neuropathy
- Autonomic
- Somatic

---

tissues and greater use of free fatty acids as a hepatic energy source. The lack of insulin favors lipolysis, beta-oxidation of free fatty acids in the liver, and hepatic formation of acetoacetate and beta-hydroxybutyrate from the excess acetyl-coenzyme A generated by fatty acid oxidation.[8] These biochemical events result in metabolic acidosis, hyperglycemia, and dehydration secondary to osmotic diuresis. Signs and symptoms of DKA include nausea, vomiting, weakness, tachypnea, hypotension, tachycardia, stupor, and acetone on the breath. The diagnosis of DKA depends on the laboratory findings of hyperglycemia, ketosis, and acidosis.[8] **Sodium-glucose cotransporter-2 inhibitors (SGLT2i)** are oral medications designed to lower blood glucose levels in patients with type 2 DM by increasing renal excretion of glucose.[9] The clinical use of SGLT2i agents has increased significantly following reports that they improve heart and kidney failure outcomes

in patients with type 2 DM.[10] Unfortunately, SGLT2i medications are occasionally associated with "euglycemic" DKA with modestly elevated glucose levels.[11] In perioperative patients using SGLT2i medications, ketoacidosis may be precipitated by preprocedural fasting.[12] During the recent COVID-19 pandemic, infection with the **SARS-CoV-2 virus** was specifically identified as an initiating event for DKA.[13]

HHS occurs predominantly in older patients with type 2 DM.[8] Laboratory findings in HHS are hyperglycemia (blood glucose level often greater than 600 mg/dL [33.3 mmol/L]), hyperosmolality (>320 mOsm/kg), and moderate azotemia (serum blood urea nitrogen [BUN] often greater than 60 mg/dL [21.4 mmol/L]), without ketonemia or significant acidosis. The absence of significant ketosis in HHS may indicate an inhibition of lipolysis by low levels of insulin.[8] There are reports of coronary, cerebral, and peripheral vascular occlusions from either vasoconstriction or thrombosis in HHS.[14,15] DKA and HHS are probably related conditions; inadequate insulin therapy and infection are the most common precipitating events for both.[16]

Hypoglycemia, defined as a blood glucose level < 70 mg/dL (3.9 mmol/L),[17] is a continuing health threat in diabetic patients, especially when they are receiving insulin therapy. Hypoglycemia results from an imbalance between insulin or oral hypoglycemic agents and available metabolic fuels. In hospitalized patients with DM, the risk factors for hypoglycemia are multifactorial, and include changes in medications or nutritional intake.[18] Symptomatic awareness of hypoglycemia and counterregulatory responses may be inadequate in diabetic patients with recurrent episodes of hypoglycemia or autonomic neuropathy.[19] Continuous glucose monitoring may decrease the incidence of hypoglycemia in these patients.[17]

In general, the rate of chronic complications increases with the duration of DM. A number of prospective clinical trials have demonstrated fewer microvascular and macrovascular complications with improved glycemic control in both type 1 and type 2 DM,[20–22] though there is controversy about the impact of tight glycemic control, particularly with macrovascular complications in type 2 DM.[23] The level of glycemic control should be individualized to balance the risk of hypoglycemia against risks of chronic complications.

Clinical Presentation and Diagnosis

Box 43.2 lists the current diagnostic criteria for DM in *nonpregnant* patients.[2] Risk factors associated with **GDM** include: (1) age > 35 years, (2) obesity (body mass index [BMI] > 30 kg/m²), (3) family history of DM, (4) male fetus, (5) prior history of GDM, (6) multiple gestation, (7) history of polycystic ovary syndrome, and (8) prior delivery of a macrosomic neonate.[4] Several observational clinical studies, including the Hyperglycemia and Adverse Pregnancy Outcome study,[24] have shown that adverse pregnancy outcomes are a continuous function of glucose intolerance in pregnancy. Box 43.3 lists the current recommendations of the American Diabetes Association (ADA) for screening and diagnosis of GDM, including one-step and two-step procedures.[2] The choice between one-step and two-step screening strategies for GDM at 24 to 28 weeks' gestation remains controversial.[2–4] As diagnostic thresholds decrease for any disease process, the apparent prevalence in the population

BOX 43.2 Criteria for the Diagnosis of Diabetes Mellitus in Nonpregnant Patients

1. Fasting plasma glucose ≥ 126 mg/dL (≥7 mmol/L). Fasting is defined as no caloric intake for at least 8 h.[a]
   OR
2. Two-hour plasma glucose ≥ 200 mg/dL (≥11.1 mmol/L) during an oral glucose tolerance test. The test should be performed as described by the World Health Organization, using an oral glucose load containing the equivalent of 75 g of anhydrous glucose dissolved in water.[a]
   OR
3. Hemoglobin A1c ≥ 6.5% (≥48 mmol/mol). The test should be performed in a laboratory using a method that is certified and standardized by the National Glycohemoglobin Standardization Program to the Diabetes Control and Complications Trial assay.[a]
   OR
4. In a patient with classic symptoms of hyperglycemia or hyperglycemic crisis, a random plasma glucose ≥ 200 mg/dL (≥11.1 mmol/L).

[a]In the absence of unequivocal hyperglycemia, diagnosis requires two abnormal test results from the same sample or in two separate test samples.
From ElSayed NA, Aleppo G, Aroda VR, et al. American Diabetes Association. 2. Classification and diagnosis of diabetes: standards of care in diabetes—2023. *Diabetes Care*. 2023;46(suppl 1):S19–S40.

BOX 43.3 Screening and Diagnostic Strategies for Gestational Diabetes Mellitus

A. One-step strategy
  1. Perform a 75-g oral glucose tolerance test, with plasma glucose measurements when the patient is fasting and at 1 and 2 h, at 24–28 weeks' gestation in women not previously diagnosed with DM.
  2. The oral glucose tolerance test should be performed in the morning after an overnight fast of at least 8 h.
  3. The diagnosis of GDM is made when any of the following plasma glucose values are met or exceeded:
  • Fasting: 92 mg/dL (5.1 mmol/L)
  • 1 h: 180 mg/dL (10 mmol/L)
  • 2 h: 153 mg/dL (8.5 mmol/L)
B. Two-step strategy
  1. Step 1:
  • Perform a nonfasting 50-g oral glucose load test, with a plasma glucose measurement at 1 h, at 24–28 weeks' gestation in women not previously diagnosed with overt DM.
  • If plasma glucose ≥130, 135, or 140 mg/dL (≥7.2, 7.5, or 7.8 mmol/L, respectively) 1 h after glucose load, then proceed to a 100-g oral glucose tolerance test (Step 2).
  2. Step 2:
  • The 100-g oral glucose tolerance test should be performed when the patient is fasting.
  • The diagnosis of GDM is made if at least two of the following four plasma glucose samples (measured fasting and at 1, 2, and 3 h during the oral glucose tolerance test) are met or exceeded (Carpenter-Coustan criteria).

Sample	Carpenter-Coustan
Fasting	95 mg/dL (5.3 mmol/L)
1 h	180 mg/dL (10.0 mmol/L)
2 h	155 mg/dL (8.6 mmol/L)
3 h	140 mg/dL (7.8 mmol/L)

DM, Diabetes mellitus; *GDM*, gestational diabetes mellitus.
From ElSayed NA, Aleppo G, Aroda VR, et al. American Diabetes Association. 2. Classification and diagnosis of diabetes: standards of care in diabetes—2023. *Diabetes Care*. 2023;46(suppl 1):S19–S40.

increases. The continuing debate over screening protocols for GDM centers on whether treatment of an expanded patient population is cost-effective and will improve outcomes.

Glycosylated hemoglobin measurements are used as time-integrated estimates of glycemic control, although both analytical and physiologic factors may affect this relationship.[25] The normal range for **hemoglobin A1c** in nondiabetic pregnant women is 4.0% to 5.5%, compared with 4.8% to 6.5% in nondiabetic nonpregnant women.[26]

Interaction With Pregnancy

How Does Pregnancy Affect Diabetes Mellitus?

Pregnancy is characterized by progressive peripheral resistance to insulin at the receptor and postreceptor levels in the second and third trimesters for all pregnant women (not only those with DM) (Fig. 43.2).[27,28] The presumed mechanism involves an increase in counterregulatory hormones from the placenta during pregnancy (e.g., lactogen, growth hormone, cortisol, progesterone, and adipokines). The change in placental lactogen is an appealing hypothesis, given that (1) a graph of serum lactogen level during pregnancy is similar in shape to that of insulin requirement in pregnant women with type 1 DM[29] and (2) placental lactogen has growth hormone–like activity.[30] Also, maternal adipokines likely have significant effects on insulin secretion and resistance in pregnancy, while facilitating the provision of maternal fuels to the fetus.[31]

GDM develops when a patient cannot mount a sufficient compensatory insulin response during pregnancy. In many patients, **GDM** can be viewed as a preclinical state of glucose intolerance that is not detectable before pregnancy. After delivery, many patients return to normal glucose tolerance, but

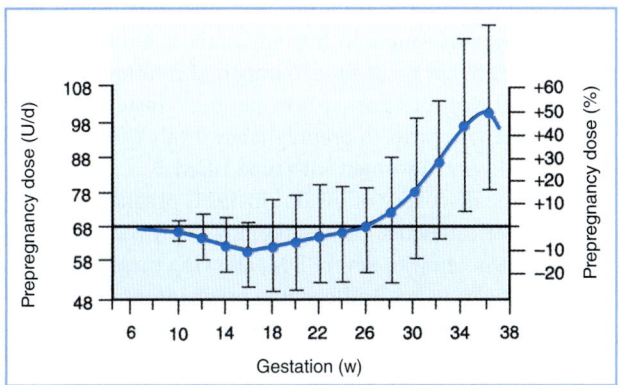

Fig. 43.2 Insulin requirements in euglycemic women with type 1 diabetes mellitus during pregnancy. From Crombach G, Siebolds M, Mies R. Insulin use in pregnancy: clinical pharmacokinetic considerations. *Clin Pharmacokinet*. 1993;24:89–100.

have a sevenfold increased risk of type 2 DM in later life.[3,4] The recurrence rate for **GDM** in a subsequent pregnancy is 41%.[32]

In patients with **pregestational DM**, insulin requirement decreases slightly between 11 and 16 weeks' gestation, and then progressively increases during pregnancy primarily because of peripheral insulin resistance.[28] At term, the daily insulin requirement is approximately 1.0 insulin unit/kg, compared with 0.7 unit/kg before pregnancy.[33] Insulin requirement may be higher in pregnancies with multiple gestation.[34] During late pregnancy in healthy patients, basal and glucose-stimulated plasma insulin levels are twice the postpartum measurements.[35] These changes reflect pregnancy-related increases in pancreatic islet cell mass and glucose sensitivity, probably secondary to the net effect of competing progesterone and lactogenic hormone stimuli in the endocrine pancreas.[36,37] Near term, maternal overnight insulin requirement may decrease, presumably as a result of a "siphoning of maternal fuels" by the growing fetus during the overnight maternal fast.[38]

Endogenous plasma insulin concentration during labor and delivery in nondiabetic parturients differs from exogenous insulin requirement in laboring diabetic women. In nondiabetic parturients, the plasma glucose concentration is only one of many factors that affect endogenous insulin secretion; glucose production and use are markedly higher during painful labor than postpartum.[39] Plasma insulin concentration remains unchanged except for a brief increase during the third stage of labor and immediately postpartum.[39,40] This finding suggests that glucose use during labor is largely independent of insulin.

In patients with type 1 DM, insulin requirement decreases with the onset of the first stage of labor.[41] These patients may require no additional insulin during the first stage of labor, although insulin requirement is modified by (1) the level of metabolic control before labor, (2) the residual effect of prior doses of subcutaneous insulin, and (3) the glucose infusion rate.[41,42] Insulin requirement increases during the second stage of labor via an unknown mechanism.[41,42] The use of epidural analgesia or oxytocin does not affect exogenous insulin requirement during the first and second stages of labor.[41] After delivery—either vaginal or cesarean—insulin requirement in women with type 1 DM decreases markedly for at least several days, although there is significant variability among individuals (Fig. 43.3).[38,43] Presumably, the decreased insulin requirement results from the loss of counterregulatory hormones produced by the placenta. Pituitary growth hormone responsiveness to hypoglycemia is blunted in late pregnancy and may contribute to impaired counterregulatory responses during the postpartum period.[44] Insulin requirement gradually returns to prepregnancy levels within several weeks of delivery in women with type 1 DM.[38]

Before the discovery of insulin in 1921, pregnancies were rare in diabetic patients. Insulin therapy improved the rate of survival in women with severe DM, allowing these women to reach childbearing age and become pregnant. Maternal outcomes improved, but fetal and neonatal morbidity and mortality remained high.[45]

Diabetic ketoacidosis. The incidence of DKA has decreased from 9% to between 1% and 3% of diabetic pregnancies,[46] probably as a result of improvements in medical care and patient education. Similarly, the incidence of perinatal and

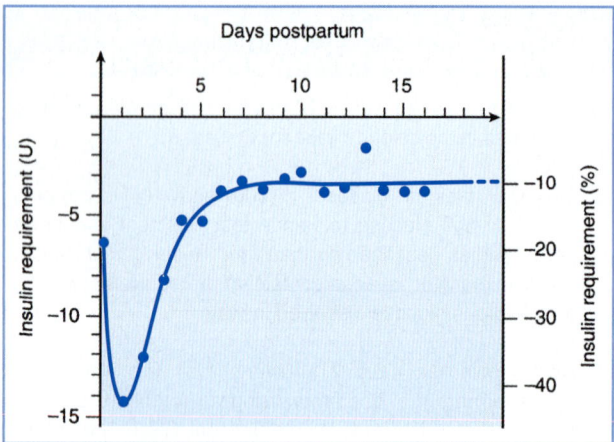

Fig. 43.3 Insulin Requirements in the Postpartum Period. From Crombach G, Siebolds M, Mies R. Insulin use in pregnancy: clinical pharmacokinetic considerations. *Clin Pharmacokinet.* 1993;24:89–100.

maternal mortality from DKA during pregnancy has decreased in the past several decades. In a large database study, pregnant patients with DKA had longer hospitalizations and a higher risk of renal damage but a lower mortality rate compared with nonpregnant DKA controls.[47] DKA occurs most commonly in the third trimester and predominantly in patients with type 1 DM (85%), but it can also occur in patients with type 2 DM (6%) or GDM (9%).[48,49] The underlying risk for DKA during pregnancy reflects some of the metabolic adaptations of pregnancy including peripheral insulin resistance.

The clinical factors most associated with DKA in pregnancy are: (1) nausea and vomiting, (2) infection, (3) poor compliance or noncompliance with insulin therapy, (4) insulin pump failure, (5) use of beta-adrenergic receptor agonists, and (6) use of glucocorticoids.[46,48–50] The infection rate is 3.2 times greater in pregnant women with pregestational type 1 DM than in nondiabetic pregnant women.[51] **COVID-19** infection may be associated with DKA in pregnant patients.[52]

Nonreassuring fetal heart rate patterns during episodes of maternal DKA, with resolution after appropriate medical management, have been described.[53] The mechanism of fetal compromise during DKA is unclear, but it may be related to changes in uterine blood flow. Blechner et al.[54] demonstrated that uterine artery blood flow is reduced by acute maternal metabolic acidosis, and Takahashi et al.[55] described reversible redistribution of fetal blood flow during an episode of maternal DKA on the basis of Doppler pulsatility indices of the umbilical and middle cerebral arteries. HHS is a rare occurrence during pregnancy.[56]

Hypoglycemia. Hypoglycemia occurs in 36% to 71% of pregnant women with pregestational type 1 DM and is a significant health risk.[57–59] This rate is 3 to 15 times greater than that in similar groups of nonpregnant patients with type 1 DM[58]; 80% to 84% of severe hypoglycemia episodes occur before 20 weeks' gestation.[57] The risk for hypoglycemia during pregnancy in patients with type 1 DM increases with tight glucose control. This pattern mirrors clinical experience in nonpregnant women with type 1 DM, in which tight insulin control was shown to be associated with a threefold increase in the occurrence of severe hypoglycemia.[60] In both pregnant and nonpregnant patients with type 1 DM, counterregulatory hormone responses to hypoglycemia are impaired after intensive insulin therapy.[61] Although not consistent in all studies, acute mild to moderate maternal hypoglycemia may be associated with adverse neonatal outcome.[62,63]

Other complications. The relationship between pregnancy and the development of macrovascular complications of DM is largely unknown. A history of GDM confers an increased lifetime risk of myocardial infarction in women with type 2 DM.[64] Patients with pregestational type 1 DM have higher systolic and diastolic blood pressure during pregnancy, and are three times more likely than nondiabetic controls to have gestational hypertension.[65] Both pregestational DM and GDM are significant risk factors for the development of **preeclampsia**.[66,67]

Pregnancy may accelerate the development of **proliferative retinopathy**, a microvascular complication of pregestational DM.[27,59,68,69] In both pregnant and nonpregnant patients with DM, abrupt control of hyperglycemia has been associated with an acute transient progression of retinopathy.[27,59]

Similar to diabetic retinopathy, the progression of diabetic **nephropathy** during pregnancy in patients with pregestational DM depends on the prepregnancy baseline of renal disease and the effectiveness of antihypertensive therapy.[59,68,70] Based on existing evidence, it is unlikely that pregnancy changes the long-term progression of **somatic** or **autonomic neuropathy** in diabetic women.[27,59,71]

How Does Diabetes Mellitus Affect the Mother and Fetus?

Both pregestational DM and GDM are associated with higher rates of gestational hypertension, polyhydramnios, preterm birth, and cesarean delivery.[3,27,72] The incidences of preterm labor and delivery and cesarean delivery are higher in women with pregestational DM than in women with GDM.[72] Trial of labor after cesarean delivery in patients with GDM is associated with higher rates of operative vaginal delivery and repeat cesarean delivery compared with that in nondiabetic controls.[73]

Box 43.4 lists the fetal complications of maternal DM during pregnancy. **Fetal macrosomia**, historically defined as a birth weight > 4000 or 4500 g, is a well-recognized complication of maternal DM.[74] Most studies suggest that both pregestational DM and GDM result in an increased incidence of fetal macrosomia.[3,27,72,74] In GDM, the HAPO study demonstrated that neonatal macrosomia is a linear function of maternal hyperglycemia.[24] In a randomized clinical trial of pregestational DM, the use of continuous glucose monitoring was associated with a lower incidence of macrosomic neonates.[75] In addition to maternal hyperglycemia, other possible factors contributing to fetal macrosomia in DM include maternal obesity, gestational weight gain, variations in maternal blood glucose, and maternal lipid levels.[76]

Macrosomia results in an increased risk for **shoulder dystocia** and **birth trauma** with vaginal delivery.[74,77] Moreover, when comparisons are made within birth weight categories above 4000 g, pregnancies in diabetic women have a higher risk for shoulder dystocia than nondiabetic women.[74] Several mechanisms have been suggested for the development of fetal macrosomia in diabetic pregnancy. Maternal

---

BOX 43.4 Fetal Complications of Maternal Diabetes Mellitus

During Pregnancy and the Puerperium
Chronic
- Macrosomia
- Shoulder dystocia
- Birth injury or trauma
- Structural malformations
  Central nervous system: anencephaly, encephalocele, meningomyelocele, spina bifida, holoprosencephaly
  Cardiac: transposition of great vessels, ventricular septal defect, situs inversus, single ventricle, hypoplastic left ventricle
  Skeletal: caudal regression
  Renal: agenesis, multicystic dysplasia
  Gastrointestinal: anal or rectal atresia, small left colon
  Pulmonary: hypoplasia

Acute
- Intrauterine or neonatal death
- Neonatal respiratory distress syndrome
- Neonatal hypoglycemia
- Neonatal hyperbilirubinemia

After Pregnancy
- Glucose intolerance
- Possible impairment of cognitive development

---

hyperglycemia can result in fetal hyperglycemia, with reactive fetal hyperinsulinemia and an anabolic response in the fetus.[78] Shoulder dystocia may reflect the excessive growth of the fetal trunk (relative to the fetal head) in response to fetal hyperinsulinemia.[79]

Women with pregestational DM are at increased risk for **fetal anomalies** (see Box 43.4). The incidence of major anomalies, estimated to be 6% to 10%, is five times higher than in nondiabetic controls.[80] Overall, cardiovascular anomalies are most common, followed by anomalies of the central nervous system (CNS). Caudal regression syndrome, though uncommon, is 200 times more likely in diabetic than in nondiabetic pregnancies.

Mechanisms that may be involved in the development of fetal structural malformations in diabetic pregnancies include embryonic apoptosis, yolk sac vasculopathy, and altered uptake of glucosamine by embryonic cells.[81–83] Most fetal structural malformations that occur during pregnancy are likely to have a multifactorial etiology. However, hyperglycemia during the period of critical organogenesis before the 8th week after conception is probably the single strongest etiologic factor in diabetic women.[27] Hemoglobin A1c levels in pregnancy correlate with the incidence of major congenital anomalies that occur in women with pregestational DM.[82,84]

Studies have suggested that patient education and strict glycemic control during the preconception period may reduce the rate of major congenital anomalies from 10% to 1% in patients with pregestational DM.[27,85] The latter figure is similar to the baseline risk for major structural malformations in the general population. Strict glycemic control initiated during the preconception period also increases the incidence of maternal hypoglycemic episodes. These studies suggest that hypoglycemia is not a significant factor in the etiology of human malformations, because the rate of anomalies decreased 10-fold despite hypoglycemic episodes.[27,85] Similarly, strict glycemic control before conception also has been associated with a threefold decrease in the incidence of spontaneous abortion in women with pregestational DM.[86] Dicker et al.[87] observed normal induced ovulation, *in vitro* fertilization, and early embryonic development in a small series of infertile patients with pregestational DM who attended a preconception diabetes clinic. However, less than one-third of women with known pregestational DM receive appropriate medical care before conception.[27]

In the past 75 years, the perinatal mortality rate in the United States has steadily decreased from 18% to 3%.[27,88,89] If the entire population is considered, the perinatal mortality rate likely remains higher in patients with pregestational DM than in nondiabetic controls. The rate in patients with GDM is intermediate between the rate in women with pregestational diabetes and the rate in nondiabetic controls.

Historically, **intrauterine fetal death** was responsible for approximately 40% of perinatal deaths in women with DM, with 68% occurring between 36 and 40 weeks' gestation.[88] In contemporary reports, the ratio of intrauterine deaths to neonatal deaths in diabetic pregnancies has varied from 0 to 1.0. Fetal macrosomia is a risk factor for intrauterine fetal demise in both diabetic and nondiabetic pregnancies. Recurrent episodes of intrauterine hypoxia can occur in diabetic pregnancies that end in stillbirth; episodes of hypoxia may reflect reduced uteroplacental blood flow and changes in fetal carbohydrate metabolism. **Congenital anomalies** have now emerged as the leading cause of perinatal mortality in diabetic pregnancies.[27,89] This change likely reflects better obstetric care during pregnancy, despite the lack of adequate glycemic control before conception in many patients.

Studies have reported a risk of **neonatal respiratory distress syndrome (RDS)** up to 5.6 times higher in diabetic pregnancies compared with nondiabetic controls.[72,90,91] In a metaanalysis, Li et al.[91] reported pooled odds ratios for the association between maternal DM and neonatal RDS of 1.57 (95% confidence interval [CI], 1.28 to 1.93) for GDM and 2.66 (95% CI, 2.06 to 3.44) for pregestational DM. However, some studies have been unable to verify a relationship between diabetic pregnancies and neonatal RDS. Potential confounding factors include more preterm and cesarean deliveries in diabetic pregnancies. Proposed mechanisms linking diabetic pregnancies to neonatal RDS include alterations in specific surfactant proteins and phospholipids.[90]

Neonatal hypoglycemia has an estimated incidence of 27% in diabetic pregnancies.[92] This occurs in both pregestational DM and GDM, with a ninefold higher risk compared with nondiabetic controls.[72,92] Glucose is freely shared between the fetal and maternal circulations, but their insulin systems are separated by the placenta. Neonatal hypoglycemia likely results from sustained fetal hyperinsulinemia in response to chronic and acute intrauterine hyperglycemia.[93] Studies have demonstrated higher fetal insulin levels and exaggerated fetal insulin responses to acute maternal hyperglycemia in diabetic

pregnancies.[94,95] An acute increase in maternal glucose concentration, as might occur if a dextrose-containing solution is used for intravenous hydration during administration of neuraxial anesthesia, can lead to reactive neonatal hypoglycemia, even in nondiabetic women.[96]

There is a fourfold higher incidence of **neonatal hyperbilirubinemia** in diabetic pregnancies compared with nondiabetic controls.[3,27,97–99] A mild elevation in neonatal serum bilirubin is a normal physiologic process, perhaps with some advantages via antioxidant effects.[97] Moderate to severe elevations require immediate clinical evaluation and probable treatment with phototherapy, to avoid the kernicterus spectrum disorder with irreversible neuronal damage.[98] Neonatal polycythemia is observed in infants of diabetic mothers, perhaps reflecting chronic intrauterine hypoxemia. Delayed clamping of the umbilical cord during delivery results in increased blood volume in all neonates. In one randomized study, delayed clamping increased the risk of newborn hyperbilirubinemia in diabetic pregnancies but not in nondiabetic pregnancies.[99] There is no evidence that newborns from diabetic pregnancies have a higher rate of kernicterus.

Children of diabetic mothers are at increased risk for development of DM, likely from a combination of genetic and intrauterine environmental factors.[100] In terms of heredity, for both type 1 and type 2 DM, the concordance rate is higher in monozygotic twins compared with dizygotic twins. The risk of a sibling developing DM is 15-fold higher for type 1 DM and 4- to 6-fold higher for type 2 DM, compared with the general population.[101]

Obstetric Management
Glycemic Control

Strict glycemic control, ideally beginning in the preconception period, is the best way to prevent fetal structural malformations in women with pregestational DM.[28,85] Determination of hemoglobin A1c concentrations may help the physician determine the adequacy of preconceptional glycemic control.[84,102]

The goal of insulin therapy is to provide plasma insulin concentrations that lead to tight glucose control without hypoglycemia.[103] The patient should frequently determine capillary blood glucose concentration using a reflectance meter or a transdermal tissue glucose measurement using a minimally invasive continuous monitoring system.[17,75,104–106] In general, insulin requirement increases progressively during the second and third trimesters of pregnancy. Table 43.1 illustrates glycemic targets recommended by the ADA for pregnant patients with either pregestational DM or GDM.[103] Of course, strict glycemic control increases the risk for maternal hypoglycemia.

Therapeutic insulin is available in several forms. Initially, insulin was isolated as a natural product from domestic animals (e.g., cattle, pigs). In the 1980s, synthetic human insulin became commercially available and has replaced beef and pork insulin in human medicine. The subsequent development of human insulin analogs, beginning in the 1990s, provides many clinical alternatives for therapeutic insulin action (Table 43.2).[107]

Because insulin requirement decreases abruptly at delivery, it is important to verify the times, doses, insulin preparations,

TABLE 43.1 American Diabetes Association: Glycemic Targets in Pregnancy for Women With Diabetes Mellitus

Parameter	Pregestational and Gestational Diabetes Mellitus[a]
Hemoglobin A1c	6%
Fasting plasma glucose	<95 mg/dL (<5.3 mmol/L)
1-h postprandial plasma glucose	<140 mg/dL (<7.8 mmol/L)

[a]Assumes patients with low risk for hypoglycemia; otherwise, targets should be adjusted higher on an individual basis.
Modified from ElSayed NA, Aleppo G, Aroda VR, et al. American Diabetes Association. 15. Management of diabetes in pregnancy: standards of care in diabetes—2023. *Diabetes Care.* 2023;46(suppl 1): S254–S266.

TABLE 43.2 Pharmacokinetics of Subcutaneous Insulin Administration in Nonpregnant Humans

Insulin Preparations	Onset	Peak	Duration
Short-Acting Class			
Regular	30–60 min	2–4 h	6–8 h
Lispro[a]	10–15 min	1–1.5 h	3–5 h
Aspart[a]	10–15 min	1–2 h	3–5 h
Glulisine[a]	10–15 min	1–2 h	3–5 h
Fast-Acting Aspart[a]	3–4 min	1 h	3–5 h
Ultra-Rapid Lispro[a]	3–4 min	1 h	3–5 h
Intermediate-Acting Class			
NPH	2.5–3 h	5–7 h	13–16 h
Long-Acting Class			
Glargine[a]	2–3 h	No peak	24 h
Detemir[a]	2–3 h	6–8 h	24 h
Degudec[a]	2–4 h	No peak	42 h

NPH, Neutral protamine Hagedorn.
[a]Insulin analog
Data from Kramer CK, Retnakaran R, Zinman B. Insulin and insulin analogs as antidiabetic therapy: a perspective from clinical trials. *Cell Metabolism.* 2021;33:740–747.

and routes of administration in the 24 hours before delivery to avoid maternal postpartum hypoglycemia.[27,68,103]

Management of **DKA** is similar in pregnant and nonpregnant women. It involves (1) intravenous hydration, (2) intravenous insulin, (3) treatment of the underlying cause of DKA, (4) careful monitoring of blood glucose and electrolyte levels, and (5) restriction of bicarbonate therapy to cases of extreme acidosis.[46,50] Initial management of the critically ill pregnant woman should focus on the effective management of DKA. Fetal compromise is likely to resolve with appropriate maternal medical management.[53,108]

Incretins are peptide hormones synthesized by specific gut epithelial cells in response to ingested nutrients, with modulatory effects on gastric emptying and pancreatic insulin secretion.[109] The major human incretins are glucagon-like peptide-1 (GLP-1) and glucose-dependent insulinotropic polypeptide. Pharmaceuticals that mimic incretin action, such as GLP-1 receptor agonists (GLP-1-RA), have been available since 2005 for the treatment of type 2 DM. GLP-1-RAs also alter appetite with significant weight loss in obese patients, irrespective of DM,[109] which has led to their widespread use.

One of the major complications of GLP-1-RA medications is gastroparesis, with an increased risk of gastric content regurgitation and pulmonary aspiration during general anesthesia.[109] The gastrointestinal changes of normal pregnancy, including decreased lower esophageal sphincter tone, when combined with the gastroparesis associated with GLP-1-RAs, may increase maternal risk of aspiration.

Data regarding the use of GLP-1-RAs during pregnancy are limited, though some studies suggest they may be safe for the fetus.[110] Nonetheless, the US Food and Drug Administration currently does not recommend their use during pregnancy or lactation, and it is recommended that they should be stopped 2 months prior to conception.[111]

Diet and exercise are the initial therapeutic approaches for glycemic control in women with GDM.[3,4] Pharmacologic therapy with oral hypoglycemic agents and/or insulin is initiated if the lifestyle changes are not clinically effective.[3,4,68,103] Concerns about the long-term health implications of GDM have resulted in clinical initiatives for postpartum metabolic surveillance.[3,4,103] The goal is to identify and treat postpartum type 2 DM, with an emphasis on lifestyle interventions.

Timing of Delivery

Timing of delivery is important in the management of diabetic pregnancies; the obstetric provider must weigh the risks of preterm delivery with the risk of late-term fetal demise. Typically, a nonstress test is performed twice weekly in patients with pregestational DM, beginning at 32 weeks' gestation.[27] A nonreactive nonstress test should prompt the performance of a fetal biophysical profile (see Chapter 6). Patients with poorly controlled GDM should probably undergo antepartum fetal surveillance similar to that in patients with pregestational DM.[3] In the presence of reassuring fetal testing, delivery can be delayed until after 38 weeks' gestation.[3,27,112] Poor glycemic control or maternal nephropathy may necessitate an earlier delivery.[3,27]

The decision regarding the method of delivery requires consideration of estimated fetal weight, fetal condition, cervical dilation and effacement, and previous obstetric history. The obstetric provider may choose elective cesarean delivery in the diabetic parturient with evidence of fetal macrosomia to decrease the risk for shoulder dystocia.

Anesthetic Management

There are a limited number of studies of the anesthetic management of pregnant women with DM. In general, neuraxial analgesia and anesthesia are the preferred techniques for labor and cesarean delivery, but in many circumstances the clinical decisions about these patients must be guided by logical extensions of studies of nonpregnant diabetic patients and nondiabetic pregnant patients.

Preanesthetic evaluation of the woman with DM should include a history and physical examination that focuses on the identification of the acute and chronic complications of DM (see Box 43.1). We are not aware of any published data on the relationship between the complications of DM and responses to anesthetic agents or on anesthetic outcomes in pregnant diabetic patients. In a study of nonpregnant diabetic patients, preoperative evidence of **autonomic cardiovascular dysfunction** was predictive of the need for a vasopressor during general anesthesia.[113] Because of the potential for hypotension during neuraxial anesthesia, noninvasive testing of autonomic function may be useful in obstetric patients with pregestational DM. For example, in nonpregnant diabetic patients, the corrected QT interval on an electrocardiogram correlates with the severity of autonomic neuropathy.[114] Patients with evidence of autonomic dysfunction may benefit from more frequent blood pressure measurement and more vigorous use of intravenous hydration and pressor agents during the administration of neuraxial anesthesia. **Gastroparesis** is a manifestation of autonomic neuropathy in diabetic patients.[115] In both nondiabetic and gestational diabetic patients having cesarean delivery, oral consumption of 300 mL of a nonparticulate carbohydrate solution 2 hours before surgery appears to be safe and well accepted by patients.[115,116] In nonpregnant diabetic patients, autonomic neuropathy is associated with a decreased cough reflex threshold and a higher incidence of obstructive sleep apnea.[117,118]

Concerns have been expressed about local anesthetic toxicity in patients with diabetic polyneuropathy undergoing neuraxial or peripheral nerve blocks because diabetic nerves may be more susceptible to injury. Nevertheless, the benefits conferred by neuraxial anesthesia make it the technique of choice for the diabetic parturient as for any parturient.[119]

Several studies have examined the maternal, fetal, and neonatal effects of **neuraxial anesthesia** for cesarean delivery in women with pregestational DM.[120–123] Datta and Brown[120] observed that in patients with pregestational DM, spinal anesthesia was associated with slightly lower umbilical cord blood pH at delivery compared with general anesthesia. Subsequently, these investigators noted an association between fetal acidosis and peripartum maternal hypotension in patients with pregestational DM who received epidural anesthesia for cesarean delivery.[121] In these studies, acute maternal hyperglycemia—secondary to intravenous hydration with 5% dextrose before administration of neuraxial anesthesia—was a potentially confounding factor.[120,121]

Neonatal acidosis is *not* likely to occur during **spinal** or **epidural anesthesia** for cesarean delivery in diabetic parturients, provided that (1) maternal glycemic control is satisfactory,

(2) the patient receives intravenous volume expansion with a non–dextrose-containing balanced salt solution, and (3) hypotension is prevented or treated promptly.[122,123]

After administration of epidural anesthesia for cesarean delivery, Ramanathan et al.[123] observed an increased incidence of neonatal hypoglycemia in patients with pregestational DM compared with nondiabetic controls (35% versus 7%, respectively). In this study, maternal glycemic control was fair (mean fasting plasma glucose level was 127 mg/dL [7.1 mmol/L]), a non–dextrose-containing solution was used for intravenous hydration, and intravenous insulin therapy was adjusted on the basis of frequent blood glucose determinations. This study illustrates the neonate's vulnerability to hypoglycemia after a diabetic pregnancy despite meticulous anesthesia care at the time of delivery.

Maternal hypoglycemia has been described following neuraxial anesthesia.[124,125] In one case, it was hypothesized to be secondary to a rapid decrease in catecholamine levels following onset of analgesia.[124] In another case, it was hypothesized to have been related to an abrupt increase in insulin sensitivity following placental delivery in a patient who had received exogenous insulin before spinal anesthesia for cesarean delivery.[125]

In a retrospective study of women with well-controlled GDM having vaginal delivery at term, epidural labor analgesia was associated with lower cord blood glucose concentration and improved neonatal acid-base status.[126]

Neonatal hypoglycemia can be avoided if there is tight control of maternal glucose levels, which should be continued into the peripartum period.[103] Maternal insulin requirements decrease with the onset of labor, increase again during the second stage of labor, and decrease markedly during the early postpartum period.[41,42] Intravenous regular insulin therapy is the most flexible method of treatment during this period of rapid change. Absorption of subcutaneous insulin may be unpredictable and may increase the risk for maternal hypoglycemia, especially during the postpartum period.[42]

Intravenous glucose and insulin infusions during the peripartum period should be titrated to maintain a maternal blood glucose concentration of 70 to 90 mg/dL (3.9 to 5 mmol/L). During active labor, the glucose requirement is 2.5 mg/kg/min or more.[39] For cesarean delivery in patients using a subcutaneous insulin pump, a preoperative strategy should be formulated for perioperative insulin pump management. This plan should identify individual, other than the patient, who are experienced and knowledgeable in adjusting the insulin pump if the patient is not able to adjust it herself during surgery. Further, the pump along with the requisite tubing must be strategically draped out of the sterile field. Some patients and obstetric providers prefer discontinuing the subcutaneous insulin pump preoperatively in favor of an intravenous insulin infusion. The preanesthetic evaluation is an excellent opportunity to discuss with the patient the expected changes in insulin requirement at the time of delivery.

Many perioperative strategies have been proposed for metabolic control in nonpregnant patients with DM.[127] No convincing evidence suggests that any clinical strategy for perioperative diabetic control is superior in terms of patient outcome. Frequent blood glucose measurements (e.g., at 30- to 60-minute intervals), followed by appropriate adjustment of glucose and insulin infusions, represent the cornerstone of optimal perioperative care in patients with DM. In nonpregnant patients, DM may be associated with challenging neuromuscular monitoring because of diabetic polyneuropathy or alterations at the neuromuscular junction.[128]

Difficult direct laryngoscopy and tracheal intubation has been reported in nonpregnant patients with DM and the **diabetic stiff-joint syndrome** or **diabetic scleredema**.[129] This syndrome occurs in patients with long-standing DM type 1 and is associated with nonfamilial short stature, joint contractures, and tight skin.[130] Fortunately, the incidence of this unusual syndrome is decreasing, perhaps because of improved medical care. During the preanesthesia evaluation of patients with DM, the anesthesia provider can screen for the stiff-joint syndrome by looking for the "prayer sign" (Fig. 43.4). There is a case report of a pregnant patient with pregestational DM and diabetic scleredema who experienced anterior spinal artery syndrome after the administration of epidural anesthesia for cesarean delivery.[131] The author suggested that spinal cord vascular compression resulted from a combination of (1) preexisting microvascular disease, (2) an epidural space that was stiff because of connective tissue disease, and (3) administration of a large volume (35 mL) of the

local anesthetic agent. In patients with a history and physical examination that suggest diabetic stiff-joint syndrome, the anesthesia provider should consider two potential problems: (1) difficult direct laryngoscopy and tracheal intubation and (2) a noncompliant epidural space.

Infection is an important cause of morbidity in pregnant women with pregestational DM[51]; therefore strict aseptic technique should be used during the administration of neuraxial anesthesia.[119]

THYROID DISORDERS

Thyroid Hormone Physiology

The follicular cells of the thyroid gland sequester iodine and synthesize thyroglobulin, an iodinated precursor protein. Thyroglobulin is secreted into the lumen of the microscopic thyroid follicles before it undergoes reuptake, proteolysis, and transfer to lysosomes, where it undergoes degradation.[132,133] This process results in the systemic release of the thyroid hormones: thyroxine (T_4) and 3,5,3'-triiodothyronine (T_3). Reverse T_3 (3,3',5'-triiodothyronine) is a structural variant with much less physiologic potency in most target organs.[133]

Thyroid hormone synthesis and release are controlled primarily by thyroid-stimulating hormone (TSH)—a trophic hormone from the pituitary gland—and the supply of iodine. The thyroid hormones normally participate in a negative feedback loop that regulates TSH secretion (Fig. 43.5) and thyrotropin-releasing hormone production in the hypothalamus.[132,134]

Thyroid hormones are highly bound to proteins in the blood. In euthyroid nonpregnant humans, the normal total serum concentrations of T_4 and T_3 are 50 to 150 nmol/L and 1.4 to 3.2 nmol/L, respectively. The unbound or free fractions of T_4 and T_3 are 0.03% and 0.3% of total circulating T_4 and T_3, respectively.[135,136] Similar proportions of T_4 and T_3 are distributed among the three major plasma proteins that bind thyroid hormones, which are (1) thyroxine-binding globulin (TBG) (70% to 80%), (2) thyroxine-binding prealbumin or transthyretin (10% to 20%), and (3) albumin (10% to 15%).[135,136] The serum concentration of unbound or free T_4 is typically the major determinant of thyroid hormone activity in target tissues. Thyroid hormones are temporarily inert while bound to plasma proteins. Changes in the concentrations of thyroxine-binding proteins can occur during various physiologic states (e.g., pregnancy) and disease processes. Thyroid hormone action does not change with fluctuations in the total concentration of T_4 as long as the concentration of free T_4 remains constant.

Thyroid hormone is an endocrine regulator in many target organs (e.g., liver, kidneys, skeletal and cardiac muscles, brain, pituitary gland, placenta).[137] The defined physiologic effects of thyroid hormones are mediated by regulation of specific gene products. These effects include (1) somatic and nervous system development, (2) calorigenesis, (3) augmented skeletal and cardiac muscle performance, (4) intermediary metabolism, and (5) feedback control.[132,137]

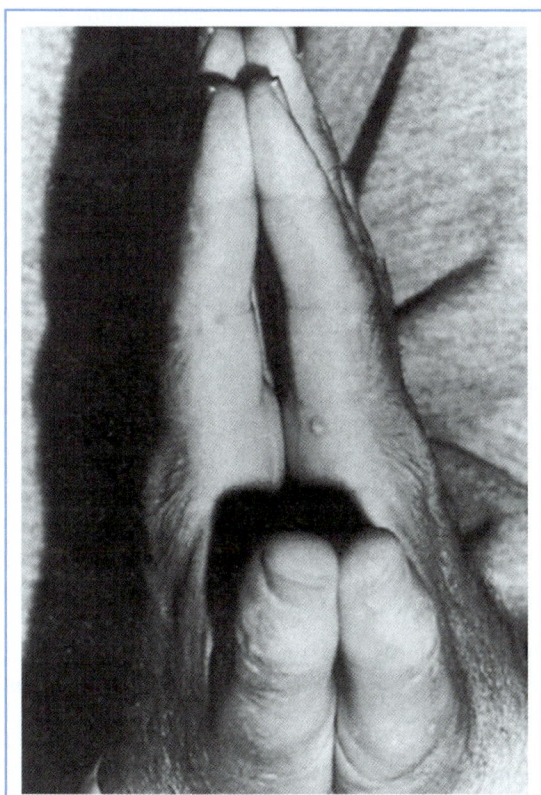

Fig. 43.4 Inability to approximate the palmar surfaces of the phalangeal joints despite maximal effort, secondary to diabetic stiff-joint syndrome. From Hogan K, Rusy D, Springman SR. Difficult laryngoscopy and diabetes mellitus. *Anesth Analg.* 1988;67:1162–1165.

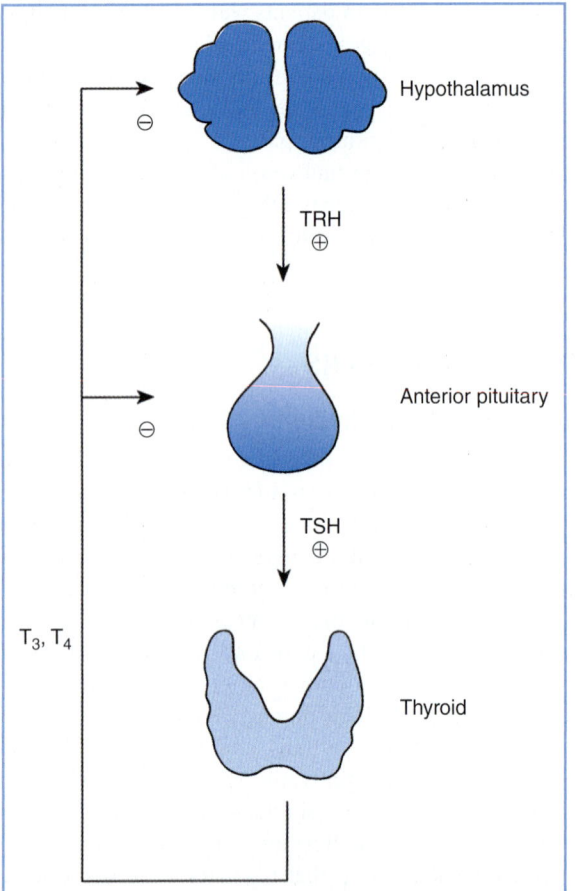

Fig. 43.5 Normal Feedback Control of Thyroid Hormone Secretion. *TRH*, Thyrotropin-releasing hormone; *TSH*, thyroid-stimulating hormone; T_3, triiodothyronine; T_4, thyroxine. From Davies PH, Franklyn JA. The effects of drugs on tests of thyroid function. *Eur J Clin Pharmacol.* 1991;40:439–451.

In the cells of target tissues, free T_4 enters via specific transport proteins.[138] The molecular actions of T_4 begin with the enzymatic deiodination of T_4 to T_3. Iodothyronine deiodinase is widely distributed in the body and occurs in three molecular forms.[139] Only 20% of the daily T_3 production is secreted by the thyroid gland; the rest is formed by peripheral deiodination. In the classic model of thyroid hormone action, T_3 enters the nuclei of target cells, binds to specific thyroid hormone receptors, and alters genomic transcription of specific proteins.[137,138] Research has now characterized other mechanisms of action for thyroid hormones, including cell-surface nontranscriptional T_4 effects through an integrin protein receptor[140] and T_3 effects on mitochondrial transcription.[141] Variations in the number and types of thyroid hormone receptors, as well as receptor linkage to development- or tissue-specific genomic expression, provide additional levels of physiologic control and vulnerability to disease processes.[137–141]

Antithyroid medications may affect single or multiple steps in thyroid hormone synthesis and release, as well as concentrations of plasma-binding proteins, deiodinase activity, and peripheral uptake of thyroid hormones.[132]

Laboratory evaluation of thyroid function consists of two measurements in most patients. First, the serum concentration of free T_4 can be directly measured or indirectly calculated. Second, the serum concentration of TSH is measured to assess the negative feedback loop that controls the thyroid gland. The TSH concentration is judged as appropriate or inappropriate in the context of the serum concentration of free T_4.

During normal human pregnancy, the serum concentration of TBG steadily increases until it reaches a plateau at 20 weeks' gestation, when it is 50% greater than the nonpregnant level. The higher concentration of TBG results from both greater synthesis and a prolonged half-life during pregnancy. The normal pregnant woman is euthyroid because the serum concentrations of free T_4 and T_3 are in the normal or low-normal range for nonpregnant individuals. However, the increased concentration of TBG means that total serum concentrations of T_4 and T_3 during pregnancy are at or above the upper limit of normal for nonpregnant women.[135]

Human chorionic gonadotropin (hCG) is a placental protein that shares some structural features with TSH. The serum concentrations of TSH and hCG have an inverse relationship during normal human pregnancy, reflecting the mild TSH-like activity that results from increased plasma concentrations of hCG during early pregnancy.[142]

Iodine deficiency is a major cause of hypothyroidism worldwide, and normal development of the fetus is dependent on availability of T_4 and T_3, with particular vulnerability in the fetal brain.[143–145] Maternal iodine availability is decreased during pregnancy because of greater fetal uptake and increased maternal renal clearance.[146] The recommended daily intake of iodine during pregnancy varies between 150 and 250 µg, but is less than 500 µg.[23,147,148] The iodine content is variable between different formulations of prenatal vitamins, and patient compliance with vitamin intake is variable.[148,149] In geographic areas with marginal environmental iodine availability, all of these factors may place mothers and fetuses at risk for hypothyroidism.

Hyperthyroidism
Definition and Epidemiology
Hyperthyroidism is defined by an abnormal increase in the serum concentration of unbound or free thyroid hormones. In iodine-replete populations, the prevalence of hyperthyroidism is 0.2% to 1.9%, with a female-to-male ratio of 10:1.[150,151] The etiology of hyperthyroidism is shown in Box 43.5. Graves' disease is responsible for 70% to 90% of cases; thyroiditis and the combined category of toxic adenoma and toxic multinodular goiter each account for approximately 5%.

Pathophysiology
Graves' disease is an autoimmune thyroid disease.[152] Its etiology is likely multifactorial and includes both **environmental** (e.g., stress, hormones) and **genetic** influences.[153] Several autoantibodies against thyroid tissue have been described

BOX 43.5 Etiology of Hyperthyroidism

Excessive TSH–receptor stimulation
- Graves' disease
- hCG–related thyrotoxicosis
    - Gestational transient thyrotoxicosis
    - Familial gestational hyperthyroidism
    - Hydatidiform mole, choriocarcinoma
- TSH-producing pituitary adenoma

Autonomous thyroid hormone secretion
- Toxic multinodular goiter
- Solitary toxic adenoma
- Familial or sporadic nonautoimmune hyperthyroidism

Destructive thyroiditis
- Subacute de Quervain thyroiditis
- Silent or painless thyroiditis; postpartum thyroiditis
- Acute suppurative thyroiditis
- Drug-induced
    - Amiodarone
    - Excess iodine intake
    - Tyrosine kinase inhibitors
    - Immune checkpoint inhibitors

Extrathyroidal source of thyroid hormone
- Thyrotoxicosis factitia
- Struma ovarii
- Metastases of differentiated thyroid cancer
- Hamburger thyrotoxicosis

hCG, Human chorionic gonadotropin; *TSH*, thyroid stimulating hormone.
Modified from Wiersinga WM, Poppe KG, Effraimidis G. Hyperthyroidism: aetiology, pathogenesis, diagnosis, management, complications, and prognosis. *Lancet Diabetes Endocrinol.* 2023;11: 282–298.

in patients with this disease. Autoantibodies known as **thyroid receptor antibodies (TRAbs)** directed against the TSH receptor in the thyroid gland may either augment or inhibit TSH action, depending on their binding specificities.[153,154] The binding specificities of TRAbs in the blood of each patient with Graves' disease determine the net thyroid-stimulating activity. Autoantibodies against thyroid peroxidase, the sodium-iodide symporter, and thyroglobulin also have been described in patients with Graves' disease and other forms of autoimmune thyroid disorders.

Clinical Presentation and Diagnosis

Hyperthyroidism presents as a physiologic state dominated by an increased metabolic rate. A hyperthyroid symptom scale has been developed on the basis of the following 10 clinical factors: nervousness, sweating, heat intolerance, hyperactivity, tremor, weakness, hyperdynamic precordium, diarrhea, appetite, and level of incapacitation.[155] This symptom scale has been useful to follow the clinical course of patients with Graves' disease. Exophthalmos or infiltrative ophthalmopathy is clinically apparent in many patients, although the reported prevalence varies from 25% to 70%.[152,156] Other physical signs may occur at low frequency, including pretibial myxedema or dermopathy (1% to 2%) and nail changes or acropachy (<1%). The thyroid-associated orbitopathy (TAO) in Graves' disease is caused by an inflammatory process with enlargement of the extraocular muscle bodies, and deposition of adipose tissue and extracellular glycosaminoglycans within the bony orbit.[156,157] In addition to hyperthyroidism and TRAbs, the risk factors for TAO include smoking and radioactive iodine treatment. The pathogenetic targets are orbital fibroblasts with a "cross-talk" mechanism between TSH receptor and insulin-like growth factor-1 (IGF-1) receptor pathways.[156,157] Traditional therapies for TAO have included conservative measures to maintain eye moisture, plus glucocorticoids, radiotherapy, or orbital decompressive surgery for severe cases.[152,156,157] Recent clinical trials with **teprotumumab**, a monoclonal antibody that blocks IGF-1 signals, have demonstrated therapeutic efficacy in TAO, but it is contraindicated in pregnancy.[158]

Hyperthyroidism stimulates the cardiovascular system in excess of the underlying increased metabolic rate, resulting in a hyperkinetic circulatory state.[159,160] Heart rate, myocardial contractility, cardiac output, ventricular size, systolic blood pressure, pulse pressure, and pulmonary vascular resistance all increase, and peripheral vascular resistance decreases.[161,162] Sinus tachycardia is the most common arrhythmia, but the incidence of atrial fibrillation is also increased.[163] Cardiomyopathy can be demonstrated during exercise in hyperthyroid patients, independent of beta-adrenergic receptors; it is reversible with normalization of thyroid function.[164]

The diagnosis of hyperthyroidism depends on increased serum concentrations of free T_4. The more common forms of hyperthyroidism (e.g., Graves' disease, toxic adenoma, toxic multinodular goiter) may be differentiated from the less common forms by a radioiodine uptake study. The identification of TSH receptor autoantibodies may have a role in distinguishing Graves' disease from toxic adenoma or multinodular goiter.[154]

Interaction With Pregnancy

Normal human pregnancy is a euthyroid state, with normal plasma concentration of free T_4 despite increased plasma concentrations of TBG and total T_4. During pregnancy, hyperthyroidism results from the same causes as in nonpregnant patients (see Box 43.5). Graves' disease is the leading cause of hyperthyroidism during pregnancy, with a prevalence of 0.2%, which is lower than in the general population.[147] The lower prevalence may reflect a beneficial effect of the immunotolerance of pregnancy on autoimmune disorders. Human pregnancy also is associated with a change in the specificity of TSH receptor antibodies between stimulatory and blocking activities.[165]

Gestational trophoblastic neoplasms (GTNs) are frequently associated with elevated serum hCG concentration. A high concentration of hCG may possess significant thyroid-stimulating bioactivity because of the structural homology between hCG and TSH.[135,142] This is the underlying mechanism for both relatively common gestational transient thyrotoxicosis[166] and rare hyperthyroidism in association with GTNs.[167] Also, hyperemesis gravidarum and gestational transient thyrotoxicosis may be parallel disease processes in pregnancy, with elevated hCG a shared mechanism.[147,168] Hyperthyroidism can, on rare occasions, result from two coincident disease processes (e.g., Graves' disease and struma ovarii) in both pregnant and nonpregnant women.[169]

The reported prevalence of thyroid nodules, currently 34% to 66% of adults, has increased because of identification of incidental asymptomatic nodules with improved diagnostic imaging modalities.[170] Pregnancy is associated with increases in the number and size of thyroid nodules.[169] Pregnancy probably does not affect the development or recurrence of thyroid carcinoma, and the effect on the progression of active disease remains controversial.[147,171] Evaluation of a thyroid nodule that presents during pregnancy should include measurement of serum TSH and free T_4 concentrations, plus ultrasonographic examination of the thyroid gland and cervical lymph nodes. Sonographic features of concern include a nodule greater than 1 to 2 cm in diameter, a solid hypoechoic nodule, irregular margins, or microcalcifications.[147,168] Suspicious thyroid nodules can be further evaluated with fine-needle aspiration or percutaneous needle biopsy. Malignant lesions, depending on the level of cellular differentiation, can be resected in the second trimester or observed until after delivery.[147,168] Radioactive iodine therapy is contraindicated during both pregnancy and lactation because it readily crosses the placenta and transfers into breast milk.

Medical and Surgical Management

Current therapies for Graves' disease in nonpregnant patients include radioactive iodine, antithyroid medications, and surgery.[150,152,172]

Radioactive iodine is administered orally as iodine-131 (^{131}I), a radionuclide that emits beta and gamma radiation. The specific dose is based on individual factors and severity of disease.[173] All forms of iodine are sequestered by the thyroid gland, with any excess excreted in the urine. ^{131}I exerts a therapeutic effect in Graves' disease, primarily through local emission of beta radiation. In most patients with Graves' disease, hypothyroidism develops after a therapeutic dose of radioactive iodine, necessitating careful follow-up and long-term thyroid hormone replacement therapy. Otherwise, in nonpregnant patients, the long-term health risks of radioactive iodine therapy are minimal. Currently recommended treatment is to delay pregnancy for 6 months to 1 year after radioactive iodine therapy,[172,173] despite ^{131}I having a half-life of only 8 days.

Propylthiouracil and **methimazole** are the antithyroid medications used to treat Graves' disease.[150,152,172] Both drugs interfere with the incorporation of iodine into thyroglobulin and with subsequent coupling reactions in the thyroid gland, and propylthiouracil inhibits iodothyronine deiodinase in peripheral tissues. Typical oral doses are 10 to 30 mg daily for methimazole and 100 to 150 mg three times daily for propylthiouracil.[150,172] The long-term clinical strategy is to adjust the

dose downward as tolerated. Some patients with Graves' disease experience remission after the administration of an antithyroid medication. Asymptomatic agranulocytosis is a rare complication of antithyroid medications, with an incidence of 0.1% to 0.3% and typical onset within 3 months of initiating therapy.[152,172] Another rare complication of both antithyroid drugs is hepatotoxicity, with an estimated incidence of less than 0.1%.[152,172] **Immunomodulation therapies** are likely to have an impact on the treatment of Graves' disease in the near future.[152,174]

Surgical therapy for Graves' disease is typically reserved for patients unable or unwilling to undergo treatment with radioactive iodine or antithyroid medications.[152,175] Total thyroidectomy is the most common procedure.[175] Perioperative complications of thyroid surgery include: (1) unilateral or bilateral vocal cord paralysis secondary to recurrent laryngeal nerve injury, (2) wound hematoma, (3) pneumothorax, (4) hypoparathyroidism, and (5) thyroid storm.[175,176] Hypocalcemia secondary to acute hypoparathyroidism may manifest as laryngospasm during the postoperative period.[176]

Thyroid storm. Thyroid storm, also known as thyroid crisis, is a life-threatening exacerbation or decompensation of a preexisting hyperthyroid state.[172,177,178] It is a clinical diagnosis based on the following signs and symptoms: (1) fever, (2) mental and emotional disturbances, (3) tachycardia, (4) tachypnea, (5) diarrhea, (6) congestive heart failure, and (7) atrial fibrillation. Without treatment, thyroid storm may progress to coma, multiorgan system failure, and death. The mortality rate approached 100% in earlier series, but improved therapy has reduced the mortality rate to 1.2% to 3.6% in hospitalized patients.[179]

In most cases, thyroid storm is associated with a precipitating event in a patient with untreated or incompletely treated hyperthyroidism (Box 43.6).[172,180] A widely utilized scoring system for thyroid storm based on symptoms was proposed by Burch and Wartofsky (Box 43.7).[177] A total score > 44 is highly suggestive of thyroid storm, and a total score < 25 makes the diagnosis unlikely.

The current incidence of thyroid storm in hyperthyroid patients is difficult to determine but appears to be much lower than in the past. Akamizu et al.[181] estimated that the incidence

---

BOX 43.6   Events Associated With Precipitation of Thyroid Storm

- Surgery
- Parturition
- Trauma
- Emotional stress
- Iodinated contrast agents
- Treatment with iodine-131
- Pulmonary embolism
- Burn injury
- Infection
- Diabetic ketoacidosis
- Hypoglycemia

Modified from Klubo-Gwiezdzinska J, Wartofsky L. Thyroid emergencies. *Med Clin North Am.* 2012;96:385–403.

BOX 43.7 Burch-Wartofsky Diagnostic Criteria for Thyroid Storm

Categories and Signs/Symptoms	Points
Thermoregulatory Dysfunction	
Temperature °F (°C)	
<99 (<37.2)	0
99–99.9 (37.2–37.7)	5
100–100.9 (37.8–38.2)	10
101–101.9 (38.3–38.8)	15
102–102.9 (38.9–39.4)	20
103–103.9 (39.5–39.9)	25
≥104 (≥40)	30
Central Nervous System Effects	
Absent	0
Agitation	10
Delirium, psychosis, or extreme lethargy	20
Seizure or coma	30
Gastrointestinal-Hepatic Dysfunction	
Absent	0
Diarrhea, nausea/vomiting, abdominal pain	10
Unexplained jaundice	20
Cardiovascular Dysfunction: Tachycardia (beats/min)	
<90	0
90–109	5
110–119	10
120–129	15
130–139	20
≥140	25
Cardiovascular Dysfunction: Congestive Heart Failure	
Absent	0
Mild	5
Moderate	10
Severe	15
Cardiovascular Dysfunction: Atrial Fibrillation	
Absent	0
Present	10
Precipitant History	
Negative	0
Positive	10

The highest point values from each category are added together to arrive at a total score.

Interpretation of the Total Score:

>44	Highly suggestive of thyroid storm
25–44	Suggestive of impending thyroid storm
<25	Unlikely to represent thyroid storm

Modified from: Burch HB, Wartofsky L. Life-threatening thyrotoxicosis: thyroid storm. *Endocrinol Metab Clin North Am.* 1993;22:263–277.

thyroid storm and its unpredictable nature make prospective clinical study extremely challenging.

The mechanism of the development of thyroid storm is unknown, although its clinical presentation is consistent with an exaggerated thyroid hormone effect. Limited data suggest that total serum concentrations of T_4 and T_3 are not increased during thyroid storm in hyperthyroid patients,[182] although one case report suggested otherwise.[183] Alternatively, the precipitating event may augment thyroid hormone action by increasing the circulating free fraction of thyroid hormones. This hypothesis is supported by data that demonstrate higher serum concentrations of free T_4 during thyroid storm as well as by observations of changes in thyroid hormone binding during fever or systemic illness.[184] It is possible that increased peripheral conversion of T_4 to T_3 in target tissues contributes to thyroid storm. Catecholamine secretion probably contributes to symptoms, although it is unclear whether this is a trigger or a by-product of the condition. The role of the sympathetic nervous system is supported by historical observations that spinal anesthesia to the fourth thoracic dermatome level is therapeutic.[185]

Box 43.8 outlines the treatment of thyroid storm. Treatment of thyroid storm has been characterized as general supportive measures plus the "5 Bs": **B**lock synthesis (propylthiouracil, iodine), **B**lock release (iodine), **B**lock conversion of T_4 to T_3 (beta-adrenergic receptor blockers, glucocorticoids, propylthiouracil), **B**eta-adrenergic receptor blockers, and **B**lock enterohepatic circulation (cholestyramine).[186] Several points merit discussion. Glucocorticoid supplementation is listed as a general supportive measure because endogenous glucocorticoid production is impaired in patients with hyperthyroidism.[187] Glucocorticoids also inhibit both thyroid hormone production and the peripheral conversion of T_4 to T_3.[188] Propylthiouracil and methimazole reduce thyroid hormone production, but only propylthiouracil inhibits the peripheral conversion of T_4 to T_3 (as discussed earlier). In addition to the relief of many symptoms of hyperthyroidism, several beta-adrenergic receptor antagonists (including propranolol, metoprolol, and atenolol) inhibit the peripheral conversion of T_4 to T_3.[189] Acute iodine administration decreases thyroid hormone production (Wolff-Chaikoff effect) and its release into the circulation. It is reasonable to delay iodine treatment until 1 hour after the administration of propylthiouracil to avoid subsequent increased iodine use by the thyroid gland.

Thyroid storm is an acute hypermetabolic state that may be difficult to distinguish clinically from malignant hyperthermia in the perioperative period. Rhabdomyolysis is one of the few features of the latter disorder that has not also been reported in thyroid storm.[190] Three cases of thyroid storm treated with dantrolene have been reported.[191-193] Two patients survived, but the third succumbed to multiorgan system failure that antedated the dantrolene therapy. In another case, a patient with known Graves' disease undergoing subtotal thyroidectomy had an intraoperative hypermetabolic crisis that was initially diagnosed and treated as thyroid storm. The correct diagnosis of malignant hyperthermia was made on the basis of subsequent blood gas analysis, and the patient

of thyroid storm in Japan was 0.2 per 100,000 hospitalized patients between 2004 and 2008. Gallindo et al.[179] reported an incidence in the United States of 4.8 to 5.6 per 100,000 hospitalized hyperthyroid patients from 2004 to 2013. The rarity of

---

BOX 43.8   Treatment of Thyroid Storm

Block Thyroid Hormone Synthesis

Antithyroid medications:

    Propylthiouracil (PTU): 600 mg loading dose, followed by
      200–250 mg orally every 4–6 h

    OR

    Methimazole: 20–30 mg orally every 4–6 h

    (Note: Propylthiouracil also inhibits peripheral conversion of
T_4 to T_3)

Block Thyroid Hormone Release

Iodine:

    Supersaturated potassium iodide solution (SSKI): five
      drops orally every 6–8 h

    OR

    Lugol's solution: 5–10 drops orally every 6–8 h

    (Note: Iodine administration should be delayed until at least
one hour after giving propylthiouracil or methimazole)

**Block Peripheral Conversion of Thyroxine (T_4) to
3,5,3'-Triiodothyronine (T_3)**

Glucocorticoid:

    Hydrocortisone 100 mg IV every 6 h

    OR

    Dexamethasone 2 mg IV every 6 h

Beta-Adrenergic Receptor Blocker:

    Propranolol 1–2 mg IV every 15 min up to maximum 10 mg

    Other beta-adrenergic receptor blockers to consider:
      metoprolol, atenolol, esmolol

Propylthiouracil: see above

Beta-Adrenergic Receptor Blocker

(see above)

Block Enterohepatic Circulation

Cholestyramine: 4 g orally every 6–12 h

General Supportive Measures

Oxygen

Cooling measures

Acetaminophen (paracetamol)

Intravenous hydration

Glucose and electrolyte replacement

Nutritional support

Glucocorticoid supplementation

Consider Other Therapies

Plasma exchange

Treatment of the Underlying Precipitating Condition

Modified from Carroll R, Matfin G. Endocrine and metabolic emergencies: thyroid storm. *Ther Adv Endocrinol Metab*. 2010;1:139–145.

---

was successfully treated with dantrolene.[194] Dantrolene therapy should not be delayed when both the diagnoses of malignant hyperthermia and thyroid storm are being considered, because it is not detrimental in patients with thyroid storm. Plasma exchange is another unusual but effective therapeutic option for thyroid storm.[195]

Preoperative preparation. Many cases of perioperative thyroid storm involve thyroid surgery. The preoperative

therapeutic goals are to inhibit thyroid hormone synthesis and secretion in patients with preexisting hyperthyroidism and to decrease the vascularity of the thyroid gland. The four main therapies used in preoperative preparation are similar to those discussed above: administration of (1) an antithyroid medication (primarily propylthiouracil), (2) a beta-adrenergic receptor antagonist, (3) a glucocorticoid, and (4) iodine.[196,197]

Beta-adrenergic receptor blockade may be sufficient to prevent perioperative thyroid storm,[197] although thyroid storm has been reported after preoperative preparation with propranolol alone.[198] One advantage of beta-adrenergic receptor antagonists over antithyroid medications is the shorter time typically required for preoperative preparation (2 weeks versus 6 to 8 weeks, respectively).[199] Some investigators have recommended preoperative preparation with a beta-adrenergic receptor antagonist, with the addition of iodine beginning 10 days before surgery.[200] The use of beta-adrenergic receptor antagonists entails a risk for hypoglycemia in hyperthyroid patients because they have reduced hepatic glucose reserves, and nonspecific beta-adrenergic receptor blockade results in a pharmacologic blunting of counterregulatory sympathetic responses.[201]

Elective surgery should not proceed without adequate preoperative preparation of hyperthyroid patients. In cases of emergency surgery, physicians should consider using the therapies discussed for the treatment of thyroid storm (as discussed earlier) (see Box 43.8).

Medical and surgical management during pregnancy. All of the therapeutic options used in nonpregnant hyperthyroid patients should be efficacious in pregnant women (Box 43.8). However, the potential effects on the fetus dictate modifications in some of the options for treatment of hyperthyroidism during pregnancy.[147,168,202,203] Radioactive iodine is contraindicated during pregnancy, as discussed above.

The mainstays of therapy for hyperthyroidism during pregnancy are the thioamide antithyroid medications, **propylthiouracil** and **methimazole**, though they cross the placenta affecting both the maternal and fetal thyroid glands. Although these agents are similar in efficacy for treatment of hyperthyroidism during pregnancy, propylthiouracil has been used more frequently than methimazole. Propylthiouracil is favored in the first trimester of pregnancy, owing to rare congenital anomalies reported with methimazole (e.g., scalp defects, choanal atresia). After the first trimester, therapy can be switched to methimazole if there are concerns for hepatotoxicity with propylthiouracil.[147,168,202,203]

Surgical therapy (e.g., subtotal thyroidectomy) is generally reserved for pregnant women in whom medical therapy has failed.[147,202] The pregnant woman should receive preoperative preparation with a beta-adrenergic receptor antagonist, a glucocorticoid, and iodine to minimize the risk for thyroid storm. Clinical data suggest that treating maternal Graves' disease with iodine does not result in fetal hypothyroidism, implying that short-term preoperative maternal treatment with iodine should be safe for the fetus.[204]

One national database study of pregnant women undergoing thyroid or parathyroid surgery demonstrated a twofold increase in surgical complications compared with age-matched nonpregnant controls.[205] In pregnant patients with Graves' disease, surgical thyroidectomy may lead to fetal hyperthyroidism through placental passage of persistent maternal TSAbs.[206]

During pregnancy, **thyroid storm** is a rare hypermetabolic event. Previous reports of a 2% to 4% incidence among pregnant patients are probably overestimates of the true incidence.[181] Most contemporary cases of thyroid storm during pregnancy occur in patients with undiagnosed or undertreated preexisting hyperthyroidism.[207,208] Precipitating events for thyroid storm during pregnancy include preeclampsia, infection, trauma, stress, intravenous radiocontrast dye, thyroid cancer, normal labor and delivery, and cesarean delivery.[46,50,209]

Treatment of thyroid storm is identical for both pregnant and nonpregnant patients (as discussed earlier) (see Box 43.8). **Esmolol** has been described for the treatment of hyperthyroidism in both pregnant and nonpregnant patients.[46,210] It may be considered when a short-acting and titratable beta-adrenergic receptor antagonist is required, for example, when there is left ventricular dysfunction, for which hyperthyroidism is a risk factor in both nonpregnant and pregnant patients.[164,211] However, care is warranted because laboratory and clinical observations suggest that maternal administration of esmolol may result in fetal bradycardia and acidosis.[212,213] Additional challenges in acute care are presented by the association between untreated hyperthyroidism and secondary pulmonary hypertension.[214]

In general, maternal and fetal interests are best served by optimal maternal therapy. When the physician opts for maternal therapy that could, in theory, adversely affect fetal well-being, the rationale should be documented in the medical record.

Obstetric Management

Hyperthyroidism during pregnancy increases the risk for preeclampsia, fetal growth restriction, and preterm birth.[168,215–218] Pregnant patients with treated hyperthyroidism have perinatal outcomes intermediate between untreated hyperthyroidism and euthyroid parturients.[219] Treatment with ^{131}I at least 6 months prior to conception is associated with normal pregnancy outcomes.[16] The presence of hyperthyroidism does not affect the obstetric management of preeclampsia.

In women with Graves' disease, the placental transfer of antithyroid medications or TRAbs may result in the development of **fetal goiter**,[168,220] which can interfere with vaginal delivery or lead to airway obstruction in the newborn. Fetal goiter can occur with either fetal hypothyroidism or hyperthyroidism.[220] Fetal goiter can be diagnosed with ultrasonography, and the etiology determined by color Doppler blood flow patterns within the fetal thyroid.[221] Appropriate intrauterine therapy depends on the cause of the fetal goiter and may include adjustments of maternal antithyroid drug doses or intraamniotic injection of levothyroxine.[220,221] In pregnant women with Graves' disease, maternal serum concentrations of TRAbs during the third trimester, and their net stimulatory or inhibitory effects, may predict neonatal thyroid function.

Normal somatic and intellectual development have been reported in the children of hyperthyroid mothers treated with antithyroid medications,[222] and such treatment does not contraindicate breastfeeding.[147]

Anesthetic Management

No prospective randomized studies have evaluated the efficacy or safety of various anesthetic techniques in patients with hyperthyroidism. The following features of hyperthyroidism may affect anesthetic management: (1) the hyperdynamic cardiovascular system and the possibility of cardiomyopathy, (2) partial airway obstruction secondary to an enlarged thyroid gland, (3) respiratory muscle weakness, and (4) the rare possibility of thyroid storm.[223]

Halpern described two patients with uncontrolled hyperthyroidism who required anesthesia for cesarean delivery and suggested that either neuraxial or general anesthesia can be safely administered in these parturients.[223] On the basis of theoretical concerns, he suggested the omission of epinephrine from epidural local anesthetic solutions and the use of an alpha-adrenergic receptor agonist (e.g., phenylephrine) for the treatment of hypotension. However, earlier clinical studies in nonpregnant subjects with spontaneous hyperthyroidism have shown normal hemodynamic responses to exogenous epinephrine, norepinephrine (noradrenaline), phenylephrine, and clonidine.[224,225] Therefore it appears safe to use epinephrine to minimize local anesthetic uptake and toxicity during the administration of epidural anesthesia in both euthyroid and hyperthyroid patients. Low-dose combined spinal-epidural anesthesia for urgent cesarean delivery in a patient with uncontrolled hyperthyroidism, thyrotoxic heart disease, and severe preeclampsia has been described.[226]

Hyperthyroid women should receive glucocorticoid supplementation because they have a relative deficiency of glucocorticoid reserves.[187] It seems prudent to avoid medications associated with tachycardia (e.g., ketamine, atropine). Patients with Graves' disease may have exophthalmos and need additional care to prevent corneal abrasions or excess pressure on the globe during general anesthesia.[227]

Adequate preoperative preparation minimizes the risk for perioperative thyroid storm; when time permits, the goal is to make the patient euthyroid. In an emergency, the hyperthyroid patient can be prepared for surgery with oral propylthiouracil, an intravenous glucocorticoid, sodium iodide, and a beta-adrenergic receptor antagonist. The anesthesia provider should be prepared to treat perioperative thyroid storm (see Box 43.8).

Hypothyroidism
Definition and Epidemiology

Hypothyroidism is defined by an abnormally low serum concentration of free T_4. The prevalence of overt hypothyroidism in the iodine-sufficient population is 1% to 2%, which is similar to that of hyperthyroidism.[151] Hypothyroidism is more common in women and the elderly.

Pathophysiology

The etiology of hypothyroidism can be divided into primary and secondary categories (Box 43.9); primary hypothyroidism is more common than secondary hypothyroidism. The

BOX 43.9 Etiology of Hypothyroidism

Primary
Autoimmune
- Hashimoto's thyroiditis
- Atrophic hypothyroidism

Iatrogenic
- Radioiodine therapy for hyperthyroidism
- Subtotal thyroidectomy

Pharmacologic
- Iodine deficiency or excess
- Lithium
- Amiodarone
- Antithyroid drugs

Congenital
- Dyshormonogenesis
- Thyroid gland dysgenesis or agenesis

Secondary
Pituitary Dysfunction
- Irradiation
- Surgery
- Neoplasm
- Sheehan's syndrome
- Idiopathic

Hypothalamic Dysfunction
- Irradiation
- Granulomatous disease
- Neoplasm

From Gain LA. The diagnostic dilemmas of hyperthyroxinemia and hypothyroxinemia. *Adv Intern Med.* 1988;33:185–203.

most common etiologies of hypothyroidism are iodine deficiency and Hashimoto's thyroiditis.[151,228]

Clinical Presentation and Diagnosis

The clinical presentation of hypothyroidism is dominated by constitutional signs and symptoms such as dry skin, decreased sweating, hoarseness, paresthesias, periorbital edema, and delayed reflexes.[228,229] The constitutional symptoms are common in the general population of patients without hypothyroidism, particularly the elderly.[230] A diagnosis of hypothyroidism may be suggested by detection of the following factors during the preanesthetic history and physical examination: (1) a history of neck irradiation or radioiodine therapy; (2) the use of lithium, iodine, amiodarone, antithyroid medications, or thyroid replacement medications; and (3) a history of thyroid surgery or the presence of a surgical scar overlying the site of the thyroid gland.

Hypothyroidism is diagnosed by measuring a decreased serum concentration of free T_4. In the presence of an intact feedback loop, the serum concentration of TSH should be increased in patients with primary hypothyroidism. Serum TSH concentration is a more sensitive indicator of primary hypothyroidism than serum T_4 concentration and is therefore

the best initial laboratory test in suspected hypothyroidism.[227,228] Patients with subclinical hypothyroidism have a normal serum concentration of free T_4, but an elevated serum concentration of TSH. The estimated prevalence of subclinical hypothyroidism in the iodine-sufficient population is 4% to 9%.[231,232] Although patients with subclinical hypothyroidism are "euthyroid," there are a number of controversial elements associated with their clinical management, including the chance of progressing to overt hypothyroidism, and the risk-benefit of levothyroxine therapy versus observation. One approach is to stratify patients with subclinical hypothyroidism and individualize levothyroxine therapy based on the magnitude of TSH elevation.[231]

Interaction With Pregnancy

In iodine-sufficient populations, the prevalences of overt and subclinical hypothyroidism during pregnancy are 0.2% to 1%, and 2% to 5%, respectively.[135,168,202,233] Overt hypothyroidism is associated with a lower fertility rate compared with euthyroid women, reflecting differences in neuroendocrine and ovarian functions.[135]

Medical Management

Hypothyroidism is treated by replacement therapy with oral thyroid hormones. The medication most commonly used in replacement therapy is **levothyroxine**, which has a half-life of 5 to 7 days.[234] Numerous studies have shown that the required replacement dose of thyroid hormone increases in most hypothyroid women during pregnancy.[135,147,168,202] Ideally, the increased dose of thyroid hormone replacement should begin as soon as pregnancy is recognized and be titrated to serum TSH levels at 4- to 6-week intervals.

Obstetric Management

Overt hypothyroidism is associated with an increased incidence of the following obstetric complications: anemia, preeclampsia, fetal growth restriction, GDM, preterm delivery, placental abruption, and postpartum hemorrhage. Observations on obstetric complications in subclinical hypothyroidism are less consistent. Recommendations on levothyroxine therapy for subclinical hypothyroidism during pregnancy are variable, even among expert organizations.[147,168,202,203,235] There is consensus that early diagnosis and treatment of overt hypothyroidism are associated with improved maternal and fetal outcomes.[203] Postpartum follow-up of subclinical hypothyroidism is important because of the significant subsequent risk of overt hypothyroidism.[236]

In most instances of maternal hypothyroidism, neonatal thyroid function is normal because fetal thyroid development is typically independent of maternal thyroid function. The fetus, however, depends on maternal thyroxine until the fetal thyroid system is fully functional at 18 to 20 weeks' gestation.[237] Therefore maternal hypothyroidism in the first half of pregnancy may affect fetal brain development.[144,145] In addition, fetal hypothyroidism during the second half of pregnancy may also affect normal maturation of the CNS. With universal screening of neonates for hypothyroidism, these neonates should be readily identified. Published data suggest that cognitive development is relatively normal in hypothyroid infants who receive timely and appropriate thyroid hormone replacement with an initial dose of 10 to 15 µg/kg/day.[238]

Anesthetic Management

The clinical manifestations of hypothyroidism that may affect anesthetic management include the following[234,239]:

- Reversible myocardial dysfunction
- Hypertension
- Bradycardia
- Coronary artery disease
- Reversible defects in hypoxic and hypercapnic ventilatory drives
- Obstructive sleep apnea
- Paresthesias
- Prolonged somatosensory-evoked potential central conduction time
- Abnormal peripheral nerve conduction
- Increased peripheral nociceptive thresholds
- Hyponatremia
- Decreased glucocorticoid reserves
- Anemia
- Abnormal coagulation factors and platelets

Hypothyroid patients may have an abnormal response to peripheral nerve stimulation, which decreases the clinical utility of a nerve stimulator during neuromuscular blockade.[240] Clinical studies of vasoactive medications in nonpregnant hypothyroid patients have shown diminished responses to **isoproterenol (isoprenaline)** and **phenylephrine**.[241,242] One case report of a pregnant patient with partially treated hypothyroidism described diminished response to intravenous phenylephrine during spinal anesthesia for cesarean delivery.[243]

Delaying elective surgery to treat mild overt hypothyroidism remains controversial in terms of improving outcomes.[244,245] For emergency procedures, anesthesia care should include intravenous glucocorticoid supplementation because 7% to 18% of hypothyroid patients have impaired cortisol production.[246] **Myxedema** (hypothyroid) coma is likely the only circumstance in which acute intravenous thyroid hormone replacement is indicated.[180,234] In most hypothyroid patients, acute intravenous replacement therapy entails a significant risk for myocardial ischemia.[247]

No prospective randomized studies have compared the safety or efficacy of different anesthetic techniques in pregnant or nonpregnant hypothyroid patients. Existing evidence suggests that overt hypothyroidism is associated with decreased coagulation and increased fibrinolysis.[248] The anesthesia provider should use findings from the history and physical examination and consider laboratory testing to verify the presence of normal coagulation before administering neuraxial anesthesia to a patient with severe untreated hypothyroidism.

PHEOCHROMOCYTOMA

Definition and Epidemiology

Pheochromocytomas arise in the adrenal medulla and belong to a heterogeneous group of tumors called paragangliomas that develop from neural crest–derived chromaffin cells.[249] Extraadrenal paragangliomas may develop from sympathetic or parasympathetic tissues, and the parasympathetic forms are relatively asymptomatic in terms of secretory products.[250] **PPGL** is the overall term that encompasses both pheochromocytomas (80% to 85%) and extraadrenal paragangliomas (15% to 20%). Pheochromocytomas occur bilaterally (e.g., in the medulla of both adrenal glands) in 7% of adult cases.[251] There are several histopathologic grading systems for PPGLs, including the Pheochromocytoma of the Adrenal Gland Scaled Score and Grading System for Adrenal Pheochromocytoma and Paraganglioma schemes.[250] Unfortunately, these histopathologic features are not reliable predictors of malignant tumor behavior in individual patients.[249,252]

PPGLs have an overall annual incidence of 5 to 7 per million adults, with a 5- to 10-fold higher prevalence in hypertensive versus normotensive adults. Men and women are affected relatively equally, and the peak incidence is in the fifth decade of life.[249,250]

Pheochromocytoma is one of the tumors found in two of the **multiple endocrine neoplasia (MEN)** syndromes: **MEN 2A** (e.g., medullary thyroid carcinoma, hyperparathyroidism, pheochromocytoma) and **MEN 2B** (e.g., medullary thyroid carcinoma, mucocutaneous neuromas, pheochromocytoma).[253] Other disease processes associated with pheochromocytoma include neurofibromatosis type 1, von Hippel–Lindau disease, Sturge-Weber syndrome, and tuberous sclerosis.[254] The genetic basis of PPGLs is an active area of basic and clinical research. Distinct genetic mutations have been identified in more than 20 specific susceptibility genes encompassing 70% of the combined hereditary and sporadic cases.[249,255] Genetic testing in patients with PPGLs has an important role in determining diagnosis, prognosis, and therapy.

Pathophysiology

The pathophysiology of pheochromocytoma is related almost entirely to the systemic effects of its endocrine secretory products, typically norepinephrine and epinephrine.[256,257] Some pheochromocytomas may, however, secrete other catecholamines (e.g., dopamine, dihydroxyphenylalanine [DOPA]), peptide hormones).[258] In an individual patient, the clinical manifestations of pheochromocytoma represent the net systemic effects of the tumor's secretory products.

Clinical Presentation and Diagnosis

Patients with pheochromocytoma can have a variety of common or uncommon symptoms. Patients typically have **paroxysmal symptoms** because of the episodic nature of hormone release by the tumor (Table 43.3). The most common symptoms are sweating, tachycardia, and headaches.[259] One study

TABLE 43.3 Symptoms of Pheochromocytoma During Paroxysmal Attacks

Symptom	Patients Affected in Previous Series (%)		Patient Affected in Ross and Griffith Series (%)
	Mean	Range	
Headache	59.9	43–80	57
Sweating	52.2	37–71	61
Palpitations	49.2	44–71	63
Pallor	42.9	42–44	43
Nausea	34.5	10–42	33
Tremor	33.5	30–38	13
Anxiety	28.9	15–72	30
Abdominal pain	25.8	5–62	14
Chest pain	25.0	19–50	0
Weakness	19.4	8–58	25
Dyspnea	17.0	15–39	23
Weight loss	16.5	14–23	7
Flushing	14.8	10–19	4
Visual disturbances	12.4	11–22	19

From Ross EJ, Griffith DN. The clinical presentation of phaeochromocytoma. *Q J Med*. 1989;71:485–496.

suggested that the diagnosis of pheochromocytoma can be excluded with 99.9% certainty if a patient does not have these symptoms. The attacks may remain the same, or the symptoms may evolve over time. Pallor is common and flushing is uncommon. Paroxysmal symptoms may be triggered by a wide variety of physical activities that patients learn to avoid. Typically, these activities directly or indirectly increase the pressure around the tumor. As the tumor grows, the attacks may last longer and occur more frequently.[260]

The ability of pheochromocytomas to mimic other diseases has frustrated and confused many generations of physicians. In one series, 76% of pheochromocytomas were not diagnosed before autopsy.[261] Reports include numerous examples of pheochromocytomas that were initially confused with other medical or psychiatric disorders.[254,258–260,262,263] In addition to their systemic endocrine effects, pheochromocytomas can occasionally cause local abdominal symptoms.[264] Some patients may have an adrenal mass identified during an imaging study for another clinical purpose. These unexpected adrenal masses are termed *adrenal incidentalomas*, 7% of which are pheochromocytomas.[265] The recommended clinical evaluation of a patient with an adrenal incidentaloma includes biochemical testing to rule out pheochromocytoma, excess cortisol secretion, and primary hyperaldosteronism, followed by imaging to exclude unenhanced computerized tomography (CT) attenuation of less than 10 Hounsfield units and tumor diameter > 4 cm.[265]

Hypertension is a common but not universal finding, occurring in 77% to 98% of patients with pheochromocytoma.[259] Although many patients have paroxysmal episodes of hypertension, half may also experience *sustained* hypertension.[260] **Orthostatic hypotension** occurs in 40% to 70% of patients,[254,259] the presumed mechanisms for which are chronic vasoconstriction with intravascular volume depletion and impaired reflex responses secondary to alpha-adrenergic receptor downregulation.[266]

The current approach to the diagnosis of pheochromocytoma involves the following four steps: (1) biochemical testing for increased catecholamine secretion, (2) anatomic imaging, (3) functional imaging, and (4) genetic testing.[249,253,255] Catecholamine secretion is evaluated by measuring concentrations of norepinephrine and epinephrine or their metabolites (normetanephrine, metanephrine, and vanillylmandelic acid) in plasma or urine. Although the relative merits of these laboratory tests have been debated for years, a consensus has emerged in favor of measuring free metanephrines in plasma or urinary fractionated metanephrines as the initial laboratory test.[267,268]

Conversion of norepinephrine and epinephrine to the respective metanephrines by catechol-O-methyltransferase occurs to a large extent (84%) within the pheochromocytoma before secretion.[256] Several medical conditions may confound the diagnosis of pheochromocytoma by altering the plasma and urinary concentrations of catecholamine metabolites. These conditions include congestive heart failure, acute myocardial infarction, stroke, cocaine use, sleep apnea, and ethanol or clonidine withdrawal.[267] Medications that alter normal catecholamine secretion and metabolism include tricyclic antidepressants, acetaminophen (paracetamol), hydralazine, and beta-adrenergic receptor antagonists.[253,267] Blood sampling for the measurement of plasma metanephrines should be in the supine position after a 20-minute rest to avoid confounding the clinical interpretation.

For patients in whom initial laboratory findings are equivocal, a clonidine suppression test can be performed.[269] The basis of the test is that clonidine fails to suppress catecholamine secretion by pheochromocytoma cells.

After the laboratory diagnosis is confirmed, the pheochromocytoma is localized with anatomic and functional imaging.[249,253,270] The major anatomic imaging modalities are CT and magnetic resonance imaging (MRI). Functional imaging relies on labeled compounds with a high affinity for pheochromocytoma cells. Meta-iodobenzylguanidine (MIBG) is an analogue of norepinephrine, and ^{123}I-MIBG has been commonly used in the past for scintigraphic localization of pheochromocytomas. Currently, positron emission tomography (PET) with either fluorine-18 (^{18}F)-fluoro-2-deoxy-D-glucose (^{18}F-FDG), ^{18}F-fluoro-L-3,4-dihydroxyphenylalanine (^{18}F-DOPA), or ^{18}F-fluoro-dopamine (^{18}F-FDA) has largely replaced MIBG scintigraphy for evaluation of pheochromocytomas.[270] PPGLs have a high expression of somatostatin receptors on their cell surfaces.[271] This finding has driven the development of somatostatin analogs linked to radioactive tracers (e.g., ^{68}Ga-DOTATATE) for PET imaging of PPGLs, particularly metastatic disease. Also, the same PET probes can be used to deliver radiotherapy directly to PPGLs.[270,271]

Interaction With Pregnancy

Pheochromocytoma is rare during pregnancy, with an estimated incidence of 0.7 per 10,000 pregnancies.[272,273] This contrasts with an overall incidence of pregnancy-associated cancer in the United States of 11 per 10,000 pregnancies.[274] Both sporadic and familial types of pheochromocytoma, as well as metastatic and nonmetastatic forms, may occur during pregnancy. There is no evidence that pregnancy accelerates the growth of PPGLs. Severe maternal complications of PPGLs during pregnancy have decreased sharply over the past 60 years to a current rate of 7%, presumably because of improved diagnosis and clinical management.[275]

Clinical signs and symptoms of pheochromocytoma are similar in pregnant and nonpregnant patients.[272,273] Noninvasive hemodynamic measurements demonstrated intense vasoconstriction and decreased cardiac output during episodes of hypertension in two pregnant patients with pheochromocytoma.[276,277] The clinical recognition of pheochromocytoma during pregnancy is especially difficult because of its rarity and its similarity to preeclampsia.[278] Clinical factors that may help distinguish PPGLs from gestational hypertensive disorders include hypertension onset prior to 20 weeks' gestation, paroxysmal hypertension, orthostatic hypotension, and the absence of peripheral edema or elevated plasma uric acid.[279] Easterling et al.[277] demonstrated that either an inverse relationship between blood pressure and heart rate or an increasing hematocrit during treatment with a beta-adrenergic receptor antagonist in a patient with suspected preeclampsia suggests the presence of pheochromocytoma. Pheochromocytoma may also manifest in the early postpartum period after an unremarkable vaginal delivery.[280,281]

Plasma concentrations of epinephrine, norepinephrine, and dopamine in normal pregnant women do not differ significantly from those in nonpregnant controls.[272,279,282] These data suggest that the same threshold levels can be used to interpret most laboratory test results for the diagnosis of pheochromocytoma in pregnant and nonpregnant patients. As discussed above, the formation of metanephrines by catechol-O-methyltransferase within PPGLs leads to a steady and nonepisodic transfer of metanephrines into the maternal circulation.[283] During pregnancy, ultrasonography and MRI are the most commonly used modalities for anatomic imaging of pheochromocytomas.[272,282] Functional imaging with radiotracers should be minimized during pregnancy whenever possible to avoid fetal radiation exposure.[272]

Medical and Surgical Management

Definitive therapy for pheochromocytoma is surgical resection of the tumor.[249,253] The greatest challenge in perioperative management is to prevent or effectively treat wide swings in hemodynamic parameters. The patient is at risk for severe hypertension during induction of anesthesia and surgical manipulation of the tumor, and severe hypotension after tumor excision following an abrupt decline in circulating concentrations of catecholamines.

Preoperative Preparation

The preanesthetic evaluation should include consideration of baseline cardiac dysfunction due to episodic exposure to blood-borne catecholamines. Three types of cardiomyopathy have been described: dilated, hypertrophic, and Takotsubo.[284] The classic approach to preoperative preparation of a patient with pheochromocytoma relies on pharmacologic therapy to return the patient to a near-normal physiologic state. Patients with a norepinephrine-dominant pheochromocytoma have intense peripheral vasoconstriction and severe intravascular volume depletion. In these patients, preoperative preparation includes alpha-adrenergic receptor blockade, intravascular volume repletion, fluid intake, and a high sodium diet, usually for a period of at least 7 days.[249,253] The most commonly used alpha-adrenergic receptor antagonist is **phenoxybenzamine**, which has noncompetitive effects at both alpha-1 and alpha-2 adrenergic receptors. The initial dose is 10 mg orally twice a day, titrated upward to 40 to 50 mg twice a day.[285] **Doxazosin**, **prazosin**, and **terazosin** are competitive, alpha-1-selective adrenergic receptor antagonists that have been used successfully for preoperative treatment of patients with PPGLs. The usual initial dose of doxazosin is 1 mg orally per day, titrated upward to 2 to 8 mg daily.[286] Beta-adrenergic receptor antagonists may be added to treat arrhythmias, but their use must be preceded by effective alpha-adrenergic receptor blockade to prevent a paradoxical hypertensive response to norepinephrine.[287] Because patients with pheochromocytoma are at risk for catecholamine-induced cardiomyopathy, the use of beta-adrenergic receptor blockade must be individualized.[284] The Roizen Criteria for adequate adrenergic preoperative medical preparation for PPGLs are shown in Box 43.10.[288] These criteria are based on expert opinion and enjoy a wide acceptance in the clinical care of these patients.

BOX 43.10 The Roizen Criteria for Adequate Preoperative Alpha-Adrenergic Receptor Blockade in Patients With Pheochromocytoma

1. No in-hospital blood pressure reading higher than 160/90 mm Hg should be evident for 24 h before surgery.
2. Orthostatic hypotension is usually present and acceptable, as long as arterial blood pressure on standing is not less than 80/45 mm Hg.
3. The electrocardiogram should be free of nonpermanent ST-segment/T-wave changes for at least 1 w.
4. No more than one premature ventricular contraction should occur every 5 min.

From Roizen MF, Schreider BD, Hassan SZ. Anesthesia for patients with pheochromocytoma. *Anesthesiol Clin North Am.* 1987;5:269–275.

In addition to adrenergic receptor blockade, calcium channel blockers such as **nicardipine** and **nifedipine** have been used successfully as part of the preoperative medical regimen with PPGLs. **Metyrosine** or **alpha-methyl tyrosine** is a competitive inhibitor of tyrosine hydroxylase, the rate-limiting step for catecholamine biosynthesis.[289] It has been used at a dose of 250 to 1000 mg orally twice a day as an adjunct to preoperative alpha-adrenergic receptor blockade.[287] Patients whose symptoms or early responses to alpha-adrenergic receptor blockade suggest an epinephrine-dominant pheochromocytoma may need carefully titrated beta-adrenergic receptor blockade as their primary preoperative medical therapy.

Many aspects of the traditional preoperative medical treatment of patients with PPGLs are under continuing investigation. In general, the existing literature is mainly retrospective because of the rare incidence of PPGLs. There are many retrospective studies comparing nonselective and selective alpha-adrenergic receptor blockers in this clinical setting, and most demonstrate minor to moderate hemodynamic differences during surgery and similar postoperative outcomes with either nonselective or selective alpha-adrenergic receptor blockade.[290–293] One prospective multicenter randomized clinical trial compared nonselective (phenoxybenzamine) and selective (doxazosin) alpha-adrenergic receptor blockade in the preparation for surgical resection of PPGLs.[294] Intraoperative hemodynamic stability was better in the phenoxybenzamine group, but both groups had similar postoperative outcomes. These studies have more than a theoretical interest for patients with PPGLs because the cost of phenoxybenzamine has increased 13-fold in the past 12 years, and this medication is not available in some countries.[295,296]

The operative mortality for surgical resection of PPGLs has decreased from 45% in 1951 to less than 1% currently.[288] It is possible that a key factor in this improvement is the development of preoperative adrenergic receptor blockade regimens. In 1986 Hull stated, "Emergency surgery to remove a phaeochromocytoma from an unprepared patient should never be contemplated."[297] However, more contemporary authors have suggested that "perioperative management may actually be more critical for achieving good clinical outcomes than administration of preoperative hypotensive drugs."[298] Three retrospective studies compared patients with or without alpha-adrenergic receptor blockade for PPGL surgery.[299–301] The results had some variability of interpretation, but there were no differences in mortality. A prospective observational study compared pheochromocytoma surgery with and without preoperative alpha-adrenergic receptor blockade.[302] There were minor hemodynamic differences between the groups, but no major complications. A small prospective pilot study of 10 patients having minimally invasive adrenalectomy without alpha-adrenergic receptor blockade found no differences in perioperative or postoperative hemodynamics compared with historical controls who received alpha-adrenergic receptor blockade.[303] Proposing the elimination of preoperative alpha-adrenergic receptor blockade in PPGL patients is controversial, with interesting points on both sides of the discussion.[304] One middle ground is to consider modifying the

preoperative medical management based on the individualized risk of a hypertensive crisis.[305] Overall, it is likely that meticulous preoperative and perioperative medical care will continue to contribute substantially to patient safety with pheochromocytoma resection.

Intraoperative Management

Intraoperative management includes the treatment of episodic **hypertension** and **tachycardia** *before* excision and treatment of profound **hypotension** *after* excision. Many medications have been used successfully to manage intraoperative hypertension and tachycardia, including calcium channel blocking agents, nitroprusside, nitroglycerin, esmolol, atenolol, metoprolol, magnesium sulfate, dexmedetomidine, and adenosine. Because of the episodic nature of catecholamine secretion and the change in cardiovascular status that occurs after tumor excision, the use of agents with a short duration of action may be advantageous. The successful use of various regimens implies that the intraoperative treatment of hypertension and tachycardia depends more on the vigilance and skill of the anesthesia provider than on the specific medications used.[286,287,306]

Intraoperative monitoring of a patient with pheochromocytoma should include the use of standard monitors, an intraarterial catheter, and a urinary catheter. Ongoing assessments of cardiac contractility and cardiac filling pressures and volumes facilitate the successful treatment of catecholamine-induced cardiomyopathy or postexcision hypotension. This information may be acquired via a pulmonary artery catheter or transesophageal echocardiography.[287,306] Minimally invasive resection of pheochromocytomas has almost completely replaced open surgical approaches, except for tumors greater than 6 cm or metastatic disease.[307–309] Three minimally invasive surgical techniques have been described: laparoscopic with either transperitoneal or retroperitoneal approaches, and robotic adrenalectomy.[308] The specific surgical technique should be decided by the patient and the surgeon. Guidance from a national professional society suggests that outcomes are improved by patient referral to an experienced adrenal surgeon, defined as someone who performs six or more adrenal resections per year.[307] The advantages of minimally invasive adrenalectomy include reduced pain, shorter hospital stay, and fewer wound complications compared with open surgery.[253,308] In a small study, patients undergoing laparoscopic resection of a pheochromocytoma were randomized to receive one of two different intraabdominal pressures during peritoneal insufflation with carbon dioxide (either 8 to 10 or 15 mm Hg).[310] Patients with lower intraabdominal pressure had less perioperative catecholamine release and fewer hemodynamic fluctuations than patients with higher intraabdominal pressure.

Hypoglycemia may be a serious problem after the resection of a pheochromocytoma.[311,312] Insulin secretion is inhibited by alpha-adrenergic receptor stimulation, and removal of the tumor may result in a rebound of insulin release.[308,313] Blood glucose concentration should be measured frequently after pheochromocytoma excision.

Medical therapy for pheochromocytoma is used only as a temporizing measure during pregnancy or in patients with inoperable or metastatic disease. Pheochromocytoma recurs in 6.5% of patients who have undergone an initial complete surgical resection.[314]

Management During Pregnancy

When pheochromocytoma presents during pregnancy, surgical resection of the tumor is the preferred therapy.[272,279] A variety of clinical strategies have been associated with successful obstetric and surgical outcomes. They include: (1) open or laparoscopic tumor resection at 16 to 23 weeks' gestation followed by vaginal or cesarean delivery at 37 to 40 weeks' gestation, (2) cesarean delivery with concurrent open tumor resection, (3) cesarean delivery with open or laparoscopic tumor resection 2 to 5 months later, and (4) vaginal delivery with laparoscopic tumor resection 6 weeks later.[282,315,316]

Successful laparoscopic resections of pheochromocytoma during pregnancy between 17 and 24 weeks' gestation with good maternal and fetal outcomes have been described.[315,316] There are four case reports of robot-assisted laparoscopic adrenalectomy at 18 to 22 weeks' gestation.[317-320] When intraabdominal space is constrained by a large gravid uterus, a robotic technique may be very useful.[309,321] The choice of surgical technique will depend upon discussions between the patient and an experienced adrenal surgeon. Additional concerns, such as surgical positioning of the pregnant patient and the plans for perioperative fetal monitoring, should be resolved with interdisciplinary planning prior to the day of surgery.[283,309,322,323] Before 24 weeks' gestation, surgery should proceed as soon as the patient is adequately prepared with adrenergic receptor blockade.[273,283,309] After 24 weeks' gestation, the gravid uterus may represent a mechanical obstruction to surgery, and consideration should be given to adrenergic receptor blockade for the remainder of the pregnancy.

Phenoxybenzamine readily crosses the placenta.[324] A case series suggested that neonates should be monitored closely in an intensive care nursery after intrauterine exposure to phenoxybenzamine.[325] Other alpha-adrenergic receptor antagonists have been used successfully in pregnant patients with pheochromocytoma, including phentolamine, prazosin, and doxazosin. Because the availability of phenoxybenzamine is limited, many clinicians will choose to substitute the alpha-1 selective adrenergic receptor antagonist doxazosin for phenoxybenzamine as the first medical therapy for pregnant patients with PPGLs.[272,326] Beta-adrenergic receptor blockade may be added if needed to control tachycardia or arrhythmias or to treat an epinephrine-dominant pheochromocytoma. Beta-adrenergic receptor antagonists that have been used successfully in pregnant patients with a pheochromocytoma include propranolol, atenolol, and metoprolol.[273,282,283] Labetalol is not recommended because its mixed alpha- and beta-adrenergic receptor blocking effects may result in a paradoxical hypertensive reaction.

Medications that have been used successfully to control intraoperative hypertension and tachycardia in pregnant patients with pheochromocytoma include phentolamine, nitroprusside, nitroglycerin, magnesium sulfate, propranolol, metoprolol, remifentanil, esmolol, and hydralazine.[327-330]

Esmolol, however, may not be an ideal medication during pregnancy (as discussed earlier).[212,213] The safety of maternal administration of nitroprusside has also been questioned because of possible fetal cyanide toxicity. Adverse effects were noted in fetal lambs when high doses of nitroprusside were administered in pregnant ewes that had developed tachyphylaxis.[331] Clinical case reports suggest that a low-dose maternal infusion of nitroprusside (approximately 1 μg/kg/min) should be safe during the peripartum period.[332,333] Nitroprusside reduces uteroplacental vascular resistance in hypertensive sheep, and it antagonizes norepinephrine-induced uterine artery vasoconstriction in humans and guinea pigs.[334-336] These data suggest theoretical advantages for the perioperative use of nitroprusside in pregnant women with pheochromocytoma.

Obstetric Management

Untreated pheochromocytoma during pregnancy is associated with an increased incidence of fetal death and fetal growth restriction. The presumed mechanism is decreased uterine blood flow secondary to catecholamine secretion by the tumor. There are high levels of monoamine oxidase and catechol-O-methyltransferase in the human placenta, forming a pharmacologic buffer zone between maternal surges of catecholamines and the fetal circulation.[337,338] When pheochromocytoma is diagnosed and effective maternal alpha-adrenergic receptor blockade is instituted before delivery, the fetal death rate declines from 50% to near zero.[272,275]

Placental abruption has been reported in patients with pheochromocytoma.[339] From a hemodynamic standpoint, this process may be analogous to the occurrence of placental abruption in patients with acute cocaine intoxication.[340] Pheochromocytoma and preeclampsia may have overlapping clinical presentations; proteinuria, for example, occasionally occurs in patients with pheochromocytoma.[273,278] To avoid the increased abdominal pressure on a pheochromocytoma that can occur during active labor, cesarean delivery is often recommended.

Anesthetic Management

Preoperative preparation and intraoperative monitoring and management are discussed above. A variety of general anesthetic agents as well as spinal and epidural anesthesia have been successfully used in nonpregnant patients with pheochromocytoma.[297,306] Perioperative management of patients with PPGLs includes a concern that administered medications could indirectly injure a patient by enhancing release of catecholamines from the tumor. Box 43.11 lists several safety recommendations for perioperative medications to minimize the possibility of provoking an avoidable pheochromocytoma crisis. However, even with careful selection of medications, a catecholamine crisis can occur during an anesthetic for resection of a pheochromocytoma and one must be prepared to intervene.[341]

Two cases have been reported of nonpregnant patients with pheochromocytoma who were incorrectly diagnosed intraoperatively with malignant hyperthermia.[342,343] Manipulation of

BOX 43.11   Recommendations for Safe Use of Perioperative Medications in Patients With Pheochromocytoma

1. Avoid medications associated with catecholamine release
   - Glucocorticoids
   - Metoclopramide
   - Glucagon
   - Succinylcholine (suxamethonium)
   - Ephedrine
2. Avoid medications associated with histamine release
   - Morphine, codeine, meperidine (pethidine)
   - Atracurium, cisatracurium
   - Vancomycin
3. Medications with uncertain effects on pheochromocytoma
   - Atropine
   - Ketamine

a pheochromocytoma during resection may result in a small increase in end-tidal carbon dioxide.[344] It is unlikely, however, that the modest magnitude of this effect would be confused with malignant hyperthermia.

Cesarean delivery is almost always the preferred mode of delivery in a woman with a pheochromocytoma, though vaginal delivery with epidural analgesia and a magnesium infusion has been described.[345] Cesarean delivery, with or without concurrent tumor resection, has been accomplished safely with **general anesthesia**, **epidural anesthesia**, and **combined epidural-general anesthesia**.[288,306,346,347] One case report of spinal anesthesia using bupivacaine for cesarean delivery in a patient with an unsuspected and undiagnosed pheochromocytoma described refractory intraoperative hypotension, but satisfactory maternal and neonatal outcomes.[348] There are no prospective randomized studies of the anesthetic management of pregnant women with pheochromocytoma. It seems reasonable to avoid abrupt hemodynamic changes and to consider the medication recommendations in Box 43.11. Either neuraxial or general anesthesia for cesarean delivery should be selected on the basis of factors other than the presence or absence of a pheochromocytoma. The care with which anesthesia is administered is probably more important than the specific technique selected.

KEY POINTS

- Pregnancy is characterized by a progressive increase in peripheral insulin resistance.
- Insulin requirement decreases during the first stage of labor, increases during the second stage, and decreases again after delivery.
- Maternal diabetes mellitus is associated with a higher incidence of polyhydramnios, preterm labor, preeclampsia, fetal macrosomia, neonatal hypoglycemia, and cesarean delivery.
- Fetal structural malformations are the leading cause of perinatal mortality in diabetic parturients; strict glycemic control before conception reduces the risk.
- Normal pregnancy is a euthyroid state because serum concentrations of unbound or free thyroid hormones are within the normal nonpregnant range.
- Thyroid storm is a rare but life-threatening disorder during pregnancy. It is best prevented by effective treatment of

- preexisting hyperthyroidism and adequate preparation of the patient for surgery.
- The required dose of thyroid hormone replacement medication increases during pregnancy; neonatal thyroid function is normal in most cases of maternal hypothyroidism.
- Maternal and fetal safety is enhanced by early diagnosis of pheochromocytoma and effective adrenergic receptor blockade before resection.
- At the time of pheochromocytoma resection, the anesthesia provider should anticipate the potential for (1) episodic hypertension and tachycardia during manipulation of the tumor and (2) severe hypotension after tumor resection.
- For pregnant women with an unresected pheochromocytoma, the mode of delivery should be individualized but is most commonly by cesarean delivery.

REFERENCES

1. Sun H, Saeedi P, Karuranga S, et al. IDF Diabetes Atlas: global, regional and country-level diabetes prevalence estimates for 2021 and projections for 2045. *Diabetes Res Clin Pract*. 2022;183:109119.
2. ElSayed NA, Aleppo G, Aroda VR, et al. 2. Classification and diagnosis of diabetes: standards of care in diabetes—2023. *Diabetes Care*. 2023;46:S19–S40.
3. American College of Obstetricians and Gynecologists. Practice Bulletin No. 190: Gestational diabetes mellitus (reaffirmed 2024). *Obstet Gynecol*. 2018;131:e49–e64.
4. Tsakiridis I, Giouleka S, Mamopoulos A, et al. Diagnosis and management of gestational diabetes mellitus: an overview of national and international guidelines. *Obstet Gynecol Surv*. 2021;76:367–381.
5. Norton L, Shannon C, Gastaldelli A, DeFronzo RA. Insulin: the master regulator of glucose metabolism. *Metabolism*. 2022;129:155142.
6. Sankar A, Khodai T, McNeilly AD, et al. Experimental models of impaired hypoglycaemia-associated counter-regulation. *Trends Endocrinol Metab*. 2020;31:691–703.
7. Shaka H, Wani F, El-Amir Z, et al. Comparing patient characteristics and outcomes in type 1 versus type 2 diabetes with diabetic ketoacidosis: a review and a propensity-matched nationwide analysis. *J Investig Med*. 2021;69:1196–1200.
8. Karslioglu French E, Donihi AC, Korytkowski MT. Diabetic ketoacidosis and hyperosmolar hyperglycemic syndrome:

review of acute decompensated diabetes in adult patients. *BMJ.* 2019;365:l1114.

9. Davidson JA, Kuritzky L. Sodium glucose co-transporter 2 inhibitors and their mechanism for improving glycemia in patients with type 2 diabetes. *Postgrad Med.* 2014;126:33–48.

10. Akiyama H, Nishimura A, Morita N, Yajima T. Evolution of sodium-glucose co-transporter 2 inhibitors from a glucose-lowering drug to a pivotal therapeutic agent for cardio-renal-metabolic syndrome. *Front Endocrinol (Lausanne).* 2023;14:1111984.

11. Yaribeygi H, Maleki M, Butler AE, et al. New insights into cellular links between sodium-glucose cotransporter-2 inhibitors and ketogenesis. *J Cell Biochem.* 2022;123:1879–1890.

12. Seki H, Ideno S, Shiga T, et al. Sodium-glucose cotransporter 2 inhibitor-associated perioperative ketoacidosis: a systematic review of case reports. *J Anesth.* 2023;37:465–473.

13. Palermo NE, Sadhu AR, McDonnell ME. Diabetic ketoacidosis in COVID-19: unique concerns and considerations. *J Clin Endocrinol Metab.* 2020;105:2819–2829.

14. Au A, Toolis M. Hyperosmolar Hyperglycaemic State (HHS) complicated by life-threatening large vessel occlusive arterial thrombosis – a mini case series and important reminder for clinicians. *Diabetes Metab Syndr.* 2022;16:102515.

15. Kweh BTS, Tan T, Morokoff A. Reversible cerebral vasoconstriction syndrome associated with hyperosmolar hyperglycaemic state: a case report and literature review. *J Clin Neurosci.* 2021;84:38–41.

16. Zhang W, Chen J, Bi J, et al. Combined diabetic ketoacidosis and hyperosmolar hyperglycemic state in type 1 diabetes mellitus induced by immune checkpoint inhibitors: underrecognized and underreported emergency in ICIs-DM. *Front Endocrinol (Lausanne).* 2022;13:1084441.

17. ElSayed NA, Aleppo G, Aroda VR, et al. 6. Glycemic targets: standards of care in diabetes—2023. *Diabetes Care.* 2023;46:S97–S110.

18. Brutsaert E, Carey M, Zonszein J. The clinical impact of inpatient hypoglycemia. *J Diabetes Complications.* 2014;28:565–572.

19. Sanchez-Rangel E, Deajon-Jackson J, Hwang JJ. Pathophysiology and management of hypoglycemia in diabetes. *Ann N Y Acad Sci.* 2022;1518:25–46.

20. Aiello LP, DCCT EDIC Research Group Diabetic retinopathy and other ocular findings in the diabetes control and complications trial/epidemiology of diabetes interventions and complications study. *Diabetes Care.* 2014;37:17–23.

21. Diabetes Control and Complications Trial (DCCT)/Epidemiology of Diabetes Interventions and Complications (EDIC) Study Research Group, Intensive diabetes treatment and cardiovascular outcomes in type 1 diabetes: the DCCT/EDIC study 30-year follow-up. *Diabetes Care.* 2016;39:686–693.

22. Stratton IM, Adler AI, Neil HA, et al. Association of glycaemia with macrovascular and microvascular complications of type 2 diabetes (UKPDS 35): prospective observational study. *BMJ.* 2000;321:405–412.

23. Rodríguez-Gutiérrez R, Montori VM. Glycemic control for patients with type 2 diabetes mellitus: our evolving faith in the face of evidence. *Circ Cardiovasc Qual Outcomes.* 2016;9:504–512.

24. HAPO Study Cooperative Research Group, Metzger BE, Lowe LP, Dyer AR, et al. Hyperglycemia and adverse pregnancy outcomes. *N Engl J Med.* 2008;358:1991–2002.

25. Shepard JG, Airee A, Dake AW, et al. Limitations of A1c interpretation. *South Med J.* 2015;108:724–729.

26. Mosca A, Paleari R, Dalfra MG, et al. Reference intervals for hemoglobin A1c in pregnant women: data from an Italian multicenter study. *Clin Chem.* 2006;52:1138–1143.

27. American College of Obstetricians and Gynecologists. Practice Bulletin No. 201: Pregestational diabetes mellitus (reaffirmed 2023). *Obstet Gynecol.* 2018;132:e228–e248.

28. Kampmann U, Knorr S, Fuglsang J, Ovesen P. Determinants of maternal insulin resistance during pregnancy: an updated overview. *J Diabetes Res.* 2019;2019:5320156.

29. Josimovich JB, Kosor B, Boccella L, et al. Placental lactogen in maternal serum as an index of fetal health. *Obstet Gynecol.* 1970;36:244–250.

30. Stern C, Schwarz S, Moser G, et al. Placental endocrine sctivity: adaptation and disruption of maternal glucose metabolism in pregnancy and the influence of fetal sex. *Int J Mol Sci.* 2021;22:12722.

31. Mallardo M, Ferraro S, Daniele A, Nigro E. GDM-complicated pregnancies: focus on adipokines. *Mol Biol Rep.* 2021;48:8171–8180.

32. Khambalia AZ, Ford JB, Nassar N, et al. Occurrence and recurrence of diabetes in pregnancy. *Diabet Med.* 2013;30:452–456.

33. Roeder HA, Moore TR, Ramos GA. Insulin pump dosing across gestation in women with well-controlled type 1 diabetes mellitus. *Am J Obstet Gynecol.* 2012;207:324.e1–e5.

34. Callesen NF, Ringholm L, Stage E, et al. Insulin requirements in type 1 diabetic pregnancy: do twin pregnant women require twice as much insulin as singleton pregnant women? *Diabetes Care.* 2012;35:1246–1248.

35. Lain KY, Catalano PM. Metabolic changes in pregnancy. *Clin Obstet Gynecol.* 2007;50:938–948.

36. Baeyens L, Hindi S, Sorenson RL, German MS. β-Cell adaptation in pregnancy. *Diabetes Obes Metab.* 2016;18(suppl 1):63–70.

37. Picard F, Wanatabe M, Schoonjans K, et al. Progesterone receptor knockout mice have an improved glucose homeostasis secondary to β-cell proliferation. *Proc Natl Acad Sci U S A.* 2002;99:15644–15648.

38. Hare JW. Insulin management of type I and type II diabetes in pregnancy. *Clin Obstet Gynecol.* 1991;34:494–504.

39. Maheux PC, Bonin B, Dizazo A, et al. Glucose homeostasis during spontaneous labor in normal human pregnancy. *J Clin Endocrinol Metab.* 1996;81:209–215.

40. Holst N, Jenssen TG, Burhol PG, et al. Plasma vasoactive intestinal polypeptide, insulin, gastric inhibitory polypeptide, and blood glucose in late pregnancy and during and after delivery. *Am J Obstet Gynecol.* 1986;155:126–131.

41. Jovanovic L, Peterson CM. Insulin and glucose requirements during the first stage of labor in insulin-dependent diabetic women. *Am J Med.* 1983;75:607–612.

42. Caplan RH, Pagliara AS, Beguin EA, et al. Constant intravenous insulin infusion during labor and delivery in diabetes mellitus. *Diabetes Care.* 1982;5:6–10.

43. Davies HA, Clark JD, Dalton KJ, Edwards OM. Insulin requirements of diabetic women who breast feed. *BMJ.* 1989;298:1357–1358.

44. Yen SS, Vela P, Tsai CC. Impairment of growth hormone secretion in response to hypoglycemia during early and late pregnancy. *J Clin Endocrinol Metab.* 1970;31:29–32.

45. Feudtner C, Gabbe SG. Diabetes and pregnancy: four motifs of modern medical history. *Clin Obstet Gynecol.* 2000;43:4–16.

46. Hamidi OP, Barbour LA. Endocrine emergencies during pregnancy: diabetic ketoacidosis and thyroid storm. *Obstet Gynecol Clin North Am.* 2022;49:473–489.

47. Rougerie M, Czuzoj-Shulman N, Abenhaim HA. Diabetic ketoacidosis among pregnant and non-pregnant women: a comparison of morbidity and mortality. *J Matern Fetal Neonatal Med.* 2019;32:2649–2652.

48. Diguisto C, Strachan MWJ, Churchill D, et al. A study of diabetic ketoacidosis in the pregnant population in the United Kingdom: investigating the incidence, aetiology, management and outcomes. *Diabet Med.* 2022;39:e14743.

49. Eshkoli T, Barski L, Faingelernt Y, et al. Diabetic ketoacidosis in pregnancy – case series, pathophysiology, and review of the literature. *Eur J Obstet Gynecol Reprod Biol.* 2022;269:41–46.

50. Goodier CG. Endocrine emergencies in obstetrics. *Clin Obstet Gynecol.* 2019;62:339–346.

51. Stamler EF, Cruz ML, Mimouni F, et al. High infectious morbidity in pregnant women with insulin-dependent diabetes: an understated complication. *Am J Obstet Gynecol.* 1990;163:1217–1221.

52. Smati S, Mahot P, Bourdiol A, et al. Euglycaemic ketoacidosis during gestational diabetes with concomitant COVID-19 infection. *Diabetes Metab.* 2021;47:101181.

53. Ng YHG, Ee TX, Kanagalingam D, Tan HK. Resolution of severe fetal distress following treatment of maternal diabetic ketoacidosis. *BMJ Case Rep.* 2018;2018:bcr-2017-221325.

54. Blechner JN, Stenger VG, Prystowsky H. Blood flow to the human uterus during maternal metabolic acidosis. *Am J Obstet Gynecol.* 1975;121:789–794.

55. Takahashi Y, Kawabata I, Shinohara A, Tamaya T. Transient fetal blood flow redistribution induced by maternal diabetic ketoacidosis diagnosed by Doppler ultrasonography. *Prenat Diagn.* 2000;20:524–525.

56. Nayak S, Lippes HA, Lee RV. Hyperglycemic hyperosmolar syndrome (HHS) during pregnancy. *J Obstet Gynaecol.* 2005;25:599–601.

57. Nielsen LR, Pedersen-Bjergaard U, Thorsteinsson B, et al. Hypoglycemia in pregnant women with type 1 diabetes: predictors and role of metabolic control. *Diabetes Care.* 2008;31:9–14.

58. Ringholm L, Pedersen-Bjergaard U, Thorsteinsson B, et al. Hypoglycaemia during pregnancy in women with Type 1 diabetes. *Diabet Med.* 2012;29:558–566.

59. Rosenn BM, Miodovnik M. Medical complications of diabetes mellitus in pregnancy. *Clin Obstet Gynecol.* 2000;43:17–31.

60. The DCCT Research Group. Epidemiology of severe hypoglycemia in the diabetes control and complications trial. *Am J Med.* 1991;90:450–459.

61. Diamond MP, Reece EA, Caprio S, et al. Impairment of counterregulatory hormone responses to hypoglycemia in pregnant women with insulin-dependent diabetes mellitus. *Am J Obstet Gynecol.* 1992;166:70–77.

62. Harrison RK, Saravanan V, Davitt C, et al. Antenatal maternal hypoglycemia in women with gestational diabetes mellitus and neonatal outcomes. *J Perinatol.* 2022;42:1091–1096.

63. Reece EA, Hagay Z, Roberts AB, et al. Fetal Doppler and behavioral responses during hypoglycemia induced with the insulin clamp technique in pregnant diabetic women. *Am J Obstet Gynecol.* 1995;172:151–155.

64. Cui Y, Marshall A, Tsaih SW, Palatnik A. Impact of prior gestational diabetes on long-term type 2 diabetes complications. *J Diabetes Complications.* 2022;36:108282.

65. Peterson CM, Jovanovic-Peterson L, Mills JL, et al. The diabetes in early pregnancy study: changes in cholesterol, triglycerides, body weight, and blood pressure. The National Institute of Child Health and Human Development – the diabetes in early pregnancy study. *Am J Obstet Gynecol.* 1992;166:513–518.

66. American College of Obstetricians and Gynecologists. Practice Bulletin No. 222: Gestational hypertension and preeclampsia (reaffirmed 2023). *Obstet Gynecol.* 2020;135:e237–e260.

67. Weissgerber TL, Mudd LM. Preeclampsia and diabetes. *Curr Diab Rep.* 2015;15:9.

68. Alexopoulos AS, Blair R, Peters AL. Management of preexisting diabetes in pregnancy: a review. *JAMA.* 2019;321:1811–1819.

69. Khong EWC, Chan HHL, Watson SL, Lim LL. Pregnancy and the eye. *Curr Opin Ophthalmol.* 2021;32:527–535.

70. Spotti D. Pregnancy in women with diabetic nephropathy. *J Nephrol.* 2019;32:379–388.

71. Airaksinen KE, Salmela PI. Pregnancy is not a risk factor for a deterioration of autonomic nervous function in diabetic women. *Diabet Med.* 1993;10:540–542.

72. Malaza N, Masete M, Adam S, et al. A systematic review to compare adverse pregnancy outcomes in women with pregestational diabetes and gestational diabetes. *Int J Environ Res Public Health.* 2022;19:10846.

73. Coleman TL, Randall H, Graves W, Lindsay M. Vaginal birth after cesarean among women with gestational diabetes. *Am J Obstet Gynecol.* 2001;184:1104–1107.

74. American College of Obstetricians and Gynecologists. Practice Bulletin N. 216: Macrosomia (reaffirmed 2023). *Obstet Gynecol.* 2020;135:e18–e35.

75. Feig DS, Donovan LE, Corcoy R, et al. Continuous glucose monitoring in pregnant women with type 1 diabetes (CONCEPTT): a multicentre international randomised controlled trial. *Lancet.* 2017;390:2347–2359.

76. McGrath RT, Glastras SJ, Hocking SL, Fulcher GR. Large-for-gestational-age neonates in type 1 diabetes and pregnancy: contribution of factors beyond hyperglycemia. *Diabetes Care.* 2018;41:1821–1828.

77. Keller JD, López-Zeno JA, Dooley SL, Socol ML. Shoulder dystocia and birth trauma in gestational diabetes: a five-year experience. *Am J Obstet Gynecol.* 1991;165:928–930.

78. Beardsall K, Diderholm BM, Dunger DB. Insulin and carbohydrate metabolism. *Best Pract Res Clin Endocrinol Metab.* 2008;22:41–55.

79. McFarland MB, Trylovich CG, Langer O. Anthropometric differences in macrosomic infants of diabetic and nondiabetic mothers. *J Matern Fetal Med.* 1998;7:292–295.

80. Reece EA. Diabetes-induced birth defects: what do we know? What can we do? *Curr Diab Rep.* 2012;12:24–32.

81. Dong D, Reece EA, Lin X, et al. New development of the yolk sac theory in diabetic embryopathy: molecular mechanism and link to structural birth defects. *Am J Obstet Gynecol.* 2016;214:192–202.

82. Loeken MR. Mechanisms of congenital malformations in pregnancies with pre-existing diabetes. *Curr Diab Rep.* 2020;20:54.

83. Wang F, Reece EA, Yang P. Advances in revealing the molecular targets downstream of oxidative stress-induced proapoptotic kinase signaling in diabetic embryopathy. *Am J Obstet Gynecol.* 2015;213:125–134.

84. Martin RB, Duryea EL, Ambia A, et al. Congenital malformation risk according to hemoglobin A1c values in a

contemporary cohort with pregestational diabetes. *Am J Perinatol.* 2021;38:1217–1222.

85. Kitzmiller JL, Gavin LA, Gin GD, et al. Preconception care of diabetes. Glycemic control prevents congenital anomalies. *JAMA.* 1991;265:731–736.

86. Rosenn B, Miodovnik M, Combs CA, et al. Pre-conception management of insulin-dependent diabetes: improvement of pregnancy outcome. *Obstet Gynecol.* 1991;77:846–849.

87. Dicker D, Ben-Rafael Z, Ashkenazi J, Feldberg D. In vitro fertilization and embryo transfer in well-controlled, insulin-dependent diabetics. *Fertil Steril.* 1992;58:430–432.

88. White P. Pregnancy complicating diabetes. *Am J Med.* 1949;7:609–616.

89. Vitoratos N, Vrachnis N, Valsamakis G, et al. Perinatal mortality in diabetic pregnancy. *Ann N Y Acad Sci.* 2010;1205:94–98.

90. Azad MB, Moyce BL, Guillemette L, et al. Diabetes in pregnancy and lung health in offspring: developmental origins of respiratory disease. *Paediatr Respir Rev.* 2017;21:19–26.

91. Li Y, Wang W, Zhang D. Maternal diabetes mellitus and risk of neonatal respiratory distress syndrome: a meta-analysis. *Acta Diabetol.* 2019;56:729–740.

92. Alemu BT, Olayinka O, Baydoun HA, et al. Neonatal hypoglycemia in diabetic mothers: a systematic review. *Curr Pediatr Res.* 2017;21:42–53.

93. Pedersen J, Bojsen-Møller B, Poulsen H. Blood sugar in newborn infants of diabetic mothers. *Acta Endocrinol (Copenh).* 1954;15:33–52.

94. Obenshain SS, Adam PA, King KC, et al. Human fetal insulin response to sustained maternal hyperglycemia. *N Engl J Med.* 1970;283:566–570.

95. Oakley NW, Beard RW, Turner RC. Effect of sustained maternal hyperglycaemia on the fetus in normal and diabetic pregnancies. *Br Med J.* 1972;1:466–469.

96. Kenepp NB, Shelley WC, Kumar S, et al. Effects of newborn of hydration with glucose in patients undergoing caesarean section with regional anaesthesia. *Lancet.* 1980;1:645.

97. Hammerman C, Kaplan M. Hyperbilirubinemia in the term infant: re-evaluating what we think we know. *Clin Perinatol.* 2021;48:533–554.

98. Hegyi T, Kleinfeld A. Neonatal hyperbilirubinemia and the role of unbound bilirubin. *J Matern Fetal Neonatal Med.* 2022;35:9201–9207.

99. Pan S, Lu Q, Lan Y, et al. Differential effects of delayed cord clamping on bilirubin levels in normal and diabetic pregnancies. *Eur J Pediatr.* 2022;181:3111–3117.

100. Burlina S, Dalfra MG, Lapolla A. Short- and long-term consequences for offspring exposed to maternal diabetes: a review. *J Matern Fetal Neonatal Med.* 2019;32:687–694.

101. Florez JC, Hirschhorn J, Altshuler D. The inherited basis of diabetes mellitus: implications for the genetic analysis of complex traits. *Annu Rev Genomics Hum Genet.* 2003;4:257–291.

102. Dude AM, Badreldin N, Schieler A, Yee LM. Periconception glycemic control and congenital anomalies in women with pregestational diabetes. *BMJ Open Diabetes Res Care.* 2021;9:e001966.

103. ElSayed NA, Aleppo G, Aroda VR, et al. 15. Management of diabetes in pregnancy: standards of care in diabetes-2023. *Diabetes Care.* 2023;46:S254–S266.

104. Ahmadian N, Manickavasagan A, Ali A. Comparative assessment of blood glucose monitoring techniques: a review. *J Med Eng Technol.* 2023;47:121–130.

105. ElSayed NA, Aleppo G, Aroda VR, et al. 7. Diabetes technology: standards of care in diabetes—2023. *Diabetes Care.* 2023;46:S111–S127.

106. Yamamoto JM, Murphy HR. Benefits of real-time continuous glucose monitoring in pregnancy. *Diabetes Technol Ther.* 2021;23:S8–S14.

107. Kramer CK, Retnakaran R, Zinman B. Insulin and insulin analogs as antidiabetic therapy: a perspective from clinical trials. *Cell Metab.* 2021;33:740–747.

108. Trochtenberg A, Spiel M. Diabetic ketoacidosis in the preterm gestation. *Neoreviews.* 2021;22:e129–e135.

109. Milder DA, Milder TY, Liang SS, Kam PCA. Glucagon-like peptide-1 receptor agonists: a narrative review of clinical pharmacology and implications for peri-operative practice. *Anaesthesia.* 2024;79:735–747.

110. Cesta CE, Rotem R, Bateman BT, et al. Safety of GLP-1 receptor agonists and other second-line antidiabetics in early pregnancy. *JAMA Intern Med.* 2024;184:144–152.

111. Oxempic Highlights of Prescribing Information. http://www.accessdata.fda.gov/drugsatfda_docs/label/2020/209637s003lbl.pdf. Accessed August 15, 2024.

112. Viteri OA, Dinis J, Roman T, Sibai BM. Timing of medically indicated delivery in diabetic pregnancies: a perspective on current evidence-based recommendations. *Am J Perinatol.* 2016;33:821–825.

113. Burgos LG, Ebert TJ, Asiddao C, et al. Increased intraoperative cardiovascular morbidity in diabetics with autonomic neuropathy. *Anesthesiology.* 1989;70:591–597.

114. Tentolouris N, Katsilambros N, Papazachos G, et al. Corrected QT interval in relation to the severity of diabetic autonomic neuropathy. *Eur J Clin Invest.* 1997;27:1049–1054.

115. Liu N, Jin Y, Wang X, et al. Safety and feasibility of oral carbohydrate consumption before cesarean delivery on patients with gestational diabetes mellitus: a parallel, randomized controlled trial. *J Obstet Gynaecol Res.* 2021;47:1272–1280.

116. Shi Y, Dong B, Dong Q, et al. Effect of preoperative oral carbohydrate administration on patients undergoing cesarean section with epidural anesthesia: a pilot study. *J Perianesth Nurs.* 2021;36:30–35.

117. Behera D, Das S, Dash RJ, Jindal SK. Cough reflex threshold in diabetes mellitus with and without autonomic neuropathy. *Respiration.* 1995;62:263–268.

118. Ficker JH, Dertinger SH, Siegfried W, et al. Obstructive sleep apnoea and diabetes mellitus: the role of cardiovascular autonomic neuropathy. *Eur Respir J.* 1998;11:14–19.

119. Levy N, Lirk P. Regional anaesthesia in patients with diabetes. *Anaesthesia.* 2021;76(suppl 1):127–135.

120. Datta S, Brown WU Jr. Acid-base status in diabetic mothers and their infants following general or spinal anesthesia for cesarean section. *Anesthesiology.* 1977;47:272–276.

121. Datta S, Brown WU Jr, Ostheimer GW, et al. Epidural anesthesia for cesarean section in diabetic parturients: maternal and neonatal acid-base status and bupivacaine concentration. *Anesth Analg.* 1981;60:574–578.

122. Datta S, Kitzmiller JL, Naulty JS, et al. Acid-base status of diabetic mothers and their infants following spinal anesthesia for cesarean section. *Anesth Analg.* 1982;61:662–665.

123. Ramanathan S, Khoo P, Arismendy J. Perioperative maternal and neonatal acid-base status and glucose metabolism in patients with insulin-dependent diabetes mellitus. *Anesth Analg.* 1991;73:105–111.

124. Crites J, Ramanathan J. Acute hypoglycemia following combined spinal-epidural anesthesia (CSE) in a parturient with diabetes mellitus. *Anesthesiology*. 2000;93:591–592.

125. Ida M, Matsumura K, Kawaguchi M. Acute hypoglycemia during cesarean delivery in a patient with type-1 diabetes mellitus. *Int J Obstet Anesth*. 2019;39:144–145.

126. Beneventi F, Locatelli E, Cavagnoli C, et al. Effects of uncomplicated vaginal delivery and epidural analgesia on fetal arterial acid-base parameters at birth in gestational diabetes. *Diabetes Res Clin Pract*. 2014;103:444–451.

127. Galway U, Chahar P, Schmidt MT, et al. Perioperative challenges in management of diabetic patients undergoing non-cardiac surgery. *World J Diabetes*. 2021;12:1255–1266.

128. Saitoh Y, Kaneda K, Hattori H, et al. Monitoring of neuromuscular block after administration of vecuronium in patients with diabetes mellitus. *Br J Anaesth*. 2003;90:480–486.

129. Salzarulo HH, Taylor LA. Diabetic "stiff joint syndrome" as a cause of difficult endotracheal intubation. *Anesthesiology*. 1986;64:366–368.

130. Rosenbloom AL. Limited joint mobility in childhood diabetes: discovery, description, and decline. *J Clin Endocrinol Metab*. 2013;98:466–473.

131. Eastwood DW. Anterior spinal artery syndrome after epidural anesthesia in a pregnant diabetic patient with scleredema. *Anesth Analg*. 1991;73:90–91.

132. Burch HB. Drug effects on the thyroid. *N Engl J Med*. 2019;381:749–761.

133. Citterio CE, Targovnik HM, Arvan P. The role of thyroglobulin in thyroid hormonogenesis. *Nat Rev Endocrinol*. 2019;15:323–338.

134. Fliers E, Unmehopa UA, Alkemade A. Functional neuroanatomy of thyroid hormone feedback in the human hypothalamus and pituitary gland. *Mol Cell Endocrinol*. 2006;251:1–8.

135. Glinoer D. The regulation of thyroid function in pregnancy: pathways of endocrine adaptation from physiology to pathology. *Endocr Rev*. 1997;18:404–433.

136. McLean TR, Rank MM, Smooker PM, Richardson SJ. Evolution of thyroid hormone distributor proteins. *Mol Cell Endocrinol*. 2017;459:43–52.

137. Bianco AC, Dumitrescu A, Gereben B, et al. Paradigms of dynamic control of thyroid hormone signaling. *Endocr Rev*. 2019;40:1000–1047.

138. Tedeschi L, Vassalle C, Iervasi G, Sabatino L. Main factors involved in thyroid hormone action. *Molecules*. 2021;26:7337.

139. Luongo C, Dentice M, Salvatore D. Deiodinases and their intricate role in thyroid hormone homeostasis. *Nat Rev Endocrinol*. 2019;15:479–488.

140. Davis PJ, Goglia F, Leonard JL. Nongenomic actions of thyroid hormone. *Nat Rev Endocrinol*. 2016;12:111–121.

141. Wrutniak-Cabello C, Casas F, Cabello G. Mitochondrial T3 receptor and targets. *Mol Cell Endocrinol*. 2017;458:112–120.

142. Yoshimura M, Nishikawa M, Yoshikawa N, et al. Mechanism of thyroid stimulation by human chorionic gonadotropin in sera of normal pregnant women. *Acta Endocrinol (Copenh)*. 1991;124:173–178.

143. Pearce EN, Zimmermann MB. The prevention of iodine deficiency: a history. *Thyroid*. 2023;33:143–149.

144. Min H, Dong J, Wang Y, et al. Maternal hypothyroxinemia-induced neurodevelopmental impairments in the progeny. *Mol Neurobiol*. 2016;53:1613–1624.

145. Prezioso G, Giannini C, Chiarelli F. Effect of thyroid hormones on neurons and neurodevelopment. *Horm Res Paediatr*. 2018;90:73–81.

146. Rodriguez-Diaz E, Pearce EN. Iodine status and supplementation before, during, and after pregnancy. *Best Pract Res Clin Endocrinol Metab*. 2020;34:101430.

147. Alexander EK, Pearce EN, Brent GA, et al. 2017 Guidelines of the American Thyroid Association for the diagnosis and management of thyroid disease during pregnancy and postpartum. *Thyroid*. 2017;27:315–389.

148. Patel A, Lee SY, Stagnaro-Green A, et al. Iodine content of the best-selling United States adult and prenatal multivitamin preparations. *Thyroid*. 2019;29:124–127.

149. Gupta PM, Gahche JJ, Herrick KA, et al. Use of iodine-containing dietary supplements remains low among women of reproductive age in the United States: NHANES 2011-2014. *Nutrients*. 2018;10:422.

150. Sharma A, Stan MN. Thyrotoxicosis: diagnosis and management. *Mayo Clin Proc*. 2019;94:1048–1064.

151. Taylor PN, Albrecht D, Scholz A, et al. Global epidemiology of hyperthyroidism and hypothyroidism. *Nat Rev Endocrinol*. 2018;14:301–316.

152. Smith TJ, Hegedus L. Graves' disease. *N Engl J Med*. 2016;375:1552–1565.

153. Razmara E, Salehi M, Aslani S, et al. Graves' disease: introducing new genetic and epigenetic contributors. *J Mol Endocrinol*. 2021;66:R33–R55.

154. Dwivedi SN, Kalaria T, Buch H. Thyroid autoantibodies. *J Clin Pathol*. 2023;76:19–28.

155. Klein I, Trzepacz PT, Roberts M, Levey GS. Symptom rating scale for assessing hyperthyroidism. *Arch Intern Med*. 1988;148:387–390.

156. Bartalena L, Tanda ML. Current concepts regarding Graves' orbitopathy. *J Intern Med*. 2022;292:692–716.

157. Lee ACH, Kahaly GJ. Pathophysiology of thyroid-associated orbitopathy. *Best Pract Res Clin Endocrinol Metab*. 2023;37:101620.

158. Kossler AL, Douglas R, Dosiou C. Teprotumumab and the evolving therapeutic landscape in thyroid eye disease. *J Clin Endocrinol Metab*. 2022;107:S36–S46.

159. Stehling LC. Anesthetic management of the patient with hyperthyroidism. *Anesthesiology*. 1974;41:585–595.

160. Spaulding SW, Lippes H. Hyperthyroidism. Causes, clinical features, and diagnosis. *Med Clin North Am*. 1985;69:937–951.

161. Fazio S, Palmieri EA, Lombardi G, Biondi B. Effects of thyroid hormone on the cardiovascular system. *Recent Prog Horm Res*. 2004;59:31–50.

162. Nabbout LA, Robbins RJ. The cardiovascular effects of hyperthyroidism. *Methodist Debakey Cardiovasc J*. 2010;6:3–8.

163. Osman F, Franklyn JA, Holder RL, et al. Cardiovascular manifestations of hyperthyroidism before and after antithyroid therapy: a matched case-control study. *J Am Coll Cardiol*. 2007;49:71–81.

164. Forfar JC, Muir AL, Sawers SA, Toft AD. Abnormal left ventricular function in hyperthyroidism: evidence for a possible reversible cardiomyopathy. *N Engl J Med*. 1982;307:1165–1170.

165. McLachlan SM, Rapoport B. Thyrotropin-blocking autoantibodies and thyroid-stimulating autoantibodies: potential mechanisms involved in the pendulum swinging from hypothyroidism to hyperthyroidism or vice versa. *Thyroid*. 2013;23:14–24.

166. Iijima S. Pitfalls in the assessment of gestational transient thyrotoxicosis. *Gynecol Endocrinol.* 2020;36:662–667.

167. De Guzman E, Shakeel H, Jain R. Thyrotoxicosis: a rare presentation of molar pregnancy. *BMJ Case Rep.* 2021;14:e242131.

168. American College of Obstetricians and Gynecologists. Practice Bulletin No. 223: Thyroid disease in pregnancy (reaffirmed 2023). *Obstet Gynecol.* 2020;135:e261–e274.

169. Kung AW, Chau MT, Lao TT, et al. The effect of pregnancy on thyroid nodule formation. *J Clin Endocrinol Metab.* 2002;87:1010–1014.

170. Uppal N, Collins R, James B. Thyroid nodules: global, economic, and personal burdens. *Front Endocrinol (Lausanne).* 2023;14:1113977.

171. Papaleontiou M, Haymart MR. Thyroid nodules and cancer during pregnancy, post-partum and preconception planning: addressing the uncertainties and challenges. *Best Pract Res Clin Endocrinol Metab.* 2020;34:101363.

172. Ross DS, Burch HB, Cooper DS, et al. 2016 American Thyroid Association guidelines for diagnosis and management of hyperthyroidism and other causes of thyrotoxicosis. *Thyroid.* 2016;26:1343–1421.

173. Piccardo A, Ugolini M, Altrinetti V, et al. Radioiodine therapy of Graves' disease. *Q J Nucl Med Mol Imaging.* 2021;65:132–137.

174. Lane LC, Cheetham TD, Perros P, Pearce SHS. New therapeutic horizons for Graves' hyperthyroidism. *Endocr Rev.* 2020;41:873–884.

175. Cohen O, Ronen O, Khafif A, et al. Revisiting the role of surgery in the treatment of Graves' disease. *Clin Endocrinol (Oxf).* 2022;96:747–757.

176. Netterville JL, Aly A, Ossoff RH. Evaluation and treatment of complications of thyroid and parathyroid surgery. *Otolaryngol Clin North Am.* 1990;23:529–552.

177. Burch HB, Wartofsky L. Life-threatening thyrotoxicosis. Thyroid storm. *Endocrinol Metab Clin North Am.* 1993;22:263–277.

178. McArthur JW, Rawson RW, et al. Thyrotoxic crisis; an analysis of the thirty-six cases at the Massachusetts General Hospital during the past twenty-five years. *J Am Med Assoc.* 1947;134:868–874.

179. Galindo RJ, Hurtado CR, Pasquel FJ, et al. National trends in incidence, mortality, and clinical outcomes of patients hospitalized for thyrotoxicosis with and without thyroid storm in the United States, 2004-2013. *Thyroid.* 2019;29:36–43.

180. Klubo-Gwiezdzinska J, Wartofsky L. Thyroid emergencies. *Med Clin North Am.* 2012;96:385–403.

181. Akamizu T, Satoh T, Isozaki O, et al. Diagnostic criteria, clinical features, and incidence of thyroid storm based on nationwide surveys. *Thyroid.* 2012;22:661–679.

182. Brooks MH, Waldstein SS, Bronsky D, Sterling K. Serum triiodothyronine concentration in thyroid storm. *J Clin Endocrinol Metab.* 1975;40:339–341.

183. Jacobs HS, Mackie DB, Eastman CJ, et al. Total and free triiodothyronine and thyroxine levels in thyroid storm and recurrent hyperthydroidism. *Lancet.* 1973;2:236–238.

184. Brooks MH. Waldstein SS. Free thyroxine concentrations in thyroid storm. *Ann Intern Med.* 1980;93:694–697.

185. Knight R. The use of spinal anesthesia to control sympathetic overactivity in hyperthyroidism. *Anesthesiology.* 1945;6:225–230.

186. Carroll R, Matfin G. Endocrine and metabolic emergencies: thyroid storm. *Ther Adv Endocrinol Metab.* 2010;1:139–145.

187. Mikulaj L, Nemeth S. Contribution to the study of adrenocortical secretory function in thyrotoxicosis. *J Clin Endocrinol Metab.* 1958;18:539–542.

188. Chopra IJ, Williams DE, Orgiazzi J, Solomon DH. Opposite effects of dexamethasone on serum concentrations of 3,3',5'-triiodothyronine (reverse T3) and 3,3'5-triiodothyronine (T3). *J Clin Endocrinol Metab.* 1975;41:911–920.

189. Perrild H, Hansen JM, Skovsted L, Christensen LK. Different effects of propranolol, alprenolol, sotalol, atenolol and metoprolol on serum T3 and serum rT3 in hyperthyroidism. *Clin Endocrinol (Oxf).* 1983;18:139–142.

190. Ellinas H, Albrecht MA. Malignant hyperthermia update. *Anesthesiol Clin.* 2020;38:165–181.

191. Bennett MH, Wainwright AP. Acute thyroid crisis on induction of anaesthesia. *Anaesthesia.* 1989;44:28–30.

192. Christensen PA, Nissen LR. Treatment of thyroid storm in a child with dantrolene. *Br J Anaesth.* 1987;59:523.

193. Stevens JJ. A case of thyrotoxic crisis that mimicked malignant hyperthermia. *Anesthesiology.* 1983;59:263.

194. Nishiyama K, Kitahara A, Natsume H, et al. Malignant hyperthermia in a patient with Graves' disease during subtotal thyroidectomy. *Endocr J.* 2001;48:227–232.

195. Tan AWK, Lim BSP, Hoe JKM, et al. Therapeutic plasma exchange for control of thyroid storm. *J Clin Apher.* 2021;36:189–195.

196. Fischli S, Lucchini B, Müller W, et al. Rapid preoperative blockage of thyroid hormone production/secretion in patients with Graves' disease. *Swiss Med Wkly.* 2016;146:w14243.

197. de Mul N, Damstra J, Nieveen van Dijkum EJM, et al. Risk of perioperative thyroid storm in hyperthyroid patients: a systematic review. *Br J Anaesth.* 2021;127:879–889.

198. Strube PJ. Thyroid storm during beta blockade. *Anaesthesia.* 1984;39:343–346.

199. Caswell HT, Marks AD, Channick BJ. Propranolol for the preoperative preparation of patients with thyrotoxicosis. *Surg Gynecol Obstet.* 1978;146:908–910.

200. Feek CM, Sawers JS, Irvine WJ, et al. Combination of potassium iodide and propranolol in preparation of patients with Graves' disease for thyroid surgery. *N Engl J Med.* 1980;302:883–885.

201. Hamilton WF, Forrest AL, Gunn A, et al. Beta-adrenoceptor blockade and anaesthesia for thyroidectomy. *Anaesthesia.* 1984;39:335–342.

202. De Groot L, Abalovich M, Alexander EK, et al. Management of thyroid dysfunction during pregnancy and postpartum: an Endocrine Society clinical practice guideline. *J Clin Endocrinol Metab.* 2012;97:2543–2565.

203. Tsakiridis I, Giouleka S, Kourtis A, et al. Thyroid disease in pregnancy: a descriptive review of guidelines. *Obstet Gynecol Surv.* 2022;77:45–62.

204. Momotani N, Hisaoka T, Noh J, et al. Effects of iodine on thyroid status of fetus versus mother in treatment of Graves' disease complicated by pregnancy. *J Clin Endocrinol Metab.* 1992;75:738–744.

205. Kuy S, Roman SA, Desai R, Sosa JA. Outcomes following thyroid and parathyroid surgery in pregnant women. *Arch Surg.* 2009;144:399–406.

206. Laurberg P, Bournaud C, Karmisholt J, Orgiazzi J. Management of Graves' hyperthyroidism in pregnancy: focus

on both maternal and foetal thyroid function, and caution against surgical thyroidectomy in pregnancy. *Eur J Endocrinol.* 2009;160:1–8.

207. Thumma S, Manchala V, Mattana J. Radiocontrast-induced thyroid storm. *Am J Ther.* 2019;26:e644–e645.

208. Peace JM, Hire MG, Peralta FM. Postpartum thyroid storm in poorly controlled Graves' disease: a case report. *A. A Pract.* 2019;13:299–302.

209. Tewari K, Balderston KD, Carpenter SE, Major CA. Papillary thyroid carcinoma manifesting as thyroid storm of pregnancy: case report. *Am J Obstet Gynecol.* 1998;179:818–819.

210. Thorne AC, Bedford RF. Esmolol for perioperative management of thyrotoxic goiter. *Anesthesiology.* 1989;71:291–294.

211. Sheffield JS, Cunningham FG. Thyrotoxicosis and heart failure that complicate pregnancy. *Am J Obstet Gynecol.* 2004;190:211–217.

212. Eisenach JC, Castro MI. Maternally administered esmolol produces fetal beta-adrenergic blockade and hypoxemia in sheep. *Anesthesiology.* 1989;71:718–722.

213. Ducey JP, Knape KG. Maternal esmolol administration resulting in fetal distress and cesarean section in a term pregnancy. *Anesthesiology.* 1992;77:829–832.

214. Gazzana ML, Souza JJ, Okoshi MP, Okoshi K. Prospective echocardiographic evaluation of the right ventricle and pulmonary arterial pressure in hyperthyroid patients. *Heart Lung Circ.* 2019;28:1190–1196.

215. Aggarawal N, Suri V, Singla R, et al. Pregnancy outcome in hyperthyroidism: a case control study. *Gynecol Obstet Invest.* 2014;77:94–99.

216. Mannisto T, Mendola P, Grewal J, et al. Thyroid diseases and adverse pregnancy outcomes in a contemporary US cohort. *J Clin Endocrinol Metab.* 2013;98:2725–2733.

217. Sheehan PM, Nankervis A, Araujo Júnior E, Da Silva Costa F. Maternal thyroid disease and preterm birth: systematic review and meta-analysis. *J Clin Endocrinol Metab.* 2015;100:4325–4331.

218. Turunen S, Vääräsmäki M, Lahesmaa-Korpinen AM, et al. Maternal hyperthyroidism and pregnancy outcomes: a population-based cohort study. *Clin Endocrinol (Oxf).* 2020;93:721–728.

219. Pillar N, Levy A, Holcberg G, Sheiner E. Pregnancy and perinatal outcome in women with hyperthyroidism. *Int J Gynaecol Obstet.* 2010;108:61–64.

220. Munoz JL. Fetal thyroid disorders: pathophysiology, diagnosis and therapeutic approaches. *J Gynecol Obstet Hum Reprod.* 2019;48:231–233.

221. Delay F, Dochez V, Biquard F, et al. Management of fetal goiters: 6-year retrospective observational study in three prenatal diagnosis and treatment centers of the Pays De Loire Perinatal Network. *J Matern Fetal Neonatal Med.* 2020;33:2561–2569.

222. Messer PM, Hauffa BP, Olbricht T, et al. Antithyroid drug treatment of Graves' disease in pregnancy: long-term effects on somatic growth, intellectual development and thyroid function of the offspring. *Acta Endocrinol (Copenh).* 1990;123:311–316.

223. Halpern SH. Anaesthesia for caesarean section in patients with uncontrolled hyperthyroidism. *Can J Anaesth.* 1989;36:454–459.

224. Aoki VS, Wilson WR, Theilen EO. Studies of the reputed augmentation of the cardiovascular effects of catecholamines in patients with spontaneous hyperthyroidism. *J Pharmacol Exp Ther.* 1972;181:362–368.

225. Del Rio G, Zizzo G, Marrama P, et al. Alpha 2-adrenergic activity is normal in patients with thyroid disease. *Clin Endocrinol (Oxf).* 1994;40:235–239.

226. Liao Z, Xiong Y, Luo L. Low-dose spinal-epidural anesthesia for Cesarean section in a parturient with uncontrolled hyperthyroidism and thyrotoxic heart disease. *J Anesth.* 2016;30:731–734.

227. Chua AW, Kumar CM, Chua MJ, Harrisberg BP. Anaesthesia for ophthalmic procedures in patients with thyroid eye disease. *Anaesth Intensive Care.* 2020;48:430–438.

228. Chaker L, Razvi S, Bensenor IM, et al. Hypothyroidism. *Nat Rev Dis Primers.* 2022;8:30.

229. Zulewski H, Müller B, Exer P, et al. Estimation of tissue hypothyroidism by a new clinical score: evaluation of patients with various grades of hypothyroidism and controls. *J Clin Endocrinol Metab.* 1997;82:771–776.

230. Jansen HI, Boelen A, Heijboer AC, et al. Hypothyroidism: the difficulty in attributing symptoms to their underlying cause. *Front Endocrinol (Lausanne).* 2023;14:1130661.

231. Biondi B, Cappola AR, Cooper DS. Subclinical hypothyroidism: a review. *JAMA.* 2019;322:153–160.

232. Evron JM, Papaleontiou M. Decision making in subclinical thyroid disease. *Med Clin North Am.* 2021;105:1033–1045.

233. Lee SY, Pearce EN. Assessment and treatment of thyroid disorders in pregnancy and the postpartum period. *Nat Rev Endocrinol.* 2022;18:158–171.

234. McDermott MT. Hypothyroidism. *Ann Intern Med.* 2020;173:ITC1–ITC16.

235. Jiao XF, Zhang M, Chen J, et al. The impact of levothyroxine therapy on the pregnancy, neonatal and childhood outcomes of subclinical hypothyroidism during pregnancy: an updated systematic review, meta-analysis and trial sequential analysis. *Front Endocrinol (Lausanne).* 2022;13:964084.

236. Li N, Yang J, Chen X, et al. Postpartum follow-up of patients with subclinical hypothyroidism during pregnancy. *Thyroid.* 2020;30:1566–1573.

237. Eng L, Lam L. Thyroid function during the fetal and neonatal periods. *Neoreviews.* 2020;21:e30–e36.

238. Hanley P, Lord K, Bauer AJ. Thyroid disorders in children and adolescents: a review. *JAMA Pediatr.* 2016;170:1008–1019.

239. Peramunage D, Nikravan S. Anesthesia for endocrine emergencies. *Anesthesiol Clin.* 2020;38:149–163.

240. Miller LR, Benumof JL, Alexander L, et al. Completely absent response to peripheral nerve stimulation in an acutely hypothyroid patient. *Anesthesiology.* 1989;71:779–781.

241. Polikar R, Kennedy B, Maisel A, et al. Decreased adrenergic sensitivity in patients with hypothyroidism. *J Am Coll Cardiol.* 1990;15:94–98.

242. Polikar R, Kennedy B, Ziegler M, et al. Decreased sensitivity to alpha-adrenergic stimulation in hypothyroid patients. *J Clin Endocrinol Metab.* 1990;70:1761–1764.

243. Mohta M, Harisinghani P, Agarwal D, Sethi AK. Vasopressor for hypothyroid patients—is phenylephrine the right choice? *Anaesth Intensive Care.* 2013;41:683–684.

244. Bennett-Guerrero E, Kramer DC, Schwinn DA. Effect of chronic and acute thyroid hormone reduction on perioperative outcome. *Anesth Analg.* 1997;85:30–36.

245. Weinberg AD, Brennan MD, Gorman CA, et al. Outcome of anesthesia and surgery in hypothyroid patients. *Arch Intern Med.* 1983;143:893–897.

246. Rodríguez-Gutiérrez R, González-Velázquez C, González-Saldívar G, et al. Glucocorticoid functional reserve in full-spectrum intensity of primary hypothyroidism. *Int J Endocrinol.* 2014;2014:313519.

247. Ellyin FM, Kumar Y, Somberg JC. Hypothyroidism complicated by angina pectoris: therapeutic approaches. *J Clin Pharmacol.* 1992;32:843–847.

248. Elbers LPB, Fliers E, Cannegieter SC. The influence of thyroid function on the coagulation system and its clinical consequences. *J Thromb Haemost.* 2018;16:634–645.

249. Neumann HPH, Young WF Jr, Eng C. Pheochromocytoma and paraganglioma. *N Engl J Med.* 2019;381:552–565.

250. Juhlin CC, Mete O. Advances in adrenal and extra-adrenal paraganglioma: practical synopsis for pathologists. *Adv Anat Pathol.* 2023;30:47–57.

251. Kittah NE, Gruber LM, Bancos I, et al. Bilateral pheochromocytoma: clinical characteristics, treatment and longitudinal follow-up. *Clin Endocrinol (Oxf).* 2020;93:288–295.

252. Mete O, Asa SL, Gill AJ, et al. Overview of the 2022 WHO classification of paragangliomas and pheochromocytomas. *Endocr Pathol.* 2022;33:90–114.

253. Mathiesen JS, Effraimidis G, Rossing M, et al. Multiple endocrine neoplasia type 2: a review. *Semin Cancer Biol.* 2022;79:163–179.

254. Kaltsas GA, Papadogias D, Grossman AB. The clinical presentation (symptoms and signs) of sporadic and familial chromaffin cell tumours (phaeochromocytomas and paragangliomas). *Front Horm Res.* 2004;31:61–75.

255. Cascón A, Calsina B, Monteagudo M, et al. Genetic bases of pheochromocytoma and paraganglioma. *J Mol Endocrinol.* 2023;70:e220167.

256. Eisenhofer G, Kopin IJ, Goldstein DS. Catecholamine metabolism: a contemporary view with implications for physiology and medicine. *Pharmacol Rev.* 2004;56:331–349.

257. Flatmark T. Catecholamine biosynthesis and physiological regulation in neuroendocrine cells. *Acta Physiol Scand.* 2000;168:1–17.

258. Mannelli M, Lenders JW, Pacak K, et al. Subclinical phaeochromocytoma. *Best Pract Res Clin Endocrinol Metab.* 2012;26:507–515.

259. Ross EJ, Griffith DN. The clinical presentation of phaeochromocytoma. *Q J Med.* 1989;71:485–496.

260. Bravo EL, Gifford RW Jr. Current concepts. Pheochromocytoma: diagnosis, localization and management. *N Engl J Med.* 1984;311:1298–1303.

261. Sutton MG, Sheps SG, Lie JT. Prevalence of clinically unsuspected pheochromocytoma. Review of a 50-year autopsy series. *Mayo Clin Proc.* 1981;56:354–360.

262. Benabarre A, Bosch X, Plana MT, et al. Relapsing paranoid psychosis as the first manifestation of pheochromocytoma. *J Clin Psychiatry.* 2005;66:949–950.

263. Winter C, Schmidt-Mutter C, Cuny R, et al. Fatal form of phaeochromocytoma presenting as acute pyelonephritis. *Eur J Anaesthesiol.* 2001;18:548–553.

264. Hatada T, Nakai T, Aoki I, et al. Acute abdominal symptoms caused by hemorrhagic necrosis of a pheochromocytoma: report of a case. *Surg Today.* 1994;24:363–367.

265. Kebebew E. Adrenal incidentaloma. *N Engl J Med.* 2021;384:1542–1551.

266. Streeten DH, Anderson GH Jr. Mechanisms of orthostatic hypotension and tachycardia in patients with pheochromocytoma. *Am J Hypertens.* 1996;9:760–769.

267. Grouzmann E, Lamine F. Determination of catecholamines in plasma and urine. *Best Pract Res Clin Endocrinol Metab.* 2013;27:713–723.

268. Därr R, Kuhn M, Bode C, et al. Accuracy of recommended sampling and assay methods for the determination of plasma-free and urinary fractionated metanephrines in the diagnosis of pheochromocytoma and paraganglioma: a systematic review. *Endocrine.* 2017;56:495–503.

269. Tsiomidou S, Pamporaki C, Geroula A, et al. Clonidine suppression test for a reliable diagnosis of pheochromocytoma: when to use. *Clin Endocrinol (Oxf).* 2022;97:541–550.

270. Marcus C, Subramaniam RM. Paragangliomas and pheochromocytomas: positron emission tomography/computed tomography diagnosis and therapy. *PET Clin.* 2023;18:233–242.

271. Patel M, Tena I, Jha A, et al. Somatostatin receptors and analogs in pheochromocytoma and paraganglioma: old players in a new precision medicine world. *Front Endocrinol (Lausanne).* 2021;12:625312.

272. van der Weerd K, van Noord C, Loeve M, et al. ENDOCRINOLOGY IN PREGNANCY: Pheochromocytoma in pregnancy: case series and review of literature. *Eur J Endocrinol.* 2017;177:R49–R58.

273. Gruber LM, Young WF Jr, Bancos I. Pheochromocytoma and paraganglioma in pregnancy: a new era. *Curr Cardiol Rep.* 2021;23:60.

274. Cottreau CM, Dashevsky I, Andrade SE, et al. Pregnancy-associated cancer: a U.S. population-based study. *J Womens Health (Larchmt).* 2019;28:250–257.

275. Bancos I, Atkinson E, Eng C, et al. Maternal and fetal outcomes in phaeochromocytoma and pregnancy: a multicentre retrospective cohort study and systematic review of literature. *Lancet Diabetes Endocrinol.* 2021;9:13–21.

276. Combs CA, Easterling TR, Schmucker BC, Benedetti TJ. Hemodynamic observations during paroxysmal hypertension in a pregnancy with pheochromocytoma. *Obstet Gynecol.* 1989;74:439–441.

277. Easterling TR, Carlson K, Benedetti TJ, Mancuso JJ. Hemodynamics associated with the diagnosis and treatment of pheochromocytoma in pregnancy. *Am J Perinatol.* 1992;9:464–466.

278. Lundholm MD, Marquard J, Rao PP. Paraganglioma in pregnancy, a mimic of preeclampsia: a case report. *J Med Case Rep.* 2023;17:124.

279. Clifton-Bligh RJ. The diagnosis and management of pheochromocytoma and paraganglioma during pregnancy. *Rev Endocr Metab Disord.* 2023;24:49–56.

280. Cermakova A, Knibb AA, Hoskins C, Menon G. Post partum phaeochromocytoma. *Int J Obstet Anesth.* 2003;12:300–304.

281. Kisters K, Franitza P, Hausberg M. A case of pheochromocytoma symptomatic after delivery. *J Hypertens.* 2007;25:1977.

282. Prete A, Paragliola RM, Salvatori R, Corsello SM. Management of catecholamine-secreting tumors in pregnancy: a review. *Endocr Pract.* 2016;22:357–370.

283. Lenders JWM, Langton K, Langenhuijsen JF, Eisenhofer G. Pheochromocytoma and pregnancy. *Endocrinol Metab Clin North Am.* 2019;48:605–617.

284. Kumar A, Pappachan JM, Fernandez CJ. Catecholamine-induced cardiomyopathy: an endocrinologist's perspective. *Rev Cardiovasc Med.* 2021;22:1215–1228.

285. Tevosian SG, Ghayee HK. Pheochromocytomas and paragangliomas. *Endocrinol Metab Clin North Am.* 2019;48:727–750.

286. Fang F, Ding L, He Q, Liu M. Preoperative management of pheochromocytoma and paraganglioma. *Front Endocrinol (Lausanne).* 2020;11:586795.

287. Araujo-Castro M, Pascual-Corrales E, Nattero Chavez L, et al. Protocol for presurgical and anesthetic management of pheochromocytomas and sympathetic paragangliomas: a multidisciplinary approach. *J Endocrinol Invest.* 2021;44:2545–2555.

288. Roizen MF, Schreider BD, Hassan SZ. Anesthesia for patients with pheochromocytoma. *Anesthesiol Clin North Am.* 1987;5:269–275.

289. Sjoerdsma A, Engelman K, Spector S, Udenfriend S. Inhibition of catecholamine synthesis in man with alpha-methyl-tyrosine, an inhibitor of tyrosine hydroxylase. *Lancet.* 1965;2:1092–1094.

290. Kong H, Li N, Yang XC, et al. Nonselective compared with selective α-blockade is associated with less intraoperative hypertension in patients with pheochromocytomas and paragangliomas: a retrospective cohort study with propensity score matching. *Anesth Analg.* 2021;132:140–149.

291. Randle RW, Balentine CJ, Pitt SC, et al. Selective versus non-selective α-blockade prior to laparoscopic adrenalectomy for pheochromocytoma. *Ann Surg Oncol.* 2017;24:244–250.

292. Yang Y, Zhang J, Fang L, et al. Non-selective alpha-blockers provide more stable intraoperative hemodynamic control compared with selective alpha1-blockers in patients with pheochromocytoma and paraganglioma: a single-center retrospective cohort study with a propensity score-matched analysis from China. *Drug Des Devel Ther.* 2022;16:3599–3608.

293. Zawadzka K, Wieckowski K, Malczak P, et al. Selective vs non-selective alpha-blockade prior to adrenalectomy for pheochromocytoma: systematic review and meta-analysis. *Eur J Endocrinol.* 2021;184:751–760.

294. Buitenwerf E, Osinga TE, Timmers H, et al. Efficacy of α-blockers on hemodynamic control during pheochromocytoma resection: a randomized controlled trial. *J Clin Endocrinol Metab.* 2020;105:2381–2391.

295. James M. The impact of changes in drug availability for hemodynamic management in pheochromocytoma: prêt-à-porter or tailor-made? *Can J Anaesth.* 2015;62:1244–1247.

296. Kuo EJ, Chen L, Wright JD, et al. Phenoxybenzamine is no longer the standard agent used for alpha blockade before adrenalectomy for pheochromocytoma: a national study of 552 patients. *Surgery.* 2023;173:19–25.

297. Hull CJ. Phaeochromocytoma. Diagnosis, preoperative preparation and anaesthetic management. *Br J Anaesth.* 1986;58:1453–1468.

298. Challis BG, Casey RT, Simpson HL, Gurnell M. Is there an optimal preoperative management strategy for phaeochromocytoma/paraganglioma? *Clin Endocrinol (Oxf).* 2017;86:163–167.

299. Groeben H, Walz MK, Nottebaum BJ, et al. International multicentre review of perioperative management and outcome for catecholamine-producing tumours. *Br J Surg.* 2020;107:e170–e178.

300. Livingstone M, Duttchen K, Thompson J, et al. Hemodynamic stability during pheochromocytoma resection: lessons learned over the last two decades. *Ann Surg Oncol.* 2015;22:4175–4180.

301. Schimmack S, Kaiser J, Probst P, et al. Meta-analysis of α-blockade versus no blockade before adrenalectomy for phaeochromocytoma. *Br J Surg.* 2020;107:e102–e108.

302. Groeben H, Nottebaum BJ, Alesina PF, et al. Perioperative α-receptor blockade in phaeochromocytoma surgery: an observational case series. *Br J Anaesth.* 2017;118:182–189.

303. Gunnesson L, Nilsson M, Larsson P, et al. α-Adrenoceptor blockers and phaeochromocytoma surgery: outdated combination? *Br J Surg.* 2022;109:887–888.

304. Castinetti F, De Freminville JB, Guerin C, et al. Controversies about the systematic preoperative pharmacological treatment before pheochromocytoma or paraganglioma surgery. *Eur J Endocrinol.* 2022;186:D17–D24.

305. Isaacs M, Lee P. Preoperative alpha-blockade in phaeochromocytoma and paraganglioma: is it always necessary? *Clin Endocrinol (Oxf).* 2017;86:309–314.

306. Ramakrishna H. Pheochromocytoma resection: current concepts in anesthetic management. *J Anaesthesiol Clin Pharmacol.* 2015;31:317–323.

307. Yip L, Duh QY, Wachtel H, et al. American Association of Endocrine Surgeons guidelines for adrenalectomy: executive summary. *JAMA Surg.* 2022;157:870–877.

308. Wiseman D, Lakis ME, Nilubol N. Precision surgery for pheochromocytomas and paragangliomas. *Horm Metab Res.* 2019;51:470–482.

309. Patel D, Phay JE, Yen TWF, et al. Update on pheochromocytoma and paraganglioma from the SSO Endocrine and Head and Neck Disease Site Working Group, Part 2 of 2: perioperative management and outcomes of pheochromocytoma and paraganglioma. *Ann Surg Oncol.* 2020;27:1338–1347.

310. Sood J, Jayaraman L, Kumra VP, Chowbey PK. Laparoscopic approach to pheochromocytoma: is a lower intraabdominal pressure helpful? *Anesth Analg.* 2006;102:637–641.

311. Akiba M, Kodama T, Ito Y, et al. Hypoglycemia induced by excessive rebound secretion of insulin after removal of pheochromocytoma. *World J Surg.* 1990;14:317–324.

312. Levin H, Heifetz M. Phaeochromocytoma and severe protracted postoperative hypoglycaemia. *Can J Anaesth.* 1990;37:477–478.

313. Lopez C, Bima C, Bollati M, et al. Pathophysiology and management of glycemic alterations before and after surgery for pheochromocytoma and paraganglioma. *Int J Mol Sci.* 2023;24:5153.

314. van Heerden JA, Roland CF, Carney JA, et al. Long-term evaluation following resection of apparently benign pheochromocytoma(s)/paraganglioma(s). *World J Surg.* 1990;14:325–329.

315. Araujo-Castro M, Nattero Chavez L, Martínez Lorca A, et al. Special situations in pheochromocytomas and paragangliomas: pregnancy, metastatic disease, and cyanotic congenital heart diseases. *Clin Exp Med.* 2022;22:359–370.

316. Donatini G, Kraimps JL, Caillard C, et al. Pheochromocytoma diagnosed during pregnancy: lessons learned from a series of ten patients. *Surg Endosc.* 2018;32:3890–3900.

317. Capella CE, Chandrasekar T, Counsilman M, et al. Robotic adrenalectomy for functional adenoma in second trimester treats worsening hypertension. *Urology.* 2021;151:67–71.

318. Champion NT, Monasterio D, Mukherjee I, Picon A. Robotic-assisted left adrenal cystic mass excision in a pregnant patient. *BMJ Case Rep.* 2022;15:e245954.

319. Chu PY, Burks ML, Solorzano CC, Bao S. Robotic paraganglioma resection in a pregnant patient. *AACE Clin Case Rep.* 2020;6:e197–e200.

320. Podolsky ER, Feo L, Brooks AD, Castellanos A. Robotic resection of pheochromocytoma in the second trimester of pregnancy. *JSLS*. 2010;14:303–308.

321. Capella CE, Godovchik J, Chandrasekar T, Al-Kouatly HB. Nonobstetrical robotic-assisted laparoscopic surgery in pregnancy: a systematic literature review. *Urology*. 2021;151:58–66.

322. Bartz-Kurycki MA, Dream S, Wang TS. Surgical treatment of adrenal tumors during pregnancy. *Rev Endocr Metab Disord*. 2023;24:107–120.

323. Pearl J, Price R, Richardson W, et al. Guidelines for diagnosis, treatment, and use of laparoscopy for surgical problems during pregnancy. *Surg Endosc*. 2011;25:3479–3492.

324. Mitchell SZ, Freilich JD, Brant D, Flynn M. Anesthetic management of pheochromocytoma resection during pregnancy. *Anesth Analg*. 1987;66:478–480.

325. Santeiro ML, Stromquist C, Wyble L. Phenoxybenzamine placental transfer during the third trimester. *Ann Pharmacother*. 1996;30:1249–1251.

326. Versmissen J, Koch BC, Roofthooft DW, et al. Doxazosin treatment of phaeochromocytoma during pregnancy: placental transfer and disposition in breast milk. *Br J Clin Pharmacol*. 2016;82:568–569.

327. Dugas G, Fuller J, Singh S, Watson J. Pheochromocytoma and pregnancy: a case report and review of anesthetic management. *Can J Anaesth*. 2004;51:134–138.

328. Hamilton A, Sirrs S, Schmidt N, Onrot J. Anaesthesia for phaeochromocytoma in pregnancy. *Can J Anaesth*. 1997;44:654–657.

329. James MF, Huddle KR, Owen AD, van der Veen BW. Use of magnesium sulphate in the anaesthetic management of phaeochromocytoma in pregnancy. *Can J Anaesth*. 1988;35:178–182.

330. Lyons CW, Colmorgen GH. Medical management of pheochromocytoma in pregnancy. *Obstet Gynecol*. 1988;72:450–451.

331. Naulty J, Cefalo RC, Lewis PE. Fetal toxicity of nitroprusside in the pregnant ewe. *Am J Obstet Gynecol*. 1981;139:708–711.

332. Shoemaker CT, Meyers M. Sodium nitroprusside for control of severe hypertensive disease of pregnancy: a case report and discussion of potential toxicity. *Am J Obstet Gynecol*. 1984;149:171–173.

333. Stempel JE, O'Grady JP, Morton MJ, Johnson KA. Use of sodium nitroprusside in complications of gestational hypertension. *Obstet Gynecol*. 1982;60:533–538.

334. Lieb SM, Zugaib M, Nuwayhid B, et al. Nitroprusside-induced hemodynamic alterations in normotensive and hypertensive pregnant sheep. *Am J Obstet Gynecol*. 1981;139:925–931.

335. Nelson SH, Suresh MS. Comparison of nitroprusside and hydralazine in isolated uterine arteries from pregnant and nonpregnant patients. *Anesthesiology*. 1988;68:541–547.

336. Weiner C, Liu KZ, Thompson L, et al. Effect of pregnancy on endothelium and smooth muscle: their role in reduced adrenergic sensitivity. *Am J Physiol*. 1991;261:H1275–H1283.

337. Saarikoski S. Metabolic inactivation of noradrenaline in human placenta, umbilical cord and fetal membranes. *Br J Obstet Gynaecol*. 1983;90:525–527.

338. Dahia PL, Hayashida CY, Strunz C, et al. Low cord blood levels of catecholamine from a newborn of a pheochromocytoma patient. *Eur J Endocrinol*. 1994;130:217–219.

339. Warner KI, Poole-Ward RL, Martinez A, et al. Postpartum transabdominal laparoscopic adrenalectomy for pheochromocytoma presenting with abruption and hypertensive emergency. *Am Surg*. 2015;81:E34–E35.

340. Hulse GK, Milne E, English DR, Holman CD. Assessing the relationship between maternal cocaine use and abruptio placentae. *Addiction*. 1997;92:1547–1551.

341. Sonntagbauer M, Koch A, Strouhal U, et al. Catecholamine crisis during induction of general anesthesia: a case report. *Anaesthesist*. 2018;67:209–215.

342. Allen GC, Rosenberg H. Phaeochromocytoma presenting as acute malignant hyperthermia—a diagnostic challenge. *Can J Anaesth*. 1990;37:593–595.

343. Crowley KJ, Cunningham AJ, Conroy B, et al. Phaeochromocytoma—a presentation mimicking malignant hyperthermia. *Anaesthesia*. 1988;43:1031–1032.

344. Asai T, Shingu K. Increased carbon dioxide during anaesthesia in patients with phaeochromocytoma. *Anaesthesia*. 2004;59:830–831.

345. Morton A, Poad D, Harms P, Lambley J. Phaeochromocytoma in pregnancy: timing of surgery, mode of delivery and magnesium. *Obstet Med*. 2010;3:164–165.

346. Yang M, Kang C, Zhu S. Effects of epidural anesthesia in pheochromocytoma and paraganglioma surgeries: a protocol for systematic review and meta-analysis. *Medicine (Baltimore)*. 2022;101:e31768.

347. Cammarano WB, Gray AT, Rosen MA, Lim KH. Anesthesia for combined cesarean section and extra-adrenal pheochromocytoma resection: a case report and literature review. *Int J Obstet Anesth*. 1997;6:112–117.

348. Johnson RL, Arendt KW, Rose CH, Kinney MA. Refractory hypotension during spinal anesthesia for Cesarean delivery due to undiagnosed pheochromocytoma. *J Clin Anesth*. 2013;25:672–674.

44

Hematologic and Coagulation Disorders

Jill M. Mhyre, MD and Ada Ezihe-Ejiofor, MBBS (Nig), DA, FWACS, FRCA

CHAPTER OUTLINE

ANEMIA

Normal Hemoglobin Morphology

Normal adult hemoglobin consists of four polypeptides (two alpha and two beta chains) and an iron-containing prosthetic group (heme or ferriprotoporphyrin IX). In the early embryo, theta (θ) and zeta (ζ) chains are present instead of the alpha (α) chains, and epsilon (ε) chains are present instead of the beta (β) chains. After early embryogenesis, pairs of alpha chains are linked with pairs of either beta, gamma (γ), or delta (δ) chains to form adult hemoglobin (Hgb A = $\alpha_2\beta_2$), fetal hemoglobin (Hgb F = $\alpha_2\gamma_2$), or hemoglobin A_2 (Hgb A_2 = $\alpha_2\delta_2$). By term gestation, the ratio of hemoglobin F to hemoglobin A is approximately 1:1. By 1 year of age, hemoglobin F typically constitutes less than 1% of total hemoglobin. Although hemoglobin A_2 is present, it constitutes less than 2.5% of total adult hemoglobin.

The sequence of amino acids (141 amino acids for alpha chains and 146 for beta chains) defines the **primary structure**, the three-dimensional shape of each chain defines the **secondary structure**, the relationship between the four chains and the heme prosthetic group defines the **tertiary structure**, and the binding of the ligands 2,3-diphosphoglycerate and oxygen defines the **quaternary structure** of the hemoglobin molecule. The physiology of oxygen transport across the placenta and in the fetus is described in Chapters 4 and 5.

Anemia in Pregnancy

During the course of normal pregnancy, plasma volume increases by approximately 50%, but red blood cell mass increases by only 30%; this differential increase results in the **physiologic anemia of pregnancy** (see Chapter 2). It is important to distinguish between physiologic and pathologic anemia. Pregnant women at sea level with hemoglobin < 11 g/dL (hematocrit < 33%) in the first and third trimesters, and < 10.5 g/dL (hematocrit < 32%) in the second trimester should be considered anemic.[1,2] The global prevalence of pathologic anemia in pregnant women is estimated to be 36.5% (95% uncertainty interval, 34.0% to 39.1%).[3,4]

Iron deficiency is the most common cause of anemia in pregnancy. It becomes more prevalent as pregnancy advances. In addition to reduced hematocrit, iron-deficiency anemia is characterized by low mean corpuscular volume (MCV) and low total serum iron, ferritin, and transferrin saturation. Serum ferritin remains the most sensitive marker for iron-deficiency anemia.

Iron-deficient mothers experience an increased incidence of preterm delivery, low birth weight, and small-for-gestational-age infants, all of which are associated with poorer neurodevelopment outcomes,[5,6] although it is uncertain the degree to which this link is causal. Low maternal hemoglobin is also associated with a range of adverse maternal outcomes, including postpartum hemorrhage, preeclampsia, transfusion, postnatal depression, and maternal mortality.[7]

In the United States, the risk for iron deficiency is increased by advanced parity, short interpregnancy interval, Mexican American ethnicity, and African-American race.[8] Daily oral iron treatment in pregnancy reduces the risk for maternal anemia, but likely only improves birth outcomes in populations with high rates of anemia and preterm birth.[9–11] A 2013 metaanalysis of randomized controlled trials identified a dose-response relationship between total daily dose of iron (up to 66 mg/day) and birth weight, but found insufficient evidence of any benefit on the incidence of preterm birth or small-for-gestational-age infants.[9] Doses of oral iron also correlate directly with side effects, including nausea, vomiting, constipation, and abdominal cramps.[12] In a 2019 metaanalysis, intravenous iron was superior to oral iron for treatment of iron-deficiency anemia in pregnancy.[13] Women receiving intravenous iron achieve desired hemoglobin targets faster and with fewer side effects. However, parenteral iron formulations that contain dextran may increase the risk for venous thrombosis and allergic reactions.

Severe antepartum anemia increases the risk of peripartum blood transfusion and postpartum hemorrhage. However, it is unclear if antepartum iron supplementation reduces the risk for postpartum maternal transfusion. In a single-center quality improvement study, implementation of a standardized treatment protocol for the management of antepartum anemia was associated with increased intravenous iron utilization and predelivery hemoglobin.[14] However, no significant difference between the pre- and postimplementation groups in blood product transfusion was observed.

High maternal hemoglobin ($\geq$13.0 g/dL) is associated with increased odds of adverse infant outcomes (very low birth weight, preterm birth, small for gestational age, and stillbirth) and adverse maternal outcomes (preeclampsia, gestational diabetes, and maternal mortality).[7] In the third trimester of pregnancy, iron overload, as demonstrated by high serum ferritin and low soluble transferrin receptor concentrations, is associated with smaller birth size; consequently, the association between polycythemia and decreased fetal growth can be explained partially, but not exclusively, by inadequate plasma expansion. Further research is needed to define optimal hemoglobin thresholds during pregnancy.

Thalassemias

The thalassemias are a group of recessively inherited hemoglobinopathies that result from the reduced synthesis or dysfunction of one or more of the polypeptide globin chains.[15] This reduced synthesis leads to (1) an imbalance in globin chain ratios, (2) defective hemoglobin, and (3) erythrocyte damage resulting from excess globin subunits. In α-thalassemia, alpha-chain production is reduced, and in β-thalassemia, beta-chain production is reduced. Clinically, thalassemia syndromes are divided into **transfusion-dependent thalassemias** and **non–transfusion-dependent thalassemias**.

Patients with transfusion-dependent thalassemia require ongoing transfusion therapy for survival, but even patients with nontransfusion-dependent thalassemia may require blood transfusions during periods of stress such as infection or pregnancy.[16]

α-Thalassemia

There are two alpha-chain loci on each chromosome 16; therefore, there are four genes that can produce alpha chains.[15] Deletions or mutations can affect any or all of these genes resulting in four types of α-thalassemia: (1) **silent carrier** (three functioning genes), (2) **α-thalassemia trait/minor** (two functioning genes), (3) **hemoglobin H disease** (one functioning gene), and (4) **α^0-thalassemia** major or hemoglobin **Bart's hydrops** (no functioning genes). As the number of functioning genes decreases from three to zero, the ratio of alpha to beta chains decreases from 0.8:1 to 0.6:1 to 0.3:1 to 0:1. The depletion of alpha chains leads to a surplus of beta or beta-like globin chains. In the fetal and early postnatal period, the surplus γ-globin chains form tetramers (hemoglobin Bart's = γ_4) later replaced by β-tetramers (hemoglobin H = β_4) as beta-globin synthesis increases after delivery.[17]

In the United States, 25% to 30% of Black women are silent carriers and have slightly smaller MCV than women without thalassemia.[18,19] Silent carriers are not at increased risk for adverse outcomes during pregnancy or surgery.

The α-thalassemia trait is common among individuals of African, Southeast Asian, West Indian, Middle East, and Mediterranean ancestry. Those of Southeast Asian descent are more likely to carry two gene deletions in *cis* or on the same chromosome (−−/αα). This is associated with an increased risk for bearing offspring with hemoglobin H disease or Bart's hydrops. α-Thalassemia trait affects 2% to 3% of Black women in the United States,[18,19] and is almost exclusively a result of deletion of a single α-globin gene on each chromosome 16 (α−/α−). Due to this gene deletion in *trans* (α−/α−), hemoglobin Bart's disease does not typically develop in fetuses of α-thalassemia carriers of African descent.[20] Women with the α-thalassemia trait typically have a mild asymptomatic microcytic anemia (MCV of 70 to 75 fL) and experience no additional risk for adverse outcomes during pregnancy or surgery.

Patients with hemoglobin H disease experience moderately severe microcytic anemia, splenomegaly, fatigue, and generalized discomfort. Hemoglobin H (β_4) constitutes 2% to 15% of the total hemoglobin in these patients. Affected patients generally do not have a decreased life span, and hospitalization for the treatment of their anemia is rarely required. However, disease severity and prognosis vary, depending on the specific mutations present. Some patients have transfusion-dependent thalassemia and require lifelong transfusion and chelation therapy.

Hemoglobin Bart's hydrops, or α^0-thalassemia, is generally incompatible with life. The disease is found predominantly in Southeast Asia, China, and the Philippines. Affected individuals die *in utero* or shortly after birth of hydrops fetalis; mothers carrying these fetuses are prone to develop hypertension or peripartum hemorrhage, or both. Intact neonatal survival has been reported with intrauterine transfusion therapy and postnatal hematopoietic stem cell transplantation.[21]

β-Thalassemias

In β-thalassemia, the production of beta chains is reduced. There are more than 400 genetic causes for ineffective beta-chain production, including gene deletion, transcription mutations, RNA-processing mutations, and mutations that affect protein stability.[15] Unlike the alpha chains, which have four genes (two on each chromosome 16), beta chains have only one gene on each chromosome 11. The disease severity depends on the combination of mutations present; there are three main clinical presentations.

β⁰-thalassemia, also called **β-thalassemia major** or **Cooley anemia**, is a transfusion-dependent thalassemia characterized by a complete absence of beta-chain formation.

In **β⁺-thalassemia or thalassemia intermedia**, there is formation of beta chains but either production or function is impaired. For example, **hemoglobin E** is a variant of β⁺-thalassemia in which a point mutation on the β-globin gene decreases mRNA transcription and decreases affinity between the resulting β-globin proteins and the α-chains. Thalassemia intermedia is a spectrum and, depending on the inherited combination of mutations, individuals may have transfusion-dependent thalassemia or nontransfusion-dependent thalassemia.

Finally, **β-thalassemia minor** refers to the heterozygous carrier of β-thalassemia and is not transfusion dependent.

β-thalassemia is found most often in persons from the Mediterranean basin, the Middle East, India, Pakistan, and Southeast Asia and less often among persons from Tajikistan, Turkmenistan, Kyrgyzstan, and China.[22]

Individuals with β-thalassemia have a relative excess of alpha chains that cumulate in red blood cell precursors. Excess alpha chains undergo autooxidation and precipitate to form inclusion bodies called α-hemocromes. Oxidized ferric iron and reactive oxidative species in the α-hemocromes trigger a cascade of events leading to ineffective erythropoiesis and splenic hemolysis.[22] In the fetus, the gamma chain is unaffected; therefore, anemia only develops as gamma-chain production ceases during the first year of life. In some patients, gamma-chain production continues to a variable extent. Thus, the persistent production of hemoglobin F (even into adulthood) may minimize the effects of decreased beta-chain production.

β-Thalassemia major. Progressively severe anemia develops beginning in the first few months of extrauterine life in patients with β-thalassemia major. Untreated anemia results in tissue hypoxia, increased intestinal absorption of iron, and increased erythropoietin production. The resulting expansion of marrow cavities causes skeletal abnormalities, extramedullary hematopoiesis, leg ulcerations, osteopenia, and pathologic fractures. Splenomegaly leads to thrombocytopenia and leukopenia. Ineffective erythropoiesis and chronic hemolysis increase the risk for thrombotic complications including venous thrombosis and pulmonary hypertension, with risk particularly elevated among those who have undergone splenectomy. Similar pathology may develop in individuals with thalassemia intermedia, particularly in cases of compound hemoglobin E/β⁰-thalassemia.[16]

Patients with β-thalassemia major who present when younger than 2 years of age often have hepatomegaly and a hemoglobin concentration as low as 2 g/dL. Patients who present later in life (2 to 12 years of age) typically have a hemoglobin concentration between 4 and 10 g/dL, with marked anisopoikilocytosis and numerous target cells, nucleated red blood cells, and inclusion bodies. Levels of hemoglobin F range from 10% to 90% of the total hemoglobin, and hemoglobin A_2 constitutes the remainder of the hemoglobin present.

The mainstay of conventional treatment is transfusion combined with **iron chelation therapy**. Patients require transfusions of red blood cells (preferably leukocyte-depleted) every 2 to 4 weeks with the goal of maintaining hemoglobin between 9.0 and 10.5 g/dL, or 11.0 and 12.0 g/dL for patients with cardiac disease.[23] Patients with transfusion-dependent thalassemia receiving regular transfusions invariably develop iron overload because the human body lacks a mechanism to excrete excess iron.

The resulting iron load accumulates, first in Kupffer's cells (noncirculating macrophages found in the liver), then in liver parenchymal cells, and finally in endocrine and myocardial cells. Clinical effects of iron overload typically present by the end of the first decade of life. Deposition of iron in endocrine tissues may result in short stature, diabetes mellitus, adrenal insufficiency, hypothyroidism, hypoparathyroidism, and infertility.[24] Pulmonary fibrosis with restrictive disease, and renal dysfunction have been attributed to iron deposition. Myocardial accumulation of iron can lead to conduction abnormalities and intractable heart failure, which are exacerbated by anemia-induced tachycardia. Heart failure and infection are the most common causes of death.

There are three iron chelators currently licensed for clinical use. **Deferoxamine** was the first available chelation agent. It has a long record of successful use but requires continuous subcutaneous infusion or intermittent intramuscular injection. **Deferiprone** and **deferasirox** are oral chelation drugs. Deferiprone may reduce cardiac iron levels more quickly than other chelation agents, but no studies have demonstrated improved clinical cardiac outcomes.[25,26]

Emerging therapies in thalassemia can be classified into three major categories based on their efforts to address different features of the underlying pathophysiology of β-thalassemia: (1) correction of the globin chain imbalance, (2) addressing ineffective erythropoiesis, and (3) improving iron overload.

The rationale for bone marrow transplantation for a patient with transfusion-dependent β-thalassemia is to restore the tissue's capability of producing functional hemoglobin. **Hematopoietic stem cell transplantation** may be curative if a human leukocyte antigen (HLA)-matched family donor without β-thalassemia major is found. The main limitations to this form of therapy include the need for a suitable donor, patient fitness, and procedure-related toxicity.[27]

Research exploring gene therapy as a mechanism for correcting globin chain imbalance is still underway. In addition, multiple clinical trials are investigating molecules that target ineffective erythropoiesis or undo iron dysregulation.[27,28]

Historically, it was unusual for patients with β-thalassemia major to become pregnant. Hypogonadotropic hypogonadism is the most frequent endocrinopathy in thalassemia major; patients are predisposed to develop pubertal failure, sexual dysfunction, infertility, and short stature.[24,29] Advances in care by optimizing transfusion and chelation regimens have improved fertility, and assisted reproductive technologies facilitate conception in women with hemosiderosis-related infertility.

The metabolic demands of pregnancy increase transfusion requirements. Mordel et al.[30] reviewed reports of these patients in 1989 and suggested that up to 8 L of transfused red blood cells may be required over the course of pregnancy to maintain the hemoglobin > 10 g/dL. Almost 20 years later, Origa et al.[31] summarized the clinical course of 46 women with thalassemia major (58 pregnancies), followed for 11 years. Multidisciplinary management led to safe pregnancies and favorable outcomes for most of the pregnancies. Chelation agents are usually discontinued in pregnancy, given evidence of teratogenicity in animal models and fetal iron depletion described in case reports.[32] However, successful pregnancies have been described despite inadvertent chelation agent use during the first trimester,[33] and some experts suggest resuming chelation therapy in the second and third trimesters in women who develop cardiac symptoms or rapid increase in ferritin.[34,35]

Historically, patients with β-thalassemia major had an increased incidence of spontaneous abortion, intrauterine fetal growth restriction, and intrauterine fetal death. A systematic review of case reports and case series over a period of 17 years identified 417 pregnancies complicated by transfusion-dependent β-thalassemia. There were two maternal deaths. Among women with normal cardiovascular function, careful transfusion therapy and multidisciplinary care appears to facilitate uneventful pregnancy.[35] Although severe skeletal defects and short stature increase the risk for cesarean delivery, a trial of labor is usually appropriate as thalassemia in itself is not an indication for operative delivery.[36]

In preparation for delivery, careful history and physical examination for the cardiac, pulmonary, hepatic, skeletal, renal, and endocrine manifestations of the disease and complications of iron overload are indicated.[37] Maternal cardiac iron deposition may be quantified using modified magnetic resonance imaging. Telemetry may be indicated for dysrhythmia surveillance.[38] Heart failure and pulmonary hypertension may be identified using echocardiography. Chronic transfusions increase the risk for alloimmunization, which prolongs the time required to identify compatible allogeneic blood products in the event of peripartum hemorrhage. Intraoperative blood salvage has been safely performed during cesarean delivery in a parturient with thalassemia.[39] Postpartum pharmacologic thromboprophylaxis is generally indicated.

Craniofacial abnormalities (e.g., maxillary hypertrophy, high arched palate) that increase the risk for difficult airway management may be evident on airway examination.[37] Extramedullary hematopoiesis can result in vertebral cortical weakening, pathologic fractures, and, rarely, paraplegia.

However, in the absence of a major pathologic process of the spine, neuraxial anesthesia can be safely administered.[40] Patients with splenomegaly may develop thrombocytopenia; therefore, anesthesia providers should exclude a history of spontaneous hemorrhage and determine the platelet count before initiating a neuraxial procedure.

β-Thalassemia intermedia and minor. The clinical course is usually benign in patients with β-thalassemia minor and β-thalassemia intermedia who are not transfusion dependent. The anemia is typically mild (hemoglobin concentration of 9 to 11 g/dL) and is characterized by microcytosis, hypochromasia, and levels of hemoglobin $A_2 > 3.5\%$.

Moderate anemia develops during periods of stress, such as pregnancy and severe infection. Most patients with nontransfusion-dependent β-thalassemia tolerate pregnancy well, although the incidences of oligohydramnios and fetal growth restriction are greater than in women without thalassemia. A 2023 study also reported a higher incidence of pregnancy-induced hypertension in the β-thalassemia trait group compared to a control group.[41] Because of an increased rate of red blood cell turnover and an increased risk for neural tube defects, high-dose folate supplementation is recommended in the first trimester. Maternal anemia influences birthweight and preterm delivery. Therefore, the aim should be to maintain maternal hemoglobin > 10 g/dL to allow normal fetal growth.

Women with nontransfusion-dependent thalassemia who have never previously been transfused or who have received only minimal transfusion therapy are at risk of severe alloimmune anemia if blood transfusions are required during pregnancy. To minimize this risk, extended genotype and antibody screening should be performed before administering any transfusions during pregnancy. If transfusion becomes necessary, fully phenotype-matched blood should be administered.[42] Infection, which can cause bone marrow suppression, must be treated promptly. Nontransfusion-dependent β-thalassemia typically does not affect anesthetic management during labor or cesarean delivery.

Antenatal Thalassemia Screening

Among populations at risk for α- or β-thalassemia, antenatal screening can identify couples at increased risk for offspring with serious hemoglobinopathy. Low maternal and paternal MCV (≤80 fL) or mean corpuscular hemoglobin (≤27 pg/cell) with normal serum iron and ferritin is an indication for a peripheral smear analysis for inclusion bodies, hemoglobin electrophoresis, or both. β-thalassemia is associated with elevated HbF and elevated HbA_2 (>3.5%) levels.[20] Decreased HbA_2 suggests hemoglobin H disease. However, hemoglobin electrophoresis cannot reliably detect individuals with α-thalassemia trait; this requires molecular genetic testing. Counseling for fetal genetic testing should be offered if both parents carry at least one abnormal hemoglobin gene.

Prenatal diagnosis can be accomplished with the use of fetal cells obtained by means of chorionic villus sampling or amniocentesis and subjected to DNA analysis. The use of noninvasive prenatal diagnosis using cell-free fetal DNA obtained from maternal plasma is still experimental and is not yet recommended.[20]

Sickle Cell Disorders

A **sickle cell disorder** refers to a state in which erythrocytes undergo sickling when they are deoxygenated.[43] Normal erythrocytes have a biconcave shape, whereas sickle cells are elongated and crescent shaped, with two pointed ends. Sickling is attributed to polymorphisms in the β-chains of the hemoglobin molecule. In hemoglobin S, valine is substituted for glutamic acid as the sixth amino acid in the β-chains.[44] This substitution results in a propensity for hemoglobin molecules to aggregate when the hemoglobin is in the deoxygenated state. The hemoglobin molecules stack on top of one another and form microtubules. Hemoglobin C, D, and E are other hemoglobin variants, all characterized by point mutations in the genes that encode the β-chains; all are less prone to sickling than hemoglobin S.

Sickle cell disease refers to disorders in which sickling results in clinical signs and symptoms; it includes hemoglobin SS disease (i.e., sickle cell anemia) and several heterozygous hemoglobinopathies (e.g., sickle cell β⁰-thalassemia, hemoglobin SC disease).[20,44]

Sickle Cell Anemia

Epidemiology. Table 44.1 lists the prevalence of sickle cell anemia and the other common hemoglobinopathies in the adult Black population in the United States. Sickle cell disease is less commonly identified among Hispanic, Middle Eastern, or Asian Indian ethnic groups.[45] The current number of individuals with sickle cell disease in the United States is estimated to approach 100,000, but high-quality surveillance data are not available.[46,47]

TABLE 44.1 Prevalence of Hemoglobinopathies in the United States in Persons of African Descent

Type	Estimated Prevalence
Traits	
Hemoglobin AS	1:12.5
Hemoglobin AC	1:33
β-Thalassemia minor	1:67
Persistent hemoglobin F	1:1000
Sickling Disorders	
Hemoglobin SS	1:625
Hemoglobin SC	1:833
Hemoglobin S–β-thalassemia	1:1667
Hemoglobin S–persistent hemoglobin F	1:25,000
Hemoglobin CC	1:4444
β-Thalassemia major	1:17,778
Hemoglobin C–β-thalassemia	1:4444

Modified from Motulsky AG. Frequency of sickling disorders in U.S. blacks. *N Engl J Med.* 1973;288:31–33.

Pathophysiology. Oxygen tension is the most important determinant in sickling; other factors that affect sickling are listed in Box 44.1. Hemoglobin S begins to aggregate at a Po_2 of less than 50 mm Hg (6.7 kPa), and all the hemoglobin S is aggregated at a Po_2 of approximately 23 mm Hg (3.1 kPa). The formation of hemoglobin S aggregates is time dependent[45]; the proportion of sickled hemoglobin increases with decreasing cardiac output and prolonged venous transit time. If an erythrocyte sickles, it can return to its normal shape once the hemoglobin becomes oxygenated.[44,45] However, repeated sickling cycles produce erythrocyte metabolic abnormalities and membrane damage, eventually leading to irreversible sickling regardless of oxygen tension.[44,45] Sickled cells are cleared rapidly from the circulation by the reticuloendothelial system; as a result, the erythrocyte life span is reduced to approximately 12 days.[44,45]

Sickled cells can form aggregates and lead to vaso-occlusive crises and end-organ injury. Repeated cycles of sickling, vaso-occlusion, reperfusion injury, and acute inflammation can lead to chronic inflammation and inflammatory vascular disease. Elevated levels of cell-free hemoglobin deplete nitric oxide, activate the endothelium, and further exacerbate inflammation.[43,44] The reduced erythrocyte life span results in anemia, jaundice, cholecystitis, and a hyperdynamic hemodynamic state.

Marked ventricular hypertrophy can occur in pregnant women with sickle cell disease secondary to increased cardiac output. This may lead to a decrease in ventricular compliance and a deterioration in ventricular diastolic function.[48] Anemia also leads to erythroblastic hyperplasia, expansion of medullary spaces, and a loss of cortex in long bones, vertebral bodies, and the skull.[44] Vaso-occlusive events can give rise to **infarctive crises** (which most often occur in the chest, abdomen, back, and long bones), **cerebrovascular accidents**, and rarely **peripheral neuropathy**.[49] Aggregate formation in the spleen can result in microinfarcts.

Functional asplenia and abnormal neutrophil responses both contribute to susceptibility to infection. Consequently, the incidence of pneumonia and pyelonephritis is higher in pregnant patients with sickle cell disease than in healthy pregnant patients. **Aplastic crises** can occur from depression of erythropoiesis secondary to infection (especially parvovirus) or from marrow failure secondary to folate deficiency during pregnancy.[44] During an aplastic crisis, the hemoglobin concentration can decrease rapidly, leading to high-output cardiac failure and potentially death. **Sequestration crises** can result from the massive pooling of erythrocytes, especially in the spleen. This event occurs more frequently in patients

BOX 44.1 Factors That Increase Sickling in Women With Sickle Cell Anemia

- Hemoglobin S > 50% of the total hemoglobin concentration
- Dehydration leading to increased blood viscosity
- Hypotension causing vascular stasis
- Hypothermia
- Acidosis

with hemoglobin SC disease or sickle cell β-thalassemia than in patients with other forms of sickle cell disease. A major sequestration crisis is one in which the hemoglobin concentration is less than 6 g/dL and has decreased more than 3 g/dL from the baseline measurement.[44]

The long-term clinical course of sickle cell disease is highly variable. Higher fetal hemoglobin expression and coincident α-thalassemia were among the first genetic modulators described.[50] Subsequent work has identified a complex network of single nucleotide polymorphisms associated with specific complications of sickle cell disease, most prominently the transforming growth factor beta family of membrane-bound receptors. These receptors play a role in fibrosis, cell proliferation, hematopoiesis, osteogenesis, angiogenesis, nephropathy, wound healing, and immune response.[50]

Diagnosis. In adults, sickle cell anemia is characterized by (1) a hemoglobin concentration of 6 to 8 g/dL, (2) an elevated reticulocyte count, and (3) the presence of sickle cells on a peripheral blood smear. The diagnosis is confirmed by electrophoresis, thin-layer isoelectric focusing, or high-pressure liquid chromatography.[44] Because most hemoglobinopathies are inherited as autosomal recessive conditions, prenatal screening for abnormal hemoglobin is recommended in couples at high risk for sickle cell disease.[20] *In utero,* the diagnosis can be made through the use of restriction endonucleases specific for the sickle mutation applied to fetal cells obtained during amniocentesis or chorionic villus sampling.

Interaction with pregnancy. Pregnancy typically exacerbates the complications of sickle cell anemia. Maternal mortality from sickle cell disease contributes to as many as 1% of all maternal deaths in the United States.[51] Thromboembolic complications, infection, cardiomyopathy, and pulmonary hypertension are the most serious maternal medical complications.[51,52] Patients with sickle cell anemia have an increased incidence of preterm labor, placental abruption, fetal growth restriction, preeclampsia, and eclampsia.[51,52] Intensive fetal surveillance may reduce the risk for intrauterine fetal death.[51]

Medical management. Sickle cell anemia is a chronic anemia; blood transfusions are given only when they are specifically indicated (e.g., acute anemia, aplastic crisis, acute chest syndrome, pneumonia with hypoxemia, before or during surgery).[44,46] The goals of transfusion are to achieve a hemoglobin concentration > 8 g/dL and to ensure that hemoglobin A represents more than 40% of the total hemoglobin present. Systematic review of cohort studies suggests that prophylactic blood transfusions during pregnancy decrease perinatal and maternal mortality, preterm birth, and maternal vaso-occlusive pain episodes, pulmonary complications, and pulmonary embolism[53]; randomized trials confirm a decrease in the frequency of maternal pain crises, but more evidence is needed to evaluate the other outcomes.[54,55] If the patient's baseline hemoglobin concentration is less than 6 to 7 g/dL, simple transfusions with buffy-coat–poor, hemoglobin S–free, washed red blood cells should be adequate to meet treatment goals. Otherwise, partial exchange transfusions may be necessary.[55,56]

Hemoglobin F does not form aggregates with hemoglobin S. Hydroxyurea enhances the production of hemoglobin F and reduces vaso-occlusive crises and other complications of sickle cell anemia.[46] It is unclear whether hydroxyurea is safe in pregnancy; the drug is known to be carcinogenic, mutagenic, and teratogenic in animals.[57] However, among a small series of pregnancies conceived at the time of maternal or paternal hydroxyurea administration, there was no evidence of abnormal pregnancy outcomes or teratogenicity among surviving offspring.[57] L-Glutamine powder was approved by the US Food and Drug Administration (FDA) in 2017 to reduce acute complications of sickle cell disease, on the basis of a trial that demonstrated decreased rates of vaso-occlusive crisis.[58] Bone marrow transplantation is a potentially curative therapy for individuals with complicated sickle cell disease, although HLA-matched donors can be difficult to locate and the procedure is associated with significant morbidity and mortality.[59,60]

Obstetric management. During prenatal visits, the obstetrician should monitor maternal weight gain, blood pressure, urine protein content, and uterine and fetal growth. Antenatal aspirin therapy reduces the risk for preeclampsia (see Chapter 35).[61] Maternal surveillance for the complications of sickle cell disease should continue throughout pregnancy,[56] and antepartum fetal surveillance begins at the time of extrauterine viability (see Chapter 6). Finally, pharmacologic thromboprophylaxis is indicated both during pregnancy and postpartum.[56]

Anesthetic management. Principles of anesthetic management include (1) close surveillance for the complications of sickle cell disease, (2) use of crystalloid to maintain intravascular volume, (3) transfusion of red blood cells to maintain oxygen-carrying capacity, (4) administration of supplemental oxygen, (5) maintenance of normothermia, (6) prevention of peripheral venous stasis, and (7) provision of appropriate venous thromboembolism prophylaxis.[43,62] Preoperative evaluation should focus on recent sickle cell disease exacerbations, the degree of anemia, and chronic end-organ injury.[43,56] Pulmonary hypertension and high-output heart failure should be excluded with echocardiography. Preoperative blood transfusion to achieve a hemoglobin concentration of 10 g/dL improves perioperative outcomes for nonobstetric patients with sickle cell disease undergoing medium-risk surgery with general anesthesia,[63] but no trial has evaluated prophylactic blood transfusion before cesarean delivery. Early preparation of cross-matched blood products should be considered because alloimmunization, and the antigen cross-matching procedures recommended to prevent its development, can prolong cross-matching procedures.[43] Pain control during labor is essential; continuous neuraxial analgesia is recommended.[43] Although general anesthesia for cesarean delivery has been associated with postoperative sickling complications, either neuraxial or general anesthesia is acceptable, and the choice of anesthetic technique ultimately depends on the time available to induce anesthesia and the patient's preference and physical status.[62]

Sickle Cell Disease Variants

If a patient carries one hemoglobin S gene and another gene for a hemoglobin that has a propensity to sickle, that patient is considered to have sickle cell disease. Patients with **hemoglobin SD disease** tend to have the mildest form, and patients with **hemoglobin SC disease** or **sickle cell β-thalassemia disease** tend to have more severe disease.[44]

As with the hemoglobin S gene, hemoglobin C is most prevalent among persons of West African descent, whereas hemoglobin D is distributed among persons of African, northern European, and Indian descent. Hemoglobin E is most prevalent among persons of Southeast Asian descent.[44] Patients with hemoglobin SC and hemoglobin SD disease tend to be asymptomatic during childhood with only mild anemia. Typically, these individuals do not develop symptoms until the second half of pregnancy. During late pregnancy, they may have severe anemia (secondary to splenic sequestration) and splenomegaly. Patients with hemoglobin SC disease also tend to develop bone marrow necrosis, which predisposes to fat emboli. The other clinical manifestations are similar to those observed in patients with sickle cell anemia.[64]

Blood transfusion is recommended only when the hemoglobin concentration is less than 7 to 8 g/dL. Obstetric and anesthetic management are similar to managing patients with sickle cell anemia.

Patients who are homozygous for hemoglobin C, D, or E typically have mild anemia. Target cells often are observed, and splenomegaly is common. The diagnosis is confirmed with electrophoresis, thin-layer isoelectric focusing, or high-pressure liquid chromatography.[44] Pregnancy typically is well tolerated, and no specific change in obstetric or anesthetic management is required.

Sickle Cell Trait

Sickle cell trait (i.e., hemoglobin SA) occurs in approximately 8% of African-American women in the United States. The red blood cells of patients with sickle cell trait do not sickle until the Po_2 decreases below 15 mm Hg (2.0 kPa); therefore, red blood cell life span is normal.[65] Patients with sickle cell trait are not at increased risk for adverse outcome during surgery or the peripartum period.[66] Nevertheless, sickle cell trait is associated with higher rates of thromboembolic complications,[67] and may contribute to long-term adverse outcomes among African-American people, including renal failure and diabetes.

Likewise, people who are heterozygous for other hemoglobin variants (i.e., one gene for hemoglobin C, D, or E and one hemoglobin A) are asymptomatic. The heterozygous state for both the thalassemias and the structural hemoglobinopathies appears to protect against malaria, which may explain their geographic distribution and continued presence in the gene pool.[43]

Autoimmune Hemolytic Anemia

Patients with autoimmune hemolytic anemia produce antibodies to their own red blood cells, resulting in hemolysis and varying degrees of anemia. The annual incidence of new cases of autoimmune hemolytic anemia is approximately 1 in 80,000 persons, but the prevalence approaches 1 in 5000.[68] Warm antibodies react with red blood cells at a temperature of 35°C to 40°C, whereas cold antibodies react optimally at a temperature < 30°C. Table 44.2 lists the characteristics of the four main types of autoimmune hemolytic anemia. Approximately one-half of cases are idiopathic, with the remainder attributed to malignancies, autoimmune diseases, infections, or drugs.[69]

TABLE 44.2 Characteristics of Autoimmune Hemolytic Anemias

Disease	Immunoglobulin (Ig)	Complement Involved	Site of Red Blood Cell Destruction	Treatment	Transfusion Requirements
Incomplete warm autoantibodies	Typically IgG Rarely IgA Rarely IgM	No No C4b and C3b	Spleen Spleen Liver	Corticosteroids, splenectomy, immune globulin	Rarely needed; if given, combined with corticosteroids
Complete warm autoantibodies					
Type 1	IgM	C4b and C3b	Liver	Corticosteroids, splenectomy	Rarely needed
Type 2	IgM	C1–C9	Intracellular	Plasma exchange, corticosteroids	Frequently needed
Cold autoagglutinins and hemolysins	IgM	No	Intracellular	Corticosteroids, keeping patient warm	Very rarely needed
Biphasic hemolysins					
Acute	IgG	Yes	Intracellular agglutination	Treatment of underlying infection	Occasionally needed
Chronic	IgG	Yes	Intracellular hemolysis	Plasmapheresis, chlorambucil	Frequently needed

IgA, Immunoglobulin A; *IgG*, immunoglobulin G; *IgM*, immunoglobulin M.
From Gibson J. Autoimmune hemolytic anemia: current concepts. *Aust NZ J Med*. 1988:18:625–637; Engelfriet CP, Overbeeke MA, von dem Borne AE. Autoimmune hemolytic anemia. *Semin Hematol*. 1992;29:3–12.

Patients with **warm-reacting antibodies** typically respond to treatment with corticosteroids; splenectomy and the anti-CD20 antibody rituximab are second-line therapies.[68] After splenectomy, relapses and blood transfusions may lead to the continued requirement for intermittent or continuous corticosteroid therapy. The presence of the antibody and the requirement for extended phenotyping may delay matched blood product availability. In acute hemorrhage, the rapid transfusion of body-temperature, ABO-compatible and Rh-negative blood can be lifesaving, with the expectation that the half-life of transfused red blood cells will be shortened; this practice will allow time to procure compatible blood products.[68]

In patients with **cold-reacting antibodies**, the anemia typically is mild, and maintenance of normal body and ambient temperatures typically is all that is required to prevent hemolysis.

COAGULATION

Thrombotic and Thrombolytic Pathways

Hemostasis depends on the normal function of vascular tissue, platelets, and coagulation factors. During the initial response to loss of vessel integrity, platelets adhere to exposed collagen, facilitated by the von Willebrand factor (vWF) (primary hemostasis). Platelet activation results in the release of substances that constrict the injured vessels and cause other platelets to adhere and form a hemostatic plug. The platelet plug is not stable, and initiation of the coagulation cascade, followed by deposition and stabilization of fibrin, is necessary for definitive hemostasis (secondary hemostasis). Most coagulation factors circulate in the blood as zymogens, which are converted to active enzymes that in turn convert other zymogens to active enzymes. For example, factor X (a zymogen) is converted to factor Xa (an enzyme), which converts prothrombin (factor II) to thrombin (factor IIa).

In its original conception, the coagulation cascade (Fig. 44.1) was believed to propagate within plasma. Subsequent work located the enzymatic reactions of the **extrinsic system** primarily to the surface of subendothelial cells and those of the **intrinsic system** to the activated platelet surface.[70] Currently, a widely used model divides the coagulation cascade into three phases: (1) an **initiation phase** (classical extrinsic pathway), in which small amounts of active coagulation factors are generated; (2) an **amplification phase**, in which the level of active coagulation factors is boosted; and (3) a **propagation phase**, in which coagulation factors bind to the membrane of activated platelets, leading to the formation of fibrin clots.[70]

In the classic extrinsic pathway, tissue damage activates tissue factor (TF) (also known as factor III or thromboplastin) on the surface of extravascular cells (e.g., fibroblasts, smooth muscle cells), which are exposed to the bloodstream after tissue damage. TF has also been identified on the surfaces of syncytiotrophoblasts,[71] adhered leukocytes, circulating monocytes, and circulating microparticle membrane vesicles released by inflammatory and tumor cells.[70] TF binds factor

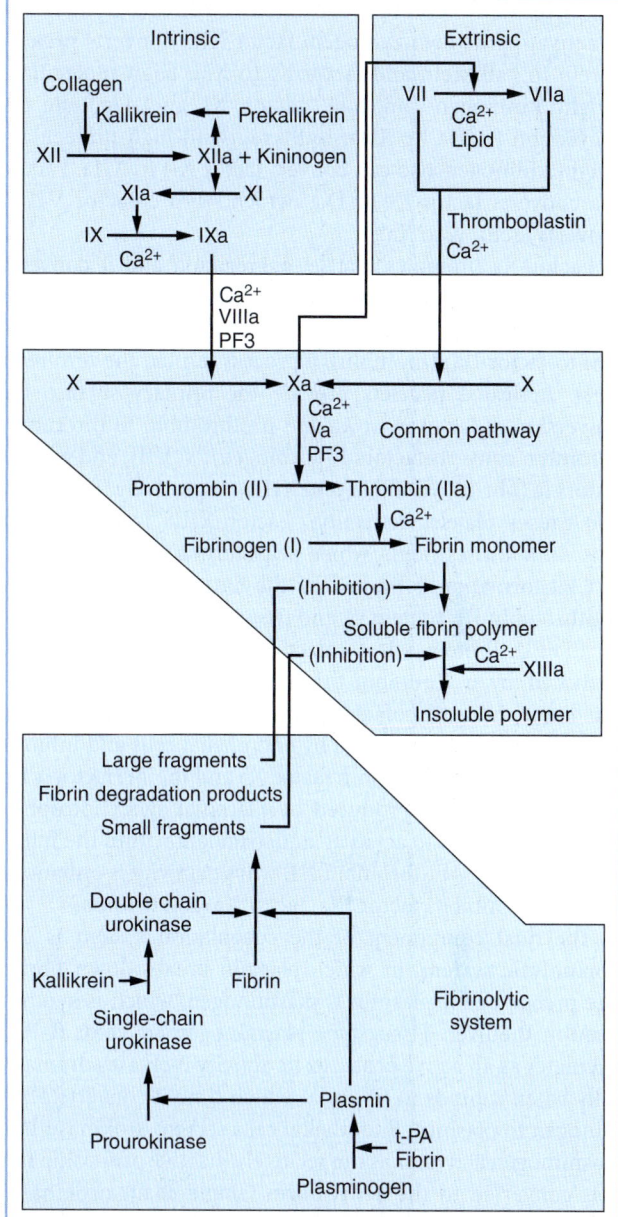

Fig. 44.1 Components of the Extrinsic, Intrinsic, and Common Pathways and the Fibrinolytic System. The term *cascade* is a misnomer that stems from the presence of positive and negative feedback loops in both the coagulation and fibrinolytic systems. *PF3,* Platelet factor 3; *t-PA,* tissue plasminogen activator.

VII and promotes proteolysis and activation to factor VIIa. On the membrane surface, the TF/VIIa complex converts factor X to Xa and small amounts of factor IX to IXa. Factor Xa amplifies conversion of factor VII to VIIa in the first of many positive feedback loops, and factor Xa forms a complex with factor Va. The membrane-bound prothrombinase complex (i.e., Xa/Va) converts small amounts of soluble prothrombin to thrombin. This thrombin diffuses to the activated platelet surface, where it amplifies the intrinsic coagulation pathway.

In the intrinsic pathway, factor XII binds to a negatively charged substrate (e.g., collagen, platelet phosphatidylserine) and may undergo autolysis to form factor XIIa, or it may be converted to XIIa by trace amounts of XIIa. In addition to activating its own zymogen, factor XIIa converts prekallikrein to kallikrein and factor XI to XIa. High-molecular-weight kininogen can bind factor XI and facilitate its conversion to XIa by XIIa. Kallikrein and high-molecular-weight kininogen also can convert factor XII to XIIa. Factor XIa converts factor IX to IXa, which, with cofactor VIIIa, converts factor X to Xa.

Factor Xa promotes platelet aggregation and it converts factors V and VIII to factors Va and VIIIa, respectively. Factor Xa, combined with cofactor Va, converts factor II (prothrombin) to factor IIa (thrombin), a process termed the *thrombin burst*. Activated platelets provide the primary surface for conversion of factor X to Xa and prothrombin to thrombin. Thrombin converts factors I (fibrinogen), V, VIII, and XIII to factors Ia (fibrin), Va, VIIIa, and XIIIa, respectively. Thrombin also causes platelet activation. Factor XIIIa is required to cross-link fibrin strands, which helps form a stable clot.

Clot formation is limited by the **natural anticoagulants** antithrombin III, protein C, and tissue factor pathway inhibitor (TFPI). Protein S is a cofactor for protein C and TFPI. Activated by a thrombin-thrombomodulin complex, activated protein C with cofactor protein S breaks down factors Va and VIIIa. TFPI is produced by endothelial cells and inhibits coagulation by binding both factor Xa and the TF/factor VIIa complex. TPFI-2 is produced by placental syncytiotrophoblasts and appears to act as an anticoagulant within the intervillous space.[72] Antithrombin III, whose activity is enhanced by heparin, inhibits factor IXa, factor Xa, and thrombin.

The final component of the coagulation system is the **fibrinolytic system**, in which plasmin breaks down fibrin. The precursor for plasmin is plasminogen, which is synthesized in the liver. Tissue-type plasminogen activator (t-PA) circulates as an active protease; its activity increases dramatically when it binds to fibrin, at which time it converts plasminogen to plasmin. Endothelial cells secrete urokinase-like plasminogen activator as the relatively inactive prourokinase; it is converted to the active form (single-chain urokinase) by plasmin. Single-chain urokinase is converted to its most active form (double-chain urokinase) by kallikrein, which is released during activation of the coagulation cascade.

Plasmin-mediated fibrinolysis is confined to the clot by the local availability of fibrin and by plasminogen activator inhibitor-1 (PAI-1), which is secreted by many cells, and by plasminogen activator inhibitor-2 (PAI-2), which is secreted primarily by the placenta. Alpha 2-antiplasmin (α2AP) is synthesized in the liver and binds circulating plasmin, but not plasmin bound to fibrin. Within immature thrombi, factor XIIIa cross-links α2AP to fibrin. Additional antifibrinolytic mechanisms protect hemostatic thrombi from early dissolution. Thrombin-activatable fibrinolysis inhibitor (TAFI) is synthesized in the liver, is activated by the thrombin-thrombomodulin complex, and inhibits fibrinolysis by eliminating the binding sites on fibrin for plasminogen and t-PA. The antifibrinolytic drugs **tranexamic acid** and **aminocaproic acid** inhibit fibrinolysis by binding to plasminogen and plasmin and preventing their binding to fibrin.

Changes in the concentrations of coagulation factors during pregnancy are outlined in Chapter 2 (see Box 2.2). The levels of most procoagulants increase during pregnancy, while anticoagulant levels remain stable or decrease.[71] Although t-PA levels decrease and antifibrinolytic proteins (i.e., PAI-1, PAI-2, TAFI, α2AP) increase, plasminogen and fibrin degradation product levels increase, suggesting that fibrinolysis continues unabated during pregnancy.

Placental syncytiotrophoblasts promote coagulation by presenting TF and phospholipids to maternal blood coursing through the intervillous space.[71] The concentrations of the thrombin-antithrombin complex and fibrin degradation products are elevated in blood from the uterine vein compared with peripheral blood, suggesting that many of the hemostatic changes of pregnancy originate in the placental bed.[73]

Deficiencies in procoagulant factors or an increase in fibrinolytic factors cause **hemorrhagic disorders**. Deficiencies in antithrombin III, protein C or S, or the fibrinolytic system cause **thromboembolic disorders**.

Assessment of Coagulation

Routine Hematology

The increase in the concentration of most coagulation factors is associated with a shortening of the prothrombin time (PT) and the activated partial thromboplastin time (aPTT) during normal pregnancy, although values remain within the nonpregnant normal limits. Similarly, fibrinogen and fibrin degradation products are increased. These changes may mask the early diagnosis of **disseminated intravascular coagulation (DIC)**, so serial laboratory parameters are indicated if the diagnosis is suspected.[71] Thrombocytopenia is a sensitive, but not specific, indicator of DIC. For women with severe preeclampsia, a platelet count is a clinically useful screening test; a result below 100,000/μL suggests the possibility of impairment of other coagulation parameters.[74,75] In the healthy parturient with no history or clinical signs of bleeding, the routine laboratory assessment of hemostasis parameters, including platelet count, is not indicated prior to the initiation of a neuraxial anesthetic procedure.[74]

Whole-Blood Viscoelastic Testing

Thromboelastography (TEG) and rotational thromboelastometry (ROTEM) measure whole-blood coagulation and provide information about the adequacy of platelet function and other coagulation factors. Both assays generate a graphic representation of clot strength (Fig. 44.2) in which specific parameters are interrelated and reflect activities of coagulation proteins, platelets, and their interaction.[76] Commonly used TEG and ROTEM parameters are defined in Table 44.3. Activators added to the whole blood can be used to accelerate clotting and to isolate specific components of coagulation (Table 44.4).

Investigations using viscoelastic monitoring confirm that pregnancy is a hypercoagulable state.[76,77] Reference ranges for normal values likely vary over the course of pregnancy and into the postpartum period.[76,77] TEG and ROTEM have been proposed to assess coagulation status in normal and high-risk

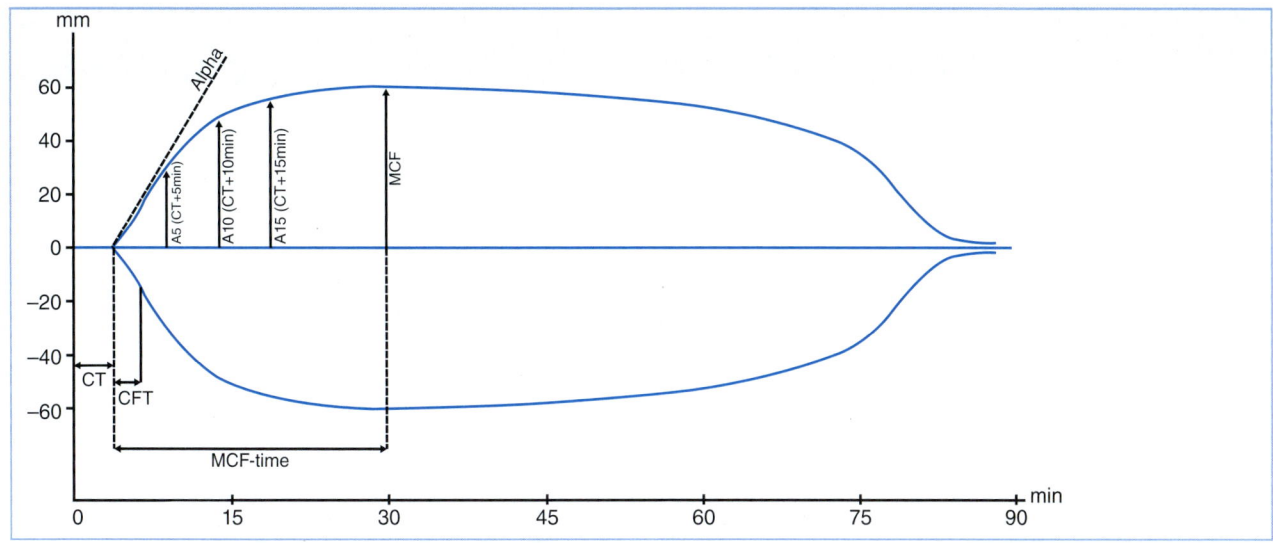

Fig. 44.2 Normal Thromboelastomeric Tracing Using the Rotational Thromboelastometry (ROTEM) Extrinsically Activated Thromboelastometric (EXTEM) Assay. *A*, Current amplitude; *Alpha*, α-angle; *A5, A10, and A15*, amplitude at specific minute interval; *CFT*, clot formation time; *CT*, clotting time; *MCF*, maximum clot firmness. From Katz D, Beilin Y. Disorders of coagulation in pregnancy. *Br J Anaesth.* 2015;115(suppl 2):ii75–ii88.

TABLE 44.3   Commonly Used Thromboelastography and Thromboelastometry Parameters

Coagulation Process	Key Components Tested	TEG	ROTEM	Definition
Clotting factor activation	Soluble coagulation factors, tissue factor	R (reaction time, min)	CT (clotting time, min)	Time to amplitude of 2 mm
Factor amplification and fibrin cross-linkage		K (kinetics time, min)	CFT (clot formation time, min)	Time for amplitude to increase from 2 to 20 mm
		α-angle (degrees)	α-angle (degrees)	Angle between the line in the middle of the graph and the tangential line of the body of the graph
Clot strength	Fibrinogen, platelets, Factor XIII	A5, A10, A15 (mm)	A5, A10, A15 (mm)	Amplitude measured at specific time points after CT or R (e.g., A5 is at 5 min)
		MA (maximum amplitude, mm)	MCF (maximum clot firmness, mm)	Maximum amplitude reached
Clot lysis	Fibrinolytic enzymes, fibrinolysis inhibitors, Factor XIII	LY30 (lysis)	LI30 (lysis index)	% of decrease in MA or MCF 30 min after MA or MCF has been reached
		EPL (estimated percent lysis)	ML (maximum lysis, %)	Maximal reduction in clot firmness after MA or MCF

ROTEM, rotational thromboelastometry; *TEG*, thromboelastography.
Modified from Katz D, Beilin Y. Disorders of coagulation in pregnancy. *Br J Anaesth.* 2015;115(suppl 2):ii75–ii88.

pregnant women,[78] to assess hemostasis before the initiation of neuraxial anesthesia in high-risk patients,[79] and to monitor the efficacy of venous thromboembolism prophylaxis.[80,81] Whether viscoelastic monitoring improves clinical outcomes in these contexts is unknown.

Observational data suggest that viscoelastic monitoring may reduce consumption of blood products when used to guide resuscitation for postpartum hemorrhage (see Chapter 37).[82] In general, deficits in clotting factor activation,

amplification, and fibrin cross-linkage may be corrected with plasma. Deficits in clot strength reflect the need for platelets or fibrinogen (either cryoprecipitate or fibrinogen concentrate). The fibrin-based thromboelastometry (FIBTEM) and functional fibrinogen assays add a platelet inhibitor (cytochalasin D or abciximab) to isolate the need for fibrinogen. For example, a FIBTEM A5 value < 10 mm corresponds to a fibrinogen concentration < 200 mg/dL. Evidence of clot lysis (LY30 > 3% or ML > 15%) supports the need for antifibrinolytic therapy.

TABLE 44.4   Additives Used in Common Viscoelastic Assays to Isolate Components of the Coagulation System

TEG-BASED TESTS		ROTEM-BASED TESTS		
Test	Activators	Test	Activator	Purpose
Kaolin-activated TEG	Kaolin	INTEM	Ellagic acid	Reveals defects in intrinsic pathway
Rapid TEG	Kaolin + tissue factor			Reveals defects in intrinsic and extrinsic pathways; tissue factor accelerates results
		EXTEM	Tissue factor	Reveals defects in intrinsic pathway; reveals platelet deficiency when compared with FIBTEM
Functional fibrinogen test	Tissue factor + abciximab	FIBTEM	Tissue factor + cytochalasin D	Addition of a platelet inhibitor reveals fibrin-based clot defects—fibrinogen deficiency
		APTEM	Tissue factor + aprotinin	Aprotinin blocks fibrinolysis; comparison with EXTEM confirms fibrinolysis

APTEM, Aprotinin-based thromboelastometry; *EXTEM*, extrinsically activated thromboelastometry; *FIBTEM*, fibrin-based thromboelastometry; *INTEM*, intrinsically activated thromboelastometry; *ROTEM*, rotational thromboelastometry; *TEG*, thromboelastography.
Modified from Solomon C, Collis RE, Collins PW. Haemostatic monitoring during postpartum haemorrhage and implications for management. *Br J Anaesth.* 2012;109:851–863.

Platelet Function Analyzer

The PFA-100 (Siemens Healthcare Diagnostics, Deerfield, IL) measures platelet function *in vitro*, especially platelet activation and aggregation. This simple test evaluates the capacity of a sodium-citrated whole-blood sample to form a platelet plug at the aperture situated on a collagen/adenosine phosphate or collagen/epinephrine surface under high-shear conditions. The time required for full occlusion of the aperture by the platelet plug is designated as the *closure time.* PFA-100 measurements do not correlate with platelet counts in healthy parturients,[83] but they may demonstrate impairment in platelet function with severe preeclampsia.[84]

THROMBOCYTOPENIC COAGULOPATHIES

Thrombocytopenia is defined as a platelet count < 150,000/μL. It affects 5% to 10% of the pregnant population, becoming more frequent as pregnancy advances.[85] **Gestational thrombocytopenia** (also known as essential thrombocytopenia) is the most common cause of thrombocytopenia in the second half of pregnancy (Table 44.5). Platelet count rarely decreases below 80,000/μL, and no changes in clinical management are indicated.[86] When platelet count decreases below 100,000/μL, pathologic thrombocytopenic conditions should be considered,[87] including: (1) primary immune thrombocytopenic purpura (ITP)[88]; (2) preeclampsia or hemolysis, elevated liver enzymes, low platelet count (HELLP) syndrome; (3) DIC; (4) thrombotic thrombocytopenic purpura (TTP) or hemolytic uremic syndrome; (5) acute fatty liver of pregnancy (AFLP); (6) secondary immune thrombocytopenia (e.g., drug-induced thrombocytopenia, antiphospholipid syndrome, systemic lupus erythematosus, viral infection); (7) posttransfusion purpura (in individuals who have received a blood transfusion in the previous 1 to 2 weeks)[89]; and (8) inherited platelet disorders (e.g., Bernard-Soulier syndrome).[85] **Pseudothrombocytopenia** is a laboratory artifact in which

chelation of calcium ions by ethylene-diamine-tetraacetic acid exposes antigenic sites that react with antibodies, causing clumping that artificially lowers the platelet count.[90] In these cases, the automated platelet count is normal if citrate anticoagulant is used.

Immune Thrombocytopenic Purpura

Although ITP (also called autoimmune thrombocytopenic purpura and idiopathic thrombocytopenic purpura) is rare, with an incidence of between 0.01% and 0.03%, it composes the majority of cases of thrombocytopenia in the first and second trimesters of pregnancy, and a sizable percentage of cases with maternal platelet counts below 80,000/μL throughout pregnancy (see Table 44.5).[91,92] In this condition, immunoglobin G (IgG) antibodies directed against platelet antigens are produced in the spleen, liver, and bone marrow, resulting in impaired platelet production and accelerated destruction.

Interaction With Pregnancy

Conservative management is typically sufficient for ITP during pregnancy. Symptoms (e.g., gingival bleeding, hematuria, gastrointestinal bleeding) suggest profound thrombocytopenia[91,93]; corticosteroids are indicated if the platelet count is less than 30,000/μL before the onset of labor or if the patient requires a procedure during pregnancy (e.g., amniocentesis, surgery).[86]

Therapy is frequently indicated in preparation for delivery,[86,88] both to achieve minimum platelet count thresholds for safe cesarean delivery (>50,000/μL) and epidural catheter placement (generally greater than 70,000/μL), and to reduce risk for postpartum hemorrhage, which appears to correlate with the degree of platelet deficit.[91]

Prednisone 10 to 20 mg per day is the initial treatment for ITP, with titration over 2 to 4 weeks to the minimum dose that achieves an adequate platelet count for delivery.[86] Unlike dexamethasone, prednisone is almost completely inactivated

TABLE 44.5 Leading Thrombocytopenia Diagnoses Based on Trimester of Presentation and Platelet Count

	First Trimester	Second Trimester	Second Trimester	Third Trimester	Third Trimester
Platelet count (per μL)		>100,000	<100,000	>100,000	<50,000
Diagnosis	ATP	GT	ATP	GT	Preeclampsia
	HT	Preeclampsia	Preeclampsia	Preeclampsia	ATP
	Other	ATP	IPD	Other[a]	Other[a]
	TTP	Other[a]	Other[a]	ATP	TTP
		IPD	GT	IPD	IPD
		TTP	TTP	TTP	GT

[a]Includes infection, disseminated intravascular coagulation, type 2B von Willebrand disease, and immune and nonimmune drug-induced thrombocytopenia.
Diagnoses are listed from most common to least common within each category. *ATP*, Autoimmune thrombocytopenic purpura; *GT*, gestational thrombocytopenia; *HT*, hereditary thrombocytopenia; *IPD*, inherited platelet disorders; *TTP*, thrombotic thrombocytopenic purpura.
Adapted from Cines DB, Levine LD. Thrombocytopenia in pregnancy. *Blood*. 2017;130:2271–2277.

by the placenta, with minimal transfer to the fetus.[92] If there is insufficient time to titrate prednisone, or there is no response to corticosteroid therapy, **intravenous immune globulin** produces a rapid but transient increase in the platelet count.[88] High-dose treatment (1000 mg/kg per day for 1 to 2 days) can achieve platelet count goals within 7 days.[86,92]

In some women with preexisting ITP who become pregnant, thrombocytopenia becomes sufficiently severe that administration of high-dose corticosteroids and immune globulin is inadequate. Splenectomy is a second-line treatment and can be accomplished safely during the second trimester of pregnancy; women who have undergone splenectomy are at increased risk for infection with encapsulated organisms.[88] Thrombopoietin-receptor agonists (e.g., romiplostim) are used in nonpregnant patients with ITP and are increasingly described in case reports and case series of pregnant women, particularly in the third trimester to prepare for delivery.[92] The drugs cross the placenta and into breastmilk; documented complications include maternal venous thrombosis and neonatal thrombocytosis. Rituximab, dapsone, azathioprine, and cyclosporine are alternative options that have been used in nonpregnant patients who have side effects with other therapies, but evidence for safe use in pregnancy is lacking.

Platelet transfusions should be reserved to treat life-threatening hemorrhage or to prepare a patient for urgent surgery, as large doses of platelets may not achieve therapeutic goals and any increase will be transient.[86,94] Standard postpartum uterotonic therapies achieve uterine contraction and minimize risk of hemorrhage related to atony. Tranexamic acid can be considered after delivery. In the days after delivery, the platelet count often returns to normal in these patients.[95]

Obstetric Management

Although maternal IgG can cross the placenta and cause fetal thrombocytopenia, severe perinatal hemorrhagic complications are rare.[86] Although there is a correlation between maternal platelet-associated IgG and fetal thrombocytopenia,

it is not possible to predict the degree of fetal thrombocytopenia based on maternal platelet count or serology.[86] Maternal ITP should not be confused with **fetal-neonatal alloimmune thrombocytopenia**, in which maternal antibodies specific to a fetal platelet antigen cause perinatal thrombocytopenia, increasing the risk for perinatal intracranial hemorrhage.

No study has demonstrated a correlation between the fetal platelet count and intrapartum fetal risk. Neonatal intracranial hemorrhage is rare, is not related to the method of delivery, and most commonly presents greater than 24 hours after delivery at the nadir of neonatal platelet count.[96] Thus, current guidelines recommend that cesarean delivery should be reserved for obstetric indications.[86,88,96] Forceps delivery, vacuum extraction, and episiotomies are frequently avoided, given the increased risk for bleeding.

Thrombotic Thrombocytopenic Purpura

The classic pentad that defines the syndrome of TTP includes (1) thrombocytopenia (platelet count as low as 10,000/μL); (2) microangiopathic hemolytic anemia; (3) fever; (4) neurologic signs such as photophobia, headache, and seizures; and (5) renal failure. Only the first two elements are essential for diagnosis.[97] Disseminated platelet aggregation is a hallmark of TTP.[97,98] Ischemic injury results from the deposition of platelet emboli and may lead to cerebral signs (headache, confusion, seizure, focal deficits, coma), renal signs (proteinuria, increased serum creatinine), splanchnic symptoms (nausea, vomiting, abdominal pain, diarrhea), or cardiac symptoms (chest pain, shortness of breath). Diseases that share some of the clinical findings of TTP include DIC, preeclampsia, HELLP syndrome, acute systemic vasculitis, and hemolytic-uremic syndrome.

TTP is associated with either a congenital or immune-mediated deficiency of the enzyme **ADAMTS13** (a disintegrin and metalloproteinase with a thrombospondin type 1 motif, member 13). ADAMTS13 is responsible for cleaving vWF multimers. These multimers promote systemic platelet aggregates and microemboli in cerebral, coronary, splenic, and renal microvasculature.[97] The presence of vWF (but not fibrinogen) in platelet aggregates helps differentiate TTP from DIC (in DIC, fibrinogen but not vWF is found in platelet aggregates).[99]

Pregnancy is a precipitating event for both initial and recurrent episodes of TTP, particularly among women with congenital ADAMTS13 deficiency, also known as Upshaw-Schulman syndrome.[97,100] While vWF increases throughout pregnancy, ADAMTS13 activity decreases by 50% between the second trimester until delivery, and then recovers to prepregnancy values by 3 weeks postpartum.[97,101] Consequently, acute TTP most often presents in the second half of pregnancy.[97]

Prompt diagnosis and effective treatment for TTP appear to improve both maternal and fetal survival,[97,100,102] although perinatal loss remains significant if the disease develops in the first and second trimesters.[97,100] Diagnosis of TTP may be delayed because of a misdiagnosis with HELLP syndrome; concurrent diagnoses have been reported.[97,100] Clinical signs that suggest TTP include microangiopathic anemia, platelet count < 30,000/µL, international normalized ratio < 1.3, MCV < 86.5 fL, creatinine < 2 g/dL, and a high ratio of lactate dehydrogenase to aspartate aminotransferase.[97,100]

In the presence of concerning laboratory findings and life-threatening neurologic or cardiac signs, daily therapeutic plasma exchange (with an exchange volume of 1.0 to 1.5 times the predicted plasma volume of the patient) is recommended while awaiting the results of ADAMTS13 activity and anti-ADAMTS13 antibody levels. Once a diagnosis of immune-mediated TTP is confirmed, plasma exchange is continued until the platelet count recovers to 150,000/µL or greater. Adjuvant immunosuppressant therapy with corticosteroids (and possibly rituximab) may be needed to reduce antibodies to ADAMTS13.[102,103] For congenital TTP, plasma exchange may be replaced by plasma infusions (10 to 15 mL/kg daily) until clinical remission, followed by maintenance infusions throughout pregnancy and puerperium.

For pregnant patients with a history of immune-mediated TTP, the International Society on Thrombosis and Haemostasis (ISTH) recommends prophylactic plasma exchange if ADAMTS13 levels decrease below 30 U/dL or 30% of normal.[104] For congenital ADAMTS13 deficiency, ADAMTS13 surveillance and regular plasma infusions limit disease recrudescence.[102] Human plasma–derived factor VIII concentrate contains variable concentrations of vWF, so plasma infusion is the preferred treatment for TTP in pregnancy.[104] Coadministered low-dose aspirin may limit the risk of placental vasculopathy and comorbid preeclampsia.

Platelet transfusions may increase morbidity due to increased platelet clumping,[105] but may be safe if administered immediately before or after plasma exchange therapy.[97] Neuraxial anesthesia is not recommended in the setting of TTP with thrombocytopenia, but may be appropriate for patients with well-managed disease, as evidenced by a normal platelet count and lactate dehydrogenase (LDH) level. One case report described spinal anesthesia administered for cesarean delivery in a woman with familial ADAMTS13 deficiency treated with fresh frozen plasma.[106]

Inherited Platelet Disorders

Inherited platelet disorders impact either platelet quantity or function or both, and can increase the risk for both peripartum and perioperative bleeding.[107]

Bernard-Soulier syndrome is a rare autosomal recessive disorder characterized by (1) thrombocytopenia, (2) large platelets on the peripheral blood smear, and (3) defects of the platelet membrane glycoprotein Ib-IX-V complex.[108] Diagnosis can be made by platelet aggregometry; PFA-100 closure time is prolonged. Due to profound functional defects that do not correlate with the platelet count, neuraxial analgesia is contraindicated.[109] Prophylactic tranexamic acid and uterotonics are recommended to limit blood loss with delivery. If bleeding develops, platelet units for transfusion should be leukocyte reduced and HLA and platelet antigen–matched in order to limit risk of platelet alloimmunization.[108,109]

Patients with **Glanzmann thrombasthenia** have a deficiency in platelet surface glycoprotein IIb/IIIa receptors, the major receptor for fibrinogen; this deficiency results in abnormal platelet aggregation.[110] These patients have a normal platelet count. The diagnosis can be made by platelet aggregometry; PFA-100 closure time is prolonged. The treatment for Glanzmann thrombasthenia during labor and delivery is similar to that for Bernard-Soulier syndrome, although platelet alloimmunization is described more commonly with Glanzmann thrombasthenia.[107,109-111] Neonates of mothers with antiplatelet antibodies may develop alloimmune thrombocytopenia, with a risk of intracranial hemorrhage.[109] Recombinant Factor VIIa (rFVIIa) 90 mg/kg is an alternative therapy when matched platelet transfusion is not possible.[109]

Drug-Induced Platelet Disorders

Drugs can accelerate platelet destruction through immunologic mechanisms.[112,113] Drugs used in obstetric patients that are known to trigger antibodies against platelet receptors include antibiotics (e.g., beta-lactam drugs, vancomycin), nonsteroidal antiinflammatory drugs (NSAIDs), abciximab, and tirofiban.[113] Most penicillins and some cephalosporins also impair platelet activity directly.[114] Likewise, heparin impairs platelet function via immunologic and nonimmunologic mechanisms. Nonimmunologic mechanisms are expected; heparin reduces thrombin production and thereby prevents thrombin from amplifying platelet activation during the thrombin burst. Heparin-induced thrombocytopenia (HIT) refers to an immunologic reaction that causes both profound platelet destruction and a prothrombotic state, usually within 5 to 10 days of starting heparin therapy.[115,116] In postoperative patients, the risk for HIT is lower with low-molecular-weight heparin (LMWH) than unfractionated heparin.[117]

Drugs that *impair* platelet function are often used in obstetric patients. Aspirin irreversibly inactivates cyclooxygenase, and *in vitro* platelet function tests can remain abnormal for as long as 1 week.[118] However, low-dose aspirin (i.e., 60 to 80 mg) does not significantly prolong the bleeding time in pregnant women.[119] Moreover, a large number of women receiving low-dose aspirin therapy for the prevention or treatment of preeclampsia have received neuraxial analgesia for labor and delivery without complications.[61] Therefore, in the absence of a coadministered anticoagulant (e.g., LMWH) or preexisting hemostatic defect (e.g., von Willebrand disease, hemophilia A, uremia) in which aspirin's effect is more pronounced,[120,121] recent ingestion of aspirin does not contraindicate the administration of neuraxial anesthesia.[122]

Other NSAIDs (e.g., ibuprofen, indomethacin, naproxen) reversibly inhibit cyclooxygenase.[123] These drugs have only a transient effect on the bleeding time[124,125] and have been given to patients with hemostatic diseases (e.g., hemophilia A) without deleterious effect.[126] Maternal ingestion of these drugs is not a contraindication for neuraxial blockade and should not affect anesthetic management for delivery.[122]

Drugs that increase platelet cyclic adenosine monophosphate (cAMP) levels decrease platelet responsiveness.[123] This increase in cAMP levels can occur after the administration of prostaglandin E_1 or prostacyclin (which stimulates adenyl cyclase) or after the administration of drugs that decrease the destruction of cAMP (e.g., caffeine, theophylline).

Dextran, which is absorbed onto platelet membranes, can reduce platelet aggregation, secretion, and procoagulant activity.[123] Because platelet membranes are a substrate for steps in the coagulation system, clot formation may also be impaired by dextran. Hydroxyethyl starch also appears to worsen platelet function.[123]

CONGENTIAL COAGULOPATHIES

von Willebrand Disease

The hemostatic disorder, von Willebrand disease, was named for Erich von Willebrand, who first described it in 1926.[127] vWF is synthesized by endothelial cells and bone marrow megakaryocytes.[128] The vWF subunit is 260 to 275 kDa. A dimer is formed by a combination of two subunits, and variable numbers of the dimers are combined to form multimers that range from 500 to 200,000 kDa. vWF plays two primary roles in coagulation: (1) it forms a complex with factor VIII, which decreases the excretion of factor VIII; and (2) it mediates platelet adhesion by binding to collagen and platelets.[128,129]

von Willebrand disease can be divided into several subtypes based on quantitative and qualitative defects in vWF (Table 44.6).[130,131] **Type 1 von Willebrand disease** is the most common congenital bleeding disorder, accounts for 80% of diagnosed von Willebrand disease, and affects up to 1% of the population. Type I disease typically is inherited as an autosomal dominant trait and is diagnosed more frequently in women than in men.[128,132] In this subtype, vWF functions normally but its levels are reduced. vWF and factor VIII increase in normal pregnancy, so antenatal bleeding is rare in women with type 1 disease[133]; however, both proteins decrease rapidly after delivery and approach baseline values at 3 weeks

TABLE 44.6	**Classification of von Willebrand Disease**
Type	Description
1	Partial quantitative deficiency of vWF
2	Qualitative vWF defects
2A	Decreased vWF-dependent platelet adhesion and a selective deficiency of high-molecular-weight vWF multimers
2B	Increased affinity for platelet glycoprotein Ib
2M	Decreased vWF-dependent platelet adhesion without a selective deficiency of high-molecular-weight vWF multimers
2N	Markedly decreased binding affinity for factor VIII
3	Virtually complete deficiency of vWF

vWF, von Willebrand factor.
From Sadler JE, Budde U, Eikenboom JC, et al. Update on the pathophysiology and classification of von Willebrand disease: a report of the Subcommittee on von Willebrand Factor. *J Thromb Haemost.* 2006;4:2103–2114.

postpartum, so the risk of delayed postpartum hemorrhage is increased.[128]

Type 2 von Willebrand disease is less common and includes a family of disorders characterized by qualitative dysfunction of vWF, with normal plasma concentrations. Although types 2A and 2M lead to decreased platelet aggregation, type 2B results from a gain-of-function mutation in which vWF increases binding between platelets, leading to accelerated platelet turnover and thrombocytopenia. Finally, **type 3 von Willebrand disease** is caused by a severe quantitative deficiency in vWF and is inherited in an autosomal recessive pattern with a population incidence of 1 per 1,000,000.

Patients with von Willebrand disease have variable levels of both vWF and factor VIII.[129] Thus, some patients with von Willebrand disease are asymptomatic. Because vWF aids in platelet binding to sites of vascular damage, symptoms of von Willebrand disease (e.g., bleeding from skin and mucosae, heavy menstrual bleeding) can mimic those of platelet disorders.[128] vWF slows the clearance of factor VIII; therefore, a deficiency can result in decreased factor VIII levels, and patients with severe disease can present with hemorrhages into muscles and joints similar to those seen in patients with classic hemophilia.

Patients with von Willebrand disease usually have decreased platelet aggregation in response to ristocetin, except for type 2B where platelet aggregation is increased. Patients with a positive bleeding screen[134] should undergo diagnostic testing as recommended by the ISTH.[135] Levels of factor VIII and vWF ristocetin cofactor should be determined during the third trimester. The risk of postpartum hemorrhage is increased for patients with a factor VIII level < 50 IU/dL.[128]

For patients with von Willebrand disease type 1, 2A, 2M, or 2N, a **desmopressin** challenge is ideally completed prior to pregnancy.[128,136] For women with evidence of benefit, 0.3 µg/kg of desmopressin (L-desamino-8-D-arginine vasopressin) is administered intravenously as labor begins, and the dose is repeated every 12 to 24 hours.[128] Desmopressin should not be administered to patients who are unresponsive to desmopressin, or who have preeclampsia, coronary artery disease, peripheral vascular disease, or increased risk of vascular thrombosis.[128,136] Instead, commercial preparations of plasma concentrates that contain both vWF and factor VIII are administered.[128] The initial dose is 40 to 80 IU/kg, with maintenance doses between 20 and 40 IU/kg every 12 hours. During labor and for at least 3 days following cesarean delivery, factor VIII and vWF ristocetin cofactor levels should each be maintained at greater than 50 IU/dL, whether with desmopressin or factor concentrates.[136] In addition, **tranexamic acid prophylaxis** appears to reduce the risk of postpartum hemorrhage in women with any type of von Willebrand disease.[136] For acute bleeding, plasma or cryoprecipitate (500 to 1500 U of factor VIII activity) may be administered.

When considering anesthetic and analgesic options, the balance between risks and benefits of a neuraxial procedure should be evaluated for each patient.[137] The ISTH recommends targeting a vWF activity level > 50 IU/dL prior to any neuraxial blockade, and maintaining that level while any neuraxial catheter remains in place and for 6 hours after removal.[136]

The factor VIII level should be checked daily during the postpartum period, and treatment should be initiated if the factor VIII level decreases below 50% of normal levels or if significant bleeding occurs.[128,138] Oral tranexamic acid is frequently prescribed for 2 weeks following delivery to prevent delayed postpartum hemorrhage.[128,136] At the same time, patients with von Willebrand disease are at increased risk for postpartum thrombosis, and prophylaxis with LMWH may be indicated.[136]

Other Coagulation Factor Deficiencies

The two most common coagulation factor deficiencies are factor VIII (**hemophilia A**) and factor IX (**hemophilia B**), which affect 1:4000 and 1:20,000 male newborns, respectively.[139] Both occur as X-linked traits. It is possible for a woman to have hemophilia if her father is a hemophiliac and her mother is a carrier for hemophilia and passes the abnormal X chromosome to her daughter.[140] Alternatively, a hemophilia carrier may develop a new mutation or an acquired factor inhibitor.[140] Finally, in early embryogenesis, half of the X chromosomes are inactivated.[141] Of the gene population, half of the abnormal genes and half of the normal genes are inactivated in females who are heterozygous for hemophilia A or B. On average, these women have half of the normal concentration of factor VIII or IX, which typically is adequate for coagulation. However, in a minority of carriers, inactivation of most of the normal genes leads to severely depressed levels of factor VIII or IX. If such a patient becomes pregnant, factor supplementation with pooled human plasma concentrate (antihemophilic factor/vWF concentrate [hemophilia A] or prothrombin complex concentrate [hemophilia B]) may be necessary before or during delivery to maintain factor levels > 50 IU/dL, both to facilitate neuraxial blockade

and to limit risk of postpartum hemorrhage.[128,142] A systematic review of case reports identified 126 people with clotting levels > 30 IU/dL who received neuraxial blockade without complications.[142]

On average, one-half of the male children of heterozygous carriers for hemophilia A or B will have hemophilia. These infants have an increased incidence of excessive bleeding after circumcision and cephalohematoma with operative vaginal delivery.[128,143] Cesarean delivery before labor reduces, but does not eliminate, the risk for cephalohematoma compared with spontaneous vaginal birth; decisions about mode of delivery should be individualized to optimally balance maternal and perinatal risk.[128,143,144] During any trial of labor and vaginal delivery, the following procedures should be avoided: (1) placement of a fetal scalp electrode, (2) fetal scalp blood pH determination, and (3) operative vaginal delivery.

Acquired hemophilia is an autoimmune disease resulting from antibodies to factor VIII and is associated with pregnancy and the postpartum period.[145] Both rFVIIa and factor VIII inhibitor bypassing activity have been used to treat bleeding in patients with acquired hemophilia, but both agents are associated with thromboembolism.[145] Immunosuppression is necessary to treat the underlying cause of the disease.

Other congenital factor deficiencies occur as autosomal recessive traits and cause symptoms only in the homozygous state.[76] Table 44.7 lists the plasma concentrations of coagulation factors that are required for hemostasis and corresponding hemostatic agents to treat each deficiency.[146] Hemostatic agent supplementation in consultation with a hematologist may facilitate safe neuraxial blockade for these patients.[147] In an emergency, factors may be rapidly replaced by administration of the appropriate pooled human plasma product or plasma (10 to 15 mL/kg). Postpartum thromboprophylaxis with LMWH should be considered when prothrombotic factors have been administered.[146]

ACQUIRED COAGULOPATHIES

Coagulopathies associated with hypertensive disorders of pregnancy and obstetric hemorrhage are discussed in Chapters 35 and 37, respectively.

Disseminated Intravascular Coagulation

DIC results from an abnormal activation of the coagulation system, which leads to (1) formation of large amounts of thrombin, (2) activation of the fibrinolytic system, and (3) depletion of coagulation factors. With upregulation of both thrombosis and fibrinolysis, the disease manifests as a continuum between hyperfibrinolytic DIC, in which hemorrhage predominates, and thrombotic DIC, in which diffuse microvascular thromboses lead to end-organ injury.[148] Laboratory findings consistent with DIC include (1) decreased platelet count, (2) decreased fibrinogen concentration, (3) variable increases in PT and aPTT, and (4) increased concentrations of D-dimer, fibrin monomer, and fibrin degradation products.[71]

TABLE 44.7 Minimum Coagulation Factor Levels

Coagulation Factor	Plasma Concentration Required for Hemostasis (IU/dL)	Sources of Deficient Protein	Adjuvant Therapies
I	10–25	Fibrinogen concentrate, cryoprecipitate, plasma	Tranexamic acid
II	40	3- or 4-factor PCC, plasma	Tranexamic acid
V	10–15	Platelet transfusion, plasma,	Tranexamic acid, rFVIIa, PCC
VII	10–20	rFVIIa concentrate, 4-factor PCC, plasma	Tranexamic acid
VIII	30	Factor VIII concentrate	Tranexamic acid, rFVIIa
IX	30	Factor IX concentrate, 3- or 4-factor PCC	Tranexamic acid, rFVIIa
X	10–15	Factor X, 3- or 4-factor PCC, plasma	Tranexamic acid
XI	20–30	Factor XI, plasma	Tranexamic acid, desmopressin, rFVIIa
XIII	1–5	Factor XIII-A2, cryoprecipitate, plasma	Tranexamic acid

PCC, Prothrombin complex concentrate; rFVIIa, recombinant factor VIIa.
Adapted from Shapiro A. The use of prophylaxis in the treatment of rare bleeding disorders. *Thromb Res.* 2020;196:590–602.

Viscoelastic monitoring confirms delayed clot activation, decreased clot strength, hypofibrinogenemia, and evidence of fibrinolysis.[76]

DIC is rare in obstetrics, developing in fewer than 1 per 1000 pregnancies.[149] The most frequent cause of DIC is placental abruption, but DIC may also complicate preeclampsia, sepsis, retained dead fetus syndrome, postpartum hemorrhage, AFLP, and amniotic fluid embolism (Fig. 44.3).[71] For women with a diagnosis that can lead to DIC, the ISTH recommends serial laboratory surveillance, with interpretation guided by a validated DIC score (Table 44.8).[150] The pregnancy-modified ISTH DIC score improves the accurate diagnosis of DIC in pregnant populations compared with the original ISTH DIC scoring system, which does not account for the hemostatic changes of pregnancy.[150] To develop the score, Erez et al.[151] analyzed laboratory values from 87 women who developed DIC, and compared them with 24,693 values from control patients to modify the thresholds of the standard ISTH score. Preliminary validation of the modified ISTH scoring system among the 684 women with abruption in the original sample demonstrated superior sensitivity and specificity to detect clinically significant DIC compared with the standard ISTH scoring system.[151] A follow-up study of 154 intensive care patients provided external validation that the pregnancy-modified ISTH DIC score improves sensitivity to detect DIC in obstetric patients compared with the standard ISTH scoring system.[152]

Therapeutic goals for these patients are to (1) treat or remove the precipitating cause, (2) replace depleted coagulation factors, (3) stop ongoing proteolytic activity (i.e., both the coagulation and fibrinolytic pathways), and (4) provide multisystem support as required.[153,154] In obstetric patients, evacuation of the uterine contents often results in removal of the precipitating cause (see Fig. 44.3). Vaginal delivery can be attempted if the mother is stable and delivery can be achieved in a timely manner. If delivery cannot be achieved quickly, cesarean delivery may be required. Rarely, cesarean delivery may be necessary to deliver a dead fetus.

Blood product transfusion is the cornerstone of hemostatic support for patients with DIC. In the presence of active bleeding or when an invasive procedure is required, the physician should transfuse plasma (15 to 30 mL/kg) to maintain the PT and aPTT within 1.5 times normal values, cryoprecipitate or fibrinogen concentrate to maintain the fibrinogen concentration > 200 mg/dL, and platelets to maintain a platelet count > 50,000/μL.[71,153,155] The laboratory turnaround time may be faster for viscoelastic monitoring with TEG or ROTEM than standard coagulation testing, and can more precisely guide hemostatic management.[148] Tranexamic acid is indicated when viscoelastic monitoring confirms the presence of fibrinolysis, but may delay resolution of microemboli in cases of thrombotic DIC.[148,155]

In a prospective, open label, randomized controlled trial of 84 women with severe postpartum hemorrhage unresponsive to uterotonic agents, human **rFVIIa** 60 μg/kg decreased the need for subsequent hemostatic surgical procedures (including intrauterine balloon insertion, uterine compression sutures, uterine or iliac artery ligation, uterine artery embolization, or peripartum hysterectomy) from 93% to 52% (RR, 0.56; 95% CI, 0.42 to 0.76).[156] Two venous thrombotic events were reported, both in the intervention arm; each recovered with anticoagulation treatment. Consequently, in 2022, the European Medicines Agency approved rFVIIa for the treatment of postpartum hemorrhage unresponsive to other therapies. The use of rFVIIa remains off-label for this purpose in the United States.

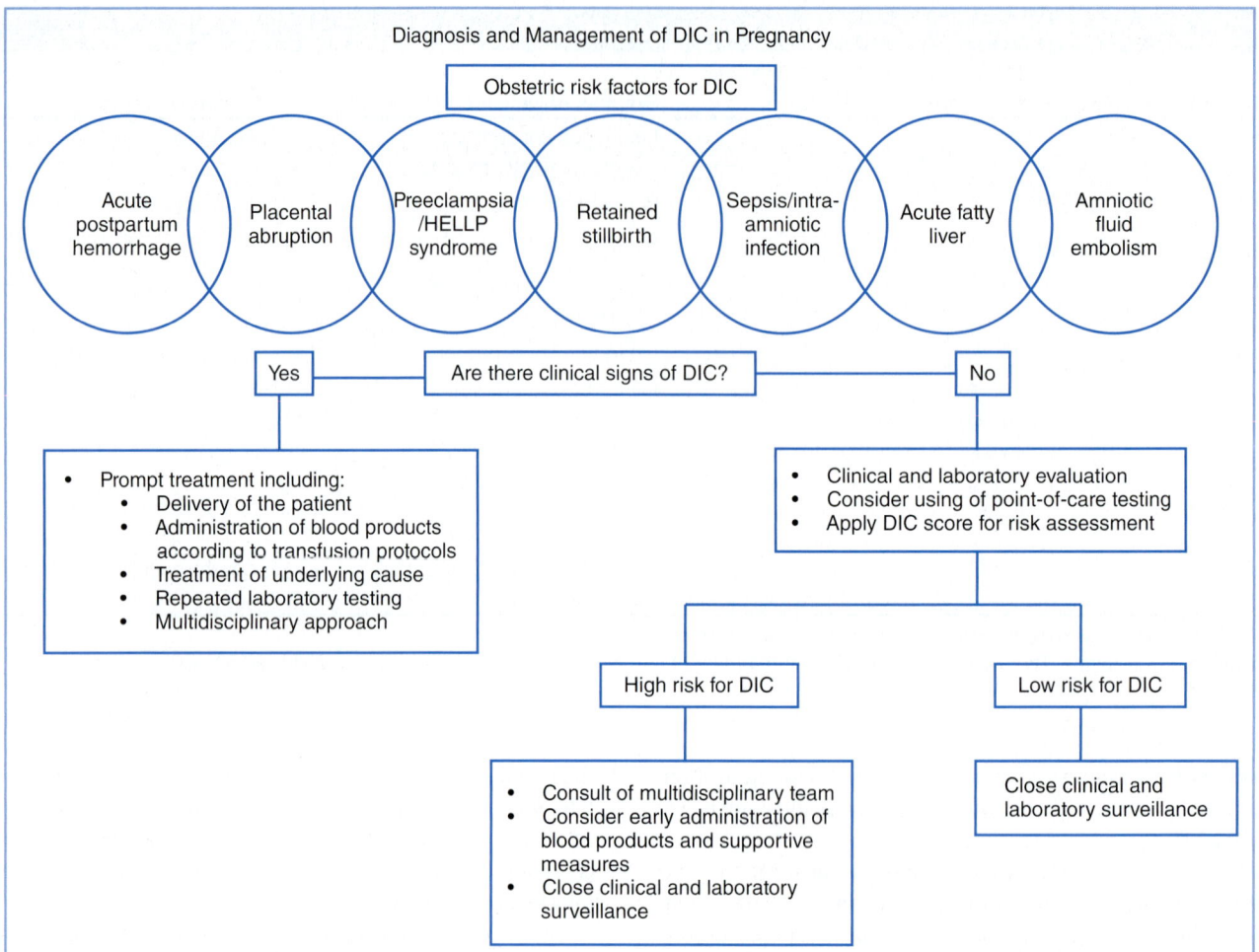

Fig. 44.3 Algorithm Summarizing Diagnosis and Treatment of Disseminated Intravascular Coagulation (DIC) During Pregnancy. *HELLP*, Hemolysis, elevated liver enzymes, and low platelet count. From Erez O. Disseminated intravascular coagulation in pregnancy—clinical phenotypes and diagnostic scores. *Thromb Res.* 2017;151(suppl 1):S56–S60.

Patients with DIC often have multiorgan system failure and require mechanical ventilatory support and care in the intensive care unit (see Chapter 53). DIC almost always mandates administration of general anesthesia in patients who require cesarean delivery or exploratory laparotomy. Given the increased risk for venous thromboembolism among patients with DIC, thromboprophylaxis with unfractionated heparin or LMWH (as soon as active bleeding is controlled), mechanical methods, or a combination of methods is indicated.[153,157]

NEURAXIAL ANESTHESIA IN THE PATIENT WITH COAGULOPATHY

Concern exists that an epidural hematoma may develop after the administration of neuraxial anesthesia in patients with coagulopathy (see Chapter 31). There are few published case reports of epidural or spinal subdural hematoma after the administration of neuraxial anesthesia in pregnant patients. Similarly, multicenter survey studies have not reported this complication in obstetric patients.[158,159] However, because of the serious consequences of an epidural hematoma, the risks

and benefits of performing neuraxial anesthesia should be carefully assessed in a patient with either clinical or laboratory evidence of coagulopathy.

Frank coagulopathy represents an absolute contraindication to the administration of neuraxial anesthesia. For patients receiving pharmacologic anticoagulation, professional societies have developed evidence-based guidelines to optimize the safety of neuraxial blockade (see Chapter 38).[122,160] For nonbleeding patients with diagnoses that increase the risk for coagulopathy (see Fig. 44.3), the anesthesia provider can use standard laboratory testing (i.e., the platelet count, PT/international normalized ratio [INR], aPTT, and fibrinogen concentration), viscoelastic testing, or both, to exclude hemostatic derangements before neuraxial blockade. If the use of a neuraxial anesthetic technique is considered in a patient with a congenital coagulopathy, the results of relevant factor assays should be greater than the minimum level required for hemostasis (see Table 44.7) before neuraxial needle placement.[130,146,147,161]

Thrombocytopenia develops in 5% to 10% of healthy women by the end of pregnancy, normally with little clinical consequence, particularly when thrombocytopenia is

TABLE 44.8 Scoring Systems to Detect Disseminated Intravascular Coagulation During Pregnancy

Parameter	ISTH Score	Pregnancy-Modified ISTH Score
Platelet count (x10³/µL)	>100 = 0	>185 = 0
	<100 = 1	101–185 = 1
	<50 = 2	51–100 = 2
		<50 = 3
Fibrin degradation products	No increase = 0	
	Moderate increase = 2	
	Strong increase = 3	
Prolonged prothrombin time (s)[a]	<3 = 0	<0.5 = 0
	3–6 = 1	0.5–1.0 = 5
	>6 = 2	1.1–1.5 = 12
		>1.5 = 25
Fibrinogen level (mg/dL)	>100 = 0	>450 = 0
	<100 = 1	400–450 = 1
		300–390 = 6
		<300 = 25
Calculated score	>5 compatible with overt DIC	>26 high probability for DIC

[a]The difference (in seconds) between the result of the patient and that of the laboratory normal control.

DIC, Disseminated intravascular coagulation; *ISTH*, International Society on Thrombosis and Haemostasis.

From Erez O. Disseminated intravascular coagulation in pregnancy—clinical phenotypes and diagnostic scores. *Thromb Res.* 2017;151(suppl 1): S56–S60.

mild (100,000 to 149,000/µL).[85] However, the combination of both quantitative and qualitative platelet deficits presents a more serious risk for epidural hematoma and may develop in women with severe preeclampsia (see Chapter 35), ITP, and congenital platelet disorders. A number of groups have reported the safe administration of neuraxial anesthesia—without any neurologic complications—in healthy pregnant women with thrombocytopenia, preeclampsia, and ITP.[162] A retrospective cohort study from the Multicenter Perioperative Outcomes Group identified no cases of epidural hematoma requiring surgical decompression among 573 parturients with a platelet count < 100,000/µL.[162] Combined with an additional 951 parturients identified by systematic review, the authors calculated an upper bound of the 95% confidence interval for risk of epidural hematoma to be 11% for a platelet count < 49,000/µL, 3% for 50,000 to 69,000/µL, and 0.2% for 70,000 to 100,000/µL.[162] A systematic review of the published literature between 1947 and 2018 identified 2413 obstetric patients who received neuraxial procedures with a platelet count < 100,000/µL, of whom 5 developed spinal epidural hematoma (platelet count range, 44,000 to 91,000/µL). One patient had an underlying arteriovenous malformation, one was coagulopathic at the time of epidural catheter removal, two had HELLP syndrome, and one had eclampsia.[163]

Multiple professional societies have published recommendations about the minimum platelet count needed to ensure safe neuraxial procedures.[164] The Society for Obstetric Anesthesiology and Perinatology published an algorithm to guide decision-making for neuraxial blockade administration in obstetric patients with thrombocytopenia (Fig. 44.4). Within this framework, neuraxial procedures are considered low risk for spinal epidural hematoma if the platelet count is greater than 70,000/µL in patients with no other risk factors.[164] Under selected circumstances, neuraxial procedures may be appropriate in a well-counseled patient with a platelet count between 50,000 and 70,000/µL.[164]

When determining whether neuraxial anesthesia is safe in a patient with thrombocytopenia, the anesthesia provider should consider the following factors: (1) clinical evidence of bleeding; (2) time interval since the platelet count was measured; (3) any recent change in the platelet count (e.g., downward trending); (4) quality of platelet function; (5) adequacy of coagulation factor level and function; and, perhaps most importantly, (6) the **risk versus benefit of performing neuraxial anesthesia**. The bleeding time measurement is *not* helpful in determining the risk for epidural hematoma. Although viscoelastic monitoring shows some promise, its usefulness in predicting the risk for epidural hematoma is unproven.

Clinical judgment represents the most important means of assessing the risk for epidural hematoma in an individual patient. Clearly, the anesthesia provider will not want to perform neuraxial anesthesia in a patient with clinical evidence of coagulopathy (e.g., bleeding from nasal or oral mucosae or venipuncture sites, presence of petechiae or ecchymoses). In contrast, a surgical patient with severe preeclampsia, severe upper airway edema, a platelet count of 60,000/µL, and no

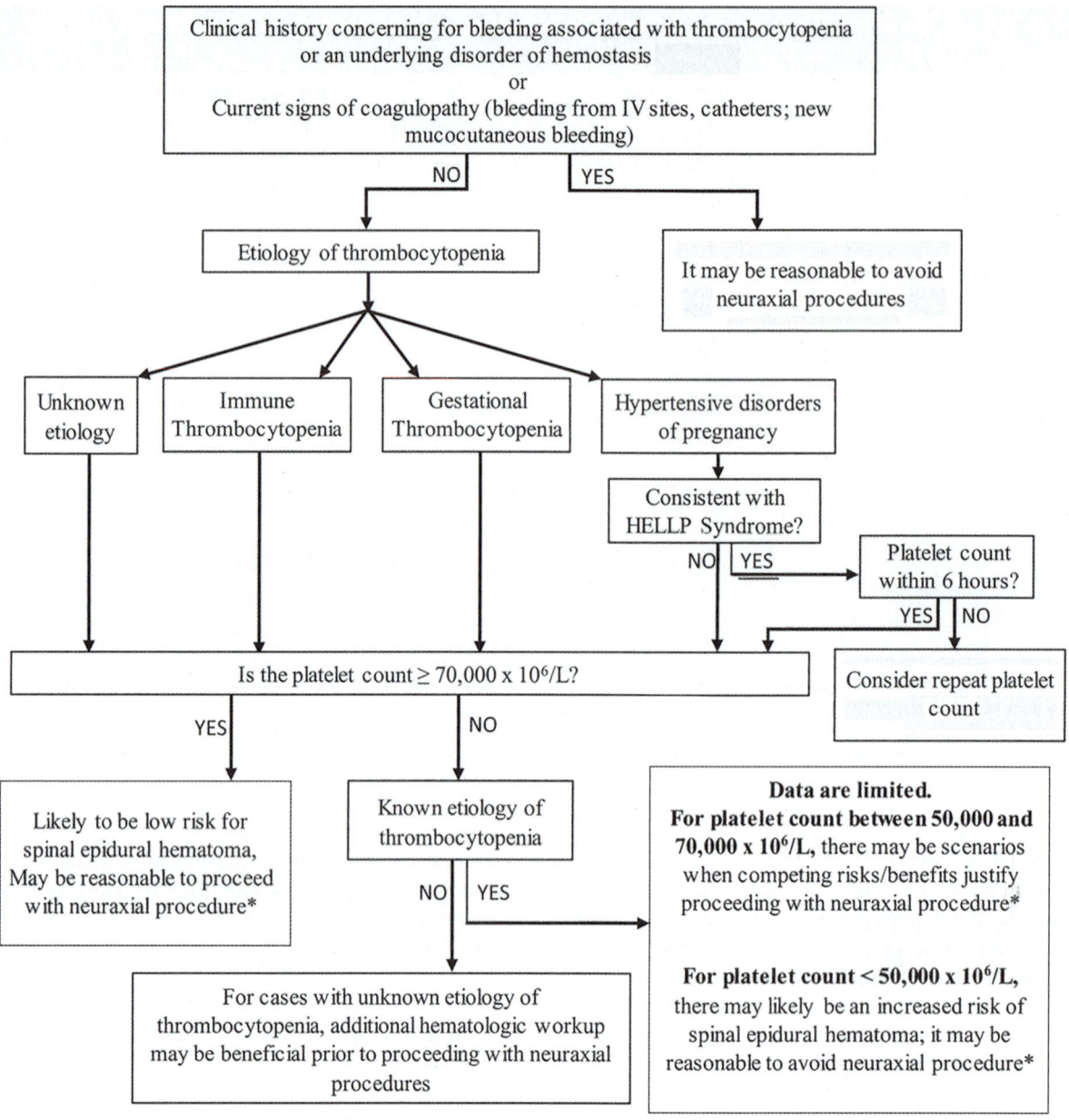

Fig. 44.4 Algorithm Summarizing Decision Making for Neuraxial Blockade in the Obstetric Patient With Thrombocytopenia. *The algorithm assumes the patient has no additional risk factors. Clinical context and competing risks might include the presence of high-risk comorbidities or difficult airway, the need for urgent general anesthesia, or the choice of neuraxial anesthetic technique (i.e., spinal versus epidural technique). *HELLP*, Hemolysis, elevated liver enzymes, low platelet count; *IV*, intravenous. From Bauer M, Arendt K, Beilin Y, Gernsheimer J, Perez Botero J, James AH, et al. The Society for Obstetric Anesthesia and Perinatology interdisciplinary consensus statement on neuraxial procedures in obstetric patients with thrombocytopenia. *Anesth Analg.* 2021;132:1531–1544.

clinical evidence of coagulopathy may be an appropriate candidate for spinal anesthesia. The risk for airway complications with general anesthesia is greater than the risk for an epidural hematoma in such a patient,[165] and spinal anesthesia may be offered after a thorough discussion of the risks and benefits. However, some anesthesia providers advocate a more conservative approach in such cases and recommend alternative methods of analgesia during labor, followed by awake laryngoscopy and tracheal intubation if cesarean delivery should become necessary.

The use of single-shot spinal anesthesia may reduce the risk for epidural vein trauma compared with epidural catheter insertion. For epidural catheter insertion, several modifications of the neuraxial technique may decrease the risk for venous injury: (1) administration of epidural analgesia early in labor before the platelet count or platelet function declines, (2) needle and catheter placement with the patient in the lateral rather than sitting position, (3) the use of a wire-embedded polyurethane rather than polyamide epidural catheter, (4) limiting catheter insertion length to 6 cm or less, and (5) administration of saline through the needle to distend the epidural space before insertion of the catheter.[166] There is no evidence that any of these recommendations reduces the likelihood of epidural hematoma in patients with platelet dysfunction or coagulopathy.

During the administration of epidural analgesia, the anesthesia provider can minimize motor blockade, which might confuse the diagnosis of epidural hematoma, by administering a dilute solution of local anesthetic with an opioid. Lower-extremity motor function should be verified at 1- to 2-hour intervals, and the epidural solution adjusted as needed to maintain lower-extremity strength. In addition, all clinical staff should be aware of the signs and symptoms of epidural hematoma, including (1) severe, unremitting backache; (2) neurologic deficit, including bowel or bladder dysfunction or radiculopathy; (3) tenderness over the spinous or paraspinous area; and (4) unexplained fever.[167] If clinical findings raise concern for epidural hematoma, immediate steps should be taken to obtain appropriate diagnostic imaging and to consult a neurosurgeon (see Chapter 31).

In some cases, severe thrombocytopenia and coagulopathy may develop *after* the placement of an epidural catheter. Epidural hematomas have been reported after epidural catheter removal in obstetric patients with coagulopathy.[163] It is possible that movement or removal of the catheter may dislodge a clot, resulting in fresh bleeding and an epidural hematoma. As such, recommended hemostatic conditions for epidural catheter removal parallel those recommended for neuraxial block administration.[164]

HYPERCOAGULABLE STATES

Effective hemostasis is maintained by an appropriate balance of procoagulant and anticoagulant activity. A congenital deficiency in anticoagulant activity occurs in more than 50% of women with pregnancy-related venous thrombosis.[168] Factor V Leiden mutation, prothrombin mutation, protein C deficiency, protein S deficiency, and antithrombin III deficiency are the most common thrombophilias diagnosed in pregnancy.[168] Venous thromboses are more common than arterial thromboses[169]; the incidence increases with surgery, pregnancy, oral contraceptive use, and immobilization. Although the results of small case-control studies have suggested that patients with thrombophilias may have an increased incidence of fetal growth restriction, intrauterine fetal death, preeclampsia, and placental abruption, these associations have not been replicated in large prospective cohorts.[168] Prophylactic anticoagulation is recommended for select thrombophilia carriers in pregnancy to reduce the risk of maternal thromboembolism (see Chapter 38), but no evidence suggests that this treatment improves pregnancy outcomes.[168,170] Commonly used anticoagulation regimens during pregnancy are listed in Table 38.2.

Factor V Leiden Mutation

Factor V Leiden is a genetic disorder attributable to genetic mutation resulting in a single amino acid substitution in the factor V protein. The mutant protein persists longer in the circulation owing to its slower degradation by activated protein C, leading to a hypercoagulable state.[168] Although heterozygous factor V Leiden affects less than 15% of the childbearing population, these women experience as many as 40% of all obstetric thromboembolic events. Among women with factor V Leiden heterozygosity, a personal history of a venous thromboembolism increases the risk of venous thromboembolism to 10% from 1% among those without previous thrombosis.[168] A homozygous state is found in 1 in 1600 individuals; these patients have at least a 25-fold higher risk for thrombosis.[168,171]

Prothrombin Gene Mutation

The prothrombin *G20210A* gene mutation results in elevated circulating prothrombin levels. This gene mutation is present in 2% to 3% of the general population and accounts for up to 17% of cases of venous thromboembolism in pregnancy.[168] For women who are heterozygous for the prothrombin mutation, a personal or family history of venous thrombosis increases the risk for a subsequent venous thromboembolism in pregnancy from less than 0.5% to approximately 10%.[168] Further, the combination of factor V Leiden and prothrombin mutations has synergistic hypercoagulable effects.[168]

Antithrombin III Deficiency

Antithrombin III is synthesized in the liver and endothelial cells. It inactivates thrombin and factors IXa, Xa, XIa, and XIIa[172]; its activity is potentiated by heparin. Deficiency of antithrombin III occurs in 0.02% to 0.4% of the general population.[168,173] The risk for thrombosis during pregnancy increases from 3% to 7% among those with antithrombin III deficiency and no prior thromboembolism to more than 40% among those with a prior venous thromboembolism.[168] Quantitative (type I) and qualitative (type II) deficiencies exist[173]; thus, both immunologic and functional assays are required to detect abnormalities.[174]

Heparin acts by potentiating the activity of antithrombin III. If antithrombin III levels are decreased, heparin may not ensure effective thromboprophylaxis. Antithrombin III replacement, with or without coadministration of heparin, has been proposed for perioperative or peripartum therapy for patients with antithrombin III deficiency and a history of venous thromboembolism.[172] Although long-term antithrombin III replacement is expensive, its use may be indicated for women who experience venous thrombosis despite thromboprophylaxis with LMWH.[175] Warfarin is an alternative option for women in the second or third trimester of pregnancy, remote from delivery.[175]

Protein C Deficiency

Protein C is produced in the liver and acts by inhibiting activated factors Va and VIIIa. Deficiency is defined by an activity level < 50%. The incidence of protein C deficiency is approximately 0.3% in the general population. Protein C levels normally increase by 35% during pregnancy, but this increase is attenuated in patients with protein C deficiency.[176] Among women with protein C deficiency, the risk for venous thromboembolism during pregnancy increases from approximately 1% among those without previous thrombosis to between 4% and 17% for those with a previous thrombosis.[168]

Protein C is a vitamin K–dependent protein with a short half-life (8 hours). If warfarin is administered without prior heparin anticoagulation, protein C levels decrease before the levels of factors II, VII, IX, and X decrease. Thrombosis with skin necrosis can result.[177]

Protein S Deficiency

Protein S acts as a cofactor for protein C. In contrast to protein C, the plasma levels of protein S normally *decrease* during pregnancy.[176] The prevalence of protein S deficiency is less than 0.1% in the general population. Protein S is also produced in the liver and depends on vitamin K for its synthesis.[177] Circulating protein S binds to C4b-binding protein (a protein of the complement system), but it is the free fraction of protein S that acts as a cofactor for protein C.[177] Immunologic assays measure total protein S concentration; therefore, a diagnosis of protein S deficiency is made either by using a functional assay (<50% activity) or by calculating the percent of protein S bound to C4b-binding protein.[177] The risk for antepartum and postpartum venous thromboembolism is low in patients with protein C or protein S deficiency; hence, thromboprophylaxis is not indicated unless the patient has a history of venous thromboembolism or additional risk factors are present.

Lupus Anticoagulant

The term *lupus anticoagulant* is a misnomer. Patients with lupus anticoagulant do *not* have coagulopathy; rather, they are at risk for thromboembolic events. The hypercoagulable state associated with lupus anticoagulant is discussed in Chapter 40.

KEY POINTS

- Blood product preparation is frequently delayed for patients with hemoglobinopathies because of high rates of alloimmunization and extended cross-matching procedures to limit future alloimmunization.
- Lifelong transfusion dependence increases the risk for hemosiderosis, causing primarily cardiac, pulmonary, and hepatic toxicity.
- Neuraxial anesthetic techniques can be used safely during labor and delivery in patients with hemoglobinopathy.
- Routine laboratory assessment of the platelet count and coagulation status is not indicated before the initiation of neuraxial procedures in healthy parturients.

- The first goal in the treatment of disseminated intravascular coagulation is to treat or remove the precipitating cause. In pregnant patients, evacuation of the uterine contents often results in removal of the precipitating cause.
- Uncorrected, frank coagulopathy represents an absolute contraindication to the administration of neuraxial anesthesia.
- In a patient with an isolated laboratory abnormality and no clinical evidence of coagulopathy, the anesthesia provider should assess the risks and benefits of performing neuraxial anesthesia.

REFERENCES

1. World Health Organization. Haemoglobin concentrations for the diagnosis of anaemia and assessment of severity; 2011. https://www.who.int/publications/i/item/WHO-NMH-NHD-MNM-11.1. Accessed January 19, 2025.
2. American College of Obstetricians and Gynecologists. Practice Bulletin No. 233: Anemia in pregnancy (reaffirmed 2024). *Obstet Gynecol*. 2021;138:e55–e64.
3. World Health Organization. World Health Statistics 2023: Monitoring health for the Sustainable Development Goals; 2023. https://www.who.int/publications/i/item/9789240074323. Accessed December 31, 2024.
4. Karami M, Chaleshgar M, Salari N, et al. Global prevalence of anemia in pregnant women: a comprehensive systematic review and meta-analysis. *Matern Child Health J*. 2022;26: 1473–1487.
5. Juul SE, Derman RJ, Auerbach M. Perinatal iron deficiency: implications for mothers and infants. *Neonatology*. 2019;115: 269–274.
6. Means RT. Iron deficiency and iron deficiency anemia: implications and impact in pregnancy, fetal development, and early childhood parameters. *Nutrients*. 2020;12:447.
7. Young MF, Oaks BM, Rogers HP, et al. Maternal low and high hemoglobin concentrations and associations with adverse maternal and infant health outcomes: an updated global systematic review and meta-analysis. *BMC Pregnancy Childbirth*. 2023;23:264.
8. Mohamed MA, Ahmad T, Macri C, Aly H. Racial disparities in maternal hemoglobin concentrations and pregnancy outcomes. *J Perinat Med*. 2012;40:141–149.
9. Haider BA, Olofin I, Wang M, et al. Anaemia, prenatal iron use, and risk of adverse pregnancy outcomes: systematic review and meta-analysis. *BMJ*. 2013;346:f3443.
10. Cantor AG, Bougatsos C, Dana T, et al. Routine iron supplementation and screening for iron deficiency anemia in pregnancy: a systematic review for the U.S. Preventive Services Task Force. *Ann Intern Med*. 2015;162:566–576.
11. Finkelstein JL, Cuthbert A, Venkatramanan S, et al. Daily oral iron supplementation during pregnancy. *Cochrane Database Syst Rev*. 2024;(8):CD004736.
12. Reveiz L, Gyte GM, Cuervo LG, Casasbuenas A. Treatments for iron-deficiency anaemia in pregnancy. *Cochrane Database Syst Rev*. 2011;(10):CD003094.
13. Govindappagari S, Burwick RM. Treatment of iron deficiency anemia in pregnancy with intravenous versus oral iron: systematic review and meta-analysis. *Am J Perinatol*. 2019;36: 366–376.
14. Hamm RF, Wang EY, Levine LD, et al. Implementation of a protocol for management of antepartum iron deficiency

anemia: a prospective cohort study. *Am J Obstet Gynecol MFM*. 2022;4:100533.

15. Tesio N, Bauer DE. Molecular basis and genetic modifiers of thalassemia. *Hematol Oncol Clin North Am*. 2023;37: 273–299.

16. Pines M, Sheth S. Clinical classification, screening, and diagnosis in beta-thalassemia and hemoglobin E/beta-thalassemia. *Hematol Oncol Clin North Am*. 2023;37:313–325.

17. Lal A, Vichinsky E. The clinical phenotypes of alpha thalassemia. *Hematol Oncol Clin North Am*. 2023;37:327–339.

18. Dozy AM, Kan YW, Embury SH, et al. Alpha-globin gene organisation in blacks precludes the severe form of alpha-thalassaemia. *Nature*. 1979;280:605–607.

19. Beutler E, West C. Hematologic differences between African-Americans and whites: the roles of iron deficiency and alpha-thalassemia on hemoglobin levels and mean corpuscular volume. *Blood*. 2005;106:740–745.

20. American College of Obstetricians and Gynecologists. Practice Bulletin No. 78: Hemoglobinopathies in pregnancy (reaffirmed 2021). *Obstet Gynecol*. 2007;109:229–237.

21. Songdej D, Babbs C, Higgs DR, Consortium BI. An international registry of survivors with Hb Bart's hydrops fetalis syndrome. *Blood*. 2017;129:1251–1259.

22. Sheth S, Thein SL. Thalassemia: a disorder of globin synthesis. In: Kaushansky K, Prchal JT, Burns LJ, et al., eds. *Williams Hematology*. 10th ed. McGraw-Hill; 2021.

23. Farmakis D, Porter J, Taher A, et al. 2021 Thalassaemia International Federation Guidelines for the management of transfusion-dependent thalassaemia. *Hemasphere*. 2022;6:e732.

24. De Sanctis V, Soliman AT, Elsedfy H, et al. Growth and endocrine disorders in thalassemia: the international network on endocrine complications in thalassemia (I-CET) position statement and guidelines. *Indian J Endocrinol Metab*. 2013;17:8–18.

25. Bollig C, Schell LK, Rucker G, et al. Deferasirox for managing iron overload in people with thalassaemia. *Cochrane Database Syst Rev*. 2017;(8):CD007476.

26. Fisher SA, Brunskill SJ, Doree C, et al. Oral deferiprone for iron chelation in people with thalassaemia. *Cochrane Database Syst Rev*. 2013;(8):CD004839.

27. Motta I, Bou-Fakhredin R, Taher AT, Cappellini MD. Beta thalassemia: new therapeutic options beyond transfusion and iron chelation. *Drugs*. 2020;80:1053–1063.

28. Paschoudi K, Yannaki E, Psatha N. Precision editing as a therapeutic approach for beta-hemoglobinopathies. *Int J Mol Sci*. 2023;24

29. Petrakos G, Andriopoulos P, Tsironi M. Pregnancy in women with thalassemia: challenges and solutions. *Int J Womens Health*. 2016;8:441–451.

30. Mordel N, Birkenfeld A, Goldfarb AN, Rachmilewitz EA. Successful full-term pregnancy in homozygous beta-thalassemia major: case report and review of the literature. *Obstet Gynecol*. 1989;73:837–840.

31. Origa R, Piga A, Quarta G, et al. Pregnancy and beta-thalassemia: an Italian multicenter experience. *Haematologica*. 2010;95:376–381.

32. Pearson HA. Iron studies in infants born to an iron overloaded mother with beta-thalassemia major: possible effects of maternal desferrioxamine therapy. *J Pediatr Hematol Oncol*. 2007;29:160–162.

33. Diamantidis MD, Neokleous N, Agapidou A, et al. Iron chelation therapy of transfusion-dependent beta-thalassemia

during pregnancy in the era of novel drugs: is deferasirox toxic? *Int J Hematol*. 2016;103:537–544.

34. Singer ST, Vichinsky EP. Deferoxamine treatment during pregnancy: is it harmful? *Am J Hematol*. 1999;60:24–26.

35. Carlberg KT, Singer ST, Vichinsky EP. Fertility and pregnancy in women with transfusion-dependent thalassemia. *Hematol Oncol Clin North Am*. 2018;32:297–315.

36. Royal College of Obstetricians & Gynaecologists. Green-top Guideline, No. 66: Management of beta thalassaemia in pregnancy; 2014. https://www.rcog.org.uk/guidance/browse-all-guidance/green-top-guidelines/management-of-beta-thalassaemia-in-pregnancy-green-top-guideline-no-66/. Accessed December 31, 2024.

37. Staikou C, Stavroulakis E, Karmaniolou I. A narrative review of peri-operative management of patients with thalassaemia. *Anaesthesia*. 2014;69:494–510.

38. Anderson LJ, Holden S, Davis B, et al. Cardiovascular T2-star (T2*) magnetic resonance for the early diagnosis of myocardial iron overload. *Eur Heart J*. 2001;22: 2171–2179.

39. Waters JH, Lukauskiene E, Anderson ME. Intraoperative blood salvage during cesarean delivery in a patient with beta thalassemia intermedia. *Anesth Analg*. 2003;97:1808–1809.

40. Butwick A, Findley I, Wonke B. Management of pregnancy in a patient with beta thalassaemia major. *Int J Obstet Anesth*. 2005;14:351–354.

41. Ruangvutilert P, Phatihattakorn C, Yaiyiam C, Panchalee T. Pregnancy outcomes among women affected with thalassemia traits. *Arch Gynecol Obstet*. 2023;307:431–438.

42. Origa R, Comitini F. Pregnancy in thalassemia. *Mediterr J Hematol Infect Dis*. 2019;11:e2019019.

43. Firth PG, Head CA. Sickle cell disease and anesthesia. *Anesthesiology*. 2004;101:766–785.

44. Sheehan VA, Gordeuk VR, Kutlar A Disorders of hemoglobin structure: sickle cell anemia and related abnormalities. In: Kaushansky K, Prchal JT, Burns LJ, et al., eds. *Williams Hematology*. 10th ed. McGraw-Hill; 2021.

45. Solanki DL, McCurdy PR, Cuttitta FF, Schechter GP. Hemolysis in sickle cell disease as measured by endogenous carbon monoxide production. A preliminary report. *Am J Clin Pathol*. 1988;89:221–225.

46. Yawn BP, Buchanan GR, Afenyi-Annan AN, et al. Management of sickle cell disease: summary of the 2014 evidence-based report by expert panel members. *JAMA*. 2014;312:1033–1048.

47. Hassell KL. Population estimates of sickle cell disease in the U.S. *Am J Prev Med*. 2010;38:S512–S521.

48. Veille JC, Hanson R. Left ventricular systolic and diastolic function in pregnant patients with sickle cell disease. *Am J Obstet Gynecol*. 1994;170:107–110.

49. Tsen LC, Cherayil G. Sickle cell-induced peripheral neuropathy following spinal anesthesia for cesarean delivery. *Anesthesiology*. 2001;95:1298–1299.

50. Steinberg MH, Sebastiani P. Genetic modifiers of sickle cell disease. *Am J Hematol*. 2012;87:795–803.

51. Villers MS, Jamison MG, De Castro LM, James AH. Morbidity associated with sickle cell disease in pregnancy. *Am J Obstet Gynecol*. 2008;199:125.e1–e5.

52. Oteng-Ntim E, Meeks D, Seed PT, et al. Adverse maternal and perinatal outcomes in pregnant women with sickle cell disease: systematic review and meta-analysis. *Blood*. 2015;125:3316–3325.

53. Malinowski AK, Shehata N, D'Souza R, et al. Prophylactic transfusion for pregnant women with sickle cell disease: a systematic review and meta-analysis. *Blood*. 2015;126: 2424–2435.

54. Koshy M, Burd L, Wallace D, et al. Prophylactic red-cell transfusions in pregnant patients with sickle cell disease. A randomized cooperative study. *N Engl J Med*. 1988;319: 1447–1452.

55. Ngo C, Kayem G, Habibi A, et al. Pregnancy in sickle cell disease: maternal and fetal outcomes in a population receiving prophylactic partial exchange transfusions. *Eur J Obstet Gynecol Reprod Biol*. 2010;152:138–142.

56. Patil V, Ratnayake G, Fastovets G. Clinical 'pearls' of maternal critical care part 2: sickle-cell disease in pregnancy. *Curr Opin Anaesthesiol*. 2017;30:326–334.

57. Ballas SK, McCarthy WF, Guo N, et al. Exposure to hydroxyurea and pregnancy outcomes in patients with sickle cell anemia. *J Natl Med Assoc*. 2009;101:1046–1051.

58. Voelker R. Sickle cell therapy drought ends. *JAMA*. 2017;318:604.

59. Smiers FJ, Krishnamurti L, Lucarelli G. Hematopoietic stem cell transplantation for hemoglobinopathies: current practice and emerging trends. *Pediatr Clin North Am*. 2010;57:181–205.

60. Vermylen C, Fernandez Robles E, Ninane J, Cornu G. Bone marrow transplantation in five children with sickle cell anaemia. *Lancet*. 1988;1:1427–1428.

61. CLASP (Collaborative Low-dose Aspirin Study in Pregnancy) Collaborative Group. CLASP: a randomised trial of low-dose aspirin for the prevention and treatment of pre-eclampsia among 9364 pregnant women. *Lancet*. 1994;343:619–629.

62. Camous J, N'da A, Etienne-Julan M, Stephan F. Anesthetic management of pregnant women with sickle cell disease—effect on postnatal sickling complications. *Can J Anaesth*. 2008;55:276–283.

63. Howard J, Malfroy M, Llewelyn C, et al. The Transfusion Alternatives Preoperatively in Sickle Cell Disease (TAPS) study: a randomised, controlled, multicentre clinical trial. *Lancet*. 2013;381:930–938.

64. Oteng-Ntim E, Ayensah B, Knight M, Howard J. Pregnancy outcome in patients with sickle cell disease in the UK—a national cohort study comparing sickle cell anaemia (HbSS) with HbSC disease. *Br J Haematol*. 2015;169:129–137.

65. Barbedo MM, McCurdy PR. Red cell life span in sickle cell trait. *Acta Haematol*. 1974;51:339–343.

66. Jans SM, de Jonge A, Lagro-Janssen AL. Maternal and perinatal outcomes amongst haemoglobinopathy carriers: a systematic review. *Int J Clin Pract*. 2010;64:1688–1698.

67. Heller P, Best WR, Nelson RB, Becktel J. Clinical implications of sickle-cell trait and glucose-6-phosphate dehydrogenase deficiency in hospitalized black male patients. *N Engl J Med*. 1979;300:1001–1005.

68. Lechner K, Jager U. How I treat autoimmune hemolytic anemias in adults. *Blood*. 2010;116:1831–1838.

69. Bass GF, Tuscano ET, Tuscano JM. Diagnosis and classification of autoimmune hemolytic anemia. *Autoimmun Rev*. 2014;13:560–564.

70. Versteeg HH, Heemskerk JW, Levi M, Reitsma PH. New fundamentals in hemostasis. *Physiol Rev*. 2013;93:327–358.

71. Thachil J, Toh CH. Disseminated intravascular coagulation in obstetric disorders and its acute haematological management. *Blood Rev*. 2009;23:167–176.

72. Kobayashi H, Matsubara S, Imanaka S. The role of tissue factor pathway inhibitor 2 in the coagulation and fibrinolysis system. *J Obstet Gynaecol Res*. 2023;49:1677–1683.

73. Higgins JR, Walshe JJ, Darling MR, et al. Hemostasis in the uteroplacental and peripheral circulations in normotensive and pre-eclamptic pregnancies. *Am J Obstet Gynecol*. 1998;179: 520–526.

74. American Society of Anesthesiologists. Task Force on Obstetric Anesthesia, Society for Obstetric Anesthesia and Perinatology. Practice guidelines for obstetric anesthesia: an updated report. *Anesthesiology*. 2016;124:270–300.

75. Leduc L, Wheeler JM, Kirshon B, et al. Coagulation profile in severe preeclampsia. *Obstet Gynecol*. 1992;79:14–18.

76. Katz D, Beilin Y. Disorders of coagulation in pregnancy. *Br J Anaesth*. 2015;115:ii75–ii88.

77. Karlsson O, Sporrong T, Hillarp A, et al. Prospective longitudinal study of thromboelastography and standard hemostatic laboratory tests in healthy women during normal pregnancy. *Anesth Analg*. 2012;115:890–898.

78. Sharma SK, Philip J, Whitten CW, et al. Assessment of changes in coagulation in parturients with preeclampsia using thromboelastography. *Anesthesiology*. 1999;90:385–390.

79. Campos CJ, Pivalizza EG, Abouleish EI. Thromboelastography in a parturient with immune thrombocytopenic purpura. *Anesth Analg*. 1998;86:675.

80. Klein SM, Slaughter TF, Vail PT, et al. Thromboelastography as a perioperative measure of anticoagulation resulting from low molecular weight heparin: a comparison with anti-Xa concentrations. *Anesth Analg*. 2000;91:1091–1095.

81. Boyce H, Hume-Smith H, Ng J, et al. Use of thromboelastography to guide thromboprophylaxis after caesarean section. *Int J Obstet Anesth*. 2011;20: 213–218.

82. Mallaiah S, Barclay P, Harrod I, et al. Introduction of an algorithm for ROTEM-guided fibrinogen concentrate administration in major obstetric haemorrhage. *Anaesthesia*. 2015;70:166–175.

83. Beilin Y, Arnold I, Hossain S. Evaluation of the platelet function analyzer (PFA-100) vs. the thromboelastogram (TEG) in the parturient. *Int J Obstet Anesth*. 2006;15:7–12.

84. Davies JR, Fernando R, Hallworth SP. Hemostatic function in healthy pregnant and preeclamptic women: an assessment using the platelet function analyzer (PFA-100) and thromboelastograph. *Anesth Analg*. 2007;104:416–420.

85. Cines DB, Levine LD. Thrombocytopenia in pregnancy. *Blood*. 2017;130:2271–2277.

86. American College of Obstetricians and Gynecologists. Practice Bulletin No. 207: Thrombocytopenia in pregnancy (reaffirmed 2022). *Obstet Gynecol*. 2019;133:e181–e193.

87. Pishko AM, Levine LD, Cines DB. Thrombocytopenia in pregnancy: diagnosis and approach to management. *Blood Rev*. 2020;40:100638.

88. Provan D, Stasi R, Newland AC, et al. International consensus report on the investigation and management of primary immune thrombocytopenia. *Blood*. 2010;115:168–186.

89. Waters AH. Post-transfusion purpura. *Blood Rev*. 1989;3: 83–87.

90. Pegels JG, Bruynes EC, Engelfriet CP, von dem Borne AE. Pseudothrombocytopenia: an immunologic study on platelet antibodies dependent on ethylene diamine tetra-acetate. *Blood*. 1982;59:157–161.

91. Care A, Pavord S, Knight M, Alfirevic Z. Severe primary autoimmune thrombocytopenia in pregnancy: a national cohort study. *BJOG*. 2017;125:604–612.

92. Bussel JB, Hou M, Cines DB. Management of primary immune thrombocytopenia in pregnancy. *N Engl J Med*. 2023;389:540–548.

93. Webert KE, Mittal R, Sigouin C, et al. A retrospective 11-year analysis of obstetric patients with idiopathic thrombocytopenic purpura. *Blood*. 2003;102:4306–4311.

94. Neunert C, Lim W, Crowther M, et al. The American Society of Hematology 2011 evidence-based practice guideline for immune thrombocytopenia. *Blood*. 2011;117: 4190–4207.

95. Kelton JG, Inwood MJ, Barr RM, et al. The prenatal prediction of thrombocytopenia in infants of mothers with clinically diagnosed immune thrombocytopenia. *Am J Obstet Gynecol*. 1982;144:449–454.

96. Payne SD, Resnik R, Moore TR, et al. Maternal characteristics and risk of severe neonatal thrombocytopenia and intracranial hemorrhage in pregnancies complicated by autoimmune thrombocytopenia. *Am J Obstet Gynecol*. 1997;177:149–155.

97. Fakhouri F, Scully M, Provot F, et al. Management of thrombotic microangiopathy in pregnancy and postpartum: report from an international working group. *Blood*. 2020;136: 2103–2117.

98. Moore JC, Murphy WG, Kelton JG. Calpain proteolysis of von Willebrand factor enhances its binding to platelet membrane glycoprotein IIb/IIIa: an explanation for platelet aggregation in thrombotic thrombocytopenic purpura. *Br J Haematol*. 1990;74:457–464.

99. Asada Y, Sumiyoshi A, Hayashi T, et al. Immunohistochemistry of vascular lesion in thrombotic thrombocytopenic purpura, with special reference to factor VIII related antigen. *Thromb Res*. 1985;38:469–479.

100. Ferrari B, Peyvandi F. How I treat thrombotic thrombo-cytopenic purpura in pregnancy. *Blood*. 2020;136: 2125–2132.

101. Mannucci PM, Canciani MT, Forza I, et al. Changes in health and disease of the metalloprotease that cleaves von Willebrand factor. *Blood*. 2001;98:2730–2735.

102. Scully M, Thomas M, Underwood M, et al. Thrombotic thrombocytopenic purpura and pregnancy: presentation, management, and subsequent pregnancy outcomes. *Blood*. 2014;124:211–219.

103. George JN. How I treat patients with thrombotic thrombocytopenic purpura: 2010. *Blood*. 2010;116: 4060–4069.

104. Zheng XL, Vesely SK, Cataland SR, et al. ISTH guidelines for treatment of thrombotic thrombocytopenic purpura. *J Thromb Haemost*. 2020;18:2496–2502.

105. Riviere E, Saint-Leger M, James C, et al. Platelet transfusion and catheter insertion for plasma exchange in patients with thrombotic thrombocytopenic purpura and a low platelet count. *Transfusion*. 2015;55:1798–1802.

106. Kato R, Shinohara A, Sato J. ADAMTS13 deficiency, an important cause of thrombocytopenia during pregnancy. *Int J Obstet Anesth*. 2009;18:73–77.

107. Orsini S, Noris P, Bury L, et al. Bleeding risk of surgery and its prevention in patients with inherited platelet disorders. *Haematologica*. 2017;102:1192–1203.

108. Peitsidis P, Datta T, Pafilis I, et al. Bernard Soulier syndrome in pregnancy: a systematic review. *Haemophilia*. 2010;16: 584–591.

109. Grainger JD, Thachil J, Will AM. How we treat the platelet glycoprotein defects; Glanzmann thrombasthenia and Bernard Soulier syndrome in children and adults. *Br J Haematol*. 2018;182:621–632.

110. Siddiq S, Clark A, Mumford A. A systematic review of the management and outcomes of pregnancy in Glanzmann thrombasthenia. *Haemophilia*. 2011;17:e858–e869.

111. Fiore M, Sentilhes L, d'Oiron R. How I manage pregnancy in women with Glanzmann thrombasthenia. *Blood*. 2022;139:2632–2641.

112. Aster RH, Curtis BR, McFarland JG, Bougie DW. Drug-induced immune thrombocytopenia: pathogenesis, diagnosis, and management. *J Thromb Haemost*. 2009;7:911–918.

113. Curtis BR. Drug-induced immune thrombocytopenia: incidence, clinical features, laboratory testing, and pathogenic mechanisms. *Immunohematology*. 2014;30:55–65.

114. Fass RJ, Copelan EA, Brandt JT, et al. Platelet-mediated bleeding caused by broad-spectrum penicillins. *J Infect Dis*. 1987;155:1242–1248.

115. Staibano P, Arnold DM, Bowdish DM, Nazy I. The unique immunological features of heparin-induced thrombocytopenia. *Br J Haematol*. 2017;177:198–207.

116. Greinacher A. Clinical practice. Heparin-induced thrombocytopenia. *N Engl J Med*. 2015;373:252–261.

117. Junqueira DR, Zorzela LM, Perini E. Unfractionated heparin versus low molecular weight heparins for avoiding heparin-induced thrombocytopenia in postoperative patients. *Cochrane Database Syst Rev*. 2017;(4):CD007557.

118. Weiss HJ, Aledort LM, Kochwa S. The effect of salicylates on the hemostatic properties of platelets in man. *J Clin Invest*. 1968;47:2169–2180.

119. Williams HD, Howard R, O'Donnell N, Findley I. The effect of low dose aspirin on bleeding times. *Anaesthesia*. 1993;48:331–333.

120. Gaspari F, Vigano G, Orisio S, et al. Aspirin prolongs bleeding time in uremia by a mechanism distinct from platelet cyclooxygenase inhibition. *J Clin Invest*. 1987;79:1788–1797.

121. Kaneshiro MM, Mielke CH Jr, Kasper CK, Rapaport SI. Bleeding time after aspirin in disorders of intrinsic clotting. *N Engl J Med*. 1969;281:1039–1042.

122. Kopp SL, Vandermeulen RD, McBane RD, Perlas A, Leffert L, Horlocker T. Regional anesthesia in the patient receiving antithrombotic or thrombolytic therapy: American Society of Regional Anesthesia and Pain Medicine evidence-based guidelines (fifth edition). *Reg Anesth Pain Med*. 2025;Epub ahead of print 25 Jan:https://doi.org/10.1136/rapm-2024-105766.

123. Levi M. Acquired qualitative platelet disorders. In: Kaushansky K, Prchal JT, Burns LJ, et al., eds. *Williams Hematology*. 10th ed. McGraw-Hill; 2021.

124. Nadell J, Bruno J, Varady J, Segre EJ. Effect of naproxen and of aspirin on bleeding time and platelet aggregation. *J Clin Pharmacol*. 1974;14:176–182.

125. Buchanan GR, Martin V, Levine PH, et al. The effects of "anti-platelet" drugs on bleeding time and platelet aggregation in normal human subjects. *Am J Clin Pathol*. 1977;68:355–359.

126. Thomas P, Hepburn B, Kim HC, Saidi P. Nonsteroidal anti-inflammatory drugs in the treatment of hemophilic arthropathy. *Am J Hematol*. 1982;12:131–137.

127. von Willebrand E. Hereditors pseudohamofile. *Finska Laeksaellsk.* 1926;68:87–122.

128. Pacheco LD, Saade GR, James AH. Von Willebrand disease, hemophilia, and other inherited bleeding disorders in pregnancy. *Obstet Gynecol.* 2023;141:493–504.

129. Mazzeffi MA, Stone ME. Perioperative management of von Willebrand disease: a review for the anesthesiologist. *J Clin Anesth.* 2011;23:418–426.

130. James AH, Kouides PA, Abdul-Kadir R, et al. Von Willebrand disease and other bleeding disorders in women: consensus on diagnosis and management from an international expert panel. *Am J Obstet Gynecol.* 2009;201:12.e1–e8.

131. Sadler JE, Budde U, Eikenboom JC, et al. Update on the pathophysiology and classification of von Willebrand disease: a report of the subcommittee on von Willebrand factor. *J Thromb Haemost.* 2006;4:2103–2114.

132. Bucciarelli P, Siboni SM, Stufano F, et al. Predictors of von Willebrand disease diagnosis in individuals with borderline von Willebrand factor plasma levels. *J Thromb Haemost.* 2015;13:228–236.

133. James AH, Konkle BA, Kouides P, et al. Postpartum von Willebrand factor levels in women with and without von Willebrand disease and implications for prophylaxis. *Haemophilia.* 2015;21:81–87.

134. Sang Medicine, Practical Haemostasis.com. Bleeding assessment: The ISTH-SSC bleeding assessment tool (BAT); 2024. https://practical-haemostasis.com/Clinical%20 Prediction%20Scores/Formulae%20code%20and%20 formulae/Formulae/Bleeding-Risk-Assessment-Score/ ISTH_BAT_score.html. Accessed January 25, 2025.

135. James PD, Connell NT, Ameer B, et al. ASH ISTH NHF WFH 2021 guidelines on the diagnosis of von Willebrand disease. *Blood Adv.* 2021;5:280–300.

136. Connell NT, Flood VH, Brignardello-Petersen R, et al. ASH ISTH NHF WFH 2021 guidelines on the management of von Willebrand disease. *Blood Adv.* 2021;5:301–325.

137. Varughese J, Cohen AJ. Experience with epidural anaesthesia in pregnant women with von Willebrand disease. *Haemophilia.* 2007;13:730–733.

138. Lipton RA, Ayromlooi J, Coller BS. Severe von Willebrand's disease during labor and delivery. *JAMA.* 1982;248:1355–1357.

139. Iorio A, Stonebraker JS, Chambost H, et al. Establishing the prevalence and prevalence at birth of hemophilia in males: a meta-analytic approach using national registries. *Ann Intern Med.* 2019;171:540–546.

140. Mori PG, Pasino M, Vadala CR, et al. Haemophilia 'A' in a 46,X,i(Xq) female. *Br J Haematol.* 1979;43:143–147.

141. Seeds JW, Cefalo RC, Miller DT, Blatt PM. Obstetric care of the affected carrier of hemophilia B. *Obstet Gynecol.* 1983;62:23S–25S.

142. Togioka BM, Burwick RM, Kujovich JL. Delivery and neuraxial technique outcomes in patients with hemophilia and in hemophilia carriers: a systematic review. *J Anesth.* 2021;35:288–302.

143. Chalmers E, Williams M, Brennand J, et al. Guideline on the management of haemophilia in the fetus and neonate. *Br J Haematol.* 2011;154:208–215.

144. Ljung R. The optimal mode of delivery for the haemophilia carrier expecting an affected infant is vaginal delivery. *Haemophilia.* 2010;16:415–419.

145. Collins PW. Management of acquired haemophilia A. *J Thromb Haemost.* 2011;9:226–235.

146. Shapiro A. The use of prophylaxis in the treatment of rare bleeding disorders. *Thromb Res.* 2020;196:590–602.

147. Singh A, Harnett MJ, Connors JM, Camann WR. Factor XI deficiency and obstetrical anesthesia. *Anesth Analg.* 2009;108:1882–1885.

148. Erez O, Othman M, Rabinovich A, et al. DIC in pregnancy—pathophysiology, clinical characteristics, diagnostic scores, and treatments. *J Blood Med.* 2022;13:21–44.

149. de Lloyd L, Jenkins PV, Bell SF, et al. Acute obstetric coagulopathy during postpartum hemorrhage is caused by hyperfibrinolysis and dysfibrinogenemia: an observational cohort study. *J Thromb Haemost.* 2023;21:862–879.

150. Rabinovich A, Abdul-Kadir R, Thachil J, et al. DIC in obstetrics: diagnostic score, highlights in management, and international registry-communication from the DIC and Women's Health SSCs of the International Society of Thrombosis and Haemostasis. *J Thromb Haemost.* 2019;17: 1562–1566.

151. Erez O, Novack L, Beer-Weisel R, et al. DIC score in pregnant women—a population based modification of the International Society on Thrombosis and Hemostasis score. *PLoS One.* 2014;9:e93240.

152. Jonard M, Ducloy-Bouthors AS, Fourrier F. Comparison of two diagnostic scores of disseminated intravascular coagulation in pregnant women admitted to the ICU. *PLoS One.* 2016;11:e0166471.

153. Wada H, Thachil J, Di Nisio M, et al. Guidance for diagnosis and treatment of DIC from harmonization of the recommendations from three guidelines. *J Thromb Haemost.* 2013.

154. Collins P, Abdul-Kadir R, Thachil J, et al. Management of coagulopathy associated with postpartum hemorrhage: guidance from the SSC of the ISTH. *J Thromb Haemost.* 2016;14:205–210.

155. Hofer S, Blaha J, Collins PW, et al. Haemostatic support in postpartum haemorrhage: a review of the literature and expert opinion. *Eur J Anaesthesiol.* 2023;40:29–38.

156. Lavigne-Lissalde G, Aya AG, Mercier FJ, et al. Recombinant human FVIIa for reducing the need for invasive second-line therapies in severe refractory postpartum hemorrhage: a multicenter, randomized, open controlled trial. *J Thromb Haemost.* 2015;13:520–529.

157. Montagnana M, Franchi M, Danese E, et al. Disseminated intravascular coagulation in obstetric and gynecologic disorders. *Semin Thromb Hemost.* 2010;36:404–418.

158. Bateman BT, Mhyre JM, Ehrenfeld J, et al. The risk and outcomes of epidural hematomas after perioperative and obstetric epidural catheterization: a report from the Multicenter Perioperative Outcomes Group Research Consortium. *Anesth Analg.* 2013;116:1380–1385.

159. Cook TM, Counsell D, Wildsmith JA. Major complications of central neuraxial block: report on the third national audit project of the Royal College of Anaesthetists. *Br J Anaesth.* 2009;102:179–190.

160. Leffert L, Butwick A, Carvalho B, et al. The Society for Obstetric Anesthesia and Perinatology consensus statement on the anesthetic management of pregnant and postpartum women receiving thromboprophylaxis or higher dose anticoagulants. *Anesth Analg.* 2018;126:928–944.

161. Dhar P, Abramovitz S, DiMichele D, et al. Management of pregnancy in a patient with severe haemophilia A. *Br J Anaesth*. 2003;91:432–435.

162. Lee LO, Bateman BT, Kheterpal S, et al. Risk of epidural hematoma after neuraxial techniques in thrombocytopenic parturients: a report from the Multicenter Perioperative Outcomes Group. *Anesthesiology*. 2017;126:1053–1063.

163. Bauer ME, Toledano RD, Houle T, et al. Lumbar neuraxial procedures in thrombocytopenic patients across populations: a systematic review and meta-analysis. *J Clin Anesth*. 2020;61: 109666.

164. Bauer ME, Arendt K, Beilin Y, et al. The Society for Obstetric Anesthesia and Perinatology interdisciplinary consensus statement on neuraxial procedures in obstetric patients with thrombocytopenia. *Anesth Analg*. 2021;132:1531–1544.

165. Goodier CG, Lu JT, Hebbar L, et al. Neuraxial anesthesia in parturients with thrombocytopenia: a multisite retrospective cohort study. *Anesth Analg*. 2015;121:988–991.

166. Mhyre JM, Greenfield ML, Tsen LC, Polley LS. A systematic review of randomized controlled trials that evaluate strategies to avoid epidural vein cannulation during obstetric epidural catheter placement. *Anesth Analg*. 2009:1232–1242.

167. Dickman CA, Shedd SA, Spetzler RF, et al. Spinal epidural hematoma associated with epidural anesthesia: complications of systemic heparinization in patients receiving peripheral vascular thrombolytic therapy. *Anesthesiology*. 1990;72:947–950.

168. American College of Obstetricians and Gynecologists. Practice Bulletin No. 197: Inherited thrombophilias in pregnancy (reaffirmed 2022). *Obstet Gynecol*. 2018;132:e18–e34.

169. Walker ID. Venous and arterial thrombosis during pregnancy: epidemiology. *Semin Vasc Med*. 2003;3:25–32.

170. Bates SM, Greer IA, Middeldorp S, et al. VTE, thrombophilia, antithrombotic therapy, and pregnancy: Antithrombotic therapy and prevention of thrombosis, 9th ed: American College of Chest Physicians evidence-based clinical practice guidelines. *Chest*. 2012;141:e691S–e736S.

171. Kujovich JL. Thrombophilia and pregnancy complications. *Am J Obstet Gynecol*. 2004;191:412–424.

172. Rodgers GM. Role of antithrombin concentrate in treatment of hereditary antithrombin deficiency. An update. *Thromb Haemost*. 2009;101:806–812.

173. Rheaume M, Weber F, Durand M, Mahone M. Pregnancy-related venous thromboembolism risk in asymptomatic women with antithrombin deficiency: a systematic review. *Obstet Gynecol*. 2016;127:649–656.

174. Patnaik MM, Moll S. Inherited antithrombin deficiency: a review. *Haemophilia*. 2008;14:1229–1239.

175. Sharpe CJ, Crowther MA, Webert KE, Donnery C. Cerebral venous thrombosis during pregnancy in the setting of type I antithrombin deficiency: case report and literature review. *Transfus Med Rev*. 2011;25:61–65.

176. Malm J, Laurell M, Dahlback B. Changes in the plasma levels of vitamin K-dependent proteins C and S and of C4b-binding protein during pregnancy and oral contraception. *Br J Haematol*. 1988;68:437–443.

177. Anderson JA, Weitz JI. Hypercoagulable states. *Crit Care Clin*. 2011;27:933–952.

45

Liver Disease

Natalie K. Smith, MD and David B. Wax, MD

LIVER DISEASES

Liver diseases can be incidental or unique to pregnancy and complicate as many as 3% of all pregnancies.[1] The more common conditions are addressed in this chapter. The hepatic aspects of preeclampsia/eclampsia and HELLP (hemolysis, elevated liver enzymes, and low platelets) syndrome are discussed in Chapter 35.

Liver Diseases Incidental to Pregnancy

Various hepatobiliary diseases are not unique to pregnancy but may affect pregnant patients. Some of these diseases may have been preexisting before pregnancy, while others may be provoked by pregnancy and may have different clinical courses during pregnancy compared with nonpregnant patients. They can lead to acute or chronic liver failure and have important implications for obstetric and anesthetic management.

Viral Hepatitis

The presentation of viral hepatitides ranges from mild, non-clinical illness to fulminant hepatic necrosis. Viral hepatitis is the most common cause of jaundice and the most frequent reason for gastroenterology consultation during pregnancy.[2] Six types—hepatitis A, B, C, D, E, and G—have been identified and are associated with specific viruses. Types A, B, and C are the most common. Infrequently, hepatitis can also be caused by herpes simplex virus (HSV), yellow fever virus, rubella virus, Epstein-Barr virus, or cytomegalovirus.

Hepatitis A virus (HAV) and **hepatitis E virus (HEV)** are typically spread by oral ingestion of food or water contaminated with feces from infected individuals. Although endemic in other countries, the current all-time low incidence of HAV of 0.4 per 100,000 in the United States is attributed to good sanitation.[3] Despite its prevalence, it has been infrequently reported among pregnant women. The incidence of HAV infection has also been reduced by vaccination for preexposure prophylaxis; immune globulin is available for postexposure prophylaxis to prevent or attenuate infection. Clinically, a preicteric phase typically occurs with nonspecific viral symptoms, followed by an icteric phase with jaundice and acholic stools. Acute treatment is supportive. Increased risk for preterm labor, premature rupture of membranes, and placental abruption have been associated with HAV during pregnancy, and vertical transmission to the fetus may occur.[4] Chronic HAV infection does not occur, but a prolonged or relapsing course occurs in up to 20% of patients, and an acute fulminant course occurs in less than 1% of patients.[5]

HEV infection may be largely asymptomatic. In symptomatic patients, the disease is usually self-limited. Pregnant women and patients already infected with another hepatitis virus, however, have more severe presentations. A mortality rate of up to 20% has been reported in pregnant women with acute HEV infection, a consequence of fulminant hepatic failure, eclampsia, and hemorrhagic complications.[6] Pregnancy complications such as premature rupture of membranes, fetal growth restriction, placenta previa, retained placenta, and preterm delivery are also more common. Chronic HEV infection may occur in immunosuppressed patients, and vertical transmission can occur.[6] **Pegylated interferon** and/or **ribavirin** treatment for chronic HEV infection has shown moderate success. An HEV vaccine was approved for use in China in 2012 but is not yet available elsewhere.[7]

Hepatitis B virus (HBV) and **hepatitis D virus (HDV)** are usually transmitted via percutaneous or permucosal exposure to infected body fluids. In high-prevalence areas, HBV infection is most commonly acquired perinatally or in early childhood. In low-prevalence areas, infection is primarily acquired in adulthood through sexual contact or intravenous drug abuse. Implementation of widespread vaccination and safety precautions in healthcare settings has reduced the incidence. Postexposure prophylaxis with HBV vaccination alone or a combination of vaccination with hepatitis B immune globulin (HBIG) is highly effective in preventing HBV transmission in adults as well as in infants of HBV-infected mothers and may prevent perinatal transmission. The majority of acute infections are asymptomatic, with only 30% of adults developing typical symptoms of hepatitis, and less than 0.5% developing fulminant hepatitis.[8] Most cases can be managed with supportive treatment, although nucleoside analog therapy may improve prognosis in severe cases. Chronic HBV develops in less than 5% of adults but in more than 20% of children, and exacerbations of chronic HBV may occur postpartum. The 5-year cumulative incidence of cirrhosis in chronic HBV may be as high as 20%, and once cirrhosis has developed the annual risk for hepatocellular carcinoma may be as high as 5%.[8] Treatment of chronic HBV aims at clearance of virus to prevent the development of cirrhosis and cancer. Vertical transmission to the fetus from hepatitis Be antigen-positive mothers can be as high as 90% without attempts to prevent transmission.[9] Vertical transmission is most likely to occur at delivery but can also occur *in utero*.[10] For patients with active disease or high viral loads, oral antiviral therapies (**lamivudine**, **telbivudine**, or **tenofovir**) reduce transmission without apparent increased risk for adverse maternal or fetal outcomes, as does cesarean delivery.[11] Interferon therapy has a finite course of treatment and an increased chance of viral clearance and reduces the risk for cirrhosis and liver cancer; however, it has more side effects and is contraindicated during pregnancy.[12] Current recommendations are to administer HBV vaccination to all neonates and to administer HBIG to all offspring of infected mothers.[10]

HDV is dependent on HBV coinfection to replicate. Acute coinfection with both viruses can be more severe than acute HBV infection alone and may result in acute liver failure. HDV superinfection in the setting of chronic HBV results in chronic HDV infection in most patients, and these patients have more rapid progression to cirrhosis.

Hepatitis C virus (HCV) transmission most commonly occurs from transfusion of infected blood products or injection of contaminated drugs (illicit or iatrogenic). Maternal-fetal and sexual transmission are less common routes of transmission; however, the rate of vertical transmission is increasing in the United States as injection drug use increases in the context of the opioid crisis, so the prevalence of HCV in pregnancy has increased.[13] Initial infection is generally asymptomatic, but up to 30% of patients develop acute hepatitis. In patients with acute HCV infection that has not cleared spontaneously within 12 weeks, treatment with pegylated interferon may be used to prevent chronic infection, with treatment success in up to 98% of patients. In most asymptomatic and untreated cases, infection persists for over 6 months and leads to chronic infection with progression to cirrhosis in up to 30% of patients within 30 years.[14] Thus, HCV is the leading cause of chronic hepatitis, cirrhosis, and liver cancer (which develops in up to 3% of patients per year) and a primary indication for liver transplantation in the developed world. Depending on the severity of liver fibrosis, therapy may be warranted to prevent these complications. Combination treatment with pegylated interferon, ribavirin, and a protease inhibitor can result in a sustained virologic response in up to 80% of patients, but it is contraindicated during pregnancy.[14] Various second-generation antiviral drugs have been introduced for single-agent or combination regimens to clear HCV infection, but there are insufficient data to endorse their use during pregnancy.[15] Maternal HCV infection is associated with an increased rate of intrauterine fetal demise, preterm delivery, fetal growth restriction, gestational diabetes, antepartum and postpartum hemorrhage, and intrahepatic cholestasis of pregnancy secondary to HCV-induced changes in hepatocytes and biliary epithelial cells.[10,16] Pregnant women with viremia have a mother-to-child transmission rate of about 5.8%, which increases to 10.8% if coinfection with human immunodeficiency virus (HIV) is present.[13,17]

Hepatitis G virus (HGV) is transmitted parenterally, sexually, or vertically. In the United States, nearly 20% of all blood preparations are infected with HGV. Although there have been reports of acute, fulminant, and chronic hepatitis and hepatic fibrosis, HGV replicates predominantly in the hematopoietic system rather than in hepatocytes. Clinical significance is mostly for those coinfected with HCV or HIV or for individuals with hematologic cancers.[18]

HSV hepatitis is a rare form of hepatitis in pregnancy; however, it is associated with a maternal mortality rate as high as 39%. The risk for disseminated HSV is high when the primary infection occurs during pregnancy. Signs and symptoms include fever, transaminitis, gastrointestinal, respiratory, neurologic, and urogenital manifestations, while only 18% present with a vesicular rash.[19] Because diagnosis can be difficult, empiric treatment with acyclovir may be indicated when pregnant women present with fulminant hepatic failure of unknown origin, as this may improve outcomes and obviate the need for liver transplantation.[20]

Cholecystitis

Cholelithiasis is present in up to 8% of pregnant women, although only 1.2% develop symptomatic disease.[21] Patients may have right upper-quadrant pain, fever, and leukocytosis, and diagnosis is generally made by ultrasonography. Serious complications include **cholangitis**, **pancreatitis**, **gangrenous cholecystitis**, and **perforation**. Conservative treatment may be considered in mild cases and includes intravenous hydration, antibiotics, opioid analgesia, bowel rest, and possibly percutaneous cholecystostomy. Although a conservative approach does not seem to be associated with poorer fetal outcomes, treatment failure or disease recurrence during pregnancy is common, so therefore surgical treatment may ultimately be required.[22] Both open and laparoscopic cholecystectomy (preferably in the second trimester) can be considered, though laparoscopic techniques offer maternal recovery advantages similar to those in the nonpregnant patient and may have slightly lower fetal complication rates. With either technique, the incidence of miscarriage or preterm labor/delivery is greater than 25%.[22,23]

Liver Abscess

Liver abscess can develop from infection by various organisms including *Entamoeba*, *Echinococcus*, *Clonorchis*, and *Ascaris*. Direct inoculation during medical instrumentation or hematogenous spread from intravenous drug abuse or endocarditis can occur. Appendicitis, diverticulitis, or other intra-abdominal infections may spread to the liver. **Fungal infections** are also possible in immunocompromised patients. Management of liver abscess includes antimicrobials, percutaneous or open drainage, and surgical resection.[24] The condition is rare during pregnancy, but treatment modalities are similar to those described for the nonpregnant patient.[25]

Autoimmune Diseases

Autoimmune hepatitis, **primary biliary cirrhosis**, and **primary sclerosing cholangitis** are conditions that may overlap and may also be associated with other extrahepatic autoimmune disorders.[26] All may lead to end-stage liver disease, and treatment with corticosteroids, other immunosuppressants, and/or ursodeoxycholic acid is aimed at preventing this progression. For advanced and intractable disease, liver transplantation may be necessary. Pregnancy in autoimmune hepatitis is associated with a 33% incidence of disease flares (mostly postpartum), one-third of which result in maternal hepatic decompensation, liver transplantation, or death. Risks for hypertensive complications of pregnancy, gestational diabetes, preterm birth, and low birth weight are also increased.[27,28] Immunosuppressive therapy during pregnancy is reportedly safe and effective for reducing disease flares. Continuation of immunosuppression with **prednisone** and **azathioprine** during pregnancy increases control of disease and decreases flares, which may lead to fulminant liver failure. **Mycophenolate mofetil** and **tacrolimus** are contraindicated in pregnancy.[29]

Vascular Syndromes

Budd-Chiari syndrome involves thrombosis of the hepatic vein or suprahepatic inferior vena cava and may be associated with pregnancy (comprising nearly half of all cases) or other hypercoagulable states. Hepatic venous congestion can also result from right-sided heart failure or other cardiopulmonary diseases that increase central venous pressure or from mechanical compression or compartment syndrome that impedes hepatic venous outflow. This congestive hepatopathy can ultimately lead to fibrosis, portal hypertension, and liver failure. **Portal vein thrombosis** may also occur and cause portal hypertension without cirrhosis. Initial therapy is anticoagulation with **low-molecular-weight heparin**, and endoscopic screening/treatment; beta-adrenergic receptor blockade (**propranolol** or **nadolol**) for prophylaxis of variceal bleeding are also recommended. Liver transplantation may ultimately be required in chronic cases. A multicenter retrospective cohort study of pregnancies in 45 women previously diagnosed with Budd-Chiari and/or portal vein thrombosis reported that 24% of first pregnancies ended in pregnancy loss[30]; two women had variceal bleeding and one developed pulmonary embolism but there were no maternal deaths. "**Shock liver**" syndrome can occur in the setting of perioperative hypotension, critical illness with septic shock or cardiac arrest, pulmonary embolism, heart failure, or heatstroke, which can cause disruption of hepatic arterial and/or portal venous inflow, resulting in acute ischemic/hypoxic hepatitis, especially in the setting of other coexisting liver disease.[31,32]

Metabolic Diseases

Wilson disease is a condition of reduced copper excretion in which gradual copper accumulation in the liver can lead to cirrhosis, while rapid accumulation may result in acute liver failure. Patients may also develop neurologic, ophthalmologic, and renal dysfunction. Fertility is generally reduced, but continuing treatment with copper-chelating agents during pregnancy can reduce the risk of spontaneous abortion and result in positive outcomes.[33] **Hemochromatosis** is a condition of iron accumulation that results in arthropathy, skin pigmentation, diabetes, hypopituitarism, hypogonadism, heart failure, and liver cirrhosis. Phlebotomy (with or without a chelating agent) to deplete iron stores markedly improves survival and prevents most of the complications.[34] **Alpha-1 antitrypsin deficiency** results in uncontrolled tissue degradation, which may lead to emphysematous changes in the lung and liver cirrhosis.[35] Pregnancy can be complicated by fetal growth restriction, preterm labor, and pneumothorax or other respiratory decompensation.[36]

Hepatotoxicity

Hepatotoxicity can result from a variety of exposures. **Acetaminophen (paracetamol)**, involved in 20% of drug overdoses during pregnancy, is metabolized by the liver into highly reactive oxides.[37] If their formation exceeds the binding capacity of glutathione, maternal and fetal hepatic injury occurs. Treatment with **N-acetylcysteine** within 16 hours of acetaminophen ingestion may bind toxic metabolites in both the mother and the fetus and improve outcomes.[37] **Alcoholic hepatitis** can result from the acute ingestion of large amounts of alcohol, and chronic alcohol ingestion may lead to cirrhosis.[38] Other agents that have the potential to cause hepatotoxicity are **antiretroviral drugs** for HIV infection, **propylthiouracil** for hyperthyroidism, **alpha-methyldopa** and **labetalol** for hypertension, **isoniazid** for tuberculosis, **statins** for antiphospholipid syndrome or hyperlipidemia, **mushrooms** and **herbal supplements**, and **industrial agents**.[39,40]

Liver Diseases Specific to Pregnancy

Liver diseases specific to pregnancy are summarized in Table 45.1.

TABLE 45.1 Liver Diseases Specific to Pregnancy

	Hyperemesis Gravidarum	Intrahepatic Cholestasis of Pregnancy	Preeclampsia/ Eclampsia	HELLP Syndrome	AFLP
Incidence	<0.3%–3%	0.3%–6%	2%–8%	0.1%–0.6%	<0.01%
Presentation	First trimester	Second or third trimester	Second or third trimester, or after delivery	Second or third trimester, or after delivery	Third trimester
Symptoms, signs, and complications	Nausea/vomiting Ketosis	Pruritus Jaundice	Hypertension Proteinuria Edema Seizures Renal failure Pulmonary edema Hepatic hematoma/ rupture	Abdominal pain Renal dysfunction Hypertension Hepatic hematoma/ rupture Liver infarction	Nausea/vomiting Abdominal pain Jaundice Hepatic failure
Laboratory findings	Elevated aminotransferase levels	Increased serum bile acid levels Hyperbilirubinemia Mild abnormalities of liver function tests	Low platelet count Proteinuria Increased uric acid level Mildly elevated aminotransferase levels	Low platelet count Hemolysis Markedly elevated aminotransferase levels	Low platelet count Hypoglycemia Mildly/moderately elevated aminotransferase levels
Treatment	Supportive management	Delivery at fetal maturity Ursodeoxycholic acid[a]	Blood pressure control Seizure control Delivery	Prompt delivery	Prompt delivery
Outcome	Benign for mother and fetus	No increase in maternal death rate Increased risk for preterm delivery and fetal loss May recur with subsequent pregnancies Increased risk for subsequent liver and biliary tract disease	Increased risk for maternal morbidity and mortality Increased risk for perinatal morbidity	Maternal death rate 1%–4% Fetal death rate 1%–30%	Maternal death rate up to 10% Fetal death rate up to 20%

AFLP, Acute fatty liver of pregnancy; *HELLP*, hemolysis, elevated liver enzymes, and low platelets.
[a]Ursodeoxycholic acid is used for symptom treatment. Its use does not change outcomes.
Adapted from Schutt VA, Minuk GY. Liver diseases unique to pregnancy. *Best Pract Res Clin Gastroenterol.* 2007;21:771–792.

Hyperemesis Gravidarum

Hyperemesis gravidarum occurs in 0.3% to 3% of pregnancies and is characterized by a severe and persistent form of nausea and vomiting that can lead to dehydration and electrolyte imbalances, as well as elevated liver transaminases, mild jaundice, and transient hyperthyroidism (see Chapter 17).[41] Obstetric ultrasonography should rule out multiple pregnancy or molar pregnancy.[42] Adverse pregnancy outcomes are rare but may occur in women who fail to gain adequate weight during pregnancy.[41]

Intrahepatic Cholestasis of Pregnancy

Intrahepatic cholestasis of pregnancy occurs with an incidence ranging from less than 2% in Europe up to 25% in some populations of South America, with the large variation possibly related to population genetics.[43] Other risk factors include multiple gestation, advanced age, and HCV infection.[16,43] Proposed causes include genetic canalicular transporter mutations that alter phospholipid or bile salt transport across hepatocyte membranes, as well as abnormal steroid hormone profiles, resulting in pruritus and elevated serum bile acid levels during the second or third trimester. Jaundice is unusual.[43]

Intrahepatic cholestasis of pregnancy has minimal impact on maternal health. Vitamin K malabsorption may lead to coagulopathy and an increased incidence of postpartum hemorrhage; however, contemporary studies have found no increased risk for obstetric bleeding or neuraxial hematoma.[44] Laboratory values should be checked before administration of neuraxial analgesia.[44] While maternal outcome is generally good, there is an increased risk for preterm delivery, fetal compromise, and intrauterine fetal death in women who have a total bile acid concentration > 100 μmol/L.[45]

Treatment with ursodeoxycholic acid or other medications does not reduce the risk of adverse outcomes and is no longer recommended.[46] Delivery before 37 weeks' gestation is recommended to minimize fetal complications.[47] Recurrence of the disease is common in subsequent pregnancies.

Acute Fatty Liver of Pregnancy

Acute fatty liver of pregnancy (AFLP), or reversible peripartum liver failure, has increased in incidence in recent decades to 28.9 per 100,000 pregnancies and is the most common cause of cirrhosis in pregnancy.[48] It is more common in twin gestations, nulliparity, and male fetuses, and it has been associated with preeclampsia and HELLP syndrome.[49,50] The disease is characterized by microvesicular fatty infiltration of the liver (and possibly kidney) believed to be caused by defective beta oxidation of fatty acids, usually in the third trimester. In AFLP, genetic enzymatic defects in the fetus (e.g., fetal long-chain 3-hydroxyacyl-CoA dehydrogenase deficiency) and placenta are thought to cause toxic free fatty acid metabolites to build up in maternal hepatocytes. Early nonspecific symptoms include anorexia, nausea, emesis, malaise, fatigue, and headache. Jaundice, edema, hypertension, hypoglycemia, diabetes insipidus, and encephalopathy may develop. Progression to fulminant hepatic and renal failure, disseminated intravascular coagulation (DIC), and acute respiratory distress syndrome (ARDS) can be rapid. AFLP may be misdiagnosed as preeclampsia or HELLP syndrome because of a similar constellation of presenting symptoms. After additional laboratory tests the definitive diagnosis can be made. AFLP is associated with lower fibrinogen levels and greater likelihood of renal dysfunction than HELLP syndrome. Rarely, percutaneous or transjugular liver biopsy to identify microvesicular fatty infiltration of hepatocytes may be needed for diagnosis in indeterminate cases.[50,51]

AFLP is a medical emergency requiring rapid evaluation and treatment. Hepatic failure and fetal death may occur within days. After diagnosis, immediate delivery of the fetus or termination of the pregnancy is recommended. Additional supportive care includes transfusion, mechanical ventilation, dialysis, plasmapheresis, antibiotics, and N-acetylcysteine. Mode of delivery is not as critical as is doing so expeditiously. Liver transplantation may be indicated in severe cases.[52] The anesthesia provider should anticipate postpartum hemorrhage, establish adequate intravenous access, and ensure that cross-matched blood is immediately available. The use of neuraxial anesthesia may be limited by coagulopathy, encephalopathy, ascites, respiratory compromise, or other contraindications. If liver function testing and clinical symptoms do not improve quickly after delivery, liver transplantation may be required.[53]

Improvements in diagnosis and management have reduced maternal mortality (once as high as 85%) to 12% to 18%. Maternal mortality most commonly occurs from liver failure, acute kidney injury, and hemorrhage.[49,54] Recovery typically occurs within 1 to 3 weeks, though it is unclear if there are significant long-term maternal sequelae. Perinatal mortality may be as high as 66% as a result of the maternal milieu as well as preterm delivery; however, outcomes are better if the disease is recognized early.[50]

Spontaneous Hepatic Rupture of Pregnancy

Hepatic rupture is a rare event that may complicate preeclampsia, eclampsia, HELLP syndrome, and AFLP, or it may be an isolated event. By definition, spontaneous hepatic rupture of pregnancy occurs in the absence of antecedent trauma. Instead, rupture is preceded by an intraparenchymal hepatic hematoma. The strong association with preeclampsia suggests that periportal hemorrhagic necrosis, hypertension, and coagulopathy may lead to hematoma formation. With expansion of the hematoma, the hepatic capsule is progressively distended and dissected from the parenchyma, leading to rupture.[55] **Primary hepatic pregnancy** with embryonic implantation on the liver is another rare condition that can result in liver hemorrhage and shock. In the early postpartum period, growth of hepatic hemangiomas, adenomas, or other potentially hemorrhagic masses may occur.

Diagnostic ultrasonography, computed tomography, magnetic resonance imaging, angiography, technetium scintigraphy, and exploratory laparotomy may demonstrate the expanding hematoma before rupture.[56] Hematomas contained within the liver may be conservatively managed with intravenous fluids and blood products. More aggressive treatments include open laparotomy, hepatic artery ligation or embolization, and compression of bleeding points with hepatic packing. Recombinant factor VIIa, although controversial, may be considered in the presence of intractable hemorrhage,[57] and liver transplantation can be considered as a last resort.[58] Maternal and fetal mortality rates with current therapy are 17% and 38%, respectively.[59]

LIVER FUNCTION AND DYSFUNCTION

Regardless of the disease state and whether it is incidental or unique to pregnancy, the signs and symptoms of acute and chronic liver diseases are similar.

Markers of Liver Dysfunction

The liver performs a variety of physiologic functions, derangements of which are characteristic of liver diseases (Box 45.1). Amino acid metabolism in the liver uses enzymes that include

BOX 45.1 Signs and Symptoms of Liver Disease

Laboratory Findings
- Increased
  - Alanine aminotransferase
  - Aspartate aminotransferase
  - Gamma glutamyl transferase
  - Bilirubin
  - Lactate
  - Prothrombin time/international normalized ratio
  - Ammonia
- Thrombocytopenia
- Hypoglycemia
- Hypoalbuminemia
- Metabolic acidosis
- Respiratory alkalosis
- Immune dysfunction
- Renal dysfunction
- Decreased systemic vascular resistance
- Portal hypertension and varices
- Pulmonary hypertension

Symptoms and Physical Findings
- Jaundice
- Pruritus
- Abdominal pain
- Decreased appetite
- Telangiectases
- Palmar erythema
- Easy bruising
- Gastrointestinal bleeding
- Ascites
- Encephalopathy

alanine aminotransferase and **aspartate aminotransferase**. Levels of these enzymes are generally normal in pregnancy, but hepatocyte injury leads to their release (commonly called *transaminitis*) into the blood, where abnormal serum levels can be detected. The liver also removes bilirubin produced from heme metabolism in the blood. Thus, liver dysfunction can lead to accumulation of bilirubin that becomes symptomatic as jaundice. Gluconeogenesis can be impaired by liver dysfunction leading to hypoglycemia and accumulation of lactate. Synthetic functions of the liver include production of albumin and coagulation factors. Although albumin concentration normally decreases during pregnancy secondary to increased maternal plasma volume, prothrombin time (PT) is unchanged during normal pregnancy; therefore, an increase in PT is an indicator of possible liver disease. Decreased thrombopoietin production in the liver, along with hypersplenism from portal hypertension, may lead to thrombocytopenia. **Alkaline phosphatase (ALP)** and **gamma glutamyl transferase (GGT)** are found in biliary tract cells. ALP is normally increased during pregnancy because of fetal and placental production, but an elevated GGT is suggestive of biliary disease. Detoxification functions

of the liver are responsible for clearance of many toxic metabolites and drugs. Failure of conversion of ammonia to urea in the liver results in accumulation of ammonia and consequent encephalopathy. Decreased clearance of estrogen and progesterone with liver disease may cause hyperventilation and other signs of a hyperestrogenic state such as telangiectases and palmar erythema, although this may occur in normal pregnancies because of increased production by the placenta. Various antigens and antibodies also show characteristic patterns of abnormalities in autoimmune and infectious forms of hepatitis and can be used for diagnosis and treatment monitoring.[60,61]

Acute Liver Failure

Acute (or fulminant) hepatic failure is an extreme complication of liver disease specific or incidental to pregnancy that manifests in profound ways that may be life threatening. Patient condition can deteriorate rapidly and unpredictably, and management in a critical care setting may be required. Treatment is mostly supportive, except in cases with specific anecdotal or proven therapies (e.g., immediate delivery for pregnancy-related causes, *N*-acetylcysteine therapy for acetaminophen toxicity, lamivudine for acute HBV infection, penicillin therapy in *Amanita phalloides* intoxication, chelating agents in Wilson disease, steroid therapy for autoimmune hepatitis). Despite advances in care, maternal mortality in women with acute liver failure is as high as 55%.[62]

Encephalopathy results from reduced hepatic ammonia metabolism that leads to astrocytic glutamine accumulation and cerebral edema. Subtle mental status changes are followed by somnolence and disorientation, incoherence, and finally by coma. The use of invasive intracranial pressure (ICP) monitoring to determine cerebral perfusion pressure (CPP) is controversial because of questionable usefulness and concerns about intracranial bleeding from the procedure. If monitored, ICP should be maintained less than 25 mm Hg, and CPP should be maintained greater than 50 mm Hg. Jugular bulb oxygen saturation can provide information about cerebral oxygen use, with levels less than 55% indicative of cerebral hypoperfusion and levels greater than 85% suggestive of cerebral hyperemia or inadequate neuronal metabolism.[63]

Patients should be kept in a quiet room with the head of the bed elevated more than 30 degrees. *N*-Acetylcysteine given early may decrease cerebral edema and improve survival. Mannitol or hypertonic saline infusion may be used to manage intracranial hypertension. Indications for tracheal intubation include (1) progressive encephalopathy; (2) ARDS; (3) pulmonary aspiration prevention; (4) sedation for agitation, which can contribute to increased ICP; and (5) hyperventilation for refractory intracranial hypertension. High tidal volumes and levels of positive end-expiratory pressure, hypercarbia, and frequent suctioning should be avoided. Hyperthermia should be actively treated, but deliberate hypothermia has not proven beneficial. **Phenytoin** or **propofol** can effectively decrease the risk for seizure activity.

Immune dysfunction is related to loss of Kupffer and other immune cell function, and complications of bacterial or fungal infections are a leading cause of mortality. Infection and sepsis have been associated with progression to high-grade encephalopathy and poorer outcomes, though prophylactic antimicrobial therapy does not appear to improve survival compared with surveillance and treatment only as needed.[63]

Coagulopathy results from impaired synthesis of coagulation factors and from thrombocytopenia, which may be caused by reduced hepatic thrombopoietin production, acute portal hypertension with splenic sequestration, and reduced marrow production. DIC may also develop. Mucocutaneous, gastrointestinal, and iatrogenic bleeding can all occur. Cholestasis leads to malabsorption of vitamin K, an important cofactor required for the synthesis of factors II, VII, IX, and X. A therapeutic trial of **vitamin K** may be attempted if malabsorption is the primary defect, but women with impaired hepatic synthesis do not respond. The routine use of fresh frozen plasma or platelet transfusion is not recommended except when there is evidence of active bleeding or an invasive procedure is planned. **Proton-pump inhibitors** may help prevent gastric stress ulcers and bleeding. Although liver failure is generally thought to be a hypocoagulable state, it can also be hypercoagulable, with clinical manifestations that are difficult to predict and that cannot be effectively prevented by prophylactic treatment with blood product transfusions.[64] Viscoelastic testing methods may be more accurate than traditional laboratory tests for selection of blood products in bleeding patients with cirrhosis and has been associated with decreased transfusion volumes and decreased use of plasma.[65]

Circulatory dysfunction is common because of low systemic vascular resistance, and subclinical myocardial injury is common. Fluid resuscitation is the initial treatment for hypotension, but fluid overload can increase the risk for cerebral edema and acute lung injury. **Norepinephrine (noradrenaline)** and **vasopressin** are preferred agents for maintaining CPP. **Corticosteroids** may be considered for patients unresponsive to vasopressors with suspected relative adrenal insufficiency.

Increased production and reduced hepatic uptake of lactate results in **metabolic acidosis**. In addition, renal function is impaired in up to 80% of patients.[66] **Renal failure**, acidemia, electrolyte disturbances, or volume overload necessitate renal replacement therapy with continuous venovenous hemofiltration with dialysis. Decreased gluconeogenesis can lead to **hypoglycemia**, whereas **hyperglycemia** may worsen neurologic outcome. Enteral feeding is preferred to parenteral nutrition, although parenteral nutrition with hypocaloric, low-glutamine, and normal protein formula appears to be safe.

For patients who are not expected to recover adequate liver function, liver transplantation may be planned. In patients with toxicity from massive liver necrosis, total hepatectomy and temporary portocaval shunting can be performed in the interim, while awaiting a donor organ. Artificial and bioartificial liver-support devices are also under development.[67]

Cirrhosis and Chronic Liver Failure

Any chronic liver disease can progress to cirrhosis, which is characterized by diffuse hepatic fibrosis. The incidence of cirrhosis in pregnancy increased from 2.5/100,000 in 2007 to 6.5/100,000 pregnancies in 2016.[68] Cirrhosis may be asymptomatic until most of the hepatic parenchyma is destroyed or until a comorbidity causes decompensation. Many manifestations are similar to those of acute liver failure, although gradual in onset and of lesser severity, whereas others are unique to cirrhosis. Pregnancy is rare in patients with cirrhosis (approximately 1 in 6000 pregnancies) because hormonal changes can cause anovulation and infertility. Risks for preeclampsia, preterm delivery, low birth weight, small-for-gestational-age, and neonatal death appear to be increased in cirrhotic parturients. Overall maternal mortality has decreased in recent years to 0.89%.[69]

Hepatic fibrosis causes increased resistance to portal blood flow, resulting in portal hypertension that promotes blood flow through portosystemic anastomoses such as esophageal, hemorrhoidal, and other intra-abdominal veins. Congestion and dilation of these vessels increase the risk for spontaneous or iatrogenic bleeding. In addition, coagulopathy of cirrhosis resulting from decreased clotting factor production and thrombocytopenia can exacerbate bleeding from many causes. **Esophageal variceal bleeding** has been reported in up to 32% of pregnant women with cirrhosis, 50% of those with known portal hypertension, and 78% of those with preexisting varices, with a mortality rate up to 50%.[70] Variceal hemorrhage is the most common cause of maternal mortality in cirrhosis.[69] It most commonly occurs later in pregnancy when maternal blood volume is expanded and fetal growth causes compression of collateral vessels. Bleeding risk theoretically increases during labor because of the repetitive intra-abdominal pressure increases, especially from pushing during the second stage, although few cases of variceal bleeding at the time of delivery have been reported. Elective cesarean delivery for women with known varices has been suggested to avoid Valsalva-related pressure and variceal bleeding, but surgical delivery also carries the risk for bleeding from abdominal wall collateral vessels. Therefore, an attempt at vaginal delivery (possibly with forceps to shorten the second stage of labor) may be considered before cesarean delivery.[29,70] Screening for varices and prophylaxis against bleeding should be considered early in the pregnancy. **Nonselective beta-adrenergic receptor antagonists** can decrease the risk for variceal bleeding by reducing portal pressure through reduction of cardiac output and splanchnic vasoconstriction, but they have been associated with fetal bradycardia, growth restriction, and hypoglycemia. Prophylactic **endoscopic band ligation** or **surgical portocaval shunting** may also be considered in high-risk parturients. Bleeding varices can be safely ligated or treated with **sclerotherapy** during pregnancy, although there is concern for shunting of toxic material to the placenta with sclerotherapy.[29,71] **Octreotide** infusion may also be considered, although its safety has not been proven in pregnant patients. **Transjugular intrahepatic portosystemic shunting** may be considered for refractory variceal bleeding (see later discussion).[72] **Surgical shunt procedures** may also be considered in extreme cases.

Splenic artery aneurysms may also develop in cirrhotic parturients with portal hypertension, and rupture in late pregnancy carries high maternal and fetal mortality rates. Management options include splenectomy, transcatheter embolization, and stent-graft placement. **Postpartum uterine hemorrhage**, a consequence of coagulopathy and varices, is another potential source of maternal morbidity and mortality, occurring in up to 5% to 45% of pregnancies in patients with cirrhosis.[71]

Encephalopathy secondary to ammonia accumulation may occur in cirrhotic patients and may be precipitated or exacerbated by sedative medications, infection, hypoglycemia, gastrointestinal hemorrhage, hypotension, or hypoxemia. Management includes correction of precipitating factors and reducing the nitrogenous load from gastrointestinal tract with oral, nonabsorbed antimicrobial agents such as **lactulose** and **neomycin**. **Flumazenil** may also improve mental status transiently, and **bromocriptine** may improve extrapyramidal symptoms, although these have not been studied extensively in cirrhotic parturients.

Massive **ascites** is uncommon in pregnancy, possibly because the increased intra-abdominal pressure from the gravid uterus opposes extravasation of fluid from splanchnic vessels and organs. If therapy is required, sodium restriction and diuretics can be used. Symptomatic ascites refractory to medical treatment may require paracentesis, although this could potentially increase the risk for bacterial peritonitis and pregnancy complications.[73]

Cardiovascular manifestations of cirrhosis include systemic vasodilation caused by reduced hepatic clearance of endogenous substances regulating vascular tone. Cardiac output is thereby increased, assuming cardiomyopathy is not present, as may occur in the settings of alcoholic cirrhosis or hemochromatosis. **Portopulmonary hypertension**, a progressive disease characterized by increased pulmonary vascular resistance caused by arteriolar medial hyperplasia, thrombosis, or fibrosis, and eventually right-sided heart failure, has been reported to result in postpartum maternal death.[74] **Hepatorenal syndrome**, renal dysfunction secondary to splanchnic and systemic vasodilation of cirrhosis, does not appear to be a common complication in cirrhotic parturients. Similarly, **hepatopulmonary syndrome** caused by intrapulmonary vasodilation and shunting resulting in hypoxemia appears to be rare during pregnancy.[73–78] An electrocardiogram and transthoracic echocardiogram to look for evidence of cirrhotic cardiomyopathy, right heart dysfunction secondary to pulmonary hypertension, and hepatopulmonary syndrome are part of the standard preanesthetic workup for patients with liver disease.[79]

LIVER SURGERY

Liver Transplantation During Pregnancy

Fulminant hepatic failure during pregnancy may necessitate liver transplantation if supportive measures prove inadequate and maternal death is likely. In second-trimester pregnancies, pregnancy following transplantation has been continued with good maternal and fetal outcomes possible. In third-trimester pregnancies, combined cesarean delivery and liver transplantation have also resulted in better maternal and fetal outcomes compared with liver transplantation followed by continued pregnancy.[80,81] In some cases, liver failure first develops or worsens postpartum and necessitates transplantation using a cadaveric organ, or, if unavailable, a living donor graft.[52,81] In patients for whom a matching organ cannot be found, artificial liver systems have been used temporarily while awaiting an organ or spontaneous recovery of the native liver.[67]

There is insufficient literature for evidence-based recommendations about specific anesthetic and surgical techniques.

Pregnancy After Liver Transplantation

The first pregnancy in a liver transplant recipient was reported in 1978.[82] Successful pregnancy outcome has even been achieved after triple organ transplantation (small intestine, liver, and pancreas).[83]

Approximately 8% of liver transplant recipients are females of reproductive age, and the hormonal changes of chronic liver disease that disrupt menstruation are usually corrected by transplantation, with 74% of women recovering regular menstrual cycles within 1 year. Still, it is recommended that pregnancy be delayed for 1 to 2 years after transplantation until graft function has stabilized on a low-dose immunosuppression regimen with low teratogenic potential.[84]

Pregnancy after liver transplantation carries an increased risk for preeclampsia, preterm birth, fetal growth restriction, and maternal graft dysfunction.[85] Cesarean delivery is commonly necessary for obstetric indications. Posttransplant thrombocytopenia has implications for administration of neuraxial anesthesia during labor and delivery as well as blood loss during cesarean delivery.

Liver Resection

Benign and malignant liver tumors occurring during pregnancy or hepatic ectopic pregnancy may require surgical resection.[86] Partial hepatectomy has been reported during pregnancy with favorable maternal outcomes. Management of the pregnancy may include termination,[87] simultaneous cesarean delivery,[88] or spontaneous vaginal delivery.[89] There are inadequate data to make specific recommendations about the intraoperative management of liver resection during pregnancy compared with nonpregnant patients.[90]

Transjugular Intrahepatic Portosystemic Shunt

Indications for a transjugular intrahepatic portosystemic shunt include variceal bleeding and massive ascites refractory to other therapies. Contraindications include right-sided heart failure, polycystic liver disease, severe hepatic failure, systemic infection, hepatic encephalopathy, hepatic tumors, and portal vein thrombosis. The procedure involves accessing a jugular vein, fluoroscopically guiding an endovascular needle into a hepatic vein, and then perforating the liver parenchyma until the needle tip reaches an intrahepatic portal vein. An endovascular stent is then placed across the liver parenchyma to maintain the shunt. The communication created between the portal and systemic venous systems decompresses the portal system, thereby decreasing the pressure that was causing bleeding and formation of ascites.[91] This procedure has been successfully performed during pregnancy and can be done with radiation-limiting techniques that minimize fetal radiation exposure allow the pregnancy to continue.[72,92,93]

ANESTHETIC CONSIDERATIONS

Anesthetic management is influenced by the extent of hepatic impairment. If hepatic synthetic and metabolic functions are intact, the patient may be managed similarly to healthy parturients. However, the parturient with evidence of severe hepatic impairment presents many challenges (Box 45.2).

For patients with underlying liver disease, ischemic or other hepatic insults may exacerbate liver dysfunction. Many retrospective analyses of various types of hepatic and nonhepatic surgery and anesthesia have focused on perioperative outcomes in patients with liver disease, although not specifically during pregnancy. Most studies have shown an association between preoperative liver disease severity and postoperative morbidity and mortality. Child-Turcotte-Pugh (CTP) scoring and, more recently, model for end-stage liver disease (MELD) scoring (based on international normalized ratio [INR], creatinine, and bilirubin) have both been used to grade severity of liver disease and associated outcomes. In cirrhotic patients undergoing elective surgery, cirrhosis has been independently associated with a 47% increased

risk for postoperative complications and an approximately 250% increased risk for in-hospital mortality.[94] Patients with a MELD score > 20 or CTP class C liver disease have a 40% risk of mortality after elective surgery, while patients with MELD score < 12 or CTP class A show a better tolerance for elective surgery, although they are still at increased risk compared with the general population. Increased duration of anesthesia also predicts poorer outcomes.[95] It is recommended that abdominal surgery be avoided or deferred, if possible, until full evaluation and optimal treatment have been completed.[96] Timing of delivery should be based on maternal and fetal considerations. If possible, it is best to fully evaluate the extent of liver disease before delivery. Early delivery should be considered if the liver disease is exacerbated by the pregnancy (e.g., AFLP or cholestasis of pregnancy) or if the pregnancy is limiting the ability to perform a full liver evaluation. Neuraxial techniques have been used safely in asymptomatic chronic hepatitis patients, as well as after liver transplantation, although data specifically on pregnant patients are lacking.[97–99]

Hepatic Effects of Anesthesia

Various studies have examined the effects of anesthetic agents on hepatic blood flow, although these investigations were not in the setting of pregnancy. Volatile halogenated anesthetic agents appear to decrease hepatic blood flow: **isoflurane**, **sevoflurane**, and **desflurane** reduce hepatic blood flow by less than 20%. **Nitrous oxide** may further decrease hepatic blood flow and may worsen pulmonary hypertension.[54] Volatile anesthetic agents also increase cerebral blood flow and may raise ICP in acute liver failure, and should be limited to less than one minimum alveolar concentration. Alternatively, **propofol** may be used in patients at risk for increased ICP.[100] **Propofol** or **ketamine** anesthesia may maintain hepatic blood flow better than inhalational anesthesia.[101–108] However, a recent randomized trial of patients undergoing pancreaticoduodenectomy revealed no difference in hepatic blood flow in patients anesthetized with propofol compared with sevoflurane, though patients anesthetized with sevoflurane required more vasopressors.[109] **Neuraxial anesthesia** also may reduce hepatic blood flow via the effects of systemic arterial hypotension secondary to sympathetic blockade.[110–112] In one study,[112] this reduction persisted during lumbar epidural anesthesia despite maintenance of normotension by infusion of colloid, but the decrease in hepatic blood flow was reversed by dopamine infusion. These findings suggest that reduced cardiac output, secondary to sympathetic blockade, may be responsible for the observed decrease in hepatic blood flow rather than hypotension. Nevertheless, judicious hydration and avoidance of systemic hypotension should minimize the chances of a clinically significant reduction in hepatic blood flow.

Pharmacokinetic Effects of Liver Failure

Liver disease can alter the normal pharmacokinetics of anesthetic agents and other drugs. Drug clearance may be decreased by hepatocyte dysfunction or reductions in liver

---

BOX 45.2   Anesthetic Guidelines for the Parturient With Liver Disease

- Evaluate the extent of hepatic impairment.
- Recognize and evaluate underlying systemic abnormalities, including coagulation and volume status.
- Assist the obstetric team with stabilization of maternal condition before delivery.
- Plan preferentially for neuraxial analgesia/anesthesia for labor, delivery, and cesarean delivery in the absence of contraindications.
- Exclude coagulopathy before administration of neuraxial anesthesia.
- Prevent further hepatic injury by optimizing hepatic blood flow and oxygenation.
- Recognize altered pharmacokinetics and pharmacodynamics.
- Prevent transmission of viral hepatitis to the healthcare team.
- Monitor the patient for evidence of postoperative hepatic dysfunction.

blood flow. Impaired hepatic synthesis of plasma proteins can lead to decreased drug binding and increased free fraction of drugs. This makes more drug available for clearance by the liver, but at the same time increases tissue availability and effective volume of distribution, which can alter drug effects and clearance. Overall, severe liver disease can decrease clearance of various agents, and repeated or continuous administration can lead to drug accumulation and adverse effects. Anesthetic agents at any concentration may cause increased sedation or decompensation in patients already compromised by hepatic encephalopathy.

Clearance of some opioids, including **morphine**, **meperidine (pethidine)**, and **alfentanil**, may be decreased in patients with advanced liver disease. Other opioids, including **fentanyl** and **sufentanil**, do not appear to have significantly impaired clearance, although repeated or continuous dosing may be problematic. **Remifentanil** pharmacokinetics are not significantly changed. **Methadone** also appears to have nearly normal disposition. **Codeine**, which requires hepatic conversion to morphine for analgesia and clearance, may not be safe or effective, and similar uncertainty exists regarding **tramadol**.[113–116] Prolonged effects can also be seen with **etomidate** and benzodiazepines including **midazolam** and **diazepam**, whereas **propofol**, **methohexital**, and **thiopental** clearances are unchanged after anesthesia induction doses.[117–121] Neuromuscular blocking agents normally cleared by the liver (**vecuronium, rocuronium**) or by liver-synthesized enzymes (**succinylcholine [suxamethonium]**), may have longer durations of action, whereas agents not dependent on liver function (**atracurium, cisatracurium**) should have normal durations of action.[122–126] The half-lives of amide local anesthetics (**lidocaine, bupivacaine, ropivacaine**) may be prolonged and potential for toxicity may be increased because of decreased liver clearance, whereas ester local anesthetics (**2-chloroprocaine**) have potentially prolonged half-lives because of decreased hepatic pseudocholinesterase synthesis.[127–129] **Acetaminophen** can be safely administered in routine doses for acute pain in patients with cirrhosis, but chronic administration can provoke hepatic injury, and reduced doses are recommended in those with decompensated liver disease. Although **ketorolac** metabolism may be normal, **nonsteroidal antiinflammatory drugs** can precipitate renal dysfunction and should be avoided.[130,131]

Neuraxial Anesthesia

Neuraxial analgesia/anesthesia is preferred for labor, vaginal delivery, and cesarean delivery and can be offered to patients with liver disease in the absence of significant intravascular volume depletion or a coagulopathy.[132] Before administration of neuraxial anesthesia, a coagulation profile and platelet count should be obtained and intravascular volume assessed. Epidural techniques in particular may have added risk in patients with portal hypertension because increased epidural venous plexus engorgement may predispose to intravascular needle/catheter placement or epidural hematoma.[133]

Encephalopathy and increased ICP may also increase the risks of neuraxial analgesia.[100]

The potential for impaired clearance of local anesthetics and opioids should also be considered, especially when repeated boluses or continuous infusions are used. No data support any local anesthetic as superior, and the authors use a standard bupivacaine/fentanyl solution. Single-shot spinal techniques with small-gauge needles may minimize the issues of drug metabolism and bleeding, although with possibly increased risk for acute hypotension and reduced liver blood flow.

General Anesthesia

Coagulopathy, obstetric hemorrhage, altered mental status, and severe fetal compromise may necessitate the use of general anesthesia for cesarean delivery. Intravascular volume should be evaluated before induction. Invasive blood pressure monitoring and pulmonary artery catheterization may be useful in the patient with cardiovascular compromise or portopulmonary hypertension. Large-bore intravenous access should be established, and blood products should be available. Gastric acid neutralization should precede rapid-sequence induction and tracheal intubation. All standard induction agents are safe, and the dose should not be altered. Delayed metabolism of succinylcholine from a reduced pseudocholinesterase concentration is of negligible clinical importance. Succinylcholine thus remains the muscle relaxant of choice for rapid-sequence induction of general anesthesia and should be administered without dose reduction. **Rocuronium** may be used if succinylcholine is contraindicated. **Sugammadex** may be considered for reversal of rocuronium; however, large doses (16 mg/kg) may worsen coagulopathy.[134] Careful gastric tube placement may be considered, even in the presence of esophageal varices.[135] For maintenance of anesthesia, agents that do not undergo significant hepatic metabolism (e.g., **isoflurane**, **desflurane**, **atracurium**, **cisatracurium**, **remifentanil**, and **nitrous oxide**) may be preferable to inhalational agents that further reduce liver blood flow or intravenous agents that may accumulate before clearance. Reversal of neuromuscular blockade must be ensured before tracheal extubation. Sugammadex may be more effective at reversing neuromuscular blockade with rocuronium in patients with liver disease compared with neostigmine.[136–138]

Postoperative Care

Although clearance is delayed in patients with severe liver disease, intravenous opioids may be administered judiciously to provide postoperative analgesia. Neuraxial opioids, especially a single dose of **morphine**, may obviate accumulation issues. Advanced liver disease can lead to hepatic encephalopathy. Neurologic deterioration in the postoperative period may result from the residual effects of anesthetic agents, acute liver decompensation, or an intracranial process. Other postoperative complications to be anticipated include paracentesis-induced circulatory dysfunction, decompensation of preexisting liver disease, cirrhotic cardiomyopathy, hepatorenal syndrome, and hepatopulmonary syndromes.

KEY POINTS

- Liver disease can be either incidental or unique to pregnancy and complicates as many as 3% of all pregnancies.
- Viral hepatitides are the most common cause of jaundice during pregnancy.
- All pregnant women should be screened for hepatitis B virus, and all neonates should be vaccinated against it.
- AFLP is a rare but life-threatening complication of pregnancy that demands rapid evaluation and prompt delivery.
- AFLP is commonly misdiagnosed as preeclampsia or HELLP syndrome because of a similar constellation of presenting symptoms.
- Hepatic rupture may complicate preeclampsia/eclampsia, HELLP syndrome, or AFLP.
- Encephalopathy may result from reduced hepatic ammonia metabolism.
- Coagulopathy may result from impaired synthesis of coagulation factors and from thrombocytopenia. Paradoxically, in some cases, liver failure may result in hypercoagulability.
- Renal failure and cardiovascular, renal, pulmonary, and immune dysfunction may accompany liver failure.

- Women with portal hypertension may develop esophageal varices that are prone to bleed during the third trimester of pregnancy, and this risk increases during labor.
- Successful pregnancy is common after liver transplantation, and pregnancy does not affect the long-term survival of hepatic allografts, although pregnancy complications are more common.
- Liver disease can alter the normal pharmacokinetics of anesthetic agents and other drugs.
- Both neuraxial and general anesthesia can be administered safely to the parturient with liver disease, with close attention to hemodynamics to preserve hepatic blood flow.
- Neuraxial analgesia/anesthesia is the preferred technique for labor, vaginal delivery, and cesarean delivery and can be offered to patients with liver disease, provided significant intravascular volume depletion and coagulopathy have been excluded.
- Hepatic, neurologic, cardiovascular, renal, and pulmonary complications should be anticipated in the postpartum period in patients with significant liver disease.

REFERENCES

1. Guntupalli SR, Steingrub J. Hepatic disease and pregnancy: an overview of diagnosis and management. *Crit Care Med.* 2005;33:S332–S339.
2. Saha S, Manlolo J, McGowan CE, et al. Gastroenterology consultations in pregnancy. *J Womens Health (Larchmt).* 2011;20:359–363.
3. Ly KN, Klevens RM. Trends in disease and complications of hepatitis A virus infection in the United States, 1999-2011: a new concern for adults. *J Infect Dis.* 2015;212:176–182.
4. Chaudhry SA, Koren G. Hepatitis A infection during pregnancy. *Can Fam Physician.* 2015;61:963–964.
5. Brundage SC, Fitzpatrick AN. Hepatitis A. *Am Fam Physician.* 2006;73:2162–2168.
6. Aslan AT, Balaban HY. Hepatitis E virus: epidemiology, diagnosis, clinical manifestations, and treatment. *World J Gastroenterol.* 2020;26:5543–5560.
7. Shata MTM, Hetta HF, Sharma Y, Sherman KE. Viral hepatitis in pregnancy. *J Viral Hepat.* 2022;29:844–861.
8. Liaw YF, Chu CM. Hepatitis B virus infection. *Lancet.* 2009;373:582–592.
9. Shepard CW, Simard EP, Finelli L, et al. Hepatitis B virus infection: epidemiology and vaccination. *Epidemiol Rev.* 2006;28:112–125.
10. Terrault NA, Levy MT, Cheung KW, Jourdain G. Viral hepatitis and pregnancy. *Nat Rev Gastroenterol Hepatol.* 2021;18:117–130.
11. Wen WH, Lai MW, Chang MH. A review of strategies to prevent mother-to-infant transmission of hepatitis B virus infection. *Expert Rev Gastroenterol Hepatol.* 2016;10:317–330.
12. Aspinall EJ, Hawkins G, Fraser A, et al. Hepatitis B prevention, diagnosis, treatment and care: a review. *Occup Med (Lond).* 2011;61:531–540.
13. Orekondy N, Cafardi J, Kushner T, Reau N. HCV in women and pregnancy. *Hepatology.* 2019;70:1836–1840.
14. Grebely J, Matthews GV, Dore GJ. Treatment of acute HCV infection. *Nat Rev Gastroenterol Hepatol.* 2011;8:265–274.
15. Spera AM, Eldin TK, Tosone G, Orlando R. Antiviral therapy for hepatitis C: has anything changed for pregnant/lactating women? *World J Hepatol.* 2016;8:557–565.
16. Wijarnpreecha K, Thongprayoon C, Sanguankeo A, et al. Hepatitis C infection and intrahepatic cholestasis of pregnancy: a systematic review and meta-analysis. *Clin Res Hepatol Gastroenterol.* 2017;41:39–45.
17. Benova L, Mohamoud YA, Calvert C, Abu-Raddad LJ. Vertical transmission of hepatitis C virus: systematic review and meta-analysis. *Clin Infect Dis.* 2014;59:765–773.
18. Reshetnyak VI, Karlovich TI, Ilchenko LU. Hepatitis G virus. *World J Gastroenterol.* 2008;14:4725–4734.
19. McCormack AL, Rabie N, Whittemore B, et al. HSV hepatitis in pregnancy: a review of the literature. *Obstet Gynecol Surv.* 2019;74:93–98.
20. Navaneethan U, Lancaster E, Venkatesh PG, et al. Herpes simplex virus hepatitis—it's high time we consider empiric treatment. *J Gastrointestin Liver Dis.* 2011;20:93–96.
21. Schwulst SJ, Son M. Management of gallstone disease during pregnancy. *JAMA Surg.* 2020;155:1162–1163.
22. Date RS, Kaushal M, Ramesh A. A review of the management of gallstone disease and its complications in pregnancy. *Am J Surg.* 2008;196:599–608.
23. Sachs A, Guglielminotti J, Miller R, et al. Risk factors and risk stratification for adverse obstetrical outcomes after

appendectomy or cholecystectomy during pregnancy. *JAMA Surg.* 2017;152:436–441.

24. Reid-Lombardo KM, Khan S, Sclabas G. Hepatic cysts and liver abscess. *Surg Clin North Am.* 2010;90:679–697.

25. Lindgren P, Pla JC, Högberg U, Tarnvik A. Listeria monocytogenes-induced liver abscess in pregnancy. *Acta Obstet Gynecol Scand.* 1997;76:486–488.

26. Westbrook RH, Yeoman AD, Kriese S, Heneghan MA. Outcomes of pregnancy in women with autoimmune hepatitis. *J Autoimmun.* 2012;38:J239–J244.

27. Chung YY, Heneghan MA. Autoimmune hepatitis in pregnancy: pearls and pitfalls. *Hepatology.* 2022;76:502–517.

28. Wang CW, Grab J, Tana MM, et al. Outcomes of pregnancy in autoimmune hepatitis: a population-based study. *Hepatology.* 2022;75:5–12.

29. Milić S, Tatalović T, Mikolašević I. Pre-existing liver disease in pregnancy: cirrhosis, autoimmune hepatitis and liver transplantation. *Best Pract Res Clin Gastroenterol.* 2020;44–45:101668.

30. Wiegers H, Hamulyák EN, Damhuis SE, et al. Pregnancy outcomes in women with Budd-Chiari syndrome or portal vein thrombosis—a multicentre retrospective cohort study. *BJOG.* 2022;129:608–617.

31. Bissonnette J, Durand F, de Raucourt E, et al. Pregnancy and vascular liver disease. *J Clin Exp Hepatol.* 2015;5:41–50.

32. Weisberg IS, Jacobson IM. Cardiovascular diseases and the liver. *Clin Liver Dis.* 2011;15:1–20.

33. Pfeiffenberger J, Beinhardt S, Gotthardt DN, et al. Pregnancy in Wilson's disease: management and outcome. *Hepatology.* 2018;67:1261–1269.

34. Aaseth J, Flaten TP, Andersen O. Hereditary iron and copper deposition: diagnostics, pathogenesis and therapeutics. *Scand J Gastroenterol.* 2007;42:673–681.

35. Atkinson AR. Pregnancy and alpha-1 antitrypsin deficiency. *Postgrad Med J.* 1987;63:817–820.

36. Gaeckle NT, Stephenson L, Reilkoff RA. Alpha-1 antitrypsin deficiency and pregnancy. *COPD.* 2020;17:326–332.

37. Wilkes JM, Clark LE, Herrera JL. Acetaminophen overdose in pregnancy. *South Med J.* 2005;98:1118–1122.

38. Choi G, Runyon BA. Alcoholic hepatitis: a clinician's guide. *Clin Liver Dis.* 2012;16:371–385.

39. Slim R, Ben Salem C, Hmouda H, Bouraoui K. Hepatotoxicity of alpha-methyldopa in pregnancy. *J Clin Pharm Ther.* 2010;35:361–363.

40. Firoz T, Webber D, Rowe H. Drug-induced fulminant hepatic failure in pregnancy. *Obstet Med.* 2015;8:190–192.

41. McParlin C, O'Donnell A, Robson SC, et al. Treatments for hyperemesis gravidarum and nausea and vomiting in pregnancy: a systematic review. *JAMA.* 2016;316:1392–1401.

42. García-Romero CS, Guzman C, Cervantes A, Cerbón M. Liver disease in pregnancy: medical aspects and their implications for mother and child. *Ann Hepatol.* 2019;18:553–562.

43. Floreani A, Gervasi MT. New insights on intrahepatic cholestasis of pregnancy. *Clin Liver Dis.* 2016;20:177–189.

44. DeLeon A, De Oliveira GS, Kalayil M, et al. The incidence of coagulopathy in pregnant patients with intrahepatic cholestasis: should we delay or avoid neuraxial analgesia? *J Clin Anesth.* 2014;26:623–627.

45. Palmer KR, Xiaohua L, Mol BW. Management of intrahepatic cholestasis in pregnancy. *Lancet.* 2019;393:853–854.

46. Girling J, Knight CL, Chappell L. Intrahepatic cholestasis of pregnancy: Green-top Guideline No. 43 June 2022. *BJOG.* 2022;129:e95–e114.

47. Wood AM, Livingston EG, Hughes BL, Kuller JA. Intrahepatic cholestasis of pregnancy: a review of diagnosis and management. *Obstet Gynecol Surv.* 2018;73:103–109.

48. Sarkar M, Djerboua M, Flemming JA. NAFLD cirrhosis is rising among childbearing women and is the most common cause of cirrhosis in pregnancy. *Clin Gastroenterol Hepatol.* 2022;20:e315–e318.

49. Nelson DB, Byrne JJ, Cunningham FG. Acute fatty liver of pregnancy. *Obstet Gynecol.* 2021;137:535–546.

50. Liu J, Ghaziani TT, Wolf JL. Acute fatty liver disease of pregnancy: updates in pathogenesis, diagnosis, and management. *Am J Gastroenterol.* 2017;112:838–846.

51. Byrne JJ, Seasely A, Nelson DB, et al. Comparing acute fatty liver of pregnancy from hemolysis, elevated liver enzymes, and low platelets syndrome. *J Matern Fetal Neonatal Med.* 2022;35:1352–1362.

52. Ringers J, Bloemenkamp K, Francisco N, et al. Auxiliary or orthotopic liver transplantation for acute fatty liver of pregnancy: case series and review of the literature. *BJOG.* 2016;123:1394–1398.

53. Reau N, Munoz SJ, Schiano T. Liver disease during pregnancy. *Am J Gastroenterol.* 2022;117:44–52.

54. Hansen JD, Perri RE, Riess ML. Liver and biliary disease of pregnancy and anesthetic implications: a review. *Anesth Analg.* 2021;133:80–92.

55. Augustin G, Hadzic M, Juras J, Oreskovic S. Hypertensive disorders in pregnancy complicated by liver rupture or hematoma: a systematic review of 391 reported cases. *World J Emerg Surg.* 2022;17:40.

56. Bural GG, Scheetz M, Laymon CM, Mountz JM. Tc-99m red blood cell bleeding scan in a pregnant woman presenting with hematemesis: a brief review of indications and guidelines for radionuclide scans during pregnancy. *Clin Nucl Med.* 2011;36:987–990.

57. Zaar M, Secher NH, Johansson PI, et al. Effects of a recombinant FVIIa analogue, NN1731, on blood loss and survival after liver trauma in the pig. *Br J Anaesth.* 2009;103:840–847.

58. Varotti G, Andorno E, Valente U. Liver transplantation for spontaneous hepatic rupture associated with HELLP syndrome. *Int J Gynaecol Obstet.* 2010;111:84–85.

59. Grand'Maison S, Sauve N, Weber F, et al. Hepatic rupture in hemolysis, elevated liver enzymes, low platelets syndrome. *Obstet Gynecol.* 2012;119:617–625.

60. Guntupalli SR, Steingrub J. Hepatic disease and pregnancy: an overview of diagnosis and management. *Crit Care Med.* 2005;33:S332–S339.

61. Koeppen B, Stanton B, Hall J, Swiatecka-Urban A. *Berne and Levy Physiology.* 8th ed. Elsevier; 2023.

62. Bhatia V, Singhal A, Panda SK, Acharya SK. A 20-year single-center experience with acute liver failure during pregnancy: is the prognosis really worse? *Hepatology.* 2008;48:1577–1585.

63. Cardoso FS, Marcelino P, Bagulho L, Karvellas CJ. Acute liver failure: an up-to-date approach. *J Crit Care.* 2017;39:25–30.

64. Lisman T, Porte RJ. Rebalanced hemostasis in patients with liver disease: evidence and clinical consequences. *Blood.* 2010;116:878–885.

65. Wei H, Child LJ. Clinical utility of viscoelastic testing in chronic liver disease: a systematic review. *World J Hepatol.* 2020;12:1115–1127.

66. Auzinger G, Wendon J. Intensive care management of acute liver failure. *Curr Opin Crit Care.* 2008;14:179–188.

67. Saliba F, Bañares R, Larsen FS, et al. Artificial liver support in patients with liver failure: a modified DELPHI consensus of international experts. *Intensive Care Med.* 2022;48:1352–1367.

68. Huang AC, Grab J, Flemming JA, et al. Pregnancies with cirrhosis are rising and associated with adverse maternal and perinatal outcomes. *Am J Gastroenterol.* 2022;117:445–452.

69. van der Slink LL, Scholten I, van Etten-Jamaludin FS, et al. Pregnancy in women with liver cirrhosis is associated with increased risk for complications: a systematic review and meta-analysis of the literature. *BJOG.* 2022;129:1644–1652.

70. Rosenfeld H, Hochner-Celnikier D, Ackerman Z. Massive bleeding from ectopic varices in the postpartum period: rare but serious complication in women with portal hypertension. *Eur J Gastroenterol Hepatol.* 2009;21:1086–1091.

71. Rahim MN, Pirani T, Williamson C, Heneghan MA. Management of pregnancy in women with cirrhosis. *United European Gastroenterol J.* 2021;9:110–119.

72. Lodato F, Cappelli A, Montagnani M, et al. Transjugular intrahepatic portosystemic shunt: a case report of rescue management of unrestrainable variceal bleeding in a pregnant woman. *Dig Liver Dis.* 2008;40:387–390.

73. Tan J, Surti B, Saab S. Pregnancy and cirrhosis. *Liver Transpl.* 2008;14:1081–1091.

74. Sigel CS, Harper TC, Thorne LB. Postpartum sudden death from pulmonary hypertension in the setting of portal hypertension. *Obstet Gynecol.* 2007;110:501–503.

75. Ramsay MA. Portopulmonary hypertension and hepatopulmonary syndrome, and liver transplantation. *Int Anesthesiol Clin.* 2006;44:69–82.

76. Steadman RH. Anesthesia for liver transplant surgery. *Anesthesiol Clin North Am.* 2004;22:687–711.

77. Heidelbaugh JJ, Bruderly M. Cirrhosis and chronic liver failure: part I. Diagnosis and evaluation. *Am Fam Physician.* 2006;74:756–762.

78. Heidelbaugh JJ, Sherbondy M. Cirrhosis and chronic liver failure: part II. Complications and treatment. *Am Fam Physician.* 2006;74:767–776.

79. Spring A, Saran JS, McCarthy S, McCluskey SA. Anesthesia for the patient with severe liver failure. *Anesthesiol Clin.* 2020;38:35–50.

80. Jarufe N, Soza A, Pérez-Ayuso RM, et al. Successful liver transplantation and delivery in a woman with fulminant hepatic failure occurring during the second trimester of pregnancy. *Liver Int.* 2006;26:494–497.

81. Romano DN, Mokuolu DC, Katz DJ, DeMaria S Jr. Orthotopic liver transplant in the pregnant recipient: a systematic review of preoperative management and maternal and fetal outcomes. *Clin Transplant.* 2021;35:e14269.

82. Walcott WO, Derick DE, Jolley JJ, Snyder DL. Successful pregnancy in a liver transplant patient. *Am J Obstet Gynecol.* 1978;132:340–341.

83. Srivastava R, Clarke S, Gupte GL, Cartmill JL. Successful pregnancy outcome following triple organ transplantation (small intestine, liver and pancreas). *Eur J Obstet Gynecol Reprod Biol.* 2012;163:238–239.

84. Jabiry-Zieniewicz Z, Dabrowski FA, Pietrzak B, et al. Pregnancy in the liver transplant recipient. *Liver Transpl.* 2016;22:1408–1417.

85. Valentin N, Guerrido I, Rozenshteyn F, et al. Pregnancy outcomes after liver transplantation: a systematic review and meta-analysis. *Am J Gastroenterol.* 2021;116:491–504.

86. Morris R, McIntosh D, Helling T, Martin JN Jr. Solid fibrous tumor of the liver: a case in pregnancy. *J Matern Fetal Neonatal Med.* 2012;25:866–868.

87. Jeng LB, Lee WC, Wang CC, et al. Hepatocellular carcinoma in a pregnant woman detected by routine screening of maternal alpha-fetoprotein. *Am J Obstet Gynecol.* 1995;172:219–220.

88. Russell P, Sanjay P, Dirkzwager I, et al. Hepatocellular carcinoma during pregnancy: case report and review of the literature. *N Z Med J.* 2012;125:141–145.

89. Gisi P, Floyd R. Hepatocellular carcinoma in pregnancy. A case report. *J Reprod Med.* 1999;44:65–67.

90. McNally SJ, Revie EJ, Massie LJ, et al. Factors in perioperative care that determine blood loss in liver surgery. *HPB (Oxford).* 2012;14:236–241.

91. Scher C. Anesthesia for transjugular intrahepatic portosystemic shunt. *Int Anesthesiol Clin.* 2009;47:21–28.

92. Savage C, Patel J, Lepe MR, et al. Transjugular intrahepatic portosystemic shunt creation for recurrent gastrointestinal bleeding during pregnancy. *J Vasc Interv Radiol.* 2007;18:902–904.

93. Chandramouli S, Lee WM, Lo J, et al. Prophylactic transjugular intrahepatic portosystemic shunt placement for cirrhosis management in pregnancy. *Hepatology.* 2020;71:1876–1878.

94. Starczewska MH, Mon W, Shirley P. Anaesthesia in patients with liver disease. *Curr Opin Anaesthesiol.* 2017;30:392–398.

95. Hickman L, Tanner L, Christein J, Vickers S. Non-hepatic abdominal surgery in patients with cirrhotic liver disease. *J Gastrointest Surg.* 2019;23:634–642.

96. de Goede B, Klitsie PJ, Lange JF, Metselaar HJK. G. Morbidity and mortality related to non-hepatic surgery in patients with liver cirrhosis: a systematic review. *Best Pract Res Clin Gastroenterol.* 2012;26:47–59.

97. Hoefnagel AL, Wissler R. Anesthetic management of vaginal delivery in a parturient with hemochromatosis induced end-organ failure. *Int J Obstet Anesth.* 2012;21:83–85.

98. Harnett MJ, Miller AD, Hurley RJ, Bhavani-Shankar K. Pregnancy, labour and delivery in a Jehovah's Witness with esophageal varices and thrombocytopenia. *Can J Anaesth.* 2000;47:1253–1255.

99. Zeyneloglu P, Pirat A, Sulemanji D, et al. Perioperative anesthetic management for recipients of orthotopic liver transplant undergoing nontransplant surgery. *Exp Clin Transplant.* 2007;5:690–692.

100. Naoum EE, Leffert LR, Chitilian HV, et al. Acute fatty liver of pregnancy: pathophysiology, anesthetic implications, and obstetrical management. *Anesthesiology.* 2019;130:446–461.

101. Frink EJ Jr, Morgan SE, Coetzee A, et al. The effects of sevoflurane, halothane, enflurane, and isoflurane on hepatic blood flow and oxygenation in chronically instrumented greyhound dogs. *Anesthesiology.* 1992;76:85–90.

102. Merin RG, Bernard JM, Doursout MF, et al. Comparison of the effects of isoflurane and desflurane on cardiovascular dynamics and regional blood flow in the chronically instrumented dog. *Anesthesiology.* 1991;74:568–574.

103. Meierhenrich R, Gauss A, Muhling B, et al. The effect of propofol and desflurane anaesthesia on human hepatic blood flow: a pilot study. *Anaesthesia.* 2010;65:1085–1093.

104. Goldfarb G, Debaene B, Ang ET, et al. Hepatic blood flow in humans during isoflurane-N$_2$O and halothane-N$_2$O anesthesia. *Anesth Analg.* 1990;71:349–353.

105. Fujita Y, Kimura K, Hamada H, Takaori M. Comparative effects of halothane, isoflurane, and sevoflurane on the liver with hepatic artery ligation in the beagle. *Anesthesiology.* 1991;75:313–318.

106. Seyde WC, Ellis JE, Longnecker DE. The addition of nitrous oxide to halothane decreases renal and splanchnic flow and increases cerebral blood flow in rats. *Br J Anaesth.* 1986;58:63–68.

107. Ray DC, Drummond GB. Halothane hepatitis. *Br J Anaesth.* 1991;67:84–99.

108. Thomson IA, Fitch W, Campbell D, Watson R. Effects of ketamine on liver blood flow and hepatic oxygen consumption. Studies in the anaesthetised greyhound. *Acta Anaesthesiol Scand.* 1988;32:10–14.

109. van Limmen J, Wyffels P, Berrevoet F, et al. Effects of propofol and sevoflurane on hepatic blood flow: a randomized controlled trial. *BMC Anesthesiol.* 2020;20:241.

110. Kennedy WF Jr, Everett GB, Cobb LA, Allen GD. Simultaneous systemic and hepatic hemodynamic measurements during high spinal anesthesia in normal man. *Anesth Analg.* 1970;49:1016–1024.

111. Kennedy WF Jr, Everett GB, Cobb LA, Allen GD. Simultaneous systemic and hepatic hemodynamic measurements during high peridural anesthesia in normal man. *Anesth Analg.* 1971;50:1069–1077.

112. Tanaka N, Nagata N, Hamakawa T, Takasaki M. The effect of dopamine on hepatic blood flow in patients undergoing epidural anesthesia. *Anesth Analg.* 1997;85:286–290.

113. Ferrier C, Marty J, Bouffard Y, et al. Alfentanil pharmacokinetics in patients with cirrhosis. *Anesthesiology.* 1985;62:480–484.

114. Tegeder I, Lötsch J, Geisslinger G. Pharmacokinetics of opioids in liver disease. *Clin Pharmacokinet.* 1999;37:17–40.

115. Haberer JP, Schoeffler P, Couderc E, Duvaldestin P. Fentanyl pharmacokinetics in anaesthetized patients with cirrhosis. *Br J Anaesth.* 1982;54:1267–1270.

116. Chauvin M, Ferrier C, Haberer JP, et al. Sufentanil pharmacokinetics in patients with cirrhosis. *Anesth Analg.* 1989;68:1–4.

117. Pandele G, Chaux F, Salvadori C, et al. Thiopental pharmacokinetics in patients with cirrhosis. *Anesthesiology.* 1983;59:123–126.

118. Duvaldestin P, Chauvin M, Lebrault C, et al. Effect of upper abdominal surgery and cirrhosis upon the pharmacokinetics of methohexital. *Acta Anaesthesiol Scand.* 1991;35:159–163.

119. van Beem H, Manger FW, van Boxtel C, van Bentem N. Etomidate anaesthesia in patients with cirrhosis of the liver: pharmacokinetic data. *Anaesthesia.* 1983;38:61–62.

120. Servin F, Desmonts JM, Haberer JP, et al. Pharmacokinetics and protein binding of propofol in patients with cirrhosis. *Anesthesiology.* 1988;69:887–891.

121. MacGilchrist AJ, Birnie GG, Cook A, et al. Pharmacokinetics and pharmacodynamics of intravenous midazolam in patients with severe alcoholic cirrhosis. *Gut.* 1986;27:190–195.

122. Lebrault C, Berger JL, D'Hollander AA, et al. Pharmacokinetics and pharmacodynamics of vecuronium (ORG NC 45) in patients with cirrhosis. *Anesthesiology.* 1985;62:601–605.

123. van Miert MM, Eastwood NB, Boyd AH, et al. The pharmacokinetics and pharmacodynamics of rocuronium in patients with hepatic cirrhosis. *Br J Clin Pharmacol.* 1997;44:139–144.

124. Duvaldestin P, Agoston S, Henzel D, et al. Pancuronium pharmacokinetics in patients with liver cirrhosis. *Br J Anaesth.* 1978;50:1131–1136.

125. Parker CJ, Hunter JM. Pharmacokinetics of atracurium and laudanosine in patients with hepatic cirrhosis. *Br J Anaesth.* 1989;62:177–183.

126. Thomas SD, Boyd AH. Prolonged neuromuscular block associated with acute fatty liver of pregnancy and reduced plasma cholinesterase. *Eur J Anaesthesiol.* 1994;11:245–249.

127. Orlando R, Piccoli P, De Martin S, et al. Cytochrome P450 1A2 is a major determinant of lidocaine metabolism in vivo: effects of liver function. *Clin Pharmacol Ther.* 2004;75:80–88.

128. Lauprecht AE, Wenger FA, El Fadil O, et al. Levobupivacaine plasma concentrations following major liver resection. *J Anesth.* 2011;25:369–375.

129. Jokinen MJ, Neuvonen PJ, Lindgren L, et al. Pharmacokinetics of ropivacaine in patients with chronic end-stage liver disease. *Anesthesiology.* 2007;106:43–55.

130. Garcia-Tsao G, Lim JK. Members of Veterans Affairs Hepatitis C Resource Center Program. Management and treatment of patients with cirrhosis and portal hypertension: recommendations from the Department of Veterans Affairs Hepatitis C Resource Center Program and the National Hepatitis C Program. *Am J Gastroenterol.* 2009;104:1802–1829.

131. Rivera-Espinosa L, Muriel P, Ordaz Gallo M, et al. Ketorolac pharmacokinetics in experimental cirrhosis by bile duct ligation in the rat. *Ann Hepatol.* 2003;2:175–181.

132. Siniscalchi A, Gamberini L, Bardi T, et al. Role of epidural anesthesia in a fast track liver resection protocol for cirrhotic patients—results after three years of practice. *World J Hepatol.* 2016;8:1097–1104.

133. Siam L, Rohde V. Varicosis of the venous epidural plexus caused by portocaval hypertension mimicking symptomatic lumbar disc herniation: case report and review of the literature. *Cent Eur Neurosurg.* 2011;72:155–158.

134. Bridion®. Whitehouse Station, NJ: Merck Sharp & Dohme Corp; 2015. https://www.google.com/aclk?sa=L&ai=DChsSEwirqMT Rw5uOAxXyEq0GHbPENjoYACICCAEQABoCcHY&co=1& ase=2&gclid=Cj0KCQjwjo7DBhCrARIsACWauSnnWVP62w UNO9XkItr8_SEipXPE3_igmad8zMzh8_6DsiCx2aGJvRYaAm mMEALw_wcB&cce=1&category=acrcp_v1_37&sig=AOD64_ 1Rf4hKYXsRphKucIenm7E4l9gO2w&q&nis=4&adurl&ved=2 ahUKEwi3ub_Rw5uOAxUEHTQIHXJjJHQQ0Qx6BAgLEAE. Accessed 1 July 2025.

135. Ritter DM, Rettke SR, Hughes RW Jr, et al. Placement of nasogastric tubes and esophageal stethoscopes in patients with documented esophageal varices. *Anesth Analg.* 1988;67:283–285.

136. Abdulatif M, Lotfy M, Mousa M, et al. Sugammadex antagonism of rocuronium-induced neuromuscular blockade in patients with liver cirrhosis undergoing liver resection: a randomized controlled study. *Minerva Anestesiol.* 2018;84:929–937.

137. Deana C, Barbariol F, D'Incà S, et al. SUGAMMADEX versus neostigmine after ROCURONIUM continuous infusion in patients undergoing liver transplantation. *BMC Anesthesiol.* 2020;20:70.

138. Fujita A, Ishibe N, Yoshihara T, et al. Rapid reversal of neuromuscular blockade by sugammadex after continuous infusion of rocuronium in patients with liver dysfunction undergoing hepatic surgery. *Acta Anaesthesiol Taiwan.* 2014;52:54–58.

46

Musculoskeletal Disorders

Roanne L. Preston, MD, FRCPC and
Jonathan P. W. Collins, MA (Oxon), BM, BCh, FRCPC

CHAPTER OUTLINE

Pregnancy commonly results in musculoskeletal complaints. Although these are typically benign and self-limiting, symptoms may be disabling in some women. In addition, preexisting musculoskeletal disorders interact with pregnancy to a variable extent, ranging from a potentially ameliorating effect of pregnancy on the course of the disease (e.g., autoimmune arthropathies) to significant and possibly life-threatening deterioration in maternal condition (e.g., uncorrected severe thoracic scoliosis). This chapter discusses the implications of the most common musculoskeletal disorders encountered in pregnant women and provides an overview of malignant hyperthermia in this population.

LUMBOPELVIC PAIN OF PREGNANCY

Lumbopelvic pain is the most common musculoskeletal complaint during pregnancy. It comprises two distinct areas of discomfort: (1) the lumbar spine area (**low back pain**) and (2) the posterior pelvic girdle area, from the sacroiliac joints radiating down into the posterior thighs (**pelvic girdle pain**).[1] Pregnancy-related lumbopelvic pain occurs at some time during gestation in more than 50% of pregnant women and impairs at least one normal activity of daily life, including sleep. The prevalence ranges from 25% to 70% and it is the most common reason for sick leave during pregnancy. Women who complain primarily of pelvic girdle pain report more disability during pregnancy than those with isolated lumbar pain.[1] Severe pelvic girdle pain is seen in less than 0.5% of women; however, differentiation between pelvic girdle pain and low back pain is important because the management differs and the disability of pelvic girdle pain is more likely to extend into the postpartum period for up to 1 to 2 years.[2] Indices developed specifically for pregnant women to assist in diagnosis and determination of the degree of disability include the Pregnancy Mobility Index and the Overall Complaints Index.[3] Risk factors for pregnancy-related lumbopelvic pain include a history of low back pain, young age, hypermobile joints, low socioeconomic class, multiparity, and spondylolisthesis; the strongest factors are prior history of lumbopelvic pain, previous non-pregnancy-related low back pain, and strenuous work.[1,4] In addition, psychological determinants may affect the development of lumbopelvic pain; women with high scores on the stress and fear domains are more likely to have significant lumbopelvic pain.[5] Women with a history of prior low back pain who test positively on a high number of pelvic pain provocation tests are at risk for long-term significant pelvic girdle pain.

The etiology of lumbopelvic pain includes hormonal and mechanical factors. The corpus luteum synthesizes and releases the peptide hormone relaxin, the maternal blood concentration of which increases 10-fold during gestation. Relaxin induces ligamentous softening and peripheral and pelvic joint laxity which cause instability of the symphysis pubis and sacroiliac joints. The extent of instability and disability may be related to the maternal concentration of relaxin; the occurrence of back pain during pregnancy correlates with serum levels of relaxin, and women with incapacitating symptoms have the greatest serum concentrations of relaxin.[6]

Mechanical changes have a later onset than hormonal changes. Women with pelvic girdle pain have increased pelvic joint motion, which increases sheer forces across the joints and likely results in pain. A kinematic study of 34 nulliparous women in the third trimester showed lumbar motion changes and erector spinae activation that may contribute to low back pain.[7] In all pregnant women, uterine enlargement results in a forward rotation of the sacrum and an increase in the lumbar lordotic curve, which tends to close the lumbar interlaminar space. This change exaggerates the mechanical load borne by both the facet joints and the posterior aspect of the intervertebral discs. These mechanical changes also may compromise nerve root foramina. Sciatica occurs in 1% of pregnant women, most cases occurring late in pregnancy. Sciatica is distinguished from pelvic girdle pain by its extension to the ankle or involvement of the foot and may be associated with neurologic changes. Disc herniation and sacral stress fractures rarely may occur in pregnancy.[8] Incapacitating pain that radiates below the knee, typically accompanied by progressive neurologic deficits or bowel and bladder dysfunction, distinguishes disc herniation from the more common and benign pregnancy-related lumbopelvic pain.[8]

In summary, hormonal changes cause sacroiliac joint dysfunction, which is responsible for the lumbopelvic pain that occurs early in pregnancy. Mechanical changes are primarily responsible for the pain that manifests during late gestation, although symphysis pubis and sacroiliac joint instability may also continue to cause pain.

Obstetric Management

Treatment is conservative in the absence of neurologic compromise. The many studies now published on various treatment modalities for lumbopelvic pain have discordant results. Moderate quality evidence from single studies supports the use of structured exercise programs, acetaminophen (paracetamol) administration, osteomanipulative therapy, pelvic belts, and acupuncture in the treatment of lumbopelvic pain.[9,10] A 2019 systematic review on prenatal exercise that included 32 studies concluded that exercise does not prevent the occurrence of lumbopelvic pain, but does reduce the severity of the pain.[11] A 2021 systematic review and metaanalysis on conservative care strategies supports muscle relaxation therapy and taping for pain, and transcutaneous electrical nerve stimulation to improve physical motion.[12] Patients with severe neurologic signs or symptoms of disc herniation should be assessed by a consultant neurosurgeon or neurologist who can provide recommendations for intrapartum and postpartum care. Because the disability associated with lumbopelvic pain, especially pelvic girdle pain, can impair the woman's ability to function postpartum, it is important to diagnose pregnancy-related lumbopelvic pain and treat it appropriately, including into the postpartum period.[11] A 2023 study looking at self-management techniques using an established self-efficacy scale for chronic medical conditions in a group of postpartum women showed that those with low self-efficacy scores were twice as likely to have ongoing pregnancy-related back pain.[4]

Anesthetic Management

No evidence suggests that epidural or spinal anesthesia is contraindicated in patients with pregnancy-related lumbopelvic pain.[13] The anesthesia provider may administer neuraxial anesthesia, even to patients with sciatica. However, neurologic signs and symptoms should be first identified, delineated, and recorded. During epidural labor analgesia it is prudent to administer local anesthetics in dilute solutions, with or without an opioid, to minimize motor block to reduce any further stress on relaxed sacroiliac joints. Women with lumbopelvic pain may be reluctant to have neuraxial anesthesia because of concern that it may aggravate symptoms. Published evidence does not support this fear and reassurance may be required.

Careful attention to the positioning of the patient with back complaints is critical. The patient must not be placed in a position that they could not tolerate before the administration of neuraxial anesthesia. The lithotomy position puts significant stress on the lower back and should be avoided whenever possible; if used, care must be taken to raise and lower both legs simultaneously to prevent injury to the lumbar spine, and extreme positions must be avoided. Finally, caregivers should avoid rotational movements of the spine during transfer of the patient between the bed and the operating table.[1]

CHRONIC LOW BACK PAIN

Approximately 50% of pregnant women with a previous history of back pain or those with chronic low back pain experience a recurrence or exacerbation of their symptoms during pregnancy.[4] Neuraxial anesthesia may be more likely to fail in patients with chronic low back pain and in those who have had back surgery,[14] although this finding is not consistent.[15]

Sharrock et al.[14] reported a 91.2% success rate for epidural anesthesia in nonobstetric patients with a history of limited spine surgery, compared with a 98.7% success rate in patients without previous back surgery. The lower success rate was postulated to be due to the distortion of surface anatomy and the tethering of the dura to the ligamentum flavum by scar formation, which renders the epidural space discontinuous or obliterated. Support for this hypothesis is provided by a description of the postlaminectomy membrane by LaRocca and Macnab,[16] who noted the postlaminectomy formation of organized fibrous tissue surrounding the dura and, at times, binding of the nerves to the posterior aspect of the disc and adjacent vertebral body. The fibrous response was proportional to the extent of surgical trauma and was more marked with greater operative exposures. Postlaminectomy spinal stenosis also may lead to attenuation or obliteration of the epidural space; the most common site of obstructive stenosis is immediately above the fusion mass.

Conversely, a prospective observational, case-controlled study that compared 42 women with a history of discectomy who had combined spinal-epidural (CSE) labor analgesia with 42 matched controls between 2007 and 2010 found no difference between groups in total bupivacaine consumption (primary outcome), duration of the neuraxial procedure, or need for epidural catheter replacement.[15] The only difference between groups was a more frequent need to attempt at more than one interspace in the discectomy group. A possible explanation for the better findings in the latter study is that surgical techniques have changed over recent decades, and newer techniques may cause less trauma and scarring in the epidural space.

Obstetric Management

It is not uncommon for obstetric providers to offer pregnant women who have had persistent chronic low back pain the option of cesarean delivery to decrease the potential for further back injury during labor. There are no data to either encourage or discourage this option.

Anesthetic Management

The anesthesia provider may offer epidural or spinal anesthesia to patients with previous lumbar spine pathology or surgery after an appropriate history and screening examination to identify any neurologic deficits. A decreased success rate for epidural anesthesia is possible, especially in patients who have had extensive surgery. Nonetheless, the experienced anesthesia provider will likely administer epidural anesthesia successfully in most patients. Spinal anesthesia may be more reliable than epidural anesthesia in these patients.

POSTPARTUM BACKACHE

Postpartum backache is a common complaint worldwide, occurring in at least 25% of women, with 5% to 7% seeking medical help. While a 2018 study using magnetic resonance imaging (MRI) found that 15% of a small cohort of women with postpartum back pain had evidence of sacroiliitis, most postpartum backache does not have underlying pathology of concern.[17]

Women have had persistent concern that labor epidural analgesia causes postpartum back pain based upon results of late postpartum postal surveys carried out in the 1990s.[18,19] However, several prospective studies provided evidence less subject to recall bias. Howell et al.[20] performed a randomized controlled trial comparing epidural with nonepidural labor analgesia in 369 nulliparous women and found no difference in the incidence or characteristics of postpartum backache at 3 and 12 months postpartum. In a follow-up study, there was no difference between the two groups in the incidence of back pain, disability, or movement restriction more than 2 years after delivery.[21]

Abbasi et al.[22] prospectively recruited 482 laboring women for postpartum follow-up interviews regarding back pain. A total of 460 women were contacted, 230 of whom received labor epidural analgesia and 230 who did not. There was no difference between groups in the incidence of back pain at 1 day (40.9% versus 40%) and 1 week (32.2% versus 35.2%), nor in the odds ratio for backache at 1 and 3 months postpartum. That notwithstanding, there is emerging evidence from large

retrospective databases and smaller prospective case-control studies that associates unintentional dural puncture and subsequent post–dural puncture headache with the development of chronic low back pain.[23–26] Prospective studies are needed to further delineate this association.

Several reports have attributed new onset back pain in the third trimester or postpartum period to osteoporosis-induced vertebral fractures.[27–29] While pregnancy-associated osteoporosis is a known entity (associated with maternal calcium loss first to the fetus and then with lactation), reports of multilevel vertebral fractures are relatively recent. Delineating features include sudden onset of new back pain in a slimmer, older pregnant, or recently postpartum woman. The fractures occur more frequently in a first pregnancy, and the mean number of vertebrae involved is four.[29] Another unusual cause of new-onset postpartum back pain is sacral stress fracture, which can occur in the absence of osteoporosis. The typical risk factors are macrosomia, rapid vaginal birth, heparin use, and pregnancy weight gain. In a literature review by Wu et al.,[8] lumbar radiculopathy occurred in up to 17% of cases of postpartum sacral fractures, highlighting the need to assess women complaining of new-onset postpartum back pain.

Acute disc herniation is rare in pregnancy, with an incidence of 1:10,000, but it is the most common indication for spinal surgery during pregnancy when neurologic compromise or incapacitating pain occurs. Special considerations include positioning of the patient in the third trimester (avoidance of the prone position), periprocedural fetal monitoring, and consideration of antecedent cesarean delivery when near term.[30] Anesthetic modality will depend upon the type and duration of procedure.[31]

Both transient and persistent postpartum backaches are common, but there is little evidence that they are related to the use of epidural labor analgesia in the absence of unintentional

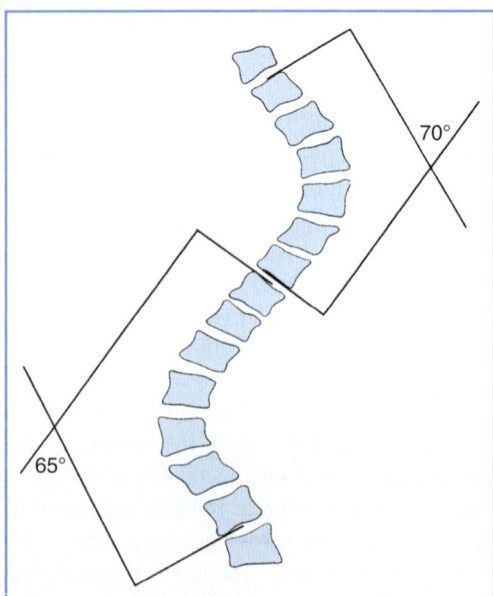

Fig. 46.1 Schematic Representation of the Cobb Angle. For each curve, a line is drawn parallel to the superior cortical plate of the proximal end vertebra and another line parallel to the inferior cortical plate of the distal end vertebra. A perpendicular line is drawn to each of these lines. The angle of intersection is the Cobb angle of the curve.

dural puncture.[22,24,26,32] Factors associated with persistent postpartum backache include: back pain before pregnancy, pregnancy-related lumbopelvic pain, prepregnancy body mass index (BMI) > 25 kg/m², depression during pregnancy, and performance of physically demanding work.[33] Some evidence supports the use of osteopathic manipulation and stabilizing exercises to help relieve postpartum backache.[34]

SCOLIOSIS

Scoliosis is a lateral deviation in the vertical axis of the spine. The severity of scoliosis is determined by measurement of the angle of spinal curves, the Cobb angle, expressed in degrees (Fig. 46.1). The prevalence of minor curves is 4 per 1000 in the North American population; larger curves occur less frequently, predominantly in females. Severe scoliosis is relatively rare in pregnant women, occurring in 0.03% to 0.07% of pregnancies.[35] Although women with moderate to severe scoliosis constitute a small proportion of obstetric patients, pregnancy in this population is common.[36] Most cases of scoliosis are idiopathic, although some are associated with other conditions, most commonly neuromuscular disorders (Box 46.1).

Scoliotic curves can be divided into structural and nonstructural varieties. **Nonstructural curves** are those seen with postural scoliosis, sciatica, and leg-length discrepancies. They do not affect the mobility of the spine and are nonprogressive. **Structural curves** are seen in patients with idiopathic scoliosis and with scoliosis resulting from the conditions listed in Box 46.1. Structural curves lead to reduced spinal mobility, and affected patients typically have a fixed prominence (rib hump) on the convex side of the curve. A rotatory component is associated with the structural scoliotic curve. The axial rotation of the vertebral body is such that the spinous processes rotate away from the convexity of the curve toward the midline of the patient (Fig. 46.2).[37] Deformation of the vertebral bodies results in shorter, thinner pedicles and laminae, and a narrower vertebral canal on the concave side. Vertebral deformation is unusual in patients with a Cobb angle < 40 degrees.

Scoliosis may interfere with the formation, growth, and development of the lungs; the occurrence of scoliosis before lung maturity may reduce the number of alveoli that ultimately form. The pulmonary vasculature develops in parallel with the alveoli; early-onset scoliosis and severe scoliosis may result in greater pulmonary vascular resistance and eventually lead to pulmonary hypertension. Musculoskeletal deformities also affect the mechanical function of the lungs; anatomic findings in scoliosis that are most commonly associated with respiratory compromise include the presence of a thoracic curve, thoracic lordosis, and rib cage deformity. The most common pulmonary function abnormality is a restrictive pattern with

---

BOX 46.1 Conditions Associated With Scoliosis

Congenital (Vertebral) Anomalies
- Hemivertebra
- Spinal dysraphism

Neurologic Disorders
- Cerebral palsy
- Polio
- Neurofibromatosis

Myopathic Disorders
- Myotonic dystrophy
- Muscular dystrophy

Connective Tissue Disorders
- Marfan syndrome
- Rheumatoid disease

Osteochondrodystrophies
- Achondroplasia/hypochondroplasia
- Osteogenesis imperfecta

Infection
- Tuberculosis

Previous Trauma

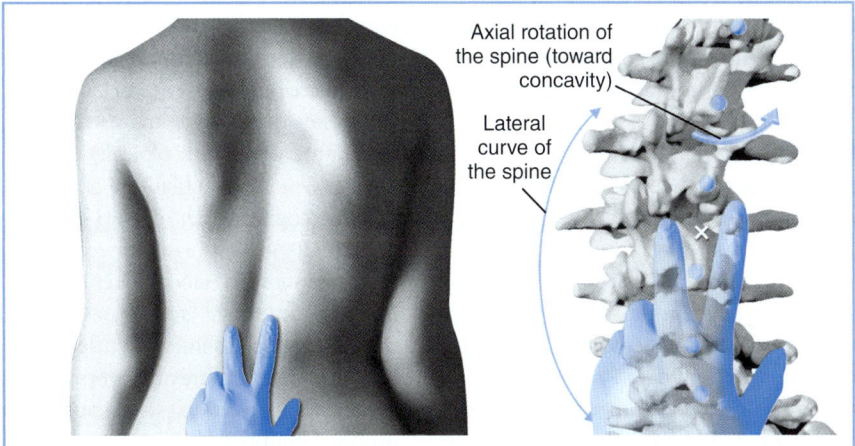

Fig. 46.2 Spinal Rotation With Scoliosis. *Left,* View of the lumbar spine in a patient with a scoliotic curve to the left demonstrating surface landmark palpation. *Right,* Skeletal anatomy at the same level in the same patient. There is a reduction in the dimensions of the interlaminar space on the concave side of the curve *(to the right)* and an expansion on the convex side. These changes are enhanced with greater severity of the curve. As the curve increases, the spinous processes rotate into the concavity of the curve, further altering the local anatomy. Surface landmark palpation from the view at left superimposed on the skeleton reveals how the palpated midline *(indicated by the white X)* is to the right of the true axial midline. Illustration by Naveen Nathan, MD, NorthShore University HealthSystem, University of Chicago Pritzker School of Medicine, Evanston, IL.

decreases in vital capacity, total lung capacity, and lung compliance. This pattern occurs in all patients with a thoracic curve > 40 degrees. The functional residual capacity is reduced and airways may close during normal tidal breathing. If the functional residual capacity is reduced to the extent that it falls below the closing capacity, atelectasis may occur in basal alveoli. The most common blood gas abnormality is an increased alveolar-to-arterial oxygen gradient, with reduced Pao_2 and a normal $Paco_2$ that result from both venoarterial shunting and altered regional perfusion. Venous admixture may lead to arterial hypoxemia. The natural history of severe, progressive scoliosis includes early death from cardiopulmonary failure.[38]

Permanent changes of the pulmonary vasculature are common in patients with a curve > 65 degrees. Pulmonary hypertension (resting mean pulmonary artery pressure exceeding 25 mm Hg [3.3 kPa]) occurs in many patients with severe deformity long before the onset of right-sided heart failure and is largely attributable to increases in vascular resistance resulting from chronic alveolar hypoxia, hypoxic pulmonary vasoconstriction, and anatomic changes in the vascular bed. Fixed pulmonary hypertension carries a grave prognosis in pregnancy and may prompt a recommendation to avoid or terminate pregnancy (see Chapter 41).

Scoliosis Associated With Neuromuscular Disease

When scoliosis develops secondary to a neurologic or myopathic disorder, abnormal respiratory function results not only from the skeletal deformity but also from abnormalities in the central control of respiration and the supraspinal innervation of the respiratory muscles, as well as from the loss of muscle function caused by the underlying disorder. Respiratory function may be further compromised by: (1) impairment of the defense mechanisms of the airways caused by loss of control of the pharynx and the larynx, (2) an ineffective cough mechanism, and (3) infrequent or reduced large breaths. Recurrent aspiration pneumonitis may result from compromised protective airway reflexes. In general, the prognosis of scoliosis caused by neuromuscular disease is poorer than that of idiopathic scoliosis and is determined predominantly by progression of the primary disorder. Affected patients typically develop irreversible respiratory failure at a younger age, and pulmonary hypertension is common.[39]

Interaction With Pregnancy

In a systematic review of 22 studies that described pregnancy outcomes in women with **adolescent idiopathic scoliosis (AIS)**, Dewan et al.[40] found that more women with AIS are likely to remain nulliparous; however, those who do have children have an equal number of children as the general population and at the same mean maternal age at time of first delivery, independent of surgery or bracing.[40] Pregnancy may exacerbate the severity of the spinal curvature, with changes of 5 to 10 degrees in 25% of patients and more than 10 degrees in 10% of patients; however, the clinical significance of these changes is not known, and some studies have not shown a curve change due to pregnancy.[41] Curve progression is more marked in those with prepregnancy curves greater than 50 degrees. The number of pregnancies is variably associated with curve progression.[36] Development of nondisabling back

pain during pregnancy is common in all patients with AIS, regardless of prior treatment and degree of curvature.[40]

The physiologic changes of pregnancy include decreases in both functional residual and closing capacities and increases in minute ventilation and oxygen demand (see Chapter 2). Thoracic cage circumference normally increases during pregnancy because of increases in both anteroposterior and transverse diameters. If the chest cage is relatively fixed by scoliosis, the diaphragm is responsible for all increments in minute ventilation. As the enlarging uterus causes elevation of the diaphragm, diaphragmatic activity is restricted and further decreases in residual and closing capacities may occur, which may result in greater ventilation-perfusion mismatch and decreased arterial oxygen content. The antepartum onset of new symptoms of respiratory compromise or the exacerbation of preexisting symptomatology is associated with higher maternal morbidity and a greater likelihood that assisted ventilation will be required after cesarean delivery.[42] Patients with a severe curve (i.e., Cobb angle > 60 degrees) but good cardiopulmonary function tolerate pregnancy well, but those with significant cardiopulmonary compromise, especially with pulmonary hypertension, have high mortality.[43]

Exertional dyspnea is uncommon in patients with scoliosis who have curves greater than 70 degrees, but it becomes more common as the deformity exceeds 100 degrees. In younger patients with a curve < 70 degrees, exercise capacity is more likely to be impaired because of the lack of regular aerobic exercise and subsequent deconditioning rather than intrinsic ventilatory impairment.[38] Although dyspnea is common in pregnancy, two features help distinguish physiologic from pathologic dyspnea.[44] First, **physiologic dyspnea** tends to occur earlier in pregnancy and often plateaus or even improves as term approaches, whereas the **pathologic dyspnea** of cardiopulmonary decompensation more often begins in the second half of pregnancy and is progressive, often becoming most severe as gestation advances and the physiologic loading is maximal. Second, physiologic dyspnea is rarely extreme, and patients can maintain most daily activities. Dyspnea that is extreme or has a limiting effect on normal activity may signal maternal cardiorespiratory decompensation. Dyspnea at rest is also rare in the absence of cardiopulmonary dysfunction, as is dyspnea that is acute in onset or progressive and intractable.

Minute ventilation typically increases by 45% during pregnancy. Minute ventilation of the unmedicated parturient increases by a further 70% to 140% in the first stage of labor and by 120% to 200% in the second stage. Oxygen consumption increases above prelabor values by 40% in the first stage and 75% in the second stage (see Chapter 2). These levels may be unattainable by the scoliotic parturient with restrictive lung disease, and respiratory failure and hypoxemia may result during labor.

Pregnant women with pulmonary hypertension have limited ability to increase cardiac output. During normal pregnancy, cardiac output increases 40% to 50% above nonpregnant measurements; during labor and delivery, even greater increases are observed (see Chapter 2). These increases are achieved by way of both larger stroke volume and higher heart rate. These demands may put an excessive burden on the cardiovascular system in parturients who had marginal cardiac reserve before pregnancy. If the right ventricle fails in the presence of pulmonary hypertension, left ventricular filling will decrease and low-output failure and sudden death may occur.[43]

Obstetric Management

Pregnant women with corrected scoliosis tolerate pregnancy, labor, and delivery well. In the absence of major lumbosacral deformity, there is little alteration of the pelvic cavity, and the incidence of malpresentation is not increased. Uterine function is normal and labor is not prolonged. Spontaneous vaginal delivery is anticipated and cesarean delivery should be reserved for obstetric indications.

The literature is conflicting as to whether the cesarean delivery rate is greater in women with corrected or uncorrected scoliosis.[35,45,46] In a retrospective study from Israel, 98 women with idiopathic scoliosis from a cohort of more than 220,000 were reviewed for birth outcomes[45]; women with scoliosis (corrected or uncorrected) were not found to have an increased risk for cesarean delivery. Conversely, Swany et al.[46] reviewed 60 female patients who underwent treatment for AIS with bracing, surgery, or observation between 1975 and 1992 and had obstetric history available. They found that the overall cesarean delivery rate of 31% for all AIS patients (operative and nonoperative) was greater than both state and national rates. Although the cesarean delivery rate was not significantly different between the operative group (35.5%) and the nonoperative (observed or braced) group (25.9%), the cesarean delivery rate was significantly higher than both state and national rates in the operative group but not in the nonoperative group. There are undoubtedly multiple confounding factors that influence the decision around mode of delivery, including patient preference, consideration of potentially difficult neuraxial anesthesia, and general obstetric preference to be "on the safe side."

Pelvic abnormalities are more common when scoliosis is associated with neuromuscular disorders and in patients with a severe, uncorrected curve. In addition, abdominal and pelvic muscle weakness predisposes parturients to problems with expulsion of the infant during the second stage of labor and may necessitate instrumental vaginal delivery. The need for instrumental or cesarean delivery is likely related to the severity of skeletal deformity, the resulting maternal compromise, and cephalopelvic disproportion.

In the second stage of labor, the diaphragm has a nonrespiratory function. With expulsive efforts, maximal isometric contractions may be sustained for 20 seconds or more; diaphragmatic fatigue has been demonstrated even in normal laboring women. In parturients whose diaphragmatic function is compromised by neuromuscular disease or severe scoliosis, the potential for fatigue and failure is greater; expulsive forces are decreased, the second stage may be prolonged, and a trial of labor may fail, necessitating instrumental or cesarean delivery. In addition, women with severe cardiopulmonary disease (especially those with gestational decompensation) may require urgent or emergency cesarean delivery because of maternal compromise or nonreassuring fetal status.

Anesthetic Management

Pregnant women who have thoracolumbar scoliosis with a Cobb angle > 30 degrees or who have undergone spinal instrumentation and fusion for scoliosis should be referred for antepartum anesthetic consultation. The anesthesia provider should (1) determine the etiology of the scoliosis as well as the severity and stability of the curve, (2) obtain a history of maternal musculoskeletal and cardiopulmonary symptoms, and (3) review prior obstetric and anesthetic experiences. For patients with scoliosis secondary to a neuromuscular disorder, the anesthesia provider should also become familiar with anesthetic considerations specific to the underlying disorder.

Women with suspected or evident pulmonary compromise should undergo evaluation by a pulmonologist, and pulmonary function studies and arterial blood gas measurements should be obtained. These patients must be reevaluated periodically to ensure that they are tolerating the increasing physiologic demands of pregnancy. Echocardiography is useful to assess right-sided heart function in patients with one or more of the following: (1) a curve ≥ 60 degrees, (2) hypoxemia on arterial blood gas measurement, (3) moderate or greater reductions in predicted lung volumes or flows, (4) pulmonary hypertension, and (5) evidence of decompensating cardiopulmonary status. Radiographic studies performed before pregnancy and operative notes describing spinal surgical procedures should be reviewed before neuraxial anesthesia is initiated in any patient with significant scoliosis or previous spinal surgery. The anesthesia provider should also examine the spine and note the surface landmarks and interspaces that are least affected by the deformity. Modes of analgesia and anesthesia for labor and delivery can be discussed during antepartum consultation.

Invasive hemodynamic monitoring is rarely indicated during labor and delivery. Pulmonary function studies that suggest significant respiratory compromise or clinical evidence of impending respiratory failure may warrant placement of an arterial catheter and serial assessment of blood gas measurements. Echocardiographic demonstration of significant right-sided heart dysfunction may warrant invasive or noninvasive cardiac function monitoring.

The anesthesia provider may offer neuraxial analgesia for labor and delivery to patients with severe thoracolumbar scoliosis. Identification of the epidural space is more difficult in these patients and the anesthesia provider should anticipate a greater incidence of complications. It is useful to remember the presence of the vertebral rotation during the performance of neuraxial anesthesia in a patient with a significant lumbar curve, which results in the spinous processes (which often may be structurally deformed) rotating into the concavity of the curve. Therefore, the midline of the epidural space is deviated toward the convexity of the curve relative to the spinous process palpable at the skin level (see Figs. 46.2 and 46.3). The extent of lateral deviation is determined largely by the severity of the deformity.[47] One method of placing an epidural or spinal needle is to direct the needle from a palpated spinous process toward the convexity of the

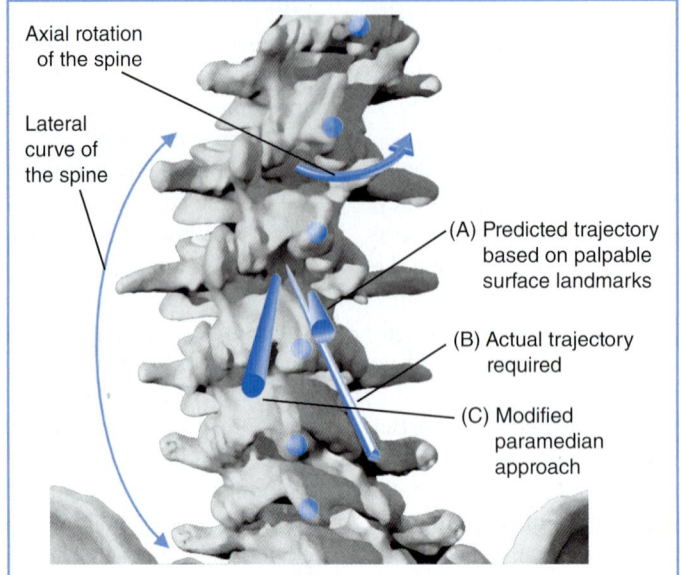

Fig. 46.3 Image of the Lumbosacral Vertebrae Affected by a Scoliotic Curve to the Left. Note the axial and lateral rotation of the vertebral bodies, and the rotation of the affected spinous processes *(blue dots)* into the concavity of the curve; these spinous processes are frequently anatomically abnormal. The apparent midline *(trajectory A)* suggested by palpated surface landmarks is to the right of the true axial midline. The figure demonstrates two approaches to enter the epidural/subarachnoid space: one where the needle is directed along the line of a spinous process toward the convexity of the curve *(trajectory B)*, and the other a modified paramedian approach where needle entry starts on the convex side of the curve and is directed perpendicular to the skin *(trajectory C)*. Illustration by Naveen Nathan, MD, NorthShore University HealthSystem, University of Chicago Pritzker School of Medicine, Evanston, IL.

curve, often at a substantial angle. Alternatively, one can use a modified paramedian approach starting at the estimated true midline of the epidural space but directing the needle perpendicular to the skin into the epidural space (see Fig. 46.3). The experienced anesthesia provider can track the resistance of both the interspinous ligament and the ligamentum flavum to maintain the correct course into the epidural space. The extent of the local anatomic distortion is the limiting factor, and the selection of spaces that are least involved with the curve is advised.

Ultrasonography is useful to facilitate administration of neuraxial anesthesia in parturients with challenging spinal anatomy, including those with scoliosis.[48,49] Asymmetry of the spine is not difficult to appreciate; learning how to use the information and determine the optimal space and needle direction requires more experience.[50] The longitudinal paramedian view may provide the best information with respect to the widest interlaminar space, and the transverse view shows presence of rotation and asymmetry.[48,51] There are a few studies on the use of preprocedural ultrasonography to identify the best space and angle of approach in parturients with difficult surface anatomy. Ekinci et al.[49] and Creaney et al.[52] randomized patients with poor palpable surface landmarks into ultrasonography-facilitated and landmark palpation-only groups. Both studies found fewer needle passes in the ultrasonography group with no increase in procedural time. Chin et al.[48] described a simplified technique for facilitating neuraxial anesthesia in patients with difficult anatomy, including scoliosis. Using a transverse view, the anesthesia provider

can visualize the rotation of the spinous process and use this information to perform essentially a paramedian approach (Fig. 46.4). Park et al.[53] randomized 44 patients with abnormal spinal anatomy to preprocedural ultrasound-assisted spinal placement or to a surface landmark–guided technique. In the ultrasound group, fewer needle passes were required (1.5 versus 6) and there was higher first-pass success (50% versus 9%) and less procedural pain.

Local anesthetic dose requirements for epidural and spinal anesthesia in the patient with scoliosis are variable. Moreover, during administration of spinal anesthesia in a patient with a severe scoliotic curve, a hyperbaric local anesthetic solution may pool in dependent portions of the spine, resulting in an inadequate block, leading some anesthesia providers to choose an isobaric local anesthetic solution.[42] It may be preferable to use a continuous technique in women with severe scoliosis so that the dose of local anesthetic agent can be titrated to the desired segmental level of anesthesia.

When offering neuraxial anesthesia to patients with a history of corrective spine surgery, the anesthesia provider must consider the following potential problems:

- Persistent back pain occurs in many patients with corrected scoliosis and correlates with both the extent of fusion and the time since surgery.[54]
- Degenerative changes occur in the spine below the area of fusion, and there is a higher incidence of both retrolisthesis and spondylolisthesis.
- MRI studies showed that 8% of patients with AIS had other neuraxial lesions, including syringomyelia (35%),

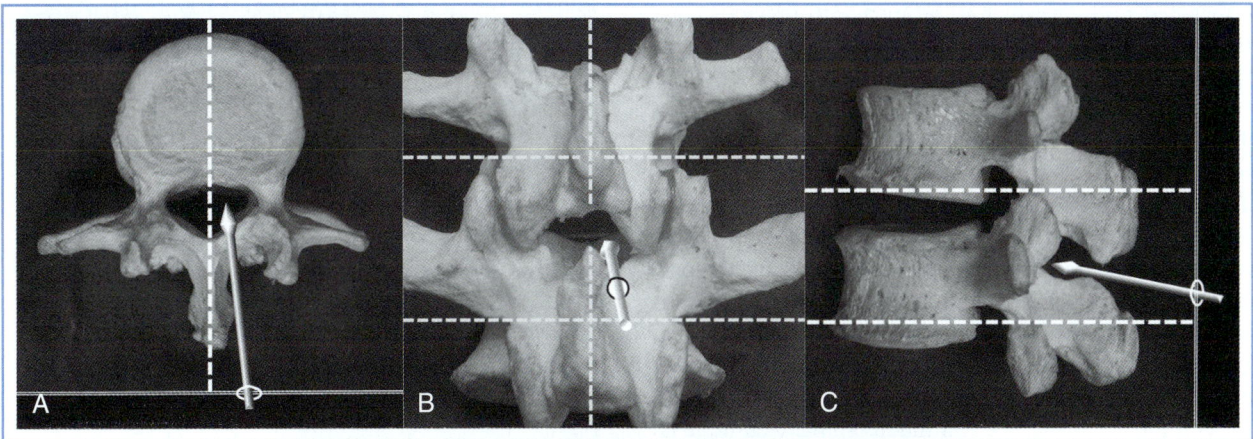

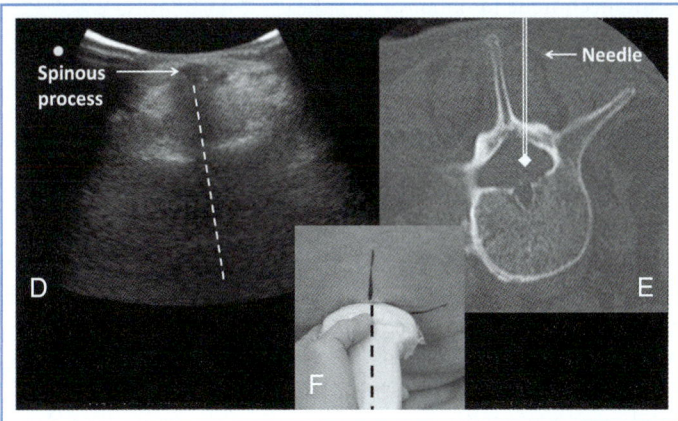

Fig. 46.4 Ultrasonography-Assisted Paramedian Approach to Neuraxial Blockade in Patients With Difficult Anatomy. An illustration of needle trajectory in the paraspinous approach in (A) the axial view, (B) the postero-anterior view, and (C) the lateral view of the spine. The white dotted lines in (B) create a rectangular shape that represents the ultrasound probe held in the transverse position as one scans for the neuraxial midline and spinous processes. Ultrasonography (D) and computed tomography (E) axial images of spine rotation in a patient with lumbar scoliosis. When the ultrasound probe is placed perpendicular to the patient's back (F), the rotation is evident from the angulation of the acoustic shadow of the spinous process. Paraspinous needle insertion should be performed 1 cm lateral to the midline (defined by the tip of the spinous process), but without medial angulation. Reprinted with permission from Chin KJ, Perlas A, Chan V. The ultrasound-assisted paraspinous approach to lumbar neuraxial blockade: a simplified technique in patients with difficult anatomy. *Acta Anaesthesiol Scand.* 2015;59:668–673.

Chiari I malformation with syrinx (28%), and isolated Chiari I malformation (25%).[55] This finding supports consideration of MRI prior to administration of neuraxial anesthesia.

- Twenty percent of patients undergo fusion to the lowest lumbar levels, limiting the potential for neuraxial anesthesia.[54,56]
- Insertion of an epidural needle in the fused area may not be possible because of the presence of instrumentation, scar tissue, and bone graft material.
- Intraoperative trauma to the ligamentum flavum may result in adhesions in or obliteration of the epidural space; these changes may interfere with the spread of injected local anesthetic.[16]
- Obliteration of the epidural space may increase the incidence of unintentional dural puncture.
- These patients often manifest a high level of anxiety about their backs and may be reluctant to have neuraxial anesthesia.

In 2009, Ko and Leffert[57] published a qualitative literature review on neuraxial anesthesia in the parturient with scoliosis. The review described 117 attempted neuraxial procedures, the majority (93) in surgically corrected patients. Overall, 71% had a successful neuraxial block; however, the corrected patients proved to be more challenging, with a 69% success rate versus 79% for the uncorrected group. The challenges in corrected patients included inability to place the needle (22%), multiple attempts (13%), patchy analgesia (10%), excessive local anesthetic dose requirement (9%), unintentional dural puncture (4%), and inadequate analgesia (4%). In the uncorrected group, the issues included patchy, asymmetric, or unilateral blocks (each 8%) and multiple attempts or failed placement (each 4%). There were also two cases of persistent low back pain of unknown etiology. Complications occurred more frequently in patients with fusion that extended to the lower lumbar and lumbosacral interspaces than in those with fusion that ended in the upper lumbar spine. These findings were corroborated by Bauchat et al.[56] in a prospective case-matched study in which 41 women with previous corrective surgery were compared with 41 healthy matched controls. The rate of neuraxial analgesia failure was higher (12% versus 0%) and the mean time to placement longer (by 41%) in the surgical correction group; however, there was no difference in local anesthetic requirement to maintain analgesia.

Thus, in patients with severe or corrected scoliosis, both the anesthesia provider and the patient should anticipate the possibility that neuraxial analgesia may fail with or without ultrasonography. Alternative modes of intrapartum analgesia include administration of single-shot spinal analgesia (which may be repeated), caudal analgesia, patient-controlled intravenous opioid analgesia, and inhalation analgesia especially with nitrous oxide.[57] A continuous spinal technique is a reasonable alternative to an epidural technique for labor or cesarean delivery in parturients who have undergone major spinal surgery with instrumentation. The dural-puncture epidural technique may also be considered as the presence of cerebrospinal fluid (CSF) confirms the epidural needle tip location and may enhance spread of epidural local anesthetic (see Chapter 24).[57,58]

SPINAL DYSRAPHISM

The term *dysraphism* refers to a neural tube closure defect; however, use of the term has expanded to include all congenital dorsal midline spinal disorders. The old and confusing terms of *spinal bifida occulta* and *spina bifida cystica* were based on clinical findings and plain film radiographs. With vastly improved neuroradiologic imaging available, a mixed clinical-neuroradiologic classification system of spinal dysraphism has been proposed that discourages use of the term *occult spinal dysraphism* for the reasons described in the following sections.[59]

Spinal dysraphisms fall into two main categories: **open spinal dysraphism (OSD)** and **closed spinal dysraphism (CSD)** (Box 46.2). OSD includes neural tube defects that are open to the environment and contain malformed spinal cord. CSD includes all midline neural tissue abnormalities that are covered by skin; they are not necessarily occult as their presence is usually suspected by cutaneous stigmata such as hairy nevi, hairy tufts, dimples, discolored patches, capillary hemangioma, and subcutaneous masses. Finally, the finding of an isolated failed fusion of the bony neural arch, found typically at L5 or S1 (80%), is sufficiently common (occurring in 5% to 36% of the population) that it can be considered a normal variant.[60] Overall, spinal dysraphism is one of the most common birth defects, with a prevalence of 0.2 to 10 per 1000 births[61]; the incidence is higher in regions that do not advocate for folate supplementation during pregnancy.

OSD is relatively uncommon, occurring in 3.7 per 10,000 births in the United States and Canada, typically at the lumbar or lumbosacral level.[62,63] Early and aggressive surgical treatment of OSD improved survival from 45% in the early 1970s to 70% to 90% by the mid-1980s. *In utero* fetal surgery, both open and fetoscopic, is now successfully normalizing

---

BOX 46.2   Clinical-Neuroradiologic Classification of Spinal Dysraphism

Open Spinal Dysraphism
- Myelomeningocele
- Myelocele
- Hemimyelomeningocele
- Hemimyelocele

Closed Spinal Dysraphism
- With a subcutaneous mass
- Without a subcutaneous mass
  - Simple dysraphic states
- Posterior spina bifida
- Intradural and intramedullary lipoma
- Filum terminale lipoma
- Tight filum terminale
- Abnormally long spinal cord
- Persistent terminal ventricle
  - Complex dysraphic states
- Dorsal enteric states
- Neurenteric cysts
- Split cord malformations
- Dermal sinus
- Caudal regression syndrome
- Segmental spinal dysgenesis

Modified from Reghunath A, Ghasi RG, Aggarwal A. Unveiling the tale of the tail: an illustration of spinal dysraphisms. *Neurosurg Rev.* 2021;44:97–114.

---

neurologic development in fetuses with identified OSD, producing a level of function that is much improved as well as decreasing need for shunting.[64] This is, however, at the cost of obstetric complications such as preterm birth, placental abruption, maternal transfusion, and uterine scar dehiscence at delivery.[64,65] With this, obstetric and anesthesia providers can expect to encounter a growing number of pregnant women with surgically closed OSD. There is now a significant amount of literature on the transition to adult healthcare for patients living with spinal dysraphism, including considerations around pregnancy in women with OSD.[66] Of interest, a 2020 cross-sectional study from Sweden found that affected individuals older than 46 years had less complex medical conditions and were more likely to be living independently compared with those aged between 18 and 30 years.[67] Better treatment options since 1985 have made it more likely that individuals with severe lesions now survive, but at the cost of higher degrees of disability.

Neurologic deficits involving the lower extremities and sphincters occur in almost all patients with open lesions, although the deficits vary in severity. Many patients have significant residual neurologic impairment and ongoing orthopedic and genitourinary complications. Hydrocephalus is present in many patients, and shunting of the ventricular system is common, with revisions often required during childhood. Hydrocephalus is associated with impaired cognitive function,[67] although by puberty, as many as 50% of patients who have received shunts no longer require them.

Kyphoscoliosis, which is common in patients with a thoracic lesion, occurs in 20% of patients with a lumbosacral defect.[68]

CSD is further divided into those with or without a subcutaneous mass. Lesions are usually in the lumbosacral region, and the skin covering these defects is frequently abnormal. Meningoceles are herniated sacs of CSF lined by dura and arachnoid; the sacs do not contain parts of the spinal cord, although nerve roots may pass through the sac.[59] CSD *without* a subcutaneous mass comprises an intermediate group of conditions in which the bony defect is associated with one or more anomalies of the spinal cord, which may be simple or complex. Complex CSD usually has cutaneous markers. Dermal sinus tracts should not be confused with pilonidal cysts; dermal cysts are frequently connected to the intradural space and therefore pose a risk for developing meningitis.[69,70]

Affected patients may have no neurologic symptoms or may have minor sensory, motor, and functional deficits of the lower limbs, bowel, and bladder; they also may have orthopedic issues such as scoliosis, limb pain, and lower extremity abnormalities.[68] Fifty percent of patients with spinal cord abnormalities have cutaneous stigmata, and 70% have a tethered spinal cord, which has implications for neuraxial anesthesia (see below).[71] The malformations may not be clinically evident at birth and present later in life with tethered cord syndrome. MRI is the preferred diagnostic imaging modality.[69]

Tethered Cord Syndrome and Chiari II Malformation

Tethered cord syndrome is characterized by neurologic deterioration secondary to traction on the conus medullaris, which typically, but not invariably, is low lying (L2–L4).[72] Congenital abnormalities of the spinal cord, such as lipoma, tight filum terminale, dermal sinus, and split cord malformations, are found in more than 50% of patients with adult-onset tethered cord syndrome.

Adult tethered cord syndrome associated with CSD is different from tethered cord syndrome occurring secondary to OSD.[73] MRI studies suggest that tethering is present in virtually all patients with OSD.[71] Although many patients with CSD do not have obvious neurologic impairment secondary to the tethering, at least 25% of adults with tethered cord syndrome have a long history of minor orthopedic, neurologic, and/or urologic issues.[72–74] Others present with acute symptoms after a precipitating event that stretched the spinal cord, such as heavy lifting, multiple pregnancies, repeated bending, or placement in the lithotomy position.[74] Of note, more than 50% of adults with tethered cord syndrome present with only a history of low back and leg pain before a precipitating event that leads to the diagnosis.[71] Menezes et al.[74] followed 24 adult patients recently diagnosed with tethered cord syndrome and found that 80% presented with nondermatomal low back or perineal pain and 87% with bladder dysfunction. The underlying dysraphic lesions were taut filum in eight patients, conus lipoma in seven, and diastematomyelia in seven. The majority had cutaneous manifestations, including dermal sinus in

six patients, hypertrichosis in five, and skin tag/cleft/dimple/subcutaneous mass in five. The common isolated finding of a defective laminar arch (spina bifida) is not associated with a low-lying or tethered cord.

Low-lying spinal cord and the possibility of undiagnosed tethered cord syndrome have come to the attention of obstetric anesthesia providers with the publication of several case reports of neurologic injury after spinal or epidural anesthesia in women subsequently diagnosed with CSD, in whom typically there was no obvious history or cutaneous stigmata.[75,76] An important feature of adult tethered cord syndrome is that the low-lying cord is located more posteriorly than a normal cord, increasing the likelihood of direct needle trauma during administration of spinal or epidural anesthesia (Fig. 46.5).[77]

OSD is usually associated with **Chiari II malformation**, which is characterized by cerebellar herniation through the foramen magnum and descent of the pons and medulla. Tethered cord from a tight filum terminale has also been deemed causal in the development of syringomyelia and subsequent Chiari II malformation.[78] Symptoms are more common if the cerebellar herniation exceeds 12 mm or if syringomyelia is present.[79,80]

Obstetric Management

As the number of patients with spinal dysraphism increases, more data are available on pregnancy-associated issues and pregnancy outcomes. Information from large US databases with more than 11,000 women with spinal dysraphism has revealed a set of complications that differs from the urinary tract infections and pressure sores that were commonly reported in the past.[81] Complications now include increased

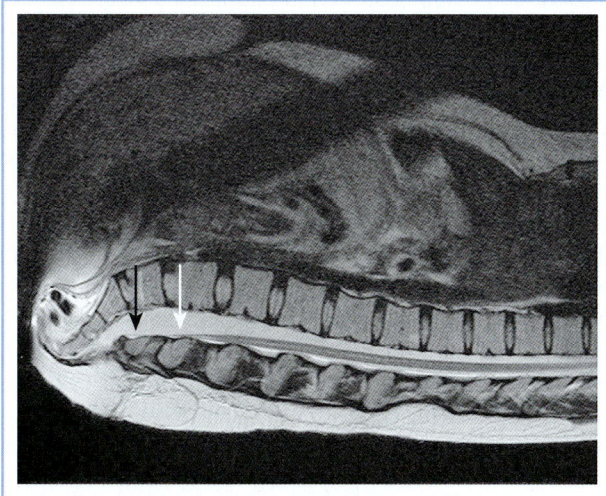

Fig. 46.5 Magnetic resonance image of the spine in a 27-y-old woman with history of a lumbar myelomeningocele excised as a neonate, with residual bladder dysfunction. A tethered spinal cord is present with a typical posterior low-lying position. The *white arrow* indicates the termination of the conus medullaris at L4 to L5, and the *black arrow* indicates the filum terminale located at L5 to S1. (This patient had a vaginal delivery at term, requiring only nitrous oxide for analgesia.)

risk for pulmonary embolism/deep venous thrombosis, seizures, and hemorrhage; patients with hydrocephalus or Chiari II malformation are more likely to suffer from the first two of these complications and are more likely to have cesarean delivery.[81] Other publications have shown that women with OSD commonly suffer from urologic and mobility issues during pregnancy and are more likely to be obese and develop diabetes.[82,83] Those with kyphoscoliosis may have rapidly compromised respiratory function as the uterus enlarges.[82] Women with known tethered cord syndrome should avoid both the squatting position and a prolonged lithotomy position for delivery.

Cesarean delivery is reserved for obstetric indications, and its incidence is increased and proportional to the severity of the underlying defect and its consequences. Vaginal delivery is more common in women who are independently mobile, is less common in wheelchair-dependent patients, and is not associated with increased complications.[84] Sterling et al.[85] reviewed the records of 32 women with spinal cord injury, 69% of whom had spinal dysraphism, and found a 60% cesarean delivery rate. Shepard et al.[84] examined 9 years of data from the National Inpatient Sample, identifying 9516 deliveries by women with spinal dysraphism. The rate of cesarean delivery was significantly higher in women with spinal dysraphism compared with those without the diagnosis (53% versus 32%), and was associated with increased maternal morbidity including preterm delivery, blood transfusion, and urinary tract infection. Those with more severe lesions and/or hydrocephalus were more likely to have cesarean delivery. Sciscent et al.[81] published similar results from another large US database in 2023 that included 11,405 women with spinal dysraphism. Similar data have recently been published from Quebec, Canada, showing higher rates of cesarean delivery, significantly increased respiratory morbidity including the need for tracheal intubation, and significantly longer hospital length of stay.[86]

Anesthetic Management

Administration of epidural or spinal anesthesia may be considered in women with various forms of spinal dysraphism and stable neurologic function. However, Sciscent et al.[81] found that patients with spinal dysraphism were only 40% as likely to receive neuraxial anesthesia compared with patients without spinal dysraphism. Imaging studies provide valuable information on neural anatomy and facilitate anesthetic management, allowing for complex collaborative planning that includes the patient and family.[87] A neurologic examination, as well as a full discussion with the patient of the risks and benefits of neuraxial anesthesia, including risk for inadequate block, should be performed and documented before the administration of neuraxial anesthesia.

An isolated laminar arch defect rarely causes issues for administration of neuraxial anesthesia. First, the lesion typically occurs at the L5 to S1 segment, below the level at which most epidural and spinal anesthetics are administered. Second, the most common anomaly is a simple midline split in the lamina, and this defect rarely seems to interfere with

either the performance or the establishment of spinal or epidural anesthesia. The epidural space may be incomplete or discontinuous across the level of an isolated laminar arch defect because of the variable formation of the ligamentum flavum at this site. An attempt to identify the epidural space at the site of this lesion may result in unintentional dural puncture.

In patients with surgically corrected OSD, the anesthesia provider should be aware that the terminal portion of the spinal cord typically lies at a vertebral level lower than normal; detethering surgery in the patient with OSD does not usually result in the conus ascending to a normal position.[72] CSD without a subcutaneous mass is of concern because of the possibility of a low-lying, posteriorly located, and tethered spinal cord, potentially with no cutaneous stigmata. A neurologic history should be taken and a screening neurologic and lower limb examination should be performed in all women known to have a defective laminar arch, preferably antenatally, to determine whether MRI for spinal dysraphism is necessary.[75,88] The presence of skin dimpling (>2.5 cm from the anal margin), hair tufts, pseudotails, and midline lumbosacral hemangiomas should raise suspicion of an underlying cord abnormality.[60] In our judgment, in women with a known low-lying cord, epidural anesthesia performed by an experienced anesthesia provider is safer than spinal anesthesia, but should be performed below the level of the cord. If spinal dysraphism is suspected but no imaging studies are available (MRI being the preferred modality), it may be prudent to avoid neuraxial anesthesia.

In the patient with an OSD lesion, the anesthesia provider should determine the level of the lesion and whether the patient has residual spinal cord function below it. Patients with a complete lesion at or above T11 are likely to experience painless labor. However, the risk for autonomic hyperreflexia should be evaluated in patients with thoracic lesions, and neuraxial anesthesia should be provided if the patient is deemed to be at risk; this issue is especially important if the lesion is between T5 and T8 (see Chapter 47). If the patient has undergone ventricular shunt placement, the current status of the shunt should be determined. Neurosurgical consultation should be obtained if questions remain about the requirement for, or function of, the shunt. Baseline renal function should be assessed as well as pulmonary function, especially in patients with scoliosis.

There are published reports of the use of epidural and spinal anesthesia in patients with OSD.[89–91] However, experience is limited, and most published series of pregnant women with OSD report neither the type of anesthesia nor complications. Tidmarsh and May[90] reported the management of intrapartum analgesia in 16 patients with spinal dysraphism, eight of whom had myelomeningocele. Five of the eight patients with OSD received epidural analgesia for labor and delivery. Three patients had a "normal" block, one patient had a sensory level that was higher than expected (T3 after the administration of 10 mL of 0.25% bupivacaine), and one patient had poor sacral analgesia. In the UK Registry of High-Risk Obstetric Anesthesia, the period from 1997 to 2002 included 23 cases of parturients with spinal dysraphisms among 102 cases of neurologic conditions.[92] Of those, the extent of the lesion was defined further in only 10 cases, and eight had only a bony arch defect. Neuraxial anesthesia was provided in eight cases. Only epidural anesthesia was used owing to concern about a low-lying or tethered cord; only five patients had MRI performed before delivery. Murphy et al.[60] published a comprehensive review of spinal dysraphism in the parturient, including a summary of reported obstetric anesthesia care. Of the 139 published cases (some only abstracts), epidural anesthesia was used in 52 cases and spinal or CSE anesthesia was used in 15 cases. There were numerous complications ranging from difficult block placement; rapid onset of anesthesia; and asymmetric, high, and failed blocks, at rates far higher than in usual obstetric patients. However, no patient had neurologic sequelae.

Asakura et al.[93] demonstrated the use of ultrasonography to detect a bony arch defect. Ultrasonographic imaging of the terminal portion of the cord is difficult, however, and although it has been shown to be feasible in children,[59] experience in neuraxial ultrasonographic imaging is insufficient for most anesthesia providers to determine the safety of neuraxial anesthesia in adults. A recent case series of four pregnant patients did show the ability to confirm other radiologic imaging results using ultrasonography, but the only patient who received neuraxial anesthesia had an isolated bony defect.[94] Spinal anesthesia should be performed below the known level of the conus medullaris or avoided in favor of epidural anesthesia. If possible, epidural analgesia should also be initiated below the level of cord termination in case of unintentional dural puncture. It should be noted that the epidural space is often abnormal, which increases the likelihood of inadequate epidural anesthesia. In women with minimal function of the lower extremities and sphincters, a detailed discussion about risks of neuraxial anesthesia in the presence of a low-lying spinal cord must take place.

Two retrospective case series described the obstetric and anesthetic management in parturients with Chiari I malformation; one reported on 95 deliveries in 63 patients[95] and one assessed 185 deliveries in 148 patients.[96] In one series, vaginal delivery was accomplished in 43% of cases and 78% had neuraxial anesthesia.[95] In the other series, 54% had a vaginal delivery and 66% had neuraxial anesthesia.[96] No patient had neurologic deterioration. The decision regarding the safety of neuraxial anesthesia in any individual patient will depend on whether the patient has signs of increased intracranial pressure and the degree of cerebellar herniation. We recommend neurologic consultation prior to delivery to aid in decision-making.

A final issue for consideration is the ongoing management of latex exposure and development of latex allergy in patients with spinal dysraphism, particularly OSD. Current guidance recommends that patients with OSD should avoid all skin contact with latex protein from birth. In addition, they should be protected from inhalation of powders that contain latex particles.[97]

CHRONIC INFLAMMATORY ARTHROPATHIES

This group of conditions includes rheumatoid arthritis (RA), psoriatic arthritis, polymyalgia rheumatica, crystal arthropathy (gout), and ankylosing spondylitis (AS). The most common arthropathies seen in pregnancy are RA and AS; RA is most affected by pregnancy and has been studied most extensively with respect to the immunologic relationship between mother and fetus.

Rheumatoid Arthritis

RA is a systemic autoimmune inflammatory disorder primarily affecting the joints. Articular features are characterized by symmetrical painful swelling of multiple joints (classically worse in the morning), ultimately progressing to joint destruction and deformity. Disease onset is typically insidious, with disease markers often evident before the onset of symptoms. Treatment should be aggressive because erosive effects are cumulative and irreversible. Extraarticular manifestations may affect multiple organ systems and are associated with high morbidity and mortality. Demonstrating substantial geographical variation, the worldwide prevalence of RA has increased by 7.4% between 1990 and 2017, with higher rates in North America, where prevalence is 0.54% to 0.63% in the United States and 0.65% to 0.78% in Canada.[98] RA occurs at least twice as frequently in women as in men, and while classically considered to be a disease of older adults, it is increasingly diagnosed in women of childbearing age.[99] Numerous risk factors for RA have been identified, implicating a combination of genetic, environmental, and infectious triggers in its pathophysiology. The diagnosis is made according to internationally agreed classification criteria.[100]

While almost any joint can be affected by RA, changes affecting the vertebral column and airway are likely to be of most interest to the obstetric anesthesia provider. While the lumbosacral spine is affected in only 5% of patients with RA, the cervical spine is commonly involved, with radiographic evidence of cervical spine deformity becoming apparent in 40% of RA patients despite optimal medical management and decreasing disease severity scores.[101] Atlantoaxial subluxation is of particular concern; it occurs secondary to disruption of the transverse ligament and erosion of the odontoid peg, allowing for dislocation of the C1 vertebra (the "atlas") on the C2 vertebra (the "axis") during neck movement. There are four subtypes of atlantoaxial subluxation: (1) anterior, occurring in 80% of patients and worsened during neck flexion; (2) posterior, occurring in 5% and worsened during neck extension; (3) vertical, occurring in 10% to 20%, causing subluxation of the odontoid peg through the foramen magnum with attendant compression of the cervico-medullary junction (cranial settling); and (4) lateral, which may lead to spinal nerve or vertebral artery compression. Subaxial subluxation (occurring at or below C3) may also occur and manifests as persistent headache or Lhermitte sign, an electric shocklike sensation that occurs with neck flexion. Atlantoaxial subluxation may be identified on lateral plain film radiographs of the cervical spine, performed in the neutral, flexed, and extended positions, on

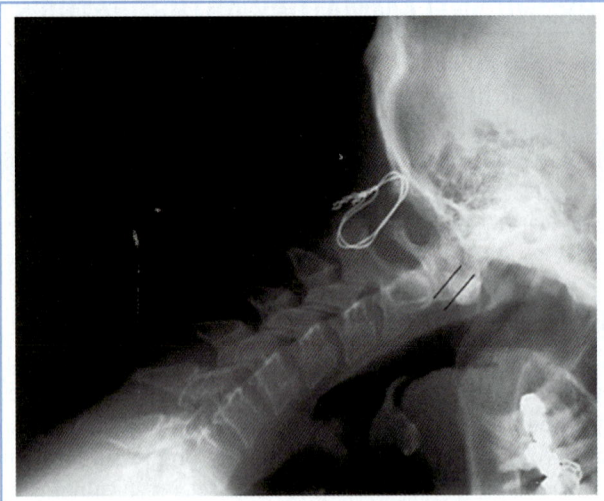

Fig. 46.6 Lateral radiographic study of the cervical spine (in flexion) in a 32-y-old woman with rheumatoid arthritis (RA). There is isolated atlantoaxial subluxation (6 mm) in the absence of other radiologic changes of RA. She presented with neck pain, and a wire was placed between the occiput and the spinous process of C2 to limit the subluxation.

BOX 46.3   Extraarticular Manifestations of Rheumatoid Arthritis

Cardiovascular
- Pericarditis
- Pericardial effusions
- Endocardial vegetations
- Myocardial nodules—conduction disturbance
- Arteritis/vasculitis

Airway
- Mandibular hypoplasia
- Cricoarytenoiditis
- Temporomandibular joint dysfunction
- Laryngeal deviation and rotation

Pulmonary
- Pleural effusion
- Pulmonary fibrosis
- Pulmonary nodules

Chest Wall
- Costochondritis

Neurologic
- Peripheral nerve compression
- Cervical nerve root compression

Hematologic
- Anemia
- Felty syndrome

Ophthalmic
- Keratoconjunctivitis

which the anterior and posterior atlantodental intervals can be measured (Fig. 46.6). Open-mouth radiographs can assess for odontoid erosion. Radiographs should be obtained in patients with clinical suspicion of cervical involvement[102]; the onset of symptoms compatible with cervical myelopathy or radiculopathy should prompt MRI and neurosurgical evaluation.

Airway management in RA may be challenging. Vertical subluxation of the odontoid process is associated with a complex scoliotic deformity of the trachea and larynx, which can make direct laryngoscopy and tracheal intubation difficult.[103] Fortunately, vertical subluxations occur primarily in older patients with severe, long-standing disease and are unlikely to be seen in women of childbearing age. Nonetheless, the cricoarytenoid and temporomandibular joints (TMJ) may be involved earlier in the disease and can complicate airway management of the parturient.[104]

Extraarticular manifestations are common in patients with RA, with severe manifestations occurring in around 40% of affected patients. Anesthesia providers have a special interest in abnormalities that affect the airway and the cardiovascular and respiratory systems (Box 46.3). Although these complications occur more typically in patients with long-standing disease, it is prudent to inquire about those associated with significant anesthetic implications. Cardiovascular mortality is especially high in patients with RA, and cardiovascular disease is often present in the absence of symptoms.

Interaction With Pregnancy

RA is associated with higher rates of infertility, preeclampsia, preterm birth, and cesarean delivery. Neonatal effects may include small-for-gestational-age infants and increased likelihood of neonatal intensive care unit (NICU) admission and stillbirth. Some of these effects may be attributable to the use of disease-modifying antirheumatic drugs (DMARDs).[99] While pregnancy

has long been held to cause an amelioration of disease activity in RA, recent studies using disease scoring systems modified to eliminate the confounding effects of the physiologic changes of pregnancy have demonstrated less benefit. Symptomatic improvement occurs in around 60% of patients, and postpartum relapse in around 47%.[105] Disease flares during pregnancy appear to be associated with interruption of DMARDs (particularly tumor necrosis factor inhibitors [TNFi]), and most respond to reinitiation of TNFi or corticosteroids.[106] It appears that most women return to a disease status comparable to their prepregnant state. Current emphasis, therefore, is on continuing appropriate medications during pregnancy.

Medical Management

The 2021 American College of Rheumatology guideline for the treatment of RA divides drug therapy into conventional synthetic DMARDs (csDMARDs), biologic DMARDs (bDMARDs), targeted synthetic DMARDs (tsDMARDs), and glucocorticoids. Symptom-modifying therapies include nonselective cyclooxygenase inhibitors (nonsteroidal antiinflammatory drugs [NSAIDs]). While for many years NSAIDs and glucocorticoids were the mainstay of therapy in RA during pregnancy, the proliferation of novel therapies has prompted European and North American societies to publish recommendations on the management of DMARDs

TABLE 46.1 Safety of Disease-Modifying Antirheumatic Drugs (DMARDs) in Pregnancy

Class	Preconception	Pregnancy	Lactation
csDMARDs Hydroxychloroquine, sulfasalazine, colchicine, azathioprine, 6-mercaptopurine, cyclosporine, tacrolimus	Continue	Continue	Continue
csDMARDs Methotrexate, mycophenolate mofetil, leflunomide, cyclophosphamide	Discontinue (teratogenic)	Discontinue (May consider cyclophosphamide for life-threatening disease in first/second trimesters)	Avoid
Nonselective NSAIDs (COX-2 inhibitors not preferred)	Safe	May be considered in first and second trimesters. *Avoid in third trimester.*	Ibuprofen preferred
Glucocorticoids Prednisone	Taper to less than 20 mg/d.	Taper to less than 20 mg/d.	Delay breastfeeding for 40 h after dose > 20 mg
bDMARDs: TNFi Certolizumab	Continue	Continue	Continue
bDMARDs: TNFi Infliximab, etanercept, adalimumab, golimumab	Continue	Continue in first and second trimesters. Discontinue prior to third trimester.	Continue
bDMARDs: TNFi Rituximab	May continue while trying to conceive. Discontinue at conception.	Consider only in severe/life-threatening disease.	Continue
bDMARDs Anakinra, belimumab, abatacept, tocilizumab, secukinumab, ustekinumab	Limited data. Discontinue and replace with known safe medication.	Limited data. Discontinue and replace with known safe medication.	No data

DMARD, Disease-modifying antirheumatic drug; *bDMARD*, biologic DMARD; *csDMARD*, conventional synthetic DMARD; *NSAID*, nonsteroidal antiinflammatory drug; *TNFi*, tumor necrosis factor inhibitor.
Modified from the American College of Rheumatology and European League Against Rheumatism guidelines (Götestam Skorpen C, Hoeltzenbein M, Tincani A, et al. The EULAR points to consider for use of antirheumatic drugs before pregnancy, and during pregnancy and lactation. *Ann Rheum Dis.* 2016;75:795–810; and Sammaritano LR, Bermas BL, Chakravarty EE, et al. 2020 American College of Rheumatology Guideline for the management of reproductive health in rheumatic and musculoskeletal diseases. *Arthritis Rheumatol.* 2020;72:529–556.)

from preconception through pregnancy to lactation (Table 46.1).[107,108] There are limited data on the use of tsDMARDs prior to and during pregnancy and lactation; these agents are likely best avoided until their safety profile is established.[107,108] While the multitude and complexity of these newer agents mandate multispecialty planning and medication management, the overarching consensus favors avoiding relapses or flares in RA disease activity by continuing therapies considered safe for use in pregnancy.

NSAIDs may be considered during pregnancy to control active disease flares but should be restricted to the first and second trimesters, and nonselective agents should be chosen. The glucocorticoids (prednisone, prednisolone) may be associated with a small increase in the rate of early pregnancy loss but do not appear to be associated with congenital malformations. Long-term corticosteroid use may increase the risk for preeclampsia, premature rupture of membranes and preterm birth, venous thromboembolism, pyelonephritis, and small-for-gestational-age neonates.[109]

Obstetric Management

Vaginal delivery is preferred for parturients with RA, and cesarean delivery should be reserved for obstetric indications. A major concern is maternal positioning during labor. Rheumatoid joints are unstable because of ligament loosening associated with chronic swelling and because of the destruction of ligaments and cartilage. It is important to determine the permissible range of motion and activity for affected joints. Special emphasis should be given to the hips, knees, and neck. Healthcare providers should be aware of the potential risks associated with forcing motion beyond the disease-imposed limits.

Anesthetic Management

The preanesthetic evaluation should include a careful evaluation of the airway. Patients with RA may have a small mandible, TMJ dysfunction, cricoarytenoid arthritis, and laryngeal deviation, all of which may complicate direct laryngoscopy.[104] In particular, these findings may be present in parturients with juvenile-onset RA. Similarly, while cervical spine involvement is not common in young patients, it may occur in patients with disease of long duration and in those with severe, deforming disease. Although there is no guideline or consensus on the need to obtain cervical spine radiographs in patients with RA, it would be reasonable even in the pregnant patient if there is severe erosive disease, neck symptoms, or disease duration ≥ 10 years.[104] The cardiac and pulmonary features of RA are not common in young patients, but signs and symptoms of pleural and pericardial effusions and pulmonary parenchymal involvement should be sought.

No evidence contraindicates the administration of spinal or epidural anesthesia in patients with RA. However, evidence in the nonpregnant population has indicated that spinal blocks rise higher than expected in patients with RA, independent of BMI.[110,111] Care should be taken to avoid excessive manipulation of the neck during administration of general anesthesia. Finally, joints should be padded and protected appropriately during labor and delivery.

Ankylosing Spondylitis

AS is a type of axial spondyloarthritis (SpA) that affects the axial skeleton. Both AS and nonradiographic axial SpA (in which there is no radiologic evidence of sacroiliitis but which may progress to AS[112]) are associated with inflammatory back pain, excess spinal bone formation proceeding to ankylosis, and a high prevalence of the HLA-B27 antigen. While the clinical spectrum is wide, and only a small proportion of patients progress to total spinal ankylosis, axial SpA can impose significant physical and social burdens on patients, many of which present during the working—and childbearing—periods of their lives.[113]

Classically held to be more common in males than females, the sex predilection appears to be decreasing, and delays in diagnosis may result in a higher disease burden in women than in men.[114] Further, and in contrast to the other inflammatory arthropathies, onset is most common during the childbearing years. Although clinically significant lesions of the cervical spine may occur early in the course of the disease, they are far more common in patients with longstanding AS (Fig. 46.7).[115] Ultimately, 21% of patients with AS develop clinically significant atlantoaxial subluxation. TMJ involvement causes limited mouth opening in 10% of patients early in the disease, increasing to 30% to 40% as the disease progresses.[116] A slower development of radiologic changes of the dorsolumbar spine occurs in women, and spinal rigidity or deformity is rare in young patients (Box 46.4).[104,117] Extraarticular manifestations, including enthesitis, inflammatory bowel disease, and psoriasis, appear more commonly in females, with the exception of anterior uveitis, which is more common in males.[114] Individuals with AS are at risk for vertebral fractures. The prevalence ranges from 10% to 17%, the most common level is C5 to C6, and the fractures are most likely to occur by the third decade.[118]

The mainstays of treatment for AS are directed physical therapy and NSAIDs. bDMARDs such as TNFi, Janus kinase inhibitors, and interleukin-17 inhibitors are recommended in patients with active disease despite continuous NSAID use.

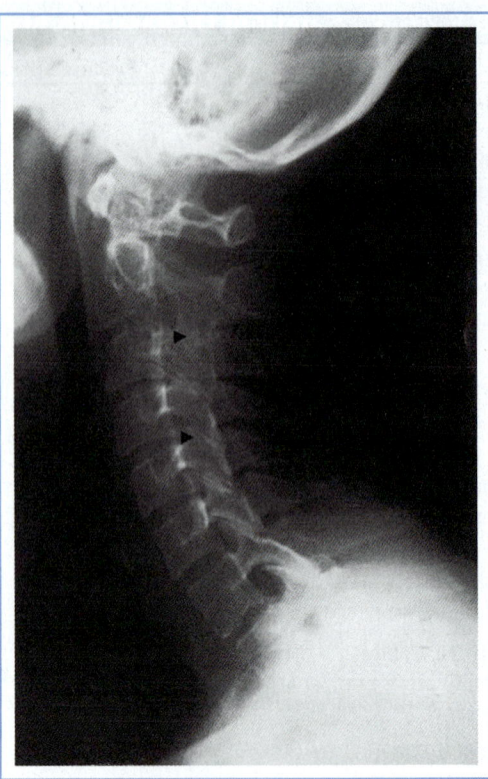

Fig. 46.7 Lateral radiographic study of the cervical spine in a 31-y-old woman with ankylosing spondylitis. There is evidence of facet joint ankylosis *(arrowheads)*, although the lordotic curve remains well preserved.

BOX 46.4 Extraarticular Manifestations of Ankylosing Spondylitis

Systemic
- Fever
- Weight loss
- Fatigue

Cardiovascular
- Aortitis
- Aortic insufficiency
- Conduction disorders—heart block

Pulmonary
- Restrictive lung disease
- Pulmonary fibrosis

Neurologic
- Cauda equina syndrome
- Vertebrobasilar insufficiency
- Peripheral nerve lesions

Hematologic
- Anemia

Urologic
- Prostatitis

Ophthalmic
- Uveitis

The csDMARDs, such as sulfasalazine and methotrexate, are reserved for situations in which these more modern drugs are unavailable[113] (Table 46.1).

Interaction With Pregnancy

AS does not appear to affect fertility. Disease flares occur in 25% to 80% of AS patients during pregnancy and in 30% to 100% of patients during the postpartum period. Active disease at the time of conception appears to predict flares during both periods, while discontinuation of TNFi during early pregnancy is associated with a threefold increased risk of disease flare during pregnancy.[119] While studies reporting pregnancy outcomes in patients with AS are typically small and heterogeneous in nature, a 2021 scoping review found increased risk of preterm and small-for-gestational-age neonates, with no increased risk of preeclampsia or cesarean delivery.[119]

Anesthetic Management

Anesthesia providers should review the patient history with respect to the duration of the disease, the presence of extraarticular features, and the recent use of analgesics. Though TMJ disorders, cervical spine involvement, and cardiopulmonary complications are rare early in the disease course, difficult tracheal intubation has been reported in parturients.[120] Severity of back symptoms is often out of proportion to the radiographic appearance of the spine, and calcification of the spinal ligaments is typically not advanced in young patients. Neuraxial anesthesia is acceptable in parturients with AS; however, even in young patients, it may be technically challenging. Calcification of the interspinous ligaments and osteophyte formation may limit the ability to flex forward, making midline needle placement difficult.[116] A paramedian approach can be considered in this instance.[121] The epidural space becomes narrowed in patients with AS, and there have been reports of unexpectedly high block,[122] as well as failed block despite confidence that the catheter was in the epidural space. After multiple failed attempts to provide epidural analgesia in a parturient with advanced AS, Hoffman et al.[123] suggested that a highly calcified posterior longitudinal ligament may limit rostral spread of local anesthetic in the epidural space. Preprocedural ultrasonography may be helpful, either to identify the best interlaminar space, or to suggest that administration of neuraxial anesthesia may be impossible.[124]

Finally, care should be taken when positioning women with AS regardless of mode of delivery, as the biomechanics of the spine are altered by decoupling of bone formation and resorption that occurs as part of the disease. Holding a flexed trunk for prolonged periods while pushing may result in vertebral fractures, as demonstrated in a case report in which a 33-year-old woman with a 5-year history of AS suffered a T12 to L1 fracture dislocation with subsequent neurologic compromise during attempted vaginal birth.[118]

ACHONDROPLASIA

Achondroplasia is a rare disorder of bone metabolism and the most common cause of disproportionate dwarfism, with a prevalence of 1 in 25,000 live births. Inherited in an autosomal dominant mode, most cases arise from spontaneous gain-of-function mutation in the fibroblast growth factor receptor 3 (FGFR3) gene.[125] Final height rarely exceeds 130 cm and almost every bone may be affected; common features include macrocephaly, midface hypoplasia, rhizomelia and brachydactyly (shortening of the limbs and digits, respectively), genu varum deformity, and joint hypermobility. While truncal length is maintained disproportionately to the limbs, the vertebral column is affected: cervical range of motion may be decreased, lumbar lordosis and thoracic kyphosis are increased, and thoracic kyphoscoliosis occurs.[126] The vertebral pedicles are short; reduced length of the neural arch leads to shortened anteroposterior and transverse diameters of the vertebral canal, resulting in stenosis of the foramen magnum and spine with attendant propensity to hydrocephalus.[127] Anesthetic management may be complicated by a tendency for upper airway obstruction, cervical spine instability, diminished functional residual capacity, and cor pulmonale.[128] Table 46.2 outlines a more detailed list of anesthetic considerations for patients with achondroplasia.

TABLE 46.2 Clinical Features and Anesthetic Considerations in Pregnant Patients With Achondroplasia

Clinical Features	Anesthetic Considerations
Craniofacial: macrocephaly, midface hypoplasia, macroglossia, short maxilla, large mandible.	Potentially difficult airway management due to narrow nasal passages and small trachea. May have limited neck extension and potential for atlantoaxial instability.
Stature and obstetric: rhizomelic dwarfism, reduced xiphoid to symphysis pubis distance, reduced likelihood of fetal head engagement.	Caution with drug dosing and equipment sizing. Likely to require cesarean delivery.
Vertebral abnormalities: lumbar hyperlordosis.	Difficulty sitting and unpredictable spread of neuraxial block.
Respiratory: narrow thorax, rib deformities, thoracolumbar kyphoscoliosis.	Restrictive lung disease. Severely reduced functional residual capacity. Central and/or obstructive sleep apnea.
Cardiac: potential for cor pulmonale.	Avoid hypoxemia, hypercarbia, acidosis, hypothermia. Caution with nitrous oxide.
Neurologic: foramen magnum stenosis, possible hydrocephalus.	Care with neck extension; avoid cervicomedullary compression. Risk of raised intracranial pressure.

From Dubiel L, Scott GA, Agaram R, et al. Achondroplasia: anaesthetic challenges for caesarean section. *Int J Obstet Anesth.* 2014;23:274–278.

Beyond neurosurgical and limb-lengthening procedures, there has previously been little in the way of specific therapy for achondroplasia. Because growth hormone (GH) levels are normal in patients with achondroplasia, GH supplementation and gonadal suppression are associated with only modest increases in height.[129] However, in 2021, the C-type natriuretic peptide analogue vosoritide was approved for the treatment of achondroplasia in children and is associated with increased linear growth. Effects on foramen magnum diameter are not yet known and, despite reassuring animal studies, the safety of vosoritide during pregnancy and lactation is unknown.[130] Additional specific therapies are in development.[131]

Obstetric Management

The uterus is an abdominal organ in the pregnant patient with achondroplasia. With advancing pregnancy, it may encroach on the small thoracic cage and lead to further decreases in the already-diminished functional residual and closing capacities; severe dyspnea may occur.[132] Back discomfort is common during pregnancy, and the reported incidence of sciatica is greater than in healthy pregnant women,[133] owing most likely to the underlying spinal abnormalities. Because cephalopelvic disproportion is highly likely, the obstetric provider should anticipate the need for cesarean delivery in most patients with achondroplasia. While the Pfannensteil incision is commonly employed, a midline incision may be required and multidisciplinary preoperative planning is indicated.[134]

Anesthetic Management

Both neuraxial and general anesthesia may be challenging in the parturient with achondroplasia. Difficult laryngoscopy and tracheal intubation (including videolaryngoscopy) must be anticipated and flexible fiberoptic bronchoscopy may be required.[135] Noninvasive blood pressure measurement may be difficult because of short limbs and placement of an arterial catheter may be necessary.[134]

Locating the epidural and subarachnoid spaces may be complicated by narrow intervertebral spaces and marked lumbar lordosis[133,136]; the use of ultrasonography may help to identify landmarks.[137] Small stature and spinal stenosis may reduce neuraxial local anesthetic requirement and, because it is difficult to estimate the appropriate dose for single-shot spinal anesthesia, a continuous epidural or CSE technique is preferable.[138] Although local anesthetic dose requirement may be anticipated to be smaller than in parturients of normal stature,[139] dose requirement has been reported to be surprisingly high,[133] further supporting the use of a titratable anesthetic technique. Transversus abdominis plane (TAP) blocks have been described for postoperative analgesia.[132]

Multidisciplinary team planning is vital, as all anesthetic options may prove challenging and time-consuming. Close attention must be paid to anesthetic drug dosing, mechanical ventilation strategies (including tracheal tube diameter), and postoperative pain management. The disproportion between truncal size and limb size may lead to under- or overestimations of doses depending on whether patient weight or age is usually used in such calculations.[132]

OSTEOGENESIS IMPERFECTA

Osteogenesis imperfecta (OI, brittle bone disease) is a genetically heterogeneous connective tissue disorder with a worldwide birth prevalence of 3 to 7 per 100,000.[140] Although at least 20 genes have been associated with OI, over 80% of cases are associated with pathogenic mutations in two genes that encode type 1 collagen: *COL1A1* and *COL1A2*. While OI is characterized by frequent fractures caused by bone fragility, it is a generalized connective tissue disorder associated with complications including middle ear hearing loss (otosclerosis), blue sclera, dentinogenesis imperfecta, and cardiopulmonary disorders. Patients with OI frequently require treatment for pain associated with their musculoskeletal abnormalities. OI does not affect fertility.[141]

Although OI may be classified according to the genetic mutation responsible, five clinically distinct subtypes are described. OI type I is a mild nondeforming condition associated with blue sclera and is the most common subtype in the general and pregnant populations.[141] OI type II is a severe (usually lethal) perinatal form. OI type III is a severe and progressively deforming syndrome. OI type IV is a common variable OI with normal sclera. OI type V is associated with progressive abnormalities of calcification.

The majority of pregnant women with OI have OI type I, although pregnancy has been reported in more severe forms of the disease.[142,143] There is considerable variability among affected patients in age at onset and frequency of fractures. Short stature is typical and kyphoscoliosis is common, as are other chest wall abnormalities. These chest and spinal abnormalities result in restrictive lung disorders (Fig. 46.8). Other abnormalities include a decreased range of motion of the shortened cervical spine; micrognathia; and malformed, brittle teeth.[143] The abnormal bleeding and early bruising seen in patients with OI is multifactorial; platelet

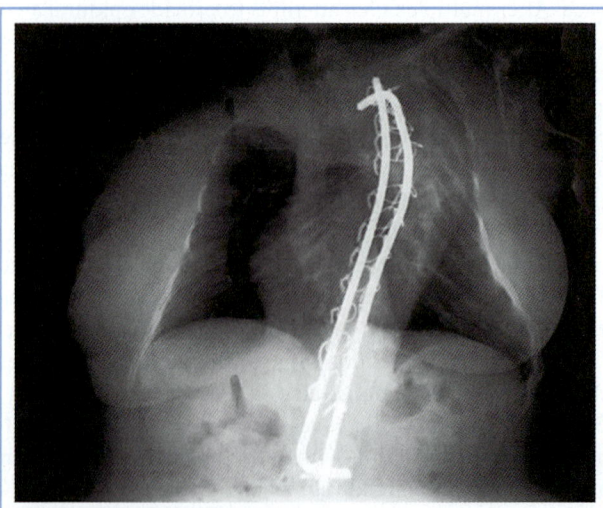

Fig. 46.8 A chest radiograph of a 30-y-old woman with osteogenesis imperfecta type I. Generalized osteoporosis, corrected thoracic kyphoscoliosis, a restricted thoracic cage, and multiple old fractures are demonstrated. (General anesthesia was provided for cesarean delivery and tubal ligation.)

dysfunction, vessel wall fragility, and reduced factor VIII are all potential contributors. Hyperthyroidism occurs in 40% of patients; an elevated concentration of thyroxine leads to increases in both oxygen consumption and heat production.[143] Although there is one published case of a patient with OI who developed malignant hyperthermia (MH), there is no clear association between the two conditions.[144] Intraoperative hyperthermia has often been reported; however, a retrospective cohort study of 49 patients with OI undergoing noncardiac surgery revealed no difference in intraoperative temperature changes compared with matched controls.[145] This information should allay ongoing concerns about risk for developing MH.

There is no cure for OI; treatment is directed at the medical prevention and surgical fixation of fractures. Bone mass and density are increased with antiresorptive and anabolic therapies such as bisphosphonates, denosumab, and teriparatide.[146] Owing to limited safety data, these agents are usually avoided prior to and during pregnancy.[147]

Obstetric Management

Normal pregnancy results in the transfer of calcium from mother to fetus; in the patient with OI, this leads to a 10% to 12% rate of maternal fracture during pregnancy. Registry studies and case series demonstrate that the incidence of cesarean delivery and pregnancy complications, including preterm birth, preeclampsia, bleeding, bone fractures, and gestational diabetes, are greater in patients with OI. Parturients with OI are also more likely to have antepartum and postpartum hemorrhage, less likely to have spontaneous vaginal birth, and less likely to receive neuraxial anesthesia. Neonates born to mothers with OI are more likely to have low or very low birthweight, more likely to require NICU admission, and have higher rates of neonatal mortality, regardless of neonatal OI status.[140,148,149] Finally, it is important to recognize the increased incidence of chronic pain, and the risk for developing acute musculoskeletal pain during pregnancy in these women.

Anesthetic Management

The anesthesia provider must be aware of the fragility of the bones, the potential for difficult tracheal intubation, and the presence and severity of restrictive lung disease. Transfers, positioning, and any invasive intervention must be accomplished with extreme care. Blood pressure cuffs and tourniquets should be applied gently to prevent fractures. Alternatives to direct laryngoscopy, such as videolaryngoscopy, may be considered to reduce the applied force necessary for laryngoscopy. While some authors have raised the theoretical concern that fasciculations following **succinylcholine (suxamethonium)** administration may be harmful, there are multiple reports of administration without incident.[145,150]

Before administration of neuraxial anesthesia, the anesthesia provider should consider the technical difficulties inherent in performing neuraxial anesthesia in patients with spinal deformities and consider preprocedural ultrasonography to facilitate needle placement. The possibility of platelet dysfunction is best evaluated by a thorough bleeding history; in the setting of a reassuring history, neuraxial anesthesia need not be withheld. Small stature and spinal abnormalities reduce local anesthetic dose requirement and increase the risk for both misplaced injection and local anesthetic systemic toxicity. It may be difficult to estimate the appropriate dose for single-shot spinal anesthesia; thus, a continuous epidural, continuous spinal, or CSE technique is preferred, barring other contraindications.[151] Nonetheless, Yeo and Paech[152] reported the successful use of both subarachnoid and epidural blocks for five cesarean deliveries in a single patient with OI type I. Dinges et al.[153] described the anesthetic management of identical twin sisters with OI type III; one twin required cesarean delivery at 32 weeks' gestation for increasing respiratory compromise and received general anesthesia because of severe corrected kyphoscoliosis and predicted difficult airway. The second twin, who had only mild scoliosis and a reassuring airway, also developed respiratory compromise and had urgent cesarean delivery under CSE anesthesia at 28 weeks' gestation for a nonreassuring fetal heart rate.

MALIGNANT HYPERTHERMIA

Epidemiology

MH is a rare condition characterized by a hypermetabolic response to **halogenated inhaled anesthetic agents** and **succinylcholine**. Presenting with otherwise inexplicable hyperthermia, tachycardia, tachypnea, increased carbon dioxide production, increased oxygen consumption, acidosis, muscle rigidity, and rhabdomyolysis after exposure to a triggering agent, MH may be associated with specific genetic mutations and/or myopathies. The prevalence of MH has been estimated at 0.18 to 0.96 per 100,000 surgical patients, with a similar prevalence reported in the obstetric population.[154] A recent decrease in the observed incidence of MH may reflect decreasing use of succinylcholine and increasing use of total intravenous anesthesia.[155]

Pathophysiology, Genetics, and Associated Disorders

MH is the result of a dysregulated entry of calcium into skeletal muscle cells. During skeletal muscle excitation-contraction coupling, the ryanodine receptor (RYR1) regulates the movement of calcium from the sarcoplasmic reticulum (SR) into the muscle cell. Numerous ryanodine receptor mutations (ryanodinopathies) have been identified, only some of which are associated with clinical MH susceptibility. Mutations in the alpha-1 subunit of the dihydropyridine-sensitive L-type voltage–dependent calcium channel receptor (CACNA1S) and the SH3 and cysteine-rich domain 3 protein (STAC3) are also associated with MH susceptibility. MH exhibits variable expression and incomplete penetrance, and associated disorders may be inherited in both dominant and recessive patterns.[156] A list of genetic mutations associated with MH may be found on the European Malignant Hyperthermia Group (EMHG) website.[157]

While not associated with MH *per se*, several other conditions have been associated with life-threatening anesthetic-associated rhabdomyolysis. Examples include the Duchenne and Becker muscular dystrophies, carnitine palmitoyl-transferase 2 deficiency, and heat- and exercise-associated rhabdomyolysis.[156]

Testing

Susceptibility to MH may be determined by genetic testing and/or a laboratory test in which freshly biopsied muscle is exposed to halothane and caffeine. In North America, the caffeine-halothane contracture test (CHCT) is available in five centers and has a sensitivity of 97% and specificity of 78%.[158] Outside North America, the EMHG developed the *in vitro* contracture test (IVCT) which has a sensitivity of 99% and specificity of 94%,[157] and the same group maintains a list of 15 accredited testing sites worldwide. Genetic testing is less invasive and less expensive than laboratory testing, and may be carried out in a wider range of locations, but CHCT or IVCT is considered to be the "gold standard" test because of the substantial false-negative rate associated with genetic testing due to incomplete characterization of the mutations responsible.[159]

Clinical Presentation and Diagnosis

The cardinal features of MH crisis are manifestations of increased skeletal muscle metabolism driven by increased intracellular calcium concentration (Box 46.5).[155] An increase in oxygen consumption and carbon dioxide production drives a sympathetic response manifesting as tachycardia, while the heat produced by muscle fiber contraction results in hyperthermia. Hypercapnia despite increasing minute volume is common. Effects on blood pressure are variable since the increased sympathetic outflow is balanced by vasodilatory effects of muscle metabolites. Clinical consequences include mixed respiratory and metabolic acidosis, cardiac arrhythmia, hyperkalemia, and rhabdomyolysis.

Symptom onset may occur in as little at 10 minutes after administration of a triggering agent, or up to several hours later. MH may present after discontinuation of a triggering agent and may present in susceptible individuals who have previously been exposed to triggers without incident. Indeed, susceptible patients may demonstrate subtle signs of myopathy, such as an exaggerated degree of the masseter muscle rigidity frequently observed after succinylcholine administration.[160]

Treatment of Malignant Hyperthermia Crisis

The cornerstone of MH crisis management is reversal of the reaction and mitigation of its metabolic consequences. The MH reaction is reversed by withdrawing the triggering agent, administering intravenous **dantrolene**, and actively cooling the patient. Multiple *aides-memoire* have been produced,[155,161] and every anesthesia provider should be drilled in recognizing and treating MH, since delay in treatment is associated with increased mortality and serious morbidity (Box 46.6).

Administration of volatile anesthetic agents and succinylcholine should be ceased immediately and any vaporizers removed from the anesthetic machine. The patient should

---

BOX 46.5   Signs and Symptoms of Malignant Hyperthermia

- Tachycardia
- Tachypnea
- Masseter spasm
- Generalized rigidity
- Elevated end-tidal CO_2 concentration
- Cyanosis
- Arrhythmias
- Acidosis
- Hyperkalemia
- Hyperpyrexia
- Myoglobinuria
- Increased creatine kinase level

BOX 46.6   Management of Malignant Hyperthermia Crisis

1. Call for help and obtain dantrolene/MH cart.
2. Notify the surgeon to finish surgery as quickly as possible.
3. Discontinue all triggering agents. If surgery needs to be continued, maintain general anesthesia with intravenous nontriggering anesthetics.
4. Hyperventilate with 100% oxygen at high gas flows ($\geq$10 L/min). If available, insert activated charcoal filters into the inspiratory and expiratory limbs of the breathing circuit.
5. Administer dantrolene 2.5 mg/kg intravenously. Repeat until signs and symptoms resolve, with decreased $ETCO_2$, muscle rigidity, and/or heart rate.
6. Perform serial blood gas measurements. Treat acidosis with sodium bicarbonate 1–2 mEq/kg.
7. Treat hyperkalemia with calcium, sodium bicarbonate, glucose, and insulin.
8. Treat dysrhythmias with standard medications, but avoid calcium channel blockers.
9. If temperature > 39°C or rising rapidly, cool patient (administration of cold intravenous solutions, removal of covers, cooling of room temperature, surface cooling with ice and/or cooling blanket, peritoneal lavage with iced saline, bladder irrigation with cold saline, use of new cooling devices).
10. Maintain urine output with fluids, mannitol, and/or furosemide.
11. Call the Malignant Hyperthermia Hotline for assistance (1-800-MH-HYPER).
12. Postoperatively, monitor patient in intensive care unit for 24–48 h. Administer maintenance dantrolene for 24 h or longer. Discontinue when metabolically stable.
13. Counsel patient and family and refer for caffeine-halothane contracture test.

Modified from Malignant Hyperthermia Association of the United States. *Emergency treatment for an acute MH event.* https://www.mhaus.org/healthcare-professionals/managing-a-crisis/. Accessed 18 July 2023.

be hyperventilated with 100% oxygen at high flows and, if available, activated charcoal filters may be inserted into the inspiratory and expiratory limbs of the breathing circuit to absorb residual vapor. Dantrolene, a postsynaptic muscle relaxant that acts on the RYR1 receptor to inhibit calcium release from the SR, should be administered intravenously at a dose of 2.5 mg/kg and repeated until clinical features subside. While doses exceeding 10 mg/kg may be required, this should prompt consideration of an alternative diagnosis. In its original formulation, dantrolene is a poorly water-soluble powder presented in 20 mg vials, each of which must be reconstituted in 60 mL sterile water, a task so labor-intensive that many guidelines recommend assigning a team to its preparation. In some jurisdictions, a newer formulation (Ryanodex) is available; this is presented in 250 mg vials and may be rapidly dissolved in 5 mL sterile water. While dantrolene crosses the placenta and might theoretically be expected to cause neonatal hypotonia if administered prior to delivery, no adverse neonatal events have been reported to date. There is one published report of postpartum uterine atony after the administration of dantrolene,[162] an effect that has subsequently been attributed to the excipient mannitol.[163] The half-life of dantrolene in breast milk is approximately 9 hours, prompting the recommendation that neonatal ingestion of breast milk is likely to be safe 2 days after maternal administration.[164]

Management of the Malignant Hyperthermia-Susceptible Parturient

Preparations for the care of an MH-susceptible pregnant patient vary little from those in the nonpregnant patient and, given similar rates of MH susceptibility in the pregnant and general populations, dantrolene should be stocked in all areas where pregnant patients might receive a triggering agent.[154] Both the EMHG and the Malignant Hyperthermia Association of the United States have published specific recommendations for the perioperative care of pregnant patients known or suspected to be MH-susceptible and for cases in which the father of the infant is similarly predisposed.[165,166] In the absence of contraindications, neuraxial anesthesia remains strongly preferred over general anesthesia for cesarean delivery in all parturients, and yet preparations must always be made for unplanned conversion to general anesthesia. Such preparations include the removal of volatile anesthetic vaporizers and succinylcholine, the known triggers of an MH event; replacement and flushing of breathing circuits and soda lime canisters; and provision of alternative muscle relaxants and reversal agents (e.g., **rocuronium** and **sugammadex**) and general anesthetic agents (e.g., total intravenous anesthesia). In the laboring MH-susceptible patient, early placement of an epidural catheter is recommended in order to facilitate urgent operative delivery if required, as all local anesthetics are safe in the patient with MH.[165]

While there remain multiple unresolved questions surrounding the management of MH in the general population,[167] it also remains unclear whether succinylcholine may be safely administered to parturients in whom the infant's father is MH-susceptible. Although succinylcholine is rapidly metabolized by maternal pseudocholinesterase and therefore crosses the placenta only to a limited extent, its avoidance would seem prudent given the widespread availability of fast-acting nondepolarizing muscle relaxants and a specific reversal agent.

KEY POINTS

- Lumbopelvic pain is the most common musculoskeletal complaint during pregnancy. It results from both hormonal and mechanical factors.
- Low back pain does not contraindicate the administration of spinal or epidural anesthesia.
- Corrected idiopathic thoracolumbar scoliosis is the most common major musculoskeletal disorder seen in pregnant women. Prepregnancy pulmonary function is a better predictor of maternal outcome than the severity of the curve.
- Neuraxial anesthesia is technically challenging in patients with scoliosis; the anesthesia provider should anticipate a greater incidence of complications and inadequate anesthesia.
- Preprocedural ultrasonography is a useful tool to facilitate neuraxial needle placement in patients with difficult surface anatomy and challenging spinal anatomy.
- Spinal dysraphism is the overall term for neural tube defects, encompassing the older terms of spina bifida occulta and spina bifida cystica.
- An isolated posterior spinal bony defect does not contraindicate the administration of spinal or epidural anesthesia.

- Adult tethered cord syndrome secondary to spinal dysraphism is important to diagnose, as it may preclude the use of spinal anesthesia.
- Pregnancy-associated disease flares are common in RA and AS, particularly if drug therapy is interrupted. Both conditions may be associated with difficult tracheal intubation and neuraxial anesthesia in addition to obstetric complications, including low birth weight and preterm delivery.
- Cephalopelvic disproportion often mandates cesarean delivery in parturients with achondroplasia or osteogenesis imperfecta. Both conditions may be associated with technically difficult neuraxial and general anesthesia. Continuous neuraxial techniques allow for careful block height titration.
- Both the obstetric and anesthesia providers should encourage early administration of neuraxial analgesia during labor in MH-susceptible patients.
- The anesthesia provider may convert epidural analgesia to epidural anesthesia for emergency cesarean delivery and thus avoid administration of general anesthesia in MH-susceptible patients.

- All local anesthetic agents are safe in MH-susceptible patients.
- If general anesthesia is indicated, the anesthesia provider should avoid succinylcholine and volatile halogenated agents in MH-susceptible patients.

- Intravenous administration of dantrolene is lifesaving treatment for a MH crisis.
- Dantrolene crosses the placenta and theoretically may result in neonatal hypotonia if administered before delivery, but no adverse neonatal events have been reported to date.

REFERENCES

1. Casagrande D, Gugala Z, Clark SM, Lindsey RW. Low back pain and pelvic girdle pain in pregnancy. *J Am Acad Orthop Surg*. 2015;23:539–549.
2. Bergström C, Persson M, Mogren I. Sick leave and healthcare utilisation in women reporting pregnancy related low back pain and/or pelvic girdle pain at 14 months postpartum. *Chiropr Man Therap*. 2016;24:7.
3. Bakker EC, van Nimwegen-Matzinger CW, Ekkel-van der Voorden W, et al. Psychological determinants of pregnancy-related lumbopelvic pain: a prospective cohort study. *Acta Obstet Gynecol Scand*. 2013;92:797–803.
4. Chunmei D, Yong C, Long G, et al. Self efficacy associated with regression from pregnancy-related pelvic girdle pain and low back pain following pregnancy. *BMC Pregnancy Childbirth*. 2023;23:122.
5. Fernando M, Nilsson-Wikmar L, Olsson CB. Fear-avoidance beliefs: a predictor for postpartum lumbopelvic pain. *Physiother Res Int*. 2020;25:e1861.
6. Aldabe D, Ribeiro DC, Milosavljevic S, Dawn Bussey M. Pregnancy-related pelvic girdle pain and its relationship with relaxin levels during pregnancy: a systematic review. *Eur Spine J*. 2012;21:1769–1776.
7. Biviá-Roig G, Lisón JF, Sánchez-Zuriaga D. Effects of pregnancy on lumbar motion patterns and muscle responses. *Spine J*. 2019;19:364–371.
8. Wu YF, Lu K, Girgis C, et al. Postpartum bilateral sacral stress fracture without osteoporosis – a case report and literature review. *Osteoporos Int*. 2021;32:623–631.
9. Franke H, Franke JD, Belz S, Fryer G. Osteopathic manipulative treatment for low back and pelvic girdle pain during and after pregnancy: a systematic review and meta-analysis. *J Bodyw Mov Ther*. 2017;21:752–762.
10. Koukoulithras I, Sr, Stamouli A, Kolokotsios S, et al. The effectiveness of non-pharmaceutical interventions upon pregnancy-related low back pain: a systematic review and meta-analysis. *Cureus*. 2021;13:e13011.
11. Davenport MH, Marchand AA, Mottola MF, et al. Exercise for the prevention and treatment of low back, pelvic girdle and lumbopelvic pain during pregnancy: a systematic review and meta-analysis. *Br J Sports Med*. 2019;53:90–98.
12. Chen L, Ferreira ML, Beckenkamp PR, et al. Comparative efficacy and safety of conservative care for pregnancy-related low back pain: a systematic review and network meta-analysis. *Phys Ther*. 2021;101(2):pzaa200.
13. Sehmbi H, D'Souza R, Bhatia A. Low back pain in pregnancy: investigations, management, and role of neuraxial analgesia and anaesthesia: a systematic review. *Gynecol Obstet Invest*. 2017;82:417–436.
14. Sharrock NE, Urquhart B, Mineo R. Extradural anaesthesia in patients with previous lumbar spine surgery. *Br J Anaesth*. 1990;65:237–239.
15. Bauchat JR, McCarthy RJ, Koski TR, et al. Prior lumbar discectomy surgery does not alter the efficacy of neuraxial labor analgesia. *Anesth Analg*. 2012;115:348–353.
16. LaRocca H, Macnab I. The laminectomy membrane. Studies in its evolution, characteristics, effects and prophylaxis in dogs. *J Bone Joint Surg Br*. 1974;56B:545–550.
17. de Winter J, de Hooge M, van de Sande M, et al. Magnetic resonance imaging of the sacroiliac joints indicating sacroiliitis according to the assessment of SpondyloArthritis International Society definition in healthy individuals, runners, and women with postpartum back pain. *Arthritis Rheumatol*. 2018;70:1042–1048.
18. MacArthur C, Lewis M, Knox EG, Crawford JS. Epidural anaesthesia and long term backache after childbirth. *BMJ*. 1990;301:9–12.
19. MacArthur C, Lewis M, Knox EG. Investigation of long term problems after obstetric epidural anaesthesia. *BMJ*. 1992;304:1279–1282.
20. Howell CJ, Kidd C, Roberts W, et al. A randomised controlled trial of epidural compared with non-epidural analgesia in labour. *BJOG*. 2001;108:27–33.
21. Howell CJ, Dean T, Lucking L, et al. Randomised study of long term outcome after epidural versus non-epidural analgesia during labour. *BMJ*. 2002;325:357.
22. Abbasi S, Hamid M, Ahmed Z, Nawaz FH. Prevalence of low back pain experienced after delivery with and without epidural analgesia: a non-randomised prospective direct and telephonic survey. *Indian J Anaesth*. 2014;58:143–148.
23. Guglielminotti J, Landau R, Li G. Major neurologic complications associated with postdural puncture headache in obstetrics: a retrospective cohort study. *Anesth Analg*. 2019;129:1328–1336.
24. Binyamin Y, Heesen P, Orbach-Zinger S, et al. Chronic pain in parturients with an accidental dural puncture: a case-controlled prospective observational study. *Acta Anaesthesiol Scand*. 2021;65:959–966.
25. Ranganathan P, Golfeiz C, Phelps AL, et al. Chronic headache and backache are long-term sequelae of unintentional dural puncture in the obstetric population. *J Clin Anesth*. 2015;27:201–206.
26. Niraj G, Mushambi M, Gauthama P, et al. Persistent headache and low back pain after accidental dural puncture in the obstetric population: a prospective, observational, multicentre cohort study. *Anaesthesia*. 2021;76:1068–1076.
27. Hardcastle SA, Yahya F, Bhalla AK. Pregnancy-associated osteoporosis: a UK case series and literature review. *Osteoporos Int*. 2019;30:939–948.
28. Jadhav A, Jadhav S, Varma A. Pregnancy- and lactation-associated osteoporotic vertebral fracture: a case report. *Cureus*. 2022;14:e31322.
29. Qian Y, Wang L, Yu L, Huang W. Pregnancy- and lactation-associated osteoporosis with vertebral fractures: a systematic review. *BMC Musculoskelet Disord*. 2021;22:926.

30. Butenschoen VM, Hitscherich H, Eicker SO, et al. Spine surgery in pregnant women: a multicenter case series and proposition of treatment algorithm. *Eur Spine J.* 2021;30:809–817.

31. Whiles E, Shafafy R, Valsamis EM, et al. The management of symptomatic lumbar disc herniation in pregnancy: a systematic review. *Global Spine J.* 2020;10:908–918.

32. Malevic A, Jatuzis D, Paliulyte V. Epidural analgesia and back pain after labor. *Medicina (Kaunas).* 2019;55:354.

33. Wiezer M, Hage-Fransen MAH, Otto A, et al. Risk factors for pelvic girdle pain postpartum and pregnancy related low back pain postpartum; a systematic review and meta-analysis. *Musculoskelet Sci Pract.* 2020;48:102154.

34. Moheboleslam Z, Mohammad Rahimi N, Aminzadeh R. A systematic review and meta-analysis of randomized controlled trials of stabilizing exercises for lumbopelvic region impact in postpartum women with low back and pelvic pain. *Biol Res Nurs.* 2022;24:338–349.

35. Chopra S, Adhikari K, Agarwal N, et al. Kyphoscoliosis complicating pregnancy: maternal and neonatal outcome. *Arch Gynecol Obstet.* 2011;284:295–297.

36. Danielsson AJ, Nachemson AL. Childbearing, curve progression, and sexual function in women 22 years after treatment for adolescent idiopathic scoliosis: a case-control study. *Spine.* 2001;26:1449–1456.

37. White A, Panjabi M. Practical biomechanics of scoliosis and kyphosis. In: White A, Panjabi M, eds. *Clinical Biomechanics of the Spine.* 2nd ed. JB Lippincott; 1990:127–168.

38. Koumbourlis AC. Scoliosis and the respiratory system. *Paediatr Respir Rev.* 2006;7:152–160.

39. Mayer OH. Scoliosis and the impact in neuromuscular disease. *Paediatr Respir Rev.* 2015;16:35–42.

40. Dewan MC, Mummareddy N, Bonfield C. The influence of pregnancy on women with adolescent idiopathic scoliosis. *Eur Spine J.* 2018;27:253–263.

41. Grabala P, Helenius I, Shah SA, et al. Impact of pregnancy on loss of deformity correction after pedicle screw instrumentation for adolescent idiopathic scoliosis. *World Neurosurg.* 2020;139:e121–e126.

42. Factor PAA, Pelaez-Crisologo MC. Obstetric management of a parturient with severe idiopathic scoliosis. *BMJ Case Rep.* 2023;16:e251405.

43. Bonnin M, Mercier FJ, Sitbon O, et al. Severe pulmonary hypertension during pregnancy: mode of delivery and anesthetic management of 15 consecutive cases. *Anesthesiology.* 2005;102:1133–1137.

44. Zeldis SM. Dyspnea during pregnancy. Distinguishing cardiac from pulmonary causes. *Clin Chest Med.* 1992;13:567–585.

45. Lebel DE, Sergienko R, Wiznitzer A, et al. Mode of delivery and other pregnancy outcomes of patients with documented scoliosis. *J Matern Fetal Neonatal Med.* 2012;25:639–641.

46. Swany L, Larson AN, Shah SA, et al. Outcomes of pregnancy in operative vs. nonoperative adolescent idiopathic scoliosis patients at mean 30-year follow-up. *Spine Deform.* 2020;8:1169–1174.

47. Liljenqvist UR, Allkemper T, Hackenberg L, et al. Analysis of vertebral morphology in idiopathic scoliosis with use of magnetic resonance imaging and multiplanar reconstruction. *J Bone Joint Surg Am.* 2002;84:359–368.

48. Chin KJ, Perlas A, Chan V. The ultrasound-assisted paraspinous approach to lumbar neuraxial blockade: a simplified technique in patients with difficult anatomy. *Acta Anaesthesiol Scand.* 2015;59:668–673.

49. Ekinci M, Alici HA, Ahiskalioglu A, et al. The use of ultrasound in planned cesarean delivery under spinal anesthesia for patients having nonprominent anatomic landmarks. *J Clin Anesth.* 2017;37:82–85.

50. Chin KJ, Perlas A, Chan V, et al. Ultrasound imaging facilitates spinal anesthesia in adults with difficult surface anatomic landmarks. *Anesthesiology.* 2011;115:94–101.

51. Boon JM, Prinsloo E, Raath RP. A paramedian approach for epidural block: an anatomic and radiologic description. *Reg Anesth Pain Med.* 2003;28:221–227.

52. Creaney M, Mullane D, Casby C, Tan T. Ultrasound to identify the lumbar space in women with impalpable bony landmarks presenting for elective caesarean delivery under spinal anaesthesia: a randomised trial. *Int J Obstet Anesth.* 2016;28:12–16.

53. Park SK, Bae J, Yoo S, et al. Ultrasound-assisted versus landmark-guided spinal anesthesia in patients with abnormal spinal anatomy: a randomized controlled trial. *Anesth Analg.* 2020;130:787–795.

54. Grabala P, Helenius I, Buchowski JM, et al. Back pain and outcomes of pregnancy after instrumented spinal fusion for adolescent idiopathic scoliosis. *World Neurosurg.* 2019;124:e404–e410.

55. Faloon M, Sahai N, Pierce TP, et al. Incidence of neuraxial abnormalities is approximately 8% among patients with adolescent idiopathic scoliosis: a meta-analysis. *Clin Orthop Relat Res.* 2018;476:1506–1513.

56. Bauchat JR, McCarthy RJ, Koski TR, Wong CA. Labor analgesia consumption and time to neuraxial catheter placement in women with a history of surgical correction for scoliosis: a case-matched study. *Anesth Analg.* 2015;121:981–987.

57. Ko JY, Leffert LR. Clinical implications of neuraxial anesthesia in the parturient with scoliosis. *Anesth Analg.* 2009;109:1930–1934.

58. Chau A, Bibbo C, Huang CC, et al. Dural puncture epidural technique improves labor analgesia quality with fewer side effects compared with epidural and combined spinal epidural techniques: a randomized clinical trial. *Anesth Analg.* 2017;124:560–569.

59. Reghunath A, Ghasi RG, Aggarwal A. Unveiling the tale of the tail: an illustration of spinal dysraphisms. *Neurosurg Rev.* 2021;44:97–114.

60. Murphy CJ, Stanley E, Kavanagh E, et al. Spinal dysraphisms in the parturient: Implications for perioperative anaesthetic care and labour analgesia. *Int J Obstet Anesth.* 2015;24:252–263.

61. Copp AJ, Stanier P, Greene ND. Neural tube defects: recent advances, unsolved questions, and controversies. *Lancet Neurol.* 2013;12:799–810.

62. Lowry RB, Bedard T, MacFarlane AJ, et al. Prevalence rates of spina bifida in Alberta, Canada: 2001-2015. Can we achieve more prevention? *Birth Defects Res.* 2019;111:151–158.

63. Mai CT, Isenburg JL, Canfield MA, et al. National population-based estimates for major birth defects, 2010–2014. *Birth Defects Res.* 2019;111:1420–1435.

64. Paslaru FG, Panaitescu AM, Iancu G, et al. Myelomeningocele surgery over the 10 years following the MOMS trial: a systematic review of outcomes in prenatal versus postnatal surgical repair. *Medicina (Kaunas).* 2021;57:707.

65. Pruthi V, Abbasi N, Ryan G, et al. Fetal surgery for open spina bifida in Canada: initial results. *J Obstet Gynaecol Can.* 2021;43:733–739.e1.

66. Fremion EJ, Dosa NP. Spina bifida transition to adult healthcare guidelines. *J Pediatr Rehabil Med*. 2019;12:423–429.

67. Bendt M, Gabrielsson H, Riedel D, et al. Adults with spina bifida: a cross-sectional study of health issues and living conditions. *Brain Behav*. 2020;10:e01736.

68. Conklin MJ, Kishan S, Nanayakkara CB, Rosenfeld SR. Orthopedic guidelines for the care of people with spina bifida. *J Pediatr Rehabil Med*. 2020;13:629–635.

69. Trapp B, de Andrade Lourenção Freddi T, de Oliveira Morais Hans M, et al. A practical approach to diagnosis of spinal dysraphism. *Radiographics*. 2021;41:559–575.

70. Bevan R, Leach P. Infected congenital cervical dermal sinuses leading to spinal cord abscess: two case reports and a review of the literature. *Childs Nerv Syst*. 2021;37:225–228.

71. Hertzler DA 2nd, DePowell JJ, Stevenson CB, Mangano FT. Tethered cord syndrome: a review of the literature from embryology to adult presentation. *Neurosurg Focus*. 2010;29:E1.

72. Singh S, Behari S, Singh V, et al. Dynamic magnetic resonance imaging parameters for objective assessment of the magnitude of tethered cord syndrome in patients with spinal dysraphism. *Acta Neurochir (Wien)*. 2019;161:147–159.

73. Yamada S, Won DJ, Pezeshkpour G, et al. Pathophysiology of tethered cord syndrome and similar complex disorders. *Neurosurg Focus*. 2007;23:E6.

74. Menezes AH, Seaman SC, Iii MAH, et al. Tethered spinal cord syndrome in adults in the MRI era: recognition, pathology, and long-term objective outcomes. *J Neurosurg Spine*. 2021;34:942–954.

75. Ahmad FU, Pandey P, Sharma BS, Garg A. Foot drop after spinal anesthesia in a patient with a low-lying cord. *Int J Obstet Anesth*. 2006;15:233–236.

76. Xue JX, Li B, Lan F. Accidental conus medullaris injury following combined epidural and spinal anesthesia in a pregnant woman with unknown tethered cord syndrome. *Chin Med J*. 2013;126:1188–1189.

77. Yamada S, Won DJ, Yamada SM, et al. Adult tethered cord syndrome: relative to spinal cord length and filum thickness. *Neurol Res*. 2004;26:732–734.

78. Royo-Salvador MB, Solé-Llenas J, Doménech JM, González-Adrio R. Results of the section of the filum terminale in 20 patients with syringomyelia, scoliosis and Chiari malformation. *Acta Neurochir (Wien)*. 2005;147:515–523.

79. Chantigian RC, Koehn MA, Ramin KD, Warner MA. Chiari I malformation in parturients. *J Clin Anesth*. 2002;14:201–205.

80. Landau R, Giraud R, Delrue V, Kern C. Spinal anesthesia for cesarean delivery in a woman with a surgically corrected type I Arnold Chiari malformation. *Anesth Analg*. 2003;97:253–255.

81. Sciscent BY, Bhanja D, Daggubati LC, et al. Pregnancy in spina bifida patients: a comparative analysis of peripartum procedures and complications. *Childs Nerv Syst*. 2023;39:625–632.

82. Sivarajah K, Ralph S, Sabaratnam R, Bakalis S. Spina bifida in pregnancy: a review of the evidence for preconception, antenatal, intrapartum and postpartum care. *Obstet Med*. 2019;12:14–21.

83. Tong CMC, Dew ME, Zimmerman KD, et al. A qualitative interview study on successful pregnancies in women with spina bifida. *J Pediatr Urol*. 2022;18:3.e1–e7.

84. Shepard CL, Yan PL, Kielb SJ, et al. Complications of delivery among mothers with spina bifida. *Urology*. 2019;123:280–286.

85. Sterling L, Keunen J, Wigdor E, et al. Pregnancy outcomes in women with spinal cord lesions. *J Obstet Gynaecol Can*. 2013;35:39–43.

86. Auger N, Arbour L, Schnitzer ME, et al. Pregnancy outcomes of women with spina bifida. *Disabil Rehabil*. 2019;41:1403–1409.

87. Katz R, McCaul CL. Anaesthetic management for caesarean section of a parturient with a known difficult airway and closed spinal dysraphism. *Int J Obstet Anesth*. 2019;38:137–142.

88. Wood GG, Jacka MJ. Spinal hematoma following spinal anesthesia in a patient with spina bifida occulta. *Anesthesiology*. 1997;87:983–984.

89. Altamimi Y, Pavy TJ. Epidural analgesia for labour in a patient with a neural tube defect. *Anaesth Intensive Care*. 2006;34:816–819.

90. Tidmarsh MD, May AE. Epidural anaesthesia and neural tube defects. *Int J Obstet Anesth*. 1998;7:111–114.

91. Kreeger RN, Hilvano A. Anesthetic options for the parturient with a neural tube defect. *Int Anesthesiol Clin*. 2005;43:65–80.

92. May AE, Fombon FN, Francis S. UK registry of high-risk obstetric anaesthesia: report on neurological disease. *Int J Obstet Anesth*. 2008;17:31–36.

93. Asakura Y, Kandatsu N, Hashimoto A, et al. Ultrasound-guided neuroaxial anesthesia: accurate diagnosis of spina bifida occulta by ultrasonography. *J Anesth*. 2009;23:312–313.

94. Doi M, Sakurai Y, Sakamaki D, et al. Ultrasonographic images of spina bifida before obstetric anesthesia: a case series. *BMC Anesthesiol*. 2023;23:134.

95. Waters JFR, O'Neal MA, Pilato M, et al. Management of anesthesia and delivery in women with Chiari I malformations. *Obstet Gynecol*. 2018;132:1180–1184.

96. Gruffi TR, Peralta FM, Thakkar MS, et al. Anesthetic management of parturients with Arnold Chiari malformation-1: a multicenter retrospective study. *Int J Obstet Anesth*. 2019;37:52–56.

97. Meneses V, Parenti S, Burns H, Adams R. Latex allergy guidelines for people with spina bifida. *J Pediatr Rehabil Med*. 2020;13:601–609.

98. Finckh A, Gilbert B, Hodkinson B, et al. Global epidemiology of rheumatoid arthritis. *Nat Rev Rheumatol*. 2022;18:591–602.

99. Sim BL, Daniel RS, Hong SS, et al. Pregnancy outcomes in women with rheumatoid arthritis: a systematic review and meta-analysis. *J Clin Rheumatol*. 2023;29:36–42.

100. Aletaha D, Neogi T, Silman AJ, et al. 2010 Rheumatoid arthritis classification criteria: an American College of Rheumatology/European League Against Rheumatism collaborative initiative. *Arthritis Rheum*. 2010;62:2569–2581.

101. Lebouille-Veldman AB, Spenkelink D, Allaart CF, Vleggeert-Lankamp CLA. The association between Disease Activity Score and rheumatoid arthritis-associated cervical deformity: radiological evaluation of the BeSt trial. *J Neurosurg Spine*. 2023;38:465–472.

102. Colebatch AN, Edwards CJ, Østergaard M, et al. EULAR recommendations for the use of imaging of the joints in the clinical management of rheumatoid arthritis. *Ann Rheum Dis*. 2013;72:804–814.

103. Keenan MA, Stiles CM, Kaufman RL. Acquired laryngeal deviation associated with cervical spine disease in erosive polyarticular arthritis. Use of the fiberoptic bronchoscope in rheumatoid disease. *Anesthesiology*. 1983;58:441–449.

104. Samanta R, Shoukrey K, Griffiths R. Rheumatoid arthritis and anaesthesia. *Anaesthesia*. 2011;66:1146–1159.

105. Jethwa H, Lam S, Smith C, Giles I. Does rheumatoid arthritis really improve during pregnancy? A systematic review and metaanalysis. *J Rheumatol*. 2019;46:245–250.

106. Littlejohn EA. Pregnancy and rheumatoid arthritis. *Best Pract Res Clin Obstet Gynaecol*. 2020;64:52–58.

107. Götestam Skorpen C, Hoeltzenbein M, Tincani A, et al. The EULAR points to consider for use of antirheumatic drugs before pregnancy, and during pregnancy and lactation. *Ann Rheum Dis*. 2016;75:795–810.

108. Sammaritano LR, Bermas BL, Chakravarty EE, et al. 2020 American College of Rheumatology Guideline for the management of reproductive health in rheumatic and musculoskeletal diseases. *Arthritis Rheumatol*. 2020;72:529–556.

109. Cai E, Czuzoj-Shulman N, Abenhaim HA. Maternal and fetal outcomes in pregnancies with long-term corticosteroid use. *J Matern Fetal Neonatal Med*. 2021;34:1797–1804.

110. Leino KA, Kuusniemi KS, Palve HK, et al. Spread of spinal block in patients with rheumatoid arthritis. *Acta Anaesthesiol Scand*. 2010;54:65–69.

111. Leino KA, Kuusniemi KS, Palve HK, et al. The effect of body mass index on the spread of spinal block in patients with rheumatoid arthritis. *J Anesth*. 2011;25:213–218.

112. Bennett AN, McGonagle D, O'Connor P, et al. Severity of baseline magnetic resonance imaging-evident sacroiliitis and HLA-B27 status in early inflammatory back pain predict radiographically evident ankylosing spondylitis at eight years. *Arthritis Rheum*. 2008;58:3413–3418.

113. Ward MM, Deodhar A, Gensler LS, et al. 2019 Update of the American College of Rheumatology/Spondylitis Association of America/Spondyloarthritis Research and Treatment Network recommendations for the treatment of ankylosing spondylitis and nonradiographic axial spondyloarthritis. *Arthritis Rheumatol*. 2019;71:1599–1613.

114. Rusman T, van Vollenhoven RF, van der Horst-Bruinsma IE. Gender differences in axial spondyloarthritis: women are not so lucky. *Curr Rheumatol Rep*. 2018;20:35.

115. Sorin S, Askari A, Moskowitz RW. Atlantoaxial subluxation as a complication of early ankylosing spondylitis. Two cases reports and a review of the literature. *Arthritis Rheum*. 1979;22:273–276.

116. Woodward LJ, Kam PC. Ankylosing spondylitis: recent developments and anaesthetic implications. *Anaesthesia*. 2009;64:540–548.

117. Giovannopoulou E, Gkasdaris G, Kapetanakis S, Kontomanolis E. Ankylosing spondylitis and pregnancy: a literature review. *Curr Rheumatol Rev*. 2017;13:162–169.

118. Mayle RE Jr, Cheng I, Carragee EJ. Thoracolumbar fracture dislocation sustained during childbirth in a patient with ankylosing spondylitis. *Spine J*. 2012;12:e5–e8.

119. Mokbel A, Lawson DO, Farrokhyar F. Pregnancy outcomes in women with ankylosing spondylitis: a scoping literature and methodological review. *Clin Rheumatol*. 2021;40:3465–3480.

120. Broomhead CJ, Davies W, Higgins D. Awake oral fibreoptic intubation for caesarean section. *Int J Obstet Anesth*. 1995;4:172–174.

121. Kumar CM, Mehta M. Ankylosing spondylitis: lateral approach to spinal anaesthesia for lower limb surgery. *Can J Anaesth*. 1995;42:73–76.

122. Batra YK, Sharma A, Rajeev S. Total spinal anaesthesia following epidural test dose in an ankylosing spondylitic patient with anticipated difficult airway undergoing total hip replacement. *Eur J Anaesthesiol*. 2006;23:897–898.

123. Hoffman SL, Zaphiratos V, Girard MA, et al. Failed epidural analgesia in a parturient with advanced ankylosing spondylitis: a novel explanation. *Can J Anaesth*. 2012;59:871–874.

124. Chin KJ, Chan V. Ultrasonography as a preoperative assessment tool: predicting the feasibility of central neuraxial blockade. *Anesth Analg*. 2010;110:252–253.

125. Dardenne E, Ishiyama N, Lin TA, Lucas MC. Current and emerging therapies for achondroplasia: the dawn of precision medicine. *Bioorg Med Chem*. 2023;87 117275.

126. Carstoniu J, Yee I, Halpern SH. Epidural anaesthesia for caesarean section in an achondroplastic dwarf. *Can J Anaesth*. 1992;39:708–711.

127. Wynne-Davies R, Walsh WK, Gormley J. Achondroplasia and hypochondroplasia. Clinical variation and spinal stenosis. *J Bone Joint Surg Br*. 1981;63B:508–515.

128. Kim JH, Woodruff BC, Girshin M. Anesthetic considerations in patients with achondroplasia. *Cureus*. 2021;13:e15832.

129. Harada D, Namba N, Hanioka Y, et al. Final adult height in long-term growth hormone-treated achondroplasia patients. *Eur J Pediatr*. 2017;176:873–879.

130. BioMarin Pharmaceutical. *Voxzogo (vosoritide) [package insert]*. U.S. Food and Drug Administration website. https://www.accessdata.fda.gov/drugsatfda_docs/label/2021/214938s000lbl.pdf. Accessed 28 July 2023.

131. Semler O, Rehberg M, Mehdiani N, et al. Current and emerging therapeutic options for the management of rare skeletal diseases. *Paediatr Drugs*. 2019;21:95–106.

132. Dubiel L, Scott GA, Agaram R, et al. Achondroplasia: anaesthetic challenges for caesarean section. *Int J Obstet Anesth*. 2014;23:274–278.

133. Beilin Y, Leibowitz AB. Anesthesia for an achondroplastic dwarf presenting for urgent cesarean section. *Int J Obstet Anesth*. 1993;2:96–97.

134. Morrow MJ, Black IH. Epidural anaesthesia for caesarean section in an achondroplastic dwarf. *Br J Anaesth*. 1998;81:619–621.

135. Huang J, Babins N. Anesthesia for cesarean delivery in an achondroplastic dwarf: a case report. *AANA J*. 2008;76:435–436.

136. Brimacombe JR, Caunt JA. Anaesthesia in a gravid achondroplastic dwarf. *Anaesthesia*. 1990;45:132–134.

137. Melekoglu R, Celik E, Eraslan S. Successful obstetric and anaesthetic management of a pregnant woman with achondroplasia. *BMJ Case Rep*. 2017;2017:bcr2017221238.

138. DeRenzo JS, Vallejo MC, Ramanathan S. Failed regional anesthesia with reduced spinal bupivacaine dosage in a parturient with achondroplasia presenting for urgent cesarean section. *Int J Obstet Anesth*. 2005;14:175–178.

139. Sharma R, Magoon R, Choudhary R, Khanna P. Anaesthesia for emergency caesarean section in a morbidly obese achondroplastic patient with PIH: feasibility of neuraxial anaesthesia? *Indian J Anaesth*. 2017;61:77–78.

140. Rao R, Cuthbertson D, Nagamani SCS, et al. Pregnancy in women with osteogenesis imperfecta: pregnancy characteristics, maternal, and neonatal outcomes. *Am J Obstet Gynecol MFM*. 2021;3:100362.

141. Zhytnik L, Simm K, Salumets A, et al. Reproductive options for families at risk of osteogenesis imperfecta: a review. *Orphanet J Rare Dis*. 2020;15:128.

142. Fiegel MJ. Cesarean delivery and colon resection in a patient with type III osteogenesis imperfecta. *Semin Cardiothorac Vasc Anesth*. 2011;15:98–101.

143. Vogel TM, Ratner EF, Thomas RC Jr, Chitkara U. Pregnancy complicated by severe osteogenesis imperfecta: a report of two cases. *Anesth Analg*. 2002;94:1315–1317.

144. Benca J, Hogan K. Malignant hyperthermia, coexisting disorders, and enzymopathies: risks and management options. *Anesth Analg.* 2009;109:1049–1053.

145. Bojanic K, Kivela JE, Gurrieri C, et al. Perioperative course and intraoperative temperatures in patients with osteogenesis imperfecta. *Eur J Anaesthesiol.* 2011;28:370–375.

146. Ralston SH, Gaston MS. Management of osteogenesis imperfecta. *Front Endocrinol (Lausanne).* 2019;10:924.

147. Pepe J, Body JJ, Hadji P, et al. Osteoporosis in premenopausal women: a clinical narrative review by the ECTS and the IOF. *J Clin Endocrinol Metab.* 2020;105:2487–2506.

148. Ruiter-Ligeti J, Czuzoj-Shulman N, Spence AR, et al. Pregnancy outcomes in women with osteogenesis imperfecta: a retrospective cohort study. *J Perinatol.* 2016;36:828–831.

149. Cozzolino M, Perelli F, Maggio L, et al. Management of osteogenesis imperfecta type I in pregnancy; a review of literature applied to clinical practice. *Arch Gynecol Obstet.* 2016;293:1153–1159.

150. Cho E, Dayan SS, Marx GF. Anaesthesia in a parturient with osteogenesis imperfecta. *Br J Anaesth.* 1992;68:422–423.

151. Murray S, Shamsuddin W, Russell R. Sequential combined spinal-epidural for caesarean delivery in osteogenesis imperfecta. *Int J Obstet Anesth.* 2010;19:127–128.

152. Yeo ST, Paech MJ. Regional anaesthesia for multiple caesarean sections in a parturient with osteogenesis imperfecta. *Int J Obstet Anesth.* 1999;8:284–287.

153. Dinges E, Ortner C, Bollag L, et al. Osteogenesis imperfecta: cesarean deliveries in identical twins. *Int J Obstet Anesth.* 2015;24:64–68.

154. Guglielminotti J, Rosenberg H, Li G. Prevalence of malignant hyperthermia diagnosis in obstetric patients in the United States, 2003 to 2014. *BMC Anesthesiol.* 2020;20:19.

155. Hopkins PM, Girard T, Dalay S, et al. Malignant hyperthermia 2020: guideline from the Association of Anaesthetists. *Anaesthesia.* 2021;76:655–664.

156. Litman RS, Griggs SM, Dowling JJ, Riazi S. Malignant hyperthermia susceptibility and related diseases. *Anesthesiology.* 2018;128:159–167.

157. European Malignant Hyperthermia Working Group. https://www.emhg.org/diagnostic-mutations. Accessed 18 July 2023.

158. Allen GC, Larach MG, Kunselman AR. The sensitivity and specificity of the caffeine-halothane contracture test: a report from the North American Malignant Hyperthermia Registry. The North American Malignant Hyperthermia Registry of MHAUS. *Anesthesiology.* 1998;88:579–588.

159. Ellinas H, Albrecht MA. Malignant hyperthermia update. *Anesthesiol Clin.* 2020;38:165–181.

160. Leary NP, Ellis FR. Masseteric muscle spasm as a normal response to suxamethonium. *Br J Anaesth.* 1990;64:488–492.

161. Riazi S, Kraeva N, Hopkins PM. Updated guide for the management of malignant hyperthermia. *Can J Anaesth.* 2018;65:709–721.

162. Weingarten AE, Korsh JI, Neuman GG, Stern SB. Postpartum uterine atony after intravenous dantrolene. *Anesth Analg.* 1987;66:269–270.

163. Shin YK, Kim YD, Collea JV, Belcher MD. Effect of dantrolene sodium on contractility of isolated human uterine muscle. *Int J Obstet Anesth.* 1995;4:197–200.

164. Fricker RM, Hoerauf KH, Drewe J, Kress HG. Secretion of dantrolene into breast milk after acute therapy of a suspected malignant hyperthermia crisis during cesarean section. *Anesthesiology.* 1998;89:1023–1025.

165. Schuster F, Johannsen S. Malignant hyperthermia and pregnancy – guidelines of the European Malignant Hyperthermia Group. *Anasthesiol Intensivmed Notfallmed Schmerzther.* 2021;56:367–372.

166. Malignant Hyperthermia Association of the United States. Parturient with an MHS partner. https://www.mhaus.org/healthcare-professionals/mhaus-recommendations/parturient-with-mhs-partner/. Accessed 18 July 2023.

167. Litman RS, Smith VI, Larach MG, et al. Consensus statement of the Malignant Hyperthermia Association of the United States on unresolved clinical questions concerning the management of patients with malignant hyperthermia. *Anesth Analg.* 2019;128:652–659.

47

Neurologic and Neuromuscular Disease

Grace Lim, MD, MS

CHAPTER OUTLINE

The choice of anesthetic technique for pregnant women with neurologic disease requires knowledge of the pathophysiology of the disorder and an understanding of controversies involved in the diagnosis and management of the disease. If a patient's neurologic condition deteriorates postpartum, the cause may be unclear, and the anesthetic technique may be blamed unfairly. There are limited published data on specific neurologic and neuromuscular disorders in pregnant women. However, few of these disorders contraindicate the use of neuraxial anesthesia. In most cases, the obstetric provider should obtain early antepartum consultation from an anesthesia provider. Early consultation allows accurate antepartum documentation of the extent and pattern of the neurologic deficit as well as discussion and formulation of the anesthetic plan with the patient, her obstetric provider, and a neurologist or neurosurgeon.

Because patients with a wide variety of neurologic disorders will present for preoperative evaluation, the following thought process will assist the clinician with completing a proper evaluation and formulating an anesthetic plan.

What is the basic pathophysiology of the neurologic disorder? Neurologic disorders may be stable, progressive, or relapsing/recurrent. It is important to understand the common disease patterns. The potential for progression of the disease after delivery will depend on the pattern of progression and underlying pathophysiology, and on the effect of pregnancy on disease progression.

What is the patient's history and current findings after neurologic examination? A history should include the onset date and current course of the disorder. Symptoms related to neurologic issues should be documented (e.g., seizure type and frequency, deficits after cerebrovascular events, cognitive deficits). A basic physical examination should be conducted to document existing deficit patterns, including cognitive dysfunction (e.g., ability to understand and cooperate), deficits involving vision, hearing, speech, and swallowing; respiratory symptoms; and weakness and sensory deficits in the head and neck, trunk, and extremities. Motor and sensory deficits are classified as mild, moderate, or severe, with a description of the affected area. Special attention should be directed to limitations in ambulatory ability (e.g., bed-bound, wheelchair, walking with assistance) or positioning.

What are the current treatments, and what testing results are available? Documentation of medical and non-medical therapies is essential. For some disorders (e.g., myasthenia gravis), documentation of the timing of treatment is also critical. In most cases, specific laboratory testing will not influence anesthetic management and outcome. However, pulmonary function testing should be considered in patients with neurologic disorders associated with respiratory compromise; the findings may assist the anesthesia provider in making recommendations about anesthetic management.

What is the impact of the neurologic disorder on other organ systems (e.g., cardiac, respiratory, airway)? The patient's neurologic disease may affect organ systems that are relevant to the anesthetic plan. For example, central core disease is associated with a risk for malignant hyperthermia. In addition, progressive neurologic disorders may significantly compromise the patient's respiratory status, thereby increasing the risks associated with neuraxial and general anesthesia.

What are the potential impacts, risks, and benefits of anesthetic options based on the disease's pathophysiology, symptoms, and treatment? Can treatment be initiated before delivery that will improve outcome? For most rare neurologic disorders, there is limited evidence on which to base decisions about anesthetic management. In these cases, the anesthesia provider should consider the disease's basic pathophysiology and its possible direct and indirect interactions with specific anesthetic techniques. Encouraging the obstetric provider to send these patients for early antepartum consultation will enable the anesthesia provider to obtain formal input from a neurologist or other consultant if necessary. A multidisciplinary discussion that includes the patient and her family may be necessary to weigh the risks and benefits of specific obstetric and anesthesia plans. A team approach to peripartum care in patients with complex neurologic disorders is essential.

What are the plans for postpartum management of the patient's disease? Will the intrapartum anesthetic **management or postpartum analgesia management influence outcomes?** Some conditions, such as multiple sclerosis, can have significant implications for the postpartum period. The anticipated progress of the disease and planned postpartum management should be discussed with the patient in the antenatal period.

In all cases, accurate documentation of the responses to the previous questions will greatly assist the team providing peripartum care for these patients. Some of the more common neurologic conditions are addressed in this chapter, and the existing literature is surveyed relative to the peripartum management. This knowledge allows the anesthesia provider an opportunity to formulate a safe and rational anesthetic plan and enables an appropriate discussion with the patient regarding the risks and benefits of anesthetic options.

MULTIPLE SCLEROSIS

Multiple sclerosis is a major cause of neurologic disability in young adults, and it is at least two to three times more common in females than in males.[1] First-time symptoms typically manifest in the second or third decade of life; therefore, the disease typically presents in females in their reproductive years.[2] The prevalence of the disorder varies with the population, and may be as high as 300 per 100,000 in some parts of North America, although the accuracy of epidemiologic estimates has been limited by heterogeneous methods for identifying people with disease and by different data analytic strategies.[1]

The disease is characterized by variable neurologic disabilities with two general patterns of presentation: (1) **exacerbating remitting**, accounting for 85% of cases, in which attacks appear abruptly and resolve over several months; and (2) **chronic progressive**, in which continued deterioration occurs over time.[3] The relapse rate varies significantly among patients, averaging approximately 0.4 attacks per year; this rate reflects the large proportion of patients with relapsing/remitting disease. The deficits tend to become more progressive and debilitating over time. Environmental factors (e.g., stress, infection, increased body temperature) may provoke a relapse. Most relapses reproduce previously experienced neurologic deficits, which can manifest as pyramidal, cerebellar, or brainstem symptoms. It is estimated that about half of affected individuals with exacerbating remitting disease will eventually convert to chronic progressive.[3]

The etiology remains unclear, although it is widely believed to be autoimmune in nature.[4] There is a clinically significant heritable component, and alleles in the human leukocyte antigen locus have been identified as risk factors for multiple sclerosis.[5] Pathologic findings include local inflammation, demyelination, gliotic scarring, and axonal loss; on magnetic resonance imaging (MRI), the formation of gray and white matter plaques is seen.[4] It is possible that the disease results from a yet undetermined combination of genetic predisposition and exposure to specific environmental factors. The more common symptoms include motor weakness, impaired vision, ataxia, bladder and bowel dysfunction, and emotional lability.

Although there is no cure, over the last two decades, relapsing/remitting multiple sclerosis has become a treatable disease as a result of advancements in disease-modifying therapies.[2] Immunosuppressive therapies may hasten recovery from a relapse, but no evidence suggests that these agents influence the progressive course of the disease. Administration of interferon-beta may significantly reduce the relapse rate and retard disability; however, an increased risk for fetal loss and low birth weight has been observed with the use of this therapy during the first trimester of pregnancy. In contrast, administration of intravenous immunoglobulin or plasmapheresis for severe relapses has no known adverse effects on pregnancy outcome.[2] Acute relapses during pregnancy are treated with short courses of high-dose corticosteroids, although longer-term use may be associated with maternal glucose intolerance, neonatal adrenal suppression, cleft palate if used in the first trimester, and an increased risk for premature rupture of membranes.[3]

Interaction With Pregnancy

The effects of multiple sclerosis and long-term use of disease-modifying therapies on fertility are poorly studied. A prospective study in Finland showed that women with multiple sclerosis were more likely to need artificial insemination to initiate pregnancy than women in general.[6] A large Danish national cohort study found that multiple sclerosis was associated with having no or fewer children[7]; however, it is not known whether this is caused by the disease itself or by altered reproductive behaviors among diseased individuals. In one study of women with multiple sclerosis undergoing assisted reproductive technology, failed assisted reproductive attempts were associated with increased annual relapse rates.[8] These findings may be explained by the stress of infertility, temporary interruption in disease-modifying therapy, and increases in inflammatory cytokines associated with hormonal therapies.

Pregnancy and obstetric outcomes in women with multiple sclerosis are likely no different from individuals without disease. One cohort study compared 198 affected women with 1584 healthy women; the number of maternal complications was not higher in women with multiple sclerosis.[9] However, infants of women with multiple sclerosis were at greater risk for meconium aspiration.[9] This finding may reflect an intrauterine environment in patients with multiple sclerosis that is more susceptible to acute hypoxic events.[7,9] A subsequent cohort study of 649 pregnancies in women with multiple sclerosis concluded that infants of these women were more likely to be small for gestational age, attributed to a suboptimal intrauterine environment.[10] Moreover, this study found that mothers with multiple sclerosis were more likely to undergo induction of labor and operative delivery, possibly as a result of neuromuscular weakness and spasticity. These findings have not been reproduced in other studies. A 2017 UK case-controlled study of 181 pregnancies in 98 mothers with multiple sclerosis and 244,573 pregnancies in 124,830 mothers without multiple sclerosis did not find any associations with neonatal birth weight, gestational age at birth,

mode of delivery, stillbirth, or neonatal death.[11] A 2011 meta-analysis did not find significant associations between multiple sclerosis and adverse obstetric and neonatal outcomes.[12] The relapse rate was lower during pregnancy than before or after pregnancy.

Data from prospective studies suggest that the rate of relapse increases during the first 3 months postpartum compared with the year before pregnancy.[13] Relapses during this period were more likely in women who had higher relapse rates in the year before pregnancy or during pregnancy. Stress, exhaustion, infection, the loss of antenatal immunosuppression, and the postpartum decline in concentrations of reproductive hormones may account for the higher postpartum relapse rate. Treatment with immunologically active agents (e.g., interferon-beta) may result in a decreased postpartum relapse rate, but data are limited.[13]

Pregnancy does not negatively affect the long-term outcome of multiple sclerosis. Data are conflicting as to whether exclusive breastfeeding is associated with a lower risk for relapse than partial or no breastfeeding.[14,15] A 2015 prospective study in 201 German women found a modestly protective effect against relapses among women with multiple sclerosis who exclusively breastfed for at least 2 months (first postpartum relapse adjusted hazard ratio, 1.70; 95% confidence interval [CI], 1.02 to 2.85; $P = .04$).[16]

Anesthetic Management

The anesthesia provider should assess the patient's level of compromise, document the pattern of deficits, and give special attention to respiratory involvement, in particular the ability to cough, clear secretions, and take vital capacity breaths. Historically, the optimal mode of anesthesia in patients with multiple sclerosis has been controversial. Most anesthesia providers have considered general anesthesia to be safe. Many anesthesia providers have been reluctant to administer neuraxial anesthesia because the effect of local anesthetic drugs on the course of the disease is unclear. Some anesthesia providers have expressed concern that neuraxial anesthesia may expose demyelinated areas of the spinal cord to potentially neurotoxic effects of local anesthetic agents. Several animal studies have investigated the histologic effects of local anesthetic agents on the normal spinal cord. In one study, subarachnoid injection of small doses of a local anesthetic agent produced no histologic changes in the spinal cord or meninges.[17] Injection of very large doses caused reversible inflammatory and degenerative changes, but all changes resolved within 14 days of injection.

Diagnostic lumbar puncture is not associated with a higher rate of relapse. Historically, two small reports implicated spinal anesthesia in the exacerbation of multiple sclerosis.[18,19] Bamford et al.[18] described one case of relapse after the administration of spinal anesthesia in nine patients, and Stenuit and Marchand[19] identified two cases of relapse after the administration of spinal anesthesia in 19 patients. Notably, there was no evidence to suggest that these relapses were related to spinal anesthesia, rather than to other factors known to exacerbate multiple sclerosis such as postoperative conditions (e.g., stress, infection, hyperpyrexia) or simply the postpartum period. Two larger observational studies have not found an association between neuraxial analgesia and anesthesia and an increased risk of postpartum relapse.[20,21] One observational cohort study found that postpartum relapse was primarily a function of disease activity, but was not associated with neuraxial procedures during labor and delivery.[22]

Available data on relapse outcomes associated with epidural analgesia and anesthesia in patients with multiple sclerosis show some cases of relapse, as would be expected. Bader et al.[23] retrospectively evaluated 32 pregnancies in women with multiple sclerosis; they observed that women who received epidural anesthesia for vaginal delivery did not have a higher incidence of relapse than those who received only local infiltration anesthesia. The Pregnancy in Multiple Sclerosis study followed 227 women who had multiple sclerosis for at least 1 year before conception, of whom 42 received epidural analgesia during labor; no adverse effect of epidural analgesia on the rate of postpartum relapse or the progression of disability was identified.[13] Similarly, a 2012 prospective study that followed 349 patients for 5 years postpartum did not find an increased risk for relapse associated with labor epidural analgesia.[24] A 2013 record linkage study from British Columbia compared 431 deliveries in women with multiple sclerosis who received peripartum epidural analgesia/anesthesia versus 2959 deliveries in women from the general population, and 128 women with multiple sclerosis who received spinal anesthesia for cesarean delivery versus 846 women in the general population; neither neuraxial technique was associated with increased disability.[25]

Although there are limited data on spinal and general anesthesia for cesarean delivery in patients with multiple sclerosis, they are both considered safe, and prior concerns over these techniques are attributable to recall bias associated with postpartum relapses after regional anesthesia.[3] No data suggest harmful effects of neuraxial opioids in women with multiple sclerosis. Considering the significant benefits of neuraxial techniques for intraoperative anesthesia and postoperative analgesia, either spinal or epidural anesthesia is the principal anesthetic technique used for cesarean delivery in patients with multiple sclerosis in many institutions.

In summary, published data do not contraindicate the use of neuraxial anesthetic techniques for labor analgesia or operative anesthesia. The patient should be aware that there is a higher incidence of relapse during the postpartum period, even without the use of neuraxial analgesia or anesthesia. In addition, when anesthetic techniques are used, the type of anesthesia selected does not appear to influence the relapse rate. Neither pregnancy nor anesthesia appears to have a negative influence on the long-term course of the disease. The willingness of anesthesia providers to use neuraxial techniques in pregnant patients with multiple sclerosis is reflected in a survey of obstetric anesthesiologists in the United Kingdom published in 2006.[26] The majority (91%) of respondents had seen fewer than 10 cases of multiple sclerosis in the past 10 years; 79% and 98% of anesthesia providers indicated they would perform a neuraxial anesthetic technique for labor and elective cesarean delivery, respectively.

HEADACHES DURING PREGNANCY

Headaches are among the most frequently observed neurologic symptoms during pregnancy (Table 47.1). Tension headaches, migraine headaches, and headaches associated with hypertensive disorders of pregnancy are commonly observed during pregnancy. *De novo* primary headaches (e.g., tension and migraine) are very common during pregnancy, particularly in the first few months of pregnancy;

TABLE 47.1	Headaches During Pregnancy		
Etiology	**Symptoms**	**Pattern**	**Treatment**
Tension headache	Dull, widespread headache	Increased incidence during peripartum period	Analgesics Tricyclic antidepressants
Migraine headache	Frontotemporal throbbing Prodrome of scotomata	Improvement in 79% of patients during pregnancy	Ergotamine contraindicated during pregnancy Promethazine Beta-adrenergic receptor antagonist for prophylaxis
Preeclampsia	Generalized headache Occasional scotomata and/or blurred vision	Occurrence during pregnancy and occasionally postpartum	Blood pressure control Delivery
Meningeal irritation (subarachnoid hemorrhage, meningitis)	Generalized headache	Increased risk for subarachnoid hemorrhage during pregnancy	Based on etiology
Brain tumor	Variable	No increase in incidence during pregnancy; possible increased growth rate	Based on etiology
Idiopathic intracranial hypertension	Generalized headache Visual symptoms	Increased incidence and worsened symptoms during pregnancy	Typically remits within 1–3 mo or after childbirth

however, new headaches in the third trimester and puerperium should prompt closer evaluation for secondary causes.[27] A pregnant patient with a history of chronic headaches who reports new or different symptoms should be closely evaluated to exclude serious causes such as preeclampsia, tumor, or intracranial vascular malformation. Features of concern include sudden onset, intense severity, altered mental status, meningeal signs, fever, vomiting, changes in vision, pulsatile tinnitus, prior malignancy or human immunodeficiency virus infection, and any localizing or lateralizing abnormality. Diagnostic neuroimaging options of computerized tomography and MRI, with or without contrast and angiography, may be used with minimal fetal radiation exposure and no association with fetal abnormalities.[27]

Tension Headaches

Tension or muscle contraction headaches are the most common type of headache observed during pregnancy. The symptoms typically consist of dull, persistent pain that extends over the entire head. The onset is usually gradual, but the symptoms may persist for long periods. Although the etiology is unknown, this type of headache is believed to be associated with stress rather than hormonal changes. These headaches are more common in women, are frequently associated with anxiety, and may be a symptom of postpartum depression.[28]

Treatment

Acetaminophen (paracetamol) should be used as a first-line analgesic in the pregnant patient. **Caffeine** and **butalbital** may be contained in some combination analgesic products. The American College of Obstetricians and Gynecologists (ACOG) has concluded that there is no clear evidence that caffeine exposure increases the risk for fetal growth restriction.[29] Because a definitive conclusion regarding high caffeine intake and the risk for miscarriage cannot be made, the ACOG recommends caffeine be limited to moderate consumption (<200 mg/day) during pregnancy. Butalbital is sometimes prescribed for treatment of migraine and tension headaches, but its appropriateness has been questioned given increased risks for abuse, overuse headache, and withdrawal. Data from the National Birth Defects Prevention Study, an ongoing case-control study, suggest that butalbital exposure in pregnancy is associated with an increased risk for congenital heart abnormalities, including tetralogy of Fallot, pulmonic stenosis, and atrial septal defect.[30] Butalbital use, however, was rare; only 73 case mothers and 15 control mothers reported periconceptional use.[31]

Ergot alkaloids (e.g., **ergotamine**) are contraindicated during pregnancy; these agents may cause marked increases in uterine tone, which may compromise placental perfusion and fetal oxygenation.[31] Use of **nonsteroidal antiinflammatory drugs (NSAIDs)** should be limited during the third trimester because of risks for premature closure of the fetal ductus arteriosus, oligohydramnios, and prolongation of pregnancy. **Opioids** have a long record of use during pregnancy, but because of escalated use and abuse and

their association with neonatal opioid withdrawal syndrome with long-term maternal exposure, their prescription during pregnancy and the puerperium is undergoing increasing scrutiny.[32] **Tricyclic antidepressants** have a record of safe use during pregnancy. Although earlier studies reported links between tricyclic antidepressant use during pregnancy and congenital malformations, most subsequent larger studies have been negative.[33]

Obstetric and Anesthetic Management

Pregnancy is not likely to reduce the frequency or severity of tension headaches because they are not hormonally mediated. Obstetric and anesthetic management are rarely affected by the presence of tension headaches, although a history of any headaches or migraines has been associated with an increased risk for placental abruption (adjusted odds ratio [aOR], 1.60; 95% CI, 1.16 to 2.20).[34] The frequency and severity of tension headaches should be assessed and documented in the preanesthetic assessment to better differentiate preexisting symptoms from new or changing symptoms in the postpartum period.

Migraine Headaches

A migraine headache is classically described as a unilateral, throbbing headache sometimes accompanied by nausea and vomiting. The duration varies from hours to days. Visual disturbances (e.g., scotomata) typically precede onset, and focal neurologic symptoms (e.g., aphasia, hemiplegia) may also occur. Most neurologists favor neurovascular vasospasm, followed by cerebral vasodilation, as a cause of these headaches; a primary vascular disorder or a disturbance in the noradrenergic nervous system also may be involved. Patients appear to be more susceptible to symptoms when serotonin levels are low.

The 1-year period prevalence of migraine headaches in the United States is 3.9% for men and 5.1% for women.[35] Prevalence is higher in middle life, between 30 and 59 years of age. Hormonal influences have a strong association with migraine headaches; estrogen withdrawal is associated with an exacerbation of symptoms. After delivery, the reduction in hormonal concentrations coincides with an increase in migraine symptoms.

Reversible cerebral vasoconstriction syndrome (RCVS), characterized by acute and severe headache secondary to multifocal cerebral artery vasoconstriction, is often misclassified as a migraine. An estimated 10% of RCVS cases occur in the peripartum period and have been associated with preeclampsia. Diagnosis is by magnetic resonance angiography with digital subtraction, and treatment involves **calcium channel blockers**, **aspirin**, and lifelong monitoring for future risk for stroke.[36-39]

Treatment

In nonpregnant patients, therapy centers around prevention, abortive treatments, and rescue treatments. Preventive medications are typically avoided during pregnancy; **beta-adrenergic receptor antagonists** (e.g., **propranolol**) may be used for prophylaxis; however, owing to their ability to cross the placenta, these agents should be used only when a patient's symptoms are severe. Antidepressants such as **selective serotonin reuptake inhibitors** can be used off-label for migraine prevention, although fetal exposure to some antidepressants has been controversially linked to congenital anomalies and adverse neonatal outcomes (see Chapters 16 and 49).[33,40,41] Abortive treatments often involve **triptans** or **ergotamine tartrate**, typically in combination with **caffeine**. However, ergot alkaloids are contraindicated during pregnancy because of associated uterotonic effects and possible (but unproven) teratogenic effects.[31,42] The use of **sumatriptan** or other selective serotonin receptor agonists is controversial. A higher incidence of congenital anomalies was observed after administration of high doses of sumatriptan in animals[42]; however, in a review of human studies, no evidence of any specific adverse effect of sumatriptan on pregnancy outcome was found.[43] A prospective study also showed no relationship between triptan use for migraine and teratogenicity.[44]

Rescue treatments are given when abortive therapies fail and include **acetaminophen**, **antiemetics**, and **NSAIDs**. In general, acetaminophen is considered the first-line treatment during pregnancy. Combination therapy with agents containing caffeine and/or butalbital should be used with caution, as should therapy with NSAIDs (see earlier discussion). Occasionally, **calcium entry–blocking agents** or **metoclopramide** are used.

Obstetric and Anesthetic Management

Women with a lifetime history of migraine have been reported to have a twofold higher risk for placental abruption. Pregnant women with migraines are at four times higher risk for developing preeclampsia, as well as at higher risk for stroke during pregnancy and the puerperium, although the data are limited.[45–48] Cerebral ischemia has been reported after the administration of **terbutaline** in pregnant patients with a migraine, although it continues to be used clinically for tocolysis.[49]

Although there are no published data on the relationship between intrapartum anesthesia and postpartum migraine headaches, one cohort study suggested that patients with a prior history of migraines may be more likely to present with atypical symptoms of post–dural puncture headache (PDPH), including nonpostural headache; cervical, thoracic, or lumbar vertebral stiffness and pain; and vertigo.[50] The association between a history of migraines and risk for PDPH is unclear.[51]

SPINAL CORD INJURY

Worldwide, there are large geographic differences in the incidence, prevalence, and lethality of spinal cord injuries.[52] Improved handling and stabilization of victims at the site of an accident and the availability of extensive rehabilitation services have resulted in more women who present for obstetric care after spinal cord injury than in the past.

Patient disability and residual function depend on the anatomic location of the injury.[53] Cord injuries below the S2 level involve mainly bladder, bowel, and sexual functions. Affected patients have relaxed perineal muscles, and women with such injuries experience labor pain. Women with a lesion above T10 do not experience labor pain. Patients with a lesion above T6 have varying levels of respiratory compromise and are at risk for autonomic hyperreflexia (see later discussion).

Spinal shock, defined as immediate and temporary areflexia/hyporeflexia and transient sensorimotor dysfunction resolving within 24 to 48 hours after injury, may develop in about half of spinal cord–injured patients.[54] Patients with injuries at or above the T6 level are at risk for **neurogenic shock** caused by loss of signals from the sympathetic nervous system. This is characterized by hemodynamic and sensorimotor abnormalities and flaccid paralysis with loss of tendon and autonomic reflexes.[54] Patients experience loss of vasomotor tone, temperature regulation, sweating, and piloerection in the parts of the body below the lesion. Pulmonary edema, hemodynamic instability, and circulatory collapse can develop in the absence of brainstem regulation of vasomotor tone. Patients are at risk for aspiration, infection, and other pulmonary complications. Paraplegic patients may have a compensatory tachycardia, whereas quadriplegic patients may have bradycardia caused by unopposed vagal tone.

After a variable period, the spinal cord–injured patient progresses to a chronic stage in which reflex activity is regained. In most cases, this return of reflex activity occurs within 1 to 6 weeks after the injury; rarely, return of reflex activity may take several months. This stage is characterized by disuse atrophy, flexor spasms, and an exaggeration of reflexes. The **mass reflex** is a phenomenon in which a stimulus that normally would cause the contraction of a few muscle units leads to the widespread spasm of entire muscle groups. It results from the absence of central inhibitory mechanisms. The mass reflex can occur with any level of spinal cord injury. It may occur with autonomic hyperreflexia in a patient with a lesion above T6.

Approximately 85% of patients with chronic spinal cord injuries at or above T6 experience the syndrome of **autonomic hyperreflexia**.[54] This is a life-threatening complication that results from the absence of central inhibition on the sympathetic neurons in the cord below the injury. Noxious stimuli, including bladder or bowel distention and uterine contractions, result in afferent transmission by means of the dorsal spinal root (Fig. 47.1).[55] These afferent neurons synapse with sympathetic neurons, and the impulse is propagated both cephalad and caudad in the sympathetic chain, without central inhibition. The propagation results in extreme sympathetic hyperactivity and severe systemic hypertension secondary to vasoconstriction below the level of the lesion. In response, the reflex arcs involving the baroreceptors of the aortic and carotid bodies lead to bradycardia and vasodilation above the level of the lesion. In patients with lesions at T6 and above, these compensatory mechanisms are insufficient to compensate for the severe vasoconstriction below the level of the lesion. Intracranial hemorrhage, arrhythmias, and myocardial infarction occur in some cases. A variety of agents with different sites of action have been used for control of the hypertension of autonomic hyperreflexia (Fig. 47.2).

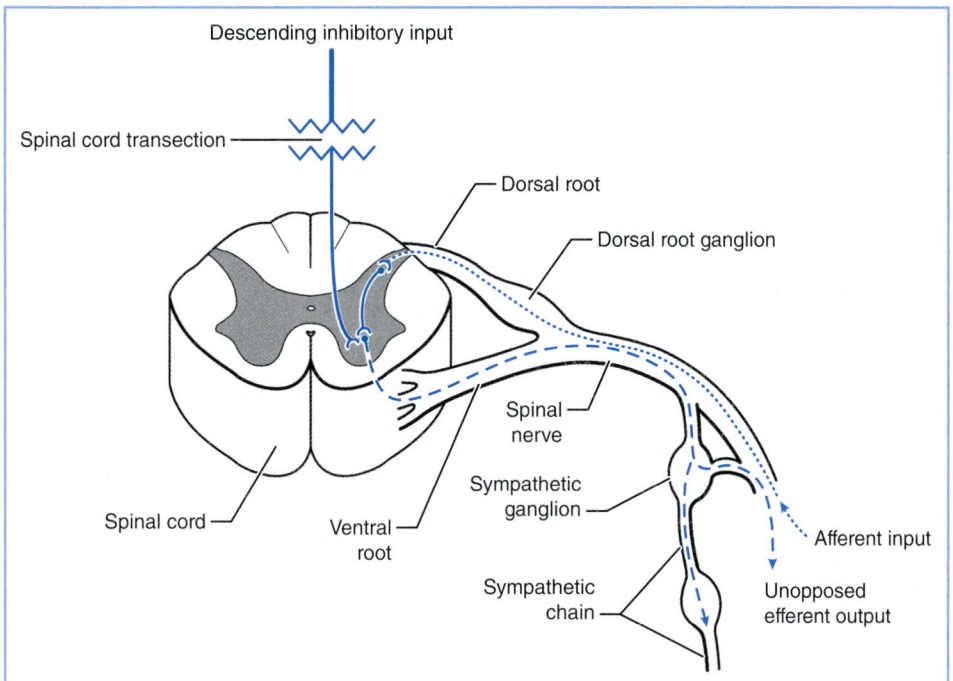

Fig. 47.1 Mechanism Involved in Autonomic Hyperreflexia. Noxious stimuli enter the dorsal horn of the spinal cord through the dorsal spinal root *(dotted line)*. These afferent neurons synapse either directly or by means of interneurons *(solid line)* with sympathetic neurons in the intermediolateral columns of the lateral horns, which then project through the anterior roots to the paraspinal sympathetic chain *(dashed line)*. The impulse is propagated peripherally at that spinal level and travels both cephalad and caudad in the sympathetic chain, exiting at multiple thoracic and lumbar levels *(dashed line)* and resulting in sympathetic hyperactivity. Illustration by Naveen Nathan, MD, NorthShore University HealthSystem, University of Chicago Pritzker School of Medicine, Evanston, IL.

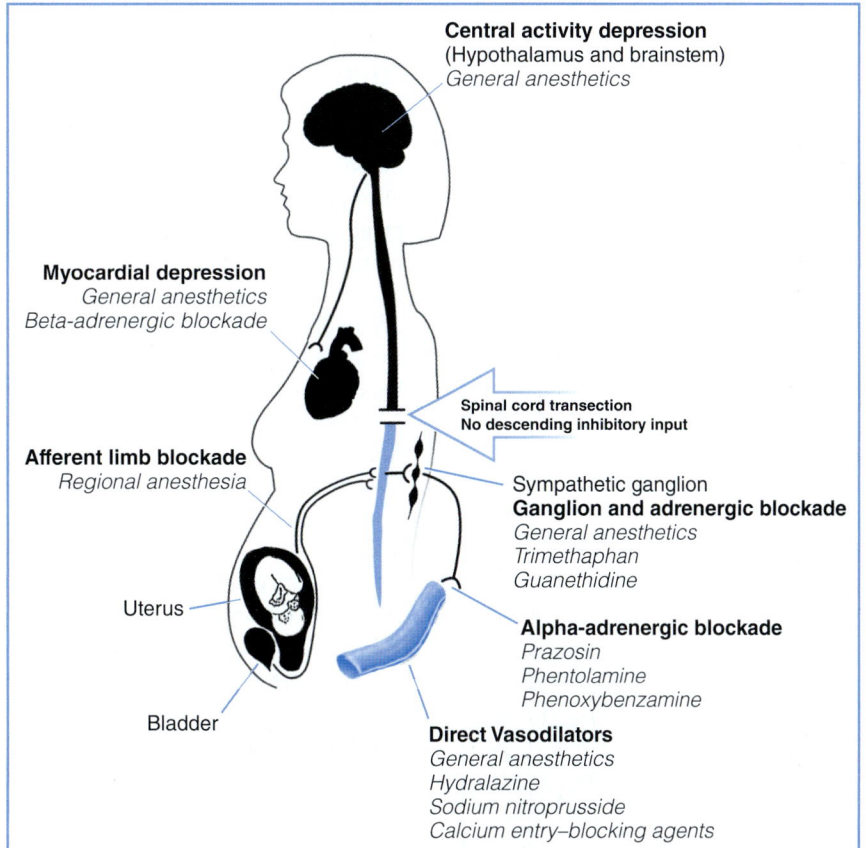

Fig. 47.2 Sites of action for agents used in the control of hypertension associated with autonomic hyperreflexia. Illustration by Naveen Nathan, MD, NorthShore University HealthSystem, University of Chicago Pritzker School of Medicine, Evanston, IL.

Obstetric Management

Although there is no estimate of the global incidence of pregnancy in women with spinal cord injury, the World Health Organization (WHO) estimates that nearly 18% of spinal cord injuries worldwide occur in women of reproductive age.[56] Pregnancy may aggravate many of the medical complications of spinal cord injury (Box 47.1).[55] The decreases in both functional residual capacity and expiratory reserve volume during pregnancy may increase the likelihood of respiratory compromise associated with spinal cord injury, with worsening of respiratory function occurring as early as 20 weeks' gestation. Patients may require tracheal intubation and mechanical ventilatory support, and cesarean delivery may be indicated to avert the fetal risks associated with maternal hypercapnia and to improve maternal respiratory mechanics. Complications of acute spinal cord injury in pregnancy include preterm birth and neonatal intensive care unit admission.[57,58]

Pregnancy increases the risks for thromboembolic complications and urinary tract infection. Loss of sympathetic tone below the level of the lesion renders pregnant patients with spinal cord injury particularly prone to orthostatic hypotension, which may result in reduced uteroplacental perfusion, necessitating careful monitoring of the fetal heart rate (FHR). In pregnant women, autonomic hyperreflexia occurs most commonly during labor; it may be triggered by uterine contractions, vaginal and cervical examinations, speculum insertion, and urethral catheterization. Autonomic hyperreflexia can be distinguished from other causes of intrapartum hypertension by the occurrence of cyclic hypertension (i.e., blood pressure increases during contractions and decreases between contractions). Symptoms of autonomic hyperreflexia are also common in the immediate postpartum period, possibly triggered by postpartum pain, urethral catheterization, and uterine contractions.[59]

Women with a lesion above T11 may be at higher risk for preterm labor.[53] Because these women do not experience labor pain, obstetric management includes weekly cervical examinations during the third trimester, and patients are instructed on uterine palpation techniques to detect contractions at home. Although vaginal delivery is preferred, the development of autonomic hyperreflexia in the second stage of labor may necessitate expedited operative vaginal delivery. Assisted vaginal delivery may also be necessary because of the inability of the mothers to push effectively during the second stage.[53] A case series of 109 births to patients with spinal cord injuries found predominantly favorable maternal and neonatal outcomes, with 37 (34%) undergoing cesarean delivery and 16 (15%) deliveries occurring preterm.[60]

Anesthetic Management

Antenatal anesthetic consultation and multidisciplinary planning are essential to optimize outcomes.[61] The ACOG recommends that a multidisciplinary team in a unit capable of intensive hemodynamic monitoring should deliver parturients with a spinal cord injury.[62] Early neuraxial anesthesia is preferred for the prevention or treatment of autonomic hyperreflexia during labor and delivery.[62] Although neuraxial labor analgesia may attenuate the risk and symptoms of autonomic hyperreflexia, it may not ablate the phenomenon entirely, particularly when low doses of local anesthetic are used.[59] Spinal anesthesia has long been reported as effective for controlling blood pressure in paraplegic patients undergoing general surgical procedures.[63] If spinal anesthesia is chosen, insertion of an intrathecal catheter and use of a continuous technique may be appropriate; this approach may allow careful titration of the resulting neuroblockade. Assessment of the level of blockade in an insensate patient may be accomplished by assessing for loss of lower extremity deep tendon reflexes and meticulous monitoring for acute hypertension and bradycardia.

Most obstetric anesthesia providers prefer the use of epidural analgesia for the prevention or treatment of autonomic hyperreflexia during labor and vaginal delivery. Consideration also should be given to providing epidural analgesia after vaginal delivery to minimize the possibility of autonomic hyperreflexia, which has been reported to occur in response to pain as late as 5 days after delivery.[64] Maintaining optimal analgesia with a transition to oral agents is important.

Case reports have historically described the successful epidural administration of 0.25% or 0.5% bupivacaine, or the administration of combined spinal-epidural (CSE) anesthesia for the mitigation of autonomic hyperreflexia.[65,66] Baraka[67] reported the successful use of epidural meperidine (pethidine), an opioid with local anesthetic properties, for controlling autonomic hyperreflexia. Abouleish et al.[68] observed that epidural fentanyl alone did not effectively treat the hypertension of autonomic hyperreflexia, but the addition of 0.25%

BOX 47.1 Medical Complications of Spinal Cord Injury Aggravated by Pregnancy

Pulmonary
- Decreased respiratory reserve
- Atelectasis and pneumonia
- Impaired cough

Hematologic
- Anemia
- Deep vein thrombosis
- Thromboembolic phenomena

Urogenital
- Chronic urinary tract infection
- Urinary tract calculi
- Proteinuria
- Renal insufficiency

Dermatologic
- Decubitus ulcers

Cardiovascular
- Hypertension
- Autonomic hyperreflexia

From Crosby E, St-Jean B, Reid D, Elliot RD. Obstetric anaesthesia and analgesia in chronic spinal cord-injured women. *Can J Anaesth.* 1992;39:487–494.

bupivacaine led to a decrease in blood pressure to baseline levels. Maehama et al.[69] described the successful use of intravenous magnesium sulfate for management of autonomic hyperreflexia during labor.

Patients with spinal cord injury often have a low baseline blood pressure and some hemodynamic instability. Placement of an intraarterial catheter before induction of anesthesia allows the continuous assessment of blood pressure and early detection and treatment of symptoms. Pulse oximetry is particularly useful in patients with respiratory compromise, and the anesthesia provider should always be available to provide ventilatory assistance if necessary.

Positioning for neuraxial block may be difficult; the anesthesia provider should consider performing the block with the patient in a lateral position because the sitting position may cause hypotension from venous pooling in the lower body. Therapeutic doses of local anesthetic should be administered cautiously with the understanding that the cephalad level of the sensory block can be fully assessed only if it is higher than the level of the spinal cord lesion. As a result, the typical epidural test dose may not identify unintentional subarachnoid injection in a patient with a spinal cord injury. Neuraxial blockade can be partially assessed by evaluating segmental reflexes below the level of the lesion. For example, the anesthesia provider can lightly stroke each side of the abdomen above and below the umbilicus, looking for contraction of the abdominal muscles and deviation of the umbilicus toward the stimulus. Reflexes are absent below the level of the block. In some patients with spastic paresis at baseline, the level of anesthesia may be confirmed by the conversion of spastic paresis to flaccid paresis.[65] A decline in blood pressure may also herald the onset of neuraxial blockade.

Alternative means of treating autonomic hyperreflexia should be available at the bedside if neuraxial analgesia or anesthesia is inadequate or not successful. Antihypertensive medications, such as **nitroglycerin**, or other vasodilators, may be effective, recognizing that hypotension can result in decreased uterine blood flow.[70] Careful titration of **sodium nitroprusside**, noting the potential for fetal/neonatal cyanide intoxication, or **beta-adrenergic receptor blockade**, may also be useful. The anesthesia provider should recognize that increased vagal activity during autonomic hyperreflexia can result in electrocardiographic changes including first- and second-degree atrioventricular block and sinus arrest.[71]

If cesarean delivery is necessary, spinal, epidural, or CSE anesthesia can be administered. Spinal anesthesia is associated with more rapid onset and more frequent need to treat hypotension.[72] The effect of neuraxial blockade on respiratory function may be less severe with epidural anesthesia than with spinal anesthesia.

Severe respiratory insufficiency or technical difficulties with neuraxial anesthesia may necessitate the use of general anesthesia.[73] If general anesthesia is required, a depolarizing muscle relaxant such as **succinylcholine (suxamethonium)** should not be given during the period of denervation injury. By a conservative definition, this period begins 24 hours after the injury and lasts for 1 year. The use of succinylcholine during this period of denervation injury may cause severe hyperkalemia.[74] Therefore, a **nondepolarizing muscle relaxant** should be used to facilitate laryngoscopy and tracheal intubation.

MYASTHENIA GRAVIS

Myasthenia gravis is an autoimmune disorder characterized by episodes of skeletal muscle weakness that are made worse by activity. Its prevalence is 150 to 250 per million.[75] Women are twice as likely to have the disease as men, and the onset is earlier. Subgroups are defined based on autoimmune and antibody disease mechanisms, skeletal muscle target molecules, thymic status, genetic characteristics, response to therapy, and disease phenotype.[75]

Myasthenia gravis results from an abnormality in autoimmune regulation, which leads to the production of antibodies against the nicotinic acetylcholine receptor or to functionally related molecules on the neuromuscular end plate of skeletal muscle. The result is receptor destruction as well as antibody-induced blockade of the remaining acetylcholine receptors.[75] Smooth muscle and cardiac muscle are not affected. The diagnosis is based on characteristic symptoms and positive antibody tests, and in the absence of antibodies, on neurophysiologic tests or response to therapy. Thymic hyperplasia is common; thymic tumors occur in approximately 10% of patients. Weakness is confined to the ocular muscles in 15% of patients. There is an association between myasthenia gravis and other autoimmune disorders, such as rheumatoid arthritis and polymyositis. In general, an early age at onset and an extended duration of purely ocular myasthenia are good prognostic signs.

Medical Management

Anticholinesterase drugs, which inhibit the breakdown of acetylcholine, are the mainstay of therapy for all subtypes of the disease. **Pyridostigmine**, a quaternary ammonium compound that does not cross the blood-brain barrier, is the preferred maintenance drug because it has less severe muscarinic side effects than other anticholinesterase drugs.[75] The treatment goal is full or nearly full remission; most patients will also require immunosuppressive therapy to meet this goal. **Prednisone** or **prednisolone** combined with **azathioprine** are the usual first-line immunosuppressants. **Mycophenolate mofetil** may also be added; other drugs include **rituximab**, **methotrexate**, **cyclosporine**, **tacrolimus**, and **cyclophosphamide**. Monotherapy with **glucocorticoids** may prevent progression of ocular myasthenia gravis to generalized disease. Thymectomy is performed in all patients with thymomas; however, there is also a benefit of total thymectomy for patients with early-onset symptoms without thymoma.[75]

Myasthenia gravis can manifest in two types of crises. A **cholinergic crisis** is rare, especially if the daily dose of pyridostigmine is less than 960 mg.[76] It results from an excess of the muscarinic effects of anticholinesterase medications combined with a poor response to anticholinesterase therapy. In contrast, a **myasthenic crisis** results from a worsening of the disease; its symptoms include worsening muscle weakness, especially muscles of respiration. Admission to an intensive care unit, ventilatory support, and rapid therapies such as plasma exchange and intravenous immune globulin are indicated.[75,76]

Many drugs can cause a worsening of myasthenic symptoms. These patients are extremely sensitive to drugs that potentiate muscle weakness. These agents include **neuromuscular blocking agents**, **quinidine**, **propranolol**, **aminoglycoside antibiotics**, and tocolytic agents such as **magnesium sulfate** and **terbutaline**. One case report noted worsened symptoms after the maternal administration of **betamethasone**.[77]

Obstetric Management

The course of myasthenia gravis during pregnancy varies. In general, approximately 30% of cases improve, 30% worsen, and 30% show no change.[78] The baseline clinical state does not predict the course of the disease during pregnancy, and the course during one pregnancy does not predict the course in a subsequent pregnancy. Because disease exacerbations occur more frequently in the first year after diagnosis of myasthenia gravis, women should be counseled to delay pregnancy for 1 to 2 years after the initial disease diagnosis.[79] There is inconsistent evidence that myasthenia gravis has adverse effects on pregnancy. One case series of 37 pregnancies with myasthenia gravis reported rates of gestational diabetes (30%), premature rupture of membranes (19%), and transient neonatal myasthenia and hyperbilirubinemia (24%), although the absence of a control group means that the specificity of risks for these conditions due to myasthenia cannot be surmised.[80]

A systematic review of 824 pregnancies with myasthenia gravis reported a 56.3% rate of vaginal delivery, an overall exacerbation risk of 33.8%, a 6.4% risk of myasthenic crisis during pregnancy, and an 8.2% risk of myasthenic crisis postpartum.[81] Complications of pregnancy and their treatment (e.g., preeclampsia) may contribute to worsening myasthenia gravis symptoms.[78] For example, magnesium therapy has been reported to precipitate a myasthenic crisis.[78,82]

The maternal physiologic changes of pregnancy, including alterations in drug absorption, increases in blood volume, and changes in renal clearance, may require adjustments in the doses of anticholinesterase drugs. Each patient should be monitored carefully for progressive respiratory compromise secondary to diaphragmatic elevation during pregnancy. Vital capacity can be measured to monitor fatigue during labor. The treatment of the myasthenic patient with preeclampsia or preterm labor is problematic because the use of magnesium sulfate for maternal seizure prophylaxis or fetal neuroprotection reduces acetylcholine release and may be associated with a significant increase in maternal and fetal muscle weakness, and even maternal death.[83] In those cases, seizure prophylaxis with anticonvulsants has been described.[84]

The uterus consists of smooth muscle; therefore, myasthenia gravis should not affect the first stage of labor. However, the second stage of labor often requires the use of striated muscle, and consequently an assisted (e.g., vacuum or forceps) vaginal delivery may be required.

Maternal IgG antibodies to the acetylcholine receptor are transferred across the placenta. Transient neonatal myasthenia gravis occurs in approximately 10% to 20% of infants of mothers with myasthenia gravis.[78] Notably, the risk and severity of neonatal myasthenia are not related to the severity of maternal disease; therefore, all neonates of mothers with myasthenia gravis must be closely monitored. The symptoms, including poor sucking, generalized hypotonia, difficulty feeding, feeble cry, ptosis, and respiratory distress, usually develop within the first 12 to 48 hours after birth and abate as the antibodies are metabolized, with resolution typically occurring within 2 to 4 weeks. **Arthrogryposis multiplex congenita** is a rare and severe disease, occurring in about 6.2 per 100,000 live births. In this condition, infants have multiple joint contractures from reduced movement *in utero*; the condition is associated with stillbirth, spontaneous abortion, and neonatal death.

Anesthetic Management

Myasthenia gravis patients should undergo early antepartum consultation with an anesthesia provider. This evaluation should assess the extent of bulbar and respiratory involvement and overall baseline muscle strength. Pulmonary function testing should be performed in patients with evidence of respiratory compromise. In a study of surgical patients, the presence of bulbar symptoms, a preoperative serum level of antiacetylcholine receptor antibody > 100 nmol/L, and intraoperative blood loss > 1000 mL were risk factors for having a postoperative myasthenic crisis.[85]

Patients with respiratory compromise may be more susceptible to opioid-induced respiratory depression, and consideration should be given to minimizing or avoiding opioids when possible. Neuraxial techniques are the preferred method for labor analgesia in patients with myasthenia gravis, and early labor neuraxial analgesia is recommended to attenuate stress and preserve maternal strength and reserve for the second stage of labor.[3] The use of anticholinesterase drugs may prolong the half-life of ester local anesthetic agents.

Neuraxial anesthetic techniques are preferred for cesarean delivery unless the patient has significant bulbar involvement or respiratory compromise. The use of bilevel positive airway pressure for ventilatory support in patients with moderate respiratory compromise may improve the safety of neuraxial anesthesia.[86]

In the patient with severe bulbar involvement or respiratory compromise, it may be prudent to secure the airway before surgery. Depolarizing muscle relaxants (e.g., **succinylcholine**) have an unpredictable effect in these patients, with affected and unaffected muscles being more sensitive and resistant to these agents, respectively.[87] However, the commonly administered dose of succinylcholine (1 to 1.5 mg/kg), which is three to five times the dose required to depress neuromuscular function by 95%, will most likely provide adequate relaxation even for resistant muscles. Anticholinesterase agents and plasmapheresis cause decreases in the activity of plasma cholinesterase and may cause delays in succinylcholine hydrolysis.

Myasthenic patients are extremely sensitive to nonde-polarizing muscle relaxants. If a nondepolarizing muscle relaxant must be given, the anesthesia provider should administer a small amount of an agent with a short half-life (e.g., **rocuronium**, **atracurium**, **vecuronium**).[87] **Mivacurium** is metabolized via plasma pseudocholinester-ase, which may be inhibited by pyridostigmine. In general, greater disease severity corresponds with enhanced sensitiv-ity to nondepolarizing muscle relaxants, necessitating the use of clinical judgment and neuromuscular monitoring to determine the amount and timing of drug doses. Myasthenia may prevent a full-strength contraction with nerve stimula-tion; therefore, a control train-of-four stimulus test should be performed before paralysis for later comparison. For nonde-polarizing agents, approximately 50% of the standard dose may be adequate, and a prolonged recovery should be antici-pated. **Sugammadex**, a cyclodextrin that works by encapsu-lating nondepolarizing neuromuscular blocking agents, may be preferred for neuromuscular blockade reversal in patients with myasthenia gravis. The limited available data on its use in pregnancy suggest that it is safe.[88,89]

After delivery, fluid shifts and decreased maternal alpha-fetoprotein concentration may necessitate an adjustment of anticholinesterase drug doses. Some patients who receive gen-eral anesthesia require postoperative ventilation. The follow-ing factors are predictive of an increased risk for postoperative ventilation: (1) female sex; (2) $FEF_{25\% \text{ to } 75\%}$ (forced expira-tory flow during the middle half of the forced vital capacity) < 3.3 L/s and less than 85% of that predicted; (3) FVC (forced vital capacity) < 2.6 L/s and less than 78% of that predicted; and (4) $MEF_{50\%}$ (maximal expiratory flow at 50% of expired vital capacity) < 3.9 L/s and less than 80% of that predicted.[90]

EPILEPSY

Epilepsy is a condition characterized by recurrent seizure activity in the absence of metabolic disorders or acute brain disease. The classification scheme for epilepsy[91] and seizure types[92] was updated in 2017 by the International League Against Epilepsy. The first level of classification is one of three seizure types: focal onset, generalized onset, and unknown onset.[92] The second level of classification is epilepsy type; these are generalized, focal, combined generalized-focal, and unknown.[91] In focal seizures, the excess neuronal discharge is limited to one hemisphere of the brain; in generalized sei-zures, the discharge occurs bilaterally and involves the entire cortex.

Medical Management

A variety of antiseizure medications are used for sei-zure therapy, depending on the type of seizure and clinical response.[93–95] A variety of adverse effects have been reported with these medications, including early-onset events (e.g., somnolence, dizziness, hypersensitivity, rash, gastrointestinal symptoms) and late-onset events (e.g., depression, leukope-nia, aplastic anemia, thrombocytopenia, megaloblastic ane-mia, hyponatremia).[94]

Prognosis for medical control of seizures is good for patients with generalized seizure disorders; as many as 20% to 40% of newly diagnosed epilepsy patients become seizure-free without or with minimal antiseizure medica-tion therapy.[96] Two in three newly treated epilepsy patients will eventually enter long-term remission (≥5 years without a seizure).[96] However, about one-third of patients will have an intermittent pattern (early remission with late recurrence or late remission). Finally, the observed number of deaths in the study compared with the general population is consis-tently increased in the first several years after the diagnosis of epilepsy.

Interaction With Pregnancy

Epilepsy is common in pregnancy, affecting about 1 in 200 parturients.[97] Maternal mortality is greater in women with epilepsy.[98] Pregnancy may increase the frequency of seizures in one in three epileptic patients; this may be secondary to increases in plasma volume and higher drug clearance, which reduces serum levels of antiepileptic drugs.[99] Women who are free of seizures for at least 9 months to 1 year before preg-nancy have a probability of 84% to 92% of remaining seizure-free during pregnancy.[100]

Optimizing antiseizure medication therapy before and during pregnancy is critical to maintain prepregnancy serum antiseizure medication levels because anticonvulsant drug levels can decrease during pregnancy, owing to decreased plasma protein binding and greater drug clearance.[101] Because of the teratogenic potential of many antiseizure medications, some physicians consider withdrawal of these drugs after 2 years without seizures and recommend waiting at least 6 addi-tional months after withdrawal before attempting to conceive. Substituting new antiseizure medications after conception is not recommended because of increased risk for teratogenicity associated with polytherapy.[99]

A variety of causes have been proposed for the increase in seizure frequency observed in some pregnant women (Table 47.2). Higher estrogen concentrations in pregnancy lower the seizure threshold.[102] Greater sodium and water retention, alkalosis secondary to hyperventilation, sleep deprivation,

TABLE 47.2 Possible Causes of Increased Seizure Frequency During Pregnancy

Mechanism	Examples
Hormonal	Changes in levels of estrogen (proconvulsant) and progesterone (anticonvulsant)
Metabolic	Increased water and sodium retention
Psychologic	Stress, sleep deprivation
Pharmacokinetic	Increase in liver metabolism, renal clearance, or volume of distribution
Physiologic	Decreased gastrointestinal absorption

and increased stress and anxiety also have been suggested as mechanisms.[103] The American Academy of Neurology and American Epilepsy Society concluded that monitoring of **lamotrigine**, **carbamazepine**, and **phenytoin** levels should be considered during pregnancy. Monitoring of **levetiracetam** and **oxcarbazepine** (and its active metabolite, monohydroxy derivative) may be considered, and monitoring of other antiepileptic agents should not be discouraged despite limited data regarding their pharmacokinetic behavior during pregnancy.[104]

Seizures in a pregnant patient can have devastating consequences. Hypoxia and acidosis that occur during a generalized seizure can result in fetal compromise or intrauterine fetal death. Placental abruption may occur. During the past three decades, the overall risk for obstetric complications in epileptic women has declined. Although some studies have suggested an increased risk for hypertension in pregnancy (including preeclampsia), bleeding, and preterm birth, a review by a panel of experts concluded that evidence is inconclusive.[100] However, women with epilepsy may have a moderately increased risk for cesarean delivery.[100]

Fetuses and neonates of women with epilepsy are more likely to have adverse pregnancy outcomes, including preterm birth, small for gestational age infant, and requirement for labor induction or cesarean delivery.[105-108] Data are insufficient to judge whether intrauterine exposure to antiseizure medications, versus epilepsy itself, increases the risk for cognitive impairment in the offspring of women with epilepsy, although there is some evidence that the risk may be increased for specific drugs.[106] Specifically, intrauterine exposure to **valproate** has been associated with maladaptive childhood behavior and autism.[31,106]

The risk for congenital malformations in women with epilepsy receiving antiseizure medication monotherapy is estimated to be 4% to 6%.[98,106] Malformations have been previously associated with antiseizure medication (e.g., cleft lip and palate, and cardiac, neural tube, and urogenital defects, specifically hypospadias).[106] A 2016 systematic review and metaanalysis of 31 studies of antiseizure medication therapies in pregnant women concluded that lamotrigine and levetiracetam carried the lowest overall risk for malformation, although data on specific malformations were insufficient.[109] Several studies have suggested that maternal folic acid supplementation before conception may decrease the risk for major congenital abnormalities in the offspring of women with epilepsy who are receiving antiseizure medications.[104]

In 2018 Tomson and Battino[110] published a review of data from the International Registry of Antiepileptic Drugs and Pregnancy and concluded that the risks of major congenital malformation associated with lamotrigine, levetiracetam, and oxcarbazepine were not different from offspring unexposed to antiepileptic drugs.

Neonates of mothers undergoing long-term antiepileptic therapy may be at risk for deficiencies in vitamin K–dependent clotting factors or other coagulation defects, despite the absence of clinically evident maternal coagulation abnormalities.[104] Enzyme-inducing antiseizure medications (e.g., **phenytoin**, **phenobarbital**, **carbamazepine**) can cross the placenta and may increase the rate of oxidative degradation of vitamin K in the fetus. Affected infants are at risk for neonatal hemorrhage and respond to typical vitamin K doses (1 mg) given intramuscularly at birth. The administration of prenatal vitamin K to epileptic women with long-term exposure to these antiseizure medications has not been conclusively shown to reduce the risk for neonatal hemorrhage.[104]

Anesthetic Management

There are significant interactions between antiseizure medications and anesthetic agents.[111] **Carbamazepine**, **phenytoin**, **phenobarbital**, and **primidone** are potent inducers of the cytochrome P450 enzymes in hepatic metabolism, which may result in decreased plasma concentrations of many medications, including neuromuscular blockers, beta-adrenergic receptor antagonists, and calcium entry–blocking agents.[94]

Serum levels of antiseizure medications should be checked if therapeutic levels are known. If the patient experiences a seizure during labor, airway protection and support of ventilation are essential. Small doses of a **benzodiazepine** or **propofol** arrest most seizures. Fetal bradycardia, typically self-limited, may necessitate immediate delivery.

Oral antiseizure medications should be continued whenever possible. Unfortunately, many of the agents are not available in parenteral forms. If oral agents cannot be taken, conversion to a parenteral agent such as **phenytoin** may be required. In general, antiseizure medications have sedating properties.

The presence of epilepsy is not a contraindication to the administration of neuraxial analgesia or anesthesia. Although antiseizure medications have been associated with adverse effects on the coagulation system, Manohar et al.[112] observed no abnormal clotting parameters or platelet counts preoperatively in a series of patients with epilepsy undergoing surgery.

If general anesthesia is necessary, it seems prudent to avoid **meperidine**, as this medication has been associated with seizures even after low to moderate doses.[101] **Sevoflurane** has stronger epileptogenic properties than **isoflurane**, but limiting the concentration to less than 1.5 minimum alveolar concentration minimizes risk, and coadministration of **nitrous oxide** and hyperventilation both counteract this effect.[113] The highest incidence of seizure activity with induction of anesthesia is believed to occur with **etomidate**. **Ketamine** may also facilitate seizures at low doses, but at high doses each of these induction agents acts as an anticonvulsant.[111]

MYOTONIA AND MYOTONIC DYSTROPHY

Myotonia is the general term used to describe a prolonged contraction of certain muscles after stimulation, which is followed by a delay in relaxation. **Myotonic dystrophies** are a genetically and phenotypically heterogeneous group of neuromuscular disorders caused by expansion defects in nucleotide sequences, principally on chromosome 19.[114] Based on clinical ascertainment, the estimated prevalence of myotonic dystrophy is about 1 in 8000; however, prevalence estimates vary widely.[114] As the most common form of myotonic disorders, myotonic dystrophies manifest in two distinct forms with different nucleotide sequences, DM1 and DM2. Both DM1 and DM2 are multisystem disorders characterized by skeletal muscle weakness and myotonia, cardiac conduction abnormalities, cataracts, hypogammaglobulinemia, and insulin resistance. DM1, also known as Steinert disease, is generally more severe and exists in congenital, juvenile, and adult forms, whereas only an adult form has been identified for DM2.[114]

Myotonias can involve specific muscles, typically the hand, facial, masseter, and pretibial muscles, which become dystrophic or wasted. The disorder is slowly progressive with continual deterioration and gradual involvement of pharyngeal and laryngeal muscles, proximal limb muscles, and the diaphragm. Uterine smooth muscle is affected and cardiac conduction abnormalities are often present. Patients typically succumb to either pulmonary or cardiac failure.

Congenital myotonic dystrophy is a severe form of myotonic dystrophy (DM1) that manifests early in infancy with hypotonia and feeding difficulties.[115] Myotonia becomes apparent during the first few years of life. In most cases, the mother has myotonic dystrophy. Sudden cardiac death is possible, due to atrioventricular block and ventricular arrhythmias.[116]

Myotonia congenita is a milder familial disorder characterized by myotonia of the skeletal muscles; multisystem involvement does not occur.[117] Unlike myotonic dystrophy, cardiac abnormalities are not present and smooth muscle is not affected. In some cases, muscle hypertrophy rather than wasting occurs. This disorder can be compatible with long life. It is distinguished from DM1 and DM2 by characteristic clinical features and an absence of significant histopathology in the muscle biopsy specimen. Myotonia congenita is characterized by dysfunction of the chloride channel.

Central core disease is a rare disorder in which muscle biopsies demonstrate the absence of oxidative enzyme activity in the longitudinal axis of the muscle fiber (i.e., the "central core").[118] Affected individuals have proximal muscle weakness and often scoliosis. This disease is caused by mutations in the skeletal muscle ryanodine receptor gene (*RYR1*) at chromosome 19q13.1, which has been associated with malignant hyperthermia.[118] Many patients with central core disease test positive for the malignant hyperthermia susceptibility trait on the caffeine-halothane contracture test (*in vitro* contracture test; see Chapter 46); these patients should be considered at risk for malignant hyperthermia and should not be exposed to triggering agents (i.e., succinylcholine, volatile halogenated agents).[118] Some patients with multiminicore and nemaline rod myopathy may also be at risk for malignant hyperthermia.[119]

Drugs such as **quinine** and **mexiletine** are most commonly used to relieve myotonic symptoms.[114,115,117] **Corticosteroids**, **phenytoin**, and **tocainide** also have been prescribed.

Obstetric Management

In pregnant patients with myotonic dystrophy, symptoms of weakness and myotonia usually remain unchanged; however, in a minority of these women, symptoms worsen during pregnancy but generally resolve after delivery.[120] Antepartum evaluation should include pulmonary function testing to assess the severity of restrictive lung disease caused by muscle wasting and an electrocardiogram, which may reveal conduction abnormalities. Patients with myotonic dystrophy type 1 should be monitored for malignant cardiac arrhythmias and peripartum cardiomyopathy.[121]

There may be a higher risk for preterm labor in patients with myotonic dystrophy. Other complications of pregnancy include polyhydramnios (secondary to reduced fetal swallowing) and an increased risk for placenta previa and accreta.[120] **Magnesium sulfate** has been reported to cause maternal respiratory compromise.[122] Poor uterine contractions may result in prolonged labor, uterine atony, and an increased risk for postpartum hemorrhage.[123] Skeletal muscle weakness increases the risk for prolonged second stage of labor and operative delivery.[120] The neonate also may have respiratory distress if affected by congenital myotonic dystrophy.

There are reports of patients with myotonia congenita who experience temporary worsening of symptoms during pregnancy.[124] Obstetric problems have not been described, most likely because this disease involves skeletal muscle only; uterine smooth muscle is not affected in these patients.

Anesthetic Management

Many reports of anesthetic management of patients with myotonic dystrophies were published before the distinction between DM1 and DM2 was appreciated, and before the era of modern anesthesia management; therefore, generalization from these reports and application to individual patients may not be valid.[125] The prolonged contractions witnessed in patients with myotonia are caused by an intrinsic muscle disorder that is not relieved by spinal or epidural anesthesia. However, infiltration with a local anesthetic may partially release contractions. Reports suggest that patients with myotonic disorders may be especially sensitive to the respiratory depressant effects of opioids and general anesthetics.[125] Sedative-hypnotic agents should be used with caution as opioids or sedatives may precipitate apnea. Neuraxial anesthesia is preferred for labor and vaginal or cesarean delivery. Both spinal and epidural anesthesia have a long history of successful use in patients with myotonic dystrophy.[126-128] Although the clinical characteristics of myotonic dystrophy DM2 are generally more benign than DM1, anesthesia providers should be aware that both may be associated with dysphagia, cardiomyopathy, and cardiac conduction abnormalities.[129] Two case reports described atrial flutter and fibrillation resulting in shock after tracheal intubation in patients with myotonic dystrophy receiving general anesthesia for cesarean delivery.[130,131]

Patients with myotonic dystrophy have a high incidence of pulmonary complications after general anesthesia.[132] Cold external temperatures and shivering are known triggers of myotonia, so the patient should be kept warm.

If general anesthesia is required, it may be prudent to limit the use of opioids and carefully titrate muscle relaxants to mitigate the risk for postoperative pulmonary complications.[133] Depolarizing agents such as **succinylcholine** should be avoided because fasciculations trigger myotonia,[134] thereby making ventilation and tracheal intubation difficult. In contrast, patients with myotonic dystrophy appear to have a normal response to **nondepolarizing muscle relaxants**.[125] Regardless, careful neuromuscular monitoring is essential, particularly in those with significant baseline muscle weakness. Reversal of neuromuscular blockade with **sugammadex** has been described.[135] In a review of dystrophic myotonias and their possible association with malignant hyperthermia, Parness et al.[136] concluded that susceptibility to malignant hyperthermia in this group of patients is similar to that of the general population. Patients with central core disease should be assumed to be susceptible to malignant hyperthermia.[118]

MUSCULAR DYSTROPHY

Muscular dystrophy is a group of disorders characterized by a progressive degeneration of skeletal muscle with intact innervation.[137] Research on the subsarcolemmal muscle fiber protein dystrophin has led to a reclassification of these disorders. Analysis of dystrophin quality and quantity can be used diagnostically before and during pregnancy and can identify carriers in some cases.

Duchenne and **Becker muscular dystrophies** are transmitted as X-linked recessive disorders and occur almost exclusively in males. However, female carriers may have electrocardiographic and/or echocardiographic abnormalities. The most common muscular dystrophies affecting females are facioscapulohumeral dystrophy and limb-girdle dystrophies. **Facioscapulohumeral dystrophy** is an autosomal dominant, slowly progressive disorder that primarily involves the muscles of the shoulders and face.[137] Over time, the pelvic and pretibial muscles may be affected. Tachycardia and arrhythmias have been infrequently reported. **Limb-girdle dystrophies** involve slow degeneration of the shoulder and pelvic muscles; exacerbations are common during pregnancy, and the risk for cesarean delivery is increased because of weakness in the trunk and pelvic muscles.[137] The inheritance pattern and severity of these diseases are variable. Cardiac conduction disorders and cardiomyopathies occur in some affected patients.

Obstetric Management

The presentations of dystrophinopathies are variable and the overall management is guided by the presence and severity of symptoms. If significant weakness is present, pulmonary function testing should be obtained to assess the extent of restrictive disease. An antepartum electrocardiogram and echocardiogram should be considered. Pregnant women with muscular dystrophies may have an increased incidence of operative delivery; the presence of severe pelvic wasting may necessitate instrumental vaginal or cesarean delivery. A study

of the course of pregnancy in women with hereditary neuromuscular disorders reported a high rate (27%) of abnormal fetal presentation in women with limb-girdle muscular dystrophy, especially in chair-bound patients. Muscle weakness worsened during and after pregnancy in one-half of patients with limb-girdle dystrophy.[120]

Anesthetic Management

Limb-girdle muscular dystrophy is associated with various cardiac abnormalities, including cardiomyopathies and conduction abnormalities. Reduced lung function and respiratory compromise can be exacerbated by the physiologic changes of pregnancy; the requirement for noninvasive positive-pressure ventilation for progression of severe restrictive pulmonary disease during the third trimester of pregnancy in a parturient with limb-girdle muscular dystrophy has been reported.[138] Neuraxial techniques are preferred for labor analgesia and cesarean delivery anesthesia. Severe disease may result in both airway abnormalities and spinal deformities, which may complicate the administration of either general or neuraxial anesthesia.

Although most female carriers of the abnormal gene for muscular dystrophies are asymptomatic, approximately 2.5% have mild symptoms of the disease.[139] Cardiac manifestations may be significant. One report described a female carrier of Becker's muscular dystrophy who had peripartum cardiomyopathy; general anesthesia was associated with intraoperative respiratory insufficiency, hemodynamic instability, and cardiac arrest.[140] There are reported cases of muscular dystrophy associated with "malignant hyperthermia–like" reactions. In a systematic review, Gurnaney et al.[141] summarized reported cases of patients with muscular dystrophy who developed hyperthermia, tachycardia, rhabdomyolysis, and hyperkalemia after exposure to **succinylcholine** and/or **volatile anesthetic agents**. However, none of these patients had other classic signs of malignant hyperthermia or evidence of hypermetabolism. The mechanism for this response may be related to the ability of these agents to exacerbate instability and permeability of dystrophin-deficient muscle membranes.[141] Although muscular dystrophy does not increase risk for **malignant hyperthermia**, volatile anesthetic agents should be used cautiously because of the risk for severe rhabdomyolysis. Succinylcholine may lead to life-threatening hyperkalemia because of upregulation of extrajunctional acetylcholine receptors or because of rhabdomyolysis and should not be administered to patients with known muscular dystrophy. In general, these patients have a normal response to **nondepolarizing muscle relaxants**, but careful neuromuscular monitoring is needed, especially in patients with severe muscle wasting.

THE PHAKOMATOSES (NEUROCUTANEOUS SYNDROMES)

The phakomatoses are congenital disorders that manifest as central nervous system (CNS) and cutaneous abnormalities.

BOX 47.2 The Congenital Neuroectodermoses

True Phakomatoses
- Tuberous sclerosis
- Neurofibromatosis

Cutaneous Angiomatosis With Abnormalities of the Central Nervous System
- Sturge-Weber syndrome
- Dermatomal hemangiomas and spinal vascular malformations
- Epidural nevus (linear sebaceous nevus) syndrome
- Osler-Rendu-Weber disease (hereditary hemorrhagic telangiectasia)
- von Hippel-Lindau disease
- Ataxia-telangiectasia (Louis-Bar disease)
- Fabry disease

Modified from Ropper AH, Samuels MA, Klein JP, Prasad S. *Adams and Victor's Principles of Neurology.* 12th ed. McGraw Hill; 2023.

Structures of ectodermal origin, such as skin, nervous system, and eyes, are commonly affected.[142] The diseases are classified into three main groups: **neurofibromatoses, tuberous sclerosis**, and **angiomatoses with CNS abnormalities** (Box 47.2).[143] The most common phakomatoses are neurofibromatosis types 1 and 2, tuberous sclerosis, **Sturge-Weber disease**, and **von Hippel-Lindau disease**. Abnormalities of the brain and spinal cord can have significant implications for anesthetic management.

Neurofibromatosis

Neurofibromatosis occurs because of excessive proliferation of neural crest elements such as Schwann cells, melanocytes, and fibroblasts. Clinical manifestations include hyperpigmented lesions (*café-au-lait* spots) accompanied by a variety of cutaneous and subcutaneous tumors. This disorder is now believed to exist in two distinct forms with gene abnormalities on two different chromosomes. Neurofibromatosis type 1, the "classic" form, has an incidence of approximately 1 in 3000.[144] The severity and progression of the disease are variable, with the neurologic symptoms depending on the location of the tumors. Intracranial tumors and paraspinal neurofibromas are a cause for concern and may require surgical excision. The risk for **pheochromocytoma** is greater in these patients.[145] Neurofibromatosis type 2 is a less common form of the disease with fewer cutaneous lesions. Acoustic neuromas as well as other cranial or spinal neurofibromas, meningiomas, and gliomas may be present.

Obstetric Management

Pregnancy may exacerbate the disease by increasing tumor growth.[145] Regression occurs after delivery in some women. A population-based cohort study of 1553 pregnancies associated with neurofibromatosis type 1 found increased risks for gestational hypertension, preeclampsia, fetal growth restriction, cerebrovascular disease, and cesarean delivery, but the risks for thromboembolic events, stillbirth, cardiac events, or maternal death were not elevated compared with the general population.[145] Pelvic neurofibromas may necessitate cesarean delivery.[145] The presence of intracranial masses may be problematic during labor and vaginal delivery, particularly with the increased intracranial pressure (ICP) that occurs with the Valsalva maneuver during the second stage of labor.

Anesthetic Management

An anesthesia provider should thoroughly assess the patient's current symptoms and known lesions, particularly if they involve neck and laryngeal tumors; these tumors are common, particularly in patients with neurofibromatosis type 1.[146] Antenatal evaluation for concomitant pheochromocytoma and potential neuraxial, intracranial, and peripheral nerve tumors should be considered.

Neuraxial anesthetic techniques can be used for labor analgesia and operative anesthesia in most patients with the disorder. However, severe kyphoscoliosis secondary to the presence of paraspinal tumors may complicate the administration of neuraxial anesthesia. The presence of asymptomatic paraspinal and intracranial tumors has prompted some anesthesia providers to suggest that neuraxial anesthesia should be administered only after careful clinical and radiographic evaluations.[147] Neurofibromas occur along the spinal nerve roots in up to 35% of patients with neurofibromatosis.[148] In neurofibromatosis type 1, the majority of these tumors are small and are found laterally in the intervertebral foramen.

The use of muscle relaxants in these patients is controversial. Both increased and decreased sensitivity to **succinylcholine** have been reported and increased sensitivity to **nondepolarizing** agents has been reported as well.[149,150] However, a number of investigators observed only minimal alterations in dose response to both depolarizing and nondepolarizing muscle relaxants in these patients and have recommended no alterations in the dose of drug.[151]

Tuberous Sclerosis

Tuberous sclerosis is characterized by epilepsy, mental disability, and adenoma sebaceum.[152] The brain shows abnormal growth of glial cells in hamartomas called tubers. Hamartomatous tumors can occur in multiple organs, including the heart, kidneys, liver, and lungs. The inheritance pattern is autosomal dominant with a variable expression, and the disease is slowly progressive.

Obstetric and Anesthetic Management

A retrospective cohort study using the Nationwide Inpatient Sample from 1998 to 2008 found that tuberous sclerosis may be associated with increased rates of preterm labor (aOR, 2.1; 95% CI, 1.3 to 3.4) and preeclampsia (aOR, 2.8; 95% CI, 1.5 to 5.2).[153] The obstetric and anesthesia providers should know the locations of lesions in an individual patient. Hemorrhage into the tumors, renal failure, and hypertension may complicate pregnancy. Renal involvement appears to represent an important prognostic factor during pregnancy, and spontaneous rupture of a renal angiomyolipoma has been reported.[154] Factors that could potentially impact anesthetic management of these patients include the presence of cardiac and renal tumors (angiomyolipomas), spinal and intracranial tubers, epilepsy, pharyngeal tumors, and pulmonary involvement.[155] Cardiac rhabdomyosarcomas have been reported to occur in over 60% of children with this disorder. These tumors generally regress with age, but arrhythmias and cardiac failure from ventricular obstruction may occur. If intracranial or spinal lesions are suspected, imaging should be considered before administration of neuraxial blockade to rule out obstructive or hemorrhagic lesions or lesions with mass effect. In addition, the airway should be assessed closely for the presence of oral tubers, which have been described in approximately 15% of these patients.

Cutaneous Angiomatosis With Central Nervous System Abnormalities

One group of phakomatoses consists of disorders in which a cutaneous vascular anomaly is accompanied by CNS abnormalities (see Box 47.2).[143] There are few reports of pregnancy in patients with these disorders. Patients may have neurologic impairment related to hemangiomas of the spinal and cranial CNS. Epidural and spinal anesthesia have been reported in only a few patients with spinal hemangiomas; epidural anesthesia may be preferable to spinal anesthesia as von Hippel-Lindau hemangioblastomas are not present in the epidural space.[156] The presence of widespread varicosities in patients with these disorders may result in a chronically low ventricular preload; if a significant increase in preload occurs during the peripartum period, cardiac overload and peripartum cardiomyopathy may occur.[157]

ACUTE IDIOPATHIC POLYNEURITIS (GUILLAIN-BARRÉ SYNDROME)

Acute idiopathic polyneuritis, also known as Guillain-Barré syndrome, is an inflammatory demyelinating illness with a reported incidence of approximately 1 case per 100,000 persons per year.[158] In 60% of patients, a viral illness precedes neurologic symptoms by 1 to 3 weeks. Zika virus is an example of an antecedent infection. Cases also have occurred after the administration of antirabies and influenza vaccines.

Patients with this disorder initially have weakness in the limbs, followed by the trunk, neck, and facial muscles. Loss of reflexes, total motor paralysis, and respiratory failure can occur. Symptoms peak at 2 to 3 weeks. The majority of patients recover completely although approximately 10% of patients have severe residual disability, and in 3% the syndrome is fatal.[158] Autonomic nervous system involvement and dysfunction may occur.

Treatment is largely supportive and may include mechanical ventilatory support. Plasmapheresis reduces the duration of illness when instituted during the evolution phase and has been used safely during pregnancy.[159]

Obstetric Management

The incidence of this syndrome appears unchanged in pregnant women, but increases in the first 3 months postpartum.[159] There is no evidence that pregnancy affects the natural history of the disease, and termination of pregnancy does not appear to improve its course.[159]

Anesthetic Management

Anesthetic management depends on patient status at the time of delivery; epidural and spinal techniques have been described in patients with Guillain-Barré syndrome.[160,161] However, some anesthesia providers have expressed concern regarding the use of neuraxial techniques in these patients, citing the theoretical potential for adverse neurologic effects as a result of anesthetic toxicity or immunologic modulation. Steiner et al.[162] implicated epidural anesthesia as a trigger of Guillain-Barré syndrome in four patients. Wiertlewski et al.[161] reported the immediate worsening of neurologic status after delivery in a pregnant patient with Guillain-Barré syndrome who had received epidural anesthesia. These authors did not establish a causal relationship between the disease and neuraxial anesthetic techniques, nor did they properly acknowledge the increased frequency of Guillain-Barré syndrome in the postpartum period.[159]

If general anesthesia is necessary, **succinylcholine** should be avoided because of the risk for hyperkalemia in patients with acute muscle wasting. Careful titration of **nondepolarizing muscle relaxants** is also necessary.

The parturient with a history of remote Guillain-Barré syndrome may have persistent diminished respiratory reserve, even in the absence of obvious residual disability. Pulmonary evaluation should be considered before the administration of anesthesia. Approximately 5% of patients experience a relapse, with a small number of cases progressing to a chronic disorder.

POLIOMYELITIS

Poliomyelitis is a disease caused by a picornavirus that is transmitted by the fecal-oral route. Most cases are asymptomatic or are accompanied by mild systemic symptoms. More severe symptoms and nervous system involvement occur in approximately 1% of patients.[163] Motor neurons in the cerebral cortex, brainstem, and spinal cord are affected. Asymmetric flaccid paralysis develops over several days. Bulbar paralysis is more common in young adults. The cerebrospinal fluid (CSF) findings are consistent with viral meningitis. Recovery occurs 3 to 4 months after onset, most likely from motor axon terminal sprouting that reinnervates the previously denervated muscle fibers; however, residual deficits often persist. A slowly progressive syndrome called **postpoliomyelitis muscular atrophy** or **postpolio syndrome** may develop as many as 40 years after the acute illness as a result of death or dysfunction of the enlarged, surviving motor neurons.[164]

Obstetric Management

Although the poliovirus vaccine has been available since the 1950s, the last phase of poliomyelitis eradication has been difficult; in 2014 the WHO declared the worldwide transmission of polio virus to formerly polio-free countries to be a public health emergency.[165] The oral form of the vaccination does not appear to have harmful effects on fetal development and can be used if vaccination is required during pregnancy.[166] A history of poliomyelitis may increase the risks for preeclampsia, maternal renal dysfunction, low-birth-weight infants, perinatal death, and cesarean delivery in poliomyelitis survivors.[167] Some of these adverse outcomes may be related to chronic pulmonary issues or mechanical obstruction during labor.

Anesthetic Management

A complete preanesthetic evaluation should be performed for the presence of respiratory impairment, sleep apnea, swallowing difficulties, and other neurologic and motor deficits in all parturients with a history of poliomyelitis. Some anesthesia providers have feared that administration of neuraxial anesthesia in patients with a history of poliomyelitis might cause reactivation of the virus or postpolio syndrome. However, there is no evidence that neuraxial analgesia or anesthesia worsens symptoms in these patients. Rezende et al.[168] reported a series of 123 patients with a history of poliomyelitis who underwent 162 surgical procedures and were observed postoperatively for 22 months. Neuraxial blockade was used in 64% of cases, with no patients exhibiting worsening of neurologic symptoms. Anesthetic considerations in these patients should include assessment for pulmonary restrictive disease as well as anatomic issues that may make neuraxial techniques difficult.[169] For the patient with postpolio syndrome in whom general anesthesia is needed, some anesthesia providers have suggested the use of a decreased dose of a short-acting **nondepolarizing muscle relaxant** rather than **succinylcholine**, which may provoke severe acute hyperkalemia.[170]

BRAIN NEOPLASMS

Intracranial neoplasms vary in incidence, histology, clinical presentation, and prognosis (Table 47.3).[171] Brain neoplasms in pregnant women appear to occur with the same relative frequency as in nonpregnant women; however, the physiologic alterations that occur during pregnancy can have profound implications for symptomatology and management.

Gliomas are the most common intracranial neoplasms, accounting for approximately 39% of all primary intracranial tumors.[172] These tumors, which result from anaplasia of astrocytes, exhibit diversity in invasive potential and include glioblastoma multiforme, astrocytomas, ependymomas, and oligodendrocytomas. Glioblastoma multiforme is the most lethal, whereas oligodendrocytomas have a better prognosis.

Meningiomas account for approximately one-third of all primary brain tumors.[172] These benign tumors originate from the dura mater or arachnoid. Surgery typically is curative.

TABLE 47.3 Classification of Primary Brain Tumors in Women Versus All Adults

Histologic Type	Percentage of All Diagnosed Tumors in Women	Percentage of All Diagnosed Tumors, General Population
Benign		
Meningioma	35	37
Schwannoma or nerve sheath tumors	7	8
Pituitary neoplasms	7	16
Other nonmalignant tumors	Data not available	7
Malignant Gliomas:		
Astrocytoma (WHO grades II–III)	11	5.5[a]
Glioblastoma (WHO grade IV)	23	15
Medulloblastoma	2	1.5[b]
Other brain neoplasms	15	10

WHO, World Health Organization.
[a]Rates are specific to diffuse astrocytoma WHO II–III.
[b]Rates are specific to oligodendroglioma WHO II–III.
Adapted from Swensen R, Kirsch W. Brain neoplasms in women: a review. *Clin Obstet Gynecol.* 2002;45:904–927; Lapointe S, Perry A, Butowski NA. Primary brain tumours in adults. *Lancet.* 2018;392(10145):432–446.

Pituitary adenomas account for 7% of diagnosed primary brain neoplasms in women.[172] Only a small fraction of these tumors cause symptoms (e.g., visual field deficits). These tumors may secrete prolactin, growth hormone, or adrenocorticotropic hormone. Tumor growth is physically limited by the sella turcica of the sphenoid bone and the hypothalamus. The resulting compression of the hypothalamus or pituitary gland may cause decreases in the production or release of vasopressin, leading to diabetes insipidus. The pituitary gland normally enlarges during pregnancy, and this additional growth may cause symptoms in a woman who was previously asymptomatic.[172] Women with known microadenomas should be carefully monitored during pregnancy to detect symptoms of pituitary compression.[173] Growth of pituitary tumors can be triggered by breastfeeding.

Bromocriptine often provides effective medical therapy for prolactin-secreting adenomas and has a track record of use during pregnancy; its continued use during breastfeeding must be balanced against its suppressive effect on lactation. Surgery is indicated for tumors that do not respond to medical management.

Schwannomas, also called **neurinomas**, account for 7% of all brain tumors in women.[172] These lesions originate in the

Schwann cells surrounding the nerve. Clinical presentation depends on the location of the tumor. Acoustic neuromas result when the eighth cranial nerve is involved; these lesions are often seen in patients with neurofibromatosis. The treatment is surgical excision.

Metastatic brain tumors are more frequent than primary brain tumors.[171] Common primary cancers include those of the lung, breast, and colon. Prognosis and therapy depend on the tumor of origin.

Brain tumors share several pathophysiologic features. Neurologic deficits can result from a mass effect or increased ICP, even if the tumor is benign. Brain edema, which may result from a combination of vasogenic and cytotoxic mechanisms, is a prominent feature of cerebral neoplasms.

The potential for brain herniation must be considered in any patient with a mass lesion. The brain is divided into three basic compartments: the falx cerebri separates the cerebrum into right and left halves, and the tentorium isolates the cerebellum. An enlarging mass can obstruct free flow of CSF or cause shifts from one compartment to another with devastating effects.

Obstetric Management

The incidence of primary brain tumors first manifesting in pregnancy does not appear to be greater than that in age-matched, nonpregnant women.[172] However, pregnancy may affect existing tumor biology; in one case series, 44% of pregnant women with an existing history of grade II or III gliomas experienced tumor progression during pregnancy or within 8 weeks postpartum.[174] Approximately 9% of patients with **choriocarcinoma** have brain metastases at the time of diagnosis.[175] A retrospective cohort study from the National Inpatient Sample reported an increased rate of maternal mortality, cesarean delivery, and preterm labor in patients with malignant brain tumors, and an increased rate of preterm labor and cesarean delivery in patients with benign brain tumors.[176] Pregnancy complications were significantly more likely to occur in patients having a neurosurgical procedure during their admission.

Although pregnancy does not affect the incidence of brain tumors, some of these lesions appear to grow faster during pregnancy. Visual field defects from pituitary adenomas worsen as a result of tumor enlargement during pregnancy, and symptoms have been observed to improve during the postpartum period. Edema and the increased blood volume may account for some of these symptoms. Pregnancy-induced hormonal changes also may play a role because estrogen and progesterone receptors are present in meningiomas and some gliomas.[172]

Diagnosis during pregnancy requires intracranial imaging. In general, MRI is preferred over other imaging modalities, if it is appropriate to the clinical case, because it avoids the use of ionizing radiation. MRI may require the use of gadolinium-based contrast agents. Gadolinium has the advantage compared with other contrast agents of not containing iodine, and studies demonstrating adverse fetal effects are lacking in humans. However, gadolinium appears rapidly in the fetal bladder and amniotic fluid, from where it may be swallowed by the fetus and absorbed from the gastrointestinal tract. Its fetal half-life is unknown. The American College of Radiology has stated that in pregnant patients, gadolinium-based contrast agents "… should only be used if their usage is considered critical and the potential benefits justify the potential unknown risk to the fetus."[177]

Management during pregnancy depends on the nature of the tumor. Surgery for benign tumors (e.g., meningiomas) with mild symptoms can often be delayed until after delivery. Women with more aggressive, malignant tumors or with tumors causing seizures or severe visual impairment may require urgent surgery during pregnancy to avoid acute neurologic deterioration. Often delivery is not necessary, or if the woman is close to full term and follow-up therapy (e.g., chemotherapy) is needed, delivery also may be recommended as soon as reasonable fetal survival can be expected. In general, pregnant and nonpregnant women with brain tumors should be considered for the same therapies with the appropriate expert consultation and shared decision-making with the patient.

In the healthy parturient, CSF pressure increases transiently with painful uterine contractions.[178] In patients with an obstructive intracranial mass lesion, this situation could result in an increased risk for brain herniation. Increased ICP from Valsalva maneuvers can further exacerbate herniation risk. The location and size of the tumor should be assessed in the individual patient so that an appropriate delivery plan can be developed with multidisciplinary input. In general, either a pain-free second stage with operative vaginal delivery to avoid the Valsalva maneuver or cesarean delivery may be appropriate.[172] If those contraindications to Valsalva include increased ICP with obstruction to intracranial CSF circulation, and/or mass effect, these patients are typically not candidates for neuraxial anesthesia.

Anesthetic Management

Many important elements should be assessed when considering the anesthetic approach for labor analgesia and cesarean delivery anesthesia in the patient with an intracranial tumor with mass effect or obstruction of CSF flow.[179] Epidural analgesia can mitigate the increase in ICP that can result with pushing during the second stage of labor,[180] and neuraxial anesthesia has a long history of successful use in pregnant women with intracranial neoplasms.[180-182] However, in pregnant women with increased ICP, unintentional dural puncture associated with an attempted epidural catheter placement may result in fatal brain herniation.[183] In cases where brain herniation is of concern, epidural procedures should be avoided as avoidance of dural puncture can never be assured. It should also be noted that epidural space expansion with medication increases ICP, although this phenomenon has not been established definitively as a cause for brain herniation. Some have favored general anesthesia for cesarean delivery in the patient with a brain neoplasm[184]; however, potential disadvantages of general anesthesia include (1) the loss of verbal and motor responses that facilitate neurologic assessment, and (2) the

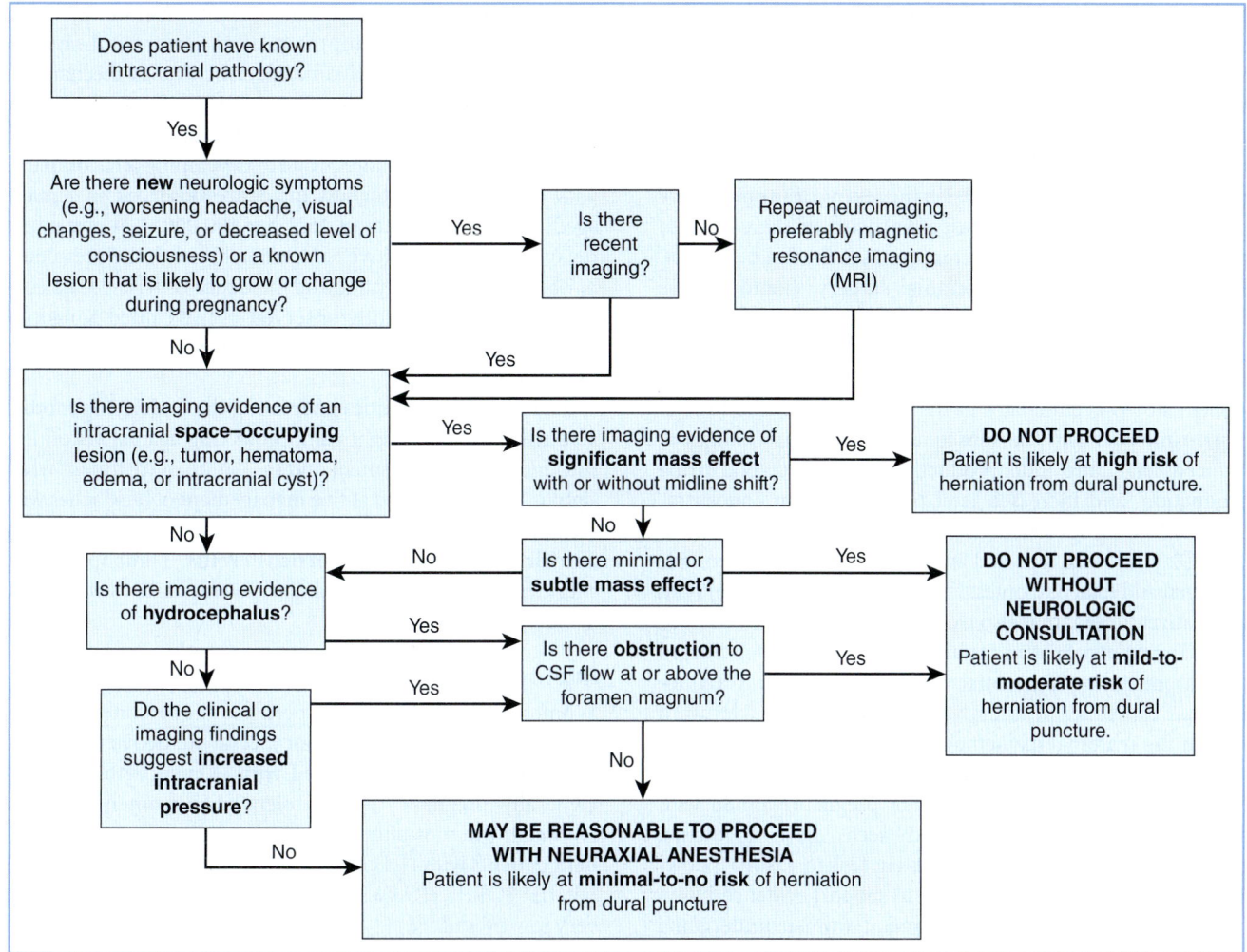

Fig. 47.3 Decision tree summarizing the critical elements for assessing the risk for neurologic deterioration from neuraxial anesthesia in patients with intracranial space–occupying lesions. *CSF,* Cerebrospinal fluid. Redrawn from Leffert LR, Schwamm LH. Neuraxial anesthesia in parturients with intracranial pathology: a comprehensive review and reassessment of risk. *Anesthesiology.* 2013;119:703–718.

risks of increased ICP with tracheal intubation and extubation. Leffert and Schwamm[179] proposed a decision tree for risk stratifying patients with intracranial space–occupying lesions for whom neuraxial anesthesia is being considered (Fig. 47.3). Generally, if an intracranial tumor does not exert mass effect or obstruct CSF flow, then neuraxial anesthesia may not present herniation risk with dural puncture. Expert consultation with neurology colleagues is prudent.

Wang and Paech[185] reviewed specific elements in the anesthetic management of the pregnant patient undergoing neurosurgery, many of which are also relevant to the patient with an intracranial tumor undergoing cesarean delivery. The induction of general anesthesia may consist of the administration of an induction dose of **propofol** or **thiopental** and either a depolarizing or a rapid-acting nondepolarizing **neuromuscular-blocking agent**. Some anesthesia providers avoid **succinylcholine** because it may cause a transient increase in ICP, but others consider this effect to be clinically insignificant.[185]

Total intravenous anesthesia, balanced intravenous and volatile anesthesia, and solely volatile anesthesia have been used for surgery during pregnancy. Nitrous oxide impairs cerebral autoregulation and increases cerebral blood flow and intracranial pressure, and therefore is likely best avoided. Propofol for anesthesia maintenance confers less confounding effects on motor evoked potentials compared with volatile agents, and it is also associated with other properties such as reduced intracranial pressure and cerebral blood volume while maintaining cerebral autoregulation. When intraoperative neuromonitoring is used, volatile anesthetics can reduce the quality of both motor and sensory evoked potentials and are therefore best avoided. For these reasons, intravenous anesthetic induction and maintenance may be preferable to volatile anesthetic agents for these procedures, considering intraoperative neuromonitoring requirements.

When appropriate, accommodations for monitoring the FHR during intracranial surgery should be made. Awake craniotomy with intraoperative FHR monitoring has been described for pregnant patients requiring neurosurgical interventions for lesions in eloquent areas of the brain, with favorable maternal and neonatal outcomes reported.[186]

To preserve cerebral and uteroplacental perfusion, hemodynamic stability should be maintained through appropriate fluid administration, avoidance of aortocaval compression, the prophylactic or early use of vasopressor drugs, and intraarterial blood pressure monitoring instituted before induction of anesthesia.[185] In general, blood pressure should be kept close to baseline measurements; in the setting of an emergency neurosurgical procedure in a patient with increased ICP, a drop in blood pressure may compromise cerebral perfusion. Fluid management for intracranial surgery should involve administration of isonatremic, isotonic, and glucose-free intravenous solutions to reduce the risk for cerebral edema and hyperglycemia.[185] Mannitol administered to a pregnant woman slowly accumulates in the fetus and can lead to fetal hyperosmolality and the subsequent physiologic changes of reduced fetal lung fluid production, decreased fetal urine production, and increased fetal plasma sodium concentration[185]; however, successful use of mannitol in doses of 0.25 to 0.5 mg/kg has been reported and is associated with favorable maternal and fetal outcomes.[185] Furosemide (frusemide) is an alternative diuretic that also can be administered.

Balancing maternal and fetal interests in cases of increased ICP in pregnancy is essential, as hyperventilation to reduce ICP may cause uterine artery vasoconstriction and a leftward shift of the maternal oxyhemoglobin dissociation curve. The maternal $Paco_2$ during normal pregnancy is 28 to 32 mmHg (3.7 to 4.3 kPa) (see Chapter 2). For pregnant women with an acute increase in ICP, Wang and Paech[185] have suggested a target $Paco_2$ range of 25 to 30 mm Hg (3.3 to 4.0 kPa); however, data are currently insufficient to support evidence-based recommendations specific to pregnant women undergoing intracranial surgery. In pregnant patients with increased ICP, maintenance of maternal $Paco_2$ in the middle or at the lower end of the normal range for pregnancy is recommended. Management should be individualized according to the clinical setting.

When the decision is made to perform a cesarean delivery and brain tumor resection sequentially during a single anesthetic, hypertension should be avoided during induction and tracheal intubation. Some authors have used combinations of high-dose **fentanyl** or **remifentanil**, **labetalol**, and **propofol** or **thiopental** with **succinylcholine**.[185,187]

Pregnant women with intracranial neoplasms may need to undergo definitive tumor resection with continuation of the pregnancy. In these women, neuraxial techniques may be considered for delivery if ICP is normal.

IDIOPATHIC INTRACRANIAL HYPERTENSION

Idiopathic intracranial hypertension (IIH), previously referred to as *pseudotumor cerebri* or *benign intracranial hypertension*, is defined by the International Headache Society as elevated intracranial pressure, headache, papilledema with or without sixth nerve palsy, and pulsatile tinnitus that is not better explained by another diagnosis. Diagnosis involves MRI with venography to exclude structural causes and dural venous sinus thrombosis, and lumbar puncture demonstrating CSF

pressure > 250 mm and CSF with normal constituents.[188] New research findings highlight the roles of hormonal dysregulation and the metabolic neuroendocrine axis as mechanisms of elevated intracranial pressure in IIH.[189] These discoveries may pave the way for innovative treatments for IIH.

Adult women are more prone to developing IIH compared with men, with the highest incidence observed in females aged 25 years, at a rate of 15.2 per 100,000.[190] A systematic review revealed a positive correlation between the prevalence of obesity in a country and the incidence of IIH.[191] This condition is more frequently observed in the United Kingdom, Italy, Israel, and the United States, whereas the incidence is lower in Asia.

IIH treatment includes addressing the underlying modifiable risk factor of weight gain, protecting against vision loss through regular assessment and escalation of treatment when sight is threatened, and active management of headaches with serial lumbar punctures and the administration of **carbonic anhydrase inhibitors** or **corticosteroids**. Lumboperitoneal shunting may be required in severe cases with visual symptoms.

Interaction With Pregnancy

Women with IIH do not experience higher rates of abortion, ectopic or molar pregnancy, cesarean delivery, preterm labor, or depression compared with women without IIH.[192] Generally, pregnancy is well tolerated in women with IIH. Although the mortality rate may be slightly higher in pregnant patients with IIH compared with pregnant patients without IIH (OR, 5.3; 95% CI, 2.9 to 9.6, $P < .0001$), it remains very low overall.[192]

Anesthetic Management

Cerebellar tonsillar herniation does not occur with lumbar puncture in IIH because of the uniform, distributed increase in ICP and the absence of obstruction to CSF flow. The reported cases of cerebellar tonsillar herniation after lumbar puncture in patients with this disorder occurred in the setting of worsening metabolic acidosis, preexisting low-lying cerebellar tonsils, severe headache and neck pain exacerbated by movement, and focal neurologic deficits at baseline suggestive of additional pathology.[193-195] In the absence of these signs and symptoms, the anesthesia provider typically can safely provide neuraxial analgesia or anesthesia.[196]

Historically, some anesthesia providers have recommended general anesthesia for cesarean delivery in patients with **lumboperitoneal shunt** because of concern that local anesthetic agents introduced into the subarachnoid space may be shunted into the peritoneum, making it difficult to achieve adequate anesthesia, and concern that the performance of neuraxial anesthesia may result in trauma to the shunt catheter. However, successful use of neuraxial anesthesia in patients with lumboperitoneal shunts has been reported.[197-199] Neuraxial anesthesia with an intrathecal catheter has been performed for both vaginal and cesarean delivery in these patients.[200,201] Placement of an intrathecal catheter also provides a therapeutic option for CSF drainage via the catheter.[200,201] Verification of the functional status of an *in situ* subarachnoid shunt should be done with neurology or neurosurgery consultation.[199] Preoperative radiographic examination may help the anesthesia provider avoid needle placement near the catheter.

MATERNAL HYDROCEPHALUS WITH SHUNT

Hydrocephalus results from a variety of conditions. The most common are certain instances of intracranial hemorrhage in preterm infants, fetal and neonatal infections, the Chiari malformations, aqueductal stenosis, and the Dandy-Walker syndrome.[202] The **Chiari malformations** consist of four classifications of extension of a portion of cerebellar tissue into the cervical canal. It is the less common, more severe forms of Chiari malformations that are more often associated with hydrocephalus. The **Dandy-Walker syndrome** occurs with failure of development of the midline of the cerebellum, with resultant hydrocephalus of the fourth ventricle.

Ventriculoatrial or ventriculoperitoneal shunt catheters are placed for the treatment of many of these disorders. Because of advances in neonatal and neurosurgical care, women with hydrocephalus and CSF shunt catheters are reaching childbearing age in increasing numbers.

Obstetric Management

Obstetric management depends on the presence of other medical and neurologic conditions. In general, although maternal shunt dependency carries a relatively high risk for complications for some patients due to shunt malfunction, proper management can lead to normal pregnancy and delivery.[203] Ventriculoperitoneal shunt is not a contraindication to pregnancy.[204] Prophylactic antibiotics to prevent shunt infection are not routinely recommended. Vaginal delivery should be attempted unless a cesarean delivery is necessary for obstetric reasons.[204]

Anesthetic Management

Anesthetic management of the patient with hydrocephalus and a functioning shunt depends on the location and function of the shunt. Both epidural and spinal anesthesia have been used in patients with lumboperitoneal, ventriculoatrial, and ventriculoperitoneal shunts (as discussed earlier).[197,198,200] A review of 24 studies that included 130 pregnancies in parturients with CSF shunts found that shunt malfunctions were common in pregnancy, that epidural analgesia is safe in women with functional shunts, and that labor anesthetic management varies in response to shunt function and clinical status.[205] A basic thought process for evaluating the use of neuraxial anesthesia in patients with hydrocephalus secondary to intracranial space occupying lesions is shown in Fig. 47.3.

INTRACRANIAL HEMORRHAGE

Cerebrovascular disease during pregnancy can result from three major mechanisms: hemorrhage, arterial infarction, and venous thrombosis. A retrospective population-based cohort study found the unadjusted incidence of subarachnoid hemorrhage (SAH) in pregnancy was 3.21 (95% CI, 2.46 to 4.13) per 100,000 deliveries.[206] Risk factors for SAH in pregnancy included smoking (OR, 3.27; 95% CI, 1.56 to 6.86), prepregnancy hypertension (OR, 12.72; 95% CI, 1.39 to 116.46), and preeclampsia or eclampsia (OR, 3.88; 95% CI, 1.00 to 15.05).

Data are conflicting as to whether the aneurysm bleeding rate is higher during pregnancy.[207] Some authors have reported a progressive increase in the incidence of aneurysm bleeding throughout gestation and up to 6 weeks postpartum, while others have found no link between pregnancy or the puerperium and increased risk for aneurysmal hemorrhage.[179,207,208] In general, asymptomatic and unruptured aneurysms in pregnancy can be managed conservatively with close monitoring and noninvasive imaging.[207] The treatment of ruptured aneurysms during pregnancy should mimic treatment of aneurysms in nonpregnant patients. The American Heart Association (AHA) guidelines for the management of aneurysmal SAH include monitoring and controlling blood pressure (avoiding sudden and profound blood pressure reduction, to balance the risk for stroke, rebleeding, and maintenance of cerebral perfusion pressure) and prompt surgical clipping or endovascular coiling to prevent rebleeding.[208] Controversy exists as to whether endovascular coiling results in better outcomes than clipping. Although the AHA has suggested that "endovascular coiling should be considered" in patients with ruptured aneurysms judged to be technically amenable to both surgical clipping and coiling, some experts argue that several factors may alter the risk-benefit ratio in pregnancy. These factors include (1) the need for exposure to ionizing radiation for coil placement, (2) the possible need for anticoagulation or use of antifibrinolytic agents, and (3) the increased rate of incomplete aneurysm occlusion associated with coiling compared with clipping.[209-211] Endovascular coiling has not been specifically studied in the pregnant population, although several cases of successful endovascular treatment of ruptured intracranial aneurysms in pregnant women have been reported.[210,212]

Bleeding from arteriovenous malformations has been reported to occur with equal or greater frequency with advancing gestational age.[209] The risk for hemorrhage from an arteriovenous malformation in pregnant women does not appear to differ from that in the general population, although the risk for bleeding appears greater during the second half of pregnancy and the first 6 weeks postpartum, corresponding to the period of high cardiac output.[209] The management of arteriovenous malformations in pregnancy does not differ from standard care of the nonpregnant patient. As with aneurysms, a multidisciplinary decision-making process allows planning based on the location of the lesion, the duration of pregnancy, and the relative risks associated with interventional and noninterventional methods of management.[179] Management of arteriovascular malformations, including those that present during pregnancy, has increasingly shifted over the past decade from a surgical to an endovascular approach.

Obstetric Management

If the lesion has been successfully treated surgically, the patient requires no related special care during labor and delivery. For an untreated aneurysm or arteriovenous malformation, the hemodynamic stress occurring during labor and delivery should be minimized. Current data do not demonstrate a definite advantage of cesarean delivery over assisted vaginal delivery.[213] The decision about the method of delivery should be based on the individual patient and their pregnancy history. For labor and vaginal delivery, neuraxial analgesia and low outlet forceps or vacuum assistance may be used to shorten the second stage of labor and attenuate fluctuations in blood pressure.

Anesthetic Management

If the parturient has undergone surgical repair of either an aneurysm or arteriovenous malformation, anesthetic management need not differ from that for other obstetric patients. Hypertension should be avoided in the parturient with an untreated lesion. If vaginal delivery is planned, epidural or CSE analgesia should be considered. For cesarean delivery, neuraxial anesthesia has been described and multidisciplinary planning with neurologic experts is important.[214]

In some cases, the neurosurgeon may ligate or excise the vascular lesion *during* pregnancy, *before* delivery. The anesthesia provider should consider the general principles of anesthetic management for pregnant women undergoing nonobstetric surgery (see Chapter 18) as well as the special considerations for pregnant women undergoing neurosurgery (as discussed earlier).[185] The risks for hypertension and intracranial bleeding, as well as the risk for pulmonary aspiration should be considered during induction of anesthesia. It is critical to maintain stable blood pressure during induction of anesthesia, laryngoscopy, tracheal intubation, and extubation. The patient should receive adequate sedation before and after arrival in the operating room. Placement of an intraarterial catheter is prudent. The anesthesia provider may attenuate the hypertensive response to laryngoscopy and tracheal intubation by intravenous administration of **esmolol**, **labetalol**, **lidocaine**, **nitroglycerin**, **nitroprusside**, and/or an opioid (e.g., **remifentanil**). **Succinylcholine** can be used for tracheal intubation.

Maintenance of anesthesia with volatile halogenated anesthetic agents is controversial for these cases.[215] Volatile anesthetic agents and nitrous oxide have undesirable cerebrovasodilation effects, whereas almost all intravenous anesthetic agents possess cerebrovasoconstrictive and cerebrodepressant properties. If sensory evoked potentials will be part of the monitoring plan, then total intravenous anesthesia may be optimal.[215] Although aggressive maternal hyperventilation may result in decreased uterine blood flow, modest hyperventilation (e.g., $Paco_2$ of 28 to 30 mm Hg [3.7 to 4.0 kPa]) may be used if needed to reduce maternal ICP. The anesthesia provider should maintain left uterine displacement in patients beyond 20 weeks' gestation. Intraoperative FHR monitoring allows assessment of the fetal response to maternal general anesthesia, hemodynamic changes, and hyperventilation, but a clear plan in case of fetal compromise that is not responding to intraoperative resuscitation efforts must be discussed with the patient, anesthesia provider, neurosurgeon, and the obstetric provider prior to surgery. At many institutions, including the author's, intraoperative FHR monitoring is used beginning at 24 weeks' gestation. Typically, an obstetric nurse monitors the FHR tracing during surgery and requests obstetric consultation if needed. An adverse change in the FHR tracing should prompt the anesthesia provider to optimize maternal oxygenation, ventilation, and perfusion. Endovascular treatment with general anesthesia avoids the need for craniotomy and deliberate hypotension. There is no consensus regarding an acceptable or safe level of hypotension in these patients, and deliberate hypotension in rarely current neuroanesthesia practice.

In some cases, the obstetric provider and neurosurgeon may perform a combined procedure (e.g., a cesarean delivery followed by ligation or excision of the neurovascular lesion). Principles of anesthetic management are then similar to those described for intracranial neurovascular surgery during pregnancy.[179,215]

CEREBRAL VEIN THROMBOSIS

Thrombosis of the cerebral veins and sinuses most often affects young adults and children; approximately 75% of the adult patients are women.[216] Thromboses commonly involve the cavernous sinus, lateral sinus, sagittal sinus, or cortical veins. Thrombosis of the cerebral veins causes venous obstruction with local effects, whereas thrombosis of the major sinuses can cause increased ICP. A prothrombotic risk factor or a direct cause can be identified in approximately 85% of patients. Pregnancy may be a precipitating factor for sinus thrombosis in a person with a genetically increased risk.[216]

Primary cerebral cortical vein thrombosis is the type of thrombosis most often seen in pregnancy. The estimated incidence of cerebral vein thrombosis during pregnancy is 1 in 2500 to 1 in 10,000 deliveries in Western countries.[217] Cerebral vein thrombosis occurs more frequently during the last trimester of pregnancy and in the first 6 postpartum weeks.[217] Although the etiology is unclear, pregnancy may predispose patients to this condition because of at least two factors. First, traumatic damage to the endothelial lining of vessels may occur during the second stage of labor. Second, pregnancy is a hypercoagulable state (see Chapters 2 and 38). Mechanical causes of sinus thrombosis may include head injury and lumbar puncture.[218] It has been postulated that low CSF pressure after a lumbar puncture with persistent CSF leaking causes the brain to shift downward, resulting in traction on the cortical veins and sinuses.

Patients with cerebral vein thrombosis may have headaches, nausea and vomiting, and blurred vision. In more severe cases, lateralizing neurologic signs, lethargy, and seizures may occur. In severe cases, transtentorial herniation caused by a focal mass effect can occur. A 2017 systematic review of cerebral vein thrombosis in pregnancy linked headache alone with favorable prognosis, while coma and obtundation predicted poor outcomes.[219]

Care should be taken to differentiate cerebral vein thrombosis from PDPH as it may manifest as a positional headache that overlaps the typical timing and treatment of PDPH in the parturient.[218] In general, the headache associated with cerebral vein thrombosis is more diffuse in location. Headache from cerebral vein thrombosis may change in quality over time and is particularly ominous if it worsens when the patient lies down (suggestive of increased ICP).

Diagnosis of cortical venous thrombosis is confirmed by contrast-enhanced magnetic resonance venography, gradient-recalled echo, or susceptibility-weighted imaging sequences.[217] The 2024 AHA/American Stroke Association guidelines for management of cerebral venous thrombosis recommend full anticoagulation with low-molecular-weight heparin (LMWH), which should continue throughout pregnancy.[217] In the postpartum period, LMWH or oral vitamin K antagonists (target international normalized ratio [INR] of 2.0 to 3.0) should be continued for at least 6 weeks, for a total minimum duration of therapy of 3 months.[217] In future pregnancies, these patients should receive LMWH prophylaxis.[217] Lumbar puncture and drainage of a large volume of CSF may be needed to treat acute elevations in ICP that stem from reduced venous drainage; the procedure must be timed with pharmacologic anticoagulation.

Obstetric and Anesthetic Management

Cerebral vein thrombosis rarely occurs before delivery, although such an occurrence may prompt an urgent delivery if associated with maternal neurologic instability and fetal deterioration. Maternal anticoagulation may complicate the decision to use or not use neuraxial anesthesia. The anesthesia provider should avoid systemic hypotension, which may reduce cerebral perfusion pressure and blood flow to injured areas already subjected to marginal perfusion. If the patient has a cerebral hematoma with mass effect, dural puncture may precipitate herniation; it is therefore preferable to administer general anesthesia for cesarean delivery, with special attention to the treatment of increased ICP. Cerebral venous thrombosis is a rare but reported complication after spinal and epidural anesthesia, presumably caused by intracranial hypotension.[218]

MOTOR NEURON DISORDERS

Motor neuron diseases are a group of disorders characterized by progressive muscular weakness and atrophy. These disorders may affect motor function alone or in conjunction with sensory deficits. There are few data on the course of these disorders in pregnant women. This discussion focuses on three of these disorders: amyotrophic lateral sclerosis (ALS) and primary spinal muscular atrophy, which are pure motor neuron disorders, and peroneal muscular atrophy, which involves both motor and sensory degeneration. Currently there is no cure for any of these degenerative disorders.

Amyotrophic Lateral Sclerosis

ALS is characterized by progressive degeneration of anterior horn cells with progressive atrophic weakness and hyperreflexia. Patients typically succumb to respiratory failure within 6 years of diagnosis. It is seen more often in patients older than 60 years, but there are several reports of this disorder in pregnant women.[220-224] Women are more likely to be diagnosed with ALS before age 60 years if they have never been pregnant or experienced their first pregnancy at or after age 30 years.[223] Physicians should assess and frequently monitor the respiratory compromise of parturients with ALS throughout the peripartum period.[222] Epidural analgesia and anesthesia have been used in these patients without evidence of worsened postoperative neurologic function.[220,221] Patients with ALS may be more sensitive to the effects of nondepolarizing muscle relaxants.[221] The physiologic changes during the late stages of pregnancy may worsen marginal respiratory status in these patients and early cesarean delivery may be warranted.[221,222]

Spinal Muscular Atrophy

Like ALS, primary spinal muscular atrophy involves degeneration of anterior horn cells. However, affected patients tend to be younger, and this disorder progresses more slowly. Some types are hereditary. Spinal muscular atrophy mainly involves the spinal cord, without involvement of the corticospinal tract. Marked kyphoscoliosis combined with truncal and limb weakness, especially involving the proximal musculature, can occur and result in significant ventilatory limitations.

Spinal muscular atrophy may be associated with an increased incidence of preterm labor and worsened muscle weakness that persists after delivery.[225] Epidural and spinal analgesia and anesthesia have been used successfully in patients with this disorder.[226] In one case, general anesthesia was used for cesarean delivery because of worsening dyspnea requiring noninvasive positive pressure ventilation.[227]

Peroneal Muscular Atrophy

Peroneal muscular atrophy, also known as *Charcot-Marie-Tooth disease*, includes several inherited peripheral motor and sensory neuropathies; it is one of the most common inherited neuromuscular diseases.[228] It involves a progressive sensory and motor degeneration of peripheral nerves and roots. The peroneal nerve is affected early. Restrictive pulmonary impairment, phrenic nerve dysfunction, diaphragmatic dysfunction, thoracic cage abnormalities, and sleep apnea have been described in association with peroneal muscular atrophy. Vocal cord dysfunction, possibly caused by laryngeal nerve involvement, can also be present. Assessment of peripartum respiratory function is essential. Approximately 30% of patients with this disorder report deterioration in overall function during pregnancy.[120]

A review of 108 deliveries in women with this disorder found increased risk for abnormal fetal presentation, emergency operative delivery, and postpartum bleeding.[229]

Both neuraxial and general anesthesia have been used for delivery.[230]

ISOLATED MONONEUROPATHIES DURING PREGNANCY

Pregnancy is associated with an increased incidence of several specific mononeuropathies: Bell's palsy, carpal tunnel syndrome, and meralgia paresthetica.

Bell's Palsy

Bell's palsy is a syndrome of acute-onset paralysis of the facial nerve; it tends to present during the third trimester and the first few weeks postpartum. The incidence is higher in women than in men and is approximately 2.5 times higher in pregnant women compared with nonpregnant women from the same age group.[231]

One study noted that pregnant women whose symptoms progressed to complete facial paralysis within 10 days of onset were less likely to experience satisfactory recovery than a comparison group of nonpregnant women.[232] Women with Bell's palsy are more likely than men to have symptoms of dry eyes, which can progress to secondary damage.[231] Although the prognosis for women with partial palsy is excellent, the authors of a 2017 review of Bell's palsy in pregnancy suggested that evidence supports early treatment with glucocorticoids, particularly in cases of complete palsy.[231]

Dorsey and Camann[233] retrospectively reviewed 36 cases of Bell's palsy associated with pregnancy. Of the 36 women,

27 received spinal or epidural analgesia or anesthesia. There were no differences in incidence or progression of the Bell's palsy or maternal and fetal outcomes in relation to the type of anesthesia given; therefore, neuraxial analgesia or anesthesia does not appear to be contraindicated in patients with Bell's palsy.

Carpal Tunnel Syndrome

Carpal tunnel syndrome is common during pregnancy; in a systematic review, the reported incidence ranged from 0.8% to 70%.[234] The disorder results from compression of the median nerve in the flexor retinaculum at the wrist. Patients typically report paresthesias and weakness in the median nerve distribution, with symptoms worse in the morning on awakening from sleep. Symptoms have been reported to persist in approximately 50% and 30% of patients after 1 and 3 years, respectively.[234] Patients may be treated with splinting of the wrists, although in severe cases, surgery may be required. In many cases, symptoms resolve spontaneously within the first 2 months postpartum and appear to correlate with losing the weight gained during pregnancy.[235]

Meralgia Paresthetica

Meralgia paresthetica involves sensory loss and paresthesias in the lateral thigh stemming from compression of the lateral femoral cutaneous nerve. Obesity and the exaggerated lordosis of pregnancy can stretch the nerve. Symptoms of meralgia paresthetica typically resolve within 3 months of delivery. This peripheral nerve palsy and other neurologic deficits are discussed in more detail in Chapter 31.

KEY POINTS

- Symptoms of multiple sclerosis may worsen postpartum, regardless of the anesthetic technique used during delivery. However, the long-term prognosis of this disease is most likely unaffected by pregnancy or anesthesia.
- Multiple sclerosis does not contraindicate the use of neuraxial (spinal or epidural) analgesia or anesthesia.
- Continuous neuraxial anesthesia is the method of choice for the prevention or treatment of autonomic hyperreflexia during labor and delivery in patients with spinal cord injury.
- Patients with myasthenia gravis require close surveillance during labor. Increasing muscle weakness may require an adjustment in the dosage of anticholinesterase drugs.

- Severe respiratory involvement may preclude the use of neuraxial anesthesia for cesarean delivery.
- The anesthesia provider should avoid succinylcholine in patients with myotonic dystrophy because fasciculations can trigger myotonia.
- Hemodynamic stability should be maintained in the parturient with an untreated intracranial aneurysm or arteriovenous malformation. Neuraxial anesthesia should be considered during labor and delivery.
- Bell's palsy, carpal tunnel syndrome, and meralgia paresthetica occur at higher rates during pregnancy. Symptoms typically resolve postpartum.

REFERENCES

1. Evans C, Beland SG, Kulaga S, et al. Incidence and prevalence of multiple sclerosis in the Americas: a systematic review. *Neuroepidemiology*. 2013;40:195–210.
2. Thone J, Thiel S, Gold R, Hellwig K. Treatment of multiple sclerosis during pregnancy—safety considerations. *Expert Opin Drug Saf*. 2017;16:523–534.
3. Hopkins AN, Alshaeri T, Akst SA, Berger JS. Neurologic disease with pregnancy and considerations for the obstetric anesthesiologist. *Semin Perinatol*. 2014;38:359–369.
4. Huang WJ, Chen WW, Zhang X. Multiple sclerosis: pathology, diagnosis and treatments. *Exp Ther Med*. 2017;13:3163–3166.
5. Hafler DA, Compston A, Sawcer S, et al. Risk alleles for multiple sclerosis identified by a genomewide study. *N Engl J Med*. 2007;357:851–862.

6. Jalkanen A, Alanen A, Airas L. Finnish Multiple Sclerosis and Pregnancy Study Group Pregnancy outcome in women with multiple sclerosis: results from a prospective nationwide study in Finland. *Mult Scler*. 2010;16:950–955.

7. Nielsen NM, Jørgensen KT, Stenager E, et al. Reproductive history and risk of multiple sclerosis. *Epidemiology*. 2011;22:546–552.

8. Hellwig K, Correale J. Artificial reproductive techniques in multiple sclerosis. *Clin Immunol*. 2013;149:219–224.

9. Mueller BA, Zhang J, Critchlow CW. Birth outcomes and need for hospitalization after delivery among women with multiple sclerosis. *Am J Obstet Gynecol*. 2002;186:446–452.

10. Dahl J, Myhr KM, Daltveit AK, et al. Pregnancy, delivery, and birth outcome in women with multiple sclerosis. *Neurology*. 2005;65:1961–1963.

11. Goldacre A, Pakpoor J, Goldacre M. Perinatal characteristics and obstetric complications in mothers with multiple sclerosis: record-linkage study. *Mult Scler Relat Disord*. 2017;12:4–8.

12. Finkelsztejn A, Brooks JB, Paschoal FM Jr, Fragoso YD. What can we really tell women with multiple sclerosis regarding pregnancy? A systematic review and meta-analysis of the literature. *BJOG*. 2011;118:790–797.

13. Vukusic S, Hutchinson M, Hours M, et al. Pregnancy and multiple sclerosis (the PRIMS study): clinical predictors of post-partum relapse. *Brain*. 2004;127:1353–1360.

14. Portaccio E, Ghezzi A, Hakiki B, et al. Breastfeeding is not related to postpartum relapses in multiple sclerosis. *Neurology*. 2011;77:145–150.

15. Langer-Gould A, Huang SM, Gupta R, et al. Exclusive breastfeeding and the risk of postpartum relapses in women with multiple sclerosis. *Arch Neurol*. 2009;66:958–963.

16. Hellwig K, Rockhoff M, Herbstritt S, et al. Exclusive breastfeeding and the effect on postpartum multiple sclerosis relapses. *JAMA Neurol*. 2015;72:1132–1138.

17. Tui A, Preiss A, Barcham I, Nevin M. Local nervous tissue changes following spinal anesthesia in experimental animals. *J Pharmacol Exp Ther*. 1944;81:209–217.

18. Bamford C, Sibley W, Laguna J. Anesthesia in multiple sclerosis. *Can J Neurol Sci*. 1978;5:41–44.

19. Stenuit J, Marchand P. Sequelae of spinal anesthesia. *Acta Neurol Psychiatr Belg*. 1968;68:626–635.

20. Harazim H, Štourač P, Janků P, et al. Obstetric anesthesia/analgesia does not affect disease course in multiple sclerosis: 10-year retrospective cohort study. *Brain Behav*. 2018;8:e01082.

21. Lavie C, Rollot F, Durand-Dubief F, et al. Neuraxial analgesia is not associated with an increased risk of post-partum relapses in MS. *Mult Scler*. 2019;25:591–600.

22. Bouvet L, Fontana M, Bouthors AS, et al. Post-partum relapse in women with multiple sclerosis after neuraxial labour analgesia or neuraxial anaesthesia: a multicentre retrospective cohort study. *Anaesth Crit Care Pain Med*. 2021;40:100834.

23. Bader AM, Hunt CO, Datta S, et al. Anesthesia for the obstetric patient with multiple sclerosis. *J Clin Anesth*. 1988;1:21–24.

24. Pasto L, Portaccio E, Ghezzi A, et al. Epidural analgesia and cesarean delivery in multiple sclerosis post-partum relapses: the Italian cohort study. *BMC Neurol*. 2012;12:165.

25. Lu E, Zhao Y, Dahlgren L, et al. Obstetrical epidural and spinal anesthesia in multiple sclerosis. *J Neurol Neurosurg Psychiatry*. 2013;260:2620–2628.

26. Drake E, Drake M, Bird J, Russell R. Obstetric regional blocks for women with multiple sclerosis: a survey of UK experience. *Int J Obstet Anesth*. 2006;15:115–123.

27. Spierings EL, Sabin TD. De novo headache during pregnancy and puerperium. *Neurologist*. 2016;21:1–7.

28. Cardona L, Klein AM. Early postpartum headache: case discussions. *Semin Neurol*. 2011;31:385–391.

29. American College of Obstetricians and Gynecologists. Committee Opinion No. 462: Moderate caffeine consumption during pregnancy (reaffirmed 2023). *Obstet Gynecol*. 2010;116:467–468.

30. Browne ML, Van Zutphen AR, Botto LD, et al. Maternal butalbital use and selected defects in the National Birth Defects Prevention Study. *Headache*. 2014;54:54–66.

31. Briggs GG, Freeman RK, Towers CV, Forinash AB. *Drugs in Pregnancy and Lactation: A Reference Guide to Fetal and Neonatal Risk*. 12th ed. Wolters Kluwer; 2021.

32. American College of Obstetricians and Gynecologists. Committee Opinion No. 711: Opioid use and opioid use disorder in pregnancy (reaffirmed 2021). *Obstet Gynecol*. 2017;130:e81–e94.

33. Ornoy A, Weinstein-Fudim L, Ergaz Z. Antidepressants, antipsychotics, and mood stabilizers in pregnancy: what do we know and how should we treat pregnant women with depression. *Birth Defects Res*. 2017;109:933–956.

34. Sanchez SE, Williams MA, Pacora PN, et al. Risk of placental abruption in relation to migraines and headaches. *BMC Womens Health*. 2010;10:30.

35. Silberstein S, Loder E, Diamond S, et al. Probable migraine in the United States: results of the American Migraine Prevalence and Prevention (AMPP) study. *Cephalalgia*. 2007;27:220–229.

36. Lee DE, Krishnan A, Collins R. Reversible cerebral vasoconstriction syndrome in the postpartum period: a case report and review of the literature. *Int J Gynaecol Obstet*. 2023;162:823–828.

37. Lucia M, Viviana M, Alba C, et al. Neurological complications in pregnancy and the puerperium: methodology for a clinical diagnosis. *J Clin Med*. 2023;12:2994.

38. Magid-Bernstein J, Omran SS, Parikh NS, et al. Reversible cerebral vasoconstriction syndrome: symptoms, incidence, and resource utilization in a population-based US cohort. *Neurology*. 2021;97:e248–e253.

39. Pacheco K, Ortiz JF, Parwani J, et al. Reversible cerebral vasoconstriction syndrome in the postpartum period: a systematic review and meta-analysis. *Neurol Int*. 2022;14:488–496.

40. Bérard A, Zhao JP, Sheehy O. Antidepressant use during pregnancy and the risk of major congenital malformations in a cohort of depressed pregnant women: an updated analysis of the Quebec Pregnancy Cohort. *BMJ Open*. 2017;7:e013372.

41. Huybrechts KF, Bateman BT, Palmsten K, et al. Antidepressant use late in pregnancy and risk of persistent pulmonary hypertension of the newborn. *JAMA*. 2015;313:2142–2151.

42. Nappi RE, Albani F, Sances G, et al. Headaches during pregnancy. *Curr Pain Headache Rep*. 2011;15:289–294.

43. Fox AW, Chambers CD, Anderson PO, et al. Evidence-based assessment of pregnancy outcome after sumatriptan exposure. *Headache*. 2002;42:8–15.

44. Spielmann K, Kayser A, Beck E, et al. Pregnancy outcome after anti-migraine triptan use: a prospective observational cohort study. *Cephalalgia*. 2018;38:1081–1092.

45. Simbar M, Karimian Z, Afrakhteh M, et al. Increased risk of pre-eclampsia (PE) among women with the history of migraine. *Clin Exp Hypertens.* 2010;32:159–165.

46. Bushnell CD, Jamison M, James AH. Migraines during pregnancy linked to stroke and vascular diseases: U.S. population based case-control study. *BMJ.* 2009;338:b664.

47. Williams MA, Peterlin BL, Gelaye B, et al. Trimester-specific blood pressure levels and hypertensive disorders among pregnant migraineurs. *Headache.* 2011;51:1468–1482.

48. Wabnitz A, Bushnell C. Migraine, cardiovascular disease, and stroke during pregnancy: systematic review of the literature. *Cephalalgia.* 2015;35:132–139.

49. Elliott JP, Morrison JC, Chauhan SP. A critical appraisal of the potential harmful effects of terbutaline sulfate use in pregnancy. *J Reprod Med.* 2013;58:123–131.

50. Loures V, Savoldelli G, Kern K, Haller G. Atypical headache following dural puncture in obstetrics. *Int J Obstet Anesth.* 2014;23:246–252.

51. Uppal V, Russell R, Sondekoppam RV, et al. Evidence-based clinical practice guidelines on postdural puncture headache: a consensus report from a multisociety international working group. *Reg Anesth Pain Med.* 2023;49:471–501.

52. Ding W, Hu S, Wang P, et al. Spinal cord injury: the global incidence, prevalence, and disability from the Global Burden of Disease Study 2019. *Spine (Phila Pa 1976).* 2022;47:1532–1540.

53. Pereira L. Obstetric management of the patient with spinal cord injury. *Obstet Gynecol Surv.* 2003;58:678–687.

54. Kang AH. Traumatic spinal cord injury. *Clin Obstet Gynecol.* 2005;48:67–72.

55. Crosby E, St-Jean B, Reid D, Elliott RD. Obstetrical anaesthesia and analgesia in chronic spinal cord-injured women. *Can J Anaesth.* 1992;39:487–494.

56. Robertson K, Ashworth F. Spinal cord injury and pregnancy. *Obstet Med.* 2022;15:99–103.

57. Mazzia C, Berndl A. Obstetric and neonatal outcomes in people who acquired a spinal cord injury during pregnancy. *J Obstet Gynaecol Can.* 2023;45:314–318.

58. McLain AB, Zhang L, Troncale J, et al. Pregnancy, labor, and delivery outcomes of women with and without spinal cord injury. *J Spinal Cord Med.* 2023;46:405–413.

59. Sharpe EE, Arendt KW, Jacob AK, Pasternak JJ. Anesthetic management of parturients with pre-existing paraplegia or tetraplegia: a case series. *Int J Obstet Anesth.* 2015;24:77–84.

60. Khalili M, Berlin M, Pettersson K, et al. Pregnancy, delivery, and neonatal outcomes among women with spinal cord injury in Sweden 1997-2015: a population-based cohort study. *Acta Obstet Gynecol Scand.* 2022;101:1282–1290.

61. Vieira I, Cunha P, Pinto M, et al. Anaesthetic management of tetraplegic pregnant patients during child delivery: a systematic review. *Rev Esp Anestesiol Reanim (Engl Ed).* 2023;70:224–230.

62. Obstetric management of patients with spinal cord injuries: ACOG Committee Opinion, Number 808 (reaffirmed 2023). *Obstet Gynecol.* 2020;135:e230–e236.

63. Hambly PR, Martin B. Anaesthesia for chronic spinal cord lesions. *Anaesthesia.* 1998;53:273–289.

64. Cross LL, Meythaler JM, Tuel SM, Cross AL. Pregnancy, labor and delivery post spinal cord injury. *Paraplegia.* 1992;30:890–902.

65. Stirt JA, Marco A, Conklin KA. Obstetric anesthesia for a quadriplegic patient with autonomic hyperreflexia. *Anesthesiology.* 1979;51:560–562.

66. Kobayashi A, Mizobe T, Tojo H, Hashimoto S. Autonomic hyperreflexia during labour. *Can J Anaesth.* 1995;42:1134–1135.

67. Baraka A. Epidural meperidine for control of autonomic hyperreflexia in a paraplegic parturient. *Anesthesiology.* 1985;62:688–690.

68. Abouleish EI, Hanley ES, Palmer SM. Can epidural fentanyl control autonomic hyperreflexia in a quadriplegic parturient? *Anesth Analg.* 1989;68:523–526.

69. Maehama T, Izena H, Kanazawa K. Management of autonomic hyperreflexia with magnesium sulfate during labor in a woman with spinal cord injury. *Am J Obstet Gynecol.* 2000;183:492–493.

70. Westgren N, Hultling C, Levi R, Westgren M. Pregnancy and delivery in women with a traumatic spinal cord injury in Sweden, 1980-1991. *Obstet Gynecol.* 1993;81:926–930.

71. Erickson RP. Autonomic hyperreflexia: pathophysiology and medical management. *Arch Phys Med Rehabil.* 1980;61:431–440.

72. Ng K, Parsons J, Cyna AM, Middleton P. Spinal versus epidural anaesthesia for caesarean section. *Cochrane Database Syst Rev.* 2004;(2):CD003765.

73. Ahmed AB, Bogod DG. Anaesthetic management of a quadriplegic patient with severe respiratory insufficiency undergoing caesarean section. *Anaesthesia.* 1996;51:1043–1045.

74. Stone WA, Beach TP, Hamelberg W. Succinylcholine—danger in the spinal-cord-injured patient. *Anesthesiology.* 1970;32:168–169.

75. Gilhus NE. Myasthenia gravis. *N Engl J Med.* 2016;375:2570–2581.

76. Bird SJ, Levine JM. Myasthenia crisis. In: Shefner JM, Parsons PE, Rabinstein AA, eds. *UpToDate.* Wolters Kluwer; 2025.

77. Catanzarite VA, McHargue AM, Sandberg EC, Dyson DC. Respiratory arrest during therapy for premature labor in a patient with myasthenia gravis. *Obstet Gynecol.* 1984;64:819–822.

78. Ferrero S, Esposito F, Biamonti M, et al. Myasthenia gravis during pregnancy. *Expert Rev Neurother.* 2008;8:979–988.

79. Varner M. Myasthenia gravis and pregnancy. *Clin Obstet Gynecol.* 2013;56:372–381.

80. Zhou Q, Yin W, Zhu J, et al. Risk factors associated with adverse pregnancy outcomes and postpartum exacerbation in women with myasthenia gravis. *Am J Reprod Immunol.* 2022;88:e13641.

81. Banner H, Niles KM, Ryu M, et al. Myasthenia gravis in pregnancy: systematic review and case series. *Obstet Med.* 2022;15:108–117.

82. Bashuk RG, Krendel DA. Myasthenia gravis presenting as weakness after magnesium administration. *Muscle Nerve.* 1990;13:708–712.

83. Ciafaloni E, Massey JM. The management of myasthenia gravis in pregnancy. *Semin Neurol.* 2004;24:95–100.

84. Lake AJ, Al Khabbaz A, Keeney R. Severe preeclampsia in the setting of myasthenia gravis. *Case Rep Obstet Gynecol.* 2017;2017:9204930.

85. Watanabe A, Watanabe T, Obama T, et al. Prognostic factors for myasthenic crisis after transsternal thymectomy in patients with myasthenia gravis. *J Thorac Cardiovasc Surg.* 2004;127:868–876.

86. Warren J, Sharma SK. Ventilatory support using bilevel positive airway pressure during neuraxial blockade in a patient with severe respiratory compromise. *Anesth Analg.* 2006;102:910–911.

87. Blichfeldt-Lauridsen L, Hansen BD. Anesthesia and myasthenia gravis. *Acta Anaesthesiol Scand.* 2012;56:17–22.

88. Soyoral L, Goktas U, Cegin MB, Baydi V. Successful use of sugammadex for caesarean section in a patient with myasthenia gravis. *Braz J Anesthesiol.* 2017;67:221–222.

89. Stourac P, Adamus M, Seidlova D, et al. Low-dose or high-dose rocuronium reversed with neostigmine or sugammadex for cesarean delivery anesthesia: a randomized controlled noninferiority trial of time to tracheal intubation and extubation. *Anesth Analg.* 2016;122:1536–1545.

90. Naguib M, el Dawlatly AA, Ashour M, Bamgboye EA. Multivariate determinants of the need for postoperative ventilation in myasthenia gravis. *Can J Anaesth.* 1996;43: 1006–1013.

91. Scheffer IE, Berkovic S, Capovilla G, et al. ILAE classification of the epilepsies: position paper of the ILAE Commission for Classification and Terminology. *Epilepsia.* 2017;58:512–521.

92. Fisher RS, Cross JH, French JA, et al. Operational classification of seizure types by the International League Against Epilepsy: position paper of the ILAE Commission for Classification and Terminology. *Epilepsia.* 2017;58: 522–530.

93. Liu G, Slater N, Perkins A. Epilepsy: treatment options. *Am Fam Physician.* 2017;96:87–96.

94. Elger CE, Schmidt D. Modern management of epilepsy: a practical approach. *Epilepsy Behav.* 2008;12:501–539.

95. Burakgazi E, French JA. Treatment of epilepsy in adults. *Epileptic Disord.* 2016;18:228–239.

96. Schmidt D, Sillanpaa M. Evidence-based review on the natural history of the epilepsies. *Curr Opin Neurol.* 2012;25: 159–163.

97. Hart LA, Sibai BM. Seizures in pregnancy: epilepsy, eclampsia, and stroke. *Semin Perinatol.* 2013;37:207–224.

98. Kinney MO, Craig JJ. Pregnancy and epilepsy; meeting the challenges over the last 25 years: the rise of the pregnancy registries. *Seizure.* 2017;44:162–168.

99. Reisinger TL, Newman M, Loring DW, et al. Antiepileptic drug clearance and seizure frequency during pregnancy in women with epilepsy. *Epilepsy Behav.* 2013;29:13–18.

100. Harden CL, Hopp J, Ting TY, et al. Practice parameter update: management issues for women with epilepsy— focus on pregnancy (an evidence-based review): obstetrical complications and change in seizure frequency: report of the Quality Standards Subcommittee and Therapeutics and Technology Assessment Subcommittee of the American Academy of Neurology and American Epilepsy Society. *Neurology.* 2009;73:126–132.

101. Patel SI, Pennell PB. Management of epilepsy during pregnancy: an update. *Ther Adv Neurol Disord.* 2016;9: 118–129.

102. Ramsay RE. Effect of hormones on seizure activity during pregnancy. *J Clin Neurophysiol.* 1987;4:23–25.

103. Yerby MS. Pregnancy and epilepsy. *Epilepsia.* 1991;32:S51–S59.

104. Harden CL, Pennell PB, Koppel BS, et al. Management issues for women with epilepsy—focus on pregnancy (an evidence-based review): III. Vitamin K, folic acid, blood levels, and breast-feeding: report of the Quality Standards Subcommittee and Therapeutics and Technology Assessment Subcommittee of the American Academy of Neurology and the American Epilepsy Society. *Epilepsia.* 2009;50:1247–1255.

105. Borthen I, Gilhus NE. Pregnancy complications in patients with epilepsy. *Curr Opin Obstet Gynecol.* 2012;24:78–83.

106. Tomson T, Battino D. Teratogenic effects of antiepileptic drugs. *Lancet Neurol.* 2012;11:803–813.

107. Hope OA, Harris KM. Management of epilepsy during pregnancy and lactation. *BMJ.* 2023;382:e074630.

108. Danielsson KC, Gilhus NE, Borthen I, et al. Maternal complications in pregnancy and childbirth for women with epilepsy: time trends in a nationwide cohort. *PLoS One.* 2019;14:e0225334.

109. Weston J, Bromley R, Jackson CF, et al. Monotherapy treatment of epilepsy in pregnancy: congenital malformation outcomes in the child. *Cochrane Database Syst Rev.* 2016;(11): CD010224.

110. Tomson T, Battino D, Bonizzoni E, et al. Comparative risk of major congenital malformations with eight different antiepileptic drugs: a prospective cohort study of the EURAP registry. *Lancet Neurol.* 2018;17:530–538.

111. Perks A, Cheema S, Mohanraj R. Anaesthesia and epilepsy. *Br J Anaesth.* 2012;108:562–571.

112. Manohar C, Avitsian R, Lozano S, et al. The effect of antiepileptic drugs on coagulation and bleeding in the perioperative period of epilepsy surgery: the Cleveland Clinic experience. *J Clin Neurosci.* 2011;18:1180–1184.

113. Iijima T, Nakamura Z, Iwao Y, Sankawa H. The epileptogenic properties of the volatile anesthetics sevoflurane and isoflurane in patients with epilepsy. *Anesth Analg.* 2000;91: 989–995.

114. Udd B, Krahe R. The myotonic dystrophies: molecular, clinical, and therapeutic challenges. *Lancet Neurol.* 2012;11: 891–905.

115. Modoni A, Silvestri G, Pomponi MG, et al. Characterization of the pattern of cognitive impairment in myotonic dystrophy type 1. *Arch Neurol.* 2004;61:1943–1947.

116. Groh WJ, Groh MR, Saha C, et al. Electrocardiographic abnormalities and sudden death in myotonic dystrophy type 1. *N Engl J Med.* 2008;358:2688–2697.

117. Heatwole CR, Moxley RT 3rd. The nondystrophic myotonias. *Neurotherapeutics.* 2007;4:238–251.

118. Jungbluth H. Central core disease. *Orphanet J Rare Dis.* 2007;2:25.

119. Klingler W, Rueffert H, Lehmann-Horn F, et al. Core myopathies and risk of malignant hyperthermia. *Anesth Analg.* 2009;109:1167–1173.

120. Awater C, Zerres K, Rudnik-Schöneborn S. Pregnancy course and outcome in women with hereditary neuromuscular disorders: comparison of obstetric risks in 178 patients. *Eur J Obstet Gynecol Reprod Biol.* 2012;162:153–159.

121. Besant G, Bourque PR, Smith IC, et al. Case report: severe peripartum cardiac disease in myotonic dystrophy type 1. *Front Cardiovasc Med.* 2022;9:899606.

122. Catanzarite V, Gambling D, Bird LM, et al. Respiratory compromise after $MgSO_4$ therapy for preterm labor in a woman with myotonic dystrophy: a case report. *J Reprod Med.* 2008;53:220–222.

123. Zagorda B, Camdessanché JP, Féasson L. Pregnancy and myopathies: reciprocal impacts between pregnancy, delivery, and myopathies and their treatments. A clinical review. *Rev Neurol (Paris).* 2021;177:225–234.

124. Gilchrist JM. Muscle disease in the pregnant woman. *Adv Neurol.* 1994;64:193–208.

125. Veyckemans F, Scholtes JL. Myotonic dystrophies type 1 and 2: anesthetic care. *Paediatr Anaesth.* 2013;23:794–803.

126. Camann WR, Johnson MD. Anesthetic management of a parturient with myotonia dystrophica: a case report. *Reg Anesth.* 1990;15:41–43.

127. Campbell AM, Thompson N. Anaesthesia for caesarean section in a patient with myotonic dystrophy receiving warfarin therapy. *Can J Anaesth.* 1995;42:409–414.

128. Cherng YG, Wang YP, Liu CC, et al. Combined spinal and epidural anesthesia for abdominal hysterectomy in a patient with myotonic dystrophy. Case report. *Reg Anesth.* 1994;19:69–72.

129. Weingarten TN, Hofer RE, Milone M, Sprung J. Anesthesia and myotonic dystrophy type 2: a case series. *Can J Anaesth.* 2010;57:248–255.

130. Chung HT, Tam AY, Wong V, et al. Dystrophia myotonica and pregnancy—an instructive case. *Postgrad Med J.* 1987;63:555–557.

131. Shirasawa Y, Ishida K, Matsumoto M. Myotonic dystrophy diagnosed after cesarean section. *J Anesth.* 2014;28:952.

132. Mathieu J, Allard P, Gobeil G, et al. Anesthetic and surgical complications in 219 cases of myotonic dystrophy. *Neurology.* 1997;49:1646–1650.

133. Owen PM, Chu C. Emergency caesarean section in a patient with myotonic dystrophy: a case of failed postoperative extubation in a patient with mild disease. *Anaesth Intensive Care.* 2011;39:293–298.

134. Paterson IS. Generalized myotonia following suxamethonium. A case report. *Br J Anaesth.* 1962;34:340–342.

135. Stourac P, Krikava I, Seidlova J, et al. Sugammadex in a parturient with myotonic dystrophy. *Br J Anaesth.* 2013;110:657–658.

136. Parness J, Bandschapp O, Girard T. The myotonias and susceptibility to malignant hyperthermia. *Anesth Analg.* 2009;109:1054–1064.

137. O'Neill GN. Inherited disorders of the neuromuscular junction. *Int Anesthesiol Clin.* 2006;44:91–106.

138. Allen T, Maguire S. Anaesthetic management of a woman with autosomal recessive limb-girdle muscular dystrophy for emergency caesarean section. *Int J Obstet Anesth.* 2007;16:370–374.

139. Molyneux MK. Anaesthetic management during labour of a manifesting carrier of Duchenne muscular dystrophy. *Int J Obstet Anesth.* 2005;14:58–61.

140. Gupta A, Hazarika A, Jain K, et al. An asymptomatic carrier of Becker's muscular dystrophy with cardiomyopathy in pregnancy: peripartum or not? *Int J Obstet Anesth.* 2017;30:77–78.

141. Gurnaney H, Brown A, Litman RS. Malignant hyperthermia and muscular dystrophies. *Anesth Analg.* 2009;109:1043–1048.

142. Lin DD, Barker PB. Neuroimaging of phakomatoses. *Semin Pediatr Neurol.* 2006;13:48–62.

143. Ropper AH, Samuels MA, Klein JP. *Adam's and Victor's Principles of Neurology.* 12th ed. McGraw-Hill; 2023.

144. Kresak JL, Walsh M. Neurofibromatosis: a review of NF1, NF2, and schwannomatosis. *J Pediatr Genet.* 2016;5:98–104.

145. Terry AR, Barker FG 2nd, Leffert L, et al. Neurofibromatosis type 1 and pregnancy complications: a population-based study. *Am J Obstet Gynecol.* 2013;209:e1–e8.

146. Hirsch NP, Murphy A, Radcliffe JJ. Neurofibromatosis: clinical presentations and anaesthetic implications. *Br J Anaesth.* 2001;86:555–564.

147. Spiegel JE, Hapgood A, Hess PE. Epidural anesthesia in a parturient with neurofibromatosis type 2 undergoing cesarean section. *Int J Obstet Anesth.* 2005;14:336–339.

148. Walsh E, Zhang Y, Madden H, et al. Pragmatic approach to neuraxial anesthesia in obstetric patients with disorders of the vertebral column, spinal cord and neuromuscular system. *Reg Anesth Pain Med.* 2021;46:258–267.

149. Mitterschiffthaler G, Maurhard U, Huter O, Brezinka C. Prolonged action of vecuronium in neurofibromatosis (von Recklinghausen's disease). *Anaesthesiol Reanim.* 1989;14:175–178.

150. Naguib M, Al-Rajeh SM, Abdulatif M, Ababtin WA. The response of a patient with von Recklinghausen's disease to succinylcholine and atracurium. *Middle East J Anaesthesiol.* 1988;9:429–434.

151. Richardson MG, Setty GK, Rawoof SA. Responses to nondepolarizing neuromuscular blockers and succinylcholine in von Recklinghausen neurofibromatosis. *Anesth Analg.* 1996;82:382–385.

152. Kohrman MH. Emerging treatments in the management of tuberous sclerosis complex. *Pediatr Neurol.* 2012;46:267–275.

153. Terry AR, Merker VL, Barker FG 2nd, et al. Pregnancy complications in women with rare tumor suppressor syndromes affecting central and peripheral nervous system. *Am J Obstet Gynecol.* 2015;213:108–109.

154. Forsnes EV, Eggleston MK, Burtman M. Placental abruption and spontaneous rupture of renal angiomyolipoma in a pregnant woman with tuberous sclerosis. *Obstet Gynecol.* 1996;88:725.

155. Causse-Mariscal A, Palot M, Visseaux H, et al. Labor analgesia and cesarean section in women affected by tuberous sclerosis: report of two cases. *Int J Obstet Anesth.* 2007;16:277–280.

156. McCarthy T, Leighton R, Mushambi M. Spinal anaesthesia for caesarean section for a woman with von Hippel Lindau disease. *Int J Obstet Anesth.* 2010;19:461–462.

157. Carta G, De Lellis V, Di Nicola M, Kaliakoudas D. Peripartum cardiomyopathy and Klippel-Trenaunay syndrome. *Clin Exp Obstet Gynecol.* 2010;37:155–157.

158. Wijdicks EF, Klein CJ. Guillain-Barré syndrome. *Mayo Clin Proc.* 2017;92:467–479.

159. Pacheco LD, Saad AF, Hankins GD, et al. Guillain-Barré syndrome in pregnancy. *Obstet Gynecol.* 2016;128:1105–1110.

160. Wipfli M, Arnold M, Luginbuhl M. Repeated spinal anesthesia in a tetraparetic patient with Guillain-Barré syndrome. *J Clin Anesth.* 2013;25:409–412.

161. Wiertlewski S, Magot A, Drapier S, et al. Worsening of neurologic symptoms after epidural anesthesia for labor in a Guillain-Barré patient. *Anesth Analg.* 2004;98:825–827.

162. Steiner I, Argov Z, Cahan C, Abramsky O. Guillain-Barré syndrome after epidural anesthesia: direct nerve root damage may trigger disease. *Neurology.* 1985;35:1473–1475.

163. Lambert DA, Giannouli E, Schmidt BJ. Postpolio syndrome and anesthesia. *Anesthesiology.* 2005;103:638–644.

164. Boyer FC, Tiffreau V, Rapin A, et al. Post-polio syndrome: pathophysiological hypotheses, diagnosis criteria, drug therapy. *Ann Phys Rehabil Med.* 2010;53:34–41.

165. Hagan JE, Wassilak SG, Craig AS, et al. Progress toward polio eradication—worldwide, 2014-2015. *MMWR Morb Mortal Wkly Rep*. 2015;64:527–531.

166. Harjulehto-Mervaala T, Aro T, Hiilesmaa VK, et al. Oral polio vaccination during pregnancy: lack of impact on fetal development and perinatal outcome. *Clin Infect Dis*. 1994;18:414–420.

167. Veiby G, Daltveit AK, Gilhus NE. Pregnancy, delivery and perinatal outcome in female survivors of polio. *J Neurol Sci*. 2007;258:27–32.

168. Rezende DPR, Rodrigues MR, Costa VV, et al. Patients with sequelae of poliomyelitis. Does the anesthetic technique impose risks? *Rev Bras Anestesiol*. 2008;58:210–219.

169. Costello JF, Balki M. Cesarean delivery under ultrasound-guided spinal anesthesia [corrected] in a parturient with poliomyelitis and Harrington instrumentation. *Can J Anaesth*. 2008;55:606–611.

170. Connelly NR, Abbott TC. Successful use of succinylcholine for cesarean delivery in a patient with postpolio syndrome. *Anesthesiology*. 2008;108:1151–1152.

171. Swensen R, Kirsch W. Brain neoplasms in women: a review. *Clin Obstet Gynecol*. 2002;45:904–927.

172. Bonfield CM, Engh JA. Pregnancy and brain tumors. *Neurol Clin*. 2012;30:937–946.

173. Araujo PB, Vieira Neto L, Gadelha MR. Pituitary tumor management in pregnancy. *Endocrinol Metab Clin North Am*. 2015;44:181–197.

174. Yust-Katz S, de Groot JF, Liu D, et al. Pregnancy and glial brain tumors. *Neuro Oncol*. 2014;16:1289–1294.

175. Soper JT, Spillman M, Sampson JH, et al. High-risk gestational trophoblastic neoplasia with brain metastases: individualized multidisciplinary therapy in the management of four patients. *Gynecol Oncol*. 2007;104:691–694.

176. Terry AR, Barker FG 2nd, Leffert L, et al. Outcomes of hospitalization in pregnant women with CNS neoplasms: a population-based study. *Neuro Oncol*. 2012;14:768–776.

177. American College of Radiology Committee on Drugs and Contrast Media. Administration of contrast media to pregnant or potentially pregnant patients. *ACR Manual on Contrast Media, Version 103*. American College of Radiology; 2017:98–101.

178. Marx GF, Zemaitis MT, Orkin LR. Cerebrospinal fluid pressures during labor and obstetrical anesthesia. *Anesthesiology*. 1961;22:348–354.

179. Leffert LR, Schwamm LH. Neuraxial anesthesia in parturients with intracranial pathology: a comprehensive review and reassessment of risk. *Anesthesiology*. 2013;119:703–718.

180. Kepes ER, Andrews IC, Radnay PA, et al. Conduct of anesthesia for delivery with grossly raised cerebrospinal fluid pressure. *N Y State J Med*. 1972;72:115–156.

181. Goroszeniuk T, Howard RS, Wright JT. The management of labour using continuous lumbar epidural analgesia in a patient with a malignant cerebral tumour. *Anaesthesia*. 1986;41:1128–1129.

182. Atanassoff PG, Alon E, Weiss BM, Lauper U. Spinal anaesthesia for caesarean section in a patient with brain neoplasma. *Can J Anaesth*. 1994;41:163–164.

183. Su TM, Lan CM, Yang LC, et al. Brain tumor presenting with fatal herniation following delivery under epidural anesthesia. *Anesthesiology*. 2002;96:508–509.

184. Chang L, Looi-Lyons L, Bartosik L, Tindal S. Anesthesia for cesarean section in two patients with brain tumours. *Can J Anaesth*. 1999;46:61–65.

185. Wang LP, Paech MJ. Neuroanesthesia for the pregnant woman. *Anesth Analg*. 2008;107:193–200.

186. Mofatteh M, Mashayekhi MS, Arfaie S, et al. Awake craniotomy during pregnancy: a systematic review of the published literature. *Neurosurg Rev*. 2023;46:290.

187. Kazemi P, Villar G, Flexman AM. Anesthetic management of neurosurgical procedures during pregnancy: a case series. *J Neurosurg Anesthesiol*. 2014;26:234–240.

188. Wakerley BR, Mollan SP, Sinclair AJ. Idiopathic intracranial hypertension: update on diagnosis and management. *Clin Med (Lond)*. 2020;20:384–388.

189. Virdee J, Larcombe S, Vijay V, et al. Reviewing the recent developments in idiopathic intracranial hpertension. *Ophthalmol Ther*. 2020;9:767–781.

190. Mollan SP, Aguiar M, Evison F, et al. The expanding burden of idiopathic intracranial hypertension. *Eye (Lond)*. 2019;33:478–485.

191. Andrews LE, Liu GT, Ko MW. Idiopathic intracranial hypertension and obesity. *Horm Res Paediatr*. 2014;81:217–225.

192. Hallan DR, Lin AC, Tankam CS, et al. Pregnancy and childbirth in women with idiopathic intracranial hypertension. *Cureus*. 2022;14:e30420.

193. Borire AA, Hughes AR, Lueck CJ. Tonsillar herniation after lumbar puncture in idiopathic intracranial hypertension. *J Neuroophthalmol*. 2015;35:293–295.

194. Hoffman KR, Chan SW, Hughes AR, Halcrow SJ. Management of cerebellar tonsillar herniation following lumbar puncture in idiopathic intracranial hypertension. *Case Rep Crit Care*. 2015;2015:895035.

195. Sullivan HC. Fatal tonsillar herniation in pseudotumor cerebri. *Neurology*. 1991;41:1142–1144.

196. Karmaniolou I, Petropoulos G, Theodoraki K. Management of idiopathic intracranial hypertension in parturients: anesthetic considerations. *Can J Anaesth*. 2011;58:650–657.

197. Bedard JM, Richardson MG, Wissler RN. Epidural anesthesia in a parturient with a lumboperitoneal shunt. *Anesthesiology*. 1999;90:621–623.

198. Kaul B, Vallejo MC, Ramanathan S, et al. Accidental spinal analgesia in the presence of a lumboperitoneal shunt in an obese parturient receiving enoxaparin therapy. *Anesth Analg*. 2002;95:441–443.

199. Heckathorn J, Cata JP, Barsoum S. Intrathecal anesthesia for cesarean delivery via a subarachnoid drain in a woman with benign intracranial hypertension. *Int J Obstet Anesth*. 2010;19:109–111.

200. Aly EE, Lawther BK. Anaesthetic management of uncontrolled idiopathic intracranial hypertension during labour and delivery using an intrathecal catheter. *Anaesthesia*. 2007;62:178–181.

201. Moore DM, Meela M, Kealy D, et al. An intrathecal catheter in a pregnant patient with idiopathic intracranial hypertension: analgesia, monitor and therapy? *Int J Obstet Anesth*. 2014;23:175–178.

202. Paciorkowski AR, Greenstein RM. When is enlargement of the subarachnoid spaces not benign? A genetic perspective. *Pediatr Neurol*. 2007;37:1–7.

203. Liakos AM, Bradley NK, Magram G, Muszynski C. Hydrocephalus and the reproductive health of women: the medical implications of maternal shunt dependency in 70 women and 138 pregnancies. *Neurol Res*. 2000;22:69–88.

204. Al-Saadi TD, Glisic M, Al Sharqi A, et al. Safety of pregnancy in ventriculoperitoneal shunt dependent women: meta-analysis

and systematic review of the literature. *Neurol India.* 2020;68: 548–554.

205. Rajagopalan S, Gopinath S, Trinh VT, Chandrasekhar S. Anesthetic considerations for labor and delivery in women with cerebrospinal fluid shunts. *Int J Obstet Anesth.* 2017;30: 23–29.

206. Korhonen A, Verho L, Aarnio K, et al. Subarachnoid hemorrhage during pregnancy and puerperium: a population-based study. *Stroke.* 2023;54:198–207.

207. Kim YW, Neal D, Hoh BL. Cerebral aneurysms in pregnancy and delivery: pregnancy and delivery do not increase the risk of aneurysm rupture. *Neurosurgery.* 2013;72:143–150.

208. Hoh BL, Ko NU, Amin-Hanjani S, et al. 2023 Guideline for the management of patients with aneurysmal subarachnoid hemorrhage: a guideline from the American Heart Association/American Stroke Association. *Stroke.* 2023;54:e314–e370.

209. Ng J, Kitchen N. Neurosurgery and pregnancy. *J Neurol Neurosurg Psychiatry.* 2008;79:745–752.

210. Liu P, Lv X, Li Y, Lv M. Endovascular management of intracranial aneurysms during pregnancy in three cases and review of the literature. *Interv Neuroradiol.* 2015;21:654–658.

211. Ladhani NNN, Swartz RH, Foley N, et al. Canadian stroke best practice consensus statement: acute stroke management during pregnancy. *Int J Stroke.* 2018;13:743–758.

212. Piotin M, de Souza Filho CB, Kothimbakam R, Moret J. Endovascular treatment of acutely ruptured intracranial aneurysms in pregnancy. *Am J Obstet Gynecol.* 2001;185: 1261–1262.

213. Agarwal N, Guerra JC, Gala NB, et al. Current treatment options for cerebral arteriovenous malformations in pregnancy: a review of the literature. *World Neurosurg.* 2014;81:83–90.

214. Carvalho CS, Resende F, Centeno MJ, et al. Anesthetic approach of pregnant woman with cerebral arteriovenous malformation and subarachnoid hemorrhage during pregnancy: case report. *Braz J Anesthesiol.* 2013;63:223–226.

215. Lin BF, Kuo CY, Wu ZF. Review of aneurysmal subarachnoid hemorrhage—focus on treatment, anesthesia, cerebral vasospasm prophylaxis, and therapy. *Acta Anaesthesiol Taiwan.* 2014;52:77–84.

216. Stam J. Thrombosis of the cerebral veins and sinuses. *N Engl J Med.* 2005;352:1791–1798.

217. Saposnik G, Bushnell C, Coutinho JM, et al. Diagnosis and management of cerebral venous thrombosis: a scientific statement from the American Heart Association. *Stroke.* 2024;55:e77–e90.

218. Lockhart EM, Baysinger CL. Intracranial venous thrombosis in the parturient. *Anesthesiology.* 2007;107:652–658.

219. Kashkoush AI, Ma H, Agarwal N, et al. Cerebral venous sinus thrombosis in pregnancy and puerperium: a pooled, systematic review. *J Clin Neurosci.* 2017;39:9–15.

220. Amjadi N, Mohammadi S, Paybast S, et al. A pregnant woman with amyotrophic lateral sclerosis from Iran: a case report. *Ann Med Surg (Lond).* 2024;86:3013–3015.

221. Hamad AA, Amer BE, Al Mawla AM, et al. Clinical characteristics, course, and outcomes of amyotrophic lateral sclerosis overlapping with pregnancy: a systematic review of 38 published cases. *Neurol Sci.* 2023;44:4219–4231.

222. Masrori P, Ospitalieri S, Forsberg K, et al. Respiratory onset of amyotrophic lateral sclerosis in a pregnant woman with a novel SOD1 mutation. *Eur J Neurol.* 2022;29:1279–1283.

223. Raymond J, Mehta P, Larson T, et al. Reproductive history and age of onset for women diagnosed with amyotrophic lateral sclerosis: data from the National ALS Registry: 2010–2018. *Neuroepidemiology.* 2021;55:416–424.

224. Wang Y, Zhang Y, Li S, et al. Transversus abdominis plane block provides effective and safe anesthesia in the cesarean section for an amyotrophic lateral sclerosis parturient: a case report. *Medicine (Baltimore).* 2021;100:e27621.

225. Frazer KL, Porter S, Goss C. The genetics and implications of neuromuscular diseases in pregnancy. *J Perinat Neonatal Nurs.* 2013;27:205–214.

226. Harris SJ, Moaz K. Caesarean section conducted under subarachnoid block in two sisters with spinal muscular atrophy. *Int J Obstet Anesth.* 2002;11:125–127.

227. Alamri LA, Foxx AM, Dwan RL, et al. Pregnancy in a patient with spinal muscular atrophy and severe restrictive lung disease. *AJP Rep.* 2023;13:e98–e101.

228. Aboussouan LS, Lewis RA, Shy ME. Disorders of pulmonary function, sleep, and the upper airway in Charcot-Marie-Tooth disease. *Lung.* 2007;185:1–7.

229. Hoff JM, Gilhus NE, Daltveit AK. Pregnancies and deliveries in patients with Charcot-Marie-Tooth disease. *Neurology.* 2005;64:459–462.

230. Greenwood JJ, Scott WE. Charcot-Marie-Tooth disease: peripartum management of two contrasting clinical cases. *Int J Obstet Anesth.* 2007;16:149–154.

231. Hussain A, Nduka C, Moth P, Malhotra R. Bell's facial nerve palsy in pregnancy: a clinical review. *J Obstet Gynaecol.* 2017;37:409–415.

232. Gillman GS, Schaitkin BM, May M, Klein SR. Bell's palsy in pregnancy: a study of recovery outcomes. *Otolaryngol Head Neck Surg.* 2002;126:26–30.

233. Dorsey DL, Camann WR. Obstetric anesthesia in patients with idiopathic facial paralysis (Bell's palsy): a 10-year survey. *Anesth Analg.* 1993;77:81–83.

234. Padua L, Di Pasquale A, Pazzaglia C, et al. Systematic review of pregnancy-related carpal tunnel syndrome. *Muscle Nerve.* 2010;42:697–702.

235. Finsen V, Zeitlmann H. Carpal tunnel syndrome during pregnancy. *Scand J Plast Reconstr Surg Hand Surg.* 2006;40: 41–45.

Obesity

Ashraf S. Habib, MBBCh, MSc, MHSc, FRCA

Obesity is a worldwide health problem, with the prevalence in the general population growing at an alarming rate. The World Obesity Federation predicts that 1 billion people globally, including one in five women, will be living with obesity by 2030, which is almost double the 2010 rate. The highest rates of obesity are found in the World Health Organization (WHO) Americas region.[1] Data from the National Health and Nutrition Examination Survey show that during 2017 to 2018, 39.7% of women of reproductive age (20 to 39 years of age) were obese, compared with a prevalence of 29.8% in 2001 to 2002.[2] Although no definition of obesity specific to pregnancy exists, a pregnant woman is generally considered overweight when her body mass index (BMI) is 25.0 to 29.9 kg/m², and obese when her BMI is greater than or equal to 30 kg/m². The WHO defines three grades of obesity: class I (BMI 30.0 to 34.9 kg/m²), class II (BMI 35.0 to 39.9 kg/m²), and class III (BMI ≥ 40 kg/m²). To allow for the weight gain of pregnancy, some groups have suggested adding 5 kg/m² to the WHO classes to define pregnancy thresholds.[3]

Obesity is associated with an increased risk for maternal morbidity and mortality.[4,5] The care of obese parturients poses significant challenges to the anesthesia provider as a result of common comorbidities, an increased cesarean delivery rate, and technical difficulties associated with both neuraxial and general anesthesia. Understanding the pathophysiologic changes and comorbidities associated with obesity and pregnancy is crucial for the safe conduct of anesthesia in these high-risk patients.

PHYSIOLOGIC CHANGES OF OBESITY

Cardiopulmonary Changes

Obesity increases the demands on the cardiopulmonary system. The effects of obesity and pregnancy on the respiratory and cardiovascular systems are summarized in Table 48.1 and Table 48.2. As energy expenditure increases in proportion to the increase in body mass,[6] oxygen consumption and carbon dioxide (CO_2) production also increase in proportion to the increase in work performed.[7] Minute ventilation is increased owing to the elevated respiratory demand, except in the 5% to 10% of obese patients with **Pickwickian syndrome**, who display a reduced sensitivity to CO_2.[8] Obesity affects the body's ability to meet these demands by changing pulmonary mechanics, altering lung volumes, and impairing oxygen consumption.

Obesity increases the weight of the chest wall; thus, greater energy expenditure is required during ventilation to move this mass. Morbidly obese patients expend a disproportionately high percentage of total oxygen consumption on respiratory work compared with lean controls, even during quiet breathing.[9] The weight gain during pregnancy further increases the work of breathing. In obese individuals, frequent shallow respirations may represent a more efficient breathing pattern than large tidal volumes. This pattern of frequent shallow respirations contrasts with the increased tidal volumes that typically accompany pregnancy.

Greater abdominal weight restricts diaphragm movement, especially in the supine or Trendelenburg positions, requiring smaller tidal volumes. Functional residual capacity (FRC) decreases at the expense of expiratory reserve volume and

TABLE 48.1 Physiologic Changes in the Respiratory System Induced by Pregnancy and Obesity

	Pregnancy	Obesity	Combined Effect
Tidal volume	↑	↓	↑
Respiratory rate	↑	↔ or ↑	↑
Minute volume	↑	↓ or ↔	↑
Expiratory reserve volume	↓	↓↓	↓
Residual volume	↓	↓ or ↔	↓
Functional residual capacity	↓↓	↓↓↓	↓↓
Vital capacity	↔	↓	↓
FEV$_1$	↔	↓ or ↔	↔
FEV$_1$/VC	↔	↔	↔
Total lung capacity	↓	↓↓	↓
Compliance	↔	↓↓	↓
Work of breathing	↑	↑↑	↑
V/Q mismatch	↑	↑	↑↑
Pao$_2$	↓	↓↓	↓
Paco$_2$	↓	↑	↓

↑, Increase; ↓, decrease, ↔, no change; more than one arrow represents the degree of intensity; *FEV$_1$*, forced expiratory volume in 1s; *VC*, vital capacity; *V/Q*, ventilation/perfusion.
Modified from Saravanakumar K, Rao SG, Cooper GM. Obesity and obstetric anaesthesia. *Anaesthesia*. 2006;61:36–48.

TABLE 48.2 Physiologic Changes in the Cardiovascular System Induced by Pregnancy and Obesity

	Pregnancy	Obesity	Combined Effect
Heart rate	↑	↑↑	↑↑
Stroke volume	↑↑	↑	↑
Cardiac output	↑↑	↑	↑↑↑
Blood volume	↑↑	↑	↑
Hematocrit	↓↓	↑	↓
Systemic vascular resistance	↓↓	↑	↔ or ↓
Mean arterial pressure	↓ or ↔	↑↑	↑↑
Systolic function	↔	↔ or ↓	↔ or ↓
Diastolic function	↔	↓	↓
Central venous pressure	↔	↑	↑↑
Pulmonary artery occlusion pressure	↔	↑↑	↑↑

↑, Increase; ↓, decrease, ↔, no change; more than one arrow represents the degree of intensity.
Modified from Saravanakumar K, Rao SG, Cooper GM. Obesity and obstetric anaesthesia. *Anaesthesia*. 2006;61:36–48.

may be less than closing capacity. Both chest wall and lung compliance decrease, but airway resistance increases as a result of reduction in lung volumes.[10]

Pulmonary diffusion typically remains normal in most women with morbid obesity. Decreased chest wall compliance and greater abdominal weight promote airway closure in the dependent portions of the lung.[11] Ventilation preferentially occurs in the more compliant, nondependent portions of the lung. In contrast, pulmonary blood flow preferentially occurs in the dependent portions of the lungs, resulting in ventilation-perfusion mismatch and hypoxemia.[11] Consistent with the positional deterioration of lung volumes, oxygenation worsens in obese individuals in the supine and Trendelenburg positions.

Blood volume and cardiac output are increased, the latter from increases in both stroke volume and heart rate. Both preload and left ventricular afterload are increased. These changes can result in both eccentric and concentric left ventricular hypertrophy. Among morbidly obese pregnant women, left atrial size, left ventricular thickness, interventricular septal thickness, and left ventricular mass are increased compared with nonobese pregnant women.[12] The increase in heart rate limits the time for diastolic filling; thus, diastolic relaxation is impaired. Pulmonary blood volume increases

in proportion to increases in cardiac output and total blood volume. Pulmonary hypertension can occur in up to 5% of obese, otherwise healthy, individuals. Aortocaval compression in the supine position may be greater in obese parturients, particularly those with a large fat panniculus.

The risks of **chronic hypertension**, **gestational hypertension**, and **preeclampsia** are also increased in women with obesity. It is estimated that the risk of preeclampsia doubles for every 5 to 7 kg/m^2 increase in BMI,[13] and is three to four times higher in those with class II or III obesity, compared with those with class I obesity.[14]

Gastrointestinal Changes

It is unclear whether obesity in pregnancy is associated with an increase in gastric volume and a decrease in gastric pH. Roberts and Shirley[15] reported that gastric volumes aspirated from obese laboring women undergoing cesarean delivery were significantly higher than those obtained from lean controls. Studies in the general surgical population, however, reported conflicting results; some confirmed these findings[16] and others reported no difference in gastric volume and pH in obese patients compared with lean patients.[17]

Similarly, data for gastric emptying in the obese population are conflicting; studies have reported delayed, unchanged, or more rapid rates of gastric emptying in obese subjects compared with lean subjects.[18] In nonobstetric obese patients, Maltby et al.[19] reported that drinking 300 mL of clear fluid

2 hours before surgery had no effect on gastric fluid volume and pH compared with fasting after midnight. Similarly, Wong et al.[20] found that gastric emptying in obese, nonlaboring term pregnant volunteers was not delayed after ingestion of 300 mL compared with 50 mL of water; gastric volume returned to baseline 60 minutes after ingestion. A study using ultrasonography to assess the gastric antrum in women undergoing elective cesarean delivery reported a positive correlation between the antral cross-sectional area and BMI, and a higher gastric volume in obese parturients with BMI ≥ 30 kg/m² compared with those with lower BMI.[21]

Both **gastroesophageal reflux** and **hiatal hernia** are more common in obese than in nonobese patients.[22] Obesity is also associated with a higher risk for difficult airway management, which is a known risk factor for pulmonary aspiration.[23] Therefore, morbidly obese patients are likely at increased risk for pulmonary aspiration of gastric contents.

Coagulation Changes

Obesity is associated with an increased risk for thromboembolic complications.[24] **Venous thromboembolism** is a leading cause of direct maternal mortality. In the United Kingdom, 72% of women who died from thromboembolic complications in 2017 to 2019 were overweight or obese.[25]

Obesity is associated with changes in coagulation, venous stasis, and endothelial injury that contribute to the pathogenesis of venous thromboembolism. For instance, adipose tissue secretes the following: (1) adipokines such as plasminogen activator inhibitor-1, which results in impaired fibrinolysis; (2) leptin, which promotes platelet aggregation; and (3) interleukin-6, which stimulates the liver to produce coagulation factors.[26,27] C-reactive protein levels are also elevated in obese women, leading to platelet activation.[28] Venous stasis is worsened in obese women by increased intraabdominal pressure, which leads to increased iliofemoral venous pressure.[29] Obesity was shown to be associated with endothelial dysfunction in the nonpregnant population.[30] Therefore, all risk factors that contribute to the pathogenesis of thromboembolic complications are likely to be exacerbated by obesity. The risk is further increased by reduced mobility, comorbidities such as preeclampsia, and an increased frequency of operative delivery.

Endocrine Changes

Gestational and nongestational diabetes mellitus occur more frequently in obese patients.[14] The pathologic process is attributed to the following: (1) peripheral insulin resistance as a result of augmentation of free fatty acids by visceral obesity,[31] (2) increased proinflammatory cytokine levels,[32] (3) relative gonadotropin resistance, and (4) low sex hormone–binding globulin concentration, which leads to hyperandrogenism and decreased insulin sensitivity.[33] The concentration of adiponectin, an adipokine with insulin-sensitizing properties, is also decreased in obesity, which leads to decreased insulin sensitivity.[26]

COMORBIDITIES ASSOCIATED WITH OBESITY

Sleep Apnea

Obesity is a significant risk factor for **obstructive sleep apnea (OSA)**, which is characterized by repeated episodes of complete or partial upper airway collapse that lead to hypoxemia and hypercarbia. Repeated periods of hypoxemia and reoxygenation lead to endocrine and metabolic disturbances, which result in increased risks for hypertension, myocardial infarction, stroke, diabetes, and metabolic syndrome.[34] It is estimated that 15% to 20% of obese pregnant women have OSA.[35] The prevalence and severity of OSA are higher among gravidas with chronic hypertension compared with BMI- and gestational age-matched normotensive pregnant women.[36]

The changes of pregnancy may both worsen and protect against OSA. For example, weight gain[37] and estrogen-induced hyperemia and edema of nasal mucosa[38] might promote OSA, whereas sleeping in the lateral position,[39] reduced rapid eye movement sleep, and the progesterone-induced increase in minute ventilation might protect against it.

OSA may adversely affect maternal and neonatal outcomes. A large in patient database study showed that pregnant women with OSA are at increased risk for **preeclampsia, eclampsia, cardiomyopathy,** and **pulmonary embolism,** and are five times more likely to die in the hospital during a pregnancy or delivery admission than women without OSA.[40] These differences were unchanged after controlling for obesity, but the associations with preeclampsia and severe cardiovascular complications were stronger in obese women. Using nationwide data, Frappaolo et al.[41] investigated outcomes associated with OSA in a sample of 76,753,013 delivery hospitalizations from 2000 to 2019. After adjusting for obesity and other clinical, demographic, and hospital characteristics, OSA was associated with increased odds for **mechanical ventilation** or **tracheostomy, acute respiratory distress syndrome, hypertensive disorders of pregnancy, stillbirth, pulmonary edema/heart failure, peripartum hysterectomy,** and **preterm birth.**

Other Comorbidities

Obesity is associated with an increased risk for a number of disease states compared with lean controls, as shown in Table 48.3.[22,24,42] These comorbidities complicate the care of obese parturients.

IMPACT OF OBESITY ON PREGNANCY

Maternal and Fetal Complications

Obesity results in greater use of healthcare resources. Chu et al.[43] reported that obese pregnant women receive significantly more prenatal tests, ultrasonographic examinations, medications, and prenatal visits with a physician, and they are at greater risk for having a high-risk pregnancy, cesarean delivery, and prolonged hospitalization compared with pregnant women of normal weight.

Obesity is associated with an increased incidence of maternal, fetal, and neonatal complications. These include a higher risk for **spontaneous abortion (miscarriage), thromboembolic complications, gestational diabetes mellitus, hypertensive disorders of pregnancy, dysfunctional labor, shoulder dystocia, operative vaginal delivery, cesarean delivery, postpartum hemorrhage (PPH), wound infection, fetal macrosomia, fetal congenital anomalies, stillbirth,** and **neonatal death** (Table 48.4).[4,44,45]

Most importantly, obesity increases the risk for **death during pregnancy.** In a French population–based case-control

TABLE 48.3 Relative Risk or Odds Ratio of Comorbidities Associated With Obesity

Comorbidity	Relative Risk	95% CI
Type 2 diabetes mellitus[a]	12.41	9.03 to 17.06
Hypertension[a]	2.42	1.95 to 3.67
Coronary artery disease[a]	3.10	2.81 to 3.43
Congestive heart failure[a]	1.78	1.07 to 2.95
Pulmonary embolism[a]	3.51	2.61 to 4.73
Stroke[a]	1.49	1.27 to 1.74
Asthma[a]	1.78	1.36 to 2.32
Gallbladder disease[a]	2.32	1.17 to 4.57
Osteoarthritis[a]	1.96	1.88 to 2.04
Chronic back pain[a]	2.81	2.27 to 3.48
	Odds Ratio	**95% CI**
Depression[b]	1.33	1.20 to 1.48
Gastroesophageal reflux disease[c]	1.73	1.46 to 2.06

CI, Confidence interval.
[a]Data from Guh DP, Zhang W, Bansback N, et al. The incidence of co-morbidities related to obesity and overweight: a systematic review and meta-analysis. *BMC Public Health.* 2009;9:88.
[b]Data from Dachew BA, Ayano G, Betts K, Alati R. The impact of pre-pregnancy BMI on maternal depressive and anxiety symptoms during pregnancy and the postpartum period: a systematic review and meta-analysis. *J Affect Disord.* 2021;281:321–330.
[c]Data from Esubi LH. Global prevalence of, and risk factors for gastro-oesophageal reflux symptoms: a meta-analysis. *Gut.* 2018;67:430–440.

TABLE 48.4 Relative Risk of Obstetric Complications in Obese Women Compared With Women With Standard BMI

Outcome	Relative Risk (95% CI)		
	Obesity Class I	Obesity Class II	Obesity Class III
Gestational diabetes mellitus	2.8 (2.3 to 3.4)	3.6 (2.8 to 4.6)	4.6 (3.6 to 5.9)
Hypertensive disorders of pregnancy	2.5 (2.1 to 3.0)	3.6 (2.9 to 4.4)	4.6 (3.4 to 6.0)
Macrosomia	2.0 (1.4 to 3.0)	2.1 (1.3 to 3.5)	2.6 (1.4 to 4.7)
Shoulder dystocia	1.2 (1.1 to 1.3)	1.3 (1.1 to 1.5)	1.3 (0.9 to 1.9)
Preterm delivery	1.2 (1.1 to 1.2)	1.2 (1.1 to 1.3)	1.2 (1.0 to 1.5)
Neonatal ICU admission	1.3 (1.2 to 1.3)	1.4 (1.3 to 1.6)	1.6 (1.4 to 1.9)
Neonatal death	1.3 (1.0 to 1.8)	1.8 (1.4 to 2.3)	1.8 (1.2 to 2.9)
Planned cesarean delivery	1.3 (1.2 to 1.5)	1.4 (1.3 to 1.6)	1.7 (1.5 to 1.8)
Unplanned cesarean delivery	1.3 (1.3 to 1.4)	1.4 (1.1 to 1.9)	1.5 (1.1 to 2.1)

Standard BMI was defined as 18.5–24.9 kg/m². Obesity classes I–III were based on the World Health Organization international classification system. Relative risk values are for the comparison with women with standard BMI. *BMI,* Body mass index; *CI,* confidence interval; *ICU,* intensive care unit. Data from D'Souza R, Horyn I, Pavalagantharajah S, et al. Maternal body mass index and pregnancy outcomes: a systematic review and metaanalysis. *Am J Obstet Gynecol MFM.* 2019;1:100041.

study that included 364 maternal deaths from the 2007 to 2012 French National Confidential Inquiry into Maternal Deaths (ENCMM, Enquête Confidentielle sur les Morts Maternelles), the adjusted odds ratio (OR) of death was 1.65 (95% confidence interval [CI], 1.24 to 2.19) in overweight women, 2.22 (95% CI, 1.55 to 3.19) in women with class I obesity, and 3.40 (95% CI, 2.17 to 5.33) in women with class II to III obesity, compared with women with normal BMI.[46] The report of the Confidential Enquiries into Maternal Deaths in the United Kingdom (MBRRACE-UK Saving Lives, Improving Mothers' Care) for 2018 to 2020 showed that 51% of women who died were overweight or obese, a trend that has been consistent for the last several reports.[47] The increased risk for death associated with obesity has been attributed to the associated comorbidities such as hypertensive disorders of pregnancy. The impact of obesity on maternal mortality is particularly evident in women who die of thromboembolism or cardiac disease.[46,47]

Anesthesia-Related Complications

Obesity has also been identified as a risk factor for anesthesia-related complications and anesthesia-related maternal mortality. A study of all maternal cardiac arrests in the United Kingdom over a 2-year period found that 24% of cases were solely as a consequence of anesthesia, three-fourths of whom were obese.[48] In the United States, Mhyre et al.[49] reported that six of eight pregnant women who died of anesthesia-related deaths in Michigan between 1985 and 2003 were obese. Because of the increased risk for complications, guidelines published both in the United

Kingdom[50] and by the American College of Obstetricians and Gynecologists (ACOG)[51] recommend a multidisciplinary approach to the care and treatment of obese pregnant women, including referral consultation with an anesthesia provider. The ACOG recommends anesthetic consultation before labor or in early labor in women with obesity to allow for adequate time to plan for care.[51] In the United Kingdom, the recommendation is to refer pregnant women with a booking BMI ≥ 40 kg/m² for antenatal anesthetic assessment and to involve a senior anesthesiologist in the care of those patients intrapartum.[50]

Progress of Labor and Method of Delivery

The progress of labor appears to be affected by obesity. A large multicenter study involving 118,978 patients whose labor management reflected current practice in the United States found that labor progressed more slowly with increasing BMI for both nulliparous and parous women.[52] The median time to progress from 4 to 10 cm cervical dilation was greater in morbidly obese women compared with lean women for both nulliparous women (7.7 versus 5.4 hours, respectively) and parous women (5.4 versus 4.6 hours, respectively). These findings were independent of gestational age and induction of labor. Entry into the active phase of labor was also delayed in parous women as a function of BMI. Possible explanations include increased fetal size, higher labor induction rates, and/or decreased responsiveness to oxytocin.[52]

Poor uterine contractility has also been demonstrated in obese parturients. Myometrium obtained from obese women at cesarean delivery contracted with less force and frequency and had less calcium flux compared with myometrium from normal-weight women.[53] This observation may be attributable to the inhibitory effect of cholesterol[53] and/or adipokines (e.g., leptin, ghrelin, apelin), which inhibit human uterine contractility *in vitro*.[54] Inadequate myometrial contractility has also been implicated in a higher rate of uterine atony and PPH, after both vaginal and operative deliveries, in obese women. However, the literature has been mixed with regard to the effect of BMI on the risk of PPH. In a large retrospective study of 30,298 pregnancies over an 8-year period,[55] the risk for PPH was significantly higher with increasing BMI (OR, 2.7; 95% CI, 2.2 to 3.4 for obesity class III versus nonobesity). Similarly, in a large cohort study involving 1,114,071 women from Sweden over a 12-year period,[56] the risk of atonic PPH was 14% higher in women with obesity class I, 47% higher in those with obesity class II, and 114% higher in those with obesity class III, compared with normal-weight women, irrespective of the mode of delivery. Conversely, a retrospective cohort study of 2,176,673 women in California reported only a modest increase in the risk of hemorrhage or atonic hemorrhage after vaginal delivery among overweight and obese women.[57] After cesarean delivery, however, women in any obesity class had up to 14% decreased odds of severe hemorrhage. Furthermore, a metaanalysis found no association between obesity and the risk of atonic PPH.[58] However, an increased dose requirement for oxytocin to achieve adequate uterine tone during scheduled cesarean delivery was reported among obese patients.[59,60]

Obesity is also associated with a higher risk for **failed medical induction of labor**. In a secondary analysis of data from a large labor induction trial involving 1273 patients, the duration of labor, oxytocin requirement, and cesarean delivery rate were significantly higher in women with a greater BMI.[61] In a large series from Sweden involving 233,887 deliveries, Cedergren[62] found a fourfold increase in the risk for cesarean delivery in parturients with a BMI > 40 kg/m² compared with parturients of normal weight, primarily because of failed or obstructed labor. Operative vaginal delivery, with its associated maternal and fetal morbidity, is also more likely in the obese parturient.[4]

Risk for **fetal macrosomia** is higher with obesity, which increases the risk for **shoulder dystocia** and its associated birth trauma, and predisposes to perineal lacerations, newborn infant injury, and PPH.[4,63] One study examining maternal anthropometric parameters associated with shoulder dystocia reported a 2.7-fold increase in the risk for shoulder dystocia in obese compared with lean parturients, even after adjustment for potential confounders such as macrosomia and diabetes.[63]

Higher BMI, increased prepregnancy weight, and excessive maternal weight gain increase the risk for both elective and emergency cesarean delivery.[64,65] This risk is further increased by obesity-related pregnancy complications such as **macrosomia, fetal growth restriction, diabetes mellitus, and hypertensive disorders of pregnancy**.[44] In a metaanalysis of 33 trials,[45] the unadjusted ORs of cesarean delivery were 1.46 (95% CI, 1.34 to 1.60), 2.05 (1.86 to 2.27), and 2.89 (2.28 to 3.79) among overweight, obese, and morbidly obese women, respectively, compared with normal-weight pregnant women.

ANESTHETIC MANAGEMENT

The high incidence of comorbid conditions among obese pregnant women necessitates careful preanesthetic assessment. A number of technical matters should be considered when caring for an obese parturient.

An appropriately sized blood pressure cuff must be used for noninvasive blood pressure measurement. Unless the length of the sphygmomanometer cuff exceeds the circumference of the arm by 20%, systolic and diastolic blood pressure measurements may overestimate true maternal blood pressure. Forearm blood pressure measurement is sometimes used if an appropriately sized blood pressure cuff is not available or if the upper arm cuff continues to slide from its position owing to the shape of the obese patient's upper arm. There is a good correlation between upper arm and forearm noninvasive measurements, but forearm pressures exceed upper arm pressures by a mean of 10 (standard deviation 10) mm Hg.[66] There is poor agreement between invasive blood pressure readings and those obtained with the currently available cylindrical blood pressure cuffs placed in various locations on the upper arm or forearm.[67] Conversely, a study that compared invasive blood pressure measurement with a conical blood pressure cuff specifically developed for forearm use showed good agreement with invasive blood pressure readings in obese patients.[68] In selected cases, such as those with hypertensive disease of pregnancy, cardiac disease, or anticipated significant bleeding, invasive monitoring of blood pressure with an intraarterial catheter may be desirable.

Intravenous access may be difficult in obese patients. Ultrasonographic guidance may be useful. If peripheral intravenous access is unsuccessful, central venous cannulation may be necessary.

Appropriately sized labor beds, transportation gurneys, and operating tables, as well as sufficient personnel to assist with patient transport, are imperative. Although standard operating tables are generally rated for persons weighing up to 500 pounds (227 kg), this rating may be insufficient for morbidly obese patients, especially when the table is articulated. Regardless of the weight rating of the table, it is critical that the obese patient be centered over the operating table pedestal at all times. Special equipment for moving and positioning the patient, such as motorized lifts, air mattresses, and longer spinal/epidural needles, may be needed (see later discussion).

Labor and Vaginal Delivery

Many of the options for labor analgesia have limitations in the obese parturient. For example, obese parturients with OSA may be more susceptible to the respiratory depressant effect of **systemic opioids**, leading to episodes of apnea and oxyhemoglobin desaturation. **Pudendal nerve block** may be technically difficult in obese patients. **Inhalation analgesia** is useful in some patients; however, **nitrous oxide** has limited effectiveness and is not available in many birthing rooms. Further, inhalation analgesia may lead to a reduced level of consciousness, which can be dangerous in an obese woman with a difficult airway.

Neuraxial analgesia is the best option for pain relief in the obese parturient. Given the greater risks for fetal macrosomia and shoulder dystocia in obese patients, adequate analgesia is often needed to facilitate an atraumatic vaginal delivery. The use of epidural analgesia during labor allows the anesthesia provider to extend epidural analgesia to surgical anesthesia for cesarean delivery and thus avoid the need for general anesthesia with its associated risks. Given the increased likelihood for cesarean delivery and the greater risk for general anesthesia in the obese parturient, the early administration of neuraxial labor analgesia is recommended in the obese parturient.

When performing neuraxial anesthesia in the obese parturient, technical difficulties may include (1) inability to palpate the spinous processes or identify the midline[69]; (2) greater depth of the epidural space,[70] which may exaggerate minor needle directional errors and increase the likelihood of identifying a lateral portion of the epidural space[71]; and (3) the presence of fat pockets as well as hormonal softening of the ligaments, which may result in a false loss of resistance and/or higher risk for unintentional dural puncture.[72] In most obese parturients, however, the epidural space can be identified with a standard-length epidural needle. Therefore, it seems prudent to use a standard-length needle first, which allows the provider better control, before considering switching to a longer needle.[73]

Observing the prominence of the seventh cervical vertebra and the gluteal cleft can facilitate identification of the midline. Asking the parturient about the perceived location of the needle during block placement (relative to the midline) can also facilitate identification of the midline. Marroquin et al.[74] reported that 77% of morbidly obese parturients who were questioned about the position of the needle during a difficult labor epidural needle placement provided useful feedback to the anesthesia provider. More objectively, ultrasonographic guidance can be used to identify the midline, image the epidural space, and measure the distance from the skin to the epidural space (see Chapter 12). Sahin et al.[75] reported that fewer attempts were needed to establish spinal anesthesia in obese parturients undergoing cesarean delivery when preprocedure ultrasonography was performed. Ultrasound image quality, which is often compromised by excessive lumbar adiposity in obese patients, may be improved with the paramedian sagittal oblique plane compared with the transverse plane.[76] Balki et al.[77] found a strong correlation between the skin-to-epidural space distance measured by ultrasonography and that measured by the epidural needle in obese parturients. However, soft tissue compression with the ultrasound probe resulted in underestimation of the depth of the epidural space in obese women.

Placing the patient in the sitting position facilitates identification of the midline and is preferred by many anesthesia providers when performing neuraxial anesthesia in obese parturients. In the lateral position, gravity may cause lateral adipose tissue to sag downward and obscure the midline. Further, the distance from the skin to the epidural space is minimized when the patient is in the sitting-flexed position.[78,79]

Care is needed to avoid dislodgement of the epidural catheter after insertion. Movement of the epidural catheter relative to the skin is most striking in obese patients. Hamilton et al.[79] demonstrated that patient movement from the sitting-flexed to the lateral decubitus position caused redistribution of the soft tissue of the back. The distance from the skin to the epidural space increases, and an unsecured catheter will appear to be drawn inward by as much as 1.0 to 2.5 cm.[79] An epidural catheter secured with tape to the back of a patient in the sitting flexed position can be unintentionally dislodged from the epidural space when the patient moves from the sitting to the lateral decubitus position. Therefore, these investigators recommended that patients be positioned in the lateral position before the epidural catheter is secured to the skin. Alternatively, when placing the block in the sitting-flexed position, the patient should be asked to sit upright before taping the catheter to the skin.

Many authors have documented technical difficulties with neuraxial techniques in obese parturients. Several studies have reported the need for more attempts to identify the epidural space[80-82] and a higher failure rate[80,83-85] of epidural catheters in obese compared with nonobese patients. A meta-analysis reported greater likelihoods of epidural failure (OR, 1.82; 95% CI, 1.23 to 2.68) and need for multiple attempts (OR, 2.21 [95% CI, 1.39 to 3.52]) in obese compared with nonobese pregnant patients.[86] Although some investigators have reported a higher incidence of unintentional dural puncture in morbidly obese parturients than in lean parturients,[87] others have not confirmed this finding.[88]

It is not clear if epidural local anesthetic dose requirements are altered in morbidly obese parturients. Hodgkinson and Husain[89] administered 20 mL of epidural bupivacaine 0.75% in the L3 to L4 interspace to women undergoing elective or emergency cesarean delivery. The patients remained supine for 40 minutes after drug injection. Twenty-seven percent of patients with BMI < 28 kg/m^2 or weight < 73 kg needed supplementation of the block at 30 minutes, whereas none of the patients with BMI > 28 kg/m^2 or weight > 73 kg required additional local anesthetic to achieve surgical anesthesia. The cephalad extent of block was associated with patient BMI and weight but not with height. Similarly, using an up-down sequential allocation study design to estimate the ED$_{50}$ (median effective dose) of epidural bupivacaine (administered in a volume of 20 mL), Panni and Columb[90] found that obese women required significantly less epidural bupivacaine for initiation of labor analgesia than lean parturients. In contrast, Milligan et al.[91] observed that neither patient position nor obesity affected the extent of sensory blockade when 12 mL of bupivacaine 0.25% was administered for epidural labor analgesia. Duggan et al.[92] found that obesity had only a weak effect in enhancing the spread of epidural local anesthetics; this effect was only observed with the largest volume and concentration used in the study (15 mL of bupivacaine 0.75%), but not with a lower volume (10 mL) and concentration (0.5%) of bupivacaine.

The goals of epidural labor analgesia should be the provision of excellent pain relief with minimal motor block (see Chapter 24). Epidural administration of a dilute solution of local anesthetic with a lipophilic opioid provides analgesia for labor while minimizing adverse effects such as hypotension and motor block. The neuraxial blockade provided to obese parturients in labor should be bilateral and provide excellent analgesia. Otherwise, the epidural catheter should be removed and replaced because an inadequate block with a frequent need for top-up doses may lead to failure should extending the block for cesarean delivery be required.[93] Regular evaluation of the parturient's neuraxial block is therefore essential to allow for early replacement of an inadequate catheter.

The **combined spinal-epidural (CSE) technique** provides a rapid onset of pain relief. In the past, some providers were concerned that an epidural catheter sited as part of a CSE technique remains untested until the spinal block has regressed. Thus, recognition of a malpositioned catheter might be delayed and result in failed epidural anesthesia should the need for emergency cesarean delivery arise. Several studies have refuted these concerns and reported a higher success rate for epidural catheters sited using a CSE technique compared with those sited using a standard epidural technique.[94,95] Presumably, the higher success rate can be attributed to observing backflow of cerebrospinal fluid (CSF) through the spinal needle, thus indirectly confirming correct epidural needle position.[94,95] Further, Booth et al.[95] found that catheter failure was more often recognized within the first 30 minutes of placement in catheters sited as part of a CSE technique compared with those sited with an epidural technique.

The **dural puncture epidural (DPE) technique** is a modification of the CSE technique in which a spinal needle is used to puncture the dura, but no intrathecal drug is injected (see Chapter 12). Some investigators have noted that the DPE technique provides improved quality of analgesia compared with the standard epidural technique, and fewer adverse effects compared with the CSE technique.[96] DPE analgesia may be a useful technique to consider in obese parturients with anticipated difficulty in identifying the epidural space. The backflow of CSF through the spinal needle confirms midline placement and that the tip of the epidural needle is located in the posterior epidural space, decreasing the risk for block failure. Furthermore, the translocation of local anesthetics administered epidurally through the dural puncture may enhance the quality and symmetry of the block. However, these potential advantages were not confirmed in a prospective study that compared the quality of labor analgesia between the DPE and standard epidural techniques in obese women with BMI ≥ 35 kg/m^2.[97] The primary outcome of the quality of labor analgesia was a composite of five

components: (1) asymmetrical block, (2) epidural top-ups, (3) catheter adjustment, (4) catheter replacement, and (5) failed conversion to epidural anesthesia, requiring general anesthesia or replacement neuraxial anesthesia for cesarean delivery. The study found no differences between the groups in the composite primary outcome or any of its individual components. It is important to note that the blocks were placed by experienced providers in this study. Conversely, a retrospective study reported that epidural catheter failure in parturients with superobesity (BMI ≥ 50 kg/m^2) was higher with the standard epidural technique (18/63, 29%) compared with a group that included catheters placed with a CSE or DPE technique (14/153, 9%).[98] Most blocks in this study were performed by residents in training, and catheter migration accounted for 29% of failures. The benefits of those techniques involving dural puncture in this patient population might therefore be more evident in the hands of inexperienced providers.

In cases of unintentional dural puncture, **continuous spinal analgesia** can be used to provide labor analgesia. In addition to providing reliable labor analgesia, continuous spinal analgesia may be converted to spinal anesthesia for emergency cesarean delivery. It is crucial, however, that the catheter be clearly labeled, and all personnel are made aware of its intrathecal location. Unintentional administration of an epidural dose of local anesthetic through the spinal catheter markedly increases the risk for high spinal block and subsequent respiratory arrest.

Some have suggested that the risk for **post–dural puncture headache (PDPH)** may be lower in the obese parturient, perhaps secondary to reduced CSF leak through the dural puncture site caused by the higher intraabdominal pressure that results from a large abdominal panniculus. However, data are conflicting. In a retrospective study of 516 women with unintentional dural puncture with a 17-gauge Tuohy needle, Peralta et al.[99] reported a significantly lower incidence of PDPH in women with BMI ≥ 31.5 kg/m^2 compared with those with BMI < 31.5 kg/m^2 (39% versus 56%, respectively), even after controlling for pushing during the second stage of labor.[99] Conversely, two other retrospective studies found no difference in the risk for PDPH between obese and nonobese parturients.[100,101] A third study found no reduction in the risk for PDPH in obese parturients compared with lean parturients, except in those with a BMI ≥ 50 kg/m^2 where the risk of PDPH was 46% compared with 72% in those with BMI < 30 kg/m^2.[102] So, while the evidence is conflicting on whether the risk of PDPH is reduced in obese compared with nonobese patients, the risk is still at least 40% following dural puncture with a Tuohy needle.

Cesarean Delivery

A thorough preanesthetic evaluation is critical to the safe care of the obese parturient undergoing cesarean delivery. Of particular importance is a thorough airway assessment. Large breasts, the greater anteroposterior diameter of the chest, airway edema, and reduced chin-to-chest distance increase the likelihood of difficult laryngoscopy and failed tracheal intubation in obstetric patients.[103] Obesity exaggerates many of the anatomic changes of pregnancy. Increased fat in the neck and shoulders increases the difficulty of positioning the patient for laryngoscopy and tracheal intubation. Excess fat deposition may also cause distorted anatomy, such as an enlarged tongue and redundant pharyngeal and palatal soft tissue. Further, the fat pads on the back of the shoulders often restrict the range of motion of the neck, exacerbating the difficulty of mask ventilation, laryngoscopy, and tracheal intubation.

All morbidly obese parturients undergoing cesarean delivery should be placed in a ramped position with left uterine displacement, regardless of the planned anesthetic technique. This position was shown to improve laryngoscopic view compared with the traditional sniffing position in morbidly obese patients undergoing elective bariatric surgery.[104] Folded blankets, a positioning pillow, or a padded ramp designed for this purpose are placed under the chest and head to achieve horizontal alignment between the external auditory meatus and the sternal notch (Fig. 48.1).[105] This position aligns the oral, pharyngeal, and tracheal axes to facilitate tracheal intubation and has been shown to improve hemodynamic and respiratory parameters during laparoscopic gastric bypass surgery.[106] Modern surgical tables can also be flexed at a number of angles and this feature can be used to optimize the patient position for laryngoscopy and tracheal intubation.

It may be difficult to position the obese patient appropriately and safely. The protuberant abdomen may shift markedly with left uterine displacement. The patient must be secured to the operating table before the table is tilted leftward; however, it is important to initiate left uterine displacement as soon as possible.

The anesthesia provider should confirm that the patient's weight does not exceed the weight limits of the operating table, consider the use of lateral table extenders, and use appropriate pads to ensure that the shoulders and arms are positioned in a horizontal plane. Correct arm position will maximize patient comfort, improve stability, and avoid neurologic injury to the upper extremity.

The anesthesia care team may be asked to participate in cephalad retraction of the large panniculus by tethering retractors to an object such as the ether screen or the head of the table. Both the obstetric and the anesthesia providers must remain cognizant of the risks for hypotension, difficulty with ventilation, and fetal compromise during cephalad retraction of the panniculus in morbidly obese patients. Hodgkinson and Husain[89] reported an intraoperative fetal death in a morbidly obese patient who had received epidural anesthesia for cesarean delivery. The death was attributed to prolonged hypotension associated with cephalad retraction of a large panniculus. A vertical and cephalad suspension of the panniculus has been suggested to avoid maternal hypotension and hypoxemia.[72] Commercially available retraction devices can also be used to retract the panniculus, but there are no data to indicate whether these devices are associated with reduced risk for hypotension or ventilation compromise compared with cephalad retraction.

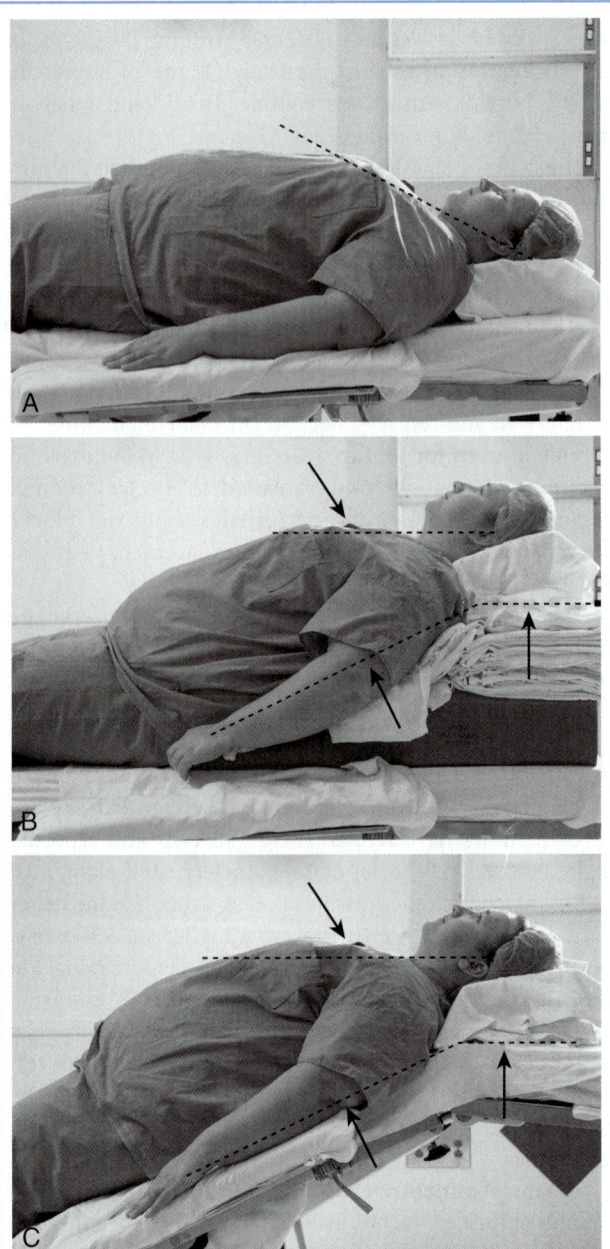

Fig. 48.1 Positioning the obese patient to facilitate intubation of the trachea. (A) Patient in the supine position using standard head support. Note that the *dashed line* (compare with B) is not parallel to the floor. (B) Elevating the patient's head with neck and shoulder supports so that an imaginary line drawn through the external auditory meatus and the sternal notch *(upper dashed line)* is parallel to the floor may facilitate tracheal intubation. (C) Similar positioning achieved by repositioning the operating table. Note the similarity of the upper and lower dashed lines with use of the second and third positioning techniques.

Pharmacologic **aspiration prophylaxis** is crucial in this patient population. Oral administration of 30 mL of a 0.3 M solution of **sodium citrate** effectively increases gastric pH within 5 minutes.[107] The anesthesia provider must be aware that the patient remains at risk for aspiration at the end of surgery; the efficacy of sodium citrate wanes 45 to 60 minutes after administration.[108] Administration of a **histamine-2**

(H$_2$)-receptor antagonist and **metoclopramide** provide additional protection (see Chapter 28).

Antibiotic Prophylaxis

Obesity is an independent predictor for **surgical site infection**.[109] The Clinical Practice Guidelines for Antibiotic Prophylaxis in Surgery recommend a dose of 3 g of **cefazolin** before cesarean delivery in women weighing more than 120 kg[110]; however, the data supporting this recommendation are inconsistent. Pevzner et al.[111] found that 2 g of cefazolin administered 30 to 60 minutes before cesarean delivery in obese and morbidly obese patients failed to achieve the targeted minimum inhibitory concentration (MIC) in 20% and 33% of patients, respectively, at the time of skin incision, and in 20% and 40% of patients, respectively, at the time of incision closure. Stitely et al.[112] randomized 20 obese patients undergoing cesarean delivery to receive 2 g or 4 g of cefazolin. The 4-g dose was associated with higher blood and tissue levels, but all collected subcutaneous and myometrial tissue samples had antibiotic concentrations above the MIC.[112] Swank et al.[113] reported that after administration of cefazolin 2 g, the target MIC was achieved in all normal and overweight parturients, but in only in 20% of women with a BMI 30 to 40 kg/m^2 and in no parturients with a BMI > 40 kg/m^2. Conversely, after cefazolin 3 g, the MIC target was achieved in all women with a BMI 30 to 40 kg/m^2 and in 71% of women with a BMI > 40 kg/m^2. Maggio et al.[114] did not find higher adipose tissue concentrations after cefazolin 3 g versus 2 g, and there was no difference in surgical site infections between the two regimens. Similarly, two retrospective studies compared surgical site infections in morbidly obese women undergoing cesarean delivery and found no difference in surgical site infections between 2-g and 3-g regimens.[115,116]

Valent et al.[117] explored another strategy; obese women undergoing cesarean delivery were randomized to receive oral **cephalexin** 500 g plus **metronidazole** 500 mg or placebo every 8 hours for 48 hours after delivery. All patients received a single 2-g intravenous dose of cefazolin before surgical incision. The rate of surgical site infection was significantly lower with the cephalexin/metronidazole regimen (6.4% versus 15.4%) (number needed to treat, 12 [95% CI, 6.7 to 33.8]).[117]

Neuraxial Techniques

Neuraxial anesthesia is the technique of choice in the obese parturient. **Single-shot spinal anesthesia** provides reliable, fast onset, and dense neuraxial blockade. However, concerns about the use of single-shot spinal anesthesia in obese patients include technical difficulties, appropriate dosing, and insufficient duration of anesthesia.

Spinal anesthesia is technically feasible in morbidly obese pregnant women, although a longer spinal needle may be required. The distribution of adipose tissue varies among obese patients. Spinal needle placement can be uneventful in women who do not have excessive adipose tissue over the midline of the back. However, in others with excessive adipose tissue at the needle placement site, identification of the intrathecal space with a small-gauge pencil-point spinal needle can be very challenging. Identification of the epidural space with a large-gauge epidural needle is often technically easier, and a needle-through-needle **CSE technique** may be easier to perform than a single-shot spinal technique in the morbidly obese parturient. Ross et al.[118] reported fewer attempts to establish the neuraxial block with a CSE technique compared with a single-shot spinal technique in morbidly obese parturients undergoing elective cesarean delivery.

The duration of surgery is often prolonged in the obese parturient[3]; therefore, single-shot spinal anesthesia may not have sufficient duration. Because intraoperative induction of general anesthesia is undesirable and potentially hazardous in morbidly obese pregnant women, a **continuous neuraxial technique** such as a CSE or epidural technique that allows the maintenance of neuraxial anesthesia with the epidural catheter is preferable to a single-shot spinal technique. **Epidural anesthesia** is preferred if the patient has a well-functioning epidural catheter *in situ*. Otherwise, a CSE technique may be preferable because it combines the reliability of the spinal block and the flexibility of epidural anesthesia. It also gives the option of initiating the block with a low dose of intrathecal local anesthetic, with the ability to increase the cephalad level of block by administering additional local anesthetic via the epidural catheter if needed (i.e., sequential CSE anesthesia). **Continuous spinal anesthesia** with a spinal catheter is also an option. Some anesthesia providers have suggested that this technique should be considered in the setting of emergency cesarean delivery for obese parturients because it may be technically easier to rapidly identify the spinal space with a large-gauge epidural needle than with a spinal needle.[109] The use of a **double-catheter technique** has been described if a high vertical supraumbilical abdominal incision is planned; a lumbar spinal catheter or CSE technique is used for intraoperative anesthesia and a thoracic epidural catheter is used for postoperative analgesia and to achieve adequate anesthesia for the upper end of the incision if needed.[119]

Local anesthetic dosing. The choice of local anesthetic dose in morbidly obese parturients is controversial. It has been a long-held belief that neuraxial local anesthetic doses should be reduced in obese patients because of fear of an unpredictable and exaggerated spread of local anesthetic, resulting in a high block. Magnetic resonance imaging (MRI) confirmed that obese patients have reduced lumbar CSF volume.[120] Engorgement of the epidural veins secondary to compression of the inferior vena cava by the gravid uterus and abdominal panniculus, as well as inward movement of soft tissue through the intervertebral foramina as a result of increased abdominal pressure, may be responsible for the reduced CSF volume in these patients. Another MRI study demonstrated an inverse correlation between the cephalad extent of block and lumbar CSF volume[121]; this finding suggests that reduced CSF volume in obese patients might increase the risk for high spinal block.

Multiple studies, however, do not support the concern of exaggerated cephalad spread of spinal anesthesia in morbidly obese women undergoing cesarean delivery. In an up-down sequential allocation dose-finding study, Lee et al.[122] reported that the estimated ED$_{95}$ (effective dose in 95% of patients) for hyperbaric bupivacaine was similar in obese and nonobese patients; no patient had an excessively high cephalad block with bupivacaine doses up to 12 mg. In another study, Carvalho et al.[123] randomized morbidly obese parturients having cesarean delivery to receive doses of hyperbaric bupivacaine ranging from 5 to 11 mg as part of a CSE technique; they found that the estimated ED$_{50}$ and ED$_{95}$ values were similar to those found in a previous study they had conducted using similar methodology in nonobese parturients. Although it was common to obtain a satisfactory initial sensory level, even with the lowest doses, few of the low-dose blocks were adequate for surgery, and many required supplementation via the epidural catheter. Thus, the findings of these studies suggest that reducing the dose of intrathecal bupivacaine is not justified in morbidly obese patients and might increase the risk for inadequate anesthesia.

Superobese parturients with a BMI > 50 kg/m^2 are rarely included in studies. Ngaka et al.[124] reported a higher block level by a median of two dermatomes but no significant differences in vasopressor requirements, hand grip strength, and peak expiratory flow rate in 25 morbidly obese parturients with a mean BMI of 51 kg/m^2 compared with nonobese parturients after intrathecal hyperbaric bupivacaine 10 mg. Another retrospective study compared the incidence of high spinal anesthesia (defined as the need to convert to general anesthesia within 20 minutes of initiation of spinal anesthesia because of high block, or a cephalad extent of anesthesia higher than T2) in nonobese; obesity class I, II, III; and superobese (BMI > 50 kg/m^2) women.[125] Anesthesia was induced with hyperbaric bupivacaine (most common dose 12 mg). The incidence of high spinal anesthesia was increased in superobese women (2.5%) compared with all other groups (≤0.71%). Vasopressor requirements were also higher in this group; unscheduled cesarean delivery was a risk factor for high spinal anesthesia.[125] A recent study found that the ED$_{90}$ of hyperbaric bupivacaine in superobese patients was 11.5 mg.[126] While this value is comparable to that found in other studies in nonobese and obese patients, success was defined as successful block for the operation up to 90 minutes, and the need for supplementation after 90 minutes was not considered a failure. Four parturients (9.5%) had a sensory level higher than T2; none was symptomatic or required general anesthesia, but the study was not designed or powered for those outcomes. Overall, these studies suggest that intrathecal dose reduction may be warranted in parturients with a BMI > 50 kg/m^2, ideally as part of a CSE technique, but not in obese women with a BMI < 50 kg/m^2. In our practice, we use a dose of hyperbaric bupivacaine 9 to 10.5 mg as part of a needle-though-needle CSE technique in superobese parturients.

Results of studies of epidural local anesthetic dosing in morbidly obese parturients are also inconsistent (see earlier discussion). Unlike single-shot spinal anesthesia in which titration of the dose is not possible, careful titration of epidural anesthesia is recommended to achieve the desired block level.

General Anesthesia

Difficult mask ventilation and tracheal intubation are associated with more rapid oxyhemoglobin desaturation during apnea in obese patients than in lean individuals. The association between obesity and a short neck can make tracheal intubation difficult in this population.[127] In a series of patients who received general anesthesia for cesarean delivery, the incidence of difficult tracheal intubation was 33% among women who weighed more than 300 lb (136.4 kg).[80] This study was performed at a time when videolaryngoscopes were not available in routine practice. Quinn et al.[128] conducted a 2-year survey of failed tracheal intubation in obstetric patients in the United Kingdom and reported that BMI was an independent predictor of failed intubation; the odds increased by 7% for each 1-kg/m^2 increase in BMI. Reale et al.[129] used data from the Multicenter Perioperative Outcomes Group from 2004 to 2019 and reported that BMI ≥ 40 kg/m^2 was associated with an increased risk of difficult intubation compared with BMI < 25 kg/m^2 (OR, 2.02; 95% CI, 1.12 to 3.64), with an estimated incidence of 1 in 28.

Airway management. The potential for failed tracheal intubation and difficult mask ventilation in the obese patient underscores the need for an experienced assistant during induction of general anesthesia. The primary anesthesia provider may fatigue rapidly with attempted mask ventilation of an obese patient. Further, the jaw-thrust maneuver may require the use of both hands, and additional personnel will be required to provide positive-pressure ventilation and cricoid pressure. A short-handled laryngoscope, assorted laryngoscope blades, various sizes of endotracheal tubes, endotracheal tube guides, supraglottic airway devices, a videolaryngoscope, a fiberoptic intubation device, and equipment suitable for emergency surgical airway (e.g., cricothyrotomy) should be readily available.[130] A **failed tracheal intubation algorithm** should be initiated and help should be called immediately in the event of a failed tracheal intubation (see Chapter 29). Supraglottic airway devices may be lifesaving in these situations. Some experts have suggested that a videolaryngoscope should be the first-line device used in obstetric patients[131]; this recommendation may be particularly relevant in the obese parturient.

Awake tracheal intubation using videolaryngoscopy or direct fiberoptic laryngoscopy is an alternative method of securing the anticipated difficult airway. However, women requiring urgent cesarean delivery may not be ideal candidates for awake tracheal intubation because of the lack of adequate time to optimally prepare the airway.

When preanesthetic assessment suggests that tracheal intubation will not be difficult, a rapid-sequence induction is indicated. The administration of general anesthesia begins with effective denitrogenation (preoxygenation), with the goal of achieving an end-tidal fractional oxygen concentration (FETO$_2$) of 90% before intravenous induction of anesthesia. During apnea, pregnant women become hypoxemic more rapidly than nonpregnant women, and obese patients become hypoxemic more rapidly than nonobese patients.[132] Therefore, adequate denitrogenation is essential before the induction of general anesthesia in obese pregnant women.

A nasal cannula insufflating oxygen 5 L/min during the period of apnea and tracheal intubation increases the time to desaturation and should be strongly considered in the obese parturient.[132] The benefit of high flow nasal oxygen (HFNO) in pregnant women, particularly among obese parturients, is not clear. Recent studies have used computer modeling to compare apneic oxygen techniques. Stolady et al.[133] showed that HFNO (with F_{ETO_2} values varying from 60% to 90% and with the airway both open and obstructed) provided longer safe apneic times (time for oxygen saturation to decrease to less than 90%) compared with preoxgenation with a face mask; however, the improvement was significantly less in obese subjects. Ellis et al.[134] found that low flow nasal oxygen (LFNO) after preoxygenation prolonged the safe apnea time to a similar degree to that with HFNO; however, the prolongation was modest with BMI > 50 kg/m². The authors suggested caution in using HFNO in patients with high BMI, because—given the risks of airway obstruction and difficult intubation—rescue bag-mask ventilation would be easier to apply with LFNO. These findings suggest that an optimal technique for periintubation oxygenation includes the use of face mask preoxygenation with gentle face mask ventilation after onset of apnea, while simultaneously administering LFNO and continuing its administration with an increase in flow rate from 5 L/min to 15 L/min during laryngoscopy.[135]

The technique of denitrogenation is important. One study demonstrated that the technique of four maximal inspirations of 100% oxygen within 30 seconds (four deep breaths [4-DB]) provides benefit similar to that provided by 3 minutes of tidal-volume breathing of 100% oxygen before rapid-sequence induction of general anesthesia for cesarean delivery.[136] However, another study reported a more rapid onset of hypoxemia in patients who used 4-DB than patients who used 3 minutes of tidal-volume breathing of 100% oxygen.[137] Goldberg et al.[138] evaluated the use of both techniques in morbidly obese nonpregnant patients undergoing gastric bypass surgery. The techniques provided similar increases in Pao_2, but patients who used the 3-minute technique showed evidence of slight retention of CO_2. The investigators speculated that a blunted ventilatory response to CO_2 contributed to the increase in $Paco_2$. Later data from a study in 20 pregnant volunteers (at 36 to 38 weeks' gestation) compared 3 minutes of tidal-volume breathing with 4-DB or eight deep breaths in 1 minute (8-DB) of 100% oxygen by measuring F_{ETO_2} after preoxygenation.[139] An F_{ETO_2} value $\geq 90\%$ was achieved in 76% of women after either the 3-minute or the 8-DB method, compared with only 18% of women after the 4-DB method.[139] The investigators concluded that for emergency cesarean delivery using general anesthesia, the 8-DB method was as effective as the 3-minute tidal volume method of preoxygenation and was more quickly performed.

It is wise to apply a tight-fitting face mask and administer 100% oxygen as soon as the patient enters the operating room; this maneuver helps achieve denitrogenation while the patient is moved to the operating table and other preparations are being made. It then seems reasonable to let circumstances dictate the selected method of denitrogenation. When the 3-minute tidal volume breathing technique is selected, the anesthesia provider should encourage the patient to take several deep breaths. In urgent situations, such as emergency cesarean delivery for maternal hemorrhage, the patient should be instructed to take eight deep breaths (8-DB) to extend the safe interval before oxyhemoglobin desaturation occurs. When time allows, the 8-DB method is preferred over the 4-DB method.

Induction and maintenance of anesthesia. The dose of intravenous induction agents should be based on lean body weight rather than total body weight.[140] This practice will avoid excessive doses of drug with subsequent adverse effects. **Propofol** 2 to 2.8 mg/kg, **thiopental (thiopentone)** 4 to 5 mg/kg, or other induction agents can be used according to availability, clinical circumstances, and anesthesia provider preference. All these agents cross the placenta and can affect the neonate.

Succinylcholine (suxamethonium) 1.0 to 1.5 mg/kg is commonly used for rapid-sequence induction and tracheal intubation in obese parturients. Lemmens and Brodsky[141] compared the efficacy of succinylcholine in dosing regimens of 1 mg/kg based on ideal body weight, lean body weight, and total body weight in morbidly obese nonpregnant patients. The third regimen (1 mg/kg total body weight) was superior for providing complete neuromuscular paralysis and predictable laryngoscopic conditions in almost every patient, whereas intubating conditions were poor in one-third of the patients dosed according to ideal body weight. The investigators also noted that "none of these dosing regimens will provide … a safe (short) duration of apnea."

Rocuronium 1 to 1.2 mg/kg provides equivalent intubating conditions to succinylcholine 1 mg/kg. However, this dose range is associated with a significantly prolonged duration of neuromuscular blockade.[142] In obese patients, the dose of rocuronium should be based on ideal body weight.[143] **Sugammadex** will effectively reverse high-dose rocuronium (1.2 mg/kg) in 2 minutes.[144] Sugammadex has been used successfully in obstetric patients with no major adverse maternal or neonatal effects.[145] The Society for Obstetric Anesthesia and Perinatology (SOAP) statement on sugammadex during pregnancy and lactation[146] recommends the judicious use of sugammadex given its unknown effects on lactation and the breastfed infant. The optimal dosing regimen in obese patients is not clear; two studies in nonpregnant obese patients suggested that sugammadex dosing can be based on ideal body weight plus 40%[147] or on corrected body weight, which is calculated as ideal body weight + 0.4 (total body weight − ideal body weight).[148] However, its use has not been specifically studied in obese parturients, and its safety in this patient population remains to be confirmed. Inadequate reversal of neuromuscular blockade in an obese parturient[149] and recurarization in another obese patient undergoing bariatric surgery[150] have been reported following administration of sugammadex for reversal of rocuronium-induced neuromuscular blockade, highlighting the importance of appropriate dosing and vigilance in ensuring adequate recovery in this patient population.

Maintenance of anesthesia is usually achieved with a volatile halogenated agent with or without **nitrous oxide**. No evidence suggests that obesity alters the minimum alveolar concentration of volatile halogenated anesthetic agents in pregnant women. In theory, the body fat reservoir could increase the threat of biotransformation of volatile halogenated agents, which would increase the risk for organ toxicity. **Isoflurane** is an appropriate choice for morbidly obese parturients owing to its limited biotransformation.[151] **Desflurane** and **sevoflurane** are associated with a shorter time to extubation than isoflurane in obese patients, although the difference may not be clinically relevant.[152,153] Although maintenance of anesthesia using total intravenous anesthesia may have potential benefits, such as causing less uterine relaxation and lower risk of postoperative nausea and vomiting compared with volatile anesthetics, there are limited data on maternal and neonatal outcomes, dosing algorithms, and pharmacokinetics, especially in obese parturients.[154,155]

Morbidly obese patients may require administration of a higher inspired oxygen concentration and may not tolerate high concentrations of nitrous oxide. Moreover, general anesthesia reduces FRC. The supine and Trendelenburg positions further decrease FRC, thus increasing the risk for intraoperative hypoxemia. The following strategies have been recommended to reduce the risk for small airway closure, atelectasis, and hypoxemia in obese patients: (1) use of inspired oxygen concentration < 0.8, (2) ventilation with tidal volumes ranging from 6 to 10 mL/kg ideal body weight, (3) increasing the respiratory rate to maintain physiologic $Paco_2$, (4) use of manual or automated periodic lung inflation (i.e., a recruitment maneuver), and (5) application of positive end-expiratory pressure (approximately 10 cm H_2O).[156]

Emergence from general anesthesia is a critical period. Indeed, maternal deaths from hypoventilation and airway obstruction have been reported during emergence and recovery from general anesthesia.[49] It is imperative that the patient is fully awake with complete reversal of neuromuscular blockade before tracheal extubation, which preferably should be performed in the semi-upright position to minimize diaphragmatic compression by abdominal viscera. Trained personnel should provide postoperative care before the discharge of the patient to the ward.

POSTOPERATIVE COMPLICATIONS

Obesity increases the risk for postoperative complications such as **endometritis, urinary tract infection, wound infection, wound dehiscence, peripheral nerve injury, hemorrhage, deep vein thrombosis, pulmonary thromboembolism, atelectasis, pneumonia, respiratory depression, hypoxemia, tracheal reintubation, myocardial infarction, cardiac arrest,** and **maternal death**.[109,157]

The combination of obesity, OSA, general anesthesia, and opioid administration may increase the risk for **opioid-induced respiratory depression**. In a report on maternal mortality in Michigan, Mhyre et al.[49] found that all anesthesia-related maternal deaths from airway obstruction or hypoventilation occurred during emergence and recovery, with obesity identified as a significant risk factor for these complications. The American Society of Anesthesiologists has issued "Practice Guidelines for the Perioperative Management of Patients with Obstructive Sleep Apnea," which include recommendations for the preoperative, intraoperative, and postoperative management of these patients (Box 48.1).[158] These recommendations are not intended specifically for pregnant women, but they do provide some guidance for the care of the obese parturient with OSA undergoing cesarean delivery.

POSTOPERATIVE CARE

Postoperative Analgesia

Adequate postoperative analgesia is crucial to facilitate early mobilization, thereby reducing the risk for thromboembolic and pulmonary complications. However, the ideal analgesic regimen in the obese parturient remains unclear. Neuraxial morphine has been shown to provide superior analgesia to that provided by parenteral and oral opioids after cesarean delivery, at the expense of increased opioid-related side effects such as pruritus and nausea.[159] There is a concern, however, that obese patients might be at greater risk for respiratory depression after neuraxial opioid administration, although few data are available. In a series of 856 patients who received intrathecal morphine 0.2 mg combined with hyperbaric bupivacaine for cesarean delivery, respiratory depression (defined as $Sao_2 \leq 85\%$ and/or respiratory rate ≤ 10 breaths/min) occurred in eight patients, all of whom were obese.[160] Conversely, a large retrospective study including 5036 parturients who received neuraxial morphine, 63% of whom were obese, did not identify any instances of respiratory depression, defined as need for naloxone or rapid response team calls for respiratory complications.[161] Another retrospective study included 11,237 women who received neuraxial morphine, 17% of whom had a BMI $\geq 40 kg/m^2$, and defined clinically significant respiratory depression as need for naloxone or rapid response team activation or tracheal intubation for respiratory events.[162] Clinically significant respiratory depression occurred in 16 cases (0.1%), with a rate of 25.7 (95% CI, 11 to 60) per 10,000 in women with a BMI $\geq 40 kg/m^2$ versus 11.7 (95% CI, 6.5 to 21) per 10,000 in women with a BMI $< 40 kg/m^2$ (OR, 2.2; 95% CI, 0.6 to 6.9; $P = .17$). Neuraxial morphine was not found causative for any event but was considered contributory in five cases. The SOAP consensus statement[163] and the guidelines from the UK National Institute for Health and Care Excellence[164] consider obesity as a risk factor warranting more frequent or continuous respiratory monitoring following neuraxial morphine administration for cesarean delivery. The risk for sedation and respiratory depression might be greater with systemic opioids compared with neuraxial opioids, although there are no data comparing the risk for respiratory depression between the two routes of opioid administration in obese parturients. In patients who have

American Society of Anesthesiologists Practice Guidelines for Perioperative Management of Patients With Obstructive Sleep Apnea

Preoperative
- Preoperative initiation of continuous positive airway pressure should be considered, particularly if OSA is severe.
- Patients with known or suspected OSA may have a difficult airway and therefore should be managed according to the American Society of Anesthesiologists "Practice Guidelines for Management of the Difficult Airway"[a] or other similar airway management guidelines.

Intraoperative
- The potential for postoperative respiratory compromise should be considered.
- Neuraxial anesthesia (spinal/epidural/combined spinal-epidural) should be considered.
- Patients at increased perioperative risk from OSA should be extubated while awake.
- Full reversal of neuromuscular blockade should be verified before tracheal extubation.
- When possible, extubation and recovery should be carried out in the lateral, semi-upright position, or other nonsupine position.

Postoperative
- Postoperative analgesia: regional analgesic techniques should be considered to reduce or eliminate the requirement for systemic opioids in patients at increased perioperative risk from OSA.
- If neuraxial analgesia is planned, the anesthesia provider should weigh the benefits (improved analgesia, decreased need for systemic opioids) and risks (respiratory depression from rostral spread) of using an opioid or opioid–local anesthetic mixture compared with a local anesthetic alone.
- If a patient-controlled systemic opioid analgesic technique is used, a continuous background infusion should be used with extreme caution or avoided entirely.
- Nonsteroidal antiinflammatory drugs and other modalities should be considered if appropriate to reduce opioid requirement.
- Concurrent administration of sedative agents increases the risk for respiratory depression and airway obstruction.
- Supplemental oxygen should be administered continuously to all patients who are at increased perioperative risk from OSA until they are able to maintain their baseline oxygen saturation while breathing room air.
- Hospitalized patients at increased risk for respiratory compromise from OSA should be monitored with continuous pulse oximetry after discharge from the postanesthesia care unit.

OSA, Obstructive sleep apnea.

Selected recommendations from American Society of Anesthesiologists. Practice guidelines for the perioperative management of patients with obstructive sleep apnea. An updated report by the American Society of Anesthesiologists Task Force on Perioperative Management of Patients with Obstructive Sleep Apnea. *Anesthesiology.* 2014;120:268–286.

[a] Apfelbaum JL, Hagberg CA, Connis RT, et al. 2022 American Society of Anesthesiologists Practice guidelines for management of the difficult airway. *Anesthesiology.* 2022;136:31–81.

not received neuraxial opioid analgesia, systemic opioids are best administered using intravenous **patient-controlled analgesia**. With all routes of opioid administration, vigilance and appropriate postoperative monitoring are essential in the obese patient who may have undiagnosed OSA and be at increased risk for opioid-induced respiratory depression. The use of sedative agents or magnesium sulfate in the postoperative period may also increase the risk for respiratory depression.[163]

A multimodal analgesic regimen including regular administration of a **nonsteroidal antiinflammatory drug** and **acetaminophen (paracetamol)** may contribute to opioid sparing and improve postoperative analgesia (see Chapter 27). A systematic review of randomized controlled trials found that **local anesthetic wound infiltration** was associated with a reduction in opioid consumption and pain scores in women undergoing cesarean delivery, but did not reduce the incidence of opioid-related side effects.[165] There are limited data on the use of this technique in women receiving neuraxial morphine, but the review suggested that opioid sparing was only achieved in women who did not receive neuraxial morphine. Analgesia was better with catheter placement below compared with above the fascia.

Similarly, a **transversus abdominis plane (TAP) block** was found to produce opioid sparing and reduce pain scores and opioid-related adverse effects in women who did not receive neuraxial morphine as part of their neuraxial anesthetic technique.[166] However, performance of a TAP block may be technically challenging in the obese parturient with a large abdominal panniculus. **Quadratus lumborum block** and **erector spinae plane block** are other truncal blocks that might have the advantage of providing more analgesia for visceral pain compared with the TAP block; however, studies are limited and have not specifically assessed the use of these blocks in obese women. It was reported that **patient-controlled epidural analgesia (PCEA)** with ropivacaine provides analgesia comparable to that provided by epidural morphine, but with more motor block, thus delaying patient mobilization.[167] PCEA techniques have not been specifically studied in obese parturients.

Thromboprophylaxis

The American College of Chest Physicians (ACCP) published guidelines for antithrombotic therapy in the parturient.[168] They used major and minor risk factors to identify women at increased risk for venous thromboembolism after cesarean delivery; obesity (BMI > 30 kg/m^2) was classified as a minor risk factor. Thromboprophylaxis was recommended in the presence of one major risk factor (risk for thromboembolism > 3%) or two minor risk factors (combined risk > 3%) (see Box 38.1). In the setting of emergency cesarean delivery (a minor risk factor), an additional minor risk factor (e.g., obesity) results in a risk > 3%, and, therefore, mechanical or pharmacologic thromboprophylaxis is recommended.

The ACOG thromboembolism guidelines do not specifically address the obese parturient.[169] They recommend perioperative **mechanical thromboprophylaxis** for all women, with the addition of **low-molecular-weight heparin (LMWH)** in selected high-risk parturients, without specifying obese women. In the United Kingdom, the guidelines of the Royal College of Obstetricians and Gynaecologists (RCOG) recommend thromboprophylaxis for at least 10 days with LMWH for all obese parturients undergoing emergency or elective cesarean delivery.[170] Further, the RCOG guidelines recommend thromboprophylaxis with LMWH for at least 10 days after vaginal delivery in all morbidly obese women. The National Partnership for Maternal Safety published a consensus bundle on venous thromboembolism in 2016.[171] Mechanical thromboprophylaxis was recommended for all women undergoing cesarean delivery, with the addition of pharmacologic prophylaxis for those with risk factors, including obesity; for vaginal delivery, it was recommended to follow the ACCP guidelines for hospitalized nonsurgical patients.[168]

KEY POINTS

- The presence of coexisting disease(s) complicates obstetric and anesthetic management of the morbidly obese pregnant woman.
- The obese pregnant woman is at increased risk for obstetric, anesthetic, neonatal, surgical, and postoperative complications.
- The obese pregnant woman should be referred to an anesthesia provider for preanesthesia consultation.
- Airway complications, which can occur during the postoperative period as well as during the induction and emergence from general anesthesia, constitute the most common cause of anesthesia-related maternal death.
- The anesthesia provider should perform a careful, thorough assessment of the airway in every obese pregnant woman and should consider securing the airway before induction of general anesthesia when a difficult airway is anticipated.

- Early administration of neuraxial labor analgesia is advised in obese parturients; anesthesia providers should critically evaluate the quality of the epidural block and replace any neuraxial catheter that does not provide excellent analgesia.
- Continuous spinal anesthesia should be considered in emergency settings involving potentially difficult tracheal intubation and in cases of unintentional dural puncture in morbidly obese patients.
- Morbidly obese parturients may be at significant risk for obstructive sleep apnea; therefore, they should be carefully monitored with continuous pulse oximetry for postoperative hypoxemia resulting from airway obstruction and/or respiratory depression after discharge from the postanesthesia care unit.

REFERENCES

1. World Obesity Federation. One billion people globally estimated to be living with obesity by 2030. *2022.* https://www.worldobesity.org/news/one-billion-people-globally-estimated-to-be-living-with-obesity-by-2030. Accessed December 2023.
2. Division of Health and Nutrition Examination Surveys. *NHANES Interactive Data Visualizations.* National Center for Health Statistics. 2021. https://www.cdc.gov/nchs/nhanes/visualization. Accessed December 2023.
3. Dennis AT, Lamb KE, Story D, et al. Associations between maternal size and health outcomes for women undergoing caesarean section: a multicentre prospective observational study (the MUM SIZE Study). *BMJ Open.* 2017;7:e015630.
4. Weiss JL, Malone FD, Emig D, et al. Obesity, obstetric complications and cesarean delivery rate – a population-based screening study. *Am J Obstet Gynecol.* 2004;190:1091–1097.
5. Lisonkova S, Muraca GM, Potts J, et al. Association between prepregnancy body mass index and severe maternal morbidity. *JAMA.* 2017;318:1777–1786.
6. Lafortuna CL, Agosti F, Galli R, et al. The energetic and cardiovascular response to treadmill walking and cycle ergometer exercise in obese women. *Eur J Appl Physiol.* 2008;103:707–717.
7. Dempsey JA, Reddan W, Balke B, Rankin J. Work capacity determinants and physiologic cost of weight-supported work in obesity. *J Appl Physiol.* 1966;21:1815–1820.

8. Lourenço RV. Diaphragm activity in obesity. *J Clin Invest.* 1969;48:1609–1614.
9. Babb TG, Ranasinghe KG, Comeau LA, et al. Dyspnea on exertion in obese women: association with an increased oxygen cost of breathing. *Am J Respir Crit Care Med.* 2008;178:116–123.
10. Parameswaran K, Todd DC, Soth M. Altered respiratory physiology in obesity. *Can Respir J.* 2006;13:203–210.
11. Holley HS, Milic-Emili J, Becklake MR, Bates DV. Regional distribution of pulmonary ventilation and perfusion in obesity. *J Clin Invest.* 1967;46:475–481.
12. Veille JC, Hanson R. Obesity, pregnancy, and left ventricular functioning during the third trimester. *Am J Obstet Gynecol.* 1994;171:980–983.
13. O'Brien TE, Ray JG, Chan WS. Maternal body mass index and the risk of preeclampsia: a systematic overview. *Epidemiology.* 2003;14:368–374.
14. D'Souza R, Horyn I, Pavalagantharajah S, et al. Maternal body mass index and pregnancy outcomes: a systematic review and metaanalysis. *Am J Obstet Gynecol MFM.* 2019;1:100041.
15. Roberts RB, Shirley MA. Reducing the risk of acid aspiration during cesarean section. *Anesth Analg.* 1974;53:859–868.
16. Mahajan V, Hashmi J, Singh R, et al. Comparative evaluation of gastric pH and volume in morbidly obese and lean patients undergoing elective surgery and effect of aspiration prophylaxis. *J Clin Anesth.* 2015;27:396–400.

17. Harter RL, Kelly WB, Kramer MG, et al. A comparison of the volume and pH of gastric contents of obese and lean surgical patients. *Anesth Analg.* 1998;86:147–152.

18. Wisen O, Hellstrom PM. Gastrointestinal motility in obesity. *J Intern Med.* 1995;237:411–418.

19. Maltby JR, Pytka S, Watson NC, et al. Drinking 300 mL of clear fluid two hours before surgery has no effect on gastric fluid volume and pH in fasting and non-fasting obese patients. *Can J Anaesth.* 2004;51:111–115.

20. Wong CA, McCarthy RJ, Fitzgerald PC, et al. Gastric emptying of water in obese pregnant women at term. *Anesth Analg.* 2007;105:751–755.

21. Amaral CK, Benevides ML, Benevides MM, et al. Ultrasound assessment of gastric antrum in term pregnant women before elective cesarean section. *Braz J Anesthesiol.* 2019;69:266–271.

22. Eslick GD. Gastrointestinal symptoms and obesity: a meta-analysis. *Obes Rev.* 2012;13:469–479.

23. Hawkins JL, Chang J, Palmer SK, et al. Anesthesia-related maternal mortality in the United States: 1979-2002. *Obstet Gynecol.* 2011;117:69–74.

24. Guh DP, Zhang W, Bansback N, et al. The incidence of co-morbidities related to obesity and overweight: a systematic review and meta-analysis. *BMC Public Health.* 2009;9:88.

25. Knight M, Bunch K, Tuffnell D, et al. *Saving Lives, Improving Mothers' Care – Lessons Learned to Inform Maternity Care From the UK and Ireland Confidential Enquiries Into Maternal Deaths and Morbidity 2017–19.* National Perinatal Epidemiology Unit, University of Oxford; 2021.

26. Guerre-Millo M. Adipose tissue and adipokines: for better or worse. *Diabetes Metab.* 2004;30:13–19.

27. Mertens I, Van Gaal LF. Obesity, haemostasis and the fibrinolytic system. *Obes Rev.* 2002;3:85–101.

28. Davi G, Guagnano MT, Ciabattoni G, et al. Platelet activation in obese women: role of inflammation and oxidant stress. *JAMA.* 2002;288:2008–2014.

29. Arfvidsson B, Eklof B, Balfour J. Iliofemoral venous pressure correlates with intraabdominal pressure in morbidly obese patients. *Vasc Endovascular Surg.* 2005;39:505–509.

30. Caballero AE. Endothelial dysfunction in obesity and insulin resistance: a road to diabetes and heart disease. *Obes Res.* 2003;11:1278–1289.

31. Boden G. Obesity, insulin resistance and free fatty acids. *Curr Opin Endocrinol Diabetes Obes.* 2011;18:139–143.

32. Farah N, Hogan AE, O'Connor N, et al. Correlation between maternal inflammatory markers and fetomaternal adiposity. *Cytokine.* 2012;60:96–99.

33. Fedorcsák P, Dale PO, Storeng R, et al. The impact of obesity and insulin resistance on the outcome of IVF or ICSI in women with polycystic ovarian syndrome. *Hum Reprod.* 2001;16:1086–1091.

34. Fung AM, Wilson DL, Barnes M, Walker SP. Obstructive sleep apnea and pregnancy: the effect on perinatal outcomes. *J Perinatol.* 2012;32:399–406.

35. Louis J, Auckley D, Miladinovic B, et al. Perinatal outcomes associated with obstructive sleep apnea in obese pregnant women. *Obstet Gynecol.* 2012;120:1085–1092.

36. Dominguez JE, Grotegut CA, Wright MC, Habib AS. Obstructive sleep apnea among gravidas with chronic hypertension compared to matched controls: a prospective cohort study. *Anesth Analg.* 2023;136:205–214.

37. Maasilta P, Bachour A, Teramo K, et al. Sleep-related disordered breathing during pregnancy in obese women. *Chest.* 2001;120:1448–1454.

38. Bende M, Gredmark T. Nasal stuffiness during pregnancy. *Laryngoscope.* 1999;109:1108–1110.

39. Oksenberg A, Dynia A, Nasser K, Gadoth N. Obstructive sleep apnoea in adults: body postures and weight changes interactions. *J Sleep Res.* 2012;21:402–409.

40. Louis JM, Mogos MF, Salemi JL, et al. Obstructive sleep apnea and severe maternal-infant morbidity/mortality in the United States, 1998-2009. *Sleep.* 2014;37:843–849.

41. Frappaolo AM, Linder AH, Wen T, et al. Trends in and outcomes associated with obstructive sleep apnea during deliveries in the United States, 2000-2019. *Am J Obstet Gynecol MFM.* 2023;5:100775.

42. Luppino FS, de Wit LM, Bouvy PF, et al. Overweight, obesity, and depression: a systematic review and meta-analysis of longitudinal studies. *Arch Gen Psychiatry.* 2010;67:220–229.

43. Chu SY, Bachman DJ, Callaghan WM, et al. Association between obesity during pregnancy and increased use of health care. *N Engl J Med.* 2008;358:1444–1453.

44. Cedergren MI. Maternal morbid obesity and the risk of adverse pregnancy outcome. *Obstet Gynecol.* 2004;103:219–224.

45. Chu SY, Kim SY, Schmid CH, et al. Maternal obesity and risk of cesarean delivery: a meta-analysis. *Obes Rev.* 2007;8:385–394.

46. Saucedo M, Esteves-Pereira AP, Pencolé L, et al. Understanding maternal mortality in women with obesity and the role of care they receive: a national case-control study. *Int J Obes (Lond).* 2021;45:258–265.

47. Knight M, Bunch K, Patel R, et al. *Saving Lives, Improving Mothers' Care Core Report – Lessons Learned to Inform Maternity Care From the UK and Ireland Confidential Enquiries Into Maternal Deaths and Morbidity 2018-20.* National Perinatal Epidemiology Unit, University of Oxford; 2022.

48. Beckett VA, Knight M, Sharpe P. The CAPS Study: Incidence, management and outcomes of cardiac arrest in pregnancy in the UK: a prospective, descriptive study. *BJOG.* 2017;124:1374–1381.

49. Mhyre JM, Riesner MN, Polley LS, Naughton NN. A series of anesthesia-related maternal deaths in Michigan, 1985-2003. *Anesthesiology.* 2007;106:1096–1104.

50. Denison FC, Aedla NR, Keag O, et al. Care of women with obesity in pregnancy: Green-top Guideline No. 72. *BJOG.* 2019;126:e62–e106.

51. Sagi-Dain L. Obesity in pregnancy: ACOG Practice Bulletin, Number 230. *Obstet Gynecol.* 2021;138:489.

52. Kominiarek MA, Zhang J, Vanveldhuisen P, et al. Contemporary labor patterns: the impact of maternal body mass index. *Am J Obstet Gynecol.* 2011;205:244.e1–e8.

53. Zhang J, Bricker L, Wray S, Quenby S. Poor uterine contractility in obese women. *BJOG.* 2007;114:343–348.

54. Hehir MP, Morrison JJ. The adipokine apelin and human uterine contractility. *Am J Obstet Gynecol.* 2012;206:359.e1–e5.

55. Scott-Pillai R, Spence D, Cardwell CR, et al. The impact of body mass index on maternal and neonatal outcomes: a retrospective study in a UK obstetric population, 2004-2011. *BJOG.* 2013;120:932–939.

56. Blomberg M. Maternal obesity and risk of postpartum hemorrhage. *Obstet Gynecol.* 2011;118:561–568.

57. Butwick AJ, Abreo A, Bateman BT, et al. Effect of maternal body mass index on postpartum hemorrhage. *Anesthesiology.* 2018;128:774–783.

58. Ende HB, Lozada MJ, Chestnut DH, et al. Risk factors for atonic postpartum hemorrhage: a systematic review and meta-analysis. *Obstet Gynecol.* 2021;137:305–323.

59. Peska E, Balki M, Maxwell C, et al. Oxytocin at elective caesarean delivery: a dose-finding study in women with obesity. *Anaesthesia.* 2021;76:918–923.

60. Tyagi A, Nigam C, Malhotra RK, et al. The minimum effective dose (ED_{90}) of prophylactic oxytocin infusion during cesarean delivery in patients with and without obesity: an up-down sequential allocation dose-response study. *Int J Obstet Anesth.* 2024;57:103962.

61. Pevzner L, Powers BL, Rayburn WF, et al. Effects of maternal obesity on duration and outcomes of prostaglandin cervical ripening and labor induction. *Obstet Gynecol.* 2009;114:1315–1321.

62. Cedergren MI. Non-elective caesarean delivery due to ineffective uterine contractility or due to obstructed labour in relation to maternal body mass index. *Eur J Obstet Gynecol Reprod Biol.* 2009;145:163–166.

63. Mazouni C, Porcu G, Cohen-Solal E, et al. Maternal and anthropomorphic risk factors for shoulder dystocia. *Acta Obstet Gynecol Scand.* 2006;85:567–570.

64. Sebire NJ, Jolly M, Harris JP, et al. Maternal obesity and pregnancy outcome: a study of 287,213 pregnancies in London. *Int J Obes Relat Metab Disord.* 2001;25:1175–1182.

65. Crane SS, Wojtowycz MA, Dye TD, et al. Association between pre-pregnancy obesity and the risk of cesarean delivery. *Obstet Gynecol.* 1997;89:213–216.

66. Pierin AM, Alavarce DC, Gusmão JL, et al. Blood pressure measurement in obese patients: comparison between upper arm and forearm measurements. *Blood Press Monit.* 2004;9:101–105.

67. Anast N, Olejniczak M, Ingrande J, Brock-Utne J. The impact of blood pressure cuff location on the accuracy of noninvasive blood pressure measurements in obese patients: an observational study. *Can J Anaesth.* 2016;63:298–306.

68. Hersh LT, Sesing JC, Luczyk WJ, et al. Validation of a conical cuff on the forearm for estimating radial artery blood pressure. *Blood Press Monit.* 2014;19:38–45.

69. Ellinas EH, Eastwood DC, Patel SN, et al. The effect of obesity on neuraxial technique difficulty in pregnant patients: a prospective, observational study. *Anesth Analg.* 2009;109:1225–1231.

70. D'Alonzo RC, White WD, Schultz JR, et al. Ethnicity and the distance to the epidural space in parturients. *Reg Anesth Pain Med.* 2008;33:24–29.

71. Clinkscales CP, Greenfield ML, Vanarase M, Polley LS. An observational study of the relationship between lumbar epidural space depth and body mass index in Michigan parturients. *Int J Obstet Anesth.* 2007;16:323–327.

72. Whitty RJ, Maxwell CV, Carvalho JC. Complications of neuraxial anesthesia in an extreme morbidly obese patient for cesarean section. *Int J Obstet Anesth.* 2007;16:139–144.

73. Patel SD, Habib AS. Anaesthesia for the parturient with obesity. *BJA Educ.* 2021;21:180–186.

74. Marroquin BM, Fecho K, Salo-Coombs V, Spielman FJ. Can parturients identify the midline during neuraxial block placement? *J Clin Anesth.* 2011;23:3–6.

75. Sahin T, Balaban O, Sahin L, et al. A randomized controlled trial of preinsertion ultrasound guidance for spinal anaesthesia in pregnancy: outcomes among obese and lean parturients: ultrasound for spinal anesthesia in pregnancy. *J Anesth.* 2014;28:413–419.

76. Sahota JS, Carvalho JC, Balki M, et al. Ultrasound estimates for midline epidural punctures in the obese parturient: paramedian sagittal oblique is comparable to transverse median plane. *Anesth Analg.* 2013;116:829–835.

77. Balki M, Lee Y, Halpern S, Carvalho JC. Ultrasound imaging of the lumbar spine in the transverse plane: the correlation between estimated and actual depth to the epidural space in obese parturients. *Anesth Analg.* 2009;108:1876–1881.

78. Hamza J, Smida M, Benhamou D, Cohen SE. Parturient's posture during epidural puncture affects the distance from skin to epidural space. *J Clin Anesth.* 1995;7:1–4.

79. Hamilton CL, Riley ET, Cohen SE. Changes in the position of epidural catheters associated with patient movement. *Anesthesiology.* 1997;86:778–784.

80. Hood DD, Dewan DM. Anesthetic and obstetric outcome in morbidly obese parturients. *Anesthesiology.* 1993;79:1210–1218.

81. Perlow JH, Morgan MA. Massive maternal obesity and perioperative cesarean morbidity. *Am J Obstet Gynecol.* 1994;170:560–565.

82. Bamgbade OA, Khalaf WM, Ajai O, et al. Obstetric anaesthesia outcome in obese and non-obese parturients undergoing caesarean delivery: an observational study. *Int J Obstet Anesth.* 2009;18:221–225.

83. Tonidandel A, Booth J, D'Angelo R, et al. Anesthetic and obstetric outcomes in morbidly obese parturients: a 20-year follow-up retrospective cohort study. *Int J Obstet Anesth.* 2014;23:357–364.

84. Dresner M, Brocklesby J, Bamber J. Audit of the influence of body mass index on the performance of epidural analgesia in labour and the subsequent mode of delivery. *BJOG.* 2006;113:1178–1181.

85. Kula AO, Riess ML, Ellinas EH. Increasing body mass index predicts increasing difficulty, failure rate, and time to discovery of failure of epidural anesthesia in laboring patients. *J Clin Anesth.* 2017;37:154–158.

86. Uyl N, de Jonge E, Uyl-de Groot C, et al. Difficult epidural placement in obese and non-obese pregnant women: a systematic review and meta-analysis. *Int J Obstet Anesth.* 2019;40:52–61.

87. Faure E, Moreno R, Thisted R. Incidence of postdural puncture headache in morbidly obese parturients. *Reg Anesth.* 1994;19:361–363.

88. Ranta P, Jouppila P, Spalding M, Jouppila R. The effect of maternal obesity on labour and labour pain. *Anaesthesia.* 1995;50:322–326.

89. Hodgkinson R, Husain FJ. Obesity and the cephalad spread of analgesia following epidural administration of bupivacaine for cesarean section. *Anesth Analg.* 1980;59:89–92.

90. Panni MK, Columb MO. Obese parturients have lower epidural local anaesthetic requirements for analgesia in labour. *Br J Anaesth.* 2006;96:106–110.

91. Milligan KR, Cramp P, Schatz L, et al. The effect of patient position and obesity on the spread of epidural analgesia. *Int J Obstet Anesth.* 1993;2:134–136.

92. Duggan J, Bowler GM, McClure JH, Wildsmith JA. Extradural block with bupivacaine: influence of dose, volume,

concentration and patient characteristics. *Br J Anaesth*. 1988;61:324–331.

93. Bauer ME, Kountanis JA, Tsen LC, et al. Risk factors for failed conversion of labor epidural analgesia to cesarean delivery anesthesia: a systematic review and meta-analysis of observational trials. *Int J Obstet Anesth*. 2012;21:294–309.

94. Pan PH, Bogard TD, Owen MD. Incidence and characteristics of failures in obstetric neuraxial analgesia and anesthesia: a retrospective analysis of 19,259 deliveries. *Int J Obstet Anesth*. 2004;13:227–233.

95. Booth JM, Pan JC, Ross VH, et al. Combined spinal-epidural technique for labor analgesia does not delay recognition of epidural catheter failures: a single-center retrospective cohort survival analysis. *Anesthesiology*. 2016;125:516–524.

96. Chau A, Bibbo C, Huang CC, et al. Dural puncture epidural technique improves labor analgesia quality with fewer side effects compared with epidural and combined spinal epidural techniques: a randomized clinical trial. *Anesth Analg*. 2017;124:560–569.

97. Tan HS, Reed SE, Mehdiratta JE, et al. Quality of labor analgesia with dural puncture epidural versus standard epidural technique in obese parturients: a double-blind randomized controlled study. *Anesthesiology*. 2022;136:678–687.

98. Arnolds D, Scavone B. Neuraxial labor analgesia failure rates in women with a body mass index ≥50 kg/m² : a single-center retrospective study. *Int J Obstet Anesth*. 2021;48:103176.

99. Peralta F, Higgins N, Lange E, et al. The relationship of body mass index with the incidence of postdural puncture headache in parturients. *Anesth Analg*. 2015;121:451–456.

100. Miu M, Paech MJ, Nathan E. The relationship between body mass index and post-dural puncture headache in obstetric patients. *Int J Obstet Anesth*. 2014;23:371–375.

101. Song J, Zhang T, Choy A, et al. Impact of obesity on post-dural puncture headache. *Int J Obstet Anesth*. 2017;30:5–9.

102. Franz AM, Jia SY, Bahnson HT, et al. The effect of second-stage pushing and body mass index on postdural puncture headache. *J Clin Anesth*. 2017;37:77–81.

103. Honarmand A, Safavi MR. Prediction of difficult laryngoscopy in obstetric patients scheduled for caesarean delivery. *Eur J Anaesthesiol*. 2008;25:714–720.

104. Brodsky JB, Lemmens HJ, Brock-Utne JG, et al. Anesthetic considerations for bariatric surgery: proper positioning is important for laryngoscopy. *Anesth Analg*. 2003;96:1841–1842.

105. Brodsky JB, Lemmens HJ, Brock-Utne JG, et al. Morbid obesity and tracheal intubation. *Anesth Analg*. 2002;94:732–736.

106. Artuso D, Wayne M, Cassaro S, et al. Hemodynamic changes during laparoscopic gastric bypass procedures. *Arch Surg*. 2005;140:289–292.

107. O'Sullivan GM, Bullingham RE. Noninvasive assessment by radiotelemetry of antacid effect during labor. *Anesth Analg*. 1985;64:95–100.

108. Dewan DM, Floyd HM, Thistlewood JM, et al. Sodium citrate pretreatment in elective cesarean section patients. *Anesth Analg*. 1985;64:34–37.

109. Soens MA, Birnbach DJ, Ranasinghe JS, van Zundert A. Obstetric anesthesia for the obese and morbidly obese patient: an ounce of prevention is worth more than a pound of treatment. *Acta Anaesthesiol Scand*. 2008;52:6–19.

110. Bratzler DW, Dellinger EP, Olsen KM, et al. Clinical practice guidelines for antimicrobial prophylaxis in surgery. *Am J Health Syst Pharm*. 2013;70:195–283.

111. Pevzner L, Swank M, Krepel C, et al. Effects of maternal obesity on tissue concentrations of prophylactic cefazolin during cesarean delivery. *Obstet Gynecol*. 2011;117:877–882.

112. Stitely M, Sweet M, Slain D, et al. Plasma and tissue cefazolin concentrations in obese patients undergoing cesarean delivery and receiving differing pre-operative doses of drug. *Surg Infect (Larchmt)*. 2013;14:455–459.

113. Swank ML, Wing DA, Nicolau DP, McNulty JA. Increased 3-gram cefazolin dosing for cesarean delivery prophylaxis in obese women. *Am J Obstet Gynecol*. 2015;213:415.e1–e8.

114. Maggio L, Nicolau DP, DaCosta M, et al. Cefazolin prophylaxis in obese women undergoing cesarean delivery: a randomized controlled trial. *Obstet Gynecol*. 2015;125:1205–1210.

115. Ahmadzia HK, Patel EM, Joshi D, et al. Obstetric surgical site infections: 2 grams compared with 3 grams of cefazolin in morbidly obese women. *Obstet Gynecol*. 2015;126:708–715.

116. Peppard WJ, Eberle DG, Kugler NW, et al. Association between preoperative cefazolin dose and surgical site infection in obese patients. *Surg Infect (Larchmt)*. 2017;18:485–490.

117. Valent AM, DeArmond C, Houston JM, et al. Effect of post–cesarean delivery oral cephalexin and metronidazole on surgical site infection among obese women: a randomized clinical trial. *JAMA*. 2017;318:1026–1034.

118. Ross VH, Dean LS, Thomas JA, et al. A randomized controlled comparison between combined spinal-epidural and single-shot spinal techniques in morbidly obese parturients undergoing cesarean delivery: time for initiation of anesthesia. *Anesth Analg*. 2014;118:168–172.

119. Polin CM, Hale B, Mauritz AA, et al. Anesthetic management of super-morbidly obese parturients for cesarean delivery with a double neuraxial catheter technique: a case series. *Int J Obstet Anesth*. 2015;24:276–280.

120. Hogan QH, Prost R, Kulier A, et al. Magnetic resonance imaging of cerebrospinal fluid volume and the influence of body habitus and abdominal pressure. *Anesthesiology*. 1996;84:1341–1349.

121. Carpenter RL, Hogan QH, Liu SS, et al. Lumbosacral cerebrospinal fluid volume is the primary determinant of sensory block extent and duration during spinal anesthesia. *Anesthesiology*. 1998;89:24–29.

122. Lee Y, Balki M, Parkes R, Carvalho JC. Dose requirement of intrathecal bupivacaine for cesarean delivery is similar in obese and normal weight women. *Rev Bras Anestesiol*. 2009;59:674–683.

123. Carvalho B, Collins J, Drover DR, et al. ED$_{50}$ and ED$_{95}$ of intrathecal bupivacaine in morbidly obese patients undergoing cesarean delivery. *Anesthesiology*. 2011;114:529–535.

124. Ngaka TC, Coetzee JF, Dyer RA. The influence of body mass index on sensorimotor block and vasopressor requirement during spinal anesthesia for elective cesarean delivery. *Anesth Analg*. 2016;123:1527–1534.

125. Lamon AM, Einhorn LM, Cooter M, Habib AS. The impact of body mass index on the risk of high spinal block in parturients undergoing cesarean delivery: a retrospective cohort study. *J Anesth*. 2017;31:552–558.

126. Tan HS, Fuller ME, Barney EZ, et al. The 90% effective dose of intrathecal hyperbaric bupivacaine for cesarean delivery under combined spinal–epidural anesthesia in parturients with super obesity: an up-down sequential allocation study. *Can J Anaesth*. 2024;71:570–578.

127. Rocke DA, Murray WB, Rout CC, Gouws E. Relative risk analysis of factors associated with difficult intubation in obstetric anesthesia. *Anesthesiology*. 1992;77:67–73.

128. Quinn AC, Milne D, Columb M, et al. Failed tracheal intubation in obstetric anaesthesia: 2 yr national case-control study in the UK. *Br J Anaesth*. 2013;110:74–80.

129. Reale SC, Bauer ME, Klumpner TT, et al. Frequency and risk factors for difficult intubation in women undergoing general anesthesia for cesarean delivery: a multicenter retrospective cohort analysis. *Anesthesiology*. 2022;136:697–708.

130. American Society of Anesthesiologists. Practice guidelines for obstetric anesthesia. An updated report by the American Society of Anesthesiologists Task Force on Obstetric Anesthesia and the Society for Obstetric Anesthesia and Perinatology. *Anesthesiology*. 2016;124:270–300.

131. Zaouter C, Calderon J, Hemmerling TM. Videolaryngoscopy as a new standard of care. *Br J Anaesth*. 2015;114:181–183.

132. Mushambi MC, Kinsella SM, Popat M, et al. Obstetric Anaesthetists' Association and Difficult Airway Society guidelines for the management of difficult and failed tracheal intubation in obstetrics. *Anaesthesia*. 2015;70:1286–1306.

133. Stolady D, Laviola M, Pillai A, Hardman JG. Effect of variable pre-oxygenation endpoints on safe apnoea time using high flow nasal oxygen for women in labour: a modelling investigation. *Br J Anaesth*. 2021;126:889–895.

134. Ellis R, Laviola M, Stolady D, et al. Comparison of apnoeic oxygen techniques in term pregnant subjects: a computational modelling study. *Br J Anaesth*. 2022;129:581–587.

135. Wong CA, Mushambi M. Peri-intubation oxygenation for Caesarean delivery: is there an optimal technique? *Br J Anaesth*. 2022;129:468–471.

136. Norris MC, Dewan DM. Preoxygenation for cesarean section: a comparison of two techniques. *Anesthesiology*. 1985;62:827–829.

137. Gambee AM, Hertzka RE, Fisher DM. Preoxygenation techniques: comparison of three minutes and four breaths. *Anesth Analg*. 1987;66:468–470.

138. Goldberg ME, Norris MC, Larijani GE, et al. Preoxygenation in the morbidly obese: a comparison of two techniques. *Anesth Analg*. 1989;68:520–522.

139. Chiron B, Laffon M, Ferrandiere M, et al. Standard preoxygenation technique versus two rapid techniques in pregnant patients. *Int J Obstet Anesth*. 2004;13:11–14.

140. Ingrande J, Lemmens HJ. Dose adjustment of anaesthetics in the morbidly obese. *Br J Anaesth*. 2010;105:i16–i23.

141. Lemmens HJ, Brodsky JB. The dose of succinylcholine in morbid obesity. *Anesth Analg*. 2006;102:438–442.

142. Perry JJ, Lee JS, Sillberg VA, Wells GA. Rocuronium versus succinylcholine for rapid sequence induction intubation. *Cochrane Database Syst Rev*. 2008:CD002788.

143. Meyhoff CS, Lund J, Jenstrup MT, et al. Should dosing of rocuronium in obese patients be based on ideal or corrected body weight? *Anesth Analg*. 2009;109:787–792.

144. Pühringer FK, Rex C, Sielenkämper AW, et al. Reversal of profound, high-dose rocuronium-induced neuromuscular blockade by sugammadex at two different time points: an international, multicenter, randomized, dose-finding, safety assessor-blinded, phase II trial. *Anesthesiology*. 2008;109:188–197.

145. Stourac P, Adamus M, Seidlova D, et al. Low-dose or high-dose rocuronium reversed with neostigmine or sugammadex for cesarean delivery anesthesia: a randomized controlled noninferiority trial of time to tracheal intubation and extubation. *Anesth Analg*. 2016;122:1536–1545.

146. Society for Obstetric Anesthesia and Perinatology statement on sugammadex during pregnancy and lactation. 2019. https://www.soap.org/assets/docs/SOAP_Statement_Sugammadex_During_Pregnancy_Lactation_APPROVED.pdf. Accessed 6 June 2025.

147. Van Lancker P, Dillemans B, Bogaert T, et al. Ideal versus corrected body weight for dosage of sugammadex in morbidly obese patients. *Anaesthesia*. 2011;66:721–725.

148. Gaszynski T, Szewczyk T, Gaszynski W. Randomized comparison of sugammadex and neostigmine for reversal of rocuronium-induced muscle relaxation in morbidly obese undergoing general anaesthesia. *Br J Anaesth*. 2012;108:236–239.

149. Kayashima K, Sozen R, Okura D. Insufficient sugammadex effect in an obese pregnant woman undergoing cesarean section under general anesthesia. *Masui*. 2014;63:188–190.

150. Le Corre F, Nejmeddine S, Fatahine C, et al. Recurarization after sugammadex reversal in an obese patient. *Can J Anaesth*. 2011;58:944–947.

151. Carpenter RL, Eger EI 2nd, Johnson BH, et al. The extent of metabolism of inhaled anesthetics in humans. *Anesthesiology*. 1986;65:201–205.

152. Torri G, Casati A, Comotti L, et al. Wash-in and wash-out curves of sevoflurane and isoflurane in morbidly obese patients. *Minerva Anestesiol*. 2002;68:523–527.

153. Juvin P, Vadam C, Malek L, et al. Postoperative recovery after desflurane, propofol, or isoflurane anesthesia among morbidly obese patients: a prospective, randomized study. *Anesth Analg*. 2000;91:714–719.

154. Metodiev Y, Lucas DN. The role of total intravenous anaesthesia for caesarean delivery. *Int J Obstet Anesth*. 2022;51:103548.

155. Paech MJ. The role of total intravenous anaesthesia for caesarean delivery. *Int J Obstet Anesth*. 2022;51:103574.

156. Pelosi P, Gregoretti C. Perioperative management of obese patients. *Best Pract Res Clin Anaesthesiol*. 2010;24:211–225.

157. Catalano PM. Management of obesity in pregnancy. *Obstet Gynecol*. 2007;109:419–433.

158. American Society of Anesthesiologists. Practice guidelines for the perioperative management of patients with obstructive sleep apnea. An updated report by the American Society of Anesthesiologists Task Force on perioperative management of patients with obstructive sleep apnea. *Anesthesiology*. 2014;120:268–286.

159. Bonnet MP, Mignon A, Mazoit JX, et al. Analgesic efficacy and adverse effects of epidural morphine compared to parenteral opioids after elective caesarean section: a systematic review. *Eur J Pain*. 2010;14:894.e1–e9.

160. Abouleish E, Rawal N, Rashad MN. The addition of 0.2 mg subarachnoid morphine to hyperbaric bupivacaine for cesarean delivery: a prospective study of 856 cases. *Reg Anesth*. 1991;16:137–140.

161. Crowgey TR, Dominguez JE, Peterson-Layne C, et al. A retrospective assessment of the incidence of respiratory depression after neuraxial morphine administration for postcesarean delivery analgesia. *Anesth Analg*. 2013;117:1368–1370.

162. Ende HB, Dwan RL, Freundlich RE, et al. Quantifying the incidence of clinically significant respiratory depression in women with and without obesity class III receiving neuraxial morphine for post-cesarean analgesia: a retrospective cohort study. *Int J Obstet Anesth*. 2021;47:103187.

163. Bauchat JR, Weiniger CF, Sultan P, et al. Society for Obstetric Anesthesia and Perinatology consensus statement: monitoring recommendations for prevention and detection of respiratory depression associated with administration of neuraxial morphine for cesarean delivery analgesia. *Anesth Analg.* 2019;129:458–474.

164. National Institute for Health and Care Excellence. *Monitoring after intrathecal or epidural opioids for caesarean birth. NICE guideline NG192.* 2021. https://www.nice.org.uk/guidance/ ng192/evidence/e-monitoring-after-intrathecal-or-epidural-opioids-for-caesarean-birth-pdf-9071941650. Accessed December 2023.

165. Adesope O, Ituk U, Habib AS. Local anaesthetic wound infiltration for postcaesarean section analgesia: a systematic review and meta-analysis. *Eur J Anaesthesiol.* 2016;33: 731–742.

166. Mishriky BM, George RB, Habib AS. Transversus abdominis plane block for analgesia after cesarean delivery: a systematic review and meta-analysis. *Can J Anaesth.* 2012;59:766–778.

167. Chen LK, Lin PL, Lin CJ, et al. Patient-controlled epidural ropivacaine as a post-cesarean analgesia: a comparison with epidural morphine. *Taiwan J Obstet Gynecol.* 2011;50: 441–446.

168. Bates SM, Greer IA, Middeldorp S, et al. VTE, thrombophilia, antithrombotic therapy, and pregnancy: antithrombotic therapy and prevention of thrombosis, 9th ed: American College of Chest Physicians evidence-based clinical practice guidelines. *Chest.* 2012;141:e691S–e736S.

169. American College of Obstetricians and Gynecologists. Practice Bulletin No. 196: Thromboembolism in pregnancy (reaffirmed 2022). *Obstet Gynecol.* 2018;132:e1–e17.

170. Royal College of Obstetricians and Gynaecologists. Reducing the risk of thrombosis and embolism during pregnancy and the puerperium. Green-Top Guideline No. 37a. http://www. rcog.org.uk/womens-health/clinical-guidance/reducing-risk-of-thrombosis-greentop37a. Accessed December 2023.

171. D'Alton ME, Friedman AM, Smiley RM, et al. National Partnership for Maternal Safety: consensus bundle on venous thromboembolism. *Obstet Gynecol.* 2016;128:688–698.

49

Psychiatric Disorders

Grace Lim, MD, MS

Psychiatric disorders occur commonly during pregnancy and can have significant effects on the mother, child, and family, and important economic costs to society. Suicide is a major cause of maternal mortality. Women have higher rates than men of many psychiatric disorders, such as anxiety, feeding and eating disorders, and depression; the reproductive years coincide with the greatest period of risk.[1] Management can be difficult and may be complicated by variable presentation of symptoms, social stigmas, confusion with normal symptoms associated with pregnancy, and inconsistent published treatment recommendations. Further, pregnant women with psychiatric disorders may resist drug treatment because of their desire to avoid fetal harm. Psychiatric disorders during pregnancy may be associated with other aspects of poor maternal health and deficient prenatal care, which may affect anesthesia care.[2] Women with a history of previous psychiatric hospitalization or an identified mental illness are at increased risk for cesarean delivery.[3]

CLASSIFICATION

Internationally, psychiatric disorders are most commonly classified according to the *International Statistical Classification of Diseases and Related Health Problems (ICD-11)*[a] produced by the WHO. In the United States, a clinical modification of *ICD* is used *(ICD-10-CM)*.[b] Although *ICD* is the official diagnostic system for mental disorders in the United States, the *Diagnostic and Statistical Manual of Mental Disorders (DSM-5)*, published by the American Psychiatric Association (APA), is widely used.[4] These classification systems provide standardized language and criteria for diagnosis and classification of mental disorders; however, definitions may not have precise boundaries and there may be considerable overlap between "mental" and "physical" disorders.[4]

EPIDEMIOLOGY

It has been estimated that more than 500,000 pregnancies each year in the United States involve women who have a psychiatric illness that either predates or emerges during pregnancy.[1] Psychiatric illness occurs in approximately 15% of pregnant women, and 10% to 13% of fetuses are exposed to psychotropic drugs.[5] The Centers for Disease Control and Prevention determined that between 2017 and 2019, mental health conditions were the leading cause (22.7%) of maternal deaths.[6] Similarly, the Confidential Enquiries into Maternal Deaths in the United Kingdom and Ireland found that psychiatric and cardiovascular disorders are the leading causes of maternal death, with each contributing to about 15% of maternal deaths; maternal suicide was the leading direct cause of death during that period.[7]

Pregnancy is widely considered a time of increased vulnerability to psychiatric disorders. However, studies suggest

[a]https://www.who.int/standards/classifications/classification-of-diseases

[b]https://www.cdc.gov/nchs/icd/icd-10/?CDC_AAref_Val=https://www.cdc.gov/nchs/icd/icd10.htm

that the prevalence is similar between pregnant and nonpregnant women.[8] A conspicuous exception is the risk for major depressive disorder, which is increased during the postpartum period and affects one in seven women.[9] Identified risk factors for developing psychiatric disorders during pregnancy include younger age, unmarried status, exposure to traumatic or stressful life events, pregnancy complications, and poor overall health. Treatment rates among pregnant women with psychiatric disorders are often low.

MOOD DISORDERS

Mood disorders include depressive disorders and bipolar disorders (BPDs) ("manic-depressive disorders").[4]

Major Depressive Disorder

The *DSM-5* has defined criteria for major depressive disorder that are based on the presence, within the same 2-week period, of specific symptoms that cause clinically significant distress or impairment in social, occupational, or other important areas of functioning; these symptoms should not be the result of the physiologic effects of a substance.[4] Although depression is recognized as being relatively common during pregnancy, many of its symptoms (e.g., weight gain, appetite changes, sleep disturbances, fatigue) must be differentiated from symptoms that may occur during normal pregnancy. Risk factors for depression during pregnancy include a history of depression or BPD, childhood mistreatment, being a single mother or having more than three children, marital problems, unwanted pregnancy, smoking, low income, age younger than 20 years, poor social support, and domestic violence.[10] The risk for major depressive illness is increased in women who have an early pregnancy loss (miscarriage); this most frequently occurs in the first month after early pregnancy loss and is more likely to occur in women who are childless or who have a prior history of major depressive disorder.[11] Depression during pregnancy is associated with an increased risk for poor obstetric outcomes, such as early pregnancy loss, preterm birth, and low birth weight.[12] To ensure timely diagnosis and treatment, the American College of Obstetricians and Gynecologists (ACOG) recommends three separate screenings for depression: at the initial prenatal visit, later in pregnancy, and postpartum.[13]

Bipolar (Manic-Depressive) Disorder

Patients with BPD have episodes of major depression with other distinct periods of mania or hypomania. A strong familial association exists. *DSM-5* diagnostic criteria for mania specify a distinct period when there is abnormally and persistently elevated, expansive, or irritable mood and persistently increased goal-directed activity or energy, which lasts at least 1 week and is present most of nearly every day or requires hospitalization.[4] Specific symptoms are listed, which should be severe enough to cause marked impairment in occupational functioning, social activities, and interpersonal relationships, and necessitate hospitalization or have psychotic features. Symptoms should not meet criteria for a mixed episode and

should not be caused by substance abuse or general medical conditions (e.g., hyperthyroidism).[4] BPD in pregnancy is particularly important because there is a strong link between discontinuation of medication and relapse of BPD and a relatively high suicide rate among patients. Treatment of BPD typically consists of mood stabilizer and antipsychotic medication, with psychotherapy as an adjunct. Electroconvulsive therapy (ECT) is very effective for patients with BPD and severe depression.[14]

Perinatal Depression

Perinatal depression is a mood disorder that affects patients during pregnancy and after childbirth. Perinatal depression includes depression that begins during pregnancy ("prenatal depression") and depression that begins after the baby is born ("postpartum depression").[4] There may be accompanying psychotic features and there is a high risk for recurrence in subsequent pregnancies.[4,15] It is important to differentiate postpartum depression from the "baby blues," which affects up to 70% of women in the first 10 days after delivery and is transient without functional impairment. It is also important to differentiate postpartum depression from delirium that arises from physical causes.[4] In a systematic review, Robertson et al.[16] showed that the strongest predictors of postpartum depression were (1) depression, anxiety, or stressful life events occurring during pregnancy or the early puerperium; (2) low levels of social support; and (3) previous history of depression. Biologic, environmental, and psychosocial effects such as hormonal changes and psychological and social role changes that occur with childbirth may increase the risk for postpartum depression.[13] Although some studies have observed associations between labor analgesia and reduced risks for postpartum depression,[17–19] others have not.[20] One study demonstrated a harmful effect for women who planned to avoid, but ended up using labor epidural analgesia.[21] These conflicting results reflect that the relationships between pain, emotion, and cognition are complex and are influenced by factors outside of physical health and interventions alone (e.g., culture, expectations, and quality of social support networks).

Postpartum Psychosis

Postpartum psychosis occurs within 2 weeks of approximately 1 to 2 per 1000 live births; a relatively high risk continues for the first 3 months postpartum. The risk is higher in patients with a history of BPD or a history of previous postpartum psychosis, as well as in women with major depression and schizophrenia. Typical features include prominence of cognitive symptoms, such as disorganization, confusion, impaired sensorium, disorientation, and distractibility. Infanticide is rare and may be associated with command hallucinations to kill the infant or delusions that the infant is possessed.[22]

ANXIETY DISORDERS

Anxiety disorders affect women twice as often as men and are the most common psychiatric disorders during pregnancy and the postpartum period.[23] There is a wide range of anxiety disorders, including **panic disorder, separation** anxiety disorder, selective mutism, specific phobia, social anxiety disorder, agoraphobia, generalized anxiety disorder, substance/medication-induced anxiety disorder, anxiety disorder due to another medical condition, other specified anxiety disorder, and unspecified anxiety disorder. Closely related to anxiety disorders are trauma- and stressor-related disorders, which include posttraumatic stress disorder (PTSD) and obsessive-compulsive disorder (OCD).[4] Clinical features of anxiety disorders in pregnant women are similar to those in nonpregnant women, but concern about the pregnancy and the fetus may be the predominant feature.[23]

Panic Disorder

Panic disorder is characterized by the occurrence of recurrent, unexpected panic attacks. Affected women experience discrete episodes of intense fear or discomfort in the absence of a true danger; these episodes are accompanied by somatic or cognitive symptoms, such as palpitations, sweating, shaking, dyspnea, choking, chest pain, nausea, paresthesias, chills, and/or flushes. Typically there is a rapid onset and peak of symptoms that may be accompanied by an urge to escape.[4] It is important to be aware of the possibility that panic attacks may occur during preparation of a patient for cesarean delivery. Panic attacks with hyperventilation may mimic local anesthetic systemic toxicity.[24] Patients with panic disorder often have comorbid major depression.[23]

Posttraumatic Stress Disorder

PTSD occurs after the experience of a traumatic event that evokes intense fear or helplessness and has been estimated to occur in 4% to 6% of women in pregnancy or postpartum.[25] PTSD may arise during the perinatal period, or preexisting PTSD can be exacerbated during pregnancy. Symptoms of PTSD are more common after emergency cesarean delivery than after other modes of delivery,[26] and PTSD has resulted from (1) awareness during general anesthesia,[27] (2) inadequate neuraxial anesthesia for cesarean delivery,[28] and (3) inadequate pain control during vaginal delivery.[29] The risk for PTSD may be increased if the pregnancy has resulted from rape or if memories of sexual trauma are triggered. It has been suggested that the childbirth experience itself can precipitate PTSD with a resulting fear of pregnancy termed tocophobia.[1] Fear of vaginal delivery may be a factor that contributes to maternal request for cesarean delivery.[30]

Obsessive-Compulsive Disorder

OCD is characterized by the presence of obsessions (intrusive thoughts or images) and compulsions (repetitive or ritualistic behaviors or thought patterns).[23] OCD is more common in pregnant and postpartum women than in the general population.[31] Obsessions most frequently center around contamination or aggression toward the child and may lead to compulsive cleaning, checking, or avoidance of the child. Care should be taken to identify infanticidal ideation.[23]

EATING DISORDERS

There are conflicting data on the effect of pregnancy in patients with feeding and eating disorders, which include anorexia nervosa and bulimia nervosa as well as pica, rumination disorder, avoidant/restrictive food intake disorder, binge-eating disorder, other specified feeding or eating disorder, and unspecified feeding or eating disorder.[4] Improvement in symptoms during pregnancy has been described, but conversely, pregnancy may result in body image preoccupations and unfavorable eating habits that may develop into a frank eating disorder. Although fertility is reduced in patients with anorexia nervosa, patients may still conceive. Patients with eating disorders have a higher risk for psychiatric comorbidity, including anxiety and postpartum depression,[1] and are at greater risk for fetal growth restriction and cesarean delivery.[23]

SCHIZOPHRENIA SPECTRUM AND OTHER PSYCHOTIC DISORDERS

These disorders include schizophrenia, other psychotic disorders, and schizotypal (personality) disorder. Defining features include abnormalities in one or more of the following areas: hallucinations, disorganized thinking, grossly disorganized or abnormal motor behavior, and negative symptoms.[4] In schizophrenia, the disorder lasts for at least 6 months, with at least 1 month of active symptoms.[4]

Limited data are available on the course of psychotic disorders in pregnancy; both deterioration and improvement have been reported. The postpartum period is thought to be a high-risk period for relapse. Compared with women without psychotic disorders, pregnant women who have psychotic disorders often receive less prenatal care; have poorer nutrition; exhibit greater use of tobacco, alcohol, and illicit drugs; and have higher rates of obstetric interventions and obstetric complications. Fear of loss of child custody may result in underreporting of symptoms.[23]

OTHER DISORDERS

Personality Disorders

Personality disorders have high prevalence rates of approximately 10% in the general population and up to 40% among psychiatric patients.[32] The *DSM-5* lists 10 specific personality disorders that are grouped into three clusters based on descriptive similarities. Patients in cluster A (paranoid, schizoid, schizotypal) appear odd or eccentric; patients in cluster B (antisocial, borderline, histrionic, narcissistic) appear dramatic, emotional, or erratic; and patients in cluster C (avoidant, dependent, obsessive-compulsive) appear anxious and fearful.[4] There is also one further category, personality disorder not otherwise specified. The *DSM-5* also provides an alternative dimensional model for personality disorders based on both personality functioning and pathologic personality traits that takes the perspective that personality disorders represent maladaptive variants of personality traits that merge into normality and into one another. This accounts for the observation that patients who meet criteria for a specific personality disorder frequently also meet criteria for other personality disorders.[4]

Pseudocyesis

Pseudocyesis is a clinical syndrome in which a woman firmly believes that she is pregnant in the absence of a true gestation. Patients may develop convincing signs and symptoms suggestive of pregnancy, including abdominal enlargement and menstrual disturbance.[33] Diagnosis can be made using a pregnancy test and ultrasonography. Physical diagnoses should be excluded. For example, tumors such as bronchogenic carcinoma may produce hormones (e.g., human chorionic gonadotrophin) that can cause secondary amenorrhea, which may be confused with pregnancy.[33]

Denial of Pregnancy

In contrast to pseudocyesis, denial of pregnancy is more common, with an estimated incidence of 1 in 400 to 516 pregnancies. It may be associated with adverse outcomes, including psychological stress, unassisted delivery, and infanticide. Patients who are identified should be referred for psychiatric assessment.[34]

Substance Abuse

Substance use during pregnancy is discussed in Chapter 52.

MANAGEMENT OF PSYCHIATRIC DISORDERS IN PREGNANCY

General Considerations

Guidelines for the management of pregnant women with psychiatric disorders have been published by the ACOG[15] and the APA,[35] and guidelines are also available from the United Kingdom[36] and Australia.[37]

Screening for anxiety and depression during pregnancy and the postpartum period is essential and recommended by the ACOG and APA for diagnosing perinatal mental health problems.[13,35] Screening can be achieved through face-to-face screening or online. Pregnant women should also be screened for substance abuse and domestic violence.[37] Positive screens require referral for support services. Patients voicing thoughts of self-harm, in any care context, must be referred for immediate support and evaluation.

Treatment options for different psychiatric disorders overlap and include nonpharmacologic and pharmacologic therapies. Data are limited on pregnancy-specific efficacy of treatments, but in general, response in pregnant patients is thought to be similar to that in nonpregnant patients.[1] A family-centered approach is recommended, and cultural and social context should be taken into account. Nonpharmacologic therapies are important because of maternal preferences and concerns about potential effects of drugs on the fetus, infant, or breast milk transfer.[15] Although there are theoretical concerns about potential harmful effects of psychotropic drugs during pregnancy and lactation, psychotropic drugs prescribed in pregnancy should be chosen for their track records of safety. The significant risks for exacerbation of illness and serious harm associated with cessation or withholding of psychotropic drugs must be balanced against these other risks.[5]

Because diabetes, obesity, smoking, and substance abuse are more common in people with psychiatric disorders, it can be difficult to separate the effects of psychiatric drugs on the fetus from the effects of these other factors. Further, some of the risks associated with psychiatric drugs may be attributable to the fact that women who take medication for psychiatric disorders are likely to have a more severe disease than women not on medication (i.e., confounding by indication).[38]

Readers are referred to published guidelines from the ACOG for the screening and diagnosis of mental health conditions during pregnancy.[13] In summary: (1) all pregnant patients should be screened for depression, anxiety, and BPD using validated instruments; (2) the screening for anxiety and depression should occur at the initial prenatal visit, later in pregnancy, and postpartum; (3) screening for BPD should occur before initiating pharmacotherapy for anxiety or depression if not already done; (4) because BPD is associated with suicide and infanticide, a mental health professional should be consulted if screening is positive for BPD; and (5) systems should be in place for effective treatment, monitoring, and follow-up of any patient who screens positive for any of the above.

A multidisciplinary approach is essential in the management of pregnant patients with psychiatric disorders, especially because many anesthesia providers may not be familiar with management of these patients. Patients who are noncooperative or violent may be challenging and require patience, compassion, and emotional support. Flexibility in management is important. For example, general anesthesia may sometimes be required if neuraxial anesthesia is considered impractical or unsafe.

Psychological and Psychosocial Therapies

Psychological and psychosocial interventions include cognitive behavioral therapy, interpersonal therapy, nondirective counseling, and peer support; these strategies are particularly effective for management of anxiety disorders and depression. Promising interventions for postpartum depression include professionally based postpartum home visits, lay- or peer-based postpartum telephone support, and interpersonal psychotherapy.[39]

Psychotropic Drugs

There is often concern about potential harmful fetal/neonatal effects of psychotropic drugs given during pregnancy and lactation. However, because of the difficulties of performing experimental studies in this area, much of the available evidence is based on observational studies that are unable to differentiate between association and causation. The decision to initiate or continue a psychotropic medication during pregnancy requires the physician and patient to carefully weigh the possible risks associated with medications versus the serious potential consequences of inadequately treated disease.

Psychiatric medications should generally be continued in pregnant women presenting for anesthesia and surgery.

Box 49.1 outlines principles for the use of psychiatric medications during pregnancy. The use of nonanesthetic drugs during pregnancy and lactation is discussed in Chapter 16.

Antidepressants are the most common psychotropic drugs prescribed in pregnancy. Previously, **tricyclic antidepressants** were commonly used and have been generally considered safe in pregnancy. These drugs may have anticholinergic side effects, including dilated pupils, agitation, seizures, delirium, hyperthermia, and arrhythmias, and they have a greater fatality risk after overdose compared with newer agents. Tricyclic antidepressants have been largely replaced by **serotonin reuptake inhibitors (SRIs)**, which are a mainstay therapy for depression and anxiety. These drugs include **selective serotonin reuptake inhibitors (SSRIs)**, such as **sertraline, paroxetine, fluoxetine**, and **citalopram**, and **serotonin-norepinephrine reuptake inhibitors (SNRIs)**, such as **desvenlafaxine, duloxetine, levomilnacipran**, and **venlafaxine**. Much research has investigated the possible association between the use of SRIs in pregnancy and an increased risk for congenital abnormalities including cardiovascular defects, persistent pulmonary hypertension, and postnatal adaptation syndrome.[40] The overall risk appears to be small and the US Food and Drug Administration advises clinicians not to change their clinical practice based on concern for heart or lung problems in the newborn.[41] The reassuring results from a large retrospective study from Sweden showed that, after accounting for confounding variables, first-trimester exposure to SRIs was associated with a small increased risk for preterm birth but no increased risk for a small-for-gestational age infant at delivery, autism spectrum disorder, or attention-deficit/hyperactivity disorder.[42] Serotonin syndrome (i.e., agitation, restlessness, hallucinations, increased body temperature, vomiting) may occur with an overdose or a combination of serotonergic drugs.[43]

Routine prescription of **benzodiazepines** for pregnant women is typically avoided, except for short-term treatment of extreme anxiety and agitation, because of concern for risks that include oral clefts, floppy baby syndrome, and neonatal withdrawal syndrome.[15]

Lithium is a foundation therapy for management of BPD. Early studies reported that use of lithium in early pregnancy was associated with an increased risk for congenital malformations, with particular concern for cardiac abnormalities, especially Ebstein's anomaly. Although the risk now appears to be less than initially thought, it has been recommended that women who are exposed to lithium in the first trimester undergo fetal echocardiography. Exposure in later gestation has been associated with fetal and neonatal diabetes insipidus, polyhydramnios (thought to occur from fetal diabetes insipidus), thyroid dysfunction, cardiac arrhythmias, hypoglycemia, preterm delivery, and floppy baby syndrome.[15] Renal clearance of lithium is increased in pregnancy; therefore serum levels should be closely monitored in pregnant women who are taking lithium. Discontinuation of lithium is associated with a high risk for recurrent illness, particularly in the postpartum period.

Anticonvulsant drugs are often used as mood stabilizers in patients with BPD. **Valproate** use in pregnancy is associated with a dose-related risk for many congenital anomalies (e.g., craniofacial, limb, cardiovascular abnormalities) and a variable risk for cognitive impairment.[1] **Fetal valproate syndrome**, which includes fetal growth restriction, facial dysmorphology, and limb and heart defects, has been described.[15] **Carbamazepine** has also been associated with congenital abnormalities, although with less frequency or severity compared with valproate.[1] **Fetal carbamazepine syndrome**, which includes facial dysmorphism and fingernail hypoplasia, has been described.[15] **Lamotrigine** appears to be associated with less fetal risk than that occurring with valproate and carbamazepine.[15] Folate supplementation should be offered to patients taking anticonvulsants to reduce the risk for neural tube defects.

Typical antipsychotic drugs (e.g., **haloperidol, thioridazine, fluphenazine, perphenazine, chlorpromazine, trifluoperazine**) have a long history of use in pregnant patients and generally have minimal teratogenic effects.[15] The phenothiazines are also used for their antiemetic effects. Fetal and neonatal toxicity after maternal exposure can include dyskinesia, extrapyramidal side effects, neonatal jaundice, and postnatal intestinal obstruction. The **neuroleptic malignant syndrome** is of particular interest to anesthesia providers because of its similarity to malignant hyperthermia. Features include hyperthermia, rigidity, mental status alteration, creatine kinase elevation, sympathetic nervous system lability, tachycardia, and tachypnea. Treatment is largely supportive and includes discontinuation of triggering agents, antipyretics, cooling, rehydration, and management of autonomic instability. The use of dantrolene, bromocriptine, and aman-tadine has been described.[43]

Atypical antipsychotic drugs (e.g., **clozapine, olanzap-ine, quetiapine, risperidone, ziprasidone, aripiprazole**) are now commonly used for treatment of schizophrenia, BPD, OCD, and resistant depression. Although these drugs are well tolerated, fewer data about reproductive safety are available when compared with older drugs.

Drug Interactions

Several drug interactions involving psychiatric drugs are rel-evant to anesthesia providers. The most important of these involve monoamine oxidase inhibitors (MAOIs), which include older irreversible drugs (e.g., phenelzine, tranyl-cypromine) and newer reversible drugs (e.g., selegiline, moclobemide). Potential interactions include (1) hyperten-sion after administration of an indirect-acting vasopressor (e.g., ephedrine, metaraminol), which results from increased norepinephrine (noradrenaline) concentration in sympa-thetic nerve endings; and (2) excitatory interactions associ-ated with serotonin toxicity. The latter are characterized by clonus, hyperreflexia, hyperthermia, and agitation, and may be precipitated by coadministration of an MAOI and an SRI. Of note, phenylpiperidine opioids, especially meperi-dine (pethidine), but also tramadol, methadone, and dex-tromethorphan, are weak SRIs and have been implicated in toxic reactions associated with MAOIs, including hyperpy-rexic coma. Irreversible MAOIs should be stopped 2 weeks before administration of anesthesia to allow regeneration of MAO and restoration of normal monoamine metabolism, and reversible MAOIs should be stopped for 24 hours before administration of anesthesia.

Electroconvulsive Therapy

ECT is considered an important treatment option in the pregnant patient with psychiatric disease, especially when balancing the risk for morbidity from psychiatric illness and the potential adverse effects of psychiatric drugs. Indications include major unipolar or bipolar depressive episodes, mania, and certain acute schizophrenia exacerbations. Acute suicide risk, poor response to medications, and patient preference may also affect the decision to use ECT. Contraindications include anticipated intolerance of associated physiologic changes that result from autonomic activation during ECT (e.g., increased intracranial pressure). Relative contraindications include hypertensive disease and impaired uteroplacental perfusion.

Emerging evidence suggests that ketamine is noninferior to ECT as therapy for treatment-resistant major depression without psychosis.[44]

There is a paucity of controlled data evaluating the use of ECT in pregnancy, with most information coming from case series. The APA has endorsed the use of ECT in all three tri-mesters of pregnancy.[35] The use of ECT in pregnancy has been considered effective, with low risk to the mother and fetus. However, one systematic review reported that adverse events such as decreased fetal heart rate, uterine contractions, and preterm labor occurred in 29% of cases.[45]

ECT for pregnant patients should be administered in a facility that can handle fetal emergencies. Anesthetic agents that have been used include thiopental (thiopentone), methohexital, propofol, succinylcholine (suxamethonium), and anticholinergics. Suggested guidelines for ECT during pregnancy are summarized in Box 49.2.[46] Perioperative coronavirus disease (COVID-19) precautions should be observed. Denitrogenation (preoxygenation), left uterine displacement, and fetal heart rate and uterine contrac-tion monitoring should be used. Pharmacologic aspiration prophylaxis and tracheal intubation should be considered in patients with symptoms of gastroesophageal reflux or advanced gestational age.[47]

BOX 49.2 Suggested Guidelines for Electroconvulsive Therapy During Pregnancy

- Obtain preoperative obstetric consultation.
- Monitor fetal heart rate and check for uterine contractions before and after the procedure.
- Ensure adequate hydration and denitrogenation (preoxygenation).
- Maintain left uterine displacement after 18–20 weeks' gestation.
- Be aware that etomidate is a superior induction agent for electroconvulsive therapy seizure quality.
- Consider pharmacologic aspiration prophylaxis and tracheal intubation in patients with symptoms of gastroesophageal reflux or advancing gestational age.
- Observe for vaginal bleeding after the procedure.

Modified from Ward HB, Fromson JA, Cooper JJ, et al. Recommenda-tions for the use of ECT in pregnancy: literature review and proposed clinical protocol. *Arch Womens Ment Health.* 2018;21:715–722.

KEY POINTS

- Psychiatric disorders occur commonly during preg-nancy, but their prevalence is often underestimated and underappreciated.
- Anxiety disorders are the most common psychiatric disor-ders in pregnant women.
- All women should be screened for depression at the first pregnant visit, again later in pregnancy, and postpartum.

- The risk for major depressive disorder is increased during the postpartum period.
- Suicide is one of the leading causes of maternal mortality.
- Psychological and psychosocial interventions are effective for many psychiatric diseases in pregnancy.
- When managing pregnant patients with psychiatric disor-ders, the risks of withholding psychiatric drugs because of

concerns for harmful fetal effects must be balanced against the potential consequences of untreated disease.

- Patients with a previous psychiatric history should be identified prenatally and frequently monitored and supported during pregnancy and the first few weeks postpartum. Psychiatric services should have priority-care pathways for pregnant and postpartum women, and care by multiple psychiatric teams should be avoided.
- A multidisciplinary approach is essential in the management of pregnant patients with psychiatric disorders,

and the partner and family should be involved with decisions.

- Awareness during general anesthesia for cesarean delivery, inadequate neuraxial anesthesia for cesarean delivery, and poor pain control during vaginal delivery may result in posttraumatic stress disorder in susceptible patients.
- Anesthesia providers should be aware of potential drug interactions with psychotropic drugs.

REFERENCES

1. Levey L, Ragan K, Hower-Hartley A, et al. Psychiatric disorders in pregnancy. *Neurol Clin.* 2004;22:863–893.
2. Vesga-López O, Blanco C, Keyes K, et al. Psychiatric disorders in pregnant and postpartum women in the United States. *Arch Gen Psychiatry.* 2008;65:805–815.
3. Wangel AM, Molin J, Moghaddassi M, Stman M. Prior psychiatric inpatient care and risk of cesarean sections: a registry study. *J Psychosom Obstet Gynaecol.* 2011;32:189–197.
4. American Psychiatric Association, *Diagnostic and Statistical Manual of Mental Disorders.* 5th ed. American Psychiatric Association; 2013.
5. Chisolm MS, Payne JL. Management of psychotropic drugs during pregnancy. *BMJ.* 2016;532:h5918.
6. Centers for Disease Control and Prevention. Pregnancy-related deaths: data from maternal mortality review committees in 36 US States, 2017–2019. https://www.cdc.gov/maternal-mortality/php/data-research/mmrc-2017-2019.html?CDC_AAref_Val=https://www.cdc.gov/reproductivehealth/maternal-mortality/erasemm/data-mmrc.html?source=email3. Accessed 27 February 2025.
7. Saving Lives, Improving Mothers' Care. *Lessons learned to inform maternity care from the UK and Ireland confidential enquiries into maternal deaths and morbidity 2018-20.* https://www.npeu.ox.ac.uk/assets/downloads/mbrrace-uk/reports/maternal-report-2022/MBRRACE-UK_Maternal_MAIN_Report_2022_UPDATE.pdf. Accessed 14 January 2024.
8. Howard LM, Molyneaux E, Dennis CL, et al. Non-psychotic mental disorders in the perinatal period. *Lancet.* 2014;384:1775–1788.
9. Moore Simas TA, Whelan A, Byatt N. Postpartum depression – new screening recommendations and treatments. *JAMA.* 2023;330:2295–2296.
10. Chaudron LH. Complex challenges in treating depression during pregnancy. *Am J Psychiatry.* 2013;170:12–20.
11. Mergl R, Quaatz SM, Lemke V, Allgaier AK. Prevalence of depression and depressive symptoms in women with previous miscarriages or stillbirths – a systematic review. *J Psychiatr Res.* 2024;169:84–96.
12. Ghimire U, Papabathini SS, Kawuki J, et al. Depression during pregnancy and the risk of low birth weight, preterm birth and intrauterine growth restriction – an updated meta-analysis. *Early Hum Dev.* 2021;152:105243.
13. American College of Obstetricians and Gynecologists. Clinical Practice Guideline No. 4: Screening and diagnosis of mental health conditions during pregnancy and postpartum. *Obstet Gynecol.* 2023;141:1232–1261.

14. Yonkers KA, Vigod S, Ross LE. Diagnosis, pathophysiology, and management of mood disorders in pregnant and postpartum women. *Obstet Gynecol.* 2011;117:961–977.
15. American College of Obstetricians and Gynecologists, Clinical Practice Guideline No. 5: Treatment and management of mental health conditions during pregnancy and postpartum. *Obstet Gynecol.* 2023;141:1262–1288.
16. Robertson E, Grace S, Wallington T, Stewart DE. Antenatal risk factors for postpartum depression: a synthesis of recent literature. *Gen Hosp Psychiatry.* 2004;26:289–295.
17. Ding T, Wang DX, Qu Y, et al. Epidural labor analgesia is associated with a decreased risk of postpartum depression: a prospective cohort study. *Anesth Analg.* 2014;119:383–392.
18. Lim G, Farrell LM, Facco FL, et al. Labor analgesia as a predictor for reduced postpartum depression scores: a retrospective observational study. *Anesth Analg.* 2018;126:1598–1605.
19. Suhitharan T, Pham TP, Chen H, et al. Investigating analgesic and psychological factors associated with risk of postpartum depression development: a case-control study. *Neuropsychiatr Dis Treat.* 2016;12:1333–1339.
20. Nahirney M, Metcalfe A, Chaput KH. Administration of epidural labor analgesia is not associated with a decreased risk of postpartum depression in an urban Canadian population of mothers: a secondary analysis of prospective cohort data. *Local Reg Anesth.* 2017;10:99–104.
21. Orbach-Zinger S, Landau R, Harousch AB, et al. The relationship between women's intention to request a labor epidural analgesia, actually delivering with labor epidural analgesia, and postpartum depression at 6 weeks: a prospective observational study. *Anesth Analg.* 2018;126:1590–1597.
22. Friedman SH, Reed E, Ross NE. Postpartum psychosis. *Curr Psychiatry Rep.* 2023;25:65–72.
23. Cantwell R. Mental disorder in pregnancy and the early postpartum. *Anaesthesia.* 2021;76(suppl 4):76–83.
24. Schulz-Stubner S. Panic attacks and hyperventilation may mimic local anesthesia toxicity. *Reg Anesth Pain Med.* 2004;29:617–618.
25. Yildiz PD, Ayers S, Phillips L. The prevalence of posttraumatic stress disorder in pregnancy and after birth: a systematic review and meta-analysis. *J Affect Disord.* 2017;208:634–645.
26. Carter J, Bick D, Gallacher D, Chang YS. Mode of birth and development of maternal postnatal post-traumatic stress disorder: a mixed-methods systematic review and meta-analysis. *Birth.* 2022;49:616–627.
27. Laurin A, Bulteau S, Dumont R, et al. Rapid and efficient treatment of post-traumatic stress disorder induced by

anaesthesia awareness with recall using reconsolidation therapy. *Br J Anaesth.* 2023;130:e483–e485.

28. Lopez U, Meyer M, Loures V, et al. Post-traumatic stress disorder in parturients delivering by caesarean section and the implication of anaesthesia: a prospective cohort study. *Health Qual Life Outcomes.* 2017;15:118.

29. Vogel TM, Homitsky S. Antepartum and intrapartum risk factors and the impact of PTSD on mother and child. *BJA Educ.* 2020;20:89–95.

30. Nieminen K, Stephansson O, Ryding EL. Women's fear of childbirth and preference for cesarean section – a cross-sectional study at various stages of pregnancy in Sweden. *Acta Obstet Gynecol Scand.* 2009;88:807–813.

31. Russell EJ, Fawcett JM, Mazmanian D. Risk of obsessive-compulsive disorder in pregnant and postpartum women: a meta-analysis. *J Clin Psychiatry.* 2013;74:377–385.

32. Zhan Yuen Wong N, Barnett P, Sheridan Rains L, et al. Evaluation of international guidance for the community treatment of 'personality disorders': a systematic review. *PLoS One.* 2023;18:e0264239.

33. Gogia S, Grieb A, Jang A, et al. Medical considerations in delusion of pregnancy: a systematic review. *J Psychosom Obstet Gynaecol.* 2022;43:51–57.

34. Chase T, Shah A, Maines J, Fusick A. Psychotic pregnancy denial: a review of the literature and its clinical considerations. *J Psychosom Obstet Gynaecol.* 2021;42:253–257.

35. Yonkers KA, Wisner KL, Stewart DE, et al. The management of depression during pregnancy: a report from the American Psychiatric Association and the American College of Obstetricians and Gynecologists. *Obstet Gynecol.* 2009;114:703–713.

36. National Institute for Health and Care Excellence. *Antenatal and postnatal mental health: clinical management and service guidance.* Updated February 11, 2020. https://www.nice.org.uk/guidance/cg192. Accessed 16 January 2024.

37. Highet NJ, the Expert Working Group. *Mental Health Care in the Perinatal Period: Australian Clinical Practice Guideline.* Centre of Perinatal Excellence (COPE); 2023.

38. Stewart DE. Clinical practice. Depression during pregnancy. *N Engl J Med.* 2011;365:1605–1611.

39. Dennis CL, Dowswell T. Psychosocial and psychological interventions for preventing postpartum depression. *Cochrane Database Syst Rev.* 2013;(2):CD001134.

40. Hanley GE, Oberlander TF. The effect of perinatal exposures on the infant: antidepressants and depression. *Best Pract Res Clin Obstet Gynaecol.* 2014;28:37–48.

41. U.S. Food and Drug Administration. Selective serotonin reuptake inhibitor (SSRI) antidepressant use during pregnancy and reports of a rare heart and lung condition in newborn babies. FDA Drug Safety Communication. https://www.fda.gov/drugs/drug-safety-and-availability/fda-drug-safety-communication-selective-serotonin-reuptake-inhibitor-ssri-antidepressant-use-during. Accessed 19 February 2024.

42. Sujan AC, Rickert ME, Öberg AS, et al. Associations of maternal antidepressant use during the first trimester of pregnancy with preterm birth, small for gestational age, autism spectrum disorder, and attention-deficit/hyperactivity disorder in offspring. *JAMA.* 2017;317:1553–1562.

43. Smith FA, Wittmann CW, Stern TA. Medical complications of psychiatric treatment. *Crit Care Clin.* 2008;24:635–656.

44. Anand A, Mathew SJ, Sanacora G, et al. Ketamine versus ECT for nonpsychotic treatment-resistant major depression. *N Engl J Med.* 2023;388:2315–2325.

45. Leiknes KA, Cooke MJ, Jarosch-von Schweder L, et al. Electroconvulsive therapy during pregnancy: a systematic review of case studies. *Arch Womens Ment Health.* 2015;18:1–39.

46. Ward HB, Fromson JA, Cooper JJ, et al. Recommendations for the use of ECT in pregnancy: literature review and proposed clinical protocol. *Arch Womens Ment Health.* 2018;21:715–722.

47. Jhaveri V, Martinez R, Trippensee A, et al. Airway complications in pregnant patients undergoing electroconvulsive therapy: a retrospective case-control study. *J ECT.* 2023;39:81–83.

50

Renal Disease

Daniel Katz, MD and Yaakov Beilin, MD

CHAPTER OUTLINE

"Children of women with renal disease used to be born dangerously or not at all—not at all if their doctors had their way."[1] This statement describes early experiences with maternal renal disease and pregnancy outcome. It remains true that renal disease may impair maternal and fetal health. Investigations during the past three decades have significantly improved both maternal and neonatal outcomes in pregnant women with renal disease.[2]

PHYSIOLOGIC CHANGES IN PREGNANCY

A review of the renal physiologic changes that occur during normal pregnancy is helpful to understand and evaluate coexisting renal disorders (see Chapter 2). Early in gestation, increased intravascular volume leads to renal enlargement. Hormonal changes result in dilation of the renal pelvis and ureters, accompanied by decreased ureteral peristalsis. Dilated uterine and ovarian veins, and the gravid uterus, may obstruct ureter drainage at the pelvic brim. Together, these changes predispose pregnant women to vesicoureteric reflux and ascending infection. Alterations in glomerular hemodynamics and tubular function also occur. Increased cardiac output and decreased intrarenal vascular resistance cause an 80% increase in renal blood flow and a 50% increase in glomerular filtration rate (GFR) during pregnancy. These

changes are somewhat less pronounced near term. Because of the increased GFR, a serum creatinine concentration > 0.6 to 0.8 mg/dL (53 to 71 μmol/L) and a blood urea nitrogen (BUN) concentration > 8 to 9 mg/dL (urea concentration > 2.9 to 3.2 mmol/L) (upper limit of normal in pregnancy) suggest renal insufficiency in the pregnant woman. Tubular sodium reabsorption and osmoregulation are reset, allowing a "physiologic hypervolemia" during gestation. Modest proteinuria, up to 300 mg/day, also occurs during pregnancy.[3]

Urinary tract infections (see Chapter 36) and renal dysfunction associated with hypertensive disorders of pregnancy (see Chapter 35) are discussed elsewhere in this text.

RENAL PARENCHYMAL DISEASE

Definition and Pathophysiology

Renal parenchymal disease consists of two general groups of disorders, **glomerulopathies** and **tubulointerstitial disease**. Glomerulopathies are further subdivided into disorders that involve inflammatory or necrotizing lesions—the **nephritic syndromes**—and disorders that involve abnormal permeability to protein and other macromolecules—the **nephrotic syndromes**. More than 20 specific glomerulopathies exist. The nomenclature for these glomerulopathies is complex, and specific diseases are not discussed in detail here.

Tubulointerstitial diseases are characterized by abnormal tubular function. They result in abnormal urine composition and concentration but are not characterized by decreased GFR until late in the disease course. The disorders in this category include interstitial nephritis, acute tubular necrosis, multiple myeloma of the kidney, and functional tubular defects such as renal tubular acidosis.

Patients with renal parenchymal disorders may remain asymptomatic for years, and they may exhibit only proteinuria and microscopic hematuria, with little if any evidence of reduced renal function. Spontaneous recovery or improvement with treatment occurs with many glomerulopathies. However, other patients exhibit progressive nephropathy, hypertension, and renal insufficiency. The incidence of chronic kidney disease (CKD) in pregnancy is as high as 3%, a stark increase from prior estimates as fertility rates in the patient population have increased.[4] In two-thirds of these patients, the disorder results from glomerulopathy, and in one-third, from tubulointerstitial disease.[5]

Diagnosis

Ideally, the severity of renal disease should be assessed by preconception GFR as classified by the National Kidney Foundation/Kidney Disease: Improving Global Outcomes organization's definition and guidelines on improving outcome, as standard GFR equations are inaccurate in pregnancy.[6] Creatinine clearance and the level of proteinuria should be determined. Urinalysis yields information about the presence of renal casts and bacteriuria. The determination of serum creatinine and BUN concentrations defines the extent of renal insufficiency. A serum creatinine concentration > 0.87 mg/dL (77 μmol/L), which may be normal in the nonpregnant woman, may represent significant renal insufficiency during pregnancy.[7] Alternatively, the obstetric provider may first detect renal dysfunction through routine prenatal screening tests as patients may otherwise be asymptomatic, because symptoms rarely develop until GFR decreases by 25%.[8] If proteinuria, hematuria, or azotemia is detected, further evaluation should be performed.

Both preeclampsia and renal disease may manifest as hypertension, proteinuria, and edema. Differentiating the two entities is complex, especially after 20 weeks' gestation. Serial blood pressure measurements define the severity of hypertension and the efficacy of current antihypertensive therapy. In cases where CKD needs to be differentiated from preeclampsia, biomarkers such as placental growth factor (PIGF) and FMS-like tyrosine kinase-1 (sFlt-1) can be obtained; in preeclampsia the sFlt-1:PIGF ratio is elevated and in CKD it is not.[9]

Although **renal tissue biopsy** is often used to establish a diagnosis in nonpregnant patients, it is rarely required to manage kidney disease in pregnancy, and may be associated with procedural complications.[10] A systematic review by Piccoli et al.[11] compared complication rates from 243 renal biopsies performed during pregnancy with 1236 performed in the postpartum period. Significant complications occurred in 7% of biopsies performed before delivery compared with 1% in the postpartum period. Most complications

were minor and included groin pain as well as hematuria. The authors did report, however, that more serious complications (e.g., bleeding and loin pain) occurred the further along in pregnancy the biopsy was performed and seemed to peak around 25 weeks' gestation. It should be noted that in 23 of the studies in the metaanalysis, kidney biopsies were performed to characterize morphologies in preeclampsia, a practice that is no longer recommended and may have influenced the subject pool substantially. Given the increased risk associated with biopsy during pregnancy, it should only be performed in patients with a high likelihood of severe glomerular disease and when a definitive diagnosis is critical to guide treatment.[10,11]

In addition to clinical information, urinalysis and inflammatory and biomarker data have also supplanted the need for renal biopsy in some cases.[12] For example, when a diagnosis is obtained through antineutrophil cytoplasmic antibodies or through double-stranded DNA antibodies, empiric treatment may begin with corticosteroids, azathioprine, or calcineurin inhibitors in lieu of a kidney biopsy.[12] Novel biomarkers at the genetic and epigenetic levels have been investigated, many of which are found in the urine and plasma/serum. The list is too extensive for the purposes of this chapter; however, one of the most robust biomarkers in kidney disease, the M-type phospholipase A2 receptor antibody, is commonly used to diagnose membranous nephropathy. It has recently gained approval from the US Food and Drug Administration for the diagnosis and monitoring of membranous nephropathy.[13]

Effect of Pregnancy on Preexisting Kidney Disease

The extent to which pregnancy affects preexisting renal disease depends on the level of renal insufficiency before pregnancy. Among women with mild antenatal renal insufficiency with well-controlled blood pressure and proteinuria < 1 g/day, pregnancy does not appear to substantially alter the natural course of renal disease.[14,15] Jungers et al.[14] evaluated the effect of pregnancy on renal function among 360 women with primary glomerulonephritis. During the study period, 171 (48%) women became pregnant. All study subjects had normal renal function at the time of entry into the study and all patients who became pregnant had normal renal function at conception. In the case-control analysis of the study, pregnancy was not identified as a risk factor for progression to end-stage renal failure. Limardo et al.[15] evaluated 223 women with biopsy-documented IgA nephropathy who had a serum creatinine level > 1.2 mg/dL (106 μmol/L), 136 of whom became pregnant. Women were observed for a minimum of 5 years (median, 10 years), and pregnancy did not seem to affect the long-term outcome of kidney disease or the onset of proteinuria or hypertension.

In contrast, Jones and Hayslett[16] analyzed the outcome of 82 pregnancies in 67 women with preexisting moderate or severe renal insufficiency (i.e., serum creatinine level > 1.4 mg/dL [124 μmol/L] before pregnancy or at the first antepartum visit). The mean ± standard deviation serum creatinine concentration increased from 1.9 ± 0.8 mg/dL (168 ± 71 μmol/L) in early pregnancy to 2.5 ± 1.3 mg/dL (221 ± 115 μmol/L) in the third trimester. The prevalence of hypertension rose from 28% at baseline to 48% during late pregnancy. Pregnancy-related deterioration of maternal renal function occurred in 43% of cases. Purdy et al.[17] also found that more than 40% of women with moderate to severe kidney disease had deterioration in renal function caused by pregnancy. Women with a serum creatinine concentration > 2.0 mg/dL (177 μmol/L) who became pregnant had a one-in-three chance of developing dialysis-dependent end-stage renal disease during or shortly after pregnancy.[18] In summary, the preponderance of evidence demonstrates that while pregnancy exacerbates renal disease, it has a greater effect on those who present with moderate to severe levels of renal dysfunction before pregnancy or in those in whom blood pressure control is difficult or there is significant proteinuria.

The pathophysiology by which pregnancy exacerbates renal disease is unknown. One hypothesis is that increased glomerular perfusion paradoxically causes further injury to the kidneys in patients with preexisting impairment of function. However, this hypothesis is unsupported by published data, which do not demonstrate evidence of hyperfiltration (i.e., an initial decline in serum creatinine concentration) during early pregnancy in patients with renal disease.[19] An alternative hypothesis is that preexisting renal disease may induce a cascade of platelet aggregation, microvascular fibrin thrombus formation, and endothelial dysfunction that leads to microvascular injury in the already tenuous kidneys.[18] In addition to general changes to renal mechanics discussed earlier, exacerbation or improvement of the initial disease process during pregnancy could also alter the long-term course of renal dysfunction.

Effect on the Mother and Fetus

Pregnant women with CKD are at an increased risk for maternal and fetal complications. Al Khalaf et al.[2] systematically reviewed all published studies of women with CKD that included a control group for comparison. They identified 31 studies between 1988 and 2021. Of these, 17 studies compared outcomes in women with and without CKD; 10 studies compared early with late stages of CKD, and 4 studies had both comparisons. Several adverse outcomes were associated with CKD, including preeclampsia, cesarean delivery, preterm birth, low birthweight, and neonatal intensive care unit (NICU) admission (Fig. 50.1). A prespecified subgroup analysis comparing early- versus late-stage CKD demonstrated similar findings, with late-stage CKD demonstrating an association with preeclampsia and very preterm birth. Other outcomes were associated as well; however, the model was not robust enough to provide risk-adjusted estimates for factors such as maternal age, smoking, body mass index, race, income, educational level, parity, and other comorbidities. Additional analyses demonstrated risk differences by the type of kidney disease, with elevated risk profiles in cases of diabetic CKD and glomerulonephritis compared with polycystic kidney disease.

Medical and Obstetric Management

During pregnancy, the nephrologist and the obstetric provider should monitor maternal renal function, blood pressure, and fetal development at frequent intervals. Monthly determination of serum creatinine concentration, creatinine clearance, and proteinuria allows the recognition of renal deterioration and establishes a baseline for the patient, which may be useful in diagnosing superimposed preeclampsia if it occurs. An antepartum consultation with the anesthesia provider should also be considered to address issues such as peripartum medication and fluid management, and to perform an overall risk assessment to discuss and develop potential plans for anesthetic technique and monitoring. Blood pressure control is important to mitigate further renal damage, and the American College of Obstetricians and Gynecologists recommends treatment for systolic blood pressure ≥ 140 mm Hg or diastolic blood pressure ≥ 90 mm Hg.[20]

Some glomerulopathies respond to corticosteroids, and corticosteroid therapy should be continued during pregnancy. Rapid deterioration of renal function that occurs before 28 weeks' gestation may require renal biopsy to exclude rapidly progressive glomerulopathies that require treatment (see earlier discussion). Up to 68% of pregnant women with CKD will have anemia.[21] These women may be treated with **iron supplementation** (oral or IV) or **erythropoietin-stimulating agents (ESAs)**. Because of its large molecular weight, recombinant erythropoietin does not appear to cross the placenta or have an adverse impact on the fetus. There is no standardized regimen; however, it should be noted that doses may need to be changed during varying stages of the pregnancy to maintain the hemoglobin target within the range of 11 to 12 g/dL, as recommended by the National Kidney Foundation for pregnant patients.

There may be a benefit to administering both iron and ESA. In a retrospective study at a single Australian institution over a 15-year period, Morton et al.[21] analyzed the impact of both iron supplementation (oral and IV) and ESA use in pregnant patients with CKD. They identified 63 pregnancies in 52 women with CKD and found that oral iron supplementation resulted in a hemoglobin higher than 10 g/dL in 9/30 (30%) of pregnancies after 12 weeks of therapy. IV iron resulted in an average increase in hemoglobin from 8.6 to 11.6 g/dL over 5 weeks. In patients receiving ESA alone, hemoglobin increased from 8.1 to 10.5 g/dL on average; when IV iron and ESA were both used, 16/18 (89%) of women had resolution of their anemia.[21] Protein restriction places the fetus at risk for growth restriction and is not advised. Deterioration of maternal renal function, the onset of preeclampsia, or evidence of fetal compromise may necessitate urgent delivery.

Hemodialysis and Long-Term Ambulatory Peritoneal Dialysis

When renal disease has progressed to end-stage renal failure (i.e., GFR < 5 mL/min), fertility is suppressed. Less than 10% of premenopausal patients undergoing dialysis have regular menses. Luteinizing hormone and follicle-stimulating

Pre—eclampsia (adjusted estimates)

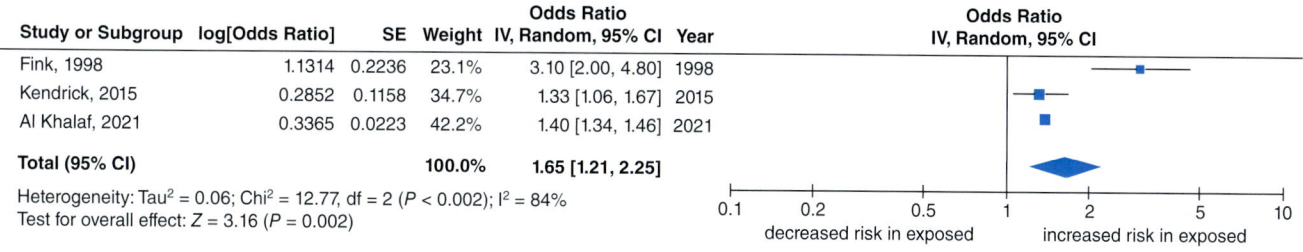

Study or Subgroup	log[Odds Ratio]	SE	Weight	Odds Ratio IV, Random, 95% CI	Year
Fink, 1998	1.9804	0.2782	23.6%	7.25 [4.20, 12.50]	1998
Jensen, 2010	1.3863	0.305	22.9%	4.00 [2.20, 7.27]	2010
Kendrick, 2015	0.1222	0.2024	25.5%	1.13 [0.76, 1.68]	2015
Al Khalaf, 2021	0.4762	0.0327	28.0%	1.61 [1.51, 1.72]	2021
Total (95% CI)			**100.0%**	**2.58 [1.33, 5.01]**	

Heterogeneity: Tau^2 = 0.41; Chi^2 = 40.77, df = 3 (P < 0.00001); I^2 = 93%
Test for overall effect: Z = 2.81 (P = 0.005)

Cesarean section (adjusted estimates)

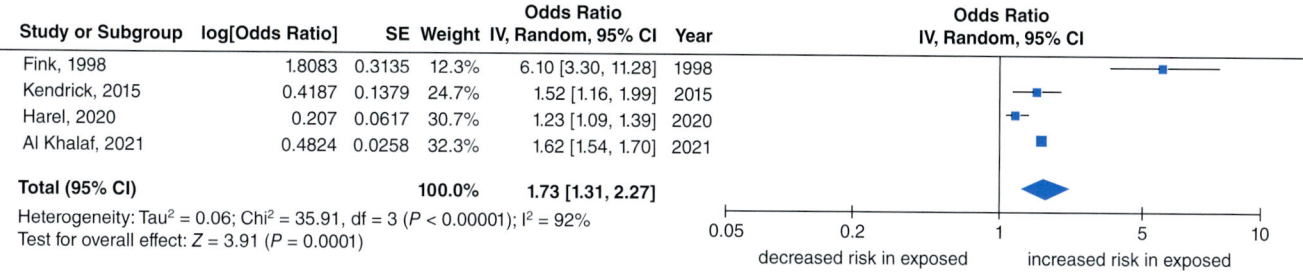

Study or Subgroup	log[Odds Ratio]	SE	Weight	Odds Ratio IV, Random, 95% CI	Year
Fink, 1998	1.1314	0.2236	23.1%	3.10 [2.00, 4.80]	1998
Kendrick, 2015	0.2852	0.1158	34.7%	1.33 [1.06, 1.67]	2015
Al Khalaf, 2021	0.3365	0.0223	42.2%	1.40 [1.34, 1.46]	2021
Total (95% CI)			**100.0%**	**1.65 [1.21, 2.25]**	

Heterogeneity: Tau^2 = 0.06; Chi^2 = 12.77, df = 2 (P < 0.002); I^2 = 84%
Test for overall effect: Z = 3.16 (P = 0.002)

Preterm birth (<37 w) (adjusted estimates)

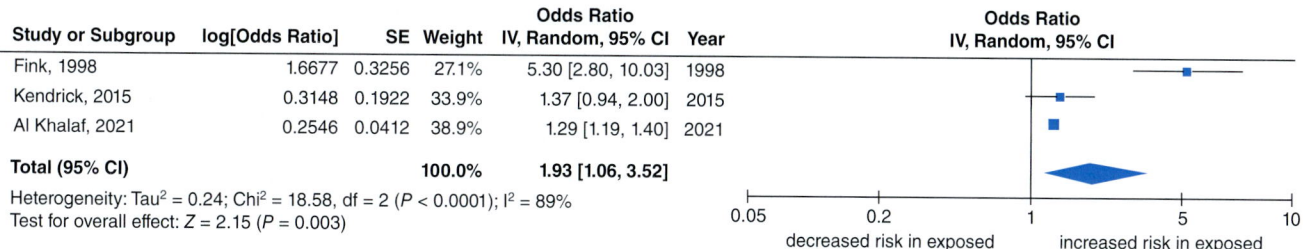

Study or Subgroup	log[Odds Ratio]	SE	Weight	Odds Ratio IV, Random, 95% CI	Year
Fink, 1998	1.8083	0.3135	12.3%	6.10 [3.30, 11.28]	1998
Kendrick, 2015	0.4187	0.1379	24.7%	1.52 [1.16, 1.99]	2015
Harel, 2020	0.207	0.0617	30.7%	1.23 [1.09, 1.39]	2020
Al Khalaf, 2021	0.4824	0.0258	32.3%	1.62 [1.54, 1.70]	2021
Total (95% CI)			**100.0%**	**1.73 [1.31, 2.27]**	

Heterogeneity: Tau^2 = 0.06; Chi^2 = 35.91, df = 3 (P < 0.00001); I^2 = 92%
Test for overall effect: Z = 3.91 (P = 0.0001)

Small for gestational age (adjusted estimates)

Study or Subgroup	log[Odds Ratio]	SE	Weight	Odds Ratio IV, Random, 95% CI	Year
Fink, 1998	1.6677	0.3256	27.1%	5.30 [2.80, 10.03]	1998
Kendrick, 2015	0.3148	0.1922	33.9%	1.37 [0.94, 2.00]	2015
Al Khalaf, 2021	0.2546	0.0412	38.9%	1.29 [1.19, 1.40]	2021
Total (95% CI)			**100.0%**	**1.93 [1.06, 3.52]**	

Heterogeneity: Tau^2 = 0.24; Chi^2 = 18.58, df = 2 (P < 0.0001); I^2 = 89%
Test for overall effect: Z = 2.15 (P = 0.003)

Fig. 50.1 Forest plots of studies of the association between CKD and fetal or neonatal outcomes. The *colored rectangles* represent the OR for each study, and the *lateral black lines* represent the 95% CI for each study. The *diamond* represents the overall OR, and the *lateral tips of the diamond* represent the 95% CI for the combined estimates. Panel A shows adjusted OR for preeclampsia, Panel B shows adjusted OR for cesarean delivery, Panel C shows adjusted OR for preterm birth, and Panel D shows adjusted OR for small for gestational age. *CI,* Confidence interval; *CKD,* chronic kidney disease; *OR,* odds ratio; *IV,* inverse variance. Modified from Al Khalaf S, Bodunde E, Maher GM, et al. Chronic kidney disease and adverse pregnancy outcomes: a systematic review and meta-analysis. *Am J Obstet Gynecol.* 2022;226: 656–670.e32.

hormone concentrations assume an anovulatory pattern, which causes 70% of affected women to be either oligo- or amenorrheic.[22] Half of all female patients undergoing dialysis exhibit hyperprolactinemia because of reduced clearance and hypothalamic disturbances.[23] Rates of conception for women on dialysis are about 1/100th of the general population.[24]

When pregnancy does occur, there are several important management considerations necessary to maximize the probability of a successful outcome. **Hemodialysis** necessitates vascular access and the need for anticoagulation of the extracorporeal circuit and may be complicated by cardiovascular instability, and large fluid and electrolyte shifts. Hypotension may compromise uteroplacental perfusion and cause fetal compromise. Even when hypotension and major fluid shifts are avoided, Doppler ultrasonographic examination of uterine and umbilical artery flow during hemodialysis suggests the occurrence of a redistribution of arterial flow away from the uteroplacental vascular bed.[25] Fetal heart rate monitoring should be considered during dialysis.[26] Rapid removal of maternal solutes and reduced oncotic pressure with attendant free-water diffusion into the amniotic cavity may lead to polyhydramnios. Live birth rates correlate positively with dialysis time, leading to changes in dialysis scheduling to shorter but more frequent runs.[27] Long-term ambulatory **peritoneal dialysis** allows less hemodynamic trespass, and the freedom to undergo dialysis at home. Complications of this modality include peritonitis and catheter difficulties.[28] With the increase in fetal survival with newer enhanced hemodialysis regimens and retrospective evidence suggesting potentially worse outcomes with peritoneal dialysis, current guidelines recommend changing from peritoneal dialysis to hemodialysis prior to conception or in the first trimester.[29]

Fetal outcomes for women on newer dialysis regimens have improved with live birth rates > 80%.[27] In a metaanalysis and systematic review of almost 550 pregnancies in patients undergoing both hemodialysis and peritoneal dialysis, Piccoli et al.[27] reported a low maternal perinatal mortality rate (0.4%), with a malformation rate of approximately 2%, which aligns with the risk in the general population. Fetal complications are most often seen in the form of respiratory distress, sepsis, and retinopathy and are likely a result of the higher incidence of preterm birth rather than related directly to dialysis. BUN levels should be kept less than 50 mg/dL (urea < 17.9 mmol/L) before dialysis and less than 30 mg/dL (urea < 10.7 mmol/L) after dialysis.[28] At birth, azotemia in the newborn is similar to that in the mother, but this quickly corrects because the newborn has normal kidney function. The long-term effects of intrauterine azotemia on newborn cognitive development are unknown; however, it appears that if the neonate survives the complications from preterm delivery, further development may be normal.[30]

Patients undergoing hemodialysis have a high rate of **viral hepatitis**; a greater frequency of active **tuberculosis**; and a higher rate of infection with **vancomycin-resistant enterococci**, **human immunodeficiency virus (HIV)**, and **methicillin-resistant** *Staphylococcus aureus*. The risk for **hepatitis C virus (HCV)** infection is particularly of concern, with reported rates as high as 36%. However, with improvement in aseptic technique and more attention to handwashing, the decline in the reuse of dialysis equipment, and the use of dedicated isolated dialysis machines for HCV-seropositive patients, the rates of infection and seroconversion can be markedly reduced.[31]

Anesthetic Management

Anesthetic management is influenced by the extent of renal dysfunction and hypertension. The parturient with stable renal disease, mild to moderate renal insufficiency, well-controlled hypertension, and euvolemia requires minimal special consideration. In contrast, the dialysis patient with end-stage renal failure presents many anesthetic challenges because renal disease may affect almost every organ system (Box 50.1). Poorly controlled hypertension may lead to left ventricular hypertrophy and dysfunction. Symptoms of cardiovascular compromise should prompt echocardiography to evaluate ventricular function. An intraarterial catheter also may aid the management of the parturient with poorly controlled hypertension, or when the continuous infusion of antihypertensive agents is required. Uremic pericarditis, cardiomyopathy, and accelerated atherosclerosis are rarely seen until advanced uremia has been present for several years.

Uremic toxins may cause functional platelet defects; these abnormalities are reversed by dialysis. Thrombocytopenia may also occur because of increased peripheral destruction of platelets. Generalized coagulopathy may result from the anticoagulation used during the dialysis process.[32] A full coagulation profile and careful bleeding history should be performed in patients on hemodialysis, especially before the initiation of neuraxial anesthesia. Hemodialysis fistulas should be padded carefully to prevent thrombosis. Blood pressure cuffs should not be placed on these extremities.

Neuraxial Anesthesia

Neuraxial anesthesia is the preferred technique for both labor analgesia and cesarean delivery, but there are some unique considerations in the parturient with renal disease. Uremic patients may be hypervolemic or hypovolemic, depending on the time elapsed since their last dialysis session. Hypovolemia and autonomic neuropathy may lead to profound hypotension during the onset of sympathetic blockade. Intravascular volume should be assessed before induction of anesthesia. Assessment of clinical signs (e.g., current body weight relative to dry body weight, skin turgor, mucous membranes, tachycardia) is generally sufficient. Transthoracic echocardiography may be useful when the volume status remains unclear. Although there are no studies in patients with CKD, a role for intravenous prehydration to prevent hypotension is unlikely because this modality is not efficacious in the healthy parturient.[33] There is insufficient evidence to recommend spinal versus epidural techniques for the patient with renal disease nor is there evidence to suggest that the practice patterns used in non-CKD parturients should be altered.

BOX 50.1 Chronic Renal Failure: Abnormalities That May Affect Anesthetic Management

Cardiovascular
- Hypertension
- Fluid overload
- Ventricular hypertrophy
- Accelerated atherosclerosis
- Uremic pericarditis
- Uremic cardiomyopathy

Pulmonary
- Increased risk for difficult airway
- Recurrent pulmonary infections
- Pleural effusion

Metabolic and Endocrine
- Hyperkalemia
- Metabolic acidosis
- Hyponatremia
- Hypocalcemia
- Hypermagnesemia
- Decreased protein binding of drugs
- Hypoglycemia

Hematologic
- Anemia
- Platelet dysfunction
- Decreased coagulation factors
- Leukocyte dysfunction

Neurologic
- Autonomic neuropathy
- Mental status changes
- Peripheral neuropathy
- Restless legs syndrome
- Seizure disorder

Gastrointestinal
- Delayed gastric emptying
- Increased gastric acidity
- Hepatic venous congestion
- Hepatitis (viral or drug-induced)
- Malnutrition

Neurologic
- Autonomic neuropathy
- Peripheral neuropathy
- Cerebrovascular insufficiency

Frequent monitoring of blood pressure and immediate treatment of hypotension is suggested.[34] Preexisting peripheral neuropathy should be documented before the administration of neuraxial anesthesia.

Local anesthetic systemic toxicity (LAST) after bupivacaine brachial plexus blockade has been reported in patients with chronic renal failure.[35] Whether LAST is related to toxic levels of local anesthetic unique to the patient with renal failure is unclear. Rice et al.[36] found no significant difference in the pharmacokinetic profile of bupivacaine after brachial plexus blockade in a group of patients with uremia compared with patients with normal renal function. There are no published data on the pharmacokinetics of epidurally administered local anesthetic agents in patients with chronic renal failure, but given the low concentration of local anesthetics used in contemporary practice, this is unlikely to be a concern.

Orko et al.[37] administered spinal anesthesia with plain bupivacaine 22.5 mg to 20 nonpregnant patients with chronic renal failure and 20 control patients. Maximal segmental anesthesia occurred more rapidly in the patients with renal disease (21 versus 35 minutes), but the duration was reduced. Further, the extent of sensory blockade was two segments higher in the patients with renal disease. There were no untoward effects in any of the patients. Potential mechanisms proposed for these findings included a difference in blood pH and potassium concentration, as well as the existence of underlying neuropathy increasing susceptibility to blockade. An alternative hypothesis suggested that the hyperdynamic state of uremia causes further distension of epidural veins, hastening onset and decreasing duration through a washout phenomenon.

General Anesthesia

Patients with chronic uremia exhibit delayed gastric emptying and hyperacidity, which may increase the risk for **aspiration pneumonitis**. In addition to sodium citrate, when time allows, the anesthesia provider also should consider administering a histamine-2 (H_2) receptor antagonist and metoclopramide. The doses should not be changed in renal failure.

All the standard induction agents are safe in patients with renal failure. **Etomidate** may have an advantage if the volume status is unknown or if there is severe left ventricular dysfunction. **Propofol** exhibits normal volume of distribution and elimination in patients with renal failure and is also commonly used. Protein binding of propofol is unaffected by renal failure.[38] The serum potassium concentration should be determined before induction of anesthesia. If the potassium concentration is greater than 5.5 mEq/L, dialysis should generally be performed before an elective procedure. **Succinylcholine (suxamethonium)** will cause a 0.5 to 0.7 mEq/L increase in potassium concentration, which is similar to the increase that occurs in patients without renal disease.[39] If the patient is already hyperkalemic, this mild elevation may be sufficient to precipitate cardiac dysrhythmias and another muscle relaxant (e.g., **rocuronium**) should be considered. Plasma cholinesterase concentrations are normal, even after dialysis, and the duration of action of succinylcholine is not prolonged.[40]

Neuromuscular blockade should be maintained with an agent that does not rely on renal elimination. **Cisatracurium** undergoes Hofmann degradation, and therefore the duration of action is not prolonged in patients with renal failure. Hypermagnesemia, commonly found in patients with kidney disease, may potentiate neuromuscular blockade.[41] Although **anticholinesterase agents** undergo renal elimination and have a prolonged duration in patients with renal insufficiency, the volume of distribution remains the same, and standard doses are used for the reversal of neuromuscular blockade. **Sugammadex** has been successfully utilized in patients undergoing cesarean delivery.[42] While it is not recommended for use in patients with end-stage renal disease as both sugammadex and the sugammadex-rocuronium complex are renally excreted and are not removed with standard forms of dialysis,[43] a large case series has documented short-term safety of its use in nonpregnant surgical patients with end-stage renal disease.[44] In this series, none of the 136 patients who received reversal with sugammadex developed symptoms of recurarization. Of note, 24 (18%) of these patients were initially reversed with neostigmine and had signs and symptoms of residual neuromuscular blockade.

Postoperative Analgesia

The principles of postoperative analgesia for the woman with renal disease are the same as for healthy women, with some important considerations because drug clearance can be altered for opioids and their metabolites (see Chapter 27). **Morphine** is generally safe as a single dose, but with longer-term use its active metabolite, morphine-6-glucuronide, may accumulate. **Meperidine (pethidine)** is of particular concern because its active metabolite, normeperidine, is neurotoxic and is renally excreted. **Hydromorphone** and **oxycodone**, and their metabolites hydromorphone-3-glucuronide and α- and β-oxycodol, respectively, are also renally excreted and may accumulate with prolonged use. **Fentanyl** and **sufentanil** are only minimally excreted in the urine, and they may be particularly useful because they are short-acting drugs. **Remifentanil** is metabolized by blood and tissue esterases and is not dependent on the kidney for excretion, making it safe for use in patients with renal failure.[45] The safest approach may be to use **neuraxial opioids** because small doses are administered. Alternative techniques that avoid opioids such as **transversus abdominis plane block** may also be considered, especially when neuraxial opioids are not administered (see Chapter 27). **Nonsteroidal antiinflammatory drugs (NSAIDs)**, although effective, are best avoided as they may worsen renal function and can interact with several renal medications, including loop diuretics.[46]

ACUTE KIDNEY INJURY

Definition and Epidemiology

Acute kidney injury (AKI) is a serious potential complication that can develop in pregnancy. The inciting disorders previously varied throughout the world; however, hypertensive disorders in pregnancy are now the leading cause of pregnancy-related acute kidney injury (PR-AKI) worldwide, followed by hemorrhage and sepsis.[47] Rapid deterioration of renal function leads to an accumulation of fluid and nitrogenous waste products with impaired electrolyte regulation. Definitions for renal dysfunction in the general population vary and have changed over time. What was previously called acute renal failure (ARF) is now included among a greater spectrum of disorders, including varying levels of kidney

dysfunction, and is now termed AKI.[48] Guidelines and recommendations (including definitions) have been maintained by the Kidney Disease: Improving Global Outcomes consortium of the International Society of Nephrologists (Table 50.1).[49] The most recent version of the recommendations are from 2012 and they are in the process of being updated. These definitions and recommendations are based on the RIFLE (risk, injury, failure, loss, and end-stage renal failure) and Acute Kidney Injury Network criteria, which have been applied to the pregnant population because no similar guidance exists for pregnant patients.

During the past five decades, the incidence of PR-AKI has decreased worldwide from 1:3000 to 1:15,000.[50] This progress has resulted from improved obstetric care and fewer septic abortions.[51] Although the overall incidence of PR-AKI is declining worldwide, it has been increasing in incidence in the United States and Canada. Shah et al.[52] reported that the incidence of AKI-related admission during pregnancy increased from 0.04% in 2006 to 0.12% in 2015. Factors associated with the increased hospitalization included older age, Black and Native American race, and diabetes mellitus. They also found that those hospitalized had a higher rate of inpatient mortality and cardiovascular events.

Pathophysiology and Diagnosis

AKI is defined by one of the following criteria: (1) increase in serum creatinine by greater than or equal to 0.3 mg/dL (26.5 μmol/L) within 48 hours, (2) increase in serum creatinine to greater than or equal to 1.5 times baseline within the last 7 days, or (3) urine volume ≤ 0.5 mL/kg/h for 6 hours.[48,53] Once the diagnosis is made, staging the level of severity of

TABLE 50.1 KDIGO Staging of Acute Kidney Injury

Stage	Serum Creatinine	Urine Output
1	1.5–1.9 times baseline or increase in serum creatinine (≥0.3 mg/dL [≥26.5 μmol/L])	<0.5 mL/kg/h for 6–12 h
2	2.0–2.9 times baseline	<0.5 mL/kg/h for greater than or equal to 12 h
3	3 times baseline or increase in serum creatinine (≥4.0 mg/dL [≥353.6 μmol/L]) or initiation of renal replacement therapy, or in patients less than 18 y, decrease in eGFR (<35 mL/min/1.73 m²)	<0.3 mL/kg/h for greater than or equal to 24 h or anuria for greater than or equal to 12 h

eGFR, Estimated glomerular filtration rate; *KDIGO*, Kidney Disease: Improving Global Outcomes.
From Kidney Disease: Improving Global Outcomes. Summary of recommendation statements. *Kidney Int Suppl.* 2012;2:8–12.

BOX 50.2 Causes of Acute Kidney Injury During Pregnancy

Prerenal
- Hyperemesis gravidarum
- Uterine hemorrhage
- Heart failure

Intrarenal
- Acute tubular necrosis
- Septic abortion
- Amniotic fluid embolism
- Drug-induced acute interstitial nephritis
- Acute glomerulonephritis
- Bilateral renal cortical necrosis
- Acute pyelonephritis
- Preeclampsia/eclampsia
- Hemolysis, elevated liver enzymes, and low platelets syndrome
- Acute fatty liver of pregnancy
- Idiopathic postpartum renal failure

Postrenal
- Urolithiasis
- Ureteral obstruction by the gravid uterus

AKI is recommended. This is an important component of management because the risk for death and renal replacement therapy increases significantly with each stage (see Table 50.1).[54] AKI is subdivided according to underlying cause (i.e., prerenal, intrarenal, and postrenal) (Box 50.2). One study examined the kidney injury molecule-1 (KIM-1) as a biomarker for the diagnosis and prediction of AKI complications in pregnancy[55]; the cohort of patients with elevated KIM-1 and endothelin-1 suffered from greater degrees of kidney injury.

Prerenal Causes

The most common prerenal causes of PR-AKI—hyperemesis gravidarum and obstetric hemorrhage—lead to hypovolemia and inadequate renal perfusion.[56,57] Urinary indices show urine osmolality > 500 mOsm/kg, urine sodium < 20 mEq/L, fractional sodium excretion < 1%, and a urine-to-plasma creatinine ratio > 40.[58] Concealed hemorrhage from placental abruption may remain unrecognized until hypotension and renal failure ensue.[59] Women with preeclampsia may be more likely to develop AKI after hemorrhage because of preexisting intravascular contraction and widespread maternal endothelial dysfunction.[2] Women who developed preeclampsia during pregnancy, with or without renal failure, are more likely to develop renal failure and other complications later in life.[60]

Intrarenal Causes

An intrarenal cause is diagnosed once prerenal and postrenal causes of AKI have been excluded. In general, oliguric intrarenal AKI is not easily reversed. Causes include acute tubular necrosis, interstitial nephritis, and acute glomerulonephritis

as well as a few causes usually only seen in pregnancy. The latter include renal cortical necrosis, acute pyelonephritis, severe preeclampsia/eclampsia, acute fatty liver of pregnancy, and idiopathic postpartum renal failure. A thorough history, review of medications, and urinalysis typically help determine the specific initiating factor.[61]

Acute tubular necrosis may result from nephrotoxic drugs, amniotic fluid embolism, rhabdomyolysis, intrauterine fetal death, and prolonged renal ischemia secondary to hemorrhage or septic shock. Urinalysis demonstrates dirty brown epithelial cell casts and coarse granular casts. Urinary indices show urine osmolality < 350 mOsm/kg, urine sodium concentration > 40 mEq/L, fractional sodium excretion > 1%, and a urine-to-plasma creatinine ratio < 20.[62]

Acute interstitial nephritis is caused by NSAIDs and various antibiotics. Patients typically exhibit fever, rash, eosinophilia, and urine eosinophils.

Acute glomerulonephritis is rare during pregnancy. It is suggested by hematuria, red cell casts, and proteinuria. Urinary indices of acute glomerulonephritis are similar to those of prerenal AKI.

Bilateral renal cortical necrosis, which is rarely observed in the nonobstetric patient, is responsible for 10% to 38% of cases of PR-AKI.[63] It may occur during early or late pregnancy. Hemorrhage is the most common precipitating event. The pathogenesis of this disorder is unclear but may involve renal hypoperfusion or endothelial damage by endotoxins imposed on the normal hypercoagulable state of pregnancy.[64] A single dose of endotoxin may precipitate bilateral renal cortical necrosis in pregnant animals and has led some investigators to view this disorder as a clinical analog of the experimental Sanarelli-Shwartzman reaction, in which thrombosis follows two intravenous injections of endotoxin given 24 hours apart.[65] Extensive microthrombi are found within the glomeruli and renal arterioles. Diagnosis is made by selective renal arteriography, which reveals absence or patchiness of blood flow in the cortex. Renal biopsy may also be performed in the absence of active coagulopathy.[66] Tranexamic acid and autoimmune disorders such as the antiphospholipid antibody syndrome have also been implicated; however, the data are limited to case reports.[67,68]

Acute pyelonephritis is one of the most common infectious complications of pregnancy (see Chapter 36). Although acute pyelonephritis rarely leads to AKI in the nongravid patient, it accounts for 5% of cases of PR-AKI, and outcome is worse if the patient is also anemic. The reason for this greater susceptibility is unclear.[69] Whalley et al.[70] noted that acute pyelonephritis causes a marked reduction of GFR in pregnant women. In contrast, pyelonephritis causes little reduction in GFR in nonpregnant patients. The kidney may be more sensitive to bacterial endotoxins during pregnancy.

Preeclampsia with severe features/eclampsia may be responsible for, or contributes to, 40% to 60% of cases of PR-AKI.[2,71] Renal failure is generally associated with severe preeclampsia or **HELLP (hemolysis, elevated liver enzymes, and low platelet count) syndrome**, where the incidence ranges from 3% to 15%.[72] However, many cases of renal dysfunction and failure may only mimic preeclampsia and may actually result from other factors.[2] Other causes of AKI should be considered before preeclampsia is determined to be the cause of renal failure.

Gul et al.[72] analyzed the maternal and fetal outcomes of 132 patients with HELLP syndrome. Despite the high rate of major complications in these patients, even when examining those with the most severe levels of renal failure (creatinine > 2.0 mg/dL [177 μmol/L]), of whom 50% required dialysis, no patient was discharged with renal impairment, and there was no maternal mortality. Perinatal mortality, however, was high (26.1%) when serum creatinine was greater than 1.2 mg/dL (106 μmol/L) and increased to 37.5% when greater than 2.0 mg/dL (177 μmol/L).

Renal histology in a woman with HELLP syndrome and renal failure demonstrated thrombotic microangiopathy and acute tubular necrosis, suggesting a possible pathogenesis of ARI associated with HELLP syndrome.[73] Of interest, Flynn et al.[74] reported the successful use of cadaveric kidneys procured from a parturient who died after HELLP syndrome and AKI. Both recipients had acceptable graft function 2 years after transplantation.

Acute fatty liver of pregnancy, a rare but life-threatening disorder of pregnancy, is associated with a 20% to 100% incidence of AKI.[75] Specific clinical features of acute fatty liver of pregnancy are discussed in Chapter 45.

The syndrome of **idiopathic postpartum renal failure** was initially described in 1968 by Robson et al.[76] Subsequently, approximately 200 cases have been reported. This syndrome is characterized by AKI, microangiopathic hemolytic anemia, and thrombocytopenia occurring 2 days to 10 weeks after an uncomplicated delivery. It appears closely related to the hemolytic-uremic syndrome. Idiopathic postpartum renal failure is typically preceded by a viral upper respiratory tract or gastrointestinal syndrome that rapidly progresses to AKI. The use of ethinyl estradiol as a contraceptive may also be causally related to this syndrome.[77] Spontaneous bleeding, congestive heart failure, hypertension, and seizures have been reported.[78] Some investigators believe that this syndrome represents a clinical analog to the generalized Shwartzman reaction, a condition induced in laboratory animals by two successive injections of endotoxin, which results in factor XII activation, thrombin generation, and fibrin deposition.[79] Others consider the platelet deposition to be the primary event that leads to microvascular thrombi.[78]

Management involves plasma exchange transfusion, dialysis, and antiplatelet therapy. The role of heparin therapy in idiopathic postpartum renal failure is controversial. The morbidity and mortality among affected patients vary by study. Reports from the 1970s and 1980s suggested a mortality rate of approximately 50%.[80] Although survival has improved with prompt diagnosis and aggressive treatment, morbidity is still high. Shrivastava et al.[81] reported three patients who had postpartum hemolytic-uremic syndrome and had initial recovery with immediate exchange transfusion; long-term follow-up was not reported. Dashe et al.[82] reported 10 patients with peripartum or postpartum hemolytic-uremic syndrome

and followed their course for a mean of 9 years. Although all 10 initially survived, one subsequently died and all had major morbidity, including recurrence of renal failure, hypertension, and seizures.

Postrenal Causes

The postrenal causes of PR-AKI include **nephrolithiasis** and ureteral obstruction by the gravid uterus.[83] The latter complication is more likely in pregnant women with polyhydramnios or multiple gestation.[84] Preexisting ureteral dilation and impaired peristalsis increase the risk for obstructive uropathy during pregnancy. Flank pain and decreased urine output during late gestation should alert the clinician to this possibility. Courban et al.[85] reported an unusual case of multiple uterine leiomyomas that caused obstructive uropathy that resulted in PR-AKI.

Effect on the Mother and Fetus

Although maternal prognosis has improved significantly in developed countries, mortality ranges between 20% and 30% in low-income countries, likely because of the lack of availability of renal replacement therapy.[86,87] Although mortality in high-income countries is very low, up to one-third of mothers do not have complete recovery and suffer long-term sequelae from their AKI episode. There is also evidence that women with recovered PR-AKI have increased rates of preeclampsia and other complications in future pregnancies even in cases where prepregnancy serum creatinine is similar.[88] The prognosis for the fetus is worse as well, with significant increases in stillbirth, perinatal death, NICU stay, lower birth weight, lower gestational age at delivery, and higher odds of cesarean delivery.[89]

Medical and Obstetric Management

Management is directed toward rapid recognition of the underlying abnormality. Reversible disorders such as hypovolemia, concealed uterine hemorrhage, urinary tract infection, ureteral obstruction, and drug-induced AKI must be excluded. Urine osmolality (>500 mOsm/kg) is a useful laboratory test to identify reversible prerenal causes. Intravascular volume should be optimized. Electrolyte and acid-base status should be monitored carefully. Hypertension and preeclampsia must be managed aggressively. Many obstetric causes of AKI also may cause disseminated intravascular coagulation; therefore, coagulation abnormalities should be excluded in pregnant women with AKI.[90]

Because urea and other metabolic products cross the placenta, hemodialysis or peritoneal dialysis should be directed toward maintaining the postdialysis BUN concentration ≤ 30 mg/dL (urea 10.7 mmol/L). Fluid shifts during hemodialysis should be minimized by short but frequent periods of dialysis. If the fetus is mature, delivery should be accomplished when the maternal condition is stabilized. The pediatrician must be alerted to the presence of high fetal BUN levels, which may lead to an osmotic diuresis and neonatal dehydration. Ertürk et al.[91] reported the first known delivery of a healthy infant during a hemodialysis session. All

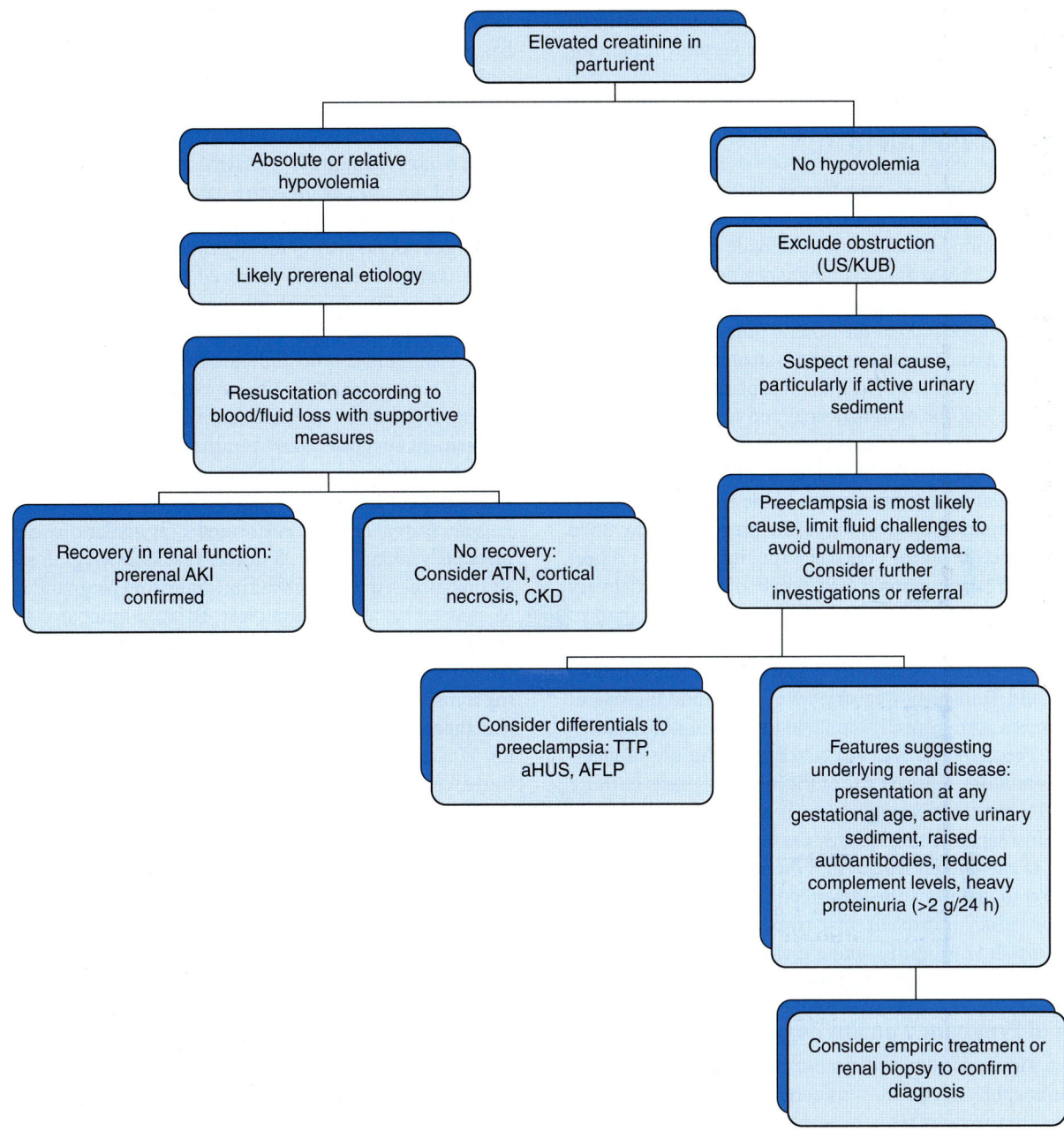

Fig. 50.2 Approach to acute kidney injury in pregnancy. *AFLP*, Acute fatty liver of pregnancy; *aHUS*, atypical hemolytic-uremic syndrome; *AKI*, acute kidney injury; *ATN*, acute tubular necrosis; *CKD*, chronic kidney disease; *KUB*, kidney, ureter, and bladder; *TTP*, thrombotic thrombocytopenic purpura; *US*, ultrasound. Modified from Hall DR, Conti-Ramsden F. Acute kidney injury in pregnancy including renal disease diagnosed in pregnancy. *Best Pract Res Clin Obstet Gynaecol.* 2019;57:47–59.

nephrotoxic drugs should be discontinued and avoided if possible. Renal dosing of medications (e.g., muscle relaxants, antibiotics, magnesium) should be considered in these patients. A flow diagram to aid in the diagnosis and management of suspected AKI is shown in Fig. 50.2[10]

Anesthetic Management

A multidisciplinary approach involving anesthesia providers, obstetric providers, and nephrologists should be employed to optimize the maternal condition before delivery in a woman with AKI. The level of azotemia, electrolyte balance, and hematologic status should be assessed. If the BUN level is greater than 80 mg/dL (urea > 28.6 mmol/L) or if the serum potassium concentration is greater than 5.5 mEq/L, dialysis should be performed before vaginal or cesarean delivery. Neuraxial anesthesia may be administered in the absence of coagulopathy, thrombocytopenia, and severe hypovolemia. Volume status may be difficult to assess, and transthoracic echocardiography may be useful.

Both spinal and epidural analgesia/anesthesia are safe and preferred to general anesthesia. As the sympathetic blockade dissipates, the mother should be monitored for evidence of volume overload and pulmonary edema. General anesthesia may be required for urgent cesarean delivery or in patients with coagulopathy or hemorrhage.

RENAL TRANSPLANTATION

Although pregnancy is uncommon in women undergoing long-term dialysis,[92] fertility is improved within months of transplantation. In a review of female renal transplant patients in the United States, a pregnancy rate of 20 per 1000 was estimated in transplanted patients in the year 2000 compared with 100 per 1000 in the general population.[93]

Although a successful obstetric outcome can be anticipated in more than 95% of kidney transplant recipients, they are at greater risk for both maternal and fetal complications than healthy women. In a systematic review of articles published between 2000 and 2010, Deshpande et al.[94] reported pregnancy-related outcome data in kidney transplant recipients. Fifty studies representing 4706 pregnancies in 3570 recipients met inclusion criteria. The incidences of preeclampsia (27%), gestational diabetes (8%), cesarean delivery (56.9%), and preterm delivery (45.6%) were greater than in the general population. In a study examining 390 postkidney transplant pregnancies from the Australia and New Zealand Dialysis and Transplant Registry, Lu et al.[95] found the rate of preeclampsia rose from 27% in 2000 to 2004 to 48% in 2018 to 2021. Preeclampsia was associated with the use of calcineurin inhibitors, however use of the inhibitor drugs in those with and without preeclampsia was high (97% versus 88%, P = .005). In a separate cohort study examining renal transplant patients in the United Kingdom, potential predictive factors for poorer outcomes were described, including more than one prior kidney transplant, first-trimester serum creatinine > 125 μmol/L (1.4 mg/dL), and a diastolic blood pressure > 90 mm Hg in both the second and third trimesters.[96]

Effect of Pregnancy on the Renal Allograft

When a kidney is removed from a donor and transplanted into an anephric recipient, it undergoes a process of hyperfiltration. In the short term, hyperfiltration attempts to bring the GFR toward the rate of a binephric system. In the long term, this hyperfiltration may lead to glomerular sclerosis and loss of renal function.[97] In normal pregnancy, the GFR increases by 30% to 50% during the first and second trimesters and subsequently decreases somewhat during the third trimester. Theoretically, this additional hyperfiltration of pregnancy predisposes the patient to a loss of renal function.

Baylis and Reckelhoff[98] allayed many of these concerns by demonstrating that gestational hyperfiltration is not associated with increased glomerular pressure because of matching afferent and efferent arteriolar vasodilation. They produced hyperfiltration in rodent kidneys by performing uninephrectomy, maintaining the animals on a high-protein diet and subjecting them to five consecutive pregnancies. The investigators observed no functional impairment or renal histologic changes in this animal model. In addition, they demonstrated that glomerular pressure is lower in female rats than in male

rats 10 months after uninephrectomy.[99] Similar sex advantage has been seen in humans after uninephrectomy.[100]

There have been numerous studies assessing graft function after pregnancy. Most studies suggest that there is no adverse effect provided renal function is normal before conception and there is no evidence of hypertension.[101–103] Levidiotis et al.[101] analyzed 40 years of outcome data from the Australian and New Zealand Dialysis and Transplant Registry and did not find any impact of pregnancy on 20-year graft or patient survival.

Rahamimov et al.[102] compared long-term graft survival, kidney function, and patient survival between women who became pregnant after renal transplantation (n = 39; 55 births) and those who did not (n = 117). Each pregnant woman was matched with three nonpregnant women for 12 factors that may affect graft survival. Graft survival (61.6%) and patient survival (84.8%) in the pregnant women did not differ from the matched nonpregnant group (68.7% graft and 78.8% patient survival) during the 15-year follow-up study.

Van Buren et al.[103] performed a systematic review and metaanalysis and found 38 studies that assessed graft loss, and 18 that assessed serum creatinine following pregnancy. Of the 38 studies that assessed graft loss, 10 had a nulliparous control group; there was no difference in graft survival between the two groups. Serum creatinine was followed for 10 years following transplantation and only in the first 2 years after pregnancy was there a slight increase in serum creatinine of 0.18 (95% CI, 0.05 to 0.32) mg/dL [16.4 (95% CI, 4.4 to 28.3) μmol/L] in those who were pregnant versus those who were not.

Effect on the Fetus

Although pregnancy seems to have minimal effect on maternal health or allograft survival in renal transplant recipients, fetal outcome is less favorable. In a Norwegian cohort study, the adjusted incidence rate ratio of patients with preterm delivery was 4.45 (95% CI, 2.13 to 9.30).[104] Likewise, the incidence of delivering an infant below the 10th percentile in birth weight was double that of the control cohort, and the risk for stillbirth or perinatal death within the first 24 hours was 10-fold greater. Despite the increases in relative risk, absolute outcomes are reassuring. For example, in a large systematic review, Deshpande et al.[94] found a 73.5% live birth rate in renal transplant patients (study publication years 2000 to 2011). In the study by Lu et al.,[95] the live birth rate was 97% (data from 2000 to 2021).

Most posttransplantation protocols consist of a primary immunosuppressant (**cyclosporine** or **tacrolimus**) and one or two adjunctive agents (**azathioprine**, **mycophenolate mofetil**, **sirolimus**, and/or **corticosteroids**).[105] All of the immunosuppressant agent appear to be nonteratogenic[106,107] except mycophenolate mofetil (see Chapter 16). Anderka et al.[108] reported on malformations in 14 offspring exposed to mycophenolate mofetil. Malformations included microtia, anotia, and cardiovascular malformations. A different immunosuppressive agent should be considered and increased fetal surveillance is needed if it is used. A thorough review of immunosuppressive drugs and their impact on pregnancy and fetal well-being after kidney transplantation is beyond the scope of this chapter, but were reviewed by Chandra et al.[109]

Intrauterine exposure to cyclosporine impairs development and function of T, B, and NK lymphocytes in neonates. This effect, as well as depressed levels of serum immunoglobulin, persists during the first year of life.[110] These factors place the infant at risk for a suboptimal immunologic response after administration of classic vaccines and for adverse effects after administration of live, attenuated vaccines.

Transplant recipients may become infected with **cytomegalovirus (CMV)** at the time of transplantation, or they may experience reactivation secondary to immunosuppression. Active CMV infection during pregnancy is associated with congenital anomalies (e.g., cerebral cysts, microcephaly, mental retardation). In addition, active neonatal CMV infection may lead to serious illness or death.

After renal transplantation, residual impairment of renal function may lead to false-positive results of biochemical screening for **trisomy 21**. Karidas et al.[111] demonstrated a significant correlation between free β-subunit human chorionic gonadotropin and BUN and creatinine concentrations. Similar alterations in alpha-fetoprotein levels were not observed. In this setting, the double-marker biochemical test may be interpreted inaccurately. In patients with altered BUN and creatinine concentrations, first-trimester nuchal translucency measurement—in combination with second-trimester ultrasonography—may be a more useful screening regimen (see Chapter 6).

Medical and Obstetric Management

Discontinuation of immunosuppressant therapy, even years after transplantation, may lead to acute rejection. Thus, the renal transplant recipient's immunosuppressant regimen must be continued during pregnancy unless toxicity results, although some practitioners discontinue mycophenolate mofetil if an alternative is available. Cyclosporine requirements increase during pregnancy, most likely because of enhanced metabolism.[112] The pregnant patient must be intensively monitored for any evidence of acute or chronic allograft rejection, infection, ureteral and renal artery obstruction, impaired renal function, hypertension, fluid volume disturbances, anemia, or any combination of these symptoms. Recombinant human erythropoietin (darbepoetin) has been successfully used to treat anemia during pregnancy (see earlier discussion). There are reports of ESA use in the post-transplant patient as well, although the degree of success and dosage regimens are highly variable.[113,114]

Initial laboratory studies in pregnant renal transplant patients include (1) complete blood cell count, (2) renal function tests, (3) serum electrolyte and glucose concentrations, and (4) viral serologic testing for CMV, hepatitis B virus, HCV, and HIV. Serial ultrasonographic assessments allow the recognition of fetal anomalies and the evaluation of fetal growth.

Cultures of the lower genital tract should be obtained in women with lesions suggestive of herpes simplex virus infection. A patient who presents in labor and with evidence of active genital herpes simplex virus infection should undergo cesarean delivery (see Chapter 36).

Vaginal examinations are minimized and always performed in a strict aseptic manner. The renal allograft is typically implanted in the extraperitoneal iliac fossa and does not impair vaginal delivery. Prophylactic antibiotics and stress-dose corticosteroids are indicated in patients who undergo cesarean delivery.

Anesthetic Management

In the absence of renal dysfunction and hypertension, anesthetic management of the parturient with a renal transplant is similar to that of the healthy parturient. Strict aseptic technique is maintained during the placement of intravascular catheters and the performance of neuraxial anesthetic techniques. In the absence of systemic infection, immunosuppression itself should not be considered a contraindication to administration of epidural or spinal anesthesia.

UROLITHIASIS

Definition and Epidemiology

Urolithiasis is characterized by the abnormal formation of calculi within the renal calyces or pelvis. Symptomatic urolithiasis occurs in 1:200 to 1:2000 pregnancies, which is no different from that in the nonpregnant population.[115,116] It is more common among White than African American women, and more common in parous women in the second and third trimesters.[116]

Pathophysiology

The presence of urolithiasis presumes an underlying physiologic abnormality that leads to persistent supersaturation of the minerals involved. During pregnancy, an elevated plasma 1,25-dihydroxyvitamin D level causes greater intestinal absorption of calcium, net mobilization of calcium from bone, and a state of absorptive hypercalciuria.[117] Ultimately, these changes provide calcium for the fetal skeleton. Because pregnant women do not develop urolithiasis at a rate greater than those in the general population, it appears that the occurrence of other physiologic changes during pregnancy offsets these factors that might promote the formation of stones. Calcium stone inhibitors such as citrate, magnesium, and glycoprotein are excreted in the urine to a greater extent during pregnancy.[118] As expected, calcium stones account for the majority of stones in both the general population (80%) as well as in pregnancy (74%). However, whereas calcium oxalate stones are more prominent in the general population, calcium phosphate stones are more common in pregnancy.[119] This difference is thought to be caused by both the renal physiologic changes of pregnancy as well as a higher pH of urine during pregnancy.

Diagnosis

As mentioned earlier, urolithiasis most commonly manifests during the second or third trimester. Only 20% of affected pregnant women recount a prior history of renal calculi. More than 80% of cases of gestational urolithiasis are diagnosed in parous women, possibly reflecting the higher incidence of this disease with advanced age.[120] Similar to that seen in nonpregnant women, stones occur with equal frequency on the right and left sides.[121] The signs and symptoms of urolithiasis during pregnancy are often nonspecific and may include flank pain, hematuria, nausea, vomiting, and fever; these symptoms must be differentiated from those occurring from ectopic pregnancy, preterm labor, appendicitis, pyelonephritis, and benign hematuria of pregnancy. A history of previous urolithiasis, recurrent urinary tract infections, or urologic surgery is suggestive. Examination may reveal costovertebral tenderness, abdominal tenderness, pyuria, and hematuria. Urolithiasis must be considered in patients with pyelonephritis who remain febrile or have continued bacteriuria despite 48 hours of parenteral antibiotics.

The initial imaging modality for the evaluation of urolithiasis during pregnancy is **transabdominal ultrasonography**, as it is often readily available and confers no ionizing radiation. Transabdominal ultrasonography is limited by its diagnostic capabilities and is very operator dependent. Burgess et al.[122] found that transabdominal ultrasonography has a sensitivity of about 54% and specificity of 78.6%.

If the ultrasonography is nondiagnostic, there is debate over which modality should be used next. Traditionally, 1.5 T (not 3 T) **magnetic resonance imaging (MRI)** has been recommended by both the American Urological Association (AUA) and the European Association of Urology (EUA).[123,124] Although there is a theoretical risk of teratogenicity because of deposition of energy in the body in the form of heat which occurs during MRI, it has not been demonstrated in several long-term studies using 1.5 T magnets.[125,126] The use of gadolinium contrast should be limited and only used if it significantly improves diagnostic performance and is expected to improve fetal or maternal outcome.[127] Several pregnancy-specific imaging protocols have been developed but the best imaging protocol for urolithiasis appears to be half-Fourier single-shot turbo-spin echo magnetic resonance urography with a diagnostic accuracy of up to 89%.[128]

Computed tomography (CT), the gold standard for detection of nephrolithiasis, has been avoided in pregnancy owing to fears of ionizing radiation delivery to the fetus. **Low-dose computed tomography (LDCT)**, however, can accomplish noninferior diagnostic accuracy compared with traditional CT.[122] The risk of fetal abnormalities is negligible at levels < 50 mSv and the dose of radiation from LDCT, depending on the protocol, can be as low as 0.65 mSv.[127,129] Head-to-head trials between modalities are lacking; however, current evidence suggests that LDCT has a higher positive predictive value compared with MR and ultrasonography, has the lowest incidence of negative ureteroscopy, and provides the best information to clinicians regarding surgical planning; therefore, it should be considered if the other modalities are inconclusive.[127,129]

Effect of Pregnancy on Urolithiasis

In an effort to determine any effect of pregnancy on the natural history of urolithiasis, Coe et al.[130] reviewed the records of 58 pregnancies in women with a preexisting diagnosis of urolithiasis. The stone recurrence rate in this group was 0.49 stones per patient-year, which was not significantly different from the rate of 0.44 stones per patient-year in the general population. The authors concluded that pregnancy does not alter the activity or severity of stone disease.

Effect on the Mother and Fetus

In a 2021 systematic review and metaanalysis of eight studies comprising 26,577 mothers with urolithiasis, Zhou et al.[131] demonstrated an association of urolithiasis with preterm birth or very preterm birth risk, preeclampsia, hypertension, cesarean delivery, and gestational diabetes mellitus. Urolithiasis was not associated with low birth weight, premature rupture of membranes, or infant death. The etiology of preterm labor and perhaps delivery is unclear but may be related to urinary tract infections that occur with a greater frequency in those with urolithiasis, increased nausea and vomiting resulting in prostaglandin production, or the presence of subclinical renal disease.[132,133] Honoré[134] suggested that there is a higher incidence of renal stones among women who have a spontaneous abortion. He hypothesized that abnormalities of calcium hemostasis may lead to myometrial hyperirritability or abnormal hormonal secretion by the corpus luteum, the placenta, or both. Rare cases of ureteral rupture[135] and obstructed labor caused by a bladder calculus[136] have been reported.

Urologic and Obstetric Management

Women with a history of urolithiasis should increase their intake of fluids. Calcium supplementation through prenatal vitamins should be avoided in women with recurrent urolithiasis. Between 70% and 90% of stones pass spontaneously; however, this is very dependent on stone size as well as the patient population selected in the study.[124] Initial management steps for expectant management include hydration, antiemetics, and appropriate analgesia with **acetaminophen (paracetamol)** and, if needed, **opioids**. Infected hydronephrosis, especially with impaired renal function or urosepsis, is an indication for more aggressive therapy. Up to 17% of women with nephrolithiasis have concomitant pyelonephritis, but the true progression rate from obstruction to infection is unclear.[137]

Medical management, commonly used for treatment of urolithiasis,[116,138] is limited during pregnancy by fetal concerns. Medical expulsive therapy with **alpha-adrenergic receptor blocking agents** has been used successfully to increase the rate of stone passage and decrease pain associated with expulsion by relaxing ureteral smooth muscle.[139] There are no randomized studies examining safety or efficacy in the pregnant population; however, a retrospective study of 207 pregnant women with renal colic showed no significant difference in spontaneous stone passage rate between 69 patients receiving **tamsulosin** and 138 controls (79% versus 75%, respectively), despite similar stone sizes and locations.[140] Additionally, there were no differences between groups in mean gestational age, birth weight, Apgar scores, length of hospital stay, or need for intervention. Other medical treatments that are used to treat urolithiasis, including **thiazide diuretics, xanthine oxidase inhibitors, and D-penicillamine**, are contraindicated during pregnancy owing to possible effects on the fetus.

Urologic intervention is indicated in the patient with persistent pyelonephritis, deterioration of renal function, massive hydronephrosis, persistent pain, or sepsis. **Ureteral stent placement** with ureteroscopy and ultrasonographic guidance, or percutaneous nephrostomy, should be considered because either can be performed without the need for anesthesia or radiation exposure. However, as many as 45% to 80% of women will require manipulation or exchange of tubes for occlusion or dislodgement.[141] **Holmium:yttrium-aluminum-garnet laser lithotripsy**, using state-of-the-art ureteroscopes, is an emerging technique for stone management in pregnancy.[142] Extracorporeal shockwave lithotripsy should be avoided during pregnancy because the shockwaves may be harmful to the fetus.[143] Given the commonness of stent migration and encrustation, as well as the need for multiple procedures for nephrostomy, current AUA guidelines state that ureteroscopy should be offered to patients who fail observation/trial of passage, and the EUA guidelines report the ureteroscopy is a reasonable alternative to stents and percutaneous nephrostomy.[124,144]

The following conditions may raise suspicion of the presence of **primary hyperparathyroidism** in a pregnant woman: (1) urolithiasis with or without pancreatitis, (2) hyperemesis beyond the first trimester, (3) a history of recurrent spontaneous abortion or intrauterine fetal death, (4) neonatal hypocalcemia or tetany, and (5) a total serum calcium concentration > 10.1 mg/dL (2.5 mmol/L) during the second trimester or > 8.8 mg/dL (2.2 mmol/L) during the third trimester.[145]

Anesthetic Management

Anesthesia providers are occasionally asked to provide analgesia for patients with renal or ureteral stones. The ureters receive sensory innervation through the renal, ovarian, and hypogastric plexuses (T11-L1 spinal segments). During conservative management of urolithiasis, **epidural analgesia** provides the patient with effective pain relief and facilitates the passage of the calculus, possibly through decreased ureteral spasm. Ready and Johnson[146] reported the use of epidural analgesia in a patient with severe renal colic at 23 weeks' gestation. Analgesia maintained for 16 hours allowed the passage of the stone. Neuraxial analgesia avoids the use of systemic opioids, which impair normal peristalsis in ureteric smooth muscle. Improved maternal pain control may also decrease endogenous catecholamine release and improve uteroplacental blood flow.

KEY POINTS

- Pregnant women with moderate or severe renal insufficiency are at increased risk for deterioration of renal function, exacerbation of hypertension, and other obstetric complications, including fetal growth restriction and preterm delivery.
- Patients requiring renal dialysis have decreased fertility and pregnancy is rare.
- Pregnancy does not affect the long-term survival of a renal allograft.
- Both preeclampsia and renal disease may manifest as hypertension, proteinuria, and edema; the distinction between the two disorders is often unclear, especially after 20 weeks' gestation.
- Renal disease affects almost every organ system, therefore a thorough history before initiation of anesthesia, with an emphasis on the cardiac and respiratory system, is critical.

- Anesthetic management is influenced by the extent of renal dysfunction and hypertension.
- Neuraxial anesthetic techniques are safe and are the preferred methods for labor analgesia and anesthesia for cesarean delivery.
- Renal transplantation improves fertility rates within a few months of transplantation. Immunosuppressive therapy must be continued during pregnancy in renal transplant patients. The anesthesia provider should maintain a strict aseptic technique during the placement of intravascular catheters and the performance of neuraxial anesthetic techniques.
- Epidural analgesia may facilitate the spontaneous passage of renal calculi.

REFERENCES

1. Pregnancy and renal disease. *Lancet*. 1975;2:801–802.
2. Al Khalaf S, Bodunde E, Maher GM, et al. Chronic kidney disease and adverse pregnancy outcomes: a systematic review and meta-analysis. *Am J Obstet Gynecol*. 2022;226: 656–670.e32.
3. Jeyabalan A, Lain KY. Anatomic and functional changes of the upper urinary tract during pregnancy. *Urol Clin North Am*. 2007;34:1–6.
4. Reynolds ML, Herrera CA. Chronic kidney disease and pregnancy. *Adv Chronic Kidney Dis*. 2020;27:461–468.
5. Levey AS, Coresh J. Chronic kidney disease. *Lancet*. 2012;379:165–180.
6. Levey AS, Eckardt KU, Tsukamoto Y, et al. Definition and classification of chronic kidney disease: a position statement from Kidney Disease: Improving Global Outcomes (KDIGO). *Kidney Int*. 2005;67:2089–2100.
7. Wiles K, Bramham K, Seed PT, et al. Serum creatinine in pregnancy: a systematic review. *Kidney Int Rep*. 2019;4:408–419.

8. Williams D, Davison J. Chronic kidney disease in pregnancy. *BMJ.* 2008;336:211–215.

9. Rolfo A, Attini R, Nuzzo AM, et al. Chronic kidney disease may be differentially diagnosed from preeclampsia by serum biomarkers. *Kidney Int.* 2013;83:177–181.

10. Hall DR, Conti-Ramsden F. Acute kidney injury in pregnancy including renal disease diagnosed in pregnancy. *Best Pract Res Clin Obstet Gynaecol.* 2019;57:47–59.

11. Piccoli GB, Daidola G, Attini R, et al. Kidney biopsy in pregnancy: evidence for counselling? A systematic narrative review. *BJOG.* 2013;120:412–427.

12. Hladunewich MA, Bramham K, Jim B, Maynard S. Managing glomerular disease in pregnancy. *Nephrol Dial Transplant.* 2017;32:i48–i56.

13. van de Logt AE, Fresquet M, Wetzels JF, Brenchley P. The anti-PLA2R antibody in membranous nephropathy: what we know and what remains a decade after its discovery. *Kidney Int.* 2019;96:1292–1302.

14. Jungers P, Houillier P, Forget D, et al. Influence of pregnancy on the course of primary chronic glomerulonephritis. *Lancet.* 1995;346:1122–1124.

15. Limardo M, Imbasciati E, Ravani P, et al. Pregnancy and progression of IgA nephropathy: results of an Italian multicenter study. *Am J Kidney Dis.* 2010;56:506–512.

16. Jones DC, Hayslett JP. Outcome of pregnancy in women with moderate or severe renal insufficiency. *N Engl J Med.* 1996;335:226–232.

17. Purdy LP, Hantsch CE, Molitch ME, et al. Effect of pregnancy on renal function in patients with moderate-to-severe diabetic renal insufficiency. *Diabetes Care.* 1996;19:1067–1074.

18. Epstein FH. Pregnancy and renal disease. *N Engl J Med.* 1996;335:277–278.

19. Baylis C. Glomerular filtration rate in normal and abnormal pregnancies. *Semin Nephrol.* 1999;19:133–139.

20. American College of Obstetricians and Gynecologists. Practice Bulletin No. 203: Chronic hypertension in pregnancy (reaffirmed 2024). *Obstet Gynecol.* 2019;133:e26–e50.

21. Morton A, Burke M, Morton A, Kumar S. Anaemia in chronic kidney disease pregnancy. *Obstet Med.* 2021;14:116–120.

22. Chakhtoura Z, Meunier M, Caby J, et al. Gynecologic follow up of 129 women on dialysis and after kidney transplantation: a retrospective cohort study. *Eur J Obstet Gynecol Reprod Biol.* 2015;187:1–5.

23. Lim VS. Reproductive function in patients with renal insufficiency. *Am J Kidney Dis.* 1987;9:363–367.

24. Oliverio AL, Hladunewich MA. End-stage kidney disease and dialysis in pregnancy. *Adv Chronic Kidney Dis.* 2020;27:477–485.

25. Krakow D, Castro LC, Schwieger J. Effect of hemodialysis on uterine and umbilical artery Doppler flow velocity waveforms. *Am J Obstet Gynecol.* 1994;170:1386–1388.

26. Malone FD, Craigo SD, Giatras I, et al. Suggested ultrasound parameters for the assessment of fetal well-being during chronic hemodialysis. *Ultrasound Obstet Gynecol.* 1998;11:450–452.

27. Piccoli GB, Minelli F, Versino E, et al. Pregnancy in dialysis patients in the new millennium: a systematic review and meta-regression analysis correlating dialysis schedules and pregnancy outcomes. *Nephrol Dial Transplant.* 2016;31:1915–1934.

28. Reddy SS, Holley JL. Management of the pregnant chronic dialysis patient. *Adv Chronic Kidney Dis.* 2007;14:146–155.

29. Wiles K, Chappell L, Clark K, et al. Clinical practice guideline on pregnancy and renal disease. *BMC Nephrol.* 2019;20:401.

30. Piccoli GB, Cabiddu G, Daidone G, et al. The children of dialysis: live-born babies from on-dialysis mothers in Italy—an epidemiological perspective comparing dialysis, kidney transplantation and the overall population. *Nephrol Dial Transplant.* 2014;29:1578–1586.

31. Hu TH, Su WW, Yang CC, et al. Elimination of hepatitis C virus in a dialysis population: a collaborative care model in Taiwan. *Am J Kidney Dis.* 2021;78:511–519.e1.

32. Kaw D, Malhotra D. Platelet dysfunction and end-stage renal disease. *Semin Dial.* 2006;19:317–322.

33. Rout CC, Akoojee SS, Rocke DA, Gouws E. Rapid administration of crystalloid preload does not decrease the incidence of hypotension after spinal anaesthesia for elective caesarean section. *Br J Anaesth.* 1992;68:394–397.

34. Tighe KE, Smith ID, Bogod DG. Caesarean section in chronic renal failure. *Eur J Anaesthesiol.* 1995;12:185–187.

35. Lucas LF, Tsueda K. Cardiovascular depression after brachial plexus block in two diabetic patients with renal failure. *Anesthesiology.* 1990;73:1032–1035.

36. Rice AS, Pither CE, Tucker GT. Plasma concentrations of bupivacaine after supraclavicular brachial plexus blockade in patients with chronic renal failure. *Anaesthesia.* 1991;46:354–357.

37. Orko R, Pitkänen M, Rosenberg PH. Subarachnoid anaesthesia with 0.75% bupivacaine in patients with chronic renal failure. *Br J Anaesth.* 1986;58:605–609.

38. Costela JL, Jiménez R, Calvo R, et al. Serum protein binding of propofol in patients with renal failure or hepatic cirrhosis. *Acta Anaesthesiol Scand.* 1996;40:741–745.

39. Miller RD, Way WL, Hamilton WK, Layzer RB. Succinylcholine-induced hyperkalemia in patients with renal failure? *Anesthesiology.* 1972;36:138–141.

40. Ryan DW. Preoperative serum cholinesterase concentration in chronic renal failure: clinical experience of suxamethonium in 81 patients undergoing renal transplant. *Br J Anaesth.* 1977;49:945–949.

41. Ghoneim MM, Long JP. The interaction between magnesium and other neuromuscular blocking agents. *Anesthesiology.* 1970;32:23–27.

42. Stourac P, Adamus M, Seidlova D, et al. Low-dose or high-dose rocuronium reversed with neostigmine or sugammadex for cesarean delivery anesthesia: a randomized controlled noninferiority trial of time to tracheal intubation and extubation. *Anesth Analg.* 2016;122:1536–1545.

43. Cammu G, Van Vlem B, van den Heuvel M, et al. Dialysability of sugammadex and its complex with rocuronium in intensive care patients with severe renal impairment. *Br J Anaesth.* 2012;109:382–390.

44. Adams DR, Tollinche LE, Yeoh CB, et al. Short-term safety and effectiveness of sugammadex for surgical patients with end-stage renal disease: a two-centre retrospective study. *Anaesthesia.* 2020;75:348–352.

45. Niscola P, Scaramucci L, Vischini G, et al. The use of major analgesics in patients with renal dysfunction. *Curr Drug Targets.* 2010;11:752–758.

46. Heleniak Z, Cieplińska M, Szychliński T, et al. Nonsteroidal anti-inflammatory drug use in patients with chronic kidney disease. *J Nephrol.* 2017;30:781–786.

47. Davidson B, Bajpai D, Shah S, et al. Pregnancy-associated acute kidney injury in low-resource settings: progress over the last decade. *Semin Nephrol.* 2022;42:151317.

48. Khwaja A. KDIGO clinical practice guidelines for acute kidney injury. *Nephron Clin Pract.* 2012;120:179–184.

49. Kidney Disease: Improving Global Outcomes (KDIGO) consortium of the International Society of Nephrologists. https://kdigo.org/. Accessed September 22, 2023.

50. van Hook JW. Acute kidney injury during pregnancy. *Clin Obstet Gynecol.* 2014;57:851–861.

51. Nwoko R, Plecas D, Garovic VD. Acute kidney injury in the pregnant patient. *Clin Nephrol.* 2012;78:478–486.

52. Shah S, Meganathan K, Christianson AL, et al. Pregnancy-related acute kidney injury in the United States: clinical outcomes and health care utilization. *Am J Nephrol.* 2020;51:216–226.

53. Mehta RL, Kellum JA, Shah SV, et al. Acute kidney injury network: report of an initiative to improve outcomes in acute kidney injury. *Crit Care.* 2007;11:R31.

54. Thakar CV, Christianson A, Freyberg R, et al. Incidence and outcomes of acute kidney injury in intensive care units: a Veterans Administration study. *Crit Care Med.* 2009;37: 2552–2558.

55. Zhou Y, Fan W, Dong J, et al. Establishment of a model to predict the prognosis of pregnancy-related acute kidney injury. *Minerva Urol Nefrol.* 2018;70:437–443.

56. Hill JB, Yost NP, Wendel GD Jr. Acute renal failure in association with severe hyperemesis gravidarum. *Obstet Gynecol.* 2002;100:1119–1121.

57. Hassan I, Junejo AM, Dawani ML. Etiology and outcome of acute renal failure in pregnancy. *J Coll Physicians Surg Pak.* 2009;19:714–717.

58. Albright RC Jr. Acute renal failure: a practical update. *Mayo Clin Proc.* 2001;76:67–74.

59. Krane NK. Acute renal failure in pregnancy. *Arch Intern Med.* 1988;148:2347–2357.

60. Reddy S, Jim B. Hypertension and pregnancy: management and future risks. *Adv Chronic Kidney Dis.* 2019;26:137–145.

61. Cavanaugh C, Perazella MA. Urine sediment examination in the diagnosis and management of kidney disease: core curriculum 2019. *Am J Kidney Dis.* 2019;73:258–272.

62. Kanbay M, Kasapoglu B, Perazella MA. Acute tubular necrosis and pre-renal acute kidney injury: utility of urine microscopy in their evaluation—a systematic review. *Int Urol Nephrol.* 2010;42:425–433.

63. Nwoko R, Plecas D, Garovic VD. Acute kidney injury in the pregnant patient. *Clin Nephrol.* 2012;78:478–486.

64. Khan RZ, Badr KF. Endotoxin and renal function: perspectives to the understanding of septic acute renal failure and toxic shock. *Nephrol Dial Transplant.* 1999;14:814–818.

65. Chahin AB, Opal JM, Opal SM. Whatever happened to the Shwartzman phenomenon? *Innate Immun.* 2018;24:466–479.

66. Kuller JA, D'Andrea NM, McMahon MJ. Renal biopsy and pregnancy. *Am J Obstet Gynecol.* 2001;184:1093–1096.

67. Ko DH, Kim TH, Kim JW, et al. Tranexamic acid-induced acute renal cortical necrosis in post-endoscopic papillectomy bleeding. *Clin Endosc.* 2017;50:609–613.

68. Vellanki VS, Parvathina S, Gondi S, et al. Post-partum bilateral renal cortical necrosis in antiphospholipid syndrome and systemic lupus erythematosus. *Saudi J Kidney Dis Transpl.* 2013;24:549–552.

69. Cunningham HM, Knochenhauer HE, Federspiel JJ, et al. Associations between anemia and outcomes of pregnant patients with pyelonephritis. *Am J Perinatol.* 2024;41(suppl 1): e2403–e2409.

70. Whalley PJ, Cunningham FG, Martin FG. Transient renal dysfunction associated with acute pyelonephritis of pregnancy. *Obstet Gynecol.* 1975;46:174–177.

71. Drakeley AJ, Le Roux PA, Anthony J, Penny J. Acute renal failure complicating severe preeclampsia requiring admission to an obstetric intensive care unit. *Am J Obstet Gynecol.* 2002;186:253–256.

72. Gul A, Aslan H, Cebeci A, et al. Maternal and fetal outcomes in HELLP syndrome complicated with acute renal failure. *Ren Fail.* 2004;26:557–562.

73. Abraham KA, Kennelly M, Dorman AM, Walshe JJ. Pathogenesis of acute renal failure associated with the HELLP syndrome: a case report and review of the literature. *Eur J Obstet Gynecol Reprod Biol.* 2003;108:99–102.

74. Flynn MF, Power RE, Murphy DM, et al. Successful transplantation of kidneys from a donor with HELLP syndrome-related death. *Transpl Int.* 2001;14:108–110.

75. Taber-Hight E, Shah S. Acute kidney injury in pregnancy. *Adv Chronic Kidney Dis.* 2020;27:455–460.

76. Robson JS, Martin AM, Ruckley V, Macdonald MK. Irreversible post-partum renal failure: a new syndrome. *Q J Med.* 1968;37:423–435.

77. Hayslett JP. Current concepts. Postpartum renal failure. *N Engl J Med.* 1985;312:1556–1559.

78. Sun NC, Johnson WJ, Sung DT, Woods JE. Idiopathic postpartum renal failure: review and case report of a successful renal transplantation. *Mayo Clin Proc.* 1975;50:395–401.

79. Grünfeld JP, Pertuiset N. Acute renal failure in pregnancy. *Adv Exp Med Biol.* 1987;212:245–250.

80. Li PK, Lai FM, Tam JS, Lai KN. Acute renal failure due to postpartum haemolytic uraemic syndrome. *Aust N Z J Obstet Gynaecol.* 1988;28:228–230.

81. Shrivastava M, Modi G, Singh RK, Navaid S. Early diagnosis and management of postpartum hemolytic uremic syndrome with plasma exchange. *Transfus Apher Sci.* 2011;44:257–262.

82. Dashe JS, Ramin SM, Cunningham FG. The long-term consequences of thrombotic microangiopathy (thrombotic thrombocytopenic purpura and hemolytic uremic syndrome) in pregnancy. *Obstet Gynecol.* 1998;91:662–668.

83. Khanna N, Nguyen H. Reversible acute renal failure in association with bilateral ureteral obstruction and hydronephrosis in pregnancy. *Am J Obstet Gynecol.* 2001;184:239–240.

84. Brandes JC, Fritsche C. Obstructive acute renal failure by a gravid uterus: a case report and review. *Am J Kidney Dis.* 1991;18:398–401.

85. Courban D, Blank S, Harris MA, et al. Acute renal failure in the first trimester resulting from uterine leiomyomas. *Am J Obstet Gynecol.* 1997;177:472–473.

86. Bentata Y, Housni B, Mimouni A, et al. Acute kidney injury related to pregnancy in developing countries: etiology and risk factors in an intensive care unit. *J Nephrol.* 2012;25: 764–775.

87. Prakash J, Niwas SS, Parekh A, et al. Acute kidney injury in late pregnancy in developing countries. *Ren Fail.* 2010;32:309–313.

88. Tangren JS, Powe CE, Ankers E, et al. Pregnancy outcomes after clinical recovery from AKI. *J Am Soc Nephrol.* 2017;28:1566–1574.

89. Liu Y, Ma X, Zheng J, et al. Pregnancy outcomes in patients with acute kidney injury during pregnancy: a systematic review and meta-analysis. *BMC Pregnancy Childbirth.* 2017;17:235.

90. Szczepanski J, Griffin A, Novotny S, Wallace K. Acute kidney injury in pregnancies complicated with preeclampsia or HELLP syndrome. *Front Med (Lausanne).* 2020;7:22.

91. Ertürk S, Akar H, Uçkuyu A, et al. Delivery of healthy infant during hemodialysis session. *J Nephrol.* 2000;13:75–77.

92. Toma H, Tanabe K, Tokumoto T, et al. Pregnancy in women receiving renal dialysis or transplantation in Japan: a nationwide survey. *Nephrol Dial Transplant.* 1999;14:1511–1516.

93. Gill JS, Zalunardo N, Rose C, Tonelli M. The pregnancy rate and live birth rate in kidney transplant recipients. *Am J Transplant.* 2009;9:1541–1549.

94. Deshpande NA, James NT, Kucirka LM, et al. Pregnancy outcomes in kidney transplant recipients: a systematic review and meta-analysis. *Am J Transplant.* 2011;11:2388–2404.

95. Lu J, Hewawasam E, Davies CE, et al. Pre-eclampsia after kidney transplantation: rates and association with graft survival and function. *Clin J Am Soc Nephrol.* 2023;18:920–929.

96. Bramham K, Nelson-Piercy C, Gao H, et al. Pregnancy in renal transplant recipients: a UK national cohort study. *Clin J Am Soc Nephrol.* 2013;8:290–298.

97. Terasaki PI, Koyama H, Cecka JM, Gjertson DW. The hyperfiltration hypothesis in human renal transplantation. *Transplantation.* 1994;57:1450–1454.

98. Baylis C, Reckelhoff JF. Renal hemodynamics in normal and hypertensive pregnancy: lessons from micropuncture. *Am J Kidney Dis.* 1991;17:98–104.

99. Baylis C, Wilson CB. Sex and the single kidney. *Am J Kidney Dis.* 1989;13:290–298.

100. Goldfarb DA, Matin SF, Braun WE, et al. Renal outcome 25 years after donor nephrectomy. *J Urol.* 2001;166:2043–2047.

101. Levidiotis V, Chang S, McDonald S. Pregnancy and maternal outcomes among kidney transplant recipients. *J Am Soc Nephrol.* 2009;20:2433–2440.

102. Rahamimov R, Ben-Haroush A, Wittenberg C, et al. Pregnancy in renal transplant recipients: long-term effect on patient and graft survival. A single center experience. *Transplantation.* 2006;81:660–664.

103. van Buren MC, Schellekens A, Groenhof TKJ, et al. Long-term graft survival and graft function following pregnancy in kidney transplant recipients: a systematic review and meta-analysis. *Transplantation.* 2020;104:1675–1685.

104. Majak GB, Sandven I, Lorentzen B, et al. Pregnancy outcomes following maternal kidney transplantation: a national cohort study. *Acta Obstet Gynecol Scand.* 2016;95:1153–1161.

105. Gaston RS. Maintenance immunosuppression in the renal transplant recipient: an overview. *Am J Kidney Dis.* 2001;38:S25–S35.

106. Bar J, Stahl B, Hod M, et al. Is immunosuppression therapy in renal allograft recipients teratogenic? A single-center experience. *Am J Med Genet A.* 2003;116A:31–36.

107. Tan PK, Tan AS, Tan HK, et al. Pregnancy after renal transplantation: experience in Singapore General Hospital. *Ann Acad Med Singapore.* 2002;31:285–289.

108. Anderka MT, Lin AE, Abuelo DN, et al. Reviewing the evidence for mycophenolate mofetil as a new teratogen: case report and review of the literature. *Am J Med Genet A.* 2009;149A:1241–1248.

109. Chandra A, Midtvedt K, Åsberg A, Eide IA. Immunosuppression and reproductive health after kidney transplantation. *Transplantation.* 2019;103:e325–e333.

110. Schen FP, Stallone G, Schena A, et al. Pregnancy in renal transplantation: immunologic evaluation of neonates from mothers with transplanted kidney. *Transpl Immunol.* 2002;9:161–164.

111. Karidas CN, Michailidis GD, Spencer K, Economides DL. Biochemical screening for Down syndrome in pregnancies following renal transplantation. *Prenat Diagn.* 2002;22:226–230.

112. Biesenbach G, Zazgornik J, Kaiser W, et al. Cyclosporin requirement during pregnancy in renal transplant recipients. *Nephrol Dial Transplant.* 1989;4:667–669.

113. Cyganek A, Pietrzak B, Kociszewska-Najman B, et al. Anemia treatment with erythropoietin in pregnant renal recipients. *Transplant Proc.* 2011;43:2970–2972.

114. Goshorn J, Youell TD. Darbepoetin alfa treatment for post-renal transplantation anemia during pregnancy. *Am J Kidney Dis.* 2005;46:e81–e86.

115. Demir M, Yagmur I, Pelit ES, et al. Urolithiasis and its treatment in pregnant women: 10-year clinical experience from a single centre. *Cureus.* 2021;13:e13752.

116. Meher S, Gibbons N, DasGupta R. Renal stones in pregnancy. *Obstet Med.* 2014;7:103–110.

117. Semins MJ, Matlaga BR. Kidney stones during pregnancy. *Nat Rev Urol.* 2014;11:163–168.

118. Loughlin KR, Ker LA. The current management of urolithiasis during pregnancy. *Urol Clin North Am.* 2002;29:701–704.

119. Meria P, Hadjadj H, Jungers P, et al. Stone formation and pregnancy: pathophysiological insights gained from morphoconstitutional stone analysis. *J Urol.* 2010;183:1412–1416.

120. Butler EL, Cox SM, Eberts EG, Cunningham FG. Symptomatic nephrolithiasis complicating pregnancy. *Obstet Gynecol.* 2000;96:753–756.

121. Parulkar BG, Hopkins TB, Wollin MR, et al. Renal colic during pregnancy: a case for conservative treatment. *J Urol.* 1998;159:365–368.

122. Burgess KL, Gettman MT, Rangel LJ, Krambeck AE. Diagnosis of urolithiasis and rate of spontaneous passage during pregnancy. *J Urol.* 2011;186:2280–2284.

123. Fulgham PF, Assimos DG, Pearle MS, Preminger GM. Clinical effectiveness protocols for imaging in the management of ureteral calculous disease: AUA technology assessment. *J Urol.* 2013;189:1203–1213.

124. Türk C, Petřík A, Sarica K, et al. EAU guidelines on diagnosis and conservative management of urolithiasis. *Eur Urol.* 2016;69:468–474.

125. Kok RD, de Vries MM, Heerschap A, van den Berg PP. Absence of harmful effects of magnetic resonance exposure at 1.5 T in utero during the third trimester of pregnancy: a follow-up study. *Magn Reson Imaging.* 2004;22:851–854.

126. Ray JG, Vermeulen MJ, Bharatha A, et al. Association between MRI exposure during pregnancy and fetal and childhood outcomes. *JAMA.* 2016;316:952–961.

127. American College of Obstetricians and Gynecologists. Committee Opinion No. 723: Guidelines for diagnostic

imaging during pregnancy and lactation (reaffirmed 2021). *Obstet Gynecol.* 2017;130:e210–e216.

128. Mullins JK, Semins MJ, Hyams ES, et al. Half Fourier single-shot turbo spin-echo magnetic resonance urography for the evaluation of suspected renal colic in pregnancy. *Urology.* 2012;79:1252–1255.

129. White WM, Johnson EB, Zite NB, et al. Predictive value of current imaging modalities for the detection of urolithiasis during pregnancy: a multicenter, longitudinal study. *J Urol.* 2013;189:931–934.

130. Coe FL, Parks JH, Lindheimer MD. Nephrolithiasis during pregnancy. *N Engl J Med.* 1978;298:324–326.

131. Zhou Q, Chen WQ, Xie XS, et al. Maternal and neonatal outcomes of pregnancy complicated by urolithiasis: a systematic review and meta-analysis. *J Nephrol.* 2021;34:1569–1580.

132. Lewis DF, Robichaux AG 3rd, Jaekle RK, et al. Urolithiasis in pregnancy: diagnosis, management and pregnancy outcome. *J Reprod Med.* 2003;48:28–32.

133. Body C, Christie JA. Gastrointestinal diseases in pregnancy: nausea, vomiting, hyperemesis gravidarum, gastroesophageal reflux disease, constipation, and diarrhea. *Gastroenterol Clin North Am.* 2016;45:267–283.

134. Honoré LH. The increased incidence of renal stones in women with spontaneous abortion: a retrospective study. *Am J Obstet Gynecol.* 1980;137:145–146.

135. Eaton A, Martin PC. Ruptured ureter in pregnancy—a unique case? *Br J Urol.* 1981;53:78–79.

136. Keepanasseril A, Nanjappa B, Prasad GV, et al. Vesical calculus: an unusual cause of labour dystocia. *J Obstet Gynaecol.* 2012;32:596–597.

137. Swartz MA, Lydon-Rochelle MT, Simon D, et al. Admission for nephrolithiasis in pregnancy and risk of adverse birth outcomes. *Obstet Gynecol.* 2007;109:1099–1104.

138. Pedro RN, Das K, Buchholz N. Urolithiasis in pregnancy. *Int J Surg.* 2016;36:688–692.

139. Parsons JK, Hergan LA, Sakamoto K, Lakin C. Efficacy of alpha-blockers for the treatment of ureteral stones. *J Urol.* 2007;177:983–987.

140. Theriault B, Morin F, Cloutier J. Safety and efficacy of Tamsulosin as medical expulsive therapy in pregnancy. *World J Urol.* 2020;38:2301–2306.

141. Khoo L, Anson K, Patel U. Success and short-term complication rates of percutaneous nephrostomy during pregnancy. *J Vasc Interv Radiol.* 2004;15:1469–1473.

142. Watterson JD, Girvan AR, Beiko DT, et al. Ureteroscopy and holmium:YAG laser lithotripsy: an emerging definitive management strategy for symptomatic ureteral calculi in pregnancy. *Urology.* 2002;60:383–387.

143. Asgari MA, Safarinejad MR, Hosseini SY, Dadkhah F. Extracorporeal shock wave lithotripsy of renal calculi during early pregnancy. *BJU Int.* 1999;84:615–617.

144. Assimos D, Krambeck A, Miller NL, et al. Surgical management of stones: American Urological Association/Endourological Society guideline, PART I. *J Urol.* 2016;196:1153–1160.

145. Schnatz PF, Curry SL. Primary hyperparathyroidism in pregnancy: evidence-based management. *Obstet Gynecol Surv.* 2002;57:365–376.

146. Ready LB, Johnson ES. Epidural block for treatment of renal colic during pregnancy. *Can Anaesth Soc J.* 1981;28:77–79.

51

Respiratory Disease

Emily E. Naoum, MD and Karen S. Lindeman, MD

CHAPTER OUTLINE

Parturients with respiratory disease present several areas of concern to the obstetric anesthesia provider, including airway hyperresponsiveness and obstruction and reactions to tracheal intubation. This chapter reviews the pathophysiology, clinical presentation, and management during the puerperium of asthma, cigarette smoking, cystic fibrosis, and respiratory failure.

ASTHMA

Definition

Asthma is defined by clinical symptoms with three characteristics: (1) reversible airway obstruction, (2) airway inflammation, and (3) airway hyperresponsiveness.[1,2] **Airway obstruction** produces the clinical manifestations of wheezing, cough, and dyspnea. **Airway inflammation** modulates the course of asthma by independently producing airway obstruction and enhancing airway hyperresponsiveness. **Airway hyperresponsiveness** is marked by exaggerated responses to a wide variety of bronchoconstrictor stimuli, including histamine, methacholine, prostaglandin $F_{2\alpha}$, hypoosmotic solutions, and cold air.

Epidemiology

From 2006 to 2018, the prevalence of asthma remained stable among adults in the United States at 7.9%.[3] There are geographic, ethnic, and socioeconomic differences in the rates of asthma with higher rates in the Northeast than in the South or West; higher prevalence in Black, Puerto Rican, and Hispanic persons; and higher prevalence in low-income populations.[3]

The prevalence of asthma in women of childbearing age continues to rise; it was approximately 3% in the 1990s and increased to approximately 8.8% in the early 2000s.[4] Flores et al.[5] found that from 2001 to 2016, the rate of asthma rose from 8.8% to 12% in women of childbearing age (18 to 44 years); during the study period, overall, 10.9% of pregnant women reported having asthma. Women with Medicaid or public health insurance, body mass index $\geq 30\,kg/m^2$, or hypertension were more likely to have asthma and/or asthma attacks.[5]

Pathophysiology

Asthma is believed to occur under a variety of environmental influences in the presence of genetic susceptibility.[6] Although in the past it was considered to be a single disease, the current view is that it is a syndrome consisting of various phenotypes. The most important potential mechanisms are (1) an enhancement of contractility or an impairment of relaxation of airway smooth muscle, (2) a neural imbalance, (3) airway inflammation, and (4) changes in the function of the airway epithelium.[1]

Airway Smooth Muscle

Contraction of airway smooth muscle is believed to be the most important factor producing acute airway obstruction. For many years, an enhancement of airway smooth muscle responsiveness to contractile agonists was assumed to be a major mechanism of asthma; however, *in vitro* and *in vivo* studies have not consistently demonstrated this pathophysiology.[7,8] Instead of an enhancement in responsiveness to contractile stimuli, a reduction in responsiveness to relaxant stimuli may contribute to airway obstruction.[9] Although the mechanism for this effect is poorly understood, a reduction in airway sensitivity to beta-adrenergic agonists could contribute to airway hyperresponsiveness by altering the balance between constricting and dilating influences.

Neural Components

A balance between constricting and dilating influences also exists with respect to the autonomic nervous system. A shift in this balance, with an increase in constricting influences, may be a mechanism of asthma.

The **parasympathetic nervous system** provides the dominant constrictor input to the airways (Fig. 51.1). Efferent cholinergic fibers travel in the vagus nerve to synapse in ganglia within the airway wall. Postganglionic fibers release acetylcholine to activate muscarinic receptors and stimulate airway smooth muscle contraction. A negative feedback system limits release of acetylcholine from nerve terminals. Muscarinic

autoreceptors, or receptors on the nerve ending, also are activated by acetylcholine and inhibit further release of acetylcholine from the nerve terminal.[10]

The importance of exaggerated cholinergic efferent activity in the pathogenesis of airway hyperreactivity has been debated extensively. The relatively limited efficacy of anticholinergic agents in relieving clinical bronchospasm and growing evidence supporting other mechanisms suggest that this pathway has a limited role in the pathophysiology of asthma. However, this mechanism appears to be very important in the perioperative management of asthmatic subjects. Reflex stimulation of airway smooth muscle during placement of a tracheal tube represents one of the most important causes of bronchospasm in the perioperative period.

An alternative mechanism by which the parasympathetic nervous system may contribute to airway hyperresponsiveness is through dysfunction of the muscarinic autoreceptors, which allows increased postganglionic release of acetylcholine after reflex stimulation.[10] This mechanism may explain the airway hyperresponsiveness that occurs for several weeks after an upper respiratory tract infection, although additional autoreceptor-independent mechanisms may also be present.[11,12] The role of this mechanism in the pathophysiology of clinical asthma is unclear.

The **sympathetic nervous system** primarily acts to decrease airway tone. In contrast to the parasympathetic nervous system, sympathetic innervation of airway smooth muscle in humans is either sparse or absent.[13] Circulating catecholamines activate beta-adrenergic receptors in airway smooth muscle and provide the primary sympathetic input to human airways. Because airways of normal human subjects do not become hyperresponsive after beta-adrenergic blockade,[14] it is unlikely that impaired catecholamine secretion contributes significantly to the pathogenesis of asthma.

The alpha-adrenergic system is thought to play a relatively minor role in determining the state of airway responsiveness. Although alpha-adrenergic receptors are present in human airways,[15] the protective effects of alpha-adrenergic antagonists have been disappointing and can be attributed to other properties, such as antihistamine activity.

In addition to cholinergic and adrenergic input, a third neural system, the **nonadrenergic noncholinergic (NANC)** system, provides efferent nerves to the airways. Both constricting and dilating pathways have been identified.[16] **Nitric oxide** serves as the inhibitory NANC neurotransmitter in human airways.[17] A relative increase in constricting influences or a decrease in dilating influences in the NANC system could potentially contribute to asthma. However, asthmatic subjects demonstrated no deficit in NANC inhibitory pathways,[18] and inhibition of NANC excitatory neurotransmission did not improve airway hyperresponsiveness.[19] Thus, current evidence does not support imbalance of the NANC system as a major mechanism of asthma.

Airway Inflammation

Airway inflammation appears to serve primarily as a modulating influence in asthma. Inflammation is certainly

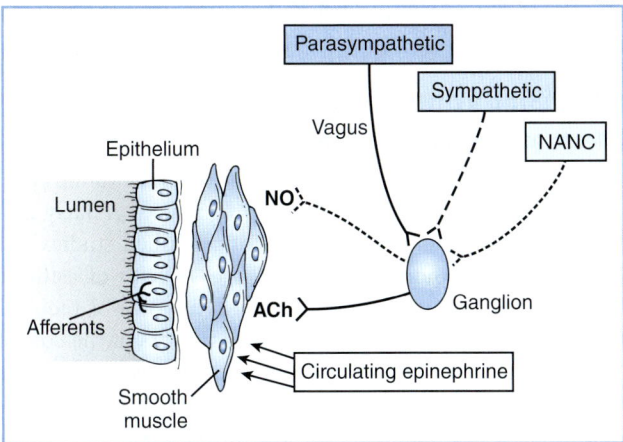

Fig. 51.1 Neural Control of the Airway. Parasympathetic, sympathetic, and nonadrenergic noncholinergic (NANC) efferents innervate ganglia within the airway wall. Postganglionic cholinergic efferents release acetylcholine (ACh) to constrict airway smooth muscle. Postganglionic NANC efferents release nitric oxide (NO) to relax airway smooth muscle. Circulating epinephrine relaxes the airway. Afferents from the airway originate in the epithelium and are activated by airway irritation, as occurs with tracheal intubation.

present in some but not all asthmatic subjects.[20] The process of inflammation involves airway wall edema and infiltration of the mucosa by a variety of inflammatory cells, including neutrophils, mast cells, helper T lymphocytes, macrophages, and eosinophils. These cells produce and release mediators of inflammation, such as histamine, leukotrienes, platelet-activating factor, prostaglandins, thromboxanes, cytokines, serotonin, and nitric oxide.[21] Airway inflammation can also reduce airway diameter. Airway hyperresponsiveness is correlated with increased baseline airway tone.[22] Although inflammation appears to modulate the course of asthma, other factors certainly contribute to the pathogenesis.

Airway Epithelium

The epithelium provides a barrier to protect the subepithelial layers against stimuli that could provoke bronchospasm. Airways of asthmatic subjects demonstrate areas of epithelial destruction,[23] and the clinical significance of this finding has been demonstrated.[24]

The epithelium not only serves as a barrier but also plays an active role in the maintenance of airway tone, producing constricting and dilating factors.[25] An alteration in the balance between these factors could alter airway responsiveness. The relative importance of alterations in epithelial function in the pathogenesis of asthma is unknown.

Diagnosis

Medical History

The classic symptoms of asthma include wheezing, cough, dyspnea, and chest tightness. A patient's medical history also should include information about the pattern and severity of the symptoms, precipitating and aggravating factors, and the duration and course of these symptoms.

Physical Examination

Physical examination is directed to the respiratory tract. Auscultation of the chest may reveal expiratory wheezing and a prolonged phase of expiration. During asthma exacerbations, wheezes may not be heard because of severely reduced air exchange.[2] The airway examination may also be notable for allergic rhinitis or nasal polyps, which are associated with asthma.[2]

Laboratory Studies

Laboratory studies that aid in the diagnosis of asthma depend on findings from the medical history and physical examination. In general, pulmonary function tests are useful to document the severity and establish the reversibility of obstruction; spirometry tests used in patients with asthma are shown in Box 51.1. Although these tests may aid the diagnosis of asthma, pulmonary function measurements often do not correlate directly with symptoms.[26] An expert working group of the National Heart, Lung and Blood Institute recommended that spirometry measurements before and after inhalation of a short-acting bronchodilator should be undertaken for patients in whom the diagnosis of asthma is being considered.[26]

> **BOX 51.1   Pulmonary Function Tests in Patients With Asthma**
>
> **Forced vital capacity**
> - The volume of gas exhaled after maximal inspiration
> - May be reduced in asthma
>
> **Forced expiratory volume in 1 s**
> - The volume exhaled in the first second after maximal inspiration
> - May be reduced in asthma
>
> **FEV_1/FVC**
> - < 0.75 in asthma
>
> **Peak expiratory flow rate**
> - Maximal flow rate that can be exhaled following a full inspiration
> - May be reduced in asthma

FEV_1, Forced expiratory volume in 1 s; FVC, forced vital capacity.

> **BOX 51.2   Factors That May Improve or Worsen Asthma During Pregnancy**
>
> **Factors that may improve asthma**
> - Progesterone-induced relaxation of airway smooth muscle
> - Increased production of bronchodilating prostaglandins
> - Higher circulating cortisol level
>
> **Factors that may worsen asthma**
> - Decreased sensitivity to beta-adrenergic agonists
> - Increased production of bronchoconstricting prostaglandins
> - Reduced sensitivity to circulating cortisol because of binding of steroid hormones (e.g., progesterone) to cortisol receptors

---

For patients in whom the diagnosis is uncertain using traditional methods, the National Asthma Education and Prevention Program (NAEPP) conditionally recommends measurement of fractional exhaled nitric oxide (FeNO) to aid the diagnosis.[26]

Interaction With Pregnancy

Effects of Pregnancy on Asthma

The overall course of asthma has been reported to improve, worsen, or remain the same during pregnancy.[27] A likely reason for the variation in the results of published studies is a difference in methods of assessing the severity of asthma. Most studies have used either clinical symptoms or requirements for pharmacologic therapy as indicators of the course of the disease. These measures do not correlate with objective measures of airway obstruction.[28] A US obstetric cohort study found that exacerbations of asthma during pregnancy occur in as many as 40% of subjects receiving standard clinical care, and risk of exacerbation correlates with severity of prepregnancy asthma.[29]

Several mechanisms may be responsible for the changes in the clinical course of asthma during pregnancy (Box 51.2). An increase in progesterone level is thought to be one mechanism that improves asthma during pregnancy. Progesterone relaxes uterine and gastrointestinal smooth muscle and may or may not have similar effects on airway smooth muscle. Conversely, progesterone may actually worsen asthma by enhancing inflammation.[30] Thus, effects of pregnancy on asthma appear to involve a number of factors other than direct effects of hormones on airway smooth muscle.

Effects of Asthma on the Parturient and Fetus

Many investigators have questioned whether maternal asthma adversely affects perinatal outcome. Variation in study design (e.g., retrospective and prospective) and differences in severity and treatment of asthma may account for differences in study results. A systematic review reported increased incidences of cesarean delivery, gestational diabetes, antepartum and postpartum hemorrhage, placenta previa and abruption, and premature rupture of membranes in patients with severe asthma. Moderate to severe asthma increased the risk for cesarean delivery and gestational diabetes compared with mild asthma.[31] Although asthma in pregnancy is associated with an increased risk for adverse perinatal outcomes, a metaanalysis of cohort studies suggested that active asthma management, which is intended to reduce the exacerbation rate, may reduce the risk for perinatal complications, particularly preterm delivery.[32] No controlled studies have documented better perinatal outcome with aggressive asthma treatment. Potential mechanisms of increased perinatal morbidity and mortality in patients with uncontrolled asthma include hypoxemia and hypocapnia, inflammation, and altered placental function from asthma-associated mediator release.[33] A prospective cohort study of nearly 80,000 parous women demonstrated that hypertensive disorders of pregnancy were associated with an increased risk for asthma, which may reflect shared mechanisms such as vascular remodeling and endothelial abnormalities.[34]

Medical Management

Pharmacologic therapy for asthma during pregnancy is directed toward avoiding acute exacerbations and episodes of status asthmaticus. Management algorithms generally rely on consensus opinions owing to a paucity of randomized controlled trials. Two of the most widely cited sources, the Global Initiative for Asthma (GINA)[2] and the NAEPP[26] in the United States, base guidelines on systematic reviews and metaanalyses in addition to individual studies. Although general principles typically dictate that unnecessary medication should be avoided during pregnancy, GINA guidelines state that risks for uncontrolled asthma exceed medication-associated risks in pregnancy.[2] Medications that are currently used to treat asthma fall into two general categories: bronchodilators and antiinflammatory agents. These agents generally are safe for the fetus.

Bronchodilators

Beta-adrenergic agonists exert beneficial effects in asthmatic patients by activation of beta$_2$-adrenergic receptors, which mediate several processes (Box 51.3). **Short-acting**

> **BOX 51.3 Mechanisms of Beneficial Effects of Beta-Adrenergic Agonists in Asthma**
>
> - Direct airway smooth muscle relaxation
> - Enhanced mucociliary transport
> - Decreased airway edema
> - Inhibition of cholinergic neurotransmission

beta-adrenergic agonists (SABAs) are frequently used for acute exacerbations of asthma. **Long-acting beta-adrenergic agonists (LABAs)**, when combined with inhaled **corticosteroids** (ICSs), are also effective in treating acute asthma and for asthma maintenance.[35] Both SABAs and LABAs may be administered as aerosols, orally, or parenterally. The aerosol route is generally preferred during pregnancy because high concentrations of the medication can be delivered directly to the site of action in the airways, with relatively less drug delivered to the uteroplacental circulation.

The limited number of human studies investigating the fetal safety of long-term administration of beta-adrenergic agonists have not shown significant adverse neonatal outcomes.[36,37] In addition, the long history of use of these agents without reports of teratogenicity suggests that their use should not be restricted because of fetal concerns (see Chapter 16).

Methylxanthines (e.g., **theophylline**, **aminophylline**) were used for many years in the long-term treatment of asthma. Although their mechanism of action is controversial, relaxation of airway smooth muscle is the most prominent effect. The ability of these agents to inhibit intracellular phosphodiesterase and increase concentrations of cyclic adenosine monophosphate (cAMP) is not the mechanism of bronchodilation, because these effects do not occur at clinically relevant concentrations *in vivo*.[38] Their use is now limited to patients whose asthma responds poorly to other forms of therapy. Methylxanthines do not appear to cause significant adverse fetal outcomes.[39] Serum concentrations of theophylline should be monitored carefully, especially in the third trimester, when theophylline clearance decreases.[40]

Bronchodilation with **anticholinergic agents** occurs through the blockade of muscarinic receptors on airway smooth muscle. Because of their limited efficacy, the NAEPP recommends only using anticholinergic medications in combination with other bronchodilators or antiinflammatory agents.[35] The quaternary anticholinergic agent **ipratropium bromide** can be delivered as an aerosol, allowing higher concentrations in the lung with reductions in systemic absorption and potential effects on the fetus. Human data on the safety of anticholinergic agents and on potential teratogenicity are lacking, but ipratropium bromide is not associated with teratogenicity in animal studies.[41]

Magnesium sulfate relaxes airway smooth muscle, most likely via its antagonism of calcium entry into airway smooth muscle cells.[42] Its use is limited primarily to acute bronchospasm.[43]

Antiinflammatory Agents

Proposed mechanisms of action for **corticosteroids** are (1) decreases in cellular infiltration and mediator release, (2) reduction in airway permeability, and (3) upregulation of the beta-adrenergic system.[44] Unlike bronchodilators, corticosteroids not only reduce airway sensitivity to a constrictor stimulus[45] but also decrease the maximal extent of airway narrowing, a feature that may predict severity of an acute asthmatic episode.[46]

Both systemic and inhaled corticosteroids serve as mainstays in acute and maintenance asthma therapy. Neither systemic nor inhaled corticosteroids have been proven to increase the risk for congenital malformations in humans, but ICSs are preferred over systemic corticosteroids because of fewer maternal side effects and reduced delivery to the fetus. Systemic corticosteroids are now limited to acute exacerbations and persistent, severe asthma. Although oral corticosteroid use is associated with an increased incidence of low-birth-weight infants,[47] ICSs do not appear to increase perinatal risk.[48]

Corticosteroids may exacerbate maternal glucose intolerance, especially in women who also receive treatment with a beta-adrenergic agonist. Thus, careful monitoring of maternal glucose concentration is indicated when corticosteroids are used. However, because corticosteroids are efficacious in controlling severe asthma during pregnancy, these agents should not be withheld from the medical regimen.

Some authorities have recommended that corticosteroid-dependent asthmatic women receive large doses of parenteral corticosteroids during labor to prevent complications related to adrenal suppression.[49] The scientific basis for this recommendation is questionable as ICSs in moderate doses do not produce adrenocortical suppression.[50] The potential for adrenal insufficiency in infants of asthmatic mothers taking systemic or inhaled corticosteroids appears to be very low, most likely owing to the widespread use of either prednisone or prednisolone. In the mother, prednisone is converted rapidly to prednisolone, which crosses the placental barrier to a very limited extent.

Cromolyn sodium and **nedocromil sodium** belong to a class of drugs that are thought to reduce inflammation and mediator release primarily by stabilizing mast cells and perhaps other inflammatory cells. These medications are no longer recommended for asthma management.[2]

Based on the observation that leukotrienes are released into the airways by immune cells and contribute to the inflammatory process, other forms of antiinflammatory therapy are **leukotriene receptor antagonists** and **leukotriene synthesis inhibitors**. Safety data for the use of these agents in pregnancy are scarce (see Chapter 16). A large, retrospective cohort analysis that included more than 1500 women who received **montelukast** during pregnancy found no difference in congenital malformations compared with women who did not have asthma.[51]

A recombinant monoclonal anti-IgE antibody, **omalizumab**, is used specifically in patients with allergic asthma that is refractory to ICSs. A prospective, observational study of 250 women who received omalizumab during pregnancy demonstrated no increased risk of major congenital malformations, preterm birth, and small-for-gestational-age babies compared with pregnant women with asthma who did not receive the medication.[52] Omalizumab may be continued in women who are already receiving therapy and become pregnant if the benefit is deemed to outweigh potential harm.[2]

Obstetric Management

The following aspects of obstetric management of the asthmatic parturient may differ from that of the nonasthmatic patient: (1) induction of labor, (2) management of postpartum hemorrhage, and (3) treatment of hypertension.

For induction of labor, prostaglandins should be administered cautiously in women with asthma. Prostaglandin $F_{2\alpha}$ constricts airways *in vivo*[53] and *in vitro*.[54] Airways of asthmatic subjects demonstrate greater sensitivity to prostaglandin $F_{2\alpha}$, and its use to induce labor is associated with bronchospasm.[55] Prostaglandin E_2 can have either dilating or constricting effects on the airways, perhaps because of its ability to activate a variety of different types of prostaglandin receptors.[56] Because of the known risk for bronchospasm after exposure to prostaglandin $F_{2\alpha}$ and the possible risk after exposure to prostaglandin E_2, alternative methods of induction of labor are preferred in asthmatic women.

Likewise, asthma represents a relative contraindication to the administration of **15-methyl prostaglandin $F_{2\alpha}$ (carboprost, Hemabate)** for the treatment of postpartum hemorrhage. **Oxytocin**, **ergot alkaloids**, and **misoprostol** are all considered safe for the treatment of postpartum hemorrhage in the parturient with asthma.

Beta-adrenergic receptor antagonists are used to treat hypertension in some pregnant women. In asthmatic women, these agents may provoke bronchospasm when used acutely and should not be used as first-line treatment.[57,58] Other antihypertensive agents, such as **hydralazine**, **nifedipine**, and **nitroglycerin**, do not seem to enhance airway responsiveness.

Anesthetic Management

Preoperative Assessment

During the preoperative evaluation, the anesthesia provider should assess the severity of the disease and whether an acute asthmatic episode is present. The medical history should include information about symptoms of wheezing, dyspnea, and cough. Further information should be sought about the frequency and severity of symptoms, the course of these symptoms during pregnancy, and the date of the most recent exacerbation, as well as any history of tracheal intubation or hospitalization. Patients who have frequent, severe attacks are at increased risk for morbidity in the peripartum period.

Physical examination should focus on the pulmonary system. Chest auscultation may demonstrate wheezing with or without a prolonged expiratory phase. However, wheezing may not be audible if air movement is markedly reduced. Additional signs of an acute exacerbation of asthma include tachypnea, exaggerated (>20 mm Hg) pulsus paradoxus, and the use of accessory respiratory muscles.

In a pregnant woman with stable asthma, laboratory tests add little to anesthetic management. However, if an acute exacerbation is suspected, chest radiographic examination, arterial blood gas measurement, and pulmonary function tests may assist with diagnosis and therapy. **Chest radiographic examination** helps diagnose precipitating or complicating conditions such as pneumonia, pneumothorax, and heart failure. During an episode of acute asthma, **arterial blood gas measurement** often shows hypoxemia and respiratory alkalosis. After a prolonged, severe episode, arterial carbon dioxide tension increases as a result of fatigue. **Spirometry** measures the volume of gas exhaled over time (see Box 51.1). The most convenient indirect measurement for assessing airway obstruction during labor is the **peak expiratory flow rate**, which can be measured at the bedside with a flowmeter.

Management During Labor and Vaginal Delivery

The goals of analgesia for labor and delivery in asthmatic women include (1) provision of pain relief, (2) reduction in the stimulus to hyperpnea, and (3) prevention or relief of maternal stress. The goal of adequate pain relief does not differ for asthmatic women. It is important to prevent hyperpnea and stress in women with a history of asthmatic episodes triggered by exercise or stress. These goals should be accomplished with minimal sedation, minimal paralysis of the muscles of respiration, and minimal depression of the fetus, and can be accomplished with a number of analgesic modalities.

Systemic opioids may provide reasonable pain relief and reduce the stimulus to hyperpnea, especially during the early part of the first stage of labor. In theory, opioids reduce the risk for bronchospasm in asthmatic subjects. Opioid receptors are believed to be present in the respiratory tract[59] and to inhibit release of excitatory neuropeptides. The clinical relevance of these findings is unknown, because moderate doses of inhaled **morphine** do not significantly alter airway tone. Conversely, high doses of some opioids (e.g., morphine) may increase the risk for bronchospasm by releasing histamine. The risk associated with using moderate doses of morphine does not seem excessive, because airway tone does not change in subjects with moderate to severe asthma after inhalation of morphine.[60] An opioid that does not release histamine (e.g., **fentanyl**, **remifentanil**) may be a better choice for the asthmatic parturient. High doses of opioids are not desirable in subjects with active wheezing because of the risks for maternal and neonatal respiratory depression (see Chapter 23).

Neuraxial analgesic techniques, including epidural or combined spinal-epidural (CSE) analgesia, provide continuous pain relief with a reduction in the stimulus to hyperventilation (see Chapter 24). These goals typically are achieved without maternal sedation or neonatal depression. Unlike other analgesic techniques, continuous lumbar epidural analgesia adds a margin of safety by providing the opportunity to extend the sensory block for cesarean delivery. The possibility of extension allows the anesthesia provider to avoid some of the risks associated with general anesthesia, particularly airway manipulation and bronchospasm. The most significant disadvantage of epidural anesthesia in an asthmatic subject is the risk of high thoracic motor block and respiratory insufficiency. Use of an appropriate epidural test dose and maintenance of sensory level at the T10 dermatome minimize this risk. In addition, the use of a dilute concentration of local anesthetic combined with a modest dose of a lipophilic opioid produces satisfactory analgesia with less motor block than local anesthetic alone.

Management During Cesarean Delivery

The choice between neuraxial anesthesia and general anesthesia for cesarean delivery depends on obstetric considerations and the respiratory status of the parturient. In general, avoidance of airway instrumentation is desirable because tracheal intubation markedly increases airway tone in asthmatic subjects.[61]

The most important advantage of neuraxial anesthesia in the asthmatic patient is the avoidance of tracheal intubation. Stable asthmatic patients can undergo either spinal or epidural anesthesia. In unstable asthmatic patients who require the use of accessory muscles of respiration, neuraxial anesthesia may be hazardous because of impaired ventilatory capacity in the presence of a high thoracic motor block. Although it has been suggested that ropivacaine and levobupivacaine may cause less motor block than bupivacaine, decreases in maternal pulmonary function tests were similar following spinal anesthesia with bupivacaine, ropivacaine, or levobupivacaine for cesarean delivery.[62]

The adrenal medulla receives innervation from preganglionic sympathetic fibers arising from the T6 to L2 spinal segments. Some authors have postulated that neuraxial anesthesia and the ensuing sympathectomy could precipitate or potentiate bronchospasm during cesarean delivery in asthmatic subjects by reducing adrenal output of epinephrine (adrenaline). This possibility seems remote. First, although epinephrine infusion can reduce airway reactivity in asthmatic subjects,[63] epinephrine concentrations do not decrease during nonobstetric surgery performed with neuraxial anesthesia that achieves high thoracic sensory levels.[64] Second, the contention that neuraxial anesthesia may prevent increases in circulating epinephrine that are required to compensate for stress-induced bronchospasm does not appear to be valid. Bronchoconstriction does not stimulate epinephrine secretion in human asthmatic subjects.[65] Thus, neuraxial anesthesia is appropriate for cesarean delivery in stable asthmatic subjects.

General anesthesia for asthmatic women undergoing cesarean delivery requires a balance between the competing considerations of pulmonary aspiration and intraoperative bronchospasm. Although airway instrumentation provides a significant stimulus for bronchospasm, the high risk for aspiration mandates tracheal intubation during administration of general anesthesia in parturients.

The main options for tracheal intubation are rapid-sequence induction and awake fiberoptic intubation, although inhalational induction of general anesthesia with sevoflurane has been described in a parturient with status asthmaticus.[66] Indications for awake intubation in asthmatic subjects are similar to those for nonasthmatic patients. Pretreatment with a local anesthetic and a beta-adrenergic agonist can attenuate reflex-induced bronchoconstriction. The benefits of topical local anesthesia and airway nerve blocks for awake intubation should be weighed against a possible increase in the risk for aspiration from the loss of protective airway reflexes. Rapid-sequence induction for cesarean delivery in asthmatic patients is most often accomplished using either **propofol** or **ketamine**, with ketamine long considered the agent of choice because of its sympathomimetic properties, which relax airway smooth muscle and inhibit neural reflexes.[67] Beneficial airway effects of propofol also appear to occur via inhibition of airway reflexes. Intravenous **lidocaine (lignocaine)**, administered prior to the induction agent, inhibits airway reflexes and attenuates irritant-induced bronchoconstriction,[68] including during tracheal intubation, and produces an additional protective effect above that of beta-adrenergic agonist pretreatment alone.[69]

Although **volatile halogenated anesthetic agents** can relax uterine tone, their use should be considered for the maintenance of anesthesia. These agents attenuate airway responsiveness through direct effects on airway smooth muscle,[70,71] inhibition of airway reflexes,[72] and effects on the epithelium.[73] If possible, the inhaled concentration should be administered at less than 0.5 minimum alveolar concentration to limit the possibility of uterine relaxation and hemorrhage. **Sevoflurane** acts as a bronchodilator in large and small airways[74] and reverses airway constriction associated with tracheal intubation.[75] **Desflurane** may have irritant effects on the airway owing to smooth muscle contraction in the airway.[76,77] Based on a systematic review, **isoflurane** and sevoflurane are considered superior to desflurane in asthmatic patients.[78]

An inhaled bronchodilator can be added if bronchospasm occurs. The potential disadvantage of this technique is that the most effective bronchodilators (i.e., the beta-adrenergic agonists) also relax uterine smooth muscle. The administration of a beta-adrenergic agonist by aerosol delivers a relatively greater dose of drug to the airways and minimizes uterine relaxation.

Emergence from general anesthesia, as with induction, requires a balance between reducing the risk for aspiration and lowering the risk for bronchospasm. Extubation of the trachea when the patient is awake minimizes the risk for aspiration, but the tracheal tube may stimulate reflexes and precipitate bronchospasm as the depth of anesthesia is reduced. If bronchospasm occurs during emergence, bronchodilators can be administered.

CIGARETTE SMOKING AND ELECTRONIC NICOTINE DELIVERY SYSTEMS

Epidemiology

Cigarette smoking is a significant, preventable cause of maternal morbidity and perinatal morbidity and mortality.[79] From 2016 to 2021 the prevalence of smoking among pregnant women in the United States declined significantly, from 7.2%

to 4.6%.[80] E-cigarettes and other electronic nicotine delivery systems (ENDS) that deliver nicotine as an inhaled aerosol have increased in popularity, especially in young adults. The Pregnancy Risk Assessment Monitoring System (PRAMS) revealed increasing use of ENDS from 2016 to 2019, to 4.3% of women just before pregnancy and 1.3% in the last trimester. This estimate may underreport true prevalence, as the US Centers for Disease Control and Prevention collect PRAMS data by mail or telephone questionnaire.[81]

Pathophysiology

Cigarette smoke contains a large number of separate components that have a variety of biologic effects. Nonrespiratory effects of cigarette smoking are described in Chapter 52.

The primary respiratory effects of cigarette smoking include small airway obstruction, altered ventilation/perfusion relationship, and impairment of ciliary transport.[82] The precise mechanisms for these effects are unknown. Smoking increases airway mucus production and reduces clearance, presumably by impairment of ciliary transport. Cigarette smoking is associated with an increase in nonspecific airway reactivity, possibly through epithelial damage, altered airway geometry caused by increased mucus secretion, or upregulation of endothelin receptors.[82] These changes lead to a marked increase in the incidence of postoperative pulmonary complications.[83]

E-cigarettes and other ENDS aerosols consist of nicotine and a multitude of other chemicals in various combinations. Acute effects of ENDS in humans include increased airway resistance, inflammation, and airway reactivity.[84] Self-reported studies of chronic effects describe the development of symptoms similar to asthma associated with ENDS use, but the pathophysiology is unclear.[85]

Interaction With Pregnancy

Few studies have documented the respiratory effects of cigarette smoking or ENDS use during pregnancy. In one study, reductions in forced expiratory flow rates suggested that pregnant women who smoke cigarettes have greater small airway resistance than those who do not smoke.[86] These and other abnormalities were similar to the changes in airway function observed in nonpregnant smokers; although further studies are needed, other respiratory effects of cigarette smoking in pregnant women are likely similar to those in nonpregnant women.

Cigarette smoking adversely affects pregnancy in a number of ways. The association between smoking and low birth weight has a genetic influence, such that the specific variation of the nicotinic acetylcholine receptor gene cluster is associated with lower newborn birth weight in smokers but not in nonsmokers.[87] Respiratory effects of maternal cigarette smoking on the fetus include impaired lung growth and pulmonary function.[88] Further details regarding adverse maternal and fetal effects of smoking are described in Chapter 52.

Evidence of respiratory effects of e-cigarettes in the fetus continues to emerge as usage increases. Animal models demonstrate defects of fetal lung development in the presence of chronic maternal exposure to e-cigarette vapor.[89]

Medical Management

Cessation of smoking is the preferred form of medical management. Smoking cessation techniques include nonpharmacologic and pharmacologic methods. Nonpharmacologic methods incur little risk, are moderately effective,[90] and are preferred to pharmacologic methods owing to a paucity of randomized controlled trials assessing risks and benefits.[91] Das et al.[92] demonstrated that smoking cessation before or early in pregnancy resulted in prompt improvement in maternal airway function, but no controlled studies have evaluated effects of smoking cessation on peripartum outcome. Despite a paucity of data, the American College of Obstetrics and Gynecology recommends cessation of e-cigarette use during pregnancy.[93]

Anesthetic Management

For vaginal delivery, any of the analgesic techniques described earlier for asthmatic parturients are acceptable. For cesarean delivery, tracheal intubation is associated with bronchospasm in smokers[94]; neuraxial anesthesia avoids airway instrumentation and is therefore preferable to general anesthesia, although no controlled studies have documented differences in peripartum morbidity. If general anesthesia is required, methods for reducing the risk for intraoperative bronchospasm described previously should be considered. One study noted that respiratory resistance did not decrease after tracheal intubation in smokers anesthetized with **desflurane**,[95] suggesting that other volatile halogenated anesthetic agents might be preferable.

CYSTIC FIBROSIS

Epidemiology

Cystic fibrosis (CF), a lethal genetic disorder that is transmitted as an autosomal recessive trait, affects approximately 1 in 5000 births in the United States.[96,97] Because of improvements in diagnosis and therapy, a growing number of women with CF survive to reproductive age. From 2005 to 2014 the pregnancy rate in CF patients in the United States decreased approximately 2% per year. This decline was consistent with the overall national trend; however, the pregnancy rate in CF patients was much lower than that in the general population.[98] In a retrospective multinational study, Shteinberg et al.[99] found that 35% of women with CF had subfertility, which was approximately three times higher than in the general population.

Pathophysiology

Clinical features of CF result from abnormalities of epithelial tissues, especially in the respiratory, digestive, and reproductive tracts. Normal epithelial cells secrete Cl^- in response to an increase in intracellular cyclic adenosine monophosphate (cAMP). In CF, a genetic mutation makes epithelial cells unable to alter Cl^- permeability in response to changes in

cyclic adenosine monophosphate (cAMP).[100,101] The responsible gene is located on chromosome 7 and encodes a protein known as the *cystic fibrosis transmembrane regulator* (CFTR),[102] which may be absent or dysfunctional as a result of multiple mutations. The CFTR acts as a Cl^- channel but also has a number of other actions. CF is characterized by impaired water flow from the interior to the exterior of epithelial cells, leading to obstruction of exocrine glands with mucus.

In the lungs, abnormalities of electrolyte transport alter the composition of airway secretions. Inflammation, with infiltration of polymorphonuclear leukocytes, also contributes to changes in airway secretions.[103] Large numbers of disintegrating neutrophils release DNA in quantities sufficient to overwhelm the ability of deoxyribonuclease I (DNAse I), an endogenously released enzyme, to digest extracellular DNA. Undigested DNA increases the viscosity of airway secretions, which causes obstruction of small airways and reduced lung volumes. The ensuing ventilation-perfusion inequalities produce arterial hypoxemia. Some patients have hyperreactive airways. Spontaneous pneumothorax occurs with an annual incidence estimated at 0.64%.[104] Chronic airway obstruction and impaired mucus clearance increase the frequency of pulmonary infection. Additional contributory factors to inflammation include tumor necrosis factor alpha (TNF-α) mutations, fatty acid metabolism abnormalities, and increased arachidonic acid and metabolites.[105] Most patients become colonized or infected with *Pseudomonas aeruginosa*. Eventually, tissue damage leads to bronchiectasis and pulmonary insufficiency. Chronic hypoxemia and lung destruction may produce pulmonary hypertension and cor pulmonale. Nonrespiratory manifestations of CF include pancreatic exocrine insufficiency, intestinal obstruction, and infertility.

Diagnosis

Clinical criteria for the diagnosis of CF include (1) the presence of chronic obstructive lung disease and colonization with *P. aeruginosa* before 20 years of age, (2) exocrine pancreatic insufficiency, and (3) a family history of CF. Laboratory findings include (1) sweat Cl^- concentration > 60 mEq/L, (2) *CFTR* genotype with two known CF mutations, and (3) detection of CFTR dysfunction by the nasal potential difference test.[106] Chest radiographs often demonstrate hyperinflation, and arterial blood gas measurement may show hypoxemia. Pulmonary function tests, which can reveal obstructive or restrictive lung patterns, are useful to assess the severity of the disease. With serial measurements, clinicians should look for evidence of an increased residual volume and a reduced FEV_1.[107]

Interaction With Pregnancy

Effect of Pregnancy on Cystic Fibrosis

The following factors may contribute to the deterioration of pulmonary function during pregnancy: (1) increased airway responsiveness and obstruction (as can occur in patients with asthma), (2) increased work of breathing, and (3) cardiovascular changes such as congestive heart failure and pulmonary hypertension associated with the increased blood volume of pregnancy.

In spite of potential negative effects of pregnancy on the course of CF, long-term maternal outcome does not appear to be affected.[108] However, temporary reductions in FEV_1 in the immediate postpartum period may occur,[109] and pre-pregnancy FEV_1 is a useful predictor of ability to tolerate pregnancy.[110]

Effect of Cystic Fibrosis on Pregnancy

CF has been associated with an increased risk for low-birth-weight infants and preterm delivery, but recent evidence suggests that improved care of these patients can mitigate these problems.[111,112] Affected women with poor pre-pregnancy FEV_1 ($\leq 50\%$ predicted) are more likely to have cesarean delivery, preterm delivery, and low-birth-weight infants compared with women with $FEV_1 > 50\%$ predicted.[111-113] Potential mechanisms for these complications include chronic hypoxemia and poor maternal nutrition. Pancreatic insufficiency, poor nutritional status, CF-related diabetes mellitus, poor cardiac function, and high bacterial burden have been associated with poorer pregnancy outcomes.[114]

Medical Management

Respiratory management of CF is primarily symptomatic. Patients with large volumes of mucus production undergo mechanical airway clearance. Some patients inhale recombinant human DNAse I to reduce viscosity of lung secretions caused by accumulating DNA. Hypertonic saline inhalation aids clearance of airway mucus.[115] Bronchodilators may help those patients who manifest a reversible component of airway obstruction. Continuous oxygen therapy may benefit patients with hypoxemia and cor pulmonale.

Long-term antibiotic therapy with inhaled **tobramycin** reduces both the incidence of recurrent pulmonary infection and the frequency of exacerbations in patients with CF.[116] Long-term administration of oral **azithromycin** also decreases exacerbations from CF[117] through either its antibiotic or its antiinflammatory properties. Effects of long-term antibiotic therapy on the fetus are unknown.

Other forms of therapy include gene therapy and lung transplantation. The goal of gene therapy is to improve function of the defective CFTR protein. **Ivacaftor** and **lumacaftor/ivacaftor** combination therapies are used for patients with certain specific mutations. With only anecdotal experience in pregnancy, the safety of these CFTR modulators for the fetus has not yet been established. Concerns regarding these medications include potential increased risk of neonatal cataracts; infants exposed to these medications *in utero* or while breastfeeding are recommended to undergo a screening ophthalmologic examination.[114]

Pulmonary deterioration sometimes necessitates double-lung transplantation, although it is unclear whether this alters survival.[118] Pregnancy following lung transplantation is associated with a high risk of prematurity, neonatal complications, and rates of rejection.[119,120]

Obstetric Management

Because of the influence of pregravid maternal health on pregnancy outcome, the primary obstetric issue centers on the advisability of pregnancy in patients with CF. Criteria for termination of pregnancy are not clearly defined. Genetic counseling regarding the risk for CF in offspring is another important component of obstetric management.

Anesthetic Management

Considerations for anesthetic management focus primarily on the pulmonary system. Because of the high incidence of hypoxemia in patients with CF, continuous monitoring of oxygen saturation and appropriate oxygen therapy are advisable. The increased cardiac output at the time of delivery is important to consider in women with right heart dysfunction, including those with pulmonary hypertension, as it may merit invasive monitoring in patients at risk of heart failure.[114]

The goals of pain relief during labor are to provide adequate analgesia and to prevent maternal hyperventilation while avoiding high thoracic motor block and respiratory depression. High thoracic motor block may impair the parturient's ability to cough and eliminate thick secretions. Hyperventilation increases the work of breathing and may cause decompensation in patients with severe pulmonary dysfunction. For pain relief during labor, parenteral opioid analgesia may worsen pulmonary function by depressing respiratory drive and inhibiting cough. Intrathecal opioids have been used successfully,[121] but patients should be monitored carefully for respiratory depression. Continuous lumbar epidural analgesia, with a sensory nerve block maintained at the level of the T10 dermatome, can provide excellent pain relief and reduce the stimulus for hyperventilation, with minimal motor block of the thorax. A dilute solution of bupivacaine, with or without a lipophilic opioid, provides sensory analgesia with minimal motor block and is therefore nearly ideal in this setting.[122] In healthy parturients, this technique actually improves respiratory function slightly.[123]

Cesarean delivery should be reserved for obstetric indications. No studies have documented differences in outcome between general anesthesia and neuraxial anesthesia in patients with CF; however, neuraxial anesthesia offers the advantage of avoiding tracheal intubation which may be associated with bronchospasm or obstruction of the tracheal tube with secretions. Neuraxial anesthesia also avoids positive-pressure ventilation, which may enlarge a preexisting pneumothorax. The primary consideration for neuraxial anesthesia during cesarean delivery is to avoid high thoracic motor block, which may impair ventilation and the ability to cough. Effective spinal anesthesia for cesarean delivery slightly decreases vital capacity.[124] Methods for reducing the risk for excessively high motor block include the use of a continuous catheter technique, which allows titration of the local anesthetic agent to achieve the desired sensory level, and the use of the lowest concentration of local anesthetic (with or without a lipophilic opioid) that provides surgical anesthesia. Both epidural and CSE anesthesia have been used.[125] Patients with severe cardiorespiratory manifestations of CF may benefit from extracorporeal membrane oxygenation (ECMO) peripartum, and consultation with an ECMO team may help optimize the patient for delivery and potential support.[122]

For general anesthesia, techniques to reduce the risk for bronchospasm, as described for patients with asthma (see earlier discussion), may be warranted. Additional considerations include (1) humidification of gases to prevent inspissation of mucus, (2) frequent suctioning to remove excess secretions, and (3) use of ventilator settings that allow an appropriately long expiratory phase to prevent air trapping and pneumothorax. It may be prudent to avoid nitrous oxide because of the risk for pneumothorax. Patients should be allowed to awaken fully before extubation of the trachea. Early chest physiotherapy and mobilization are recommended in the immediate postoperative period to reduce the risk of venous thromboembolism, infection, and deconditioning.[126]

RESPIRATORY FAILURE

Epidemiology

The prevalence of acute respiratory failure during pregnancy is thought to be as high as 1 in 500 with an estimated 0.1% to 0.3% of pregnancies affected.[127–129] While the most common obstetric causes are hypertensive disease and hemorrhage,[130] a significant number of patients suffer from **acute respiratory distress syndrome (ARDS)**. A large database analysis of more than 55 million pregnancies from 2006 to 2012 revealed that the number of pregnant patients requiring mechanical ventilation as a result of ARDS increased from 36.5 cases per 100,000 live births in 2006 to 59.6 cases per 100,000 live births in 2012, with an in-hospital mortality rate of 9%.[131]

Pregnancy may predispose women to the development of ARDS secondary to the physiologic changes that occur during pregnancy, including increased blood volume, reduced oncotic pressure, upregulation of the inflammatory response, increased capillary leak, decreased lower esophageal sphincter tone, and increased intraabdominal pressure.[132] A study that compared pregnant and nonpregnant women with ARDS found that pregnant women were younger and had greater severity of ARDS and higher driving pressures than nonpregnant women; maternal and perinatal mortality were high at 18.5% and 37%, respectively.[133] Notably, mortality in the latter study was not significantly different between the pregnant and the nonpregnant cohort.

Pathophysiology

The pathophysiology of respiratory failure depends on the underlying disorder. ARDS results from a group of predisposing conditions, but a common final pathway leads to similar manifestations.[134] Damage to the alveolar and capillary membranes initiates a cascade of events leading to fluid transudation that often is accompanied by pulmonary venoconstriction. Direct injury to the alveolar and capillary membranes can result from pulmonary aspiration of gastric contents and perhaps oxygen toxicity. Indirect toxicity

can result from humoral and cellular mechanisms caused by triggers such as sepsis and amniotic fluid embolism. Transudation of fluid leads to atelectasis, airway obstruction, reduced lung compliance, and altered ventilation-perfusion relationship. Both physiologic dead space and shunt fractions are increased.

Diagnosis

A variety of disorders can cause acute respiratory failure during pregnancy (Box 51.4). Specific diagnostic criteria depend on the disorder.

The diagnosis of ARDS requires the exclusion of other disorders and can be made with reference to the **Berlin Criteria**. Prominent characteristics include arterial hypoxemia, radiographic evidence of bilateral pulmonary opacities, and nonhydrostatic pulmonary edema within 1 week of a recognized predisposing condition (see Chapter 53).[135]

BOX 51.4 Etiology of Respiratory Failure During Pregnancy

Acute Respiratory Distress Syndrome
- Infection
  - Bacterial, viral, or fungal pneumonia
  - Endometritis
  - Pyelonephritis
  - Skin and/or soft tissue infection
  - Sepsis
- Preeclampsia
- Hemorrhage
  - Multiple transfusions/transfusion-related acute lung injury
  - Disseminated intravascular coagulation
- Aspiration of gastric contents
- Embolism
- Trauma
- Burns
- Drowning
- Intracranial hemorrhage
- Reperfusion injury
- Inhalational injury
- Pancreatitis
- Drugs
  - Salicylates
  - Opioids
- Fat embolization

Asthma

Pulmonary Embolism
- Thromboembolism
- Amniotic fluid embolism
- Venous air embolism

Cystic Fibrosis

Pulmonary Edema
- Beta-adrenergic receptor agonists (e.g., ritodrine, terbutaline)
- Transfusion-associated acute circulatory overload
- Preeclampsia/eclampsia
- Magnesium
- Cardiogenic

Interaction With Pregnancy

Pregnancy is not known to alter the overall course of respiratory failure. However, differences in outcome between pregnant and nonpregnant patients have been observed in subsets of patients with respiratory failure. In a series of patients with **severe acute respiratory syndrome**, pregnant patients had greater morbidity and mortality.[136] The **coronavirus disease 2019 (COVID-19)** pandemic was associated with substantially increased risks of ARDS, critical illness-related morbidity, and mortality across all patients affected, including pregnant women.[137,138] A cross-sectional study demonstrated a 33.3% increase in maternal deaths after the onset of the COVID-19 pandemic, with a shift to indirect causes of death, including viral and respiratory disease, and a 41% increase in late maternal mortality.[139]

Although delivery of the infant has been suggested as a method to improve maternal respiratory status in patients with ARDS, evidence indicates that improvement in ventilator parameters depends on the gestational age and may not result in a clinically significant reduction in airway pressures or increase in oxygenation.[140,141] The most significant effect of respiratory failure on pregnancy is a reduction in oxygen delivery to the fetus. This reduction results most commonly from maternal arterial hypoxemia or maternal hypotension, which often accompanies respiratory failure. Hypotension may result from associated underlying conditions or from elevated mean airway pressures during mechanical ventilation. High rates of prenatal complications with or without preterm delivery have been reported.[133,142,143]

Medical Management

Therapeutic strategies for managing respiratory failure during pregnancy do not differ qualitatively from those in nonpregnant patients. The primary goals of medical management are to (1) eliminate predisposing conditions, (2) limit fluid transudation, and (3) maintain maternal oxygen delivery. Fluid restriction and diuretics help limit fluid transudation, although this therapy must be used cautiously when the underlying cause of respiratory failure is associated with intravascular fluid depletion. The goals for maintenance of oxygen delivery may differ quantitatively during pregnancy. Oxygen delivery to the fetus worsens significantly when Pao_2 decreases to less than 70 mm Hg (9.3 kPa) or oxygen saturation (Sao_2) falls below 95%.[132] Standard methods of maintaining oxygen delivery include (1) administration of a higher inspired concentration of oxygen, (2) administration of bronchodilators in the presence of reversible airway obstruction, (3) administration of pharmacologic agents to support the circulation as needed, and (4) mechanical ventilation. A higher inspired oxygen concentration, delivered by face mask, is safe during pregnancy and may obviate the necessity of tracheal intubation and associated risks for aspiration and difficult airway management. Bronchodilator therapy can also be used for respiratory failure, as described earlier for asthma. Pharmacologic agents for circulatory support include drugs with both alpha- and beta-adrenergic receptor activity.

Indications for tracheal intubation and mechanical ventilation are similar for pregnant and nonpregnant patients with respiratory failure.[136,144] Maternal and fetal effects of current approaches to mechanical ventilation, including use of low tidal volumes and permissive hypercapnia, have not been studied in pregnant patients. Positive end-expiratory pressure may be used if cardiac output is maintained to allow sufficient blood flow to the uterus.

Some pregnant patients with respiratory failure do not show adequate response to conventional methods of treatment. For these patients, treatment options include ECMO,[145] high-frequency oscillatory ventilation,[146] and inhaled **nitric oxide**.[147] Nitric oxide relaxes vascular smooth muscle. Rapid inactivation of nitric oxide by binding to hemoglobin in the circulation allows inhaled nitric oxide to produce pulmonary vasodilation without systemic vascular effects. Selective pulmonary vasodilation in well-ventilated areas of the lung presumably improves oxygen delivery. The safety of these alternative forms of treatment in pregnancy is unknown because reports of their use are anecdotal.

Obstetric Management

Pregnant women with ARDS have increased risks for preterm delivery, low-birth-weight infants, and neonatal intensive care unit stay.[129,148] Fetal heart rate monitoring practices vary across institutions ranging from once every several days to continuous, owing to lack of evidence-based consensus guidelines. The frequency of monitoring should be determined based on multidisciplinary input on an individual basis, considering the gestational age, etiology of illness, and patient wishes.[149,150] Because the beneficial effects of delivery on the course of respiratory failure have not been proven, indications for induction of labor or cesarean delivery in this setting are not well defined. Observational studies have not clearly shown an association between delivery and improved respiratory status in pregnant women with respiratory failure.[134,151–153] In general, prolonging the pregnancy up to 32 weeks' gestation is favored to avoid the morbidity of preterm delivery, to allow the fetus to grow and to reduce neonatal complications.[154,155]

Data to support decisions regarding mode of delivery are limited. The majority of women with severe ARDS have cesarean delivery; however, vaginal delivery is possible during mechanical ventilation[141,154,156–158] and may avoid complications of major intraabdominal surgery in a critically ill woman. If the plan is to pursue an induction of labor, fluid restriction and optimization of oxygenation and hemodynamics are of paramount importance.

Anesthetic Management

The anesthetic management of patients with respiratory failure requires appropriate medical management. During labor, analgesia for mechanically ventilated patients can be achieved with intravenous opioids, which are often used for sedation during mechanical ventilation. Lumbar epidural analgesia provides pain relief without the neonatal respiratory depression associated with high doses of opioids. Labor epidural analgesia also reduces oxygen consumption,[159] which may be beneficial in hypoxemic patients. The use of labor epidural analgesia in patients with respiratory failure depends on underlying conditions and ongoing therapy. Close attention should be paid to intravascular volume, adequacy of coagulation, and presence or absence of infection. For women receiving ECMO, it may be necessary to withhold systemic anticoagulation and assess coagulation

function before administration of neuraxial analgesia or anesthesia to reduce the risk of spinal epidural hematoma.[160,161]

In mechanically ventilated patients, general endotracheal anesthesia is often the most convenient choice for cesarean delivery. Aside from the issues of medical management (see earlier discussion), the techniques and pharmacologic agents do not differ substantially from those used in patients without respiratory failure.

KEY POINTS

- Patients with asthma, infection, respiratory failure, or cystic fibrosis and patients who smoke cigarettes may have reversible airway obstruction.
- In patients with airway hyperresponsiveness, tracheal intubation provides one of the greatest stimuli for bronchospasm during the perioperative period.
- Inhaled beta$_2$-adrenergic agonists are the most effective therapy for perioperative bronchospasm.
- Most bronchodilators also produce uterine relaxation. However, their administration by aerosol minimizes their effects on uterine tone.

- Neuraxial anesthesia is often the anesthetic technique of choice in patients with respiratory disease because it does not require tracheal intubation.
- Techniques of neuraxial anesthesia should be modified to reduce the likelihood of a high thoracic motor block in patients with significant respiratory disease.
- Pregnant women with acute respiratory failure may be managed with standard therapies as well as rescue measures for refractory hypoxemia to maintain the pregnancy; however, in some cases delivery may be considered.

REFERENCES

1. Guidelines for the diagnosis and management of asthma 2007 (EPR-3). National Heart, Lung, and Blood Institute; 2007. https://www.epa.gov/sites/default/files/2014-09/documents/asthgdln.pdf. Accessed September 14, 2023.
2. Global initiative for asthma: global strategy for asthma management and prevention. Updated 2023. https://ginasthma.org/wp-content/uploads/2023/07/GINA-2023-Full-report-23_07_06-WMS.pdf. Accessed September 14, 2023.
3. Pate CA, Zahran HS, Qin X, et al. Asthma surveillance—United States, 2006-2018. *MMWR Surveill Summ*. 2021; 70:1–32.
4. Kwon HL, Triche EW, Belanger K, Bracken MB. The epidemiology of asthma during pregnancy: prevalence, diagnosis, and symptoms. *Immunol Allergy Clin North Am*. 2006;26:29–62.
5. Flores KF, Bandoli G, Chambers CD, et al. Asthma prevalence among women aged 18 to 44 in the United States: national health and nutrition examination survey 2001–2016. *J Asthma*. 2020;57:693–702.
6. Melén E, Pershagen G. Pathophysiology of asthma: lessons from genetic research with particular focus on severe asthma. *J Intern Med*. 2012;272:108–120.
7. Vincenc KS, Black JL, Yan K, et al. Comparison of in vivo and in vitro responses to histamine in human airways. *Am Rev Respir Dis*. 1983;128:875–879.
8. Armour CL, Lazar NM, Schellenberg RR, et al. A comparison of in vivo and in vitro human airway reactivity to histamine. *Am Rev Respir Dis*. 1984;129:907–910.
9. Skloot G, Permutt S, Togias A. Airway hyperresponsiveness in asthma: a problem of limited smooth muscle relaxation with inspiration. *J Clin Invest*. 1995;96:2393–2403.
10. Pincus AB, Fryer AD, Jacoby DB. Mini review: neural mechanisms underlying airway hyperresponsiveness. *Neurosci Lett*. 2021;751:135795.

11. Fryer AD, Jacoby DB. Parainfluenza virus infection damages inhibitory M2 muscarinic receptors on pulmonary parasympathetic nerves in the guinea-pig. *Br J Pharmacol*. 1991;102:267–271.
12. Sorkness R, Clough JJ, Castleman WL, Lemanske RF Jr. Virus-induced airway obstruction and parasympathetic hyperresponsiveness in adult rats. *Am J Respir Crit Care Med*. 1994;150:28–34.
13. van der Velden VH, Hulsmann AR. Autonomic innervation of human airways: structure, function, and pathophysiology in asthma. *Neuroimmunomodulation*. 1999;6:145–159.
14. Tattersfield AE, Leaver DG, Pride NB. Effects of beta-adrenergic blockade and stimulation on normal human airways. *J Appl Physiol*. 1973;35:613–619.
15. Spina D, Rigby PJ, Paterson JW, Goldie RG. Alpha 1-adrenoceptor function and autoradiographic distribution in human asthmatic lung. *Br J Pharmacol*. 1989;97:701–708.
16. Krishnakumar S, Holmes EP, Moore RM, et al. Non-adrenergic non-cholinergic excitatory innervation in the airways: role of neurokinin-2 receptors. *Auton Autacoid Pharmacol*. 2002;22:215–224.
17. Belvisi MG, Stretton CD, Yacoub M, Barnes PJ. Nitric oxide is the endogenous neurotransmitter of bronchodilator nerves in humans. *Eur J Pharmacol*. 1992;210:221–222.
18. Lammers JW, Minette P, McCusker MT, et al. Capsaicin-induced bronchodilation in mild asthmatic subjects: possible role of nonadrenergic inhibitory system. *J Appl Physiol*. 1989; 67:856–861.
19. Kraan J, Vink-Klooster H, Postma DS. The NK-2 receptor antagonist SR 48968c does not improve adenosine hyper-responsiveness and airway obstruction in allergic asthma. *Clin Exp Allergy*. 2001;31:274–278.
20. Hogg JC, James AL, Pare PD. Evidence for inflammation in asthma. *Am Rev Respir Dis*. 1991;143:S39–S42.
21. Tattersfield AE, Knox AJ, Britton JR, Hall IP. Asthma. *Lancet*. 2002;360:1313–1322.

22. Bergner A, Kellner J, Kemp da Silva A, et al. Bronchial hyperreactivity is correlated with increased baseline airway tone. *Eur J Med Res.* 2006;11:77–84.

23. Hogg JC. Pathology of asthma. *J Allergy Clin Immunol.* 1993;92:1–5.

24. Knight DA, Holgate ST. The airway epithelium: structural and functional properties in health and disease. *Respirology.* 2003;8:432–446.

25. Qin XQ, Xiang Y, Liu C, et al. The role of bronchial epithelial cells in airway hyperresponsiveness. *Sheng Li Xue Bao.* 2007;59:454–464.

26. Expert Panel Working Group of the National Heart, Lung, and Blood Institute (NHLBI) administered and coordinated National Asthma Education and Prevention Program Coordinating Committee (NAEPPCC), Cloutier MM, Baptist AP, et al. 2020 focused updates to the Asthma Management Guidelines: a report from the National Asthma Education and Prevention Program Coordinating Committee Expert Panel Working Group. *J Allergy Clin Immunol.* 2020; 146:1217–1270.

27. Schatz M, Dombrowski MP, Wise R, et al. Asthma morbidity during pregnancy can be predicted by severity classification. *J Allergy Clin Immunol.* 2003;112:283–288.

28. Teeter JG, Bleecker ER. Relationship between airway obstruction and respiratory symptoms in adult asthmatics. *Chest.* 1998;113:272–277.

29. Stevens DR, Perkins N, Chen Z, et al. Determining the clinical course of asthma in pregnancy. *J Allergy Clin Immunol Pract.* 2022;10:793–802.e10.

30. Hellings PW, Vandekerckhove P, Claeys R, et al. Progesterone increases airway eosinophilia and hyper-responsiveness in a murine model of allergic asthma. *Clin Exp Allergy.* 2003;33:1457–1463.

31. Wang G, Murphy VE, Namazy J, et al. The risk of maternal and placental complications in pregnant women with asthma: a systematic review and meta-analysis. *J Matern Fetal Neonatal Med.* 2014;27:934–942.

32. Murphy VE, Namazy JA, Powell H, et al. A meta-analysis of adverse perinatal outcomes in women with asthma. *BJOG.* 2011;118:1314–1323.

33. Murphy VE, Gibson PG, Smith R, Clifton VL. Asthma during pregnancy: mechanisms and treatment implications. *Eur Respir J.* 2005;25:731–750.

34. Wang YX, Varraso R, Dumas O, et al. Hypertensive disorders of pregnancy and risk of asthma and chronic obstructive pulmonary disease: a prospective cohort study. *Lancet Reg Health Am.* 2023;23:100540.

35. Chipps BE, Murphy KR, Oppenheimer J. 2020 NAEPP guidelines update and GINA 2021—asthma care differences, overlap, and challenges. *J Allergy Clin Immunol Pract.* 2022;10:S19–S30.

36. Bonham CA, Patterson KC, Strek ME. Asthma outcomes and management during pregnancy. *Chest.* 2018;153:515–527.

37. Eltonsy S, Forget A, Beauchesne MF, Blais L. Risk of congenital malformations for asthmatic pregnant women using a long-acting β_2-agonist and inhaled corticosteroid combination versus higher-dose inhaled corticosteroid monotherapy. *J Allergy Clin Immunol.* 2015;135:123–130.

38. Bukowskyj M, Nakatsu K, Munt PW. Theophylline reassessed. *Ann Intern Med.* 1984;101:63–73.

39. Gluck JC, Gluck PA. Asthma controller therapy during pregnancy. *Am J Obstet Gynecol.* 2005;192:369–380.

40. Carter BL, Driscoll CE, Smith GD. Theophylline clearance during pregnancy. *Obstet Gynecol.* 1986;68:555–559.

41. Barsky HE. Asthma and pregnancy. A challenge for everyone concerned. *Postgrad Med.* 1991;89:125–132.

42. Gourgoulianis KI, Chatziparasidis G, Chatziefthimiou A, Molyvdas PA. Magnesium as a relaxing factor of airway smooth muscles. *J Aerosol Med.* 2001;14:301–307.

43. Rowe BH, Camargo CA Jr. The role of magnesium sulfate in the acute and chronic management of asthma. *Curr Opin Pulm Med.* 2008;14:70–76.

44. Barnes PJ. Molecular mechanisms and cellular effects of glucocorticosteroids. *Immunol Allergy Clin North Am.* 2005;25:451–468.

45. Berry M, Morgan A, Shaw DE, et al. Pathological features and inhaled corticosteroid response of eosinophilic and non-eosinophilic asthma. *Thorax.* 2007;62:1043–1049.

46. Bel EH, Timmers MC, Zwinderman AH, et al. The effect of inhaled corticosteroids on the maximal degree of airway narrowing to methacholine in asthmatic subjects. *Am Rev Respir Dis.* 1991;143:109–113.

47. Namazy JA, Murphy VE, Powell H, et al. Effects of asthma severity, exacerbations and oral corticosteroids on perinatal outcomes. *Eur Respir J.* 2013;41:1082–1090.

48. Schatz M, Dombrowski MP, Wise R, et al. The relationship of asthma medication use to perinatal outcomes. *J Allergy Clin Immunol.* 2004;113:1040–1045.

49. Greenberger PA. Asthma during pregnancy. *J Asthma.* 1990;27:341–347.

50. Barnes NC. The properties of inhaled corticosteroids: similarities and differences. *Prim Care Respir J.* 2007;16: 149–154.

51. Nelsen LM, Shields KE, Cunningham ML, et al. Congenital malformations among infants born to women receiving montelukast, inhaled corticosteroids, and other asthma medications. *J Allergy Clin Immunol.* 2012;129:251–254.e1–e6.

52. Namazy JA, Blais L, Andrews EB, et al. Pregnancy outcomes in the omalizumab pregnancy registry and a disease-matched comparator cohort. *J Allergy Clin Immunol.* 2020;145: 528–536.e1.

53. Mathe AA, Hedqvist P. Effect of prostaglandins F2 alpha and E2 on airway conductance in healthy subjects and asthmatic patients. *Am Rev Respir Dis.* 1975;111:313–320.

54. Ishimura M, Kataoka S, Suda M, et al. Effects of KP-496, a novel dual antagonist for leukotriene D4 and thromboxane A2 receptors, on contractions induced by various agonists in the guinea pig trachea. *Allergol Int.* 2006;55:403–410.

55. Kreisman H, Van de Weil W, Mitchell CA. Respiratory function during prostaglandin-induced labor. *Am Rev Respir Dis.* 1975;111:564–566.

56. Tilley SL, Hartney JM, Erikson CJ, et al. Receptors and pathways mediating the effects of prostaglandin E2 on airway tone. *Am J Physiol Lung Cell Mol Physiol.* 2003;284:L599–L606.

57. American College of Obstetrician and Gynecologists. Practice Bulletin No. 222: Gestational hypertension and preeclampsia (reaffirmed 2023). *Obstet Gynecol.* 2020;135:e237–e260.

58. Leff AR. Endogenous regulation of bronchomotor tone. *Am Rev Respir Dis.* 1988;137:1198–1216.

59. Belvisi MG, Rogers DF, Barnes PJ. Neurogenic plasma extravasation: inhibition by morphine in guinea pig airways in vivo. *J Appl Physiol.* 1989;66:268–272.

60. Otulana B, Okikawa J, Linn L, et al. Safety and pharmacokinetics of inhaled morphine delivered using the AERx system in patients with moderate-to-severe asthma. *Int J Clin Pharmacol Ther.* 2004;42:456–462.

61. Groeben H, Schlicht M, Stieglitz S, et al. Both local anesthetics and salbutamol pretreatment affect reflex bronchoconstriction in volunteers with asthma undergoing awake fiberoptic intubation. *Anesthesiology.* 2002;97:1445–1450.

62. Lirk P, Kleber N, Mitterschiffthaler G, et al. Pulmonary effects of bupivacaine, ropivacaine, and levobupivacaine in parturients undergoing spinal anaesthesia for elective caesarean delivery: a randomised controlled study. *Int J Obstet Anesth.* 2010;19:287–292.

63. Knox AJ, Campos-Gongora H, Wisniewski A, et al. Modification of bronchial reactivity by physiological concentrations of plasma epinephrine. *J Appl Physiol.* 1992;73:1004–1007.

64. Pflug AE, Halter JB. Effect of spinal anesthesia on adrenergic tone and the neuroendocrine responses to surgical stress in humans. *Anesthesiology.* 1981;55:120–126.

65. Emerman CL, Cydulka RK. Changes in serum catecholamine levels during acute bronchospasm. *Ann Emerg Med.* 1993;22:1836–1841.

66. Que JC, Lusaya VO. Sevoflurane induction for emergency cesarean section in a parturient in status asthmaticus. *Anesthesiology.* 1999;90:1475–1476.

67. Brown RH, Wagner EM. Mechanisms of bronchoprotection by anesthetic induction agents: propofol versus ketamine. *Anesthesiology.* 1999;90:822–828.

68. Groeben H, Schwalen A, Irsfeld S, et al. Intravenous lidocaine and bupivacaine dose-dependently attenuate bronchial hyperreactivity in awake volunteers. *Anesthesiology.* 1996;84:533–539.

69. Groeben H, Silvanus MT, Beste M, Peters J. Combined intravenous lidocaine and inhaled salbutamol protect against bronchial hyperreactivity more effectively than lidocaine or salbutamol alone. *Anesthesiology.* 1998;89:862–868.

70. Mercier FJ, Naline E, Bardou M, et al. Relaxation of proximal and distal isolated human bronchi by halothane, isoflurane and desflurane. *Eur Respir J.* 2002;20:286–292.

71. Duracher C, Blanc FX, Gueugniaud PY, et al. The effects of isoflurane on airway smooth muscle crossbridge kinetics in Fisher and Lewis rats. *Anesth Analg.* 2005;101:136.

72. Warner DO, Vettermann J, Brichant JF, Rehder K. Direct and neurally mediated effects of halothane on pulmonary resistance in vivo. *Anesthesiology.* 1990;72:1057–1063.

73. Park KW, Dai HB, Lowenstein E, Sellke FW. Epithelial dependence of the bronchodilatory effect of sevoflurane and desflurane in rat distal bronchi. *Anesth Analg.* 1998;86:646–651.

74. Burburan SM, Xisto DG, Ferreira HC, et al. Lung mechanics and histology during sevoflurane anesthesia in a model of chronic allergic asthma. *Anesth Analg.* 2007;104:631–637.

75. Rooke GA, Choi JH, Bishop MJ. The effect of isoflurane, halothane, sevoflurane, and thiopental/nitrous oxide on respiratory system resistance after tracheal intubation. *Anesthesiology.* 1997;86:1294–1299.

76. Satoh J, Yamakage M. Desflurane induces airway contraction mainly by activating transient receptor potential A1 of sensory C-fibers. *J Anesth.* 2009;23:620–623.

77. Satoh JI, Yamakage M, Kobayashi T, et al. Desflurane but not sevoflurane can increase lung resistance via tachykinin pathways. *Br J Anaesth.* 2009;102:704–713.

78. Bayable SD, Melesse DY, Lema GF, Ahmed SA. Perioperative management of patients with asthma during elective surgery: a systematic review. *Ann Med Surg (Lond).* 2021;70:102874.

79. Cnattingius S. The epidemiology of smoking during pregnancy: smoking prevalence, maternal characteristics, and pregnancy outcomes. *Nicotine Tob Res.* 2004;6:S125–S140.

80. Martin JA, Osterman MJK, Driscoll AK. Declines in cigarette smoking during pregnancy in the United States, 2016–2021. *NCHS Data Brief.* 2023(458):1–8.

81. Head SK, Zaganjor I, Kofie JN, et al. Patterns and trends in use of electronic nicotine delivery systems before and during pregnancy: pregnancy risk assessment monitoring system, United States, 2016-2019. *J Community Health.* 2022;47:351–360.

82. Carrick MA, Robson JM, Thomas C. Smoking and anaesthesia. *BJA Educ.* 2019;19:1–6.

83. Grønkjær M, Eliasen M, Skov-Ettrup LS, et al. Preoperative smoking status and postoperative complications: a systematic review and meta-analysis. *Ann Surg.* 2014;259:52–71.

84. Tsai M, Byun MK, Shin J, Crotty Alexander LE. Effects of e-cigarettes and vaping devices on cardiac and pulmonary physiology. *J Physiol.* 2020;598:5039–5062.

85. Xie W, Tackett AP, Berlowitz JB, et al. Association of electronic cigarette use with respiratory symptom development among U.S. young adults. *Am J Respir Crit Care Med.* 2022;205:1320–1329.

86. Das TK, Moutquin JM, Parent JG. Effect of cigarette smoking on maternal airway function during pregnancy. *Am J Obstet Gynecol.* 1991;165:675–679.

87. Tyrrell J, Huikari V, Christie JT, et al. Genetic variation in the 15q25 nicotinic acetylcholine receptor gene cluster (CHRNA5-CHRNA3-CHRNB4) interacts with maternal self-reported smoking status during pregnancy to influence birth weight. *Hum Mol Gen.* 2012;21:5344–5358.

88. McEvoy CT, Spindel ER. Pulmonary effects of maternal smoking on the fetus and child: effects on lung development, respiratory morbidities, and life long lung health. *Paediatr Respir Rev.* 2017;21:27–33.

89. Ozekin YH, Saal ML, Pineda RH, et al. Intrauterine exposure to nicotine through maternal vaping disrupts embryonic lung and skeletal development via the Kcnj2 potassium channel. *Dev Biol.* 2023;501:111–123.

90. Gould GS, Havard A, Lim LL, et al. Exposure to tobacco, environmental tobacco smoke and nicotine in pregnancy: a pragmatic overview of reviews of maternal and child outcomes, effectiveness of interventions and barriers and facilitators to quitting. *Int J Env Res Public Health.* 2020;17:2034.

91. Claire R, Chamberlain C, Davey MA, et al. Pharmacological interventions for promoting smoking cessation during pregnancy. *Cochrane Database Syst Rev.* 2020;(3):CD010078.

92. Das TK, Moutquin JM, Lindsay C, et al. Effects of smoking cessation on maternal airway function and birth weight. *Obstet Gynecol.* 1998;92:201–205.

93. American College of Obstetricians and Gynecologists. Committee Opinion N. 807: Tobacco and nicotine cessation during pregnancy (reaffirmed 2023). *Obstet Gynecol.* 2020;135:e221–e229.

94. Kim ES, Bishop MJ. Endotracheal intubation, but not laryngeal mask airway insertion, produces reversible bronchoconstriction. *Anesthesiology*. 1999;90:391–394.

95. Goff MJ, Arain SR, Ficke DJ, et al. Absence of bronchodilation during desflurane anesthesia: a comparison to sevoflurane and thiopental. *Anesthesiology*. 2000;93:404–408.

96. Knapp EA, Fink AK, Goss CH, et al. The Cystic Fibrosis Foundation patient registry. Design and methods of a national observational disease registry. *Ann Am Thorac Soc*. 2016;13:1173–1179.

97. Stephenson AL, Swaleh S, Sykes J, et al. Contemporary cystic fibrosis incidence rates in Canada and the United States. *J Cyst Fibros*. 2023;22:443–449.

98. Heltshe SL, Godfrey EM, Josephy T, et al. Pregnancy among cystic fibrosis women in the era of CFTR modulators. *J Cyst Fibros*. 2017;16:687–694.

99. Shteinberg M, Lulu AB, Downey DG, et al. Failure to conceive in women with CF is associated with pancreatic insufficiency and advancing age. *J Cyst Fibros*. 2019;18:525–529.

100. Hwang TC, Lu L, Zeitlin PL, et al. Cl⁻ channels in CF: lack of activation by protein kinase C and cAMP-dependent protein kinase. *Science*. 1989;244:1351–1353.

101. Li M, McCann JD, Liedtke CM, et al. Cyclic AMP-dependent protein kinase opens chloride channels in normal but not cystic fibrosis airway epithelium. *Nature*. 1988;331:358–360.

102. Riordan JR, Rommens JM, Kerem B, et al. Identification of the cystic fibrosis gene: cloning and characterization of complementary DNA. *Science*. 1989;245:1066–1073.

103. Konstan MW, Hilliard KA, Norvell TM, Berger M. Bronchoalveolar lavage findings in cystic fibrosis patients with stable, clinically mild lung disease suggest ongoing infection and inflammation. *Am J Respir Crit Care Med*. 1994;150:448–454.

104. Flume PA, Strange C, Ye X, et al. Pneumothorax in cystic fibrosis. *Chest*. 2005;128:720–728.

105. Freedman SD, Blanco PG, Zaman MM, et al. Association of cystic fibrosis with abnormalities in fatty acid metabolism. *N Engl J Med*. 2004;350:560–569.

106. Farrell PM, White TB, Ren CL, et al. Diagnosis of cystic fibrosis: consensus guidelines from the cystic fibrosis foundation. *J Pediatr*. 2017;181S:S4–S15.e1.

107. Kerem E, Reisman J, Corey M, et al. Prediction of mortality in patients with cystic fibrosis. *N Engl J Med*. 1992;326:1187–1191.

108. Ahluwalia M, Hoag JB, Hadeh A, et al. Cystic fibrosis and pregnancy in the modern era: a case control study. *J Cyst Fibros*. 2014;13:69–73.

109. Renton M, Priestley L, Bennett L, et al. Pregnancy outcomes in cystic fibrosis: a 10-year experience from a UK centre. *Obstet Med*. 2015;8:99–101.

110. Geake J, Tay G, Callaway L, Bell SC. Pregnancy and cystic fibrosis: approach to contemporary management. *Obstet Med*. 2014;7:147–155.

111. Reynaud Q, Rousset Jablonski C, Poupon-Bourdy S, et al. Pregnancy outcome in women with cystic fibrosis and poor pulmonary function. *J Cyst Fibros*. 2020;19:80–83.

112. Ashcroft A, Chapman SJ, Mackillop L. The outcome of pregnancy in women with cystic fibrosis: a UK population-based descriptive study. *BJOG*. 2020;127:1696–1703.

113. Padoan RF, Quattrucci S, Amato A, et al. Perinatal outcomes in women with cystic fibrosis: data from the Italian Cystic Fibrosis Registry. *Acta Obstet Gynecol Scand*. 2021;100:1439–1444.

114. Gur M, Pollak M, Bar-Yoseph R, Bentur L. Pregnancy in cystic fibrosis—past, present, and future. *J Clin Med*. 2023;12:1468.

115. Reeves EP, Molloy K, Pohl K, McElvaney NG. Hypertonic saline in treatment of pulmonary disease in cystic fibrosis. *ScientificWorldJournal*. 2012;2012:465230.

116. Ramsey BW, Pepe MS, Quan JM, et al. Intermittent administration of inhaled tobramycin in patients with cystic fibrosis. Cystic Fibrosis Inhaled Tobramycin Study Group. *N Engl J Med*. 1999;340:23–30.

117. McArdle JR, Talwalkar JS. Macrolides in cystic fibrosis. *Clin Chest Med*. 2007;28:347–360.

118. Liou TG, Adler FR, Cox DR, Cahill BC. Lung transplantation and survival in children with cystic fibrosis. *N Engl J Med*. 2007;357:2143–2152.

119. Gyi KM, Hodson ME, Yacoub MY. Pregnancy in cystic fibrosis lung transplant recipients: case series and review. *J Cyst Fibros*. 2006;5:171–175.

120. Shaner J, Coscia LA, Constantinescu S, et al. Pregnancy after lung transplant. *Prog Transpl*. 2012;22:134–140.

121. Hyde NH, Harrison DM. Intrathecal morphine in a parturient with cystic fibrosis. *Anesth Analg*. 1986;65:1357–1358.

122. Franklin Dos Santos T, Rabassa A, Aljure O, Zbeidy R. Perioperative management and preemptive ECMO cannulation of a parturient with cystic fibrosis undergoing cesarean delivery. *Case Rep Anesthesiol*. 2020;2020:8814729.

123. von Ungern-Sternberg BS, Regli A, Bucher E, et al. The effect of epidural analgesia in labour on maternal respiratory function. *Anaesthesia*. 2004;59:350–353.

124. von Ungern-Sternberg BS, Regli A, Bucher E, et al. Impact of spinal anaesthesia and obesity on maternal respiratory function during elective caesarean section. *Anaesthesia*. 2004;59:743–749.

125. Deighan M, Ash S, McMorrow R. Anaesthesia for parturients with severe cystic fibrosis: a case series. *Int J Obstet Anesth*. 2014;23:75–79.

126. Jain R, Kazmerski TM, Zuckerwise LC, et al. Pregnancy in cystic fibrosis: review of the literature and expert recommendations. *J Cyst Fibros*. 2022;21:387–395.

127. Lapinsky SE. Management of acute respiratory failure in pregnancy. *Semin Respir Crit Care Med*. 2017;38:201–207.

128. Lapinsky SE. Acute respiratory failure in pregnancy. *Obstet Med*. 2015;8:126–132.

129. Watts A, Duarte AG. Acute respiratory distress syndrome in pregnancy: updates in principles and practice. *Clin Obstet Gynecol*. 2023;66:208–222.

130. Pollock W, Rose L, Dennis CL. Pregnant and postpartum admissions to the intensive care unit: a systematic review. *Intensive Care Med*. 2010;36:1465–1474.

131. Rush B, Martinka P, Kilb B, et al. Acute respiratory distress syndrome in pregnant women. *Obstet Gynecol*. 2017;129:530–535.

132. Cole DE, Taylor TL, McCullough DM, et al. Acute respiratory distress syndrome in pregnancy. *Crit Care Med*. 2005;33:S269–S278.

133. Muthu V, Agarwal R, Dhooria S, et al. Epidemiology, lung mechanics and outcomes of ARDS: a comparison between pregnant and non-pregnant subjects. *J Crit Care*. 2019;50:207–212.

134. Ware LB, Matthay MA. The acute respiratory distress syndrome. *N Engl J Med.* 2000;342:1334–1349.

135. ARDS Definition Task Force, Ranieri VM, Rubenfeld GD, et al. Acute respiratory distress syndrome: the Berlin Definition. *JAMA.* 2012;307:2526–2533.

136. Lam CM, Wong SF, Leung TN, et al. A case-controlled study comparing clinical course and outcomes of pregnant and non-pregnant women with severe acute respiratory syndrome. *BJOG.* 2004;111:771–774.

137. Ko JY, DeSisto CL, Simeone RM, et al. Adverse pregnancy outcomes, maternal complications, and severe illness among US delivery hospitalizations with and without a coronavirus disease 2019 (COVID-19) diagnosis. *Clin Infect Dis.* 2021;73:S24–S31.

138. Villar J, Ariff S, Gunier RB, et al. Maternal and neonatal morbidity and mortality among pregnant women with and without COVID-19 infection: the INTERCOVID multinational cohort study. *JAMA Pediatr.* 2021;175:817–826.

139. Thoma ME, Declercq ER. All-cause maternal mortality in the US before vs during the COVID-19 pandemic. *JAMA Netw Open.* 2022;5:e2219133.

140. Lapinski SE, Rojas-Suarez JA, Crozier TM, et al. Mechanical ventilation in critically-ill pregnant women: a case series. *Int J Obstet Anesth.* 2015;24:323–328.

141. Péju E, Belicard F, Silva S, et al. Management and outcomes of pregnant women admitted to intensive care unit for severe pneumonia related to SARS-CoV-2 infection: the multicenter and international COVIDPREG study. *Intensive Care Med.* 2022;48:1185–1196.

142. Mabie WC, Barton JR, Sibai BM. Adult respiratory distress syndrome in pregnancy. *Am J Obstet Gynecol.* 1992;167:950–957.

143. Catanzarite V, Willms D, Wong D, et al. Acute respiratory distress syndrome in pregnancy and the puerperium: causes, courses, and outcomes. *Obstet Gynecol.* 2001;97:760–764.

144. Deblieux PM, Summer WR. Acute respiratory failure in pregnancy. *Clin Obstet Gynecol.* 1996;39:143–152.

145. Nari P, Davies AR, Beca J, et al. Extracorporeal membrane oxygenation for severe ARDS in pregnant and postpartum women during the 2009 H1N1 pandemic. *Intensive Care Med.* 2011;37:648–654.

146. Raphael JH, Bexton MD. Combined high frequency ventilation in the management of respiratory failure in late pregnancy. *Anaesthesia.* 1993;48:596–598.

147. Huang S, DeSantis ER. Treatment of pulmonary arterial hypertension in pregnancy. *Am J Health Syst Pharm.* 2007;64:1922–1926.

148. Naoum EE, Chalupka A, Haft J, et al. Extracorporeal life support in pregnancy: a systematic review. *J Am Heart Assoc.* 2020;9:e016072.

149. American College of Obstetricians and Gynecologists. Practice Bulletin No. 211: Critical care in pregnancy (reaffirmed 2025). *Obstet Gynecol.* 2019;133:e303–e319.

150. Cypher RL. A standardized approach to electronic fetal monitoring in critical care obstetrics. *J Perinat Neonatal Nurs.* 2018;32:212–221.

151. Collop NA, Sahn SA. Critical illness in pregnancy. An analysis of 20 patients admitted to a medical intensive care unit. *Chest.* 1993;103:1548–1552.

152. Tomlinson MW, Caruthers TJ, Whitty JE, Gonik B. Does delivery improve maternal condition in the respiratory-compromised gravida? *Obstet Gynecol.* 1998;91:108–111.

153. Vasquez DN, Giannoni R, Salvatierra A, et al. Ventilatory parameters in obstetric patients with COVID-19 and impact of delivery: a multicenter prospective cohort study. *Chest.* 2023;163:554–566.

154. Aissi James S, Guervilly C, Lesouhaitier M, et al. Delivery decision in pregnant women rescued by ECMO for severe ARDS: a retrospective multicenter cohort study. *Crit Care.* 2022;26:312.

155. Resende MHF, Yarnell CJ, D'Souza R, et al. Clinical decision analysis of elective delivery vs expectant management for pregnant individuals with COVID-19-related acute respiratory distress syndrome. *Am J Obstet Gynecol MFM.* 2022;4:100697.

156. Jenkins TM, Troiano NH, Graves CR, et al. Mechanical ventilation in an obstetric population: characteristics and delivery rates. *Am J Obstet Gynecol.* 2003;188:549–552.

157. Pacheco LD, Gei AF, VanHook JW, et al. Burns in pregnancy. *Obstet Gynecol.* 2005;106:1210–1212.

158. Fatnic E, Blanco NL, Cobiletchi R, et al. Outcome predictors and patient progress following delivery in pregnant and postpartum patients with severe COVID-19 pneumonitis in intensive care units in Israel (OB-COVICU): a nationwide cohort study. *Lancet Respir Med.* 2023;11:520–529.

159. Ackerman WE 3rd, Molnar JM, Juneja MM. Beneficial effect of epidural anesthesia on oxygen consumption in a parturient with adult respiratory distress syndrome. *South Med J.* 1993;86:361–364.

160. Meng ML, Arendt KW, Banayan JM, et al. Anesthetic care of the pregnant patient with cardiovascular disease: a scientific statement from the American Heart Association. *Circulation.* 2023;147:e657–e673.

161. Leffert L, Butwick A, Carvalho B, et al. The Society for Obstetric Anesthesia and Perinatology consensus statement on the anesthetic management of pregnant and postpartum women receiving thromboprophylaxis or higher dose anticoagulants. *Anesth Analg.* 2018;126:928–944.

52

Substance Use Disorders

Roulhac D. Toledano, MD, PhD and Lisa R. Leffert, MD

CHAPTER OUTLINE

Substance use disorder describes a continuum of mild, moderate, or severe dependence on one or more licit or illicit substances. Estimates of the prevalence of maternal substance use vary depending on the specific substance, the maternal age group and other demographics, the extent of use, and the data source. According to the US National Survey on Drug Use and Health in 2022, 5.5% of pregnant women smoked cigarettes, 11.0% used alcohol, and 9.6% used illicit drugs in the past month, compared with 14.9%, 52.9%, and 21.0%, respectively, among nonpregnant women 15 to 44 years of age.[1] While the overall prevalence of substance use disorder during pregnancy has remained relatively stable over the past several years, the use of alternative forms of tobacco (e.g., e-cigarettes or vaping products) and marijuana has increased with increasing availability and legalization, and opioid use has increased fivefold, in parallel with the national opioid crisis.[2]

Anesthesia providers may encounter pregnant patients with substance use disorder during the peripartum period or during the administration of anesthesia for nonobstetric procedures during pregnancy. Depending on the substance, pregnant women may experience little to no acute or chronic adverse effects, or, alternatively, they may manifest systemic (e.g., cardiovascular, pulmonary, neurologic) and/or obstetric complications (e.g., intrauterine growth restriction, preterm labor, placental abruption, fetal death).[3–7] Patients with substance use disorder may also have heightened sensitivity to pain and/or tolerance to opioid analgesics,[8–11] which may impact acute postoperative pain management. Neonates of mothers with an opioid substance use disorder may experience neonatal opioid withdrawal syndrome.

DRUG DETECTION

Optimal care of patients with substance use disorder requires developing a therapeutic bond and identifying which substances have been taken.[12] Ideally, screening and testing for substance use should be integrated into prenatal care; those patients with a known untreated disorder should ideally be referred for antenatal anesthesiology consultation. Providers should ask questions in a respectful and nonjudgmental manner. It is vital to respect patient confidentiality, which may require speaking to the patient without family or friends present. Self-reporting typically underrepresents the true prevalence of drug use.[13–15] Therefore, healthcare providers should be familiar with the characteristic signs and symptoms associated with acute and chronic intoxication and withdrawal. Although analysis of urine, meconium, and hair are the most common methods to test pregnant patients and their infants for the presence of illicit drugs, analysis of saliva, umbilical cord tissue, amniotic fluid, and neonatal gastric aspirate can also be performed (Tables 52.1 and 52.2).[13–18] It is vital to understand which compounds a particular drug test identifies before interpreting the results. Caution should be used when interpreting toxicology test results after initiation of neuraxial labor analgesia with fentanyl; maternal neuraxial fentanyl may lead to positive toxicology tests, including maternal liquid chromatography specimens and neonatal urine screens.[19,20] Caregivers should also be aware that the immunoassays used in drug testing can have false-positive or false-negative results in the presence of structurally related drugs or additives. Gas chromatography with mass spectrometry ideally should be used to provide confirmation of positive results, when feasible.[15]

TABLE 52.1 Drug Detection: Overview

Specimen	Advantages	Limitations
Urine	Detection of diverse group of illicit substances (except volatile alcohols) Specimen and test readily available Short turnaround time (30 min at point of care; 2 h for laboratory specimens) More sensitive test (compared with meconium and hair) for cannabis	Underrepresents most illicit drug use Significant false-positive rate for phencyclidine Narrow detection window compared with that for meconium and hair Specimen can more easily be adulterated
Blood	Most commonly used for volatile alcohols (can detect other illicit substances) Specimen and test readily available	Invasive Narrow detection window compared with that for urine, meconium, and hair
Meconium	Highly sensitive (compared with urine testing) for cocaine and opioids Wide detection window No false-positive results for cocaine Noninvasive	Report may be delayed (days) Low sensitivity and specificity for detecting cannabinoids, heroin, and amphetamines via immunoassay
Hair	Highly sensitive test for detecting cocaine (3 times that of urine) and opioids Wide detection window (reflects chronic cumulative use) Samples can be stored at room temperature Samples can be analyzed remote from collection	Multiple hairs required; harvested close to scalp Environmental contamination may cause false-positive result Low sensitivity for detecting tetrahydrocannabinol and alcohol
Umbilical cord blood	Comparable to meconium with more rapid results May reflect a wide window of detection Ability to detect codeine, morphine, 6-MAM (heroin metabolite), and meconium Noninvasive	Specimen not available before delivery Lower sensitivity to methadone, cocaine, and opioids compared with meconium
Oral fluid	Highly sensitive for methamphetamine and other basic drugs Easy, noninvasive Primarily detects parent compound	If mouth is dry, salivary stimulation may be associated with a decreased drug concentration in oral fluid

6-MAM, 6-Monoacetylmorphine.
Data from references 13, 14, 16, 153, 244–248.

LICIT SUBSTANCES

Alcohol

Epidemiology

Since 1981, official advisories have warned against the use of alcohol by pregnant women or women considering pregnancy.[21] Yet the 2022 National Survey on Drug Use and Health noted that 11.0% of pregnant women 15 to 44 years of age reported past-month alcohol use; of those, 5.3% reported binge drinking.[22] Not all of these people have alcohol use disorder or are drinking alcohol recklessly. Some may not be aware that they are pregnant or may not be knowledgeable of the adverse effects of alcohol on their pregnancy.

Pharmacology

Alcohol is absorbed through the gastrointestinal tract, primarily within the small intestine, and is then metabolized by alcohol and acetaldehyde dehydrogenases.[23–25] This process leads to the production of acetaldehyde and the reduction of nicotinamide adenine dinucleotide (NAD^+) to NADH. The intracellular accumulation of NADH relative to NAD^+ contributes to metabolic derangements, including the inhibition of fatty acid oxidation (which may result in fatty liver) and the inhibition of gluconeogenesis (which can lead to hypoglycemia or lactic acidosis).

Systemic Effects

Legally defined "intoxication" implies a blood alcohol ≥ 80 mg/dL, although behavioral, cognitive, and psychomotor changes can occur at levels of 20 to 30 mg/dL (after one to two drinks) (Table 52.3).[23–25]

Alcohol has complex effects on the central nervous system (CNS); it acts as both a depressant and a stimulant through a variety of neurotransmitter pathways.[25] Consuming alcohol in conjunction with barbiturates or benzodiazepines compounds these effects. Endogenous opioids interact with alcohol to "reinforce" further alcohol use; this effect is blunted by opioid antagonists such as naltrexone, which can be used in the treatment of alcohol use disorder.

Alcohol and its metabolites (e.g., acetaldehyde) can be directly toxic to brain tissue.[23,24] Chronic alcoholism is associated with brain atrophy that results in impairment of memory, abstract problem-solving, verbal learning, and visual-spatial processing. Additional adverse neurologic effects result from vitamin (e.g., thiamine, vitamin B_{12}) deficiencies.

Heavy alcohol consumption can result in hepatic cirrhosis, which, in turn, can lead to encephalopathy, coagulopathy, and esophageal varices (Table 52.4). Gastrointestinal mucosal injury, pancreatitis, and cardiomyopathy may also occur.[7,24,26,27] In a retrospective cohort study of the Nationwide Inpatient Sample database in the United States, women with

TABLE 52.2	Drug Detection Window in Urine[a]	
Drug[b]	Analyte	Detection Window
Tobacco	Cotinine	19 h (urine $T_{1/2}$)
	Nicotine	2 h (urine $T_{1/2}$)
Cocaine	Cocaine	3–6 h
	Benzoylecgonine	IV use: 1–2 d
		Intranasal use: 2–3 d
Amphetamines	Amphetamine	1–3 d
	Methamphetamine	Smoked: 60 h
MDMA (ecstasy)	MDMA	1–3 d
Cannabis	Tetrahydrocannabinol	Smoked: 10 h
	11-Nor-9-carboxy-delta-9-tetrahydrocannabinol	Up to 25 d
LSD	LSD	24 h
	2-Oxo-3-OH-LSD	96 h
Heroin	6-Monoacetyl morphine	IV use: 2–4.5 h
	Morphine	19–54 h
Prescription opioids	Oxycodone	2–4 d
	Fentanyl	24–72 h
	Hydrocodone	2–4 d
Benzodiazepines	Flunitrazepam: 7-aminoflunitrazepam	<72 h
		Chronic use: 4–6 w
γ-Hydroxybutyric acid	Rapidly metabolized to CO_2 and H_2O	<12 h

IV, Intravenously; *LSD,* lysergic acid diethylamide; *MDMA,* methylenedioxymethamphetamine; $T_{1/2}$, half-life.

[a]Average values based on recent use; precise values may vary according to method of ingestion, assay employed, and duration of use.

[b]Detection of methadone, buprenorphine, oxycodone, and oxymorphone typically requires an additional screening test.

Data from references 4, 18, 94, 121, 249.

a diagnosis of alcohol use disorder undergoing cesarean delivery were twice as likely as women without alcohol use disorder to develop a hospital-acquired infection, including urinary tract infection or sepsis.[28] The underlying pathophysiology was not reported but could be attributable to an immunocompromised state.

Symptoms of acute alcohol withdrawal (e.g., nausea, vomiting, tachycardia, hypertension, arrhythmias, tremors, hallucinations, agitation, seizures) usually occur within 6 to 48 hours after cessation of chronic consumption (Table 52.5). Pharmacologic therapy to minimize the signs and symptoms of alcohol withdrawal includes the use of benzodiazepines and alpha$_2$-adrenergic receptor agonists (e.g., clonidine).[7]

Dexmedetomidine, a potent alpha$_2$-adrenergic receptor agonist, has also been investigated as an adjunct therapy.[29] The most severe condition associated with alcohol withdrawal, delirium tremens, manifests as agitation, disorientation, hallucinations, and fever combined with autonomic instability. Delirium tremens, though rare in pregnant women, can lead to maternal and fetal death if untreated.[7]

Effects on Pregnancy and the Fetus

Intrauterine alcohol exposure is the leading cause of preventable birth defects in the United States.[30,31] No safe level of alcohol consumption by pregnant women has been identified, as studies investigating minimal to moderate prenatal alcohol exposure during pregnancy have been limited by confounding variables.[32,33] *Fetal alcohol spectrum disorder* describes the range of effects that can occur in an individual whose mother drank alcohol during pregnancy. These effects include physical, mental, behavioral, and/or learning disabilities with possible lifelong implications.[34] *Fetal alcohol syndrome* (FAS) is a clinical diagnosis based on the presence of particular neonatal facial features (e.g., small palpebral fissures; flat mid-face with a short, upturned nose; thin upper lip) and significant impairment in neurodevelopment and physical growth.[30,35] A range of complications that occur with a high prevalence in children affected by FAS include disorders of conduct and language, chronic serous otitis media, and peripheral nerve abnormalities.[36] Education and screening for prenatal alcohol exposure can facilitate treatment and improve pregnancy outcomes by encouraging cessation of alcohol consumption as soon as pregnancy is recognized.

Anesthetic Management

Alcohol-intoxicated parturients are at increased risk for behavioral problems, electrolyte abnormalities, greater gastric acid secretion, and cointoxication with other substances.[7,26] Determining whether the patient can protect her airway is of paramount importance because acute intoxication increases the risk for pulmonary aspiration of gastric contents. In addition, these patients may have intravascular volume depletion secondary to vomiting, inadequate oral intake, diuresis, and hypoalbuminemia. Significant alcohol ingestion in the setting of poor oral intake may also manifest as severe hypoglycemia.[24,27,37]

Neuraxial analgesia or anesthesia can be safely administered for labor or cesarean delivery in patients with alcohol use disorder provided that (1) the patient is cooperative, (2) there is no evidence of coagulopathy (as a result of liver disease), (3) the patient is volume replete, and (4) baseline neurologic deficits (e.g., peripheral neuropathy, cognitive deficits) are assessed and documented.[7]

If emergency delivery is required and the patient is either uncooperative or too sedated to protect their airway, general anesthesia will be necessary. The patient should receive pharmacologic aspiration prophylaxis (e.g., nonparticulate antacid, histamine-2 [H$_2$]-receptor antagonist, metoclopramide) and should undergo a rapid-sequence induction of general anesthesia with tracheal intubation (see Chapter 26).

TABLE 52.3 Acute Intoxication and Organ Dysfunction

Substance	Neurologic	Cardiovascular	Pulmonary	Gastrointestinal	Hematologic	Other
Alcohol	↓ Cognition	–	↑ Risk for aspiration	–	–	↑ Cortisol ↓ Glucose
Tobacco	–	↑ HR, BP, myocardial work	↓ Tissue oxygenation secondary to ↑ carboxyhemoglobin ↓ Mucociliary clearance ↑ Airway irritability	–	–	Impaired wound healing
Caffeine	–	Mild ↑ BP in low doses	–	–	–	Diuresis
Cannabis	↓ Cognitive and motor performance	Biphasic autonomic effect ST-segment and T-wave changes on ECG	↑ HR If smoked: effects similar to those of tobacco	Appetite stimulation	–	Conjunctival vasodilation and reddening
Cocaine	Subarachnoid or intracranial hemorrhage Cerebral infarct Seizures	Hemodynamic instability, arrhythmias Acute myocardial infarction Aortic dissection	If free based: pulmonary edema and pulmonary hemorrhage If smoked: see "Tobacco" If snorted: nasal septal injury and epistaxis	↑ AST and ALT	↓ Platelets (?)	Infection ↑ Temperature ↑ Cortisol ↑ Glucose
Amphetamines	Seizures Stroke Paranoia Hallucinations	Similar to effects associated with cocaine	–	–	–	Proteinuria ↑ Temperature
Hallucinogens	Hallucinations Paranoia Intracerebral hemorrhage (rare) Seizures (rare)	Supraventricular tachycardia (rare) Acute myocardial infarction (rare)	–	–	–	–
Opioids	–	↓ HR ↓ BP Tachyarrhythmia Bradyarrhythmia	Respiratory depression	–	–	–
Volatile substances	Encephalopathy Seizures	Arrhythmias Acute myocardial infarction	Hypoxemia Bronchospasm Acute respiratory distress syndrome	Mucosal injury		Ethylene glycol ingestion Metabolic acidosis Renal failure

ALT, Alanine aminotransferase; AST, aspartate aminotransferase; BP, blood pressure; ECG, electrocardiogram; HR, heart rate; ↑, increase in; ↓, decrease in; ?, questionable.

TABLE 52.4	Organ System Effects of Chronic Substance Use Disorder					
Substance	**Neurologic**	**Cardiac**	**Pulmonary**	**Gastrointestinal**	**Hematologic**	**Other**
Alcohol	Peripheral neuropathy Brain atrophy Encephalopathy	Cardiomyopathy	—	Hepatitis Cirrhosis Gastric mucosal injury Pancreatitis	Anemia (± leukopenia, thrombocytopenia) Coagulopathy	↑ Cortisol
Tobacco	—	Atherosclerosis	Diffusion capacity abnormalities ↓ Pulmonary immune function ↑ Incidence of bronchitis, COPD ↑ Airway irritability ↑ Risk for lung cancer	—	—	—
Caffeine	Cessation may produce withdrawal headache	Does *not* negatively affect cardiac health at moderate dose	—	—	—	↑ Risk for bladder dysfunction with high dose
Cannabis	↓ Attention, memory ↓ Ability to process complex information	—	*If smoked:* effects similar to those associated with tobacco	↑ Rare forms of oropharyngeal cancer	—	—
Cocaine	Brain atrophy	Cardiomyopathy Myocarditis Blood vessel occlusion	*If smoked:* effects similar to those associated with tobacco *If snorted:* mucosal and nasal septal injury	Gastrointestinal ischemia/ulceration ↑ AST and ALT	↓ Platelets (?)	Renal failure
Amphetamines	Paranoid psychosis Impaired memory	—	—	—	—	↑ Tooth decay ("meth mouth")
Hallucinogens (episodic use)	Delayed hallucinations	—	—	—	—	—
Opioids	Abnormal pain sensitivity	Infective endocarditis	—	—	—	Hepatitis or HIV infection with exposure to contaminated needles
Volatile substances	Visual loss Cranial neuropathy Peripheral neuropathy Autonomic dysfunction Ataxia Brain atrophy Encephalopathy	Cardiomyopathy Acute myocardial infarction	—	Nonviral hepatitis Hepatocellular carcinoma	Aplastic anemia	"Glue-sniffer's" rash Renal failure

ALT, Alanine aminotransferase; *AST,* aspartate aminotransferase; *COPD,* chronic obstructive pulmonary disease; *HIV,* human immunodeficiency virus; ↑, increase in; ↓, decrease in; ?, questionable.

TABLE 52.5   Symptoms of and Treatment for Substance Use Withdrawal

Substance	Symptoms	Therapy
Alcohol (ethanol)	Nausea Vomiting Tachycardia Hypertension Tremor Hallucinations Agitation	Benzodiazepines and alpha$_2$-adrenergic agonist (e.g., clonidine)
	Delirium tremens: Autonomic instability/arrhythmias Seizures Severe tremors Disorientation Fever	Benzodiazepines and alpha$_2$-adrenergic receptor agonists (e.g., clonidine) Antiarrhythmics Anticonvulsants (e.g., phenytoin)
Tobacco	Cravings Irritability Headache Cough Insomnia	Nicotine replacement therapies, including patch, gum, and inhalers
Caffeine	Headache Anxiety Depressed mood Fatigue	Supportive care Caffeine ingestion
Cannabis	Mild abstinence syndrome Headache Restlessness Tremor Anxiety Autonomic effects	Supportive care
Cocaine	Prolonged sleep phase Hunger Anxiety Weakness Headache Tremors and seizures	Supportive care Reintroduction of drug, if necessary, with slow taper
Amphetamines	Fatigue Depression Hunger Intense cravings	Tricyclic antidepressants, dopaminergic agents (e.g., bromocriptine), and amino acid therapy (no therapy has proved to be successful)
Hallucinogens (e.g., phencyclidine, lysergic acid diethylamide)	No clearly associated withdrawal symptoms, although psychological dependence can occur	Not applicable
Opioids (e.g., heroin)	Flu-like symptoms, such as fatigue, weakness, restlessness, rhinorrhea, perspiration, fever, diarrhea	Supportive therapy Alpha$_2$-adrenergic agonists (e.g., clonidine) Doxepin Reintroduction of drug, if necessary, with slow taper
Volatile substances (e.g., ethylene glycol, toluene, glue)	Not applicable	Not applicable

Evidence from published reports is inconclusive about predictable differences in anesthetic requirements in patients with acute and chronic alcohol use.[38] Acute alcohol intoxication is believed to decrease anesthetic requirements, in part because of the additive effect of alcohol and other CNS depressants. Findings from two small studies suggest that the propofol dose required to induce anesthesia in chronic alcoholic patients is higher than in patients who drink alcohol socially.[39,40] However, no large population studies have assessed dose requirements for volatile anesthetic agents or hypnotic agents in patients who chronically drink alcohol.

Short-term consumption of alcohol inhibits the metabolism of drugs by the liver through competition for cytochrome P450, which results in higher plasma concentrations of hepatically metabolized drugs. *Long-term* consumption of alcohol increases the activity of cytochrome P450, resulting in decreased levels of medications such as diazepam and labetalol and increased levels of toxic metabolites from hepatic degradation of illicit drugs such as cocaine (see Chapter 16).[24] Both pregnancy and liver disease can lead to decreased plasma concentrations of pseudocholinesterase; however, this does not seem to have a clinically significant effect on the degradation of succinylcholine or ester local anesthetic agents.[38]

Pregnant women who regularly consume large amounts of alcohol and undergo general anesthesia for cesarean delivery may be at high risk for awareness under anesthesia.[41] The high doses of volatile anesthetic agents often recommended in nonpregnant, chronic alcohol-using patients can lead to significant uterine atony and potential increased blood loss. Therefore, a balanced anesthetic technique with a generous dose of hypnotic agent and optimal neuromuscular blockade (e.g., with succinylcholine) for induction, followed by maintenance with a volatile anesthetic agent (limited to 0.5 MAC [minimum alveolar concentration] after delivery to prevent uterine atony), nitrous oxide, and an opioid and benzodiazepine (for analgesia and amnesia) should be considered. For postoperative pain management, a transversus abdominis plane (TAP) block or alternative regional anesthetic technique (e.g., erector spinae plane block, quadratus lumborum block) may be performed, in conjunction with the administration of systemic nonopioid analgesic medications, to reduce or eliminate the use of opioids (see Chapter 27). Withholding additional muscle relaxation after induction and adding a brain function monitor if the circumstance permits may help identify patients who could benefit from additional anesthesia.[42]

Caffeine

Epidemiology

On a daily basis, 80% to 98% of women drink caffeine-containing beverages.[7,43] Dietary caffeine consumption during pregnancy is common in the United States, although the quantity appears to decrease after pregnancy recognition.[44]

Pharmacology

Caffeine (1,3,7-trimethylxanthine) is a naturally occurring alkaloid found in coffee, tea, cocoa, caffeinated soft drinks and energy drinks, and medicines.[43,45] The primary sources of caffeine in the adult diet are coffee (56 to 100 mg/100 mL if brewed) and tea (20 to 73 mg/100 mL). Caffeine is readily absorbed through the gastrointestinal tract and reaches maximum blood concentrations 1 to 1.5 hours after ingestion. Caffeine undergoes hepatic metabolism and is excreted in the urine.[43,45] In pregnancy, the half-life increases from 4 hours in the first trimester to 11.5 to 18 hours by the third trimester.[46] Caffeine crosses the placenta and can also be found in breast milk. The half-life in the neonate is prolonged compared with

that in children and in nonpregnant women. Habitual use of caffeine at levels greater than 500 to 600 mg/day is defined in some studies as abuse.[47,48]

Systemic Effects

Caffeine acts as an antagonist to the adenosine receptor. In the absence of the inhibitory effects of adenosine, the neurotransmitters norepinephrine, dopamine, and serotonin are released in increased concentrations.[43,49] Systemic effects of caffeine include CNS stimulation, changes in blood pressure and metabolic rate, and diuresis (see Table 52.3).[45] The side effects attributed to caffeine vary among individuals, in part related to the dose ingested and the chronicity of use. Studies of the effects of caffeine on alertness, vigilance, mood, and memory have produced inconsistent results.[43]

Moderate caffeine intake for nonpregnant women is defined as less than 400 mg/day (3 to 5 cups/day), whereas moderate consumption during pregnancy is defined as less than 200 mg/day (1 to 2 cups/day). In general, moderate consumption does not seem to negatively affect cardiovascular health in most people. Although some people who ingest caffeine report tachycardia and palpitations, doses < 450 mg/day do not appear to increase significant cardiac arrhythmias in healthy people or those with ischemia or ventricular ectopy. Caffeine doses as low as 250 mg have been reported to have a hypertensive effect after acute ingestion (an increase in systolic blood pressure of 5 to 15 mm Hg and an increase in diastolic blood pressure of 5 to 10 mm Hg), particularly in caffeine-naïve individuals; however, epidemiologic studies have produced inconsistent results. Caffeine appears to affect bladder function; moderate caffeine intake may exacerbate preexisting bladder symptoms, and excessive intake (>400 mg/day) may increase the risk for bladder dysfunction.[43]

Evidence suggests that caffeine is not a human carcinogen.[45] The lethal dose of caffeine in humans is estimated to be 10 g; however, only a few such cases have been reported.[43]

Caffeine withdrawal is associated with headache, anxiety, depressed mood, and fatigue (see Table 52.5). Typically, symptoms begin 12 to 24 hours after cessation of use, peak at 20 to 48 hours, and last up to 7 days. The severity and likelihood of symptoms are not predictable.[43]

Effects on Pregnancy and the Fetus

Caffeine readily crosses the placenta and in lower doses (i.e., 8 mg/kg) does not appear to cause a decrease in uterine blood flow or fetal oxygenation.[50] Whereas animal studies have shown a teratogenic effect with very high doses, moderate doses of less than 200 mg/day in pregnancy do not appear to result in teratogenesis in humans.[43,47,51] A 2021 study[52] and a 2023 systematic review and metaanalysis[53] reported an association between maternal caffeine consumption, even in amounts less than 200 mg/day, and intrauterine growth restriction and decreased birth weight. Moderate caffeine intake (<200 mg/day) during pregnancy does not appear to be a major contributing factor in spontaneous abortion or preterm birth.[54] Weng et al.[55] found an increased risk of miscarriage with increasing caffeine consumption, with an adjusted hazard ratio of 2.23 (95% confidence interval [CI], 1.34 to 3.69) for consumption greater than 200 mg/day, but other studies have reached contradictory conclusions.

Moderate first-trimester caffeine intake was found to have either no significant effect or to have a protective effect on the development of maternal gestational diabetes mellitus, depending on the population studied.[48] Moderate intake of caffeine in lactating women does not appear to adversely affect postnatal development.[43,45]

Anesthetic Management

Perhaps of greatest significance to the anesthesia provider is the potential for **caffeine withdrawal headache** from abrupt caffeine cessation during the peripartum period. Caffeine withdrawal should be considered in a postpartum patient with a nonspecific, nonpositional headache without associated lateralizing neurologic findings (see Chapter 30). There is no compelling evidence that caffeine is effective in the treatment of post–dural puncture headache (see Chapter 30).

Nicotine and Other Chemicals in Tobacco and Electronic Cigarettes

Epidemiology

As public awareness has grown regarding the hazards of smoking during pregnancy, the prevalence of cigarette smoking during pregnancy has declined. An estimated 13.6% of pregnant women reported past-month smoking in 2015,[56] compared to 5.5% in 2022.[22] However, the use of electronic cigarettes (e-cigarettes), which have been marketed as a safe alternative to cigarette smoking, has been steadily increasing. Studies estimate the prevalence of "vaping" during pregnancy between 0.6% and 15%.[57] As the dose of nicotine consumed by patients who use e-cigarettes is thought to be comparable to that consumed by cigarette smokers,[57] the US Food and Drug Administration ruled in 2016 that electronic nicotine delivery systems should be subject to the same regulations as cigarettes.

Pharmacology

More than 4000 chemicals are found in tobacco, including nicotine, carbon monoxide, and cyanides.[25] Tobacco is most often smoked, but it can also be chewed or sniffed. Nicotine, the principal component of tobacco, can be extracted from tobacco and administered electronically via e-cigarettes, vaporizers, vape pens, hookah pens, mod or pod systems, and e-pipes. Nicotine acts at peripheral and central nicotinic (acetylcholine) receptors throughout the body to affect the release of catecholamines. Its effects begin immediately upon exposure, and the half-life is typically a few hours; it is metabolized in the liver and the lungs and excreted by the kidneys. Nicotine's acute effects are of a shorter duration in heavy smokers than in light smokers.

Carbon monoxide, which is formed by the incomplete combustion of tobacco and charcoal in cigarettes and water pipes (i.e., hookahs), interferes with oxygen delivery to the cells by competitively binding to hemoglobin, decreasing the latter's oxygen-binding capacity and shifting the oxyhemoglobin dissociation curve to the left.[58] Depending on the extent of smoke inhalation, carbon monoxide may occupy 3% to 15% (or more) of the oxygen-carrying capacity of the blood.[59]

Electronic nicotine delivery systems contain solvent carriers (e.g., propylene glycol, glycerol) to produce aerosols that resemble cigarette smoke, and may contain flavoring. The health consequences of these substances on the mother and fetus are largely unknown.

Systemic Effects

Peripherally, nicotine increases sympathetic tone, thereby increasing maternal heart rate, blood pressure, and cardiac work (see Table 52.3).[60] Nicotine affects neurotransmitter release in different areas of the brain, producing feelings of alertness, euphoria, and, ultimately, dependence.[25,60]

Increased production of carboxyhemoglobin is thought to be a major factor in the impaired wound healing observed in smokers.[58] Smoking also promotes atherosclerosis. The pulmonary effects of tobacco smoking include increased volume of mucus, impaired mucociliary clearance, and an increased incidence of bronchitis and chronic obstructive pulmonary disease (see Table 52.4).[60]

Tobacco is addictive, and cessation of its use produces withdrawal symptoms of cravings, irritability, headache, cough, and insomnia (see Table 52.5). Smoking cessation interventions include counseling and therapy, hypnosis, acupuncture, and pharmacologic therapy. There is insufficient evidence to recommend nicotine replacement therapy (e.g., nicotine patch) in pregnancy; the American College of Obstetricians and Gynecologists (ACOG) recommends that it be used only after a detailed discussion with the patient of the possible risks of pharmacotherapeutic smoking cessation agents, the known risks of continued smoking, and the need for close supervision.[61]

Effects on Pregnancy and the Fetus

Significant perinatal risks are associated with cigarette smoking and alternative nicotine delivery products during pregnancy. Nicotine has a low molecular weight and readily crosses the placenta, eventually yielding higher fetal than maternal nicotine concentrations.[3] Nicotine intake in any form during pregnancy has known adverse effects on fetal lung and brain tissue.[57,62,63] Smoking cigarettes may result in decreased fetal oxygenation because of increased concentrations of carboxyhemoglobin and reduced uteroplacental perfusion. This compromised state can lead to decreased uptake of nourishing amino acids by the placenta.[64] Smoking also adversely affects fetal growth.[64-66] Smoking cessation in early pregnancy has been associated with a greater reduction in risk for intrauterine growth restriction compared with cessation later in pregnancy.[67]

Cigarette smoking during pregnancy is also associated with orofacial clefts, low birth weight, spontaneous fetal loss, preterm premature rupture of membranes, placenta previa, placental abruption, ectopic pregnancy, and increased perinatal mortality.[61,68–70] Children born to mothers who smoke during pregnancy have a higher incidence of asthma and respiratory infections.[71–74] Paradoxically, smoking has been associated with a reduced risk for preeclampsia, although this may be related to the higher rates of early pregnancy loss among pregnant smokers (see Chapter 35).[75,76]

Although the negative impact of fetal tobacco exposure on growth appears to resolve by 2 years of age,[77] there may be other long-term effects. A growing number of studies indicate that prenatal tobacco exposure may be associated with an increased risk for attention deficit/hyperactivity disorder, although it is not clear whether the relationship is causal. Holz et al.[78] examined offspring exposed to prenatal cigarette smoking using functional magnetic resonance imaging in a prospective 25-year study. After controlling for confounders, including adversity and sex, prenatal smoking exposure appeared to have long-term effects on neural activity and development. A study by Quinn et al.[79] suggested this association may be caused by confounding effects of other lifestyle and genetic issues; when cousins and siblings discordant on prenatal smoking and severe mental illness were compared, increased risk for severe mental illness in the smoking-exposed newborns was not observed.

Limited studies have reported that infants born to women who use smokeless tobacco during pregnancy have comparable rates of low birth weight, stillbirth, shortened gestational age, and neonatal apnea to those infants born to women who smoked cigarettes during pregnancy.[80,81] Data derived from animal studies suggest that the nicotine exposure from e-cigarette use during pregnancy appears to have similar harmful effects on lung development and offspring lung health as conventional cigarettes.[63] More research is needed to quantify the perinatal effects of alternative nicotine and tobacco delivery products.

Anesthetic Management

Cigarette smoking is a risk factor for several perioperative complications, including respiratory sequelae and impaired wound healing.[58,60] Smoking results in increased airway secretions, decreased ciliary motility, and impaired gas exchange.[60] Smoking is also associated with an increase in nonspecific airway reactivity; tracheal intubation may provoke bronchospasm. Smokers may be more likely to cough following emergence from general anesthesia, but the data are mixed and may be related to the specific volatile anesthetic agent used.[82,83]

The physiologic benefits of smoking cessation are progressive. Even brief smoke-free intervals can result in a reduction in the carboxyhemoglobin concentration, some improved ciliary function, and decreased small airway obstruction.[84] However, 6 months of abstinence may be required before the function of alveolar macrophages and pulmonary cytokines during and after general anesthesia in former smokers is similar to that of nonsmokers.[84] Neuraxial anesthesia avoids airway manipulation and is typically preferred in parturients who smoke.

Emerging evidence suggests that the inhaled agents and byproducts from e-cigarettes with and without nicotine may increase the risk of perioperative complications. Like combustible tobacco products, e-cigarette use results in increased airway reactivity and, with chronic use, reversible obstructive lung disease. General surgical patients are advised to abstain from e-cigarette use for 6 weeks prior to elective procedures and may benefit from administration of a short-acting beta-adrenergic agonist, such as albuterol.[85,86] E-cigarette users may also present with elevated blood pressure and tachycardia, which are known effects of nicotine. New-onset hypertension in pregnancy resulting from recent nicotine intake must be distinguished from preeclampsia. Inhalation of vaping aerosols from e-cigarettes with or without nicotine may increase platelet aggregation, resulting in an increased risk of thrombosis. Nicotine from e-cigarettes impairs wound healing because of decreased blood flow to the surgical site and impaired inflammatory response.

ILLICIT SUBSTANCES, RESTRICTED SUBSTANCES, AND PRESCRIPTION DRUG MISUSE

Amphetamines and "Club" Drugs

Amphetamines have historically been prescribed as components of nasal decongestants, bronchodilators, weight-loss drugs, and therapies for narcolepsy and attention deficit/hyperactivity disorder.[87] However, because of their high potential for misuse, amphetamines have been categorized by the US Drug Enforcement Agency (DEA) as Schedule II stimulants since 1971.[88] Methamphetamine and MDMA (3,4-methylenedioxymethamphetamine) ("ecstasy") are thought to be the most widely misused illicit amphetamines.[88]

Epidemiology

Women of reproductive age may use methamphetamines for a variety of reasons, including appetite suppression, weight loss, and a means of coping with stress. According to the 2021 National Survey on Drug Use and Health, 0.9% of pregnant women reported past-month methamphetamine use compared with 0.6% of nonpregnant women aged 15 to 44 years.[22] In endemic areas, however, the estimated prevalence ranges from 0.7% to 5%.[89] Survey data from 2021 reported 0.2% past-month MDMA use among pregnant women compared with 0.4% among nonpregnant women 15 to 44 years of age.[22] Polydrug use in women who use methamphetamine and MDMA appears to be common.[88,90]

Pharmacology

Amphetamines (and related compounds) are amines that exist as either salts of various acids or free bases. Used illicitly, they can be ingested orally, inhaled, or, less commonly, injected, resulting in significant CNS penetration.[25] The plasma half-life ranges from 5 to 30 hours. Metabolism is variable; up to 30% of the parent compound can be found in the urine. Detection of these compounds and their metabolites in the urine is possible up to several days after ingestion.[4]

Methamphetamine ("speed," "meth," "ice," or "crystal") is a congener of amphetamine that contains a methyl radical.[88] This white, odorless, bitter-tasting powder can be smoked, snorted, ingested orally, or administered rectally.[90] Its availability is facilitated by production in low-cost home laboratories. Methamphetamine is more potent than amphetamine and has a longer half-life; 50% of the drug is cleared in 12 hours. When it is smoked or injected intravenously, the "flash" from this drug is intense and of short duration. Snorting produces euphoria within 5 minutes, while oral ingestion takes approximately 20 minutes.[87]

The use of MDMA during pregnancy is increasingly common in the United States.[91,92] MDMA has a methylenedioxy group attached to the aromatic ring of the amphetamine molecule that confers some of its hallucinogenic effects (see later discussion).[93] The effects of MDMA typically begin approximately 20 minutes after ingestion and last approximately 6 hours; large doses have effects for up to 2 days. MDMA is metabolized by the liver and excreted by the kidneys.[4]

The "club" drug, gamma-hydroxybutyric acid (GHB), also known as liquid ecstasy or liquid X, is derived from gamma-aminobutyric acid (GABA), which readily enters the brain when ingested, producing hallucinogenic, anxiolytic, euphoric, and sedative effects.[94] Severe cardiorespiratory depression, coma, and seizures can occur at high doses. Overdose is common, owing in part to the variable individual responses to the drug.[94,95] Chronic use may be associated with a downregulation of GABA receptors, and withdrawal manifests as insomnia, tachycardia, hypertension, and nausea/vomiting.[94]

Another designer drug of the phenethylamine class is 3,4-methylenedioxypyrovalerone, also known as "bath salts." Typically sold in crystal or powder form that can be snorted, smoked, or injected, this substance acts as a norepinephrine and dopamine reuptake inhibitor.[96] It is not detected by common drug screening tests. Adverse effects resemble those of amphetamines (e.g., agitation, hypertension, tachycardia), and dependence and withdrawal can occur.[97] In rare instances, it can cause severe hyperthermia or hyponatremia. The DEA banned the active ingredients in bath salts after several deaths were reported.[98]

Systemic Effects

Acute amphetamine ingestion leads to indirect sympathetic activation through the release of norepinephrine, dopamine, and serotonin from adrenergic nerve terminals (see Table 52.3).[4,99] The physiologic effects of amphetamines are similar to those of cocaine and other stimulants, with two important differences: (1) amphetamines and their derivatives lack local anesthetic properties and (2) amphetamine can inhibit monoamine oxidase activity, leading to decreased degradation of catecholamines.[4]

Long-term, unrestricted use of high doses of amphetamines can have a number of adverse maternal effects, including damage to the cardiovascular and neurologic systems as well as behavioral changes such as hostility, violence, hallucinations, and paranoid psychosis (see Table 52.4).[90]

Methamphetamine is slow to metabolize and has a much longer duration of action than cocaine.[87]

The **cardiovascular** effects of amphetamines and their derivatives are similar to those of cocaine[4]: vasoconstriction, tachycardia, and labile blood pressure.[27] Patients are typically hypertensive, although catecholamine depletion can result in hypotension. Arrhythmias, myocardial ischemia, endothelial damage, dilated cardiomyopathy, and acceleration of atherosclerosis can also occur. Indeed, cardiovascular disease-related mortality is the leading cause of death among chronic methamphetamine users.[89] Recommendations for the management of cardiovascular complications include resuscitation using intravenous fluids or judicious use of phenylephrine for hypotension. If pharmacotherapy is needed to treat hypertension, then labetalol, an alpha- and beta-adrenergic receptor antagonist, may be preferred over a pure beta-adrenergic receptor antagonist. Direct vasodilators (e.g., nitrates or hydralazine) can be used but may exacerbate tachycardia.[4] Acute amphetamine intoxication may result in severe headache, hypertension, and seizures, and can mimic the signs and symptoms of severe preeclampsia or eclampsia.[100]

The pleasurable effects of methamphetamine and the deleterious **neurologic** sequelae are believed to be the result of high levels of dopamine in the brain. In addition to positive feelings, patients who have taken methamphetamine may experience anxiety, mood disturbances, paranoia, and hallucinations. Severe intracranial hypertension[5] and hemorrhagic stroke[101] have been reported in the setting of acute use. Chronic use has been associated with impairment of motor function and verbal learning, as well as with significant changes in the areas of the brain associated with memory and emotion (see Table 52.4).[87] Volkow et al.[102] observed that prolonged abstinence (12 to 17 months) resulted in significant recovery of brain dopamine transporters, although performance on neuropsychologic tests did not improve to the same extent. In addition, psychotic features of long-time amphetamine use may be precipitated by stress in former users after months or even years of abstinence.[87]

MDMA use has been associated with numerous adverse effects, including hyperthermia, hyponatremia, and seizures.[9] Healthy volunteers given MDMA in experimental settings have demonstrated CNS effects that include enhanced mood and heightened awareness, as well as a dose-dependent moderate increase in blood pressure.[103,104] Recreational MDMA use has also been associated with neurohormonal changes, including increased cortisol and oxytocin.[105]

Psychostimulant withdrawal causes fatigue, depression, hunger, and intense cravings (see Table 52.5). Pharmacologic therapy for stimulant withdrawal (e.g., tricyclic antidepressants, dopaminergic agents [e.g., bromocriptine], amino acid replacement therapy) has not been particularly successful.[106] Seizures, severe hypertension, and hyperthermia from methamphetamine overdose can be fatal. Treatment goals include provision of a calm environment (with or without a benzodiazepine) and airway protection. Active cooling, antihypertensive agents, and anticonvulsants should be used as needed.[93,106]

Effects on Pregnancy and the Fetus

Further research is needed to evaluate the long-term effects of prenatal exposure to supratherapeutic doses of amphetamines. Amphetamine ingestion results in high levels of circulating catecholamines, which may lead to vasoconstriction and decreased uteroplacental blood flow. Animal studies have suggested that intrauterine exposure to methamphetamine is associated with an increased incidence of retinal defects, cleft palate, and rib malformations as well as a decreased overall rate of growth and motor development.[90,107] Results from a retrospective cohort study indicate that methamphetamine use in pregnant women was associated with an increased risk for gestational hypertension, preeclampsia, fetal death, abruption, preterm birth, neonatal death, and infant death.[108] A 2018 metaanalysis of retrospective, case-controlled studies found that methamphetamine use during pregnancy resulted in lower neonatal birth weight, head circumference, and body length compared to control pregnancies, but found no difference in the incidence of maternal hypertension or preeclampsia.[109] Studies of the potential long-term effects on neonatal neurodevelopment and cardiovascular outcomes are limited by a small sample size and confounding factors. Findings from the Infant Development, Environment and Lifestyle study and the National Institute on Drug Abuse suggest that children prenatally exposed to methamphetamine appear to be at a higher risk for impaired executive function, attention deficit/hyperactivity disorder, and increased aggressive behavior, although early adversity (e.g., abuse or neglect) is a likely confounding variable.[110–113] Effects on language and cognition and gross motor development appear to be transient or negligible, respectively.

Anesthetic Management

Amphetamines cause indirect sympathetic activation. Intoxicated patients are at risk for dangerous cardiovascular events, including hemodynamic instability and cardiac arrest.

Recommendations for anesthetic management of patients with amphetamine and cocaine toxicity are similar.[4] A cooperative patient may be a candidate for neuraxial analgesia or anesthesia, although refractory hypotension has been reported in a long-time amphetamine user who received neuraxial anesthesia with intravenous propofol sedation.[114] The authors attributed the response to downregulation of beta-adrenergic receptors and catecholamine depletion. As with cocaine, phenylephrine may be a better choice for the treatment of hypotension than ephedrine; as an indirect-acting agent, ephedrine may cause an exaggerated hemodynamic response if circulating catecholamines are high or, alternatively, be ineffective if catecholamines are depleted.

Parturients who use amphetamines may be at increased risk for urgent cesarean delivery requiring general anesthesia. Evidence from animal studies suggests that acute ingestion of amphetamines increases the MAC for volatile halogenated anesthetic agents, whereas chronic ingestion of amphetamines decreases the MAC of volatile agents.[115,116] There is a well-recognized association between methamphetamine

use and severe tooth decay (i.e., "meth mouth"), which can present a significant hazard during laryngoscopy. The airway assessment should include attention to fragile or loose teeth that might be dislodged during laryngoscopy as well as to the possibility of burns throughout the airway. High doses of MDMA can cause rhabdomyolysis.[93]

Cocaine

Although the use of cocaine dates back to CE 600,[117] cocaine was formally introduced into clinical practice as a local anesthetic in the 1880s. During this period, Sigmund Freud also experimented with cocaine's ability to combat hunger, fatigue, and opiate addiction.[117,118] Cocaine has both vasoconstrictive and local anesthetic properties as a result of its ability to block sodium channels during depolarization.

Epidemiology

The prevalence of cocaine use during pregnancy is difficult to estimate as 60% to 90% of pregnant cocaine users engage in polysubstance use, including tobacco.[119,120] Survey data in 2021 reported the prevalence of past-month cocaine use in pregnant women 15 to 44 years of age as 0.2%.[22]

Pharmacology

Cocaine is an ester of benzoic acid and the base ecgonine, which is the parent compound of atropine and scopolamine.[118,121] When dissolved in hydrochloric acid to form a water-soluble powder (cocaine hydrochloride), cocaine can be chewed, administered intravenously ("mainlined"), or taken intranasally ("snorted"). Intrarectal and intravaginal use has also been reported.[122] When cocaine is processed with either sodium bicarbonate ("crack") or ammonia and ether ("free base"), the resulting cocaine alkaloid can be smoked.[118,121,123] The amount and duration of exposure are more important determinants of cocaine's effects than the chemical formulation. Smoked cocaine ("crack" or free base) is rapidly absorbed through the lungs and reaches the brain in 6 to 8 seconds; intravenous cocaine reaches the brain in 12 to 16 seconds; and snorted cocaine reaches the brain in 3 to 5 minutes.[124] The typical half-life of cocaine is 30 to 90 minutes, although its effects can last as long as 6 hours.[118]

Cocaine is metabolized to ecgonine esters and benzoylecgonine (biologically inactive) by plasma and hepatic cholinesterases and to norcocaine (biologically active) by nonenzymatic hydrolysis. Only small amounts of cocaine are excreted unchanged in the urine. In the presence of alcohol, cocaine is transesterified to cocaethylene, which has a longer half-life and greater physiologic effects than cocaine.[123,124]

Systemic Effects

Cocaine has complex actions on the central and peripheral nervous systems and on nerve conduction. The powerful sympathomimetic effects of cocaine are caused by the drug's inhibition of the reuptake of norepinephrine, dopamine, and serotonin, which allows these neurotransmitters to accumulate at the synaptic clefts and produce sustained stimulation.[117,123,124] This process can result in as much as a fivefold increase in circulating concentrations of catecholamines,[4] which, in turn, may lead to feelings of euphoria, increased energy, and decreased fear.[117,124] Repetitive use of cocaine eventually leads to depletion of neurotransmitter stores, upregulation of receptors, and a higher dose requirement to achieve the desired euphoric effects.[118]

The peripheral nervous system effects of cocaine and its derivatives result from binding to tissue receptors involved in monoamine reuptake, which results in hypertension and/or labile blood pressure and tachycardia. Cocaine produces widespread small- and large-vessel occlusion through vasospasm, thrombosis, and endothelial injury, which may result in significant end-organ damage.[118]

Cocaine has profound effects on the **cardiovascular** system, and pregnancy appears to enhance them. Acute administration of cocaine increases peripheral vascular resistance, cardiac contractility, and myocardial oxygen demand (see Table 52.3).[118,125] Coronary vasoconstriction also occurs; a greater effect occurs in diseased vessel segments than in nondiseased segments.[123] Studies in vitro indicate that cocaine can have a procoagulant effect in small and large vessels.[4] This may lead to thrombus formation and coronary plaque rupture in the setting of cocaine-induced hypertension.[118,126]

Cocaine-induced chest pain is a common complaint among young people presenting to the emergency department.[127] Mittleman et al.[126] found that cocaine use was associated with a significant, abrupt, and transient increase in the risk for acute myocardial infarction in patients who were otherwise at low risk.[128] The occurrence of cocaine-induced electrocardiographic changes is fairly common and is not necessarily associated with true ischemia.[123,129] If ischemia is suspected, treatment with supplemental oxygen, aspirin, and vasodilators, with or without reperfusion therapy,[127] as well as measurement of troponin levels,[128] is indicated. Although cocaine users who suffer a myocardial infarction have fewer postinfarction sequelae than the general population, the incidence of major cardiovascular complications is not trivial; 5% to 7% have congestive heart failure, 4% to 17% have ventricular arrhythmias, and up to 2% die.[123] Prompt recognition of acute cocaine-induced cardiovascular toxicity facilitates management.

Not all cocaine-induced hypertension in pregnant women requires immediate intervention, but if pharmacotherapy is used, it is important to understand the potential undesired consequences. **Beta-adrenergic receptor blockade** may result in unopposed alpha-adrenergic receptor–mediated vasoconstriction that can lead to coronary artery vasoconstriction and myocardial failure. Labetalol, an alpha- and beta-adrenergic receptor antagonist, may be preferred, although it does not fully ameliorate cocaine-induced coronary artery vasoconstriction. Direct vasodilators (e.g., nitrates, hydralazine) can be used but may cause further tachycardia and, in the case of hydralazine, may not restore uterine blood flow.[4,123,130] Calcium entry-blocking agents, such as nifedipine and nimodipine, have been found to potentiate the toxic effects of cocaine in animal models, although the mechanism has not been determined.[4,131,132] Based on a 2016

systematic review, benzodiazepines and other GABA-active agents are among the pharmacologic treatments that may at least partially mitigate tachycardia, hypertension, dysrhythmia, and coronary vasospasm associated with acute cocaine toxicity. High-quality randomized prospective studies are needed to further elucidate the optimal treatment.[133]

Other acute cardiovascular effects of cocaine include QT prolongation, bradycardia, and arrhythmias, including supraventricular or ventricular tachycardia and ventricular fibrillation.[118] Severe bradycardia can be treated with atropine or electrical pacing. Stable supraventricular tachycardia (SVT) can be treated with vagal maneuvers or with adenosine. In the unstable patient with SVT, direct current (DC) cardioversion may be required.[134,135]

In a retrospective multicenter study, Shih et al.[136] found that the therapeutic use of lidocaine in nonpregnant patients with cocaine-induced myocardial infarction did not potentiate the cardiovascular or CNS effects of cocaine. Although amiodarone therapy for maternal and fetal arrhythmias has been described as having only minor adverse effects in some patients, there are reports of associated fetal hypothyroidism and fetal growth restriction (see Chapter 41).[134,137,138] Thus, amiodarone in pregnant women is reserved for malignant arrhythmias that are refractory to other therapies.

Long-time cocaine use can cause left ventricular hypertrophy or dilated cardiomyopathy with accompanying systolic dysfunction (see Table 52.4).[118,123] Aortic dissection has also been reported.[123] Intravenous use of cocaine and other injectable drugs increases the risk for development of infective endocarditis. Noncardiogenic pulmonary edema, pulmonary hypertension, and right-sided heart failure can also occur in the setting of cocaine use.[4,118]

The **neurologic** complications of cocaine may be transient or permanent. Morbidity and mortality may result from subarachnoid hemorrhage, intracerebral hemorrhage, cerebral vasculitis, transient ischemic attacks, and/or cerebral infarcts, particularly in the setting of additional risk factors, such as hypertension, alcohol, or smoking.[6,101,139] Cocaine-induced seizures, if self-limited, are typically treated with supportive care and benzodiazepines.[139]

Respiratory complications occur in 25% of cocaine users. Smoking cocaine can have profound respiratory effects, which include bronchospasm, chronic cough, and diffusion capacity abnormalities.[122,124] Pregnant women who use cocaine are at increased risk for peripartum wheezing.[6] Inhaled cocaine vapor can produce thermal airway burns. "Snorting" cocaine can lead to epistaxis, oral ulcers, and nasal septal injury. The intense pulmonary and bronchial arterial vasoconstriction produced by cocaine can cause interstitial and alveolar hemorrhage. Pneumothorax, pneumomediastinum, and pneumopericardium have also been reported.[118]

Cocaine ingestion can result in serious **gastrointestinal** complications, such as ischemia, ulceration, and perforation.[124] Cocaine's anticholinergic effects include delayed gastric emptying and an increased risk for aspiration.[118] Although some cocaine users have abnormal liver enzyme levels, cocaine is not clearly hepatotoxic.[124]

Hematologic consequences of cocaine exposure during pregnancy may, in rare instances, include thrombocytopenia.[9,140,141] Whereas Kain et al.[140] found the rate of thrombocytopenia to be higher in the cocaine group than in the drug-free group (6.7% versus 1.5%, respectively), Gershon et al.[142] found that in pregnant women who tested positive for cocaine, only 2.5% had a platelet count < 140,000/µL, compared with 4.7% in the cocaine-negative group.

Renal failure can result from cocaine use secondary to rhabdomyolysis, renal infarction, or impaired immunologic function.[118] Cocaine-using patients have a higher prevalence of syphilis, human immunodeficiency virus (HIV) infection, and other **infectious diseases** compared with noncocaine-using patients, even after controlling for intravenous drug use.[124,143] Studies of the **endocrine system** in gravid ewes have shown that cocaine exposure results in increases in maternal adrenocorticotropic hormone and cortisol, as well as maternal and fetal plasma glucose and lactate.[144,145] Cocaine also impairs cutaneous vasodilation and sweating. The lethal effects of cocaine are related, in part, to the drug's tendency to produce **hyperthermia**, particularly in hot weather.[146] Cocaine use has been associated with **sudden death** from several of the factors discussed earlier, including cardiac arrhythmias, respiratory arrest, status epilepticus, and impaired thermoregulation.

Cocaine withdrawal can be difficult to recognize because of its nonspecific signs and symptoms: extreme fatigue followed by hunger, anxiety, weakness, headache, tremors, and seizures (see Table 52.5). Recommended therapy involves supportive care and a slow taper over days to weeks.[27]

Effects on Pregnancy and the Fetus

Pregnant women metabolize cocaine to norcocaine to a greater extent than their nonpregnant counterparts, exposing both mother and fetus to this more potent metabolite.[117,121] With its low molecular weight and high lipophilicity, it is mostly un-ionized at physiologic pH and readily crosses the placenta.[6,117] Generalized vasoconstriction from cocaine and its metabolites may result *in utero* placental insufficiency, acidosis, and fetal hypoxia.[91]

In a 2011 metaanalysis, Gouin et al.[147] found that cocaine use during pregnancy was associated with significantly higher risk for preterm birth, low birthweight, and small-for-gestational-age infants. Obstetric complications associated with maternal cocaine use include a higher incidence of placental abruption and preterm labor; the latter occurs in 17% to 29% of pregnant women who use cocaine.[148] Several small studies and case reports also suggest an increased risk of spontaneous abortion, stillbirth (likely related to placental abruption), and uterine rupture.[91,149–151] Acute cocaine toxicity can mimic preeclampsia or eclampsia when pregnant women present with severe hypertension, hyperreflexia, headache, blurred vision, and/or seizures, but it can be differentiated through a positive urine test result for cocaine, the presence of normal laboratory measurements, and rapid resolution of symptoms without delivery.[152] There is also an association between cocaine use and an increased risk for sexually transmitted diseases and failure to obtain prenatal care.[153]

The impact of maternal use of cocaine (particularly "crack") on the fetus has been the subject of intense legal, political, and scientific debate since the 1980s.[154] Initial animal data and retrospective human studies suggested an increased risk for major congenital anomalies (e.g., genitourinary and abdominal wall defects) in fetuses exposed to cocaine. However, these reports are confounded by concurrent use of other drugs and low statistical power.[155] Subsequent studies found no significant difference in type or number of congenital anomalies between infants with exposure to cocaine *in utero* and infants without exposure, after accounting for confounding variables.[156,157]

Frank et al.[158] reviewed studies published between 1984 and 2000 to assess the possible relationships between maternal cocaine use during pregnancy and childhood outcomes. After controlling for possible confounding factors, they found no consistent negative association with physical growth, developmental test scores, or expressive or receptive language skills. They observed less optimal motor performance up to 7 months of age, after which the differences between cocaine-exposed and nonexposed infants disappeared.

Studies investigating trajectories of motor, mental, or behavioral development in infants with prenatal cocaine exposure have had conflicting results, in part related to confounding risk factors such as exposure to adverse postnatal environments.[159–161] In a 15-year follow-up study of adolescents prenatally exposed to cocaine, Richardson at al.[162] noted that exposure to violence partially mediated the impact on (self-reported) delinquent behaviors by the adolescents. In addition, the first-trimester-exposed adolescents had poorer performance on tests related to problem solving and abstract thinking. Definitive assessment of long-term outcomes of children exposure to cocaine *in utero* remain elusive.

In terms of other health consequences, Bauer et al.[156] found that infectious complications, such as hepatitis, syphilis, and, to a lesser extent, HIV infection, were more common in infants of women who ingest cocaine.

Anesthetic Management

Pregnant women who use cocaine are at risk for acute and chronic multiorgan system dysfunction[143] and the need for urgent cesarean delivery. During labor, early administration of neuraxial anesthesia should be encouraged if the patient is cooperative and has a platelet count above the threshold recommended by professional society guidelines.[163] Neuraxial anesthesia can reduce circulating levels of catecholamines and mitigate some of the systemic effects of cocaine.[6] Also, an epidural catheter placed for labor analgesia can usually be used to provide anesthesia for an intrapartum cesarean delivery, if needed. Treatment of hypotension should include volume resuscitation and, if needed, careful titration of a direct-acting vasopressor, such as phenylephrine.[9,164]

When an ester local anesthetic agent (or succinylcholine) is administered to a patient who has ingested cocaine, these medications may compete with cocaine for available plasma cholinesterase[6,121]; however, the clinical significance of these effects, if any, is unknown. Despite the theoretical risk for altered metabolism of succinylcholine, a standard intubating dose should be administered.[120] Changes in mu- and kappa-opioid receptors and altered baseline endorphin levels may result in an increased perception of pain in cocaine-using patients despite the presence of an apparently satisfactory level of neuraxial anesthesia.[9] Ross et al.[165] observed a reduced duration of intrathecal sufentanil analgesia during labor in parturients who used cocaine, although the quality of analgesia was not diminished.

Patients who ingest cocaine and receive general anesthesia are at greater risk for hypertension and tachycardia during and after laryngoscopy and tracheal intubation.[6,7] If general anesthesia is required, premedication with a benzodiazepine may help attenuate the acute physiologic effects of cocaine. As the anticholinergic effects of cocaine can delay gastric emptying and may also increase the risk for pulmonary aspiration, pharmacologic prophylaxis and a rapid-sequence induction of general anesthesia are indicated. Propofol may be well tolerated, whereas ketamine may potentiate the CNS vasoconstrictive effects of cocaine, potentially increasing the risk for cerebrovascular morbidity.[9] Both etomidate and cocaine can result in disinhibition of CNS control of extrapyramidal activity, and their effects may be additive.[7] Dexmedetomidine, an alpha$_2$-adrenergic receptor agonist, has been shown in animal studies to delay the onset of cocaine-induced seizures and may be useful in selected patients.[166] Early studies in dogs demonstrated that acute cocaine ingestion can cause hyperthermia in both laboratory animals and humans[118,146]; therefore, the core temperature should be monitored in patients with acute cocaine intoxication. However, given the propensity for nasal septal defects in these patients, temperature probes (and other tubes and monitors) should *not* be inserted intranasally. Active warming should be used only if the patient is hypothermic.

Cannabis

Cannabis is the restricted drug used most commonly in pregnancy, with 7.2% of pregnant women between 15 and 44 years of age reporting past-month use in 2021.[22] Although cannabis use is lower in the pregnant than in the nonpregnant population (18.8%),[22] its use in pregnancy is increasing, particularly among young, urban, and socioeconomically disadvantaged women. Contributing factors are thought to include the legalization of medical marijuana, the decriminalization of recreational marijuana, and the drug's antiemetic properties.

Pharmacology

Cannabis contains more than 400 compounds, including more than 60 cannabinoids. Most of the psychotropic effects are caused by 9-tetrahydrocannabinol (THC).[9,167] Noncannabinoid constituents of cannabis are similar to those in tobacco, but without the nicotine. Inhaled THC is absorbed through the lungs and reaches the brain within minutes. Oral ingestion of cannabis results in blood THC concentrations that are 25% to 30% lower than those obtained by smoking, but with a delayed onset of up to 2 hours. The lipid-soluble cannabinoids are sequestered in fatty tissues and gradually released into other tissues. A single ingestion can have an elimination half-life of up to 7 days; complete elimination of the inactive metabolite 11-nor-9-carboxy-delta-9-tetrahydrocannabinol takes as long as 25 to 30 days. Metabolism occurs in the liver, with excretion in the urine. Measured concentrations of metabolites in the blood and urine correlate poorly with the degree of intoxication.[167] Synthetic cannabinoids feature the primary psychoactive component of cannabis and are not detected on routine urine assays for THC.[168]

Systemic Effects

Cannabis interacts with specific cannabinoid receptors in the brain and peripheral nerves. Psychoactive effects include anxiolysis, analgesia, appetite stimulation, euphoria, and, sometimes, dysphoria (see Table 52.3).[167] Cannabis intoxication impairs cognitive and psychomotor function. Impairment of memory, attention, and the ability to process complex information can occur with long-time heavy use (see Table 52.4). It is unclear whether these effects are reversible.

Acute intoxication with cannabis appears to have a biphasic effect on the autonomic nervous system: low doses cause tachycardia and higher cardiac output from increased sympathetic and decreased parasympathetic tone; high doses produce sympathetic inhibition and parasympathetic stimulation, resulting in bradycardia and hypotension.[4,9] Although ventricular ectopy can occur, life-threatening arrhythmias in patients without preexisting cardiac disease are rare, and autonomic disturbances are generally well tolerated. Reversible ST-segment and T-wave abnormalities may occur, perhaps as a result of the higher heart rate associated with cannabis use.[4] Synthetic cannabinoids may produce more exaggerated physiologic effects. Although large studies are lacking, two cases have been reported of otherwise healthy women who developed ischemic stroke after first-time use.[169]

Cannabis smoke contains many of the same toxins as tobacco smoke, often in higher concentrations. As with tobacco, the respiratory consequences of smoking cannabis include mucociliary dysfunction, increased susceptibility to bronchitis, and chronic obstructive pulmonary disease (see Table 52.4). Acute intoxication may cause conjunctival vasodilation and visible reddening of the eyes. Although high doses of cannabis can cause hallucinations and psychosis, fatal overdose has not been documented.[5,167]

Withdrawal from long-time cannabis use may produce a mild abstinence syndrome that includes headache, restlessness, tremor, anxiety, and autonomic effects, similar to those of withdrawal from benzodiazepines and hypnotic drugs (see Table 52.5).[4,170]

Effects on Pregnancy and the Fetus

It is difficult to ascertain the specific effects of cannabis on pregnancy and the developing fetus, in part because of potential confounding exposures (e.g., polysubstance use, adverse socioeconomic conditions). Due to concerns for impaired fetal neurodevelopment and for maternal and fetal exposure to toxins in cannabis smoke, the ACOG discourages the use of any cannabis during pregnancy and lactation.[171]

Prenatal cannabis exposure does not appear to result in major fetal structural anatomic defects,[172–174] although studies have reported smaller head circumferences, lower birth weights, and smaller birth lengths among neonates exposed to cannabis *in utero*, particularly with heavier exposure early in gestation.[175,176] Some studies have shown cannabis use in pregnancy to be associated with an increased risk for stillbirth and preterm birth, but the validity of these findings may be limited by confounding factors such as concomitant cigarette smoking.[177–179] A 2016 metaanalysis of 31 observational (including cohort and case-control) studies comparing neonatal outcomes in women who used cannabis during pregnancy with women who did not found that maternal cannabis use does not appear to be an independent risk factor for low birth weight or preterm birth.[180]

Exposure to exogenous cannabinoids *in utero* may negatively affect brain development and function. Long-term effects in children with prenatal cannabis exposure include inattention and impulsivity, deficits in problem solving, academic underachievement, and a predisposition to smoking cannabis and tobacco.[181–183]

Anesthetic Management

Neuraxial analgesia is typically preferred during labor and delivery and can be safely performed in patients who use cannabis, in the absence of contraindications. Drug-related changes in heart rate and blood pressure are usually well tolerated in otherwise healthy patients with acute cannabis intoxication. However, the administration of atropine and ketamine can exacerbate existing tachycardia.[9]

Long-time cannabis smokers are at risk for similar respiratory complications during and after general anesthesia as tobacco smokers, including increased airway secretions, impaired mucociliary clearance, and potentially increased airway reactivity.[60,167] Persistent postextubation laryngospasm in a patient with a history of heavy cannabis smoking has been reported.[184]

Acute intoxication with cannabis can have additive effects with sedative agents and volatile anesthetic agents, including myocardial depression[9,27]; careful titration to clinical effect is recommended. The effect of cannabis on pain perception has been explored in an experimental model of human pain. Wallace et al.[185] found that smoked cannabis had a differential effect on pain scores; a low dose had no effect, a medium dose reduced pain, and a high dose significantly increased pain. The clinical implications of these findings are unclear.

Hallucinogens

Hallucinogens include lysergic acid diethylamide (LSD), phencyclidine (PCP), psilocybin, ayahuasca, and mescaline.[106] MDMA also has hallucinogenic effects (see earlier discussion).

Epidemiology

Hallucinogen use in pregnancy is thought to be uncommon.[7,186] Survey data from 2021 reported a 0.2% prevalence of past-month hallucinogen use in pregnant women compared with 1.3% in nonpregnant women ages 15 to 44 years.[22]

Pharmacology

The hallucinogens are a diverse group of drugs notable for their complex mechanism of actions that include agonist, partial agonist, and antagonist effects at serotonergic, dopaminergic, and adrenergic receptors. Overall, the adrenergic effects of these drugs are mild compared with those of cocaine and amphetamines.[4]

Both **psilocybin**, the hallucinogen in some wild mushrooms, and the synthetic compound **LSD** are indole derivatives that chemically resemble serotonin.[4,106] When smoked or taken orally, intranasally, intravenously, or rectally, they evoke auditory, visual, and tactile hallucinations. Clinical effects usually develop over 15 to 60 minutes and last for 6 to 12 hours.[7,106] LSD is 100 times more potent than psilocybin and can be detected in urine or plasma for up to 3 days. LSD is metabolized by the liver and has a plasma half-life of 100 minutes.[4] The potency of individual samples of psilocybin varies; physiologic effects typically occur at doses of 20 to 60 mg. Most of the drug is excreted in the first 8 hours, although small amounts are excreted for up to 1 week.[106]

Ayahuasca is a psychoactive brew used in ritual healing ceremonies and is composed primarily of two Amazonian plants; the key ingredients are beta-carboline and tryptamine derivatives.[187,188] Its potency and effects depend on the relative concentrations of each of its constituents. **PCP**, initially developed as a general anesthetic agent, was removed from the legal market in 1978. **Ketamine**, a related compound, is an anesthetic agent that is also a drug of abuse. Both PCP and ketamine bind to the *N*-methyl-D-aspartate (NMDA) receptor. The psychological effects of PCP typically last 12 to 48 hours, while ketamine has a shorter duration of action.[106]

Unlike the phenylethylamines MDMA and liquid ecstasy (GHB), which also have properties of amphetamines, **mescaline** is exclusively hallucinogenic. Found as the active ingredient in peyote cactus buttons, mescaline is typically eaten or drunk as tea. The effects of mescaline, which last approximately 12 hours, include visual hallucinations, nausea, and vomiting.[106]

Systemic Effects

Ingestion of hallucinogens causes activation of the sympathetic nervous system, which results in hypertension, tachycardia, dilated pupils, and increased core body temperature (see Table 52.3).[7] The **cardiovascular effects** of these drugs are rarely serious, although some instances of supraventricular tachycardia and acute myocardial infarction have been reported. Myocardial infarction may result from vasospasm and increased platelet aggregation.[4]

Carotid artery occlusion has been reported after the use of LSD. PCP use has been associated with seizures, delayed hypertensive crisis, and intracerebral hemorrhage.[5] Overdose with PCP can be associated with confusion and combativeness, which may progress to seizures and catatonia.

Some users of LSD experience a "bad trip," which is likely to be a manifestation of an acute anxiety reaction. Other users report "flashbacks" or systemic effects of these drugs that occur months or even years after ingestion. Some of these episodes are likely a result of delayed release of small amounts of drug from fatty tissue.

The psychological effects of psilocybin include giddiness, visual hallucinations, and gastrointestinal dysfunction. Morbidity is associated primarily with inadvertent ingestion of toxic species of mushrooms.[106] Although psychological dependence on these drugs has been observed, withdrawal symptoms are not associated with abstinence (see Table 52.5).[7]

A direct causal relationship between use of hallucinogens and death has not been documented; however, these drugs can cause feelings of paranoia and panic that can lead to accidents or fatalities.[5,7]

Effects on Pregnancy and the Fetus

There is conflicting evidence as to whether intrauterine PCP exposure has deleterious fetal effects. Mvula et al.[189] found that PCP-positive women had smaller and more preterm infants compared with non–PCP-positive women. The PCP-positive women were also more likely to have syphilis and diabetes and to use tobacco, alcohol, and cannabis. Early reports of chromosomal damage secondary to LSD were not confirmed by later studies.[5] The potential effects of prenatal exposure to ayahuasca has led to active discussion in the literature without a definitive conclusion.[187,188]

Anesthetic Management

Management of a hallucinogen-intoxicated patient is primarily supportive and noninterventional.[4] Stressful situations can provoke panic attacks, which in turn can intensify the physiologic effects of these drugs. Specific recommendations include provision of a quiet, supportive environment and administration of a benzodiazepine, if needed. Neuroleptic medications are relatively contraindicated as they can intensify toxic reactions.[4,7]

Hemodynamic perturbations are usually relatively mild and well tolerated.[9] Occasionally, patients experience supraventricular tachycardia, hypertension, and myocardial ischemia.[4] The acutely intoxicated patient may have an exaggerated response to ephedrine[7]; phenylephrine is preferable and should be titrated to effect. LSD may have some intrinsic anticholinesterase activity, but the clinical significance is unclear. Hallucinogens may also prolong opioid-induced analgesia and respiratory depression.[9]

Either neuraxial or general anesthesia can be administered for vaginal or cesarean delivery in the usual fashion, as the clinical situation warrants.

Opioids

Opioids refer to the class of naturally occurring, semisynthetic, and synthetic drugs that are structurally and functionally related to morphine. The term *opiate* specifically describes any of the natural derivatives of poppy plants, including opium, morphine, heroin, and codeine (see Chapter 13).[25]

Epidemiology

As in the general population, opioid use disorder in pregnant women has increased dramatically. A large population-based study revealed a 127% increase in prevalence (from 0.17% in 1998 to 0.39% in 2011 in the 20 to 34 years age group), as well as an increased risk for in-hospital mortality.[190] Opioid-related maternal deaths more than doubled from 2010 to 2016,[191] and over the past two decades opioid overdose has emerged as a leading cause of pregnancy-associated mortality.[192] Risk factors for maternal opioid use disorder include untreated psychiatric disorders, such as anxiety and depression, and chronic pain. In a 2021 interview study of single women on Medicaid insurance with opioid use disorder, all reported experience with intimate partner violence.[193] The biologic, psychiatric, and social influences that affect known gender and sex differences in the risk of developing opioid use disorder and/or opioid overdose continue to be investigated.[194]

Historically, opioids were thought to be safe for pregnant women and were liberally prescribed for treatment of headache and back and abdominal pain.[195,196] However, there is emerging evidence that increases in prescription opioid use among pregnant women have resulted in a sharp increase in opioid use disorder among these patients, as well as an increase in admissions to substance use treatment facilities during pregnancy.[197] Using data from commercial insurance beneficiaries, Bateman et al.[198] estimated that approximately 1 in 300 previously opioid naïve pregnant women become persistent prescription opioid users after cesarean delivery.

Pharmacology

The naturally occurring opioids are metabolized to morphine, which has a plasma half-life of 2 to 3 hours. Morphine then undergoes rapid metabolism in the liver and is excreted in the urine, where both active and inactive metabolites can be detected for up to 2 days in occasional users, and longer in chronic users.[4,25]

Heroin (diacetylmorphine or diamorphine) is a commonly used and highly addictive semisynthetic analog of morphine that has no legal use in the United States. It can be smoked, snorted, or injected intravenously or intramuscularly. The speed of onset varies from less than 1 to 15 minutes, depending on the delivery method. Outside the United States, diamorphine is administered via the epidural or intrathecal route to provide postcesarean delivery analgesia (see Chapter 27). Heroin's elimination half-life is typically 1 to 2 hours. Heroin is more lipid soluble than other opioids and rapidly crosses the blood-brain barrier, resulting in significant and toxic CNS effects.[199] It is metabolized by cytochrome P450 in the liver and excreted in the urine.[4,25,27,199] The concomitant use of drugs such as omeprazole or amitriptyline can inhibit clearance, while anticonvulsants may increase clearance.[200] Street heroin has increased potency and an increased lethal overdose potential, as it is now often mixed with the semisynthetic or synthetic opioids (e.g., fentanyl).

Oxycodone, **hydromorphone**, and **hydrocodone** are rapidly acting semisynthetic opioids that are often prescribed legitimately and used illicitly. The oral bioavailability of oxycodone is higher than that of morphine, and its potency with oral ingestion is greater.[25] Hydromorphone is roughly five times more potent than morphine when administered orally and nine times more potent when given intravenously.

Methadone is a synthetic compound that is structurally unrelated to the other opioids but has similar effects.[25] It is formulated as a racemic mixture of two enantiomers: R-methadone, which is a potent mu- and delta-opioid receptor agonist, and S-methadone, which is a noncompetitive NMDA antagonist that prevents the reuptake of 5-hydroxytryptamine and norepinephrine.[201] Available in powder form, methadone can be reconstituted for oral, rectal, or intravenous use.[202] Oral bioavailability of methadone is roughly three times that of morphine.[201,202] There is significant interindividual variability in its clinical effect and duration of action, with the peak effect occurring approximately 3 hours after oral ingestion, and its half-life varying from 15 to 40 hours.[25,27,201–203] Life-threatening complications can result from the cumulative effects of successive doses[201] or from prolongation of the cardiac QTc interval prompting the lethal arrhythmia, *torsades de pointes.*

Unlike morphine, methadone undergoes biotransformation (rather than conjugation) in the liver and is excreted primarily by the fecal route. Methadone has been used since the 1960s for medication-assisted therapy for patients suffering from opioid-use disorders and since the 1970s for this indication in pregnant patients. Methadone must be dispensed daily from a certified clinic when used for medication-assisted therapy. Methadone is also used as an analgesic in patients with chronic pain and as a perioperative analgesic and anesthetic adjuvant.[201,203] Pregnancy is associated with greater methadone metabolism and reduced bioavailability because of greater maternal blood volume and changes in hepatic enzymatic activity and glomerular filtration rate.[25,203,204]

Buprenorphine (Subutex) is a semisynthetic opioid that acts as a partial mu-opioid receptor agonist (with low intrinsic opioid activity) and kappa-opioid receptor antagonist that can also be used as medication for patients suffering from opioid use disorders.[205–207] **Suboxone,** one of the two sublingual formulations of this drug, is a combination of buprenorphine and naloxone (which is biochemically active only if the user attempts to snort, inject, or cook the drug).[206] Buprenorphine binds to the mu-opioid receptor with an affinity up to 1000 times greater than that of morphine, with a slow dissociation half-life of approximately 166 minutes.[206] Primary metabolism of buprenorphine occurs in the liver with excretion in the bile.[208] Like methadone, buprenorphine can prolong the QTc interval. Buprenorphine has a ceiling effect at 24 to 32 mg, which decreases the risk for respiratory depression compared with other mu-opioid agonists.[206,209] The ACOG preferentially supports the use of buprenorphine for medication for opioid use disorder (MOUD) during pregnancy because of its several practical advantages over methadone, including a lower likelihood of overdose, fewer drug interactions, fewer required dose adjustments throughout pregnancy, and ease of treatment as an outpatient.[210] However, because of significant concerns for precipitating withdrawal, pregnant patients who are successfully receiving MOUD therapy with methadone should not transition to buprenorphine.

Fentanyl is a highly potent synthetic opioid that can be delivered by intravenous, transmucosal, intranasal, buccal, transdermal, epidural, intrathecal, or inhalational routes.[211] Though fentanyl has a rapid speed of onset, its duration of action is limited by redistribution (half-life ranging from 3.1 to 7.9 hours). Highly lipid soluble, fentanyl is primarily metabolized by the liver, with 10% excreted by the kidneys.[212] Fentanyl has increasingly become a drug of misuse, as its components are easy and inexpensive to obtain and its effects are powerful. Work is underway to develop a fentanyl vaccine to protect against its lethal effects.[213] Fentanyl, carfentanil (an elephant tranquilizer that is 100 times more potent than fentanyl)[214] and other fentanyl derivatives are being surreptitiously integrated into many other drugs of misuse, resulting in substantial morbidity and mortality.[215]

Systemic Effects

Opioids mimic the activity of endogenous peptides and exert their effects through binding to mu-, delta-, and kappa-opioid receptors. Morphine and heroin exert their euphoric, analgesic, and reinforcing effects primarily through stimulation of the mu-opioid receptor. Long-time opioid misuse causes neuroadaptations in the brain that may explain the manifestations of withdrawal.[25,199]

Opioids act in the CNS to reduce sympathetic activity and increase parasympathetic activity. The resulting cardiovascular effects include bradycardia, hypotension, and, in some cases, potentially lethal tachyarrhythmias and bradyarrhythmias (see Table 52.3). Noncardiogenic pulmonary edema has been observed in some cases of overdose and is believed to be caused by hypoxia, intense pulmonary vasoconstriction, and, in some cases, the use of reversal agents (e.g., naloxone).[4] Opiates, such as morphine, promote histamine release from mast cells.

Opioid-induced respiratory depression occurs through a direct effect on the brainstem that reduces the ventilatory response to hypercarbia.[199] Opioid overdose can progress from miosis and respiratory depression to obtundation and death.[5] As opioid overdose deaths in the general population have increased by almost threefold (2002 to 2015), one aspect of the public health response has been a proliferation of more easily accessible, opioid antagonist (i.e., naloxone) therapy.[216] Treatment of overdose also includes maintenance of a patent airway and provision of hemodynamic support as needed.[4]

People who use opioids or other drugs intravenously are at risk for infective endocarditis (usually affecting right-sided valves), HIV infection, viral hepatitis, septic emboli, and pulmonary abscess formation.[4,27] In addition, hilar adenopathy may develop as a result of ingestion of additives such as quinine and starch. Opioid-dependent patients may have additional end-organ damage and may exhibit opioid tolerance, physical dependence, and withdrawal.[200]

Studies have found an association between opioid administration and abnormal pain sensitivity, including opioid-induced hyperalgesia and allodynia (see Table 52.4).[8,217] Opioid tolerance develops with chronic use and is related to the amount and duration of drug exposure; tolerance results from changes in drug distribution and metabolism (pharmacokinetics) and in receptor density and activity (pharmacodynamics).[200] However, tolerance to side effects such as sedation does not develop to the same degree.[217] Both hyperalgesia and tolerance can lead to challenges in pain management in the peripartum period, particularly after cesarean delivery.

Acute opioid withdrawal results from sympathetic hyperactivity, resulting in flulike signs and symptoms such as fatigue, weakness, restlessness, rhinorrhea, perspiration, fever, and diarrhea (see Table 52.5).[5,27] These manifestations can persist for several days if not treated. The onset and duration of withdrawal symptoms vary with the opioid taken; morphine or heroin withdrawal symptoms typically begin within 6 to 18 hours after the last dose, reach their peak intensity by 3 days, and last for 7 to 10 days. Methadone withdrawal symptoms are delayed, with onset within 24 to 48 hours, peak intensity within 3 to 21 days, and duration up to 6 to 7 weeks.[200] Clonidine, an alpha$_2$-adrenergic receptor agonist, can modulate these effects, although postural hypotension may result.[27] Acute withdrawal can also be treated by administration of a short-acting opioid and initiation of a gradual dose taper.[7]

Whereas medically supervised opioid detoxification during pregnancy is reported, it is generally not recommended primarily because of the high rate of relapse.[210] Instead, the ACOG recommends MOUD in combination with behavior modification therapy.[210] Several studies have shown that MOUD promotes better medical and prenatal care,[218] fewer unplanned pregnancies,[11] decreased symptoms of neonatal opioid withdrawal, and less maternal illicit drug use at delivery.[202,204] MOUD with buprenorphine has also shown favorable results with particular advantages regarding neonatal outcomes.[10,209,219] A 2022 cohort study of pregnant women with opioid use disorder who were insured by Medicaid from 2000 through 2018 found that buprenorphine use during pregnancy was associated with fewer adverse neonatal outcomes (e.g., neonatal abstinence syndrome, preterm birth, low birth weight, and small size for gestational age) compared to methadone. However, the risk of maternal adverse events, such as cesarean delivery or life-threatening complications, was similar between the two opioids.[220]

Effects on Pregnancy and the Fetus

Unrestricted opioid use during pregnancy increases the risk of respiratory depression, overdose, and death.[221] In addition, individuals who inject opioids are at increased risk of skin infections, including cellulitis and abscess formation, endocarditis, and osteomyelitis. Sharing needles also places these people at risk for hepatitis B, hepatitis C, and HIV infection. Pregnant women with untreated opioid use disorder may engage in high-risk behaviors, such as prostitution, and suffer related consequences, including incarceration or loss of child custody.[210] Finally, opioid use disorder during pregnancy is associated with coexisting mental health conditions that predispose the expectant mothers to polysubstance use, poor nutrition, and inadequate social support systems. Specifically, posttraumatic stress disorder, anxiety, and depression are more widespread among pregnant women with opioid use disorder than in healthy counterparts; in one study, more than 30% of pregnant women receiving MOUD reported moderate to severe depression.[209,222]

The effects of opioid use on pregnancy and pregnancy outcomes have been evaluated in several retrospective and observational studies. Two retrospective population-based studies showed an association between maternal therapeutic use of opioid medications early in pregnancy and spina bifida, cardiac defects, and gastroschisis,[223,224] but data were obtained retrospectively via maternal interviews and did not control for dose, therapeutic indication, duration, or frequency of opioid exposure. A subsequent metaanalysis concluded that there was uncertainty as to whether opioid use was linked to congenital defects.[225] A separate large population-based study showed an increased risk for several adverse pregnancy outcomes in women with opioid misuse or dependence, including preterm labor, fetal growth restriction, transfusion, and in-hospital mortality.[190]

Evidence is increasing that prenatal opioid use has a negative impact on neonatal brain development.[194] Opioid exposure appears to adversely affect developing oligodendrocytes and the process of myelinization, the size of certain brain structures, and the connectivity between parts of the brain.[226] It is challenging to separate the long-term impact of these effects from that of structural determinants of health. Close follow-up into childhood is suggested.[227]

Heroin use during pregnancy is associated with first-trimester spontaneous abortion, preterm delivery, and fetal growth restriction, in part as a result of poor maternal nutrition.[3,202,218,228] Maternal and neonatal infection and neonatal opioid withdrawal syndrome have also been described. Children born to women using heroin were found to have normal development at the time of entry into school.[3] *In utero* heroin exposure may be associated with a high rate of attention deficit/hyperactivity disorder.

A common neonatal effect of chronic *in utero* opioid exposure is the development of withdrawal symptoms. **Neonatal opioid withdrawal syndrome**, which occurs in neonates repeatedly exposed to opioids, is characterized by irritability, poor feeding, abnormal sleep patterns, diarrhea, fever, and seizures. Affected neonates may also have autonomic symptoms such as yawning and mottling. If prolonged and untreated, neonatal opioid withdrawal syndrome can result in death.[3,228]

Anesthetic Management

Preanesthesia assessment and communication. Establishing trust and effective communication is critical in the care of opioid-tolerant or methadone- or buprenorphine-maintained patients and may improve the ability to elicit a more complete drug history. Ideally, the anesthesia provider can meet the patient before she presents for delivery and develops a mutually agreeable strategy for pain management with appropriate goals for pain intensity scores. Providers, family, and patients may express concern that exposure to opioids or other sedatives will prompt cravings or a frank relapse. Although withholding appropriate analgesic and anxiolytic medications from such a patient is not justified, patient monitoring (e.g., drug screens, pill counts) may be necessary.[200]

Opioid maintenance requirements. Chronic opioids or MOUD should be continued throughout hospitalization and postpartum,[158,200–202] with additional therapies for acute pain management. For those patients receiving methadone maintenance therapy, the precise dose must be confirmed with the drug's dispenser because improper dosing can result in inadequate analgesia, withdrawal, or life-threatening overdose.[201] Any methadone or buprenorphine dose adjustments during pregnancy or postpartum must be done in close consultation with the prescribing physician.[210] The recommendation is to maintain buprenorphine therapy throughout the delivery period to minimize the risk for maternal or fetal withdrawal or relapse.[210] Buprenorphine or methadone doses can be divided (e.g., buprenorphine three times daily) to maximize the analgesic properties of the medication.[206] However, administration of the correct total dose must be ensured. In all cases, the use of multimodal pain management techniques (see later discussion and Chapter 27) is crucial.

Anesthetic technique and dose requirements. The peripartum anesthetic goals for chronic opioid-using parturients or those receiving methadone or buprenorphine MOUD include, as for all patients, provision of a safe environment that maximizes maternal comfort and bonding with the neonate. Neuraxial analgesia or anesthesia is the technique of choice for women undergoing vaginal or cesarean delivery, assuming that the patient is cooperative and has no evidence of coagulopathy or other contraindication. In a review of relevant publications, Cassidy and Cyna[229] cataloged the needs of opioid-dependent patients across a broad range of anesthetic techniques and modes of delivery. The proportion of women that required general anesthesia for cesarean delivery and the number who requested epidural labor analgesia did not differ compared with non–opioid-dependent women. However, a high incidence of pain management challenges was observed, particularly after cesarean delivery; 26% of the patients required consultation for in-patient pain management in addition to usual labor analgesia, and 74% of the patients had difficulties with postcesarean analgesia. These women also had significant vascular access problems and generated more emergency calls for fainting and collapse.

Labor analgesia. Meyer et al.[10,11] noted that pregnant women on methadone or buprenorphine maintenance therapy had similar pain scores and analgesia requirements during labor and vaginal delivery compared with matched controls. It is therefore reasonable to expect that patient reports of inadequate labor epidural analgesia should be treated as they would be in patients without opioid use disorder. Epidural catheter replacement should be promptly offered as needed. Although not studied in this patient population, it seems reasonable to consider the addition of nonopioid adjuvants such as clonidine for labor analgesia, particularly for the treatment of breakthrough pain (see Chapter 24). In contrast, mixed

opioid agonist/antagonist drugs (e.g., nalbuphine) that are commonly employed for labor analgesia or for treatment of neuraxial opioid-induced pruritus should be avoided in patients with a history of opioid use disorder because they can precipitate withdrawal. If neuraxial techniques are contraindicated or provide insufficient pain relief for labor, inhaled nitrous oxide or intravenous patient-controlled analgesia with opioid agonists can also be used, acknowledging that the opioid requirement is likely to be considerably higher (see Chapter 23). Multimodal therapy, including a fixed schedule of nonsteroidal antiinflammatory drugs (NSAIDs) and acetaminophen (paracetamol), should be used after vaginal delivery.[200]

Cesarean delivery anesthesia. Whenever feasible, neuraxial anesthesia (spinal, epidural, or combined spinal-epidural anesthesia) should be utilized for cesarean delivery anesthesia. The potential for decreased MAC in a patient with acute opioid intoxication or, alternatively, the potential for cross-tolerance with CNS depressants in a patient with a history of chronic opioid use, may occur during general anesthesia.[7] However, given that obstetric patients are, in general, a group at high risk for awareness under general anesthesia, it is prudent to prioritize an adequate depth of anesthesia.[230]

Postoperative analgesia. Postoperative pain management can be particularly challenging in patients with a history of chronic opioid use. Both methadone- and buprenorphine-maintained women consistently demonstrate higher pain scores and higher postoperative opioid requirements after cesarean delivery.[10,11] For cesarean delivery, multimodal analgesia with a fixed schedule of NSAID and acetaminophen therapy is highly recommended. Although perioperative use of gabapentin, an NMDA receptor antagonist, has not produced significant additional benefits with neuraxial opioids in the general obstetric population,[231] it is possible that these high-risk patients may benefit from gabapentin administration. However, cumulative increased risk for respiratory depression with high-dose neuraxial morphine, gabapentin, and any additional opioids has been reported in the nonpregnant population.[232,233] Alternatively, women who ingest opioids chronically or those using MOUD may benefit from the higher neuraxial opioid-dosing strategy described by Booth et al.[234] (spinal morphine 300 μg and acetaminophen 1 g every 6 hours for 24 hours). Low-dose ketamine, another NMDA antagonist, has also been used as a single intraoperative dose or as a low-dose postoperative infusion to augment analgesia.[235,236] Other strategies include using patient-controlled epidural analgesia (consider placing a low thoracic epidural catheter), a regional block (e.g., TAP block, quadratus lumborum block), or intravenous patient-controlled opioid analgesia (see Chapter 27).

Volatile Substances

Volatile substances are chemically diverse and readily available and can be sniffed, aerosolized, or ingested to produce feelings of euphoria, excitement, and invulnerability.[237–239]

The five classes of these substances include aromatic hydrocarbons (e.g., toluene), halocarbons (e.g., trichloroethylene), aliphatic hydrocarbons (e.g., propane), inhaled anesthetics (e.g., halogenated ethers and nitrous oxide), and alkyl nitrites (e.g., amyl nitrite).[239]

Epidemiology

The 2021 National Survey on Drug Use and Health reported that 0.2% of nonpregnant women 15 to 44 years of age used inhalants in the past month[22]; the prevalence of use in pregnant women is unknown.

Pharmacology

Volatile substances act by diverse mechanisms, although they commonly have low vapor pressure and high volatility at room air, which facilitates rapid absorption. Excretion is primarily through the lungs.[239] Typically, exposure is to very high concentrations for short periods (e.g., 15 minutes). Detection, although difficult, can be enhanced by the presence of the "glue sniffer's" facial rash[27] or the odor of the inhalant.[238] Laboratory assays can detect many solvents in the blood within 10 hours of exposure. Urine assays are available only for certain volatile substances (e.g., toluene, chlorinated solvents), but may provide a longer window of detection.[4]

Toluene, a primary component of household paint and cleaning agents, is sniffed or ingested orally for its transient euphoric effects.[9] Whereas animal studies suggest that only a small fraction of the original vapor reaches the brain, the effects on GABA, glutamate, and other neurotransmitter systems are profound.[239] **Ethylene glycol**, a bittersweet-tasting component of antifreeze, brake fluids, and industrial solvents, is sometimes used as an inexpensive substitute for alcohol. It is rapidly absorbed via the gastrointestinal tract, reaching maximal blood concentrations within 1 to 4 hours, and metabolized to four toxic organic acids by the hepatic enzyme alcohol dehydrogenase. Primary screening for ethylene glycol intoxication includes serum anion-gap metabolic acidosis, high urine osmolality with an osmol gap, and the presence of calcium oxalate crystals in the urine.[240,241]

Systemic Effects

Typically, the user of volatile substances feels an initial sense of euphoria followed by a brief period of disinhibition and impulsivity. Intoxication can be prolonged through repeated inhalation. As the dose increases, dizziness, diplopia, and disorientation manifest, followed by headache, nausea, vomiting, drowsiness, and sleep.[238]

Mucous membrane irritation can result in rhinorrhea, epistaxis, excessive salivation, and conjunctival redness. Nausea, vomiting, and diarrhea can also occur.[238] Ingestion of volatile substances can lead to potentially lethal tachyarrhythmias, likely secondary to sympathetic stimulation, or bradyarrhythmias from decreased sinoatrial node automaticity or direct vagal stimulation and myocardial depression (see Table 52.3).[4] Hypoxemia may occur as a result of carboxyhemoglobinemia, methemoglobinemia, or suffocation.[4,238,242]

Chronic inhalant use can cause multiorgan system disease, with **cardiac** (e.g., cardiomyopathy, arrhythmias, myocardial infarction), **pulmonary** (e.g., wheezing, acute respiratory distress syndrome, pulmonary hypertension), **central and peripheral nervous system** (e.g., cognitive impairment, ataxia, muscle weakness, peripheral neuropathy), and **autonomic dysfunction** (see Table 52.4).[4,5] Renal toxicity, aplastic anemia, and hepatocellular carcinoma have also been reported.[106,238] Imaging studies have demonstrated loss of brain mass, white matter degeneration, and subcortical abnormalities in long-term users. Significant methemoglobinemia with attendant cyanosis can also occur from exposure to some compounds.[4,238,242]

Cessation of chronic use can lead to reversal of many of the pathophysiologic changes, although the CNS effects may persist. Death from inhalant use typically occurs from suffocation, aspiration, or accidental injury. **Sudden sniffing death syndrome**, likely secondary to a fatal arrhythmia in the setting of a sensitized myocardium, electrolyte abnormalities, and hypoxemia, has been reported in both new and long-term users.[238]

With ingestion of ethylene glycol, the accumulation of toxic metabolites (glycolic and oxalic acid) can result in CNS depression, seizure activity, severe acidosis, organ (primarily kidney) failure, and death. Fatal cardiopulmonary manifestations may occur 12 to 24 hours after ingestion; **renal failure** is likely to occur 24 to 72 hours after ingestion in survivors. The estimated lethal dose of undiluted ethylene glycol is 1.4 mL/kg. Treatment of ethylene glycol ingestion may require the induction of emesis with ipecac or the use of gastric lavage. The conversion of ethylene glycol to its toxic metabolites can be prevented with the use of the antidote **fomepizole** or **ethanol**. Hemodialysis may be warranted.[241]

Ingestion of toluene can cause cardiac arrhythmias, acute respiratory distress syndrome, hepatic failure, cerebral edema, and death.[9]

Effects on Pregnancy and the Fetus

In animal studies, acute and chronic toluene exposure during pregnancy results in the presence of toluene in the fetal brain.[243] Volatile substance use has been associated with human intrauterine fetal growth restriction, preterm delivery, and perinatal mortality.[7]

Ethylene glycol intoxication can present with hypertension, seizures, and coma and may be misdiagnosed as eclampsia.[240] Hemodynamic instability, severe metabolic acidosis, and acute renal failure should prompt suspicion of intoxication. Ethylene glycol poisoning can be successfully treated with hemodialysis and intravenous ethanol; an exposed neonate may require diuresis and replacement transfusion.

Anesthetic Management

Identification of volatile substance use in the parturient is critical to safe anesthesia care.[242] Decontamination of skin and clothing is required.[238] A careful physical examination, including the oropharynx, and documentation of preexisting neurologic deficits should be undertaken, and electrolyte abnormalities should be corrected.[7]

If the patient is cooperative and able to protect her airway, neuraxial labor analgesia can be administered. Initial treatment of hypotension should include intravenous fluids first, followed by phenylephrine if necessary, given the propensity toward arrhythmias. Atropine should be readily available but used with caution. In a stable patient with sustained

tachyarrhythmias, selective beta-adrenergic receptor antagonists should be the first-line therapy.[4]

In intoxicated or otherwise uncooperative patients, rapid-sequence induction of general anesthesia for cesarean delivery may be indicated.[7] Propofol or etomidate may be preferred induction agents to ketamine, as the latter may exacerbate tachyarrhythmias. Oxygenation and ventilation can be complicated by preexisting pulmonary complications.

KEY POINTS

- Licit and illicit substance use by pregnant women may result in significant maternal and fetal risks.
- Anesthesia providers often care for pregnant women with substance use disorders during the peripartum period and when administering anesthesia for nonobstetric surgery during pregnancy.
- Maternal self-reporting underestimates the true incidence of substance use. Drug testing (e.g., urine, blood, oral fluid, hair, meconium) should be performed if substance use disorder is suspected.
- Optimal care of patients with substance use disorder requires a therapeutic bond and an explicit pain management plan. Anesthesia providers should ask patients questions in a respectful and nonjudgmental manner.
- Neuraxial anesthetic techniques are the preferred methods for labor analgesia and cesarean delivery anesthesia for most patients with a history of substance use disorder, provided that the patient is cooperative, able to protect their airway, and does not have a coagulopathy or a platelet count below the threshold suggested by anesthesia professional society guidelines.
- Although patients with opioid or other substance use disorder may have abnormal pain sensitivity, providers should not assume that the etiology of inadequate neuraxial labor analgesia is solely a result of the patient's disorder. Opioid-tolerant patients can have inadequate or failed neuraxial analgesia and anesthesia just like their opioid-naïve counterparts.
- Smoking during pregnancy negatively affects fetal growth. Pregnant women who smoke are more likely to suffer respiratory complications and impaired wound healing.
- There is an association between moderate maternal caffeine intake during pregnancy and decreased birth weight, but further research is warranted. Moderate caffeine intake

during pregnancy (<200 mg/day) does not appear to contribute significantly to spontaneous abortion or preterm birth.
- Cannabis is the most common restricted substance used by pregnant women. Smoking cannabis increases maternal respiratory comorbidities. There may be long-term effects on exposed offspring, including inattention and impulsivity, deficits in problem solving, and academic underachievement.
- Cocaine use has been associated with sudden death from a variety of factors, including cardiac arrhythmias, respiratory arrest, status epilepticus, and impaired thermoregulation. Maternal cocaine use increases the likelihood of placental abruption and urgent cesarean delivery.
- Acute cocaine intoxication can mimic preeclampsia, eclampsia, or malignant hyperthermia.
- Evidence is conflicting as to whether intrauterine hallucinogen exposure has deleterious effects on the fetus.
- Volatile substance use can lead to severe maternal hypoxemia and potentially lethal arrhythmias.
- Ingestion of amphetamines results in high levels of circulating catecholamines, leading to hemodynamic instability and, in some cases, cardiac arrest.
- Care of the opioid-dependent patient should involve maintenance of long-term opioid requirements, multimodal management of acute pain, and avoidance of opioid antagonists and mixed agonist/antagonist agents outside of MOUD (unless the patient shows signs of overdose).
- Buprenorphine is increasingly becoming the opioid of choice for MOUD in patients who use heroin or have other opioid use disorders. Goals of care in these and methadone-maintained patients include continuing their methadone or buprenorphine treatment, adding multimodal acute pain therapy, and avoiding opioid antagonists.

REFERENCES

1. Substance Abuse and Mental Health Services Administration. *2022 National Survey on Drug Use and Health.* U.S. Department of Health & Human Services; 2023. https://www.samhsa.gov/data/sites/default/files/reports/rpt42728/NSDUHDetailedTabs2022/NSDUHDetailedTabs2022/NSDUHDetTabsSect8pe2022.htm#tab8.27b. Accessed July 26, 2024.

2. Polak K, Kelpin S, Terplan M. Screening for substance use in pregnancy and the newborn. *Semin Fetal Neonatal Med.* 2019;24:90–94.
3. Huestis MA, Choo RE. Drug abuse's smallest victims: in utero drug exposure. *Forensic Sci Int.* 2002;128:20–30.
4. Ghuran A, Nolan J. Recreational drug misuse: issues for the cardiologist. *Heart.* 2000;83:627–633.
5. Brust JC. Neurologic complications of substance abuse. *J Acquir Immune Defic Syndr.* 2002;31:S29–S34.

6. Kain ZN, Mayes LC, Ferris CA, et al. Cocaine-abusing parturients undergoing cesarean section. A cohort study. *Anesthesiology.* 1996;85:1028–1035.

7. Kuczkowski KM. Anesthetic implications of drug abuse in pregnancy. *J Clin Anesth.* 2003;15:382–394.

8. Mao J. Opioid-induced abnormal pain sensitivity: implications in clinical opioid therapy. *Pain.* 2002;100: 213–217.

9. Hernandez M, Birnbach DJ, Van Zundert AA. Anesthetic management of the illicit-substance-using patient. *Curr Opin Anaesthesiol.* 2005;18:315–324.

10. Meyer M, Paranya G, Keefer Norris A, Howard D. Intrapartum and postpartum analgesia for women maintained on buprenorphine during pregnancy. *Eur J Pain.* 2010;14: 939–943.

11. Meyer M, Wagner K, Benvenuto A, et al. Intrapartum and postpartum analgesia for women maintained on methadone during pregnancy. *Obstet Gynecol.* 2007;110:261–266.

12. Keegan J, Parva M, Finnegan M, et al. Addiction in pregnancy. *J Addict Dis.* 2010;29:175–191.

13. Ostrea EM Jr, Knapp DK, Tannenbaum L, et al. Estimates of illicit drug use during pregnancy by maternal interview, hair analysis, and meconium analysis. *J Pediatr.* 2001;138:344–348.

14. Montgomery D, Plate C, Alder SC, et al. Testing for fetal exposure to illicit drugs using umbilical cord tissue vs meconium. *J Perinatol.* 2006;26:11–14.

15. Lester BM, Andreozzi L, Appiah L. Substance use during pregnancy: time for policy to catch up with research. *Harm Reduct J.* 2004;1:5.

16. Lester BM, ElSohly M, Wright LL, et al. The maternal lifestyle study: drug use by meconium toxicology and maternal self-report. *Pediatrics.* 2001;107:309–317.

17. Musshoff F, Madea B. Review of biologic matrices (urine, blood, hair) as indicators of recent or ongoing cannabis use. *Ther Drug Monit.* 2006;28:155–163.

18. Verstraete AG. Detection times of drugs of abuse in blood, urine, and oral fluid. *Ther Drug Monit.* 2004;26:200–205.

19. Siegel MR, Mahowald GK, Uljon SN, et al. Fentanyl in the labor epidural impacts the results of intrapartum and postpartum maternal and neonatal toxicology tests. *Am J Obstet Gynecol.* 2023;228:741.e1–e7.

20. Novikov N, Melanson SEF, Ransohoff JR, Petrides AK. Rates of fentanyl positivity in neonatal urine following maternal analgesia during labor and delivery. *J Appl Lab Med.* 2020;5:686–694.

21. United States Centers for Disease Control and Prevention. Alcohol consumption among pregnant and childbearing-aged women—United States, 1991 and 1995. *MMWR Morb Mortal Wkly Rep.* 1997;46:346–350.

22. Substance Abuse and Mental Health Services Administration. *2021 National Survey of Drug Use and Health (NSDUH): Detailed Tables.* Center for Behavioral Health Statistics and Quality; 2023. https://www.samhsa.gov/data/report/2021-nsduh-detailed-tables. Accessed July 26, 2024.

23. Spampinato MV, Castillo M, Rojas R, et al. Magnetic resonance imaging findings in substance abuse: alcohol and alcoholism and syndromes associated with alcohol abuse. *Top Magn Reson Imaging.* 2005;16:223–230.

24. Lieber CS. Medical disorders of alcoholism. *N Engl J Med.* 1995;333:1058–1065.

25. Reynolds EW, Bada HS. Pharmacology of drugs of abuse. *Obstet Gynecol Clin North Am.* 2003;30:501–522.

26. Khan H, Nagda J. Substance abuse. In: Pian-Smith M, Leffert L, eds. *Obstetric Anesthesia.* Cambridge University Press; 2007.

27. Wood PR, Soni N. Anaesthesia and substance abuse. *Anaesthesia.* 1989;44:672–680.

28. de Wit M, Goldberg A, Chelmow D. Alcohol use disorders and hospital-acquired infections in women undergoing cesarean delivery. *Obstet Gynecol.* 2013;122:72–78.

29. Rayner SG, Weinert CR, Peng H, et al. Dexmedetomidine as adjunct treatment for severe alcohol withdrawal in the ICU. *Ann Intensive Care.* 2012;2:12.

30. Floyd RL, O'Connor MJ, Sokol RJ, et al. Recognition and prevention of fetal alcohol syndrome. *Obstet Gynecol.* 2005;106:1059–1064.

31. Wright A, Walker J. Management of women who use drugs during pregnancy. *Semin Fetal Neonatal Med.* 2007;12: 114–118.

32. McCarthy FP, O'Keeffe LM, Khashan AS, et al. Association between maternal alcohol consumption in early pregnancy and pregnancy outcomes. *Obstet Gynecol.* 2013;122:830–837.

33. Nykjaer C, Alwan NA, Greenwood DC, et al. Maternal alcohol intake prior to and during pregnancy and risk of adverse birth outcomes: evidence from a British cohort. *J Epidemiol Community Health.* 2014;68:542–549.

34. Bertrand J, Floyd L, Weber MK, et al. *Fetal Alcohol Syndrome: Guidelines for Referral and Diagnosis.* Centers for Disease Control and Prevention; 2004.

35. Jones K, Smith D. Recognition of the fetal alcohol syndrome in early infancy. *Lancet.* 1973;302:999–1001.

36. Popova S, Lange S, Shield K, et al. Comorbidity of fetal alcohol spectrum disorder: a systematic review and meta-analysis. *Lancet.* 2016;387:978–987.

37. Ackland GL, Smith M, McGlennan AP. Acute, severe hypoglycemia occurring during general anesthesia in a nondiabetic adult. *Anesth Analg.* 2007;105:553–554.

38. Bruce DL. Alcoholism and anesthesia. *Anesth Analg.* 1983;62:84–96.

39. Fassoulaki A, Farinotti R, Servin F, Desmonts JM. Chronic alcoholism increases the induction dose of propofol in humans. *Anesth Analg.* 1993;77:553–556.

40. Liang C, Chen J, Gu W, et al. Chronic alcoholism increases the induction dose of propofol. *Acta Anaesthesiol Scand.* 2011;55:1113–1117.

41. Ghoneim MM. Awareness during anesthesia. *Anesthesiology.* 2000;92:597–602.

42. Robins K, Lyons G. Intraoperative awareness during general anesthesia for cesarean delivery. *Anesth Analg.* 2009;109: 886–890.

43. Nawrot P, Jordan S, Eastwood J, et al. Effects of caffeine on human health. *Food Addit Contam.* 2003;20:1–30.

44. Chen L, Bell EM, Browne ML, et al. Exploring maternal patterns of dietary caffeine consumption before conception and during pregnancy. *Matern Child Health J.* 2014;18: 2446–2455.

45. Higdon JV, Frei B. Coffee and health: a review of recent human research. *Crit Rev Food Sci Nutr.* 2006;46:101–123.

46. Grosso LM, Triche E, Benowitz NL, Bracken MB. Prenatal caffeine assessment: fetal and maternal biomarkers or self-reported intake? *Ann Epidemiol.* 2008;18:172–178.

47. Browne ML, Bell EM, Druschel CM, et al. Maternal caffeine consumption and risk of cardiovascular malformations. *Birth Defects Res A Clin Mol Teratol.* 2007;79:533–543.

48. Hinkle SN, Laughon SK, Catov JM, et al. First trimester coffee and tea intake and risk of gestational diabetes mellitus: a study within a national birth cohort. *BJOG*. 2015;122:420–428.

49. Bech BH, Obel C, Henriksen TB, Olsen J. Effect of reducing caffeine intake on birth weight and length of gestation: randomised controlled trial. *BMJ*. 2007;334:409.

50. Conover WB, Key TC, Resnik R. Maternal cardiovascular response to caffeine infusion in the pregnant ewe. *Am J Obstet Gynecol*. 1983;145:534–538.

51. Browne ML. Maternal exposure to caffeine and risk of congenital anomalies: a systematic review. *Epidemiology*. 2006;17:324–331.

52. Gleason JL, Tekola-Ayele F, Sundaram R, et al. Association between maternal caffeine consumption and metabolism and neonatal anthropometry: a secondary analysis of the NICHD fetal growth studies-singletons. *JAMA Netw Open*. 2021;4:e213238.

53. Soltani S, Salari-Moghaddam A, Saneei P, et al. Maternal caffeine consumption during pregnancy and risk of low birth weight: a dose-response meta-analysis of cohort studies. *Crit Rev Food Sci Nutr*. 2023;63:224–233.

54. American College of Obstetricians and Gynecologists. Committee Opinion No. 462: Moderate caffeine consumption during pregnancy (reaffirmed 2023). *Obstet Gynecol*. 2010;116:467–468.

55. Weng X, Odouli R, Li DK. Maternal caffeine consumption during pregnancy and the risk of miscarriage: a prospective cohort study. *Am J Obstet Gynecol*. 2008;198:279.e1–e8.

56. Substance Abuse and Mental Health Services Administration. *Results From the 2015 National Survey on Drug Use and Health: Detailed Tables*. Center for Behavioral Health Statistics and Quality; 2016. https://www.samhsa.gov/data/sites/default/files/NSDUH-DetTabs-2015/NSDUH-DetTabs-2015/NSDUH-DetTabs-2015.pdf. Accessed June 29, 2025.

57. Whittington JR, Simmons PM, Phillips AM, et al. The use of electronic cigarettes in pregnancy: a review of the literature. *Obstet Gynecol Surv*. 2018;73:544–549.

58. Hlastala MP, McKenna HP, Franada RL, Detter JC. Influence of carbon monoxide on hemoglobin-oxygen binding. *J Appl Physiol*. 1976;41:893–899.

59. Klausen K, Andersen C, Nandrup S. Acute effects of cigarette smoking and inhalation of carbon monoxide during maximal exercise. *Eur J Appl Physiol Occup Physiol*. 1983;51:371–379.

60. Warner DO. Perioperative abstinence from cigarettes: physiologic and clinical consequences. *Anesthesiology*. 2006;104:356–367.

61. American College of Obstetricians and Gynecologists. Committee Opinion No. 807: Tobacco and nicotine cessation during pregnancy (reaffirmed 2023). *Obstet Gynecol*. 2020;135:e221–e229.

62. Centers for Disease Control and Prevention. *E-Cigarettes and Pregnancy*. Centers for Disease Control and Prevention; 2024. https://www.cdc.gov/maternal-infant-health/pregnancy-substance-abuse/e-cigarettes.html?CDC_AAref_Val=https://www.cdc.gov/reproductivehealth/maternalinfanthealth/substance-abuse/e-cigarettes-pregnancy.htm. Accessed July 26, 2024.

63. Spindel ER, McEvoy CT. The role of nicotine in the effects of maternal smoking during pregnancy on lung development and childhood respiratory disease. Implications for dangers of e-cigarettes. *Am J Respir Crit Care Med*. 2016;193:486–494.

64. Sastry BV. Placental toxicology: tobacco smoke, abused drugs, multiple chemical interactions, and placental function. *Reprod Fertil Dev*. 1991;3:355–372.

65. Bada HS, Das A, Bauer CR, et al. Low birth weight and preterm births: etiologic fraction attributable to prenatal drug exposure. *J Perinatol*. 2005;25:631–637.

66. Salihu HM, Aliyu MH, Pierre-Louis BJ, Alexander GR. Levels of excess infant deaths attributable to maternal smoking during pregnancy in the United States. *Matern Child Health J*. 2003;7:219–227.

67. Baba S, Wikstrom AK, Stephansson O, Cnattingius S. Changes in snuff and smoking habits in Swedish pregnant women and risk for small for gestational age births. *BJOG*. 2013;120:456–462.

68. Moore E, Blatt K, Chen A, et al. Relationship of trimester-specific smoking patterns and risk of preterm birth. *Am J Obstet Gynecol*. 2016;215:109.e1–e6.

69. Kistin N, Handler A, Davis F, Ferre C. Cocaine and cigarettes: a comparison of risks. *Paediatr Perinat Epidemiol*. 1996;10:269–278.

70. U.S. Department of Health and Human Services. *The Health Consequences of Smoking: 50 Years of Progress. A Report of the Surgeon General*. U.S. Department of Health and Human Services, Centers for Disease Control and Prevention, National Center for Chronic Disease Prevention and Health Promotion, Office on Smoking and Health; 2014. https://www.ncbi.nlm.nih.gov/books/NBK179276/. Accessed July 26, 2024.

71. Li YF, Langholz B, Salam MT, Gilliland FD. Maternal and grandmaternal smoking patterns are associated with early childhood asthma. *Chest*. 2005;127:1232–1241.

72. Ding Z, Pang L, Chai H, et al. The causal association between maternal smoking around birth on childhood asthma: a Mendelian randomization study. *Front Public Health*. 2022;10:1059195.

73. Brand JS, Hiyoshi A, Cao Y, et al. Maternal smoking during pregnancy and fractures in offspring: national register based sibling comparison study. *BMJ*. 2020;368:l7057.

74. Riedel C, Schonberger K, Yang S, et al. Parental smoking and childhood obesity: higher effect estimates for maternal smoking in pregnancy compared with paternal smoking—a meta-analysis. *Int J Epidemiol*. 2014;43:1593–1606.

75. Klonoff-Cohen H, Edelstein S, Savitz D. Cigarette smoking and preeclampsia. *Obstet Gynecol*. 1993;81:541–544.

76. Lisonkova S, Joseph KS. Left truncation bias as a potential explanation for the protective effect of smoking on preeclampsia. *Epidemiology*. 2015;26:436–440.

77. Fried PA, Watkinson B, Gray R. Growth from birth to early adolescence in offspring prenatally exposed to cigarettes and marijuana. *Neurotoxicol Teratol*. 1999;21:513–525.

78. Holz NE, Boecker R, Baumeister S, et al. Effect of prenatal exposure to tobacco smoke on inhibitory control: neuroimaging results from a 25-year prospective study. *JAMA Psychiatry*. 2014;71:786–796.

79. Quinn PD, Rickert ME, Weibull CE, et al. Association between maternal smoking during pregnancy and severe mental illness in offspring. *JAMA Psychiatry*. 2017;74:589–596.

80. Hurt RD, Renner CC, Patten CA, et al. Iqmik—a form of smokeless tobacco used by pregnant Alaska natives: nicotine exposure in their neonates. *J Matern Fetal Neonatal Med*. 2005;17:281–289.

81. Gupta PC, Subramoney S. Smokeless tobacco use, birth weight, and gestational age: population based, prospective cohort study of 1217 women in Mumbai, India. *BMJ*. 2004;328:1538.

82. Wilkes AR, Hall JE, Wright E, Grundler S. The effect of humidification and smoking habit on the incidence of adverse airway events during deepening of anaesthesia with desflurane. *Anaesthesia*. 2000;55:685–689.

83. Kim ES, Bishop MJ. Cough during emergence from isoflurane anesthesia. *Anesth Analg*. 1998;87:1170–1174.

84. Kotani N, Kushikata T, Hashimoto H, et al. Recovery of intraoperative microbicidal and inflammatory functions of alveolar immune cells after a tobacco smoke-free period. *Anesthesiology*. 2001;94:999–1006.

85. Dimitriadis K, Narkiewicz K, Leontsinis I, et al. Acute effects of electronic and tobacco cigarette smoking on sympathetic nerve activity and blood pressure in humans. *Int J Env Res Public Health*. 2022;19:3237.

86. Hobson A, Arndt K, Barenklau S. Vaping: anesthesia considerations for patients using electronic cigarettes. *AANA J*. 2020;88:27–34.

87. American College of Obstetricians and Gynecologists. Committee Opinion No. 479: Methamphetamine abuse in women of reproductive age (reaffirmed 2021). *Obstet Gynecol*. 2011;117:751–755.

88. Arria AM, Derauf C, Lagasse LL, et al. Methamphetamine and other substance use during pregnancy: preliminary estimates from the Infant Development, Environment, and Lifestyle (IDEAL) Study. *Matern Child Health J*. 2006;10:293–302.

89. Sankaran D, Lakshminrusimha S, Manja V. Methamphetamine: burden, mechanism and impact on pregnancy, the fetus, and newborn. *J Perinatol*. 2022;42: 293–299.

90. Wouldes T, LaGasse L, Sheridan J, Lester BM. Maternal methamphetamine use during pregnancy and child outcome: what do we know? *N Z Med J*. 2004;117:U1180.

91. Smid MC, Metz TD, Gordon AJ. Stimulant use in pregnancy: an under-recognized epidemic among pregnant women. *Clin Obstet Gynecol*. 2019;62:168–184.

92. Ho E, Karimi-Tabesh L, Koren G. Characteristics of pregnant women who use ecstasy (3, 4-methylenedioxymethamphetamine). *Neurotoxicol Teratol*. 2001;23: 561–567.

93. Kalant H. The pharmacology and toxicology of "ecstasy" (MDMA) and related drugs. *CMAJ*. 2001;165:917–928.

94. Rodgers J, Ashton CH, Gilvarry E, Young AH. Liquid ecstasy: a new kid on the dance floor. *Br J Psychiatry*. 2004;184: 104–106.

95. Ludlow J, Christmas T, Paech MJ, Orr B. Drug abuse and dependency during pregnancy: anaesthetic issues. *Anaesth Intensive Care*. 2007;35:881–893.

96. Smith C, Cardile AP, Miller M. Bath salts as a "legal high". *Am J Med*. 2011;124:e7–e8.

97. Antoniou T, Juurlink DN. Five things to know about…"bath salts". *CMAJ*. 2012;184:1713.

98. Falgiani M, Desai B, Ryan M. "Bath salts" intoxication: a case report. *Case Rep Emerg Med*. 2012;2012:976314.

99. Samuels SI, Maze A, Albright G. Cardiac arrest during cesarean section in a chronic amphetamine abuser. *Anesth Analg*. 1979;58:528–530.

100. Kuczkowski KM. Postpartum convulsions and acute hemodynamic instability in the parturient with recent amphetamine intake. *Arch Gynecol Obstet*. 2009;280: 1059–1061.

101. Westover AN, McBride S, Haley RW. Stroke in young adults who abuse amphetamines or cocaine: a population-based study of hospitalized patients. *Arch Gen Psychiatry*. 2007;64: 495–502.

102. Volkow ND, Chang L, Wang GJ, et al. Loss of dopamine transporters in methamphetamine abusers recovers with protracted abstinence. *J Neurosci*. 2001;21:9414–9418.

103. Vollenweider FX, Gamma A, Liechti M, Huber T. Psychological and cardiovascular effects and short-term sequelae of MDMA ("Ecstasy") in MDMA-naïve healthy volunteers. *Neuropsychopharmacology*. 1998;19:241.

104. Clark CM, Frye CG, Wardle MC, et al. Acute effects of MDMA on autonomic cardiac activity and their relation to subjective prosocial and stimulant effects. *Psychophysiology*. 2015;52:429–435.

105. Parrott AC. Oxytocin, cortisol and 3,4-methylenedioxymethamphetamine: neurohormonal aspects of recreational 'ecstasy'. *Behav Pharmacol*. 2016;27:649–658.

106. Sajo E. Pharmacology of substance abuse. *Lippincotts Prim Care Pract*. 2000;4:319–335.

107. Oro AS, Dixon SD. Perinatal cocaine and methamphetamine exposure: maternal and neonatal correlates. *J Pediatr*. 1987;111:571–578.

108. Gorman MC, Orme KS, Nguyen NT, et al. Outcomes in pregnancies complicated by methamphetamine use. *Am J Obstet Gynecol*. 2014;211:429.e1–e7.

109. Kalaitzopoulos DR, Chatzistergiou K, Amylidi AL, et al. Effect of methamphetamine hydrochloride on pregnancy outcome: a systematic review and meta-analysis. *J Addict Med*. 2018;12:220–226.

110. Eze N, Smith LM, LaGasse LL, et al. School-aged outcomes following prenatal methamphetamine exposure: 7.5-year follow-up from the Infant Development, Environment, and Lifestyle Study. *J Pediatr*. 2016;170:34–38.e1.

111. Kiblawi ZN, Smith LM, LaGasse LL, et al. The effect of prenatal methamphetamine exposure on attention as assessed by continuous performance tests: results from the Infant Development, Environment, and Lifestyle Study. *J Dev Behav Pediatr*. 2013;34:31–37.

112. Smith LM, Diaz S, LaGasse LL, et al. Developmental and behavioral consequences of prenatal methamphetamine exposure: a review of the Infant Development, Environment, and Lifestyle (IDEAL) Study. *Neurotoxicol Teratol*. 2015;51:35–44.

113. National Institute on Drug Abuse. *What Are the Risks of Methamphetamine Misuse During Pregnancy?* National Institute on Drug Abuse; 2021. www.drugabuse.gov/publications/research-reports/methamphetamine/what-are-risks-methamphetamine-misuse-during-pregnancy. Accessed July 26, 2024.

114. Hanzawa S, Nemoto M, Etoh S, et al. A case of amphetamine-induced down-regulation of beta-adrenoceptor [Japanese]. *Masui*. 2001;50:1242–1245.

115. Johnston RR, Way WL, Miller RD. Alteration of anesthetic requirement by amphetamine. *Anesthesiology*. 1972;36: 357–363.

116. Michel R, Adams AP. Acute amphetamine abuse. Problems during general anaesthesia for neurosurgery. *Anaesthesia*. 1979;34:1016–1019.

117. Fajemirokun-Odudeyi O, Lindow SW. Obstetric implications of cocaine use in pregnancy: a literature review. *Eur J Obstet Gynecol Reprod Biol*. 2004;112:2–8.

118. Shanti CM, Lucas CE. Cocaine and the critical care challenge. *Crit Care Med*. 2003;31:1851–1859.

119. Bauer CR, Langer JC, Shankaran S, et al. Acute neonatal effects of cocaine exposure during pregnancy. *Arch Pediatr Adolesc Med.* 2005;159:824–834.

120. Kuczkowski KM. Peripartum care of the cocaine-abusing parturient: are we ready? *Acta Obstet Gynecol Scand.* 2005;84:108–116.

121. Fleming JA, Byck R, Barash PG. Pharmacology and therapeutic applications of cocaine. *Anesthesiology.* 1990;73:518–531.

122. Ettinger NA, Albin RJ. A review of the respiratory effects of smoking cocaine. *Am J Med.* 1989;87:664–668.

123. Lange RA, Hillis LD. Cardiovascular complications of cocaine use. *N Engl J Med.* 2001;345:351–358.

124. Warner EA. Cocaine abuse. *Ann Intern Med.* 1993;119:226–235.

125. Feng Q. Postnatal consequences of prenatal cocaine exposure and myocardial apoptosis: does cocaine in utero imperil the adult heart? *Br J Pharmacol.* 2005;144:887–888.

126. Mittleman MA, Mintzer D, Maclure M, et al. Triggering of myocardial infarction by cocaine. *Circulation.* 1999;99:2737–2741.

127. Hollander JE, Henry TD. Evaluation and management of the patient who has cocaine-associated chest pain. *Cardiol Clin.* 2006;24:103–114.

128. Livingston JC, Mabie BC, Ramanathan J. Crack cocaine, myocardial infarction, and troponin I levels at the time of cesarean delivery. *Anesth Analg.* 2000;91:913–915.

129. Kuczkowski KM. More on the idiosyncratic effects of cocaine on the human heart. *Emerg Med J.* 2007;24:147.

130. Vertommen J, Hughes S, Rosen M, et al. Hydralazine does not restore uterine blood flow during cocaine-induced hypertension in the pregnant ewe. *Anesthesiology.* 1992;76:580–587.

131. Ansah T-A, Wade LH, Kopsombut P, Shockley DC. Nifedipine potentiates the toxic effects of cocaine in mice. *Prog Neuropsychopharmacol Biol Psychiatry.* 2002;26:357–362.

132. Derlet RW, Albertson TE. Potentiation of cocaine toxicity with calcium channel blockers. *Am J Emerg Med.* 1989;7:464–468.

133. Richards JR, Garber D, Laurin EG, et al. Treatment of cocaine cardiovascular toxicity: a systematic review. *Clin Toxicol (Phila).* 2016;54:345–364.

134. Gowda RM, Khan IA, Mehta NJ, et al. Cardiac arrhythmias in pregnancy: clinical and therapeutic considerations. *Int J Cardiol.* 2003;88:129–133.

135. Mason BA, Ricci-Goodman J, Koos BJ. Adenosine in the treatment of maternal paroxysmal supraventricular tachycardia. *Obstet Gynecol.* 1992;80:478–480.

136. Shih RD, Hollander JE, Burstein JL, et al. Clinical safety of lidocaine in patients with cocaine-associated myocardial infarction. *Ann Emerg Med.* 1995;26:702–706.

137. Widerhorn J, Bhandari AK, Bughi S, et al. Fetal and neonatal adverse effects profile of amiodarone treatment during pregnancy. *Am Heart J.* 1991;122:1162–1166.

138. Schleich JM, Bernard Du Haut Cilly F, Laurent MC, Almange C. Early prenatal management of a fetal ventricular tachycardia treated in utero by amiodarone with long term follow-up. *Prenat Diagn.* 2000;20:449–452.

139. Spivey WH, Euerle B. Neurologic complications of cocaine abuse. *Ann Emerg Med.* 1990;19:1422–1428.

140. Kain ZN, Mayes LC, Pakes J, et al. Thrombocytopenia in pregnant women who use cocaine. *Am J Obstet Gynecol.* 1995;173:885–890.

141. Orser B. Thrombocytopenia and cocaine abuse. *Anesthesiology.* 1991;74:195–196.

142. Gershon RY, Fisher AJ, Graves WL. The cocaine-abusing parturient is not at an increased risk for thrombocytopenia. *Anesth Analg.* 1996;82:865–866.

143. Kain ZN, Rimar S, Barash PG. Cocaine abuse in the parturient and effects on the fetus and neonate. *Anesth Analg.* 1993;77:835–845.

144. Owiny JR, Jones MT, Sadowsky D, et al. Cocaine in pregnancy: the effect of maternal administration of cocaine on the maternal and fetal pituitary-adrenal axes. *Am J Obstet Gynecol.* 1991;164:658–663.

145. Owiny JR, Sadowsky D, Jones MT, et al. Effect of maternal cocaine administration on maternal and fetal glucose, lactate, and insulin in sheep. *Obstet Gynecol.* 1991;77:901–904.

146. Crandall CG, Vongpatanasin W, Victor RG. Mechanism of cocaine-induced hyperthermia in humans. *Ann Intern Med.* 2002;136:785–791.

147. Gouin K, Murphy K, Shah PS. Effects of cocaine use during pregnancy on low birthweight and preterm birth: systematic review and metaanalyses. *Am J Obstet Gynecol.* 2011;204:340.e1–e12.

148. Little BB, Snell LM, Trimmer KJ, et al. Peripartum cocaine use and adverse pregnancy outcome. *Am J Hum Biol.* 1999;11:598–602.

149. Ness RB, Grisso JA, Hirschinger N, et al. Cocaine and tobacco use and the risk of spontaneous abortion. *N Engl J Med.* 1999;340:333–339.

150. Bingol N, Fuchs M, Diaz V, et al. Teratogenicity of cocaine in humans. *J Pediatr.* 1987;110:93–96.

151. Gonsoulin W, Borge D, Moise KJ Jr. Rupture of unscarred uterus in primigravid woman in association with cocaine abuse. *Am J Obstet Gynecol.* 1990;163:526–527.

152. Towers CV, Pircon RA, Nageotte MP, et al. Cocaine intoxication presenting as preeclampsia and eclampsia. *Obstet Gynecol.* 1993;81:545–547.

153. Kline J, Ng SK, Schittini M, et al. Cocaine use during pregnancy: sensitive detection by hair assay. *Am J Public Health.* 1997;87:352–358.

154. Shankaran S, Lester BM, Das A, et al. Impact of maternal substance use during pregnancy on childhood outcome. *Semin Fetal Neonatal Med.* 2007;12:143–150.

155. Richardson GA, Hamel SC, Goldschmidt L, Day NL. Growth of infants prenatally exposed to cocaine/crack: comparison of a prenatal care and a no prenatal care sample. *Pediatrics.* 1999;104:e18.

156. Bauer CR, Shankaran S, Bada HS, et al. The maternal lifestyle study: drug exposure during pregnancy and short-term maternal outcomes. *Am J Obstet Gynecol.* 2002;186:487–495.

157. Behnke M, Eyler FD, Garvan CW, Wobie K. The search for congenital malformations in newborns with fetal cocaine exposure. *Pediatrics.* 2001;107:E74.

158. Frank DA, Augustyn M, Knight WG, et al. Growth, development, and behavior in early childhood following prenatal cocaine exposure: a systematic review. *JAMA.* 2001;285:1613–1625.

159. Mayes L, Snyder PJ, Langlois E, Hunter N. Visuospatial working memory in school-aged children exposed in utero to cocaine. *Child Neuropsychol.* 2007;13:205–218.

160. Eiden RD, Coles CD, Schuetze P, Colder CR. Externalizing behavior problems among polydrug cocaine-exposed children: indirect pathways via maternal harshness and

self-regulation in early childhood. *Psychol Addict Behav.* 2014;28:139–153.

161. Dennis T, Bendersky M, Ramsay D, Lewis M. Reactivity and regulation in children prenatally exposed to cocaine. *Dev Psychol.* 2006;42:688–697.

162. Richardson GA, Goldschmidt L, Larkby C, Day NL. Effects of prenatal cocaine exposure on adolescent development. *Neurotoxicol Teratol.* 2015;49:41–48.

163. Bauer ME, Arendt K, Beilin Y, et al. The Society for Obstetric Anesthesia and Perinatology interdisciplinary consensus statement on neuraxial procedures in obstetric patients with thrombocytopenia. *Anesth Analg.* 2021;132:1531–1544.

164. Bloomstone JA. The drug-abusing parturient. *Int Anesthesiol Clin.* 2002;40:137–150.

165. Ross VH, Moore CH, Pan PH, et al. Reduced duration of intrathecal sufentanil analgesia in laboring cocaine users. *Anesth Analg.* 2003;97:1504–1508.

166. Whittington RA, Virag L, Vulliemoz Y, et al. Dexmedetomidine increases the cocaine seizure threshold in rats. *Anesthesiology.* 2002;97:693–700.

167. Ashton CH. Pharmacology and effects of cannabis: a brief review. *Br J Psychiatry.* 2001;178:101–106.

168. Gunderson EW. Synthetic cannabinoids: a new frontier of designer drugs. *Ann Intern Med.* 2013;159:563–564.

169. Bernson-Leung ME, Leung LY, Kumar S. Synthetic cannabis and acute ischemic stroke. *J Stroke Cerebrovasc Dis.* 2014;23:1239–1241.

170. Hatch EE, Bracken MB. Effect of marijuana use in pregnancy on fetal growth. *Am J Epidemiol.* 1986;124:986–993.

171. American College of Obstetricians and Gynecologists. Committee Opinion No. 722: Marijuana use during pregnancy and lactation (reaffirmed 2021). *Obstet Gynecol.* 2018;131:164.

172. Astley SJ, Clarren SK, Little RE, et al. Analysis of facial shape in children gestationally exposed to marijuana, alcohol, and/or cocaine. *Pediatrics.* 1992;89:67–77.

173. van Gelder MM, Reefhuis J, Caton AR, et al. Maternal periconceptional illicit drug use and the risk of congenital malformations. *Epidemiology.* 2009;20:60–66.

174. Warshak CR, Regan J, Moore B, et al. Association between marijuana use and adverse obstetrical and neonatal outcomes. *J Perinatol.* 2015;35:991–995.

175. Gray TR, Eiden RD, Leonard KE, et al. Identifying prenatal cannabis exposure and effects of concurrent tobacco exposure on neonatal growth. *Clin Chem.* 2010;56:1442–1450.

176. El Marroun H, Tiemeier H, Steegers EA, et al. Intrauterine cannabis exposure affects fetal growth trajectories: the Generation R Study. *J Am Acad Child Adolesc Psychiatry.* 2009;48:1173–1181.

177. Varner MW, Silver RM, Rowland Hogue CJ, et al. Association between stillbirth and illicit drug use and smoking during pregnancy. *Obstet Gynecol.* 2014;123:113–125.

178. Saurel-Cubizolles MJ, Prunet C, BB. Cannabis use during pregnancy in France in 2010. *BJOG.* 2014;121:971–977.

179. Fried PA. Marijuana use during pregnancy: consequences for the offspring. *Semin Perinatol.* 1991;15:280–287.

180. Conner SN, Bedell V, Lipsey K, et al. Maternal marijuana use and adverse neonatal outcomes: a systematic review and meta-analysis. *Obstet Gynecol.* 2016;128:713–723.

181. Goldschmidt L, Richardson GA, Larkby C, Day NL. Early marijuana initiation: the link between prenatal marijuana exposure, early childhood behavior, and negative adult roles. *Neurotoxicol Teratol.* 2016;58:40–45.

182. Huizink AC. Prenatal cannabis exposure and infant outcomes: overview of studies. *Prog Neuropsychopharmacol Biol Psychiatry.* 2014;52:45–52.

183. Smith AM, Mioduszewski O, Hatchard T, et al. Prenatal marijuana exposure impacts executive functioning into young adulthood: an fMRI study. *Neurotoxicol Teratol.* 2016;58:53–59.

184. White SM. Cannabis abuse and laryngospasm. *Anaesthesia.* 2002;57:622–623.

185. Wallace M, Schulteis G, Atkinson JH, et al. Dose-dependent effects of smoked cannabis on capsaicin-induced pain and hyperalgesia in healthy volunteers. *Anesthesiology.* 2007;107:785–796.

186. Scott K, Lust K. Illicit substance use in pregnancy—a review. *Obstet Med.* 2010;3:94–100.

187. dos Santos RG. Safety and side effects of ayahuasca in humans—an overview focusing on developmental toxicology. *J Psychoact Drugs.* 2013;45:68–78.

188. Labate BC. Consumption of ayahuasca by children and pregnant women: medical controversies and religious perspectives. *J Psychoact Drugs.* 2011;43:27–35.

189. Mvula MM, Miller JM Jr, Ragan FA. Relationship of phencyclidine and pregnancy outcome. *J Reprod Med.* 1999;44:1021–1024.

190. Maeda A, Bateman BT, Clancy CR, et al. Opioid abuse and dependence during pregnancy: temporal trends and obstetrical outcomes. *Anesthesiology.* 2014;121: 1158–1165.

191. Gemmill A, Kiang MV, Alexander MJ. Trends in pregnancy-associated mortality involving opioids in the United States, 2007-2016. *Am J Obstet Gynecol.* 2019;220:115–116.

192. Sanjanwala AR, Lim G, Krans EE. Opioids and opioid use disorder in pregnancy. *Obstet Gynecol Clin North Am.* 2023;50:229–240.

193. Pallatino C, Chang JC, Krans EE. The intersection of intimate partner violence and substance use among women with opioid use disorder. *Subst Abus.* 2021;42:197–204.

194. McHugh RK. The importance of studying sex and gender differences in opioid misuse. *JAMA Netw Open.* 2020;3:e2030676.

195. Bateman BT, Hernandez-Diaz S, Rathmell JP, et al. Patterns of opioid utilization in pregnancy in a large cohort of commercial insurance beneficiaries in the United States. *Anesthesiology.* 2014;120:1216–1224.

196. Desai RJ, Hernandez-Diaz S, Bateman BT, Huybrechts KF. Increase in prescription opioid use during pregnancy among Medicaid-enrolled women. *Obstet Gynecol.* 2014;123: 997–1002.

197. Krans EE, Patrick SW. Opioid use disorder in pregnancy: health policy and practice in the midst of an epidemic. *Obstet Gynecol.* 2016;128:4–10.

198. Bateman BT, Franklin JM, Bykov K, et al. Persistent opioid use following cesarean delivery: patterns and predictors among opioid-naive women. *Am J Obstet Gynecol.* 2016;215: 353.e1–e18.

199. Sporer KA. Acute heroin overdose. *Ann Intern Med.* 1999;130:584–590.

200. Mitra S, Sinatra RS. Perioperative management of acute pain in the opioid-dependent patient. *Anesthesiology.* 2004;101:212–227.

201. Peng PW, Tumber PS, Gourlay D. Review article: perioperative pain management of patients on methadone therapy. *Can J Anaesth*. 2005;52:513–523.

202. Fajemirokun-Odudeyi O, Sinha C, Tutty S, et al. Pregnancy outcome in women who use opiates. *Eur J Obstet Gynecol Reprod Biol*. 2006;126:170–175.

203. Kandall SR, Doberczak TM, Jantunen M, Stein J. The methadone-maintained pregnancy. *Clin Perinatol*. 1999;26:173–183.

204. McCarthy JJ, Leamon MH, Parr MS, Anania B. High-dose methadone maintenance in pregnancy: maternal and neonatal outcomes. *Am J Obstet Gynecol*. 2005;193:606–610.

205. Back SA, Craig A, Luo NL, et al. Protective effects of caffeine on chronic hypoxia-induced perinatal white matter injury. *Ann Neurol*. 2006;60:696–705.

206. Bryson EO, Lipson S, Gevirtz C. Anesthesia for patients on buprenorphine. *Anesthesiol Clin*. 2010;28:611–617.

207. Jones HE, Kaltenbach K, Heil SH, et al. Neonatal abstinence syndrome after methadone or buprenorphine exposure. *N Engl J Med*. 2010;363:2320–2331.

208. Gevirtz C, Frost EA, Bryson EO. Perioperative implications of buprenorphine maintenance treatment for opioid addiction. *Int Anesthesiol Clin*. 2011;49:147–155.

209. Alto WA, O'Connor AB. Management of women treated with buprenorphine during pregnancy. *Am J Obstet Gynecol*. 2011;205:302–308.

210. American College of Obstetricians and Gynecologists. Committee Opinion No. 711: Opioid use and opioid use disorder in pregnancy (reaffirmed 2021). *Obstet Gynecol*. 2017;130:e81–e94.

211. Nelson L, Schwaner R. Transdermal fentanyl: pharmacology and toxicology. *J Med Toxicol*. 2009;5:230–241.

212. Peng PW, Sandler AN. A review of the use of fentanyl analgesia in the management of acute pain in adults. *Anesthesiology*. 1999;90:576–599.

213. Bremer PT, Kimishima A, Schlosburg JE, et al. Combatting synthetic designer opioids: a conjugate vaccine ablates lethal doses of fentanyl class drugs. *Angew Chem Int Ed Engl*. 2016;55:3772–3775.

214. George AV, Lu JJ, Pisano MV, et al. Carfentanil—an ultra potent opioid. *Am J Emerg Med*. 2010;28:530–532.

215. Health Alert Network. *Rising Numbers of Deaths Involving Fentanyl and Fentanyl Analogs, Including Carfentanil, and Increased Usage and Mixing With Non-opioids*. Centers for Disease Control and Prevention; 2018. https://emergency.cdc.gov/han/han00413.asp. Accessed April 26, 2023.

216. National Institute on Drug Abuse. Overdose death rates; 2024. https://www.drugabuse.gov/related-topics/trends-statistics/overdose-death-rates. Accessed July 26, 2024.

217. Hayhurst CJ, Durieux ME. Differential opioid tolerance and opioid-induced hyperalgesia: a clinical reality. *Anesthesiology*. 2016;124:483–488.

218. Fischer G. Treatment of opioid dependence in pregnant women. *Addiction*. 2000;95:1141–1144.

219. Rausgaard NLK, Ibsen IO, Jorgensen JS, et al. Management and monitoring of opioid use in pregnancy. *Acta Obstet Gynecol Scand*. 2020;99:7–15.

220. Suarez EA, Huybrechts KF, Straub L, et al. Buprenorphine versus methadone for opioid use disorder in pregnancy. *N Engl J Med*. 2022;387:2033–2044.

221. Virginia Department of Health. *Pregnancy-Associated Deaths From Drug Overdose in Virginia, 1999-2007: A Report From the Virginia Maternal Mortality Review Team*. Virginia Department of Health; 2015. https://www.vdh.virginia.gov/content/uploads/sites/18/2016/04/Final-Pregnancy-Associated-Deaths-Due-to-Drug-Overdose.pdf. Accessed July 26, 2024.

222. Holbrook A, Kaltenbach K. Co-occurring psychiatric symptoms in opioid-dependent women: the prevalence of antenatal and postnatal depression. *Am J Drug Alcohol Abuse*. 2012;38:575–579.

223. Broussard CS, Rasmussen SA, Reefhuis J, et al. Maternal treatment with opioid analgesics and risk for birth defects. *Am J Obstet Gynecol*. 2011;204:314.e1–e11.

224. Yazdy MM, Mitchell AA, Tinker SC, et al. Periconceptional use of opioids and the risk of neural tube defects. *Obstet Gynecol*. 2013;122:838–844.

225. Lind JN, Interrante JD, Ailes EC, et al. Maternal use of opioids during pregnancy and congenital malformations: a systematic review. *Pediatrics*. 2017;139

226. Caritis SN, Panigrahy A. Opioids affect the fetal brain: reframing the detoxification debate. *Am J Obstet Gynecol*. 2019;221:602–608.

227. Mactier H, Hamilton R. Prenatal opioid exposure—increasing evidence of harm. *Early Hum Dev*. 2020;150:105188.

228. Sinha C, Ohadike P, Carrick P, et al. Neonatal outcome following maternal opiate use in late pregnancy. *Int J Gynaecol Obstet*. 2001;74:241–246.

229. Cassidy B, Cyna AM. Challenges that opioid-dependent women present to the obstetric anaesthetist. *Anaesth Intensive Care*. 2004;32:494–501.

230. Pandit JJ, Andrade J, Bogod DG, et al. The 5th National Audit Project (NAP5) on accidental awareness during general anaesthesia: summary of main findings and risk factors. *Anaesthesia*. 2014;69:1089–1101.

231. Monks DT, Hoppe DW, Downey K, et al. A perioperative course of gabapentin does not produce a clinically meaningful improvement in analgesia after cesarean delivery: a randomized controlled trial. *Anesthesiology*. 2015;123:320–326.

232. Gomes T, Juurlink DN, Antoniou T, et al. Gabapentin, opioids, and the risk of opioid-related death: a population-based nested case–control study. *PLoS Med*. 2017;14:e1002396.

233. Cavalcante AN, Sprung J, Schroeder DR, Weingarten TN. Multimodal analgesic therapy with gabapentin and its association with postoperative respiratory depression. *Anest Analg*. 2017;125:141–146.

234. Booth JL, Harris LC, Eisenach JC, Pan PH. A randomized controlled trial comparing two multimodal analgesic techniques in patients predicted to have severe pain after cesarean delivery. *Anesth Analg*. 2016;122:1114–1119.

235. Jouguelet-Lacoste J, La Colla L, Schilling D, Chelly JE. The use of intravenous infusion or single dose of low-dose ketamine for postoperative analgesia: a review of the current literature. *Pain Med*. 2015;16:383–403.

236. Haliloglu M, Ozdemir M, Uzture N, et al. Perioperative low-dose ketamine improves postoperative analgesia following cesarean delivery with general anesthesia. *J Matern Fetal Neonatal Med*. 2016;29:962–966.

237. Kuczkowski KM. Ethylene glycol and other solvent use in pregnancy: a new phenomenon and a new diagnostic dilemma. *Acta Anaesthesiol Scand*. 2006;50:1037.

238. Williams JF, Storck M. Inhalant abuse. *Pediatrics*. 2007;119:1009–1017.

239. Beckley JT, Woodward JJ. Volatile solvents as drugs of abuse: focus on the cortico-mesolimbic circuitry. *Neuropsychopharmacology*. 2013;38:2555–2567.

240. Kralova I, Stepanek Z, Dusek J. Ethylene glycol intoxication misdiagnosed as eclampsia. *Acta Anaesthesiol Scand*. 2006;50:385–387.

241. Leth PM, Gregersen M. Ethylene glycol poisoning. *Forensic Sci Int*. 2005;155:179–184.

242. Kuczkowski KM. Solvents in pregnancy: an emerging problem in obstetrics and obstetric anaesthesia. *Anaesthesia*. 2003;58:1036–1037.

243. Bowen SE, Hannigan JH, Irtenkauf S. Maternal and fetal blood and organ toluene levels in rats following acute and repeated binge inhalation exposure. *Reprod Toxicol*. 2007;24:343–352.

244. Gray TR, LaGasse LL, Smith LM, et al. Identification of prenatal amphetamines exposure by maternal interview and meconium toxicology in the Infant Development, Environment and Lifestyle (IDEAL) Study. *Ther Drug Monit*. 2009;31:769–775.

245. Concheiro M, González-Colmenero E, Lendoiro E, et al. Alternative matrices for cocaine, heroin, and methadone in utero drug exposure detection. *Ther Drug Monit*. 2013;35:502–509.

246. Launiainen T, Nupponen I, Halmesmäki E, Ojanperä I. Meconium drug testing reveals maternal misuse of medicinal opioids among addicted mothers. *Drug Test Anal*. 2013;5:529–533.

247. Lendoiro E, González-Colmenero E, Concheiro-Guisán A, et al. Maternal hair analysis for the detection of illicit drugs, medicines, and alcohol exposure during pregnancy. *Ther Drug Monit*. 2013;35:296–304.

248. Jones JT, Jones M, Jones B, et al. Detection of codeine, morphine, 6-monoacetylmorphine, and meconin in human umbilical cord tissue: method validation and evidence of in utero heroin exposure. *Ther Drug Monit*. 2015;37:45–52.

249. Haufroid V, Lison D. Urinary cotinine as a tobacco-smoke exposure index: a minireview. *Int Arch Occup Env Health*. 1998;71:162–168.

53

Trauma and Critical Care

Kaitlyn Brennan, DO, MPH, Edward R. Sherwood, MD, PhD, and Luis D. Pacheco, MD

CHAPTER OUTLINE

The management of critically ill obstetric patients most commonly involves treatment of disease processes that occur as a direct consequence of pregnancy. Although sometimes life-threatening, these conditions are usually reversible. Delivery of the infant often attenuates or ablates the disease process, and the mother typically recovers with supportive and resuscitative measures. Primary obstetric disorders account for 50% to 80% of intensive care unit (ICU) admissions for pregnant patients; approximately 80% of these admissions result from preeclampsia, sepsis, and/or hemorrhage (Box 53.1).[1,2] The estimated ICU admission rate for obstetric patients is 0.5% to 1% in the United States; the mortality rate among this population is 12% to 20%.[2]

Trauma accounts for 45% to 50% of all maternal deaths in the United States, and it is the most common nonobstetric cause of maternal death.[2,3] Other common nonobstetric causes of ICU admission are respiratory failure, endocrine disorders, preexisting autoimmune disease, and thromboembolic disorders.[2,3] Ethnic minorities and women with low socioeconomic status have the highest rates of morbidity and mortality. Modern medicine has allowed women with complex medical problems such as congenital heart disease and cystic fibrosis to survive into childbearing age, and these patients are at increased risk for complications during pregnancy and have a higher incidence of ICU admission. Among critically ill obstetric patients admitted to an ICU, the most common cause of death is acute respiratory distress syndrome (ARDS), which can complicate both obstetric and nonobstetric disease processes.[4]

Critical maternal illness places the fetus at significant risk for morbidity and mortality. Important fetal risk factors include maternal shock, transfusion of blood products, and early gestational age at the time of critical maternal illness.[2-4]

TRAUMA DURING PREGNANCY

Epidemiology

Trauma affects 5% to 8% of pregnancies in the United States and is a leading nonobstetric cause of maternal death; as many as 20% of affected women require emergency surgery.[5,6] It is likely that the reported incidence of maternal trauma is underestimated due to underreporting, especially in cases of domestic violence.[7] Motor vehicle crashes are the most common cause of injury-related maternal deaths (49% to 70%), followed by domestic violence (11% to 25%) and falls (9% to 23%).[8] Not using a seat belt is a major risk factor for maternal and fetal injury in motor vehicle trauma.[9] Penetrating trauma and burns are less common than blunt mechanisms of injury.[8] Regardless of the mechanism of injury, trauma is a threat to the life of the mother and fetus. The rate of maternal trauma admission to an ICU increases with each trimester: 8% occur in the first trimester, 40% in the second trimester, and 52% in the third trimester.[10] Most women are able to continue their pregnancy at home, but up to 38% are hospitalized until delivery.

Risk factors for maternal trauma include age < 25 years, low socioeconomic status, minority race, use of illicit drugs or alcohol, and domestic violence.[10,11] It is important to remember that any female patient of reproductive age who is a victim of trauma could be pregnant at the time of injury.

Complications and Outcomes

As in the general population, hemorrhagic shock and brain injury are the most common mechanisms of death in pregnant trauma victims.[12] Pelvic and acetabular fractures also pose a significant risk, with pelvic fractures being the most common maternal injury contributing to fetal death. Injuries

BOX 53.1 Causes of Critical Illness in Pregnancy

Obstetric Causes
- Acute fatty liver of pregnancy
- Amniotic fluid embolism
- Cardiomyopathy
- Chorioamnionitis
- HELLP syndrome
- Hemorrhage
- Pelvic septic thrombophlebitis
- Placental abruption
- Preeclampsia/eclampsia
- Puerperal sepsis

Nonobstetric Causes
- Acute renal failure
- Autoimmune disorders
- Chronic respiratory disease
- Diabetic ketoacidosis
- Substance use disorder
- Pneumonia
- Pulmonary thromboembolism
- Trauma
- Urinary tract infection

HELLP, Hemolysis, elevated liver enzymes, low platelet count.

and complications that are unique to pregnant trauma victims include uterine rupture, placental abruption, preterm labor, and direct fetal injury. Although rare (0.6% of injuries), uterine rupture is a major threat to the life of both the mother (10% mortality) and the fetus (near 100% mortality).[13] Placental abruption complicates 1% to 5% of minor injuries and 20% to 60% of major trauma and usually occurs from 16 weeks' gestation onward.[14] Placental abruption can cause major overt and occult hemorrhage and coagulopathy and should be considered as a possible source of bleeding in the unstable pregnant trauma patient. Preterm labor is a common (25%) complication of trauma and can be precipitated even in cases of apparently minor injury.[15] Premature rupture of membranes increases the risk for both preterm labor and infection. Amniotic fluid embolism is a rare complication of maternal trauma, but it should be considered as part of the differential diagnosis in patients who are refractory to resuscitation.

Fetal-maternal (transplacental) hemorrhage can occur after trauma and result in maternal isoimmunization with the D antigen of the fetal red blood cell (RBC) Rhesus protein complex ($Rh_0[D]$) in the Rh-negative mother. The **Kleihauer-Betke test** is used to identify fetal blood in the maternal circulation after maternal injury. Acid applied to a peripheral maternal blood smear eliminates adult hemoglobin, while fetal hemoglobin is resistant. Subsequent staining lights up the intact fetal cells against a background of pale maternal cells, and the ratio of fetal to maternal cells can be used to calculate the total volume of fetal RBCs in the maternal circulation. When fetal-maternal hemorrhage is present, treatment with $Rh_0(D)$ **immune globulin** (RhoGAM) is generally indicated. In a study performed at the R. Adams

Cowley Shock Trauma Center of the University of Maryland, more than 50% of evaluated pregnant trauma victims were positive for fetal-maternal hemorrhage as determined by a positive Kleihauer-Betke test.[16] Essentially all patients with a positive test had uterine contractions, whereas patients with a negative Kleihauer-Betke test did not have contractions. The investigators concluded that the Kleihauer-Betke test was a sensitive and specific predictor of preterm labor in pregnant trauma patients and should be performed in all victims regardless of blood Rh phenotype.

Fetal Trauma and Outcome

The fetal mortality rate after maternal blunt trauma has been reported to range from 3.4% to 38.0%; placental abruption, uterine rupture, maternal shock, and maternal death are the most frequent factors associated with fetal demise (Box 53.2).[11,17] The risk for direct fetal trauma increases with gestational age because the bony pelvis protects the uterus and fetus before 13 weeks' gestation. Pregnant women who sustain blunt trauma have a lower risk for bowel injury than nonpregnant patients because the uterus acts as a shield and pushes the abdominal contents into the upper abdomen.[18] Maternal pelvic fractures are associated with uteroplacental injury and fetal skull fractures. A skull fracture is the most common direct fetal injury and has a reported fetal mortality rate of 42%.[19]

The relationship between the Injury Severity Score (ISS) (see later discussion) and fetal outcome is controversial. Analysis of outcomes from 1075 pregnant trauma victims showed that an ISS > 15 was associated with increased risk for fetal demise.[20] In contrast, a study using data from the state of Washington found no correlation between ISS and pregnancy outcomes.[21] Fetal demise occurred even in women with low ISS. Evidence suggests that decreased serum bicarbonate, an indicator of systemic hypoperfusion, is associated with fetal demise after maternal trauma. Altered maternal mental status and the presence of head trauma have also been linked to adverse fetal outcomes.

It is crucial to preserve maternal cardiac output, blood pressure, and oxygen delivery to optimize maternal recovery and protect fetal well-being. However, fetal loss can occur

BOX 53.2 Factors Associated With Fetal Demise After Trauma

- Ejection from vehicle
- Maternal pelvic fracture
- High maternal Injury Severity Score (>15)
- Maternal death
- Maternal hypotension
- Uterine rupture
- Uterine tenderness
- Placental abruption
- Vaginal bleeding
- Abnormal fetal heart rate pattern
- Amniotic fluid on pelvic examination
- Maternal history of alcohol use
- Maternal history of smoking

even if the mother has not incurred serious injuries. Thus, all pregnant women should be evaluated in a medical setting after trauma, regardless of the apparent severity of injury. The fetus remains at risk for delayed complications after maternal discharge from the hospital. Delayed complications include a twofold increase in the risk for preterm delivery and a ninefold increase in the risk for fetal death.[21] Late complications of trauma, such as cerebral palsy, have also been reported in children born to mothers who experienced trauma during pregnancy.[22]

Initial Assessment and Resuscitation

The initial assessment and resuscitation should focus on the mother; it is axiomatic that maternal resuscitation typically facilitates fetal resuscitation. A systematic approach to initial resuscitation and stabilization should be used (Fig. 53.1).[23] Immediate interventions are initiated to identify and treat life-threatening conditions based on the principles of Advanced Trauma Life Support.[24] The initial, **primary survey** should focus on ensuring adequate airway protection, ventilation (breathing), and circulation (the "ABCs"

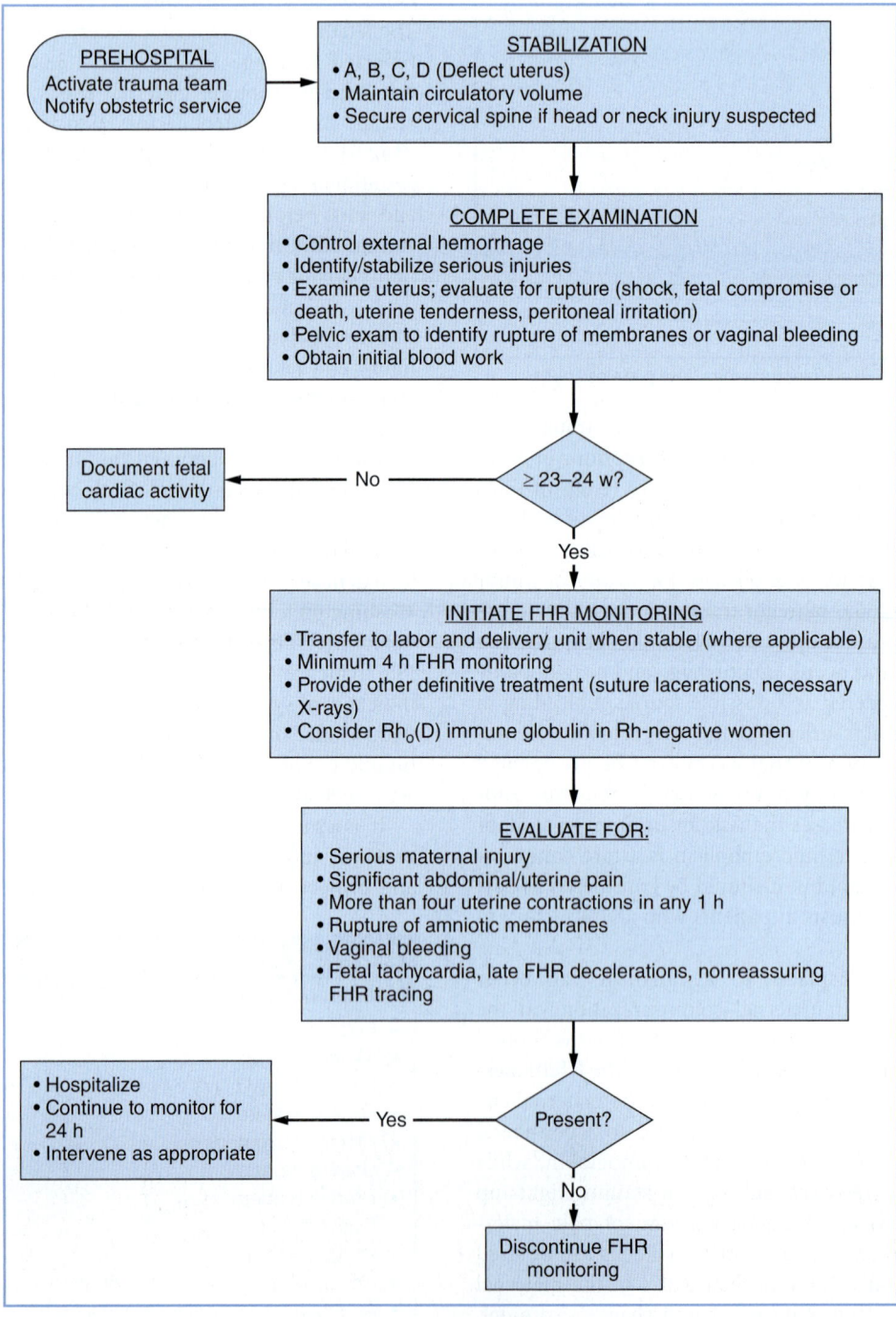

Fig. 53.1 Algorithm for Management of the Pregnant Woman After Trauma. *A, B, C,* Airway, breathing, circulation; *FHR,* fetal heart rate. Modified from Chames MC, Pearlman MD. Trauma during pregnancy: outcomes and clinical management. *Clin Obstet Gynecol.* 2008;51:398–408.

of resuscitation). Pregnant women experience significant changes in cardiopulmonary and metabolic function that must be considered during resuscitation (Table 53.1).

Airway

Airway patency, stabilization, and protection should be ensured as quickly as possible in all critically injured patients, including those who are pregnant. The status of the patient's airway can be quickly assessed by eliciting a verbal response. The inability to speak is an indication of severely impaired mental status or the inability to move adequate air to mediate phonation, either of which should prompt interventions to secure and protect the airway. Additional means of assessing airway patency include auscultation of the chest, assessment of chest movement, and assessment of air movement at the mouth and nose. Immediate interventions to establish airway

TABLE 53.1 Physiologic Changes of Pregnancy That May Affect Trauma Management

Parameter	Effect of Pregnancy	Implications
Airway		
Functional residual capacity	Decreased by 20%	More rapid oxyhemoglobin desaturation during periods of apnea
Oxygen consumption	Increased by 15%–20%	
Airway edema	May be present	Tracheal intubation more difficult
Lower esophageal sphincter tone	Decreased	Increased risk for aspiration
Gastric emptying	Decreased during labor	
Breathing		
Diaphragm	Displaced cephalad	Place chest tubes at higher intercostal space
Respiratory rate	No change	
Tidal volume	Increased 35%–45%	
pH	7.42–7.46, partially compensated respiratory alkalosis	
$Paco_2$	28–32 mm Hg	Reflects normal hyperventilation
HCO_3^-	19–22 mEq/L	Reduced buffering capacity
Base deficit	2–3 mEq/L	
Pao_2	100–107 mm Hg	
Circulation		
Blood volume	Increased by 40%–50%	Significant blood loss may occur before onset of symptoms and hypotension
Cardiac output	Increased by 40%–50%	
Heart rate	Increased by 15%–25%	Early diagnosis of hypovolemia more difficult
Systolic blood pressure	Decreased by 5–15 mm Hg (more pronounced during mid-pregnancy)	
Diastolic blood pressure	Decreased by 5–15 mm Hg (more pronounced during mid-pregnancy)	
Hemoglobin	10–12 g/dL	Physiologic anemia
Gravid uterus	Aortocaval compression	Decreased cardiac output in the supine position; left uterine displacement required
Other		
Coagulation factors	Increased	Hypercoagulable state
BUN, creatinine	Decreased	Abnormal measurements often overlooked[a]
Symphysis pubis/sacroiliac joints	Widened	May alter radiographic interpretations

BUN, Blood urea nitrogen.

[a]The reported measurements may fall within the normal range for the hospital laboratory, but the measurements may actually be abnormally high for a pregnant patient.

patency include head-tilt and jaw-thrust maneuvers, as well as placement of an oral or nasopharyngeal airway to facilitate bag-and-mask ventilation and oxygenation.

It is essential to consider the possibility of cervical spine injury, facial fractures, and skull base injuries. Excessive head-tilt maneuvers can worsen injury if a cervical spine fracture is present. Patients who have sustained severe trauma should be suspected of having a cervical spine injury until proven otherwise. Cervical spine injury must be ruled out by radiographic and physical examination criteria.[24] The cervical spine should be stabilized with a hard collar and in-line stabilization until the severity of injury has been established. In cases of documented cervical spine injury, great care must be taken not to worsen spinal cord injury. A nasopharyngeal airway should not be placed in patients with suspected facial or skull base fractures to avoid further trauma and worsening of preexisting conditions.

Most patients who require interventions to open or support the airway, as just described, will ultimately require tracheal intubation. Indications for tracheal intubation include impaired mental status, airway obstruction, inability to clear secretions or blood from the airway, inadequate spontaneous ventilation, and hypoxemia that is refractory to supplemental oxygen administration.[25] Tracheal intubation of pregnant patients is complicated by changes in respiratory system structure and function (see Table 53.1) (see Chapter 29).[14] Among the most prominent alterations are airway (including vocal cord) edema, decreased functional residual capacity, and increased oxygen consumption. Airway edema impairs vocal cord visualization, thus complicating laryngoscopy and tracheal intubation. Decreased functional residual capacity and increased oxygen consumption result in more rapid oxyhemoglobin desaturation during periods of apnea. These factors increase the risk for failed tracheal intubation and hypoxemia.

Gastric emptying is normal in pregnant women before the onset of labor (see Chapter 28). However, lower esophageal sphincter tone is commonly decreased in pregnant women (see Table 53.1). Thus, pregnant women are at increased risk for regurgitation and pulmonary aspiration of gastric contents and, similar to all trauma victims, are considered to have a full stomach on arrival in the emergency department or operating room. Therefore, in most cases, rapid-sequence induction of general anesthesia is performed to facilitate tracheal intubation. However, the specific tracheal intubation technique will depend on the practitioner's skills and resources, as well as on the location of the patient's injuries. Alternative approaches to rapid-sequence induction include awake tracheal intubation and tracheostomy.

Several factors can complicate tracheal intubation in the trauma patient. The patient may be combative, which complicates awake tracheal intubation strategies. Blood in the airway can limit the use of a fiberoptic bronchoscope and impair visualization of the glottis when using a standard or video laryngoscope. The presence of facial fractures, direct airway injuries, trauma-induced airway edema, and tracheal deviation can limit access to the airway.

Finally, airway management, including tracheal intubation, is more challenging in the presence of cervical spine injury. If cervical spine injury is present or suspected, it is crucial to avoid flexion, extension, or lateral movement of the neck. The spine is protected using in-line stabilization and/or a hard cervical collar. Airway management devices such as a gum elastic bougie, a video laryngoscope, a lighted intubating stylet, and/or an intubating supraglottic airway (SGA), among others, should be available for use if standard laryngoscopy is difficult or impossible. An SGA such as a laryngeal mask airway can be used to temporarily provide ventilation in cases in which mask ventilation and tracheal intubation have failed, but an SGA will not provide protection from aspiration and should be replaced by a secure airway device as soon as possible. In some cases, cricothyroidotomy or tracheostomy may be necessary to provide a secure airway.

Breathing

Adequate ventilation and oxygenation should be ensured for the benefit of both the mother and the fetus. Supplemental oxygen should be administered immediately, even if the patient is breathing spontaneously. Mechanical ventilation is often necessary after tracheal intubation in patients with respiratory failure and/or hypoxemia. Ventilation can be compromised by trauma-associated factors such as pneumothorax, hemothorax, lung contusion, mediastinal compression, and chest wall injuries. These problems must be identified during the primary survey[24] and treated to optimize ventilation and oxygenation. In women with advanced pregnancy, it may be necessary to place chest tubes in a more cephalad location than normal owing to the cephalad displacement of the diaphragm and intraabdominal structures by the gravid uterus. Pregnant trauma patients should be ventilated to maintain $Paco_2$ at a level that is normal for pregnancy (28 to 32 mm Hg) (see Table 53.1). Positive end-expiratory pressure (PEEP) may be added to improve oxygenation, if indicated; however, PEEP should be titrated carefully in the hypovolemic patient because it may impair venous return and worsen cardiac output and organ perfusion.

Circulation

Once respiratory stabilization has been achieved, it is essential to assess cardiovascular function and to determine whether the patient is in shock. Two large-bore peripheral intravenous catheters should be placed in the upper extremities to facilitate resuscitation. Central venous access facilitates rapid resuscitation but may be difficult to obtain. Intraosseous cannulation should be considered if it is difficult or impossible to obtain peripheral or central venous access.

Fluid resuscitation should be initiated using crystalloid solution, but blood transfusion should be considered if significant blood loss is apparent or suspected. Left uterine displacement should be initiated immediately to prevent or minimize aortocaval compression by the gravid uterus. The adverse effects of aortocaval compression may be exacerbated during periods of trauma-associated hypovolemia. The use of the pneumatic antishock garment to stabilize fractures or control hemorrhage is relatively contraindicated in pregnant women owing to its adverse effects on venous return.

The hallmark clinical signs of shock are listed in Box 53.3. The presence of these signs indicates a need for timely and appropriate fluid resuscitation. A rapid assessment of sources of blood loss should be performed. In trauma victims, the most common locations of exsanguinating blood loss are the chest, abdomen, retroperitoneum, long bones, and external sites. In the pregnant trauma patient, placental abruption and uterine rupture are also potential sources of hemorrhage. A brief physical examination will identify fractures of the long bones and external sites of bleeding. Thoracic blood loss and pelvic fractures can be identified by chest and pelvic radiographs, respectively. Focused abdominal sonography in trauma (FAST) or diagnostic peritoneal lavage can be used to identify intraabdominal bleeding. However, diagnostic peritoneal lavage may be difficult to perform safely in advanced pregnancy. FAST can be rapidly performed to assess the hepatorenal, splenorenal, and pelvic spaces, which are the most common sites of major hemorrhage in trauma patients. FAST can also be used to assess uteroplacental integrity and the presence of intrauterine bleeding. Finally, ultrasonography facilitates assessment of cardiac filling and recognition of cardiac tamponade in patients with thoracic trauma.

It is important to recognize that pregnant trauma patients may lose a significant amount of blood before the development of hypotension. Pregnant patients have a 40% to 50% increase in blood volume by the third trimester. Classic signs of hypovolemia, such as tachycardia, hypotension, and poor capillary refill, may not be evident until blood loss approaches 1.5 to 2 L. Therefore, it is likely that a pregnant trauma victim will have lost significantly more blood volume and oxygen-carrying capacity than a comparable nonpregnant patient when signs of cardiovascular deterioration become evident. Resuscitation should be guided by apparent blood loss to maintain adequate maternal cardiac output and uteroplacental perfusion. Because of the physiologic anemia of pregnancy, oxygen-carrying capacity may be significantly impaired at the time that hypovolemia becomes evident. In addition, maternal perfusion of vital organs is often sustained at the expense of uteroplacental perfusion. Uterine blood flow may decrease by as much as 30% before the mother shows signs of hypovolemia. Therefore, a nonreassuring fetal heart rate (FHR) pattern may be the first sign of significant intravascular volume loss. Fluids should be warmed to minimize the risk for hypothermia, which can contribute to coagulopathy, arrhythmias, and altered drug responses.

Fluid resuscitation. Current practice supports the use of crystalloid solutions to resuscitate the hypovolemic trauma victim during the early phases of resuscitation, with the caveat that recent studies show the benefits of early damage control resuscitation using blood products.[26] Furthermore, the benefits and harm of crystalloid versus colloid have yet to be fully resolved. The Saline versus Albumin Fluid Evaluation (SAFE)[27] did not show any difference in survival in nonpregnant trauma patients randomized to receive resuscitation with colloid or crystalloid, with the exception of patients with head trauma, who had poorer outcomes when resuscitated with albumin. The CRISTAL trial also did not demonstrate differences in 28-day mortality when comparing crystalloid to colloid, but 90-day mortality was lower in patients who received colloid.[28] However, the authors considered the results exploratory and cautioned against conclusions about the efficacy of colloid solutions until further investigations are completed.

Balanced salt solutions (lactated Ringer's solution, PlasmaLyte) are typically preferred over normal saline in patients without closed head injury. Balanced salt solutions have significant buffering properties and are less likely than normal saline solution to cause hyperchloremic metabolic acidosis during high-volume resuscitation. A 2018 trial showed that the use of balanced crystalloids for resuscitation of critically ill patients was associated with a lower incidence of the composite outcome (death, need for renal-replacement therapy, or renal dysfunction) compared with normal saline.[29] Other buffered salt solutions, such as Ringer's ethyl pyruvate and Ringer's hydroxybutyrate, also may have value. Currently, no evidence supports the use of one buffered isotonic crystalloid solution over another.

The use of **hypertonic crystalloid solutions** such as 3% sodium chloride is controversial; currently, no evidence supports their routine use in pregnant trauma victims who did not suffer traumatic brain injury (TBI). Hypernatremia is a risk in patients resuscitated with hypertonic saline, and some studies have shown increased mortality in patients resuscitated with hypertonic crystalloid solutions.[30] In a 2017 systematic review, Wu et al.[31] did not identify significant survival or complication risk associated with hypertonic saline resuscitation compared with isotonic saline in patients with hemorrhagic shock.[31] In contrast, Asehnoune et al.[32] reported improved adjusted 90-day survival in trauma patients with TBI and intracranial hypertension treated with continuous hyperosmolar therapy.[32] Metaanalyses from 2020[33] and 2022[34] showed that treatment of trauma patients suffering TBI and intracranial hypertension with hypertonic saline results in decreased intracranial pressure (ICP) and secondary brain injury. The use of 3% saline was most effective and provided more sustained decreases in ICP and improvement in

---

BOX 53.3 Clinical Signs of Shock in the Trauma Patient

- Agitation
- Confusion
- Poor capillary refill
- Mottled appearance
- Cool extremities
- Diaphoresis
- Tachypnea
- Tachycardia
- Weak distal pulses
- Hypotension
- Decreased pulse pressure
- Decreased urine output
- Lactic acidosis

cerebral perfusion compared to mannitol. In general, hypertonic resuscitation does not appear to be beneficial to trauma patients without TBI but likely benefits patients with TBI and elevated ICP.

Some practitioners have advocated **hypovolemic resuscitation** in patients with major hemorrhage after trauma.[35] This technique employs **permissive hypotension** (systolic blood pressure of 80 to 90 mm Hg) until hemorrhage can be controlled in the operative setting. The underlying premise of hypovolemic (hypotensive) resuscitation is that overresuscitation worsens ongoing blood loss because of higher perfusion pressure and dilution of clotting factors. Small boluses of fluids are administered to maintain perfusion in patients without evidence of closed head injury. The use of hypotensive resuscitation is likely detrimental in patients with closed head injury because it is crucial to maintain adequate cerebral perfusion pressure (CPP) in patients with elevated ICP.[36] (CPP is the difference between mean arterial pressure [MAP] and ICP.) No definitive published data support the use of hypotensive resuscitation in pregnant trauma patients. Current guidelines do not support this approach because it may compromise uteroplacental perfusion.

The resuscitative endovascular balloon occlusion of the aorta (REBOA) catheter is a large-vessel occlusion device that is typically deployed into the aorta during periods of severe intraabdominal and pelvic hemorrhage, and is becoming increasingly utilized in cases of major trauma.[37] A proximal pressure transducer is used to titrate balloon inflation to maintain central pressures and limit downstream bleeding as reparative procedures are executed. The device is a less invasive alternative to emergency department thoracotomy and aortic cross-clamping to temporize noncompressible torso hemorrhage. In patients without penetrating thoracic injury, Brenner et al.[38] reported a survival benefit for REBOA compared with patients who received resuscitative thoracotomy.[38] A 2023 randomized clinical trial among trauma victims with hemorrhagic shock in the United Kingdom found increased mortality with the use of REBOA (odds ratio, 1.58; 95% credible interval 0.72 to 3.52).[39] Thus, the efficacy of using the REBOA during trauma resuscitation remains to be fully determined in all subsets of trauma patients with hemorrhage. The effectiveness and safety of the REBOA catheter remain to be established in critically injured pregnant patients.

Damage control principles and resuscitation. The traditional approach to treatment of traumatic life-threatening injuries has been definitive operative repair. However, some patients experience progressive physiologic decline during long surgical procedures and develop severe derangements such as hypothermia, metabolic acidosis, and coagulopathy, a combination that has become known as the deadly triad.[40] These pathologic alterations require rapid and effective treatment to prevent severe morbidity and death. More recently, practitioners have advocated the use of a more targeted surgical approach, termed damage control surgery, which is initiated to control hemorrhage without providing early definitive repair of injuries.[41] Major surgical bleeding is controlled, and the thoracic and abdominal cavities are packed to provide hemostasis. Gastrointestinal diversion is performed, and body cavities are temporarily closed, often using vacuum-type closure systems. Active volume resuscitation is performed using blood products rather than crystalloids, an approach known as damage control resuscitation, to achieve metabolic homeostasis. Once stable hemodynamic and acid-base status, coagulation function, and temperature are achieved, the patient is returned to the operating room for definitive repair of injuries.

Blood products. All trauma centers should have rapid access to type O, Rh-negative blood for emergency use before type-specific or cross-matched blood is available. Trauma specialists advocate for damage-control resuscitation using packed RBCs, platelets, and plasma units mixed in equal proportions (1:1:1). Several investigators have reported the value of this approach in military practice, and they have specifically observed that this approach results in more effective resuscitation, less coagulopathy, and improved survival than more traditional approaches utilizing crystalloids.[42] Based on experience over the last few years, damage-control resuscitation is also considered to be the optimal strategy for managing civilian patients with exsanguinating trauma.[43] The Pragmatic, Randomized, Optimal Platelet and Plasma Ratios (PROPPR) trial showed that damage-control surgery and balanced blood product resuscitation (1:1:1 ratio) is associated with improved hemostasis at 3 hours after intervention and a decreased incidence of death by exsanguination at 24 hours after injury, although overall mortality at 24 hours and 30 days after injury was not improved compared with patients receiving damage-control surgery with blood products in a 1:1:2 ratio.[44] Based on current evidence, the Eastern Association for the Surgery of Trauma recommends the use of balanced blood product resuscitation in exsanguinating trauma patients.[45]

Despite implementation of damage-control resuscitation, coagulopathy remains a significant problem for trauma patients requiring large-volume resuscitation. Damage-control resuscitation provides clotting factors via transfused plasma and direct administration of platelets. However, tissue injury and release of endogenous anticoagulants often result in sustained alterations in coagulation. Consequently, some practitioners advocate adopting a goal-directed approach to treat trauma-induced coagulopathy based on viscoelastic monitoring, either with thromboelastography or rotational thromboelastometry (see Chapter 44).[46] Gonzalez et al.[47] reported that goal-directed treatment of trauma-associated coagulopathy, compared with standard assessment of coagulation status, was associated with lower mortality and decreased use of plasma and platelets during the acute phase of resuscitation. However, the study had limitations, and further work is needed to define the benefits of goal-directed treatment of coagulopathy in the trauma patient suffering large-volume hemorrhage.

Secondary Survey

As in all trauma cases, it is crucial to evaluate the mother for significant abdominal, thoracic, orthopedic, and neurologic injuries. A head-to-toe examination should be performed to determine the presence of injuries and the need for intervention. A more detailed evaluation of neurologic function, as well as examination of the head and neck, should be performed. This survey includes examination of posterior structures that may be obscured by the supine position and the presence of a cervical collar. The torso should be examined to identify thoracic and abdominal injuries. The thoracic examination should include chest auscultation, inspection, and palpation. Palpation of the abdomen should be performed to evaluate abdominal tenderness, and a rectal examination should be performed to identify evidence of intraluminal bleeding. The extremities must be examined to identify deformities, and each joint should be manipulated. Distal perfusion of the extremities must be continuously monitored, especially in limbs that show signs of significant injury. This is accomplished by evaluation of distal pulses and capillary refill. In cases of penetrating injury, the sites of entry and exit should be identified. It is especially important to carefully examine the areas that are difficult to access such as the oral cavity, perineum, axilla, scalp, and back. Once the secondary survey has been performed, more targeted assessments of suspected injuries can be performed using radiologic imaging.

Fetal survey. After initial stabilization of the mother, information about the pregnancy should be gathered through a focused history and physical examination. The history should include the date of the last menstrual period, expected date of delivery, and status of the pregnancy. In cases in which there is uncertainty regarding fetal age, an approximate determination can be made by measuring fundal height. The fetal age is estimated to be 1 week for each centimeter of fundal height above the symphysis pubis. In addition to the assessment of fundal height, the abdominal examination should include an assessment of uterine tenderness and consistency, the presence or absence of uterine contractions, and fetal position and movement.

A pelvic examination should be performed to evaluate cervical dilation and effacement, fetal station, and the presence of amniotic fluid and blood. The FHR is assessed by Doppler auscultation or ultrasonography. If maternal stability permits, ultrasonography facilitates estimation of fetal age and assessment of uteroplacental injury.

If no fetal cardiac activity is identified, fetal resuscitation should not be attempted (see Fig. 53.1). In a series of 441 pregnant trauma patients, the absence of a detectable FHR was associated with fetal death in all cases.[6] When an FHR is detected, an assessment of fetal viability should be performed. An estimated gestational age of 23 to 24 weeks and an estimated fetal weight of 500 g are common thresholds for extrauterine fetal viability. The FHR should be monitored in cases in which the fetus is determined to be viable. In cases in which a nonviable fetus is present, the importance of FHR monitoring is unclear. However, alterations in FHR and FHR variability may signal maternal deterioration and serve as a good monitor of the effectiveness of maternal resuscitation.

FHR monitoring is generally performed with external Doppler auscultation, and a tocodynamometer is used to assess uterine contractions. Adverse fetal outcomes are unlikely in cases with a reassuring FHR tracing (see Chapters 6 and 8) and no early-warning signs of uteroplacental injury (bleeding, abdominal pain).[48] In contrast, an abnormal FHR tracing or evidence of uteroplacental injury (vaginal bleeding, uterine contractions, uterine tenderness, presence of amniotic fluid on vaginal examination) predicts poor fetal outcome in approximately 50% of cases.[49]

Fetal Monitoring

Continuous electronic FHR monitoring is the current standard of care for pregnant trauma victims with a viable fetus.[6,10] FHR monitoring should be initiated as soon as maternal stabilization allows because placental abruption can occur early during the course of resuscitation. Continuous electronic FHR monitoring is more sensitive for placental abruption than ultrasonography, physical examination, or Kleihauer-Betke testing. Occasional uterine contractions are common after trauma and are usually not associated with poor fetal outcome.[49–51] Random uterine contractions usually resolve within a few hours of the trauma. However, regular and prolonged uterine contractions (eight contractions per hour for more than 4 hours) are associated with placental abruption, which has a high fetal mortality rate.[52] The diagnosis of placental abruption should trigger immediate cesarean delivery for both fetal and maternal indications; a large percentage of viable fetuses can be rescued if expedited delivery is performed, and placental abruption will exacerbate maternal hemorrhage and coagulopathy. The presence of fetal bradycardia and/or frequent late FHR decelerations should also prompt delivery if the mother is stable and adequately resuscitated.

The ideal duration of FHR monitoring has not been determined. However, a common practice, based on a prospective study of 60 pregnant trauma patients at more than 20 weeks' gestation, is to monitor the FHR for 4 hours.[53] If maternal-fetal abnormalities are not detected within 4 hours, it is generally considered safe to discontinue FHR monitoring because a normal FHR tracing has a negative predictive value of 100% when combined with a normal maternal physical examination. However, the presence of abnormalities such as vaginal bleeding, spontaneous rupture of membranes, category II and III FHR patterns (see Box 8.3), persistent uterine contractions, uterine tenderness, abdominal pain, and/or need for maternal analgesia should prompt further FHR monitoring. The sensitivity of ultrasonography for placental abruption ranges from 50% to 80%, but ultrasonography is a safe and effective means of assessing fetal viability, FHR, placental location, gestational age, and amniotic fluid volume. It is particularly valuable in the presence of maternal tachycardia, when it can be difficult to differentiate maternal and FHRs using Doppler auscultation.

Laboratory Studies

Laboratory evaluation in pregnant trauma patients does not differ from the evaluation for nonpregnant patients, with a few exceptions. As for all trauma patients, the laboratory evaluation will be driven by the type and severity of injury.

For most patients with significant injury, standard analysis includes a complete blood cell count, coagulation studies, serum electrolyte measurements, blood glucose and lactate levels, liver function tests, arterial blood gas analysis, urinalysis, and toxicology screening, as well as sending a blood sample for typing and cross-matching for compatible blood products (Box 53.4).

The presence of disseminated intravascular coagulation (DIC) and low blood bicarbonate levels is associated with poor fetal outcome.[54,55] Both abnormalities reflect severe maternal injury and should prompt aggressive maternal resuscitation. Of special consideration in pregnant trauma patients is maternal-fetal hemorrhage. The Kleihauer-Betke test is used to detect the entry of fetal blood into the maternal circulation.[16] Although typically performed in $Rh_0(D)$ antigen–negative mothers to detect transplacental hemorrhage and the potential for developing $Rh_0(D)$ sensitization, this test may help predict adverse fetal outcomes in all pregnant trauma patients (see earlier discussion).

Imaging Studies

The pregnant trauma patient often requires imaging to evaluate orthopedic, head, thoracic, and abdominal injuries. Although many patients and physicians are concerned about the fetal effects of ionizing radiation, the risks for teratogenesis, malignancy, and gene mutation are small with a radiation exposure < 5 to 10 rads (see Chapter 18).[56,57] Less than 1% of trauma patients receive more than 3 rads of radiation exposure. Shielding of the fetus with lead is no longer recommended as this provides negligible benefits and may negatively affect the efficacy of the examination.[58] Intravenous pyelography subjects the fetus to as much as 1.4 rads of exposure, but the test can be invaluable in diagnosing injuries to the kidneys, ureters, and bladder. Computed tomography (CT) is associated with greater radiation exposure than plain radiography, but exposure levels are generally below that considered to be dangerous to the fetus. Modern multidetector (multislice) CT results in higher fetal radiation exposure, but it has significant advantages in speed and image resolution. Overall, the small risk for fetal radiation exposure is outweighed by the benefits to the injured mother and, by extension, the fetus.

Injury Scoring

Several injury scoring scales have been developed over the past 40 years. The scoring systems provide a framework for standardizing clinical management, benchmarking outcomes, and planning research. Presently, no reliable scoring tool exists for predicting maternal or fetal outcome after trauma. Currently used scoring systems include (1) anatomic injury scales that rely on physical examination and diagnostic procedures, (2) physiologic injury scales that rely on assessment of physiologic responses and function, and (3) combination injury scales.

One of the first anatomy-based injury scales was the **Abbreviated Injury Scale (AIS)** developed by the Association for the Advancement of Automotive Medicine.[59] Each of nine body regions is given an ISS that ranges from 1 (minor) to 6 (maximal [currently untreatable]). Although the AIS effectively describes the severity of injuries at specific locations, it provides a limited assessment of the overall pathophysiologic impact of all injuries. The **ISS**, which was developed to address this issue, is obtained by summing the square of the three highest severity scores from the AIS. The ISS ranges from 1 to 75. Minor injuries are classified as an ISS of less than 9; moderate, from 9 to 15; serious, from 16 to 25; and severe, greater than 25. The ISS correlates with the risk for preterm delivery after trauma, but its value in predicting fetal death, placental abruption, and other adverse outcomes is controversial.[11] The American Association for the Surgery of Trauma developed the **Organ Injury Scale**[60]; this organ-based severity scale is designed to facilitate clinical investigation and outcomes research.

The value of injury scoring scales in predicting adverse maternal and fetal outcomes remains to be established. Distelhorst et al.[61] reported improved birth outcomes in pregnant patients treated at dedicated trauma centers. However, after controlling for the ISS, the level of trauma designation was not associated with any differences in most birth outcomes, with the exception of *higher* risk for preterm labor and meconium-stained amniotic fluid at level 1 and 2 centers compared with level 3 and 4 centers.[62] It is not known whether trauma-level designation correlates with level of maternal care designation (see Chapter 11) or whether level of maternal care designation predicts trauma outcomes during pregnancy.[63]

Anatomic scoring systems have value in describing the extent and severity of injuries to specific organ systems. However, physiologic scoring systems may add prognostic value. The **Glasgow Coma Scale (GCS)**, which is among the most widely used physiologic scoring systems, evaluates the neurologic status of the trauma patient. The GCS evaluates eye opening, verbal response, and motor activity; scores range from 3 to 15, with 3 indicating the absence of neurologic activity and 15 representing intact neurologic function. A GCS score < 9 reflects severe impairment, whereas a score of 9 to 12 reflects moderate disability. However, concerns

---

BOX 53.4   Initial Laboratory Analysis for the Pregnant Trauma Patient

- Blood type and cross-match
- Complete blood cell count
- Prothrombin (INR) and partial thromboplastin times
- Fibrinogen
- Serum electrolytes, BUN, creatinine, glucose
- Liver function tests
- Serum amylase level
- Blood lactate
- Arterial blood gas measurement
- Toxicology screen
- Kleihauer-Betke assay
- Urinalysis

BUN, Blood urea nitrogen; *INR,* international normalized ratio.

have been raised about interrater reliability and lack of prognostic utility for the GCS. Some researchers have proposed that a simplified motor score would be more reliable. Evidence suggests that the GCS score has a poor correlation with fetal outcome.[11]

Traumatic Brain Injury

Brain injury is common in patients who suffer from motor vehicle crashes, and it is a major cause of mortality among pregnant trauma victims.[64] It is important to perform a thorough neurologic examination with particular attention to level of consciousness. Altered mental status may be an indicator of evolving intracranial pathology, intoxication, hypoperfusion, and/or metabolic disturbances. Mental status should be reevaluated frequently because intracranial pathologic processes may not be apparent on initial evaluation and may evolve during resuscitation.

Elevated ICP is a common finding in patients with TBI and may be a significant threat to life. A head CT is the imaging study of choice for identifying the site and severity of intracranial pathologic processes in trauma patients, and it should be performed within 1 hour of arrival in the emergency department.[24]

Crystalloid or damage control resuscitation using blood products should be used for resuscitation in patients with TBI; resuscitation with albumin is deleterious in patients with TBI (see earlier discussion).[27] Evidence indicates that selective use of 3% hypertonic saline in patients with TBI and intracranial hypertension may be beneficial.[33,34] Hypotensive resuscitation is contraindicated in patients with TBI and elevated ICP. It is crucial to maintain MAP and CPP to minimize the risk for brain ischemia and permanent brain injury. The extent of brain injury will worsen if CPP is not maintained. It is also important to maintain cerebral oxygen delivery by optimizing maternal cardiac output and blood oxygen-carrying capacity.

It may be necessary to intubate the trachea of patients with deteriorating mental status for airway protection and provision of ventilatory support. Hypoventilation should be avoided because it increases ICP. Hyperventilation to a $Paco_2$ between 25 and 30 mm Hg will provide a transient decrease in ICP and may be useful until definitive treatment can be initiated. However, hyperventilation can be disadvantageous for the fetus because it can decrease uteroplacental blood flow by decreasing maternal cardiac output and blood pressure, and perhaps by causing uteroplacental vasoconstriction. Therefore, it is prudent to maintain $Paco_2$ at levels that are normal in pregnant women (28 to 32 mm Hg). Additional maneuvers to decrease ICP include treatment with a diuretic such as mannitol or furosemide and elevation of the head 30 to 45 degrees. Treatment with hypertonic saline can also decrease intracranial volume and ICP, and may improve outcomes in patients with TBI.[32]

Corticosteroids are no longer recommended for patients with TBI because their administration in this setting is associated with increased mortality. Barbiturates decrease cerebral oxygen use and blood flow and may provide cerebral

protection in patients with severe impairment. Both mannitol and furosemide cross the placenta and could cause alterations in fetal plasma osmolality and decrease fetal intravascular volume. However, concern regarding adverse fetal effects should be overridden by the needs of the mother in cases of TBI.

Cardiopulmonary Resuscitation

The incidence of cardiac arrest in pregnancy is reported to be 1:20,000 to 1:40,000 patients in industrialized countries.[65,66] Cardiac arrest during hospitalization for delivery is more common because it includes postpartum cardiac arrest.[66,67] The most frequent causes are trauma, peripartum hemorrhage, embolic phenomena, stroke, preeclampsia/eclampsia, sepsis, status asthmaticus, and anesthesia-related complications.[67,68]

Cardiopulmonary resuscitation should be initiated immediately (see Chapter 41). The 2020 American Heart Association (AHA) guidelines highlight the importance of initiating high-quality chest compressions to facilitate circulation.[69] Guidelines have simplified the list of modifications to cardiopulmonary resuscitation during pregnancy (Box 53.5)[70]; pregnant women benefit from standard high-quality cardiopulmonary resuscitation similar to that performed in nonpregnant patients. Hands should be placed in the usual location on the center of the victim's chest; there is no scientific evidence to support changing the hand position from that used to resuscitate nonpregnant patients.[69,70] Chest compressions should be performed at a rate of 100 per minute at a depth of at least 5 cm. Interruptions should be minimized. Cardiac arrest in the pregnant patient is complicated by the physiologic changes of pregnancy, particularly the effect of the gravid uterus on aortocaval blood

---

BOX 53.5 Modification of Cardiopulmonary Resuscitation During Pregnancy

- Perform manual left uterine displacement (see Fig. 53.2).
- Anticipate difficult airway management.
- Obtain intravenous access above the diaphragm.
- If patient is receiving magnesium sulfate, discontinue magnesium infusion and administer calcium chloride or calcium gluconate.
- Remove all fetal monitors before delivery; internal fetal monitors may be cut externally. Fetal monitor removal should not delay defibrillation.
- If spontaneous circulation does not return with usual resuscitative measures, resuscitative hysterotomy or cesarean delivery should be performed if gestational age is 20 w or greater, aiming for delivery within 5 min of cardiac arrest.[a]
- Continue all resuscitation efforts during and after cesarean delivery.

[a]Do not transfer patient to the operating room if the cardiac arrest occurred outside of the operating room.
Summarized from Jeejeebhoy FM, Zelop CM, Lipman S, et al. Cardiac arrest in pregnancy: a scientific statement from the American Heart Association. *Circulation.* 2015;132:1747–1773; Lipman S, Cohen S, Einav S, et al. The Society for Obstetric Anesthesia and Perinatology consensus statement on the management of cardiac arrest in pregnancy. *Anesth Analg.* 2014;118:1003–1016.

flow. Well-performed chest compressions in the nonpregnant patient typically result in cardiac output that is approximately 30% of normal. In pregnant patients, aortocaval compression reduces the cardiac output that results from chest compressions. Therefore, the AHA guidelines advocate **manual left uterine displacement** with the patient in the supine position (Fig. 53.2).[69,70]

Due to the increased propensity for pregnant patients to become hypoxic, if an arrest occurs in the hospital setting, the airway should be quickly secured and the mother ventilated with 100% oxygen.[69] Chest impedance is unchanged during pregnancy; therefore, the usual voltage levels for defibrillation should be used in pregnant patients.[70] Electric cardioversion during pregnancy appears to be safe for the fetus (see Chapter 41); removal of fetal scalp electrodes should not delay maternal defibrillation. Intravenous or intraosseous access should be secured to facilitate resuscitation. Advanced Cardiac Life Support guidelines should be followed to identify and treat causes of cardiopulmonary arrest. The use of transthoracic echocardiography (TTE) to identify causes of cardiac arrest in pregnancy may prove difficult, as the traditional subxiphoid view may be impossible in a pregnant patient at term. Chest compressions should not be delayed for TTE. Important etiologies of maternal cardiac arrest, such as pulmonary embolism and amniotic fluid embolism, may reveal profound right heart dysfunction on bedside exam, while cardiac arrest due to hypovolemic shock may reveal an underfilled left ventricle.

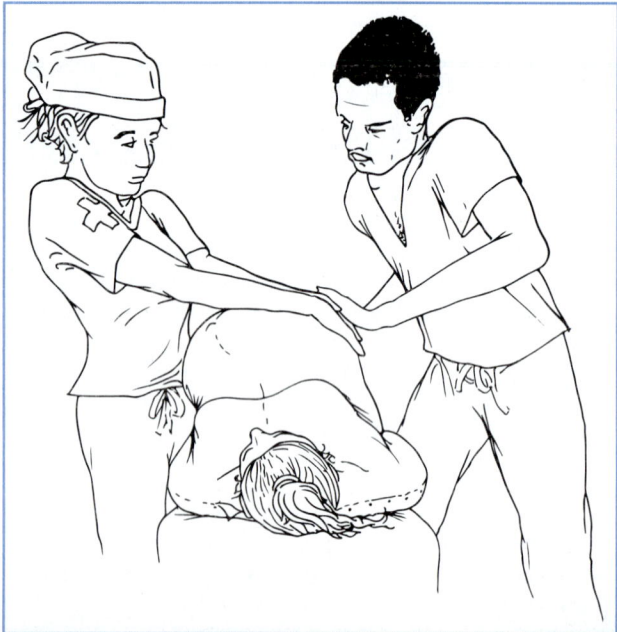

Fig. 53.2 Manual left uterine displacement (LUD) should be performed for any woman in cardiac arrest in whom the uterus can be palpated at or above the umbilicus. LUD can be performed from the right or left side. From the left side, the uterus is cupped and lifted off the major vessels to the left. From the right side, the uterus is pushed upward and to the left. Illustration by Naveen Nathan, MD, NorthShore University HealthSystem, University of Chicago Pritzker School of Medicine, Evanston, IL.

If the return of spontaneous circulation does not occur with the usual resuscitative measures, and if the fundal height is at or above the umbilicus (approximately 20 weeks' gestation), the AHA recommends that cesarean delivery (**resuscitative hysterotomy**) should be performed within 5 minutes of cardiac arrest.[69] Timely delivery facilitates successful resuscitation of both the mother and the infant.[70] If possible, preparations for perimortem cesarean delivery should occur while resuscitative measures are initiated.[69,71] The patient should not be moved to the operating room for the procedure, but rather it should be performed at the location of the cardiac arrest.[65,71] Early uterine evacuation optimizes maternal resuscitation, even if the fetus has already died.

A 2012 systematic review of case reports identified 54% survival to hospital discharge among 94 women suffering cardiac arrest during pregnancy; increased survival was associated with decreased time to cesarean delivery.[72] In a prospective descriptive study performed in the United Kingdom, Beckett et al.[66] reported a 42% mortality rate for women suffering cardiac arrest during pregnancy. Survival was lowest among women who arrested at home, for whom timely cesarean delivery was not available. After 24 weeks' gestational age, delivery improved perinatal survival. In the UK cohort, 79% (46/58) of infants delivered during maternal cardiac arrest survived, including the offspring of 14 women who did not survive.[66]

The 2020 AHA guidelines recommend targeted temperature management for post–cardiac arrest care in the pregnant patient.[69] However, targeted temperature management for out-of-hospital cardiac arrest in nonpregnant patients has recently been challenged.[73,74] Therefore, it should be considered on a case-by-case basis in the pregnant population; if pregnant patients are therapeutically cooled, continuous fetal monitoring is warranted.

Management of the Brain-Dead Patient

Brain death in the pregnant patient is a rare occurrence; however, several summaries of case reports have been published. Esmaeilzadeh et al.[75] summarized 30 cases published between 1982 and 2010. Nontraumatic brain injury, primarily intracranial hemorrhage, was the cause of death in 26 of 30 cases. The mean gestational ages at times of injury and delivery were 22 and 30 weeks, respectively. Twelve viable infants survived beyond the neonatal period.

In cases of maternal brain death, care providers should focus on saving the life of the fetus; maternal organ preservation for harvest and donation is a secondary consideration. Maintenance of vital functions in mothers with catastrophic brain injury is justified to meet these two goals, but in many cases ethical and legal concerns must be addressed. Consideration must be given to gestational age and the chance for fetal survival. Before 23 weeks' gestation, the chance for extrauterine fetal survival is small. In general, management should follow current guidelines for organ preservation therapy.

The question of whether to preserve maternal circulation and organ function to facilitate fetal development is an ethical, legal, and social dilemma. A fundamental issue relates to the support of the brain-dead mother as an incubator for the unborn fetus. It is important to recognize that, in the case of maternal brain death, the primary patient is no longer the pregnant woman, but the fetus. In many cases, the mother's wishes are not known, but it in most cases it is ethically permissible to consider corporeal support to allow for delivery at a later gestational age.[76–78] Currently, there is no generally accepted lower limit of gestational age for maintenance of maternal support. A systematic review by Dodaro et al.[79] specifically examined cases of brain death in pregnancy in which attempts were made at maternal somatic support to maximize fetal outcomes. The researchers found, much like previously published case reports, a predominance of brain death due to intracranial hemorrhage, subarachnoid hemorrhage, and hematoma. A predominance of fetuses were born via cesarean, and most (77%) survived, with increasing survival at later gestational ages.[79] While these data may help to frame the decision-making process around maternal somatic support, each case must be addressed on an individual basis, with close communication among the family, a cohort of care providers, and the hospital ethics committee.

CRITICAL CARE DURING PREGNANCY

Stroke

Ischemic Stroke

Pregnant women are at increased risk for ischemic stroke compared with their nonpregnant counterparts.[80] This risk increases with the presence of hypertensive disorders of pregnancy.[81] New data suggest that the presence of infection on the delivery admission is an important risk factor for peripartum stroke.[82] Pregnancy is a hypercoagulable state characterized by decreased fibrinolysis, increased levels of clotting factors, and decreased levels of certain natural anticoagulants (e.g., protein S). The increased preload associated with pregnancy can combine with a hypercoagulable state to increase the risk of stroke due to a patent foramen ovale.[83]

Clinical manifestations of ischemic stroke are similar to those seen in the young, nonpregnant population and include focal neurologic symptoms, seizures, decreased level of consciousness, and abnormal cranial nerve function. Once the diagnosis is suspected, and initial evaluation and therapy—including airway protection—have been addressed, a non–contrast-enhanced CT should follow immediately.[84] The fetal radiation exposure from this test is less than 1 rad.[57] If the CT shows no evidence of hemorrhagic stroke, the patient is assumed to have an ischemic stroke. Magnetic resonance imaging (MRI) is more sensitive in detecting early ischemic events; however, the test is more time-consuming and may not be emergently available. Consideration of thrombolytic therapy should follow, including evaluation of contraindications for thrombolytic therapy (Box 53.6). Thrombolytic therapy with recombinant tissue plasminogen activator (r-tPA) has been reported during pregnancy and appears to be safe for the fetus; transplacental passage of r-tPA is minimal.

However, retroplacental bleeding with pregnancy loss has been reported.[85–87] A consultation with an experienced neurologist is recommended.

The r-tPA is administered intravenously at a dose of 0.9 mg/kg (maximum, 90 mg) over 1 hour (10% of the dose is commonly administered as an initial bolus over the first minute).[84] The therapeutic window (i.e., time from onset of symptoms to administration of the agent) is 4.5 hours. Patients who are candidates for this therapy should be watched closely in an ICU environment that includes fetal surveillance by a maternal-fetal medicine specialist. Blood pressure should be maintained below 180/105 mm Hg during r-tPA therapy with the use of agents such as labetalol or nicardipine.[84] Neurologic deterioration during thrombolytic infusion should raise the suspicion of **hemorrhagic transformation**; the infusion should be stopped immediately and the head CT should be repeated. If hemorrhagic transformation is present, reversal of r-tPA is achieved with administration of cryoprecipitate (10 units) with the goal of maintaining a serum fibrinogen level above 150 mg/dL. The added benefit of platelet transfusion is not clear. If cryoprecipitate or fibrinogen concentrate is not available, tranexamic acid 1 g intravenously may be administered.[88]

Patients with ischemic stroke who are not candidates for r-tPA therapy should receive aspirin (162 to 325 mg/day) for 1 to 2 weeks; subsequently, the dose may be decreased to 100 mg/day.[89] Deep vein thrombosis prophylaxis with unfractionated heparin or low-molecular-weight heparin should also be started on admission unless contraindicated.

BOX 53.6 Major Contraindications for Thrombolysis in Ischemic Stroke Patients

- History of a previous intracranial hemorrhage
- Genitourinary or gastrointestinal bleeding in the previous 3 w
- Closed head trauma in the previous 3 mo
- Major surgery in the previous 2 w
- Blood pressure > 185/110 mm Hg despite antihypertensive therapy
- Acute active bleeding
- Evidence that symptoms are clearing spontaneously
- Hemorrhagic transformation on initial imaging
- Massive ischemic stroke (hypodensity affecting more than one-third of the cerebral hemisphere)
- Platelet count < 100,000/μL
- Concurrent heparin or warfarin therapy with prolonged PT or aPTT
- Blood glucose < 50 mg/dL (symptoms may be caused by hypoglycemia)
- Evidence of a seizure with postictal residual neurologic impairment

aPTT, Activated partial thromboplastin time; *PT*, prothrombin time. Summarized from Powers WJ, Rabinstein AA, Ackerson T, et al. 2018 guidelines for the early management of patients with acute ischemic stroke: a guideline for healthcare professionals from the American Heart Association/American Stroke Association. *Stroke.* 2018;49:e46–e110.

Outcome data related to blood pressure management in patients with acute ischemic stroke are inconsistent. In 2018 the AHA and the American Stroke Association recommended that in patients who are not receiving thrombolytic therapy, emergency antihypertensive medication should be withheld unless the blood pressure is higher than 220/120 mm Hg.[84] This recommendation does not apply to women with ischemic stroke in the presence of preeclampsia, in whom current guidelines recommend treatment with antihypertensive agents if the blood pressure is greater than 160/110 mm Hg. If the patient has received thrombolytic therapy, aspirin and prophylactic doses of heparin should be withheld for 24 hours after completion of the infusion. Fever should be aggressively treated to achieve normothermia. Blood glucose control with a target between 140 and 180 mg/dL is recommended in the setting of ischemic stroke. Intravenous insulin may be used as needed. Seizure prophylaxis in ischemic stroke is not recommended.[84]

Cerebral sinus and vein thrombosis may occur during pregnancy and the puerperium, but most cases occur postpartum. The practitioner should suspect cerebral sinus thrombosis in the presence of severe headache, focal neurologic signs, and/or papilledema. The diagnostic test of choice is magnetic resonance venography (MRV). Most cases involve the transverse sinuses. Initial imaging reveals concomitant areas of hemorrhage in as many as 40% of these cases. Despite the latter, treatment involves immediate therapeutic anticoagulation with unfractionated heparin or low-molecular-weight heparin unless a massive hemorrhage is present.[89,90]

Hemorrhagic Stroke

Pregnancy typically is accompanied by a 40% to 50% increase in both cardiac output and effective blood volume. These changes, coupled with hormone-induced increased fragility of vessel wall structures (secondary to increased levels of estrogen, progesterone, matrix metalloproteinases, and relaxin), may render pregnant patients more susceptible to hemorrhagic stroke resulting in intracerebral and subarachnoid hemorrhage.[91] Half of strokes in pregnancy are hemorrhagic.[92]

Intracerebral hemorrhage. Intracerebral hemorrhage is usually a secondary complication of hypertensive emergencies (e.g., preeclampsia, hypertensive encephalopathy). Clinical presentation is similar to that in nonpregnant individuals. The diagnosis is confirmed with non–contrast-enhanced CT.

As in any other stroke victim, initial management involves securing the airway and facilitating oxygenation and ventilation. ICP monitoring should be considered in patients with a GCS score < 8, clinical evidence of transtentorial herniation, or evidence of significant intraventricular hemorrhage or hydrocephalus.[93]

Blood pressure control in the setting of intracerebral hemorrhage is controversial. Past evidence suggested that acute blood pressure control with the aim of reducing systolic pressure to 140 mm Hg is safe and could be associated with improved functional outcomes.[93,94] However, evidence from recent clinical trials does not support benefit from strict blood pressure control (systolic blood pressure goal below 140 mm Hg) compared with traditional management (systolic blood pressure goal below 180 mm Hg).[95] In some studies, patients randomized to strict blood pressure control had a higher risk for acute kidney injury.[95] Blood pressure control is currently recommended in patients with intracerebral hemorrhage and a systolic blood pressure >160 to 200 mm Hg.[96] In cases of intracerebral hemorrhage associated with preeclampsia, most practitioners recommend maintenance of systolic and diastolic blood pressures between 140 and 160 mm Hg and 90 to 110 mm Hg, respectively, to maintain uteroplacental perfusion pressure (see Chapter 35). Blood pressure should be monitored invasively and treated with a titratable intravenous agent such as labetalol or nicardipine.

In the setting of intracerebral hemorrhage associated with warfarin use, rapid reversal of the anticoagulation effect is of paramount importance. Vitamin K (10 mg intravenously over a minimum of 20 minutes) should be administered, along with **prothrombin complex concentrate**, which contains the vitamin K–dependent clotting factors II, VII, IX, and X.[96] Prothrombin complex concentrate can be infused over 15 to 30 minutes. The role of recombinant activated factor VII in this setting is limited, and its use is not recommended at this time.[96]

The risk for seizures after intracerebral hemorrhage is higher in cases of lobar hemorrhage; the risk is small if hemorrhage is localized to the basal ganglia, and even less if limited to the posterior fossa. Unless clinical seizures are observed or nonconvulsive activity is noted on the electroencephalogram (EEG), routine seizure prophylaxis in patients with intracerebral hemorrhage is not recommended; therapy may be associated with poorer long-term functional outcome.[93] The exception is intracerebral hemorrhage in the setting of preeclampsia, for which magnesium is indicated for seizure prophylaxis. As with most brain injuries, glucose control is paramount in the management of intracerebral hemorrhage. Blood glucose should be maintained between 140 and 180 mg/dL in critically ill patients with brain injuries.[93,96] Once bleeding cessation is documented by repeat imaging, deep vein thrombosis prophylaxis with unfractionated heparin or low-molecular-weight heparin should be initiated (usually 1 to 4 days after the intracerebral hemorrhage). Patients should also receive mechanical prophylaxis with sequential compression devices.

Subarachnoid hemorrhage. Subarachnoid hemorrhage may be traumatic or nontraumatic. The most common cause of nontraumatic subarachnoid hemorrhage is rupture of a cerebral aneurysm. The clinical presentation varies from the complaint of the "worst headache in my life" to profound coma. The diagnosis is made by CT followed by cerebral angiography to locate the source of the bleeding; CT angiography detects aneurysms as small as 2 mm. Once the aneurysm is located, two management options exist. Craniotomy with clipping of the aneurysm has been the traditional treatment. More recently, coiling of the aneurysm has emerged as a less invasive option. Endovascular coiling is currently the preferred treatment option as it has been associated with better long-term neurologic outcomes and less mortality.[97] Coiling has not been specifically studied in the pregnant population, although several cases of successful endovascular treatment of ruptured intracranial aneurysms in pregnant women have been reported.

Regardless of the treatment modality, it is crucial to secure the aneurysm as early as possible. Before the aneurysm is secured, blood pressure control should target a systolic blood pressure < 160 mm Hg.[97]

Delayed vasospasm is one of the most serious complications of subarachnoid hemorrhage. The onset is usually 3 to 5 days after the hemorrhage and manifests as worsening of the neurologic examination (either new focal symptoms or decreased level of consciousness). If a change in the neurologic status is noted, an immediate CT should be performed to rule out rebleeding or hydrocephalus; if absent, vasospasm is likely. Vasospasm is confirmed with cerebral angiography. All patients should be treated with nimodipine (60 mg orally every 4 hours for 21 days) as prophylaxis against delayed-onset ischemia secondary to cerebral vasospasm.[97] Nimodipine is the only agent that has shown improved outcomes in the treatment of delayed cerebral ischemia. Data do not lend support to the efficacy of magnesium sulfate[98] or statins.[99]

Once surgical or endovascular treatment is completed, blood pressure control may be less rigorous because hypertension may be a compensatory mechanism to maintain CPP in the setting of vasospasm. During pregnancy, extremely high blood pressure may lead to placental abruption and should be avoided. Maintaining a systolic blood pressure < 160 mm Hg may be reasonable during pregnancy after securing the aneurysm.

Historically, patients presenting with symptomatic delayed cerebral vasospasm have been treated with "triple H therapy." Triple H therapy consists of inducing *hypervolemia* (through administration of crystalloids or colloids), leading to *hemodilution*, accompanied by induced *hypertension* (by using vasopressors) in an attempt to increase cerebral perfusion. Evidence of the efficacy of triple H therapy is limited.[100] The use of hypervolemia and subsequent hemodilution may even be detrimental as a result of a decrease in arterial oxygen content.[101] Instead, many practitioners recommend induced hypertension with intravenous infusion of norepinephrine, phenylephrine, or dopamine, and titration of systolic blood pressure to measurements higher than 180 mm Hg (MAP > 120 mm Hg). However, during pregnancy, the use of high-dose vasopressors to induce hypertension may lead to uteroplacental vasoconstriction and hypoperfusion and subsequent fetal demise. Additionally, the hypertension may increase the risk for placental abruption. Pregnant patients requiring induced hypertension for delayed vasospasm present a significant clinical dilemma. If the fetus is sufficiently mature (e.g., more than 32 weeks' gestation), it may be advisable to deliver the fetus before initiation of induced hypertension. If delivery is not an option, balloon angioplasty of the constricted vessels by an interventional radiologist may be considered in lieu of induced hypertension.

Subarachnoid hemorrhage may also lead to extracerebral manifestations, most commonly hyponatremia, cardiac

dysfunction, and neurogenic pulmonary edema. **Hyponatremia** may occur from several causes. The most common is the syndrome of **inappropriate antidiuretic hormone secretion**; however, it may also be secondary to increased secretion of atrial and ventricular natriuretic **peptides—cerebral salt-wasting syndrome**.[102,103] Hyponatremia after subarachnoid hemorrhage increases the likelihood of vasospasm and seizure, and is a poor prognostic indicator.[104,105] Treatment with normal saline usually suffices. Hypertonic saline may be required but should be used with caution in patients with subarachnoid hemorrhage.[104]

The massive liberation of catecholamines that accompanies subarachnoid hemorrhage is believed to cause subendocardial ischemia, leading to "**cardiac stunning**" with concomitant arrhythmias and decreased cardiac output. Patients may require inotropic support and antiarrhythmic therapy. **Neurogenic pulmonary edema** usually occurs within hours of the bleeding event and has both a hydrostatic component (from cardiac stunning and pulmonary venous constriction as a result of increased catecholamine secretion) and a noncardiogenic component (from endothelial injury owing to activation of the inflammatory cascade secondary to the presence of severe brain injury). Treatment of neurogenic pulmonary edema is supportive and requires low tidal volume ventilation strategies and the use of PEEP to improve oxygenation.

Subarachnoid hemorrhage may also occur secondary to rupture of brain **arteriovenous malformations**.[106] General intensive care provided to these patients is similar to that used in aneurysmal subarachnoid hemorrhage with a few exceptions. The risk for vasospasm after subarachnoid hemorrhage from arteriovenous malformations is lower and rarely warrants therapy. Once removed (surgically), adjacent brain tissue will be exposed to increased cerebral blood flow, leading to cerebral edema. Localized cerebral edema may be prevented by the avoidance of severe hypertension. The decision to surgically treat a ruptured arteriovenous malformation is controversial and depends on the location and type of venous drainage (superficial or deep).[106] The risk for rebleeding during pregnancy is increased and treatment (e.g., surgical resection, embolization) is commonly recommended for accessible lesions.[107]

As with intracerebral hemorrhage in general, normothermia should be maintained and the maximum blood glucose level should be maintained between 140 and 180 mg/dL. Seizure prophylaxis in the setting of subarachnoid hemorrhage is controversial. Prolonged use of phenytoin has been associated with poor neurologic outcomes and should be avoided.[108] A systematic review suggested that 3 days of seizure prophylaxis therapy provides similar seizure prevention with more favorable outcomes compared with longer-term treatment.[108] In general, widespread use of seizure prophylaxis in subarachnoid hemorrhage is not recommended.

Status Epilepticus

Status epilepticus is defined as a continuous, generalized seizure lasting more than 5 minutes or two or more seizures with no return to baseline consciousness between the seizures.[109]

Status epilepticus can be either convulsive or nonconvulsive in nature, with the latter being more difficult to diagnose, and more resistant to antiepileptic drugs. Status epilepticus may be caused by noncompliance with antiepileptic medications, stroke, brain tumor, central nervous system infection, head trauma, metabolic derangements (e.g., uremia, hepatic encephalopathy, electrolyte abnormalities), cerebral hypoxia, and hypoglycemia/hyperglycemia. Rarely, eclamptic seizures may progress to status epilepticus.

Treatment should start at 5 minutes of seizure activity, as prolonged seizure can lead to irreversible neurologic damage. Intravenous access should be obtained and hypoglycemia ruled out promptly. Seizure-induced muscle breakdown may lead to myoglobin-induced kidney injury.[109] Initial pharmacologic therapy includes an intravenous benzodiazepine (e.g., lorazepam 0.1 mg/kg, diazepam 0.15 mg/kg).[110] Second-line agents include phenytoin, valproate, lacosamide, and levetiracetam. Importantly, valproate may pose a risk of impaired cognitive development in children exposed *in utero*. This, combined with its teratogenic effects, makes other antiepileptic drugs more attractive choices for status epilepticus.[111] If intravenous access is difficult, intramuscular drug administration is an option. Intramuscular midazolam (10 mg) is at least as effective as intravenous lorazepam in the prehospital management of status epilepticus.[112] If seizure control is not achieved, general anesthesia may be required with a continuous infusion of propofol, ketamine, or phenobarbital.[110] Many practitioners recommend 24 to 48 hours of seizure control documented by EEG before slowly weaning the infusion.

Acute Respiratory Distress Syndrome

ARDS is a severe form of noncardiogenic pulmonary edema; it is a common cause of mortality in the critically ill obstetric patient. ARDS is defined as the acute onset (within 7 days of known clinical insult) of noncardiogenic pulmonary edema (usually secondary to an inflammatory insult) with bilateral pulmonary infiltrates and a partial pressure of oxygen to inspired fraction of oxygen ratio (P/F ratio) < 300 with PEEP of at least 5 cm H_2O.[113] Mild ARDS is defined as a P/F ratio between 200 and 300, moderate ARDS between 100 and 200, and severe ARDS as a ratio below 100. The term *acute lung injury* is no longer used. The mortality rate from severe ARDS is approximately 45%.[113]

ARDS may occur secondary to a pulmonary or extrapulmonary pathologic process. The common denominator is activation of the inflammatory cascade, leading to inflammation-induced endothelial/epithelial injury in the lung with subsequent leaking of protein-rich fluid into the alveoli. Direct (pulmonary) insults that may lead to ARDS include pneumonia, aspiration pneumonitis, pulmonary contusion, and smoke inhalation during burns. Indirect (extrapulmonary) causes include sepsis, pancreatitis, trauma, and massive transfusion. Similar to the nonobstetric population, the most common cause of ARDS in pregnant women is sepsis.[114] Certain obstetric conditions (e.g., placental abruption, amniotic fluid embolism, preeclampsia) may also cause ARDS because these conditions are associated with inflammation

and subsequent diffuse endothelial injury. Pregnant patients with severe placental abruption or amniotic fluid embolism complicated by DIC and massive transfusion of blood products are also at increased risk for ARDS.

Initial treatment for the patient with acute hypoxemic respiratory failure of noncardiac origin falls into ventilatory and nonventilatory strategies (Box 53.7). Of vital importance, the underlying cause of the ARDS must be addressed simultaneously with the institution of supportive measures (e.g., broad-spectrum antibiotics and surgical drainage if indicated in cases of sepsis-related ARDS; immediate delivery in patients with chorioamnionitis).

Ventilatory Strategies

The only intervention that has convincingly decreased mortality in ARDS is **lung-protective mechanical ventilation**.[115]

BOX 53.7   Management Strategies in Patients With Acute Respiratory Distress Syndrome During Pregnancy

Ventilatory Strategies
- Lung-protective mechanical ventilation
  - Limit tidal volume to 6 to 8 mL/kg (ideal body weight[a]). If possible, maintain $Paco_2$ < 60 mm Hg. Limit plateau pressures to 30 to 35 cm H_2O.
- Oxygenation goals
  - Maintain Pao_2 ≥ 55 mm Hg and Spo_2 ≥ 88% as long as the electronic FHR tracing is reassuring. A higher Pao_2 may be required in patients with nonreassuring fetal status.
- Provide adequate PEEP
  - Titrate according to oxygen requirements.
- Rescue therapies
  - Prone ventilation, extracorporeal membrane oxygenation, airway pressure release ventilation, recruitment maneuvers.

Nonventilatory Strategies
- Limit fluid administration
  - Avoid excessive fluids, especially after the initial phase of resuscitation.
- Neuromuscular blockade (cisatracurium)
  - May consider early use of cisatracurium for 48 h. Avoid coadministration of corticosteroids and aminoglycosides.
- Corticosteroids (no consistent evidence of improved survival)
  - Methylprednisolone 1 mg/kg bolus over 30 min followed by a continuous infusion of 1 mg/kg/d for 14 d. The dose is then decreased by half for 1 w, then decreased by half again for 4 d, and finally decreased by half one last time for 3 d.
- Inhaled prostacyclin/nitric oxide
  - Despite improvements in oxygenation, data on survival benefit are lacking. Avoid intravenous vasodilators (e.g., epoprostenol) because these drugs may worsen oxygenation by increasing the shunt fraction.

[a]Ideal body weight in kilograms (females) = 45.5 + 0.91 (height in centimeters − 152.4).

FHR, Fetal heart rate; *PEEP*, positive end-expiratory pressure.

ARDS is a heterogeneous disease in which some areas of the lung are affected (consolidated with edema) and others are not. During tidal volume delivery, gas flow is predominantly distributed to unaffected portions of the lung. If large tidal volumes are used, these "normal" areas of the lung are exposed to excessive volumes and pressures that lead to **volutrauma** and **barotrauma**, respectively. Overdistention of the lung provokes a local inflammatory response that further injures the lung parenchyma; locally produced inflammatory mediators (i.e., cytokines) may translocate to the systemic circulation and provoke worsening multiorgan failure **(biotrauma)**.[116] If large tidal volumes are used with low PEEP, the constant opening and closing of the recruited alveoli **(atelectrauma)** will also worsen lung inflammation. These four insults (volutrauma, barotrauma, biotrauma, and atelectrauma) constitute what is known as **ventilator-induced lung injury**.[117]

In a randomized clinical trial involving 861 patients with ARDS, patients randomized to receive mechanical ventilation with a small tidal volume (6 mL/kg ideal body weight) and a limitation of plateau pressure to less than 30 cm H_2O had a mortality of 31% compared with 40% in the group randomized to receive a larger tidal volume (12 mL/kg ideal body weight).[115] Since the publication of this trial, intensivists have adopted strategies that limit tidal volumes to decrease ventilator-induced lung injury and improve outcomes in patients with ARDS. By limiting tidal volumes, minute ventilation is invariably decreased, leading to hypercarbia and respiratory acidemia. To improve minute ventilation, the intensivist may increase the respiratory rate up to 35 breaths per minute to maintain, ideally, an arterial pH above 7.3.[117]

Significant maternal hypercarbia may result in decreased removal of carbon dioxide from the fetus, leading to fetal acidemia. Tidal volumes from 6 to 8 mL/kg (ideal body weight) can be used to ventilate pregnant women with ARDS; attempts should be made to maintain maternal $Paco_2$ below 60 mm Hg. Because of decreased compliance of the chest wall during pregnancy, plateau pressures of up to 35 cm H_2O may be tolerated. Continuous electronic FHR monitoring is recommended because abnormal FHR patterns may occur during periods of fetal acidemia.

The use of low tidal volumes to limit ventilator-induced lung injury must be accompanied by adequate levels of PEEP to recruit alveolar units. A discussion of optimization of PEEP is beyond the scope of this chapter, but the reader may access Fio_2-PEEP tables that titrate PEEP according to oxygen requirements.[118] Alternatively, PEEP may be increased gradually provided it does not result in increased plateau pressures (as this indicates overdistention as opposed to recruitment). The oxygenation goal is to achieve a Pao_2 of at least 55 mm Hg or higher with an Sao_2 (as measured by pulse oximetry) of at least 88% or higher.[118] A 2020 trial of patients with ARDS compared conservative oxygenation (target Pao_2 between 55 and 70 mm Hg and Sao_2 88% to 92%) with a liberal approach (target Pao_2 90 to 105 mm Hg and Sao_2 above 96%).[119] While there was no difference in the primary outcome of mortality at 28 days, the conservative approach had more cases of

mesenteric ischemia and a harm signal with higher mortality at 90 days. An editorial accompanying the study suggested a target Sao_2 of 90% may be favored.[120] The use of high PEEP (levels up to 15 cm H_2O or higher) is associated with decreased mortality in the subset of patients with the most severe forms of ARDS.[121]

When patients with ARDS are turned from the supine to the prone position, oxygenation often greatly improves, likely secondarily to anterior displacement of the heart with resultant recruitment of the posterior lung segments and improved ventilation-perfusion matching. Decreased mortality from ARDS was observed in patients with P/F ratios < 150 when prone ventilation was applied early in the course of the disease and for at least 16 hours per day.[122] The use of prone ventilation during the second half of pregnancy is obviously technically demanding (but achievable) because of the enlarged gravid uterus.

Other ventilatory strategies that may be used in ARDS, but have not been associated with reduced mortality, include the use of recruitment maneuvers, airway pressure release ventilation, high-frequency oscillatory ventilation (HFOV), and extracorporeal membrane oxygenation (ECMO).[118,123,124] HFOV is not recommended as it has been associated with either no benefit or increased mortality.[125] The largest clinical trial to date evaluating venovenous ECMO for ARDS did not find a difference in mortality compared with lung protective mechanical ventilation; however, there was a 28% crossover rate to the ECMO arm.[126] A subsequent metaanalysis has found a survival benefit with venovenous ECMO among carefully selected patients with severe ARDS refractory to conventional mechanical ventilation and prone positioning.[127]

While delivery of the fetus has been shown to improve maternal oxygenation (without improvements in survival), no changes in lung compliance or any other significant ventilator parameters (PEEP, driving pressure, plateau pressure) have been identified following delivery.[128] Thus, delivery should not occur for the sole purpose of improving the maternal respiratory status. However, in cases of life-threatening hypoxemia with a viable fetus and nonreassuring fetal status (especially after 32 weeks' gestation), delivery to prevent stillbirth may be warranted.

Nonventilatory Strategies

Nonventilatory strategies play an important role in the management of patients who suffer ARDS (see Box 53.7). The early use of neuromuscular blockade does not improve the survival in patients with ARDS and is not recommended.[129]

Because ARDS occurs secondary to inflammation-mediated lung injury, interest has risen regarding the possible benefits of **corticosteroid therapy**. Theoretically, low-dose corticosteroids could be immunomodulatory (not immunosuppressive), leading to downregulation of excessive inflammation, and thus limiting acute lung injury.[130] Overall, published evidence indicates that low-dose corticosteroids reduce systemic inflammation, improve oxygenation, reduce multiorgan dysfunction, and decrease the duration of mechanical ventilation and ICU stay in patients with ARDS.[130] If used, low-dose corticosteroids (see Box 53.7) should be initiated before day 14 of the disease; after day 14, corticosteroid therapy is not recommended. The effect on survival is controversial, although some evidence suggests that corticosteroids decrease mortality in patients with ARDS.[131] Of interest, the use of these low doses has not been associated with an increased risk for gastrointestinal hemorrhage, nosocomial infection, or myopathy.[130] A study using dexamethasone in patients with moderate to severe ARDS and PEEP ≥ 10 cm H_2O found decreased mortality with the use of corticosteroids.[132] An association between corticosteroids and congenital facial clefts has been suggested[133]; however, this association is mainly based on animal data. Corticosteroid therapy should not be withheld during pregnancy, if indicated. If used in pregnancy for ARDS, the use of methylprednisolone in lieu of dexamethasone is suggested, as the former is inactivated by placental enzymes, exposing the fetus to minimal concentrations.

Management of fluid balance is fundamental to the care of patients with ARDS. A randomized trial found that conservative fluid management (mean fluid balance in the first 7 days, -136 mL) was associated with a shorter duration of mechanical ventilation and a shorter length of stay in the ICU than liberal fluid management (mean fluid balance, $+6992$ mL).[134] At the time of enrollment, most patients had been fluid resuscitated and were hemodynamically stable. The incidence of adverse effects (e.g., shock, need for renal dialysis) did not differ between groups.

Fluid restriction in patients with ARDS is usually initiated on day 2 to 3 of the disease process; the first several days are commonly associated with hypotension and shock that invariably requires fluid resuscitation. Provided shock has resolved and vasopressors are not required to support blood pressure, fluids should be restricted to the amount required to maintain hemodynamic stability. Enteral feeding should be the main source of fluids in lieu of intravenous "maintenance fluids." If a diuretic is used to achieve a negative fluid balance, judicious use is recommended. Continuous electronic FHR monitoring is recommended to assess the adequacy of uteroplacental perfusion.

Right ventricular failure may be seen in up to 25% of patients with ARDS. Alveolar "flooding" limits oxygenation with resultant hypoxic pulmonary vasoconstriction. The increase in pulmonary vascular resistance may lead to acute cor pulmonale and right ventricular failure, accompanied by a severe decrease in cardiac output (from both right-sided failure and left ventricular diastolic dysfunction secondary to left sided interventricular septum deviation). The administration of an inhaled pulmonary vasodilator such as nitric oxide or prostacyclin often leads to improved oxygenation and right ventricular function. However, there is no evidence that these interventions improve survival.[135] Pregnancy is not a contraindication for pulmonary vasodilator therapy. Pharmaconutritional therapy for ARDS (e.g., omega-3 fatty acids, linolenic acid, antioxidants) has not been shown to be beneficial and is not recommended.[136]

Nutrition and Glucose Control

Critically ill patients require nutrition to heal. **Enteral nutrition** is of paramount importance and should be implemented within 24 to 48 hours of admission to the ICU.[137] Enteral nutrition (either through a nasogastric tube or a Dobhoff tube with the tip placed in the duodenum) helps maintain gut barrier integrity, thus preventing bacterial and cytokine translocation from the intestine. Enteral nutrition should be discontinued in patients requiring high doses of vasopressors because of a possible increase in the risk for bowel ischemia.[137]

The total amount of calories needed during critical illness is unknown.[138] More than 200 formulas exist to calculate daily energy requirements while in the ICU; many of these formulas align with a simple calculation of 25 kcal/kg/day (ideal body weight).[137] Recent guidelines for nonpregnant individuals suggest the administration of 12 to 25 kcal/kg/day during critical illness.[137] An extra 300 kcal/day should be added during pregnancy (500 kcal/day in patients with multiple gestation). Overfeeding should be avoided because it may lead to fatty liver, volume overload, excessive carbon dioxide production, hyperglycemia, infection, and immunosuppression. Protein delivery should not be restricted, and critically ill patients should receive 1.2 to 2.0 g/kg/day of protein.[137] Most available enteral feeding formulas do not contain sufficient protein; it may be necessary to add additional protein to standard formulas. In the setting of ARDS, either trophic feeding or full-calorie feeding is acceptable during the first week of the disease.

Stress hyperglycemia refers to the elevation in blood glucose concentration associated with critical illness. Stress hyperglycemia is caused by multiple factors, including massive catecholamine release and systemic inflammation. Hyperglycemia is commonly worsened with initiation of nutritional support. Hyperglycemia worsens oxidative injury and potentiates inflammation and clotting. A 2001 study suggested that tight glycemic control during critical illness (achieved using an intravenous insulin infusion to maintain blood glucose level between 80 and 110 mg/dL) was associated with decreased mortality and other benefits.[139] These findings were not replicated in later studies; the largest available randomized controlled trial actually found that tight glucose control led to a 2.6% increase in mortality compared with less stringent glucose control.[140] Maintaining the blood glucose between 80 and 110 mg/dL commonly leads to episodes of iatrogenic hypoglycemia, which may worsen outcome.[140] Current guidelines recommend a target blood glucose level between 140 and 180 mg/dL in ICU patients.[137] The same targets are suggested for critically ill pregnant individuals.

Transfusion Triggers

Most RBC transfusions in the ICU are used to treat anemia in hemodynamically stable patients who are not actively bleeding.[141] Anemia in the critically ill patient commonly results from inflammation-induced inhibition of erythropoiesis and excessive phlebotomy.[141] Administration of RBCs theoretically leads to an increase in arterial blood oxygen content, oxygen delivery, and, ultimately, oxygen consumption. Unfortunately, no clear evidence indicates that RBC transfusions improve oxygen consumption.[142,143] In reality, significant risks are associated with the transfusion of blood products in the ICU (Table 53.2).[143]

The largest published trial to date evaluating the role of RBC transfusion in hemodynamically stable ICU patients found no difference in outcome between patients randomized to a liberal transfusion strategy (transfuse to maintain hemoglobin > 10 g/dL) or a restrictive strategy (transfuse to maintain a hemoglobin > 7 g/dL).[144] A subgroup analysis revealed that mortality was *increased* with the liberal transfusion strategy in the subgroup of patients younger than 50 years of age and with less severe disease (Acute Physiology and Chronic Health Evaluation II score < 20). Based on these findings, most intensivists do not transfuse hemodynamically stable patients in the ICU until the hemoglobin level is less than 7 g/dL. (In patients with acute coronary syndrome, the threshold may be higher at 8 g/dL.[141]) Although each case should be individualized, it seems reasonable to apply these guidelines to critically ill pregnant patients. Plasma, cryoprecipitate, and platelets should not be transfused for the sole purpose of correcting laboratory measurements in patients who are not actively bleeding and are not undergoing an invasive procedure.

Sepsis

Sepsis occurs as the result of a maladaptive systemic inflammatory response to an infectious insult.[145] It is the leading cause of mortality in ICUs in developed countries, and the incidence is increasing worldwide. Sepsis is also one of the leading causes of maternal mortality (see Chapter 36).[146] The incidence of death from sepsis in obstetric patients is lower than that in nonobstetric patients. This likely reflects the fact that pregnant women are younger and have fewer coexisting medical pathologic processes.

Management

Of pivotal importance in the management of sepsis is achieving early infection source control and instituting adequate antibiotic therapy and resuscitation. Infected fluid collections or tissues should be drained/excised if clinically indicated.[147,148] Broad-spectrum antibiotics should be initiated quickly (ideally after cultures have been obtained); narrow-spectrum antibiotic administration should follow once culture results are available.

TABLE 53.2 **Potential Complications Associated With Transfusion of Blood Products**

Transfusion-related acute lung injury	Noncardiogenic pulmonary edema that occurs within 6 hours of transfusion Risk higher after platelet and plasma transfusions Supportive treatment
Transfusion-related circulatory overload	Hydrostatic pulmonary edema secondary to volume overload
Transfusion-related immunomodulation	After transfusion, decreased immunity with increased risk for nosocomial infections
Infectious complications	Viral (hepatitis B and C, HIV, cytomegalovirus, parvovirus B19, West Nile virus, human T-lymphotropic virus) or bacterial (*Staphylococcus* species, *E. coli*, *Pseudomonas* species, *Yersinia*) Bacterial infections are more common
Febrile reactions	Secondary to leukocytes and cytokines accumulated during storage May decrease with leukoreduction
Allergic nonhemolytic reactions	Urticaria and pruritus, secondary to soluble antigens in the donor plasma
Hemolytic reactions	Secondary to preexisting recipient alloantibodies against donor erythrocytes Sudden onset of fever and chills, back pain, hypotension, dyspnea, renal injury, and DIC
Posttransfusion purpura	Purpura and bleeding manifestations after transfusion of blood products Usually seen in patients with antibodies that react against the human platelet antigen-1 from donor platelets Treat with intravenous immunoglobulin
Increased risk for multiorgan system failure	Likely secondary to cytokines contained in stored blood products
Graft-versus-host reaction	Lymphocytes transfused to patient not recognized as foreign; such cells react against host tissues, leading to pancytopenia, rash, hepatitis, and diarrhea Mainly seen in patients with profound immunosuppression or in patients receiving blood products from close relatives who share human leukocyte antigens May be prevented with leukoreduction and gamma radiation of blood products.

DIC, Disseminated intravascular coagulation; *HIV*, human immunodeficiency virus.
Modified from Gilliss BM, Looney MR, Gropper MA. Reducing noninfectious risks of blood transfusion. *Anesthesiology*. 2011;115:635–649.

Fluid management. The cornerstone of resuscitation in sepsis is early fluid therapy. Current guidelines recommend the early administration of 30 mL/kg of crystalloid solution; vasopressors are indicated if a mean arterial blood pressure of at least 65 mm Hg is not achieved.[148] The placenta should be regarded as the maternal end organ that is most sensitive to hypoperfusion. For this reason, FHR decelerations are often an early sign of maternal hypoperfusion.

Fluid resuscitation improves tissue perfusion by increasing driving pressure and modulating early inflammation by decreasing concentrations of proinflammatory cytokines. Crystalloids (normal saline, lactated Ringer's solution, PlasmaLyte) have an intravascular half-life of 30 to 60 minutes compared with 16 hours for colloids such as albumin. Theoretically, the use of colloid leads to a more efficient resuscitation. The largest published trial comparing the use of crystalloids and colloids in critically ill patients found no difference in outcomes between groups.[27] However, a subgroup analysis suggested that patients with sepsis might benefit from albumin administration.[27] A 2024 editorial concluded that the optimal approach to fluid management of patients with sepsis, including the question of benefits and harms of crystalloid versus colloid solutions, remains unclear.[149] Currently, there is no evidence that colloids (mainly albumin) are superior to crystalloids for fluid resuscitation in patients with sepsis. The use of balanced crystalloid solutions (e.g., lactated Ringer's solution, PlasmaLyte) is currently recommended; normal saline is associated with increased adverse renal effects among critically ill patients.[29]

The use of hydroxyl ethyl starch in patients with sepsis is associated with increased rates of kidney injury and mortality, and is not recommended.[150,151]

In the past, early goal-directed therapy (defined as "adjustments in cardiac preload, afterload, and contractility to balance oxygen delivery with oxygen demand" to achieve a normal central venous mixed oxygen concentration) was advocated. More recent evidence shows that this approach does not improve outcomes and may be harmful as it introduces the risks associated with central venous line insertion.[152,153]

Excessive fluid resuscitation and a positive fluid balance have consistently been associated with increased mortality in critically ill patients. A trial in patients with ARDS showed that *after* the initial phase of resuscitation, patients who were randomized to receive a conservative fluid regimen had improved lung function and a shorter duration of mechanical ventilation and ICU stay compared with patients who received a liberal fluid regimen.[134] The study did not have sufficient power to identify a difference in 60-day mortality.

Thus, it appears that early in sepsis (the first 6 hours), patients benefit from aggressive initial fluid resuscitation. Later, a conservative fluid strategy may be beneficial, with fluid administration guided by *dynamic* rather than static measurements of preload.[154] For example, in mechanically ventilated patients with sinus rhythm and who are not triggering the ventilator, pulse pressure variation above 13% accurately predicts fluid responsiveness.[155] Similarly, in nonintubated patients or

patients not in sinus rhythm, an increase in stroke volume (usually 10% to 15%) as assessed by transthoracic echocardiography or noninvasive cardiac output monitoring during passive leg raising (or after administration of a fluid bolus) accurately predicts fluid responsiveness.[154] Bedside ultrasonographic evaluation of changes in the inferior vena cava (IVC) diameter induced by the respiratory cycle is also useful in titrating fluid administration. Patients with an enlarged IVC that does not vary in size with the respiratory cycle are very unlikely to improve with further fluid boluses.

Vasopressors and inotropes. If MAP > 65 mm Hg is not achieved with fluid therapy alone, vasopressors are indicated.[148] The vasopressor of choice in septic shock is norepinephrine. Norepinephrine increases blood pressure primarily by increasing systemic vascular resistance.

Obstetricians have traditionally expressed concern regarding the potential adverse effects of vasopressors on uteroplacental perfusion. However, in the setting of septic shock, restoration of maternal organ perfusion pressure is essential for fetal survival. Multiple case reports have described improved fetal status with the use of vasopressors to increase MAP. Guidelines from the Society for Maternal-Fetal Medicine recommend norepinephrine as the vasopressor of choice for the treatment of septic shock during pregnancy.[147]

Vasopressin is a peptide hormone synthesized in the hypothalamus and stored in the pituitary gland. A relative deficiency of vasopressin has been described during septic shock. Vasopressin causes direct vascular smooth muscle constriction via stimulation of V_1 receptors. It also increases the response to catecholamines, likely by increasing cortisol secretion through its action on V_3 receptors in the pituitary gland. Additionally, vasopressin causes vasoconstriction by closing ATP-dependent potassium channels. Observational studies have shown that the addition of low-dose vasopressin (0.03 U/min) to traditional vasopressor therapy can raise blood pressure in vasopressor-refractory septic shock. A large randomized clinical trial reported no difference in mortality in patients with vasopressor-dependent septic shock who were randomized to receive either vasopressin or norepinephrine in addition to open-label vasopressor therapy.[156] However, the trial did not address the use of vasopressin as rescue therapy for septic shock that is resistant to conventional vasopressors. Vasopressin is commonly used in catecholamine-refractory septic shock and in patients who experience significant tachyarrythmias with the use of catecholamines.

No good data exist regarding the use of vasopressin during septic shock in pregnant women. Theoretically, it may activate uterine V_{1a} receptors, leading to uterine contractions. Caution is recommended if this agent is used during pregnancy.

Myocardial contractility is compromised in septic shock (see earlier discussion). **Septic cardiomyopathy** may be "unmasked" when vasopressors are used to increase systemic vascular resistance. An assessment of cardiac output (e.g., bedside transthoracic echocardiography) is beneficial when vasopressors (primarily norepinephrine and vasopressin) are used without concomitant inotropic support. If worsening cardiac output is noted after initiating vasoconstrictor therapy, inotropic support (e.g., dobutamine, milrinone) may be beneficial.

Anecdotal data suggest that catecholamines may not be effective in patients with severe acidemia. However, data do not support the use of sodium bicarbonate therapy during resuscitation. In patients with sepsis, bicarbonate therapy is not indicated if the pH is above 7.15.[148] If the pH is less than 7.15, the use of sodium bicarbonate should be individualized. Particular care should be taken if the practitioner chooses to use bicarbonate during pregnancy because bicarbonate does not cross the placenta, but the carbon dioxide generated from its administration crosses the placenta to the fetal compartment, leading to potential fetal acidemia. A recent trial found no benefit with the use of sodium bicarbonate in patients with severe metabolic acidemia in the ICU, although decreased mortality was suggested in a subgroup analysis of patients with a pH < 7.2 and acute kidney injury.[157]

Corticosteroids. Approximately 50% to 75% of patients with sepsis/septic shock have critical illness–related corticosteroid insufficiency. Cytokines lead to a dysfunctional hypothalamic-pituitary-adrenal axis with a consequent decrease in cortisol secretion. Cortisol plays a pivotal role in the upregulation of catecholamine receptors at the vascular level (leading to an increased response to endogenous and exogenous catecholamines).

The use of corticosteroid therapy in patients with septic shock has long been controversial. In the past, large doses of corticosteroids were used; however, more recent studies suggest that low-dose corticosteroids (hydrocortisone 200 mg/day) may be beneficial.[158] Currently, physiologic doses of corticosteroids are recommended in patients who fail to respond to catecholamine therapy.[148,159] A 2018 study demonstrated improved survival with corticosteroids among patients with "catecholamine resistant shock," defined as the inability to achieve a MAP of 65 mm Hg despite norepinephrine above 0.25 µg/kg/min.[159] Given the lack of definitive evidence, this is a reasonable threshold to identify candidates for corticosteroid therapy in pregnancy. The agent of choice is hydrocortisone (50 mg bolus intravenously every 6 hours or a continuous intravenous infusion at 10 mg/h) together with oral fludrocortisone 50 µg daily.[147] This low dose of glucocorticoid is believed to be immunomodulatory; the excessive inflammatory response that leads to shock is downregulated without causing immunosuppression. Once begun, treatment should be maintained for 7 days; tapering is not necessary. The adrenocorticotropic hormone stimulation test or measurement of random cortisol levels is not necessary to identify patients with septic shock who should receive glucocorticoids.

Monitoring resuscitation. Traditionally, the main goal of resuscitation efforts in sepsis has been to achieve "normal" vital signs (MAP > 65 mm Hg, urine output > 0.5 mL/kg/h, normal heart rate).[148] Unfortunately, clinical signs and symptoms lack sensitivity for detection of tissue hypoperfusion. Patients may have normal vital signs and still have organ hypoperfusion and anaerobic metabolism. Different strategies have been proposed to detect these patients with "occult shock." Resuscitation may be guided by blood lactate levels. Patients with persistent lactic acidosis, despite apparently normal vital signs, may require further resuscitation to increase tissue oxygen delivery.

Another option is to optimize hemodynamic support using central ($Sc\bar{v}o_2$) and mixed venous ($S\bar{v}o_2$) oxyhemoglobin saturation monitoring. Patients with tissue hypoperfusion will extract more oxygen in an attempt to increase aerobic metabolism. The increased extraction will lead to a decrease in the oxygen saturation of hemoglobin returning to the central circulation. $S\bar{v}o_2$ is the saturation of hemoglobin obtained from blood sampled from the pulmonary artery. It requires placement of a pulmonary artery catheter; a normal value is greater than 65%. Pregnancy does not alter the $S\bar{v}o_2$.[160]

$Sc\bar{v}o_2$ is the oxyhemoglobin saturation of a blood sample obtained from the junction of the superior vena cava and the right atrium. This measurement is readily achieved by obtaining a blood sample from a central venous catheter. The normal value is greater than 70%. To our knowledge, normal values for $Sc\bar{v}o_2$ during pregnancy have not been described.

The Fetus During Critical Maternal Illness

In almost all cases, therapeutic interventions in the critically ill pregnant patient should not be withheld because of fetal concerns.[71] When the alternative is death or severe injury, very few drugs or diagnostic or therapeutic maneuvers are contraindicated. Most medications (sedatives, neuromuscular blocking agents, corticosteroids, vasopressors, inotropes, antibiotics) may be used safely (or with minimal risks that are commonly outweighed by the benefits) during pregnancy. Some of the common agents used in the ICU setting and the associated fetal risks are listed in Table 53.3.

Imaging studies should be performed as needed (see Chapter 18). Abdominal shielding is not necessary. When possible, ultrasonography and MRI are preferred because no ionizing radiation is used. Radiation exposure from common studies, such as a chest or abdominal radiography or CT of the head or chest, are all below the upper limit of safety (5 rads) recommended by the American College of Obstetricians and Gynecologists.[57] Similarly, the use of radiopaque (iodide containing) or paramagnetic contrast media (e.g., gadolinium) during pregnancy is acceptable, provided the study is considered fundamental to the care of the patient.[57]

Critically ill pregnant patients should receive continuous electronic FHR monitoring after 24 weeks' gestation (lower age limit of viability) to continuously evaluate fetal well-being. The presence of fetal bradycardia, tachycardia, or persistent FHR decelerations may signal uterine hypoperfusion that requires improved resuscitation efforts. Each case should be evaluated individually with the aid of a maternal-fetal medicine specialist. Pregnant women beyond 20 weeks' gestation should be positioned either in the left or right decubitus position to avoid uterine compression of the IVC, which results in a decrease in cardiac preload.

TABLE 53.3	**Common Medications Used During Critical Illness**
Medication	**Comments**
Norepinephrine	Uterine vessels are very sensitive to vasoconstriction because they are rich in alpha-adrenergic receptors. As with any vasopressor, this agent may be used after adequate volume resuscitation and with continuous electronic FHR monitoring. Norepinephrine is the preferred agent in sepsis.
Dopamine	Dopamine is associated with more tachyarrhythmias than norepinephrine. As with norepinephrine, it should be used after adequate fluid resuscitation and with continuous electronic FHR monitoring. Not currently recommended as a first-line pressor in critical care.
Vasopressin	Low doses used for the treatment of diabetes insipidus have not been associated with fetal harm. No data exist on its use as a continuous infusion for septic shock in pregnancy. Potentially, vasopressin may lead to activation of V_{1a} receptors and uterine contractions; thus, caution is recommended if used during pregnancy. Continuous electronic FHR monitoring is highly desirable.
Dobutamine	Provides inotropic support
Milrinone	Provides inotropic support
Phenylephrine	Pure vasopressor, no inotropic support
Epinephrine	Both vasopressor and inotropic support
Hydrocortisone	Some data suggest an association between corticosteroid use during the first trimester and fetal cleft lip/palate. However, if required to improve maternal outcomes, use should not be deferred.
Midazolam	No clear correlation between the use of midazolam and fetal anomalies has been described. Use of any sedative close to the time of delivery is associated with neonatal depression.
Lorazepam	Limited data have associated prolonged use with fetal anomalies. It is unlikely that its use during a few days of critical illness outside the first trimester is teratogenic.
Propofol	May result in hypotension
Dexmedetomidine	This agent crosses the placenta, but no published studies link dexmedetomidine to fetal malformations.
Cisatracurium	May have antiinflammatory properties (beneficial in treatment of ARDS)
Vecuronium	Accumulates in renal and/or liver failure
Morphine	Histamine release may result in hypotension
Fentanyl	Minimal hemodynamic disturbances
Hydromorphone	Minimal hemodynamic disturbances
Haloperidol	Commonly used to treat agitated delirium

ARDS, Acute respiratory distress syndrome; *FHR*, fetal heart rate.

KEY POINTS

- Trauma is the most common nonobstetric cause of maternal death.
- Head injury and hemorrhagic shock are the most common causes of death in the pregnant trauma victim.
- Even minor trauma increases the risk for placental abruption and preterm labor.
- Resuscitation of the critically ill or injured obstetric patient should be based on the premise that optimized maternal resuscitation will be most beneficial to the fetus.

- Care of the pregnant trauma patient should be based on Advanced Trauma Life Support principles. Additional attention should be given to complications that are specific to pregnancy, such as uterine rupture and placental abruption.
- In addition to standard Advanced Cardiac Life Support guidelines for cardiac arrest, considerations for resuscitation of the pregnant patient include maintenance of left uterine displacement and evacuation of the uterus. If the return of spontaneous circulation does not occur with the

usual resuscitative measures, and if the fundal height is at or above the umbilicus (approximately 20 weeks' gestation), cesarean delivery (resuscitative hysterotomy) should be performed within 5 minutes of cardiac arrest.

- Neurologic emergencies during pregnancy require prompt intensive care to avoid secondary brain injury caused by hypoxia, hypercarbia, seizures, hyponatremia, hyperglycemia, and rebleeding episodes.

- Patients with acute respiratory distress syndrome should receive lung-protective mechanical ventilation. When possible, excessive fluid administration should be avoided.

- Early enteral nutrition and glucose control are basic tenants of contemporary critical care.

- A transfusion of blood products in critically ill patients should follow a restrictive strategy.

- Prompt diagnosis, infection source control, adequate antibiotic therapy, and early fluid resuscitation are fundamental principles of the early management of sepsis.

- Fetal heart rate monitoring is indicated in pregnant trauma victims and critically ill obstetric patients beginning at 24 weeks' gestation; altered fetal heart rate patterns can serve as a valuable indicator of inadequate resuscitation.

REFERENCES

1. Leovic MP, Robbins HN, Foley MR, Starikov RS. The "virtual" obstetrical intensive care unit: providing critical care for contemporary obstetrics in nontraditional locations. *Am J Obstet Gynecol.* 2016;215:e1–e4.

2. Guntupalli KK, Hall N, Karnad DR, et al. Critical illness in pregnancy: part I: an approach to a pregnant patient in the ICU and common obstetric disorders. *Chest.* 2015;148:1093–1104.

3. Guntupalli KK, Karnad DR, Bandi V, et al. Critical illness in pregnancy: part II: common medical conditions complicating pregnancy and puerperium. *Chest.* 2015;148:1333–1345.

4. Zieleskiewicz L, Chantry A, Duclos G, et al. Intensive care and pregnancy: epidemiology and general principles of management of obstetrics ICU patients during pregnancy. *Anaesth Crit Care Pain Med.* 2016;35:S51–S57.

5. Jacob S, Bloebaum L, Shah G, Varner MW. Maternal mortality in Utah. *Obstet Gynecol.* 1998;91:187–191.

6. Rogers FB, Rozycki GS, Osler TM, et al. A multi-institutional study of factors associated with fetal death in injured pregnant patients. *Arch Surg.* 1999;134:1274–1277.

7. Petrone P, Talving P, Browder T, et al. Abdominal injuries in pregnancy: a 155-month study at two level 1 trauma centers. *Injury.* 2011;42:47–49.

8. Petrone P, Jimenez-Morillas P, Axelrad A, Marini CP. Traumatic injuries to the pregnant patient: a critical literature review. *Eur J Trauma Emerg Surg.* 2017;45:383–392.

9. Metz TD, Abbott JT. Uterine trauma in pregnancy after motor vehicle crashes with airbag deployment: a 30-case series. *J Trauma.* 2006;61:658–661.

10. Curet MJ, Schermer CR, Demarest GB, et al. Predictors of outcome in trauma during pregnancy: identification of patients who can be monitored for less than 6 hours. *J Trauma.* 2000;49:18–24.

11. Aboutanos SZ, Aboutanos MB, Dompkowski D, et al. Predictors of fetal outcome in pregnant trauma patients: a five-year institutional review. *Am Surg.* 2007;73:824–827.

12. Chesnut RM. Care of central nervous system injuries. *Surg Clin North Am.* 2007;87:119–156.

13. El-Kady D, Gilbert WM, Anderson J, et al. Trauma during pregnancy: an analysis of maternal and fetal outcomes in a large population. *Am J Obstet Gynecol.* 2004;190:1661–1668.

14. Grossman NB. Blunt trauma in pregnancy. *Am Fam Physician.* 2004;70:1303–1310.

15. Melamed N, Aviram A, Silver M, et al. Pregnancy course and outcome following blunt trauma. *J Matern Fetal Neonatal Med.* 2012;25:1612–1617.

16. Muench MV, Baschat AA, Reddy UM, et al. Kleihauer-Betke testing is important in all cases of maternal trauma. *J Trauma.* 2004;57:1094–1098.

17. Brown HL. Trauma in pregnancy. *Obstet Gynecol.* 2009;114:147–160.

18. Richards JR, Ormsby EL, Romo MV, et al. Blunt abdominal injury in the pregnant patient: detection with US. *Radiology.* 2004;233:463–470.

19. Morgan JA, Marcus PS. Prenatal diagnosis and management of intrauterine fracture. *Obstet Gynecol Surv.* 2010;65:249–259.

20. Wall SL, Figueiredo F, Laing GL, Clarke DL. The spectrum and outcome of pregnant trauma patients in a metropolitan trauma service in South Africa. *Injury.* 2014;45:1220–1223.

21. Schiff MA, Holt VL. The Injury Severity Score in pregnant trauma patients: predicting placental abruption and fetal death. *J Trauma.* 2002;53:946–949.

22. Hayes B, Ryan S, Stephenson JB, King MD. Cerebral palsy after maternal trauma in pregnancy. *Dev Med Child Neurol.* 2007;49:700–706.

23. Chames MC, Pearlman MD. Trauma during pregnancy: outcomes and clinical management. *Clin Obstet Gynecol.* 2008;51:398–408.

24. American College of Surgeons Committee on Trauma. *ATLS®: Advanced Trauma Life Support Student Course Manual.* 10th ed. American College of Surgeons; 2018.

25. Oxford CM, Ludmir J. Trauma in pregnancy. *Clin Obstet Gynecol.* 2009;52:611–629.

26. Petrosoniak A, Pavenski K, da Luz LT, Callum J. Massive hemorrhage protocol: a practical approach to the bleeding trauma patient. *Emerg Med Clin North Am.* 2023;41:51–69.

27. SAFE Study Investigators, Australian and New Zealand Intensive Care Society Clinical Trials Group, Australian Red Cross Blood Service, et al. Saline or albumin for fluid resuscitation in patients with traumatic brain injury. *N Engl J Med.* 2007;357:874–884.

28. Annane D, Siami S, Jaber S, et al. Effects of fluid resuscitation with colloids vs crystalloids on mortality in critically ill patients presenting with hypovolemic shock: the CRISTAL randomized trial. *JAMA.* 2013;310:1809–1817.

29. Semler MW, Self WH, Wanderer JP, et al. Balanced crystalloids versus saline in critically ill adults. *N Engl J Med.* 2018;378:829–839.

30. Brasel KJ, Bulger E, Cook AJ, et al. Hypertonic resuscitation: design and implementation of a prehospital intervention trial. *J Am Coll Surg.* 2008;206:220–232.

31. Wu MC, Liao TY, Lee EM, et al. Administration of hypertonic solutions for hemorrhagic shock: a systematic review and meta-analysis of clinical trials. *Anesth Analg.* 2017;125:1549–1557.

32. Asehnoune K, Lasocki S, Seguin P, et al. Association between continuous hyperosmolar therapy and survival in patients with traumatic brain injury—a multicentre prospective cohort study and systematic review. *Crit Care.* 2017;21:328.

33. Shi J, Tan L, Ye J, Hu L. Hypertonic saline and mannitol in patients with traumatic brain injury: a systematic and meta-analysis. *Medicine (Baltimore).* 2020;99:e21655.

34. Gharizadeh N, Ghojazadeh M, Naseri A, et al. Hypertonic saline for traumatic brain injury: a systematic review and meta-analysis. *Eur J Med Res.* 2022;27:254.

35. Lippi G, Favaloro EJ, Cervellin G. Massive posttraumatic bleeding: epidemiology, causes, clinical features, and therapeutic management. *Semin Thromb Hemost.* 2013;39:83–93.

36. Fowler R, Pepe PE. Fluid resuscitation of the patient with major trauma. *Curr Opin Anaesthesiol.* 2002;15:173–178.

37. Gamberini E, Coccolini F, Tamagnini B, et al. Resuscitative endovascular balloon occlusion of the aorta in trauma: a systematic review of the literature. *World J Emerg Surg.* 2017;12:42.

38. Brenner M, Inaba K, Aiolfi A, et al. Resuscitative endovascular balloon occlusion of the aorta and resuscitative thoracotomy in select patients with hemorrhagic shock: early results from the American Association for the Surgery of Trauma Aortic Occlusion in Resuscitation for Trauma and Acute Care Surgery Registry. *J Am Coll Surg.* 2018;226:730–740.

39. Jansen JO, Hudson J, Cochran C, et al. Emergency department resuscitative endovascular balloon occlusion of the aorta in trauma patients with exsanguinating hemorrhage: the UK-REBOA randomized clinical trial. *JAMA.* 2023;330:1862–1871.

40. Arul GS, Pugh HE, Mercer SJ, Midwinter MJ. Optimising communication in the damage control resuscitation—damage control surgery sequence in major trauma management. *J R Army Med Corps.* 2012;158:82–84.

41. Curry N, Davis PW. What's new in resuscitation strategies for the patient with multiple trauma? *Injury.* 2012;43:1021–1028.

42. Cohen MJ. Towards hemostatic resuscitation: the changing understanding of acute traumatic biology, massive bleeding, and damage-control resuscitation. *Surg Clin North Am.* 2012;92:877–891.

43. Undurraga Perl VJ, Leroux B, Cook MR, et al. Damage-control resuscitation and emergency laparotomy: findings from the PROPPR study. *J Trauma Acute Care Surg.* 2016;80:568–574.

44. Holcomb JB, Tilley BC, Baraniuk S, et al. Transfusion of plasma, platelets, and red blood cells in a 1:1:1 vs a 1:1:2 ratio and mortality in patients with severe trauma: the PROPPR randomized clinical trial. *JAMA.* 2015;313:471–482.

45. Cannon JW, Khan MA, Raja AS, et al. Damage control resuscitation in patients with severe traumatic hemorrhage: a practice management guideline from the Eastern Association for the Surgery of Trauma. *J Trauma Acute Care Surg.* 2017;82:605–617.

46. Stensballe J, Henriksen HH, Johansson PI. Early haemorrhage control and management of trauma-induced coagulopathy: the importance of goal-directed therapy. *Curr Opin Crit Care.* 2017;23:503–510.

47. Gonzalez E, Moore EE, Moore HB, et al. Goal-directed hemostatic resuscitation of trauma-induced coagulopathy: a pragmatic randomized clinical trial comparing a viscoelastic assay to conventional coagulation assays. *Ann Surg.* 2016;263:1051–1059.

48. Weinberg L, Steele RG, Pugh R, et al. The pregnant trauma patient. *Anaesth Intensive Care.* 2005;33:167–180.

49. Connolly AM, Katz VL, Bash KL, et al. Trauma and pregnancy. *Am J Perinatol.* 1997;14:331–336.

50. Drost TF, Rosemurgy AS, Sherman HF, et al. Major trauma in pregnant women: maternal/fetal outcome. *J Trauma.* 1990;30:574–578.

51. Shah S, Miller PR, Meredith JW, Chang MC. Elevated admission white blood cell count in pregnant trauma patients: an indicator of ongoing placental abruption. *Am Surg.* 2002;68:644–647.

52. Atkinson AL, Santolaya-Forgas J, Blitzer DN, et al. Risk factors for perinatal mortality in patients admitted to the hospital with the diagnosis of placental abruption. *J Matern Fetal Neonatal Med.* 2015;28:594–597.

53. Pearlman MD, Tintinalli JE, Lorenz RP. A prospective controlled study of outcome after trauma during pregnancy. *Am J Obstet Gynecol.* 1990;162:1502–1507.

54. Scorpio RJ, Esposito TJ, Smith LG, Gens DR. Blunt trauma during pregnancy: factors affecting fetal outcome. *J Trauma.* 1992;32:213–216.

55. Baerga-Varela Y, Zietlow SP, Bannon MP, et al. Trauma in pregnancy. *Mayo Clin Proc.* 2000;75:1243–1248.

56. McCollough CH, Schueler BA, Atwell TD, et al. Radiation exposure and pregnancy: when should we be concerned? *Radiographics.* 2007;27:909–917.

57. American College of Obstetricians and Gynecologists. Committee Opinion No. 723: Guidelines for diagnostic imaging during pregnancy and lactation (reaffirmed 2021). *Obstet Gynecol.* 2017;130:933–934.

58. American Association of Physicists in Medicine. AAPM position statement on the use of patient gonadal and fetal shielding; 2019. https://www.aapm.org/org/policies/details.asp?id=468. Accessed January 11, 2025.

59. Association for the Advancement of Automotive Medicine. Abbreviated injury scale. Available at: https://www.aaam.org/abbreviated-injury-scale-ais/. Accessed December 31, 2024.

60. Esposito TJ, Tinkoff G, Reed J, et al. American Association for the Surgery of Trauma organ injury scale (OIS): past, present, and future. *J Trauma Acute Care Surg.* 2013;74:1163–1174.

61. Distelhorst JT, Krishnamoorthy V, Schiff MA. Association between hospital trauma designation and maternal and neonatal outcomes after injury among pregnant women in Washington state. *J Am Coll Surg.* 2016;222:296–302.

62. Distelhorst JT, Soltis MA, Krishnamoorthy V, Schiff MA. Hospital trauma level's association with outcomes for injured pregnant women and their neonates in Washington state, 1995-2012. *Int J Crit Illn Inj Sci.* 2017;7:142–149.

63. American College of Obstetricians and Gynecologists, Society for Maternal-Fetal Medicine. Obstetric Care Consensus No. 9: Levels of maternal care (reaffirmed 2021). *Obstet Gynecol.* 2019;134:e41–e55.

64. Berry C, Ley EJ, Mirocha J, et al. Do pregnant women have improved outcomes after traumatic brain injury? *Am J Surg.* 2011;201:429–432.

65. Lipman S, Cohen S, Einav S, et al. The Society for Obstetric Anesthesia and Perinatology consensus statement on the management of cardiac arrest in pregnancy. *Anesth Analg.* 2014;118:1003–1016.

66. Beckett VA, Knight M, Sharpe P. The CAPS study: incidence, management and outcomes of cardiac arrest in pregnancy in the UK: a prospective, descriptive study. *BJOG.* 2017;124:1374–1381.

67. Mhyre JM, Tsen LC, Einav S, et al. Cardiac arrest during hospitalization for delivery in the United States, 1998-2011. *Anesthesiology.* 2014;120:810–818.

68. Jeejeebhoy FM, Zelop CM, Windrim R, et al. Management of cardiac arrest in pregnancy: a systematic review. *Resuscitation.* 2011;82:801–809.

69. Merchant RM, Topjian AA, Panchal AR, et al. Part 1: Executive Summary: 2020 American Heart Association guidelines for cardiopulmonary resuscitation and emergency cardiovascular care. *Circulation.* 2020;142:S337–S357.

70. Jeejeebhoy FM, Zelop CM, Lipman S, et al. Cardiac arrest in pregnancy: a scientific statement from the American Heart Association. *Circulation.* 2015;132:1747–1773.

71. American College of Obstetricians and Gynecologists. Practice Bulletin No. 211: Critical care in pregnancy (reaffirmed 2021). *Obstet Gynecol.* 2019;133:e303–e319.

72. Einav S, Kaufman N, Sela HY. Maternal cardiac arrest and perimortem caesarean delivery: evidence or expert-based? *Resuscitation.* 2012;83:1191–1200.

73. Dankiewicz J, Cronberg T, Lilja G, et al. Hypothermia versus normothermia after out-of-hospital cardiac arrest. *N Engl J Med.* 2021;384:2283–2294.

74. Taccone FS, Dankiewicz J, Cariou A, et al. Hypothermia vs normothermia in patients with cardiac arrest and nonshockable rhythm: a meta-analysis. *JAMA Neurol.* 2024;81:126–133.

75. Esmaeilzadeh M, Dictus C, Kayvanpour E, et al. One life ends, another begins: management of a brain-dead pregnant mother—a systematic review. *BMC Med.* 2010;8:74.

76. Barr JJ. When death Is not the end: continuing somatic care during postmortem pregnancy. *Linacre Q.* 2019;86:275–282.

77. Manninen BA. Sustaining a pregnant cadaver for the purpose of gestating a fetus: a limited defense. *Kennedy Inst Ethics J.* 2016;26:399–430.

78. Cartolovni A, Habek D. Guidelines for the management of the social and ethical challenges in brain death during pregnancy. *Int J Gynaecol Obstet.* 2019;146:149–156.

79. Dodaro MG, Seidenari A, Marino IR, et al. Brain death in pregnancy: a systematic review focusing on perinatal outcomes. *Am J Obstet Gynecol.* 2021;224:445–469.

80. Wiebers DO. Ischemic cerebrovascular complications of pregnancy. *Arch Neurol.* 1985;42:1106–1113.

81. Leffert LR, Clancy CR, Bateman BT, et al. Hypertensive disorders and pregnancy-related stroke: frequency, trends, risk factors, and outcomes. *Obstet Gynecol.* 2015;125:124–131.

82. Miller EC, Gallo M, Kulick ER, et al. Infections and risk of peripartum stroke during delivery admissions. *Stroke.* 2018;49:1129–1134.

83. Miller EC, Leffert L. Stroke in pregnancy: a focused update. *Anesth Analg.* 2020;130:1085–1096.

84. Powers WJ, Rabinstein AA, Ackerson T, et al. 2018 guidelines for the early management of patients with acute ischemic stroke: a guideline for healthcare professionals from the American Heart Association/American Stroke Association. *Stroke.* 2018;49:e46–e110.

85. Wiese KM, Talkad A, Mathews M, Wang D. Intravenous recombinant tissue plasminogen activator in a pregnant woman with cardioembolic stroke. *Stroke.* 2006;37:2168–2169.

86. Li Y, Margraf J, Kluck B, et al. Thrombolytic therapy for ischemic stroke secondary to paradoxical embolism in pregnancy: a case report and literature review. *Neurologist.* 2012;18:44–48.

87. Vaid U, Baram M, Marik PE. Thrombolytic therapy in a patient with suspected pulmonary embolism despite a negative computed tomography pulmonary angiogram. *Respir Care.* 2011;56:336–338.

88. French KF, White J, Hoesch RE. Treatment of intracerebral hemorrhage with tranexamic acid after thrombolysis with tissue plasminogen activator. *Neurocrit Care.* 2012;17:107–111.

89. Lansberg MG, O'Donnell MJ, Khatri P, et al. Antithrombotic and thrombolytic therapy for ischemic stroke: antithrombotic therapy and prevention of thrombosis, 9th ed: American College of Chest Physicians evidence-based clinical practice guidelines. *Chest.* 2012;141:e601S–e636S.

90. Stam J. Thrombosis of the cerebral veins and sinuses. *N Engl J Med.* 2005;352:1791–1798.

91. Karnad DR, Guntupalli KK. Neurologic disorders in pregnancy. *Crit Care Med.* 2005;33:S362–S371.

92. Leffert LR, Clancy CR, Bateman BT, et al. Patient characteristics and outcomes after hemorrhagic stroke in pregnancy. *Circ Cardiovasc Qual Outcomes.* 2015;8:S170–S178.

93. Flower O, Smith M. The acute management of intracerebral hemorrhage. *Curr Opin Crit Care.* 2011;17:106–114.

94. Grise EM, Adeoye O. Blood pressure control for acute ischemic and hemorrhagic stroke. *Curr Opin Crit Care.* 2012;18:132–138.

95. Bosel J. Blood pressure control for acute severe ischemic and hemorrhagic stroke. *Curr Opin Crit Care.* 2017;23:81–86.

96. Hemphill JC 3rd, Greenberg SM, Anderson CS, et al. Guidelines for the management of spontaneous intracerebral hemorrhage: a guideline for healthcare professionals from the American Heart Association/American Stroke Association. *Stroke.* 2015;46:2032–2060.

97. Connolly ES Jr, Rabinstein AA, Carhuapoma JR, et al. Guidelines for the management of aneurysmal subarachnoid hemorrhage: a guideline for healthcare professionals from the American Heart Association/American Stroke Association. *Stroke.* 2012;43:1711–1737.

98. Leijenaar JF, Dorhout Mees SM, Algra A, et al. Effect of magnesium treatment and glucose levels on delayed cerebral ischemia in patients with subarachnoid hemorrhage: a substudy of the Magnesium in Aneurysmal Subarachnoid Haemorrhage trial (MASH-II). *Int J Stroke.* 2015;10:108–112.

99. Kirkpatrick PJ, Turner CL, Smith C, et al. Simvastatin in aneurysmal subarachnoid haemorrhage (STASH): a multicentre randomised phase 3 trial. *Lancet Neurol.* 2014;13:666–675.

100. Muroi C, Seule M, Mishima K, Keller E. Novel treatments for vasospasm after subarachnoid hemorrhage. *Curr Opin Crit Care*. 2012;18:119–126.

101. Rabinstein AA. Vasospasm and statin therapy: yet another cautionary tale. *Neurocrit Care*. 2010;12:310–312.

102. Wartenberg KE. Critical care of poor-grade subarachnoid hemorrhage. *Curr Opin Crit Care*. 2011;17:85–93.

103. Benvenga S. What is the pathogenesis of hyponatremia after subarachnoid hemorrhage? *Nat Clin Pract Endocrinol Metab*. 2006;2:608–609.

104. Marupudi NI, Mittal S. Diagnosis and management of hyponatremia in patients with aneurysmal subarachnoid hemorrhage. *J Clin Med*. 2015;4:756–767.

105. Mount DB. The brain in hyponatremia: both culprit and victim. *Semin Nephrol*. 2009;29:196–215.

106. van Beijnum J, van der Worp HB, Buis DR, et al. Treatment of brain arteriovenous malformations: a systematic review and meta-analysis. *JAMA*. 2011;306:2011–2019.

107. Friedlander RM. Clinical practice. Arteriovenous malformations of the brain. *N Engl J Med*. 2007;356:2704–2712.

108. Lanzino G, D'Urso PI, Suarez J. Seizures and anticonvulsants after aneurysmal subarachnoid hemorrhage. *Neurocrit Care*. 2011;15:247–256.

109. Marik PE, Varon J. The management of status epilepticus. *Chest*. 2004;126:582–591.

110. Lee SK. Diagnosis and treatment of status epilepticus. *J Epilepsy Res*. 2020;10:45–54.

111. Gedzelman E, Meador KJ. Antiepileptic drugs in women with epilepsy during pregnancy. *Ther Adv Drug Saf*. 2012;3:71–87.

112. Silbergleit R, Durkalski V, Lowenstein D, et al. Intramuscular versus intravenous therapy for prehospital status epilepticus. *N Engl J Med*. 2012;366:591–600.

113. Ranieri VM, Rubenfeld GD, Thompson BT, et al. Acute respiratory distress syndrome: the Berlin definition. *JAMA*. 2012;307:2526–2533.

114. Cole DE, Taylor TL, McCullough DM, et al. Acute respiratory distress syndrome in pregnancy. *Crit Care Med*. 2005;33:S269–S278.

115. The Acute Respiratory Distress Syndrome Network. Ventilation with lower tidal volumes as compared with traditional tidal volumes for acute lung injury and the acute respiratory distress syndrome. *N Engl J Med*. 2000;342:1301–1308.

116. Kuiper JW, Groeneveld AB, Slutsky AS, Plotz FB. Mechanical ventilation and acute renal failure. *Crit Care Med*. 2005;33:1408–1415.

117. Kolobow T. Acute respiratory failure. On how to injure healthy lungs (and prevent sick lungs from recovering). *ASAIO Trans*. 1988;34:31–34.

118. Haas CF. Mechanical ventilation with lung protective strategies: what works? *Crit Care Clin*. 2011;27:469–486.

119. Barrot L, Asfar P, Mauny F, et al. Liberal or conservative oxygen therapy for acute respiratory distress syndrome. *N Engl J Med*. 2020;382:999–1008.

120. Angus DC. Oxygen therapy for the critically ill. *N Engl J Med*. 2020;382:1054–1056.

121. Walkey AJ, Del Sorbo L, Hodgson CL, et al. Higher PEEP versus lower PEEP strategies for patients with acute respiratory distress syndrome. A systematic review and meta-analysis. *Ann Am Thorac Soc*. 2017;14:S297–S303.

122. Gattinoni L, Tognoni G, Pesenti A, et al. Effect of prone positioning on the survival of patients with acute respiratory failure. *N Engl J Med*. 2001;345:568–573.

123. Park PK, Napolitano LM, Bartlett RH. Extracorporeal membrane oxygenation in adult acute respiratory distress syndrome. *Crit Care Clin*. 2011;27:627–646.

124. Maung AA, Kaplan LJ. Airway pressure release ventilation in acute respiratory distress syndrome. *Crit Care Clin*. 2011;27:501–509.

125. Ferguson ND, Cook DJ, Guyatt GH, et al. High-frequency oscillation in early acute respiratory distress syndrome. *N Engl J Med*. 2013;368:795–805.

126. Combes A, Hajage D, Capellier G, et al. Extracorporeal membrane oxygenation for severe acute respiratory distress syndrome. *N Engl J Med*. 2018;378:1965–1975.

127. Wang J, Wang Y, Wang T, et al. Is extracorporeal membrane oxygenation the standard care for acute respiratory distress syndrome: a systematic review and meta-analysis. *Heart Lung Circ*. 2021;30:631–641.

128. Vasquez DN, Giannoni R, Salvatierra A, et al. Ventilatory parameters in obstetric patients with COVID-19 and impact of delivery: a multicenter prospective cohort study. *Chest*. 2023;163:554–566.

129. National Heart, Lung, and Blood Institute PETAL Clinical Trials Network, Moss M, Huang DT, et al. Early neuromuscular blockade in the acute respiratory distress syndrome. *N Engl J Med*. 2019;380:1997–2008.

130. Marik PE, Meduri GU, Rocco PR, Annane D. Glucocorticoid treatment in acute lung injury and acute respiratory distress syndrome. *Crit Care Clin*. 2011;27:589–607.

131. Tang BM, Craig JC, Eslick GD, et al. Use of corticosteroids in acute lung injury and acute respiratory distress syndrome: a systematic review and meta-analysis. *Crit Care Med*. 2009;37:1594–1603.

132. Villar J, Ferrando C, Martinez D, et al. Dexamethasone treatment for the acute respiratory distress syndrome: a multicentre, randomised controlled trial. *Lancet Respir Med*. 2020;8:267–276.

133. Briggs GG, Freeman RK, Tower CV, Forinash AB. *Drugs in Pregnancy and Lactation: A Reference Guide to Fetal and Neonatal Risk*. 12th ed. Lippincott Williams & Wilkins; 2021.

134. Wiedemann HP, Wheeler AP, Bernard GR, et al. Comparison of two fluid-management strategies in acute lung injury. *N Engl J Med*. 2006;354:2564–2575.

135. Puri N, Dellinger RP. Inhaled nitric oxide and inhaled prostacyclin in acute respiratory distress syndrome: what is the evidence? *Crit Care Clin*. 2011;27:561–587.

136. Rice TW, Wheeler AP, Thompson BT, et al. Enteral omega-3 fatty acid, gamma-linolenic acid, and antioxidant supplementation in acute lung injury. *JAMA*. 2011;306:1574–1581.

137. Compher C, Bingham AL, McCall M, et al. Guidelines for the provision of nutrition support therapy in the adult critically ill patient: the American Society for Parenteral and Enteral Nutrition. *JPEN J Parenter Enteral Nutr*. 2022;46:12–41.

138. Heyland DK, Cahill N, Day AG. Optimal amount of calories for critically ill patients: depends on how you slice the cake! *Crit Care Med*. 2011;39:2619–2626.

139. van den Berghe G, Wouters P, Weekers F, et al. Intensive insulin therapy in critically ill patients. *N Engl J Med*. 2001;345:1359–1367.

140. Finfer S, Chittock DR, Su SY, et al. Intensive versus conventional glucose control in critically ill patients. *N Engl J Med*. 2009;360:1283–1297.

141. Napolitano LM, Kurek S, Luchette FA, et al. Clinical practice guideline: red blood cell transfusion in adult trauma and critical care. *J Trauma*. 2009;67:1439–1442.

142. Vincent JL, Sakr Y, De Backer D, Van der Linden P. Efficacy of allogeneic red blood cell transfusions. *Best Pract Res Clin Anaesthesiol.* 2007;21:209–219.

143. Marik PE, Corwin HL. Efficacy of red blood cell transfusion in the critically ill: a systematic review of the literature. *Crit Care Med.* 2008;36:2667–2674.

144. Hebert PC, Wells G, Blajchman MA, et al. A multicenter, randomized, controlled clinical trial of transfusion requirements in critical care. *N Engl J Med.* 1999;340:409–417.

145. Nduka OO, Parrillo JE. The pathophysiology of septic shock. *Crit Care Clin.* 2009;25:677–702, vii.

146. World Health Organization, GBD 2015 Maternal Mortality Collaborators. Global, regional, and national levels of maternal mortality, 1990-2015: a systematic analysis for the Global Burden of Disease Study 2015. *Lancet.* 2016;388:1775–1812.

147. Society for Maternal-Fetal Medicine, Shields AD, Plante LA, et al. Society for Maternal-Fetal Medicine Consult Series #67: Maternal sepsis. *Am J Obstet Gynecol.* 2023;229:B2–B19.

148. Rhodes A, Evans LE, Alhazzani W, et al. Surviving Sepsis Campaign: international guidelines for management of sepsis and septic shock: 2016. *Intensive Care Med.* 2017;43:304–377.

149. Huang D, Chen JT. Early choices, lasting impact: the colloid versus crystalloid decision in early sepsis. *Crit Care Med.* 2024;52:1646–1648.

150. Estrada CA, Murugan R. Hydroxyethyl starch in severe sepsis: end of starch era? *Crit Care.* 2013;17:310.

151. Patel A, Waheed U, Brett SJ. Randomised trials of 6% tetrastarch (hydroxyethyl starch 130/0.4 or 0.42) for severe sepsis reporting mortality: systematic review and meta-analysis. *Intensive Care Med.* 2013;39:811–822.

152. Yealy DM, Kellum JA, Huang DT, et al. A randomized trial of protocol-based care for early septic shock. *N Engl J Med.* 2014;370:1683–1693.

153. Peake SL, Delaney A, Bailey M, et al. Goal-directed resuscitation for patients with early septic shock. *N Engl J Med.* 2014;371:1496–1506.

154. Preau S, Saulnier F, Dewavrin F, et al. Passive leg raising is predictive of fluid responsiveness in spontaneously breathing patients with severe sepsis or acute pancreatitis. *Crit Care Med.* 2010;38:819–825.

155. Michard F, Boussat S, Chemla D, et al. Relation between respiratory changes in arterial pulse pressure and fluid responsiveness in septic patients with acute circulatory failure. *Am J Respir Crit Care Med.* 2000;162:134–138.

156. Russell JA, Walley KR, Singer J, et al. Vasopressin versus norepinephrine infusion in patients with septic shock. *N Engl J Med.* 2008;358:877–887.

157. Jaber S, Paugam C, Futier E, et al. Sodium bicarbonate therapy for patients with severe metabolic acidaemia in the intensive care unit (BICAR-ICU): a multicentre, open-label, randomised controlled, phase 3 trial. *Lancet.* 2018;392:31–40.

158. Annane D, Bellissant E, Bollaert PE, et al. Corticosteroids in the treatment of severe sepsis and septic shock in adults: a systematic review. *JAMA.* 2009;301:2362–2375.

159. Annane D, Renault A, Brun-Buisson C, et al. Hydrocortisone plus fludrocortisone for adults with septic shock. *N Engl J Med.* 2018;378:809–818.

160. Hankins GD, Clark SL, Uckan E, Van Hook JW. Maternal oxygen transport variables during the third trimester of normal pregnancy. *Am J Obstet Gynecol.* 1999;180:406–409.

Page numbers followed by "*f*" indicate figures, "*t*" indicate tables, and "*b*" indicate boxes.